Digestive Tract Surgery

A Text and Atlas

HOLLY R. FISCHER, MFA, ILLUSTRATOR

With 58 Contributors

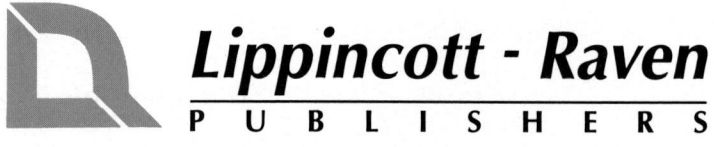
Lippincott - Raven
PUBLISHERS

Digestive Tract Surgery

A Text and Atlas

EDITED BY

RICHARD H. BELL, JR., MD

Professor and Vice Chairman
Department of Surgery
University of Washington School of Medicine
Chief, Surgical Service
Department of Veterans Affairs Medical Center
Seattle, Washington

LAYTON F. RIKKERS, MD

M.M. Musselman Professor of Surgery
Chairman, Department of Surgery
University of Nebraska College of Medicine
University of Nebraska Hospital and Clinics
Omaha, Nebraska

MICHAEL W. MULHOLLAND, MD, PhD

Professor and Associate Chairman
Department of Surgery
University of Michigan School of Medicine
University of Michigan Medical Center
Ann Arbor, Michigan

Acquisitions Editor: Lisa McAllister
Associate Editor: Paula Callaghan
Associate Managing Editor: Grace R. Caputo
Production Manager: Caren Erlichman
Senior Production Coordinator: Kevin P. Johnson
Assistant Art Director: Doug Smock
Indexer: Sandra King
Compositor: Tapsco, Inc.
Prepress: Jay's Publisher's Service, Inc.
Printer/Binder: Quebecor/Kingsport
Color Insert Printer: Walsworth Publishing Company

Library of Congress Cataloging-in-Publication Data

Digestive tract surgery: a text and atlas/edited by Richard H.
  Bell, Jr., Layton F. Rikkers, Michael W. Mulholland.
      p.   cm.
    Includes bibliographical references and index.
    ISBN 0-397-51344-5 (alk. paper)
    1. Digestive organs—Surgery.   2. Digestive organs—Diseases.
  3. Digestive organs—Surgery—Atlases.   I. Bell, Richard H., 1946–
    II. Rikkers, Layton F.   III. Mulholland, Michael W.
    [DNLM: 1. Digestive System Diseases—surgery.   2. Digestive System
  Diseases—surgery—atlases.   WI 900 D572 1996]
  RD540.D54   1996
  617.4'3—dc20
  DNLM/DLC
  for Library of Congress   95-981
                                                                               CIP

9   8   7   6   5   4   3   2   1

Contributors

Kareem Abu-Elmagd, MD, PhD
Assistant Professor of Surgery
University of Pittsburgh School of Medicine
University of Pittsburgh Medical Center
Presbyterian-University Hospital
Pittsburgh, Pennsylvania

Richard H. Bell, Jr., MD
Professor and Vice Chairman
Department of Surgery
University of Washington School of Medicine
Chief, Surgical Service
Department of Veterans Affairs Medical Center
Seattle, Washington

Scott J. Boley, MD
Professor of Surgery and Pediatrics
Albert Einstein College of Medicine
Chief, Pediatric Surgical Services
Montefiore Medical Center
Bronx, New York

Howard Bourdages, MD
University of Minnesota Medical School—Minneapolis
Minneapolis, Minnesota

Henry Buchwald, MD, PhD
Professor of Surgery and Biomedical Engineering
University of Minnesota Medical School—Minneapolis
Minneapolis, Minnesota

Jon M. Burch, MD
Professor of Surgery
University of Colorado School of Medicine
Associate Director of Surgery
Chief of General Surgery
Denver General Hospital
Denver, Colorado

Christian T. Campos, MD
Harvard Medical School
Boston, Massachusetts

Lisa M. Colletti, MD
Assistant Professor of Surgery
University of Michigan Medical School
University of Michigan Hospitals
Ann Arbor, Michigan

Lillian G. Dawes, MD
Assistant Professor of Surgery
Northwestern University Medical Center
Chicago, Illinois

Frederic E. Eckhauser, MD
Professor of Surgery
University of Michigan Medical School
Chief, Division of Gastrointestinal Surgery
Director, Multidisciplinary Gastrointestinal Oncology Clinic
University of Michigan Medical Center
Ann Arbor, Michigan

Mark K. Ferguson, MD
Associate Professor of Surgery
University of Chicago Pritzker School of Medicine
Chief, Section of Thoracic Surgery
University of Chicago Medical Center
Chicago, Illinois

John J. Fung, MD, PhD
Associate Professor of Surgery
University of Pittsburgh School of Medicine
Chief, Division of Transplant Surgery
University of Pittsburgh Medical Center
Pittsburgh, Pennsylvania

John B. Hanks, MD
C. Bruce Morton Professor of Surgery
Chief, Division of General Surgery
University of Virginia Health Sciences Center
Charlottesville, Virginia

William L. Hasler, MD
Assistant Professor of Internal Medicine
Division of Gastroenterology
University of Michigan Medical School
University of Michigan Medical Center
Ann Arbor, Michigan

W. Scott Helton, MD
Assistant Professor of Surgery
University of Washington School of Medicine
University of Washington Medical Center
Seattle, Washington

J. Michael Henderson, MB, ChB
Chairman
Division of General Surgery
The Cleveland Clinic Foundation
Cleveland, Ohio

Ronald A. Hinder, MD, PhD
Professor and Stuchenhoff Chair of Surgery
Creighton University School of Medicine
St Joseph Hospital
Omaha, Nebraska

Roger L. Jenkins, MD
Associate Professor of Surgery
Harvard Medical School
Chief, Division of Hepatobiliary Surgery and Liver
   Transplantation
New England Deaconess Hospital
Boston, Massachusetts

Gregory J. Jurkovich, MD
Professor of Surgery
University of Washington School of Medicine
Chief of Trauma
Director, Emergency Surgical Services
Harborview Medical Center
Seattle, Washington

Kim U. Kahng, MD
Associate Professor of Surgery
Vice Chairman, Administrative Affairs
Medical College of Pennsylvania
Hahnemann University School of Medicine
Philadelphia, Pennsylvania

Ronald N. Kaleya, MD
Associate Professor of Surgery
Albert Einstein College of Medicine
Associate Attending Physician
Department of Surgery and Medical Oncology
Montefiore Medical Center
Bronx, New York

Michael Kimmey, MD
Associate Professor of Medicine
University of Washington School of Medicine
Seattle, Washington

James A. Knol, MD
Associate Professor of Surgery
University of Michigan Medical School
University of Michigan Hospitals
Ann Arbor, Michigan

Alan N. Langnas, MD
Associate Professor of Surgery
University of Nebraska College of Medicine
University of Nebraska Medical Center
Omaha, Nebraska

Keith D. Lillemoe, MD
Associate Professor of Surgery
Johns Hopkins University School of Medicine
Johns Hopkins Hospital
Baltimore, Maryland

D. Scott Lind, MD
Assistant Professor of Surgery
University of Florida College of Medicine
Shands Teaching Hospital
Gainesville, Florida

Alex G. Little, MD
Professor and Chairman
Department of Surgery
University of Nevada School of Medicine
Chief of Surgery
University Medical Center of Southern Nevada
Las Vegas, Nevada

Robert D. Madoff, MD
Clinical Assistant Professor of Surgery
Director of Research
Division of Colon and Rectal Surgery
University of Minnesota Medical School
Minneapolis, Minnesota

David W. McFadden, MD
Associate Professor and Chief
Division of General Surgery
University of California, Los Angeles, UCLA School of Medicine
Los Angeles, California
Chief, General Surgery
Sepulveda Department of Veterans Affairs Medical Center
North Hills, California

Dan M. Meyer, MD
Assistant Professor of Thoracic and Cardiovascular Surgery
University of Texas Southwestern Medical Center at Dallas
Parkland Memorial Hospital
Dallas, Texas

William G. Meyers, MD
Professor and Chief
Division of Gastrointestinal Surgery
Duke University School of Medicine
Duke University Medical Center
Durham, North Carolina

Fabrizio Michelassi, MD
Associate Professor of Surgery
Chief, Section of General Surgery
University of Chicago Pritzker School of Medicine
Chicago, Illinois

Jeffrey F. Moley, MD
Associate Professor of Surgery
Washington University School of Medicine
Barnes Hospital
St Louis Department of Veterans Affairs Medical Center
St Louis, Missouri

Ernest E. Moore, MD
Professor and Vice Chairman of Surgery
University of Colorado Health Sciences Center
Chief, Department of Surgery
Denver General Hospital
Denver, Colorado

Michael W. Mulholland, MD, PhD
Professor and Associate Chairman
Department of Surgery
University of Michigan School of Medicine
University of Michigan Hospital
Ann Arbor, Michigan

Sean J. Mulvihill, MD
Associate Professor of Surgery
Chief, Division of General Surgery
University of California, San Francisco, School of Medicine
San Francisco, California

David L. Nahrwold, MD
Loyal and Edith Davis Professor and Chairman
Department of Surgery
Northwestern University Medical School
Surgeon-in-Chief
Northwestern Memorial Hospital
Chicago, Illinois

Jeffrey A. Norton, MD
Professor of Surgery
Chief of Endocrine and Oncologic Surgery
Washington University School of Medicine
Barnes Hospital
St Louis, Missouri

Michael S. Nussbaum, MD
Assistant Professor of Surgery
University of Cincinnati College of Medicine
University of Cincinnati Medical Center
Cincinnati, Ohio

Henry A. Pitt, MD
Professor and Vice-Chairman
Department of Surgery
Johns Hopkins Medical Institutions
Baltimore, Maryland

Joe B. Putnam, Jr., MD
Associate Professor of Thoracic and Cardiovascular Surgery
Associate Surgeon
University of Texas M.D. Anderson Cancer Center
Houston, Texas

Steven E. Raper, MD
Associate Professor of Surgery
Institute for Human Gene Therapy
University of Pennsylvania School of Medicine
Philadelphia, Pennsylvania

David W. Rattner, MD
Associate Professor of Surgery
Harvard Medical School
Associate Visiting Surgeon
Massachusetts General Hospital
Boston, Massachusetts

Howard A. Reber, MD
Professor of Surgery
University of California, Los Angeles, UCLA School of Medicine
Chief of Surgery
Sepulveda Department of Veterans Affairs Medical Center
Los Angeles, California

R. Lawrence Reed II, MD
Associate Professor of Surgery and Anesthesiology
Duke University School of Medicine
Director, Trauma Center
Director, Surgical Intensive Care Unit
Duke University Medical Center
Durham, North Carolina

Layton F. Rikkers, MD
M.M. Musselman Professor of Surgery
Chairman, Department of Surgery
University of Nebraska College of Medicine
University of Nebraska Hospital and Clinics
Omaha, Nebraska

Lynn K. Rosenlof, MD
University of Virginia School of Medicine
Charlottesville, Virginia

Joel J. Roslyn, MD
Professor and Chairman
Department of Surgery
Medical College of Pennsylvania
Hahnemann University School of Medicine
Philadelphia, Pennsylvania

Jack A. Roth, MD
Professor and Chairman
Department of Thoracic and Cardiovascular Surgery
Professor of Tumor Biology
University of Texas M.D. Anderson Cancer Center
Houston, Texas

David A. Rothenberger, MD
Director and Clinical Professor
Division of Colon and Rectal Surgery
Department of Surgery
University of Minnesota Medical School
University of Minnesota Hospital and Clinic
Minneapolis, Minnesota

Byers W. Shaw, Jr., MD
Shackleford-Marischal Professor of Surgery
University of Nebraska College of Medicine
Chief, Division of Transplantation
University of Nebraska Medical Center
Omaha, Nebraska

Nathaniel J. Soper, MD
Associate Professor of Surgery
Washington University School of Medicine
Barnes Hospital
St Louis, Missouri

Wiley W. Souba, MD, ScD
Professor of Surgery
Harvard Medical School
Chief, Division of Surgical Oncology
Massachusetts General Hospital
Boston, Massachusetts

Robert J. Stratta, MD
Associate Professor of Surgery
University of Nebraska College of Medicine
University of Nebraska Medical Center
Director of Pancreas Transplantation
University Hospital and Clarkson Hospital
Omaha, Nebraska

Rodney J. Taylor, MD
Professor of Surgery
Chief, Section of Urology
Chief of Kidney Transplantation
University of Nebraska Medical Center
Omaha, Nebraska

Jon S. Thompson, MD
Professor and Vice-Chairman
Department of Surgery
University of Nebraska Medical Center
University of Nebraska Hospital and Clinics
Omaha, Nebraska

Sean Tierney, FRCSI
 Johns Hopkins Medical Institutions
 Baltimore, Maryland

Satoru Todo, MD
 Professor of Surgery
 Pittsburgh Transplantation Institute
 University of Pittsburgh School of Medicine
 Pittsburgh, Pennsylvania

Anthony M. Vernava III, MD
 Associate Professor of Surgery
 St Louis University School of Medicine
 Chief, Section of Colon and Rectal Surgery
 St Louis University Health Sciences Center
 St Louis, Missouri

Andrew L. Warshaw, MD
 Harold and Ellen Danser Professor of Surgery
 Harvard Medical School
 Chief, Division of General Surgery
 Associate Chief, Division of Surgical Services
 Massachusetts General Hospital
 Boston, Massachusetts

Gerald B. Zelenock, MD
 Professor of Surgery
 Division of Vascular Surgery
 University of Michigan School of Medicine
 University of Michigan Hospitals
 Ann Arbor, Michigan

Preface

Textbooks are created for the purpose of education. All who have been educated as surgeons and those of us who have participated in the education of future surgeons are keenly aware that the best surgeons display a combination of technical skill and clinical judgment. Operative technical ability springs from a firm understanding of the process of surgery—a comprehension both of the objectives of an operation and of the individual steps required to meet the objectives. Clinical judgment develops partly from experience, but it also stems from knowledge of disease and from a clear understanding of the role of surgical therapy in management of a given disease. Such knowledge and understanding cannot be gathered entirely firsthand; they depend on a command of the surgical literature and the experience of others.

In view of the need for surgeons to acquire both technical skills and detailed clinical knowledge, it is surprising that textbooks in general surgery have traditionally emphasized one or the other, but not both. Many atlases of gastrointestinal surgery have been written, but few contain more than minimal information about the diseases for which the operations are intended, the indications for the operation, or the possible adverse consequences of operative therapy. On the other hand, many comprehensive didactic textbooks of surgery lack satisfying detail about operative procedures and rarely answer the practical technical questions surgeons face before entering the operating room.

In bringing forth a new book in the field of digestive tract surgery, we were motivated by the desire to create a textbook that would be both comprehensive in its discussion of gastrointestinal diseases *and* detailed in its presentation of operative technique.

Digestive Tract Surgery: A Text and Atlas is unique in this regard, and this singularity is reflected in its format. The seven parts of the book each focus on one of the major organs in the digestive tract (esophagus, stomach, liver, biliary tract, pancreas, small intestine, and colorectum). Within each part, comprehensive chapters on the major diseases of that organ are followed by a detailed atlas of the operations performed in their treatment. The seven atlases are easily located by color-tabbed pages that allow the reader to move quickly from the informational text to the operative figures.

To make the atlases valuable to surgeons, we believed that they should be comprehensive and that the illustrations should be created by a single artist. Many textbooks contain illustrations culled from a number of previous works. This approach often results in differing presentation styles and conceptual inconsistencies, making it difficult to follow the steps of an operation. In *Digestive Tract Surgery,* procedures are presented in a uniform fashion, enabling the reader to visualize them from beginning to end.

Both the text chapters and the atlases in *Digestive Tract Surgery* are sufficiently comprehensive to be of use to experienced practitioners of surgery as well as to senior trainees, who may be seeking detailed and sophisticated information about a given operation or disease. At the same time, the book will be useful to students who wish to go beyond standard textbook information and acquire detailed information about gastrointestinal surgery.

Gastrointestinal surgery has changed significantly in the past few years. We have endeavored to include up-to-date technical information on laparoscopic surgery, both for accepted procedures, such as laparoscopic cholecystectomy, and for procedures likely to become a standard part of the surgical repertoire, such as laparoscopic fundoplication. We have also made a conscious decision to include a significant amount of information about transplantation of digestive tract organs. Although most general surgeons do not perform these procedures, knowledge of the indications for transplantation is critical for surgical decision making in areas such as portal hypertension. The field of transplantation is moving forward rapidly and is likely to interface more and more with traditional surgery in the years to come.

In choosing the contributors for *Digestive Tract Surgery,* we sought surgeons who had meaningful and significant clinical experience with the diseases and operations described. The text chapters and atlases were created by surgeons who, we believe, have anticipated the needs of the practicing gastrointestinal surgeon and provided useful and practical information to the reader. In addition, the authors chosen are making significant contributions to new clinical knowledge.

In summary, we believe that *Digestive Tract Surgery: A Text and Atlas* is a truly new book—new in concept and new in scope. We hope our readers find that it combines the unique elements of surgery in a way that will be genuinely educational.

Richard H. Bell, Jr., MD
Layton F. Rikkers, MD
Michael W. Mulholland, MD, PHD

Acknowledgments

The creation of a book with the scope of *Digestive Tract Surgery: A Text and Atlas* is a group effort, and we have enjoyed the support and collaboration of a number of able and enthusiastic individuals. We would like to thank all the contributing authors, who devoted considerable time and effort to ensuring that the book would be comprehensive, up-to-date, readable, and authoritative.

A very special acknowledgment must be made to Holly Fischer, who took on the immense task of creating an entirely new and exhaustive visual depiction of gastrointestinal surgery. Holly's imagination, ingenuity, understanding of surgical anatomy, and artistic skill have combined to produce what we believe is the definitive rendering of today's digestive tract operations.

Since the beginning, we have benefited from the experience and counsel of the staff at Lippincott–Raven Publishers, including Lisa McAllister, Senior Editor, who sustained us with her enthusiasm for the project; Paula Callaghan, Associate Editor, who helped us with innumerable questions and decisions along the way; and Grace Caputo, Associate Managing Editor, who brought the final product to life.

We would finally like to acknowledge Ann Ruder, Patricia Thompson, and Steve Wiesner, who helped us immeasurably with our editorial tasks and who deserve much of the credit for keeping the project moving forward.

Contents

Digestive Tract Surgery

A Text and Atlas

PART I
Esophagus

Digestive Tract Surgery: A Text and Atlas, edited by Richard H. Bell, Layton F. Rikkers, and Michael W. Mulholland. Lippincott-Raven Publishers, Philadelphia, © 1996.

1

Gastroesophageal Reflux Disease

Ronald A. Hinder

EPIDEMIOLOGY

Gastroesophageal reflux is a common condition. Even in normal people, a certain amount of acid reflux occurs under physiologic conditions, mainly after meals, and is of no pathologic consequence. About 44% of Americans experience the symptom of heartburn at least once a month, and 18% of these people regularly take some form of nonprescription medication for the problem.[1] Most of these people treat themselves with antacids and have not discussed these symptoms with their physicians.[2] Esophagitis is present in 19% of patients undergoing endoscopy for upper abdominal symptoms[3] and is thought to be present in 1.1% of the population at large[4] (Fig. 1-1). Gastroesophageal reflux disease (GERD) is a condition of relatively young people with a peak incidence at 30 to 40 years of age. However, the mean age of patients with severe esophagitis is over 60 years, and more than half of patients presenting with Barrett's esophagus are older than 70 years of age. It therefore seems that the severity of the disease increases with age.[5] The sex incidence is about equal, with some series reporting more males and others reporting more females.[6-11] However, Barrett's esophagus has a slight male predominance.[12,13] GERD appears to be a disease of the Western world, with low incidence reported in Africa and Asia. Because of the high incidence of reflux in patients with hiatal hernias, it was first believed that the presence of the hiatal hernia was responsible for the gastroesophageal reflux. More recently, it was established that the basic problem in GERD is a defective lower esophageal sphincter (LES). Hiatal hernias have been reported in up to 15% of the normal population, compared with 63% to 94% of patients with esophagitis.[14,15]

Most GERD does not result in any significant sequelae, but complications such as ulceration, strictures, hemorrhage, Barrett's esophagus, and, rarely, Barrett's adenocarcinoma occasionally ensue. The adult annual mortality rate for GERD was estimated to be as low as 0.1 per 100,000 population from 1957 to 1961.[6] The incidence must be higher because these figures do not take into account deaths from operative complications or adenocarcinoma. Most GERD is treated by intermittent therapy aimed at acid reduction. When this fails, or in the presence of complications, surgery may be indicated.

PATHOPHYSIOLOGY

Gastroesophageal reflux disease occurs when the gastric content is allowed access to the esophageal lumen, resulting in symptoms and esophageal mucosal damage. The severity of disease depends on the amount of acid refluxed into the esophagus, the length of time that the acid is allowed to remain in contact with the esophageal mucosa, and the susceptibility of the esophageal mucosa to acid. Enzymes such as pepsin and trypsin may play a significant part in esophageal mucosal damage. Alkaline secretions from the duodenum and bile acids have also been implicated in esophageal disease, particularly in Barrett's esophagus and strictures.

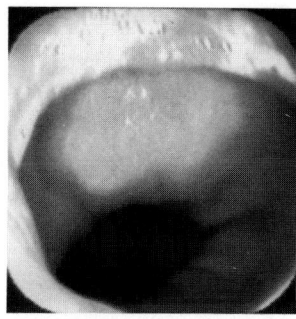

Figure 1-1 Endoscopic appearance of grade I esophagitis in distal esophagus. (See Color Fig. 1-1.)

Lower Esophageal Sphincter

The LES forms the most important part of the physiologic barrier between the esophagus and stomach. The LES is a thickening of the esophageal musculature in the lower 5 cm of the esophagus.[16] This is composed of a thickening of the circular muscle layer, particularly on the greater curvature side of the sphincter. Below this, oblique muscle fibers run from the angle of His toward the lesser curvature (Fig. 1-2). The sphincter lies partly within the chest and partly within the abdomen. This area of the esophageal musculature has a higher density of neuronal plexuses than is found in the esophageal body.[17] Muscle from this region is more responsive to gastrin and has a heightened sensitivity to cholinergic and adrenergic compounds compared with the surrounding smooth muscle. The LES has a resting pressure that can be measured in the interprandial period by obtaining pressure measurements within the lumen of the esophagus. Studies of the LES in normal people have shown that the 2.5th percentile of normal is 6 mmHg pressure with a total length of over 2 cm and with an intraabdominal component measuring more than 1 cm in length. Gastroesophageal reflux is likely to occur if the pressure or length of the sphincter falls below these lower limits of normal. Failure of the LES mechanism can be due to any number of events, including primary weakness of the smooth muscle, short length of the sphincter, defective control mechanisms, an abnormally high number of transient relaxations, and dislocation of the LES into the chest (Fig. 1-3). It is not clear whether esophageal mucosal inflammation has a negative influence on LES pressure.[18,19] Not all gastroesophageal reflux events are related to impaired LES pressure; a defective sphincter is only found in 60% of patients with GERD.[20] Only 18% to 23% of all reflux episodes can be explained by deficient esophageal sphincter pressures.[21] An effective way of representing the overall antireflux ability of the LES is the expression of *vector volume.* This calculation expresses the pressure

and length of the sphincter around its circumference as a vector volume. This gives a single value to be compared with a normal range.[22]

Controlling Mechanisms

The LES is under various neural and hormonal control mechanisms in addition to the influence of the crura and the surrounding intraabdominal or intrathoracic pressures. The resting pressure shows large variations and can reach values of about 100 mmHg. The highest values are seen during phase III of the migrating motor complex in the stomach, which suggests that there is a direct influence of gastric motility on the LES.[23] Hormones that are known to increase the tone in the LES are motilin and gastrin, whereas cholecystokinin, secretin, and vasoactive intestinal peptide cause a decrease in LES tone.[24–27] Other hormones, such as substance P, are implicated in maintaining LES tone. In patients with GERD, the LES shows a poor response to stimulants such as gastrin and bethanechol.[28] Patients with GERD have significantly lower basal levels of motilin and an impaired postprandial cholecystokinin response.[29] It is not clear whether these are primary or secondary events. Nitric oxide has also been found to play a role in the control of LES pressure.

Intrathoracic Lower Esophageal Sphincter

The resting LES pressure is contributed to by the surrounding crura and the intraabdominal pressure. If the LES is translocated into the chest, such as occurs with hiatal hernia, these factors are ineffective, and reflux can occur. The crura play a part in producing LES pressure; increases in pressure can be recorded even when the sphincter muscle is relaxed. Intraabdominal

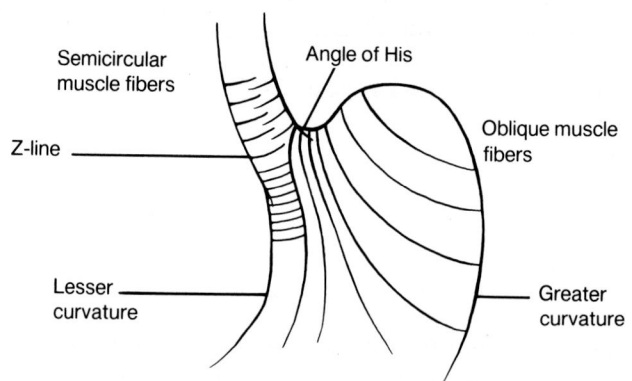

Figure 1-2 Anatomy of the lower esophageal sphincter. (After Liebermann-Meffert, D, Allgower M, Schmid P, Blum AL. Muscular equivalent of the lower esophageal sphincter. Gastroenterology 1979;76:31)

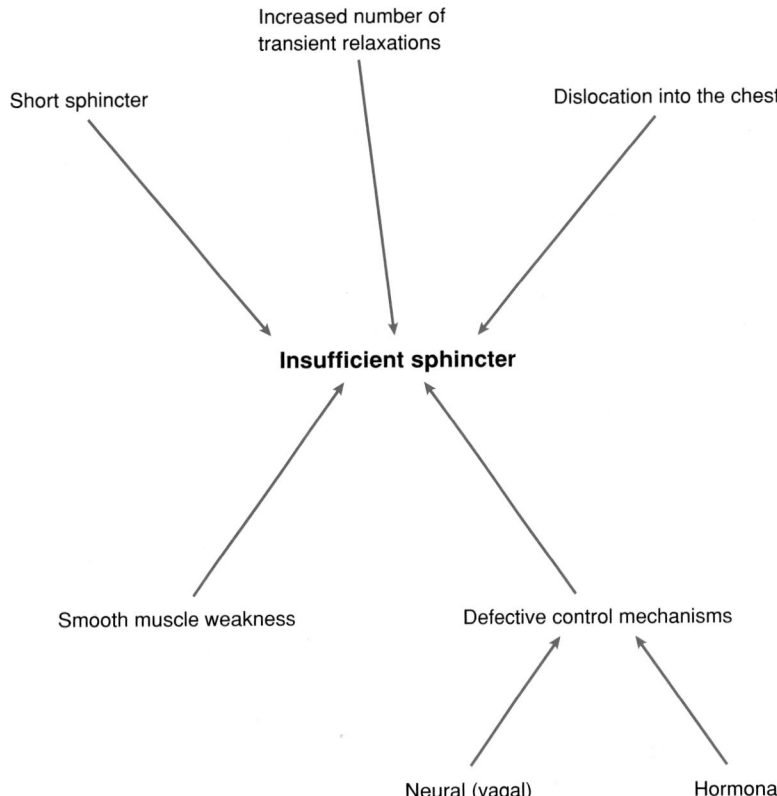

Figure 1-3 Reasons for failure of the lower esophageal sphincter.

pressure may increase the pressure at the LES by direct pressure on the sphincter or by inducing active contractions in the LES, resulting in pressures much higher than the intraabdominal pressure.

Dislocation of the LES into the chest can be identified by recording a high pressure zone at a level located anatomically in the chest. Occasionally a "double-hump" phenomenon can be identified manometrically with two high-pressure zones in the distal esophagus.[30] The lower high-pressure zone is created by the diaphragmatic crura and the upper by the LES, which has been dislocated into the chest. The pressure that the LES can generate in the chest is lower than normal but is able to prevent reflux under most conditions. Under straining conditions, this can be more easily overcome than when the crura contribute to the pressure.[31]

Transient Relaxations

Relaxation of the LES normally occurs with swallowing. Sphincter relaxation is also an interprandial even.... These so-called transient relaxations of the LES may play a role in GERD but are probably more significant during normal physiologic events, such as belching.

The clinical importance of transient relaxations of the LES is not known. Transient relaxations appear to account for more than 90% of reflux episodes in healthy controls, but whether this is of importance in pathologic reflux is not clear.[21,32] Contradictory evidence exists regarding the number of transient relaxations of the LES in patients with GERD. Pharyngeal electromyographic activity without induction of swallows has been observed at the same time as transient relaxations of the LES. This indicates that subthreshold swallows may produce transient relaxations of the LES. It is thought that mechanoreceptors in the upper stomach initiate vagal reflexes that result in sphincter relaxation. These mechanoreceptors are thought to be stimulated by gastric distention; indeed, balloon distention leads to sphincter relaxation. The observation of an increased number of reflux episodes postprandially supports this hypothesis. It is believed that constriction of the hernial sac by the diaphragm may create high pressures on the upper stomach, leading to stimulation of mechanoreceptors with an increased number of transient relaxations of the LES. This hypothesis is unproved and requires further investigation.[33]

Esophageal Body Acid Clearance

An important part of esophageal mucosal damage associated with GERD is the length of time that the refluxate remains in contact with the esophageal mucosa. Instillation of radiolabeled 0.1N HCl has shown that most acid is cleared during the first peristaltic wave on swallowing.[34] The pH in the esophageal lumen then slowly falls in a stepwise fashion with each subsequent peristaltic wave. A small amount of retained acid is able to maintain a low esophageal pH. Swallowed saliva is responsible for the neutralization of much refluxed acid. About 7 mL of saliva is able to neutralize 1 mL of 0.1N HCl, and stimulation of salivary secretion results in accelerated acid clearance from the esophagus.[35] Esophageal pain produces an increase in salivary secretion. Saliva production is inhibited during sleep, and if reflux occurs during sleep, this mechanism of clearance and neutralization of acid is markedly impaired. About one swallow per minute occurs in the awake state, but the rate is markedly reduced at night when this protective mechanism is needed. Secondary peristaltic waves to acid reflux are less effective than primary waves induced by swallowing.

The effectiveness of peristaltic contractions is important in the clearance of acid from the esophagus. A peristaltic pressure of 30 mmHg is necessary in the distal esophagus to achieve good acid clearance. The severity of reflux esophagitis is related to the loss of peristaltic activity in the esophagus; one fourth of patients with mild esophagitis had weak peristalsis, whereas half of those with severe esophagitis had weak peristaltic waves.[36] Half of patients with GERD have disturbed clearance function in the esophageal body. It is unclear whether this impairment is primary or secondary, nor is it known whether peristaltic clearance improves after therapy for reflux. Some studies have shown an improvement of esophageal clearance function after therapy, whereas others have been unable to demonstrate this. Three fourths of patients with hiatal hernias show re-reflux of material in and out of the esophagus.

Influence of Delayed Gastric Emptying

Gastric distention associated with delayed emptying of food from the stomach may result in stretching of the stomach and taking up of the LES, with resultant shortening. These mechanisms probably play a role in GERD, since reflux is a common event after meals. Delayed gastric emptying of liquids or solids occurs in patients with GERD.[37] About 40% of patients with GERD have abnormally delayed gastric emptying.[38] The degree of esophagitis is often less in patients with delayed gastric emptying. This suggests that the prolonged presence of food in the stomach may buffer the acid, resulting in a bland refluxate.

Gastric Acid Secretion

Gastric acid secretion appears to play only a minor role in GERD because 95% of all patients have normal gastric acid secretion. Despite this fact, a small subset of patients with gastric acid hypersecretion and normal LES function appear to have increased exposure of the esophagus to acid. It is possible that a small amount of acid reflux of a concentrated nature or frequent acid reflux can result in abnormal esophageal acid exposure. These patients may be well served by highly selective vagotomy.

Mucosal Resistance

Esophageal mucosal integrity is maintained by several local factors, including the following:

- Production of bicarbonate by submucosal glands
- Hydrophobic mucosal surface
- Resistance to transmucosal ion diffusion
- Cellular mechanisms
- Epidermal growth factor

The human esophagus is capable of secreting large amounts of bicarbonate.[39] This secretion may be important in the prevention of acid injury during sleep and in the supine position.

Hydrophobic properties of the gastric and esophageal mucosa are induced by phospholipids and contribute to resistance to damage. Tight junctions in the upper cell layer of the intercellular space form a barrier to transmucosal ion diffusion.

Cellular mechanisms of resistance maintain the intercellular milieu and, during cellular damage, provide integrity of the esophageal mucosa. Cellular sodium uptake is markedly increased after acid injury. Glutathione levels in the lower esophageal mucosa of rats are higher than in the upper regions of the esophagus. In rats, both acid and gastroduodenal secretions produce damage that can be ascribed to free radical injury. This damage can be prevented by superoxide dismutase and other free radical scavengers, suggesting that esophagitis is a free radical event. Esophageal mucosal glutathione production is increased by damaging agents.

Increased cell turnover occurs in the presence of esophageal damage. The role of zinc has been studied in the normal activity of enzymes such as DNA and RNA polymerase, reverse transcriptase, and thymidine kinase, which are essential for cell proliferation and esophageal mucosal healing.

The ability of the esophageal mucosa to regenerate after having been damaged plays a part in GERD. This may be influenced by substances such as epidermal growth factor, which is both secreted in the saliva and found in the esophageal mucosa. Epidermal growth factor is known to increase the mucus content of the esophageal mucosa, to alter intracellular pH, and to stimulate DNA synthesis. Patients with Barrett's esophagus have impaired epidermal growth factor secretion in the saliva.[40] Furthermore, they have an increase in epidermal growth factor receptors in the esophageal mucosa, which could be interpreted as a reaction to low epidermal growth factor levels in the saliva and mucosa.

Alkaline Reflux

Esophagitis may persist even under intensive antacid therapy. This suggests that damage may be caused by agents other than acid, such as enzymes or alkaline secretions. The alkaline secretions in the foregut that are known to cause damage to both the gastric and esophageal mucosa originate in the lumen of the duodenum. The term *alkaline esophagitis* suggests that a high pH level by itself causes esophageal injury. However, the constituents of the alkaline refluxate are more important in causing mucosal damage because the esophageal pH seldom rises above 7.5, which is not damaging in its own right. Many components of duodenal juice have been implicated in the development of mucosal injury, such as bile acids, pancreatic enzymes, and lysolecithin. Esophagitis can be produced experimentally by both bile and pancreatic secretions. A mixed refluxate, composed of gastric juice and duodenal content, is more harmful than pure acid reflux. Bile acids have been extensively studied in this regard. Their main action on mucosal membranes appears to be their ability to produce hydrogen ion back-diffusion into the mucosa. Deconjugated and secondary bile acids are more harmful than conjugated or primary bile acids.[41] Different bile acids are active at different pH levels. Deconjugated and glycine-conjugated bile acids are active at pH levels between 4.0 and 5.0, and taurine-conjugated bile acids are soluble down to a pH of 1.2. At low pH, damage appears to be mediated by the direct uptake of bile acids, whereas at higher pH, the damage is mediated by the dissolution of membrane lipids.

Lysolecithin is present in the duodenogastric refluxate and has been implicated in mucosal injury. It is derived from biliary lecithin by the action of pancreatic phospholipase A. This reaction is accelerated by trypsin and bile acids. Lysolecithin has been shown to increase mucosal permeability, to increase hydrogen ion back-diffusion, to decrease the transmural electrical potential difference, and to produce microscopic injury.[42]

Pancreatic enzymes, such as trypsin, lipase, and carboxypeptidase, have all been shown to produce mucosal changes when incubated with esophageal mucosa. These enzymes are thought to be inactivated in the stomach. Trypsin is active in an alkaline environment (pH 5.0 to 8.0), and pepsin is more active in an acid environment (pH 2.0 to 5.0). Trypsin is inactivated by pepsin at pH less than 3.5; but in the absence of pepsin, trypsin is stable in an acid environment. Furthermore, active trypsin has been found in the stomach at pH levels between 3.5 and 7.0 after a meal.[43] When active, these proteolytic enzymes damage the mucosa by digesting surface tissue protein. Bile salts also interact with these enzymes. Soluble deconjugated bile salts significantly enhance mucosal injury caused by trypsin and in the alkaline environment, whereas taurodeoxycholate diminishes the damage caused by trypsin.

Pathogenetic mechanisms of duodenogastroesophageal reflux include alterations in antroduodenal motility promoting duodenogastric reflux, previous cholecystectomy, and delayed gastric emptying. In patients with proven duodenogastric reflux, antroduodenal motility is disturbed. There is a decrease in the number of antral contractions and a diminution in the propulsive activity in the distal duodenum. These motility events promote duodenogastric reflux. Impaired antroduodenal motility has been observed in patients after cholecystectomy. In addition, after cholecystectomy, there is increased duodenogastric reflux. Duodenogastric reflux may be pathologic in these patients for two reasons. First, because of the loss of the gallbladder, there is a constant flow of bile into the duodenum, which is not commonly seen in the fasting state. Second, the bile composition that exists after cholecystectomy may change to a more noxious form. The amount of technetium-99m HIDA in the stomach is increased in patients both before and after cholecystectomy compared with normal subjects without gallstones. This suggests that there may be a generalized foregut motility disorder in these patients that promotes duodenogastric and even gastroesophageal reflux. After laparoscopic cholecystectomy, there are a greater number of alkaline events in the stomach. The rate of gastric emptying is delayed in some patients with duodenogastric reflux. The hypothesis that poor antroduodenal motility leads to a nonphysiologic common cavity between the duodenum and stomach, resulting in increased reflux, poor clearance of the refluxate, and possibly altered gastric emptying, is attractive and requires further research.

Alkaline esophageal exposure can be identified in 30% of patients with GERD. Nevertheless, pure alkaline esophageal reflux is rare in patients with an intact pylorus. Most cases with pure alkaline reflux are related to gastric resectional surgery. The gastric remnant appears not to produce enough acid to neutralize the duodenal

Dual probe pH monitoring

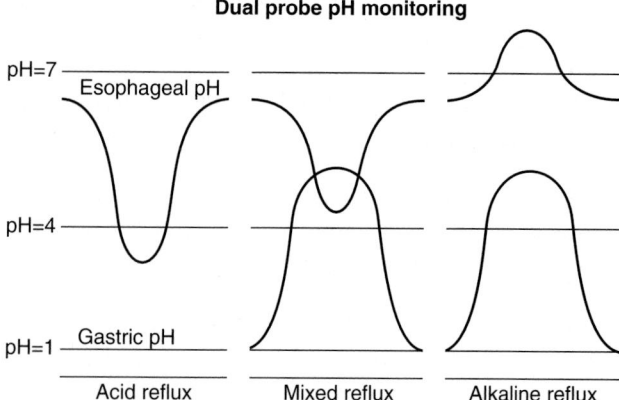

Figure 1-4 Types of alkaline reflux as measured by simultaneous gastric and esophageal pH levels. (After Fiorucci S, Santucci L, Chiucchia S, Morelli A. Gastric acidity gastroesophageal reflux patterns in patients with esophagitis. Gastroenterology 1992;103:855)

fluid, and the esophagus is exposed to almost pure duodenal content.

The evaluation of patients with duodenogastric reflux is difficult. Specific tests may have to be carried out to diagnose both duodenogastric and duodenoesophageal reflux. These tests may include endoscopy and biopsy of the stomach, esophageal and gastric pH monitoring, radionuclide scanning studies, gastric aspiration studies, provocation testing, gastric acid analysis, and gastric emptying studies. Simultaneous dual-probe pH monitoring, with one pH electrode in the esophagus and the other in the stomach, may be of value. Under these circumstances, pure acid reflux, mixed reflux, or pure alkaline reflux may be identified. Gastric pH monitoring may be employed to identify an abnormal alkaline environment in the stomach[44] (Fig. 1-4). The gastric environment in patients with Barrett's esophagus is more alkaline, suggesting that this disease is associated with duodenogastric reflux. In association with this finding, the esophageal environment was found to be more alkaline in Barrett's esophagus, particularly in patients with the complications of stricture, dysplasia, or ulceration.

The symptoms of alkaline esophageal exposure may be similar to those of acid esophageal exposure. However, patients may give a history of epigastric pain, nausea, and bilious vomiting, which should alert the clinician to the possibility of alkaline gastric exposure. This may be confirmed at endoscopy with biopsy. Care should be taken to differentiate between symptoms produced from the esophagus or the stomach before therapy is initiated. Mucosal protective agents may be of value in the treatment of patients with gastric mucosal damage.

CLINICAL EVALUATION

The full evaluation of patients with GERD should include a carefully taken history, endoscopy, radiology, esophageal manometry, 24-hour esophageal pH measurement, and studies of gastric acid secretion and motility. A scheme of when to order these tests is shown in Figure 1-5.

The symptoms of GERD may mimic those of several other foregut conditions. The most common symptom is heartburn, which is seen in about 80% of patients. This usually occurs after meals, when it may be related to gastric distention and to the action of gastrointestinal peptides on the LES. Patients may also experience heartburn when they are in the recumbent position. This is partly due to the effect of gravity and the less efficient clearing of acid from the esophagus in this position. The ability of the esophagus to carry out normal peristaltic activity is also decreased during sleep. Bending over, wearing tight clothing, and exercising may result in a rise in intraabdominal pressure with resultant reflux.

The next most common symptom of GERD is regur-

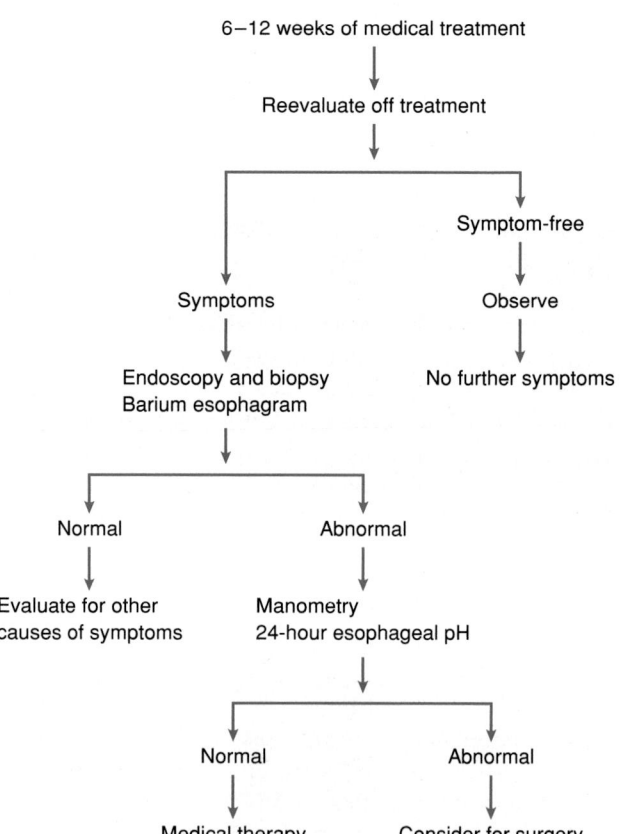

gitation, which is the effortless return of gastric contents into the pharynx or mouth. This needs to be distinguished from vomiting, which is associated with nausea or forcible abdominal contractions. Patients usually describe a burning sensation in the throat at the time of acid regurgitation. In some cases, patients may be able to differentiate between the burning sensation of acid and the bitter sensation of bile.

A troublesome symptom is dysphagia. This is often defined as difficulty in swallowing but is more accurately described as a sensation of slowed or blocked passage of food through the esophagus. There are various degrees of dysphagia. The most common is that which is not related to a stricture or obstructing ring but is the feeling of slow passage of food through the esophagus that commonly occurs in patients with severe esophagitis or severe Barrett's esophagus. This may be related to poor esophageal motility associated with these complications. The most benign form of narrowing is the frequently observed lower esophageal constriction known as *Schatzki's ring,* which is present in up to 5% of the population (Fig. 1-6). It is believed that the irrita-

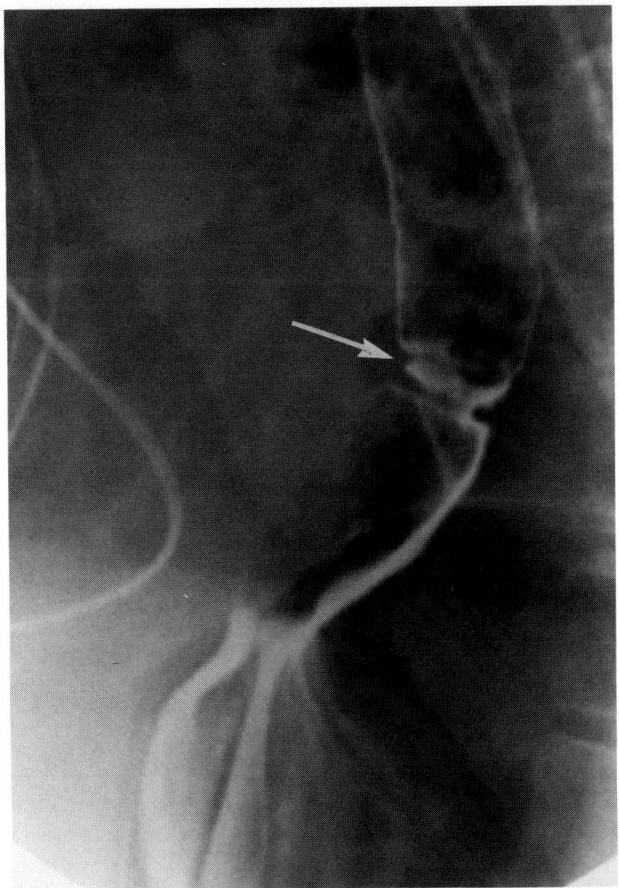

Figure 1-6 Radiograph of Schatzki's ring appearance on barium swallow.

tion and inflammation of GERD leads to submucosal fibrosis. Schatzski's rings are usually easily treated by a single dilation, which is successful in about half of cases.[45] Patients with Schatzski's ring are more likely to have GERD than is the general population.[45] A long history of reflux symptoms, together with progressive dysphagia, first to solids and later to softer foods and liquids, implies a peptic stricture due to scarring. All patients with the symptom of dysphagia should have endoscopy and biopsies to exclude a malignant stricture. This may occur in Barrett's esophagus with esophageal adenocarcinoma.

Odynophagia, which is painful swallowing, is not common, but occurs with mucosal disease such as erosive esophagitis or ulceration. It is more usually associated with esophageal candidiasis, which may be secondary to a severe motor disorder such as scleroderma.

Angina-like symptoms may occur as a result of chronic GERD. Many patients with symptoms that appear to be due to angina have negative cardiac workups. In these patients, esophageal testing may indicate a spastic abnormality of the esophagus or the presence of GERD. However, microvascular angina may also produce symptoms of this nature, and careful testing must be carried out to ensure that the correct diagnosis for the chest pain is made.

Water brash is due to excessive salivation. Reflux of acid into the lower esophagus stimulates salivary production, which induces swallowing and aids in acid clearance. In some patients, this may produce a feeling of fullness in the throat, which is described as the *globus sensation.* The globus sensation is more commonly found in patients with gastric acid hypersecretion, possibly resulting in acid gastroesophageal reflux.

Various respiratory symptoms can occur with GERD. Patients may complain of nighttime cough, recurrent pneumonia, asthma, or unexplained fevers. Respiratory complications are frequently encountered in patients with esophageal motility disorders, such as scleroderma, preventing effective clearance of the refluxate.[46] Not all patients with pulmonary symptoms due to GERD have typical esophageal symptoms. It may be necessary to carry out manometry and 24-hour esophageal pH studies to establish this link, which can sometimes be confirmed by the disappearance of symptoms on adequate antireflux therapy. It is not certain whether these symptoms are due to reflex bronchospasm caused by esophageal vagal stimulation by acid or whether the bronchial spasm is induced by aspiration.[47]

Other symptoms that may be associated with GERD are bloating, early satiety, nausea, belching, and hiccups. These are commonly seen in GERD, but their etiology in relation to this disease is obscure. It is possible that they coexist as part of a generalized gut disorder related to GERD. Significant bleeding is a rare complication of GERD, but chronic blood loss may lead to iron deficiency anemia. This is particularly true in paraesophageal hernias. A careful evaluation should be made for other bleeding disorders in the gut.

Symptoms of GERD are not specific for the disease, and relying on symptoms alone for making the diagnosis can be misleading. The absence of symptoms, however, usually is sufficient to exclude the diagnosis of GERD.

COMPLICATIONS

As the severity of GERD increases, so does the risk of complications. These complications include severe esophagitis, Barrett's esophagus, ulceration, and stricture. A simple classification of the severity of endoscopic esophagitis is shown in Table 1-1.

Barrett's Esophagus

Barrett's esophagus is diagnosed when a columnar lining to the esophagus is recognized more than 2 to 3 cm above the LES area (Fig. 1-7). This is not unusual and has been recognized in up to 2% of the population. It has a bimodal age distribution in late childhood and the sixth decade and is now known to be the result of chronic GERD with metaplasia of the squamous lining to a columnar lining. Reflux is thought to result in destruction and desquamation of the squamous epithelium, with replacement by the inherently more acid-resistant columnar epithelium. Patients with Barrett's esophagus have been found to have a more defective LES than other patients with GERD.[48] These patients

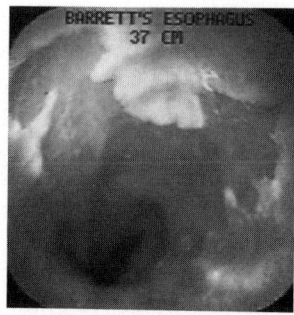

Figure 1-7 Endoscopic appearance of Barrett's esophagus. (See Color Fig. 1-7.)

also have decreased amplitude of contractions in the distal esophagus. Increased duodenogastric reflux has been reported in patients with Barrett's esophagus.[49] Combined esophageal and gastric pH monitoring have shown that esophageal exposure to pH over 7.0, together with evidence of abnormal duodenogastric reflux, occurs in patients with Barrett's esophagus. These patients have a higher incidence of gastric and esophageal alkalinization than other patients with esophagitis (Fig. 1-8). The treatment of patients with Barrett's esophagus is controversial because prolonged therapy against acid may be contraindicated in a disease that may be potentially produced by alkaline exposure. Experiments in rats have indicated that damage to the esophageal mucosa by alkaline reflux is worsened by the addition of acid suppression with omeprazole or by vagotomy. Continued medical therapy, however, has not been associated with a significant increase in the

Table 1-1   Savary-Miller Classification of Reflux Esophagitis

Grade	Endoscopic Features
I	One or more supravestibular nonconfluent mucosal lesions with or without exudate or superficial erosions; may be accompanied by erythema
II	Confluent erosive, exudative lesions
III	Circumferential erosive, exudative lesions with mural inflammatory infiltration
IV	Chronic mucosal disease: ulcers, mural fibrosis, strictures, scarring with columnar epithelium, or short esophagus

(After Ollyo JB, Fantolliet C, Brossard E, Long F. Savary's new endoscopic classification of reflux esophagitis. Act Endosc 1992;22:307)

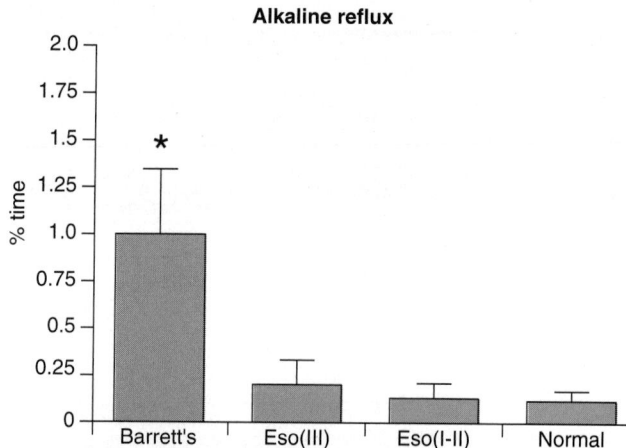

Figure 1-8 Patients with Barrett's esophagus have a higher exposure to alkali than normal subjects and other patients with reflux disease and varying degrees of esophagitis. Eso(III), grade III esophagitis; Eso(I–II), grade I or II esophagitis. *$P < .01$.

level of columnar epithelium in the esophagus. These patients, however, should undergo regular surveillance for dysplastic or malignant change.

Surgical therapy for Barrett's esophagus is advised in patients who are resistant to medical therapy and in those who develop complications such as ulceration, stricture, or severe dysplasia. Antireflux procedures, such as the Nissen fundoplication,[50] relieve symptoms and may even prevent extension of the columnar epithelium.[51] It is unclear whether the progression to dysplasia or malignancy is arrested by surgery, but some evidence suggests that dysplastic changes may stop or even reverse.[52] However, reports have been made of adenocarcinoma developing in Barrett's esophagus after antireflux surgery.

Ulceration

Esophageal mucosal ulceration due to severe GERD usually occurs at the squamocolumnar junction and is sometimes associated with stricture formation. Solitary ulcers are seen in Barrett's esophagus and are typically found in the middle of the columnar epithelium. Ulcers are an indication of severe disease and may heal by stricture formation. About two thirds of ulcers may be healed with medical therapy; however, this may take some months to achieve. Patients should be carefully interrogated to obtain a history of ingestion of pills, such as nonsteroidal antiinflammatory drugs, iron, and potassium, which are known to damage the esophageal mucosa.

Esophageal Stricture

Reflux patients with stricture are generally older, have a longer duration of reflux symptoms, have significantly reduced LES pressures, and more frequently display abnormal esophageal motility. Conditions that predispose to stricture formation include scleroderma, Zollinger-Ellison syndrome, and achalasia after balloon dilation. The morbidity of peptic strictures includes the increased risk of food impaction, the propensity for pulmonary aspiration, frequent coexistence of Barrett's esophagus, and the need for esophageal dilation with the occasional complication of perforation. Patients with esophageal strictures have a higher frequency of esophageal body dysmotility than patients without strictures (64% versus 32%). The most common abnormality is simultaneous or repetitive contractions. Complete aperistalsis may eventually occur and has a poor prognosis. It is not known whether the peristaltic dysfunction results from esophagitis or reflects a primary motor disorder predisposing to stricture formation. Patients with esophageal strictures tend to have higher acid secretion than patients with uncomplicated reflux. In addition, significant alkaline exposure occurs in Barrett's esophagus patients with the complication of stricture. Hiatal hernia is a common finding in patients with stricture; 42% of reflux patients without endoscopic esophagitis, 63% of those with endoscopic esophagitis, and 85% of patients with a peptic stricture have hiatal hernias.[53]

Peptic strictures are usually located near the squamocolumnar junction and are usually 1 or 2 cm long. Only occasionally are more extensive strictures found

Table 1-2 Differential Diagnosis of Benign Esophageal Strictures

Peptic and Miscellaneous Strictures	Infections	Drugs
Acid or alkaline reflux	*Monilia* (*Candida*)	Antibiotics such as doxycycline
Caustic injection	Tuberculosis	Potassium chloride
Nasogastric tube or trauma	Crohn's disease	Quinidine
Rings or webs	Typhoid	Salicyclates and nonsteroidal antiinflammatory
Postoperative	Cytomegalovirus	drugs
Epidermolysis bullosa	Herpes	Ascorbic acid
Esophageal atresia		Oral contraceptives
Down's syndrome		Parasulfate
Sclerotherapy		Phenytoin
Radiation		Clinitest
Eosinophilic esophagitis		Emperonium bromide
Sarcoidosis		
Amyloidosis		
Submucosal tumors		

(After Marks RD, Richter JE. Peptic strictures of the esophagus. Am J Gastroenterol 1993;88:1160)

Table 1-3 Indications for Surgical Treatment of Esophageal Strictures

Inability to adequately dilate a stricture
Frequent recurrence of stricture
Inability to control gastroesophageal reflux disease
Extraesophageal manifestations such as recurrent aspiration
    pneumonia
Prohibitive cost or noncompliance with long-term medical
    treatment

in reflux disease. Predisposing conditions should be sought and identified. These include a history of an indwelling nasogastric tube, pill esophagitis, or Zollinger-Ellison syndrome. The differential diagnosis of benign esophageal strictures includes infections and drug-induced strictures (Table 1-2). Congenital causes include tracheoesophageal fistula.

Patients usually present with dysphagia, chest pain, or chronic cough. Symptoms of GERD occur in most patients; however, 25% deny antecedent symptoms. Forty-four percent of strictures are associated with Barrett's esophagus.

Most strictures can be treated by antacid medication and esophageal dilation. Three types of dilators are used:

- Mercury-filled rubber bougies (eg, Maloney and Hurst)
- Fixed-size dilators passed over an endoscopically placed guide wire (eg, Eder-Puestow, Celestin, Buess, and Savary-Gilliard)
- Balloon dilators passed over an endoscopically placed guide wire and inflated at the site of the stricture

Relief from dysphagia is usually provided by creating a lumen diameter larger than 14 mm (44F). The success rate for dilation is over 90%, with a complication rate of 0.4% to 0.6%. Dilation might be expected to increase gastroesophageal reflux, but this has not been found to be the case on pH testing.[54] In patients who require frequent dilation, have strictures complicated by bleeding or ulceration, or have continued reflux symptoms despite medical therapy, antireflux surgery should be considered. About one fourth of patients eventually require surgery, which has a 70% to 90% success rate in controlling symptoms. A biliary diversion procedure may be added to the antireflux operation if there is clear evidence of alkaline disease. The main indications to proceed with surgical intervention are shown in Table 1-3.

Patients who have undergone surgical therapy re-

quire fewer subsequent dilations than those on medical therapy. Surgical patients required an average of 1.6 subsequent dilations, versus an average of 3.1 subsequent dilations after medical therapy. Some patients with severe strictures or with absent or poor esophageal body motility may be considered for esophagectomy and esophageal replacement by an interposed segment of colon or small bowel. A Thal fundic patch[55] or diversion of duodenal content with vagotomy and antrectomy or the "duodenal switch"[56] should be considered in patients with obvious alkaline reflux disease.

PARAESOPHAGEAL HIATAL HERNIA

Hiatal hernias have been classified into three types. The most common is the *sliding hiatal hernia*, in which the gastroesophageal junction migrates into the chest through the esophageal hiatus (Fig. 1-9). This is associated with GERD. The second is the *paraesophageal hernia*,

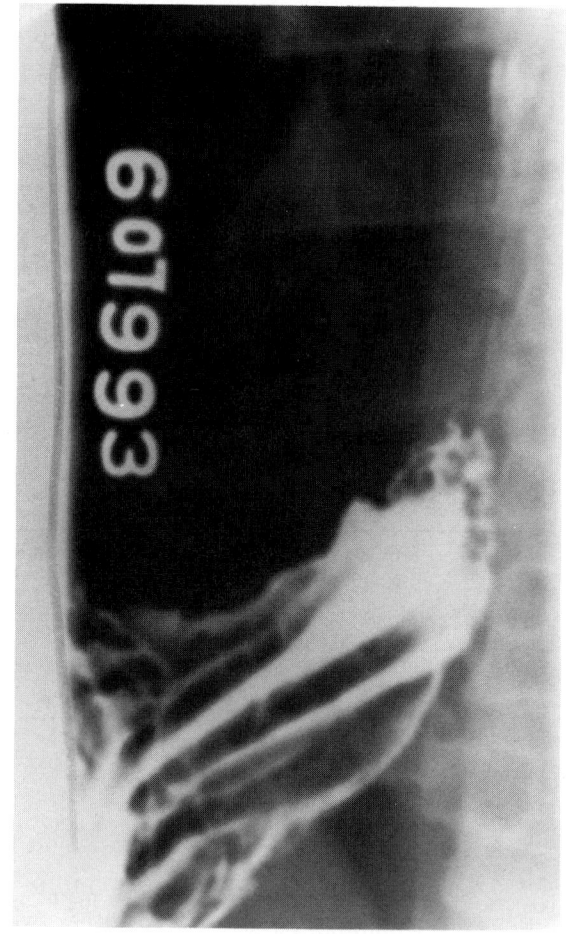

Figure 1-9 Typical sliding hiatal hernia.

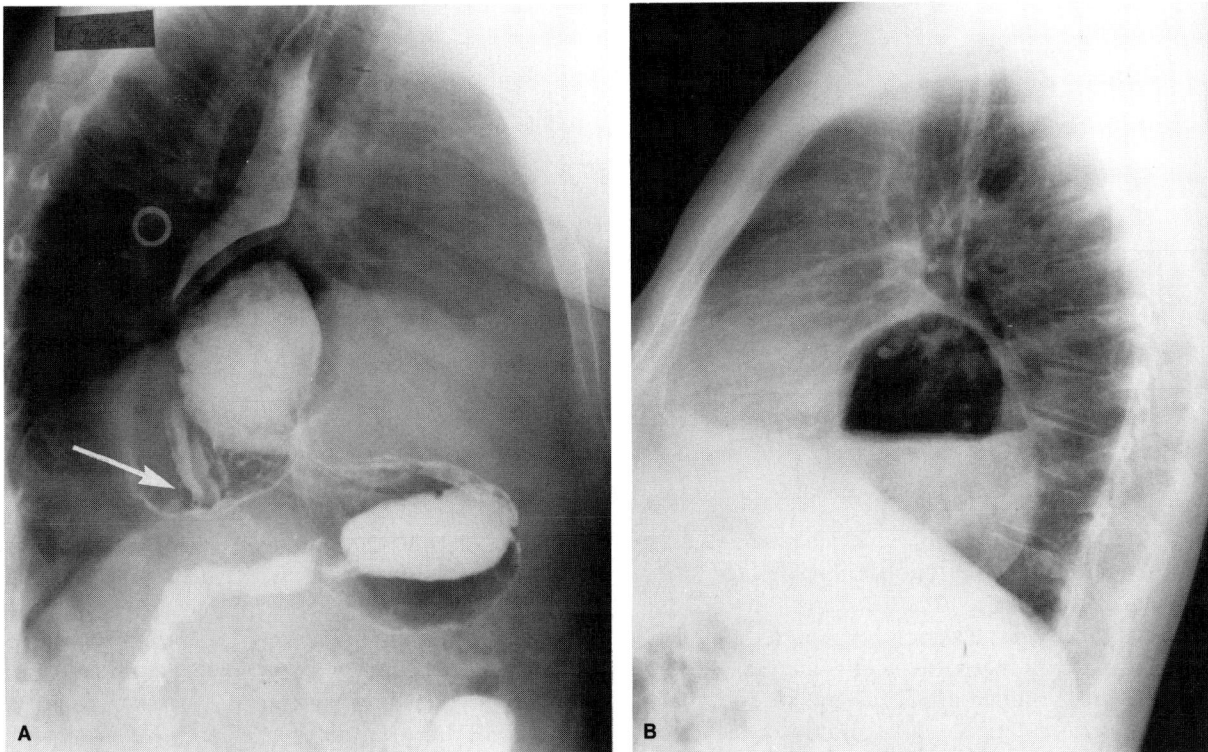

Figure 1-10 (**A**) Paraesophageal, or rolling, hiatal hernia. Lower esophageal sphincter (*arrow*) is in normal position. (**B**) Lateral chest radiograph of paraesophageal hernia with gas- and fluid-filled stomach.

in which the fundus of the stomach herniates into the thorax in association with a normally positioned gastroesophageal junction (Fig. 1-10). These hernias are rare and are not usually associated with GERD symptoms but present with obstructive symptoms or bleeding. The third type is the *mixed hernia,* in which both the gastroesophageal junction and the fundus of the stomach herniate into the thorax (Fig. 1-11). These may be regarded as a variant of the true paraesophageal hernia.

The incidence of paraesophageal hernia varies from 3.5% to 33% of all hiatal hernias, depending on the criteria for diagnosis. The condition occurs in older patients, with a median age of 61 years, as opposed to patients with sliding hernias, whose median age is 48 years. A widened hiatus anterior to the esophagus, possibly congenital in origin, is often found in patients with a paraesophageal hernia. Occasionally, the left bundle of the right crus of the diaphragm is absent, and the defect extends into the left leaf of the diaphragm. It is most common for the fundus to rotate up into the chest along the longitudinal axis of the stomach (organoaxial volvulus; Fig. 1-12). Rotation may also occur

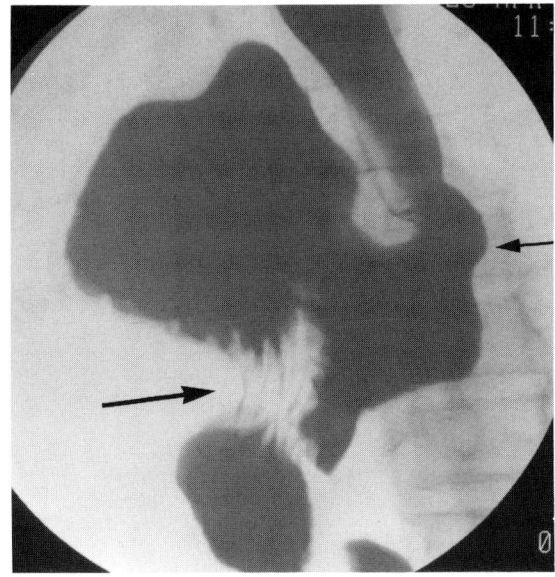

Figure 1-11 Sliding and rolling, or mixed, hiatal hernia. Upper arrow indicates lower esophageal sphincter; lower arrow indicates diaphragm.

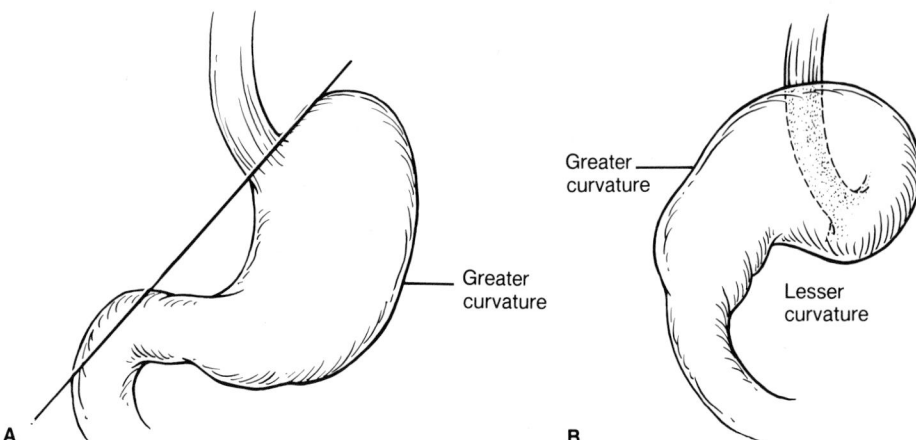

Figure 1-12 Organoaxial paraesophageal hernia. (After Menguy R. Surgical management of large parasophageal hernia with complete intrathoracic stomach. World J Surg 1988;12:415)

around the transverse axis (mesentericoaxial volvulus; Fig. 1-13), but this is less common. Paraesophageal hernia may occur after antireflux procedures in which the esophageal hiatus is not adequately reapproximated after dissection. Other mechanisms include surgical disruption of the phrenoesophageal membrane, postoperative gastric dilation, and failure to recognize esophageal shortening or an existing hiatal defect at surgery. A study in children indicated a 16.8% incidence of paraesophageal hernia after Nissen fundoplication.[57] This was frequently seen in patients in whom the esophageal hiatus had not been formally closed during the operative procedure. This indicates the need for this maneuver during surgical therapy.

The most common symptom is dysphagia and fullness after meals. Symptoms of GERD are uncommon. Some patients present with anemia due to chronic blood loss. The bleeding may be due to gastritis, ulcer-

ation, or vascular engorgement caused by venous obstruction at the hiatus. Gastric ulceration may occur at the point of constriction or within the herniated stomach. Twenty-three percent of patients with paraesophageal hernias have been reported to have gastric ulceration.[58] Twenty percent of patients with paraesophageal hernias present as surgical emergencies with excessive bleeding, incarceration, volvulus, strangulation, or perforation.

The condition is usually easily diagnosed on barium roentgenography, and the entire stomach may be found to lie within the chest cavity (see Fig. 1-11). Endoscopy can confirm the presence of a paraesophageal hernia, although the gastroscopic picture may be confusing in the presence of a paraesophageal hernia because of the distortion of the stomach. It is often difficult to intubate or identify the pylorus.

The presence of a paraesophageal hernia is usually

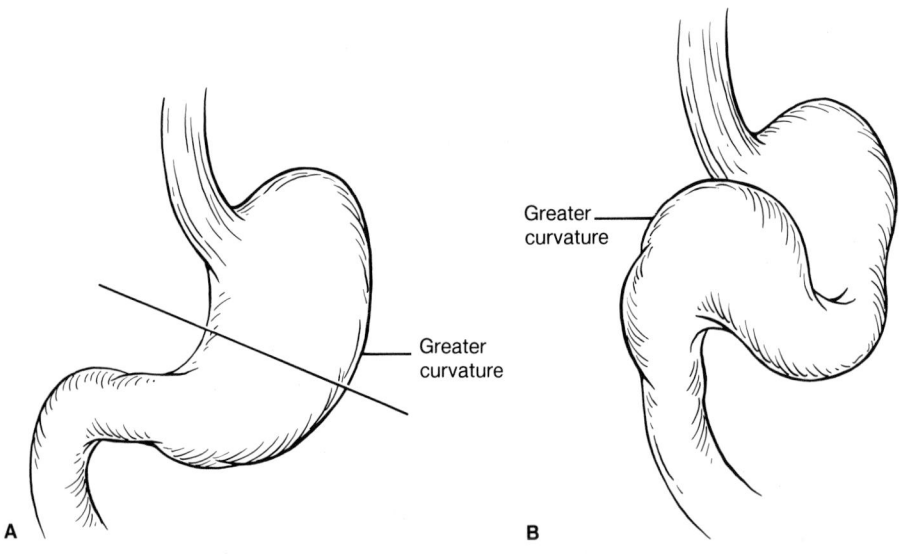

Figure 1-13 Mesentericoaxial paraesophageal hernia. (After Menguy R. Surgical management of large paraesophageal hernia with complete intrathoracic stomach. World J Surg 1988;12:415)

an indication for surgical repair. In one series of 21 patients treated conservatively,[59] 6 died of complications of strangulation, perforation, severe hemorrhage, or acute dilation of the herniated stomach. During surgical therapy, the stomach should be replaced in the abdomen, the sac dissected out of the mediastinum and excised, the hiatal defect closed, and usually an antireflux procedure added. If the LES is in good position and the phrenoesophageal membrane appears to be intact, an antireflux procedure may not be necessary. If the gastroesophageal junction is mobile, some have suggested the use of a posterior gastropexy in the form of a Hill procedure.

MEDICAL MANAGEMENT

Once the diagnosis of GERD has been made, patients should be advised on life-style modifications. These should include elevation of the head of the bed, weight reduction, avoidance of tight clothing, diet modification including the avoidance of late evening meals, cessation of smoking, and avoidance of drugs that decrease the LES pressure. These patients usually obtain relief by over-the-counter antacids taken as required. In patients with more severe disease, prokinetic agents, such as metoclopramide and cisapride, may be of use. These patients usually are treated with histamine-2 (H$_2$) receptor antagonists and mucosal coating drugs such as sucralfate. Drugs such as Gaviscon create a floating barrier on the gastric content to protect the esophageal mucosa from gastroesophageal reflux. Those with severe esophagitis may require high-dose H$_2$-receptor antagonists or powerful suppression of acid secretion with proton pump inhibitors such as omeprazole. A scheme for the medical therapy of GERD is shown in Table 1-4.

Antacids are commonly used to treat symptoms of GERD. Antacids may temporarily neutralize gastric acid and provide relief from symptoms, but they have a short duration of action, do not control nocturnal acid secretion, and may cause rebound acid secretion. They are an inexpensive form of therapy and remain important in controlling mild symptoms. Aluminum-containing antacids bind bile acids, decreasing the damaging effect of these substances on the esophageal mucosa. Certain prokinetic drugs have been used to improve LES pressure, enhance esophageal peristalsis, and augment gastric emptying. These include bethanechol, metoclopramide, domperidone, cisapride, and erythromycin. None of these drugs has a pronounced effect in decreasing GERD or in improving healing. They are usually used in combination with antacid medications.

The most commonly used inhibitors of acid secretion that are prescribed are the H$_2$-receptor antagonists, which work at the histamine receptor sites on the parietal cells in the stomach. They have been found to decrease gastric acid secretion by 60% to 70%.[60] The efficacy of these agents depends on the duration of therapy and the severity of mucosal damage before instituting therapy.[61] In patients with mild esophagitis, there is a 65% to 70% healing rate at 6 weeks, which can be increased to 80% to 90% at 12 weeks. However, in patients with moderate esophagitis, these figures fall to 40% to 45% healing at 6 weeks and 60% to 65% healing at 12 weeks. In patients with severe reflux esophagitis, the healing rate at 6 weeks is only 20% to 30% and 30% to 50% at 12 weeks. Treatment with high doses of H$_2$-receptor blockers has been found to increase the rate of healing. Despite this, most patients have a relapse of their disease when treatment is stopped. After 1 year of treatment, over 75% of patients have recurrence of GERD. This has led to the use of low-dose H$_2$-receptor blockers in long-term therapy. The long-term effect of medical therapy for GERD is disappointing, however, and many patients experience relapse unless they are on high-dose antacid therapy. Resistance to these drugs may also occur, and some patients who have initially gained relief from their symptoms may eventually get recurrence of their disease. The use of low-dose H$_2$-receptor blockers or weakened omeprazole shows a steady rise in relapse of the disease with time, with only 50% to 60% remaining healed after 6 months of therapy.

The advent of drugs able to poison the proton pump has somewhat improved the healing rate on medical therapy. A single daily dose of omeprazole can inhibit

Table 1-4 Medical Therapy of Gastroesophageal Reflux Disease

MILD ESOPHAGITIS
Elevation of the head of the bed
Weight reduction
Diet modification, avoidance of late-evening meals
Cessation of smoking
Avoidance of drugs that decrease lower esophageal sphincter pressure
Antacids
Antacids and alginates

MODERATE ESOPHAGITIS
Prokinetic agents
Mucosal coating agents
H$_2$-receptor antagonists (standard dose)

EROSIVE ESOPHAGITIS
H$_2$-receptor antagonists (high dose)
Omeprazole (standard dose)

REFRACTORY ESOPHAGITIS
Omeprazole (high dose)
Combination therapy

acid secretion by more than 90%. In a controlled randomized trial, esophagitis was healed in 57% to 74% of patients after 4 weeks of omeprazole therapy and in 78% to 97% after 8 weeks.[62] This was significantly greater than in patients treated with H_2-receptor antagonists. About 10% of patients with severe esophagitis do not heal, even on high-dose omeprazole therapy. This suggests that there may be other factors in addition to acid reflux in the pathogenesis of their disease. A likely candidate is alkaline duodenal secretions. Experiments in rats have shown that with duodenoesophageal reflux, esophageal damage is worsened by administration of acid blockers. At this time, omeprazole has only been released for short-term therapy because of the dangers of hypergastrinemia, which occurs with long-term acid suppression. This potentially can cause overgrowth of the gastric and esophageal mucosa and has been associated with carcinoid tumors in rats. Acid suppression by omeprazole or vagotomy in rats increases esophageal and gastric mucosal weight and DNA content. A metaanalysis of patients on medical therapy has shown that the best response to long-term medical therapy is achieved in patients with mild to moderate esophagitis, older patients, and those with minimal symptoms of regurgitation. This indicates the generally poor value of medical therapy in severe disease. Further predictors of a poor outcome include heartburn, regurgitation, and the number of symptoms. The success of surgical therapy is less dependent on the severity of disease.

SURGICAL THERAPY

Surgical therapy has evolved from the Allison repair,[63] in which the hiatal hernia was reduced and the esophageal hiatus was narrowed. In view of the fact that this procedure did little to restore LES function, the results were poor. As an understanding of the pathogenetic mechanisms in GERD emerged, effective surgical procedures were developed aimed at improving these defects. Surgical therapy revolves around the goals shown in Table 1-5. In addition, highly selective vagotomy may be added to decrease gastric acid secretion in patients with preexisting ulcer disease or gastric acid hypersecretion. Similarly, in those in whom clear evidence for alkaline GERD has been established, biliary diversion may be employed. This may take the form of a Roux-en-Y anastomosis or the duodenal switch procedure.[56]

Indications

Surgery should only be contemplated in patients who have failed medical therapy and who have definite evidence of a weak LES in the presence of reasonably good

Table 1-5 Objectives of Surgical Therapy for Gastroesophageal Reflux Disease

Reduction of the hiatal hernia and replacement of the lower esophageal sphincter into the abdomen

Establishment of an adequate intraabdominal portion of esophagus

Re-creation of the esophagogastric angle at the hiatus to act as a nonrefluxing valve

Support of the lower esophageal sphincter area with a fundic wrap to assist in increasing resting lower esophageal sphincter pressure

Approximation of the crura to hold the fundoplication in the abdomen and to assist in creating adequate sphincter pressure

esophageal body motility. Care must be taken to exclude secondary forms of the disease, such as those related to gastric acid hypersecretion, gastroparesis caused by metabolic disorders such as diabetes mellitus, and primary disturbances of esophageal clearance function, as occur in systemic sclerosis. Because the symptoms of GERD are often nonspecific, other functional foregut disorders with similar symptoms should be excluded, such as diffuse esophageal spasm, nutcracker esophagus, achalasia, and primary duodenogastric reflux. It is also important to consider and exclude ischemic heart disease as a cause of chest pain.

Surgery is indicated in all patients with severe reflux esophagitis (grades III and IV), particularly in patients who fail to respond to medical therapy. These patients are at high risk for developing complications, and long-term medical therapy is not often successful. Medical therapy fails in a high proportion of patients with severe reflux esophagitis.[64,65] Surgery should also be considered in patients with low-grade esophagitis (grades I and II) who have symptoms while taking medication. Patients with complications such as ulceration, stricture, and severe Barrett's esophagus are also good candidates for surgery. In all patients being considered for surgical therapy, the presence of a mechanically defective sphincter should be verified. This is defined as a sphincter with a resting pressure below 6 mmHg, an intraabdominal sphincter length of less than 1 cm, or a total sphincter length of less than 2 cm. These all would predispose to persistent reflux disease.[66] The response to medical therapy over more than one decade is less than satisfactory under these conditions.[64] GERD may also present with respiratory symptoms, such as chronic laryngitis, pulmonary aspiration, recurrent pneumonia, and even asthma. Only about half of these patients have a history of heartburn or show endoscopic evidence of severe reflux esophagitis. These patients should undergo pulmonary function studies and 24-hour esophageal pH monitoring in an attempt to confirm the relation between acid reflux and respiratory symptoms. A positive reflux score on 24-hour pH testing with reflux-induced chronic wheezing or asthma attacks, in addition to an incompetent sphincter diagnosed by manometry, presents a strong indication for surgical intervention. In some patients, the presence of a large hiatal hernia may result in severe dysphagia, which may in its own right demand surgical therapy.[67]

Methods

The most commonly performed surgical procedures for GERD are the Nissen fundoplication[50] (Fig. 1-14), the Hill procedure,[68] the Toupet procedure,[69] and the Belsey operation.[70]

Nissen Fundoplication

See Section III of Atlas Chapter 5 for a step-by-step description of the Nissen fundoplication.

The Nissen fundoplication (see Fig. 1-14*A*) was first described in 1956 and, with a 90% success rate at 10 years, has been demonstrated to be an effective procedure for GERD.[50,71] The original technique, using the anterior and posterior wall for the construction of the wrap, was associated with considerable side effects that have encouraged modifications. Subsequently, a technique of fundoplication was developed that relies on wrapping only the anterior wall of the fundus around the distal esophagus.[72] This technique is considered to allow a more precise formation of the fundic wrap. Most recently, techniques for performance of the

"floppy" Nissen fundoplication have been developed, which has become the standard procedure in many centers.[73]

FLOPPY NISSEN FUNDOPLICATION, TRANSAB-DOMINAL APPROACH. The approach is through an upper midline laparotomy with exposure of the esophageal hiatus. The gastrohepatic ligament is divided. Care should be taken to avoid damaging the hepatic branches of the vagus nerve, an aberrant left hepatic artery, or the left gastric artery. The incision of the gastrohepatic ligament is then continued over the anterior surface of the esophagus with division of the parietal peritoneum over the esophagus. The fat pad that usually covers the anterior surface of the cardia and esophagus is removed. Special care must be taken because this tissue contains large blood vessels and the anterior trunk of the vagus nerve adherent to the esophagus. Bleeding in this area leads to poor visualization and difficulty in the identification of anatomic structures. After blunt finger dissection of the esophagus, the posterior trunk of the vagus is identified, and a sling is passed around the esophagus, excluding the posterior nerve. Retraction on the sling opens the space behind the esophagus, allowing identification of the right and left crura of the esophageal hiatus.

The next step is to mobilize the gastric fundus. The short gastric vessels are divided starting at a point about 10 cm aboral from the angle of His. It is important to the success of the operation that the gastric fundus is completely mobilized to allow a tension-free fundoplication around the esophagus without including the gastric corpus. Blood vessels passing from the greater cur-

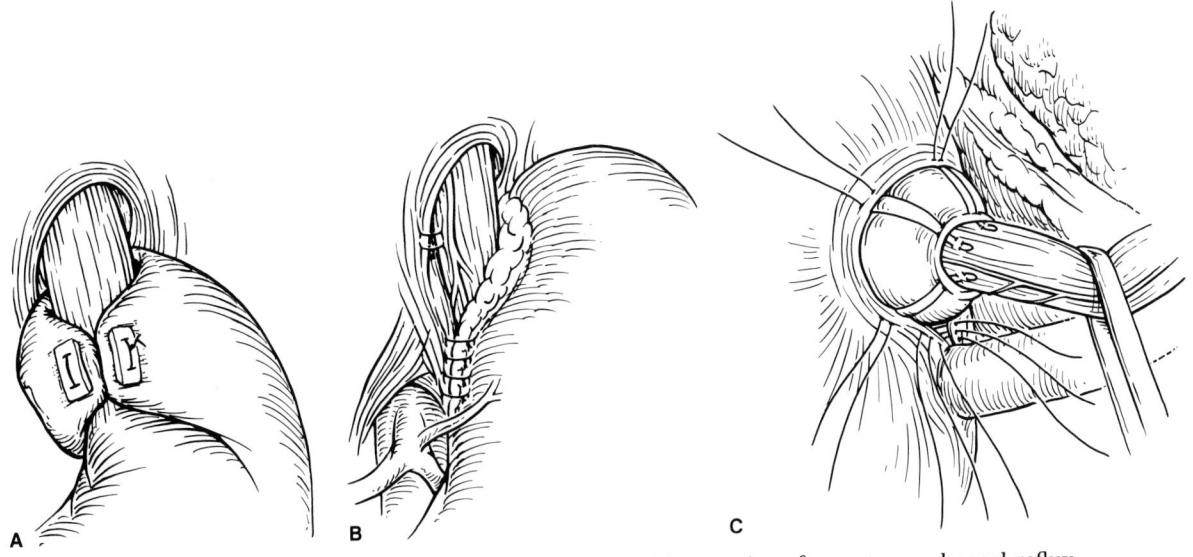

Figure 1-14 The Nissen (**A**), Hill (**B**), and Belsey (**C**) operations for gastroesophageal reflux disease.

vature of the stomach to the retroperitoneum should also be divided. These are mainly found on the most superior part of the greater curvature.

It is then possible to proceed with the repair. The first step is approximation of the crura. A 56F to 60F Maloney bougie is passed into the esophagus by the anesthesiologist, and the left and right crura are approximated with three or four nonabsorbable sutures behind the dilator. The mobilized fundus is grasped with a Babcock tissue forceps at a point about 5 to 6 cm from the angle of His measured along the greater curvature and brought behind the esophagus. This is fixed around the esophagus to a more distal part of the fundus so that they snugly approximate over a size 56F to 60F Maloney bougie placed in the esophageal lumen. For the approximation of the left and right fundal wrap around the esophagus, a U-shaped 2-0 Prolene suture is used. This suture also includes the muscle wall of the esophagus to hold the wrap in place and to prevent the stomach from slipping up through the fundoplication. The suture is buttressed using two Teflon felt pledgets, one on each side of the fundic wrap. When the suture is tied, it should be possible to insert the index finger between esophagus and fundic wrap. A second simple suture may be added either above or below this to snug the fundoplication to the desired tension around the esophagus. The wrap is made no longer than 2 cm in length.

SUMMARY OF IMPORTANT COMPONENTS OF THE OPERATION

1. The wrap should be loose. This is achieved by using a 56F to 60F Maloney bougie in the esophagus to size the tightness of the wrap. Furthermore, the wrap should be no longer than 2 cm to ensure a persistent postoperative dysphagia rate of less than 3%.[74]
2. The gastric fundus must be completely mobilized to avoid torsion of the esophagus, tension of the wrap, or inclusion of gastric corpus in the wrap, which may lead to incomplete swallowing-induced relaxations of the sphincter with delayed esophageal clearance function.[74] The same effect may occur if a distal portion of the stomach is chosen for the construction of the fundoplication. The ideal point is about 5 to 6 cm distal to the angle of His, measured along the greater curvature.
3. The gastric fundus must be wrapped around the esophagus and not around the upper stomach. This would result in dysphagia and failure to control reflux.
4. The crural repair is important because it helps to hold the fundoplication in the abdomen. Because the diaphragmatic crura are also part of

the barrier against reflux, the approximation of the crura supports the effect of the fundal wrap, especially under straining conditions.

Taking these issues into account, the floppy Nissen fundoplication provides a success rate of about 90% during a follow-up period of 10 years.[74] The LES resting pressure is significantly increased, with a substantial increase in intraabdominal length. Persistent dysphagia was decreased from 21% to 3% and temporary swallowing problems from 83% to 39% by following these principles. In addition, the incidence of complete sphincter relaxation after swallowing was increased from 31% to 71%.

A common failure of the Nissen fundoplication is slippage or disruption of the wrap. Various radiologic types of disruption have been demonstrated (Fig. 1-15). Type I represents complete, or almost complete, disruption of the wrap, with recurrence of the hiatal hernia in most cases. Type II involves slippage of part of the stomach above the diaphragm. An hourglass defect is created with part of the stomach above and part below the esophageal hiatus in the diaphragm. This is frequently caused by the wrap having been incorrectly placed around the upper stomach rather than around the esophagus. Type III may also be associated with an hourglass defect, since part of the stomach lies above and part lies below the fundoplication. This is the so-called slipped Nissen. This may occur as a result of slippage of the stomach through the wrap or incorrect placement of the wrap around the stomach at the time of surgery. Type IV occurs when the intact wrap herniates through the esophageal hiatus into the chest.

LAPAROSCOPIC NISSEN FUNDOPLICATION. The laparoscopic Nissen fundoplication has become our standard surgical procedure for GERD.[75] We elect to perform this operation in almost all cases regardless of the weight of the patient or whether there have been previous abdominal operations. If the esophagus is shortened, as evidenced by a fixed hernia measuring more than 5 cm, the laparoscopic technique is not used, and the repair is carried out by the thoracic approach. The laparoscopic procedure is performed in the same manner as for the conventional repair, with similar emphasis on the important points described earlier.

The preferred position for the patient is in steep reverse Trendelenburg. After establishing the pneumoperitoneum, 10-mm trocars are introduced into the abdominal cavity (Fig. 1-16). To obtain access to the hiatus, the left lobe of the liver is retracted with a liver retractor. Division of the triangular ligament is not recommended because the left liver lobe would drop into the operative field of view.

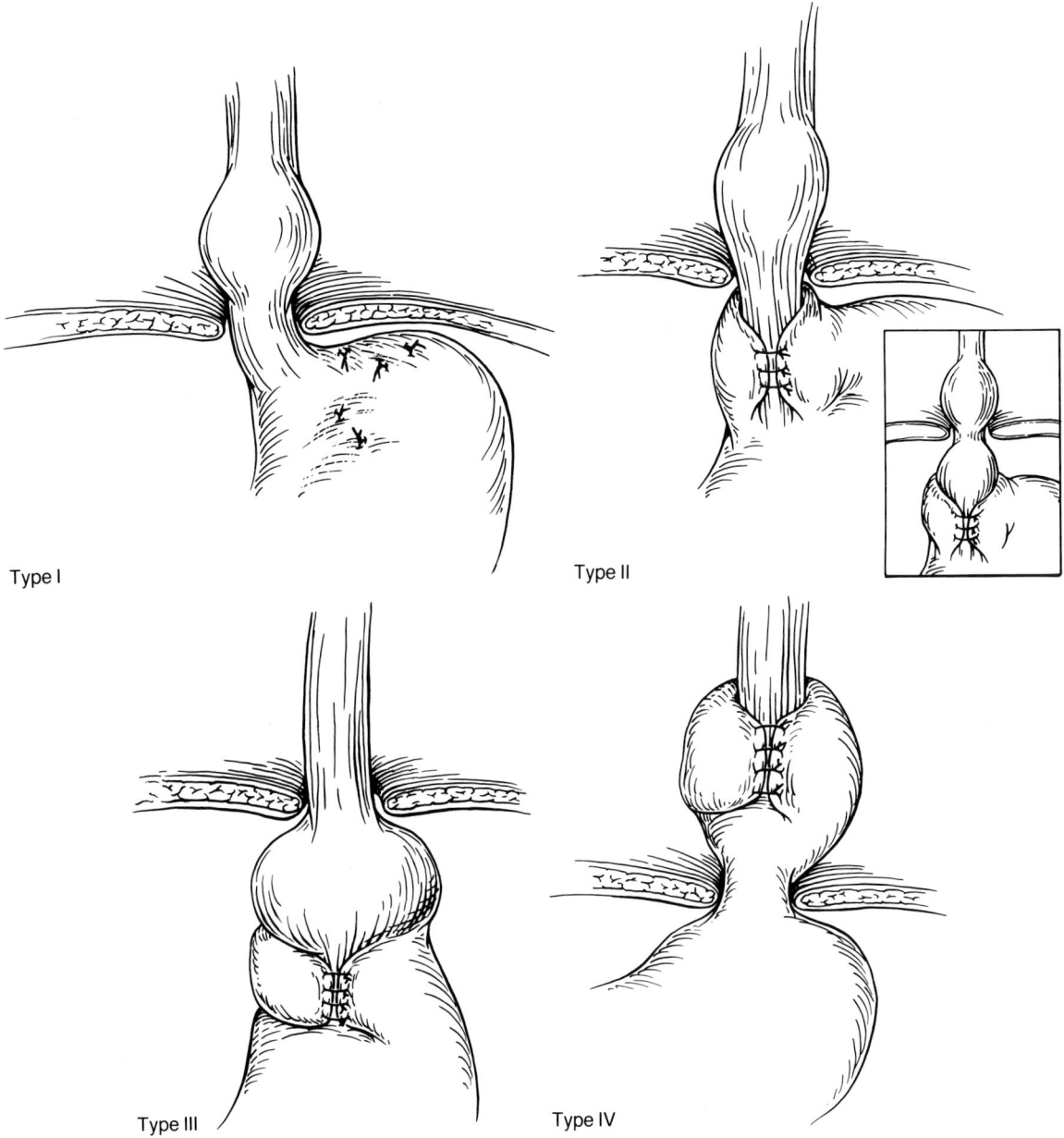

Type I

Type II

Type III

Type IV

Figure 1-15 Types of surgical failure of Nissen fundoplication.

The next step of the operation is the division of the gastrohepatic omentum superior to the hepatic branches of the vagus nerve. These can be seen passing through the omentum in thin patients. Damage to the left gastric artery or an aberrant hepatic artery must be avoided. The anterior edge of the right crus can then be seen and dissected off the right-hand side of the esophagus. Once the esophagus is identified, the posterior trunk of the vagus nerve can easily be separated from the esophagus. The fat pad over the gastric cardia and distal esophagus is then incised. This must be performed carefully to avoid damage to the esophagus and

the fairly large blood vessels frequently encountered. Bleeding from these vessels may lead to impaired visualization and can necessitate conversion to the open procedure.

Dissection of the crura is continued to establish the point where the left and right crura join anterior to the esophagus. The anterior part of the left crus can usually be separated from the esophagus without difficulty. The posterior portion of the left crus should be mobilized off the left side of the esophagus. To create a window behind the esophagus, it is necessary to elevate the esophagus from its right-hand side and to separate loose tis-

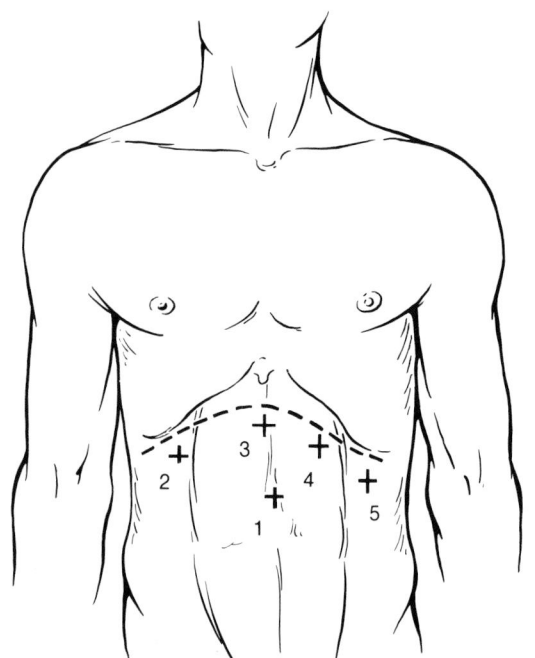

Figure 1-16 Placement of ports for laparoscopic Nissen fundoplication.

sue behind the esophagus. Dissection too far superiorly should be avoided because it may result in damage to the left pleura. Dissection too far inferiorly may result in muscle fibers of the esophagus or stomach being misidentified as crural fibers, resulting in perforation of these organs. Once this window is established, the crura are approximated as in the open procedure, with one or two nonabsorbable sutures placed in the crura behind the esophagus with a 56F to 60F Maloney bougie in place. The suture material used is 2-0 Prolene. The operation is continued with mobilization of the greater curvature in preparation for the fundoplication. This is performed in the same way as described for the open procedure. The short gastric vessels are double clipped. The repair can then be commenced. Choosing the part of the fundus for the wrap is carried out using the same criteria as for the open procedure. The fundus of the stomach is brought posteriorly behind the esophagus and approximated in exactly the same way as for the open procedure.

TRANSTHORACIC APPROACH TO NISSEN FUNDOPLICATION. The usual indication for the transthoracic approach is that the transabdominal approach is not possible. In very obese patients, the transabdominal procedure gives poor exposure, whereas the transthoracic approach allows for better visualization and a more accurate repair. This indication is now less clear,

however, because the laparoscopic technique provides good exposure even in obese patients. I have operated laparoscopically on patients weighing more than 300 pounds without difficulty. Shortening of the esophagus is indicated by a sliding hiatal hernia of more than 5 or 6 cm that does not reduce below the diaphragm in the upright position or under stretch during endoscopy or radiography. To allow placement of the fundoplication below the diaphragm without tension, maximal mobilization of the esophagus is required. This can best be achieved by the thoracic approach. In addition, it allows for a Collis gastroplasty to be used to gain extra length of the esophagus if the esophagus is still too short after extended mobilization.[76] In patients with a slipped fundoplication located in the chest, the thoracic approach allows for safe dissection, and if necessary, a circumferential incision in the diaphragm can be made, allowing simultaneous dissection from the abdominal side of the diaphragm. Patients with concomitant esophageal spasm or vigorous achalasia who require a long myotomy are best treated using the thoracic approach, as are patients with undefined pulmonary pathology on the left side, which requires operative evaluation.

After a posterolateral left-sided thoracotomy in the sixth intercostal space, mobilization of the esophagus is commenced from the diaphragm up to the aortic arch. Care has to be taken not to damage the thoracic duct or the trunks of the vagus nerve. In the presence of a previous hiatal hernia repair, the thoracotomy can be performed in the seventh intercostal space, which allows for better access to the abdomen through a circumferential incision in the diaphragm. The diaphragmatic incision is made about 3 cm from the chest wall and is about 10 to 15 cm in length. After extensive esophageal mobilization, the hernial sac can be dissected off the diaphragm. This can be achieved through the hiatus or through the circumferential diaphragmatic incision. After division of all attachments, the gastric fundus is pulled into the chest. A few short gastric vessels must be divided. The fat pad on the anterior surface of the distal esophagus and cardia is dissected, taking care to avoid damage to the anterior trunk of the vagus nerve. The posterior trunk must be identified and dissected off the esophagus. The next step is to place the sutures for the approximation of the diaphragmatic crura. Four to six sutures are usually necessary. They are not tied at this time. The fundoplication is then constructed. The fundus is wrapped around the distal esophagus proximal to the angle of His. The U-shaped suture for the fixation of the wrap is placed by the same technique as in the abdominal procedure, except that it is located more posteriorly. Before placing this suture, a 56F to 60F Maloney bougie is passed through the esophagus into the stomach by the anesthesiologist. The fundoplication is placed in the abdomen. If the tension on the esophagus is not too great, the fundoplication will remain in the abdominal cavity even when the diaphragm is gently manipulated. The crural sutures can then be tied. If the fundoplication tends to slide back into the chest, the esophagus should be further mobilized, which can be accomplished by division of the branches of the posterior vagus trunk to the left pulmonary plexus. If this maneuver fails, a Collis gastroplasty[76] or colon interposition has to be considered. This is only necessary in rare cases, particularly if the wrap is kept short.

Belsey Mark IV Operation

The Belsey Mark IV operation (see Fig. 1-14*C* and Section III of Atlas Chap. 5) is in principle a similar procedure to the transthoracic Nissen fundoplication. The thoracotomy is performed at the same site, and the mobilization of the esophagus is done in the same way. After mobilization of the esophagus, starting from the diaphragm and extending up to the aortic arch, the hernial sac is freed from all its attachments. The posterior trunk of the vagus nerve is protected, and the gastric fundus is pulled into the chest. A few short gastric vessels must be divided. The sutures for approximation of the diaphragmatic crura are placed as described earlier. The fundus is wrapped anteriorly around the esophagus. This lies at a 90-degree angle to the fundoplication achieved in the transthoracic Nissen fundoplication and comes to lie only around the anterior two thirds of the distal esophagus. The fundus is fixed to the esophagus with two rows of three U-shaped sutures each. The first row is placed about 1.5 cm above the gastroesophageal junction. The sutures grasp the esophageal muscle but do not traverse the entire wall. One of these sutures is placed on the anterior side of the esophagus, the other two on the right and left side. To place the suture on the right side, the esophagus has to be rotated. It is important that this suture is not placed too far anteriorly, which would result only in an anterolateral fundoplication of lower efficiency. The second row of U-shaped sutures is placed 1 or 2 cm above the first row, and these are carefully tied without strangulating the tissue. The tails of the sutures are not cut off; they are passed through the diaphragm from the abdominal to the thoracic surface about 1.5 cm apart on the edge of the hiatus. These sutures are placed at the 4-, 8-, and 12-o'clock positions. It is important to place the right lateral suture at exactly the 4-o'clock position and not too far anteriorly to avoid the creation of an anterolateral fundoplication. The fundoplication is placed into the abdomen, where it should remain if the esophagus

has been correctly mobilized as described earlier. The three diaphragmatic sutures are tied so that there is close apposition between the fundoplication and the diaphragm. Finally, the crural sutures are tied.

Hill Repair

The Hill repair depends on fixing the LES in the abdomen and on creating an angulation in the lower esophagus to prevent reflux (see Fig. 1-14*B* and Section III of Atlas Chap. 5). Through an upper midline abdominal incision, the liver is retracted in the same way as described for the abdominal approach to the Nissen fundoplication. The gastrohepatic ligament is divided, preserving the hepatic branches of the vagus nerve. The dissection is continued over the anterior surface of the esophagus. The loose fat pad anterior to the esophagus is dissected, taking care not to damage the anterior trunk of the vagus nerve. The right and left diaphragmatic crura are prepared as described for the Nissen procedure. The crura are dissected posteriorly to the point where they decussate over the aorta, and the preaortic fascia is identified and defined. The gastric fundus is mobilized along the greater curve in the same way as for the Nissen fundoplication. After identification of the posterior trunk of the vagus nerve, the esophagus is rotated clockwise when viewed from the abdomen, and both the anterior and posterior bundles of the phrenoesophageal ligament are visualized.

The first step of the repair is, as in all other procedures, the approximation of the crura. Five sutures are then placed through the anterior and posterior bundles of the phrenoesophageal ligament so that it is plicated at the right-hand side of the esophagus. These sutures also pass through the preaortic fascia. To do this safely, a finger has to be inserted into the hiatus beneath the preaortic fascia. The sutures may be buttressed by Teflon pledgets. These sutures can be tied over a 56F to 60F bougie in the esophagus or, as Hill originally described, by manometric control.[77] Hill ties the upper three sutures with a single throw and measures the sphincter resting pressure, which should be in the range of 35 to 45 mmHg. If this pressure level is obtained, all sutures are tied completely.

Other Techniques of Antireflux Surgery

Other fundoplication techniques are the Toupet repair[69] (see Section III of Atlas Chap. 5), which involves a 270-degree posterior fundoplication, and the Dor operation,[78] which is an anterior fundoplication. In the Toupet procedure, the diaphragmatic crura are sutured to the posterior fundic wrap, which restores their supporting effect on the LES and also prevents the wrap from slipping into the chest. Few data have been published about the efficacy of these procedures and their effect on the LES. In a randomized study, it was stated that the Toupet procedure is superior to the Nissen fundoplication.[69] In this study, the recent modifications of the Nissen procedure[74] were not employed. These include adequate fundic mobilization, crural repair, and a wrap of no more than 2 cm. The Toupet procedure has not yet been compared with a properly conducted Nissen repair.

The Angelchik prosthesis[79] is an ineffective technique for antireflux surgery and should no longer be used. It results in a high rate of persistent, severe dysphagia and does not control GERD effectively.[80] Complications such as migration of the prosthesis into the chest or erosion into the lumen of the esophagus or stomach have been described.

Evaluation of Various Antireflux Procedures

A metaanalysis of 1152 collected patients from 17 studies evaluating outcome after the open Nissen, Belsey, Rossetti, and Toupet operations was recently carried out by McCloy (personal communication). Eighty-seven percent of patients had esophagitis, 8% stricture, and 17% Barrett's esophagus before operation. Four patients died, giving an operative mortality of 0.35%. Splenectomy was required in 0.8%, and an esophageal

Table 1-6 Evaluation of Surgical Therapy for Gastroesophageal Reflux: Analysis of 1152 Procedures

	Occurrence (%)	
	Before Surgery	After Surgery
ESOPHAGITIS		
None	13	85–99
Mild to moderate	49	1–7
Severe	38	0–4
HEARTBURN		
None	0–10	82–94
Mild to moderate	10–50	6–18
Severe	40–90	0
REGURGITATION		
None	2–21	94
Mild to moderate	48–70	6
Severe	16–50	0
DYSPHAGIA		
None	68	69
Mild to moderate	28	29
Severe	4	2

Table 1-7 Long-Term Results (1–12 Years) After 1141 Open Nissen Fundoplication Procedures

Outcome	Occurrence (%)
Good result	87
Mild dysphagia	8
Gas bloat	8
Reflux recurrence	7
Death	1

(After Stein HJ, Delleester TR, Hinder RA. Outpatient physiologic testing and surgical management of foregut motility disorders. Curr Probl Surg 1992;29:521)

tear occurred in 0.4%. Four percent had an additional cholecystectomy for gallstones or vagotomy for peptic ulcer. Early postoperative results showed that 5% had pneumonia, 2% wound infections, and 1.2% incisional hernias. The global assessment of the surgical result at 5 years was considered to be excellent or good in 84% to 90% of cases and fair to poor in 10% to 16%. There was a 5% relapse rate at 5 years. A detailed analysis of the results is shown in Tables 1-6 and 1-7. Of significance is the fact that, unlike with medical therapy, there was no deterioration in the success of surgical therapy beyond the first year.

Lerut reported on the outcome of the transthoracic Belsey repair (personal communication). Evaluation at 1 year revealed the presence of mild esophagitis (grade 1) in 13.2% of patients. When globally evaluated, 77.5% were found to have a very good result, 7.5% had a good result, and 15% had a bad outcome. Dysphagia was seen in 2.8%, gas bloat occurred in 2.8%, and 8.8% complained of pain at the thoracotomy site.

Generally, the results of the Belsey operation are similar to those of the Nissen operation. Success rates of nearly 90% are reported.[71] The influence on the LES resting pressure and on the intraabdominal length is reported to be somewhat less after the Belsey operation than after the Nissen fundoplication. Side effects, such as temporary dysphagia, persistent dysphagia, and inability to belch or vomit, appear about as often as after the floppy Nissen operation. The frequency of temporary diarrhea appears to be less. Pulmonary complications are more commonly noted after the Belsey operation than after the transabdominal Nissen fundoplication.[81]

Although some have reported that the Nissen operation is superior to the Hill operation in controlling GERD symptoms, Hill demonstrated a success rate of nearly 90% in an early series without intraoperative manometry and 96% in a later series in which he evaluated the efficiency of the repair by intraoperative manometric measurements.[77] Temporary and persistent dysphagia is reported to occur more often after the Hill operation than after the floppy Nissen or Belsey fundoplication, but the inability to belch or vomit appears to occur less frequently.[71]

Results of Laparoscopic Nissen Fundoplication

At my center, we performed 154 laparoscopic Nissen fundoplications between July 1991 and July 1993. The median operative time was 2.5 hours. In 6 of the first 33 cases, the laparoscopic operation had to be converted to open laparotomy (Table 1-8). In the next 121 cases, only one patient required conversion, because of too severe adhesions from previous surgery. This indicates the long learning curve for the procedure, but once mastered, the technique becomes routine. In 6 cases, intraoperative complications occurred. These included bleeding from a short gastric artery necessitating conversion to open laparotomy, pneumothorax in three patients who did not require a chest drain or conversion to the open procedure, one gastric perforation treated by laparoscopic repair, and two perforations during dissection successfully treated by open repair. A duodenal perforation presented in an elderly patient on the fourth postoperative day. This patient died from intraabdominal sepsis and was the only mortality. Two patients had breakdown of the crural repair on postoperative days 3 and 5, associated with gastric distention and herniation of the stomach into the mediastinum. These were easily repaired by laparoscopy in one case and laparotomy in the other.

The length of postoperative hospital stay was 1 to 3 days in 63% of patients, and most of the remainder left the hospital by the fourth postoperative day. In more recent experience, few patients remain in hospital longer than 2 days.

Early postoperative complaints include transient dysphagia in most patients, bloating, early satiety, nausea, diarrhea, and chest pain. Most of these symptoms settle within 1 month. Long-term (4 to 24 months) complications are shown in Table 1-9. One patient had severe dysphagia due to a tight wrap, which necessitated reoperation. The long-term outcome has been excellent, with 83% of patients symptom-free at 4 to 24 months after surgery.

A comparison of preoperative and postoperative manometric findings showed that the total length of the LES did not change significantly, but there was an increase in intraabdominal length with elevation of the resting LES pressure similar to that seen after the open procedure.

Experience with laparoscopic Nissen fundoplication is accumulating in several centers, with series of 50 to 350 patients being reported by at least 10 surgeons. The mortality rate is less than 1%, with an acceptable morbidity. There have been reports of gastric or esophageal perforation (0.5% to 2%), bleeding (1% to 2%), pneumothorax (0% to 3%), pneumomediastinum (0% to 5%), small bowel perforation (0.5%), pulmonary complications (2% to 4%), pulmonary embolism (0% to 4%), herniation at a trocar site (0% to 2%), and wrap necrosis (one case). Follow-up over 3 months to 2.5 years has shown the presence of dysphagia (1% to 8%), regurgitation (2%), vomiting (1%), chest pain (3%), weight loss (1% to 45%), early satiety (0% to 15%), recurrent heartburn (0% to 5%), diarrhea (0% to 3%), and epigastric pain (0% to 2%). These are similar results to those seen after open surgery (see Tables 1-6 and 1-7).

Antireflux Surgery in Patients With Poor Esophageal Body Function

Several studies have reported esophageal body peristaltic disorders in reflux esophagitis.[82] Control of the reflux disease either medically or surgically does not substantially improve these motility disturbances. It might be expected that in patients with very poor esophageal body function (amplitudes in the distal esophagus be-

Table 1-9 Long-Term (4–24 Months) Outcome After 100 Laparoscopic Nissen Fundoplication Procedures

Outcome	Occurence (%)
No symptoms	83
Dysphagia (7 mild, 1 required reoperation)	8
Chest pain	4
Recurrent heartburn	2
Diarrhea	2
Return of asthma	1
Incisional hernia	1

Table 1-8 Reasons for Conversion of Laparoscopic Nissen Fundoplication to the Open Procedure

Difficulty in adequately exposing anatomy
Gastric or esophageal perforation
Bleeding
Adhesions from previous surgery

low 30 mmHg), antireflux surgery would result in an increased frequency of dysphagia. The frequency of postoperative dysphagia after the Belsey operation is in fact significantly increased in patients with poor esophageal body function.[81] It is not clear what the most suitable procedure is in such a situation, but it seems that it is best not to perform a 360-degree wrap in patients with poor esophageal function and to reserve the Belsey or Toupet procedure for these circumstances. Postoperative dysphagia is significantly more frequent after the Hill repair and least frequent after the Belsey fundoplication.[71] When the Nissen operation was modified as mentioned earlier (floppy Nissen operation), there was a dramatic decrease in early postoperative dysphagia from 83% to 39% and persistent dysphagia from 21% to 3%.[74] After an esophageal myotomy for achalasia or spastic conditions of the esophagus, I favor the Toupet partial fundoplication (see Section III of Atlas Chap. 5). The Dor antireflux procedure, in which only an anterior flap fundoplication is carried out, can also be used.

Analysis of Failures of Antireflux Surgery

Failure to control gastroesophageal reflux, persistent dysphagia, inability to belch or vomit, and gas bloat is frequently the result of a technical error in surgery or poorly indicated surgery. Inappropriate indications for surgery result from insufficient preoperative diagnostic testing. Surgery should only be considered in patients with a mechanically weak LES with symptoms clearly related to GERD confirmed on 24-hour pH testing. Primary motility disorders of the esophageal body with disturbance of clearance function are not an indication for antireflux surgery. Moreover, in patients with reflux esophagitis caused by gastric hypersecretion without evidence of an insufficient antireflux barrier, attention should be focused on the control of gastric acid secretion. Esophagitis caused by medication in pill form must be identified.

A common technical mistake in antireflux surgery is the failure to perform an adequate crural closure. The diaphragmatic crura are an important part of the antireflux mechanism and are responsible for the pressure increase during straining-induced reflex contractions of the sphincter. An inadequate crural repair, therefore, results in ineffective control of reflux. Furthermore, the reconstruction of the hiatus is necessary to retain the fundoplication in the abdomen. Failure to perform a crural repair causes slippage of the fundoplication into the chest, resulting in severe dysphagia and failure to prevent reflux. The same may occur when the esophagus is too short and not adequately mobilized. In patients with fixed hernias, therefore, I prefer the trans-

thoracic approach. A fundoplication that is too tight or too long (more than 2 cm) is a common reason for persistent dysphagia. On the other hand, a wrap that is too loose is inadequate to prevent gastroesophageal reflux. Hill prefers to evaluate the correct pressure level by intraoperative manometry.[77]

Positioning of the fundic wrap around the stomach rather than the esophagus occurs when the surgeon does not identify the angle of His accurately or after a correctly placed fundoplication slips because of a breakdown of the fundoplication. This usually arises when the U-shaped suture is tied too tightly, squeezing and breaking out of the esophageal tissue, or when Teflon felt pledgets are not used. The slipped fundoplication not only fails to control gastroesophageal reflux but also may result in dysphagia and can cause gastric ulceration in the obstructed pouch in about 30% of cases. The same errors in technique can lead to a complete disruption of the fundoplication with consequent recurrence of the reflux disease.

Gastroesophageal reflux disease is a common condition that can usually be controlled by medical therapy. Severe complications may result, however, and can be avoided by timely surgical therapy in carefully selected patients. The long-term outcome after surgery is excellent, and surgical repair has proved to be durable over many years of follow-up.

REFERENCES

1. Jamieson GC, Duranceau A. Gastroesophageal reflux. Philadelphia, WB Saunders, 1988:65.
2. Gallup Survey on Heartburn Across America. Princeton, Gallup Organization, March 28, 1988.
3. Ainley CC, Forgacs IC, Keeling PWN, et al. Outpatient endoscopic survey of smoking and peptic ulcers. Gut 1986;27:648.
4. Khuroo MS, Mahajan R, Zargor SA, et al. Prevalence of peptic ulcers in India: an endoscopic and epidemiological study in urban Kashmir. Gut 1989;30:930.
5. Khoury GA, Bolton J. Age: an important factor in Barrett's oesophagus. Ann R Coll Surg Eng 1989;71:50.
6. Brunner PI, Karmondy AM, Needham CD. Severe peptic oesophagitis. Gut 1969;10:831.
7. Postlethwaite RW, Musser AW. Changes in the esophagus in 1000 autopsy specimens. J Thorac Cardiovasc Surg 1974;68:953.
8. Wesdorps ICE, Bartelsman JF, den Hartog Jager FCA, et al. Results of conservative treatment of benign esophageal strictures: a follow up study in 100 patients. Gastroenterology 1982;82:487.

9. Palmer ED. The hiatus hernia-esophagitis-esophageal stricture complex: twenty-year prospective study. Am J Med 1968;44:566.

10. Koelz HR, Birchler R, Bretholz A, et al. Healing and relapse of reflux esophagitis during treatment with ranitidine. Gastroenterology 1986;91:1198.

11. Dawson J, Bernard J, Delattre M. Cimetidine 800 mg at bedtime in reflux esophagitis: a multicenter trial. In: Stewart JR, Holschcer AH, eds. Diseases of the esophagus. New York, Springer-Verlag, 1987;1116.

12. Parrilla P, Ortiz A, Martineez de Haro LF, et al. Evaluation of the magnitude of gastroesophageal reflux in Barrett's oesophagus. Gut 1990;31:964.

13. Polepalle SC, McCallum RW. Barrett's esophagus: current assessment and future perspectives. Gastroenterol Clin North Am 1990;19:733.

14. Berstad A, Weberg R, Froyshor LI, et al. Relationship of hiatal hernia to reflux esophagitis: a prospective study of coincidence using endoscopy. Scand J Gastroenterol 1986;21:55.

15. Ott DJ, Gelford DW, Chen YM, et al. Predictive relationship of hiatal hernia to reflux esophagitis. Gastrointest Radiol 1985;10:317.

16. Liebermann-Meffert D, Allgower M, Schmid P, Blum AL. Muscular equivalent of the lower esophageal sphincter. Gastroenterology 1979;76:31.

17. Sengupta A, Paterson WG, Goyal RK. Atypical localization of myenteric neurons in the opossum lower esophageal sphincter. Am J Anat 1987;180:352.

18. Biancani P, Barwick K, Selling J, McCallum R. Effects of acute experimental esophagitis on mechanical properties of the lower esophageal sphincter. Gastroenterology 1984;87:8.

19. Eastwood GL, Castell DO, Higgs RH. Experimental esophagitis in cats impairs lower esophageal sphincter pressure. Gastroenterology 1975;69:146.

20. Zaninotto G, DeMeester TR, Schqizer W, Johansson KE, Cheng SC. The lower esophageal sphincter in health and disease. Am J Surg 1988;155:104.

21. Dodds WJ, Dent J, Hogan WJ, et al. Mechanisms of gastroesophageal reflux in patients with reflux esophagitis. N Engl J Med 1982;307:1547.

22. Stein HJ, DeMeester TR, Naspetti R, Jamieson J, Perry RE. Three-dimensional imaging of the lower esophageal sphincter in gastroesophageal reflux disease. Ann Surg 1991;214:374.

23. Dent J, Dodds WJ, Sekiguchi T, Hogan WJ, Arndorfer RC. Interdigestive phasic contractions of the human lower esophageal sphincter. Gastroenterology 1983;83:453.

24. Goyal RK, McGuigan JE. Is gastrin a major determinant of basal lower esophageal sphincter pressure? A double-blind controlled study using high titer gastrin antiserum. J Clin Invest 1976;57:291.

25. Biancani P, Walsh JH, Behar J. Vasoactive intestinal peptide: a neurotransmitter for lower esophageal sphincter relaxation. J Clin Invest 1984;73:963.

26. Goyal RK, Said SI, Rattan S. Vasoactive intestinal peptides as a possible neurotransmitter of noncholinergic, noradrenergic neurons. Nature 1988;288:378.

27. Yamashita Y, Kako N, Homma K, et al. Neuropeptide release from isolated perfused, lower esophageal sphincter region of the rabbit and the effect of vasoactive intestinal peptide on the sphincter. Surgery 1992;112:227.

28. Grossman MI. What is physiological? Gastroenterology 1973;65:994.

29. Perdikis G, Wilson P, Hinder RA, et al. Gastroesophageal reflux disease is associated with enteric hormone abnormalities. Am J Surg 1994;167:186.

30. Kaul BK, DeMeester TR, Oka M, et al. The cause of dysphagia in uncomplicated sliding hiatal hernia and its relief by hiatal herniorrhaphy: a roentgenographic, manometric, and clinical study. Ann Surg 1990;211:406.

31. Mittal RK, Rochester DF, McCallum RW. Sphincteric action of the diaphragm during a relaxed esophageal sphincter. Am J Physiol 1989;256:G139.

32. Mittal RK, McCallum RW. Characteristics and frequency of transient relaxations of the lower esophageal sphincter in patients with reflux esophagitis. Gastroenterology 1988;95:593.

33. Holloway RH, Dent J. Pathophysiology of gastroesophageal reflux: lower esophageal sphincter dysfunction in gastroesophageal reflux disease. Gastroenterol Clin North Am 1990;19:517.

34. Helm JF, Dodds WJ, Pelc LR, Palmer DW, Teeter BC. Effect of esophageal emptying and saliva on clearance of acid from the esophagus. N Engl J Med 1984;310:284.

35. Helm JF, Dodds WJ, Riedel DR, Teeter BC, Hogan WJ, Arndorfer RC. Determinants of esophageal acid clearance in normal subjects. Gastroenterology 1983;85:607.

36. Kahrilas PJ, Dodds WJ, Hogan WJ, Kern M, Arndorfer RC, Reece A. Esophageal peristaltic dysfunction in peptic esophagitis. Gastroenterology 1986;91:897.

37. McCallum RW, Berkowitz DM, Lerner E. Gastric emptying in patients with gastro-esophageal reflux. Gastroenterology 1981;80:285.

38. Schwitzer W, Hinder RA, DeMeester TR. Does delayed gastric emptying contribute to gastroesophageal reflux disease? Am J Surg 1989;157:74.

39. Sarosiek J, Hetzel DP, Yu Z, et al. Evidence on secretion of epidermal growth factor by the esophageal mucosa in humans. Am J Gastroenterol 1993;88:1081.

40. Gray MR, Donnelly RJ, Kingsnorth AN. Role of salivary epidermal growth factor in the pathogenesis of Barrett's columnar lined oesophagus. Br J Surg 1991;78:1461.

41. Ritchie WP Jr, Felger TX. Differing ulcerogenic potential of dihydroxy and trihydroxy bile salts in canine gastric mucosa. Surgery 1981;89:342.

42. Kivilaakso E, Fromm D, Silen W. Effects of lysolecithin on isolated gastric mucosa. Surgery 1978;84:616.

43. Wenger J, Trowbridge CG. Bile and trypsin in the stomach after a test meal. South Med J 1971;64:1063.

44. Fuchs KH, DeMeester TR, Hinder RA, Stein HJ, Barlow AP, Gupta NC. Computerized identification of pathologic duodenogastric reflux using 24-hr gastric pH monitoring. Ann Surg 1991;213:13.

45. Jamieson J, Hinder RA, DeMeester TR, Litchfield D, Barlow A, Bailey RT Jr. An analysis of 32 patients with Schatzki's ring. Am J Surg 1989;158:563.

46. Johnson DA, Drane WE, Curran J, et al. Pulmonary disease in progressive systemic sclerosis: a complication of gastroesophageal reflux and occult aspiration? Arch Intern Med 1989;149:589.

47. Goldman J, Bennett JR. Gastroesophageal reflux and respiratory disorders in adults. Lancet 1988;2:493.

48. Iascone C, DeMeester TR, Little AG, et al. Barrett's esophagus: functional assessment, proposed pathogenesis, and surgical therapy. Arch Surg 1983;118:543.

49. Attwood SE, DeMeester TR, Bremner CG, et al. Alkaline gastroesophageal reflux: implications in the development of complication in Barrett's columnar-lined lower esophagus. Surgery 1989;106:764.

50. Nissen R. Gastropexy and "fundoplication" in surgical treatment of hiatus hernia. Am J Dig Dis 1961;6:954.

51. Brand DL, Ylvisaker JT, Gelfard M, et al. Regression of columnar esophageal (Barrett's) epithelium after anti-reflux surgery. N Engl J Med 1980;302:844.

52. Sjogren RW Jr, Johnson LF. Barrett's oesophagus: a review. Am J Med 1983;74:313.

53. Marks RD, Richter JE. Peptic strictures of the esophagus. Am J Gastroenterol 1993;88:1160.

54. Penagini R, Al Dabbagh M, Misiewicz JJ, et al. Effect of dilatation of peptic esophageal strictures on gastroesophageal reflux, dysphagia and stricture diameter. Dig Dis Sci 1988;33:389.

55. Hatafuku T, Maki T, Thal AP. Fundic patch operation in the treatment of advanced achalasia of the esophagus. Surg Gynecol Obstet 1972;134:617.

56. Albertucci M, Smyrk TC, Marcus JN. Experimental and clinical results with proximal end-to-end duodenojejunostomy for pathologic duodenogastric reflux. Ann Surg 1987;206:414.

57. Alrabeeah A, Giacomantonio M, Gillis DA. Paraesophageal hernia after Nissen fundoplication: a real complication in pediatric patients. J Pediatr Surg 1988;23:766.

58. Rakic SR, Pesko P, Dunjic M, Gerzic Z. Healing of gastric ulcer associated with para-esophageal hernia after hernial reduction. Am J Surg 1992;163:443.

59. Skinner DB, Belsey RHR. Surgical management of esophageal reflux and hiatus hernia: long-term results with 1030 patients. J Thorac Cardiovasc Surg 1967;53:33.

60. Jones DB, Howden CW, Burget DW, et al. Acid suppression in duodenal ulcer: a meta-analysis to define optimal dosing with antisecretory drugs. Gut 1987;28:1120.

61. Meuwissen SG, Klinkengerg-Knol EC. Management of gastro-oesophageal reflux disease: are there alternatives to omeprazole? Digestion 1989;44:54.

62. Johnson DA. Medical therapy for gastroesophageal reflux disease. Am J Med 1992;92:88.

63. Allison PR. Reflux esophagitis, sliding hiatus hernia, and the anatomy of repair. Surg Gynecol Obstet 1951;92:419.

64. Lieberman DA, Keeffee EB. Treatment of severe esophagitis with cimetidine and metoclopramide. Ann Intern Med 1986;104:21.

65. Spechler SJ, VA Study Group. Comparison of medical and surgical therapy for complicated gastroesophageal reflux disease in veterans. N Engl J Med 1992;326:786.

66. Zaninotto G, DiMario F, Costantini M, et al. Oesophagitis and pH of refluxate: an experimental and clinical study. Br J Surg 1992;79:161.

67. Kaul BK, DeMeester TR, Oka M, et al. The cause of dysphagia in uncomplicated sliding hiatal hernia and its relief by hiatal herniorrhaphy: a roentgenographic, manometric, and clinical study. Ann Surg 1990;211:406.

68. Hill LD, Tobias JA. An effective operation for hiatal hernia: an eight-year appraisal. Ann Surg 1967;166:681.

69. Thor KBA, Silander T. Long-term randomized prospective trial of the Nissen procedure versus a modified Toupet technique. Ann Surg 1989;210:719.

70. Baue AE, Belsey RHR. The treatment of sliding hiatus hernia and reflux esophagitis by the Mark IV technique. Surgery 1967;62:396.

71. DeMeester TR, Johnson LF, Kent AH. Evaluation of current operations for the prevention of gastroesophageal reflux. Ann Surg 1974;180:511.

72. Rossetti M, Hell K. Fundoplication for the treatment of gastroesophageal reflux in hiatal hernia. World J Surg 1977;1:439.

73. Donahue PE, Bombeck CT. The modified Nissen fundoplication-reflux prevention without gas bloat. Chir Gastroenterol 1977;11:15.

74. DeMeester TR, Bonavina L, Albertucci M. Nissen fundoplication for gastroesophageal reflux disease: evaluation of primary repair in 100 consecutive patients. Ann Surg 1986;204:9.

75. Hinder RA, Filipi CJ. The technique of laparoscopic Nissen fundoplication. Surg Laparosc Endosc 1991;2:265.

76. Pearson FG, Cooper JD, Nelems JM. Gastroplasty and fundoplication in the management of complex reflux problems. J Thorac Cardiovasc Surg 1978;76:665.

77. Hill LD. Intraoperative measurement of lower esophageal sphincter pressure. J Thorac Cardiovasc Surg 1978;75:378.

78. Dor J, Humbert P, Paoli JM, et al. Traitement du reflux par la technique dite de Heller-Nissen modifiée. Presse Med 1967;75:2563.

79. Angelchik JP, Cohen R. A new surgical procedure for the treatment of gastroesophageal reflux and hiatal hernia. Surg Gynecol Obstet 1979;148:246.

80. Stuart RC, Dawson K, Keeling P, Byrne PJ, Hennessy TPJ. A prospective randomized trial of Angelchik prosthesis versus Nissen fundoplication. Br J Surg 1989;76:86.

81. Stipa S, Fegiz G, Iascone C, et al. Belsey and Nissen operations for gastroesophageal reflux. Ann Surg 1989;210:583.

82. Olsen AM, Schlegel JF. Motility disturbances caused by esophagitis. J Thorac Cardiovasc Surg 1965;50:607.

Digestive Tract Surgery: A Text and Atlas, edited by Richard H. Bell,
Layton F. Rikkers, and Michael W. Mulholland.
Lippincott-Raven Publishers, Philadelphia, © 1996.

2

Motility Disorders of the Esophagus

Alex G. Little

The esophagus is a muscular tube lined with squamous epithelium. Although saliva and the scant amount of mucus produced by the esophageal submucosal glands make a modest contribution to early digestion, the principal function of the esophagus is transportation rather than digestion. Accordingly, alterations in motor function or motility reflect a breakdown in the primary function of the esophagus that is quickly and strongly perceived by the patient. The most typical or common symptom of esophageal dysmotility is dysphagia, which can be related to difficulty in clearing the oropharynx (oropharyngeal dysphagia) or which can occur while the food bolus is within the esophagus (esophageal dysphagia). Patients may also have signs of aspiration, such as cough or hoarseness. Aspiration can be due to the diversion of oral contents into the larynx when the upper esophageal sphincter (UES) malfunctions during a swallow or can be related to regurgitation of esophageal contents through the UES. The final symptom caused by esophageal motility disorders is chest pain. This symptom can be frustrating to patients and physicians, because the pathophysiology is sometimes unclear and, accordingly, the results of treatment unpredictable.

When motility dysfunction is the result of a primary esophageal disease, it is referred to as a *primary motility disorder.* When the dysfunction is consequent to a systemic process or disease of another organ, it is referred to as a *secondary motility disorder.* Both these categories are considered in this chapter.

The understanding of normal physiology allows appreciation of abnormal function and enables the surgeon to devise and carry out corrective surgery for the abnormal function. In this context, the esophagus must be understood as a specific organ, but its role within and interactions with the rest of the gastrointestinal tract must also be appreciated. Factors that are particularly relevant to understanding of esophageal motility and dysmotility are the relations to pharyngeal function and to the motor and secretory activities of the gastroduodenal complex.

Esophageal manometry is the most helpful tool for evaluation of esophageal motor function. This test is performed by passing a catheter assembly through the nose and on through the esophagus into the stomach. As the catheter is withdrawn, pressures are recorded from three or more sites simultaneously, either by using small transducers in the catheter system or by measuring resistance to flow as the catheter is perfused. Figure 2-1 depicts a normal series of motor events as recorded during a motility evaluation. This depiction complements the description of normal function given later and can be used for comparison to the manometric findings associated with specific motility disorders.

Entry into the esophagus is through the UES. This sphincter, or upper esophageal high-pressure zone, is created by the cricopharyngeal muscle. As shown in Figure 2-2, this muscle is in continuity with, and can even be considered the lowest of, the pharyngeal constrictors. This implies physiologically that this muscular complex normally works in a coordinated fashion. During the swallowing process, the muscles of the pharynx contract to propel food into the esophagus. Simultaneously, the UES relaxes its normal tone to allow pas-

27

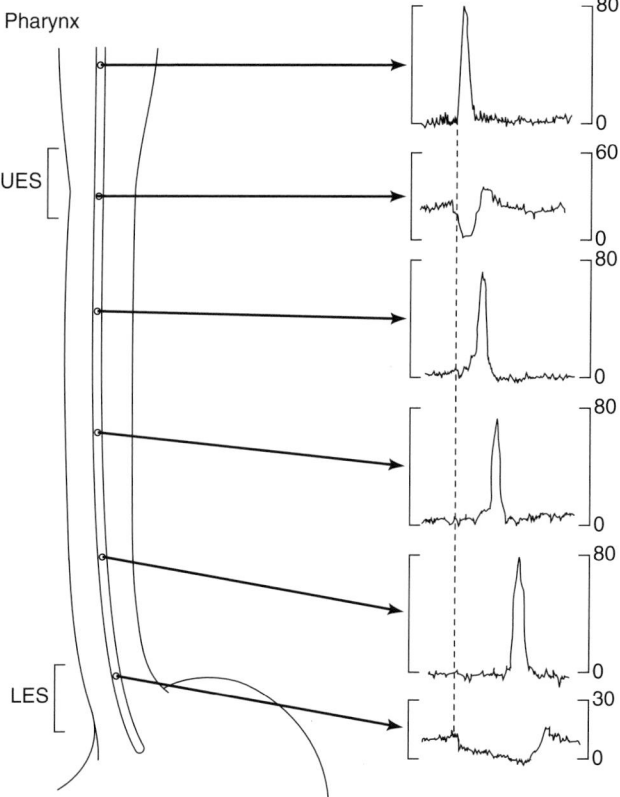

Figure 2-1. Depiction of motor events during a normal manometric or motility examination. (*Left*) The technique involves placing a catheter into the esophagus and detecting and recording pressures at various levels, including the upper esophageal sphincter (UES) and the lower esophageal sphincters (LES). (*Right*) Motility events are depicted as they would be displayed on a motility tracing. The pressure scale is in mmHg. A swallow is indicated by a spike in pharyngeal pressure. Simultaneously, the UES relaxes to allow the food bolus to be propelled into the cervical esophagus without resistance. The swallow also initiates a series of sequential contractions in the esophageal body. This peristaltic wave transports the bolus to the lower esophagus. Under gravitational effects, liquids may travel more rapidly than the bolus. The LES relaxes at the same time as the swallow, presumably to let any liquids that precede the arrival of the peristaltic wave to pass unimpeded into the stomach. The LES remains relaxed until the peristaltic wave has terminated. Both sphincters regain their resting tone after completion of this sequence.

sage of the bolus.[1] Once the bolus has passed, the sphincter contracts and regains its normal resting tone, keeping the upper esophagus closed. This state of tonic contraction prevents air from entering the esophagus and ensures that esophageal contents are not allowed to regurgitate passively into the pharynx.

A swallow initiates a peristaltic sequence of esophageal contractions that begins at the time of UES relax-

ation. Under normal circumstances, this wave of sequential contraction of both the inner circular and outer longitudinal muscles progresses aborally and transports the bolus to the lower esophageal sphincter (LES). A peristaltic wave that is initiated by a swallow is called a *primary peristaltic sequence of contractions. Secondary peristalsis,* on the other hand, is initiated by esophageal distension. This response protects the esophagus from refluxed gastric contents and can be elicited by inflation of a balloon within the esophageal lumen. *Tertiary peristalsis* represents a spontaneous, unprovoked motor event. Physiologic esophageal contractions are peristaltic or sequential; normally, less than 10% are simultaneous. Repetitive and nontransmitted contractions are uncommon in younger people, but their frequency increases with advancing age.

The LES can be easily and reliably demonstrated manometrically as a high-pressure zone, typically 15 to 25 mmHg higher than resting gastric pressure. Swallows initiate LES relaxation, which persists until the esophageal body peristaltic wave arrives at the LES. The benefit of this seemingly early relaxation relates to the fact that liquids traverse the upright esophagus faster than does the wave of contractions. If LES relaxation did not occur until the peristaltic wave reached the

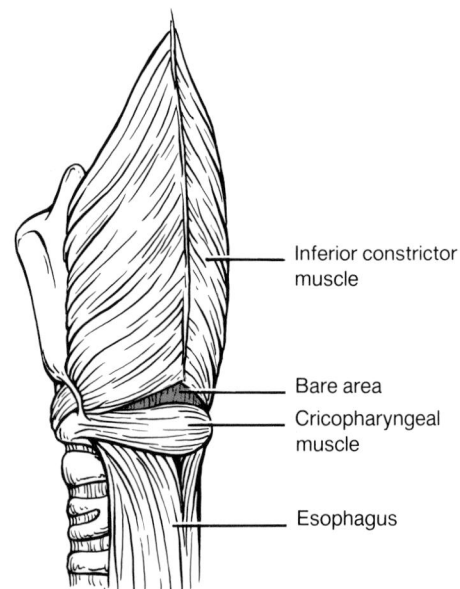

Figure 2-2 Depiction of posterior anatomy of the pharynx and upper esophagus. The cricopharyngeal muscle, which constitutes the upper esophageal sphincter, is really in series with the pharyngeal constrictor muscles. This anatomic relation is reflected in the physiologic need for coordination between pharyngeal contraction and cricopharyngeal relaxation during swallowing. The bare area between the muscles is where a Zenker's diverticulum arises.

sphincter, liquids might encounter a closed sphincter. Interestingly, the anatomic counterpart of the sphincter is difficult to identify. There is no hypertrophied band of muscle, such as is found at the pylorus, nor is there a distinct muscular entity, such as the cricopharyngeus in the upper esophagus. Rather, microscopic dissection shows that the sphincter is created in part by the geometry of muscular fiber arrangement that results in a gastroesophageal, muscular sling.[2] Another interesting feature of the LES is its unique array of neuromuscular receptors. As a result, the musculature of the lower esophagus responds differently to both agonist and antagonist challenges than does muscle more proximal in the esophagus or muscle in the stomach.[3] There is surely an LES, but its structure is unique in the gastrointestinal tract.

UPPER ESOPHAGUS

Oropharyngeal and UES function can be objectively evaluated radiographically and manometrically. Cine swallow radiographic studies often provide definitive information about the function of the oral and pharyngeal phases of swallowing. In contrast, radiographic assessment of the UES is rarely helpful. As discussed later, identification of Zenker's diverticulum is diagnostic of UES dysfunction; however, a posterior indentation, presumably caused by cricopharyngeal contraction, is not a diagnostic finding. In fact, most patients with this so-called cricopharyngeal bar on barium swallow (Fig. 2-3) are free of any symptoms.[4]

Manometric evaluation of the oropharyngeal–UES axis is, unfortunately, neither accurate nor reproducible enough to be a reliable diagnostic tool.[4,5] Major limitations include the speed with which motor events occur, the movement of the UES during swallowing, and the asymmetry of the UES, which is ovoid rather than circular. Both the quantitation of UES contractions and the evaluation of the coordination of its relaxation and contraction with pharyngeal events are difficult.

Motility disorders of the upper esophagus are essentially dysfunctions of the UES and must be appreciated within the context of the interrelation and dependence of the sphincter on oropharyngeal function. The process of swallowing is typically described as consisting of three stages: (1) the voluntary preparatory or oral stage, (2) the involuntary pharyngeal stage, and (3) the esophageal stage. During the oral stage, food is chewed and mixed with saliva and positioned as a bolus on the anterior surface of the tongue. During the pharyngeal phase, food is transferred from the pharynx, through the UES, and into the esophagus. This complex process is initiated by voluntary activity, but it becomes invol-

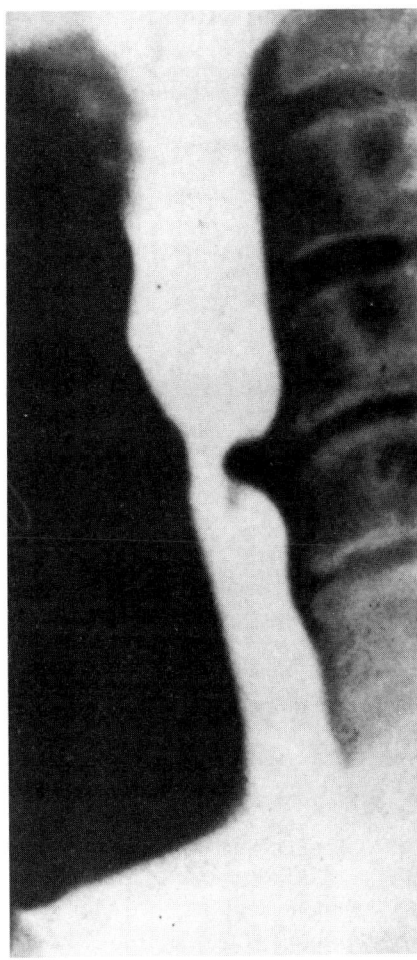

Figure 2-3 Barium swallow radiograph showing a posterior indentation in the barium column at the level of the cricopharyngeal muscle. This cricopharyngeal bar or impression is presumably caused by contraction of this muscle. This finding is usually not associated with symptoms and is a nonspecific finding.

untary when the food bolus encounters and activates the sensory receptors in the oropharynx. Patients with cricopharyngeal or UES dysfunction typically present with oropharyngeal dysphagia or difficulty in clearing food from the mouth and oropharynx. Dysfunction of the pharynx can also cause symptoms of oropharyngeal dysphagia. The conditions enumerated in Table 2-1 produce a clinical picture identical to UES malfunction and constitute the differential diagnoses of oropharyngeal dysphagia.

Oropharyngeal Dysphagia Due to Nervous System Causes

A cerebrovascular accident (CVA) frequently causes oropharyngeal dysphagia by affecting the involuntary initiation of the pharyngeal swallowing reflex, by dis-

Table 2-1   Causes of Oropharyngeal Dysphagia

NERVOUS SYSTEM
Central Nervous System
Cerebrovascular accident
Multiple sclerosis
Amyotrophic lateral sclerosis
Parkinson's disease
Wilson's disease
Brain tumors
Peripheral Nervous System
Myasthenia gravis
Poliomyelitis
Peripheral neuropathies

MUSCULAR SYSTEM
Primary myositis
Muscular dystrophy
Collagen vascular diseases
Metabolic myopathy

UPPER ESOPHAGEAL SPHINCTER
Hypertension
Hypotension
Premature closure
Delayed relaxation
Incomplete relaxation

rupting pharyngeal peristalsis, or by interfering with the coordination of UES relaxation. Like other CVA sequelae, the dysphagia may persist or may resolve. In one report,[6] about half of patients experienced dysphagia after a CVA, but this symptom resolved in 86% of affected patients within 2 weeks. Aspiration can also follow a CVA and has been documented in up to 30% of patients.[6] Surgical intervention directed at the UES for patients with persistent dysphagia is not beneficial and may even be harmful by further impairing pharyngeal function and increasing the amount of aspiration.

Other nervous system causes of oropharyngeal dysphagia are listed in Table 2-1. Effective surgical treatment for these conditions does not exist. When oropharyngeal dysfunction in a patient without esophageal dysfunction is found, consultation with a neurologist is appropriate.

Oropharyngeal Dysphagia Caused by Muscular Diseases

Diseases of muscle diminish the effectiveness of pharyngeal muscular contraction. Polymyositis and dermatomyositis result in inflammation of pharyngeal striated muscle, which weakens their contractile force. Myotonic dystrophy and oculopharyngeal muscular dystrophy can cause oropharyngeal dysphagia. The latter disease is characterized by abnormalities of ampli-

tude, duration, and frequency of pharyngeal contractions with apparently normal UES function. The pharyngeal muscles and their function can also be affected by metabolic disorders, such as thyrotoxicosis, and by collagen vascular diseases, such as systemic lupus erythematosus.

Oropharyngeal Dysphagia Caused by Upper Esophageal Sphincter Dysfunction

The possible abnormalities of UES function are listed in Table 2-1. However, because of the intrinsic limitations of UES manometry, identification of any of these specific abnormalities is uncommon. More frequently encountered is the patient who complains of oropharyngeal dysphagia but has normal oropharyngeal function according to a cine swallow study and no identifiable UES abnormality. The question then arises about the advisability of performing a cricopharyngeal myotomy on clinical grounds alone. This may be a reasonable solution, but it requires a careful and comprehensive evaluation to show that oropharyngeal function is normal and a strong clinical impression that an organic abnormality is present. When patients are carefully selected based on these criteria, results of a cricopharyngeal myotomy are satisfactory.[7,8]

By far the most common disorder of the upper esophagus is the UES dysfunction that is associated with Zenker's diverticulum, the radiographic appearance of which is shown in Figure 2-4. Patients with this disorder are thought to have dyscoordination between pharyngeal contraction and UES relaxation. It is not possible to document this abnormality in every patient, but the manometric tracing shown in Figure 2-5 is typical and shows the UES exhibiting premature relaxation and closure. In this patient, the UES is in the process of contracting rather than being fully relaxed during the time of pharyngeal contraction. Consequently, there is resistance, a functional obstruction, to pharyngeal emptying. When this occurs, the patient experiences dysphagia. Because there is difficulty in achieving food entry into the esophagus, aspiration can occur as food particles are diverted toward the larynx. Over time, the posterior mucosa between the pharyngeal constrictors and UES is exposed to an elevated intraluminal pressure, and Zenker's diverticulum is literally blown out. This takes place through Killian's triangle, which is the aspect of the posterior pharynx between the lower border of the inferior pharyngeal constrictor muscle and the upper border of the cricopharyngeus, where the muscular buttress of the posterior pharynx is the least substantial (Fig. 2-6). The diverticulum is a result of UES dysfunction; it is not the basic problem.[9]

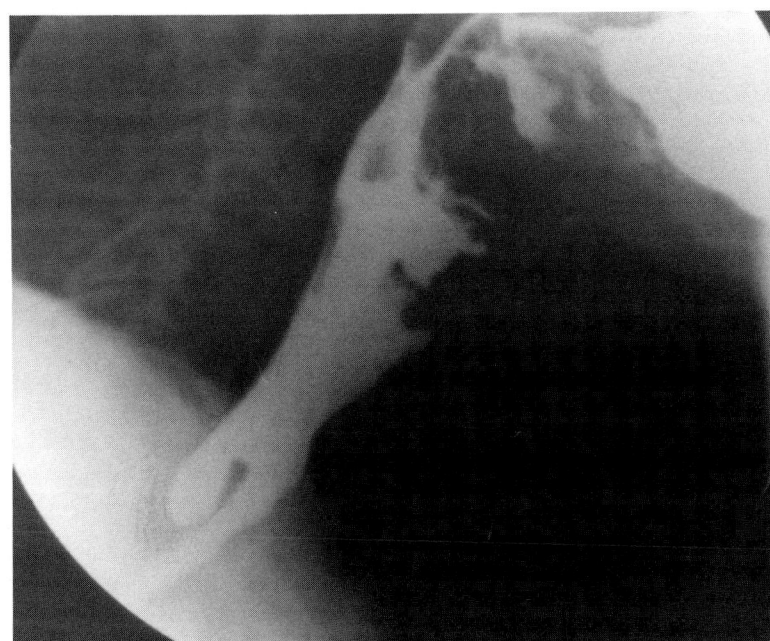

Figure 2-4 Barium swallow radiograph showing a typical, moderate-size Zenker's or pharyngoesophageal diverticulum. Although it originates in the posterior midline, as shown here, most diverticula diverge to the left as they enlarge.

Surgical treatment is routinely indicated to relieve dysphagia and prevent aspiration. Both symptoms are common. Restoring the ability to swallow without difficulty improves the patient's quality of life. Eliminating aspiration protects these patients, who are often elderly, from such devastating complications as aspiration pneumonia. The essential feature of operative repair is performing a cricopharyngeal myotomy, an action that effectively reduces UES resistance and, therefore, addresses the principal feature of the pathophysiology.[10] As depicted in Section II of Atlas Chapter 5, the myotomy should extend from the diverticulum for a distance of 3 to 5 cm distally onto the esophagus. The diverticulum can be handled in several ways. If small, it can become simply a mucosal bulge after the myotomy has released the esophageal mucosa and require no specific handling. Usually, the diverticulum remains as a distinct entity, in which case the surgeon can either resect (diverticulectomy) or suspend it from the prevertebral fascia (diverticulopexy). Both alternatives can be successful, one by anatomically removing the diverticulum, the other by functionally separating it from the food stream. Section II of Atlas Chapter 5 depicts both these techniques. Diverticulopexy has the advantage of avoiding an esophageal suture line; however, with modern stapling instruments, suture line disruption is uncommon, and the risk is minimal.[9] Accordingly, either diverticulectomy or diverticulopexy are acceptable as long as an adequate myotomy is always performed.

As documented by several reports,[10–12] the mortality rate associated with operative intervention is low,

averaging less than 1% even in the typical population of elderly patients. Some morbidity does occur, but it usually is minimal and involves superficial and deep wound infections. Long-term results include complete resolution of symptoms in about 80% of patients and improvement in most of the rest.[10–12]

An endoscopic alternative to the traditional open method is available and is depicted in Figure 2-7. Under endoscopic control, one limb of a gastrointestinal anastomosis stapler is placed in the diverticulum and one limb is placed in the esophagus. When the stapler is fired, the back of the esophagus is stapled to the diverticulum, and the common wall, which includes the UES, is divided. Experience with this technique is limited, and it does leave a remnant of the diverticulum that could trap food.[13] Accordingly, this approach should be reserved for occasional patients who are not candidates for open operation.

ESOPHAGEAL BODY AND LOWER ESOPHAGEAL SPHINCTER

Few disorders affect only the esophageal body or only the LES. Most affect function of both the body and the LES, presumably by either directly impairing the smooth muscle of the distal esophagus and the LES or by affecting the neural control of this region.

Achalasia

Achalasia is the most common disorder that produces dysfunction of the esophageal body and the LES. This is an idiopathic condition that histopathologically is asso-

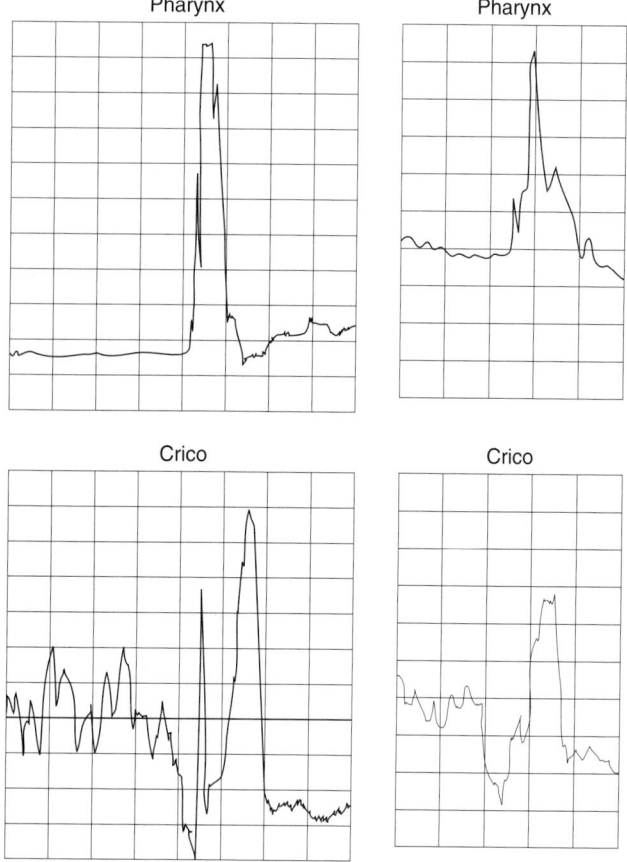

Pharynx   Pharynx

Crico   Crico

Figure 2-5 Manometric representations of the functional defect responsible for Zenker's diverticulum. (*Left*) A normal motility sequence. The simultaneous recordings show that cricopharyngeal relaxation coincides exactly with pharyngeal contraction. (*Right*) Manometric tracing obtained from a patient with a Zenker's diverticulum. The cricopharyngeal or upper esophageal sphincter has relaxed prematurely and is actually in the process of contracting when the pharyngeal muscles exert their maximal contraction force. Accordingly, the sphincter produces a functional resistance to pharyngeal emptying. This process causes the patient's symptoms and is responsible for the development of the diverticulum.

ciated with a reduction in the number or even absence of the ganglion cells of Auerbach's myenteric plexus.[14] In addition, there is hypertrophy of both the circular and longitudinal esophageal muscles and hypertrophy of esophageal nerves. The esophagus behaves as though it has become denervated, which can be demonstrated by a hypersensitivity response to cholinergic stimulation. A pathophysiologically similar condition, Chagas' disease, is seen in South America and is caused by the parasite *Trypanosoma cruzi*. In this condition, the parasite invades the nervous system and produces the achalasia-like condition. Based on this observation, it is speculated that achalasia is secondary to a viral or

autoimmune process affecting either the central or peripheral nervous system. This etiologic theory is supported by experimental evidence in animals that surgical creation of a defect along the neural visceromotor axis can produce the same esophageal dysfunction seen in achalasia.[15-17] Thus, an acquired central or peripheral nervous system lesion, such as a viral infection, could cause achalasia, but this putative etiology has not been proved in humans.

Clinical Presentation

Achalasia is seen equally in both sexes and has a typical onset in the third or fourth decade of life, although it can occur both earlier and later in life. All patients with achalasia have a history of dysphagia. This symptom typically is insidious in its development. The patient may have learned to accommodate to difficulty in swallowing by chewing more thoroughly and taking more liquids with meals. Nonetheless, all patients sense that solid foods, particularly meats and breads, tend to either stick or not pass normally. With time, the esophagus enlarges and dilates in response to the holdup of food, and the sensation of dysphagia may subside and even disappear as the esophagus becomes a reservoir organ.[18] In this situation, regurgitation of esophageal contents is extremely common. Regurgitation during sleep results in aspiration manifested by nocturnal cough or pneumonitis.

The diagnosis of achalasia is suggested by a clinical presentation featuring the symptoms of dysphagia and regurgitation and is supported by the radiographic appearance shown in Figure 2-8. Typically, the esophagus is dilated and tapers smoothly distally, producing the characteristic "bird's beak" appearance. Depending on the severity and duration of the disease, the esophagus may be only mildly dilated or may be markedly enlarged with a sigmoid configuration.

The ultimate diagnosis of achalasia rests on the manometric findings illustrated in Figure 2-9. The first abnormality of significance is absent or incomplete relaxation of the LES. The second important diagnostic manometric finding is the complete absence of peristalsis in the smooth muscle portion of the esophagus; that is, all contractions are simultaneous. This means that the poorly relaxing sphincter produces a functional distal obstruction, and the condition is worsened by the absence of peristaltic esophageal contractions. To empty the esophagus, the patient must accumulate a food column that exerts enough hydrostatic pressure at its bottom to force food through the tonically contracted sphincter. Other manometric abnormalities that are frequently but not always present include a high

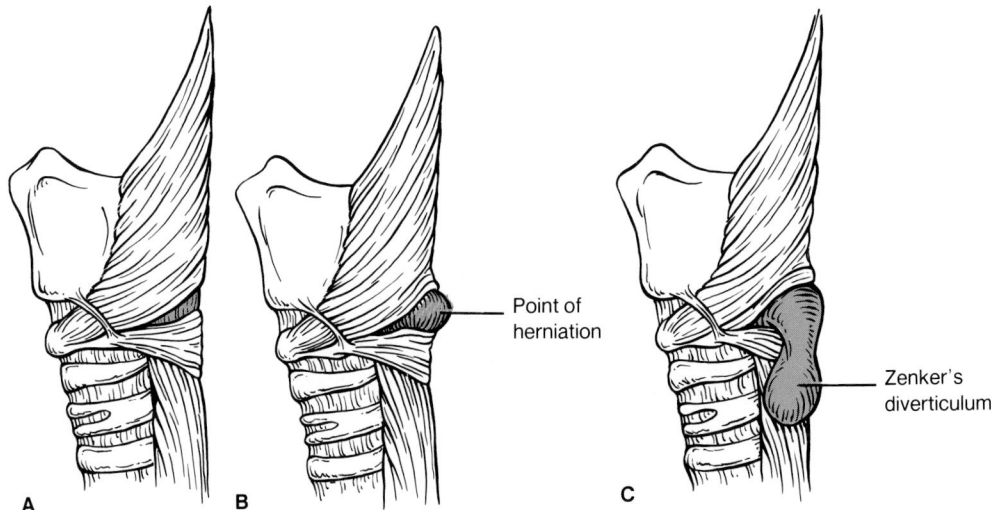

Figure 2-6 Pathogenesis of Zenker's diverticulum. As a result of contraction of the upper esophageal sphincter during swallowing, the posterior mucosa between the pharyngeal constrictor muscles and the upper esophageal sphincter is exposed to an elevated intraluminal pressure. The diverticulum occurs where the muscular buttress of the posterior pharynx is weakest.

resting pressure in the LES and low-amplitude esophageal contractions.

At endoscopy, the esophageal mucosa is usually normal, but retained food is frequently encountered. Accordingly, it is helpful to cleanse the esophagus by irrigation before endoscopy so that the complete mucosal surface can be seen. Endoscopic examination is necessary to rule out carcinoma of the distal esophagus–gastroesophageal junction. These tumors, which can be primary adenocarcinomas or metastatic, can produce a clinical and manometric picture indistinguishable from primary achalasia.[19] This condition is called *pseudoachalasia.* Endoscopy is also important because achalasia predisposes to development of squamous cell carcinoma of the middle esophagus.[20] Because the enlarged lumen allows a cancer to grow for a significant period

before it produces obstructive symptoms, careful endoscopic analysis is particularly important. An example of this type of finding is shown in Figure 2-10. At the lower end of the esophagus, there may be evidence of retention esophagitis, and the esophageal sphincter is noted to be closed at all times. The endoscope, however, usually passes easily because this is not a fixed obstruction.

Treatment

Treatment of achalasia is directed at the LES which, in addition to demonstrating incomplete or no relaxation, may also be hypertensive. Medical management includes the use of smooth muscle relaxants, such as nitrates, or, more popularly, calcium-channel blocking

Figure 2-7 Endoscopic approach to treatment of Zenker's diverticulum. One limb of a gastrointestinal anastomosis stapler is placed in the diverticulum and the other within the esophagus. When the instrument is fired, the common wall is stapled together and divided between the staples, creating a common channel and opening the upper sphincter.

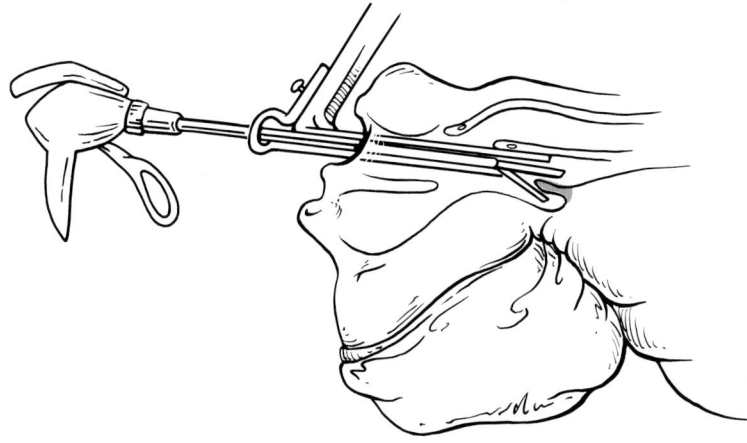

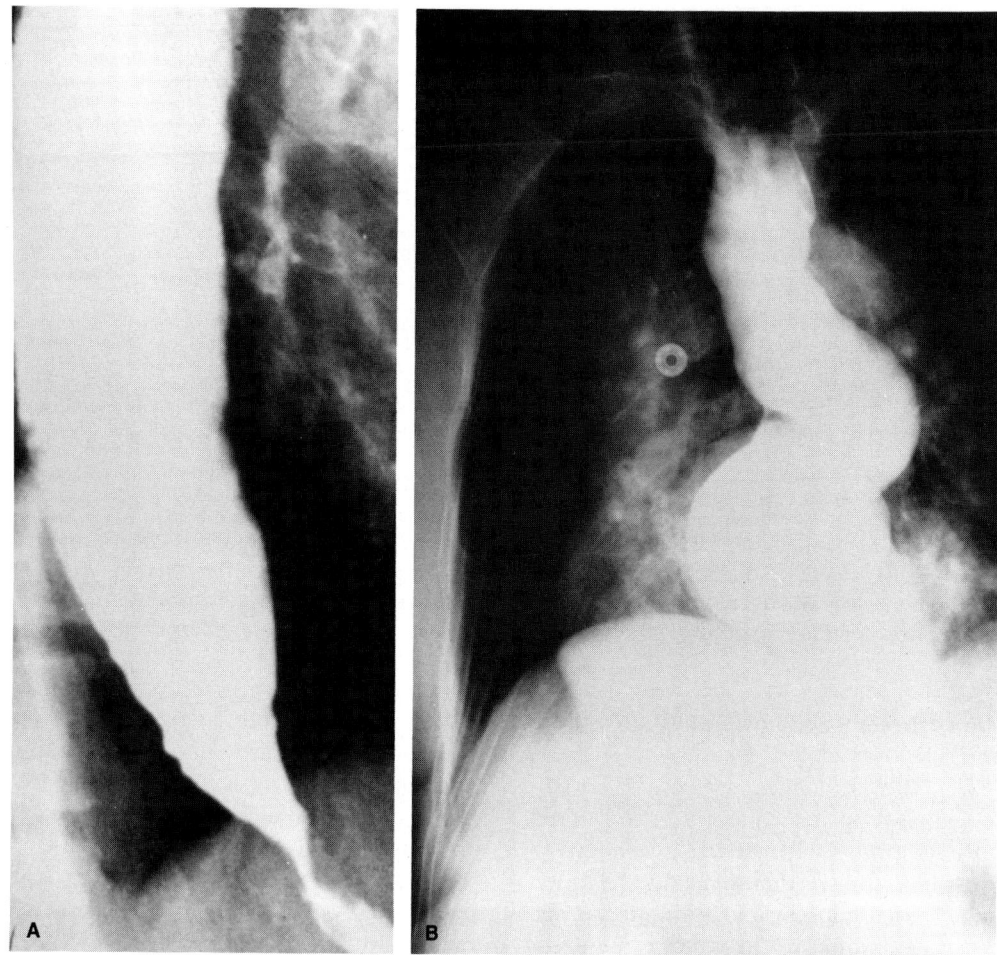

Figure 2-8 Typical radiographic appearances of patients with achalasia. **(A)** Radiograph of the typical findings in relatively early achalasia. The esophageal body is clearly dilated but retains its normal configuration. Distally, at the gastroesophageal junction, there is a smooth, tapered narrowing, which is frequently described as resembling a bird's beak. **(B)** Radiograph of a patient with advanced achalasia. The esophagus is enormously dilated and has assumed a sigmoid, convoluted shape. At this stage, the esophagus has become a reservoir organ.

agents.[21,22] Slow calcium-channel blockers, such as nifedipine, usually decrease LES pressure by 10% to 30%. This unfortunately usually does not result in a significant clinical improvement for the average patient. The most effective treatment choices are pneumatic dilation of the LES, open surgical myotomy, or a minimally invasive surgical approach with laparoscopic or thoracoscopic esophageal myotomy.

Pneumatic dilation of the LES is a reasonable initial therapeutic choice for most patients. This technique involves placement of a balloon catheter across the lower sphincter, using fluoroscopic or endoscopic control.[23–25] The balloon is inflated to a designated pressure and to a diameter of 3 to 4 cm. This sequence of balloon placement and inflation is shown in Figure 2-11. Typically, the patient experiences chest or epigastric pain

during the procedure, and when the balloon is removed, it has blood on it. This picture suggests that balloon dilation results in forceful rupture of the musculature of the lower esophagus. Despite this, perforation is relatively uncommon and occurs in only 3% to 5% of patients.[24] Long-term results, with up to two dilation sessions, show significant improvement in swallowing in about two thirds of patients.[23–25] Late complications, such as gastroesophageal reflux, are uncommon. Since this procedure can be performed in the outpatient setting without the need for general anesthesia or an operation, it is the initial therapeutic choice for most patients. Patients who are not good candidates for dilation include patients with a very dilated esophagus, patients in whom it is difficult to pass the balloon through the LES, patients with so-called vigorous achalasia and rel-

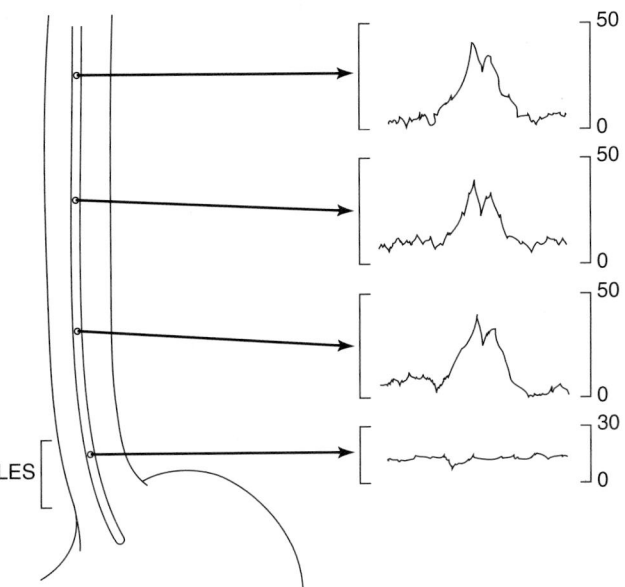

Figure 2-9 Manometric tracing showing the typical findings in achalasia. The lower esophageal sphincter (LES) remains contracted during all swallows; this functional distal obstruction is probably the most important aspect of the pathophysiology. In addition, all esophageal contractions are simultaneous, so there is no peristaltic stripping wave to help the esophagus empty.

atively high-pressure contractions who appear to be at a somewhat higher risk for perforation, and younger patients, such as those in the second or third decade of life, who require a more definitive approach.

Surgical myotomy can be performed through either an open or a minimally invasive approach. The technique of open myotomy, which was first described by Heller,[26] has evolved so that a single rather than the original double myotomy is performed through a left thoracotomy. This operation is illustrated in Section II of Atlas Chapter 5. The optimal length of the proximal extent of the myotomy is undefined, but it appears to be relatively unimportant, except in some patients with vigorous achalasia in whom the frequent swallows that occur while eating a meal seem to trigger a rapid-fire, almost fibrillatory pattern of esophageal body repetitive contractions. This motility pattern, shown in Figure 2-12, can be demonstrated when manometry is performed in an ambulatory setting with the patient consuming a normal meal.[27] This motility pattern is associated with intraesophageal shuttling of a food bolus and contributes to the patient's dysphagia. The myotomy should therefore be extended up to the aortic arch in these patients. However, the key to the operation for all patients is clearly extending the myotomy along the distal esophagus, through the lower sphincter, and onto the stomach. Some surgeons who frequently perform

this operation believe that a carefully performed myotomy alone is sufficient treatment for achalasia. Results in experienced hands show that dysphagia is consistently relieved in over 80% of patients.[28-30] Development of postoperative gastroesophageal reflux occurs with variable frequency, with reports ranging from 5% to 25% of patients.[28-32]

An alternative surgical approach is based on the belief that a complete myotomy is more likely if the stomach and gastroesophageal junction are freed by complete dissection of the hiatus. When this is done, and the fat pad is excised from the anterior part of the gastroesophageal junction, the myotomy can be performed with ideal exposure. This helps to ensure complete division of the muscle. Once the myotomy is completed, it is necessary to reconstruct both the hiatus and the gastroesophageal junction to prevent iatrogenic reflux. This is best accomplished by closing the hiatus posteriorly and performing a Belsey Mark IV antireflux procedure, as shown in Sections II and III of Atlas Chapter 5. This operation is simplified by the thick esophageal muscle found in patients with achalasia, which greatly improves the surgical conditions for constructing the Belsey fundoplication. This combined operation addresses the two reasons for failure of simple myotomy: inadequate division of the fibers of the LES and iatrogenic gastroesophageal reflux. An inadequate myotomy results in persistent dysphagia, while an exorbitant myotomy leads to an incompetent cardia. The combined procedure relieves dysphagia in over 80% of patients and incorporates features designed to prevent

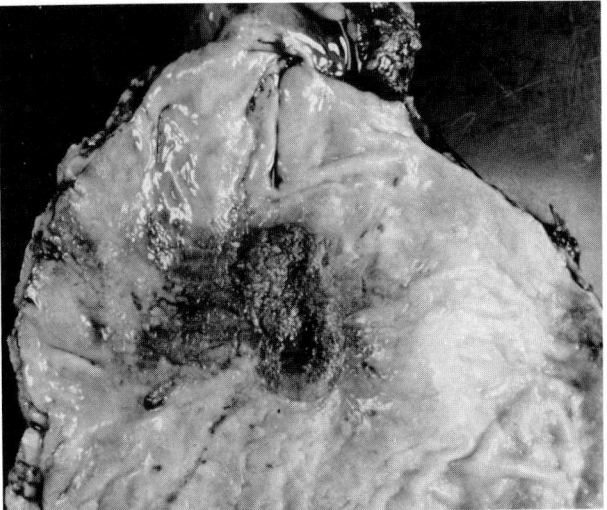

Figure 2-10 Development of carcinoma in a patient with achalasia. The squamous cell carcinoma of the esophageal body was detected on endoscopy. Barium swallow did not detect this early cancer, which would have been missed without a careful endoscopic examination.

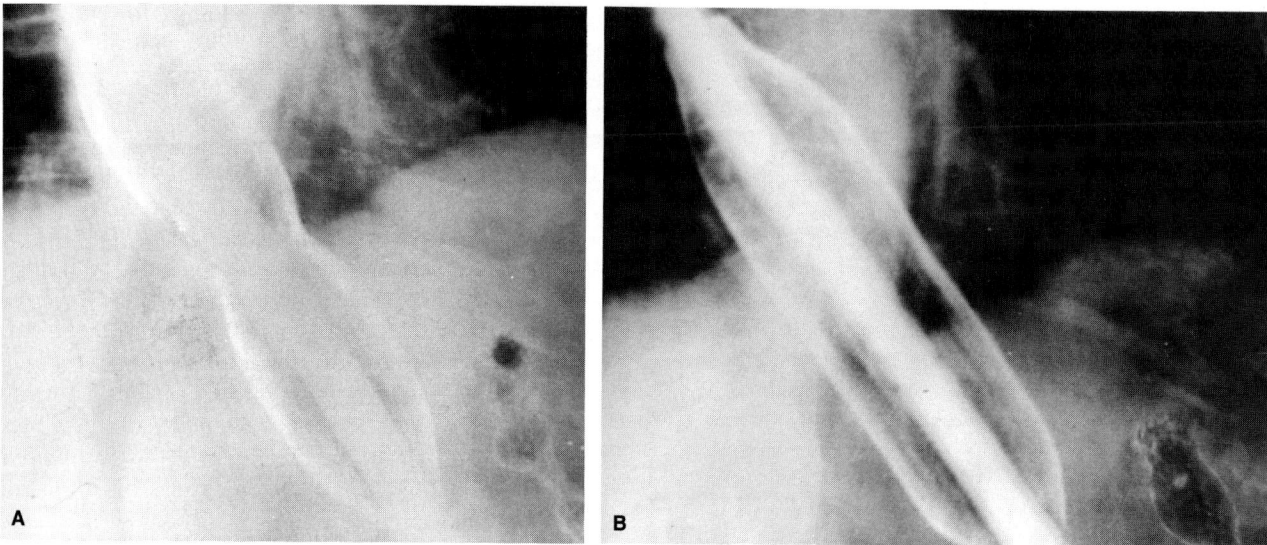

Figure 2-11 Pneumatic dilation of achalasia. (**A**) The pneumatic balloon dilator is positioned across the gastroesophageal junction, which is causing a waistlike indentation in the partially inflated balloon. (**B**) The dilator is now fully inflated, and the waist in the balloon has disappeared, indicating that the muscular squeeze of the lower esophageal sphincter has been overcome.

the development of reflux.[33,34] Although alternative surgical antireflux options have been used, the Belsey technique appears to provide the best results because it does not rely on raising LES pressures to achieve reflux control and, therefore, does not cause dysphagia.[35–37]

Finally, experienced thoracic surgeons have been able to accomplish esophageal myotomy using a video-assisted approach. This has been carried out both through abdominal and thoracic exposures,[38,39] as illustrated in Section II of Atlas Chapter 5. The thoracic route more closely approximates the approach that thoracic surgeons are accustomed to using and allows the surgeon the option of converting to a standard, open thoracic approach if necessary. Using the thoracoscope and an endoscope positioned within the esophagus to provide countertraction and to recognize when the myotomy has crossed the gastroesophageal junction, the technique really is not different from the open procedure. It does require experience with minimally invasive surgical techniques and the capability of handling complications. Long-term results are not yet available. Whether this approach will complement or replace pneumatic dilation and the open procedures remains undetermined.

Diffuse Esophageal Spasm

Spasm is a nonspecific term that connotes involuntary muscular contractions. Historically, the term *diffuse esophageal spasm* (DES) was used to describe vari-

able nonspecific motor disorders of the esophageal body.[40–42] Implied in its use was the suggestion of an increased force of contractions as well as an abnormal contraction pattern. Manometry has brought the condition into sharper focus, and DES now is defined as an esophageal motor disorder diagnosed by the manometric finding of frequent simultaneous esophageal contractions. This pattern (Fig. 2-13) is not the same as in achalasia, since some normal peristalsis must also be present in DES.[43–45] UES and LES function is usually normal.[44] The minimal required frequency of simultaneous contractions for the diagnosis of DES is more than 10% to 20% of all esophageal contractions in response to wet swallow challenges. The emphasis of the manometric criteria for the diagnosis of DES is the pattern rather than the force of the esophageal contractions.

The radiographic appearance of DES shown in Figure 2-14 makes it obvious why this disorder has been referred to as a *corkscrew esophagus*. This radiographic appearance, however, is seen in only about 30% of DES patients and can occur in patients with no symptoms.[46] Thus, the diagnostic accuracy of radiographic examination is limited because it is neither sufficiently sensitive nor specific. Manometry, therefore, is the essential diagnostic modality.

The symptoms of DES are dysphagia, substernal chest pain, or both. The symptoms usually are episodic rather than constant. The pathogenesis of the symp-

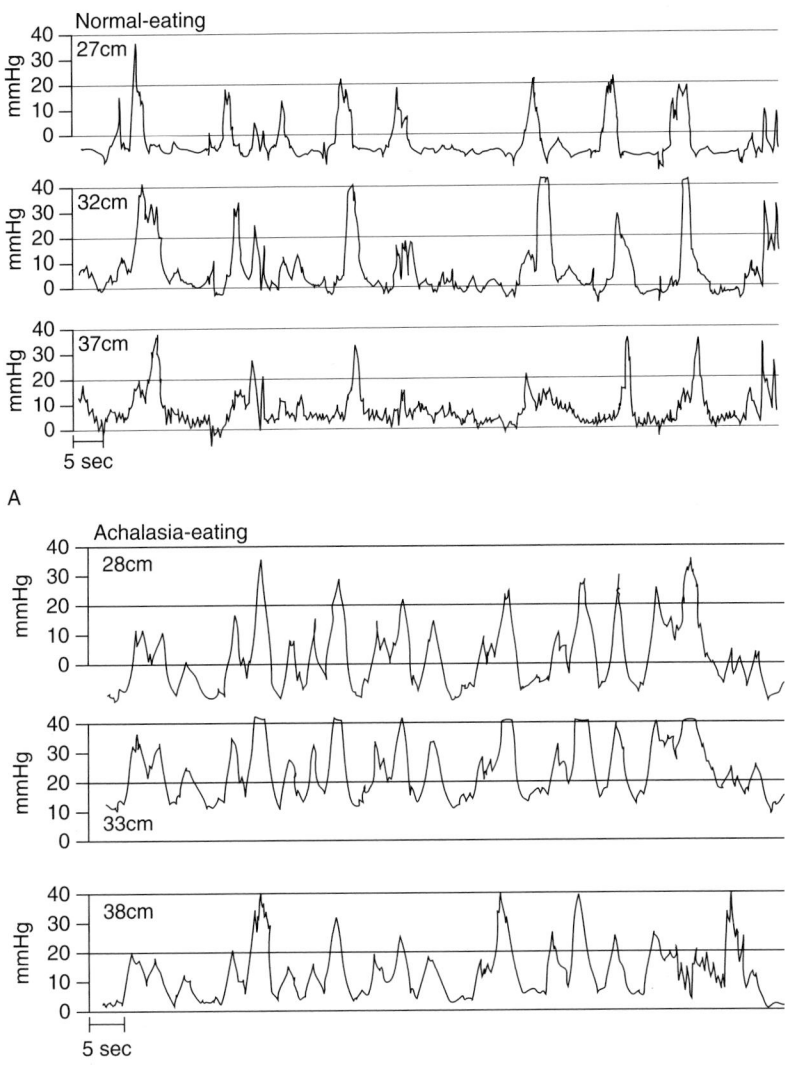

Figure 2-12 (**A**) Manometric tracing obtained from a normal volunteer who is eating a meal. All contractions are peristaltic, and there are only three or four contraction waves per minute. (**B**) Manometric tracing obtained from a patient with achalasia who is eating a meal. The motility pattern here is nearly fibrillatory, with a rapid-fire sequence of simultaneous contractions.

toms is not clear. In some patients with dysphagia, delay in esophageal transit is thought to be due to ineffective peristalsis. The pathophysiology of the chest pain, typically described as crushing or squeezing, which is usually the dominant symptom, is far less well defined. It may be due to abnormal esophageal sensitivity rather than abnormal function because the pain and the simultaneous contractions are not usually temporally related.

Further confounding our understanding of DES are two additional considerations. The first is that some patients have the motility abnormality but have absolutely no symptoms. It is doubtful that manometric differences from normal in the absence of symptoms constitutes a disease. The other interesting but confusing observation is that some patients with gastroesophageal reflux disease (GERD) have a manometric picture identical to that of patients with DES. Most GERD pa-

tients can be distinguished easily from patients with primary DES. The former have heartburn, not crushing or squeezing chest pain, and reflux is demonstrated by esophageal pH manometry. They respond to appropriate medical or surgical treatment of their primary disorder, which is pathologic reflux.[47]

Initial treatment for patients with symptomatic DES should be supportive; explanation and reassurance have been said to be the most important elements in the management of these patients.[48] This emphasis is based on the observed relation between DES and psychiatric disturbances, such as chronic emotional states.[49] Smooth muscle relaxants, including nitrates and calcium-channel blocking agents, such as nifedipine, can be effective and should be the second line of medical therapy.[48] Operative treatment should be used infrequently and only for carefully selected patients. A long myotomy can relieve dysphagia if that is a significant

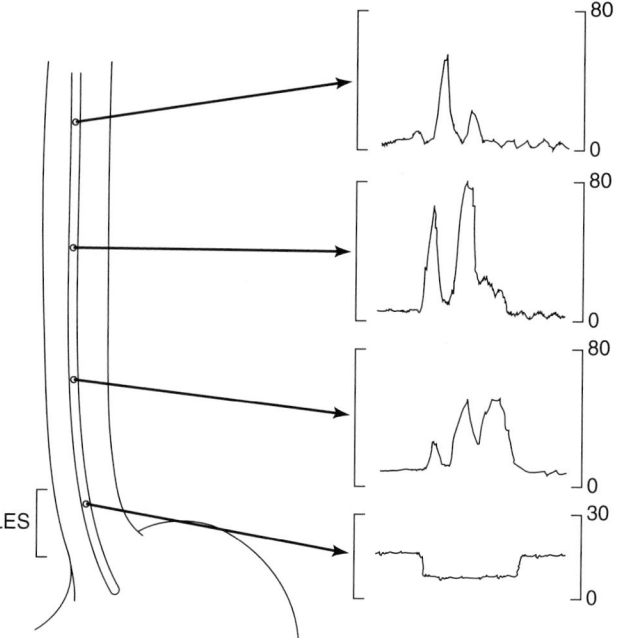

Figure 2-13 Manometric tracing from a patient with diffuse esophageal spasm. Shown here is the hallmark abnormality, which is the presence of simultaneous contractions. These contractions are often repetitive. In addition, there is always some normal peristalsis that distinguishes this manometric abnormality from achalasia. As shown here, the lower esophageal sphincter (LES) usually functions normally.

component of the patient's symptom complex. Unfortunately, myotomy for pain, the more common and troublesome symptom, produces unpredictable results and consequently should be infrequently performed.[50-52] When myotomy is carried out, it must be long enough to encompass all areas of abnormal motility identified by manometry.

High-Amplitude Peristaltic Contractions

Some patients have high-amplitude peristaltic contractions (HAPC) identified by esophageal manometry, usually as part of an evaluation for chest pain and frequently after an extensive cardiac evaluation.[53] In addition to the high-pressure contractions, there are frequently interspersed normal-pressure contractions. In contrast to DES, this is a motor disorder defined by the force or amplitude of esophageal contractions rather than their pattern. The high-pressure contractions have led to the use of the term *nutcracker esophagus* for this disorder.[54] An example of the manometric findings is shown in Figure 2-15. As is the case with asymptomatic patients with manometric features of DES, some patients with manometric HAPC have no symp-

toms. The motility findings should not be treated in the absence of symptoms.

Patients with HAPC have angina-like chest pain and only occasionally complain of dysphagia. In fact, the esophageal disorder is usually suspected and identified only after a cardiac evaluation has been completed without a diagnosis of ischemic myocardial disease. The way in which these high-pressure contractions produce chest pain is not clear. In fact, it is not even certain that the abnormal contractions are the cause of the chest pain. Patients may have pain when esophageal motility is normal and conversely may be resting comfortably when an extremely high-pressure contraction occurs on the manometric tracing. Patients with motor disorders and chest pain have a high prevalence of psychiatric disturbances that are believed to affect their perception of pain.[55]

With the lack of understanding of the pathophysiology of this disorder, it is not surprising that results of both medical and surgical therapy directed at the esoph-

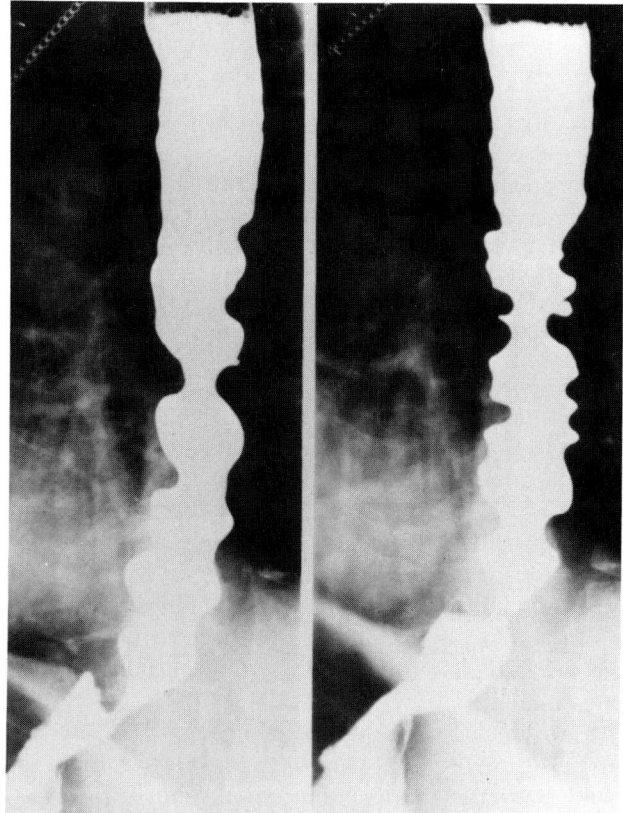

Figure 2-14 Radiographic appearance of a patient with diffuse esophageal spasm. The multiple simultaneous contractions are responsible for the segmentation phenomenon depicted here. Unfortunately, this appearance is nonspecific and can be seen in presumably normal subjects and in patients with gastroesophageal reflux disease.

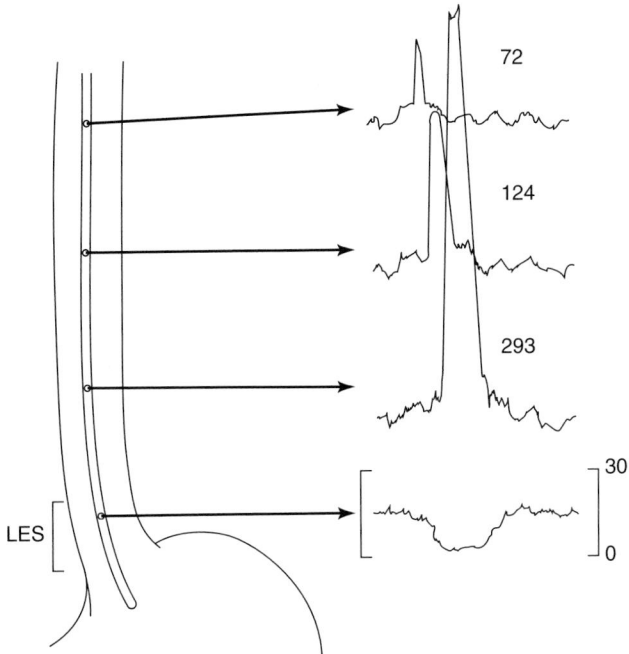

Figure 2-15 A typical manometric tracing from a patient with high-amplitude peristaltic contractions. The pattern is normal as the contractions are sequential and peristaltic; however, the pressure amplitude approaches 300 mmHg in the distal esophagus. Lower esophageal sphincter (LES) function is normal.

agus are unpredictable and frequently ineffective. Although one study found that patients treated with the smooth muscle relaxant nifedipine had symptomatic improvement, this was believed to be due more to the supportive patient–doctor relationship than to the smooth muscle relaxant properties of the drug.[56] Pain relief did not correlate with changes in contraction pressure. Therapy for these patients, therefore, should be selective. Only a small number of patients are reasonable candidates for surgery. A long myotomy effectively reduces the pressure or amplitude of esophageal contractions and usually produces at least a reduction in the chest pain, but operative intervention should be reserved for those patients whose symptoms resist maximal medical and supportive care.[53]

Esophageal Diverticulum

Epiphrenic and mid-esophageal diverticula are relatively uncommon in the general population. These esophageal body diverticula are found primarily in patients with achalasia. The pathophysiology of diverticula in this disease is presumably similar to that which causes the development of colonic diverticula; that is, the diverticulum is the result of the increased pressure

within the esophageal body. They do not represent a separate pathologic condition and are typically resected at the time of definitive surgical treatment for the achalasia.

Epiphrenic and mid-esophageal diverticula are much less frequently encountered in patients without achalasia. Coinciding with a decrease in the United States in the incidence of inflammatory diseases of the mediastinum, such as tuberculosis, the incidence of traction diverticula has waned, and most of these cases are now pulsion diverticula. They are the result of motor disorders of the LES or the esophageal body.[57] Patients with diverticula are usually symptomatic, with the most common symptom being dysphagia. Regurgitation, with or without pulmonary aspiration, also is common. Barium swallow radiograph identifies the diverticulum (Fig. 2-16).

Manometric examination of patients with esophageal body diverticula and achalasia shows the typical motility pattern of achalasia. Manometric examination

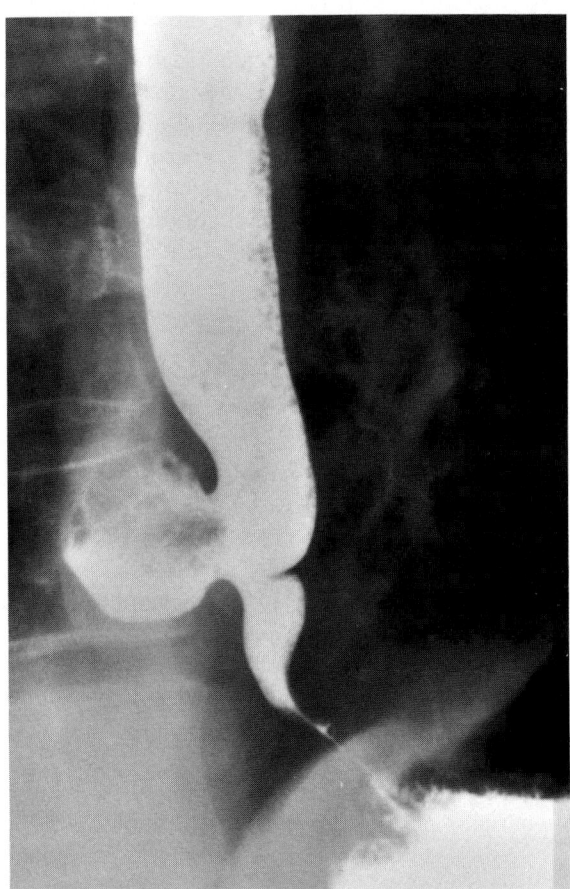

Figure 2-16 Radiographic appearance of a diverticulum of the distal esophagus. This epiphrenic diverticulum was associated with dysphagia and the manometric findings displayed in Figure 2-17*A*.

in patients with a diverticulum but without achalasia usually reveals motor dysfunction distal to the diverticulum.[57-60] In some patients, this disorder involves high-pressure contractions; in others, spontaneous, simultaneous, or repetitive contractions are observed. These are nonspecific findings in the sense that the abnormal motility pattern does not fit any specific, named esophageal motor abnormality. Nonetheless, they are the cause both of the patient's symptoms and of the diverticulum.

Representative examples of the types of motor dysfunction seen are provided in Figure 2-17. Surgical therapy must address the motor dysfunction, which should be documented manometrically before surgery. If the LES is completely normal, diverticulectomy combined with distal myotomy of the esophageal body is sufficient. If there is any question about the LES playing an etiologic role, the patient should be treated by a myotomy across the LES region. Following the principles for treatment of achalasia, reconstruction with a Belsey Mark IV fundoplication prevents the development of reflux without causing dysphagia.[57] This operation is illustrated in Sections II and III of Atlas Chapter 5. Diverticulectomy alone is insufficient treatment for a pulsion diverticulum. The patient remains symptomatic without a myotomy of all the muscle shown by manometry to be abnormal. In addition, a diverticulectomy closure site is more likely to leak postoperatively if a distal obstruction—the abnormally functioning segment of the esophagus—is allowed to remain.

Collagen Vascular Diseases

The degree of esophageal dysfunction in patients with collagen vascular disease is determined by the extent of smooth muscle involvement. Scleroderma is the most common of the collagen vascular diseases to disrupt esophageal function.[61] In patients with scleroderma, the distal esophagus and the LES, which are constituted completely by smooth muscle, have diminished tone and function. The degree of the impairment is variable, but many patients have a nearly flaccid distal esophagus. Consequently, there is no barrier to gastroesophageal reflux, which therefore occurs freely across the patulous LES.[61,62] Mucosal injury is potentiated by ineffective esophageal clearance of the refluxed material by the noncontracting lower esophagus. In essence, these patients suffer from a virulent form of GERD.

When both symptoms and esophagitis can be controlled with medical management, that course should be followed. Persistent esophagitis is worrisome because of the likelihood of progressive damage and is a strong relative indication for a surgical antireflux procedure.[62] Despite the increased risk of perioperative

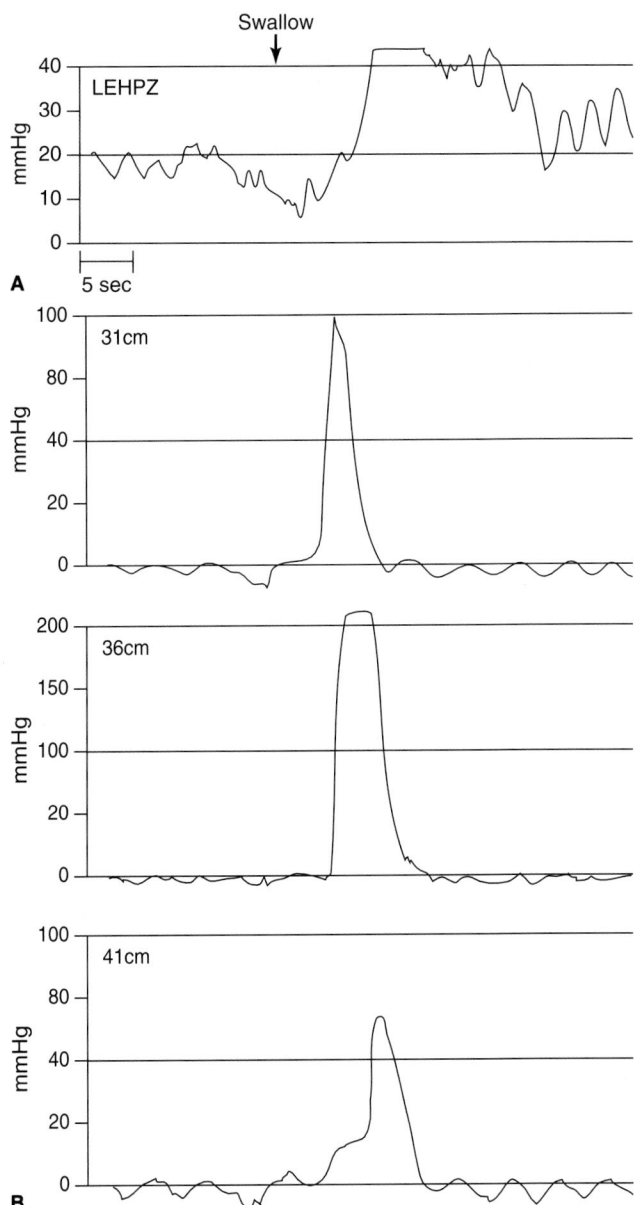

Figure 2-17 Manometric tracings obtained in patients with diverticula of the distal esophagus. (**A**) Manometric tracing from the patient whose barium swallow radiograph was shown in Figure 2-16. The abnormal motor function present is an extremely elevated lower esophageal sphincter high-pressure zone (LEHPZ) after the normal swallowing-induced relaxation of the sphincter. The sphincter pressure exceeds 40 mmHg for several seconds, and about 15 seconds elapse before pressure returns to baseline. (**B**) This motility tracing is normal at 31 and 41 cm from the incisor teeth but reveals high-pressure contractions in the mid-esophagus at 36 cm. This patient had dysphagia and a diverticulum of the middle esophagus.

morbidity because of the systemic disease, this must be balanced against the high probability of stricture development due to florid reflux. In fact, in the presence of esophagitis but before stricture development, antireflux surgery is safe and effective in these patients.[62] This elective, controlled approach is greatly preferred to delaying until development of a fibrous stricture necessitates a more extensive surgical procedure, such as resection and colon interposition.[63] When antireflux surgery is performed, the surgeon must remember and account for the diminished propulsive strength of the esophageal body. This means either choosing an operation that does not feature a complete gastric wrap or simply being sure that a Nissen-type complete wrap fulfills the requirements of being loose and having a suture line length of no more than 1.5 to 2 cm.

REFERENCES

1. Winans CS. The pharyngoesophageal closure mechanism: a manometric study. Gastroenterology 1972;63:768.
2. Liebermann-Meffert D, Allgower M, Schmid P, Blum AL. Muscular equivalent of the lower esophageal sphincter. Gastroenterology 1979;76:31.
3. Christensen J. Pharmacologic identification of the lower esophageal sphincter. J Clin Invest 1970;49:681.
4. Nelson JB, Richter JE. Upper esophageal motility disorders. Gastroenterol Clin North Am 1989;18:195.
5. Christensen J. Motor functions of the pharynx and esophagus. In: Johnson LR, ed. Physiology of the gastrointestinal tract, ed 2. New York, Raven, 1987;595.
6. Gordon C, Hewer BL, Wade DT. Dysphagia in acute stroke. Br Med J 1987;295:411.
7. Ellis FH, Crozier RE. Cervical esophageal dysphagia: indications for and results of cricopharyngeal myotomy. Ann Surg 1981;194:279.
8. Orringer MB. Extended cervical esophagomyotomy for cricopharyngeal dysfunction. J Thorac Cardiovasc Surg 1980;80:669.
9. Little AG, Skinner DB. The management of Zenker's diverticulum: cricopharyngeal myotomy and diverticulopexy. In: Kittle CF, ed. Current controversies in thoracic surgery. Philadelphia, WB Saunders, 1986;3:15.
10. Skinner DB, Altorki N, Ferguson M, Little AG. Zenker's diverticulum: clinical features and surgical management. Dis Esophagus 1988;1:19.
11. Duranceau A, Rheault MG, Jamieson GG. Physiologic response to cricopharyngeal myotomy and diverticulum suspension. Surgery 1983;94:655.
12. Ellis FH, Schlegel JF, Lynch VP, Payne WS. Cricopharyngeal myotomy for pharyngoesophageal diverticulum. Ann Surg 1969;170:340.
13. Collard JM, Otte JB, Kestens PJ. Endoscopic stapling technique of esophago-diverticulostomy for Zenker's diverticulum. Ann Thorac Surg 1993;56:573.
14. Cassella RR, Brown AL, Sayre GP. Achalasia of the esophagus: pathologic and etiologic considerations. Am J Surg 1964;160:474.
15. Burgess JN, Schlegel JF, Ellis FH. The effect of denervation on feline esophageal function and morphology. J Surg Res 1972;12:24.
16. Goto S, Grosfeld JL. The effect of a neurotoxin (benzalkonium chloride) on the lower esophagus. J Surg Res 1989;47:117.
17. Higgs B, Kerr FWL, Ellis FH. The experimental production of esophageal achalasia by electrolytic lesions in the medulla. J Thorac Cardiovasc Surg 1968;50:613.
18. Chakkaphak S, Chakkaphak K, Ferguson MK, Little AG. Disorders of esophageal motility. Surg Gynecol Obstet 1991;172:325.
19. Herrera AF, Colon J, Valdes-Dapena A, Roth JLA. Achalasia or carcinoma? The significance of the mecholyl test. Dig Dis 1970;15:1073.
20. Carter R, Brewer LA III. Achalasia and esophageal carcinoma. Am J Surg 1975;130:114.
21. Orlando RC, Bozymski EM. Clinical and manometric effects of nitroglycerin in diffuse esophageal spasm. N Engl J Med 1973;289:23.
22. Traube M, Hongo M, Magyar L, McCallum RW. Effects of nifedipine in achalasia and in patients with high-amplitude peristaltic esophageal contractions. JAMA 1984;252:1733.
23. Elta GH, Nostrant TT, Wilson JAP. Treatment of achalasia with the Witzel pneumatic dilator. Gastrointest Endosc 1987;2:101.
24. Heimlich HJ, O'Conner TW, Flores DC. Case for pneumatic dilatation in achalasia. Ann Otol 1978;87:519.
25. Vantrappen G, Hellemans J, Deloof W, Valembois DP, Vandenbroucke J. Treatment of achalasia with pneumatic dilations. Gut 1971;12:268.
26. Payne WS. Heller's contribution to the surgical treatment of achalasia of the esophagus. Ann Thorac Surg 1989;48:876.
27. Little AG, Chen W, Ferguson MK, Skinner DB, Evander A, Krzystek M. Physiologic evaluation of esophageal function in patients with achalasia and diffuse esophageal spasm. Ann Surg 1986;203:500.
28. Ellis FH, Crozier RE, Watkins E. Operation for esophageal achalasia. J Thorac Cardiovasc Surg 1984;88:344.
29. Ellis FH, Gibb SP, Crozier RE. Esophagomyotomy for achalasia of the esophagus. Ann Surg 1980;192:157.
30. Okike N, Payne WS, Neufeld DM, Bernatz PE, Pairolero PC, Sanderson DR. Esophago-myotomy versus forceful dilation for achalasia of the esophagus: results in 899 patients. Ann Thorac Surg 1979;28:119.
31. Yon J, Christensen J. An uncontrolled comparison of treatments for achalasia. Ann Surg 1975;182:672.
32. Thomson D, Shoenut JP, Trenholm BG, Teskey JM. Reflux patterns following limited myotomy without fundoplication for achalasia. Ann Thorac Surg 1987;43:550.
33. Little AG, Soriano A, Ferguson MK, Winans CS, Skinner DB. Surgical treatment of achalasia: results with esopha-

gomyotomy and Belsey repair. Ann Thorac Surg 1988;45:489.

34. Altorki NK, Little AG. Achalasia and diffuse spasm of the esophagus. In Nyhus LM, Baker RJ, eds. Mastery of surgery, ed 2. Boston, Little, Brown, 1992:494.

35. Donahue PE, Schlesinger PK, Samelson S. Achalasia of the esophagus. Ann Surg 1986;203:505.

36. Duranceau A, LaFontaine ER, Vallieres B. Effects of total fundoplication on function of the esophagus after myotomy for achalasia. Am J Surg 1981;143:22.

37. Stipa S, Gegiz G, Iascone C, et al. Heller-Belsey and Heller-Nissen operations for achalasia of the esophagus. Surg Gynecol Obstet 1990;170:212.

38. Pellegrini C, Wetter LA, Patti M, et al. Thoracoscopic esophagomyotomy: initial experience with a new approach for the treatment of achalasia. Ann Surg 1992;216:291.

39. Ancona E, Peracchia A, Zaninotto G, Rossi M, Bonavina L, Segalin A. Heller laparo-scopic cardiomyotomy with antireflux anterior fundoplication (DOR) in the treatment of esophageal achalasia. Surg Endosc 1993;7P:459.

40. Gillies M, Nicks R, Skyring A. Clinical, manometric, and pathological studies in diffuse oesophageal spasm. Br Med J 1967;2:527.

41. Gonzalez G. Diffuse esophageal spasm. AJR 1973;117:251.

42. Henderson RD, Ryder C, Marryatt G. Extended esophageal myotomy and short total fundoplication hernia repair in diffuse esophageal spasm: five-year review in 34 patients. Ann Thorac Surg 1987;43:25.

43. Cohen S. Classification of esophageal motility disorders. Gastroenterology 1983;84:1050.

44. Dalton CB, Castell DO, Hewson EG, Wu WC, Richter JE. Diffuse esophageal spasm. Dig Dis Sci 1991;36:1025.

45. Richter JE, Castell DO. Diffuse esophageal spasm: a reappraisal. Ann Intern Med 1984;100:242.

46. Little AG, Bandt PD. Are there specific radiographic features of diffuse esophageal spasm? In: Giuli R, ed. Primary esophageal motility disorders. Berlin, Springer-Verlag, 1991:643.

47. Little AG. What is the incidence of associated hiatal hernia or gastroesophageal reflux in patients with diffuse esophageal spasm? In: Giuli R, ed. Primary esophageal motility disorders. Berlin, Springer-Verlag, 1991:662.

48. Scarpignato C, Franze A. What is the role of smooth muscle relaxants in the treatment of diffuse esophageal spasm? In: Giuli R, ed. Primary esophageal motility disorders. Berlin, Springer-Verlag, 1991:701.

49. Schuster MM. Esophageal spasm and psychiatric disorder. (Editorial) N Engl J Med 1983;309:1382.

50. Eypasch EP, DeMeester TR, Klingman RR, Stein HJ. Physiologic assessment and surgical management of diffuse esophageal spasm. J Thorac Cardiovasc Surg 1991;104:859.

51. Little AG. Motor disturbances of the esophagus. In: Skinner DB, Moody F, eds. Surgical treatment of digestive disease. Chicago, Year Book Medical Publishers, 1989:122.

52. Ellis FS. How long should the esophagomyotomy be in patients with diffuse esophageal spasm? In: Giuli R, ed. Primary esophageal motility disorders. Berlin, Springer-Verlag, 1991:718.

53. Ferguson MK, Little AG. Angina-like chest pain associated with high-amplitude peristaltic contractions of the esophagus. Surgery 1988;104:713.

54. Orr WC, Robinson MG. Hypertensive peristalsis in the pathogenesis of chest pain: further exploration of the "nutcracker" esophagus. Am J Gastroenterol 1982;77:604.

55. Clouse RE, Lustman PJ. Psychiatric illness and contraction abnormalities of the esophagus. N Engl J Med 1983;309:1337.

56. Richter JE, Dalton CB, Bradley LA, Castell BO. Oral nifedipine in the treatment of non-cardiac chest pain in patients with the nutcracker esophagus. Gastroenterology 1987;93:21.

57. Evander A, Little AG, Ferguson MK, Skinner DB. Diverticula of the mid- and lower esophagus: pathogenesis and surgical management. World J Surg 1986;10:820.

58. Altorki NK, Sunagawa M, Skinner DB. Thoracic esophageal diverticula. J Thorac Cardiovasc Surg 1993;105:260.

59. Debas HT, Payne WS, Cameron AJ, Carlson HC. Physiopathology of lower esophageal diverticulum and its implications for treatment. Surg Gynecol Obstet 1980;151:593.

60. Benacci JC, Deschamps C, Trastek VF, Allen MS, Daly RC, Pairolero PC. Epiphrenic diverticulum: results of surgical treatment. Ann Thorac Surg 1993;55:1109.

61. Zamost BJ, Hirschberg J, Ippoliti AF, Furst DE, Clements PJ, Weinstein WM. Esophagitis in scleroderma. Gastroenterology 1987;92:421.

62. Orringer MB, Dabich L, Zarafonetis CJD, Sloan H. Gastroesophageal reflux in esophageal scleroderma: diagnosis and implications. Ann Thorac Surg 1976;22:120.

63. McLaughlin JS, Roig R, Woodruff MFA. Surgical treatment of strictures of the esophagus in patients with scleroderma. J Thorac Cardiovasc Surg 1971;61:641.

Digestive Tract Surgery: A Text and Atlas, edited by Richard H. Bell, Layton F. Rikkers, and Michael W. Mulholland. Lippincott-Raven Publishers, Philadelphia, © 1996.

3

Neoplasms of the Esophagus

Joe B. Putnam, Jr. | *Jack A. Roth*

The virulence of esophageal neoplasms reflects the late stage at diagnosis, the patients' poor general health, and a paucity of effective therapies for regional and distant metastases. Neoplasms of the esophagus accounted for 11,300 of estimated new cancer cases in the United States in 1993. More men (8100) than women (3200) acquired the disease, and more than 10,200 deaths were attributed to esophageal neoplasms in 1993 (7600 men, 2600 women). The 5-year relative survival for whites has increased only slightly from 5% (1974 to 1976) to 9% (1983 to 1988); for blacks, the 5-year survival has remained essentially unchanged (4% in 1974 to 1976; 6% in 1983 to 1988).[1]

The spectrum of esophageal neoplasms is changing in the United States. In the past, squamous cell carcinoma of the esophagus was common and generally associated with black race, male gender, smoking, alcohol abuse, and poor socioeconomic environment. Now, adenocarcinoma of the esophagus is increasing in comparison to squamous cell carcinoma,[2,3] occurring more frequently in middle-aged white men. Adenocarcinoma can arise from severely dysplastic columnar epithelium within the esophagus (Barrett's esophagus) or from gastric cardia neoplasms that extend into the distal esophagus. The risk of adenocarcinoma is also increased in patients who smoke (2.3 times), former smokers (1.9 times), and patients who use alcohol (2.3 times greater for patients consuming more than 4 oz of alcohol per day). The age-adjusted annual incidence rate for combined esophageal and gastric cardia adenocarcinoma is 5.8 per 100,000 population; this incidence places adenocarcinoma of the esophagus and gastroesophageal junction as one of the top 15 neoplasms among white men in the United States.[4]

EPIDEMIOLOGY AND PREDISPOSING CONDITIONS

The initiating event in esophageal carcinogenesis may be exposure to *N*-nitrosamines through diet (food preparation or storage) or in vivo exposure (produced in the stomach). The carcinogenic effects are enhanced by alcohol (seen in Europe and the United States), dietary deficiencies (lack of fresh fruits and vegetables and of vitamin A, C, and riboflavin, seen in China and Southwest Asia) and mycotoxins (seen in South Africa).[5–8] Pickled vegetables and a preference for consuming beverages or soups at high temperature in the diet of Hong Kong Chinese are associated with an increased risk of esophageal cancer. This provides credible evidence for the carcinogenicity of *N*-nitroso agents for esophageal carcinoma in humans and the high risk of cancer development in the Chinese.[9]

Tylosis, a genetic syndrome manifested by hyperkeratosis and esophageal papillomas, which is inherited in an autosomal dominant pattern, is associated with an increased risk of squamous cell carcinoma of the esophagus.[8] Achalasia may also predispose to squamous cell carcinoma. The tumor usually appears at the air–fluid interface—the site of most severe inflammation. Even after correction of achalasia, the risk of carcinoma may persist,[10] and patients may benefit from annual or biannual endoscopy.

Barrett's esophagus (columnar-lined epithelium beyond the gastroesophageal junction) is often associated with gastroesophageal reflux and may progress through various grades of dysplasia: mild, moderate, or severe. Severe dysplasia is synonymous with adenocarcinoma in situ, and these patients should undergo esophagectomy.

Caustic burns to the esophagus can result in squamous cell carcinoma 40 to 50 years later. Patients who ingested caustics at an early age are more prone to the development of squamous cell carcinoma than other patients.[11] Three fourths of all these tumors are located in the middle third of the esophagus.[11,12] Survival after resection is about 13% at 5 years. Because of the increased risk, patients with a prior history of caustic ingestion should be routinely screened, particularly when the time from injury exceeds 20 years.[12]

In 1919, D.R. Patterson[13] and A.B. Kelly[13a] independently described a syndrome consisting of dysphagia from an esophageal web, iron deficiency anemia, and glossitis. This syndrome typically occurs in edentulous middle-aged women. The condition is premalignant; about 10% of patients develop neoplasms of the esophagus or hypopharynx.

Infection by certain microorganisms has been associated with the development of esophageal neoplasms. These microorganisms may act indirectly on the esophageal epithelium by forming carcinogens or other products to enhance carcinogenesis or by directly affecting the esophagus.[14] Human papillomavirus DNA is associated with squamous cell carcinoma in Japan; patients with papillomavirus infection have poorer survival than patients not infected.[15] This virus has been noted in almost half of patients with squamous cell carcinoma in China.[16]

Patients at high risk for gastric carcinoma and potentially for neoplasms involving the gastroesophageal junction have a high incidence of *Helicobacter pylori* infection. In one recent study of 5908 Japanese American men at high risk for gastric carcinoma,[17] 94% of patients with gastric carcinoma also had *H pylori* antibodies, while 76% of matched control patients had *H pylori* antibodies. Although most patients with *H pylori* infection do not develop gastric carcinoma, associated factors in combination with *H pylori* infection may predispose to carcinogenesis.[17] In one study,[18] over 15% of patients with Barrett's esophagus were infected with *H pylori*, and all patients who were infected also had chronic inflammatory reactions. Colonization by *H pylori* without inflammation did not occur. The role of *H pylori* infection in the subsequent development of esophageal carcinoma remains to be described.

ANATOMY

The esophagus begins at the cricoid cartilage at the level of the cricopharyngeus muscle and topographically at the level of the sixth cervical vertebrae. The cervical esophagus is about 5 cm long, extends to the thoracic inlet, and lies just to the left of midline. The thoracic esophagus begins at the thoracic inlet and extends to the diaphragmatic esophageal hiatus. The intrathoracic esophagus is 20 to 25 cm long.

During endoscopy, lesions are localized in the esophagus by measuring the distance to the abnormality from the central incisor teeth. By this measure, the esophagus begins about 15 to 18 cm from the incisors at the cricopharyngeus muscle and terminates at the gastroesophageal junction, 38 to 40 cm distally. The thoracic inlet begins about 20 cm from the central incisors (at the level of T-1).

The esophagus lies dorsal to the left main-stem bronchus at its junction with the trachea. Tracheoesophageal fistulas usually occur at this point. The carina is 23 to 25 cm from the incisors (angle of Louis, anteriorly; T4-5, posteriorly). The arch of the aorta passes in front of the esophagus at this level and may produce a visible pulsation during esophagoscopy.

The American Joint Committee for Cancer Staging and End Results Reporting[19] divides the esophagus into the *cervical esophagus,* from the cricoid cartilage to the thoracic inlet; the *upper thoracic esophagus,* extending from the thoracic inlet to the tracheal bifurcation; the *middle thoracic esophagus,* which is the proximal half of the esophagus from the tracheal bifurcation to the esophagogastric junction; and the *lower thoracic esophagus,* which is the distal half of the esophagus between the tracheal bifurcation and the esophagogastric junction, including the abdominal esophagus.

In common use, lesions within the esophagus are described as being in the *upper third,* between the cricopharyngeus and the aortic arch; the *middle third,* between the superior portion of the aortic arch and the inferior pulmonary vein; and the *lower* or *distal third,* between the inferior pulmonary vein and the stomach. About 15% of all esophageal cancers occur in the upper third of the esophagus, 50% in the middle, and 35% in the lower third. Adenocarcinomas occur most frequently in the lower third of the esophagus.

The blood supply to the esophagus consists of branches from the inferior thyroid artery, the bronchial arteries, the left gastric artery, and the inferior phrenic artery. These arteries branch just before entry into the esophagus. This vascular network extends into the esophagus and supplies the submucosal area with the richest vascular supply.[20] The veins from the thoracic esophagus drain into the azygous and hemiazygous system and into the intercostal veins, which are tributaries of the azygous system.

The lymphatic supply of the esophagus is extensive. A dense network of lymphatic vessels within the mucosa and the submucosa communicate freely with lymphatic channels in the muscular layers of the esophagus and with those that extend through the esophagus into the thoracic nodes. Neoplasms from any portion of the esophagus can travel to any other portion of the esophagus through the lymphatic channels. Tumors may spread to the supraclavicular or cervical lymph nodes. A thorough examination of both supraclavicular fossae and the area behind the sternocleidomastoid muscles and the clavicular heads can yield positive results to the careful examiner. A histologic diagnosis can be obtained by fine-needle aspiration and cytologic examination[21] or by lymph node excision. A positive result demonstrates systemic spread of the disease and modifies subsequent treatment. Although lymphatic flow may be unpredictable, the lymphatic drainage favors longitudinal rather than circumferential spread.

Lymph drains to the internal jugular, cervical, and supraclavicular areas for the upper third; the peritracheal, hilar, subcarinal, periesophageal, periaortic, and pericardial nodes for the upper and middle thirds; and the lesser curvature, left gastric, and celiac axis nodes for the distal third. Metastases to the celiac nodes occur in 10% of esophageal cancers located in the cervical and upper thoracic esophagus. Middle-third esophageal tumors have celiac nodal involvement in up to 44% of patients.[22] Most commonly, the distal esophagus drains to these beds. Optimally, 10 cm of esophagus beyond the tumor must be treated or resected. Because the length of the esophagus is only 20 to 25 cm in the chest, a total esophagectomy is often needed for optimal surgical control. A lesser resection can be performed, but "skip areas" can increase the risk of local recurrence.[23,24]

CLINICAL PRESENTATION

Patients with esophageal cancer are usually men between 55 and 65 years of age with a long-standing history of cigarette abuse and heavy alcohol intake. The initial symptoms are dysphagia and weight loss in 90% of patients. Difficulty in swallowing occurs when the diameter of the esophagus is narrowed to less than 13 mm (40F) because the esophagus is distensible. Most patients complain of food sticking at some point within the thorax. Occasionally, the onset of dysphagia is sudden, but most patients complain of a vague difficulty in swallowing for the preceding 3 to 6 months. Patients with cancers of the middle of lower third of the esophagus may complain of food sticking in the epigastrium. Odynophagia (painful swallowing) is seen in about half of patients with cancer of the esophagus. Regurgitation of undigested food, retrosternal or epigastric pain, or aspiration pneumonia may be present. More advanced lesions may present with hematemesis, melena, cough from a tracheoesophageal fistula, hemoptysis, or signs

related to nerve involvement, such as Horner's syndrome or paralysis of the recurrent laryngeal nerve (Table 3-1). Patients with tumors of the esophagus may present with superior vena cava syndrome, but this is rare in the absence of dysphagia. Erosion of the esophagus into the aorta can result in exsanguinating hemorrhage. Other signs of unresectability include malignant pleural effusion and malignant ascites. Palpable supraclavicular or cervical lymph nodes should be excised to exclude metastases. Metastasis to the bones can produce a paraneoplastic syndrome from hypercalcemia. Bone pain suggests metastases, particularly when point tenderness is identified.

DIAGNOSIS

All patients with dysphagia require a plain chest roentgenogram and a barium swallow. Rarely do other lesions present with the characteristic barium swallow appearance of cancer of the esophagus (Fig. 3-1). All patients should undergo esophagoscopy (Fig. 3-2) for histologic diagnosis of the tumor and for evaluation of intramural metastases. Both flexible and rigid esophagoscopy can be used. Intramural metastases can be identified in up to 11% of patients, and up to 70% of these can be detected proximal to the tumor by esophagoscopy.[24]

All lesions seen at the time of the esophagoscopy must be excised for biopsy and brushed. Brushings of the tumor are diagnostic in 90% of cases; only 70% of biopsies are diagnostic.[25,26] When both techniques are used, a neoplasm (true-positive) is confirmed in more than 95% of patients.

Early diagnosis of esophageal carcinoma or a premalignant lesion can enhance survival because treatment could attenuate or cure the disease. Screening for early-stage carcinoma or premalignant lesions can reduce the death rate from esophageal carcinoma in areas of high incidence. The Linxian County Hospital in the

Table 3-1 Signs and Symptoms Produced by Advanced Carcinoma of the Esophagus

Dysphagia
Weight loss
Hoarseness from recurrent laryngeal nerve paralysis
Dyspnea from diaphragm paralysis (phrenic nerve)
Cough (tracheoesophageal fistula)
Superior vena cava syndrome
Palpable supraclavicular lymphadenopathy
Malignant effusion (pleural or peritoneal)
Bone pain

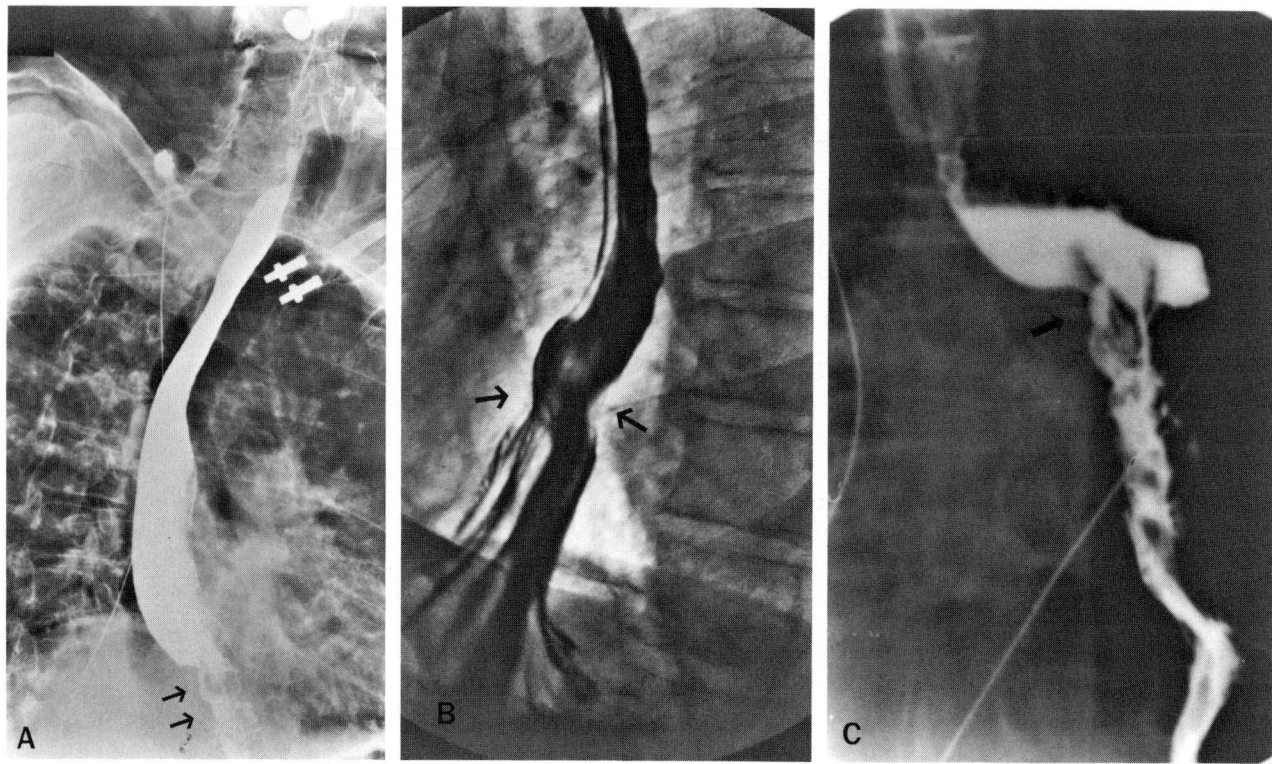

Figure 3-1 (A) Barium swallow radiograph in a patient with dysphagia from distal esophageal carcinoma (*arrows*). (B) Severe dysplasia in Barrett's esophagus was noted at the gastroesophageal junction (*arrows*) in a patient with long-standing reflux. The esophagus was shortened from the chronic esophagitis. Transhiatal esophagectomy was performed. A perigastric lymph node was positive for metastatic carcinoma. (C) Larger tumors may produce a "shelf" of tumor from a circumferential narrowing of the esophageal lumen (*arrow*). The esophagus dilates proximal to the obstruction.

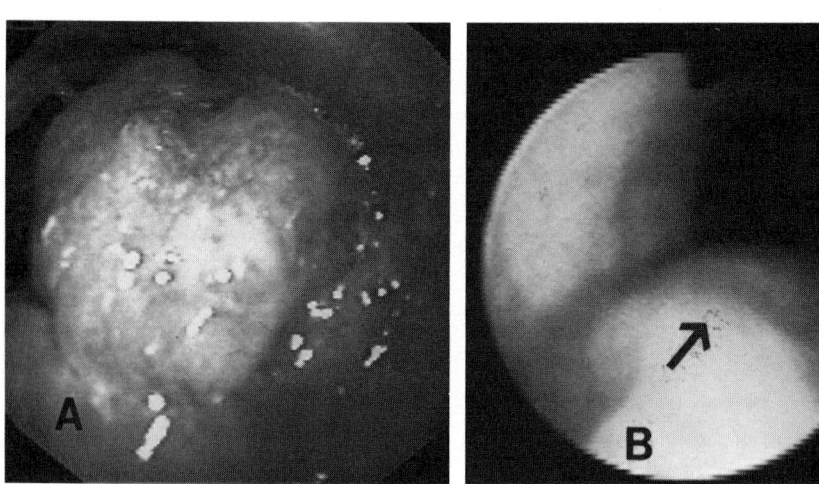

Figure 3-2 (A) Esophagoscopy demonstrates a tumor at a level 25 cm from the incisors. The tumor extends from 25 to 30 cm. No evidence of proximal or distal esophageal intramural metastases was seen. (B) Bronchoscopy in the same patient revealed a bulge of the membranous trachea just above the carina (*arrow*). The area was excised for histology and brushed for cytology. All specimens were negative for tumor. (See Color Fig. 3-2.)

Hunan Province of China has developed a technique of abrasive cytology using a catheter with a balloon covered with cotton to scrape loose esophageal mucosal cells. Cytology is 90% accurate in patients with very early cancer of the esophagus.[27]

STAGING

Clinical staging of esophageal carcinoma (1) identifies patients who may benefit from definitive treatment of their primary carcinoma, (2) excludes patients with metastases from surgery because their survival is short (about 6 months), and (3) assesses response to treatment. Accurate clinical staging of esophageal carcinoma is difficult because of its location deep within the thorax. Many esophageal cancers treated with preoperative irradiation or chemotherapy can be staged only clinically because postsurgical pathologic evaluation may not accurately define the stage of the initially diagnosed cancer. The TNM staging system for the cervical and thoracic esophagus is outlined in Tables 3-2 and 3-3.

Clinical staging for esophageal carcinoma includes a chest roentgenogram, a barium swallow, and computed tomographic (CT) scans of the chest and abdomen (with particular attention to the liver and adrenal glands; Fig. 3-3). CT scans of the chest can accurately identify tracheal or aortic invasion by tumor. CT scanning, however, is a relatively poor way to detect small abdominal lymph node metastases or small liver metastases. In patients with complaints of bone pain, a plain

Table 3-2 TNM Staging for Esophageal Cancer

PRIMARY TUMOR

TX	Primary tumor cannot be assessed
T0	No evidence of primary tumor
Tis	Carcinoma in situ
T1	Tumor invades lamina propria or submucosa
T2	Tumor invades muscularis propria
T3	Tumor invades adventitia
T4	Tumor invades adjacent structures

REGIONAL LYMPH NODES

NX	Regional nodes cannot be assessed
N0	No regional node metastasis
N1	Regional node metastasis

DISTANT METASTASIS

MX	Presence of distant metastasis cannot be assessed
M0	No distant metastasis
M1	Distant metastasis

(After Beahrs OH, Henson DE, Hutter RVP, Myers MH. Manual for staging of cancer, ed 3. Philadelphia, JB Lippincott, 1988:63)

Table 3-3 Stage Grouping for Esophageal Cancer

Stage 0	Tis	N0	M0
Stage I	T1	N0	M0
Stage IIA	T2	N0	M0
	T3	N0	M0
Stage IIB	T1	N1	M0
	T2	N1	M0
Stage III	T3	N1	M0
	T4	Any N	M0
Stage IV	Any T	Any N	M1

(After Beahrs OH, Henson DE, Hutter RVP, Myers MH. Manual for staging of cancer, ed 3. Philadelphia, JB Lippincott, 1988:63)

film of the bone and a bone scan should be obtained. A bronchoscopy is mandatory for patients with a middle- or upper-third tumor (Fig. 3-4). Both bone scans and bronchoscopy can identify metastases not evident on CT scan.[28] Pulmonary function studies assess physiologic reserve and ability to tolerate surgery.

NATURAL HISTORY AND PATTERNS OF SPREAD

Esophageal cancers are rarely found when still small and easily treated. Patients with esophageal carcinoma may have no symptoms until the tumor is large and partial obstruction occurs. The patient frequently presents late because the distensible esophagus compensates for tumor partially obstructing the lumen. Patients with in situ carcinoma may have no symptoms for 3 or 4 years, until advanced cancer develops.[29] The length of the esophagus involved by the neoplasm correlates with the extent of involvement of adjacent structures and inversely relates to curability. The unique lymphatic drainage of the esophagus and the long interval during which the tumor is asymptomatic account for the extensive nodal involvement or invasion into structures adjacent to the esophagus. In one series of 117 patients with esophagectomy and extensive lymph node dissection,[30] lymphatic metastases were identified in the neck in 32% of patients and in about half of the lymph nodes in the chest and abdomen.

Distant metastases are less often identified when patients present with dysphagia. Autopsies have shown that widespread distant metastases are almost always present at death.[31] Esophageal carcinoma can spread to virtually any organ (liver, lung, pleura, stomach, peritoneum, kidney, adrenal gland, brain, and bone), and metastases may be present as subclinical disease when the patient is first diagnosed.[32]

Synchronous or metachronous malignancies of the

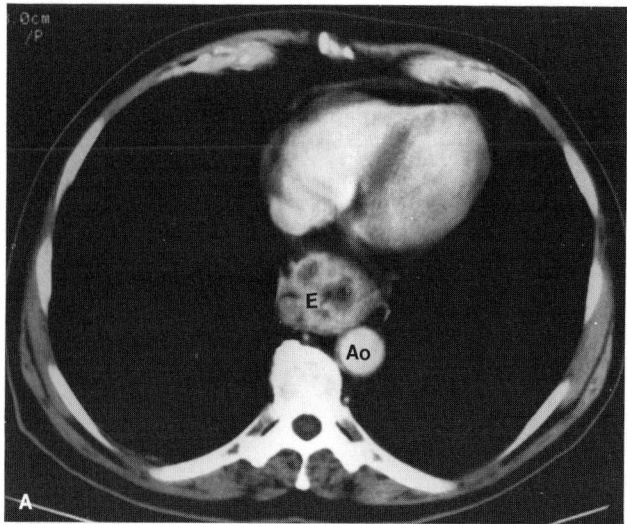

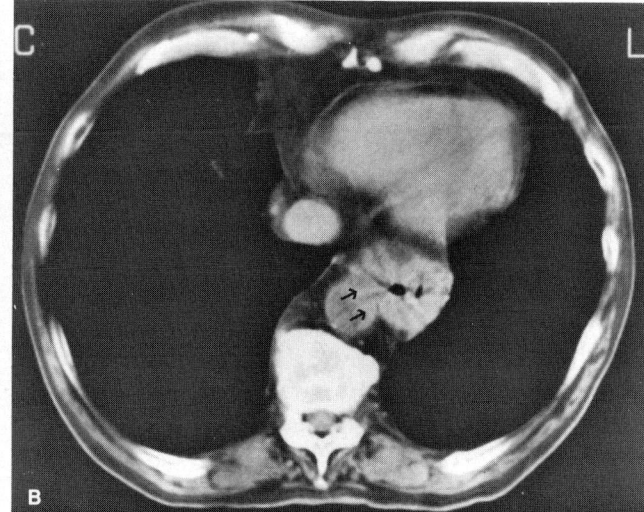

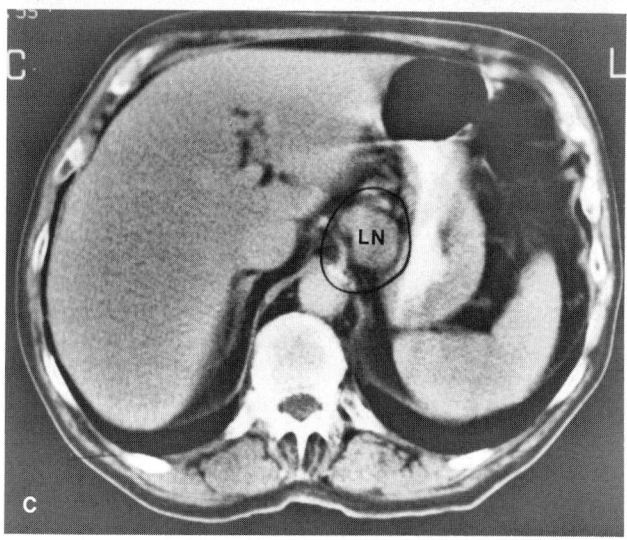

Figure 3-3 CT scan of the chest and abdomen provides an assessment of the tumor's location and its involvement with other structures. **(A)** The esophageal tumor (E) is free from the vertebral fascia but abuts the aorta (Ao). **(B)** The tumor appears to involve the aortic adventitia (*arrows*). At operation, however, the tumor was separable from the adventitia of the aorta. **(C)** Celiac lymphadenopathy. Involved celiac lymph nodes (LN) may not always be visualized by CT. At celiotomy, a thorough examination of the celiac axis should be undertaken for assessment of regional or extraregional metastases.

aerodigestive tract occur in 5% to 12% of patients with esophageal carcinoma. About half can be found in the oral cavity, pharynx, larynx, and lung. Oral and pharyngeal cancers are particularly associated with esophageal carcinoma; laryngeal cancers are most often associated with lung carcinoma. Direct laryngoscopy, bronchoscopy, and esophagoscopy in patients with primary head and neck cancer reveal that 5% of patients have synchronous lung cancer, esophageal cancer, or both. Most of these synchronous malignancies are asymptomatic.[33,34]

TREATMENT OF CARCINOMA OF THE ESOPHAGUS

The diagnostic and therapeutic approaches to squamous cell carcinoma and adenocarcinoma are similar. In early stages of the disease (no lymph node metasta-

ses), surgery can provide a cure for the patient. Up to 70% of patients with stage I carcinoma of the esophagus survive 5 years after resection[35]; gender, age, site, and histologic type have little impact on subsequent survival. In later stages of esophageal carcinoma (positive lymph node metastases or invasion into thoracic structures), resection may provide the best palliation for dysphagia yet not improve survival. In patients with locally advanced disease, chemotherapy or chemotherapy plus radiation therapy given as adjuvant or primary therapy can improve control of the local tumor and distant metastases and potentially improve survival.

Clinical Evaluation

Patients require various examinations to evaluate the extent of their tumor and their ability or fitness to tolerate the treatment proposed (Fig. 3-5). Any patient

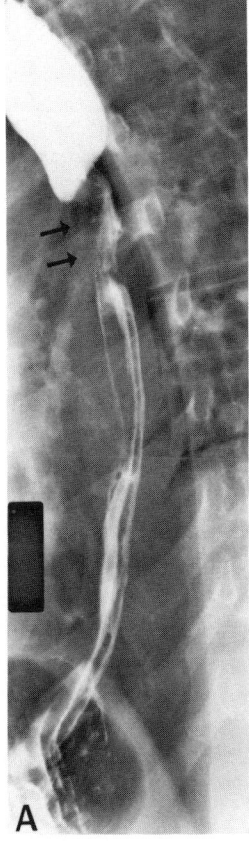

Figure 3-4 The potential for resectability of middle-third neoplasms that abut the trachea may be assessed by thoracotomy before celiotomy. (**A**) Barium swallow demonstrated a high middle-third tumor just above the carina. Preoperative bronchoscopy did not reveal any mucosal abnormalities; biopsy and brushings of the carina were negative for tumor. (**B**) An exploratory right thoracotomy was performed, and the tumor was completely separated from the trachea. No invasion occurred. A mediastinal lymph node dissection completed the pathologic staging. LMSB, left mainstem bronchus; RMSB, right mainstem bronchus; T, tumor. (See Color Fig. 3-4*B*.)

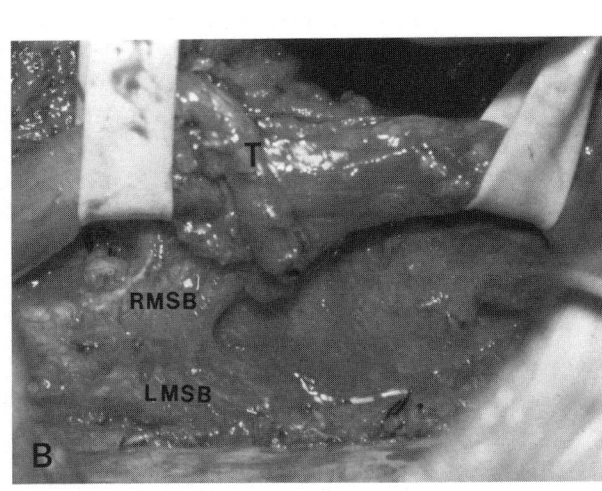

who presents with dysphagia and weight loss must be considered to have esophageal carcinoma until this diagnosis is excluded. The patient must be evaluated for the extent of disease and to determine whether an operation can be safely performed. A thorough history and examination can yield important clues to the extent of the tumor and potential for metastases. Symptoms produced by advanced esophageal cancers may indicate unresectable disease. Patients without evidence of extraregional spread of the disease, on the other hand, may be excellent candidates for surgical resection or for multimodality treatment of carcinoma of the esophagus.

Radiographic staging assists the physician and the patient in determining the best treatment options. In patients who have locally resectable tumors without distant metastases, surgery provides excellent palliation. Tumors that invade the distal posterior membranous trachea or that cause a tracheoesophageal fistula are not surgically resectable. Both barium swallow and esophagoscopy provide information on tumor length, circumferential extent, and character (eg, bleeding, fungating, polypoid). Patients with metastases from

esophageal carcinoma have shortened life expectancies, and surgical resection is not usually justified.[36]

Endoscopic ultrasonography has been used to assess circumferential involvement of the esophageal carcinoma with the surrounding structures, particularly for clinical staging of tumors of the upper and middle third of the esophagus. The length of the tumor, infiltration into adjacent organs, and involvement of lymph nodes can be assessed by this technique.[37–40]

CT scans of the thorax and abdomen assist in identifying the location and extent of the primary tumor. Metastases to the lung, celiac axis lymph nodes, liver, adrenal glands, or other thoracic and abdominal abnormalities may be noted.[28,41–43] CT scanning underestimates tumor length and is inaccurate in assessing the degree of periesophageal lymph node involvement or adjacent tissue invasion. Lesion width greater than 3 cm and the presence of extraesophageal spread of tumor are associated with poorer survival.[44] Magnetic resonance imaging (MRI) is infrequently used. MRI can, however, evaluate the involvement of esophageal cancer with vascular structures, such as the aorta, or with the membranous trachea, better than CT scanning.

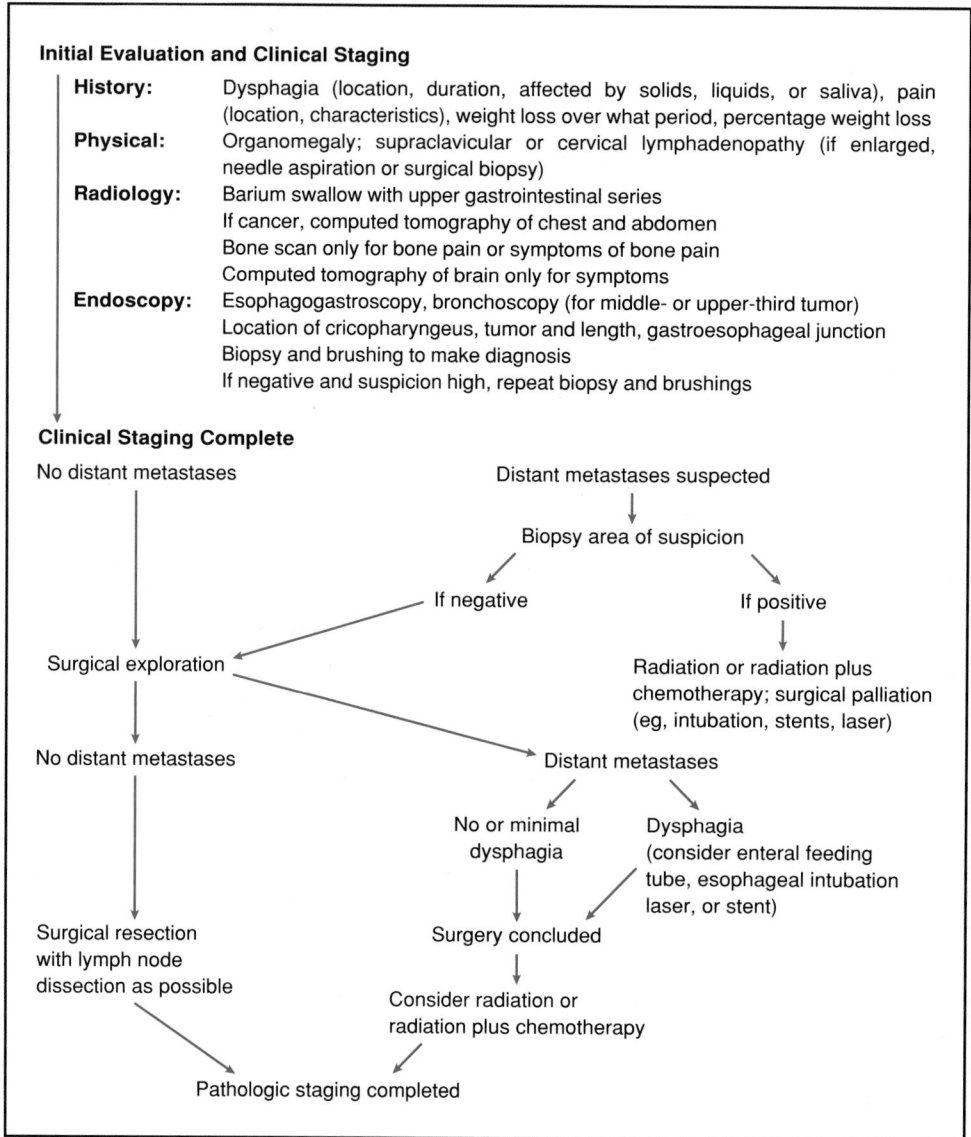

Initial Evaluation and Clinical Staging

History: Dysphagia (location, duration, affected by solids, liquids, or saliva), pain (location, characteristics), weight loss over what period, percentage weight loss

Physical: Organomegaly; supraclavicular or cervical lymphadenopathy (if enlarged, needle aspiration or surgical biopsy)

Radiology: Barium swallow with upper gastrointestinal series
If cancer, computed tomography of chest and abdomen
Bone scan only for bone pain or symptoms of bone pain
Computed tomography of brain only for symptoms

Endoscopy: Esophagogastroscopy, bronchoscopy (for middle- or upper-third tumor)
Location of cricopharyngeus, tumor and length, gastroesophageal junction
Biopsy and brushing to make diagnosis
If negative and suspicion high, repeat biopsy and brushings

Clinical Staging Complete

No distant metastases

Distant metastases suspected

Biopsy area of suspicion

If negative

If positive

Surgical exploration

Radiation or radiation plus chemotherapy; surgical palliation (eg, intubation, stents, laser)

No distant metastases

Distant metastases

No or minimal dysphagia

Dysphagia (consider enteral feeding tube, esophageal intubation laser, or stent)

Surgical resection with lymph node dissection as possible

Surgery concluded

Consider radiation or radiation plus chemotherapy

Pathologic staging completed

Figure 3-5 Evaluation of a patient with suspected esophageal carcinoma. Distant metastases are considered to be sites of tumor beyond the locoregional area. Any lymph nodes may be considered distant disease, but locoregional lymph node metastases may be resected with the primary tumor, with subsequent survival benefit and palliation of dysphagia. Patients with middle-third or cervical tumors and positive celiac nodes are most like patients with distant metastases; therefore, esophagectomy is not generally recommended. Patients with esophageal tumors and supraclavicular lymph node metastases should not be considered surgical candidates.

Endoscopy, rigid or flexible, is ideal for evaluating the mucosal extent of esophageal cancers. Patients with tumors of the upper- or middle-third esophagus can benefit from rigid esophagoscopy and bronchoscopy to assess tumor extent and the mobility of the esophagus and trachea.

Because of the high frequency of other malignancies within the aerodigestive tract, a careful exam-

ination of the mouth, pharynx, larynx, and tracheo-bronchial tree must be performed (particularly with upper- and middle-third lesions). Bronchoscopy is not required in patients with a distal-third tumor who have a normal chest roentgenogram and a normal CT scan of the chest. In patients with an upper- or middle-third tumor, flexible bronchoscopy is required. The esophagus lies just posterior to the membranous trachea. Rigid bronchoscopy helps to evaluate fixation of the posterior membranous trachea to the tumor. Bulging of the distal posterior membranous trachea or proximal left mainstem bronchus suggests tumor abutting these structures. Biopsy and brushings of this area are essential.

Patients with distal esophageal tumors and clinically enlarged celiac nodes or resectable histologically positive celiac nodes may be suitable for surgery. However, patients with cervical or middle-third esophageal carcinoma and histologically confirmed celiac axis nodal metastases can be considered as having incurable carcinoma. In the absence of significant dysphagia, nonsurgical treatment may be most beneficial. Biopsy of the celiac and lesser curvature lymph nodes is valuable in planning therapy and providing prognostic data. These nodes are resected separately or en bloc with the primary tumor. Celiac node involvement occurs in 10% of patients with upper esophageal malignancies. With lower esophageal cancers, the incidence increases at least five-fold.[22] If the patient has liver or bony metastases or extensive unresectable regional lymphadenopathy, he or she should be palliated by other methods. Patients with histologic evidence of distant metastases (eg, liver) have shortened survival (6 months) and frequently do not benefit from surgery.

Surgical Therapy

Surgery alone palliates dysphagia, although it rarely provides cure except in cases of carcinoma in situ or stage I carcinoma. Combined modality therapy can improve palliation and survival in patients with esophageal carcinoma.[45-48] The presence of metastases (bone, liver, brain, extensive and unresectable regional nodal metastases) precludes any attempt at resection for cure. Surgeons should not routinely undertake palliative esophageal resection or ''bypass'' the unresectable esophageal tumor because the risk of the procedure is greater than the anticipated survival benefit.

Various techniques of esophagectomy have been proposed. Ideally, esophagectomy should relieve dysphagia, minimize operative mortality (under 10%), minimize hospitalization (less than 2 weeks), and minimize late complications and morbidity (eg, infection, stricture, reflux, aspiration).[49] Patients with local or locoregional carcinoma of the esophagus are usually considered suitable candidates for resection of the esophagus and reestablishment of gastrointestinal continuity. Adequate cardiac and pulmonary reserves are needed. Age is not a contraindication for resection. Patients older than 70 years have a postoperative mortality (13%) similar to other age groups.[50] Abdominal venous varicosities from alcoholic cirrhosis or portal hypertension may preclude any attempt at resection.

Preparation of the Patient for Surgery

Proper evaluation of the patient and planning of the operation make the postoperative course of the esophagectomy patient stable and predictable. Patients are not permitted to smoke for a minimum of 2 weeks before surgery. Otherwise, increased mucus production (bronchorrhea) within the first few days after cessation of cigarette smoking can compound the problem of adequate postoperative pulmonary hygiene with thick secretions and can lead to prolonged intubation, atelectasis, poor pulmonary function, and pneumonia. Reintubation may be required. Incentive spirometry begun before surgery and continued throughout the perioperative course minimizes atelectasis.

Physically active patients with a normal electrocardiogram do not require further evaluation of cardiac function before surgery. Advanced age (60 years or older), known heart disease, or abnormal electrocardiogram indicates further cardiac evaluation.

The patient's nutritional status is optimized before surgery with either enteral or intravenous alimentation.[51,52] In the past, it was suggested that patients with at least 5 days of preoperative nutritional support had fewer complications.[53] Recent studies, however, have shown benefits of preoperative total parenteral nutrition only in patients who were severely malnourished before surgery.[54] Weight loss of over 10% of body weight impacts negatively on subsequent survival. Patients with weight loss of less than 10% of body weight responded better to chemotherapy and did better overall than patients with over 10% weight loss, implying less advanced disease.[45] Correction of weight loss before surgery unfortunately does not necessarily improve prognosis.[45,55] Enteral feedings are preferred over parenteral alimentation if supplemental preoperative nutrition is given. Soft Silastic nasogastric feeding tubes can be placed blindly or under fluoroscopic guidance even in patients with severe obstruction. Percutaneous gastrostomy may be required if several weeks of enteral nutrition is planned. Patients with esophageal cancer are prone to dehydration, even those with good oral intake. All patients should therefore be admitted to the hospital at least one night before surgery for intravenous hydration. All patients should have a dental examination before surgery. Virulent mediastinitis from periodontal infections and synergistic oral bacterial contamination can be fatal; dental work should precede esophageal resection. Perioperative antibiotics (second-generation cephalosporin) are routinely used. Patients with esophageal obstruction may require coverage for anaerobic bacteria.

All patients should receive deep venous thrombosis and pulmonary embolus prophylaxis. Subcutaneous heparin, 5000 U every 8 to 12 hours, is inexpensive and well tolerated. Elastic hose or intermittent compression stockings can also be effective.

In the operating room, a radial artery catheter and at least two large-bore intravenous lines are placed to provide fluids and blood products. A central venous line can be helpful in older patients or in patients with underlying cardiac dysfunction. A Foley catheter is inserted. Unless previously performed by the surgeon, esophagoscopy is always performed in the operating room before resection to define the location of the tumor and to determine the presence of secondary tumors. Flexible or rigid bronchoscopy is also performed by the surgeon in patients with esophageal carcinoma of the middle or upper third to evaluate tumor involvement of the posterior membranous trachea.

Approaches to Esophageal Resection

Esophagectomy for carcinoma of the esophagus poses considerable technical challenges to the surgeon and physiologic challenges to the patient. Despite this, esophagectomy provides excellent palliation from dysphagia and is not surpassed by any other modality. Surgery remains the primary treatment of esophageal tumors confined to the esophagus and periesophageal tissues.

The choice of technique of esophagectomy incorporates many factors into a single clinical decision:

- Intent of the surgeon, for example, operation for complete resection or palliation
- Location of the tumor (cervical, middle, or lower third)
- Suitability for multimodality treatment (various regimens of perioperative chemotherapy, or radiation therapy)[56]
- Extent of disease (abutting aorta or esophagus)
- Location of the anastomosis—cervical or thoracic
- Choice and suitability of conduit
- Pyloromyotomy, pyloroplasty, or no drainage procedure
- Experience of the surgeon

The esophagus can be resected using a transthoracic approach or an extrathoracic approach (see Section IV of Atlas Chap. 5). The fitness of the patient, the location and clinical stage of the tumor, and the technical factors involved in esophagectomy (Table 3-4) all affect the choice of resection (Table 3-5). Transthoracic esophagectomies such as the Lewis procedure[57] (right thoracotomy with intrathoracic anastomosis) and the total thoracic esophagectomy[58] (Akiyama procedure: retrosternal gastric interposition with cervical anasto-

Table 3-4 Technical Considerations

VARIABLES
Extent of resection
Level of anastomosis—cervical or thoracic
Transthoracic versus transhiatal resection
Conduit choice for establishment of gastrointestinal continuity
Location of tumor within the esophagus

OPERATION
Transthoracic esophagectomy
Transhiatal esophagectomy
Total thoracic esophagectomy

CHOICE OF CONDUIT
Stomach
Colon
  Left colon
  Transverse colon
  Right colon
Jejunum
  Only for tumors isolated to the hypopharynx or high cervical esophagus

SITES OF CONDUIT
Posterior mediastinum
Retrosternal
Subcutaneous

mosis followed by right thoracotomy for esophagectomy) are commonly performed. The left thoracotomy with esophagectomy and intrathoracic anastomosis is less often performed because the potential to maximize the length of esophageal resection is limited. In transhiatal esophagectomy, the esophagus is resected bluntly through the thoracic hiatus or "inlet" and the diaphragmatic esophageal hiatus.[59,60] The radical esophagectomy (en bloc esophagectomy)[61] carries no better survival value than transhiatal esophagectomy—a more palliative procedure. The benefits and risks vary with the technique used for resection (Table 3-6).

In all procedures, an exploratory laparotomy is performed for an initial assessment of resectability (see Sections I and IV of Atlas Chap. 5). The abdomen is examined, and in particular, the liver and celiac nodes are assessed for the presence of metastases. If a middle-third tumor is present and celiac lymph node metastases are identified, esophagectomy is not routinely recommended. However, with near or complete obstruction, consideration should be given to a complete regional lymph node dissection with esophagectomy. This decision must be individualized. The hiatus is briefly explored to determine the tumor's extent and relation to the spine, the aorta, and other thoracic structures. If no metastases are identified, the stomach is mobilized with its attached blood supply (right gastro-

Table 3-5 Types of Resection

TRANSTHORACIC ESOPHAGECTOMY
Laparotomy and preparation of conduit (stomach preferred)
Assessment of resectability
Right thoracotomy for esophageal mobilization and resection
Intrathoracic anastomosis

TOTAL THORACIC ESOPHAGECTOMY
Laparotomy and preparation of conduit (stomach preferred)
Assessment of resectability
Neck exploration and mobilization of esophagus
Resection of head of left clavicle to widen thoracic inlet
Retrosternal placement of conduit
Cervical anastomosis
Right thoracotomy for esophageal mobilization and resection

TRANSHIATAL ESOPHAGECTOMY
Laparotomy and preparation of conduit (stomach preferred)
Assessment of resectability
Neck exploration and mobilization of esophagus
Transhiatal resection
Cervical anastomosis

RADICAL EN BLOC ESOPHAGECTOMY
Laparotomy and preparation of conduit (colon)
Thoracoabdominal exploration with en bloc resection of:
    Thoracic esophagus
    Mediastinal lymph nodes
    Stomach
    Spleen
    Celiac and thoracic lymph nodes

epiploic and right gastric arteries). Nodes within the gastrohepatic ligament are taken with specimen.

Further mobilization of the stomach is obtained by a wide Kocher maneuver to free the duodenum. If cholelithiasis is identified, the gallbladder is removed. A pyloromyotomy or pyloroplasty should be performed to decrease the risk of gastric outlet obstruction and the complications of gastric stasis.[62] Some surgeons use no drainage procedure; however, postoperative problems with gastric drainage cannot be predicted.[63] Complications of pyloroplasty or pyloromyotomy are minimal.[62,63] A jejunostomy feeding tube is placed 20 cm distal to the ligament of Treitz.

ESOPHAGECTOMY WITH THORACOTOMY. In the Lewis procedure, a right posterolateral thoracotomy incision is used, and the chest is entered through the fifth intercostal space. After the esophagus is removed, a mediastinal node dissection is performed. The thoracic anastomosis (hand-sewn or mechanical) is placed above the azygous vein. A nasogastric tube is placed under direct guidance by the surgeon. Two chest tubes are placed for drainage. (See Sections IV and VI of Atlas Chap. 5.)

In the total thoracic esophagectomy, the gastric conduit is placed retrosternally. Resection of the left clavicle, a portion of the manubrium, and the medial portion of the first rib is performed to enlarge the thoracic inlet. A cervical esophagogastrostomy is performed. A nasogastric tube is placed under direct vision before completing the anastomosis. A right thoracotomy is then performed for esophagectomy. The esophagus, stapled closed at its proximal and distal end, is resected with the tumor. A mediastinal lymph node dissection is performed.

In patients with an extensive middle-third tumor, a transthoracic approach using right thoracotomy can be performed before celiotomy to assess resectability and to mobilize the esophagus. Should the mass be unresectable, the risk of the proposed esophagectomy is avoided.

ESOPHAGECTOMY WITHOUT THORACOTOMY. Transhiatal esophagectomy has potential advantages over esophagectomy with thoracotomy. A thoracotomy is avoided, and the operation can be performed with the patient in one position. A cervical anastomosis is used. The cervical esophagus is mobilized through an oblique incision in the neck to the level of the left main-stem bronchus. Care is taken to stay lateral and posterior to the tracheoesophageal groove and the recurrent laryngeal nerve. The abdominal exploration and mobilization of the stomach are performed as previously described. The hiatus is exposed, and the esophagus is mobilized posteriorly and anteriorly. Care is taken to avoid injury to the bronchial branches off the aorta, the aorta itself, the membranous trachea, and the azygous vein. If the tumor is adherent to the prevertebral fascia or to the aorta, a right thoracotomy may be necessary to free the tumor. Mediastinal blood loss is usually less than 600 to 800 mL. The esophagus is pulled through the posterior mediastinum with a Penrose drain as a guide to the tunnel.

The mediastinum is inspected for bleeding. Pleural entry occurs in more than half of patients, and chest tubes are placed when the pleural tear is discovered. The stomach is divided with at least a 5-cm radial margin from the gastroesophageal junction on the lower curvature. A long gastric tube is created with five or six loads of a surgical stapling device. The gastric conduit is placed into the posterior mediastinum, advanced to the neck, and secured to the prevertebral fascia. The abdomen is closed, and then the cervical esophagogastrostomy is created. A nasogastric tube is placed through the nose and through the anastomosis under direct vision. The nasogastric tube is left above the pyloromyotomy. A nasogastric tube does not prevent a leak but decompresses the conduit. A chest radiograph

Table 3-6   Advantages and Disadvantages of Specific Types of Esophageal Resection

Procedure	Advantages	Disadvantages
Transthoracic esophagectomy	Standard resection Good visualization for esophageal resection and lymph node dissection	Requires repositioning the patient Requires thoracotomy Less than maximal resection of thoracic esophagus Thoracic anastomosis Resectability not determined until thoracotomy performed
Transhiatal esophagectomy	No thoracotomy Cervical anastomosis Maximal resection	Learning curve Less complete mediastinal lymph node dissection Intraoperative thoracic complications may require thoracotomy
Total thoracic esophagectomy	Cervical anastomosis Gastrointestinal continuity established early in the procedure Maximal esophagus resected Good visualization for resection and lymph node dissection Posterior mediastinum free of conduit for adjuvant radiation if needed	Requires repositioning patient Requires thoracotomy Resectability not determined until thoracotomy performed

is obtained in the operating room at the conclusion of the procedure to assess the position of the chest tubes and nasogastric tube. (See Sections IV and VI of Atlas Chap. 5.)

Esophageal neoplasms in the cervical esophagus may involve the posterior membranous trachea or the cricopharyngeus muscle. Tumors in the hypopharynx may extend to the cervical esophagus. Resection of the larynx and the esophagus is often required.[64–67] An anterior cervical tracheostomy with gastric interposition or jejunal interposition is commonly performed when the tumor does not extend past the thoracic inlet. When the tumor involves more of the trachea, an anterior mediastinal tracheostomy can be constructed after removal of the breast plate. A minimum of 5 cm of normal trachea above the carina is required for safe construction of an anterior mediastinal tracheostomy. The esophagus is mobilized with a transhiatal approach.[68,69] Laryngoesophagectomy with gastric interposition offers the best chance for cure or palliation of advanced hypopharyngeal and laryngeal tumors. Patients who underwent prior radiation therapy can also be resected safely, although healing may be poor. In one study,[65] 41 patients with squamous cell carcinoma of the cervical esophagus were treated with laryngectomy, esophagectomy, and gastric interposition.

Twenty-one patients had undergone prior radiation therapy. Complications included one operative death (2.5%) and anastomotic leaks in 9 patients (22%). All 9 had received previous radiation therapy, and 3 patients required flap reconstruction. The average postoperative stay was 31 days. The overall 2-year survival rate was 35%. In another study of 42 patients,[70] the mortality rate was 19%, and the complication rate was 40%. Average length of hospitalization ranged from 23 days (without complications) to 44 days (with complications). Patients with head and neck neoplasms involving the larynx and cervical esophagus only, without extension past the thoracic inlet, benefit from jejunal interposition as a free flap. Hypoparathyroidism is the most morbid complication and is best prevented by preserving at least one parathyroid gland. If all parathyroid glands must be removed, a diligent effort must be made to find one or two normal glands in the specimen and reimplant them into a forearm muscle.

After esophagectomy, the nasogastric tube is irrigated with saline and placed on low continuous suction to maintain patency. Patients require more fluids than would be expected from the usual thoracic procedure because of the mediastinal dissection. After extubation, the patient should be placed in the semi-Fowler position to decrease the risk of aspiration of bile and gastric secretions. Jejunostomy tube feedings are begun 12 to 24 hours after surgery and increased as tolerated. A barium swallow is performed 7 to 10 days after surgery (Fig. 3-6). The cervical anastomosis is examined for location, patency, and evidence of anastomotic leak. The pyloromyotomy or pyloroplasty is examined for patency, leak, and adequacy of drainage.

Establishment of Conduits

The stomach is the conduit of choice for the reestablishment of gastrointestinal continuity after esophagectomy. Patients with prior gastric resection often do not have sufficient remaining stomach to serve as a conduit. Colon or jejunum can also be used to reestablish gastrointestinal continuity. Blood supply to the colon is well known and can be easily discerned on preoperative angiography or intraoperatively with finger palpation or Doppler probe. The use of colon for a conduit adds time and morbidity because additional anastomoses are required. The blood supply to the jejunum provides less length than the colon. (See Section VI of Atlas Chap. 5.)

COLON. The colon is the second organ of choice for esophageal replacement after the stomach. The right colon is usually used in an isoperistaltic position and the left colon in an antiperistaltic position. The quality of the colon and the character and anatomy of the vascular supply of the desired segment often assist the surgeon in determining the best portion to use as a conduit. The blood supply to the colon is not always constant (left side vascular supply is more constant than the right side); for this reason, a preoperative angiogram is valuable in planning the blood supply to be preserved during mobilization of the colon.

The right colon can be mobilized by dividing the ileocolic and right colic arteries and basing the blood supply on the middle colic artery. If the length is not sufficient, the left colon may be preferable. The transverse colon can also be used in a peristaltic fashion. The right colic artery and the middle colic artery are divided, and the colon pedicle is based on the left colic artery. The left colon has a more consistent blood supply than the right colon. The left colon and sigmoid can be mobilized and the left colic artery divided.

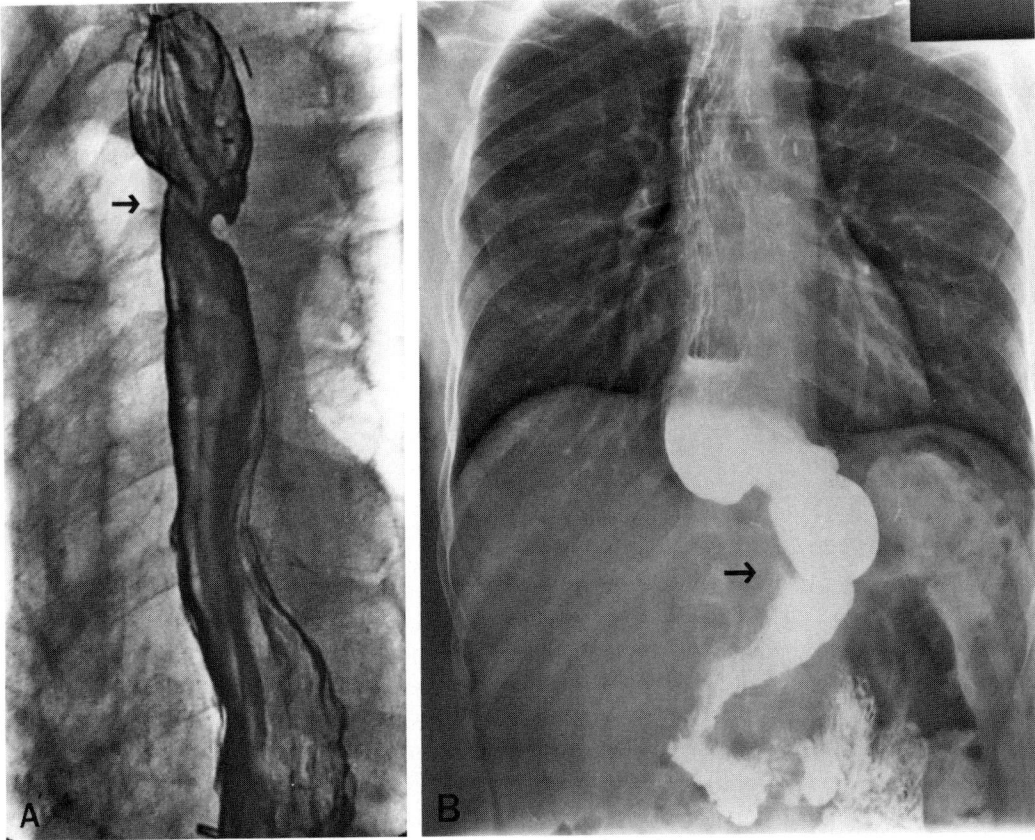

Figure 3-6 (**A**) Cervical anastomosis after transhiatal esophagectomy. (**B**) Excellent drainage of the gastric conduit by gravity.

Branches from the inferior mesenteric artery can also be divided to further mobilize the sigmoid colon. At least 2 cm of mesentery are needed to protect the marginal artery. The colon pedicle is positioned through the mesentery behind the colocolostomy. If a portion of the stomach exists, the colon pedicle can be brought behind the stomach through the lesser sac before it is positioned in the posterior or anterior mediastinum. In the abdomen, the cologastrostomy or colojejunostomy is fashioned with an end colon to side stomach or side jejunum (antimesenteric) anastomosis. A cervical or thoracic esophagocolostomy is created.

In one study,[71] complications occurred in up to 35.7% of patients who underwent left colon interposition (mortality, 11.9%). Functional results were good to excellent in more than two thirds of patients. Cervical anastomotic leakage was encountered in 13.5% of patients and accounted for all the poor functional results. In another study,[72] 21 patients had left colon interposition; three patients required reoperation for empyema, ischemia, and subphrenic abscess. No patient had a leak, and the 30-day operative mortality was 4.5%. Functional results were rated as good.

JEJUNUM. Free jejunal interposition has been used successfully after resection for carcinoma of the upper cervical esophagus or hypopharynx that does not extend past the thoracic inlet. Once the esophagus is resected, the proximal and distal anastomoses are completed to stabilize the graft. Vascular corrections are made to the external carotid artery and the internal jugular vein. Fifteen to 20 cm of jejunum can be used as a free graft. Jejunum is useful for reconstruction of the cervical esophagus[73]; the leak rate is low,[74] and viability can be monitored by a portion of jejunum outside the incision.[75] Infrequently, jejunum is used after esophagogastrectomy for gastroesophageal junction tumors. This may not be advisable because adequate esophageal margins may not be obtained, and local recurrence may occur (Fig. 3-7).

Results of Esophagectomy

Although overall survival after esophageal resection has remained fairly constant, operative mortality has slowly decreased during the past 30 years. Five-year survival after esophagectomy is about 20% (Fig. 3-8). Major problems of inadequate staging, intrathoracic extension of tumor, reestablishment of gastrointestinal continuity, location and construction of the esophageal–conduit anastomosis, anastomotic leak, and postoperative respiratory compromise[76] have been identified and various solutions proposed. Each technique of esophagectomy has particular advantages and

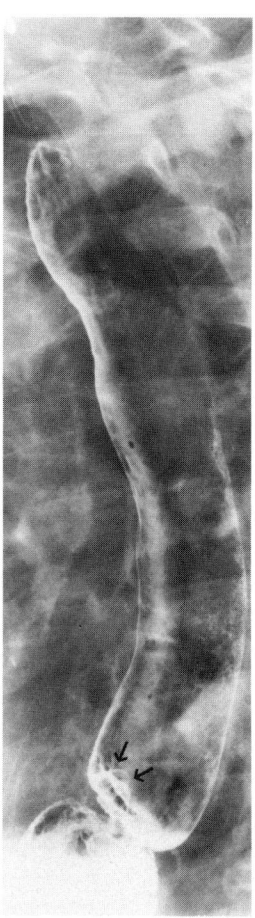

Figure 3-7 Recurrent adenocarcinoma of esophagojejunal anastomosis (*arrows*) after gastrectomy and distal esophagectomy with transabdominal creation of an esophagojejunostomy. Esophageal resection margins 3 cm from the original tumor were negative for malignancy. A completion esophagectomy and left colon interposition were performed.

disadvantages. Most surgeons develop expertise and emphasize a single technique of esophagectomy. However, this may not be optimal. Differing clinical situations may dictate that a particular technique is preferable. The well-trained thoracic surgeon should be facile with all techniques of esophageal resection. The decrease in operative mortality reflects refinement in surgical technique resulting from experience in operative and perioperative care, and a defined interest by specialists in the surgical treatment of esophageal carcinoma.

In one report of the results of surgery for esophageal cancer,[77] 275 patients underwent resection, with a 30-day mortality rate of only 2.2%. Intrathoracic esophagogastrostomy was performed in 196 patients and cervical anastomosis in 61 patients (53 had transhiatal

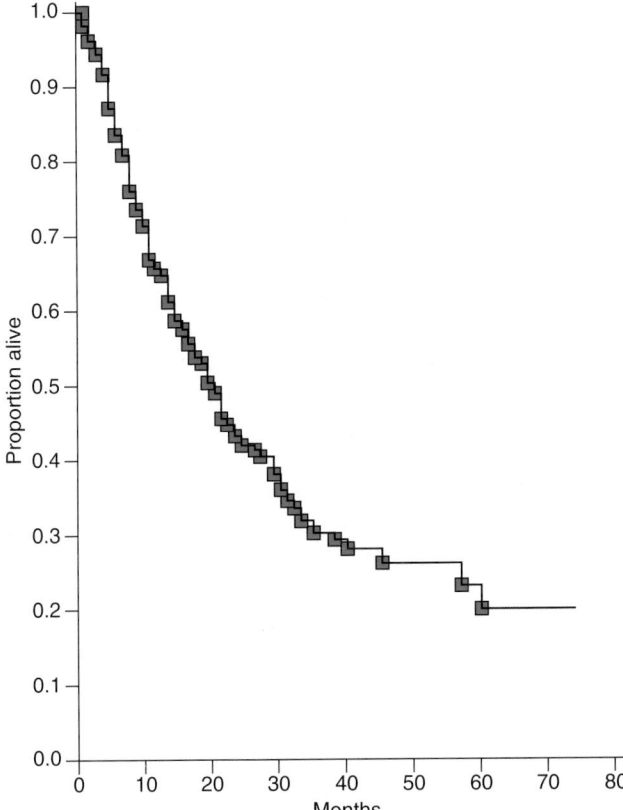

Figure 3-8 Actuarial survival rate after esophagectomy in 221 patients with esophageal carcinoma. The 5-year survival rate was 19%; the median survival was 22 months. (After Putnam JB, Suell DA, Natarajan G, et al. A comparison of three techniques of esophagectomy within a residency training program. Ann Thorac Surg 1994;57:319)

esophagectomy). Major complications (prolonged hospital stay) occurred in 40 patients (14.5%). Stage was the most important determinant of long-term survival. The actuarial 5-year survival rate was 20.8% for all patients and 23.3% when an apparently curative resection was performed. In another reported experience,[78] 104 patients with intrathoracic anastomoses after esophagectomy for carcinoma of the esophagus had no anastomotic leaks; 64 patients had a left thoracoabdominal incision, and 40 patients had a Lewis transthoracic esophagectomy. All anastomoses were constructed using a two-layer inverting technique with interrupted silk sutures. Operative mortality was 2.9% (3 patients); 5 patients required one to three dilations (5%). Major complications included pneumonia (12 patients, 12%) and reexploration for bleeding (2 patients, 2%). Positive lymph node metastases were identified in 75% of patients. Anastomotic recurrence was documented in 6 patients (6%). In a review of 6123 cases of carcinoma of the gastric cardia and esophagus,[79] the resectability rate was 89.9%. The overall mortality rate was 3%, and the complication rate was 10.3%. The 5-year survival rate was 36.8%, and the 10-year survival rate was 17.2%.

In one recent series of 100 patients treated with laparotomy and right thoracotomy,[80] postoperative complications occurred in 27 (including pulmonary complications in 11 and anastomotic leak in 9). The operative mortality rate (at 30 days) was 3%. The 5-year survival rate was 85% for stage I, 34% for stage II, and 15% for stage III carcinoma. Thirty-one patients required dilations for some degree of dysphagia after operation. In another series of 100 patients,[81] 70 were cured and 30 palliated. The operative mortality rate was 4%, and the morbidity rate was 7% (due to anastomotic leakage). Fifteen patients had pulmonary complications. The 3-year survival rate was 25% and was better in early-stage disease (stages I and II, 68.4%) than in later-stage disease (stage III, 23%).

Radical resection for esophageal cancer can be compared with radical resection for breast cancer. The value of surgical resection is local control of the neoplasm. Although surgery may be considered curative for early-stage disease in either instance, surgery cannot control the systemic spread or wide local extent of lymphatic spread in either disease. For this reason, it might be predicted that stage-specific survival after radical en bloc esophagectomy[61] is no greater than that of transhiatal esophagectomy.[82] Extended en bloc resection of esophageal carcinoma consisting of en bloc thoracic esophagectomy, mediastinal lymph node dissection, and gastrectomy with abdominal (celiac) lymph node dissection has been evaluated. Gastrointestinal continuity was reestablished using the left colon. The operative mortality rate was 7%, and the actuarial survival rates were 53% at 5 years (stages I and II).[83] In another series of 111 patients treated with en bloc esophagectomy,[84] the operative mortality rate was 11%, and complications occurred in 49 patients (44%). Survival again depended on stage. Some evidence for a role for extended surgery was seen in a series of 198 patients who underwent resection of esophageal carcinoma during 15 years.[85] Pathologic staging and close follow-up revealed improved survival in patients with positive lymph nodes when radical lymph node dissection was performed. The operative mortality rate was 3% in the last 2 years of the study.

A total thoracic esophagectomy as described by Akiyama and colleagues[58] consists of laparotomy for mobilization of the stomach or colon with retrosternal placement of the conduit and cervical anastomosis. A right thoracotomy is performed for esophageal resection. Total thoracic esophagectomy (21 patients) was compared with the Lewis procedure (25 patients). The overall mortality rate was 22% but decreased to 5% during the last 3 years of the study. The 5-year survival rate was 20%. No differences in long-term survival between the two groups were noted, but there was better reflux control after total thoracic esophagectomy.[86]

Transhiatal esophagectomy has been proposed by various surgeons as an alternative to transthoracic esophagectomy. Critics of transhiatal esophagectomy suggest that the operation is subjective, dangerous (because it is done "blind"), and an inadequate cancer operation. Proponents suggest that transhiatal esophagectomy minimizes physiologic trauma to the patient, pulmonary complications, operative time, and hospitalization and maximizes palliation. Even with middle-third tumors, operative mortality is similar to the transthoracic approach.[87] A learning curve for transhiatal esophagectomy is apparent because surgeons with less experience have more complications than surgeons with more experience. Orringer and colleagues[60] reported the results of transhiatal esophagectomy in 583 patients, including 417 patients with carcinoma. The operative mortality rate for patients with carcinoma was 5%. The anastomotic leak rate was 9%. For all patients, complications included pleural entry (74%), left recurrent laryngeal nerve injury (59 patients, 9%; 40 resolved, 19 had permanent paralysis), chylothorax (2%), tracheal laceration (4 patients), splenectomy (4%), and bleeding (4 patients required intraoperative thoracotomy for control; 3 other patients were explored after surgery).

In contrast, other authors[88] described transhiatal esophagectomy performed in 40 patients with a 30-day mortality rate of 12%. Complications included intraoperative pneumothorax in 71% treated by tube thoracostomy, transient hoarseness in 19%, leak in 17%, and pulmonary complications in 7%. In another report of 54 patients after transhiatal esophagectomy,[89] respiratory complications were common (41%) and caused all six postoperative deaths (11%). Atrial fibrillation occurred in 26%, and transient recurrent laryngeal nerve palsy occurred in 11%. The overall 3-year survival rate was 10%. All patients had normal swallowing, but 11 had strictures requiring dilation (20%) at some point after surgery.

Local recurrence of esophageal neoplasms may occur after transhiatal esophagectomy.[90] Patterns of recurrence were examined in 35 patients. Thirteen patients (37%) were free of disease after 18 months. Recurrent esophageal cancer developed in 22 patients (63%) within 14 months. Eleven patients (32%) experienced local recurrence. Metastatic spread was usually outside the conduit, and CT was better than barium studies in detecting recurrence.[91]

Comparison of Techniques of Esophagectomy

The results of three techniques of esophagectomy performed at the University of Texas M.D. Anderson Cancer Center between 1986 and 1992 were reviewed.[92] Transthoracic esophagectomy (134 patients), transhiatal esophagectomy (42 patients), or total thoracic esophagectomy (45 patients) was performed on 221 patients (adenocarcinoma, 146; squamous cell carcinoma, 72; other, 3). During this period, the overall resectability rate was 89.1% (221 of 248). Different operations had different complications, although operating room time, transfusion requirements, and days of hospitalization were similar. The operative mortality rate was 6.3% (14 of 221; transthoracic esophagectomy 9.6%, 10 of 134; transhiatal esophagectomy 4.8%, 2 of 42; total thoracic esophagectomy 4.4%, 2 of 45). Patients with cervical anastomoses had a higher leak rate (11%) than those with intrathoracic anastomoses (6%). Median survival was 22 months (19% 5-year survival rate; see Fig. 3-8) and did not differ by type of operation (Fig. 3-9). Rates of local and distant recurrence were also similar (9% to 15% all local; 31% to 34% all distant). Survival for resection of carcinoma of the esophagus reflected stage of disease, not the technique used.

Transthoracic esophagectomy and transhiatal esophagectomy have been compared in other studies. In one study,[93] 52 patients underwent transthoracic esophagectomy, and 26 patients underwent transhiatal esophagectomy. Five anastomotic leaks occurred in the transhiatal group (only 1 required longer than a 14-day hospitalization). Three leaks occurred in the transthoracic group, with hospitalization stay extended by several weeks. The overall morbidity rate was high: transthoracic, 75%; transhiatal, 85% (P = ns). The overall mortality rate was similar: transthoracic, 6% (3 of 52); transhiatal, 8% (2 of 26). Transhiatal esophagectomy was as effective as transthoracic esophagectomy without causing significant increase in hospitalization, mortality, or morbidity. Another comparison was made between transhiatal and transthoracic esophagectomy in 72 patients.[94] Transthoracic esophagectomy was performed in 43 patients and transhiatal esophagectomy in 29. Demographics between the two groups were similar. The incidence of complications in the transhiatal group was 48%; in the transthoracic group, it was 86% ($P < .05$). Transhiatal esophagectomy was favored over transthoracic in mortality rate (7% versus 14%; $P < .05$), intraoperative blood loss (1187 mL versus 2150 mL; $P < .05$), and postoperative hospitalization (12.3 days versus 22.2 days; $P < .05$). There was no difference in survival. In another series,[95] 210 patients with middle or distal esophageal carcinoma underwent resection with

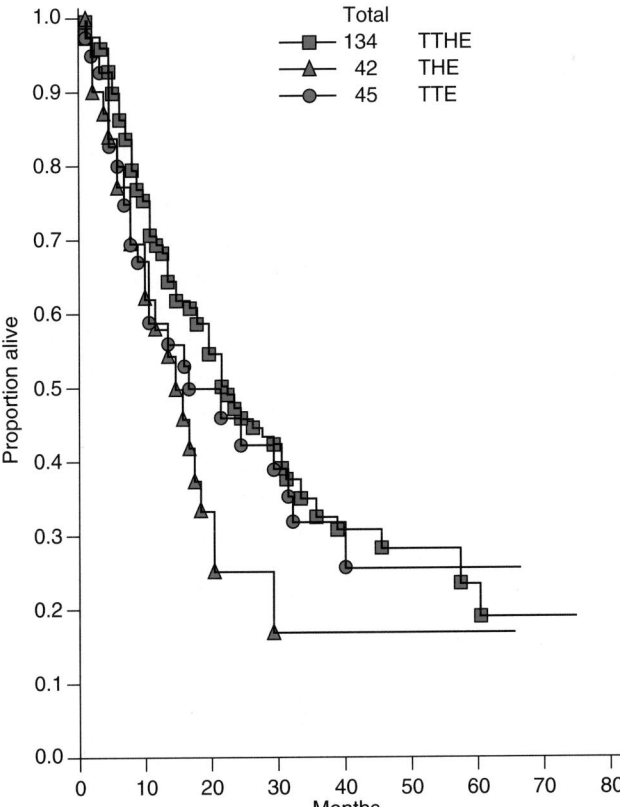

Figure 3-9 Overall survival rates for esophageal carcinoma by technique of surgery. No differences in survival rates were attributed to the technique of esophagectomy used. TTHE, transthoracic esophagectomy (Lewis procedure); THE, transhiatal esophagectomy; TTE, total thoracic esophagectomy (Akiyama) procedure. (After Putnam JB, Suell DA, Natarajan G, et al. A comparison of three techniques of esophagectomy within a residency training program. Ann Thorac Surg 1994;57:319)

transhiatal (38 patients) or transthoracic (172 patients) esophagectomy. More complications occurred in the transhiatal group (excessive bleeding and perforation of the esophagus at the tumor in seven patients, 18%; and recurrent laryngeal nerve injury in five patients, 13%). Survival was better in the transthoracic group. The transhiatal approach was infrequently used in this study, which may account for the increase in complications.

The left thoracotomy approach has been used for esophagectomy, but the resection is hampered by the aortic arch. In 110 patients treated by left thoracotomy, the postoperative mortality rate was 2.7%, and morbidity was caused by respiratory complications, which occurred in 21 patients (19%).[96] Similar results were noted in a series of 115 patients,[97] with a perioperative mortality rate of 8.7% (10 of 115), a leakage rate of 1.7% (2

of 115), and benign stricture in 16 patients (14%). The survival rate at 3 years was 22.1%.

Other techniques for esophagectomy have been advocated. Endothoracic endoesophageal pull-through "cores" out the mucosa of the esophagus with the tumor, theoretically eliminating bleeding, chylothorax, and membranous tracheal injury. In a study of 68 patients,[98] there were no intraoperative deaths and the operative mortality rate was 13.2% (9 patients). Overall leaks occurred in 8 patients (13.3%). Stomach was preferred as conduit; however, left colon (isoperistaltic) was used for reconstruction if stomach was not suitable. Other techniques for improving on the visualization or dissection of the intrathoracic esophagus without thoracotomy have been proposed. A ring dissector has been used to encircle the esophagus and, with gentle manual pressure, blindly remove the attachments of the esophagus to the mediastinum. This technique can decrease the trauma associated with transhiatal esophagectomy.[99] An endoscopic technique with a rigid scope to assist in dissection of the intrathoracic esophagus, particularly the area around the carina, has been described. Recurrent laryngeal nerve injury and pulmonary complications were less frequent with endoscopic dissection than with transhiatal esophagectomy.[100]

Intrathoracic dissection and resection of the esophagus can be performed with video-assisted thoracic surgery (VATS) techniques. The limitations of these techniques are related to limitations of movement and working with instruments through the rigid thorax. Still, esophageal and regional thoracic node dissection with thoracoscopy can provide staging information comparable to other open techniques.[101] Transhiatal or blunt esophagectomy is the least invasive means of esophagectomy; VATS techniques would provide better visualization of the esophagus and the tumor and better staging with nodal dissection. Initial staging with VATS can better enable physicians to select patients for prospective trials; the cost-effectiveness of such staging is not known. Preoperative or nonoperative treatment modalities and protocols can be appropriately recommended when the stage is known.

The lack of a uniform operation for esophagectomy reflects the myriad presentations of the neoplasm and its involvement with adjacent thoracic structures. The best choice of operation considers the potential for complete resection of local and regional disease, the patient's physiologic status, the complications unique for the technique of esophagectomy proposed, and the experience and training of the surgeon.

Complications of Surgery

Complications of esophageal surgery are best avoided because their consequences can be fatal (Table 3-7).

The reported incidence of anastomotic leak after

Table 3-7 Causes of Morbidity After Esophageal Resection

Anastomotic leak (cervical or thoracic)
Anastomotic stricture
Respiratory insufficiency (pneumonia, aspiration, chronic obstructive pulmonary disease)
Congestive heart failure
Pulmonary embolism
Cardiac arrhythmia
Obstruction at hiatus, pyloromyotomy
Wound infection or dehiscence
Ruptured spleen or splenectomy
Phlebitis
Abscess (subphrenic)
Torsion, gangrene, or rupture of gastrointestinal replacement
Hemorrhage

esophagectomy ranges from 0% to 25%. A leak most often occurs at the esophageal anastomosis but can also occur from the gastric suture line (along the lesser curve used to lengthen the stomach). The thoracic approach to the esophagus is transpleural, and a leak drains from the mediastinum into the pleural space. An intrathoracic leak can be lethal but occurs less frequently than after a cervical anastomosis. A cervical leak is less morbid because mediastinitis is infrequent. The stomach fills the posterior mediastinum and prevents any infection from the cervical anastomosis from spreading to the mediastinum. Any patient with a fever of 38.3°C (101°F) or higher 48 hours or more after esophageal resection has a leak with mediastinitis until proved otherwise. A sip of meglumine diatrizoate (Gastrografin) excludes a gross disruption; thin barium excludes a small leak.

Techniques and results for various anastomotic constructions were evaluated in 221 anastomoses,[102] 122 sutured and 99 stapled. Leaks occurred in 21 sutured anastomoses (17.2%) and 7 stapled anastomoses (7.1%; $P < .05$). Strictures were more common in the stapled group (13 of 99, 13%) compared with the hand-sewn group (2 of 122, 1.6%; $P < .01$). The overall mortality rate was 20%, and the leakage-related mortality rate was 4.7%. Benign strictures occurred in 22% of patients who underwent operations; the strictures were dilated.[103]

Cervical and thoracic anastomosis for esophagectomy were compared in a prospective trial.[104] Forty-nine patients underwent laparotomy and right thoracotomy with intrathoracic anastomosis, and 43 patients underwent laparotomy, right thoracotomy, and cervical anastomosis. Anastomotic leak was more frequent after cervical anastomosis (26%) than after intrathoracic anastomosis (4%; $P < .002$). Respiratory complica-

tions were not significantly different between the two procedures. The 30-day mortality rates were similar for the two groups (14.3% intrathoracic versus 9.3% cervical). Strictures occurred in 14% of intrathoracic and 23% of cervical anastomoses. Another study examined single-layered versus double-layered cervical anastomoses for esophagogastrostomy.[105] The single-layered anastomosis was superior to the double-layered anastomosis because the incidence of fibrotic strictures was lower. The rates of cervical anastomotic leak were similar.

An anastomotic leak in the chest is life-threatening. Improvements in techniques for hand-sewn anastomoses and better mechanical stapling devices may eventually eliminate this complication. In one series, hand-sewn anastomoses and single-layer anastomoses were more likely to leak than mechanical or stapled anastomoses and double-layered suturing.[106]

Mobilization of middle-third tumors through a transhiatal approach requires a careful preoperative evaluation and a careful assessment of the extent of the tumor at the time of exploration with flexible or rigid bronchoscopy and flexible or rigid esophagoscopy. When malignant cells are identified on bronchoscopy, the patient is unresectable. When malignant cells are not identified and the patient is at an acceptable risk for resection, the surgeon can proceed with operation. In mobilizing the tumor off the trachea, a tracheal tear may occur laterally at the junction of the membranous and cartilaginous trachea. The balloon of the endotracheal tube is deflated and then guided by the surgeon into the left main-stem bronchus past the tear. The balloon is then inflated, and the tear is repaired using right thoracotomy with fine interrupted sutures of Prolene and then patched or reinforced with pleura, pericardial fat, or intercostal muscle.

The azygous vein may be adherent to tumors of the middle third of the esophagus so that avulsion of the azygous vein with resultant hemorrhage can occur during transhiatal esophagectomy. The location above the right main-stem bronchus precludes an attempt at definitive control of this bleeding from the abdomen or the neck; therefore, a right thoracotomy is required. Temporary control of the bleeding is obtained by packing sponges into the upper mediastinum from the neck and into the posterior mediastinum from the abdomen. The abdomen is closed, and a right thoracotomy is performed to control the bleeding. The esophagus is then mobilized if possible.

Chylothorax occurs in 5% of patients after extensive lymph node dissection. The risk of chylothorax can be reduced by elective ligation of the thoracic duct (2.1%), compared with no ligation (9%; $P < .02$).[107]

ADENOCARCINOMA OF THE ESOPHAGUS

The term *gastroesophageal junction tumor* is applied to any adenocarcinoma arising in that location. Many of these tumors arise in Barrett's esophagus (columnar-lined esophagus). The treatment and survival of patients with neoplasms of the distal esophagus and the gastric cardia (extending into the esophagus) are similar.

Primary adenocarcinoma of the esophagus is not as rare as was once thought. Some studies have shown that adenocarcinoma accounts for 34% of all esophageal cancers and 60% of lower-third tumors of the esophagus.[108] More recently, rates of adenocarcinoma have increased from 4% to 10% per year in contrast to declining rates of adenocarcinoma in the more distal portions of the stomach.[3,109-111] The Surveillance, Epidemiology, and End Results (SEER) program also noted that the incidence of adenocarcinoma (0.4 per 100,000 people overall incidence) increased by more than 74% in white men between 1973 and 1982, most (79%) arising in the lower third of the esophagus.[111] Adenocarcinoma primarily affects white men,[111,112] perhaps because these patients have a high frequency of hiatal hernia (40%), smoking, and alcohol use. *H pylori* infection has been associated with an increased risk of gastric carcinoma,[17,113-115] although its role in the pathogenesis of esophageal adenocarcinoma is not known.

Adenocarcinoma can arise from three sources: superficial and deep glands of the esophagus, embryonic remnants of glandular epithelium in the esophagus, or metaplastic glandular epithelium. The superficial and deep glands of the esophagus are mucus-secreting cells that are indistinguishable in appearance from the cardiac glands of the stomach. The origin of these glands may be congenital, or they may arise from Barrett's esophagus (columnar-lined epithelium). Secretions from the superficial glands located within the mucosa enter the lumen of the esophagus through ducts lined by a single layer of mucus cells. The terminal portion of the ducts from these glands is lined with squamous cells. The deep esophageal glands may give rise to the mucoepidermoid carcinomas occasionally found in the esophagus.[116,117]

Barrett's Esophagus

Barrett's esophagus is found in up to 20% of patients undergoing esophagoscopy for esophagitis. The relation between Barrett's esophagus and adenocarcinoma is not completely known, but 59% to 86% of all adenocarcinomas arise in Barrett's esophagus. Thus, an etiology common to both Barrett's and adenocarcinomas may exist.[118,119]

Why Barrett's mucosa occurs is not clear. Repetitive chemical trauma from reflux can damage the squamous mucosa of the esophagus, which is then replaced by glandular epithelium growing up from the stomach. Submucosal esophageal glands within the esophagus may proliferate and cover the injured esophageal surface.

The natural history of Barrett's mucosa has been studied. It may never resolve, and medical or surgical management may have little influence on the subsequent development of malignancy. Routine screening should be performed for all patients with Barrett's esophagus. Patients with severe dysplasia should undergo esophageal resection.[120] In 241 patients evaluated with Barrett's mucosa, the prevalence of adenocarcinoma was 27% (65 patients). Seventy-two patients (30%) were operated on for adenocarcinoma arising from Barrett's mucosa. In 8 patients, the carcinoma was discovered on routine endoscopy, with an incidence of 3.3%, and in 4 others, disease progression from Barrett's mucosa to adenocarcinoma was documented. Most patients were resectable (61 of 65, 94%). The operative mortality rate was 3.3%, and the actuarial 5-year survival rate was 23.7%. Adenocarcinoma occurred in 6 patients who underwent prior antireflux surgery. Antireflux surgery does not protect against the development of carcinoma in patients with a previous diagnosis of Barrett's, and surveillance must be continued for life.[121]

Incidence of Adenocarcinoma in Barrett's Esophagus

Numerous investigators have examined the clinical and molecular changes that occur as Barrett's esophagus mucosa evolves from mild dysplasia to severe dysplasia and carcinoma in situ to invasive malignancy. Barrett's esophagus is frequently identified at the tumor periphery, suggesting that adenocarcinoma originates from Barrett's mucosa. Not all patients have Barrett's mucosa identified. This absence of Barrett's mucosa by histology may relate to overgrowth of adenocarcinoma in all areas previously occupied by the Barrett's mucosa, or it may occur because the neoplasm arises in an area uninvolved by Barrett's esophagus.

Clinical Changes

In 50 patients with Barrett's esophagus, 12 (24%) had superficial adenocarcinoma. High-grade dysplasia was identified in 6 of the 12 patients and later evolved to carcinoma.[122] In one study,[123] 16 patients who had adenocarcinoma arising in Barrett's esophagus were compared with 34 patients with adenocarcinoma but without Barrett's esophagus. Marked male predominance was noted in malignant Barrett's, and most were located at the gastroesophageal junction. The 4-year survival rate in patients with non–Barrett's adenocarcinoma was 35%, compared with 60% in those with Barrett's adenocarcinoma.

Molecular Changes

As a premalignant lesion, Barrett's mucosa has been studied intensively for particular histologic and molecular changes that may predispose it to malignancy. Abnormalities have been demonstrated in Barrett's mucosa histologically and by flow cytometry.[124,125] Electron microscopic examination of cytoplasmic organelles has revealed an abnormal depletion of organelles required for mucus biosynthesis. These observations can assist in identifying patients at risk for developing adenocarcinoma of the esophagus.[126]

Ornithine decarboxylase is the rate-limiting enzyme in polyamine biosynthesis and is usually induced during the G1 phase of the cell cycle. An increase in cellular polyamine synthesis is a general characteristic of growing cells. Ornithine decarboxylase activity in Barrett's mucosa is elevated when compared with adjacent gastric or small intestinal epithelium,[127,128] suggesting that the regulation of polyamine metabolism by this enzyme can be altered in this premalignant tissue. Treatment with the differentiating agent 13-*cis*-retinoic acid produced no change in the extent of the lesion in 11 patients.[124,129]

Molecular techniques can probe for changes in the *ras* oncogene or *P53* tumor suppressor gene. c-Ha-*ras* protooncogene expression was undetectable in Barrett's esophagus. No amplification of c-Ha-*ras* or six other protooncogenes was detected.[130] However, *P53* mutations occurred in four of seven samples of Barrett's epithelium with little or no dysplasia adjacent to esophageal adenocarcinoma. *P53* mutations can be a marker for premalignant change in Barrett's mucosa. Other molecular events may be required to develop carcinoma because *P53* mutations are not always present in developing cancer.[131]

Management of Barrett's Esophagus

Medical Management

In one prospective randomized study, 67 patients with Barrett's esophagus were followed for 36 months. Medical management (histamine-2 blockers) did not result in consistent reduction in the extent of Barrett's epithelium during a 3-year period. Eighty-two percent of patients had less than a 1 cm change in length of the lesion per year.[132] Omeprazole, 20 mg/d, reduced the percentage of time with pH below 4.0 and the number of reflux episodes longer than 5 minutes and lowered intragastric acidity but had no effect on acid clearance in the esophagus.[133]

Surgical Management

Surgery is the treatment of choice for Barrett's esophagus with severe or high-grade dysplasia.[120,134–136] A single biopsy of severe dysplasia in suitable patients warrants esophagectomy.[136] Esophagectomy for high-grade or severe dysplasia without evidence of invasive carcinoma raises concerns of risk and benefits. The management of high-grade dysplasia was examined in nine patients without evidence of carcinoma who had columnar-lined esophagus extending orad from the cardia. Eight patients underwent resection and colon interposition. One patient had sleeve resection of the cervical esophagus. Multifocal carcinoma was found in three patients, and one patient had microinvasive carcinoma. No carcinoma was found in the remaining four patients. Esophagectomy is indicated for severe dysplasia because 45% of patients have adenocarcinoma and long-term survival is high.[137]

Antireflux Procedures for Treatment of Barrett's Esophagus

The role of gastroesophageal reflux in the genesis of Barrett's esophagus is unknown, although the two are associated. Routine surveillance (esophagogastroscopy) in patients with Barrett's esophagus permits early detection of severe dysplasia or carcinoma in situ and presumably improves patient selection for esophagectomy and long-term survival. Patients should be followed with esophagoscopy at least once every 2 years with serial longitudinal biopsies and brushings.

An antireflux surgical procedure can correct the reflux and reverse the changes associated with Barrett's esophagus, although this reversal is not consistent.[138] Regression of Barrett's epithelium has been noted after antireflux surgery. Thirty-seven patients with Barrett's mucosa were identified from 241 patients who had an antireflux procedure.[139] Four patients (11%) had partial regression of their Barrett's changes, but carcinoma developed in 3 (8%) during the 16-year study period. Good reflux control was obtained in 92%. The authors recommended antireflux procedures for gastroesophageal reflux in patients with Barrett's esophagus with mild or moderate dysplasia. Yearly endoscopic and histologic surveillance was recommended.

Surveillance for Patients With Barrett's Esophagus

The sensitivity and optimal frequency of screening endoscopy in patients with Barrett's esophagus is not known. In a study of 19 patients under surveillance by periodic endoscopy (median interval, 6 months), all but one had esophagectomy when carcinoma or severe dysplasia was diagnosed.[139a] The survival rate for patients under surveillance was 62% at 5 years, compared with 20% in a group of patients not under surveillance (*P* = .007). Stage of disease was earlier for patients under surveillance than patients not under surveillance (58% stage 0 and I versus 21%, respectively; *P* = .006). Routine surveillance can permit earlier detection of adenocarcinoma at an earlier stage with the most potential for long-term survival.

In 32 patients under surveillance for Barrett's esophagus,[139b] cancer developed in 3 during 166 patient-years. Dysplasia was found in 2 of these patients 6 and 15 months before the diagnosis of carcinoma. Frank adenocarcinoma developed in 1 patient. Barrett's epithelium was unchanged in all but 3 patients despite the surgery or medical treatment for 3 to 12 years. In another study,[140] 62 cases of Barrett's esophagus were identified among 707 patients with hiatal hernia (8.7%). Ten carcinomas were associated with Barrett's changes, with a prevalence of 13.8%. Fifty-one patients had antireflux procedures, and 11 underwent resection. Six patients who underwent resection had carcinoma, and 5 patients had severe dysplasia. The incidence of adenocarcinoma was one new case per 274 patient-years (1.72%). Some authors suggest that annual screening for patients with Barrett's esophagus is not effective because the incidence of cancer in their study population was 1 in 170 patient-years and the overall survival of patients with Barrett's esophagus was not different from that of an age- and sex-matched control population.[141] Others recommend endoscopic surveillance every 2 years as a better use of resources.[142]

ALTERNATIVES AND ADJUVANTS TO SURGICAL THERAPY FOR ESOPHAGEAL CARCINOMA

Long-term survival after esophagectomy is limited to patients with early stages of the disease in whom all tumor and lymphatic extension can be resected. Surgery alone effectively palliates dysphagia; however, patients frequently succumb to distant metastases,[143,144] which often are present subclinically at diagnosis. Alternatives to surgery include chemotherapy and radiation therapy, alone or in combination. Systemic chemotherapy can enhance survival when combined with locoregional therapy. Single-agent chemotherapy has minimal effect on esophageal carcinoma; combination chemotherapy (more than one drug) or chemoradiation therapy can yield significant response rates and enhanced survival when compared with single agents.

Radiation therapy often controls the primary tumor and adjacent regional lymph node drainage areas without the risk of surgery; however, for most patients, dysphagia is better palliated with surgery. After treatment with radiation therapy, dysphagia recurs in more than half of patients.

Various trials are ongoing to examine the results of adjuvant therapy, for example, chemotherapy followed by surgery, chemotherapy and radiation therapy followed by surgery, or chemotherapy and radiation therapy only. Definitive phase III trials are underway to evaluate multimodality therapy.[145]

Presurgical adjuvant therapy has theoretic advantages over surgery alone:

1. Patient tolerance of the therapy is satisfactory.
2. Micrometastases can be eliminated, preventing distant failure.
3. Blood supply to the tumor is intact (for chemotherapy).
4. Tumor response to the therapy can be assessed, and postoperative therapy can be based on this response or lack thereof.
5. The rate of resectability can be increased.
6. Radiation therapy can be omitted to reduce the cumulative toxicity and maximize treatment efficacy when required.

Radiation Therapy

Preoperative radiation therapy when given as definitive treatment (50 to 60 Gy, modified by various chemotherapy drugs used as radiation-sensitizing agents) can produce scar or adhesions and preclude esophagectomy. Smaller doses of radiation therapy (30-Gy range, split-dose) are insufficient for definitive treatment, and survival advantages are rare. If the initial esophageal carcinoma is bulky and preoperative radiation therapy is used, any locally residual disease or locally recurrent carcinoma has limited postoperative treatment options. Preoperative radiation therapy (30 Gy) for patients with advanced disease produces no survival benefit over surgery alone.[146] The response of local tumor to chemotherapy plus radiation therapy is better than with radiation therapy alone. Survival trends suggest an enhanced 5-year survival rate with chemotherapy plus radiation therapy (16%) than with radiation therapy alone (6%; *P* = .16).[147] A prospective trial evaluating primary radiation therapy for esophageal carcinoma versus esophagectomy alone has not been performed.

Postoperative radiation therapy in patients with residual disease in the thorax after esophagectomy can limit local recurrence and enhance survival. In one prospective trial,[148] the efficacy of postoperative radiation therapy after esophagectomy for squamous cell carcinoma was evaluated. Patients with complete resection were randomly assigned to postoperative radiation therapy or no therapy. Local recurrence rates were similar between the two groups (10% versus 13%, respectively). Survival was not improved by the addition of radiation therapy. Intrathoracic recurrence and tracheobronchial obstruction were significantly reduced for patients with partial resection and radiation therapy when compared with partial resection only. Complications occurred in the intrathoracic gastric conduit after radiation therapy. These complications can be minimized by placing the gastric conduit in a retrosternal position, away from the radiation field, and by performing a cervical anastomosis when postoperative radiation therapy is planned.

Chemotherapy and Combined Chemotherapy and Radiation Therapy

Chemotherapy given before surgery may be more effective than after surgery because blood supply is intact in the local or regional area of primary tumor, chemotherapy-resistant clones are reduced, and reduced primary tumor size can facilitate surgery. In an early study[45] of perioperative chemotherapy (cisplatin, vindesine, and bleomycin) plus surgery versus surgery alone in the treatment of esophageal carcinoma, chemotherapy responders had prolonged survival after surgery compared with patients who had surgery alone. In another trial,[149] the effects of etoposide, 5-fluorouracil (5-FU), and cisplatin for perioperative treatment of patients with adenocarcinoma were evaluated. Patients were given two courses of chemotherapy preoperatively (Fig. 3-10), and those who responded with tumor size reduction preoperatively received three or four additional courses beginning 1 to 2 months after surgery. Twenty-eight patients completed therapy, and 17 patients had a major response. One patient had a complete pathologic response. Thirty-two patients underwent exploration, and 25 patients underwent complete resection. Median survival was 23 months. No intraoperative deaths occurred.

Chemotherapy given concurrently with radiation therapy acts synergistically in enhancing local control. Twenty to 30% of patients so treated have no neoplasm in their resected specimen, and their survival is excellent. One author questioned the need for esophagec-

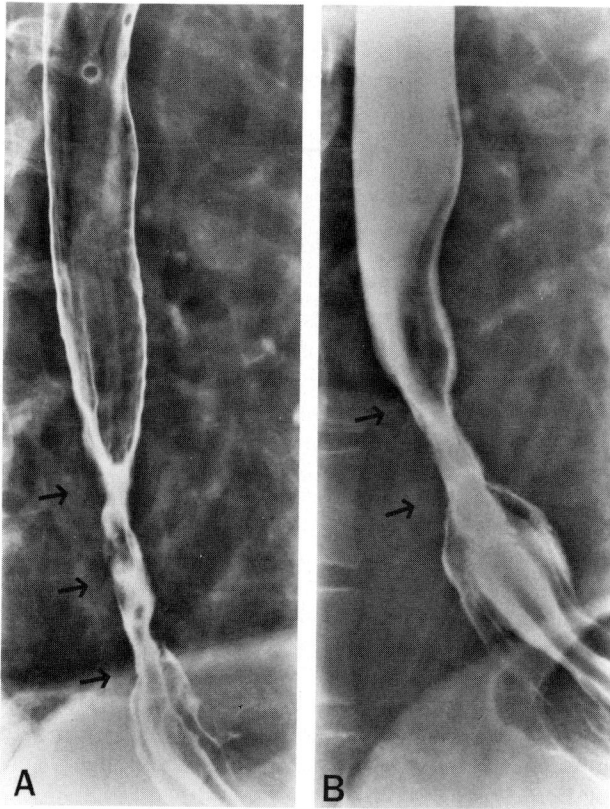

Figure 3-10 Barium esophagrams from before (**A**) and after (**B**) chemotherapy. The patient, a 78-year-old man with distal esophageal adenocarcinoma (*arrows*), was treated with three cycles of combination chemotherapy before transhiatal esophagectomy. Partial response to the chemotherapy was noted with regression of tumor. Postoperative chemotherapy was also given.

tomy because nonsurgical treatment provided a median survival of 18 to 24 months.[150] The results of treating patients with combination chemotherapy and radiation therapy for esophageal carcinoma were recently reviewed.[151] Combinations of 5-FU or mitomycin C with radiation therapy with or without surgery have been effective. Mitomycin C produces a response in up to 40% of patients with squamous cell carcinoma, although its efficacy in adenocarcinoma is not known. The use of 5-FU with radiation therapy or combination 5-FU plus mitomycin C with radiation reflects the increased efficacy of radiation therapy with additional chemotherapy. The potential synergism between 5-FU and mitomycin C or 5-FU and cisplatin with radiation therapy (30 Gy) is reflected in a pathologic complete response rate of about 25% and median survival of 12 to 19 months. Patients with squamous cell carcinoma treated with chemoradiation who refused surgery had a 5-year survival rate of about 18%.[152] In another study, patients with stage I and II disease were treated definitively with radiation therapy (60 Gy) for 6 to 7 weeks and with continuous-infusion 5-FU. Mitomycin C was infused on day 2. Median survival was 18 months, 3-year survival was 29%, and 5-year survival was 18%.[153]

In a phase III prospective, randomized, and stratified trial,[154] combined chemotherapy and radiation therapy was compared with radiation therapy alone in patients with cancer of the esophagus. Concurrent therapy with cisplatin, 5-FU, and radiation was superior to radiation therapy alone (median survival of 12.5 months versus 8.9 months, respectively; 2-year survival rate of 38% versus 10%, respectively). Patients with combined treatment had fewer local and distant recurrences but had more complications of the therapy. This study supports treating patients with combined chemotherapy and radiation therapy when a nonsurgical treatment is desired.

In a phase II study,[155] survival after preoperative chemotherapy (cisplatin, vinblastine, and continuous-infusion mitomycin C) and radiation was improved. Patients who underwent the prescribed therapy followed by transhiatal esophagectomy had a 46% 3-year survival, compared with 23% for historical control patients treated with surgery alone. Over 27% of patients had complete responses (no identifiable tumor) after esophagectomy, and their 5-year survival rate was 70%. In another series,[156] 47 patients were treated with radiation therapy (30 or 36 Gy) and chemotherapy (5-FU, cisplatin) during a 5-week period. Twenty-one percent of resectable patients (8 of 39) had no tumor in the resected specimen. The survival rate was improved at 3 years and was significantly different from historical controls. Seven patients who refused surgery after obtaining excellent relief from their dysphagia had survival results similar to patients undergoing esophagectomy.

Other studies have examined the role of combination chemotherapy alone and with radiation therapy before surgery. In a single-arm study[157] of preoperative chemotherapy (cisplatin, 5-FU, and bolus vinblastine) concurrent with radiation (45 Gy), followed by transhiatal esophagectomy, 84% of patients were resectable, and 24% had no tumor in the resected specimen. Survival for resectable patients was 44 months for squamous cell carcinoma and 32 months for adenocarcinoma; the 5-year survival rates were estimated at 43% and 36%, respectively. Long-term survival was noted after esophagectomy in 32% of patients with residual tumor in the resected specimen, supporting the role of esophagectomy in patients treated with preoperative therapy. Other groups have not noted an improvement in local control in patients treated with preoperative chemotherapy and radiation therapy and surgery.[158] A

survival advantage was not identified because distant metastases were not as well controlled as the local tumor. Postoperative chemotherapy and radiation therapy have been proposed,[159] but most studies suggest that treatment before surgery is well tolerated and effective. Perioperative adjuvant therapy has the most potential to enhance survival and to control local and regional disease.

A large intergroup trial (Cancer and Leukemia Group B, Eastern Cooperative Oncology Group, North Central Cancer Treatment Group, Radiation Therapy Oncology Group, and the Southwest Oncology Group) is evaluating treatment results in patients with carcinoma of the esophagus. Potentially resectable patients are randomly assigned to undergo immediate surgery or preoperative chemotherapy followed by surgery and postoperative chemotherapy. Preoperatively, cisplatin, 100 mg/m^2, bolus, and 5-FU, 1000 mg/m^2, infusion days 1 through 5, are given beginning on days 1, 29, and 58. Surgery is performed about 1 month after the last chemotherapy. Additional chemotherapy (two cycles) is given after surgery.

PALLIATION FOR ESOPHAGEAL CARCINOMA

Patients with esophageal carcinoma may be surgically unresectable because of the extent of the tumor locally or metastases distally. These patients require some relief from dysphagia and pain. Numerous modalities are available for palliation of dysphagia, including external-beam radiation therapy, intraluminal brachytherapy, intubation through the tumor with various prostheses, placement of stents, use of laser for reopening the occluded esophagus, and simple dilation[160] (Table 3-8).

Patients with unresectable esophageal carcinoma

Table 3-8 Procedures for Palliation for Carcinoma of the Esophagus

Simple dilation
Intraluminal intubation
Stent placement
Laser ablation of obstruction
Brachytherapy
Surgery
    Resection and reconstruction or bypass
        Placement of conduit
            Right side of chest
            Retrosternal
            Presternal

can be initially treated with external-beam radiation therapy (with and without chemotherapy) for local control of the tumor and for palliation. If dysphagia persists, treatment should be individualized. Laser ablation of obstructing lesions may carry less morbidity than esophageal intubation. Brachytherapy can also be considered after laser ablation.

External-Beam Radiation Therapy

External-beam radiation therapy alone for local control of esophageal cancer is used less frequently as combined radiation therapy and chemotherapy proves its effectiveness. Combined radiation therapy and chemotherapy has benefit for inoperable patients. In one study of 16 inoperable patients, a response occurred in 56% overall and in 70% of patients with locoregional disease. The 1-year survival rates were 31% overall and 40% for patients with locoregional disease.[161]

Intraluminal Brachytherapy

Patients with symptomatic esophageal carcinoma not amenable to surgical resection and previously treated with external-beam radiation therapy may be candidates for intraluminal brachytherapy. In this procedure, a radioactive bead is placed through a catheter prepositioned through the area to be irradiated. The bead passes through the area in a given amount of time to provide a finite and controlled radiation dose to the local tissues. The depth of penetration of the radiation rarely exceeds 2 to 3 cm. Intraluminal brachytherapy after completion of external-beam radiation therapy resulted in local control of the esophageal carcinoma in 31% of patients.[162] In another study,[163] 9 patients with advanced squamous cell carcinoma of the middle third of the esophagus with intraluminal brachytherapy were all alive after 9 months. Even without prior external-beam irradiation, intraluminal brachytherapy can be effective. One study[164] showed that 9 of 10 patients with advanced esophageal cancer treated with intraluminal brachytherapy achieved palliation equivalent to that of external-beam irradiation. Most patients had already failed other palliative modalities. Intraluminal brachytherapy was used in 16 of 45 patients (previously treated with laser), with prolongation of palliation.[165] In patients unsuitable for surgery, a combination of external-beam radiation therapy and intraluminal brachytherapy can be considered to palliate dysphagia. Generally, external-beam radiation therapy is used first, and brachytherapy is used later if necessary. In one study of 70 patients,[166] swallowing was restored in 92%, but half required dilation. Fistula occurred in 4 patients; the actuarial survival rate was 42% at 1 year.

Surgery

Because of the high attendant mortality and morbidity,[167,168] resection or bypass of unresectable esophageal carcinoma should not be considered as a means of palliation. General contraindications to surgical procedures for palliation of the esophagus are outlined in Table 3-9. The survival of patients with metastatic esophageal carcinoma is poor.[169] To subject such patients, already debilitated from malnutrition and tumor burden, to a lengthy operative resection is ill advised. Although some advocate such an approach, most surgeons do not support bypass procedures for palliation of esophageal carcinoma. When bypass rather than esophagectomy is performed, anastomotic leak rates can reach 42.7%, compared with 18.3% for resection.[74] In 37 patients who underwent gastric bypass for palliation of esophageal carcinoma,[36] operative mortality was 24% (9 patients), and anastomotic leaks occurred in 19% (7 patients). Only 25% of patients (7 of 28 patients) achieved good palliation. The average survival in patients leaving the hospital alive was 5.9 months.

Other groups have examined the value of esophageal bypass alone or in comparison with another mode of palliation. In 124 patients who underwent esophageal bypass for unresectable disease,[167] hospital mortality was 10% (13 deaths). Median survival was 5 months and was improved by radiation therapy. Eighty-two percent of surviving patients had complete and lasting palliation from dysphagia after the surgery. In another study,[165] 71 patients were palliated with either surgery (26 patients) or endoscopic laser palliation (45 patients). Survival rates were the same in both groups. The stenosis-free interval was longer in the surgery group (24 weeks), and local reocclusion was more common in the group treated with laser therapy. The hospital mortality rate was 19%, and complications occurred

Table 3-9 Contraindications to Palliative Esophagectomy for Esophageal Neoplasms

Poor medical condition
Inadequate cardiopulmonary function
Visceral (extraregional) metastases
Malignant pleural effusion
Malignant ascites
Recurrent laryngeal, phrenic, or sympathetic nerve involvement
Superior vena cava obstruction
Tracheoesophageal fistula
Extension into aorta or spinal column

in 31%. In a group of patients treated with bypass, intubation, or laser ablation,[170] the overall mortality rate was 9.6% and the 1-year survival rate 29.1%. Excellent or good results were obtained in 78% of patients. In 49 patients undergoing bypass, the mortality rate was 20.4% (median survival, 6.2 months). Intubation was performed in 254 patients, with a 30-day mortality of 10.2% (median survival, 4 months). Laser therapy was performed in 50 patients, with no operative mortality but with no survival advantage (median survival, 4.1 months).

Cervical esophagostomy and gastrostomy are not palliative for patients with esophageal carcinoma. The stoma is difficult to manage, and patients are social outcasts. Oral alimentation is not possible.

Dilation

Simple dilation is inconsistently effective in the treatment of esophageal carcinoma. The neoplasm continues to grow to narrow the lumen despite frequent dilations. In 41 patients,[171] dysphagia recurred in all, and most dilations were repeated at 4-week intervals. Most patients required no more than three dilations during their remaining life-span. The complication rate (perforation) was low (5%).

Esophageal Intubation

For many years, tubes of various sorts have been forced through obstructing tumors in an attempt to relieve dysphagia. Complication rates from placement of tubes are high (10% or greater), as are hospital mortality rates (10% or greater). In one study, 71 patients treated with pulsion intubation (pushed from above) experienced a 15.5% mortality rate (11 deaths); 39 patients treated by traction intubation (pulled from below) had a 15.4% mortality rate (6 deaths).[172] Mortality rates were similar in other studies.[173] Esophageal intubation can be helpful in patients with tracheoesophageal fistula to prevent or limit soiling of the tracheobronchial tree.[174]

Various tubes are available for palliation, including Celestin tubes implanted by laparotomy and traction, Procter-Livingston tubes implanted by pulsion with laparotomy for staging, and Atkinson tubes placed by pulsion. Patients treated with the Atkinson tube had few complications and only a 6% mortality rate compared with the others (42%). Patients undergoing laparotomy had an associated 41% hospital mortality rate.[175]

Several studies have compared intubation with laser therapy for palliation. Most suggest that laser therapy has lower rates of mortality and morbidity. Survival is equivalent.[176,177] In 116 patients treated by intubation and 28 patients by laser therapy,[178] the morbidity

rates were 13.8% for intubation and 3.6% for laser ablation. Mortality rates were 4.3% for intubation and 0% for laser ablation. Forty-three patients treated with laser therapy and 30 patients treated with intraluminal intubation were compared in a prospective, nonrandomized, two-center trial.[179] Relief of dysphagia (80%) and survival (5 to 6 months) were similar. Laser-treated patients did better for the remainder of their lives but required more procedures.

Metallic expandable stents can be used with some success for short-term palliative management of unresectable esophagogastric neoplasms.[180]

Laser Ablation

Laser ablation of obstructing lesions is effective in palliating dysphagia from obstructing esophageal carcinoma in over 80% of patients in most series.[181–185] As noted, laser therapy has been shown to result in a lower mortality rate and fewer complications than tube insertion. Of 69 patients treated with laser therapy and 27 patients treated with esophageal tube insertion, those who underwent laser ablation had no fatal complications, an overall complication rate of 8.7%, and a 1-year survival rate of 12%. Patients treated with tube insertion had a 30-day mortality rate of 11%, a complication rate of 48%, and no survivors at 1 year.[186] Laser therapy followed by intubation was not significantly better than laser therapy alone.[177] A prospective randomized trial examined esophageal intubation alone (10 patients), intubation plus radiation (8 patients), and laser ablation plus radiation (9 patients). Eighty percent of patients who underwent tube insertion had complications. Survival rates were not significantly different among groups.

Several factors can affect improved long-term outcome after laser ablation, including initial tumor length less than 6 cm,[176,187] improvement after the initial laser treatment, and histology (adenocarcinoma).[176]

Chemotherapy and Radiation Therapy

Chemotherapy given concurrently with radiation therapy acts synergistically to enhance local control, palliate dysphagia, and increase survival. Complete pathologic response was found in 20% to 30% of patients after treatment, and their survival was the best of all groups examined. Median survival can reach 18 to 24 months.[150] In one study, continuous-infusion 5-FU and radiation therapy (50 Gy) was used for palliation. Mitomycin C was infused on day 2 of treatment. Median survival was 9 months for patients in stage III and 7 months for those in stage IV. Seventy-seven percent of patients were rendered free of dysphagia, and 60% of these patients remained free of dysphagia until death.[153]

OTHER TUMORS OF THE ESOPHAGUS

Adenocarcinoma and squamous cell carcinoma constitute 98% to 99% of all esophageal neoplasms. Benign smooth muscle tumors occur infrequently; the mucosa overlying the tumor appears normal. Simple enucleation can be performed. Small cell carcinoma, melanoma, sarcoma, or carcinosarcomas occur in 1% to 2% of patients. Distant metastases occur in 75% of patients with these unusual neoplasms.[188] Surgical resection for palliation of dysphagia and local control for patients without metastases can be undertaken, with a small percentage of patients having long-term benefit.

Benign Tumors

Leiomyoma of the esophagus is rare yet is the most common benign tumor of the esophagus.[189] Although occurring most frequently in the middle third of the esophagus, leiomyomas can develop at any level.[190] Presenting symptoms include dysphagia or pain. The lesion, identified on barium swallow as an extrinsic mass, appears as a smooth, rounded filling defect. CT can assist in distinguishing the relations of the mass with surrounding structures. Esophagoscopy can reveal a bulge but normal mucosa. The yield of a biopsy of the mass through a normal mucosa is low, and the risk of perforating the mucosa increases the difficulty of enucleation. Biopsy should not be performed if the mucosa is normal.

Esophageal ultrasonography provides a clear image of intramural abnormalities and assists in determining the extent of submucosal lesions.[191] Ultrasonography is better than CT and endoscopy in detection, staging, and follow-up of leiomyomas.[192]

Transthoracic enucleation provides excellent local control (Fig. 3-11). A right or left thoracotomy incision can be used, depending on the location of the tumor. Tumors of the middle- or upper-third esophagus may extend inferiorly and superiorly more than expected; a right thoracotomy facilitates exposure and avoids the anatomic limitations imposed by the aortic arch. Surgical results after resection of leiomyoma are excellent, with minimal morbidity and no mortality.[189,193] VATS techniques have been used for enucleation of leiomyomas, thus avoiding open thoracotomy.[194] Few patients have been treated in this manner, and no long-term follow up is available.

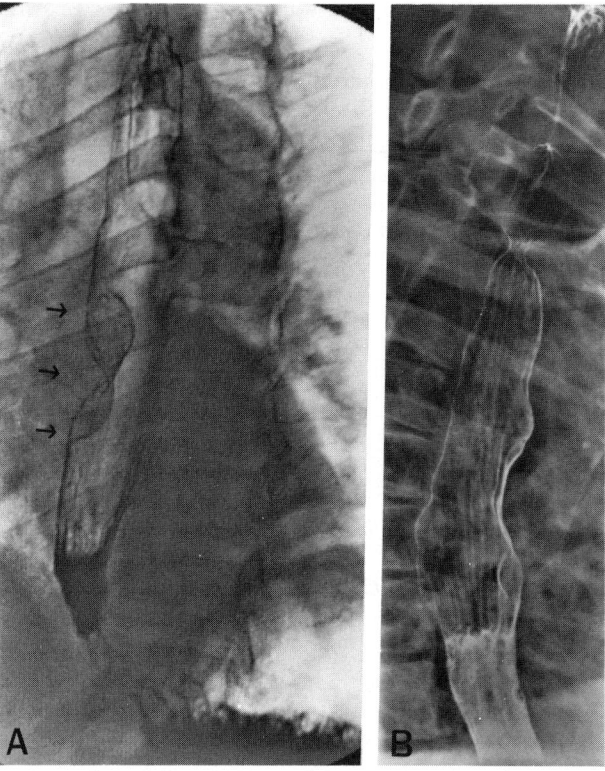

Figure 3-11 **(A)** An esophegeal leiomyoma was identified in the middle third of the esophagus (*arrows*). Endoscopy revealed a bulge at the appropriate location and normal mucosa. A biopsy specimen was not obtained. A right transthoracic approach was used for enucleation of the tumor from the esophageal musculature and mucosa. The muscle layer was repaired loosely. **(B)** Postresection barium swallow demonstrated no residual defect and normal outflow of barium into the stomach.

Small Cell Carcinoma

Small cell carcinomas of the esophagus are rare neoplasms, occurring in only 1% of all patients presenting with esophageal tumors during a 17-year period.[195] The tumors are characterized by an aggressive biology, frequently with spread beyond the local area at diagnosis. These tumors show evidence of neurosecretory granules and multidifferentiation.[196] Surgical resection is infrequently performed because prognosis is poor.[197] In one series,[188] 3 of 11 patients had surgical resection; median survival was 5 months. Death results most frequently from distant metastases. Palliation of dysphagia can be accomplished with chemotherapy and external-beam radiation therapy. The therapeutic approach to patients with small cell carcinoma of the esophagus parallels the treatment of small cell carcinoma of the lung.[198]

Melanoma

Primary melanoma of the esophagus usually has an aggressive biologic behavior and extensive submucosal spread. Surgery with generous resection margins has been advocated by some authors in the absence of metastases (5-year survival, 4.2%). Radiation and chemotherapy are reserved for palliative treatment.[199] Median survival after esophagectomy is 5 months.[188]

Sarcomatoid Tumors

Patients with sarcomatoid tumors of the esophagus may have both bulky sarcomatous and carcinomatous elements. Survival depends on the degree of biologic aggressiveness.[200] After resection of primary sarcomas of the esophagus, patients have a 5-year survival rate of about 23% (median, 20 months).[188]

The best treatment for neoplastic diseases of the esophagus is yet to be determined. The etiology is variable and prevention is difficult. Once symptoms occur, the disease is often locally advanced. Surgery offers immediate palliation and good control of local disease, with modern series reporting acceptable rates of mortality (less than 6%) and morbidity. Radiation therapy, like surgical therapy, treats local and regional disease. Most patients however, succumb to distant metastases. Chemotherapy before and after surgery can minimize distant metastases and enhance survival. Studies that are evaluating various chemotherapeutic agents and schedules of chemotherapy combined with radiation therapy with or without surgery should better define the role of these therapies in the treatment of esophageal neoplasms. The results of these studies will yield a foundation for future multimodality treatment of esophageal carcinoma.

REFERENCES

1. Boring CC, Squires TS, Tong T. Cancer statistics, 1992. Cancer 1991;43:7.
2. Powell J, McConkey CC. The rising trend in oesophageal adenocarcinoma and gastric cardia. Eur J Cancer Prev 1992;1:265.
3. Blot WJ, Devesa SS, Kneller RW, Fraumeni JF Jr. Rising incidence of adenocarcinoma of the esophagus and gastric cardia. JAMA 1991;265:1287.
4. Blot WJ, Devesa SS, Fraumeni JF. Continuing climb in rates of esophageal adenocarcinoma: an update. (Abstract) JAMA 1993;270:1320.
5. Craddock VM. Aetiology of oesophageal cancer: some operative factors. Eur J Cancer Prev 1992;1:89.
6. Muir CS, McKinney PA. Cancer of the oesophagus: a global overview. Eur J Cancer Prev 1992;1:259.
7. Hsia CC, Wu JL, Lu XQ, Li YS. Natural occurrence and clastogenic effects of nivalenol, deoxynivalenol, 3-acetyl-deoxynivalenol, 15-acetyl-deoxynivalenol, and zearalenone in corn from a high-risk area of esophageal cancer. Cancer Detect Prev 1988;13:79.
8. Ghadirian P, Vobecky J, Vobecky JS. Factors associated with cancer of the oesophagus: an overview. Cancer Detect Prev 1988;11:225.
9. Cheng KK, Day NE, Duffy SW, Lam TH, Fok M, Wong J. Pickled vegetables in the aetiology of oesophageal cancer in Hong Kong Chinese. Lancet 1992;339:1314.
10. Aggestrup S, Holm JC, Sorensen HR. Does achalasia predispose to cancer of the esophagus? Chest 1992;102:1013.
11. Hopkins RA, Postlethwait RW. Caustic burns and carcinoma of the esophagus. Ann Surg 1981;194:146.
12. Isolauri J, Markkula H. Lye ingestion and carcinoma of the esophagus. Acta Chir Scand 1989;155:269.
13. Patterson DR. Clinical type of dysphagia. J Laryngol Rhinol Otol 1919;34:289.
13a. Kelly AB. Spasm at the entrance of the oesophagus. J Laryngol Rhinol Otol 1919;34:285.
14. Chang F, Syrjanen S, Wang L, Syrjanen K. Infectious agents in the etiology of esophageal cancer. Gastroenterology 1992;103:1336.
15. Furihata M, Ohtsuki Y, Ogoshi S, Takahashi A, Tamiya T, Ogata T. Prognostic significance of human papillomavirus genomes (type-16, -18) and aberrant expression of p53 protein in human esophageal cancer. Int J Cancer 1993;54:226.
16. Chang F, Syrjanen S, Shen Q, Wang L, Wang D, Syrjanen K. Human papillomavirus involvement in esophageal precancerous lesions and squamous cell carcinomas as evidenced by microscopy and different DNA techniques. Scand J Gastroenterol 1992;27:553.
17. Nomura A, Stemmermann GN, Chyou PH, Kato I, Perez-Perez GI, Blaser MJ. *Helicobacter pylori* infection and gastric carcinoma among Japanese Americans in Hawaii. N Engl J Med 1991;325:1132.
18. Borhan Manesh F, Farnum JB. Study of *Helicobacter pylori* colonization of patches of heterotopic gastric mucosa (HGM) at the upper esophagus. Dig Dis Sci 1993;38:142.
19. Beahrs OH, Henson DE, Hutter RVP, Myers MH. Manual for staging of cancer, ed 3. American Joint Committee on Cancer. Philadelphia, JB Lippincott, 1988;63.
20. Liebermann-Meffert DMI, Luescher U, Neff U, Ruedi TP, Allgower M. Esophagectomy without thoracotomy: is there a risk of intramediastinal bleeding? Ann Surg 1987;206:184.
21. van Overhagen H, Lameris JS, Zonderland HM, Tilanus HW, van Pel R, Schutte HE. Ultrasound and ultrasound-guided fine needle aspiration biopsy of supraclavicular

lymph nodes in patients with esophageal carcinoma. Cancer 1991;67:585.

22. Guernsey JM, Knudsen DF. Abdominal exploration in the evaluation of patients with carcinoma of the thoracic esophagus. J Thorac Cardiovasc Surg 1970;59:62.

23. Watson WL, Goodner JT, Miller TP, et al. Torek esophagectomy: the case against segmental resection for esophageal cancer. J Thorac Cardiovasc Surg 1956;32:347.

24. Takubo K, Sasajima K, Yamashita K, Tanaka Y, Fujita K. Prognostic significance of intramural metastasis in patients with esophageal carcinoma. Cancer 1990;65:1816.

25. Kobayashi S, Kasugai T. Brushing cytology for the diagnosis of gastric cancer involving the cardia of the lower esophagus. Acta Cytol 1978;22:155.

26. Winaiwer SJ, Sherlock P, Belladonn JA, et al. Endoscopic brush cytology in esophageal cancer. JAMA 1975;232:1358.

27. Wu YK, Juang GJ, Shao LF, et al. Progress in the study and surgical treatment of cancer of the esophagus in China, 1940–1980. J Thorac Cardiovasc Surg 1982;84:325.

28. Inculet RI, Keller SM, Dwyer A, Roth JA. Evaluation of noninvasive tests for the preoperative staging of carcinoma of the esophagus: a prospective study. Ann Thorac Surg 1985;40:561.

29. Guanrei Y, He H, Sunghong Q, et al. Endoscopic diagnosis of 115 cases of early esophageal carcinoma. Endoscopy 1982;14:157.

30. Isono K, Ochiai T, Okuyama K, Onoda S. The treatment of lymph node metastasis from esophageal cancer by extensive lymphadenectomy. Jpn J Surg 1990;20:151.

31. Mantravadi R, Ladd T, Briele H, et al. Carcinoma of the esophagus: sites of failure. Int J Radiat Oncol Biol Phys 1982;8:1897.

32. Arbitol A, Straus M, Granklin G, et al. Infusional chemotherapy and cyclic chemotherapy for inoperable esophageal and gastric cardia carcinoma. Am J Clin Oncol 1983;6:195.

33. Shibuya H, Tahogi M, Horiuchi J, et al. Carcinomas of the esophagus with synchronous or metachronous primary carcinoma in other organs. Acta Radiol Oncol 1982;21:39.

34. Shons AR, McQuarrie DG. Multiple primary epidermoid carcinomas of the upper aerodigestive tract. Arch Surg 1985;120:1007.

35. Moghissi K. Surgical resection for stage I cancer of the oesophagus and cardia. Br J Surg 1992;79:935.

36. Orringer MB. Substernal gastric bypass of the excluded esophagus: results of an ill-advised operation. Surgery 1984;96:467.

37. Halvorsen RA Jr, Thompson WM. Primary neoplasms of the hollow organs of the gastrointestinal tract: staging and follow-up. Cancer 1991;67:1181.

38. Rice TW, Boyce GA, Sivak MV. Esophageal ultrasound and the preoperative staging of carcinoma of the esophagus. J Thorac Cardiovasc Surg 1991;101:536.

39. Siewert JR, Holscher AH, Dittler HJ. Preoperative staging and risk analysis in esophageal carcinoma. Hepatogastroenterology 1990;37:382.

40. Tio TL, Coene PP, Luiken GJ, Tytgat GN. Endosonography in the clinical staging of esophagogastric carcinoma. Gastrointest Endosc 1990;36:S2.

41. Sharma OP, Subnani S. Role of computerized tomography imaging in staging oesophageal carcinoma. Semin Surg Oncol 1989;5:355.

42. Duignan JP, McEntee GP, O'Connell DJ, Bouchier Hayes DJ, O'Malley E. The role of CT in the management of carcinoma of the oesophagus and cardia. Ann R Coll Surg Engl 1987;69:286.

43. Salonen O, Kivisaari L, Standertskjold Nordenstam CG, Somer K, Virkkunen P. Computed tomography in staging of oesophageal carcinoma. Scand J Gastroenterol 1987;22:65.

44. Lefor AT, Merino MM, Steinberg SM, et al. Computerized tomographic prediction of extraluminal spread and prognostic implications of lesion width in esophageal carcinoma. Cancer 1988;62:1287.

45. Roth JA, Pass HI, Flanagan MM, Graeber GM, Rosenberg JC, Steinberg S. Randomized clinical trial of preoperative and postoperative adjuvant chemotherapy with cisplatin, vindesine, and bleomycin for carcinoma of the esophagus. J Thorac Cardiovasc Surg 1988;96:242.

46. Whittington R, Coia LR, Haller DG, Rubenstein JH, Rosato EF. Adenocarcinoma of the esophagus and esophagogastric junction: the effects of single and combined modalities on the survival and patterns of failure following treatment. Int J Radiat Oncol Biol Phys 1990;19:593.

47. Orringer MB, Forastiere AA, Perez Tamayo C, Urba S, Takasugi BJ, Bromberg J. Chemotherapy and radiation therapy before transhiatal esophagectomy for esophageal carcinoma. Ann Thorac Surg 1990;49:348.

48. Roth JA, Ajani JA, Rich TA. Multidisciplinary therapy for esophageal cancer. Adv Surg 1990;23:239.

49. Orringer MB. Transthoracic versus transhiatal esophagectomy: what difference does it make? Ann Thorac Surg 1987;44:116.

50. Muehrcke DD, Kaplan DK, Donnelly RJ. Oesophagogastrectomy in patients over 70. Thorax 1989;44:141.

51. Burt ME, Gorschboth CM, Brennan MF. A controlled prospective randomized trial evaluating the metabolic effects of enteral and parenteral nutrition in the cancer patient. Cancer 1982;49:1092.

52. Jensen S. Clinical effects of enteral and parenteral nutrition preceding cancer surgery. Med Oncol Tumor Pharmacother 1985;2:225.

53. Daly JM, Massar E, Giacco G, et al. Parenteral nutrition in esophageal cancer patients. Ann Surg 1982;196:203.

54. The Veterans Affairs Total Parenteral Nutrition Cooperative Study Group. Perioperative total parenteral nutrition in surgical patients. N Engl J Med 1991;325:525.

55. Pedersen H, Hansen HS, Cederquist C, et al. The prognostic significance of weight loss and its integration in

stage grouping of oesophageal cancer. Acta Chir Scand 1982;148:363.

56. Sugarbaker DJ, DeCamp MM. Selecting the surgical approach to cancer of the esophagus. Chest 1993;103:410S.

57. Lewis I. The surgical treatment of carcinoma of the esophagus with special reference to a new operation for growth of the middle third. Br J Surg 1946;2:18.

58. Akiyama H, Hiyama M, Hashimoto C. Resection and reconstruction for carcinoma of the thoracic oesophagus. Br J Surg 1976;63:206.

59. Orringer MB, Sloan H. Esophagectomy without thoracotomy. J Thorac Cardiovasc Surg 1978;76:643.

60. Orringer MB, Marshall B, Stirling MC. Transhiatal esophagectomy for benign and malignant disease. J Thorac Cardiovasc Surg 1993;105:265.

61. Skinner DB. En bloc resection for neoplasms of the esophagus and cardia. J Thorac Cardiovasc Surg 1983;85:59.

62. Mannell A, McKnight A, Esser JD. Role of pyloroplasty in the retrosternal stomach: results of a prospective, randomized, controlled trial. Br J Surg 1990;77:57.

63. Cheung HC, Siu KF, Wong J. Is pyloroplasty necessary in esophageal replacement by stomach? A prospective, randomized controlled trial. Surgery 1987;102:19.

64. Mansour KA, Picone AL, Coleman JJ III. Surgery for high cervical esophageal carcinoma: experience with 11 patients. Ann Thorac Surg 1990;49:597.

65. Goldberg M, Freeman J, Gullane PJ, Patterson GA, Todd TR, McShane D. Transhiatal esophagectomy with gastric transposition for pharyngolaryngeal malignant disease. J Thorac Cardiovasc Surg 1989;97:327.

66. Grillo HC, Mathisen DJ. Cervical exenteration. Ann Thorac Surg 1990;49:401.

67. Orringer MD, Sloan H. Anterior mediastinal tracheostomy: indications, techniques, and clinical experience. J Thorac Cardiovasc Surg 1979;78:85.

68. Lam KH, Choi TK, Wei WI, Lau WF, Wong J. Present status of pharyngogastric anastomosis following pharyngolaryngo-oesophagectomy. Br J Surg 1987;74:122.

69. Baker JW Jr, Schechter GL. Management of panesophageal cancer by blunt resection without thoracotomy and reconstruction with stomach. Ann Surg 1986;203:491.

70. Ujiki GT, Pearl GJ, Poticha S, Sisson GA, Shields TW. Mortality and morbidity of gastric "pull-up" for replacement of the pharyngoesophagus. Arch Surg 1987;122:644.

71. Huang MH, Sung CY, Hsu HK, Huang BS, Hsu WH, Chien KY. Reconstruction of the esophagus with the left colon. Ann Thorac Surg 1989;48:660.

72. Lundell L, Olbe L. Colonic interposition for reconstruction after resection of cancer in the esophagus and gastroesophageal junction. Eur J Surg 1991;157:189.

73. Carlson GW, Schusterman MA, Guillamondegui OM. Total reconstruction of the hypo-pharynx and cervical esophagus: a 20-year experience. Ann Plast Surg 1992;29:408.

74. Lorentz T, Fok M, Wong J. Anastomotic leakage after resection and bypass for esophageal cancer: lessons learned from the past. World J Surg 1989;13:472.

75. Bafitis H, Stallings JO, Ban J. A reliable method for monitoring the microvascular patency of free jejunal transfers in reconstructing the pharynx and cervical esophagus. Plast Reconstr Surg 1989;83:896.

76. Byth PL, Mullens AJ. Peri-operative care for oesophagectomy patients. Aust Clin Rev 1991;11:45.

77. Ellis FH Jr. Treatment of carcinoma of the esophagus or cardia. Mayo Clin Proc 1989;64:945.

78. Mathisen DJ, Grillo HC, Wilkins EW Jr, Moncure AC, Hilgenberg AD. Transthoracic esophagectomy: a safe approach to carcinoma of the esophagus. Ann Thorac Surg 1988;45:137.

79. Shao LF, Gao ZG, Yang NP, Wei GQ, Wang YD, Cheng CP. Results of surgical treatment in 6,123 cases of carcinoma of the esophagus and gastric cardia. J Surg Oncol 1989;42:170.

80. King RM, Pairolero PC, Trastek VF, Payne WS, Bernatz PE. Ivor Lewis esophago-gastrectomy for carcinoma of the esophagus: early and late functional results. Ann Thorac Surg 1987;44:119.

81. Lozach P, Topart P, Etienne J, Charles JF. Ivor Lewis operation for epidermoid carcinoma of the esophagus. Ann Thorac Surg 1991;52:1154.

82. Orringer MB. Transhiatal esophagectomy without thoracotomy for carcinoma of the esophagus. Adv Surg 1986;19:1.

83. DeMeester TR, Zaninotto G, Johansson KE. Selective therapeutic approach to cancer of the lower esophagus and cardia. J Thorac Cardiovasc Surg 1988;95:42.

84. Altorki NK, Skinner DB. En bloc esophagectomy: the first 100 patients. Hepatogastroenterol 1990;37:360.

85. Lerut T, De Leyn P, Coosemans W, Van Raemdonck D, Scheys I, LeSaffre E. Surgical strategies in esophageal carcinoma with emphasis on radical lymphadenectomy. Ann Surg 1992;216:583.

86. Plukker JT, van Slooten EA, Joosten HJ. The Akiyama procedure in the surgical management of oesophageal cardiacarcinoma. Eur J Surg Oncol 1988;14:33.

87. Hurley JP, Keeling P. Transhiatal oesophagectomy: its role for tumours of the middle third of the intrathoracic oesophagus. Isr Med J 1990;83:23.

88. Gupta NM. Transhiatal esophagectomy. Acta Chir Scand 1990;156:149.

89. Gotley DC, Beard J, Cooper MJ, Britton DC, Williamson RC. Abdominocervical (transhiatal) oesophagectomy in the management of oesophageal carcinoma. Br J Surg 1990;77:815.

90. Forastiere AA, Orringer MB, Perez Tamayo C, et al. Concurrent chemotherapy and radiation therapy followed by transhiatal esophagectomy for local-regional cancer of the esophagus. J Clin Oncol 1990;8:119.

91. Becker CD, Barbier PA, Terrier F, Porcellini B. Patterns of recurrence of esophageal carcinoma after transhiatal esophagectomy and gastric interposition. AJR 1987;148:273.

92. Putnam JB, Suell DA, McMurtrey MJ, et al. A compari-

son of three techniques of esophagectomy within a residency training program. Ann Thorac Surg 1994;57:319.

93. Hankins JR, Attar S, Coughlin TR Jr, et al. Carcinoma of the esophagus: a comparison of the results of transhiatal versus transthoracic resection. Ann Thorac Surg 1989;47:700.

94. Goldfaden D, Orringer MB, Appelman HD, Kalish R. Adenocarcinoma of the distal esophagus and gastric cardia: comparison of results of transhiatal esophagectomy and thoracoabdominal esophagogastrectomy. J Thorac Cardiovasc Surg 1986;91:242.

95. Fok M, Siu KF, Wong J. A comparison of transhiatal and transthoracic resection for carcinoma of the thoracic esophagus. Am J Surg 1989;158:414.

96. Pradhan GN, Eng JB, Sabanathan S. Left thoracotomy approach for resection of carcinoma of the esophagus. Surg Gynecol Obstet 1989;168:49.

97. Page RD, Khalil JF, Whyte RI, Kaplan DK, Donnelly RJ. Esophagogastrectomy via left thoracophrenotomy. Ann Thorac Surg 1990;49:763.

98. Saidi F, Abbassi A, Shadmehr MB, Khoshnevis Asl G. Endothoracic endoesophageal pull-through operation: a new approach to cancers of the esophagus and proximal stomach. J Thorac Cardiovasc Surg 1991;102:43.

99. Gertsch P, Vauthey N, Maddern G. Transhiatal esophagectomy using a ring dissector. Surg Gynecol Obstet 1993;176:389.

100. Bumm R, Holscher AH, Feussner H, Tachibana M, Bartels H, Siewert JR. Endodissection of the thoracic esophagus: technique and clinical results in transhiatal esophagectomy. Ann Surg 1993;218:97.

101. Fiocco M, Krasna MJ. Thoracoscopic lymph node dissection in the staging of esophageal carcinoma. J Laparoendosc Surg 1992;2:111.

102. McManus KG, Ritchie AJ, McGuigan J, Stevenson HM, Gibbons JR. Sutures, staplers, leaks and strictures: a review of anastomoses in oesophageal resection at Royal Victoria Hospital, Belfast 1977–1986. Eur J Cardiothorac Surg 1990;4:97.

103. Smirniotis V, Morritt GG. EEA stapler in oesophagogastrectomies. Int Surg 1990;75:36.

104. Chasseray VM, Kiroff GK, Buard JL, Launois B. Cervical or thoracic anastomosis for esophagectomy for carcinoma. Surg Gynecol Obstet 1989;169:55.

105. Zieren HU, Muller JM, Pichlmaier H. Prospective randomized study of one- or two-layer anastomosis following oesophageal resection and cervical oesophagogastrostomy. Br J Surg 1993;80:608.

106. Peracchia A, Bardini R, Ruol A, Asolati M, Scibetta D. Esophagovisceral anastomotic leak: a prospective statistical study of predisposing factors. J Thorac Cardiovasc Surg 1988;95:685.

107. Dougenis D, Walker WS, Cameron EW, Walbaum PR. Management of chylothorax complicating extensive esophageal resection. Surg Gynecol Obstet 1992;174:501.

108. Wang HH, Antonioli DA, Goldman H. Comparative features of esophageal and gastric adenocarcinomas: recent changes in type and frequency. Hum Pathol 1986;17:482.

109. Powell J, McConkey CC. Increasing incidence of adenocarcinoma of the gastric cardia and adjacent sites. Br J Cancer 1990;62:440.

110. Lund O, Hasenkam JM, Aagaard MT, Kimose HH. Time-related changes in characteristics of prognostic significance in carcinomas of the oesophagus and cardia. Br J Surg 1989;76:1301.

111. Yang PC, Davis S. Incidence of cancer of the esophagus in the US by histologic type. Cancer 1988;61:612.

112. Rogers EL, Goldkind SF, Iseri OA, et al. Adenocarcinoma of the lower esophagus: a disease primarily of white men with Barrett's esophagus. J Clin Gastroenterol 1986;8:613.

113. Parsonnet J, Friedman GD, Vandersteen DP, et al. *Helicobacter pylori* infection and the risk of gastric carcinoma. N Engl J Med 1991;325:1127.

114. Loffeld RJ, Willems I, Flendrig JA, Arends JW. *Helicobacter pylori* and gastric carcinoma. Histopathology 1990;17:537.

115. Correa P, Fox J, Fontham E, et al. *Helicobacter pylori* and gastric carcinoma: serum antibody prevalence in populations with contrasting cancer risks. Cancer 1990;66:2569.

116. Ming SC. Tumors of the esophagus and stomach. In: Atlas of tumor pathology, series 2, fascile 7. Washington, DC, Armed Forces Institute of Pathology.

117. Barrett N. The lower esophagus lined by columnar epithelium. Surgery 1957;41:881.

118. Rosenberg JC, Budev H, Edwards RC, et al. Analysis of adenocarcinoma in Barrett's esophagus utilizing a staging system. Cancer 1985;55:1353.

119. Kalish RJ, Clancy PE, Orringer MB, et al. Clinical, epidemiologic and morphologic comparison between adenocarcinomas arising in Barrett's esophageal mucosa and in the gastric cardia. Gastroenterology 1984;86:461.

120. Dent J. Approaches to oesophageal columnar metaplasia (Barrett's oesophagus). Scand J Gastroenterol 1989;168(Suppl):60.

121. Streitz JM Jr, Ellis FH Jr, Gibb SP, Balogh K, Watkins E Jr. Adenocarcinoma in Barrett's esophagus: a clinicopathologic study of 65 cases. Ann Surg 1991;213:122.

122. De Baecque C, Potet F, Molas G, Flejou JF, Barbier P, Martignon C. Superficial adeno-carcinoma of the oesophagus arising in Barrett's mucosa with dysplasia: a clinico-pathological study of 12 patients. Histopathology 1990;16:213.

123. Duhaylongsod FG, Wolfe WG. Barrett's esophagus and adenocarcinoma of the esophagus and gastroesophageal junction. J Thorac Cardiovasc Surg 1991;102:36.

124. Garewal HS, Sampliner RE, Fennerty MB. Flow cytometry in Barrett's esophagus: what have we learned so far? Ann Thorac Surg 1991;36:548.

125. Haggitt RC, Reid BJ, Rabinovitch PS, Rubin CE. Barrett's esophagus: correlation between mucin histochemistry,

flow cytometry, and histologic diagnosis for predicting increased cancer risk. Am J Pathol 1988;131:53.

126. Levine DS, Reid BJ, Haggitt RC, Rubin CE, Rabinovitch PS. Correlation of ultrastructural aberrations with dysplasia and flow cytometric abnormalities in Barrett's epithelium. Gastroenterology 1989;96:355.

127. Garewal HS, Gerner EW, Sampliner RE, Roe D. Ornithine decarboxylase and polyamine levels in columnar upper gastrointestinal mucosae in patients with Barrett's esophagus. Cancer Res 1988;48:3288.

128. Yoshida M, Hayashi H, Taira M, Isono K. Elevated expression of the ornithine decarboxylase gene in human esophageal cancer. Cancer Res 1992;52:6671.

129. Garewal HS, Sampliner R. Barrett's esophagus: a model premalignant lesion for adeno-carcinoma. Prevent Med 1989;18:749.

130. Meltzer SJ, Zhou D, Weinstein WM. Tissue-specific expression of c-Ha-ras in premalignant gastrointestinal mucosae. Exp Mol Pathol 1989;51:264.

131. Bai SX. Primary esophageal adenocarcinoma: report of 19 cases. Chung Hua Chung Liu Tsa Chih 1989;11:383.

132. Sampliner RE, Garewal HS, Fennerty MB, Aickin M. Lack of impact of therapy on extent of Barrett's esophagus in 67 patients. Dig Dis Sci 1990;35:93.

133. Fiorucci S, Santucci L, Farroni F, Pelli MA, Morelli A. Effect of omeprazole on gastro-esophageal reflux in Barrett's esophagus. Am J Gastroenterol 1989;84:1263.

134. Altorki NK, Skinner DB, Segalin A, Stephens JK, Ferguson MK, Little AG. Indications for esophagectomy in nonmalignant Barrett's esophagus: a 10-year experience. Ann Thorac Surg 1990;49:724.

135. Palley SL, Sampliner RE, Garewal HS. Management of high-grade dysplasia in Barrett's esophagus. J Clin Gastroenterol 1989;11:369.

136. Williamson WA, Ellis FH, Gibb SP, et al. Barrett's esophagus: prevalence and incidence of adenocarcinoma. Arch Intern Med 1991;151:2212.

137. Altorki NK, Sunagawa M, Little AG, Skinner DB. High-grade dysplasia in the columnar-lined esophagus. Am J Surg 1991;161:97.

138. Starnes VA, Adkins RB, Ballinger JG, et al. Barrett's esophagus: a surgical entity. Arch Surg 1984;119:563.

139. Williamson WA, Ellis FH Jr, Gibb SP, Shahian DM, Aretz HT. Effect of antireflux operation on Barrett's mucosa. Ann Thorac Surg 1990;49:537.

139a. Streitz JM Jr, Andrews CW Jr, Ellis FH Jr. Endoscopic surveillance of Barrett's esophagus: does it help? J Thorac Cardiovasc Surg 1993;105:383.

139b. Ovaska J, Miettinen M, Kivilaakso E. Adenocarcinoma arising in Barrett's esophagus. Dig Dis Sci 1989;34:1336.

140. Ribet M, Mensier E, Pruvot FR. Barrett's esophagus and adenocarcinoma. Eur J Cardiothorac Surg 1987;1:29.

141. Van der VeenAH, Dees J, Blankensteijn JD, Van Blankenstein M. Adenocarcinoma in Barrett's oesophagus: an overrated risk. Gut 1989;30:14.

142. Achkar E, Carey W. The cost of surveillance for adeno-

carcinoma complicating Barrett's esophagus. Am J Gastroenterol 1988;83:291.

143. Finley RJ, Inculet RI. The results of esophagogastrectomy without thoracotomy for adeno-carcinoma of the esophagogastric junction. Ann Surg 1989;210:535.

144. Jobsen JJ, van Andel JG, Eijkenboom WMH, et al. Carcinoma of the esophagus: treatment results. Radiother Oncol 1986;5:101.

145. Kelsen D. Neoadjuvant therapy of esophageal cancer. Can J Surg 1989;32:410.

146. Fujita H, Kakegawa T, Kawahara H, et al. Preoperative radiation for carcinoma of the thoracic esophagus involving adjacent organs: a comparative and multivariate analysis of prognosis. Kurume Med J 1992;39:175.

147. Araujo CM, Souhami L, Gil RA, et al. A randomized trial comparing radiation therapy versus concomitant radiation therapy and chemotherapy in carcinoma of the thoracic esophagus. Cancer 1991;67:2258.

148. Fok M, Sham JS, Choy D, Cheng SW, Wong J. Postoperative radiotherapy for carcinoma of the esophagus: a prospective, randomized controlled study. Surgery 1993;113:138.

149. Ajani JA, Roth JA, Ryan B, et al. Evaluation of pre- and postoperative chemotherapy for resectable adenocarcinoma of the esophagus or gastroesophageal junction. J Clin Oncol 1990;8:1231.

150. Coia LR. Esophageal cancer: is esophagectomy necessary? Oncology 1989;3:101.

151. Coia LR. The use of mitomycin in esophageal cancer. Oncology 1993;50(Suppl 1):53.

152. Wolfe WG, Vaughn AL, Seigler HF, Hathorn JW, Leopold KA, Duhaylongsod FG. Survival of patients with carcinoma of the esophagus treated with combined-modality therapy. J Thorac Cardiovasc Surg 1993;105:749.

153. Coia LR, Engstrom PF, Paul AR, Stafford PM, Hanks GE. Long-term results of infusional 5-FU, mitomycin-C and radiation as primary management of esophageal carcinoma. Int J Radiat Oncol Biol Phys 1991;20:29.

154. Herskovic A, Martz K, Al-Sarraf M, et al. Combined chemotherapy and radiotherapy compared with radiotherapy alone in patients with cancer of the esophagus. N Engl J Med 1992;326:1593.

155. Orringer MB. Multimodality therapy for esophageal carcinoma: update. Chest 1993;103:406S.

156. Naunheim KS, Petruska P, Roy TS, et al. Preoperative chemotherapy and radiotherapy for esophageal carcinoma. J Thorac Cardiovasc Surg 1992;103:887.

157. Forastiere AA, Orringer MB, Perez-Tamayo C, Urba SG, Zahurak M. Preoperative chemo-radiation followed by transhiatal esophagectomy for carcinoma of the esophagus: final report. J Clin Oncol 1993;11:1118.

158. Kavanagh B, Anscher M, Leopold K, et al. Patterns of failure following combined modality therapy for esophageal cancer, 1984–1990. Int J Radiat Oncol Biol Phys 1992;24:633.

159. Saito T, Shigemitsu Y, Kinoshita T, et al. Cisplatin, vindesine, pepleomycin and concurrent radiation therapy

following esophagectomy with lymphadenectomy for patients with an esophageal carcinoma. Oncology 1993;50:293.

160. Buset M, Cremer M. Endoscopic palliation of malignant dysphagia. Acta Gastroenterol Belg 1992;55:264.

161. Saito T, Kinoshita T, Shigemitsu Y, et al. Cisplatin, vindesine, pepleomycin and combined radiation therapy for inoperable esophageal carcinoma. Jpn J Clin Oncol 1993;23:123.

162. Hareyama M, Nishio M, Kagami Y, Narimatsu N, Saito A, Sakurai T. Intracavitary brachytherapy combined with external-beam irradiation for squamous cell carcinoma of the thoracic esophagus. Int J Radiat Oncol Biol Phys 1992;24:235.

163. Sur RK, Kochhar R, Singh DP, et al. High dose rate intracavitary therapy in advanced carcinoma esophagus. Indian J Gastroenterol 1991;10:43.

164. Fleischman EH, Kagan AR, Bellotti JE, Streeter OE Jr, Harvey JC. Effective palliation for inoperable esophageal cancer using intensive intracavitary radiation. J Surg Oncol 1990;44:234.

165. Holting T, Friedl P, Schraube N, Fritz P, Schlag P, Herfarth C. Palliation of esophageal cancer: operative resection versus laser and afterloading therapy. Surg Endosc 1991;5:4.

166. Agrawal RK, Dawes PJ, Clague MB. Combined external beam and intracavitary radiotherapy in oesophageal carcinoma. Clin Oncol 1992;4:222.

167. Mannell A, Becker PJ, Nissenbaum M. Bypass surgery for unresectable oesophageal cancer: early and late results in 124 cases. Br J Surg 1988;75:283.

168. Hambraeus GM, Walther BS. Oesophagectomy without thoracotomy: experiences from 30 cases. Scand J Thorac Cardiovasc Surg 1988;22:216.

169. Skinner DB. Esophageal malignancies: experience with 110 cases. Surg Clin North Am 1976;56:137.

170. Segalin A, Little AG, Ruol A, et al. Surgical and endoscopic palliation of esophageal carcinoma. Ann Thorac Surg 1989;48:267.

171. Lundell L, Leth R, Lind T, Lonroth H, Sjovall M, Olbe L. Palliative endoscopic dilatation in carcinoma of the esophagus and esophagogastric junction. Acta Chir Scand 1989;155:179.

172. Pattison CW, Griffin SC, Coker C, Townsend ER, Fountain SW. Palliative intubation of malignant oesophageal strictures. Scand J Thorac Cardiovasc Surg 1990;24:153.

173. Unruh HW, Pagliero KM. Pulsion intubation versus traction intubation for obstructing carcinomas of the esophagus. Ann Thorac Surg 1985;40:337.

174. Storms P, Pagliero KM. Self adjusting stent in the management of malignant tracheo-oesophageal fistula. Acta Chir Belg 1990;90:9.

175. Kratz JM, Reed CE, Crawford FA, Stroud MR, Parker EF. A comparison of endoesophageal tubes: improved results with the Atkinson tube. J Thorac Cardiovasc Surg 1989;97:19.

176. Alderson D, Wright PD. Laser recanalization versus endoscopic intubation in the palliation of malignant dysphagia. Br J Surg 1990;77:1151.

177. Barr H, Krasner N, Raouf A, Walker RJ. Prospective randomised trial of laser therapy only and laser therapy followed by endoscopic intubation for the palliation of malignant dysphagia. Gut 1990;31:252.

178. Buset M, des Marez B, Baize M, et al. Palliative endoscopic management of obstructive esophagogastric cancer: laser or prosthesis. Gastrointest Endosc 1987;33:357.

179. Loizou LA, Grigg D, Atkinson M, Robertson C, Bown SG. A prospective comparison of laser therapy and intubation in endoscopic palliation for malignant dysphagia. Gastroenterology 1991;100:1303.

180. Song HY, Choi KC, Cho BH, Ahn DS, Kim KS. Esophagogastric neoplasms: palliation with a modified Gianturco stent. Radiology 1991;180:349.

181. Isaac JR, Sim EK, Ngoi SS, Goh PM. Safe and rapid palliation of dysphagia for carcinoma of the esophagus. Am Surg 1991;57:245.

182. Siegel HI, Laskin KJ, Dabezies MA, Fisher RS, Krevsky B. The effect of endoscopic laser therapy on survival in patients with squamous-cell carcinoma of the esophagus: further experience. J Clin Gastroenterol 1991;13:142.

183. Schulze S, Fischerman K. Palliation of oesophagogastric neoplasms with Nd:YAG laser treatment. Scand J Gastroenterol 1990;25:1024.

184. Ahmed ME, Gustavsson S. Current palliative modalities for esophageal carcinoma: clinical review. Acta Chir Scand 1990;156:95.

185. Brennan FN, McCarthy JH, Laurence BH. Endoscopic Nd-YAG laser therapy for palliation of upper gastrointestinal malignancy. Med J Aust 1990;153:27.

186. Hahl J, Salo J, Ovaska J, Haapiainen R, Kalima T, Schroder T. Comparison of endoscopic Nd:YAG laser therapy and oesophageal tube in palliation of oesophagogastric malignancy. Scand J Gastroenterol 1991;26:103.

187. Naveau S, Chiesa A, Poynard T, Chaput JC. Endoscopic Nd-YAG laser therapy as palliative treatment for esophageal and cardial cancer: parameters affecting long-term outcome. Dig Dis Sci 1990;35:294.

188. Caldwell CB, Bains MS, Burt M. Unusual malignant neoplasms of the esophagus: oat cell carcinoma, melanoma, and sarcoma. J Thorac Cardiovasc Surg 1991;101:100.

189. Solomon MP, Rosenblum H, Rosato FE. Leiomyoma of the esophagus. Ann Surg 1993;199:246.

190. Murata Y, Yoshida M, Akimoto S, Ide H, Suzuki S, Hanyu F. Evaluation of endoscopic ultrasonography for the diagnosis of submucosal tumors of the esophagus. Surg Endosc 1988;2:51.

191. Yasuda K, Nakajima M, Kawai K. Endoscopic ultrasonography in the diagnosis of submucosal tumor of the upper digestive tract. Scand J Gastroenterol 1986;123(Suppl):59.

192. Tio TL, Tytgat GN, den Hartog Jager FC. Endoscopic ultrasonography for the evaluation of smooth muscle tu-

mors in the upper gastrointestinal tract: an experience with 42 cases. Gastrointest Endosc 1990;36:342.

193. Rendina EA, Venuta F, Pescarmona EO, et al. Leiomyoma of the esophagus. Scand J Thorac Cardiovasc Surg 1990;24:79.

194. Bardini R, Segalin A, Ruol A, Pavanello M, Peracchia A. Videothoracoscopic enucleation of esophageal leiomyoma. Ann Thorac Surg 1992;54:576.

195. Nichols GL, Kelsen DP. Small cell carcinoma of the esophagus: the Memorial Hospital experience 1970 to 1987. Cancer 1989;64:1531.

196. Mori M, Matsukuma A, Adachi Y, et al. Small cell carcinoma of the esophagus. Cancer 1989;63:564.

197. Beyer KL, Marshall JB, Diaz Arias AA, Loy TS. Primary small-cell carcinoma of the esophagus: report of 11 cases and review of the literature. J Clin Gastroenterol 1991;13:135.

198. Tennvall J, Johansson L, Albertsson M. Small cell carcinoma of the oesophagus: a clinical and immunohistopathological review. Eur J Surg Oncol 1990;16:109.

199. Sabanathan S; Eng J. Primary malignant melanoma of the esophagus. Scand J Thorac Cardiovasc Surg 1990;24:83.

200. Weidner N. Sarcomatoid carcinoma of the upper aerodigestive tract. Semin Diagn Pathol 1987;4:157.

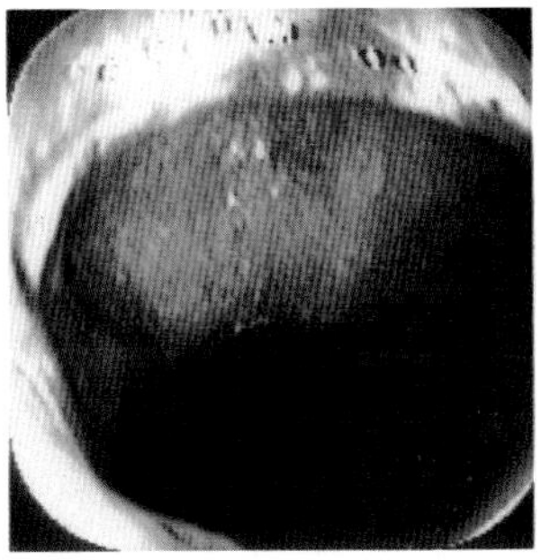

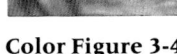

Color Figure 1-1

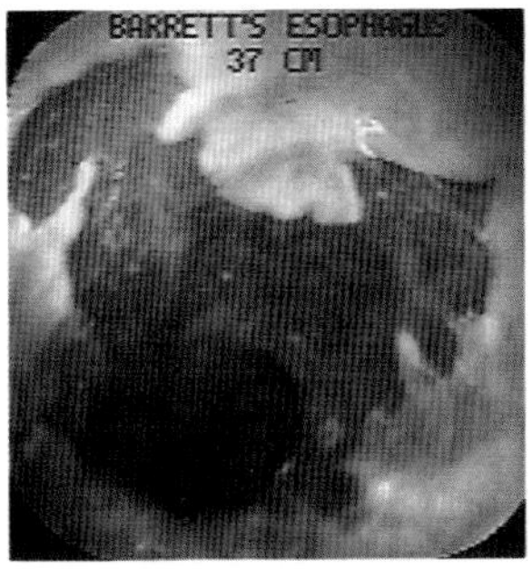

Color Figure 1-7

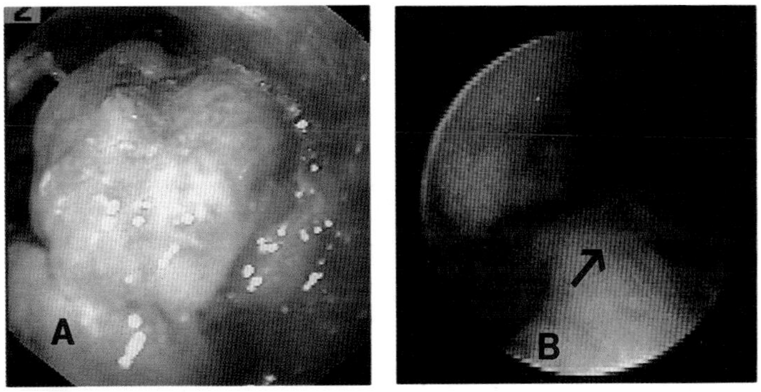

Color Figure 3-2

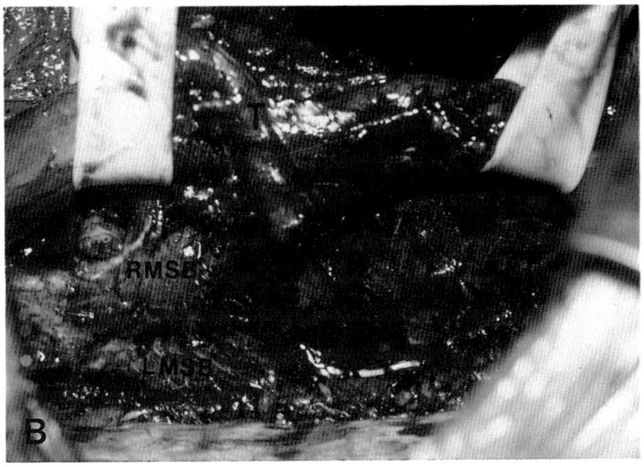

Color Figure 3-4

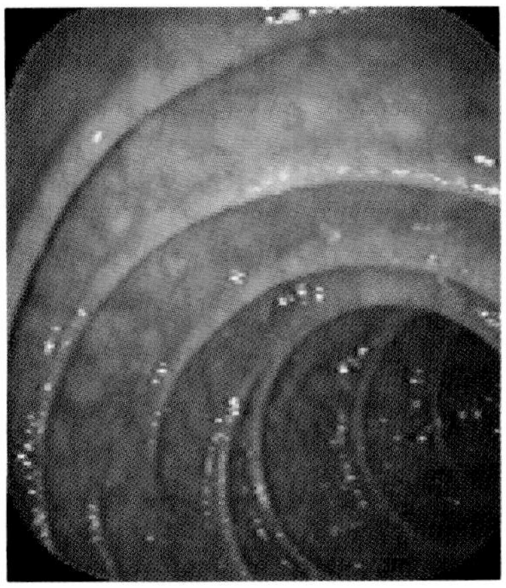

Color Figure 6-6

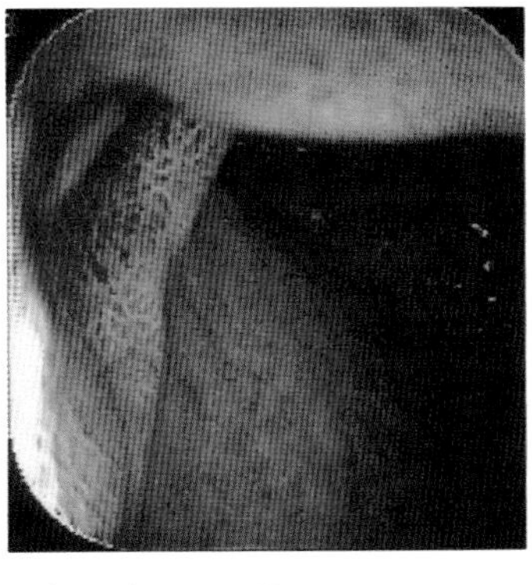

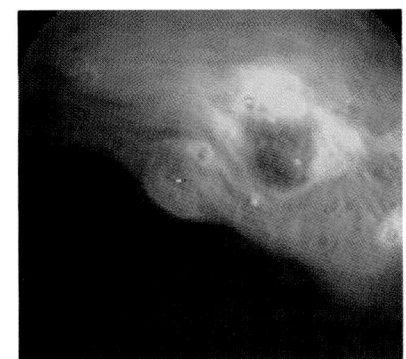

Color Figure 6-7

Color Figure 6-24

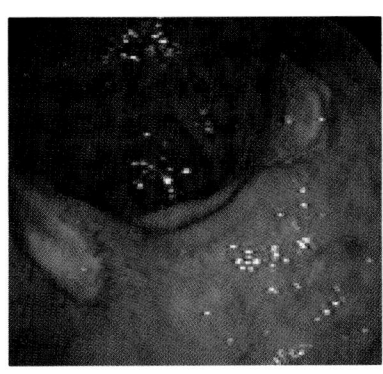

Color Figure 6-29

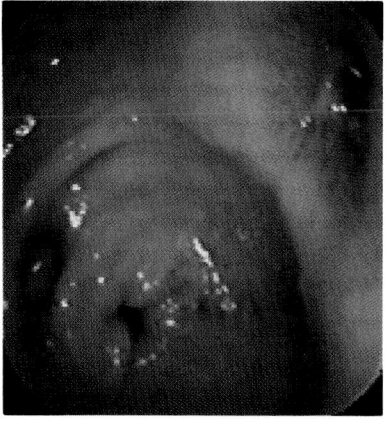

Color Figure 6-30

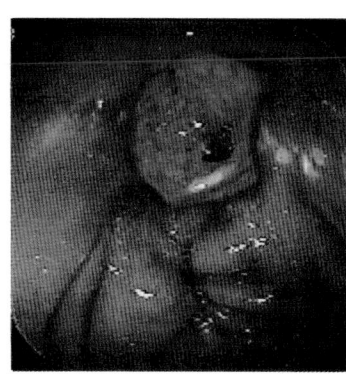

Color Figure 6-31

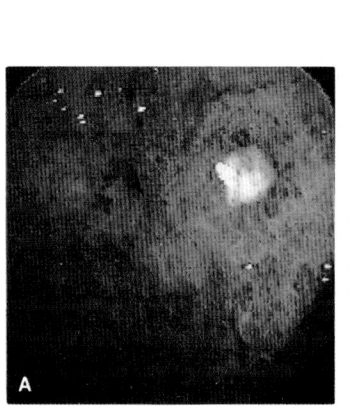
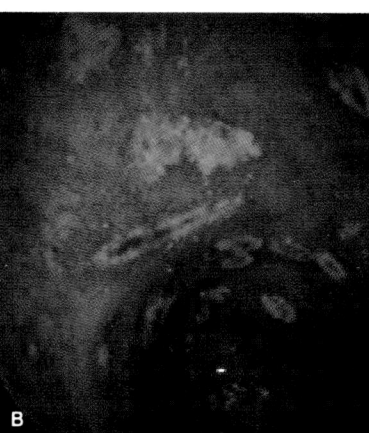
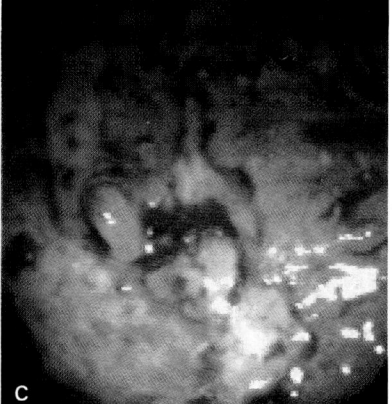

Color Figure 6-33

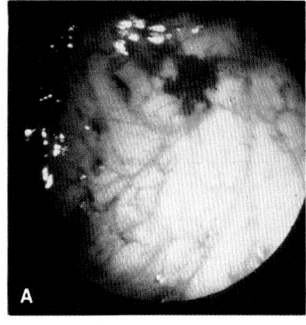
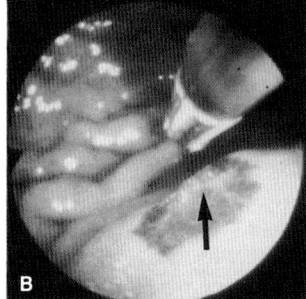

Color Figure 8-18

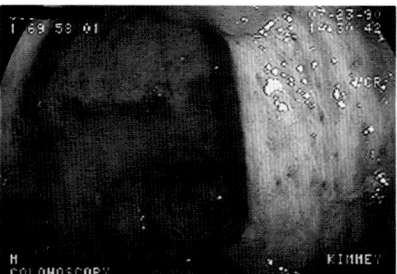

Color Figure 8-19

Digestive Tract Surgery: A Text and Atlas, edited by Richard H. Bell,
Layton F. Rikkers, and Michael W. Mulholland.
Lippincott-Raven Publishers, Philadelphia, © 1996.

4

Esophageal Trauma

Dan M. Meyer

Traumatic injuries of the esophagus are relatively uncommon, making an individual surgeon's or institution's experience with this injury limited. Therefore, recommendations regarding the diagnosis and management are varied. Most esophageal injuries are secondary to penetrating trauma,[1] either due to extrinsic injury or the result of intrinsic perforation caused by manipulation of the esophagus with esophagoscopes, endotracheal tubes, or other devices. Most are iatrogenic[2-8] (Table 4-1).

Diagnosis and management of esophageal injuries are guided by anatomic features and by consideration of the mechanism of injury. The cervical esophagus is the most commonly injured segment. Trauma to this portion is rarely an isolated event because of its proximity to other cervical structures. Thoracic esophageal wounds are uncommon and are usually the result of missile injuries. Nonpenetrating esophageal injuries are rare[9] and occur after trauma to the chest or upper abdomen or as the result of accidental insufflation of air under pressure into the esophagus.[10] Blunt traumatic injuries frequently involve the cervical region and are usually associated with tracheal or laryngeal trauma. Barogenic injuries, such as Boerhaave's syndrome, occur most frequently in the distal thoracic esophagus and typically are diagnosed late. Corrosive injuries may involve a large segment of thoracic and intraabdominal esophagus and are often devastating. Finally, retained foreign bodies require endoscopic retrieval and esophageal surveillance to ensure against mucosal or more extensive esophageal injury. The overall mortality rate of esophageal trauma patients is 20% to 25%.

ANATOMIC CONSIDERATIONS

The esophagus is anatomically divided into cervical, thoracic, and abdominal regions (Fig. 4-1). The cervical esophagus extends from the cricopharyngeus muscle (C-6) to the thoracic inlet (suprasternal notch), about 18 cm from the upper incisors. As it enters the posterior mediastinum, it becomes the thoracic esophagus. The thoracic esophagus extends 18 cm to 40 cm from the incisors. This region of the esophagus can be further divided anatomically into upper, middle, and distal. The upper thoracic esophagus extends from the thoracic inlet to the level of the tracheal bifurcation, about 24 cm from the upper incisor teeth. The middle thoracic esophagus starts at the tracheal bifurcation and extends to a level about 32 cm from the upper incisors. The distal or lower thoracic esophagus is 8 cm in length and ends at the esophagogastric junction about 40 cm from the upper incisors. The thoracic esophagus exits the thorax at the esophageal hiatus to terminate in the gastric cardia a variable distance within the abdomen (4 to 8 cm). The intraabdominal portion of the esophagus starts at the esophageal hiatus and ends in the union with the stomach. In normal adults, the distance from the inferior alveolar ridge to the gastroesophageal junction varies between 38 and 43 cm (Table 4-2).

Management of esophageal trauma is directly influenced by anatomic factors. The fact that esophageal injuries constitute "the most rapidly fatal and most serious perforation of the gastrointestinal tract"[11] relates to two important features of esophageal anatomy—its vascular supply and its somatic composition. In the cervical portion, the blood supply of the esophagus is from the inferior thyroid artery. In the thoracic esophagus, the supply comes directly from the aorta by way of the bronchial arteries; in the abdominal region, the left gastric artery is the primary vascular source. The cervical portion, therefore, is expected to have a superior capacity for healing because the inferior thyroid artery has a broad distribution. Conversely, the thoracic esophagus,

Table 4-1 Causes of Esophageal Perforation and Types of Instrumental Perforation

Iatrogenic and Instrumental (51%)
    Intraluminal
        Esophagoscopy (35%)
        Bougienage (20%)
        Pneumatic dilation (25%)
        Sclerosis of esophageal varices (2%)
        Intraesophageal tube placement (18%); nasogastric,
            Sengstaken-Blakemore, prosthetic
        Endotracheal tube placement
    Extraluminal
        Mediastinoscopy
        Intraoperative injury
            Thyroid resection
            Leiomyoma enucleation
            Proximal gastric vagotomy
            Pneumonectomy
            Decortication
        Radiation therapy
Traumatic (19%)
    Penetrating
    Nonpenetrating
    Corrosive
Barogenic (16%)
    Postemetic
    Miscellaneous
Retained foreign body (7%)
Tumor (4%)
Other (3%)

(Data from references 2–8)

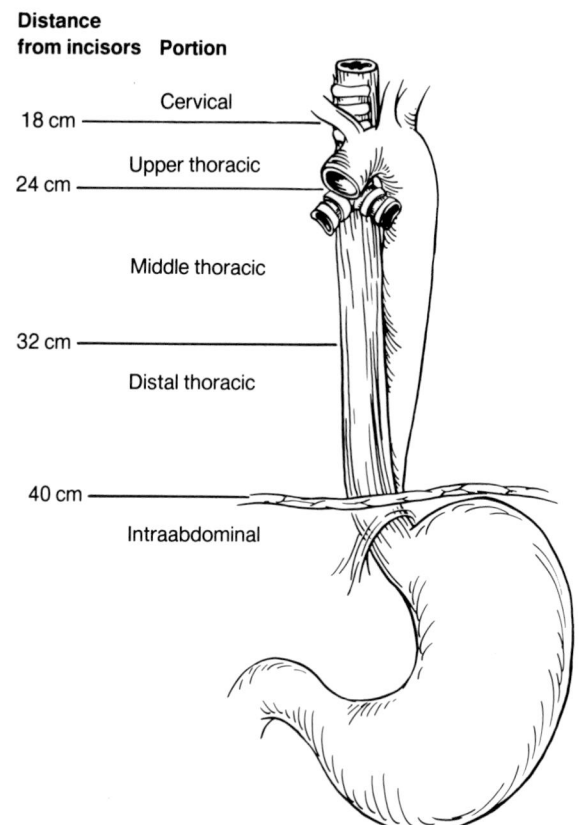

Figure 4-1 Anatomic and endoscopic landmarks of the esophagus.

with a strictly segmental distribution, has a more tenuous vascular supply.

The layers that compose the esophageal wall are the mucosa, submucosa, an inner circular muscular layer, and an outer longitudinal muscular layer. The reasons for the high failure rate of anastomotic healing in the esophagus are not precisely known, but leaks and dehiscence are more common than in other parts of the gastrointestinal tract. This may be due to tenuous vascular supply, a weaker muscular wall, the absence of a serosal layer, the negative intrathoracic pressure that dissipates contaminated materials into the mediastinum, or other unidentified factors.

Cervical perforations usually occur posteriorly, where the esophageal wall is thin. Dissection through the retroesophageal space allows spread of contamination to the mediastinum. The prevertebral fascia can limit lateral spread. Thoracic esophageal perforation, conversely, results in direct mediastinal contamination and more rapid development of pneumomediastinum and mediastinitis than after cervical perforation. The thin mediastinal pleura is frequently ruptured, producing contamination of the pleural space. Gastric contents and fluids are drawn into pleural space by negative intrathoracic pressure, resulting in further inflammation and fluid sequestration, hypovolemia, and early appearance of tachycardia and systemic sepsis. Similarly, perforation of the abdominal esophagus occurs directly into the free peritoneal cavity and results in peritonitis. These anatomic features directly influence the symptom complex and clinical course of these patients.

Cervical esophageal injury must be suspected in

Table 4-2 Endoscopic Measurements of Important Anatomic Landmarks

| | Distance From Upper Incisors (cm) | | | |
	1 y	6 y	14 y	Adulthood
Cricopharyngeus	9	11	14	16
Aorta	14	16	21	23
Left bronchus	15	18	24	27
Hiatus	18	24	33	38
Cardia	19	25	34	40
Greater curvature	27	33	43	53

any patient suffering penetration to the neck. Past practice was to recommend mandatory operative exploration for all patients whose wounds penetrated the platysma muscle. However, trends in trauma management have expanded both the diagnostic repertoire and management themes to include both operative and expectant or nonoperative management. The platysma muscle is the first structure encountered beneath the skin; it covers the entire anterior triangle and the anteroinferior aspect of the posterior triangle. The muscle is thin, is covered by a superficial fascia, and overlies the deep cervical fascia (Fig. 4-2). The deep cervical fascia helps support the muscles, vessels, and viscera of the neck. It is divided into three parts—the investing layer, the pretracheal layer, and the prevertebral layer. The pretracheal layer is in proximity to the esophagus; it adheres to the thyroid and cricoid cartilage and extends into the thorax, where it fuses with the pericardium.

MECHANISMS OF INJURY

Iatrogenic injury is usually caused by instrumental esophageal perforation. It occurs in about 1 in every 10,000 upper endoscopic procedures.[1] A survey in 1974

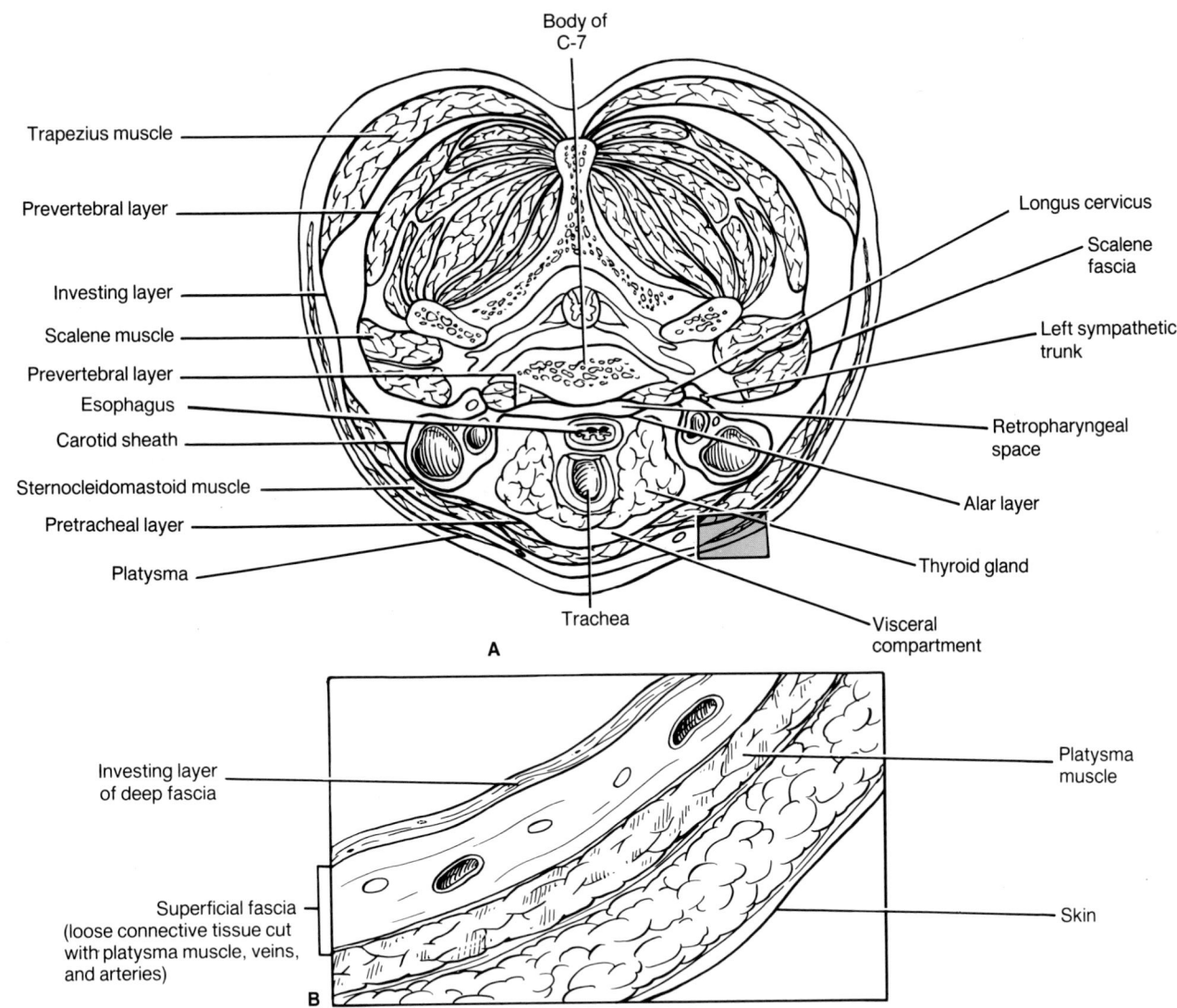

Figure 4-2 (**A**) Cross-sectional depiction of the cervical fascial planes. (**B**) Enlarged view of colored area in **A**. (After Gray SW, Skandalakis JE, McClusky DA. Atlas of surgical anatomy. Baltimore, Williams & Wilkins, 1985:15)

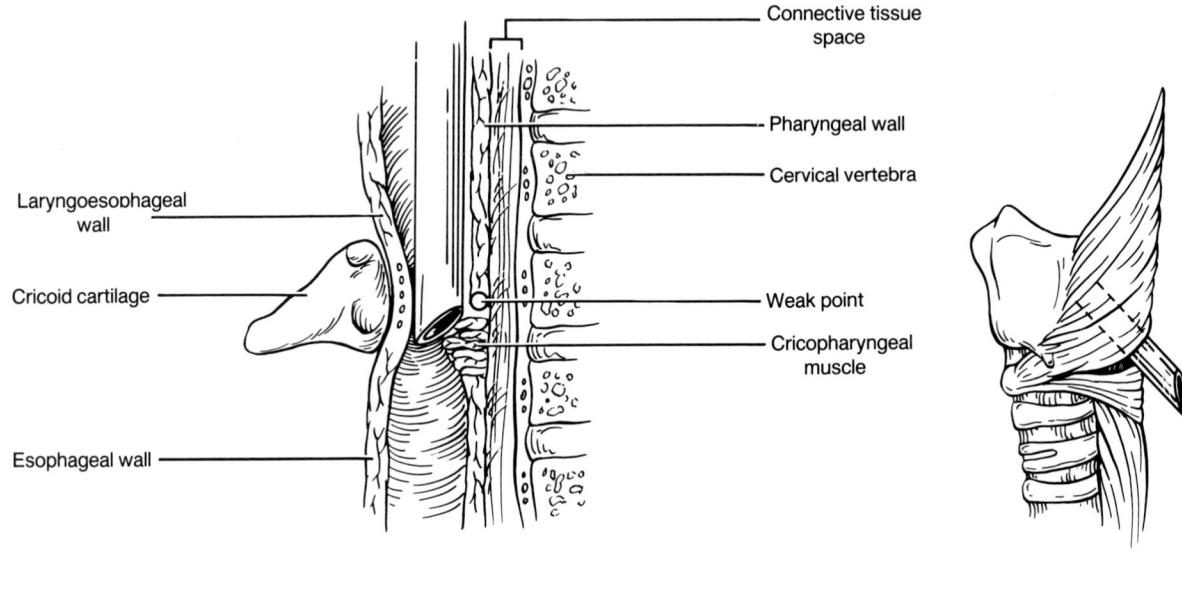

A **B**

Figure 4-3   Area at risk for high instrumental perforation. Relaxation of the cricopharyngeus muscle is necessary for safe passage of an instrument, allowing the cricoid cartilage to move anteriorly away from the cervical spine. (**A**) The weak spot in the posterior cervical esophagus is indicated. (**B**) Forceful passage of the endoscope in this area may result in perforation. (After Terracol J, Sweet RH. Diseases of the esophagus. Philadelphia, WB Saunders, 1958)

showed the incidence of perforation to be 0.03% in simple upper endoscopic procedures and 0.25% in those procedures involving bougienage.[12] With more aggressive manipulation, the risk of perforation understandably increases. Pneumatic dilation for achalasia has a much higher risk of perforation (1% to 10%),[13] as does endoscopic sclerosis of esophageal varices (1% to 4%).[14] Esophageal perforation can also occur during placement of a nasogastric tube,[15] Sengstaken-Blakemore tube,[16] endoesophageal prostheses,[17] or endotracheal tubes.[18]

The anatomic area at greatest risk for instrumental injury is the cricopharyngeal region of the cervical esophagus. At Lannier's triangle, formed by the constrictor pharyngeus and cricopharyngeus muscles at the level of the C-5 and C-6 vertebrae, the posterior esophageal mucosa is covered only by fascia (Fig. 4-3). Risk of perforation is also increased by hyperextension of the neck and the presence of kyphosis or cervical vertebral spurs. The next most common site of perforation during instrumentation is the narrow and fixed region of the distal esophagus just proximal to the hiatus. The middle thoracic esophagus near the aortic arch and left main bronchus are also possible sites of perforation (Fig. 4-4). Other areas at risk include the esophagus just proximal to an obstructive process, areas with extensive involvement by carcinoma, and biopsy sites.

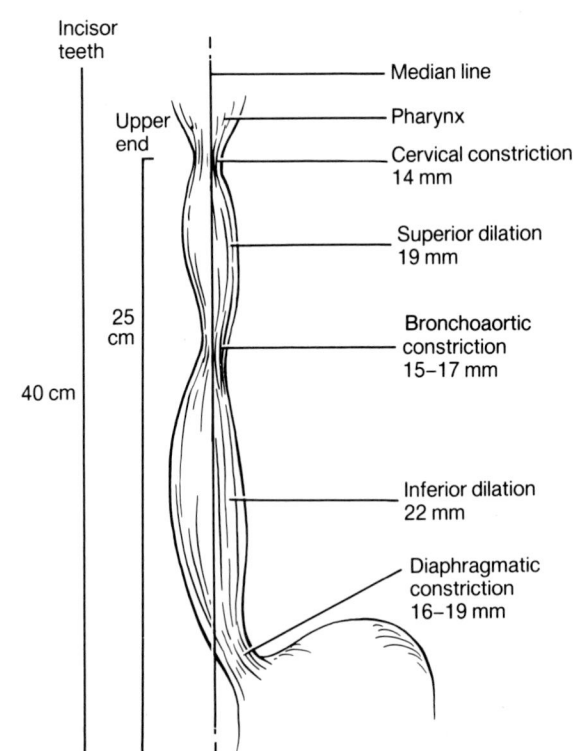

Figure 4-4   Areas of regional narrowing in the esophagus. (After Boies LR, Hilger JA, Priest RE. Fundamentals of otolaryngology, ed 4. Philadelphia, WB Saunders, 1964)

Penetrating injuries to the esophagus usually involve the cervical region and are due to either stab wounds or gunshot wounds, although other instruments may be responsible. Injury to the cervical esophagus, while not immediately life threatening, can have a devastating end result if the injury is missed. The most common cause of death and disability relates to the associated vascular injuries with exsanguination, stroke secondary to embolism or vascular occlusion, or neurologic injury secondary to spinal cord involvement. Similarly, because of close apposition of the aorta and spinal column, exsanguination and associated neurologic complications constitute the common causes of mortality and morbidity in penetrating injuries to the thoracic and abdominal esophagus.

One of the major problems associated with the management of penetrating neck trauma is the assessment of apparently small or innocuous wounds. A consideration of the kinetics of the wounding agent is important in assessing tissue destruction. Based on the definition of kinetic energy, $KE = \frac{1}{2}mv^2$, as the velocity of a missile doubles, the potential energy released increases by a factor of four. Therefore, the extent of injury can be affected by the type of weapon used (low-versus high-velocity missile) and by qualities of the projectile (mass, expansion, and fragmentation qualities). Moreover, the velocity of the projectile at impact and the subsequent rate of deceleration of the bullet determines the energy that is released to the target area. The blast effect is associated with the release of a large amount of energy, which causes significant cavitation and tissue damage, often in an apparently superficial wound. This occurs because of the missile's ability to produce both a temporary and permanent cavity, the latter being formed by the actual path of the bullet (Fig. 4-5). The cavitation effect is proposed to be due to elastic recoil of the tissue, which causes air to be trapped by negative pressure.[19] With an increase in the velocity of the missile, the size of the cavity and the formed pressure wave increase, potentially causing damage out of proportion to the bullet diameter. The higher the energy, the greater the cavitation and associated tissue damage.[19,20] Therefore, missile wounds can penetrate more deeply than stab wounds and produce an area of damage extending beyond the actual projectile tract, secondary to the cavitation effect. In these situations, concern over a potential blast injury must be considered during diagnostic evaluation.

Nonpenetrating trauma to the esophagus is frequently due to an increase in intraluminal pressure. Blunt abdominal trauma may increase intraabdominal pressure and, in the event of a closed glottis, can result in perforation of the distal thoracic or abdominal esophagus. A combination of penetrating and nonpen-

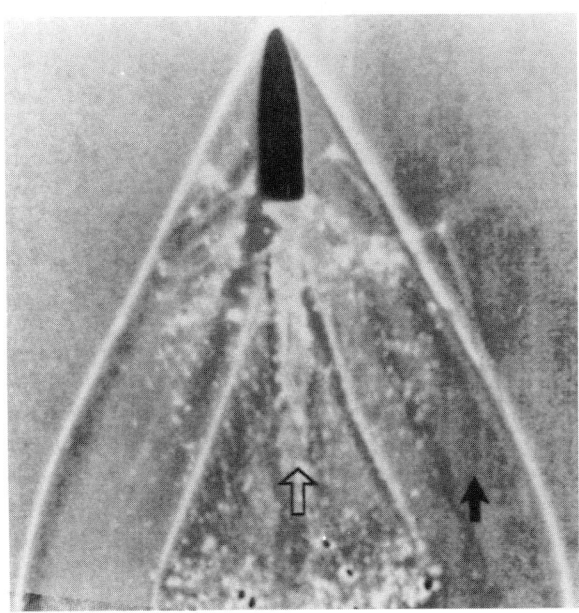

Figure 4-5 Cavitation effect of missiles. Open arrow denotes permanent cavity; closed arrow indicates temporary cavity. (Barach E, Tomlanovich M, Nowak R. Ballistics: a pathophysiologic examination of the wounding mechanisms of firearms. Part 1. J Trauma 1986;26:231)

etrating mechanisms can occur during a single injury. For example, a blunt cervical hyperextension injury can be sufficiently severe to cause esophageal perforation from adjacent bony fragments of the cervical esophagus. Close scrutiny of the injury on physical and radiographic examination usually elucidates these processes.

Even more uncommon is the compressed air injury to the thoracic esophagus. One case report describes esophageal rupture from an accidental discharge of gas from a compressed air tank into the oral cavity.[10] Pressure required for experimental rupture of esophagus is about 5 psi.[21,22] The lower end of esophagus is anatomically the weakest portion of this organ, and consequently, most spontaneous ruptures occur in the distal third. Pressure rupture of the upper part of esophagus has, however, been reported.[23] Similar barogenic mechanisms are present in postemetic injuries (Boerhaave's syndrome). Forceful vomiting, childbirth, weight lifting, or blunt abdominal trauma can cause longitudinal full-thickness perforation of all esophageal layers to occur on the left wall of the distal supradiaphragmatic esophagus, extending into the pleural cavity in more than 60% of cases.[24] The acute increase in pressure in the lower esophagus, rather than the amount of pressure generated, appears to be an important feature.

Corrosive injury of the esophagus is an increasingly significant problem since the introduction of liquid drain cleaners. Access to these products has increased, and the severity of caustic injury to the esophagus has also become greater. The extent of caustic burn is determined in part by the concentration and quantity of the agent, the state of the material (liquid or solid), amount of gastric content at time of caustic ingestion, and the anatomic integrity of stomach and esophagus. Solid lye adheres to the oropharyngeal and proximal esophageal mucosa. These agents cause liquefaction necrosis, involving the dissolution of protein, collagen, saponification of fats, dehydration of tissue, and thrombosis of blood vessels. Deep tissue injury results, which may affect adjacent organs. Solid lye inflicts burns in a patchy or linear rather than a diffuse circumferential distribution. Rarely is there gastric involvement with solid lye ingestion because it is unlikely for sufficient quantity of substance to reach the stomach. Liquid corrosives, conversely, are highly viscous, affect large areas of the esophagus and stomach, and inflict more extensive damage than solid agents. Because strong alkali, when ingested, combine with gastric acid to make a vigorous exothermic reaction, extensive esophagogastric necrosis can occur. Acids, in contrast, cause an immediate coagulation necrosis, with the coagulum hindering further tissue penetration. The greater destructive capacity of alkali over acids was noted in one series of ingestion patients in which esophageal injury was more common with alkali injuries (all of 15 patients) than with acid ingestion (3 of 5 patients).[25] Early detection and intervention is critical because these injuries are immediate and cause significant destruction on contact with the esophageal wall. There is a necrotic phase followed by a healing phase. If the injury is limited to the mucosa, healing occurs within 3 to 4 weeks. Submucosal involvement requires 3 to 4 months for healing.

Foreign bodies in the esophagus can cause problems both acutely and subacutely. In the United States, about 1500 people a year die as a result of foreign-body ingestion.[26] Most foreign bodies enter the gastrointestinal tract (80%); less than 20% enter the tracheobronchial tree. In the latter case, acute airway obstruction can occur. The subacute problems occurring with retained foreign objects are pressure necrosis of the esophageal wall and the formation of a mass lesion, as would occur with prolonged meat impaction. Foreign bodies lodge in three main locations: the cervical area, just below the cricopharyngeal sphincter; the level of the aortic arch; and the esophageal hiatus at the level of the gastric cardia (see Fig. 4-4). Most objects (80% to 90%) pass spontaneously, but the remainder require endoscopic retrieval.

DIAGNOSTIC MODALITIES

History

History is an important aspect of the evaluation of patients with suspected iatrogenic injuries, although symptoms are often nonspecific. Pain, however, is commonly present, and its manifestation depends on the location of the perforation. Thoracic perforation manifests as chest pain and subcutaneous emphysema, and dyspnea is often prominent even in the absence of pneumothorax. Abdominal perforation is evidenced by dull retrosternal ache and by epigastric pain radiating to the shoulders, characteristic of diaphragmatic irritation. The cause of the perforation, as well as the interval between perforation and diagnosis, may also be important. Therefore, information regarding procedures and timing should help raise suspicion of a possible perforation. For example, the presence of neck, chest, or abdominal pain after upper endoscopy necessitates further study to exclude the possibility that perforation has occurred. Most endoscopic injuries, however, are noted by the endoscopist. Somatic complaints of neck stiffness and aching or a history of regurgitation of bloody material can all help focus further evaluation toward the esophagus.

The key point in evaluating patients with traumatic perforation is to maintain a high index of suspicion. Penetrating wounds to the esophagus are notoriously difficult to diagnose because patients are often asymptomatic early in the course, and frequently associated injuries demand more attention or cause more symptoms. Unless esophageal injury is suspected in patients with penetrating wounds to the neck or chest, the diagnosis can be missed, leading to increased morbidity and mortality. A high index of suspicion is necessary to diagnose esophageal injury from gunshot wounds, and esophagography is recommended for all stable patients who present with a missile wound in immediate proximity to the esophagus or in any patient with transmediastinal penetration.[27]

In evaluating patients with nonpenetrating injury of the esophagus, a high index of suspicion and early diagnosis are also critical. Any patient with sudden onset of dyspnea and chest pain after any episode that could cause an unusual increase in intrathoracic or intraabdominal pressure should be evaluated. Patients with postemetic injuries usually give a distinct history of overeating and drinking, then vomiting, followed by severe chest pain and dyspnea. Those with corrosive injuries and retained foreign bodies typically give a history of intentional or unintentional ingestion of a caustic substance or foreign object.

Physical Examination

A thorough physical examination must focus beyond the surface injury. Investigation into the possibility of associated cervical, thoracic, or abdominal esophageal injury must be considered. Pneumothorax and hemothorax particularly should be excluded. The size of the wound is usually a poor indicator of the extent of underlying injury. Physical examination is reported to have a sensitivity of 80%, a specificity of 64%, and an accuracy of 72% in the diagnosis of esophageal injuries.[28] Clinical findings associated with upper aerodigestive injuries include decreased ventilatory exchange, stridor, change in pitch of voice, bubbling wound or subcutaneous emphysema, dysphagia, hemoptysis, epistaxis, hematemesis or blood in nasogastric tube, or cervical hematoma. Occasionally, tenderness in the area of the injury is the only clue to the presence of significant injury.

Cervical perforation may manifest as local tenderness, subcutaneous emphysema, and cervical rigidity. Posterior perforation results in suppuration, first in the retrovisceral space and then in the fascial planes leading into the mediastinum. Perforation of the anterior or lateral walls of the cervical esophagus may cause mediastinitis by fascial attachments between the pretracheal space and the pericardium. Inflammatory changes in the cervical region may not develop for many hours, with signs of systemic sepsis often not presenting for up to 24 hours.

Perforation of the thoracic esophagus may cause mediastinal emphysema presenting as Hamman's sign, a loud crunching sound synchronous with the heartbeat. As esophageal contents enter the mediastinum because of negative intrathoracic pressure, caustic digestive fluids, food, and bacteria contaminate the periesophageal spaces, leading to an inflammatory response and eventual suppuration. Subsequent pneumothorax, subcutaneous emphysema in the cervical region, and mediastinitis may ensue. Perforations of the proximal and mid-thoracic esophagus may communicate with the right pleural cavity, and perforation of the distal thoracic esophagus ordinarily involves the left pleural space. Lower intrathoracic or intraabdominal esophageal perforation may cause signs of intraabdominal peritonitis.

Systemic signs, such as tachycardia, tachypnea, and fever, may develop early, with progression to sepsis and shock occurring within hours (Fig. 4-6). In patients with Boerhaave's syndrome, however, many of these signs may not be present. In many cases of spontaneous perforation of the esophagus, the diagnosis is not initially evident.[29] Mackler's triad (vomiting, lower thoracic pain, and subcutaneous emphysema, to which

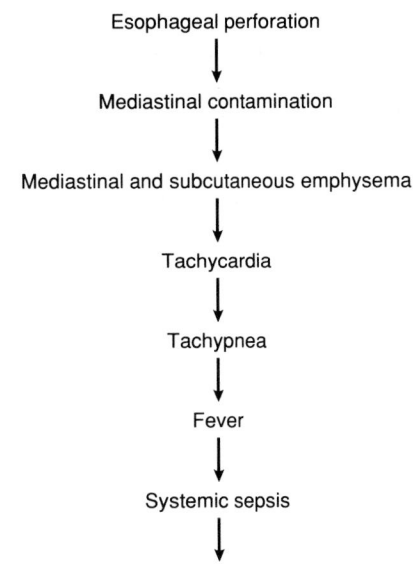

Figure 4-6 Sequence of symptoms and signs that follow esophageal perforation.

pneumomediastinum and an air–fluid level in pleural cavity can be added) is the classic presentation of the syndrome. Table 4-3 lists unusual clinical features of Boerhaave's syndrome, and Table 4-4 lists examples of initial misdiagnoses.

Radiographic Studies

After a thorough history and physical examination, the diagnostic and therapeutic plan should be based on the stability of the patient and the location of the injury. Because esophageal injury is rarely an isolated event, an associated vascular injury is more often the cause of acute hemodynamic instability. Frequently, the esophageal injury is appreciated only after exploration for a major vascular or airway injury.

The findings on plain radiographs vary depending on the location and cause of perforation as well as on the time interval between the injury and radiographic examination. Cervical injuries may show an increased distance between the trachea and vertebrae (prevertebral shadow) and paraesophageal air. Also, retained foreign bodies can be identified. In cases of nonpenetrating injuries of the cervical esophagus, lateral cervical spine roentgenograms may show retropharyngeal or subcutaneous emphysema. Thoracic esophageal perforation may show widening of the entire mediastinum, emphysema of the mediastinum or cervical area, hydrothorax, or pneumothorax (Fig. 4-7). Mediastinal air may be seen, especially along the paravertebral stripes, the aortic arch, or the base of the neck. Radiographs

Table 4-3 Boerhaave's Syndrome: Atypical Clinical History and Features

ATYPICAL CLINICAL HISTORY
Absence of vomiting
Absence of pain
Asthma
Carbachol injection
Childbirth
During sleep
Binge eating
Heimlich maneuver
Hyperemesis gravidarum
Infancy
Laughter
Lifting
Prolonged coughing and hiccups
Straining at stool
Asymptomatic

ATYPICAL CLINICAL FEATURES
Cold water polydipsia
Change in voice
Extreme swelling of face and neck
Pericarditis
Pneumopericardium
Pneumoperitoneum
Proptosis
Rupture of herniated gastric cardia
Low pleural fluid amylase

(Henderson JAM, Peloquin AJM. Boerhaave revisited: spontaneous esophageal perforation as a diagnostic masquerader. Am J Med 1989;86:559)

Table 4-4 Initial Misdiagnoses of Boerhaave's Syndrome

Aspiration pneumonia
Appendicitis
Dissecting aneurysm
Esophagitis
Lung abscess
Mesenteric thrombosis
Myocardial infarction
Pancreatitis
Perforated peptic ulcer or other abdominal viscus
Pericarditis
Pneumomediastinum
Pneumoperitoneum
Pneumothorax
Pulmonary embolism
Ureteral stone or colic
Acute pyelonephritis
Ruptured subphrenic abscess
Incarcerated diphragmatic hernia
Esophageal or gastric ulcer
Splenic bleeding

(Henderson JAM, Peloquin AJM. Boerhaave revisited: spontaneous esophageal perforation as a diagnostic masquerader. Am J Med 1989;86:559)

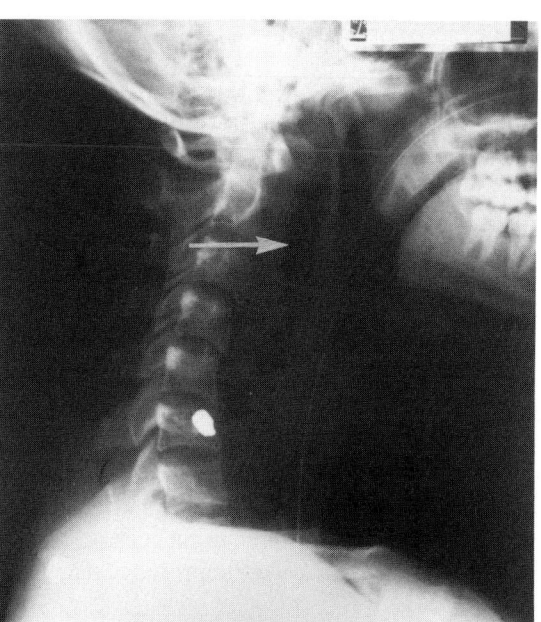

Figure 4-7 Radiograph of the neck demonstrating retropharyngeal air (*arrow*) in a patient with a gunshot wound of the cervical esophagus.

should be obtained in all patients with penetrating neck injuries if no other studies are indicated. In Boerhaave's syndrome, a chest radiograph may show mediastinal and subcutaneous emphysema, a paraspinal mass, or evidence of pneumothorax or hydrothorax (more commonly in the left pleural space). Overall, a diverse array of radiographic signs are all suggestive of perforated esophagus and require further diagnostic study with contrast esophagogram (Fig. 4-8).

Barium esophagography is the gold standard for the diagnosis of esophageal perforation, although false-negative findings occur in up to 10% of cases.[29] In evaluating the cervical esophagus, a report found that barium swallow, using biplane cineradiography, had a sensitivity of 89%, a specificity of 100%, and an accuracy of 94%.[28] Most radiologists recommend an initial bolus of water-soluble contrast medium, then a repeat study with a small amount of barium if no leak is appreciated. This latter step is important because there is a 30% to 50% false-negative rate with meglumine diatrizoate (Gastrografin) alone.[30] Water-soluble contrast medium is rapidly absorbed and is less irritating than barium should substantial extravasation occur. When requesting a contrast study, a biplane cineesophagogram is necessary to ensure optimal visualization of the esophagus.

Computed tomography (CT) has been used to detect changes after penetrating esophageal injury.[31] Findings suggestive of esophageal injury include air in the soft tissues of the mediastinum surrounding the esophagus,

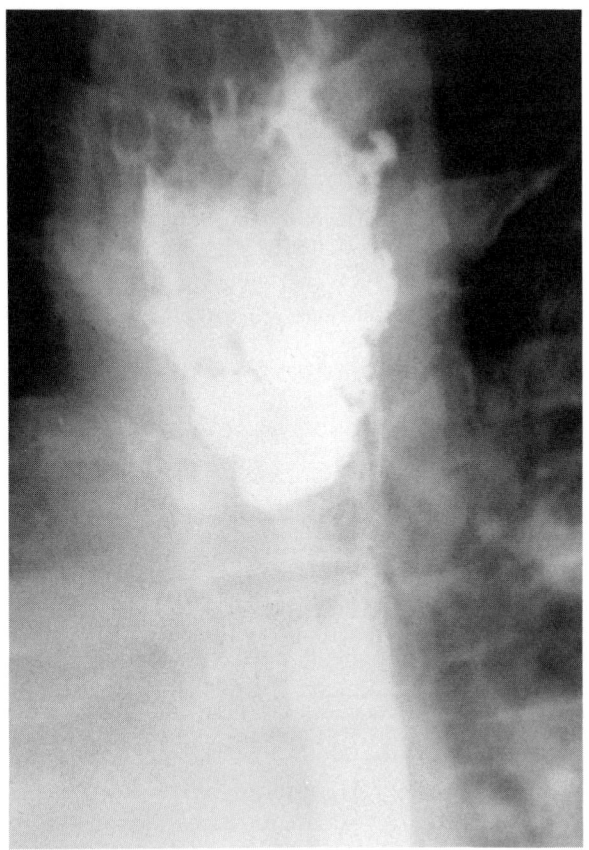

Figure 4-8 Contrast esophagogram showing region of cervical esophageal perforation.

abscess cavities adjacent to esophagus in either the pleural space or mediastinum, and the demonstration of an actual communication between the air-filled esophagus and an adjacent mediastinal or paramediastinal air–fluid collection. In the follow-up setting, CT has been used to evaluate the response to therapy as well as to guide percutaneous drainage of loculated pleural fluid collections in the postoperative period or during nonoperative therapy.

Endoscopy

Endoscopy is indicated in the evaluation of patients with suspected esophageal injury, particularly those with a negative or equivocal contrast study, transmediastinal wounds, or equivocal operative findings. Rigid esophagoscopy can be more reliable than flexible endoscopy. In a prospective study of 118 hemodynamically stable patients with penetrating zone II and III neck trauma,[28] using a combination of barium swallow plus flexible and rigid esophagoscopy, five of eight esophageal injuries were missed with flexible endoscopy. In contrast, rigid endoscopy detected eight of nine

esophageal injuries, with a sensitivity of 89%, a specificity of 95%, and an accuracy of 94%. The combination of cineradiography and rigid esophagoscopy missed no esophageal injuries. Overall, there were no false-positive results, but there was one false-negative on barium swallow and one false-negative on rigid endoscopy (not in the same patient). If esophagography is equivocal, rigid esophagoscopy should be performed to rule out esophageal injury. Although the combination of barium swallow and rigid esophagoscopy missed no injuries, these studies are time-consuming and costly. In addition, rigid endoscopy usually requires general anesthesia. In contrast to this study, other reports found flexible esophagoscopy to be highly accurate in localizing as well as directly visualizing perforations.[32] Results of esophagoscopy can help direct mode of therapy, especially in cases considered for conservative management. The use of endoscopy for trauma must be performed cautiously by experienced operators because once blood or clot is encountered, further attempts to visualize the injury may complete a partial-thickness injury or extend a full-thickness injury.

One area in which the role of endoscopy is fully accepted is in the evaluation of corrosive injuries. Many studies support the advantage of early, aggressive diagnosis and management in the care of these patients.[33–35] In one report,[34] endoscopy was performed within 12 hours of admission. Care was taken to avoid passage of the rigid endoscope past the region of severe circumferential injury. The findings at endoscopy immediately and directly affected further management. In this report and others, the endoscopic appearance of the injured esophagus was used to classify the extent of burn (Table 4-5). A modified classification system of esophageal burns was developed from experience with 381 endoscopic examinations of 81 patients with corrosive ingestion[36] (Table 4-6). The use of a specific grading system not only facilitates accurate communication of information regarding the injury but also has prognostic and therapeutic significance.

Both rigid and flexible endoscopes have a role in evaluating and treating patients with retained foreign bodies. Not only is retrieval of the object critical, but evaluation of the esophageal mucosa after removal is important to detect wall injury from pressure necrosis.

Thoracentesis

Thoracentesis is usually performed in situations in which the diagnosis of esophageal perforation has not yet been entertained. Pleural effusion may be acidic from regurgitated gastric juice, unless large amounts of blood dilute it. Pleural fluid with food particles, a pH value below 6.0, or an elevated amylase level is virtu-

Table 4-5 Endoscopic Grading and Pathologic Findings After Corrosive Injury to the Esophagus and Stomach

Grade	Endoscopic Findings	Pathologic Findings
0	Normal examination	No injury
I	Mucosal hyperemia and edema Occasional superficial mucosal desquamation and exudate	Superficial mucosal involvement Minimal or no loss of mucosa
II	Mucosal sloughing Hemorrhage, exudate, ulceration, pseudomembrane formation, and granulation tissue Deep discrete or circumferential ulceration	Transmucosal involvement with or without muscularis affected No extension into periesophageal or perigastric tissue
III	Sloughing of tissue with deep ulcerations Complete obliteration of esophageal lumen by massive edema; charring and eschar formation; full-thickness necrosis with perforation	Full-thickness injury with extension into periesophageal or perigastric tissue Mediastinal or intraperitoneal organs may be involved Penetration or perforation
IV		As in grade III with disseminated intravascular coagulation and metabolic acidosis

(Estrera A, Taylor W, Mills LJ, Platt MR. Corrosive burns of the esophagus and stomach: a recommendation for an aggressive surgical approach. Ann Thorac Surg 1986;41:276)

ally diagnostic of esophageal perforation. Lower esophageal lesions have a greater propensity to develop pleural effusions, more commonly on the left.

Diagnostic Algorithm

Complete assessment of esophageal trauma is based on the interpretation of the diagnostic studies described earlier. This information directs the therapeutic path

Table 4-6 Modified Endoscopic Grading System for Corrosive Injuries of the Esophagus and Stomach

Grade	Endoscopic findings
0	Normal examination
1	Edema and hyperemia of the mucosa
2a	Friability, hemorrhages, erosions, blisters, whitish membranes, exudates, and superficial ulcerations
2b	Same as grade 2a, plus deep discrete or circumferential ulceration
3a	Multiple ulcerations and small, scattered areas of necrosis
3b	Extensive areas of necrosis

(Adapted from Zargar SA, Kochar R, Mehta S, Mehta SK. The role of fiberoptic endoscopy in the management of corrosive ingestion and modified endoscopic classification of burns. Gastrointest Endosc 1991;37:165)

necessary for successful management of patients with cervical, thoracic, and abdominal esophageal injuries. Some authors argue that for zone II cervical injuries, routine exploration without numerous diagnostic tests is a more time- and cost-efficient method of managing patients. However, trends favor nonoperative management of penetrating trauma, mandating a full diagnostic evaluation.

Controversy regarding aggressive surgical exploration versus selective nonoperative management are based on early studies comparing the morbidity and mortality from these approaches in patients with cervical vascular injuries. Studies in the 1950s initially confirmed the efficacy of early operative therapy, showing a mortality rate of 6% in patients operated on early versus 35% in patients in whom surgery was either deferred or omitted.[37] The most common causes of death were hemorrhage, sepsis, and pulmonary dysfunction. Subsequent studies have confirmed these findings, with the emphasis focused on early detection of carotid artery injuries.[38,39] Proponents of aggressive exploration of all cervical injuries with platysmal penetration cite the low morbidity and mortality from early exploration when compared with later exploration.[38] One study reviewed 246 patients with penetrating neck injuries.[39] A policy of mandatory exploration resulted in negative findings in 156 (63%) patients, with a morbidity rate of less than 1%, no deaths, and a mean duration of hospitalization of 3 days. In the 90 patients with positive results on neck explorations, the morbidity rate was 8%, the mortality rate was 9%, and mean hospitalization was 8.5 days. A normal physical examination did not always predict the operative findings, and 13 (14.4%) of the 90 patients with a clinically negative physical examination had positive findings on exploration. These injuries included two hypopharyngeal injuries and one esophageal injury and a variety of major vascular injuries. In contrast, others successfully treated patients selectively based on the absence of physical signs of injury and recommended specific approaches based on the anatomic zone of injury[40] (Fig. 4-9). For injuries in zone I, chest radiograph and fluoroesophagography were recommended. For zone II injuries, clinically asymptomatic patients were treated expectantly, whereas those with clinical suspicion of injury underwent exploration. Zone III injuries to the aerodigestive tract were so infrequent that full endoscopy was thought to be of little benefit. Rather, fiberoptic laryngopharyngoscopy can be performed to evaluate such injuries.

With numerous reports touting the efficacy of selective, nonoperative management of asymptomatic patients with penetrating cervical trauma,[40–44] more demand is placed on diagnostic studies, including the more widespread use of endoscopy and esophagography. One group of surgeons selectively treated 110 patients with gunshot wounds of the neck.[45] Twelve patients were operated on immediately because of physical findings. Thirty-five patients were observed without further diagnostic work-up. The remaining intermediate group of 63 patients was evaluated with arteriography, esophagoscopy, or esophagography. Forty-eight patients underwent esophagography, 15 of whom had positive examinations; esophagoscopy

was positive in all 15 patients. This overall approach resulted in a low mortality rate of 2.7% in the entire group of patients. Thus, some surgeons advocate a selective approach, recommending investigation in patients exhibiting dysphagia, hemoptysis, hematemesis, or subcutaneous emphysema.[46] The evaluation includes a complete cervical spine series, meglumine diatrizoate swallow, followed by barium if negative. If necessary, esophagoscopy can be performed. Moreover, because of the difference in kinetic energy released between gunshot and stab wounds, mandatory exploration is recommended in patients suffering high-velocity gunshot wounds, buckshot or birdshot wounds from an effective range of less than 5 m, and shrapnel wounds. A selective approach can be taken for evaluation of patients with low-velocity bullets or with buckshot or birdshot wounds from more than 5 m.

Another study reviewed 193 patients with penetrating neck trauma.[47] Fifty-seven patients were selectively observed, 76 patients had mandatory exploration, and the remaining 60 patients underwent exploration because symptoms or signs prompted various diagnostic studies that in turn suggested the need for surgery. As shown by a 50% rate of negative exploration in the latter two groups, physical signs and symptoms proved to be unreliable indicators of injury. Conversely, arteriography (100%), bronchoscopy and laryngoscopy (100%), esophagography (90%), and esophagoscopy (86%) appeared to be accurate predictors of injury when compared with routine surgery. For nine esophageal and seven hypopharyngeal injuries, esophagography had a sensitivity of 80% and a specificity of 94%. Esophagoscopy had a sensitivity of 67% and a specificity of 89%. The length of hospitalization was shortest in patients undergoing selective management (2.8 days), whereas that of the negative and positive ex-

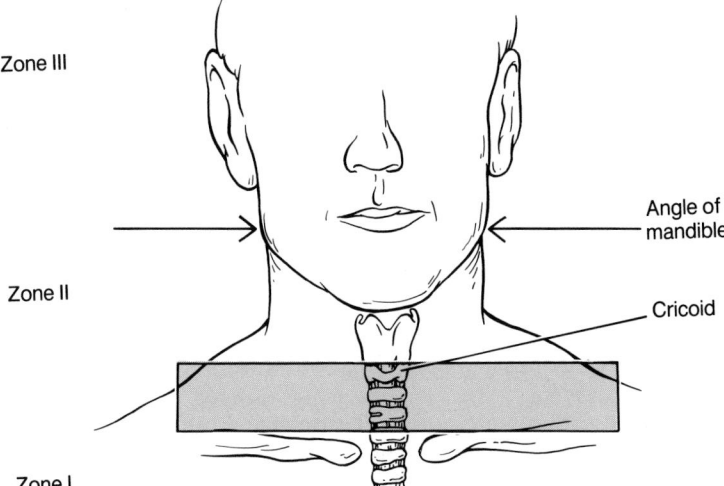

Zone III

Zone II

Zone I

Angle of mandible

Cricoid

Figure 4-9 Clinical zones of the neck. The colored area refers to zone II in some classifications. (After Jurkovich GJ. The neck. In: Moore EE, ed. Early care of the injured patient, ed 4. Philadelphia, BC Decker, 1990:127)

ploration groups was 4.2 days and 9.5 days, respectively. The cost of a negative nonoperative evaluation was not significantly different from the cost of a negative exploration. In the absence of specific signs of injury, such as hematemesis or air exiting the wound, it was concluded that arteriography and panendoscopy were as safe and appropriate as mandatory exploration.

The final algorithm to be discussed involves the diagnosis and management of transmediastinal gunshot wounds, an injury that exposes the esophagus to risk at various locations. One group described a management plan for 76 such patients.[48] Thirty-three of the patients were hemodynamically unstable and therefore underwent immediate thoracotomy or median sternotomy. An average of 2.7 major structures were injured per patient, and 8 of 33 patients had esophageal injuries. The remaining 43 patients, who were stable on admission, underwent an evaluation consisting of aortography, esophagography, esophagoscopy, and bronchoscopy, the latter two procedures performed under general anesthesia. Nine of these patients were found to have esophageal injuries. There were two false-negative esophagoscopic procedures and one false-negative esophagogram, but the combination of the two studies successfully diagnosed all esophageal injuries.

In summarizing the proper management of patients with penetrating cervical trauma, one must consider the zone of injury involved. Management of zone I and II injuries often is dictated by radiographic or endoscopic findings. If the aerodigestive tract can be cleared, a nonoperative approach may be selected. Zone III injuries rarely involve the esophagus but rather affect the pharynx or hypopharynx. Care of these injuries depends primarily on the findings at fiberoptic laryngopharyngoscopy. Zone II injuries, because of the surgical accessibility, are often treated by direct exploration, but this approach is dictated by the individual surgeon.

The diagnosis of thoracic and intraabdominal esophageal rupture is also difficult, requiring the astute clinician to recognize the organs at risk for injury in those regions and assess the patient appropriately. It is usually necessary to exclude esophageal injury specifically when suspected. Definitive diagnosis of esophageal injury is made by esophagography, esophagoscopy, or both. At the time of surgery, if no injury can be identified, instillation of methylene blue or air through a nasogastric tube can be helpful in locating an occult injury.

PERIOPERATIVE CARE

Resuscitation

Care of the patient with potential esophageal injury, as in all cases of trauma management, demands primary attention to airway control. Laryngeal or esophageal injuries may cause progressive cervical swelling that can jeopardize airway patency. Therefore, when these injuries are suspected, precautions for controlling the airway should be taken. After the airway is secured, evaluation of breathing is performed. In patients with penetrating chest or lower cervical trauma, inadequate ventilation may be caused by a tension pneumothorax or hemopneumothorax. Immediate attention to these conditions is critical. Cervical injuries mandate spinal cord precautions to prevent further injuries or deterioration of a known cervical spine injury.

Another important aspect of resuscitation focuses on evaluation of the hemodynamic status of the patient. Although isolated esophageal injuries do not independently cause early instability, the frequently associated vascular or airway injury can lead to hemodynamic compromise. Major vascular injuries, when located in the neck, can be controlled by local pressure. Thoracic vascular injuries may require sternotomy or thoracotomy for rapid control. Airway problems causing significant hemodynamic compromise may require needle or tube thoracostomy as the initial step in the management algorithm. It is in the later period of evaluation that an esophageal injury can cause cardiovascular collapse from a volume-losing or septic process.

Anesthetic Considerations

Patients sustaining potential esophageal trauma must be treated with anesthetic techniques applied to all severely injured patients. Additionally, those with suspected cervical injuries require the anesthetic management specific to this patient population. First, immobilization of the cervical spine is required unless its integrity has been ensured. For intubation, an oral intubation route using manual in-line axial support is preferred. Second, the technique of induction is important; a modified rapid sequence induction is generally used.[49] This entails mask ventilation followed by cricoid pressure while the intubation is performed. If difficulties are encountered during this procedure, the operating team must be prepared for surgical control of the airway, although this is rarely indicated. Other important points during anesthetic induction include the prevention of aspiration and the evaluation and management of comorbid medical conditions, such as coronary artery disease, metabolic problems, and conditions that can modify pharmacologic agents often used for intubation. Finally, the anesthesiologist must adjust for abnormal pulmonary physiology often present after chest trauma.

Rapid control intubation is only one of the techniques used to gain access to the airway in the trauma patient, with awake intubation and fiberoptic intubation the alternatives. Moreover, in patients with suspected thoracic esophageal injury, the use of a double-lumen endotracheal tube is often helpful. With rapid control intubation, the patient is preoxygenated with 100% oxygen while awake. It is important that during the preoxygenation period and before intubation, no positive pressure ventilation is given through the mask. This lessens the risk of inflation of the stomach and subsequent regurgitation. After pretreatment with d-tubocurarine, succinylcholine is administered, followed by immediate intubation.

Awake intubation is used frequently in patients with airway and cervical injuries. The primary advantage of this technique is that the patient voluntarily controls his or her own airway and thereby has the benefit of maintaining intact protective reflexes. Before intubation, the patient is anesthetized topically using lidocaine, followed by intravenous sedation. Awake intubation can be accomplished using either the oral or the nasal route. However, for cervical trauma, direct visualization using an oral route is preferable. Most of the maneuvers before intubation are concerned with maintenance of a low level of stimulation until control of the injury is obtained. Therefore, the cooperation of a particular patient can influence the decision to use this technique, especially in the trauma population. Fiberoptic intubation is reserved for difficult or failed intubation attempts and for positioning a double-lumen endotracheal tube.

Antibiotic Management

The choice of antibiotic coverage for patients with esophageal injuries is dictated by the indication for its use. For prophylactic use, the indication for most acute trauma, first- or second-generation cephalosporin coverage is adequate. If it is known preoperatively that there is isolated esophageal trauma, penicillin is a good choice, especially for cervical injuries. However, with the possibility of associated airway or pulmonary injury, better gram-negative coverage is indicated, and a second-generation cephalosporin is preferred. For medical management of localized esophageal perforations, broad-spectrum coverage, such as penicillin, clindamycin, and an aminoglycoside, is adequate.[50] The important issue is to cover the commonly seen pathogens and to tailor antimicrobial agents subsequently to culture and sensitivity data.

Intraoperative Monitoring

Once the diagnosis of esophageal injury is made or suspected, immediate intervention is begun. Efforts are taken to limit further contamination of the mediastinum, to maintain fluid and electrolyte balance, and to adequately control infection. Intraoperative hemodynamic monitoring should be routinely used in most trauma situations. If the operation is performed early in the posttrauma period when intravascular volume shifts are minimal, in the absence of preexisting conditions, no specific intraoperative monitoring is indicated. In patients diagnosed later in the course of the perforation, signs of early or established sepsis may be present. These patients require invasive monitoring intraoperatively, with intraarterial and central venous pressure monitoring. A subgroup of these patients with fulminant sepsis or with associated adult respiratory distress syndrome can benefit from pulmonary artery catheter placement for hemodynamic and oxygenation monitoring.

Postoperatively, supportive care with antibiotic and intravenous fluid therapy is required. Once extubated, aggressive respiratory therapy is required to prevent atelectasis and subsequent pneumonia, as can occur after thoracotomy. Intermittent positive pressure breathing treatments should be avoided, however, because of the potential pressure placed on the esophageal suture line. Finally, attention should be directed to maintaining chest tube patency to ensure complete drainage of potentially injurious material.

MANAGEMENT

Treatment of esophageal perforation is based on many factors, including the cause of the perforation, the location, the presence or absence of underlying esophageal disease, and the interval between perforation and diagnosis. Moreover, the age and physiologic status of the patient, the condition of esophagus, the extent of soilage, and injury to adjacent organs and tissues at the time of surgery are critical factors. The goals of treatment, independent of the means to achieve this end, are to prevent further soilage from the perforation, eliminate the infection produced by soilage, restore integrity and continuity of gastrointestinal tract, and maintain adequate nutrition. Treatment options are either medical (nonoperative) or surgical.

Nonoperative management of esophageal perforations is limited to a few distinct indications. These include instrumental perforation, small perforations after bougienage of peptic strictures or achalasia, or perforation after sclerosis of esophageal varices. Successful medical treatment depends on limited local contamination, as might be expected in patients with peptic or motility disorders, which typically lead to periesophageal fibrosis limiting contamination of the mediastinum. Similarly, patients with cervical esophageal per foration, because of a limited area of contamination, are candidates for attempted nonoperative therapy. Patients with esophageal perforation diagnosed several days after injury who exhibit minimal symptoms can be treated medically. Early recognition, however, is usually critical for successful medical management.

When deemed suitable for a trial of medical therapy, the patient is kept NPO, intravenous antibiotics are begun and maintained for 7 to 14 days, total parenteral nutrition is started, and a nasogastric tube is placed. If an area of fluid collection is present, this is drained by either tube thoracostomy or CT-directed catheter placement. One group of surgeons reported their experience with nonoperative management of esophageal perforations.[50] Their criteria for nonoperative therapy included an early or well-encapsulated perforation, or, if seen late, an esophageal perforation that was well contained within the mediastinum or between the mediastinum and visceral lung pleura with no free pleural extravasation. If a cavity was present, it must have been well drained back into the esophagus with minimal pleural soilage. The patient must not have eaten between the time of injury and diagnosis. Moreover, the perforation must not have been present in the area of a tumor, in the abdomen, or in an area proximal to an obstructive process. Finally, these patients must have demonstrated minimal symptoms or signs of physiologic abnormalities or sepsis.

If medically treated patients fail to show signs of improvement within 24 hours or develop progression of symptoms, surgical exploration is mandatory. Delay in embarking on surgical therapy can allow progression of mediastinitis and subsequent death. Overall, conservative management for minimal esophageal perforation has a limited and distinct role that requires close surveillance to prevent delays of surgical exploration and drainage if indicated.

Another area in which medical management has as an important role is in caustic injury of the esophagus. In a controlled, randomized study evaluating the efficacy of corticosteroid use in patients with corrosive injury,[51] 131 children with significant caustic burns of the esophagus were prospectively evaluated. Acting on the hypothesis that steroids inhibit the inflammatory response and thus would prevent the development of stricture, patients underwent endoscopy within 24 hours of injury, with the scope passed only to the area of the first serious burn. Subjects were then randomly assigned to receive either steroids or placebo. A dose of 2.5 mg/kg/d of prednisone was given for a total of 3 weeks and subsequently tapered over 2 to 3 weeks. Intravenous ampicillin was also given. Strictures were classified as mild, moderate, or severe. Treatment involved antegrade dilation for mild and moderate in-

volvement and retrograde dilation for the severe cases. Of the 131 patients, all had oral or pharyngeal burns, and 60 patients had esophageal burns on endoscopy. Strictures developed in 10 of the 31 steroid-treated patients and in 11 of the 29 control patients, a nonsignificant difference. Furthermore, the need for esophageal resection and replacement, which correlated with the degree of injury, was not significantly different between the two groups.

Retained foreign bodies, such as coins, are usually removed in infants and children using general endotracheal anesthesia and rigid endoscopy. Objects smaller than 20 mm can be pushed into the stomach and usually pass without incident. Alternative techniques include Foley catheter placement for retrieval of an object. This method allows no control for prevention of aspiration of the object as it is removed, however, and so is not recommended. Only 1% of foreign bodies require surgical removal; children are involved in 80% of these cases.

Button batteries are probably the most dangerous foreign bodies commonly ingested. Children younger than 5 years of age are most commonly involved. Most battery systems contain an alkali, a substance strong enough to cause rapid liquefaction necrosis of the esophageal wall. Injury induced by battery ingestion includes direct corrosive action, low-voltage burns, and pressure necrosis. Therefore, a button battery lodged in the esophagus should be considered an acute emergency.

Radiographically, a coin and a battery can be distinguished by the presence of a double density shadow with the latter. From a technical standpoint, grasping a battery can be difficult. The use of a through-the-scope balloon under direct visualization can be helpful. Occasionally, the battery reacts with the esophageal wall, making removal difficult and necessitating endoscopic dissection. The battery can be pushed into the stomach, then removed with a Dormia basket or polypectomy snare. If retrieval is not possible in the stomach, batteries often pass distally and are evacuated without complications. Close follow-up of the esophagus after battery removal is mandatory, with a barium swallow obtained 24 to 36 hours and 10 to 14 days after endoscopic removal to exclude stricture or late fistula formation.

Sharp and pointed foreign bodies, such as toothpicks, nails, needles, bones, safety pins, and dental prostheses, are also commonly ingested. Objects longer than 5 cm and wider than 2 cm rarely pass into the stomach and require endoscopic removal. Open safety pins must be pushed into the stomach using the flexible endoscope, turned around, grasped at the hinged end and pulled out in that direction. Another option to manage sharp objects, such as a safety pin or a dental plate with sharp clips or points, is to grasp the spring with a rotating forceps and to carry the pin with its point trailing into the stomach. With fluoroscopic guidance, inversion of the pin is accomplished, and the pin is withdrawn with the point trailing. Alternative procedures, such as sheathing the sharp point with the esophagoscope and closure of the pin, are more difficult to accomplish. Although fewer than 1% of ingested foreign bodies perforate the gastrointestinal tract, all sharp and pointed objects should be removed before they pass from the stomach because of a 15% to 35% incidence of intestinal perforation, usually in the area of the ileocecal valve.[52] When the foreign body has already passed into the small bowel, daily radiographs are necessary to follow progression for 3 consecutive days. Failure to progress through the small bowel during this time indicates the need for surgical intervention.

Impacted meat is a commonly retained substance that does not typically require surgical intervention. If the patient is able to swallow the oral secretions and the diagnosis is confirmed on barium swallow, emergency endoscopy is not needed. However, if clearing of secretions is a problem, an urgent endoscopy should be performed to prevent aspiration and airway obstruction. Because meat impaction is usually seen in adults, general anesthesia is usually not necessary. Flexible endoscopic removal is accomplished with an endoscopic loop device. After the removal of the foreign body, it is important to assess the esophageal wall for evidence of pressure necrosis and for underlying esophageal pathology. Alternative therapy for meat impaction has included the use of papain or glucagon. However, these agents have a success rate of about 50% and are recommended only when flexible endoscopy is not available or is contraindicated. Morbidity of foreign-body removal with either a flexible or rigid endoscope should be less than 1%. There is, however, a small but real risk of perforation (0.34%) and mortality (0.05%) with these procedures.

Surgical Technique and Exposure

The goal of operative management of esophageal injury is to provide adequate drainage at the site of perforation and to obtain secure closure of the affected esophagus. Often, this also involves débridement of infected and necrotic tissue. Moreover, depending on the extent of injury, correction or elimination of distal obstruction may be indicated. The surgeon should plan for the postoperative period, often choosing to place a jejunostomy tube in anticipation of a prolonged recovery phase.

The techniques by which the perforated esophagus

can be repaired are listed in Table 4-7. Primary closure of the injured esophagus is the most frequently used and preferred method. Débridement of nonviable tissue and closure of mucosa and muscle in separate layers are basic principles employed. It is important to expose the mucosal perforation fully and to perform an exact repair, even if myotomy is required to achieve this end. A two-layer closure of the perforation is recommended, with a continuous 4-0 absorbable suture for the mucosal layer and interrupted 4-0 silk sutures for the more superficial muscular layer. Because of the unique anatomy of the esophagus with the lack of serosal covering, only the mucosa and submucosa can reliably hold sutures. Therefore, most surgeons recommend reinforcement of the suture line with parietal pleura, a local muscle flap such as strap muscles, or a tissue pedicle flap (see Section V in Atlas Chap. 5). This is particularly true in cases in which the interval between injury and treatment exceeds more than a few hours. Regardless of the method employed, secure closure requires suturing the reinforcing tissue closely, as for an anastomosis, rather than simply tacking it.

A variety of incisions are available to provide exposure for esophageal trauma (Fig. 4-10), with selection guided by zone of potential or known injury. Cervical esophageal injuries are best treated by early exploration, primary closure, nasogastric suction, and extensive wound drainage in proximity to the site of repair. For these injuries, an incision along the anterior border of the sternocleidomastoid muscle gives excellent exposure for zone II and III injuries (Fig. 4-11). Al-

---

Table 4-7   Techniques for Repair of a Perforated Esophagus

Primary closure and wide drainage
Reinforced primary closure and wide drainage
    Pleural flap[56]
    Primary muscle flap closure[6]
Thal patch[57]
Serosal buttress[58]
Diaphragmatic pedicle flap[59]
Primary repair, nasogastric suction, drainage, gastrostomy tube, jejunostomy tube
Resection[63]
Drainage alone
T-tube drainage[60]
Tube esophagostomy[53]
Intraluminal stent
Exclusion and diversion
    Nasogastric suction, gastrostomy tube above and below gastric staple line[54]
    Cervical loop esophagostomy, gastrostomy tube[55]
    Cervical esophagostomy in continuity, drainage, esophageal band, gastrostomy[61]

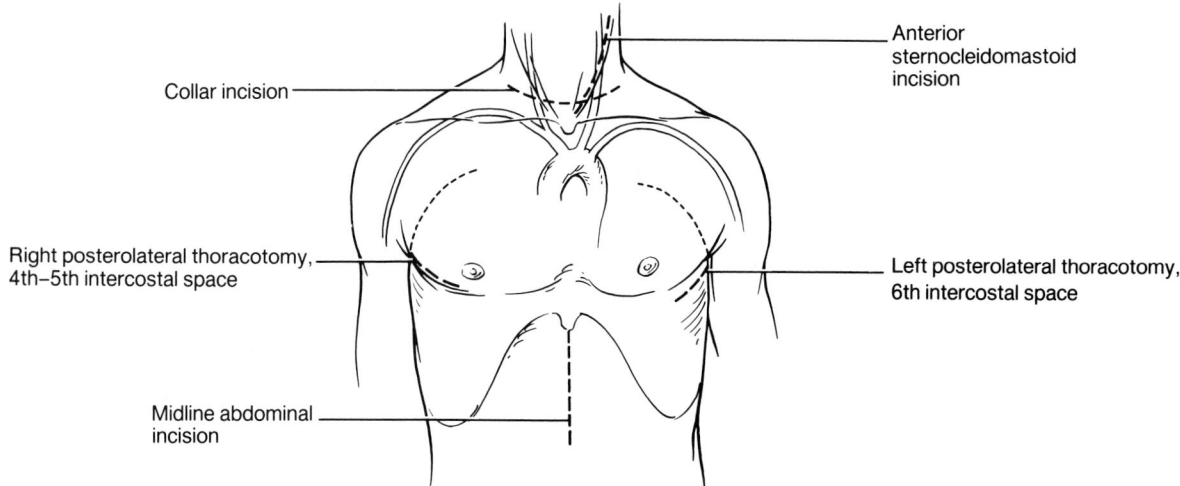

Figure 4-10 Incisions used for operative exposure of injuries to the esophagus. The collar incision is used for zone I esophageal injuries; the right thoracotomy for proximal and middle thoracic injuries; the midline abdominal incision for intraabdominal esophageal injuries; the anterior sternocleidomastoid incision for zone II and III esophageal injuries; and the left posterolateral thoracotomy for distal thoracic esophageal injuries.

ternatively, a collar incision can also provide this exposure as well as visualization for bilateral injuries or those affecting zone I. After excluding injuries to the vascular and respiratory structures, exploration of the cervical esophagus is easily performed. The omohyoid is divided or retracted, the deep cervical fascia is incised, the connection of the anterior cervical vein into the internal jugular is divided, and the plane between the esophagus and prevertebral fascia is bluntly dissected. Primary repair is recommended; however, because of the excellent blood supply to the esophagus in this region, simple drainage is the critical aspect of the treatment plan. After repair, drains are placed in the retroesophageal space and brought out through the neck.

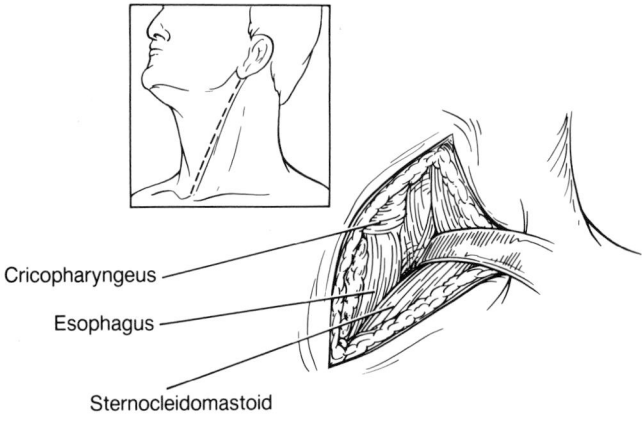

Figure 4-11 Surgical exposure of the cervical esophagus.

Perforations in the proximal or middle thoracic esophagus can be approached through a right posterolateral thoracotomy in the fourth or fifth intercostal space (see Section I in Atlas Chap. 5). Injuries in the distal thoracic esophagus are best approached through a left posterolateral thoracotomy in the sixth intercostal space. Intraabdominal esophageal injuries are usually diagnosed and approached through an upper midline laparotomy incision. Once the esophagus is exposed, air or methylene blue instillation may be required to demonstrate the perforation. After identifying the injury, mobilization of a limited region of the esophagus is important to provide complete visualization of the anterior and posterior surfaces of the esophagus and to ensure against missing an exit wound (see Section V in Atlas Chap. 5). Full mobilization of the esophagus is contraindicated because of the segmental nature of the blood supply.

One of the most successful series describing management of thoracic esophageal perforations used the pleural wrap procedure.[3] Eighteen patients were treated between 4 hours and 14 days after perforation. The patient population included perforations from trauma (2), iatrogenic causes (7), and barotrauma (9). In 11 (61%), the diagnosis was not made for more than 24 hours, a situation traditionally associated with a 25% to 40% mortality rate. In 14 patients, the perforation was sutured, then buttressed with a circumferential wrap of parietal pleura[56] (see Section V in Atlas Chap. 5). All 14 patients recovered and were discharged from the hospital after a median stay of 20 days. Other forms of treatment, including resection and diversion procedures, had poor results: 3 of 4 patients died from sepsis after long periods of hospitalization. The overall mortality rate in the series was 17%. Significantly, the pleural wrap was equally effective with both early and delayed perforations. Based on their data, the authors advocate routine use of a pleural wrap. For extensive perforations that cannot be closed primarily, they recommend resection and drainage, followed by staged esophageal reconstruction. Their review of the literature supported their thesis (Table 4-8).

The conclusions of the authors support our practice of reinforcing all suture repairs with autogenous tissue. Moreover, the successful results with a buttress of autogenous pleural tissue challenge the role of primary repair alone. The authors also conclude that there is no role for simple drainage as definitive treatment, stating that either closure of the perforation should be done with sutures and buttressed with autogenous tissue or an alternative procedure should be employed. I do not agree fully with the latter statement because some cervical esophageal perforations will heal with adequate drainage alone due to the excellent blood supply in this region. The other point emphasized in this report is that there is no fixed period beyond which primary débridement and repair is contraindicated. In this series, the longest repair was performed at 8 days. In conclusion, débridement, primary closure, reinforcement with autologous tissue, and wide drainage are the key steps in the management of esophageal perforation.

Alternative Methods

In patients suffering more extensive esophageal injuries or in those presenting with a significant delay, primary closure of the perforation can be technically impossible. Aggressive débridement, esophageal diversion or exclusion, and even resection have been described. Moreover, if the perforation occurs in an abnormal esophagus, morbidity and mortality can rise even further. A variety of procedures can be attempted, depending on the extent of involvement, the condition of the patient, and the preference of the surgeon.

Primary repair of an esophageal perforation with buttressing is the procedure of choice in most situations. However, other procedures are available to achieve similar ends. A gastric patch can be used when the distal 4 cm of the esophagus is injured.[57] After closure and buttressing of the perforation, wide drainage of the mediastinum from the apex to the chest to the diaphragm is imperative. A large chest tube positioned posteriorly at the level of the repair (secured in place with an absorbable suture) and a smaller one placed anteriorly supply satisfactory drainage. The Thal patch, the serosal buttress,[58] and the diaphragmatic pedicle flap[59] are among the viable options if simpler repairs are not available (Figs. 4-12 and 4-13).

On rare occasions, such as cases of diffuse inflammation, drainage alone is the only therapeutic alternative. Another option involves closure of the perforation around a T-tube.[60] This maneuver creates a controlled esophagocutaneous fistula. It is a useful technique when the security of an attempted repair is in doubt or when adequate tissue to reinforce the closure is not available. Like many of the alternative procedures, the experience has been limited (13 cases in 18 years), and the mortality rate is high (36%).

Esophageal diversion and exclusion is a technique used in a select group of patients who have thoracic or intraabdominal esophageal perforation diagnosed late in its course and extensive destruction of this region. Based on the theory that gastric reflux into the esophagus aggravates inflammation and interferes with healing, an operative approach was developed that involves exclusion of the esophagus by ligation of the cardia to prevent gastroesophageal reflux, diversion in continuity of oral secretions by cervical esophagostomy, primary closure of the perforation, drainage of the mediastinum and pleura, tube gastrostomy, antibiotic therapy, and nutritional support.[61]

The actual technique (see Section V in Atlas Chap. 5) includes suture closure of the perforation and drainage of the mediastinal and pleural spaces. Two absorbable 0-0 sutures and a Teflon felt are placed below the perforation, above the cardia, and deep to the vagus nerves. Diversion is accomplished using a cervical esophagostomy in continuity sutured to subcutaneous tissue and skin. This can be closed later when the thoracic esophagus is addressed. The use of absorbable suture instead of the originally described umbilical tape for the exclusion avoids the need for a second major surgery because the gastroesophageal junction simply can be dilated to break the suture. At times, reconstruc-

Table 4-8 Review of 10 Published Reports of Simple and Buttressed Repairs for Esophageal Perforation

Method	Patients	Fistulas (%)	Mortality Rate (%)
Simple repair	158	39	25
Repair with autogenous tissue buttress	99	13	6

(After Gouge TH, Depan HJ, Spencer FC. Experience with the Grillo pleural wrap procedure in 18 patients with perforation of the thoracic esophagus. Ann Surg 1989;209:612)

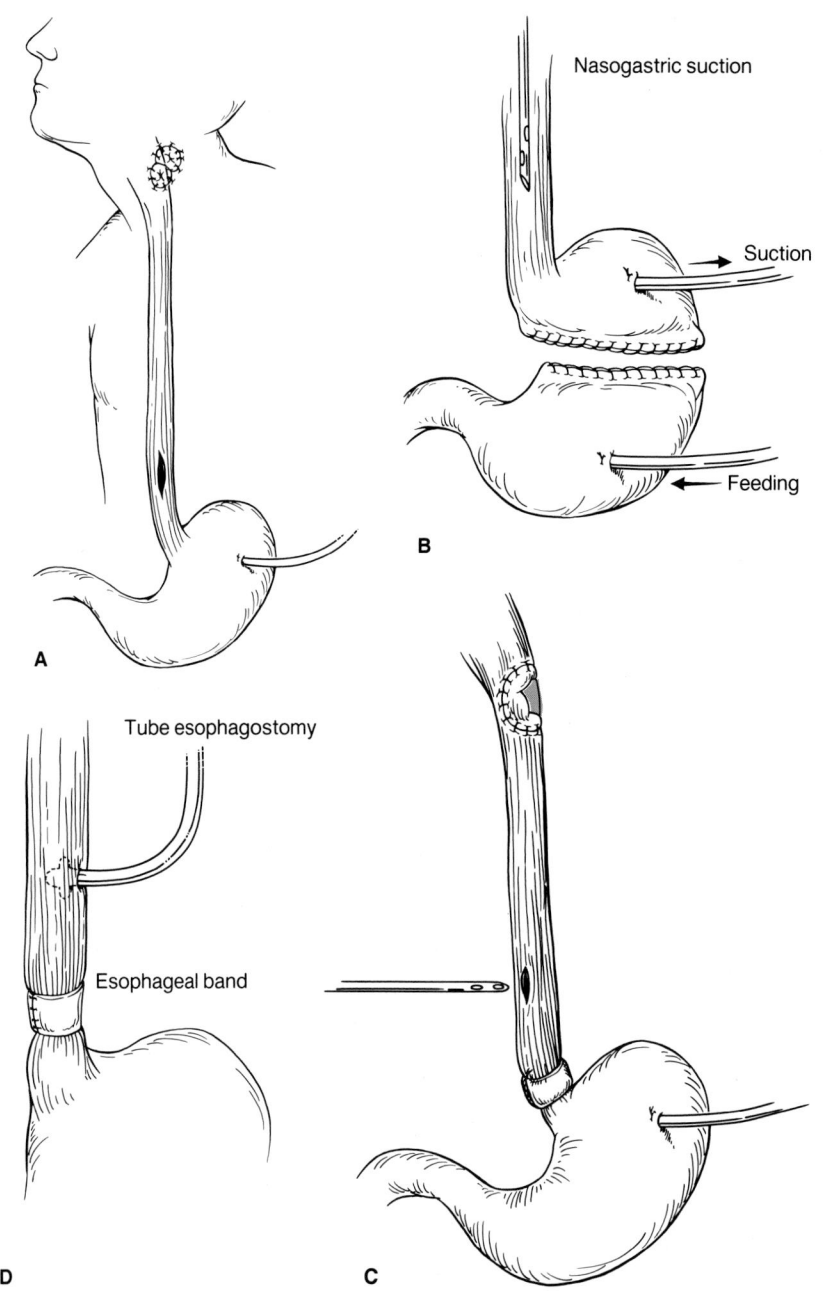

Figure 4-12 Surgical options in the management of complicated esophageal perforations.

tion of the thoracic esophagus is necessary, with the particular procedure dependent on the original injury.

The diversion procedure has evolved since its inception. The current technique does not mandate later operation for removal of Teflon felt. Rather, a #2 polypropylene suture is doubled through a Rumel plastic tourniquet and brought out alongside the gastrostomy. The esophagus is protected by material such as artificial dura or pericardium to keep the sutures from cutting through. Three or 4 weeks later, the suture can be re-

moved, and a Maloney bougie can be passed to open the esophagus. Alternatively, temporary closure of the cervical and intraabdominal esophagus using absorbable staples made from a lactide–glycolic copolymer has been reported.[62] Although controversy exists as to which method of treatment is preferable, esophageal diversion or exclusion are options when more conservative methods are not available. Regardless of the procedure selected, care must be taken during mobilization of the esophagus to preserve the surrounding blood sup-

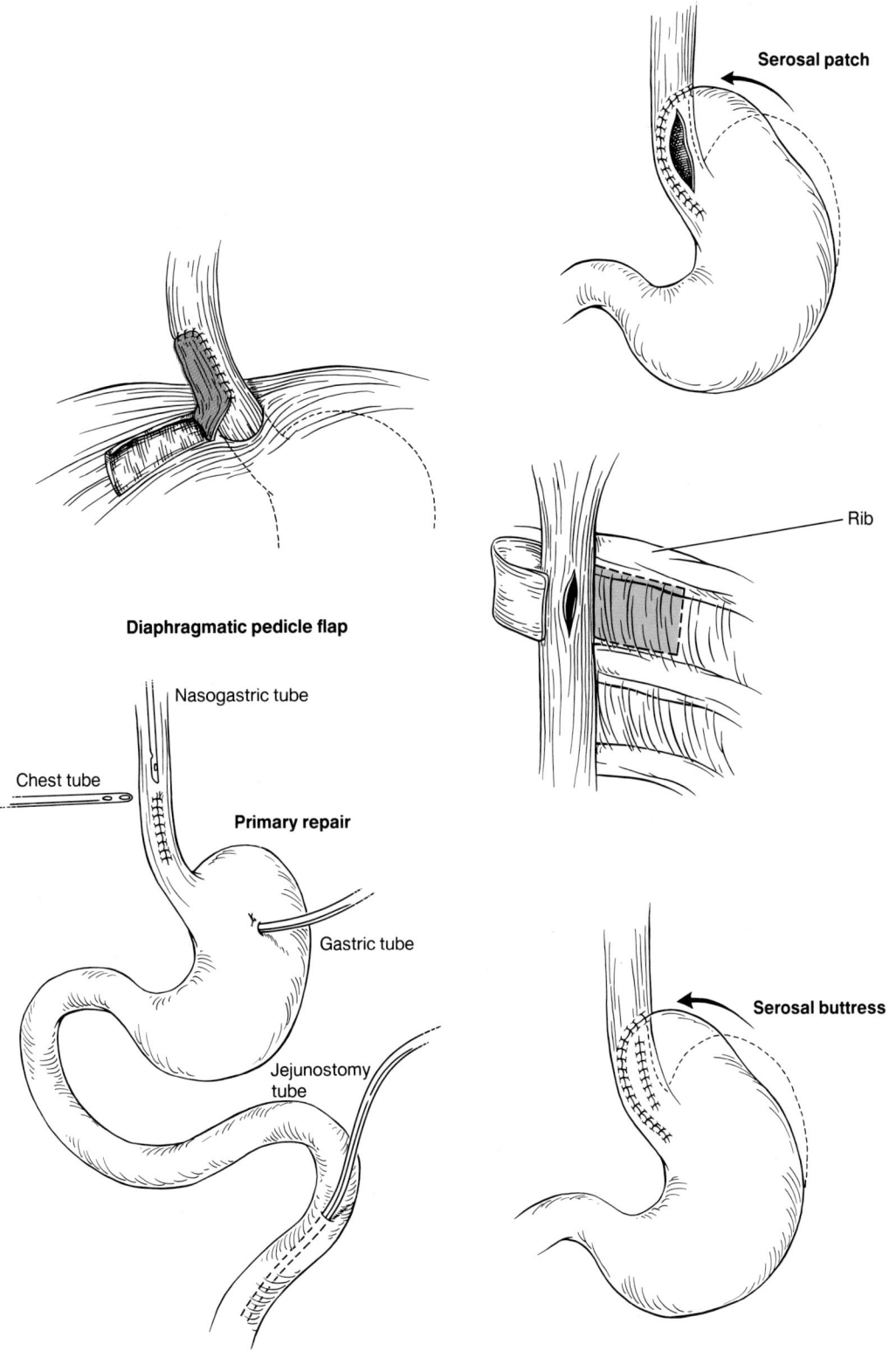

Figure 4-13   Alternative repairs of esophageal perforation.

ply and prevent injury to the recurrent laryngeal nerves. Reconstruction can be accomplished at a later date when the patient's condition has stabilized and the nutritional status is optimal.

The last technique for perforation to be addressed is that of resection. The results of resection were reported in one group of 24 patients with complicated esophageal perforation.[63] The decision favoring resection over primary repair is based on presence of one or more of the following: distal obstruction, other intrinsic esophageal disease, severe mediastinal contamination and sepsis, or severe fluid and electrolyte imbalance. The mortality rate in this series was 12.5%. Sixty-two percent underwent transhiatal esophagectomy, with 13 of 24 having primary reconstruction. The average time between esophagectomy and delayed reconstruction was 8.6 weeks. The staged procedure was deemed safer because of the risk of anastomotic disruption in the presence of sepsis. The technique (transthoracic or transhiatal) and staging (immediate or delayed reconstruction) of the operation depended on the condition of patient and the degree of contamination. (See Section IV in Atlas Chap. 5.)

Intraluminal stent placement is used primarily after corrosive injuries to the esophagus in patients who do not require esophagogastrectomy. In adults, the stent consists of a silicone tube (47 cm long) with an outer diameter of $\frac{5}{8}$ inch (Fig. 4-14). In preparation for placement, an 18F nasogastric tube is first placed transnasally and then withdrawn through a gastrotomy. The nasogastric tube is then secured to the stent, and in a

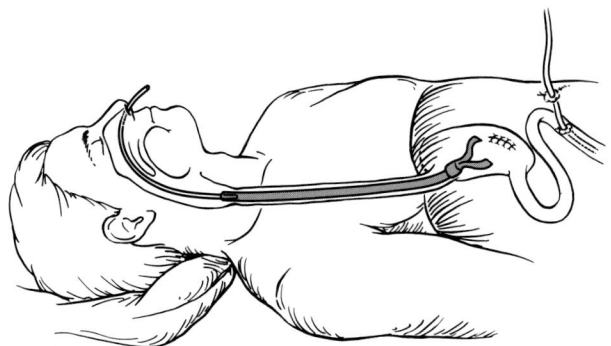

Figure 4-15 Intraluminal stent placement for corrosive injury of the esophagus.

retrograde fashion, the stent is pulled up into the esophagus to above the cricopharyngeal junction. The distal end of the tube extends through the esophagogastric junction (Fig. 4-15). After about 21 days, it is removed under general anesthesia, with endoscopy performed at that time to assess healing.

In situations in which esophageal dilation is not an option for management of stricture formation after caustic injury, many other conduit options are available[64] (see Section VI in Atlas Chap. 5). These include small intestine, gastric tube, colon, total stomach, colic patch, free patch of intestine, or free or pedicled patch of pericardium. Although interposed colon is the most common means of reconstruction, the procedure can be difficult because of manipulation of the vascular pedicle. Complications of colon interposition grafts include anastomotic stricture, late redundancy and stasis, and growth retardation. Free grafts of small intestine are also possible, although these require exacting microvascular techniques and are subject to thrombosis. Gastric mobilization is another technique used often, with anastomosis possible in the high cervical or base of tongue region. The colon, small intestine, and stomach all are acceptable, although no conduit is a completely adequate substitute for the native esophagus.

Incision of stricture instead of resection with patch reconstruction has been described. A colic patch (Fig. 4-16) consists of a segment of colon based on the right branch of the middle colic artery. The esophageal stricture is incised longitudinally until normal esophagus is reached at each end of the stenosis. The measured colic segment is opened on its antimesenteric border. The patch is fashioned while still in the abdomen to facilitate control of any bleeding during formation of the patch. When fashioned, the patch is passed behind the stomach and through the esophageal hiatus into the chest. The patch should fit without redundancy and is sewn in place. A 10-year follow-up study revealed excellent results in six patients and good results in three

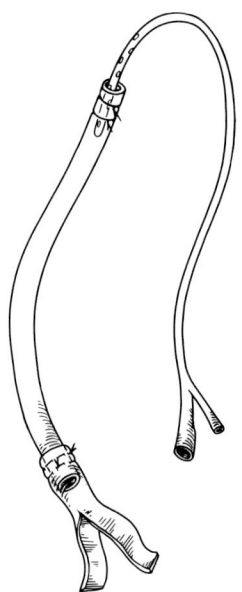

Figure 4-14 Intraluminal esophageal stent.

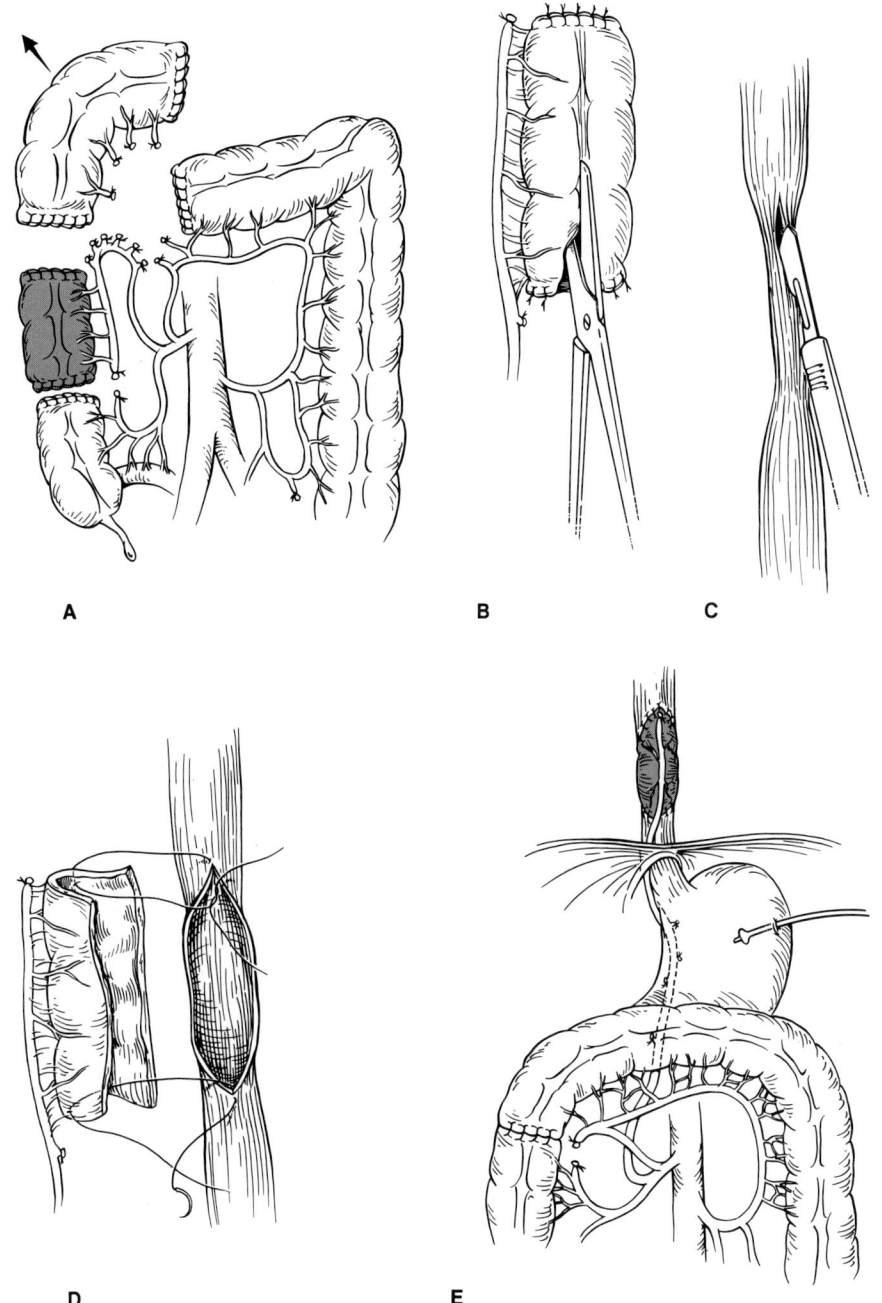

Figure 4-16 Colic patch esophagoplasty for management of corrosive stricture.

patients.[65] No major complications occurred, but in three patients, there was a tendency for the patch to bulge, producing a pseudodiverticulum. Functional results were good, however. When the patch was perfectly tailored to the defect, no bulging or redundancy was found.

Esophageal resection has also been suggested for management of some caustic strictures. In one series,[66] 75 patients with severe caustic esophageal strictures (65

patients) or emergency postcaustic esophageal resections (10 patients) were reviewed. Indications for reconstruction included complete obstruction or significant narrowing of the esophagus. Operations ranged from elective reconstruction (bypass) in 81.3%, elective esophagectomy and replacement of esophagus in 5.3%, and emergency resection and elective reconstruction in the remaining patients. The authors preferred reconstruction with the transverse and left colon or jejunum, positioned either in the posterior mediastinum or substernally. The substernal route was often easier than the posterior mediastinal path because of the severe fibrosis often present in the latter area. With bypass procedures, the esophagus is left in continuity, decreasing the intraoperative blood loss and operating time. Partial resection of the manubrium and clavicular head was required for patients with a narrow thoracic outlet. Acceptable morbidity and no mortality were reported in this series, with results described as good in almost 90%, fair in 5.3%, and poor in the remaining patients. Morbidity included anastomotic leaks in 8% and cervical anastomotic strictures in 4% of patients. Leakage from the cervical anastomosis usually stopped spontaneously, and strictures were managed by dilation or revision. Long-term follow-up averaged 6 months (range, 2 months to 15 years).

ASSOCIATED INJURIES AND COMPLICATIONS

Airway and Tracheoesophageal Fistula

The trachea is at risk of injury with penetrating or blunt trauma to the esophagus. Acute airway compromise is a common cause of death in these patients. One series reported on 24 patients with combined tracheal and esophageal injuries.[66] Commonly, the tracheal injury was the more apparent, with the associated esophageal lesion detected because of proximity, aspiration, or blood in the nasogastric tube. Diagnostic tests employed included rigid esophagoscopy, flexible esophagoscopy, contrast esophagography, and direct operative exploration of the potentially involved areas.

In tracheoesophageal fistula due to penetrating trauma, most in a series of 23 patients had clinical evidence of significant injury, primarily referable to the tracheal perforation.[67] Only 2 patients had no evidence of significant injury at the time of exploration. Most surgeons recommend placement of a muscle flap interposition graft between tracheal and esophageal repairs and over any associated carotid artery repair. Anterior placement of drains is recommended to avoid crossing over the carotid artery. When an ipsilateral carotid artery injury is present, drainage should be directed through the opposite side of neck. In cases of extensive esophageal trauma, initial consideration should be given to construction of a side or end esophagostomy to avoid precipitating associated problems such as tracheoesophageal fistula, mediastinal abscesses, wound infection, and carotid artery rupture.

The morbidity rate in the series of patients described earlier was significant at 74%, including eight cases of pneumonia, eight esophageal leaks, six tracheoesophageal fistulas, five mediastinal abscesses, four wound infections, and two carotid artery ruptures.[67] The most common associated major injuries were to the cervicothoracic spinal cord, lung, heart, or vascular structures. In patients without tracheostomies, there were no deaths, and the morbidity rate was 50%. In contrast, patients with tracheostomies had higher rates of mortality (17.9%) and morbidity (92%). Because the addition of a tracheostomy to a simple tracheal repair can actually lead to a higher incidence of infection-related morbidity, such as pneumonia, mediastinal abscesses, and wound infections, the authors recommended limiting the use of tracheostomy to conditions of extensive tracheal destruction and those requiring end-to-end anastomoses. Late recognition of a traumatic tracheoesophageal fistula can result in significant inflammatory changes, making the repair difficult. Occasionally, esophageal diversion is necessary before definitive repair. Severe mediastinitis may accompany late detection of these injuries as well.

Postintubation injuries, a fairly common problem in this age of increasing critical care management, can also affect the esophagus. Although the complications of prolonged intubation are well known to effect the trachea, tracheoesophageal fistula formation can also occur. The mechanism of formation of this condition may be simply prolonged overinflation of the endotracheal tube cuff and subsequent erosion or, more commonly, the combination of prolonged intubation in the presence of a nasogastric tube. This combination allows constant irritation of the adjacent tracheal and esophageal walls, allowing for fistula formation.

Postintubation tracheoesophageal fistula is manifested by progressive ventilatory difficulty, gastric distention, and copious secretions. To prevent this problem, endotracheal tube or tracheostomy tube cuff pressures should be maintained below 20 mmHg. This should help prevent the destruction of the columnar epithelium that can occur with elevated intratracheal pressures (50 mmHg for 15 minutes). Efforts to limit excessive tension and motion on the tracheostomy or endotracheal tube apparatus and to prevent infection are also of value.

Isolated esophageal fistula formation after repair of an injured esophagus is another complication associated with esophageal trauma. In a review of 46 patients with cervical esophageal injuries,[68] esophageal fistulas developed in 4 (9%), all of whom had gunshot wounds as their mechanism of injury. Three were in shock at the time of presentation. The association between shock and fistula formation was statistically significant, but that of gunshot wounds and fistula formation was not. Although one might suspect that the blast effect of a gunshot wound have a direct effect on the repair or on healing, this was not supported by the data. Because of the low percentage of patients with devastating injuries or combined tracheoesophageal injuries, the use of esophageal diversion is not recommended. Instead, management should include careful débridement, a two-layer closure, and closed suction drainage. Postoperatively, barium esophagography should be performed before beginning oral intake or removing the cervical drain. This is an important point because half of esophageal fistulas are initially asymptomatic.

Adult Respiratory Distress Syndrome

Adult respiratory distress syndrome (ARDS) is defined as ventilatory dependence for longer than 96 hours, with no other specific cause of the respiratory failure. The timely correction of a tracheoesophageal fistula may allow rapid reversal of respiratory failure before this more prolonged ventilator dependency occurs. The syndrome includes two or three of the following: Pao_2 ($Fio_2 = 100\%$) less than 250 mmHg, pulmonary venoarterial shunt more than 25%, and a chest radiograph demonstrating diffuse interstitial edema.[69] The primary lung dysfunction may be multifactorial. Direct parenchymal injuries may be related to the original trauma. Similarly, injury to the lung may be related to a period of relative hypoperfusion. Indirect lung injury may be due to gastric aspiration or aspiration of blood from the esophageal injury. The mode of ventilatory management and the level of oxygen required can cause injury to the lungs. On a microscopic level, a lung exposed to a significant period of hemorrhagic shock may demonstrate leukostasis, endothelial swelling, perivascular edema, and dispersed fat globules. With progressive pulmonary compromise, interstitial and alveolar edema occurs along with interstitial and intraalveolar migration of polymorphonucleocytes. Partial functional impairment is present at this level. Late in the course of posttraumatic ARDS, interstitial and intraalveolar fibrosis leads to a total functional impairment. Restrictive pulmonary function develops, often requiring challenging ventilatory and oxygenation strategies.

Treatment of ARDS requires aggressive ventilator management, constant assessment of ventilatory pressures and oxygen consumption, and patience. Limiting the inspired oxygen concentration to 50% is attempted because of concern for oxygen toxicity. This is usually accomplished by increasing the patient's mean airway pressure and functional residual capacity, usually by means of the addition of positive end-expiratory pressure. Alternatively, newer ventilatory modes, such as pressure control ventilation with or without inverse ratio, can increase Pao_2 and decrease the extent of the venoarterial shunt. The use of prophylactic positive end-expiratory pressure has been shown in one prospective study to decrease the incidence of ARDS and pulmonary mortality in patients at high risk for developing the syndrome.[70] Others have presented data disputing this practice, although study design differed in the two reports.[71] Corticosteroids have also been suggested as part of the treatment for ARDS, but there is no firm basis for their use.[72] Aggressive ventilatory and general supportive care continue to form the core management of these patients.

Infections

In general, cervical infections do not occur acutely but rather several days after injury. One should consider missed injuries to the respiratory or gastrointestinal tracts when soft tissue or fascial infections develop. Meningitis due to spinal fluid contamination may occur. Cervical osteomyelitis is occasionally seen after gunshot wounds, especially if the missile has traversed the gastrointestinal tract.[73,74] Although abscesses are generally confined to fascial planes, on rare occasion, they erode into normal or repaired vascular structures, causing major hemorrhage.

In a review of 38 cases of civilian gunshot wounds to the cervical spine,[75] none of the 16 patients treated nonoperatively had infectious complications. However, in the operative group, a spinal fluid infection developed in 1 patient and a superficial wound infection in another. A lower incidence of infections occurs after low-velocity missile injuries than with those produced by higher-velocity, fragmenting missiles typical of military use. In a report of 4 patients with cervical osteomyelitis after transpharyngeal gunshot wounds,[76] delayed operative intervention and inadequate débridement of devitalized soft tissue and bone were common features. It was concluded that thorough débridement of soft tissue and bone, adequate drainage, broad-spectrum antibiotics, and rigid immobilization of the cervical spine were crucial elements in the care of these patients.

RESULTS

Iatrogenic perforations of the esophagus usually have the best therapeutic results because of the typically early recognition that follows the injury. The trend toward nonoperative therapy includes the use of intravenous antibiotics, CT drainage, and total parenteral nutrition. In a limited series,[50] excellent results were obtained in a select group of eight patients. In an extensive review of the literature,[1] nonoperative management resulted in an overall mortality rate of 22%. In two large series,[7,16] one with 900 patients, and the other with 428 patients, the mortality rates were 25% and 38%, respectively. These retrospective data are subject to scrutiny because it is difficult to determine whether nonoperative therapy was chosen because it was the best therapy or because of the inability of patients to tolerate or consent to operative therapy.

Focusing on the etiology of the perforation, a combined review of 450 patients with iatrogenic and instrumental injuries showed a mortality rate of 19%, whereas spontaneous ruptures of the esophagus had a mortality rate of 39%.[1,4,5,7,8,29,32,75,76] A comparison between two individual series,[77,78] one with iatrogenic perforations and the other with spontaneous perforations, did not demonstrate a significant difference between the groups. Series of traumatic perforations had a mortality rate of 9%,[1,4,5,7,8,32,33,75,76] probably due to early diagnosis and treatment in the setting of multiple injury.[8]

Location of the injury is important in determining outcome. In 439 patients with cervical esophageal lacerations, the mortality rate was 6%.[1,4,5,8,32,78] In the thoracic and abdominal esophagus, the mortality rates were 34% and 29%, respectively.

Mortality figures are affected by the time between injury and diagnosis. A delay in treatment of greater than 24 hours after perforation is associated with higher rates of complications and mortality. When treatment is initiated within 24 hours, the mortality rate decreases from 26% to 11.4%.[5]

In examining the results of operative treatment of esophageal perforation in 325 patients in 13 published series between 1980 and 1990,[3,4,7,8,16,29,32,68,75,76,79,80] the mortality rate ranged from 0% to 54%, averaging 15%. Mortality rates were improved with reinforced primary repair when compared with primary closure alone (6% versus 25%, respectively).[3] Similarly, fistula formation decreased from 39% to 13% when esophageal closure was reinforced. Other mortality data include the results from exclusion and diversion (39%), drainage only (34%), and resection and drainage (29%). These increased mortality rates no doubt reflect the complexity of disease involved.

One individual experience with iatrogenic injuries consisted of 47 patients treated for instrumental perforation of the esophagus.[29] The distribution of injuries was cervical in 38%, mid-thoracic in 25%, and distal thoracic in 37%. Most perforations occurred during dilation for primary esophageal disorders; they rarely occurred during dilation of primary strictures. Most cervical perforations were treated by drainage only, and thoracic perforations were managed by primary repair and drainage. Resection and reanastomosis were used

for distal esophageal perforations, some of which were associated with benign or malignant strictures. The overall mortality rate was 13% for those treated nonsurgically, with a morbidity rate of 50%. For those undergoing surgical treatment, the mortality rate was 10% and the morbidity rate was 38%. Three of four deaths occurred in patients undergoing esophageal resection.

A similar experience was reported in 14 perforations (0.7%) among 1831 endoscopic procedures for benign disease.[81] The perforation rate was 0.35% for flexible esophagoscopy, 0.38% for Maloney dilator, and 6.67% for rigid esophagoscopy. Eleven of 14 perforations were intrathoracic, and all three deaths were in this group. Surgical treatment included primary repair and correction of the underlying esophageal condition. Although optimal management was believed to be surgical closure and drainage, a trial of nonoperative therapy was recommended for patients with limited cervical perforations and for poor surgical risk patients. Early diagnosis (within 6 hours) was shown to reduce the morbidity and mortality rates.

A classic report described 68 patients with esophageal perforation secondary to external trauma, instrumentation, and Boerhaave's syndrome.[58] The management pattern favored primary two-layer closure, with occasional use of gastric fundus or pleural flap. In unstable patients, wide drainage was the primary mode of therapy. Nonoperative treatment was reserved for selected patients with minimal injuries and no significant leak. Decreased morbidity and mortality rates were observed in patients repaired primarily with buttress compared with those without buttress (morbidity, 15.4% versus 72%; mortality, 0% versus 36%). The overall mortality rate was 23%, with intraoperative esophageal injury having the highest mortality rate (43%), followed by instrumental perforation (24%), postemetic injuries (18%), and external trauma (17%).

Others have emphasized the importance of individualization of therapy and effect of the site of injury.[78] In a series of 90 patients, factors associated with the lower morbidity and mortality rates of cervical perforations included the confined area of potential contamination, the excellent blood supply in this region of esophagus, and therefore the more effective control by antibiotics in this region. Drainage of the laceration was deemed the most important aspect of treatment in this group of perforations, and the mortality rate was reported to be 5%. Thoracic esophageal perforations were more serious because there is greater potential for contamination of the mediastinum and pleural cavity, often leading to severe sepsis. Critical steps in the management include early operation, débridement of nonviable tissue, a two-layer reinforced closure, and wide drainage. More extensive procedures are often necessary for operations occurring more than 24 hours after perforation. The mortality rate in this group was 18%. Nonoperative therapy is reserved for very small, contained leaks.

In a comprehensive review of 75 patients with esophageal perforations secondary to trauma, anastomotic leaks, and spontaneous or iatrogenic causes, treatment was dictated by the rapidity of diagnosis.[6] Esophageal injuries recognized early were preferentially repaired by reinforced two-layer closure. Large defects not amenable to primary suture closure were managed using primary muscle flap coverage to obtain defect closure. Wide drainage was critical in all cases and served as the hallmark of therapy for injuries recognized late or for cases of anastomotic leak. Additionally, injuries at high risk for leak (inherent esophageal disease or tenuous closure because of extent of disease) were managed with gastrostomy and feeding jejunostomy. Loculated collections were managed using CT-directed needle aspiration. In instances of failed healing, cervical esophagostomy was used to decrease persistent drainage and was followed by muscle flap closure as necessary for definitive closure.

In a series of 48 patients with gunshot wounds of the cervical (24), thoracic (17), and abdominal (7) esophagus, associated injuries of significance included tracheoesophageal fistula (8) and major vascular injuries (12).[27] The most common surgical procedure was primary closure and wide mediastinal drainage. The specific operation, however, was dictated by the location and extent of injury. Injuries to the cervical esophagus were managed by primary repair and plication with a well-vascularized sternocleidomastoid or omohyoid muscle flap. The thoracic esophagus was repaired primarily and buttressed with a pleural flap. If concomitant tracheal injury was present, additional pleural flap was imperative. For esophageal injuries below the aortic arch, concomitant gastrostomy and jejunostomy were deemed useful. Exteriorization proximal to injury and distal esophageal ligation were reserved for injuries with significant loss of esophageal wall. Injuries of the abdominal esophagus were managed by primary repair with gastric fundoplication. The overall mortality rate was 20.8%. None of the 7 patients with reinforced primary repair and drainage died or leaked at the suture line.

Another report dedicated to the management of esophageal gunshot wounds described 20 patients with perforations to the cervical (9), thoracic (10), and abdominal (1) esophagus.[82] Early operation (average time to operation, 3.8 hours) and primary repair with or without reinforcement were the operative principles. Two exclusions were performed: one for a transected and shredded cervical esophagus, and another for an intraabdominal perforation associated with massive hemorrhage. Associated injuries were significant in 18 patients and included pulmonary (12), vascular (9), tracheal (6), recurrent laryngeal nerve (3), and hepatic (3) injuries. These associated injuries were directly related to postoperative morbidity in the form of bilateral vocal cord paralysis, tracheocutaneous fistula, and pneumonia and atelectasis. Esophageal leak occurred in only 1 patient (5%) with a cervical injury. The total morbidity rate was 70%. The overall mortality rate was 15%. The high incidence of associated major organ involvement in patients suffering gunshot wounds to the esophagus was emphasized in this report. If sepsis from esophageal breakdown is avoided, mortality and major morbidity are related to associated vascular and neurologic injuries rather than to the esophageal injury.

In a review of nonpenetrating perforation of the cervical esophagus,[9] 11 patients were treated by operative or nonoperative methods. The nonoperative group received nasogastric drainage tubes, intravenous fluids, antibiotics, and parenteral nutrition. The operative group underwent débridement, primary surgical closure, and retroesophageal drainage. Small injuries in the pharynx (less than 2 cm) were managed medically, but surgical repair and drainage were recommended for lacerations greater than 2 cm or involving the cervical esophagus.

Results with management of spontaneous rupture of the esophagus are compromised primarily because of the delay in diagnosis and treatment. Prompt surgical repair, regardless of the time after onset, remains the only indicated therapy. In a review of 34 patients during a 30-year period,[24] all received intravenous antibiotics, nasogastric tubes, and surgical exploration. Primary surgical repair was performed in 26 patients and buttressed in 20 of these patients. Despite the use of reinforced repairs, the mortality rate was significant (41%) and was independent of the timing of surgery. Conversely, the morbidity rate of 75% in the 20 survivors was directly related to delay in surgical intervention. This finding is not supported by another study in which there was no correlation between results and timing of repair.[83] In a series of 10 patients, 5 were seen within 24 hours of onset of symptoms, and 5 were seen after 24 hours or later. No significant difference was observed between the presentation or subsequent clinical course in each group. Nine patients underwent primary repair and drainage, and 1 required resection. the mortality rate for the series was 10%, appreciably lower than the range present in the literature (26% to 51%). The morbidity rate for this group of patients was 40%, with 30% developing leaks. Regardless of timing of diagnosis and treatment, primary closure combined with wide drainage appears to be the optimal treatment of perforated intrathoracic esophagus.

Aggressive operative intervention has improved results in caring for burn injuries of the esophagus. In a report of 11 patients with third-degree burns,[33] 3 patients were treated with early operation and esophagogastrectomies, and all survived. Conversely, of the patients treated without early surgical intervention, 3 of 11 died. Therefore, an aggressive operative approach in patients with full-thickness caustic injury to the esophagus was recommended.

This shift in management of corrosive injuries was well demonstrated in a report comparing one group of patients treated conservatively to a second group later in the surgeons' experience treated with an aggressive surgical approach.[34] The latter protocol included routine endoscopy within 12 hours, with no advancement of the endoscope past the area of most severe circumferential injury. Patients with first-degree burns were observed for 24 to 48 hours and released without specific therapy. Emergency exploratory celiotomy was reserved for patients with at least a second-degree esophageal burns. Esophageal stent placement was performed in patients with second-degree burns and in those with a third-degree injury without extensive full-thickness necrosis. The stent was left in place for at least

21 days (Fig. 4-17). In patients with extensive full-thickness involvement, immediate esophagogastric resection was performed. This procedure included total esophagogastrectomy, cervical esophagostomy, jejunostomy, and resection of any involved adjacent organs. Staged reconstruction, usually with a colon interposition, was performed at 6 to 8 weeks. Using this protocol, 62 patients were evaluated. Results showed lower morbidity and mortality rates in patients treated with the aggressive surgical approach than in patients treated conservatively. Specifically, there was less stricture formation in the surgical group and a lower mortality rate for third-degree injuries. The authors credited early endoscopy as the critical factor in improving results, both to confirm the diagnosis and to classify the extent of burn injury.

The importance of endoscopy for evaluating caustic injury was reiterated in another study that reviewed 41 patients, 12 of whom required invasive treatment.[35] As shown in Table 4-5, burns were classified as grades 0 through 3. Esophagoscopy accurately predicted the probability of esophageal stricture, with all patients of grade 2 or 3 injuries developing stricture. Grade 1 and 2 injuries were treated conservatively, but grade 3 lesions generally required resection. Strictures developed in 9 patients, and 3 responded to dilation; 6 required esophageal reconstruction. When necessary, surgical options include oversewing and draining the distal esophagus, in conjunction with a diverting cervical esophagostomy, or anastomosis of the inflamed but viable esophagus to a Roux-en-Y jejunal limb. The latter treatment avoids the risk of a blind distal esophagus and the need for cervical esophagostomy. Definitive intervention for stricture can be made after 2 to 3 weeks with the aid of a barium esophagogram.

In a prospective study of 81 patients with corrosive injuries to the esophagus using a modified endoscopic grading system[36] (see Table 4-6), patients with grade 0, 1, or 2a injuries all recovered without incident. Those with grade 2b injuries and all survivors with grade 3 injuries had esophageal and gastric strictures requiring endoscopic or surgical treatment. Early death was confined to patients with grade 3 burns. Marked increases in morbidity and mortality rates were noted in grade 3b lesions compared with grade 3a lesions. The authors therefore recommended prompt surgical therapy with primary or delayed esophageal reconstruction in an attempt to reduce the morbidity and mortality in the latter group. Grade 3a burns can be managed without surgery in the acute phase, with later elective resection, if necessary, for stenosis refractory to medical therapy. No perforation or other complication occurred as a result of endoscopy performed within hours of corrosive ingestion, or between weeks 3 and 10. The authors con-

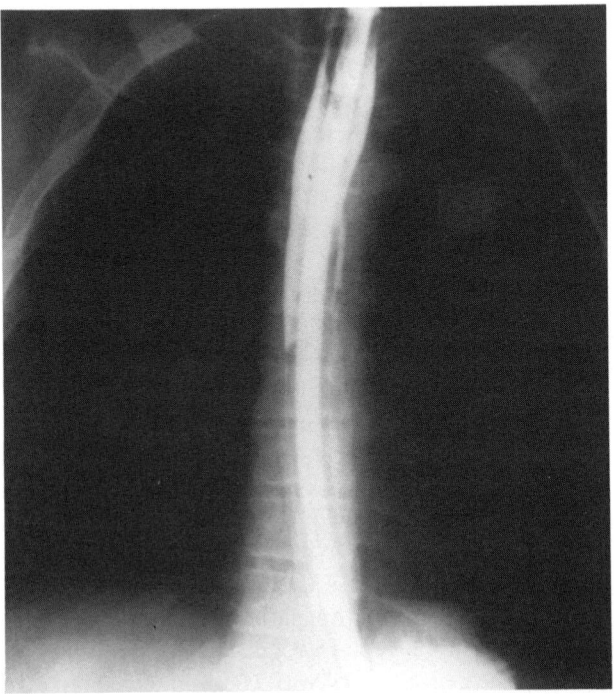

Figure 4-17 Barium esophagogram performed 3 weeks after intraluminal stent placement for corrosive esophageal injury. Free flow of contrast through a widely patent esophagus is demonstrated.

cluded that early endoscopy is not only safe and accurate but also critical for proper management of caustic injuries to the esophagus.

Proper care of patients with injury to the esophagus is founded on maintaining a high index of suspicion for this injury during the initial evaluation. Even the most innocuous-appearing wounds should demand complete attention. After a thorough history and physical examination, the diagnostic algorithm must include biplane cine-esophagography and often esophagoscopy. The evaluation is dictated in part by the mechanism of injury and by the anatomic location of the suspected injury.

The management of the injured patient is based on the physiologic status of the patient and on the result of diagnostic evaluation. Factors to be considered include the etiology and location of the injury, the condition of the esophagus, and the presence or absence of intrinsic esophageal disease. Specific anesthetic and perioperative management is critical. Asymptomatic or hemodynamically stable patients can be evaluated in an organized format. Management of the perforated esophagus in this situation consists of exploration and primary repair of the injury. Simple reinforcement of the repair is also recommended. Nonoperative management is considered only in the most contained injuries. The symptomatic or hemodynamically unstable patient mandates exploration, and the specific operative intervention depends on the patient's general condition as well as the degree of soilage and the presence of injury to adjacent organs. In all situations, wide cervical or mediastinal drainage constitutes the foundation for treatment of this group of patients. Primary esophageal closure is attempted, with reinforcement using a wide variety of available techniques. Diversion and exclusion techniques, primary resection, and staged reconstruction of the injured esophagus are other possibilities that are less frequently required. Corrosive injuries require an equally aggressive diagnostic and therapeutic regimen.

Associated injuries and complications can influence the course of the condition to a greater extent than the primary esophageal injury, with support often requiring intensive respiratory and medical intervention. These conditions, as well as the primary esophageal lesion, must be detected and addressed early to prevent the significant morbidity and mortality commonly associated with the injured esophagus. In all cases, effective therapy demands prevention of further contamination and infection, restoration of gastrointestinal integrity, and maintenance of adequate nutrition.

REFERENCES

1. Jones WG II, Ginsberg RJ. Esophageal perforation: a continuing challenge. Ann Thorac Surg 1992;53:534.
2. Bladergroen MR, Lowe JE, Postlethwait RW. Diagnosis and recommended management of esophageal perforation and rupture. Ann Thorac Surg 1986;42:235.
3. Gouge TH, Depan HJ, Spencer FC. Experience with the Grillo pleural wrap procedure in 18 patients with perforation of the thoracic esophagus. Ann Surg 1989;209:612.
4. Attar S, Hankins JR, Suter CM, Coughlin TR, Sequeira A, McLaughlin JS. Esophageal perforation: a therapeutic challenge. Ann Thorac Surg 1990;50:45.
5. Nesbitt JC, Sawyers JL. Surgical management of esophageal perforation. Am Surg 1987;53:183.
6. Richardson JD, Martin LF, Borzotta AP, Polk HC. Unifying concepts in treatment of esophageal leaks. Am J Surg 1985;149:157.
7. Goldstein LA, Thompson WR. Esophageal perforations: a 15 year experience. Am J Surg 1982;143:495.
8. Flynn AE, Verrier ED, Way LW, Thomas AN, Pellegrini CA. Esophageal perforation. Arch Surg 1989;124:1211.
9. Niezgoda JA, McMenamin P, Graeber GM. Pharyngoesophageal perforation after blunt neck trauma. Ann Thorac Surg 1990;50:615.
10. Guth AA, Gouge TH, Depan HJ. Blast injury to the thoracic esophagus. Ann Thorac Surg 1991;51:837.
11. Sealy WC. Rupture of the esophagus. Am J Surg 1963;105:505.
12. Silivis SE, Nebel O, Rogers G, Sugava C, Mandelstam P. Endoscopic complications: result of the 1974 American Society of Gastrointestinal Endoscopy survey. JAMA 1976;235:928.
13. Okike N, Payne WS, Neufeld DM, Bernatz PE, Pairolero PC, Sanderson DR. Esophago-myotomy versus forceful dilation for achalasia of the esophagus: results in 899 patients. Ann Thorac Surg 1979;28:119.
14. Perino LE, Gholson CF, Goff JS. Esophageal perforation after fiberoptic variceal sclero-therapy. J Clin Gastroenterol 1987;9:286.
15. Jackson RH, Payne K, Bacon BR. Esophageal perforation due to nasogastric intubation. Am J Gastroenterol 1990;85:439.
16. Larsen K, Skov Jensen B, Axelsen F. Perforation and rupture of the esophagus. Scand J Thorac Cardiovasc Surg 1983;17:311.
17. Michel L, Grillo HC, Malt RA. Operative and nonoperative management of esophageal perforations. Ann Surg 1981;194:57.
18. Dubost C, Kaswin D, Durante A, Jehanno C, Kaswin R.

Esophageal perforation during attempted endotracheal intubation. J Thorac Cardiovasc Surg 1979;78:44.

19. Ordog GJ, Wasserberger J, Balasubramaniam S. Shotgun wound ballistics. J Trauma 1988;28:624.

20. Ordog GJ, Wasserberger J, Prakash A, Balasubramaniam S. Civilian gunshot wounds: determinants of injury. J Trauma 1987;27:943.

21. Kinsella TJ, Morse RW, Hertzog AJ. Spontaneous rupture of the esophagus. J Thorac Surg 1984;17:613.

22. Mackler SA. Spontaneous rupture of the esophagus: an experimental and clinical study. Surg Gynecol Obstet 1952;95:345.

23. Bates M. Pressure rupture of the mid thoracic esophagus. Br J Surg 1969;56:327.

24. Pate JW, Walker WA, Cole FH Jr, Owen EW, Johnson WH. Spontaneous rupture of the esophagus: a 30-year experience. Ann Thorac Surg 1989;47:689.

25. Sugawa C, Lucas CE. Caustic injury of the upper gastrointestinal tract in adults: a clinical and endoscopic study. Surgery 1989;106:802.

26. Webb WA. Management of foreign bodies of the upper gastrointestinal tract. Gastroenterol 1988;94:204.

27. Symbas PN, Hatcher CR, Vlasis SE. Esophageal gunshot injuries. Ann Surg 1980;191:703.

28. Weigelt JA, Thal ER, Snyder WH, Fry RE, Meier DE, Kilman WJ. Diagnosis of penetrating cervical esophageal injuries. Am J Surg 1987;154:619.

29. Sarr MG, Pemberton JH, Payne WS. Management of instrumental perforations of the esophagus. J Thorac Cardiovasc Surg 1982;84:211.

30. Spenler CW, Benfield JR. Esophageal disruption from blunt and penetrating external trauma. Arch Surg 1976;111:663.

31. Backer CL, LoCicero J III, Hartz RS, Donaldson JS, Shields T. Computed tomography in patients with esophageal perforation. Chest 1990;98:1078.

32. Moghissi K, Pender D. Instrumental perforations of the oesophagus and their management. Thorax 1988;43:642.

33. Kirsh MM, Peterson A, Brown JW, Orringer MB, Ritter F, Sloan H. Treatment of caustic injuries of the esophagus: a ten-year experience. Ann Surg 1978;188:675.

34. Estrera A, Taylor W, Mills LJ, Platt MR. Corrosive burns of the esophagus and stomach: a recommendation for an aggressive surgical approach. Ann Thorac Surg 1986;41:276.

35. Ferguson MK, Migliore M, Staszak VM, Little AG. Early evaluation and therapy for caustic esophageal injury. Am J Surg 1989;157:116.

36. Zargar SA, Kochhar R, Mehta S, Mehta SK. The role of fiberoptic endoscopy in the management of corrosive ingestion and modified endoscopic classification of burns. Gastrointest Endosc 1991;37:165.

37. Fogelman MJ, Stewart RD. Penetrating wounds of the neck. Am J Surg 1956;91:581.

38. Bishara RA, Pasch AR, Douglas DD, Schuler JJ, Lim LT, Flanigan DP. The necessity of mandatory exploration of penetrating zone II neck injuries. Surgery 1986;100:655.

39. Saletta JD, Lowe RJ, Lim LT, et al. Penetrating trauma of the neck. J Trauma 1976;16:579.

40. Jurkovich GJ, Zingarelli W, Wallace J, Curreri PW. Penetrating neck trauma: diagnostic studies in the asymptomatic patient. J Trauma 1985;25:819.

41. Dunbar LL, Adkins RB, Waterhouse G. Penetrating injuries to the neck: selective management. Am Surg 1984;50:198.

42. Narrod JA, Moore EE. Selective management of penetrating neck injuries. Arch Surg 1984;119:574.

43. Ayuyao AM, Kaledzi YL, Parsa MH, Freeman HP. Penetrating neck wounds: mandatory versus selective exploration. Ann Surg 1985;202:563.

44. Wood J, Fabian TC, Mangiante EC. Penetrating neck injuries: recommendations for selective management. J Trauma 1989;29:602.

45. Ordog GJ, Albin D, Wasserberger J, Schlater TL, Balasubramaniam S. 110 bullet wounds to the neck. J Trauma 1985;25:238.

46. Ordog GJ. Penetrating neck trauma. J Trauma 1987;27:543.

47. Noyes LD, McSwain NE, Markowitz IP. Panendoscopy with arteriography versus mandatory exploration of penetrating wounds of the neck. Ann Surg 1986;204:21.

48. Richardson JD, Flint LM, Snow NJ, Gray LA, Trinkle JK. Management of transmediastinal gunshot wounds. Surgery 1981;90:671.

49. Grande CM, Stene JK, Bernhard WN. Airway management: considerations in the trauma patient. Crit Care Clin 1990;6:37.

50. Cameron JL, Kieffer RF, Hendrix TR, Mehigan DG, Baker RR. Selective nonoperative management of contained intrathoracic esophageal disruptions. Ann Thorac Surg 1979;27:404.

51. Anderson KD, Rouse TM, Randolph JG. A controlled trial of corticosteroids in children with corrosive injury of the esophagus. N Engl J Med 1990;323:637.

52. Maleki M, Evans WE. Foreign body perforation of the intestinal tract. Arch Surg 1970;101:475.

53. Ergin MA, Wetstein L, Griepp RB. Temporary diverting cervical esophagostomy. Surg Gynecol Obstet 1980;151:97.

54. Shor-Pinsker E, Silva-Cuevas A, Franco-Vazquez R, Pedroza-Martinez L, de Lachica Mere M. Gastrotomy with double gastrostomy in the perforation of the esophagus. Arch Surg 1970;101:433.

55. Menguy R. Near-total esophageal exclusion by cervical esophagostomy and tube gastrostomy in the management of massive esophageal perforation: report of a case. Ann Surg 1971; 173:613.

56. Grillo HC, Wilkins EW. Esophageal repair following late diagnosis of intrathoracic perforation. Ann Thorac Surg 1975;20:387.

57. Thal AP. A unified approach to surgical problems of the esophagogastric junction. Ann Surg 1968;168:542.

58. Rosoff L Sr, White EJ. Perforation of the esophagus. Am J Surg 1974;128:207.

59. Jara FM. Diaphragmatic pedicle flap for treatment of

Boerhaave's syndrome. J Thorac Cardiovasc Surg 1979;78:931.

60. Abbott OA, Mansour KA, Logan WD Jr, Hatcher CR, Symbas PN. Atraumatic so-called "spontaneous" rupture of the esophagus. J Thorac Cardiovasc Surg 1970;59:67.

61. Urschel HC, Razzuk MA, Wood RD, Galbraith N, Pockey M, Paulson DL. Improved management of esophageal perforation: exclusion and diversion in continuity. Ann Surg 1974;179:587.

62. Bardini R, Bonavina L, Pavanello M, Asolati M, Peracchia A. Temporary double exclusion of the perforated esophagus using absorbable staples. Ann Thorac Surg 1992;54:1165.

63. Orringer MB, Stirling MC. Esophagectomy for esophageal disruption. Ann Thorac Surg 1990;49:35.

64. Othersen HB Jr, Parker EF, Smith CD. The surgical management of esophageal stricture in children. Ann Surg 1988;207:590.

65. Othersen HB Jr, Smith CD. Colon-patch esophagoplasty in children: an alternative to esophageal replacement. J Pediatr Surg 1986;21:224.

66. Kelly JP, Webb WR, Mouldin PV, et al. Management of airway trauma II: combined injuries of the trachea and esophagus. Ann Thorac Surg 1989;43:160.

67. Feliciano DV, Bitondo CG, Mattox KL, et al. Combined tracheoesophageal injuries. Am J Surg 1985;150:710.

68. Winter RP, Weigelt JA. Cervical esophageal trauma: incidence and cause of esophageal fistulas. Arch Surg 1990;125:849.

69. Weigelt JA. Current concepts in the management of the adult respiratory distress syndrome. World J Surg 1990;11:161.

70. Weigelt JA, Mitchell RA, Snyder WH III. Early positive end-expiratory pressure in the adult respiratory distress syndrome. Arch Surg 1979;114:497.

71. Pepe PE, Hudson LD, Carrico CJ. Early application of positive end-expiratory pressure in patients at risk for the adult respiratory distress syndrome. N Engl J Med 1984;311:281.

72. Weigelt JA, Norcross JF, Borman KB, et al. Early steroid therapy for respiratory failure. Arch Surg 1985;120:536.

73. Heiden JS, Weiss MH, Rosenberg AW, et al. Penetrating gunshot wounds of the cervical spine in civilians. J Neurosurg 1975;42:575.

74. Jones RE, Bucholz RW, Schaefer SD, et al. Cervical osteomyelitis complicating trans-pharyngeal gunshot wounds to the neck. J Trauma 1979;19:630.

75. Skinner DB, Little AG, DeMeester TR. Management of esophageal perforation. Am J Surg 1980;139:760.

76. Ajalat GM, Mulder DG. Esophageal perforations: the need for an individualized approach. Arch Surg 1984;119:1318.

77. Triggiani E, Belsey R. Oesophageal trauma: incidence, diagnosis, and management. Thorax 1977;32:241.

78. Brewer LA III, Carter R, Mulder GA, Stiles QR. Options in the management of perforations of the esophagus. Am J Surg 1986;152:62.

79. Radmark T, Sandberg N, Pettersson G. Instrumental perforation of the oesophagus: a ten-year study from two ENT clinics. J Laryngol Otol 1986;100:461.

80. Borgeskov S, Brynitz S, Siemenssen O. Perforation of the esophagus: experience from a department of thoracic surgery. Scand J Thorac Cardiovasc Surg 1984;18:93.

81. Nashef SAM, Pagliero KM. Instrumental perforation of the esophagus in benign disease. Ann Thorac Surg 1987;44:360.

82. Pass LJ, LeNarz LA, Schreiber JT, Estrera AS. Management of esophageal gunshot wounds. Ann Thorac Surg 1987;44:253.

83. Ohri SK, Liakakos TA, Pathi V, Townsend ER, Fountain SW. Primary repair of iatrogenic thoracic esophageal perforation and Boerhaave's syndrome. Ann Thorac Surg 1993;55:603.

Digestive Tract Surgery: A Text and Atlas, edited by Richard H. Bell, Layton F. Rikkers, and Michael W. Mulholland. Lippincott-Raven Publishers, Philadelphia, © 1996.

5

Atlas of Esophageal Surgery

Mark K. Ferguson

PREOPERATIVE PREPARATION

Most patients who are to undergo an esophageal operation should receive perioperative systemic antibiotic therapy. Although the likelihood of opening the alimentary tract is small during elective operations for benign disease, such as myotomy or fundoplication, the risks of antibiotic administration are outweighed by the potential harm of an intrathoracic or intraabdominal infection. A first-generation cephalosporin typically is used unless there is concern about a penicillin allergy. Broad-spectrum antibiotic coverage is indicated for patients who have high-grade esophageal obstructions or in whom colon interposition is a possibility.

Patients are routinely evaluated for pulmonary functional status. All patients are required to stop smoking for at least 2 weeks preoperatively. If their status is compromised, pharmacotherapy, including bronchodilators, oxygen, and possibly steroids, is instituted preoperatively. Postoperative pulmonary care includes chest physical therapy, administration of oxygen and bronchodilators when indicated, routine use of incentive spirometers and breathing exercises, and early ambulation.

Although nutritional consequences of esophageal disease are often severe, perioperative nutritional repletion is not always feasible. When possible, this is accomplished with oral formula supplements, enteral feedings, or parenteral nutrition. Perioperative nutritional needs are also important. If oral intake is to be delayed for more than a few days, a jejunostomy feeding tube is placed and enteral feedings are started in the early postoperative period.

SECTION I   *Operative Approaches*

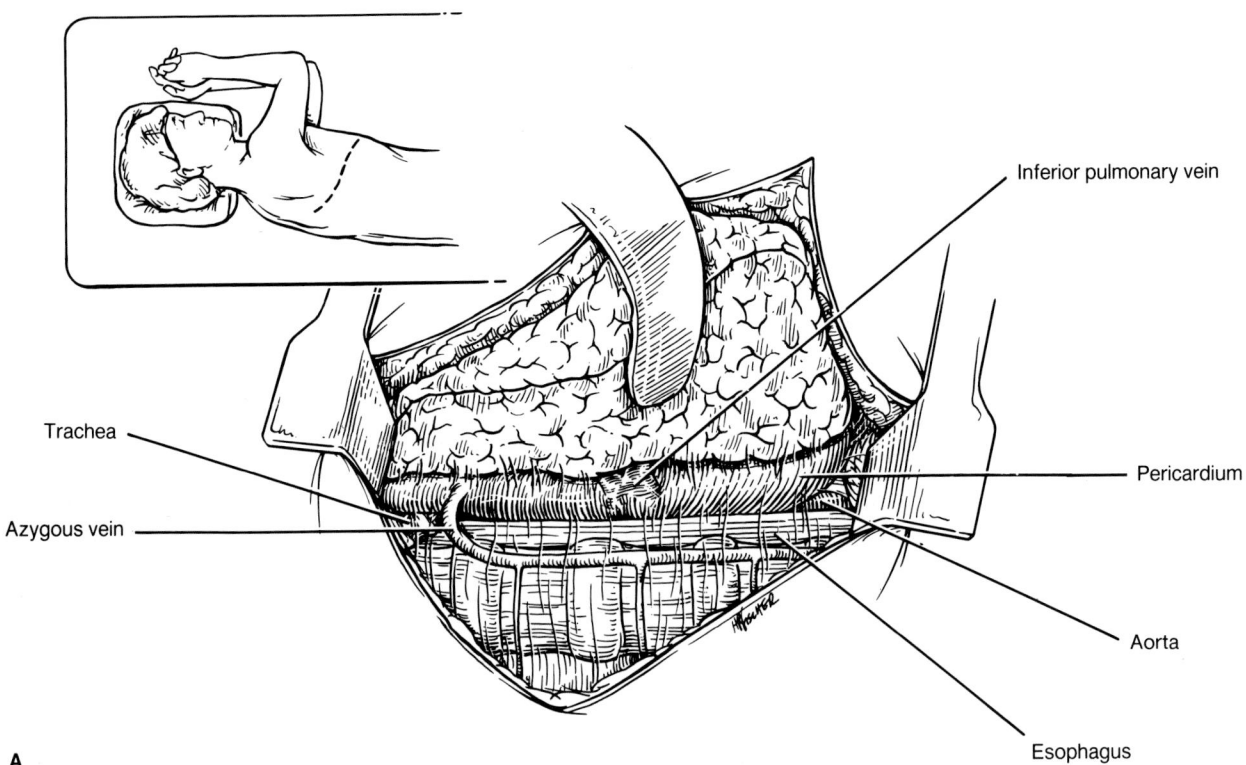

A

Figure 5-I-1

Right Thoracotomy

(**A**) The most common approach to the esophagus is through a right thoracotomy. The patient is placed in a true lateral position, and a lateral or posterolateral thoracotomy is performed in the fifth or sixth intercostal space. If simultaneous access to the abdomen is necessary, an anterolateral thoracotomy is used with the patient in a semirecumbent position. The esophagus lies medial to the azygos vein, between the vertebral bodies and the aorta.

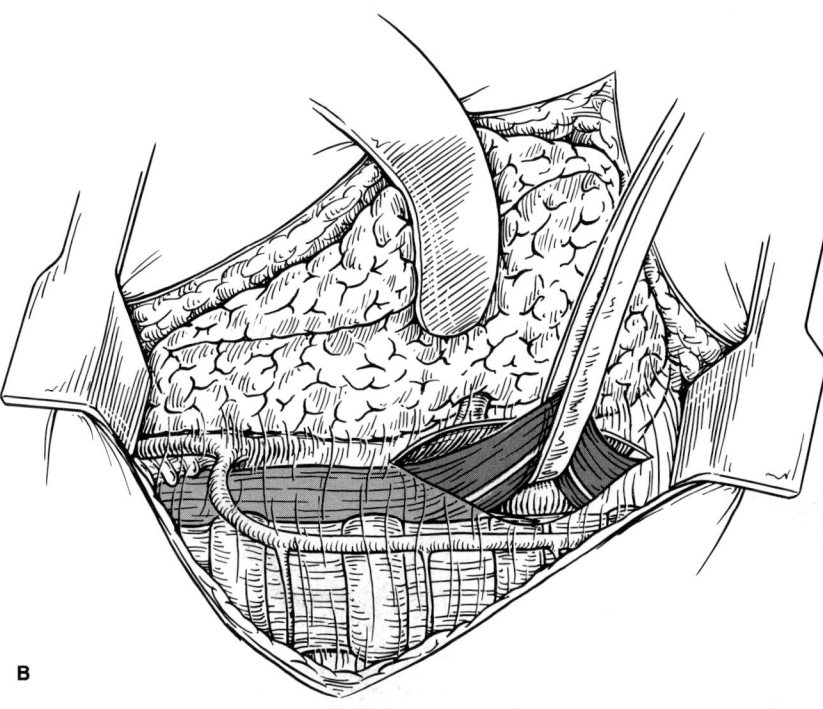

B

Figure 5-I-1 *(Continued)*

(B) The extent of esophageal mobilization and the amount of surrounding tissue mobilized en bloc with the esophagus vary greatly depending on the underlying pathology and the objectives of the operation. The distal esophagus (highlighted) is easily mobilized by incising the overlying mediastinal pleura after dividing the pulmonary ligament. The esophagus is freed from surrounding tissue with a combination of blunt and sharp dissection. Care is taken to control direct arterial branches from the aorta to the esophagus. Mobilization of the middle and superior esophagus is often facilitated by dividing the azygos vein. Care must be taken in separating the esophagus from the membranous portion of the trachea, which is susceptible to injury in the presence of adjacent inflammation or a contiguous neoplastic process.

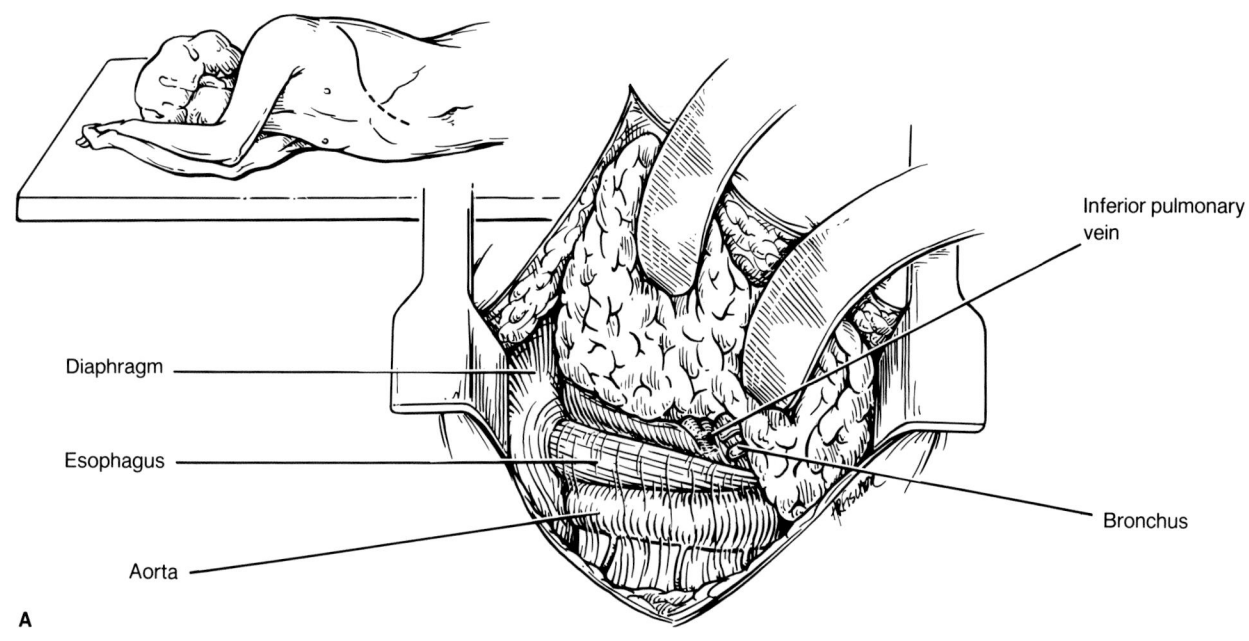

Inferior pulmonary vein

Diaphragm

Esophagus

Aorta

Bronchus

A

Figure 5-I-2

Left Thoracotomy

(**A**) A left thoracotomy can be used to gain access to the distal esophagus and, through a peripheral incision in the diaphragm, the upper abdomen. The patient is placed in a true lateral position or is rolled slightly posteriorly to permit access to the left upper quadrant if necessary. A lateral or posterolateral thoracotomy is performed, entering the chest in the seventh intercostal space. The incision can be converted into a thoracoabdominal approach by extending it across the costal margin and through the rectus muscle to the midline of the abdomen. The esophagus lies anteromedial to the aorta and anterolateral to the vertebral bodies.

(**B**) The esophagus is mobilized by first dividing the pulmonary ligament, permitting retraction of the lung in a superior direction. As with a right thoracotomy approach, the extent of mobilization and the amount of paraesophageal tissue included en bloc depend on the underlying disease process and the objectives of the operation. The esophagus (highlighted) is exposed by dividing the overlying mediastinal pleura. Using a combination of blunt and sharp dissection, the esophagus is freed from surrounding tissues. Care must be taken to control direct arterial branches from the aorta to the esophagus. The upper limit of mobilization in continuity under direct vision is the aortic arch.

(**C**) The upper abdomen can be exposed through a left thoracotomy by incising the diaphragm peripherally, sparing its innervation by the phrenic nerve. The incision is started near the diaphragmatic insertion on the sternum 1 to 2 cm from the chest wall (**inset**). A 1- to 2-cm cuff of diaphragm is left peripherally to facilitate closure at the conclusion of the operation. The posterior extent of the incision is marked by the tip of the spleen. This incision permits excellent exposure of the stomach, spleen, transverse colon, splenic flexure, left lobe of the liver, and pylorus.

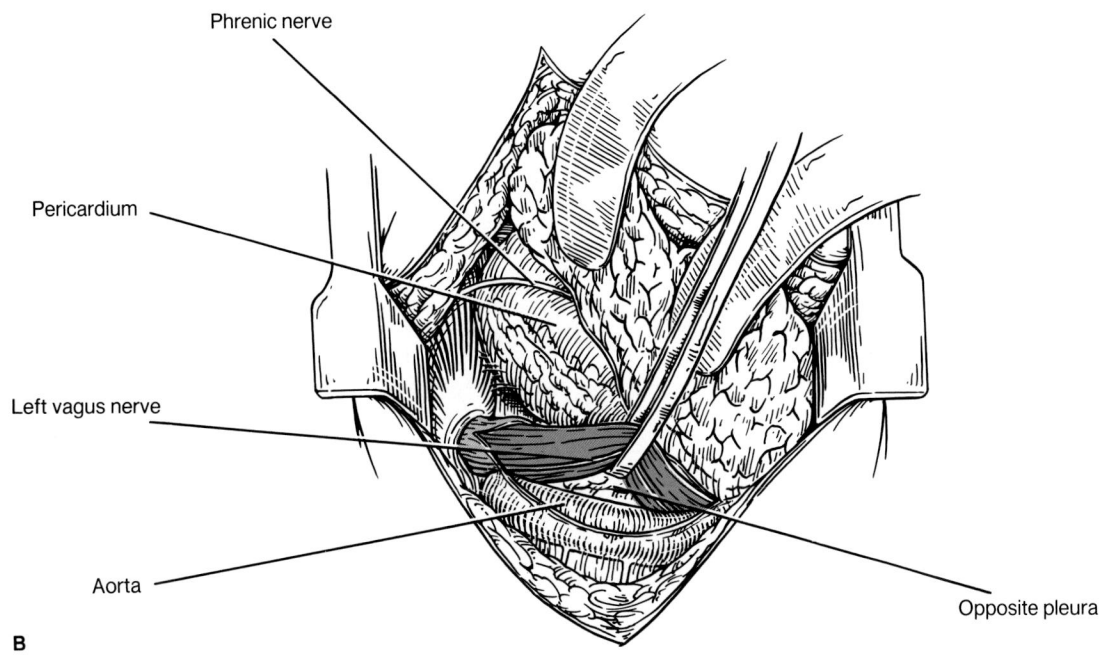

Phrenic nerve

Pericardium

Left vagus nerve

Aorta

Opposite pleura

B

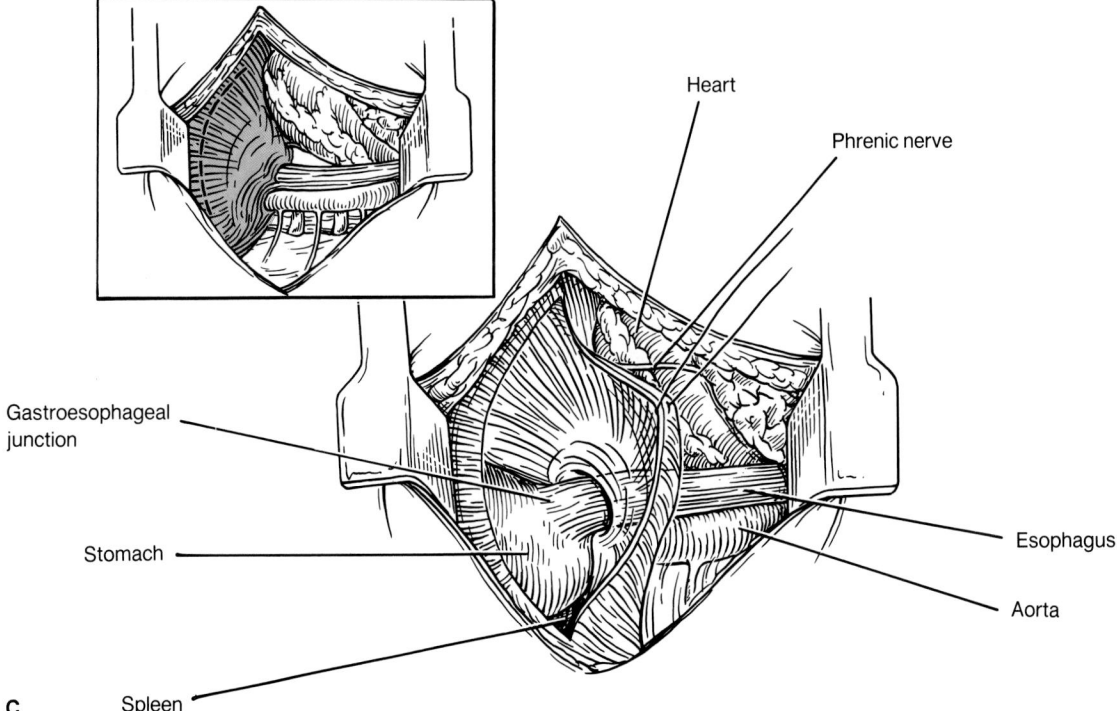

Heart

Phrenic nerve

Gastroesophageal junction

Stomach

Esophagus

Aorta

Spleen

C

Figure 5-I-2 *(Continued)*

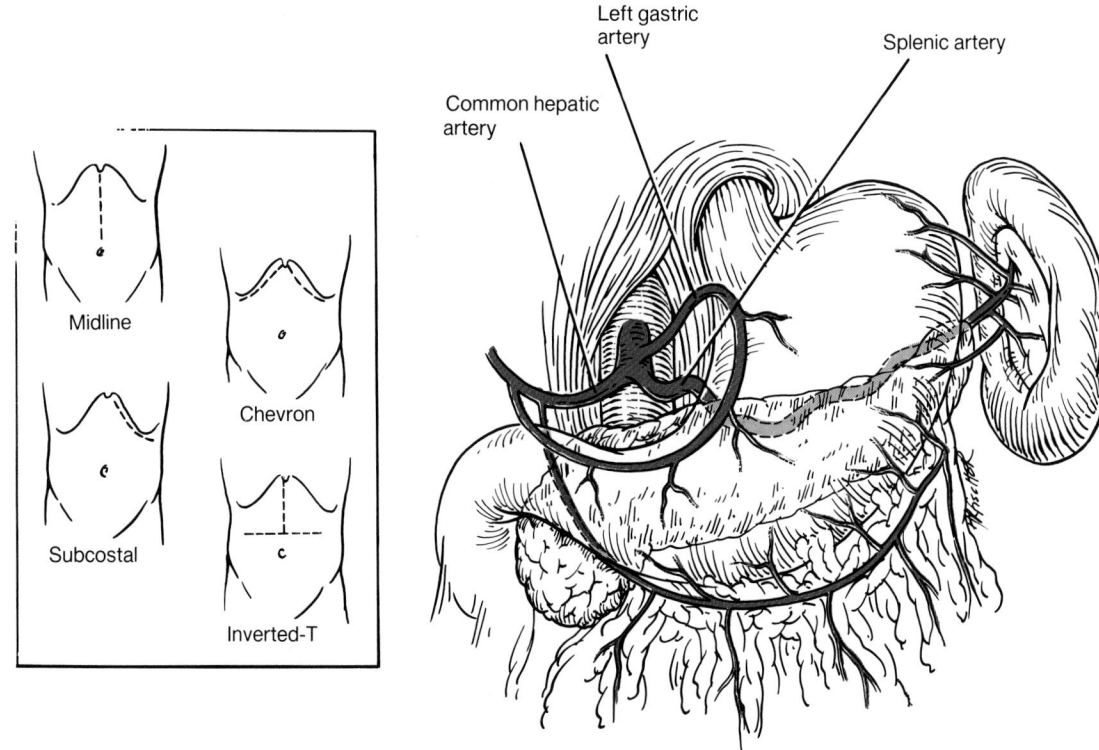

Figure 5-I-3

Abdominal Approach

A variety of incisions provide excellent access to the esophagogastric junction and stomach (**inset**). Important anatomic landmarks include the esophageal hiatus and the aortic hiatus. The celiac axis gives off the splenic artery, left gastric artery, and the common hepatic artery (*highlighted*). The right gastroepiploic artery is most commonly a branch of the common hepatic artery and supplies much of the greater curvature of the stomach.

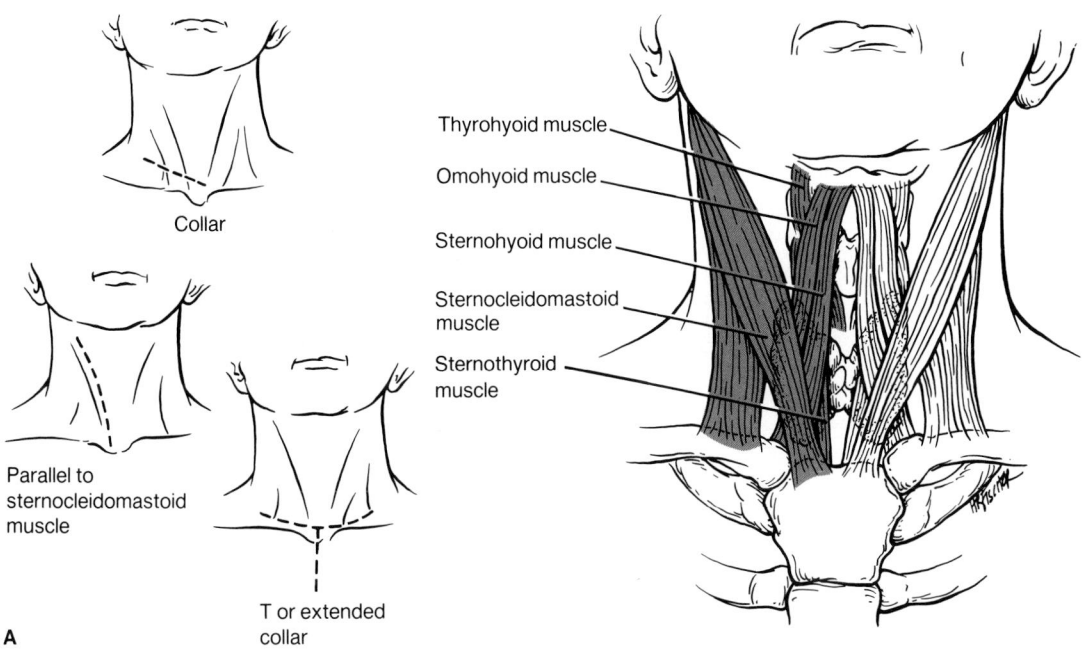

Thyrohyoid muscle
Omohyoid muscle
Sternohyoid muscle
Sternocleidomastoid muscle
Sternothyroid muscle

Collar

Parallel to sternocleidomastoid muscle

T or extended collar

A

Figure 5-I-4

Cervical Approach

(**A**) A variety of incisions give excellent access to the cervical and upper thoracic esophagus. An approach that suffices for most operations is provided by a limited collar incision or an incision made parallel to the sternocleidomastoid muscle. Dissection is carried medial to the carotid sheath, and the esophagus is exposed in the prevertebral space posterior to the trachea. The extended collar incision is used for bilateral approaches to the esophagus. The T incision, which includes partial sternotomy, is useful for exposure of the esophagus as it passes through the thoracic inlet.

(Continued)

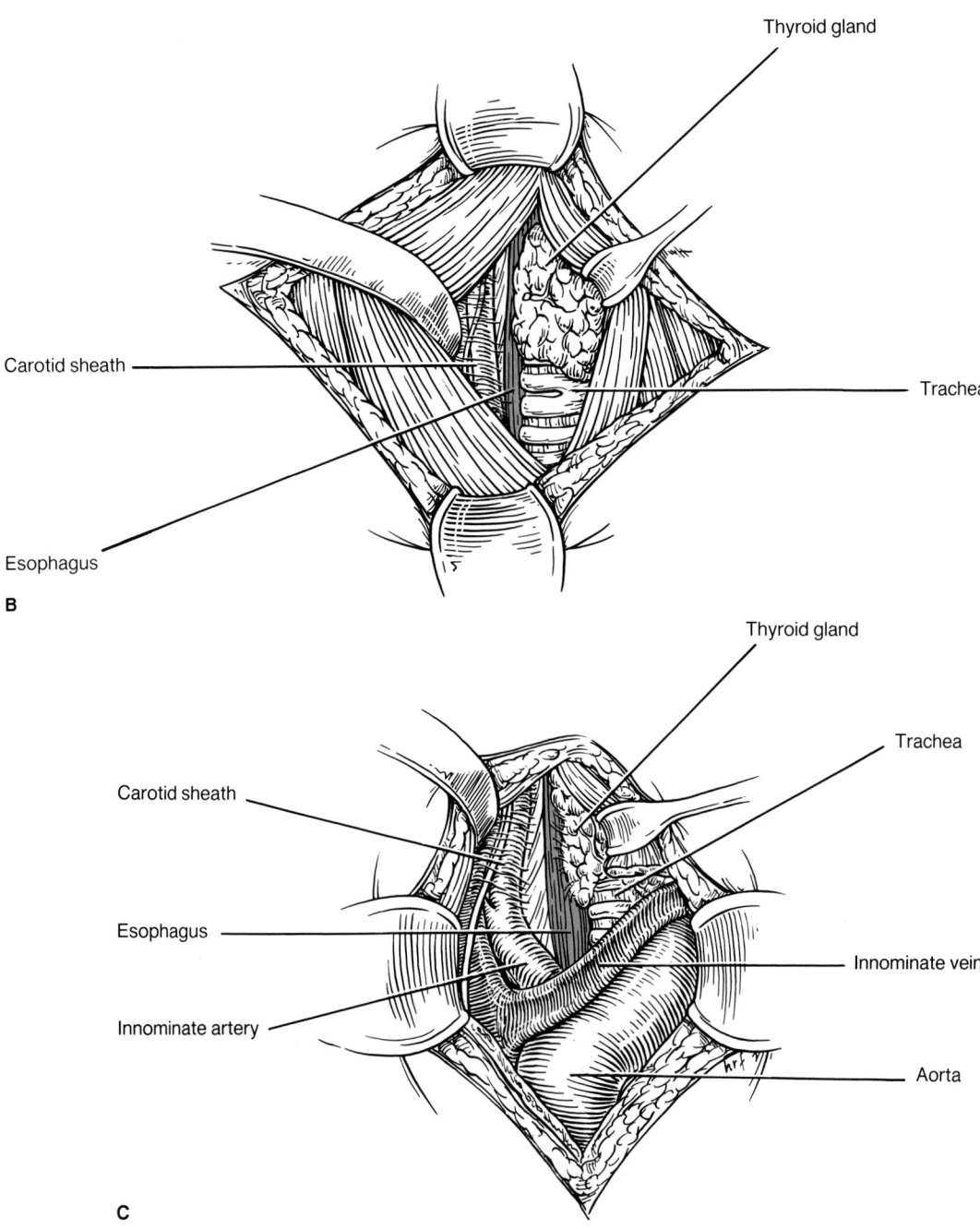

Figure 5-I-4 *(Continued)*

(B) The sternocleidomastoid muscle and carotid sheath are reflected laterally, and the strap muscles with the underlying trachea and thyroid gland are reflected medially. The esophagus is seen in the prevertebral space posterior to the trachea. It is sometimes necessary to divide the middle thyroid vein to provide this exposure. It is not necessary to divide any of the illustrated muscles to obtain this degree of exposure.

(C) The T incision with partial sternotomy permits an extended dissection of the esophagus at the level of the thoracic inlet. The innominate vein is mobilized and retracted inferiorly, and the innominate artery is retracted laterally. Retraction of the trachea to the left side permits exposure of the proximal esophagus, and additional dissection under direct vision can be performed posterior to the aortic arch.

SECTION II *Motility Disorders*

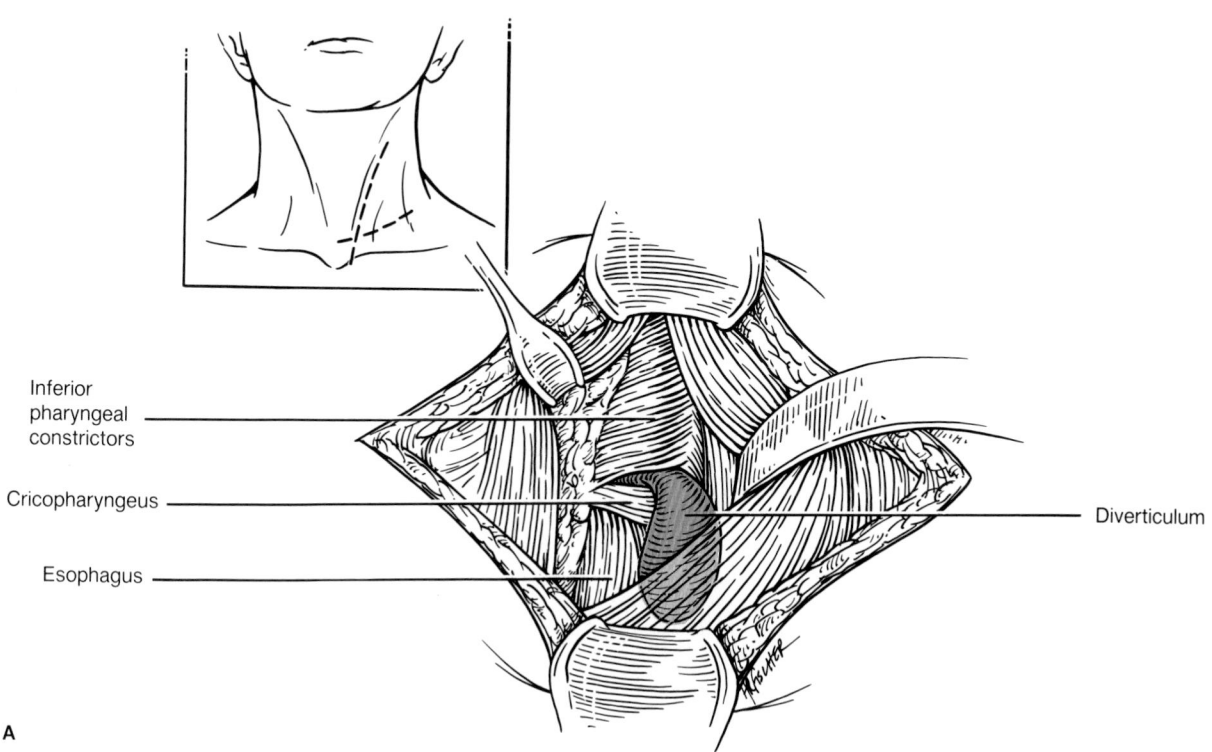

Inferior pharyngeal constrictors

Cricopharyngeus

Esophagus

Diverticulum

A

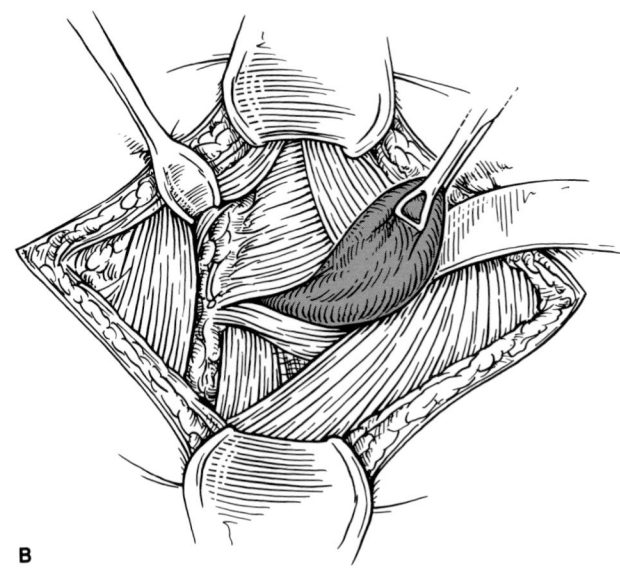

B

Figure 5-II-1

Cricopharyngeal Myotomy, Diverticulopexy, and Diverticulectomy

(**A**) The surgical approach to a cricopharyngeal diverticulum (or cricopharyngeal bar) is usually through the left side of the neck, because the diverticulum typically presents to the left. A collar incision or incision parallel to the sternocleidomastoid muscle is used. The diverticulum is easily identified in the prevertebral space.

(**B**) The diverticulum is mobilized to the level of its neck, which is superior to the cricopharyngeal muscle. An investing layer of adventitia is excised so that the mucosal layer is exposed. Diverticula sometimes extend well into the mediastinum. Large diverticula such as these are usually mobilized easily through the cervical approach illustrated.

(Continued)

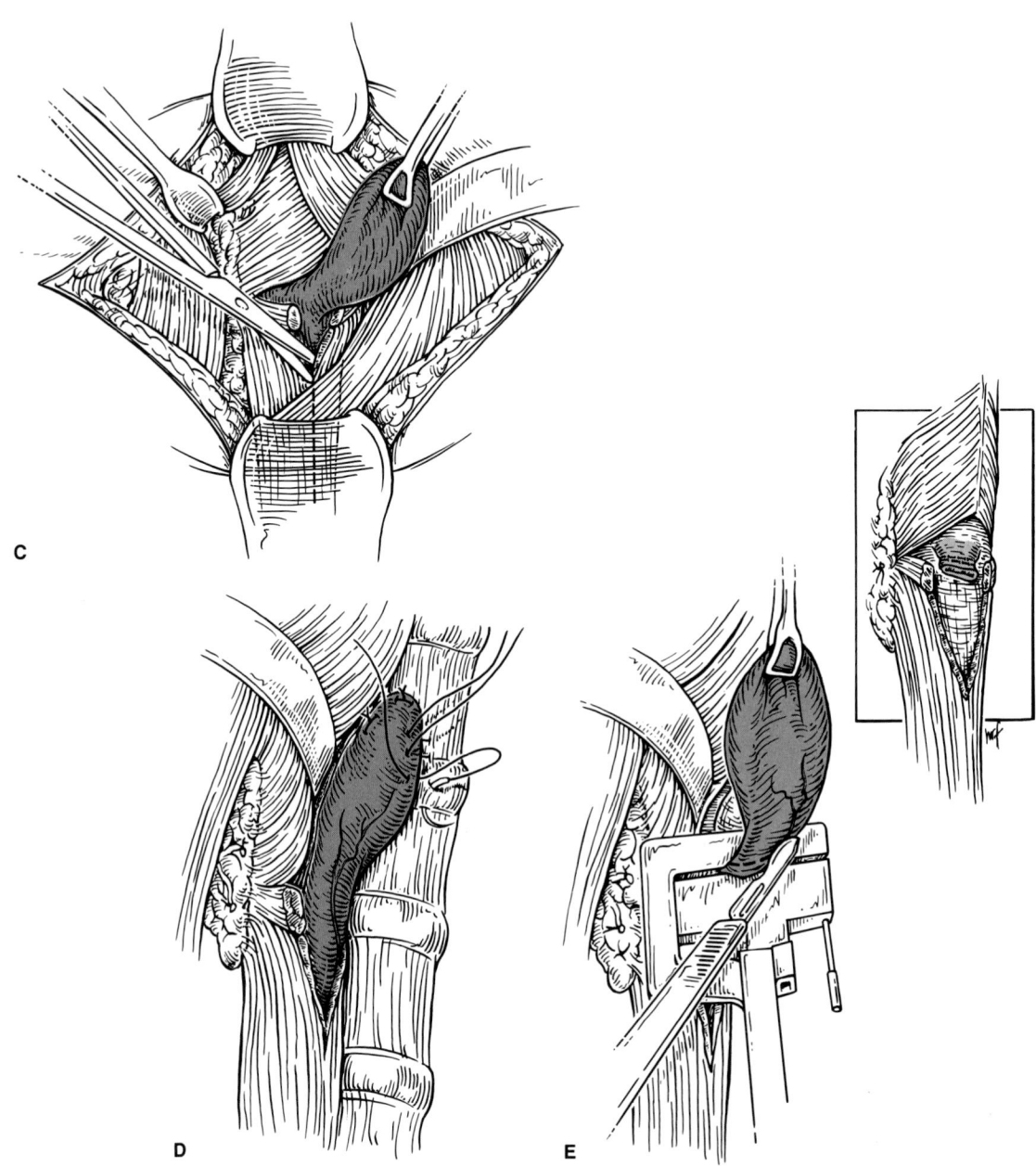

Figure 5-II-1 *(Continued)*

(**C**) A crucial part of the procedure is the cricopharyngeal myotomy. A vertical incision is made through the cricopharyngeal muscle from the neck of the diverticulum inferiorly for a distance of 4 to 5 cm. The muscle edges are bluntly dissected from the esophageal mucosa to prevent them from healing together by secondary intention.

(**D**) The diverticulum can be managed using one of several techniques. Small diverticula are inverted and sewn to the prevertebral fascia using plicating mattress sutures (diverticulopexy). This eliminates entry into the mucosa, a source of potential fistula formation after diverticulectomy. Small diverticula (less than 2 cm) require no special therapy other than myotomy.

(**E**) Moderate to large diverticula can be excised after completion of the myotomy. Current stapling devices provide a secure closure. Care is taken not to excise mucosa beyond the neck of the diverticulum, which would cause narrowing of the pharyngoesophageal lumen.

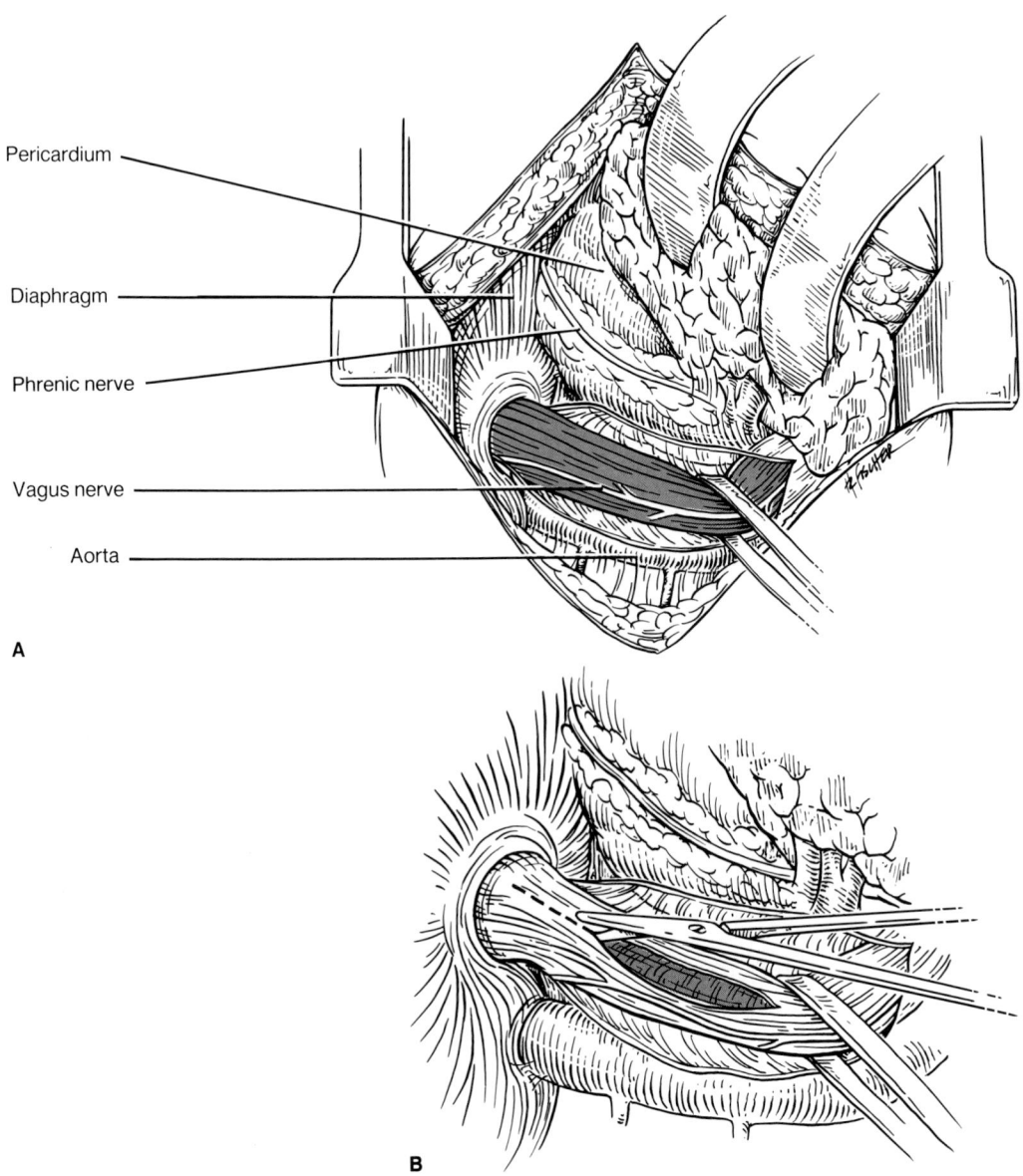

Pericardium

Diaphragm

Phrenic nerve

Vagus nerve

Aorta

A

B

Figure 5-II-2

Myotomy With Fundoplication

(**A**) Myotomy for achalasia or diffuse esophageal spasm is most commonly performed through a left thoracotomy, entering the chest through the seventh intercostal space. For a limited myotomy, minimal dissection at the hiatus is necessary. Traction on the mobilized esophagus permits visualization of the esophagogastric junction, and the myotomy is performed over a distance of at least 5 cm, the distal extent terminating at the inferior margin of the lower esophageal sphincter. Because of uncertainties surrounding identification of the inferior margin of the lower esophageal sphincter, many surgeons use a more extensive myotomy, which requires mobilization of the esophagus and dissection of the hiatus.

(**B**) For a long myotomy extending onto the stomach, the muscle layers of the esophagus are incised sharply from the level of the inferior pulmonary vein and extending 1 to

(Continued)

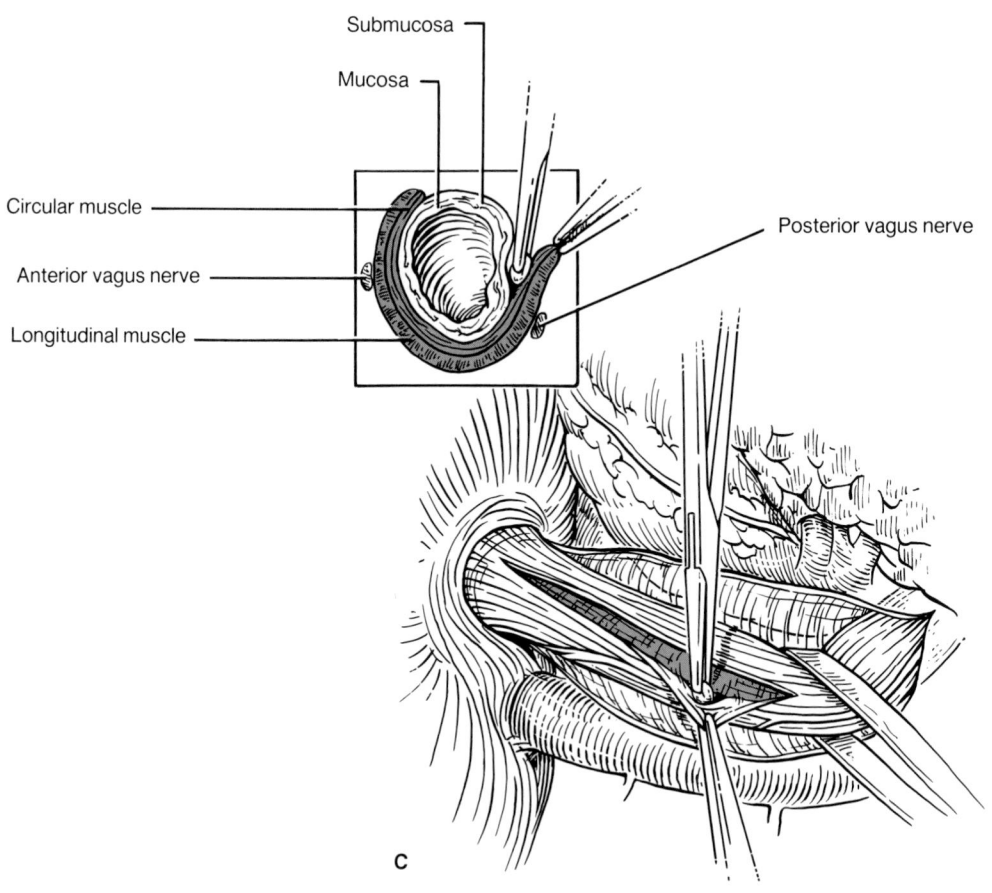

Figure 5-II-2 *(Continued)*

2 cm onto the stomach. Dissection can be performed with a blade or scissors. The myotomy is performed midway between the two vagus nerves.

(C) After the myotomy is completed, the muscularis propria is bluntly dissected from the submucosa to prevent healing together of the cut muscle edges. The lateral extent of mobilization is usually the vagus nerves. This frees up 30% to 50% of the esophageal circumference.

(D) When an extended myotomy and complete mobilization of the hiatus are performed, modified fundoplication is necessary to prevent postoperative gastroesophageal reflux. A common antireflux operation performed under these circumstances is a modified Belsey Mark IV partial fundoplication. Heavy sutures are placed through the left and right crura to enable partial closure of the esophageal hiatus. These are left untied until the fundoplication is finished. In contrast to the standard Belsey Mark IV fundoplication, only two mattress sutures are placed in the first layer, omitting the center stitch.

(E) After tying the first layer of mattress sutures, the second layer of sutures is placed, imbricating an additional 1 cm of esophagus and stomach at the level of the esophagogastric junction. These sutures are brought through the diaphragm so that, when they are tied, the wrap is anchored beneath the diaphragm.

(F) Once the esophagogastric junction is manually reduced below the diaphragm, the second row of sutures is tied down. The crural stitches are then tied, with care taken to preserve space at the esophageal hiatus posteriorly that will easily admit a fingertip. This ensures that there will be no undue obstruction at the hiatus. The completed fundoplication wrap thus encompasses about 270 degrees of the esophageal circumference (**inset**).

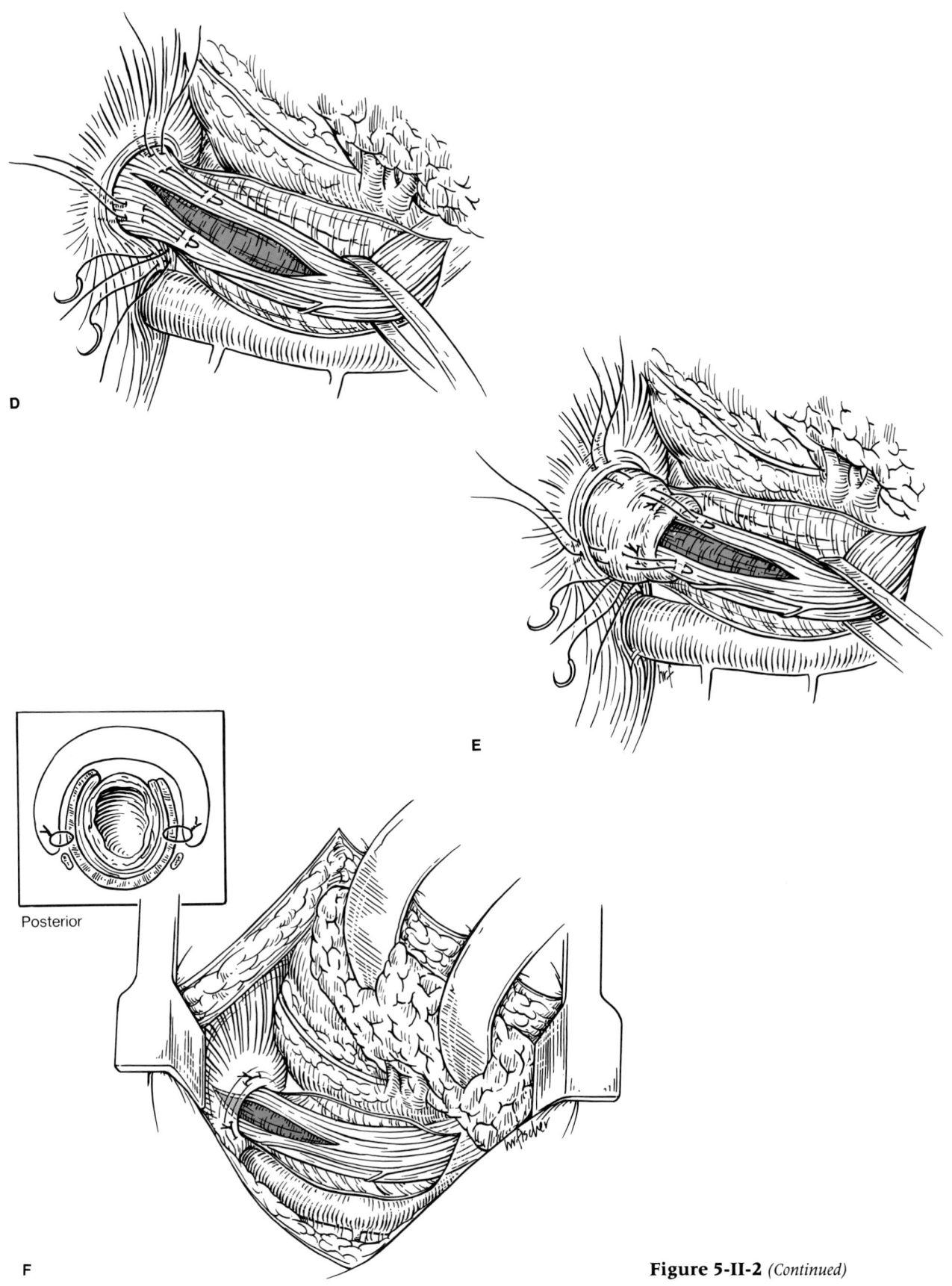

D

E

Posterior

F

Figure 5-II-2 *(Continued)*

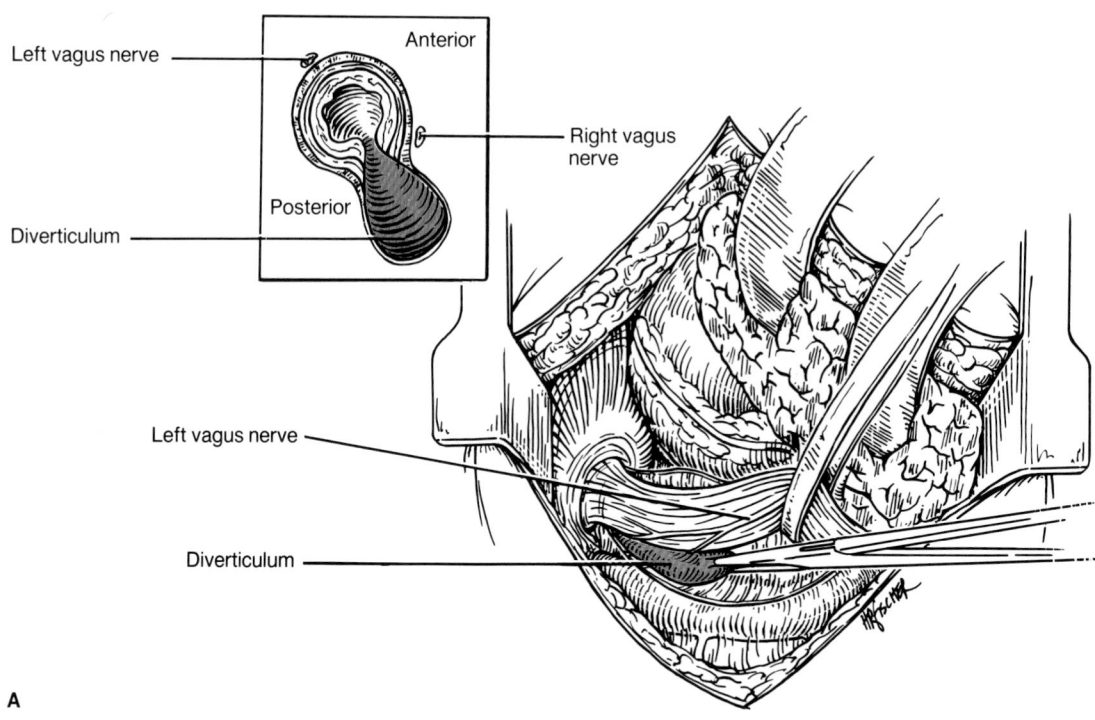

A

Figure 5-II-3

Esophageal Myotomy and Diverticulectomy

(**A**) The open approach to resection of an epiphrenic diverticulum is usually through the left side of the chest in the seventh intercostal space. The diverticulum typically presents posteromedially. This necessitates mobilization of the esophagus and dissection of the diverticulum from the mediastinum. The esophagus is then rotated slightly to expose the neck of the diverticulum.

(**B**) The submucosa is removed from the diverticulum to the level of its neck, revealing the mucosa. This is done with a combination of blunt and sharp dissection.

(**C**) The diverticulum is excised after placing a large bougie (50F to 60F) down the esophageal lumen to prevent removal of too much mucosa. Closure is performed either with a stapling device (shown) or manually.

(**D**) The remaining defect in the esophageal musculature is closed over the mucosal repair.

(**E**) The esophagus is rotated back to its normal position, and a longitudinal myotomy is performed from just above the level of the neck of the diverticulum distally. Considerations about the distal extent of myotomy and the need for subsequent fundoplication are similar to those described previously (see Fig. 5-II-2*A*).

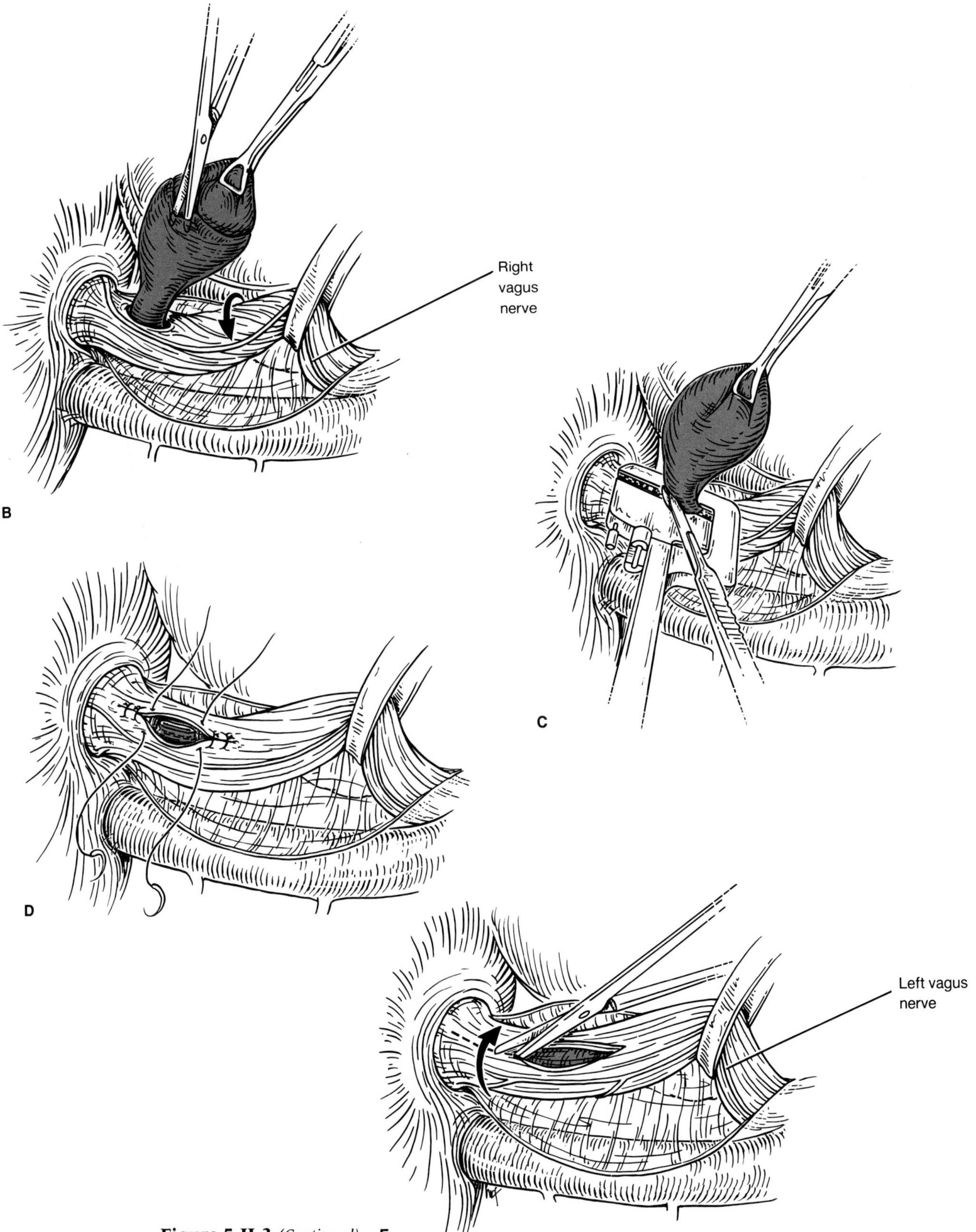

Right
vagus
nerve

B

C

D

Left vagus
nerve

Figure 5-II-3 *(Continued)* **E**

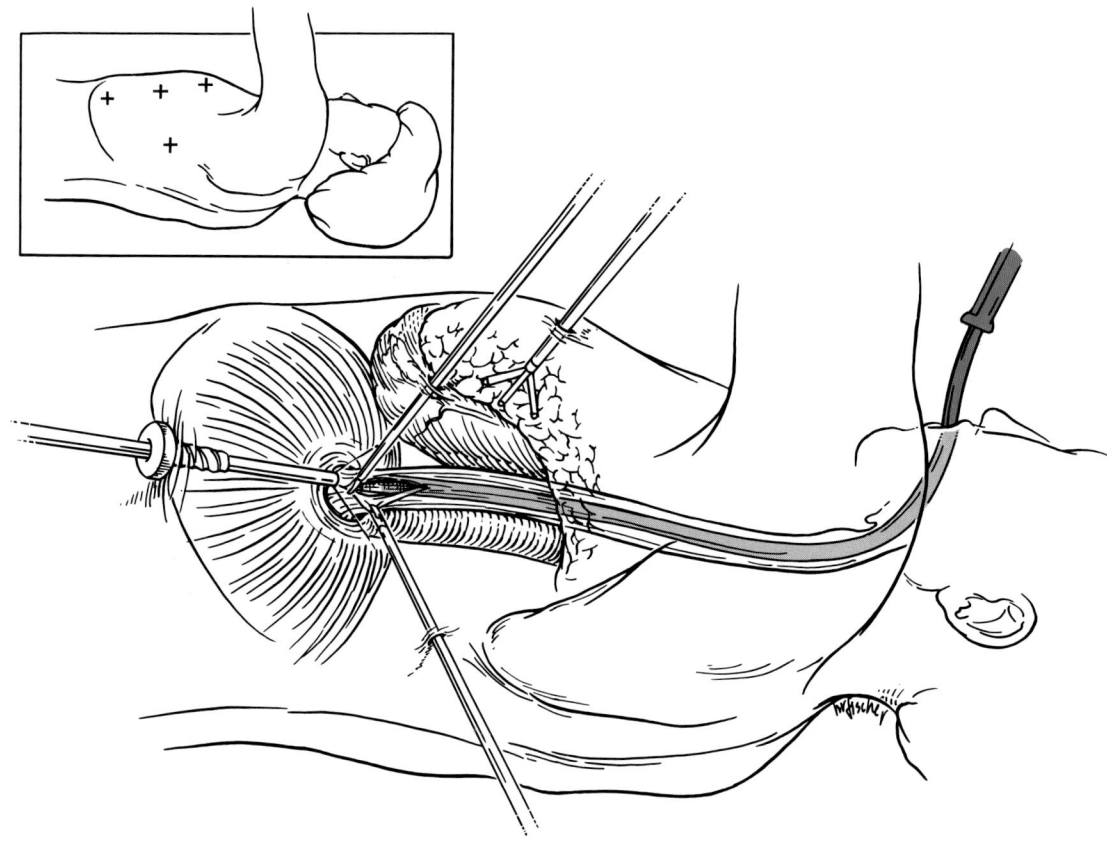

Figure 5-II-4

Thoracoscopic Myotomy

The patient is placed in the lateral position, and the left lung is collapsed. The camera port is placed laterally near the eighth intercostal space, and working ports are placed two interspaces higher, both anterior and posterior to the camera port (**inset**). Additional ports are placed to elevate the lung superiorly and to retract the diaphragm inferiorly (latter not shown). The myotomy is begun 5 cm above the esophagogastric junction and extended distally until the lower esophageal sphincter has been completely divided. An indwelling esophagoscope is used to determine the appropriate distal extent of myotomy and to insufflate air to ascertain whether mucosal injury has occurred during myotomy. The muscularis propria is dissected from the mucosa as described in Figure 5-II-2*C*.

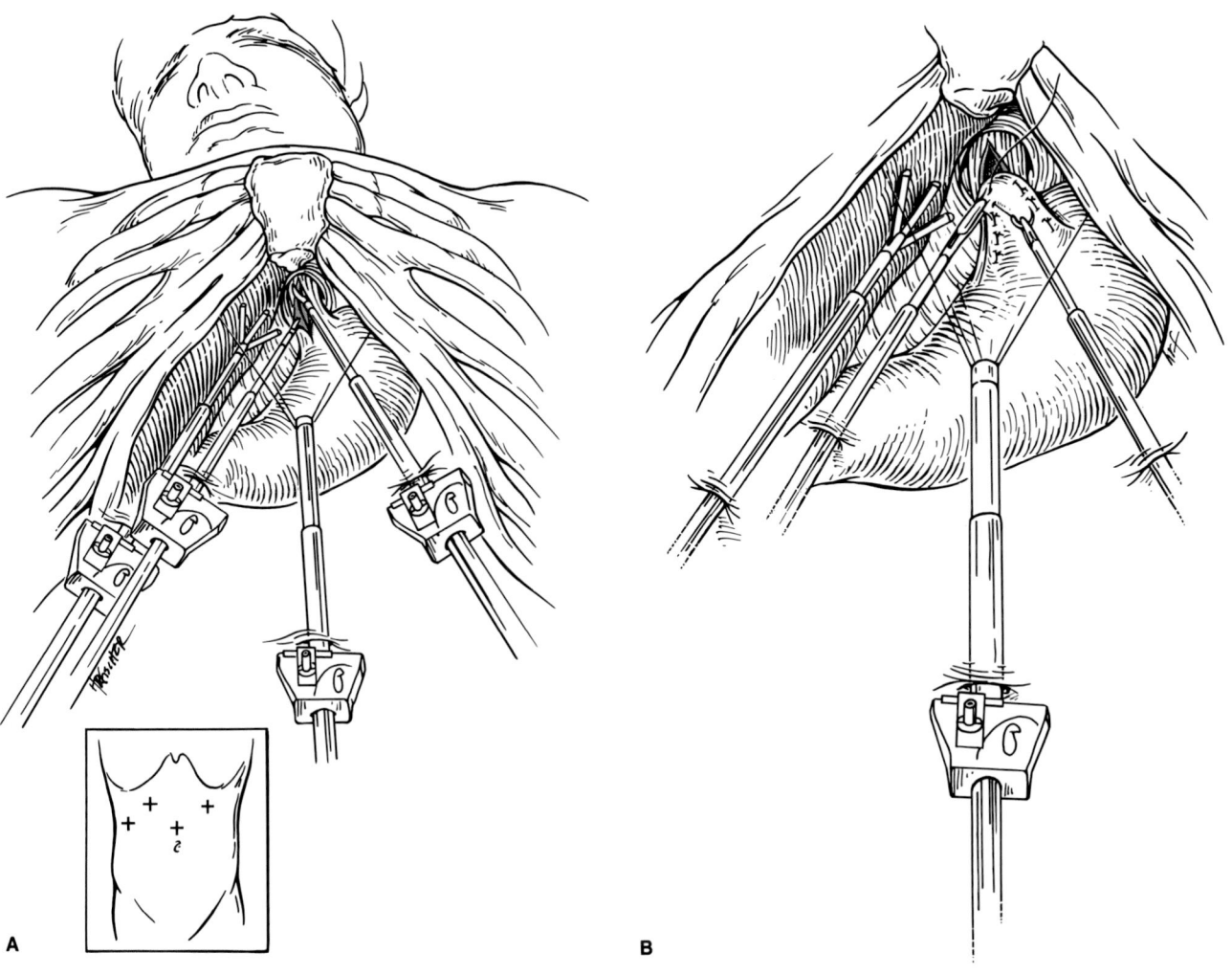

A   B

Figure 5-II-5

Laparoscopic Myotomy and Fundoplication

(**A**) The patient is placed in the lithotomy position, and the surgeon stands at the foot of the table between the patient's legs. After intraabdominal insufflation of carbon dioxide, the camera port is placed in a supraumbilical site, and operating ports are placed superiorly on either side of it. Additional ports are placed for retraction of the liver and to assist in the dissection of the gastroesophageal junction if necessary (**inset**). The myotomy is performed from a point 1 to 2 cm distal to the esophagogastric junction and is extended superiorly for 5 cm. The muscularis propria is dissected from the mucosa as described in Figure 5-II-2C.

(**B**) Abdominal approaches to myotomy for achalasia result in a high incidence of gastroesophageal reflux unless a modified fundoplication is added to the procedure. A portion of the gastric fundus is sutured to the cut edges of the esophageal muscle and overlies the myotomy. This partial wrap is performed with interrupted sutures and covers up to 180 degrees of the esophageal circumference.

SECTION III   *Gastroesophageal Reflux*

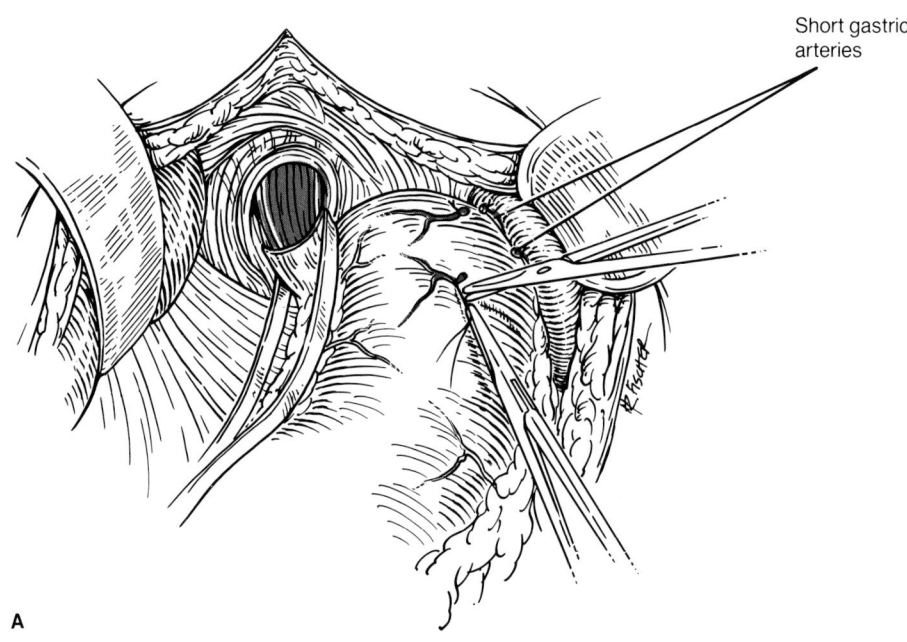

Short gastric
arteries

A

Figure 5-III-1

Total Fundoplication: Abdominal Approach (Nissen)

(**A**) The abdominal esophagus is mobilized and encircled with a small rubber drain. Several proximal short gastric vessels are divided to facilitate mobilization of the gastric fundus.

(**B**) The esophagus is retracted laterally, exposing the diaphragmatic crura. Heavy, nonabsorbable crural stitches are placed to calibrate the esophageal hiatus to an appropriate size. The hiatus should admit the tip of one finger alongside the esophagus when the appropriate size calibration is accomplished.

(**C**) After removing the fat pad covering the esophagogastric junction, the esophagus is retracted caudally and the gastric fundus is manually passed posterior to it.

(**D**) Nonabsorbable stitches are placed between the gastric fundus to the left of the esophagus, through the esophagus, and through the gastric fundus that has been passed posteriorly and to the right of the esophagus. The figure illustrates three stitches in place, each separated by 1 cm from the next, creating a 2-cm wrap. The wrap is usually performed with a large rubber bougie in the esophagus (50F to 60F).

(**E**) The fundoplication sutures are tied, and the bougie is removed. The wrap rests without tension in its intraabdominal location. Sufficient redundancy of the wrap permits passage of a finger within the wrap alongside the esophagus.

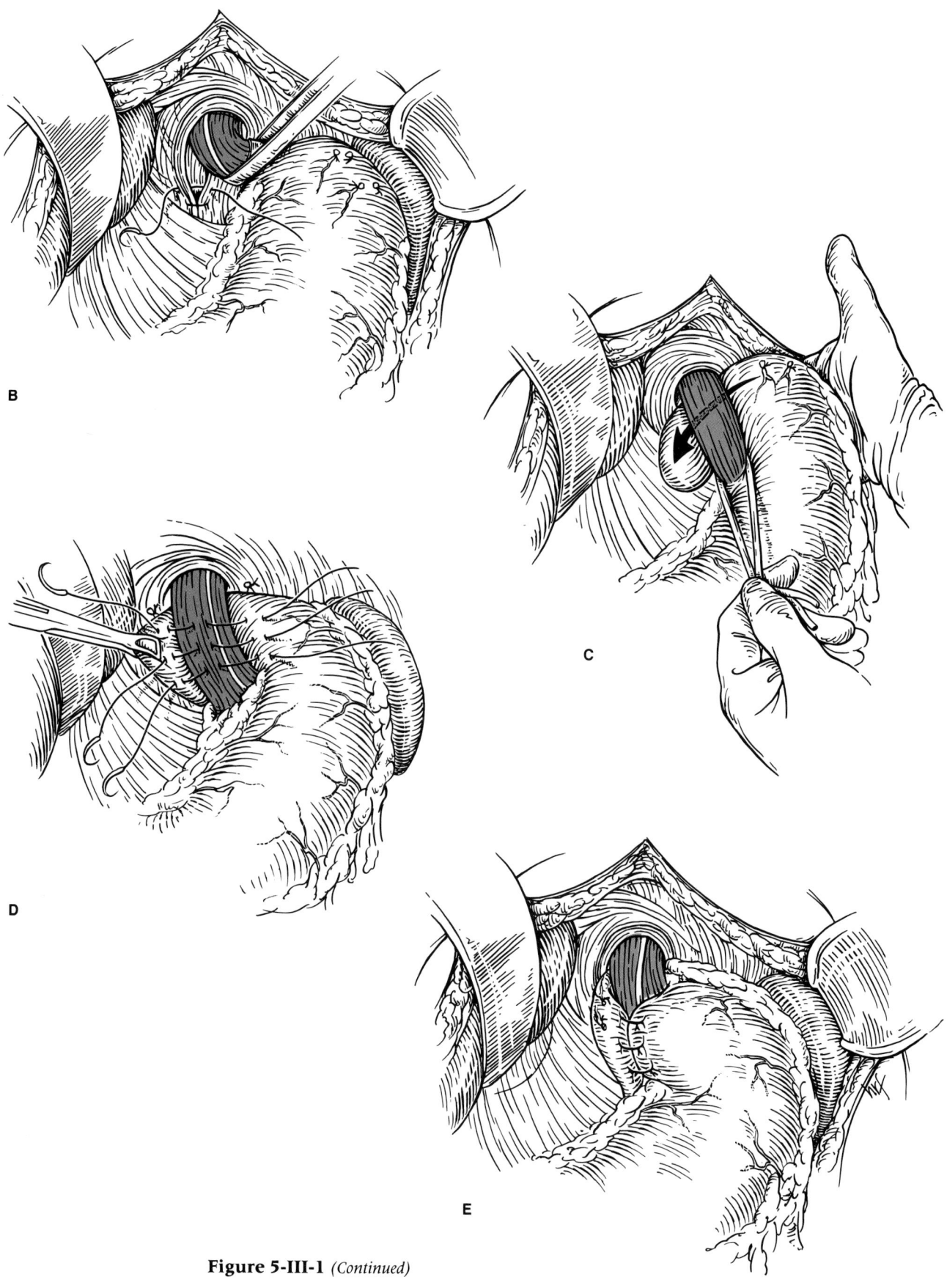

Figure 5-III-1 *(Continued)*

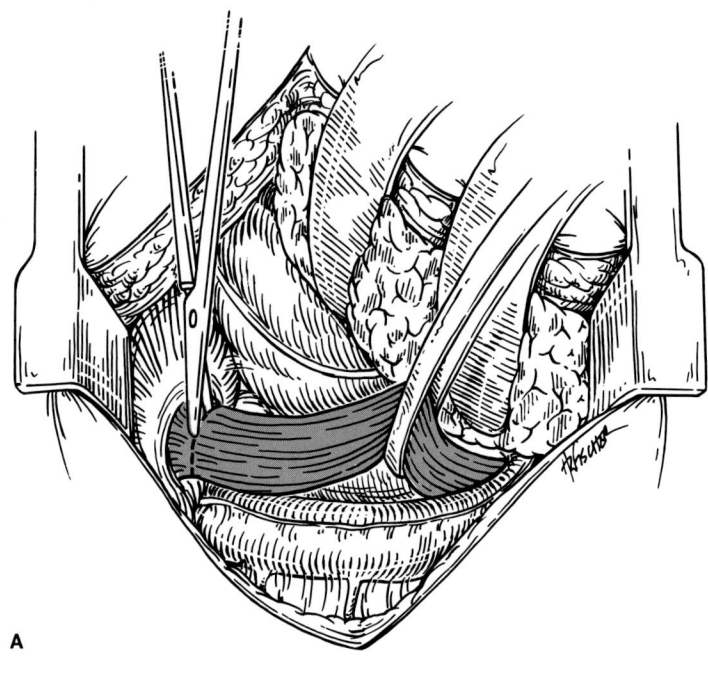

A

Figure 5-III-2

Total Fundoplication: Thoracic Approach

(**A**) The chest is entered through the seventh intercostal space, the pulmonary ligament is divided, and the distal esophagus is mobilized from its bed. The phrenoesophageal membrane is divided near its insertion on the esophagus to enable entry into the abdomen through the esophageal hiatus.

(**B**) The phrenoesophageal membrane is divided posteriorly to permit entry into the retrocrural space, where a large branch of the inferior phrenic artery (Belsey's artery) is often found. A complete dissection in this region exposes both crura, the free retroperitoneal space, and the left lobe of the liver.

(**C**) The fat pad overlying the esophagogastric junction is excised to permit apposition of the gastric serosa to the esophagus.

(**D**) Crural stitches are placed but not tied until the completion of the fundoplication. Several short gastric vessels are divided, and the gastric fundus is wrapped posteriorly around the esophagus.

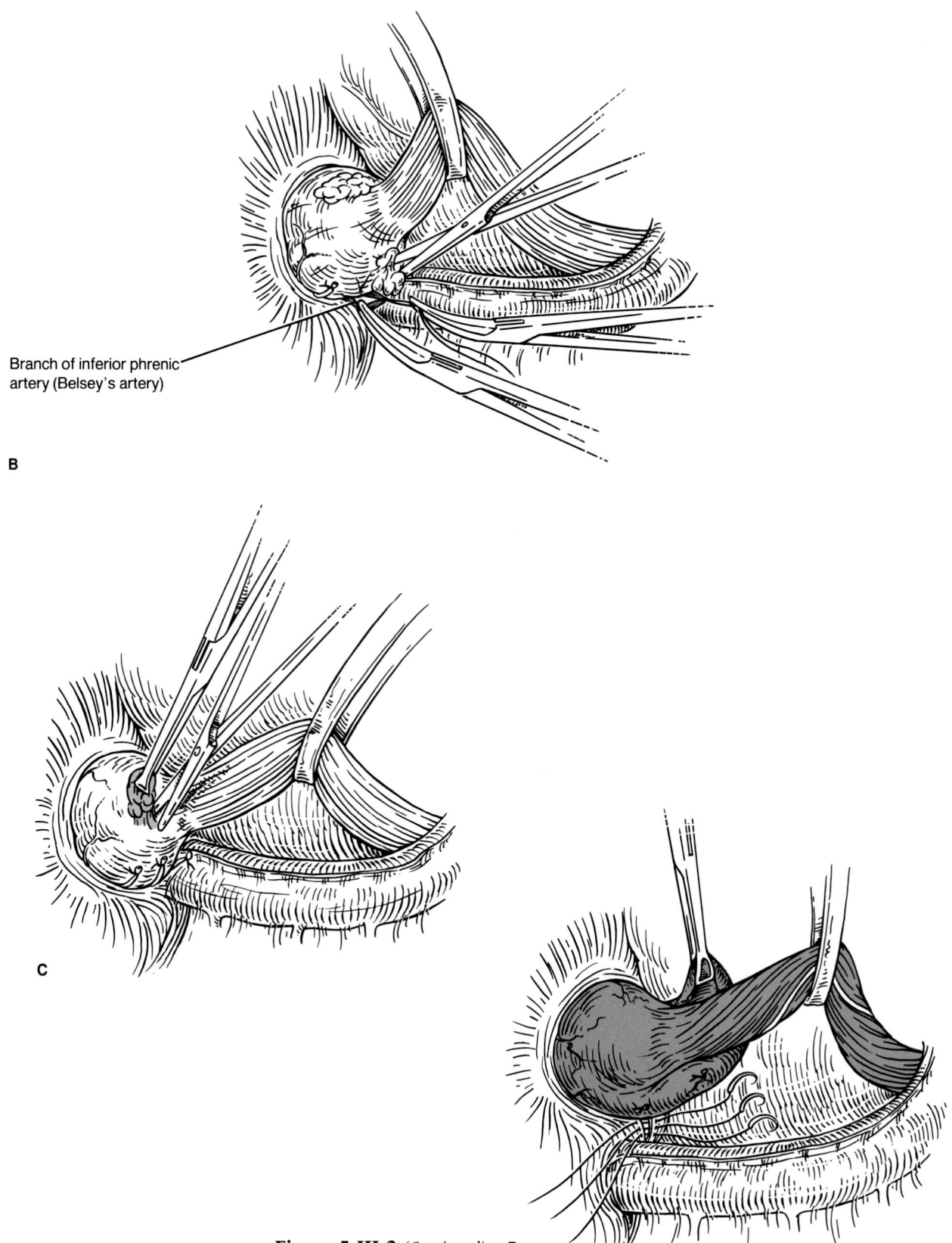

Branch of inferior phrenic
artery (Belsey's artery)

B

C

Figure 5-III-2 *(Continued)* **D**

(Figure continues on page 128)

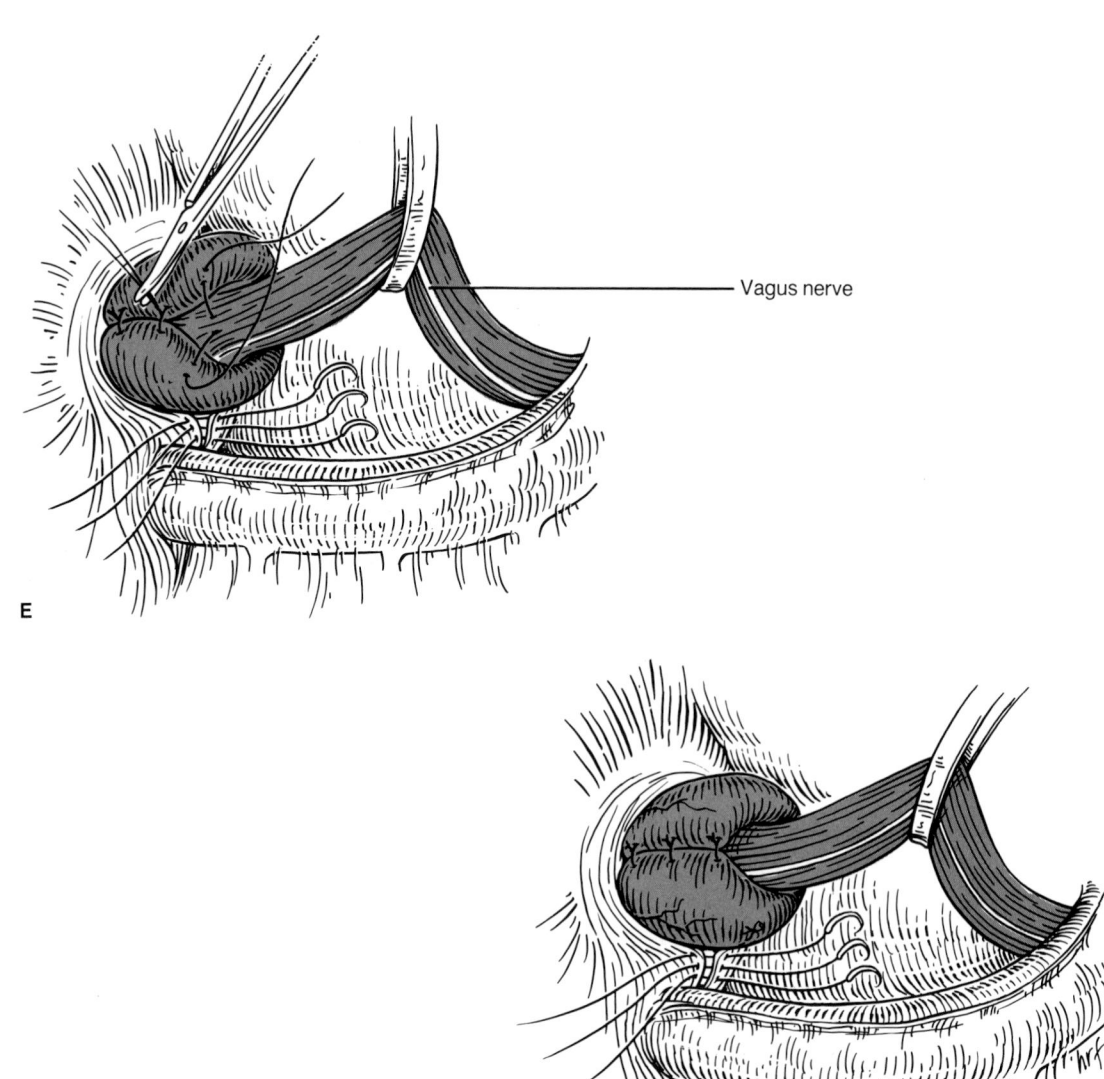

Figure 5-III-2 *(Continued)*

(E) Three interrupted sutures are placed through the gastric fundus to the left of the esophagus, through the esophagus, and again through the gastric fundus lying to the right of the esophagus. These are separated by 1 cm, providing a 2-cm wrap on completion of the fundoplication.

(F) The fundoplication sutures are tied. The wrap is manually reduced into the abdomen, where it should rest without tension. The crural stitches are then tied to calibrate the esophageal hiatus so that it easily admits a single finger alongside the esophagus.

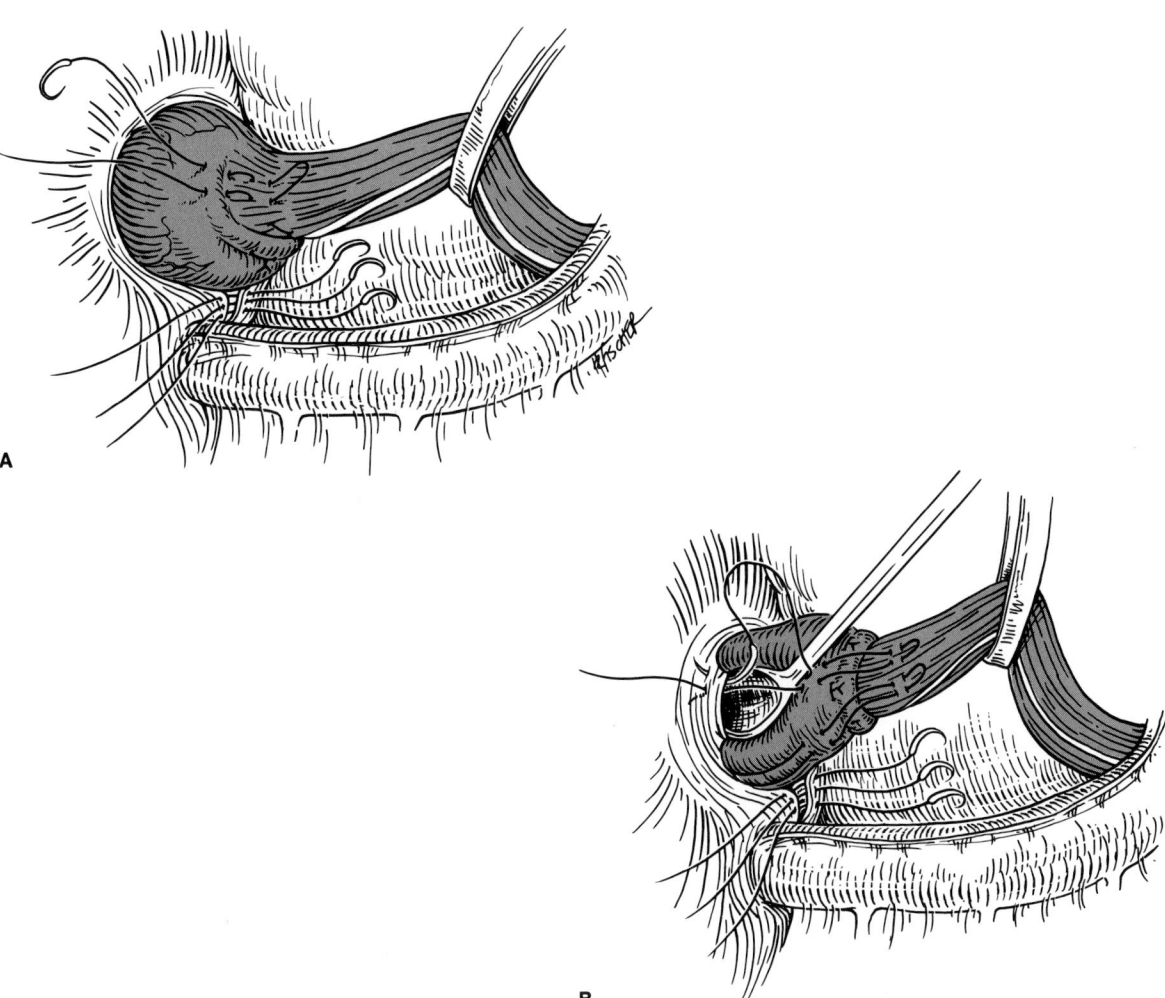

Figure 5-III-3

Partial Fundoplication (Belsey Mark IV)

(**A**) A Belsey Mark IV partial fundoplication is performed using a transthoracic approach, entering the chest in the seventh interspace. The pulmonary ligament is divided, and the distal esophagus and stomach are mobilized. Crural stitches are placed but not tied until the completion of the fundoplication. The fat pad overlying the esophagogastric junction is removed. The partial fundoplication wrap is begun by placing a mattress suture through the stomach 1 cm distal to the esophagogastric junction and through the esophagus 1 cm proximal to the esophagogastric junction. Similar stitches are placed alongside the anterior and posterior vagus nerves so that the wrap will encompass 240 to 270 degrees of the esophageal circumference.

(**B**) The first row sutures have been tied, creating the initial portion of the partial fundoplication. A second row of sutures is placed in the same position as the first, encompassing an additional 1 cm of the esophagus proximally and an additional 1 cm of the stomach distally. The ends of the suture are brought through the diaphragm close to the margin of the central tendon.

(Continued)

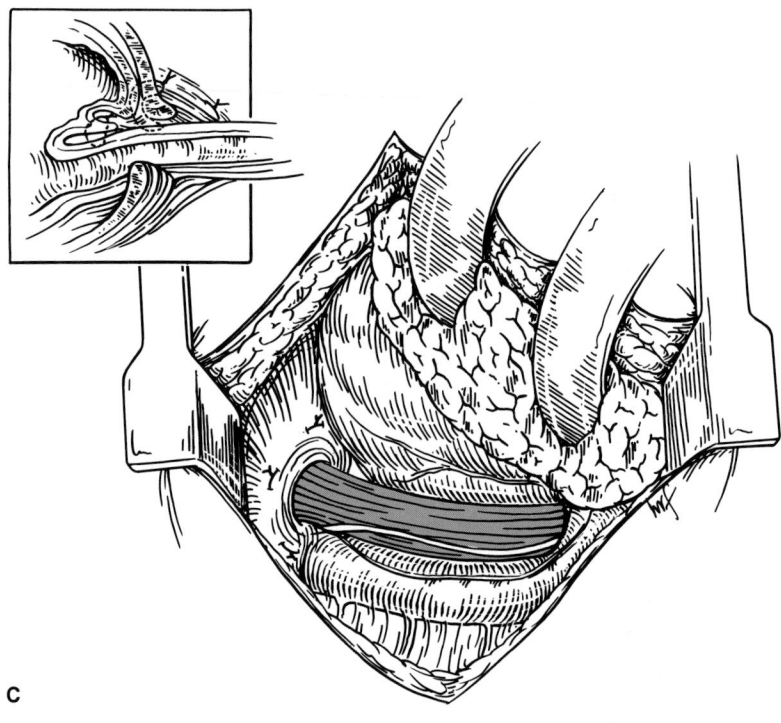

c

Figure 5-III-3 *(Continued)*

(**C**) The wrap is reduced below the diaphragm, and the fundoplication sutures in the second row are tied, anchoring the stomach to the underside of the diaphragm (**inset**). The crural sutures are then tied to calibrate the esophageal hiatus.

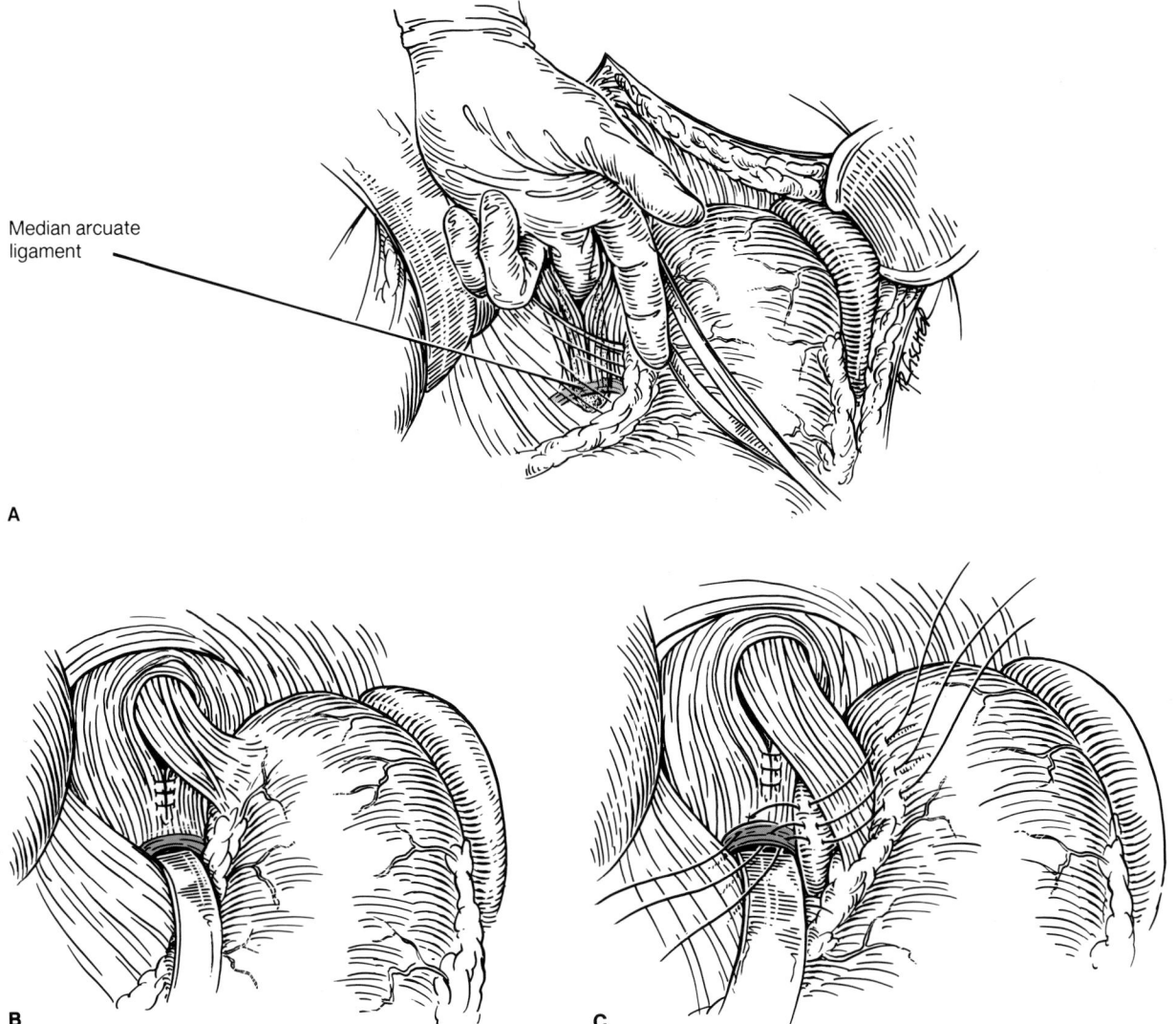

Median arcuate
ligament

A

B

C

Figure 5-III-4

Partial Fundoplication (Hill)

(**A**) A Hill partial fundoplication is illustrated as performed through an abdominal approach. The abdominal esophagus is mobilized, encircled with a flat rubber drain, and retracted laterally. The diaphragmatic crura are identified, and dissection is carried down posteriorly to the median arcuate ligament as it crosses the abdominal aorta.

(**B**) Crural stitches are placed and tied to calibrate the esophageal hiatus. A flat retractor or dilator is placed under the lip of the median arcuate ligament to elevate the ligament and protect the aorta.

(**C**) Division of the proximal short gastric vessels is sometimes necessary. The tip of the gastric fundus is passed posteriorly behind the esophagus. Nonabsorbable sutures are placed between the gastric fundus to the left of the esophagus, through the gastric fundus on the right of the esophagus, and through the median arcuate ligament.

(Continued)

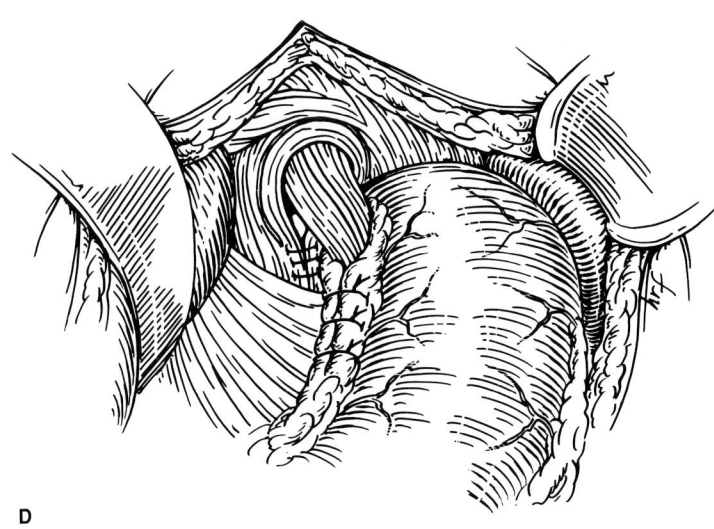

D

Figure 5-III-4 *(Continued)*

(**D**) The sutures are tied to complete the fundoplication.

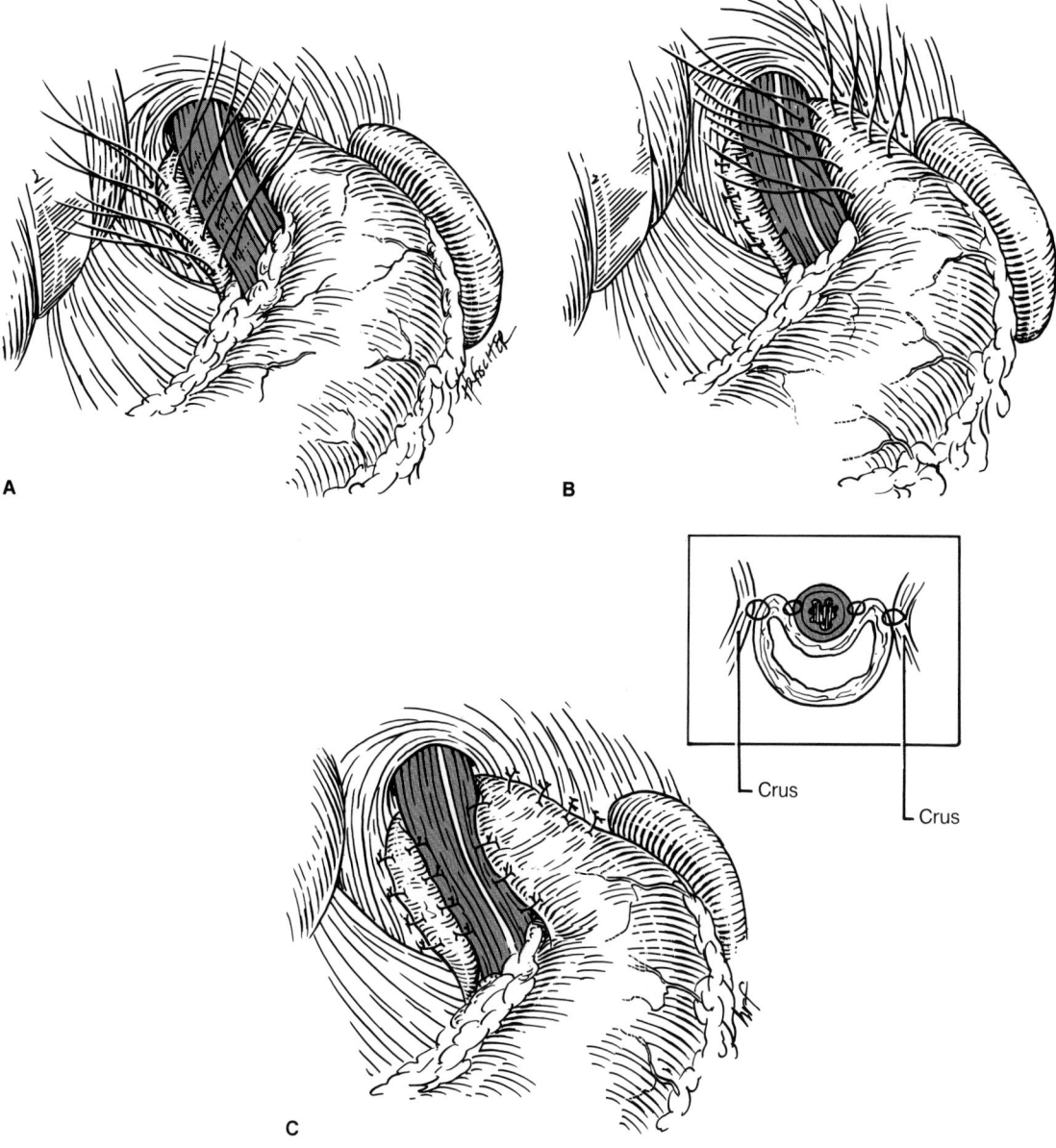

Crus

Crus

Figure 5-III-5

Partial Fundoplication (Toupet)

(**A**) A Toupet partial fundoplication performed through an abdominal approach is illustrated. The gastric fundus and abdominal fundus are mobilized, and the tip of the gastric fundus is passed posteriorly around the esophagus. Interrupted, nonabsorbable sutures are used to tack the wrapped portion of the fundus to the esophagus just anterior to the anterior vagus nerve. Similar sutures are used to stitch the wrapped portion of the fundus to the diaphragm near the edge of the right crus.

(**B**) The left side of the esophagus is stitched to the gastric fundus just anterior to the posterior vagus nerve. Similar sutures are used to stitch the gastric fundus to the diaphragm lateral to the left crus.

(**C**) The partial posterior fundoplication is complete, creating a 180- to 210-degree wrap around the esophagus (**inset**).

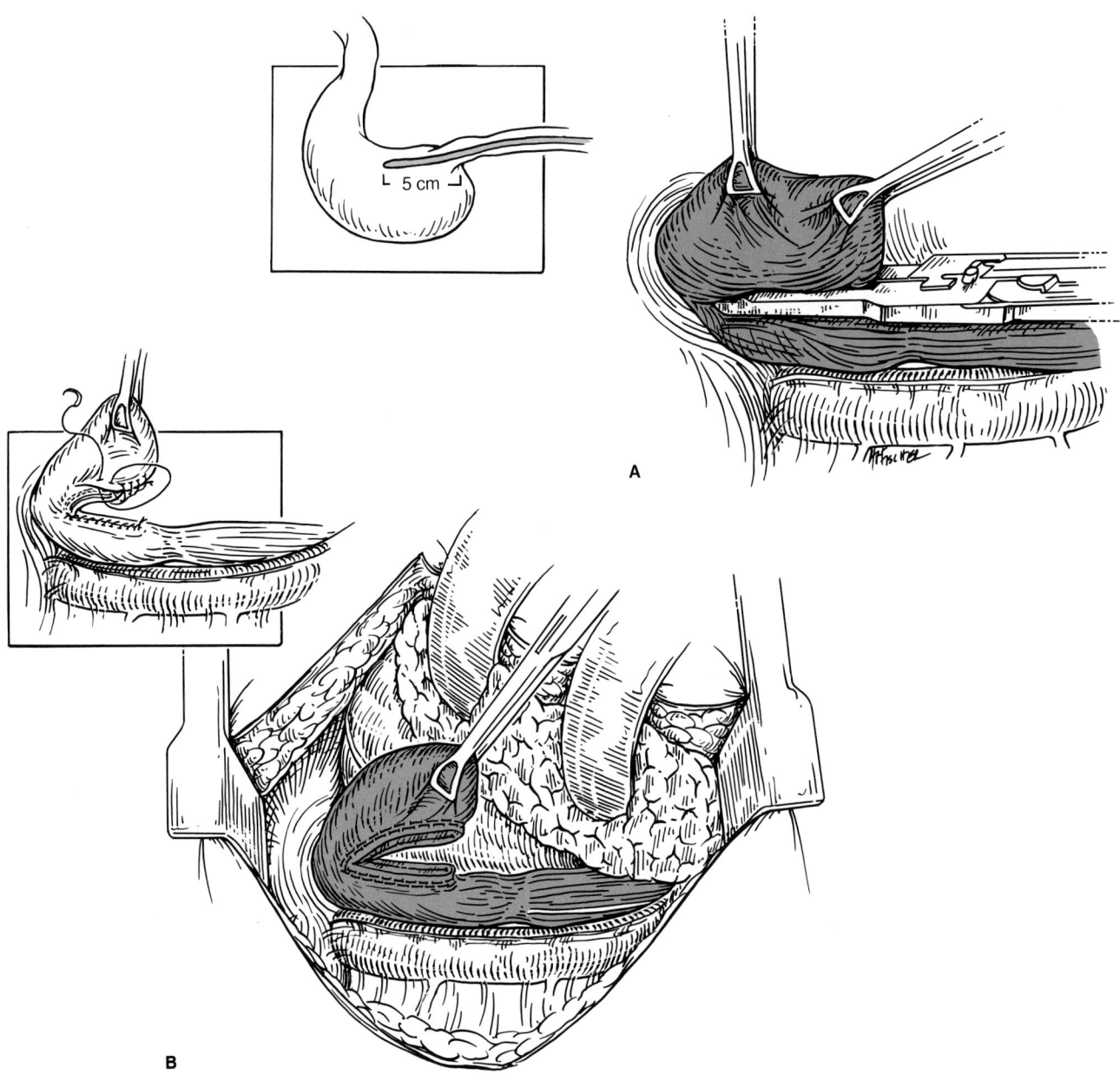

Figure 5-III-6

Esophageal Lengthening (Gastroplasty) and Fundoplication

(**A**) When esophageal shortening is present, and a fundoplication wrap that will rest comfortably in an intraabdominal location cannot be fashioned, an esophageal lengthening procedure (Collis gastroplasty) can be performed. This is best approached through a left thoracotomy that enters the chest in the seventh interspace. The esophagus and stomach are completely mobilized. A large dilator is passed down the esophagus and into the stomach. A linear cutting stapler is placed parallel to the dilator, beginning at the esophagogastric junction and extending inferiorly parallel to the lesser curvature, preserving all of the gastric fundus.

(**B**) The stapler is fired, and the stapled margins are oversewn (**inset**). This creates a neoesophagus and an enlarged gastric fundus with increased mobility.

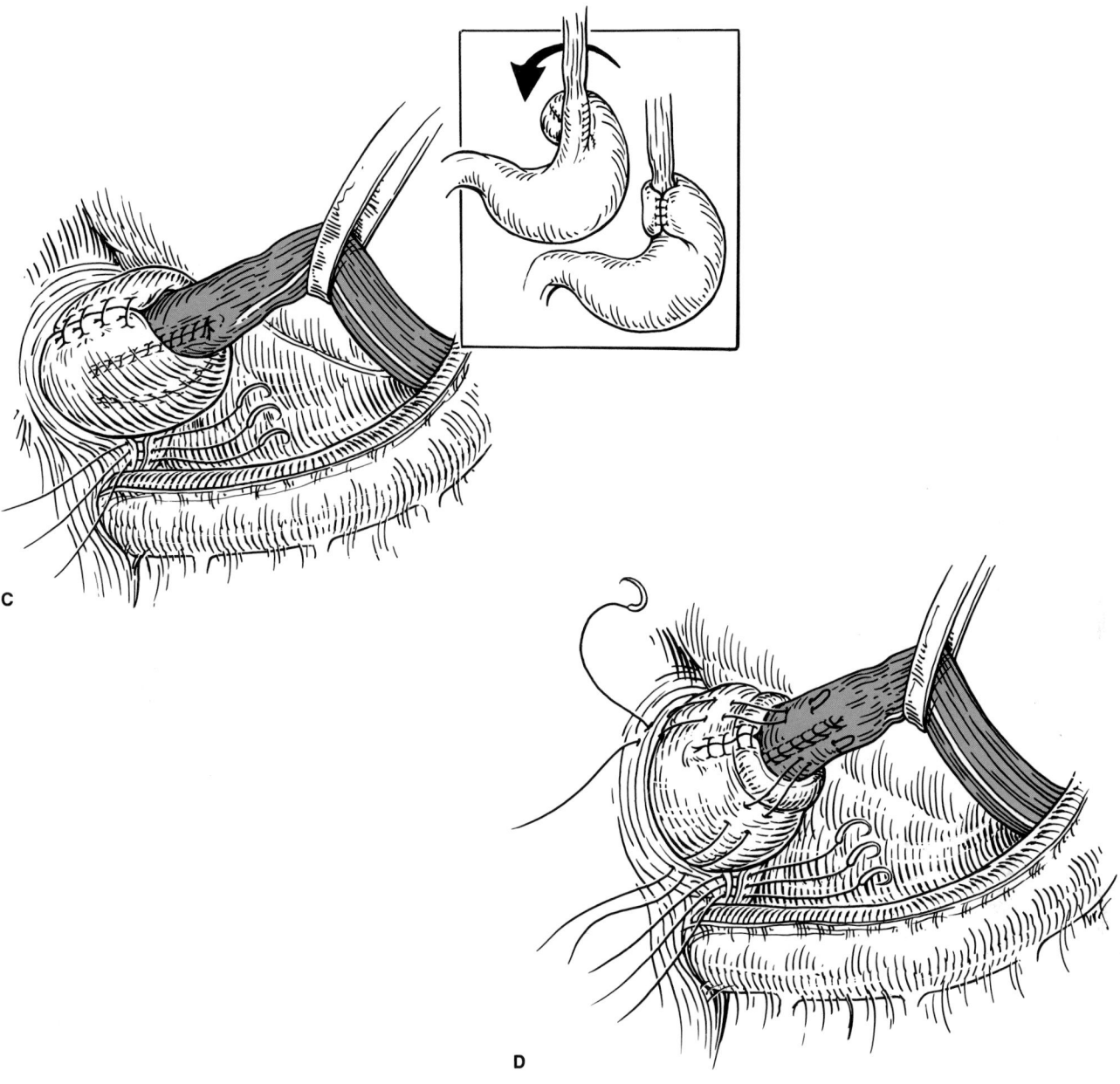

Figure 5-III-6 *(Continued)*

(**C**) The gastric fundus is used here to create either a partial or total fundoplication. This illustration depicts a total (Nissen) fundoplication in which the gastric fundus is wrapped posteriorly around the neoesophagus (**inset**) and sutured in place. After reduction of the fundoplication into the abdomen, the crural sutures are tied to calibrate the esophageal hiatus.

(**D**) The gastric fundus is used to create a partial (Belsey Mark IV) fundoplication. The first row of sutures is placed and tied. The second row of sutures is placed, which enables the fundoplication to be anchored below the diaphragm. After reduction of the fundoplication and tying of the fundoplication sutures, the crural stitches are tied to calibrate the esophageal hiatus.

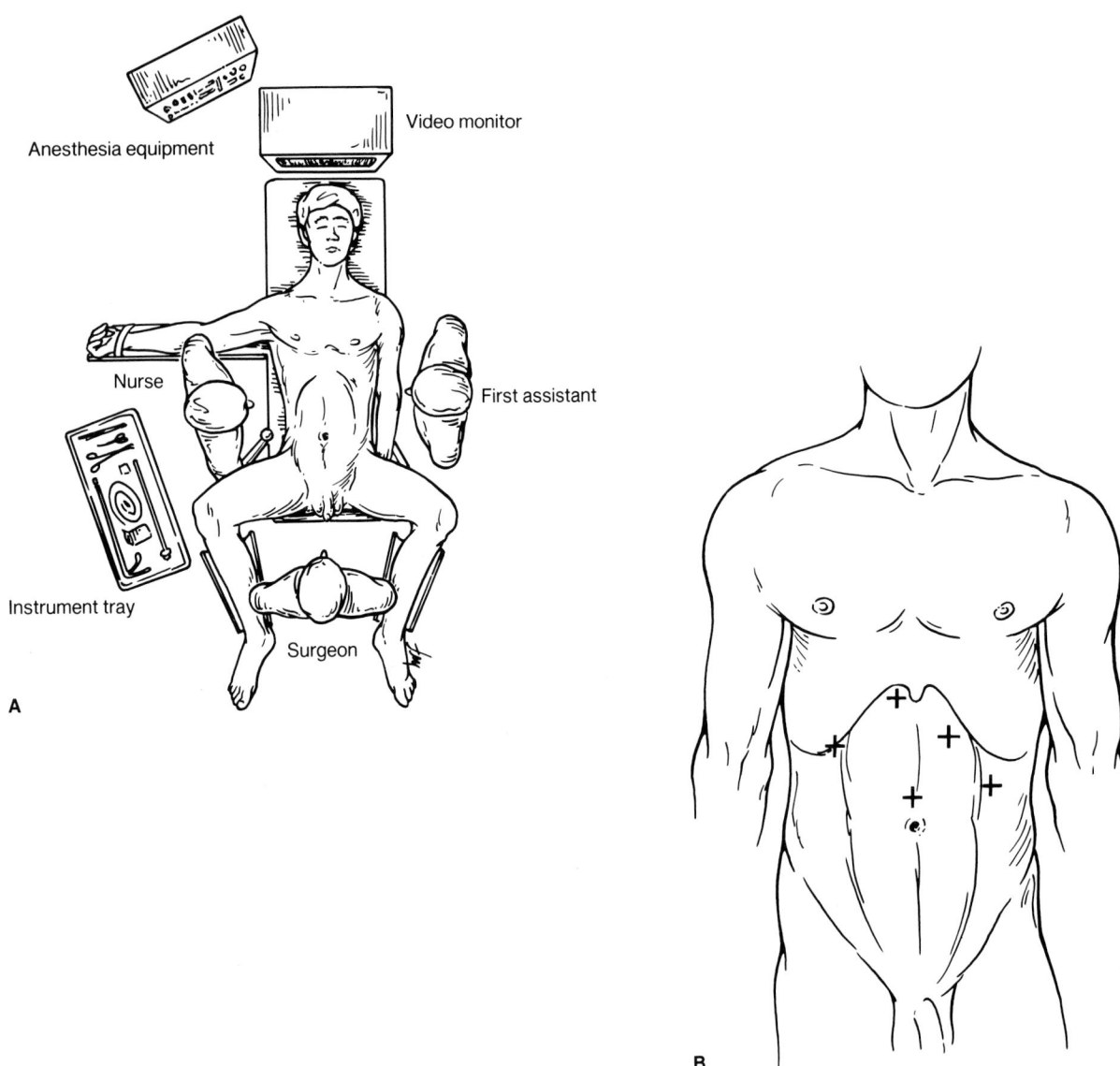

Figure 5-III-7

Laparoscopic Total Fundoplication

(**A**) The patient is positioned supine, with the legs in stirrups and the knees elevated and slightly bent. The first assistant stands at the patient's left, and a video monitor is placed near the head of the table.

(**B**) The camera port (10 to 12 mm) is placed in a supraumbilical position and retraction and operating ports (10 to 12 mm) are placed near the right and left costal margins, as indicated.

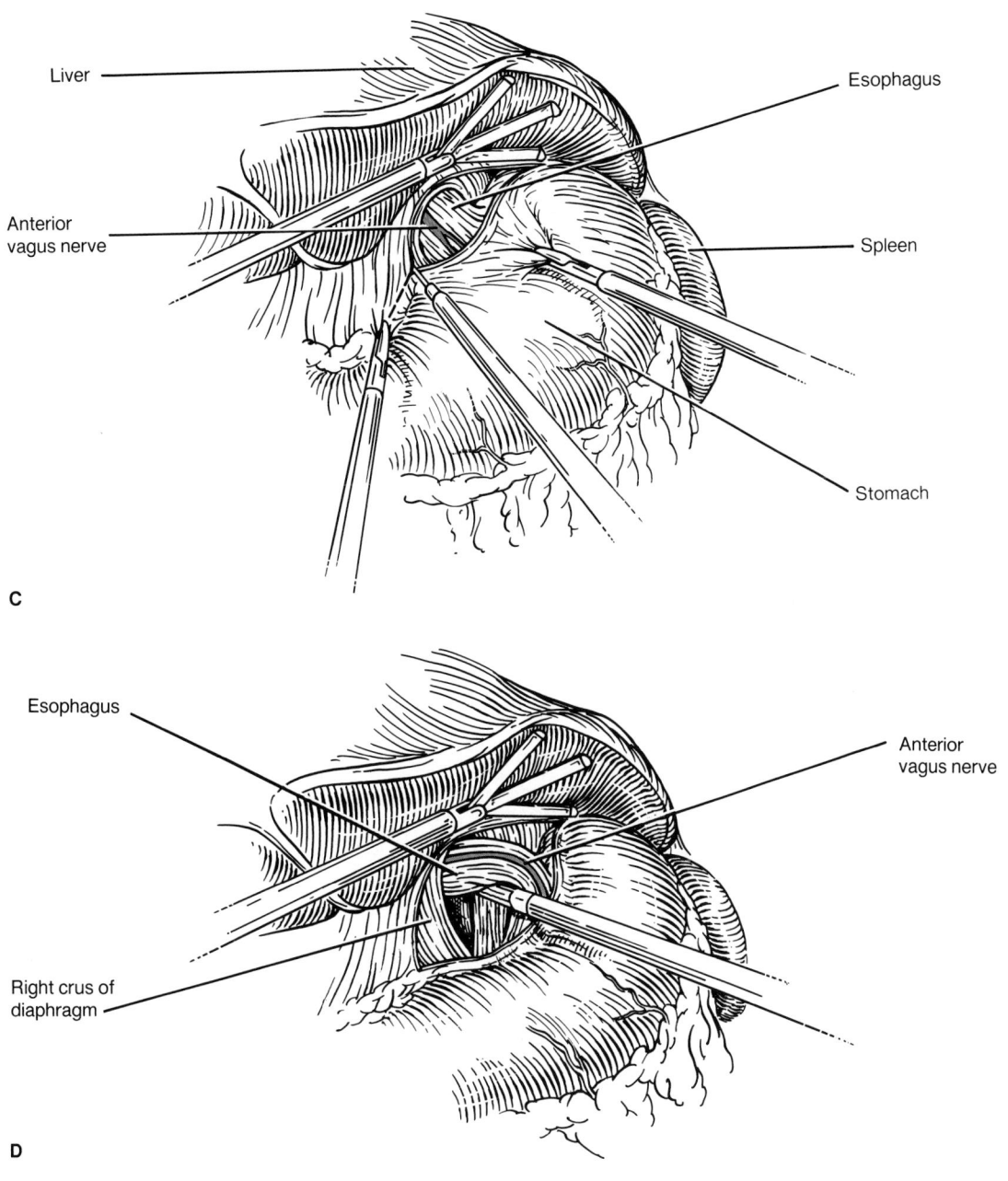

Figure 5-III-7 *(Continued)*

(C) The superior right and left subcostal ports are used for retraction of the liver and stomach, respectively. The surgeon uses the remaining two ports to begin mobilization of the esophagogastric junction by dividing the gastrohepatic omentum.

(D) The anterior surface of the esophagus is exposed, and dissection is carried along the right crus of the diaphragm, elevating the esophagus from its bed. The anterior vagus nerve is identified on the anteromedial side of the esophagus.

(Continued)

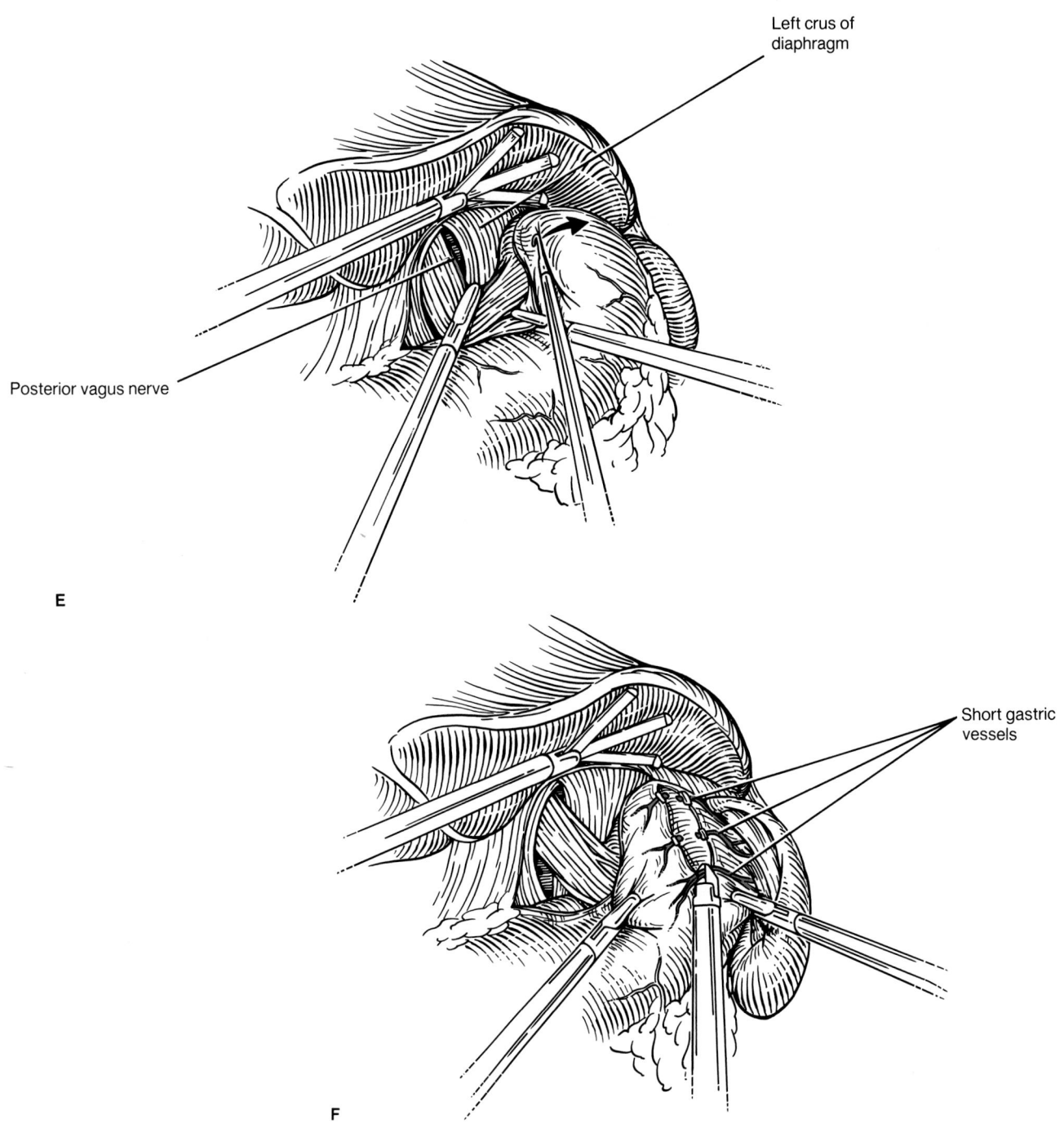

Figure 5-III-7 *(Continued)*

(**E**) Using a 30-degree angled telescope, the left crus is identified and the esophagus is dissected from it to again reveal the posterior aspect of the esophagus and the posterior vagus nerve. The stomach is retracted caudally to facilitate this exposure.

(**F**) The stomach is retracted inferomedially and, with the operative field visualized using the 30-degree angled telescope, several proximal short gastric vessels are clipped and divided to mobilize the gastric fundus.

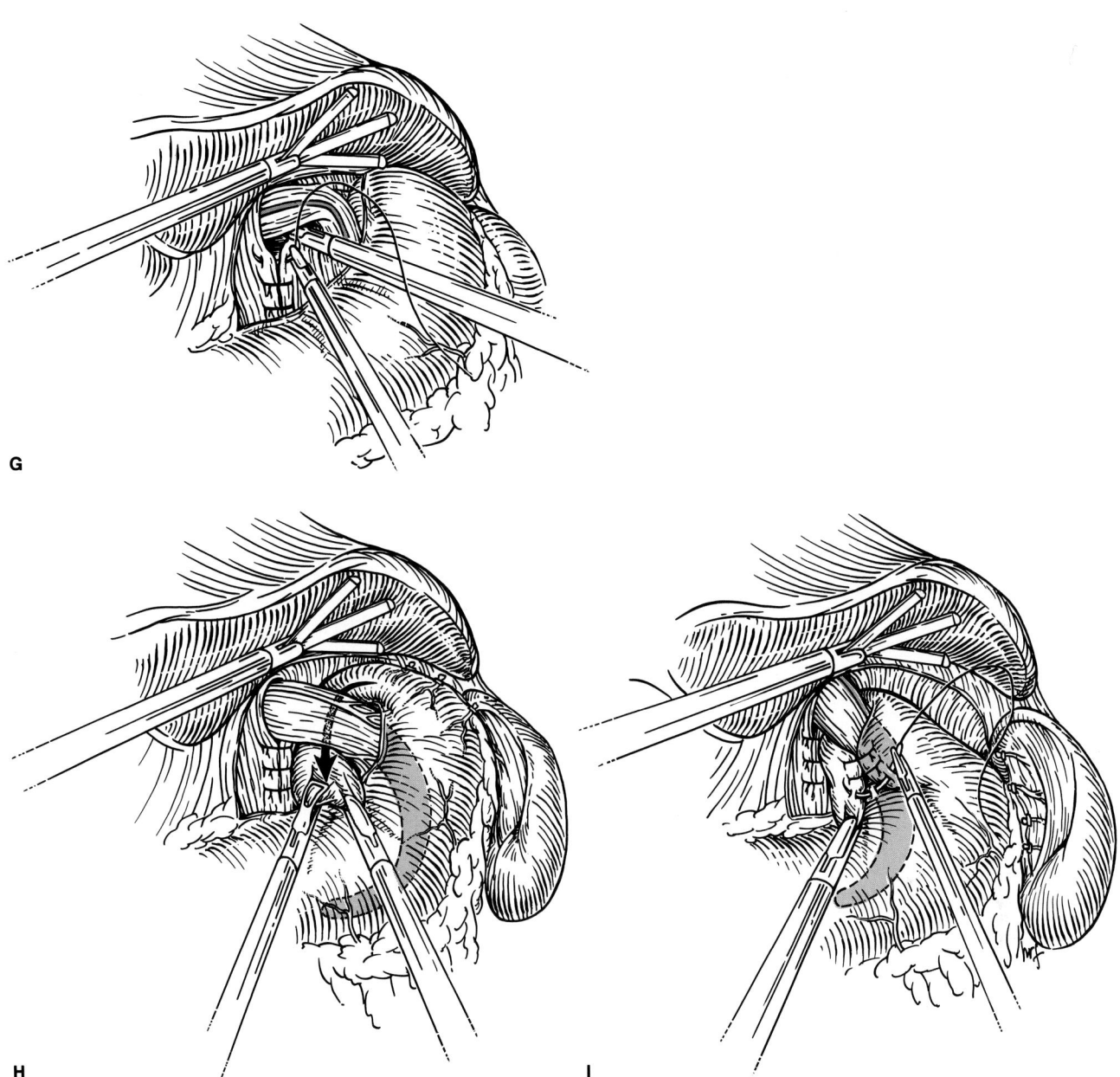

Figure 5-III-7 *(Continued)*

(G) Heavy crural sutures are placed and tied to calibrate the esophageal hiatus.

(H) The esophagogastric fat pad is removed. A large bougie is placed through the esophagus once the fundus has been wrapped posteriorly. Placement of the bougie before wrapping the fundus makes the latter maneuver difficult.

(I) Fundoplication sutures are placed through the lateral fundus, through the esophagus, and through the wrapped portion of fundus, then tied. The bougie is removed.

SECTION IV *Neoplasms*

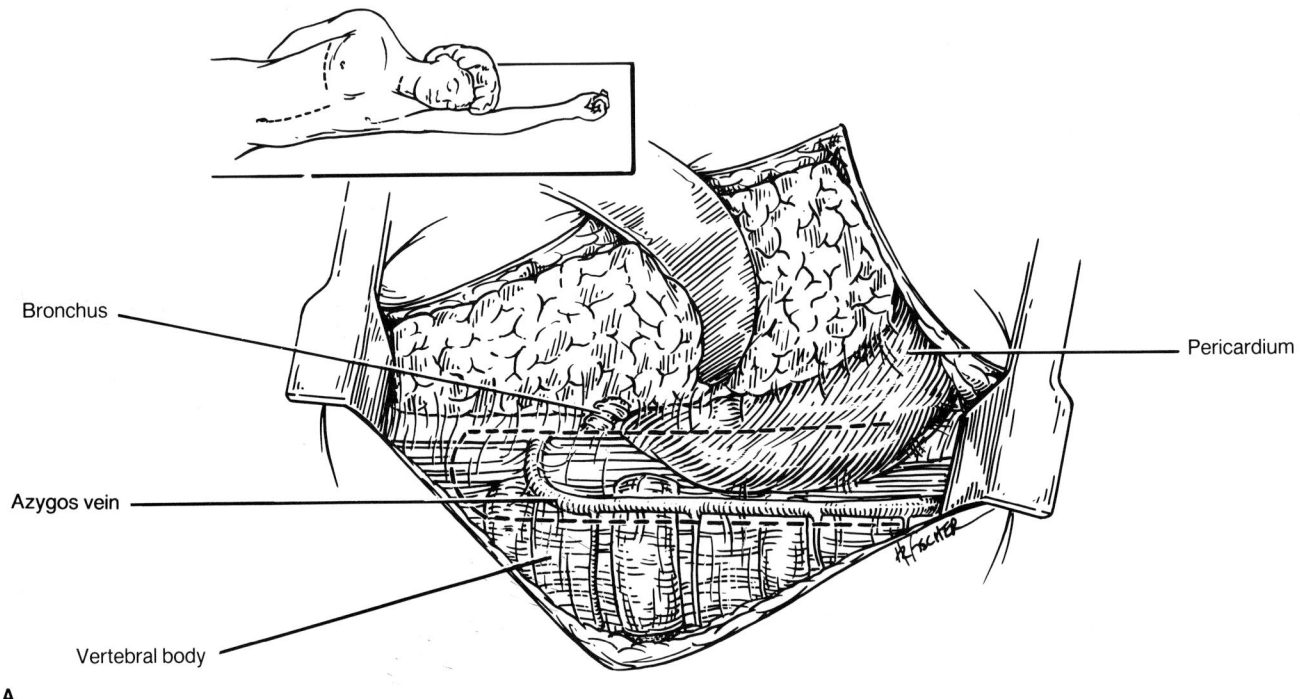

Bronchus

Pericardium

Azygos vein

Vertebral body

A

Figure 5-IV-1

Total Thoracic Esophagectomy: Open Approach

(**A**) A near-total thoracic esophagectomy is most commonly performed using a modified Ivor Lewis approach that includes a laparotomy, a thoracotomy, and in some cases, a cervical incision. (**Inset**) The patient can be placed in a semilateral position (assistant's view), in which case no repositioning is necessary to complete the operation. A true lateral position can also be used for the thoracotomy, but this requires repositioning the patient to perform the laparotomy and cervical incision (if included). The chest is opened through the fifth or sixth interspace. The typical extent of dissection is shown by the dashed line.

(**B**) Standard esophageal resection is begun by incising the mediastinal pleura posterior and anterior to the esophagus. The esophagus is mobilized at a distance of at least 5 cm from the gross extent of tumor and encircled with a tape or rubber drain to provide traction. All adventitial tissue surrounding the esophagus is included in the dissection. The pericardium and contralateral pleura remain intact. For middle and upper thoracic esophageal cancers, a segment of the azygos vein is resected with the esophagus, as illustrated. Some surgeons routinely resect the entire azygos vein and thoracic duct as part of this dissection.

(**C**) Once the thoracic esophagus is completely mobilized, dissection is carried through the phrenoesophageal membrane and into the abdomen. For low-lying tumors, a ring of diaphragm 1 cm wide is resected en bloc with the esophagus.

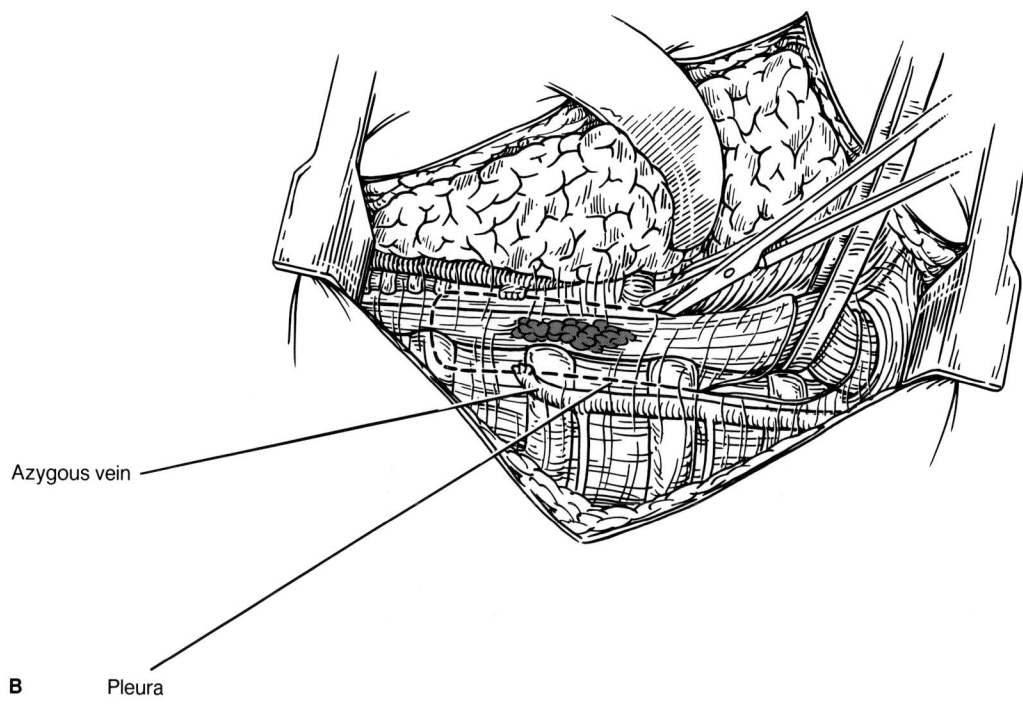

Azygous vein

B Pleura

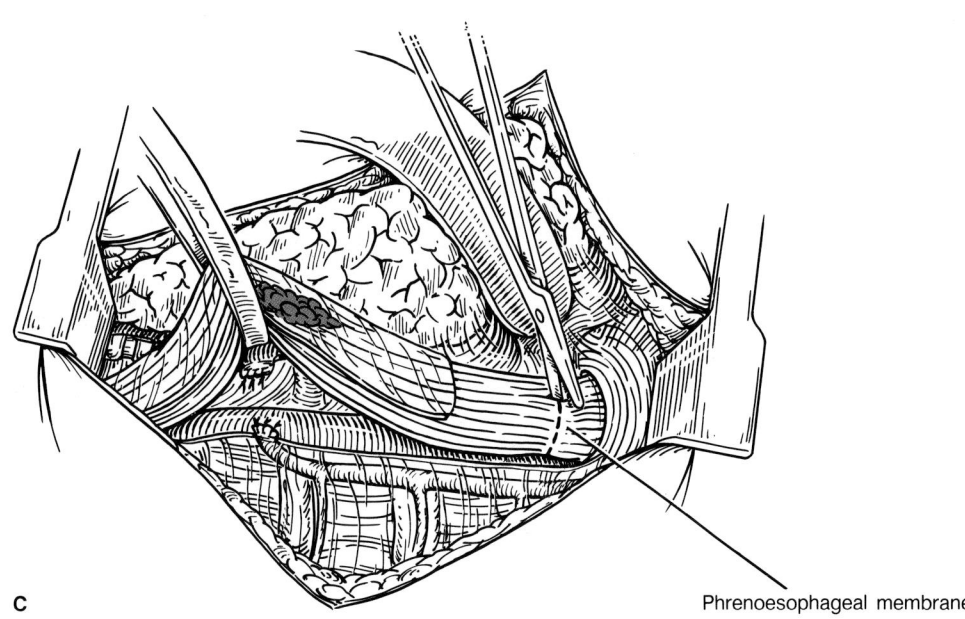

C

Phrenoesophageal membrane

Figure 5-IV-1 *(Continued)*

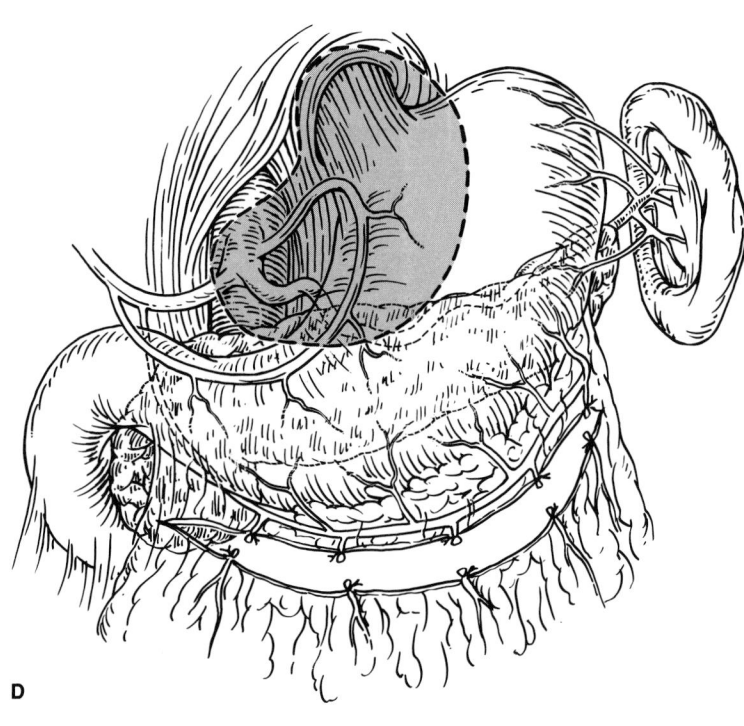

D

Figure 5-IV-1 *(Continued)*

(**D**) The extent of partial gastrectomy and abdominal dissection is illustrated. Reconstruction is most often accomplished using a gastric tube, the blood supply of which is provided by the right gastroepiploic artery. The greater omentum is divided peripheral to this arcade, with care taken to preserve the origin of the right gastroepiploic artery.

(**E**) After division of the short gastric vessels, the stomach is reflected superiorly, and the left gastric artery is divided at the level of its origin from the celiac axis. The coronary vein is similarly divided. All accompanying lymph nodes are dissected with the specimen.

(**F**) The gastrohepatic omentum is divided close to the liver, and the resection is carried through to the lesser curvature of the stomach four or five vascular arcades distal to the esophagogastric junction. Using a linear cutting stapler, a tube is created from the stomach by resecting the esophagogastric junction and the lesser curvature of the stomach at a minimum distance of 5 cm from gross tumor. An emptying procedure (pyloroplasty or pyloromyotomy) can be performed.

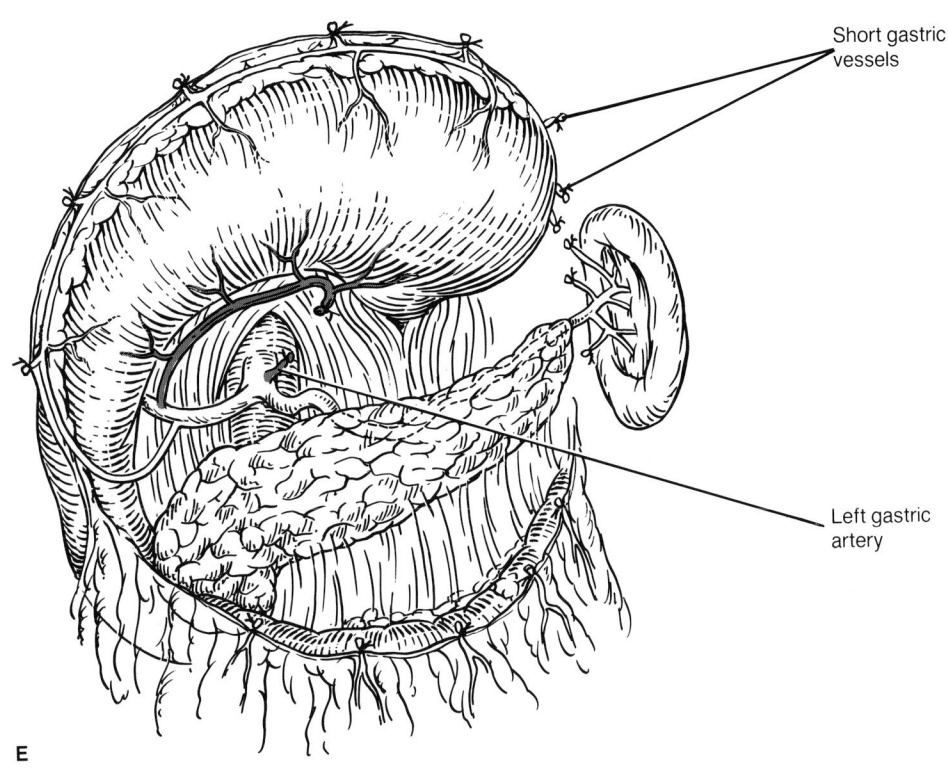

Short gastric
vessels

Left gastric
artery

E

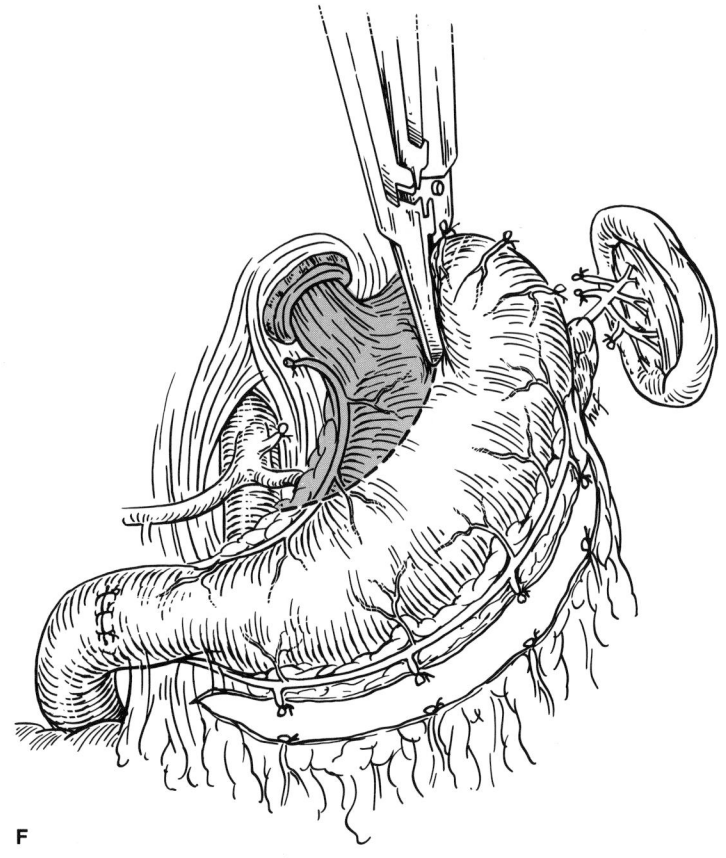

F

Figure 5-IV-1 *(Continued)*

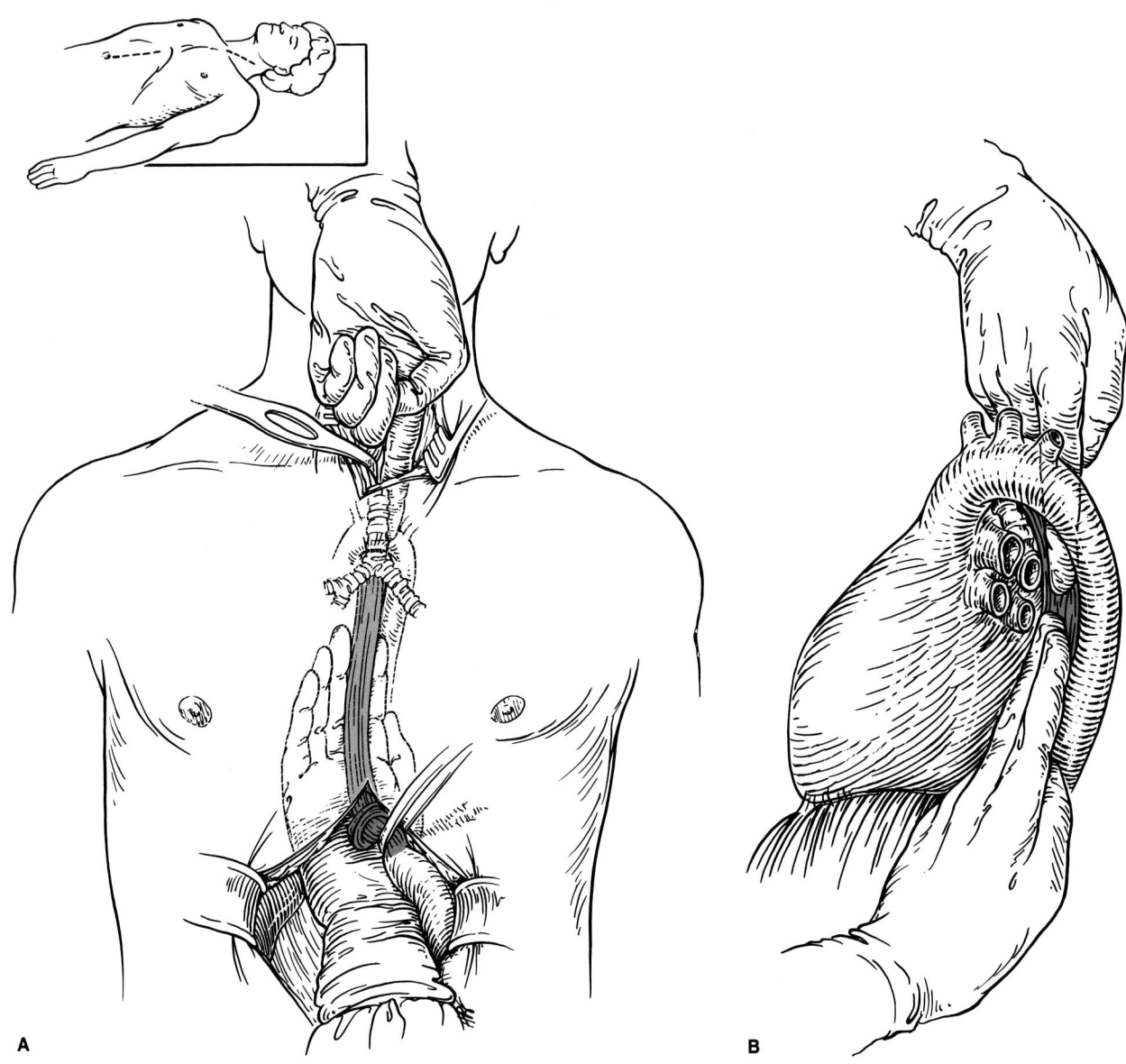

A

B

Figure 5-IV-2

Total Thoracic Esophagectomy: Transhiatal Approach

(**A**) Transhiatal esophagectomy is performed through a laparotomy and cervical incision. After the stomach is completely mobilized, the abdominal esophagus is dissected and encircled with tape or a rubber drain for use in retracting. The xiphisternum is elevated, and the mediastinal dissection on the esophagus is begun under direct vision by sharply or bluntly dividing esophageal attachments to the prevertebral fascia posteriorly and the pericardium anteriorly. The dissection is extended manually to the level of the carina or aortic arch. The cervical esophagus is mobilized, and circumferential dissection is carried to the level of the aortic arch.

(**B**) When the surgeon's hands meet through the two incisions near the level of the aortic arch, two fingers of the lower hand are used to strip lateral attachments from the esophagus along its anterolateral surfaces.

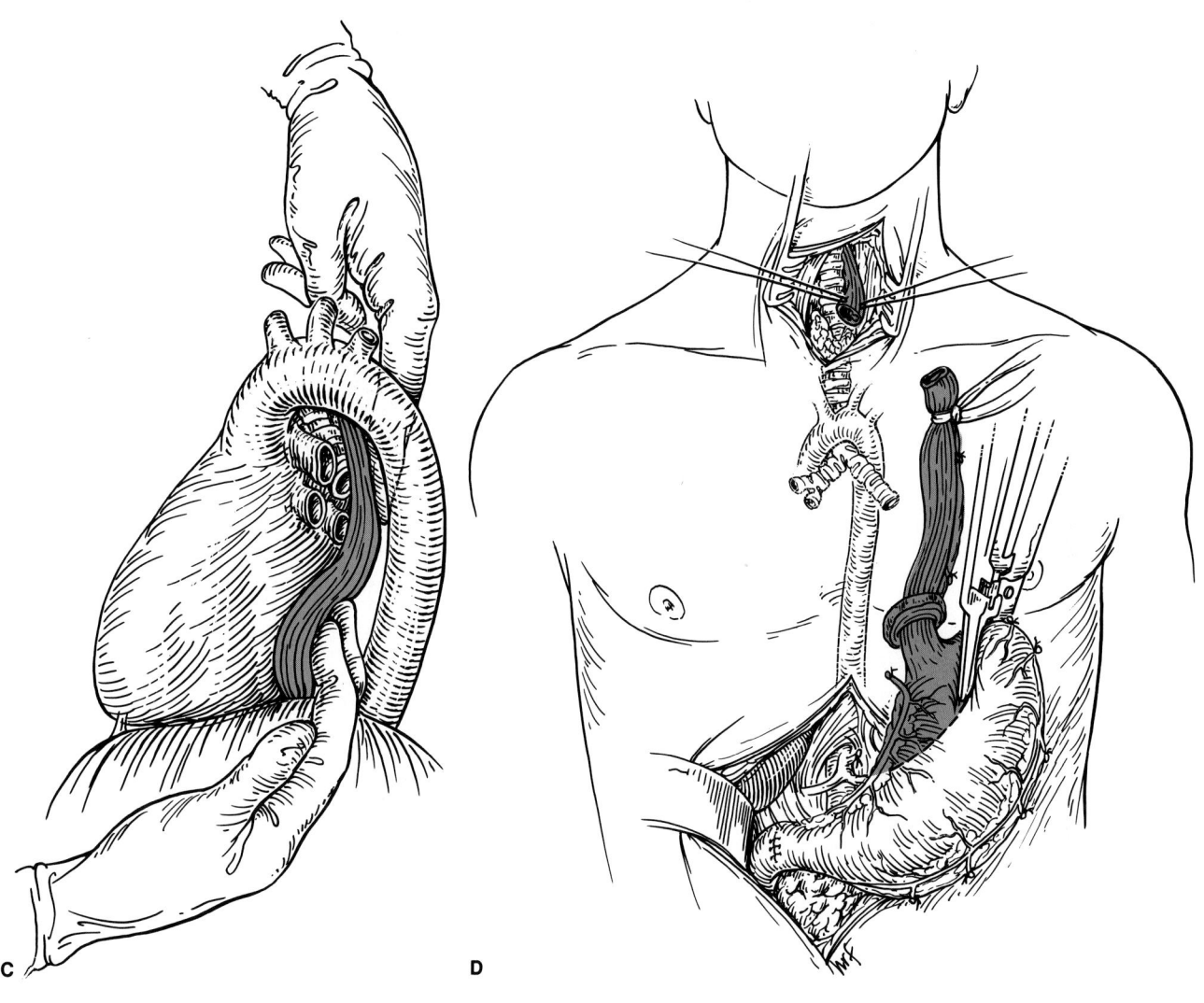

C

D

Figure 5-IV-2 *(Continued)*

(C) A similar blunt dissection of the lateral attachments is performed from posterior using two fingers of the surgeon's lower hand to complete the mobilization of the esophagus.

(D) The esophagus is divided and then withdrawn through the abdominal incision, where the resection is completed by excising the esophagogastric junction and lesser curvature of the stomach en bloc.

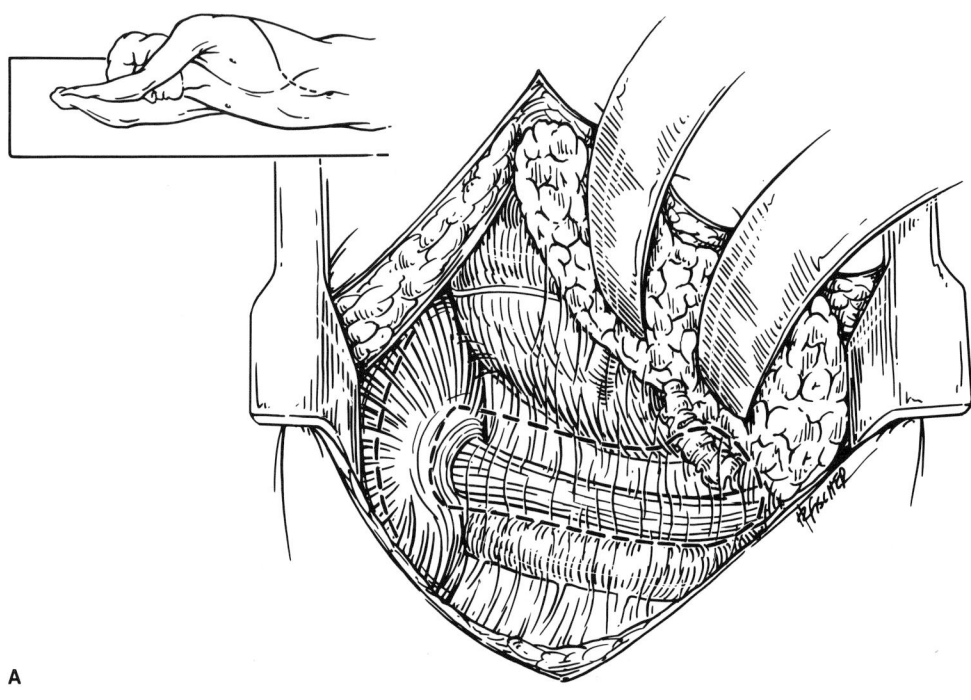

A

Figure 5-IV-3

Partial Esophagectomy: Left Thoracotomy Approach

(**A**) Tumors of the distal esophagus or esophagogastric junction can be approached exclusively through a left thoracotomy or left thoracoabdominal incision (**inset**). The chest is entered through the sixth or seventh interspace. The extent of standard dissection is illustrated by the dashed line over the mediastinum. Exposure of the upper abdominal contents is attained through a peripheral incision in the diaphragm made 1 to 2 cm from its insertion in the chest wall, extending from near the sternum to the tip of the spleen.

(**B**) The thoracic portion of the dissection is accomplished by incising the mediastinal pleura posterior and anterior to the esophagus. Mobilization of the esophagus and the surrounding adventitial tissues is begun at least 5 cm from the proximal gross extent of tumor. The pericardium and contralateral pleura are left intact. After completion of the abdominal and thoracic portions of the dissection, a rim of diaphragm 1 to 2 cm wide is resected en bloc with the specimen. Blunt dissection beneath the aortic arch can be performed and extended superior to the arch into the neck if a total esophagectomy is indicated.

(**C**) Exposure of upper abdominal organs through the transdiaphragmatic approach is illustrated. The stomach is reflected superiorly after mobilization from the omentum (preserving the right gastroepiploic vessels) and division of the short gastric vessels. The left gastric artery is divided at its origin from the celiac axis, and associated lymph nodes are resected with the specimen.

(**D**) After the retroperitoneal dissection is completed, the gastrohepatic omentum is divided along the liver to meet the lesser curvature of the stomach four or five vascular arcades distal to the esophagogastric junction. After all dissection is completed, the stomach is fashioned into a tube by resecting the esophagogastric junction and lesser curvature using a linear cutting stapler following a line at least 5 cm from gross distal extent of tumor. A gastric emptying procedure can be performed (*not shown*).

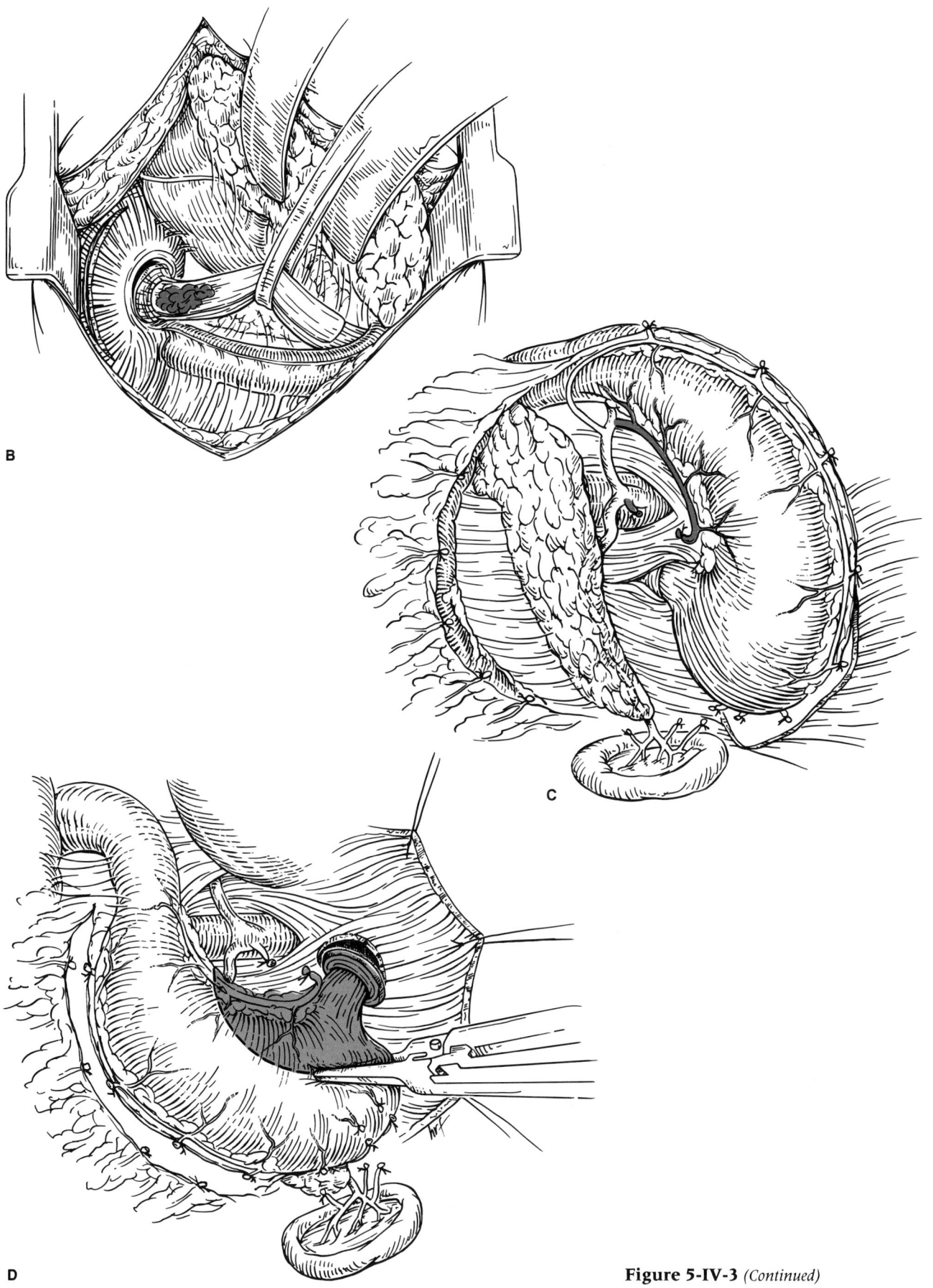

B

C

D

Figure 5-IV-3 (Continued)

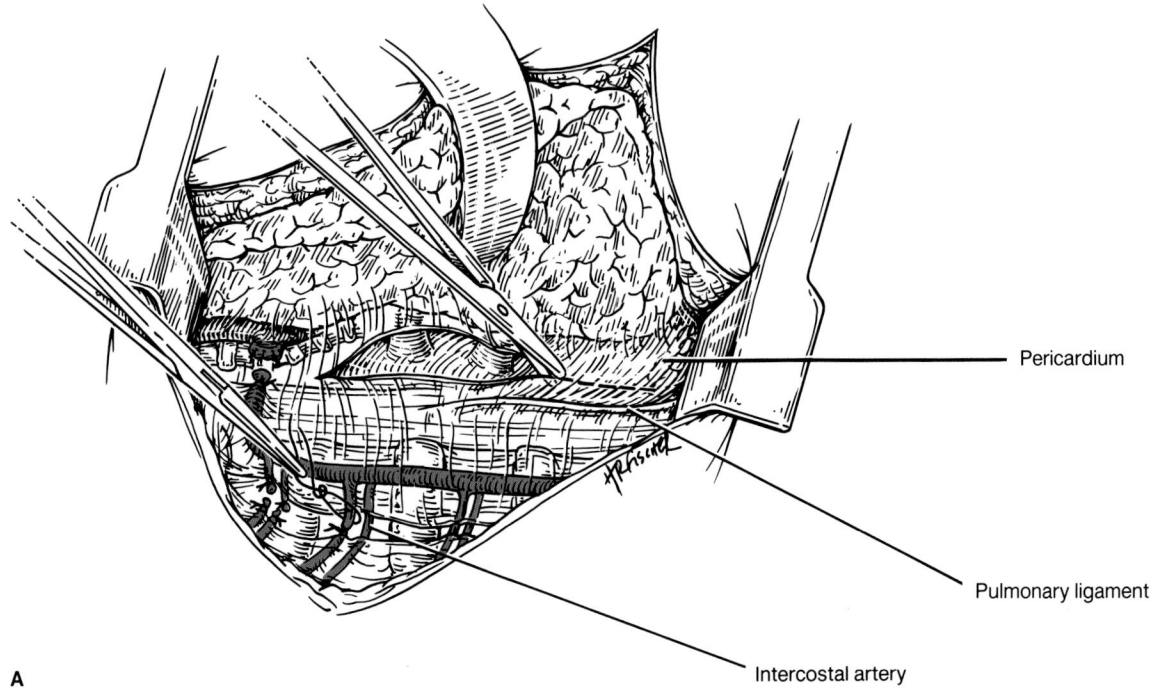

Pericardium

Pulmonary ligament

Intercostal artery

A

Figure 5-IV-4

Radical (En Bloc) Esophagectomy: Right Thoracotomy Approach

(**A**) Radical en bloc esophagectomy for tumors of the middle- and upper-thoracic esophagus is performed through a right lateral or posterolateral thoracotomy. The right intercostal vessels are divided lateral to the azygos vein, and the azygos vein is divided at its junction with the superior vena cava. The mediastinal pleura is entered anterior to the esophagus, and the posterior pericardium is divided from the level of the diaphragm, extending superiorly just medial to the pulmonary veins.

(**B**) The esophagus is mobilized from the prevertebral fascia, and the intercostal arteries are divided at their origin from the aorta. The contralateral pleura is resected in continuity with the specimen after completion of the resection of the posterior pericardium to a level opposite the contralateral pulmonary veins. En bloc dissection of the subcarinal and paratracheal nodes is performed, preserving the right and left recurrent laryngeal nerves. The superior and inferior margins of dissection are 10 cm from the gross extent of the tumor.

(**C**) The abdominal portion of an en bloc dissection includes omentectomy and preservation of the right gastroepiploic arcade. The splenic artery and associated lymph nodes are dissected from the superior surface of the pancreas, and the artery is divided at its origin from the celiac axis. Common hepatic artery nodes are also dissected. The spleen is taken en bloc with the specimen. The remainder of the gastric dissection is performed in a standard fashion. The stomach is transected at a point at least 10 cm distal to the distal extent of gross tumor, often including portions of the left gastroepiploic arcade in the specimen. This extent of dissection limits reconstructive possibilities using the stomach.

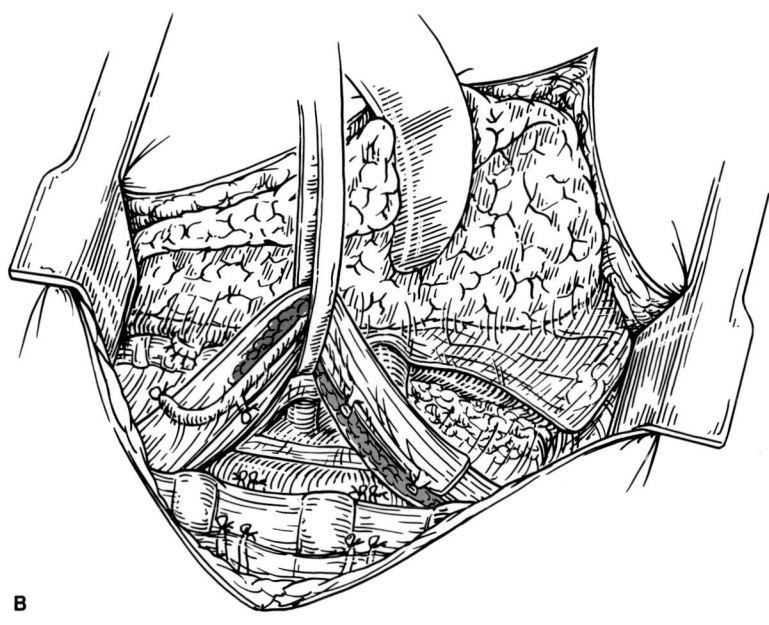

B

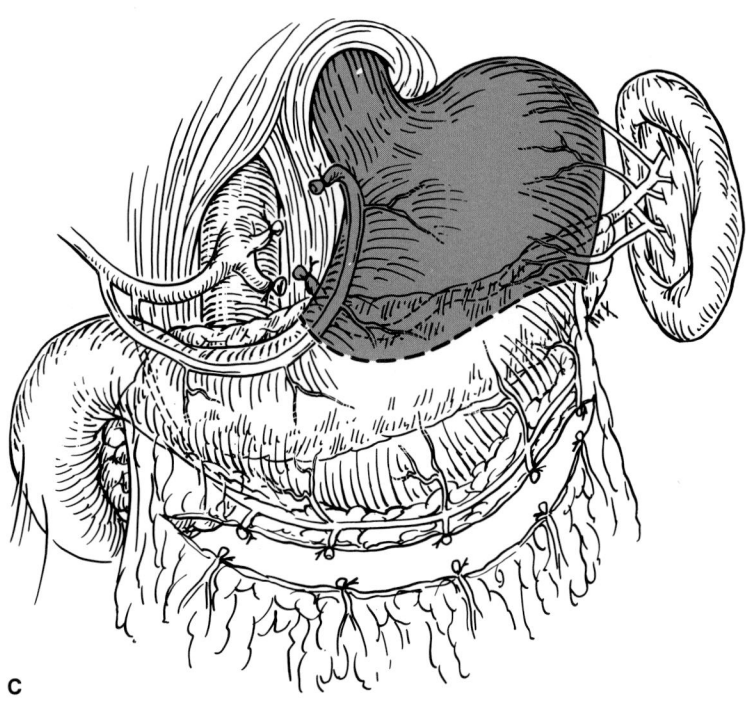

C

Figure 5-IV-4 *(Continued)*

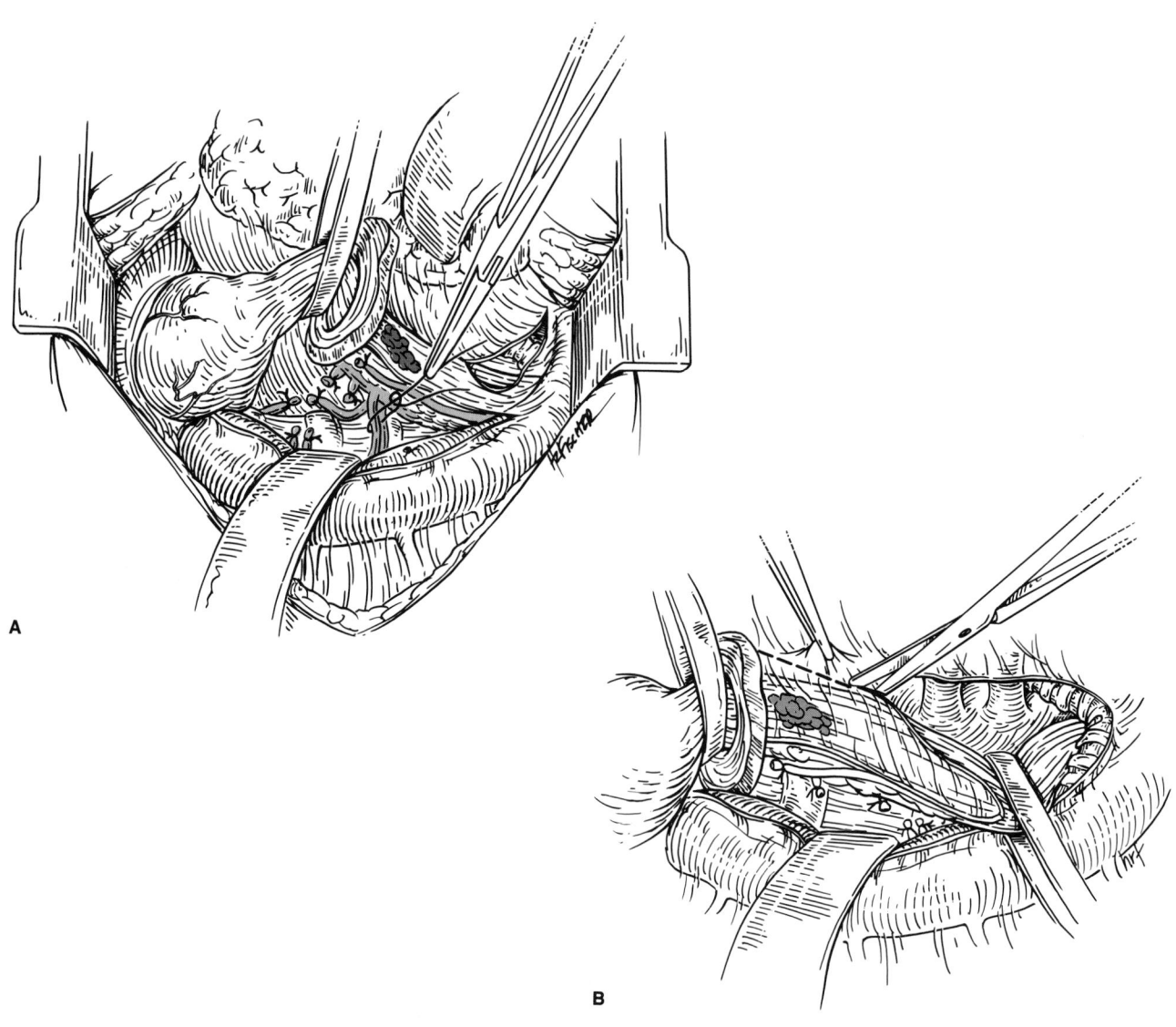

A

B

Figure 5-IV-5

Radical (En Bloc) Esophagectomy: Left Approach

(**A**) Radical en bloc esophagectomy through an exclusive left thoracotomy is used for tumors of the distal esophagus and gastroesophageal junction. The mediastinal pleura is incised anterior to the esophagus, and the posterior pericardium is taken en bloc with the specimen from the level of the inferior pulmonary veins to the diaphragm. Contralateral parietal pleura is included. The right intercostal vessels are divided at their origin from the aorta and again just beyond the azygos vein. The azygos vein and thoracic duct are taken en bloc with the specimen.

(**B**) A generous rim of diaphragm is included with the specimen. The anterior portion of the dissection is completed, including the posterior pericardium en bloc with the specimen. The ligated azygos vein, thoracic duct, and intercostal vessels are evident deep to the esophagus. If total esophagectomy is necessary, the dissection can be continued bluntly beneath the aortic arch and in the superior mediastinum up into the neck under direct vision.

SECTION V *Trauma*

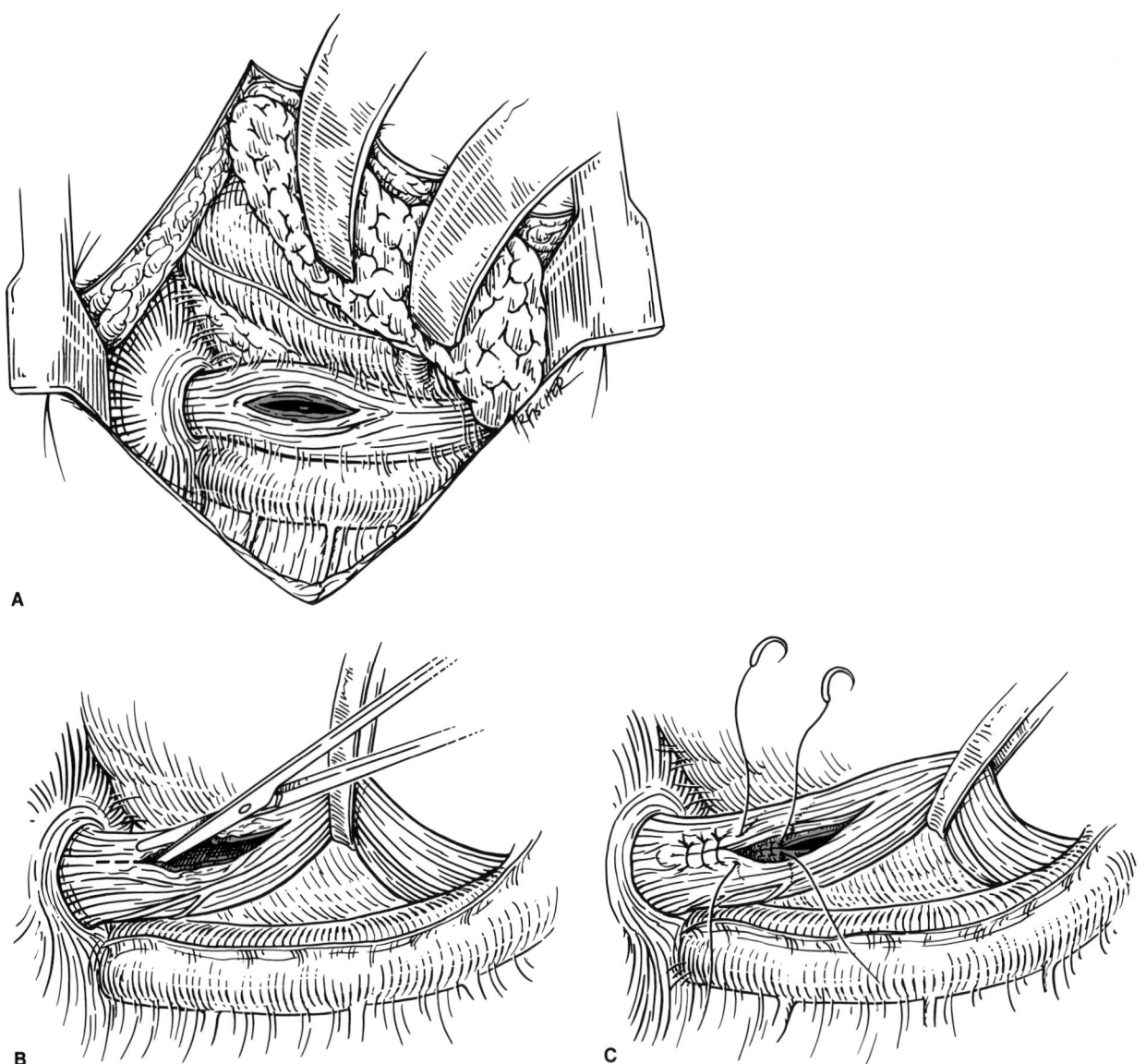

A

B

C

Figure 5-V-1

Primary Closure of Perforation

(**A**) The site of an esophageal perforation is exposed after mobilization of the pulmonary ligament and division of the mediastinal pleura.

(**B**) It is sometimes necessary to mobilize the esophagus to facilitate exposure of the site of perforation. The underlying mucosal defect is frequently larger than that in the smooth muscle layers, often necessitating extension of the smooth muscle defect to reveal the edges of the mucosal injury.

(**C**) A two-layer closure is performed, reinforcing the mucosal repair by reapproximating the overlying smooth muscle.

(Continued)

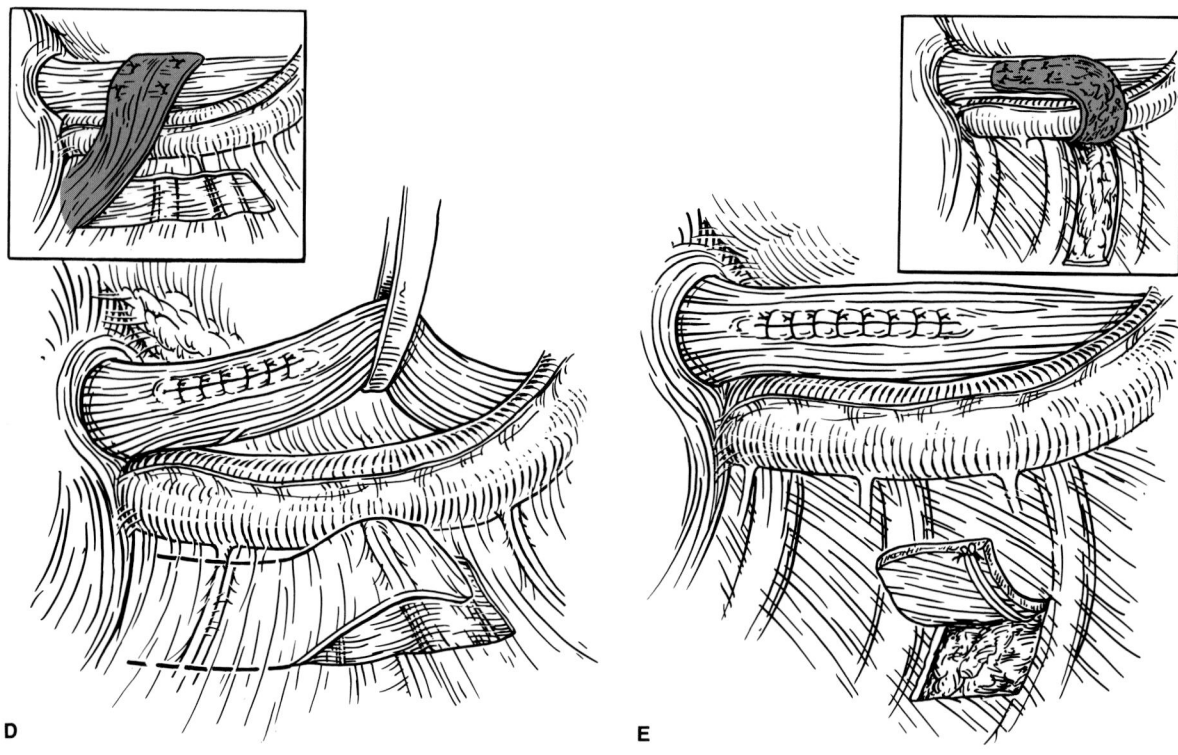

D   E

Figure 5-V-1 *(Continued)*

(**D**) It is often useful to reinforce primary repair of an esophageal perforation using a pedicled flap of pleura or other vascularized tissue. The pleural flap should be based at a distance from the line of division of the parietal pleura created to mobilize the esophagus so as not to compromise the blood supply to the pleural flap. This is tacked over the esophagus to completely cover the original defect (**inset**).

(**E**) If the parietal pleura is inadequate to cover the original defect, a vascularized pedicle of intercostal muscle can be raised en bloc with intercostal vessels. For larger flaps, a segment of rib is removed, preserving the intercostal pedicle and creating a double width of intercostal muscle pedicle with a dual blood supply.

(**F**) The pericardial fat pad provides excellent vascularized coverage for esophageal defects. The blood supply originates superiorly. Its long length and mobility make it suitable for all but the most distally located defects.

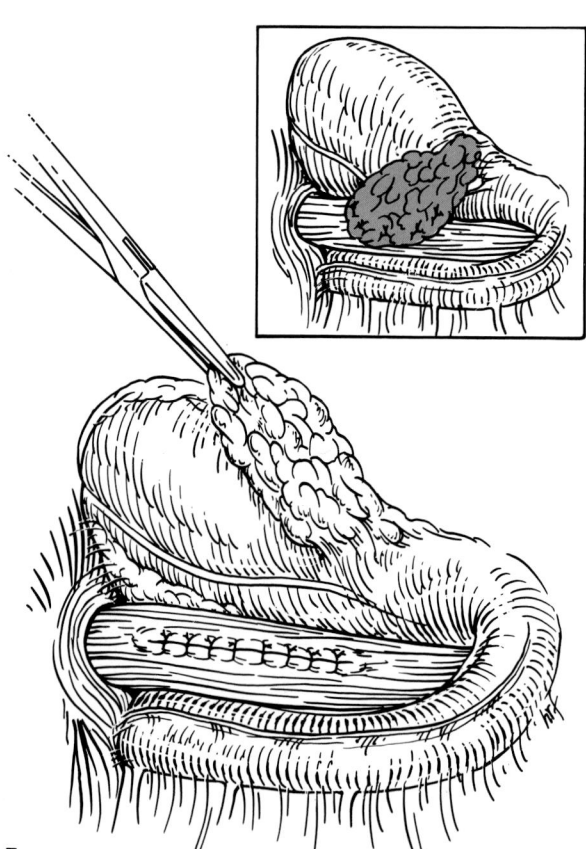

F

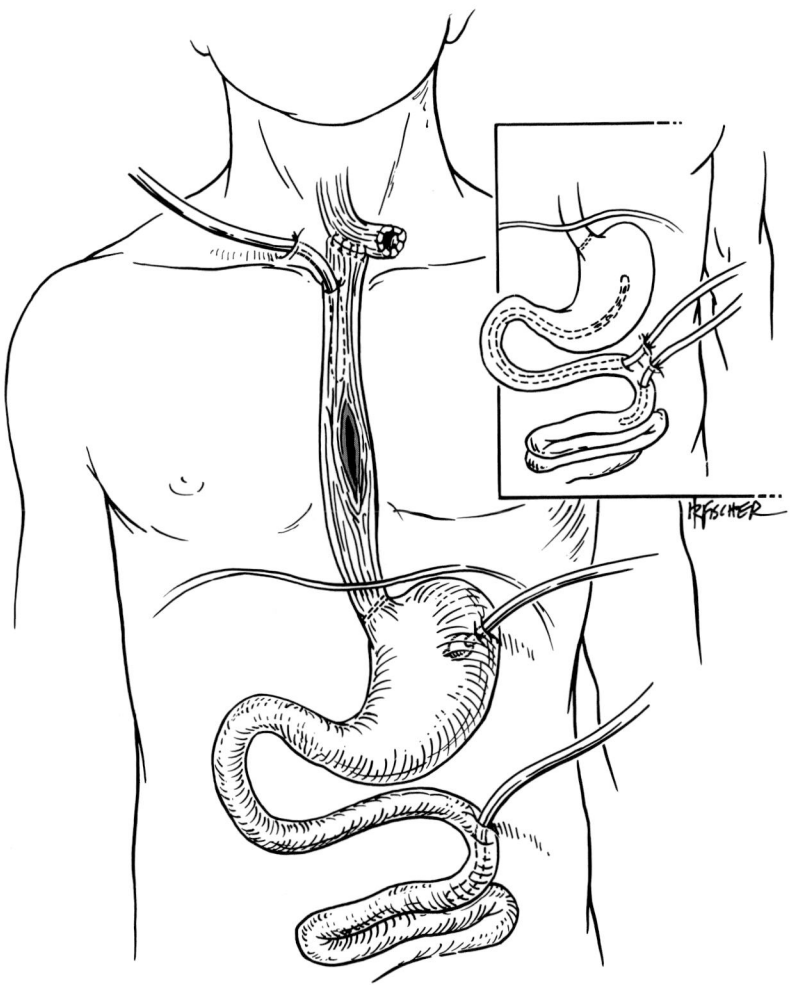

Figure 5-V-2

Exclusion and Diversion

In instances in which esophageal exclusion is necessary, an end-cervical esophagostomy is performed. The distal end of the cervical esophagus is closed and is sewn to the lateral wall of the proximal cervical esophagus to prevent retraction into the mediastinum and to facilitate subsequent reanastomosis. If drainage of the perforated segment is necessary, it can be accomplished percutaneously, entering the side wall of the intrathoracic esophagus. A tube is placed for jejunal feedings, and a separate gastric drainage tube is placed, either directly into the stomach or retrograde to the duodenum and pylorus (**inset**), to decompress the stomach and prevent gastroesophageal reflux. A stapling device or ligature can be used at the esophagogastric junction to further exclude the esophagus from the stomach temporarily.

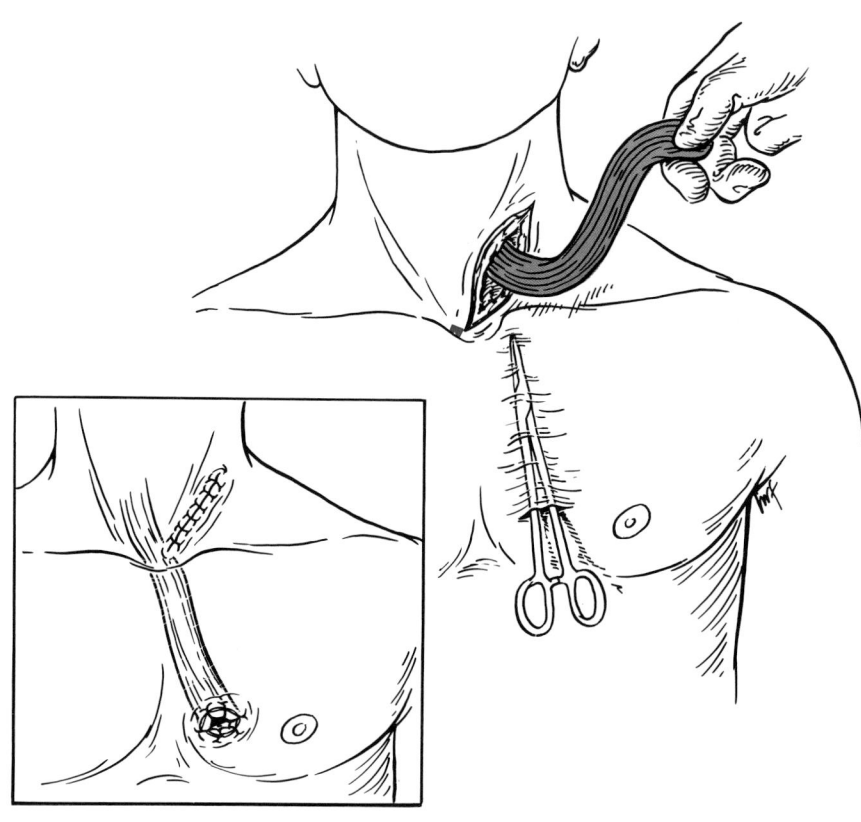

Figure 5-V-3

Esophagostomy

In situations in which the esophagus cannot be salvaged and is removed, all viable esophagus proximal to the injury is preserved and is tunneled subcutaneously from the cervical incision. An esophagostomy on the anterior chest wall is easily fitted with a stomal appliance.

SECTION VI *Esophageal Reconstruction*

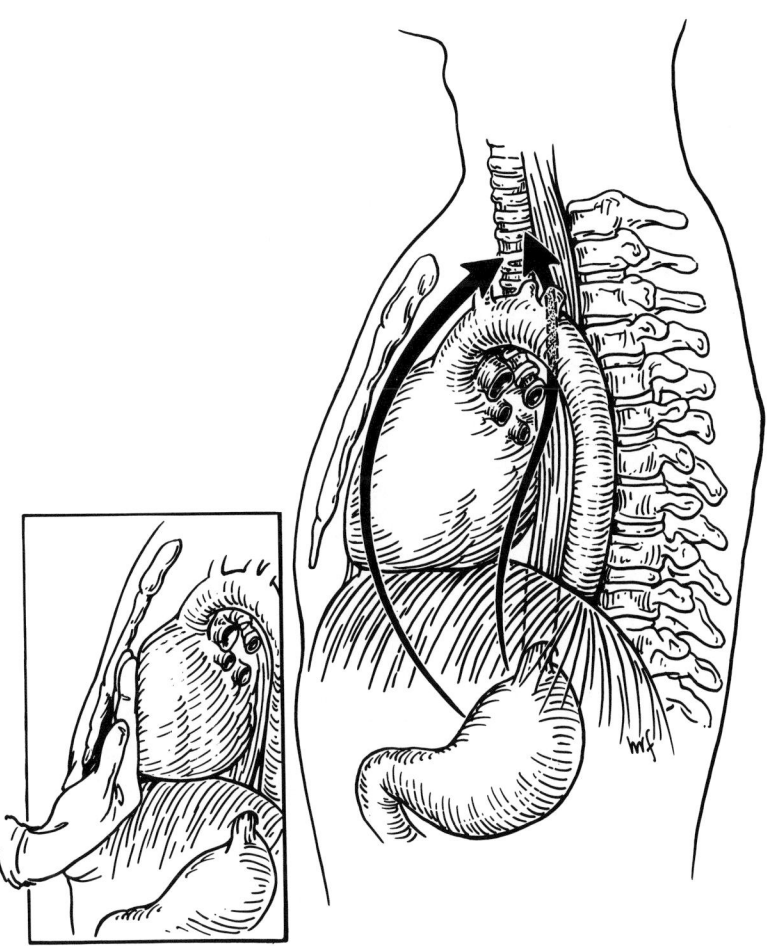

Figure 5-VI-1

Routes for Reconstruction

The two most common routes for reconstruction are in the posterior mediastinum through the bed of the resected esophagus and through the anterior mediastinum in the retrosternal space. This latter potential space is bluntly dissected between the surfaces of the parietal pleura laterally, the posterior surface of the sternum anteriorly (between the internal mammary vessels), and the pericardium posteriorly (**inset**).

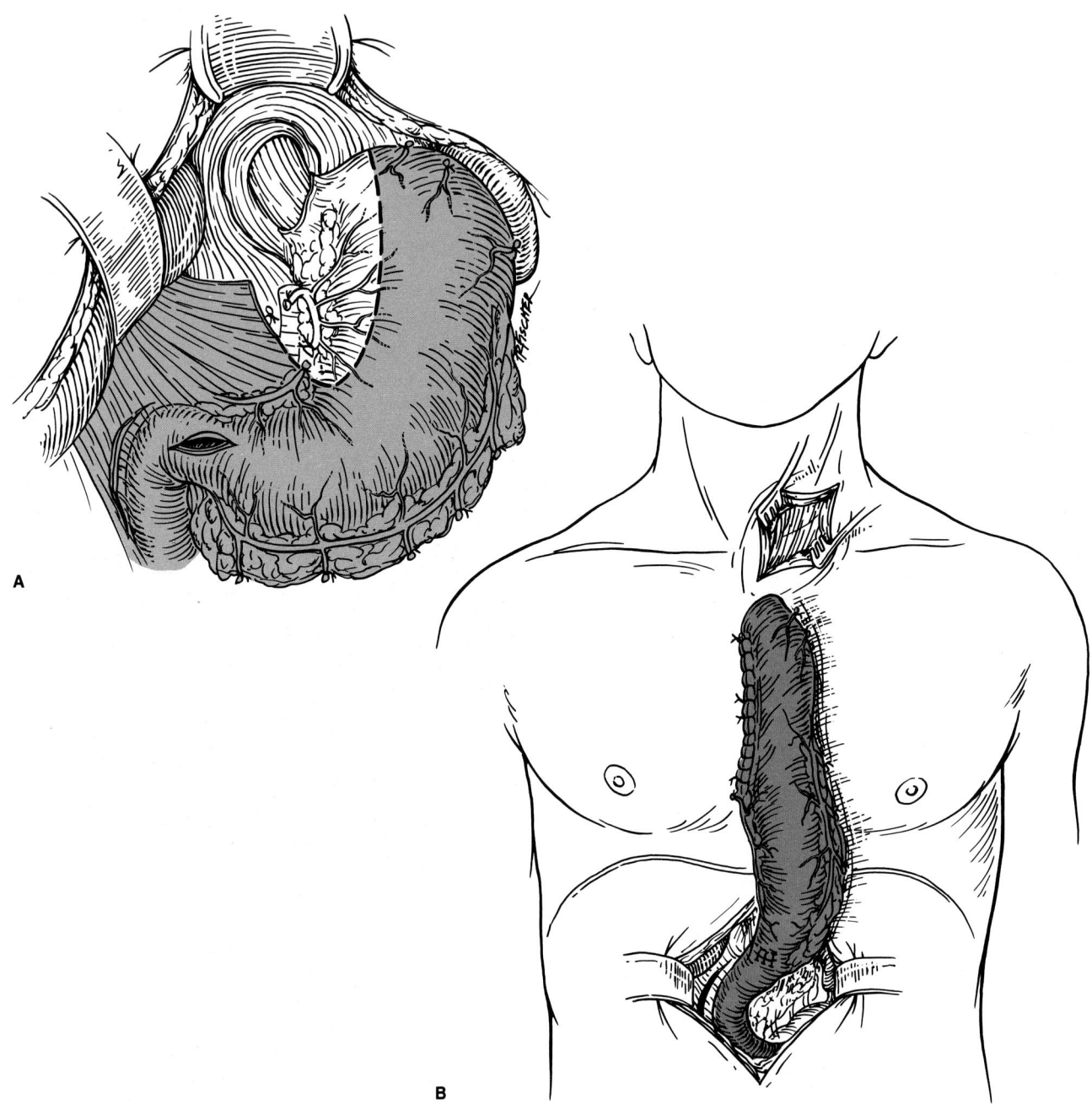

Figure 5-VI-2

Stomach Pull-Up

(**A**) The organ used most commonly for reconstruction is the stomach. Although the whole stomach can be used as a reconstructive organ, it is often best to create a large tube of the stomach by resecting the esophagogastric junction and lesser curvature. This does not compromise the vascular supply to the stomach or the overall length of the stomach, but it can reduce gastric acid production and improve emptying through the interposed organ.

(**B**) After resection of the lesser curvature using a linear cutting stapler and performance of a complete Kocher maneuver, the stomach easily reaches the hyoid bone without tension. The adequacy of gastric length can be assessed by laying the stomach on the chest wall before passing it through the mediastinal tunnel.

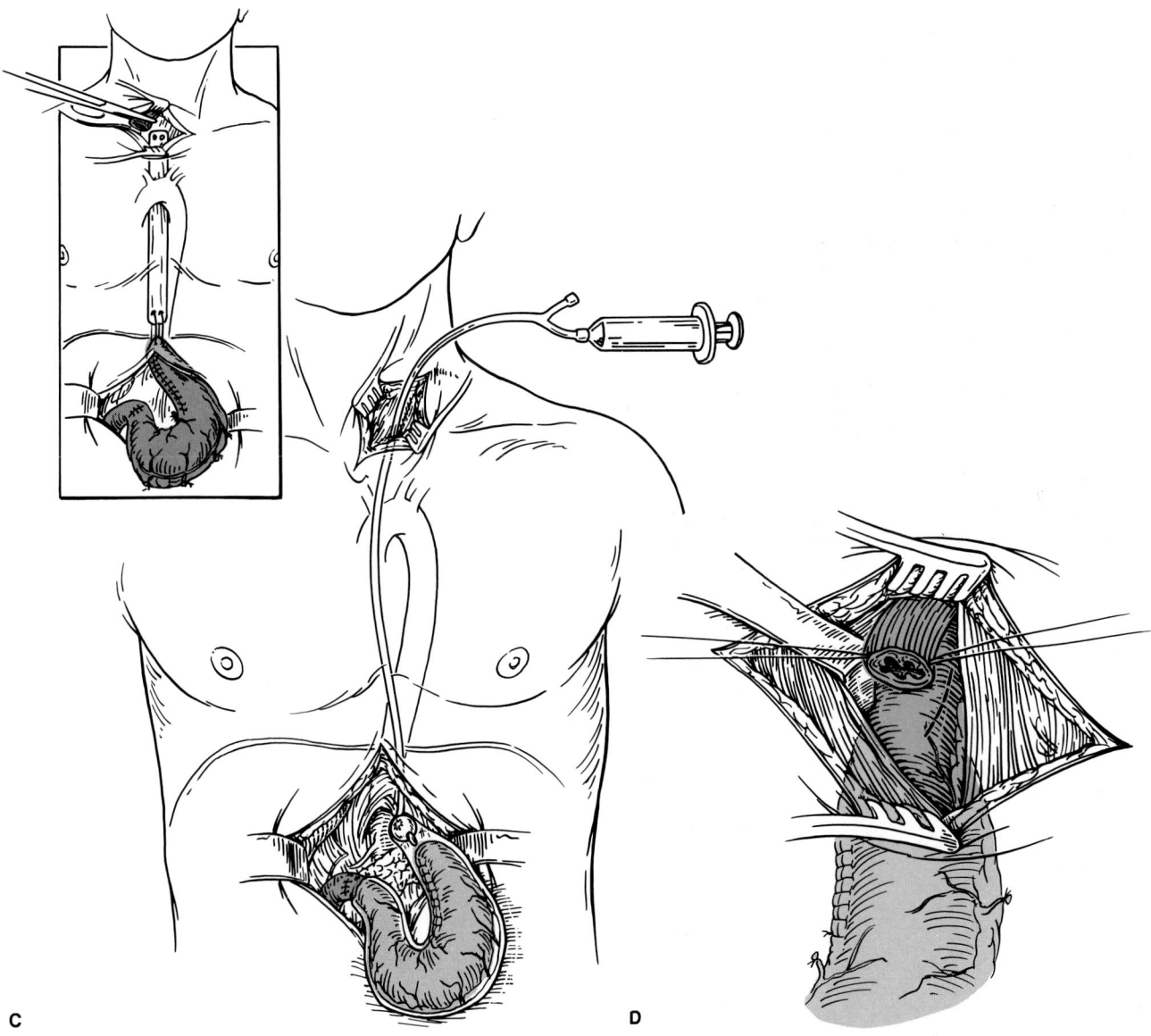

Figure 5-VI-2 *(Continued)*

(C) The stomach is sometimes passed manually through the mediastinal tunnel. A malleable retractor with predrilled holes also can be passed through the tunnel and attached to the gastric fundus by sutures to facilitate passage of the stomach through the mediastinum (**inset**). Alternatively, a large Foley catheter can be passed through the mediastinal tunnel into the abdomen. The stomach tube is placed in a cylindrical plastic bag, the tip of the catheter is passed through a small hole in the tip of the bag, and the balloon is inflated. Suction is applied to the drainage lumen of the catheter to approximate the plastic bag to the stomach tube, permitting traction to be exerted on all surfaces of the stomach rather than just at the tip of the fundus. The catheter is withdrawn through the mediastinum, followed closely by the gastric tube.

(D) A gastrotomy is performed opposite the lesser curvature suture line and an end-to-side esophagogastrostomy is performed. The tip of the stomach can be sutured to the prevertebral fascia to prevent excess tension from developing on the anastomosis.

(Continued)

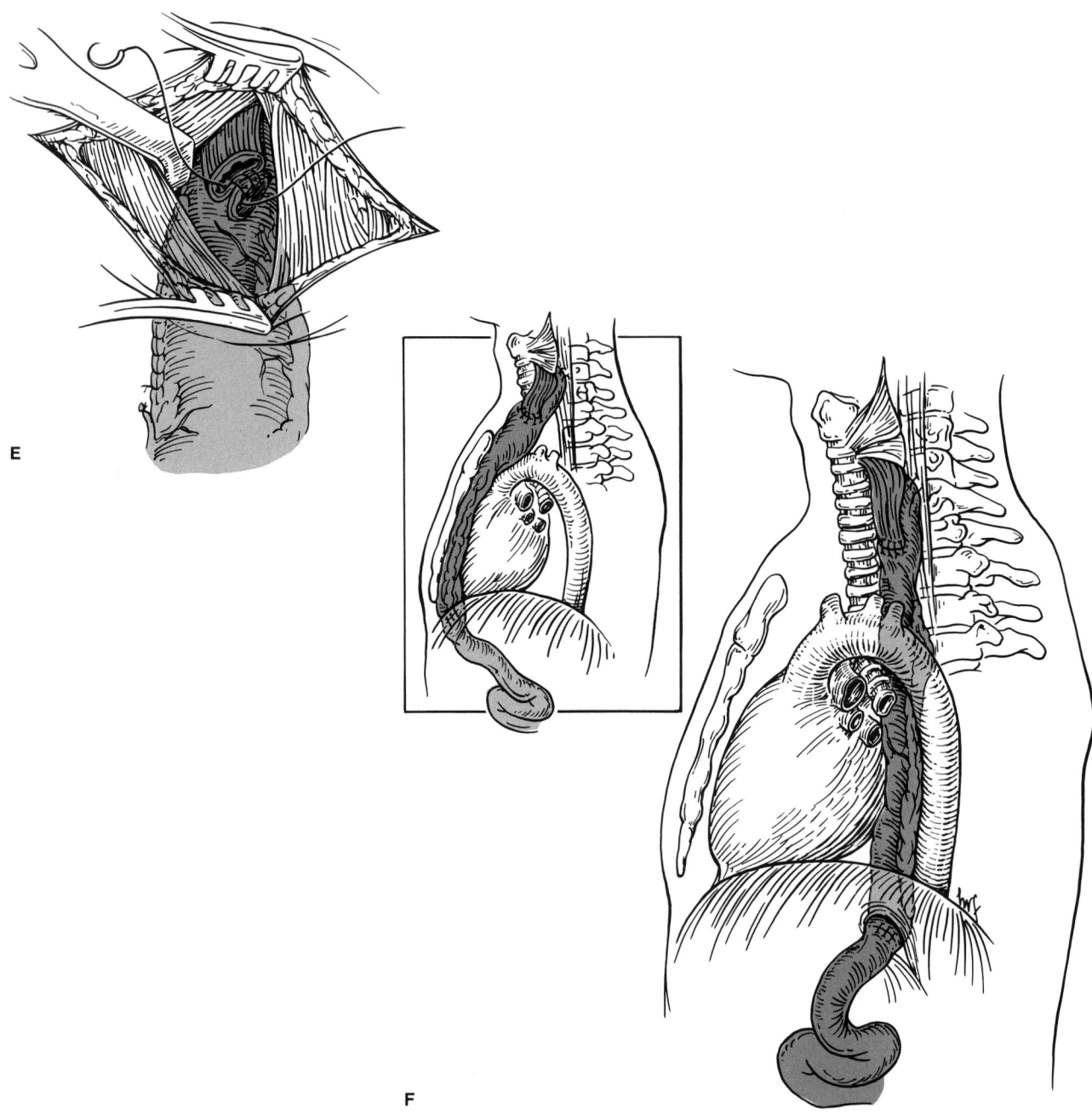

Figure 5-VI-2 *(Continued)*

(**E**) An anastomosis can be performed in two layers, but a single layer using interrupted sutures through the full thickness of stomach and esophagus is equally effective. A naso-enteral tube is typically placed across the anastomosis to drain the stomach in the early postoperative period.

(**F**) The completed gastric pull-up in the posterior mediastinal space. Its relatively straight course is evident, and the mobility of the first three portions of the duodenum is clear from the position of the pyloroplasty at the level of the esophageal hiatus. The retrosternal route is also satisfactory for use in reconstruction but creates some angulation of the esophagus near the esophagogastrostomy (**inset**).

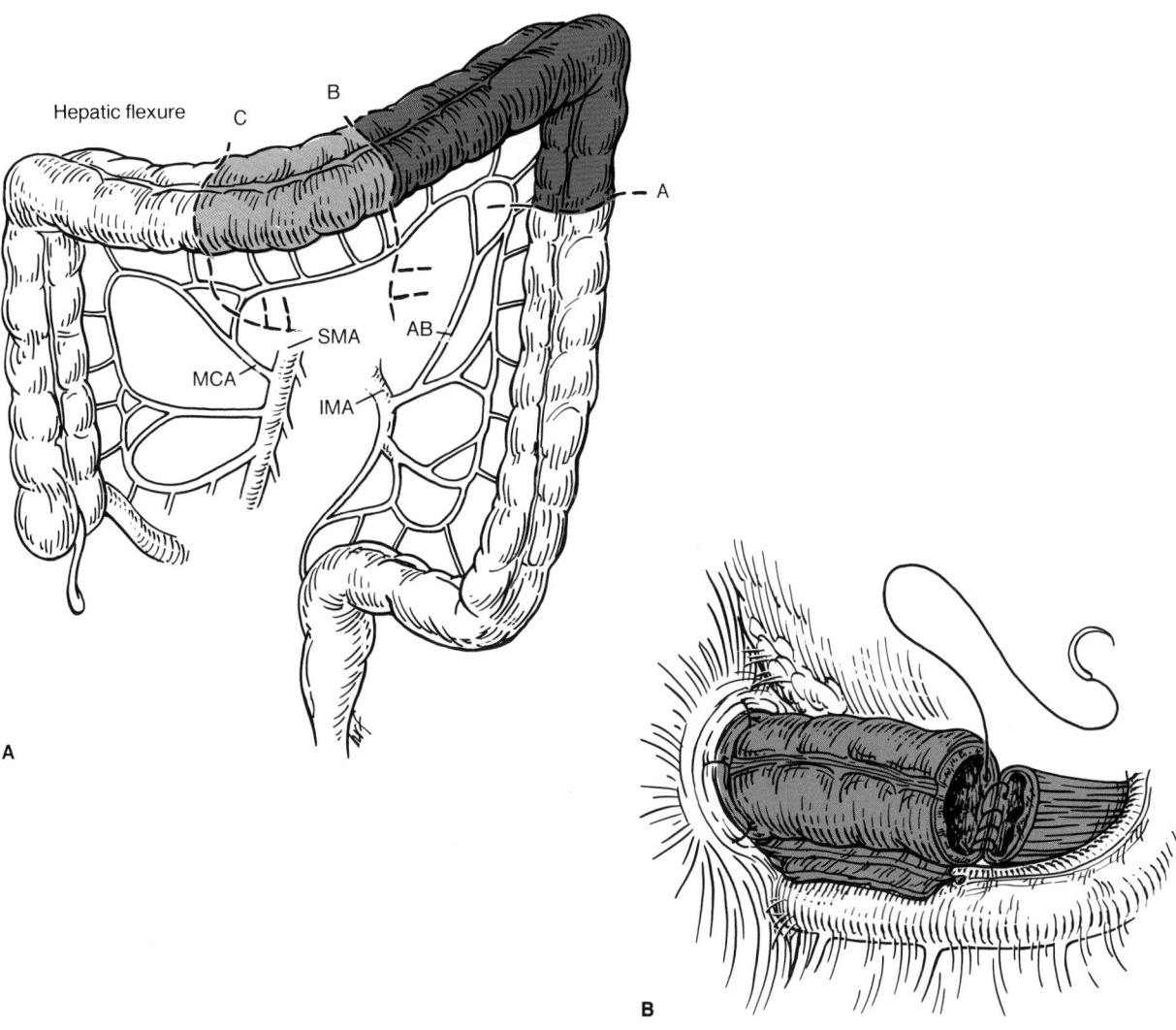

A

B

Figure 5-VI-3

Colon Interposition

(**A**) An isoperistaltic colon interposition is typically performed with a segment of the transverse and descending colon. The usual anatomy of the arterial supply is illustrated. Blood supply to the interposition segment is provided by the ascending branch (AB) of the left colic artery (a branch of the inferior mesenteric artery [IMA]) and its anastomoses to the marginal artery (of Drummond). The division line for short segment interpositions is indicated (A to B). Long segment interpositions (A to C) sometimes require inclusion of the middle colic artery (MCA; divided from the superior mesenteric artery [SMA]) to maintain blood supply to the proximal end of the interposition segment. Use of the right colon as an isoperistaltic reconstructive segment is also possible, but the blood supply is less constant and the size discrepancy between the esophagus and proximal right colon is more pronounced.

(**B**) The short segment is mobilized and brought through the esophageal hiatus. An end-to-end anastomosis is performed using a running or interrupted suture technique. Care is taken to enlarge the esophageal hiatus so there is no impingement on the venous return of the colon segment.

(Continued)

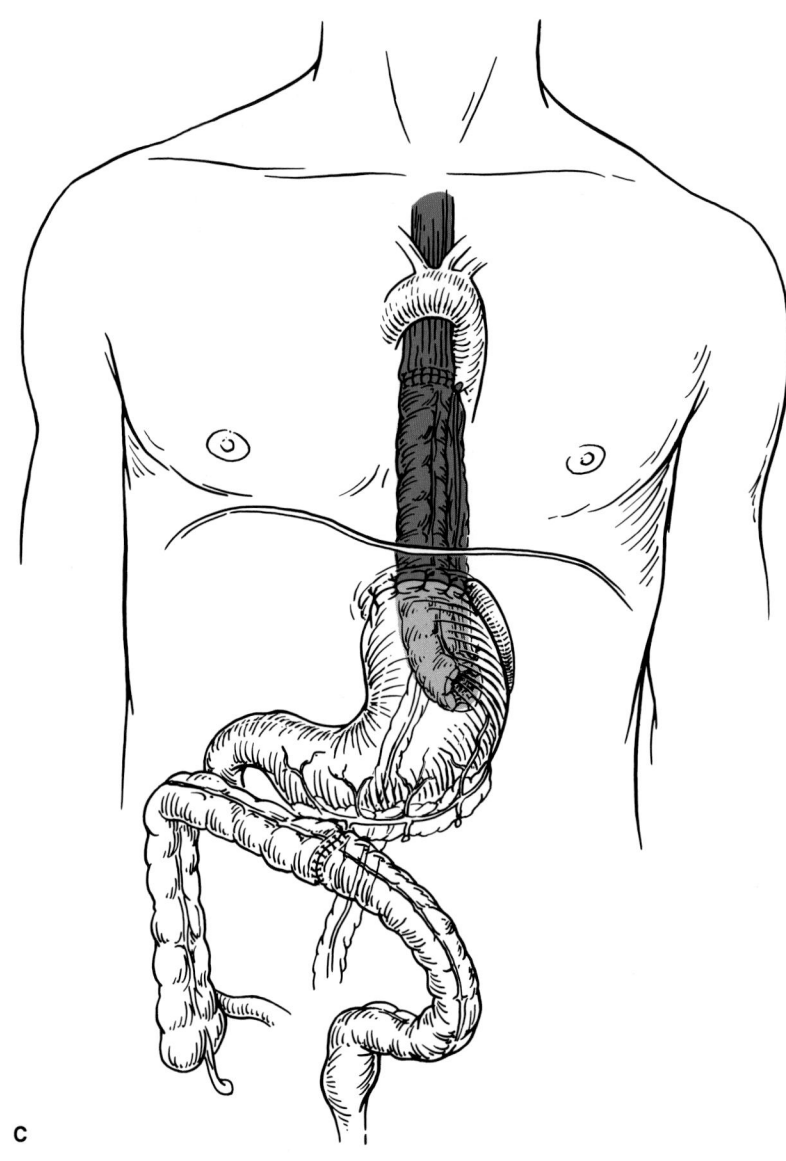

c

Figure 5-VI-3 *(Continued)*

(C) After completion of the proximal anastomosis, the interposition segment is retracted into the abdomen to eliminate redundancy of the interposition and is sutured to the posterior wall of the stomach. The vascular pedicle thus passes through the retrogastric space. Tissues at the margin of the esophageal hiatus are loosely stitched to the colon serosa to prevent herniation of abdominal contents into the mediastinum. Loosely suturing the stomach to the diaphragm in a horseshoe fashion anterior to the esophageal hiatus creates a partial antireflux barrier.

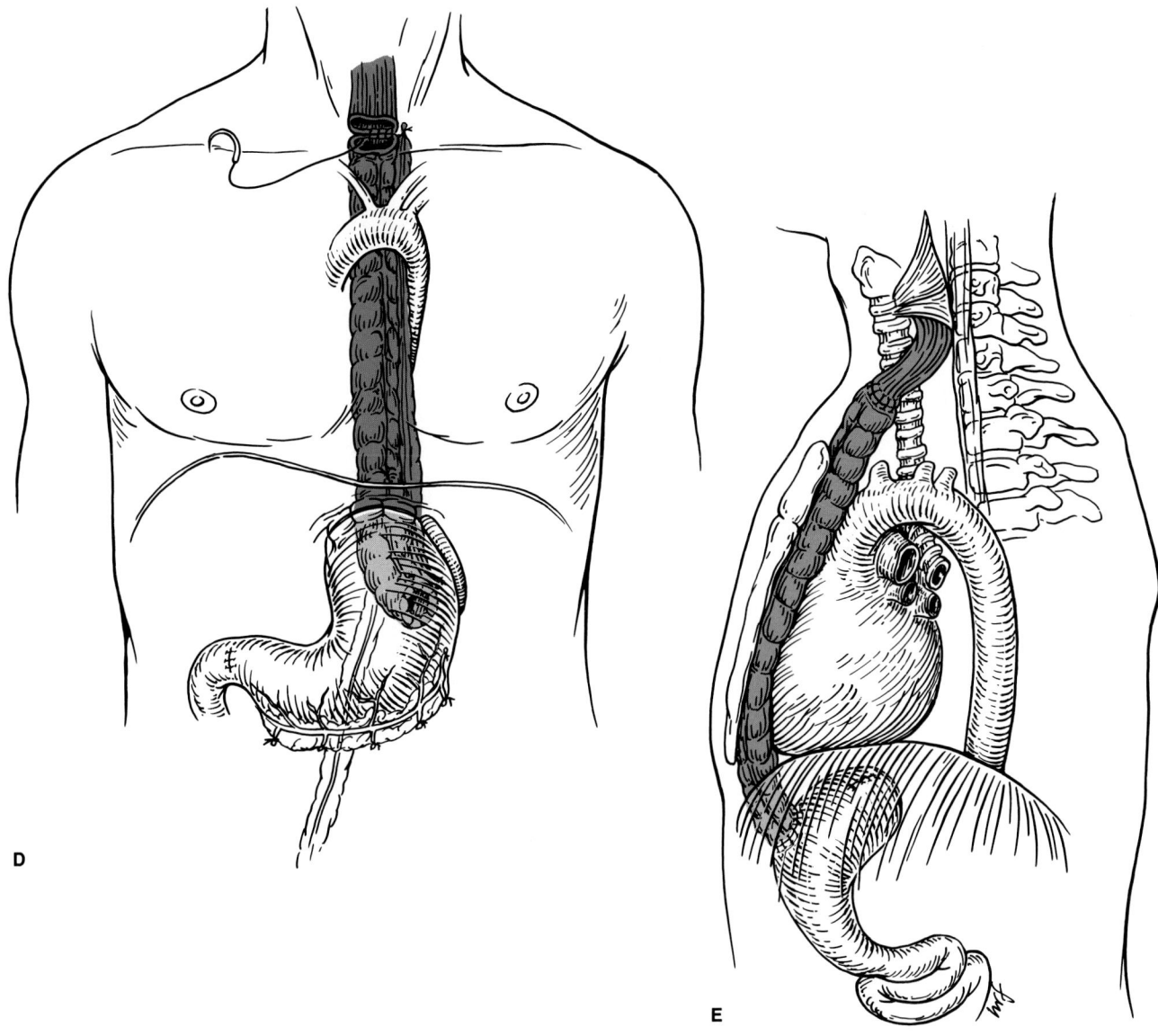

Figure 5-VI-3 *(Continued)*

(**D**) A long-segment colon interposition is shown, with the interposed segment passing beneath the arch of the aorta in the bed of the esophagus. The aortic arch helps maintain the position of the interposed segment and avoid redundancy.

(**E**) Placing a colon interposition in the retrosternal space necessitates a cologastrostomy positioned on the anterior surface of the stomach. Angulation of the esophagus proximal to its junction with the interposed segment sometimes causes mild dysphagia.

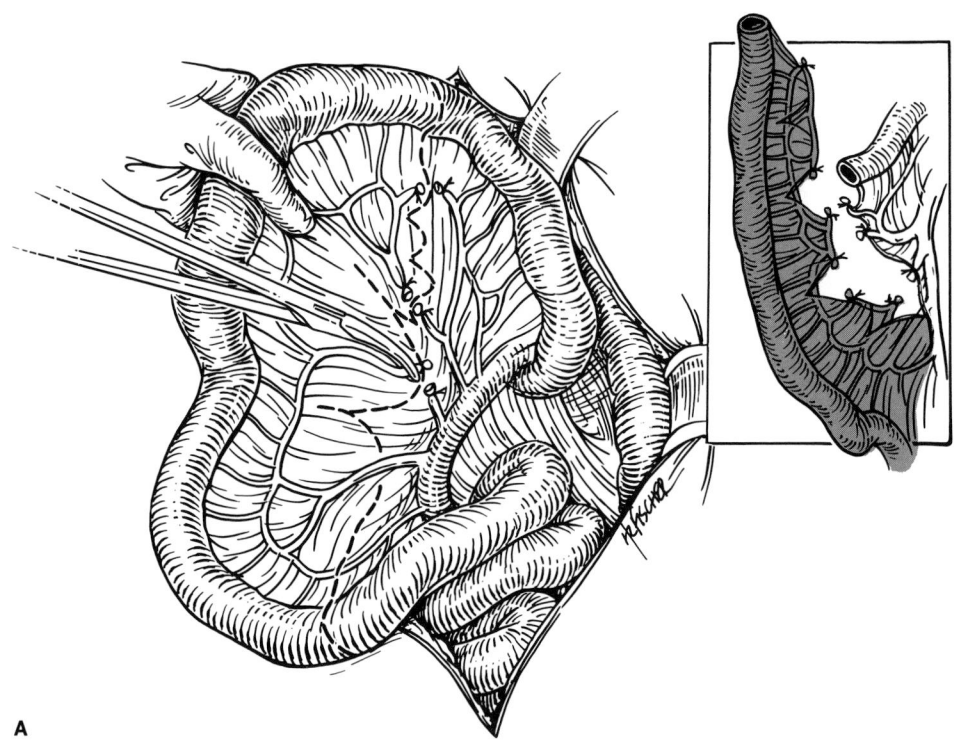

A

Figure 5-VI-4

Jejunal Interposition

(**A**) Preparation of a jejunal segment for esophageal reconstruction is facilitated by trans-illumination of the small bowel mesentery. The vascular arcades of the first two or three loops of the jejunum are typically short, and using a loop of jejunum further distal in the alimentary tract is advisable. An arterial trunk off the superior mesenteric artery that supplies the necessary length of jejunum is identified and left intact until the remainder of the vascular dissection is completed. Several notch incisions in the mesentery are sometimes required to permit straightening of the interposition segment.

(**B**) The jejunal segment is brought through the transverse mesocolon to be anastomosed in an isoperistaltic fashion between the distal esophagus and the posterior wall of the stomach. The remaining ends of the jejunum are anastomosed, and the jejunal mesenteric defect is closed if technically feasible.

(**C**) The completed jejunal interposition is sometimes more redundant than other organ reconstructions of the esophagus. An end-to-side esophagojejunostomy, rather than an end-to-end esophagojejunostomy (shown), is sometimes necessitated by the shape of the vascular arcade of the jejunum.

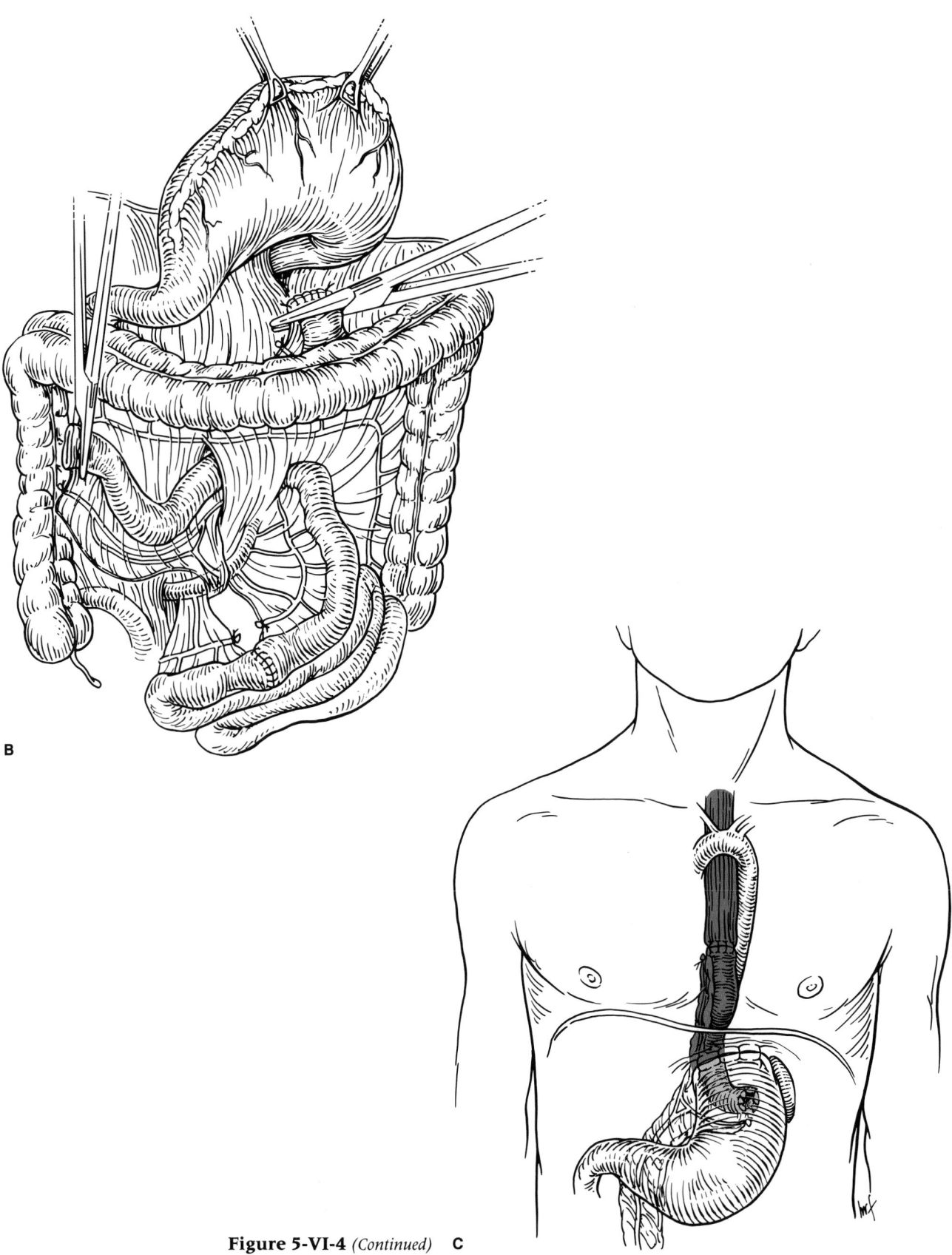

Figure 5-VI-4 *(Continued)* **C**

PART II
Stomach and Duodenum

Digestive Tract Surgery: A Text and Atlas, edited by Richard H. Bell,
Layton F. Rikkers, and Michael W. Mulholland.
Lippincott-Raven Publishers, Philadelphia, © 1996.

6

Peptic Ulcer Disease

Michael W. Mulholland

DUODENAL ULCER

Epidemiology

Peptic ulceration is a common disease in Western societies, with major public health implications. Although hospitalization rates, numbers of operations for peptic ulcer, and disease-related mortality decreased in the two decades before 1980, continued progress has been frustratingly slow. In the United States, 300,000 new cases of peptic ulcer are diagnosed each year, and because of the high rate of recurrent disease, 4 million people are estimated to receive treatment for peptic ulcer annually. Peptic ulceration occurs most commonly between 45 and 65 years of age, although in recent years, the incidence has increased appreciably in elderly patients. Men are affected more often than women.

Although hospitalization for uncomplicated peptic ulcer has been dramatically reduced, the incidence of perforation and bleeding as complications of peptic ulceration has not been changed by the introduction of newer antisecretory medications[1] (Fig. 6-1). Surgeons are treating an older population with frequent comorbid illness and with ulcer disease of greater chronicity. Surgical treatment deals increasingly with the complications of peptic ulceration. Hemorrhage is the most common complication requiring hospitalization and the most frequent ulcer-related cause of death. Although overall ulcer mortality has declined during the past 20 years, it has risen significantly in patients older than 75 years of age. In the United States, about 10,000 deaths per year list peptic ulceration as a contributing cause.

Pathogenesis

A number of factors have been implicated in the pathogenesis of peptic ulceration. These factors can be categorized as environmental or as disturbances of gastric acid secretion or gastric mucosal defense. In population studies, the disease often appears multifactorial and complex. In individual patients, subtle defects in acid–pepsin secretion or in resistance of mucosa to peptic injury can predispose to duodenal ulceration. Because multiple factors are necessary to maintain gastroduodenal health, it is not surprising that a single pathogenic mechanism has not been identified as the cause of ulceration (Table 6-1).

Environmental Factors

Cigarette smoking is an important environmental factor in the development of peptic ulceration, and peptic ulcer morbidity and mortality rates parallel smoking rates. The decline in smoking rates in American men after 1960 was matched by declining rates of peptic disease; increased cigarette use by young and middle-aged women has been reflected in increased rates of ulceration in women. The mechanisms by which smoking contributes to peptic ulceration are unknown but may include stimulation of gastric acid secretion, decreased duodenal mucosal bicarbonate secretion, altered mucosal prostaglandin production, or changes in mucosal blood flow or gastric motility. Smoking increases the risk of ulcer in patients taking nonsteroidal antiinflammatory drugs (NSAIDs). Smoking is a major risk factor for recurrence of duodenal ulcer and is associated with delayed ulcer healing and increased complication rates.[2] Although treatment with histamine-2 (H_2) recep-

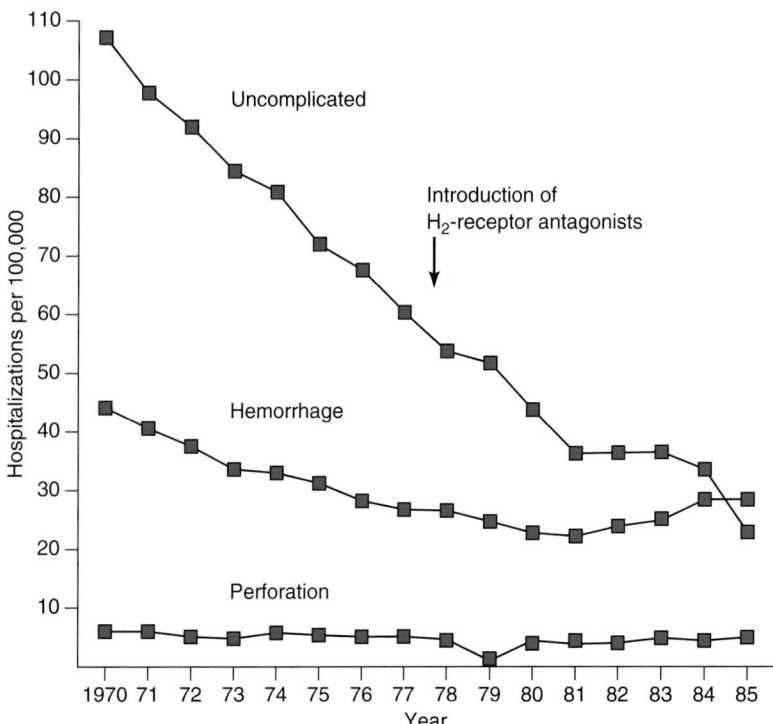

Figure 6-1 Hospitalization rates for duodenal ulcer. (After Kurata JH, Corboy ED. Current peptic ulcer time trends: an epidemiological profile. J Clin Gastroenterol 1988;10:259)

tor antagonists can reduce the risk of recurrent ulcer in patients who continue to smoke, cessation of smoking is a more important intervention.

A persuasive case can be made that infestation of gastric mucosa by the microorganism *Helicobacter pylori* contributes to the development of duodenal ulceration. A strong association exists between the presence of *H pylori* in gastric mucosa and the development of duodenal ulceration.[3,4] In over 90% of duodenal ulcer cases, the organism can be demonstrated in biopsy specimens

---

**Table 6-1   Factors Associated
With the Development of Duodenal Ulcer**

ENVIRONMENTAL
Smoking
Helicobacter pylori
Nonsteroidal antiinflammatory drug use

GASTRIC ACID SECRETION
Increased basal acid output
Increased nocturnal acid secretion
Increased pentagastrin-stimulated maximal acid output
Increasd meal-stimulated acid secretion
Increased sensitivity to gastrin
Accelerated gastric emptying

MUCOSAL DEFENSE
Decreased bicarbonate secretion
Decreased mucosal responsiveness to prostaglandins

---

of gastric mucosa. *H pylori* recognizes binding sites on antral cells, and it is widely accepted that the organism causes antral gastritis. Antral biopsy specimens from patients who harbor the organism reveal epithelial damage and an inflammatory response in the underlying lamina propria. Although *H pylori* cannot bind to normal duodenal epithelium, gastric metaplasia is almost always found in the mucosa surrounding duodenal ulcers, and metaplastic epithelium can be colonized by *H pylori*. Importantly, mucosal infestation with *H pylori* appears to predate the development of ulceration. In a prospective, longitudinal study covering 10 years, duodenal ulcer developed in 11% of patients with *H pylori*–associated gastritis and in fewer than 1% of *H pylori*–negative patients.[5]

A role for *H pylori* in the development of duodenal ulcers is also supported by the effects of eradication of the organism on ulcer recurrence. Standard therapeutic regimens have no effect on *H pylori* and are followed, after cessation of treatment, by a recurrence rate no different from untreated controls. When patients are treated with a bismuth compound plus an antibiotic (metronidazole), *H pylori* is eradicated in up to 75% of patients.[6] Elimination of the organism is followed by resolution of gastritis. Ulcer recurrence is substantially lower in patients in whom the organism is eradicated than in patients in whom *H pylori* persists.

The association of *H pylori* with duodenal ulcer is not specific, however. There is an age-related prevalence in asymptomatic controls, and the organism has been isolated from patients with gastric ulcer or nonulcer dyspepsia. Human-to-human transmission is presumed. Transmission through endoscope and biopsy equipment has been demonstrated, and gastroenterologists have a higher than expected rate of infestation.[7] Potential virulence factors that allow *H pylori* to escape the bacteriocidal action of gastric acid, adhere to epithelial cells, and cause mucosal damage are an area of intense investigation. *H pylori* possesses urease activity, which can promote adherence and protect the organism from the effects of luminal acid.

NSAIDs are a major cause of gastroduodenal mucosal damage because of their systemic suppression of prostaglandin production. A large number of experimental models have demonstrated that NSAIDs injure the gastroduodenal mucosa, producing a variety of lesions, ranging from superficial mucosal erosions to invasive, perforating ulcers.[8,9] Associated hemorrhage is common. Similar lesions can be produced by antibodies directed against prostaglandins, and damage due to NSAIDs can be prevented or reversed by administration of prostaglandin analogues. Experimental ulcers heal rapidly when the drug is withdrawn, with a time course corresponding to reversal of antiprostaglandin effects.

The use of NSAIDs is surprisingly widespread in society, with about 3 million people using NSAIDs on a daily basis in the United States. All available NSAIDs possess risks of gastroduodenal ulceration. Clinically important ulceration is estimated to occur at a rate of 2% to 4% per patient-year of use.[10]

Although an association has been unequivocally demonstrated between gastric ulcer formation and NSAID use, the implication that NSAIDs cause duodenal ulcer has been controversial. Instead of inciting duodenal ulcer formation, it appears more likely that NSAID use increases the frequency of peptic complications for patients with preexisting duodenal ulceration.[11] A significant association between NSAID use and duodenal ulcer perforation or hemorrhage has been demonstrated, especially in patients older than 65 years of age. These complications carry a two- to threefold increase in mortality in NSAID users relative to age-matched controls.[12]

A number of chronic diseases have been associated with duodenal ulceration (Table 6-2). In most cases, the mechanisms responsible for these relations are not known. Alcohol is a common agent used to induce gastric mucosal damage in animal models. At concentrations relevant to human consumption, acute ethanol exposure is a modest stimulant to acid secretion but does not appear to cause significant mucosal injury. Although the direct effects of chronic alcohol exposure are less well studied, hepatic cirrhosis is associated with

Table 6-2　Diseases Associated With Duodenal Ulcer

Gastrinoma
Multiple endocrine neoplasia type I
Chronic pulmonary disease
　Smoking
　α1-Antitrypsin deficiency
Systemic mastocytosis
Chronic renal failure
Cirrhosis

a five-fold increased risk of duodenal ulcer. There is a clear association between chronic obstructive pulmonary disease and peptic ulcer.[13] The relation cannot be solely attributed to smoking because ulcer risk is also increased in patients with lung disease due to α_1-antitrypsin deficiency. Associations with chronic renal failure, use of corticosteroids, chronic psychological stress, or various foods are poorly substantiated.

Gastric Acid Secretion

The development of duodenal ulceration depends critically on the presence of gastric acid and pepsin activity in luminal secretions. Duodenal ulcers do not form in the presence of anacidity, and suppression of acid secretion is the foundation of most therapeutic regimens that treat duodenal ulcers. Although clear abnormalities in acid secretion can be demonstrated in groups of patients with duodenal ulceration, individual patients are frequently within the normal range. With the exception of unusual conditions, such as the Zollinger-Ellison Syndrome (see Chap. 26), gastric acid hypersecretion is rarely proved, as an isolated abnormality, to cause duodenal ulceration.

Human gastric acid secretion follows a diurnal pattern, with highest rates of secretion occurring during nighttime and early morning hours. Basal acid secretion, most commonly measured by nocturnal collection of gastric juice, is elevated in groups of patients with duodenal ulcer[14] (Fig. 6-2). Vagal overactivity has been postulated to cause elevation of basal acid output. Basal acid output is, in part, reflective of total parietal cell mass, and a subset of patients with duodenal ulcers appears to have a greater total parietal cell mass than normal subjects. Treatment of duodenal ulcer with nocturnal dosing of antisecretory drugs is designed to suppress basal acid secretion.

Acid secretory capacity is also increased, relative to normal subjects, in groups of duodenal ulcer patients. Maximal acid secretory capacity can be elicited by administration of exogenous pentagastrin or histamine

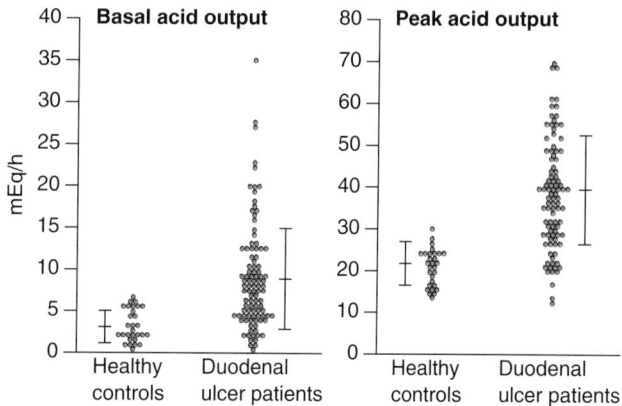

Figure 6-2 Basal and peak stimulated gastric acid secretion rates for healthy control patients and duodenal ulcer patients. Solid lines represent normal limits. Duodenal ulcer patients demonstrate elevations of both basal and stimulated acid secretion. (After Corinaldesi R, Stanghellini V, Paparo GF, et al. Gastric acid secretion and gastric emptying of liquids in 99 male duodenal ulcer patients. Dig Dis Sci 1989;34:251)

and is expressed as maximal acid output. The maximal acid output of normal adult men approximates 20 mEq/h; with histamine stimulation, duodenal ulcer patients secrete a mean of 40 mEq/h. As with basal acid secretion, the range of maximal acid output measurements for ulcer patients shows considerable overlap with normal subjects, and the values for most patients with duodenal ulcers fall within the range of those for normal subjects.

Meal-stimulated acid output is the net result of a large number of neural and hormonal signals, both stimulatory and inhibitory. Reports of meal-stimulated acid secretion in ulcer patients have been contradictory. Most studies have reported increased meal responses in duodenal ulcer patients; a recent study failed to demonstrate increased peak meal-stimulated acid secretion, although pentagastrin-stimulated maximal acid output was elevated.[15]

Because acid secreted into the gastric lumen exerts its harmful effects within the duodenum, defects in gastroduodenal motility and gastric emptying have been postulated to be part of the pathogenesis of duodenal ulceration. An extremely steep pH gradient normally exists within the duodenal bulb. In the presence of a mean fasting gastric pH of 1.9, the pH in the proximal duodenal bulb has been demonstrated to be 3.3, increasing to 4.2 in the midpoint of the bulb and to 5.1 at the apex.[16] Accelerated emptying of gastric contents or altered inhibitory feedback from the acidified duodenum can result in exposure of duodenal mucosa to decreased pH for prolonged periods. Studies supporting and refuting a role for abnormal gastric emptying have

been reported[17,18] (Fig. 6-3). It appears likely that a subset of ulcer patients exhibit abnormalities of gastric emptying.

Endocrine abnormalities do not appear to be important in the pathogenesis of duodenal ulceration. Excluding patients with Zollinger-Ellison syndrome, there is no strong evidence that abnormalities in circulating gastrin exist in peptic ulcer patients. A subset of patients have an increased sensitivity to endogenous gastrin or its analogue, pentagastrin, in terms of acid responsiveness. Tissue levels of the inhibitory peptide somatostatin and the effects of administered somatostatin appear to be normal.

Mucosal Defense

Because many patients with duodenal ulcer secrete normal amounts of acid and pepsin, defects in the ability of the duodenal mucosa to resist injury have been sought. In addition, a number of agents have been used to treat duodenal ulcer that do not affect acid secretion. Drugs that protect the mucosa from injury at doses lower than those needed to inhibit acid secretion are termed *cytoprotective*. Mucosally secreted mucus and bicarbonate and mucosal prostaglandins appear to be endogenous cytoprotective factors.

Acidic gastric secretions are neutralized in the proximal duodenum by alkaline pancreatic juice and by bicarbonate secreted by duodenal surface epithelial cells. Mucosal bicarbonate secretion is probably as important as pancreatic secretion in neutralizing acid in the proximal duodenum because pancreatic juice can

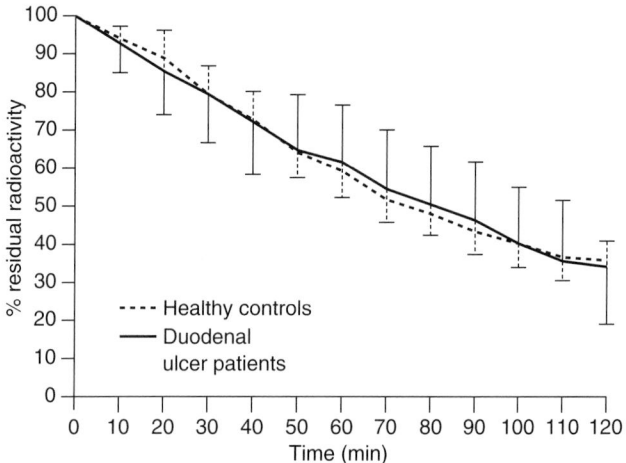

Figure 6-3 Gastric emptying of liquids of duodenal ulcer patients and normal control patients. (After Corinaldesi R, Stanghellini V, Paparo GF, et al. Gastric acid secretion and gastric emptying of liquids in 99 male duodenal ulcer patients. Dig Dis Sci 1989;34:251)

reach the bulb only through antiperistaltic movement. In healthy subjects, basal bicarbonate secretion by the proximal duodenal mucosa is similar in magnitude to basal pancreatic secretion. Epithelial secretion of bicarbonate creates a pH gradient within the overlying mucus layer, near neutrality at the mucosal surface (Fig. 6-4). Exposure of the duodenal mucosa to solutions of reduced pH increases bicarbonate secretion. Prostaglandins A and E are also potent agonists for bicarbonate secretion. Conversely, epithelial bicarbonate secretion is suppressed by cyclooxygenase inhibitors (NSAIDs).

Studies have indicated that both basal and acid-stimulated duodenal mucosal bicarbonate secretion are lower in duodenal ulcer patients than in normal subjects.[19] In response to acidification of the duodenal bulb, ulcer patients had about 40% of the bicarbonate response of controls (Fig. 6-5). These findings suggest a mechanism by which duodenal mucosa could be susceptible to injury even in the presence of normal amounts of gastric acid.

Mucosal prostaglandins have a number of properties that could protect gastroduodenal mucosa from injury or accelerate healing of ulcers. Prostaglandins increase mucosal proliferation, increase mucus secretion and nutrient blood flow, and promote lysosome stability. Prostaglandins stimulate mucosal bicarbonate secretion. Abnormalities in mucosal prostaglandin synthesis and action have been postulated to exist in subsets of duodenal ulcer patients. Prostaglandin synthesis in duodenal biopsy specimens from patients with ulcer disease has generally been normal, but some reports suggest that mucosal bicarbonate response to prostaglandin E_2 is impaired in duodenal ulcer patients.[20,21]

Diagnosis

The hallmark of duodenal ulcer is epigastric pain. The pain is described as burning or piercing and nonradiating. Classically, the pain is most intense in the early morning hours, and patients may complain of being awakened at night. Food or ingestion of antacids usually brings relief. Unfortunately, this symptom complex is not specific for duodenal ulcer. Although 90% of ulcer patients have epigastric pain, similar symptoms are seen in up to 80% of patients with nonulcer dyspepsia. The mechanism of ulcer pain is not understood. During treatment, relief of symptoms usually precedes ulcer healing. Provocative tests, involving dripping of acidic solutions onto ulcer craters, do not reliably reproduce symptoms. About 10% of ulcer patients have hemorrhage or perforation as their first sign of ulcer disease, without preexisting pain.

Histologic examination of duodenal ulcers reveals evidence of chronicity. The luminal surface is usually covered by fibrinopurulent debris overlying granulation tissue infiltrated by inflammatory cells. A collagenous scar forms the base of the ulcer. Variable amounts of edema, with thickening of muscularis mucosa and submucosa, surround the ulcer. Repeated cycles of ulceration and healing result in increased deposition of collagen, causing a permanent scar and distortion of the proximal duodenum. Deeper extension of the ulcer into the duodenal wall can result in perforation or penetration into another organ, most commonly the pancreas.

Duodenal ulcers can be diagnosed by endoscopy or contrast radiography. When direct comparisons were made, upper gastrointestinal endoscopy and double-contrast barium meals had equivalent diagnostic accuracy.[22] Single-contrast radiographs should be considered obsolete. Radiographically, duodenal ulcers are characterized by retention of barium in the ulcer crater. When viewed in profile, the ulcer can be seen to project beyond the duodenal lumen. Distortion of the duodenal bulb by chronic scarring is a secondary sign of prior ulceration. The development of smaller endoscopes, incorporation of video equipment, and the ability to perform endoscopic biopsies have caused endoscopy largely to supplant radiography as the diagnostic preference. About half of endoscopically diagnosed duodenal ulcers are located on the anterior wall. The small diameter of the duodenal lumen almost always requires that the ulcer be viewed tangentially (Figs. 6-6 and

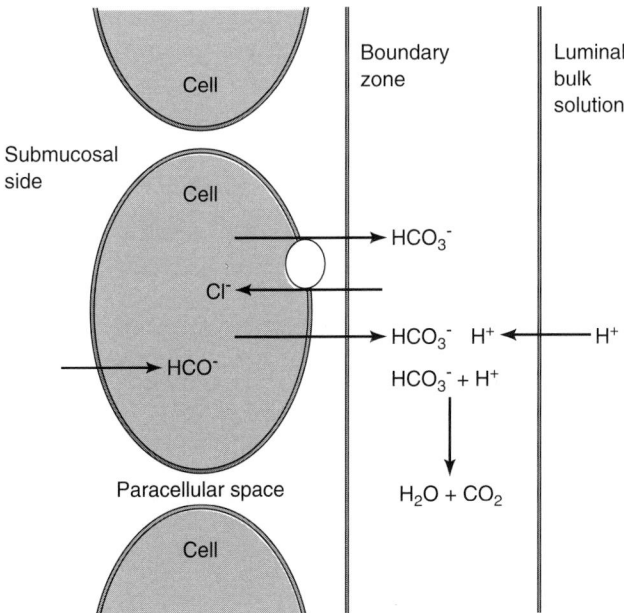

Figure 6-4 Schematic representation of gastric mucosal bicarbonate secretion.

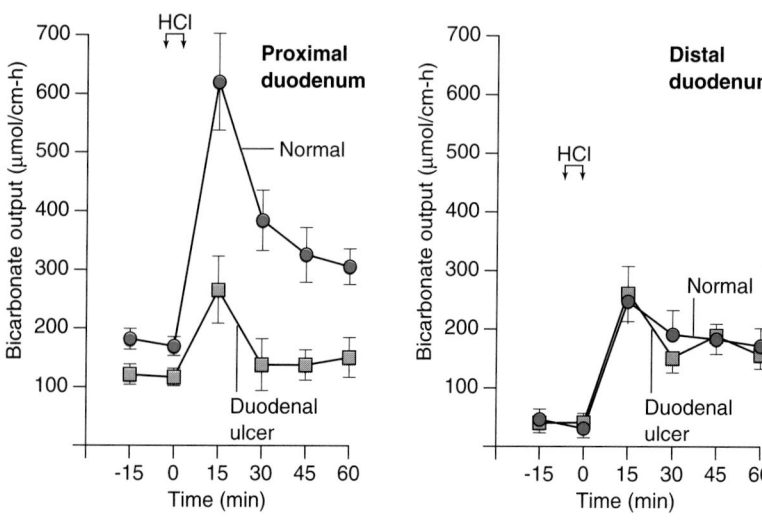

Figure 6-5 Proximal and distal duodenal bicarbonate secretion in normal subjects compared with patients with duodenal ulcers. (After Isenberg JI, Selling JA, Hogan DL, et al. Impaired proximal duodenal mucosal bicarbonate secretion in patients with duodenal ulcer. N Engl J Med 1987;316:374)

6-7). The ulcer base should be examined for signs associated with recent hemorrhage (discussed later). Duodenal ulcers with typical endoscopic morphology do not require biopsy.

Medical Therapy

All gastric surgeons must have a working knowledge of the drugs available to treat peptic ulceration because (1) the agents are among the most common drugs employed in surgical practice; (2) the widespread use of such drugs has profoundly altered the indications for surgery in peptic ulceration; and (3) the power and the limitations of drug treatment can affect the choice of operation performed.

Drugs used to treat peptic ulcer can be grouped as those that suppress acid secretion by the parietal cell and those that protect gastroduodenal mucosa without affecting acid secretion. The parietal cell has surface receptors for histamine, gastrin, and acetylcholine (Fig. 6-8). Histamine receptor occupation increases intracellular levels of cyclic adenosine monophosphate (cAMP); gastrin and acetylcholine act through pathways that mobilize intracellular calcium. Subsequent to receptor occupation, a series of intracellular reactions involving protein phosphorylation eventuates in activation of the parietal cell proton pump. This pump, localized to the plasma membrane that lines the parietal cell secretory canaliculus, exchanges H^+ ions for K^+. Energy for this reaction is derived from the hydrolysis of adenosine triphosphate. Because histamine activates a different signal pathway from acetylcholine or gastrin, combining histamine with either acetylcholine or gastrin produces a response greater than the sum of responses to the individual agonists. This increased acid secretion is called *potentiation*. Conversely, blockade of

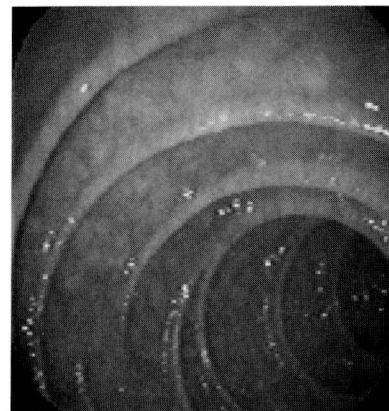

Figure 6-6 Endoscopic appearance of normal duodenal mucosa. (See Color Fig. 6-6.)

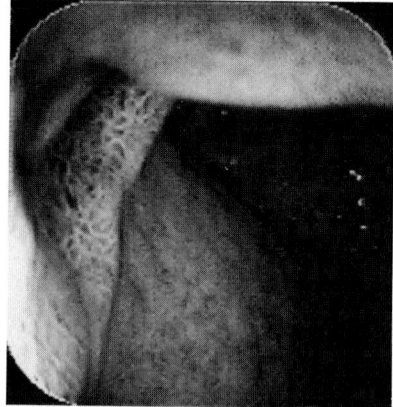

Figure 6-7 Tangential endoscopic view of pyloric channel ulcer (10-o'clock position). (See Color Fig. 6-7.)

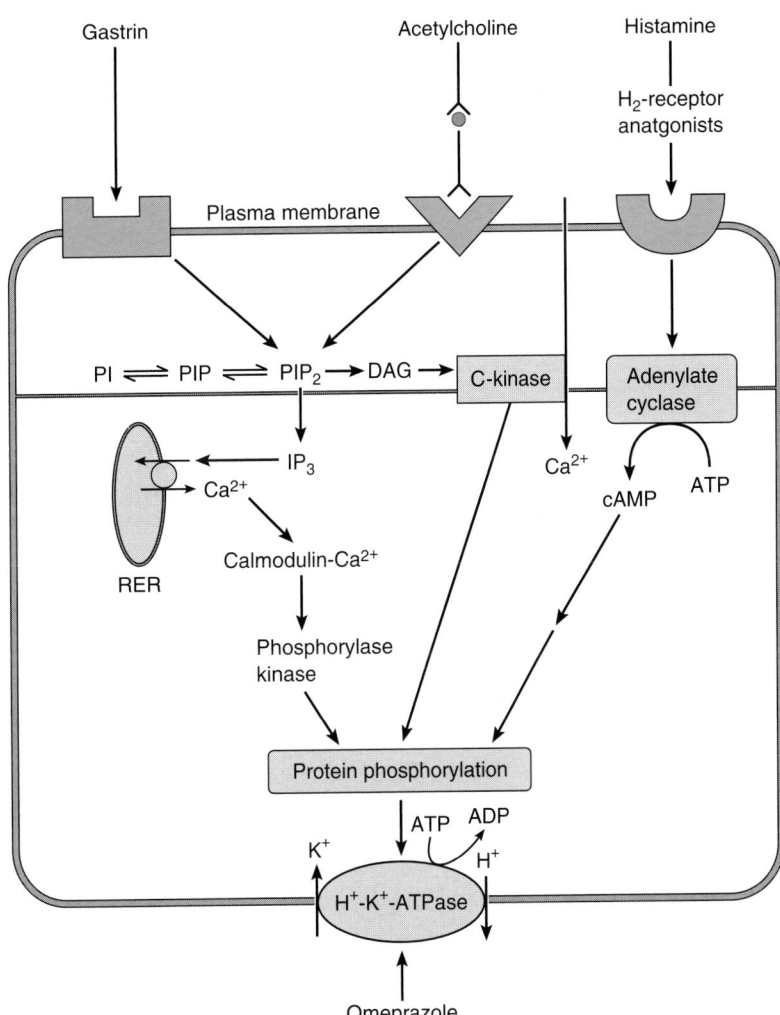

Figure 6-8 Schematic representation of gastric parietal cell demonstrating cellular mechanisms operative in secretion of acid and sites of action of antisecretory drugs.

histamine receptors inhibits responsiveness to either acetylcholine or gastrin.

Histamine-2 Receptor Antagonists

Four H_2-receptor antagonists are approved by the Food and Drug Administration for use in the United States—cimetidine, ranitidine, famotidine, and nizatidine. Their structures and relation to histamine are shown in Figure 6-9. These four agents bind to the histamine receptor in a reversible, competitive manner. In addition to inhibiting histamine-stimulated acid secretion, the H_2-receptor antagonists inhibit basal, meal-stimulated, and pentagastrin-stimulated acid secretion. The observation that H_2-receptor antagonists can potently inhibit vagus- and gastrin-stimulated secretion attests to potentiation by histamine of gastrin- or acetylcholine-stimulated gastric acid responses. This observation has practical consequences in terms of noc-

turnal dosing to suppress vagally dependent basal secretion or treatment of Zollinger-Ellison syndrome.

All H_2-receptor antagonists are absorbed rapidly from the small intestine, with peak blood levels 1 to 3 hours after oral ingestion.[23] Bioavailability is not affected by food but can be decreased by antacids or sucralfate. All four agents are eliminated by renal excretion and hepatic degradation. The serum half-lives of all four agents are increased by renal insufficiency, which may require dose adjustment. Although the drugs are metabolized by the liver, hepatic dysfunction has no significant impact on pharmacokinetics, and dose adjustments are not necessary in patients with liver disease. H_2-receptor clearance decreases with advancing age, principally becuase of declines in renal function.

On a molar basis, ranitidine is 4 to 8 times more potent than cimetidine; famotidine is 20 to 50 times more potent than cimetidine. Equipotent oral doses are: famotidine 40 mg, ranitidine 300 mg, nizatidine 300 mg, and cimetidine 1200 mg.[24] Increases in potency do

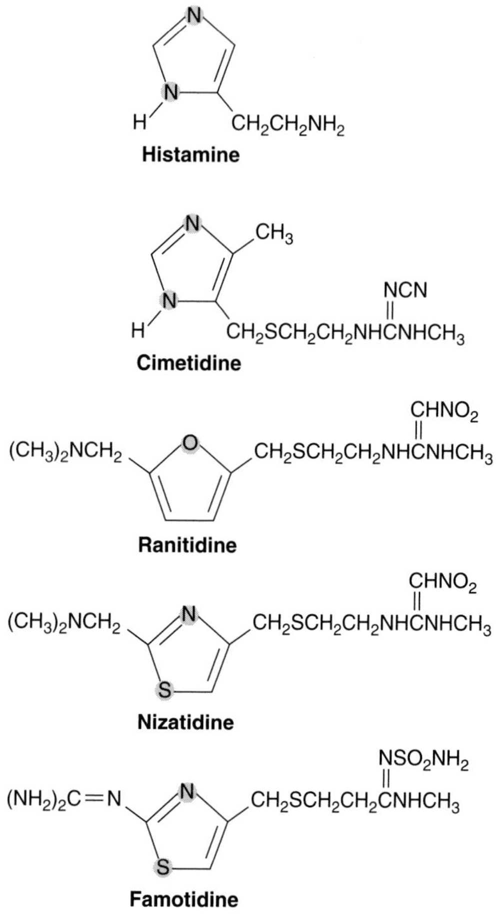

Figure 6-9 Chemical structures of histamine and H_2-receptor antagonists.

not have clinical significance. The drugs can be administered in doses that produce equivalent acid suppression without toxicity (Table 6-3).

Although a large number of side effects have been reported for the various H_2-receptor antagonists, all are remarkably well tolerated and safe. The incidence of drug reactions approximates 3%, not significantly different from placebo-treated patients.[25] There is no convincing evidence that any of the available agents has a superior safety profile. Central nervous system reactions, such as confusion or lethargy, occur in about 1% of patients receiving intravenous cimetidine. Elderly patients, especially those with renal impairment, appear to be particularly vulnerable. Central nervous system toxicity responds to dose reduction. Cimetidine and, to a lesser degree, ranitidine bind to the microsomal cytochrome P-450 oxidase system. Famotidine and nizatidine have no significant interaction with this system. Because of interactions with the cytochrome P-450 system, cimetidine can interfere with the metabolism of drugs that also use this system. The pharmaco-

kinetics of theophylline, phenytoin, lidocaine, and warfarin, all of which have narrow therapeutic ranges, are affected, and when cimetidine is used, drug level monitoring and dose adjustment may be needed. A simpler alternative often is to prescribe famotidine or nizatidine.

Proton Pump Inhibitors

Omeprazole is a substituted benzimidazole derivative that acts as a proton pump inhibitor (Fig. 6-10). Omeprazole is a weak base with a pK of 4.0. In an acidic environment, such as the parietal cell secretory canaliculus, omeprazole becomes protonated and highly reactive. Covalent bonds are formed with the H^+–K^+ adenosine triphosphatase, resulting in permanent inhibition of the enzyme and a prolonged duration of drug action. Because protonated omeprazole cannot diffuse through plasma membranes, the drug becomes concentrated at its site of action. Although other proton pumps are distributed throughout the body, the parietal cell enzyme is structurally unique and is the only target for omeprazole, providing exquisite specificity.

Omeprazole inhibits basal acid secretion as well as secretion stimulated by pentagastrin, histamine, cholinergic agonists, or a meal. Acid suppression is dose dependent; total anacidity (98% suppression) is achieved at a single dose of 80 mg.[26] At 24 hours after drug administration, 60% to 70% of acid suppression persists. Greater degrees of acid inhibition occur with repeated doses because of increased absorption of drug.

Omeprazole is unstable in an acidic environment and is supplied in an enteric-coated formulation. Bioavailability is increased during 3 to 5 days of administration because increasing acid suppression decreases gastric degradation of the native compound. Antacids do not interfere with omeprazole absorption, but the drug should not be ingested with food. Absorbed omeprazole has a rapid distribution and is extracted by the liver and the gastric mucosa. When examined by autoradiography, radiolabeled omeprazole is detected only in the stomach at 48 hours.

Omeprazole that is not concentrated in gastric parietal cells is rapidly metabolized by the liver. Known metabolites have no antisecretory activity. In contrast to H_2-receptor antagonists, renal excretion is not important, and dose adjustments are not necessary in patients with renal insufficiency. No recommendations for drug dosing in hepatic disease are available.

Clinical experience with omeprazole is much smaller than with H_2-receptor antagonists, and information regarding its safety record are less secure. Nonetheless, side effects have been reported to occur no more frequently than in placebo- or H_2-receptor antag-

Table 6-3   Pharmacology of Histamine-2 Receptor Antagonists

	Cimetidine	*Ranitidine*	*Nizatidine*	*Famotidine*
Relative potency	1	4–8	4–8	20–50
Equivalent dose	1600 mg	300 mg	300 mg	40 mg
Bioavailability	60%–80%	50%–60%	90%–100%	40%–50%
Peak serum concentration (h)	1–2	1–3	1–3	1–3
Serum half-life (h)	1.5–2.5	2–3	1–2	2.5–4
Urinary excretion	50%	30%	>90%	30%
Doses for acute duodenal ulcer	300 mg qid	150 mg qid	150 mg bid	20 mg bid
	400 mg bid	300 mg hs	300 mg hs	40 mg hs
	800 mg hs			
Doses for acute gastric ulcer	300 mg qid	150 mg bid		40 mg hs
	400 mg bid	300 mg hs		
	800 mg hs			
Maintenance dose	400 mg hs	150 mg hs	150 mg hs	20 mg hs

(After Isenberg JI, McQuaid KR, Laine L, Rubin W. Acid-peptic disorders. In: Yamada T, ed. Textbook of gastroenterology. Philadelphia, JB Lippincott, 1991:1270)

onist–treated controls. Omeprazole inhibits the cytochrome P-450 system and can prolong metabolism of drugs using this pathway. In addition, omeprazole can interfere with absorption of drugs that require an acidic gastric environment, the most important being ketoconazole.

Repeated dosing with omeprazole results in increased levels of circulating gastrin; elevation of serum gastrin correlates with the degree of acid suppression produced. In humans, prolonged hypergastrinemia secondary to achlorhydria (atrophic gastritis) or Zollinger-Ellison syndrome is associated with increased risk of gastric carcinoid tumors (see Chap. 9). Concerns about the long-term use of omeprazole have arisen for this reason. In rats, prolonged high-dose omeprazole causes sustained hypergastrinemia, which leads secondarily to enterochromaffin-like (ECL) cell hyperplasia.[27] Gastric carcinoid tumors have developed from ECL cell hyperplasia in this model. The risk of ECL cell hyperplasia in humans is unclear and appears to be low, but because of these safety concerns, long-term uninterrupted use of omeprazole has not been approved for patients with peptic ulcer.

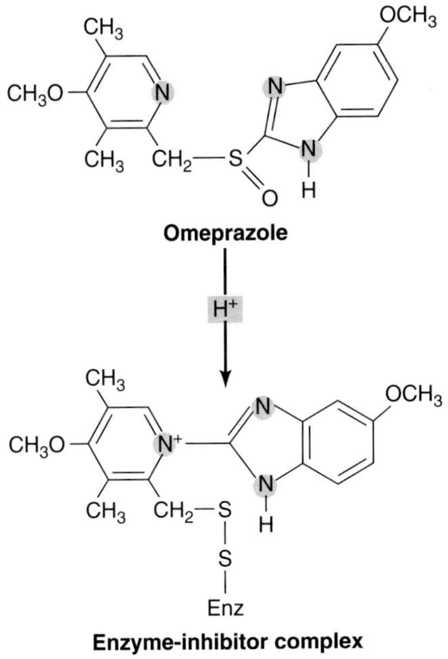

Sucralfate

Sucralfate is the aluminum salt of sulfated sucrose (Fig. 6-11). Sucralfate has no buffering capacity, so neutralizing actions are not the mechanism of its therapeutic effects. In the presence of acid, the aluminum moieties dissociate, and sucralfate binds to positively charged proteins exposed in the base of the ulcer. It has

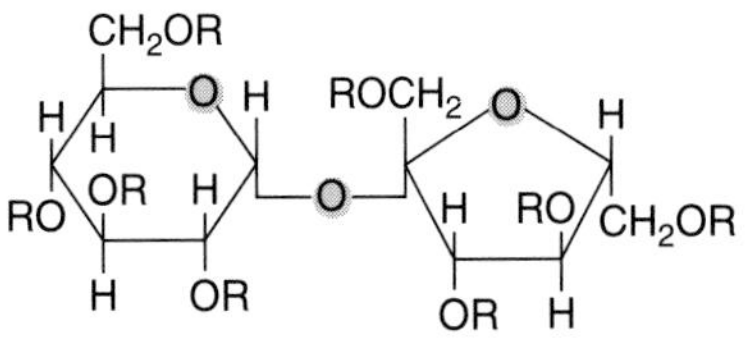

Figure 6-10 Chemical structure of omeprazole. Within the acidic environment of the parietal cell secretory canaliculus, omeprazole becomes protonated and highly reactive. A disulfide complex forms with a cysteine group of the hydrogen ion pump, resulting in permanent inactivation.

$R = SO_3Al_2(OH)_5$

Figure 6-11 Chemical structure of sucralfate.

been widely reported that binding of sucralfate to the ulcer base impedes contact of luminal pepsin and bile salts with the ulcer. Other cytoprotective activities may be more important. Sucralfate stimulates mucosal prostaglandin E_2 production and increases mucus and bicarbonate secretion.[28] Sucralfate binds epidermal growth factor (EGF) secreted from saliva and protects it from destruction by gastric acid.[29] The drug stimulates epithelial proliferation at the ulcer margin, perhaps by delivery of undegraded EGF to the site of ulceration.

Sucralfate is administered in the absence of food two to four times daily. Systemic absorption is less than 5%, making sucralfate an attractive choice in pregnant patients. Aluminum absorption is less than 0.01%, and aluminum accumulation during short-term therapy is not clinically significant.[30]

Sucralfate has virtually no systemic toxicity. Constipation is reported in 2% of patients. Sucralfate can impair the absorption of warfarin and phenytoin.

Prostaglandin Derivatives

Prostaglandins are 20-carbon oxygenated fatty acids derived from arachidonic acid, which is present in cell membranes. Arachidonic acid is converted by cyclooxygenase to endoperoxides with eventual formation of prostacyclin, prostaglandins E and F, or thromboxane. Prostaglandins do not function as classic hormones, instead acting locally in a paracrine fashion. Native prostaglandins have an extremely short biologic half-life. Prostaglandin derivatives, such as misoprostol, a synthetic methylated analogue of prostaglandin E_1, combine many of the biologic properties of the parent compound with a prolonged half-life (Fig. 6-12). Misoprostol has been approved by the Food and Drug Administration for human use.

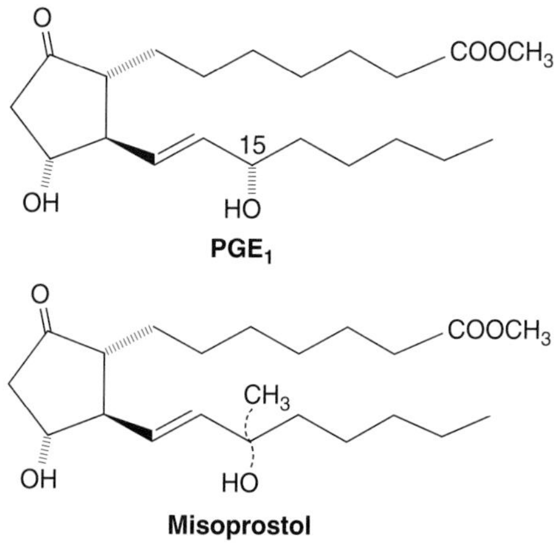

Figure 6-12 Chemical structures of prostaglandin E_1 and misoprostol.

The mechanisms by which prostaglandin analogues protect against drug-induced gastric mucosal damage or accelerate ulcer healing are not fully understood. Prostaglandins have a number of properties that could be contributory. Prostaglandin analogues stimulate both mucus and bicarbonate secretion. The agents increase mucosal blood flow, an important element in animal models of ulcer healing.[31] Misoprostol also inhibits gastric acid secretion at doses used to treat ulcer disease, although the drug is less potent than H_2-receptor antagonists or omeprazole. Misoprostol suppresses acid secretion by inhibiting cAMP production in parietal cells. There are no effects on gastrin release.

Misoprostol is absorbed in the small intestine. Metabolites of the drug are excreted in the urine, with more than 80% eliminated by 24 hours. Drug half-life is 1.5 hours.[32] There is no known interaction of misoprostol with the hepatic P-450 drug metabolizing system.

The most common side effects associated with prostaglandin analogues are a consequence of actions on intestinal fluid and electrolyte transport and effects on gastrointestinal and uterine smooth muscle. Secondary to stimulation of cAMP production in intestinal epithelial cells, prostaglandin analogues increase intestinal sodium, potassium, chloride, and water secretion. Diarrhea occurs in 20% of patients treated with prostaglandin derivatives but can be ameliorated in most cases by dose reduction. Diarrhea is significantly more common than with H_2-receptor antagonists, omeprazole, or sucralfate. Increases in uterine smooth muscle contractility may cause increased uterine bleeding; this contravenes use of prostaglandin analogues in pregnant women or in women planning pregnancy.

Colloidal Bismuth Subcitrate

Bismuth compounds in the form of colloidal bismuth subcitrate and subsalicylate have been used to treat patients with duodenal ulceration with increasing frequency since the association of duodenal ulcers with *H pylori* was recognized. The therapeutic effects of colloidal bismuth compounds do not relate solely to their antimicrobial actions. Colloidal bismuth compounds precipitate in the acidic environment of the stomach and form a coating over the ulcer crater. This coating has been postulated to prevent diffusion of hydrogen ions and to protect against peptic digestion. Colloidal bismuth stimulates mucosal prostaglandin E_2 production with secondary increases in mucosal bicarbonate secretion.[33] Colloidal bismuth binds EGF, and in experimental studies, causes accumulation of EGF within the ulcer.[34] The compound has no antisecretory or buffering activity.

Colloidal bismuth is available in liquid form and as chewable or coated tablets. Most ingested drug is excreted in the feces in the form of bismuth sulfide. Trace amounts are absorbed systemically where bismuth is excreted in the urine. Tissue accumulation of bismuth can be demonstrated in the kidneys with long-term administration; chronic toxicity risks are unknown. Few adverse reactions have been reported with colloidal bismuth, in part because of its poor absorption. The solution has an unpleasant smell. Chewable tablets cause staining of the teeth and tongue; the stool is blackened and can be confused with melena.

Antacids

Antacids were the mainstay of ulcer treatment before the introduction of H_2-receptor antagonists (Table 6-4). Most commercially available antacids contain calcium carbonate, magnesium hydroxide, or aluminum hydroxide, either singly or in combination. At high doses (over 500 mmol/d), antacids act primarily as neutralizing agents for luminal acid. The greatest benefit is realized in the hour after a meal. Studies have indicated that lower-dose antacid regimens (below 200 mmol/d) can also promote ulcer healing.[35,36] This lower dose has only modest buffering capacity, implying that some other mechanism of healing must be activated.

The major side effects of antacid therapy are diarrhea caused by magnesium-containing compounds and constipation due to aluminum-containing compounds. Most preparations contain a mix of aluminum hydrox-

Table 6-4 Comparison of Antacids

Antacid	Composition	Acid-Neutralizing* Capacity
Delcid	Mg, Al	42.0
Maalox TC	Mg, Al	28.3
Mylanta II	Mg, Al	25.4
Gelusil II	Mg, Al	24.0
Basaljel	Al	22.0
Titralac	Ca	19.0
Camalox	Mg, Al, Ca	18.0
Alternagel	Al	16.0
Riopan	Mg, Al	15.0
Riopan Plus	Mg, Al	15.0
Aludrox	Mg, Al	14.0
Maalox Plus	Mg, Al	13.5
Gelusil	Mg, Al	12.0
Kolantyl Gel	Mg, Al	10.5
Amphojel	Al	6.5
Phosphaljel	Al	1.5

* Milliequivalent of acid neutralized per 5 mL of liquid or per tablet.

Table 6-5 Histamine-2 Receptor Antagonists in Duodenal Ulcer Therapy

Drug	Dosage	4-Week Healing (%)	Suppression of 24-Hour Acidity (%)
Cimetidine	400 mg bid	72	37
Cimetidine	300 mg qid	74	65
Cimetidine	800 mg hs	80	48
Ranitidine	150 mg hs	75	45
Ranitidine	300 mg hs	84	68
Famotidine	40 mg hs	82	64

(After Jones DB, Howden CW, Burget DW, et al. Acid suppression in duodenal ulcer: a meta-analysis to define optimal dosing with antisecretory drugs. Gut 1987;28:1120)

ide and magnesium hydroxide to minimize alterations in bowel function. In patients with renal failure, elevation of serum magnesium and aluminum can occur.

Treatment of Acute Ulceration

Three goals have been established for the treatment of acute duodenal ulceration—relief of pain, acceleration of ulcer healing, and prevention of complications during the healing process. Given the number of effective agents available for clinical use, the choice depends on dose frequency, cost, patient acceptance and compliance, and occurrence of unwanted side effects. Treatment of duodenal ulceration can be guided by information available from the large number of prospective randomized therapeutic trials available (Table 6-5).

H_2-receptor antagonists are highly effective in promoting ulcer healing. Ranitidine, 150 mg twice daily, or cimetidine, 400 mg twice daily, heals 60% to 75% of duodenal ulcers at 4 weeks and 85% to 90% at 8 weeks.[37] As the importance of nocturnal acid secretion in the pathogenesis of peptic ulcer has been realized, a number of trials have demonstrated that ranitidine, 300 mg at bedtime, or cimetidine, 800 mg at bedtime, produces similar healing rates to twice-daily dosing regimens.[38] Famotidine, 40 mg, or nizatidine, 300 mg, with supper are equally effective.[39,40] When H_2-receptor antagonists are stopped, ulcer recurrence has been demonstrated in as many as half of patients within 1 year. Maintenance therapy with nocturnal H_2-receptor antagonists reduces the risk of recurrence to 10% to 30%.

Omeprazole has been compared with ranitidine or cimetidine in a number of trials (Table 6-6). Omeprazole, 20 mg/d, produces superior ulcer healing at 2 or 4 weeks, with equivalent rates of healing (90% or more) after 8 weeks of therapy. Omeprazole provides superior

Table 6-6 Omeprazole in Duodenal Ulcer Therapy

Drug	Dosage	4-Week Healing (%)	8-Week Healing (%)	Suppression of 24-Hour Acidity (%)
Omeprazole	20 mg qd	70–80	85–95	90
Omeprazole	40 mg qd	80	95	98

pain relief during the first 2 weeks of treatment when compared with H$_2$-receptor antagonists.

Sucralfate is an acceptable alternative to H$_2$-receptor antagonists or omeprazole for the treatment of acute ulceration, with healing rates of 85% to 95% at 8 weeks when administered at 1 g four times daily or 2 g twice daily.[41] Colloidal bismuth is of clinical interest because of its efficacy and reduced rate of ulcer recurrence; however, because long-term toxicity data are missing, bismuth compounds must be considered second-line choices. Antacids and prostaglandin E derivatives are not commonly used as primary therapy for duodenal ulcer, antacids because of large volumes needed, frequent dosing, and alteration of bowel habits, and prostaglandins because diarrhea and abdominal cramps are frequent at doses needed to suppress acid production.

Operative Treatment

Operative therapy is reserved for the complications of peptic ulcer. Classically, indications for operation have included intractability, perforation, hemorrhage, and obstruction. When operative treatment is employed, the first goal should be alteration of the underlying ulcer diathesis so that ulcer healing is promoted and recurrences minimized. A second surgical goal is correction of associated anatomic defects, such as pyloric stenosis or perforation. The final objective should be safety in the immediate postoperative period and long-term freedom from undesirable side effects. In modern practice, the surgeon treating the complications of peptic ulcer can select from medicinal, endoscopic, radiologic, and operative approaches. Appropriate treatment often requires a combination of more than one method.

Although a number of operations have been used to treat peptic ulcer historically, three procedures—proximal gastric vagotomy, truncal vagotomy and drainage, and truncal vagotomy and antrectomy—are employed currently. Operations such as gastroenterostomy or subtotal gastrectomy without vagotomy have been discarded as ineffective or inappropriate. Selective vagotomy, an operation in which extragastric vagal branches are spared but the entire stomach is denervated, has no advantage over proximal gastric vagotomy and should be considered obsolete.

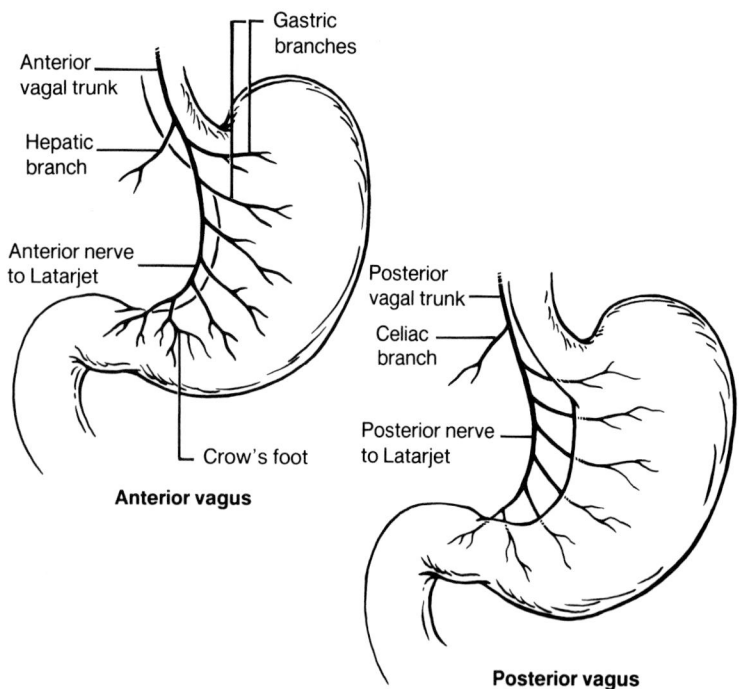

Figure 6-13 Normal vagal anatomy.

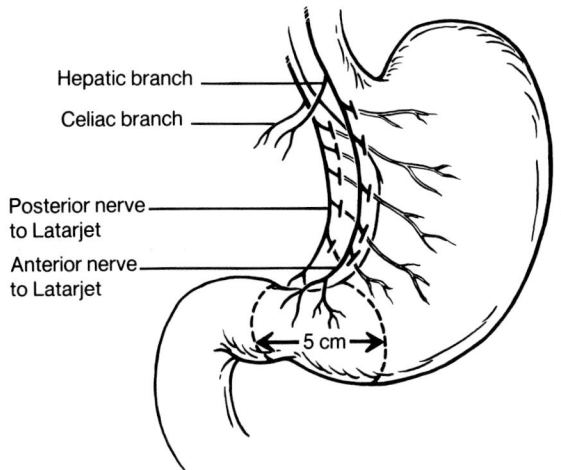

Figure 6-14 Proximal gastric vagotomy.

Proximal gastric vagotomy involves division of nerve fibers to the acid-secreting gastric fundus (Figs. 6-13 and 6-14). Vagal fibers to the antrum and pylorus remain intact. The hepatic branch of the anterior vagus and the celiac branch of the posterior vagus are not transected. The dissection along the lesser curvature of the stomach begins 5 cm proximal to the pylorus. The distal 5 to 7 cm of esophagus is skeletonized to interrupt vagal fibers that reach the gastric fundus by traveling intramurally within the esophagus. Proximal gastric vagotomy has also been called *highly selective vagotomy* and *parietal cell vagotomy.*

In procedures that include truncal vagotomy, both vagal nerves are divided at the esophageal hiatus (Fig. 6-15). By division at this level, parasympathetic inner-

vation is eliminated for the entire stomach and for all digestive organs to the level of the transverse colon. Denervation of the antropyloric region of the stomach may result in uncoordinated pyloric relaxation and gastric retention of solids and liquids. Gastric drainage is ensured by division of the pyloric sphincter through performance of pyloroplasty. A Heineke-Mikulicz pyloroplasty, the most common variant, is performed by making a longitudinal incision through the pylorus and then closing the incision transversely (Fig. 6-16). Variants of this procedure include the Finney pyloroplasty and the Jaboulay procedure.

A more pronounced reduction in acid production may be achieved when truncal vagotomy is combined with antrectomy. Removal of the antral source of gastrin augments the parasympathetic denervation of the gastric fundus. The duodenum is divided at the pylorus and along a line from the lesser curvature proximal to the incisura angularis to the midpoint of the greater curvature (Fig. 6-17). Reconstruction can be through gastroduodenostomy (Billroth I) or gastrojejunostomy

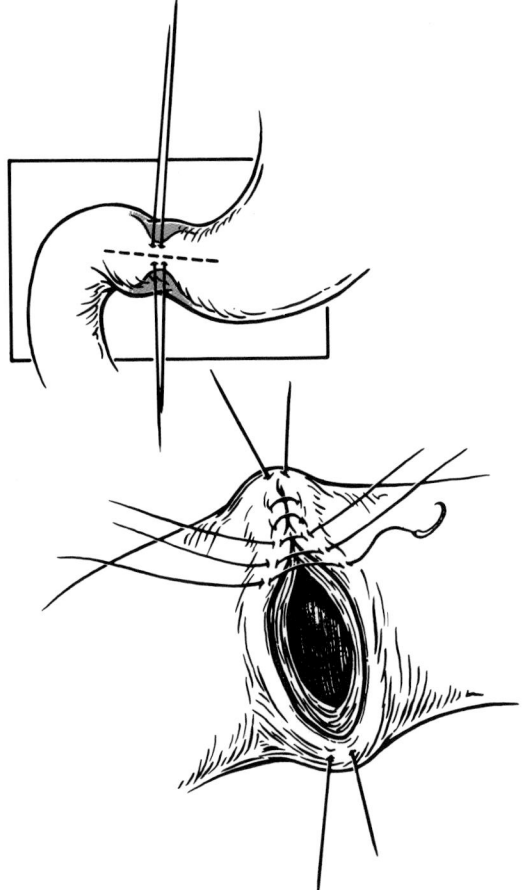

Figure 6-16 Pyloroplasty formation. The Heineke-Mikulicz pyloroplasty involves a longitudinal incision through the pylorus followed by transverse closure.

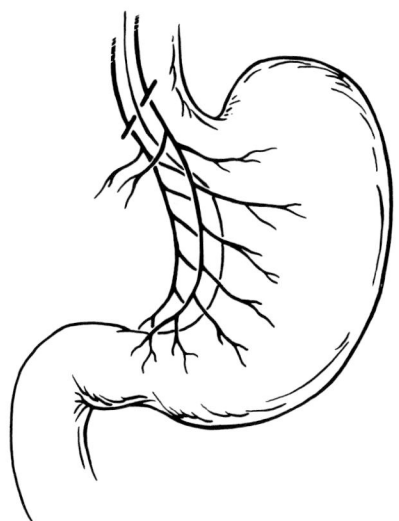

Figure 6-15 Level of division of vagal nerves in truncal vagotomy.

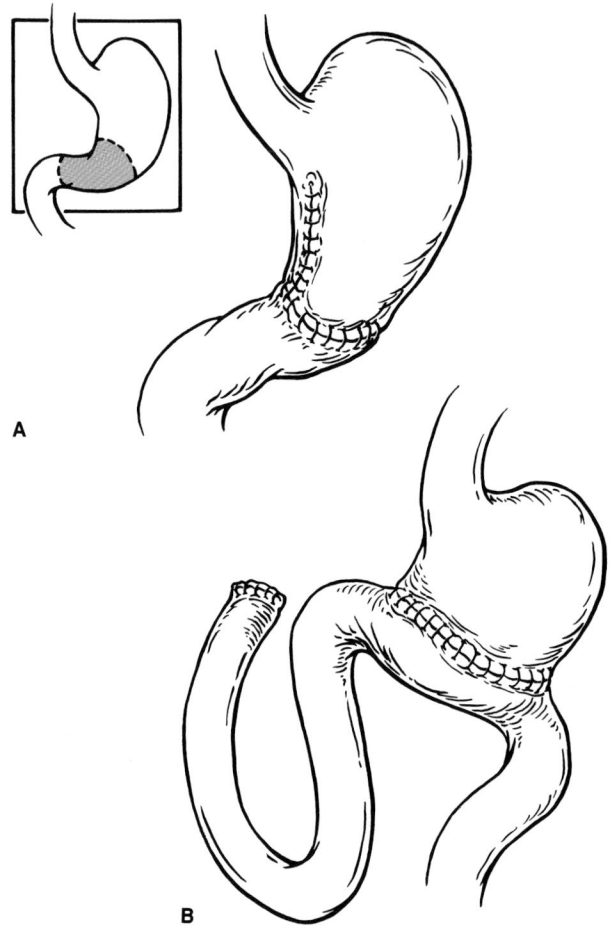

Figure 6-17 Antrectomy with Billroth I reconstruction (**A**) or Billroth II gastrojejunostomy (**B**).

(Billroth II). Details of these operative procedures are presented in Section V of Atlas Chapter 11.

Physiologic Results of Duodenal Ulcer Surgery

Some form of vagotomy is incorporated in virtually every operation performed for treatment of duodenal ulcer. Vagotomy reduces acid production by interrupting cholinergic input of parietal cells from efferent secretory fibers contained in the vagus nerves (Table 6-7). Truncal vagotomy reduces basal acid secretion by about 80%. Alterations in acid secretion are noted in the immediate postoperative period and are permanent. Maximal acid output in response to pentagastrin is reduced by about half. Meal-stimulated acid output is decreased by 60% to 70% relative to preoperative values. Basal and stimulated pepsin secretion parallel acid secretion; reductions in pepsin output after vagotomy are similar to those in acid secretion. Reductions in acid secretion

after proximal gastric vagotomy are similar to those produced by truncal vagotomy.

Both truncal vagotomy and proximal gastric vagotomy are associated with a state of postoperative hypergastrinemia. Fasting basal serum gastrin levels are elevated two to three times normal, and the postprandial response is exaggerated. Loss of inhibitory feedback to gastrin release from luminal acid and removal of inhibitory vagal fibers have been postulated to cause hypergastrinemia in the immediate postoperative period. Chronic hypergastrinemia is sustained by these factors and by the development of gastrin cell hyperplasia.[42]

The addition of antrectomy to truncal vagotomy results in postoperative reduction in circulating gastrin. The major source of circulating gastrin after antrectomy is the duodenum; gastrin 34 is the predominant circulating form.

Vagal efferent secretory fibers account for only 2% to 3% of all fibers in the vagi. The remainder are afferent fibers or motor-efferent fibers. Both these nonsecretory fiber types are important in regulating motor function of the stomach, and both truncal vagotomy and proximal gastric vagotomy cause alterations in gastric emptying. Interruption of the vagal innervation of the proximal stomach abolishes receptive relaxation. Receptive relaxation is a vagally mediated process by which the proximal stomach relaxes on ingestion of food so that increasing volume is accommodated without increasing intragastric pressure. Thus, after vagotomy, for any given volume ingested, rises in intragastric pressure are greater than normal. As a result, the gastroduodenal pressure gradient, which is the primary determinant of the rate of liquid emptying, is higher

---

Table 6-7 Physiologic Alterations Caused by Truncal Vagotomy

GASTRIC
Reduced basal acid secretion
Reduced maximal acid output
Reduced basal and stimulated pepsin secretion
Fasting and stimulated hypergastrinemia
Loss of receptive relaxation
Loss of pyloric relaxation
Defective antral motor function

SMALL INTESTINE
Loss of regulation of motor, secretory, absorptive activity

GALLBLADDER
Defective contraction

PANCREAS
Decreased basal enzyme secretion
Loss of cephalic and gastric phases of pancreatic secretion

than normal. Emptying of liquids is accelerated after truncal or proximal gastric vagotomy.

Because the distal stomach innervation is not disturbed with proximal gastric vagotomy, antral grinding and mixing of solid food is not disturbed with this operation[43] (Fig. 6-18). Truncal vagotomy impairs pyloric sphincter relaxation, causing potential gastric retention. Destruction of the pyloric sphincter by performance of a pyloroplasty is usually followed by increased rates of solid and liquid emptying.

Truncal vagotomy also affects a number of extragastric functions because of loss of parasympathetic innervation (see Table 6-7). Both basal and postprandial pancreatic enzyme secretion are decreased. Although fecal fat content doubles after truncal vagotomy, clinically recognized steatorrhea does not occur. Postprandial bile flow is diminished, and gallbladder volume is increased due to reduced gallbladder contractility. The release of a number of gastrointestinal peptide hormones is impaired. Failure of sham feeding to increase circulating levels of pancreatic polypeptide has been used as a test of completeness of truncal vagotomy.

Intractable Duodenal Ulcer

Intractability is an indication for duodenal ulcer surgery. In the past, the term *intractability* referred to ulcers that caused chronic pain because of failure to heal or because of frequent relapse. Defined in this way, intractability is seldom now a reason for operation because newer antisecretory agents, such as omeprazole, can provide relief of pain in up to 90% of patients within 2 weeks of beginning therapy (Fig. 6-19). However, absence of pain cannot be equated with ulcer healing, and ulcer complications can occur in the absence of symptoms. A more useful definition of intractability

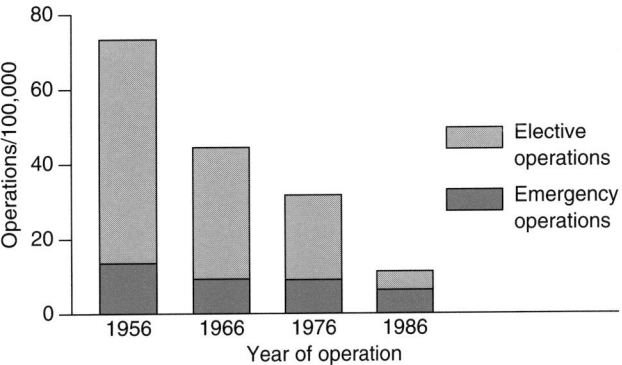

Figure 6-19 Rates for elective and emergent operations for duodenal ulcer over four decades. (After Gustavsson S, Nyren O. Time trends in peptic ulcer surgery, 1956 to 1986. Ann Surg 1989;210:704)

focuses on the state of mucosal healing. Ulcers should be considered intractable in the following instances: (1) initial healing is not achieved, so ulceration persists at 3 months in the presence of active therapy; (2) ulcers recur within 1 year despite active H_2-receptor therapy with intervening maintenance therapy; or (3) ulcer disease is characterized by cycles of prolonged activity that interfere with occupation or life-style. Special consideration for operation should also be given to H_2-receptor antagonist–resistant ulcers that are larger than 2 cm (giant duodenal ulcer) or associated with a prior history of complication (perforation or hemorrhage).

Intractability is the major indication for elective operation in duodenal ulcer. Because a number of potential procedures are available, attempts have been made to select patients for specific operations based on preoperative characteristics, especially acid secretory status. Unfortunately, stratification of patients as high or low acid secretors does not predict postoperative ulcer recurrence. Instead, the choice for operation should focus on operative safety, the rate of recurrent ulceration, and the occurrence of undesirable side effects. Because elective gastric operations are associated with low mortality rates, the decision often involves a trade-off between ulcer recurrence and postoperative side effects.

Proximal gastric vagotomy has much to recommend it as the preferred operation for intractable duodenal ulcer. Proximal gastric vagotomy has the lowest reported operative mortality rate of procedures used to treat duodenal ulcer, less than 0.5% worldwide. This impressive safety record may reflect the fact that the gastrointestinal tract is not entered and gastric suture lines are not created, lessening the risk of postoperative infection or anastomotic dehiscence.

Chronic postoperative symptoms are uncommon after proximal gastric vagotomy and are usually easily

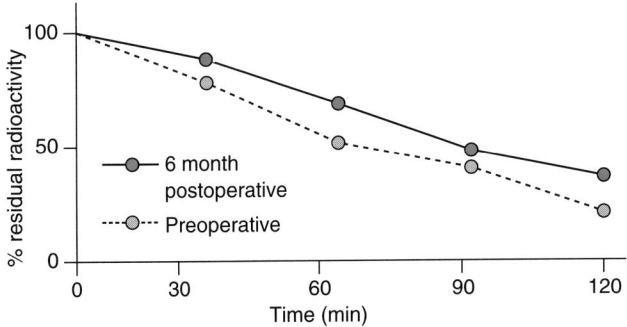

Figure 6-18 Preoperative and postoperative rates of gastric emptying of solids in patients undergoing proximal gastric vagotomy. (After Mistiaen W, Van Hee R, Blockx P, et al. Gastric emptying for solids in patients with duodenal ulcer before and after highly selective vagotomy. Dig Dis Sci 1990;35:310)

controlled. Dumping is a postprandial symptom complex of abdominal discomfort, sweating, dizziness, and weakness that occurs after abdominal vagotomy. Dumping occurs in 2% to 5% of patients after proximal gastric vagotomy.[44-47] Most affected patients improve with time, and dumping symptoms are rarely disabling. After truncal vagotomy and pyloroplasty, significant dumping is present in about 10% to 15% of patients initially and is persistent in 1%. Postoperative dumping is reported by 10% to 20% of patients who undergo truncal vagotomy and antrectomy.

Postoperative diarrhea occurs in about 5% of patients who undergo proximal gastric vagotomy and, like dumping, is usually not severe. The incidence of postoperative diarrhea parallels dumping rates in patients who undergo truncal vagotomy and pyloroplasty or antrectomy. Like dumping, chronic postvagotomy diarrhea persists in about 1% to 2% of patients after the latter operations.

Mild dysphagia is occasionally present in the early postoperative period after proximal gastric vagotomy, perhaps as a resultof the periesophageal dissection, but it is not persistent. Bile reflux with bilious vomiting, anemia, weight loss, and hypocalcemia is another side effect reported after truncal vagotomy and gastric resection that is not encountered after proximal gastric vagotomy.

An overall assessment of gastrointestinal complaints is provided by a standard grading system called the *Visick classification* (Table 6-8). In a recent review of more than 25 operative series, Visick I or II scores were reported in 85% to 95% of patients who had undergone proximal gastric vagotomy.[48] Visick I and II scores after truncal vagotomy and pyloroplasty or truncal vagotomy and antrectomy averaged 70%.

The low rate of postoperative side effects after proximal gastric vagotomy is obtained at the cost of a relatively high, and variable, rate of recurrent ulcer. A compilation of reports of proximal gastric vagotomy, published after 1984, is presented in Table 6-9. When proximal gastric vagotomy is performed by experienced gastric surgeons, recurrences range from 5% to 15%. Incomplete vagotomy is unequivocally the major cause of recurrent ulcer, and variability in recurrence rates among series reflects differences in surgical skill and technique. Recurrent ulcer occurs in 8% to 12% of patients after truncal vagotomy and pyloroplasty.[49] The lowest rate of recurrent ulcer, about 1%, is observed after truncal vagotomy and antrectomy.

Three caveats apply when considering recurrence rates after proximal gastric vagotomy. First, ulcer recurrences are cumulative, and follow-up times of less than 5 to 10 years may be misleading. Second, the methods used to detect recurrences vary widely among series; when routine endoscopy is used, reported recurrence rates are higher. Third, series that include prepyloric and pyloric channel ulcers with duodenal ulcers may have higher than expected recurrence rates.[50] Prepyloric ulcers are defined as those occurring within 3 cm of the pylorus. The reason for reduced efficacy of proximal gastric vagotomy when used for ulcers in this position is unclear.

Recurrent ulcers that develop after proximal gastric vagotomy often respond to medical management. More than half of patients with recurrent ulcers heal with H$_2$-receptor therapy.[51] In contrast, most recurrent ulcers after truncal vagotomy and drainage or antrectomy eventually require reoperation.

Table 6-9 Ulcer Recurrnce After Proximal Gastric Vagotomy

Investigator	Follow-Up (y)	Recurrence Rate (%)
Gorey (1984)	12	7.0
Stoddard (1984)	8	8.8
Marceau (1986)	3–12	12.0
Clark (1986)	1–15	17.4
Enskog (1986)	1–10	13.8
Stael von Holstein (1987)	10	18.0
Jordan (1987)	8–10	10.0
Hoffman (1987)	14–18	30.0
Herrington (1987)	6–13	9.2
Goodman (1987)	2–7	4.4
Meisner (1988)	15	27.0
Braghetto (1988)	3	3.0
Soper (1989)	5–13	14.0
Raab (1989)	16	29.7
Valen (1991)	3–14	13.0
Macintyre (1991)	15	18.5
Johnston (1991)	10–20	15.0
Emas (1992)	1–16	23.0

Table 6-8 Visick Symptom Scoring System

Visick Rating	Criteria
I	Excellent results; no symptoms
II	Good results; patient volunteers no complaints on interview; questioning reveals mild complaints that are easily controlled
III	Poor results; mild to moderate symptoms not prevented by care but not interfering seriously with life or work
IV	Failure; ulcer recurrence or symptoms or complications that interfere with life or work

Perforation

Although the overall rate of duodenal ulcer perforation has not declined, evidence indicates that the demographic profile of patients who present with perforation has changed (Fig. 6-20). Increasingly, older patients with coexisting diseases are affected. In one series,[52] 63% were over 60 years old, and 44% were more than 70 years of age. More than half of perforations occur in previously undiagnosed ulcers; in two thirds of cases, perforation is the first symptom of disease. The lifetime risk of perforation in untreated patients can be as high as 10%.

Typically, the patient experiences sudden, incapacitating epigastric pain, followed shortly by generalized abdominal pain. Chemical irritation of the peritoneum by gastric contents causes symptoms to reach peak intensity quickly. Subphrenic collection of gastric contents can result in scapular radiation of pain; spread along the right pericolic gutter can cause symptoms in the right lower quadrant. Respiration and movement exacerbate discomfort. The expected clinical signs may

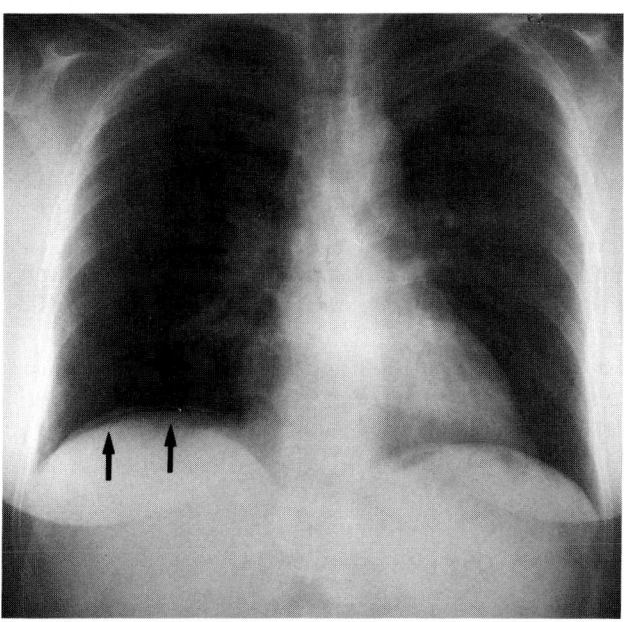

Figure 6-21 Upright abdominal radiograph demonstrating pneumoperitoneum (*arrows*).

be significantly muted in elderly patients and in those receiving corticosteroids.

Low-grade fever and tachycardia are frequent, but hypotension is unusual early after perforation. Leukocytosis and elevation of serum amylase are common and nonspecific. Pneumoperitoneum is visible on 80% of plain abdominal films (Fig. 6-21) but is less frequently present in elderly patients. When perforation is suspected but pneumoperitoneum absent, water-soluble contrast can be administered to demonstrate extravasation.

The septic consequences of duodenal perforation relate both to bacterial colonization of the stomach before perforation and to the chronicity of perforation. Although the empty, acid-secreting human stomach may be sterile, 100 to 1000 organisms are normally present in each milliliter. Lactobacilli and aerobic streptococci predominate. Hypochlorhydria, both spontaneous and iatrogenic, and gastric stasis cause increases in total bacterial counts and proliferation of coliform species. If peritoneal fluid samples are obtained 6 to 12 hours after clinical perforation, only 45% are culture-positive; at 12 to 24 hours, 67% become positive. Initial antibiotic choices should be broadly directed against a mixed enteric flora.

Occasional reports have advocated nonoperative management of perforated duodenal ulcer. Stringent exclusion criteria and the potentially serious consequences of operative delay limit nonsurgical therapy to the small proportion of patients with already-sealed

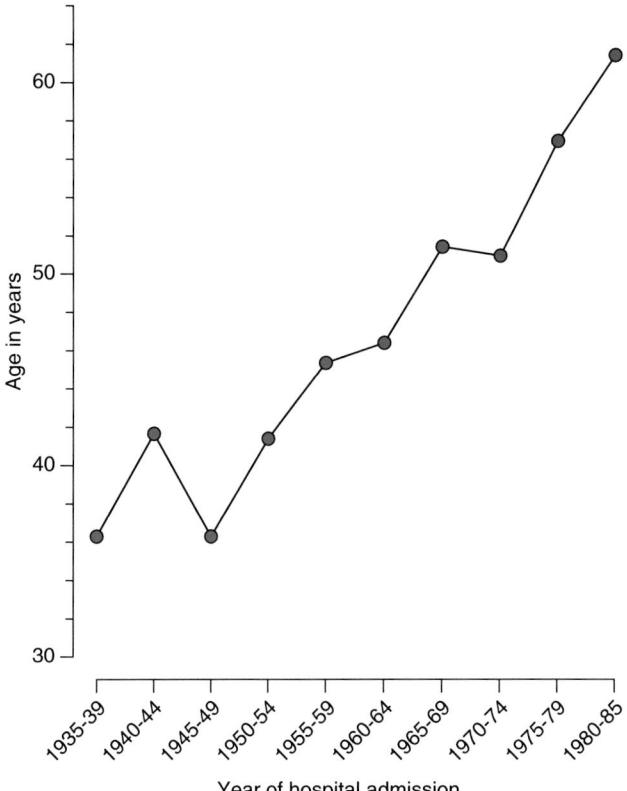

Figure 6-20 Changes in median patient age for perforated gastroduodenal ulcer from 1935 to 1985. (After Svanes C, Salveson H, Espehaug B, et al. A multifactorial analysis of factors related to lethality after treatment of perforated gastroduodenal ulcer, 1935–1985. Ann Surg 1989;209:418)

perforations that are clinically stable at the time of diagnosis. Advocates of nonoperative management have excluded patients with a history of gastric ulcer, serious coexisting medical diseases, and perforation of greater than 24 hours' duration with clinical deterioration, associated shock, or diagnostic uncertainty.[53] Treatment with intravenous fluid resuscitation, nasogastric aspiration, and intravenous antibiotics is followed at 4 to 6 hours by meglumine diatrizoate (Gastrografin) contrast radiography to exclude free intraperitoneal extravasation of gastric contents. Contrast leakage or lack of clinical improvement is an indication for immediate operation. In one series,[54] 28% of patients treated nonoperatively had clinical deterioration within 24 hours and required operation. Perforated gastric and colonic carcinomas were discovered in 3 of 11 patients who failed conservative management. Hospital stay was 35% longer in the group treated nonoperatively; complication rates were not lower. Patients older than 70 years of age were less likely to respond to nonoperative treatment than younger patients.

All operations for perforated duodenal ulcer should have three goals: patient safety, peritoneal cleansing, and closure of the perforation. A fourth goal, which can be achieved in most patients, is alteration of the ulcer diathesis so that the risk of recurrent ulceration is minimized.

Operative risk factors for patients with perforated ulcer have been defined prospectively.[55] Concurrent medical illness, preoperative shock, and perforations of greater than 48 hours' duration were features that increased mortality. Importantly, older age, gross peritoneal soiling, and the length of antecedent ulcer history did not affect mortality rates. When these factors were used to guide patient selection, definitive operation could be performed as safely as patch closure.[56] In patients without these risk factors, definitive ulcer surgery produced neither mortality nor serious morbidity. Hospital stay was not prolonged. These findings provide a framework for patient selection for definitive operation. Perforated duodenal ulcer patients with preoperative shock, concurrent serious medical illness (eg, recent myocardial infarction), or long-standing perforation should undergo expeditious peritoneal irrigation and omental patch closure of the defect (Fig. 6-22). Postoperative management of the ulcer diathesis for patients treated in this manner should include antisecretory medication and perhaps delayed, reoperative definitive ulcer surgery. Patients without these risk factors are candidates for closure of the perforation combined with definitive ulcer operation.

Standard teaching has been that simple omental patch closure of duodenal perforation in patients with chronically symptomatic disease is not adequate ther-

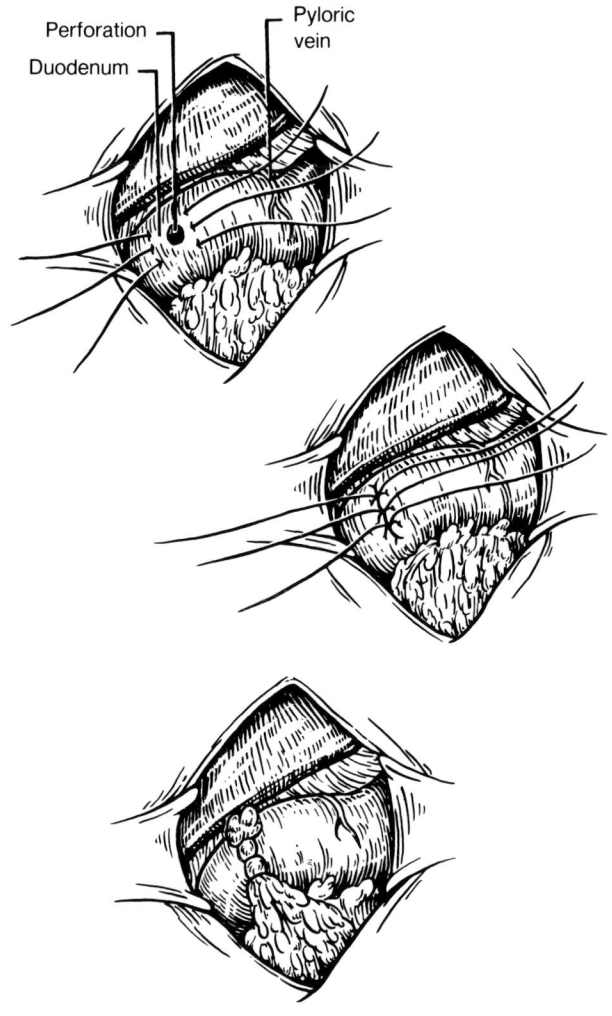

Figure 6-22 Omental patch closure of perforated duodenal ulcer.

apy. Some 60% to 80% of patients treated in this manner develop recurrent ulceration; 85% of recurrences are symptomatic. A second operation is required in half, often emergently. Up to 10% of patients experience repeated perforation. Alternatively, it has been argued that definitive ulcer treatment in patients with acute ulceration unnecessarily subjects patients with a low risk of recurrent disease to chronic postoperative symptoms.

Unfortunately, although it is possible to determine chronicity and thus likelihood of ulcer relapse in groups of patients based on clinical characteristics, this prediction cannot be made with certainty in individual cases. In addition, the favorable long-term outcome of acute perforations may have been overstated. By 5 to 6 years after patch closure, symptomatic recurrence rates in patients with acute ulcer perforation approximate those

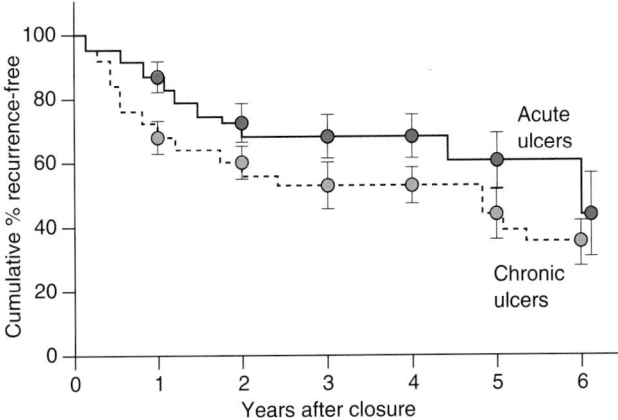

Figure 6-23 Long-term follow-up of patients with perforated chronic and acute duodenal ulcers treated with omental patch closure only. The early favorable results associated with acute ulcers begins to diminish with longer observation. (After Boey J, Branicki FJ, Alagaratnam TT, et al. Proximal gastric vagotomy: the preferred operation for perforations in acute duodenal ulcer. Ann Surg 1988;208:169)

for patients with chronic ulcers[57] (Fig. 6-23). Antiulcer drug therapy confers protection for patients treated with patch closure alone, but this choice often means a commitment to lifelong therapy. These considerations argue in favor of performing a definitive ulcer procedure for all patients with perforated duodenal ulcer, both acute and chronic. The argument becomes stronger if the operation chosen is associated with a low rate of postoperative side effects. An exception exists for patients who develop perforation in clear association with ingestion of NSAIDs. These patients should be treated by omental patch closure only and permanent discontinuation of the drug.

Omental patch closure of the perforation, combined with proximal gastric vagotomy, is an attractive choice for patients with perforated duodenal ulcer. The procedure is both safe and effective in preventing ulcer recurrence. In a prospective trial comparing simple closure, truncal vagotomy and drainage, and patch closure plus proximal gastric vagotomy for perforated chronic duodenal ulcer, there was no mortality and only minor postoperative complications. At 39 months, cumulative recurrence rates were 63%, 12%, and 4%, respectively.[56] These encouraging results have been confirmed in two other trials for perforated chronic ulcers and in a separate trial limited to patients with perforated acute duodenal ulcers[57-59] (Table 6-10). Ninety percent of patients with perforated acute duodenal ulcers treated with proximal gastric vagotomy had Visick I scores after operation. There were no instances of symptomatic dumping or gastroesophageal reflux.[57]

Hemorrhage

About 125,000 patients are hospitalized annually in the United States because of bleeding from peptic ulceration, and hemorrhage remains the leading cause of death associated with duodenal ulcer. The incidence of bleeding has not decreased since the introduction of H_2-receptor antagonists; most patients are not receiving active treatment at the time of hemorrhage.[60,61]

The mortality from upper gastrointestinal bleeding has remained at about 10% during the past 5 decades despite great advances in medical and surgical care, the introduction of endoscopy, improvements in blood products, and intensive patient monitoring. The lack of improvement in survival statistics relates in large part to the increasing proportion of patients older than 60

Table 6-10   Proximal Gastric Vagotomy in Perforated Duodenal Ulcer

Investigator	Patients	Ulcer Type	Recurrence Rate (%)
Boey et al (1982)[56]			
Simple closure	35	Chronic	63.3
Closure plus PGV	34		3.8
Christiansen et al (1987)[58]			
Simple closure	25	Chronic	52
Closure plus PGV	25		16
Ceneviva et al (1986)[59]			
Simple closure	38	Chronic	58
Closure plus PGV	38		5
Boey et al (1988)[57]			
Simple closure	41	Acute	36.6
Closure plus PGV	37		10.6

PGV, proximal gastric vagotomy.

Table 6-11 Associated Diseases and Mortality Rates From Ulcer Hemorrhage

	Mortality Rate (%)	
	With Disease	Without Disease
Renal	29.4	9.4
Hepatic	24.6	6.9
Neoplastic	24.3	9.6
Central nervous system	23.5	8.7
Pulmonary	22.6	8.2

(After Gilbert DA. Epidemiology of upper gastrointestinal bleeding. Gastrointest Endosc 1990;36:S8)

years of age. In one series,[62] about 45% of patients were older than 60 years of age. In about half of bleeding patients, serious comorbid illnesses are reported.

The prognosis for massive bleeding is primarily determined by patient risk factors, the nature of therapeutic procedures used being of secondary importance (Table 6-11). In patients older than 60 years of age, concomitant medical illness, ulcer size greater than 1 cm, and transfusion requirements in excess of five units are associated with increased mortality risk.[63] Although most patients with upper gastrointestinal hemorrhage stop bleeding spontaneously, up to 30% do not or experience recurrent hemorrhage soon after admission. Active or recurrent hemorrhage impacts transfusion requirements, the need for surgery, and overall mortality (Table 6-12).

Most patients with bleeding from duodenal ulceration present with hematemesis with or without melena. Loss of consciousness or signs of hypovolemic shock are present in only 20% at the time of presentation. Resuscitation begins during the initial evaluation. A large-bore nasogastric tube should be inserted to

Table 6-12 Ulcer Bleeding Status During Endoscopy and Clinical Outcome

	Patients	Mortality Rate (%)	Transfusion >5 Units (%)	Surgery (%)
DUODENAL ULCER				
Active	142	10.6	43.7	41.6
Inactive	333	3.0	21.3	12.9
GASTRIC ULCER				
Active	102	11.8	38.2	24.5
Inactive	352	6.8	21.3	12.2

(After Gilbert DA. Epidemiology of upper gastrointestinal bleeding. Gastrointest Endosc 1990;36:S8)

evacuate blood. Gastric lavage with warm saline is performed to estimate the rapidity of ongoing blood loss and to prepare for endoscopic examination. The time-honored use of cold saline lavage should be abandoned because it is not helpful in arresting bleeding and results in systemic hypothermia with resultant coagulopathy.

Upper endoscopy is the preferred diagnostic method for bleeding duodenal ulcer. Endoscopic examination requires a conscious, cooperative, hemodynamically stable patient and thus should not be undertaken before adequate restoration of intravascular volume. Endoscopic findings have importance in predicting continuing or recurrent hemorrhage and have been correlated with the need for emergency operation.[64] Endoscopic stigmata of recent hemorrhage are listed in Table 6-13. At one extreme, arterial spurting seen at endoscopy is associated with an 85% chance of continued bleeding and requires immediate therapeutic intervention. At the other end of the spectrum, a clean ulcer base without any stigmata of recent hemorrhage is a reliable sign that the ulcer will not rebleed. A visible vessel is defined as a protruding red, blue, or white mound in the base of a peptic ulcer that has recently bled (Fig. 6-24). Although originally thought to represent the artery itself, the "visible vessel" is actually an organized clot adherent to a side hole in the bleeding vessel located beneath the ulcer base. Bleeding vessels are typically large, with an average diameter of 0.7 mm.

Stigmata are found more frequently when endoscopy is performed early than when delayed for 1, 2, or 3 days, and for this reason, upper endoscopy should be performed at the time of admission.[65] Recurrent bleeding is most apt to occur within 72 hours of the index bleed. Endoscopic stigmata of recent hemorrhage are not sufficiently accurate to be used alone as indications for operation. Instead, they serve as a warning that aggressive therapy and careful follow-up are necessary.

The ability to visualize duodenal ulcers endoscopically has led to the development of methods that treat hemorrhagic complications endoscopically. Most endo-

Table 6-13 Endoscopic Stigmata of Hemorrhage

Stigmata	Rebleeding Risk
Arterial bleeding	High
Visible vessel with oozing or clot	Moderate
Oozing without visible vessel	Moderate
Clot without visible vessel	Moderate
Visible vessel alone	Low
Older stigmata but no vessel	Low
No stigmata	None

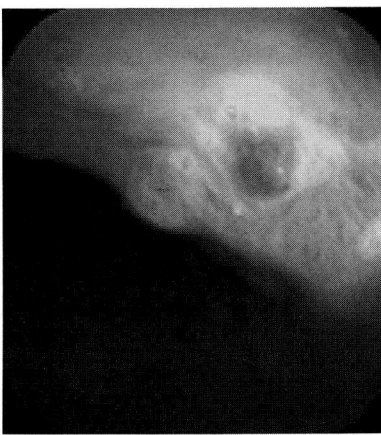

Figure 6-24 Gastric ulcer with visible vessel protruding from its base. (See Color Fig. 6-24.)

scopic methods rely on thermal hemostasis. Local heating causes collagen to denature and contract so that the bleeding artery is welded closed. To optimize heat delivery to tissues, two principles apply.[66] First, the vessel must be coapted during energy delivery to eliminate dissipation of heat by continuing flow of blood within the artery. Second, the peak temperature of the target tissue must not be so high that tissue evaporation re-

sults. If peak temperatures are too high, risks of perforation or exacerbation of bleeding are increased.

A number of methods to deliver heat to duodenal ulcers endoscopically have been devised. Laser photocoagulation and monopolar electrocoagulation have not achieved widespread acceptance. The Nd:YAG laser has a favorable tissue penetration profile, but contact tips for most laser systems do not allow vessel coaptation. In addition, the systems are expensive, require a high level of technical skill, and lack the portability of nonlaser systems. Monopolar electrocautery delivers electric current to tissues close to the probe tip, which then passes through the body to a grounding plate. Improper current intensities can cause sparking and temperature bursts up to several thousand degrees Celsius with immediate tissue evaporation.

Bipolar electrocoagulation operates by completion of a circuit between two electrodes on a probe surface. The probes are portable, are inexpensive, and contain an irrigation system to wash the bleeding site.[67] Importantly, the probes can be applied tangentially; most duodenal ulcers are difficult to view en face (Fig. 6-25). The maximal temperature achieved with bipolar electrocoagulation is 100°C, the temperature at which tissue water boils. Forceful application

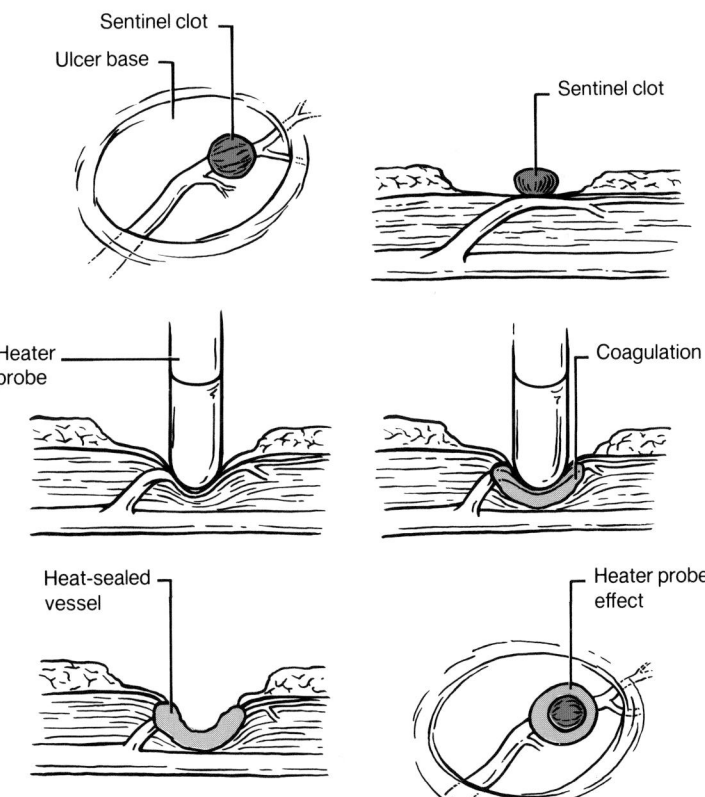

Figure 6-25 Tangential application of endoscopic electrocautery or heater probe to bleeding duodenal ulcer. The probe must be applied with sufficient force to coapt the walls of the bleeding artery. With walls apposed, heating welds shut the vessel walls.

of the probe is important because apposition increases the area and depth of coagulation and the hemostatic weld strength.

The heat probe is capped with a hollow metallic cylinder with a silicon diode heating element that monitors energy delivery.[68] The metallic tip distributes heat uniformly, with a maximal temperature of 250°C. The probe has an irrigation system and allows vessel tamponade and tangential application.

Both bipolar electrocoagulation and heat probes are effective in acutely arresting hemorrhage from duodenal ulcers. Initial cessation of bleeding has been reported in about 90% of patients (Table 6-14). Rebleeding rates are variable but have been reported in up to 20% of treated patients. A large number of trials have reported long-term outcomes after endoscopic hemostasis, with variable success. A metaanalysis indicated significant decreases in rebleeding, transfusion requirements, and need for surgery in patients treated with endoscopic hemostasis.

A National Institutes of Health Consensus Development Conference has recommended endoscopic hemostasis in selected high-risk patients.[69] Clinical features indicating high risk for rebleeding or death, and thus justifying endoscopic hemostasis, include hemodynamic instability, continuing transfusion requirement, red hematemesis or stool, age older than 60 years, and coexisting serious medical diseases. Patients who begin to bleed while in the hospital or who rebleed after hospitalization are at increased risk. The endoscopic finding of a visible vessel or oozing beneath an adherent clot are also indications for endoscopic hemostasis.

Each of the clinical features listed previously is also an indication for operation if endoscopic treatment is not possible or successful. Massive exsanguination requires immediate operation without attempts at endoscopic therapy. Because elderly patients are less toler-

ant of recurrent hemorrhage and hypotension than younger patients, operation should be undertaken earlier. There are two goals for emergency surgery in bleeding duodenal ulcer: control of hemorrhage and performance of a definitive antiulcer procedure.

The operation should begin by performance of a Kocher maneuver and opening of the duodenum (Fig. 6-26). The bleeding ulcer is sutured directly. Attempts to control bleeding by ligation of the gastroduodenal artery above the duodenum are futile because of the rich collateral supply to this area. If chronic ulcer disease has resulted in foreshortening of the first portion of the duodenum, the common bile duct can be endangered by sutures placed deeply in the ulcer bed. Intraoperative cholangiography should be used if this complication is suspected.

After bleeding has been controlled, the choices for subsequent definitive ulcer operation include truncal vagotomy and pyloroplasty, truncal vagotomy and antrectomy, and proximal gastric vagotomy. When used for acute bleeding, each procedure has a mortality rate of 5% to 10%. Most deaths occur in elderly patients and are associated with inadequate transfusion and operative delay. Recurrent bleeding in the immediate postoperative period has been reported in 15% to 20% of patients after truncal vagotomy and pyloroplasty and in 5% or less after truncal vagotomy and antrectomy.[70] Experience with proximal gastric vagotomy after control of bleeding through a duodenotomy is encouraging, although much more limited than with the other procedures. Rebleeding in the immediate postoperative period has been reported in as few as 4% of patients after proximal gastric vagotomy.[71] Vagotomy and pyloroplasty is appropriate when massive hemorrhage or shock requires a short operation as a safety factor. In patients who are stable after control of hemorrhage, proximal gastric vagotomy is preferred.

Obstruction

Gastric outlet obstruction is the least frequent complication of peptic ulcer disease, occurring in 2% to 5% of patients. Pyloric obstruction is the result of recurrent ulceration in the pyloric channel, increasing cicatrization occurring with each cycle of ulceration. Edema associated with active ulceration can also cause obstruction but usually denotes underlying, nearly critical stenosis. Early satiety and vomiting of undigested food are usual symptoms. Weight loss is common. Insertion of a nasogastric tube results in evacuation of large volumes of gastric fluid, which may be feculent. In the setting of prolonged vomiting, serum electrolytes reveal a hypochloremic, hypokalemic alkalosis due to loss of H^+ and Cl^- in the vomitus and compensatory renal secre-

Table 6-14 Results With Multipolar Electrocoagulation, Heater Probe, and No Endoscopic Treatment in Ulcer Hemorrhage

	Control	Multipolar Electrocoagulation	Heater Probe
Hemostasis	20%	90%	93%
Rebleeding	72%	44%	22%
Surgery	41%	33%	3%
Transfused units	3.5	3.7	1.3
Mortality	9%	3%	3%

(After Laine L. Bipolar/multipolar electrocoagulation. Gastrointest Endosc 1990;36:S38)

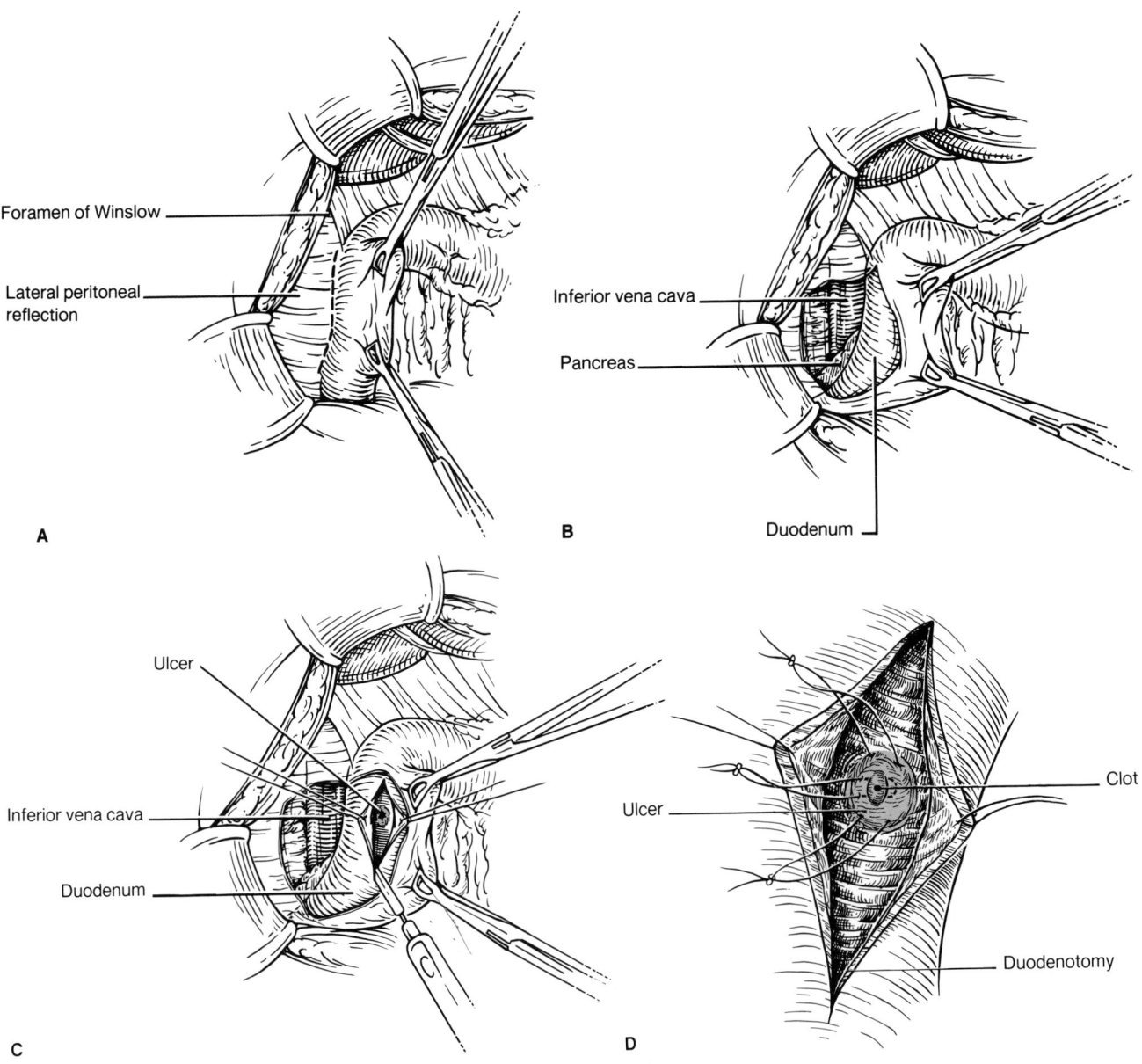

Foramen of Winslow

Lateral peritoneal reflection

A

Inferior vena cava

Pancreas

Duodenum

B

Ulcer

Inferior vena cava

Duodenum

C

Ulcer

Clot

Duodenotomy

D

Figure 6-26 Initial maneuvers in operative management of bleeding duodenal ulcer. (**A**) The duodenum is mobilized from the retroperitoneum by a Kocher maneuver. (**B**) As the duodenum is reflected forward, the retroperitoneal duodenum, posterior aspect of the pancreatic head, and inferior vena cava are visualized. (**C**) A longitudinal duodenotomy permits direct visualization of the ulcer. Vessels entering the ulcer base peripherally are controlled by circumferential sutures. (**D**) Vessels entering perpendicularly are controlled by use of a U-stitch.

tion of K^+ in exchange for H^+. A positive saline load test indicates a fixed stenosis. At 30 minutes after instillation of 750 mL of saline through the nasogastric tube, retrieval of 300 mL of fluid constitutes a positive test.

Initial management should consist of nasogastric decompression, correction of electrolyte abnormalities, and institution of H_2-receptor therapy and parenteral nutritional support. Endoscopy is performed to confirm the nature of the stenosis and to obtain biopsy specimens. About 85% of pyloric stenoses are amenable to endoscopically guided dilation. Immediate symptomatic improvement is reported in 80% of patients treated with balloon dilation. Unfortunately, only 40% sustain improvement beyond 3 months.[72]

Operative treatment of gastric outlet obstruction begins with inspection of the pyloroduodenal region. If severe scarring make excision of the antrum and pylorus unsafe, then the operation of choice becomes truncal vagotomy and gastrojejunostomy. In most instances, the area can be safely mobilized and resected, and the choice becomes truncal vagotomy and pyloroplasty or truncal vagotomy and antrectomy. The incidence of recurrent ulcer and postoperative symptoms for these two operations is similar to that presented for intractable ulcer. An initial enthusiasm for proximal gastric vagotomy and pyloric dilation has declined.[73] Two problems hinder the use of this procedure for obstruction—inadvertent pyloric rupture during dilation in as many as 15% of cases and increased rates of ulcer recurrence.[74]

GASTRIC ULCER

Pathogenesis

Although great progress has been made in elucidating the pathogenesis of duodenal ulcer, the causes of gastric ulcer remain much less clearly defined. Benign gastric ulcers can be divided into four types (Fig. 6-27). Type I ulcers occur in the body of the stomach and are not associated with any other gastroduodenal disease. Type II gastric ulcers occur in the body of the stomach and are associated with duodenal ulceration, either active or in remission. Type III ulcers are located in the prepy-loric area of the stomach. Physiologic abnormalities associated with type II and type III gastric ulcers are similar to those identified in duodenal ulcer patients (see earlier). High gastric ulcers, occurring proximally along the lesser curvature of the stomach, have been classified as type IV ulcers; their pathologic features most closely resemble type I ulcers.[75,76]

Gastric Mucosal Barrier

The normal gastric mucosa constitutes a "barrier" resistant to the back-diffusion of hydrogen ions from the gastric lumen (Fig. 6-28). The resistance to hydrogen ion back-diffusion is both anatomic and functional as a result of tight junctions between cells, efficient mechanisms of intracellular pH maintenance, the buffering capacity of mucosal blood flow, surface mucus, epithelial bicarbonate secretion, and many other factors. In animal models and in humans, when this barrier is disrupted, epithelial damage and ulceration can result. In experimental models, a number of agents (NSAIDs, ethanol, acidified bile salts) disturb barrier function; each can cause ulceration. In humans, the most clearly documented cause of gastric mucosal damage is NSAIDs. A statistically significant association exists between NSAID ingestion and the development of gastric ulcer and its complications of bleeding or perfo-

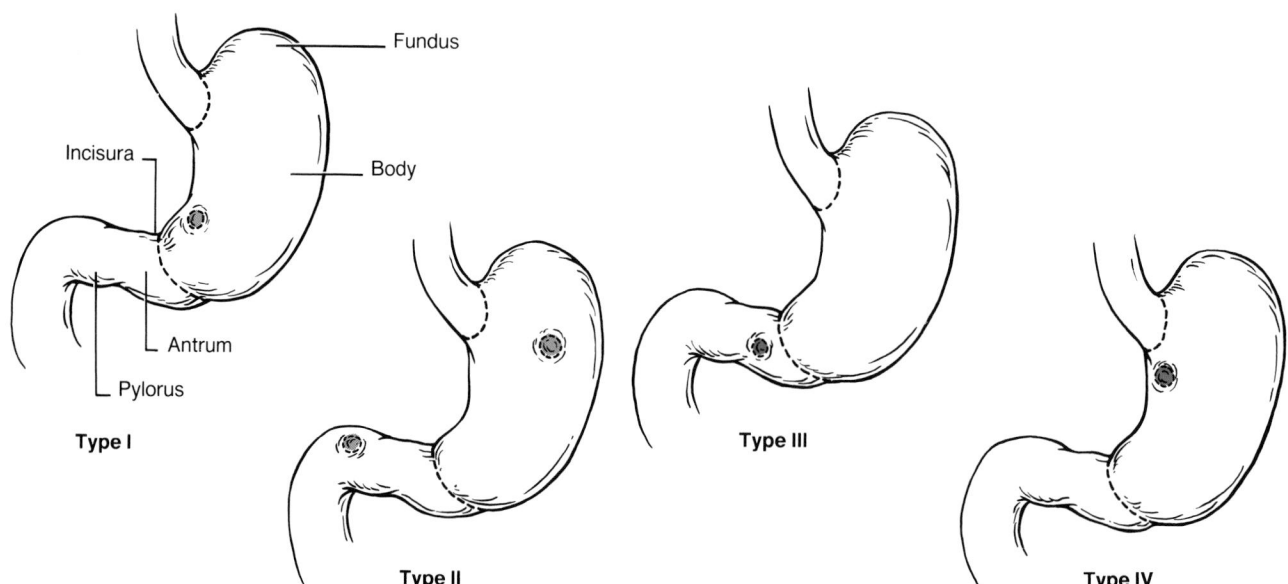

Figure 6-27 Locations of gastric ulcers with associated conditions. Type I ulcers are located in the gastric body, usually along the lesser curvature; they are associated with normal or low acid secretion. Type II ulcers include those in the gastric body and duodenal ulcers; they are associated with hypersecretion of acid. Type III ulcers are prepyloric in location and are also associated with hypersecretion of acid. Type IV ulcers are located high on the lesser curvature, in proximity to the esophagogastric junction; they are associated with low acid secretion.

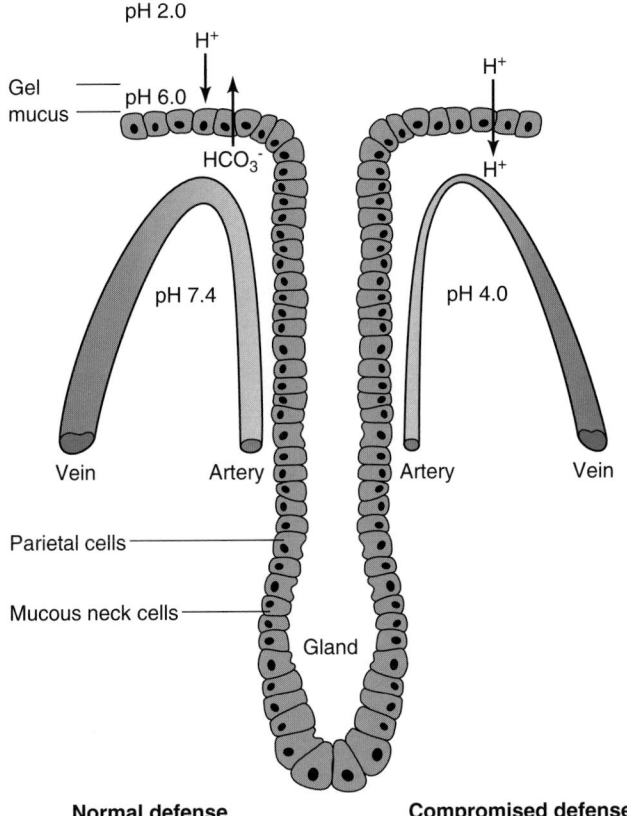

Figure 6-28 Schematic diagram of the gastric epithelium with the components of the normal gastric mucosal barrier. Hydrogen ions diffusing from the lumen are neutralized by bicarbonate ions secreted by gastric surface cells, creating a microenvironment at the surface near neutrality.

ration. In the following discussion, *gastric ulcer* is defined as ulceration that does not develop in association with ingestion of NSAIDs.

Gastric Acid Secretion

Gastric ulcers can develop in the presence of minute amounts of luminal acid, and there are no convincing data that abnormalities of gastric acid secretion play a role in gastric ulceration. Basal and stimulated acid secretion are within normal limits in gastric ulcer patients as a group. In fact, hypochlorhydria is common in type I gastric ulcer. In duodenal ulcer, a threshold of acid secretion appears to be necessary; duodenal ulcers heal and do not recur when acid secretion is less than 10 mmol/h. No minimal acid secretory response exists for gastric ulceration. Thus, although treatment with antisecretory drugs is standard for gastric ulcer, this approach lacks as substantial a physiologic rationale as for duodenal ulcer. A metaanalysis of drug therapy in

gastric ulcer showed no significant correlation between the magnitude of the antisecretory effect and healing rates.[77]

Gastritis and Ulceration

Most gastric ulcers develop along the lesser curvature of the stomach, on the antral side of the junction of the antral and oxyntic mucosae. Chronic superficial gastritis is nearly universal in the area immediately surrounding the ulcer and in the antrum. Gastritis can extend for a variable distance into the fundic mucosa.

The causes of antral gastritis in gastric ulcer are not fully understood. Abnormal pyloric function with reflux of duodenal contents has been postulated to initiate antral injury. Duodenogastric reflux can be assessed with the radiopharmaceutical technetium-99m HIDA, an agent that is concentrated and then secreted by the liver. With a gamma camera, bile reflux can be monitored quantitatively without instrumentation of the patient. Using this test, duodenogastric reflux of bile has been demonstrated to be similar among patients with gastric ulcer, duodenal ulcer, and age-matched controls. Although refluxed bile salts and lysolecithin promote ulceration in experimental models, the bile-chelating agent cholestyramine does not promote ulcer healing; and although bile reflux is universal after antrectomy with Billroth I reconstruction, postoperative gastric ulceration is rare.

The demonstration that *H pylori* can cause antral gastritis and that eradication of the organism by bismuth subcitrate correlates with resolution of gastritis strengthens its association with gastric ulcer.

Motility and Mucosal Blood Flow

A variety of motility disturbances have been linked to gastric ulcers, none definitively. Resting and nutrient-stimulated pyloric sphincter pressures have been reported to be lower than normal in small subsets of patients with gastric ulcer.[78] Gastric emptying of solids has also been reported to be impaired.[79] High-amplitude gastric contractions have been observed in gastric ulcer patients, and sustained contractions in the area of the incisura angularis have been postulated to cause localized mucosal ischemia.

Diagnosis

Gastric ulcers are associated with epigastric pain similar to that described for duodenal ulcers. The symptoms, nonspecific and often vague, are common to a number of diseases, from nonulcer dyspepsia to early gastric cancer. Because of the ready availability of highly

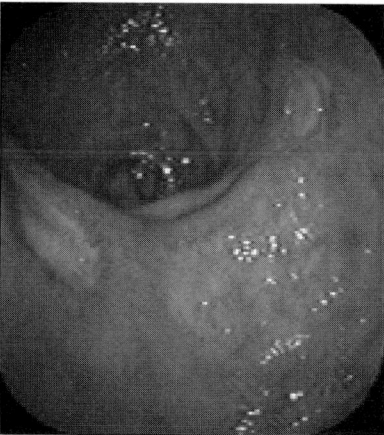

Figure 6-29 Two benign gastric ulcers in the body of the stomach. They have sharply defined margins and clean ulcer bases. Despite the appearance of benign ulcer, biopsy is necessary to exclude malignancy. (See Color Fig. 6-29.)

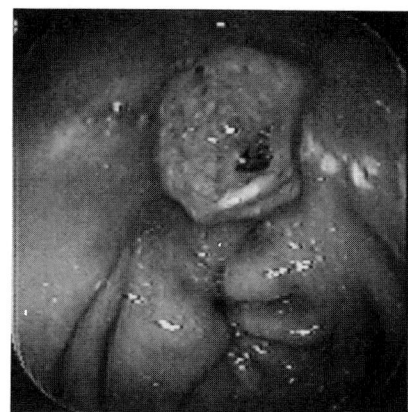

Figure 6-31 Deeply penetrating prepyloric antral gastric ulcer with small adherent clot in its base. (See Color Fig. 6-31.)

effective antisecretory drugs, treatment is instituted before diagnosis in many symptomatic patients. This policy of treating first is appropriate only for patients younger than 40 years with mild symptoms and no complication of ulcer disease. For older patients, or for those with chronic symptoms, signs of systemic illness, or signs suggesting another disease process (ie, biliary tract or pancreatic disease), a diagnosis must be established initially. Upper endoscopy is preferred because it has 95% accuracy for distinguishing benign gastric ulcer from gastric cancer when endoscopic appearance, endoscopic biopsy, and brush cytology are combined[80] (Figs. 6-29 through 6-31). All gastric ulcers observed by endoscopy should undergo biopsy to exclude malignancy.

Medical Therapy

Because most patients with type I gastric ulcers have normal or reduced rates of gastric acid secretion, treatment of gastric ulcers with antisecretory agents may seem paradoxical. Nonetheless, further reduction of gastric acid secretion with such agents is associated with accelerated ulcer healing. Unlike duodenal ulcers, healing rates in gastric ulcers treated with antisecretory medications are correlated with duration of therapy rather than with degree of acid suppression.[77]

H_2-receptor antagonists have well-established efficacy in treatment of acute gastric ulcers. Healing rates for gastric ulcers treated with H_2-receptor antagonists are summarized in Table 6-15. Cumulative healing rates are equivalent to those reported for duodenal ulcer, but time to complete healing averages 2 weeks longer for gastric ulcer. Risk factors that predict failure of medical therapy include continued smoking, ulcers larger than 2 cm, and multiple ulcerations.[81]

Omeprazole also has demonstrated benefit in the acute treatment of gastric ulcers. Omeprazole at doses of 20 to 40 mg/d is equivalent or superior to H_2-receptor

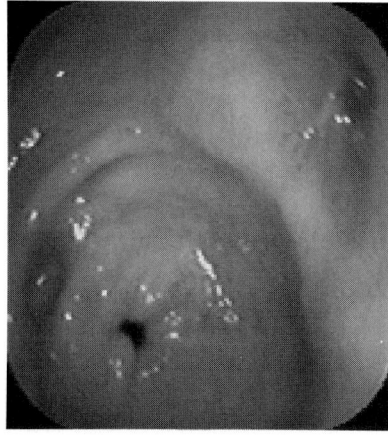

Figure 6-30 Gastric ulcers in the antrum. The pylorus is located centrally in this view. Areas of gastritis surrounding the ulcer appear erythematous. (See Color Fig. 6-30.)

Table 6-15 Treatment of Gastric Ulcer With Antisecretory Medications

Drug	Dosage	Healing Rate (%)	
		4 Weeks	8 Weeks
Omeprazole	20 mg/d	75	90
Omeprazole	40 mg/d	80	95
Ranitidine	150 mg bid	65	85
Cimetidine	400 mg bid	60	75

antagonists in terms of pain relief and 4-week healing rates (see Table 6-15). The efficacy of high-dose omeprazole confirms the importance of gastric acid—even low amounts—in the formation of gastric ulcers.

A number of studies have compared synthetic analogues of prostaglandin E with H_2-receptor antagonists. When given at doses high enough to suppress acid secretion, most studies suggest that prostaglandin analogues are superior to placebo but less effective than H_2-receptor antagonists at 8 weeks. These observations would suggest that lower doses of prostaglandins, doses that might have cytoprotective but not antisecretory effects, would not be as effective as H_2-receptor antagonists. Although misoprostol is approved in the United States for gastric ulcer, it is most useful in selected patients with NSAID-associated ulceration who must continue NSAID treatment.

Sucralfate, a drug believed to augment mucosal defense mechanisms, is effective in promoting healing of gastric ulcer. Comparable healing rates have been reported for sucralfate, 2 g given twice daily, and cimetidine, 400 mg given twice daily, at 4 and 8 weeks.[82] Data regarding efficacy of colloidal bismuth in healing of gastric ulcers are less secure than for the other agents listed. Experience suggests that colloidal bismuth is significantly better than placebo and equivalent to established H_2-receptor antagonists. The long-term safety profile of colloidal bismuth has not been established.

Operative Treatment

Intractable Gastric Ulcer

When gastric ulcers fail to heal completely with standard medical management, the possibility of malignancy must be reassessed. Scattered reports of partial healing of malignant ulcers with H_2-receptor treatment have appeared. Other causes of nonhealing include Crohn's disease, gastric lymphoma, eosinophilic gastroenteritis, tuberculosis, and gastric cytomegalovirus infection. If these other diagnoses are confidently excluded, omeprazole, 40 mg/d for 12 weeks, has been shown to result in healing in 95% of cases. Elective surgical treatment for gastric ulcer should be considered when a newly diagnosed ulcer does not heal after 12 weeks of active therapy, with recurrent disease after initial complete healing, when ulcer biopsies demonstrate mucosal dysplasia, and when malignancy can not be excluded.

Although the presence of gastric acid is necessary for gastric ulcers to develop, mucosal defects are more important in the pathogenesis. As a result, gastric ulcer procedures that reduce acid secretion are less reliable than those that remove the susceptible mucosa. A consideration of the four types of gastric ulcer, associated duodenal ulcer, and acid secretory status is vital in making an appropriate choice.

TYPE I ULCERS. Type I gastric ulcers are best treated by antrectomy, performed in a manner that includes the ulcer. Gastroduodenal reconstruction (Billroth I) is more physiologically sound than gastrojejunal anastamosis. The operative mortality rate averages 1% to 2%, as do 5-year ulcer recurrence rates. Anastomotic leaks or obstruction and external duodenal fistulas are uncommon after antrectomy for type I gastric ulcers because the duodenum is usually normal.[83,84] About 90% of patients are in the Visick I or II category postoperatively. Truncal vagotomy is not necessary because type I ulcer patients are rarely hypersecretors of acid. There is no strong evidence that ulcer cure rates are improved by the addition of truncal vagotomy, and the incidence of postoperative symptoms is slightly increased.

Truncal vagotomy plus pyloroplasty has no advantage when used for type I gastric ulcers. Operative mortality rates and postoperative sequelae are not significantly decreased, and postoperative ulcer recurrences are higher than with antrectomy. For selected patients, excision of the ulcer, combined with proximal gastric vagotomy, is a second choice. Ulcer excision excludes malignancy, but recurrence rates are four to six times higher (average 15%) for proximal gastric vagotomy than for antrectomy.

TYPE II ULCERS. Type II ulcers that have both gastric and duodenal components should be treated by an operation that reduces acid secretion and removes the mucosa at risk. Truncal vagotomy plus antrectomy has a 1% to 2% operative mortality rate when performed electively. If duodenal inflammation or scarring preclude gastroduodenal anastomosis, gastrojejunostomy should be performed. Postoperative ulcer recurrence rates of 5% or less are reported. Secondary choices include truncal vagotomy and pyloroplasty or proximal gastric vagotomy, both combined with ulcer excision for histologic confirmation.

TYPE III ULCERS. Patients with pyloric or prepyloric ulcers (type III) tend to have high rates of gastric acid secretion and therapeutic responses resembling duodenal ulcer patients. The elective procedure of choice is truncal vagotomy and antrectomy to include the ulcer. Operative morbidity rates and ulcer recurrences are similar to those reported for type II gastric ulcers. Proximal gastric vagotomy is less effective for ulcers located in this region, with recurrence rates up to 40% reported.

TYPE IV ULCERS. High gastric ulcers (type IV) are defined as those in which the upper border of the ulcer is within 2 cm of the gastroesophageal junction. Type IV ulcer patients tend to be older, with 20% older than 75 years of age; 45% have significant medical comorbidity that increases operative risk.[85] The ulcer is larger than 2 cm in two thirds of patients. Ulcers in this location can usually be excised by antrectomy, in which the resection is extended along the lesser curvature of the stomach to include the ulcer (Pauchet maneuver). The procedure has the advantage that the ulcer-bearing area of the stomach is removed, but a large gastric reservoir along the greater curvature is preserved. The ulcer recurrence rate approximates 5%.

Emergency Operation

Acute hemorrhage is a more serious complication in gastric ulcer than in duodenal ulcer because an older age group is affected and because spontaneous cessation is less likely. Risk factors for bleeding include NSAID use and ulcer size equal to or greater than 3 cm.[86] Initial resuscitation and endoscopic evaluation are similar to those employed for duodenal ulcer; attempts at endoscopic hemostasis are warranted. In the presence of hemorrhage, the preferred operation for type I, II, or III ulcers is antrectomy with Billroth I reconstruction. Truncal vagotomy should also be performed for type II and III ulcers.

For acutely bleeding high (type IV) gastric ulcers, antrectomy with lesser curvature extension to include the ulcer is preferred. Occasionally, the ulcer lies so close to the esophagogastric junction that its excision would distort the esophagus, thus precluding resection. In this instance, the bleeding ulcer can be treated by vessel transfixion and ulcer oversewing. Ulcer oversewing alone is not a definitive operation, and recurrence rates of 40% are expected. Proximal gastric vagotomy can be added if lesser curvature edema and fibrosis are not severe. Truncal vagotomy and pyloroplasty after ulcer oversewing is a secondary option.

Perforation of gastric ulcer is associated with a mortality rate about twice that of perforated duodenal ulcer. This increased risk is explained, in part, by the increased age of affected patients and by disease-related changes in gastric bacteriology. Operative treatment of perforated gastric ulcers is accomplished by distal gastrectomy that encompasses the site of perforation. In unstable patients, excision of the ulcer and patch closure can be used as an expeditious alternative.

STRESS GASTRITIS

The term *stress gastritis* denotes a clinical syndrome in which gastric mucosal erosions occur in the setting of trauma, sepsis, or other severe physiologic stress. *Erosive gastritis* and *stress ulcer* are frequently used synonyms. The gastric injury is confined to the epithelium in the form of shallow, well-demarcated ulcers. The lesions usually do not extend below the level of the muscularis mucosae, and signs of chronicity, such as collagen deposition, are absent. Erosions are usually localized to the acid-secreting fundus, less common in the antrum, and rare in the duodenum.

Pathogenesis

Some form of severe physiologic challenge can be identified in virtually all patients who develop stress gastritis. Trauma, especially when associated with shock, is a common antecedent to stress gastritis. Intraabdominal injuries are more often associated with the development of stress erosions than injuries confined to the extremities or soft tissues. Sepsis is frequently associated with stress ulceration; patients with unresolved intraperitoneal or pulmonary infection are at highest risk. Patients with thermal injury that involves more than 35% of total body surface area demonstrate stress-related gastric mucosal damage in up to 85% of cases.[87] The development of secondary organ dysfunction, which manifests as jaundice, uremia, or respiratory failure, greatly increases the risk for stress gastritis.

A special form of gastroduodenal ulcer can also develop in patients with head injury, intracranial tumor, or intracranial surgery that results in increased intracranial pressure. The lesion, termed *Cushing's ulcer*, tends to be deeply penetrating and can involve the duodenum as well as the stomach. Perforation is a complication of Cushing's ulcer that is rarely observed in other forms of stress gastritis. Hypergastrinemia and hypersecretion of acid, while common in patients with Cushing's ulcer, are distinctly unusual in patients with other forms of stress gastritis.

The development of stress gastritis is commonly depicted as an imbalance between aggressive, injurious luminal factors and gastric mucosal defenses (Fig. 6-32). Both clinical and experimental observations indicate that a necessary precondition for the development of stress gastritis is gastric mucosal ischemia. Most patients with stress gastritis have an antecedent episode of shock from hemorrhage, sepsis, or cardiac dysfunction.[88] In dogs, hemorrhagic shock induces lesions nearly identical to those observed in human disease. Using ex vivo models, the degree of mucosal ischemia produced correlates directly with the magnitude of mucosal injury. Conversely, infusion of vasoactive peptides that cause mucosal hyperemia has been shown to prevent mucosal injury.[89]

Strong evidence also exists that the presence of some luminal acid is necessary for the development of

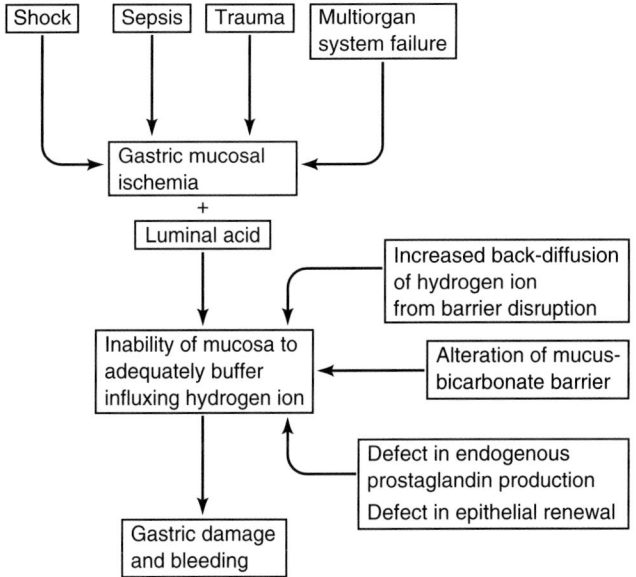

Figure 6-32 Schematic representation of various factors thought to be responsible for the pathogenesis of stress gastritis. (After Miller TA. Mechanisms of stress-related mucosal damage. Am J Med 1987;83:14)

stress gastritis. However, with the exception of Cushing's ulcers, increased rates of gastric acid secretion are not observed in association with stress gastritis. In health, luminal acid does not diffuse back into the gastric epithelium to any measurable degree. When the normal gastric mucosal barrier is disrupted, luminal hydrogen ions diffuse into the gastric epithelium, with reciprocal loss of sodium, potassium, and protein into the gastric lumen. Reduction of gastric mucosal blood flow can impair delivery of energy substrates to the mucosa and interfere with buffering or removal of intramural hydrogen ions, exacerbating the effects of back-diffusing acid.

Other potential pathogenetic influences are less well established. In experimental models, duodenogastric reflux of bile has been shown to cause gastric mucosal damage. Because stress ulcers in animals can be prevented by administration of exogenous prostaglandins, it is tempting to speculate that the processes that cause stress gastritis deplete endogenous prostaglandins. Similarly, defects in epithelial renewal have been sought in humans with stress gastritis. Agents such as epidermal growth factor and pentagastrin, which stimulate mucosal protein and DNA production, prevent the formation of experimental stress gastritis.

Clinical Presentation

Symptoms caused by stress gastritis are related to bleeding. Perhaps because the erosions are so superficial, epigastric pain is distinctly uncommon and should suggest a different diagnosis. Perforation is rare. The most sensitive and specific method of diagnosis is endoscopy. When endoscopy was performed as surveillance, lesions were reported in 70% to 100% of susceptible patients, often within 12 to 24 hours of the precipitating event. Stress gastritis and ulceration are localized predominantly to the fundus of the stomach. The endoscopic appearance varies from discrete, superficial ulcers to areas of confluent mucosal loss (Fig. 6-33). Untreated lesions are progressive over 3 to 5 days but usually heal without residual scarring within 2 weeks if the causative factors have resolved.

Prophylactic Treatment

Prophylactic treatment should be instituted early in all susceptible patients to prevent the formation of stress gastritis and the potentially serious sequelae of hemor-

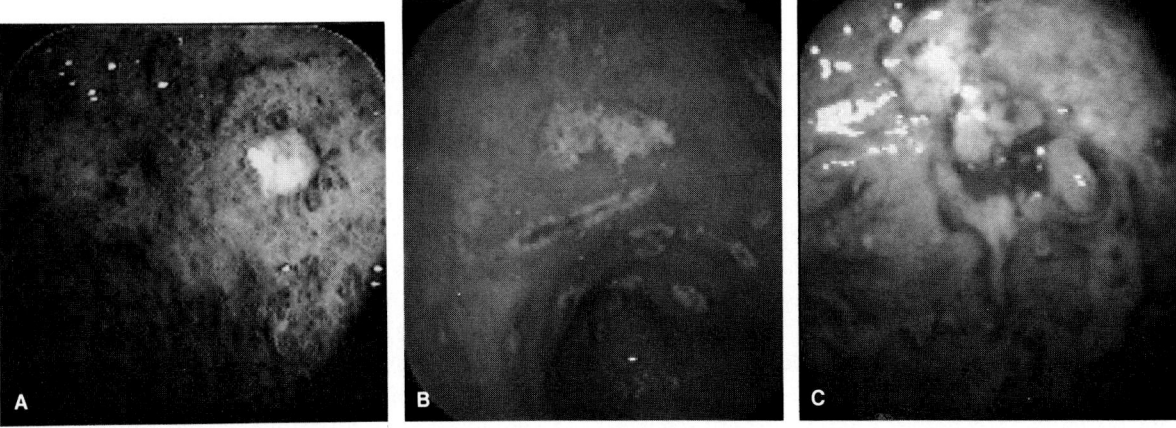

Figure 6-33 Stress ulcerations may vary from single, superficial lesions (**A**); to multiple, diffuse ulcers (**B**); to confluent loss of mucosa (**C**). (See Color Fig. 6-33.)

rhage. To be successful, the prophylaxis of stress gastritis must be based on the following clinical goals:

- Correction of any state of systemic hypoperfusion
- Control of sepsis, including institution of appropriate antibiotic therapy and drainage of surgical sites of infection
- Provision of adequate nutritional support
- Correction of systemic acid–base abnormalities

Prophylaxis of stress gastritis usually also emphasizes reduction of intragastric acidity. A large body of clinical evidence indicates that neutralization of intragastric acidity both prevents ulcer formation and reduces the incidence of bleeding from stress gastritis. The goal of prophylactic treatment should be to keep intragastric pH above 5.0. At this level, the proteolytic enzyme trypsin is irreversibly denatured. Debate has centered around the optimal method of maintaining elevated intragastric pH, with most attention focused on antacids and H_2-receptor antagonists.

A large number of studies are available that demonstrate that antacids are effective in preventing stress gastritis bleeding. The use of topical antacids requires that a nasogastric tube be in place. The pH of gastric secretions is periodically checked, and antacids are administered in a quantity sufficient to maintain optimal pH. Between antacid administrations, the nasogastric tube is clamped. Despite proven efficacy, the use of antacids is associated with a number of problems. The need for an indwelling nasogastric tube increases the risk of aspiration. Continual monitoring of pH to ensure that target pH is met increases nursing demands. Diarrhea, hypermagnesemia, and hypophosphatemia may develop.

Because of the inconvenience and occasional metabolic disturbances associated with antacid therapy, H_2-receptor antagonists have been extensively evaluated for prophylaxis of stress gastritis. Because a nasogastric tube is not necessary, the ability to monitor efficacy in the form of pH control or occult blood loss is absent, but when overt bleeding is used as an end point, there is little doubt that H_2-receptor antagonists are effective prophylaxis for stress gastritis. Intermittent dosing with cimetidine has been approved since 1977 and has had the most extensive evaluation. A collected review comparing antacids with cimetidine, usually 300 to 400 mg every 4 to 6 hours, reported comparable results.[90] Equivalent doses of ranitidine for bolus administration are 50 mg every 6 to 8 hours.

When fixed bolus doses of cimetidine are used, intragastric pH varies widely over time. Because stress gastritis bleeding is related to intragastric pH, efficacy can be improved by continuous intravenous administration of H_2-receptor antagonists. Continuous infusion of cimetidine at 50 mg/h, after a 300-mg priming dose, has been shown to be equivalent to an antacid drip in maintaining intragastric pH above 4.0. The equivalent dose of ranitidine is 6 to 8 mg/h by continuous intravenous infusion after a priming dose of 50 mg.

Several reports have demonstrated that sucralfate, administered through a nasogastric tube, prevents bleeding from stress gastritis with the same efficacy as antacids or H_2-receptor antagonists.[91] The proven ability of sucralfate to prevent stress-related bleeding is interesting in view of its lack of effect on intragastric acidity, suggesting that another mechanism for cytoprotection must exist. As a potentially important secondary issue in sucralfate therapy, some investigators have noted an association between elevated intragastric pH and the development of gastric bacterial colonization and nosocomial pneumonia. In one study,[92] patients treated with sucralfate prophylactically had significantly lower numbers of gram-negative bacteria in gastric aspirates, pharyngeal swabs, and tracheal aspirates than patients treated with a combination of antacids and H_2-receptor antagonists. The rate of pneumonia was half as high in the sucralfate-treated group. These intriguing findings require confirmation.

Treatment of Active Bleeding

Prophylactic measures prevent clinically significant bleeding in more than 95% of patients at risk from stress gastritis. Overt bleeding most commonly occurs between 3 and 7 days after injury and may present as a slow fall in the hematocrit or may be massive and exsanguinating. It is imperative that a specific diagnosis precede treatment. In most instances, endoscopic visualization is possible; if massive bleeding prevents endoscopic examination, visceral angiography is the next choice. Initial treatment includes transfusion, correction of coagulation defects and thrombocytopenia, and elimination of septic foci. Few data suggest that antacids or H_2-receptor antagonists are effective in stopping active hemorrhage. Endoscopic treatment is occasionally successful if bleeding is confined to discrete, punctate lesions. Diffuse gastritis or confluent ulceration are poorly treated by endoscopic methods. Hemorrhage ceases with these initial measures in about four fifths of patients.

In patients who continue to bleed with conservative management, angiographic therapy should be attempted before operative intervention. If the left gastric artery is selectively cannulated, infusion of vasopressin at a continuous rate of 0.2 to 0.4 U/min controls bleeding in 80% of patients. The infusion should be continued for 48 hours and then slowly tapered. An alternative angiographic approach involves selective embolization of the bleeding vessel through the left gastric artery with autologous blood clots, metal coils, or Gelfoam. Vasopressin infusion or embolization would appear to be irrational if one accepts that mucosal ischemia is integral to the pathogenesis of stress gastritis. These treatments should be considered temporizing measures, and vigorous efforts to identify and treat underlying causes of stress gastritis, especially intraperitoneal infection, should be pursued.

A small subset of patients continue to bleed from stress gastritis despite aggressive nonoperative treatment. The best operative procedure to control hemorrhage is controversial, and there are no prospective or randomized trials to guide selection. Operations less than total gastrectomy are associated with high rates of rebleeding (20% to 30%), but few of these critically ill patients can tolerate a procedure of this magnitude. The operative mortality rate approaches 40% for total gastrectomy. Miller and colleagues[88] advocate vagotomy and pyloroplasty combined with oversewing of bleeding stress ulcers. A longitudinal anterior gastrotomy allows evacuation of clots and visualization of the epithelium. If the mucosal surface is diffusely ulcerated, partial gastric resection is combined with truncal vagotomy. Recurrent bleeding is treated by reoperation with total gastrectomy.[88]

REFERENCES

1. Kurata JH, Corboy ED. Current peptic ulcer time trends: an epidemiological profile. J Clin Gastroenterol 1988; 10:259.
2. Piper DW, Nasiry R, McIntosh J, et al. Smoking, alcohol, analgesics, and chronic duodenal ulcer. Scand J Gastroenterol 1984;19:1015.
3. Megraud F, Lamouliatte H. *Helicobacter pylori* and duodenal ulcer: evidence suggesting causation. Dig Dis Sci 1992;37:769.
4. Peterson WL. *Helicobacter pylori* and peptic ulcer disease. N Engl J Med 1991;324:1043.
5. Sipponen P, Varis K, Fraki O, et al. Cumulative 10-year risk of symptomatic duodenal and gastric ulcer in patients with or without chronic gastritis. Scand J Gastroenterol 1990;25:966.
6. O'Riordan T, Mathai E, Tobin E, et al. Adjuvant antibiotic therapy in duodenal ulcers treated with colloidal bismuth subcitrate. Gut 1990;31:999.
7. Mitchell HM, Lee A, Carrick J. Increased incidence of *Campylobacter pylori* infection in gastroenterologists: further evidence to support person-to-person transmission of *C. pylori*. Scand J Gastroenterol 1989;24:396.
8. Rainsford KD. Mechanisms of gastrointestinal ulceration by non-steroidal anti-inflammatory/analgesic drugs. In: Rainsford KD, Velo GP, eds. Advances in in-

flammation research: side effects of anti-inflammation/analgesic drugs, vol 6. New York, Raven, 1984.
9. Flemstrom G, Turnberg LA. Gastroduodenal defence mechanisms. Clin Gastroenterol 1984;13:327.
10. FDC reports, vol 8. Washington, DC, US Government Printing Office, November 29, 1987.
11. Langman MJS. Epidemiologic evidence on the association between peptic ulceration and antiinflammatory drug use. Gastroenterology 1989;96:640.
12. Armstrong CP, Blower AL. Non-steroidal anti-inflammatory drugs and life threatening complications of peptic ulceration. Gut 1987;28:527.
13. Stemmerman GN, Marcus EB, Buist AS, et al. Relative impact of smoking and reduced pulmonary function on peptic ulcer risk. Gastroenterology 1989;96:1419.
14. Lam SK. Pathogenesis and pathophysiology of duodenal ulcer. Clin Gastroenterol 1984;13:447.
15. Blair AJ III, Feldman M, Barnett C, et al. Detailed comparison of basal and food-stimulated gastric acid secretion rates and serum gastrin concentrations in duodenal ulcer patients and normal subjects. J Clin Invest 1987;79:582.
16. Rhodes J, Prestwich CJ. Acidity at different sites in the proximal duodenum of normal subjects and patients with duodenal ulcer. Gut 1966;7:509.
17. Corinaldesi R, Stanghellini V, Paparo GF, et al. Gastric acid secretion and gastric emptying of liquids in 99 male duodenal ulcer patients. Dig Dis Sci 1989;34:251.
18. Eriksen CA, Sadek SA, Cuschieri A. 24-hour ambulatory dual gastroduodenal pH monitoring: the role of acid in duodenal ulcer disease. Ann Surg 1988;208:702.
19. Isenberg JI, Selling JA, Hogan DL, et al. Impaired proximal duodenal mucosal bicarbonate secretion in patients with duodenal ulcer. N Engl J Med 1987;316:374.
20. Bukhave K, Rask-Madsen J, Hogan DL, et al. Proximal duodenal prostaglandin E_2 release and mucosal bicarbonate secretion are altered in patients with duodenal ulcer. Gastroenterology 1990;99:951.
21. Hogan DL, Koss MA, Isenberg JI. Impaired proximal duodenal mucosal bicarbonate secretion in duodenal ulcer patients involves a prostaglandin-mediated cellular defect. (Abstract) Gastroenterology 1990;98:A60.
22. Cotton PB, Shorvon PJ. Analysis of endoscopy and radiography in the diagnosis, follow-up and treatment of peptic ulcer disease. Clin Gastroenterol 1984;13:383.
23. Feldman M, Burton ME. Histamine$_2$-receptor antagonists: standard therapy for acid-peptic diseases. N Engl J Med 1990;323:1672.
24. Isenberg JI, McQuaid KR, Laine L, et al. Acid-peptic disorders. In: Yamada T, ed. Textbook of gastroenterology. Philadelphia, JB Lippincott, 1991:1267.
25. Sontag SJ. Current status of maintenance therapy in peptic ulcer disease. Am J Gastroenterol 1988;83:607.
26. Holt S, Howden CW. Omeprazole: overview and opinion. Dig Dis Sci 1991;36:385.
27. Tielemans Y, Hakanson R, Sundler F, et al. Proliferation of enterochromaffinlike cells in omeprazole-treated hypergastrinemic rats. Gastroenterology 1989;96:723.

28. Rees WDW. Mechanisms of gastroduodenal protection by sucralfate. Am J Med 1991;91(Suppl 2A):58S.

29. Konturek SJ, Brzozowski T, Bielanski W, et al. Epidermal growth factor in the gastroprotective and ulcer-healing actions of sucralfate in rats. Am J Med 1989;86(Suppl 6A):32.

30. Haram EM, Weberg R, Berstad A. Urinary excretion of aluminum after ingestion of sucralfate and an aluminum-containing antacid in man. Scand J Gastroenterol 1987;22:615.

31. Rees WDW, Turnberg LA. Mechanisms of gastric mucosal protection: a role for the "mucus–bicarbonate" barrier. Clin Sci 1982;62:343.

32. Schoenhard G, Opperman J, Kohn FE. Metabolism and pharmacokinetic studies of misoprostol. Dig Dis Sci 1985;30(Suppl 11):126S.

33. Wagstaff AJ, Benfield P, Monk JP. Colloidal bismuth subcitrate: a review of its pharmacodynamic and pharmacokinetic properties, and its therapeutic use in peptic ulcer disease. Drugs 1988;36:132.

34. Slomiany BL, Bilski J, Sarosiek J, et al. Colloidal bismuth subcitrate (De-Nol) inhibits peptic degradation of epidermal growth factor. (Abstract) Gastroenterology 1988;94:A431.

35. Peterson WL, Sturdevant RAL, Frankl HD, et al. Healing of duodenal ulcer with an antacid regimen. N Engl J Med 1977;297:341.

36. Berstad A, Weberg R. Antacids for peptic ulcer: do we have anything better? Scand J Gastroenterol 1986;21(Suppl 125):32.

37. Thomas JM, Misiewicz G. Histamine H-2 receptor antagonists in the short- and long-term treatment of duodenal ulcer. Clin Gastroenterol 1984;13:501.

38. Lee FI, Reed PI, Crowe JP, et al. Acute treatment of duodenal ulcer: a multicentre study to compare ranitidine 150 mg twice daily with ranitidine 300 mg once at night. Gut 1986;27:1091.

39. Langtry HD, Grant SM, Goa KL. Famotidine: an updated review of its pharmacodynamic and pharmacokinetic properties, and therapeutic use in peptic ulcer disease and other allied diseases. Drugs 1989;38:551.

40. Price AH, Brogden RN. Nizatidine: a preliminary review of its pharmacodynamic and pharmacokinetic properties, and its therapeutic use in peptic ulcer disease. Drugs 1988;36:521.

41. Hunt RH. Treatment of peptic ulcer disease with sucralfate: a review. Am J Med 1991;91(Suppl 2A)102S.

42. Mulholland MW, Bonsack M, Delaney JP. Proliferation of gastric endocrine cells after vagotomy in the rat. Endocrinology 1985;117:1578.

43. Mistiaen W, Van Hee R, Blockx P, et al. Gastric emptying for solids in patients with duodenal ulcer before and after highly selective vagotomy. Dig Dis Sci 1990;35:310.

44. Humphrey CS, Johnston D, Walker BE, et al. Incidence of dumping after truncal and SVW pyloroplasty and HSV without drainage procedure. Br Med J 1972;3:785.

45. Amdrup E, Andersen D, Hostrup H. The Aarhus County vagotomy trial. I. An interim report on preliminary results and the incidence of sequelae following parietal cell vagotomy and selective gastric vagotomy in 748 patients. World J Surg 1978;2:85.

46. Enskog L, Rydberg B, Adami HO, et al. Clinical results 1-10 years after highly selective vagotomy in 306 patients with prepyloric and duodenal ulcer disease. Br J Surg 1986;73:357.

47. Stoddard CJ, Vassilakis JS, Duthie HL. Highly selective vagotomy or truncal vagotomy and pyloroplasty for chronic duodenal ulcer: a randomized prospective clinical study. Br J Surg 1978;65:793.

48. Schirmer BD. Current status of proximal gastric vagotomy. Ann Surg 1989;209:131.

49. Mulholland M, Morrow C, Dunn DH, et al. Surgical treatment of duodenal ulcer: a prospective randomized study. Arch Surg 1982;117:393.

50. Hollinshead JW, Smith RC, Gillett DJ. Parietal cell vagotomy: experience with 144 patients with prepyloric or duodenal ulcer. World J Surg 1982;6:596.

51. Knight CD Jr, Van Heerden JA, Kelly KA. Proximal gastric vagotomy: update. Ann Surg 1983;197:22.

52. Gunshefski L, Flancbaum L, Brolin RE, et al. Changing patterns in perforated peptic ulcer disease. Am Surg 1990;56:270.

53. Cocks JR. Perforated peptic ulcer: the changing scene. Dig Dis 1992;10:10.

54. Crofts TJ, Park KGM, Steele RJC, et al. A randomized trial of nonoperative treatment for perforated peptic ulcer. N Engl J Med 1989;320:970.

55. Boey J, Wong J, Ong GB. A prospective study of operative risk factors in perforated duodenal ulcers. Ann Surg 1982;195:265.

56. Boey J, Lee NW, Koo J, et al. Immediate definitive surgery for perforated duodenal ulcers: a prospective controlled trial. Ann Surg 1982;196:338.

57. Boey J, Branicki FJ, Alagaratnam TT, et al. Proximal gastric vagotomy: the preferred operation for perforations in acute duodenal ulcer. Ann Surg 1988;208:169.

58. Christiansen J, Andersen OB, Bonnesen T, at al. Perforated duodenal ulcer managed by simple closure versus closure and proximal gastric vagotomy. Br J Surg 1987;74:286.

59. Ceneviva R, de Castro e Silva O, Castelfranchi PL, et al. Simple suture with or without proximal gastric vagotomy for perforated duodenal ulcer. Br J Surg 1986;73:427.

60. Gustavsson S, Nyren O. Time trends in peptic ulcer surgery, 1956 to 1986. Ann Surg 1989;210:704.

61. Christensen A, Bousfield R, Christiansen J. Incidence of perforated and bleeding peptic ulcers before and after the introduction of H2-receptor antagonists. Ann Surg 1988;207:4.

62. Gilinsky NH. Peptic ulcer disease in the elderly. Gastroenterol Clin North Am 1990;19:255.

63. Branicki FJ, Boey J, Fok PJ, et al. Bleeding duodenal ulcer: a prospective evaluation of risk factors for rebleeding and death. Ann Surg 1990;211:411.

64. Johnston JH. Endoscopic risk factors for bleeding peptic ulcer. Gastrointest Endosc 1990;36:S16.

65. Gilbert DA. Epidemiology of upper gastrointestinal bleeding. Gastrointest Endosc 1990;36:S8.

66. Jiranek GC, Silverstein FE. Introduction to endoscopic therapy for bleeding peptic ulcer. Gastrointest Endosc 1990;36:S25.

67. Laine L. Bipolar/multipolar electrocoagulation. Gastrointest Endosc 1990;36:S38.

68. Jensen DM. Heat probe for hemostasis of bleeding peptic ulcers: techniques and results of randomized controlled trials. Gastrointest Endosc 1990;36:S42.

69. Consensus conference. Therapeutic endoscopy and bleeding ulcers. JAMA 1989;262:1369.

70. Kelley HG, Grant GN, Elliott DW. Massive gastroduodenal hemorrhage: changing concepts of management. Arch Surg 1963;87:6.

71. Hoffman J, Devantier A, Koelle T, et al. Parietal cell vagotomy as an emergency procedure for bleeding peptic ulcer. Ann Surg 1987;206:583.

72. Hogan RB, Hamilton JK, Polter DE. Preliminary experience with hydrostatic balloon dilation of gastric outlet obstruction. Gastrointest Endosc 1986;32:71.

73. Dunn DC, Thomas WEG, Hunter JO. Highly selective vagotomy and pyloric dilatation for duodenal ulcer with stenosis. Br J Surg 1981;68:194.

74. Rossi RC, Dial DF, Georgi B, et al. A five to ten year followup study of parietal cell vagotomy. Surg Gynecol Obstet 1986;162:301.

75. Csendes A, Braghetto I, Smok G. Type IV gastric ulcer: a new hypothesis. Surgery 1987;101:361.

76. Soll AH. Pathogenesis of peptic ulcer and implications for therapy. N Engl J Med 1990;322:909.

77. Howden CW, Jones DB, Peace KE, et al. The treatment of gastric ulcer with antisecretory drugs: relationship of pharmacological effect to healing rates. Dig Dis Sci 1988;33:619.

78. Fisher R, Cohen S. Physiological characteristics of the human pyloric sphincter. Gastroenterology 1973;64:67.

79. Miller LJ, Malagelada JR, Longstreth GF, et al. Dysfunctions of the stomach with gastric ulceration. Dig Dis Sci 1980;25:857.

80. Podolsky I, Storms P, Richardson C, et al. Gastric adenocarcinoma masquerading endoscopically as benign gastric ulcer. Dig Dis Sci 1988;33:1057.

81. Buckner JW III, Austin JC, Steinberg JB, et al. Factors predicting failure of medical therapy for gastric ulcers. Am J Surg 1989;158:570.

82. McCarthy DM. Sucralfate. N Engl J Med 1991;325:1017.

83. Rossi JA, Sollenberger LL, Rege RV, et al. External duodenal fistula: causes, complications, and treatment. Arch Surg 1986;121:908.

84. Ahmad W, Harbrecht PJ, Polk HC. Leaks and obstruction after gastric resection. Am J Surg 1986;152:301.

85. Jensen HE, Hoffman J, Wille-Jorgensen P. High gastric ulcer. World J Surg 1987;11:325.

86. Chua CL, Jeyaraj PR, Low CH. Relative risks of complications in giant and nongiant gastric ulcers. Am J Surg 1992;164:94.

87. Czaja AJ, McAlhany JG, Pruitt BA Jr. Acute gastroduodenal disease after thermal injury: an endoscopic evaluation of incidence and natural history. N Engl J Med 1974;291:925.

88. Miller TA, Tornwall MS, Moody FG. Stress erosive gastritis. Curr Probl Surg 1991;28:459.

89. Mercer DW, Sullivan T, Milner R, et al. Do capsaicin-sensitive neurons in the gastric mucosa mediate adaptive cytoprotection by increasing endogenous prostaglandins? Surg Forum 1991;48:182.

90. Shuman RB, Schuster DP, Zuckerman GR. Prophylactic therapy for stress ulcer bleeding: a reappraisal. Ann Intern Med 1987;106:562.

91. Jensen SL, Jensen PF. Role of sucralfate in peptic disease. Dig Dis 1992;10:153.

92. Driks MR, Craven DE, Celli BR. Nosocomial pneumonia in intubated patients given sucralfate as compared with antacids or histamine type 2 blockers. N Engl J Med 1987;317:1376.

Digestive Tract Surgery: A Text and Atlas, edited by Richard H. Bell,
Layton F. Rikkers, and Michael W. Mulholland.
Lippincott-Raven Publishers, Philadelphia, © 1996.

7

Postgastrectomy Syndromes and Motility Disorders

Frederic E. Eckhauser | *Lisa M. Colletti* | *William L. Hasler*

The surgical treatment of peptic ulcer disease has changed dramatically during the past 40 years, with a much greater emphasis on tissue preservation and limited gastric denervation. Nonetheless, any type of gastric surgery alters anatomy and physiology of the upper gastrointestinal tract and can cause some patients to develop postcibal symptoms that are distressing, persistent, and often disabling. These pathophysiologic conditions are referred to collectively as *postgastrectomy syndromes.* Although several clearly defined clinical patterns have been identified and can be effectively treated, frequently syndromes coexist, with one symptom complex dominating. These patients are among the most perplexing and challenging whom clinicians are asked to evaluate and treat.

The true incidence of postgastrectomy syndromes and motility disturbances is unknown. Some authors suggest that 25% of patients who undergo gastric surgery develop one or more postgastrectomy syndromes and that only 1% develop severe or uncontrolled symptoms that warrant remedial operation.[1] It is incumbent on the treating surgeon to pursue an accurate diagnosis vigorously because inappropriate remedial surgery can lead to residual or worsened symptoms, analgesic drug dependence, and nutritional deficiencies. With proper patient selection, remedial procedures can be expected to yield satisfactory results in about 80% of patients.

Postgastrectomy symptoms result from perturbations of normal gastric anatomy and physiology. Gastric emptying is a complex and highly coordinated process subject to a variety of neural and hormonal influences. The development of electrophysiologic

techniques and radioisotope-labeled test meals has expanded the capacity to quantify gastric dysfunction and to implement therapeutic trials based on objective data. This chapter is subdivided into three sections that review the normal physiology of gastric emptying, disorders of gastric emptying, and postgastrectomy syndromes.

PHYSIOLOGY OF GASTRIC EMPTYING

Motor activity of the stomach serves distinct roles under fasting and fed conditions. Interdigestive patterns clear the stomach of undigested debris. After meal ingestion, the stomach accommodates the ingested bolus, with little change in intragastric pressure, and then grinds and disperses the meal into fine particles that are delivered to the duodenum at a rate optimal for digestion. The stomach can be divided into three regions based on function: (1) the proximal stomach, including the cardia, fundus, and proximal body; (2) the distal stomach, including the distal body and antrum; and (3) the pylorus. Coordinated actions of these regions with feedback control from the small intestine regulate emptying of gastric contents into the duodenum. Gastric emptying is also dependent on nutritive and physical characteristics of the ingested material.

Regional Patterns of Gastric Motor Activity

Each region of the stomach possesses distinct electromechanical properties that correspond to its function. The proximal stomach generates tonic motor activity for accommodation and storage of food, regulation of intragastric pressure, and gradual propulsion of chyme into the distal stomach. The distal stomach exhibits phasic contractile activity, which grinds and triturates solids and propels undigested contents. The pylorus serves as a sieve to regulate outflow of intraluminal contents from the stomach.

The proximal stomach exhibits two distinct patterns of contraction.[2] Slow, sustained contractions up to 6 minutes in duration constitute 80% of fundic motor activity and determine basal intragastric pressure. Superimposed on these slow changes in tone are more rapid, intense phasic contractions up to 30 seconds in duration. The proximal stomach maintains a stable intragastric pressure after meal ingestion. This function is mediated by two neural reflexes: receptive relaxation and gastric accommodation. Receptive relaxation is the reduction in proximal gastric tone that occurs with swallowing. As a result, the stomach can accommodate more than a liter of fluid with less than a 10-mmHg increase in intragastric pressure. Transfer of the swallowed bolus into the stomach is not required to activate receptive relaxation because the reflex occurs with a dry swallow or mechanical stimulation of the pharynx. Gastric accommodation and reflex relaxation of the proximal stomach in response to gastric distention are mediated by stimulation of mechanoreceptors in the gastric wall. Unlike receptive relaxation, accommodation does not require stimulation of the pharynx or esophagus.

In contrast to the fundus, the distal stomach exhibits predominantly phasic contractions, which can be intense and often exceed 100 mmHg. The phasic motor activity of the distal stomach propagates as a coordinated ring contraction, increasing in amplitude and velocity as it approaches the distal antrum. Because of modulating neural and hormonal inputs, not all ring contractions traverse the entire distal stomach, with some contractions dying out before they reach the pylorus.

The distal stomach exhibits characteristic patterns under fasting and meal-stimulated conditions. The migrating motor complex (MMC) is the stereotypical fasting pattern that clears the stomach of undigested food particles, mucus, and sloughed epithelial cells. Loss of the MMC in certain diseases leads to stasis and bezoar formation. The human MMC consists of four distinct phases with a combined duration of 84 to 112 minutes[3] (Fig. 7-1). Phase I is a period of motor quiescence that lasts 40% to 60% of the total cycle length. Phase II, which occupies 20% to 30% of the cycle length, is a period of increasing but irregular contractions. Phase III is a 5- to 10-minute period of intense, rhythmic contractions that propagate aborally, with complete oblit-

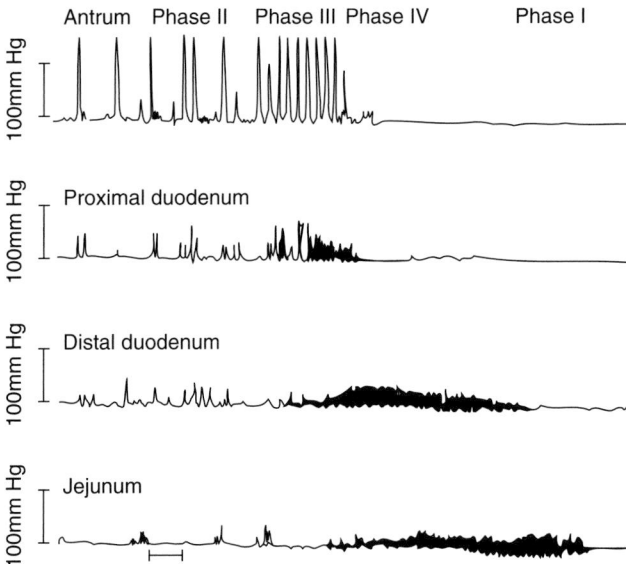

Figure 7-1 The migrating motor complex from a healthy human consists of four phases: phase I, a quiescent period; phase II, a period of irregular contractile activity; phase III, a brief complex of intense rhythmic contractions that propagate from the distal stomach into the small intestine; and phase IV, a transitional phase back to quiescence. (After Rees WDW, Malagelada JR, Miller LJ, et al. Human interdigestive and postprandial gastrointestinal motor and gastrointestinal hormone patterns. Dig Dis Sci 1982;27:321)

eration of the antral and intestinal lumens. Seventy-one percent of phase III complexes originate in the stomach, with 28% beginning in the duodenum and 1% in the proximal jejunum.[4] Phase IV is a brief period of transitional motor activity from the intense motility of phase III to the quiescence of phase I. The propulsive characteristics of interdigestive motor activity vary depending on the phase of the MMC. Emptying of inert liquids or endogenous secretions is more rapid during phase III than during phases I and II.

Induction of gastric phase III motor complexes is thought to result from release of the hormone motilin from specific duodenal mucosal cells. Phase III complexes correlate temporally with elevations in plasma motilin. Premature antral phase III activity is inducible by intravenous infusion of motilin. The most convincing evidence that motilin is a physiologic mediator of gastric phase III activity comes from studies using antibodies to motilin that suppress circulating motilin levels.[5] After infusion of motilin antisera in dogs, gastric phase III activity is abolished for several hours and is replaced by irregular phasic motor activity. The importance of motilin as a physiologic regulator of the MMC is supported by observations that duodenectomy, which removes most of the motilin-secreting tissue, alters interdigestive motility.

After a meal, the MMC is replaced by a fed pattern of intermittent phasic contractions of varying amplitude. The fed pattern begins 5 to 10 minutes after ingestion and persists as long as food remains in the stomach. Fluoroscopic studies show that fed antral contractions propel the ingested material distally, only to be repelled into the proximal stomach, thus serving to mix and grind the solid food.[6] Contractile amplitudes during the fed state depend both on the consistency and the composition of the ingested material, with large particles inducing more intense antral contractions than homogenized food. Highly viscous intragastric contents prolong the duration of the fed pattern for several hours. The duration of the fed period is proportional to the type of nutrient consumed, with fats inducing a more prolonged fed pattern than proteins or carbohydrates.

Pyloric smooth muscle is composed of two circumferential loops that coalesce over the lesser curvature of the stomach. The thinner proximal muscular loop is detected only with fine dissection, whereas the thicker distal loop, consisting of circular muscle with reinforcing fibers from the longitudinal layer of the antrum, represents the visible sphincter. A septum of connective tissue electrically isolates the pyloric circular muscle from the duodenal bulb. Because of its thickness, the pylorus acts as a mechanical stricture to passage of large particles, even in the absence of active contraction. The sphincteric properties of the pylorus are aided by a highly folded mucosa, which narrows the luminal diameter. In the dog, the pylorus has a resting pressure of 10 mmHg and exhibits intermittent spontaneous contractions. In humans, resistance to flow is also aided by phasic activity.[7]

The pylorus exhibits characteristic motor patterns under fasting and fed conditions. During phase III of the MMC, the pylorus remains open, and fasting gastric contents exit into the duodenum. Under fed conditions, the pylorus exhibits prolonged periods of closure interrupted by brief intervals, about twice per minute, during which antral contents are expelled into the intestine. After a meal, large particles do not traverse the pylorus.

Patterns of Gastric Electrical Activity

The resting membrane potential of gastric smooth muscle shows a gradient decreasing from −48 mV in the proximal stomach to −71 mV in the distal stomach. Muscle from the proximal stomach does not exhibit oscillations in membrane potential. The electrical threshold for contraction is −50 mV; thus, under basal condi-

tions, the proximal stomach is in a state of tonic contraction, which can be modulated by neural or hormonal input.[8] Because of the steep character of the contractile response to membrane potential changes in the proximal stomach, minor membrane depolarizations or hyperpolarizations result in significant increases or decreases in tone.

Superimposed on the resting potential is a rhythmic depolarization, known as the *pacesetter potential* or *slow wave*, which consists of an initial rapid depolarization followed by a prolonged plateau potential[9] (Fig. 7-2). Although slow waves can be spontaneously generated from any site in the distal stomach, muscle cells along the greater curvature in the gastric body exhibit the highest frequency and act as the dominant pacemaker to entrain the rest of the stomach. In humans, the dominant pacesetter potential oscillates at 3 cycles per minute (cpm). The pacesetter potential propagates both distally and circumferentially through the muscle layers. Unlike the heart, there are no specialized conduction pathways for pacemaker activity. Conduction is faster circumferentially than longitudinally, ensuring distal propagation as rings of membrane depolarization. The pacesetter potential of the pylorus is entrained to the same frequency as the adjacent antrum (3 cpm), but because of the thick fibrous septum, most slow waves are not propagated into the duodenum.

For contraction to occur, the slow wave must achieve a threshold level of depolarization. Under quiescent conditions, the plateau potential is more negative than this threshold, and little or no contraction re-

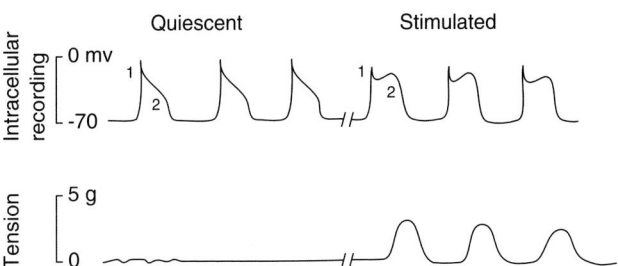

Figure 7-2 The intracellular electrical activity of distal gastric smooth muscle and the resultant contractile response are displayed under quiescent conditions and after stimulation with a contractile agonist. In the unstimulated state, distal gastric smooth muscle exhibits rhythmic electrical activity with an initial upstroke (1) followed by a plateau potential (2). Because the amplitude of this electrical depolarization does not reach a critical threshold, no contraction occurs. With stimulation, there is prolongation and enhancement of the plateau such that a threshold depolarization is achieved, resulting in phasic contractions in the distal stomach. (After Kim CH. Electrical activity of the stomach: clinical implications. Mayo Clin Proc 1986;61:205)

sults (see Fig. 7-2). The presence of a contractile agonist increases the duration and amplitude of the plateau potential and induces action potentials, which are brief, intense depolarizations superimposed on the plateau potential. These events provide the additional depolarization necessary to exceed the contractile threshold. In contrast, relaxing agents reduce plateau potential amplitude or duration or prevent the stimulatory effects of contractile agonists. Because the contractile threshold is exceeded only during each plateau potential, the slow wave determines the maximal frequency of contractions. Thus, unlike the tonic activity of the proximal stomach, the distal stomach exhibits phasic contractions with a maximal frequency of 3 cpm.

Gastric Emptying of Liquids

Emptying of inert liquids, such as water or isotonic saline, follows a single exponential curve, termed *first-order kinetics*[10] (Fig. 7-3). In other words, the volume of

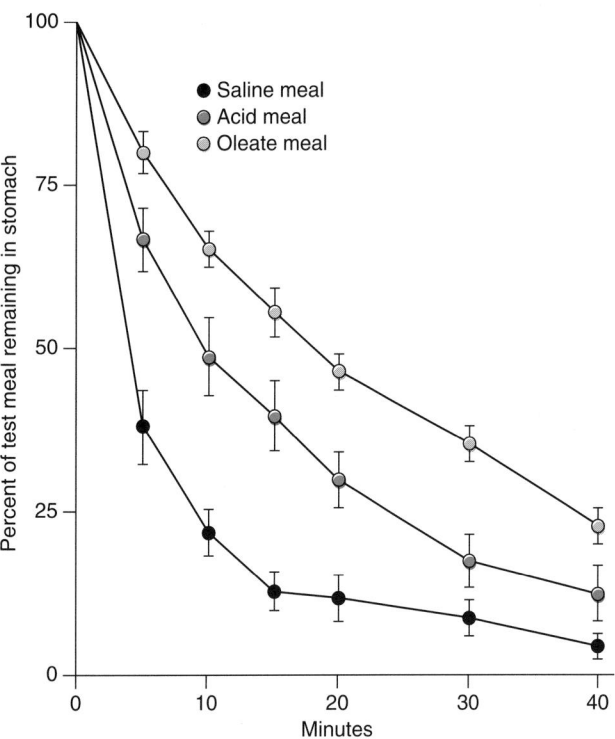

Figure 7-3 Gastric emptying of an inert liquid (0.9% NaCl) exhibits first-order kinetics in which the amount of liquid leaving the stomach remains a constant fraction of the fluid that remains in the stomach. With addition of acid or nutrients (oleate) to an inert liquid meal (0.9% NaCl), emptying from the stomach is slowed owing to feedback inhibition from small intestinal factors. (After Dooley CP, Reznick JB, Valenzuela JE. Variations in gastric and duodenal motility during gastric emptying of liquid meals in humans. Gastroenterology 1984;87:1114)

liquid that is emptied into the duodenum in a given time is a constant fraction of the volume remaining in the stomach. Thus, 300 mL of saline empties at twice the rate of a 150-mL load. In humans, inert liquids empty rapidly, with a time to 50% emptying ranging from 8 to 18 minutes.

In contrast to inert liquids, the gastric emptying of nutrient-containing liquids follows a curvilinear function, with an initial rapid phase lasting 5 to 30 minutes followed by a slower phase in which the nutrient is emptied at a constant rate for up to 2 hours[10] (see Fig. 7-3). Because of the linearity of liquid nutrient emptying, 300 mL of 11% glucose empties at the same rate as 150 mL. Liquids with high caloric density empty more slowly than liquids with fewer calories per unit volume. In general, liquid emptying is controlled at a rate that delivers 200 kcal/h to the duodenum. Thus, 0.25 mol of glucose empties four times as fast as 1 mol of glucose.

Other characteristics of the nutrient are important regulators of liquid emptying as well.[11] Carbohydrates and most amino acids modulate intestinal delivery by action on intestinal osmoreceptors. L-Tryptophan is distinguished from other amino acids in that it can delay liquid emptying in isotonic solutions, leading investigators to postulate specific intestinal L-tryptophan receptors. Isocaloric amounts of starch, disaccharides, and monosaccharides are equipotent at delaying liquid emptying, as are isocaloric quantities of protein and amino acids, suggesting that the digestive products of carbohydrate and protein hydrolysis are major regulators of emptying. Fatty acids, rather than complete triglycerides, are also important regulators. Medium-chain fatty acids of 12 to 14 carbons are more potent than longer or shorter fatty acids.

Physicochemical factors modulate the rate of liquid gastric emptying.[12] Titratable acid delivery to the duodenum is constant regardless of the pH or lipid solubility of acids in the gastric lumen. Thus, a large amount of a weak acid can be a more potent inhibitor of liquid emptying than a trivial amount of a strong acid, such as hydrochloric acid. Emptying of hypertonic or hyperviscous liquids is slower than emptying of compounds of normal tonicity or viscosity. Gravity has minimal effect on liquid emptying of carbohydrate or acidic solutions.

Gastric Emptying of Digestible Solids

The delivery of digestible solid foods to the duodenum is much slower than that of liquids, with a time for 50% emptying of about 2 hours[13] (Fig. 7-4). Solid-phase emptying exhibits an initial lag phase, which persists for up to 1 hour, during which little or no duodenal delivery occurs. Cinefluoroscopic studies show extensive mixing and retropulsion during this phase, in

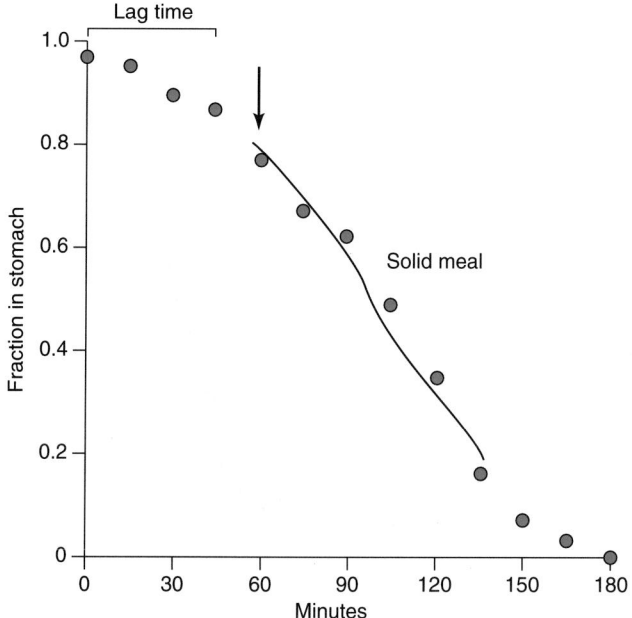

Figure 7-4 The gastric emptying of digestible solids is characterized by an initial lag phase in which little chyme is delivered to the duodenum, followed by a linear emptying phase with a fixed rate of emptying. (After Camilleri M, Malagelada JR, Brown ML, et al. Relation between antral motility and gastric emptying of solids and liquids in humans. Am J Physiol 1985;249:G580)

Gastric Emptying of Fats and Indigestible Solids

The stomach exhibits characteristic emptying patterns for fats and indigestible solid foods. Many fats are solid or semisolid before ingestion; after being warmed to body temperature in the stomach, they are converted to a liquid phase. Liquid fats are emptied more slowly than aqueous liquids.[11] Fats possess a specific gravity of less than 1 g/cm^3, float on top of aqueous liquids in the stomach, and tend to be emptied last. Because of poor aqueous solubility, fats coalesce into large globules, and despite antral motor activity, fats do not disperse into fine particles as do most solids. Fluid fats also adhere to solid food particles, further delaying their emptying. Fats are potent inducers of enterogastric inhibition of emptying.

Indigestible solids, the nonnutritive fibrous remnants of a meal, are usually not emptied with the dispersible, digestible solids. Indigestible solids exit the stomach with the phase III activity of the MMC after completion of the fed motor pattern. Indigestible spheres less than 1 mm in diameter freely pass into the intestine during the fed period, often at rates faster than solid nutritive food. Larger spheres pass more slowly, usually after an initial lag period, with the calorie-containing components of a solid meal.[15] Undigested materials as large as 2 cm in diameter have been demonstrated to pass into the intestine under normal conditions.

Neural Regulation of Gastric Emptying

The stomach receives a rich innervation from the vagus and splanchnic nerves. The nerves contain efferent fibers that modulate gastric motility and afferent fibers that transmit sensory information from the gut. The gastric wall also possesses intrinsic nerves, which provide the neural programming necessary for many of the functions of the stomach. The myenteric plexus, located between the longitudinal and circular muscle layers, provides most of the intrinsic nerve supply.

Only a few thousand vagal efferent fibers project from the brain stem to the stomach, and only selected neurons in the myenteric plexus receive input from the central nervous system. There are two types of vagal efferent fibers—those that respond with a low threshold to electrical stimulation, and those with a high threshold.[16] Low-threshold activity is excitatory to gastric and pyloric motor function and is mediated by cholinergic pathways. High-threshold fibers are inhibitory to gastric and pyloric contractile activity, most likely through release of vasoactive intestinal peptide and nitric oxide. Most of the efferent sympathetic neural

which solid food is crushed and dispersed into fine particles.[5] A linear emptying phase of 1 or more hours follows, during which the dispersed particles are slowly delivered to the duodenum. After ingestion of digestible solids, 95% of particles delivered to the proximal intestine are less than 0.5 mm in diameter, demonstrating the efficacy of gastric trituration.

Solid meals possess several properties that modify their rate of delivery to the intestine. Particulate size affects the rate of solid emptying.[14] Physical characteristics of the meal alter the function of the stomach to retain large particles. If meal viscosity is increased, particles much larger than 1 mm can be delivered to the duodenum. The caloric content and character of a meal also determine the rate of solid-phase emptying. Addition of fats, triglycerides, or carbohydrates to a solid meal delays emptying by prolonging the initial lag phase. In contrast, if a low-calorie substance, such as lettuce, is added to a solid meal to enhance its volume but not nutritive value, emptying is accelerated. The amount of liquid consumed with solid food alters the duodenal delivery of solid nutrients. In a mixed solid and liquid meal, liquids are emptied more rapidly than solids, suggesting that the stomach can distinguish the two phases when presented simultaneously.

activity to the stomach projects through the celiac ganglia. The sympathetic nerve supply inhibits gastric contractile activity by reducing cholinergic transmission.

Afferent nerve fibers greatly outnumber efferent fibers in the vagus and splanchnic nerves.[17] Vagal afferent fibers from the stomach terminate in the nucleus solitarius, where second-order neurons then project to other brain-stem nuclei. Gastric sensory information also is transmitted through the splanchnic nerves to the dorsal horn of the spinal cord, where second-order neurons project to the brain stem and cerebral cortex. A number of gastric receptors respond to intragastric stimulation. Mucosal receptors respond to mechanical stroking or to chemical stimuli, such as hydrochloric acid. Smooth muscle mechanoreceptors are activated by distention, antral contractions, or exposure to hot or cold temperatures. Receptors in the mesentery and serosa respond to tension on the viscera or to forceful contraction and can mediate perception of visceral pain.

The innervation of the stomach plays an important role in the modulation of motor activity in the different gastric regions. The vagus nerves contain both the afferent and efferent limbs of receptive relaxation and accommodation in the proximal stomach. Both reflexes are thought to be mediated by release of vasoactive intestinal peptide.[18] Truncal or proximal gastric vagotomy decreases gastric distensibility and increases intragastric pressure after bolus ingestion. Changes in vagal innervation can modulate fasting motility in the stomach. Bilateral vagotomy increases the threshold for induction of the fed pattern and shortens its duration. Acute vagal cooling converts the fed pattern to one of intermittent phase III activity.

The pylorus is subject to neural control that is distinct from the adjacent duodenum and antrum. Vagally mediated pyloric contractions are blocked by naloxone, indicating mediation by opiate pathways.[19] Electrical stimulation of duodenal muscle increases pyloric contraction, whereas antral activation relaxes the pylorus. Intact neural pathways are essential for normal gastric emptying of both solids and liquids. Truncal or proximal vagotomy results in rapid delivery of liquids into the duodenum. Truncal vagotomy also slows emptying of digestible and indigestible solids and can lead to bezoar formation in susceptible patients.

Finally, neural input from the central nervous system is a potent regulator of gastric motor activity and gastric emptying. Induction of stress alters normal fasting and fed gastric motility, with resultant delays in gastric emptying. Multiple neural pathways appear to be involved as these stress responses are blocked by truncal vagotomy or by antagonism of adrenergic or opiate receptors.

Hormonal Regulation of Gastric Emptying

Numerous hormones and paracrine factors have motor effects on the stomach. Hormonal factors are responsible for inducing the fed pattern in the distal stomach. If a meal is infused into an extrinsically denervated autotransplanted loop of small intestine, the gastric MMC is interrupted. Similarly, when blood from a recently fed animal is perfused in an isolated stomach preparation, motor complexes resembling the fed pattern are observed. Although many hormones are released postprandially, no known hormone clearly reproduces all the motor effects seen after a meal; the hormone or hormones responsible for inducing the fed pattern remain unknown.

Integrated Responses

Control of gastric emptying requires the concerted action of the distinct physiologic regions of the stomach. The integrated responses include the coordination of antral and pyloric activity after meal ingestion, propagation of antral and duodenal motor complexes under fasting and fed conditions, and inhibition of gastric motor activity and emptying by small intestinal feedback.

Terminal Antral Contractions

The integrated function of the distal stomach and pylorus has been best characterized by cinefluoroscopic evaluation.[6,11] In these studies, a minor ring contraction in the gastric body is followed 2 to 3 seconds later by an intense propagating contractile ring that obliterates the lumen. The minor contraction reaches the pylorus, inducing pyloric closure as the larger contraction approaches the mid-portion of the antrum. The intense contractile ring further propagates into the distal antrum, propelling trapped food material against the occluded pylorus, resulting in grinding and mixing, followed by retropulsion of the bolus into the more proximal stomach as the second contractile wave reaches the pylorus (Fig. 7-5). It has been hypothesized that the shear forces induced by the sudden change in velocity of the intragastric contents and the squeezing action by the antral walls are responsible for dispersion of large particles into smaller ones.

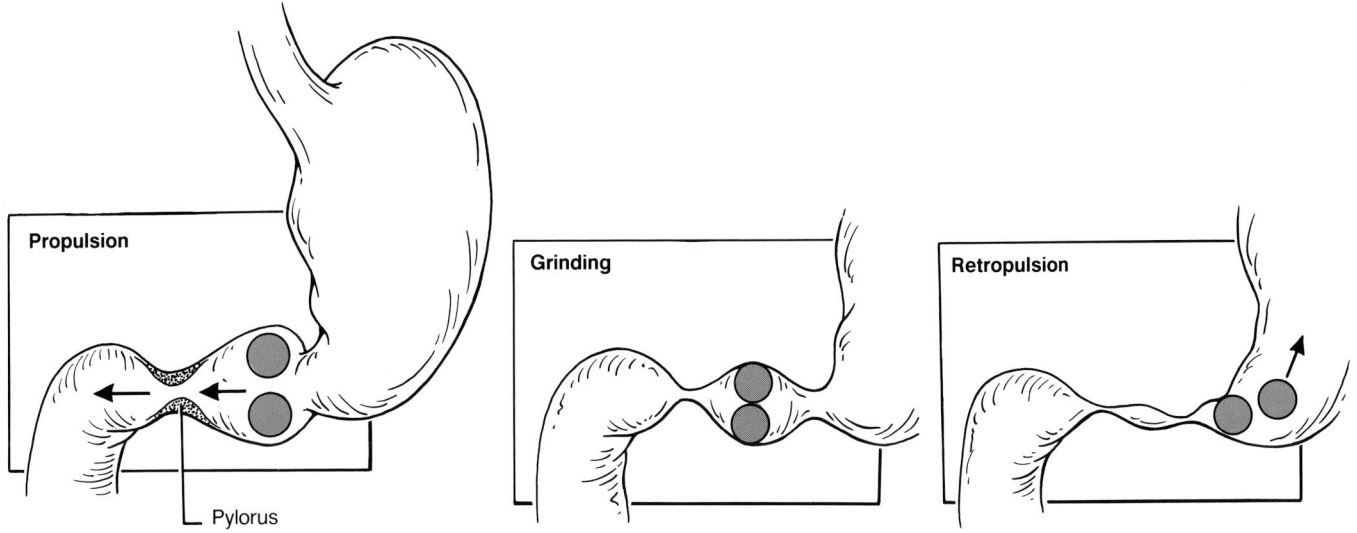

Figure 7-5 Cinefluoroscopic studies demonstrate a stereotyped motor pattern of ring contractile events in the distal stomach and pylorus that result initially in aboral propulsion of the solid food bolus, followed by mixing and grinding, and finally retropulsion of the mixed bolus into the proximal stomach due to the presence of pyloric closure. (After Meyer JH. Motility of the stomach and gastroduodenal junction. In: Johnson LR, ed. Physiology of the gastrointestinal tract, ed 2. New York, Raven, 1987:613)

Gastroduodenal Coordination

The duodenum exhibits a pacemaker distinct from the distal stomach with a frequency of 11 to 12 cpm. Because of the fibrous septum between the duodenum and pylorus, most gastric electrical activity is not propagated into the small intestine. However, some conduction occurs, resulting in intermittent coordination of antroduodenal electrical activity, with one gastric pacesetter potential firing in phase with every three to four duodenal cycles.[20]

The duodenum exhibits other contractile patterns in addition to propagated antroduodenal contractions. After a meal, isolated contractions in the duodenum segment and mix the food particles with pancreaticobiliary secretions. Under some conditions, strong retroperistaltic contractions in the duodenum propel intestinal contents orally, inducing duodenogastric reflux. Perturbation of gastric motor function can alter small intestinal motor patterns. Distention of the stomach slows small intestinal transit in a phenomenon known as the *gastroenteric reflex*. In contrast, the *gastroileal reflex* is characterized by an increase in propulsive ileal motor activity after ingestion of a meal. Finally, decreases in ileocecal pressure have been described in response to nutrient ingestion.

Intestinal Feedback Inhibition

Motor activity in each of the regions of the stomach is subject to feedback inhibition by the small intestine.[21] Balloon distention of the duodenum or colon re-duces fundic tone and decreases antral contractions. Additional enterogastric reflexes that inhibit proximal gastric tone and distal phasic activity are induced by intraduodenal perfusion of acid, proteins, or fat. Intraduodenal fat perfusion also reduces phasic motor activity in the denervated stomach, indicating that hormonal pathways are involved as well.

Protein or amino acid perfusates that contain L-tryptophan are the most potent inhibitors of antral motor activity. Similarly, long-chain triglycerides are more effective inhibitors of distal contractions than are short- or medium-length lipids. Infusion of fats, amino acids, hypertonic glucose, or hydrochloric acid into the duodenum produces a decrease in transpyloric flow that is associated with pyloric closure.

Feedback control by the small intestine is one of the most important regulators of gastric emptying. Duodenal perfusion of amino acids can nearly abolish gastric emptying of solids and can also delay delivery of liquids. Intestinal perfusion with nutrients slows emptying of solids by prolonging the duration of the lag phase. A number of agents delay gastric emptying through effects on small intestinal osmoreceptors. Special receptors appear to exist for pH, fats, and certain amino acids (especially L-tryptophan). Inhibition of gastric emptying by lipids also requires the presence of component fatty acids.

Intestinal feedback inhibition of gastric emptying is dependent on the length of intestine exposed to a stimulus. Osmoreceptors that mediate inhibition by hypertonic salts are localized to the duodenum. In contrast, acids and nutrients have inhibitory properties over a much longer segment of small bowel. Maximal inhibition of liquid emptying is seen with exposure of the proximal 150 cm of small intestine to acid, glucose, or oleic acid, although perfusion of only the most proximal 15 cm of duodenum delays delivery of liquids into the intestine. Regions other than the proximal intestine can also modulate gastric emptying. Balloon distention of the rectum reduces emptying of solids. Gastric emptying of solids is more strongly inhibited by perfusion of the ileum with glucose than perfusion of more proximal bowel segments. This phenomenon, known as the *ileal brake,* has been described for other nutrients as well. Ileal oleic acid perfusion results in 62% gastric retention of solids and 34% retention of liquids at 4 hours compared with control values of 25% and 4%, respectively.[22]

Diagnostic Tests for Assessing Gastric Motility

Intraluminal Manometry

Manometric techniques for the measurement of phasic motor activity in the stomach and small intestine are available in specialized referral centers. Gastrointestinal manometry requires fluoroscopic placement of a water-perfused or solid-state polyvinyl catheter with four to six antral pressure ports and two to four duodenal ports. Specialized catheters can be designed to measure pyloric motility. A standard gastrointestinal manometric study requires 6 to 8 hours. The initial 4 to 5 hours are used to record motility under fasting conditions. During this time, the clinician should observe one or more cycles of the MMC. After the fasting period, gastric and intestinal motor activity is stimulated by a nutrient meal and measured for 1 to 2 hours. Repeated measurements of gastroduodenal motility also afford the clinician the opportunity to test the effects of prokinetic agents, such as metoclopramide, erythromycin, or cisapride. Advances in miniaturization have provided the capability of recording 24-hour motor activity in an ambulatory setting.

Gastroduodenal manometry should be considered in patients with unexplained nausea and delayed gastric emptying who have not responded to prokinetic agents and in patients with motility disorders who are being considered for remedial surgery. The absence of normal MMC activity or reduction in the amplitude or number of postprandial phasic contractions is consistent with gastroparesis. Reduced motor activity in both the stomach and small intestine is a myopathic pattern seen in a diverse group of diseases, including scleroderma, visceral myopathies, and amyloidosis.[23] In contrast, intense uncoordinated phasic bursts in the stomach and duodenum suggest visceral neuropathy, neuropathic forms of scleroderma, or myotonic dystrophy. A pattern known as the *minute rhythm,* a regular pattern of intestinal bursts occurring about once a minute, is seen with mechanical obstruction or some visceral neuropathies. Some patients with irritable bowel syndrome exhibit short periods of intestinal bursts or the minute rhythm; however, irritable bowel syndrome does not disrupt the MMC or fed motor pattern.

Electronic Barostat

Intraluminal manometry is the most sensitive means of assessing phasic motor activity in the distal stomach, but it cannot be used to quantitate tonic changes in the fundus. The electronic barostat was developed to measure changes in tone in capacious viscera, such as the proximal stomach and rectum, using fluoroscopic placement of highly compliant balloons.[24] The barostat measures changes in intragastric volume by infusing or withdrawing air under computer control to maintain intragastric pressure at the minimal level necessary to distend the balloon. Generally, measurement of fundic tone remains a research tool; however, the barostat has been used on one group of patients with gastroparesis after gastric surgery. These patients were found to exhibit larger intragastric volumes for given pressures, signifying impaired tone in the residual gastric pouch.[24]

Electrogastrography

Phasic motor activity in the distal stomach is controlled by rhythmic electrical oscillations known as the pacesetter potential or slow wave. The technique of electrogastrography (EGG) has made possible the measurement of gastric slow-wave activity in a noninvasive fashion. Although early studies employed electrodes fixed either endoscopically or fluoroscopically to the gastric mucosa, bandpass filtering has allowed investigators to record pacesetter potential signals from electrodes placed cutaneously on the abdomen overlying the stomach. Most EGG filters allow high-fidelity recording of electrical activity in the frequency range occupied by normal and abnormal slow waves.[25] EGG typically is performed in a darkened, quiet, warm environment to minimize motion artifact. Studies are done under fasting conditions for 15 to 30 minutes; the patient is then given water or a nutrient meal, and postprandial recording continues for 45 to 90 minutes. The raw signal is analyzed by fast Fourier transformation to produce a frequency spectrum of the dominant frequencies as a function of time. Under fasting conditions, the slow wave typically is present at low amplitude at 3 cpm. After a meal, the frequency transiently decreases, and the amplitude of the signal increases markedly (Fig. 7-6).

A number of slow-wave disturbances have been described in association with nausea and other upper gut symptoms in clinical conditions such as gastroparesis, nonulcer dyspepsia, nausea of pregnancy, motion sickness, and eating disorders, including anorexia nervosa. The most commonly described abnormalities are disturbances of the EGG rhythm, including tachygastria (Fig. 7-7) and bradygastria (Fig. 7-8). Some patients exhibit several dominant peaks across the frequency spectrum and are characterized as having gastric tachybradyarrhythmia. All these dysrhythmias result in inefficient gastric contraction. Tachygastric waves are of low amplitude and do not reach the electrical threshold necessary to induce contraction, resulting in an atonic stomach. Bradygastria leads to infrequent, poorly coordinated contractions. The other main abnormality described is an absence of the signal amplitude increase after a meal, which is often seen in patients with underlying motor abnormalities, such as gastroparesis.[26]

Although many patients with delayed gastric emptying exhibit EGG abnormalities, patients with abnormal scintigraphy may have completely normal EGG tracings. Conversely, some patients with normal gastric emptying results have markedly abnormal EGG findings. The two tests identify distinct patient populations and are complementary. A major focus of ongoing investigation is to develop drugs that act as gastric slow-wave antiarrhythmics. Drugs such as the dopamine antagonist domperidone or the newly approved prokinetic agent cisapride appear to exhibit this effect. However, no controlled trials have yet shown that the antiemetic effects of a given drug result from its antiarrhythmic effects.

EGG is a clinical tool that should be limited to major referral centers specializing in the evaluation of patients with gastric dysmotility. EGG should also be considered for diagnosis in patients with unexplained upper abdominal symptoms and normal gastric scintigraphy and in patients with delayed gastric emptying who fail to respond to standard prokinetic agents. The finding of a slow-wave disturbance on EGG rules out most cases of psychogenic vomiting. The presence of a dysrhythmic recording also should direct the clinician to consider medications that have slow-wave stabilizing effects, such as domperidone or cisapride, and to avoid prokinetics, such as erythromycin, which have been shown to induce gastric dysrhythmias.

GASTRIC MOTILITY DISORDERS

Common gastrointestinal symptoms, such as abdominal pain, early satiety, nausea, vomiting, and bloating, are frequently attributed to gastric motility disorders. These disorders involve complex myogenic and neuro-

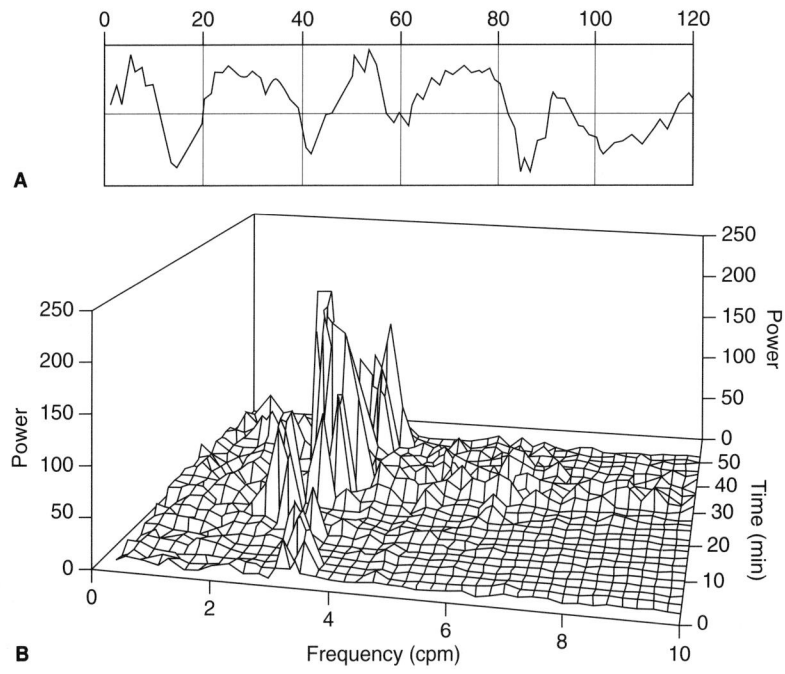

Figure 7-6 Results from an electrogastrographic study of a healthy volunteer. (**A**) The raw slow-wave signal after meal ingestion appears as a regular sinusoidal wave with a period of about 20 seconds. The raw signal can be analyzed by power spectral analysis to determine the dominant slow-wave frequency at any given time. (**B**) Pseudo–three-dimensional plotting from the power spectral analysis. With fasting, the slow wave was regular at 3 cpm, but of low intensity. With meal ingestion (at 15 minutes), there was a transient decrease in slow-wave frequency and a prolonged increase in signal amplitude at 3 cpm.

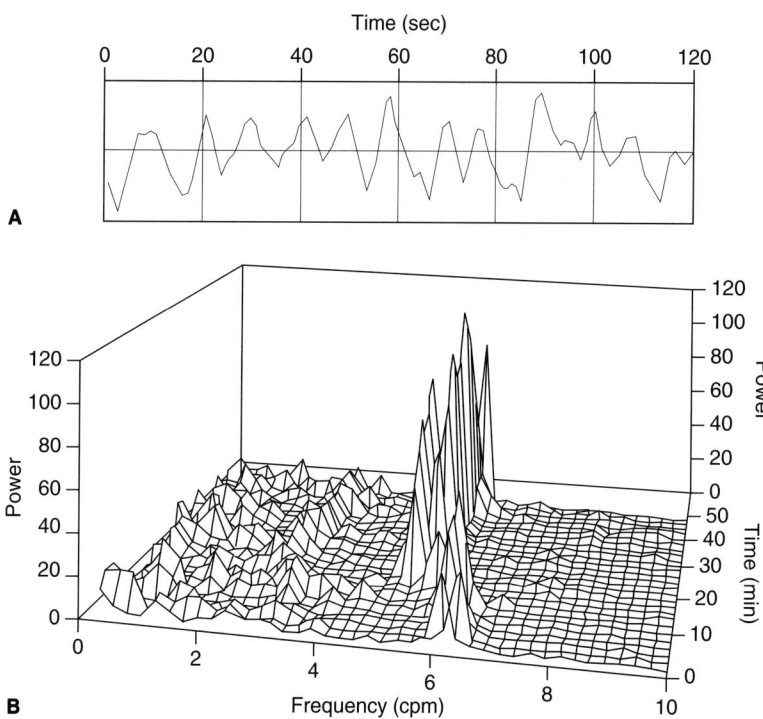

Figure 7-7 Electrogastrography (EGG) was used to evaluate a patient with persistent nausea, bloating, and fullness who had previously demonstrated a normal solid-phase gastric emptying scan. (**A**) Low-amplitude raw EGG signal with a period of about 10 seconds. (**B**) Pseudo–three-dimensional plotting demonstrates the presence of a dominant slow-wave frequency that is much higher (5 to 6 cpm) than normal. This patient had EGG evidence of tachygastria.

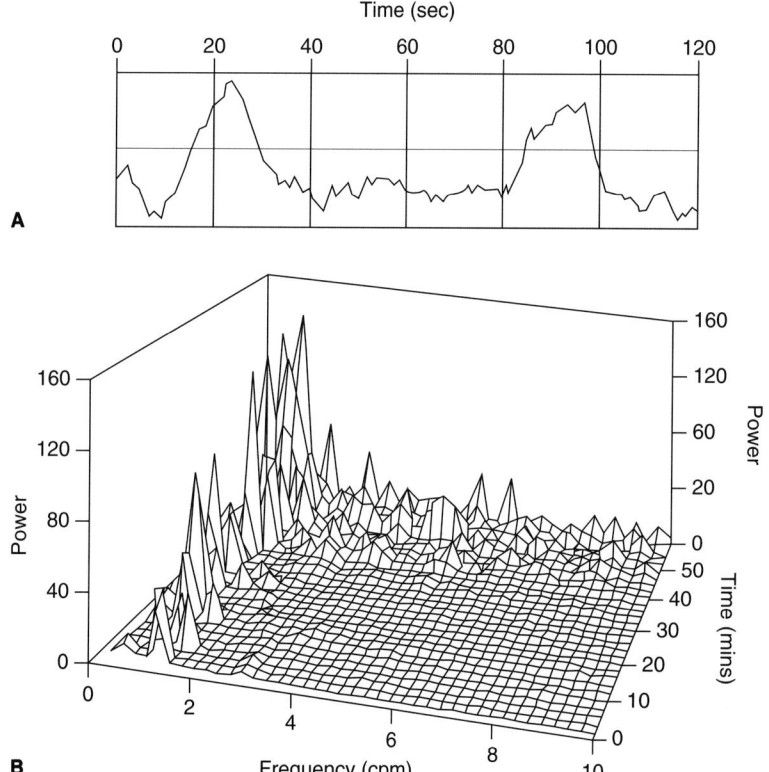

Figure 7-8 Electrogastrography was performed on a 22-year-old woman in the 11th week of pregnancy. (**A**) Intense but infrequent slow waves are seen on the raw tracing. (**B**) Pseudo–three-dimensional plotting of the power spectral analysis demonstrates that the bulk of the slow-wave signal is in the frequency range of 0.75 to 2 cpm. Thus, this pregnant patient exhibited bradygastria in association with first-trimester nausea.

humoral mechanisms that normally control gastric motility. They can be further subclassified according to the type of transit disorder and the affected region of the gastrointestinal tract.[27] This section focuses on delayed gastric transit due to defective propulsion (gastroparesis) and does not address disorders due to mechanical obstruction, such as pyloric or duodenal stenosis.

Pathophysiology and Symptoms

As indicated earlier, the proximal stomach includes the cardia and upper portion of the corpus and acts as a reservoir that allows food to be accommodated without an excessive increase in intragastric pressure. Disorders of receptive relaxation can result clinically in dumping symptoms or dyspepsia, depending on whether the response is exaggerated or delayed.

The distal stomach includes the distal corpus, antrum, and antroduodenal region. This portion of the stomach grinds and mixes gastric contents and regulates expulsion of chyme into the duodenum. These actions are controlled by peristaltic contractions that begin in the corpus and progress aborally toward the pylorus. Continued antegrade and retrograde propulsion of gastric contents grinds and reduces solids to progressively smaller particles. Once particle size has been reduced to 1 to 2 mm, coordinated peristalsis of the antroduodenal region propels gastric contents into the duodenum. Periodically, powerful rhythmic contractions of the stomach sweep indigestible solids into the duodenum. These contractions occur during late phase II and phase III of the MMC.

Delayed gastric emptying can result from a variety of motility disorders, including weak antral contractions, discoordination of antroduodenal peristalsis, and increased functional resistance at the gastric outlet. Accelerated gastric emptying can result from decreased resistance at the gastric outlet due to pyloroplasty. Gastric arrhythmia can also contribute to altered gastric emptying. Such arrhythmias frequently are initially confined to the interdigestive period and disappear in response to meal ingestion. However, they can become dominant over time and result in delayed gastric emptying. Abnormalities of interdigestive motility, especially absence of phase III gastric motility, are commonly observed in patients with diabetic and idiopathic forms of gastroparesis and also occur after truncal vagotomy and partial gastric resection.[28]

Postsurgical Gastroparesis

Postsurgical gastroparesis syndrome is a complex motility disorder characterized by postprandial nausea, vomiting, pain, and gastric atony without evidence of mechanical gastric obstruction. In patients with a prior history of gastric surgery, it is important to differentiate this syndrome from mechanical or inflammatory causes of delayed gastric emptying because the treatment and outcomes differ greatly. The reported incidence of this complication varies from 1.6% to 30%, depending on the indication for operation and the type of procedure performed.[29,30]

Postsurgical gastroparesis is a diagnosis of exclusion. Well-recognized causes of gastric hypomotility, including advanced diabetes, neuromuscular disorders, electrolyte abnormalities, and drug toxicities, must be excluded. One must then distinguish between mechanical and functional disorders of gastric emptying. Mechanical causes include stomal stenosis or edema, kinking or entrapment of the efferent limb in an internal hernia, and postsurgical adhesions. When these findings are encountered at reoperation, the diagnosis is clearcut. However, operative findings are frequently more subtle, leading to confusion in diagnosis and inappropriate surgery. This can lead to residual or worsened symptoms, analgesic drug dependence, and nutritional deficiencies.

The incidence of gastroparesis appears to be highest among patients who undergo ulcer surgery for obstructive symptoms and can be exacerbated by concomitant vagotomy.[30,31] In one study,[32] investigators demonstrated gastric atony in 25% of patients who underwent vagotomy and drainage for obstructing duodenal ulcer. Sex- and age-matched patients who underwent vagotomy and drainage for nonobstructing duodenal ulcers were also evaluated, and none exhibited delayed gastric emptying after operation. Postoperative gastric retention was not observed in patients who underwent subtotal gastric resection for obstructing duodenal ulcer.

Some have hypothesized that preoperative gastric decompression can offset the effects of vagotomy by allowing the stomach to regain its intrinsic muscle tone. Unfortunately, there is little concrete evidence to support this notion. In fact, one large retrospective study of patients operated on for obstructing peptic ulcers[33] demonstrated no correlation between the development of postoperative gastric atony and the length of preoperative gastric decompression, the use of preoperative nutritional support, or the type of surgical procedure performed.

Evidence also suggests that highly selective vagotomy can cause gastric hypomotility in patients with preoperative gastric stasis.[34] One study reported on marked disturbances in gastric myoelectric and manometric activity after highly selective vagotomy among patients with delayed preoperative gastric emptying.[35] The observed myoelectrical disturbances were associated with impaired antral peristaltic activity. By comparison, a group of patients with normal preoperative gastric emptying experienced only sporadic and transient disturbances of gastric myoelectric activity after operation.

Diagnosis

Conventional barium contrast studies and fiberoptic endoscopy are useful for documenting the presence of associated pathology. Liquid loading tests using either physiologic saline or water are performed by instilling a fixed volume into the stomach and withdrawing whatever remains 30 minutes later. Residual volumes exceeding 200 mL with a loading volume of 750 mL are reported to indicate delayed gastric emptying.[35] These studies are difficult to standardize, lack sensitivity, and have limited value because they measure only the liquid component of gastric emptying.

Radioisotopic scans are a reliable, noninvasive means of assessing both liquid and solid phases of gastric emptying if one recognizes the inherent limitations of the methodology. The results of liquid-phase emptying scans can be markedly affected by intragastric dilution due to swallowed secretions or duodenogastric reflux. Solid-phase scans are affected by dissociation of the isotope from the ingested meal, variable rates of mucosal absorption, and the effects of "phase changes" resulting from liquefaction of solids by the stomach. The development of reproducible test standards has greatly reduced variability in results.[36]

The diagnosis of gastric emptying disorders should never be based on clinical findings alone. In one study,[37] 48 patients suspected of having gastroparesis were investigated with quantitative solid-phase gastric emptying studies. Nearly 45% of patients exhibited radionuclide evidence of delayed gastric emptying despite barium and endoscopic studies that were normal or showed nonspecific pathologic changes. Institution of treatment resulted in positive clinical responses and correlated with changes in gastric emptying.

Medical Therapy

In the past, the medical treatment of gastroparesis was limited to diet and behavior modification along with avoidance of drugs such as opiates, anticholinergics, β-agonists, and tricyclic antidepressants. Several classes of drugs have since been introduced for treatment of gastroparesis.

Bethanechol is a cholinergic agent that is similar structurally and pharmacologically to acetylcholine. The drug mimics parasympathetic nervous system activity and causes contraction of the stomach and urinary bladder. Therapeutic doses in humans of 10 to 50 mg orally or 2.5 to 10 mg subcutaneously three or four times daily produce relatively few systemic side effects. In one study,[38] effective gastric contractions were produced in six postvagotomy patients after subcutaneous administration of bethanechol. Subsequent oral administration of bethanechol maintained symptomatic improvement during the treatment period, but two patients (33%) in whom the drug was discontinued required retreatment several weeks later for recurrent symptoms. Both of the restimulated patients were rendered symptom free after retreatment and remained so thereafter.

Metoclopramide is structurally related to procainamide but has no anesthetic activity. Metoclopramide possesses both central nervous system and peripheral gastrointestinal effects. Centrally, the drug is a powerful antiemetic, primarily because of antidopaminergic activity. Peripherally, metoclopramide increases lower esophageal sphincter tone and gastric emptying and shortens small bowel transit time through cholinergic and antidopaminergic mechanisms.[39]

The efficacy of metoclopramide for treatment for postsurgical gastroparesis is unproved.[28,40] In one study,[40] improved gastric emptying of a radionuclide-labeled test meal was noted in 17 of 20 patients (85%) with postvagotomy gastric atony treated with intravenous metoclopramide administered at a dose of 0.3 mg/kg. However, several authors have questioned the efficacy of metoclopramide for these patients. One author treated 19 gastroparetic patients with metoclopramide (of whom 9 had undergone previous gastric surgery) and observed an objective response rate of only 22%.[37] Data from other institutions suggest that metoclopramide and other gastrokinetic agents have little proven benefit in patients with well-documented postsurgical gastroparesis.[41] Investigators have hypothesized that the absence of the antrum limits the ability of the remaining stomach remnant to respond to the drug. Although metoclopramide has been shown to increase fundic motility, the proximal gastric remnant that remains after distal hemigastrectomy may be either too small or hypomuscular to generate sufficient pressure to affect gastric emptying.

Other drugs have been used to enhance gastric emptying, with varied results. Domperidone is a dopaminergic antagonist that stimulates gastrointestinal motility but has no central nervous system effects because it does not cross the blood–brain barrier.[39] The lack of adverse central effects, particularly dystonic extrapyramidal symptoms, makes domperidone an attractive alternative to metoclopramide. Although this drug appears to be promising in patients with diabetic or idiopathic forms of gastroparesis, no clinical data support its efficacy in patients with postsurgical gastroparesis.

Cisapride is a relatively new prokinetic agent that appears to act on the gut by facilitating release of acetylcholine at the level of the myenteric plexus. Cisapride differs from domperidone and metoclopramide in that it does not exhibit antidopaminergic activity. Limited comparative clinical trials have shown that both cisapride and metoclopramide enhance gastric emptying, intensify antral contractions, and shorten intestinal transit time.[42] Cisapride appears to be equally effective for idiopathic and diabetic forms of gastroparesis as well as for postsurgical gastric atony, but multicenter trials are needed to fully evaluate its efficacy.

Erythromycin increases postprandial motility by inducing powerful peristaltic antral contractions and improving antroduodenal coordination. This effect results from binding of erythromycin to motilin receptors on gastrointestinal smooth muscle and is proportional to receptor affinity.[43] Several clinical studies in normal volunteers and patients with diabetic gastroparesis have shown that intravenously administered erythromycin has a dose-related effect on the interdigestive motility of the stomach and the small intestine.[44] High doses of erythromycin (350 mg given intravenously) have an especially strong postprandial stimulatory effect on antral contractility in normal subjects and diabetics, suggesting possible therapeutic benefit in patients with antral hypomotility due to other causes. This observation is especially intriguing in patients with postsurgical gastroparesis. In one study,[45] intravenous administration of 250 mg of erythromycin 30 minutes before each meal to a patient with postvagotomy gastroparesis resulted in an excellent clinical and radiologic response. Gastric emptying, measured by a radionuclide solid-phase gastric emptying study, improved markedly, and preexisting symptoms of nocturnal and postprandial regurgitation, nausea, and heartburn were completely alleviated. The same authors showed that oral erythromycin also improved postvagotomy gastric motor dysfunction and indicated that timing the oral 250-mg dose before meals is critical to ensuring an optimal response.

Surgical Treatment

The surgical approach to patients with postsurgical gastric emptying disorders is controversial. Early postsurgical gastroparesis appears to respond favorably to prolonged nasogastric decompression and nutritional support using either enteral or parenteral routes. In the absence of a demonstrable mechanical cause of gastric outlet obstruction, reoperation is rarely necessary in this setting.

Postsurgical gastroparesis can occur after vagot-

omy combined with either a gastric drainage procedure or distal gastric resection. Conservatism is important in the treatment of patients who exhibit early postoperative gastric atony. In one study,[46] 46 patents who experienced delayed gastric emptying after distal gastric resection with or without vagotomy were evaluated. Of this group, 10 patients (22%) underwent reoperation an average of 30 days after the initial procedure. At reoperation, stomal patency was demonstrated in 8 patients (80%). Additional findings included perianastomotic adhesions and kinking, which was corrected in 4 patients, and minimal or no abnormal findings in 2 patients. Despite correction of the suspected mechanical causes of delayed gastric emptying, resumption of normal gastric function was no different in patients with or without abnormal findings at reoperation (22 versus 16 days).

Upper gastrointestinal endoscopy, barium contrast radiography, or both should be obtained to exclude mechanical causes of delayed gastric emptying. A solid-phase radionuclide gastric emptying scan should be obtained to document objectively the degree of gastroparesis and to evaluate the response to gastrokinetic agents. Finally, a dedicated small bowel radiographic study should be obtained to rule out the possibility of distal bowel pathology and the possible presence of a more generalized motor disorder of the gastrointestinal tract.

In patients who have undergone a previous vagotomy and drainage procedure, it is reasonable to consider a conservative distal hemigastrectomy with either Billroth I or Billroth II reconstruction. Alternatively, a 40- to 50-cm Roux-en-Y limb of jejunum can be used to establish gastroenteric continuity after hemigastrectomy.

A potential disadvantage of Roux-en-Y reconstruction is the possibility of worsening gastric stasis during the early postoperative period.[47] Roux limb motility can be affected by transection of the jejunum and bypass of the duodenal pacemaker. These effects may alter myoelectrical coordination, resulting in a dystonic Roux limb. In one study, recordings from electrodes implanted at the time of Roux-en-Y limb reconstruction showed dysfunctional or absent MMC activity, accompanied in some instances by postprandial high-amplitude contractions, that correlated with symptoms of pain.[48] Despite these findings, many authorities believe that construction of a Roux-en-Y limb has no constant, predictable effect on gastric emptying. Of 11 patients with alkaline reflux gastritis treated with Roux-en-Y limb diversion, 3 (27%) had delayed gastric emptying complicated by bezoar formation, and 8 exhibited no change or accelerated emptying.[49] There were no technical features of the operation or mechanical abnormalities that predicted which patients would develop delayed gastric emptying.

Patients with documented gastroparesis after multiple previous gastric operations, including hemigastrectomy or distal subtotal gastrectomy, have limited alternatives. The reservoir capacity of the stomach has already been compromised by previous surgery. Simple revision of the anastomosis or limited reresection may be ineffective, especially in patients with a small gastric remnant. Near-completion or completion gastrectomy with Roux-en-Y reconstruction appears to provide the best palliation in such patients. In one study,[41] 13 of 15 patients (87%) with postsurgical gastroparesis refractory to prokinetic agents and diet and behavior modification therapy achieved a satisfactory clinical outcome after completion gastrectomy. Completion gastrectomy in this setting can be accomplished with virtually no mortality, and complications related to the esophageal anastomosis can be minimized by strict attention to the technical details of the procedure.

Gastric pacing has been attempted as an alternative therapy for postsurgical gastroparesis. Smooth muscle cells of the human stomach spontaneously change membrane potential, creating slow waves or pacemaker potentials, with the proximal gastric corpus acting as the pacemaker. Pacemaker potentials spread distally through the gastric wall, initiating action potentials, which trigger the onset of contractions. The strength of contractions is proportional to the amplitude and frequency of the action potentials. Without action potentials, gastric emptying is slow or absent. Action potentials are abolished during postoperative ileus, probably in response to release of inhibitory neurotransmitters, such as norepinephrine and vasoactive intestinal polypeptide.[50]

Alterations in gastric rhythm have been identified after gastric operations, but it is unclear whether such dysrhythmias contribute to postoperative gastroparesis. In one study,[51] gastric myoelectric activity, gastric emptying, and clinical course were studied in a series of patients at high risk for developing gastroparesis after gastric surgery. Gastric dysrhythmias persisted beyond the first postoperative day in 35% of patients. Delayed gastric emptying was documented by a radionuclide meal in 88% of patients, but only 40% had symptoms of gastroparesis. Pacing suppressed ectopic pacemakers and restored normal gastric rhythm (pacesetter potentials) in two thirds of patients but did not improve gastric emptying.

Failure of pacing to normalize gastric emptying in the setting of postoperative gastroparesis is not entirely surprising. Although pacing can abolish abnormal gastric rhythms and restore normal pacesetter potentials,

it has no apparent stimulatory effect on action potentials or contractions. One potential application might be to combine pacing and administration of gastrokinetic agents with different sites of action on gastric smooth muscle. Despite the somewhat discouraging preliminary results with gastric pacing for gastroparesis, additional studies are warranted to assess its potential more completely.

Postgastrectomy Syndromes

Dumping

Dumping syndrome results from ablation, resection, or bypass of the pyloric sphincter and is characterized by postcibal vasomotor and gastrointestinal symptoms. Vasomotor manifestations include dizziness, lethargy, sweating, pallor, and palpitations that occur within minutes of ingesting a meal. Patients frequently experience an intense desire to lie down. Gastrointestinal symptoms occur later and consist of colicky abdominal pain, distention, and explosive diarrhea.

The pathogenesis of early dumping has not been fully elucidated. Rapid emptying of chyme into the small intestine causes fluid shifts from the extracellular compartment into the intestinal lumen to restore and maintain isotonicity. The resulting contraction of the intravascular volume is partly responsible for the vasomotor symptoms of acute dumping. Elaboration of vasoactive peptides, such as bradykinin, serotonin, neurotensin, and vasoactive intestinal polypeptide, can also contribute to vasomotor instability.[52] Late dumping can occur in association with early dumping or as a discrete entity. Late dumping is characterized by vasomotor symptoms and is relieved by ingestion of carbohydrates. Intestinal distention with release of enteroglucagon, resulting in excess insulin production and hypoglycemia, is implicated in the pathogenesis of this condition.[53] Gastrointestinal symptoms are not prominent with late dumping.

Dumping symptoms are fairly common after resection, bypass, or ablation of the pyloric sphincter. Fortunately, adaptation occurs over time, and most patients experience subsidence of their symptoms. In most cases, dietary measures, including avoidance of carbohydrates and restriction of fluid intake with meals, are successful. Intractable symptoms develop in less than 1% of patients but can cause severe disability resulting in weight loss, fear of eating, and inability to maintain gainful employment.

One promising form of nonoperative treatment is the use of octreotide, an analogue of somatostatin that slows gastric emptying, prolongs intestinal transit, and reduces splanchnic blood flow.[54] The beneficial effects of somatostatin infusion in small numbers of patients with dumping syndrome were reported in the mid-1980s. The native peptide is not useful clinically because of its limited stability and short half-life (about 2 minutes), requiring administration by continuous intravenous infusion. The development of a long-acting octapeptide analogue of somatostatin (octreotide) proved beneficial because a longer half-life (75 to 90 minutes) enables administration by subcutaneous route. In one study,[55] 62 patients with dumping syndrome received single doses of 50 or 100 μg of octreotide 15 to 60 minutes before meal provocation. Marked improvement was seen in symptoms of early and late dumping, together with suppressed changes in insulin and glucose, gastrointestinal peptide levels, pulse rate, systolic blood pressure, and packed red cell volume. Beneficial control of symptoms has been reported with long-term treatment.

The goal of remedial surgery to relieve the dumping syndrome is to slow the rate of gastric emptying. Procedures should be individualized according to the nature of the previous surgery. In patients with vagotomy and gastroenterostomy, take-down of the gastroenterostomy can yield satisfactory results.[56] Although some postcibal distention is common, significant gastric retention is unusual. Reconstruction of the pylorus has yielded promising results in patients after vagotomy and pyloroplasty.[57] This procedure effectively reduces the rate of gastric emptying and ameliorates vasomotor symptoms but not gastrointestinal complaints.

The most difficult group of patients includes those who have undergone previous gastric resection. Interposition of a 10- to 15-cm isoperistaltic jejunal segment between the gastric remnant and the duodenum has been advocated by some authors as a method for slowing gastric emptying.[55] Other investigators have not been able to confirm the effectiveness of this procedure and have documented satisfactory results in only a minority of patients. In one study,[1] investigators compared the efficacy of isoperistaltic jejunal segments, double jejunal limb pouches, and antiperistaltic jejunal segments in 55 patients undergoing remedial surgery for dumping syndrome. Satisfactory results were observed in only 20% of patients with an isoperistaltic jejunal segment. By comparison, 94% of patients with an antiperistaltic jejunal segment obtained satisfactory results. Theoretic risks of the procedure include obstruction, worsened duodenogastric reflux, and ulceration and stenosis of the gastroenteric anastomosis, but these were not observed in this study. Cineradiographic studies obtained postoperatively showed that reversed segments functioned effectively for up to 15 years. The authors recommended using a 10-cm antiperistaltic segment to avoid obstruction of the gastric remnant

and advocated reexploration of the esophageal hiatus with truncal vagotomy to prevent jejunal ulceration (Fig. 7-9).

Roux-en-Y gastroenterostomy has been used in some centers to treat dumping[58] (Fig. 7-10). Transection of the jejunum to prepare a Roux limb alters its contractility and delays gastric emptying. Although this rationale is appealing, use of a Roux limb for dumping has produced mixed results. The Roux limb procedure effectively decreases dumping symptoms in most patients, but up to 30% develop complaints referred to as the *Roux stasis syndrome.*[59] The syndrome manifests with abdominal pain, epigastric fullness, nausea, and food vomiting and has been attributed to defective peristalsis in the Roux limb. Possible solutions include the use of an uncut Roux limb to discourage development of ectopic pacemakers and antegrade pacing of the Roux limb.[60,61] Although these approaches are promising, further studies are necessary before they can be advocated for widespread clinical use.

Postvagotomy Diarrhea

The cause of postvagotomy diarrhea is not known. Diverse etiologies have been postulated, including gastric stasis and hypoacidity causing bacte-

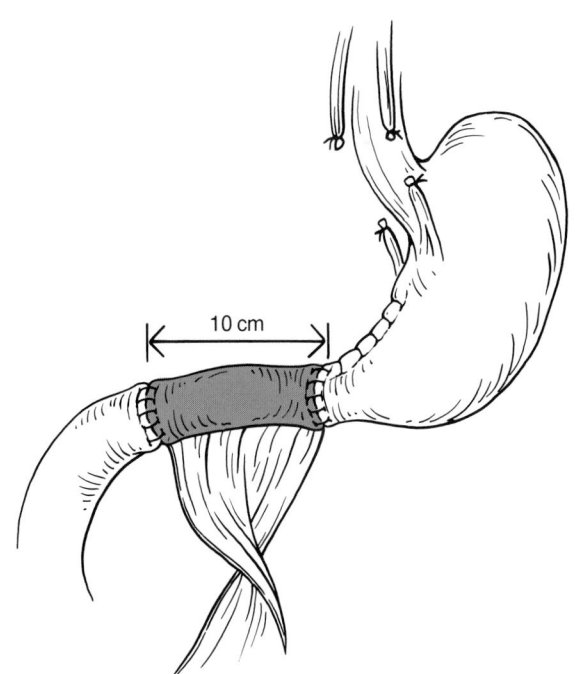

Figure 7-9 The remedial operation of choice for dumping syndrome consists of interposing an antiperistaltic 10-cm segment of jejunum between the gastric remnant and the duodenum. (After Sawyers JL, Herrington JL Jr. Treatment of postgastrectomy syndromes. Am Surg 1980;46:202)

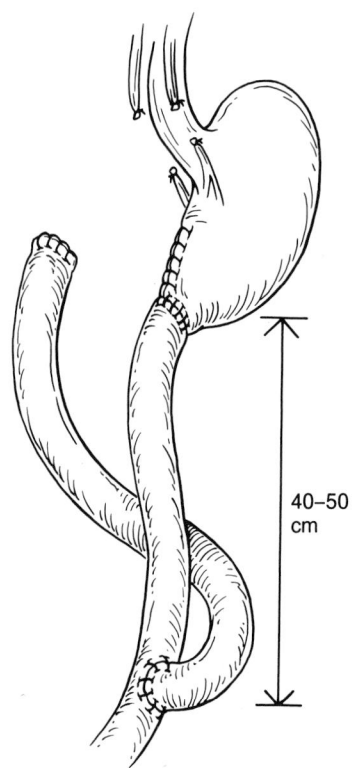

Figure 7-10 Roux-en-Y gastroenterostomy has also been advocated for treatment of dumping syndrome. However, a small percentage of patients experience gastric stasis secondary to altered peristalsis in the Roux limb. The enteroenterostomy should be constructed 40 to 50 cm distal to the gastric pouch to prevent bile reflux. A vagotomy should be performed routinely to prevent marginal ulceration. This procedure is also effective treatment for alkaline reflux gastritis. (After Sawyers JL, Herrington JL Jr. Treatment of postgastrectomy syndromes. Am Surg 1980;46:206)

ter meals. Antidiarrheal and antispasmodic agents, such as codeine or loperamide, can be useful for persistent symptoms. If evaluation shows evidence of bacterial overgrowth and malabsorption, a trial of antibacterial drugs, such as metronidazole, is warranted. Cholestyramine, an ion-exchange resin that binds unconjugated bile acids, can also be effective.

Intractable diarrhea that is refractory to conservative management is uncommon and occurs in about 1% of patients after vagotomy. Several types of remedial operations, all designed to prolong intestinal transit, have been tried with varying results. Investigators have recommended using a 10-cm antiperistaltic jejunal segment placed 100 cm distal to the ligament of Treitz[63] (Fig. 7-11). Of 10 patients treated with this procedure, 7 were judged to have excellent results, 2 were improved, and 1 had a fair result. Long-term relief of symptoms for up to 11 years was achieved in most patients, and none of the patients developed evidence of

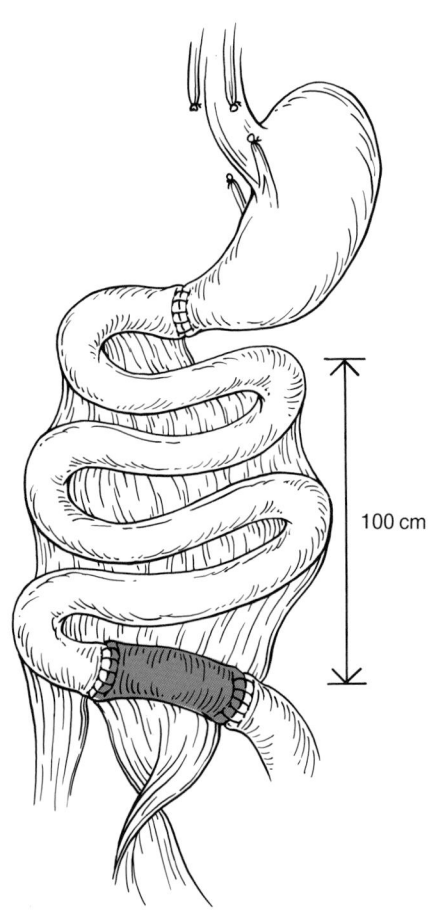

Figure 7-11 The remedial operation for patients with postvagotomy diarrhea is reversal of a 10-cm jejunal segment about 100 cm distal to the ligament of Treitz. (After Sawyers JL, Herrington JL Jr. Treatment of postgastrectomy syndromes. Am Surg 1980;46:203)

rial overgrowth and malabsorption, altered pancreaticobiliary function, decreased mesenteric blood flow, alterations in mucosal villi, and rapid transit of unconjugated bile salts into the colon, with resulting inhibition of water absorption.[62]

Although diarrhea can occur as a component of dumping syndrome, it can also occur as a discrete condition. Patients have episodic bouts of copious, watery stools. The diarrhea is usually explosive, frequently awakens patients from sleep, and can occur without warning. Patients may be unable to distinguish between the urge to pass flatus and a bowel movement and are frequently incontinent of feces. In a minority of patients, diarrhea is severe enough to cause malnutrition, weight loss, and incapacitation.

Medical treatment consists of avoiding carbohydrates and milk products, restricting liquid intake with meals, and lying supine for 20 to 30 minutes af-

intestinal obstruction. However, other investigators[56] have indicated dissatisfaction with this procedure, citing frequent obstructive symptoms and bacterial overgrowth severe enough to warrant reversal. The use of a distal onlay reversed graft to create a nonpropulsive segment of distal small bowel has been reported. This procedure, described originally in dogs, uses a 10-cm segment of mid-ileum, which is carefully isolated on its vascular pedicle, reversed, split along its antimesenteric border, and anastomosed to an equivalent-length enterotomy made in an adjacent segment of ileum[64] (Fig. 7-12). Clinical results were excellent in seven of eight patients followed for 3 to 6 months, with no radiographic evidence of proximal bowel dilation, metabolic evidence of bacterial overgrowth, or symptoms of obstruction. Although intriguing, these results must be considered experimental.

Small Gastric Remnant Syndrome

The small gastric remnant syndrome occurs after extensive distal gastrectomy in which 80% to 90% of the stomach is removed. Addition of vagotomy abolishes receptive relaxation, which normally allows the stomach to accommodate a given volume without a marked increase in pressure. Such patients frequently exhibit postcibal abdominal fullness, early satiety, weight loss, iron deficiency anemia, and various nutritional deficits. Medical treatment can be valuable, but complete rehabilitation cannot be achieved without the use of parenteral nutrition and, frequently, remedial surgery. The purpose of all remedial procedures is to increase gastric reservoir function by constructing a pouch below the small gastric remnant (Fig. 7-13). The various pouch procedures yield satisfactory results in about half of patients. Stasis and ulceration may de-

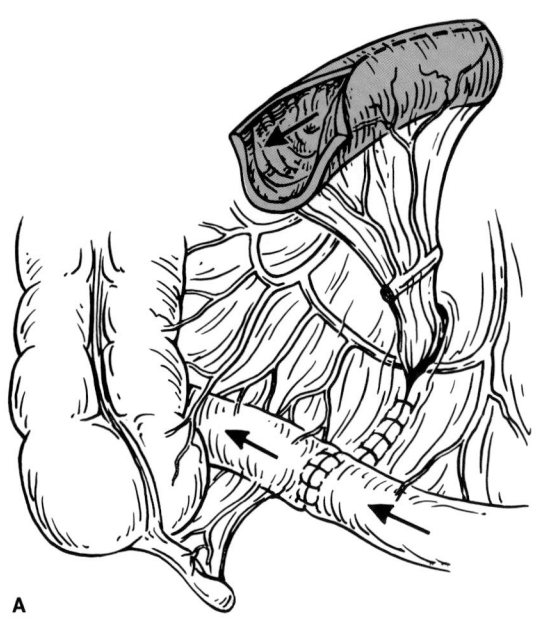
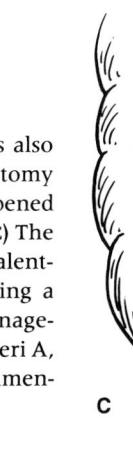
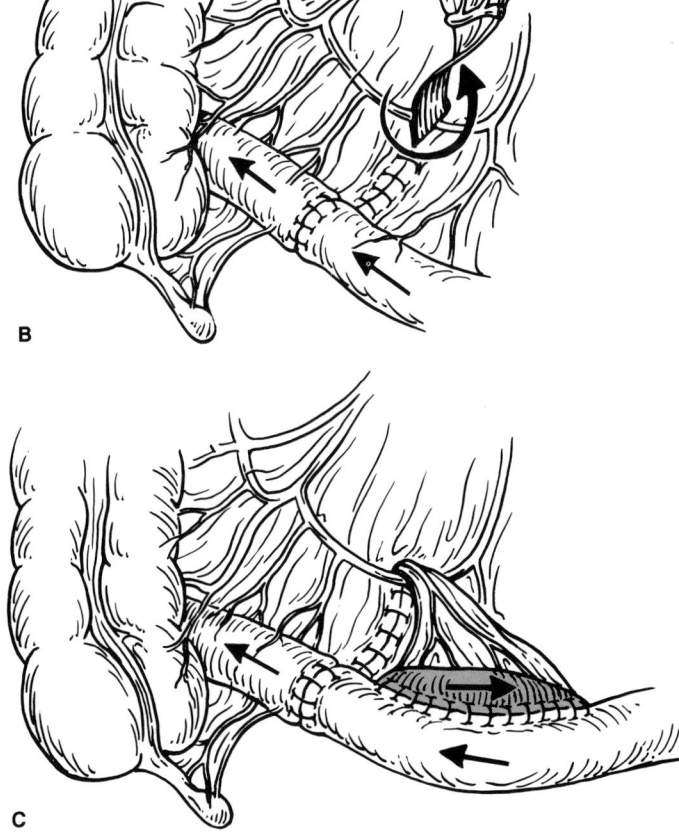

Figure 7-12 The distal onlay reversed graft has also been advocated for treatment of severe postvagotomy diarrhea. (**A** and **B**) A 10-cm segment of bowel is opened longitudinally along the antimesenteric border. (**C**) The open bowel segment is anastomosed to an equivalent-length enterotomy in the adjacent ileum, creating a nonpropulsive segment. (After Cuschieri A. Management of postgastric surgery syndromes. In: Cuschieri A, Skinner DB, eds. Reconstructive surgery of the alimentary tract. London, Butterworth, 1985:93)

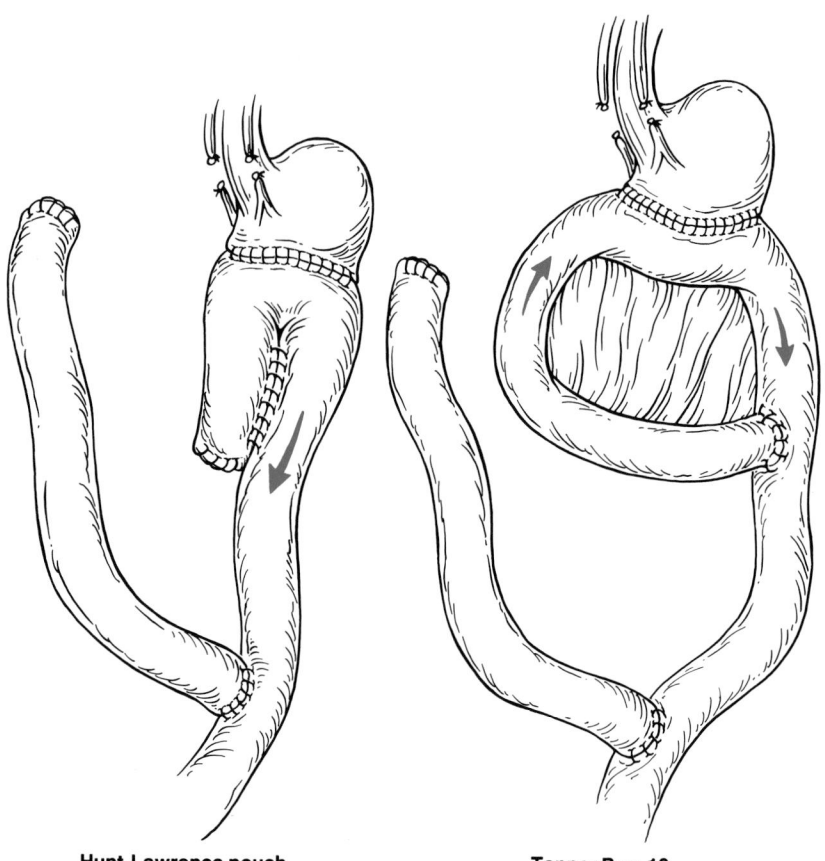

Hunt-Lawrence pouch

Tanner Rue-19

Figure 7-13 Multiple remedial operations have been proposed for treatment of small gastric pouch syndrome. The clinical results from these procedures are comparable. (After Sawyers JL, Herrington JL Jr. Treatment of postgastrectomy syndromes. Am Surg 1980;46:204)

velop over time as the jejunal pouches elongate and become more saccular. These procedures should be recommended only in patients with severe and disabling symptoms.

Afferent Loop Syndrome

The afferent loop syndrome is uncommon and occurs after Billroth II gastrojejunostomy. This procedure creates a short segment of bowel consisting of duodenum and proximal jejunum in which stasis can develop if there is partial or complete obstruction. Anatomic factors that contribute to obstruction include internal small bowel herniation, intussusception, kinking due to adhesions, volvulus of the afferent loop, and stomal stenosis secondary to anastomotic ulceration. The incidence of this condition increases if the afferent loop is too long (greater than 10 to 15 cm), incorrectly positioned along the lesser curvature of the stomach, or antecolic in location.

If afferent loop obstruction occurs in the early postoperative period, it can lead to dehiscence of the duodenal stump. Afferent loop obstruction that occurs months or years after the initial operation characteristically presents with postcibal epigastric fullness associated with nausea and projectile vomiting of bile containing little or no food. The association of symptoms with eating causes patients to limit food intake, with resulting weight loss and inanition. In some patients, an epigastric mass is palpable shortly after meals. Obstruction of the afferent loop may result in symptoms that mimic other upper abdominal conditions, such as pancreatitis, intestinal obstruction, or a perforated viscus. Serum amylase and lipase can be elevated if intraluminal pressure in the afferent loop exceeds pancreatic ductal secretory pressure. Similarly, jaundice can occur secondary to obstruction of biliary outflow.

Afferent loop obstruction causes accumulation of biliary and pancreatic secretions in the afferent loop during a meal. The resulting increase in intraluminal pressure causes nausea and vomiting. Sudden evacuation of the afferent loop results in copious vomiting of bilious material containing little food or particulate matter. If the obstruction is complete, pain may be severe and unrelenting, bile vomiting may not occur, and pancreatic enzymes and liver function tests may be abnormally elevated. This condition must be considered a form of closed-loop obstruction, and prompt surgical intervention is necessary to prevent perforation.

Chronic afferent loop syndrome is a mechanical problem for which there is no satisfactory medical therapy. Although the diagnosis can usually be made on the basis of clinical history, further studies are warranted. Plain radiographs and barium studies of the upper gastrointestinal tract are usually nondiagnostic. Computed tomography and ultrasound have been used successfully to make the diagnosis, and provocative studies can be useful in patients with equivocal findings.[65] Fiberoptic endoscopy should be routinely employed to exclude other conditions, such as alkaline reflux gastritis, carcinoma, and marginal ulceration.

The best treatment of chronic afferent loop syndrome is prevention. Ideally, the gastrojejunostomy should be constructed 5 to 15 cm distal to the ligament of Treitz and should be retrocolic in position. The gastroenterostomy stoma should lie in a horizontal plane with the patient upright, and the afferent limb should be positioned along the greater curvature of the stomach (isoperistaltic). The defect in the mesocolon created to accommodate a retrocolic anastomosis should be carefully approximated to reduce the likelihood of internal herniation.

Several methods have been developed for treating afferent loop syndrome. Simply shortening, suspending, or reanchoring the dilated afferent limb provides unsatisfactory results. In critically ill patients with a markedly distended afferent loop, a simple enteroenterostomy between the two limbs of the gastrojejunostomy should be considered (Fig. 7-14). In most instances, the operation of choice is a Roux-en-Y anastomosis. This procedure can be performed with low operative risk and excellent clinical results.[66] A vagot-

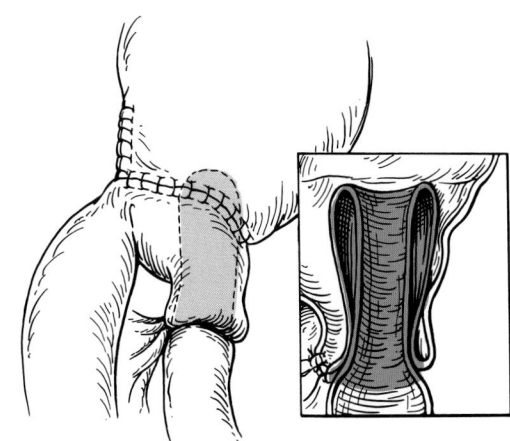

Figure 7-15 Jejunogastric intussusception is a rare complication of Billroth II gastrojejunostomy. In most cases, the efferent limb intussuscepts into the stomach. Operative treatment consists of reducing the intussusception if feasible and anchoring the limb to the transverse mesocolon. Alternative forms of treatment include converting the gastroenterostomy to a gastroduodenostomy or fashioning a new retrocolic gastroenterostomy and anchoring both limbs to the transverse mesocolon. (After McClelland RN. Peptic ulcer surgery: postoperative care and immediate complications. In: Sleisenger MH, ed. Gastrointestinal disease: pathophysiology, diagnosis, management. Philadelphia, WB Saunders, 1973:802)

omy should be performed to reduce the risk of anastomotic ulceration, and the Roux limb should be at least 45 cm long to prevent subsequent bile reflux.

Efferent Loop Syndrome

The efferent loop syndrome is less common than obstruction of the afferent loop and most frequently is associated with retroanastomotic internal hernias. Obstruction due to adhesions or jejunogastric intussusception have been described. Symptoms of uncomplicated efferent limb obstruction are similar to small bowel obstruction with colicky abdominal pain, abdominal distention, and vomiting of bile and intestinal contents. Treatment is primarily surgical and should be dictated by findings at operation.

Jejunogastric intussusception is a rare cause of efferent loop obstruction and usually occurs after an antecolic Billroth II gastrojejunostomy.[67] Most cases occur years after initial operation, and fewer than 10% present within 1 month of surgery. In most cases, the efferent limb intussuscepts into the stomach (Fig. 7-15). Diagnosis of the chronic form can be difficult because contrast studies are positive only at the time of actual intussusception.[68] With acute intussusception, barium contrast studies can demonstrate a classic "coiled-spring" sign within the gastric remnant. Fiberoptic gastroscopy can be useful in patients

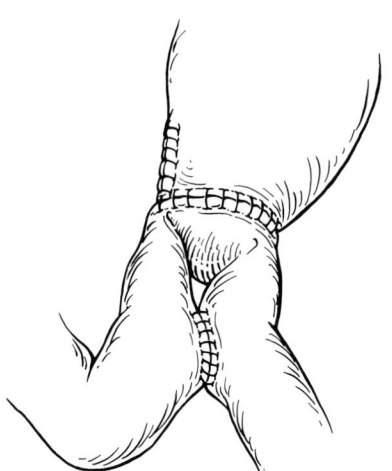

Figure 7-14 Emergency procedure for acute afferent loop syndrome with impeding bowel perforation. An enteroenterostomy is created between the two limbs of the gastroenterostomy, decompressing the dilated afferent limb. (After McClelland RN. Peptic ulcer surgery: postoperative care and immediate complications. In: Sleisenger MH, ed. Gastrointestinal disease: pathophysiology, diagnosis, management. Philadelphia, WB Saunders, 1973:802)

with suggestive symptoms but nondiagnostic radiographic studies. If gastroscopy is performed, the patient should be placed in the Trendelenburg position to avoid missing an intussusception that might not be apparent with the patient supine or upright.

Acute jejunogastric intussusception can be managed conservatively in most patients; about one third of patients require operation. Two thirds of operated patients require bowel resection because the intussusception cannot be reduced. Once the intussuscepted loop has been reduced or resected, it should be anchored to the transverse mesocolon. Chronic forms of this condition can be treated by converting a gastroenterostomy to a gastroduodenostomy or by fashioning a new retrocolic gastroenterostomy and suturing the efferent loop to the transverse mesocolon.

Alkaline Reflux Gastritis

Alkaline reflux gastritis is the postgastrectomy syndrome for which surgical remediation is most often recommended. Symptomatic reflux can occur after ablation, resection, or bypass of the pylorus and is most common after Billroth II gastrojejunostomy. The potentially adverse effects of bile, pancreatic juice, and duodenal contents on gastric mucosa are well known. Virtually all patients experience enterogastric reflux after major gastric surgery, but only 3% have symptoms severe enough to seek medical attention. Patients complain of burning epigastric pain that is exacerbated by eating, frequent nausea, and bilious vomiting that does not relieve the pain. Symptoms of gastroesophageal reflux can coexist. Aversion to eating develops in many patients, and weight loss is common.

Endoscopy is essential to establish the diagnosis and to rule out other conditions that might produce similar symptoms. Endoscopic findings include mucosal erythema of the gastric remnant, bile staining, and mucosal friability. It is not unusual to evoke bleeding from the mucosal surfaces with minor scope trauma. Characteristic histologic findings include intestinalization of gastric glands, inflammatory changes, loss of parietal cells, and ulceration. Unfortunately, endoscopic findings do not always correlate with symptoms.

Most patients are achlorhydric or hypochlorhydric. Gastric acid analysis should be performed to eliminate the possibility of hyperchlorhydria caused by Zollinger-Ellison syndrome, retained antrum, incomplete vagotomy, or inadequate gastric resection.

A technetium scintiscan can be obtained to document objectively the presence of enterogastric reflux. Provocative testing in which the stomach is perfused with either physiologic saline, bile, or an alkaline solution can be used to correlate symptoms with the presence of bile in the stomach.[69] The latter study has also been successfully used to predict patient response to bile diversion.[70]

Medical treatment for patients with documented alkaline reflux gastritis consists of prokinetic agents to enhance gastric emptying and thereby decrease contact time between alkaline pancreaticobiliary secretions and the gastric mucosa and aluminum-containing antacids or cholestyramine to bind bile salts. Sucralfate has been used because of its cytoprotective effects. Multiple-drug regimens, such as metoclopramide combined with cholestyramine, have not provided any added benefit compared with single-drug therapy.[71]

Remedial operations to treat alkaline reflux gastritis all have as their goal diversion of bile away from the stomach or gastric remnant. The operation of choice is the Roux-en-Y procedure, with diversion of alkaline duodenal secretions 45 to 55 cm distal to the gastric pouch (see Fig. 7-10). This procedure is technically easy and is about 85% effective in relieving symptoms. Because this operation is ulcerogenic, vagotomy should also be performed. The 15% to 20% of patients with alkaline reflux gastritis who fail to improve after bile diversion represent a particularly difficult group of patients. Patients with preoperative evidence of delayed gastric emptying appear to be at highest risk. Therefore, a solid-phase radionuclide gastric emptying study should be obtained routinely in patients with alkaline reflux gastritis who are being considered for reoperation. In patients with delayed gastric emptying, bile diversion should be combined with near-total gastric resection, leaving a 10% to 20% gastric remnant.

A duodenal switch operation has been described for treatment of alkaline reflux gastritis.[72] The duodenum is divided several centimeters beyond the pylorus, and the distal end is closed. A 55-cm Roux-en-Y limb is constructed and anastomosed to the proximal duodenum in an end-to-end fashion. In one study,[72] most patients treated with this operation had improvement of their symptoms; however, the number of patients treated was small, and no long-term follow-up was available. Further studies are needed to confirm this procedure's efficacy.

REFERENCES

1. Sawyers JL, Herrington JL. Treatment of postgastrectomy syndromes. Am Surg 1980;46:201.
2. Lind JF, Duthie HI, Schlegel JF, et al. Motility of the gastric fundus. Am J Physiol 1961;201:197.
3. Rees WDW, Malagelada JR, Miller LJ, et al. Human interdigestive and postprandial gastrointestinal motor and gastrointestinal hormone patterns. Dig Dis Sci 1982;27:321.
4. Dooley CP, DiLorenzo C, Valenzuela JE. Variability of

migrating motor complex in humans. Dig Dis Sci 1992;37:723.

5. Lee KY, Chang TM, Chey WY. Effect of rabbit antimotilin serum on myoelectric activity and plasma motilin concentrations in fasting dog. Am J Physiol 1983;245:G547.

6. Cannon WB. The movements of the stomach studied by means of roentgen rays. Am J Physiol 1898;1:359.

7. Schulze-Delrieu K, Ehrlein HJ, Blum AL. Mechanics of the pylorus. In: Akkermans LMA, Johnson AG, Read NW, eds. Gastric and gastroduodenal motility. New York, Praeger, 1984:87.

8. Szurszewski JH. Electrical basis of gastrointestinal motility. In: Johnson LR, ed. Physiology of the gastrointestinal tract. New York, Raven, 1981:1435.

9. Kim CH. Electrical activity of the stomach: clinical implications. Mayo Clin Proc 1986;61:205.

10. Dooley CP, Reznick JB, Valenzuela, JE. Variations in gastric and duodenal motility during gastric emptying of liquid meals in humans. Gastroenterology 1984;87:1114.

11. Meyer JH. Motility of the stomach and gastroduodenal junction. In: Johnson LR, ed. Physiology of the gastrointestinal tract, ed 2. New York, Raven, 1987:613.

12. Miller J, Kauffman G, Elashoff J, et al. Search for resistances controlling gastric emptying of liquid meals. Am J Physiol 1981;241:G403.

13. Camilleri M, Malagelada JR, Brown ML, et al. Relation between antral motility and gastric emptying of solids and liquids in humans. Am J Physiol 1985;249:G580.

14. Weiner K, Graham LS, Reedy T, et al. Simultaneous gastric emptying of two solid foods. Gastroenterology 1981;81:257.

15. Meyer JH, Elashoff J, Porter-Fink V, et al. Human postprandial gastric emptying of 1–3 millimeter spheres. Gastroenterology 1988;94:1315.

16. Roman C, Gonella J. Extrinsic control of digestive tract motility. In: Johnson LR, ed. Physiology of the gastrointestinal tract. New York, Raven, 1981:289.

17. Grundy D, Scratcherd T. The role of the vagus and sympathetic nerves in the control of gastric motility. In: Akkermans LMA, Johnson AG, Read NW, eds. Gastric and gastroduodenal motility. New York, Praeger, 1984:21.

18. Fahrenkrug J, Haglund U, Jodal M. Nervous release of vasoactive intestinal polypeptide in the gastrointestinal tract: possible physiological implications. J Physiol 1978;284:291.

19. Edin R, Lundberg J, Terenius L, et al. Evidence for vagal enkephalinergic neural control of the feline pylorus and stomach. Gastroenterology 1980;78:492.

20. Lederer PC, Lauterbach H, Schmitt W, Domschke W, Lux G. Coordination of gastric and duodenal interdigestive motility and the effect of metoclopramide. In: Labo G, Bortolotti M, eds. Gastrointestinal motility. Verona, Cortina International, 1983:109.

21. Raybould HE. Capsaicin-sensitive vagal afferents and CCK in inhibition of gastric motor function induced by intestinal nutrients. Peptides 1991;12:1279.

22. Dreznik Z, Brocksmith D, Meininger TA, et al. Inhibitory effect of ileal oleate on postprandial motility of the upper gut. Am J Physiol 1991;261:G458.

23. Malagelada JR, Camilleri M, Stranghellini V. Manometric diagnosis of gastrointestinal motility disorders. New York, Thieme, 1986.

24. Azpiroz F, Malagelada JR. Gastric tone measured by an electronic barostat in health and postsurgical gastroparesis. Gastroenterology 1987;92:934.

25. Hasler W, Owyang C. Peptide-induced gastric dysrhythmias: a new cause of gastroparesis. Regul Pept Lett 1990;2:6.

26. Geldof H, van der Schee EJ, van Blankenstein M, et al. Electrogastrographic study of gastric myoelectrical activity in patients with unexplained nausea and vomiting. Gut 1986;27:799.

27. Wingate DL. Synopsis of clinical syndromes. In: Christensen J, Wingate DL, eds. A guide to gastrointestinal motility. Bristol, UK, Wright-PSG, 1983:230.

28. Malagelada JR, Rees WD, Mazzotta LJ, et al. Gastric motor abnormalities in diabetic and postvagotomy gastroparesis: effect of metoclopramide and bethanacol. Gastroenterology 1980;78:286.

29. Jordan GL, Walker LL. Severe problems with gastric emptying after gastric surgery. Ann Surg 1973;177:660.

30. Kraft RO, Fry WJ, DeWeese MS. Postvagotomy gastric atony. Arch Surg 1964;88:865.

31. Latchis KS, Canter JW, Shorb PE. Delayed gastric emptying following operations for peptic ulcer. Am J Surg 1972;38:181.

32. Bergin WF, Jordan PH. Gastric atonia and delayed gastric emptying after vagotomy for obstructing ulcer. Am J Surg 1959;98:612.

33. Hunt JL. Postoperative gastric atony in obstructing peptic ulcers. Am J Surg 1979;138:835.

34. Bortolotti M, Labo G, Serantoni C, et al. Effect of highly selective vagotomy on gastric motor activity of duodenal ulcer patients. Digestion 1978;17:108.

35. Goldstein H, Boyle JD. The saline load test: a bedside evaluation of gastric retention. Gastroenterology 1965;49:375.

36. Minami H, McCallum RW. The physiology and pathophysiology of gastric emptying in humans. Gastroenterology 1984;86:1592.

37. Pellegrini CA, Broderick WC, Van Dyke D, et al. Diagnosis and treatment of gastric emptying disorders: clinical usefulness of radionuclide measurements of gastric emptying. Am J Surg 1983;145:143.

38. Sheiner HJ, Catchpole BN. Drug therapy for postvagotomy gastric stasis. Br J Surg 1976;63:608.

39. Minami H, McCallum RW. The physiology and pathophysiology of gastric emptying in humans. Gastroenterology 1984;86:1592.

40. McClelland RN, Horton JW. Relief of acute, persistent postvagotomy atony by metoclopramide. Ann Surg 1978;188:439.

41. Eckhauser FE, Knol JA, Raper SA. Completion gastrectomy for postsurgical gastroparesis: preliminary results with 15 patients. Ann Surg 1988;208:345.

42. Baeyens R, Reyntijens A, Verlinden M. Cisapride accelerates gastric emptying and mouth to cecum transit of a barium meal. Eur J Pharmacol 1984;27:315.

43. Peeters TL, Matthijs G, Depoortere I, et al. Erythromycin is a motilin receptor agonist. Am J Physiol 1989;257:G470.

44. Tack J, Janssens J, Vantrappen G, et al. Effect of erythromycin on gastric motility in controls and diabetic gastroparesis. Gastroenterology 1992;103:729.

45. Mozwecz H, Pavel D, Pitrak D, et al. Erythromycin stearate as prokinetic agent in postvagotomy gastroparesis. Dig Dis Sci 1990;35:902.

46. Cohen AM, Ottinger LW. Delayed gastric emptying following gastrectomy. Ann Surg 1976;184:689.

47. Hocking MP, Vogel SB, Falasca CA, et al. Delayed gastric emptying of liquids and solids following Roux-en-Y biliary diversion. Am J Surg 1985;150:166.

48. Mathias JR, Fernandez A, Sninsky CA, et al. Nausea, vomiting and abdominal pain after Roux-en-Y anastomosis: motility of the jejunal limb. Gastroenterology 1985;88:101.

49. Pelligrini CA, Patti MG, Lewin M, et al. Alkaline reflux gastritis and the effect of biliary diversion on gastric emptying of solid food. Am J Surg 1985;150:166.

50. Smith JR, Kelly KA, Weinshilboum RM. Pathophysiology of postoperative ileus. Arch Surg 1977;112:203.

51. Hocking MP, Vogel SB, Sninsky CA. Human gastric myoelectric activity and gastric emptying following gastric surgery and with pacing. Gastroenterology 1992;103:1811.

52. Lawaetz O, Blackburn AM, Bloom S, et al. Gut hormone profile and gastric emptying in the dumping syndrome: a hypothesis concerning the pathogenesis. Scand J Gastroenterol 1983;18:73.

53. Schultz KT, Neelon FA, Nilson LB, et al. Mechanism of postgastrectomy hypoglycemia. Arch Intern Med 1971;128:240.

54. Reichlin S. Somatostatin. N Engl J Med 1983:309:1495.

55. Lamers CBHW, Bijlstra AM, Harris AG. Octreotide, a long-acting somatostatin analog, in the management of postoperative dumping syndrome. Dig Dis Sci 1993;38:359.

56. Cuschieri A. Management of postgastrectomy syndromes. In: Cuschieri A, Skinner DB, eds. Reconstructive surgery of the gastrointestinal tract. London, Butterworths, 1985:81.

57. Cheadle WG, Baker PR, Cuschieri A. Pyloric reconstruction for severe vasomotor dumping after vagotomy and pyloroplasty. Ann Surg 1985;202:568.

58. Kelly KA, Becker JM, van Heerden JA. Reconstructive gastric surgery. Br J Surg 1981;68:687.

59. Mathias JR, Fernandez A, Sninsky CA, et al. Nausea, vomiting and abdominal pain after Roux-en-Y anastomosis: motility of the jejunal limb. Gastroenterology. 1985;88:101.

60. Van Stiegmann G, Goff JS. An alternative to Roux-en-Y for treatment of bile reflux gastritis. Surg Gynecol Obstet 1988;166:69.

61. Karlstrom L, Kelly KA. Ectopic jejunal pacemakers and gastric emptying after Roux gastrectomy: effect of intestinal pacing. Surgery 1989;106:867.

62. Delcore R, Cheung LY. Surgical options in postgastrectomy syndromes. Surg Clin North Am 1991;71:57.

63. Herrington JL Jr, Edwards WH, Carter JH, et al. Treatment of severe postvagotomy diarrhea by reversed jejunal segment. Ann Surg 1968;168:522.

64. Sadowski J. Experimental investigations on improvement of intestinal absorption in dogs subjected to massive resection of small intestine combined with the use of an onlay reversed segment of intestine. Polish Med Sci Hist 1967;10:85.

65. Brown CD, Kraus JW. Afferent loop syndrome revisited: new emphasis on ultrasound and computerized tomography. South Med J 1981;74:599.

66. Brook-Cowden GL, Braasch JW, Gibb SP, et al. Postgastrectomy syndromes. Am J Surg 1976;131:464.

67. Caudell WS, Lee ML Jr. Acute and chronic jejunogastric intussusception. N Engl J Med 1955;253:655.

68. Dolan KD, Hockman RE. Jejunogastric intussusception ten years after gastric surgery. JAMA 1968;295:128.

69. Warshaw AL. Intragastric alkaline infusion: a simple accurate provocative test for the diagnosis of symptomatic alkaline reflux gastritis. Ann Surg 1981;194:297.

70. Rutledge PL, Warshaw AL. Diagnosis of symptomatic alkaline reflux gastritis and prediction of response to bile diversion by intragastric alkali provocation. Am J Surg 1988;155:82.

71. Meshkinpour H, Elashoff J, Stewart HJ, et al. Effect of cholestyramine on the symptoms of reflux gastritis. Gastroenterology 1977;73:441.

72. DeMeester TR, Fuchs KH, Ball CS, et al. Experimental and clinical results with proximal end-to-end duodenojejunostomy for pathologic duodenogastric reflux. Ann Surg 1987;206:414.

Digestive Tract Surgery: A Text and Atlas, edited by Richard H. Bell, Layton F. Rikkers, and Michael W. Mulholland. Lippincott-Raven Publishers, Philadelphia, © 1996.

8

Gastrointestinal Hemorrhage

W. Scott Helton | *Michael Kimmey*

The management of gastrointestinal (GI) bleeding should follow three general principles: hemodynamic stabilization and resuscitation of the patient, diagnosis and control of the site of bleeding, and long-term prevention of recurrent bleeding. This chapter focuses on diagnostic and therapeutic approaches to patients with upper and lower GI bleeding. Salient aspects of patient history are discussed, followed by methods of resuscitation. The appropriate selection and application of diagnostic tests and the use of endoscopic and angiographic techniques for controlling bleeding are discussed in detail as they apply to specific causes of bleeding. Although diagnostic and therapeutic algorithms are provided and discussed in detail, the treatment of upper and lower GI bleeding involves a multidisciplinary approach that must be selectively applied to each patient.

INITIAL ASSESSMENT AND RESUSCITATION

The initial management of patients with GI bleeding simultaneously involves taking a brief history, performing a primary physical survey, and implementing resuscitative measures. While pertinent historical facts are solicited about the nature and extent of bleeding, the patient is rapidly assessed for an adequate airway, oxygenation, and hemodynamic stability. Vital signs are taken, and the patients' skin and mucous membranes are examined for signs of insufficient perfusion. If a patient is obtunded and vomiting blood, strong consideration should be given to placing an endotracheal tube to ensure an adequate airway and to prevent aspiration. Supplemental oxygen should be administered by nasal prongs or mask to all patients with GI bleeding to max-

imize oxygen delivery to the tissues. Adequate intravascular volume resuscitation with large-bore intravenous access for infusion of crystalloid and blood products should be established as the airway and oxygenation are being secured. Two 16-gauge peripheral catheters are preferred. If peripheral veins are of insufficient quality, central venous access should be rapidly instituted, preferably by the internal jugular or subclavian veins. Monitoring of the central venous pressure also provides useful information for resuscitation in elderly patients with cardiovascular or pulmonary insufficiency. Normal saline or lactated Ringer solution should be administered initially with the rate dictated by the patient's volume status. Blood is drawn for complete blood count, platelet count, prothrombin time, and routine blood chemistry. If the patient has any evidence of significant blood loss, such as hypotension, continuing hematemesis, or hematochezia, or a low hematocrit, an emergent type and crossmatch for whole blood or packed red blood cells is requested.

The rate of bleeding guides the urgency and selection of further tests and treatment and dictates where the patient should be resuscitated and further evaluated. Unstable patients should be resuscitated in the emergency department or intensive care unit; patients who have no active signs of bleeding and a history more suggestive of subacute or chronic GI blood loss can be worked up on the general ward.

The Need for Transfusion

The decision to perform a transfusion should be based primarily on physiologic signs of inadequate tissue perfusion and oxygen delivery. Patients with a low hematocrit (less than 25%) who also manifest poor tissue ox-

223

ygenation (eg, angina or altered sensorium) should be emergently transfused. Patients who continue to bleed despite therapy or who are in shock and have initial low hematocrit should also undergo emergency transfusion. Additional factors should be considered in stable patients and in patients with less severe bleeding. What is the probability of the patient losing additional blood or having recurrent bleeding? If bleeding is continuing slowly or the probability of rebleeding is high and the hematocrit is low, transfusion is appropriate. If the patient has underlying coronary artery disease or congestive heart failure, further bleeding can cause myocardial ischemia or can impair the patient's capacity to compensate for additional bleeding.

What To Transfuse

Patients with active bleeding should receive transfusions with whole blood, whereas those without signs of active bleeding should receive packed red blood cells. In addition to receiving blood to increase oxygen-carrying capacity, patients with GI bleeding should be investigated for deficits in coagulation. Patients should be asked whether they take aspirin or any anticoagulants. If there is a history of a coagulation disorder, the appropriate blood component should be administered to correct the underlying coagulation defect. Table 8-1 lists common coagulation problems and the appropriate component therapy needed to correct the deficit. Fresh frozen plasma or platelets should be administered when there is a deficiency of clotting factors or severe thrombocytopenia (less than 50,000 platelets/μL) or when the patient has received more than 10 units of blood be-

cause of dilutional coagulopathy, which occurs with massive transfusion.

History

After the initial steps of management have been performed, the physician focuses on gathering a more detailed history from all possible sources. The importance of a detailed and thorough history cannot be overemphasized in the evaluation of GI bleeding because it can significantly narrow the differential diagnosis in most cases as well as expedite and direct therapy. Evaluation of the rate of bleeding starts by asking the patient, ambulance personnel, or other observers about the nature and volume of hematemesis or hematochezia. Was the vomitus massive, bright red, or like coffee grounds? How many episodes of hematemesis or hematochezia have occurred? Large amounts of bright red vomitus (hematemesis) or persistent passage of bright red blood, clots, or maroon blood from the rectum (hematochezia) are indicative of potentially life-threatening bleeding.[1] Patients with both hematemesis and red hematochezia have the most massive bleeding. Hematochezia usually is a result of colonic bleeding but may originate from an upper intestinal site if the bleeding is brisk. A history of tarry, foul-smelling stools (melena) indicates that a component of the blood loss is slower because there must be time for colonic bacteria to degrade hemoglobin. Melena can result from bleeding in the upper GI tract or right colon. The clinician should also inquire about a history of orthostasis, fatigue, and dyspnea because these can reflect chronic GI blood loss.

Serial vital signs and the patient's response to fluid resuscitation provide the best indication of a patient's stability regardless of the hematocrit. A flow sheet is useful to document resuscitative measures and the patient's responses. Persistent postural hypotension or tachycardia despite fluid resuscitation suggests significant ongoing bleeding. Serial hematocrit determinations provide additional information about the amount of bleeding that has occurred as well as the amount of ongoing bleeding.

Inquiry should be made about previous episodes of GI bleeding, and the patient should be asked to recall the specific diagnosis, treatment, and outcome. When available, the medical record should always be reviewed for any previously documented episodes of bleeding and for medical conditions predisposing to GI bleeding, such as cirrhosis, cancer, coagulopathies, and connective tissue disorders.

A careful medication history should be taken from each patient with GI bleeding. The most important medications associated with GI bleeding are the nonsteroidal antiinflammatory drugs (NSAIDs). These in-

---

Table 8-1 Resuscitation for Massive Gastrointestinal Bleeding

Factor	Indication
Whole blood	Hypovolemic shock or active bleeding
Packed red cells	Increased oxygen-carrying capacity, slow or chronic bleeding
Fresh frozen plasma	Liver disease, DIC, massive transfusion with packed red cells
Cryoprecipitate	Factor VIII deficiency (hemophilia, DIC, von Willebrand's disease)
Platelets	Thrombocytopenia (<50,000/μL), DIC and hemorrhage, abnormal function: uremia, cirrhosis, aspirin, nonsteroidal antiinflammatory drugs
Vitamin K	Antibiotic therapy, obstructive jaundice, fat malabsorption

DIC, disseminated intravascular coagulation.

clude prescription medications, over-the-counter ibuprofen, and aspirin. These medications can cause bleeding by inhibiting prostaglandin synthesis or platelet function. Series of patients with GI hemorrhage showed that about 80% had taken NSAIDs or had platelet functional abnormalities due to recent aspirin ingestion. Aspirin can continue to inhibit platelet function for up to 1 week after ingestion. A three- to four-fold increased risk of ulcer bleeding exists in patients taking NSAIDs.[2,3] Patients who take oral anticoagulants also have a three- to four-fold increased risk of ulcer hemorrhage. Patients taking NSAIDs, oral corticosteroids, or a combination of NSAIDs and oral anticoagulants have about a 15-fold increased risk of significant upper GI bleeding.[4,5]

A number of medical illnesses are associated with increased risk of GI hemorrhage (Table 8-2). Immunocompromised patients, such as those with organ transplants, human immunodeficiency virus (HIV), or acquired immunodeficiency syndrome (AIDS), or patients who recently completed or are actively receiving chemotherapy and radiation can bleed from causes not commonly seen in healthy populations (Table 8-3). Patients in the intensive care unit with sepsis, multiple organ failure, burns, or neurologic injury are at increased risk for stress ulceration and acute duodenal ulcer. Patients undergoing cardiac surgery are most likely

Table 8-2   Medical Conditions Predisposed to Bleeding

BLEEDING DISEASES
von Willebrand's disease
Idiopathic thrombocytopenic purpura
Factor X deficiency

SKIN DISEASES
Olser-Weber-Rendu syndrome
Kaposi's sarcoma
Pseudoxanthoma elasticum
Ehlers-Danlos syndrome

ANTICOAGULATION
Sodium warfarin (Coumadin)
Heparin
Aspirin
Nonsteroidal antiinflammatory drugs

CHRONIC ILLNESSES
Aortic stenosis
Chronic renal failure
Cirrhosis

LYMPHOPROLIFERATIVE DISORDERS

CARDIAC SURGERY

ACQUIRED IMMUNODEFICIENCY SYNDROME

Table 8-3   Bleeding in Immunocompromised Patients*

BONE MARROW TRANSPLANT RECIPIENTS
Esophagitis and ulcers (cytomegalovirus, candidiasis, herpes)
Graft-versus-host disease—small bowel and gastric mucosal bleeding

ORGAN TRANSPLANT RECIPIENTS
Colonic cytomegalovirus ulcers
Esophagitis
Lymphoma
Colitis

ACQUIRED IMMUNODEFICIENCY SYNDROME
Kaposi's sarcoma—any site of gastrointestinal tract
Cytomegalovirus

* In these situations, it is important to establish the exact pathogen because the pharmacologic treatment is specifically directed at the offending agent, eg, candidiasis (amphotericin ± fluconazole) versus herpes simplex (acyclovir) versus cytomegalovirus (gancyclovir).

to be bleeding from an acute duodenal ulcer.[6] Table 8-4 illustrates a number of potential iatrogenic causes of GI bleeding secondary to interventional measures.

Physical Examination

Examination begins by obtaining vital signs and assessing the patient's volume and cardiovascular status. Warmth of the peripheral extremities, capillary refill, mucous membrane color, and moisture are noted. The sclera are examined for evidence of jaundice. Stigmata of cirrhosis (spider angiomas, caput medusae, gynecomastia, ascites, asterixis, testicular atrophy, palmar erythema) are sought. The skin is examined for perioral telangiectasia, suggesting a hereditary vascular anomaly such as Osler-Weber-Rendu syndrome. Abnormal tendons and hyperflexible joints may suggest the presence of Ehlers-Danlos syndrome. Vascular nodules sug-

Table 8-4   Iatrogenic Gastrointestinal Bleeding

Procedure Performed	Site of Bleeding
Biopsy	Site performed
Balloon dilation	Site performed
Sphincterotomy	Site performed
Polypectomy	Site performed
Sclerotherapy	Recurrent variceal bleed, Sclerosant-induced esophageal ulcer
Intestinal resection	Anastomotic bleeding
Percutaneous biliary procedure	Hemobilia
Percutaneous pancreatic drainage	Hemosuccus pancreaticus

gestive of Kaposi's sarcoma should be looked for in AIDS patients with GI bleeding. Abdominal examination should determine whether there is splenomegaly or ascites (evidence of cirrhosis and portal hypertension), masses (cancer), and tenderness (enteritis or peptic ulcer). Evidence of lymphadenopathy may suggest underlying malignancy or AIDS. Direct inspection and digital examination of the anal canal and rectum should be performed to detect fissures, fistulas, and masses. Examination of the lungs and heart for signs of aspiration pneumonia, congestive heart failure, or valvular heart disease guides further testing and monitoring during resuscitation.

Identification of the general location of GI bleeding is important for selecting appropriate diagnostic and therapeutic procedures. A history of hematemesis suggests an upper GI bleeding source. In the absence of hematemesis, an oral or nasogastric tube should be placed immediately to check for the presence of intragastric blood. The presence of a bloody aspirate confirms an upper GI source, whereas a nonbloody aspirate usually excludes active bleeding from the esophagus or stomach.[7] A nonbloody gastric aspirate, even if it is bile stained, does not absolutely exclude a bleeding duodenal lesion because up to 20% of bleeding duodenal ulcers have a negative gastric aspirate due to a closed pylorus or intermittent bleeding.[8] Gastric lavage with saline that demonstrates ongoing red discoloration suggests active bleeding. Coffee-ground–like aspirate usually reflects old blood or slow blood loss and usually clears with lavage. Bright red hematochezia is most often the result of a colonic source, unless bleeding from the upper GI tract is severe and intestinal transit is rapid. Signs of significant intravascular volume depletion are usually present if an upper source of bleeding is the cause of hematochezia. Less specific findings suggestive of an upper GI site of bleeding include hyperactive bowel sounds, intestinal cramping, and an elevated blood urea nitrogen/creatinine ratio resulting from volume depletion and absorbed blood proteins.[9]

UPPER GASTROINTESTINAL BLEEDING

The three most common causes of massive upper GI bleeding are posteriorly penetrating duodenal ulcers, large gastric ulcers, and esophageal or gastric varices (Table 8-5). Patients with stigmata of chronic liver disease, known cirrhosis, or a history of varices should be suspected of having bleeding varices. The presence of significant abdominal pain before hematemesis is suggestive of a nonvariceal source of bleeding, such as esophagitis, peptic ulcer disease, or tumor.

Table 8-5 Causes of Upper Gastrointestinal Bleeding

Lesion	Range (%)	Average (%)
Duodenal ulcer	15–25	20
Gastric ulcer	20–25	20
Acute gastric erosions	12–25	15
Esophagogastric varices	10–30	20
Mallory-Weiss tear	8–15	12
Esophagitis	5–10	8
Other	5	5

Diagnostic Endoscopy

Endoscopy is the initial procedure for all patients with a history, physical examination, or gastric aspirate suggestive of upper GI bleeding because it is the most sensitive and rapid method for identifying the source of bleeding.[6,10] Establishing a prompt diagnosis aids in subsequent management of the patient.[11] In addition, endoscopy often allows specific therapy directed at the site of bleeding. In the 1970s and early 1980s, controlled trials investigating the influence of endoscopic diagnosis in patients with upper GI bleeding demonstrated that early diagnosis had no impact on patient outcome or mortality.[12] However, endoscopic therapy was limited during these trials. Advances in endoscopic techniques now permit immediate control of bleeding in most conditions. In addition, endoscopic therapy has been shown to reduce the incidence of rebleeding, decrease transfusion requirements, and improve survival in specific patient populations.[13] Endoscopic diagnosis and the response to endoscopic therapy help determine the level of hospital care required and can provide a reasonable estimate of the duration of hospitalization. For example, patients with bleeding varices or with duodenal or gastric ulcers with stigmata of recent hemorrhage should be followed in the intensive care unit for a minimum of 24 hours because the probability and severity of recurrent bleeding is significant. In contrast, patients with gastric erosions or Mallory-Weiss tears or ulcers with clean bases have a low probability of recurrent bleeding and can be safely treated on the general medical floor or discharged from the hospital.[14]

Timing of the Procedure

The urgency of endoscopy is contingent on the patient's clinical condition. If active bleeding is present or hypotension existed at any time, emergent endoscopy is indicated as soon as the patient is hemodynamically stable. In contrast, if the amount of upper GI bleeding is judged to be minor, endoscopy can be performed within the next 24 hours. If the patient is actively bleeding, endoscopy is best performed at the patient's bedside in the intensive care unit or in the emergency department. An occasional patient with massive bleeding requires endoscopy in the operating room after endotracheal intubation while preparation is being made for surgery. Hemodynamically stable patients can be examined in the endoscopy suite. Patients should not receive any antacids, sucralfate, or barium contrast before endoscopy, because these agents can interfere with visualization of the mucosa.

Technique

Gastric lavage is mandatory to cleanse the stomach before emergent endoscopy. The patient should be provided with nasal oxygen and rolled into the left lateral decubitus position in a slight Trendelenburg position. Continuous electrocardiogram and oxygen saturation monitoring are required. Adequate nursing support and suctioning equipment should be present. The oropharynx is anesthetized with a topical anesthetic spray. The nasogastric tube is removed, and a large-bore (34F to 40F) orogastric tube is placed. Aliquots of room-temperature tap water (500 to 1000 mL) are instilled and removed by gravity and manual suction. There is no benefit in the use of iced solutions or the addition of the vasoconstrictor norepinephrine (Levarterenol) to the lavage fluid.[15,16] When the blood in the gastric aspirate has cleared or decreased, endoscopy is performed. Administration of short-acting intravenous sedatives (meperidine, morphine, midazolam, or diazepam) is useful in most patients. Naloxone and flumazenil should be available in case of narcotic- or benzodiazepine-induced respiratory suppression. The endoscopist should always be prepared to perform endoscopic therapy for controlling bleeding.

The esophagus, stomach, and duodenum are inspected briefly in that order. If bleeding is encountered in the distal esophagus or stomach, an attempt should still be made to visualize the duodenum to exclude a more distal bleeding lesion. After inspection of the duodenum, the endoscope is withdrawn into the stomach for a more thorough inspection. A retroflexed view of the cardia, fundus, and gastroesophageal junction should always be performed to exclude proximal sites of bleeding that may have been missed on introduction of the endoscope. If the fundus is obscured by a dependent pool of blood, the patient should be rolled onto the back or opposite side so that a clear view of the entire stomach wall is achieved. A large blood clot can prevent complete visualization of the stomach or duodenum. In this circumstance, additional attempts at gastric lavage should be performed and endoscopy repeated.

Occasionally, bleeding can be so massive that it is not possible to clear the stomach or esophagus of blood, and endoscopy cannot be safely or satisfactorily performed. If esophageal varices are seen and believed to be the source of bleeding, the patient should be treated accordingly. Once variceal hemorrhage is controlled, the patient can be reexamined, and sclerotherapy or banding can be performed. If varices are not seen or suspected in a patient with exsanguinating upper GI hemorrhage, the patient should go directly to the operating room or to angiography for diagnosis and control of the bleeding.

The diagnostic accuracy of upper endoscopy approaches 95% when the site of bleeding is the esophagus, stomach, or duodenum, and most forms of endoscopic therapy have greater than 90% success at short-term control of hemorrhage.

Complications

Serious complications of diagnostic panendoscopy with modern endoscopes should be rare, provided the endoscopist is fully trained.[17] Overall complication rates for diagnostic and therapeutic endoscopies should be less than 1%.[18] However, significant complications can occur when endoscopy is undertaken in inappropriate settings with inadequate staff, monitoring, or resuscitation equipment. Death attributable to emergent upper endoscopy is rare but can be the result of pulmonary aspiration, respiratory arrest, and esophageal tears or rupture.[17,19]

Therapeutic Endoscopy

Significant technologic advances have been made in endoscopic techniques for treating GI bleeding. Although these techniques were originally developed to treat bleeding gastric and duodenal ulcers, they can be safely used to control bleeding from almost all mucosal sources of GI bleeding within reach of the endoscope (Table 8-6). Endoscopic control of bleeding is the definitive therapy for many lesions, including bleeding tumors, ulcers, vascular malformations, and Mallory-Weiss tears. For lesions ultimately requiring surgery, such as large gastric and duodenal ulcers or tumors, endoscopic hemostasis can allow stabilization of the patient and an elective operation under more favorable circumstances. Surgical consultation should be obtained when using endoscopic hemostatic techniques in the event that bleeding is not controlled, recurs, or a complication from the technique (worsened bleeding or perforation) results.

Table 8-6   Endoscopic Techniques for Controlling Gastrointestinal Bleeding

LASER PHOTOCOAGULATION
Nd:YAG
Argon

MULTIPOLAR ELECTROCOAGULATION

HEATER PROBE

INJECTION THERAPY
Epinephrine
Polidocanal plus thrombin
Epinephrine 1:10,000 or 1:20,000 plus thrombin
Saline (normal or 3%)
Absolute ethanol
Sclerosants

BANDING
Varices of esophagus, stomach, stomas, colon, rectum

Endoscopic hemostatic techniques can be divided into thermal, injection, and banding techniques. Thermal techniques include the neodymium-yttrium aluminum garnet (Nd:YAG) laser, monopolar electrocoagulation, multipolar electrocoagulation, and heater probe. Injection techniques involve placing a variety of chemical solutions through a needle catheter into the bleeding lesion. The coagulation probes, lasers, or injection catheters are passed through the working channel of the endoscope and are directly applied to the bleeding lesion under direct vision (Fig. 8-1). Endoscopic band-ing involves placing a rubber band onto the base of a varix, similar to hemorrhoidal banding.[20] Although individual trials have failed to demonstrate a significant improvement in survival in patients with bleeding ulcers controlled with endoscopic hemostatic techniques, metaanalysis that pools the results of several large studies has documented an improvement in mortality rate using endoscopic therapy.[13,21]

Laser therapy with either an Nd:YAG or argon laser significantly reduces the need for urgent surgery for bleeding ulcers.[21] However, laser units are expensive, are not portable, require more technical expertise, and have a potential risk of perforation because of transmural tissue injury. Laser therapy is not the endoscopic technique of choice for most bleeding mucosal lesions. Laser therapy is primarily used to control bleeding in patients with multiple vascular malformations or bulky tumors.

Monopolar electrocoagulation has been shown to be highly effective in achieving hemostasis in actively bleeding ulcers.[22] However, like laser therapy, monopolar electrocoagulation causes significant depth of tissue injury and is no longer recommended.

Multipolar electrocoagulation probes and heater probes are the two most widely used thermal methods of endoscopic therapy. With either device, forceful tamponade of the bleeding vessel to produce temporary cessation of bleeding is the first step (see Fig. 8-1A). Next, the probe is heated to 100°C, causing coagulation of the bleeding vessel. With bipolar electrocoagulation, heat

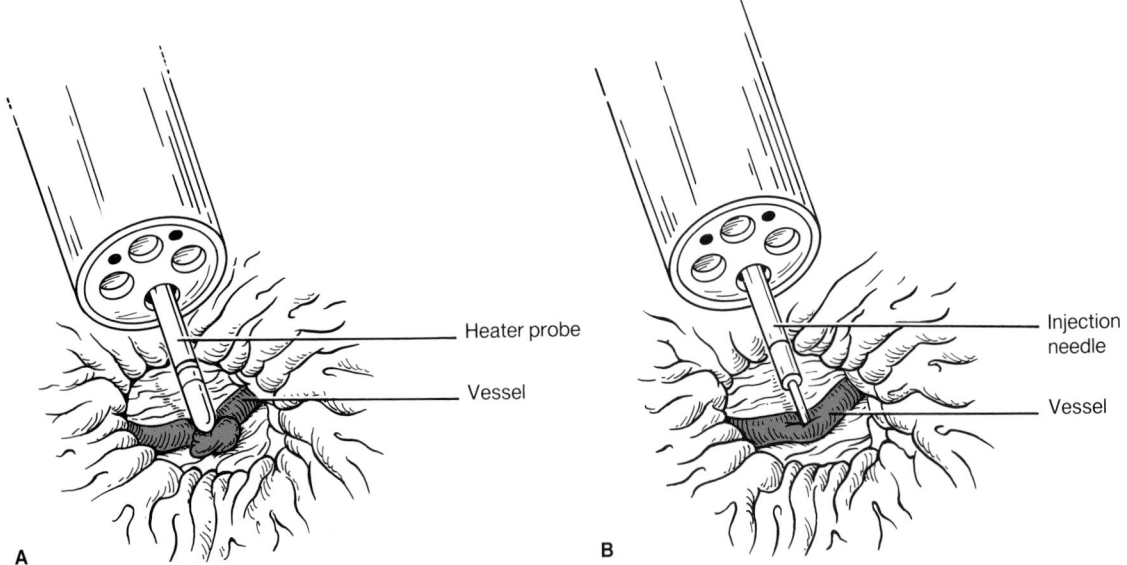

A   B

Figure 8-1 **(A)** Endoscopic heater probe. A heater probe is pushed against a visible vessel in the base of a peptic ulcer to tamponade bleeding. A jet of water is used to wash away any clot, and then the tamponaded vessel is coagulated. **(B)** Endoscopic injection therapy. An endoscopic needle is used to inject epinephrine around the base and into the center of an ulcer.

is generated by an electrical current passing through tissue connecting electrodes on the probe tip to cause coagulation of the vessel. Both these techniques are relatively inexpensive, are portable, and cause less tissue injury than laser or monopolar electrocoagulation. Clinical trials demonstrate that both the multipolar and heater probes[23] are highly successful in achieving hemostasis and in preventing rebleeding in actively bleeding patients and in patients with visible vessels in peptic ulcers.[23-25] Endoscopic hemostatic therapy also shortens hospital stay, decreases the number of blood transfusions and the need for emergency surgery, and lowers overall hospital costs in patients with upper GI bleeding from ulcers and Mallory-Weiss tears.[24]

Proper multipolar electrocoagulation technique is essential for achieving good hemostasis of bleeding peptic ulcers and includes tamponade of the lesion, use of a large probe, a low-energy setting, and prolonged coagulation.[26] Therapeutic efficacy of the heater probe is also dependent on proper technique, which includes forceful tamponade, a setting of 25 to 30 J, and repeated application.

Injection Therapy

Hemostatic injection therapy is possibly the most cost-effective and simple method of endoscopic hemostasis (see Fig. 8-1*B*). The only equipment required is an injection catheter. Prospective trials have demonstrated that injection therapy is as efficacious as thermal methods for achieving hemostasis in bleeding ulcers.[27] Injected agents include epinephrine, absolute ethanol, sodium tetradecyl sulfate, hypertonic saline, 50% dextrose, and polidocanol. The solutions are injected around the periphery of a visible or bleeding vessel, followed by injection centrally at the site of fibrin clot. It is unclear if any agent or combination of agents is best for injection therapy because all appear to be highly efficacious.[23] Some reports suggest that epinephrine followed by a sclerosant is associated with a lower rebleeding rate.[28] A total of 8 to 10 mL of adrenaline (1/10,000) is injected in depots of 0.5 to 1 mL into and around the bleeding point. Alcohol is injected in aliquots of 0.1 to 0.5 mL in a similar fashion. Repeat endoscopic therapy or surgery is indicated if persistent or recurrent bleeding occurs within the next 48 hours.

Endoscopic Banding

The technique of endoscopic banding is becoming more popular in the acute and chronic control of bleeding esophageal varices. The technique involves loading a rubber band onto the end of the endoscope, which is then introduced into the esophagus. A varix is sucked into an adaptor on the end of the endoscope and the rubber band discharged off of the endoscope onto the varix (Fig. 8-2). Application of multiple bands requires that the endoscope be removed, loaded with another rubber band, and reintroduced. The use of an overtube placed into the esophagus at the beginning of the procedure facilitates multiple withdrawals and reintroductions. Clinical trials have demonstrated that variceal banding is as effective as emergency sclerotherapy.[20,29] Deep ulcers and esophageal strictures appear to be less frequent with banding than with endoscopic sclerotherapy.[20,29]

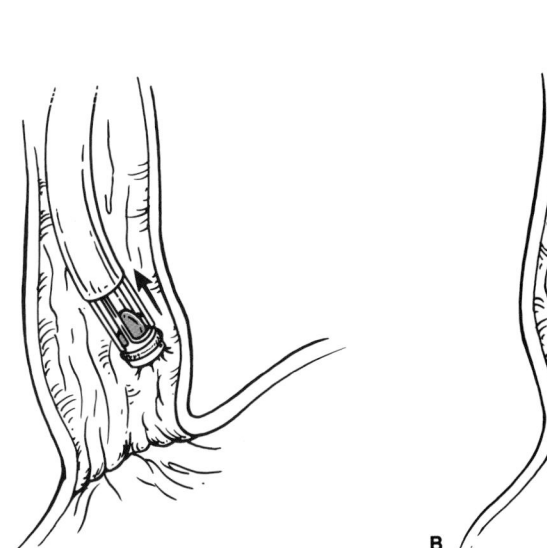

Figure 8-2   Endoscopic banding.   **A**   **B**

Table 8-7   Angiographic Control of Intestinal Bleeding: Sites of Origin

Colonic diverticula
Varices of any site
Mallory-Weiss tears refractory to injection therapy
Dieulafoiy's ulcers
Vascular ectasias
Arteriovenous malformations
Ruptured pseudoanuerysms
Posttraumatic or intervention-induced bleeding
Bleeding into a pancreatic pseudocyst
Hemobilia
Hemosuccus pancreaticus

Complications

Complications, including mortality, can accompany endoscopic therapeutic procedures, such as injection sclerotherapy and emergency coagulation of massively bleeding sites. The risk of injection sclerotherapy is dependent on the experience of the endoscopist and the amount of sclerosant administered. Sclerotherapy can result in esophageal ulcers, strictures, fever, esophageal perforation, portal vein thrombosis, and increased bleeding. Injection therapy of gastric ulcers with alcohol may rarely cause gastric infarction. Esophageal tears have been reported secondary to overtube placement. Endoscopic coagulation inappropriately applied can cause more bleeding and gastric or duodenal perforation. The incidence of gastric perforation from endoscopic thermal techniques is reported to be less than 1%.[25] The overall complication rates for endoscopic techniques compare favorably with those associated with alternative operative procedures for the same sources of bleeding.

Mesenteric Angiography

Selective visceral angiography is an important diagnostic and therapeutic tool in the evaluation and treatment of patients with upper and lower GI hemorrhage. For some patients, angiographic control of bleeding can be more expeditious and less morbid than operative attempts. Table 8-7 lists conditions for which angiography is useful as the primary mode of diagnosis and therapy. There are several conditions, including ruptured mesenteric pseudoaneurysms, hemobilia, and hemosuccus pancreaticus, in which operation has a poor chance of adequately controlling the site of bleeding. These conditions are associated with an excessive operative morbidity and mortality. Diagnostic and therapeutic angiography is the procedure of first choice in these situations.

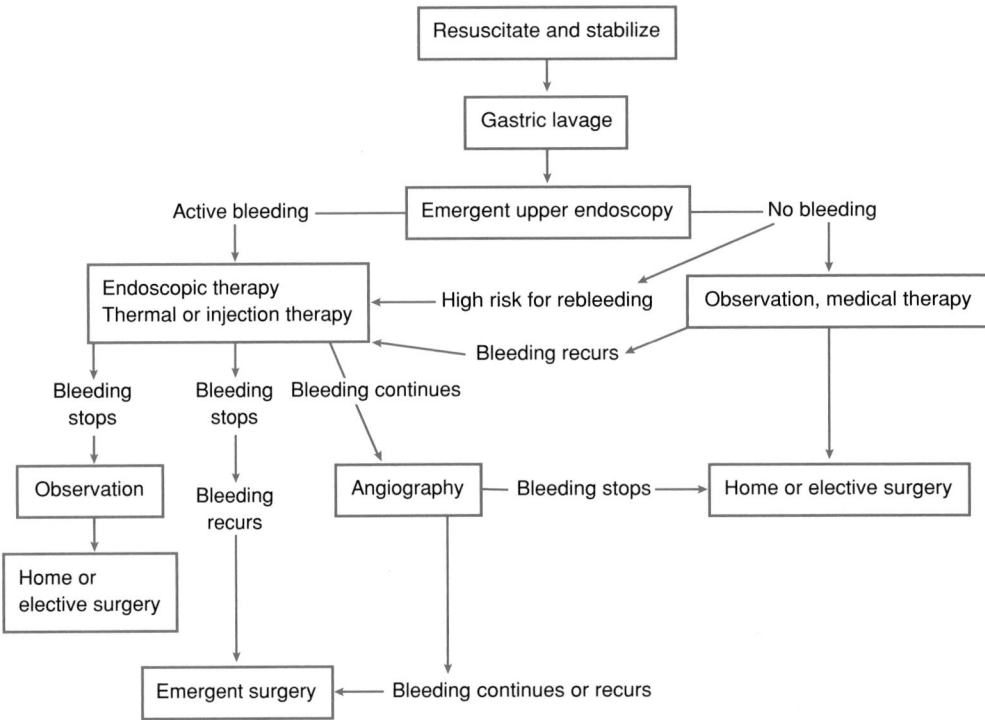

Figure 8-3 Diagnostic and therapeutic algorithm for upper gastrointestinal bleeding.

When patients have rapid bleeding (more than 1 mL/min), they should proceed directly to angiography after nondiagnostic endoscopy (Fig. 8-3). Once a bleeding site is identified by angiography, intraarterial vasopressin infusion is initiated at 0.2 to 0.4 U/min for 20 minutes, after which a second arteriogram is performed[30] (Fig. 8-4). If bleeding persists, the dose of vasopressin (Pitressin) is increased up to 1 U/min for another 10 minutes. If hemorrhage persists, embolization techniques should be considered to control the bleeding, provided superselective catheterization of the feeding vessel is possible. This method is highly effective for controlling bleeding from duodenal and gastric ulcers, Dieulafoy's ulcers, vascular malformations, ruptured pseudoaneurysms, and posttraumatic or intervention-induced bleeding.[31]

Angiographic localization of bleeding is sensitive when the rate of bleeding is greater than 1 mL/min, but the diagnostic yield is low when the rate of bleeding is less than 0.5 mL/min. Selective mesenteric angiography localizes the site of bleeding in 40% to 86% of rapidly bleeding patients.[32,33] When the site of bleeding is identified, angiographic embolization controls bleeding in 86% to 100% of patients[30,31,34] (Fig. 8-5). Temporary angiographic control approaches 100% for many conditions. Long-term control is less successful. Patients who continue to bleed or who bleed again after angiography should undergo emergent operation.

The superior mesenteric artery, inferior mesenteric artery, and celiac arteries are sequentially injected, with the order determined by the most likely site of bleeding. The results of endoscopy direct angiography to the most likely location of bleeding in cases of massive bleeding, whereas scintigraphy is useful in localizing the most likely site in patients with low to moderate rates of bleeding. Failure of a site of bleeding to be identified by angiography is often due to the episodic nature of the bleeding or vasoconstriction of the vessel supplying the bleeding site. Intravenous administration of a vasodilator such as tolazoline (Priscoline), 25 mg, or pa-

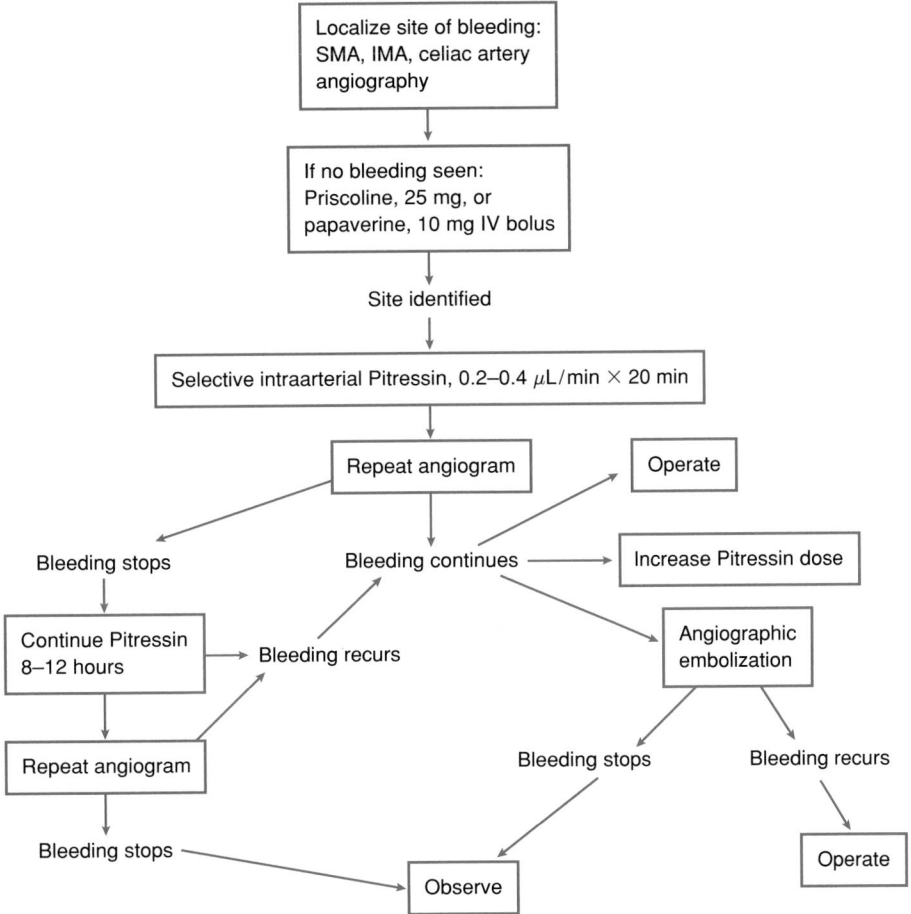

Figure 8-4 Diagnostic and therapeutic algorithm for angiographic control of upper and lower gastrointestinal bleeding.

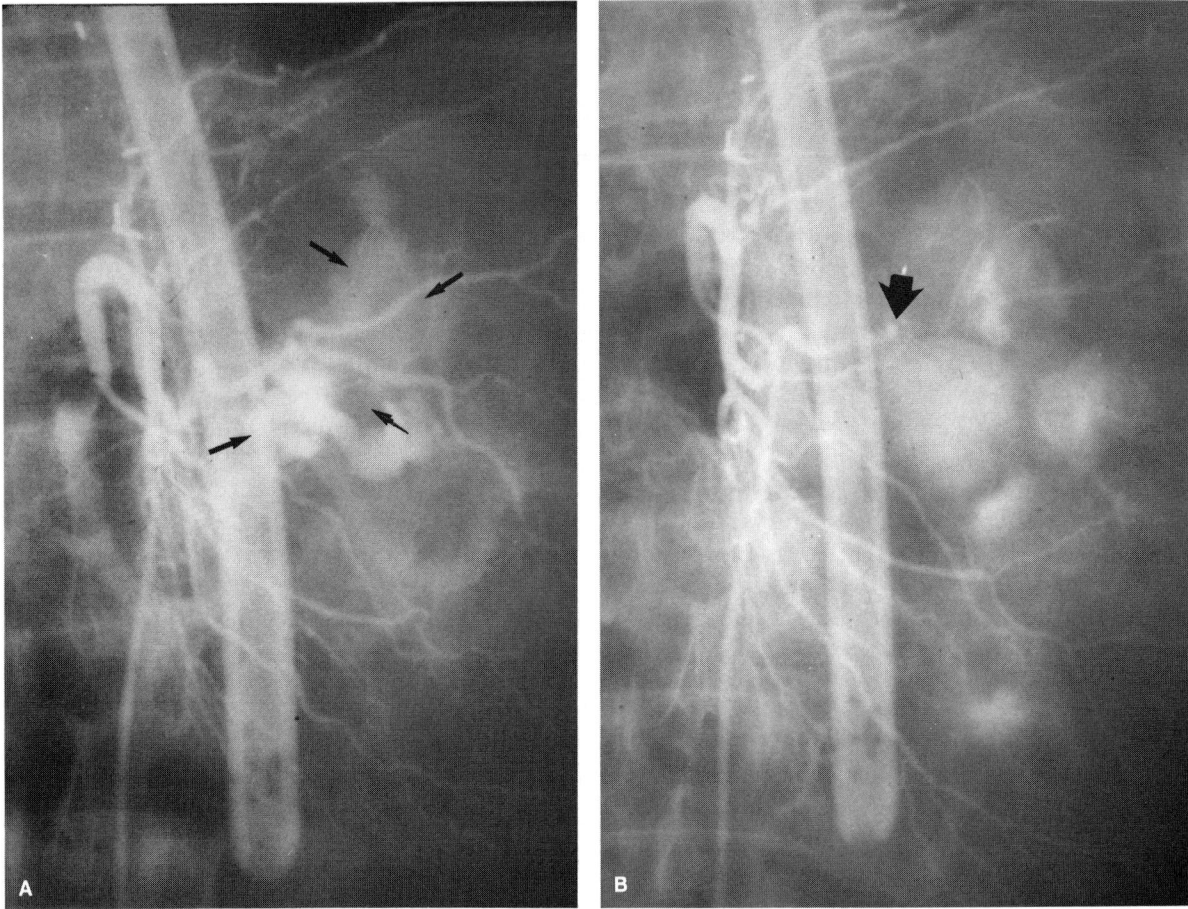

Figure 8-5 (**A**) Selective angiogram of left gastric artery reveals bleeding from a branch of the left gastric vessel along the lesser curvature of the stomach as evidenced by contrast pooling in the stomach (*arrows*). (**B**) After selective embolization (*arrow*), bleeding stopped. (Courtesy of H. Ricketts Radiology Library, University of Washington, Seattle)

paverine, 10 mg, before repeating selective angiography can delineate the site (see Fig. 8-4).

Advances in angiographic technique allow skilled angiographers to thread catheters into third-order arterial branches, such as the pancreaticoduodenal, gastroepiploic, first jejunal, or ileocolic artery. This distal cannulation allows selective embolization with lessened chance of ischemia to other areas. Because of the rich anastomotic arterial network of the upper GI tract, many bleeding lesions are fed from more than one vascular arcade. For this reason, embolotherapy for massive duodenal hemorrhage requires embolization of more than one feeding blood vessel[34] (Fig. 8-6). A variety of embolic materials can be used for occluding bleeding vessels, including polyvinyl alcohol, flexible coils, methyl-methacrylate, cyanoacrylate, and absorbable gelatin sponge. When a bleeding lesion cannot be controlled by angiography, the infusion of arterial va-

soconstrictors, such as vasopressin or epinephrine, can significantly slow the bleeding while the patient is being prepared for surgery.

Angiography is not without hazard or side effects. In large series,[30,35] the overall complication rate of diagnostic and therapeutic angiography was 9% to 13%. Patients with compromised renal function are at risk from contrast, and efforts should be made to hydrate the patient before angiography and to establish diuresis. Patients with a history of contrast allergy can be studied but should be premedicated with intravenous methylprednisolone, 1 g, and intravenous diphenhydramine (Benadryl), 50 mg.

Arterial embolization for control of bleeding, although highly effective, is associated with a risk of ischemic mucosal necrosis, perforation, and late stenosis.[31,34] The risk for ischemic complications is increased in patients with lower GI bleeding, because of limited

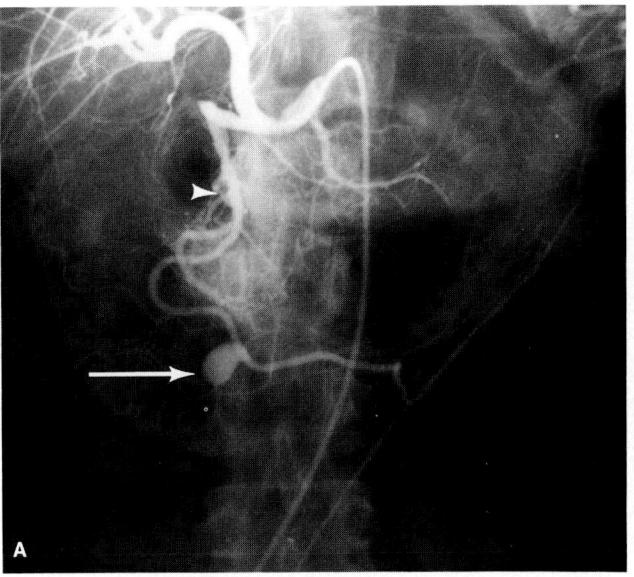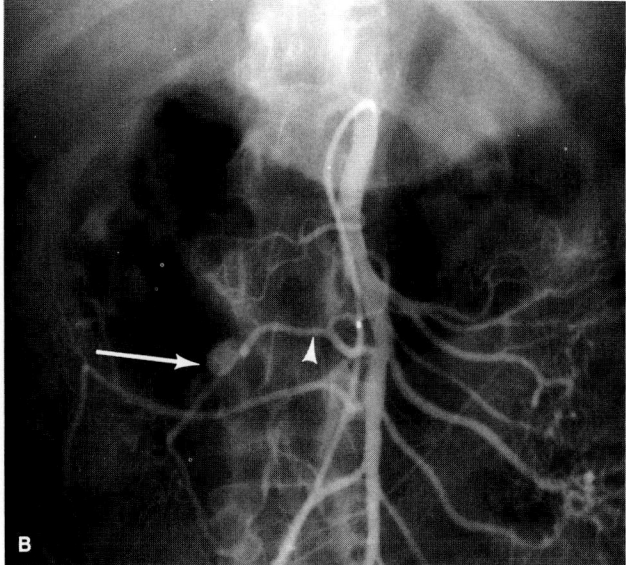

Figure 8-6 Angiograms demonstrating a bleeding duodenal ulcer (*arrows*) supplied from both the gastroduodenal artery (*arrowhead* in **A**) and the inferior pancreaticoduodenal arcade (*arrowhead* in **B**). Control of bleeding required superselective catheterization and embolization of both feeding vessels. (Courtesy of Dr. D. Coldwell, University of Washington, Seattle)

arterial collaterals in the distal small bowel and colon, and in patients with previous GI operations or significant visceral atherosclerosis.

Other Diagnostic Procedures

There is no role for radionuclide imaging or barium contrast studies in patients with hemodynamically significant upper GI bleeding. Radionuclide imaging by dynamic scintigraphy can be useful in patients with episodic, recurrent, occult upper GI bleeding or in patients suspected of having hemobilia, bleeding into the pancreatic duct, or a pseudocyst. Figure 8-3 illustrates a diagnostic algorithm for patients with upper GI bleeding.

Operative Exploration for Unknown Sites of Upper Gastrointestinal Bleeding

The principles of operating on patients with GI bleeding can be summarized as follows:

1. Attempt to localize the site of bleeding before operation.
2. Do not delay operation if the patient continues to bleed or has recurrent bleeding even when a bleeding site is not known.
3. Perform intraoperative endoscopy in all patients in whom a confirmed site is not identified preoperatively and after brief intraabdominal exploration.

4. Do not perform undirected intestinal resection unless intraoperative attempts at localization have failed and an area of potential pathology (eg, colonic diverticula) can be confirmed.

Less than 2.5% of all patients who present with upper GI bleeding require emergency operation, and most have a preoperative diagnosis.[36] Hence, it is unusual to operate on a patient with uncontrolled and undiagnosed upper GI hemorrhage.

A generous midline incision is made that extends from the xiphoid to just below the umbilicus. A self-retaining retractor is placed, and wide exposure of the stomach and duodenum is achieved. Brief inspection determines whether the stomach and duodenum are filled with blood and whether there is cirrhosis or portal hypertension. If the stomach is distended with blood, a 10-cm vertically oriented gastrotomy is placed in the mid-gastric body about 4 cm medial to the lesser curve using the electrocautery. This incision allows rapid evacuation of clot and inspection of the entire lesser curve (the most common site for ulcer or tumor) proximally up to the gastroesophageal junction. Through the same incision, the body and entire antrum can be inspected. If a bleeding site is identified, the gastrotomy incision can be extended in the direction of the lesion to allow ligation or resection of the site of bleeding. If no bleeding site is identified and fresh blood appears to be coming from within the stomach, careful bimanual palpation of the entire stomach is performed. If there is no apparent source for bleeding in the stomach and fresh blood is seen coming from the pylorus, a duodenal ulcer should be suspected. A wide Kocher maneuver is performed and the duodenum carefully inspected and palpated. If there is no evidence of duodenal ulcer disease, an endoscope can be placed through the gastrotomy and pylorus and the duodenum inspected. An intestinal clamp should be placed across the small bowel just distal to the ligament of Treitz to minimize air introduced into the small bowel.

ACUTE LOWER GASTROINTESTINAL BLEEDING

History and Physical Examination

Tables 8-8 and 8-9 illustrate the common causes and locations of lower GI bleeding. Constipation, altered bowel habits, pain, and diarrhea are all symptoms that can be caused by serious large bowel disorders, including carcinoma, polyps, diverticular disease, and inflammatory bowel disease. Patients presenting with acute bloody diarrhea may be experiencing an episode of ischemic colitis, self-limited infectious colitis, antibiotic-associated colitis, Crohn's disease, or ulcerative colitis. Patients should be asked about the presence of abdominal pain, mucous stools, abdominal distention, weight loss, fatigue, and a family history of colon cancer or inflammatory bowel disease. Perianal or rectal pain with or without defecation may reflect perirectal disease, such as anal fissure, ulcers, tumors, or hemorrhoids. A history of diverticulosis should be sought and any previous barium enema inspected to localize the site of diverticula. Previous intestinal operations, colon resections, or polypectomies are important clues to possible underlying pathology. Peripheral vascular disease, a history of atrial fibrillation, congestive heart failure, embolic disease, and ingestion of digitalis all increase the likelihood of ischemic enteritis or colitis. Immuno-

Table 8-8 Causes of Massive Hematochezia

Cause	Frequency (%)
Angiodysplasia	30
Diverticulosis	17
Neoplasm	11
Colitis, ulcers	9
Other colonic or rectal	5
Small bowel lesion	9
Missed upper gastrointestinal source	11
Undiagnosed	6

Table 8-9 Locations of Lower Gastrointestinal Bleeding

Location	Frequency (%) All Patients (No Prescreening)	Excluding Anorectal Lesions
Anorectal	13	
Colon	55	74
Small bowel	29	11
Stomach	0	9
Unknown	3	6

(After Jensen DM, Machicado GA, Kovacs TOG, et al. Controlled, randomized study of heater probe and BICAP for hemostasis of severe ulcer bleeding. [Abstract] Gastroenterology 1988;94:A208)

suppressed patients have an expanded differential diagnosis that includes unusual pathogens and lesions that can cause colonic bleeding (see Table 8-3). A history of anal intercourse or rectal trauma should be sought in patients with bright red blood originating in the rectal vault. If hematochezia is the presenting complaint and there has been no hematemesis, the probability is that bleeding is originating from the colon. Physical examination in patients with lower GI bleeding proceeds similarly to that described for patients with upper GI bleeding, followed by directed examination of the anus, rectum, and colon.

Anoscopy and Sigmoidoscopy

Anoscopy and rigid or flexible sigmoidoscopy should be performed immediately after digital examination to exclude lesions such as hemorrhoids, anal fissure, rectal ulcers, trauma, colitis, and rectal cancers. A retroflexed view can be the best way to visualize bleeding internal hemorrhoids. If a low-lying colorectal lesion is identified, a decision should be made regarding treatment in the emergency room. Bleeding hemorrhoids can usually be directly banded or injected in the emergency room. Significant arterial bleeding from other perianal lesions can be temporarily controlled by injection with epinephrine and compression. Definitive control for bleeding rectal carcinomas or ulcers should probably be performed in the operating room with good lighting and adequate anesthesia. Bleeding lesions identified higher in the rectum can often be managed colonoscopically by laser, contact probes, or injection therapy.

Diagnostic and Therapeutic Colonoscopy

Colonoscopy is the procedure of choice in patients with lower GI hemorrhage when no site of bleeding has been identified on anoscopy or sigmoidoscopy.[37] Colonoscopy is the most sensitive and specific means of identifying a site of colonic bleeding. If there is active bleeding, precolonoscopic bowel purge with a nonabsorbable electrolyte solution increases the chances of identifying a site of bleeding. The purge should be room temperature and administered by nasogastric tube at 1 L/h, until rectal effluent is clear of stool and clots, and then immediately followed by colonoscopy. In 80 consecutive patients with hematochezia treated in this fashion, diagnostic sensitivity was 86%.[37] Four percent of patients given a normal saline purge experienced fluid overload, and there were no technical complications related to the colonoscopy. The purge should not be administered if there is suspicion of an obstructing colon lesion.

Colonoscopy should be performed in cooperative patients at the bedside in the intensive care unit or in the endoscopy suite. Patients should have supplemental oxygen and continuous electrocardiogram monitoring. Midazolam administered in 1- to 2-mg increments with or without an intravenous narcotic is useful for sedation and analgesia. The use of fluoroscopy is sometimes helpful in determining the exact location of the colonoscope if a bleeding lesion is found and cannot be coagulated. Experienced colonoscopists can usually enter the terminal ileum, gaining important diagnostic information about involvement of this area with Crohn's disease, or detecting fresh blood coming from a more proximal site. If a site of bleeding is not identified by colonoscopy and blood has been visualized in the right colon, it is prudent to perform upper endoscopy while the patient is sedated.

The endoscopist should be prepared to perform colonoscopic therapy should an appropriate lesion be identified, including polypectomy, multipolar or heater probe coagulation, and injection therapy. The most commonly diagnosed lesions causing hematochezia are listed in Table 8-8 and include angiodysplasia, diverticulosis, polyps, tumors, and colitis.

Hemodynamically unstable patients with hematochezia should rapidly undergo upper endoscopy if brief inspection of their anorectum does not reveal a source. If the upper endoscopy is negative, these patients should proceed directly to mesenteric angiography. In patients with less severe bleeding, dynamic scintigraphy should be performed and, if positive, followed immediately by mesenteric angiography.

With adequate training and modern instruments, serious complications of diagnostic colonoscopy should be less than 1 in 1000 procedures.[38] Rates of perforations range from 0.06% to 0.57%; hemorrhage, 0.01% to 0.04%; and mortality, 0.01% to 0.15%. Complications during therapeutic colonoscopy should be less than 0.1%, and the serious complications of bleeding or perforation should be less than 2%.

Angiography

Angiography for suspected lower GI bleeding has three goals: to locate and define the nature of bleeding, to stop the bleeding, and to direct the surgeon to the correct location for the correct operation should bleeding continue or recur.[39] About 75% of all lower GI hemorrhages can be permanently or temporarily controlled angiographically.[30,33,40] Preoperative angiographic localization and control of colonic bleeding significantly diminish operative morbidity and mortality in patients ultimately requiring operation.[33] In a review of more than 247 patients,[33] angiography localized bleeding in 69% and controlled bleeding by the use of vasopressin in 82%. By providing accurate preoperation, localization resulted in a recurrent bleeding rate of 6% in 167 patients after segmental colon resection.

Angiography is particularly useful in the diagnosis and treatment of lower GI bleeding when hemorrhage is massive, the site of bleeding is unknown, and colonoscopy cannot be performed. If colonic bleeding is slow and intermittent, an attempt to localize the bleeding site by radionuclide imaging is often helpful and necessary in directing the angiographic approach[41] (Fig. 8-7). The blood supply to the lower small bowel and colon does not have the rich anastomotic network that exists in the upper GI tract. Hence, transcatheter embolization of particulate material directly into the bleeding artery is associated with higher rates of bowel ischemia and infarction and should be reserved for patients with excessive operative risk.

Scintigraphy

Radionucleotide (technetium-99m [^{99m}Tc]) tagged red cell scanning is the most sensitive method for detecting low-level (0.1 mL/min) bleeding, particularly when dynamic images are displayed over time. The ability of scintigraphy to detect GI bleeding is dependent on several factors, including the rate of bleeding, the transit time of blood along the GI tract, and the manner in which the scans are obtained. Rapid transit of blood along the small bowel decreases the accumulation of activity at the point of bleeding, resulting in misleading sites of bleeding. The use of computerized cinematic acquisition and display of scintigrams in real time significantly corrects this problem and improves localization of GI bleeding when compared with the use of static displays. Patients are scanned at 15-second acquisitions during a 90-minute run. Each 15-second image provides a static image (similar to a single frame of a

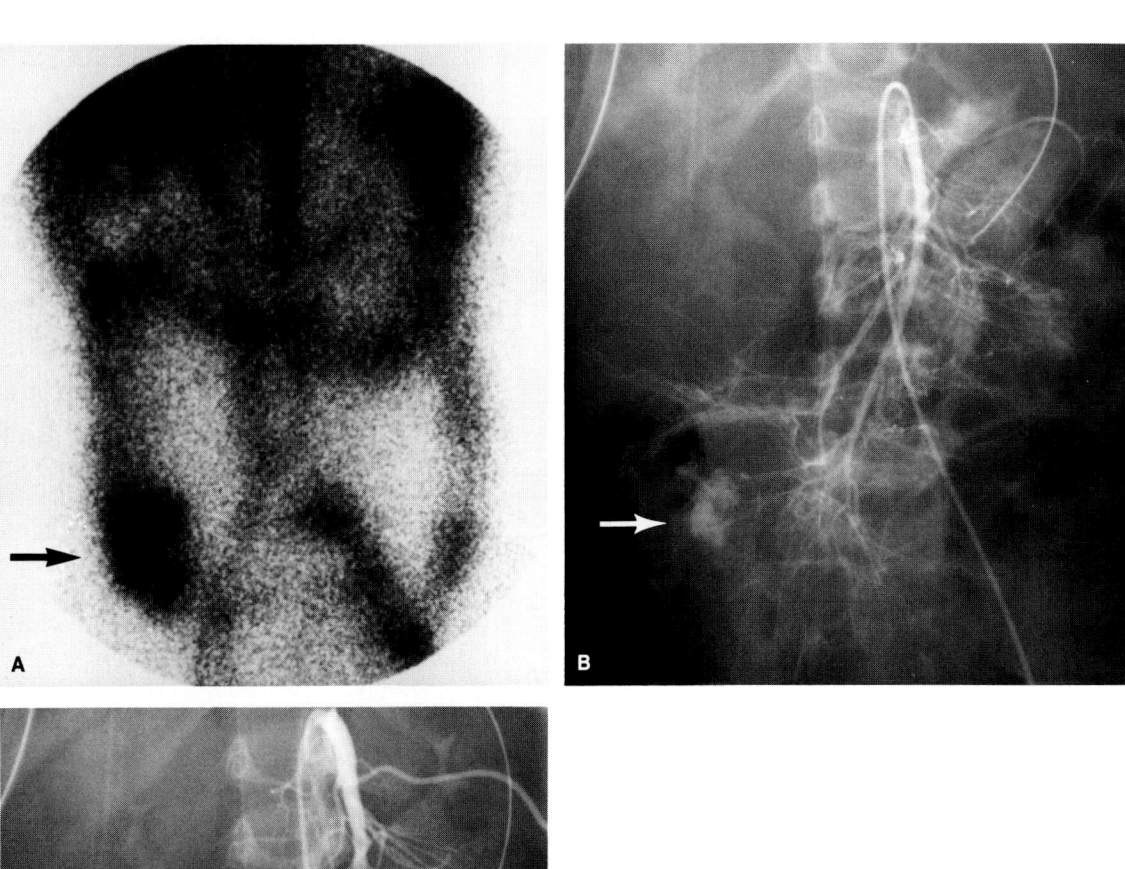

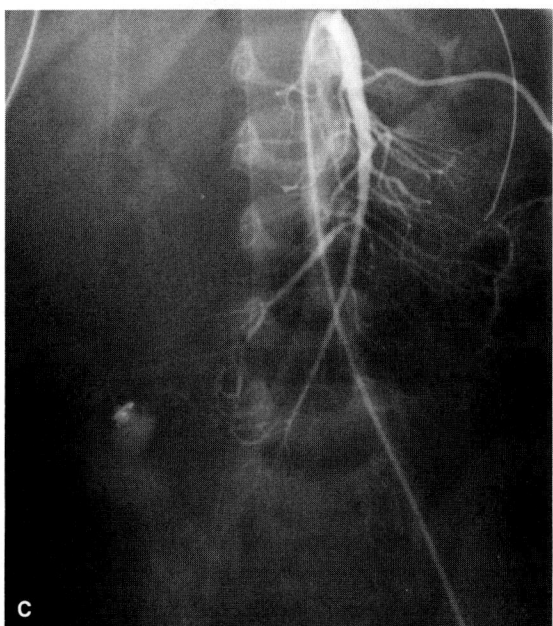

Figure 8-7 (**A**) Positive ^{99m}Tc red cell scan demonstrating radionuclide accumulation in the right lower quadrant (*arrow*) indicative of either right colon or small bowel bleeding. (**B** and **C**) Selective visceral angiograms in the same patient shown in **A** demonstrate contrast extravasation into the lumen of the cecum (*arrow*), localizing the site of bleeding to the right colon. **C** demonstrates decreased bleeding into the cecum after intraarterial vasopressin. Note vasoconstriction of arterioles compared with **B**. (Courtesy of Dr. C. Rohrmann, University of Washington, Seattle)

movie), and all the static images are rerun on a computer screen in real time. The sensitivity of scintigraphy to detect bleeding is significant (about 79%) if the patient is being scanned while actively bleeding. When a patient is repeatedly scanned during the course of a day, sensitivity of the bleeding can be increased, but localization of the bleeding is less reliable. If the scan does not detect any evidence of bleeding, the patient should be rescanned. The half-life of technetium allows scanning to be performed during a 24-hour period.

Performing surgery solely on the basis of static red blood cell scintigraphy in patients with lower GI bleed-

ing has undesirable results in as many as 40% of patients.[42,43]

Intraoperative Scintigraphy

Intraoperative scintigraphy has been used to localize bleeding of small intestinal origin in patients without preoperative localization by endoscopy or angiography. If a standard preoperative ^{99m}Tc red blood cell scan is positive and the patient previously had nondiagnostic endoscopy or angiography, laparotomy and intraoperative scintigraphy can be performed. When there is no obvious pathology identified on abdominal exploration, consideration should be given to performing intraoperative scintigraphy before intraoperative enteroscopy. Clamps are placed at 30-cm intervals along the small bowel and colon, and the segments are imaged sequentially with a mobile gamma camera. This technique is rapid and easily performed and can effectively identify sites of active small intestinal bleeding. If the patient did not have a recent ^{99m}Tc red cell scan and had a nondiagnostic endoscopy and angiography, 5 to 7 mL of blood is labeled with ^{99m}Tc and injected just before laparotomy.

Barium Studies

Barium contrast studies have no role in the diagnosis of patients with acute upper or lower GI bleeding. Contrast within the bowel lumen obscures endoscopic visu-

alization as well as angiographic localization. The major role for barium contrast studies is in the evaluation of patients with chronic, recurrent GI bleeding of obscure origin (Figs. 8-8 and 8-9). The most common causes of GI bleeding diagnosed by contrast studies include inflammatory bowel disease, small bowel tumors, and metastasis. Figure 8-10 illustrates a patient with small bowel bleeding identified by angiography and contrast examination.

Surgical Localization of Lower Gastrointestinal Bleeding

Ideally, patients with lower GI bleeding should have the site of bleeding localized before operation. However, in about 6% of all patients, a cause of bleeding cannot be identified by either colonoscopy or angiogra-

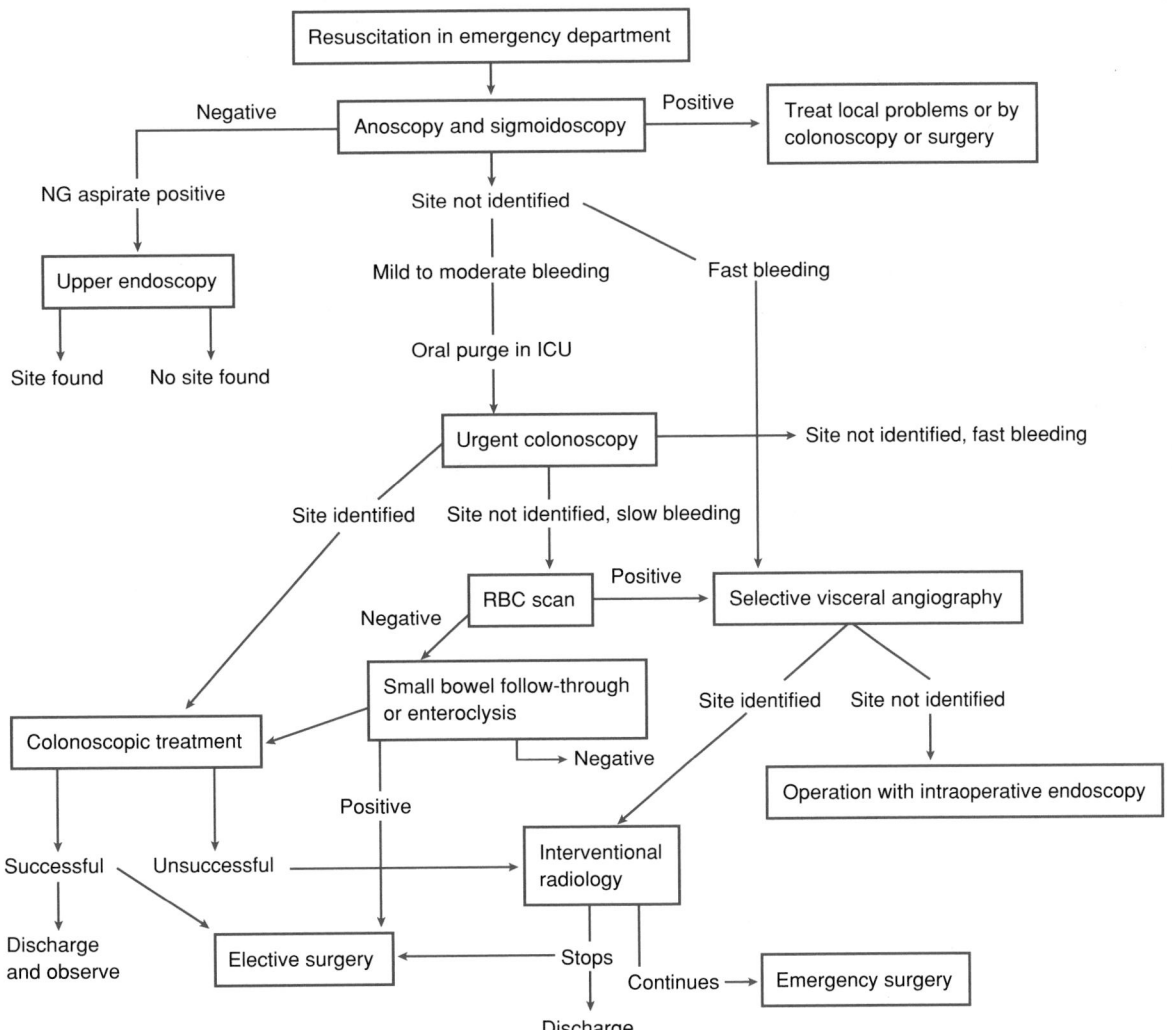

Figure 8-8 Diagnostic and therapeutic algorithm for hematochezia.

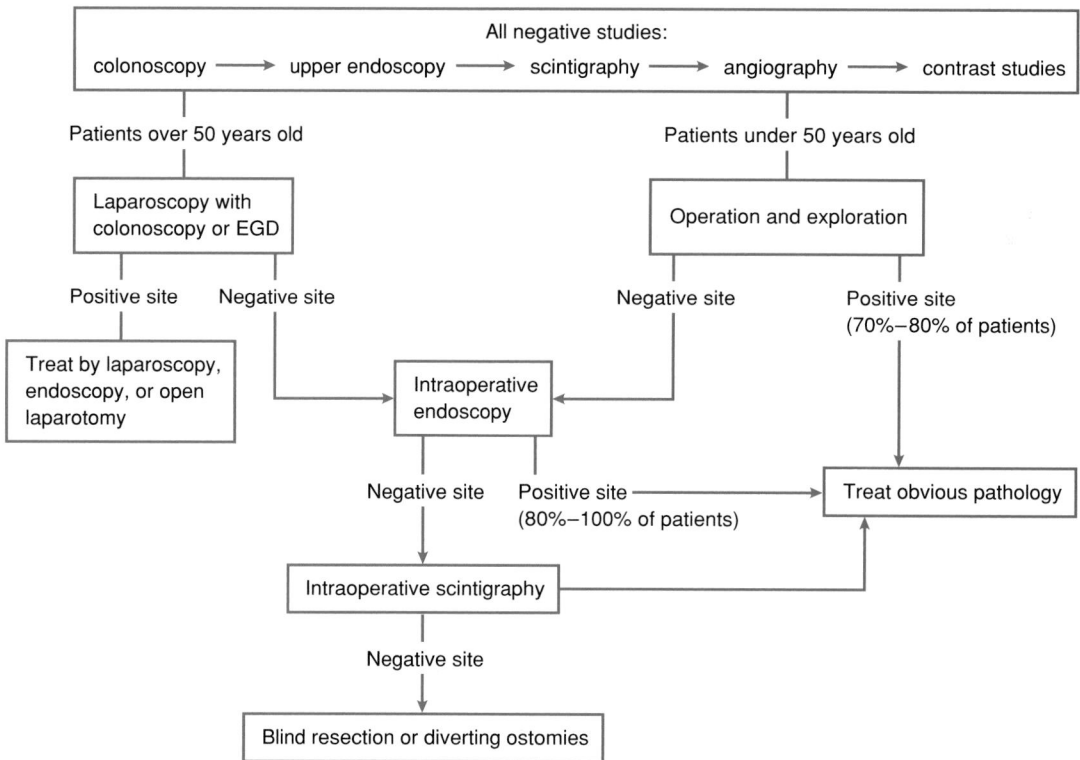

Figure 8-9 Diagnostic and therapeutic algorithm for occult gastrointestinal bleeding.

phy.[44,45] At laparotomy, additional diagnostic measures can be performed if a source of bleeding is not evident. The availability of intraoperative colonoscopy and transabdominal endoscopy significantly increases the chances of identifying the source of bleeding. Patients should be placed in a low modified Sims position with the buttocks barely over the edge of the operating table to facilitate on-table colonic lavage and transrectal introduction and passage of the colonoscope.

On entering the abdominal cavity, the surgeon should immediately look for evidence of proximal GI bleeding and bimanually palpate the entire stomach, duodenum, small bowel, and large bowel. If there is evidence of bleeding from the stomach or duodenum, endoscopy should be performed.

Videoendoscopy is preferable to fiberoptic endoscopy in the operating room so that the operating surgeons can also view the mucosa. In the presence of massive colonic bleeding, the colonoscope can be advanced proximally with the surgeon's assistance. If intraluminal blood obscures endoscopic visualization, rapid colonic lavage can be performed through a colotomy placed in the appendix. Lavage fluid should be administered at 0.3 L/min for 10 minutes, and a large rectal tube (40 F) should be placed to facilitate evacuation of the colonic effluent. After colonic purge, the colonoscope can be reintroduced. Occluding the colon with

atraumatic intestinal clamps at the mid-transverse colon and mid-descending colon can facilitate insufflation as well as contain and localize the bleeding to a particular segment of colon.

If diverticular bleeding is suspected but cannot be localized and there is a previous barium enema documenting the location of diverticula, resection of all involved segments of colon should be performed. If there is no clearly identified site of bleeding in the opened resected specimen, careful inspection of the entire small bowel is in order, and the patient should also undergo upper endoscopy. If the site of bleeding is still unidentified, the patient should have a temporary enterostomy so that postoperative hemorrhage can be readily investigated by transstomal enteroscopy.

Patients with a suspected or diagnosed Meckel's diverticulum may benefit from laparoscopic resection. Laparoscopy can also aid in the diagnosis of occult GI bleeding when combined with simultaneous upper or lower endoscopy. Dieulafoy's ulcers can be visualized laparoscopically with transillumination of the stomach wall and then oversewn or clipped. The laparoscopic surgeon can clip the feeding vessels from the left gastric artery or oversew the bleeding lesion by passing a needle through the stomach wall to the endoscopist, who then passes the needle back out. The endoscopist also views the bleeding vessel to be certain that adequate

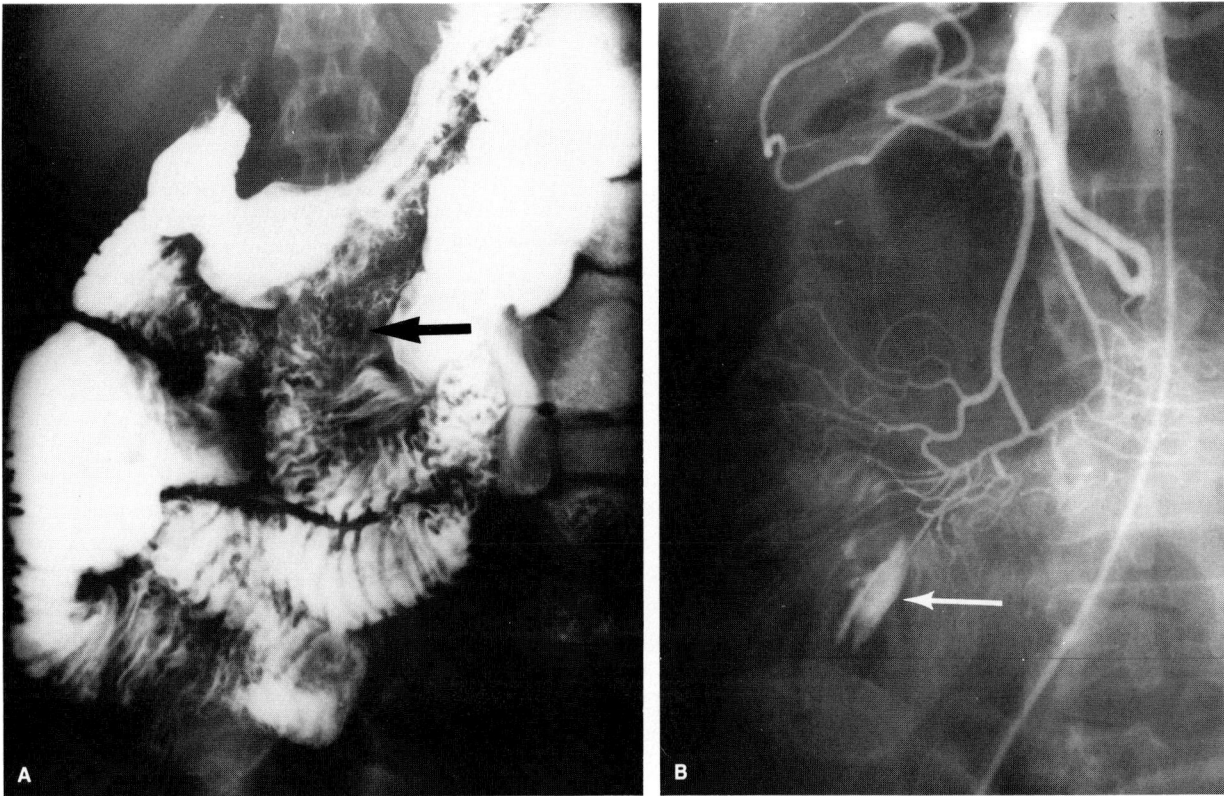

Figure 8-10 (**A**) Small bowel contrast examination of the jejunum demonstrates mucosal filling defect (*arrow*) consistent with metastatic disease. (**B**) Superselective angiogram reveals contrast extravasation (*arrow*) into the same jejunal loop with mucosal filling defect. The patient had metastatic malignant melanoma. (Courtesy of Dr. C. Rohrmann, University of Washington, Seattle)

hemostasis has been accomplished. This approach can also be used for oversewing vascular lesions in the proximal small bowel. Combined endoscopic and laparoscopic treatment of bleeding lesions on the stomach wall also benefits other selected patients.[46]

SPECIFIC CAUSES OF UPPER GASTROINTESTINAL HEMORRHAGE

Peptic Ulcer

Peptic ulceration accounts for about half of all cases of upper GI bleeding (see Table 8-5). In 70% to 80% of cases, bleeding from peptic ulcers ceases spontaneously without subsequent rebleeding.[25] However, in about 25% of cases, rebleeding occurs,[47] with an overall mortality rate of about 10%.[12] Both clinical and endoscopic features identify patients at risk for recurrent or persistent bleeding from peptic ulcers. Clinical features include coagulopathy, onset of bleeding in patients al-

ready hospitalized, and hypotension on initial presentation.[25] Endoscopic features predictive of rebleeding are listed in Table 8-10. Figure 8-11 schematically illustrates a bleeding and visible vessel. Patients who presented initially with hypotension and were found at endoscopy to have a nonbleeding visible vessel in the ulcer base had an 80% predicted incidence of rebleeding in one study.[48]

Patients with an actively bleeding ulcer and those

Table 8-10 Endoscopic Features Predicting Recurrent Bleeding in Patients With Gastric and Duodenal Ulcers

Endoscopic Finding	Prevalence (%)	Risk of Rebleeding (%)
Active bleeding	15	100
Visible vessel	25	50
Oozing	15	30
Spot or clot	20	15
Clean ulcer base	25	2

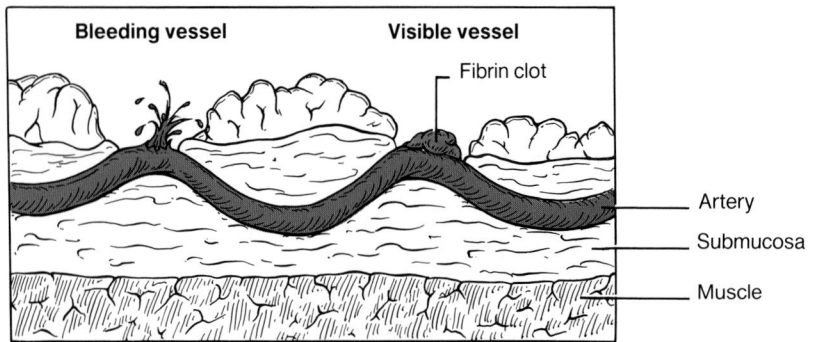

Figure 8-11   The visible vessel sign usually represents a clot adherent to a submucosal artery at the base of an ulcer. A spurting vessel is usually from an erosion in the side of a penetrating submucosal vessel traversing the base of an ulcer.

at high risk for recurrent bleeding should undergo emergent endoscopic hemostatic therapy.[25] To ensure optimal visualization, patients should not be administered antacids or sucralfate before endoscopy. Endoscopic hemostatic therapy (both injection and thermal techniques) significantly decreases the risk of rebleeding (69% relative reduction), need for emergency surgery (62% decrease), and hospital mortality rate (30% decrease). These patients should have a surgeon involved in their care from the outset because the need for emergent surgery despite endoscopic therapy approaches 10%.[25] Prospective trials have delineated predictive factors for recurrent bleeding after hemostatic therapy. Size and location of an ulcer are highly predictive of recurrent bleeding. Large (more than 2 cm) ulcers, ulcers located high on the lesser curve of the stomach close to the left gastric artery, and posterior inferior ulcers in the duodenum close to the gastroduodenal artery have about a 20% to 40% incidence of recurrent bleeding after endoscopic therapy.[49]

Angiographic embolization achieves short-term hemostasis in bleeding duodenal ulcers in about 90% of patients[31] (Table 8-11). However, recurrent bleeding and long-term complications, particularly duodenal stenosis, are not insignificant.

For bleeding gastric ulcers, partial gastric resection is the procedure of choice. Biopsy is essential to rule out malignancy. Laparoscopic resection of bleeding gastric lesions is technically feasible[46] but should not be performed in hemodynamically unstable patients. The technique requires intraoperative upper gastroscopy to guide the surgeon in placing the linear GI stapling device to ensure complete excision of the ulcer.

Two types of operations have been proposed for acutely bleeding duodenal ulcers: (1) oversewing of the ulcer plus vagotomy and drainage, or (2) gastric resection with excision of the ulcer. The results of the first randomized controlled trial[50] comparing these two operations for acutely bleeding peptic ulcers are presented in Table 8-12. Briefly, 120 patients with acutely bleeding duodenal ulcers were randomized to undergo vagotomy and oversewing or gastric resection with or without vagotomy. The high mortality rate (23%) in this study should be noted because none of the patients received endoscopic hemostatic therapy before operation. The gastric resection group was further randomized to receive a Billroth I or Billroth II reconstruction. Postoperative rebleeding was less in patients undergoing gastric resection, but complications (duodenal leak) were much higher when patients had a Billroth II anastomosis. Death in this study was more common in patients who were older than 60 years of age, had massive bleeding on presentation, had preoperative transfusion of more than three units, and had posterior location of the ulcer.

The most common cause of recurrent ulcer hemorrhage in the postoperative period is inadequate suture ligation of the initial bleeding point. Less severe bleeding may be from the suture line and can be investigated endoscopically and treated using injection therapy.

When properly performed, secondary hemorrhage from ligated bleeding duodenal ulcers occurs in less than 4%.[51] When recurrent bleeding occurs, the bleeding vessel should be directly visualized and then resutured to ensure that control has been achieved. If recurrent ulcer bleeding originates from a previously ligated gastric ulcer, gastrectomy plus vagotomy should be the secondary operation.

Table 8-11   Angiographic Embolization of Bleeding Duodenal Ulcer

	Initial Success (%)	Long-Term Success (%)	Duodenal Stenosis (%)
Terminal muscular branch occlusion	96	53*	7
Gastroduodenal artery occlusion	86	27	25

* Long-term success was 90% in patients embolized with cyanoacrylate.

Table 8-12   Emergent Operation for Bleeding Peptic Ulcer

	Postoperative Bleeding (%)	*Duodenal Leak (%)*	*Mortality Rate (%)*
VAGOTOMY AND OVERSEWING	17	12	22
Artery ligation*	0	0	12
No ligation	20	4	24
GASTRIC RESECTION†	3‡	13	23
Billroth I	4	0	21
Billroth II	3	22‡	25

* Artery ligation refers to ligation of the gastroduodenal trunk and right gastroepiploic artery.
† Patients in the gastric resection group were randomly assigned to receive a Billroth I or Billroth II procedure.
‡ $P < .05$ versus vagotomy and oversewing group.
(After Millat B, Hay JM, Valleur P, Fingerhut A, Fagniez PL. Emergency surgical treatment for bleeding duodenal ulcer: oversewing plus vagotomy versus gastric resection, a controlled randomized trial. World J Surg 1993;17:568)

Gastric Erosions

Gastric erosions are not a major cause of GI hemorrhage. Erosions are superficial lesions that by definition do not extend into the submucosa where large arteries are present that can result in significant bleeding. A prospective study[52] of 445 patients found gastric erosions to account for only 3% of cases of major upper GI bleeding. Most gastric and duodenal erosions are caused by NSAID ingestion. Only if an erosion deepens and becomes an ulcer is there a significant bleeding risk.

Stress Ulcer

Stress-related gastric mucosal damage occurs in critically ill patients with sepsis, extensive burns, head injury, and multiple organ failure. With attention to treatment of sepsis, adequate mechanical ventilation, nutrition, and other supportive care, the incidence of significant stress ulceration in the intensive care unit has fallen to less than 5%.[53] The incidence of stress ulcer is reduced by antisecretory drugs and sucralfate. When significant upper GI hemorrhage occurs in these settings, upper endoscopy is indicated to exclude other causes of bleeding. Stress-related mucosal damage has the characteristic appearance of multiple, bleeding, superficial erosions. Aggressive medical and pharmacologic therapy and attention to treatment of the patient's underlying illness usually stop the bleeding.

Esophagitis and Esophageal Ulcer

Reflux-induced esophagitis and bleeding should be treated by vigorous medical antireflux measures and acid suppression after endoscopic diagnosis. Refractory bleeding can usually be controlled acutely with endoscopic hemostatic injection therapy, but long-term control may require an antireflux operation. Other causes of esophageal bleeding include ulceration arising in Barrett's esophagus, malignant ulcer, postsclerotherapy ulcer, infectious ulcer (herpes simplex or cytomegalovirus), and pill ulcers (quinidine, iron, NSAIDs, potassium, tetracycline). Bleeding from any of these causes can usually be controlled medically or endoscopically. It is rare that a patient with bleeding of esophageal origin requires emergent or even elective operation. A particularly difficult situation can be bleeding from an esophageal ulcer secondary to injection sclerotherapy in patients with portal hypertension. If medical therapy fails, endoscopic injection therapy or heater probe may be successful. Vasoconstrictors and balloon tamponade should be instituted if endoscopic therapy fails, and semiemergent portosystemic shunting or transjugular intrahepatic portosystemic shunting (TIPS) should be undertaken as a last resort.

Varices

Bleeding esophagogastric varices are caused by portal hypertension, usually due to cirrhosis. In North America, 90% of bleeding esophagogastric varices are due to chronic alcoholism, whereas in Asia and developing countries, varices arise primarily as the consequence of hepatitis B–induced postnecrotic cirrhosis or schistosomiasis. The risk of bleeding from varices is related to the severity of the patient's underlying liver disease,[54] a corrected portal pressure exceeding 12 mmHg, variceal size,[55] and specific endoscopic signs,[54,56] including diffuse redness on top of varices; hematocystic spots; large, tortuous varices; proximal extension in the esophagus; and esophagitis. Recent heavy alcoholic intake can acutely increase portal pressure and thus precipitate variceal bleeding. Bleeding esophagogastric varices account for between 10% and 30% of all episodes of GI bleeding, depending on the patient population. A minority of cases of portal hypertension and bleeding esophagogastric varices arise from occlusion of the portal or splenic vein.[57]

Diagnosis

All patients with suspected variceal bleeding should undergo emergent upper endoscopy. Endoscopy should document the number, size, and length of varices; the location of bleeding, if present; and signs of recent bleeding. About 90% of bleeding esophagogastric varices arise near the gastroesophageal junction.[58] Occasionally, bleeding originates from gastric varices or portal hypertensive gastropathy. Rarely, bleeding results from duodenal, stomal, or rectal varices.[57] Nonvariceal causes of upper GI hemorrhage are present in 20% to 50% of patients with known varices.[59]

Management

Figure 8-12 illustrates a treatment algorithm for bleeding esophagogastric varices.[57] All patients require immediate resuscitation, correction of coagulation defects, and admission to the intensive care unit. Transfusion is required in most patients. Pharmacologic reduction of portal pressure can temporarily arrest variceal hemorrhage (Table 8-13). Intravenous vasopressin is the most widely used vasoconstrictor. Side effects of mesenteric and myocardial ischemia with this drug can be reduced by simultaneous infusion of nitroglycerin. Studies suggest that octreotide and metoclopramide are also effective.

Endoscopic sclerotherapy or variceal banding is highly effective at acutely stopping variceal bleeding (about a 90% success rate).[20,57,60,61] Variceal banding is a new technique that appears to be as efficacious as sclerotherapy and is associated with fewer complications of deep ulcers and stricture.[20,29] When a delay in

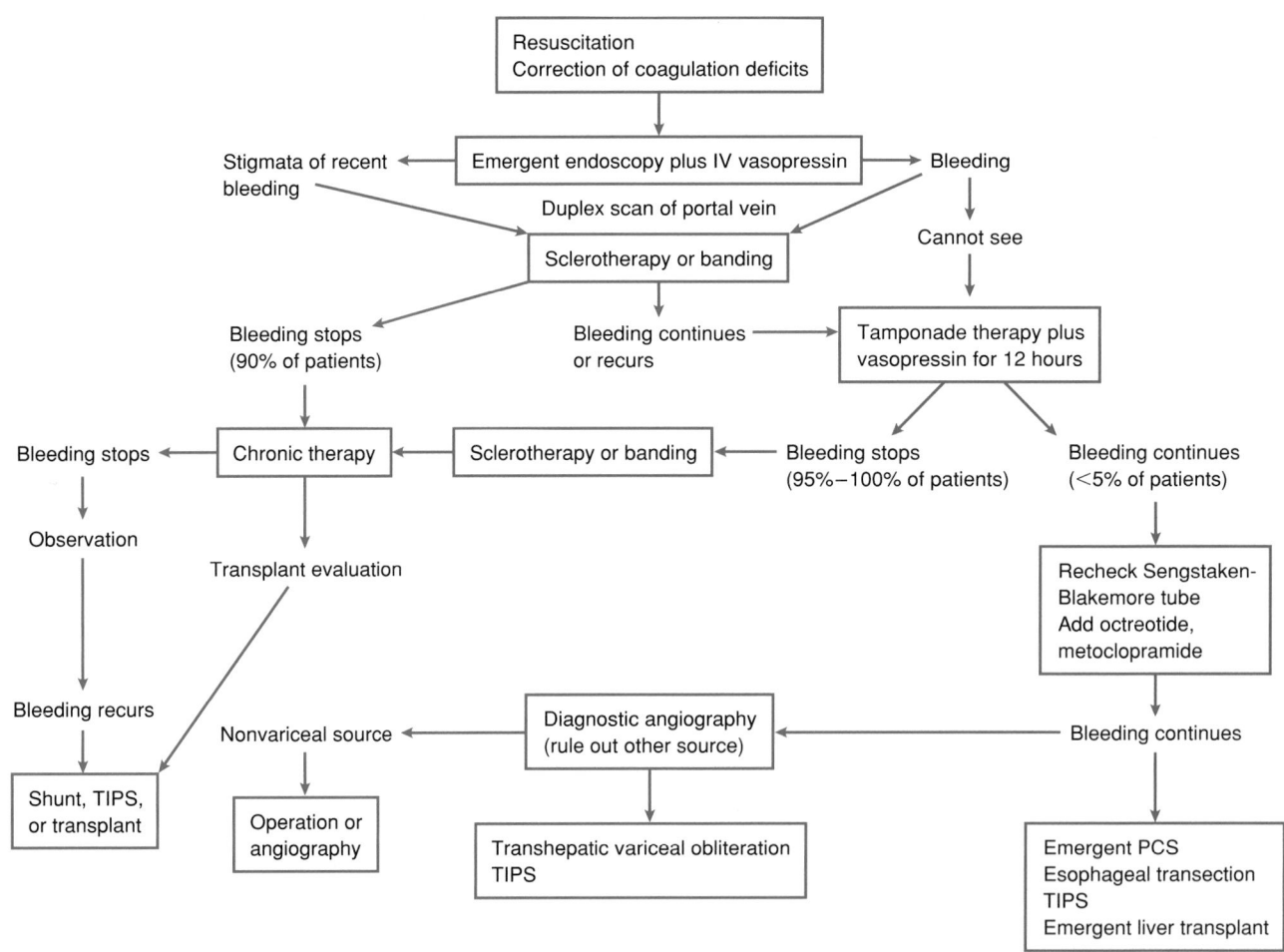

Figure 8-12 Diagnostic and therapeutic algorithm for bleeding esophagogastric varices. TIPS, transjugular intrahepatic portosystemic shunt; PCS, portacaval shunt.

Table 8-13   Pharmacologic Control of Bleeding Varices

Drug	Dosage	Efficacy (%)	Complications
Vasopressin	0.4–0.6 U/min	30–70 (acute)	High
Nitroglycerin	40–400 μg/min IV, keep blood pressure >100 syst		Low
Somatostatin	50 μg/h IV infusion	50–70 (acute)	Low
Metoclopramide	20 mg IV push	80–90 (acute)	Low

emergent endoscopy is unavoidable, pharmacologic therapy alone or in combination with balloon tamponade is indicated until endoscopy can be performed. Exsanguinating patients should be emergently intubated, followed by placement of a tamponade tube (Fig. 8-13). This approach controls up to 95% of all bleeding esophagogastric varices.[57] If bleeding continues, the physician should recheck the position and force of the tamponade tube and consider the possibility that the bleeding is coming from a nonvariceal source.

All physicians who treat patients with esophagogastric varices should be familiar with the proper use of esophageal tamponade devices. Improper use of these tubes is associated with high patient mortality secondary to pulmonary aspiration and esophageal rupture. Patients should have their airway protected by endotracheal intubation before placement of these tubes. After sedation, the well-lubricated tube is placed through the mouth and on through the esophagus into the stomach. The tube should slide easily and never be forced. The tube is then aspirated, and air is injected into the gastric port to document its position in the stomach. Tube position in the stomach should be confirmed by an abdominal radiograph after placement of 50 mL of air into the gastric balloon, to avoid injury to the esophagus. Next, an additional 300 mL of air is insufflated, and the tube is retracted with 1 to 2 kg of force and then secured to the face guard of a football helmet or catcher's mask. When bleeding is not controlled with inflation of the gastric balloon, the esophageal balloon should be inflated to no more than 40 mmHg. The esophagus above the gastric or esophageal balloon should be continuously suctioned to evacuate oral secretions.

The mortality rate from bleeding varices is about 50% per episode.[57] Early rebleeding occurs in a high percentage of patients, and definitive therapy should be planned at the first hospitalization. Duplex sonography is imperative to identify patients with portal or splenic vein occlusion because noncirrhotic patients with esophageal or gastric varices secondary to portal vein or splenic vein thrombosis are cured by splenorenal shunt and splenectomy, respectively.[62] Long-term therapy for portal hypertension and bleeding esophageal and gas-

tric varices in cirrhotic patients includes β-blockers, chronic sclerotherapy or banding, portosystemic shunting, devascularization operations, and liver transplantation. These approaches are discussed in Chapter 20.

Mallory-Weiss Tear

Mallory-Weiss tears, linear lacerations in the mucosa of the gastroesophageal junction, account for 8% to 16% of upper GI bleeding (see Table 8-5). The classic history is one of forceful vomiting, retching, or coughing that precedes hematemesis in an alcoholic patient.[63] In fact, most patients who present with Mallory-Weiss tears have no history of prior emesis.[59] Most Mallory-Weiss tears are located on the gastric side of the gastroesophageal junction, with fewer than 20% involving the esophagus. Bleeding from Mallory-Weiss tears stops spontaneously without any form of therapy in 80% to 90% of patients,[64,65] and rebleeding is uncommon. For patients who have persistent or significant bleeding, endoscopic injection or thermal techniques are highly effective. When endoscopic therapy is available, the need to oversew a Mallory-Weiss tear should be rare. If endoscopic therapy is unsuccessful, a vertically oriented gastrotomy is placed in the stomach to within 4 cm of the cardioesophageal junction to facilitate oversewing the gastroesophageal junction with absorbable sutures.

Dieulafoy's Ulcer

Patients who present with massive, recurrent, and obscure upper GI bleeding should be suspected of harboring an ectatic submucosal artery within the stomach that has erupted into the lumen.[66] Significant ulceration is not seen in these patients. Lesions typically occur within 10 cm of the gastroesophageal junction, generally along the lesser curvature of the stomach.[67] These lesions bleed intermittently and appear as spurting submucosal vessels. Endoscopic therapy with injection or electrocoagulation may stop the bleeding.[67,68] When endoscopy is not definitive, the patient should undergo laparoscopy[69] or laparotomy with wedge re-

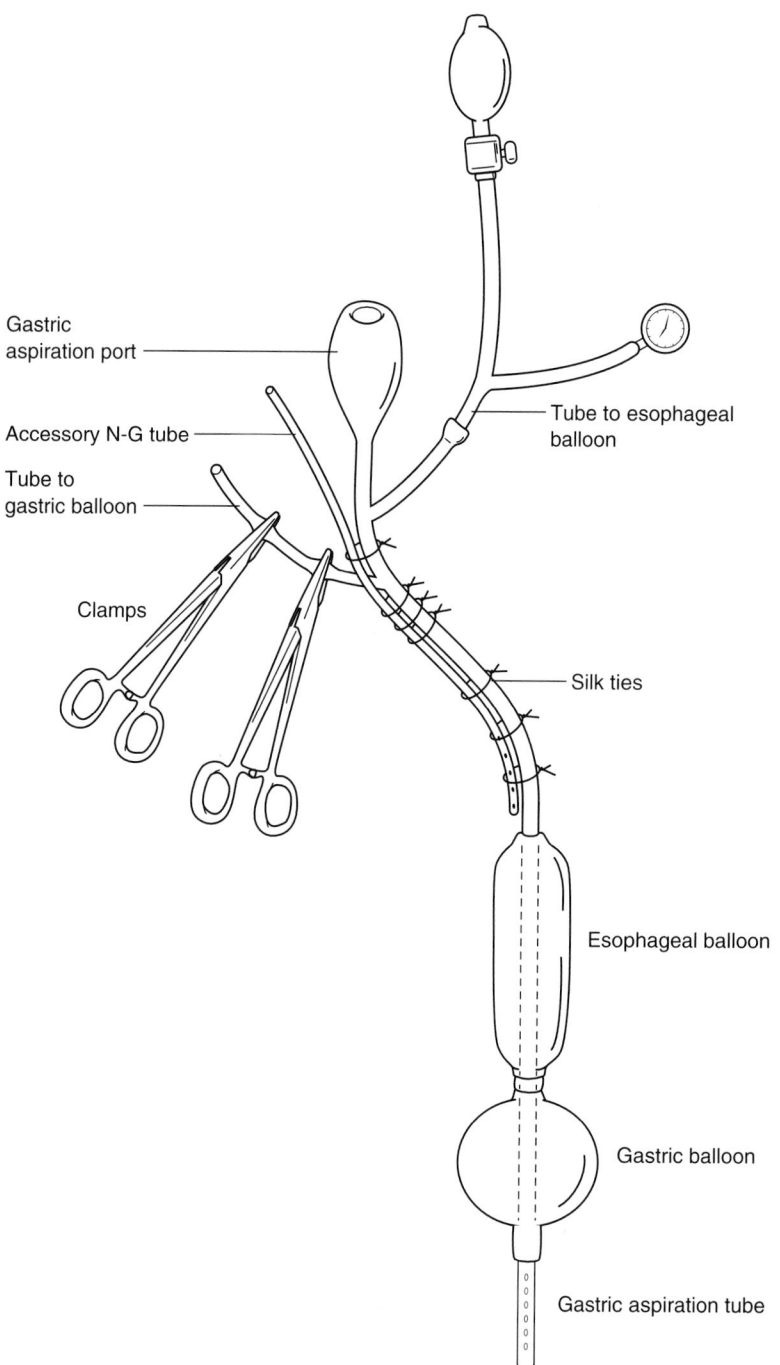

Gastric
aspiration port

Accessory N-G tube

Tube to
gastric balloon

Clamps

Tube to esophageal
balloon

Silk ties

Esophageal balloon

Gastric balloon

Gastric aspiration tube

Figure 8-13 Sengstaken-Blakemore tube.

section of the lesion.[67,68] Laparoscopic wedge resection with a linear stapling device requires simultaneous endoscopy to ensure that the resection includes the mucosal site of bleeding.

Dieulafoy's lesions were initially thought to occur only in the stomach and in elderly patients with atherosclerotic vascular disease. Reports have demonstrated, however, that this vascular lesion also occurs in the nonelderly[67] and in the duodenum and jejunum.[70,71] Le-

sions in the duodenum can be successfully treated by endoscopic injection hemostatic therapy,[70] but recurrent bleeding is an indication for operation.

Hemobilia

The term *hemobilia* describes hemorrhage into the biliary tract. In 1972, most cases of hemobilia were secondary to liver trauma (48%), biliary infection (28%), gallstones (10%), pseudoaneurysms of the hepatic artery (7%), and primary or metastatic tumors (5%).[72] Today, hemobilia is usually iatrogenic, due to percutaneous liver biopsy and interventional manipulations of the liver, portal system, and biliary tree.[73] Up to 4% of percutaneous cholangiograms[74] and 9% of percutaneously placed transhepatic biliary drains result in hemobilia.[75] Hemobilia also results when the hepatic artery or one of its branches ruptures or is eroded by an adjacent inflammatory process (eg, gallstones, intrahepatic and biliary infections), pressure necrosis from biliary stents, infiltrating tumors (hepatomas and cholangiocarcinomas), or rupture of pseudoaneurysms resulting from blunt or penetrating hepatic trauma. Iatrogenic injury to the bile duct or branches of the hepatic artery during upper abdominal operations, particularly open cholecystectomy, common bile duct exploration, and liver resection, can result in hemobilia. Pancreatitis or pseudocysts can erode into the splenic or gastroduodenal arteries, resulting in pseudoaneurysm rupture into the bile duct.

Diagnosis

Hemobilia should be strongly suspected in any patient with a history of hepatic trauma, recent hepatobiliary surgery, or percutaneous hepatic interventional procedure who has hematemesis, melena, or GI blood loss of undetermined origin. GI bleeding associated with right upper quadrant pain, biliary colic, and jaundice suggests hemobilia. Hemobilia may be obvious when a T-tube or percutaneous biliary catheter drains blood. In the absence of a catheter in the biliary tree, hemobilia is diagnosed most commonly by direct visualization of blood coming from the ampulla of Vater, by hepatic arteriography, or by a ^{99m}Tc-labeled red cell scan. Cholangiography can reveal filling defects from blood clots within the bile ducts. If hemobilia is intermittent, the ^{99m}Tc-labeled red cell scan is possibly the most sensitive diagnostic test. Patients with hemodynamically significant bleeding should undergo emergent mesenteric angiography before any other diagnostic test because angiographic embolization of the bleeding site is the treatment of choice[76] (Fig. 8-14).

Treatment and Outcome

Angiographic embolization is the procedure of choice for all causes of hemobilia and has a success rate approaching 100%.[77] Superselective embolization is not only more successful in identifying the site of bleeding but also has lower mortality and morbidity rates than does surgery in patients with hemobilia.[78] The mortality rate from hemobilia was previously signifi-

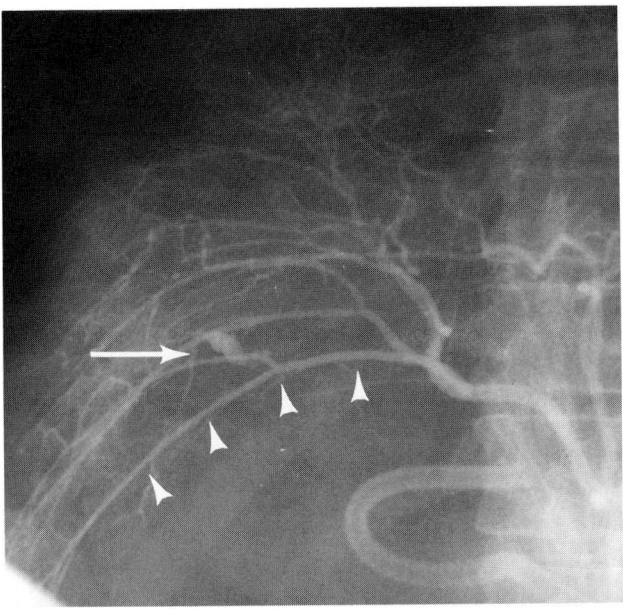

Figure 8-14 Hepatic angiogram in a patient with massive hemobilia after common bile duct exploration. There is bleeding (contrast extravasation; *arrow*) from a branch of the right hepatic artery. Cephalic displacement of the vessels (*arrowheads*) by a large subhepatic hematoma is visible. (Courtesy of Dr. C. Rohrmann, University of Washington, Seattle)

cant, ranging between 10% and 20% in large series.[79] High mortality is related to delay in diagnosis and depends on the underlying cause of the disease and condition of the patient. With prompt diagnosis and treatment using angiographic techniques, the mortality rate from hemobilia is low.

Meckel's Diverticulum

Meckel's diverticulum should be suspected in any patient with significant GI bleeding presenting as melena or hematochezia in whom colonoscopy, upper endoscopy, and angiography are negative. Bleeding is the most common problem associated with Meckel's diverticulum and occurs in about half of patients when the diverticulum contains ectopic gastric mucosa.[80] Bleeding tends to be pronounced and is associated with mortality rates as high as 6%.[81]

Because gastric mucosa concentrates technetium, a ^{99m}Tc-pertechnetate scan detects a bleeding Meckel's diverticulum in 50% to 90% of cases[81]—even when it is not actively bleeding (Fig. 8-15). Small bowel enteroclysis can also reveal a Meckel's diverticulum. When suspected, laparoscopy should be performed to confirm the diagnosis. If a Meckel's diverticulum is identified, segmental small bowel resection is indicated.[82] Extracorporeal small bowel resection is performed by bring-

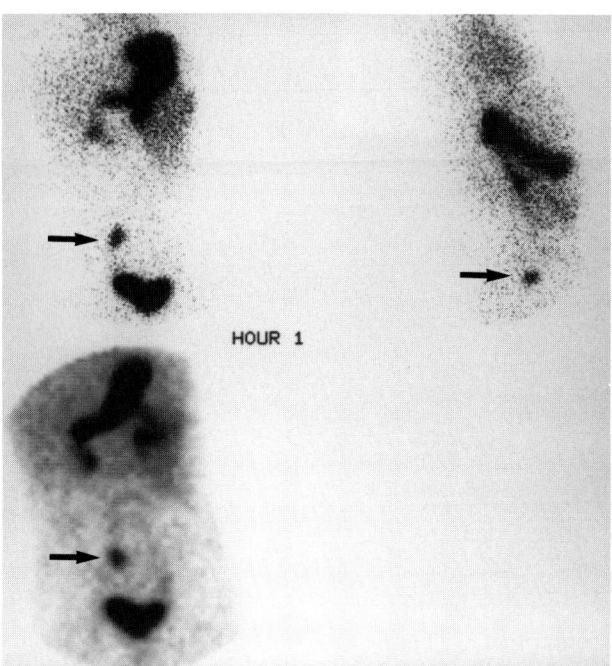

Figure 8-15 Positive ^{99m}Tc pertechnetate scan showing a typical Meckel's diverticulum with ectopic gastric epithelium imaged by scintigraphy (*arrows*). (Courtesy of Dr. M. Graham, University of Washington, Seattle)

ing the ileum up through a muscle split incision placed in the right lower quadrant.

Neoplasms

Benign and malignant tumors of the GI tract are common causes of chronic, occult bleeding but do not usually present as acute or life-threatening bleeding. When located in the esophagus, stomach, duodenum, colon, or rectum, tumors are usually identified by endoscopy. Immediate control of bleeding usually can be achieved by endoscopic therapy, whereas surgical resection is the treatment of choice for long-term control. When bleeding tumors are located in the small bowel, diagnosis can be more difficult. Small bowel follow-through radiographs can demonstrate mucosal lesions anatomically associated with bleeding lesions shown by superselective angiography or red blood cell scan. The small bowel contrast study in Figure 8-10*A* demonstrates multiple mucosal metastases secondary to melanoma, and the selective angiogram reveals the site of bleeding by contrast pooling in the same loop of small bowel.

Vascular Enteric Fistula

Aortoenteric fistula is a rare but lethal cause of GI hemorrhage. The most common site of aortoenteric fistula is between the third portion of the duodenum and the proximal aortic suture line after reconstructive abdominal aortic surgery. Patients may have occult, intermittent, or exsanguinating hemorrhage as the initial manifestation of an aortoenteric fistula. A so-called herald bleed occurs in a number of patients in whom a brief episode of bleeding spontaneously stops but is followed by massive hemorrhage several days or weeks later. Signs and symptoms of bacteremia and sepsis can accompany the GI bleeding and may be the only evidence of fistula.

All patients with a history of previous intraabdominal vascular surgery presenting with hematochezia, melena, hematemesis, or occult guaiac-positive stool should be considered to have a vascular enteric fistula. Visualization of vascular graft material or bleeding from the distal portion of the duodenum are usually diagnostic but present in less than 40% of patients.[83] Abdominal computed tomography with intravenous and oral contrast usually shows direct apposition of the duodenum to the aorta without any fat plane between the two structures.[84] Graft infection, demonstrable on computed tomographic scan as fluid surrounding the graft, should also raise suspicion of an enteric fistula. Angiography and bowel contrast studies are not indicated, because they have a high false-negative rate. Less than one third of aortoenteric fistulas are diagnosed without an operation.[85] Hence, if a site of bleeding cannot be identified in a patient who has an aortic graft, abdominal exploration is indicated to exclude the presence of a fistula. The treatment of choice for any vascular enteric fistula is extraanatomic bypass, removal of the infected graft, closure of the intestinal fistula, and buttressing of the vascular stump with vascularized healthy tissue. The overall mortality rate is high in these patients (about 80%), and death is usually secondary to exsanguinating hemorrhage through the fistula preoperatively or to a delayed ''blow-out'' of the aortic stump closure occurring weeks to months after reconstruction. A nontraditional form of intraabdominal bypass has been reported with good palliation and reasonable long-term survival.[86]

Postoperative Gastrointestinal Bleeding

Life-threatening GI hemorrhage in the early postoperative period can present as an unexplained fall in hematocrit, hypovolemia or hypotension, hematemesis, melena, or hematochezia. The three most common causes of postoperative GI hemorrhage are bleeding from anastomotic suture lines, inadequately treated peptic ulcers, and missed coexistent pathology.[51] The patient's history is the most important clue to the nature of the bleeding. For example, cardiac surgery patients with upper GI hemorrhage have acute duodenal ulcer as the most common cause of bleeding.[6] Patients should be promptly resuscitated and adequate intravenous access ensured. Coagulation status must be checked and corrected. Anticoagulants and NSAIDs should be stopped. If the patient has received aspirin, platelet transfusion may be indicated.

Stable patients with upper intestinal bleeding should undergo gastric lavage and emergent endoscopy. The presence of a recently created gastric or intestinal anastomosis does not eliminate endoscopic examination, although care must be taken with air insufflation and manipulation of the scope. If a bleeding site is identified, endoscopic hemostasis should be attempted. If hemostasis cannot be achieved, the patient should be promptly returned to the operating room. Hemodynamically unstable patients should not undergo endoscopy but should proceed directly to the operating room.

Suture Line Bleeding

If bleeding originates from the suture line of a gastroenterostomy, the stomach should be opened longitudinally at least 4 cm above the anastomosis rather than dismantling the suture line (Fig. 8-16). The stomach is evacuated of clot, and the suture line is inspected. Identified points of suture line bleeding can be directly oversewn. If no site of bleeding is identified, the entire stomach and distal esophagus are inspected to exclude coexistent pathology, including gastric ulcer, gastritis, varices, esophagitis, or esophageal tear. The lesser sac should be entered to allow complete mobilization of the stomach and palpation and exposure of the posterior

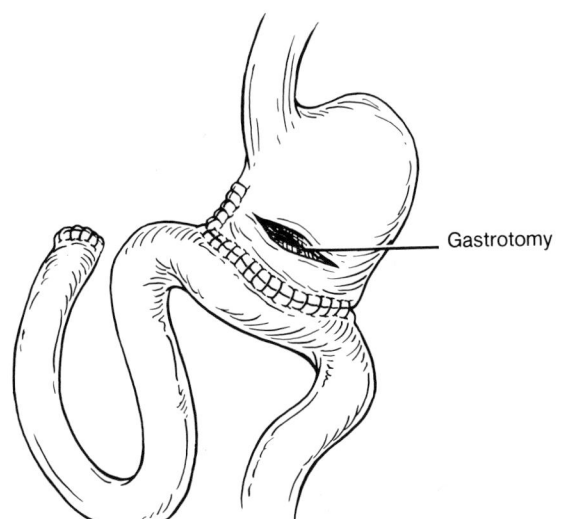

Figure 8-16 Placement of a gastrotomy incision to inspect suspected suture line bleeding.

stomach wall. If thorough exploration of the entire stomach is not achieved directly, the gastrotomy is closed and the duodenum occluded. This maneuver allows the stomach to be insufflated for an endoscopic examination.

Postpolypectomy Bleeding

Postpolypectomy bleeding can be immediate or delayed up to 14 days. Immediate bleeding occurs when the stalk of a polyp is cut before sufficient coagulation of the stalk vessels occurs. Repeat colonoscopy is indicated to control the bleeding. If the amount of bleeding is too great to allow identification of the polypectomy site, the patient should be taken to the angiography suite for angiographic control of bleeding or to the operating room. If a remnant stalk can be identified, it should be grasped with a snare and held for 10 minutes without use of cautery. If rebleeding occurs on release, careful electrocoagulation or injection of the stalk with epinephrine should be performed. When blood obscures the polypectomy site, the patient's position should be shifted to drain the blood away from the area.

SPECIFIC CAUSES OF LOWER GASTROINTESTINAL BLEEDING

Diverticular Bleeding

Bleeding from colonic diverticula is generally seen in elderly patients (older than 65 years) with asymptomatic diverticulosis and not in those with diverticulitis. Bleeding is usually abrupt in onset, often massive, and usually painless. Diverticular bleeding accounts for about 20% of causes of bleeding in patients presenting with massive hematochezia. Diverticular bleeding stops spontaneously in most patients. In one report,[18] about 5% of patients with diverticular bleeding required operation. Others[33,37] reported that the need for operation for persistent or recurrent diverticular bleeding is between 41% and 47%. Diverticular bleeding can usually be localized by colonoscopy after bowel preparation with lavage.[37] Colonoscopic diagnosis is based on visualizing active bleeding from a diverticulum or adherent clot within a diverticulum without evidence of bleeding from other sites in the colon. When bleeding is massive or colonoscopy is unavailable, angiography should be used. Diagnosis is made by seeing contrast pooling in a segment of colon known to have diverticula (Fig. 8-17). Angiographically administered vasopressin has been reported to control 92% of cases of acutely bleeding diverticula, although recurrent bleeding is not uncommon. Angiographic localization and hemostasis of di-

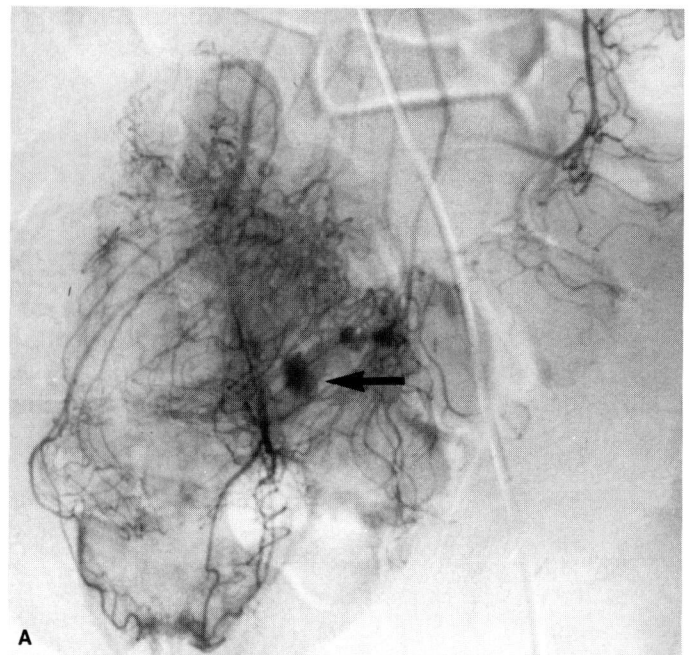

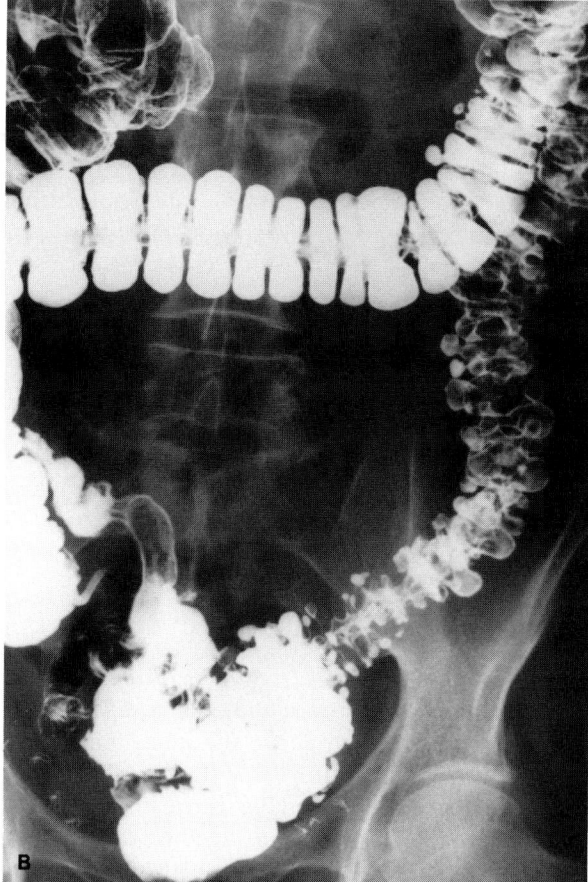

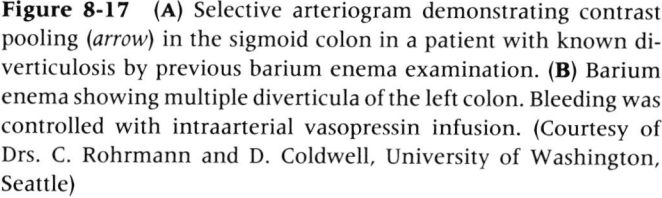

Figure 8-17 (**A**) Selective arteriogram demonstrating contrast pooling (*arrow*) in the sigmoid colon in a patient with known diverticulosis by previous barium enema examination. (**B**) Barium enema showing multiple diverticula of the left colon. Bleeding was controlled with intraarterial vasopressin infusion. (Courtesy of Drs. C. Rohrmann and D. Coldwell, University of Washington, Seattle)

verticular bleeding leads to hemodynamic stabilization of the patient and directs segmental colon resection for persistent bleeders, with an operative mortality rate of 11%.[87] Preoperative localization and segmental colon resection lead to about a 6% incidence of recurrent diverticular bleeding, compared with a 33% incidence after undirected hemicolectomy.[88] Mortality in these patients is related to advanced patient age and comorbid illness, delay in diagnosis, hypotension, and large transfusion requirements. Undirected subtotal colectomy should be performed only when intraoperative colonoscopy is nondiagnostic and bleeding proximal to the cecum has been excluded.

Vascular Anomalies

A number of acquired and congenital vascular anomalies can lead to acute, recurrent, or chronic bleeding from the upper and lower GI tracts. Some of the vascular malformations of the gut are associated with cutaneous disorders, including hereditary hemorrhagic telangiectasia (Osler-Weber-Rendu syndrome),[89] elastic tissue disorders (pseudoxanthoma elasticum and Ehlers-Danlos syndrome),[90] CREST syndrome, and blue rubber bleb syndrome.[91] Vascular lesions in all these conditions are benign, found throughout the GI tract, and usually detectable by endoscopy. Bleeding is usually intermittent, recurrent, and mild. Endoscopic thermal ablation is the treatment of choice if the lesions can be seen.[37,92] When lesions are diffuse, extensive, or in the small bowel, surgical resection is usually required. Vascular lesions in patients with Osler-Weber-Rendu syndrome may regress with estrogen–progesterone therapy.[93]

Angiodysplasia

Angiodysplasia is a microvascular abnormality of the mucosa and submucosa of the colon that can rupture or ulcerate and cause chronic, intermittent, or acute colonic bleeding. The pathogenesis of angiodysplasia is believed to be related to chronic obstruction of small veins passing through a hypertrophied muscularis propria. Obstruction results in capillary dilation and the formation of arteriovenous malformations. The most common site of angiodysplasia is in the large-diameter cecum and proximal right colon where transmural bowel wall tension is greatest.[94] Angiodysplasia is most commonly seen in elderly patients and is associated with renal failure and aortic stenosis.[94,95] The prevalence of angiodysplasia ranges from 1.4% to 53% of elderly patients with no symptoms and accounts for about 30% of episodes of massive hematochezia.[34] About 11% of patients with colonic angiodysplasia also have small bowel lesions.[96] Bleeding from angiodysplastic lesions is usually slower than bleeding from diverticula and stops spontaneously in 80% of patients; recurrent and chronic bleeding is not uncommon. When a patient bleeds a second time, the risk of future hemorrhage increases to 50%.[97]

Diagnosis

Colonoscopy is the first choice for diagnosing angiodysplasia of the colon, with a reported specificity approaching 99% and sensitivity of 68%.[98] Sensitivity increases to 81% with adequate bowel preparation. Mucosal involvement by angiodysplasia is requisite for colonoscopic diagnosis. Angiodysplastic lesions are typically 4 to 8 mm in diameter, cherry red, flat, or slightly raised (Fig. 8-18). The edges appear scalloped, and larger draining veins may be visible.[98] Lesions can occur singly or in groups. Larger lesions may appear superficially eroded and can be confused with inflammatory bowel disease or radiation-induced telangiectasia. Angiographic criteria for diagnosis include clusters of small arteries, visualization of a vascular tuft, and early and prolonged opacification of a draining vein, usually the ileocolic. Angiography detects only 36% to 70% of cases.[99] If angiography is performed while bleeding occurs, detection rates approach 86%. Colonoscopic diagnosis of acute bleeding may not be safe or possible when bleeding is massive. Under these circumstances, angiography is warranted for both diagnosis and temporary control of bleeding by superselective vasopressin infusion.[33]

Treatment

Treatment of angiodysplasia is indicated when it is identified as the site of bleeding or when recurrent colonic bleeding requires transfusion and no other lesions in the lower or upper GI tract are identified. As recently as 1986, subtotal colectomy was recommended as the procedure of choice for angiodysplasia of the colon.[33] Angiographic infusion of vasopressin can temporarily control nearly all patients with bleeding angiodysplasia, but the incidence of recurrent bleeding is high (about 33%).[33] Nevertheless, temporary angiographic hemostasis allows postponement of surgery until the patient is in a more stable condition, permits segmental resection, and reduces postoperative mortality. Even with preoperative angiographic localization, 10% of patients with angiodysplasia experience rebleeding after operation because of the multifocal nature of the disease. Angiographic embolization of bleeding angiodysplastic lesions with Gelfoam is effective but is associated with an 18% recurrence rate and 40% hospital mortality rate related to colonic ischemia.[100]

The preferred therapy for angiodysplastic lesions is eradication by endoscopic thermal techniques—Nd:YAG laser, multipolar coagulation, or heater probe.[92,101] If colonoscopy cannot be performed because of a rapid rate of bleeding, angiographic control of the bleeding is obtained by superselective intraarterial vasopressin infusion. This maneuver almost always provides hemodynamic stabilization and allows adequate bowel preparation and then semielective colonoscopic therapy. Success rates with this approach range between 86% and 90% using the argon or Nd:YAG laser, with an ac-

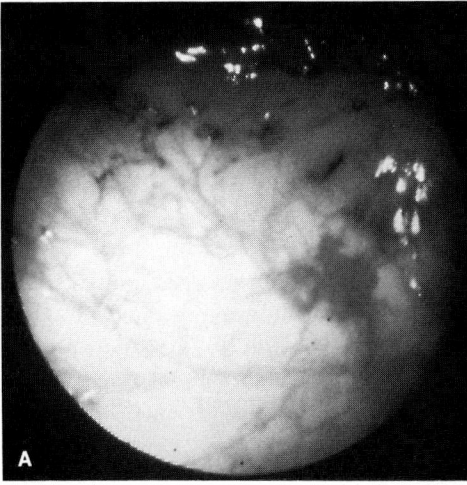
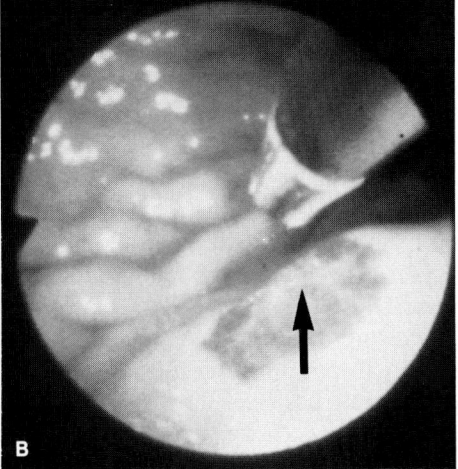

Figure 8-18 Angiodysplastic lesion of the right colon before (**A**) and after (**B**) endoscopic electrocoagulation. (See Color Fig. 8-18.) (Courtesy of Dr. M. Kimmey, University of Washington, Seattle)

ceptably low complication rate of 0% to 6%.[92,95] Like surgery, failures are usually related to missed lesions in other parts of the bowel. Electrocoagulation of the right colon requires caution because of the risk of perforation. Emergency surgery for bleeding angiodysplasia should be reserved for young patients, patients with intractable bleeding, and patients who have numerous or extensive lesions.

Varices

Rectal and colonic varices may occur in portal hypertension. The latter usually occur at colostomy sites. The varices tend to run longitudinally, are often tortuous, and are blue in color. Care must be taken not to mistake varices for a colonic polyp. Endoscopic Doppler or ultrasound can distinguish varices from solid lesions. Bleeding rectal and sigmoid varices are best treated by endoscopic banding or injection sclerotherapy, which also can be used on stomal varices. Rectal varices can also be oversewn through an operating anoscope.

Vasculitis

Vasculitis of the colon and rectum as a cause of lower GI bleeding is rare. These lesions can occur in patients with Henoch-Schönlein syndrome and polyarteritis nodosa or can be secondary to radiation enteritis. Treatment depends on the severity and extent of the vasculitis and can be pharmacologic (intravenous and transrectal steroids), colonoscopic (laser), or surgical resection.

Massive Hematochezia in Immunosuppressed Patients

Immunosuppressed patients, bone marrow and solid organ transplant recipients, AIDS patients, or patients who recently underwent chemotherapy may have hematochezia secondary to an infectious etiology. Massive lower GI bleeding may be the presenting manifestation of cytomegalovirus colitis, usually arising from an ulcer in the right colon[102] (Fig. 8-19). This lesion also occurs in patients with chronic renal failure. Bleeding in bone marrow transplant recipients is usually due to radiation- and chemotherapy-induced mucositis, acute graft-versus-host disease, infection-related colitis, or neutropenic enterocolitis. Management of diffuse bleeding is almost always nonsurgical.[103] Surgery for nonlocalized GI bleeding has been shown to be highly ineffective in bone marrow transplant recipients and is associated with a high mortality rate.

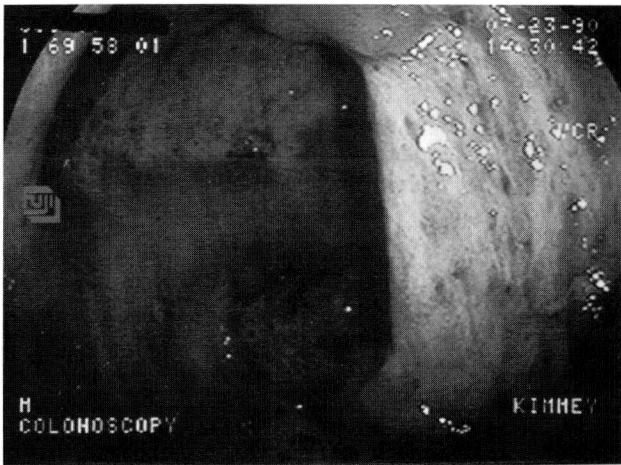

Figure 8-19 Cytomegalovirus ulcers of the colon. (See Color Fig. 8-19.) (Courtesy of Dr. M. Kimmey, University of Washington, Seattle)

Inflammatory Bowel Disease

Gastrointestinal hemorrhage in patients with inflammatory bowel disease accounts for up to 10% of patients presenting with severe hematochezia.[37,44] Most patients with ulcerative colitis and significant bleeding also have a history of prolonged diarrhea and other manifestations of inflammatory bowel disease. In more than two thirds of these patients, bleeding is controlled by medical management of the ulcerative colitis.[37] Occasionally, patients require subtotal colectomy for continued bleeding and active disease. Patients with Crohn's disease can bleed significantly from an ulcer that has eroded into an intestinal artery. The most common sites of bleeding are the right colon and ileum or at an ileocolic anastomosis.

OCCULT GASTROINTESTINAL BLEEDING

Over 95% of patients with GI bleeding have a site identified in the upper or lower GI track accessible to endoscopy. For patients in whom a site of bleeding is not identified by standard upper and lower endoscopy, the most likely sources of bleeding are vascular ectatic lesions of the small bowel, malignant and benign tumors of the small bowel, ulcerative disease, and congenital anomalies.[104,105] Diagnostic work-up in these patients requires an organized approach involving several disciplines: nuclear medicine, interventional radiology, gastroenterology, and surgery. Figure 8-9 illustrates a diagnostic and therapeutic algorithm for patients with occult GI bleeding.

Extended upper endoscopy with a long endoscope (enteroscopy) to visualize the proximal jejunum, selective mesenteric angiography, ^{99m}Tc-labeled red cell scintigraphy, and small bowel enteroclysis allow successful localization of a bleeding site in most patients.[106] All these tests, however, can be nondiagnostic in patients with intermittently recurrent bleeding. Some clinicians argue that in patients younger than 50 years, extensive preoperative localization procedures should not be performed as long as intraoperative enteroscopy is available.[45,105] In patients older than 50 in whom the incidence of vascular ectasia increases, preoperative ^{99m}Tc-labeled red blood cell scintigraphy followed by angiography is advised.[106]

Algorithms such as the one displayed in Figures 8-3 and 8-8, which employ a combination of modern techniques, have significantly increased the preoperative localization of GI bleeding in patients with occult GI bleeding. Investigators reported a 100% diagnostic yield in patients with occult GI bleeding using such an approach.[45] In this series, patients had previously undergone upper GI endoscopy, colonoscopy, small bowel barium series, small bowel scintigraphy, enteroclysis, and angiography. The authors used preoperative small bowel enteroscopy, followed by intraoperative enteroscopy and intraoperative scintigraphy, significantly enhancing diagnostic yield.[107]

Vascular abnormalities constitute 34% to 40% of small bowel lesions that cause occult GI bleeding.[45,105] Small bowel enteroscopy is helpful in identifying vascular ectasia.[45,108] The lesions are usually nonpalpable. In one study,[45] only 1 of 26 arteriovenous malformations of the small bowel was identified by gross inspection and palpation, whereas 24 of 26 arteriovenous malformations were identified with small bowel enteroscopy. The therapeutic options for treating small bowel vascular ectasia include laser photocoagulation, transmural oversewing of the lesion, and intestinal resection. No data suggest that any one of these modalities is superior to the others. Unfortunately, the postoperative rebleeding rate ranges from 21% to 52%.[45,105,107]

Intraoperative enteroscopy ideally requires two teams at the operating room table: the surgical team and the endoscopic team. After thorough abdominal exploration and complete inspection and transillumination of the small bowel, enteroscopy is performed. A long endoscope or colonoscope can be introduced orally by the endoscopist and advanced distally by the surgeon. This approach has the potential for mural trauma, creating iatrogenic mucosal injury and making identification of potential bleeding lesions more difficult.[105] It is preferable to introduce the endoscope through an enterotomy made at the midpoint of the small intestine. Antegrade inspection is performed from the mid-intestine proximally, eliminating the problem of iatrogenic injury of the small bowel. Advancement of the endoscope is much easier and requires less force because of elimination of the need to negotiate the esophagus, stomach, and duodenum. Videoendoscopy allows everyone in the operating room to view the endoscopic field. The surgeon facilitates small bowel insufflation with air by compressing the intestine a short distance in front of the endoscope.

ACQUIRED IMMUNODEFICIENCY SYNDROME

Surgeons are increasingly asked to consult and treat patients with AIDS who develop life-threatening GI hemorrhage. HIV-positive patients may have GI hemorrhage originating from any of the sites seen in the general patient population. In addition, AIDS patients may have bleeding from lesions associated with other immunocompromised patients. One longitudinal study[109] demonstrated that the cumulative probability of acute GI bleeding in a group of AIDS patients was 6% at 14 months. Bleeding in these patients was associated with significantly reduced survival. In 60% of bleeding patients, the lesion was associated with AIDS, but in the remainder, the source of bleeding was not a direct consequence of HIV infection. Because many of the causes are potentially treatable, a complete diagnostic approach is indicated. The most common AIDS-associated causes of GI hemorrhage are listed in Table 8-3. Readily treated lesions include isolated cytomegalovirus ulcers, intestinal lymphoma, Kaposi's sarcoma, or cytomegalovirus enteritis. Bleeding from large Kaposi's sarcomas of the intestinal tract can be controlled with endoscopic sclerotherapy.

REFERENCES

1. Wara P, Stodkilde H. Bleeding pattern before admission as guideline for emergency endoscopy Scand J Gastroenterol 1985;20:72.
2. Griffin MR, Piper JM, Daugherty JR, Snowden M, Ray WA. Nonsteroidal anti-inflammatory drug use and increased risk for peptic ulcer disease in elderly persons. Ann Intern Med 1991;114:257.
3. Gabriel SE, Jaakkimainen L, Bombardier C. Risk for serious gastrointestinal complications related to use of nonsteroidal anti-inflammatory drugs. Am Coll Physicians 1991;115:787.
4. Carson JL, Strom BL, Schinnar R, Duff A, Sim E. The low risk of upper gastrointestinal bleeding in patients dispensed corticosteroids. Am J Med 1991;91:223.

5. Shorr RI, Ray WA, Daugherty JR, Griffin MR. Concurrent use of nonsteroidal anti-inflammatory drugs and oral anticoagulants places elderly persons at high risk for hemorrhagic peptic ulcer disease. Arch Intern Med 1993;153:1665.

6. Lebovics E, Lee SS, Dworkin BM, et al. Upper gastrointestinal bleeding following open heart surgery: predominant findings of aggressive duodenal ulcer disease. Dig Dis Sci 1991;6:757.

7. Luk GD, Bynum TE, Hendrix TR. Gastric aspiration in localization of gastrointestinal hemorrhage. JAMA 1979;241:576.

8. Cuellar RE, Gavaler JS, Alexander JA, et al. Gastrointestinal tract hemorrhage. Arch Intern Med 1990;150:1381.

9. Richards RJ, Donica MB, Grayer D. Can the blood urea nitrogen/creatinine ratio distinguish upper from lower gastrointestinal bleeding? J Clin Gastroenterol 1990;12:500.

10. Cowen AE, Macrae FA. Gastrointestinal endoscopy: an accurate and safe primary diagnostic and therapeutic modality. Med J Aust 1992;157:52.

11. Dooley C, Larson A, Stace N, et al. Double contrast barium meal and upper gastrointestinal endoscopy: a comparative study. Ann Intern Med 1984;101:538.

12. Peterson WL, Barnett CC, Smith HJ, Allen MH, Corbett DB. Routine early endoscopy in upper-gastrointestinal tract bleeding: a randomized, controlled trial. N Engl J Med 1981;304:925.

13. Sacks HS, Chalmers TC, Blum AL, Berrier J, Pagano D. Endoscopic hemostasis: an effective therapy for bleeding peptic ulcers. JAMA 1990;264:494.

14. Laine L, Cohen H, Brodhead J, et al. Prospective evaluation of immediate versus delayed rebleeding and prognostic value of endoscopy in patients with upper gastrointestinal hemorrhage. Gastroenterology 1992;102:314.

15. Ponsky JL, Hoffman M, Swyangim DS. Saline irrigation in gastric hemorrhage: the effect of temperature. J Surg Res 1980;28:204.

16. Waterman NG, Walker JL. Effect of a topical adrenergic agent on gastric blood flow. Am J Surg 1973;127:241.

17. Hart R, Classen M. Complications of diagnostic gastrointestinal endoscopy. Endoscopy 1990;22:229.

18. Gostout CJ, Wang KK, Ahlquist DA, et al. Acute gastrointestinal bleeding. J Clin Gastroenterol 1992;14:260.

19. Daneshmend TK, Bell GD, Logan RF. Sedation for upper gastrointestinal endoscopy: results of a nationwide survey. Gut 1991;32:12.

20. Stiegmann G, Goff JS, Michaletz-Onody PA, et al. Endoscopic sclerotherapy as compared with endoscopic ligation for bleeding esophageal varices. N Engl J Med 1992;326:1527.

21. Cook DJ, Guyatt GH, Salena BJ, Laine L. Endoscopic therapy for acute non-variceal upper gastrointestinal hemorrhage: a meta-analysis. Gastroenterology 1992;102:139.

22. Moreto M, Zaballa M, Ibanez S, Setien F, Figa M. Efficacy of monopolar electrocoagulation in the treatment of bleeding gastric ulcer: a controlled trial. Endoscopy 1987;19:54.

23. Lin HJ, Lee FY, Kang WM, et al. Heat probe thermocoagulation and pure alcohol injection in massive peptic ulcer haemorrhage: a prospective, randomised controlled trial. Gut 1990;31:753.

24. Laine L. Multipolar electrocoagulation in the treatment of active upper gastrointestinal tract hemorrhage: a prospective controlled trial. N Engl J Med 1987;316:1613.

25. Therapeutic endoscopy and bleeding ulcers. NIH Consensus Development Conference Statement. JAMA 1989;262:1369.

26. Laine L. Determination of the optimal technique for bipolar electrocoagulation treatment: an experimental evaluation of the BICAP and Gold probes. Gastroenterology 1991;100:107.

27. Chung SCS, Leung JWC, Steele RJC, Crofts TJ, Li AKC. Endoscopic injection of adrenaline for actively bleeding ulcers: a randomised trial. Br Med J 1988;296:1631.

28. Lin H-J, Prng C-L, Lee S-D. Is sclerosant injection mandatory after an epinephrine injection for arrest of peptic ulcer haemorrhage? A prospective, randomised, comparative study. Gut 1993;34:1182.

29. Laine L, E-Newibi HM, Migikovsky B, et al. Endoscopic ligation compared with sclerotherapy for the treatment of bleeding esophageal varices. Ann Intern Med 1993;119:1.

30. Feldman L, Greenfield AJ, Waltman AC, et al. Transcatheter vessel occlusion: angiographic results vs. clinical success. Radiology 1983;147:1.

31. Lang EK. Transcatheter embolization in management of hemorrhage from duodenal ulcer: long-term results and complications. Radiology 1992;182:703.

32. Fiorito JJ, Brandt LJ, Kozicky O, Grosman IM, Sprayragen S. The diagnostic yield of superior mesenteric angiography: correlation with the pattern of gastrointestinal bleeding. Am J Gastroenterol 1989;84:878.

33. Browder W, Cerise EJ, Litwin MS. Impact of emergency angiography in massive lower gastrointestinal bleeding. Ann Surg 1986;204:530.

34. Okazaki M, Higashihara H, Ono H, et al. Embolotherapy of massive duodenal hemorrhage. Gastrointest Radiol 1992;17:319.

35. Jensen DM, Machicado GA, Kovacs TOG, et al. Controlled, randomized study of heater probe and BICAP for hemostasis of severe ulcer bleeding. (Abstract) Gastroenterology 1988;94:A208.

36. Sugawa C, Steffes CP, Nakamura R, et al. Upper GI bleeding in an urban hospital. Ann Surg 1990;212:521.

37. Jensen M, Machicado G. Diagnosis and treatment of severe hematochezia: the role of urgent colonoscopy after purge. Gastroenterology 1988;95:1569.

38. Macrae FA, Tan K, Williams CB. Towards safer colonoscopy: complications of 5,000 diagnostic and therapeutic colonoscopies. Gut 1983;24:376.

39. Clark RA, Colley DP, Eggen FM. Acute arterial gastroin-

testinal hemorrhage: efficacy of transcatheter control. AJR 1981;136:1185.

40. Gomes AS, Lois JF, McCoy RD. Angiographic treatment of gastrointestinal hemorrhage: comparison with vasopressin infusion and embolization. AJR 1986;146: 1031.

41. Smith R, Copely DJ, Bolen FH. 99m Tc RBC scintigraphy: correlation of gastrointestinal bleeding rates with scintigraphic findings. AJR 1987;148:869.

42. Voeller GR, Bunch G, Britt LG. Use of technetium-labelled red blood cell scintigraphy in the detection and management of gastrointestinal hemorrhage. Surgery 1991;110:799.

43. Hunter JM, Pezim MD. Limited value of technetium 99m–labelled red cell scintigraphy in localization of lower gastrointestinal bleeding. Am J Surg 1990;159: 504.

44. Wagner HE, Stain SC, Gilg M, Gertsch P. Systematic assessment of massive bleeding of the lower part of the gastrointestinal tract. Surgery 1992;175:445.

45. Szold A, Katz LB, Lewis BS. Surgical approach to occult gastrointestinal bleeding. Am J Surg 1992;163:90.

46. Abercrombie JF, McAnena OJ, Rogers J, Williams NS. Laparoscopic resection of a bleeding gastric tumour. Br J Surg 1993;80:373.

47. Maleka J, Haukipuro K, Laitinen S, Kairaluoma MI. Endoscopy for the diagnosis of acute upper gastrointestinal bleeding. Scand J Gastroenterol 1991;26:1082.

48. Bornman PC, Theodorou NA, Shuttleworth RD, et al. Importance of hypovolaemic shock and endoscopic signs in predicting recurrent haemorrhage from peptic ulceration: a prospective evaluation. Br Med J 1985;291:245.

49. Brullet E, Campo R, Bedos G, et al. Site and size of bleeding peptic ulcer: is there any relation to the efficacy of hemostatic sclerotherapy? Endoscopy 1991;23:73.

50. Millat B, Hay JM, Valleur P, Fingerhut A, Fagniez PL. Emergency surgical treatment for bleeding duodenal ulcer: oversewing plus vagotomy versus gastric resection, a controlled randomized trial. World J Surg 1993;17: 568.

51. Taylor White T, Debas HT, Mulholland MW. Gastric surgery. In: Taylor White T, Mulholland MW, Harrison RC, eds. Reoperative gastrointestinal surgery. Norwalk, CT, Appleton & Lange, 1989:101.

52. Laine L. Upper gastrointestinal hemorrhage. West J Med 1991;155:274.

53. Reusser P, Gyr K, Scheudegger D, et al. Prospective endoscopic study of stress erosions and ulcers in critically ill neurosurgical patients: current incidence and effect of acid-reducing prophylaxis. Crit Care Med 1991;19: 446.

54. Beppu K, Inokuchi K, Koyanagi N, et al. Prediction of variceal hemorrhage by esophageal endoscopy. Gastrointest Endosc 1981;27:213.

55. Garcia-Tsao G, Groszmann R, Fisher R, et al. Portal pressure, presence of gastroesophageal varices and variceal bleeding. Hepatology 1985;5:419.

56. North Italian Endoscopic Club for the Study and Treatment of Esophageal Varices. Prediction of the first variceal hemorrhage in patients with cirrhosis of the liver and esophageal varices: a prospective multicenter study. N Engl J Med 1988;319:983.

57. Johansen K, Helton WS. Portal hypertension and bleeding esophageal varices. Ann Vasc Surg 1992;6:553.

58. Burroughs AK. The management of bleeding due to portal hypertension. I. The management of acute bleeding episodes. Q J Med 1988;67:447.

59. Sutton FM. Upper gastrointestinal bleeding in patients with esophageal varices: what is the most common source? Am J Med 1987;83:273.

60. Paquet KJ, Feussner H. Endoscopic sclerosis and esophageal balloon tamponade in acute hemorrhage from esophageal varices: a prospective controlled randomized trial. Hepatology 1985;5:580.

61. Larson AW, Cohen H, Zweiban B, et al. Acute esophageal variceal sclerotherapy: results of a prospective randomized controlled trial. JAMA 1986;255:497.

62. Warren WD, Henderson JM, Millikan WJ, Galambos JT, Bryan FC. Management of variceal bleeding in patients with noncirrhotic portal vein thrombosis. Ann Surg 1988;207:623.

63. Mallory GK, Weiss W. Hemorrhages from lacerations of the cardiac orifice of the stomach due to vomiting. Am J Med Sci 1929;278:506.

64. Knauer CM. Mallory-Weiss syndrome: characterization of Mallory-Weiss lacerations in 528 patients with upper gastrointestinal hemorrhage. Gastroenterology 1976; 71:5.

65. Sugawa C, Benishek D, Walk AJ. Mallory-Weiss syndrome: a study of 224 patients. Am J Surg 1983;145:30.

66. Dieulafoy G. Exulcerratio simplex: l'intervention chirurgicale dans les hematemeses foudrooyantes consecutives a l'exulceration simple de l'estomac. Bull Acad Natl Med (Paris) 1898;49:49.

67. Arora A, Mehrotra R, Patnaik PK, et al. Dieulafoy's lesion: a rare cause of massive upper gastrointestinal haemorrhage. Trop Gastroenterol 1991;12:25.

68. Bech-Knudsen F, Toftgaard C. Exulceratio simplex Dieulafoy. Surg Gynecol Obstet 1993;176:139.

69. Mixter C, Sullivan C. Control of proximal gastric bleeding: combined laparoscopic and endoscopic approach. J Laparoendosc Surg 1992;2:105.

70. Goldenberg SP, DeLuca VA Jr, Marignani P. Endoscopic treatment of Dieulafoy's lesion of the duodenum. Am J Gastroenterol 1990;85:1201.

71. Vetto JT, Richman PS, Kariger K, Passaro E Jr. Cirsoid aneurysms of the jejunum: an unrecognized cause of massive gastrointestinal bleeding. Arch Surg 1989;124: 1460.

72. Sandblom P. Hemobilia (biliary tract hemorrhage). Springfield, IL, Charles C Thomas, 1972.

73. Merrell SW, Schneider PD. Hemobilia: evolution of current diagnosis and treatment. West J Med 1991;155: 621.

74. Savader SJ, Trerotola SO, Merine DS, Venbrux AC, Os-

terman FA. Hemobilia after percutaneous transhepatic biliary drainage: treatment with transcatheter embolotherapy. J Vasc Intervent Radiol 1992;3:345.

75. Meuller PR, van Sonnenberg E, Ferruci JT. Percutaneous biliary drainage: technical and catheter related problems and 200 procedures. AJR 1982;138:17.

76. Okazaki M, Ono H, Higashihara H, et al. Angiographic management of massive hemobilia due to iatrogenic trauma. Gastrointest Radiol 1991;16:205.

77. Zajko A, Chablani V, Bron K, Jungreis C. Hemobilia complicating transhepatic catheter drainage in liver transplant recipients: management with selective embolization. Cardiovasc Intervent Radiol 1990;13:285.

78. Lygidakis NJ, Okazaki M, Damtsios G. Iatrogenic hemobilia: how to approach it. Hepatogastroenterology 1991;38:454.

79. Sandblom P. Iatrogenic hemobilia. Am J Surg 1986;151:754.

80. Mackey WC, Dineen P. A fifty year experience with Meckel's diverticulum. Surg Gynecol Obstet 1983;156:56.

81. Brown CK, Olahaker JS. Meckel's diverticulum. Am J Emerg Med 1988;6:157.

82. Echenique M, Dominguez AS, Echenique I, Rivera V. Laparoscopic diagnosis and treatment of Meckel's diverticulum complicated by gastrointestinal bleeding. J Laparoendosc Surg 1993;3:145.

83. Kleinman LH, Towne JB, Bernhard VM. A diagnostic and therapeutic approach to aortoenteric fistulas: clinical experience with 20 patients. Surgery 1979;86:868.

84. Low R, Wall S, Jeffrey R, et al. Aortoenteric fistula and perigraft infection: evaluation with CT. Radiology 1990;175:157.

85. Goldstone J, Cunningham C. Diagnosis, treatment and prevention of aorto-enteric fistulas. Acta Chir Scand 1990;555(Suppl):165.

86. Robinson J, Johansen K. Aortic sepsis: is there a role for in situ graft reconstruction? J Vasc Surg 1991;13:677.

87. Setya V, Singer JA, Minken SL. Subtotal colectomy as a last resort for unrelenting, unlocalized, lower gastrointestinal hemorrhage: experience with 12 cases. Am Surg 1992;58:295.

88. McGuire H, Haynes B. Massive hemorrhage from diverticulosis of the colon: guidelines for therapy based on bleeding patterns observed in fifty cases. Ann Surg 1972;175:847.

89. Vase P, Grove O. Gastrointestinal lesions in hereditary hemorrhagic telangiectasia. Gastroenterology 1986;91:1079.

90. McCreedy A, Zimmerman TJ, Webster SF. Management of upper gastrointestinal hemorrhage in patients with pseudoxanthoma elasticum. Surgery 1989;105:170.

91. Jennings M, Ward P, Maddocks JL. Blue rubber bleb naevus disease: an uncommon cause of gastrointestinal tract bleeding. Gut 1988;29:1408.

92. Lanthier P, d'Harveng B, Vanheuverzwyn R, et al. Colonic angiodysplasia: follow-up of patients after endoscopic treatment for bleeding lesions. Dis Colon Rectum 1989;32:296.

93. Van Cutsem E, Rutgeerts P, Vantrappen G. Treatment of bleeding gastrointestinal vascular malformations with oestrogen-progesterone. Lancet 1990;355:953.

94. Boley SJ, Sammartano R, Adams A, et al. On the nature and etiology of vascular ectasion of colon. Gastroenterology 1977;72:650.

95. Richter JM, Christensen MR, Colditz GA, Nishioka NS. Angiodysplasia: natural history and efficacy of therapeutic interventions. Dig Dis Sci 1989;34:1542.

96. Cello J, Grendell J. Endoscopic laser treatment for gastrointestinal ectasias. Ann Intern Med 1986;104:352.

97. Nath R, Sequeir F, Wertzman A, et al. Lower gastrointestinal bleeding: diagnostic approach and management conclusion. Am J Surg 1981;141:478.

98. Richter J, Hedberg S, Christos A, et al. Angiodysplasia: clinical presentation and colonoscopic diagnosis. Dig Dis Sci 1984;29:481.

99. Hutchheon D, Kabelin J, Bulkley B, et al. Effect of therapy on bleeding rates in gastrointestinal angiodysplasia. Am Surg 1987;53:6.

100. Sinderman K, Franklin J, Sos T. Successful transcatheter Gelfoam embolization of a bleeding vascular ectasia. AJR 1978;131:157.

101. Foutch PG. Angiodysplasia of the gastrointestinal tract. Am J Gastroenterol 1993;88:807.

102. Foucar E, Miukai K, Foucar K, Sutherland DER, Van Buren CT. Colon ulceration in lethal cytomegalovirus infection. Ann Surg 1981;76:788.

103. McDonald G, Shulman H, Sullivan KM, Spencer G. Intestinal and hepatic complications of human bone marrow transplantation. Gastroenterology 1986;90:460.

104. Spechler S, Schimmel E. Gastrointestinal tract bleeding of unknown origin. Arch Intern Med 1982;142:236.

105. Ress AM, Benacci JC, Sarr MG. Efficacy of intraoperative enteroscopy in diagnosis and prevention of recurrent, occult gastrointestinal bleeding. Am J Surg 1992;163:94.

106. Bowden TA. Endoscopy of the small intestine. Surg Endosc 1989;69:1237.

107. Lewis BS, Wenger JS, Waye JD. Small bowel enteroscopy and intraoperative enteroscopy for obscure gastrointestinal bleeding. Am J Gastroenterol 1991;86:171.

108. Lau WY, Wong SY, Yuen WK, Wong KK. Intraoperative enterology for bleeding angiodysplasias of small intestine. Surg Gynecol Obstet 1989;168:341.

109. Lazzarin A, Bianchi-Porro G. Acute upper gastrointestinal bleeding in patients with AIDS: a relatively uncommon condition associated with reduced survival. Gut 1991;32:987.

Digestive Tract Surgery: A Text and Atlas, edited by Richard H. Bell,
Layton F. Rikkers, and Michael W. Mulholland.
Lippincott-Raven Publishers, Philadelphia, © 1996.

9

Neoplasms of the Stomach

Sean J. Mulvihill

Worldwide, gastric neoplasms are health problems of special importance to the surgeon. Most neoplasms of the stomach arise from the epithelial lining, and most of these are adenocarcinomas. Important advances have been made in understanding the epidemiology and risk factors for certain types of gastric cancer. It is still unclear how these factors conspire to induce neoplasia. Unlike the case with colon cancer, the molecular events underlying the development of gastric cancer remain largely unexplored. A better understanding of the pathogenesis of these tumors is expected when these underlying molecular changes are defined. In some countries with high incidence of gastric cancer, screening programs have been valuable in identifying patients with early lesions. This is not an efficient strategy in the United States, and most patients in this country present with advanced lesions. Surgical resection remains the mainstay of therapy for gastric cancer. Surgery is curative for most patients with early lesions and can palliate symptoms such as pain, bleeding, or obstruction in patients with advanced cancer. Effective chemotherapy for gastric cancer remains to be developed.

GASTRIC POLYPS

Overview and Clinical Presentation

Gastric mucosal polyps are rare, especially compared with the frequency of colonic polyps. Most are incidentally discovered during endoscopic or radiologic evaluation of patients with upper gastrointestinal (GI) tract symptoms. Usually, symptoms cannot be attributed to the polyps. Occasionally, however, gastric polyps are

the source of occult GI blood loss or, if located at the pylorus, can cause intermittent symptoms of gastric outlet obstruction. Polyps should be distinguished from mucosal abnormalities secondary to submucosal tumors, such as leiomyomas or lipomas. These later conditions are discussed separately in the section, Gastric Mesenchymal Tumors. Similarly, gastric carcinoid tumors are a special type of lesion arising from enterochromaffin cells and are considered separately.

Classification

Historical autopsy series suggested that the prevalence of gastric polyps was 0.4% to 0.7% of the population at the time of death. More recent endoscopic surveys, however, suggest that gastric polyps are found in 2% to 3% of examinations. This higher figure is likely attributable to selection of patients with GI symptoms for endoscopic evaluation. The most common type of polyp is the *hyperplastic polyp* (Fig. 9-1*A*). This is not a true neoplasm but a regenerative reaction of normal epithelium to injury. Hyperplastic polyps account for about 75% of all gastric polyps. These polyps are small, usually sessile, and have no particular predilection for site of occurrence within the stomach. They are commonly associated with atrophic gastritis. *Adenomatous polyps* (see Fig. 9-1*B*) are true neoplasms and account for 5% to 10% of gastric polyps. These lesions are most commonly sessile or pedunculated, but flat and depressed lesions have been described. The microscopic pattern is usually tubular or tubulovillous. Frank villous adenomas are unusual in the stomach. Adenomatous polyps are associated with atrophic gastritis and polyposis syndromes, such as familial polyposis coli and Gardner's syndrome. Adenomatous polyps have a distinct malig-

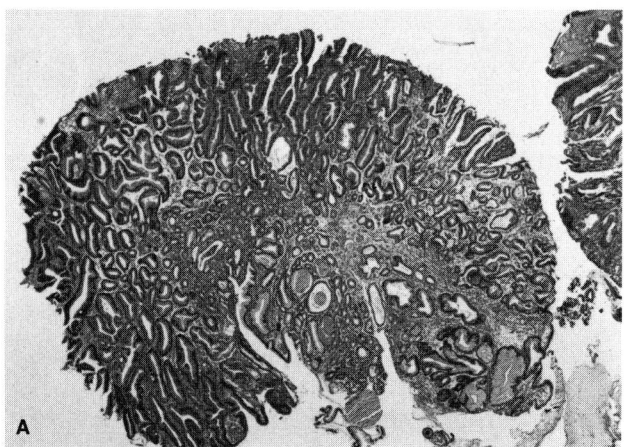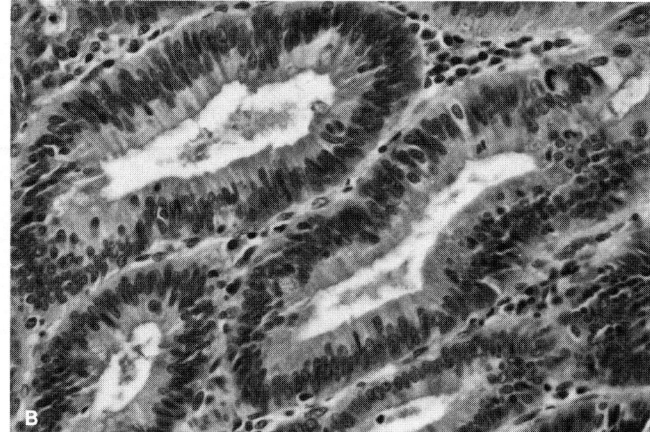

Figure 9-1 Histologic appearance of gastric polyps. **(A)** A hyperplastic polyp at low power. This lesion is usually a regenerative reaction to epithelial injury. **(B)** An adenomatous polyp at higher power. Adenomatous polyps have malignant potential. (Courtesy of Noel Weidner, MD, University of California, San Francisco)

nant potential. The risk of developing cancer is proportional to the size of the adenoma, with larger adenomas (particularly those greater than 2 cm in diameter) presenting greatest risk. The reported incidence of associated carcinoma in adenomatous polyps less than 2 cm in diameter is 24%, whereas the incidence is 4% in polyps less than 2 cm in diameter.[1] *Inflammatory polyps*, also known as *eosinophilic granulomas,* are small lesions, usually located in the antrum. Inflammatory polyps have the appearance of pyogenic granulomas. Microscopically, these tumors are composed of fibroblasts proliferating in a whorl-like pattern. Within the fibroblast matrix are numerous thin-walled blood vessels and an inflammatory infiltrate of eosinophils, lymphocytes, plasma cells, and histiocytes.

Treatment

Symptomatic polyps require excision. This can usually be accomplished with endoscopic polypectomy. Large symptomatic polyps not amenable to endoscopic resection should undergo biopsy in six to eight sites to exclude malignancy. If no cancer is identified by biopsy, the lesion should be locally excised at operation. Frozen section histologic examination of the specimen should be performed, and if carcinoma is present, appropriate gastric resection should be undertaken. Small asymptomatic adenomatous polyps should be managed with endoscopic polypectomy when identified. Asymptomatic adenomatous polyps larger than 2 cm are not usually amenable to endoscopic resection and, because of their risk for malignant transformation, should be completely excised by operative wedge resection. Small hy-

perplastic polyps can be safely monitored with yearly endoscopic examinations.

Polyposis Syndromes

Familial Polyposis Coli

This autosomal dominant syndrome is characterized by the presence of numerous sessile and pedunculated adenomatous polyps within the colon. The polyps may carpet the entire colonic mucosal surface. Polyps arise in childhood and usually become clinically evident in early adult life. Carcinoma of the colon uniformly occurs in untreated patients, most commonly by the end of the third decade of life. Sixty to 90% of these patients have asymptomatic gastric polyps in addition to the colonic lesions. When multiple gastric polyps are identified in patients with familial polyposis coli, representative biopsies should be performed. All adenomatous polyps should be excised endoscopically. In some patients, this requires multiple endoscopic sessions. Surveillance to identify new polyps should be repeated at 6-month intervals. If no adenomatous polyps are present at the initial screening examination, the surveillance interval can be safely lengthened to 3 years.[2]

Gardner's Syndrome

Gardner's syndrome is an autosomal dominant syndrome manifested by the presence of multiple colonic adenomatous polyps. In addition, these patients have bony and soft tissue lesions as well as a characteristic hypertrophy of retinal epithelial pigment, which can be detected on fundoscopic examination. As in patients with familial polyposis coli, gastric polyps are frequently present. Treatment is similar to that for patients with familial polyposis coli.

Peutz-Jeghers Syndrome

Peutz-Jeghers syndrome is characterized by the presence of hamartomatous polyps throughout the GI tract as well as perioral or mucosal melanotic pigmented lesions. Polyps are most commonly found in the small intestine but can occur in the stomach or colon. Histologically, the polyps typically show prominent branching bands of smooth muscle within the lamina propria. The clinical manifestations of Peutz-Jeghers syndrome usually arise during adolescence. The syndrome is familial and is often associated with periampullary cancer and nongastrointestinal cancer.

Cowden's Disease

Cowden's disease is an autosomal dominant disorder also known as *disseminated hereditary GI polyposis* with orocutaneous hamartomatosis.[3] These patients have multiple hamartomas in diverse tissues, including the GI tract. All sites from the esophagus to the rectum are involved with roughly equal frequency. Most of the gastric polyps are small hyperplastic lesions. Cowden's disease is the most protean of the polyposis syndromes. There is a high frequency of associated malignant tumors of various organ systems.

Juvenile Polyposis

Juvenile polyposis represents an inherited syndrome of multiple GI polyps. Although most polyps arise in the colon, in some patients, they are confined to the stomach. Unlike in familial polyposis coli, in which the histologic appearance of the polyps is uniform, the polyps in juvenile polyposis are varied. They may be hyperplastic, hamartomatous, or, occasionally, adenomatous. The natural history of these lesions is also varied: some regress spontaneously, others autoamputate. The polyps have some malignant potential.

Cronkhite-Canada Syndrome

Cronkhite-Canada syndrome is a rare, acquired, nonfamilial cause of GI polyposis that was first described in 1955.[4] The original description was of two adult patients (42 and 75 years of age) with extensive GI polyposis, especially in the stomach, associated with pigmented epidermal lesions, alopecia, and onycho-

trophia. This syndrome often has a fulminant course with GI protein loss and malnutrition.

Gastropathies

Ménétrier's Disease

This syndrome describes patients with diffuse gastric rugal hypertrophy associated with gastric carcinoma. In afflicted patients, the hypertrophic rugae are so thickened that they have been compared to cerebral convolutions. Other organs, such as the esophagus and duodenum, are uninvolved. Grossly and radiographically, the disorder can be confused with pseudolymphoma. Ménétrier's disease appears to be an acquired, not a familial, disorder, but the cause is unknown. There are no clearcut associations with other illnesses. It has been hypothesized that the disorder is due to the influence of abnormal secretion of mitogenic factors. This hypothesis, however, is unproved. Unlike gastrinoma, there is no associated parietal cell hypertrophy, nor is gastric acid hypersecretion present. About 75% of patients are male, usually 30 to 50 years of age. The main symptoms are usually nonspecific abdominal pain, occult GI blood loss, weight loss, and diarrhea. Physical examination is usually unrevealing, except for mild upper abdominal tenderness and evidence of recent weight loss. In advanced cases, edema may be present. The gastropathy is associated with paracellular leakage of protein-rich fluid, leading to hypoproteinemia. In severe cases, this results in depletion of coagulation factors, immunoglobulins, and albumin. Pathologically, the hypertrophic rugae are confined to the fundus and body in some patients. In others, however, abnormal mucosa is seen throughout the stomach. Microscopic features include hyperplasia of the surface compartment of the gastric mucosa with concomitant atrophy of the glandular component. In many patients, the gastric mucosa is involved with interstitial round cell inflammation. Cystic dilation of the basilar portion of the gastric glands is a typical finding.[5]

Treatment of patients with Ménétrier's disease is controversial because of the somewhat uncertain natural history of the disease, especially regarding the risk of carcinoma. Remission has occurred spontaneously, after treatment with histamine-2 receptor antagonists, and after vagotomy. Recurrence, however, is common. For patients with symptoms related to the hypoproteinemia, such as infections, coagulopathy, or pulmonary edema, total gastrectomy is indicated. Complete relief of symptoms and restoration of normal serum protein concentrations is seen in nearly all surgically treated patients. If resection is considered, all involved stomach must be removed, otherwise anastomotic dehiscence is a significant problem. Gastrectomy is also warranted in patients with Ménétrier's disease complicated by gastric carcinoma. Total gastrectomy is the procedure of choice if metastases are not present. Whether resection should be advised in other patients with Ménétrier's disease depends on the general health and age of the patient, the degree of the mucosal changes, and the availability of close endoscopic surveillance.

Hypertrophic, Hypersecretory Gastropathy

This rare syndrome has many of the gross features of Ménétrier's disease. A major difference, however, is the presence of parietal cell hyperplasia and acid hypersecretion. Only a few cases have been reported,[6] and the cause is unknown.

GASTRIC CARCINOMA

Epidemiology

Until 1950, gastric cancer was the leading cause of cancer death in men in the United States. The incidence of gastric cancer has fallen in the United States during the past 30 years by about 65% (Fig. 9-2). Today, gastric

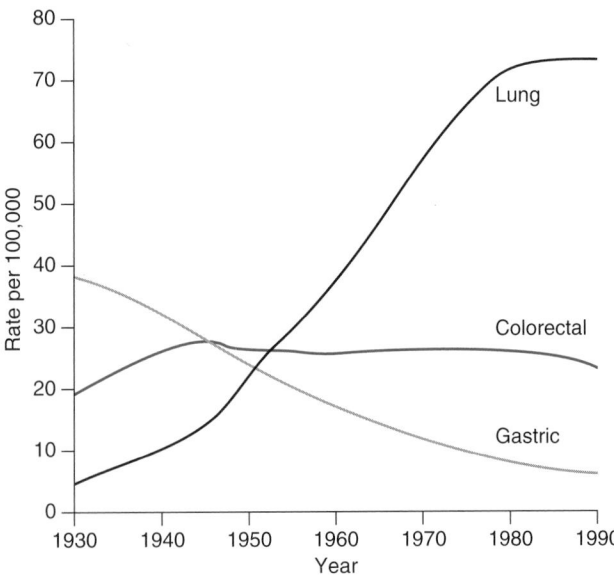

Figure 9-2 Yearly death rate from common malignancies in men in the United States. The mortality rate for patients with gastric cancer has declined significantly since 1930. That for lung cancer has risen dramatically, whereas the death rates for other tumors, such as colorectal cancer, have remained constant. (After Boring CC, Squires TS, Tong T. Cancer statistics, 1993. Cancer 1993;43:7)

cancer is the sixth most common cause of death from cancer in men and the eighth most common cause of death from cancer in women.[7] These decreases in incidence and death rate have not been completely explained. Most of the decline has been observed in the so-called intestinal-type of gastric cancer (a pathologic description is given later). Curiously, in recent years, there has been a small, unexplained increase in the incidence of gastric cancer in the United States. Gastric cancer remains a major health problem in other countries, including Japan, Chile, and Argentina. Costa Rica has the highest reported death rate from gastric cancer in the world, at 66.9 and 34.1 deaths per 100,000 per year for males and females, respectively. In the United States, 24,400 new cases of gastric cancer and 13,300 deaths from this tumor are observed yearly. The population death rates from gastric cancer in the United States are 7.4 and 3.4 per 100,000 per year for males and females, respectively.[7]

Overall, gastric cancer is twice as common in men as in women. This difference is limited to cancers located in the proximal stomach, where there is a four- to five-fold male predominance. The gender distribution of antral lesions is about equal. The risk of gastric cancer increases dramatically with age. The incidence is greater in lower socioeconomic groups than in upper-class patients. Racial differences have been observed, with blacks having the highest incidence. A distinct trend has been observed in the United States toward an increase in the number of tumors in the proximal stomach and a decline in distal tumors.

Etiology

The cause of gastric carcinoma remains puzzling, although strides have been made in recent years in identifying etiologic factors. Analysis has focused mainly on dietary and environmental factors, genetic factors, the development of precursor lesions, and, most recently, the role of the bacterium *Helicobacter pylori*. The relative importance of each of these factors in a given patient with gastric cancer is uncertain.

Environmental Factors

Environmental factors figure strongly in the pathogenesis of gastric carcinoma. Migration studies suggest that these environmental factors have special influence early in life. Studies of adult Japanese immigrants to Hawaii showed that the risk of gastric cancer was only minimally less than that of residents of Japan. Successive generations of Hawaiian-born Japanese, however, had significantly reduced risk of gastric cancer. The risk in Hawaiians of Japanese heritage is now indistinguishable from that of native Hawaiians.[8] Similar findings have been reported in Polish immigrants to the United States, European immigrants to Australia, and Puerto Rican immigrants to New York.

Dietary differences are believed to account for the geographic variations in incidence and for the differences in gastric cancer risk found in migration studies. Foods associated with gastric cancer include barbequed, smoked, or brine-cured fish or meat, starch, and pickled vegetables.[9] A strong correlation has been observed between increased salt consumption and gastric cancer.[10] A reduced risk of development of gastric cancer is present in people with diets high in fresh fruits and vegetables, vitamin C, and whole milk as well as in those with access to refrigeration. These dietary factors appear relevant to the development of a particular histologic form of gastric cancer termed *intestinal-type.* The likely link among these dietary factors is the conversion of foodstuff nitrates to nitrites and then to nitrosamines during digestion.[11] Although unproved in humans, several lines of evidence link these compounds to the development of gastric cancer. Nitrosamines have been shown to cause gastric cancer in animal models. Geographic areas with high environmental nitrate concentrations also have high rates of gastric cancer. High-risk diets, including pickled, barbequed, and smoked foods, are high in nitrates. Conversely, refrigeration inhibits the conversion of nitrates to nitrites. Similarly, vitamin C inhibits nitrosamine formation. Some bacteria resident in the stomach are capable of converting nitrates to nitrites. These bacteria are present in increased concentrations in achlorhydric patients with atrophic gastritis, a strong predisposing condition for cancer formation. Increased concentrations of nitroso compounds have also been found in the gastric juice of patients after gastric resection for benign peptic ulcers. These patients are statistically at increased risk for the future development of cancer in the remaining gastric stump.

Other environmental factors believed to increase the risk of development of gastric cancer include cigarette smoking and asbestos. These factors, however, are much less strongly correlated with gastric cancer than the previously discussed dietary influences. Ethanol and caffeine consumption do not appear to confer increased risk. A moderate reduction in risk has been observed with increased dietary fiber intake.

Genetic Factors

It has long been suspected that genetic factors influence the development of gastric cancer. People with blood group A are at increased risk, implying some genetic linkage.[12] A similar risk association has not been identified with specific human leukocytic antigens. Anecdotal papers have reported gastric cancer occurring in monozygotic twins, occasionally simultaneously. A two- to three-fold increased risk has been reported for first-degree relatives of patients with gastric cancer, and families have been reported with unusual clustering of gastric tumors.

At the molecular level, less is known of the factors leading to gastric cancer than in other systems, such as colon cancer. Mutations of the *P53* tumor suppressor gene have been reported in up to half of all patients.[13] Induction of c-*myc* and *ras* protooncogenes has been reported to occur in less than 10% of gastric cancers. One report suggests unusually high expression of tyrosine kinase, a rate-limiting enzyme in cell replication, in gastric carcinomas.[14] In a minority of patients, amplification of receptors for epidermal growth factor and transforming growth factor-α, or the related protein c-*erb*-B2 have been demonstrated.[15] No unifying molecular pathology has been identified in patients with gastric cancer, and further work is required to establish the molecular events leading to gastric carcinogenesis.

Precursor Lesions

Several precursor lesions increase the risk for development of gastric cancer, including adenomatous polyps, chronic atrophic gastritis, gastric ulcer, Ménétrier's disease, and a history of prior gastric resection. These factors relate to the development of intestinal-type cancer but have no clear relation to the development of diffuse-type cancer. As in the colon, adenomatous polyps appear to be a precursor lesion for the development of gastric cancer. The polyp–cancer sequence has not been as clearly established in the stomach as it has in the colon. An important aspect of the risk of cancer from polyps is the opportunity to intervene with endoscopic polypectomy and interrupt the process. For this reason, the value of treatment of adenomatous gastric polyps should not be minimized.

Chronic atrophic gastritis is a common, associated lesion in patients with gastric cancer, particularly the intestinal type.[16] The pathophysiology of development of carcinoma in the setting of chronic atrophic gastritis is not well understood, but hypotheses have been generated.[17] The leading view is that environmental factors, such as diet and *H pylori*, lead to a multifocal, superficial gastritis, beginning at the antral–corpus junction. The initial hyperplastic response converts to an intestinal metaplasia over time. As the metaplasia progresses, involved cells assume a colonic intestinal cell phenotype and begin to secrete sulfated mucins. Under the influence of luminal carcinogens, such as nitroso compounds, dysplastic foci develop, which progress to carcinoma. The risk factors for gastric cancer can be accounted for within this model (Fig. 9-3). Animal models of gastric carcinogenesis also support this view of stepwise progression.

Chronic inflammatory changes associated with gastric ulcer have been proposed to play a role in the development of gastric cancer, but it is difficult to separate the effects of gastric ulcer from those of other processes, such as *H pylori* infestation and chronic atrophic gastritis, because they commonly coexist. Gastric carcinomas often present as ulcerated tumors, but there is little evidence to support the idea that benign ulcers progress to malignancy.

Ménétrier's disease appears to be associated with increased risk for the development of gastric carcinoma. Follow-up studies of patients afflicted with Ménétrier's disease suggest that at least 10% develop carcinoma during observation. Although Ménétrier's disease is uncommon, its discovery offers an opportunity for early intervention, such as gastrectomy, which eliminates the risk of cancer.

Patients who previously underwent partial gastrectomy for benign peptic ulcer disease have a small, but statistically significant, increased risk for the subsequent development of gastric cancer.[18] The risk appears to be about two-fold above matched controls. For practical purposes, this level of risk is not high enough to warrant screening efforts in this patient population.[19] A history of cigarette smoking, in some series, accounts for the observed excess mortality in patients with a history of gastric surgery for ulcer disease.[20] A similar excess mortality related to cigarette smoking has been observed in ulcer patients treated with histamine-2 receptor antagonists. However, the excess mortality from gastric cancer attributed to prior gastric surgery may be due instead to other confounding risk factors, such as smoking or *H pylori*.

Helicobacter pylori

Several lines of evidence support the concept that infection of the gastric mucosa with *H pylori* plays a role in the development of gastric carcinoma.[21] First, epidemiologic studies show that the prevalence of *H pylori* infection parallels that of gastric cancer. This association has been observed both geographically and temporally. In populations with a high incidence of gastric cancer, such as Peru and Mexico, infection with the bacteria is almost universal. In the United States, the decline in incidence of gastric cancer over time is paralleled by an apparent decline in seroprevalence rates for *H pylori*. Second, *H pylori* is associated with precursor lesions that lead to the development of gastric cancer. This association has been most convincingly observed with chronic atrophic gastritis, but there is also evidence that *H pylori* may be associated with intestinal metaplasia. Third, case-control studies demonstrate a moderately increased risk of development of gastric carcinoma in patients infected with *H pylori* (Table 9-1). This risk is especially clear for intestinal-type gastric cancer. Finally, the biologic sequence of chronic inflammation leading to cell proliferation, dysplasia, and cancer has been demonstrated in models, such as ulcer-

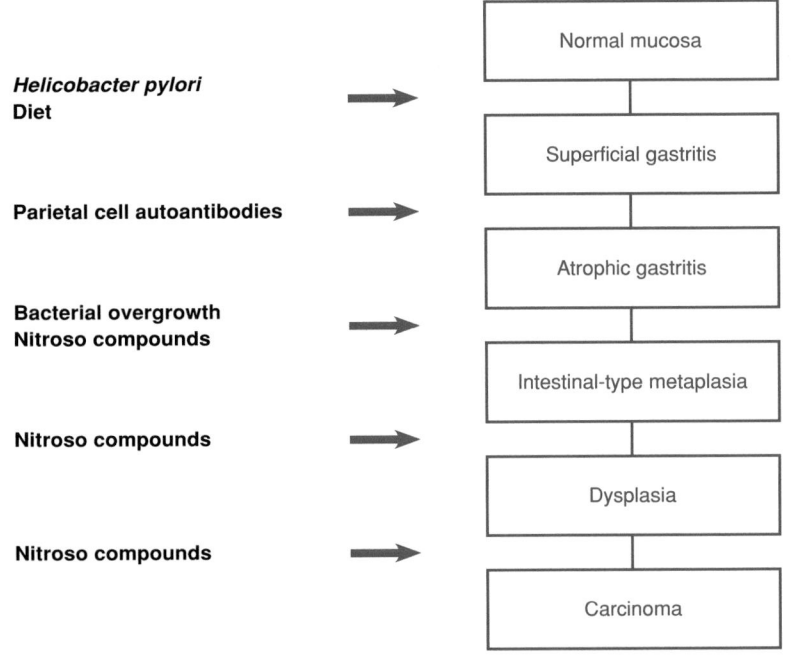

Figure 9-3 Proposed multistep process leading from atrophic gastritis to gastric carcinoma. The most important factors appear to be dietary influences and infection with the bacterium *Helicobacter pylori*. Reduction in acid secretion with chronic gastritis promotes bacterial overgrowth and the conversion of dietary nitrates into carcinogenic nitroso compounds. (After Correa P. A human model of gastric carcinogenesis. Cancer Res 1988;48:3554)

Table 9-1 Case-Control Studies Suggesting a Link Between *Helicobacter pylori* **and Gastric Carcinoma**

Study	Infected Cancer Cases	Infected Controls	Odds Ratio (95% CI)
Forman et al, 1991[76]	10/29 (69%)	54/116 (47%)	2.8 (1–8)
Nomura et al, 1980[35]	103/109 (94%)	83/109 (76%)	6.0 (2.1–17.3)
Parsonnet, 1993[83]	92/109 (84%)	66/109 (66%)	3.6 (1.8–7.3)
Hansson et al, 1993[78]	90/112 (80%)	63/103 (61%)	2.6 (1.3–5)

ative colitis and colon cancer, and chronic osteomyelitis and squamous cell carcinoma. Some features of *H pylori* infection parallel these processes. *H pylori* induces a gastric inflammatory response, including, in experimental models, cell proliferation.

The data regarding the role of *H pylori* infection in the development of gastric carcinoma remain open to interpretation, and although the epidemiologic evidence strongly suggests a link between the two conditions, causality has not been established. It is possible that the same circumstances that lead to gastric carcinoma also predispose to *H pylori* infestation as a secondary event. Further studies examining the effect of *H pylori* on molecular changes in the gastric epithelium and clinical trials evaluating the risk of development of gastric cancer after eradication of the organism remain to be performed.

Pathology

In the United States, about 40% of gastric cancers are located in the antrum or distal stomach, 25% in the body, and 35% in the fundus or cardia. Around the world, distal lesions tend to be more prevalent in regions of high incidence, whereas proximal lesions tend to be more frequent in regions of low incidence. Numerous pathologic classifications for gastric cancer have been described. Some are based on gross or endoscopic appearance of tumors, others are based on microscopic anatomy. Unfortunately, no uniformity in pathologic classification has been achieved in the literature on gastric cancer.

Macroscopic Classification

On gross inspection, several different patterns of tumor growth are evident. Historically, four types were outlined: type I (polypoid lesions), type II (ulcerating lesions with distinct borders and elevated edges), type III (ulcerating lesions with indistinct borders), and type IV (diffuse, infiltrating lesions with indistinct borders). Type IV lesions have also been referred to as *linitis plastica* because the infiltrating tumor produces a thick-

ened, rigid, nondistensible gastric wall. Some have compared the gross appearance of these stomachs to stiff leather bottles. The features of the gross tumor types can usually be appreciated preoperatively with either endoscopy or barium contrast radiographic examination. Figure 9-4 illustrates these major gross forms of gastric cancer.

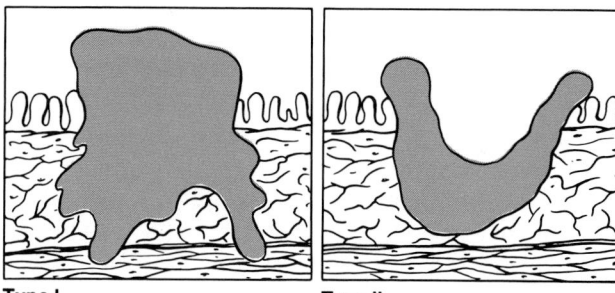

Type I   Type II

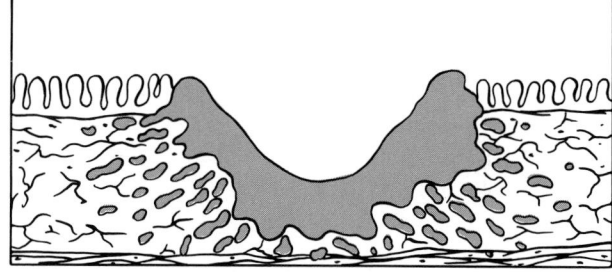

Type III

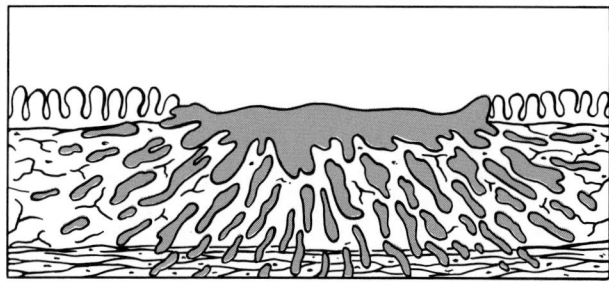

Type IV

Figure 9-4 Gross classification of types of gastric cancer according to Borrmann. Type I lesions are exophytic, polypoid, and fungating. Type II and III lesions are ulcerating and have either elevated, distinct (II) or indistinct (III) borders. Type IV lesions are diffusely infiltrating and are also known as *linitis plastica.*

Five morphologic types of gastric cancer have been described: fungating (about 36% of tumors), diffuse (26%), ulcerating (25%), polypoid (7%), and superficial (6%). In this classification, the fungating tumors are defined as large, intraluminal masses that project into the gastric lumen, perhaps associated with superficial ulceration. In the diffuse form, the tumor is found to extend throughout the gastric wall without forming a discrete mass. The wall of the stomach is usually thickened and nondistensible. Other tumors have a predominantly ulcerated appearance with a deeply excavated, large ulcer with irregular margins and base. The gastric rugae usually extend up to the ulcer margins (Fig. 9-5). Polypoid tumors are unusual and have the appearance of a large sessile polyp. These tumors have a cauliflower appearance and usually have a well-defined base. Superficial tumors are those with irregular, raised or depressed mucosal patches without mass or infiltration. These superficial gastric cancers have been termed *early gastric cancer*. Because of their special importance, they are discussed separately in more detail.

Other terms have also been used to describe unusual forms of gastric cancer. *Colloid carcinoma*, for example, refers to tumors that secrete large amounts of mucin, giving the tumor mass a gelatinous consistency. *Medullary tumors* are described as those with solid bands of tumor cells. Several problems have made these morphologic classifications of gastric cancer unreliable. Many tumors have characteristics of more than one type, making categorization problematic. Second, no clear relation has been identified between the gross appearance of the tumors and outcome, thus no useful prognostic information can be gained from the categorization. These problems led to the development of histologic classification systems.

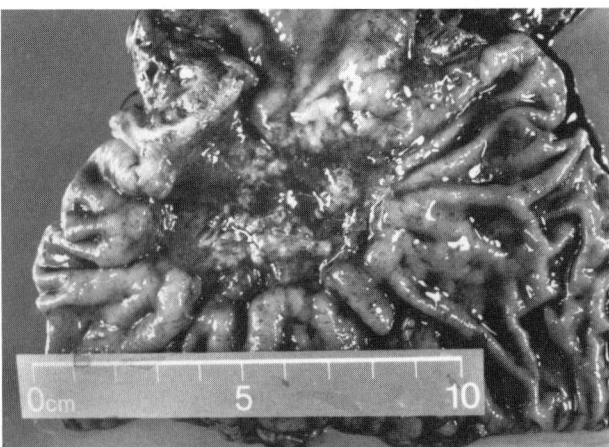

Figure 9-5 Gross appearance of an ulcerating gastric adenocarcinoma. The base is irregular, and thickened folds are visible at the lesion margin.

Histologic Classification

One of the commonly used histologic classifications of gastric cancers was developed by the World Health Organization (WHO) in an attempt to provide a uniform nomenclature for the various tumor types.[22] In this system, tumors are divided into papillary, tubular, mucinous, signet ring cell, and undifferentiated types. Histologically, papillary tumors demonstrate multiple finger-like projections within a bulky intraluminal mass. Tubular cancers have branching glands embedded in a fibrous stroma. Mucinous tumors show large amounts of mucin, which sometimes is secreted extracellularly. When the intracellular mucus pushes the cell nucleus eccentrically to the periphery, the cells have a "signet ring" appearance. All these various types can also be categorized according to the degree of cellular differentiation. Some are highly undifferentiated and have lost cellular and glandular architecture. At the other end of the spectrum are well-differentiated tumors in which cellular and glandular architecture is preserved. The WHO system is problematic in that some tumors are difficult to classify, and like the gross morphologic systems, no clear relation between histologic classification and biologic behavior has been found.

To simplify the histologic staging and provide prognostic information, investigators divided gastric cancers into two types: intestinal and diffuse. *Intestinal-type* tumors have a histologic appearance similar to colon cancer with a glandular pattern and surrounding intestinal metaplasia. These tumors are usually well circumscribed and have a polypoid or ulcerated macroscopic appearance (Fig. 9-6*A*). Intestinal-type tumors are most commonly seen in geographic areas with high incidence of gastric cancer, are related to dietary influences, and usually arise in elderly men. Compared with the diffuse form, intestinal-type tumors have a better prognosis. When advanced, they tend to spread hematogenously. *Diffuse-type* tumors lack cell cohesion and do not form glands. They tend to infiltrate transmurally and are often associated with lymphatic metastases and carcinomatosis (see Fig. 9-6*B*). Diffuse-type tumors are more commonly seen in geographic areas with a low incidence of gastric cancer and are more common in younger patients and women. They tend to be poorly differentiated and have a worse prognosis than the intestinal type of gastric cancer. Less common histologic types include squamous, carcinosarcoma, and adenoacanthoma.[23] In the United States, about 50% of all gastric cancers are of the diffuse type, 40% are of the intestinal type, and 10% are either mixed or show a rarer histologic pattern. The macroscopic and microscopic types of gastric cancer are summarized in Table 9-2.

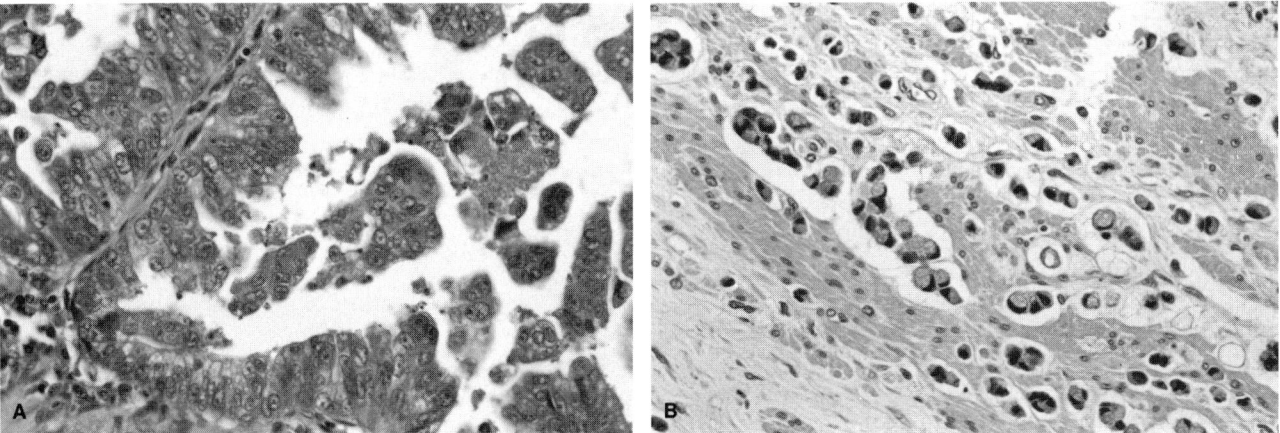

Figure 9-6 (**A**) Histologic section from the stomach of a patient with intestinal-type gastric cancer, demonstrating a glandular pattern reminiscent of colon cancer. (**B**) Similar histologic section from the stomach of a patient with diffuse-type cancer. In this tumor, the cells are not cohesive, do not form glands, and infiltrate widely through the gastric wall. (Courtesy of Noel Weidner, MD, University of California, San Francisco)

Early Gastric Cancer

Early gastric cancer is a special problem notable for the improved outcome in afflicted patients compared with other forms of gastric cancer. Early gastric cancer is defined as a tumor limited in depth of invasion to the mucosa or submucosa of the gastric wall, irrespective of the presence or absence of lymph node metastases. As such, early gastric cancer is a pathologic diagnosis and does not relate to the time course of the lesion, as the name suggests. Early gastric cancer accounts for 5% to 10% of gastric cancer patients in the United States, 10% to 15% of European patients, and 35% to 40% of patients in Japan. It is unclear whether these geographic differences reflect the results of aggressive screening programs in Japan or if there are intrinsic differences in the tumors in these populations. The average age of patients with early gastric cancer in the United States is 65 years, whereas it is 55 years in Japan. Most patients have vague upper GI symptoms suggestive of peptic ulcer disease. Weight loss in patients with early gastric cancer is unusual, unlike the cachexia commonly ob-

served in advanced lesions. The mean duration of symptoms in patients with early lesions is between 2 and 3 years but is only 6 to 8 months in patients with advanced lesions.

Staging

The preferred staging system for patients with gastric cancer is the TNM system[24] (Table 9-3). This system represents a consensus of several national and international cancer societies, including the American Joint Committee on Cancer, the Unio Internationalis Contra Cancrum, and the Japanese Committee on Cancer, and represents an effort to achieve worldwide standardization of reporting of staging. The system is pathologically oriented and has a disadvantage in that patients cannot be staged preoperatively. The factors in the system include depth of tumor invasion in the gastric wall, the presence and extent of nodal metastases, and the presence of distant metastases. Staging in this system has direct usefulness in predicting prognosis.

Only 10% to 20% of patients with primary tumors limited to the mucosa or submucosa have lymph node metastases at the time of presentation, compared with 50% of patients with tumors penetrating the muscularis and 75% of patients with transmural lesions.[25] Five-year survival in the absence of nodal metastases is about 80%, but this falls to 40% with involvement of N1 (perigastric) nodes and to 20% with involvement of N2 (regional) nodes.[26]

Tumor size has an effect that, in general, parallels that of depth of invasion. The gross appearance of the

---

Table 9-2   Types of Gastric Cancer

GROSS APPEARANCE	HISTOLOGIC APPEARANCE
Superficial	Intestinal
Polypoid	Diffuse
Ulcerative	Mixed
Infiltrative	Squamous
	Carcinosarcoma
	Adenoacanthoma

Table 9-3   TNM Staging of Gastric Cancer

Designation	Description
PRIMARY TUMOR	
TX	Primary tumor cannot be assessed
T0	No evidence of primary tumor
Tis	Noninvasive carcinoma-in-situ
T1	Extension to submucosa
T2	Extension to serosa
T3	Extension through serosa
T4	Invasion of adjacent organs
REGIONAL LYMPH NODES	
NX	Regional nodes cannot be assessed
N0	No regional nodal metastases
N1	Involvement of perigastric nodes within 3 cm of primary tumor
N2	Involvement of perigastric nodes more than 3 cm from primary tumor
DISTANT METASTASES	
MX	Distant metastases cannot be assessed
M0	No distant metastases
M1	Distant metastases present

Stage	Primary Tumor	Nodal Status	Distant Metastases
0	Tis	N0	M0
IA	T1	N0	M0
IB	T1	N1	M0
II	T1	N2	M0
	T2	N1	M0
	T3	N0	M0
IIIA	T2	N2	M0
	T3	N1	M0
	T4	N0	M0
IIIB	T3	N2	M0
	T4	N1	M0
IV	T4	N2	M0
	Any T	Any N	M1

lesion is also important. In advanced lesions (see Fig. 9-4), the stage predicts outcome, with polypoid (type I) and ulcerating (type II) lesions having better prognoses than those with an infiltrating component (types III and IV). A similar effect of gross tumor appearance has been reported.[27] Histologic appearance of the tumor has an appreciable effect on prognosis. Intestinal-type lesions have better outcomes than diffuse lesions. Similarly, patients with well-differentiated tumors in the WHO classification survive longer than those with poorly differentiated lesions. A pronounced host response of lymphocytic or plasma cell infiltration into the tumor has been reported to be a good prognostic sign. No uniform gender effects on survival of patients with gastric cancer have been reported, although in some reports, women have somewhat better survival. Age appears to have some effect, with patients older than 60 years having worse prognoses. In general, factors such as the histologic appearance of the tumor, host response, and age have secondary importance compared with the extent of invasion of the gastric wall and the presence of lymph node metastases when predicting outcome.

Clinical Presentation

The clinical presentation of patients with gastric carcinoma depends on the location of the primary tumor, tumor extent, and the presence of ulceration. Studies suggest that the diagnosis of gastric carcinoma is being made with less delay than in years past, yet there has been no corresponding improvement in outcome.[28] Early gastric cancer, the type with the best prognosis, commonly presents without symptoms, hence the rationale for screening programs in populations at high risk. The most common symptoms in patients with gastric cancer are abdominal pain and weight loss (Table 9-4). The abdominal pain is usually indistinguishable from that due to peptic ulcer disease, and commonly initial symptoms are attributed to the latter disorder. Proximal lesions at the cardia can infiltrate submucosally into the lower esophagus and produce dysphagia. Occasionally, the disease in these patients is confused with achalasia. Lesions at the pylorus are more likely to cause symptoms of gastric outlet obstruction. Ulcerative lesions commonly cause GI blood loss, manifested chronically by weakness and iron-deficiency anemia, or more acutely with melena or hematemesis. The weight loss associated with gastric cancer is usually not due to inability to eat secondary to gastric outlet obstruction. Patients report loss of appetite and vague postprandial discomfort. The decrease in food intake in many patients does not always correlate with the degree of weight loss and muscle wasting. It has been hypothesized that gastric carcinoma secretes substances that induce catabolic metabolic changes. A likely mediator

Table 9-4   Symptoms of Patients With Gastric Cancer: Results of Two Representative Series

Symptom	Frequency (%)	
	Meyers et al[28] (n = 255)	Weed et al[29] (n = 298)
Abdominal pain	51	66
Weight loss	72	50
Nausea, vomiting	40	32
Anorexia	35	25
Dysphagia	22	23
Bleeding	31	23
Perforation	1	Not stated

is tumor necrosis factor, which has been identified in increased amounts in the serum of some cancer patients.[30]

The physical findings commonly observed in patients with gastric cancer are listed in Table 9-5. Early lesions reveal no findings on physical examination, and physical findings are signs of advanced disease. The presence of hepatomegaly may represent liver metastases. Ascites, present in less than 5% of patients at the time of diagnosis, is an important sign of carcinomatosis and inoperability. A palpable anterior rectal mass (Blumer's shelf), representing pelvic metastases, is present in 2% to 5% of patients. Ovarian metastases occur uncommonly at initial presentation but can be detected by the presence of adnexal enlargement, usually bilateral, on pelvic examination (Krukenberg tumor). The thoracic duct carries abdominal lymph to the systemic circulation, usually through the left subclavian or jugular vein. The smaller right lymphatic duct drains to the right subclavian or jugular veins. About 5% of gastric cancer patients have supraclavicular or cervical lymphadenopathy as a manifestation of widespread lymph node metastases. The classic description of this sign in the left supraclavicular fossa carries the eponym *Virchow's node*. Gastric carcinoma can metastasize to the umbilicus, producing a palpable mass. This finding is usually associated with carcinomatosis. An epigastric mass or fullness is present in 15% to 20% of patients. Although this finding may suggest the presence of a bulky primary tumor, there is little relation to resectability.

Unusual patients with gastric cancer present with skin manifestations, such as acanthosis nigricans, metastatic skin nodules, warty keratoses, or dermatomyositis. Gastric carcinoma induces a propensity for venous thrombosis, and an occasional patient presents with thrombophlebitis. Rare reported patients have presented with signs and symptoms of gastrocolic fistula from erosion of the primary tumor into the transverse colon.

Table 9-5   Physical Findings in Patients With Gastric Cancer

Finding	Approximate Frequency (%)
Guaiac-positive stool	35
Obvious weight loss	25
Abdominal mass or fullness	20
Epigastric tenderness	15
Hepatomegaly	5
Rectal shelf	3
Lymphadenopathy	3
Ascites	2

Table 9-6   Serum Markers in the Detection of Gastric Cancer

Marker	Sensitivity (%)	References
CEA	40	35, 80, 81
CA 19-9	40	35, 78, 81
CA 72-4	94	35
CA 242	44	82
CA 195	50	81
CA 50	48	78
TATI	46	83

CEA, carcinoembryonic antigen; TATI, tumor-associated trypsin inhibitor.

Diagnostic Evaluation

Role of Screening Programs

In areas of high prevalence, screening programs have been valuable in identifying early lesions. In Japan, for example, mass screening programs have a diagnostic yield of about 0.1% of all patients examined.[31] Roughly half of these patients have early gastric cancer and are curable. Screening appears to have been less effective in Chile, with early cancers detected in only 15% of patients with malignancy in the screened population.[32] Because of the low incidence of gastric cancer in the United States, screening programs are not cost-effective.[33] An argument can be made for screening certain groups at higher risk in the United States, such as patients with chronic atrophic gastritis, pernicious anemia, Ménétrier's disease, adenomatous polyps, and a prior history of partial gastrectomy. In Scandinavia, however, planned endoscopic follow-up of gastrectomy patients has failed to reduce the mortality from gastric cancer, compared with unscreened control patients.[34]

Laboratory Investigation

No laboratory investigation is specific for gastric cancer. Although the efficacy of a large number of serum markers in the detection of gastric cancer has been studied, the results have been disappointing (Table 9-6). Overall, the sensitivity of commonly used cancer markers, such as carcinoembryonic antigen (CEA), is less than 50%. Patients with elevated CEA levels are more likely to have advanced lesions, especially liver metastases, than early, curable lesions. Serum CEA levels are not useful in either the diagnostic evaluation of patients with symptoms or the screening of those without. One report suggests that a new marker, CA 72-4, is elevated in 94% of patients with gastric cancer.[35] Further studies are required to confirm these results and to assess this marker's practical usefulness as a screening tool in high-risk populations.

Because chronic atrophic gastritis is commonly associated with gastric cancer, several strategies have been devised to identify these high-risk patients. Serum pepsinogen levels are decreased in chronic atrophic gastritis. In one study, low serum pepsinogen levels were found in 31% of gastric cancer patients, compared with 6% of matched controls.[36] Similarly, about two thirds of patients with gastric cancer have achlorhydria due to chronic atrophic gastritis, compared with about 20% of age-matched control patients. Achlorhydria can be identified through gastric analysis, although the test is uncommonly performed and can be misinterpreted if the patient has been taking antisecretory agents.

Patients with chronic blood loss may be anemic, with hypochromic, microcytic indices suggestive of iron deficiency. In the presence of chronic atrophic gastritis, anemia can also be due to vitamin B_{12} deficiency. Liver function tests are normal unless metastases are present. Elevation of alkaline phosphatase or lactic dehydrogenase is the most sensitive indicator of mass lesions in the liver.

Endoscopy

Endoscopy should be performed in patients with symptoms suspicious for carcinoma, including unexplained epigastric pain, postprandial discomfort, GI bleeding, or unexplained weight loss. Endoscopic biopsy should be performed on all gastric ulcers except those that are clearly superficial, because it is difficult to differentiate benign and malignant ulcers accurately by gross endoscopic appearance alone. The number of biopsies performed correlates directly with the diagnostic accuracy.[37] At a minimum, four quadrant biopsies should be performed. When eight or more biopsy specimens are taken, the chance of missing an underlying carcinoma in a gastric ulcer is nearly zero. Brush cytology complements biopsy and increases diagnostic accuracy. Endoscopy appears to be more sensitive than contrast radiography in detecting small gastric carcinomas. The ability to biopsy suspicious lesions and excise small polyps through the endoscope are additional factors that have made upper GI endoscopy the preferred initial approach to patients with suspicious symptoms in many centers.

Endoscopy is limited in certain situations. Small tumors near the cardia may be missed, especially by inexperienced operators. Occasionally, diffusely infiltrative gastric carcinomas have only subtle mucosal signs. The experienced endoscopist can recognize, however, that the stomach is not distensible. In the setting of acute hemorrhage, an ulcerating carcinoma may be mistaken for benign gastric ulcer because of an inability to view the lesion adequately.

Radiologic Examination

Historically, radiographic examination of the upper GI tract was the primary technique in patients with symptoms suggestive of gastric malignancy. Compression and double-contrast techniques have increased the sensitivity of radiography in these patients. Several features distinguish malignant gastric ulcers from their benign counterparts (Fig. 9-7). In carcinoma with ulceration, the ulcer cavity arises from a heaped-up margin and does not penetrate into the wall of the stomach. In contrast, benign ulcers have no associated mass, and the crater usually penetrates into the gastric wall. The gastric rugae in malignant ulcers maintain their contour up to and beyond the lesion, whereas in benign ulcers, the rugae typically radiate outward from the center of the crater. Finally, malignant ulcers are usually larger than 1 cm in diameter, whereas benign ulcers can be of any size.

Although radiologic contrast examination of the stomach has, in some ways, been superceded by endos-

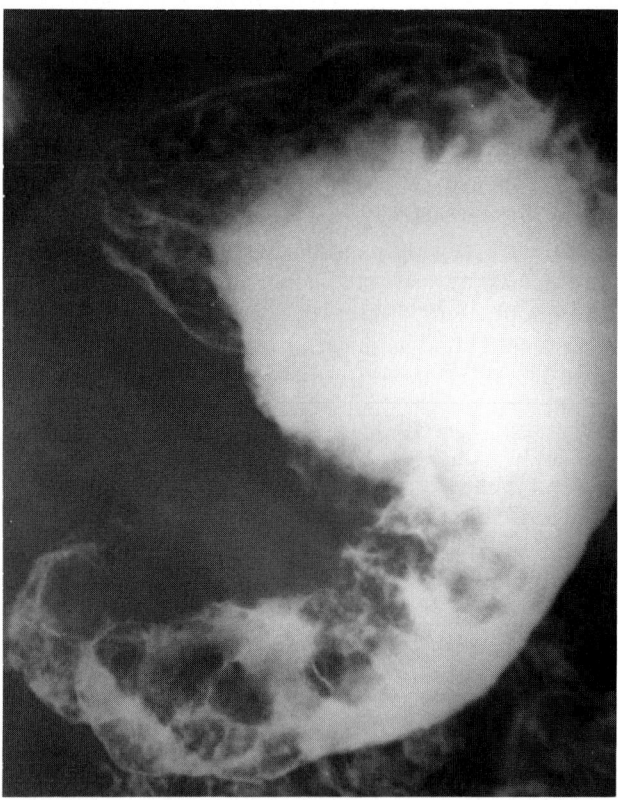

Figure 9-7 Radiographic appearance of gastric adenocarcinoma with use of an oral contrast medium.

copy, it still has a role in patients for whom surgery is considered. Air contrast barium radiography delineates gastric anatomy and also provides a reference for the surgeon regarding the location of the tumor. This information can aid in operative planning. Computed tomography (CT) of the upper abdomen is also useful for preoperative staging in selected patients (Fig. 9-8). CT can detect advanced lesions with direct local invasion of the pancreas or liver. Additionally, it is sensitive in detecting liver metastases and regional lymphadenopathy. Depending on the overall condition of the patient, the findings of CT can lead one to avoid surgery. Staging with CT is unnecessary in patients for whom gastrectomy is planned to palliate symptoms because it does not provide useful information beyond that obtained at exploratory laparotomy.[38]

Endoscopic ultrasonography is a new technique that has become possible through the development of miniaturized probes adaptable to flexible endoscopes. This is a demanding technique and requires close cooperation between the endoscopist and the ultrasonographer. Early results suggest that this technique provides accurate staging of the depth of gastric wall invasion and the presence or absence of lymph node metastases.[39,40] This technique is likely to have special importance in the pretreatment staging evaluation of patients considered for preoperative (neoadjuvant) chemotherapy or immunotherapy.

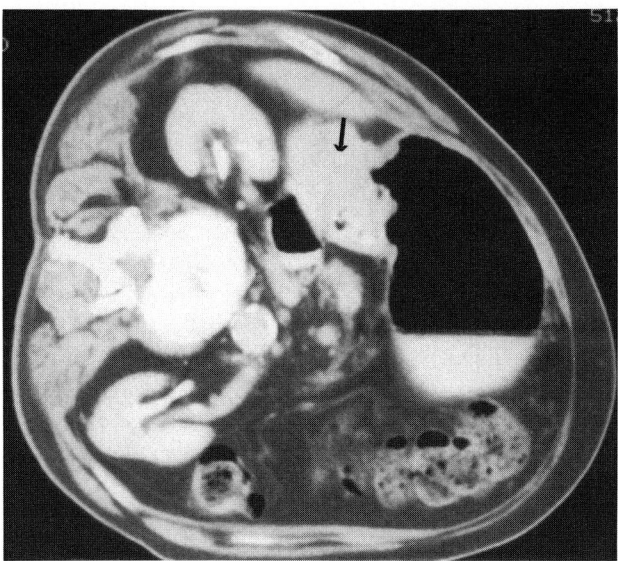

Figure 9-8 Obstructing antral carcinoma as seen by CT. The patient was put in the left lateral decubitus position for study. The interface between the tumor (*arrow*) and air in the stomach and duodenal bulb assists in characterizing the local extent of the tumor. CT is also valuable in identifying regional lymphadenopathy, liver metastasis, and carcinomatosis.

Treatment and Outcome

Surgery

APPROACH TO THE PATIENT. The main therapy for patients with gastric cancer is surgical resection. Although some advances in chemotherapy and radiation therapy have improved the outlook for certain patient groups, for the average patient, surgery offers the only chance of cure. Once a patient with gastric cancer has been identified, the clinical, pathologic, and radiographic staging criteria described earlier should be evaluated. In the absence of metastatic disease, an exploratory laparotomy should be undertaken. During exploration, the nature and extent of the primary tumor and the status of regional lymph nodes should be assessed. Careful attention should be paid to the liver to exclude metastases, and the possibility of carcinomatosis should be excluded by evaluation of visceral and parietal peritoneal surfaces. If metastases are absent, a curative resection should be performed. The principle guiding operative resection for cure of gastric cancer is to remove both the primary tumor and associated involved lymph nodes completely. The magnitude of the operation required to achieve this goal has been the subject of controversy. The main discussion has focused on the extent of gastric resection required to achieve local control and the role of radical lymphadenectomy.

Some patients thought to have curable lesions preoperatively are found to have occult metastases at the time of abdominal exploration. In most cases, these patients benefit from a palliative resection, with the goal of excising the primary tumor completely but leaving behind grossly evident liver, nodal, or peritoneal metastases. In these patients undergoing exploratory laparotomy, little additional risk is undertaken by resecting the primary lesion, and future bleeding or obstruction from growth of the primary tumor is avoided.

Other patients are known to have metastases from findings on radiographic screening procedures. A surgical approach to these patients must be carefully individualized. The surgeon should consider factors such as the extent of metastases, the overall condition of the patient, and the presence of complications of the primary tumor, including bleeding or obstruction, before deciding on a course of action. If the burden of tumor outside the stomach is small, the patient is in good condition, and the primary tumor has caused bleeding or obstruction, palliative gastrectomy usually is beneficial. On the other hand, if extensive metastases are present, or if the patient is in poor condition with an asymptomatic primary tumor, gastrectomy is not warranted.

EXTENT OF GASTRECTOMY. In planning a curative operation for gastric cancer, knowledge of the extent of disease within the stomach is required. Although the gross tumor margins can usually be determined intraoperatively through careful inspection and bimanual palpation of the stomach, pathologic studies show that microscopic submucosal tumor extension is common in gastric cancer. Intramural metastasis can occur up to 6 cm proximal to the grossly evident tumor and up to 3 cm into the duodenum.[41,42] Thus, the minimal requirements to ensure complete microscopic gastric resection are gross margins of 4 to 6 cm around the primary tumor. In practical terms, this translates to subtotal gastrectomy for the usual distal carcinoma and total gastrectomy for proximal lesions.

Some controversy exists over the use of subtotal and total gastrectomy for gastric carcinoma. In some centers, total gastrectomy is used routinely rather than distal subtotal gastrectomy, even for distal lesions. Supporters of this approach cite the benefit of wider excision of the primary tumor and potentially improved cure rates. This claim has not been borne out in controlled trials,[43] in which the survival rates of patients undergoing subtotal gastrectomy for distal lesions are not significantly different from those of patients undergoing total gastrectomy. Furthermore, in most series, total gastrectomy carries a somewhat higher risk in terms of mortality and morbidity than subtotal gastrectomy. For these reasons, subtotal gastrectomy appears to be a superior approach for the average patient with a distal lesion, particularly if the lesion has intestinal-type histology. Surveys in both the United States and Europe suggest that this is the standard in practice on both continents.[44,45] Reconstruction of GI continuity in patients after subtotal gastrectomy is ordinarily achieved with a Billroth II gastrojejunostomy. The functional result is probably better when the jejunal loop is brought through the transverse mesocolon, which allows for a short afferent limb. For patients with retroperitoneal or mesocolic lymphadenopathy, the reconstruction should be antecolic to avoid potential obstruction by tumor.

Total gastrectomy is indicated mainly for localized lesions of the mid-body or fundus and for linitis plastica–type lesions. Other indications for total gastrectomy include Ménétrier's disease complicated by cancer, gastric stump cancer after distal resection for benign disease, and cancer associated with multiple, diffuse, gastric polyps. Concomitant en bloc splenectomy is warranted for patients with greater curvature lesions. Reconstruction after total gastrectomy is best achieved by a 45-cm Roux-en-Y limb performed in an end-to-side fashion. The most direct route for the Roux limb to the esophagus is retrocolic, and this is preferred for most patients. An antecolic approach is warranted for patients with bulky residual retroperitoneal lymphadenopathy. In the past, reconstruction using a loop esophagojejunostomy was commonly performed, and

although it has an advantage over the Roux-en-Y reconstruction in that only one anastomosis is required, its use has been abandoned by most surgeons because of the frequent problem of bile reflux esophagitis. In some centers, a reservoir is constructed as a pouch of jejunum in the hope of improving the long-term nutritional status of patients undergoing total gastrectomy. This maneuver appears unnecessary because the average patient tolerates total gastrectomy with Roux-en-Y reconstruction well.

For cardia lesions near the gastroesophageal junction, esophagogastrectomy is required to achieve clear proximal margins. In patients with these lesions, total gastrectomy with extended esophageal resection does not add in any beneficial way to the distal margin and eliminates the distal stomach as an option for reconstruction. Instead, these patients are best approached through a left thoracoabdominal incision, with division of the diaphragm to expose the distal thoracic esophagus. At least a 10-cm margin of esophagus should be taken proximal to the tumor, and frozen section examination of this margin is advisable to ensure absence of microscopic infiltration of tumor. The distal margin is usually not problematic and should include about 6 cm of normal stomach. The right gastroepiploic vessels should be preserved to ensure adequate blood supply to the distal stomach. The vagal nerve trunks should be divided in the chest at the proximal margin to aid in mobilization of the distal esophagus. Reconstruction of GI continuity is through an esophagogastrostomy in an end-to-side fashion in the left chest. A pyloroplasty or pyloromyotomy is performed to improve postoperative gastric emptying. Alternatively, a two-cavity approach, beginning with laparotomy and mobilization of the stomach and tumor followed by a right posterolateral thoracotomy for esophagectomy, can be considered. The treatment strategies for patients with cardiac, midbody, and pyloric cancers are illustrated in Figure 9-9.

The optimal extent of resection for patients with early gastric cancer is unclear. Most patients with early gastric cancer are cured with complete surgical excision. Limited excision or endoscopic resection of these potentially curable lesions should be reserved for patients who are otherwise not suitable operative candidates or should be performed in the context of carefully controlled clinical trials.

ROLE OF LYMPHADENECTOMY. All patients undergoing curative resection of gastric cancer should have en bloc resection of the lymph node groups draining the region of the primary tumor. This dissection should include at the least omental, pyloric, and lesser curvature nodes. For lesions of the proximal stomach along the greater curvature, splenectomy should be in-

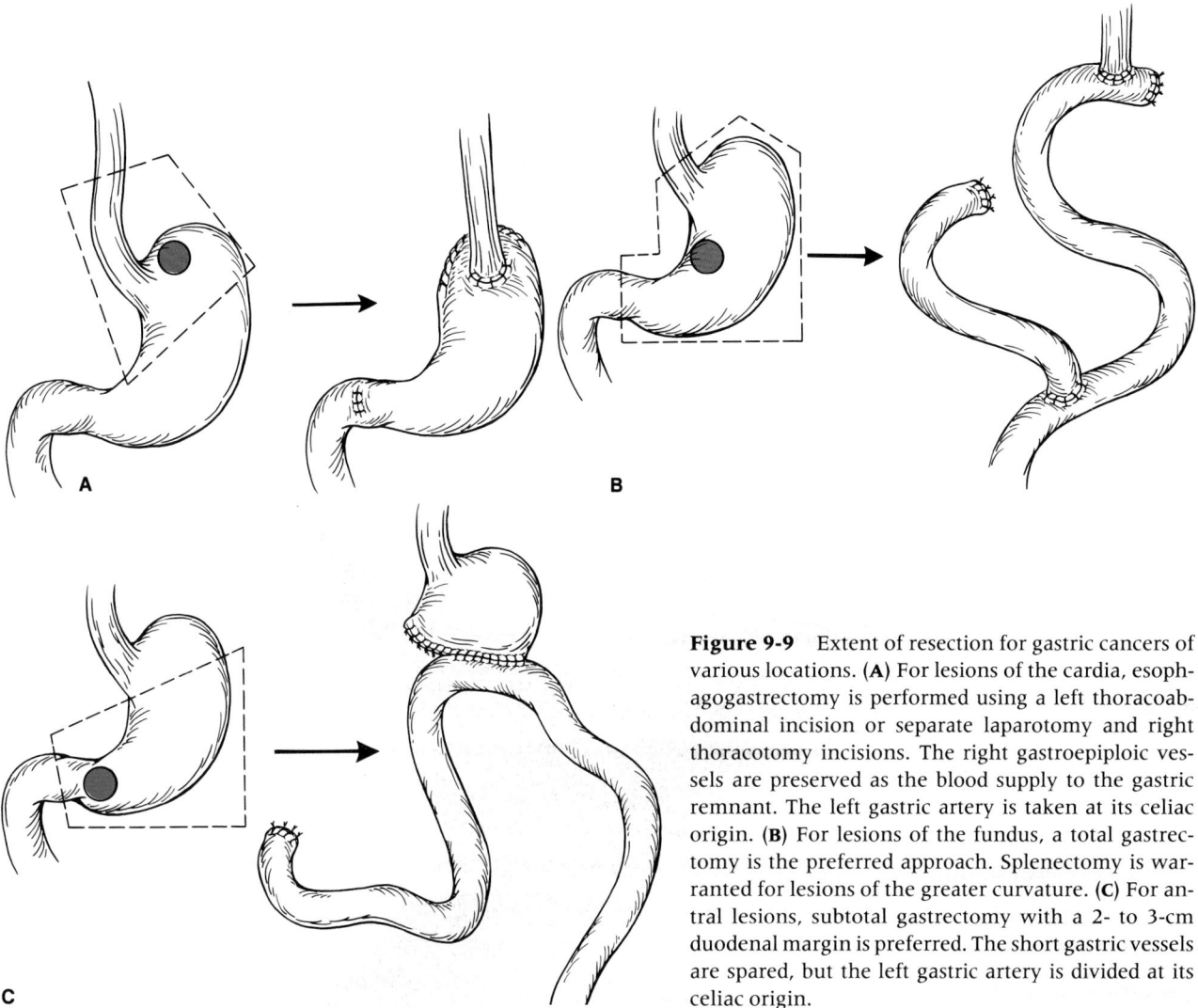

Figure 9-9 Extent of resection for gastric cancers of various locations. (**A**) For lesions of the cardia, esophagogastrectomy is performed using a left thoracoabdominal incision or separate laparotomy and right thoracotomy incisions. The right gastroepiploic vessels are preserved as the blood supply to the gastric remnant. The left gastric artery is taken at its celiac origin. (**B**) For lesions of the fundus, a total gastrectomy is the preferred approach. Splenectomy is warranted for lesions of the greater curvature. (**C**) For antral lesions, subtotal gastrectomy with a 2- to 3-cm duodenal margin is preferred. The short gastric vessels are spared, but the left gastric artery is divided at its celiac origin.

cluded to incorporate splenic hilar nodes. In the Japanese experience, improvements in outcome have been attributed, at least in part, to the more widespread application of radical lymphadenectomy in patients with gastric cancer. To provide uniformity of reporting in gastric cancer trials, the Japanese have developed standards for nodal dissection. The nodal groups referred to in many of these trials include the following: N1 (perigastric nodes), N2 (splenic, left gastric, and celiac axis nodes), N3 (hepatoduodenal and root of mesentery nodes), and N4 (periaortic and middle colic nodes). In Japan, resection of N1 and N2 nodal groups is performed in all patients with invasive gastric cancer, including those with early lesions. For advanced lesions with full-thickness gastric wall penetration, an N3 dissection is included. This extensive lymphadenectomy is not the standard in Europe or the United States, and it remains unclear whether outcome in Western patients can be improved by more radical surgery. Although the overall outcome of patients treated for gastric cancer in Japan is superior to the outcome observed in the United States and Europe, it remains to be seen whether this is due to differences in the operative approach or more fundamental differences in the biology of the tumors seen in the different parts of the world. In Japan, a higher proportion of patients with good prognostic features, such as early gastric cancer and intestinal-type histology, are seen than in patients treated in the West.

Enthusiasm for radical lymphadenectomy in patients with gastric cancer should be tempered with the perspective that, for all other tumors, more radical surgery does not increase survival but does increase operative complication rates. Thus, for melanoma, as well as colon, lung, breast, and thyroid cancer, the trend has been toward more conservative surgery. For some tumors, such as prostate, cervical, and ovarian cancer, the presence of distant nodal metastases is used as a contra-indication to radical resection because the salvage rate with initial surgery is low. A multinational clinical trial is underway to test the hypothesis that more radical lymphadenectomy improves survival in patients with gastric cancer. A small completed trial showed no benefit in survival but did reveal increased postoperative complication rates in patients undergoing the more extensive operations.[46]

RESULTS OF SURGERY. In the United States, the overall survival rate at 5 years of patients undergoing gastrectomy for gastric cancer is 15% to 20%. In Japan, overall survival is about 50%. The results of treatment of gastric cancer in the United States are significantly worse than for other tumors, such as colon and breast cancer. Survival is stage dependent. In the United States, overall 5-year survival rate for patients with stage I lesions is 65%. This decreases to 30% for stage II lesions and to 10% for stage III lesions. In general, no 5-year survival is expected in patients presenting with stage IV lesions. Stage-dependent survival of patients in one large, representative, single-institution report is given in Table 9-7. Patients undergoing resection for cure have improved survival over patients undergoing palliative resection. In Japan, results of surgery have improved over time (Fig. 9-10), whereas in the West, no major improvement in surgical cure rates has been observed.

The operative risk of gastrectomy for gastric cancer has improved significantly in recent years. Before 1970, the mean operative mortality rate for gastrectomy for gastric cancer was 16%. The operative mortality rate declined to 12% in the decade from 1979 to 1980. In the following decade, the overall reported mortality rate in the English language literature decreased to 5%.[47] Many series report operative mortality rates between 0% and 2%. Although the reasons for this improvement have not been clearly defined, it is likely that improvements in operative technique, anesthetic care, and postoperative treatment have all played a role.

Table 9-7   Survival Rate of Patients With Gastric Cancer

Stage	5-Year Survival Rate (%)
I	65
II	22
III	5
IV	0

(Diehl JT, Hermann RE, Cooperman AM, Hoerr SO. Gastric carcinoma: a ten-year review. Ann Surg 1983;198:9)

Adjuvant Chemotherapy

Given that only a minority of patients with gastric cancer, at least in the West, are cured by resection of their tumors, interest has focused on developing effective adjuvant chemotherapy with the goal of improving survival. To date, adjuvant chemotherapy for patients undergoing complete resection of gastric carcinoma has not made a significant impact on long-term survival.[48,49] Most trials have used combination chemotherapy, with the FAM regimen (5-fluorouracil [5-FU], doxorubicin [Adriamycin], and mitomycin C), or 5-FU and semustine being the standards. The toxicity of these regimens appears to outweigh any benefit, and today adjuvant chemotherapy has little role outside the confines of controlled clinical trials.

Because of the lack of efficacy of standard forms of adjuvant chemotherapy in patients with resectable gastric cancer, novel approaches have been considered. Neoadjuvant chemotherapy is under study, in which patients are treated with chemotherapy before operation. Initial reports in small numbers of patients appear promising,[50] but further evaluation is required before this approach can be recommended outside of clinical trials. Other novel approaches under development include intraperitoneal chemotherapy, hormonal therapy, and the use of biologic response modifiers.

Treatment of Advanced Disease

The options for patients with advanced disease are limited.[51,52] Cytotoxic chemotherapy has limited response rates and no significant benefit on overall survival. The best-studied single agent, 5-FU, elicits responses in about 20% of patients. Combination therapy with FAM is the most popular regimen, with partial responses evident in 30% to 40% of treated patients. No clearcut survival advantage has been demonstrated, however. A modification of the FAM regimen with the addition of methotrexate (the FAMtx regimen) has been found to improve both response rates and survival, compared with FAM alone, in early trials. A German group reported results of a new combination therapy consisting of etoposide, doxorubicin, and cisplatin (the EAP regimen). Overall response to this combination was 70%, the highest of any reported therapy. The toxicity of this treatment is high, and other investigators have not matched the initial promising results.

GASTRIC CARCINOID TUMORS

Gastric carcinoids are rare tumors that arise from enterochromaffin cells of the gastric epithelium. They represent only 2% to 3% of all carcinoid tumors and only

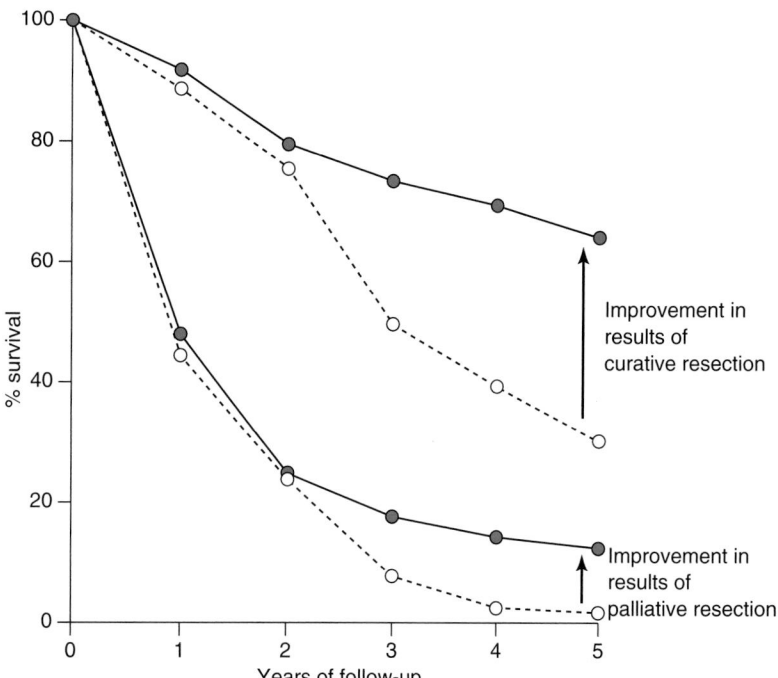

Figure 9-10 Survival in patients undergoing resection for gastric cancer in Japan during 1957 through 1963 (*dashed lines*) and 1966 through 1975 (*solid lines*). Improvement in outcome in patients undergoing both curative and palliative resection has been observed. This improvement has been attributed to the development of screening programs allowing detection of early-stage lesions. (After Yamada E, Miyaishi S, Nakazato H, et al. The surgical treatment of cancer of the stomach. Int Surg 1980;65:387)

0.3% of all tumors of the stomach. Unlike the more common mid-gut carcinoids, gastric carcinoid tumors only rarely cause the carcinoid syndrome. The reason for this observation may relate to fundamental biologic differences between the tumors arising from the foregut and mid-gut. Foregut tumors do not contain serotonin, one of the putative causative agents of the flushing, diarrhea, and bronchoconstriction typical of the carcinoid syndrome. Mid-gut tumors, conversely, are rich in serotonin. This difference is manifested in the histologic staining patterns of the tumors. Serotonin has strong silver-reducing properties, thus mid-gut tumors react avidly with silver stains (argentaffin positive), whereas foregut tumors require additional reducing agents before staining is evident (argyrophilic).

Microscopically, gastric carcinoid tumors are composed of uniform round or polygonal cells arranged in sheets with centrally located nuclei. Carcinoid tumors contain a number of vasoactive substances and peptides, some of which have important biologic actions. Immunochemical staining of gastric carcinoid tumors shows nearly universal presence of chromogranin A and neuron-specific enolase and occasional presence of other peptides, such as human chorionic gonadotrophin-α and somatostatin.

Gastric carcinoid tumors arise in three clinical settings: (1) in association with chronic atrophic gastritis, pernicious anemia, achlorhydria, and hypergastrinemia; (2) in association with the hyperplastic gastropathy and hypergastrinemia of Zollinger-Ellison syndrome; and (3) rare sporadic cases in the absence of

hypergastrinemia. The first is by far the most common setting. The proposed pathophysiology of pernicious anemia and gastric carcinoid tumor formation in patients with chronic atrophic gastritis is outlined in Figure 9-11. Serum gastrin levels are elevated in patients with chronic atrophic gastritis limited to the fundus and body of the stomach. Hypergastrinemia is likely due to loss of the normal inhibitory feedback inhibition of gastrin release by antral acidification. Gastrin has known mitogenic effects on enterochromaffin cells in vitro and in vivo. Animal models of sustained hypergastrinemia due to acid suppression by proton pump inhibitors or gastric corpectomy lead to enterochromaffin cell hyperplasia and multiple gastric carcinoid tumors. Gastric carcinoid tumors in this setting appear to have an indolent course, and several reports indicate that regression of these tumors can be seen with correction of the hypergastrinemia by antrectomy.[53]

Gastric carcinoid tumors in the setting of Zollinger-Ellison syndrome are rare, with some 27 reported cases.[54] No gender preference has been identified, and the mean age of these patients is 45 years. In 12% of cases, metastases were reported. Most cases of gastric carcinoid tumor and gastrinoma have been in the setting of a multiple endocrine neoplasia (MEN) syndrome. Loss of an MEN-1 antioncogene located on chromosome 11 underlies the development of insulinoma in patients with the MEN-1 syndrome, and it is possible that similar molecular events are present in patients with MEN-1 syndrome, gastrinoma, and multiple gastric carcinoid tumors.

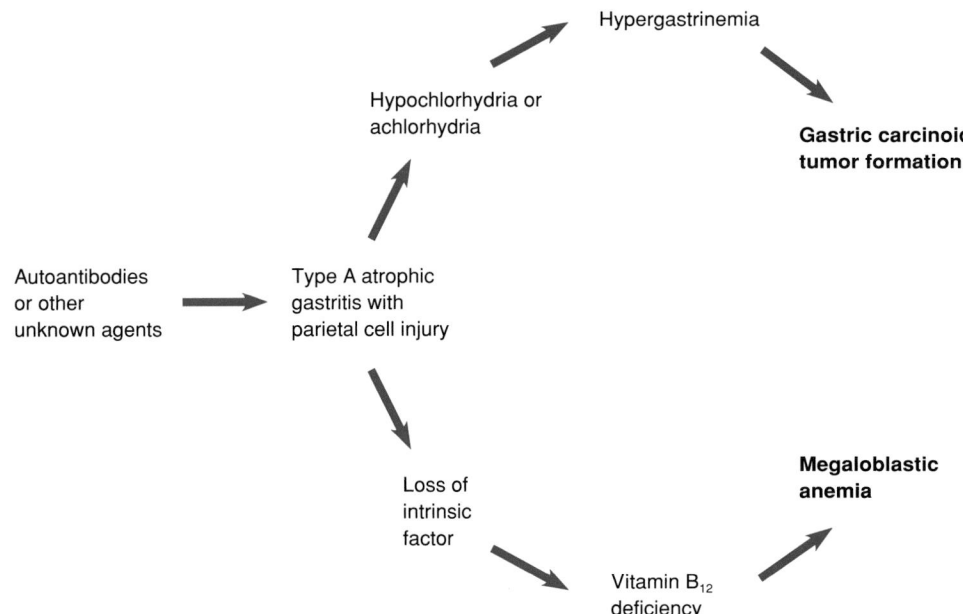

Figure 9-11 Pathophysiology of gastric carcinoid formation and pernicious anemia in patients with chronic atrophic gastritis. Autoantibodies or other agents lead to parietal cell destruction and atrophic gastritis. Loss of parietal cell function results in hypochlorhydria or achlorhydria and loss of intrinsic factor secretion. The latter results in vitamin B_{12} malabsorption and megaloblastic anemia. The reduced acid secretion causes loss of the normal feedback inhibitory mechanisms that restrain gastrin release, and hypergastrinemia results. Prolonged gastrin stimulation promotes enterochromaffin cell hyperplasia in the gastric body and fundus, which, over time, is transformed into multiple gastric carcinoid tumors.

The clinical presentation of patients with gastric carcinoid tumors is varied. Symptoms, if present, are nonspecific. Features of the carcinoid syndrome are rarely present. Most tumors are discovered during endoscopy for vague upper GI symptoms, with the finding of small, often multiple, polyps in the body or fundus in association with atrophic gastritis. Endoscopic biopsy usually confirms the diagnosis. Measurement of basal serum gastrin levels is useful to identify hypergastrinemia because this can influence subsequent management. Gastric secretory responses in the basal state and to pentagastrin stimulation can distinguish hypergastrinemia due to atrophic gastritis from gastrinoma.

Treatment of gastric carcinoid tumors is controversial. In the most common situation, in which the tumors are multiple and associated with chronic atrophic gastritis and hypergastrinemia, elimination of the gastrin drive by antrectomy may result in complete tumor regression. Antrectomy is becoming the preferred approach, but continued endoscopic surveillance of the remaining stomach is required to exclude malignancy. If the carcinoid is solitary, local excision plus antrectomy is the preferred approach. This removes the gastrin drive but also allows complete histologic evaluation of the tumor to exclude the presence of a

concomitant adenocarcinoma. For patients with multiple diffuse tumors, total gastrectomy is another acceptable option. In the setting of metastases, chemotherapy with 5-FU, streptozocin, or doxorubicin is the preferred approach. Symptoms from the carcinoid syndrome, if present, can be effectively palliated with the somatostatin analogue octreotide.

GASTRIC MESENCHYMAL TUMORS

Leiomyoma

Leiomyomas of the GI tract occur frequently but seldom attain a size that draws them to clinical attention. Leiomyomas are mesenchymal tumors and usually arise from smooth muscle cells of the muscularis propria, but they can arise from similar cells in the muscularis mucosae or even the smooth muscle cells of blood vessels. On gross examination, tumors range from a few millimeters to 5 to 6 cm in diameter. Typically, leiomyomas are well-circumscribed, firm to palpation, and white to tan in color. A prominent central indentation may be present, which is pathognomonic on radiologic imaging. Although usually arising in the gastric wall, as they enlarge, leiomyomas can bulge into the gastric lumen or out to the serosa. The former pattern appears to be more common. Microscopically, the tumors are composed of uniform, spindle-shaped cells arranged in interlacing bundles. Mitoses and nuclear atypia are absent, and if present, these features are more consistent with a diagnosis of leiomyosarcoma.

Most leiomyomas are clinically silent, but when symptomatic, they usually cause GI bleeding. Hemorrhage has been attributed to tumor propensity for central mucosal ulceration. When bleeding is present, it is usually occult or manifested by melena. Massive hemorrhage leading to hematemesis is unusual.

The diagnosis of gastric leiomyomas is usually established by upper GI tract endoscopy. Typically, a 2- to 3-cm submucosal tumor with a central, reddish puckering is identified. The overlying mucosa is smooth, and endoscopic biopsy, unless deep, may not reveal the underlying pathology. Radiographic examination of the stomach with barium and gas contrast may show a filling defect. Radiographs are less sensitive than endoscopic examination. Although not usually required for the diagnosis of gastric leiomyomas, selective arteriography has proved useful in the diagnosis of similar lesions distal to the pylorus and should be considered in the evaluation of patients with occult GI blood loss.

The treatment of leiomyomas of the stomach is surgical resection. For most lesions, local excision with a few-millimeter margin of normal tissue is all that is required. Because benign and malignant lesions cannot always be accurately differentiated preoperatively or even at the time of operation, larger lesions should be resected with a wider margin of normal tissue.

Leiomyoblastoma

Leiomyoblastoma is a variant of gastric smooth muscle tumors with characteristic "bizarre" histologic features.[55] These tumors have polyhedral, rather than elongated, cells but in other respects are similar to smooth muscle cells. They are also known as *epithelioid leiomyomas.* In young women, Carney[56] described a syndrome of multiple gastric leiomyoblastomas, pulmonary chondromas, and functioning extraadrenal paragangliomas. The biologic behavior of these tumors has generally mimicked that of benign leiomyomas, however some aggressive tumors have been reported. Treatment is resection.

Leiomyosarcoma

Leiomyosarcomas are uncommon tumors of the stomach and represent the malignant subtype of gastric smooth muscle tumors. Leiomyosarcomas account for

only about 3% of all gastric neoplasms. Because of rarity, no single institution has a large contemporary experience with this tumor and controlled trials examining treatment strategies are not available. The prognosis of patients with these tumors is, in general, better than that for those with adenocarcinoma of the stomach. Microscopically, leiomyosarcomas are distinguished from their benign counterparts by the presence of mitotic activity. Staging of malignant tumors is dependent largely on the number of mitoses observed microscopically. Unfortunately, there is not uniform correlation between mitotic activity and clinical behavior, thus it is prudent to approach all gastric smooth muscle tumors as if they were malignant.

Abdominal pain and GI bleeding are the most common presenting symptoms, with each occurring in 40% to 50% of patients. Symptoms of obstruction caused by a mass-occupying lesion, including nausea and vomiting, are seen in about 10% of patients. A palpable abdominal mass is present in 15%. Ascites is uncommon, even in advanced disease. Either endoscopy or upper GI barium contrast studies generally identify the lesion. CT of the upper abdomen is useful for staging. A chest radiograph should be obtained to exclude pulmonary metastases.

Most gastric leiomyosarcomas are located in the body of the stomach. About one third are found in the cardia and a minority are located in the antrum. The average tumor size at presentation approximates 10 cm in diameter. Lymph node metastases are present in only 5% of patients. Like other intraabdominal sarcomas, metastases to the liver occur in 10% to 15%.

Treatment is surgical resection. The extent of resection for gastric leiomyosarcoma has been controversial. The guiding principle is to achieve microscopically tumor-free resection margins. This can usually be accomplished by local excision with gross margins of 2 to 3 cm. Radical lymphadenectomy or omentectomy, unlike the case in gastric adenocarcinoma, appears to have little influence on cure, as only a small fraction of patients have lymph node metastases. The major prognostic factors in large series are tumor grade, tumor size, and local extent of the tumor.[57] Nearly all patients with tumors less than 5 to 6 cm in diameter are cured by resection. Similarly, survival is proportional to tumor grade. Few patients with local invasion of adjacent organs are cured by radical en bloc resection; they may benefit from palliation of symptoms related to the primary tumor.

The overall patient survival rate after curative surgical resection is 60% at 5 years. Few unresectable patients or patients who undergo palliative resection survive more than 2 years. No effective adjuvant chemotherapy has been reported after curative resection.

Systemic chemotherapy for advanced disease is not effective at significantly reducing tumor burden, and there is little evidence that any regimen prolongs survival. Doxorubicin-containing multidrug regimens appear to have the greatest response rates.

Kaposi's Sarcoma

Kaposi's sarcoma is an unusual tumor that arises from the lymphatic endothelial cell. Although it was first reported in elderly Mediterranean men, this lesion has assumed new importance because of its frequency as a manifestation of the acquired immunodeficiency syndrome. Kaposi's sarcoma also occurs at higher than expected frequency in transplantation patients requiring immunosuppression. In acquired immunodeficiency syndrome, the pathophysiology probably involves stimulation of lymphatic endothelial cell proliferation by both cytokine products of the immune system and human immunodeficiency virus protein products, such as *tat*.[58] Most tumors are cutaneous, but the GI tract is commonly involved.[59] In transplantation patients with Kaposi's sarcoma, visceral tumors are present in about half of cases. Most tumors are asymptomatic, but occasional patients present with bleeding or, less commonly, obstruction. The lesions are identifiable endoscopically as multiple, flat, reddish or bluish-tinted plaques or as umbilicated nodules. Usually, the lesions are submucosal, and superficial mucosal biopsy specimens show normal overlying epithelium.

Treatment is predicated on the clinical situation and the condition of the patient. Fortunately, most gastric lesions are silent and require no symptomatic treatment. Bleeding lesions can be managed with endoscopic coagulation, and surgery is rarely required. Cytotoxic chemotherapy produces responses in a significant minority of patients and should be considered if the patient's general condition permits. Immunomodulatory agents, such as interferon, have had some limited benefit. In patients with transplants, alteration of the immunosuppressive regimen can result in rapid regression of the tumors.

GASTRIC LYMPHOMA

Lymphoma

Primary gastric lymphoma is the second most common malignant gastric tumor but with an incidence far lower than adenocarcinoma. Between 2% and 5% of gastric malignancies are lymphomas, and about 95% are carcinomas. Evidence suggests that the incidence of primary gastric lymphoma is rising.[60,61] The average patient with gastric lymphoma is 50 to 60 years of age. Most series reveal a slight male gender dominance. Although the cause of gastric lymphoma is unknown, it has been suggested that, like gastric adenocarcinoma, infection with the bacteria *H pylori* can play a role. Evidence to support this hypothesis includes the presence of mucosal lymphoid follicles and epithelial B-cell infiltrates in patients with *H pylori* gastritis as well as the greater than 90% frequency of *H pylori* in patients with gastric lymphoma.[62] Whether the association is causal or incidental remains to be determined.

Classification

Gastric lymphomas are usually primary to the stomach but occasionally are a secondary manifestation of systemic lymphoma. Table 9-8 shows two of the most common classification systems. The Rappaport system divides subtypes of tumors on the basis of architecture and historically was an important advance. As knowledge of the immune system increased, a National Institutes of Health–sponsored conference proposed a "working formulation" that acknowledged the prognostic influence of grade of lesion. Other classification systems are also in use.[63] It has been suggested that most primary gastric lymphomas arise from mucosa-associated lymphoid tissue.[64] These are relatively low-grade lesions with better prognoses than high-grade lymphomas.

Table 9-8   Comparison of the Rappaport and Working Formulation Classifications of Lymphomas

Rappaport	Working Formulation
	LOW GRADE
Well-differentiated lymphocytic	A. Small lymphocytic
Nodular, poorly differentiated lymphocytic	B. Follicular, predominantly small cleaved cell
Nodular mixed cell	C. Follicular, mixed, small cleaved and large cell
	INTERMEDIATE GRADE
Nodular histiocytic	D. Follicular, predominantly large cell
Diffuse, poorly differentiated lymphocytic	E. Diffuse, small cleaved cell
Diffuse, mixed cell type	F. Diffuse, mixed, small and large cell
Diffuse, histiocytic	G. Diffuse, large cell
	HIGH GRADE
Diffuse, histiocytic	H. Large cell, immunoblastic
Lymphoblastic	I. Lymphoblastic
Diffuse, undifferentiated	J. Small noncleaved cell

Staging

A number of staging systems have been devised for extranodal non-Hodgkin's lymphoma, and none is entirely satisfactory. The most commonly used staging is a modification of the Ann Arbor system[65] (Table 9-9). In stage IE, only the stomach is involved. Stage IE and stage II1E, in which the stomach and contiguous lymph nodes are involved, have the best prognoses. Occasionally, in stage III and IV patients, it is difficult to determine if the tumor arose primarily in the stomach or if the gastric disease is a manifestation of metastases from a diffuse lymphoma.

Clinical Features

The symptoms of patients with gastric lymphoma largely mimic those of patients with adenocarcinoma of the stomach, and it is not usually possible to distinguish patients with the two tumors on clinical grounds. The most common symptoms are epigastric pain, early satiety, and weight loss. Occasionally, other constitutional symptoms, such as fevers and night sweats, are present. Less than 10% of patients have no symptoms when detected. A significant minority of patients present urgently with hemorrhage, perforation, or obstruction. Physical examination does not usually reveal systemic adenopathy. A palpable mass is present in half of patients.

Diagnostic Evaluation

Most gastric lymphomas are detected by upper GI endoscopy and biopsy. The lesions have variable appearance, ranging from small, superficial, stellate ulcers to bulky masses with diffuse rugal thickening. Multiple deep biopsies may be required to diagnose the lesion accurately if the overlying mucosa is still intact. Overall, a combination of endoscopic biopsy and cytology correctly diagnoses 75% to 90% of patients with gastric lymphoma preoperatively. Barium contrast studies are useful to reveal the anatomic location of the lesion within the stomach and to aid operative planning. Staging of gastric lymphoma includes CT to assess the extent of the tumor within the gastric wall, to identify regional or distant lymphadenopathy, and to assess splenic or hepatic involvement. Endoscopic ultrasonography has proved useful in staging gastric wall involvement.[39] Bone marrow biopsy is useful in selected patients to exclude disseminated lymphoma. Chest radiography should be performed to exclude mediastinal involvement.

Treatment

Treatment of primary gastric lymphoma remains controversial, mainly because of the lack of controlled trials directly comparing treatment options on a stage-for-stage basis. Gastrectomy, chemotherapy, and radiation therapy each have advantages and disadvantages in the treatment of these patients. Because no conclusive data exist, treatment recommendations are necessarily biased, based on the observer's experience with outcome of various treatment strategies, analysis of imperfect literature, and value judgments of the impact of a treatment plan on the patient's quality of life. Gastrectomy is the preferred approach for patients with stage 1E or II1E disease in most centers. Postoperative adjuvant chemotherapy is probably not warranted for patients with stage 1E disease who have undergone successful resection with no gross or microscopic evidence of tumor at surgical margins. There are better rationale and data to support adjuvant chemotherapy for patients with stage II1E disease, although no randomized trials have been performed. Patients with stage II2E are treated with combination chemotherapy and radiation therapy. Patients with stage IIIE or IV tumors are best treated with chemotherapy alone. Patients who present emergently with perforation or significant hemorrhage require palliative resection, if their general condition permits. Occasionally, palliative gastrectomy is also required for patients who develop bleeding or perforation during chemotherapy; however, the risk of this occurrence has probably been overstated in the literature.

The strategy for surgical management of early stage gastric lymphoma is to clear all gross disease. Ordinarily, this can be accomplished with a distal gastrectomy, incorporating the primary nodal drainage groups en bloc in the resection. The spleen is rarely involved in primarily gastric lymphoma, except by direct extension.[66] If this is the case, splenectomy is warranted, but in most patients, splenectomy confers no improvement in outcome. Liver biopsy should be performed to exclude visceral hepatic involvement, and any suspicious distant lymph nodes should undergo biopsy. If the tu-

Table 9-9 Staging of Primary Gastric Lymphoma

Stage	Description
1E	Involvement of the stomach only
II1E	Involvement of stomach and contiguous lymph nodes
II2E	Involvement of stomach and noncontiguous, subdiaphragmatic lymph nodes
IIIE	Involvement of stomach, nodes on both sides of the diaphragm, or spleen
IV	Diffuse involvement of stomach and extralymphatic sites (liver, bone marrow)

mor extends significantly into the duodenum or esophagus, resection is not warranted. These patients are unlikely to be cured by resection and are probably better treated with chemotherapy. Similarly, nodal disease beyond the primary gastric drainage groups portends poor prognosis, and resection is not indicated except to palliate symptoms of bleeding, perforation, or obstruction.

Chemotherapy is indicated, both as adjuvant therapy after successful resection and as primary treatment for advanced gastric lymphoma.[67] The most commonly used regimens include the CHOP regimen (cyclophosphamide, hydroxydoxorubicin, vincristine, and prednisone) and the C-MOPP regimen (cyclophosphamide, methotrexate, vincristine, procarbazine, and prednisone). More intensive regimens have been devised, including the MACOP-B regimen (methotrexate, doxorubicin, cyclophosphamide, vincristine, and prednisone) and the pro-MACE-MOPP regimen (cyclophosphamide, etoposide, doxorubicin, nitrogen mustard, procarbazine, high-dose methotrexate with citrovorum rescue, and prednisone). Some small studies suggest a satisfactory outcome of patients with early-stage gastric lymphoma treated with a combination of chemotherapy and radiation therapy.[22]

Radiation therapy has two main roles in the treatment of patients with primary gastric lymphoma. Some evidence suggests that postoperative radiation therapy improves local control and survival in patients after gastrectomy.[68,69] Other series have failed to confirm a beneficial effect of adjuvant radiation, and it is not the standard approach in most centers for patients with early lesions.[66,70] Radiation has been successfully used as primary treatment for localized gastric lymphoma in small numbers of patients.[71] Most evidence suggests, however, that surgery is superior to radiation therapy in localized gastric lymphoma. In advanced lymphoma, radiation may have a role in achieving local control, but no randomized trials have directly compared this approach with chemotherapy alone. The minimum effective dose appears to be greater than 40 Gy.[72] Whole abdominal irradiation is not required.

Prognosis

Survival of patients with primary gastric lymphoma is stage dependent.[64,66,69,73] Treatment of patients with stage IE lesions results in 5-year survival rates of 75% to 80% in most series. Patients with stage IIE lesions have an average survival rate of 40% at 5 years. The outcome of patients with stage IIIE or IV lesions is poor, with rare 5-year survivors. Factors other than stage that appear to influence outcome include tumor size, with lesions less than 5 cm in diameter having better outcome, and gastric wall invasion, with transmural le-

sions having poorer outcome. Histologic subtype has a weak association with prognosis; the best outcome is in well-differentiated, small cell tumors.

Pseudolymphoma

Gastric pseudolymphoma is a rare condition composed of an exaggerated infiltrate of benign-appearing lymphocytes within the gastric wall. The pattern of the lymphocytic infiltrate resembles, in some ways, that of a follicular lymphoma. Distinguishing features include the presence of reactive germinal centers and mixed populations of lymphocytes, including plasma cells.[74] Regional lymph nodes are not involved. Immunotyping reveals the lymphocytic infiltrate to be polyclonal, unlike lymphoma, in which a monoclonal pattern is present. Pseudolymphoma is usually associated with inflammatory lesions such as gastric ulcer, and has been thought, until recently, to represent a benign immune response to chronic injury. Several recent reports have suggested that pseudolymphoma is a risk factor for gastric lymphoma and may represent low-grade lymphoma or a clonal precursor lesion. Evidence supporting this view includes the relatively frequent association of pseudolymphoma with focal malignant lymphoma and a few reported cases of progression of pseudolymphoma to lymphoma. In some cases, immunochemical and molecular identity of the lymphocytes from the pseudolymphoma and the malignant component have been established. Treatment of pseudolymphoma is generally surgical resection.[75]

TUMORS METASTATIC TO THE STOMACH

The stomach is occasionally the site of metastasis from other malignancies. In autopsy series, tumors metastatic to the upper gut from extraabdominal primary sites have a prevalence of about 1%. Any tumor manifested by carcinomatosis, for example, can involve the serosal surface of the stomach. Typical tumors include ovarian, colonic, and pancreatic carcinoma. Other tumors can involve the stomach by direct local extension. The most common tumors of this type are pancreatic carcinoma and hepatocellular carcinoma, especially in segments II and III of the left hepatic lobe. Finally, the stomach can be the site of hematogenous metastases. Melanoma, adenocarcinoma of the breast, and squamous cell carcinoma of the lung appear to be the most common primary tumors.[76] Curiously, in some reports, the stomach is the only site of metastasis.

Most patients with metastatic tumors to the stomach have no symptoms directly referable to that site. If symptoms are present, they are usually related to either acute bleeding with hematemesis or melena or to chronic blood loss with anemia. An occasional patient presents with symptoms of gastric outlet obstruction. Evaluation by means of an upper GI contrast series or endoscopy usually identifies the problem. Some metastatic tumors, such as melanoma, can be readily identified by their gross appearance at endoscopy. Biopsy is confirmatory. CT of the upper abdomen may be warranted to define the extent of disease, if surgical resection is considered.

Treatment of these lesions is predicated on the extent of tumor present, the patient's general condition, the severity of symptoms, and the predicted natural history. For fit patients with symptomatic tumors limited to the stomach, resection can provide significant palliation. Most patients, however, are less appropriate surgical candidates, and comfort care is indicated.

REFERENCES

1. Tomasulo J. Gastric polyps, histologic types, and their relationship to gastric carcinoma. Cancer 1971;27:346.
2. Sarre RG, Frost AG, Jagelman DG, Petras RE, Sivak MV, McGannon E. Gastric and duodenal polyps in familial adenomatous polyposis: a prospective study of the nature and prevalence of upper gastrointestinal polyps. Gut 1987;28:306.
3. Gorensek M, Matko I, Skralovnik A, Rode M, Satler J, Jutersek A. Disseminated hereditary gastrointestinal polyposis with orocutaneous hamartomatosis (Cowden's disease). Endoscopy 1984;16:59.
4. Cronkhite LW Jr, Canada WJ. Generalized gastrointestinal polyposis: an unusual syndrome of polyposis, pigmentation, alopecia and onychotrophia. N Engl J Med 1955;252:1011.
5. Scharschmidt BF. The natural history of hypertrophic gastropathy (Menetrier's disease). Am J Med 1977;63:644.
6. Overholt BF, Jeffries GH. Hypertrophic, hypersecretory protein-losing gastropathy. Gastroenterology 1970;58:80.
7. Boring CC, Squires TS, Tong T. Cancer statistics, 1993. CA 1993;43:7.
8. Haenzel W, Kurihara M, Segi M, Lee RKC. Stomach cancer among Japanese in Hawaii. JNCI 1972;49:969.
9. Risch HA, Jain M, Choi NW, et al. Dietary factors and the incidence of cancer of the stomach. Am J Epidemiol 1985;122:947.
10. Chen VW, Abu-Elyazeed RR, Zavala DE, et al. Risk factors of gastric precancerous lesions in a high-risk Colombian population. I. Salt. Nutr Cancer 1990;13:59.
11. Chen VW, Abu-Elyazeed RR, Zavala DE, et al. Risk factors of gastric precancerous lesions in a high-risk Colombian population. II. Nitrate and nitrite. Nutr Cancer 1990;13:67.
12. Aird I, Bentall HH, Roberts JAF. A relationship between cancer of the stomach and the ABO blood groups. Br Med J 1953;1:799.
13. Imazeki F, Omata M, Nose H, Ohto M, Isono K. p53 Gene mutations in gastric and esophageal cancers. Gastroenterology 1992;103:892.
14. Iwase T, Tanaka M, Suzuki M, Maito Y, Sugimura H, Kino I. Identification of protein-tyrosine kinase genes preferentially expressed in embryo stomach and gastric cancer. Biochem Biophys Res Commun 1993;194:698.
15. Wright PA, Quirke P, Attanoos R, Williams GT. Molecular pathology of gastric carcinoma: progress and prospects. Hum Pathol 1992;23:848.
16. Sipponen P, Kekki M, Siurala M. Atrophic gastritis and intestinal metaplasia in gastric cancer: comparisons with a representative population sample. Cancer 1983;52:1062.
17. Correa P. A human model of gastric carcinogenesis. Cancer Res 1988;48:3554.
18. Stalnilowicz R, Benbassat J. Risk of gastric cancer after gastric surgery for benign disorders. Arch Intern Med 1990;150:2022.
19. Schafer LW, Larson DE, Melton III J, Higgins JA, Ilstrup DM. The risk of gastric carcinoma after surgical treatment for benign ulcer disease: a population-based study in Olmsted County, Minnesota. N Engl J Med 1983;309:1210.
20. Tersmette AC, Offerhaus GJ, Giardiello FM, et al. Long-term prognosis after partial gastrectomy for benign conditions: survival and smoking-related death of 2633 Amsterdam postgastrectomy patients followed up since surgery between 1931 and 1960. Gastroenterology 1991;101:148.
21. Parsonnet J, Friedman GD, Vandersteen DP, et al. *Helicobacter pylori* infection and the risk of gastric carcinoma. N Engl J Med 1991;325:1127.
22. Maor MH, Velasquez WS, Fuller LM, Silvemintz KB. Stomach conservation in stages IE and IIE gastric non-Hodgkin's lymphoma. J Clin Oncol 1990;8:266.
23. Lauren P. The two histological main types of gastric carcinoma: diffuse and so-called intestinal type carcinoma. Acta Pathol Microbiol Scand 1965;64:31.
24. Kennedy BJ. The unified international gastric cancer staging classification system. Scand J Gastroenterol 1987;22(Suppl):11.
25. Yamada E, Miyaishi S, Nakazato H, et al. The surgical treatment of cancer of the stomach. Int Surg 1980;65:387.
26. Miwa K. Cancer of the stomach in Japan. Gann Monograph on Cancer Research 1979;22:61.
27. Haraguchi M, Okamura T, Sugimachi K. Accurate prognostic value of morphovolumetric analysis of advanced carcinoma of the stomach. Surg Gynecol Obstet 1987;164:335.
28. Meyers WC, Damiano RJ Jr, Postlethwait RW, Rotolo FS. Adenocarcinoma of the stomach: changing patterns over the last 4 decades. Ann Surg 1987;205:1.
29. Weed TE, Nuessle W, Ochsner A. Carcinoma of the stom-

ach: why are we failing to improve survival? Ann Surg 1981;193;407.

30. Tracey KJ, Vlassar H, Cerami A. Peptide regulatory factors: cachectin/tumour necrosis factor. Lancet 1989;5: 1122.

31. Hisamichi S. Screening for gastric cancer. World J Surg 1989;13:31.

32. Llorens P. Gastric cancer mass screening in Chile. Semin Surg Oncol 1991;7:339.

33. Sonnenberg A. Endoscopic screening for gastric stump cancer: would it be beneficial? A hypothetical cohort study. Gastroenterology 1984;87:489.

34. Stael-von-Holstein C, Ericksson S, Huldt B, Hammar E. Endoscopic screening during 17 years for gastric stump carcinoma: a prospective clinical trial. Scand J Gastroenterol 1991;26:1020.

35. Byrne DJ, Browning MC, Cushieri A. CA72-4: A new tumour marker for gastric cancer. Br J Surg 1990;77:1010.

36. Nomura AM, Stemmermann GN, Samloff IM. Serum pepsinogen I as a predictor of stomach cancer. Ann Intern Med 1980;93:537.

37. Graham DY, Schwartz JT, Cain GD, Gyorky F. Prospective evaluation of biopsy number in the diagnosis of esophageal and gastric cancer. Gastroenterology 1982; 82:228.

38. Andaker L, Morales O, Hojer H, Backstrand B, Borch K, Larsson J. Evaluation of preoperative computed tomography in gastric malignancy. Surgery 1991;109:132.

39. Caletti G, Ferrari A, Brocchi E, Barbara L. Accuracy of endoscopic ultrasonography in the diagnosis and staging of gastric cancer and lymphoma. Surgery 1993;113:14.

40. Nicholson DA, Shorvan PJ. Endoscopic ultrasound of the stomach. (Review) Br J Surg 1993;66:487.

41. Bozzetti F, Bonfanti G, Bufalino R, et al. Adequacy of margins of resection in gastrectomy for cancer. Ann Surg 1982;196:685.

42. Zinninger MM. Extension of gastric cancer in the intramural lymphatics and its relation to gastrectomy. Am Surg 1954;20:920.

43. Gouzi JL, Huguier M, Fagniez PL, et al. Total versus subtotal gastrectomy for adenocarcinoma of the antrum: a French prospective controlled study. Ann Surg 1989; 209:162.

44. Heberer G, Teichmann RK, Kramling HJ, Gunther B. Results of gastric resection for carcinoma of the stomach: the European experience. World J Surg 1988;12:374.

45. Wanebo HJ, Kennedy BJ, Chmiel J, Steele G Jr, Winchester D, Osteen R. Cancer of the stomach: a patient care study by the American College of Surgeons. Ann Surg 1993;218:583.

46. Dent DM, Madden MV, Price SK. Randomized comparison of R1 and R2 gastrectomy for gastric carcinoma. Br J Surg 1988;75:110.

47. MacIntyre IMC, Akoh JA. Improving survival in gastric cancer: review of operative mortality in English language publications from 1970. Br J Surg 1991;78:773.

48. Bleiberg H, Gerard B, Deguiral P. Adjuvant therapy in resectable gastric cancer. Br J Cancer 1992;66:987.

49. Hermans J, Bonekamp JJ, Boon MC, et al. Adjuvant therapy after curative resection for gastric cancer: meta-analysis of randomized trials. J Clin Oncol 1993;11:1441.

50. Yonemura Y, Sawa T, Kinoshita K, et al. Neoadjuvant chemotherapy for high-grade advanced gastric cancer. World J Surg 1993;17:256.

51. Saini A, Waxman J. Chemotherapy for gastric cancer. Gut 1992;33:1153.

52. Venook AP. The current state of chemotherapy for gastric cancer. Postgrad Gen Surg 1992;4:233.

53. Hirschowitz B, Griffith J, Pellegrin D, Cummings OW. Rapid regression of enterochromaffinlike cell gastric carcinoids in pernicious anemia after antrectomy. Gastroenterology 1992;102:1409.

54. Rindi G, Luinetti O, Cornaggia M, Capella C, Solcia E. Three subtypes of gastric argyrophil carcinoid and the gastric neuroendocrine carcinoma: a clinicopathologic study. Gastroenterology 1993;104:994.

55. Stout AP. Bizarre smooth muscle tumors of the stomach. Cancer 1962;15:400.

56. Carney JA. The triad of gastric epithelioid leiomyosarcoma, pulmonary chondroma, and functioning extraadrenal paraganglioma: a five-year review. Medicine (Baltimore) 1983;62:159.

57. Grant CS, Kim CH, Farrugia G, Zinsmeister A, Goeliner JR. Gastric leiomyosarcoma: prognostic factors and surgical management. Arch Surg 1991;126:985.

58. Ensoli B, Barillari G, Salahuddin SZ, Gallo RC, Wong-Staal F. Tat protein of HIV-1 stimulates growth of cells derived from Kaposi's sarcoma lesions of AIDS patients. Nature 1990;345:84.

59. Friedman S, Wright T, Altman D. Gastrointestinal manifestations of Kaposi's sarcoma in acquired immunodeficiency syndrome: endoscopic and autopsy findings. Gastroenterology 1985;89:102.

60. Hayes J, Dunn E. Has the incidence of primary gastric lymphoma increased? Cancer 1989;63:2073.

61. Severson RK, Davis S. Increasing incidence of primary gastric lymphoma. Cancer 1990;66:1283.

62. Wotherspoon AC, Ortiz-Hidalgo C, Falzon MR, Isaacson PG. Helicobacter pylori–associated gastritis and primary B-cell gastric lymphoma. Lancet 1991;338:1175.

63. Ersboll J, Schulz HB, Hougaard P, et al. Comparison of the working formulation of non-Hodgkin's lymphoma with the Rappaport, Kiel, and Lukes-Collins classifications. Cancer 1985;55:2442.

64. Cogliatti SB, Schmid U, Schumacher U, et al. Primary B-cell gastric lymphoma: a clinicopathological study of 145 patients. Gastroenterology 1991;101:1159.

65. Carbone PP, Kaplan HS, Musshoff K, Smithers DW, Tubiana M. Report of a committee of Hodgkin's disease staging classification. Cancer Res 1971;31:1860.

66. Rosen CB, van Heerden JA, Martin JK, Wold LE, Ilstrup DM. Is an aggressive surgical approach to the patient with gastric lymphoma warranted? Ann Surg 1987;205: 634.

67. Solidoro A, Payet C, Sanchez-Lihon J, Montalbetti JA.

Gastric lymphomas: chemotherapy as a primary treatment. Semin Surg Oncol 1990;6:218.

68. Hockey MS, Powell J, Crockert J, Fieldings WL. Primary gastric lymphoma. Br J Surg 1987;74:483.

69. Shiu MH, Karas M, Nisce L, Lee BJ, Filippa DA, Lieberman PH. Management of primary gastric lymphoma. Ann Surg 1982;195:196.

70. Schwarz RJ, Conners JM, Schmidt N. Diagnosis and management of stage IE and IIE gastric lymphoma. Am J Surg 1993;165:561.

71. Burgers JM, Taal BG, van Heerde P, Somers R, den-Hartog-Jager FC, Hart AA. Treatment results of primary stage I and II non-Hodgkin's lymphoma of the stomach. Radiother Oncol 1988;11:319.

72. Shimm DS, Dosoretz DE, Anderson T, Linggood RM, Harris NL, Wang CC. Primary gastric lymphoma: an analysis with emphasis on prognostic factors and radiation therapy. Cancer 1983;52:2044.

73. Talamonti MS, Dawes LG, Joehl RJ, Nahrwold DL. Gastrointestinal lymphoma: a case for primary surgical resection. Arch Surg 1990;125:972.

74. Brooks JJ, Enterline HT. Gastric pseudolymphoma: its three subtypes and relation to lymphoma. Cancer 1983;51:476.

75. Orr RK, Lininger JR, Lawrence W Jr. Gastric pseudolymphoma: a challenging clinical problem. Ann Surg 1984;200:185.

76. Kadakia SC, Parker A, Canales L. Metastatic tumors to the upper gastrointestinal tract: endoscopic experience. Am J Gastroenterol 1992;87:1418.

77. Forman D, Newell DG, Fullerton F, et al. Association between infection with *Helicobacter pylori* and risk of gastric cancer: evidence from a prospective investigation. Br Med J 1991;302:1302.

78. Haglund C, Roberts PJ, Jalanko H, Kunsela P. Tumour markers CA 19.9 and CA 50 in digestive tract malignancies. Scand J Gastroenterol 1992;27:169.

79. Hansson LE, Engstrand L, Nyrén O. *Helicobacter pylori* infection: independent risk indicator of gastric adenocarcinoma. Gastroenterology 1993;105:1098.

80. Ikeda Y, Mori M, Adachi Y, Matsushima T, Sigimachi K, Saku M. Carcinoembryonic antigen (CEA) in stage IV gastric cancer as a risk factor for liver metastasis: a univariate and multivariate analysis. J Surg Oncol 1993;53:235.

81. Kornek G, Depisch D, Temsch EM, Scheithauer W. Comparative analysis of cancer-associated antigen CA-195, CA 19-9 and carcinoembryonic antigen in diagnosis, follow-up and monitoring of response to chemotherapy in patients with gastrointestinal cancer. J Cancer Res Clin Oncol 1991;117:493.

82. Kuusela P, Haglund C, Roberts PJ. Comparison of a new tumour marker CA 242 with CA 19-9, CA 50 and carcinoembryonic antigen (CEA) in digestive tract diseases. Br J Cancer 1991;63:636.

83. Loizate-Toricaguena A, Lamiquiz-Vallejo A. Tumor-associated trypsin inhibitor (TATI) in benign and malignant gastric disease. Scand J Clin Lab Invest 1991;207(Suppl):59.

84. Parsonnet J. *Helicobacter pylori* and gastric cancer. Gastroenterol Clin North Am 1993;22:89.

Digestive Tract Surgery: A Text and Atlas, edited by Richard H. Bell,
Layton F. Rikkers, and Michael W. Mulholland.
Lippincott-Raven Publishers, Philadelphia, © 1996.

10

Surgery for Obesity

Christian T. Campos | *Henry Buchwald* | *Howard Bourdages*

Obesity, defined as exceeding of the ideal body weight as outlined on the Metropolitan Life Insurance Company height and weight tables,[1] has a relatively high prevalence, affecting nearly 26% of Americans aged 20 to 75 years.[2] The incidence of obesity has increased during the past two decades, and the prevalence of this disorder is disproportionately high in women, the poor, and certain ethnic groups.

Morbid obesity, defined as being 100 lb (45.5 kg) or 100% above ideal body weight according to these actuarial tables,[3] is estimated to affect between 3% and 5% of the US adult population and, by definition, is associated with the development of life-threatening complications. Numerous therapeutic approaches to this problem have been advocated, including low-calorie diets, anorectic drugs, behavior modification, and exercise therapy, but the only treatment proven to be effective in the long-term management of morbid obesity is surgical intervention.[4]

The pathogenesis of morbid obesity is poorly understood. The balance between caloric intake and overall energy expenditure constitutes a remarkably precise but poorly defined process of physiologic regulation that ultimately determines body mass. In general, humans tend to maintain a set weight, with minor fluctuations.[5] In obese persons, this set-point of stored energy is too high. Whether this results from a low metabolic rate with low energy expenditure, from excessive caloric intake, or from a combination of both remains unclear.[6] Animal and human data suggest that obesity may be an inherited characteristic; however, neither the specific genetic abnormality nor the degree of genetic influence has been defined. Epidemiologic studies show that less than 10% of children of lean parents are obese. If one parent is obese, 50% of the children will be obese; if both parents are obese, nearly 80% of their offspring will be obese.[7] In light of the available data, it is best to regard morbid obesity as multifactorial in origin, the result of various genetic, psychological, environmental, social, and cultural influences that interact to result in a complex disorder of both appetite regulation and energy metabolism. The view that morbid obesity results simply from a lack of self control by the patient is a gross and callous oversimplification that is encountered too frequently within the medical profession and society at large.

MEDICAL, PSYCHOLOGICAL, AND SOCIOECONOMIC CONSEQUENCES OF MORBID OBESITY

Morbid obesity is clearly associated with a significantly reduced life expectancy. In a compilation of 16 cases of extraordinary obesity (average weight, 811 lb [369 kg]), the mean age at death was 35 years (range, 22 to 59 years).[8] The mortality rate of obesity rises geometrically as a function of the percent increase in weight above the ideal body weight. The mortality rate accelerates steeply once patients are 40% to 50% overweight, and patients who are more than 100% above their ideal body weight are at markedly increased risk of premature death.[3]

The principal causes of the excessive early mortality rate among obese persons are heart disease, stroke, and diabetes.[9] Hypertension is the most common cardiovascular complication. In the Framingham study, the incidence of sudden death increased significantly in men who were over 30% above their ideal body weight.[10] Stroke is considerably more common in obese persons.[11] Obesity results in cardiac hypertrophy and can lead to congestive heart failure even in the absence of other cardiac disease.[12] Venous disease also is more prevalent among the morbidly obese, with chronic venous insufficiency and thrombophlebitis being the most common manifestations.

Increased body weight is associated with a greater incidence of diabetes mellitus. Adult-onset diabetes mellitus is at least 3 to 4 times more common in the obese.[13] Other endocrine abnormalities observed in obese patients include virilization secondary to elevated serum adrenocorticotropic hormone levels causing increased cortisol and androgenic steroid production by the adrenal glands in women. Massively obese men have low serum testosterone levels and elevated estrogen levels resulting from enhanced conversion of androgens to estrogens by adipose tissue. Menstrual irregularities and secondary amenorrhea are more common in obese women.[14]

Morbidly obese patients have decreased pulmonary function, primarily because of a reduction in expiratory reserve volume. Dyspnea is common. Chest wall bulk and insensitivity to chronic hypercarbia can lead to alveolar hypoventilation with drowsiness and episodic involuntary sleep, a condition known as the pickwickian syndrome. Although uncommon, the pickwickian syndrome has a mortality rate approaching 30%.[15]

Chronic cholelithiasis and cholecystitis have been observed in 30% to 40% of morbidly obese persons.[16] Altered liver function has been reported, and many patients have some degree of fatty metamorphosis of the liver. Cirrhosis of the liver is 2.5 times more common in obese men and 1.5 times more common in obese women.[17]

Obesity can be positively correlated with carcinoma of the stomach.[18] Endometrial carcinoma is more common in obese women, perhaps because of enhanced peripheral conversion of excess androgens to estrogens by adipose tissue.[19] Breast carcinoma also is more frequent in obese women.[19,20]

Orthopedic problems occur frequently in morbidly obese persons, particularly osteoarthritis of the lumbar spine, herniation of intervertebral disks, and degenerative osteoarthritis of the hips and knees.[21] Skin disorders are more common in obese patients, with intertriginous dermatitis and venous stasis ulceration encountered most often.

Morbid obesity is not simply a physical problem. This condition also has significant psychological and socioeconomic consequences.[22] In Western society, obesity is an undesirable social attribute. The belief that the morbidly obese are responsible for their physical plight through an inherent character flaw or moral weakness is deeply rooted. Severely overweight persons experi-

ence great difficulty with interpersonal relationships, courtship, marriage, employment, and community acceptance. The morbidly obese tend to isolate themselves from society and withdraw from exposure to ridicule. Employers are reluctant to hire obese persons, and they often fall into lower income brackets. Unemployment is common among the morbidly obese, and many are sustained by the welfare system. Greater health hazards can be associated with employing obese workers.[23] Employers often believe that morbidly obese workers cannot cope with their jobs, are unsightly to customers, and, most important, are prohibitively expensive to insure. A summary of the major medical, psychological, and socioeconomic consequences of morbid obesity is presented in Table 10-1.

NONSURGICAL APPROACHES TO MORBID OBESITY

In March 1992, the National Institutes of Health Technology Assessment Conference on Methods for Voluntary Weight Loss concluded that nonsurgical methods

---

Table 10-1 Major Medical, Psychological, and Socioeconomic Consequences of Morbid Obesity

MEDICAL
Hypertension
Myocardial infarction
Cerebrovascular accident
Congestive heart failure
Diabetes mellitus
Gout
Virilization
Menstrual abnormalities
Carcinoma of the uterus and breast
Dyspnea
Pickwickian syndrome
Sleep apnea
Cholelithiasis
Hepatic steatosis and cirrhosis
Degenerative joint disease
Degenerative back and intervertebral disk disease
Intertriginous dermatitis
Varicose veins
Venous stasis ulceration
Thromboembolism

PSYCHOLOGICAL
Passive-dependent or passive-aggressive personality
Distortion of body image
Interpersonal relationship, courtship, and marriage difficulties
Sexual dysfunction

SOCIOECONOMIC
Limited educational opportunity
Reduced socioeconomic mobility
Job discrimination
Uninsurability
Reliance on social and economic support programs

of weight loss are not effective in the long term, except in rare instances. Data reviewed at that time showed that nearly all participants in any nonsurgical weight loss program regained their lost weight within 5 years.[4] In a randomized prospective study comparing surgery for weight loss with dietary caloric restriction alone, investigators followed up 128 patients between 1979 and 1981.[24] They found a maximum weight loss of 57 lb (26 kg) in patients who underwent horizontal gastroplasty compared with 48 lb (22 kg) in patients who were treated with diet alone. This difference was not statistically significant. However, at 2 years of follow-up, the diet-treated patients had regained all their lost weight, whereas the surgically treated patients maintained a 26-lb (12-kg) weight reduction ($P < .05$). With the further development of more effective surgical procedures to induce and maintain weight loss, even greater sustained weight loss is anticipated in morbidly obese patients undergoing surgery compared with patients treated with dietary caloric restriction alone.

Although prescription and nonprescription medications are available to induce weight loss, there is no role for long-term pharmacologic therapy in the management of morbid obesity. Anorectic drugs, when added to low-calorie diets, can result in 11- to 22-lb (5- to 10-kg) weight reduction.[25] However, weight regain is rapid once pharmacologic support is withdrawn, and a weight loss of this magnitude is trivial in the morbidly obese population.

Behavior modification techniques, in conjunction with low-calorie diets and increased physical activity, are used by various lay and professional weight loss programs. Weekly weight losses of 1 to 2 lb (0.5 to 1 kg) have been reported; however, nearly all lost weight is regained after 5 years.[26]

INDICATIONS FOR SURGICAL MANAGEMENT

Guidelines for selecting patients for operative management of morbid obesity vary among surgeons and are in the process of evolution. The National Institutes of Health Consensus Development Conference on Surgical Treatment of Morbid Obesity[27] advocated operative intervention for obese patients who are at least 100 lb (45 kg) or 100% above their ideal body weight, have serious physical or psychosocial problems because of their obesity, have failed adequate trials of nonsurgical therapy, or have repeatedly regained lost weight after transient periods of successful weight loss. The following guidelines have been established[28]:

1. Patients should exceed ideal body weight by at least 100 lb (45 kg) or 100%.

2. They should have no known causative and correctable metabolic or endocrine etiology for their morbid obesity.
3. They should have an objectively measurable complication (physical, psychological, social, or economic) that might benefit from weight reduction.
4. They should be intelligent enough to comprehend the full import of the proposed surgical procedure, including all known and unknown risks.
5. They should be willing to be observed for a prolonged period.
6. They should have attempted weight reduction using conservative treatment modalities without success.

In rare circumstances, patients who are not quite 100 lb (45 kg) or 100% above their ideal body weight are candidates for operative intervention. These patients must clearly manifest complications of obesity (eg, degenerative joint disease, diabetes, hypertension) that would be significantly improved after successful weight loss, and must meet all other established guidelines for obesity surgery.

Age is not an absolute barrier to consideration for obesity surgery. Although obesity procedures are performed infrequently on patients older than 60 years, they are done in certain circumstances (ie, severe degenerative joint disease). Obesity surgery also can be offered, after careful screening, to young patients between the ages of 10 and 18 years.

Patients with morbid obesity are best served at centers with a multidisciplinary team approach and commitment to the care of this particular patient population. All patients should be screened carefully before surgery, and a thorough history should be obtained, with particular attention to previous weight loss attempts, obesity-related illnesses, psychological and economic issues, and long-term expectations. The surgical staff should provide patients with complete information regarding the available surgical options and their lifelong consequences. Nursing and dietary issues should be explained in detail by dedicated nursing and dietary professionals. Active participation by patients and their families in a long-term follow-up program that includes medical, psychological, and nutritional/dietary support should be stressed. If patients wish to proceed after this preoperative evaluation, they are admitted to the hospital for the operative phase of a long-term management program for the treatment of morbid obesity.

SURGICAL APPROACHES TO MORBID OBESITY

No discussion of surgical approaches to morbid obesity would be complete without mention of the jejunoileal bypass operation, first reported in 1954.[29] In its final form, the proximal 40 cm of jejunum was anastomosed to the distal 4 cm of ileum. This operation was extremely popular in the 1960s and 1970s, during which time it is estimated that more than 200,000 of these procedures were performed in the United States. In terms of weight loss, the jejunoileal bypass was an excellent operation. In one series of more than 700 patients,[30] the mean weight loss achieved during the first year was 88 lb (40 kg), representing 65% of the excess body weight in these patients. The maximum weight loss occurred between 1 and 2 years after operation, with stabilization between 3 and 4 years. Thereafter, most patients regained 10 to 20 lb (4.5 to 9 kg), finally achieving a weight 20% to 40% above their ideal body weight.

Jejunoileal bypass has been abandoned as a primary therapy for morbid obesity. The demise of this operation was due primarily to its metabolic consequences, of which liver failure was the most significant.[31] Other serious side effects included diarrhea, electrolyte disturbances, gas-bloat syndrome, arthralgia and arthritis, and nephrolithiasis. In one experience, about 25% of patients who underwent this operation had serious late complications, and 8% had progressive liver function abnormalities requiring takedown of the jejunoileal bypass. Because of this high rate of complications and, most important, because of the comparable success of gastric restrictive procedures in producing significant, sustained weight loss with relative freedom from late complications, jejunoileal bypass now is rarely performed and gastric restrictive operations are the preferred surgical approach to the management of morbid obesity.[32]

Gastrointestinal Bypass

Clinical Antecedents and Early Development

The origins of gastric bypass for morbid obesity are found in the 60% Billroth II gastrectomy with retrocolic gastroenterostomy for the treatment of peptic ulcer disease. Although this procedure was effective in preventing ulcer recurrence, patients were unable to gain and frequently lost weight. Discouraged with the results of jejunoileal bypass, investigators hypothesized that a small proximal gastric pouch anastomosed to the upper small intestine would induce weight loss if the procedure was not ulcerogenic. After confirming that a small gastric pouch did not produce sufficient acid to cause an ulcer at the gastrojejunostomy, surgeons reported results with transection of the stomach and creation of a nearly 100-mL proximal pouch drained into a retrocolic loop gastrojejunostomy with a 2-cm stoma.[33] To in-

crease the weight reduction, modifications narrowing the stoma to 8 to 12 mm and reducing the pouch volume to less than 60 mL were introduced.[34]

The stomach also can be stapled rather than transected, creating an antecolic loop gastrojejunostomy to the anterior surface of the proximal gastric pouch.[35] To prevent the occasional problems of symptomatic bile reflux with gastritis and esophagitis, investigators introduced the Roux-en-Y gastrojejunostomy, first with transection of the stomach and then with simple stapling to create a 30-mL upper pouch.[36] This modification rapidly became the standard gastric restrictive operation. More recently, this technique has been modified by the placement of a vertical staple line between the lesser curvature and the angle of His, with drainage of this 30-mL pouch into the Roux-en-Y jejunal limb along the lesser curve of the stomach. The gastrojejunostomy is fashioned with an EEA stapler, creating a 1-cm stoma.[37]

Operative Technique

Patients undergo a standard mechanical and antibiotic bowel preparation on the day before surgery, often at home after having received detailed instructions during their preoperative clinic visit. On the day of surgery, patients are positioned supine and pneumatic compression stockings are placed on the lower extremities. After wide preparation of the skin, a midline incision is made from the xiphoid process to just above the umbilicus. The subcutaneous tissue is divided by manual retraction. On entering the abdomen, the round ligament of the liver is divided to facilitate exposure and a plastic wound protector drape is inserted. The xiphoid can be partially split to gain additional exposure superiorly. A needle biopsy of the liver is routinely performed and, if cholelithiasis is present, the gallbladder is removed.

The ligament of Treitz is identified, and the jejunum is divided about 25 cm distal to this point using a GIA stapling device. The staple lines are reinforced with interrupted nonabsorbable sutures. The Roux-en-Y limb is fashioned by performing a side-to-side jejunojejunostomy 70 cm distal to the point of initial jejunal division using the GIA stapling device, reinforcing the entire anastomosis with interrupted nonabsorbable sutures (Fig. 10-1). The rotational mesenteric defect is closed carefully to prevent internal herniation.

After the Roux-en-Y limb is completed, patients are placed in steep Trendelenburg position and abdominal retractors are situated below both costal margins. When the retractors have been secured, patients are placed in steep reverse Trendelenburg position, bringing the upper abdominal contents caudally into the operating field. Because of the sheer mass of the abdomi-

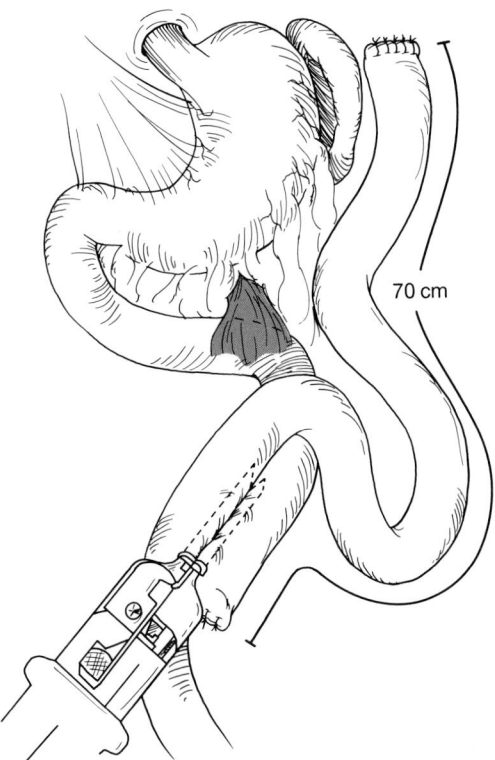

70 cm

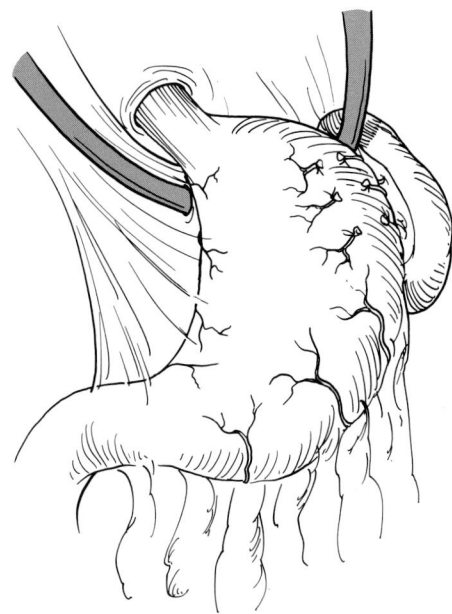

Figure 10-3 A small opening is made along the lesser curvature below the first set of feeding vessels of the gastroesophageal junction and is used to pass a Penrose drain around the stomach toward the greater curvature.

Figure 10-1 The Roux-en-Y limb is created with a GIA stapler, reinforced throughout its circumference with interrupted 5-0 nonabsorbable sutures, and measured to 70 cm.

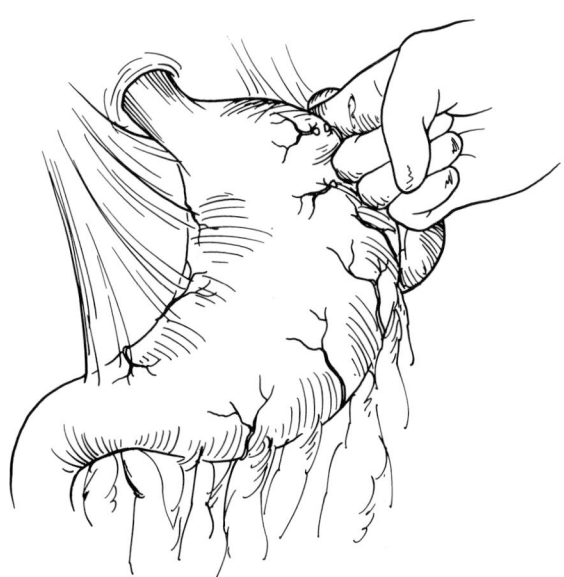

Figure 10-2 The upper portion of the greater curvature of the stomach is mobilized by division of several short gastric vessels. Downward retraction of the stomach, as well as placement of the hand in the lesser sac, is essential to expose vessels for sequential ligation and division.

nal wall, the upper quadrants of the peritoneal cavity can be difficult to reach. The importance of having adequate retraction of the abdominal wall cannot be overemphasized: it is one of the key points in performing any type of morbid obesity surgery. Whatever type of retraction system is used, a large amount of force generally is required to gain proper exposure. Patients commonly experience some rib discomfort after surgery because of the intraoperative tension placed on the thoracic cage. However, this discomfort usually is transient.

The left triangular ligament of the liver is divided with cautery, and the left lateral segment of the liver is retracted to the patient's right to facilitate exposure. The upper greater curvature of the stomach is mobilized to the gastroesophageal junction by dividing the first three or four short gastric vessels (Fig. 10-2). A retrogastric plane is developed in the lesser peritoneal sac. A small opening is made in the lesser omentum below the first set of feeding vessels, and a Penrose drain is passed through this opening around the stomach (Fig. 10-3).

The previously fashioned Roux-en-Y limb is brought to the stomach in an antecolic manner (Fig. 10-4) and anastomosed just below the esophagogastric junction on the greater curvature using a side-to-side technique, facilitated by use of the GIA stapling device (Fig. 10-5). A 1-cm orifice is created. The nasogastric tube is passed into the Roux limb under direct vision,

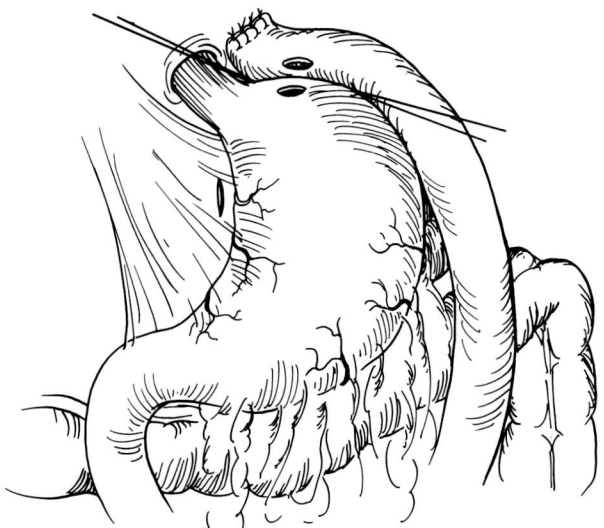

Figure 10-4 The gastrojejunostomy is created and tacking sutures applied. Cautery is used to create two openings for the GIA stapler.

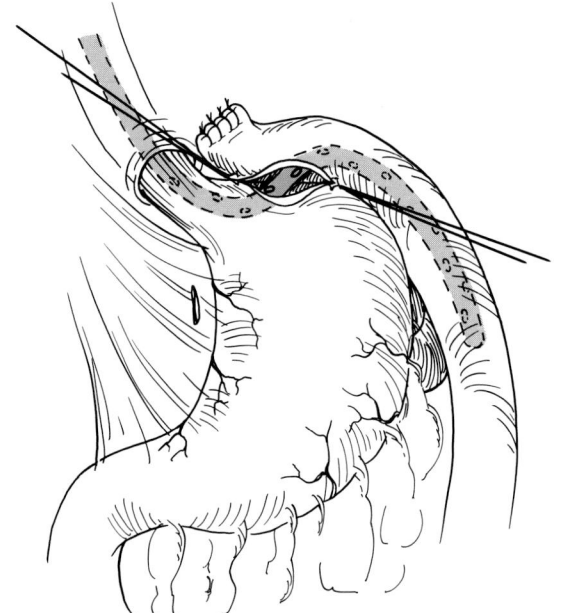

Figure 10-6 The nasogastric tube is passed into the Roux-en-Y limb under direct vision.

with suction holes positioned in the stomach as well as the jejunum (Fig. 10-6). The anastomosis is completed (Fig. 10-7) and circumferentially reinforced with interrupted nonabsorbable sutures (Fig. 10-8). A 70-cm Roux-en-Y limb generally reaches the stomach with ease. When undue tension is apparent, incising the peritoneum overlying the jejunal mesentery or dividing the greater omentum provides additional length. Only rarely must the jejunal limb be brought to the stomach in a retrocolic fashion.

Next, the Penrose drain is removed and the TA-90 stapler is inserted from the greater curvature of the

stomach, just below the gastrojejunostomy, to the previously created opening on the lesser curvature (Fig. 10-9). The stapler is fired to create the smallest possible gastric pouch. A cartridge is used that places four rows of staples 1 mm apart with a single application of the stapler. The volume of the gastric pouch need not be measured as previously reported,[38] because these measurements are of questionable reproducibility and reliability. The Roux-en-Y limb of jejunum is tacked to the

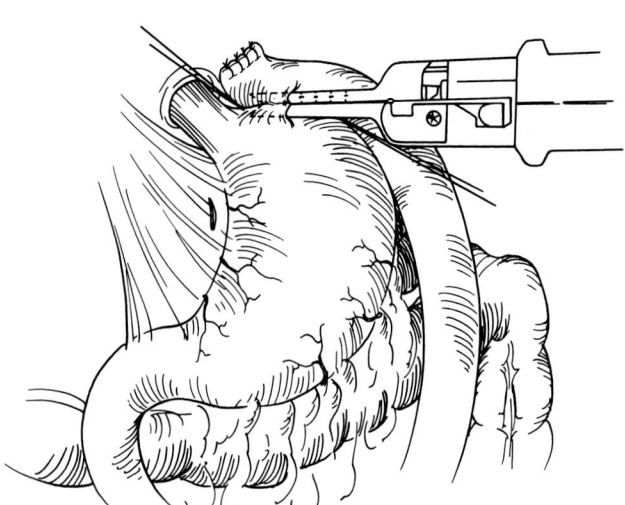

Figure 10-5 The GIA stapler is inserted.

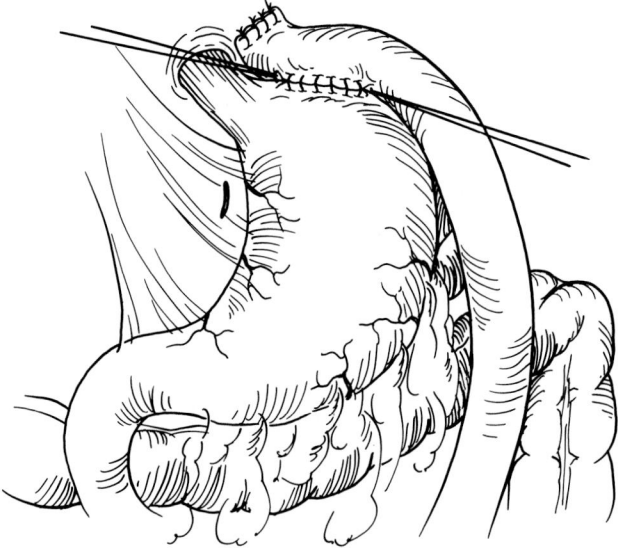

Figure 10-7 The anterior row of sutures is placed.

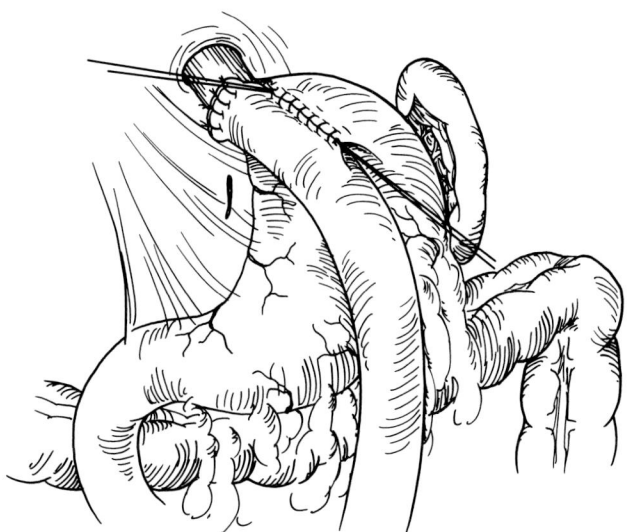

Figure 10-8 A posterior row of sutures along the back wall completes the gastrojejunostomy.

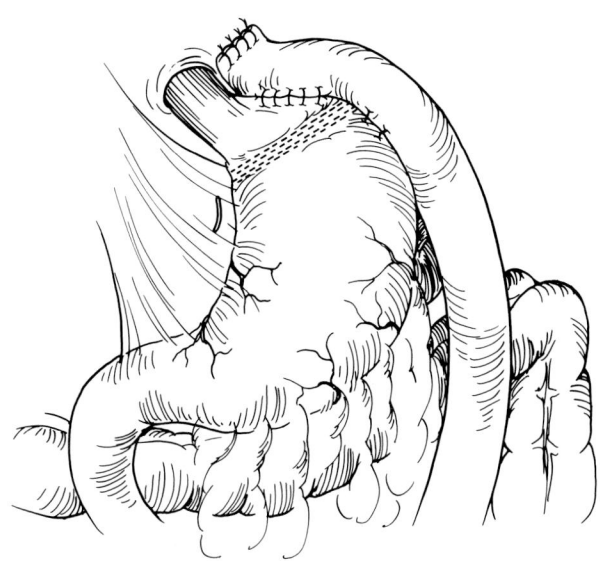

Figure 10-10 The completed staple line has four rows of staples. The Roux-en-Y limb is tacked along the greater curvature to prevent kinking.

stomach below the anastomosis along the greater curvature to prevent kinking (Fig. 10-10).

At this point, the abdomen is irrigated with saline containing either a first-generation cephalosporin or 0.25% neomycin. The retractors and the wound protector drape are removed, and patients are returned to a horizontal position for closure. The surgical team changes gowns and gloves, and new instruments are used for closure. The midline fascia is closed with interrupted nonabsorbable sutures. The abdominal wall

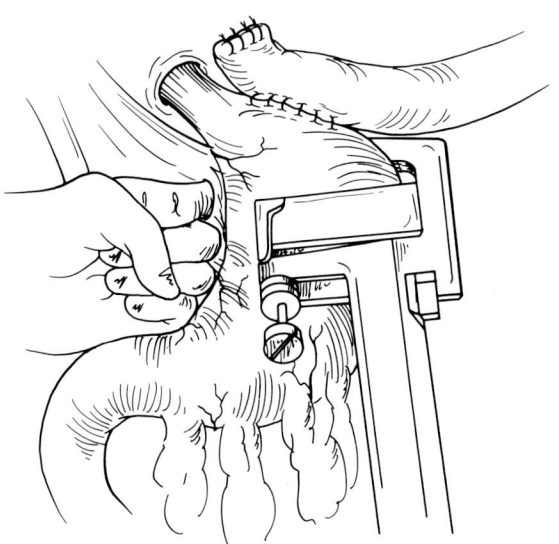

Figure 10-9 A finger is used to guide placement of a TA-90 stapler from the greater curvature to the lesser curvature underneath the completed gastrojejunostomy.

must be closed meticulously in these patients to minimize the incidence of postoperative incisional hernia. A large drain is placed above the fascial closure and brought out through a lateral stab incision. The large mass of adipose tissue tends to drain copiously. Seromas and wound infections are more common in undrained wounds. The subcutaneous tissues and Scarpa's fascia are closed over the drain with interrupted absorbable sutures. The skin edges are reapproximated with metal clips. Patients are extubated in the operating room, and early postoperative ambulation and vigorous pulmonary toilet are stressed. The subcutaneous drain is removed when its daily output falls below 20 mL. The nasogastric tube is removed when bowel motility returns, generally on the third or fourth postoperative day.

The success of the gastrointestinal bypass operation depends on the creation of a small gastric pouch and a small gastric outlet that maintain their size over a long period. Although pouch volume does not need to be measured routinely, it should be about 30 to 35 mL and not exceed 50 mL. The problem of gastric staple line disruption is minimized by placing four parallel rows of staples. Because of the abundant blood supply of the stomach, this does not result in vascular compromise. It also is important to reinforce the gastrojejunal anastomosis, because dilation could result in weight regain. Generally, the stoma of a gastric bypass gastrojejunostomy should measure 0.75 to 1.2 cm to obtain and maintain adequate weight loss.

Gastroplasty

Clinical Antecedents and Early Development

In 1971, transection gastrointestinal bypass was modified by partially dividing the stomach from the lesser curvature, leaving a channel along the greater curvature.[39] This novel procedure, designated a gastroplasty, restricted the gastric reservoir but preserved the normal digestive function of the distal stomach and the normal digestive and absorptive functions of the duodenum. Gastroplasty was believed to be more physiologic than gastrointestinal bypass. By creating a small upper pouch and a narrow stoma, it was hoped that caloric intake would be sufficiently restricted to achieve successful weight loss.

In 1977, horizontal gastroplasty was modified further by stapling rather than dividing the stomach, and by reinforcing the stoma with mesh or a running suture.[40] However, the results of this technique were disappointing, with unacceptably high rates of weight regain after initial loss, and horizontal gastroplasty no longer is advocated as an effective procedure for the management of morbid obesity.[41]

In 1980, the vertical-banded gastroplasty was introduced.[42] In this procedure, a window is created in the mid-stomach, close to the lesser curvature, using a 28-mm EEA stapling device. With a 30F or 32F dilator held in place along the lesser curvature, a vertically oriented staple line is placed between this window and the angle of His using a TA-90 stapler, creating an upper gastric pouch with a volume of about 30 mL. The stoma is reinforced by wrapping a 6 cm by 1.5 cm Marlex band around the lesser curvature channel through the gastric window.

A modification of the vertical-banded gastroplasty was described in 1981[43] and advocated subsequently.[44,45] In the Silastic ring vertical gastroplasty procedure, no gastric window is created. A 24F dilator is held along the lesser curvature, and a modified TA-90 stapler with a notch constructed in the heel to accommodate the dilator is positioned vertically along the lesser curvature up to the angle of His. By firing this stapler, a gastric pouch with a capacity of about 30 mL is created. The lesser curvature outlet then is reinforced with a 44-mm length of 3-mm hollow silicone elastomer (Silastic) tubing sutured around the outlet, with a 2-0 polypropylene suture placed through the tubing and twice through both walls of the stomach at the end of the staple line, and finally tied to itself over the dilator. The Silastic ring vertical gastroplasty and the vertical-banded gastroplasty are the two gastroplasty procedures with acceptable long-term weight loss results that are used in the management of morbid obesity.

Operative Technique

The Silastic ring vertical gastroplasty is simpler to perform than the vertical-banded gastroplasty; does not require creation of a gastric window using the EEA stapler; does not involve the use of the highly reactive Marlex band, which has been reported to erode into the stomach; and produces equivalent weight loss. As for a gastrointestinal bypass, patients receive a mechanical and antibiotic bowel preparation on the day before surgery, generally at home. At the time of surgery, patients are placed in a supine position on the operating table with pneumatic compression stockings wrapped around the lower extremities. An upper midline incision is made from the xiphoid process to just above the umbilicus. After the abdomen has been entered, the round ligament of the liver is divided to facilitate exposure. A plastic wound protector drape is inserted, and a needle biopsy of the liver is performed routinely. If cholelithiasis is present, the gallbladder is removed.

Patients then are placed in steep Trendelenburg position and abdominal retractors are situated below both costal margins. After the retractors have been secured, patients are placed in steep reverse Trendelenburg position, bringing the abdominal contents caudally into the operating field. The left triangular ligament of the liver is partially divided, and the free edge of the lateral segment of the liver is retracted to the right to expose the esophageal hiatus and the upper stomach. A small

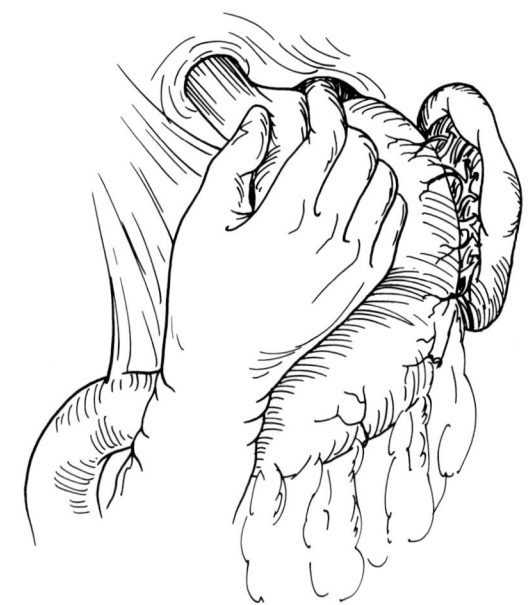

Figure 10-11 Mobilization is not as extensive as for gastrointestinal bypass, and greater curvature dissection is limited to freeing the angle of His above any of the short gastric vessels.

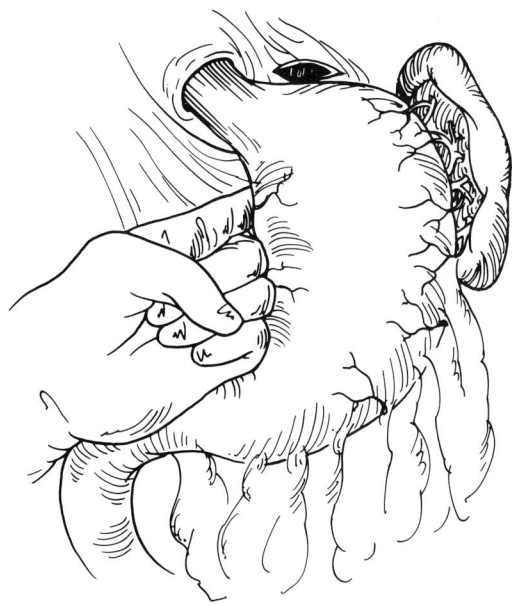

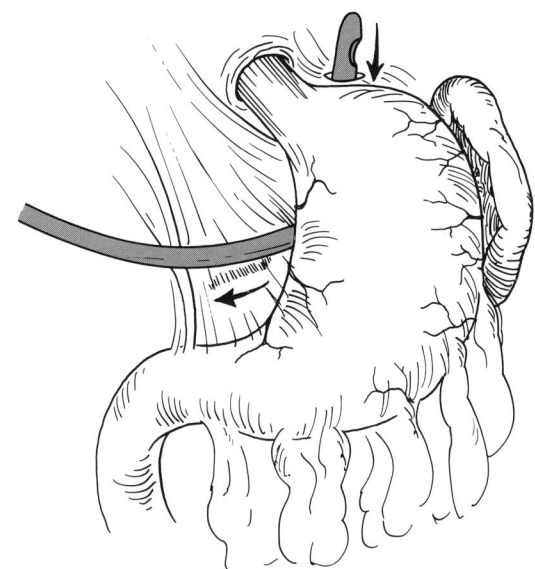

Figure 10-13 A red Robinson catheter is placed behind the stomach from the angle of His to the opening in the lesser omentum.

Figure 10-12 A small opening is created along the lesser curvature further down than for gastrointestinal bypass, midway between the esophagogastric junction and the crow's foot of vessels. A finger is passed behind the stomach to the angle of His.

opening in the gastrosplenic ligament is created high on the greater curvature at the angle of His, generally without requiring the division of short gastric vessels (Fig. 10-11). A similar, small opening is made in the lesser omentum along the lesser curvature below the first set of feeding vessels, and a retrogastric plane is developed manually between these two openings within the lesser peritoneal sac (Fig. 10-12). A red Robinson catheter is passed through these openings behind the stomach (Fig. 10-13).

A 24F dilator then is passed through the mouth and into the stomach by the anesthesiologist. Using the red Robinson catheter as a guide, a specially modified TA-90 stapler with a notch constructed in the heel to accommodate the dilator (TA-90B) is positioned vertically (Fig. 10-14). The dilator is held in place along the lesser curvature up to the angle of His (Fig. 10-15). When the stapler is fired, a gastric pouch with a capacity of about 30 mL is created. The lesser curvature gastroplasty outlet then is reinforced with a 44-mm length of 3-mm Silastic tubing, with a 2-0 polypropylene suture placed through the tubing, placed twice through both walls of the stomach at the end of the staple line, and tied to itself over the 24F dilator (Fig. 10-16). It is secured with a single 5-0 nonabsorbable suture taken in a Lembert manner. The Silastic ring is not covered with serosal bites of stomach because erosion of the ring into the stomach has been reported with covered rings. The di-

lator is removed and replaced with a nasogastric tube to complete the gastroplasty procedure.

The postoperative dietary care of patients who have undergone gastroplasty requires careful attention, and considerable dietary retraining and support are necessary before these patients are discharged from the hos-

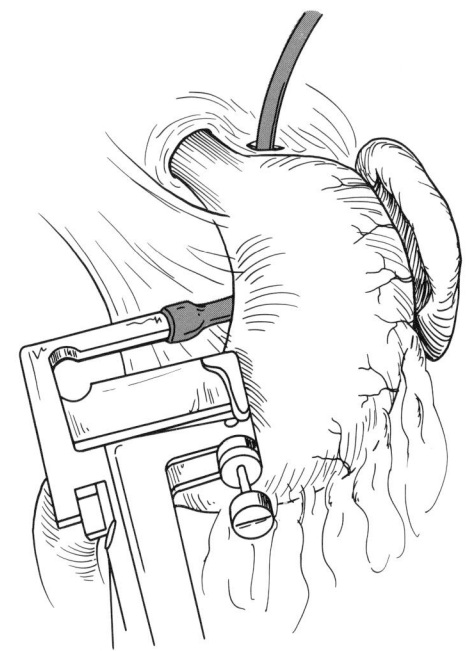

Figure 10-14 The notched TA-90B stapler is passed using the red Robinson catheter to guide the instrument upward.

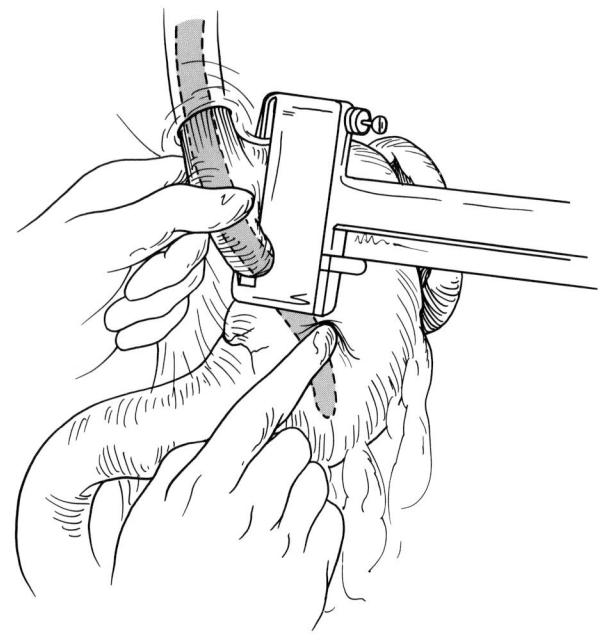

Figure 10-15 The gastric pouch is created by firing the TA-90B stapler alongside a 24F dilator held along the lesser curvature.

pital. Whereas patients who have undergone gastrointestinal bypass are discharged eating a soft-solid diet that is almost uniformly well tolerated, patients who have had gastroplasty may not be able to tolerate soft-solid food for the first 4 to 6 weeks after surgery. Pa-

tients who have undergone gastroplasty may require a liquid diet for a longer period and are discharged from the hospital eating pureed foods. If vomiting occurs after the diet is advanced to include soft solids, pureed foods are reinstituted. As anticipated, dietary indiscretion remains a frequent problem in this population, and patients have been readmitted to the hospital soon after discharge with intractable vomiting caused by impaction of an inadequately chewed food bolus in the gastroplasty outlet. If persistent vomiting occurs after gastroplasty, upper gastrointestinal endoscopy is performed to examine the gastroplasty outlet. If a food bolus is impacted, this can be cleared using the endoscope. If food impaction is not identified and the gastroplasty outlet is swollen closed, spontaneous passage or expulsion of the food bolus is presumed to have occurred, and a nasogastric tube is placed under direct vision. Edema of the gastroplasty outlet usually resolves after 1 to 4 days. Resolution of the gastroplasty outlet obstruction is confirmed radiographically with a barium swallow before the nasogastric tube is removed and a liquid diet is allowed. This postoperative scenario has been observed in about 2% to 3% of patients. Its occurrence can be minimized by thorough postoperative dietary counseling that is reinforced during the first few postoperative outpatient clinic visits. However, occasional intolerance of soft solid food distinguishes patients who have undergone gastroplasty from those who have had gastrointestinal bypass during the first 6 to 12 months after operation.

Other Surgical Approaches

The use of jaw wiring to treat obesity was based on the observation that patients with mandibular fractures lost weight as a result of fixation of the maxilla to the mandible. Problems with oral hygiene, aspiration after emesis, and uniform weight regain after discontinuation of fixation proved this to be an unacceptable long-term therapy for morbid obesity.[46] Rarely, preliminary jaw wiring followed by a definitive gastric weight loss procedure with removal of the jaw fixation is performed in extremely obese patients.

Gastric balloons, placed into the stomach using the endoscope and inflated, were felt to increase satiety and lead to modification of eating habits in morbidly obese patients. Uniform weight regain after initial limited weight loss has led to the abandonment of gastric balloon therapy for morbid obesity.[47]

Some investigators have advocated wrapping the entire stomach in a restrictive Marlex sac,[48] and others have proposed banding the entire stomach to create a small upper gastric pouch and a restrictive stoma.[49] Un-

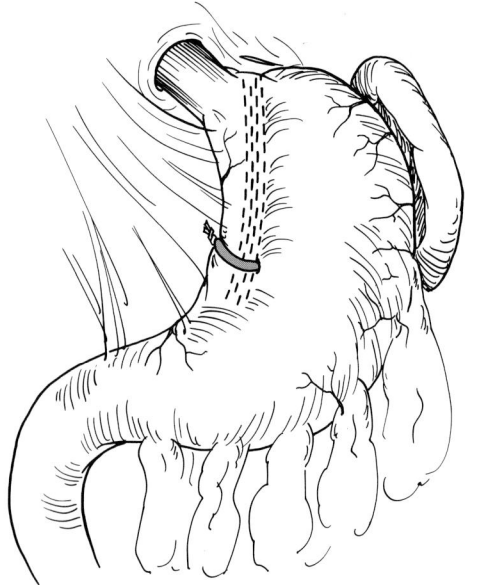

Figure 10-16 The Silastic ring with Prolene suture has been placed to reinforce the gastric pouch outlet to prevent dilation.

acceptably high complication rates and almost uniform weight regain have discredited both these procedures.

In 1979, the biliopancreatic bypass was introduced,[50] a complicated procedure that led to sustained weight loss through selective, rather than indiscriminate, malabsorption. Biliopancreatic bypass consists of a distal, 70% gastrectomy with diversion of biliopancreatic secretions into the terminal ileum with a long Roux-en-Y gastroenterostomy. The gastric remnant is drained by dividing the ileum 250 cm proximal to the ileocecal valve and connecting the distal segment into the gastric pouch. The proximal segment, containing the biliary and pancreatic secretions, is anastomosed to the terminal ileum 50 cm proximal to the ileocecal valve. This divides the gastrointestinal tract into three regions: (1) the alimentary tract from the gastroenterostomy to the enteroenterostomy, (2) the biliopancreatic tract from the duodenal stump to the enteroenterostomy, and (3) the common tract from the enteroenterostomy to the ileocecal valve. Water, electrolytes, and water-soluble vitamins, which do not require digestion by biliopancreatic secretions, are absorbed in the alimentary tract. Fats and carbohydrates, the major dietary caloric sources, are digested and only minimally absorbed in the short common tract. There is no blind loop, and bile acids are absorbed in the common tract, minimizing diarrhea.

The loss of excess body weight after biliopancreatic bypass has been 50% to 70% after 1 year in uncontrolled series.[51] Anemia and severe protein deficiency requiring intensive oral protein supplementation and occasional intravenous parenteral nutrition have been reported occasionally after this procedure. Most patients have two or three loose stools per day and produce a moderate amount of foul-smelling flatus.

Biliopancreatic bypass is not widely performed in the United States. It is a technically involved operation, and normal gastrointestinal continuity cannot be restored if patients request reversal of the procedure. Failure to achieve successful weight loss with a technically adequate gastrointestinal bypass or gastroplasty due to continued consumption of a high-fat, high-carbohydrate diet may be an indication for biliopancreatic bypass.[52] However, gastrointestinal bypass and vertical-banded or Silastic ring vertical gastroplasty are less complex and more physiologic alternatives with proven long-term efficacy and minimal morbidity.

RESULTS OF GASTROINTESTINAL BYPASS AND GASTROPLASTY

Operative Mortality and Morbidity

With current surgical and anesthetic management, gastrointestinal bypass and gastroplasty can be performed with an operative mortality rate of less than 1% and a major morbidity rate of less than 10%.[53] In one series,[54] only one postoperative death occurred in 364 consecutive patients (0.3%). Postoperative pneumonia developed in 3.3% of patients, pulmonary embolism in 0.9%, bacteriuria in 4.9%, gastrointestinal bleeding in 1.5%, and wound infection in 0.8%. The National Bariatric Surgery Registry has reported an operative mortality rate of 0.1% in 5178 patients.[55] The median hospital stay was 4 days, and 89.7% of patients had no postoperative morbidity. The most frequently occurring complications were respiratory dysfunction (4.5%), gastrointestinal tract leak (0.6%), and deep venous thrombosis (0.3%).

Weight Loss

The weight loss results of gastrointestinal bypass are the standard to which all surgical procedures for morbid obesity are compared. In a prospective randomized comparison with jejunoileal bypass,[36] a 112-lb (51-kg) weight loss 1 year after gastrointestinal bypass was reported, and other studies have described 44%, 50%, and 51% reductions in excess body weight 1, 2, and 3 years, respectively, after gastrointestinal bypass.[56] In another series of 106 patients,[54] a 62% loss of excess body weight 1 year after gastrointestinal bypass was observed. This was maintained over 3 years and was comparable to the weight loss achieved in 205 patients undergoing jejunoileal bypass during the same period.

Randomized, prospective comparisons of vertical gastroplasty and gastrointestinal bypass have shown that the latter procedure leads to somewhat greater weight loss with an increased incidence of nutritional deficiencies. In one report,[52] vertical-banded gastroplasty resulted in a 43% loss of excess body weight after 1 year, significantly less than the 66% loss achieved by gastrointestinal bypass. Similar results also were seen 2 and 3 years after operation. Other investigators have reported a success rate of 67% for gastrointestinal bypass versus 48% for vertical-banded gastroplasty in 310 patients over a 3-year follow-up period during which success was defined as the loss of over 50% of excess body weight or a current pregnancy.[57] In another report,[58] a success rate of 58% for gastrointestinal bypass versus 39% for vertical-banded gastroplasty ($P = .08$) was noted in 106 patients, with success defined as a body mass index of less than 77 lb/m² (35 kg/m²). In a retrospective review of 35 consecutive patients undergoing either gastrointestinal bypass or Silastic ring vertical gastroplasty,[59] investigators noted a 91.7-lb (41.7-kg) weight loss 1 year after the former and a 86.7-lb (39.4-kg) weight loss 1 year after the latter (P = not significant). A much higher incidence of feeding problems, including inability to eat solid food and vomiting, was seen in the gastroplasty group. At 1-year follow-up, 93% of patients who had undergone gastrointestinal bypass could eat a diet of solid food compared with only 62% of those who had undergone Silastic ring vertical gastroplasty. Only 7% of the gastrointestinal bypass group reported vomiting, whereas 76% of the gastroplasty group reported at least occasional vomiting.

Complications

Complications after gastrointestinal bypass are uncommon and essentially limited to transient nausea and vomiting, gastric staple line failure, dumping syndrome, and peptic ulcer disease. Of 106 consecutive patients undergoing gastrointestinal bypass, 11 experienced transient nausea or vomiting that resolved as they adapted to severe restriction of their gastric reservoir capacity.[54] In another analysis, only 7% of patients who had undergone gastrointestinal bypass reported any vomiting after 1 year of follow-up.[59]

Gastric staple line disruption occurs in about 5% of patients and is manifested by weight regain after successful weight loss, and by loss of satiety after eating small meals. Reoperation with revision of the gastric staple line is required.[60] Failure of gastrointestinal bypass, with inadequate weight loss or weight regain, also can be caused by pouch or anastomotic dilation. These problems require operative revision for correction.[60]

The dumping syndrome may occur after gastrointestinal bypass but responds favorably to dietary restriction of simple sugars and avoidance of idiosyncratically provocative food items. Gastritis in the excluded stomach and frank peptic ulcer disease with bleeding or perforation are extremely rare but troublesome complications in these patients. Endoscopic evaluation of the excluded stomach and duodenum is impossible. Persistent upper gastrointestinal pain responding to a trial of histamine receptor antagonist therapy may be the only confirmatory evidence for gastritis. Rare cases of upper gastrointestinal bleeding or perforation from a duodenal ulcer have been reported.[61] Stomal ulcer also is rare and responds to antacids and histamine receptor antagonist therapy. With persistent or recurrent upper abdominal pain, or with bleeding that is unresponsive to histamine receptor antagonist therapy, near-total 90% gastrectomy can have good results. Bile reflux gastritis and esophagitis were eliminated by adoption of the Roux-en-Y gastrojejunostomy rather than the loop gastrojejunostomy reconstruction. Because the duodenum, the principal site of iron absorption, is excluded from the food stream after gastrointestinal bypass, iron-deficiency anemia occasionally develops. This responds well to oral iron supplementation, and parenteral iron administration only rarely is necessary. Because intrinsic factor is lacking after gastrointestinal bypass, vitamin B_{12} deficiency is anticipated. The administration of intramuscular vitamin B_{12} every 4 to 6 weeks is recommended to prevent the development of pernicious anemia.

The use of vertical-banded or Silastic ring vertical gastroplasty avoids many of the complications associated with gastrointestinal bypass. Vitamin B_{12} deficiency, iron deficiency, and the dumping syndrome do not develop after gastroplasty. The most frequently observed problem is persistent nausea or vomiting and solid food intolerance due to the small gastric pouch and the reinforced, banded gastroplasty outlet. The evaluation and treatment of problems related to solid food intolerance or impaction of inadequately chewed food have been discussed (see Gastroplasty: Operative Technique). After Silastic ring vertical gastroplasty, patients ingest a pureed diet for at least 4 to 6 weeks and must be instructed to chew foods well to prevent obstruction of the gastroplasty outlet. In a review of 35 patients,[59] 76% of those undergoing Silastic ring vertical gastroplasty experienced at least occasional vomiting. About 2% to 3% of patients in one series required readmission to the hospital for intractable vomiting due to swelling of the gastroplasty orifice or impaction of a food bolus within the gastroplasty outlet.

Amelioration of Secondary Complications of Morbid Obesity

Significant loss of excess body weight, whether achieved by gastrointestinal bypass or by Silastic ring vertical gastroplasty, leads to improvement in nearly all the secondary complications of morbid obesity. Hypertension generally improves or resolves. In one report,[62] hypertension was noted in 26% of morbidly obese patients before surgery. After surgery, hypertension resolved in 66% of these patients. Loss of excess body weight results in increased exercise tolerance and greater cardiac reserve. The risk of coronary artery disease and cerebrovascular disease is reduced through control of major risk factors such as hypertension, diabetes, and hyperlipidemia. Non–insulin-dependent and insulin-dependent diabetes are significantly improved after surgery for morbid obesity. In a series of 515 morbidly obese patients undergoing gastrointestinal bypass,[63] 41.2% were euglycemic and 55.9% were either diabetic or had glucose intolerance before surgery. After surgery, 88.7% were euglycemic and only 5.8% remained diabetic, and two thirds of the latter patients had markedly improved glucose control and reduced daily insulin requirements. Significant improvements are observed in many of the other secondary complications of morbid obesity outlined in Table 10-1 after successful weight loss surgery. The quality of life for most patients undergoing gastrointestinal bypass, vertical-banded gastroplasty, or Silastic ring vertical gastroplasty, though difficult to measure, appears to be greatly improved. Over 90% of patients who have undergone gastrointestinal bypass and have achieved successful weight loss without significant postoperative sequelae experience a greater sense of well-being.

> Morbid obesity is a disease of multifactorial etiology with significant medical, psychological, and socioeconomic consequences that is associated with a markedly reduced life expectancy. Only surgical intervention has been shown to result in effective, sustained weight loss in these patients. Malabsorption procedures, of which the jejunoileal bypass was the prototype, have been essentially abandoned because of their frequent, and occasionally severe, side effects. Gastric restrictive procedures have become the standard for the surgical treatment of morbid obesity. Roux-en-Y gastrointestinal bypass and either vertical-banded gastroplasty or Silastic ring vertical gastroplasty lead to significant, sustained reductions in excess body weight with minimal morbidity and, in experienced centers, low operative and perioperative mortality rates. After successful surgically induced weight loss, many of the secondary complications of morbid obesity improve or completely resolve, and it is reasonable to expect an improvement in overall survival.

REFERENCES

1. Metropolitan Life Insurance Company. 1983 Height and weight tables. Stat Bull Metrop Insur Co 1983;64:2.
2. Kuczmarski RJ. Prevalence of overweight and weight gain in the United States. Am J Clin Nutr 1992;55(Suppl):495S.
3. Van Itallie TB. Morbid obesity: a hazardous disorder that resists conservative treatment. Am J Clin Nutr 1980;33(Suppl):358.
4. National Institutes of Health Consensus Development Conference Statement. Gastrointestinal surgery for severe obesity. Am J Clin Nutr 1992;55(Suppl):615S.
5. Hirsch J, Leibel RL. New light on obesity. N Engl J Med 1988;318:509.
6. Ravussin E, Lillioja S, Knowler WC, et al. Reduced rate of energy expenditure as a risk factor for body-weight gain. N Engl J Med 1988;318:467.
7. Menguy R. Morbid obesity. In: Schwartz SI, Ellis H, eds. Maingot's abdominal operations, ed 9. Norwalk, CT, Appleton & Lange, 1990:771.
8. Bray GA. The obese patient. Philadelphia, WB Saunders, 1976.
9. Howard L, Jenks JS. Medical aspects of morbid obesity. In: Linner JH, ed. Surgery for morbid obesity. New York, Springer-Verlag, 1984:1.
10. Kannel WB, Gordon T. Physiologic and medical concomitants of obesity: the Framingham study. In: Bray GA, ed. Obesity in America. Bethesda, MD, US Department of Health, Education, and Welfare, NIH publication no. 79-359, 1979:125.
11. Heyden S, Hames CG, Bartel A, et al. Weight and weight history in relation to cerebrovascular and ischemic heart disease. Arch Intern Med 1971;128:956.
12. Amad KH, Brennan JC, Alexander JK. The cardiac pathology of chronic exogenous obesity. Circulation 1965;32:740.
13. Jeanrenaud B. Insulin and obesity. Diabetologia 1979;17:133.
14. Glass AR, Burman KD, Dahms WT, Boehm TM. Endocrine function in human obesity. Metabolism 1981;30:89.
15. Burwell CS, Robins ED, Whaley RD, Bickelman AG. Extreme obesity associated with alveolar hypoventilation: a pickwickian syndrome. Am J Med 1956;21:811.
16. Marks HH. Influence of obesity on morbidity and mortality. Bull NY Acad Med 1960;36:296.
17. Buchwald H, Lober PH, Varco RL. Liver biopsy findings in seventy-seven consecutive patients undergoing jejunoileal bypass for morbid obesity. Am J Surg 1974;127:48.
18. Zacho A, Larsen V, Christensen J. Body weight and cancer of the stomach. Acta Chir Scand 1965;130:125.
19. National Institutes of Health Consensus Development Panel on the Health Implications of Obesity. Health complications of obesity. Ann Intern Med 1985;103:1073.
20. Willett WC, Browne ML, Bain C, et al. Relative weight and risk of breast cancer among premenopausal women. Am J Epidemiol 1985;122:731.
21. Bray GA. Complications of obesity. Ann Intern Med 1985;103:1052.
22. Wadden TA, Stunkard AJ. Social and psychological consequences of obesity. Ann Intern Med 1985;103:1062.
23. Drenick EJ, Bale GS, Seltzer F, Johnson DG. Excessive mortality and causes of death in morbidly obese men. JAMA 1980;243:443.
24. Andersen T, Backer OG, Stokholm KH, Quaade F. Randomized trial of diet and gastroplasty compared with diet alone in morbid obesity. N Engl J Med 1984;310:352.
25. Garrow JS. Treatment of morbid obesity by nonsurgical means: diet, drugs, behavior modification, exercise. Gastroenterol Clin North Am 1987;16:443.
26. National Institutes of Health Technology Assessment Conference Panel. Methods for voluntary weight loss and control. Ann Intern Med 1992;116:942.
27. Van Itallie TB, Burton BT. National Institutes of Health Consensus Development Conference on Surgical Treatment of Morbid Obesity. Ann Surg 1979;189:455.
28. O'Leary JP. Historical perspective on intestinal bypass

procedures. In: Griffen WO Jr, Printen KJ, eds. Surgical management of morbid obesity. New York, Marcel Dekker, 1987:1.

29. Kremen AJ, Linner JH, Nelson CH. An experimental evaluation of the nutritional importance of proximal and distal small intestine. Ann Surg 1954;140:439.

30. Rucker RD Jr, Chan EK, Horstmann J, et al. Searching for the best weight reduction operation. Surgery 1984;96:624.

31. Andersen T, Juhl E, Quaade F. Fatal outcome after jejunoileal bypass for obesity. Am J Surg 1981;142:619.

32. Buchwald H, Rucker RD Jr. The rise and fall of jejunoileal bypass. In: Nelson RL, Nyhus LM, eds. Surgery of the small intestine. New York, Appleton-Century-Crofts, 1987:529.

33. Mason EE, Ito C. Gastric bypass. Ann Surg 1969;170: 329.

34. Mason EE, Printen KJ, Bloomers TJ, et al. Gastric bypass for obesity after ten years' experience. Int J Obes 1978;2: 197.

35. Alden JF. Gastric and jejunoileal bypass: a comparison in the treatment of morbid obesity. Arch Surg 1977;112: 799.

36. Griffen WO Jr, Young VL, Stevenson CC. A prospective comparison of gastric and jejunoileal bypass procedures for morbid obesity. Ann Surg 1977;186:500.

37. Torres JC, Oca CF, Garrison RN. Gastric bypass: Roux-en-Y gastrojejunostomy from the lesser curvature. South Med J 1983;76:1217.

38. Linner JH. Gastric operations: specific techniques. In: Linner JH, ed. Surgery for morbid obesity. New York, Springer-Verlag, 1984:70.

39. Printen KJ, Mason EE. Gastric surgery for relief of morbid obesity. Arch Surg 1973;106:428.

40. Gomez CA. Gastroplasty in the surgical treatment of morbid obesity. Am J Clin Nutr 1980;33(Suppl):406.

41. Linner JH. Comparative effectiveness of gastric bypass and gastroplasty. Arch Surg 1982;117:695.

42. Mason EE. Vertical banded gastroplasty for obesity. Arch Surg 1982;117:701.

43. Laws HL. Standardized gastroplasty orifice. Am J Surg 1981;144:393.

44. Eckhout GV, Willbanks OL, Moore JT. Vertical ring gastroplasty for morbid obesity. Am J Surg 1986;152:713.

45. Willbanks OL. Long-term results of silicone elastomer ring vertical gastroplasty for the treatment of morbid obesity. Surgery 1987;101:606.

46. Kark AE. Jaw wiring. Am J Clin Nutr 1980;33(Suppl): 420.

47. Geliebter A, Melton PM, Gage D, McCray RS, Hashim SA. Gastric balloon to treat obesity: a double-blind study in nondieting subjects. Am J Clin Nutr 1990;51:584.

48. Wilkinson LH. Reduction of gastric reservoir capacity. Am J Clin Nutr 1980;33(Suppl):515.

49. Granstrom L, Backman L. Technical complications and related operations after gastric banding. Acta Chir Scand 1987;153:215.

50. Scopinaro N, Gianetta E, Civalleri D, Bonalumi U, Bachi V. Biliopancreatic bypass for obesity. II. Initial experience in man. Br J Surg 1979;66:618.

51. Scopinaro N, Gianetta E, Civalleri D, et al. Biliopancreatic bypass. In: Griffen WO Jr, Printen KJ, eds. Surgical management of morbid obesity. New York, Marcel Dekker, 1987:93.

52. Sugerman HJ, Starkey JV, Birkenhauer R. A randomized prospective trial of gastric bypass versus vertical banded gastroplasty for morbid obesity and their effects on sweets versus non–sweets eaters. Ann Surg 1987;205: 613.

53. Griffen WO Jr. Gastric bypass. In: Griffen WO Jr, Printen KJ, eds. Surgical management of morbid obesity. New York, Marcel Dekker, 1987:35.

54. Rucker RD Jr, Horstmann J, Schneider PD, Varco RL, Buchwald H. Comparisons between jejunoileal and gastric bypass operations for morbid obesity. Surgery 1982;92:241.

55. Mason EE, Renquist KE, Jiang D. Perioperative risks and safety of surgery for severe obesity. Am J Clin Nutr 1992;55(Suppl):573S.

56. Buckwalter JA. Clinical trial of jejunoileal and gastric bypass for the treatment of morbid obesity: four-year progress report. Am Surg 1980;46:377.

57. Hall JC, Watts JM, O'Brien PE, et al. Gastric surgery for morbid obesity: the Adelaide study. Ann Surg 1990;211: 419.

58. MacLean LD, Rhode BM, Sampalis J, Forse RA. Results of the surgical treatment of obesity. Am J Surg 1993;165: 155.

59. Zimmermann V, Campos CT, Buchwald H. Weight loss comparison of gastric bypass and Silastic ring vertical gastroplasty. Obesity Surg 1992;2:47.

60. Buchwald H, Campos CT. Remedial operations following surgery for morbid obesity. In: McQuarrie DG, Humphrey EW, eds. Reoperative general surgery. St Louis, Mosby–Year Book, 1992:270.

61. Printen KJ, LaFave JW, Alden JF. Bleeding from the bypassed stomach following gastric bypass. Surg Gynecol Obstet 1983;156:65.

62. Foley EF, Benotti PN, Borlase BC, Hollingshead J, Blackburn GL. Impact of gastric restrictive surgery on hypertension in the morbidly obese. Am J Surg 1992;163:294.

63. Pories WJ, MacDonald KG Jr, Morgan EJ, et al. Surgical treatment of obesity and its effect on diabetes: 10-y follow-up. Am J Clin Nutr 1992;55(Suppl):582S.

Digestive Tract Surgery: A Text and Atlas, edited by Richard H. Bell,
Layton F. Rikkers, and Michael W. Mulholland.
Lippincott-Raven Publishers, Philadelphia, © 1996.

11

Atlas of Gastric Surgery

Michael W. Mulholland

PREOPERATIVE PREPARATION

All patients undergoing gastric resection should receive perioperative systemic antibiotics. Achlorhydria and long-standing gastric outlet obstruction are associated with increased numbers of enteric organisms within the gastric lumen, so antibiotic coverage should be broadened in these circumstances.

As with all major abdominal operations, anemia and coagulation deficits should be corrected before operation. Because gastric operations require upper abdominal incision with resultant pulmonary compromise, attention to bronchial toilet is mandatory. Cigarettes smoking should be terminated; bronchodilators and chest physical therapy may be helpful in selected cases.

Gastric outlet obstruction is associated with hypokalemic alkalosis. Vomiting or nasogastric aspiration of stomach secretions results in loss of hydrogen and chloride ions. Renal attempts to correct alkalosis cause loss of potassium in urine. Electrolyte abnormalities must be corrected before operation. Retained food and gastric bezoars may require lavage through a large-bore evacuation tube for complete removal.

295

SECTION I *Surgical Anatomy*

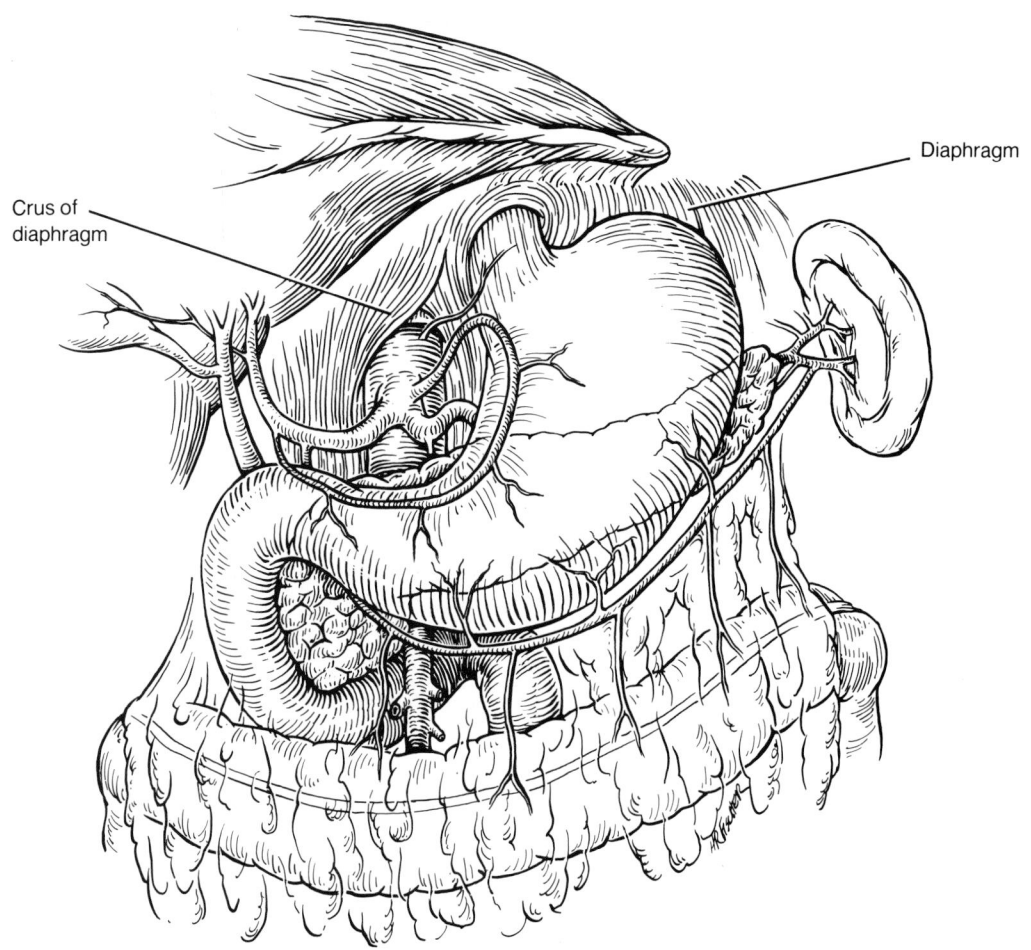

Figure 11-I-1

Topographic Anatomy of the Stomach

The stomach is located in the upper abdomen, in apposition to a number of structures that may be affected by gastric diseases and that must be considered in performing gastric operations. The lower end of the esophagus terminates in the stomach immediately after penetrating the diaphragm at the esophageal hiatus. The stomach can be divided into the fundus, body, and antrum based on differences in mucosal histology, but no external landmarks delineate these regions, and surgically defined anatomy is somewhat arbitrary. The fundus lies to the left and superior to the esophagogastric junction. The junction of the body and antrum can be defined approximately by a line running from a point 6 to 8 cm proximal to the pylorus along the lesser curvature to a point one third of the distance from the pylorus to the esophagogastric junction along the greater curvature.

Anteriorly and superiorly, the stomach is in contact with the left lobe of the liver and, when distended, with the parietal peritoneum. Posteriorly, the stomach relates to the undersurface of the diaphragm, the left adrenal gland, and the pancreatic neck, body, and tail. The spleen lies to the left and posterior to the gastric fundus. The greater omentum hangs from the inferior edge of the stomach and is in contact with the transverse colonic mesentery and the transverse colon.

(Continued)

Figure 11-I-1 *(Continued)*

The first portion of the duodenum is covered by peritoneum; the remaining portions are retroperitoneal. The first portion of the duodenum is related to the neck of the gallbladder superiorly and to the common bile duct, gastroduodenal artery, and portal vein posteriorly. The second portion is usually covered anteriorly by the transverse colonic mesentery. The right kidney and inferior vena cava are posterior; the medial border encompasses the pancreas. The third portion of the duodenum passes horizontally and lies inferior to the transverse mesentery. The inferior vena cava is posterior to the third portion of the duodenum, and the superior mesenteric artery and vein cross anteriorly. The fourth portion of the duodenum passes upward and to the left, anterior to the aorta. The duodenum becomes the jejunum at the level of the second lumbar vertebra by passing the ligament of Treitz.

Figure 11-I-2

Gastric Arterial Supply

Five major arteries supply the stomach. The left gastric artery is derived from the celiac trunk and travels along the lesser curvature of the stomach. The right gastric artery, derived from the common hepatic artery, also supplies the lesser curvature. The greater curvature receives arterial supply from the right gastroepiploic artery, a branch of the gastroduodenal artery, and from the left gastroepiploic artery, a branch of the distal splenic artery. The short gastric arteries, variable in number, supply the greater curvature opposite the spleen. The distal esophagus and posterior fundus may receive additional blood supply by a small, and variable, branch derived from the splenic artery.

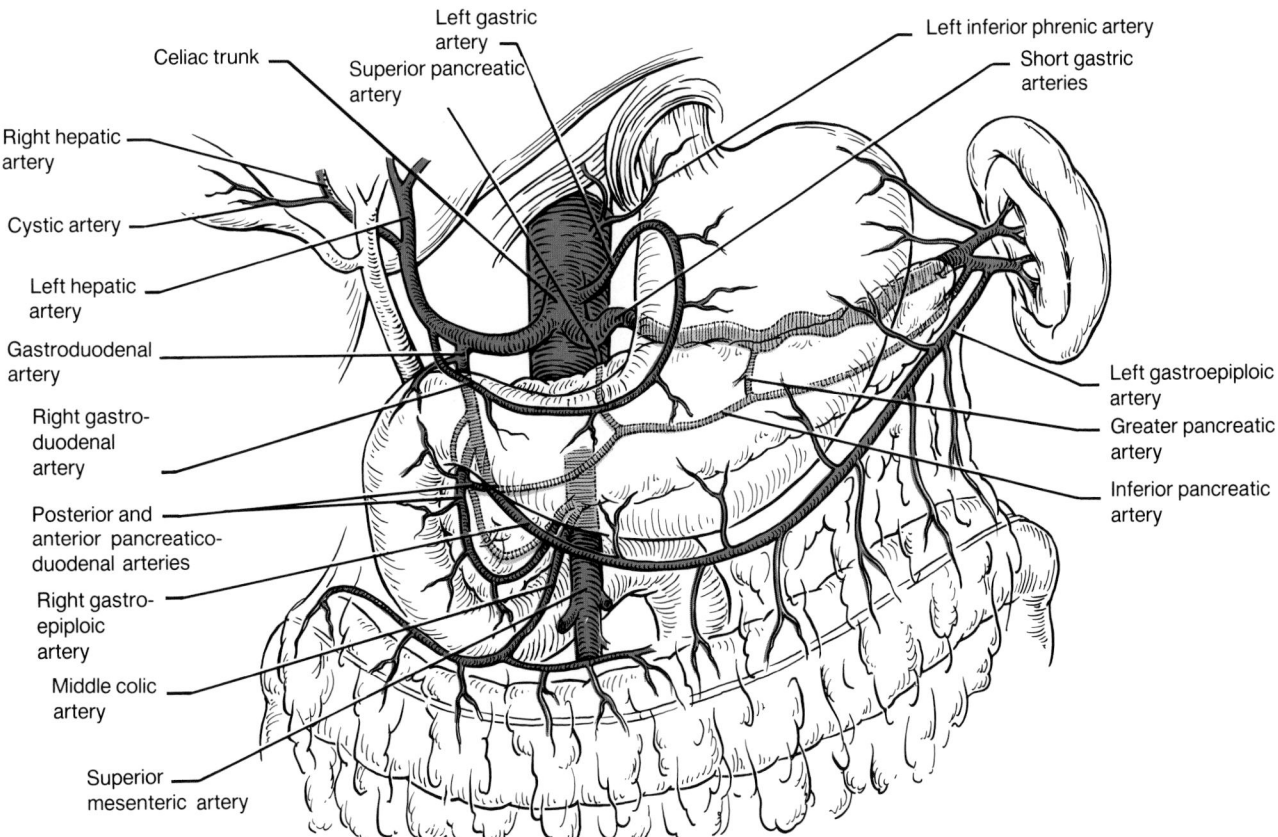

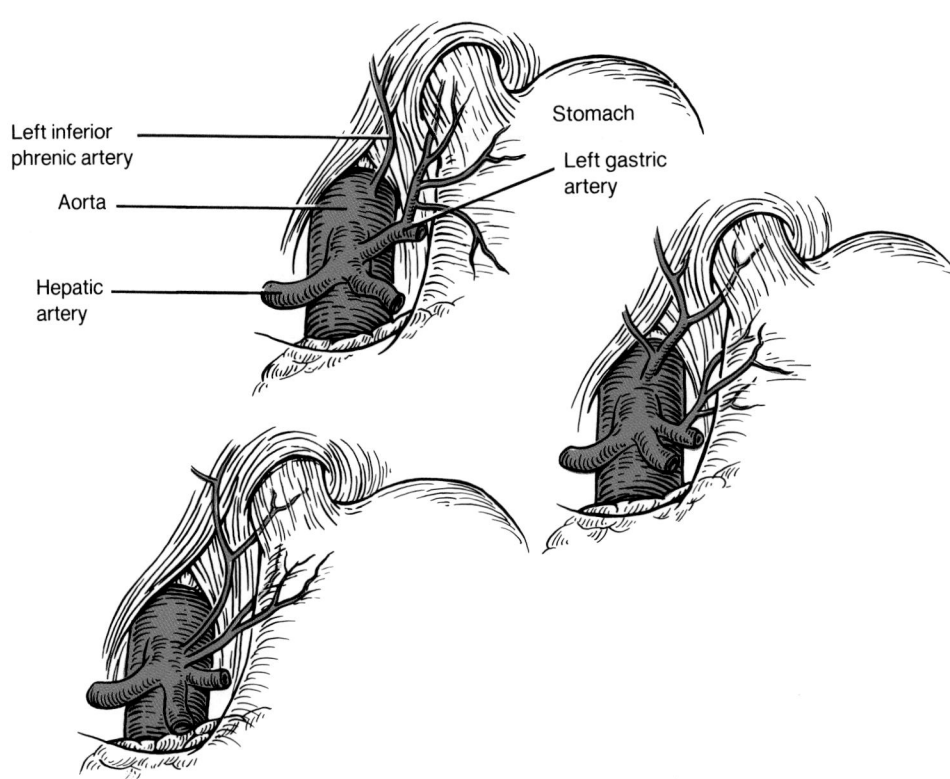

Figure 11-I-3

Arterial Supply to the Esophagogastric Junction

The arterial supply to the esophagogastric junction can be provided by the left gastric artery or the left inferior phrenic artery, occasionally by branches of both vessels.*

* Skandalakis JE, Gray SW, Rowe JS. Anatomical complications in general surgery. New York, McGraw-Hill, 1983.

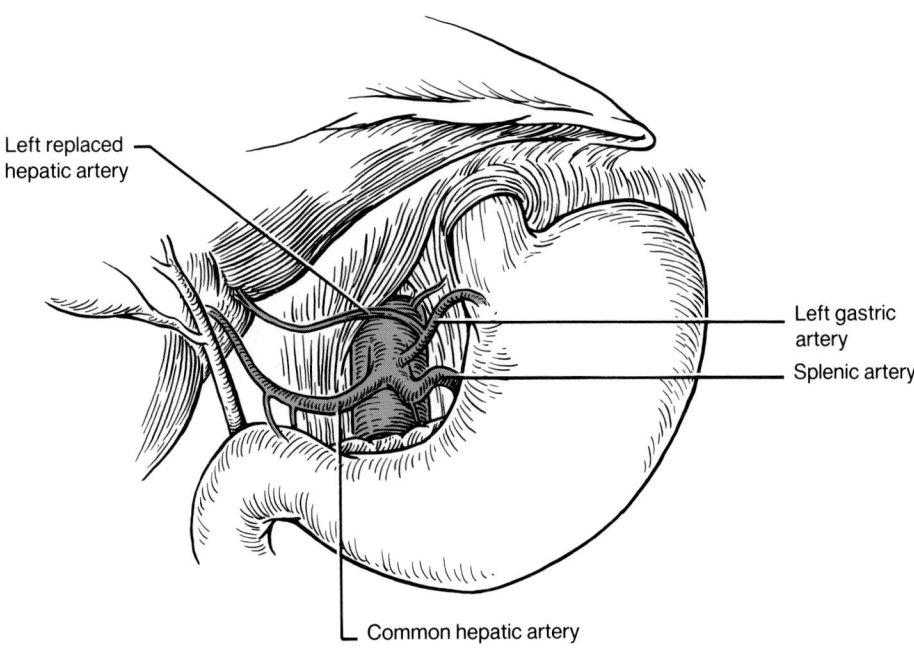

Left replaced
hepatic artery

Left gastric
artery

Splenic artery

Common hepatic artery

Figure 11-I-4

Aberrant Left Hepatic Artery

The left hepatic artery has an aberrant origin from the left gastric artery and is the sole blood supply to the left hepatic lobe in approximately 8% of individuals. An aberrant left hepatic artery can be appreciated by inspection of the pars flaccida of the gastrohepatic omentum along the lesser curvature of the stomach. An aberrant left hepatic artery must be carefully preserved if the left gastric artery is ligated during the course of gastric resection.

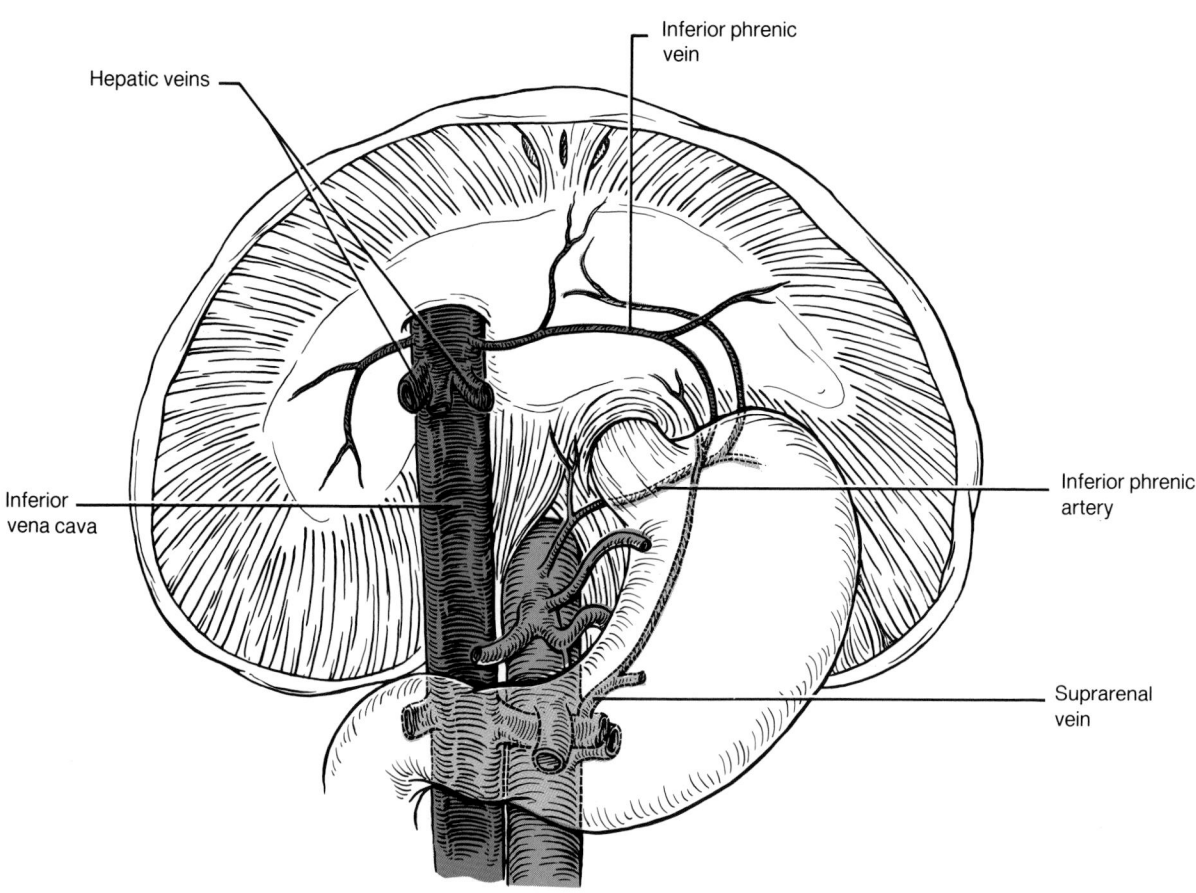

Figure 11-I-5

Blood Supply to the Diaphragm

The left diaphragm is supplied by the left inferior phrenic artery, which arises from the celiac trunk or the aorta in an equal proportion of cases. The left inferior phrenic vein passes anterior to the esophageal hiatus and courses medially to drain into the inferior vena cava. The inferior phrenic vein is vulnerable to injury when the triangular ligament of the left hepatic lobe is divided to gain exposure for the area of the esophagogastric junction.

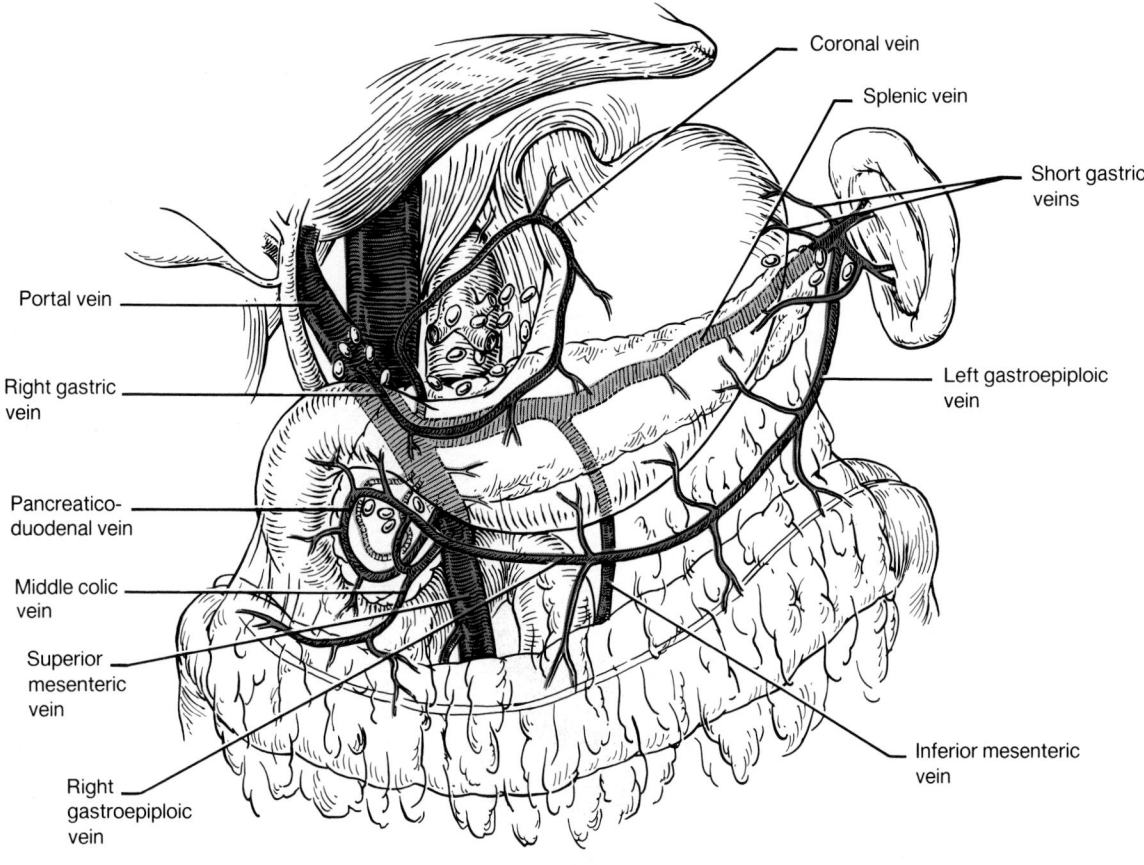

Coronal vein
Splenic vein
Short gastric veins
Portal vein
Right gastric vein
Left gastroepiploic vein
Pancreatico-duodenal vein
Middle colic vein
Superior mesenteric vein
Right gastroepiploic vein
Inferior mesenteric vein

Figure 11-I-6

Venous Drainage of the Stomach

The venous drainage of the stomach parallels the arterial supply. The left gastric vein, also termed the *coronary vein,* travels along the lesser curvature to a point 3 or 4 cm distal to the esophagogastric junction, where it courses obliquely downward and to the right to enter the portal vein (75% of cases) or the splenic vein (25%).

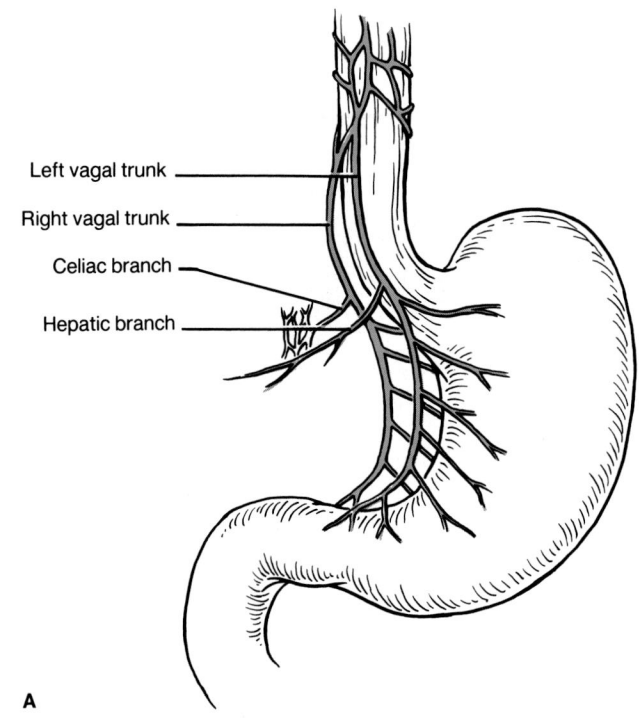

Left vagal trunk

Right vagal trunk

Celiac branch

Hepatic branch

A

Figure 11-I-7

Vagal Anatomy

(A) The vagal nerves form a plexus surrounding the intrathoracic esophagus but coalesce into two major trunks before entering the abdomen through the esophageal hiatus of the diaphragm. The anterior (left) vagus nerve assumes a position in immediate contact with the anterior wall of the esophagus. The position of the posterior vagal trunk exhibits greater variability but is usually found between the posteromedial wall of the esophagus and the right diaphragmatic crus.

(B) The hepatic division of the anterior vagal nerve separates from the anterior trunk at the level of the esophagogastric junction and passes between the avascular leaflets of the gastrohepatic ligament. Fibers within the hepatic division innervate the gallbladder, biliary ducts, and liver.

(C) The celiac division of the posterior vagal trunk crosses the right diaphragmatic crus, often paralleling the left gastric artery. The celiac division is usually larger than the hepatic division. Branches of the celiac division pass to the celiac ganglion. The anterior and posterior gastric divisions of the vagal trunks are contained within the gastrohepatic omentum, approximately 0.5 to 1 cm from and paralleling the lesser curvature. Small gastric branches terminate in the gastric fundus, body, and antrum.

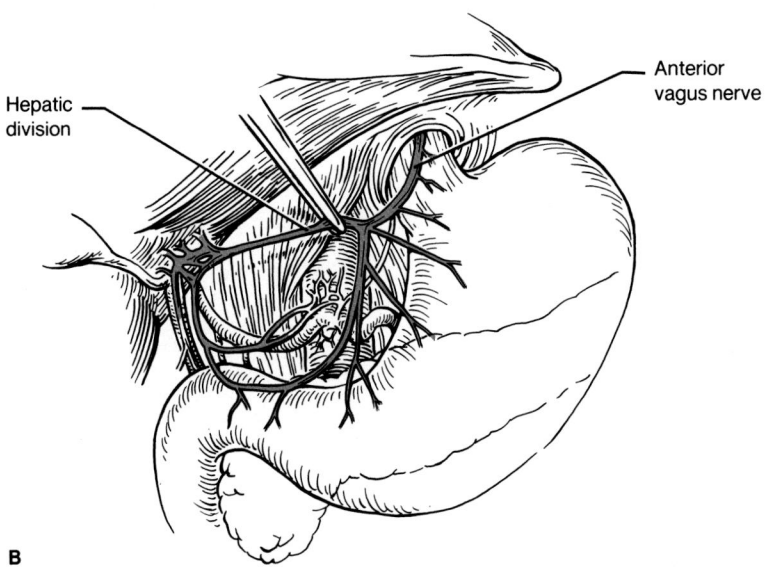

Hepatic
division

Anterior
vagus nerve

B

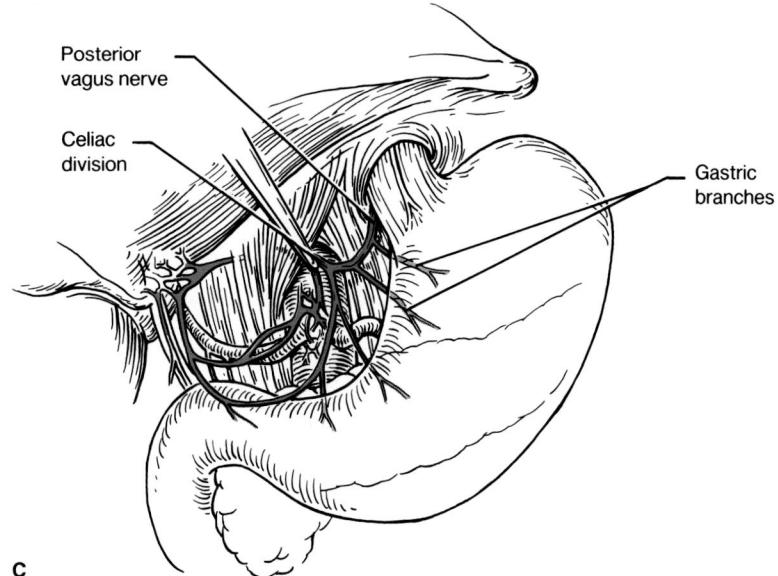

Posterior
vagus nerve

Celiac
division

Gastric
branches

C

Figure 11-I-7 *(Continued)*

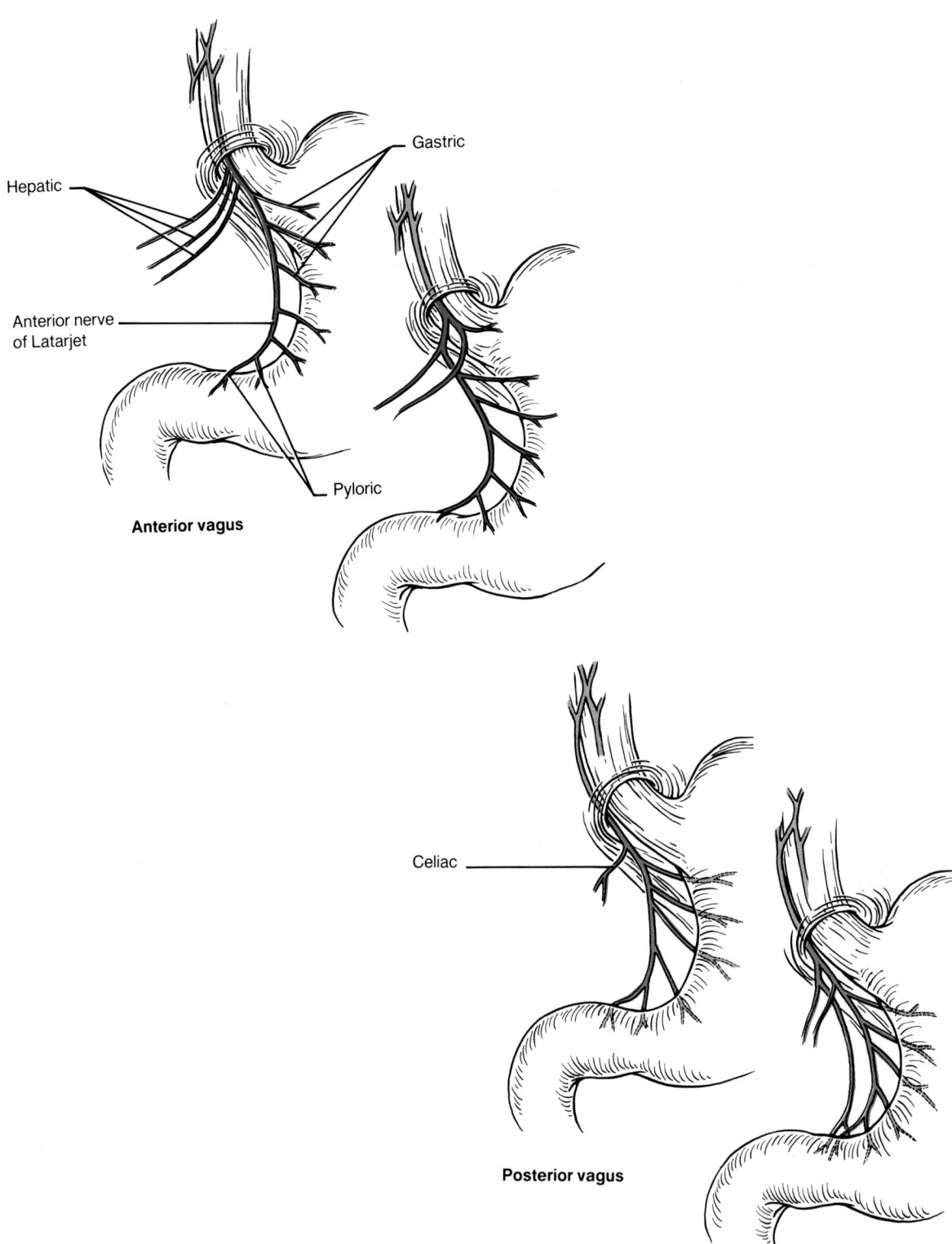

Figure 11-I-8

Variations in Vagal Anatomy

Variations in vagal anatomy, more frequently observed with the anterior vagus nerve, are of surgical importance.

SECTION II *Truncal Vagotomy and Drainage*

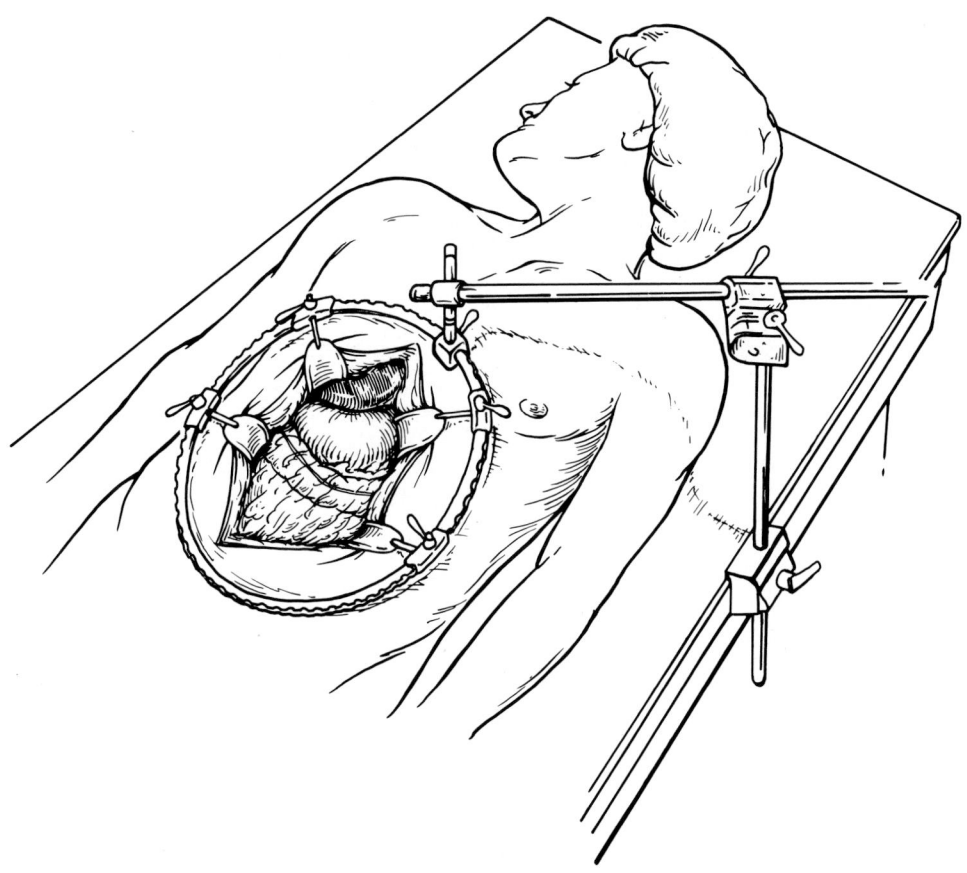

Figure 11-II-1

Incision

A long vertical midline incision extending to the xyphoid provides superior exposure of the upper abdomen for performance of truncal vagotomy. Exposure is provided by a self-retaining ring-type retractor. The costal margins should be retracted superiorly and elevated. Tilting the operating table to achieve a modest degree of reverse Trendelenberg position is often helpful.

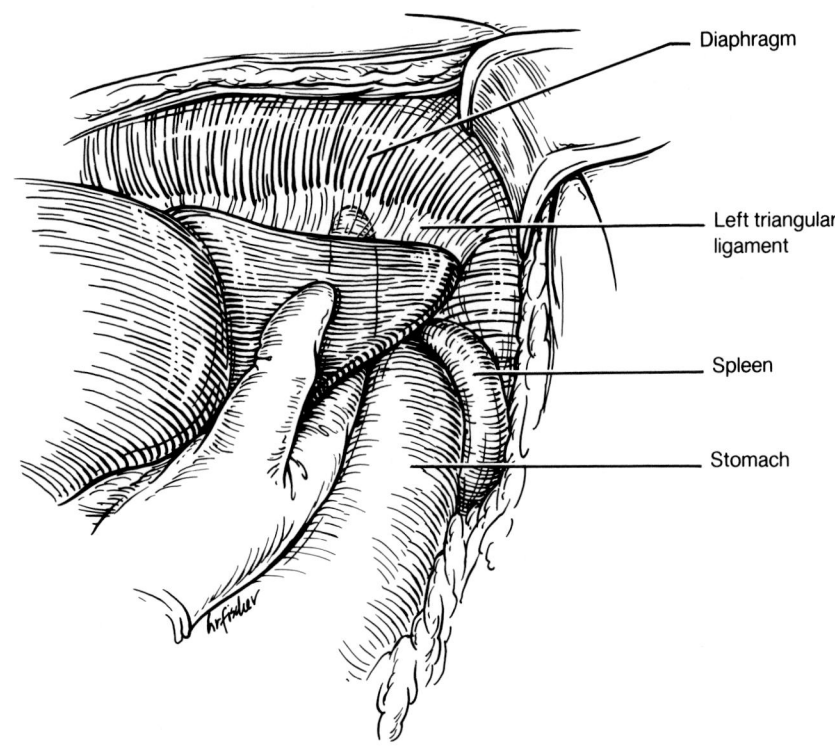

Diaphragm

Left triangular ligament

Spleen

Stomach

Figure 11-II-2

Mobilization of the Left Lateral Segment of the Liver

Mobilization of the left lateral segment of the liver improves exposure of the intraabdominal esophagus. The operating surgeon places the right hand under the left lateral segment, palm upward, and retracts the liver inferiorly. The edge of the left triangular ligament is thin and translucent; the surgeon's gloved fingers are usually visible through the peritoneum. If the greater curvature of the stomach and attached omentum impede visibility, a rolled, moistened pack can be placed laterally and behind the right hand to improve exposure.

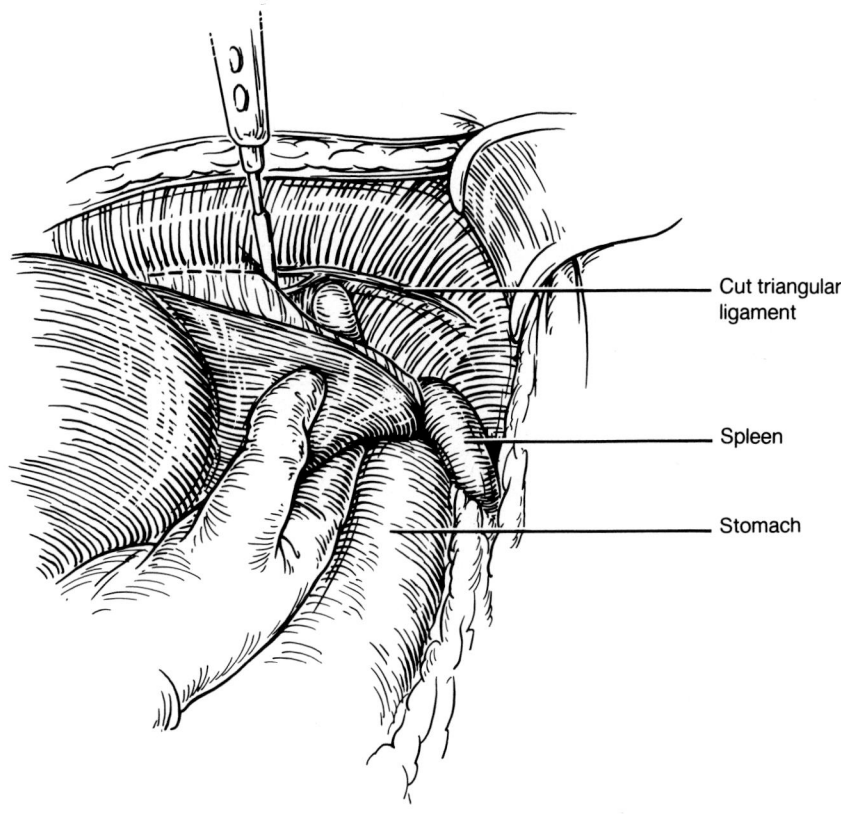

Cut triangular
ligament

Spleen

Stomach

Figure 11-II-3

Division of the Triangular Ligament

The left triangular ligament can be divided with cautery. As division progresses medially, care must be taken to expose separately the anterior and posterior leaves of the triangular ligament. Both peritoneal layers and interposed areolar tissue should be divided individually. The inferior phrenic vein is often in proximity to the posterior peritoneal edge of the triangular ligament and can be injured if proper exposure is not maintained. Mobilization of the left triangular ligament need not extend to the right of the midline.

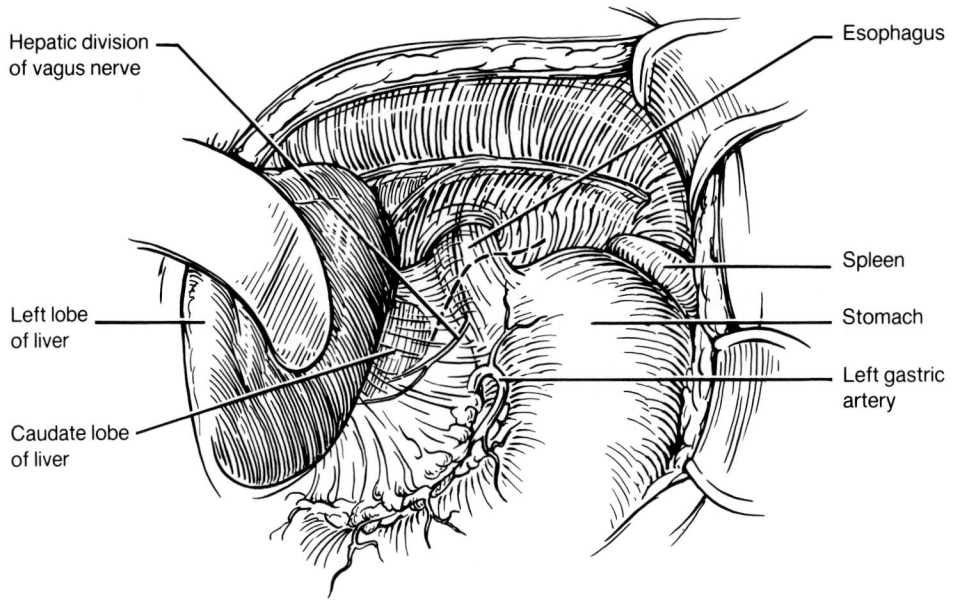

Figure 11-II-4

Exposure of the Esophagogastric Junction

The left lateral segment of the liver is folded inferiorly, protected with a moistened pad, and gently retracted to the patient's right. The area of the intraabdominal esophagus can be appreciated visually or by palpation of a previously placed nasogastric tube. The peritoneum overlying the esophagogastric junction is divided transversely using cautery. The hepatic branch of the anterior vagus nerve is usually visible within the leaves of the gastrohepatic ligament and should be preserved.

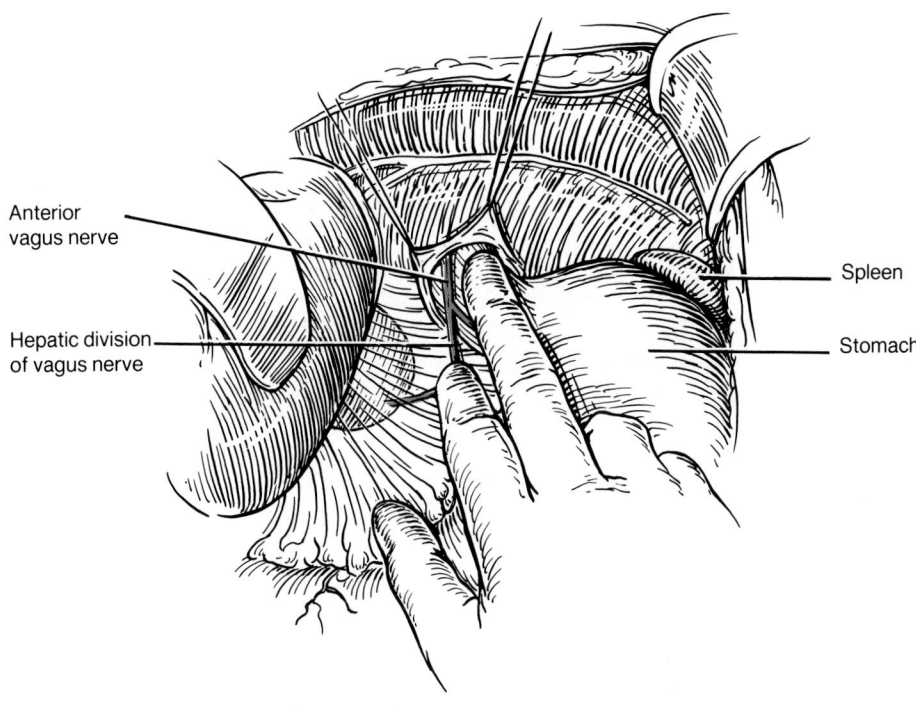

Figure 11-II-5

Exposure of Anterior Vagus Nerve

After division of the peritoneum overlying the esophagogastric junction, the anterior vagal nerve can be seen on the anterior surface of the esophagus. The nerve can be palpated by passing the index finger over the anterior surface of the esophagus. Retraction of the stomach aids in palpation of the vagal trunk. If the location of the anterior vagal nerve is difficult to confirm, the position of the nerve can be accentuated by hooking the right index finger over the hepatic branch of the anterior vagus and gently retracting it caudally. The vagal trunk is tensed by this maneuver and can be felt by the middle finger of the right hand.

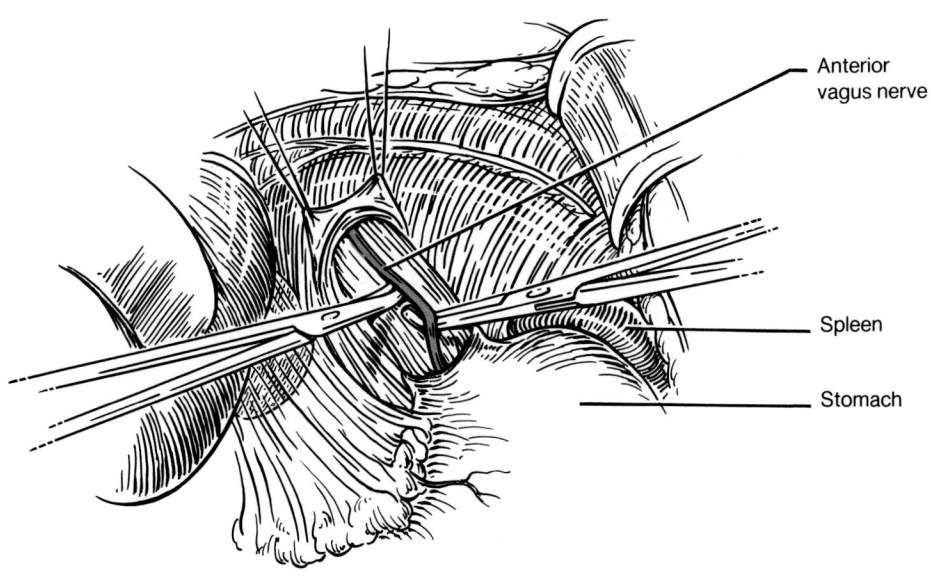

Anterior
vagus nerve

Spleen

Stomach

Figure 11-II-6

Isolation of the Anterior Vagal Trunk

The anterior vagal trunk is encircled using a nerve hook or a right angle clamp and dissected sharply from the underlying esophageal musculature.

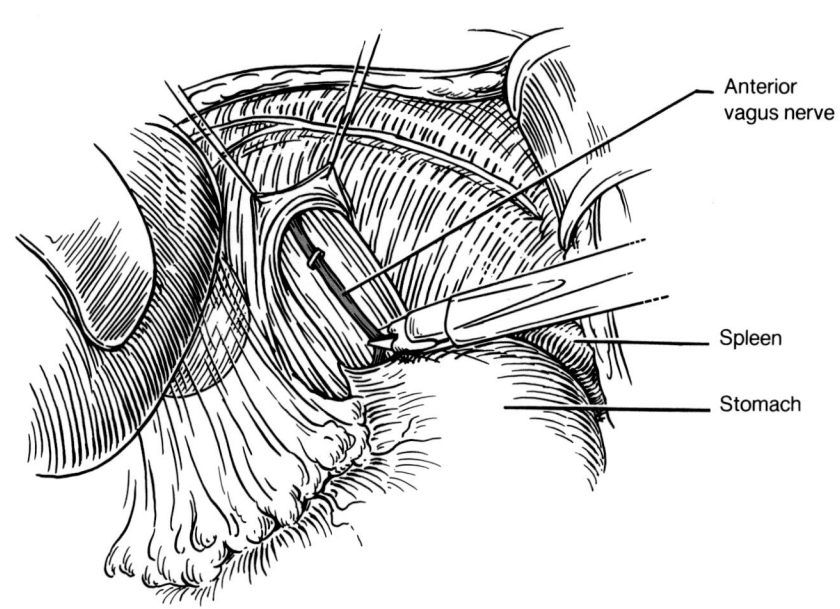

Anterior
vagus nerve

Spleen

Stomach

Figure 11-II-7

Ligation of the Nerve Trunk

The nerve trunk is ligated proximally and distally using surgical clips, and a segment approximately 2 cm long is excised. All nerve tissue must be sent for histologic confirmation.

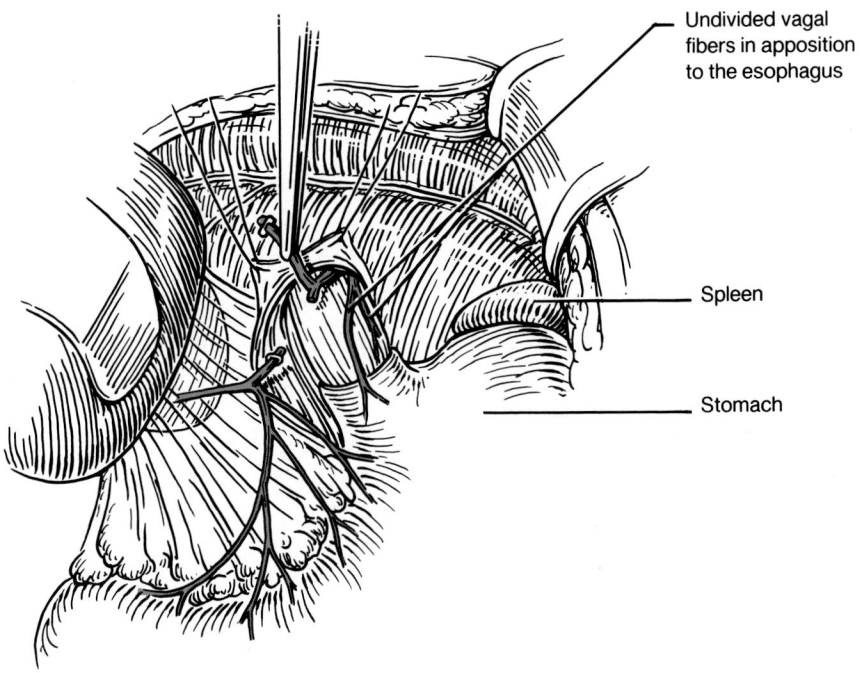

Undivided vagal
fibers in apposition
to the esophagus

Spleen

Stomach

Figure 11-II-8

Division of Esophageal Branches

After division of the main vagal trunk, small vagal fibers traversing the esophagus to reach the proximal stomach must be sought. The proximal end of the divided vagal trunk is grasped with a hemostat and retracted superiorly and to the right. As the vagal trunk is traced proximally into the posterior mediastinum, vagal fibers entering the distal esophagus are exposed and divided.

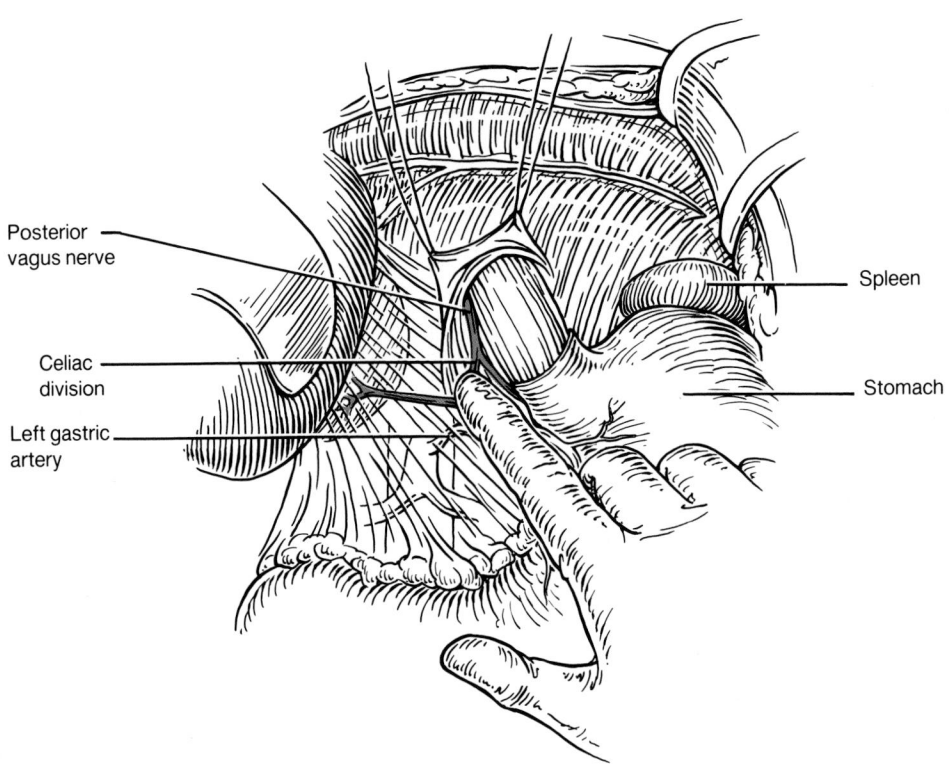

Posterior vagus nerve

Celiac division

Left gastric artery

Spleen

Stomach

Figure 11-II-9

Exposure of the Posterior Vagal Trunk

The surgical assistant retracts the esophagus to the left, allowing the operating surgeon to expose the right diaphragmatic crus. The posterior vagal trunk can be identified visually or by palpation in the space defined by the posteromedial wall of the esophagus and the right crus. The position of the posterior vagal trunk can be verified by retraction of the celiac division. The index finger of the right hand is placed over the celiac division of the posterior nerve. Because the celiac division travels in proximity to the left gastric artery, this pulse can also be used as a landmark. Gentle inferior pressure will bring the posterior trunk into greater prominence so that its position can be sensed by the middle finger of the examining hand.

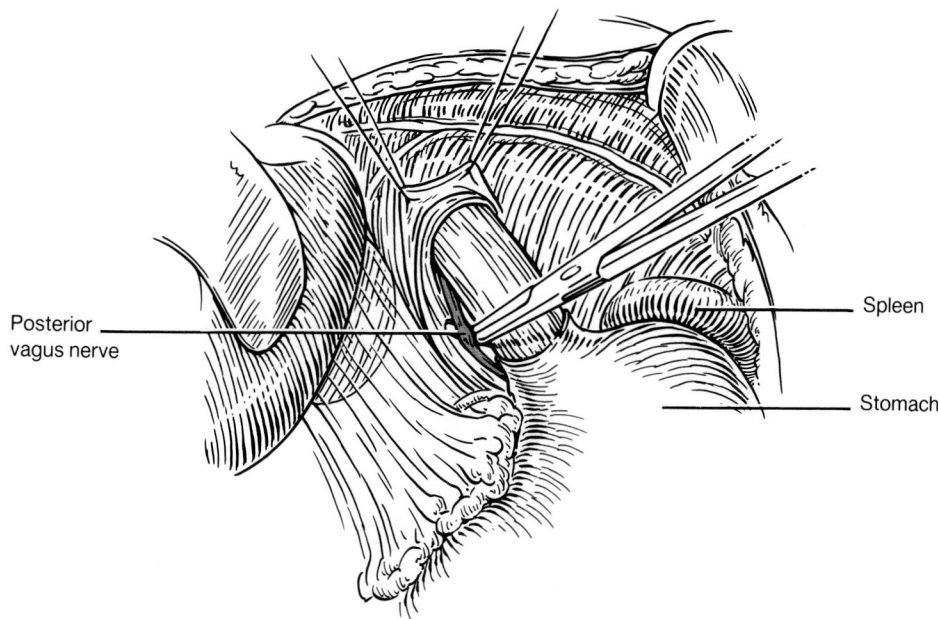

Figure 11-II-10

Isolation of the Posterior Vagal Trunk

The posterior vagal trunk is isolated from surrounding structures using a nerve hook or right angle clamp.

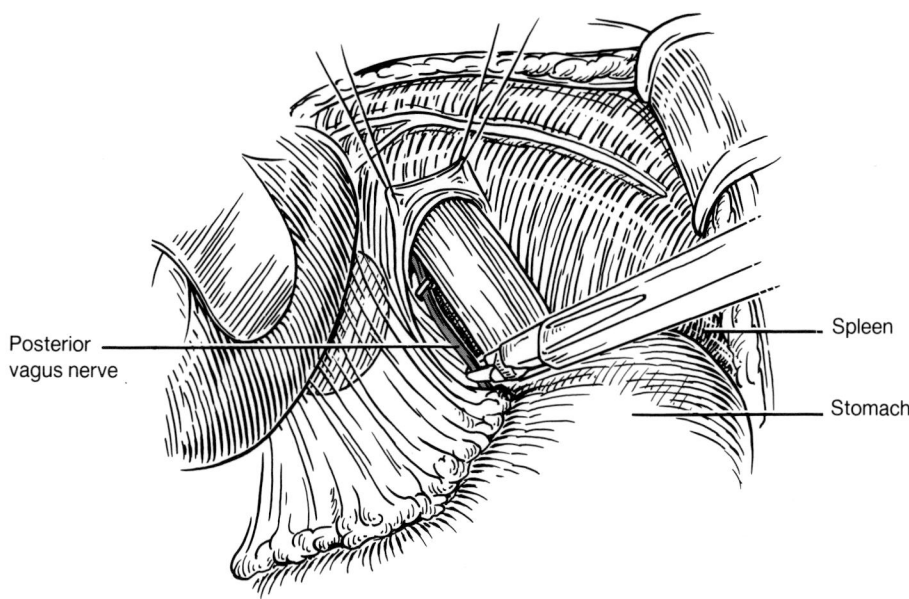

Figure 11-II-11

Nerve Division

A segment of the posterior trunk is ligated with surgical clips in preparation for division.

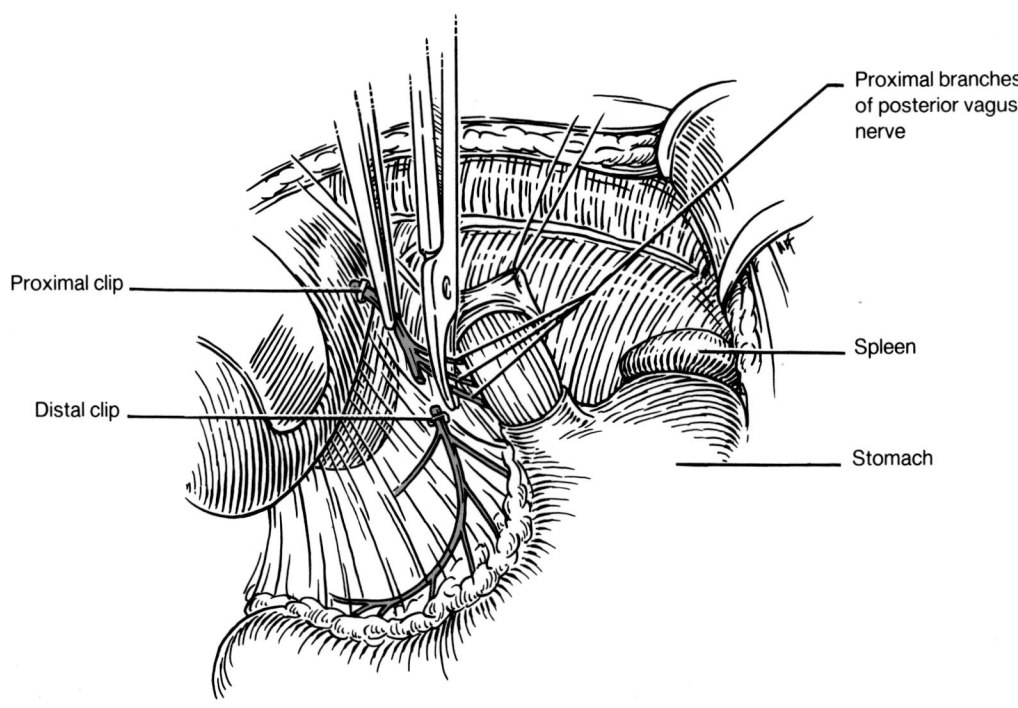

Figure 11-II-12

Division of Esophageal Branches

The proximal divided end of the posterior vagal trunk is grasped and retracted superiorly. As the nerve trunk is traced back into the posterior mediastinum, small branches entering the distal esophagus are divided.

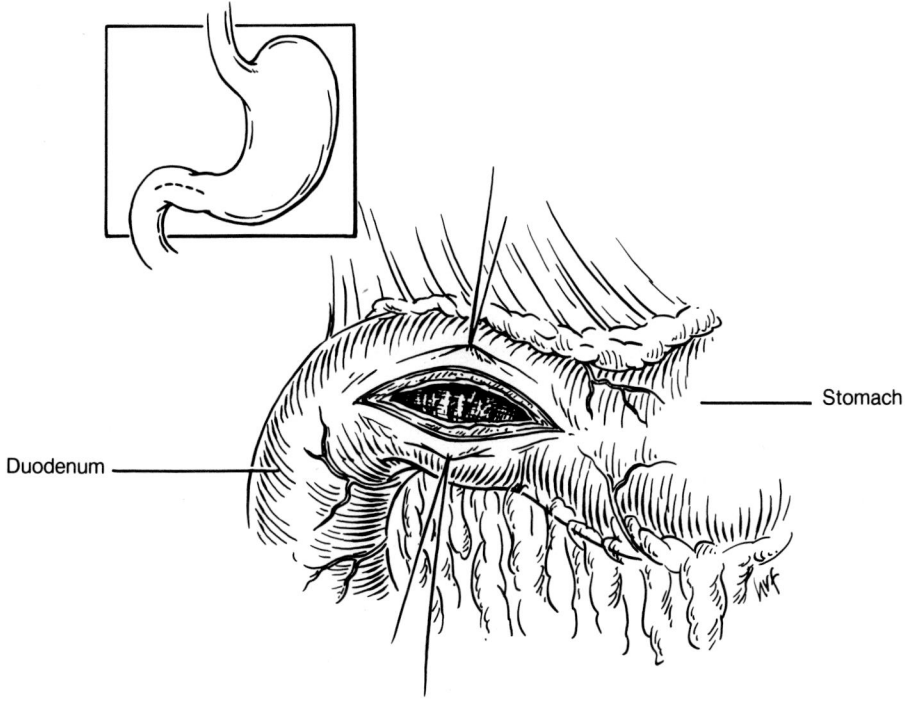

Duodenum

Stomach

Figure 11-II-13

Heineke-Mikulicz Pyloroplasty Incision

A Heineke-Mikulicz pyloroplasty can be performed if inflammation has not caused scarring of the pylorus or foreshortening of the proximal duodenum. The muscular ring of the pylorus permits its identification by palpation; the pyloric vein, crossing the sphincter anteriorly, is another constant landmark. The pylorus is divided, with the incision extending into the distal stomach and proximal duodenum for a distance approximately 3 cm each direction. Stay sutures are placed at the pyloric ring superiorly and inferiorly.

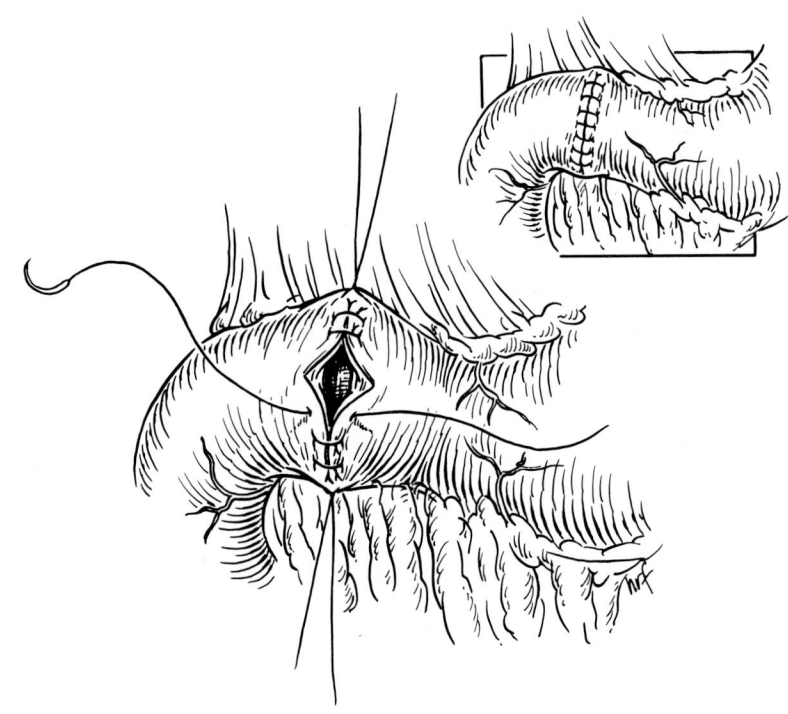

Figure 11-II-14

Closure of Pyloroplasty Incision

Traction on stay sutures superiorly and inferiorly converts the longitudinal incision into a transverse closure. The incision is closed using interrupted permanent sutures.

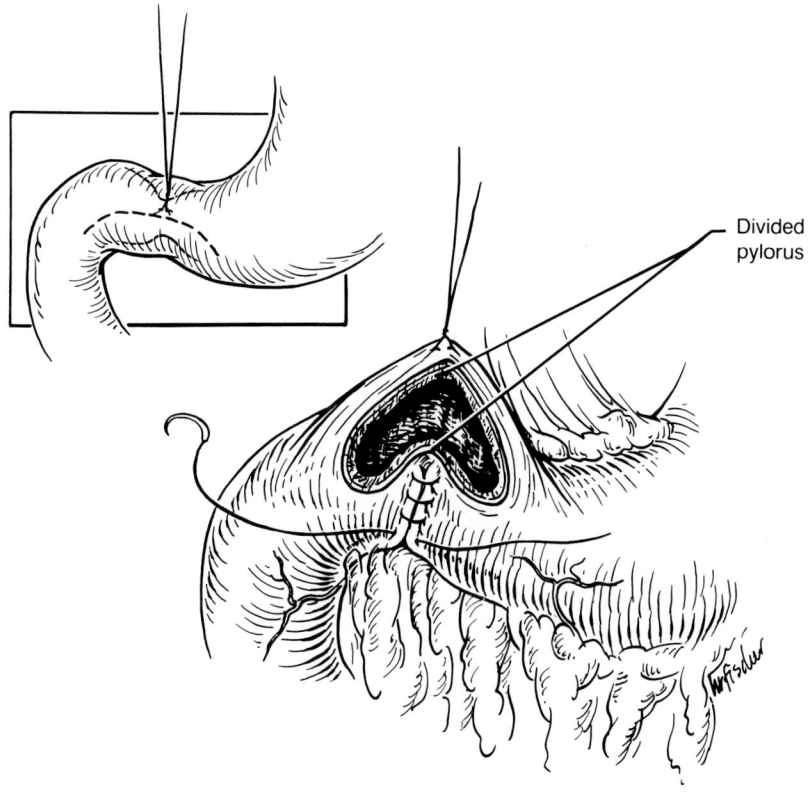

Divided
pylorus

Figure 11-II-15

Finney Pyloroplasty Incision

A Finney pyloroplasty uses an extended, curved gastroduodenal incision, centered on the pylorus. A single stay suture is placed at the pyloric ring and retracted superiorly. Beginning at the inferior point of division of the pyloric sphincter, 3-0 nonabsorbable seromuscular sutures are used to approximate the inferior wall of the gastric antrum and the medial wall of the proximal duodenum.

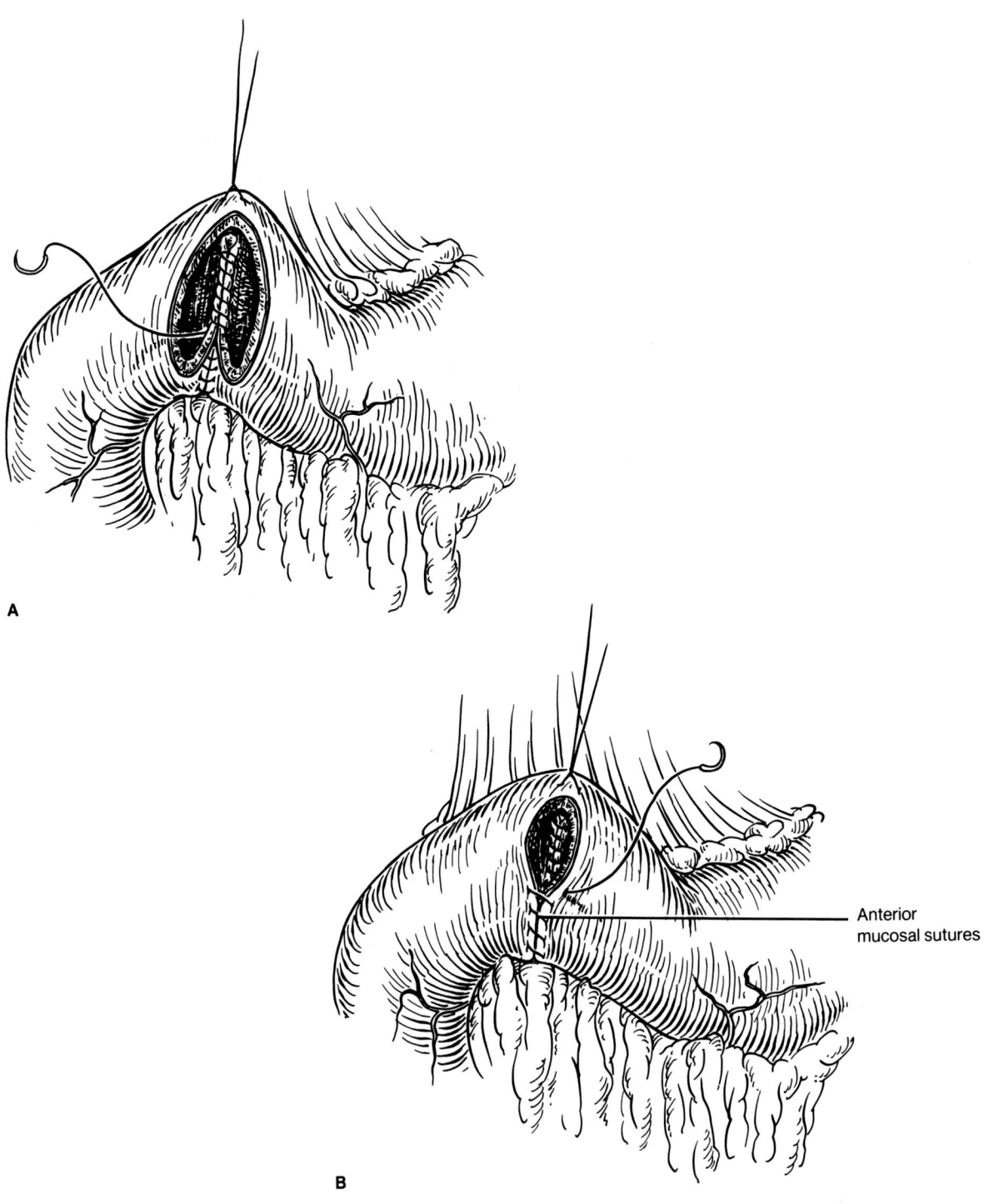

Anterior
mucosal sutures

Figure 11-II-16

Posterior Mucosal Suture

(**A**) Continuous absorbable suture is used to approximate gastric and duodenal mucosae. The suture line begins at the superior end of the back wall and proceeds inferiorly. All layers of the gastric and duodenal wall are included.

(**B**) The mucosal suture is continued anteriorly to the apex of the incision.

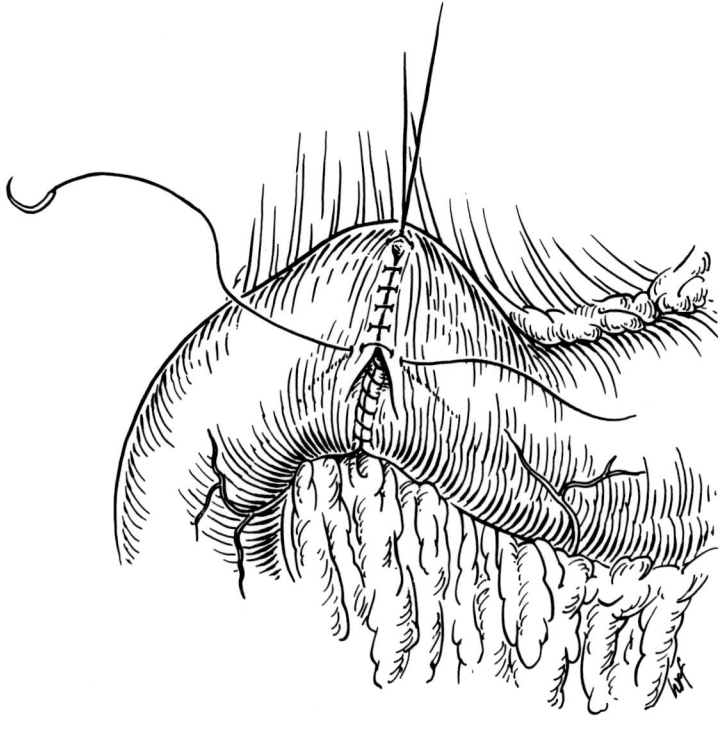

Figure 11-II-17

Completion of the Anastomosis

The anterior portion of the anastomosis is reinforced with interrupted seromuscular 3-0 nonabsorbable sutures.

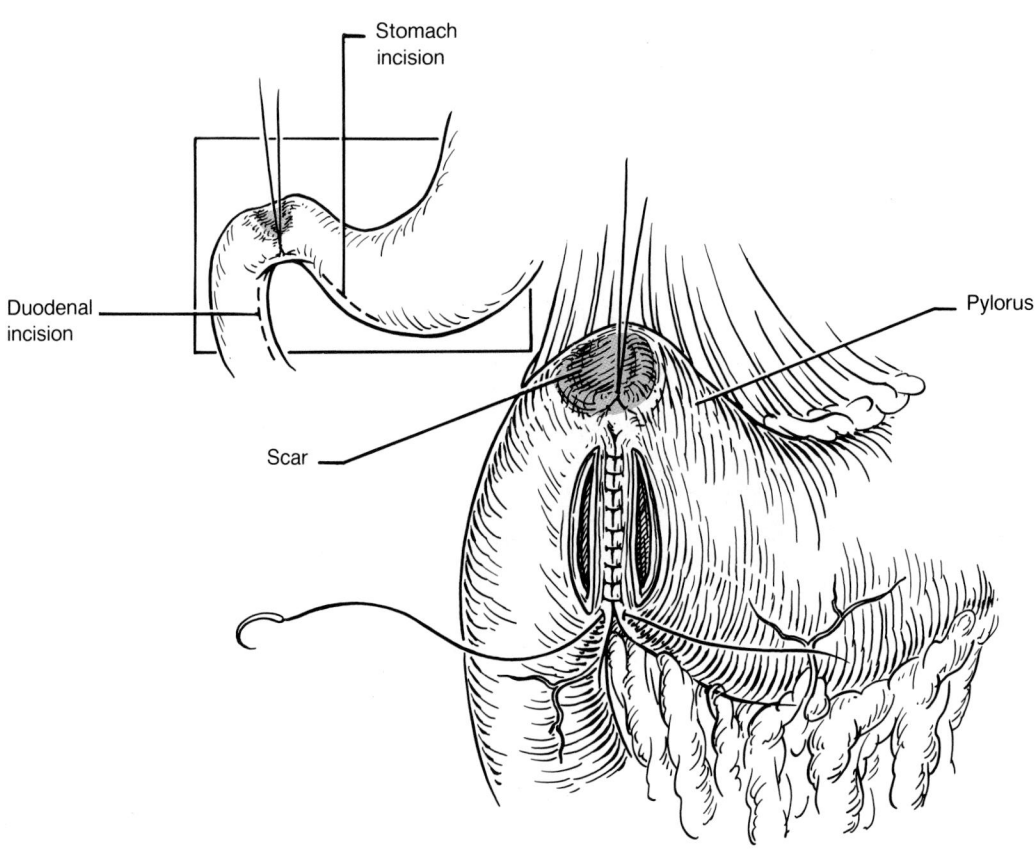

Figure 11-II-18

Jaboulay Pyloroplasty

If severe scarring precludes safe division of the pylorus, a Jaboulay pyloroplasty can be used as an alternative to the Finney procedure. Parallel incisions are made on the inferior wall of the antrum and the medial wall of the proximal duodenum, approaching but not traversing the pylorus. Interrupted 3-0 nonabsorbable sutures are placed in a seromuscular fashion.

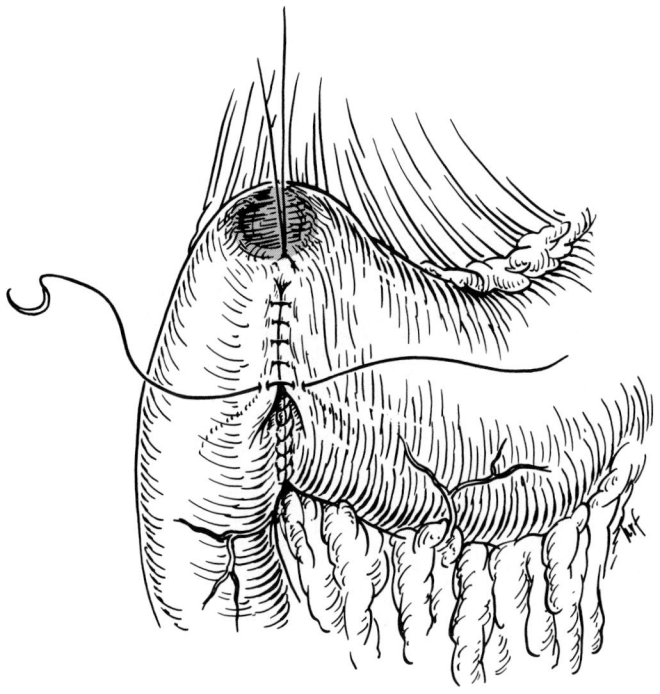

Figure 11-II-19

Completion of Jaboulay Anastomosis

After placement of a continuous absorbable mucosal suture, the anterior aspect of the anastomosis is reinforced using interrupted 3-0 nonabsorbable sutures.

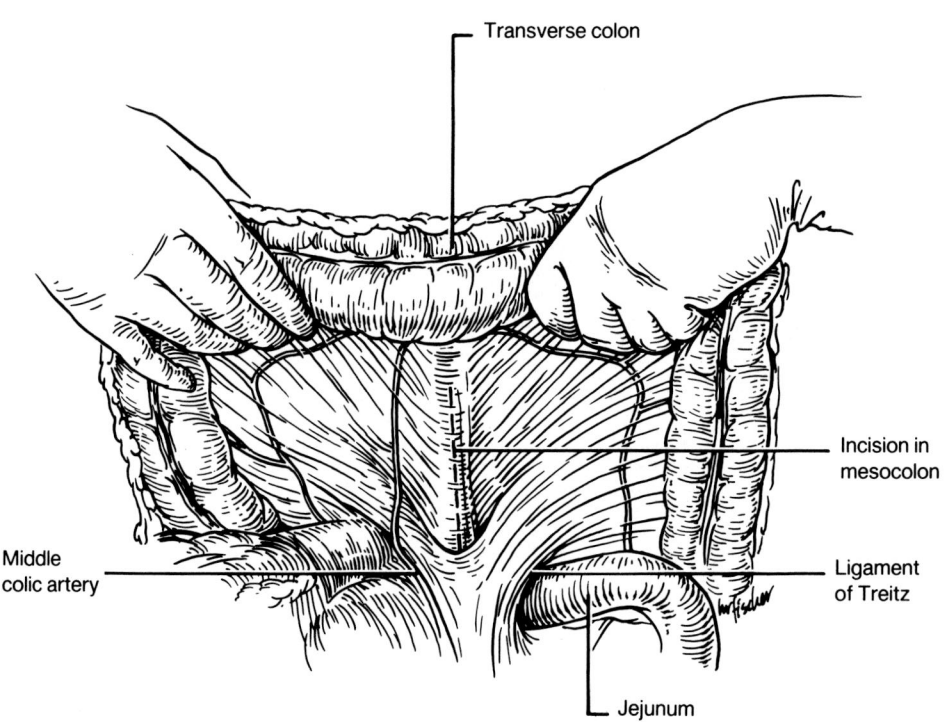

Figure 11-II-20

Drainage via Gastrojejunostomy

Occasionally, severe scarring of the pyloric area makes pyloroplasty difficult or unsafe. In selected instances, gastrojejunostomy can be used as an alternative. For benign disease, retrocolic positioning is preferred. The transverse colon is retracted upward and the vascular arcades within the transverse mesentery are inspected. An avascular area to the left of the middle colic vessels is chosen; an incision large enough to deliver the jejunum to the antrum is created.

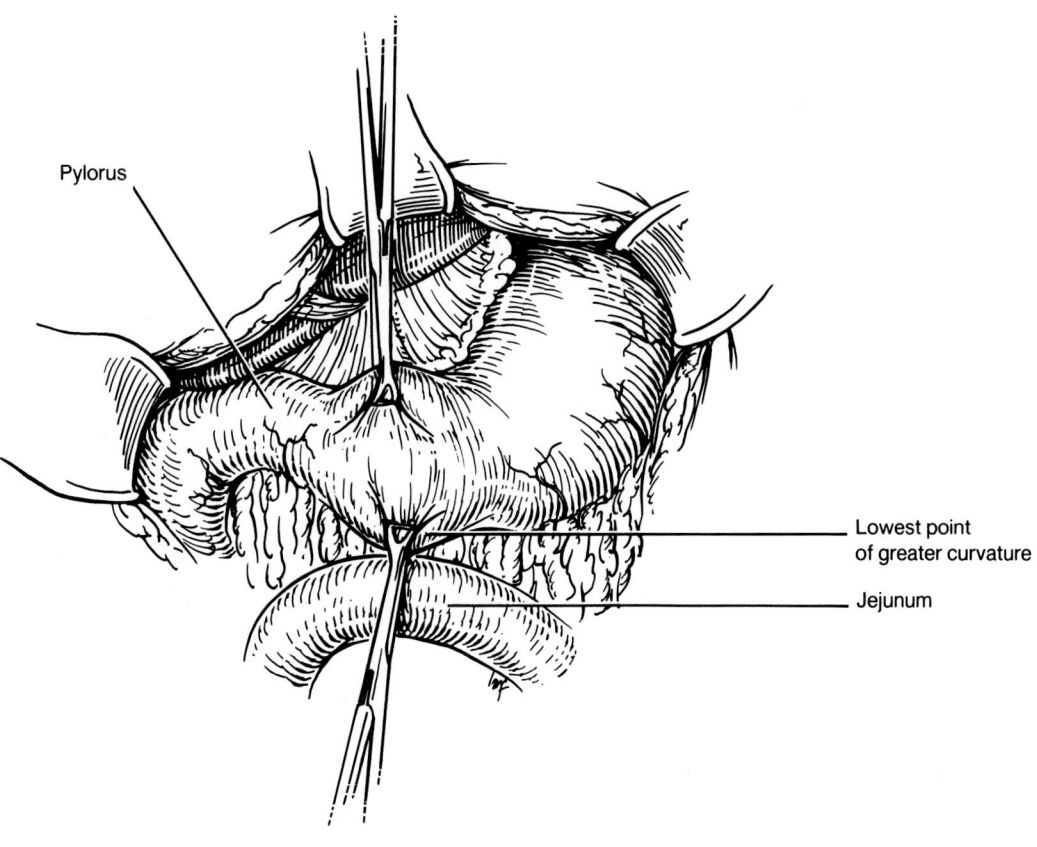

Pylorus

Lowest point
of greater curvature

Jejunum

Figure 11-II-21

Anastomotic Site

The first loop of jejunum that will reach without tension is approximated to the gastric antrum. A site on the gastric antrum—distal, dependent, and free of large serosal vessels—is chosen for anastomosis.

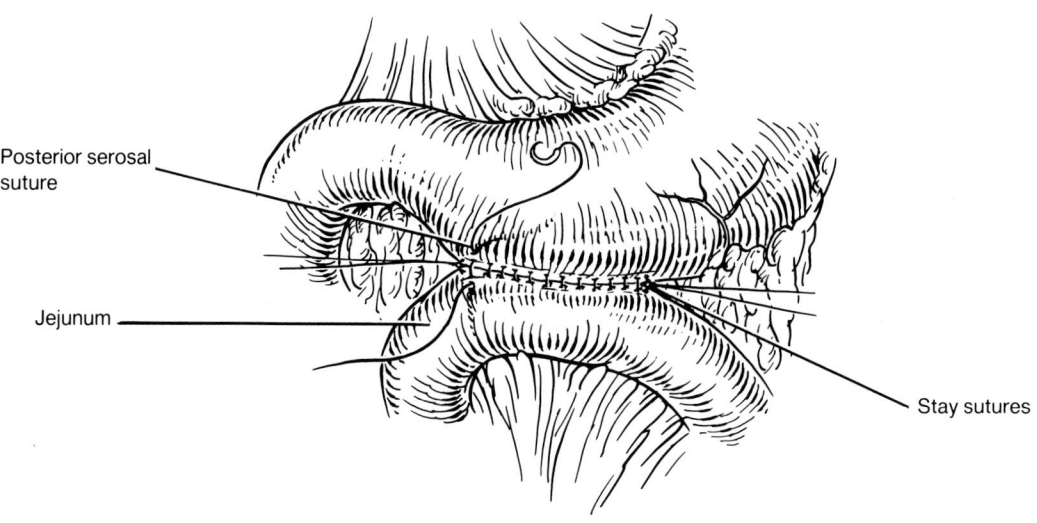

Figure 11-II-22

Posterior Serosal Sutures

Stay sutures, including the antrum and jejunum, orient the anastomosis. Seromuscular sutures of 3-0 are placed and tied.

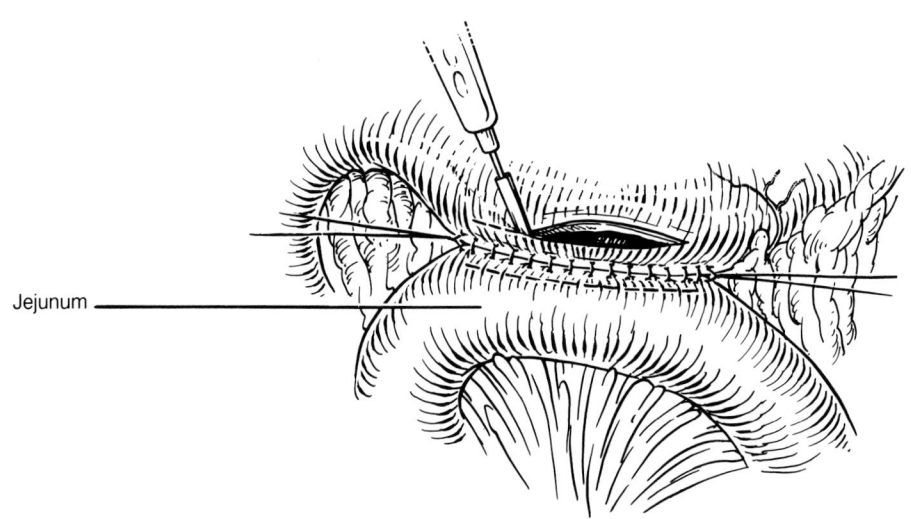

Figure 11-II-23

Gastric Incision

Electrocautery is used to create equal length gastric and jejunal incisions. Care must be exerted not to thermally injure the bowel wall opposite the incision while creating the opening.

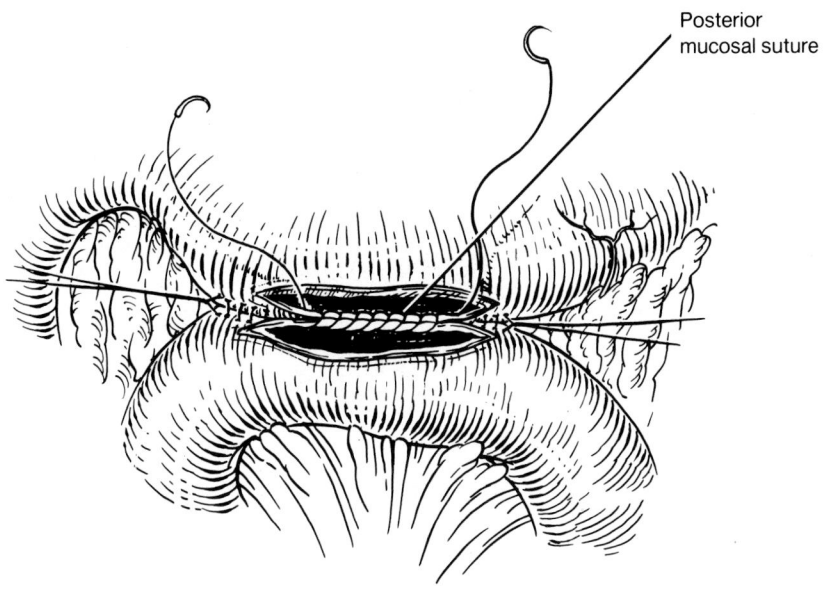

Posterior
mucosal suture

Figure 11-II-24

Posterior Mucosal Suture

A continuous mucosal suture of absorbable material is begun posteriorly and continued along the anterior portion of the anastomosis. Use of double-armed suture permits the surgeon to move in both directions.

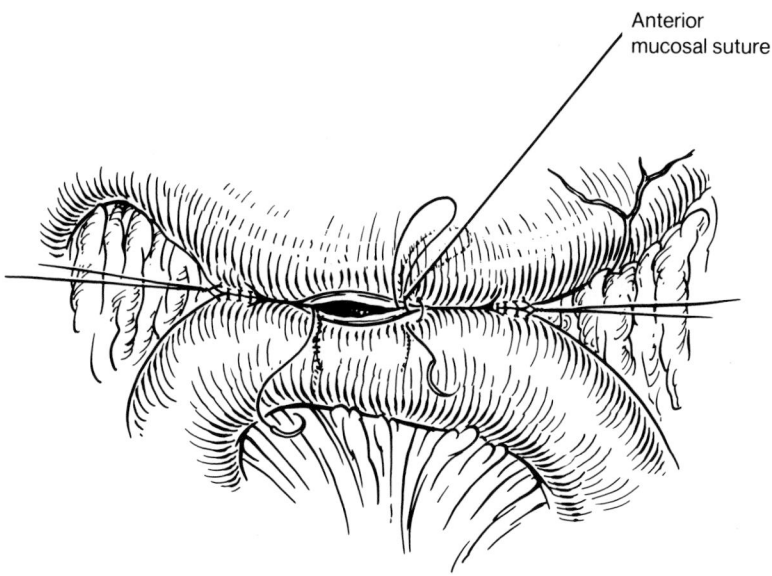

Anterior
mucosal suture

Figure 11-II-25

Anterior Mucosal Suture

The anterior mucosal suture line can be completed as a whip stitch or as a running mattress suture (Connell stitch).

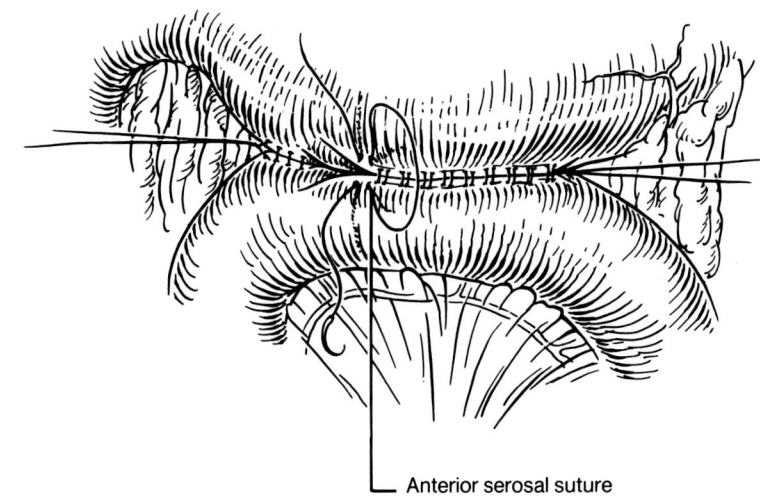

Anterior serosal suture

Figure 11-II-26

Completion of Anastomosis

Interrupted seromuscular sutures are used to complete the double-layer anastomosis.

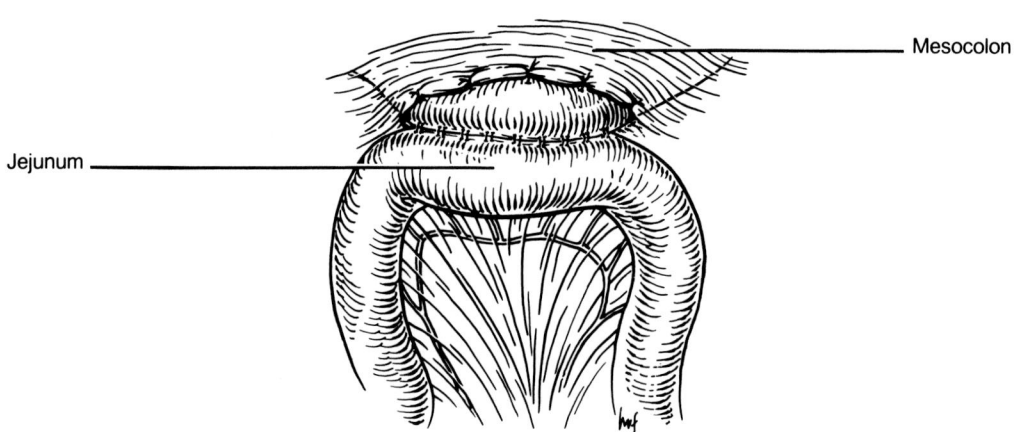

Mesocolon

Jejunum

Figure 11-II-27

Closure of Mesenteric Defect

The completed gastrojejunal anastomosis should be delivered beneath the transverse mesentery to prevent angulation or obstruction of efferent or afferent jejunal limbs. The mesenteric defect is closed with sutures to the gastric wall.

SECTION III *Proximal Gastric Vagotomy*

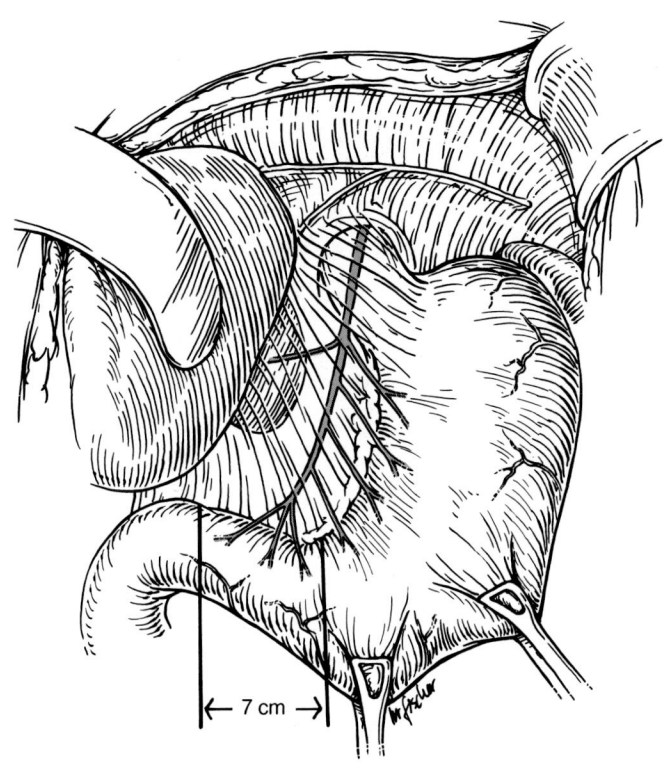

Figure 11-III-1

Anterior Gastric Division of Vagus Nerve

In proximal gastric vagotomy, the innervation of the distal 7 cm of the stomach is maintained by preservation of the nerve of Latarjet. Terminal vagal branches can be seen as fine white fibers accompanying vessels that enter the lesser curvature of the stomach, and the main bundle of the gastric division lies parallel to the gastric wall.

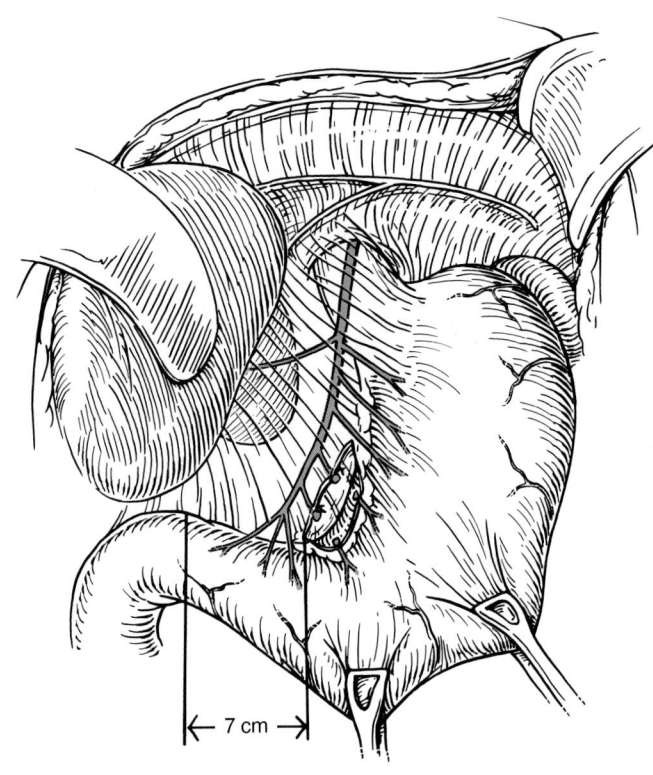

← 7 cm →

Figure 11-III-2

Beginning Dissection

The dissection is begun in the anterior layer of the gastrohepatic omentum 7 cm proximal to the pylorus. The dissection is confined to the area between the gastric wall and the anterior nerve of Latarjet. Ligatures must be placed so that they neither include a portion of the gastric wall nor compromise the innervation of the antrum.

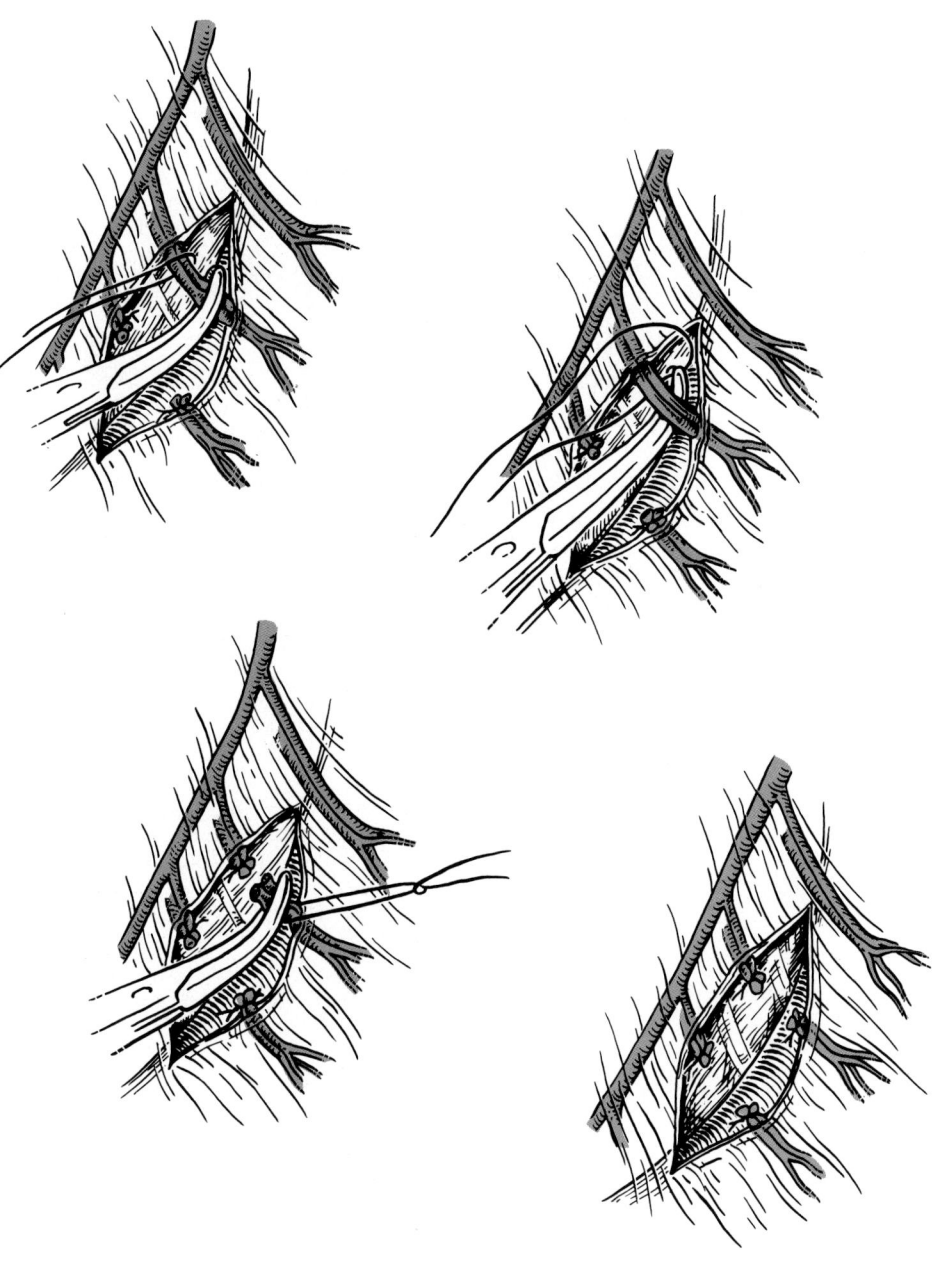

Figure 11-III-3

Neurovascular Ligation

The anterior leaf of the gastrohepatic omentum is divided between clamps; nerve fibers are divided as the small vessels they accompany are ligated. Meticulous dissection of the neurovascular arcade along the lesser curvature is crucial. Hematoma formation within the omental leaflets obscures the needed anatomic detail.

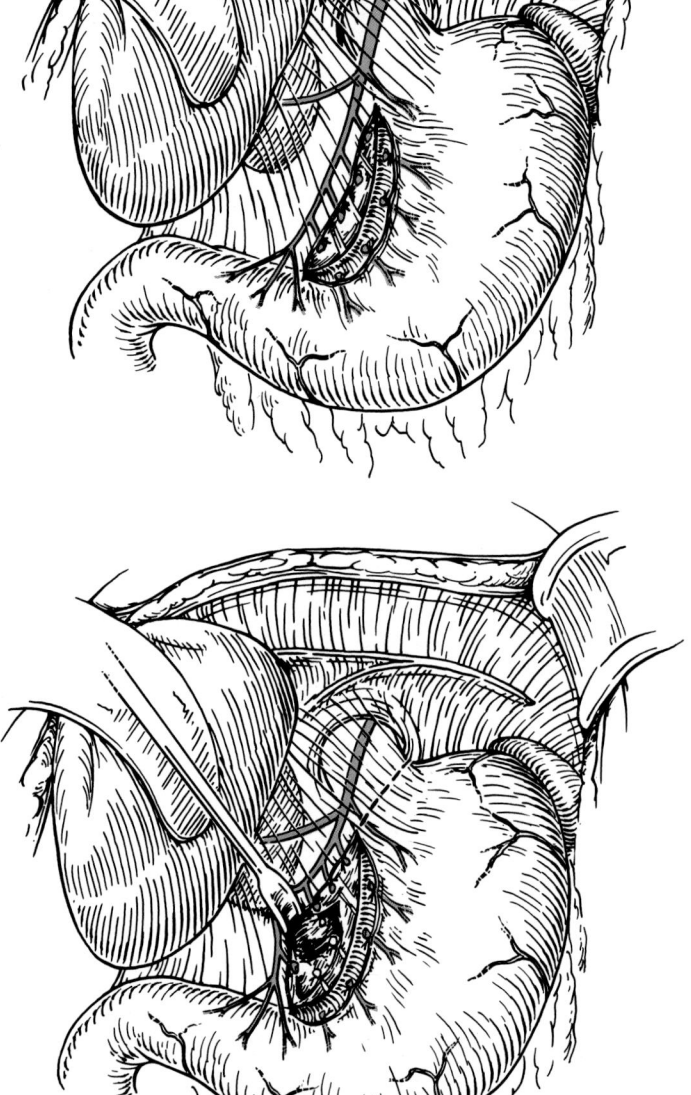

Figure 11-III-4

Continuing Dissection of Anterior Omental Leaflet

Dissection of the anterior leaflet of the gastrohepatic omentum continues proximally along a line directly toward the right edge of the esophagogastric junction.

Figure 11-III-5

Dissection of Lesser Curvature Posteriorly

The posterior layer of the gastrohepatic omentum is also divided, beginning 7 cm proximal to the pylorus. Between the anterior and posterior layers of omentum exists a loose, almost avascular, layer of areolar tissue. Exposure of the posterior layer of the gastrohe-

(Continued)

Figure 11-III-5 *(Continued)*

patic omentum can be improved by rotating the gastric wall anteriorly and gently retracting the anterior and posterior gastric vagal divisions superiorly with a vein retractor. As the dissection approaches the gastroesophageal junction, the anterior peritoneum overlying the cardioesophageal junction is divided, with the incision directed toward the angle of His. It is often helpful to encircle the distal esophagus with a soft Penrose drain at this point. In passing the drain behind the esophagus, care must be taken not to encircle the posterior vagus nerve.

Figure 11-III-6

Periesophageal Incision

An incision is made in the peritoneum and areolar tissue to the left of the esophagus and is extended superiorly to the undersurface of the diaphragm.

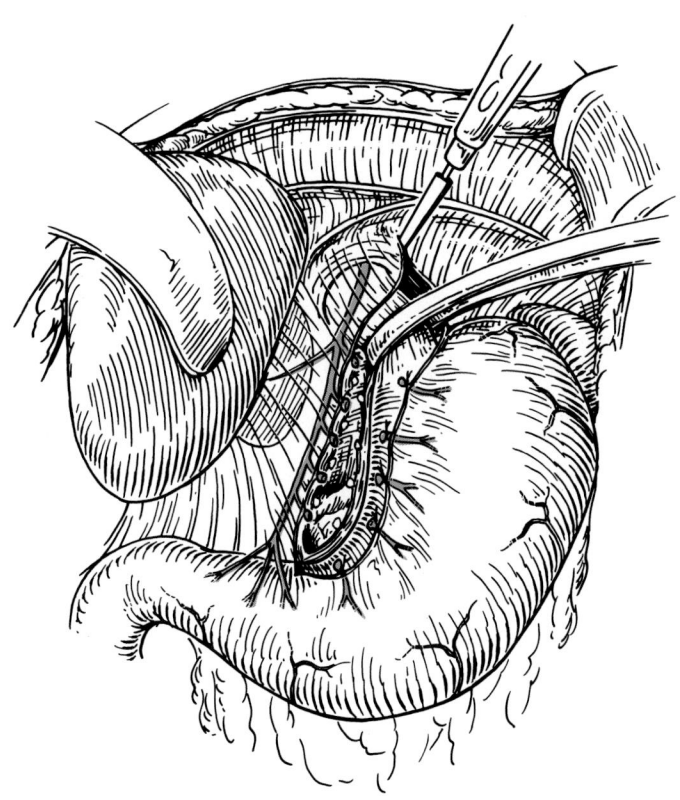

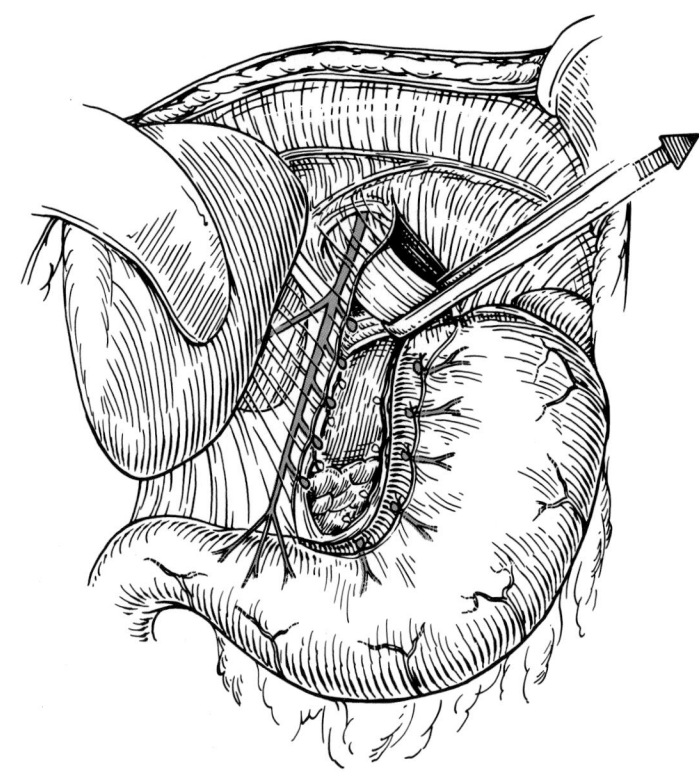

Figure 11-III-7

Esophageal Dissection

A variable number of branches of the vagal trunks enter the esophagus and pass intra-murally to innervate the proximal stomach. To ensure their division, a portion of distal esophagus 5 to 7 cm long must be skeletonized. The Penrose drain is retracted slightly anteriorly and to the left. The connective tissue that contains the vagal trunks is reflected away from the distal esophagus by dissecting directly on the longitudinal muscle layer. The course of the dissection proceeds from inferior to superior and from the left to the right. It is not necessary to encircle the vagal trunks, and care should be taken not to grasp them directly with forceps.

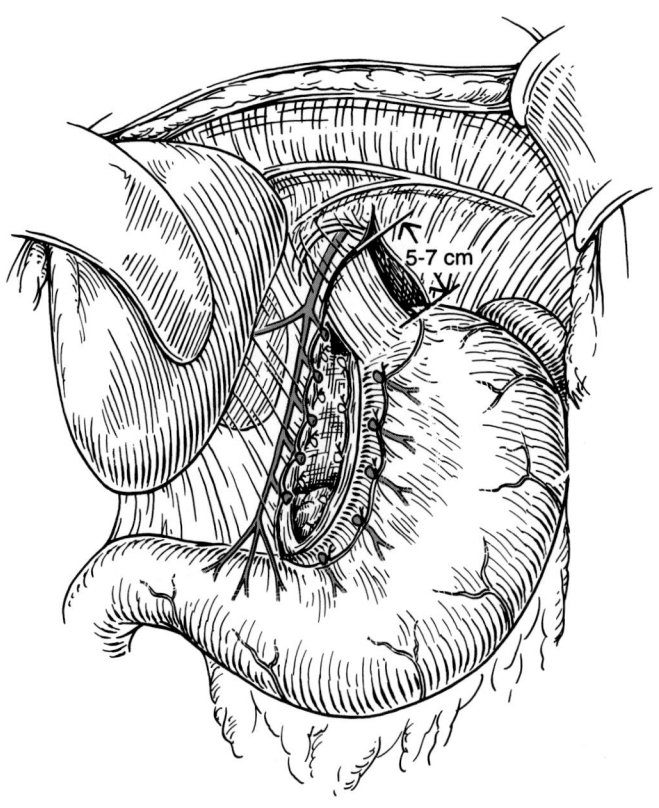

5-7 cm

Figure 11-III-8

Completed Dissection

It is not necessary to reperitonealize the lesser curvature of the stomach at the completion of the dissection.

SECTION IV *Laparoscopic Vagotomy*

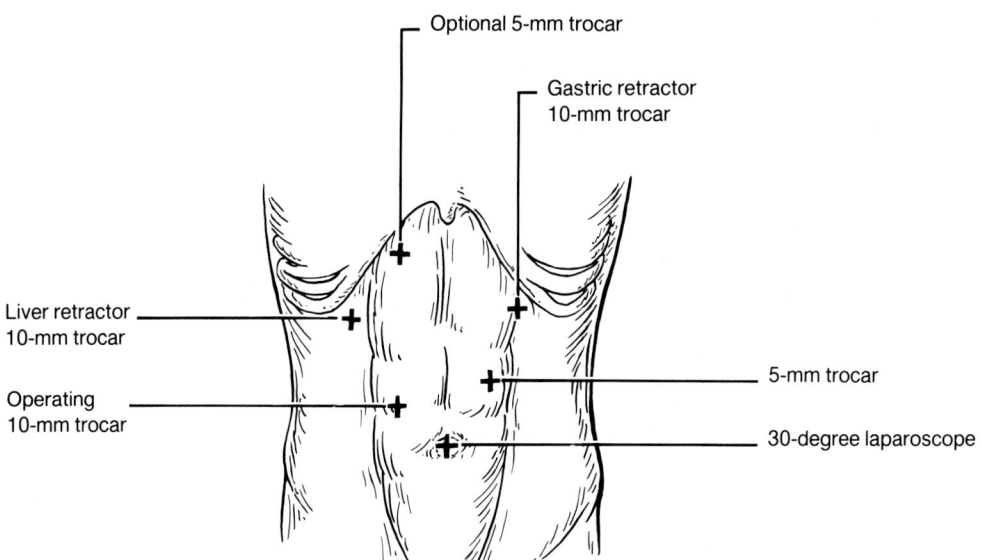

Figure 11-IV-1

Port Placements and Positioning

Pneumoperitoneum is established in standard fashion. An angled (30 to 45 degrees) camera is introduced by means of a laparoscope placed infraumbilically. A modest degree of reverse Trendelenburg position is useful in exposing the upper abdomen.

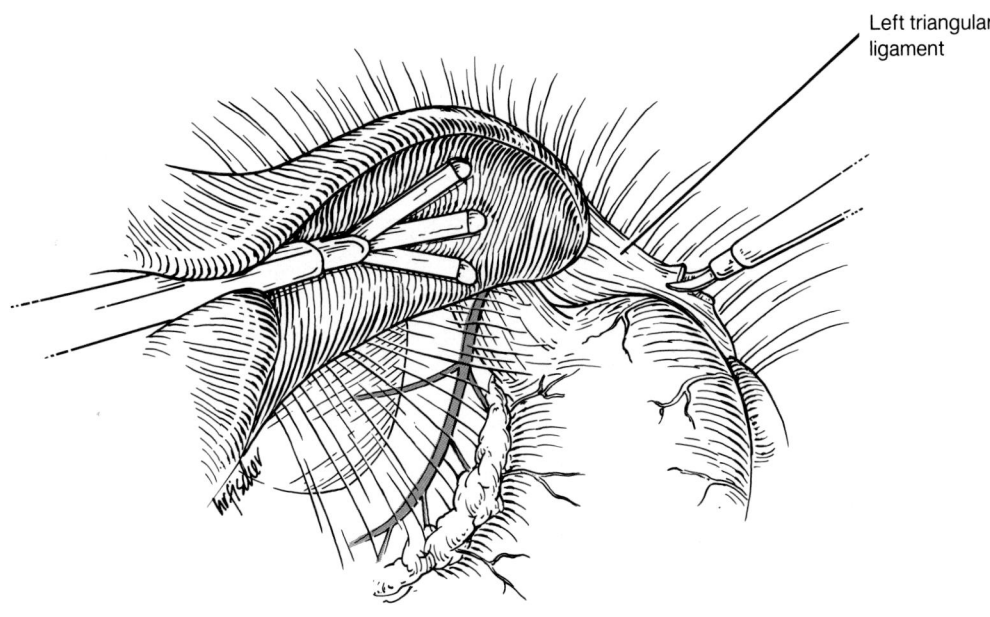

Left triangular
ligament

Figure 11-IV-2

Liver Retraction

A fan-type retractor is inserted through the right subcostal port and used to retract the
left lobe of the liver upward and toward the patient's right. A portion of the left triangular
ligament is divided using curved laparoscopic scissors to gain additional exposure of the
gastroesophageal junction.

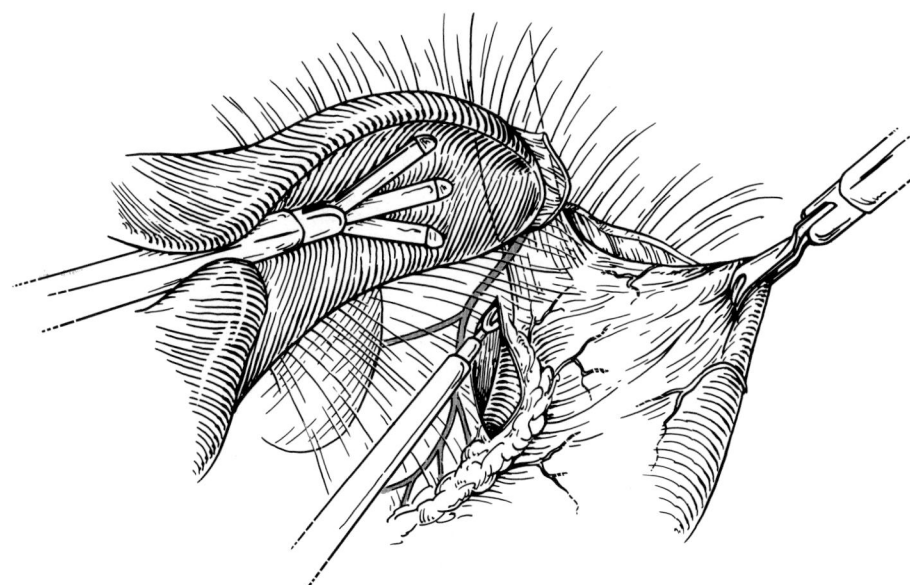

Figure 11-IV-3

Division of Gastrohepatic Omentum

An atraumatic grasping forceps is inserted through the left subcostal port and used to
retract the greater curvature of the stomach to the left. A window is made in the avascular
portion of the gastrohepatic omentum parallel to the lesser curvature to facilitate approach to the posterior aspect of the distal esophagus.

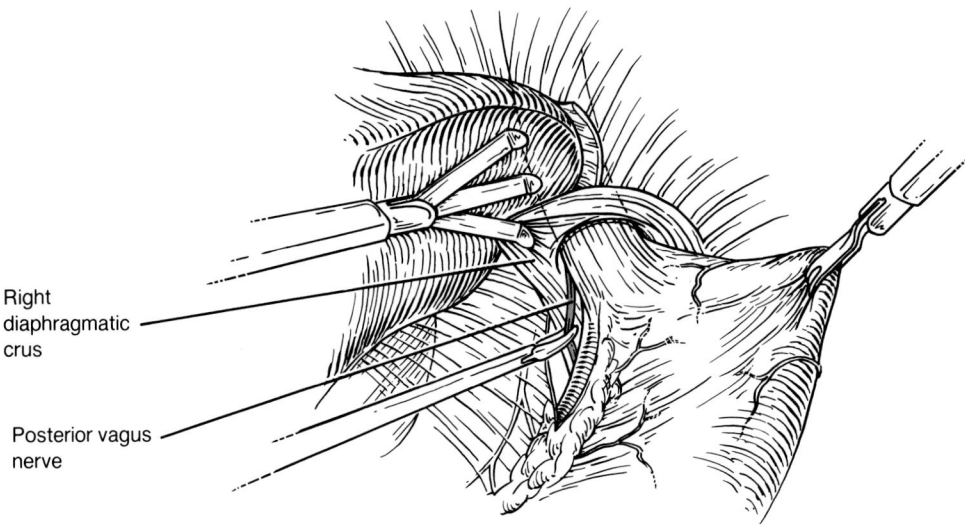

Right
diaphragmatic
crus

Posterior vagus
nerve

Figure 11-IV-4

Identification of Posterior Vagus

The right crus of the diaphragm is identified and retracted to the right, opening up the space between the posterior esophagus and the right crus. A curved dissecting forceps, introduced through the operating port, is used to identify and isolate the posterior vagus nerve. The nerve is gently grasped and retracted to the right.

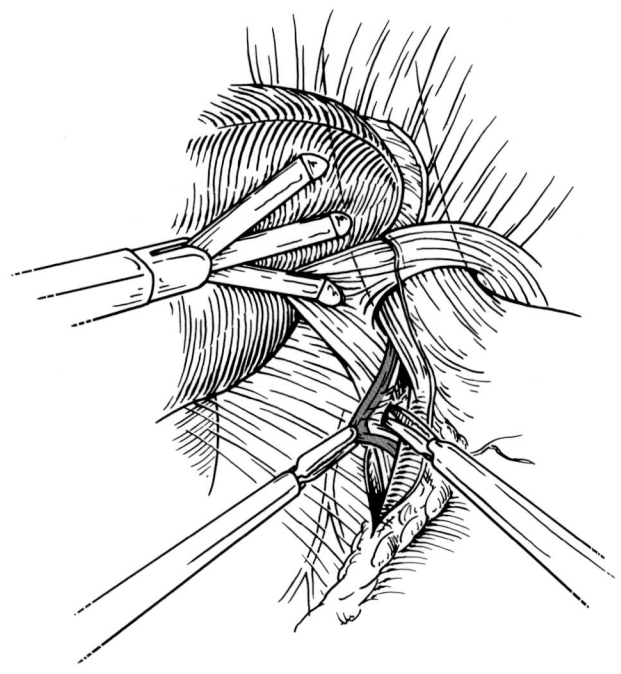

Figure 11-IV-5

Dissection of Vagal Length

Using a dissector inserted through a left abdominal port, a length of posterior vagus nerve is cleared of adherent tissue.

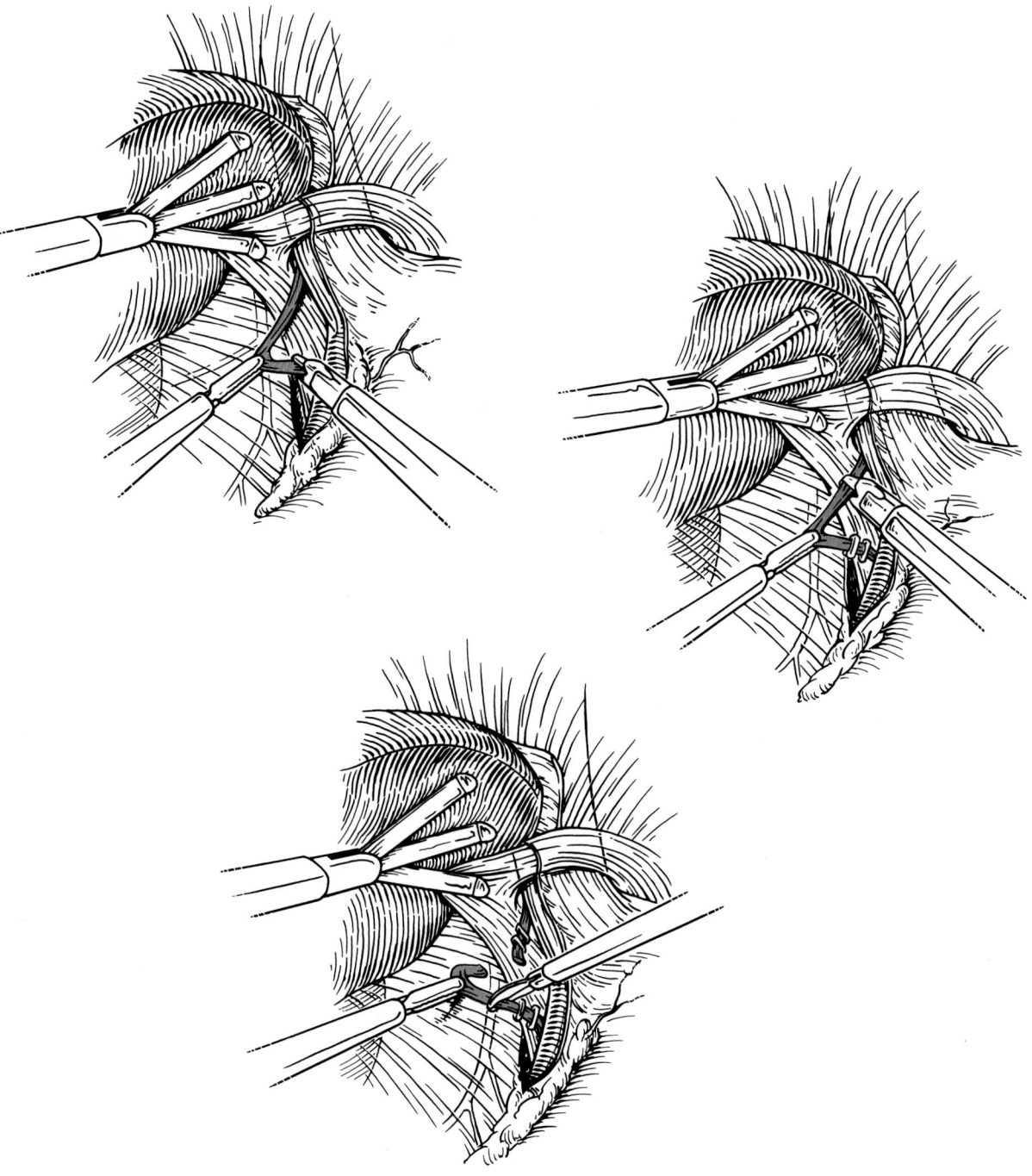

Figure 11-IV-6

Division of Posterior Trunk

The posterior vagal trunk is ligated proximally and distally with clips before excision of a segment for histologic examination. The proximal division should be at the level of the esophageal hiatus.

Hepatic
division

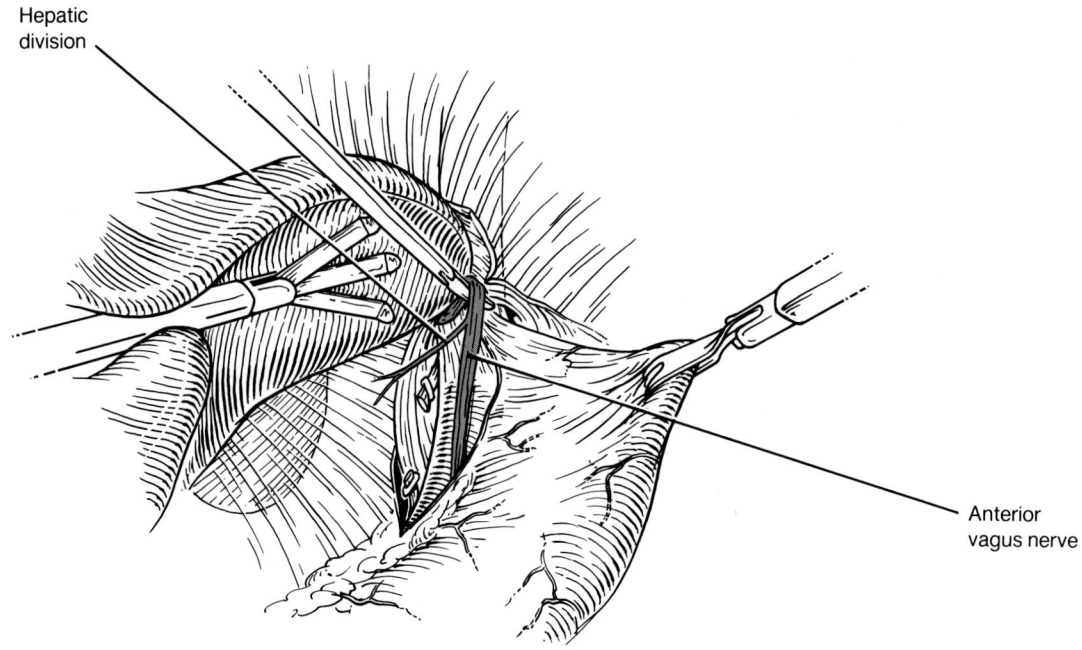

Anterior
vagus nerve

Figure 11-IV-7

Identification of Anterior Vagus Nerve

The peritoneum overlying the esophagogastric junction anteriorly is divided, exposing
the anterior vagus nerve. The anterior vagus nerve is elevated by a curved dissecting
forceps passed through the operating port. Using a dissector passed through the left abdominal port, a 5-cm segment of anterior vagus is dissected free from the surrounding
esophageal and proximal gastric tissues.

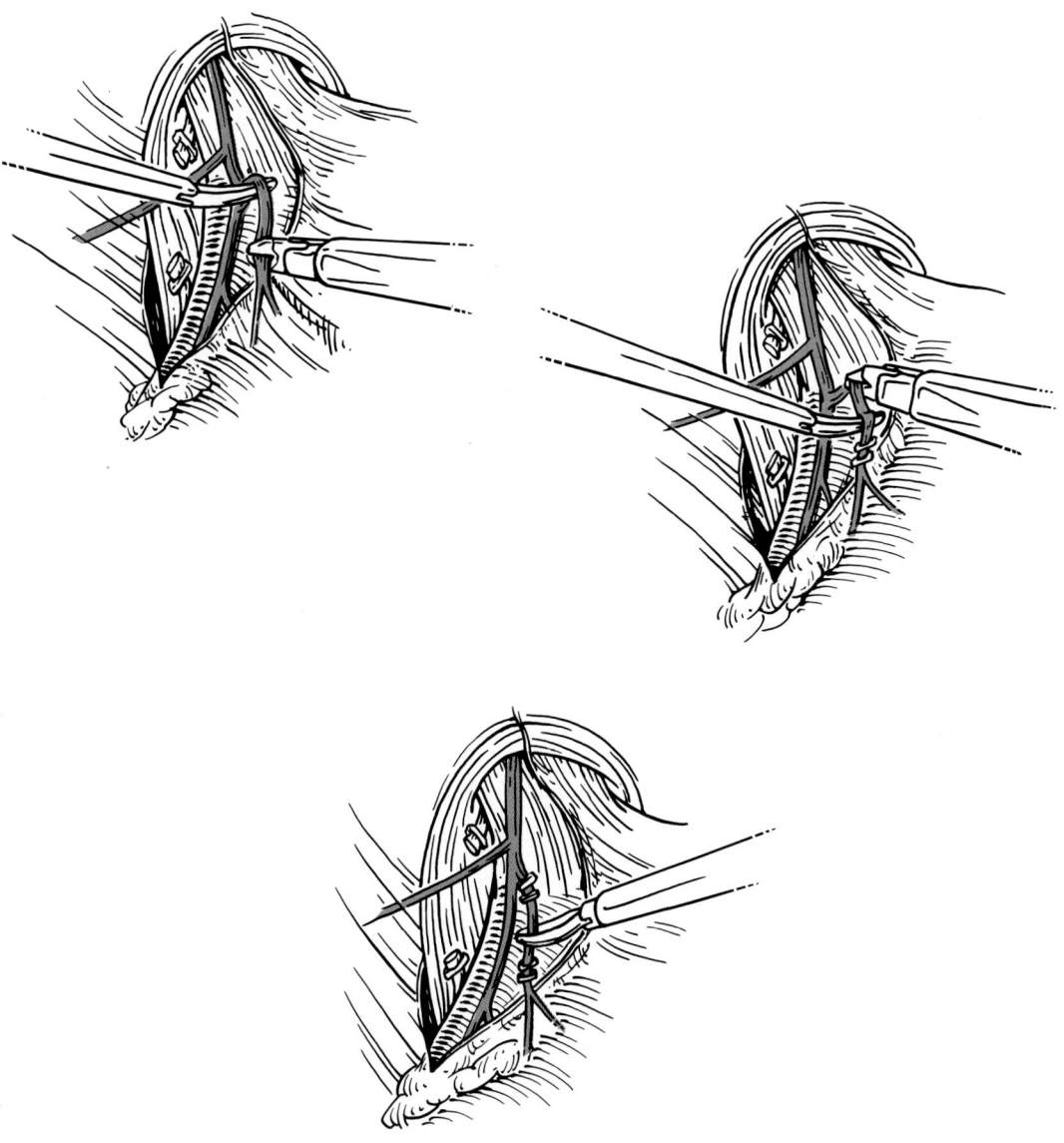

Figure 11-IV-8

Division of Vagal Branches

Any small anterior vagal branches entering the distal esophagus or proximal stomach are individually ligated with clips and divided.

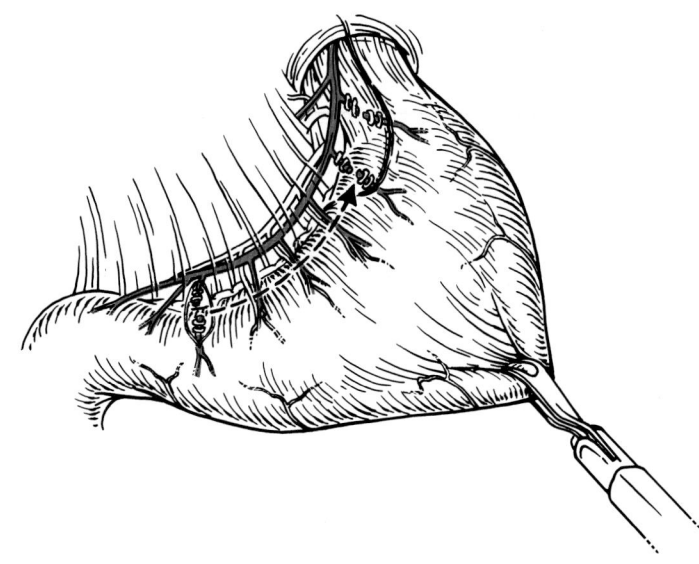

Figure 11-IV-9

Distal Extent of Dissection

The distal dissection should extend to within 7 cm of the pylorus, sparing the anterior nerve of Latarjet. The left-sided retracting forceps is shifted distally to gain proper exposure. Each neurovascular bundle is individually dissected, ligated with clips, and divided with scissors. Dissection proceeds in a distal to proximal direction.

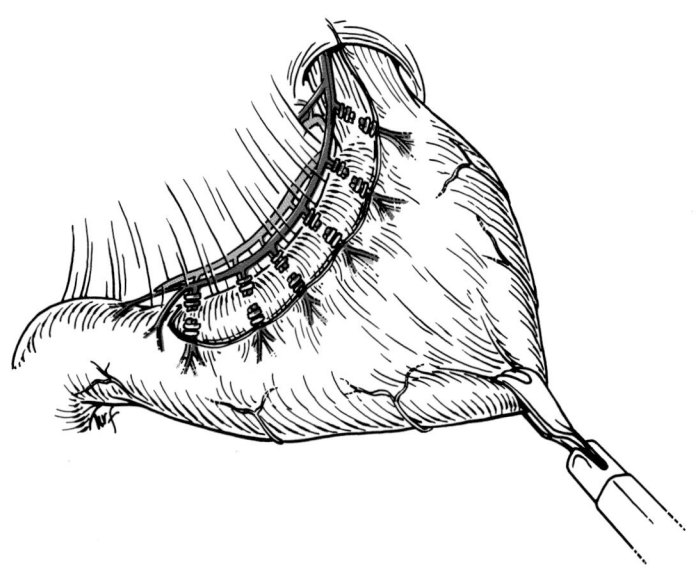

Figure 11-IV-10

Completed Dissection

The completed dissection is inspected for hemostasis. Fascial defects at 10-mm trocar sites are closed with sutures.

SECTION V *Partial Gastrectomy*

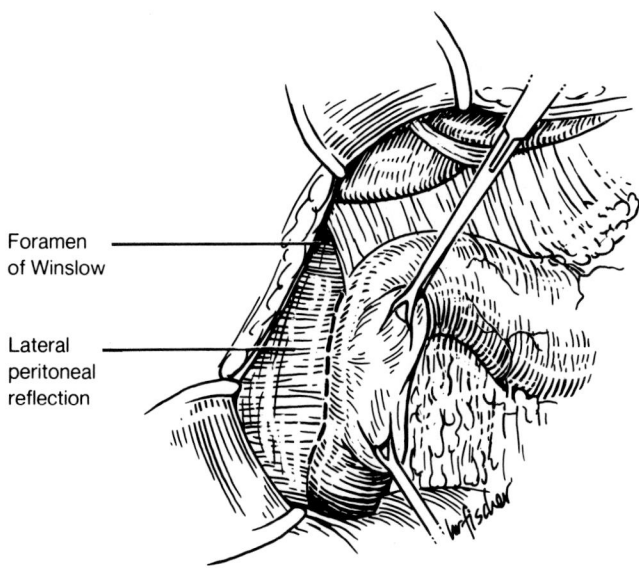

Figure 11-V-1

Kocher Maneuver

When partial gastrectomy is to be combined with gastroduodenal reconstruction, mobilization of the duodenum is necessary to assess the suitability of the duodenum for anastomosis. The hepatic flexure of the colon is reflected inferiorly. The surgical assistant retracts the duodenum medially, exposing the reflection of the peritoneum from the duodenum onto the retroperitoneum. An incision in the retroperitoneum paralleling the second portion of the duodenum can be made with cautery.

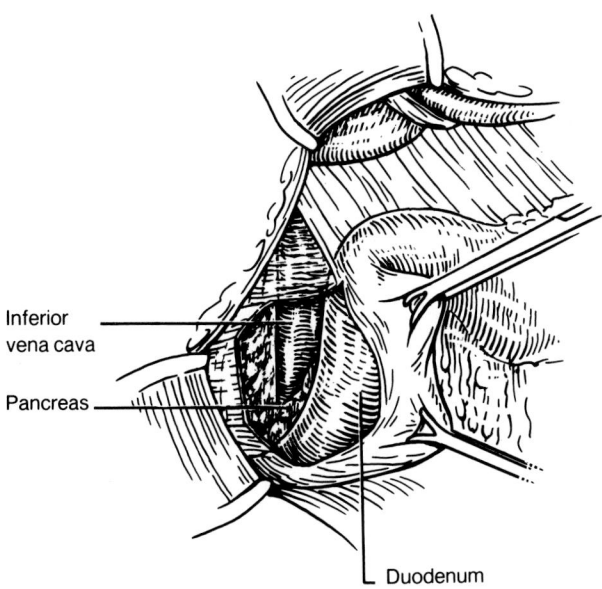

Figure 11-V-2

Exposure of Inferior Vena Cava

The duodenum is retracted medially and slightly anteriorly. Development of the avascular plain behind the duodenum exposes the inferior vena cava and right gonadal vein. The posterior aspect of the duodenal sweep and the pancreatic head are visualized and easily palpated.

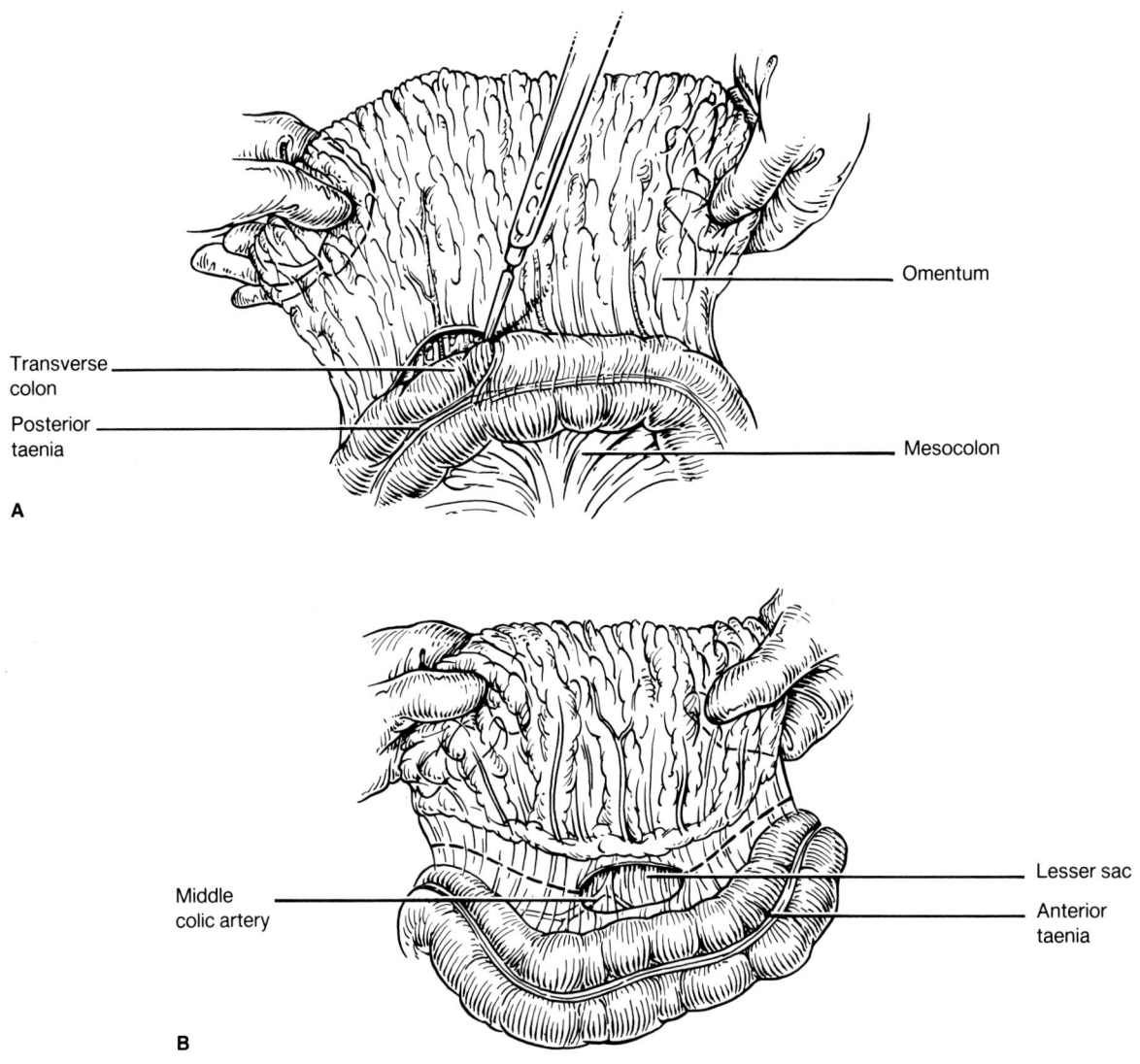

Figure 11-V-3

Entry Into the Lesser Sac

(A) The posterior wall of the stomach should be inspected to evaluate possible inflammatory or neoplastic involvement of retrogastric structures. The lesser sac can be entered by dividing the attachment of the greater omentum to the transverse colon. An avascular plane can be developed immediately adjacent to the transverse colon.

(B) The lesser sac can often be identified most easily by beginning the dissection somewhat to the left of midline. Care must be taken not to injure the middle colic vessels in separating omental and transverse mesenteric layers.

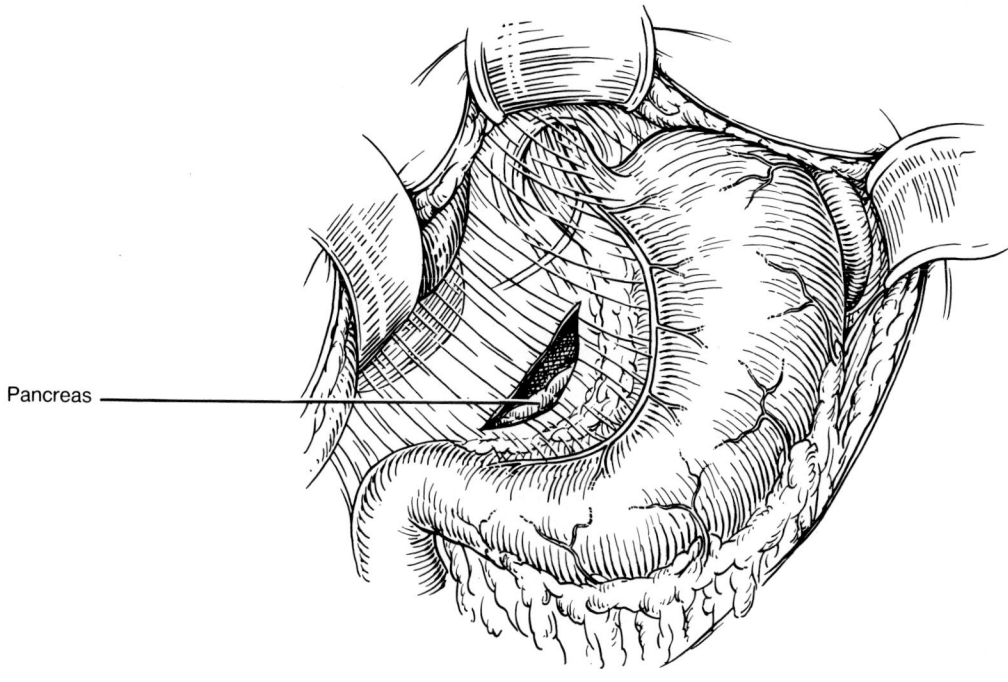

Pancreas

Figure 11-V-4

Incision of Gastrohepatic Ligament

An alternative approach to the retrogastric space can be obtained by division of the avascular superior portion of the gastrohepatic omentum.

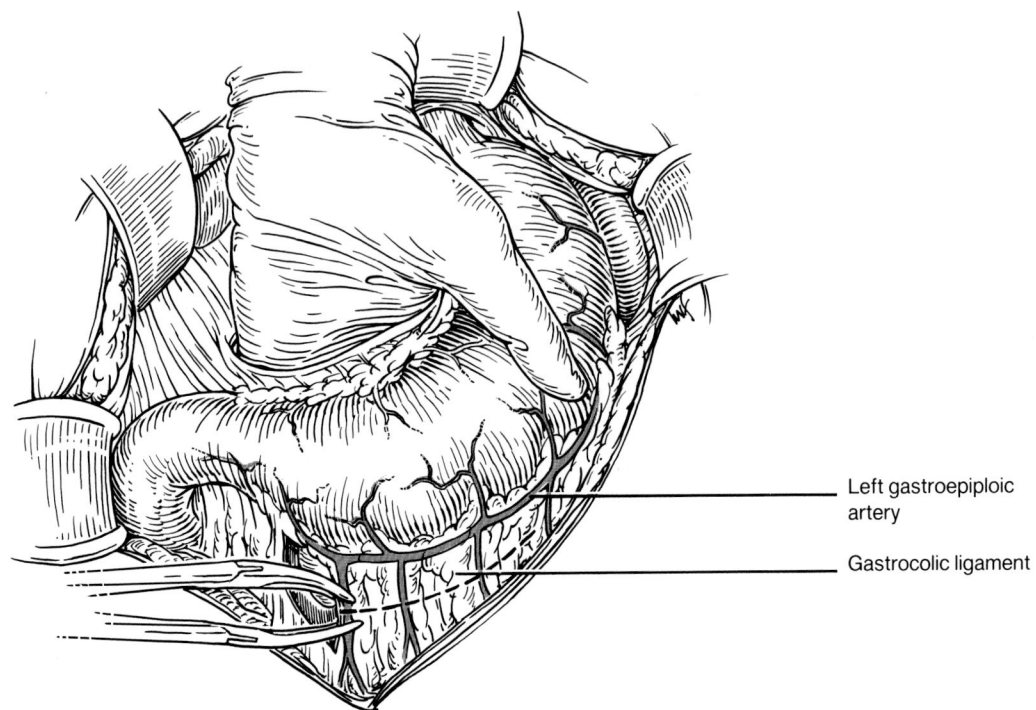

Left gastroepiploic
artery

Gastrocolic ligament

Figure 11-V-5

Division of Gastrocolic Omentum

Using this alternative approach, the surgeon's left hand is introduced into the retrogastric space to guide the initial division of the gastrocolic omentum and to protect against injury to the middle colic vessels. If gastric resection is performed for benign disease and omental resection is not necessary, gastroepiploic vessels can be preserved. Because the omentum receives its blood supply from both right and left gastroepiploic arteries, division of small vessels along the greater curvature will not lead to omental infarction.

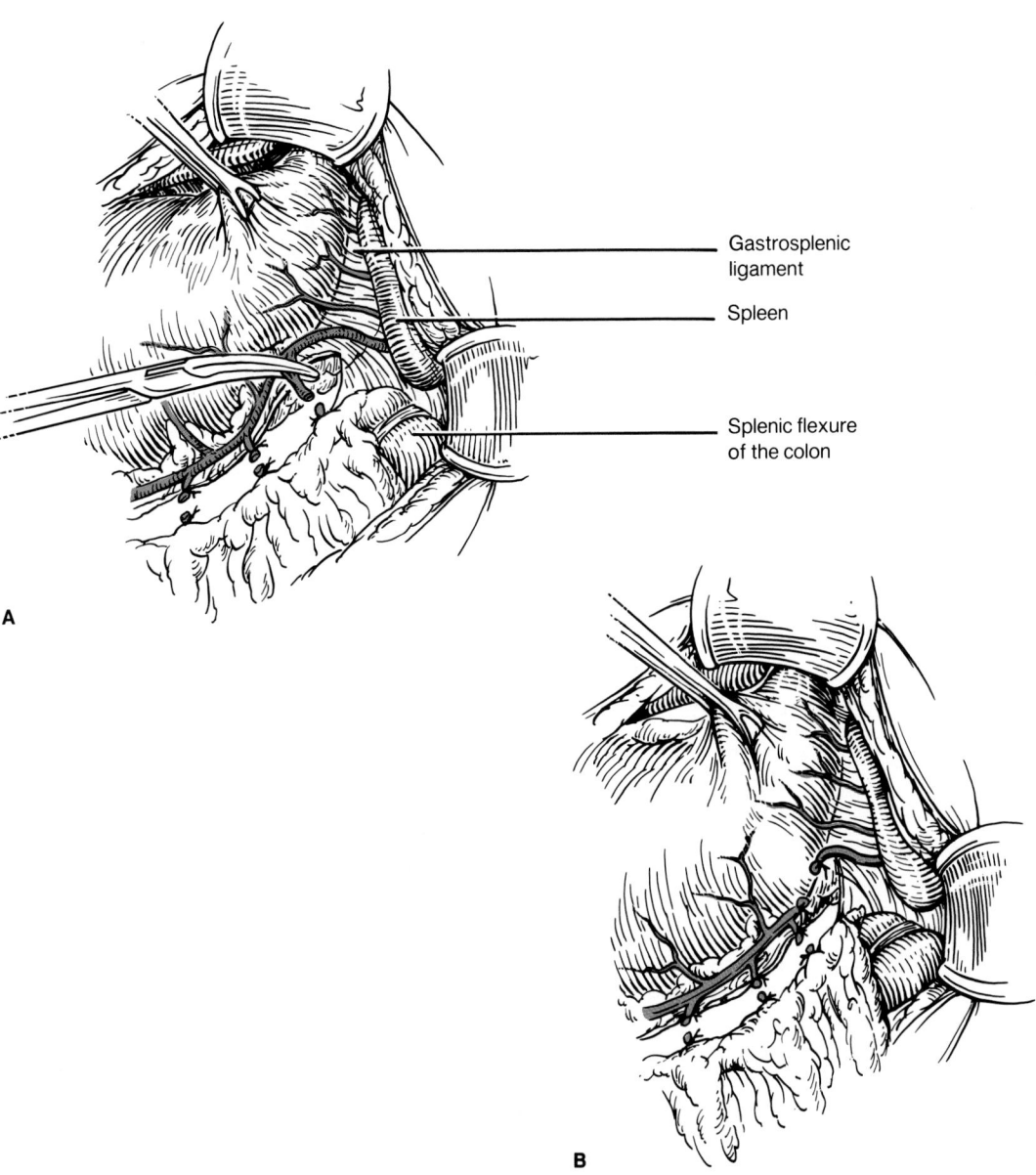

Gastrosplenic
ligament

Spleen

Splenic flexure
of the colon

A

B

Figure 11-V-6

Preparation of Greater Curvature for Hemigastrectomy

(**A**) Preparation for a 50% gastric resection involves division of the gastrocolic ligament to a point about halfway between the pylorus and the esophagogastric junction. This point often corresponds to the transition from right to left gastroepiploic vessels.

(**B**) The gastric wall should be cleared of omental fat for a short distance in preparation for subsequent resection and anastomosis.

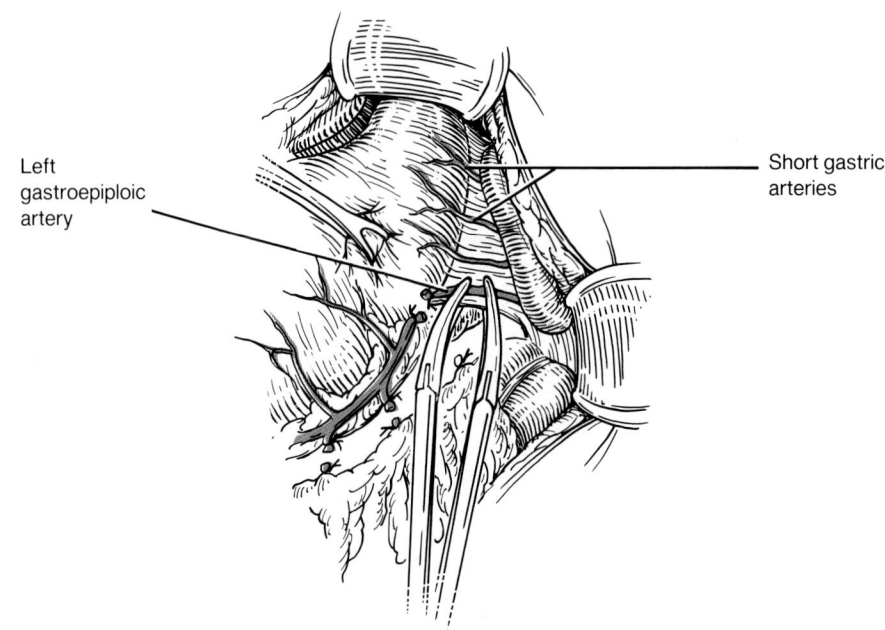

Left
gastroepiploic
artery

Short gastric
arteries

Figure 11-V-7

Preparation for Subtotal Gastrectomy

Performance of subtotal gastrectomy requires division of left gastroepiploic vessels and lower short gastric vessels. Omental resection is usually necessary if these vessels are divided.

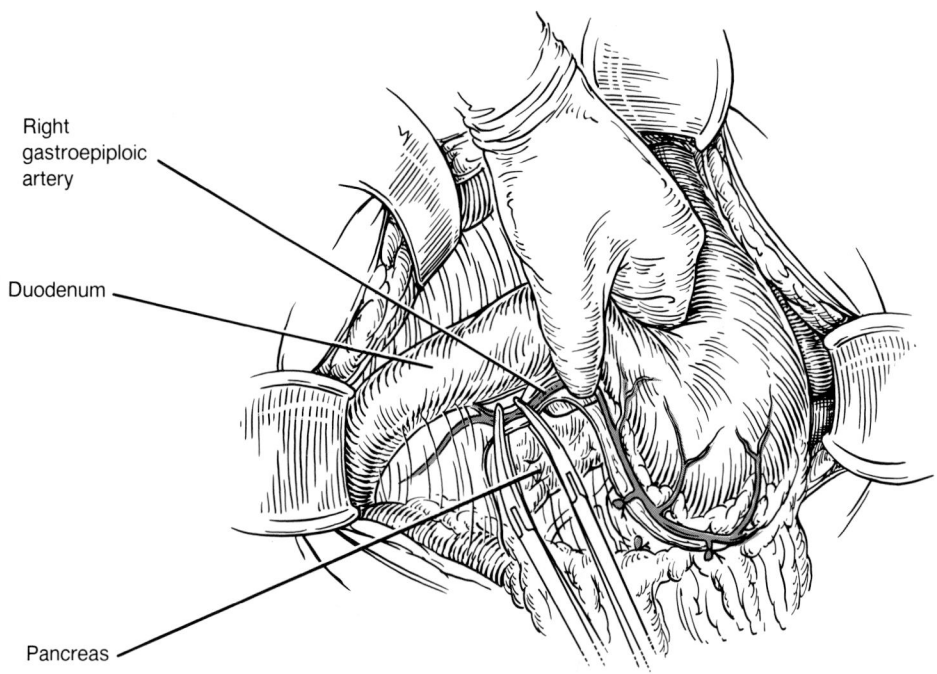

Right
gastroepiploic
artery

Duodenum

Pancreas

Figure 11-V-8

Division of Right Gastroepiploic Vessels

The right gastroepiploic vessels are exposed by retracting the stomach cephalad. The right gastroepiploic artery is divided close to its origin from the gastroduodenal artery. Fine connective tissue between the posterior antropyloric region and the anterior surface of the pancreas can be divided sharply.

346

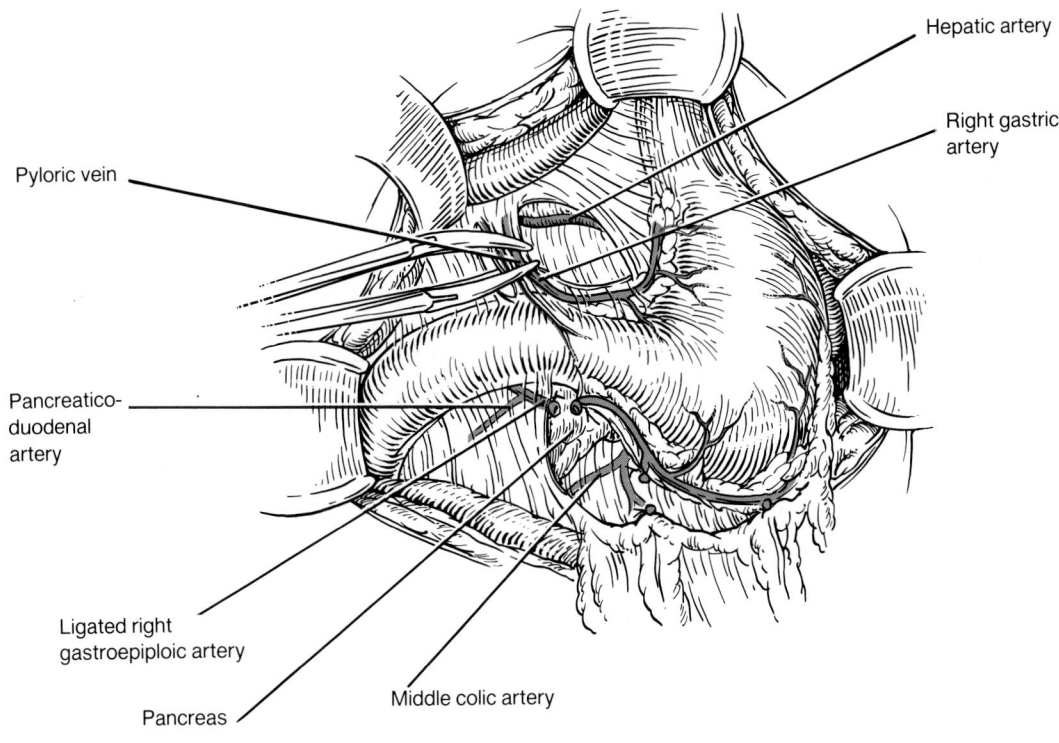

Hepatic artery

Right gastric artery

Pyloric vein

Pancreatico-duodenal artery

Ligated right gastroepiploic artery

Pancreas

Middle colic artery

Figure 11-V-9

Ligation of Right Gastric Vessels

The right gastric vessels will be identified at the superior border of the proximal duodenum. The vessels should be divided close to the duodenal wall. Care must be taken not to injure the common hepatic artery or common bile duct if inflammation or tumor has distorted the first portion of the duodenum.

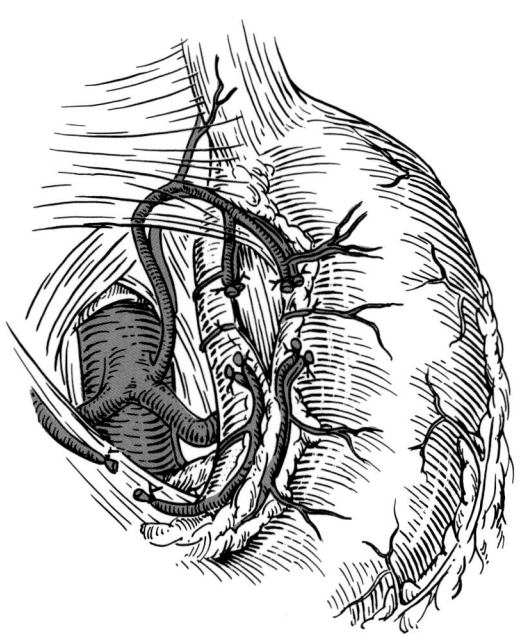

Figure 11-V-10

Dissection of Lesser Curvature

An area along the lesser curvature is selected for division and anastomosis. Branches of the left gastric artery supply the lesser curvature as paired vessels to the anterior and posterior surfaces. These branches should be ligated separately and the loose connective tissue between them cleared from the gastric wall.

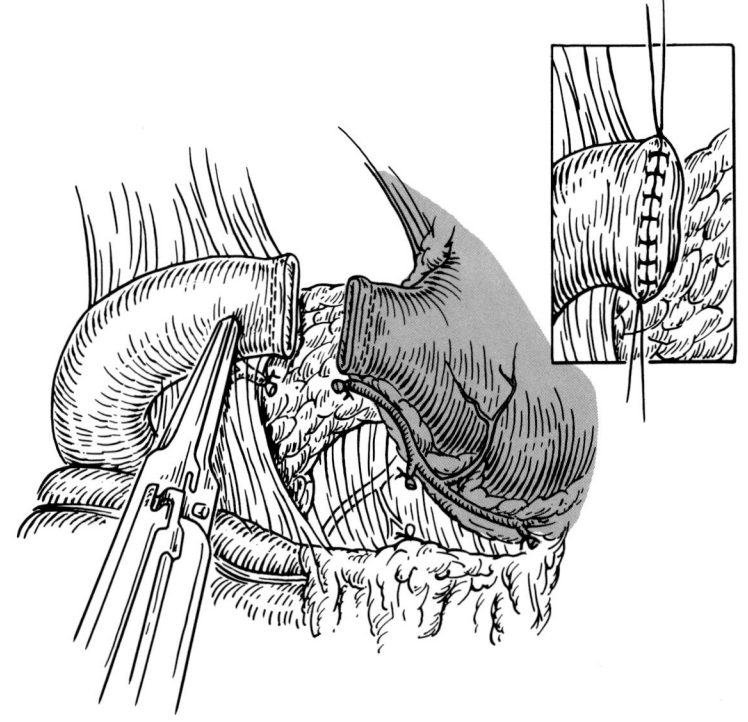

Figure 11-V-11

Division of the Duodenum

The proximal duodenum is divided using a GIA stapler for ease of closure. The double staple line closure of the divided duodenum can be reinforced, at the surgeon's preference, with interrupted 3-0 nonabsorbable sutures.

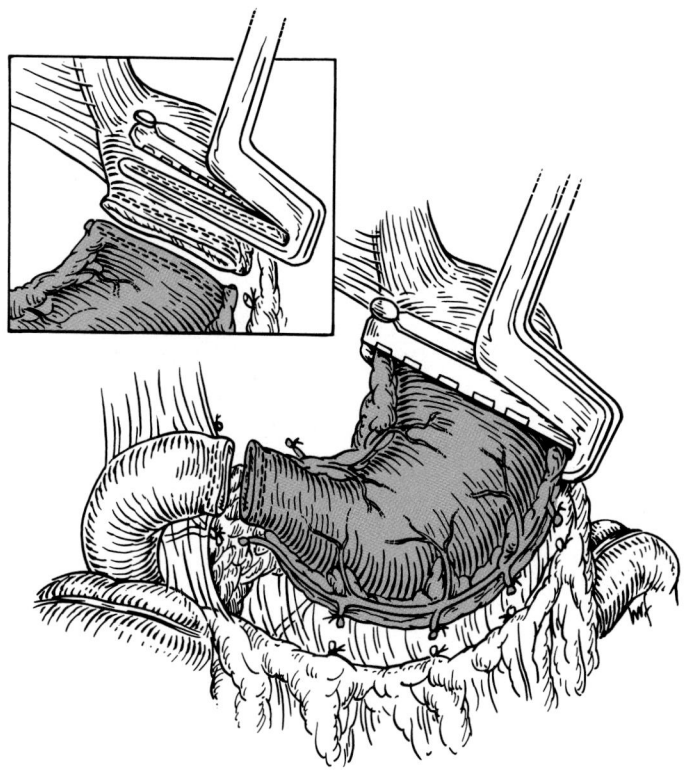

Figure 11-V-12

Division of the Proximal Stomach

A TA-90 stapler can be used to close the gastric remnant with a double row of staples. An occlusive clamp can be placed distally to prevent spillage of gastric contents, or the resected specimen can be closed by a second application of the TA-90 stapler. Alternatively, long-length GIA staplers can be used to staple and divide the stomach. A second application of the GIA staples will be necessary if the stomach is too broad.

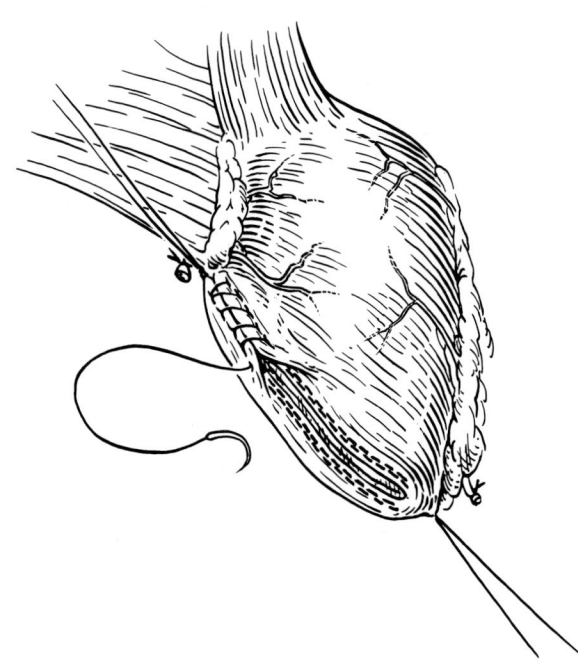

Figure 11-V-13

Oversewing of Gastric Suture Line

Some oozing of blood may occur between staples but usually stops spontaneously. The superior portion of the gastric staple line is inverted with interrupted nonabsorbable sutures or a continuous monofilament suture. Traction sutures, placed at either end of the stapled closure, are useful in preventing retraction of the gastric remnant from the operative field.

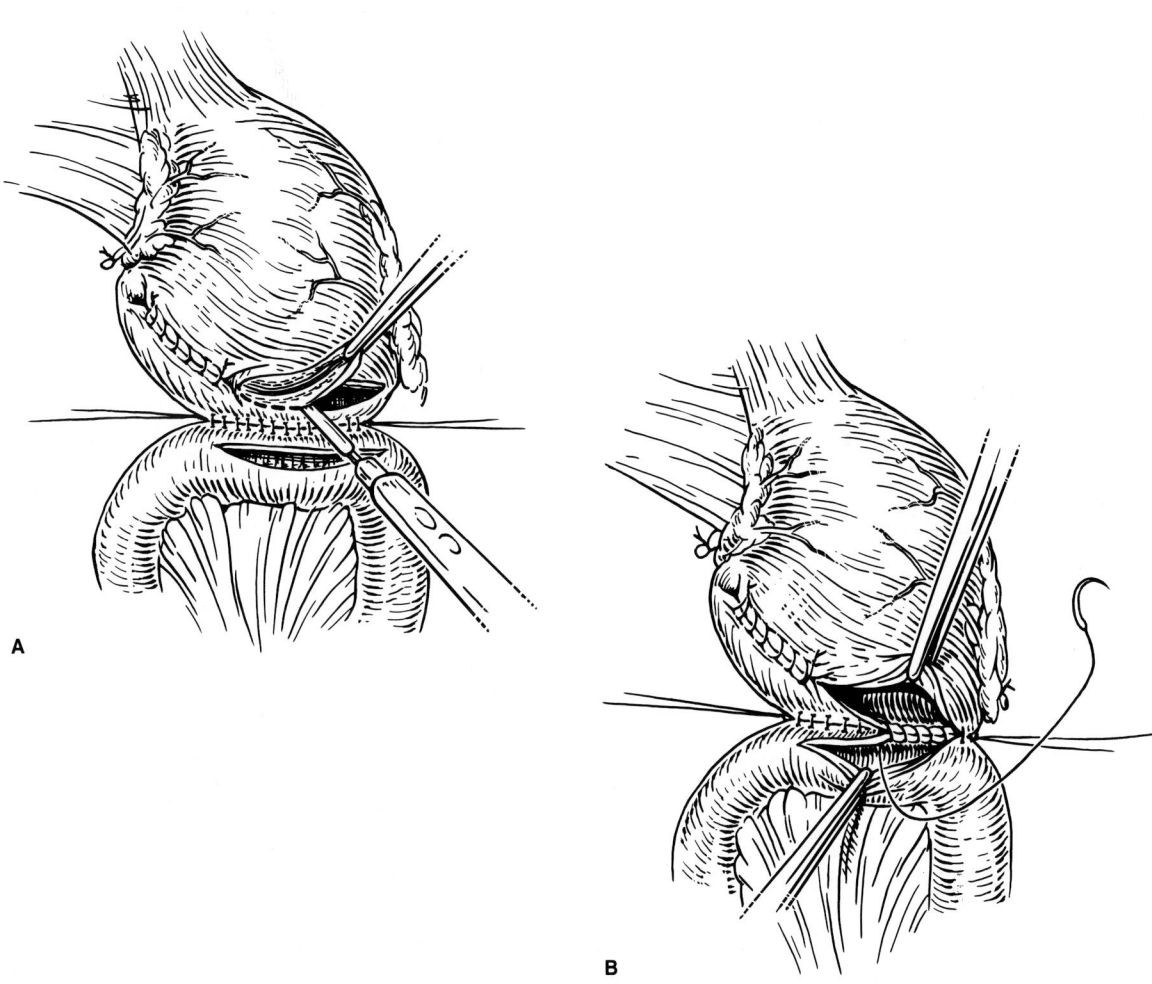

A

B

Figure 11-V-14

Gastrojejunostomy: Sutured Technique

(**A**) A proximal loop of jejunum is brought through an incision in the transverse meso-colon to lie in apposition to the stomach. Interrupted nonabsorbable sutures are placed in seromuscular fashion from the posterior gastric wall to the antimesenteric border of the jejunum. An incision in the jejunum is created with electrocautery. A gastrotomy of equal length is created by partial excision of the stapled gastric closure.

(**B**) The posterior mucosal closure is created using a continuous absorbable suture. The transition from posterior anastomosis to anterior anastomosis involves suturing three structures—the posterior gastric wall, the jejunal apex, and the anterior gastric wall. Gastrojejunostomy can also be performed in Roux-en-Y fashion. Creation of a Roux limb is illustrated in Figures 11-VI-8 and 11-VI-9.

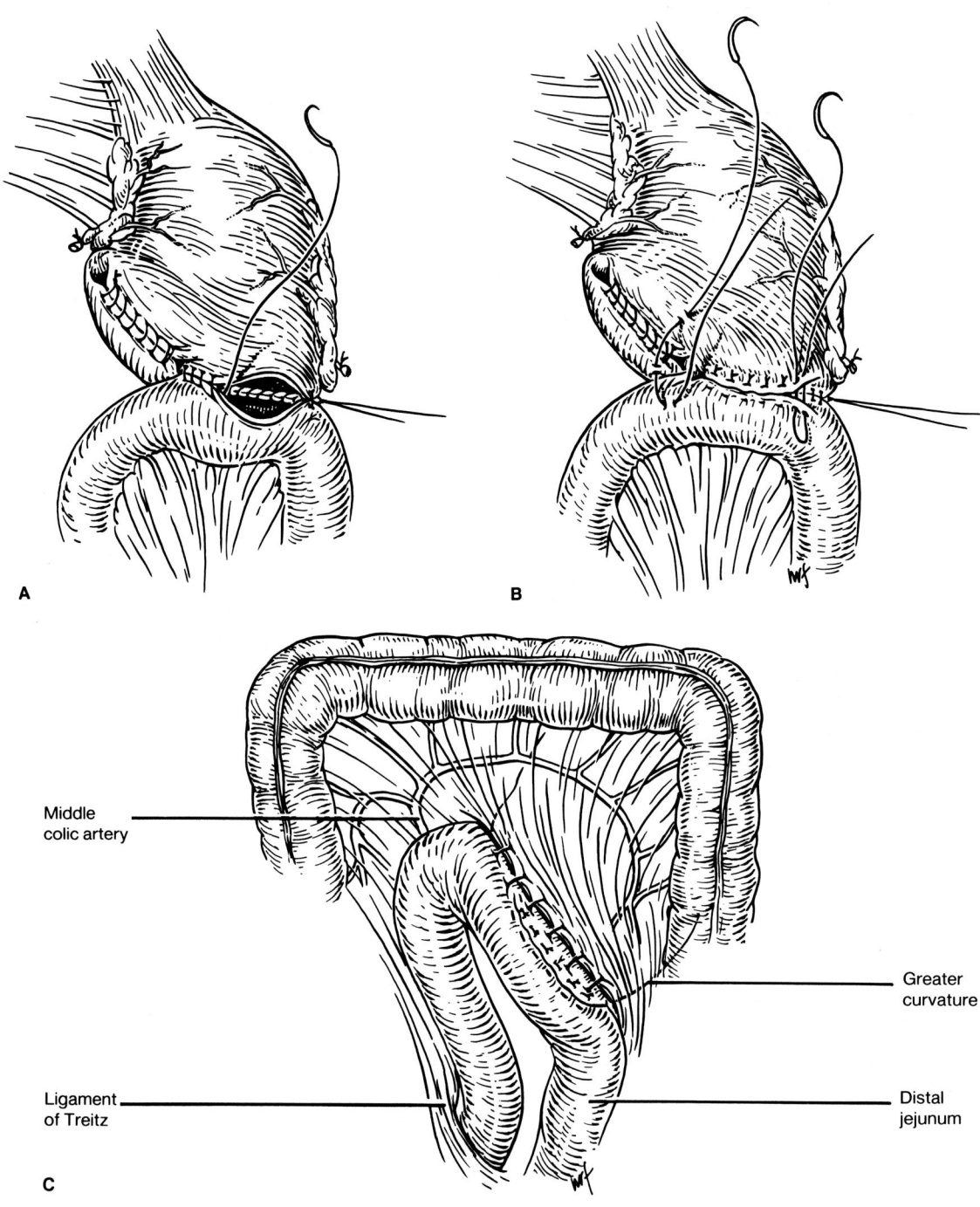

Middle
colic artery

Greater
curvature

Ligament
of Treitz

Distal
jejunum

Figure 11-V-15

Anterior Anastomosis

(**A**) The mucosal suture is continued along the length of the anterior aspect of the anastomosis.

(**B**) A layer of interrupted 3-0 nonabsorbable sutures completes the anterior anastomosis. Corner stitches must include anterior the gastric wall, posterior gastric wall, and jejunum.

(**C**) The gastrojejunal anastomosis is delivered beneath the transverse mesentery and is secured in this position by sutures form the mesentery to the gastric wall.

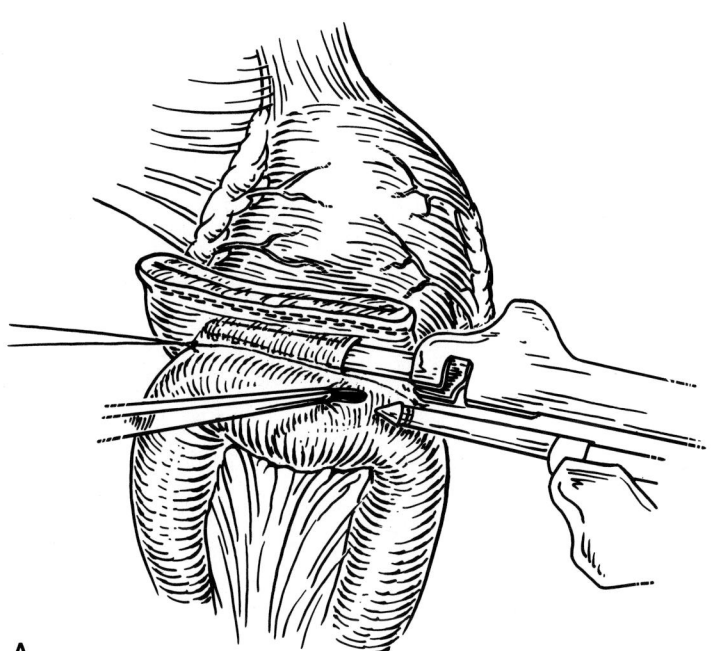

A

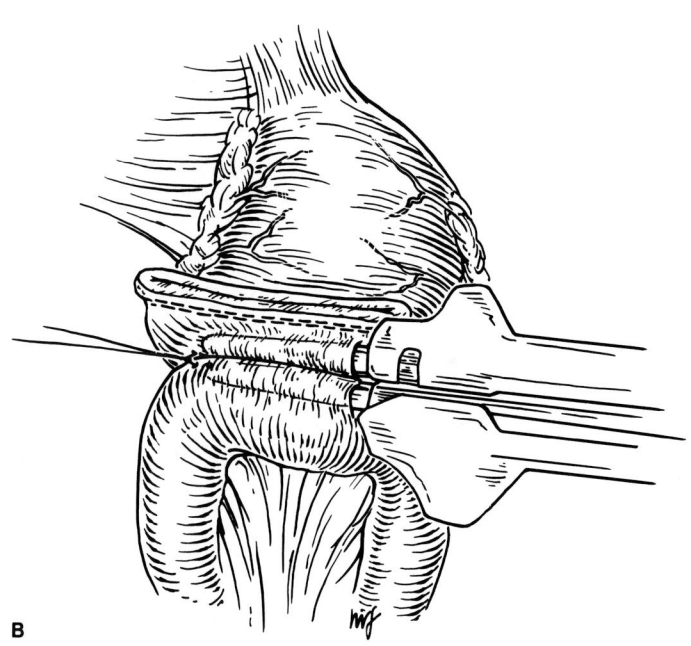

B

Figure 11-V-16

Gastrojejunostomy: Stapled Technique

(**A**) Using a GIA-type instrument, a stapled gastrojejunostomy can be created. The back wall of the stomach and the antimesenteric surface of the jejunum are approximated by traction sutures. Using electrocautery, an incision is created in the stomach 2.5 to 3 cm from the stapled closure. A similar wound is made in the jejunum along the antimesenteric border, and each fork of the stapling instrument is inserted separately.

(**B**) The instrument is closed and fired, creating an anastomosis with two staggered rows of staples. Placement of the anastomosis 2.5 to 3 cm from the transected gastric edge ensures adequate blood flow to the gastric wall distal to the staple line. The instrument is withdrawn, and the staple line is inspected for hemostasis.

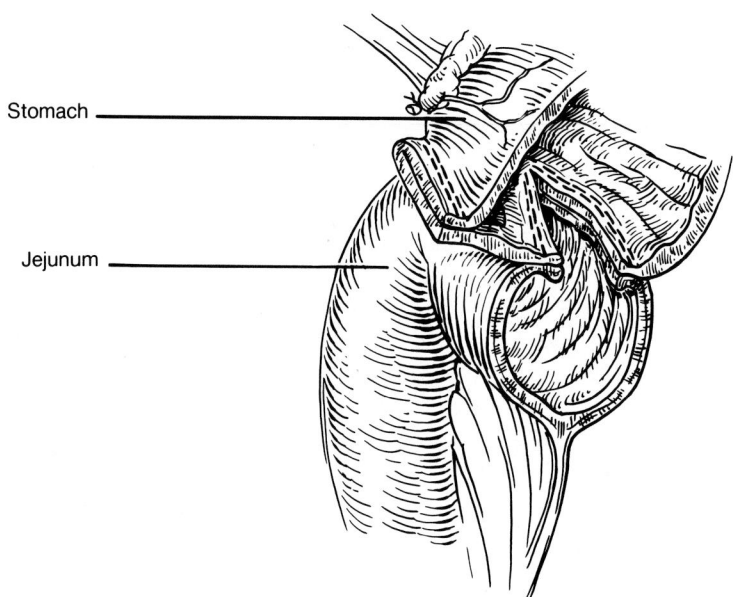

Stomach

Jejunum

Figure 11-V-17

Completed Anastomosis

The stapled gastrojejunal anastomosis.

Figure 11-V-18

Closure of Residual Defect

The defect left by insertion of the GIA stapler is closed by application of a TA stapling device.

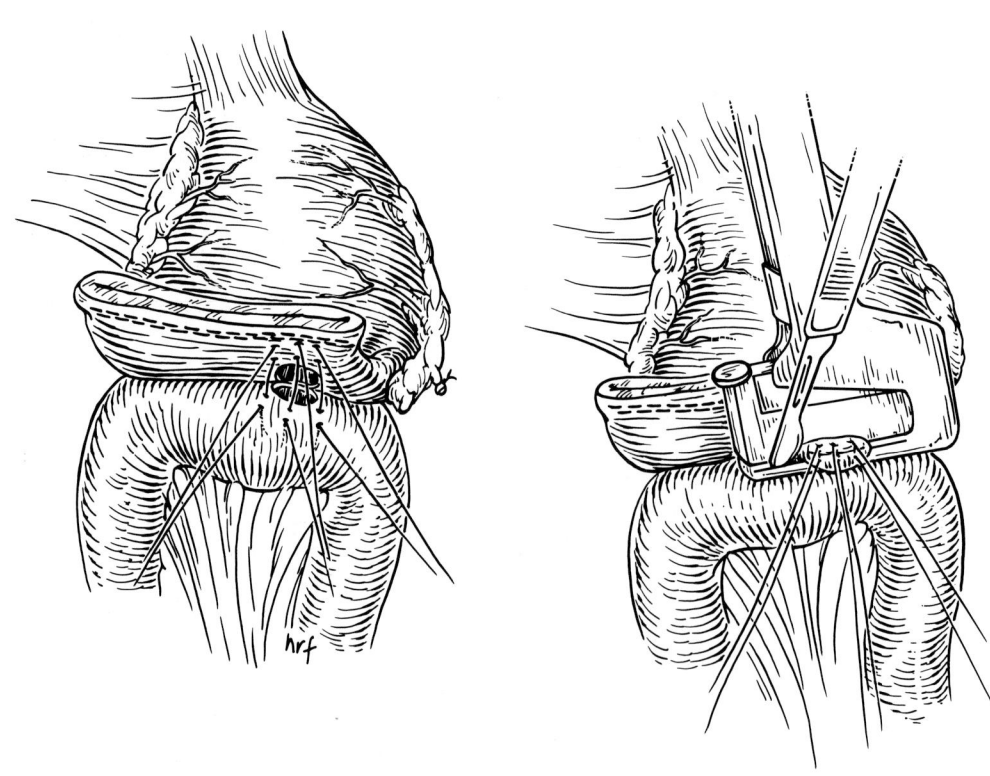

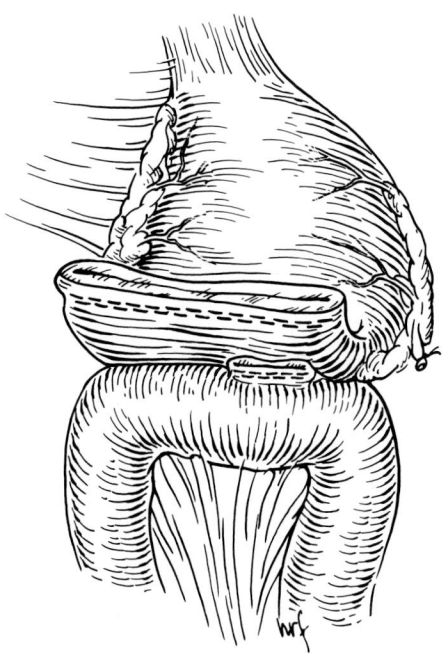

Figure 11-V-18 *(Continued)*

Figure 11-V-19

Gastroduodenostomy: Sutured Technique

(**A**) The posterior wall of the first portion of the duodenum and the posterior surface of the stomach are approximated with interrupted sutures. The stapled closure of the duodenum and a portion of the gastric staple line are then excised using electrocautery.

(**B**) An inner mucosal closure, incorporating all layers of duodenum and stomach, is begun with a continuous absorbable suture.

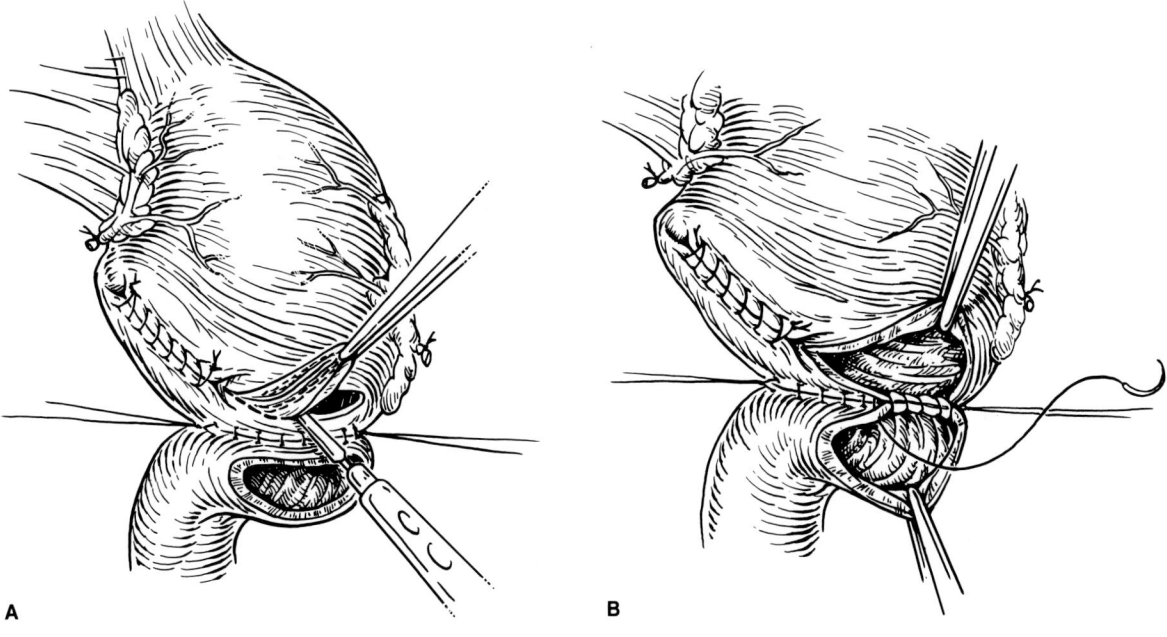

A   B

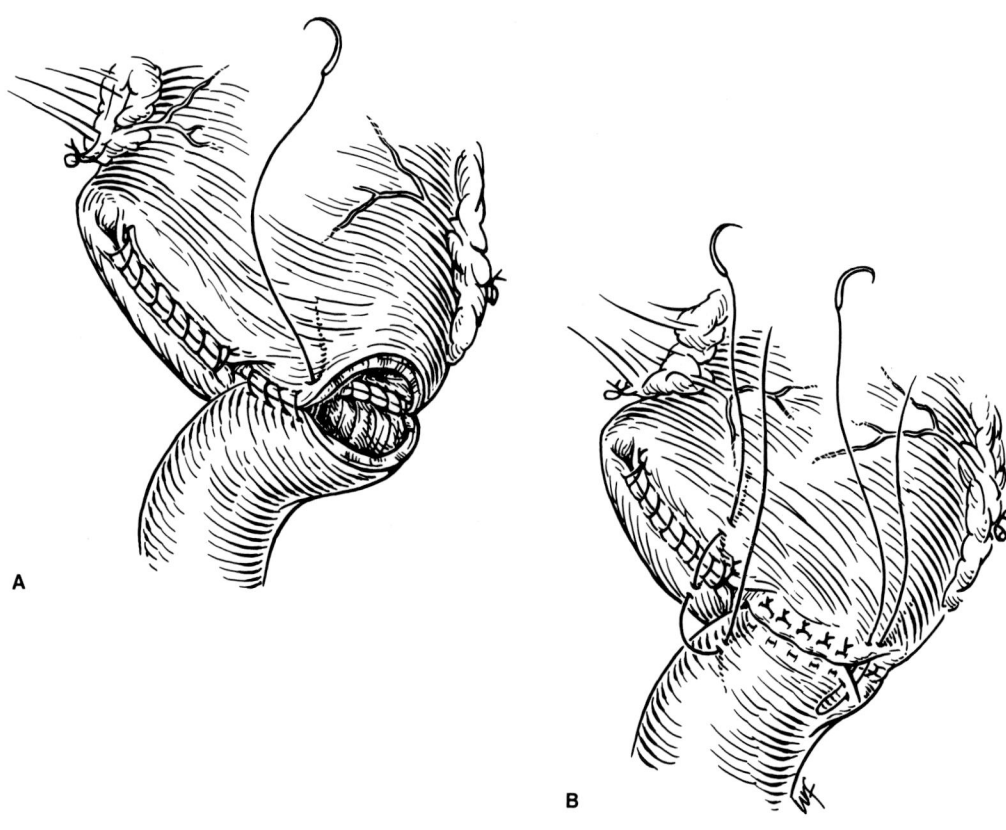

Figure 11-V-20

Anterior Gastroduodenal Anastomosis

(**A**) The mucosal suture is continued anteriorly.

(**B**) Interrupted 3-0 nonabsorbable seromuscular sutures are used to complete the anastomosis anteriorly. At the superior corner of the anastomosis, the suture should include both the anterior and posterior gastric walls as well as the superior duodenal wall.

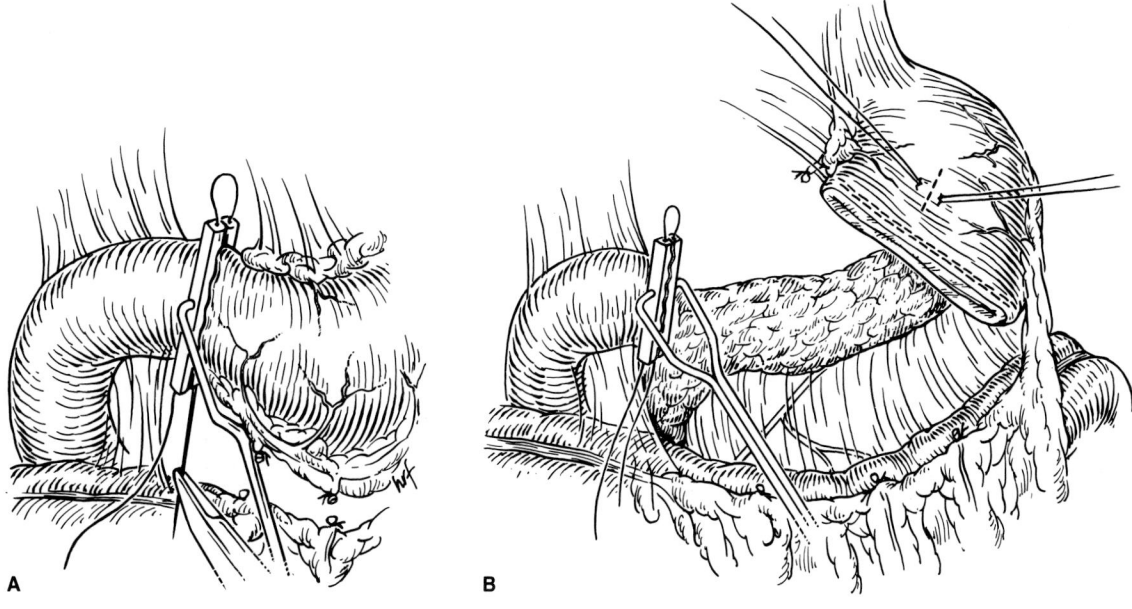

A   **B**

Figure 11-V-21

Gastroduodenal Anastomosis: Stapled Technique

(**A**) If a stapled technique is selected, a pursestring clamp is placed across the proximal duodenum. A 3-0 monofilament suture on a straight needle is passed through the clamp to create a pursestring. A double-armed suture is most convenient.

(**B**) The pylorus is transected proximal to the clamp. Two traction sutures are placed in the anterior wall of the gastric remnant in preparation for a longitudinal gastrotomy.

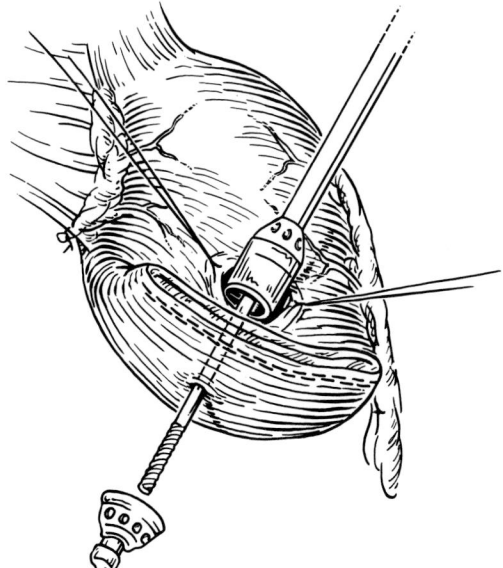

Figure 11-V-22

Placement of EEA Stapler

An EEA stapler is used to create the anastomosis. The instrument, without the anvil, is introduced into the stomach. At a point 3 cm proximal to the stapled gastric closure, the rod of the instrument is advanced through the posterior gastric wall. The anvil is reattached.

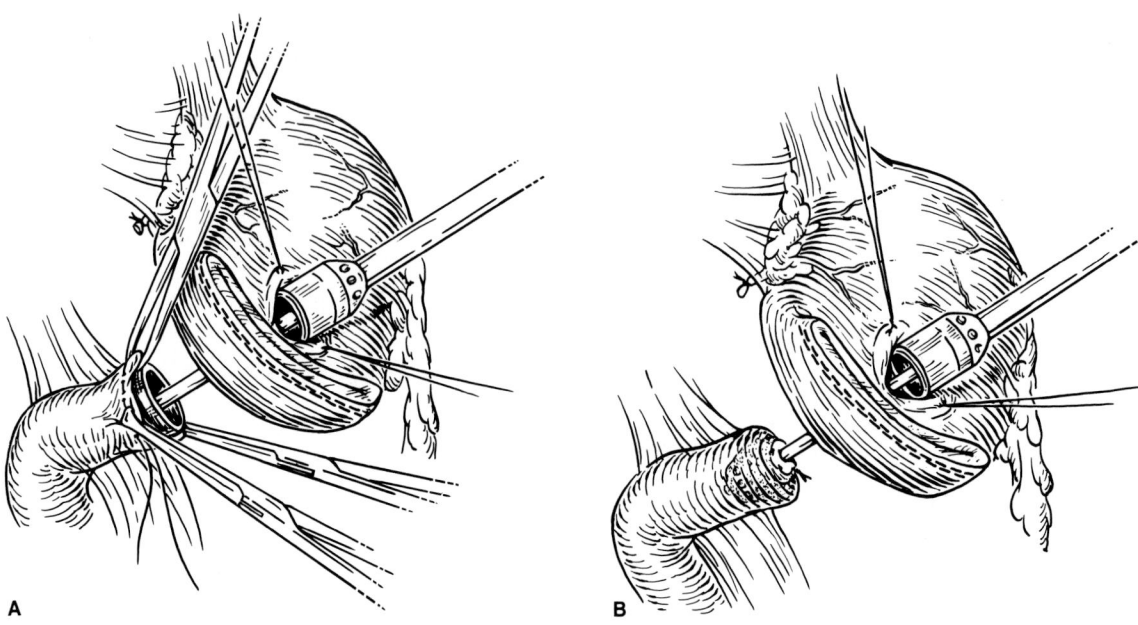

A   B

Figure 11-V-23

Duodenal Positioning

(**A**) The EEA anvil is passed into the proximal duodenum.

(**B**) The duodenal pursestring suture is tied.

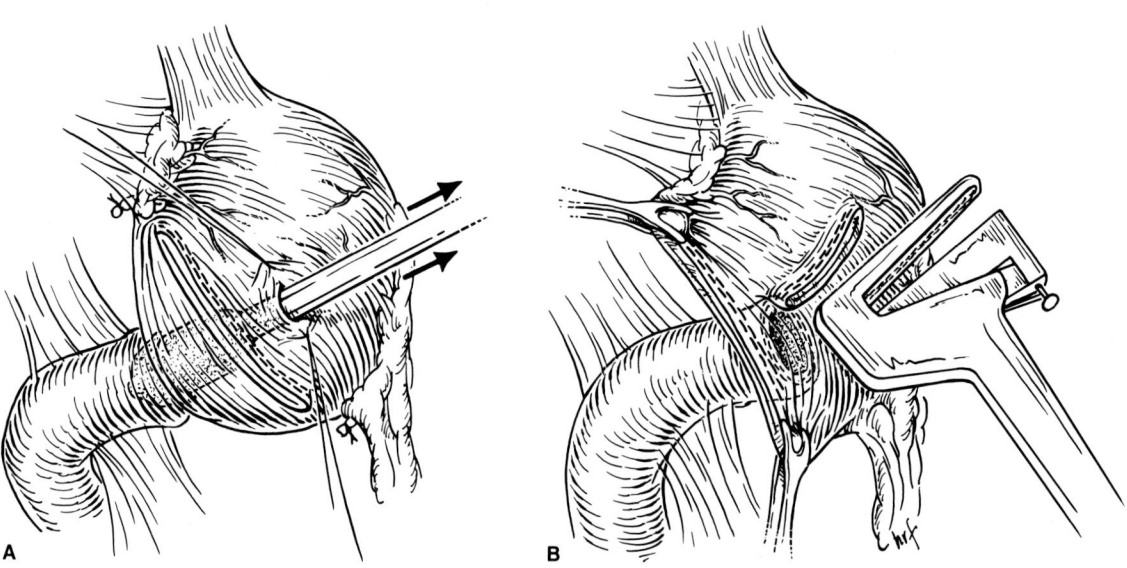

A   B

Figure 11-V-24

Creation of Anastomosis

(**A**) The EEA instrument is closed, fired, and gently withdrawn. The anastomosis is inspected for hemostasis.

(**B**) The anterior gastrotomy, created to introduce the EEA instrument, is closed by application of a TA-type stapler.

SECTION VI   *Total Gastrectomy*

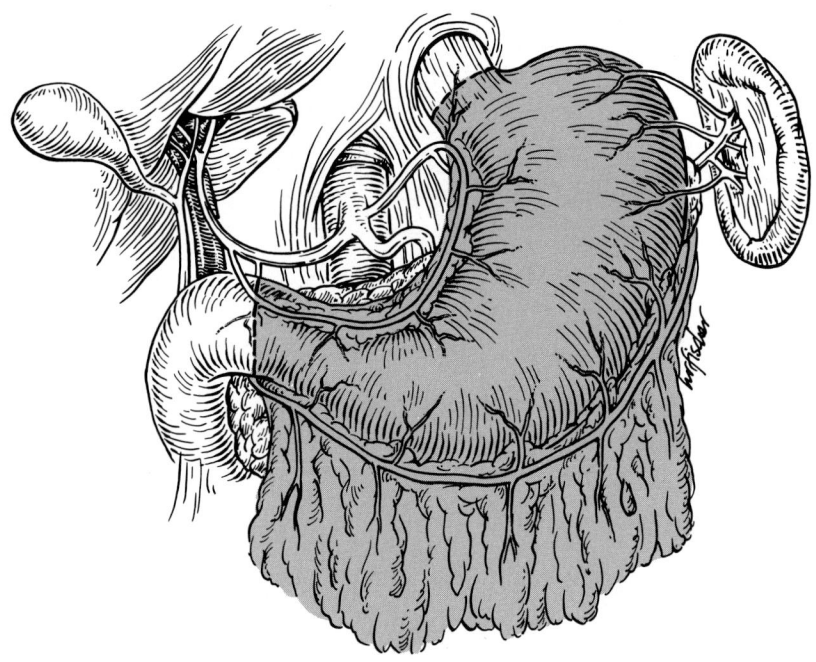

Figure 11-VI-1

Initial Dissection

The initial steps in total gastrectomy are similar to those outlined for partial gastrectomy. Total gastrectomy requires concomitant omentectomy.

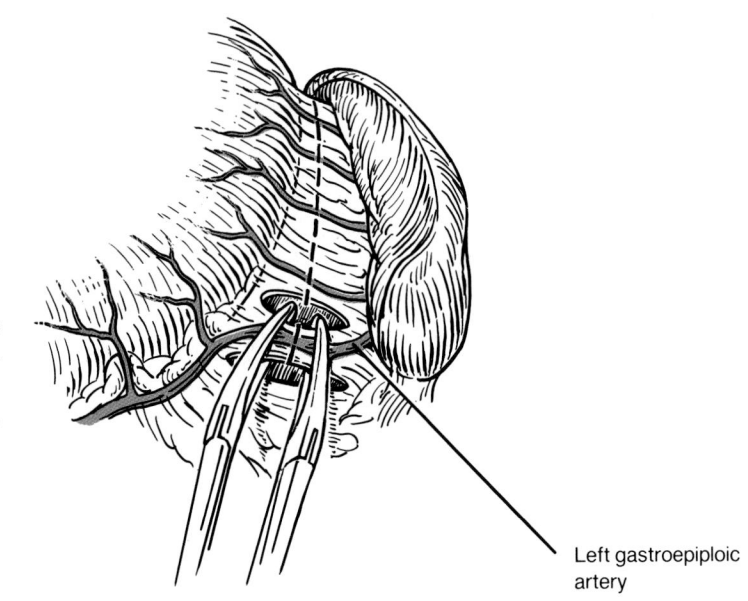

Figure 11-VI-2

Division of Short Gastric Vessels

When gastric neoplastic disease does not involve the adjacent spleen, dissection of the greater curvature should continue by division of the left gastroepiploic and short gastric vessels. The posterior fundus is often supplied by a retroperitoneal arterial branch. This vessel is found medial to the most superior short gastric artery and can be exposed by rotating the gastric fundus anteriorly and to the right.

Left gastroepiploic artery

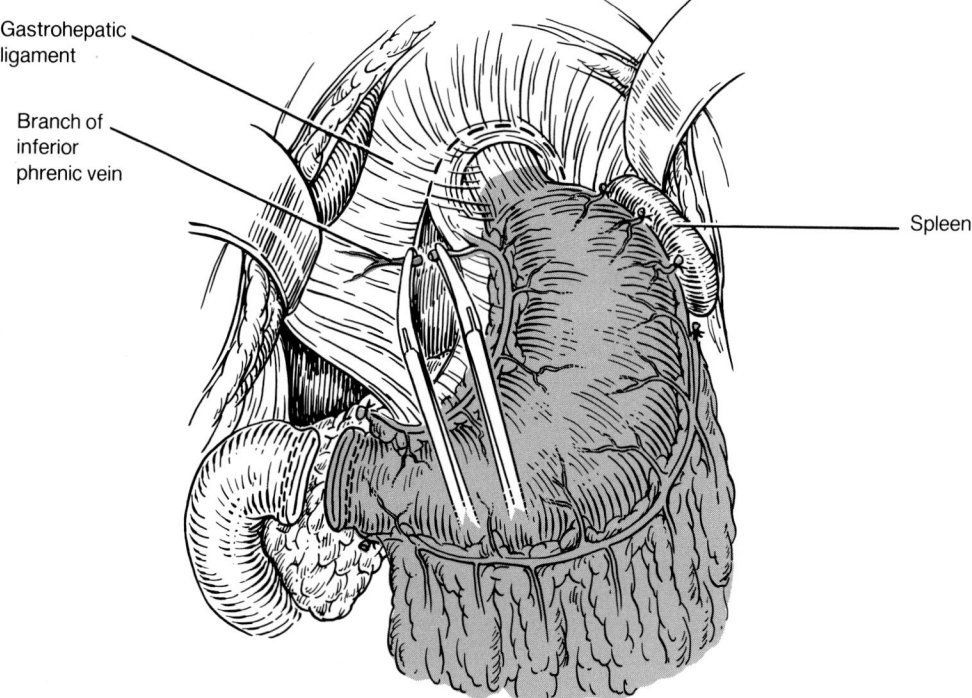

Gastrohepatic ligament

Branch of inferior phrenic vein

Spleen

Figure 11-VI-3

Division of Gastrohepatic Ligament

Division of the gastrohepatic ligament continues superiorly to the level of the esophageal hiatus. If neoplastic involvement requires a wide dissection, a branch of the inferior phrenic vein may be encountered and can be controlled with clamps. The dissection then continues by dividing the peritoneum overlying the esophagus transversely. Exposure can often be improved by encircling the esophagus with a Penrose drain and retracting anteriorly and to the left.

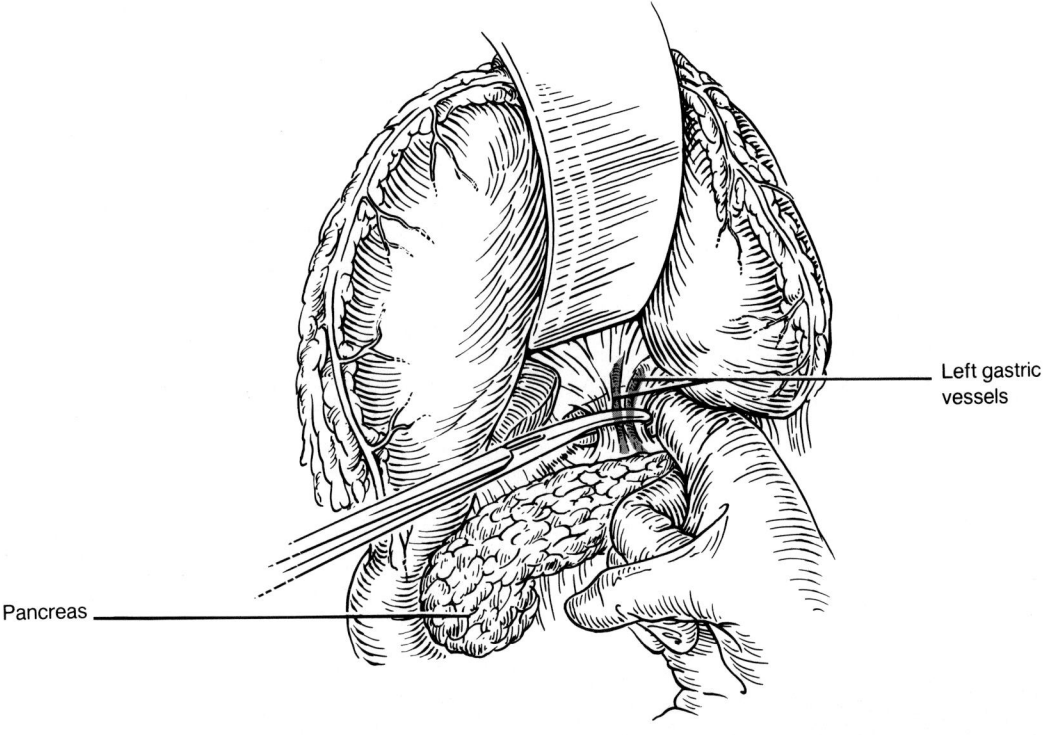

Left gastric vessels

Pancreas

Figure 11-VI-4

Division of Left Gastric Artery

Dissection of the left gastric artery and associated lymph nodes is best approached with the stomach reflected cephalad. The surgeon can encircle the vascular pedicle with a finger to guide dissection and placement of clamps. Care must be exercised that the nearby pancreas is not injured by retractors or inappropriately placed ligatures.

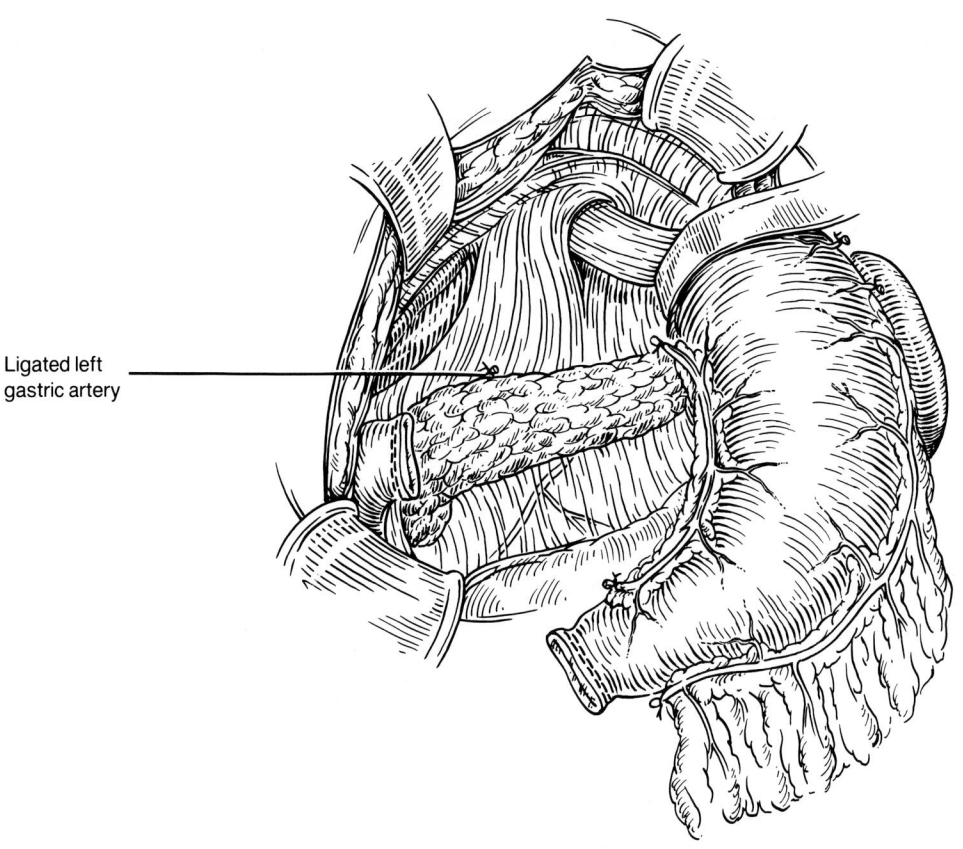

Ligated left
gastric artery

Figure 11-VI-5

Completed Dissection

With the stomach completely mobilized, the distal esophagus can be inspected; if additional length is required, mobilization from the posterior mediastinum can be performed.

Esophagus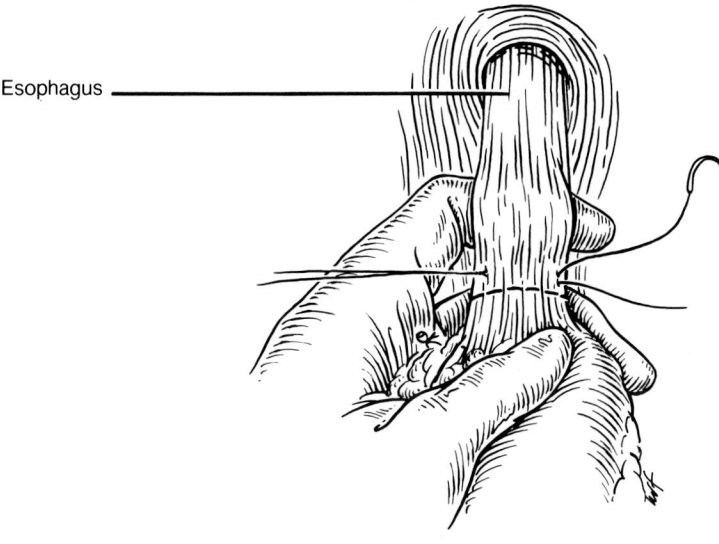

Figure 11-VI-6

Esophageal Division

Two stay sutures are placed in the esophagus laterally to prevent retraction, and the esophagus is transected.

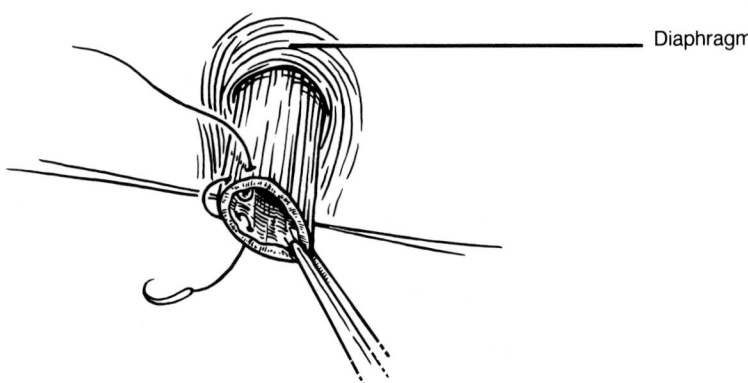 Diaphragm

Figure 11-VI-7

Pursestring Suture

In preparation for a stapled esophagojejunal anastomosis, a pursestring suture of 3-0 monofilament material is placed in the distal esophagus.

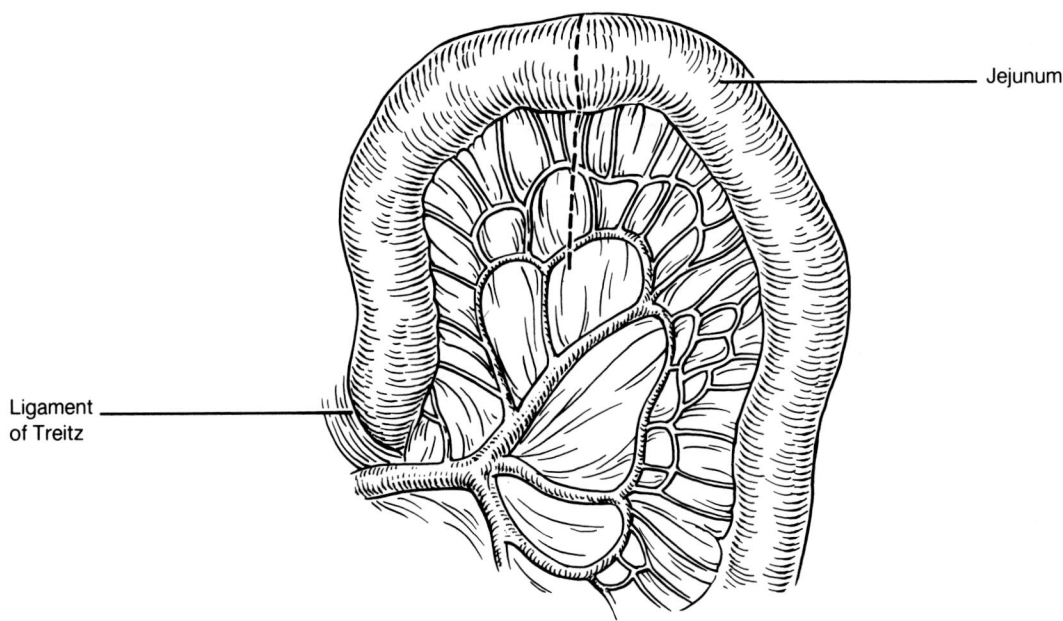

Jejunum

Ligament of Treitz

Figure 11-VI-8

Creation of Roux-en-Y Limb

The proximal jejunum is fanned out, and the vascular arcades are observed by transillumination. Two or more vascular arcades may need to be divided to provide a length of bowel to reach the esophagus without tension. The bowel is divided with a GIA stapler.

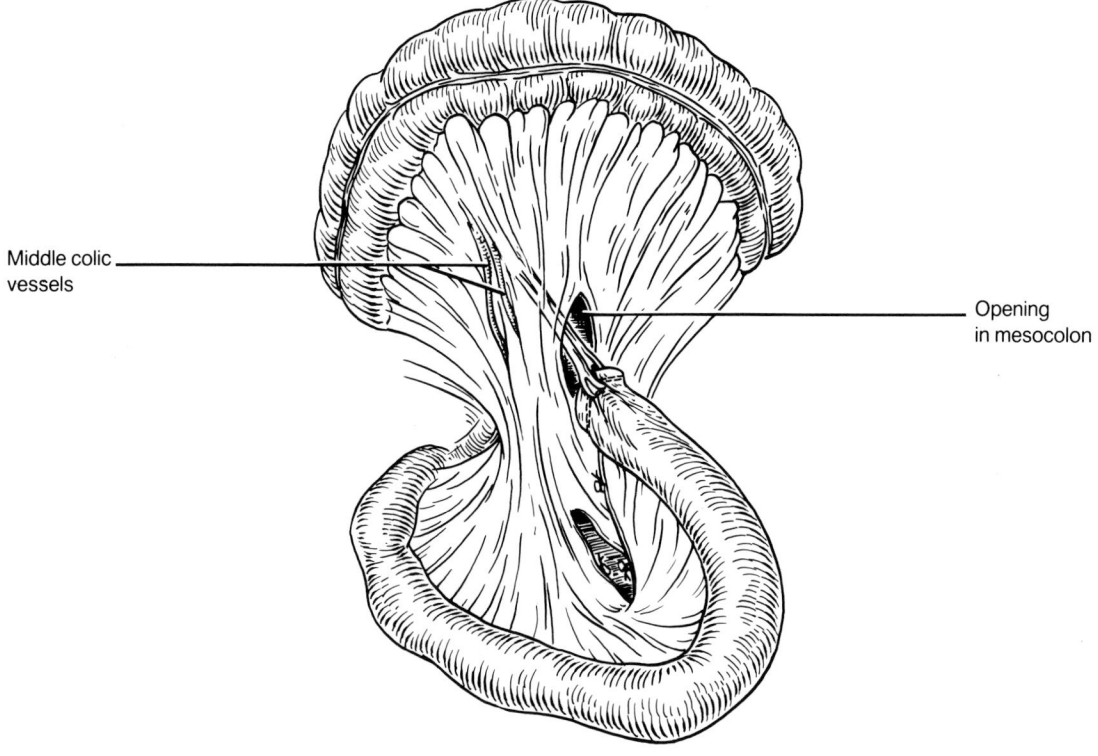

Middle colic vessels

Opening in mesocolon

Figure 11-VI-9

Retrocolic Passage of Roux Limb

An opening is made in the transverse mesentery to the left of the middle colic vessels and above the ligament of Treitz. The distal end of the transected jejunum is passed retrocolically to the area of the distal esophagus.

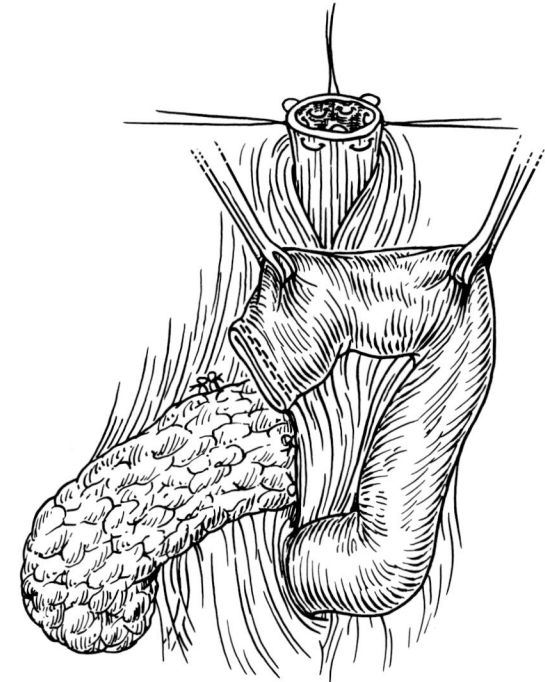

Figure 11-VI-10

Orientation of Jejunum

The jejunal limb must be approximated to the esophagus without angulation or tension. The stapled jejunal closure is excised to permit introduction of an EEA-type stapling device.

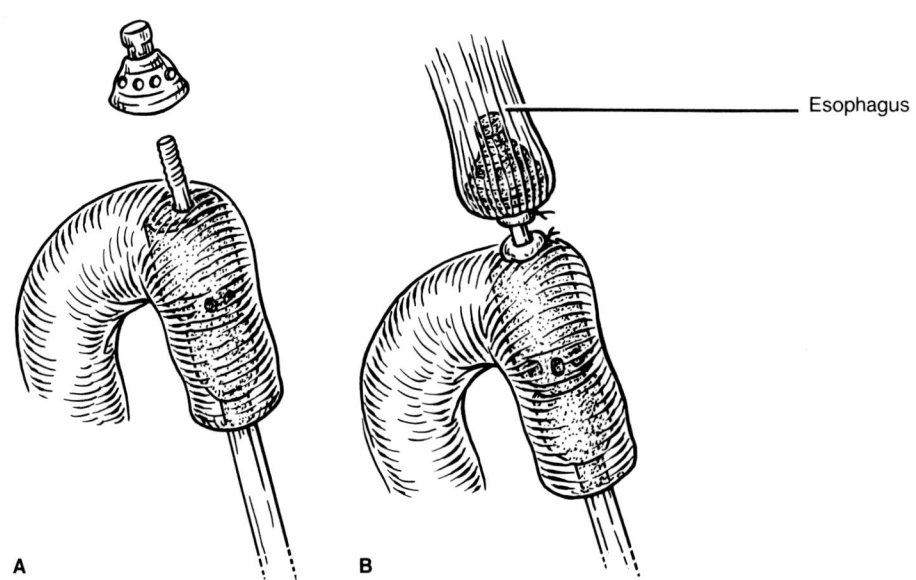

Esophagus

A   **B**

Figure 11-VI-11

EEA Anastomosis

(**A**) An EEA stapling device, without anvil, is introduced through the open end of the Roux-en-Y limb and positioned so that the post exits the antimesenteric border of the jejunum 3 to 4 cm distally. The anvil is reattached.

(**B**) The anvil is inserted into the distal esophagus, and the previously placed esophageal pursestring suture is tied. The EEA device is fired, creating an end-to-side esophagojejunal anastomosis. The EEA is opened, and the contained rings of tissue are inspected. A complete and uninterrupted ring of esophageal tissue must be present to ensure a leak-free anastomosis.

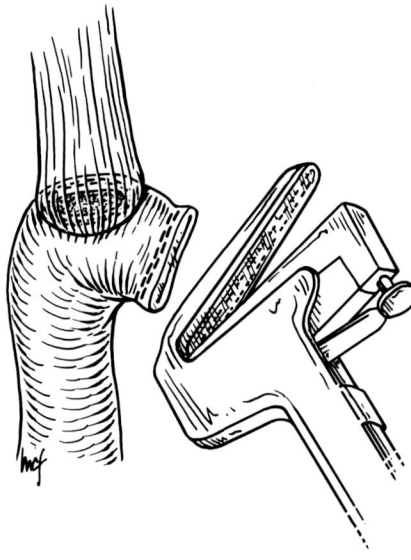

Figure 11-VI-12

Completion of Anastomosis

After withdrawal of the EEA stapler, the open end of the jejunal limb is closed with a TA stapler. With the surgeon's guidance, a nasogastric tube is placed across the anastomosis. Integrity of the anastomosis is ensured by watching for bubbles in the saline-filled operative field as air is insufflated through the nasogastric tube with the jejunum manually occluded distally.

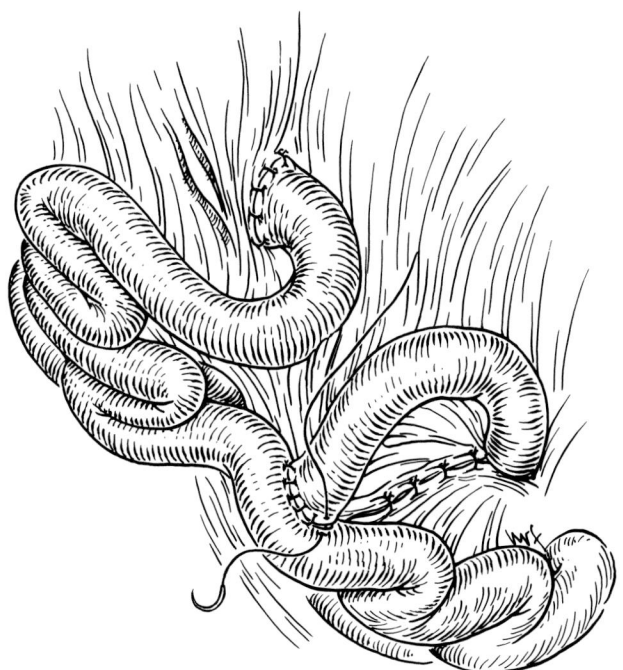

Figure 11-VI-13

Roux-en-Y Reconstruction

Intestinal continuity is restored by an end-to-side enteroenterostomy 40 cm distal to the esophagojejunal anastomosis. The transverse mesentery is approximated to the jejunal limb with interrupted sutures. The mesenteric defect created by division of the vascular arcades is closed to prevent internal herniation. A feeding jejunostomy is a useful adjunct.

SECTION VII   Gastrostomy

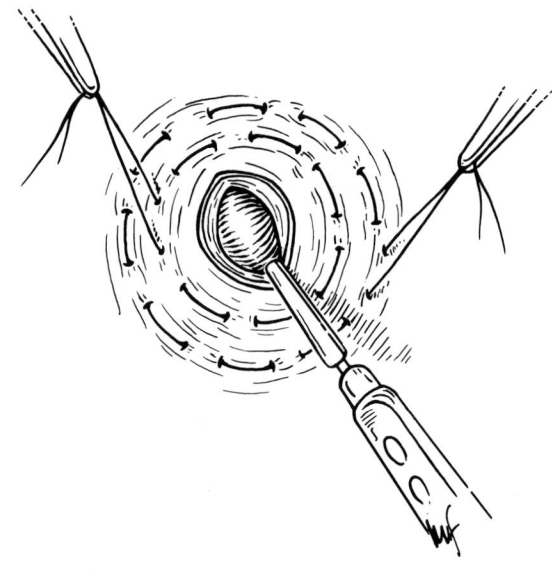

Figure 11-VII-1

Stamm Gastrostomy

Open gastrostomy can be performed in conjunction with laparotomy for other intraabdominal pathology or as a separate procedure. The gastric corpus is delivered to the operative field. Two concentric 2-0 or 3-0 nonabsorbable pursestring sutures are placed, and a small full-thickness gastric wound is created using electrocautery.

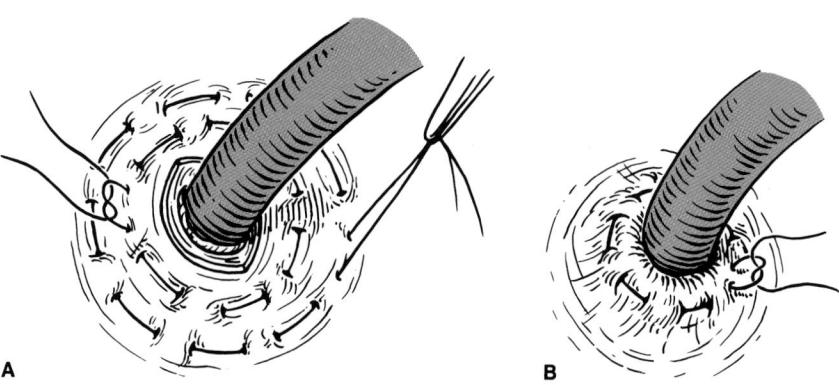

A   B

Figure 11-VII-2

Tube Placement

(**A**) A large (20F) mushroom-tipped catheter is placed, and the inner suture is tied.

(**B**) The gastrostomy tube is pushed inward as the second suture is tied, creating an inverted valve of gastric wall.

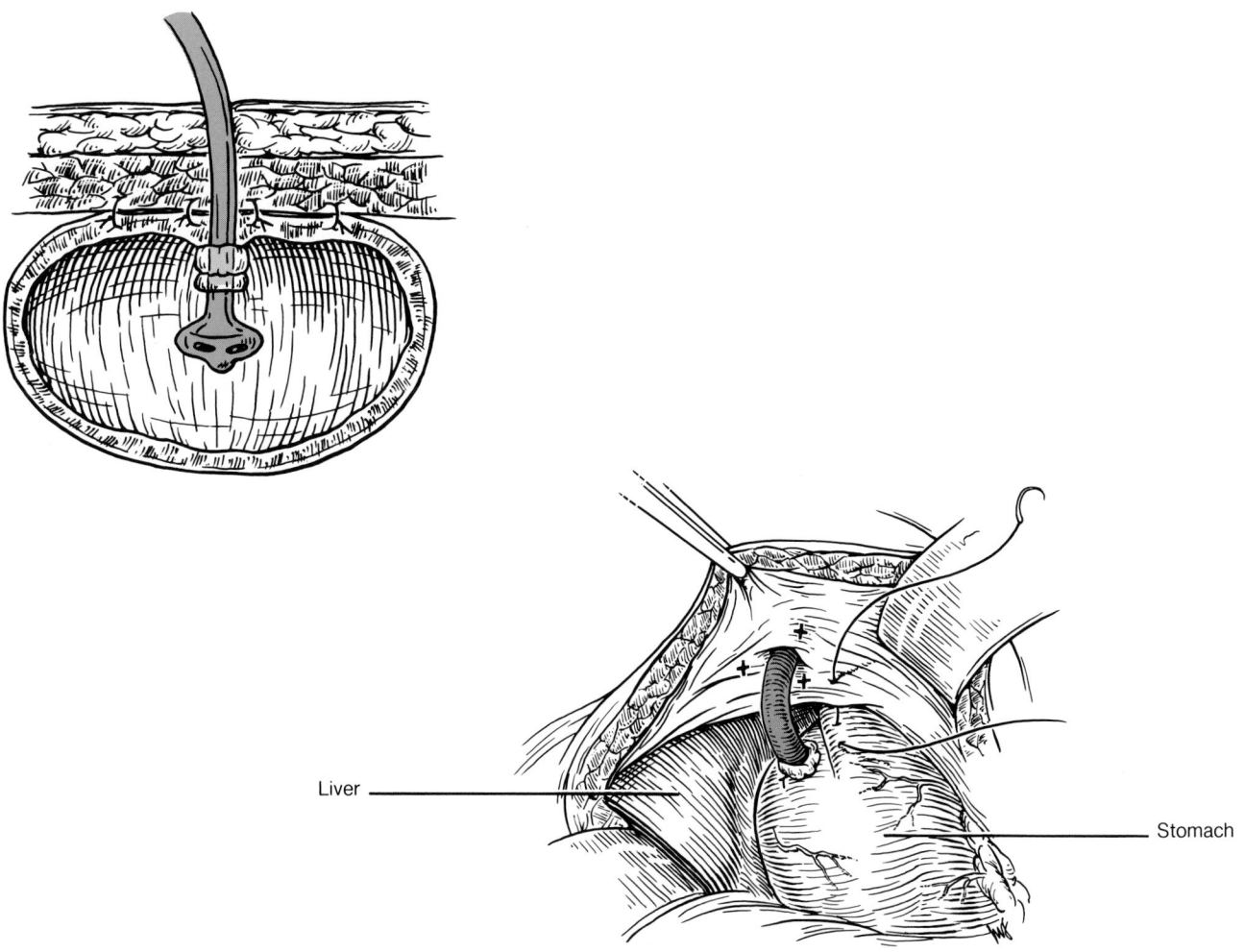

Figure 11-VII-3

Anchoring Sutures

Sutures passed through the parietal peritoneum and the seromuscular surface of the stomach are used to anchor the stomach to the anterior abdominal wall. The stomach must reach the anterior peritoneum without tension for a secure seal.

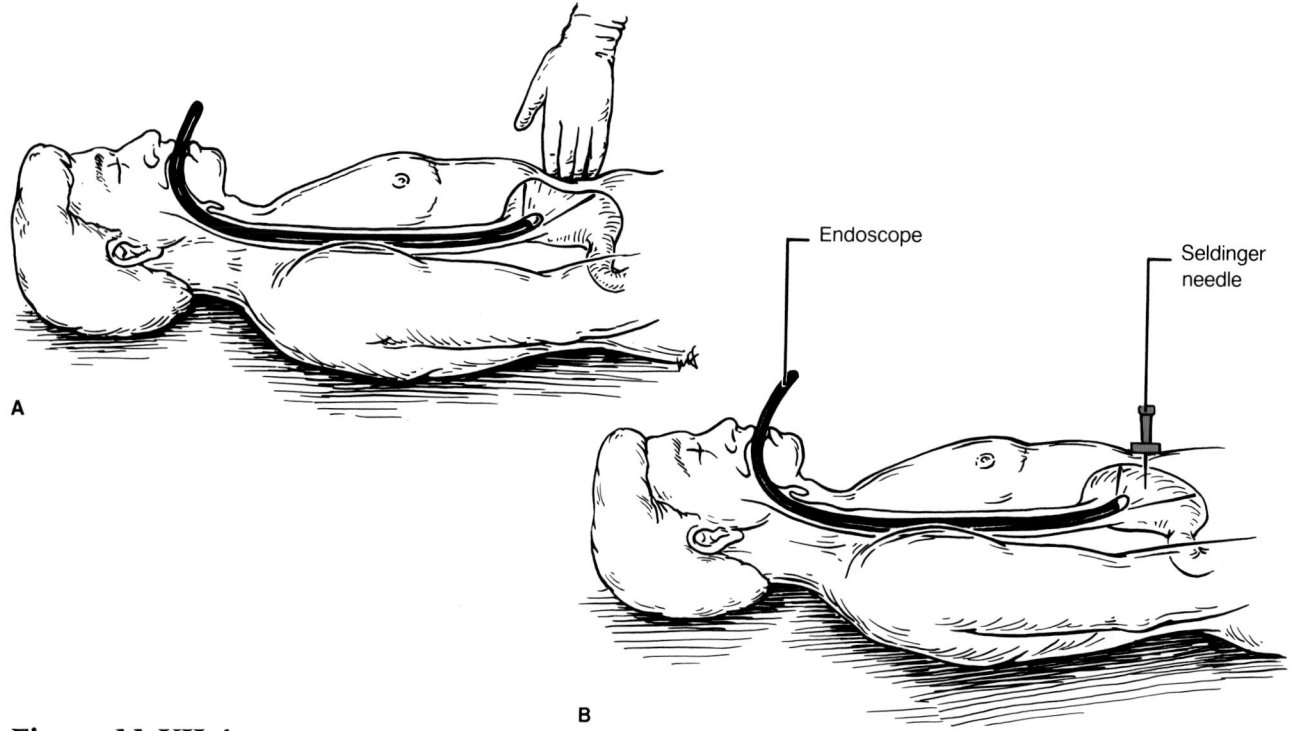

A

B

Endoscope

Seldinger needle

Figure 11-VII-4

Percutaneous Endoscopic Gastrostomy

Percutaneous endoscopic gastrostomy is performed under intravenous sedation, with local anesthetic supplementation for the pharynx and abdominal wall. The procedure is contraindicated in the presence of oral obstruction, as with large oral cancers. Prior abdominal operation does not automatically exclude percutaneous endoscopic gastrostomy, although adhesions can limit mobility of the stomach and thereby prevent its apposition to the anterior abdominal wall, an absolute requirement for the procedure.

(**A**) With the patient supine, the gastroscope is introduced and the stomach is distended by insufflation of air. The endoscopic view is directed toward the anterior gastric wall in the mid-body of the stomach. An assistant presses lightly in the left upper quadrant. If the stomach is properly distended and contacts the anterior abdominal wall freely without interposition of other structures, a clear imprint of the finger should be visible endoscopically.

(**B**) Under direct vision, a Seldinger needle is passed into the stomach.

(**C**) Through this introducer needle, a flexible guide wire is passed into the stomach. An endoscopic polypectomy snare is passed through the endoscope and is used to grasp the flexible guide wire.

(**D**) The endoscope is withdrawn with the snare grasping the guide wire. After removal of the gastroscope, the flexible guide wire exits the mouth and the left upper quadrant abdominal wall.

(**E**) The narrowly tapered end of the gastrostomy tube is passed over the guide wire until this end appears at the level of the abdominal skin. The gastrostomy tube is grasped and "pulled" through the esophagus and into position. The motion of the tube is arrested when the flanged gastric end of the tube brings the gastric wall into contact with the undersurface of the abdominal peritoneum. The guide wire is removed.

(**F**) A retention disk or bar is applied externally to prevent retraction of the gastrostomy tube, the appliance is trimmed to an appropriate length, and a cap is provided. Gastroscopy is repeated to ensure that the tube is properly positioned and that no mucosal injury has occurred.

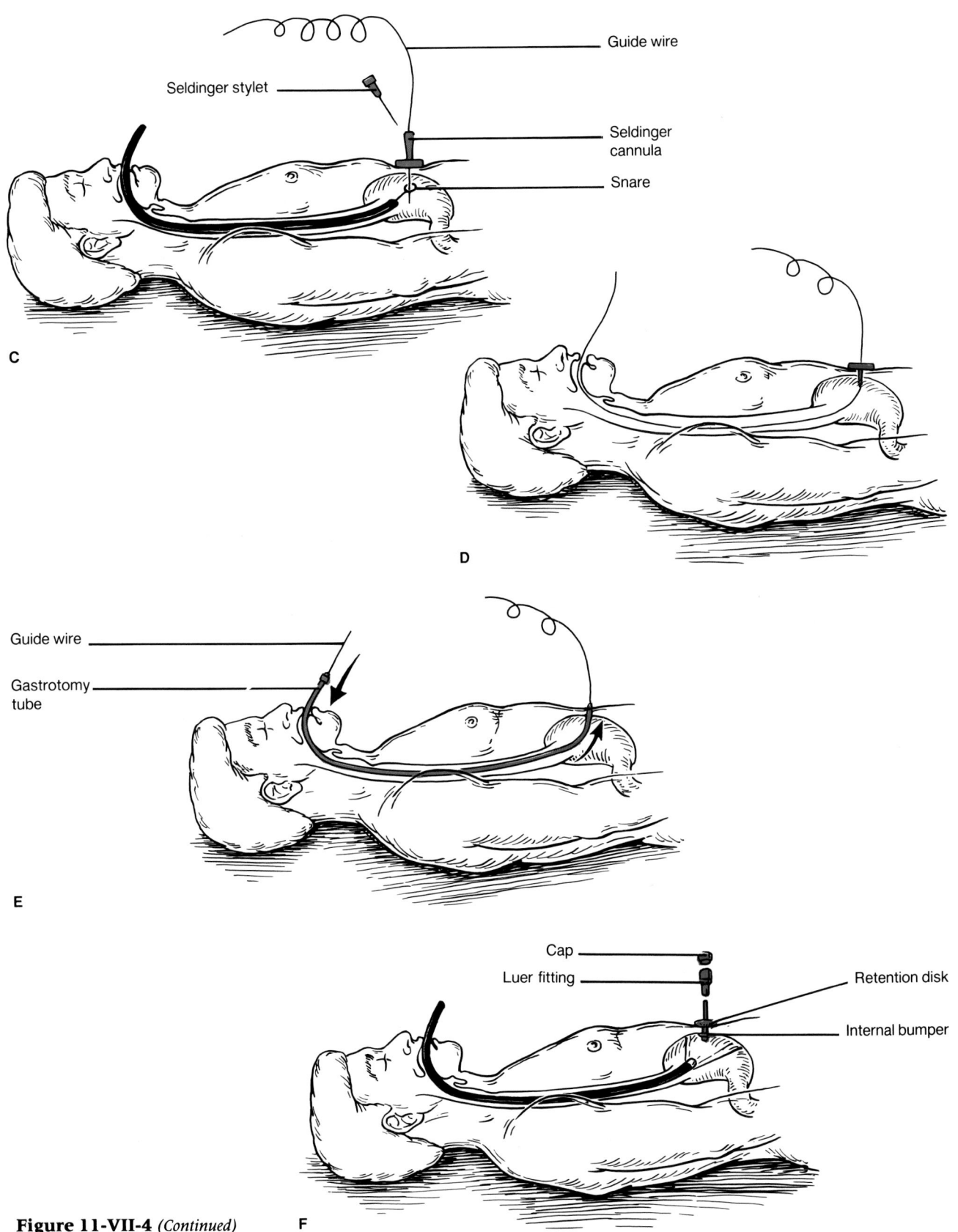

Figure 11-VII-4 *(Continued)*

SECTION VIII *Gastric Bypass and Gastroplasty*

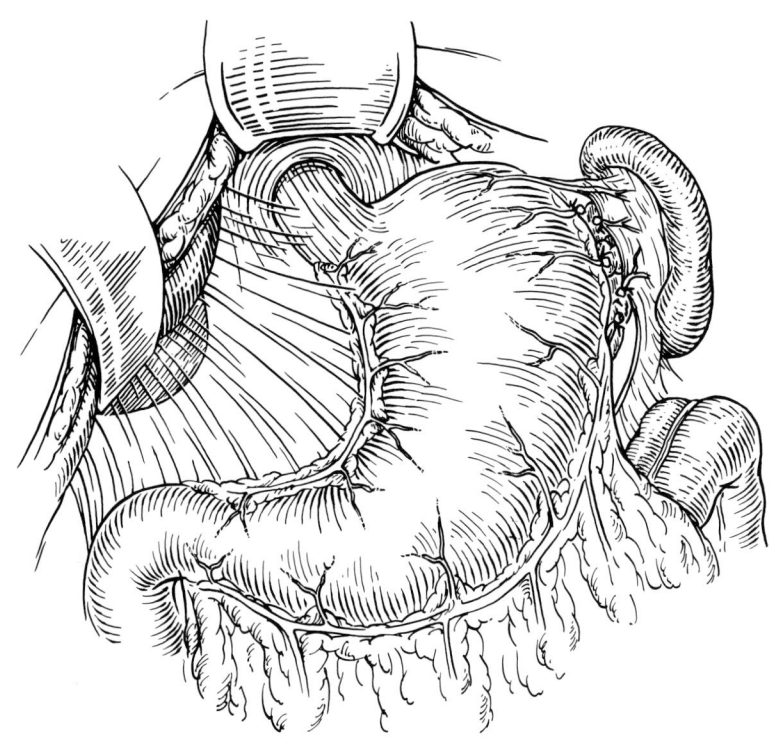

Figure 11-VIII-1

Gastric Bypass

Gastric bypass is performed through a vertical upper abdominal incision. Self-retaining retractors are used to provide exposure. The short gastric vessels are ligated and divided to mobilize the gastric fundus.

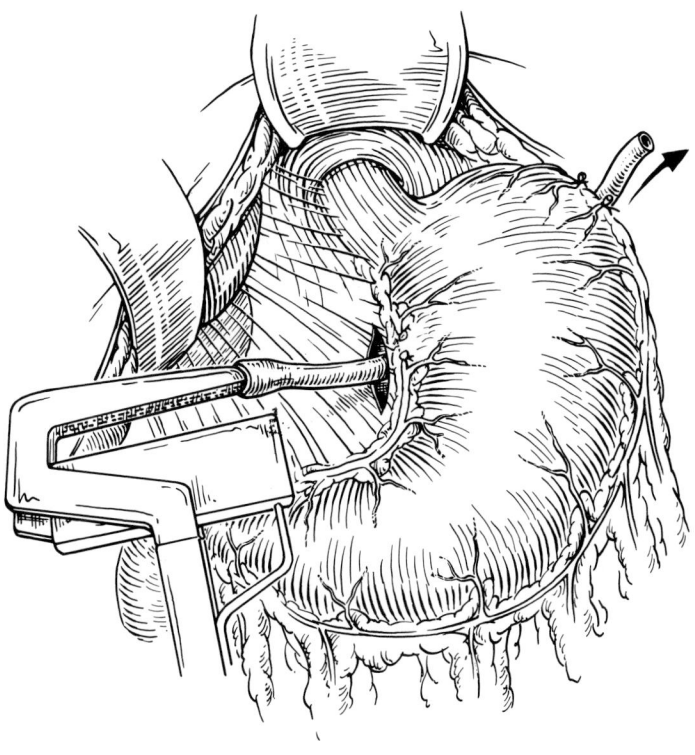

Figure 11-VIII-2

Stapler Positioning

A window in the gastrocolic omentum is created immediately adjacent to the lesser curvature. The dissection should be close to the gastric wall so that the nerves of Latarjet are not injured. One branch of the left gastric artery to the proximal stomach must be preserved superior to the area of dissection. A soft catheter is passed through the window, behind the stomach, to exit at the greater curvature. A TA-90 stapler is inserted into the end of the catheter to ensure atraumatic passage behind the proximal stomach.

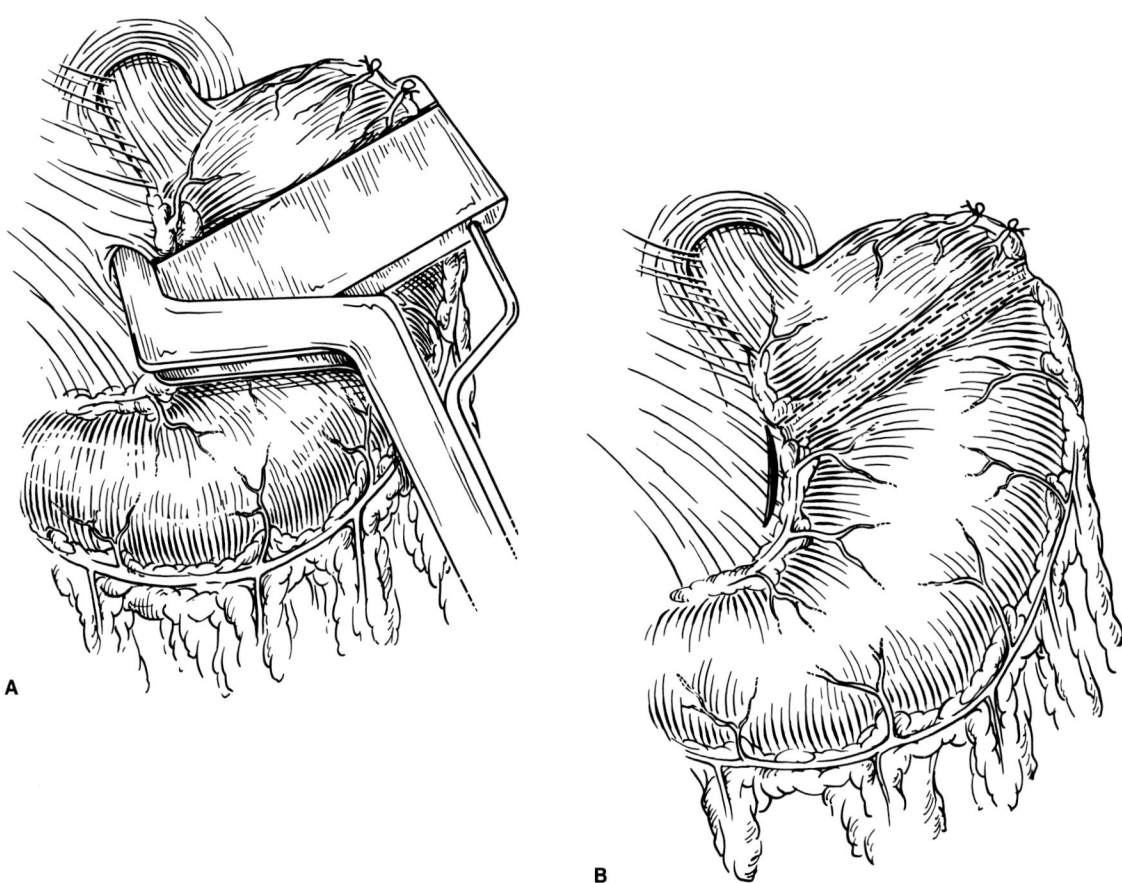

Figure 11-VIII-3

Stapler Application

(**A**) The stapler is positioned to achieve a proximal gastric pouch volume of 50 to 60 mL. The TA stapler is fired, reloaded, and repositioned within 5 mm of the first staple line.

(**B**) A second firing of the stapler provides a partition of four staggered rows of staples.

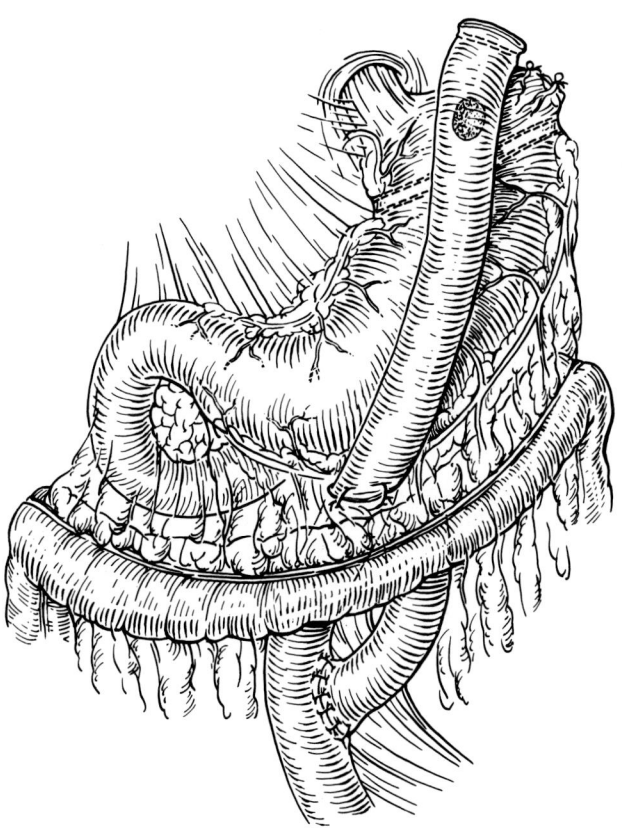

Figure 11-VIII-4

Gastrojejunostomy

A retrocolic Roux-en-Y limb 40 cm long is constructed as outlined in Section VI. Gastro-intestinal continuity is restored by construction of a two-layer gastrojejunostomy. The inner diameter of the anastomosis should be 10 mm to prevent rapid emptying of the gastric pouch.

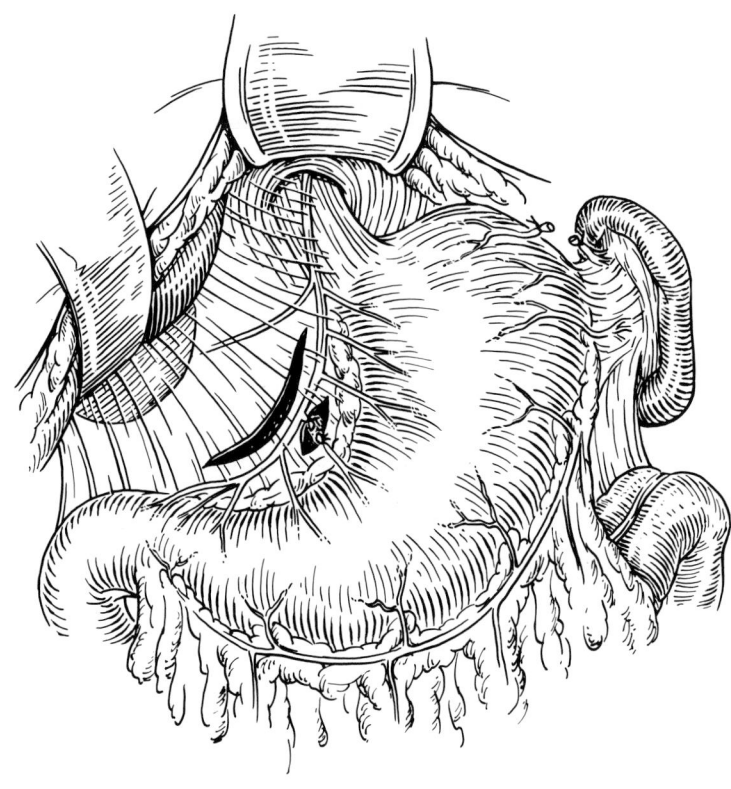

Figure 11-VIII-5

Vertical Banded Gastroplasty

The upper aspect of the greater curvature is mobilized for a distance of 7.5 to 10 cm by division of the uppermost short gastric vessels. An incision is made in the gastrohepatic ligament to gain access to the retrogastric space. Care must be taken not to injure the vagal divisions contained within this layer. A small window is created along the lesser curvature midway between the esophagogastric junction and the pylorus.

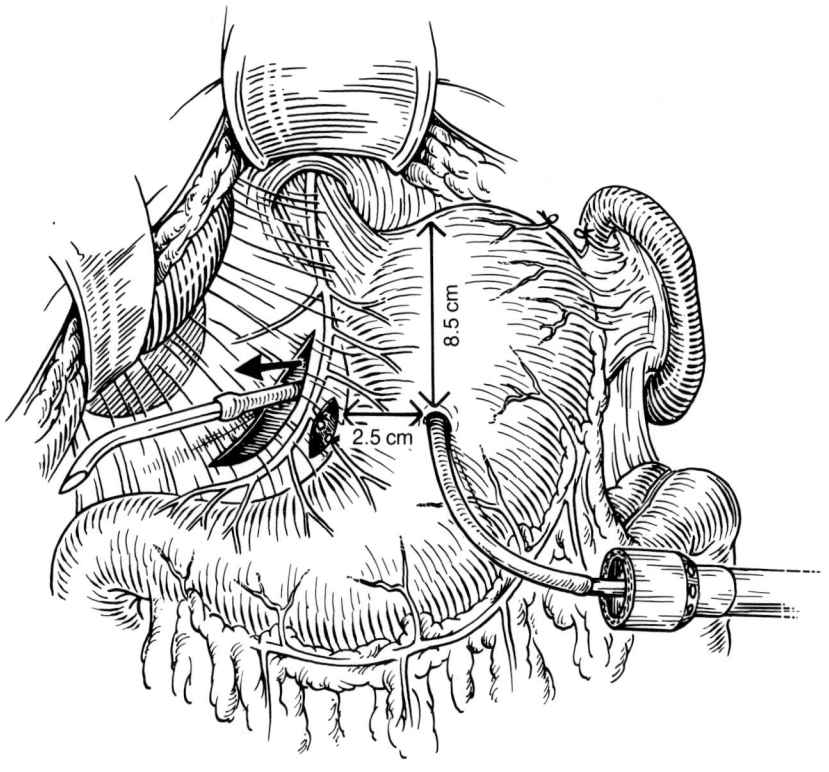

Figure 11-VIII-6

Transgastric Passage of EEA Stapler

A trocar is used to pierce the anterior and posterior walls of the stomach. The point of entry is 8 cm distal to the angle of His along the lesser curvature and 2.5 cm from the lesser curvature. The trocar is connected, by means of a soft catheter, to a 24-mm EEA stapler.

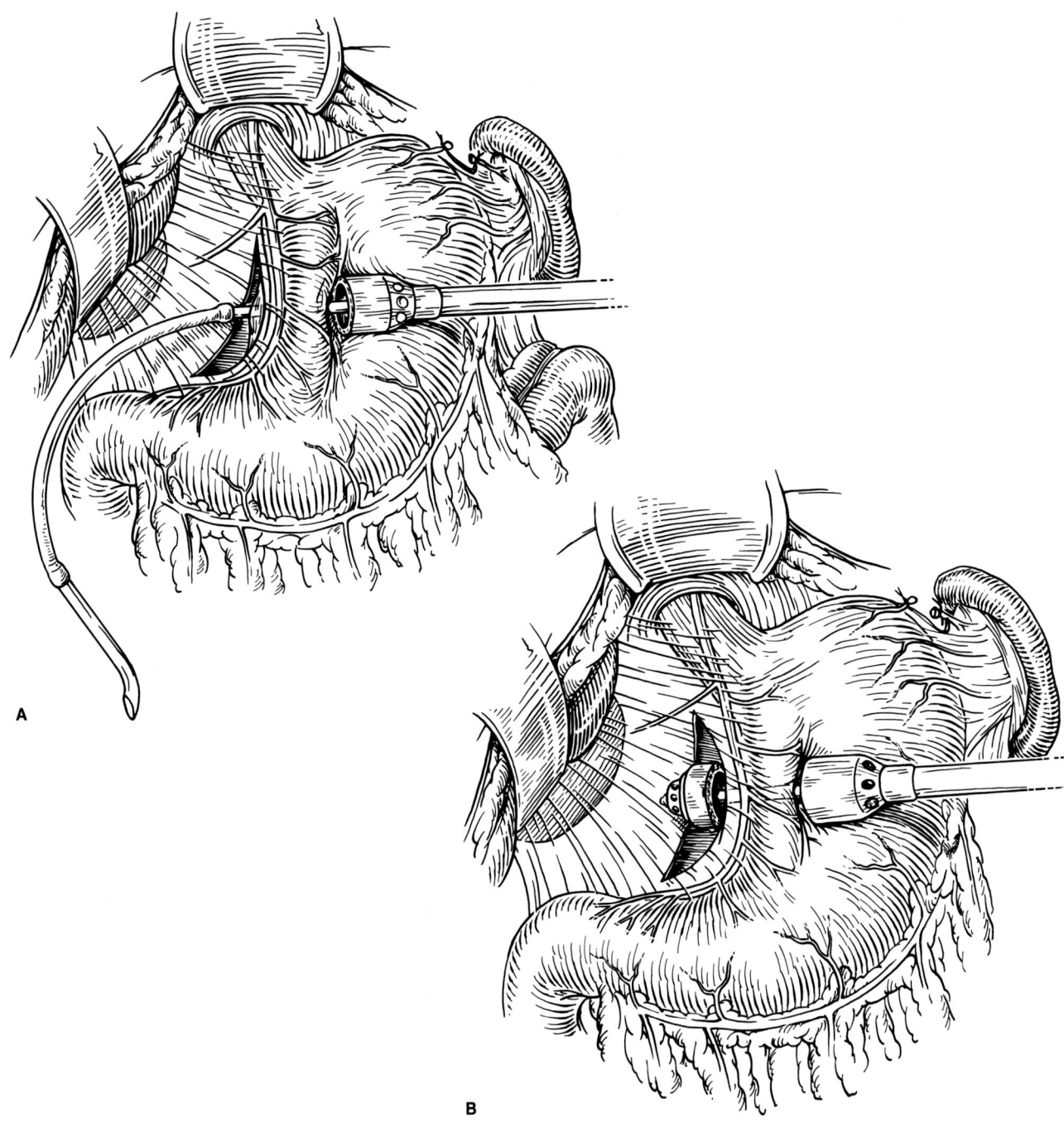

Figure 11-VIII-7

Positioning of EEA Stapler

(**A**) An alternative method for positioning the EEA stapler is to pass a 32F esophageal dilator into the stomach. The dilator is held along the lesser curvature, and the trocar is passed through both gastric walls laterally. Care must be taken not to injure the pancreas or vagal nerves in the passage of the trocar.

(**B**) The trocar is removed, and the 24-mm anvil is attached to the stapler. Firing the stapler creates a circular aperture in the mid-stomach.

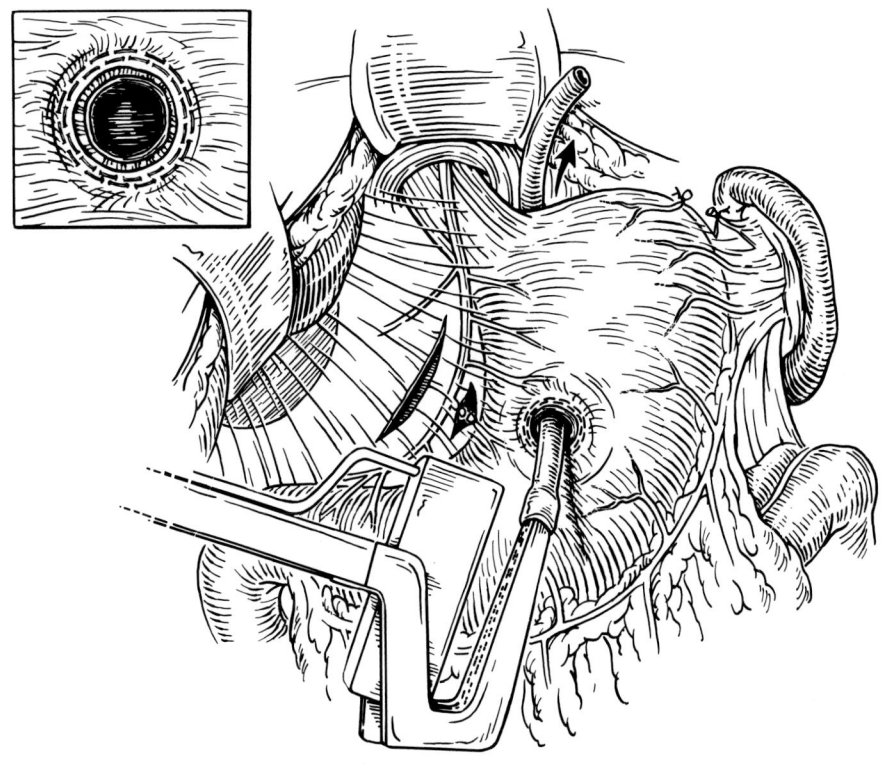

Figure 11-VIII-8

Passage of TA Stapler

A soft catheter is used to pass one jaw of a TA-90 stapler through the EEA-created hole and into position paralleling the lesser curvature of the stomach.

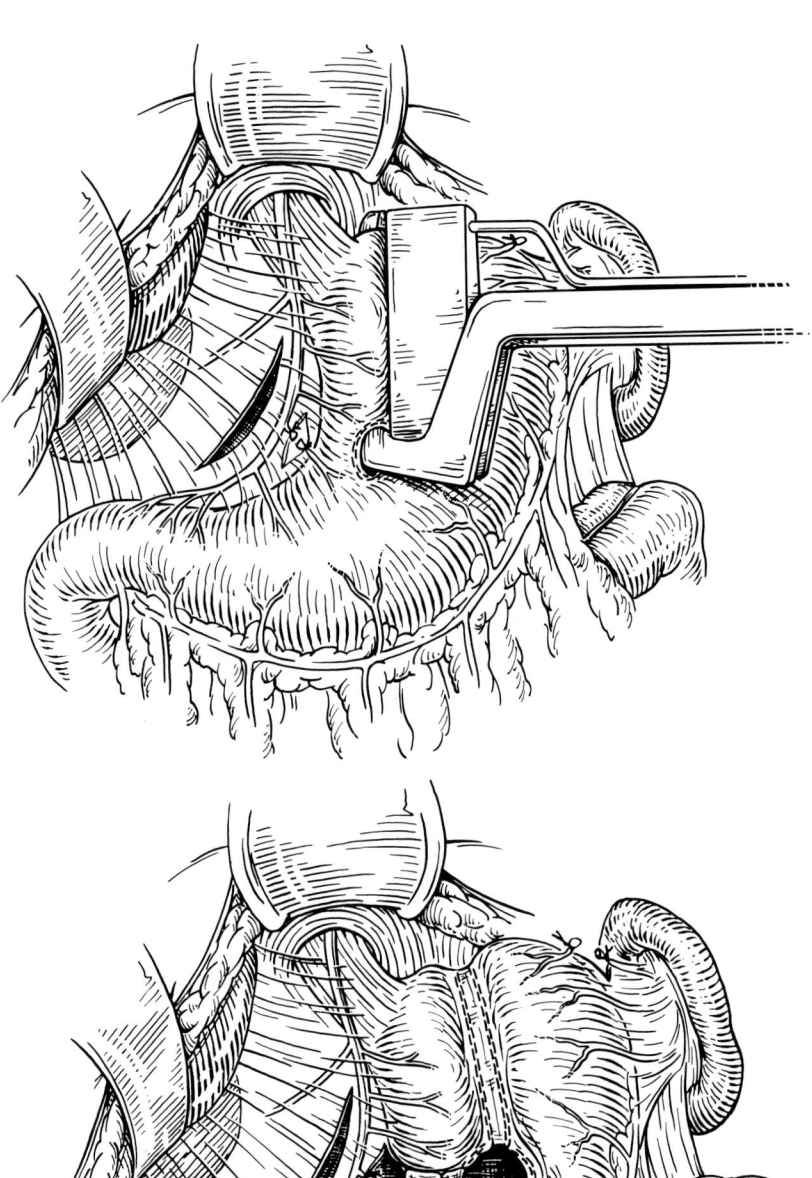

Figure 11-VIII-9

Creation of Gastric Partition

The stapler is fired twice, creating a partition of four rows of staples.

Figure 11-VIII-10

Pouch Outlet Band

A 32F esophageal dilator is positioned to ensure that the gastric pouch outlet is 1.2 cm in diameter. A band of Marlex 1.5 cm in diameter is wrapped around the outlet and sutured to itself.

PART III
Biliary System

Digestive Tract Surgery: A Text and Atlas, edited by Richard H. Bell, Layton F. Rikkers, and Michael W. Mulholland. Lippincott-Raven Publishers, Philadelphia, © 1996.

12

Calculous Gallbladder Disease

Joel J. Roslyn | *Kim U. Kahng*

Calculous disease of the gallbladder continues to be one of the more common maladies afflicting humanity. The first recognized case of cholelithiasis was reported more than 1500 years ago. Over the centuries, the clinical management of gallstone disease has been influenced by our evolving understanding of the pathogenesis of gallstones (Table 12-1). In the Middle Ages, it was not uncommon for the affluent aristocracy suffering from biliary colic to be referred by the local alchemists to spas whose waters were rich in magnesium sulfate.[1] Although perhaps not appreciated at the time, magnesium sulfate is a potent stimulant of gallbladder contraction and emptying. Given that altered gallbladder motor activity with consequent stasis is critical to the formation of gallstones,[2] this ancient remedy may well have had a pathophysiologic basis. In the late 1800s, cholecystostomy was considered to be the treatment of choice for patients with symptomatic gallstone disease.[3] The current era for the treatment of gallstones was heralded in 1882 by Carl Langenbuch when he performed the first successful cholecystectomy.[4] For the past 100 years, open cholecystectomy has remained the gold standard for the management of gallstone disease. In recent years, considerable attention has been focused on the development of nonoperative or minimally invasive techniques for the management of symptomatic cholelithiasis. The oral dissolution of gallstones, which for many years remained merely a dream, has become a reality. Unfortunately, the efficacy of these drugs has been disappointing, and their clinical utility is limited. Biliary lithotripsy appears to be safe and effective in carefully selected patients. The reported high rate of stone recurrence, however, has curtailed the broad application of this technology. Similarly, recurrent stone formation, as well as complica-tions of catheter placement, has diminished the enthusiasm for the percutaneous intraluminal instillation of contact dissolution agents, such as methyl tert-butyl ether (MTBE).

The introduction and development of laparoscopic techniques have revolutionized the operative treatment of gallstone disease. In many parts of the world, laparoscopic cholecystectomy has become the preferred treatment for patients with symptomatic gallstone disease. Since the initial reports of laparoscopic cholecystectomy,[5,6] the literature has become replete with numerous series detailing the efficacy and benefits of this procedure. Although some concerns linger about the ultimate cost, the incidence of bile duct injury, and appropriate credentialing mechanisms, laparoscopic cholecystectomy is emerging as the new standard of care.

GALLSTONE CLASSIFICATION

Gallstones are classified based on composition, location, and site of origin. Insights into the various etiologies of the heterogeneous array of disorders that are grouped as gallstone disease and into the differing factors responsible for the formation of these stones provide a rational basis for the selection of appropriate therapeutic strategies.

Gallstone Composition

Gallstones are found within the gallbladder, extrahepatic biliary tract, or intrahepatic ductal system. Most Western patients have gallbladder stones, whereas intrahepatic stone disease is endemic to parts of Southeast Asia. Despite the wide variance in color, size, shape,

383

**Table 12-1   Status of Cholecystectomy:
Historical Perspective**

Year	Status
1700s	Drinking waters rich in magnesium sulfate
1867	Cholecystolithotomy—Bobbs
1882	Cholecystectomy—Langenbuch
1937	Oral dissolution—Rewbridge
1972	Chenodeoxycholic acid—Danzinger
1986	Electrohydraulic shock-wave lithotripsy—Paumgartner, Sauerbruch
1987	Contact dissolution—Thistle
1988	Laparoscopic cholecystectomy

and configuration of gallbladder stones, these calculi are often simplistically grouped as either cholesterol or pigment stones. Pure cholesterol gallstones are actually uncommon, and most patients in the United States have mixed gallstones. These calculi often contain small amounts of calcium salts, bile pigments, bile acids, proteins, and lipids in addition to cholesterol. In the United States, patients with cholesterol and mixed gallstones account for about 60% to 70% of all patients with gallstones. The critical step in the formation of cholesterol and mixed gallstones is the failure to maintain biliary cholesterol in solution. It has become apparent that the pathogenesis of cholesterol gallstones is multifactorial. Depending on the clinical situation, numerous etiologic factors may be present in varying degrees and act in concert to promote the hepatic secretion of cholesterol-saturated bile, gallbladder stasis, and altered gallbladder absorptive and secretory function. The presence of cholesterol-saturated bile and increased amounts of mucus in a poorly emptying gallbladder provides an excellent milieu for nucleation and stone growth.

The term *pigment gallstone disease* refers to a heterogeneous group of conditions with various etiologies characterized by formation of gallstones containing high concentrations of bilirubin and low amounts of cholesterol (less than 10%). Although some of these stones are composed purely of pigments, most contain significant amounts of calcium bilirubinate. *Black pigment gallstones* are typically tarry in appearance and form exclusively in the gallbladder. They are common in patients with cirrhosis or hemolytic disorders. *Brown pigment gallstones* are soft, earthy, and easily crushable. These stones form in association with endemic biliary infections.

Location and Site of Origin

In the United States and most other parts of the world, most patients with calculous disease have gallstones within the gallbladder. These stones can be either cho-

lesterol, mixed, or pigment. Common bile duct stones are generally classified as either primary (those formed de novo in the common bile duct) or secondary (those that arise in the gallbladder and pass through the cystic duct into the choledochus). Although some authors have suggested otherwise,[7,8] most epidemiologic evidence suggests that most common bile duct stones are of gallbladder origin.[9-11] Most ductal stones that are proved to be cholesterol calculi are formed in the gallbladder. Calcium bilirubinate or pigment stones can form anywhere in the biliary tract and therefore constitute the largest fraction of primary common bile duct stones. Several factors are important in the pathogenesis of primary ductal stones, including biliary bacterial infection and stasis of bile. Whereas intrahepatic stones are uncommon in Western countries, the incidence of hepatolithiasis is high in Southeast Asia. The clinical features of this entity are discussed in greater detail in Chapter 13.

EPIDEMIOLOGY

Incidence

The incidence of biliary calculous disease varies widely throughout the world. In the United States, about 10% of the population have gallstones, and a million new cases are diagnosed each year. Autopsy series performed in the United States suggest that gallstones are present in at least 20% of women and in 8% of men older than 40 years of age. Similar findings were reported in a population-based study that examined the incidence of gallstones in Hispanics residing in the United States.[12] In Europe, the incidence of gallstones ranges from 8.4% to 33.7% in women and from 5% to 13.1% in men.[13-15] Gallstones are even more common in parts of Asia, although these are primarily pigment stones. The incidence of cholesterol gallstones in Pima Indians, a tribe living in the southwest part of the United States, has been well characterized. In this group, the incidence of gallstones in women between the ages of 25 and 34 years is over 70%.[16] In contrast, the incidence of gallstones is reported to be less than 5% in parts of Africa.[17]

Factors Predisposing to Gallstone Formation

Age

In all populations studied, the incidence of gallstones increases with age[18-20] (Table 12-2). Gallstones occasionally occur in children, but when present in this age group, they are typically associated with hemolytic

Table 12-2 Incidence of Gallbladder Disease by Age

Patient Age (y)	Patients With Stones (%)	
	Women	Men
10–39	5	1
40–49	12	4
50–59	16	6
60–69	25	10
70–79	29	15
80–89	31	18
≥90	35	24

disorders, congenital anomalies, ileal disorders, short bowel syndrome, or long-term total parenteral nutrition. Although the physiologic basis for the increasing incidence of gallstones with aging is not completely understood, several potential contributing factors have been identified. With advancing age, cholesterol saturation of bile increases. This appears to be secondary to decreased activity of 7α-hydroxylase and increased activity of 3-hydroxy-3-methylglutaryl coenzyme A (HMG-CoA) reductase.[21] These hepatic enzymes are critical in cholesterol biosynthesis. Changes in the ratio of androgen to estrogen can initiate these alterations in hepatic enzyme function. In addition to these effects on hepatobiliary metabolism, changes in biliary motility can also contribute to the higher incidence of gallstones with aging. Gallbladder sensitivity to cholecystokinin (CCK), the primary hormonal stimulus for gallbladder contraction, decreases with age, although this can be partially offset by a compensatory increase in circulating levels of CCK.[22]

Hereditary and Ethnic Factors

The most striking evidence of genetic factors predisposing to gallstone formation occurs in the Pima Indian population. The prevalence of gallstones in Pima women 15 to 24 years of age is 12% and increases to over 70% in women between the ages of 25 and 34 years.[16] In this population, extremely high lithogenic indices are present before the development of gallstones. This impressive propensity to develop gallstones appears to be related to an increase in hepatic biliary cholesterol secretion and a concomitant decrease in bile acid secretion.[23] In other populations, data about familial factors in gallstone formation conflict. One study demonstrated a two-fold higher incidence of gallstones in the first-degree relatives of the gallstone-bearing primary cohort.[24] In contrast, investigations of identical twins have failed to demonstrate a strong genetic in-

fluence. Better definition of the specific relation between hereditary and ethnic factors and gallstone formation requires additional study.

Gender and Hormonal Milieu

The classic adage that the typical patient with gallstones is female, overweight, and in the later childbearing years still has clinical relevance. The basis for this axiom has become clearer as our understanding of the influence of gender and hormonal factors on the formation of cholesterol gallstones has advanced. A four-fold greater incidence of cholesterol gallstones among women compared with men was suggested by early data. More recent studies from Europe suggest that, at least in this population, this gender-based difference is not nearly as great.[19,20,25] No such difference in prevalence is seen when considering pigment gallstones.[26]

The link between hormonal changes, pregnancy, and gallstone formation was recognized more than 100 years ago. Contemporary epidemiologic studies indicate that multiple pregnancies increase the risk of gallstone formation.[12,20] The effect of exogenous estrogen therapy on the risk of gallstone formation remains unclear. A large cooperative study reported that the administration of exogenous estrogen to premenopausal and postmenopausal women[27,28] or to men[29] significantly increases the risk of cholesterol gallstone formation. In contrast, two separate studies from Europe were unable to identify any difference in gallstone risk in women using oral contraceptives.[19,20] Considerable data now suggest that the increased risk of stone formation in these clinical settings is due to hormonally induced alterations in gallbladder motility and hepatic biliary metabolism.

A physiologic basis for pregnancy-related gallstone formation has been provided by ultrasonographic evaluation of gallbladder kinetics. During the second and third trimesters, both absolute gallbladder volume and residual volume after contraction are increased. In addition, the rate of emptying and percentage of initial volume emptied are diminished. Thus, it appears that incomplete gallbladder emptying and stasis of bile are significant contributing factors for gallstone formation during pregnancy.[30] Experimental studies indicate that estrogen administration results in decreased synthesis and secretion of bile acids as well as a secondary decrease in lecithin secretion.[31] In addition, conversion of cholesterol to bile acids is decreased.[32] The net effect of these changes in biliary metabolism is a relative increase in cholesterol secretion and cholesterol saturation of bile, the prerequisite for subsequent gallstone formation.

Obesity

Epidemiologic studies suggest that the morbidly obese have an increased incidence of cholelithiasis.[33] An analogous observation is that over 25% of obese patients who undergo vertical-banded gastroplasty previously required cholecystectomy.[34] Because of the association between obesity and cholelithiasis, cholecystectomy, if not already done, is routinely recommended at the time of vertical-banded gastroplasty.[35,36] Metabolic studies in obese patients have demonstrated an increase in hepatic secretion of cholesterol, both absolute and relative to the secretion of bile and lecithin.[37,38] Of note, obese patients are more resistant to oral dissolution therapy than normal-weight patients.[39]

Numerous studies indicate that cholelithiasis can be a complication of both nonoperative and operative treatment of morbid obesity. Rapid weight loss, as part of either a physician-supervised or commercial program, has been associated with secretion of cholesterol-saturated bile and gallstone formation.[40,41] The precise mechanisms that account for the development of stones in these settings remains obscure.[42]

Other Conditions

An increased risk of gallstone formation has been reported in a number of diverse clinical settings. The common bonds these disorders share include alterations in biliary metabolism and decreased gallbladder motility. Hyperlipidemia, diabetes mellitus, cystic fibrosis, and disease or resection of the terminal ileum have all been associated with an increased prevalence of gallstones. Although a causal relation between truncal vagotomy and gallstones has long been suspected based on clinical observations, experimental models have failed to substantiate this hypothesis. Several studies have shown an increased incidence of gallstones in both children and adults receiving total parenteral nutrition.[43–45] These stones are composed primarily of calcium bilirubinate and probably form as a consequence of biliary stasis.

GALLSTONE PATHOGENESIS

Cholesterol Gallstones

Despite considerable investigations, the pathogenesis of cholesterol gallstones is still not completely understood. For years, the formation of cholesterol gallstones has been conveniently separated into three stages—cholesterol saturation, nucleation, and stone growth. Since the documentation of the physicochemical basis of cholesterol gallstone formation[46] (Fig. 12-1), the hepatic secretion of cholesterol-saturated bile has generally been accepted as a prerequisite for gallstone formation. Until recently, disturbance in mixed micelle formation was considered a key factor in determining cholesterol solubility in bile (Fig. 12-2). This concept has been challenged by the demonstration that much of biliary cholesterol exists in a vesicular form.[47] Furthermore, nucleation by cholesterol monohydrate crystal formation occurs from aggregation of vesicles[48] (Fig. 12-3). Considerable evidence suggests the existence of a *nucleation defect* in patients with cholesterol gallstones. The exact nature of this abnormality has yet to be defined. Some authors have suggested that antinucleating factors are absent in the bile of patients with gallstones,[49] but others suggest that pronucleating factors are the cause of this nucleation defect.[50] Apolipoproteins AI and AII appear to be antinucleating factors, and nonmucin and mucin glycoproteins have been identified as potential pronucleating factors. Fractionation experiments have identified both nucleation-promoting and nucleation-inhibiting biliary proteins. The balance of promoting to inhibiting activity appears to shift in favor of nucleation in bile samples obtained from gallstone patients.[51] Nucleation and at least the early phases of crystal agglomeration probably occur in the mucin gel layer.

In addition to altered hepatic metabolism, changes in gallbladder function are significant factors in the pathogenesis of cholesterol gallstones. Stasis of bile within the gallbladder is a critical link between the hepatic secretion of cholesterol-saturated bile and stone

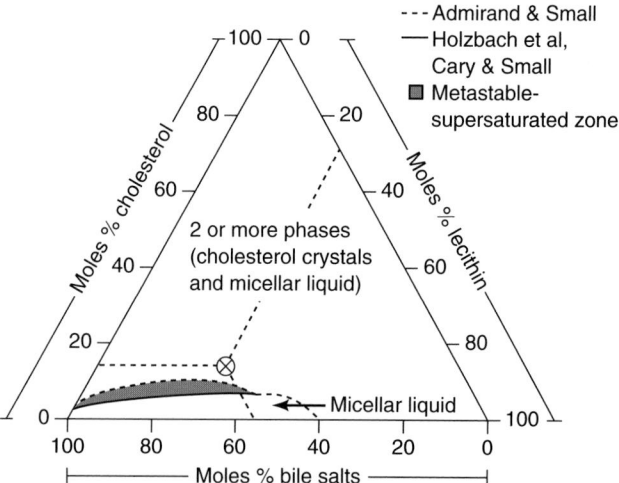

Figure 12-1 Relation among major lipid components in bile that define cholesterol saturation. These triangular coordinates have been modified as our understanding of the pathogenesis of cholesterol gallstone formation has evolved.

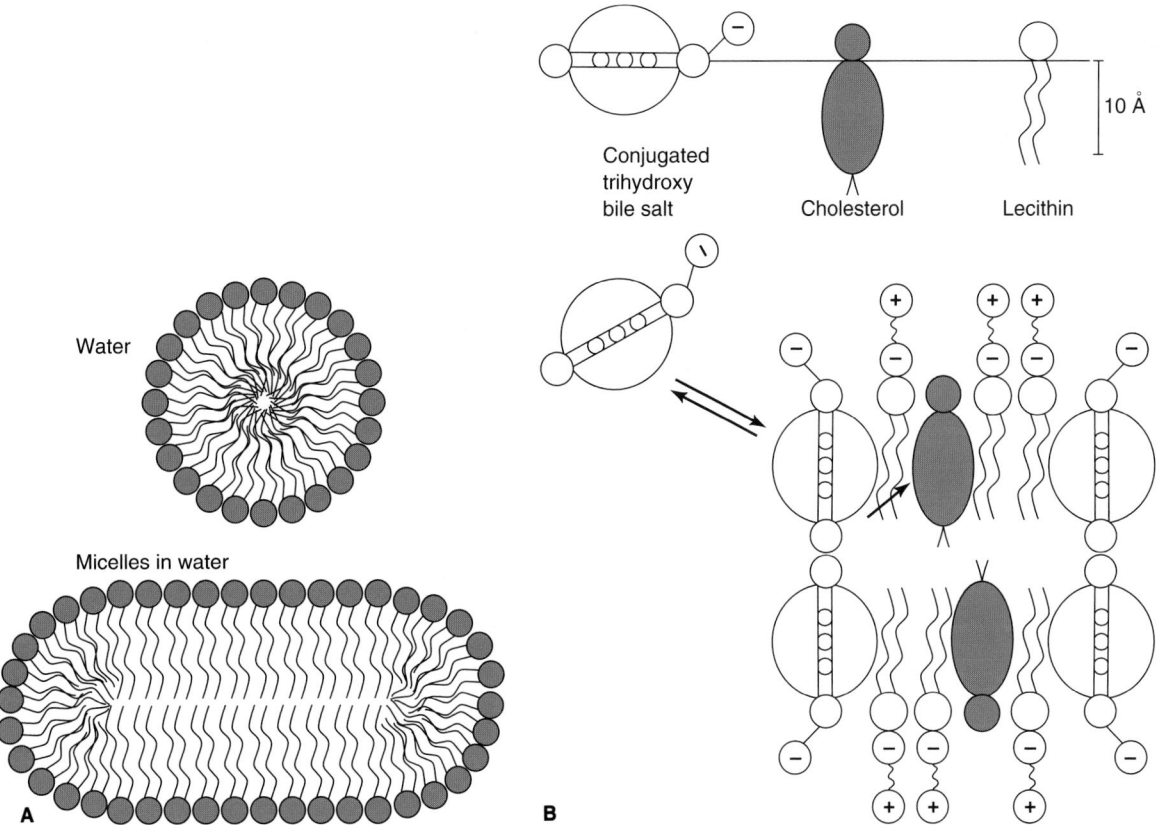

Figure 12-2 (**A**) Micelles are amphipathic compounds with hydrophobic ends oriented inward and hydrophilic ends pointed outward. (**B**) Bile acid micelle formation is key to cholesterol solubilization. Incorporation of lecithin into the micellar structure induces micellar swelling, which facilitates transport of cholesterol.

formation. Experimental studies using animal models of diet-induced cholesterol gallstone formation have identified specific motor defects, including decreased gallbladder emptying and increased cystic duct resistance.[52-54] Stasis of bile within the gallbladder appears to provide an ideal milieu for the precipitation of specific factors present in gallbladder bile. Other elements of gallbladder function that can contribute to cholesterol gallstone formation include calcium metabolism,[55,56] prostaglandin activity,[57] changes in mucosal absorptive and secretory function,[58,59] and an unexplained defect in acidification.[60]

Biliary sludge has been identified as a precursor of cholesterol gallstones. Initially thought to be an innocuous ultrasonographic finding composed of amorphous crystalline material, sludge is now generally recognized to contain cholesterol–lecithin crystals, cholesterol monohydrate crystals, calcium bilirubinate, and mucin.[61] These findings may explain the clinical observation that many cholesterol stones contain a central nidus of calcium bilirubinate. Sludge has been shown to progress to gallstones in clinical studies and is a com-

mon finding in specific settings that predispose to biliary stasis and gallbladder hypomotility, including the postoperative state, burns, total parenteral nutrition, and pregnancy.

The etiologic role of bacteria in the pathogenesis of pigment stones has been well established for more than 25 years. Only recently, however, have bacteria been implicated as a causative factor in cholesterol gallstone formation.[62]

Pigment Gallstones

It was suggested in 1966 that β-glucuronidase released by *Escherichia coli* induced the enzymatic hydrolysis of bilirubin glucuronide into free bilirubin and glucuronic acid, and that this was the basis for all pigment gallstone formation[63] (Fig. 12-4). More recently, a number of studies have shown that, in addition to bacterial infection, excessive bilirubin production, disorders of bile acid and calcium metabolism, and gallbladder stasis are all factors that can contribute to the formation of pigment stones. The multifactorial concept for pigment

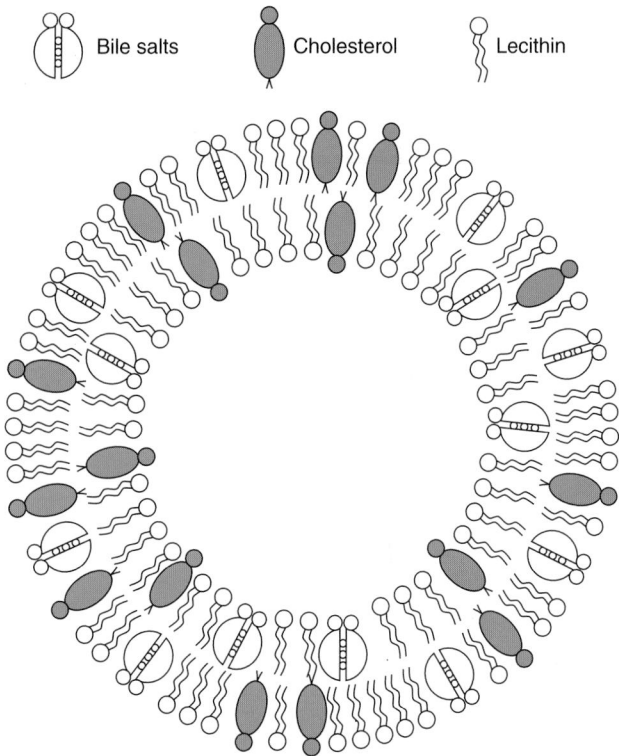

Figure 12-3 Unilamellar bile acid–lecithin vesicle. The amphipathic molecules of lecithin and bile acids form a lipid bilayer, and cholesterol is solubilized within the nonpolar portion of the bilayer.

gallstone formation is underscored by the recognition that these calculi occur in a number of diverse clinical settings, including hemolytic disorders, cirrhosis, biliary infections, and ileal resection, as well as during the administration of long-term parenteral nutrition.

CLINICAL FEATURES OF GALLSTONES

Natural History

The natural history of gallstone disease has assumed greater importance because of new and innovative treatment modalities as well as evolving perspectives focusing on health care reform. The economic significance of the clinical management of patients with gallstones is underscored by the frequency with which this disease occurs in the United States and throughout the world. Longitudinal studies indicate that the rate at which gallstones become symptomatic is low and that during a 20-year period, less than 20% of asymptomatic patients require surgery based on symptoms or complications of cholelithiasis. Therefore, cholecystectomy

for asymptomatic stones is difficult to justify.[64,65] Similarly, there is no support for nonoperative therapy of asymptomatic gallstones.[66] An expectant approach to asymptomatic stones is further supported by data from a single institutional study showing that death is rarely the outcome of the index presentation for patients with previously asymptomatic stones.[67] Once symptoms occur, however, the clinical course is not predictable. Minor episodes of biliary colic can resolve or can be superseded by complications such as biliary pancreatitis. Because of the uncertain course of symptomatic stones, intervention is widely advocated once symptoms develop. The management of diabetic patients with asymptomatic gallstones has been particularly controversial. For many years, it was generally accepted that cholecystectomy was indicated for the asymptomatic diabetic with gallstones. This principle was based on the belief that this subset of patients was more susceptible to septic complications. Studies have challenged this axiom, and the role of elective cholecystectomy in this setting remains poorly defined.

Diagnosis

Several diagnostic studies are available to evaluate the patient with symptoms suggestive of cholelithiasis. Recognition of the sensitivity, specificity, and limitations of these studies has helped to define the utility that each has in establishing the correct diagnosis. This is particularly significant in the development of cost-effective strategies for patient care.

Plain Abdominal Radiography

Supine and upright abdominal films are frequently obtained for patients presenting with acute abdominal pain. These films are usually considered part of the initial data base and can be useful in excluding diagnoses other than gallstone disease. On occasion, they provide enough information to establish a diagnosis of biliary stone disease. Plain films visualize only gallstones con-

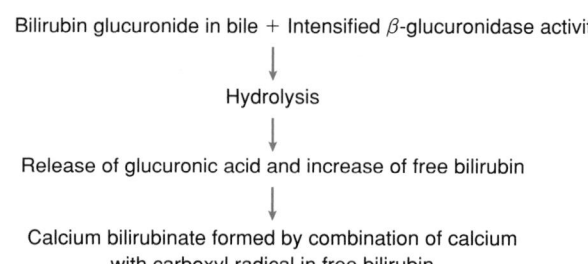

Figure 12-4 Summary of key steps involved in formation of calcium bilirubinate stones.

taining significant amounts of calcium, which occur in 10% to 25% of patients. The characteristic appearance is an incomplete ring density in the right upper quadrant (Fig. 12-5). Rarely, a tense, distended gallbladder results in a mass effect on plain films. The diagnosis of emphysematous cholecystitis can be made by the finding of air within the gallbladder wall or within the lumen. The calcified silhouette of a gallbladder is pathognomonic of a porcelain gallbladder (Fig. 12-6). Air within the biliary tract is evidence of a cholecystoenteric fistula.

Oral Cholecystography

Oral cholecystography was developed more than 70 years ago.[68] Hepatic excretion of halogenated contrast material into bile and subsequent concentration in the gallbladder results in opacification of a normally functioning gallbladder. Filling defects within the opacified gallbladder indicate the presence of gallstones (Fig. 12-7). Nonvisualization of the gallbladder suggests gallbladder disease. In ideal circumstances, the accuracy of oral cholecystography approaches 95%. However, because of poor patient compliance, hepatic dys-

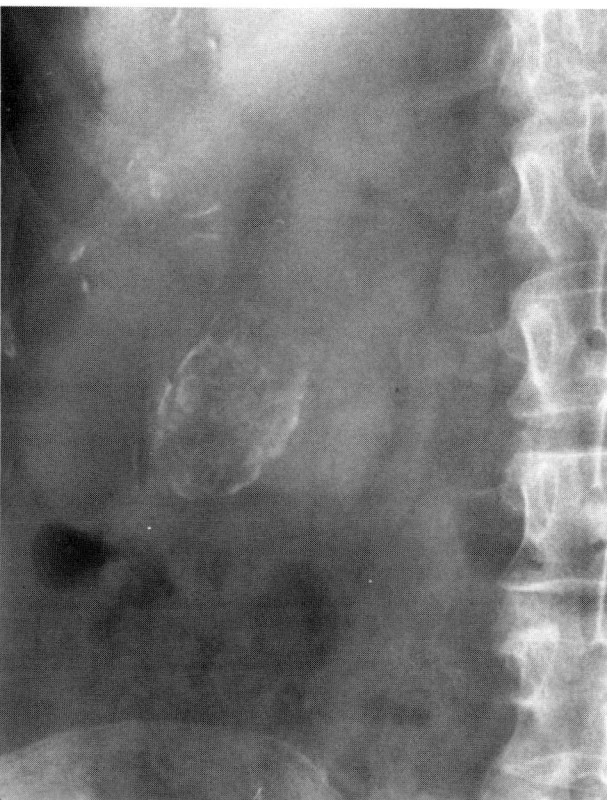

Figure 12-6 Plain abdominal radiograph demonstrating classic finding of porcelain gallbladder.

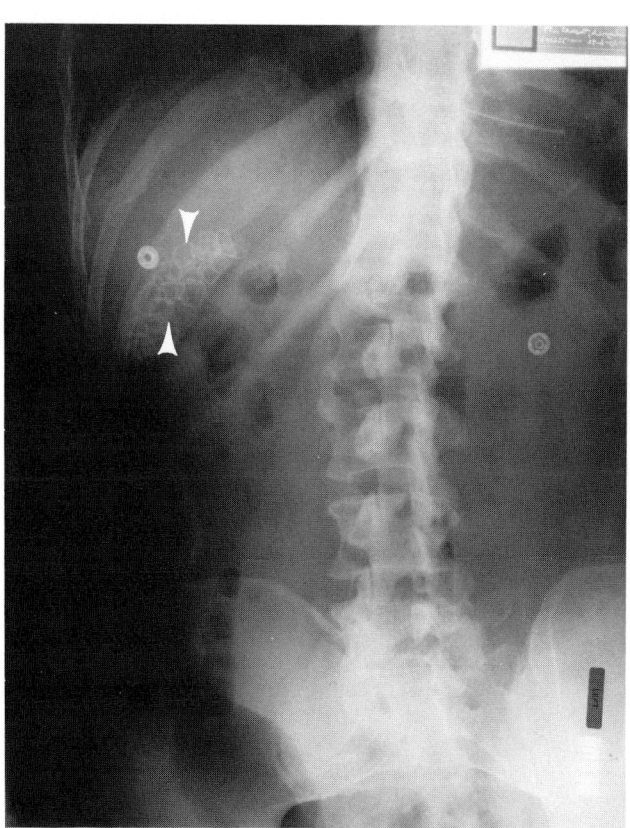

Figure 12-5 Plain abdominal radiograph demonstrating calcified gallstones (*arrows*).

function, or lack of absorption of the contrast tablets due to emesis, malabsorption, or diarrhea, inconclusive or false-positive results are not infrequent.

Abdominal Ultrasonography

During the past 15 years, ultrasonography has emerged as the test of choice in patients with symptomatic gallstone disease. Advantages over oral cholecystography include ease of performance, independence from patient compliance or gastrointestinal function, and avoidance of radiation exposure. Ultrasonography also evaluates the common bile duct, pancreas, and liver. The accuracy of identifying gallbladder stones using real-time ultrasonography exceeds 95%.[69] The classic ultrasonographic findings that indicate the presence of gallstones are intraluminal echogenic foci with acoustic shadowing that move as the patient changes position (Fig. 12-8). Information can be provided about number and size of stones, gallbladder shape and size, and gallbladder wall thickness. When the clinical diagnosis is acute cholecystitis, the specific ultrasonographic findings that support the diagnosis are gallblad-

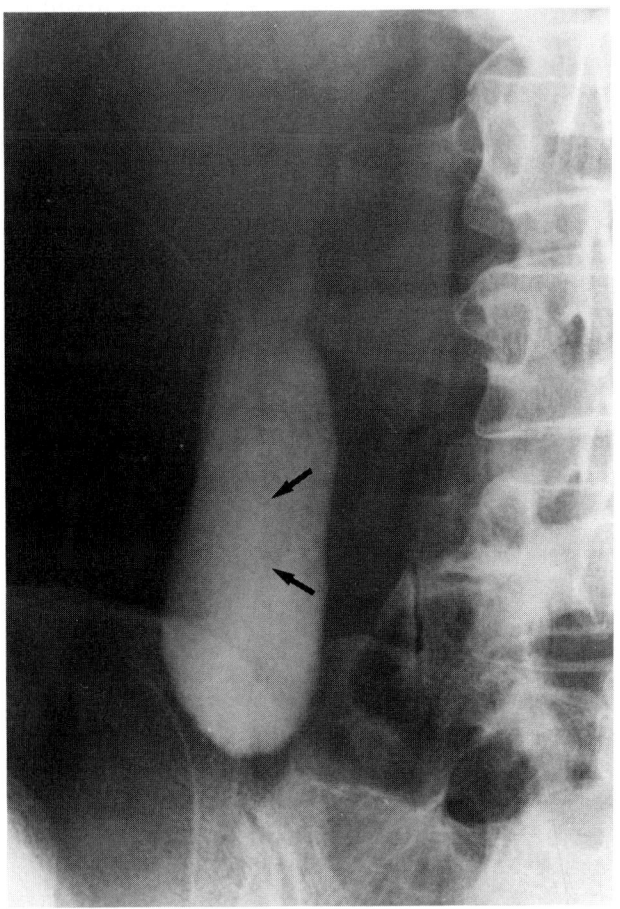

Figure 12-7 Oral cholecystogram demonstrating multiple filling defects (*arrows*) indicative of small gallstones in an opacified gallbladder.

der wall thickening, pericholecystic fluid, and a sonographic Murphy's sign.[70]

Computed Tomography

The characteristic appearance of calcified gallstones allows the specificity of computed tomographic (CT) scans in detecting the presence of calcified gallstones to approach 100% (Fig. 12-9). The overall sensitivity of CT, however, does not approach that of ultrasonography because most stones do not contain significant amounts of calcium.[71] The low sensitivity, coupled with the radiation exposure and the cost of the study, indicates that there is no justification for CT as a routine study to evaluate the patient with uncomplicated gallstone disease.

Biliary Scintigraphy

The intravenous injection of radionuclides, such as technetium-99m–substituted iminodiacetic acid derivatives, results in imaging of the hepatobiliary tract as these agents are cleared from the circulation and excreted by hepatocytes into the biliary tree. The newer radiopharmaceuticals with shortened half-lives provide improved visualization with less radiation exposure, even in the face of significantly elevated serum bilirubin levels. Biliary scintigraphy can indicate the presence of focal hepatic masses, parenchymal dysfunction, and gallbladder dysmotility. Although cholelithiasis cannot be detected by biliary scintigraphy, cystic duct

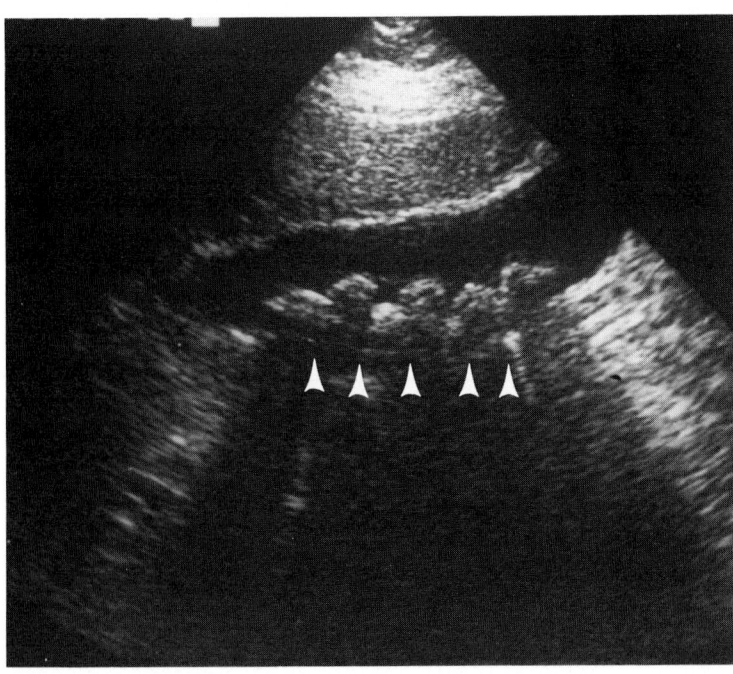

Figure 12-8 Abdominal ultrasound, sagittal section, showing multiple rolling stones (*arrows*).

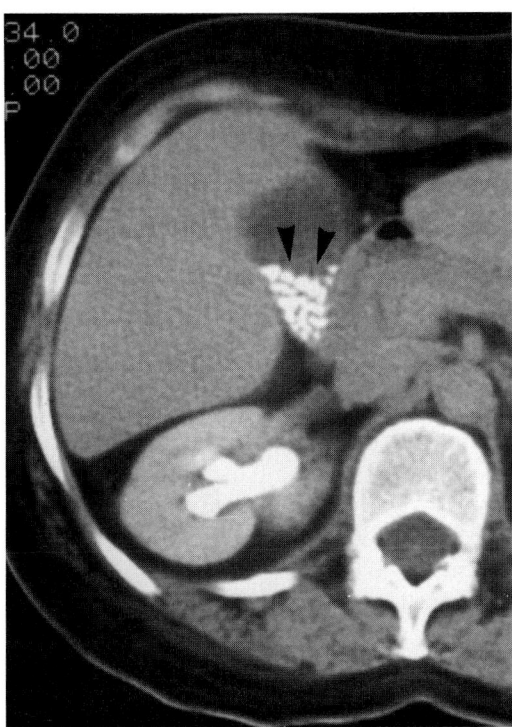

Figure 12-9 Multiple calcified gallstones (*arrows*) are visible on this CT scan.

obstruction can be reliably ascertained in the clinical setting of acute cholecystitis (Fig. 12-10).

Biliary Drainage and Cholecystokinin Cholescintigraphy

In the patient with classic symptoms of biliary colic who has no evidence of gallstones on either oral cholecystography or abdominal ultrasonography, duodenal aspiration of bile in conjunction with CCK cholecystography can be useful in detecting stones too small to see by conventional means as well as in the identification of cholesterolosis, or biliary dyskinesia. A tube is placed under fluoroscopic control into the second portion of the duodenum, CCK is administered intravenously, and bile is collected from the duodenum. Scintigraphic images are obtained at 5- to 10-minute intervals. The development of pain after the injection of CCK, the failure of the gallbladder to empty, or the presence of cholesterol or bilirubinate crystals in the duodenal aspirates suggests the presence of gallbladder disease. Cholecystectomy performed on the basis of these criteria results in pain improvement in 80% of patients.[72]

Common Clinical Manifestations

Biliary Colic

The classic symptom of patients with cholelithiasis is intermittent right upper quadrant pain. This characteristic pain, referred to as biliary colic, is generally abrupt in onset and resolves within minutes to several hours. The pain results from cystic duct obstruction and distention of a hollow viscus, the gallbladder. In contrast to the waxing and waning pattern of pain that is so typical of other colicky syndromes, biliary colic is often described as the sudden onset of pain that builds in intensity to a peak. The pain then plateaus for a period before its gradual diminution (Fig. 12-11). Although the classic site is in the right upper quadrant, the pain of biliary colic can localize to the midepigastrium, the back, or the inferior edge of the scapula. Biliary colic typically occurs postprandially, particularly in the evening after a large meal. Clinical lore suggests that fatty foods are poorly tolerated; however, ingestion of any type of meal can precipitate an attack of biliary colic.

Chronic Cholecystitis

The mere presence of gallstones often leads to inflammation of the gallbladder wall. In addition, repeated bouts of acute or subacute cholecystitis can lead to histologic findings consistent with chronic cholecystitis. Associated symptoms are biliary colic with recurring bouts of postprandial pain. Ultrasound findings often include cholelithiasis and a thickened gallbladder wall. Depending on the severity of the inflammatory process, as well as the chronicity, this diagnosis can be suggested by a small, shrunken gallbladder.

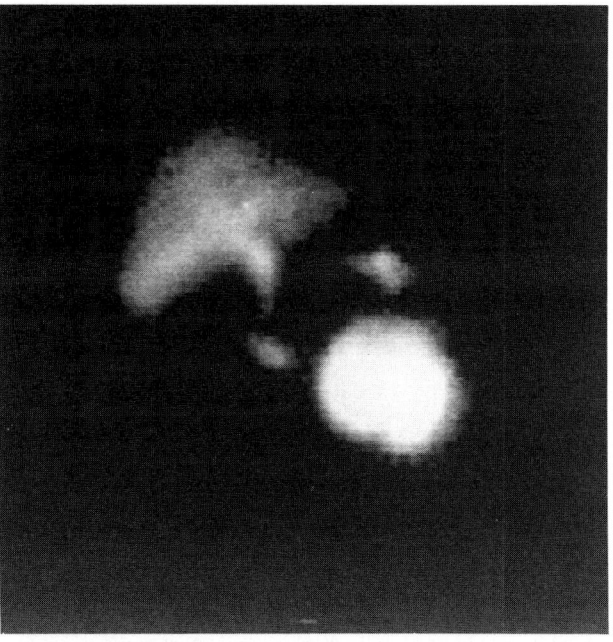

Figure 12-10 HIDA scan in a patient with clinical evidence of acute cholecystitis. Scan confirms diagnosis by failure to visualize gallbladder due to cystic duct obstruction.

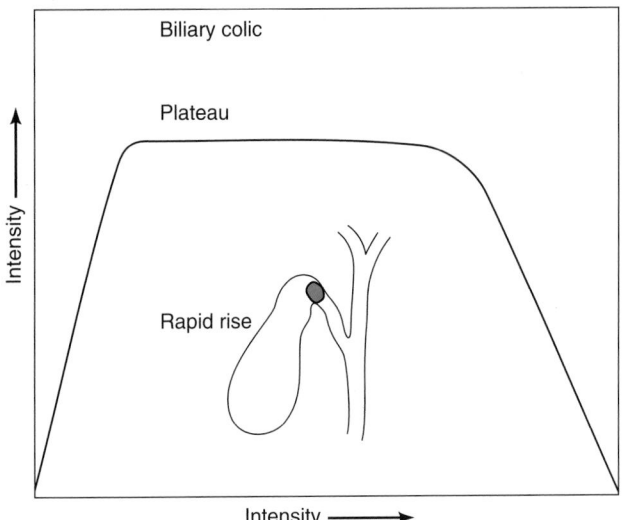

Figure 12-11 Representation of severity of pain over time in patients with biliary colic. (After Schoenfield LJ. Diseases of the gallbladder and biliary system. New York, John Wiley & Sons, 1977:118)

Acute Cholecystitis

PATHOGENESIS. The initial event leading to the development of acute cholecystitis is cystic duct obstruction. This is usually due to a stone impacted in the duct or, less commonly, to a stone lodged in Hartmann's pouch (Fig. 12-12). The pathogenesis of cholecystitis remains poorly defined. Mechanical, chemical, and infectious mechanisms are thought to be interrelated contributing factors. Gallbladder distention eventually leads to ischemia, chemical irritation secondary to local release of lysolecithin and other factors. The finding that bile cultures are positive in 75% of cases indicates that infection is a major component of acute

cholecystitis. The organisms most frequently cultured from patients with acute cholecystitis include *E coli*, *Klebsiella* sp, and enterococci. Current opinion, however, is that bacterial infection is a consequence rather than a cause of the acute inflammation.

INCIDENCE. Acute cholecystitis has traditionally accounted for 20% of all patients undergoing cholecystectomy.[73] The incidence of cholecystitis may be rising.[74,75] In an analysis of 42,474 cholecystectomies performed in a 12-month period, 35% were performed for acute cholecystitis.[76] This trend is particularly notable in hospitals that provide care for the indigent. In one such institution, the proportion of all patients requiring cholecystectomy that had acute cholecystitis increased from 33% to 49% in an 8-year period. Possible explanations for the growing incidence of acute cholecystitis include alterations in reimbursement strategies, reallocation of resources, limited access to health care for an increasing segment of the population, and physician attitudes about surgery, especially in the geriatric population.[77]

CLINICAL MANIFESTATIONS. The pain of acute cholecystitis is similar to biliary colic; however, distinguishing features include duration and localization of pain. Rather than spontaneously resolving, as with biliary colic, the pain of acute cholecystitis can persist several days. As the gallbladder becomes progressively more distended, the contiguous parietal peritoneum becomes inflamed, resulting in the perception of well-localized pain. Associated symptoms include anorexia, nausea, emesis, and low-grade fever. Most patients with acute cholecystitis have an elevated temperature, but fever may be conspicuously absent in elderly or immunocompromised patients. Abdominal examination

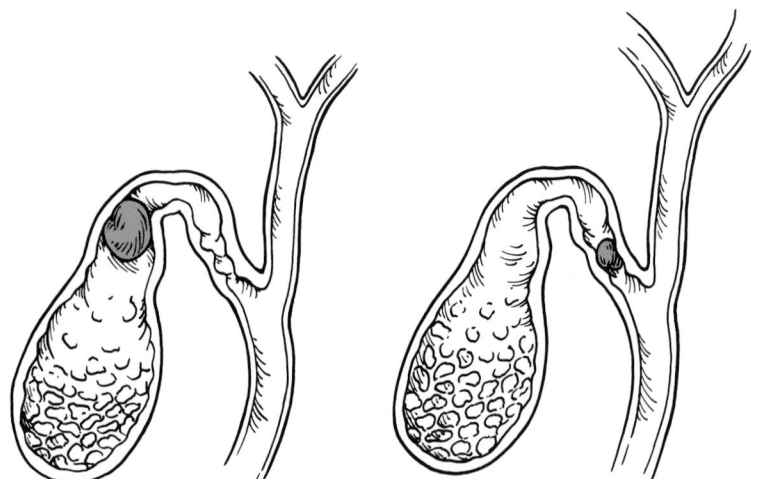

Figure 12-12 Stone obstructing the cystic duct or gallbladder infundibulum depicted as a factor in the pathogenesis of acute cholecystitis.

reveals tenderness with guarding over the fundus of the gallbladder in the right upper quadrant. A palpable mass in the right upper quadrant can be appreciated in 20% of patients with acute cholecystitis. This finding may be due to a distended gallbladder or to omentum that becomes adherent to the inflamed gallbladder. Arrest of the inspiratory effort due to increasing pain as the descent of the diaphragm moves the gallbladder against the examining hand, called Murphy's sign, is a classic indication of acute cholecystitis. Jaundice is generally not a major component of acute cholecystitis and, in the absence of choledocholithiasis, is present in less than 15% of patients with acute cholecystitis. Although the specificity of this remains unclear, jaundice in this setting probably results from contiguous inflammation.

DIAGNOSTIC EVALUATION. The combination of right upper quadrant pain and tenderness, fever, and leukocytosis is highly suggestive of acute cholecystitis. Additional laboratory and radiologic studies serve to confirm the clinical diagnosis. Modest abnormalities in serum liver function test results are not unusual. Marked elevations of alkaline phosphatase and bilirubin suggest that the diagnosis of cholangitis, rather than acute cholecystitis, should be entertained. The study with the highest specificity for acute cholecystitis is hepatobiliary scintigraphy. Hepatobiliary scintigraphy has a diagnostic accuracy for acute cholecystitis that approaches 98%. Limitations of the study include potential false-positive results, exposure of the patient to radioactive material, and the length of time required to demonstrate nonvisualization of the gallbladder. Because the presence of cholelithiasis is the only other required information in the patient with a straightforward clinical presentation of acute cholecystitis, ultrasonography has emerged as the diagnostic procedure of choice in this clinical setting. Hepatobiliary scintigraphy should be reserved for cases in which the diagnosis remains unclear after ultrasonography.

Diseases that can mimic acute cholecystitis include duodenal ulcer disease, acute appendicitis, gastric ulcer, acute pancreatitis, viral hepatitis, acute alcoholic hepatitis, pneumonia, and myocardial ischemia, all of which can cause right upper quadrant pain.

TREATMENT. Treatment of acute cholecystitis has evolved during the past 20 years. Traditionally, initial therapy consisted of hospitalization, intravenous hydration, and antimicrobial therapy. Cholecystectomy was deferred for 6 to 8 weeks to allow all inflammation to subside. This approach was challenged by a number of prospective randomized studies that compared delayed with early cholecystectomy for acute cholecystitis. Although operative morbidity and mortality rates were similar, advantages of early cholecystectomy included a reduction in length of hospitalization and the avoidance of recurrent episodes of acute cholecystitis.[78,79] Furthermore, morbidity and mortality rates were significantly increased for patients who failed to respond to nonoperative therapy and required emergency cholecystectomy several days after the onset of their symptoms. These findings, coupled with the ease of cholecystectomy early in the course of acute cholecystitis, has led to the widespread adoption of early cholecystectomy as the standard of care for acute cholecystitis.

Recommendations for the care of patients with acute cholecystitis include rapid diagnosis, intravenous hydration, institution of broad-spectrum antibiotic therapy, and urgent cholecystectomy within 24 to 48 hours after hospitalization. Bile cultures are positive in about 75% to 80% of patients with acute cholecystitis. The organisms most commonly found include *E coli, Klebsiella* sp, enterococci, and anaerobic streptococci. Either a second-generation cephalosporin or, in very ill patients, triple-drug therapy consisting of an aminoglycoside, ampicillin, and metronidazole (Flagyl) or clindamycin, can be used. The potential nephrotoxicity of aminoglycosides and the associated costs of these agents diminish their attractiveness in this setting. The administration of a second-generation cephalosporin has become the mainstay of treatment for most patients with acute, uncomplicated cholecystitis.

Because 75% of patients with acute cholecystitis quickly improve with antibiotic therapy, one might be lulled into relaxing the time frame for early cholecystectomy. Cholecystectomy in the subacute phase, however, can be difficult. In place of the edema that facilitates dissection in early acute cholecystitis, the subacute phase is characterized by increased vascularity and early fibrosis, which make the dissection more difficult. Although "early" can be difficult to define precisely, avoidance of operating in the subacute phase is most easily achieved by prompt, semielective cholecystectomy once the diagnosis of acute cholecystitis has been established. Occasionally, cholecystectomy may be ill-advised, as in the case of the extremely high-risk patient who has acute cholecystitis. In this clinical setting, cholecystostomy (performed under local anesthesia) or percutaneous catheter drainage of the gallbladder[80] can be life-saving.

Choledocholithiasis

About 10% to 15% of patients with cholelithiasis have stones in the common bile duct. The incidence of ductal stones increases with age and has been reported to be as high as 50% in patients more than 65 years of age. Most common duct stones form in the gallbladder and pass into the choledochus through the cystic duct. Unfortunately, 1% to 5% of patients who undergo cholecystectomy have stones left behind in the bile duct that require removal at a later date. Depending on the individual circumstances, this can be accomplished endoscopically, percutaneously with radiologic assistance, by lithotripsy, by direct instillation of specific agents into the bile duct, or surgically. Common bile duct stones can be asymptomatic, or they can cause obstructive jaundice, cholangitis, or biliary pancreatitis.

Gallstone Pancreatitis

The causal relation between ductal stones and pancreatitis was first recognized nearly 100 years ago.[81] It has only recently been demonstrated that the transient blockage of the ampulla of Vater by a migrating stone initiates the cascade of events culminating in pancreatitis.[82] Factors predisposing to biliary pancreatitis include the presence of multiple small stones and a patent cystic duct. The pathogenesis and pathophysiology of this complication of gallstone disease has been the subject of considerable investigation in recent years. Strategies have been developed for a rational approach to the patient with biliary pancreatitis. These issues are more formally discussed in subsequent chapters.

Nonspecific Symptoms

Atypical presentations of gallstone disease are not uncommon. Rather than the symptoms of classic biliary colic, complaints include chronic upper abdominal discomfort, dyspepsia, flatulence, eructation, and heartburn. There is no physiologic or anatomic basis to explain how gallbladder disease causes these nonspecific symptoms. Nonetheless, cholecystectomy often results in relief or symptoms.

Complications of Cholecystitis

Perforation

Perforation of the gallbladder is not an uncommon complication of acute cholecystitis. Most reports suggest that it occurs in 3% to 10% of patients with acute gallbladder inflammation. Traditionally, gallbladder perforation is classified as acute, subacute, or chronic. The clinical setting in which these entities occur and their presentation tend to be different.

Acute, free perforation is uncommon (although not rare) and typically occurs in patients who are immune suppressed or have some evidence of systemic vascular disease. A 20% incidence of severe atherosclerotic heart disease or diabetes has been reported in patients with acute gallbladder perforation.[83,84] The fundus is the least vascularized portion of the gallbladder and is the most common site of free perforation. These patients often present with an acute abdomen, and aggressive treatment and urgent operative intervention is essential. Precise preoperative diagnosis is unusual, and the situation is often clarified at the time of surgery.

The pathophysiology of subacute and chronic perforations appears to be similar. In both situations, longstanding gallstone disease and repeated episodes of inflammation lead to scarring, fibrosis, and adhesions between the gallbladder and contiguous structures. Perforation with contained sepsis usually results as diffuse contamination is minimized by the adhesive process. Gallbladder perforation with pericholecystic fluid or abscess formation is often suspected on ultrasonography or CT scan. Optimal treatment includes cholecystectomy, if technically feasible, and wide drainage of the area.

Chronic perforation with formation of either a cholecystoenteric or a cholecystocutaneous fistula represents the most common type of gallbladder perforation. Fistulization into the duodenum is most common. A cholecystoduodenal fistula occurs when a stone erodes through the gallbladder and passes directly into the adherent duodenum. This process is often silent, and the patient may have no symptoms. Small stones traverse the length of the gastrointestinal tract without complication and pass unnoticed in the feces. Stones 2 cm or larger may be asymptomatic until they become impacted in the terminal ileum. The mechanical small bowel obstruction that results is referred to as a *gallstone ileus* (Fig. 12-13). This complication should be suspected in elderly women who present with small bowel obstruction, absence of prior laparotomies, an intact gallbladder, and the presence of pneumobilia in the right upper quadrant. Appropriate treatment includes resuscitation, nasogastric decompression, and early operation. The primary goal of an operation for these patients is to correct the bowel obstruction by removal of the stone. This is often best accomplished by "milking" the stone in a retrograde manner, creating an enterotomy over the stone, removing it, and then repairing the bowel wall. Because most of these patients are elderly and frail, definitive management of the biliary enteric fistula can be delayed to another time or, in some cases, not undertaken at all. In stable patients with definable anatomy, cholecystectomy and closure of the duodenal fistula can be accomplished at the same time that the bowel obstruction is relieved.

Empyema

Empyema of the gallbladder is a variant of acute cholecystitis and occurs primarily in the elderly.[85] The main distinction between empyema and uncompli-

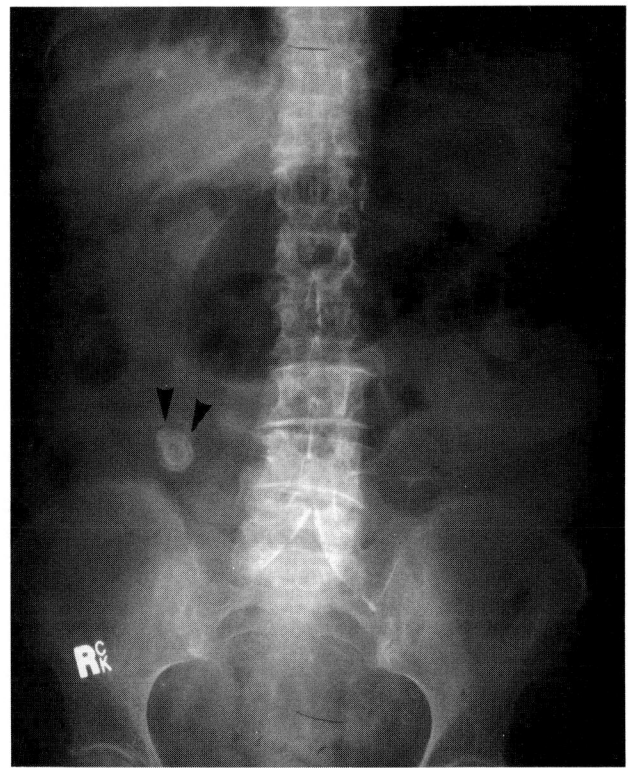

Figure 12-13 Plain abdominal radiograph demonstrating gallstone (*arrows*) in right lower quadrant in elderly woman with gallstone ileus.

cated, acute cholecystitis is the presence of pus within the gallbladder lumen in the former. In addition to complaining of right upper quadrant pain, these patients appear to be in toxic conditions, with high fever and marked leukocytosis. Early cholecystectomy is mandatory after adequate resuscitation to prevent gram-negative sepsis or perforation.

Emphysematous Cholecystitis

The presence of gas within the wall of the gallbladder represents an unusual but interesting complication of acute cholecystitis. This entity occurs most often in elderly men, with diabetes being present in 40%. The classic finding of gas within the gallbladder wall results from infection with gas-producing organisms, usually *Clostridium perfringens*. These patients are in extremely toxic states and have evidence of severe sepsis. Urgent intervention is required.

Hydrops

Whereas acute obstruction of the cystic duct typically results in acute cholecystitis, obstruction of a more chronic nature is often associated with the curious en-

tity of hydrops of the gallbladder. It is generally believed that the slow, insidious obstruction of the duct leads to slow distention of the gallbladder as a result of continuous secretion of sterile mucus or a clear transudate. What converts the gallbladder epithelium from its usual absorptive state to one of secretion continues to be a mystery. These patients often present with massively distended gallbladders and minimal or no pain. The diagnosis may be suggested on plain film by the presence of a shadow in the right upper quadrant. Cholecystectomy is curative.

MANAGEMENT OF GALLSTONES

The cost of treating gallstone disease exceeds $3 billion and is estimated to approach $5 billion by the year 2000. Despite extensive efforts to identify nonoperative treatment modalities, the mainstay of therapy for symptomatic gallstone disease remains the surgical removal of the gallbladder—either laparoscopically or with the standard open technique.

Open Cholecystectomy

Because gallbladder disease is widely prevalent, cholecystectomy is a commonly required procedure. Between 500,000 and 700,000 cholecystectomies are performed each year in the United States. Indications for cholecystectomy include biliary colic, acute and chronic cholecystitis, and other complications of gallstone disease. Specific issues regarding the role of cholecystectomy for asymptomatic gallstones have been previously addressed.

Patients scheduled for elective cholecystectomy are admitted to the hospital on the day of surgery. A number of studies have shown that same-day admittance policies have not adversely affected complication rates or outcome. The safety of same-day admittance, combined with a shortened length of stay, has improved the cost-effective manner in which cholecystectomy is performed.[86–88]

Open cholecystectomy continues to be a safe and effective procedure. The technical aspects have not changed appreciably during the past 25 years. Outcome after cholecystectomy depends on age, underlying disease status, and comorbid conditions. Cardiovascular disease is the most frequent cause of mortality after cholecystectomy.[89] Early data spanning several decades indicated that cholecystectomy had a 1% mortality rate.[90] Experience over a more limited time span indicates an overall mortality rate of 0.5%.[91] Contemporary experience suggests that mortality rates continue to improve. A population-based study was conducted of

42,474 cholecystectomies done in 1989, representing 8% of the total number of cholecystectomies done in the United States that year.[76] The overall mortality rate was 0.17%. The mortality rate was 0.03% in patients younger than 65 years of age, and 0.5% in those older than 65 (Table 12-3).

Laparoscopic Cholecystectomy

Perspective

Although laparoscopic cholecystectomy was first reported only in 1988,[5] it has rapidly emerged as the preferred procedure in many parts of the world for the management of patients with symptomatic gallstone disease. It has been suggested that less than 25% of all cholecystectomies being performed are done using the traditional open technique, and the remaining 75% are being accomplished laparoscopically. Theoretic advantages of laparoscopic removal of the gallbladder include reduced postoperative pain and discomfort, improved recovery, faster recuperation, better cosmetic result, shortened hospital stay, and lower cost. Although this procedure has been embraced by both the medical and lay communities, lingering questions remain. Unresolved issues include accreditation and credentialing processes, indications and contraindications for the procedure, incidence of bile duct injuries, and cost-effectiveness. Old controversies have reemerged, including the role of intraoperative cholangiography, the timing of cholecystectomy for patients with acute cholecystitis, and the optimal management of patients with abnormal liver function tests. New and intriguing questions will undoubtedly continue to surface as skills are developed in laparoscopic surgical techniques.

Technique

From a technical viewpoint, the key to performing laparoscopic cholecystectomy is the creation of a satisfactory pneumoperitoneum. Once the laparoscope is introduced, the principles for safe laparoscopic cholecystectomy are the same as those for open cholecystectomy. The cystic duct and cystic artery must be clearly visualized. The recognition of the common variations in ductal and arterial structures is crucial to avoid ductal injury and vascular compromise or hemorrhage. Initial recommendations included routine cholangiography to define the ductal anatomy better. As experience with laparoscopic cholecystectomy has accumulated, selective cholangiography has been advocated instead. The indications for cholangiography during either open or laparoscopic cholecystectomy are the same.[92] These include common bile duct dilation, history of jaundice or hyperamylasemia, abnormal liver function tests, and palpable ductal stones. It is essential that surgeons performing laparoscopic cholecystectomy be expert in intraoperative cholangiography. Cholangiography performed laparoscopically is more challenging than the open technique. Indications to convert to open cholecystectomy include inability to identify key anatomic structures, significant inflammation with adhesions to adjacent viscera, hemorrhage, bile duct injury, or the discovery of unexpected pathology, such as gallbladder carcinoma. Conversion to an open procedure occurs in about 3% to 6% of elective cases and in up to 26% of procedures performed for acute cholecystitis.

Indications and Contraindications

The indications for cholecystectomy should remain constant whether a laparoscopic or open procedure is being contemplated. Issues related to the treatment of asymptomatic stones were discussed earlier, and the same guidelines should be applied for laparoscopic surgery as for the open procedure. The most frequent indication for laparoscopic cholecystectomy is recurrent biliary colic. Absolute contraindications for laparoscopic cholecystectomy are similar to those for the open procedure and include inability to tolerate general anesthesia and uncorrectable coagulopathy. During the early days of laparoscopic surgery, prior surgery or the presence of acute cholecystitis were viewed as contraindications to this approach. As more experience has been obtained, perspectives regarding these issues have evolved. It has become clear that, although the presence of postoperative or inflammatory adhesions provides for a more challenging situation, it does not preclude attempts at laparoscopic removal of the

Table 12-3 Effect of Age on Outcome

	Age (y)	
	<65	>65
Number	30,059	12,415
Percentage of group	70.8	29.2
Morbidity rate (%)	10.2	25.7*
Number of deaths	9	62
Mortality rate (%)	0.03	0.50*
Length of stay (d)	4.7	7.3*
Charges ($)	5980	9728*

* P < .0001 versus age below 65 years.
(Roslyn JJ, Binns GS, Hughes EX, Saunders KD, Cates JA, Zinner MJ. Open cholecystectomy: a contemporary analysis of 42,474 patients. Ann Surg 1993;218:129).

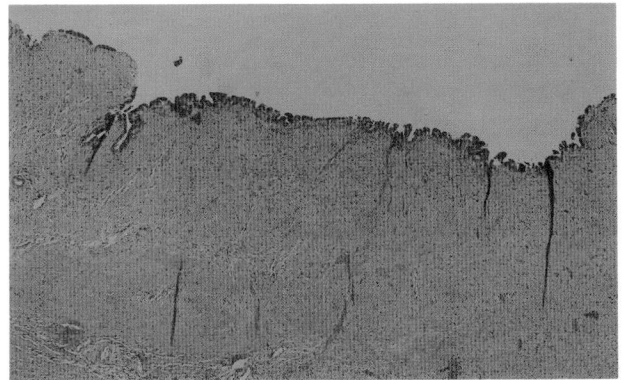

Color Figure 14-2

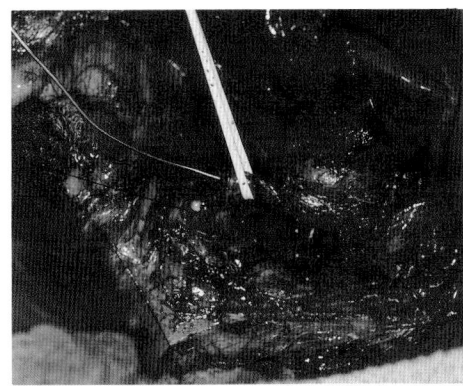

Color Figure 14-10

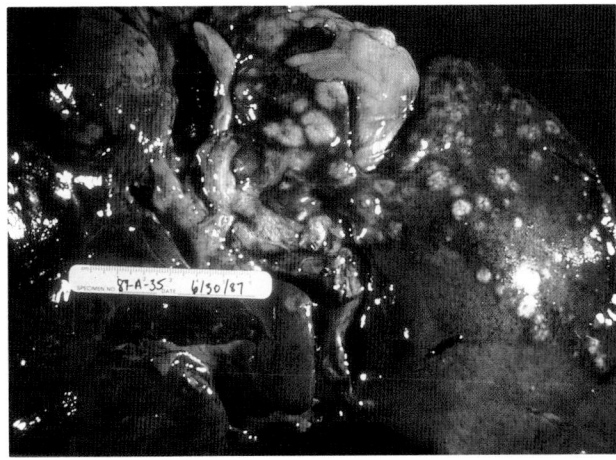

Color Figure 16-1

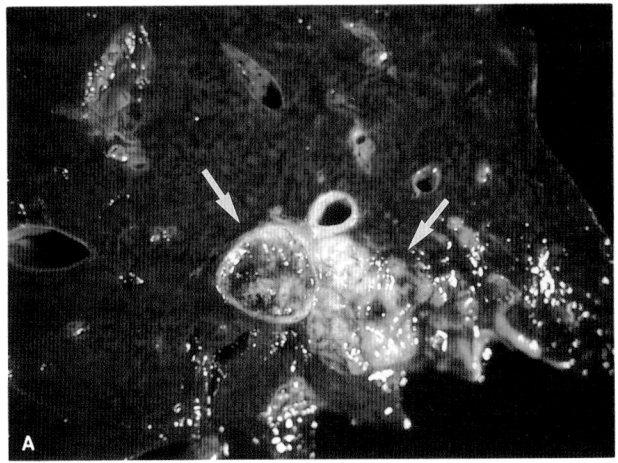

Color Figure 16-6

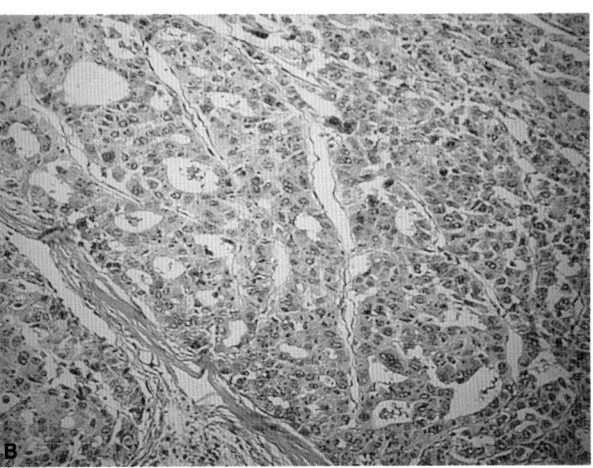

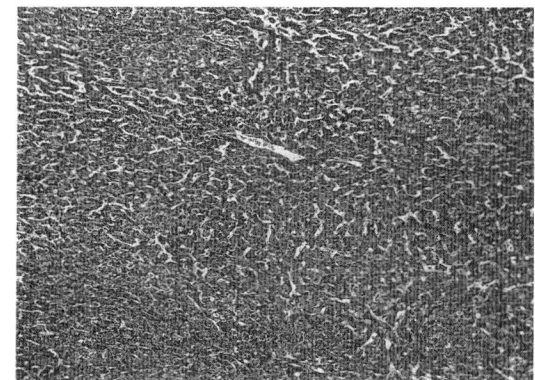

Color Figure 18-7

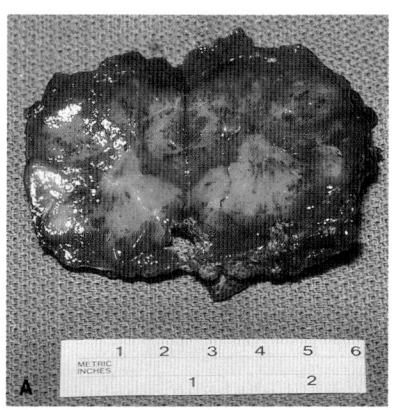

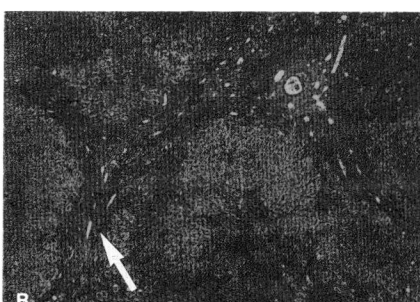

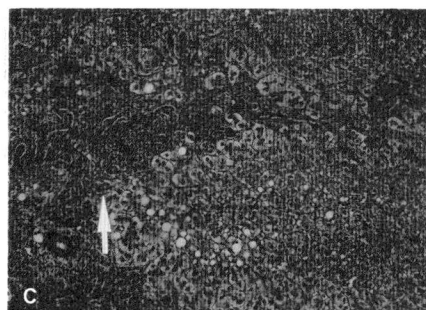

Color Figure 18-9

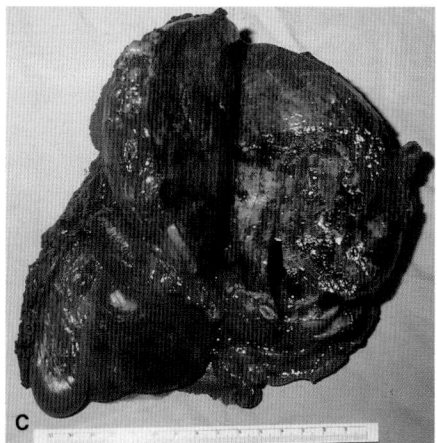

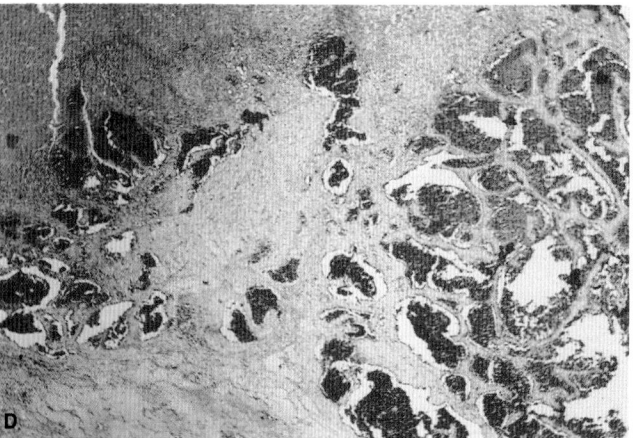

Color Figure 18-10

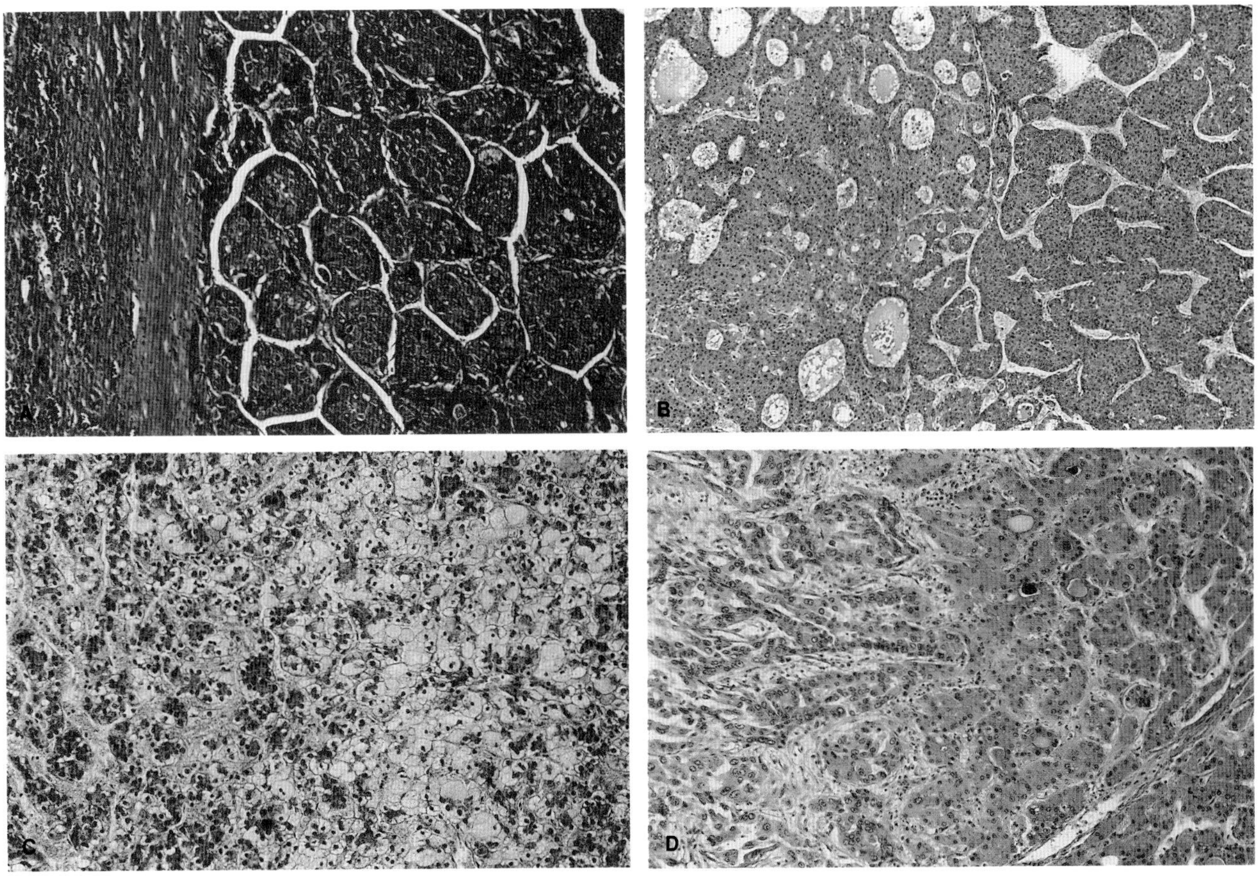

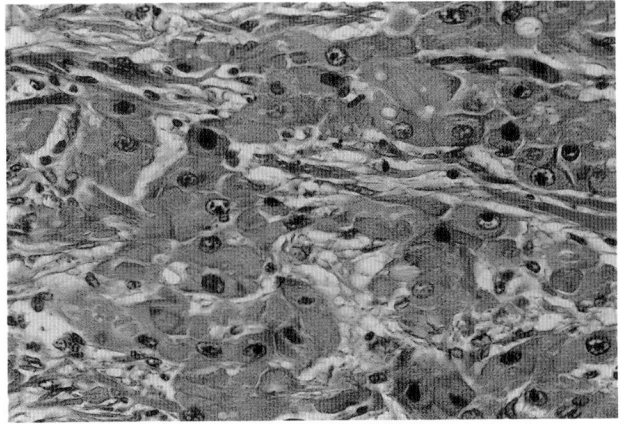

Color Figure 19-3

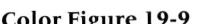

Color Figure 19-9

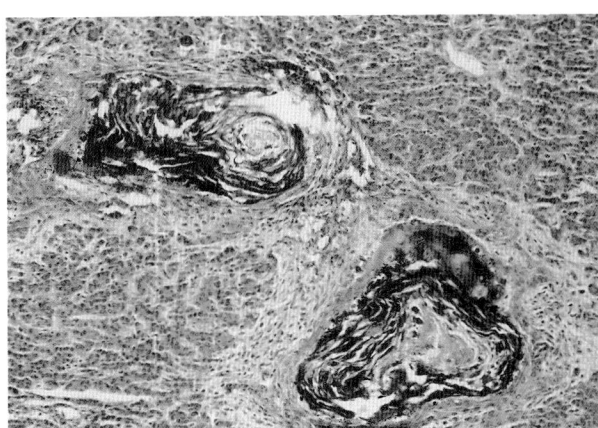

Color Figure 19-11

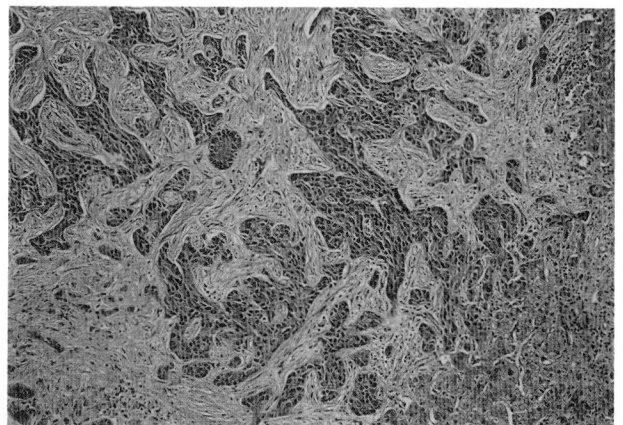

Color Figure 19-12

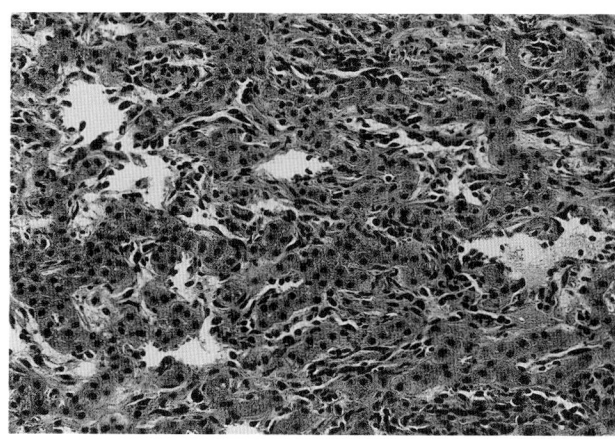

Color Figure 19-15

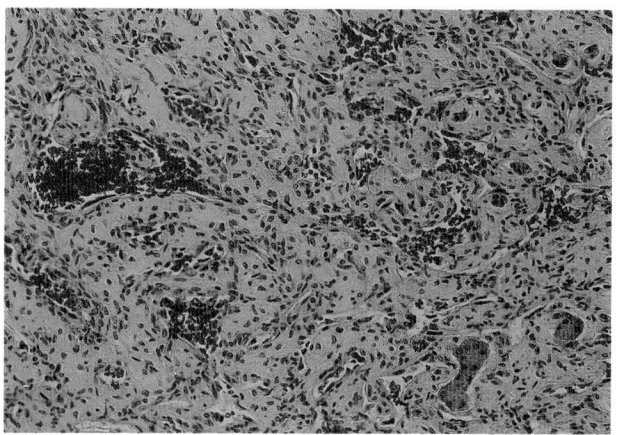

Color Figure 19-17

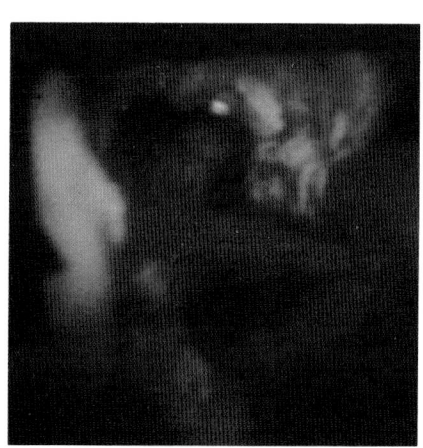

Color Figure 20-4

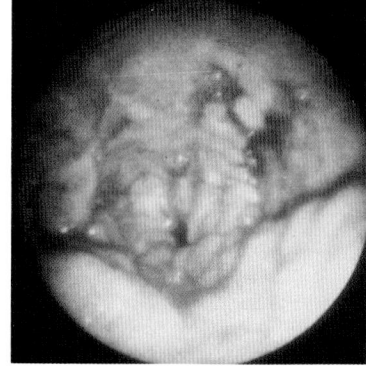

Color Figure 20-5

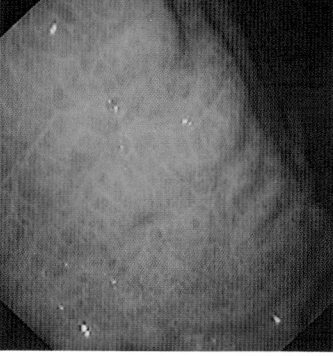

Color Figure 20-6

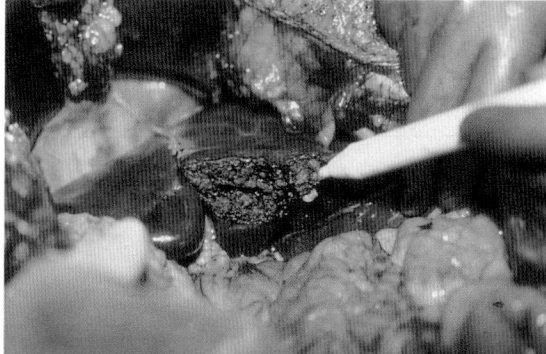

Color Figure 22-12

gallbladder. Moreover, there is considerable evidence that in selected patients with acute cholecystitis, laparoscopic cholecystectomy can be safely performed. The role of this procedure in patients with common duct stone disease remains controversial but undoubtedly will be clarified during the next several years. Other clinical settings in which caution and judgment must be exercised include cirrhosis, portal hypertension, and pregnancy.

Morbidity and Mortality

Potential complications associated with laparoscopic cholecystectomy include problems secondary to development of a pneumoperitoneum, technical difficulties resulting from catheter placement, and all the pitfalls that have been well documented with open cholecystectomy.

Insufflation of carbon dioxide gas has been associated with hypotension, bradycardia, cardiac arrhythmia, and hypercarbia. Although the pathophysiology of these disturbances has not been completely elucidated, these complications are likely related to gas emboli, vasovagal reaction, and direct absorption of carbon dioxide. Awareness of these potential complications is particularly important in patients with coexisting cardiopulmonary disease. Careful intraoperative monitoring is clearly mandated; however, the true incidence of complications from pneumoperitoneum remains indeterminate.[93] Complications related to trocar placement include subcutaneous emphysema, abdominal wall bleeding and hematoma, and bowel, bladder, or vascular injury.

In general, complications associated with laparoscopic removal of the gallbladder are similar to open cholecystectomy. The major complications that have been the focal point of discussion include bleeding, bile leakage from the cystic duct stump, and bile duct injury. The true incidence with which major hemorrhage occurs is indeterminate because most such cases can now be effectively managed laparoscopically, without need for conversion. Perhaps the most controversial and elusive issue related to laparoscopic surgery has been the identification of the incidence with which bile duct injury occurs. Numerous reports in the literature have suggested that the risk of bile duct injury during open cholecystectomy is between 0.1% and 0.2%. Early experience with laparoscopic cholecystectomy suggested that the incidence of bile duct injury was perhaps 10 times as great. There is a learning curve associated with this technology, and more recent reports indicate that the incidence of bile duct injury associated with this procedure approximates 0.5%.[94–96] The number of re-

cent reports focusing on this issue suggest that the reported incidence is underestimating this problem.[97–99]

Gallbladder spillage is a common occurrence during laparoscopic cholecystectomy. Although efforts should be spent to prevent this from happening, considerable experience suggests that this rarely is the source of significant morbidity. If spillage of bile and stones does occur, the field should be thoroughly irrigated and attempts made to retrieve the stones as completely as possible.

Role in Acute Cholecystitis

The presence of acute cholecystitis was generally viewed during the early years of laparoscopic cholecystectomy as a contraindication to the procedure. With greater experience, surgeons have come to recognize that this procedure can be performed safely in carefully selected patients. The principles that have evolved over the last several years regarding the timing of open cholecystectomy should be applied to patients being considered for a laparoscopic approach. Practice suggests that patients with a presumptive diagnosis of acute cholecystitis should be admitted to the hospital, with initiation of intravenous hydration and appropriate antibiotics, and operation should be performed within the first 24 to 72 hours. There is little question that laparoscopic cholecystectomy is more difficult to perform in the presence of acute inflammation. Specifically, the combination of adhesions, distention of the gallbladder, and limited visualization of the vascular and ductal structures makes this procedure more challenging in this setting. The available literature focusing on the safety of laparoscopic cholecystectomy for patients with acute cholecystitis represents a selected population, and some caution needs to be exercised in extrapolation of data. Surgeons performing this procedure in the setting of acute cholecystitis should be experienced in this technique, should recognize that the procedure takes longer to complete, and should be prepared to convert to an open procedure. The conversion rate to open cholecystectomy for patients with acute cholecystitis approaches 26%, as compared with 5% in patients with chronic cholecystitis. Nonetheless, laparoscopic cholecystectomy can be safely performed with minimal morbidity and mortality in patients with acute inflammation if care and judgment are exercised. Laparoscopic cholecystectomy should not be undertaken in the setting of acute cholecystitis until the surgeon has had sufficient experience with more routine cases. Regardless of the experience of the individual surgeon, one should have a relatively low threshold for conversion to an open procedure.

Role of Preoperative Endoscopic Retrograde Cholangiopancreatography

Common bile duct stones are present in 8% to 15% of all patients with cholelithiasis who undergo cholecystectomy. In patients older than 65 years of age, the incidence of choledocholithiasis increases to 50%. For many years, the management of these patients was straightforward, with common bile duct exploration and stone extraction being performed at the time of cholecystectomy. The advent of endoscopic retrograde cholangiopancreatography (ERCP) has revolutionized our approach to these patients, and many such persons have been treated primarily with endoscopic stone removal and sphincterotomy.

Common bile duct stones can be documented preoperatively, at the time of surgery, or after an operative procedure. Considerable controversy exists regarding the optimal perioperative management of a patient with suspected common bile duct stones. In this era of laparoscopic cholecystectomy, many surgeons have opted for preoperative ERCP and stone extraction. The rationale for this approach is based on the difficulty of laparoscopic stone extraction. Preoperative ERCP and stone removal can be performed safely with minimal morbidity and mortality and can obviate the need for a protracted operation.[100,101] Additional data suggest that this approach can be more cost-effective than conventional management strategies. A disadvantage of this approach is the performance of an unnecessary procedure with some risk, albeit minimal, in a large number of patients. In addition, the long-term effects of sphincterotomy remain unclear.

Medical Dissolution

For centuries, physicians have been intrigued by the prospect of definitively managing symptomatic gallstones without resorting to operative intervention. Genuine progress in this quest required a clearer understanding of the pathogenesis of this disorder. The description of the physicochemical basis of gallstone disease paved the way for a group of investigators in the early 1970s to develop agents effective in cholesterol gallstone dissolution.[102,103] The first agent used was the primary bile acid, chenodeoxycholic acid (CDCA). The efficacy of CDCA is based on its ability to reduce lithogenicity and the degree of cholesterol saturation of bile by selectively inhibiting HMG-CoA reductase (rate-limiting enzyme in cholesterol biosynthesis). The efficacy of CDCA was defined by data published in 1981 by the National Cooperative Gallstone Study Group.[104] In this controlled, prospective, randomized study of more than 900 patients, complete gallstone dissolution

was achieved in only 14%, and partial response in an additional 28%. The utility of this drug is further limited by the need for at least 9 months of intensive therapy in most cases, propensity for stone recurrence when therapy is discontinued, adverse effect of dietary cholesterol, potential toxicity and side effects, and high cost. CDCA therapy is often associated with diarrhea, and about 25% of patients experience a transient elevation of hepatic transaminases.

In the early 1970s, serendipity led to the discovery that an over-the-counter drug widely used in Japan for its tonic effects was effective in dissolving cholesterol gallstones. Ursodeoxycholic acid (UDCA), now commercially available (Actigal), was initially thought to be a more effective dissolution agent than CDCA. Its mechanism of action differs from CDCA and probably relates to specific effects on micellar stability, nucleation, and cholesterol absorption from the gut. Although uncontrolled studies suggested that gallstone dissolution occurred in up to 75% of patients treated with UDCA, more recent experience suggests that the rate of dissolution in selected patients approaches 50%. The toxicity and side effects associated with UDCA administration are significantly less than with CDCA. Unfortunately, stone recurrence occurs at the rate of 10% per year for the first 5 years after discontinuation of either CDCA or UDCA. Thus, the clinical indications for these drugs are limited.

Lovastatin, a potent inhibitor of HMG-CoA reductase, is effective in reducing both biliary cholesterol levels and bile lithogenicity in patients with hypercholesterolemia. These findings led to a preliminary study in which the efficacy of lovastatin in achieving gallstone dissolution was assessed in a dietary animal model of cholesterol gallstones. The results of this study indicated that, despite an ongoing lithogenic stimulus, this agent induced gallstone dissolution in 28% of animals.[105] Further studies are needed to define the efficacy and role of these agents in the management of patients with gallstones. It has been estimated that only 10% of all patients in the United States with gallstones are suitable candidates for oral dissolution therapy. The clinical utility of these agents is particularly limited by cost (about $1500 per year) and recurrence rates (50% in 5 years). To date, medical dissolution of gallstones has been limited to stones composed of cholesterol. Studies are underway to identify agents capable of dissolving pigment gallstones.

Contact Dissolution

Percutaneous transhepatic cholangiography provided the basis and rationale for the development of direct contact dissolution. This procedure, also known as percutaneous transhepatic cholecystolitholysis, was introduced in the 1980s as a nonoperative alternative for the management of patients with symptomatic gallstones.[106] Under local anesthesia, a pigtail catheter is placed percutaneously through the parenchyma of the liver into the gallbladder (Fig. 12-14). This can be done using fluoroscopic or ultrasonographic guidance. Appropriate agents can then be infused directly into the gallbladder and affect dissolution. The efficacy of this invasive procedure is limited in part by catheter-related complications, including bleeding and bile leakage.

The drug of choice for contact dissolution is MTBE. This agent is an aliphatic ether, which is a potent solvent for cholesterol and can rapidly induce dissolution. It is important to aspirate the contents of the gallbladder at a defined time after infusion of this drug. Failure to minimize the amount of drug escaping from the gallbladder into the duodenum has been associated with transient abdominal pain, emesis, and duodenitis. Patient selection is essential for a satisfactory outcome, and specific criteria include the presence of cholesterol gallstones and a patent cystic duct. In carefully selected patients, MTBE can be particularly effective, although multiple treatments may be required (Fig. 12-15). Unfortunately, stones recur at a rate of about 10% per year, reaching a plateau at 60% at 5 years.

Biliary Lithotripsy

Based on a large and satisfactory experience in patients with nephroureterolithiasis, electrohydraulic shock-wave lithotripsy (ESWL) was hailed by many as a potential panacea for the nonoperative management of patients with symptomatic gallstone disease. Shock waves, composed of high and low frequencies, are generated by electromagnetically produced deflections of a membrane, underwater spark discharges, or piezoelec-tric crystals. It is these shock waves that are able to cause fragmentation. Potential advantages of ESWL include high patient compliance and acceptance, avoidance of surgical incision and associated pain and disability, and avoidance of potential surgical complications.

Practical concerns have focused on the potential for small fragments to cause biliary colic, acute cholecystitis, or gallstone pancreatitis and the inability to increase bile flow significantly (analogous to hydration affecting increased urine output). Numerous studies have attempted to define specific criteria for patient selection based on stone composition, size, number, volume, and amount of calcium.[107,108] Based on available selection criteria (Table 12-4), studies performed in the United States and in Europe suggest that only about 20% of patients with gallstones are suitable candidates for ESWL.[109,110]

Fragmentation can be achieved in most carefully selected patients. Clearance of fragments can require considerable time, and data suggest that 90% of patients need up to 18 months to achieve complete stone and fragment disappearance.[111] Treatment outcome in these patients is enhanced by adjuvant therapy with oral dissolution agents. Because the gallbladder remains intact, it is not surprising the reported recurrence rate after successful ESWL is comparable to other nonoperative modalities, 50% at 5 years. The role of biliary lithotripsy is poorly defined at this time. In 1992, a National Institutes of Health Consensus Conference was convened to examine treatment strategies for the management of gallstone disease. The conclusions were that open cholecystectomy remains the gold standard of therapy and that laparoscopic cholecystectomy is safe and effective (Table 12-5). The charge for the future is to maximize safety and cost-effectiveness of the laparoscopic approach.

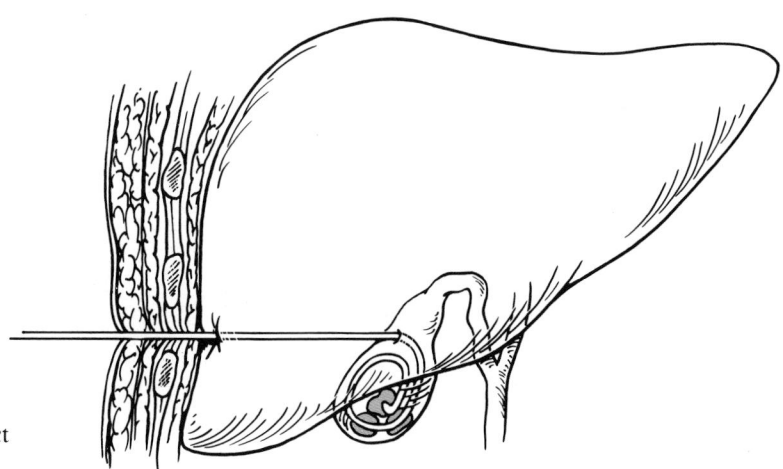

Figure 12-14 Technique employed for contact dissolution with instillation of MTBE.

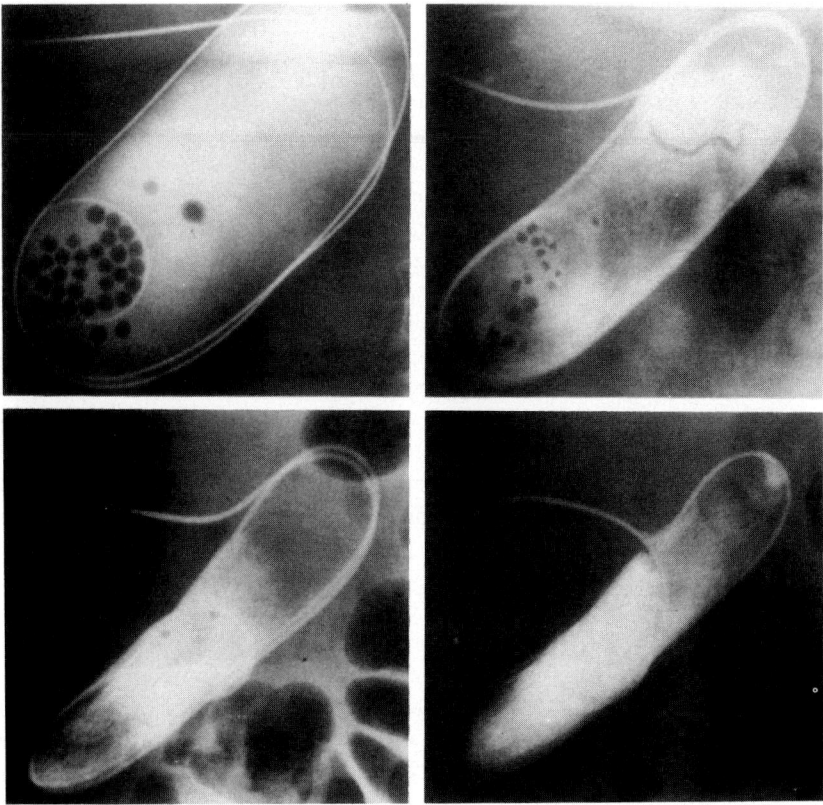

Figure 12-15 Dissolution of small stones by instillation of MTBE. (After Thistle JL, May GR, Bender CE, et al. Dissolution of cholesterol gallbladder stones by methyl tert-butyl ether administered by percutaneous transhepatic catheter. N Engl J Med 1989;320:633)

GALLSTONE DISEASE IN SPECIFIC CLINICAL SETTINGS

Acalculous Cholecystitis

Acute acalculous cholecystitis accounts for less than 5% of all patients undergoing surgery on the biliary tract. This interesting clinical entity is most commonly observed in patients in the intensive care unit after trauma, burns, or surgery. The precise pathogenesis of this disorder is unclear, although a number of etiologies have been proposed. Current dogma suggests that this is a multifactorial disease, with different factors playing a greater or lesser role, based on the specific clinical setting. The two most significant factors appear to be biliary stasis as a consequence of decreased gallbladder

stimulation, ampullary spasm or obstruction, or cystic duct obstruction, and increased viscosity of bile due to dehydration or multiple transfusions. The combination of these factors probably leads to altered metabolism of unidentified substances that initiate a cascade of events resulting in acute inflammation of the gallbladder.

The diagnosis of acalculous cholecystitis is challenging and often elusive. The key to expeditious diagnosis is a high index of suspicion. In the proper clinical setting, development of abdominal pain or a picture of sepsis should trigger consideration of this diagnosis.

Table 12-4   Exclusion Criteria for Electrohydraulic Shock-Wave Biliary Lithotripsy

More than three stones
Very large or calcified stones
Nonfunctioning gallbladder
Complications from gallstone disease

Table 12-5   Conclusions About Gallstones and Laparoscopic Cholecystectomy: National Institutes of Health Consensus Conference, September 14–16, 1992

Open cholecystectomy remains the standard.
Oral bile acid therapy, with or without electrohydraulic shock-wave lithotripsy, is less effective.
Contact dissolution has limited clinical applicability.
Laparoscopic cholecystectomy is safe and effective.
Efforts should be spent to maximize safety and cost-effectiveness of laparoscopic cholcystectomy.

Because many of these patients have had a recent operative procedure or have sustained a major insult, physical examination can be difficult to assess. Ultrasonography can be helpful in providing further support for the clinician's impression.[112] Conventional biliary scintigraphy has not proved to be of particular benefit in patients suspected of acalculous disease. In a series of reports, the use of indium-labeled leukocyte imaging and morphine-augmented cholescintigraphy has been advocated in the evaluation of patients suspected of having acalculous disease.[113,114] Ultimately, cholecystectomy may be required to establish or refute the diagnosis of acalculous cholecystitis. Most reports indicate that the mortality rate for this disease is significant. This probably relates to the underlying disorders and the delay in diagnosis leading to a more acute and complex situation. After stabilization, definitive management can be accomplished by cholecystectomy, open cholecystostomy, or percutaneous cholecystostomy, depending on the condition of the patient and the presence or absence of gangrene of the gallbladder wall.

Cholecystitis in the Elderly

The incidence of acute cholecystitis appears to be increasing in all groups of patients, particularly in those older than 70 years of age. It remains unclear whether this trend is due to an evolution in the disease process or merely to an evolving health care system. The clinical presentation of the elderly with acute cholecystitis is much more varied than in younger patients. The atypical presentation that so often occurs in this age group mandates a high index of clinical suspicion. Although abdominal pain is the most constant complaint in these patients, many present with fever, nausea and emesis, palpable abdominal mass, or jaundice. Perhaps most alarming is the report suggesting that up to 12% of elderly patients with acute cholecystitis present in septic shock.[115] Considerable data suggest that the incidence of severe complications of cholecystitis, such as choledocholithiasis, gallbladder perforation, emphysematous cholecystitis, and septic problems in general, is greater in the elderly than in younger patients. The mortality rate for cholecystectomy is higher in elderly patients than younger patients and is especially increased in the group undergoing urgent or emergent cholecystectomy. Whether these findings are due to differences in disease presentation or reflect delays in operation because of physician reluctance to refer elderly patients for elective surgery remains unclear. In general, elderly patients with acute cholecystitis are best treated by rapid resuscitation and evaluation followed by timely cholecystectomy.

Cirrhosis and Gallstones

Although moderate consumption of alcohol can have a relative protective effect in terms of cholesterol gallstone formation, cirrhosis of the liver has been associated with a significant increased incidence of pigment gallstones.[116,117] The exact cause of these stones is unclear, but altered bile acid metabolism has been implicated as an important factor. Regardless of the type of gallstones present, cholecystectomy in cirrhotic patients has been associated with significant morbidity and mortality rates. In most cases, the difficulties arise from hemorrhage as a consequence of portal hypertension and coagulopathy. A prolonged prothrombin time is a major risk factor in most series. Indications for operative intervention should be stringent, and careful consideration should be given to the perioperative risk in each individual patient. Operation should be undertaken only in patients who have symptoms and who are reasonable operative risks. Cirrhosis is not an absolute contraindication to laparoscopic cholecystectomy, although appropriate judgment should be exercised in patient selection. Much of the operative bleeding problems can be obviated by partial cholecystectomy, in which the posterior wall of the gallbladder is cauterized and left in situ. This avoids inadvertent dissection into the substance of the liver.

Gallstones and Diabetes

Adults with diabetes mellitus have an increased prevalence of cholesterol gallstones. This presumably results from specific alterations in biliary metabolism, leading to hepatic secretion of cholesterol-saturated bile, and perhaps to some extent from gallbladder dysmotility and biliary stasis. For many years, it had been generally agreed that elective cholecystectomy was indicated in the asymptomatic diabetic with gallstones on the basis of an increased risk of significant septic complications. Clinical experience suggests that emphysematous and gangrenous cholecystitis are much more common among diabetic males than the general population. In contrast, the incidence of gallbladder perforation, wound infection, and overall morbidity and mortality rates were not significantly different in a review of 175 diabetic and nondiabetic patients undergoing cholecystectomy.[118] The role of prophylactic cholecystectomy in the diabetic with asymptomatic gallstones remains unclear.

OTHER GALLBLADDER DISORDERS

Porcelain Gallbladder

Although porcelain gallbladder is believed to be a complication of recurrent attacks of gallstone disease, most of these patients have no symptoms when they come to the attention of a physician. Often, the evaluation is prompted by a suspicious mass noted on physical examination or the incidental discovery of a calcified gallbladder (see Fig. 12-6). Regardless of symptoms, cholecystectomy is strongly recommended because of the reported 25% to 50% risk of adenocarcinoma.[119]

Hyperplastic Cholecystoses

Hyperplastic cholecystoses refers to a family of disorders, of which adenomyomatosis and cholesterolosis are the two most common, characterized by proliferation of normal components of the gallbladder wall. Lesions of multiple origins may be present in the same patient, and the distribution can be localized or generalized throughout the gallbladder. Gallstones are present in about half of patients with hyperplastic cholecystoses.

Adenomyomatosis represents a spectrum of disorders in which there is either localized or generalized hyperplasia of the mucosa and muscular layers of the gallbladder. Adenomyomas are typically sessile lesions located in the fundus.

Cholesterolosis is an interesting clinical entity of unknown etiology that is characterized by deposition of cholesterol esters and lipids in the gallbladder epithelium. Although there is no link with systemic disorders of cholesterol metabolism, most of these patients have a significantly increased amount of cholesterol in bile as compared with normal patients without gallstones. Although these lesions may be focal, the classic example of cholesterolosis is the "strawberry gallbladder," in which there are yellowish protrusions laden with cholesterol covering the surface of the gallbladder.

The frequency with which symptoms exist in patients with hyperplastic cholecystoses remains poorly defined. Most authors think that any symptoms are in fact due to the presence of gallstones. There is little evidence that oral dissolution agents are of any benefit in these patients, and cholecystectomy is generally reserved for patients with demonstrable symptoms and gallstones.

REFERENCES

1. Glen F, Grafe WR Jr. Historical events in biliary tract surgery. Arch Surg 1966;93:848.
2. LaMorte WW, Schoetz DJ Jr, Birkett DH, et al. The role of the gallbladder in the pathogenesis of cholesterol gallstones. Gastroenterology 1979;77:580.
3. Hermann RE. Surgery for acute and chronic cholecystitis. Surg Clin North Am 1990;70:1263.
4. Langenbuch C. Ein fall von Exstirpation der Gallenblase wegen Chroniser Cholelithiasis. Berl Clin Wochenschr 1882;19:725.
5. DuBois F, Icard P, Berthelot G, Levard H. Coelioscopic cholecystectomy: preliminary report of 36 cases. Ann Surg 1990;211:60.
6. Reddick EA, Olsen DO. Laparoscopic laser cholecystectomy: a comparison with mini-lap cholecystectomy. Surg Endosc 1989;3:131.
7. Madden JL, Vanderheyden L, Kandalaft S. The nature and surgical significance of common duct stones. Surg Gynecol Obstet 1968;126:3.
8. Madden JL. Primary common bile duct stones. World J Surg 1978;2:465.
9. Saharia PC, Zuidema GD, Cameron JL. Primary common bile duct stones. Ann Surg 1977;185:598.
10. Way LW, Admirand WH, Dunphy JE. Management of choledocholithiasis. Ann Surg 1973;176:347.
11. Girard RM, Legros G. Stones in the common bile duct: surgical approaches. In: Blumgart LH, ed. Surgery of the liver and biliary tract. New York, Churchill Livingstone, 1988:577.
12. Maurer KR, Everhart JE, Ezzati TM, et al. Prevalence of gallstone disease in Hispanic populations in the United States. Gastroenterology 1989;96:487.
13. Acalovschi M, Dumitrascu D, Caluser I, Ban A. Comparative prevalence of gallstone disease at 100-year interval in a large Romanian town, a necropsy study. Dig Dis Sci 1987;32:354.
14. Balzer K, Goebell H, Breuer N, Ruping KN, Leder LD. Epidemiology of gallstones in a German industrial town (Essen) from 1940–1975. Digestion 1986;33:189.
15. Sama C, Morselli Labate AM, Taroni F, Barbara L. Epidemiology and natural history of gallstone disease. Semin Liver Dis 1990;10:149.
16. Sampliner RE, Bennett PH, Comess LJ, et al. Gallbladder disease in Pima Indians: demonstration of high prevalence and early onset by cholecystography. N Engl J Med 1970;283:1358.
17. Biss K, Ho KJ, Mikkelson B, et al. Some unique biologic characteristics of the Masai of East Africa. N Engl J Med 1971;284:694.
18. Friedman GD, Kannel WB, Dawber TR. The epidemiology of gallbladder disease: observations in the Framingham Study. J Chronic Dis 1966;19:273.
19. GREPCO. Prevalence of gallstone disease in an Indian adult female population. Am J Epidemiol 1984;119:796.
20. Barbara L, Festi D, Frabboni R, et al. Incidence and risk factors for gallstone disease: the "Sirmione Study." Hepatology 1988;8:1256.
21. Bowen JC, Brenner HI, Ferrante WA, Maule WF. Gallstone disease: pathophysiology, epidemiology, natural history, and treatment options. Med Clin North Am 1992;76:1143.
22. Khalil T, Walker JP, Wiener I, et al. Effect of aging on gallbladder contraction and release of cholecystokinin-33 in humans. Surgery 1985;98:423.
23. Bell CC Jr, McCormick WC III, Gregory DH, et al. Rela-

tionship of bile acid pool size to the formation of litho-genous bile in male Indians of the Southwest. Surg Gynecol Obstet 1972;134:473.

24. Gilat T, Feldman C, Halpern Z, Dan M, Bar-Meir S. An increased familial frequency of gallstones. Gastroenterology 1983;84:242.

25. Jorgensen T, Kay L, Schultz-Larsen K. The epidemiology of gallstones in a 70-year-old Danish population. Scand J Gastroenterol 1990;25:335.

26. Trotman BW, Soloway RD. Pigment vs. cholesterol cholelithiasis: clinical and epidemiologic aspects. Am J Dig Dis 1975;20:735.

27. Boston Collaborative Drug Surveillance Program. Oral contraceptives and venous thromboembolic disease, surgically confirmed gallbladder disease and breast tumors. Lancet 1973;1:1399.

28. Boston Collaborative Drug Surveillance Program. Surgically confirmed gallbladder disease, venous thromboembolism and breast tumors in relation to postmenopausal estrogen therapy. N Engl J Med 1974;190:15.

29. Coronary Drug Project Research Group. Gallbladder disease as a side effect of drugs influencing lipid metabolism: experience in the coronary drug project. N Engl J Med 1977;296:1185.

30. Braverman DZ, Johnson ML, Kern F Jr. Effects of pregnancy and contraceptive steroids on gallbladder function. N Engl J Med 1980;302:362.

31. Nilsson S, Schersten T. Importance of bile acids for phospholipid secretion into human hepatic bile. Gastroenterology 1969;57:525.

32. Bonorris GG, Coyne MJ, Chung A, et al. Mechanism of estrogen-induced saturated bile in the hamster. J Lab Clin Med 1977;90:963.

33. Rim AA, Werner LH, Yserloo VB, et al. Relationship of obesity and disease in 73,532 weight-conscious women. Public Health Rep 1975;90:40.

34. Deitel M, Petrov I. Incidence of symptomatic gallstones after bariatric operations. Surg Gynecol Obstet 1987;164:397.

35. Calhoun R, Willbanks O. Coexistence of gallbladder disease and morbid obesity. Am J Surg 1987;154:655.

36. Schmidt JH, Hocking MP, Rout WR, et al. The case for prophylactic cholecystectomy concomitant with gastric restriction for morbid obesity. Am Surg 1988;54:269.

37. Freeman JB, Meyer PD, Printen KJ, et al. Analysis of gallbladder bile in morbid obesity. Am J Surg 1975;129:163.

38. Mabee TM, Meyer P, DenBesten L, et al. The mechanism of increased gallstone formation in obese human subjects. Surgery 1976;79:460.

39. Iser JH, Maton PN, Murphy GM, et al. Resistance to chenodeoxycholic acid (CDCA) treatment in obese patients with gallstones. Br Med J 1978;1:1509.

40. Yang H, Petersen GM, Roth MP, Schoenfield LJ, Marks JW. Risk factors for gallstone formation during rapid weight loss. Dig Dis Sci 1992;37:912.

41. Shiffman ML, Sugerman HJ, Kellum HJ, Moore EW. Changes in the composition of gallbladder bile following weight reduction and gallstone formation. Gastroenterology 1992;103:214.

42. Shiffman ML, Shamburek RD, Schwartz CC, Sugerman HJ, Kellum JM, Moore EW. Gallbladder mucin, arachidonic acid, and bile lipids in patients who develop gallstones during weight reduction. Gastroenterology 1993;105:1200.

43. Roslyn JJ, Pitt HA, Mann LL, Ament ME, DenBesten L. Gallbladder disease in patients on long-term parenteral nutrition. Gastroenterology 1983;84:148.

44. Roslyn JJ, Berquist WE, Pitt HA, et al. Increased risk of gallstones in children on total parenteral nutrition. Pediatrics 1983;91:784.

45. Pitt HA, King W III, Mann LL, et al. Prolonged parenteral nutrition increases the risk of cholelithiasis. Am J Surg 1983;145:106.

46. Admirand WH, Small DM. The physicochemical basis of cholesterol gallstone formation in man. J Clin Invest 1968;47:1043.

47. Somjen GJ, Gilat T. Contribution of vesicular and micellar carriers to cholesterol transport in human bile. J Lipid Res 1985;26:699.

48. Peled Y, Halpern Z, Baruch R, Goldman G, Gilat T. Cholesterol nucleation from its carriers in human bile. Hepatology 1988;8:914.

49. Holzbach RT, Kibe A, Theil E, et al. Biliary proteins: unique inhibitors of cholesterol crystal nucleation in human gallbladder bile. J Clin Invest 1984;73:35.

50. Burnstein MJ, Ilson RG, Petrunka CN, et al. Evidence for a potent nucleating factor in the gallbladder bile of patients with cholesterol gallstones. Gastroenterology 1983;85:801.

51. Groen AK, Stout JPJ, Drapers JAG, Hoek FJ, Grijm R, Tytgat GNJ. Cholesterol nucleation-influencing activity in T-tube bile. Hepatology 1988;8:347.

52. Doty JE, Pitt HA, Kuchenbecker SL, DenBesten L. Impaired gallbladder emptying before gallstone formation in the prairie dog. Gastroenterology 1983;85:168.

53. Fridhandler TM, Davison JS, Shaffer EA. Defective gallbladder contractility in the ground squirrel and prairie dog during early stages of cholesterol gallstone formation. Gastroenterology 1983;85:830.

54. Pitt HA, Roslyn JJ, Kuchenbecker S, DenBesten L. The role of increased cystic duct resistance in the pathogenesis of cholesterol gallstones. J Surg Res 1981;30:508.

55. Shiffman ML, Moore EW. Defective acidification leads to $CaCO_3$ supersaturation of gallbladder bile in patients with all types of gallstones. Gastroenterology 1988;94:591.

56. Dawes LG, Rege RV. Calcium and calcium binding in human gallstone disease. Arch Surg 1990;125:1606.

57. LaMorte WW, Booker ML, Scott TE, et al. Increases in gallbladder prostaglanding synthesis before the formation of cholesterol gallstones. Surgery 1985;98:445.

58. Nahrwold DL, Rose RC, Ward SP. Abnormalities in gallbladder morphology and function in patients with cholelithiasis. Ann Surg 1976;184:415.

59. LaMont JT, Turner BS, DiBenedetto D, Handin R,

Schafer AI. Arachidonic acid stimulates mucin secretion in prairie dog gallbladder. Am J Physiol 1983;245:G92.

60. Knyrim K, Vakil N. Bile composition, microspheroliths, antinucleating activity, and gallstone calcification. Gastroenterology 1992;103:552.

61. Lee SP, Maher K, Nicholls JF. Origin and fate of biliary sludge. Gastroenterology 1988;94:170.

62. Vitetta L, Sali A, Moritz V, Shaw A, Carson P, Little P. Bacteria and gallstone nucleation. Aust N Z J Surg 1989;59:571.

63. Maki T. Pathogenesis of calcium bilirubinate gallstones: role of *E. coli*, β-glucuronidase and coagulation by inorganic ions, polyelectrolytes, and agitation. Ann Surg 1966;164:190.

64. Gracie WA, Ransohoff DF. The natural history of silent gallstones: the innocent gallstone is not a myth. N Engl J Med 1982;307:798.

65. McSherry CK, Ferstenberg H, Calhoun WF, et al. The natural history of diagnosed gallstone disease in symptomatic and asymptomatic patients. Ann Surg 1985;202:59.

66. Ransohoff DF, Gracie WA. Management of patients with symptomatic gallstones: a quantitative analysis. Am J Med 1990;88:154.

67. Cuccihiaro G, Watters CR, Rossitch JC, Meyers WC. Deaths from gallstone, incidence and associated clinical factors. Ann Surg 1989;209:149.

68. Graham EA, Cole WH. Roentgenologic examination of the gallbladder, preliminary report of a new method utilizing the intravenous injection of tetrabromophenolphthalein. JAMA 1924;82:613.

69. Cooperberg PL, Burhenne HJ. Real-time ultrasonography: diagnostic technique of choice in calculous gallbladder disease. N Engl J Med 1980;302:1277.

70. Ralls PW, Halls J, Lapin SA, et al. Prospective evaluation of the sonographic Murphy sign in suspected acute cholecystitis. JCU 1982;10:113.

71. Barakos JA, Rawls PW, Lapin SA, et al. Cholelithiasis: evaluation with CT. Radiology 1987;162:415.

72. Burnstein MJ, Vassal KP, Strasberg SM. Results of combined biliary drainage and cholecystokinin cholecystography in 81 patients with normal oral cholecystograms. Ann Surg 1982;196:627.

73. Hermann RE. The spectrum of biliary stone disease. Am J Surg 1989;158:171.

74. Diettrich NA, Cacioppo JC, Davis RP. The vanishing elective cholecystectomy: trends and their consequences. Arch Surg 1988;123:810.

75. Reiss R, Nudelman I, Gutman C, Deutsch AA. Changing trends in surgery for acute cholecystitis. World J Surg 1991;14:567.

76. Roslyn JJ, Binns GS, Hughes EX, Saunders KD, Cates JA, Zinner MJ. Open cholecystectomy: a contemporary analysis of 42,474 patients. Ann Surg 1993;218:129.

77. Saunders-Kirkwood KD, Aizen B, Thompson JE Jr, et al. Cholecystectomy: the impact of socioeconomic change. Ann Surg 1992;215:318.

78. Norrby A, Herlin P, Holmin T, et al. Early or delayed cholecystectomy in acute cholecystitis? A clinical trial. Br J Surg 1983;70:163.

79. van der Linden W, Sunzel H. Early versus delayed operation for acute cholecystitis: a controlled clinical trial. Am J Surg 1970;120:7.

80. McGahan JP, Lindfors KK. Percutaneous cholecystostomy: an alternative to surgical cholecystomy for acute cholecystitis? Radiology 1989;173:481.

81. Opie EL. The etiology of acute hemorrhagic pancreatitis. Bull Johns Hopkins Hosp 1901;12:182.

82. Acosta JM, Ledesma CL. Gallstone migration as a cause of acute pancreatitis. N Engl J Med 1974;290:484.

83. Abu-Dalu J, Urca I. Acute cholecystitis with perforation into the peritoneal cavity. Arch Surg 1971;102:108.

84. Williams NF, Scobie TK. Perforation of the gallbladder: analysis of 19 cases. Can Med Assoc J 1976;115:1223.

85. Thornton JR, Heaton KW, Espiner HJ, Eltringham WK. Empyema of the gallbladder: reappraisal of a neglected disease. Gut 1983;24:1183.

86. Reder VA, Fineberg HY, Rosoff CB, White LS. Shorter length of stay for simply cholecystectomy: cost-effectiveness of alternative strategies. Med Care 1983;21:745.

87. Moss G. Discharge within 24 hours of elective cholecystectomy: the first 100 patients. Arch Surg 1986;121:1159.

88. Hall RC. Short hospital stay: two hospital days for cholecystectomy. Am J Surg 1987;154:510.

89. McSherry CK, Glenn F. The incidence and causes of death following surgery for nonmalignant biliary tract disease. Ann Surg 1980;191:271.

90. Glenn F. Trends in surgical treatment of calculous disease of the biliary tract. Surg Gynecol Obstet 1975;140:877.

91. Ganey JB, Johnson PA Jr, Prillaman PE, McSwain GR. Cholecystectomy: clinical experience with a large series. Am J Surg 1986;151:352.

92. Soper NJ, Dunnegan DL. Routine versus selective intraoperative cholangiography during laparoscopic cholecystectomy. World J Surg 1992;16:1133.

93. Wittgen CM, Andrus CH, Fitzgerald SD, et al. Analysis of the hemodynamic and ventilatory effects of laparoscopic cholecystectomy. Arch Surg 1991;126:997.

94. Peters JH, Ellison CE, Innes JT, et al. Safety and efficacy of laparoscopic cholecystectomy: a prospective analysis of 100 initial patients. Ann Surg 1991;213:3.

95. Schirmer BD, Edge SB, Dix J, et al. Laparoscopic cholecystectomy: treatment of choice for symptomatic cholelithiasis. Ann Surg 1991;213:665.

96. Perissat J, Collet D, Belliard R, et al. Laparoscopic cholecystectomy: the state of the art. A report of 700 consecutive cases. World J Surg 1992;16:1074.

97. Davidoff AM, Pappas TN, Murray EA, et al. Mechanisms of major biliary injury during laparoscopic cholecystectomy. Ann Surg 1992;215:196.

98. Moosa AR, Easter DW, van Sonnenberg E, et al. Laparoscopic injuries to the bile duct: a cause for cancer. Ann Surg 1992;59:243.

99. Cates JA, Kallman C, Busuttil R, et al. Biliary complications of laparoscopic cholecystectomy. Am Surg 1993;59:243.

100. Steigmann GV, Pearlman NW, Goff JS, Sun JH, Norton LW. Endoscopic cholangiography and stone removal prior to cholecystectomy. Arch Surg 1989;124:787.

101. Boulay J, Schellenberg R, Brady PG. Role of ERCP and therapeutic biliary endoscopy in association in laparoscopic cholecystectomy. Am J Gastroenterol 1992;87:837.

102. Thistle JL, Schoenfield LJ. Induced alterations in the composition of bile of persons having cholelithiasis. Gastroenterology 1971;61:488.

103. Danzinger RG, Hoffmann AE, Schoenfield LJ, et al. Dissolution of cholesterol gallstones by chenodeoxycholic acid. N Engl J Med 1972;288:1.

104. Schoenfield LJ, Lachin JM, the Steering Committee and the National Gallstone Study Group. Chenodiol (chenodeoxycholic acid) for dissolution of gallstones: the National Cooperative Gallstone Study. Ann Intern Med 1981;95:257.

105. Saunders KD, Cates JA, Abedin MZ, Roslyn JJ. Lovastatin and gallstone dissolution: a preliminary study. Surgery 1993;113:28.

106. Thistle JL, May GR, Bender CE, et al. Dissolution of cholesterol gallbladder stones by methyl tert-butyl ether administered by percutaneous transhepatic catheter. N Engl J Med 1989;320:633.

107. Arends T, Nemcek AA, Rege RV, et al. The effect of volume and number on fragmentation of gallstones by lithotripsy. J Surg Res 1990;48:279.

108. Sackmann M, Delius M, Sauerbruch T, et al. Shock wave lithotripsy of gallbladder stones: the first 175 patients. N Engl J Med 1988;318:393.

109. Magnuson TH, Lillemoe KD, Pitt HA. How many Americans will be eligible for biliary lithotripsy? Arch Surg 1980;124:1185.

110. Bass EB, Steinbert EP, Pitt HA, et al. Cost-effectiveness of extracorporeal shock-wave lithotripsy versus cholecystectomy for symptomatic gallstones. Gastroenterology 1991;101:189.

111. Burnett D, Ertan A, Jones R, et al. Use of external shock-wave lithotripsy and adjuvant ursoliol for treatment of radiolucent gallstones: a national multicenter study. Dig Dis Sci 1989;34:1011.

112. Imhof M, Raunest J, Ohmann CH, Roher HD. Acute acalculous cholecystitis complicating trauma: a prospective sonographic study. World J Surg 1992;16:1160.

113. Fink-Bennett D, Clarke K, Tsai D, et al. Indium-111 leukocyte imaging in acute cholecystitis. J Nucl Med 1991;32:803.

114. Fink-Bennett D, Balan H, Robbins T, Tsai D. Morphine-augmented cholescintigraphy: its efficacy in detecting acute cholecystitis. J Nucl Med 1991;32:1231.

115. Hafif A, Gutman M, Kaplan O, Winkler E, Rozin RR, Skornick Y. The management of acute cholecystitis in elderly patients. Am Surg 1991;57:648.

116. Bouchier IAD. Postmortem study of the frequency of gallstones in patients with cirrhosis of the liver. Gut 1969;10:705.

117. Nicholas P, Rinaudo PA, Conn HO. Increased incidence of cholelithiasis in Laennec's cirrhosis: a postmortem evaluation of pathogenesis. Gastroenterology 1972;63:112.

118. Walsch DB, Eckhauser FE, Ramsburg SR, et al. Risk associated with diabetes mellitus in patients undergoing gallbladder surgery. Surgery 1982;91:254.

119. Berk RN, Armbuster T, Salzstein S. Carcinoma of the gallbladder associated with the porcelain gallbladder. Radiology 1972;106:29.

Digestive Tract Surgery: A Text and Atlas, edited by Richard H. Bell,
Layton F. Rikkers, and Michael W. Mulholland.
Lippincott-Raven Publishers, Philadelphia, © 1996.

13

Choledocholithiasis and Cholangitis

Sean Tierney | *Henry A. Pitt*

CHOLEDOCHOLITHIASIS

The percentage of patients with gallstones who also have common duct stones increases with age. The incidence of associated choledocholithiasis is below 5% in patients who are in their third decade but over 80% in patients who are in their ninth decade. Choledocholithiasis historically has been the most common cause of cholangitis in Western societies, whereas hepatolithiasis is the most frequent cause of so-called Oriental cholangitis in East Asia. This chapter discusses the pathogenesis and management of choledocholithiasis, cholangitis, and intrahepatic stones.

Pathogenesis and Classification

Source

Common bile duct stones can be classified as either primary or secondary. Primary duct stones develop within the biliary ductal system, whereas secondary stones are formed within the gallbladder and subsequently pass into the ducts. The distinction between primary and secondary stones is important because significant differences exist in their pathogenesis and management. In the United States, about 50% to 85% of common duct stones are secondary and only a small percentage form primarily in the bile ducts.[1]

Primary Duct Stones

In Western populations, primary bile duct stones typically occur in patients with sphincter of Oddi dysfunction, benign biliary strictures, sclerosing cholan-

gitis, or cystic dilatation of the bile ducts. These conditions are characterized by bile stasis, which promotes the overgrowth of bacteria. The results of bile cultures are positive in up to 90% of patients with primary brown pigment stones.[2] The bacteria produce the enzymes phospholipase A_1, which releases free fatty acids from biliary phospholipids, β-glucuronidase, which deconjugates bilirubin glucuronide, and hydrolase, which deconjugates bile acids.[3] Free fatty acids and deconjugated bilirubin and bile acids are poorly soluble at typical biliary pH levels and precipitate, forming insoluble calcium salts. Cholesterol also is rendered insoluble because of the loss of bile acids and phospholipid from bile.

Insoluble biliary lipids and calcium salts form sludge, to which is added mucin and dead bacterial cytoskeletons, promoting stone growth (Fig. 13-1). The result is the formation of brown pigment stones, which characteristically contain significant amounts of fatty acids as calcium palmitate, and more cholesterol than black pigment stones (Fig. 13-2). Brown pigment stones are uncommon in Western populations, accounting for as little as 1% of gallbladder stones,[2] but are considerably more prevalent in Asian populations, where they often are found in the intrahepatic ducts.

Secondary Stones

Secondary bile duct stones, which form in the gallbladder, represent the typical spectrum of cholesterol and black pigment stones. In the United States, about 75% of gallbladder stones are cholesterol stones, whereas 20% to 25% are black pigment stones.[4] Bacte-

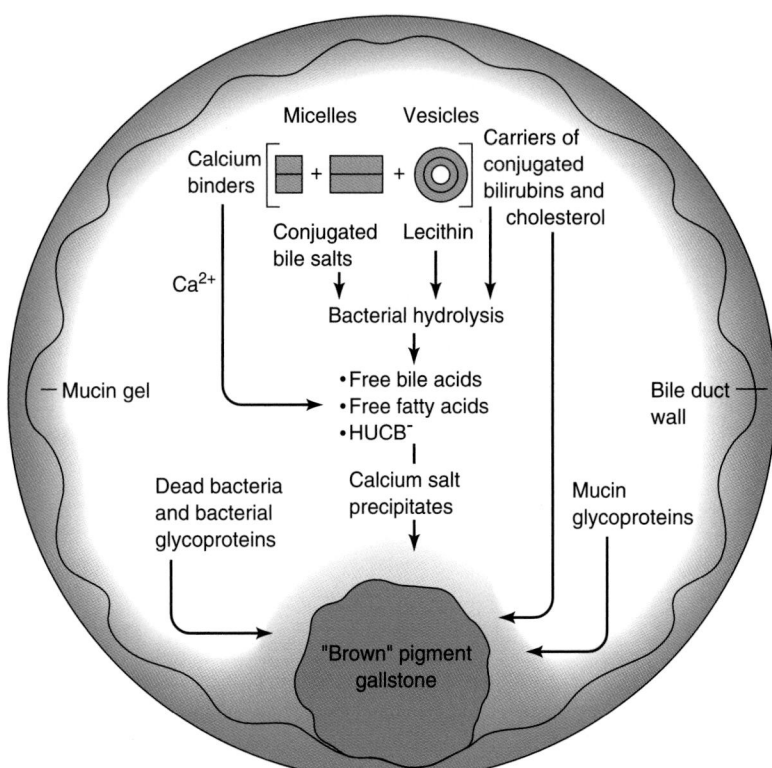

Figure 13-1 Pathogenesis of brown pigment stones in the common bile duct. (After Carey MC. Pathogenesis of gallstones. Recent Prog Med 1992;83:379)

ria have been identified on the surface, but not in the core, of both cholesterol and black pigment stones formed in the gallbladder.[2] Thus, infection does not play a pivotal role in the formation of these two stone types. The three prerequisites for cholesterol gallstone formation are unphysiologic cholesterol supersaturation, biliary stasis, and accelerated crystal nucleation.[3]

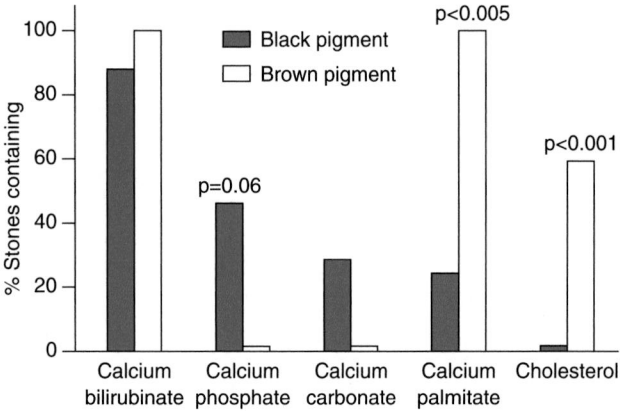

Figure 13-2 Relative proportions of different calcium salts in pigment stones. (After Kaufman HS, Magnuson TH, Lillemoe KD, Frasca P, Pitt HA. The role of bacteria in gallbladder and common duct stone formation. Ann Surg 1989;209: 584)

Gender, parity, obesity, weight loss, and, perhaps, genetics also are important risk factors. Black pigment stones develop in patients in whom bilirubin excretion is increased as a result of hemolytic disorders, in patients with ileal disorders, in patients with cirrhosis, and in patients with profound gallbladder stasis such as occurs during prolonged fasting or long-term parenteral nutrition.[5]

Diagnosis

The overall incidence of gallstones in the United States is estimated at 10% to 20%, and increases to 40% in the elderly.[6] Most patients with stones in the gallbladder do not have symptoms. Asymptomatic individuals have a 1% to 3% risk of developing symptoms and complications each year. Surprisingly, patients with choledocholithiasis also may not have symptoms for a long time. In one autopsy series of 615 patients older than 60 years, stones were found in the bile duct in 1% of patients.[7] These stones also may pass through the sphincter of Oddi and be evacuated without causing symptoms.

Clinical Findings

Common duct stones usually cause symptoms when they create obstruction. The clinical presentation depends on the level and degree of obstruction, and on the presence or absence of biliary infection. Simple obstruction of the common duct results in right upper quadrant abdominal pain and jaundice. Typically, jaundice and pain due to common duct stones are more transient or intermittent than when biliary obstruction is due to malignancy. The principal findings on physical examination are tenderness in the right upper quadrant and jaundice. Cholangitis supervenes if obstruction of bile flow occurs in the presence of infected bile. The presentation of cholangitis is discussed in detail later.

Pancreatitis develops when gallstones cause temporary or sustained obstruction of the ampulla of Vater. Opie,[8] a pathologist, first identified the fact that gallstones cause pancreatitis. At autopsy, he found the ampulla of a patient to be obstructed by an impacted gallstone. In most patients, however, gallstone pancreatitis is precipitated by transient obstruction of the ampulla by a migratory stone. Pancreatitis also may result from transient ampullary obstruction by cholesterol crystals or sludge from the gallbladder.[9]

Gallstones are responsible for up to 50% of all cases of pancreatitis, and 4% to 8% of patients with gallstones have gallstone pancreatitis.[10,11] Most patients with gallstone pancreatitis experience a mild, self-limited attack from which they recover in a few days. However, a few have severe pancreatitis with peripancreatic necrosis, infection, or pseudocyst formation. Patients with gallstone pancreatitis also are likely to have a recurrent attack within a few months[10]; therefore, early intervention in the form of surgical or endoscopic therapy is indicated for these severely ill patients.

Laboratory Results

Common bile duct stones are present in 10% to 15% of patients with gallstones. The incidence varies with age and is about 5% in younger patients and 20% in older patients with gallstones. Accurate identification of these patients is essential to prevent unnecessary common duct exploration and to reduce the incidence of retained stones after cholecystectomy. The diagnosis may be apparent when patients have cholangitis or pancreatitis. However, in many patients undergoing cholecystectomy, the presence of common duct stones may not be apparent from the signs and symptoms. Several studies have attempted to identify specific factors that predict the presence of silent common duct stones in patients undergoing cholecystectomy[12–14] (Table 13-1).

The results of liver function tests and pancreatic enzyme determinations may be normal in patients with common bile duct stones.[12] However, elevation of the serum bilirubin level can be a useful indicator of the presence of choledocholithiasis. The likelihood of finding stones in the common duct increases as the level of serum bilirubin rises. Stones are found in one third of patients when the preoperative serum bilirubin level is greater than 1.3 mg/dL,[14] in two thirds of patients when it is greater than 3 mg/dL,[13] and in almost all patients when it is greater than 6.7 mg/dL.[12]

An elevated serum alkaline phosphatase level also is a useful predictor of choledocholithiasis. The incidence of common duct stones is 46% when the alkaline phosphatase level is above 200 IU/L, and 58% when it is above 250 IU/L.[13] In one study,[14] common duct stones were found in 40% of patients when both bilirubin and alkaline phosphatase levels were elevated, and in less than 5% of patients when both these parameters were normal.

The white blood cell count, serum amylase level, and liver transaminase levels are of no help in identifying patients with silent common duct stones,[13,14] even though these may be elevated in patients with cholangitis or pancreatitis. A history of jaundice and a dilated common bile duct are important factors to be considered in detecting otherwise silent common duct stones (see Table 13-1). The characteristic laboratory findings among patients with cholangitis are discussed later.

Radiologic Findings

Although abnormal laboratory test results may be suggestive, the most reliable means of detecting a common duct stone is cholangiography. However, the cost and morbidity of invasive cholangiography preclude its use as a screening test. Several radiologic techniques are available as alternatives for the diagnosis of common duct stones. Some of these techniques also offer the opportunity for treatment of choledocholithiasis, allowing therapy to be tailored for each individual patient.

PREOPERATIVE

ULTRASOUND. Ultrasound is an inexpensive, noninvasive, and readily available method for investigating the biliary tree. Ultrasound is about 97% accurate in diagnosing gallstones in the gallbladder in the elective setting, and 80% to 85% accurate in the presence of acute cholecystitis. Similarly, ultrasound can predict common bile duct dilatation with an accuracy of about 90%.[15] Several studies have shown that common bile duct dilatation is a useful predictor of choledocholithiasis,[14] but others have reported that stones are found in only 14% to 20% of patients when all other predictors are excluded.[12] Ultrasound is not as successful in directly demonstrating common duct stones. Several fac-

Table 13-1   Predictors of Common Bile Duct Stones

Percentage With Stones	Bilirubin (>1.3 mg/dL)	Alkaline Phosphatase (>39 IU/L)	History of Jaundice	Common Bile Duct Diameter (>12 mm)
5	−	−	−	−
33	+	−	−	−
40	+	+	−	−
100	+	+	−	+
100	+	+	+	+

+, feature present; −, feature absent.
(Adapted from Lacaine F, Corlette MB, Bismuth H. Preoperative evaluation of the risk of common bile duct stones. Arch Surg 1980;115:1114)

tors militate against the detection of small stones in the common bile duct by ultrasound[16]:

1. Gas in the duodenum can obscure the distal common bile duct.
2. The sound beam can be reflected and refracted by the curved wall of the duct.
3. The common duct may lie beyond the optimal focal zone of the high-frequency transducers needed to visualize small stones.

Most series report the sensitivity of sonography in detecting common duct stones to be in the range of 15% to 30%.

The sensitivity of ultrasound in detecting common duct stones is increased to between 80% and 100% when the ultrasonic transducer is introduced into the duodenum using the endoscope.[17] A high-frequency (7.5- to 12-MHz) ultrasonic probe is passed into the duodenum under endoscopic guidance, and a water-filled balloon is used to enhance acoustic coupling. The high frequency limits the effective imaging range of the transducer to 6 cm. The distal bile duct is visualized by positioning the transducer at the level of the ampulla, and the proximal common bile duct and hepatic duct are visualized through the wall in the first part of the duodenum. In one series of 52 patients, 17 (33%) of whom had choledocholithiasis, endoscopic ultrasound was found to have a sensitivity and specificity of 100% in the detection of common bile duct stones.[18] In a preliminary report, 3 of 4 patients with choledocholithiasis, and all 16 patients with stone-free ducts were correctly identified.[17]

COMPUTED TOMOGRAPHY. Computed tomography (CT) also is an excellent technique for detecting bile duct obstruction by demonstrating dilatation of the intrahepatic or extrahepatic ducts.[19] CT is a more sensitive detector of common duct stones (75% to 90%) than

is ultrasound.[20,21] It has been proposed that the sensitivity of CT scanning for ductal stones can be improved by administering intravenous or oral biliary contrast,[22] but this technique has not been widely applied. CT also is an important tool in the evaluation of patients with jaundice by identifying the level of biliary obstruction and the presence or absence of a pancreatic mass.

CHOLANGIOGRAPHY. Cholangiography remains the gold standard in the diagnosis of choledocholithiasis. Several routes have been used to introduce contrast into the common bile duct for preoperative cholangiography. Formerly, intravenous cholangiography was the only method available for preoperative assessment of the bile duct. However, low diagnostic accuracy, poor visualization of the ductal system, concerns about allergic reactions, and the availability of percutaneous and endoscopic cholangiography have rendered intravenous cholangiography obsolete.[23] Endoscopic retrograde cholangiopancreatography (ERCP) and percutaneous transhepatic cholangiography (PTC) are the most accurate means of detecting stones in the common bile duct (Fig. 13-3).

Since its introduction in the early 1970s, ERCP has revolutionized the diagnosis and treatment of choledocholithiasis. Prophylactic antibiotics should be administered for this procedure, particularly to patients with duct obstruction or recent cholangitis. Expert endoscopists can successfully cannulate the common bile duct in about 90% to 95% of patients.[24] However, previous Billroth II gastroenterostomy may make the procedure technically impossible, particularly in patients with an antecolic anastomosis or a long afferent limb. The most common complication of ERCP is hyperamylasemia, which occurs in 30% to 75% of patients,[25] but only 1% have severe pancreatitis.[26] Cholangitis occurs in 1% of patients, and those who have a previous history of cholangitis are at greatest risk. Severe bleeding

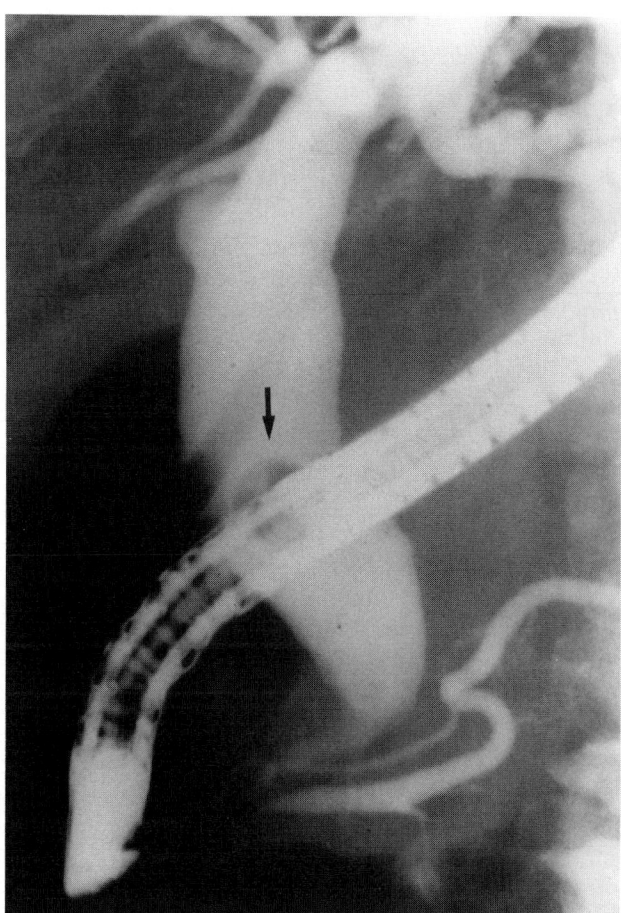

Figure 13-3 Endoscopic retrograde cholangiopancreatography demonstrating a common bile duct stone (*arrow*) in a patient who underwent cholecystectomy.

catheter can be positioned in the bile duct over a guide wire.

INTRAOPERATIVE

ULTRASOUND. Ultrasound can be used during cholecystectomy for the detection of common bile duct stones.[27,28] One study compared intraoperative ultrasound with intraoperative cholangiography during open cholecystectomy.[28] Using 7-MHz transducers, the ductal system was successfully visualized in 123 of 131 patients. Ductal stones were correctly identified in 12 of 13 patients using ultrasound, but were clearly seen on cholangiography in only 6 of these patients. Overall, in expert hands, intraoperative ultrasound has a positive predictive value of 72% to 79%.

Intraoperative ultrasound can be a particularly useful adjunct to laparoscopic surgery. A technique of intraluminal biliary ultrasonography that can be performed during laparoscopic cholecystectomy has been described.[29] A high-frequency ultrasonic probe in a 6F sheath is introduced into the abdomen through an operating port and passed into the bile duct through the cystic duct. Preliminary data suggest that this technique is as sensitive as cholangiography. However, these probes are no smaller than the newest choledochoscopes that are available for laparoscopic common duct exploration. These choledochoscopes can be used for stone identification and removal under direct vision. Other disadvantages of intraoperative ultrasound as a diagnostic test for common duct stones are that the technique is highly operator dependent and that bile duct anatomy is not adequately demonstrated.

and duodenal perforation typically occur only in patients who require endoscopic sphincterotomy and not in those who undergo diagnostic ERCP alone.

ERCP is the modality of choice in most patients in whom common duct stones are suspected. However, if previous gastric surgery or other conditions make endoscopic access to the biliary tree impossible, a percutaneous approach may be used. PTC is particularly appropriate in patients with extensive intrahepatic stone disease or Oriental cholangiohepatitis, but also may be useful in the diagnosis and drainage of patients with biliary sepsis due to distal common duct stones when ERCP is technically impossible. PTC is contraindicated in patients with an uncorrected coagulopathy and may be technically difficult in the presence of normal-caliber intrahepatic bile ducts. After the administration of antibiotic prophylaxis, a narrow-bore needle is introduced through the skin into an intrahepatic bile duct, and cholangiography is performed. If percutaneous stone extraction is planned or biliary drainage is indicated, a

OPERATIVE CHOLANGIOGRAPHY. The debate over the usefulness and cost-effectiveness of routine intraoperative cholangiography has continued for decades and has been further fueled by the introduction of laparoscopic cholecystectomy.[30,31] Advocates of routine intraoperative cholangiography argue that asymptomatic common duct stones can be identified and common duct injuries prevented by defining biliary anatomy early in the procedure. Critics of this approach suggest that the incidence of retained stones in patients is no greater when cholangiography is performed selectively on the basis of clinical and laboratory criteria. They also suggest that the greatest risk of bile duct injury occurs early in the procedure and is not likely to be reduced by the use of routine cholangiography.[30,32] However, operative cholangiography always should be performed before the common bile duct is explored during open or laparoscopic cholecystectomy. Even if stones have been proven to be present before surgery, operative cholangiography demonstrates ductal anatomy and shows the distribution of the stones in the biliary tree at the time of surgery.

The same technical principles apply whether the procedure is performed during open or laparoscopic cholecystectomy. Fluoroscopy greatly facilitates operative cholangiography and should be used whenever possible. When fluoroscopy is unavailable and conventional x-ray equipment is used, the patient's left side should be elevated to rotate the distal common bile duct away from the spine. The use of dilute contrast (less than 50%) aids in the detection of small stones, particularly when the ductal system is dilated.

Cannulation of the cystic duct is facilitated during open cholecystectomy by applying traction on the gallbladder to stabilize the cystic duct while a small transverse incision is made. A probe can be used to dilate or disrupt the valves of Heister to allow cannulation of the cystic duct, but care should be taken not to force the probe through the posterior wall of the duct. The cholangiocatheter is introduced through the cystic duct and secured with a ligature or clip.

Many recent reports describe the technique of laparoscopic cholangiography.[33–35] A cholangiocatheter, a ureteric catheter,[34,35] or a self-retaining balloon-tipped catheter can be used to perform cholangiography. The catheter is introduced through a lateral operative port or through a 14-gauge polyethylene intravenous catheter that is inserted laterally in the right upper quadrant, grasped with a forceps, and guided into the cystic duct. Upward and lateral traction on the gallbladder facilitates introduction of the catheter into the cystic duct. The catheter is fixed in the duct with a hemoclip. Alternatively, a cholangioclamp,[35] with a hollow center through which a 4F or 5F ureteric catheter is passed, can be used. The instrument is introduced through the right upper quadrant port and then used to guide the catheter into the duct. The jaws of the grasper then are closed around the cystic duct, which keeps the catheter in position and provides a watertight seal. If the valves of Heister prevent passage of the catheter, a soft guide wire can be passed initially, over which the catheter is introduced into the duct.

All air should be excluded from the injection system before the cholangiocatheter is inserted, because air bubbles may mimic stones and result in an unnecessary exploration of the common duct. Saline then is injected to ensure that there are no leaks and that contrast will flow freely into the duct. When fluoroscopy is used, contrast is injected slowly, and frequent spot exposures are taken. Alternatively, a plain radiograph is taken after the injection of 7 mL of contrast, and a second film is taken after about 20 mL has been injected. This technique should prevent a small stone in a large duct from being overlooked, illustrate the anatomy of the intra-

hepatic ducts, and demonstrate the patency of the sphincter of Oddi (Fig. 13-4).

If contrast fails to enter the duodenum, spasm of the sphincter of Oddi due to opiate administration may be responsible. The intravenous administration of naloxone to relax the sphincter, followed by repeated cholangiography, may prevent an unnecessary duct exploration. If no narcotics have been used, glucagon can be given to relieve sphincter spasm. Alternatively, contrast may flow freely into the duodenum and fail to fill the intrahepatic ducts. If this occurs, the patient should be placed in the Trendelenburg position or, in rare circumstances, the distal bile duct can be occluded using a well-padded vascular clamp.

POSTOPERATIVE. Retained common bile duct stones are identified in 2% to 10% of patients who have undergone common duct exploration. Most retained common bile duct stones in these patients are diagnosed on routine T-tube cholangiography 7 to 10 days after operation. However, retained stones may be suspected in patients with persistently large volumes of postoperative bile drainage from the T-tube. The potential for retained stones and the need for diagnosis is a

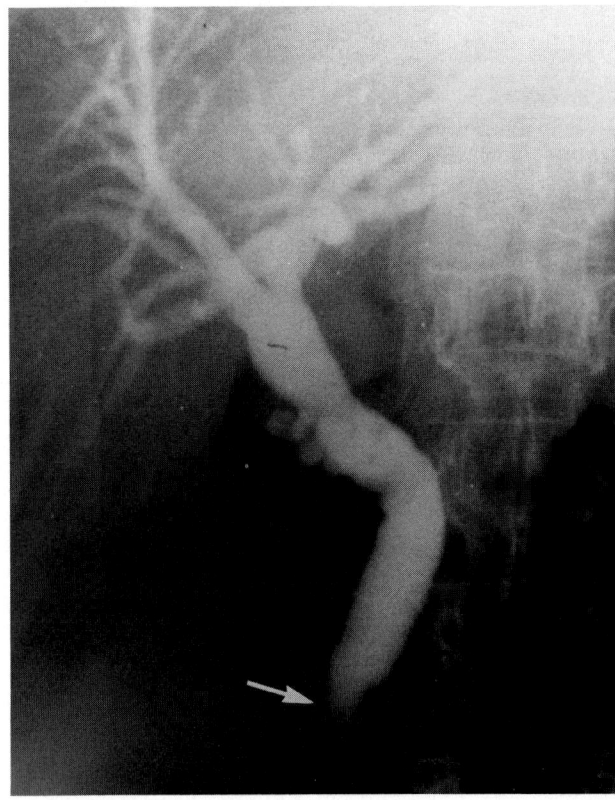

Figure 13-4 Intraoperative cholangiogram demonstrating a stone (*arrow*) obstructing the distal bile duct.

primary reason for the routine use of a postoperative T-tube after common bile duct exploration.

Choledocholithiasis also may present, or be detected for the first time, in patients who have undergone cholecystectomy either recently or months to years earlier. ERCP is the method of choice for the diagnosis and treatment of such patients. Alternatively, transhepatic cholangiography may be useful, particularly if the stones are within the liver, or if previous gastrointestinal surgery makes ERCP difficult or impossible.

T-TUBE CHOLANGIOGRAPHY. As with other forms of cholangiography, care should be taken during T-tube cholangiography to prevent the introduction of air bubbles, which may mimic retained stones. Residual blood clots also may be confused with stones. When filling defects are seen on a postoperative T-tube cholangiogram (Fig. 13-5), the tube should be left in position and the cholangiogram repeated after 7 to 10 days. If re-

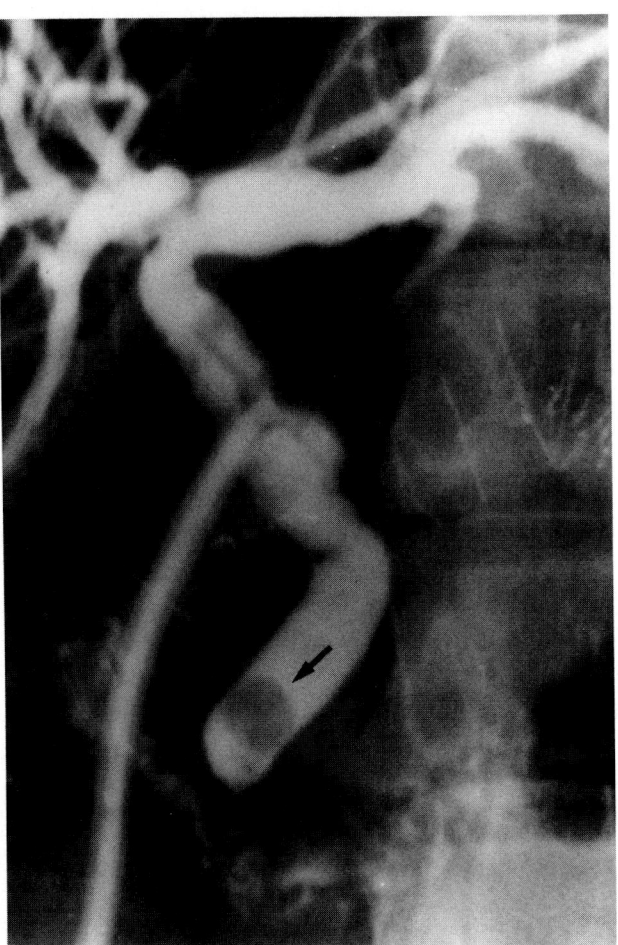

Figure 13-5 T-tube cholangiogram demonstrating a retained common duct stone (*arrow*).

tained stones are confirmed, the T-tube can be clamped and left in position for 6 weeks, provided there is no obstruction or infection. Small stones (less than 0.5 cm) may pass spontaneously in 5% to 10% of patients during this period, which allows the tract to mature for nonoperative techniques of stone extraction (see later).

Treatment

Nonoperative

ENDOSCOPIC SPHINCTEROTOMY. A diagnostic ERCP is performed initially to confirm the presence of stones, as described previously. It may be possible to retrieve one or two small stones using a basket through an intact papilla, or after balloon dilatation of the papilla. However, sphincterotomy is necessary in most patients who require endoscopic stone extraction. After sphincterotomy, most stones smaller than 1 cm in diameter pass spontaneously within a few days. Alternatively, a balloon catheter or a Dormia basket can be used to extract the stones. Stones larger than 2 cm may require additional measures, such as lithotripsy or the use of dissolution agents instilled through a nasobiliary cannula. Stones can be removed successfully in 85% to 90% of patients.[36] If clearance is incomplete, a nasobiliary drain or endoscopic stent should be placed in the bile duct to maintain biliary drainage.

Endoscopic sphincterotomy is contraindicated in patients with a coagulopathy or a long distal bile duct stricture. Even in expert hands, complications of ERCP combined with endoscopic sphincterotomy occur in about 10% of patients. Potential problems include bleeding severe enough to require transfusion (2% to 3%), duodenal perforation (1%), severe pancreatitis (2%), and significant cholangitis (1% to 2%).[26] The mortality rate after endoscopic sphincterotomy is about 1%.[26]

PERCUTANEOUS STONE EXTRACTION. In selected circumstances, common duct stones can be removed using a percutaneous approach.[37] However, these techniques usually are reserved for the treatment of patients with extensive intrahepatic stone disease. Catheters are placed in the biliary tree at the time of percutaneous cholangiography, and the tract is progressively enlarged over several weeks until it will accommodate a 14F to 16F catheter. If the tract is large enough, stones can be retrieved using either a Dormia basket under fluoroscopic guidance or a small choledochoscope under direct vision. Alternatively, it may be easier to trap stones or fragments in a basket and push them into the duodenum.[37,38] Electrohydraulic or laser lithotripsy probes, stone dissolution agents, and repeated procedures may be required to achieve complete clearance of the ductal system.

EXTRACORPOREAL SHOCK WAVE LITHOTRIPSY. Extracorporeal shock wave lithotripsy (ESWL) also has been used as a less invasive means of treating common bile duct stones.[39,40] In a multicenter trial involving a selected group of 42 patients,[39] ESWL was successful in fragmenting common bile duct stones in 95% of patients. Additional procedures, including endoscopic fragment extraction or stent placement, biliary lavage, and open surgery, were required to clear the duct in 50% of patients, and 74% of patients were free of stones on discharge from the hospital. The principal biliary complications were biliary pain (15%), hemobilia (5%), and biliary sepsis (5%). In addition, ESWL-related pulmonary or renal complications occurred in 13% of patients and ileus occurred in 2.5%. Similar results were reported in a group of 62 patients.[40] Both studies concluded that ESWL may play a useful adjunctive role in the management of large common bile duct stones.

Surgery

OPEN COMMON DUCT EXPLORATION. Open choledochostomy is the gold standard against which other methods for removing common duct stones must be measured. Adequate exposure is important, and an incision made for cholecystectomy may only need to be extended to allow adequate exploration of the duct. Kocherization of the duodenum and gentle palpation of the intrapancreatic bile duct should be the first step in common duct exploration (Fig. 13-6). This maneuver may dislodge an impacted stone in the lower end of the

bile duct, reducing the need for instrumentation and the risk of trauma to the duct. The duct should be opened with a longitudinal incision in the anterior wall between two fine stay sutures. Rigid instruments should not be used to remove stones from the common duct because they can injure the delicate ductal epithelium. It is more prudent to begin by passing a soft rubber catheter (8F or 10F) and gently irrigating the duct. This catheter often will pass through the sphincter of Oddi into the duodenum. A Fogarty balloon catheter then can be passed both distally and proximally while the balloon is inflated and withdrawn, and the procedure is repeated until all stones and debris have been removed.

Adequate clearance of the duct should be confirmed visually using choledochoscopy, which has been shown to reduce the incidence of retained stones to between 2% and 4% without increasing the morbidity associated with common duct exploration.[41] Either a rigid or a flexible choledochoscope can be used, but the latter is preferred when the distance between the choledochostomy and the duodenum is greater than 6 cm (Fig. 13-7). The scope is passed distally toward the duodenum and proximally into the hepatic ducts. Any remaining stones or debris are removed by irrigation or the use of instruments such as stone forceps, Dormia baskets, and Fogarty catheters. Ultrasonic or laser lithotripsy may be useful in clearing stones in difficult cases.[42]

Placement of a T-tube at the end of the exploration decompresses the system and allows subsequent access to the biliary tree to retrieve retained stones. The T-tube needs to be large (greater than 14F) to facilitate subsequent procedures. If the duct is too small, a Whelan-

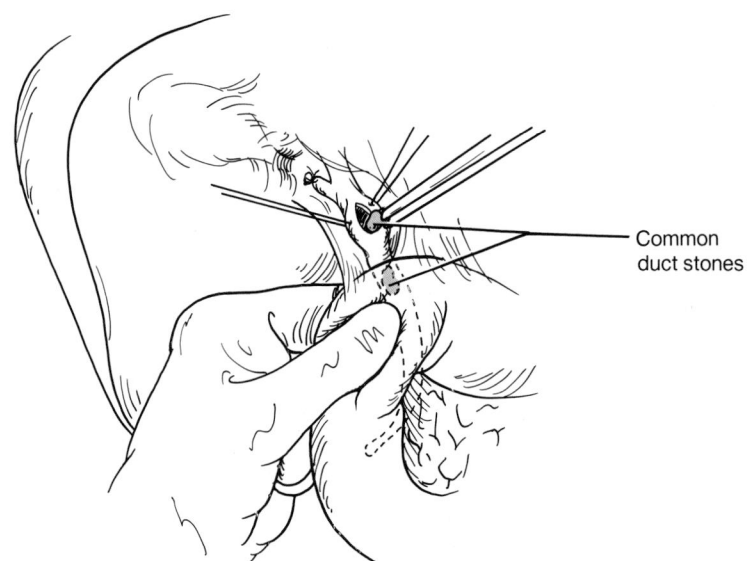

— Common duct stones

Figure 13-6 The first step in common duct exploration is kocherization of the duodenum and gentle palpation of the distal common bile duct, which may dislodge a stone impacted in the ampulla.

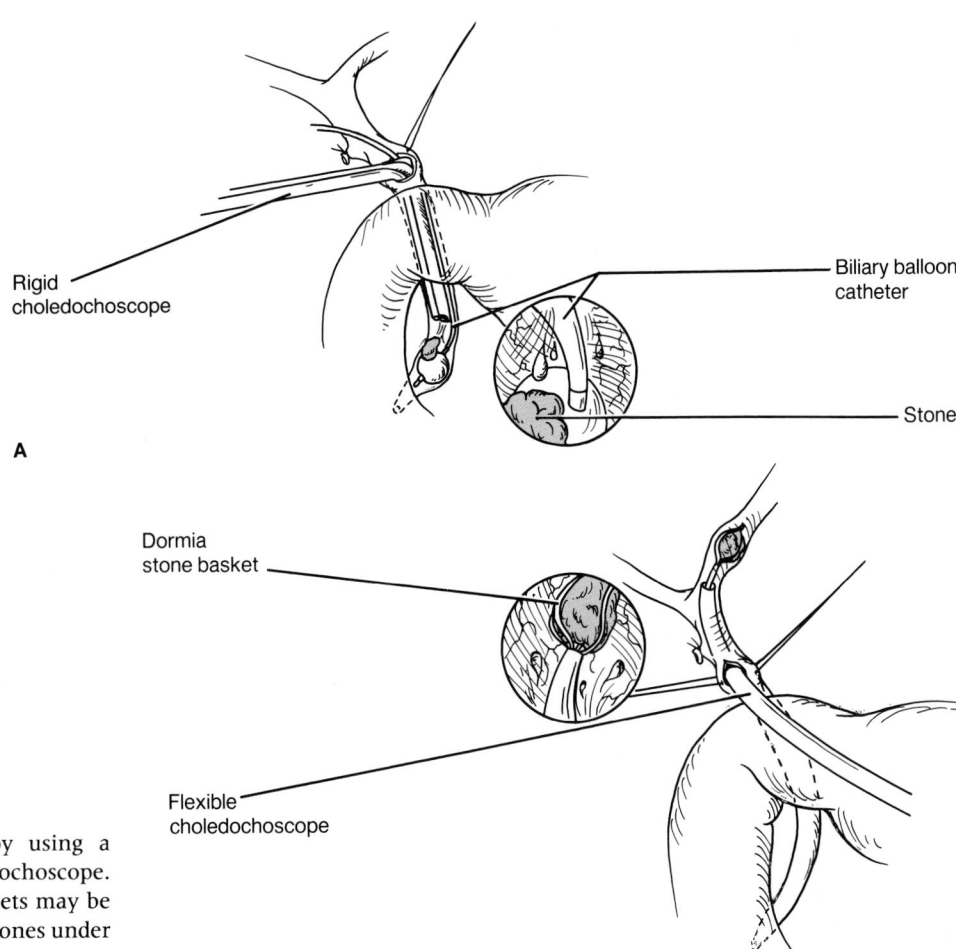

Rigid
choledochoscope

Biliary balloon
catheter

Stone

A

Dormia
stone basket

Flexible
choledochoscope

B

Figure 13-7 Choledochoscopy using a rigid (**A**) or flexible (**B**) choledochoscope. Balloon catheters or stone baskets may be used to retrieve common duct stones under direct vision.

Moss tube, in which the base of the T is of smaller bore than the stem, can be used. The T-tube should exit directly, allowing some slack for postoperative abdominal distention, and laterally, to facilitate radiologically guided procedures if these should prove necessary. Completion cholangiography should be performed before closure of the abdomen, because this step has been shown to reduce the incidence of retained stones by 75%. Precautions must be taken to exclude air bubbles, and it may be necessary to administer glucagon to reverse spasm of the sphincter of Oddi or naloxone to reverse the effects of opiates if the contrast medium fails to flow into the duodenum. If stones are demonstrated, the duct should be reexplored.

In certain situations, the technique may be modified. When the cystic duct is large, the common duct can be explored through it. However, if the angle with the common duct is particularly acute, access to the proximal ducts may be restricted. The use of a T-tube is not mandatory after such an exploration. When the common bile duct is small, the risk of late stricture after exploration may be increased. In these circumstances,

the duct can be explored from below, avoiding the need for a choledochostomy and a T-tube.[43] In this procedure, a Fogarty catheter is introduced through the cystic duct and passed into the duodenum to help identify the ampulla. A sphincteroplasty is performed through a small duodenotomy, with care taken to prevent injury to the pancreatic duct, and the common duct is explored from below. Choledochoscopy also can be performed through the sphincteroplasty. Completion cholangiography is performed through the cystic duct, which then is ligated.

LAPAROSCOPIC COMMON DUCT EXPLORATION. When common duct stones are identified on cholangiography during laparoscopic cholecystectomy, several procedures have been described for removing them without resorting to open choledochostomy. A Fogarty catheter can be introduced through the 14-gauge intravenous cannula sleeve used for cholangiography[34] and passed into the common duct through the cystic duct. The catheter may push stones in front of it as it is advanced into the duodenum. Alternatively,

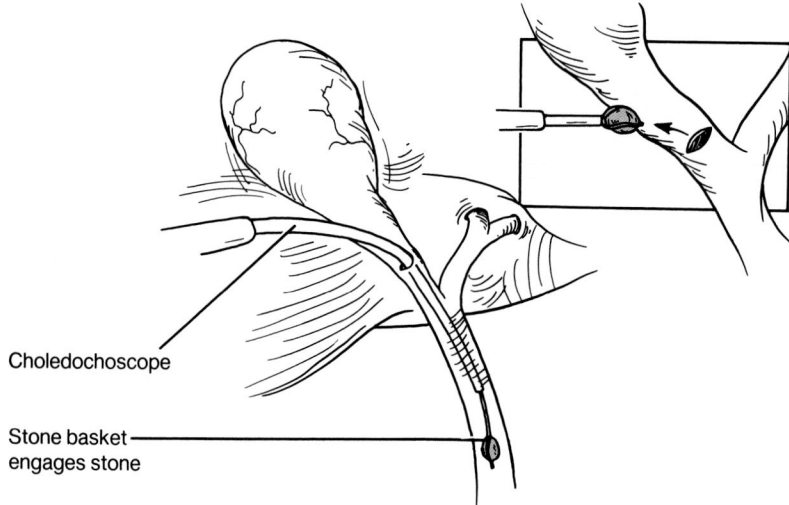

Choledochoscope

Stone basket engages stone

Figure 13-8 A Dormia basket introduced into the abdomen through a 14-gauge cannula may be used to extract stones from the common duct under fluoroscopic guidance. **(Inset)** The basket and stone are withdrawn, along with the choledochoscope. (After Bailey RW, Zucker KA. Laparoscopic cholangiography and management of choledocholithiasis. In: Zucker KA, ed. Surgical laparoscopy. St Louis, Quality Medical, 1991:201)

stones can be retrieved through the cystic duct by withdrawing the catheter with the balloon inflated. Frequently, however, stones fail to pass into the cystic duct and must be retrieved by other means. Contrast material can be instilled into the duct, and a Dormia basket, introduced through the same 14-gauge cannula, can be used under fluoroscopic guidance to capture and retrieve stones[44] (Fig. 13-8).

A flexible choledochoscope also can be introduced through the midclavicular port and passed into the common duct through the cystic duct, which may need to be gently dilated. Small, flexible scopes of 11F typically are used, but smaller (9.4F or less) scopes are available to facilitate the procedure in smaller ductal systems.[45] These scopes are flexible and, at least theoretically, can be manipulated into the proximal ducts. Stones can be captured using a Dormia basket passed through the operating channel. The whole ensemblage is removed from the duct, and the stones are grasped in a forceps and withdrawn from the abdomen. The procedure is made easier if a second camera is attached to the endoscope, and the image is displayed on a second monitor or mixed into the operative picture.

If the cystic duct cannot be dilated sufficiently to accommodate a choledochoscope, the scope can be introduced through a standard choledochostomy. However, a T-tube is indicated after choledochostomy, and suturing using the laparoscope remains a slow, tedious process. Many experienced laparoscopic surgeons prefer to proceed to open choledochostomy or to consider postoperative endoscopic sphincterotomy in these circumstances. The presence of many stones in the common bile duct or of stones in the hepatic duct is a relative contraindication to laparoscopic exploration of the ducts. Flexible choledochoscopes and the availability of small-diameter electrohydraulic and laser lithotripsy probes allow lithotriptic clearance of large numbers of common duct stones within a reasonable period using the laparoscope.[45] However, these patients are more likely to have retained or recurrent stones and may be better served with a drainage procedure.

In the largest series reported,[34] laparoscopic common bile duct exploration was attempted in 77 of 1000 patients undergoing cholecystectomy and was accomplished successfully in 960 of these patients. Three patients were converted to an open procedure because common duct stones were inaccessible using laparoscopic techniques. Postoperative endoscopic cholangiography was required in 20 patients and revealed retained stones in 5 (0.5% of all patients undergoing laparoscopic cholecystectomy). This figure included 2 patients who had stones identified at intraoperative cholangiography that could not be removed using the laparoscope.

The most common complication of transcystic bile duct exploration is hyperamylasemia, but clinical pancreatitis is uncommon. Other complications include cholangitis, bile leaks, common duct injury (primarily caused by the guide wire), and entrapment of the basket in the duodenum requiring open removal.[46]

DRAINAGE PROCEDURES. Up to 30% of patients undergoing open choledochostomy require some form of biliary drainage procedure.[26] The options are transduodenal sphincteroplasty, choledochoduodenostomy, and choledochojejunostomy. Sphincteroplasty is indicated in patients with any of the following:

- Sphincter stenosis or dysfunction
- Possible ampullary tumor (where it represents an opportunity to perform a biopsy)
- Recurrent pancreatitis

- Multiple stones in a nondilated system
- Choledochocele

Anastomosis of the duct to the duodenum or a loop of jejunum is indicated when the duct is dilated to more than 2 cm in the presence of any of the following:

- Primary common duct stones
- Multiple stones
- A long distal inflammatory stricture
- Perivaterian duodenal diverticulum

Many surgeons prefer drainage into the jejunum rather than the duodenum because of the risk of recurrent cholangitis, pancreatitis, or duodenal fistula, and the rare, but well-documented, sump syndrome[47] associated with side-to-side choledochoduodenostomy.

SPHINCTEROPLASTY. When sphincteroplasty is indicated, kocherization of the duodenum and common duct exploration, including choledochoscopy, should be performed before a duodenotomy is made. The ampulla is best identified by passing a Fogarty catheter through the choledochostomy into the duodenum (Fig. 13-9A). A small transverse duodenotomy is made directly over the ampulla. Two stay sutures placed on each side of the ampulla are lifted forward, and a small incision is made at the 11-o'clock position, staying well away from the pancreatic duct, which usually is situated at the 4-o'clock position (see Fig. 13-9B). Interrupted absorbable sutures are placed along each side of the incision, which is progressively extended until a Bakes dilator the size of the common duct passes easily. A final suture placed at the apex is important to protect against a duodenal leak (see Fig. 13-9C). The duodenotomy should be closed transversely to preserve an adequate duodenal lumen.

CHOLEDOCHODUODENOSTOMY. In choledochoduodenostomy, the common duct can be anastomosed to the duodenum in either a side-to-side or an end-to-side fashion. Side-to-side anastomosis is performed by making a longitudinal choledochostomy just above the upper border of the first part of the duodenum and opening the duodenum longitudinally. A transverse choledochostomy parallel to the duodenotomy also is acceptable and may be less likely to become obstructed. The anastomosis can be performed using a double-layer technique of interrupted sutures, although many surgeons prefer a single-layer technique (see Fig. 13-10B and C). A side-to-side anastomosis leaves the distal bile duct in continuity and can lead to the sump syndrome.[47] In this situation, food debris from the duodenum can enter and accumulate in the distal limb of the duct and act as a nidus for bacterial growth. Eventually,

the anastomosis or the pancreatic duct orifice can become obstructed by this debris, leading to cholangitis or pancreatitis. Complete division and oversewing of the common duct and end-to-side anastomosis of the proximal duct to the duodenum prevents the development of the sump syndrome (Fig. 13-10). In either case, supporting the anastomosis with a T-tube decompresses the system and provides drainage should a duodenal leak occur. Closed suction drains are placed near, but not directly on, the anastomosis.

CHOLEDOCHOJEJUNOSTOMY. Choledochojejunostomy can be performed using either a jejunal loop in continuity or a Roux-en-Y limb, but the latter is preferable. In either case, the common duct should be divided and the anastomosis performed end-to-side to prevent the sump syndrome. If a loop in continuity is used, the anastomosis should be defunctionalized by performing a side-to-side jejunojejunostomy. A Roux-en-Y limb, preferably brought up behind the colon, provides defunctionalized isoperistaltic drainage of the bile duct with a low-tension anastomosis and protects against intestinal reflux and cholangitis (Fig. 13-11). Increased gastric acid production can be a problem with a Roux-en-Y loop[48] but is easily managed with H_2 blockers.

Stenting the anastomosis decompresses the biliary tract in the early postoperative period and can provide access for cholangiography or the removal of retained stones. A T-tube can be used as a stent if the length of bile duct above the anastomosis is adequate. When the anastomosis lies close to the bifurcation of the hepatic ducts, preoperative or intraoperative placement of a transhepatic stent is a better option. Recurrent stones can be a problem in patients with intrahepatic stones and strictures, and long-term stent placement should be considered in these patients to maintain access to the biliary tree.[49] Alternatively, percutaneous techniques can be used later in these patients to remove recurrent stones.[50]

Postoperative

T-TUBE STONE EXTRACTION. Retained common duct stones can be extracted through the T-tube tract, when the tract is fully mature, using the Burhenne technique.[51] The T-tube is removed after passing a guide wire through it, and a steerable catheter is passed along the tract. Special stone retrieval baskets are used to capture and remove the stone under fluoroscopic guidance. Small-caliber choledochoscopes can be passed along the tract to retrieve stones under direct vision[52] (Fig. 13-12). Stones that are too large to pass along the tract can be fragmented using electrohydraulic, laser, or ultrasonic lithotripsy devices under vision.[53] Fragments can be re-

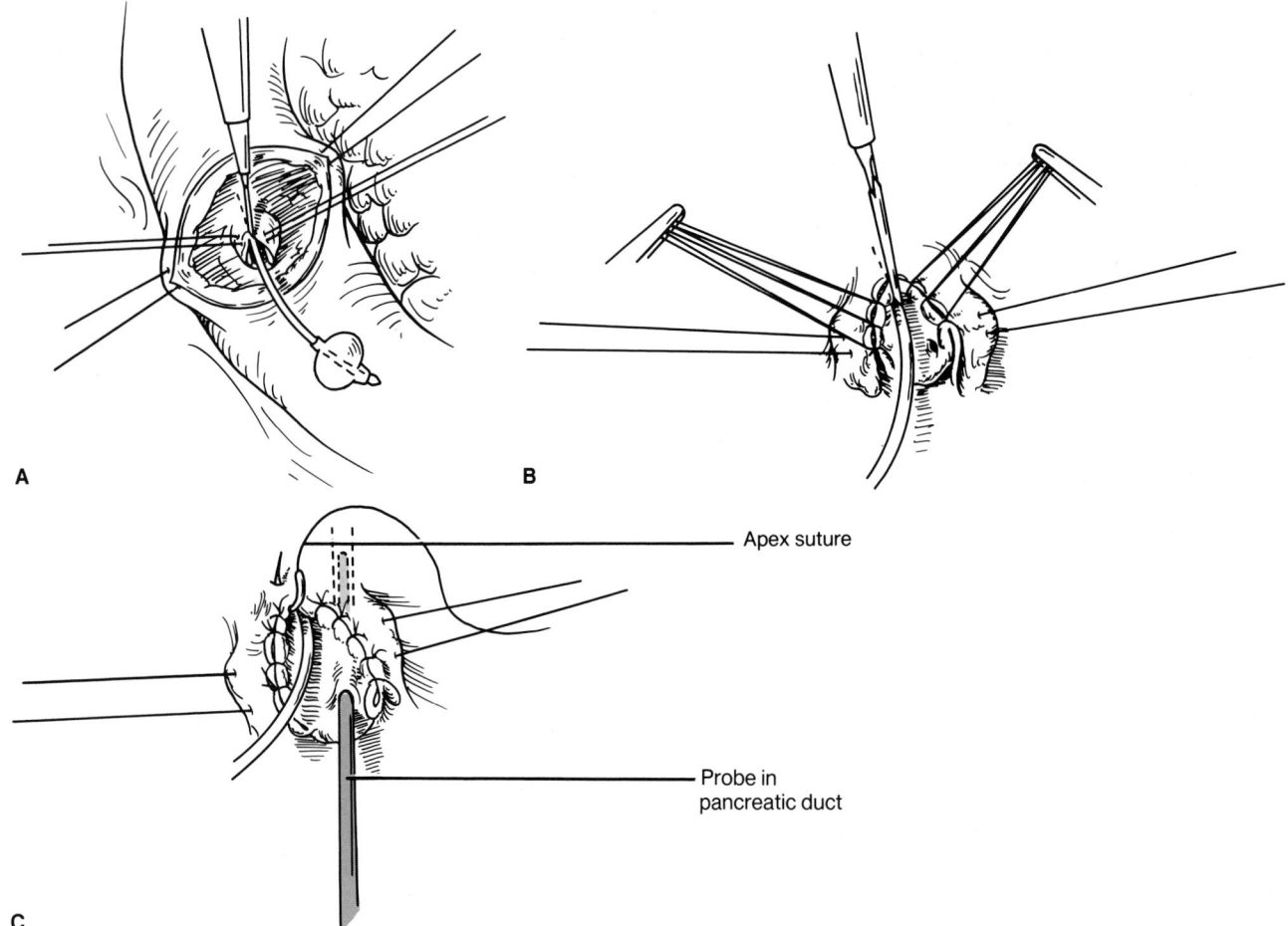

A

B

Apex suture

Probe in
pancreatic duct

C

Figure 13-9 Transduodenal sphincteroplasty. (**A**) Duodenotomy, using a balloon catheter to identify the common bile duct, and initial sphincterotomy. (**B**) Extension of sphincterotomy and initial suture placement. (**C**) Pancreatic duct identified with a probe, and the important, final, apical suture.

trieved piecemeal or pushed into the duodenum. Stone clearance can be achieved in 90% of patients using these techniques, although repeated procedures are needed in some cases.[52] Stone clearance should be confirmed by completion cholangiography; if stones remain or the cholangiogram is inadequate, a catheter should be left in position to facilitate further procedures and to ensure adequate biliary drainage.

GALLSTONE DISSOLUTION. Some authors have used gallstone dissolution agents successfully in the management of retained cholesterol stones in patients with T-tubes.[54] Several agents have been used in this setting. The infusion of saline alone, or of saline combined with heparin, has a success rate of about 20%, which is equal to the spontaneous passage rate.[55] Sodium cholate also has been used, but is associated with considerable morbidity.[56] Monooctanoin, a medium-

chain diglyceride, dissolves 50% to 86% of retained stones when it is administered at a rate of 3 to 7 mL/h in buffer at a pH of 7.4 over 5 days.[54] Monooctanoin causes minor gastrointestinal disturbances in 10% to 50% of patients, and precautions should be taken to maintain intrabiliary pressure below 12 cm H_2O to prevent systemic absorption, which causes respiratory distress and right upper quadrant pain.

Situational Management

Traditionally, open choledochostomy and common bile duct exploration has been viewed as the gold standard for the treatment of common duct stones. However, with the advent of laparoscopic cholecystectomy and the refinement of nonoperative techniques, the treatment of patients with choledocholithiasis should be individualized. Although most would agree that

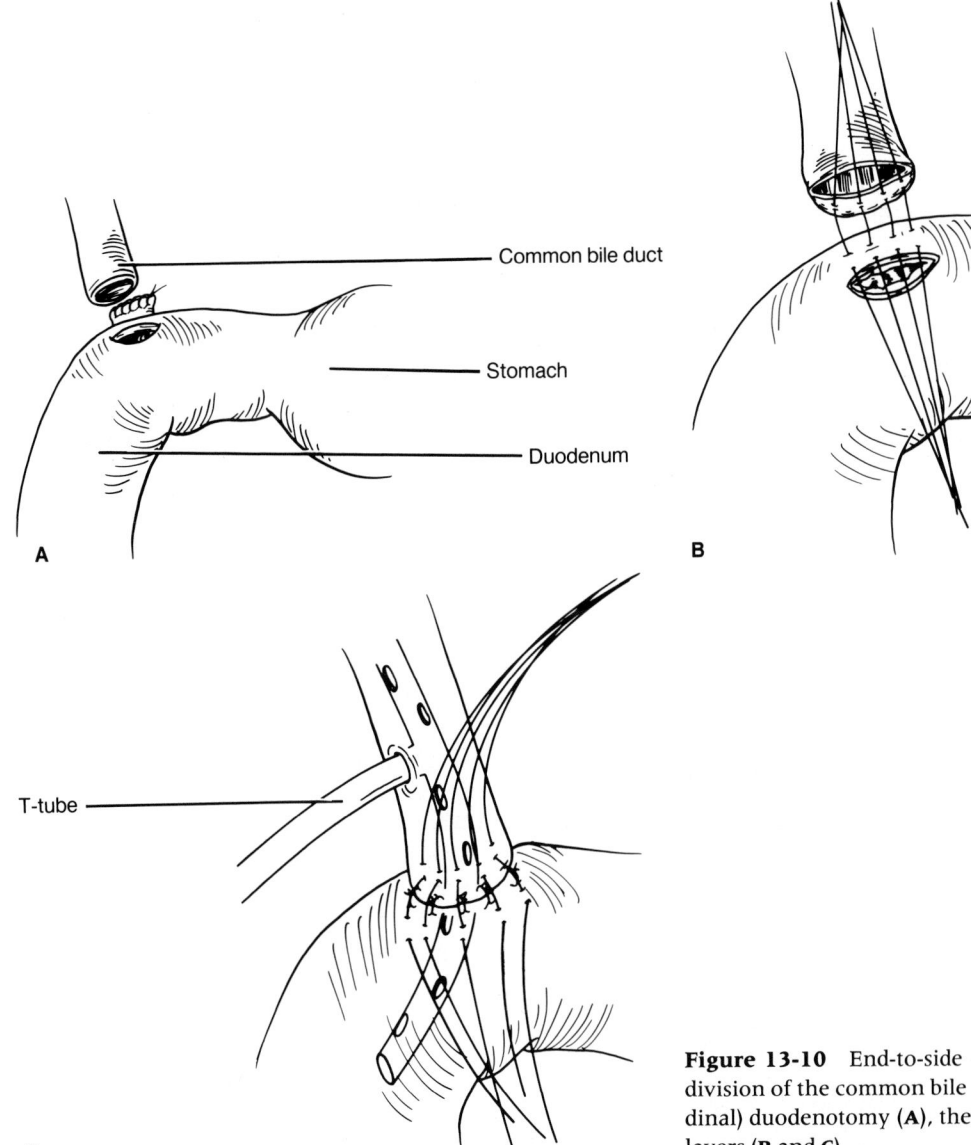

Common bile duct

Stomach

Duodenum

A

B

T-tube

C

Figure 13-10 End-to-side choledochoduodenostomy. After division of the common bile duct and a transverse (or longitudinal) duodenotomy (**A**), the anastomosis is performed in two layers (**B** and **C**).

symptomatic common duct stones should be removed, the timing and choice of procedure remains a topic of considerable debate. Factors to be considered in choosing the most appropriate therapeutic modality include the following:

- The degree of local endoscopic, radiologic, and laparoscopic expertise
- The severity and nature of the presenting symptoms
- The presence or absence of the gallbladder

LOCAL EXPERTISE. The choice of which procedure to perform for an individual patient is determined, to a large extent, by the local expertise in laparoscopic common duct exploration and endoscopic sphinctero-

tomy. Most patients with common duct stones who are undergoing laparoscopic cholecystectomy are treated successfully with preoperative ERCP combined with sphincterotomy, when necessary, and followed within a few days by laparoscopic cholecystectomy. Postoperative ERCP and endoscopic stone extraction, when necessary, also can be used when retained common duct stones are suspected.

Surgeons at one institution have reported their experience using this approach in 400 consecutive patients.[30] Preoperative ERCP was performed in 11% of all patients, of whom 7.8% had clinical indications of choledocholithiasis. Common duct stones were identified before surgery in 3.5% of patients and were removed successfully using the endoscope. Only 1.6% of patients required postoperative cholangiography be-

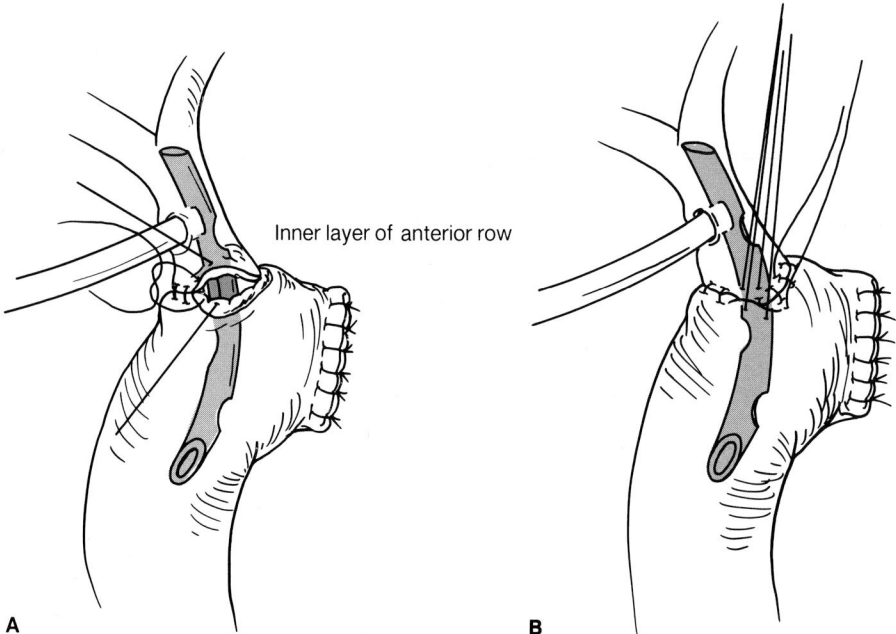

Inner layer of anterior row

A   B

Figure 13-11 Roux-en-Y choled-ochojejunostomy. A Roux-en-Y loop is brought up behind the colon, and the anastomosis is performed end-to-side over a T-tube, as illustrated here, or over a single transhepatic stent. A jejuno-jejunostomy is performed 60 cm distally.

cause of symptoms suggestive of retained stones, and stones were identified on these postoperative cholangiograms in only 0.8% of patients.

A group from Canada reported the results of a similar approach in a series of 1300 patients undergoing laparoscopic cholecystectomy.[32] Seventy-three patients (5.6%) had common duct stones. Common duct stones were identified in 50 patients using preoperative ERCP and were removed by either endoscopic sphinctero-

tomy (45 patients) or open common duct exploration (5 patients). Intraoperative cholangiography was performed in only 4.2% of patients, and stones were identified in 6 of these patients (0.5% of the total). These patients, and 11 others who had retained stones in the postoperative period, were treated successfully with postoperative endoscopic sphincterotomy.

The successful management of common duct stones using laparoscopic common duct exploration

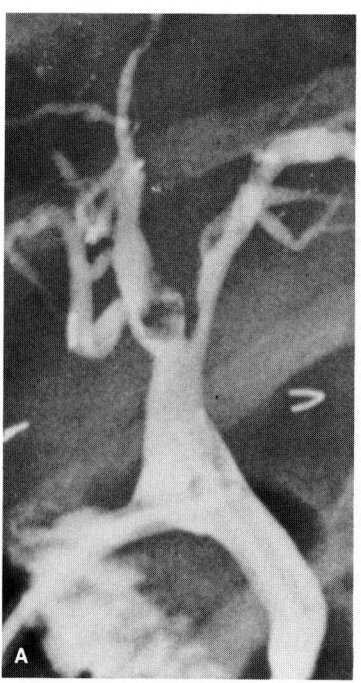
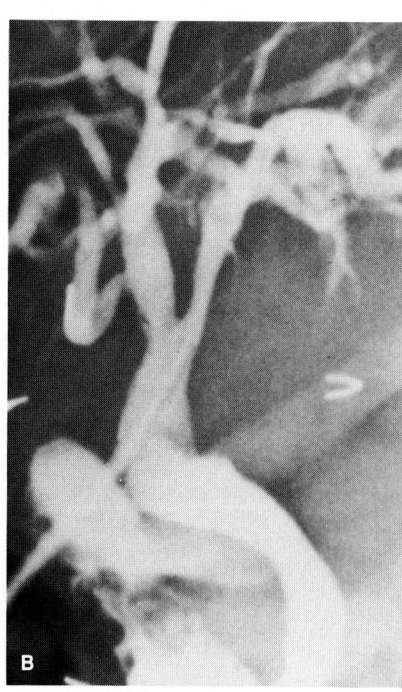

A   B

Figure 13-12 T-tube cholangiogram before (**A**) and after (**B**) extraction of a right hepatic duct stone through a T-tube tract.

during laparoscopic cholecystectomy has been reported in several series, with stone clearance rates of 57% to 98%.[34] Thus, laparoscopic exploration of the common duct is likely to play a substantial role in the management of choledocholithiasis in the future. In those institutions where surgeons are experienced in laparoscopic common bile duct exploration and expert endoscopists are available, a reasonable approach might include liberal use of intraoperative cholangiography, laparoscopic removal of common duct stones where possible, and postoperative endoscopic sphincterotomy when stones cannot be removed using the laparoscope.

SEVERITY AND NATURE OF PRESENTATION. Most patients with symptoms caused by stones in the common duct have transient pain and jaundice. These individuals can be investigated as outpatients and treated electively. The treatment of patients with cholangitis is discussed later. Most patients with gallstone pancreatitis have a mild attack and recover fully within a few days with supportive treatment. The offending stone usually causes only transient obstruction and passes through the sphincter of Oddi into the duodenum spontaneously. However, some patients have severe pancreatitis, with significant morbidity and mortality. Early surgical intervention may prevent the progression to severe pancreatitis and thereby reduce the morbidity and mortality rates in these patients. However, a prospective randomized trial of 165 patients demonstrated that the mortality rate actually is higher in patients who undergo surgery within 48 hours than in those in whom surgery is delayed until the initial episode has resolved[57] (Table 13-2).

Two prospective randomized trials indicate that early endoscopic cholangiography with selective sphincterotomy may improve outcome in patients with severe gallstone pancreatitis.[58,59] One study compared urgent ERCP, with sphincterotomy and stone extraction when necessary, with conventional management of pancreatitis in 121 patients who were stratified according to the severity of pancreatitis.[58] Common duct stones were found in 63% of patients with severe pancreatitis and in only 26% of those with mild attacks. The overall incidence of complications was reduced from 34% to 17% (P < .03) in the endoscopically treated group. The hospital stay also was shorter for these patients, but the difference was significant only among those with severe pancreatitis (9.5 days versus 17 days, P < .05). In addition, mortality rates were lower in the endoscopically treated group (2% versus 8%), but this difference was not statistically significant (Table 13-3).

A Hong Kong investigation similarly found that both the morbidity rate (57% versus 22%) and the mor-

Table 13-2 Urgent Versus Delayed Surgery for Gallstone Pancreatitis

	Early Surgery (<48 h)	Late Surgery (>48 h)
NUMBER OF PATIENTS		
Mild pancreatitis*	60	65
Severe pancreatitis*	23	17
TOTAL	83	82
MORBIDITY RATE (%)		
Mild pancreatitis	7	3
Severe pancreatitis	83	18†
TOTAL	30	5†
MORTALITY RATE (%)		
Mild pancreatitis	3	0
Severe pancreatitis	48	12
TOTAL	15	2

* Pancreatitis was defined as mild if patients had three or fewer of Ranson's criteria,[103] and as severe if four or more criteria were present.
† P < .05 versus early surgery.
(Adapted from Kelly TR, Wagner DS. Gallstone pancreatitis: a prospective randomized trial of the timing of surgery. Surgery 1988;104:600)

tality rate (22% versus 12%) were lower in patients with severe gallstone pancreatitis who were treated using the endoscope.[59] However, there was no difference in outcome among patients with milder pancreatitis (see Table 13-3). These studies suggest that, in patients with severe pancreatitis believed to be caused by gallstones, emergency ERCP, sphincterotomy, and stone extraction when necessary is the treatment of choice.

PRESENCE OF THE GALLBLADDER. Patients who have common duct stones early after cholecystectomy often are treated best using nonoperative approaches such as T-tube extraction, endoscopic sphincterotomy, or percutaneous stone extraction. Open surgery should be reserved for patients in whom these methods are inappropriate or impossible. The optimal treatment of patients with intact gallbladders and common duct stones remains controversial.

Published reports indicate that, after endoscopic sphincterotomy, between 9% and 28% of patients subsequently require cholecystectomy for acute or chronic cholecystitis.[60] Although endoscopic sphincterotomy alone may be appropriate therapy in elderly or high-risk patients, a strong argument can be made for removing the gallbladder in younger patients who have stones in both the gallbladder and the common bile duct.[26] Retrospective studies comparing endoscopic sphincterotomy alone with common bile duct exploration in patients with intact gallbladders indicate that morbidity and mortality rates are similar,[61] but the incidence of

Table 13-3   Urgent Endoscopy Versus Conservative Treatment of Pancreatitis

	Leicester[58]		Hong Kong[59]	
	ERCP ± ES	Conservative Therapy	ERCP ± ES	Conservative Therapy
NUMBER OF PATIENTS				
Mild*	34	34	56	58
Severe*	25	28	41	40
TOTAL	59	62	97	98
MORBIDITY RATE (%)				
Mild	12	12	14	10
Severe	24	61†	22	57
TOTAL	17	34†	18	29‡
MORTALITY RATE (%)				
Mild	0	0	0	0
Severe	4	18	12	22
TOTAL	2	8	5	9
HOSPITAL STAY (DAYS)				
Mild	9	11		
Severe	9	17†		

ERCP, endoscopic retrograde cholangiopancreatography; ES, endoscopic sphincterotomy.
* Pancreatitis was defined as mild if patients had three or fewer of Ranson's criteria,[103] and as severe if four or more criteria were present.
† $P < .05$.
‡ $P = .07$ versus endoscopic group.

retained stones requiring additional procedures may be lower after open exploration.[62] In addition, there are concerns about the long-term effects of sphincterotomy on the biliary tract in young patients. Sphincterotomy results in gallbladder stasis, bacterial overgrowth, and an increase in secondary bile acids, all factors that may cause gallbladder cancer after 10 to 20 years.

Two randomized controlled studies attempted to determine whether endoscopic sphincterotomy before open cholecystectomy offers any advantage over open cholecystectomy and common bile duct exploration.[63,64] One trial found that rates of stone clearance, morbidity, and mortality were similar for each method.[63] Another investigation observed that the open approach was more effective than the endoscopic method in clearing the duct of stones[64] (Table 13-4). Both studies concluded that routine endoscopic sphincterotomy before open cholecystectomy is not worthwhile. Similar studies have not been performed, however, in the era of laparoscopic cholecystectomy.

Results

Cholangiography remains the gold standard in the diagnosis of common duct stones. In expert hands, the accuracy of both endoscopic and intraoperative cholangiography is about 95%, and routine operative cholangiography during cholecystectomy reveals otherwise unsuspected stones in 5% to 7% of patients. The widespread use of preoperative and intraoperative cholangiography has reduced the incidence of negative common duct exploration to less than 20%.[41] The incidence of retained stones after common duct exploration may be as high as 10%. However, the routine use of choledochoscopy after common duct exploration dramatically reduces the incidence of retained stones to between 2% and 4%. Open common duct exploration also is a safe procedure, and the operative mortality rate varies from 0% to 2.7% in reported series.[26]

It is against this standard that the success and complication rates of other methods of common duct stone retrieval must be compared. Early reports indicate that laparoscopic common duct stone extraction is feasible in selected patients with satisfactory results.[34] The operative mortality rate among patients undergoing drainage procedures is similar to that seen with choledochostomy alone. Nonoperative treatment of common duct stones by endoscopic and T-tube stone extraction is successful in selected patients in 85% to 95% of cases. However, endoscopic sphincterotomy carries a mortality rate of 1%, and significant morbidity occurs in about 10% of patients.

Table 13-4 Preoperative Endoscopic Sphincterotomy (ES) Versus Open Common Bile Duct Exploration (CBDE)

	Leicester Royal[63]		Los Angeles County[64]	
	ES + Cholecystectomy	Cholecystectomy CBDE	ES + Cholecystectomy	Cholecystectomy CBDE
Number of patients	55	60	26	26
Morbidity rate (%)	60	8	11	11
Mortality rate (%)	4	2	0	0
Retained stone rate (%)	9	8	35	12*

* $P < .05$ versus after endoscopic sphincterotomy.

CHOLANGITIS

Pathophysiology

Obstruction

Cholangitis is an acute bacterial infection within the biliary ductal system. Charcot[65] was the first to identify the importance of biliary obstruction in the pathogenesis of cholangitis when he described the clinical entity in 1877. Normal bile duct pressures are between 9 and 15 cm H_2O, but obstruction results in an elevation of bile duct pressures to between 18 and 29 cm H_2O. In experimental animals, an increase in bile duct pressure above 20 cm H_2O results in reflux of biliary bacteria into lymphatics,[66] and bacteria appear in the hepatic vein when the pressure rises above 25 cm H_2O.

Microbiology

Obstruction alone, however, is not sufficient; bacteria also must be present in the bile for cholangitis to develop. Bile in the gallbladder and common bile duct normally is sterile. However, results of bile cultures are positive in 30% to 50% of patients with gallstones,[67] and in 75% to 90% of patients with choledocholithiasis.[68] Results of bile cultures also are positive in 25% to 50% of patients with complete biliary obstruction, such as that seen with malignant disease.[69] Other risk factors for bactibilia include age greater than 60 years, bilioenteric anastomosis, and invasive biliary procedures.[70]

Several potential mechanisms exist for bacterial contamination of the biliary tree. Reflux of intestinal contents into the bile duct is an important cause of bactibilia in patients with a bilioenteric anastomosis and in those in whom the sphincteric mechanism has been disrupted by prior sphincterotomy.[71] However, the importance of duodenal reflux among patients with an intact sphincter is unclear. Experimental studies indicate that bacteria may travel in the portal vein and be excreted into the bile by the liver.[72] Portal bacteremia is not common in humans, but has been demonstrated in patients with inflammatory bowel disease and in those with Oriental cholangiohepatitis.[73] It also has been suggested that a chronically infected gallbladder may be the source of biliary bacteria in some patients with cholangitis.[74] In addition, hepatic arterial bacteremia and lymphatic transmission from the gut have been proposed as sources of bactibilia, but are largely unsupported by experimental data. Invasive procedures such as endoscopic and transhepatic cholangiography, and the use of biliary stents and endoprostheses have become some of the most important causes of bacterial contamination of the biliary tree.[75,76]

The organisms most commonly cultured from bile are *Escherichia coli, Klebsiella pneumoniae,* and *Enterococcus* sp.[77] The finding of *Enterobacter* and *Pseudomonas* sp, identified in 24% to 34% of patients,[78] may reflect the presence of indwelling stents or represent selection by previous antibiotic therapy.[79] Anaerobes, principally *Bacteroides fragilis,* are found in the bile of as many as 50% of patients with choledocholithiasis.[80] One study found that 60% of patients had more than one organism in their biliary tree,[81] and polymicrobial cultures also have been identified in several other series.[77,82] Similar organisms have been identified in the blood of 30% to 50% of patients with cholangitis.[77,82]

Etiology

Obstruction of the biliary tree usually is caused by common duct stones, benign biliary strictures, malignancy, or obstruction of a biliary–intestinal anastomosis. In past series,[78] choledocholithiasis has been the most common cause of cholangitis, accounting for 70% of all cases. In more recent series,[83] with increasing use of cholangiography, biliary stents, and endoprostheses in the treatment of malignant disease of the biliary

Table 13-5   Changing Etiology of Cholangitis at Johns Hopkins Hospital

Etiology (%)	1952–1974 (n = 76)	1976–1978 (n = 40)	1983–1985 (n = 48)	1986–1989 (n = 96)
Choledocholithiasis	70	70	32	28
Benign duct stricture	13	18	14	12
Malignant stricture	17	10	30	57
Sclerosing cholangitis	0	3	24	3

(Lipsett PA, Pitt HA. Acute cholangitis. Surg Clin North Am 1990; 70:1297)

tract, malignancy has accounted for 57% of all cases of cholangitis (Table 13-5).

Diagnosis

Clinical Findings

The clinical presentation of cholangitis ranges from a mild self-limiting illness that does not require treatment to a toxic condition in which patients are obtunded and hypotensive. The typical clinical features of fever, jaundice, and abdominal pain were first described more than 100 years ago.[65] In a series from one institution, fever was present in 92% of patients, jaundice in 65%, and abdominal pain in only 42%. About 5% of patients in most series have septic shock (Table 13-6). Physical findings in cholangitis are variable. Patients may have jaundice and mild right upper quadrant tenderness, but marked tenderness is unusual and should raise the suspicion of an alternative diagnosis, such as acute cholecystitis.

Laboratory Results

Laboratory investigations may be helpful in confirming the clinical diagnosis of acute cholangitis. Most patients with cholangitis have leukocytosis, but leuko-

Table 13-6   Presentation of Patients With Cholangitis

Symptom	Incidence (%)
Fever	92
Jaundice	67
Chills	65
Abdominal pain	42
Charcot's triad	19
Shock	4

(Adapted from Pitt HA, Couse NE. Biliary sepsis and toxic cholangitis. In: Moody FG, Carey LC, Jones RS, et al, eds. Surgical treatment of digestive disease. Chicago, Mosby–Year Book, 1990;337)

penia can occur in patients with severe sepsis. Serum bilirubin and alkaline phosphatase levels are elevated in 80% of patients with cholangitis, and are higher in patients with malignant obstruction. Liver transaminase levels also are elevated in most patients, with higher levels associated with benign disease. The serum amylase level is markedly increased in about one third of patients with cholangitis,[81] suggesting that the cholangitis is caused by benign, rather than malignant, biliary tract disease. It also has been shown that levels of the tumor marker CA19-9 are elevated in acute cholangitis and return to normal after successful treatment.[84] The results of blood cultures are positive in 30% of patients with cholangitis, and are useful in identifying the causative organism and guiding the choice of antibiotics.

Radiologic Findings

Ultrasound and CT scanning are useful in the evaluation of patients with suspected cholangitis.[81] Both modalities are excellent for detecting intrahepatic and extrahepatic bile duct dilatation, but CT scanning is better than ultrasound at demonstrating common duct stones and periampullary tumors. Cholangiography is required in most patients to define biliary pathology and the nature of bile duct obstruction before definitive treatment. Either endoscopic retrograde cholangiography or PTC can be used.

Treatment

General Support

The initial treatment of patients with cholangitis is supportive. Fluid and electrolyte imbalances should be corrected and antibiotic therapy commenced. Severely ill patients may require admission to the intensive care unit for invasive monitoring. Pressor support may be required if hydration is insufficient to maintain blood pressure. When a pressor is indicated, low-dose dopamine should be used to preserve renal blood flow because these patients are at particularly high risk for the development of renal failure.

Antibiotic Therapy

The choice of antibiotic should reflect the likely pathogens, the severity of the illness, the response to therapy, and the results of sensitivity tests when these become available. Traditionally, an aminoglycoside has been used to provide coverage of gram-negative organisms,[69] ampicillin to provide additional protection against *Enterococcus*,[78] and metronidazole or clindamycin to treat anaerobic organisms such as *B fragilis.* Piperacillin or mezlocillin may be as effective as combined therapy with an aminoglycoside and ampicillin,[85,86] as well as being less nephrotoxic. In addition to their activity against gram-negative organisms, certain third-generation cephalosporins or penicillins combined with β-lactamase inhibitors also may be effective against anaerobes.

Many studies have focused on the relevance of biliary excretion and bile–serum ratios of different antibiotics to the therapeutic efficacy of these agents. One investigator[87] found that rifamide, an antibiotic that achieves high biliary concentrations, was less effective than gentamicin, which is poorly excreted in bile, in the prevention of septic complications after elective biliary surgery. Adequate serum and tissue concentrations and an appropriate antibacterial spectrum, as determined by blood and bile cultures, are more important factors to be considered in choosing an antibiotic regimen than are differences in the biliary concentrations of these agents.

Patients with mild illness can be treated on an outpatient basis with oral antibiotics. Prolonged aminoglycoside therapy is inappropriate in these patients, and the newer penicillins or third-generation cephalosporins may be more useful. When aminoglycoside therapy is used in patients with cholangitis, serum antibiotic levels and renal function must be monitored closely because of the increased risk of renal dysfunction associated with aminoglycoside use in these patients.

Biliary Decompression

About 70% of patients respond to supportive measures and antibiotic therapy alone. Cholangiography can be performed when patients have been afebrile for 24 hours, and definitive treatment of the obstructing lesion may be carried out during the same hospital stay. Patients who do not demonstrate clinical and laboratory evidence of improvement within 12 to 24 hours, and those who have septic shock (5%), require emergency cholangiography and urgent biliary decompres-

sion. However, the optimal approach to draining the duct in these severely ill patients has been the subject of considerable debate.

One group addressed this question in a prospective randomized study comparing endoscopic biliary decompression with open choledochotomy[88] (Table 13-7). Eighty-two patients with severe cholangitis were randomly assigned after emergency endoscopic cholangiography to have a nasobiliary drain positioned after a small sphincterotomy (less than 0.5 cm) was performed, or to undergo common bile duct exploration and placement of a T-tube. Patients undergoing surgical drainage required ventilatory support for a longer period (80 hours versus 51 hours, $P < .05$) and were more likely to have complications (66% versus 34%, $P < .05$) and retained stones (23% versus 7%, $P < .03$). The mortality rate also was significantly greater in the group that received surgical treatment (32% versus 7%, $P < .03$). The results of this study indicate that, in the few patients who have severe cholangitis, including septic shock, early endoscopic drainage is preferable to emergency surgery.

Many patients with cholangitis already have indwelling biliary catheters or endoprostheses. In these patients, all external catheters should be placed on external drainage, and supportive and antibiotic therapy should be initiated. In some cases, the catheters are occluded by sludge and must be changed to provide adequate biliary drainage. Cholangitis can be prevented in this group of patients by changing the catheters at regular intervals (every 3 months) to prevent occlusion.

Patients without biliary tubes in whom endoscopic access is contraindicated because of a previous Billroth II gastrectomy can be treated using a percutaneous approach. PTC and drainage are preferable in patients with proximal obstruction by malignant disease or benign bile duct stricture, but are contraindicated in pa-

Table 13-7 Endoscopic Sphincterotomy Versus Open Common Duct Exploration for Severe Cholangitis

	Endoscopic Sphincterotomy	Open Choledochotomy
Number of patients	41	41
Ventilator support (h)	47	80*
Fasting (h)	51	80*
Morbidity rate (%)	34	66
Retained stone rate (%)	7	29*
Mortality rate (%)	7	32*

* $P < .05$ versus endoscopic sphincterotomy.
(Adapted from Lai ECS, Mok FPT, Tan ESY, et al. Endoscopic biliary drainage for severe acute cholangitis. N Engl J Med 1992;326:1582)

tients with ascites, uncorrected coagulopathy, or non-dilated intrahepatic bile ducts. It is preferable to avoid the use of excessive volumes of contrast media during cholangiography, because any increase in biliary pressure may promote cholangiovenous reflux and result in bacteremia. At the initial procedure, the catheter should be positioned in the proximal biliary tree. The catheter can be advanced through the obstructing lesion electively when the initial sepsis has resolved.

Results

Acute renal failure and intrahepatic abscess formation are the most common complications of acute cholangitis. Acute renal failure occurs in as many as 33% of patients with cholangitis.[69] The etiology of renal failure occurring in association with cholangitis is multifactorial. Ischemia may result from hypoperfusion in patients with sepsis and hypovolemia.[89] In addition, elevated levels of bile pigments may sensitize the renal parenchyma to ischemic injury, because the risk of renal failure is related directly to the serum bilirubin concentration.[90] Renal damage produced by circulating endotoxin also may play an important role in the production of renal failure in patients with cholangitis.[90] Intrahepatic abscess formation occurs less commonly but should be considered in patients with toxic cholangitis and in those who fail to respond to adequate supportive treatment. Ultrasonography or CT scanning may reveal multiple hepatic abscesses in these patients, which can be drained through the skin or at operation.

Most patients respond well to initial supportive measures and antibiotics, and 70% were cured by these measures in one series.[85] Alterations in antibiotic regimens or biliary drainage procedures are necessary in 25% of cases. The mortality rate associated with cholangitis is about 5%.[79] Poor prognostic factors include toxic cholangitis, malignant biliary obstruction, cirrhosis, renal failure, and liver abscess.

INTRAHEPATIC STONES

Although intrahepatic stones (or hepatolithiasis) are relatively uncommon in Western countries, they are prevalent in Asia and represent a difficult management problem for physicians in that region. Both surgical and nonoperative therapies have been suggested, but the optimal approach is to combine both modalities in a multidisciplinary team approach.[49]

Pathogenesis

Stone Composition

The stones found in hepatolithiasis are predominantly soft brown pigment stones that consist primarily of calcium bilirubinate and calcium palmitate, but have a relatively high cholesterol content (see Fig. 13-2). The mechanism of formation of brown pigment stones and the reasons for their unique composition were discussed earlier.

Underlying Pathology

Intrahepatic stones typically occur in association with diseases characterized by prolonged partial bile duct obstruction, such as sclerosing cholangitis, benign or malignant biliary strictures, cystic dilatation of the biliary tree, and even choledocholithiasis itself. In addition, in Asian populations, stones may form in the intrahepatic biliary tree as part of the syndrome of Oriental cholangiohepatitis. In this condition, infestation of the biliary tract with the parasites *Ascaris lumbricoides* and *Clonorchis sinensis* is thought to promote biliary stasis either by directly causing mechanical obstruction or by producing duct wall damage that leads to secondary stricture formation. Bactibilia also is common, possibly as a result of episodic portal bacteremia. Some authors believe that pigment stone formation is primarily a result of this bactibilia,[73] and suggest that the parasitic infection, which is endemic in these populations, is coincidental.

Diagnosis

Clinical Findings

Most patients with hepatolithiasis have had previous biliary surgery. These patients usually have cholangitis, pain, or jaundice.[49] Cholangitis is the most frequent presentation, occurring in about two thirds of patients. Typically, cholangitis is recurrent, and it may be severe and associated with abscess formation and significant destruction of hepatic parenchyma. Pain occurs in over 60% of patients and may be episodic or persistent.[91] Jaundice is noted in 39% to 60% of patients at presentation.[49,91] The findings on physical examination often are nonspecific and may include hepatomegaly, right upper quadrant tenderness, and jaundice.

Laboratory Results

The laboratory investigation of patients with cholangitis caused by intrahepatic stones was discussed earlier. In patients with septic complications, leukocytosis is usual. Many of these patients are found to have elevated levels on liver function testing. The results of blood cultures are positive in 47% of these patients at presentation and, when available, the results of bile cultures are positive in almost 90%.[91] However, particularly in patients without cholangitis, liver function test results may be normal and are not a reliable indicator of the extent of disease.

Radiologic Findings

Ultrasound and CT are useful noninvasive techniques for detecting dilated ducts and intrahepatic stones lying within them. These modalities also may demonstrate complications such as intrahepatic abscess formation and parenchymal destruction. However, neither ultrasound nor CT is sensitive for detecting stone disease in nondilated ducts. Radionuclide imaging using iminodiacetic acid derivatives may show delayed emptying of affected ducts or complete absence of uptake in severely damaged segments, but it is not useful in the routine assessment of these patients.

Cholangiography, either percutaneous or endoscopic, is the most valuable technique in the evaluation of patients with hepatolithiasis. The indications for choosing the most appropriate route were discussed previously. In most of these patients, the percutaneous route is preferable because it allows direct access to the intrahepatic biliary tree for later therapeutic procedures, if necessary. Biliary decompression can be performed as an emergency procedure in the treatment of

patients with severe toxic cholangitis, or of those whose cholangitis fails to respond to conservative measures.

Treatment

Percutaneous

After a percutaneous catheter has been placed under ultrasound or fluoroscopic guidance, the tract is enlarged gradually using successively larger catheters until it can accommodate at least a 16F catheter, then it is allowed to mature for 5 to 6 weeks.[92] At that time, stones can be removed either under fluoroscopic guidance using a conventional or steerable stone retrieval basket, or under direct vision using a choledochoscope passed along the catheter tract[93,94] (Fig. 13-13). Several of these procedures may be required to effect complete stone removal. These techniques can be combined with electrohydraulic lithotripsy in the treatment of stones that are too large to be removed intact.[95]

In selected patients, percutaneous balloon dilatation of intrahepatic ductal strictures can be performed through the tract, thus alleviating the underlying pathology.[96,97] Stents can be left in place to allow repeated procedures, and to exclude the possibility of cholangiocarcinoma. Brushings can be obtained through the tract for cytologic diagnosis, or a choledochoscope can be used to survey and biopsy the ductal mucosa directly. In some patients, particularly those with sclerosing cholangitis, the biliary stents are left in position indefinitely. When stents are left in place, they should be changed electively every 3 months over a guide wire to

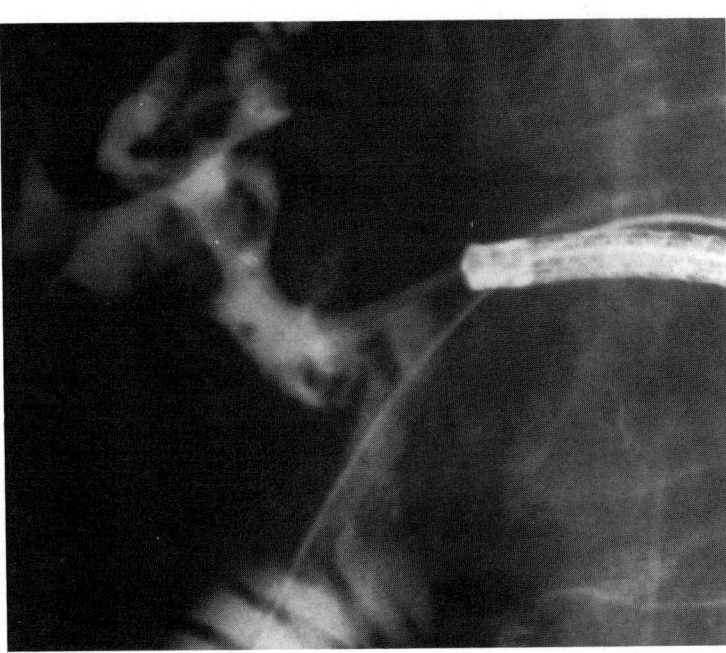

Figure 13-13 Percutaneous choledochoscopy performed through transhepatic stent tracts demonstrating extensive intrahepatic stone disease in a patient who had a previous choledochojejunostomy. (Pitt HA, Venbrux AC, Coleman J, et al. Intrahepatic stones: the transhepatic team approach. Ann Surg 1994;219:527)

prevent stent occlusion and cholangitis. Complications of percutaneous techniques include cholangitis, bleeding that may be severe enough to require transfusion or emergency surgery, and pancreatitis.

Because of the relatively high cholesterol content of these stones, pharmacologic therapy using ursodeoxycholic acid is of benefit in some patients, either as primary therapy or as an adjunct to percutaneous or operative clearance. Ros and colleagues[98] reported successful clearance of hepatolithiasis in 12 adults with underlying Caroli's disease using ursodeoxycholic acid. These patients remained free of stones on maintenance therapy 48 months after initial treatment.

Surgery

Some patients with intrahepatic stone disease are treated successfully using percutaneous techniques alone. However, surgery remains an important part of therapy for many patients with hepatolithiasis. Surgical options include choledochostomy, choledochoduodenostomy, sphincteroplasty, choledochojejunostomy or hepaticojejunostomy with or without a transhepatic stent, hepaticocutaneous jejunostomy, and liver resection. Formerly, many patients were treated with surgical duct exploration and stone removal, together with either a sphincteroplasty or a choledochoduodenostomy to drain the duct. More recently, the need for long-term access to the intrahepatic biliary tree has been appreciated. Some authors recommend draining the hepatic duct into a Roux-en-Y loop of jejunum and creating a cutaneous fistula between the Roux loop and the skin (hepaticocutaneous jejunostomy), allowing long-term percutaneous access to the hepatic duct for later stone removal.[99] Alternatively, a hepaticojejunostomy can be performed and long-term percutaneous access to the biliary tree maintained using transhepatic stents.[49]

In many patients, particularly those in Asia, the disease process is confined to one lobe, more commonly the left lobe, or even to a single segment. For patients with localized hepatolithiasis associated with extensive intrahepatic strictures, chronic infection, and extensive parenchymal destruction, some authors have proposed hepatic resection as the most appropriate surgical treatment.[100] Hepatic resection also is indicated if there is a suspicion that cholangiocarcinoma may exist in the diseased segment.[101] Resection can be combined with stone clearance, hepaticojejunostomy, and either a cutaneous fistula or a transhepatic stent when mild disease exists on the contralateral side. However, resection of one lobe is of little benefit when there is extensive disease in the residual liver tissue.

Combined Approach

In practice, treatment must be tailored to individual patients. One report highlighted the importance of a multidisciplinary team approach to the treatment of patients with hepatolithiasis.[49] This approach, which combines percutaneous techniques, surgery alone, or surgery followed by percutaneous extraction of residual or recurrent stones, has been used successfully in several centers.[93,94]

Results

In selected patients, percutaneous techniques alone are adequate therapy for hepatolithiasis. In a series of 54 patients, 14 (26%) were treated exclusively using percutaneous techniques, 40 (74%) underwent surgery, and 18 of the latter (33%) required postoperative percu-

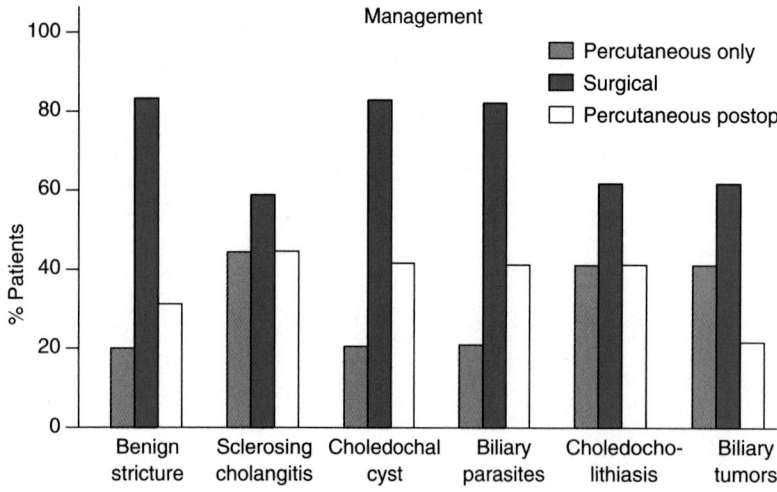

Figure 13-14 Percentage of patients treated only percutaneously (26% overall), surgically (74% overall), and by postoperative percutaneous techniques (33% overall). (After Pitt HA, Venbrux AC, Coleman J, et al. Intrahepatic stones: the transhepatic team approach. Ann Surg 1994;219:527)

taneous procedures[49] (Fig. 13-14). At a mean follow-up of 60 months, successful stone clearance had been obtained in 94% of patients, and 87% were free of symptoms. Twenty percent of patients had recurrent stones and 19% had recurrent strictures, which were managed successfully using percutaneous techniques in all but one case. The procedure-related morbidity was 35% and there were no in-hospital deaths in this series.

These data compare favorably with the results of several large series from Asia, which have reported a stone clearance and recurrence rates of 90%[93,102] and 16%,[93] respectively. These centers also have used segmental hepatic resection in many patients, with similar success rates. In this setting, hepatic resection is associated with an operative mortality rate of 2% and a morbidity rate of 32%.[101] In summary, hepatolithiasis is a difficult clinical problem requiring prolonged therapy. The most successful method is a multidisciplinary team approach involving radiologists and surgeons, using both percutaneous and operative techniques to achieve stone clearance in most patients.

REFERENCES

1. Lillemoe KD, Pitt HA, Gadacz TR. Retained common bile duct stones. In: Sawyer JL, Williams LF, eds. Difficult problems in general surgery. Chicago, Year Book, 1989:155.
2. Kaufman HS, Magnuson TH, Lillemoe KD, Frasca P, Pitt HA. The role of bacteria in gallbladder and common duct stone formation. Ann Surg 1989;209:584.
3. Carey MC. Pathogenesis of gallstones. Am J Surg 1993;165:410.
4. Magnusson TH, Lillemoe KD, Pitt HA. How many Americans will be eligible for biliary lithotripsy? Arch Surg 1989;124:1195.
5. Roslyn JJ, Pitt HA, Mann LL, et al. Gallbladder disease in patients on long-term parenteral nutrition. Gastroenterology 1983;84:148.
6. NIH consensus conference statement on gallstones and laparoscopic cholecystectomy. Am J Surg 1993;165:390.
7. Johnson G, Sprinkle PN. Autopsy incidence of cholelithiasis in a general hospital. N C Med J 1962;23:107.
8. Opie EL. The etiology of acute hemorrhagic pancreatitis. Johns Hopkins Hosp Bull 1901;121:182.
9. Lee SP, Nicholls JF, Park HZ. Biliary sludge as a cause of acute pancreatitis. N Engl J Med 1992;326:589.
10. Patti MG, Pellegrini CA. Gallstone pancreatitis. Surg Clin North Am 1990;70:1277.
11. Armstrong CP, Taylor TV, Jeacock J. The biliary tract in patients with acute gallstone pancreatitis. Br J Surg 1985;72:551.
12. Way LW, Admirand WH, Dunphy JE. Management of choledocholithiasis. Ann Surg 1972;176:347.
13. Saltzstein EC, Peacock JB, Thomas MD. Preoperative bilirubin, alkaline phosphatase and amylase levels as predictors of common duct stones. Surg Gynecol Obstet 1982;154:381.
14. Lacaine F, Corlette MB, Bismuth H. Preoperative evaluation of the risk of common bile duct stones. Arch Surg 1980;115:1114.
15. Goldstein LI, Sample WF, Kadell BM, Weiner M. Grey-scale ultrasonography and thin needle cholangiography. JAMA 1977;238:1041.
16. Einstein DM, Lapin SA, Ralls PW, Halls JM. The insensitivity of sonography in the detection of choledocholithiasis. AJR 1984;142:725.
17. Edmundowicz SA, Aliperti G, Middleton WD. Preliminary experience using endoscopic ultrasonography in the diagnosis of choledocholithiasis. Endoscopy 1992;24:774.
18. Amouyal P, Amouyal G, Mompoint D. Endosonography: promising method for diagnosis of extrahepatic cholestasis. Lancet 1989;2:1195.
19. Pedrosa CS, Casanova R, Rodriguez R. Computed tomography in obstructive jaundice. Radiology 1981;139:627.
20. Baron RL, Stanley RJ, Lee KJT, Koehler RE, Levitt RG. Computed tomographic features of biliary obstruction. AJR 1983;140:1173.
21. Jeffrey RB, Federle MP, Laing FC, Wall S, Rego J, Moss AA. Computed tomography of choledocholithiasis. AJR 1983;140:1179.
22. Mitchell SE, Clark RA. A comparison of computed tomography and sonography in choledocholithiasis. AJR 1984;142:729.
23. Eubanks B, Martinez CR, Mehigan D, Cameron JL. Current role of intravenous cholangiography. Am J Surg 1982;143:731.
24. Siegel JH, Pullano W. Two new methods for selective bile duct cannulation and sphincterotomy. Gastrointest Endosc 1987;33:438.
25. Cotton PB, Lehman G, Vennes J, et al. Endoscopic sphincterotomy complications and their management: an attempt at consensus. Gastrointest Endosc 1991;37:383.
26. Pitt HA. Is endoscopic sphincterotomy a safe and effective method for the management of stones in the distal bile duct? In: Gitnick G, ed. Controversies in gastroenterology. New York, Churchill Livingstone, 1984:97.
27. Jakimowicz JJ, Rutten H, Jurgens PJ, Carol EJ. Comparison of operative ultrasonography and radiography in screening of the common bile duct for calculi. World J Surg 1987;11:628.
28. Mosnier H, Roullet Audy J-C, Bouche O, Guivarc'h M. Intraoperative sonography during cholecystectomy for gallstones. Surg Gynecol Obstet 1992;174:469.
29. Thompson H, Kisslo K, Farouk M, Chung K, Saperstein LA, Meyers WC. Technique of intraluminal biliary ultrasonography during laparoscopic cholecystectomy. Laparoscopy 1992;165:265.

30. Lillemoe KD, Yeo CJ, Talamini MA, Wang BH, Pitt HA, Gadacz TR. Selective cholangiography: current role in laparoscopic surgery. Ann Surg 1992;215:669.

31. Phillips EH. Routine versus selective intraoperative cholangiography. Am J Surg 1993;165:505.

32. Barkun JS, Fried GM, Barkun AN, et al. Cholecystectomy without operative cholangiography. Ann Surg 1993;218:371.

33. Berci G, Sackier JM, Paz-Partlow M. Routine or selected intraoperative cholangiography during laparoscopic cholecystectomy. Am J Surg 1991;161:355.

34. Petelin JB. Laparoscopic approach to common duct pathology. Am J Surg 1993;165:487.

35. Sackier JM, Berci G, Phillips E, Carroll B, Schapiro S, Paz-Partlow M. The role of cholangiography in laparoscopic cholecystectomy. Arch Surg 1991;126:1021.

36. Cotton PB, Vallon JA. British experience with duodenoscopic sphincterotomy for removal of bile duct stones. Br J Surg 1981;68:373.

37. Groen JN, Lock MT, Lamers JS, et al. Removal of common bile duct stones by the combination of percutaneous transhepatic dilatation and extracorporeal shock-wave lithotripsy. Gastroenterology 1989;87:202.

38. Stokes KR, Falchuk KR, Clouse ME. Biliary duct stones: update on 54 cases after percutaneous transhepatic removal. Radiology 1989;179:999.

39. Bland KI, Jones RS, Maher JW, et al. Extracorporeal shock-wave lithotripsy of bile duct calculi: an interim report of the Dornier U.S. bile duct lithotripsy prospective study. Ann Surg 1989;209:742.

40. den Toom R, Nijs HGT, van Blankenstein M, et al. Extracorporeal shock wave treatment of common bile duct stones: experience with two different lithotripters at a single institution. Br J Surg 1991;78:809.

41. DenBesten L, Berci G. The current status of biliary tract surgery: an international study of 1072 patients. World J Surg 1986;10:116.

42. Motson RW, Wetter LA. Operative choledochoscopy: common bile duct exploration is incomplete without it. Br J Surg 1990;77:975.

43. Ratych RE, Sitzman JV, Lillemoe KD, Yeo CJ, Cameron JL. Transduodenal exploration of the common bile duct in patients with nondilated ducts. Surg Gynecol Obstet 1991;173:49.

44. Hunter JG. Laparoscopic transcystic common bile duct exploration. Am J Surg 1992;163:53.

45. Smith PC, Clayman RV, Soper NJ. Laparoscopic cholecystectomy and choledochoscopy for the treatment of cholelithiasis and choledocholithiasis. Surgery 1990;111:230.

46. Hunter JG, Soper NJ. Laparoscopic management of bile duct stones. Surg Clin North Am 1992;72:1077.

47. Tompkins RK, Lai ECS. Reoperative surgery. Philadelphia, JB Lippincott, 1988:178.

48. Tompkins RK, Johnson J, Strom FK, et al. Operative endoscopy in the management of biliary tract neoplasms. Am J Surg 1976;132:174.

49. Pitt HA, Venbrux AC, Coleman J, et al. Intrahepatic stones: the transhepatic team approach. Ann Surg 1994;219:527.

50. Russell E, Yrizarry H, et al. Percutaneous transjejunal biliary dilatation: alternate management for benign strictures. Radiology 1985;159:209.

51. Burhenne HJ. Nonoperative retained biliary tract stone extraction: a new roentgenological technique. AJR 1973;117:388.

52. Chen MF, Chou FF, Wang CS, Yang YI. Experience with and complications of postoperative choledochofiberoscopy for retained biliary stones. Acta Chir Scand 1982;148:503.

53. Ponsky JL. Alternative methods in the management of bile duct stones. Surg Clin North Am 1992;72:1099.

54. Thistle JL, Carlson GL, Goldfarb S, et al. Monooctanoin, a dissolution agent for retained cholesterol bile duct stones: physical properties and clinical applications. Gastroenterology 1980;78:1016.

55. Gardner B, Dennis CR, Patti J. Current status of heparin dissolution of gallstones: experimental and clinical observations. Am J Surg 1975;130:293.

56. Pitt HA, Cameron JL. Sodium cholate dissolution of retained biliary stones: mortality rate following intrahepatic infusion. Surgery 1979;85:457.

57. Kelly TR, Wagner DS. Gallstone pancreatitis: a prospective randomized trial of the time of surgery. Surgery 1988;104:600.

58. Neoptolemos JP, Carr-Locke DL, London NJ, Bailey JA, James D, Fossard DP. Controlled trial of urgent endoscopic retrograde cholangiopancreatography and endoscopic sphincterotomy versus conservative treatment for acute pancreatitis due to gallstones. Lancet 1988;2:979.

59. Fan S, Lai ECS, Ok FP, Lo CM, Zheng SS, Wong J. Early treatment of acute biliary pancreatitis by endoscopic papillotomy. N Engl J Med 1993;328:228.

60. Neoptolemos JP, Carr-Locke DL, Fraser I, Fossard DP. The management of common duct calculi by endoscopic sphincterotomy in patients with gallstones. Br J Surg 1984;71:69.

61. Miller BM, Kozarek RA, Ryan JA, Ball TJ, Traverso LW. Surgical versus endoscopic management of common bile duct stones. Ann Surg 1988;207:135.

62. Schwab G, Pointner R, Wetscher G, Glasser K, Foltin E, Bodner E. Treatment of calculi of the common bile duct. Surg Gynecol Obstet 1992;175:115.

63. Neoptolemos JP, Carr-Locke DL, Fossard DP. Prospective randomized trial of preoperative endoscopic sphincterotomy versus surgery alone for common bile duct stones. BMJ 1987;294:470.

64. Stain SC, Cohen H, Tsuishoysha M, Donovan AJ. Choledocholithiasis: endoscopic sphincterotomy or common bile duct exploration. Ann Surg 1991;213:627.

65. Charcot JM. Lecons sur les maladies du foi des voies biliares et des rins. Paris, Faculte de Medecin de Paris, 1877.

66. Mallet-Guy P. Value of preoperative manometric and

roentgenographic examination in the diagnosis of pathologic changes and functional disturbances of the biliary tract. Surg Gynecol Obstet 1952;165:385.

67. Fukunga FH. Gallbladder bacteriology, histology and gallstones. Arch Surg 1973;106:169.

68. Keighley MR, Flinn R, Alexander-Williams J. Multivariate analysis of clinical and operative findings associated with biliary sepsis. Br J Surg 1976;63:528.

69. Pitt HA, Postier RG, Cameron JL. Bacteremia after tube cholangiography. Ann Surg 1980;191:30.

70. Neoptolemos JP, Carr-Locke DL, Fossard DP. Prospective randomized study of preoperative endoscopic sphincterotomy versus surgery alone for common bile duct stones. BMJ 1987;294:470.

71. Kracht M, Thompson JN, Bernhoft RA, et al. Cholangitis after endoscopic sphincterotomy in patients with stricture of the biliary duct. Surg Gynecol Obstet 1986;163:324.

72. Sung JY, Shaffer EA, Olson ME, et al. Bacterial invasion of the biliary system by way of the portal-venous system. Hepatology 1991;14:313.

73. Ong GB. A study of recurrent pyogenic cholangitis. Arch Surg 1962;84:199.

74. Edlund YA, Mollstedt BO, Ouchterlony O. Bacteriological investigation of the biliary system and liver in biliary tract disease correlated to clinical data and microstructure of the gallbladder and liver. Acta Chir Scand 1959;116:461.

75. Lai EC, Lo CMC, Choi TK, et al. Urgent biliary decompression after endoscopic retrograde cholangiopancreatography. Am J Surg 1989;157:121.

76. Blenkharn JI, Benjamin IS. Infection during percutaneous transhepatic biliary drainage. Surgery 1989;105:239.

77. Gigot JF, Leese T, Dereme T, Coutinho J, Castaing D, Bismuth H. Acute cholangitis: multivariate analysis of risk factors. Ann Surg 1989;209:435.

78. Pitt HA, Zuidema GD. Factors influencing mortality in the treatment of pyogenic hepatic abscess. Surg Gynecol Obstet 1975;140:228.

79. Lipsett PA, Pitt HA. Acute cholangitis. Surg Clin North Am 1990;70:1297.

80. Kosowski K, Karczewska E, Kasprowicz A, et al. Bacteria in bile of patients with bile duct inflammation. Eur J Clin Microbiol 1987;6:575.

81. Saharia PC, Cameron JL. Clinical management of acute cholangitis. Surg Gynecol Obstet 1976;142:369.

82. Boey JH, Way LW. Acute cholangitis. Ann Surg 1980;191:264.

83. Stewart L, Pellegrini CA, Way LW. Cholangiovenous reflux pathways as defined by corrosion casting and scanning electron microscopy. Am J Surg 1988;155:23.

84. Albert MA, Steinberg WM, Henry JP. Elevated serum levels of tumor marker CA 19-9 in acute cholangitis. Dig Dis Sci 1988;33:1223.

85. Thompson JE Jr, Pitt HA, Doty JE, et al. Broad spectrum penicillin as an adequate therapy for acute cholangitis. Surg Gynecol Obstet 1990;67:325.

86. Gerecht WB, Henry NK, Hoffman WW, et al. Prospective randomized comparison of mezlocillin therapy alone with combined ampicillin and gentamycin therapy for patients with cholangitis. Arch Intern Med 1989;149:1279.

87. Keighley MR, Baddely RM, Burdon DW, et al. A controlled trial of parenteral prophylactic gentamycin therapy in biliary surgery. Br J Surg 1975;62:215.

88. Lai ECS, Mok FPT, Tan ESY, et al. Endoscopic biliary drainage for severe acute cholangitis. N Engl J Med 1992;326:1582.

89. Gubern JM, Sancho JJ, O'Sim J, et al. A randomized trial on the effect of mannitol on postoperative renal function in patients with obstructive jaundice. Surgery 1988;103:39.

90. Pain JA, Cahill CJ, Bailey ME. Preoperative complications in obstructive jaundice: therapeutic considerations. Br J Surg 1985;73:775.

91. Fan ST, Lai ECS, Mok FPT, Choi TK, Wong J. Acute cholangitis secondary to hepatolithiasis. Arch Surg 1991;126:1027.

92. Venbrux AC, Robbins KV, Savader SJ, et al. Endoscopy as an adjuvant to biliary radiologic intervention. Radiology 1991;180:355.

93. Fan ST, Choi TK, Lo CM, Mok FPT, Lai ECS, Wong J. Treatment of hepatolithiasis: improvement of result by a systematic approach. Surgery 1991;109:474.

94. Choi TK, Fok M, Lee MJR, Lui R, Wong J. Postoperative flexible choledochoscopy for residual intrahepatic stones. Ann Surg 1986;203:260.

95. Yoshimoto H, Ikeda S, Tanaka M, Matsumoto S, Juroda Y. Choledochoscopic electrohydraulic lithotripsy and lithotomy for stones in the common bile duct, intrahepatic ducts, and gallbladder. Ann Surg 1990;210:576.

96. Hutson DG, Russell E, Schiff E, Levi JJ, Zeppa R. Balloon dilatation of biliary strictures through a choledochojejuno-cutaneous fistula. Ann Surg 1984;199:637.

97. Tanaka M, Yoshimoto H, Ikeda S, et al. Two approaches for electrohydraulic lithotripsy in the common bile duct. Surgery 1985;98:313.

98. Ros E. Ursodeoxycholic acid treatment of primary hepatolithiasis in Caroli's syndrome. Lancet 1993;342:404.

99. Fan ST, Mok F, Zheng SS, Lai ECS, Lao CM, Wong J. Appraisal of hepaticocutaneous jejunostomy in the management of hepatolithiasis. Am J Surg 1993;165:332.

100. Choi TK, Wong J. Partial hepatectomy for intrahepatic stones. World J Surg 1986;10:281.

101. Fan ST, Lai ECS, Wong J. Hepatic resection for hepatolithiasis. Arch Surg 1993;128:1070.

102. Yamakama T. Percutaneous cholangioscopy for management of retained biliary tract stones and intrahepatic stones. Endoscopy 1989;21:333.

103. Ranson JHC. Etiologic and prognostic factors in human acute pancreatitis: a review. Am J Gastroenterol 1982;77:633.

104. Pitt HA, Couse NF. Biliary sepsis and toxic cholangitis. In: Moody FG, Carey LC, Jones RS, et al, eds. Surgical treatment of digestive disease, ed 2. Chicago, Mosby–Year Book, 1990:337.

Digestive Tract Surgery: A Text and Atlas, edited by Richard H. Bell,
Layton F. Rikkers, and Michael W. Mulholland.
Lippincott-Raven Publishers, Philadelphia, © 1996.

14

Cystic Disease of the Biliary Tract

Nathaniel J. Soper

Cystic lesions of the biliary tract are uncommon problems that can appear in various forms and combinations. Nonbiliary hepatic cysts, which can be distinguished from biliary cysts by the combination of noninvasive imaging and cholangiography, are not discussed in this chapter. Choledochal cysts are unusual congenital dilations of the bile duct that can be confined to either the extrahepatic or intrahepatic biliary tree or can affect both simultaneously. Choledochal cysts are more common in women and in Asians. Although initially thought to be rare, modern imaging technology has facilitated identification of choledochal cysts, leading to an apparent increase in their incidence. Establishing the diagnosis of choledochal cysts is important because they predispose to cholangitis, gallstones, jaundice, portal hypertension, and cholangiocarcinoma, and nonsurgical management usually fails.

The first anatomic description of a choledochal cyst was in 1723,[1] and the first case report was published in 1852.[2] Because choledochal cysts are relatively rare in Western countries, it was not until 1959 that the first large series was reported in English by Alonzo-Lej and colleagues.[3] In their review, a classification system for the cysts was detailed, which has subsequently been modified.[4,5] Alonzo-Lej and colleagues[3] also described various modes of treatment of choledochal cysts, depending on the type of anomaly. The preferred operative therapy for choledochal cysts has subsequently been modified as the natural history and long-term outcome has been clarified.

ANATOMIC CLASSIFICATION

Choledochal cysts are localized dilations of the bile duct and thus are not true cysts. As opposed to diffuse dilation of the proximal biliary tree seen in acquired obstruction of the distal bile duct, the bile ducts above and below the cyst and the gallbladder are usually of normal caliber or are slightly dilated proximally. However, choledochal cysts can be associated with fusiform dilation of both extrahepatic and intrahepatic bile ducts. Several classifications for bile duct cysts have been proposed, but the scheme described by Alonzo-Lej and colleagues[3] is the basis for the most commonly used system (Fig. 14-1).

Type I, or cystic dilation of the common bile duct, is by far the most common variety, constituting between 65% and 90% of the reported cases. Type I cysts can be further divided into those that are saccular (Ia), localized (Ib), or fusiform (Ic). Most commonly, type I cysts are large and saccular and involve most of the extrahepatic biliary system. The common bile duct is usually narrow distal to the cyst but on occasion can be of normal caliber or dilated down to its ampullary orifice. With type I cysts, the cystic duct can enter the dilated region directly or can enter a normal common bile duct uninvolved by the cyst.

Type II choledochal cysts are isolated diverticula of the common bile duct. Type II cysts are rare, comprising less than 3% of all cases. Type III cysts, also known as *choledochoceles*, are characterized by dilation of the intraduodenal portion of the common bile duct. The rela-

433

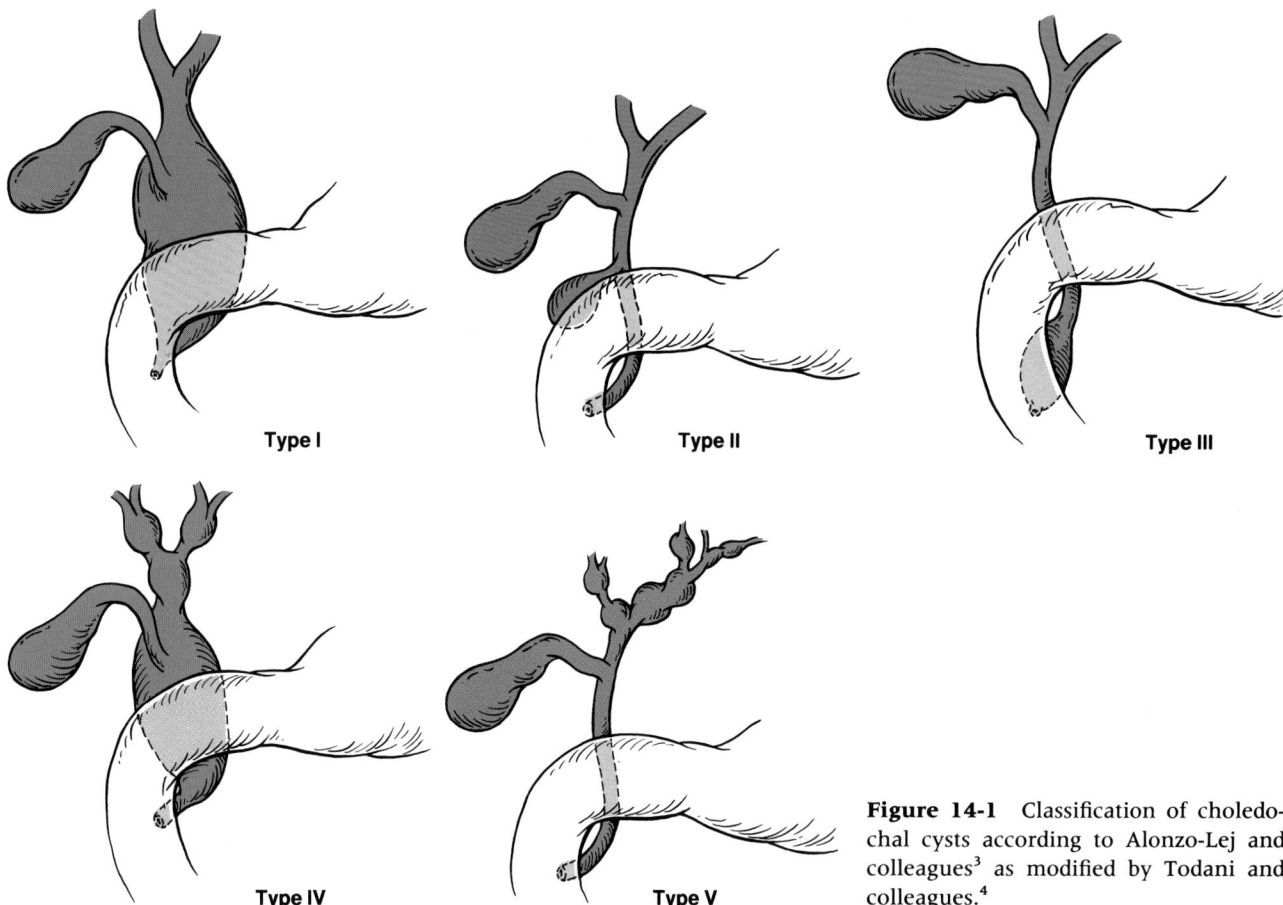

Figure 14-1 Classification of choledochal cysts according to Alonzo-Lej and colleagues[3] as modified by Todani and colleagues.[4]

tive frequency of type III cysts varies from 2% to 20% of cases in different series. In these cases, the cystic portion can also be intrapancreatic. Usually, both the common bile duct and main pancreatic duct enter the choledochocele separately; the choledochocele then empties into the duodenal lumen through a narrow opening.

Types IV and V were added to Alonzo-Lej's classification system by Todani and colleagues in 1977.[4] Type IV consists of multiple cysts, either intrahepatic and extrahepatic (IVa) or extrahepatic only (IVb), whereas type V forms of the anomaly are single or multiple intrahepatic cysts only. These isolated intrahepatic cysts, which can be associated with hepatic fibrosis, are referred to as *Caroli's disease.*[6] Caroli's disease is managed differently than other forms of choledochal cysts and is discussed separately later.

PATHOLOGY

Histologically, the wall of extrahepatic choledochal cysts consists of a thick (4- to 5-mm) fibrotic mass of dense collagenous connective tissue interlaced with strands of smooth muscle.[7,8] There is generally some degree of inflammatory reaction in the wall, and typical biliary mucosal lining is usually absent (Fig. 14-2). Sparse islands of columnar epithelium are usually seen. The size of the cysts varies from small cysts less than 1 cm in diameter to giant cysts more than 10 cm in diameter (Fig. 14-3). In infants, there may be complete obstruction of the distal common bile duct, suggesting a form of biliary atresia. The findings on liver biopsy vary with the age of the patient and generally reflect chronic biliary obstruction, ranging from normal to advanced biliary cirrhosis. Patients with Caroli's disease usually have significant periductal fibrosis. Neoplasia can develop in choledochal cysts and is usually adenocarcinoma. In patients with choledochocele, the cyst may be lined either by duodenal mucosa or biliary mucosa.[9]

Intraoperative culture of the fluid contained within choledochal cysts is usually sterile, but there may be superinfection by a variety of bacteria, most commonly gram-negative rods. When there is significant distal obstruction or pigment stones within the cyst, cholangitis can develop, with associated periportal inflammation. Congenital choledochal cysts contain stones much

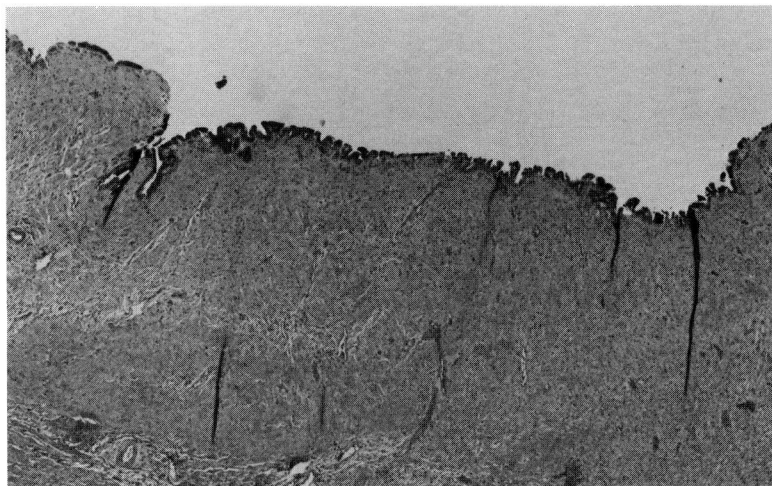

Figure 14-2 Typical histologic cross section of the lining of a choledochal cyst. Some columnar epithelium remains, but many areas are denuded, and there is a moderate inflammatory reaction throughout the wall of the duct. (See Color Fig. 14-2.)

less frequently than do acquired biliary dilations, which develop proximal to primary or secondary biliary strictures.

ETIOLOGY

Numerous theories have been proposed and subsequently discarded to explain the pathogenesis of choledochal cysts. Because there is no good animal model of this disease entity, little experimental evidence has been published to support any of the theories.

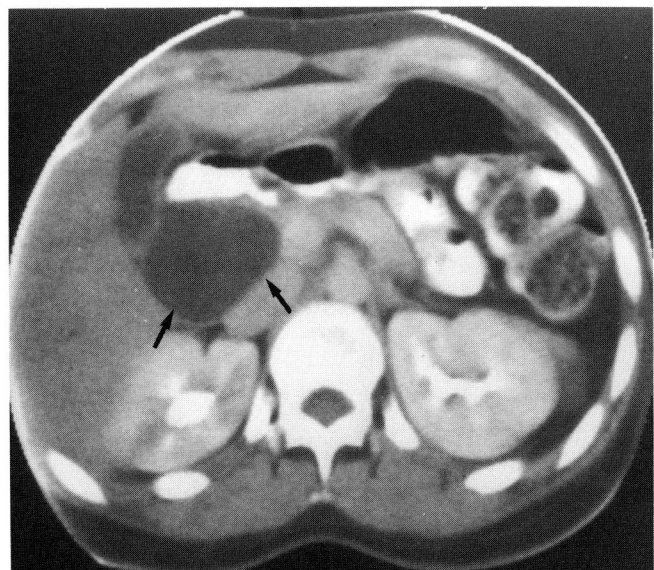

Figure 14-3 CT scan of a large choledochal cyst (*arrows*) seen anterior to the right kidney and posterior to the duodenum near the head of the pancreas.

It is likely that the different forms of choledochal cysts arise from differing pathogenetic mechanisms. The classic embryologic theory for type I cysts proposes that cystic abnormalities result from abnormal canalization of the biliary passages.[10] The bile ducts develop from an outgrowth on the ventral aspect of the foregut, which is initially a solid core of cells that subsequently recanalizes, a process that is not complete until the fifth month of gestation. Types II and III choledochal cysts are likely developmental anomalies similar to diverticula of the duodenum or small bowel.

The greatest debate focuses on the etiology of type I cysts because these cysts are considerably more common than the other varieties. Early theories suggested a congenital weakness of the bile duct or a combination of distal obstruction and an intrinsic structural defect of the bile duct.[3,11] Another theory suggests that choledochal cysts result from an unequal proliferation of the epithelial cells of the extrahepatic bile ducts during the stage when the primitive choledochus was still a solid core of cells.[10] This theory proposes that choledochal cysts are derived from excessive localized proliferation with subsequent vacuolization during the recanalization phase. Although this hypothesis is reasonable, it has no experimental support.

The most likely explanation for the pathogenesis of choledochal cysts relates to an abnormal junction of the pancreatic and bile ducts within the pancreas, which is often seen on cholangiography.[12] Normally, the common channel of the pancreatic and bile ducts is shorter than 10 mm in adults, and these ducts join within the muscular segment of the sphincter of Oddi, preventing reflux of pancreatic juice into the common bile duct. In most patients with choledochal cysts, the common pancreaticobiliary channel is much longer (more than

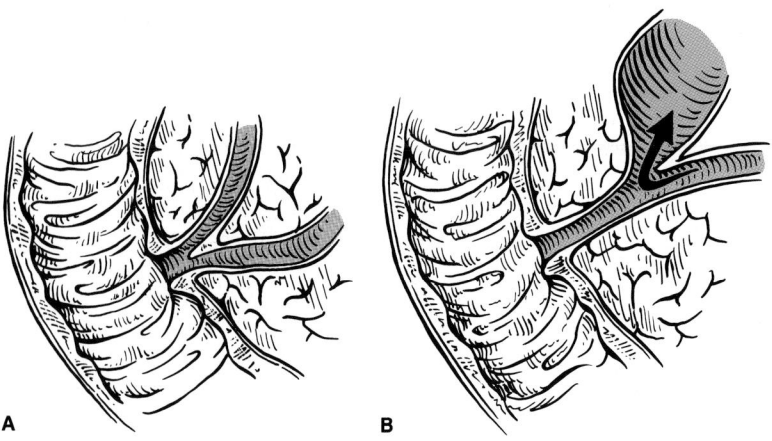

Figure 14-4 Proposed etiologic mechanism in the formation of choledochal cysts. (**A**) Normal relation of distal bile and pancreatic ducts. (**B**) Abnormally high junction of the pancreatic and bile ducts allows reflux of pancreatic juice into the bile duct, leading to destruction of the duct wall with subsequent dilation.

20 mm; Fig. 14-4). This anomalous junction of the pancreatic and bile ducts outside the influence of the sphincter of Oddi allows reflux of pancreatic juice into the choledochus because of the higher pressure in the pancreatic duct than the bile duct. Reflux of pancreatic enzymes into the bile duct can cause damage to the duct wall. The potential results are inflammation, ductal dilation, and biliary absorption of amylase (false pancreatitis), all of which occur with choledochal cysts.[13] In one study,[14] the bile of eight patients with choledochal cysts and anomalous junction of the pancreatic and bile ducts was analyzed, and markedly elevated levels of amylase, phospholipase A$_2$, and lysophosphatidylcholine were found. The latter is a cytotoxic biliary phospholipid produced from phosphatidylcholine by phospholipase A$_2$. These findings support the theory of aberrant junction of the pancreatic and bile ducts leading to type I choledochal cysts.

Not all patients with choledochal cysts, however, have an abnormal pancreaticobiliary junction, and destruction of bile duct epithelium alone does not cause choledochal cysts. Increased intraluminal pressure can also be important; ligation of the distal common bile duct in fetal lambs has produced cystic biliary dilation.[15] Therefore, although the common-channel theory remains attractive, developmental factors can also play a role. It has been postulated that abnormal distal bile and pancreatic duct anatomy is only one manifestation of a disordered embryology that affects the entire extrahepatic biliary ductal system.[16]

CLINICAL PRESENTATION

The incidence of choledochal cysts in Western countries is between 1:100,000 and 1:150,000 live births, but it is more common in Japan. The female/male ratio in both Occidental and Japanese series is 3:1 to 4:1. About 60% of cases are diagnosed before 10 years of age, but choledochal cysts are being discovered more commonly in adults as imaging studies are becoming more sophisticated and widely applied. The classic triad—right upper quadrant pain, jaundice, and a palpable abdominal mass—is now the exception rather than the rule, as reported in older series (Table 14-1). Publications from 1975,[20] 1991,[21] and 1993[33] reported that 38%, 15%, and 15% of patients, respectively, had this triad of diagnostic findings. Also, fewer patients now present with late complications of the disease, such as cirrhosis, cholangitis with sepsis, or peritonitis secondary to cyst rupture.

The pain from choledochal cysts often mimics biliary colic or acute cholecystitis, and jaundice is usually mild and may be intermittent. If a mass is present, it is usually soft, nontender, and mobile. Symptoms differ in children of varying ages. Neonates usually present with complete biliary obstruction, and older children often have abdominal pain and jaundice. Patients with choledochoceles (type III choledochal cysts) may present with recurrent acute pancreatitis, biliary colic, cholangitis, or duodenal obstruction with nausea and vomiting.[17,18]

Table 14-1 Presentation of Choledochal Cysts

Investigator	Jaundice (%)	Pain (%)	Mass (%)	Triad (%)
Alonzo-Lej et al (1959)[3]	73	65	60	21
Flanigan (1975)[20]	64	55	58	38
Chijiwa & Koga (1993)[33]	43	78	33	15

DIAGNOSIS

Before the widespread availability of accurate imaging modalities, the correct diagnosis of choledochal cysts was infrequently made before operation. Currently, laboratory studies in these cases are used to determine the clinical condition rather than to make the diagnosis. Because jaundice is the most common presenting sign of choledochal cysts, the primary laboratory findings are conjugated hyperbilirubinemia and an increased level of serum alkaline phosphatase. Jaundice may be intermittent and mild in adults, whereas in infants it is often severe and unrelenting. When biliary obstruction has been present for a long time or when early cirrhosis has developed, abnormalities in other liver enzymes and in the coagulation profile can be present. Patients with choledochoceles may have hyperamylasemia and pain from pancreatitis, and those with type I choledochal cysts can manifest hyperamylasemia as a result of increased absorption of pancreatic amylase from the bile duct. When cholangitis is present, evidence of cholestasis is present along with leukocytosis.

The specific diagnosis of choledochal cysts, however, depends on accurate imaging rather than physical examination and blood analysis. Historically, radiographic studies were not particularly helpful because standard contrast studies (eg, upper gastrointestinal series, intravenous cholangiography) were seldom diagnostic until choledochal cysts grew to large sizes. Abdominal ultrasonography is now the most helpful initial screening study for choledochal cysts. This modality is used routinely to evaluate the patient with any of the three classic signs of choledochal cysts—jaundice, pain, and a right upper quadrant abdominal mass. Once a thick-walled cyst in the right upper quadrant is demonstrated by ultrasound, its relation to the bile ducts can be investigated with more invasive contrast studies. Computed tomography can complement the findings on ultrasound, particularly when the diagnosis is in doubt, and can identify associated mass lesions (Fig. 14-5). Biliary scintigrams with an iminodiacetic acid derivative (eg, DISIDA) should be obtained in patients presenting with acute symptoms to exclude acute cholecystitis; they demonstrate filling of both the gallbladder and large common bile duct, with slow emptying into the intestine.

Accurate delineation of the biliary tree should be performed with either endoscopic retrograde cholangiopancreatography (ERCP) or percutaneous transhepatic cholangiography (PTC). These two studies are complementary, with ERCP more accurately visualizing the distal duct (Fig. 14-6) and PTC delineating the proximal ductal system. Prophylactic antibiotics should be administered immediately before ERCP or PTC to minimize the risk of superinfection and cholangitis. Cholangiograms are useful to exclude other causes of a dilated common bile duct (eg, stricture, tumor, or stone disease) and to establish the anatomic relations necessary to formulate an appropriate operative plan. ERCP is usually performed initially because it visualizes the ampulla, allowing demonstration of a choledochocele, and also defines abnormalities of the pancreaticobiliary junction.[19] The ampulla can be cannulated in over 90%

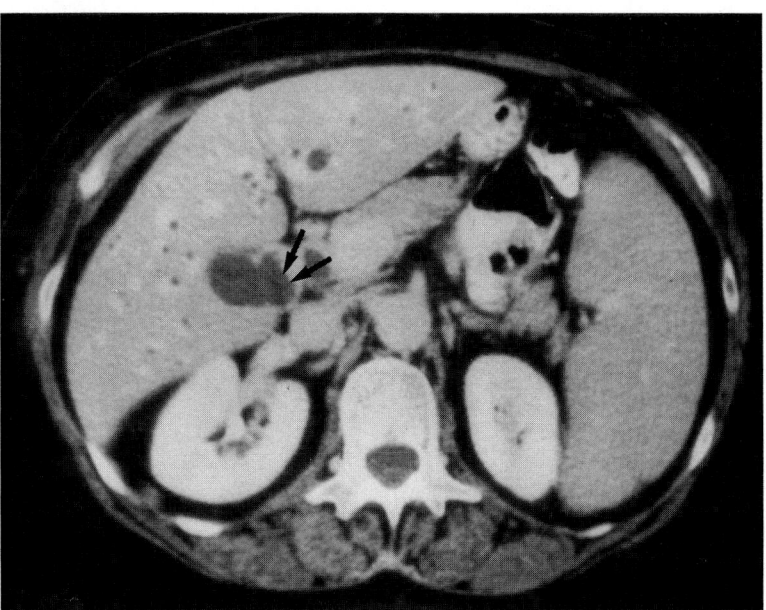

Figure 14-5 CT scan revealing a choledochal cyst with an associated mass lesion in its medial wall, which subsequently was diagnosed as cholangiocarcinoma (*arrows*).

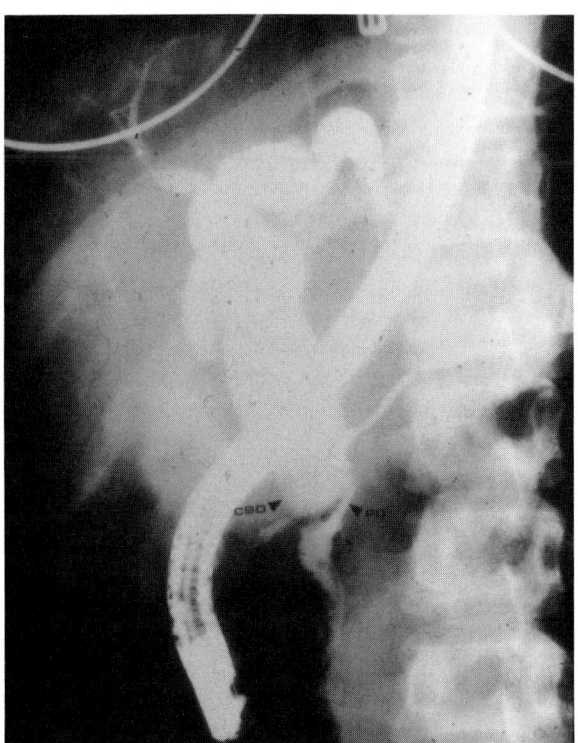

Figure 14-6 Endoscopic retrograde cholangiopancreatogram revealing anomalous pancreatobiliary junction and type IV choledochal cyst. CBD, common bile duct; PD, pancreatic duct.

of cases, and the proximal biliary system is opacified in most patients because there is seldom complete obstruction of the bile duct. PTC is successful in 75% to 90% of cases and is mandatory in patients in whom ERCP has been unsuccessful or in whom the intrahepatic biliary system has not been visualized adequately. Additionally, percutaneously placed catheters can aid in the operative identification of the bile ducts and can be used for postoperative stenting. Using these various imaging modalities, preoperative diagnosis of choledochal cysts has increased from fewer than 40% of patients in the 1970s to greater than 80% of cases in the 1990s.[20,21] In the rare patient whose entire biliary tree has not been demonstrated preoperatively by PTC or ERCP, operative cholangiography should be performed to define precise anatomic detail.

COMPLICATIONS

Choledochal cysts may be complicated by recurrent cholangitis, pancreatitis, common bile duct stones, acute cholecystitis, cyst rupture with diffuse peritonitis,

biliary cirrhosis, portal hypertension, and cholangiocarcinoma. Common duct stones are seen in up to 8% of cases and are probably secondary to biliary stasis. Liver histology reveals cirrhosis in 32% of patients and congenital hepatic fibrosis in 4% of patients with choledochal cysts.[22] After decompressive surgery, however, milder forms of hepatic fibrosis may regress with recovery of normal liver histology and disappearance of portal hypertension.[23] The incidence of cholangiocarcinoma in untreated choledochal cysts ranges from 2.5% to 28%.[24,25] The female/male ratio of malignant change is 3:1, and the average age is 34 years, which is much younger than the age at which primary cholangiocarcinoma usually occurs. Carcinoma may occur within the cystic segment (Fig. 14-7), within normal intrahepatic ducts, or even after extrahepatic cyst excision.[26] The histology of these neoplasms is usually adenocarcinoma, but adenosquamous, squamous, and carcinoid tumors have also been reported.[27]

SURGICAL MANAGEMENT

When diagnosed, choledochal cysts should be treated operatively. Expectant observation and medical treatment of biliary cysts are both almost uniformly fatal; in one report,[28] 29 of 30 patients treated nonoperatively died from the disease. External drainage is associated

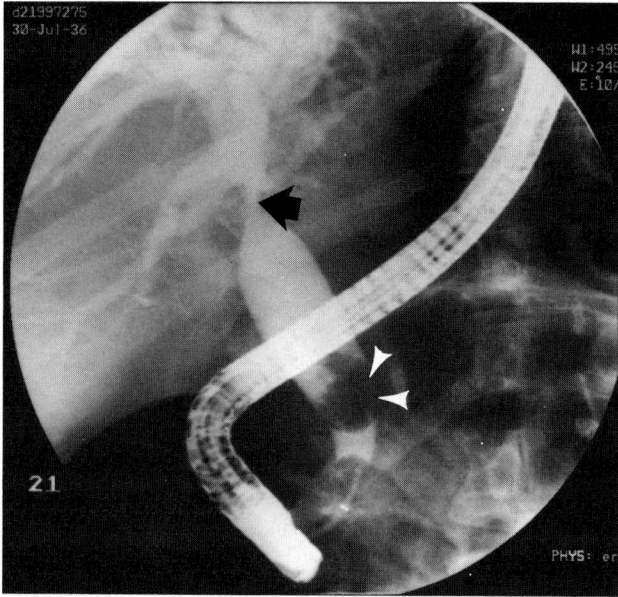

Figure 14-7 Cholangiocarcinoma arising in a type I choledochal cyst. Contained within the bile duct are two separate foci with a papillary carcinoma distally (*white arrows*) and a scirrhous carcinoma at the bifurcation (*black arrow*).

with a mortality rate of up to 80%.[20] Patients who are severely ill from sepsis can be temporized by external drainage, but there is no other role for this therapy. Historically, many operative approaches to choledochal cysts have been described, but consensus has been reached for managing types I, II, and IV choledochal cysts: cyst excision followed by Roux-en-Y hepaticojejunostomy (Fig. 14-8).

In their 1959 report, Alonzo-Lej and colleagues[3] analyzed the various historical approaches used to treat choledochal cysts. Excision of the cyst with anastomosis of the common hepatic duct to the duodenum was first reported in 1924, but excision was technically difficult, and subsequent mortality rates were 15% to 30%.[29] The procedure of choice through the 1950s was cyst duodenostomy. Long-term follow-up, however, revealed the rate of reoperation and other morbidity to be 30% to 50%.[3,8,30] Reflux of duodenal contents into the biliary tree resulted in recurrent cholangitis, and patients frequently developed biliary cirrhosis and portal hypertension. Roux-en-Y choledochal cyst jejunostomy was next performed as an alternative to avoid reflux of the duodenal contents into the biliary tract. This was the preferred treatment from the 1950s to the 1970s.[5,8,20] Postoperative cholangitis, however, was still seen with this approach as a result of stenosis of the anastomosis. These strictures were presumably caused by the presence of inflammation in the wall of the cyst. These problems with cystic and enteric bypass therapy,

along with the growing appreciation of carcinoma associated with biliary cysts, led to cyst excision with Roux-en-Y hepaticojejunostomy as the procedure of choice for types I and IV choledochal cysts.[20]

When excising a choledochal cyst that is adherent to the underlying portal vein, it may be preferable to develop a plane between the lining of the cyst and its serosa to excise the epithelium while leaving the serosa in place[31] (Fig. 14-9). This technique avoids injury to the surrounding tissue. Whenever a choledochal cyst operation is performed, the gallbladder should be removed because it subsequently becomes defunctionalized and prone to develop acute cholecystitis. The detailed biliary anatomy, including the junction of pancreatic duct and common bile duct, usually has been ascertained preoperatively by ERCP or PTC. If there is any doubt, however, an intraoperative cholangiogram should be performed by direct puncture of either the gallbladder or the cyst after aspirating the bile contained within it. After excising the cyst and exposing an adequate length of normal proximal bile duct, a direct anastomosis is performed with a defunctionalized Roux-en-Y limb of jejunum.

Management of types II and III choledochal cysts varies from this approach. For the rare type II cyst, the diverticulum should be excised, with reconstruction of the common bile duct over a T-tube exiting the duct through a separate choledochotomy. For the type III choledochal cyst or choledochocele, complete excision is not necessary because the choledochocele rarely is covered with biliary ductal epithelium. Therefore, the risk of subsequent cholangiocarcinoma is low. Indeed, only two cases of carcinoma complicating a choledochocele have been reported.[18] The usual treatment recommended for large choledochoceles that obstruct the duodenum is surgical excision of the cyst with sphincteroplasty while taking care to avoid the pancreatic duct.[4] A number of reports,[17,18] however, document the safety and efficacy of endoscopic sphincterotomy alone for unroofing the bile duct. Occasionally, pancreatic duct sphincterotomy or sphincteroplasty is also needed to decompress the pancreas.

Operative Technique

Preoperatively, the patient's condition must be optimized by correcting intravascular volume abnormalities, treating cholangitis with broad-spectrum antibiotics, and normalizing coagulation parameters by administering vitamin K. Preoperative placement of biliary catheters may be necessary to decompress the biliary system; the presence of the catheters can facilitate intraoperative identification of the bile ducts. The

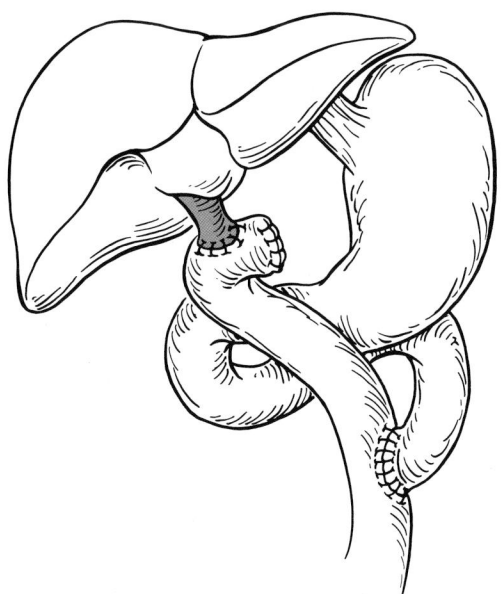

Figure 14-8 The mainstay of surgical treatment of type I and IV choledochal cysts is excision of the cyst and reconstruction by Roux-en-Y hepaticojejunostomy.

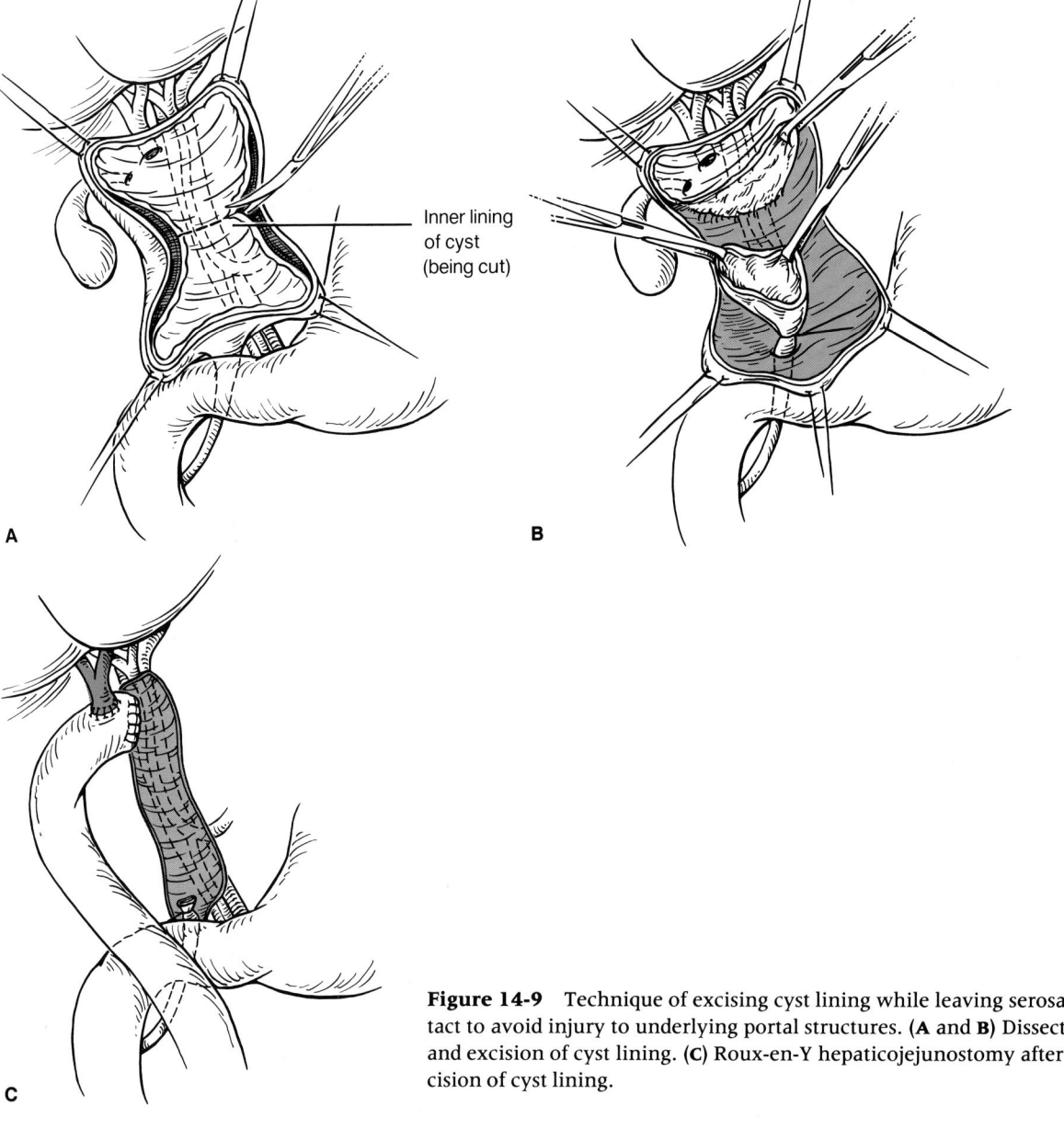

Inner lining
of cyst
(being cut)

A

B

C

Figure 14-9 Technique of excising cyst lining while leaving serosa intact to avoid injury to underlying portal structures. (**A** and **B**) Dissection and excision of cyst lining. (**C**) Roux-en-Y hepaticojejunostomy after excision of cyst lining.

abdomen can be approached either through a bilateral subcostal incision or a vertical upper midline incision. The ascending colon and hepatic flexure are reflected inferiorly and medially, and an extensive Kocher maneuver is performed. This permits exposure of the entire biliary tree and allows manipulation of the duodenum and the head of the pancreas. If needed, a wedge biopsy of the liver is performed after placing horizontal mattress sutures of chromic catgut through the capsule of the liver at the biopsy site. An operative cholangiogram is performed if the biliary anatomy is unclear. Intraoperative ultrasound examination can also clarify

anatomic relations when the cyst has displaced the structures contained within the porta hepatis and liver hilum. Combining the results of cholangiography and operative exploration, the extent of the cyst and its relation to the proximal biliary tree and pancreatic duct can be ascertained.

The entire cyst can be excised in most patients. An exception is when significant fibrosis and inflammation surround the biliary structures. Before dissecting the cyst, all the hilar structures, including the right and left hepatic ducts, the hepatic artery, and the portal vein, should be exposed and isolated from the surrounding tissue. The gallbladder is dissected from its bed in an antegrade fashion beginning at the fundus and progressing to the cystic duct. The cyst is mobilized down to where the common bile duct passes behind the posterior aspect of the pancreas and at that point is encircled (Fig. 14-10). The anterior wall of the distal common bile duct is divided transversely, and if percutaneous transhepatic catheters were placed preoperatively, they are extracted through the end of the duct. The posterior wall of the biliary tree is then divided, and the defunctionalized distal common bile duct is oversewn with interrupted silk sutures. Occasionally, the distal bile duct is still dilated where it passes into the pancreas. It is preferable in this case to amputate the cyst and close the wide-mouthed ductal opening to avoid injuring the pancreatic duct.

Once the cyst has been divided distally, it is reflected in a cephalad direction and dissected free from the hepatic artery and portal vein. The dissection is carried up to the bifurcation of the hepatic ducts. If the choledochal cyst involves the bifurcation or if there is stricture at the bifurcation, the right and left hepatic ducts must be dissected and divided so that the bifurcation can be resected with the specimen. If the dilation extends up into the liver (type IV choledochal cyst), the hepatic duct is divided just distal to the bifurcation.

A Roux-en-Y limb 50 to 60 cm long is constructed and its proximal end brought up through an opening in the transverse mesocolon so that it lies in the hilum of the liver without tension. A small incision about three quarters the length of the bile duct diameter is made in the antimesenteric wall of the jejunum several centime-

ters distal to its blind end. A hepaticojejunostomy is created using a single layer of interrupted 4-0 monofilament synthetic absorbable sutures. After placing the posterior row, the transhepatic catheters are placed down into the Roux limb, and the anterior row of sutures is placed. The posterior sutures are tied with the knots inside the lumen, whereas the anterior row is placed with the knots outside the lumen. The transhepatic catheters are left in place for 4 to 8 weeks to decompress the anastomosis and to provide access for postoperative cholangiograms to document adequate healing.

The end of the Roux-en-Y limb is tacked to the undersurface of the hepatic capsule using interrupted sutures, and the mesocolon is closed with interrupted absorbable sutures. A soft suction catheter is placed behind the anastomosis and is removed in the early postoperative period if no bile is seen in the drain output. After bowel function has returned, a cholangiogram is performed, and the percutaneous transhepatic catheters are capped. Patients are taught to irrigate the catheters on a daily basis. These are removed 4 to 8 weeks after surgery after a repeat cholangiogram documents the absence of leak or stricture.

When significant pericyst inflammation is encountered, it may be unwise to dissect the entire cyst wall away from the underlying structures in the porta hepatis. Rather, an intramural resection can be performed[31] (see Fig. 14-9). The cyst is entered in its midportion laterally, and an intramural resection of the lining is performed. Eventually, the medial and inferior portions of the cyst wall remain in place to avoid dan-

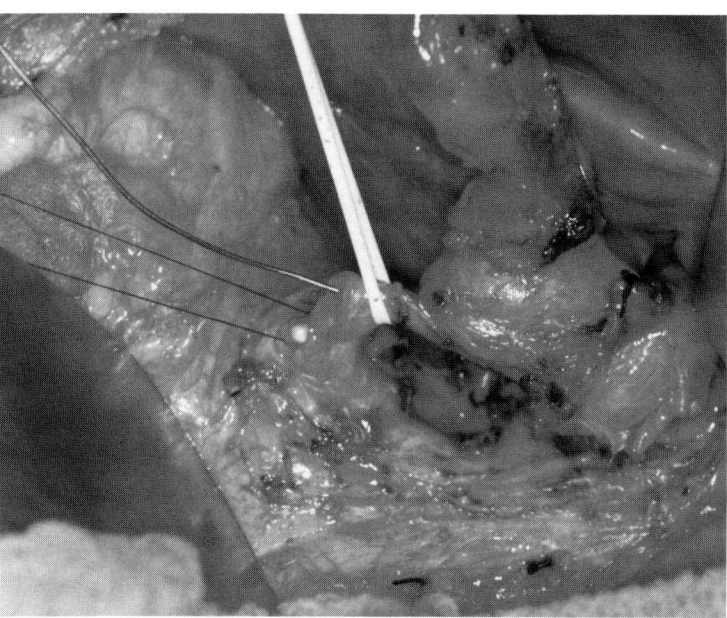

Figure 14-10 During excision of a choledochal cyst, the distal bile duct is encircled with a sling. The choledochal cyst and gallbladder are seen to the right, with the liver edge elevated by a retractor seen in the right portion of the photograph. (See Color Fig. 14-10.)

gerous posterior dissection associated with blood loss from the hepatic artery and portal vein. Demonstration of this submucosal plane can be facilitated by injecting saline solution into the cyst wall or by entering the plane by following the course of the cystic duct as it enters the cyst.[32]

Choledochoceles (type III cysts) are approached by exposing the duodenum and porta hepatis as described earlier. Traction sutures are placed in an antimesenteric position in the second portion of the duodenum, and a longitudinal duodenotomy is made. The choledochocele is then directly visualized and is unroofed beginning at the aperture that drains its contents into the duodenum (Fig. 14-11). After opening the cyst, probes are placed into the common bile duct and into the duct of Wirsung, and the entire choledochocele is resected. If the duct orifices are tiny, it is preferable to perform a sphincteroplasty and reapproximate the mucosa using multiple interrupted 4-0 absorbable sutures. Once hemostasis of the edges of the unroofed choledochocele has been obtained, the duodenotomy is closed transversely to avoid luminal narrowing.

Complications and Results

Recent series report excellent early results with cyst excision for patients with types I, II, and IV choledochal cysts.[8,20,21,33–35] Operative deaths are rare, but reoperations are necessary in up to 10% of patients for hemorrhage, leak or stenosis of the anastomosis.[36] When cysts

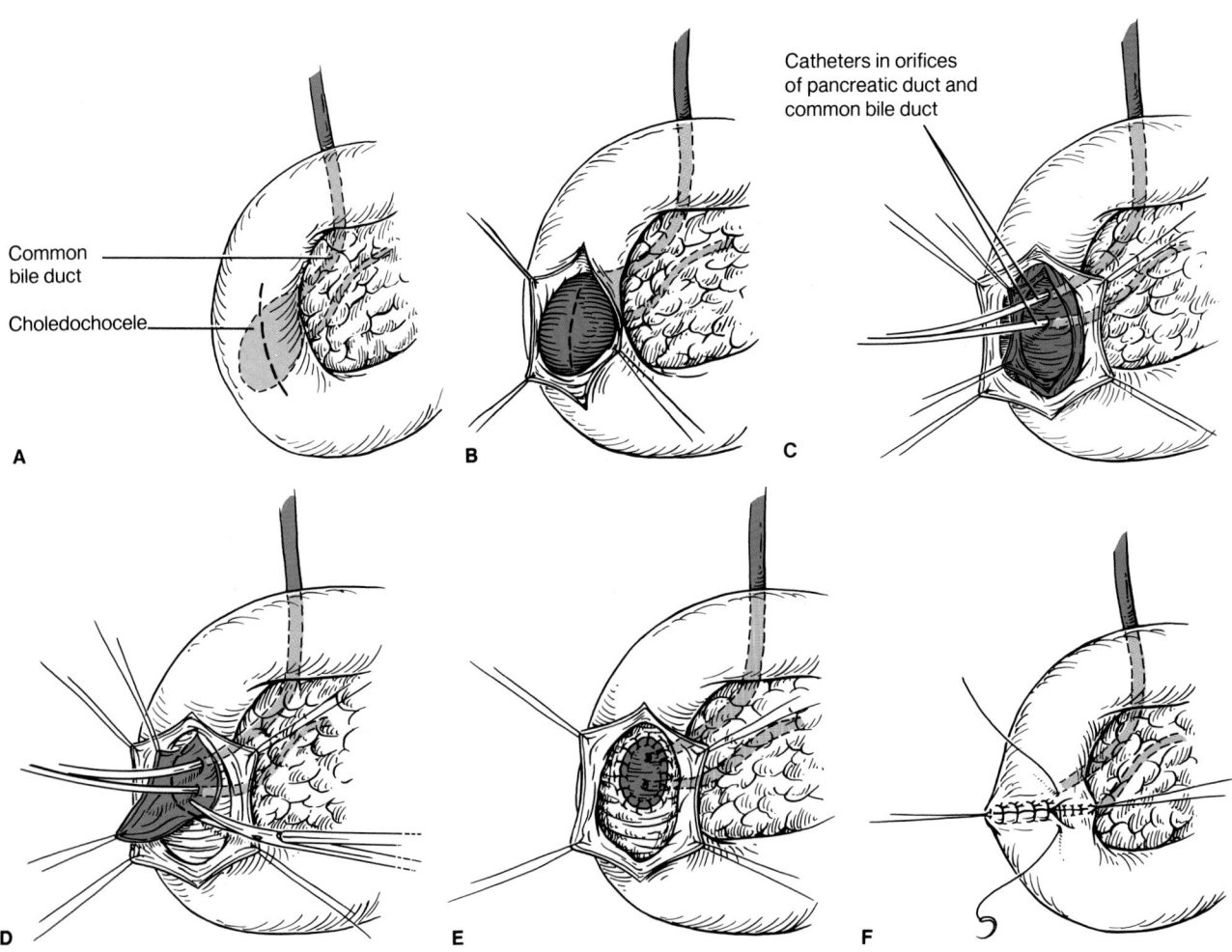

Figure 14-11 Technique for resection of an obstructing choledochocele. (**A**) Duodenotomy at the level of the choledochocele. (**B**) Incision into the choledochocele. (**C** and **D**) Excision of choledochocele after identification of common bile duct and pancreatic duct orifices. (**E**) Suture approximation of duodenal mucosa to remaining choledochocele. (**F**) Transverse suture closure of duodenotomy in two layers.

of the extrahepatic bile duct are combined with cystic dilation extending into the liver (type IV), simple excision of the extrahepatic portion leads to regression of the intrahepatic dilation within 3 to 5 years after operation.[34] In contrast, a large percentage of patients undergoing bypass procedures alone need reoperation, either for anastomotic stricture and cholangitis or development of bile duct carcinoma.[33–37] The lifetime risk of cholangiocarcinoma can be as high as 50% if nonresectional surgery is carried out.[20,25] Bile stasis and continued pancreatic reflux with subsequent chronic inflammation are thought causally relevant. It is likely that the cancer risk is higher in patients presenting as adults (5% to 40%).[37] Carcinoma can arise in areas of the biliary tree not involved with cystic dilation at the time of original operation.[26,37] Cholangiocarcinoma that develops in previously normal bile ducts after excision of a type II choledochal cyst has led some to suggest that excision of the entire extrahepatic tree may be more appropriate than limited resection, even in the presence of an isolated bile duct diverticulum.[24] However, this aggressive approach to surgical treatment has not been embraced by many surgeons. Because of the high incidence of cholangiocarcinoma after bypass operations, it is unclear whether all patients previously treated by nonexcisional means should have elective resection of the cyst. Most authors recommend elective excision only for those patients with documented bouts of cholangitis, with close monitoring of patients who have had an uneventful course.

CAROLI'S DISEASE

Congenital cystic malformations involving only the intrahepatic bile ducts (or type V choledochal cysts) received little attention until the 1958 report by Caroli and colleagues.[6] Caroli's disease is a relatively rare entity and is usually divided into a *simple* type and a *periportal fibrosis* type. Simple Caroli's disease can be complicated by recurring inflammation, infection, and pain but is not associated with hepatic fibrosis leading to cirrhosis and portal hypertension. Type V choledochal cyst is rare, with fewer than 200 cases in the world literature. The etiology is unknown, although a hereditary component is supported by a report of the condition in two siblings.[38] Caroli's disease may masquerade as hydatid liver disease.[39] However, the diagnosis can be made by the sonographic demonstration of intracystic vascular tracts (Marchal's sign).[40] The saccular cystic dilations are usually bilateral, but when unilateral, they more commonly affect the left lobe. Patients with the periportal fibrosis type of Caroli's disease usually present in childhood with cirrhosis and portal hypertension, whereas simple Caroli's disease may present later in life as recurrent episodes of cholangitis.

The treatment of patients with type V choledochal cysts depends on the anatomic characteristics in the individual patient, the presence or absence of associated liver disease, and the extent of infection. When the disease is unilobular, a hepatic lobectomy should be considered.[41] Bilateral ductal dilation can be best managed by the insertion of long-term indwelling transhepatic catheters that can be used to flush the ducts and ensure access to the biliary tree for cholangioscopes or balloons for stone removal or balloon dilation of stenotic areas.[42] In patients with severe cirrhosis or recurrent cholangitis, orthotopic hepatic transplantation should be considered. The prognosis for patients with intrahepatic choledochal cysts depends on the anatomic variety. The outcome for those associated with extrahepatic cysts (type IV) or unilateral disease amenable to resection is usually good. Long-term prognosis for patients with bilateral intrahepatic cysts (type V) has traditionally been poor. It is hoped that with aggressive treatment and the option of transplantation, the outlook can be improved. However, the specter of cholangiocarcinoma in this disease has also recently been raised.[42,43] It appears that the risk of cholangiocarcinoma developing can be as high as 7% in these patients, suggesting that Caroli's disease is also a premalignant lesion.

Modern imaging techniques have allowed precise delineation of choledochal cyst anatomy and have suggested an etiologic mechanism for type I and IV cysts. It is likely that these cysts result from pancreatic reflux into the biliary tree due to an anomalous junction of the main pancreatic duct with the common bile duct. Although in the past, surgical bypass of the cyst was practiced, the subsequent development of anastomotic stenosis or cancer has led most surgeons to abandon this approach. The recommended treatment of types I and IV cysts is total cyst excision with Roux-en-Y hepaticojejunostomy or choledochojejunostomy. This provides an excellent long-term result with few complications. Other forms of choledochal cysts require different modes of treatment. The rare type II diverticulum can often be simply excised. Choledochoceles (type III) can usually be managed by endoscopic sphincterotomy, but if the cyst obstructs the duodenum, it may be preferable to perform a transduodenal cyst excision. Patients with Caroli's disease are treated as dictated by the anatomy. Those with unilobar disease can be treated by hepatic lobectomy, but the ultimate treatment for those with bilateral disease is liver transplantation.

REFERENCES

1. Vater A. Dissertation in auguralis medica, poes diss. qua Scirris viscerum dissert, c.s. ezlerus, volume 70. Edinburgh, University Library, 1723:19.
2. Douglas AH. Case of dilatation of the common bile duct. Monthly J Med Sci (Lond) 1852;14:97.
3. Alonzo-Lej F, Raver WB, Pessagno DJ. Congenital choledochal cysts, with a report of two, and an analysis of 94 cases. Int Abstr Surg 1959;108:1.
4. Todani T, Watanabe Y, Narusue M, Tabuchi K, Okajima K. Congenital bile duct cysts: classification, operative procedures, and review of 37 cases including cancer arising from choledochal cysts. Am J Surg 1977;134:263.
5. Longmire WP, Madiola SA, Gordon HE. Congenital cystic disease of the liver and biliary system. Am Surg 1971;174:711.
6. Caroli J, Soupalt R, Kossakowski J, et al. La dilatation polykystique congenitale des voies biliares intrahepatiques: essai de classificacion. Semin Hop Paris 1958;34:488.
7. Oguchi Y, Okada A, Nakamira T, et al. Histopathologic studies of congenital dilatation of the bile ducts as related to an anomalous junction of the pancreaticobiliary ductal system: clinical and experimental studies. Surgery 1988;103:168.
8. O'Neill JA Jr. Choledochal cyst. Curr Probl Surg 1992;29:363.
9. Sarris GE, Tsang D. Choledochocele: case report, literature review and a proposed classification. Surgery 1989;105:408.
10. Yotsuyanagi S. Contribution to aetiology and pathology of idiopathic cystic dilatation of the common bile duct with report of three cases. Gann 1935;30:601.
11. Glenn F, McSherry CK. Congenital segmental cystic dilatation of the biliary ductal system. Ann Surg 1973;177:705.
12. Babbitt DP. Congenital choledochal cysts: new etiological concept based on anomalous relationships of common bile duct and pancreatic bulb. Ann Radiol 1969;12:231.
13. Todani T, Urushihara N, Watanabe Y, et al. Pseudopancreatitis in choledochal cysts in children: intraoperative study of amylase levels in the serum. J Pediatr Surg 1990;25:303.
14. Shimada K, Yanagisiwa J, Nachiama F. Increased lysophosphatidylcholine and pancreatic enzyme content in bile of patients with anomalous pancreatobiliary ductal junction. Hepatology 1991;13:438.
15. Spitz L. Experimental production of cystic dilatation of the common bile duct in neonatal lambs. J Pediatr Surg 1977;12:39.
16. Lilly JR. Surgery of coexisting biliary malformations in choledochal cyst. J Pediatr Surg 1979;14:643.
17. Venu RP, Geenen JE, Hogan WJ, et al. Role of endoscopic retrograde cholangiopancreatography in the diagnosis and treatment of choledochocele. Gastroenterology 1984;87:1144.
18. Martin RF, Biber BP, Bosco JJ, Howell DA. Symptomatic choledochoceles in adults: endoscopic retrograde cholangiopancreatography recognition and management. Arch Surg 1992;127:536.
19. Wiedmeyer DA, Stewart ET, Dodds WV, et al. Choledochal cysts: findings on cholangiopancreatography with emphasis on ectasia of the common channel. AJR 1989;153:969.
20. Flanigan DP. Biliary cysts. Ann Surg 1975;182:635.
21. Lopez RR, Penson CW, Campbell JR, Harrison M, Katon RM. Variation in management based on type of choledochal cyst. Am J Surg 1991;161:612.
22. Kim SH. Survey by the surgical section of the American Academy of Pediatrics. J Pediatr Surg 1981;16:402.
23. Yeong ML, Nicholson GI, Lee SP. Regression of biliary cirrhosis following choledochal cyst drainage. Gastroenterology 1982;82:332.
24. Yamaguchi M. Congenital choledochal cysts: analysis of 1,433 patients in the Japanese literature. Am J Surg 1980;140:653.
25. Rossi RL, Silverman ML, Braasch JW, et al. Carcinomas arising in cystic conditions of the bile duct. Am Surg 1987;205:377.
26. Coyle KA, Bradley III EL. Cholangiocarcinoma developing after simple excision of a type II choledochal cyst. South Med J 1992;85:540.
27. Ueyama T, Ding J, Hashimoto H, Tsuneyoshi M, Enjoji M. Carcinoid tumor arising in the wall of a congenital bile duct cyst. Arch Pathol Lab Med 1992;116:291.
28. Tsardakas E, Robnett AH. Congenital cystic dilatation of the common bile duct. Arch Surg 1956;72:311.
29. McWhorter GL. Congenital cystic dilatation of the common bile duct: report of a case with cure. Arch Surg 1924;8:604.
30. Gross RE. The surgery of infancy and childhood. Philadelphia, WB Saunders, 1953:524.
31. Lilly JR. Total excision of choledochal cyst. Surg Gynecol Obstet 1978;146:254.
32. Todani T, Watanabe Y, Mizuguchi, et al. Hepaticoduodenostomy at the hepatic hilum after excision of choledochal cyst. Am J Surg 1981;142:584.
33. Chijiiwa K, Koga A. Surgical management and long term follow-up of patients with choledochal cysts. Am J Surg 1993;165:238.
34. Joseph VT. Surgical techniques and long term results in the treatment of choledochal cysts. J Pediatr Surg 1990;25:782.
35. Nagorney DM, McIlrath DC, Adson MA. Choledochal cysts in adults: clinical management. Surgery 1984;96:656.
36. Todani T, Watanabe Y, Toki A, Urushihara N, Sato Y. Re-

operation for congenital choledochal cyst. Ann Surg 1988;207:142.

37. Todani T, Watanabe Y, Toki A, Urushihara N. Carcinoma related to choledochal cysts with internal drainage operations. Surg Gynecol Obstet 1987;164:61.

38. Hogland M, Muran C, Schmidt D. Caroli's disease in two sisters: diagnosis by ultrasonography and computed tomography. Acta Radiol 1989;30:459.

39. Akoglus M, Davidson BR. Missed diagnosis: Caroli's disease misdiagnosed as hydatid liver cysts. Postgrad Med J 1991;67:60.

40. Toma P, Lucigrai G, Pelizza A. Sonographic patterns of Caroli's disease: report of 5 new cases. J Clin Ultrasound 1991;19:155.

41. Mercadier M, Chigot JP, Clot JP, Langlois P, Lansiaux P. Caroli's disease. World J Surg 1984;8:22.

42. Dayton MT, Longmire WP Jr, Tompkins RK. Caroli's disease: a premalignant condition? Am J Surg 1983;145:41.

43. Rogstad K, Freeman J, Moorghen M, Record CO. Difficulty in diagnosing complications of Caroli's disease. J Clin Gastroenterol 1986;8:582.

Digestive Tract Surgery: A Text and Atlas, edited by Richard H. Bell,
Layton F. Rikkers, and Michael W. Mulholland.
Lippincott-Raven Publishers, Philadelphia, © 1996.

15

Benign Biliary Strictures

Keith D. Lillemoe

Benign biliary strictures represent one of the most difficult challenges that a surgeon faces. Despite numerous technologic developments that have facilitated diagnosis and management, bile duct strictures remain a significant clinical problem. If the strictures are unrecognized or managed improperly, life-threatening complications such as biliary cirrhosis, portal hypertension, and cholangitis can develop. To avoid these complications, virtually every patient with a bile duct stricture should undergo evaluation and be treated with the goal of relieving the obstruction to bile flow and its associated hepatic injury.

Benign bile duct strictures have numerous causes (Table 15-1). Most biliary strictures occur after primary operations on the gallbladder or biliary tree. With the introduction of laparoscopic cholecystectomy, bile duct injuries and associated strictures have been seen with an increased frequency. Operative injury to the bile ducts can also occur during nonbiliary operations or as a result of penetrating or blunt abdominal trauma. Inflammatory conditions, including chronic pancreatitis, gallstones within the gallbladder or the bile duct, stenosis of the sphincter of Oddi, duodenal ulcers, and biliary tract infections, can all cause benign bile duct strictures. Finally, primary sclerosing cholangitis, a rare disease of unknown etiology, can result in multiple strictures of the intrahepatic and extrahepatic bile ducts.

A bile duct stricture complicating a cholecystectomy can represent a devastating injury with emotional overtones for both the patient and surgeon. Prompt recognition and treatment is essential to ensure optimal results. This chapter, therefore, focuses primarily on postoperative biliary strictures and their management.

POSTOPERATIVE BILIARY STRICTURES

Pathogenesis

Most benign bile duct strictures occur after injury to the bile duct during cholecystectomy. The bile duct can also be injured during exploration of the common bile duct or during other upper abdominal operations, including gastrectomy, portacaval shunt, and hepatic and pancreatic procedures. In all these cases, the strictures are associated with an iatrogenic injury to the biliary tree. The exact incidence of bile duct injury is unknown because many cases go unreported in the literature. Data from Scandinavia during the pre–laparoscopic cholecystectomy years of 1975 to 1981 suggest that the incidence of bile duct injury during open cholecystectomy is about 1 in 1000 (0.1%).[1,2] A more recent analysis from the United States of 42,474 open cholecystectomies performed in 1989 found the incidence of bile duct injury to be 0.2%.[3]

The incidence of bile duct injury after laparoscopic cholecystectomy is higher. During the initial reports with this procedure, the incidence of major ductal injury was about 1%, reflecting the learning curve associated with the procedure.[4–6] Although a number of centers have reported large numbers of laparoscopic cholecystectomies without a bile duct injury,[7–10] the most accurate data of the true incidence of such injuries will likely come from surveys encompassing thousands of patients. These reports reflect the results from a large number of surgeons and hospitals in both the community and teaching centers. Two such studies are available. One smaller series,[11] focusing on 4640 patients in a single state, found the incidence of biliary injury to be 0.39%. A second national survey,[12] including 77,604

Table 15-1   Causes of Benign Bile Duct Strictures

POSTOPERATIVE STRICTURES
Injuries occuring at primary biliary operations:
    Laparoscopic cholecystectomy
    Open cholecystectomy
    Common bile duct exploration
Injuries at other operative procedures:
    Gastrectomy
    Hepatic resection
    Portacaval shunt
    Pancreatic procedures
Strictures of a biliary enteric anastomosis
Blunt or penetrating trauma

STRICTURES DUE TO INFLAMMATORY CONDITIONS
Chronic pancreatitis
Cholelithiasis and choledocholithiasis
Primary sclerosing cholangitis
Sphincter of Oddi stenosis
Duodenal ulcer
Crohn's disease
Viral infections
Toxic drugs

cases performed by 5358 surgeons in more than 1100 hospitals, found the incidence of bile duct injury to be 0.6%. Finally, the dramatic increase in the number of referrals seen at tertiary centers with bile duct injuries secondary to laparoscopic cholecystectomy[13–16] suggests that the true incidence is even higher than that reported in the literature.

A number of factors are associated with bile duct injury during open cholecystectomy, including inadequate exposure and lighting, surgical inexperience, and failure to identify structures before clamping, ligating, or dividing them. More specific causes of bile duct injury also exist. Bleeding from the cystic or hepatic arteries can lead to bile duct injury during an attempt to gain hemostasis. The generous application of Ligaclips to hilar areas, not well visualized, can result in placing a clip on or across a bile duct, with resultant injury (Fig. 15-1). The so-called difficult cholecystectomy during operations for acute cholecystitis is often cited as contributing to bile duct injury. Acute inflammation can distort tissue planes, and a tense, distended gallbladder can make exposure in the hilum difficult. Despite these potential technical problems, reviews of iatrogenic bile duct injury during cholecystectomy have shown that inflammation and bleeding play a small role.[1,17]

Failure to recognize congenital anomalies of the bile ducts, such as insertion of the right hepatic duct into the cystic duct or a long common wall between the cystic duct and the common bile duct, can also lead to injury (Fig. 15-2). Variations from the commonly described anatomic pattern of the extrahepatic biliary tree

and adjacent hepatic arteries occur in more than half of patients.[18] Many of these involve an abnormal termination of the cystic duct with the common hepatic duct. Attempts to ligate the cystic duct flush with the common bile duct in such cases can result in bile duct injury. Excessive traction of the cystic duct can also lead to an avulsion injury or to inclusion of a portion of the common bile duct wall in the cystic duct stump ligature. In the Scandinavian review,[1] an anatomic anomaly was recognized only after injury had occurred in 16 of 55 cases.

The factors associated with bile duct injury during laparoscopic cholecystectomy are similar to those associated with the open procedure. Several studies[3,10,11,19,20] have noted a correlation between the surgeon's experience with laparoscopic cholecystectomy and the risk of injury to the bile duct. In the

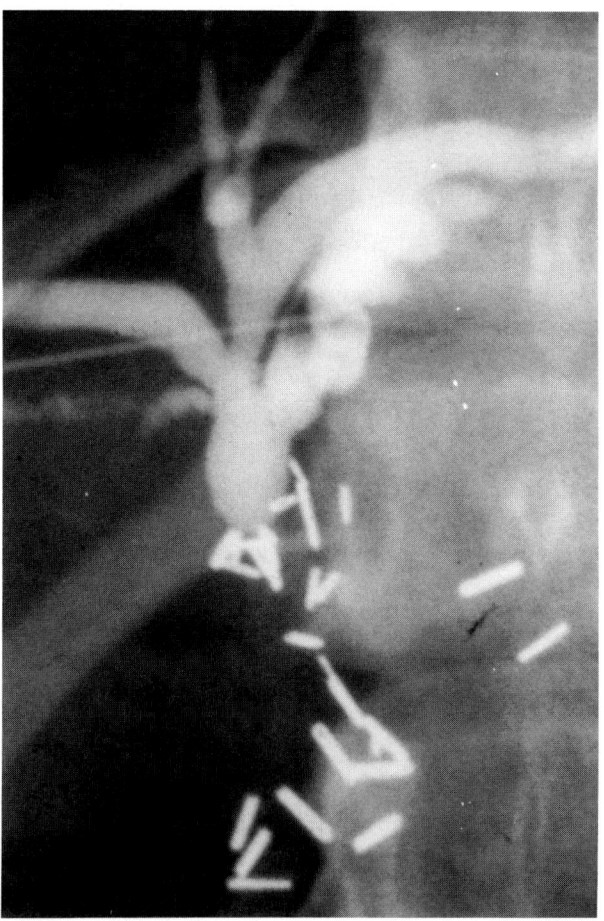

Figure 15-1 Percutaneous transhepatic cholangiogram in a patient with a bile duct stricture secondary to iatrogenic injury during cholecystectomy. A large number of Ligaclips are visible in the area of the stricture. (Lillemoe KD, Pitt HA, Cameron JL. Postoperative bile duct strictures. Surg Clin North Am 1990;70:1355)

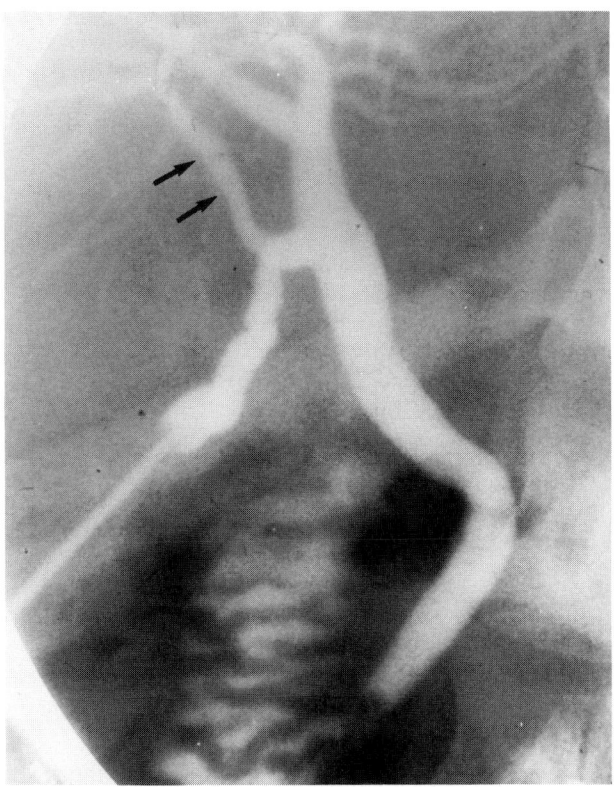

Figure 15-2 Operative cholangiogram demonstrating a right lobe segmental bile duct (*arrows*) entering the cystic duct. Division of the cystic duct proximal to this insertion can result in a bile leak or obstruction of bile flow from a significant segment of the liver. (Lillemoe KD, Pitt HA, Cameron JL. Current management of benign bile duct strictures. Adv Surg 1992;25:119)

multicenter study reported by the Southern Surgeon's Club,[3] bile duct injury occurred in 2.2% of patients during the surgeon's initial 13 procedures but declined to 0.1% during subsequent procedures. In a national survey,[12] the incidence of injury fell from 0.65% in hospitals performing 100 or fewer cases to 0.42% at institutions with more than 100 cases. Finally, in a series of 11 ductal injuries reported by Rossi and associates,[21] 10 of the laparoscopic procedures were associated with factors that increased the technical difficulty of the operative dissection, including the presence of acute or chronic inflammation, bleeding, and excess fat in the porta hepatis.

A number of technical factors can increase the risk of common bile duct injury during the performance of a laparoscopic cholecystectomy. The use of an end-viewing (zero-degree) laparoscope alters the surgeon's perspective of the operative field because the portal structures are viewed from their inferior aspect rather than from directly above, as in an open cholecystec-

tomy. This change in visual orientation can result in misidentifying the common bile duct as the cystic duct. The cephalad displacement of the gallbladder fundus required for adequate retraction of the liver causes the cystic duct and the common bile duct to be become aligned in the same plane. Viewed through the laparoscope, the common bile duct can easily be mistaken for the cystic duct and inadvertently ligated or divided—the so-called classic injury (Fig. 15-3). The cephalad retraction of the gallbladder can also place the cystic duct parallel and in proximity to the common hepatic and right hepatic ducts. Failure to recognize the closeness of these structures can result in injury to the hepatic ducts during dissection of the cystic duct and artery. Tenting of the common bile duct can also occur from cephalad displacement of the gallbladder. This creates an especially hazardous situation in the patient with a short cystic duct, in whom a clip may be inadvertently placed across a portion of the common bile duct.

In series describing the management of major biliary complications after laparoscopic cholecystectomy, the most common mechanism of injury involved dissection of the common bile duct as if it were the cystic duct. The common bile duct is then clipped and divided. The surgeon, thinking that he or she has divided the cystic duct, dissects the common bile duct proximally into the hilum, and at some point transects the proximal biliary system. Therefore, the surgeon actually removes a portion of the biliary tree. In addition, the right hepatic artery is often injured because of its proximity. In one report,[19] this injury occurred in 9 of 12 patients. Similarly, in a larger series,[14] this injury—or a variant—occurred in 24 of 38 patients with major bile duct injuries.

Prevention of bile duct injuries is dependent on proper exposure of the porta hepatis and accurate identification of the structures within Calot's triangle. A number of measures to prevent bile duct injuries during laparoscopic cholecystectomy have been recommended:

- Use of a 30-degree laparoscope
- Cephalad retraction of the gallbladder fundus
- Lateral retraction of the infundibulum of the gallbladder
- Initial dissection of the neck of the gallbladder
- Visualization of the junction of the gallbladder neck and cystic duct, with application of clips only after positive identification of this junction
- No attempt to completely mobilize the cystic duct–common bile duct junction
- Avoidance of blind clip application or cautery to control bleeding in the porta hepatis

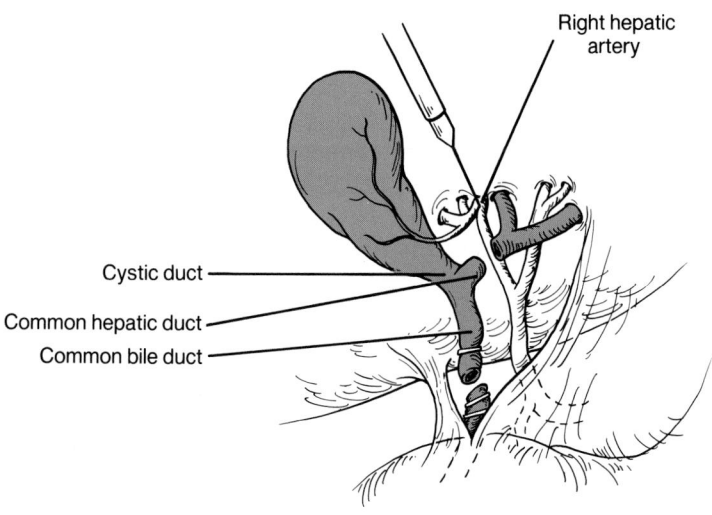

Figure 15-3 Classic laparoscopic bile duct injury. The common bile duct is mistaken for the cystic duct and transected. A variable extent of the extrahepatic biliary tree is resected with the gallbladder. The right hepatic artery, in background, is also often injured. (Branum G, Schmidt C, Baile J, et al. Management of major biliary complications after laparoscopic cholecystectomy. Ann Surg 1993; 217:532)

- Early conversion to an open procedure if anatomy is unclear

Although application of such measures and experience are key to safe performance of the laparoscopic procedure, the most important factor in preventing injuries to the common bile duct is early conversion to an open cholecystectomy if the anatomy cannot be clearly defined. Some investigators[22,23] have recommended that operative cholangiography be performed routinely during laparoscopic cholecystectomy to reduce the possibility of injury to the extrahepatic biliary tree. Advocates of this approach argue that cholangiography provides the surgeon with anatomic information critical for preventing inadvertent ductal injury, including the length and course of the cystic duct and the presence of associated biliary anomalies. There is no convincing evidence, however, that operative cholangiography prevents or reduces the incidence of ductal injuries during laparoscopic cholecystectomy. Bile duct injuries have occurred despite the routine performance of operative cholangiography and can be associated with the actual performance of the cholangiographic procedure. Finally, there appears to be no difference in the incidence of bile duct injury in series reporting routine versus selective cholangiography.[10,23–26]

The importance of ischemia of the bile duct in the development of postoperative strictures has been emphasized.[27,28] Unnecessary dissection around the bile duct can divide or injure the major arteries of the bile duct, which run in the 3- and 9-o'clock positions (Fig. 15-4). These axial arteries provide the nutrient blood supply of the supraduodenal bile duct, with flow coming from below in about 60% of patients and from above in 38% of patients. In 2% of patients, the common duct is supplied directly from the common hepatic artery in a nonaxial fashion. Thus, the portion of the supraduodenal bile duct proximal to the locus of transection or damage is vulnerable to ischemia, which can contribute to fibrosis and stricture formation during the healing process.

Another important contributing factor to the development of a stricture after bile duct injury is the intense connective tissue response that can occur and result in fibrosis and scarring. Experimental work in the canine model has provided insight into the morphologic, ultrastructural, and biochemical consequences of bile duct injury.[29] In this model, bile duct ligation causes immediate and sustained elevation of bile duct pressure and progressive increase in bile duct diameter. Histologic changes at 1 month after ligation have shown that the bile duct wall is thickened five times normal, with a reduction of mucosal folds and loss of surface microvilli, associated with a well-defined epithelial degeneration. Biochemical analysis of connective tissue response to ligation has demonstrated that collagen synthesis and proline hydroxylase activity is increased within 2 weeks in the obstructed bile duct and is sustained throughout the period of observation. Moreover, the presence of bile can predispose to the development of bile duct strictures because bile diversion can minimize experimental fibrosis in a canine model.[30] Bile is thought to provide a constant irritating effect on the healing process, which promotes excessive collagen scar formation. Finally, a marked local inflammatory response can develop in the adjacent tissues in association with bile leakage, which occurs with most bile duct injuries. The leakage of bile can cause inflammation, which is intensified in the face of infection, as in the development of a phlegmon or abscess. This inflammation results in more pronounced fibrosis and scar-

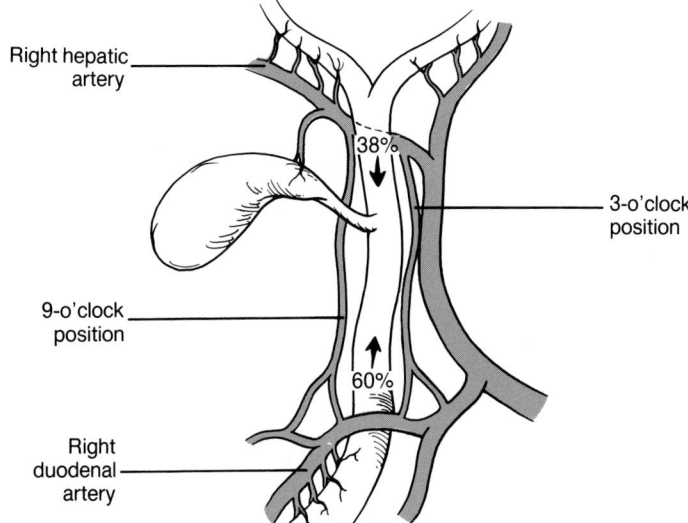

Figure 15-4 Anterior view of the blood supply of the human bile duct. The blood supply to the bile ducts in the hilum of the liver (**above**) and the retropancreatic bile duct (**below**) from adjacent arteries is profuse. The supraduodenal bile duct blood supply is axial and tenuous, with 60% from below and 38% from above. The small main axial vessels (arteries in the 3- and 9-o'clock positions) are vulnerable and easily damaged. (After Terblanche J, Allison HF, Northover JMA. An ischemic basis for biliary strictures. Surgery 1983;94:52)

ring in the periductal tissue, further contributing to stricture formation. This may be a major contributing factor to bile duct strictures that follow laparoscopic cholecystectomy.

Bile duct injury can also occur during common duct exploration. Excessive instrumentation or dilation of the distal bile duct during attempts at stone extraction or sphincter manipulation can result in bile duct injury. Moreover, exploration and T-tube insertion in a small bile duct can lead to a stricture. In this setting, passage of a Fogarty biliary catheter through the cystic duct and transduodenal sphincteroplasty may be safer than supraduodenal duct exploration. Reports of laparoscopic common bile duct exploration have been made.[31,32] Both transcystic duct exploration and actual choledochotomy have been employed. Although bile duct strictures have not been observed in these preliminary reports, further experience will be necessary to document the safety of these techniques.

After cholecystectomy and common bile duct exploration, the two most common operations associated with bile duct injury are gastrectomy and hepatic resection. The most common situation resulting in biliary injury during the course of a gastrectomy involves dissection of the pyloric region and the first portion of the duodenum in the face of inflammation from peptic ulcer disease. The injury usually occurs during mobilization of the duodenum either for creation of a Billroth I gastroduodenostomy or for closure of the duodenal stump. Biliary injury during liver resection is most likely to occur during dissection of the hilum. Management of a bile duct injury after a partial hepatectomy can be extremely difficult and can result in significant complications if the re-

maining lobe atrophies. Operative cholangiography can be helpful to identify anatomy and avoid injury in difficult cases.

In addition to iatrogenic bile duct injury occurring during cholecystectomy or other operations, postoperative bile duct strictures can also occur at previous biliary anastomoses. Such strictures can occur at a biliary enteric anastomosis performed for reconstruction after resection for benign or malignant disease of the pancreaticobiliary system, after end-to-end repair of a traumatic injury, or after liver transplantation. Ischemia of the anastomosis due to excessive skeletonization of the duct in preparation for the anastomosis is most likely an important factor in many such strictures.

Unfortunately, the recurrence of bile duct strictures after an initial attempt at end-to-end repair is common.[17,33] A number of factors have been evaluated in patients who developed a recurrent bile duct stricture, including the length of follow-up, the influence of previous operations, the type of operation performed, the type of sutures used, and the use of and the duration of postoperative stenting.[17] Previous attempts at repair and a procedure other than choledochojejunostomy or hepaticojejunostomy appear to be associated with a higher incidence of recurrent stricture. The type of suture material used for repair does not influence the outcome. When postoperative bile duct stents are used, a longer period of stenting appears to be favorable. Another report[33] confirmed the advantage of a biliary enteric anastomosis but could not show a correlation with previous attempts at repair or an advantage to postoperative stenting. Both authors stress the importance of long-term follow-up of bile duct anastomoses because stric-

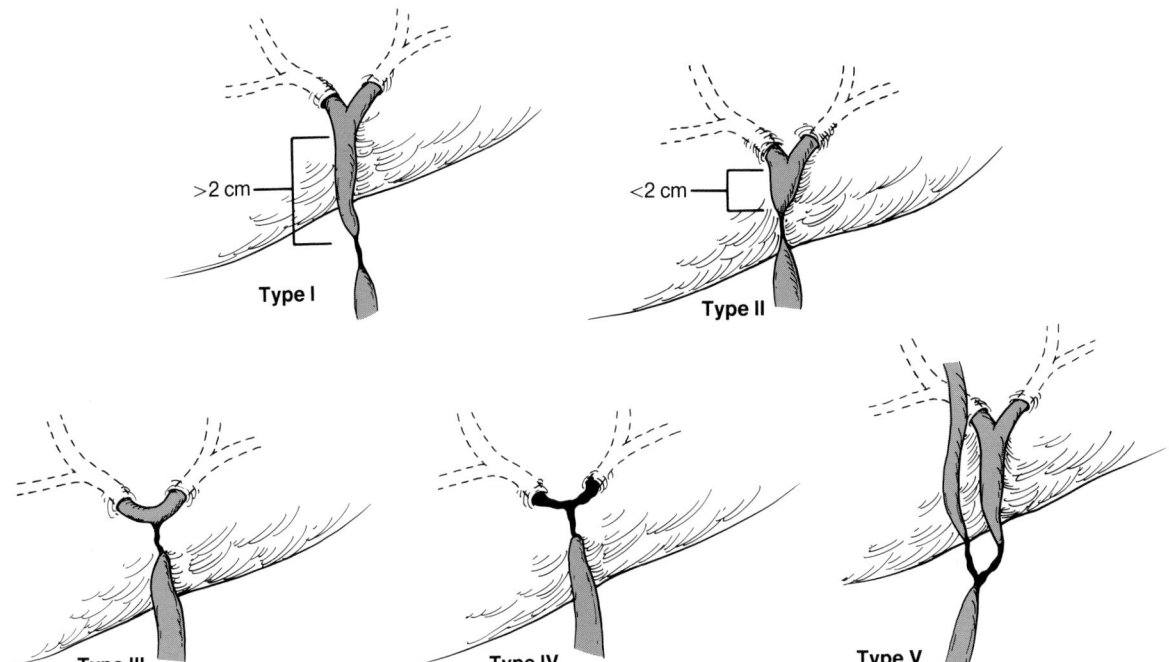

Figure 15-5 Classification of bile duct strictures based on the level of the stricture related to the confluence of the hepatic ducts. Types I and II are below the bifurcation, more than and less than 2 cm, respectively. In type III, the stricture extends to an intact bifurcation, while a type IV stricture involves the bifurcation. Type V strictures involve an accessory right hepatic duct. The common bile duct may or may not be involved. (After Bismuth H. Postoperative strictures of the bile duct. In: Blumgart LH, ed. The biliary tract. Clinical surgery international, vol 5. Edinburgh, Churchill Livingstone, 1982:209)

tures can develop years after the anastomosis is constructed.

Location and Classification

The location of a bile duct stricture is of primary importance in dictating management and predicting outcome. In recognition of this, a classification of benign bile duct strictures based on the anatomic pattern of involvement has been developed[34] (Fig. 15-5). This classification not only defines postoperative strictures in a specific manner but also permits comparison of various treatment modalities with respect to the extent of involved bile duct. The distribution of strictures from the open cholecystectomy era based on this classification is shown in Table 15-2. The distribution of bile duct injuries after laparoscopic cholecystectomy has not been clearly defined but appears dependent on the mechanism of injury. In the classic injury, the initial bile duct transection occurs below the insertion of the cystic duct (Bismuth type I). Unfortunately, the injury is usually not recognized until a segment of bile duct is resected and the hepatic duct is divided at or near the bifurcation (Bismuth type II or III). Although a Bismuth classifica-

tion of the bile duct injuries was not provided, one report confirmed this observation by noting multiple ducts involved in the injury in 31 of 38 patients.[14] In this series, three or more bile ducts were involved in 23 of 38 patients. Injuries associated with a lateral wall thermal injury or clip application tend to be lower (Bismuth type I).

Table 15-2 Distribution of Bile Duct Strictures Based on Bismuth Classification

Type	Description	Incidence (%)
1	Low common hepatic or bile duct (common hepatic duct > 2 cm)	18–26
2	Middle common hepatic duct (common hepatic duct < 2 cm)	27–38
3	Hilar stricture	20–33
4	Destruction of hilar confluence (right and left hepatic ducts separated)	14–16
5	Involvement of right hepatic branch alone or with common duct	0–7

(Lillemoe KD, Pitt HA, Cameron JL. Current management of benign bile duct strictures. Adv Surg 1992;25:119)

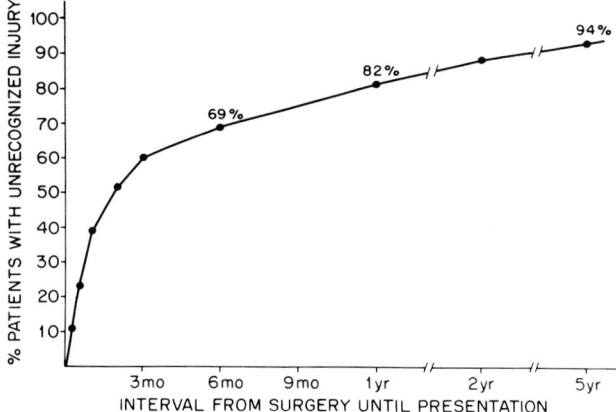

Figure 15-6 The cumulative percentage of patients developing strictures is shown with respect to the time interval from the procedure during which the injury occurred until the presentation of symptoms. (After Pitt HA, Miyamoto T, Parapatis SK, et al. Factors influencing outcome in patients with postoperative biliary strictures. Am J Surg 1982;144:14)

Clinical Presentation

Most patients with benign postoperative bile duct strictures present early after their initial operation (Fig. 15-6). After open cholecystectomy, only about 10% of postoperative strictures are actually suspected within the first week after cholecystectomy; however, nearly 70% of patients are diagnosed within the first 6 months and over 80% within 1 year of surgery.[17] In the remaining patients, presentation can be delayed for many years after the initial operative procedure. In the few series reporting bile duct injuries after laparoscopic cholecystectomy, the recognition typically occurs either during the procedure or, more commonly, in the early postoperative period.

Patients suspected of having postoperative bile duct strictures within days to weeks of the initial operation usually present in one of two ways. One mode of presentation is the progressive elevation of liver function tests, particularly total bilirubin and alkaline phosphatase. These changes can be seen as early as the second or third postoperative day. The development of jaundice may be associated with biliary sepsis. The second mode of early presentation is bile drainage from operatively placed drains or through the wound. The amount of bile drainage may represent the entire bile production and can be associated with development of fluid and electrolyte abnormalities. In patients without drains or in whom drains have been removed, the bile may leak freely into the peritoneal cavity or may loculate as a subhepatic or a subphrenic collection. This mode of presentation appears to be common in patients with bile duct injuries that occurred during laparoscopic cholecystectomy. The free accumulation of bile into the peritoneal cavity results in either bile ascites or bile peritonitis. Similarly, a loculated bile collection can result in a sterile biloma (Fig. 15-7) or in an infected subhepatic or subdiaphragmatic abscess. In all bile leaks, whether controlled through a drain or with free or loculated intraabdominal bile accumulation, prompt investigation is warranted.

Patients with postoperative bile duct strictures who present months to years after the initial operation frequently have evidence of cholangitis. Fever, chills, abdominal pain, and jaundice are present in most of these

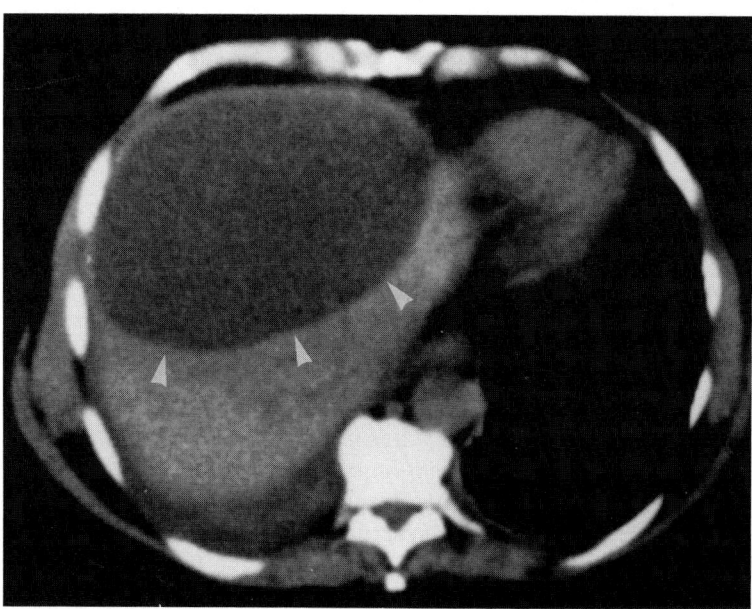

Figure 15-7 Large bile collection (biloma; *arrows*) occurring after bile duct injury. (After Lillemoe KD, Pitt HA, Cameron JL. Current management of benign bile duct strictures. Adv Surg 1992;25:119)

patients. The episodes of cholangitis are frequently mild and respond to antibiotic therapy. Repetitive episodes usually occur before the definitive diagnosis. Less commonly, patients present with painless jaundice and no evidence of sepsis. Finally, in cases with a markedly delayed diagnosis, the patients present with advanced biliary cirrhosis and portal hypertension.

Late Manifestations

Chronic, unrelieved biliary obstruction can lead to secondary biliary cirrhosis and its complications.[35] In such cases, high local concentrations of bile salts at the canalicular membrane initiate pathologic changes in the biliary system.[36] Bile thrombi form within dilated centrilobular bile canaliculi, and secondary changes are seen in adjacent hepatocytes. An inflammatory exudate follows with deposition of collagen and eventual fibrosis and scarring around the bile ducts and smaller ductules. These changes further impair bile flow. Fibrosis is followed by liver cell hyperplasia. The complications of portal hypertension and ascites can develop as early as 2 years after the onset of obstruction. In such cases, severe cholangitis and a history of unsuccessful attempts at repair are often present. Such advanced liver changes can be documented on preoperative liver biopsy. Nevertheless, surgeons should proceed with evaluation and consideration of definitive treatment because many patients still benefit from surgical relief of obstruction.[37,38]

A final late complication of long-standing biliary obstruction due to benign bile duct strictures is the development of liver atrophy.[39] Segmental or lobar liver atrophy can result from segmental bile duct or portal venous occlusion. This complication occurs most frequently with proximal duct obstruction, either benign or malignant. If unilobar atrophy occurs, the contralateral lobe hypertrophies, presenting diagnostic and operative difficulties because of rotation of hilar structures. Moreover, the bile ducts within an atrophic segment are often grossly dilated and may be filled with infected bile. Drainage or resection of such segments can prevent repeated episodes of cholangitis or liver abscess.

Laboratory Investigations

Liver function tests usually show evidence of cholestasis. The serum bilirubin level can fluctuate and may even be normal on occasion. When elevated, the serum bilirubin level usually ranges from 2 to 6 mg/dL unless secondary biliary cirrhosis has developed. Increases in bilirubin are often associated with cholangitis and may represent obstruction of the narrow bile duct lumen by biliary sludge that forms proximal to the stricture. The serum alkaline phosphatase level is usually elevated. Serum transaminase levels are normal or minimally elevated; during episodes of cholangitis, transaminase levels may be transiently elevated. If advanced liver disease exists with impaired hepatic synthetic function, the serum albumin level and prothrombin time may also be abnormal.

Radiologic Examinations

The imaging techniques of abdominal ultrasound and computed tomography (CT) play an initial role in the evaluation of patients with benign postoperative biliary strictures. In patients who present in the early postoperative period with evidence of a bile leak or biliary sepsis, these studies are useful to rule out the presence of intraabdominal collections that might require drainage (see Fig. 15-7). Moreover, in patients who present with jaundice months or years after the operation, both ultrasound and CT can confirm biliary obstruction by demonstrating a dilated biliary tree. CT is especially useful in localizing the site of obstruction based on the extent of dilation of the extrahepatic bile ducts. Finally, in patients whose presentations are remote from the operation, CT can help to rule out biliary or pancreatic neoplasms as a cause of jaundice.

In patients suspected of having an early postoperative bile duct injury, a radionucleotide biliary scan with iminodiacetic acid can confirm a bile leak. Such studies can quickly and noninvasively confirm the presence of a biliary fistula but may lack the sensitivity to delineate anatomy or the actual site of a leak (Fig. 15-8). Radionucleotide studies can be useful, however, in the postoperative evaluation of patients after stricture repair. In patients with postoperative external bile fistulas, injection of water-soluble contrast media through the drainage tract (sinography) can often define the site of leakage and the anatomy of the biliary tree.

The gold standard for patients with bile duct strictures is cholangiography. Either percutaneous transhepatic cholangiography (PTC) or endoscopic retrograde cholangiography (ERC) can define the site of the injury or stricture. ERC is most often the initial route of cholangiography for early bile duct injuries because the biliary tree is often not dilated, making PTC technically more difficult. ERC, however, is often limited in that the discontinuity of the extrahepatic bile duct usually prevents adequate filling of the proximal biliary tree (Fig. 15-9). In many cases, especially after laparoscopic bile duct injury, ERC demonstrates a normal-size distal bile duct up to the site of the obstruction. PTC is more useful because it defines the anatomy of the proximal biliary tree that is to be used in the surgical reconstruction (Fig. 15-10). Moreover, PTC can be followed by

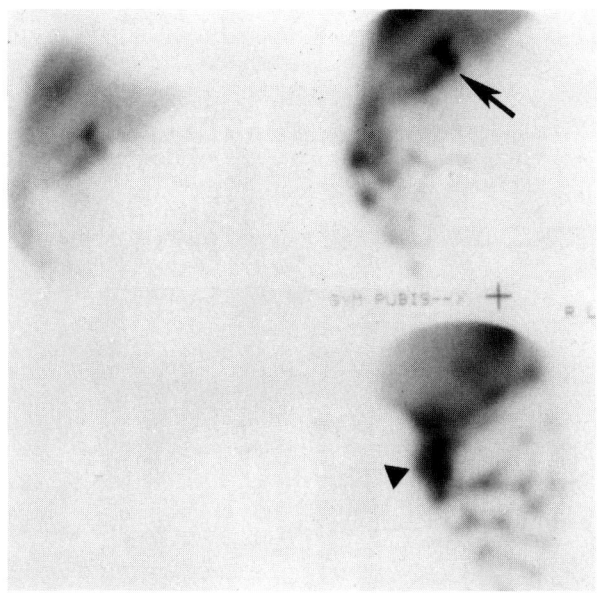

Figure 15-8 Radionucleotide scan obtained after laparoscopic cholecystectomy showing abnormal radiotracer accumulation in the subhepatic space (*arrow*) and right paracolic gutter (*arrowhead*). The site of the leak ultimately proved to be a cystic duct leak.

placement of transhepatic catheters, which can be useful in decompressing the biliary system to treat or prevent cholangitis or to control a bile leak. These catheters can also be of assistance in surgical reconstruction[40] and can provide access to the biliary tree for nonoperative dilation. Regardless of which technique is chosen, patients should receive prophylactic antibiotic coverage before cholangiography because of the high incidence of procedure-associated cholangitis.

The diagnosis of a benign postoperative stricture early after cholecystectomy is often easy. In a significant percentage of patients, however, presentation is so remote from past surgery as to raise suspicion of malignant biliary obstruction. CT is useful as a first step to rule out the presence of a pancreatic mass as a cause of biliary obstruction. In other cases, the cholangiographic pattern suggests malignant obstruction. In cases in which the hepatic duct bifurcation is involved, distinguishing cholangiocarcinoma from a benign stricture can be difficult. Significant experience has been gained in establishing a preoperative diagnosis using either bile cytology or cytologic brushings or biopsies obtained through transhepatic catheters. One report suggested that if multiple brushings of the bile duct epithelium for cytologic analysis are negative for malignancy, the probability of bile duct carcinoma is nearly zero.[41] In patients with a late presentation, a segment of the bile duct stricture should be re-

sected at the time of repair and submitted for pathologic frozen section diagnosis to rule out the presence of cholangiocarcinoma.

Preoperative Management

The preoperative management of a patient with bile duct stricture depends primarily on the timing of the presentation. Patients who present in the early postoperative period may be septic, with either cholangitis or intraabdominal bile collections. Sepsis must be controlled first with broad-spectrum parenteral antibiotics, percutaneous or endoscopic biliary drainage, percutaneous or operative drainage of bile leaks, or a combination of these. Once biliary drainage has been achieved and sepsis controlled, there is no hurry in proceeding with surgical reconstruction. Attention should be paid to correcting fluid and electrolyte abnormalities, anemia, and nutritional deficits. The combination of proximal biliary decompression and external drainage allows most biliary fistulas to be controlled or even

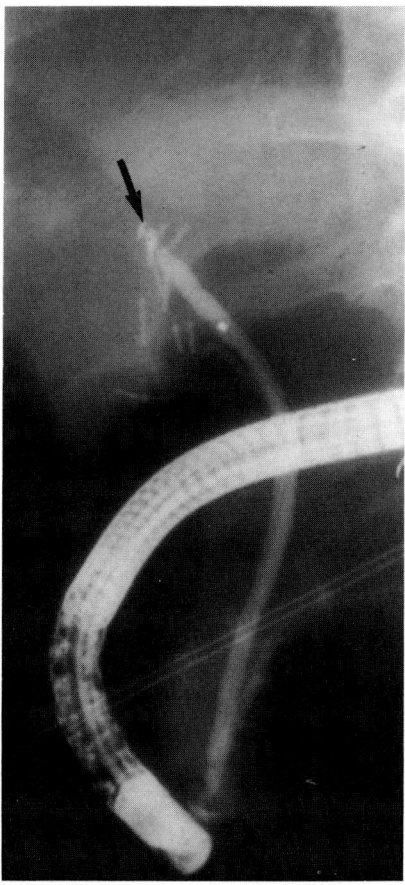

Figure 15-9 Endoscopic retrograde cholangiogram showing that the common bile duct does not fill beyond the large Ligaclip, which appears to be placed across the duct (*arrow*).

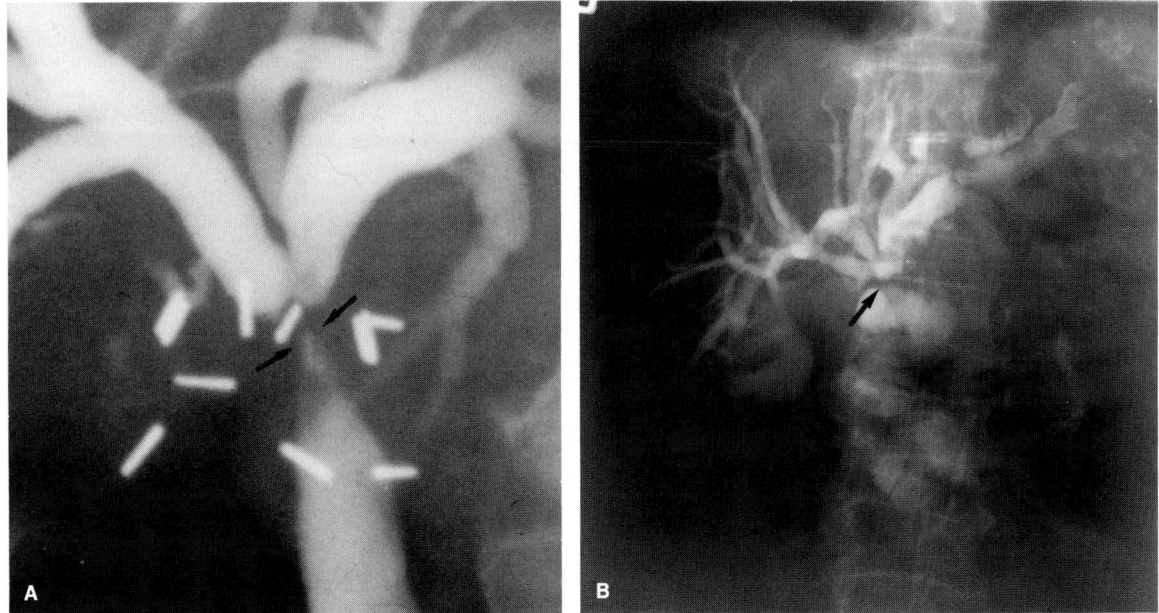

Figure 15-10 (**A**) Percutaneous transhepatic cholangiogram (PTC) demonstrating bile duct stricture (*arrows*) at hepatic duct bifurcation with proximal duct dilation. (**B**) PTC demonstrating stricture at a hepaticojejunostomy anastomosis (*arrows*). (Lillemoe KD, Pitt HA, Cameron JL. Current management of benign bile duct strictures. Adv Surg 1992;25:119)

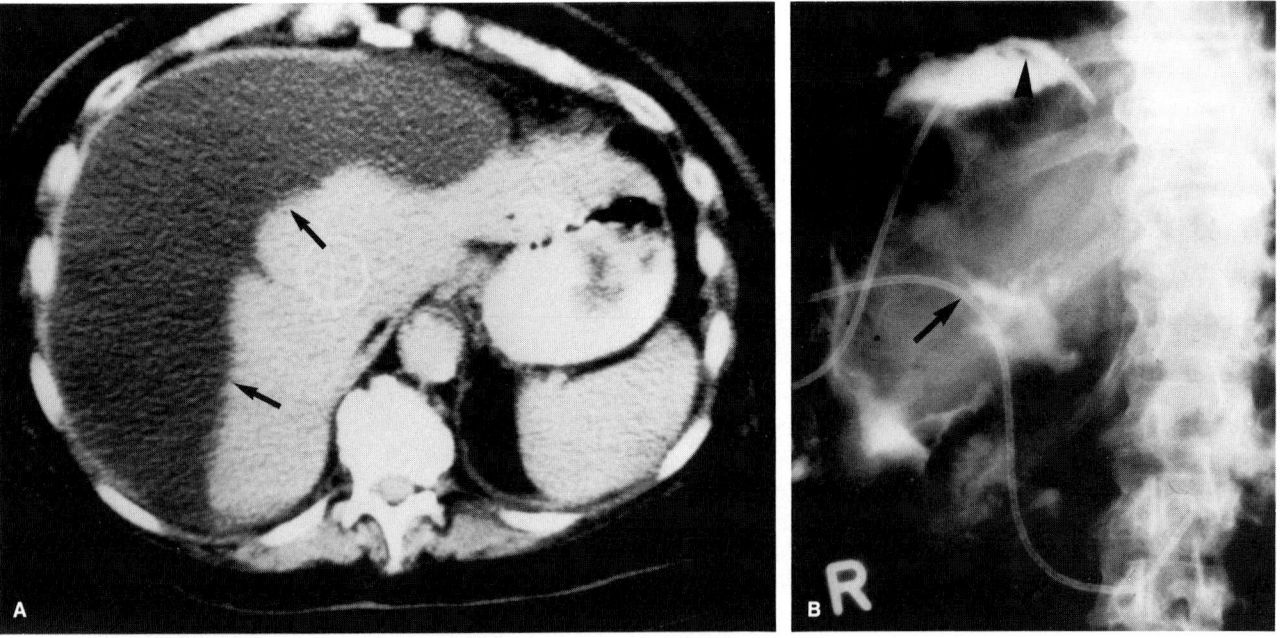

Figure 15-11 (**A**) CT of a patient with a large postoperative bile collection (*arrows*). (**B**) Percutaneous transhepatic cholangiogram showing a bile leak at the site of operative injury and a biliary drainage catheter passed through the area of injury (*arrow*). A percutaneous drainage catheter is draining the subdiaphragmatic bile collection (*arrowhead*). (Lillemoe KD, Pitt HA, Cameron JL. Postoperative bile duct strictures. Surg Clin North Am 1990;70:1355)

closed[14,42,43] (Fig. 15-11). The patient can then be discharged home to allow several months to elapse for resolution of the inflammation in the periportal region and for recovery of overall health status.[44]

In patients who present with a biliary stricture remote from the initial operation, symptoms of cholangitis can necessitate urgent cholangiography and biliary decompression after delineation of the anatomic pathology. Biliary drainage is best accomplished using the transhepatic method, although endoscopic stent placement can also be successful. Parenteral antibiotics and biliary drainage should be continued until sepsis is controlled. In patients who present with jaundice but without cholangitis, cholangiography should be performed to define the anatomy. The use of preoperative biliary stenting in these patients is controversial. In such patients with benign bile duct strictures, preoperative biliary decompression has not been demonstrated to improve outcome.[45]

Surgical Management

The goal of operative management of a bile duct stricture is the establishment of bile flow into the proximal gastrointestinal tract in a manner that prevents cholangitis, sludge or stone formation, restricture, and biliary cirrhosis. This goal is best accomplished with a tension-free anastomosis between healthy tissues that are free of scar tissue.

Immediate Repair of Intraoperative Bile Duct Injury

In many cases, proper management of a bile duct injury recognized at the time of cholecystectomy can avoid the development of a bile duct stricture. Unfortunately, bile duct injury during open cholecystectomy is recognized at the original surgery in only 12% to 46% of patients.[46-49] Recognition of laparoscopic bile duct injuries at the time of the original laparoscopic operation is also uncommon. In the initial 12 patients with major bile duct injuries seen at one center, none was recognized at the original operation.[19] This likely represents the inexperience of the laparoscopic surgeons because most of the injuries occurred within the first 11 procedures of each of the surgeons.

In almost all cases in which an injury occurs and is recognized, repair is best performed at that time. If a bile duct injury is suspected at laparoscopic cholecystectomy, immediate conversion to an open procedure should occur. Operative cholangiography should be performed early to delineate the existing anatomy. If a segmental or accessory duct smaller than 3 mm has been injured and cholangiography demonstrates segmental or subsegmental drainage of the injured ductal system, simple ligation of the injured duct is adequate.[50] However, if the injured duct is 4 mm or larger, it is likely to drain multiple hepatic segments or the entire right or left lobe, and thus the injury requires operative repair.

The aims of all repairs should be to maintain ductal length and not sacrifice tissue as well as to prevent postoperative bile leakage. To accomplish these goals, all repairs at the time of initial operation should involve some form of external bile drainage. Although lateral injuries without significant loss of length are unusual, they must be recognized and repaired to avoid a bile leak. If such a defect is small, as with an avulsion injury of the cystic duct, direct repair over a T-tube can often be accomplished without the development of a late stricture. Unfortunately, in most cases, the bile duct is transected with or without excision of a length of the injured duct. If the injured segment of the bile duct is short (generally less than 1 cm) and the two ends can be opposed without tension, an end-to-end anastomosis can be performed with placement of a T-tube through a separate choledochotomy either above or below the anastomosis. Generous mobilization of the duodenum out of the retroperitoneum (Kocher maneuver) can be useful to help approximate the ends of the bile ducts. An end-to-end repair, however, should be avoided if the ductal injury is near the hepatic duct bifurcation.

In proximal injuries and in those in which the injured segment of bile duct is longer than 1 cm, an end-to-end bile duct anastomosis should be avoided because of the excessive tension that usually results. In these circumstances, the distal bile duct should be oversewn, and the proximal bile duct should be debrided of injured tissue and anastomosed in an end-to-side fashion to a Roux-en-Y loop of jejunum. The Roux-en-Y limb should be at least 40 cm long to avoid the reflux of intestinal contents into the anastomosis. The use of a Roux-en-Y jejunal limb is also preferable to anastomosis to the duodenum because, in the latter case, an anastomotic leak results in a duodenal fistula. Regardless of the type of anastomosis, the area should be drained externally with a closed suction drain.

The long-term results of immediate repair of common bile duct injuries is uncertain. Most injuries occur away from major centers, and the patients with a successful outcome are unlikely to be reported in the literature. In reports from Sweden and Chile,[2,51] the results of immediate repair are poor. In the Swedish report,[2] early primary repair with end-to-end anastomosis resulted in good results in only 22% of patients. Anastomotic leak requiring reoperation occurred in 32% of patients. A late stricture occurred in another 37% of patients. In patients who underwent immediate repair with a biliary enteric anastomosis, good results were seen in 54% of patients, with restricture occurring in only 12% of patients. Similarly poor late results were also noted in another series,[51] in which 29 of 36 patients with primary end-to-end repair developed postoperative strictures within 4 years. In contrast, a report from the United States demonstrated excellent results in eight patients who underwent an intraoperative repair.[49] Two early bile fistulas developed, but both closed spontaneously. Moreover, although end-to-end anastomosis was performed in seven of the eight patients, none of the patients had developed a bile duct stricture during a limited follow-up (3 months to 6 years; mean, 2.5 years). A German publication also reported successful long-term results in 13 of 14 patients undergoing immediate repair of an immediately recognized bile duct injury (follow-up, 7 years).[10] These results reflect those of a major center and are unlikely to be extended to the entire surgical community.

Elective Repair of Established Strictures

Several principles are associated with successful repair of a biliary stricture:

- Exposure of healthy proximal bile ducts that provide drainage of the entire liver
- Preparation of a suitable segment of intestine that can be brought to the area of the stricture without tension, most frequently a Roux-en-Y jejunal limb
- Creation of a direct biliary enteric mucosa-to-mucosa anastomosis

A number of surgical alternatives exist for primary repair of bile duct strictures, including end-to-end repair, Roux-en-Y hepaticojejunostomy or choledochojejunostomy, choledochoduodenostomy, and mucosal grafting. The choice of repair depends on a number of factors, including the extent and location of the stricture; the history of previous, unsuccessful attempts at repair; the experience of the surgeon; and the timing of the repair. Simple excision of a bile duct stricture and end-to-end bile duct anastomosis or repair of the damaged duct can rarely be accomplished because of invariable loss of duct length as a result of fibrosis associated with the injury. Similarly, anastomosis of the proximal bile duct to the duodenum as a choledochoduodenostomy is not suitable for most postcholecystectomy strictures because an adequate length of bile duct for creating a tension-free anastomosis to the duodenum usually cannot be obtained. Thus, in almost all cases, a hepaticojejunostomy constructed to a Roux-en-Y limb of jejunum is the preferable procedure.

Adequate exposure is essential for reconstruction of the biliary tree. The abdomen can be reexplored through a right subcostal incision; however, extension to the left side as a bilateral subcostal incision is usually necessary. In patients with a narrow costal margin or with a prior midline incision, a midline approach usually provides excellent exposure.

EXPOSURE OF THE PROXIMAL BILE DUCT. Exposure of the porta hepatis usually requires division of adhesions of the duodenum and hepatic flexure of the colon to Glisson's capsule and the gallbladder fossa. Identification of the proximal biliary segment is difficult and can be aided by the presence of a transhepatic biliary catheter placed at the time of preoperative PTC.[40] Once the proximal bile duct has been identified, it should be encircled with a vessel loop. The bile duct is then divided at the lowermost extent of the stricture and dissected proximally. A segment of the strictured duct should be resected and submitted for pathologic examination to rule out cholangiocarcinoma. The distal duct should be oversewn, and the bile duct proximal to the stricture should then be carefully dissected circumferentially in a cephalad direction for a distance of about 5 mm. Excessive dissection should be avoided to prevent vascular compromise of this segment of duct, which will be used for the anastomosis.

BILIARY ANASTOMOSIS WITH TRANSHEPATIC STENTS. Although a number of alternatives for repair of bile duct strictures exist, the best results have been achieved with Roux-en-Y choledochojejunostomy or hepaticojejunostomy.[2,17,33,52,53] Although the role of transanastomotic stenting remains controversial, there are several potential advantages to this approach. In the early postoperative period, a stent is useful to decompress the biliary tree and to provide access for cholangiography or removal of retained intrahepatic stones. If the injury has involved the common bile duct or the common hepatic duct at least 2 cm distal to the bifurcation and adequate, proximal bile duct mucosa can be defined (Bismuth type I), the use of long-term biliary stents is not necessary. In these situations, the preoperatively placed percutaneous transhepatic catheter or an operatively placed T-tube is used to decompress the biliary enteric anastomosis for 4 to 6 weeks after reconstruction. However, when adequate proximal bile duct is not available for a good mucosa-to-mucosa anastomosis, as is often the case when there were prior attempts at repair, long-term stenting of the biliary enteric anastomosis with a Silastic transhepatic stent, usually for at least 12 months, is favored.

Silastic transhepatic biliary stents can be inserted by a number of methods, including use of either preoperatively placed percutaneous transhepatic catheters,

Randall stone forceps, or a long Bakes dilator.[54] The simplest approach involves the use of percutaneously placed transhepatic catheters. For strictures of the common hepatic duct just distal to the hepatic duct bifurcation (Bismuth type II), only one transhepatic stent is needed. However, for higher strictures involving the hepatic duct bifurcation (Bismuth type III or IV), both the right and left main hepatic ducts should be preoperatively stented.

After mobilization and division of the bile duct, the biliary catheters protrude through the proximal end. A radiologic guide wire is then placed through these catheters. A 14F coudé catheter, with its smallest diameter end oriented toward the hepatic hilum, is then passed over the guide wire and sutured to the biliary catheter (Fig. 15-12A). The long arteriography guide wire is recommended because the sutures occasionally break, resulting in loss of the established tract. The coudé catheter is pulled upward through the preexisting catheter track into the hepatic parenchyma by withdrawing the preoperatively placed catheter upward through the liver. Progressively larger coudé catheters are passed, dilating the intrahepatic tract. Finally, a Silastic biliary stent is passed over the guide wire and sutured into the widened end of the coudé catheter. The Silastic stent is then positioned within the previously formed transhepatic tract as the coudé catheter is pulled forward through the liver.

If a transhepatic biliary catheter has not been placed preoperatively, a Randall stone forceps or a long Bakes dilator can be introduced into either the right or left hepatic duct and used to assist the placement of the Silastic transhepatic stents (see Fig. 15-12B). After advancing the instrument as far as possible, generally to within 1 to 2 cm of the surface of the liver, Glisson's capsule is incised with the cautery, and the instrument is advanced out the superior aspect of the liver. The Silastic catheter is then secured to the instrument and is pulled into position as the instrument is withdrawn downward out of the hepatic hilus. Alternatively, a heavy suture can be passed and sutured to a coudé catheter and, subsequently, to the Silastic stent as described earlier.

After stent placement, a Roux-en-Y jejunal limb is prepared for the biliary enteric anastomosis. The use of the defunctionalized Roux-en-Y limb minimizes the risk associated with anastomotic leak and prevents reflux of intestinal contents into the biliary tree. The Roux-en-Y limb should be at least 40 to 60 cm long, with its closed end brought up to the hepatic hilus in a tension-free retrocolic position. The anastomosis is then performed as an end-to-side hepaticojejunostomy (see Fig. 15-12C). If an acceptable proximal biliary segment is available with an adequate circumferential ring

of healthy bile duct mucosa, a mucosa-to-mucosa biliary enteric anastomosis can be performed over a preoperatively placed percutaneous transhepatic catheter or an operatively placed T-tube. This anastomosis can be done in one or two layers, usually with 4-0 or 5-0 synthetic absorbable sutures. In this situation, the use of a larger Silastic transhepatic stent for long-term stenting is not necessary.

If adequate healthy bile duct mucosa is not present, particularly in cases with prior attempts at repair, the side of the Roux-en-Y jejunal limb is sutured circumferentially with interrupted 4-0 or 5-0 synthetic absorbable sutures to the ductal tissue at the exit site of the Silastic stent from the hepatic hilum. In cases in which two Silastic transhepatic stents are necessary, bilateral hepaticojejunostomies are performed separately to the Roux-en-Y loop. After completion of the biliary enteric anastomoses, the Roux-en-Y jejunal loop is tacked to the undersurface of the liver to avoid tension on the anastomosis (see Fig. 15-12D). Fluorocholangiography can then be performed to check the position of the transhepatic stents. The defect in the transverse mesocolon, through which the retrocolic Roux-en-Y limb was placed, is closed to prevent small bowel herniation. Closed suction drains are left near the biliary enteric anastomosis. The sites where the Silastic stents exit the liver are also drained.

The Silastic stents are 70 cm long and come in 12F to 22F sizes. Multiple side holes are present along 40% of the length of the stent. These side holes are left to reside within the intrahepatic biliary tree and the portion of the Roux-en-Y jejunal limb used for the biliary anastomosis. The ends of the stents without the side holes exit through the hepatic parenchyma and are brought out through stab wounds in the upper anterior abdomen. The stents are fixed to the skin with wire sutures and are attached initially to a bile bag for dependent gravity drainage.

BILIARY ANASTOMOSIS WITHOUT STENTS. A number of other techniques have been described for management of bile duct strictures involving the bifurcation of one or both of the hepatic ducts. The left hepatic duct always has an extrahepatic course at the base of the quadrate lobe (segment IV). A long opening along the anterior surface of the left hepatic duct is anastomosed to the side of the Roux-en-Y limb 2 to 3 cm distal to its closed end[55,56] (Fig. 15-13). Because it is possible to dissect a long length of the anterior surface of the left hepatic duct, this procedure permits anastomosis to normal mucosa, even though there may be fibrosis and stricture at the bifurcation of the ducts and within the distal portion of the hepatic ducts. Obviously, there must be some communication between

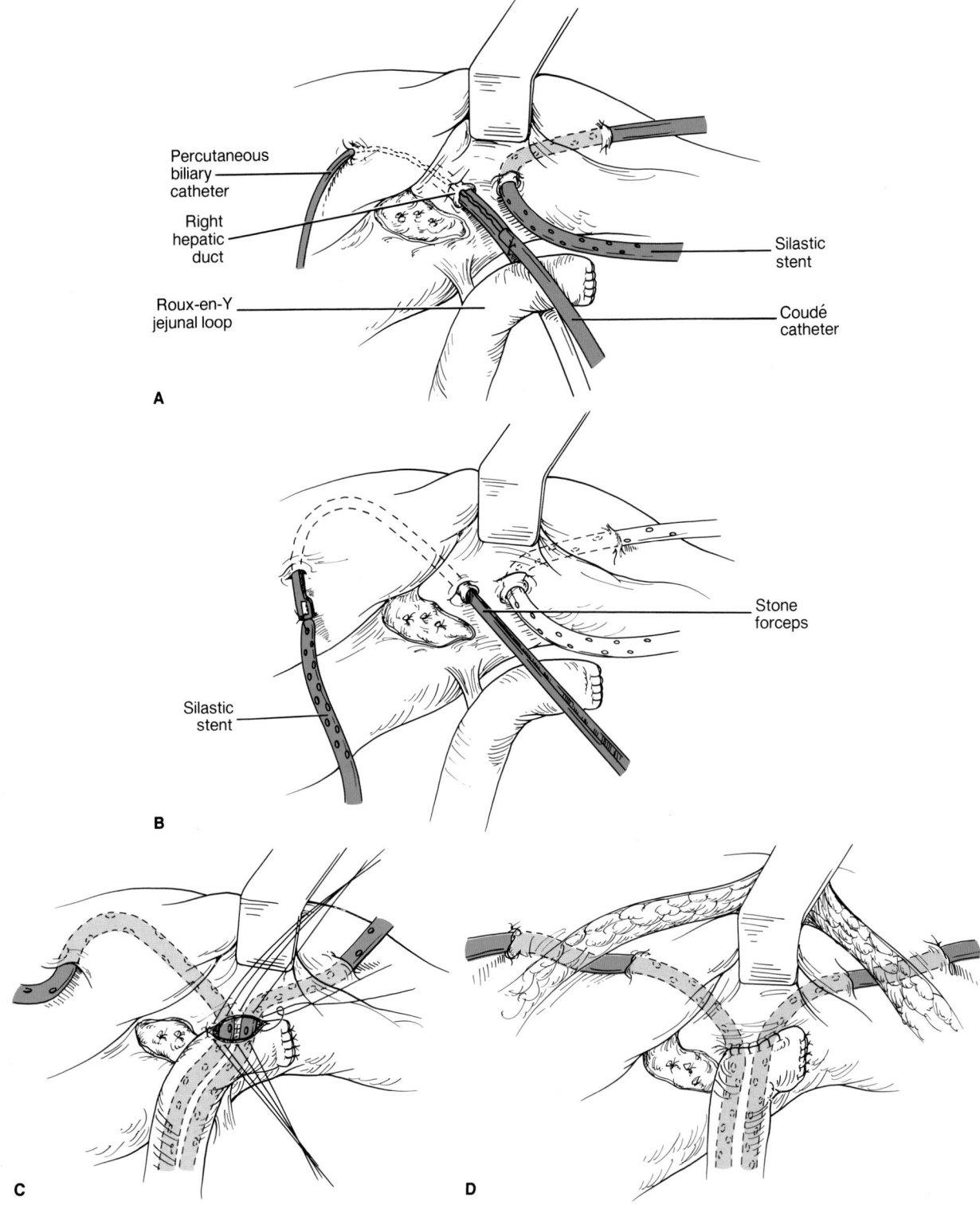

Percutaneous
biliary
catheter

Right
hepatic
duct

Roux-en-Y
jejunal loop

Silastic
stent

Coudé
catheter

A

Silastic
stent

Stone
forceps

B

C

D

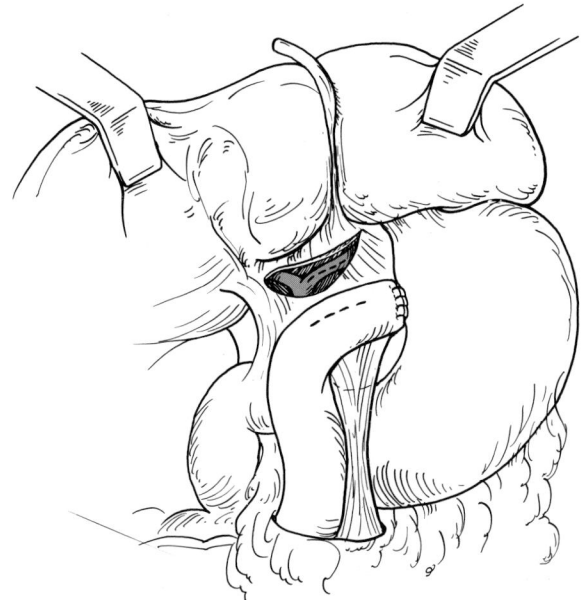

Figure 15-13 Exposure of the left hepatic duct and the confluence by incision of the peritoneal reflection at the base of the quadrate lobe. A Roux-en-Y loop has been prepared. The dotted lines on the duct and jejunum indicate the lines of incision. (After Blumgart LH, Thompson JN. The management of benign strictures of the bile ducts. Curr Probl Surg 1987;24:1)

the right and left ducts for this procedure to drain the right lobe effectively.

When the bifurcation is strictured and excised, there is no communication between the right and left ducts. The alternatives then include anastomosis of the two bile ducts to each other, thereby creating a new confluence that can be anastomosed as a single unit to the Roux-en-Y limb, and the creation of two separate anastomoses to the jejunal limb. Advocates of these techniques do not usually use biliary stents.

One technique designed to gain exposure of the proximal ducts in high strictures (Bismuth type III) involves incising Glisson's capsule at the junction of the quadrate lobe (segment IV) and the left lateral segment (segment III) where the falciform ligament joins the liver. This incision exposes a branch of the left intrahepatic duct. This maneuver allows dissection of an adequate length of proximal hepatic duct for creation of a side-to-side, mucosa-to-mucosa anastomosis.[55]

MUCOSAL GRAFT TECHNIQUE. The jejunal mucosal graft technique involves a sutureless anastomosis in which a circular portion of the seromuscular wall of the Roux-en-Y jejunal limb is removed and a transhepatic catheter is placed in the jejunal limb through a small incision in the pouting jejunal mucosa.[57,58] The mucosa is then anchored to the catheter, and the catheter and the tented mucosa are pulled proximally into the lumen of the bile duct, where they adhere to the bile duct mucosa. The seromuscular surface of the jejunal limb is sutured to the scar around the duct in the hilum of the liver to reduce tension and to hold the mucosal graft into position. Although results have been satisfactory with this technique,[59] it is not based on the principle of a precise mucosa-to-mucosa apposition of normal ductal tissues to the jejunum. Therefore, this technique should be reserved for cases in which it is impossible to define normal duct tissue.

INTRAHEPATIC CHOLANGIOJEJUNOSTOMY (LONGMIRE PROCEDURE). A final alternative for patients with multiple previous operations in the hilus is the Longmire procedure, which involves mobilization of the left lobe of the liver and division of the left lateral segment, exposing the segment III hepatic duct and, occasionally, a segment II bile duct.[60] A Roux-en-Y jejunal loop can then be anastomosed to the surface of the exposed liver as an alternative to direct anastomosis to the

◀ **Figure 15-12** **(A)** A coudé catheter is sutured to the preoperatively placed transhepatic catheter, which protrudes through the transected right hepatic duct. The coudé catheter and subsequently the silastic stent can then be pulled through the catheter tract in the hepatic parenchyma. **(B)** Alternatively, a Stone forceps can be passed into the hepatic duct, advanced through the intrahepatic biliary tree, and forced out through the parenchyma on the anterior surface of the liver. A Silastic biliary stent is then sutured to the end of the forceps so that it can be drawn back into the intrahepatic biliary tree and out the hepatic duct. **(C)** A Roux-en-Y jejunal loop is then anastomosed to the hepatic duct, liver capsule, and other structures at the egress site of the Silastic stent in the hilum of the liver. The portion of the stent that passes through the liver and into the jejunum contains multiple side holes. **(D)** The completed biliary–enteric anastomosis over bilateral Silastic biliary stents is tacked to the undersurface of the liver. (After Cameron JL, Gayler BW, Zuidema GD. The use of Silastic transhepatic stents in benign and malignant biliary strictures. Ann Surg 1978;188:552)

bile duct. A similar procedure can also be performed to a segment IV branch that lies deep to the gallbladder bed on the right. These procedures, however, are associated with greater blood loss and provide less effective biliary drainage than can be obtained by most other methods.

Role of Postoperative Biliary Stenting

The role of biliary stenting and the length of time that the stent is employed remain controversial. Some authors favor at least short-term stenting of all bile duct stricture repairs; however, a number of authors disagree with stenting even in the early postoperative period.[61–63] As stated previously, when a large bile duct with circumferential mucosa is available, only a short period of stenting is necessary. In cases in which the anastomosis is performed high in the hilum to a bile duct or ducts of questionable quality, transhepatic Silastic stents should be left for at least a year after operation. Transhepatic Silastic stents with one end left in the jejunum (J-tube) are preferred. However, other authors have described the use of transhepatic U-tubes.[64,65] U-tubes, like Silastic J-stents, exit through the anterior surface of the liver and the anterior abdominal wall on one end, but the other end is brought through the Roux-en-Y limb as a Witzel enterostomy and then brought through the anterior abdominal wall. Although it has been suggested that U-tubes are more easily changed, J-tubes can easily be replaced over guide wires. Additionally, when bilateral stents are necessary, U-tubes require four tube exit sites versus two with the J-tubes. Moreover, the jejunal exit sites are prone to bile leakage.

The duration of stenting is also controversial, with recommended intervals ranging from 2 months to 2 years. Those supporting long-term stenting believe that the stent ensures a stable biliary anastomosis during the period of healing and scar contracture. Significantly better results were obtained in patients whose stents were in place for more than 1 month than in patients in whom the stent was removed in less than 1 month.[17] In patients stented for more than 9 months, results were significantly better if Silastic, changeable stents were employed. The likelihood of stenting having benefit in a large mucosa-to-mucosa anastomosis with normal duct tissue (Bismuth type I) is relatively small. However, a long-term stent can keep a small anastomosis to scar tissue open and prevent late fibrosis and restricture.

Postoperative Management

Postoperatively, the transhepatic catheter or Silastic biliary stent is placed to dependent gravity drainage for 5 to 7 days. Cholangiography is then performed to docu-

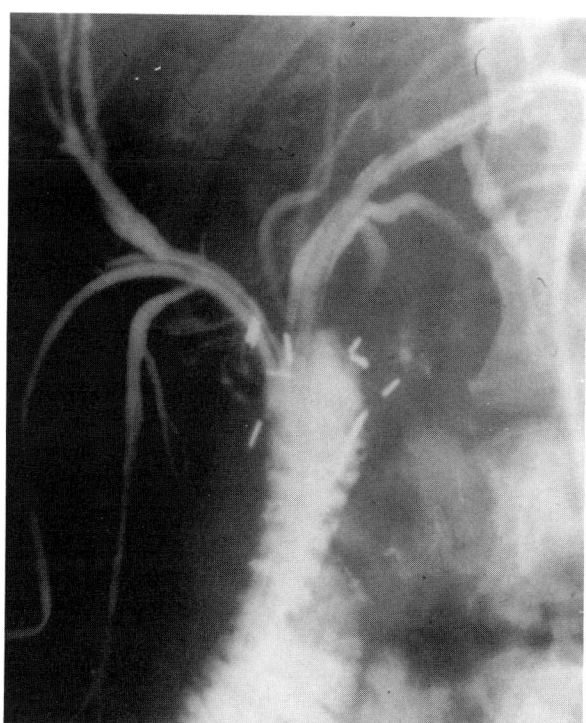

Figure 15-14 Postoperative cholangiogram performed through Silastic biliary stents showing no evidence of anastomotic leak. (Lillemoe KD, Pitt HA, Cameron JL. Postoperative bile duct strictures. Surg Clin North Am 1990;70:1355)

ment anastomotic integrity and the absence of a bile leak (Fig. 15-14). If no evidence of a leak is apparent on the postoperative cholangiogram, the stents can be internalized. The operatively placed drains can be removed 1 or 2 days later if no bile leaks after the stents have been internalized.

After hospital discharge, routine periodic stent changes are recommended because the side holes of the transhepatic stents can become occluded by biliary sludge and secretions. The stents should be exchanged fluoroscopically over guide wires every 3 to 4 months. This procedure can usually be performed on an outpatient basis, although prophylactic antibiotics are recommended to prevent cholangitis. Before stent removal, a Whitaker test,[66] which assesses biliary pressure in response to increased flow, should be performed to ensure that the anastomosis is patent and will accept a reasonable bile flow. Finally, the stent can be pulled back above the anastomosis and left in place for a 2- to 3-week clinical trial before ultimate removal.

Results

Morbidity and Mortality

Even though most repairs of bile duct strictures are performed in major medical centers by experienced surgeons, these operations are still associated with significant morbidity and mortality. In 1982, a review of 38 series published since 1900, including more than 7643 procedures performed on 5586 patients, reported an overall operative mortality rate of 8.3%.[53] In the past decade, however, most series have reported mortality rates below 5%.[10,17,52,63,64,67,68] Factors frequently associated with increased operative mortality include advanced age, comorbid disease, and a history of major biliary tract infection. The state of underlying liver disease, however, is the most important determinant of operative morbidity and mortality.[68] In patients with advanced biliary cirrhosis and portal hypertension, operative mortality rates can approach 30%, and most deaths are due to liver failure. Proximal bile duct strictures, which are more difficult to repair, are generally associated with more frequent postoperative complications.

In most series, postoperative morbidity rates range from 20% to 30%. Specific complications related to the repair of bile duct strictures include bile leaks at the site of the biliary enteric anastomosis or at the hepatic exit sites of the transhepatic stents, cholangitis, hepatic insufficiency from preexisting biliary cirrhosis, and hemobilia. Most anastomotic leaks, documented by postoperative cholangiography or by bile drainage from intraoperatively placed drains, can be successfully managed nonoperatively. Transhepatic stents divert bile externally and are advantageous if a leak develops. In most of these cases, bile leaks heal with no long-term consequences.

Long-Term Results

Excellent long-term results can be achieved in 70% to 90% of patients undergoing repair of bile duct strictures[10,17,33,52,63,67,69] (Table 15-3). The definition of satis-

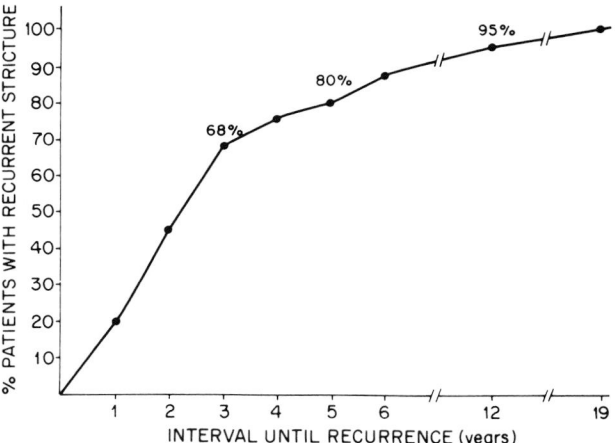

Figure 15-15 The cumulative percentage of patients with recurrent strictures is shown with respect to the time interval from the initial repair until the next repair. (After Pitt HA, Miyamoto T, Parapatis SK, et al. Factors influencing outcome in patients with postoperative biliary strictures. Am J Surg 1982;144:14)

factory results in most series requires patients to have no symptoms and no jaundice or cholangitis. Length of follow-up is important in analyzing final results, because restenosis can occur up to 20 years after the initial procedure[17,33] (Fig. 15-15). About two thirds of recurrent strictures are evident within 2 years, and 90% are seen within 7 years.[17] The percentage of patients with good results is also inversely related to the number of previous repairs. Other factors that favor a good outcome include young age at the time of stricture repair, use of a Roux-en-Y biliary enteric anastomosis, absence of infection and hepatic fibrosis, and use of transhepatic stents.[16]

One report described the experience in the treatment of 25 consecutive patients with benign postoperative strictures using long-term transhepatic stents.[52] Thirty-five percent of these patients were classified as Bismuth type II, and 40% were Bismuth type III or IV. Long-term stenting was employed for a mean of 13.8 months after operation. Three failures occurred, with two of these patients having failed multiple previous attempts at surgical repair. Thus, 88% of patients had a successful long-term outcome. No hospital mortalities occurred, and the operative morbidity was 20%.

The possibility of late restricturing requires that patients be followed indefinitely. Serum bilirubin, transaminases, and alkaline phosphatase should be monitored. Radionucleotide scanning provides good physiologic information concerning bile flow and can be useful in follow-up evaluation. Ultrasound or CT scanning to look for biliary dilation and intrahepatic stones can also be helpful.

Table 15-3   Results of Surgical Management of Bile Duct Stricutres

Year	Institution	Patients	Success Rate (%)	Follow-Up (mo)
1982	UCLA[17]	66	86	60
1984	UCSF[33]	60	78	102
1986	Cleveland Clinic[67]	105	82	60
1988	Ohio State[63]	22	95	72
1988	St George's[69]	163	72	133
1989	Johns Hopkins[52]	25	88	57
1993	Mannheim Clinic[10]	64	75	99

(Modified from Lillemoe KD, Pitt HA, Cameron JL. Postoperative bile duct strictures. Surg Clin North Am 1990;70:1355)

Nonoperative Management

Operative repair of bile duct strictures is technically difficult and continues to be associated with significant postoperative morbidity. Furthermore, the psychological trauma to the patient caused by the need for reoperation has led many to support a nonoperative approach to bile duct strictures. The technical advances in the fields of therapeutic radiology and endoscopy have led to the development of these nonoperative techniques.

Percutaneous Balloon Dilation

The largest nonoperative experience in the management of benign bile duct strictures is through the percutaneous transhepatic route. In this technique, access to the proximal biliary tree is gained, and the stricture is traversed with a guide wire under fluoroscopic guidance. At this point, dilation of the stricture is performed using angioplasty-type balloon catheters, chosen on the basis of the location of the stricture and the diameter of the normal duct. Balloons 5 to 8 mm in diameter are used for strictures at or above the common hepatic duct bifurcation. Balloons 6 to 10 mm in diameter are used for common bile duct strictures, and larger balloons (8 to 12 mm) are chosen for biliary enteric anastomotic strictures. The balloon is inflated to 10 to 12 atmospheric pressure for at least 30 seconds, and the process is repeated until no "waist deformity" is noted during inflation (Fig. 15-16). After the procedure, a transhepatic stent is left in place across the stricture to allow access to the biliary tree for follow-up cholangiography and repeat dilation and to maintain a lumen during the healing process. In most series, numerous dilations are required. The procedure in many cases can be performed with a combination of local anesthesia and intravenous sedation. However, many patients find the procedure painful, and general anesthesia has been necessary in a significant percentage of patients.

The early results of balloon dilation in a number of series have been encouraging (Table 15-4). In one multicenter review,[70] 3-year follow-up showed a 67% patency rate for anastomotic strictures and a 76% patency rate for iatrogenic primary bile duct strictures, yielding an overall 70% success rate. Patency was based

Table 15-4 Results of Transhepatic Balloon Dilation of Bile Duct Strictures

Year	Institution	Patients	Success Rate (%)	Follow-Up (mo)
1985	University of Florida[72]	13	85	24
1986	Multiple institutions[70]	61	70	36
1987	Mayo Clinic[71]	64	78	28
1987	Duke[73]	18	83	33
1989	Johns Hopkins[52]	20	55	59

(Modified from Lillemoe KD, Pitt HA, Cameron JL. Postoperative bile duct strictures. Surg Clin North Am 1990;70:1355)

on the absence of symptoms and normal serum bilirubin and alkaline phosphatase levels. In another report,[71] successful dilation was achieved in 87.5% of patients with primary ductal strictures and in 72.5% of patients with biliary enteric anastomotic strictures, for an overall success rate of 78%. In this series, success was defined as absence of symptoms after stent removal at a mean follow-up of 28 months (range, 1 to 50 months). Similar results in smaller series have also been reported.[72,73] However, in a report with one of the longest follow-up periods available, the success rate was only 55%.[51]

Complications of balloon dilation are frequent. In one report,[71] 29% of patients lost 2 g or more of hemoglobin after the procedure, and 7 of 65 patients (11%) who underwent transhepatic procedures required blood transfusion. Arteriobiliary fistulas were present in six of eight patients who did not stop bleeding spontaneously. Treatment by embolization in one case resulted in a left hepatic lobe infarction and abscess that required surgical drainage. Sepsis with positive blood cultures occurred in 24% of patients despite antibiotic prophylaxis. Pancreatitis occurred in two patients, and a catheter-related duodenal perforation, which required surgery, occurred in one patient. Sepsis and significant bleeding did not occur in patients dilated through a T-tube tract, suggesting that much of the morbidity is due to traversing the hepatic parenchyma by the large percutaneously placed catheters. In an-

Figure 15-16 (A) Transhepatic cholangiogram demonstrating stricture (*arrow*) at a previous choledochojejunostomy. (B) Progressive dilation of the strictured anastomosis with an angioplasty balloon catheter. (C) Postdilation stenting of the anastomotic stricture for prolonged periods. (D) Subsequent cholangiography demonstrating resolution of the anastomotic stricture. (After Pitt HA, Kaufman SL, Coleman J, et al. Benign postoperative biliary strictures: operate or dilate? Ann Surg 1989;210:417)

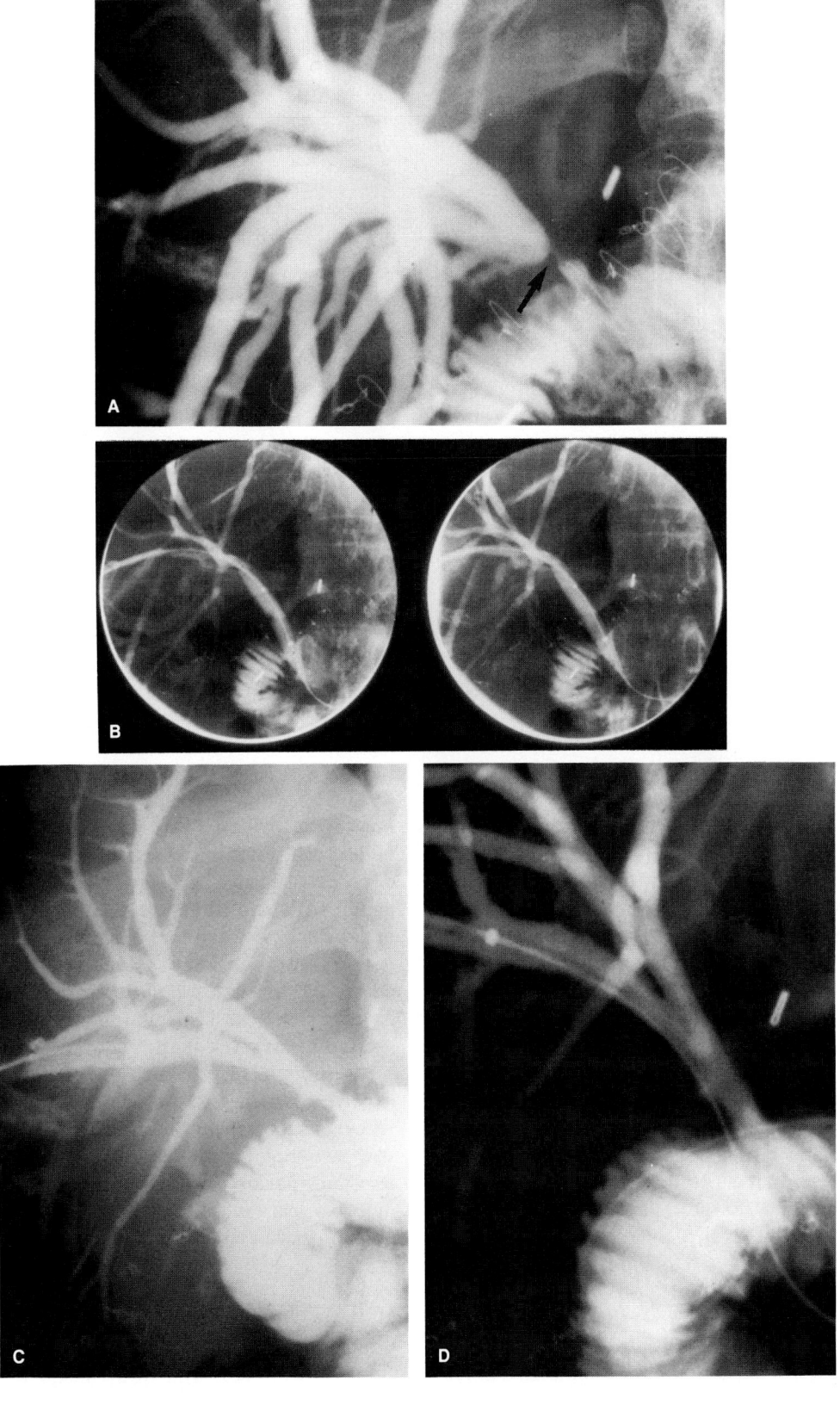

other series,[52] significant hemobilia also occurred in 20% of patients. In a multicenter review,[70] however, the morbidity was less, and septicemia developed in less than 5% of patients. No bleeding was reported, and no deaths were noted in this series.

A final route for percutaneous management of anastomotic biliary strictures is retrograde using a subcutaneous modified Roux-en-Y jejunal limb. In the largest experience with this procedure,[74] 23 patients with benign strictures were managed with this technique. Of these 23 patients, 15 had primary sclerosing cholangitis, whereas 8 patients had postoperative benign strictures. In all these patients, the jejunal limb was easily accessed, and successful dilation was performed on repeated occasions with minimal morbidity. In a more recent study,[75] nonmodified Roux-en-Y limbs were percutaneously catheterized, and strictures were dilated. The authors reported a successful result in 11 patients in whom a previous biliary enteric anastomosis had been constructed for a number of indications, including sclerosing cholangitis. This latter technique is advantageous in that it can be applied to all patients with Roux-en-Y biliary reconstruction even without special modification. Although these techniques avoid the use of biliary stents, they often require multiple procedures, and no long-term follow-up studies have been reported.

Endoscopic Dilation

The experience with endoscopic balloon dilation is somewhat more limited. This technique is technically possible only in patients with primary bile duct strictures or in strictures at a choledochoduodenal anastomosis. If long-term stenting with an endoprosthesis is indicated, repeat endoscopy is necessary to change occluded stents. This technique begins with ERC and endoscopic sphincterotomy. The stricture is traversed retrograde with an atraumatic guide wire. Sequential dilation with 4- to 10-mm balloons is employed. A large channel (4.2 mm), side-viewing duodenal scope is employed for most primary bile duct strictures. An end-viewing scope may be more useful in dilation of a strictured choledochoduodenostomy. Reevaluation with cholangiography is performed every 3 to 6 months, and redilation is performed as necessary. In most cases, an endoprosthesis is left in place for at least 6 months after dilation.

In the largest experience with this technique,[76] 66 patients underwent an initial attempt at endoscopic management of a bile duct stricture (Table 15-5). Successful stent placement was achieved in 62 of 66 patients (94%). The stricture location was defined as Bismuth type I in 45% of patients and Bismuth type II or

Table 15-5   Results of Endoscopic Balloon Dilation of Bile Duct Strictures

Year	Institution	Patients	Success Rate (%)	Follow-Up (mo)
1985	Cleveland Clinic[78]	9	55	6
1986	Amsterdam[76]	46	72	42
1989	Milwaukee[77]	25	88	48

(Modified from Lillemoe KD, Pitt HA, Cameron JL. Postoperation bile duct strictures. Surg Clin North Am 1990;70:1355)

higher in the remaining 55%. Complications occurred within 30 days of the procedure in 8% of patients, including one death (1.5%) due to sequelae of acute pancreatitis. Stents were removed at a mean of 360 days (range, 91 to 725 days) in 46 patients. During this period, a mean of five endoscopic retrograde cholangiopancreatography (ERCP) procedures were performed on each patient. Complications in the period of stenting occurred in 27% of the patients during a mean follow-up of 42 months. Excellent results, defined as having no symptoms and normal or stable liver enzyme levels, were achieved in 72% of the patients.

In a similar experience with endoscopic treatment of strictures,[77] 18 of 25 strictures were postoperative in nature. Strictures were located at the cystic duct junction in 17 patients and in the distal bile duct in the remaining 8 patients. Twenty-two of 25 patients (88%) had significant clinical benefit from the therapy. Only two complications occurred—one case each of mild pancreatitis and cholangitis. This series provides some of the longest follow-up available for this technique, ranging from 6 months to 7 years (mean, 4 ± 0.3 years). Of the 23 patients, 8 had no symptoms for more than 2 years since the last dilation, and 8 patients had no symptoms for more than 5 years.

Although these results are excellent, a great deal of expertise is necessary to achieve such results. In one report,[78] success was obtained in only 58% of patients, with two major complications in 9 patients: a common bile duct perforation and a respiratory arrest. Moreover, two patients died within 1 month because of complications of liver disease.

Comparative Data

Comparison of results of balloon dilation with those of surgery have been difficult because few centers have a significant experience with both operative and nonoperative management. Furthermore, the definition of a successful procedure, the reporting of complications, and the length of follow-up have not been consistent in the literature. Two such comparative retrospective studies exist—one comparing surgical with percutaneous management and one comparing surgical and endoscopic treatment. A retrospective review of results at one institution between 1979 and 1987 was completed, comparing percutaneous dilation and surgery.[52] In this report, 42 patients underwent 45 procedures for benign postoperative biliary strictures. Twenty-five patients underwent surgical repair with Roux-en-Y choledochojejunostomy or hepaticojejunostomy with postoperative transhepatic stenting for a mean of 13 ± 1.3 months. Twenty patients had balloon dilation, an average of 3.9 times, and were stented transhepatically for a mean of 13.3 ± 2 months. Three patients were treated with both surgery and balloon dilation.

The two groups in this analysis were similar with respect to multiple parameters that may have influenced outcome, including age, sex, secondary biliary cirrhosis, intrahepatic stones, and presentation with either obstructive jaundice or biliary fistulas. Fifty-six percent of the surgical patients and 65% of the balloon dilation patients had undergone one or more previous surgical attempts at stricture repair. In the surgical group, nine patients had undergone a previous biliary enteric anastomosis, whereas five had undergone a previous end-to-end surgical reconstruction. In the balloon dilation group, all previous repairs consisted of a biliary enteric anastomosis. Mean length of follow-up was 57 ± 7 months and 59 ± 6 months for surgery and balloon dilation, respectively.

No patient died after any of the procedures. Procedure-related morbidity occurred in 20% of surgical patients and in 35% of the patients undergoing balloon dilation. Although the overall complication rate was not different, the incidence of significant hemobilia after surgery and balloon dilation were 4% and 20%, respectively ($P < .02$). For both groups, a successful outcome was defined as no evidence of cholangitis or jaundice requiring another procedure more than 12 months from the onset of treatment. A failed treatment was defined as the need for crossover to the other treatment modality, either operation or dilation, or late death from liver failure, biliary sepsis, or portal hypertension. A successful repair was achieved in 88% of the surgical patients and in only 55% of the balloon dilation patients ($P < .02$; Fig. 15-17). The overall late mortality rate in this series was 10%. One late death occurred in the surgical group, whereas three late deaths followed balloon dilation (4% versus 15%; $P < .02$). None of the deaths, however, was attributed to liver failure, biliary sepsis, or portal hypertension associated with the bile duct stricture. Factors influencing outcome are shown in Table 15-6.

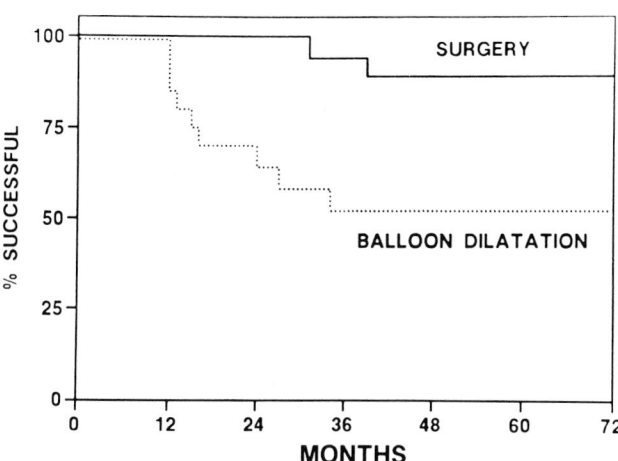

Figure 15-17 Actuarial success rates over 72 months for surgery (89%) and balloon dilatation (52%). The difference is statistically significant ($P < .01$). (After Pitt HA, Kaufman SL, Coleman J, et al. Benign postoperative biliary strictures: operate or dilate? Ann Surg 1989;210:417)

To further define the relative benefit of the two procedures, total hospital stay and total procedural costs were determined. As expected, initial hospitalization was longer for surgery than for balloon dilation. However, when rehospitalization for further dilations, complications, or recurrences was considered, total hospital stay did not differ significantly between the two groups. Mean hospital stay for surgery was 26.4 ± 2.5 days, and for balloon dilation, it was 21.4 ± 1.7 days (Fig. 15-18). Moreover, since 1984, the mean total hospital stay for surgery decreased to 17.9 ± 1.5 days, compared with 21.2 ± 1.7 days for balloon dilation. Cost data paralleled

Table 15-6 Factors Influencing Outcome of the Management of Postoperative Bile Duct Strictures

Factor	Successful Outcome (%)
TYPE OF STRICTURE	
Primary	86
Anastomotic	61
LEVEL OF STRICTURE	
Bismuth type I	100‡
Bismuth type II	59
Bismuth type III	87
Bismuth type IV	71
Bismuth type V	33

* $P < .05$ versus anastomotic strictures.
‡ $P < .05$ versus types II through V.
(Adapted from Pitt HA, Kaufman SL, Coleman J, et al. Benign postoperative biliary strictures: operate or dilate? Ann Surg 1989;210:417)

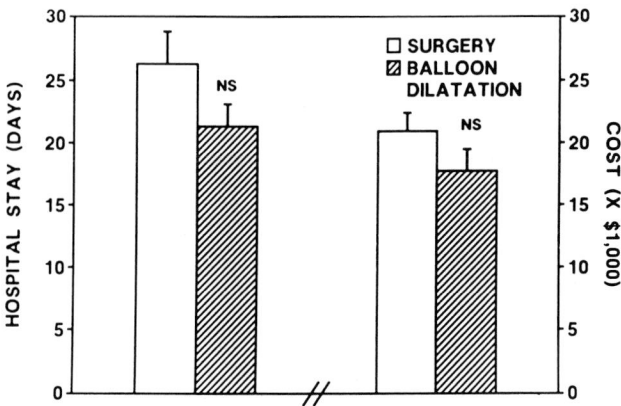

Figure 15-18 Total hospital stay and cost for surgery and balloon dilatation. Differences are not statistically significant. (After Pitt HA, Kaufman SL, Coleman J, et al. Benign postoperative biliary strictures: operate or dilate? Ann Surg 1989;210:417)

hospitalization data and did not differ significantly between the groups. Estimated total cost for surgery was $20,988 ± $1376 and for balloon dilation was $17,728 ± $1688. It was concluded from this study that until properly designed, randomized, prospective controlled trials can be performed, surgical repair for benign postoperative strictures appears to be associated with fewer problems and a greater success rate. Surgery is not associated with increased morbidity or mortality. Moreover, the total hospitalization and the cost of surgery compare favorably with those for balloon dilation.

In a second study,[76] endoscopic treatment was compared with surgical repair of benign bile duct strictures. Thirty-five patients were treated surgically and 66 were treated by endoscopic stenting. Patient characteristics, initial injury, previous repairs, and the level of obstruction were comparable in both groups. Surgical therapy consisted primarily of a Roux-en-Y hepaticojejunostomy. Endoscopic therapy consisted of placement of an endoprosthesis, with trimonthly elective exchanges for a 1-year period. Successful stent placement was accomplished in 94% of patients treated endoscopically. Six of the 66 endoscopic patients, however, underwent surgical reconstruction, either for failed stent placement or other reasons. Early complications occurred more frequently in the surgically treated group (26% versus 8%; $P < .03$). However, the only procedure-related death occurred in a patient who developed severe pancreatitis after endoscopic stent placement. Late complications, mainly episodes of cholangitis, occurred only in the endoscopic group (27%). The overall complication rates, therefore, were similar: 26% for surgical patients, and 35% for endoscopic patients. In addition,

six patients died during the period of endoscopic stenting. Although the authors state that these deaths were due to nonbiliary causes, five of the six appeared to be acute events, including a myocardial infarction (in three patients), a cerebrovascular accident, and urosepsis.

The mean follow-up was 50 months after surgery and 46 months after endoscopic stent removal. A successful result was defined as the patient having no symptoms and normal or stable liver enzymes. A good result was recorded when the patient had experienced only a single episode of cholangitis. A poor result was defined as two or more episodes of cholangitis or a recurrent stricture. After surgery, excellent results were observed in 83% of patients. Six patients (17%) had stricture recurrence at a mean of 40 months after the initial operation, with all undergoing a second surgical reconstruction with good results. After endoscopic stenting, results were excellent in 72% of patients. Eight patients (18%) had recurrent strictures at a mean of 3 months after stent removal. Six of these patients underwent surgery, and two other patients were restented.

No length-of-stay data, either for the initial procedure or total hospitalization during the entire period, were provided. In addition, no cost analysis was performed. The endoscopic patients, however, did require a mean of five endoscopic stent changes during the course of the 1 year of stenting.

The authors concluded from this study that surgery and endoscopy for benign biliary strictures have similar early results and long-term success rates. It would appear that, in environments where local expertise exists, endoscopic biliary stenting can be successfully employed in a substantial percentage of patients. Use of this procedure is limited, however, to patients in whom the biliary tree is still accessible, and the procedure is not applicable in patients who have undergone biliary reconstruction to a loop of jejunum.

BILE DUCT STRICTURES SECONDARY TO CHRONIC PANCREATITIS

Chronic pancreatitis causes a distal bile duct stricture in about 10% of patients. These strictures are secondary to the inflammation and pancreatic parenchymal fibrosis, which involves the intrapancreatic portion of the common bile duct.[35] Like strictures elsewhere, the resultant bile duct obstruction can lead to advanced biliary cirrhosis. Another important clinical feature of distal bile duct obstruction due to chronic pancreatitis is the differentiation of benign strictures from carcinoma of the pancreas.

Pathogenesis and Incidence

Transient partial obstruction of the distal common bile duct due to inflammation and edema frequently occurs in patients with acute pancreatitis. The serum bilirubin, which is usually minimally elevated, promptly returns to normal after the pancreatitis has resolved. In cases of chronic pancreatitis, the distal bile duct obstruction is due to chronic inflammation, with resultant fibrosis of the gland. These strictures classically involve only the 2- to 4-cm intrapancreatic segment of the common bile duct, with associated dilation of the entire proximal biliary tree (Fig. 15-19). In almost all cases, the cause of chronic pancreatitis is alcoholism.

Common bile duct strictures have been reported to occur in 3% to 29% of patients with chronic alcoholic pancreatitis.[79-82] In a review of a number of clinical series, the overall incidence of common bile duct stricture in patients with chronic pancreatitis was 5.7%.[83] However, the exact incidence of strictures due to chronic pancreatitis is not known because cholangiography is not routinely performed in such patients. In a series of 79 consecutive patients with moderately severe chronic pancreatitis who underwent ERCP, 36 (46%) were found to have radiographic stenosis in the intrapancreatic common bile duct.[84]

Clinical Presentation

The clinical presentation of patients with common bile duct strictures secondary to chronic pancreatitis is variable. Many patients have no symptoms, and the diagnosis of bile duct stricture is suggested only by abnormal liver function tests. The serum alkaline phosphatase appears to be the most sensitive laboratory finding and is elevated in over 80% of patients.[83] The elevation of alkaline phosphatase is persistent and usually two to three times normal values. The serum bilirubin level is usually minimally to moderately elevated and is characterized by a rising and falling pattern. The disproportionate increase in the alkaline phosphatase compared with bilirubin is compatible with benign obstruction of the distal common bile duct due to pancreatitis. Moreover, these biochemical abnormalities are highly predictive of a bile duct stricture because elevations of serum alkaline phosphatase and bilirubin are uncommon in uncomplicated chronic pancreatitis.

Abdominal pain with or without jaundice is another common presentation. In some cases, the abdominal pain of biliary origin is difficult to distinguish from the pain associated with chronic pancreatitis. Yet, recognition and treatment for a bile duct stricture is essential to prevent failure of operative procedures for relief of pain of chronic pancreatitis. Patients with a bile duct stricture due to chronic pancreatitis often have advanced disease. The incidence of pancreatic calcifications, diabetes, and malabsorption are all increased in patients with chronic pancreatitis with jaundice, compared with patients without jaundice.[79]

Cholangitis is a potentially life-threatening complication of a bile duct stricture secondary to chronic pancreatitis. Bacteria can be cultured from the bile in more than half of patients with bile duct strictures, and most organisms are gram-negative bacilli.[85,86] Despite this high incidence of bacterial infection, cholangitis is uncommon. In a review of 18 series,[83] the incidence of cholangitis was only 9%. In another series,[86] although 60% of patients had positive bile cultures, cholangitis was present in only 10% of patients.

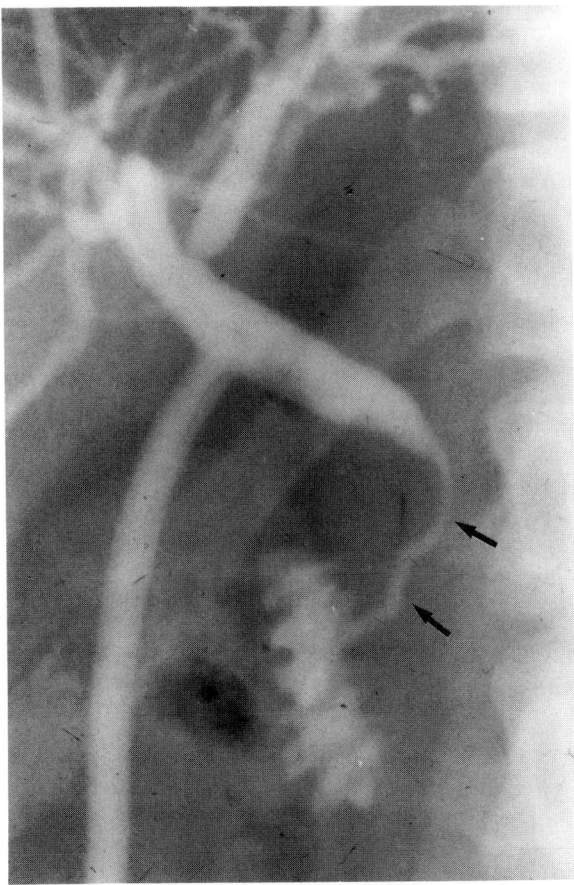

Figure 15-19 T-tube cholangiogram of a patient with a long distal common bile duct stricture (*arrows*) due to chronic pancreatitis. (Lillemoe KD, Pitt HA, Cameron JL. Current management of benign bile duct strictures. Adv Surg 1992; 25:119)

Differential Diagnosis

The differential diagnosis in patients with common bile duct strictures due to chronic pancreatitis includes a number of other important entities. The development of jaundice in alcoholics is often attributed to hepatocellular disease, such as cirrhosis or alcoholic hepatitis. Abdominal pain, jaundice, or cholangitis suggests common bile duct stones. The most important differentiation, however, is whether biliary obstruction is due to chronic pancreatitis or an underlying pancreatic malignancy. A number of clinical features can suggest one diagnosis over the other (Table 15-7); however, at times, the distinction can be virtually impossible.

In one review,[87] patients with chronic pancreatitis as the cause of biliary obstruction were significantly younger than patients with pancreatic carcinoma (average age, 47 versus 62 years). Serum bilirubin was much lower in patients with chronic pancreatitis (5.6 ± 1.5 mg/dL versus 18.5 ± 2.1). Moreover, the pattern of bilirubin elevation was different. In patients with pancreatic carcinoma, bilirubin rose steadily until biliary decompression was achieved. In patients with chronic pancreatitis, the bilirubin tended to fluctuate. Patients with biliary obstruction due to chronic pancreatitis also tend to have a history of chronic abdominal and back pain, which often precedes the development of jaundice for months or years. In comparison, patients with carcinoma frequently experience no pain or have pain only for a brief interval before the relentless increase in bilirubin. Finally, it is extremely uncommon for jaundice to be the initial presentation of chronic pancreatitis, especially in older patients. Preoperatively, these historical observations and laboratory findings, combined with radiologic evaluation, can usually differentiate most cases of benign stricture from carcinoma.

Diagnosis

The initial diagnostic step in any patient with presumed biliary obstruction is noninvasive imaging of the hepatobiliary tree. Either ultrasonography or CT is a suitable technique for this evaluation because each can easily demonstrate the presence of a dilated biliary tree, including both the common bile duct and intrahepatic bile ducts. CT is preferable because it can better define the pancreas, including the presence of a mass and pancreatic ductal dilation. The increased ability to delineate pancreatic pathology is the primary reason that CT is considered more useful in the evaluation of patients with obstructive jaundice. A well-defined pancreatic mass suggests malignancy; however, in some patients with periampullary malignancy, especially those most likely to be resectable for cure, a large mass is not present. Moreover, diffuse enlargement of the pancreatic head may be consistent with either pancreatitis or malignancy (Fig. 15-20).

The definitive evaluation of patients with biliary obstruction is cholangiography. Either ERCP or PTC

Table 15-7   Clinical Features and Characteristics Distinguishing Biliary Obstruction Due to Chronic Pancreatitis From Pancreatic Cancer

Clinical Feature	Pancreatic Carcinoma	Chronic Pancreatitis
History and physical examination	Persistent jaundice	Intermittent jaundice
	Weight loss	Alcohol abuse
	Older patient	Younger patient
	Palpable gallbladder (Courvoisier's sign)	Frequent attacks of pancreatitis
	Evidence of metastasis	Steatorrhea
Laboratory data	Markedly elevated bilirubin	Minimally elevated bilirubin
	Prolonged prothrombin time	Elevated alkaline phosphatase
	Decreased serum albumin	
Plain abdominal radiographs	Normal	Pancreatic calcification
Endoscopic retrograde cholangiopan creatography	Ductal cutoff (common bile duct and pancreatic duct)	Long, tapered stricture of intrapancreatic bile duct
		"Chain of lakes" appearance
		Pancreatic calculi
		Secondary and tertiary pancreatic ducts
CT scan	Mass in the head of the pancreas	Diffuse pancreatic enlargement
	Dilated biliary tree	Dilated common bile duct
	Metastasis	Pseudocysts

(Lillemoe KD, Cameron JL. Complications of chronic pancreatitis. In: Zuidema GD, ed. Surgery of the alimentary tract, vol 13. Philadelphia, WB Saunders, 1991:46)

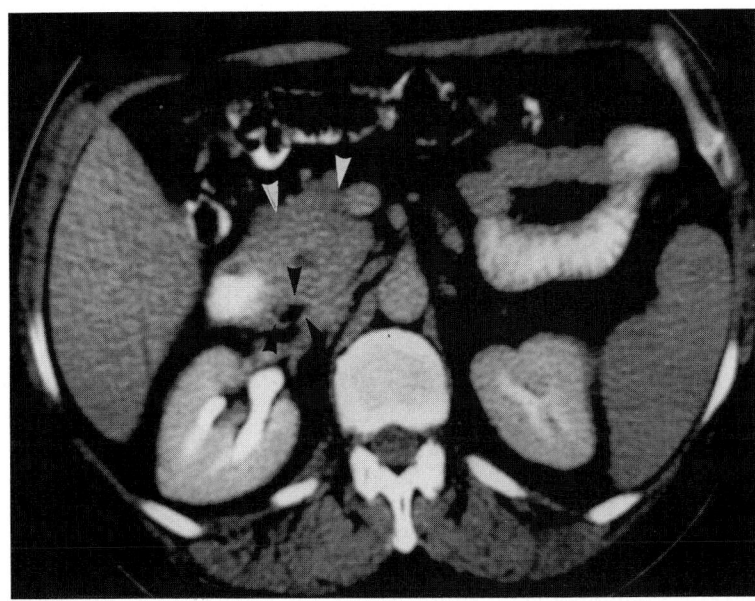

Figure 15-20. CT scan of a patient with diffuse enlargement of the head of the pancreas (*white arrowheads*). A dilated common bile duct is seen within the mass (*black arrowheads*). The patient was found to have chronic pancreatitis at resection. (Lillemoe KD, Cameron JL. Complications of chronic pancreatitis. In: Zuidema GD, ed. Surgery of the alimentary tract, vol 3. Philadelphia, WB Saunders, 1991:46)

can be useful. ERCP offers the advantage of demonstrating pathology of the pancreatic ductal system, which is essential in the optimal surgical management of chronic pancreatitis. Endoscopic examination and biopsy during ERCP can also be useful in identifying tumors of the ampulla or periampullary duodenum. Both techniques can allow decompression of the obstructed biliary tree for patients with cholangitis or severe jaundice. A long (usually 2- to 4-cm), smooth, gradual tapering of the common bile duct is most compatible with a benign stricture due to chronic pancreatitis (see Fig 15-19). In patients with carcinoma, cholangiography demonstrates an abrupt cutoff or a tumor meniscus of the common bile duct, usually located at the knee of the common bile duct where it is in close approximation to the pancreatic duct. Tumors of the distal bile duct most often present with apple-core strictures, which are usually not as long as benign strictures. Finally, ampullary and duodenal malignancies frequently cause obstruction at the most distal aspect of the common bile duct.

Management

The indications for surgical management of common bile duct strictures due to chronic pancreatitis are clear in patients with significant pain, jaundice, or cholangitis. Controversy exists, however, concerning the necessity for biliary decompression in patients with an asymptomatic elevation of serum alkaline phosphatase. Biliary bypass was first suggested when chronic changes of obstructive biliary cirrhosis were seen in liver biopsy specimens obtained from three of four patients with long-standing, functionally significant biliary obstruction due to chronic pancreatitis.[88] Another study supported this finding in 24 patients who were primarily asymptomatic and anicteric but had chronic elevation of serum alkaline phosphatase.[80] Seventy-nine percent of these patients showed obstructive liver histopathology, with secondary cirrhosis in 29%. These authors suggest that surgical biliary decompression should be considered in any patient with persistent common bile duct stricture from chronic pancreatitis to avoid biliary cirrhosis. In contrast, other authors failed to demonstrate this high incidence of biliary cirrhosis and also noted a relatively low frequency of cholangitis.[81–83,89] These authors suggest that surgical intervention be reserved only for patients with acute cholangitis, established biliary cirrhosis, or persistent jaundice. A retrospective study of 20 patients with distal bile duct strictures managed without surgery for an average of 3.8 years showed no increased morbidity when compared with 18 similar patients who had undergone biliary drainage.

Choledochoduodenostomy and Roux-en-Y choledochojejunostomy are acceptable methods of biliary bypass in patients with bile duct strictures due to chronic pancreatitis. Cholecystojejunostomy should be avoided because of problems with long-term patency when applied to benign conditions. Choledochoduodenostomy is preferred by many surgeons because it does not divert bile from the duodenum, is technically easier to perform, and leaves the jejunum intact for any associated procedures required for decompression of an obstructed gastrointestinal tract or pancreatic duct. The results of surgical management of distal bile duct strictures due to chronic pancreatitis are excellent. If the common bile duct is significantly dilated, a biliary anastomosis is technically easy to perform and has a low rate of complications. The successful relief of bile duct obstruction is achieved in most patients; however, the long-term management of abdominal pain in these patients can remain a difficult problem.

Transduodenal sphincteroplasty is not recommended in the management of common bile duct strictures due to chronic pancreatitis because the stricture is too long to be adequately managed by this technique. Similarly, endoscopic sphincterotomy has no role in the management of biliary obstruction due to chronic pancreatitis. Limited experience has been reported with endoscopic balloon dilation and short-term stenting of distal bile duct strictures due to pancreatitis.[77] These results remain preliminary, and long-term follow-up is not available. It is unlikely, however, that temporary improvement would persist in the face of ongoing chronic inflammation and fibrosis.

In many patients with chronic pancreatitis, a common bile duct stricture is not the only clinical problem. Intractable pain may also be present, and it may be necessary to perform a simultaneous procedure to alleviate this pain. In patients with a dilated pancreatic duct, a side-to-side pancreaticojejunostomy (Puestow procedure) is usually the procedure of choice. If a Roux-en-Y choledochojejunostomy was required, it is preferable to use a separate intestinal loop for decompression of the pancreatic duct to avoid continuous bathing of the pancreaticojejunostomy by bile. No evidence suggests that simple decompression of the dilated pancreatic duct in chronic pancreatitis provides long-term relief of a concomitant common bile duct stricture. Thus, in the presence of both pancreatic and bile duct obstruction, simultaneous decompression of both systems should be performed. However, prophylactic biliary bypass is not necessary in patients with a normal biliary tract and serum alkaline phosphatase who are undergoing pancreaticojejunostomy for pain.[90]

Finally, the diagnosis of pancreatic cancer must be considered in all patients undergoing laparotomy for distal bile duct obstruction. The pancreas should be carefully palpated and examined throughout the entire gland to rule out the possibility of an underlying malignancy. Transduodenal core needle biopsy specimens can be obtained. When a mass is present, however, a negative biopsy or the finding of pancreatitis does not rule out the presence of carcinoma. Although such procedures are worthwhile, the final decision rests on the clinical impression of the surgeon. With operative morbidity and mortality rates improving after pancreaticoduodenectomy,[91] it is far better to proceed with pancreatic resection than to perform a biliary and pancreatic bypass in a patient who is later found to have a malignancy. Fortunately, this situation is rare. In one review,[92] only 3 of 100 patients undergoing pancreaticojejunostomy for presumed chronic pancreatitis died of pancreatic cancer within 1 year. Moreover, in patients with pain due to chronic pancreatitis primarily of the head and in those with a small pancreatic duct, pancreaticoduodenectomy may offer the best surgical option for both managing pain and relieving bile duct obstruction.

BILE DUCT STRICTURES DUE TO CALCULUS DISEASE

Benign strictures of the bile duct can result from the chronic inflammation associated with gallstones in either the gallbladder or common bile duct. This is an uncommon cause of bile duct stricture and a rare complication of cholelithiasis or choledocholithiasis. In one series, the occurrence of a bile duct stricture in association with cholelithiasis accounted for only 4 of 134 cases (3%).[93] Nevertheless, awareness of this potential problem is important so that when a stricture is encountered during cholecystectomy or common bile duct exploration, appropriate surgical management can be carried out at the initial operation.

Bile duct strictures due to cholelithiasis are usually associated with a narrowing at the level of the common hepatic duct caused by a stone impacted in the infundibulum of the gallbladder. The narrowing can be related to two factors. First, simple compression may occur from a large stone lying adjacent to the common hepatic duct. Second, chronic or acute inflammation arising from the gallbladder or cystic duct may extend to the contiguous bile duct, resulting in stricture formation. Biliary obstruction associated with either of these conditions has become known as *Mirizzi's syndrome*. This syndrome was originally described in 1948 in patients with gallstones and the following features: an anatomic variant of a long parallel cystic duct, a gallstone impacted in the neck of the gallbladder or cystic duct, partial bile duct compression, recurrent cholangitis, and spasm of the circular fibers of the hepatic duct.[94] Mirizzi postulated that a functional sphincter developed secondary to the inflammation. He described seven cases of this syndrome from 4000 patients (0.2%) undergoing an operation for gallstones. However, in a review from Chile,[95] the incidence was estimated to be 1.3% in more than 17,000 patients operated on in an 11-year period. These authors proposed that a spectrum exists—from external compression to the development of a cholecystobiliary fistula. The fistula develops from the inflammation of the adjacent cystic and common bile duct walls, with eventual pressure necrosis and erosion by the stone (Fig. 15-21).

The clinical presentation of a bile duct stricture due to cholelithiasis is often that of acute cholecystitis with hyperbilirubinemia, usually in the range of 2 to 6 mg/ dL. If hyperbilirubinemia is present and urgent cholecystectomy is not indicated, preoperative ERC or PTC can be useful in delineating biliary anatomy. However, because most cases are associated with acute cholecystitis, most strictures are recognized at the time of cholecystectomy and operative cholangiography. When duct compression is associated with acute inflammation, the size of the common hepatic duct almost always returns to normal after the offending stone has been removed by cholecystectomy and the inflammatory process has resolved. Care must be taken during the dissection, however, to avoid creation of a defect in the common hepatic duct. If this situation is recognized at the time of surgery, the defect can usually be managed by placement of a T-tube in the duct through the defect and closure of the duct with interrupted nonabsorbable sutures

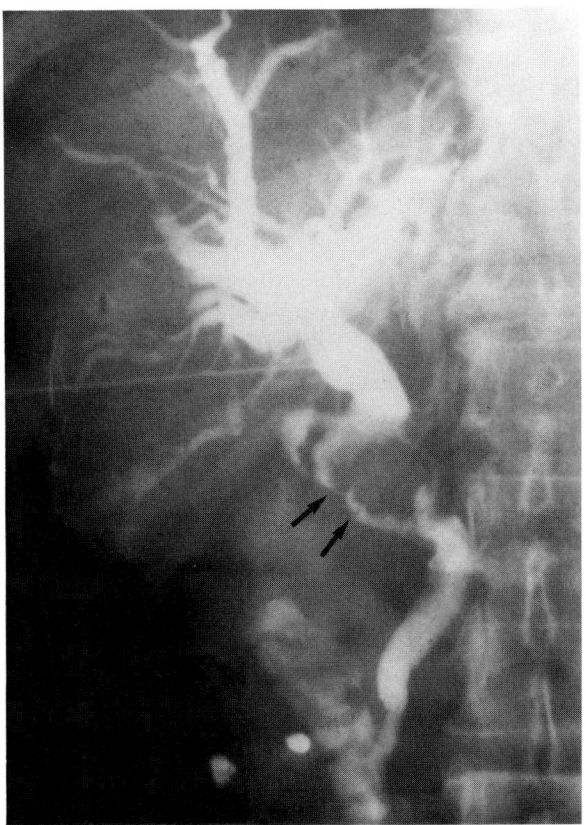

Figure 15-21 Cholangiogram demonstrating a large gallbladder stone (*arrows*) compressing and eroding into the common bile duct. (Lillemoe KD, Pitt HA, Cameron JL. Current management of benign bile duct strictures. Adv Surg 1992;25:119)

around the T-tube. The T-tube should be left in place for at least 2 to 3 months after operation. Rarely, the acute episode resolves without a biliary leak or evidence of a stricture only to again present months to years after the acute episode as a well-established bile duct stricture. In such cases, management by Roux-en-Y hepaticojejunostomy, as described previously for postoperative strictures, is appropriate.

Strictures due to choledocholithiasis are also rare. The presumed mechanism is erosion of the epithelium of the distal duct, creating inflammation with subsequent fibrosis and stricture formation. Because of the anatomic tapering of the common bile duct, nearly all stones are entrapped in the intrapancreatic portion of the duct. Often, stones in this location can be difficult to remove through the supraduodenal route. Moreover, excessive intraoperative manipulation at the time of bile duct exploration with forceps, scoops, and catheters can create additional trauma to an already friable distal duct. In some patients with difficult impacted stones, operative trauma can be reduced by transduodenal sphincteroplasty.

After the stone has been removed, the distal bile duct should be gently sized with a soft rubber catheter to ensure that no stricture exists. If a stricture persists after stone removal, it may not be recognized until the time of postoperative T-tube cholangiography. If recognized in the postoperative period, time should be allowed for resolution of inflammation before considering stricture repair. If a distal bile duct stricture does persist, a biliary enteric anastomosis with either Roux-en-Y choledochojejunostomy or choledochoduodenostomy is the treatment of choice. If the proximal duct is adequately dilated (greater than 2 cm) to allow a large choledochoduodenal anastomosis, this procedure is usually the preferable one because of its technical ease and excellent results. Transduodenal sphincteroplasty for chronic strictures of this nature are not indicated because the stricture is usually too long to be opened adequately by this technique.

PRIMARY SCLEROSING CHOLANGITIS

Primary sclerosing cholangitis is an idiopathic cholestatic liver disease characterized by inflammatory, fibrous strictures of the intrahepatic and extrahepatic bile ducts. The causes of primary sclerosing cholangitis (PSC) are unknown. Most evidence supports immunologic factors in the pathogenesis of PSC because it is often associated with other autoimmune diseases, such as ulcerative colitis, retroperitoneal fibrosis, and Riedel's thyroiditis. Specific immunologic evidence, including increased levels of circulating immune complexes,[96] and genetic associations[97] have been identified. However, it is likely that a number of causes, including viral or bacterial infections, toxic drug reactions, or congenital anomalies, can all produce the same end-stage injury that is categorized as PSC.

As noted previously, PSC is associated with a number of diseases (Table 15-8). The most common associated condition is inflammatory bowel disease. Although patients with PSC and Crohn's disease have been reported, most patients with PSC and inflammatory bowel disease have ulcerative colitis. Patients with PSC and ulcerative colitis have been compared with patients without inflammatory bowel disease.[98] The latter group is more likely to be male and to present with abnormal liver function tests as the first manifestation of the disease. The location of the bile duct involvement is also different; both intrahepatic and extrahepatic diseases are found more frequently in patients with inflammatory bowel disease (82%) than in those without it (46%). Despite these findings, there appears to be no difference in the natural history of PSC in patients with and without inflammatory bowel disease.

The usual clinical presentation of patients with PSC involves intermittent jaundice, which begins insidiously in the third to fifth decades of life. Right upper quadrant pain, pruritus, fever, weight loss, and fatigue can also occur. The disease is characterized by cyclic remissions and exacerbations. Despite the term *sclerosing cholangitis*, acute cholangitis is uncommon without previous biliary manipulation or surgery.

The diagnosis is suspected by the clinical presentation and cholestatic liver function test abnormalities. Alkaline phosphatase and serum bilirubin can fluctuate widely, depending on the status of the disease. Alkaline phosphatase is usually elevated out of proportion to the serum bilirubin. The diagnosis is confirmed by cholangiography. The cholangiographic appearance usually consists of multiple dilations and strictures (beading) of the intrahepatic and extrahepatic bile ducts (Fig. 15-22). ERC is the preferred procedure because of difficulties in cannulation of the intrahepatic ducts by the percutaneous transhepatic route because they are usually nondilated and fibrotic. The disease should be followed closely by cholangiography and liver biopsy to provide appropriate management before the development of biliary cirrhosis. The noninvasive technique of radionucleotide cholescintigraphy can also be used to follow patients with PSC.

No known specific, effective medical therapy is available for PSC, although numerous approaches with various drug therapies alone and in combination have been tried. The most encouraging results, from a prospective randomized, placebo-controlled trial,[99] suggest that ursodeoxycholic acid significantly improves serum liver function tests and liver histologic appearance. Nonoperative dilation and stenting, as discussed earlier, by either the transhepatic or endoscopic route, has been used for dominant biliary strictures. A multicenter review of nonoperative, percutaneous dilation in patients with PSC found that only 42% of patients had successful long-term results.[70] More favorable results were reported with endoscopic dilation and stenting.[100]

Because of the lack of effective medical therapy, an aggressive surgical approach has been advocated for most patients with PSC who experience symptoms. There are two primary surgical options—a direct approach to the biliary tract by resection and long-term stenting, or hepatic transplantation. The first approach employs resection of the hepatic duct bifurcation and long-term transhepatic stenting in patients with predominantly extrahepatic or bifurcation disease. This mode of therapy has been reported in 31 patients.[101] Indications for operation included persistent jaundice in 29 patients and recurrent cholangitis in 2 patients. Five of the 31 patients had secondary biliary cirrhosis before surgery, and the remaining 26 had varying degrees of fibrosis without cirrhosis. Only one postoperative death occurred in the noncirrhotic group, whereas two of five patients with cirrhosis died in the postoperative period. The 1- and 5-year actuarial survival rates for patients with fibrosis but no cirrhosis were 92% and 71%, respectively, and the actuarial survival rate at both 1 and 5 years was 20% in patients with established biliary cirrhosis (Fig. 15-23). Four patients in the noncirrhotic group, however, eventually underwent hepatic transplantation. The results for the noncirrhotic patients compare favorably

Table 15-8   Associated Diseases

Disease	Frequency
Ulcerative colitis	50%–70%
Pancreatitis	15%–25%
Diabetes mellitus	5%–10%
Retroperitoneal fibrosis	Rare
Crohn's disease	Rare
Histiocytosis X	Rare
Sicca complex	Rare
Rheumatoid osteoarthropathy	Rare
Hypertrophic osteoarthropathy	Rare
Sarcoidosis	Rare
Angioimmunoblastic lymphadenopathy	Rare
Acquired immunodeficiency syndrome	Rare

(Lillemoe KD, Pitt HA, Cameron JL. Sclerosing cholangitis. Adv Surg 1988; 21:65)

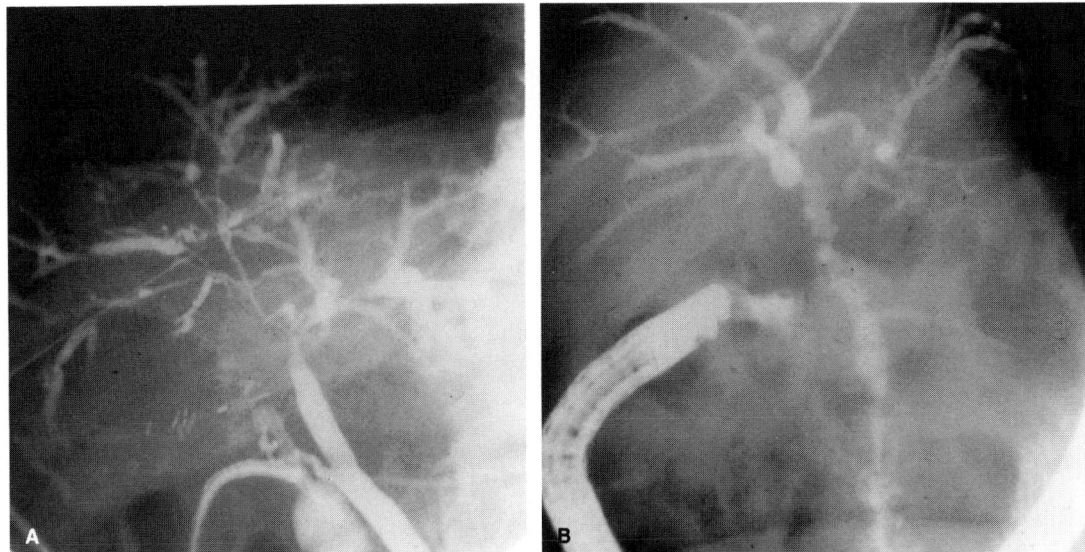

Figure 15-22 (**A**) Cholangiogram of a patient with primary sclerosing cholangitis. Note multiple irregular strictures and dilation (beading) of intrahepatic bile ducts. (**B**) Endoscopic retrograde cholangiogram showing extensive involvement of extrahepatic bile duct with primary sclerosing cholangitis. (**A**, Lillemoe KD, Pitt HA, Cameron JL. Primary sclerosing cholangitis. Surg Clin North Am 1990;70:1381; **B**, Lillemoe KD, Pitt HA, Cameron JL. Sclerosing cholangitis. Adv Surg 1988;21:65)

with the predicted survival in patients who did not undergo surgery.[102]

The other primary option for symptomatic PSC is liver transplantation. In general, most transplantation centers consider transplantation for advanced cases of PSC in which any of the following indications exist:

- Significant esophageal varices with hypersplenism
- Persistent bilirubin elevation (greater than 10 mg/dL)
- History of variceal bleeding even with normal liver synthetic function
- History of spontaneous bacterial peritonitis
- History of repeated bouts of cholangitis
- Loss of liver synthetic function.

In the largest published series of liver transplantation for PSC (55 patients),[103] the 1- and 2-year actuarial survivals were 71% and 57%, respectively. These actuarial survival rates were similar to those reported for hepatic transplantation for all patients during that time period. Another report had better results, with actuarial survival of 88% at 4 years after transplantation.[104] Concern has been raised, however, about the possibility of recurrent PSC in the transplanted liver. Although this development was uncommon in one series, a comparison of patients undergoing liver transplantation for

both PSC and primary biliary cirrhosis at another institution revealed that diffuse biliary strictures occurred more frequently in patients with PSC, as did chronic ductopenic rejection.[105] Survival and retransplantation rates, however, were not different.

The results of both biliary reconstruction and liver transplantation lead to the conclusion that, in patients with symptomatic PSC without cirrhosis and primarily hilar or extrahepatic strictures, resection of the hepatic

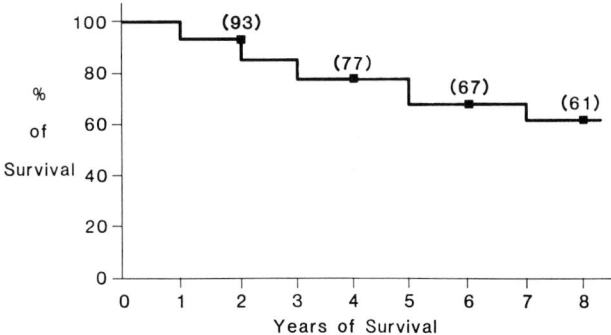

Figure 15-23 Actuarial survival among 31 noncirrhotic patients with primary sclerosing cholangitis undergoing resection of the hepatic bifurcation and long-term transhepatic stenting at the Johns Hopkins Hospital. (After Lillemoe KD, Pitt HA, Cameron JL. Primary sclerosing cholangitis. Surg Clin North Am 1990;70:1381)

bifurcation and long-term transhepatic stenting is an acceptable option. Although a theoretical concern, present data do not support the view that prior biliary tract surgery affects the long-term outcome of liver transplantation in these patients. In patients with primary intrahepatic disease or with advanced cirrhosis, liver transplantation is the preferred treatment. A real concern in these patients, however, is the 10% to 15% incidence of cholangiocarcinoma in patients with long-standing PSC. Finally, in patients with PSC and ulcerative colitis, there has been no beneficial effect on the biliary disease after colectomy.[106]

MISCELLANEOUS CAUSES OF BILE DUCT STRICTURES

A number of miscellaneous causes of benign bile duct strictures have been reported. Sphincter of Oddi stenosis or papillitis is a benign intrinsic obstruction of the outlet of the common bile duct usually associated with inflammation, fibrosis, or muscular hypertrophy. Sphincter stenosis can result in three clinical conditions—common bile duct obstruction due to fibrotic stenosis of the papilla, recurrent pancreatitis, or recurrent right upper quadrant pain without jaundice or pancreatitis.

The pathogenesis of the sphincter stenosis is unclear. In many cases, the problem is thought to be due to the trauma of the passage of multiple small stones from the common duct through the ampulla. This trauma results in inflammation, scarring, and stricture formation. Many patients with papillary stenosis, however, have no gallstones. Other potential mechanisms include primary bile duct and sphincter motility disorders and congenital anomalies.

The clinical presentation is usually either jaundice or cholangitis. In some cases, an impacted common bile duct stone is present. The diagnosis can be made with cholangiography by either the percutaneous transhepatic or endoscopic route. This condition can be managed by division of the sphincter of Oddi, performed endoscopically or operatively. If cholecystectomy was performed previously, endoscopic papillotomy is usually preferable to surgical sphincterotomy.

Duodenal pathology can rarely cause a common bile duct stricture. Inflammation, due to either duodenal ulcer disease or Crohn's disease, is a rare cause of obstructive jaundice. In most cases, the inflammation of the ulcer or the enteritis is located at or near the ampulla, resulting in distal biliary obstruction. In one review,[107] jaundice due to inflammation from peptic ulcer disease occurred in only 0.14% of 4250 patients with jaundice. In most of these cases, gastric outlet obstruc-

tion was also present, demonstrating the severity of the ulcer disease. Finally, perivaterian duodenal diverticula have been associated with low sphincter of Oddi pressures, reflux of duodenal contents, and an increased incidence of gallbladder and common duct stones. These patients may also have distal bile duct strictures.

Upper gastrointestinal series often provide information useful in diagnosing duodenal conditions. Endoscopic examination is also critical in making the diagnosis because the appearance of Crohn's disease or a duodenal diverticulum should be apparent by this examination. In some of these cases, ERCP is impossible because of the difficulty in cannulating the ampulla endoscopically. In such cases, PTC should be performed. The placement of a percutaneous transhepatic stent can allow preoperative biliary decompression and is useful in treating cases in which cholangitis is present. The management of these conditions centers around the appropriate management of the specific inflammatory process. The biliary obstruction usually resolves as either the ulcer disease or Crohn's disease improves, and biliary bypass is seldom necessary. Some patients with a perivaterian duodenal diverticulum and a distal biliary stricture can be helped by a biliary drainage procedure.

Oriental cholangiohepatitis is an unusual infection of the biliary tree frequently associated with *Clonorchis sinensis* and other parasites. These infections are most commonly seen in natives of Asian countries. Most patients present with recurrent episodes of acute cholangitis. Cholangiography may demonstrate multiple strictures of both the intrahepatic and extrahepatic biliary tree, with the bile ducts filled with sludge and stones (Fig. 15-24). The left ductal system is more often involved than the right for reasons that remain obscure. Surgical management consists of cholecystectomy and improved biliary drainage using either Roux-en-Y choledochojejunostomy or choledochoduodenostomy. Access to the biliary tree for postoperative management of intrahepatic stones or sludge should be maintained with either transhepatic biliary stents or a choledochojejunocutaneous or subcutaneous fistula. No appropriate medical management is available for this condition.

Finally, rare cases of benign intrahepatic and extrahepatic bile duct strictures have been reported secondary to intrahepatic arterial infusion of 5-fluorouracil deoxyribonucleoside, used in the treatment of hepatic metastases from colorectal carcinoma.[108] The clinical picture closely resembles that of PSC but usually can be managed by simple discontinuation of infusion and, in some cases, percutaneous transhepatic drainage. Surgery should be reserved for patients with persistent evidence of biliary obstruction and a stable tumor burden. A similar cholangiographic appearance was reported in patients with acquired immunodeficiency syndrome.[109]

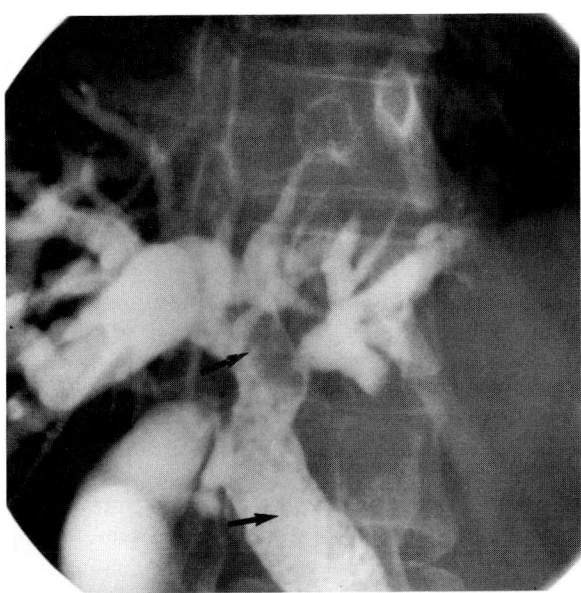

Figure 15-24 Cholangiogram in a patient with Oriental cholangiohepatitis with diffuse bile duct dilation. The biliary tree is filled with sludge and stones (*arrows*). (Lillemoe KD, Pitt HA, Cameron JL. Current management of benign bile duct strictures. Adv Surg 1992;25:119)

The pathogenesis of this injury is thought to be infectious in nature and related to cytomegalovirus or cryptosporidiosis. Little experience in the surgical management of this condition has been reported.

Benign bile duct strictures remain one of the most difficult problems encountered by the hepatobiliary surgeon. Most bile duct strictures occur as a complication of cholecystectomy. The patients may present early in the postoperative period with evidence of biliary leak or months to years later with the development of jaundice or cholangitis. The essential first step of management consists of delineation of the proximal biliary anatomy. Management techniques include either operative biliary reconstruction or nonoperative balloon dilation by either the percutaneous transhepatic or endoscopic route. The best form of surgical reconstruction of the biliary tree is a biliary enteric anastomosis from the proximal bile duct to a Roux-en-Y limb of jejunum. Long-term postoperative biliary stenting using Silastic stents can optimize results. Retrospective, nonrandomized results appear to favor this surgical technique over nonoperative dilation.

PSC is a rare cause of biliary strictures. The etiology of sclerosing cholangitis is unknown, but its association with ulcerative colitis and other diseases suggest an autoimmune condition. The diagnosis is confirmed by typical cholangiographic findings of multiple areas of stricture and dilation. No medical management has been proved to be successful. Surgical treatment for patients with symptoms includes resection of the hepatic bifurcation, with long-term transhepatic stenting of the biliary tree for patients with primarily extrahepatic or hilar disease and with no evidence of cirrhosis, and liver transplantation for the remaining patients.

Benign strictures due to other causes, such as chronic pancreatitis, calculous biliary disease, sphincter of Oddi stenosis, duodenal Crohn's disease, peptic ulcer, and perivaterian duodenal diverticula, can usually be managed by choledochoduodenostomy or choledochojejunostomy without long-term stenting. The management of other rare benign biliary strictures is dependent on their extent and underlying etiology.

REFERENCES

1. Andrén-Sandberg A, Alinder G, Bengmark S. Accidental lesions of the common bile duct at cholecystectomy: pre- and perioperative factors of importance. Ann Surg 1985;201:328.
2. Andrén-Sandberg A, Johansson S, Bengmark S. Accidental lesions of the common bile duct at cholecystectomy. II. Results of treatment. Ann Surg 1985;201:452.
3. Roslyn JJ, Binns GS, Hughes EFX, et al. Open cholecystectomy: a contemporary analysis of 42,474 patients. Ann Surg 1993;218:129.
4. Southern Surgeons Club. A prospective analysis of 1,518 laparoscopic cholecystectomies. N Engl J Med 1991;324:1073.
5. Peters JH, Ellison EC, Innes JT, et al. Safety and efficacy of laparoscopic cholecystectomy: a prospective analysis of 100 initial patients. Ann Surg 1991;213:3.
6. Zucker KA, Bailey RW, Gadacz TR, et al. Laparoscopic-guided chole-cystectomy. Am J Surg 1991;161:36.
7. Baird DR, Wilson JP, Mason EM, et al. An early review of 800 laparoscopic cholecystectomies at a university affiliated community teaching hospital. Am Surg 1991;58:206.
8. Voyles CR, Petro AB, Mecka AL, et al. A practical approach to laparoscopic cholecystectomy. Am J Surg 1991;161:365.
9. Spaw AT, Reddick EJ, Olsen DO. Laparoscopic laser cholecystectomy: analysis of 500 procedures. Surg Laparosc Endosc 1991;1:2.
10. Raute M, Podlech P, Jaschke W, et al. Manageqment of bile duct injuries and strictures following cholecystectomy. World J Surg 1993;17:553.

11. Orlando R, Russell JC, Lynch J, et al. Laparoscopic cholecystectomy: a statewide experience. Arch Surg 1993;128:494.

12. Deziel DJ, Millikan KW, Economou SG, et al. Complications of laparoscopic cholecystectomy: a national survey of 4,292 hospitals and an analysis of 77,604 cases. Am J Surg 1993;165:9.

13. Asbun HJ, Rossi RL, Lowell JA, et al. Bile duct injury during laparoscopic cholecystectomy: mechanism of injury, prevention, and management. World J Surg 1993;17:547.

14. Branum G, Schmitt C, Baillie J, et al. Management of major biliary complications after laparoscopic cholecystectomy. Ann Surg 1993;217:532.

15. Ress, AM, Sarr MG, Nagorney DM, et al. Spectrum and management of major complications of laparoscopic cholecystectomy. Am J Surg 1993;165:655.

16. Soper NJ, Flye MW, Brunt LM, et al. Diagnosis and management of biliary complications of laparoscopic cholecystectomy. Am J Surg 1993;165:663.

17. Pitt HA, Miyamoto T, Parapatis SK, et al. Factors influencing outcome in patients with postoperative biliary strictures. Am J Surg 1982;144:14.

18. Northover JMA, Terblanche J. Applied surgical anatomy of the biliary tree. Clin Surg Int 1982;5:1.

19. Davidoff Am, Pappas TN, Murray EA, et al. Mechanisms of major biliary injury during laparoscopic cholecystectomy. Ann Surg 1992;215:196.

20. Larson GM, Bitale GC, Casey J, et al. Multipractice analysis of laparoscopic cholecystectomy in 1,983 patients. Am J Surg 1992;163:221.

21. Rossi RL, Schirmer WJ, Braasch JW, et al. Laparoscopic bile duct injuries: risk factors, recognition, and repair. Arch Surg 1992;127:596.

22. Berci G, Sackier JM, Paz-Partlow M. Routine or selective intraoperative cholangiography during laparoscopic cholecystectomy? Am J Surg 1991;161:355.

23. Hunter JG. Avoidance of bile duct injury during laparoscopic cholecystectomy. Am J Surg 1991;162:71.

24. Bailey RW, Zucker KA, Flowers JL, et al. Laparoscopic cholecystectomy: experience with 375 consecutive cases. Ann Surg 1991;214:531.

25. Lillemoe KD, Yeo CJ, Talamini MA, et al. Selective cholangiography: current role in laparoscopic cholecystectomy. Ann Surg 1992;215:669.

26. Barkun JS, Fried GM, Barkun AN, et al. Cholecystectomy without operative cholangiography: implications for common bile duct injury and retained common bile duct stones. Ann Surg 1993;218:371.

27. Northover JMA, Terblanche J. A new look at the arterial supply of the bile duct in man and its surgical implications. Br J Surg 1979;66:379.

28. Terblanche J, Allison HF, Northover JMA. An ischemic basis for biliary strictures. Surgery 1983;94:52.

29. Carlson E, Zukoski CF, Campbell J, et al. Morphological, biophysical, and biochemical consequences of ligation of the common biliary duct in the dog. Am J Pathol 1977;86:301.

30. Douglas TC, Lounsbury BF, Cutter WW, et al. An experimental study of healing of the common bile duct. Surg Gynecol Obstet 1950;91:301.

31. Sackier JM, Verci G, Paz-Partlow M. Laparoscopic transcystic choledochotomy as an adjunct to laparoscopic cholecystectomy. Am Surg 1991;57:323.

32. Petelin JB. Laparoscopic approach to common duct pathology. Am J Surg 1993;165:487.

33. Pelligrini CA, Thomas MJ, Way LW. Recurrent biliary stricture: patterns of recurrent and outcome of surgical therapy. Am J Surg 1984;147:175.

34. Bismuth H. Postoperative strictures of the bile duct. In Blumgart LH, ed. The biliary tract. Edinburgh, Churchill Livingstone, 1982:209.

35. Way LW, Bernholt RA, Thomas MJ. Biliary stricture. Surg Clin North Am 1981;61:963.

36. Schaffner F, Bacchin PG, Hutterer F, et al. Mechanisms of cholestasis. IV. Structural and biochemical changes in the liver and serum in rats after bile duct ligation. Gastroenterology 1971;60:888.

37. Blumgart LH. Biliary tract obstruction: new approaches to old problems. Am J Surg 1978;135:19.

38. Weinbren HK, Hadjis NS, Blumgart LH. Structural aspects of the liver in patients with biliary disease and portal hypertension. J Clin Pathol 1985;38:1013.

39. Czerniak A, Soreide O, Gibson RN, et al. Liver atrophy complicating benign bile duct strictures: surgical and interventional radiologic approaches. Am J Surg 1986;152:294.

40. Crist DW, Kadir S, Cameron JL. The value of preoperatively placed percutaneous biliary catheters in reconstruction of the proximal part of the biliary tract. Surg Gynecol Obstet 1987;165:421.

41. Rabinovitz M, Zajko AB, Hassanein T, et al. Diagnostic value of brush cytology in the diagnosis of bile duct carcinoma: a study in 65 patients with bile duct strictures. Hepatology 1990;12:747.

42. Zuidema GD, Cameron JL, Sitzmann JV, et al. Percutaneous transhepatic management of complex biliary problems. Ann Surg 1983;197:584.

43. Kaufman SL, Kadir S, Mitchell SE. Percutaneous transhepatic biliary drainage for bile leaks and fistulas. AJR 1985;144:1055.

44. Czerniak A, Thompson JN, Soreide O, et al. The management of fistulas of the biliary tract after injury to the bile duct during cholecystectomy. Surg Gynecol Obstet 1988;167:33.

45. Pitt HA, Gomes AS, Juan LF, et al. Does preoperative percutaneous biliary drainage reduce operative risk or increase hospital cost? Ann Surg 1985;201:545.

46. Hillis TM, Westbrook KC, Caldwell FT, et al. Surgical injury of the common bile duct. Am J Surg 1977;134:712.

47. Castrini G, Pappalardo G. Iatrogenic strictures of the bile ducts: our experience with 66 cases. World J Surg 1981;5:753.

48. Kune G. Bile duct injury during cholecystectomy:

causes, prevention and surgical repair in 1979. Aust N Z J Surg 1979;49:35.

49. Browder IW, Dowling JB, Koontz KK, et al. Early management of operative injuries of the extrahepatic biliary tract. Ann Surg 1987;205:649.

50. Hadjis NS, Blumgart LH. Injury to segmental bile ducts: a reappraisal. Arch Surg 1988;123:351.

51. Csendes A, Díaz JC, Burdiles P, et al. Late results of immediate primary end to end repair in accidental section of the common bile duct. Surg Gynecol Obstet 1989;168:125.

52. Pitt HA, Kaufman SL, Coleman J, et al. Benign postoperative biliary strictures: operate or dilate? Ann Surg 1989;210:417.

53. Warren KW, Christophi C, Armendari ZR. The evolution and current perspectives of the treatment of benign bile duct strictures: a review. Surg Gastroenterol 1982;1:141.

54. Cameron JL, Gayler BW, Zuidema GD. The use of Silastic transhepatic stents in benign and malignant biliary strictures. Ann Surg 1978;188:552.

55. Hepp J, Couinaud C. L'aboud et l'utilisation du canal hepatique gauche dans les reparations de la voie biliare principale. Presse Med 1956;64:947.

56. Blumgart LH, Kelley CJ. Hepaticojejunostomy in benign and malignant high bile duct stricture: approaches to the left hepatic ducts. Br J Surg 1984;71:257.

57. Smith R. Strictures of the bile ducts. Proc R Soc Med 1969;62:131.

58. Smith R. Injuries of the bile ducts. In Smith R, Sherlock S, eds. Surgery of the gallbladder and bile ducts, ed 2. London, Butterworths, 1981:361.

59. Smith R. Obstruction of the bile ducts. Br J Surg 1979;66:69.

60. Longmire WP Jr, Sandford MC. Intrahepatic cholangiojejunostomy with partial hepatectomy for biliary obstruction. Surgery 1948;128:330.

61. Aust JB, Root HD, Urdaneta L, et al. Biliary stricture. Surgery 1967;42:601.

62. Bismuth H, Franco D, Corlete MB, et al. Long-term results of Roux-en-Y hepaticojejunostomy. Surg Gynecol Obstet 1978;146:161.

63. Innes JT, Ferrara JJ, Carey LC. Biliary reconstruction without transanastomotic stent. Am Surg 1988;54:27.

64. Parker GA, Halloran LG. Reconstruction of the bile duct with transanastomotic U tubes. Surg Gynecol Obstet 1986;162:433.

65. Millikan KW, Gleason TG, Deziel DJ, et al. The current role of U tubes for benign and malignant biliary obstruction. Ann Surg 1993;218:621.

66. van Sonnenberg E, Ferrucci JT, Neff CC. Biliary pressure: manometric and perfusion studies at percutaneous transhepatic cholangiography and percutaneous biliary drainage. Radiology 1983;148:41.

67. Genest JF, Nanon E, Grundfest-Broniatowski S, et al. Benign biliary strictures: an analytic review (1970 to 1984). Surgery 1986;99:409.

68. Blumgart LH, Kelley CJ, Benjamin IS. Benign bile duct stricture following cholecystomy: critical factors in management. Br J Surg 1984;71:836.

69. Pain JA, Knight M, Smith RS. Long-term results of the mucosal graft operation for benign bile duct strictures. (Abstract) Neth J Surg 1988:170.

70. Mueller PR, van Sonnenberg E, Ferrucci T Jr, et al. Biliary stricture dilatation: multicenter review of clinical management in 73 patients. Radiology 1986;160:17.

71. Williams HJ, Bender CE, May GR. Benign postoperative biliary strictures: dilatation with fluoroscopic guidance. Radiology 1987;163:629.

72. Vogel SB, Howard RJ, Caridi J. Evaluation of percutaneous transhepatic balloon dilatation of benign biliary strictures in high-risk patients. Am J Surg 1985;149:73.

73. Moore AV Jr, Illescas FF, Mills SR, et al. Percutaneous dilatation of benign biliary strictures. Radiology 1987;163:625.

74. Russell E, Yrizarry JM, Huber JS, et al. Percutaneous transjejunal biliary dilatation: alternate management for benign strictures. Radiology 1986;159:209.

75. Maroney TP, Ring EJ. Percutaneous transjejunal catheterization of Roux-en-Y biliary–jejunal anastomoses. Radiology 1987;164:151.

76. Davids PHP, Tanka AKF, Rauws EAJ, et al. Benign biliary strictures: surgery or endoscopy? Ann Surg 1993;217:237.

77. Geenen DJ, Geenen JE, Hogan WJ, et al. Endoscopic therapy for benign bile duct strictures. Gastrointest Endosc 1989;35:367.

78. Foutsch PG, Sivak MV Jr. Therapeutic endoscopic balloon dilatation of the extrahepatic biliary ducts. Am J Gastroenterol 1985;80:575.

79. Hollands MJ, Little JM. Obstructive jaundice in chronic pancreatitis. HPB Surg 1989;1:263.

80. Afroudakis A, Kaplowitz N. Liver histopathology in chronic common bile duct stenosis due to chronic alcoholic pancreatitis. Hepatology 1981;1:65.

81. Scott J, Summerfield JA, Elias E. Chronic pancreatitis: a cause of cholestasis. Gut 1977;18:196.

82. Yadegar J, Williams RA, Passare E Jr, et al. Common duct stricture from chronic pancreatitis. Arch Surg 1980;115:582.

83. Stahl TJ, O'Connor A, Ansel M, et al. Partial biliary obstruction caused by chronic pancreatitis: an appraisal of indications for surgical biliary drainage. Ann Surg 1988;207:26.

84. Wisloff F, Jakobsen J, Osnes M. Stenosis of the common bile duct in chronic pancreatitis. Br J Surg 1982;69:52.

85. Prinz RA, Aranha GV, Greenlee HB, et al. Common duct obstruction in patients with intractable pain of chronic pancreatitis. Am Surg 1982;48:373.

86. Littenberg G, Afroudakis A, Kaplowitz N. Common bile duct stenosis from chronic pancreatitis: a clinical and pathological spectrum. Medicine 1979;58:385.

87. Wapnick S, Hadas N, Purow E, et al. Mass in the head of the pancreas in cholestatic jaundice: carcinoma or pancreatitis? Ann Surg 1979;190:587.

88. Warshaw AL, Schapiro RH, Ferrucci JT Jr, et al. Persis-

tent obstructive jaundice, cholangitis, and biliary cirrhosis due to common bile duct stenosis in chronic pancreatitis. Gastroenterology 1976;70:562.

89. Sarles H, Sahel J. Cholestasis and lesions of the biliary tract in chronic pancreatitis. Gut 1978;19:851.

90. Bradley EL. Parapancreatic biliary and intestinal obstruction in chronic pancreatitis: is prophylactic bypass necessary? Am J Surg 1985;151:256.

91. Cameron JL, Pitt HA, Yeo CJ, et al. One hundred and forty-five consecutive pancreaticoduodenectomies without mortality. Ann Surg 1993;217:447.

92. Prinz RA, Greenlee HB. Pancreatic duct drainage in 100 patients with chronic pancreatitis. Ann Surg 1981;194:313.

93. Blumgart LH, Thompson JW. The management of benign strictures of the bile ducts. Curr Probl Surg 1987;24:1.

94. Mirizzi PL. Sidrome del coducto hepatico. J Int Circ 1948;18:737.

95. Csendes A, Díaz JC, Burdiles P. Mirizzi syndrome and cholecystobiliary fistula: a unifying classification. Br J Surg 1989;76:1139.

96. Bodenheimer HC, LaRusso NF, Thayer WR, et al. Elevated circulating immune complexes in primary sclerosing cholangitis. Hepatology 1983:;3:150.

97. Chapman RW, Varghese Z, Gaul R, et al. Close association between HLA-B8 and primary sclerosing cholangitis. Gut 1981;22:A871.

98. Rabinovitz M, Gavaler JS, Schade RR, et al. Does primary sclerosing cholangitis occurring in association with inflammatory bowel disease differ from that occurring in the absence of inflammatory bowel disease? Study of 66 subjects. Hepatology 1990;11:7.

99. Beurs U, Spengler U, Kruis W, et al. Ursodeoxycholic acid for the treatment of primary sclerosing cholangitis: a placebo-controlled trial. Hepatology 1992;16:707.

100. Johnson GK, Gechen JE, Venu RS, et al. Endoscopic treatment of biliary tract strictures in sclerosing cholangitis: a large series and recommendation for treatment. Gastrointest Endosc 1991;37:38.

101. Cameron JL, Pitt HA, Zinner MJ, et al. Resection of hepatic duct bifurcation and transhepatic stenting for sclerosing cholangitis. Ann Surg 1988;207:614.

102. Weisner RH, Grambsch PM, Dickson ER, et al. Primary sclerosing cholangitis: natural history, prognostic factors and survival analysis. Hepatology 1989;10:430.

103. Marsh JW Jr, Iwatsuki S, Makowka L, et al. Orthotopic liver transplantation for primary sclerosing cholangitis. Ann Surg 1988;207:21.

104. Langnas AN, Grazi GL, Stratta RJ, et al. Primary sclerosing cholangitis: the emerging role for liver transplantation. Am J Gastroenterol 1990;85:1136.

105. McEntec G, Wisner RH, Rosen C, et al. A comparative study of patients undergoing liver transplantation for primary sclerosing cholangitis and primary biliary cirrhosis. Transplant Proc 1991;23:1563.

106. Cangemi JR, Wiesner RH, Beaver SJ, et al. Effect of proctocolectomy for chronic ulcerative colitis on the natural history of primary sclerosing cholangitis. Gastroenterology 1989;96:790.

107. Onstad GR, Christensen N, Smith LA. Jaundice as a complication of duodenal ulcer. Surg Clin North Am 1971;51:885.

108. Kemeny MM, Battifora H, Blayney DW, et al. Sclerosing cholangitis after continuous hepatic artery infusion of FUDR. Ann Surg 1985;202:176.

109. Margulis SJ, Honig CL, Soave R, et al. Biliary tract obstruction in the acquired immunodeficiency syndrome. Ann Intern Med 1986;105:207.

Digestive Tract Surgery: A Text and Atlas, edited by Richard H. Bell, Layton F. Rikkers, and Michael W. Mulholland. Lippincott-Raven Publishers, Philadelphia, © 1996.

16

Neoplasms of the Biliary Tract

Lillian G. Dawes | *David L. Nahrwold*

Biliary neoplasms, tumors of the gallbladder and bile ducts, are uncommon. Because of their relative rarity, defining optimal therapy remains a challenge. Even though distant metastases are infrequent, the local invasiveness and anatomic location of gallbladder and bile duct carcinomas result in a poor prognosis for both these tumors. Their proximity to vital structures makes surgical resection difficult and often impossible. However, surgical removal is the only means of curing these tumors and offers reasonable palliation in some cases. The results of chemotherapy and radiation therapy have been dismal. The extent of surgical resection necessary to attain optimal results is a subject of continuing controversy. The challenges for the future are earlier diagnosis and better adjuvant therapy. In this chapter, the general characteristics of biliary neoplasms are outlined and their treatment is discussed.

BENIGN TUMORS OF THE GALLBLADDER AND BILE DUCTS

Gallbladder Tumors

Although rare, benign tumors of the gallbladder are recognized more often now than in the past because of the frequent use of diagnostic ultrasound and computed tomography (CT). The estimated incidence of benign tumors in patients who have undergone cholecystectomy is less than 3%, with a reported range of 0.5% to 3%.[1] They most commonly present as polyps or polyploid lesions. Polyps can be pseudotumors or hyperplastic growths (thought to result from inflammation), or they can be adenomas, which may be premalignant. Adenomyosis is an interesting benign lesion. Heterotopia and

tumors of the supporting tissues of the gallbladder are rare.

Pseudotumors

Cholesterolosis of the gallbladder appears grossly as yellow spots on the surface of the mucosa. Histologically, there is a proliferation of foamy macrophages filled with cholesterol in the lamina propria. The term *strawberry gallbladder* is used to denote cholesterolosis involving the entire gallbladder. The most common nonneoplastic lesion of the gallbladder is the cholesterol polyp, a small, yellow polypoid structure filled with lipid-laden macrophages. Cholesterol polyps protrude into the gallbladder lumen and are attached to the mucosa by a narrow stalk. They constitute up to 52% of all polypoid lesions.[2] Although usually less than 1 cm in size, they can be visualized on ultrasound and occasionally on CT. They are thought to form as a result of a disturbance in cholesterol metabolism and do not have a malignant potential.

Inflammatory polyps are pseudotumors believed to result from chronic inflammation. They do not have a malignant potential. Inflammatory polyps have a chronic inflammatory cell infiltrate with a single layer of columnar epithelial cells and a vascular connective tissue stalk. They also can be identified by ultrasound or CT, and are commonly associated with gallstones.

Adenomyosis

Proliferation of the mucosal epithelium and hypertrophy of the muscular layers of the gallbladder can result in focal intramural thickening of the gallbladder. Adenomyosis consists of muscular hypertrophy and

481

sometimes invagination of the epithelial mucosa between muscle layers manifested by the presence of Rokitansky-Aschoff sinuses and Luschka crypts.[3] These histologic changes also are present in chronic cholecystitis. Because most of these rare tumors occur in the fundus, it has been postulated that functional cystic duct obstruction or biliary dyskinesia is responsible for the muscular hypertrophy and subsequent development of adenomyosis. The cause of this condition is unknown. Several cases of gallbladder cancer in areas of adenomyosis have been reported, suggesting the possibility that this is a premalignant lesion.[4]

Adenomas

Adenomas of the epithelial layer of the gallbladder can be tubular or papillary. Papillary adenomas sometimes are called *papillomas,* and the condition of multiple papillomas is known as *papillomatosis.* There also are reports of cystadenomas of the gallbladder, tumors with inner layers of mucin-secreting epithelium, a mesenchymal stroma, and an outer layer of hyalinized fibrous tissue.[5] Extrahepatic cystadenomas occur more often in the bile ducts than in the gallbladder.[6] Carcinoma in situ has been reported in adenomas of the gallbladder; hence, they are thought to be premalignant lesions. In a review of 1605 gallbladder specimens, one group found 11 benign adenomas, 7 adenomas with malignant change, and 79 invasive gallbladder cancers.[7] Others also have reported a low incidence of adenomatous polyps in large series of cholecystectomies.[8] Although these lesions probably have a malignant potential, their rarity (less than the incidence of gallbladder cancer) suggests that they do not play a major role in the pathogenesis of gallbladder cancer. The cause of adenomas of the gallbladder is unknown. The role of gallstones in the formation of adenomas also is unclear; most (67% of 51 gallbladder adenomas reviewed in one series[9]) are not associated with the presence of gallstones.

Other Benign Gallbladder Tumors

Other types of benign tumors are rare. The term *heterotopia* is used to denote the presence of ectopic tissue in the gallbladder. Nodules of intestinal, pancreatic, or gastric epithelium have been found. Tumors of the supporting tissues of the gallbladder also occur, such as hemangiomas, lipomas, leiomyomas, and granular cell tumors.

BENIGN BILE DUCT TUMORS

Benign bile duct tumors are much less common than are gallbladder tumors. Only two cases of benign bile duct tumors were found among 5200 biliary tract surgeries in one series.[10] Only four cases were found in 20,000 consecutive patients who underwent biliary tract operations at another institution (0.02%).[11] Papillomas, adenomas, or cystadenomas can occur in the extrahepatic bile ducts, as can multiple polyps or papillomatosis. Reports of these adenomatous lesions in association with adenocarcinoma suggest that they may be premalignant.[12] The rare tumors of the supporting tissues found in the gallbladder also occur in the bile ducts, and include fibromas, leiomyomas, angioleiomyomas, and carcinoid tumors.

Clinical Findings

The symptoms associated with benign gallbladder tumors are similar to those of cholelithiasis. Right upper quadrant pain and discomfort, fatty food intolerance, nausea, vomiting, and an increase in flatulence are common complaints in patients with benign gallbladder tumors. Because many benign tumors are an incidental finding during cholecystectomy for symptomatic gallstones, it is difficult to separate symptoms of benign tumors from those of gallstones.

Benign tumors of the bile ducts may present with the symptoms of bile duct obstruction. Obstruction of the bile duct results in jaundice or cholangitis, and evaluation of these clinical findings leads to the diagnosis of most of these tumors. The jaundice typically is intermittent, and the only finding may be an elevated serum alkaline phosphatase level. Nonspecific symptoms of dyspepsia or anorexia also are associated with bile duct tumors.

Diagnosis and Treatment

When gallbladder tumors are identified before operation, they usually are detected by ultrasonography. Occasionally, they are found on CT or oral cholecystography, although the latter test is rarely used. The characteristic finding is a filling defect that does not move when patients change position. Patients with symptoms who have gallbladder lesions should undergo cholecystectomy. Because no diagnostic imaging procedure can distinguish benign from malignant lesions, all gallbladders that contain polypoid masses should be removed. Small polypoid lesions, a few millimeters in diameter, that are most likely cholesterol polyps or mucosal folds can be followed up with periodic ultrasound examinations if they are not associated with cholelithiasis or symptoms.[2] Any thickening or irregularity of the gallbladder wall or increase in size should prompt surgical intervention. This is important if gallbladder cancers are to be treated in earlier stages.

The initial step in the evaluation of jaundice usually is an ultrasound examination of the right upper quadrant. This may show hepatic ductal dilatation, but a bile duct tumor is rarely delineated. Endoscopic retrograde cholangiography or percutaneous transhepatic cholangiography is required to diagnose a bile duct tumor. Whenever a benign tumor in the bile duct is demonstrated, surgical excision is indicated to relieve jaundice or cholangitis. Resection of the tumor with a primary reanastomosis of the bile duct may be possible. When the length of duct that must be removed precludes a tension-free anastomosis, the biliary tree can be reconstructed with a choledochoduodenostomy or, more commonly, a Roux-en-Y choledochojejunostomy. Multiple polypoid lesions or papillomatosis of the bile ducts can be difficult to treat. When biliary papillomatosis is limited to one segment of the biliary tree, radical excision is preferable because recurrence is common with lesser therapies. These hyperplastic lesions can extend throughout the biliary ductal system,[12] limiting treatment options, but resection should be performed whenever possible.

GALLBLADDER CANCER

A locally invasive tumor, gallbladder cancer continues to have a poor prognosis because of its usual late stage at diagnosis (Fig. 16-1). First described in 1777, gallbladder cancer is relatively rare, accounting for 3% to 4% of all gastrointestinal malignancies (about 2.5 per 100,000).[13] Optimal therapy has not been defined, and recommended surgical treatments range from simple cholecystectomy to hepatic resection. When found in-

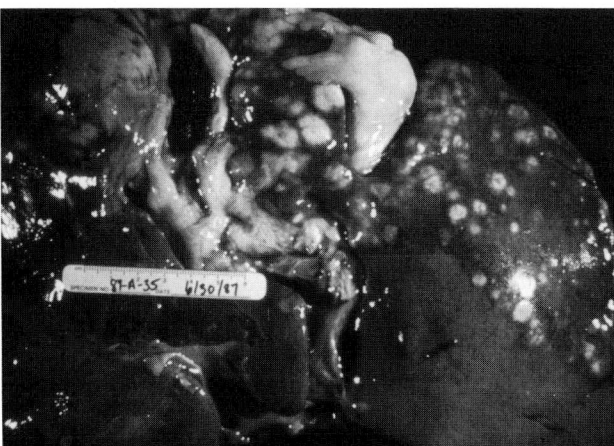

Figure 16-1 Gallbladder cancer often presents late with extensive disease. The gallbladder cancer shown extends into the liver, and there are multiple liver metastases. (See Color Fig. 16-1.)

cidentally at the time of cholecystectomy for symptomatic gallstones, it can be treated effectively by surgical removal. Often, gallbladder cancer is detected after surrounding structures have been invaded, making complete resection impossible. In its advanced stages, the dismal outlook is compounded by the lack of effective adjuvant therapy. For decades, there has been little progress in improving survival, which is measured in months. Recently, there have been some encouraging reports with more aggressive surgical therapy, at least in a subset of patients with this disease. The challenge of the future is earlier diagnosis and better adjuvant therapy.

Incidence

About 6500 people die each year of gallbladder cancer.[14] Only 2% of all biliary tract procedures are performed for this rare malignancy. The average age of onset is in the sixth or seventh decade. Women are afflicted more frequently than men, with a female/male ratio of 3:1.[14] Certain populations also have a higher incidence of this cancer. Southwest Native Americans, Alaskans, Mexicans, and Hispanics living in the United States have an estimated five to six times greater incidence of gallbladder cancer than the general population. In contrast, gallbladder cancer is much less common in blacks and is extremely rare in certain Bantu tribes in whom cholelithiasis also is infrequent.

Gallstones are commonly seen in patients with gallbladder cancer, and populations at risk for cholelithiasis have a higher incidence of gallbladder cancer. Gallstones are present in 70% to 90% of all patients with gallbladder cancer. However, only about 1.2% to 3% of all patients with symptomatic gallstones have gallbladder cancer.[15] The association of gallstones with cancer may be related to gallstone size; larger stones are associated with a greater cancer risk. A 10-fold increase in the incidence of gallbladder cancer in patients with gallstones larger than 3 cm in diameter has been reported.[16] It has been postulated that larger gallstones have been present in the gallbladder for longer periods, causing chronic irritation of the gallbladder wall, which predisposes to the development of carcinoma. Experimental models of gallbladder cancer have supported the role of chronic irritation in promoting the development of gallbladder carcinoma. The presence of cholesterol pellets in the gallbladder increased the incidence of gallbladder carcinoma from 6% to 68% in hamsters fed the carcinogen dimethylnitrosamine.[17] The higher incidence of gallbladder cancer in chronic typhoid carriers also is thought to result from chronic irritation. In addition, an anomalous junction of the pancreatic and bile ducts has been reported to be associated with gallbladder cancer, although the pathogenesis of this is unclear.[18]

The potential risk of cancer in patients with gallstones is of concern, because patients who do not have symptoms receive no treatment. The 20-year risk of gallbladder carcinoma in patients with gallstones has been estimated to be about 0.13% in the general population and as high as 1.5% in high-risk populations (ie, American Indians).[19] This small risk does not warrant routine cholecystectomy in all patients with gallstones. Patients who have calcification of the wall of the gallbladder (porcelain gallbladder) are an exception. This condition is associated with a 12.5% to 60% incidence of gallbladder cancer.[20,21] Calcification of the gallbladder wall (Fig. 16-2) should alert physicians to the high probability of malignancy, and cholecystectomy should be undertaken unless contraindicated for other reasons.

Pathology

Most gallbladder cancers are well-differentiated adenocarcinomas. Adenocarcinomas of the gallbladder can be subdivided into various types, including papil-

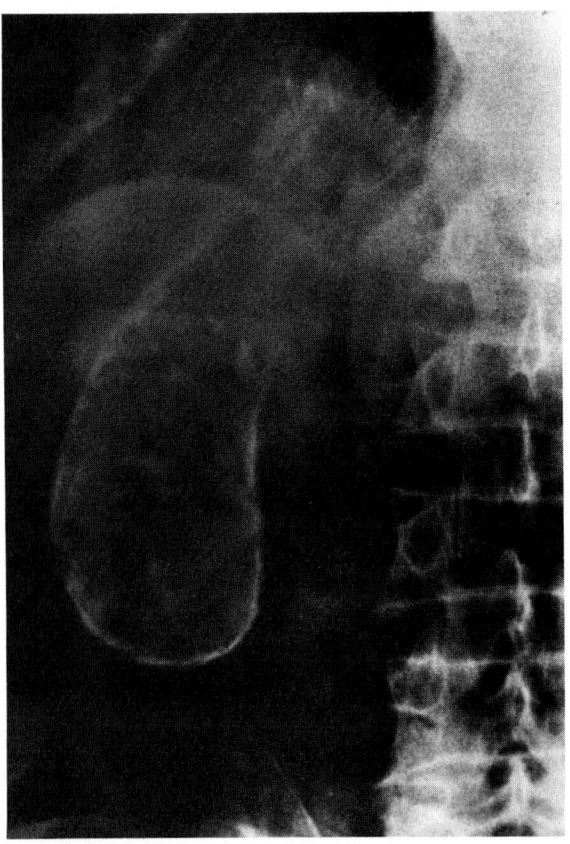

Figure 16-2 Calcification of the gallbladder wall, or a "porcelain gallbladder," is a risk factor for gallbladder cancer. Cholecystectomy should be considered for patients with this finding.

lary, serous, colloid, tubular, and glandular carcinomas. A small percentage of gallbladder cancers are squamous cell in origin, but these account for only 5% of the total. A mixture of adenomatous and squamous features, known as adenosquamous carcinoma, also has been reported. The remainder of these cancers, about 10%, are anaplastic neoplasms. More rare histologic types of gallbladder cancer include sarcomas, melanomas, carcinoid tumors, and signet ring cell carcinomas.

In a review of 3038 gallbladder cancers, one group reported that papillary adenocarcinomas had the most favorable prognosis of the various histologic types, with a 2-year survival rate of 47%.[22] This type also was associated less frequently with gallstones in another series, and showed little gender preponderance. Tubular adenocarcinoma and undifferentiated carcinomas were associated with chronic cholecystitis and epithelial metaplasia, and were more common in women. This suggests that these cancers may have different mechanisms of pathogenesis, accounting for the observed differences in biologic behavior.

The development of gallbladder cancer has been postulated to be the result of progressive changes in the gallbladder epithelium from intestinal metaplasia and hyperplasia to dysplasia and, finally, carcinoma. A review of 162 gallbladder specimens after cholecystectomy for cholelithiasis found 58.1% with intestinal metaplasia, 46.9% with hyperplasia, 16% with dysplasia, and 2.5% with carcinoma in situ.[23] These epithelial changes were either focal abnormalities or partially confluent, making single random histologic sections likely to identify less than one third of these lesions. In addition, these changes were found in areas of flat mucosa and not in adenomas. These observations are consistent with the hypothesis that inflammatory conditions predispose patients to cancer of the gallbladder and with the fact that most gallbladder cancers do not arise in polypoid lesions.

Gallbladder cancer tends to be locally invasive. The venous drainage of the gallbladder is into the adjacent liver. The most common mode of spread of gallbladder cancer is directly into the liver, particularly liver segments IV and V. The lymphatic drainage of the gallbladder is to the cystic duct lymph node, then to pericholedochal nodes and to hilar lymph nodes. Parapancreatic nodes and periduodenal nodes also can harbor metastases. The lymphatic flow also drains to the celiac and superior mesenteric lymph nodes (Fig. 16-3). In addition to spread to the liver and lymph nodes, gallbladder cancer can invade surrounding structures, most often the common bile duct or duodenum. Distant metastasis is infrequent.

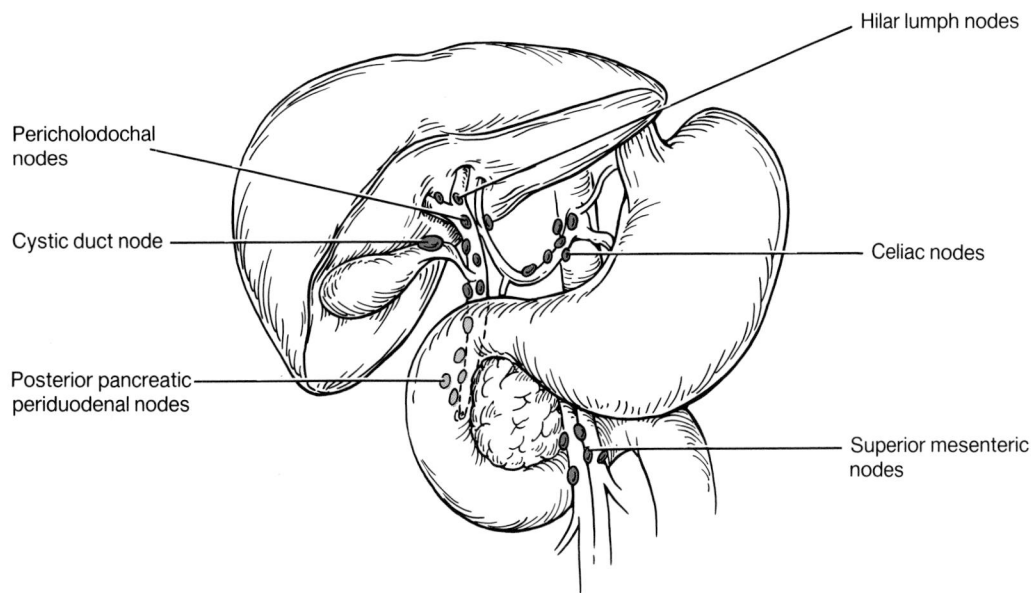

Figure 16-3 Regional lymph node metastasis is of prognostic importance in gallbladder cancer. The lymphatic drainage of the gallbladder is to the regional lymph nodes.

Staging

Based on the lymphatic and venous drainage of the gallbladder, a staging system for gallbladder cancer has been developed.[24] This system is commonly used to describe the extent of gallbladder carcinoma and has been shown to be of prognostic value (Table 16-1). Stage I disease is limited to the mucosa of the gallbladder. In stage II, the mucosa and muscularis layers are penetrated. In stage III, the subserosa is infiltrated, and stage IV includes involvement of all the layers of the gallbladder wall, as well as cystic duct lymph node metastasis. Stage V includes distant spread into either the liver or adjacent organs. Unfortunately, most patients with gallbladder carcinoma have stage V disease.

More recently, the tumor, nodes, metastasis (TNM) system has been adopted for staging biliary cancers (Table 16-2). The designation T1 reflects disease in the mucosa (T1a) or the muscle (T1b). T2 tumors extend into perimuscular connective tissue, and T3 tumors extend into serosa or one organ (if the liver is involved, there is less than 2 cm of extension into the parenchyma of the liver). T4 tumors involve more than 2 cm of extension into the liver, or two or more adjacent organs. Nodal metastasis is described as either N1a, with involvement of nodes in the hepatoduodenal ligament (cystic duct node, pericholedochal or hilar nodes), or N1b, with parapancreatic, periduodenal, periportal, celiac, or superior mesenteric lymph node metastases. The stage groupings for this system are shown in Table 16-2.[25]

Diagnosis

The signs and symptoms of gallbladder cancer are similar to those of gallstones. The symptoms of concomitant gallstones and those of gallbladder carcinoma may be difficult to distinguish in patients with small tumors. Right upper quadrant pain, discomfort, and dyspepsia can result from both. Patients with gallbladder cancer frequently have advanced disease and nonspecific signs such as weight loss and anorexia. Obstructive jaundice is common (Fig. 16-4). A mass may be present in the right upper quadrant. Tumor invasion may cause cystic duct obstruction and result in acute cholecystitis. Jaundice occurs when the tumor extends into the common bile duct. The diagnosis often is not suspected before operation, and the disease is diagnosed at laparotomy or laparoscopy in more than half of cases. Tumors with the best prognosis are those that are found incidentally at the time of cholecystectomy for symptomatic gallstone disease.

Table 16-1   Nevin's Classification for Gallbladder Cancer

Stage	Extent of Tumor
I	Mucosa only
II	Muscularis and mucosa
III	Subserosa, muscularis, and mucosa
IV	Cystic duct lymph node involvement and layers of the gallbladder wall
V	Distant spread

Table 16-2   TNM Classification for Gallbladder Carcinoma

Stage	Primary Tumor	Lymph Nodes	Metastasis
0	Tis	N0	M0
I	T1	N0	M0
II	T2	N0	M0
III	T1	N1	M0
	T2	N1	M0
	T3	N0	M0
	T3	N1	M0
IVA	T4	N0	M0
	T4	N1	M0
IVB	any T	N2	M0
	any T	any N	M1

Classification	Extent
PRIMARY TUMOR	
Tis	Carcinoma in situ
T1	Tumor invades muscosa or muscle
T1a	Mucosa
T1b	Muscle
T2	Tumor invades perimuscular connective tissue
T3	Tumor perforates serosa or invades into one adjacent organ (less than 2 cm into liver)
T4	Tumor extends more than 2 cm into liver or into 2 or more adjacent organs
REGIONAL LYMPH NODES	
N0	No regional lymph node metastasis
N1	Metastasis to cystic duct, pericholedochal, or hilar lymph nodes
N2	Metastasis to peripancreatic, periduodenal, periportal, celiac, or superior mesenteric lymph nodes

The difficulty in establishing the diagnosis of gallbladder cancer early in the course of the disease is a major factor in its poor prognosis. A reliable diagnostic test to screen for early gallbladder cancer is not available. Although there have been reports of gallbladder cancers secreting α-fetoprotein[26] and carcinoembryonic antigen, there is no reliable tumor marker for this disease. Furthermore, the standard test for right upper quadrant abdominal symptoms, ultrasonography, is not a sensitive test for early gallbladder cancer. Gallbladder polyps and carcinomas have echogenicity similar to that of normal gallbladder wall. When detected by ultrasound, a gallbladder cancer usually appears as an area of wall thickening or, less commonly, as a polypoid mass. The extent of disease is difficult to delineate on ultrasound examination because the tumor usually cannot be differentiated from surrounding liver parenchyma. In cases of cholecystitis caused by gallbladder cancer, the diagnosis is even more difficult because gall-

bladder wall irregularities or thickening may not be distinguishable from changes resulting from the inflammatory process.

CT is useful in determining extension of disease into the liver parenchyma or adjacent organs, and in demonstrating biliary obstruction. One investigation found diffuse or focal gallbladder wall thickening in 95% of patients with gallbladder cancer, an intraluminal mass in 90%, direct liver invasion in 90%, dilated bile ducts in 50%, noncontiguous liver metastases in 12%, and gastrointestinal tract invasion in 8%.[27] Yet, the sensitivity of CT in detecting early cancer of the gallbladder is limited. CT does not reliably demonstrate all histologically positive lymph nodes,[28] although lymph nodes larger than 10 mm with ring-like or heterogeneous contrast enhancement are likely to harbor metastatic disease. Preliminary results comparing CT and magnetic resonance imaging (MRI) suggest that the two modalities determine the extent of disease in gallbladder cancer with equal accuracy.[29] Endoscopic ultrasound is under investigation with respect to its accuracy in determining the extent of disease.

Surgery

The only proven effective therapy for gallbladder cancer is complete surgical removal of the tumor. Unfortunately, this is possible in only a minority of patients, about 25% of operative cases in one report.[13] More radical operations have been proposed to increase the pro-

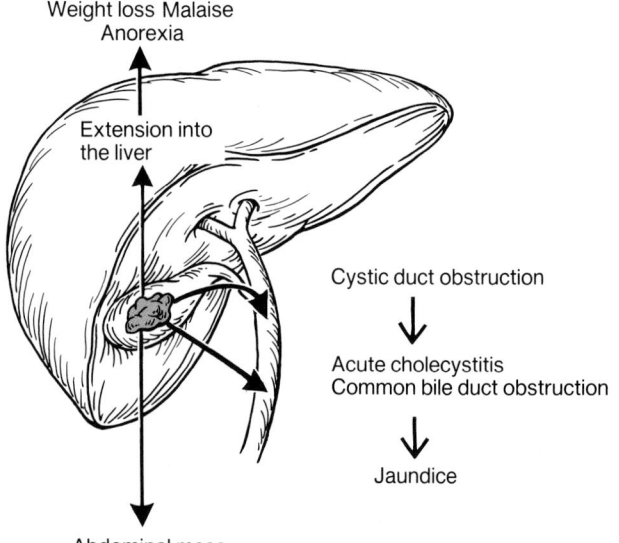

Figure 16-4 Gallbladder cancer spreads by local invasion of surrounding structures. The common symptoms of gallbladder cancer are related to the involvement of adjacent structures.

portion of patients with surgically resectable disease. However, the optimal extent of resection is controversial. Although it has been shown that more extensive operations for gallbladder cancer—including pancreaticoduodenectomy, bile duct resection, and major hepatic resection—are possible, it is unclear whether more radical procedures will lead to improved survival.

When gallbladder cancer is limited to the mucosa, it is generally accepted that cholecystectomy is the best treatment. Cholecystectomy alone results in a long-term survival rate of nearly 100% when the cancer is an incidental finding at the time of surgery for presumed benign disease.[30,31] Once the cancer involves the deeper layers of the gallbladder wall, the prognosis worsens. In one study, patients who had carcinoma confined to the mucosa and submucosa had a 5-year survival rate of 64%, whereas none of the patients who had cancer involving all layers of the gallbladder wall survived longer than $2\frac{1}{2}$ years.[32] The precise survival statistics for tumors extending into the muscularis or to the serosa are difficult to determine because most series group these together because of the small number of patients who have early stage gallbladder cancer. However, many of these patients die of recurrent gallbladder cancer after cholecystectomy alone.

Because the spread of gallbladder cancer is mainly by local extension to adjacent liver or to regional lymph nodes, several authors[33-37] have advocated wedge resection of the gallbladder bed along with regional lymphadenectomy of the hepatoduodenal ligament. This procedure has been termed *radical cholecystectomy* and has been advocated as the treatment of choice for early gallbladder cancer that extends beyond the mucosa. Of 11 patients who underwent reoperation for early gallbladder cancer, 5 were found to have lymph node involvement and 3 also had extension of the cancer into the liver.[38] A retrospective review of a 12-year period in one institution found 22 patients who underwent cholecystectomy for cure and compared them with 18 patients who underwent radical cholecystectomy for cure.[37] Although the median survival was better after the more radical procedure (3.6 years compared with 0.8 years), the 5-year survival rates were similar (32% and 33%, respectively). Another review of radical gallbladder resection found a 5-year survival rate of 40% for pT2 tumors treated with cholecystectomy, compared with a rate of 90% for pT2 tumors treated with radical resection.[31] A prospective randomized trial to evaluate radical cholecystectomy has not been performed. However, it has been shown that reoperation and radical cholecystectomy can be done with low morbidity and mortality and may affect survival. Therefore, for patients with invasive but resectable disease, a wedge resection of the liver with a 2- to 3-cm margin around the gallbladder, together with cholecystectomy and lymph node dissection, is recommended. The lymph node dissection should include all the lymph nodes and the surrounding areolar tissue from the bifurcation of the common hepatic ducts to the distal common bile duct, as well as lymph nodes along the hepatic artery to its origin from the celiac axis.

There has been renewed interest in more extensive resection than radical cholecystectomy for gallbladder cancer. In the past, partial hepatectomy, either right hepatic lobectomy or extended right hepatic lobectomy, was shown to have little effect on survival, although there had been a few reports of long-term survivors.[39,40] These survival statistics, along with the high morbidity of these procedures, led to the impression that hepatic resection was not effective therapy. Because the operative morbidity and mortality rates for major liver resections have decreased, the effect of these extensive operations on the long-term outlook for patients with gallbladder cancer is being assessed.

When gallbladder cancer recurs, it most often does so locally, frequently in liver segments IV, V, or VIII. This correlates with the common pathways for venous drainage of the gallbladder. Venous drainage is into intrahepatic portal branches of the right lobe in about two thirds of gallbladders, into the left lobe in 6%, and into both the right and left lobes in 28%.[41] This observation explains the limited effect that right hepatic lobectomy has on survival. With the frequent extension of gallbladder cancer into segments IV, V, and VIII, a medial hepatectomy (resection of segments IV, V, and VIII) has been proposed by some.[42] A median survival of 50 months has been reported for five patients treated with cholecystectomy, lymph node dissection, and medial hepatectomy.

A review of 1686 resected cases of gallbladder cancer found survival rates of 83% when disease was limited to the mucosa, 73% when it extended to the muscle layer, 37% when it extended to the subserosal layer, 15% when there was serosal involvement, and 8% when there was invasion into adjacent organs.[43] Fifty-seven percent of these patients were treated with radical procedures. Extended cholecystectomy was performed in 659 patients. Cholecystectomy was combined with bile duct resection in 163 patients and with pancreaticoduodenectomy in 64 patients. Major liver resection was performed in 302 patients (18%), and was associated with an 18% operative mortality rate.

Others, however, have not seen a dramatic change in survival rates with hepatic resection or other radical procedures.[44-46] In one large series of 724 patients,[44] there was no difference in survival between those who underwent extended resections and those who underwent radical cholecystectomy.

Laparoscopy and Gallbladder Cancer

Symptomatic cholelithiasis is treated routinely by laparoscopic cholecystectomy. Because many gallbladder cancers are found only at the time of cholecystectomy for symptomatic gallstones, the appropriate course of action when gallbladder cancer is found needs to be defined. Recent reports have demonstrated metastasis of gallbladder cancer within laparoscopic trocar sites.[47,48] Some of these cases were deemed resectable at reoperation until the metastatic implants were found. If the gallbladder is removed using the laparoscope, tumor dissemination is possible. Therefore, when gallbladder cancer is suspected at the time of laparoscopy, the surgeon should either proceed with an open operation or terminate the procedure and reoperate after further diagnostic work-up and consultation with the patient.

Laparoscopic examination before laparotomy for gallbladder carcinoma may be useful in assessing resectability. If liver or peritoneal metastases are found, laparotomy can be avoided.

Radiation Therapy

Local extension of gallbladder carcinoma often makes surgical resection impossible; even when surgical resection is successfully achieved, local recurrence is common. To improve survival and reduce recurrence rates, radiation therapy has been advocated, in the form of either intraoperative radiation therapy, brachytherapy, or postoperative radiation therapy. The benefit of radiation therapy in the treatment of gallbladder cancer is difficult to assess because most series include fewer than 10 cases, radiation doses vary, and heterogeneous lesions are compared. Given the rarity of the disease, it is not surprising that prospective randomized studies have not been done. Seven patients treated with postoperative external beam irradiation after complete resection of their gallbladder cancer have been described.[49] A dose of 4600 cGy was delivered with a boost dose of 900 cGy to the gallbladder bed. Five patients were alive with no evidence of disease after 5, 9, 11, 31, and 58 months. Although brachytherapy, which consists of the intraluminal administration of radiation using an iridium wire, has been used in patients with gallbladder cancer, experience is limited.[50] For patients with stage IV gallbladder cancer (TNM classification), 3-year survival rates of 10% for surgical resection with intraoperative radiation therapy (17 patients) and 0% for surgical resection alone (9 patients) have been reported.[51]

Chemotherapy

Results of chemotherapy for the treatment of advanced gallbladder cancer or as an adjuvant treatment after resection have been disappointing. 5-Fluorouracil (5-FU) has been used most frequently, with response rates of only 10% to 20%. The Eastern Cooperative Oncology Group conducted a randomized trial of three chemotherapy regimens for inoperable disease (5-FU alone, 5-FU and streptozocin, and 5-FU and methyl-CCNU).[52] There were no differences in survival among groups, and only 5 of 53 patients with gallbladder cancer had an objective response. Other agents that have been used for gallbladder carcinoma include mitomycin C, doxorubicin, and nitrosoureas. No agent has been noted to be effective. Intraarterial administration of 5-FU or mitomycin C also has failed to improve survival.[53]

BILE DUCT CARCINOMA

Although the best prognosis is obtained with complete surgical resection of bile duct carcinoma, there have been few long-term survivors. The optimal therapy for this tumor is still debated. Conservative operations as well as extensive radical surgical procedures have been advocated. Because few cases are cured regardless of the treatment, better adjuvant therapy is needed to improve survival in this disease.

Incidence

Malignant bile duct tumors are uncommon. Their incidence in autopsy series ranges from 0.01% to 0.20%. For the proximal bile ducts, their frequency ranges from 1 in 40,000 to 4.4 in 100,000.[54] Unlike the female predominance of gallbladder cancer, bile duct cancers have a slight male predominance. The age range is from 50 to 70 years.

Although there is an association between bile duct cancer and gallstones, it is not as striking as for gallbladder cancer. Twenty-five to 57% of patients with bile duct cancer have gallstones. Similar to gallbladder cancer, biliary tract infection is associated with these tumors. Chronic typhoid carriers and patients with *Clonorchis sinensis* infection have a higher incidence of bile duct cancer than do members of the general population. There is evidence that chemicals used in the rubber industry may increase the risk of developing cholangiocarcinoma.[55] Other conditions that are associated with bile duct cancer include choledochal cysts, congenital hepatic fibrosis, primary sclerosing cholangitis, and ulcerative colitis. The association is most striking in patients with ulcerative colitis. This predisposition is in-

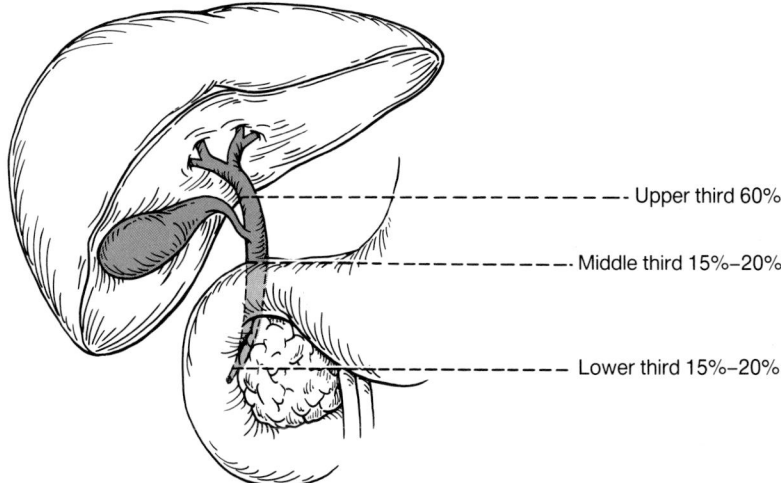

Figure 16-5 Bile duct tumors are classified by their location in the biliary tree into upper, middle, or lower third lesions. About 10% of tumors are diffuse.

dependent of whether patients have had adequate therapy for their colonic disease.[56] Bile duct tumors in patients with ulcerative colitis tend to have a more aggressive course.

Pathology

Bile duct cancer is classified according to its location within the ductal system. As proposed by Longmire, the tumors generally are classified based on three locations—upper third, middle third, and lower third (Fig. 16-5). About 60% of tumors are in the upper third of the ductal system (Fig. 16-6), which includes the confluence of the hepatic ducts. Hilar bile duct tumors have been called *Klatskin's tumors* after Gerald Klatskin, who first described 13 patients with tumors at the bifurca-

tion of the hepatic ducts.[57] The middle third tumors are located between the cystic duct and the upper border of the duodenum. The lower third lesions are located between the upper border of the duodenum and up to, but not including, the ampulla of Vater. In as many as 7% of cases, bile duct tumors are multicentric or exhibit diffuse growth.[58]

Other classifications have been used. Tumor stage is not mentioned by many authors, although some have used the TNM classification[59] (Table 16-3). Upper third or hilar bile duct tumors have been classified further into four types, as shown in Figure 16-7.[60] Type I involves the common hepatic duct, type II extends to the confluence of the hepatic ducts, type III extends into either the right or the left hepatic duct, and type IV extends into both the right and left hepatic ducts.

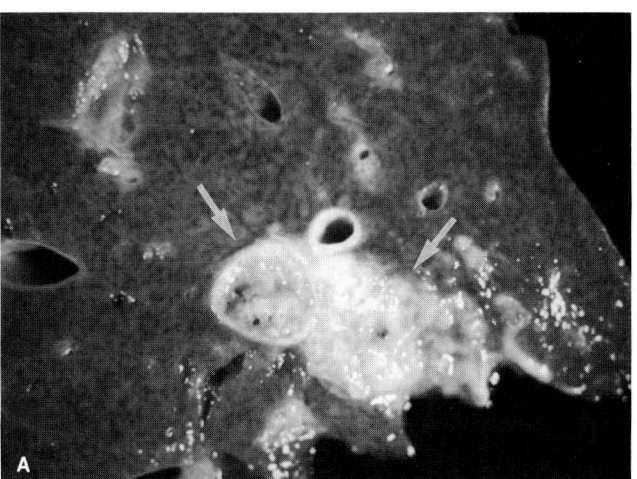
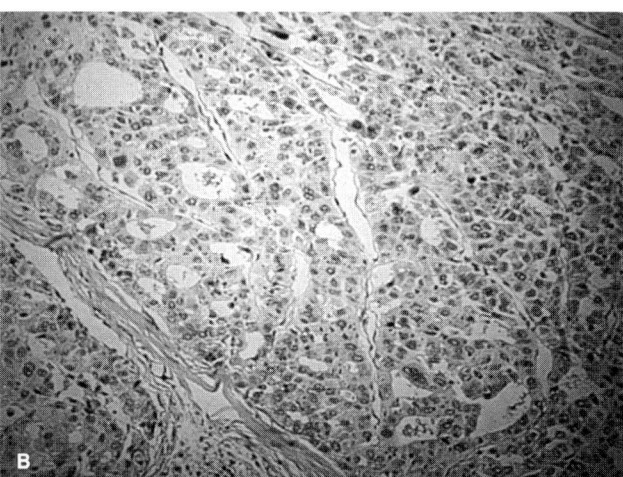

Figure 16-6 (**A**) A right hilar bile duct tumor can be seen filling the hepatic duct and invading surrounding liver parenchyma (*arrows*). (**B**) Histologically, this tumor is a well-differentiated adenocarcinoma. (See Color Fig. 16-6.)

Table 16-3 TNM Classification for Bile Duct Tumors

Stage	Primary Tumor	Lymph Nodes	Metastasis
0	Tis	N0	M0
I	T1	N0	M0
II	T2	N0	M0
III	T1	N1	M0
	T1	N2	M0
	T2	N1	M0
	T2	N2	M0
IVA	T3	any N	M0
IVB	any T	any N	M1

Classification	Extent
PRIMARY TUMOR	
Tis	Carcinoma in situ
T1	Tumor invades the mucosa or muscle layer
T1a	Mucosa
T1b	Muscle
T2	Tumor invades perimuscular connective tissue
T3	Tumor invades into adjacent structures
REGIONAL LYMPH NODES	
N0	No regional lymph node metastasis
N1	Metastasis to cystic duct, pericholedochal, or hilar lymph nodes
N2	Metastasis to peripancreatic, periduodenal, periportal, celiac, superior mesenteric, or posterior pancreaticoduodenal lymph nodes

Bile duct cancers, like gallbladder cancer, tend to be locally invasive. They often grow slowly, and distant metastases are seen less frequently than in other cancers. Morphologically, they are described as nodular, scirrhous, diffusely infiltrating, or papillary, with the first type being the most frequent. Histologically, over 95% of proximal bile duct tumors are adenocarcinomas. Because they arise from ductal epithelial cells, they also are termed *cholangiocarcinomas*. Histologic types can be described further as acinar, ductular, trabecular, alveolar, and papillary. Rarer types of bile duct tumors include mucoepidermoid cancers, cystadenocarcinomas, malignant hemangioendotheliomas, botryoid rhabdomyosarcomas, and apudomas of the bile duct.

Clinical Findings

Bile duct tumors are locally invasive. Because of the proximity of the bile ducts to the branches of the portal vein and hepatic arteries, these cancers often are unresectable. Jaundice, the most frequent presenting symptom, occurs in about 90% of cases. Tumors that obstruct the common bile duct present earlier than do hepatic ductal tumors, because bilateral ductal obstruction is required to produce jaundice. Abdominal pain occurs in 30% to 50% of patients and cholangitis is the initial finding in 10% to 30% of cases. Other initial findings are pruritus and anemia. Weight loss, anorexia, and ascites are late findings. Laboratory findings in addition to increased serum bilirubin include elevated serum alkaline phosphatase and γ-glutamyl transferase levels. An elevated alkaline phosphatase level may be the only laboratory abnormality.

Diagnosis

The diagnostic work-up usually begins with an ultrasound examination for the evaluation of jaundice. Ultrasound examination generally demonstrates intrahepatic ductal dilatation and, depending on the site of the tumor, variable degrees of extrahepatic bile duct dilatation. Although ultrasonography and CT almost always demonstrate ductal dilatation, the tumor itself is rarely seen because it tends to infiltrate along the wall of the bile duct rather than to form a mass. CT is useful for delineating both the extent of tumor invasion into the liver and the nature of any metastases. MRI also has been evaluated, and results show that CT is superior for diagnosing dilated bile ducts and MRI is better for visualizing the tumor because of improved tissue characterization.[29] MR angiography may be helpful for delineating vascular involvement.

When biliary obstruction is confirmed by ultrasonography or CT, further visualization of the biliary tree is necessary using either percutaneous transhepatic cholangiography or endoscopic retrograde cholangiopancreatography. Percutaneous transhepatic cholangiography is preferred for proximal lesions because endoscopic retrograde cholangiopancreatography may fail to visualize adequately the proximal portion of the biliary tree (Fig. 16-8). For lower bile duct lesions, endoscopic retrograde cholangiopancreatography is advantageous because brushing for cytologic diagnosis can be performed concomitantly and the possibility of bile leak from a liver puncture is avoided. Successful use of both techniques has been reported, and the optimal method depends on the expertise available. Selective celiac angiography is helpful to determine whether major adjacent vascular structures, such as the portal vein or hepatic artery, are involved, and to define vascular anatomy should resection be deemed possible.

At the time of cholangiography, a biliary stent can be placed for preoperative biliary drainage. This approach has been advocated by some to decrease the morbidity and mortality of surgical resection, and to serve as a guide for the placement of biliary stents at the

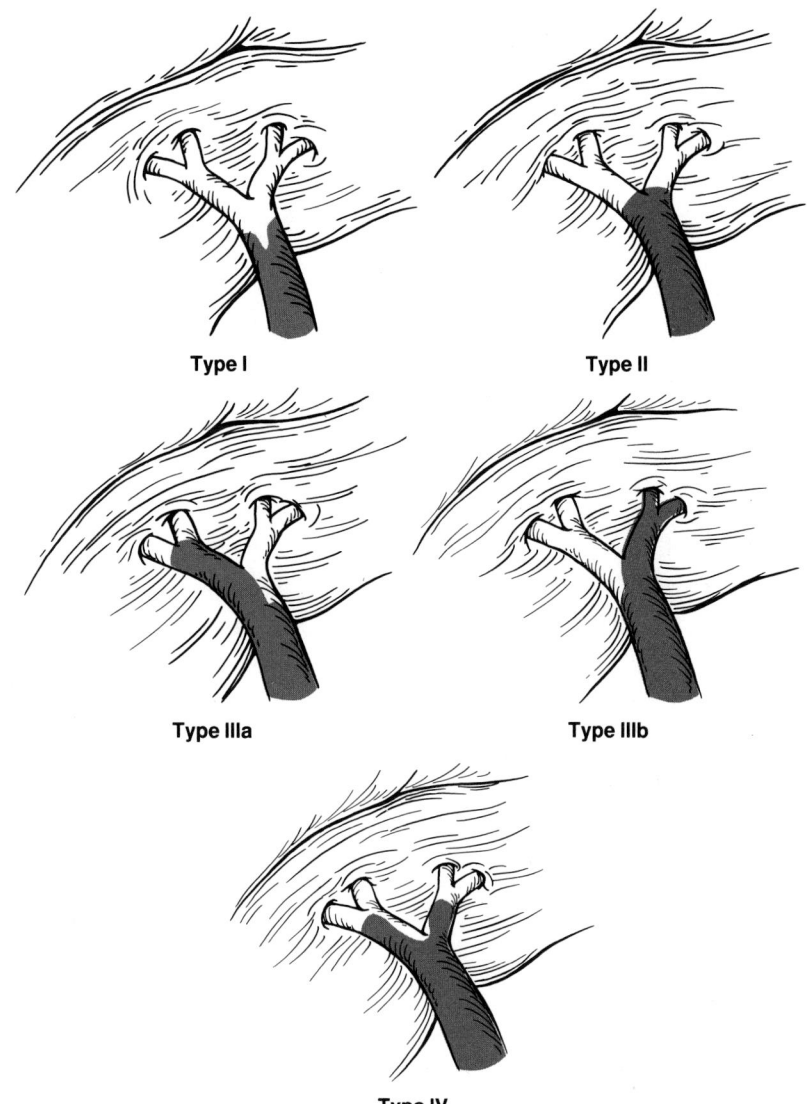

Type I

Type II

Type IIIa

Type IIIb

Type IV

Figure 16-7 Hilar bile duct tumors can be classified into four types as described by Bismuth and Corlette.[60]

time of operation.[61] Others have not shown an improvement in results with the preoperative placement of stents.[62,63]

Surgical Therapy

Middle and Lower Bile Duct Tumors

Although resection with reanastomosis of the common bile duct occasionally is possible, nearly all lesions require reconstruction with a biliary–enteric anastomosis, usually a Roux-en-Y choledochojejunostomy. For lower third lesions, a Whipple procedure (pancreaticoduodenectomy) is a potentially curative operation. Overall, both middle and lower third lesions have a better prognosis than do tumors in the hilum. This is more likely the result of higher resectability rates than of a difference in the biologic behavior of the tumors. In a series of 171 bile duct tumors in one institution, the

frequency of curative resection was 56% for distal tumors, 33% for mid-ductal tumors, and only 15% for proximal tumors.[64] Curative resection resulted in comparable survival rates regardless of the tumor's location in the biliary tract.

Hilar Bile Duct Tumors

Hilar bile duct tumors can be considered a regional rather than a local disease because, by the time of presentation, they usually have invaded adjacent liver and other periductal tissues, such as vascular and lymphatic structures. Their locally invasive nature and proximity to vital structures make curative resection difficult and infrequent. Only 15% to 30% of all hilar bile duct cancers are amenable to resection. After resection, these tumors frequently recur, leading some to advocate a conservative surgical approach. One group has pro-

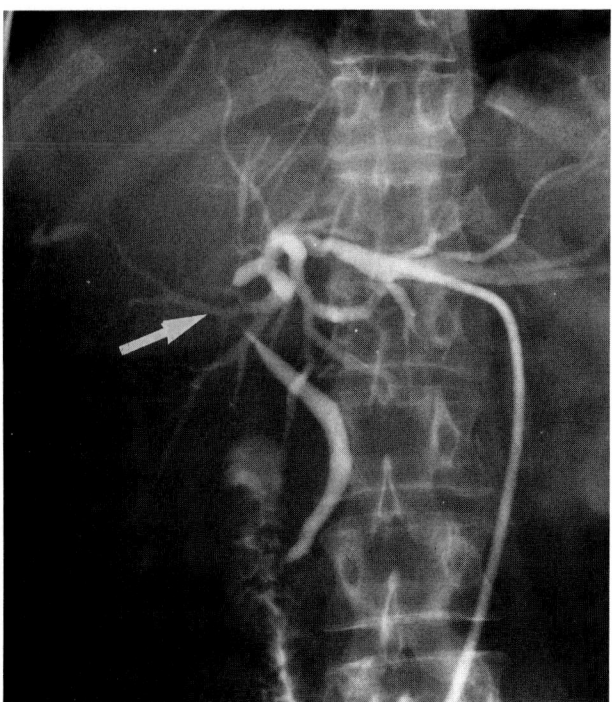

Figure 16-8 A transhepatic cholangiogram can be used to demonstrate the location of a bile duct tumor. This study demonstrates a proximal third (Klatskin's) tumor (*arrow*).

posed U-tube stent placement followed by radiation therapy. They have achieved a median survival of 33 months with this approach,[65] which is comparable to the survival achieved in many series after major hepatic resection. Others have recommended surgical placement of transhepatic stents or biliary bypass for tumors extending into the liver.[66,67] Hilar bile duct resection combined with either resection of a central core of liver around the tumor[68] or resection of segment IV and the caudate lobe[69] is performed by some surgeons. Major hepatic resection, with right or left hepatic lobectomy, has been advocated by others.[70–72] Because the caudate lobe often is invaded by bile duct cancer, caudate lobe resection has been added to anterior segmentectomy[73] or to right or left hepatic lobectomy.[74,75] These radical procedures have been extended to include vascular reconstructions when there is portal or hepatic arterial involvement,[76] with higher associated morbidity and mortality rates. Hepatic transplantation also has been performed for these tumors, but it is followed by a high rate of recurrence. Transplantation is not a recommended therapy for hilar bile duct tumors.[77]

Although controversy still exists regarding the optimal surgical procedure, it is clear that complete resection remains the only chance for long-term survival. In a review of 581 resections of hilar bile duct carcinoma, one group reported a better 5-year survival rate when major hepatic resection was added (17%) than when lo-

cal excision with or without quadrate lobe resection was performed (7%).[78] However, the operative mortality rate was higher with concomitant liver resection (15%) than with hilar resection alone (8%). Many other reports have described long-term survivors after radical resection.[75,79,80] In addition to the possibility for long-term survival, an improved quality of life has been reported when all gross tumor can be resected. One group reported a 3-year survival rate of 21% for patients undergoing curative resection.[81] In another series, 30% of patients who underwent resection lived for more than 5 years.[82] However, only a relatively small fraction of patients are eligible for resection in all series.

Unless contraindicated for other reasons, surgical exploration should be performed in all patients whose tumors are potentially resectable. If hepatic lobectomy is required to achieve complete tumor excision, it should be done only in centers with low operative morbidity and mortality rates. Bile duct resection alone may be possible if the tumor is confined to the common hepatic bile duct (type I). Local excision also should be done when the tumor involves the bifurcation but does not extend into the right or left hepatic ducts (type II). If there is extension into either the right or the left hepatic duct (type III), hepatic lobectomy along with hilar resection is warranted in selected cases. For type IV lesions that extend into both ductal systems, palliative stent placement with or without radiation therapy probably is the best treatment. Vascular reconstructions to improve resectability should be performed with caution because of the higher associated morbidity and mortality rates, as well as the questionable survival benefit.

Determination of Resectability

Often, surgical exploration is the only method of definitively determining whether a bile duct tumor is resectable. If one of the following is found either on diagnostic testing or at the time of surgery, the tumor is considered unresectable: (1) metastatic disease; (2) extensive vascular invasion (ie, tumor invading the main portal vein or involving both the right and left portal veins or the hepatic arteries); or (3) tumor within the second-order biliary radicles of both hepatic lobes. Preoperative CT is helpful to delineate the extent of local invasion. Cholangiography not only is the gold standard for diagnosis, but also is helpful in determining resectability: if both the right and left hepatic ducts are involved beyond secondary biliary radicles, the tumor is unresectable. Surgical exploration should be considered for all good-risk patients whose tumors are potentially resectable.

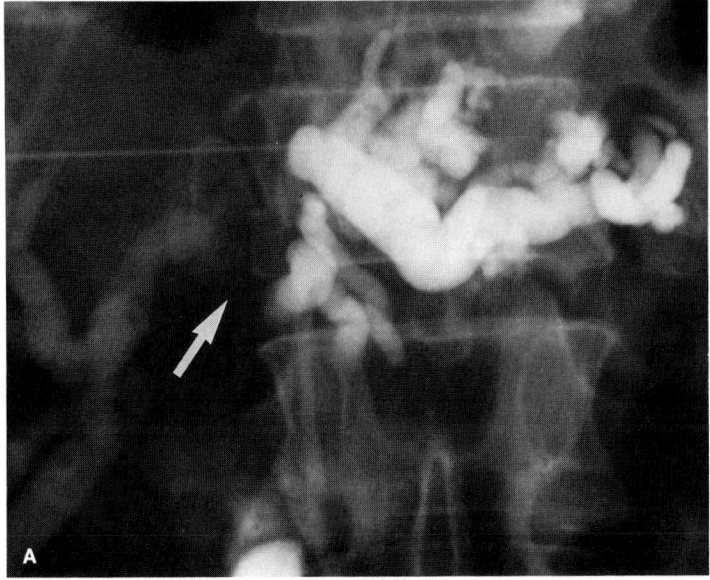

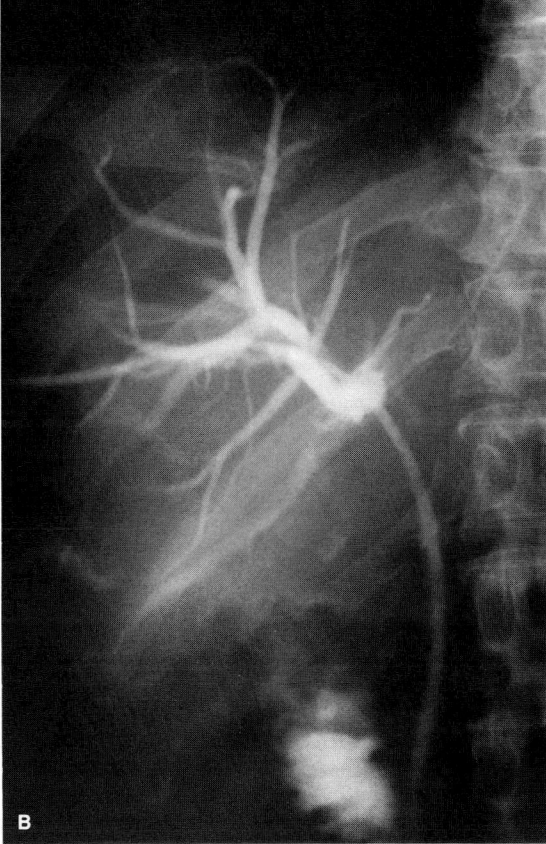

Figure 16-9 (**A**) Transhepatic cholangiogram through the left ductal system was performed for the evaluation of jaundice. A hilar bile duct tumor was found with delayed filling of the right ductal system (*arrow*). (**B**) A transhepatic stent was placed into the right ductal system for relief of jaundice.

Treatment of Unresectable Tumors

Patients with advanced unresectable disease can obtain palliation with nonoperative percutaneous or endoscopic stent placement. Stents can be placed across an obstructing, unresectable bile duct cancer either at the time of endoscopic retrograde cholangiopancreatography or through the percutaneous transhepatic approach (Fig. 16-9). Both procedures are associated with the potential complications of cholangitis, bleeding, bile leakage, and recurrent obstruction from catheter occlusion.[83] Endoprostheses have the advantage of improved patient comfort, no loss of electrolytes, and a reduced incidence of cholangitis and infection. However, they are technically more difficult to place in proximal bile duct lesions, cannot be used for cholangiography, and are not easily changed. For proximal ductal lesions, the transhepatic approach usually is required. Iridium-192 wires can be placed through external catheters for the administration of intracavitary radiation therapy. Because percutaneous drains are used for palliation, drainage of one ductal system may be sufficient. Although drainage of one ductal system usually relieves jaundice, bilateral stent placement may be necessary for control of biliary infection.

Stent placement for bile duct tumors may provide useful palliation,[84,85] but the stents become obstructed in most patients. The incidence of stent occlusion has been reduced by the use of metallic, expandable stents.[86] The 30-day mortality rate for percutaneous or endoscopic stent placement ranges from 15% to 33%.[83] Cholangitis, bleeding, and bile leaks are frequent complications. This high mortality rate in part reflects the advanced stage of disease at the time of stent placement. Similar operative mortality rates (18% to 33%) have been reported for surgical bypass.[83] Patients with bile duct tumors that are metastatic or unresectable should undergo percutaneous or endoscopic stent placement, rather than laparotomy. However, if surgical exploration is undertaken to determine resectability and the tumor is found to be unresectable, a surgical drainage procedure should be performed if possible.

Surgical bypass for palliation of bile duct cancers has been reported to result in fewer episodes of cholangitis and may provide an improved quality of life. For lower bile duct tumors, choledochojejunostomy or hepaticojejunostomy can be performed. Several methods are available to provide palliative surgical biliary drainage for hilar tumors. The Longmire procedure, which consists of transection of the left lateral liver segment and anastomosis of the dilated left hepatic duct to a loop of jejunum, is seldom used today because of the availability of other surgical alternatives and percutaneous stent placement. A preferred method of decompressing the left hepatic ductal system is by the round ligament approach to the left hepatic duct in segment III.[87] The bridge of tissue just beneath the ligamentum teres is opened to expose the dilated left hepatic duct and an anastomosis with a loop or Roux-en-Y limb of jejunum is constructed.

U-tube stent placement also can be accomplished at the time of operation.[88] A Silastic tube is placed through the abdominal wall that extends through the liver, across the bile duct tumor, out through the bile duct, and again through the abdominal wall, making a U shape. To prevent problems with leakage around the site of exit from the common bile duct, a Roux-en-Y limb of jejunum should be used as a conduit for this tube from the common duct to the abdominal wall. Some surgeons place palliative Silastic stents through the liver and the tumor or debulked hilum into a loop or segment of jejunum.[66] Percutaneous stents are placed before operation to serve as a guide for hilar duct dissection and to facilitate the placement of operative stents.

A combined radiologic–endoscopic–laparoscopic method of left hepaticogastrostomy for bypass of malignant biliary tumors has been described.[89] There was no acute mortality, and all seven patients had good relief of jaundice with this approach.

Radiation Therapy and Chemotherapy

Intraoperative, external beam, and intracavitary radiation therapy have been used for the treatment of bile duct tumors. Most reported series are small because this tumor is rare. Thus, the role of adjuvant or therapeutic radiation therapy is unclear. Some authors have reported an improvement in survival with radiation therapy but others have not. One group showed a benefit for adjuvant radiation therapy in patients with microscopic residual disease after surgical resection.[90] With resection alone, the median survival was 11 months; it increased to 21.5 months with conventional radiation therapy and to 61 months with particle helium or neon radiation therapy. Radiation therapy also improved survival from a median of 2.2 months to a median of 12.2 months in patients without metastatic disease who had palliative procedures.[91] Others have not shown prolongation of survival by the addition of radiation therapy.[90]

Radiation therapy can be associated with significant side effects, including hepatic fibrosis and duodenitis. To limit the effects of radiation therapy on surrounding structures, localized intracavitary brachytherapy has been proposed in the treatment of bile duct cancers.[92] An iridium-192 wire can be placed through transhepatic stents to deliver concentrated radiation therapy at the site of the tumor. Further studies are needed to define the role of any type of radiation therapy in the treatment of bile duct cancers.

The most commonly used chemotherapeutic agent for bile duct cancer is 5-FU, but the results of treatment with this and other agents have been poor. 5-FU and mitomycin C as single agents, and combinations of 5-FU with adriamycin and mitomycin C have resulted in a collective response rate of 29%.[93] Regional infusion therapy in one series was associated with a 39% response rate.[93]

> Unless they are discovered in their early stages, gallbladder and bile duct cancers have poor prognoses. Although more aggressive surgical therapy may improve survival in subsets of patients, controlled clinical trials are nonexistent. The extent to which radical operations should be performed and the patients who will benefit from them are not known. Because surgical resection provides the only opportunity for long-term survival, it is indicated in good-risk patients when curative resection is possible and predicted surgical morbidity and mortality are acceptable. When resection is not possible or is contraindicated, surgical bypass or biliary stent placement can offer effective palliation. Radiation therapy in conjunction with surgical therapy may improve results. Better chemotherapeutic agents are needed to treat unresectable disease and to serve as adjuvant therapy. These rare tumors are best treated at institutions where significant experience can accumulate and trials of various therapies can be carried out.

REFERENCES

1. Nahrwold DL. Benign tumors and pseudotumors of the biliary tract. In: Way LW, Pellegrini CA, eds. Surgery of the gallbladder and bile ducts. Philadelphia, WB Saunders, 1987:459.
2. Koga A, Watanabe K, Fukuyama T, et al. Diagnosis and operative indications for polypoid lesions of the gallbladder. Arch Surg 1988;123:26.
3. Reubner BH, Montgomery CK. Pathology of the liver and biliary tract. New York, Wiley Medical, 1982:325.
4. Aldridge MC, Gruffaz R, Castaing D, Bismuth H. Adenomyomatosis of the gallbladder: a premalignant lesion? Surgery 1991;109:107.
5. Ishak KG, Willis GW, Cummins SD, Bullock AA. Biliary

cystadenoma and cystadenocarcinoma: report of 14 cases and review of the literature. Cancer 1977;38:322.

6. Albores-Saavedra J, Vardaman CJ, Vuitch F. Non-neoplastic polypoid lesions and adenomas of the gallbladder. Pathol Annu 1993;28:145.

7. Kozuka S, Tsubone M, Yasui A, Hachisuka K. Relation of adenoma to carcinoma in the gallbladder. Cancer 1982;50:2226.

8. Aldridge MC, Bismuth H. Gallbladder cancer: the polyp-cancer sequence. Br J Surg 1990;77:363.

9. Christensen AH, Ishak KG. Benign tumors and pseudotumors of the gallbladder: review of 180 cases. Arch Pathol Lab Med 1970;90:423.

10. Hulten O. On precancerous bile duct tumors. Acta Chir Scand 1960;119:122.

11. Marshall JM. Tumors of the bile ducts. Surg Gynecol Obstet 1932;54:6.

12. Neumann RD, LiVolsi VA, Rosenthal NS, Burrell M, Ball TJ. Adenocarcinoma in biliary papillomatosis. Gastroenterology 1976;70:779.

13. Piehler JM, Crichlow RW. Primary carcinoma of the gallbladder. Surg Gynecol Obstet 1978;147:929.

14. Adson MA. Carcinoma of the gallbladder. Surg Clin North Am 1973;53:1203.

15. Hart J, Modan B, Shani M. Cholelithiasis in the aetiology of gallbladder neoplasms. Lancet 1971;1:1151.

16. Diehl AK. Gallstone size and risk of gallbladder cancer. JAMA 1983;250:2323.

17. Kowalewski K, Todd EF. Carcinoma of the gallbladder induced in hamsters by insertion of cholesterol pellets and feeding dimethylnitrosamine (35293). Proc Soc Exp Biol Med 1971;136:482.

18. Tseng L, Chen J, Yang K. Anomalous junction of pancreaticobiliary duct with carcinoma of the gallbladder: report of two cases. J Formos Med Assoc 1993;92:178.

19. Lowenfels AB, Lindstom CG, Conway MJ, Hastings PR. Gallstones and risk of gallbladder cancer. J Natl Cancer Inst 1985;75:77.

20. Berk RN, Armbuster TG, Saltzstein SL. Carcinoma of the porcelain gallbladder. Radiology 1973;106:29.

21. Polk HC. Carcinoma and the calcified gallbladder. Gastroenterology 1966;50:582.

22. Henson DE, Albores-Saavedra J, Corle D. Carcinoma of the gallbladder: histologic types, stage of disease, grade, and survival rates. Cancer 1992;70:1493.

23. Duarte I, Llanos O, Domke H, Harz C, Valdivieso V. Metaplasia and precursor lesions of gallbladder carcinoma. Cancer 1993;72:1878.

24. Nevin JE, Moran TJ, Kay S, King R. Carcinoma of the gallbladder: staging, treatment, and prognosis. Cancer 1976;37:141.

25. Gall FP, Kockerling F, Scheele J, Schneider C, Hohenberger W. Radical operations for carcinoma of the gallbladder: present status in Germany. World J Surg 1991;15:328.

26. Watanabe M, Hori Y, Nojima T, et al. Alpha-fetoprotein producing carcinoma of the gallbladder. Dig Dis Sci 1993;38:561.

27. Thorsen MK, Quiroz R, Lawson TL, et al. Primary biliary carcinoma: CT evaluation. Radiology 1984;152:479.

28. Ohtani T, Shirai Y, Tsukada K, Hatakeyava K, Muta T. Carcinoma of the gallbladder: CT evaluation of lymphatic spread. Radiology 1993;189:875.

29. Kersting-Sommerhoff B, Helmberger H. Radiologic diagnosis and staging of gallbladder and bile duct tumors. Endoscopy 1993;25:86.

30. Yamaguchi K, Tsuneyoshi M. Subclinical gallbladder carcinoma. Am J Surg 1992;163:382.

31. Shirai Y, Yoshida K, Tsudada K, Muto T. Inapparent carcinoma of the gallbladder: an appraisal of a radical second operation after simple cholecystectomy. Ann Surg 1992;215:326.

32. Bergdahl L. Gallbladder carcinoma first diagnosed at microscopic examination of gallbladders removed for presumed benign disease. Ann Surg 1980;191:19.

33. Fahim RB, McDonald JR, Richards JC, Ferris DO. Carcinoma of the gallbladder: a study of its modes of spread. Ann Surg 1962;156:114.

34. Glenn F, Hays DM. The scope of radical surgery in the treatment of malignant tumors of the extrahepatic biliary tract. Surg Gynecol Obstet 1954;99:529.

35. Morrow CE, Sutherland DER, Florack G, Eisenberg MM, Grage TB. Primary gallbladder carcinoma: significance of subserosal lesions and results of aggressive surgical treatment and adjuvant chemotherapy. Surgery 1983;94:709.

36. Wanebo HJ, Vezeridis MP. Carcinoma of the gallbladder. J Surg Oncol 1993;Suppl 3:134.

37. Donohue JH, Nagorney DM, Grand CS, Tsushima K. Carcinoma of the gallbladder: does radical resection improve outcome? Arch Surg 1990;125:237.

38. de Aretxabala X, Roa I, Araya JC, et al. Operative findings in patients with early forms of gallbladder cancer. Br J Surg 1990;77:291.

39. Brasfield RD. Right hepatic lobectomy for carcinoma of the gallbladder: a five-year cure. Ann Surg 1961;153:563.

40. Pack GT, Miller TR, Brasfield RD. Total right hepatic lobectomy for cancer of the gallbladder: report of three cases. Ann Surg 1955;142:6.

41. Ouchi K, Owada Y, Matsumo S. Prognostic factors in the surgical treatment of gallbladder carcinoma. Surgery 1987;101:731.

42. Torterolo E, Aizen B, Silva C, Bergalli L, Misa C, Beltran R. An approach to histologically diagnosed gallbladder carcinoma following cholecystectomy for presumed benign disease. J Surg Oncol 1993;Suppl 3:175.

43. Ogura Y, Mizumoto R, Isaji S, Kusada T, Matsuda S, Tabata M. Radical operations for carcinoma of the gallbladder: present status in Japan. World J Surg 1991;15:337.

44. Cubertafond P, Gainant A, Cucchiaro G. Surgical treatment of 724 carcinomas of the gallbladder: results of the French Surgical Association Survey. Ann Surg 1994;219:275.

45. Gagner M, Rossi RL. Radical operations for carcinoma of the gallbladder: present status in North America. World J Surg 1991;15:344.

46. Chao TC, Greager JA. Primary carcinoma of the gallbladder. Surgery 1989;106:467.

47. Fong Y, Brennan MF, Turnbull A, Colt DG, Blumgart LH. Gallbladder cancer discovered during laparoscopic surgery: potential for iatrogenic tumor dissemination. Arch Surg 1993;128:1054.

48. Clair DG, Lautz DB, Brooks DC. Rapid development of umbilical metastases after laparoscopic cholecystectomy for unsuspected gallbladder carcinoma. Surgery 1993; 113:355.

49. Bosset JF, Mantion G, Gillet M, et al. Primary carcinoma of the gallbladder: adjuvant postoperative external irradiation. Cancer 1989;64:1843.

50. Kurisu K, Hishikawa Y, Taniguchi M, et al. High-dose-rate intraluminal brachytherapy for postoperative residual tumor of the gallbladder carcinoma: a case report. Radiat Med 1991;9:241.

51. Todoroki T, Iwasaki Y, Orii K, et al. Resection combined with intraoperative radiation therapy (IORT) for stage IV (TNM) gallbladder carcinoma. World J Surg 1991;15: 357.

52. Falkson G, MacIntyre JM, Moertel CG. Eastern Cooperative Oncology Group experience with chemotherapy for inoperable gallbladder and bile duct cancer. Cancer 1984;54:965.

53. Makela JT, Kairaluoma MI. Superselective intra-arterial chemotherapy with mitomycin for gallbladder cancer. Br J Surg 1993;80:912.

54. Maram ES, Ludwig J, Kurland LT, Brian DD. Carcinoma of the gallbladder and extrahepatic bile ducts in Rochester, Minnesota, 1935–1971. Am J Epidemiol 1979;109: 152.

55. Gallinger S, Gluckman D, Langer B. Proximal bile duct cancer. Adv Surg 1990;23:89.

56. Akwari OE, van Heerden JA, Foulk WT, et al. Cancer of the bile ducts associated with ulcerative colitis. Ann Surg 1975;181:303.

57. Klatskin G. Adenocarcinoma of the hepatic duct at its bifurcation within the porta hepatis. Am J Med 1965;38: 241.

58. Saunders K, Longmire W Jr, Tompkins R, Chavez M, Cates J, Roslyn J. Diffuse bile duct tumors: guidelines for management. Am Surg 1991;57:816.

59. Beahrs OH, Henson DE, Hutter RVP, Kennedy BJ, eds. American Joint Committee on Cancer manual for staging of cancer, ed 4. Philadelphia, JB Lippincott, 1992:99.

60. Bismuth H, Nakache R, Diamond T. Management strategies in resection for hilar cholangiocarcinoma. Ann Surg 1992;215:31.

61. Nakayama T, Ikeda A, Okuda K. Percutaneous transhepatic drainage of the biliary tract: technique and results in 104 cases. Gastroenterology 1978;74:554.

62. McPherson GAD, Benjamin IS, Habib NA, Bowley NB, Blumgart LH. Percutaneous transhepatic drainage in obstructive jaundice: advantages and problems. Br J Surg 1982;69:261.

63. Pitt HA, Gomes AS, Lois JF, Mann LL, Deutsch LS, Longmire Jr WP. Does preoperative percutaneous transhe- patic biliary drainage reduce operative risk or increase hospital cost. Ann Surg 1985;201:545.

64. Nagorney DM, Donohue JH, Farnell MB, Schleck CD, Ilstrup DM. Outcomes after curative resections of cholangiocarcinoma. Arch Surg 1993;128:871.

65. Terblanche J. Carcinoma of the proximal extrahepatic biliary tree: definitive and palliative treatment. Surg Annu 1979;11:249.

66. Cameron JL, Broe P, Zuidema GD. Proximal bile duct tumors: surgical management with Silastic transhepatic biliary stents. Ann Surg 1982;196:412.

67. Lai ECS, Tompkins RK, Roslyn JJ, Mann LL. Proximal bile duct cancer: quality of survival. Ann Surg 1987;205: 111.

68. White TT. Skeletization resection and central hepatic resection in the treatment of bile duct cancer. World J Surg 1988;12:48.

69. Launois B, Maddern G. New facts in the surgical treatment of Klatskin tumours. J Surg Oncol 1993;Suppl 3: 147.

70. Baer HU, Stain SC, Dennison AR, Eggers B, Blumgart LH. Improvements in survival by aggressive resections of hilar cholangiocarcinoma. Ann Surg 1993;217:20.

71. Bengmark S, Ekberg H, Evander A, Klofver-Stahl B, Tranberg KG. Major liver resection for hilar cholangiocarcinoma. Ann Surg 1988;207:120.

72. Hadjis NS, Blenkharn JI, Alexander N, Benjamin IS, Blumgart LH. Outcome of radical surgery in hilar cholangiocarcinoma. Surgery 1990;107:597.

73. Shimada H, Izumi T, Note M, Seki H, Nakagawara G. Anterior segmentectomy with caudate lobectomy for hilar cholangiocarcinoma. Hepatogastroenterology 1993;40: 61.

74. Ogura Y, Mizumoto R, Tabata M, Matsuda S, Kusuda T. Surgical treatment of carcinoma of the hepatic duct confluence: analysis of 55 resected carcinomas. World J Surg 1993;17:85.

75. Tashiro S, Tsuji T, Kanemitsu K, Kanimoto Y, Hiraoka T, Miyauchi Y. Prolongation of survival for carcinoma at the hepatic duct confluence. Surgery 1993;113:270.

76. Lygidakis NJ, van der Heyde MN, van Dongen RJAM, Kromhout JG, Tytgat GNJ, Huibregtse K. Surgical approaches for unresectable primary carcinoma of the hepatic hilus. Surg Gynecol Obstet 1988;166:107.

77. Iwatsuki S, Gordon RD, Shaw BW, Starzl TE. Role of liver transplantation in cancer therapy. Ann Surg 1985;202: 401.

78. Boerma EJ. Research into the results of resection of hilar bile duct cancer. Surgery 1990;108:572.

79. Langer JC, Langer B, Taylor BR, Zeldin R, Cummings B. Carcinoma of the extrahepatic bile ducts: results of an aggressive surgical approach. Surgery 1985;98:752.

80. Beazley RM, Hadjis N, Benjamin IS, Blumgart LH. Clinicopathological aspects of high bile duct cancer: experience with resection and bypass surgical treatments. Ann Surg 1984;199:623.

81. Cameron JL, Pitt HA, Zinner MJ, Kaufman SL, Coleman J. Management of proximal cholangiocarcinomas by sur-

gical resection and radiotherapy. Am J Surg 1990;159:91.

82. Pinson CW, Rossi RL. Extended right hepatic lobectomy, left hepatic lobectomy and skeletonization resection for proximal bile duct cancer. World J Surg 1988;12:52.

83. Ottow RT, August DA, Sugarbaker PH. Treatment of proximal biliary tract carcinoma: an overview of techniques and results. Surgery 1985;97:251.

84. Gibson RN, Yeung E, Hadjis N, et al. Percutaneous transhepatic endoprostheses for hilar cholangiocarcinoma. Am J Surg 1988;156:363.

85. Gray R. Percutaneous biliary drainage with emphasis on hilar lesions. Can J Gastroenterol 1990;4:579.

86. LaBerge JM, Doherty M, Gordon RL, Ring EJ. Hilar malignancy: treatment with an expandable metallic transhepatic biliary stent. Radiology 1990;177:793.

87. Blumgart LH, Kelley CJ. Hepaticojejunostomy in benign and malignant high bile duct stricture: approaches to the left hepatic ducts. Br J Surg 1984;71:257.

88. Terblanche J, Kahn D, Bornman PC, Werner D. The role of U tube palliative treatment in high bile duct carcinoma. Surgery 1988;103:624.

89. Soulez G, Gagner M, Therasse E, et al. Malignant biliary obstruction: preliminary results of palliative treatment with hepaticogastrostomy under fluoroscopic, endoscopic, and laparoscopic control. Radiology 1994;192:241.

90. Schoenthaler R, Phillips TL, Castro J, Efird JT, Better A, Way LW. Carcinoma of the extrahepatic bile ducts: the University of California at San Francisco experience. Ann Surg 1994;219:267.

91. Grove MK, Hermann RE, Vogt DP, Broughan TA. Role of radiation after operative palliation in cancer of the proximal bile ducts. Am J Surg 1991;161:454.

92. Myers WC, Jones RS. Internal radiation for bile duct cancer. World J Surg 1988;12:99.

93. Oberfield RA, Rossi RL. The role of chemotherapy in the treatment of bile duct cancer. World J Surg 1988;12:105.

Digestive Tract Surgery: A Text and Atlas, edited by Richard H. Bell,
Layton F. Rikkers, and Michael W. Mulholland.
Lippincott-Raven Publishers, Philadelphia, © 1996.

17

Atlas of Biliary Surgery

William C. Meyers

Preoperative Preparation

Most patients who are to undergo an operation on the biliary tract should receive perioperative systemic antibiotics. Broad-specturm coverage is important when the biliary tract is obstructed or contains indwelling stents. A first- or second-generation cephalosporin is sufficient for uncomplicated gallstone disease.

It is important to image the obstructed biliary tract before an operation. Imaging should be done by the percutaneous transhepatic route for proximal lesions and by endoscopic retrograde cholangiography for distal lesions. If preoperative cholangitis is present, biliary decompression by either a transhepatic or endoscopic stent should be accomplished when possible. There is no evidence that routine preoperative biliary decompression decreases postoperative morbidity or mortality in the uninfected patient. However, preoperatively placed stents can be helpful in operative identification of previously injured bile ducts and in other situations in which biliary anatomy is unclear.

Upper abdominal incisions can cause postoperative pulmonary compromise. Therefore, preoperative attention to bronchial toilet and to optimization of lung function is important in patients with pulmonary diseases. Consideration should also be given to placement of an epidural catheter for postoperative pain control. A nasogastric tube and Foley catheter should be placed before laparoscopic biliary surgery to minimize the potential of stomach or bladder injury during trocar insertion.

=====

SECTION I   *Laparoscopic Cholecystectomy*

The laparoscopic approach is used for over 80% of patients undergoing cholecystectomy. The advantages of laparoscopic cholecystectomy over open cholecystectomy are less postoperative pain and a more rapid recovery. A significant disadvantage is a higher incidence of bile duct injuries. A major emphasis of this presentation is the avoidance of injury to the biliary tract during performance of a laparoscopic cholecystectomy. The principles for exposing and dissecting important anatomic structures during laparoscopic cholecystectomy are the same as those used for the open operation.

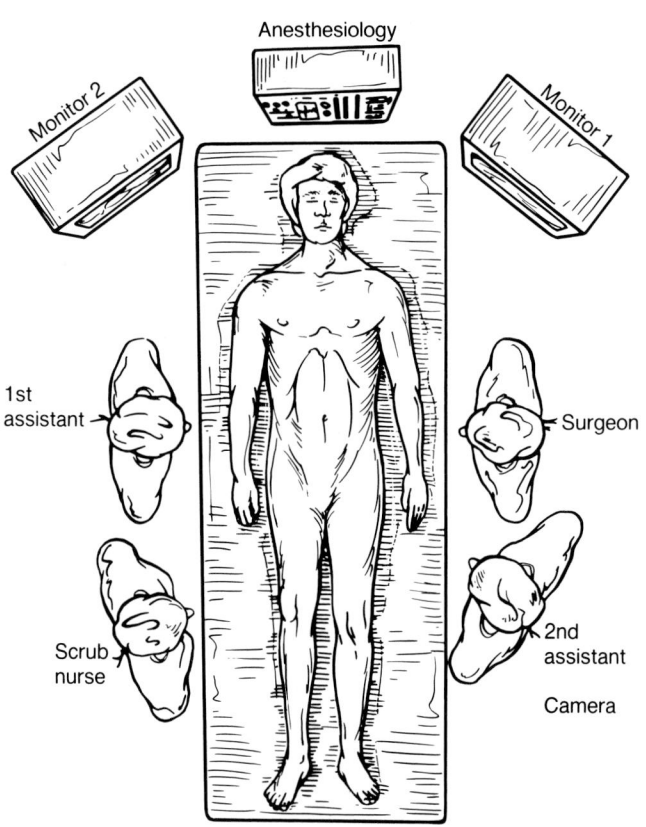

Figure 17-I-1

Operating Room Set-Up

The primary surgeon operates from the patient's left side. The assistant stands directly opposite him or her. The second assistant stands to the surgeon's left and operates the camera; the scrub nurse stands to the first assistant's right. The anesthesiologist is at the head of the table, with television monitors, cautery, and insufflator at the sides. Various mechanical devices can serve as retractors or robotic arms and can be placed on either side of the table. In the best arrangement, the monitors are suspended from the ceiling and are capable of being maneuvered into different positions. A nasogastric tube and Foley catheter are placed before the operation is begun.

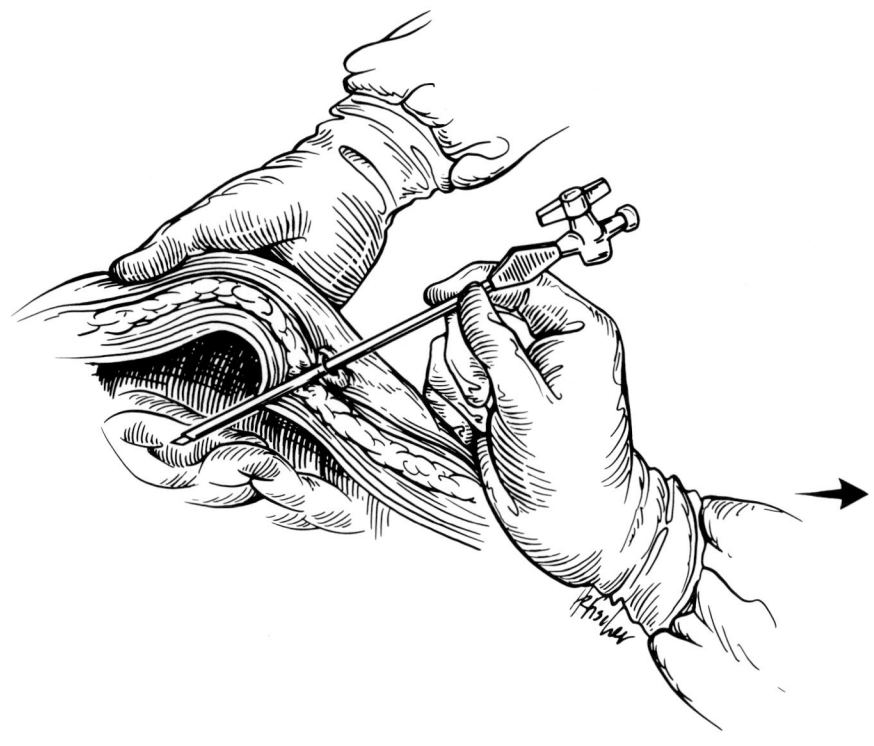

Figure 17-I-2

Blind Entry of the Abdomen

Two methods for initial entry into the abdomen can be used—the blind technique and the Hassan (open) technique. In the blind method, a Veress needle is inserted without the position of the intraabdominal viscera being known. The patient is placed in steep Trendelenburg position. A small incision is made at the inferior aspect of the umbilicus, and the needle is inserted through the fascia and peritoneum while the skin is retracted superiorly with towel clips or the fascia is retracted with Kocher clamps. Two pops are noticed as the needle enters the abdomen. It is important to aim the Veress needle directly toward the pelvic cul-de-sac and not at the aortoiliac vessels. Carbon dioxide insufflation is then begun at low flow volumes. When the insufflation pressure (in millimeters of mercury) is in single digits, it is likely that there is free flow into the peritoneal cavity, and carbon dioxide insufflation can be converted to high flow. Pressures often initially fluctuate with changes in position of the needle because of proximity to the omentum or other abdominal structures. Several liters of carbon dioxide are required to distend the abdomen of a normal-sized adult patient. After the abdomen becomes evenly distended and tympanitic, a 10-mm trocar is inserted at the umbilical site. The trocar is inserted toward the pelvis with a twisting motion rather than forceful pushing. Entrance into the free peritoneal cavity is suggested by free movement of the tip of the trocar after the stylet has been removed; it is confirmed by insertion of the camera. Some surgeons use ''grips'' to hold each trocar in place. Peak insufflation pressure is usually maintained at 15 mmHg except in pediatric or obese patients. In children, less pressure is required; in obese persons, an insufflation pressure of 18 to 20 mmHg may be necessary.

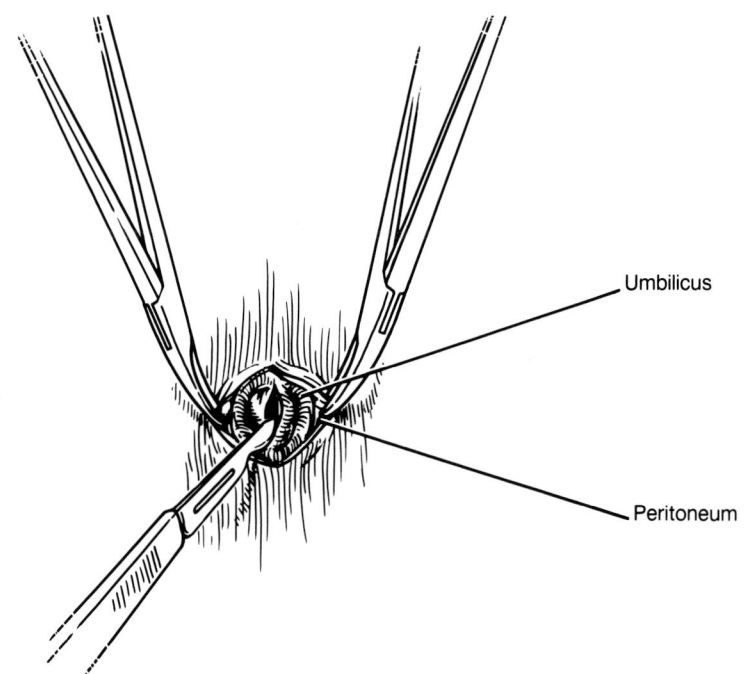

Umbilicus

Peritoneum

Figure 17-I-3

Hassan Technique

Most surgeons prefer the Hassan technique of introducing the trocar into the abdomen. A skin incision only slightly longer than the one used with the closed technique is made directly through the umbilicus or slightly below it. Kocher clamps grasp each side of the fascia, which is divided by cautery. The peritoneum can be incised after grasping it with tonsil clamps or can be bluntly entered with the finger. The exact location of the skin incision may vary when other abdominal incisions are present.

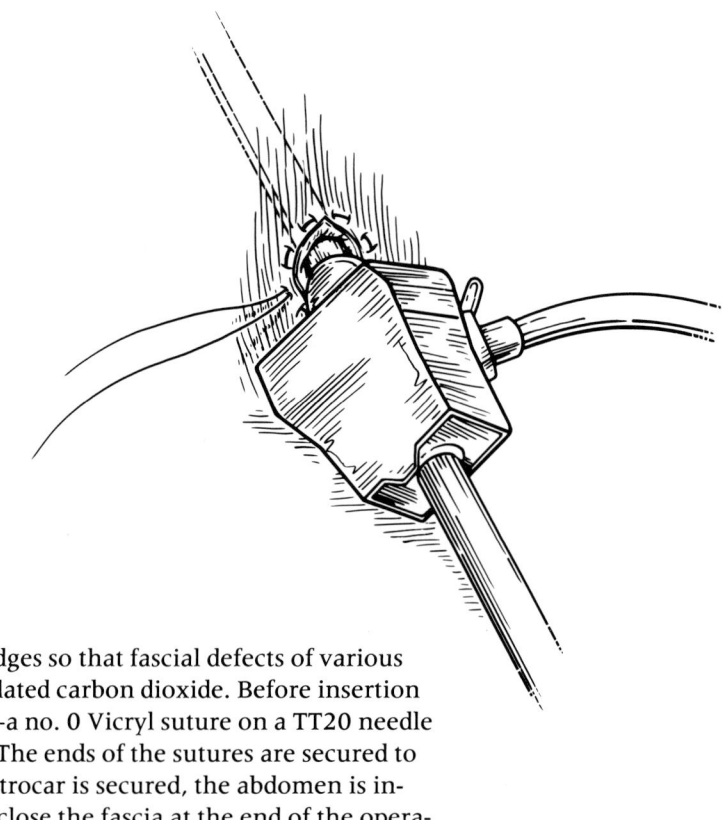

Figure 17-I-4

Trocar Placement

Most Hassan-type trocars are cone shaped with ridges so that fascial defects of various sizes can be accommodated without leak of insufflated carbon dioxide. Before insertion of the trocar, two pursestring sutures are placed—a no. 0 Vicryl suture on a TT20 needle in the fascia and a no. 1 nylon suture in the skin. The ends of the sutures are secured to the trocar to prevent it from dislodging. After the trocar is secured, the abdomen is insufflated. The fascial pursestring suture is used to close the fascia at the end of the operation. The nylon skin suture is removed.

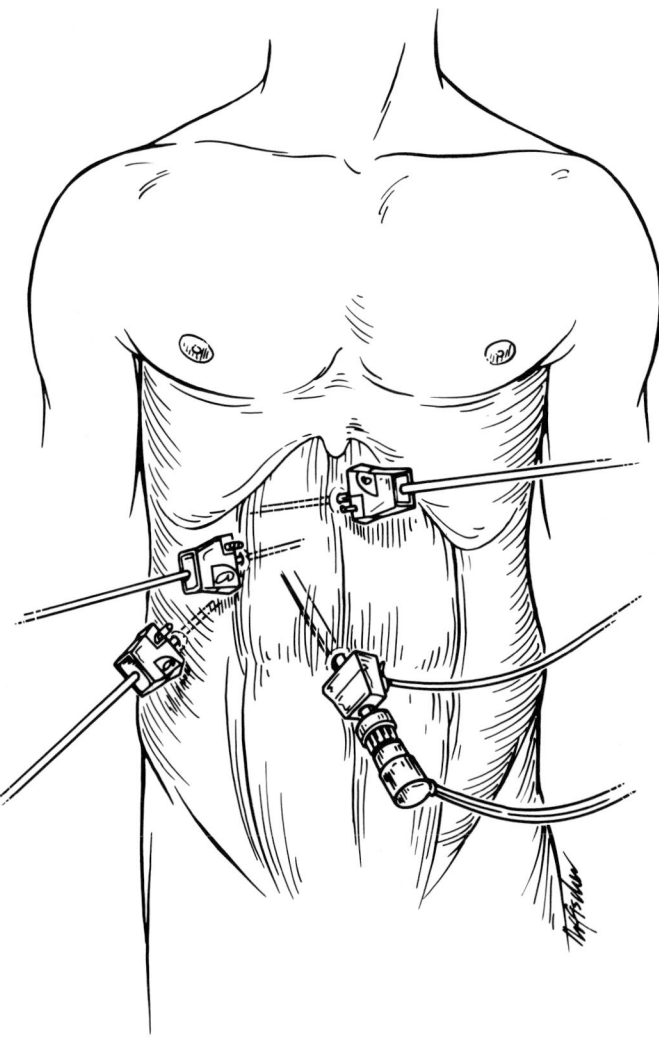

Figure 17-I-5

Trocar Ports

The umbilical port is used for the camera. The other three ports are placed in a line where a standard Kocher incision would be made if conversion to an open operation is necessary. A 10-mm trocar is inserted in the subxiphoid position, and 5-mm trocars are inserted at the two subcostal sites. The middle subcostal trocar is placed slightly closer to the subxiphoid trocar if the surgeon wishes to operate with two hands. More often, the first assistant serves as the surgeon's second hand. Each trocar is inserted under direct vision with a twisting rather than a pushing motion. The camera operator must visualize both the trocar site and underlying viscera to avoid injury to the patient. The subxiphoid trocar is directed to the right during insertion so that it penetrates the anterior aspect of the falciform ligament. A high position of this trocar is preferable, since it assists in subsequent dissection of the triangle of Calot.

After the trocars are in place, the peritoneal cavity is inspected, using both the Trendelenburg and the reverse Trendelenburg positions, to rule out other abnormalities. Laparoscopic exploration is not as sensitive as open exploration for detecting incidental abdominal pathology.

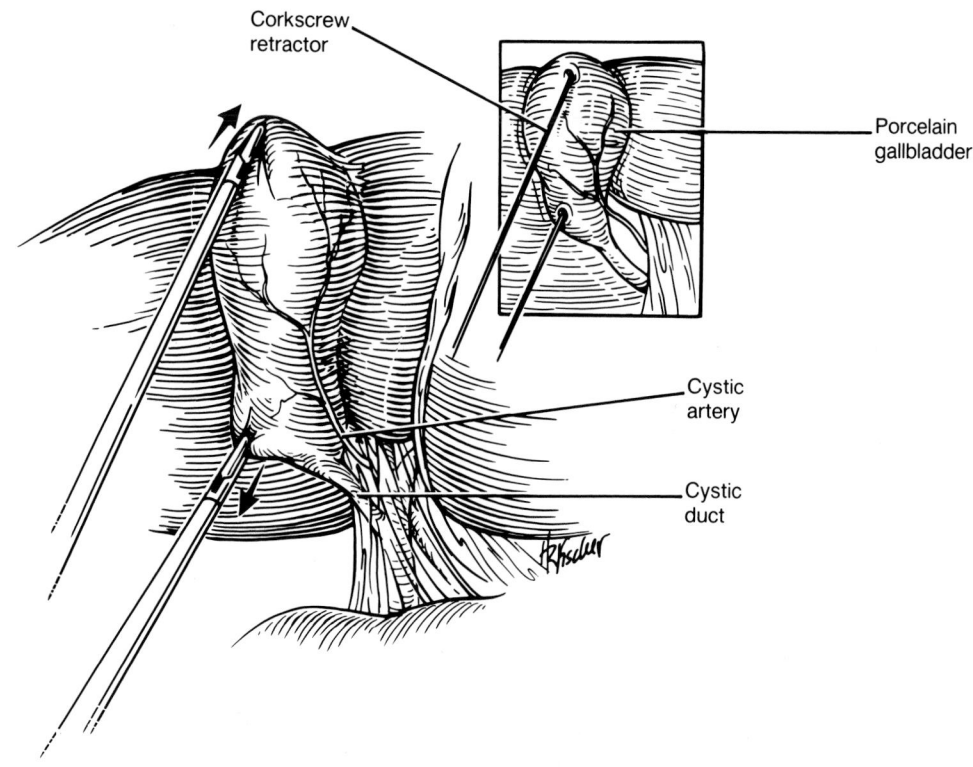

Figure 17-I-6

Gallbladder Removal

After the patient is placed in a reverse Trendelenburg position with the right side rotated slightly upward, adhesions to the gallbladder, if present, are bluntly or sharply dissected. The precise method of gallbladder removal depends on the abnormality. For example, a markedly distended gallbladder from acute cholecystitis is decompressed with a suction trocar before dissection of the vessels or gallbladder bed.

Through the lateral port, the fundus of the gallbladder is grasped with ratcheted forceps and retracted upward toward the diaphragm. This maneuver elevates the liver so that the triangle of Calot can be visualized. Through the middle port, the ampulla (infundibulum) of the gallbladder is grasped and retracted laterally and inferiorly. The cystic artery can often be seen on the gallbladder. The cystic duct is initially seen where it enters the gallbladder.

A variety of retractors can be used depending on the abnormality. For example, in acute cholecystitis, the gallbladder wall may be friable and easily torn with a grasper. A balloon-type catheter can be inserted into the gallbladder and used for retraction. A screw-type retractor (**inset**) may be required for a calcified (porcelain) gallbladder.

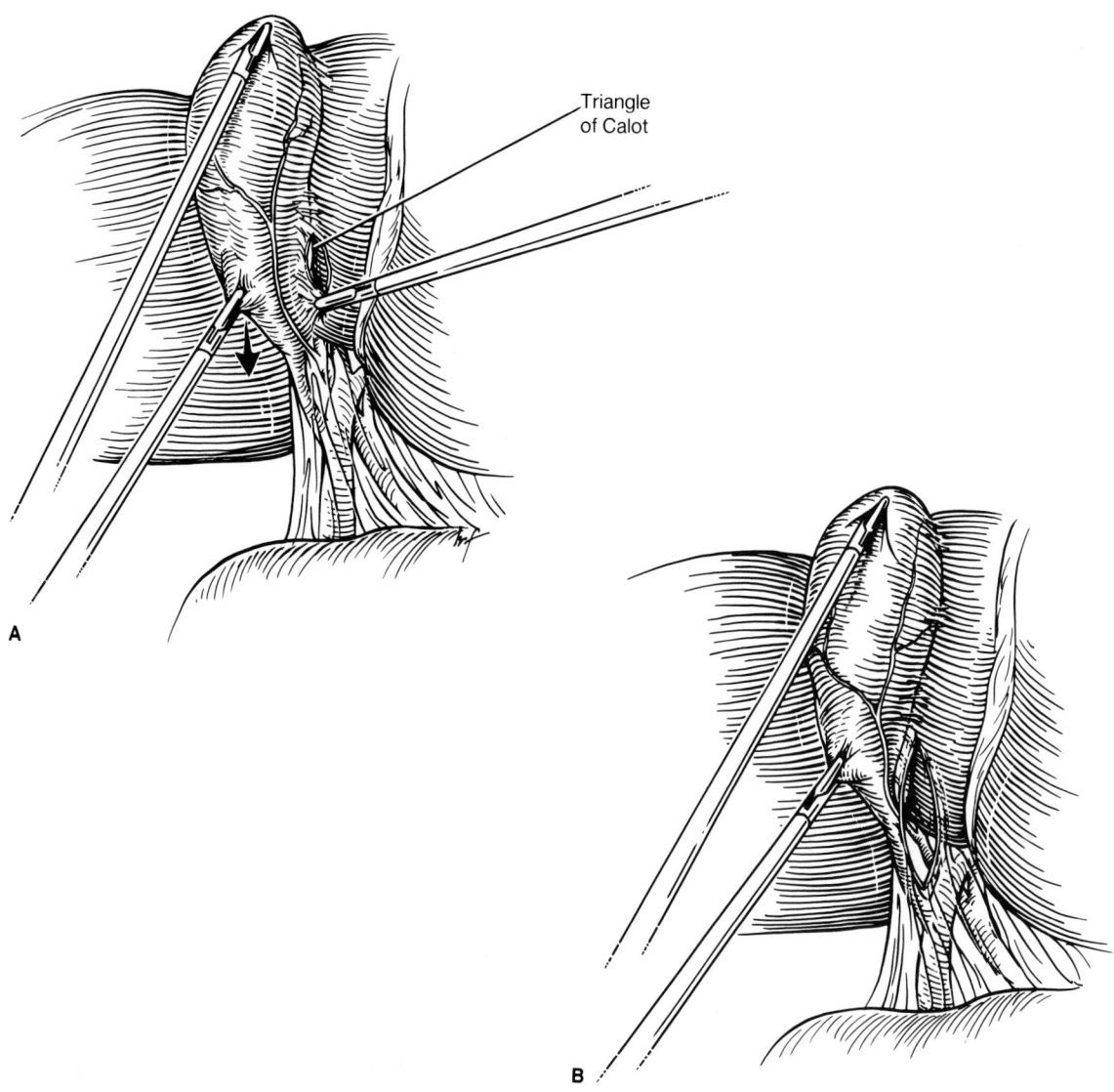

Triangle
of Calot

Figure 17-I-7

Peritoneal Incision

(**A**) Before any dissection other than adhesiolysis, a peritoneal incision is made in the triangle of Calot, which is bordered by the inferior edge of the liver, the cystic duct, and the common hepatic duct. The entire triangle of Calot is not dissected because that would include dissection of the hepatic duct area, which should be avoided.

(**B**) However, the superior border of the gallbladder needs to be visualized to identify the origin of the cystic duct.

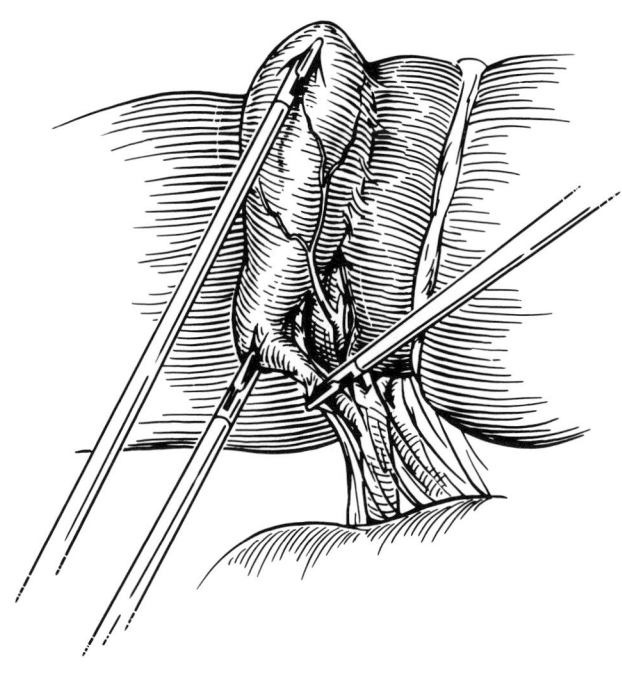

Figure 17-I-8

Dissection of the Inferior Aspect of the Gallbladder

The infundibulum of the gallbladder can be moved alternately anteriorly and posteriorly to visualize its posterior aspect. Dissection of this entire area is completed before clips are placed on either the cystic artery or the cystic duct.

Dissection is done primarily through the subxiphoid port, using a straight, blunt instrument. Fine instruments are not necessary and can be damaged during these maneuvers. Cautery should be used sparingly. In experienced hands, endoshears are useful for much of the dissection, including dissection of the gallbladder bed. However, in inexperienced hands, this technique can be dangerous. The correct direction of dissection is from the gallbladder toward the liver hilum. The cystic artery is identified as it enters the gallbladder, and after verification that it is not the right hepatic artery, it is doubly clipped proximally, singly clipped on the gallbladder side, and divided with endoshears. The use of cautery or laser is inappropriate for division of the cystic duct or artery. Heat transference to the common hepatic duct can result in a stricture, which may not be identified for months or even years later. The cystic duct is completely dissected where it enters the gallbladder, but dissection is not carried to its junction with the common bile duct.

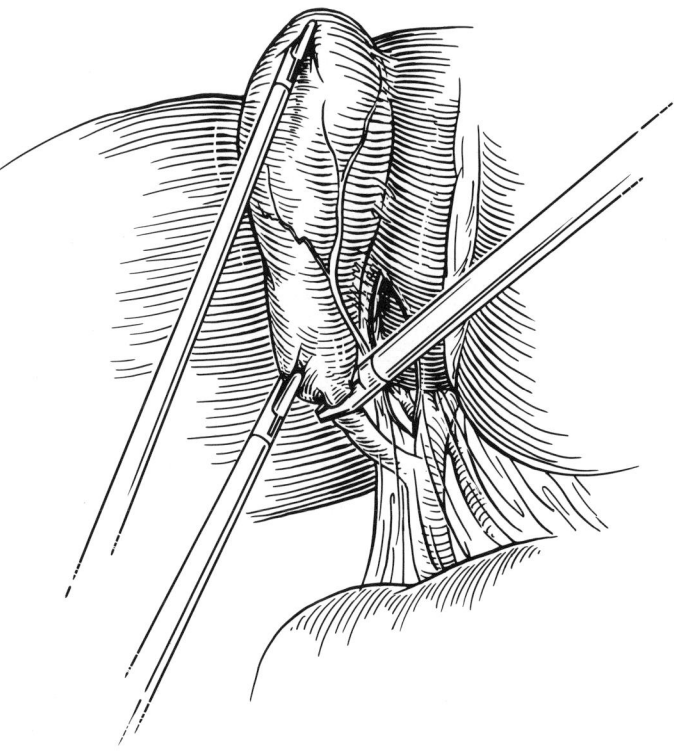

Figure 17-I-9

Selective Cholangiography

Selective cholangiography rather than routine cholangiography, which is used liberally, is practiced. Depending on the circumstances, the study may be helpful to identify common duct pathology or aberrant biliary anatomy to prevent injury. One clip is placed on the proximal cystic duct as close to the gallbladder as possible, so that it does not interfere with subsequent dissection. Before this clip is placed, the cystic duct should be milked toward the gallbladder with the dissector to dislodge a cystic duct stone if present so that it is not pushed into the common bile duct during insertion of the cholangiographic catheter.

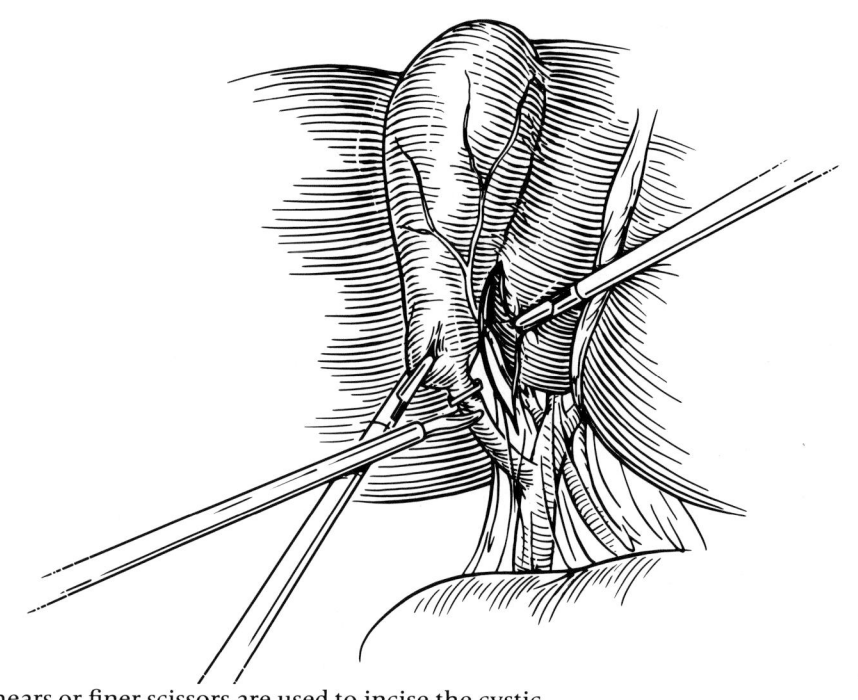

Figure 17-I-10

Incision of the Cystic Duct

After the proximal clip is placed, endoshears or finer scissors are used to incise the cystic duct across about half of its diameter. Total division of the cystic duct makes cholangiography considerably more difficult. The incision should be placed just distal to the clip.

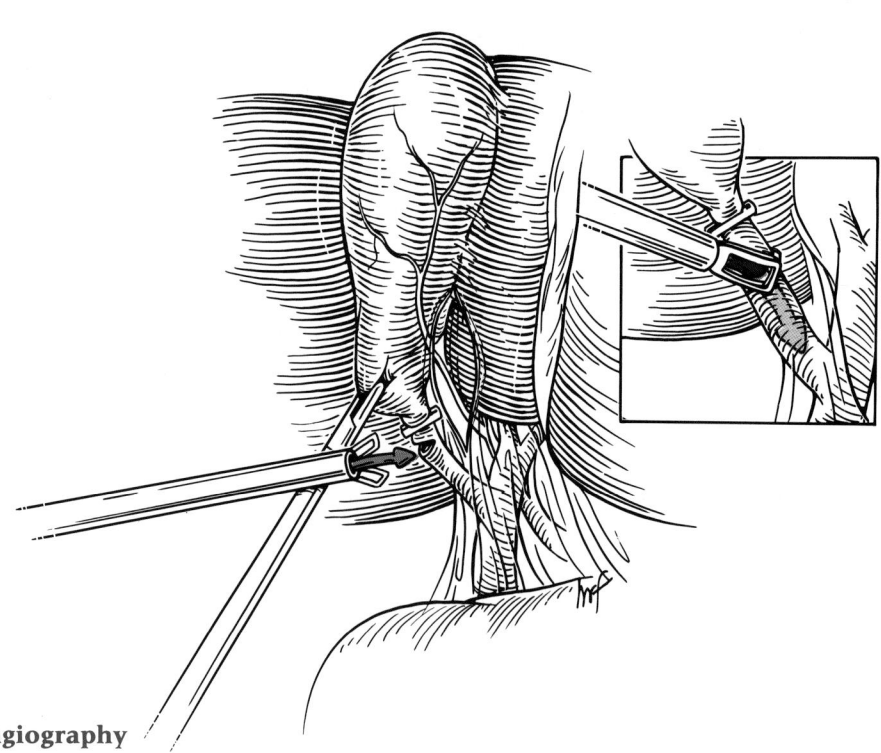

Figure 17-I-11

Taut Catheterization and Cholangiography

A taut catheter is inserted into the cystic duct after irrigation of the site of insertion if debris or blood is present. A special clamp secures the catheter within the duct. Cholangiography should be performed using fluoroscopy. Fluoroscopy is rapid and efficient, helps to distinguish air bubbles from questionable lesions, and ensures complete filling of the duct in real time. If a stone is identified, laparoscopic common duct exploration (see Section II) can be done while the fluoroscope is still in the room.

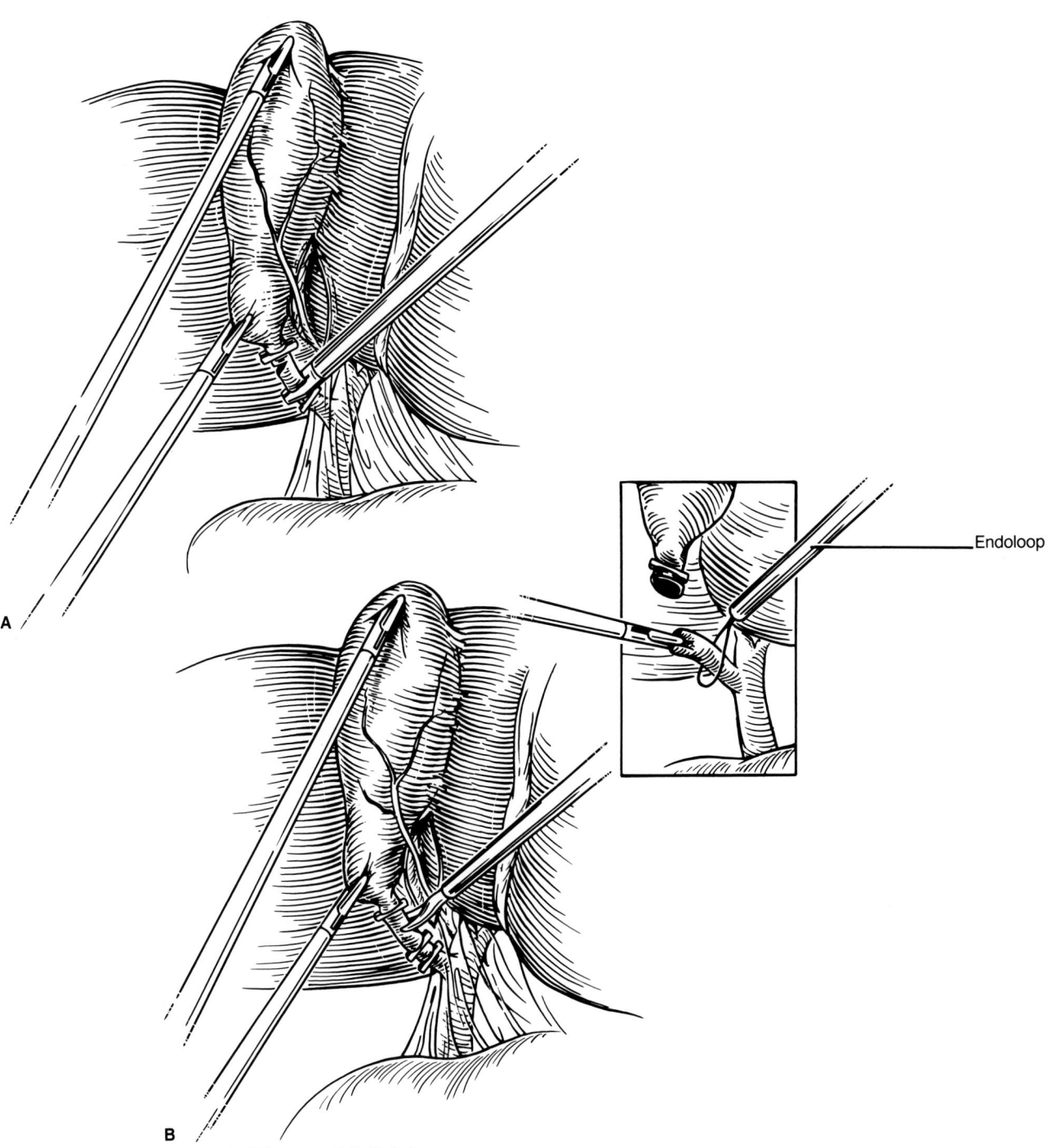

Endoloop

Figure 17-I-12

Cystic Duct and Artery Division

(**A**) After cholangiography, the catheter is removed and two clips are placed on the cystic duct proximal to the incision.

(**B**) The cystic duct is then divided with scissors. When the duct is friable or a retained stone is suspected, an endoloop (*inset*) should be used instead of, or in addition to, clips. Clips may shear through a friable duct in a patient with acute cholecystitis or can be dislodged during performance of postoperative endoscopic retrograde cholangiography.

(Continued)

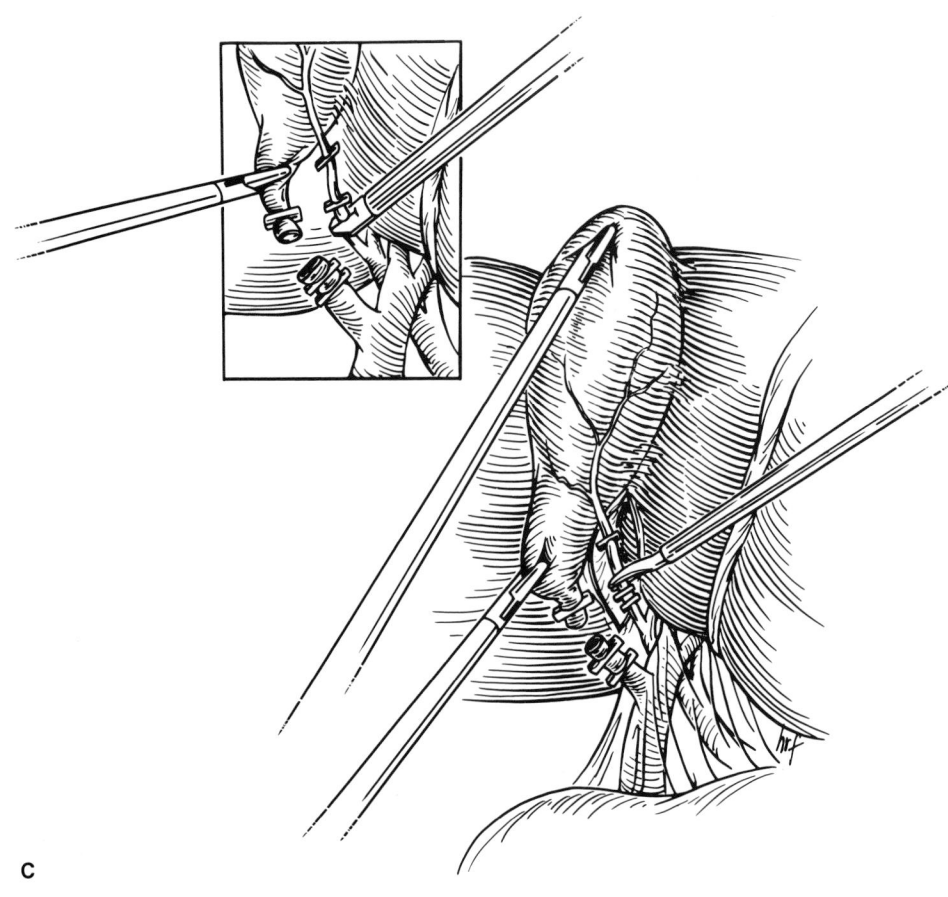

C

Figure 17-I-12. *(Continued)*

(C) After the cystic duct and artery are divided, the gallbladder infundibulum is retracted with enough tension to expose the space behind it (the inferior aspect of the triangle of Calot).

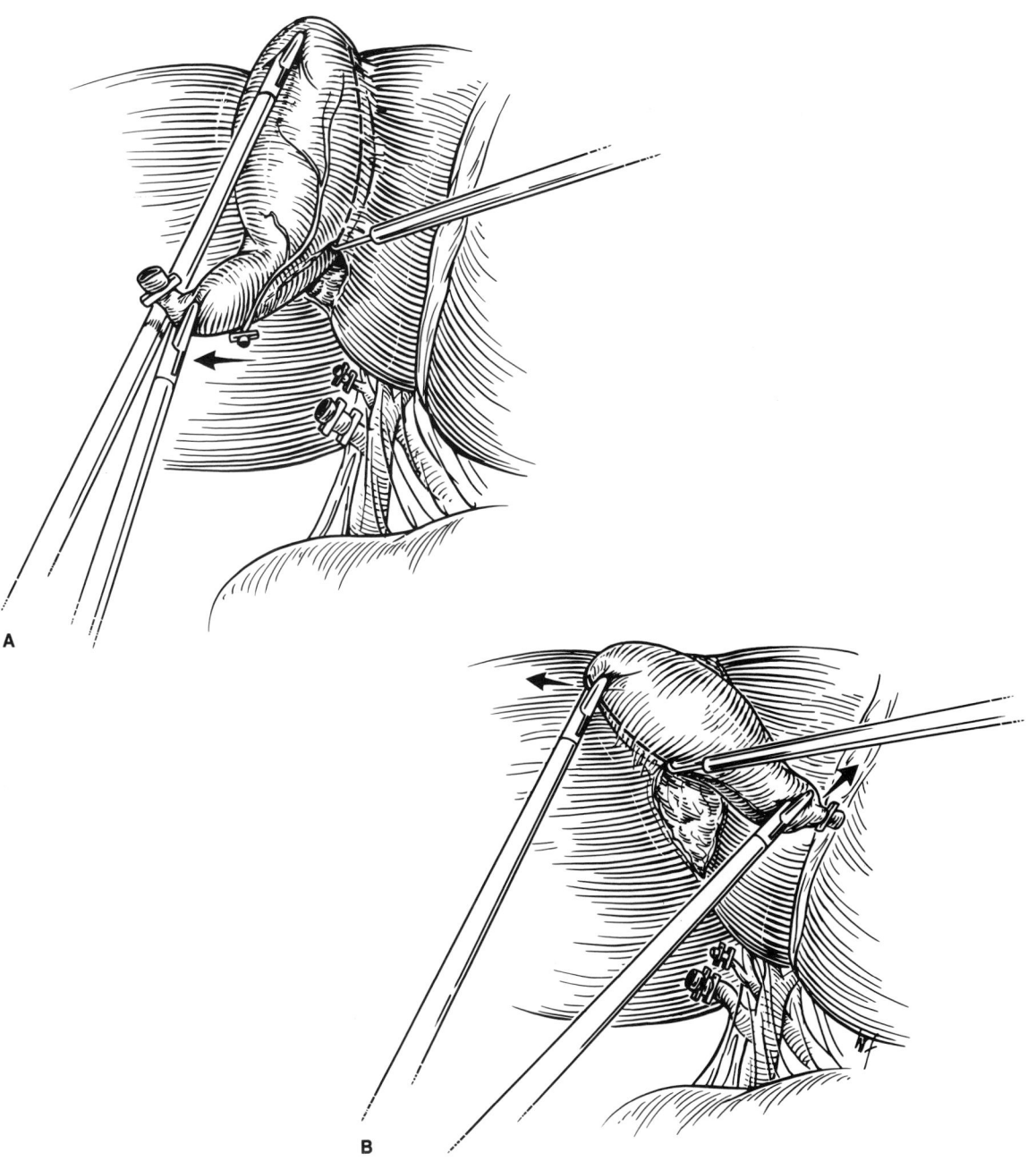

Figure 17-I-13

Gallbladder Dissection

(**A**) Small vessels are cauterized before they are divided, and minute ducts are identified and clipped. Clues to ductal injury include a large cystic duct, persistent bile drainage from an unidentified source, or accessory structures within the gallbladder bed. The ampulla or body of the gallbladder is retracted with plain or ratcheted forceps, the position of which is intermittently changed to avoid perforation of the gallbladder. A hook cautery or endoshears is used for most of this dissection, which is carried out close to the gallbladder wall to minimize bleeding from the liver.

(**B**) The posterior aspect of the gallbladder dissection.

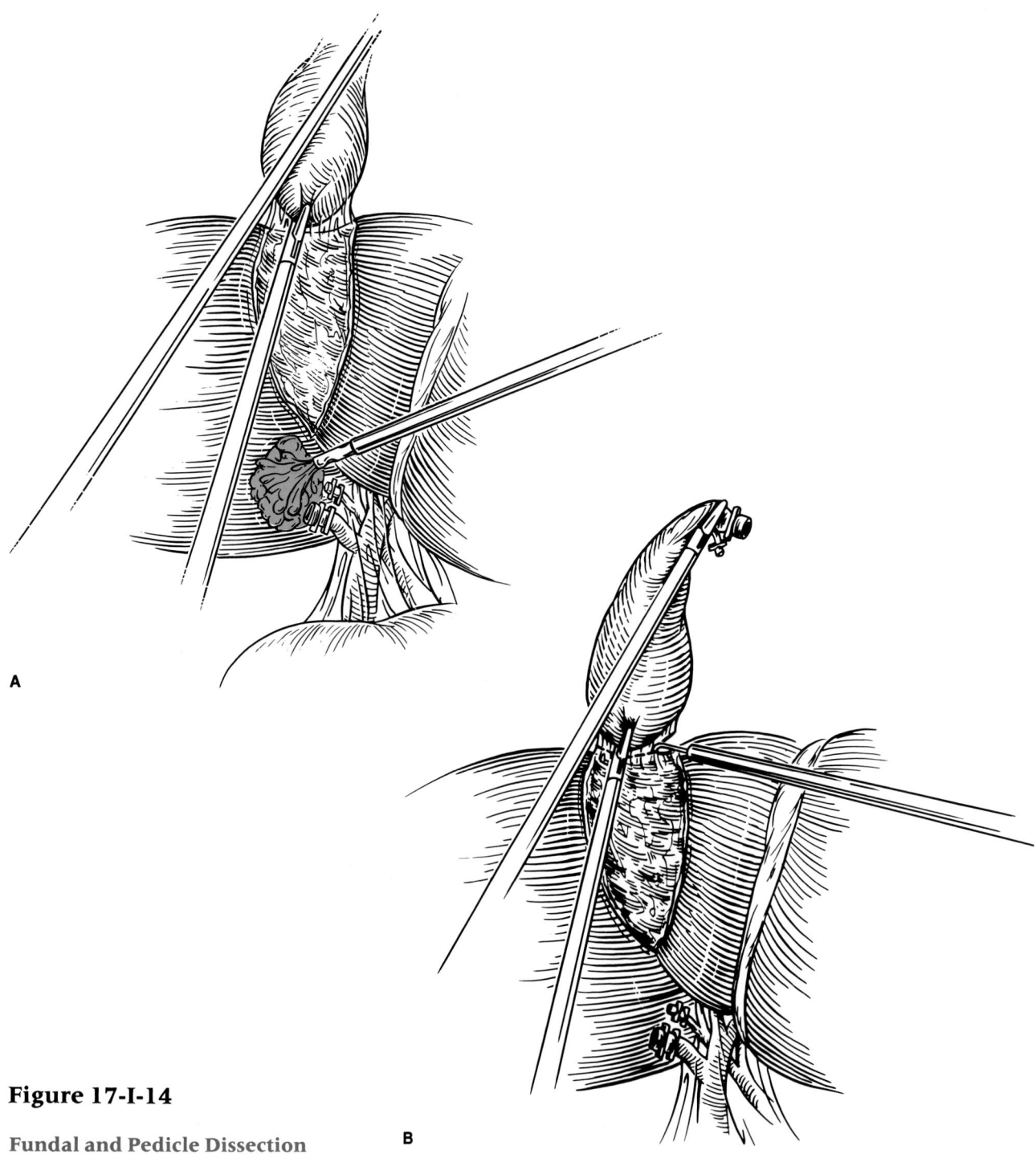

Figure 17-I-14

Fundal and Pedicle Dissection

(**A**) The most difficult part of the dissection is usually at the fundus. It is often necessary to reposition the retractors to complete this dissection. The repositioning creates the appropriate countertension for identification of the correct plane. It is best to irrigate and inspect the hilum of the liver while the gallbladder is still attached by a pedicle and can be used for retraction. Most of the irrigating solution gravitates to the right gutter, where it is easily aspirated.

(**B**) The remaining pedicle to the gallbladder is divided.

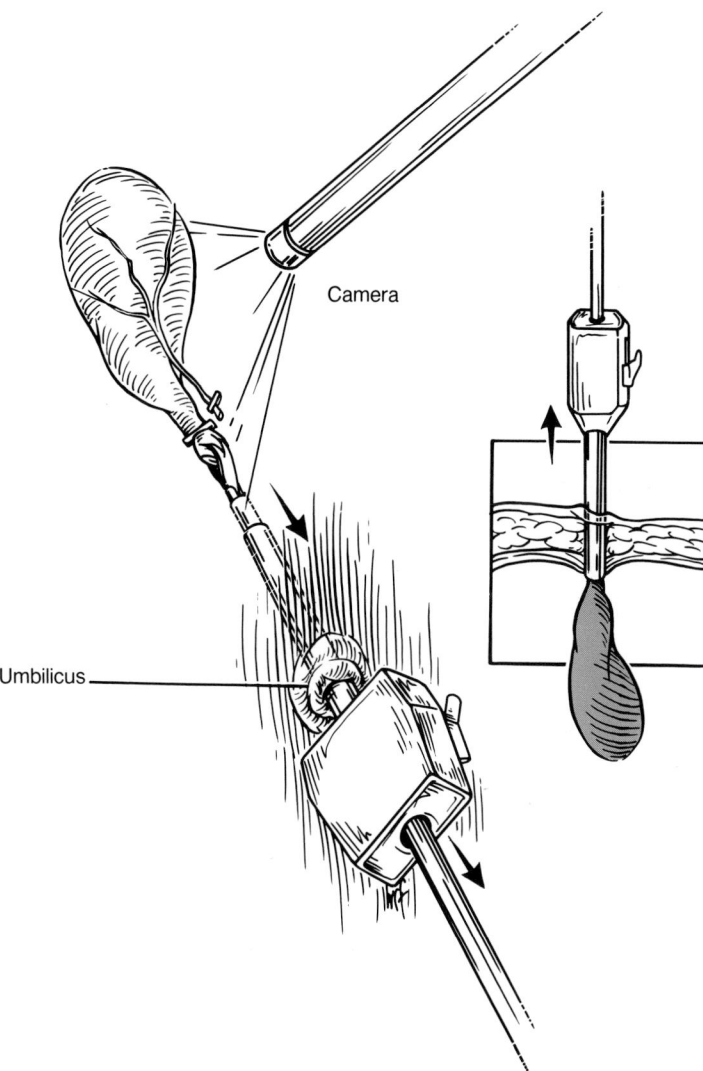

Camera

Umbilicus

Figure 17-I-15

Removal of the Gallbladder

The gallbladder is usually removed through the umbilical port, after the camera is changed to the subxiphoid port. The gallbladder is grasped at the cystic duct end by a ratcheted instrument that has been inserted through the umbilical port and is removed. An alternative is the use of the epigastric port to remove the gallbladder. Small gallbladders can be removed easily that way without necessitating a change in the position of the camera.

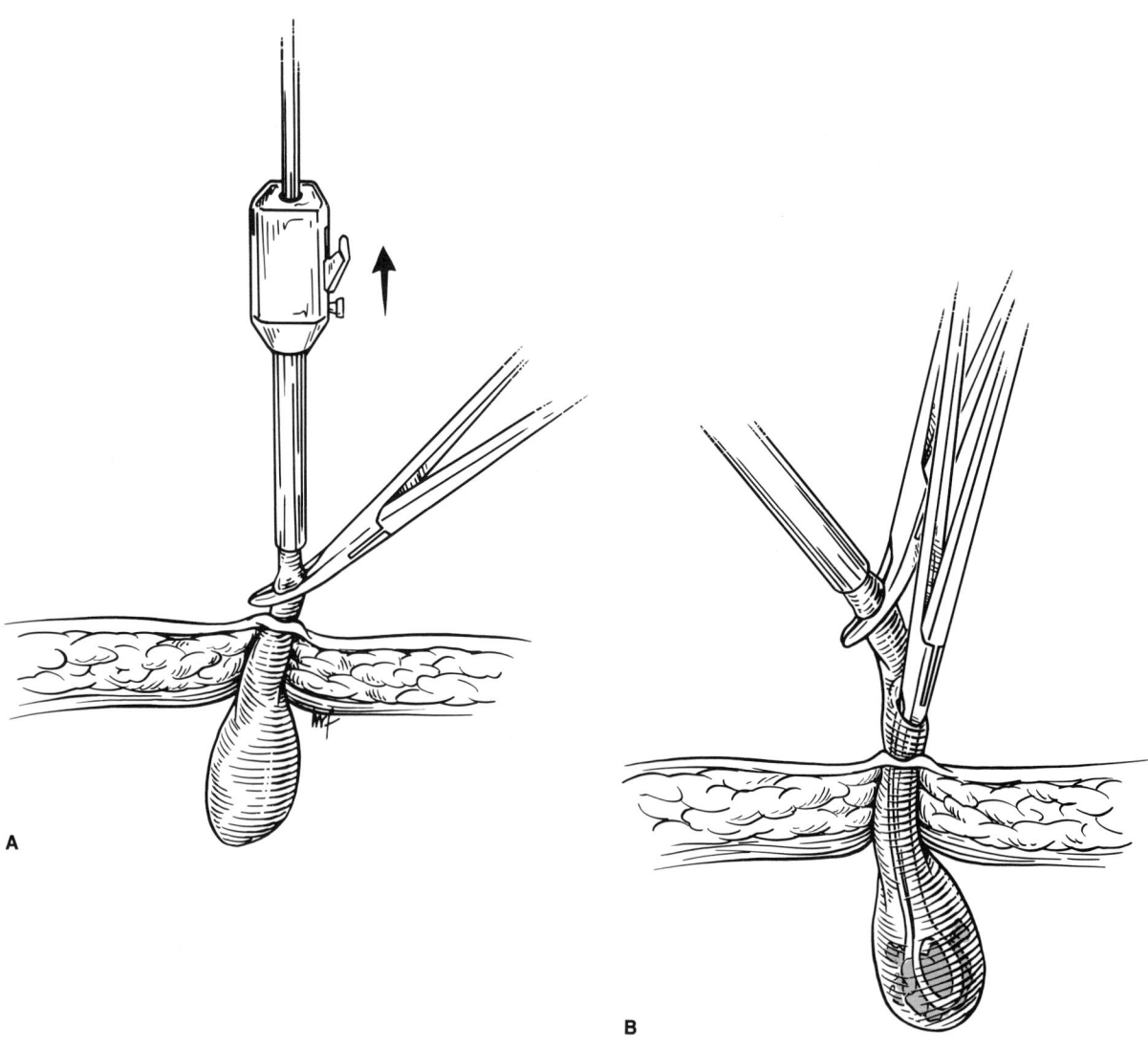

Figure 17-I-16

Volume Reduction

(**A**) It is often necessary to reduce the volume of the gallbladder contents before it can be removed.

(**B**) Bile can be aspirated and stones crushed by either a sucker or a stone forceps. Occasionally, the fascial incision must be extended to remove the gallbladder. If the Hassan technique is used, this necessitates replacing the fascial pursestring suture.

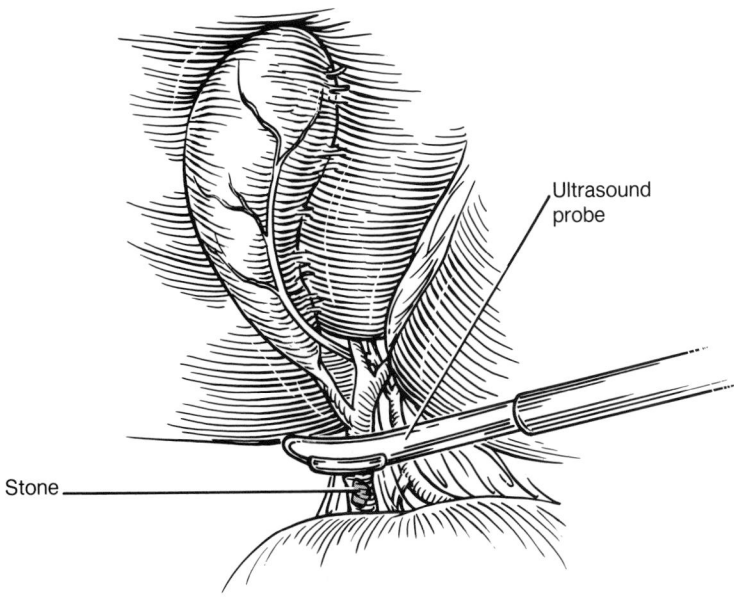

Figure 17-I-17

Laparoscopic Ultrasonography

An alternative to cholangiography is laparoscopic ultrasonography. Its accuracy depends on the operator, and comparative studies of its effectiveness are ongoing.

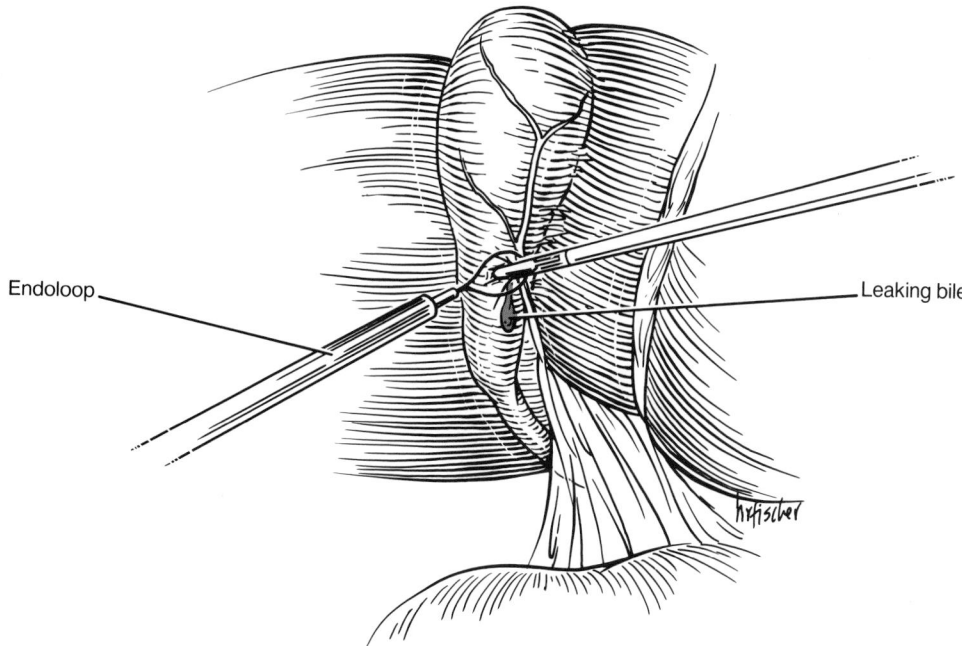

Figure 17-I-18

Repair of Perforation

Gallbladder perforations secondary to retraction can be repaired with endoloops, patched with clips, or temporarily closed with grasper retractors to avoid bile and stone spillage during the dissection. Spilled stones should be removed, since they can lead to complications.

SECTION II   *Open Cholecystectomy*

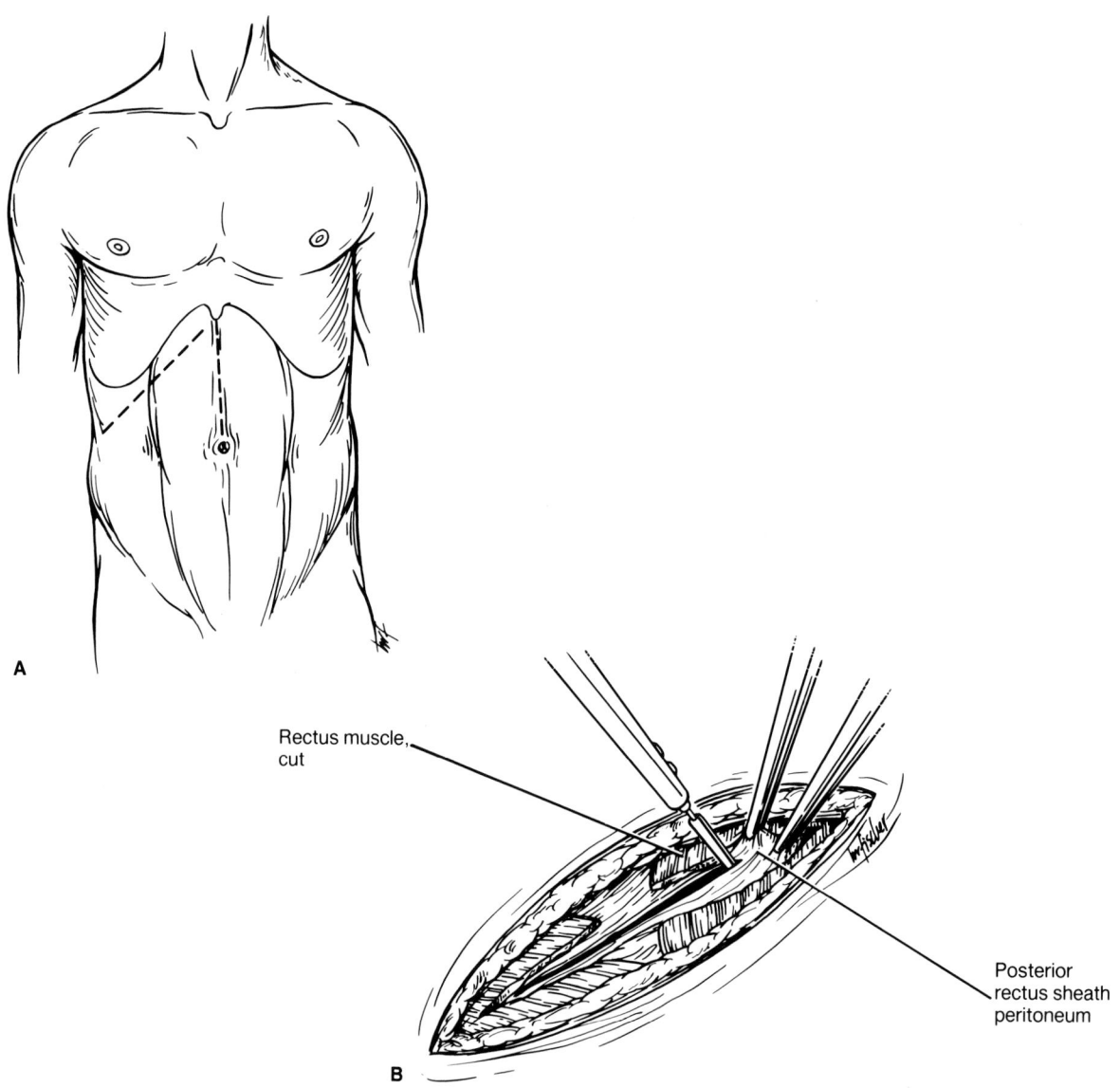

Figure 17-II-1

Incision

(**A**) A right subcostal (Kocher) incision is most commonly used for an open cholecystectomy. This incision is made two fingerbreadths below the right costal margin. Alternatively, a midline incision can be used.

(**B**) The incision is carried through the anterior fascia, the rectus muscle, and the posterior fascia, and is extended just beyond the midline. The surgeon stands to the patient's right side, although it may be easier to perform the operation from the patient's left side when a midline incision is used.

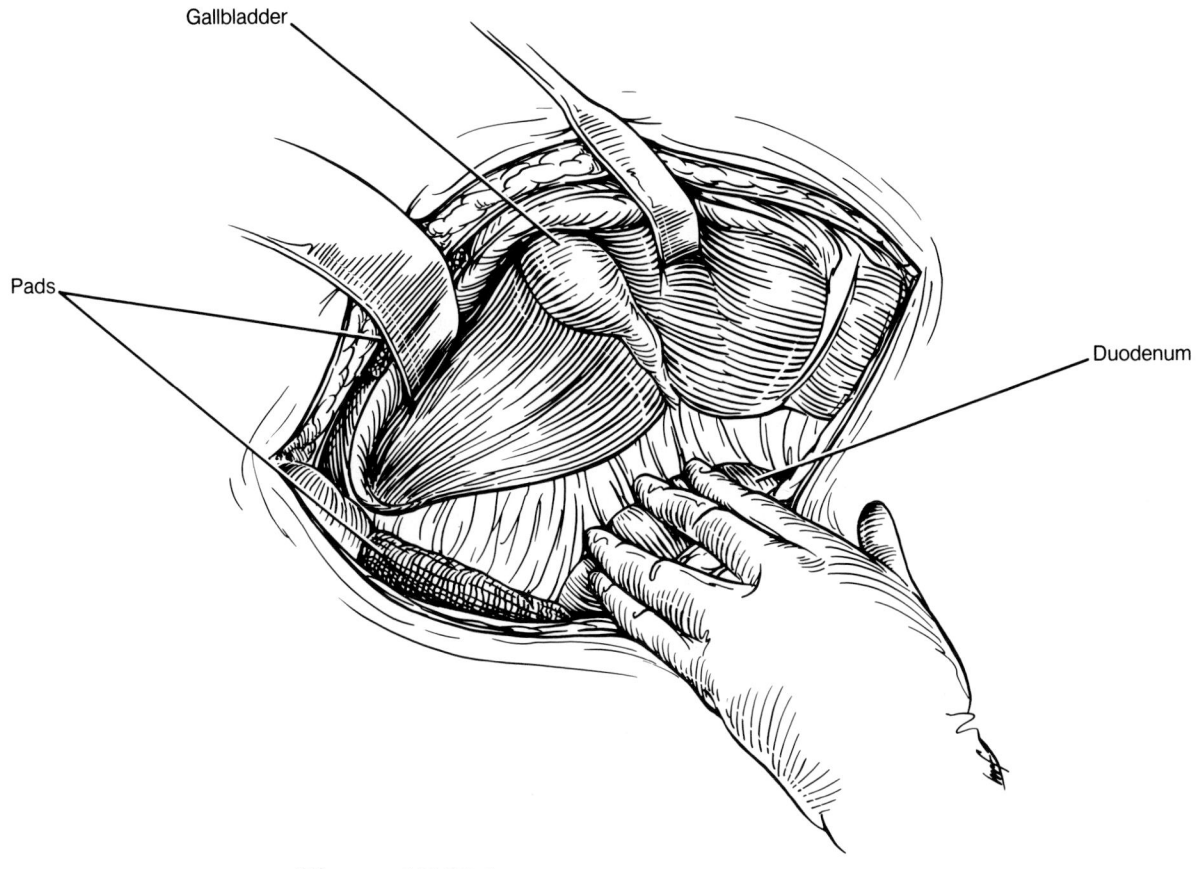

Gallbladder

Pads

Duodenum

Figure 17-II-2

Retractor Placement

After the abdomen is explored manually, adhesions are taken down from the gallbladder, and packs are placed above the liver and in the right gutter to retract the right colon. Retractors are placed on the costal margin and on the quadrate lobe just to the left of the gallbladder.

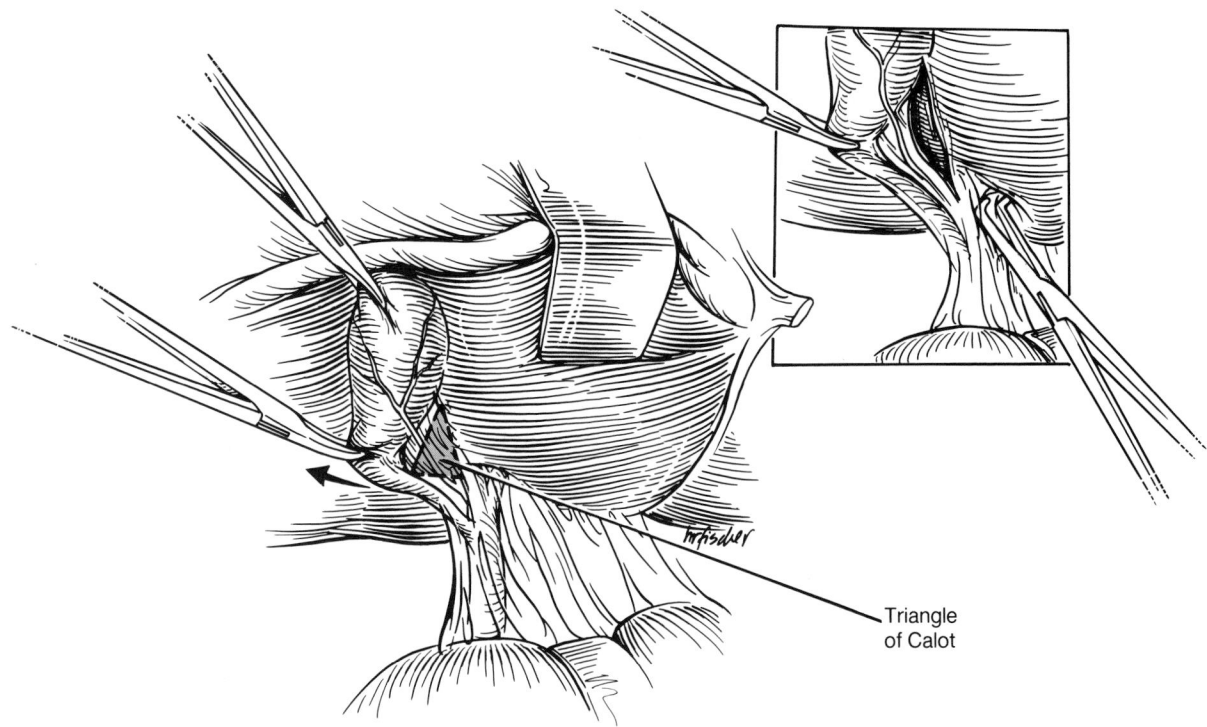

Triangle
of Calot

Figure 17-II-3

Beginning the Dissection

Kelly clamps are placed on the gallbladder, which is retracted to expose the triangle of Calot. As described for laparoscopic cholecystectomy, lateral and downward traction on the infundibulum opens the triangle. As in laparoscopic cholecystectomy, the dissection is begun with a peritoneal incision in the triangle along the superior edge of the gallbladder. The cystic artery and duct and the junction of the gallbladder and cystic duct are identified. The cystic duct is carefully followed to its junction with the common bile duct. The cystic duct stump is shorter with open cholecystectomy, because its full dissection is safer with the open technique than with the laparoscopic approach.

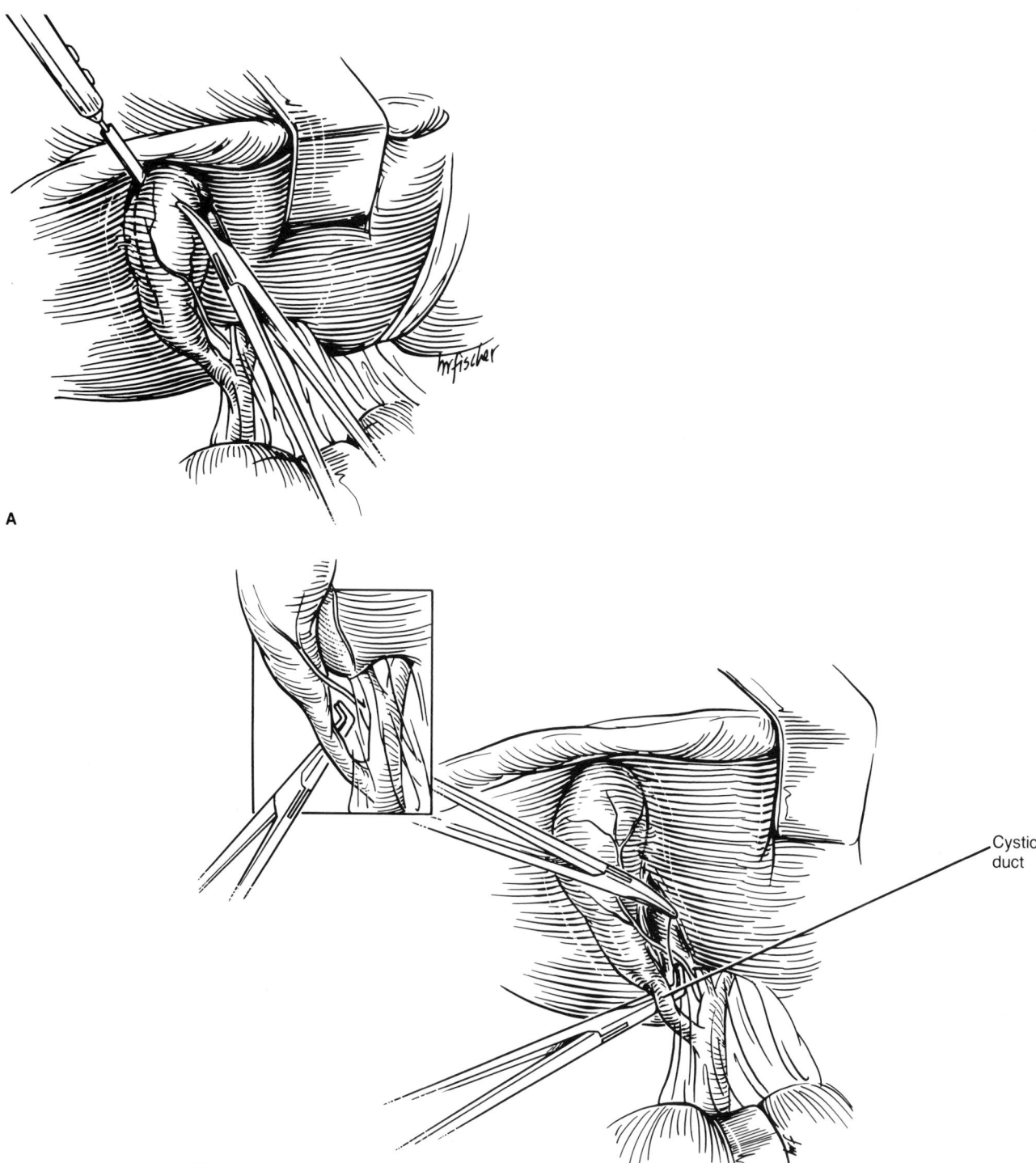

A

B

Cystic
duct

Figure 17-II-4

Retrograde Dissection Technique

(A) The safest technique is to dissect the gallbladder from its bed in a retrograde fashion from the fundus down.

(B) If possible, a Potts (double-encircling) ligature is placed on the cystic duct to prevent stones from passing into the common bile duct during dissection. This should not be done if the anatomy is not clear. A careful retrograde dissection ensures proper identification of biliary anatomy before any structures are divided. This is particularly important when anatomy is obscured because of inflammation (as in acute cholecystitis).

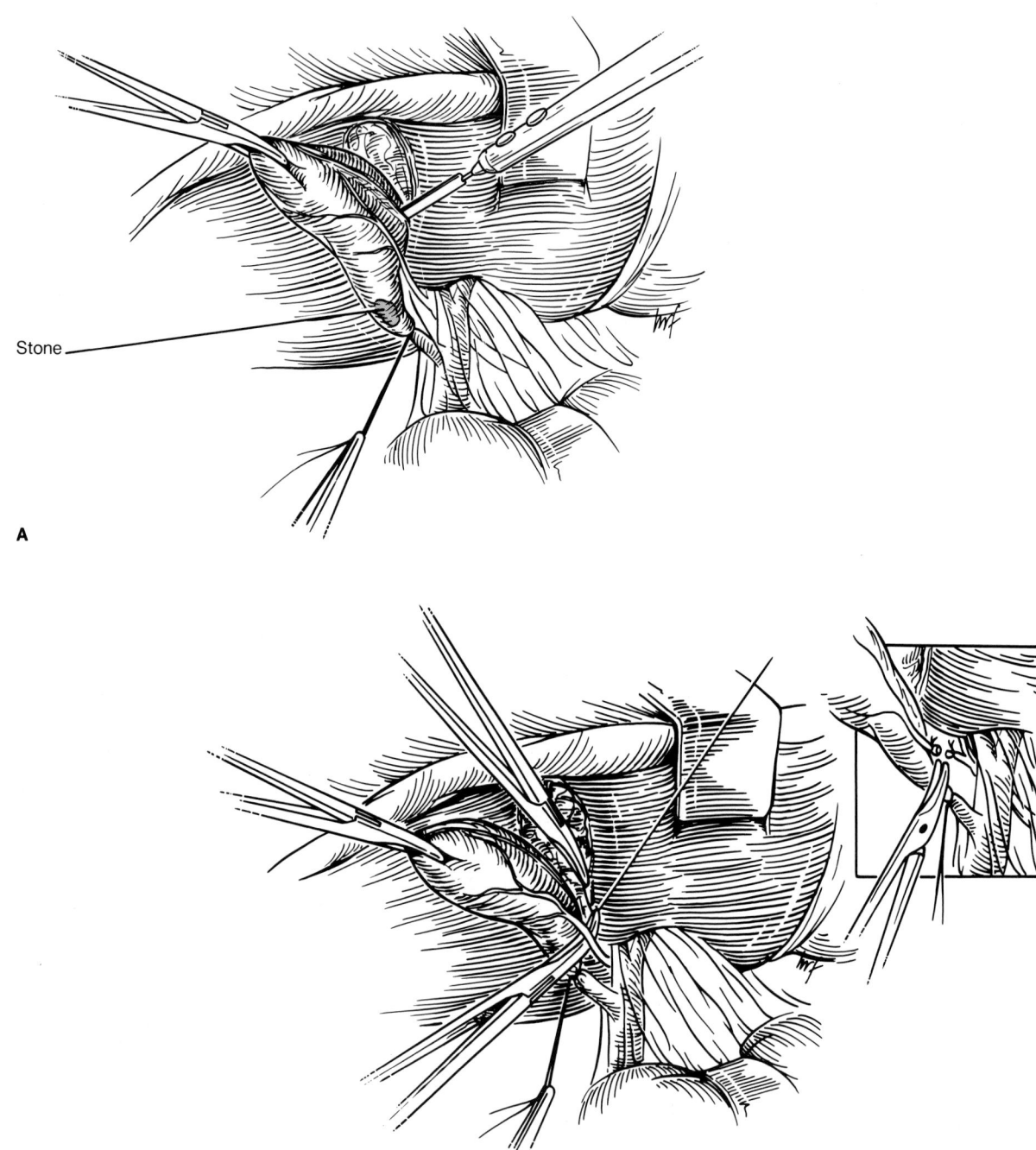

Stone

A

B

Figure 17-II-5

Retrograde Dissection of Gallbladder

(**A**) Retrograde dissection using the cautery.

(**B**) The cystic artery can be ligated and divided before or during dissection.

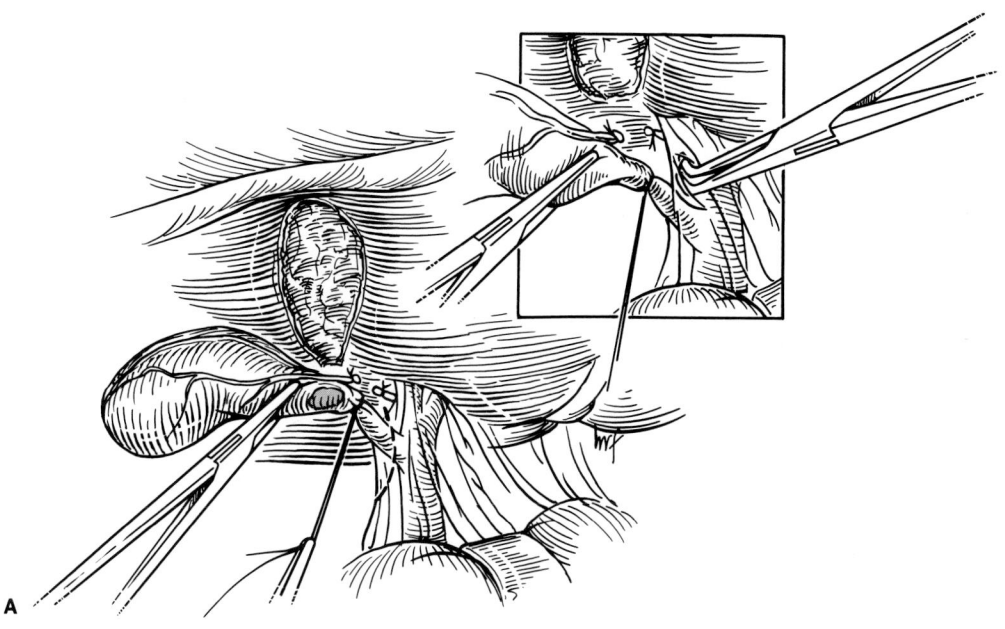

A

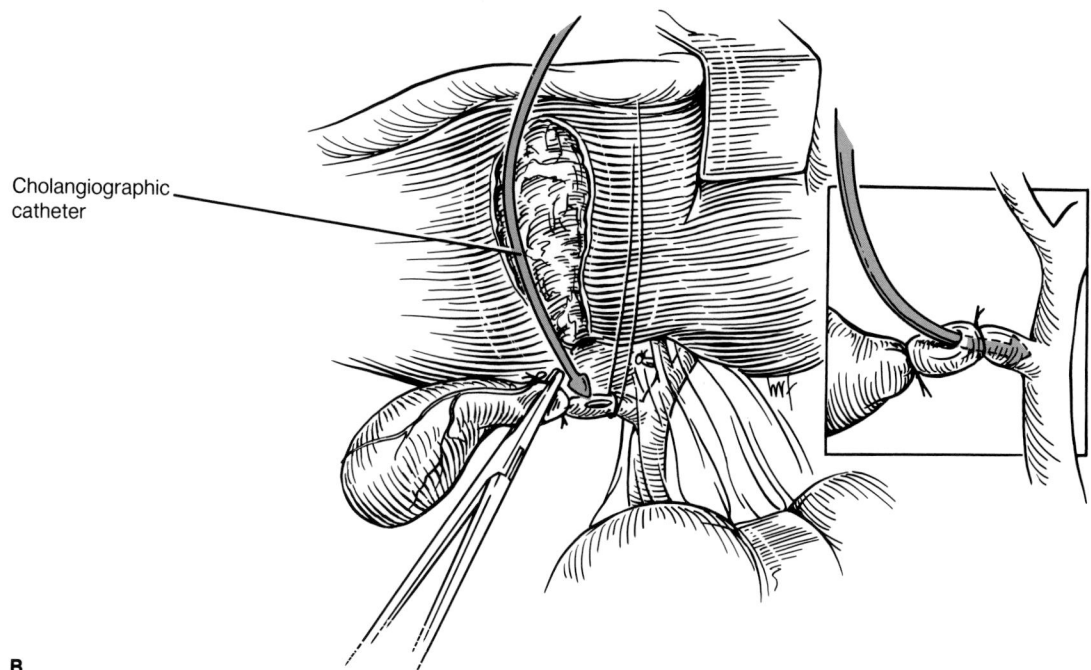

Cholangiographic catheter

B

Figure 17-II-6

Gallbladder Removal

(**A**) The gallbladder, dissected from its bed, is retracted as the cystic duct dissection is completed.

(**B**) After an incision is made in the cystic duct, a catheter is placed for cholangiography. A taut catheter or a small ureteral catheter can be used. A fluoroscopic cholangiogram is preferred.

(Continued)

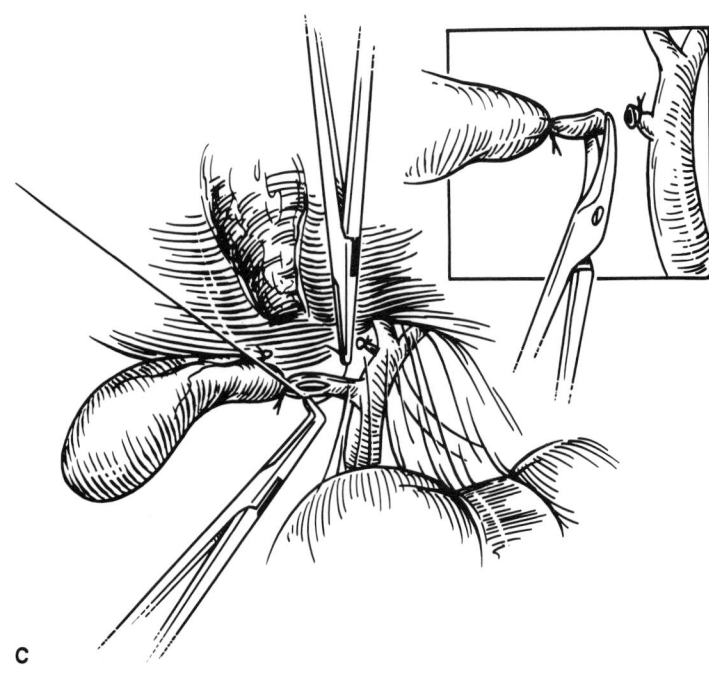

c

Figure 17-II-6 *(Continued)*

(C) After the cholangiographic catheter is removed, a ligature is placed distal to the cystic duct incision and secured 0.5 to 1 cm from its junction with the common duct. The gallbladder is removed.

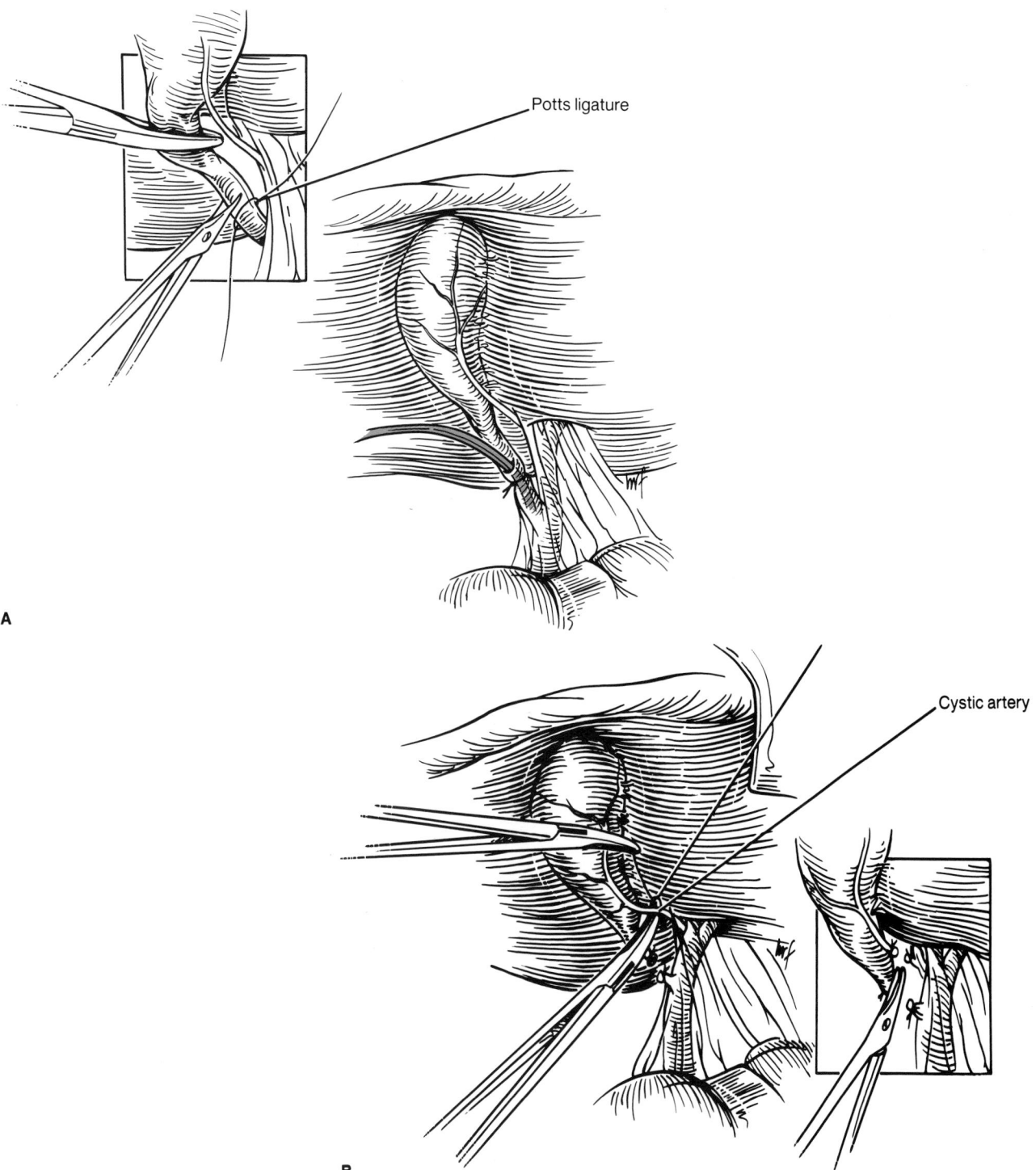

Potts ligature

Cystic artery

A

B

Figure 17-II-7

Alternative Approach

(A) When anatomy is easily defined, the cystic duct can be dissected and cholangiography performed before the gallbladder is dissected from its bed.

(B) After cholangiography is performed, the cystic duct and artery are each ligated and divided before prograde dissection from the cystic duct to the fundus is initiated.

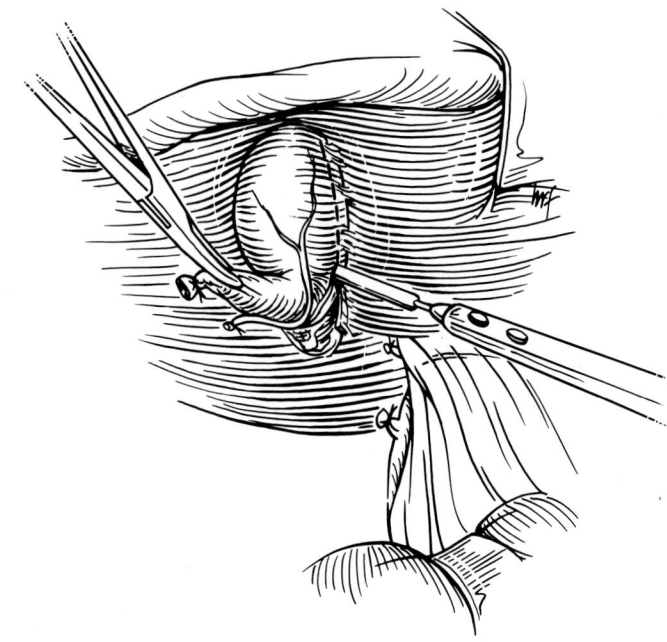

Figure 17-II-8

Prograde Dissection Technique

The gallbladder is being dissected in a prograde fashion, as it is during laparoscopic cholecystectomy. The prograde dissection is often quicker but is also riskier in inexperienced hands.

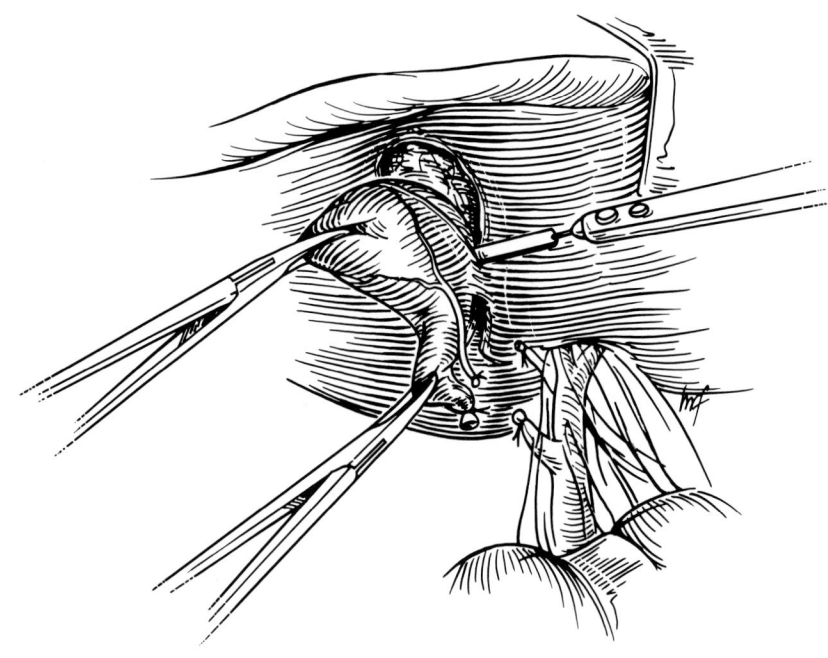

Figure 17-II-9

Combined Prograde and Retrograde Technique

During prograde removal of the gallbladder, it may be advantageous to do some of the dissection in a retrograde fashion.

SECTION III   *Laparoscopic Common Bile Duct Exploration*

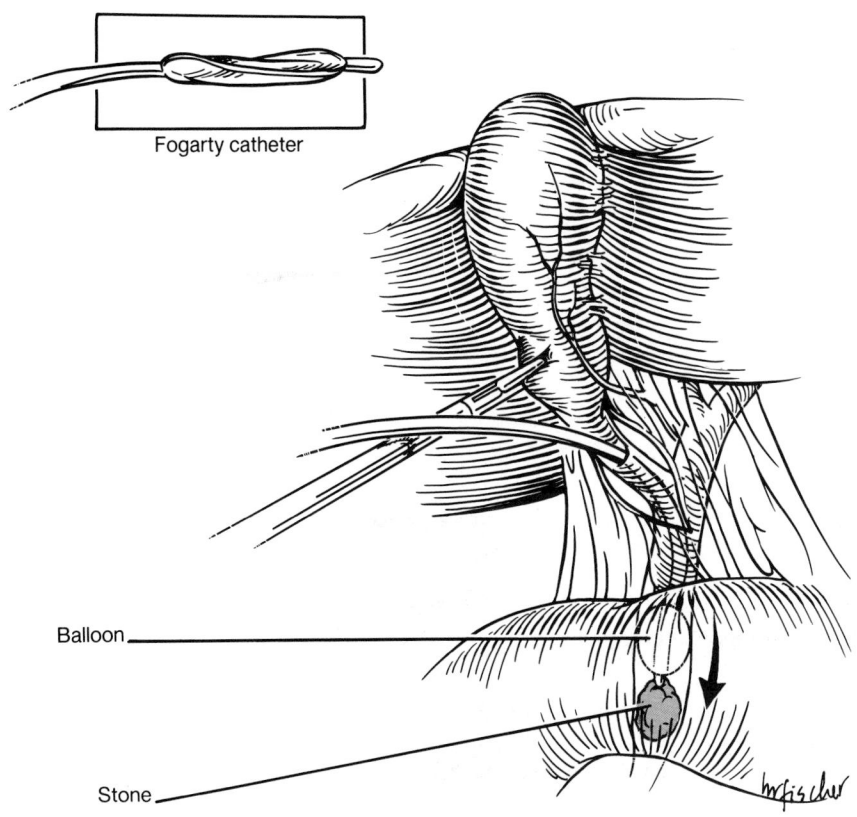

Fogarty catheter

Balloon —————————

Stone ————

Figure 17-III-1

Balloon Catheter Insertion

The technique of laparoscopic exploration of the common bile duct is only slightly different from the open method. A clip is placed on the proximal cystic duct, which is then incised. After dilation of the cystic duct under fluoroscopy, a Fogarty balloon catheter is inserted. The initial maneuver is an attempt to push the stone through the ampullary sphincter under fluoroscopic guidance.

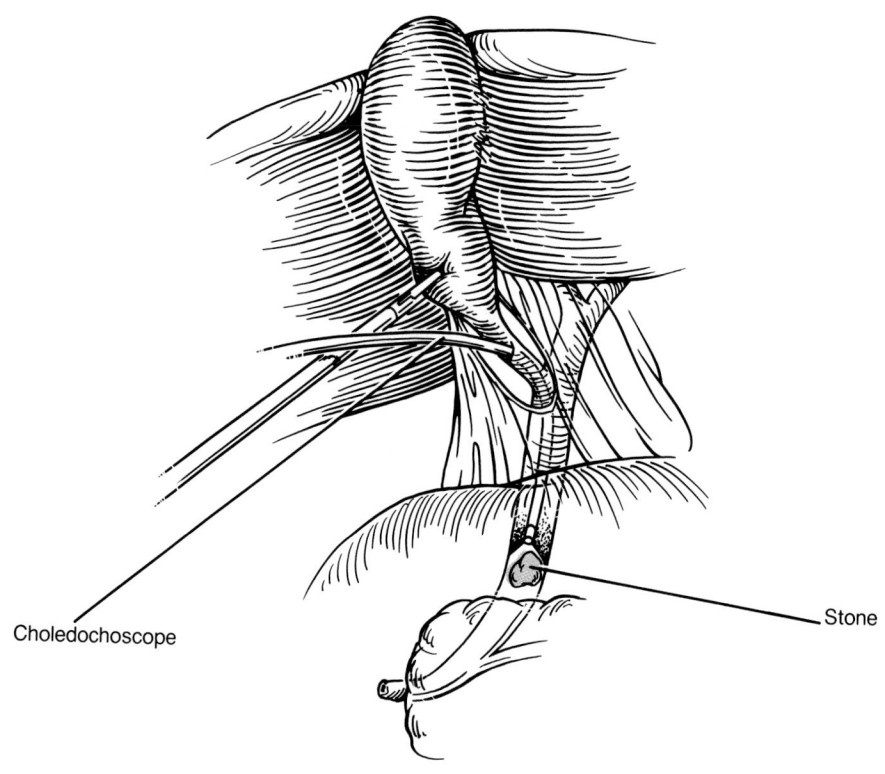

Choledochoscope

Stone

Figure 17-III-2

Choledochoscope Insertion

If necessary, a 2- to 3-mm choledochoscope is inserted to visualize the common bile duct all the way to the duodenum. This is facilitated by first placing a guide wire over which the choledochoscope is passed.

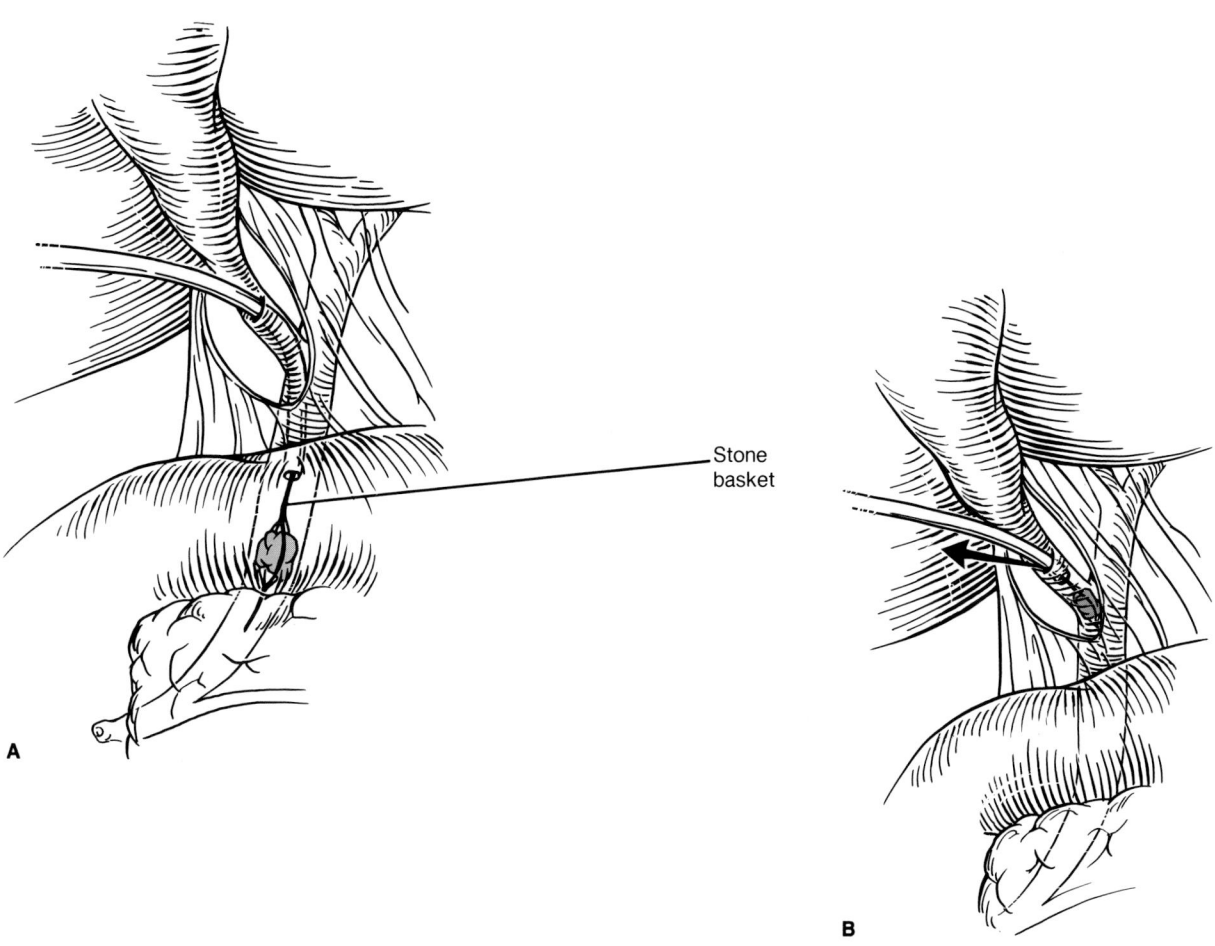

Figure 17-III-3

Stone Removal

(**A**) This stone is being removed by means of a basket, but stones can also be pushed or fragmented. The distal biliary tract is more readily visualized than the proximal bile ducts. After thorough choledochoscopic exploration, repeated cholangiography confirms the successful extraction of stones. Laparoscopic exploration of the common bile duct can also be performed by opening the common duct itself.

(**B**) However, hospital stay and morbidity are reduced if exploration and removal can be accomplished through the cystic duct.

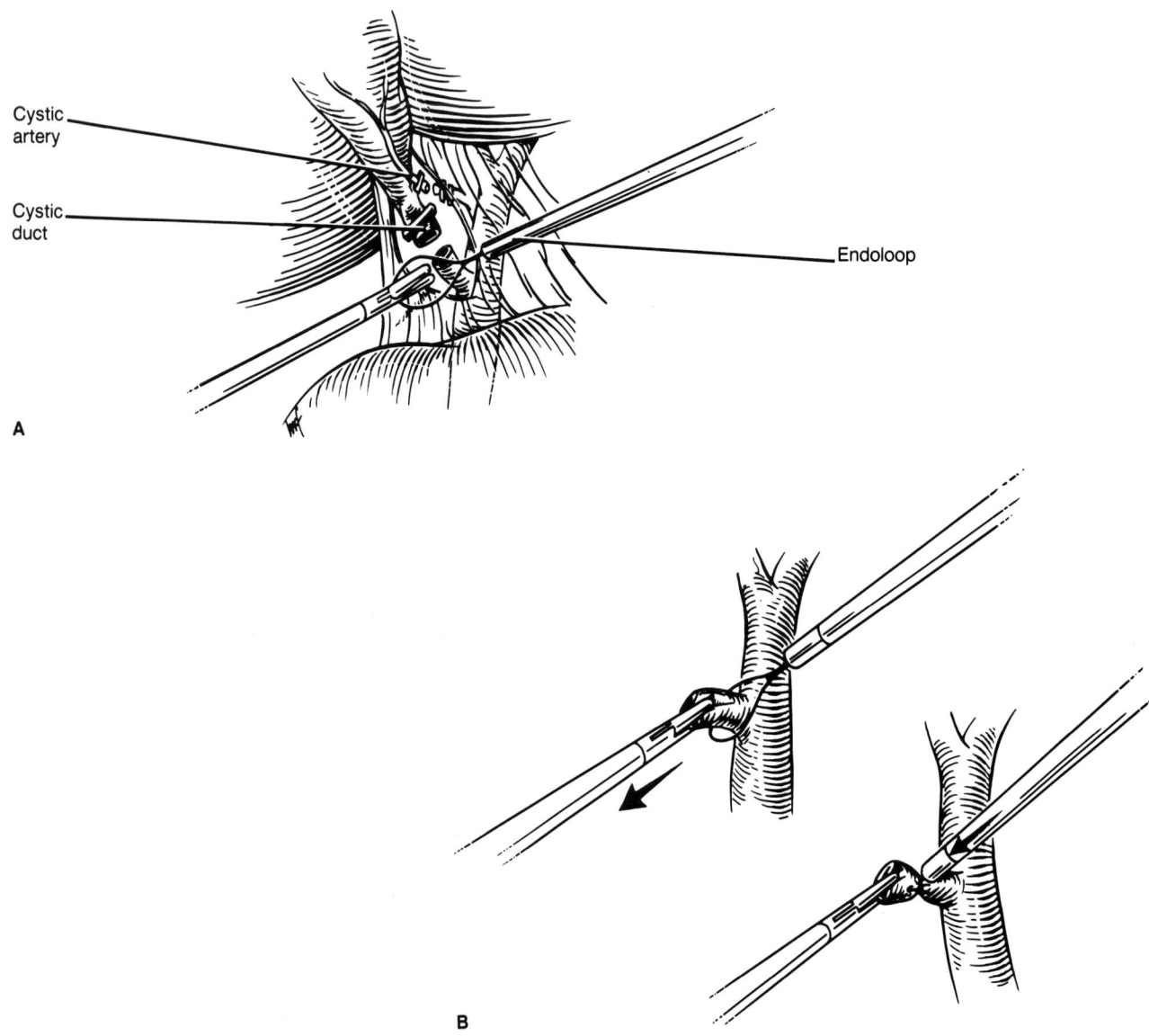

Cystic artery

Cystic duct

Endoloop

A

B

Figure 17-III-4

Ligation and Retraction of Cystic Duct Stump

(**A**) After completion of a transcystic duct exploration, the cystic duct stump is ligated with an endoloop.

(**B**) The cystic duct stump is gently retracted during application of the endoloop.

SECTION IV   *Open Common Bile Duct Exploration*

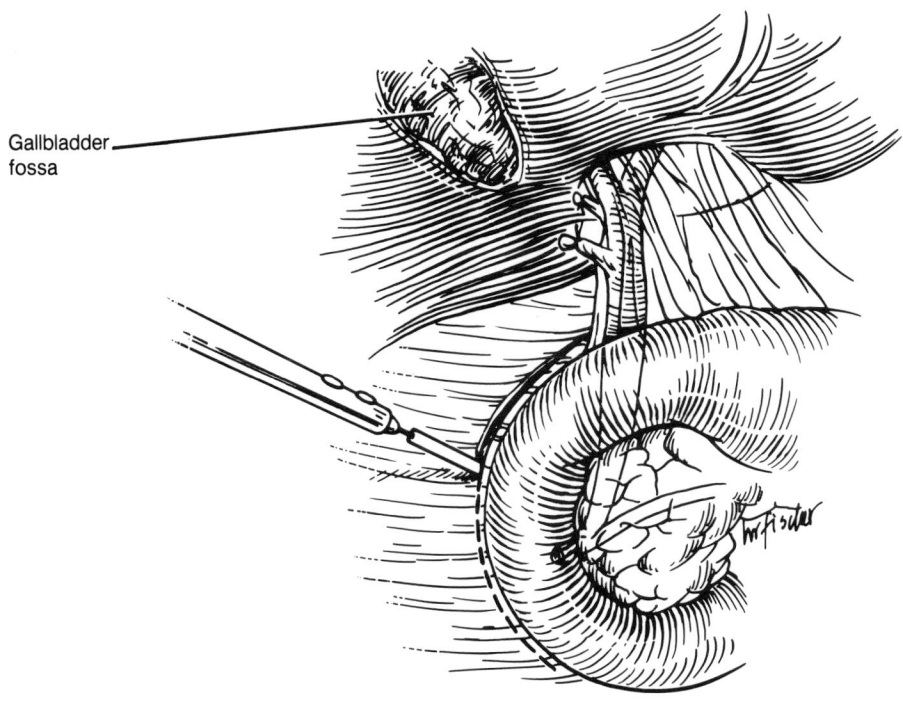

Gallbladder
fossa

Figure 17-IV-1

Kocher Maneuver

Open exploration of the common bile duct is done after the cystic duct has been ligated and divided and the gallbladder removed. A Kocher maneuver helps to expose most of the distal common duct and allows palpation for detection of stones.

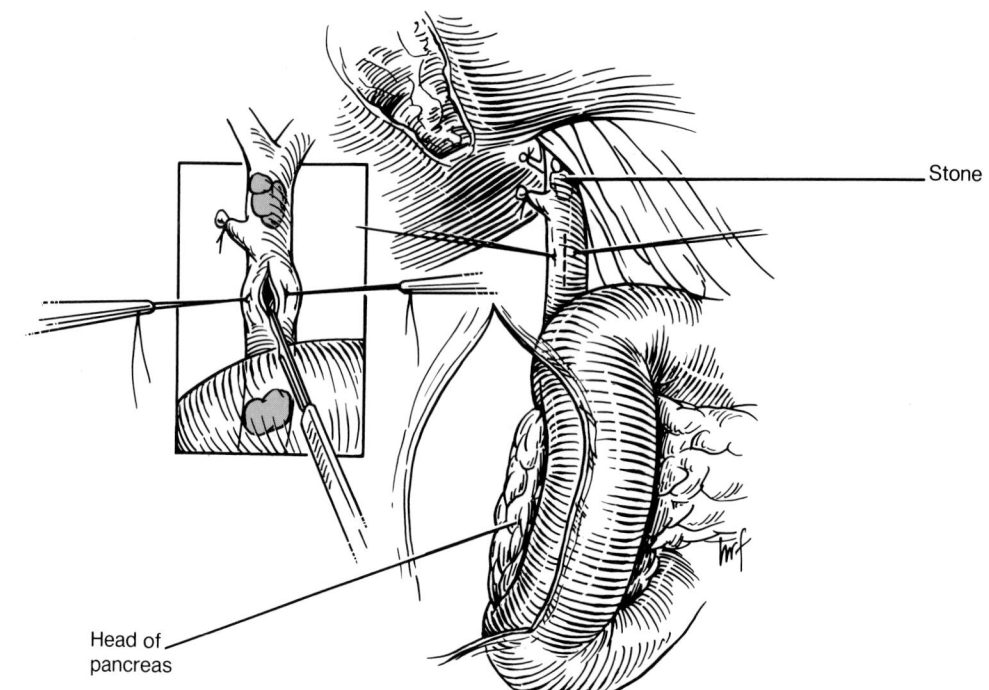

Stone

Figure 17-IV-2

Head of pancreas

Incision

A 2- to 3-cm incision is made in the mid–common bile duct, usually just distal to the cystic duct junction. The cystic duct can be attached parallel to the common bile duct for a variable distance. When this occurs, it is important to avoid opening the cystic duct rather than the common duct. Traction sutures in the common duct facilitate the initial incision and all subsequent maneuvers. Several steps are required to complete a thorough common bile duct exploration.

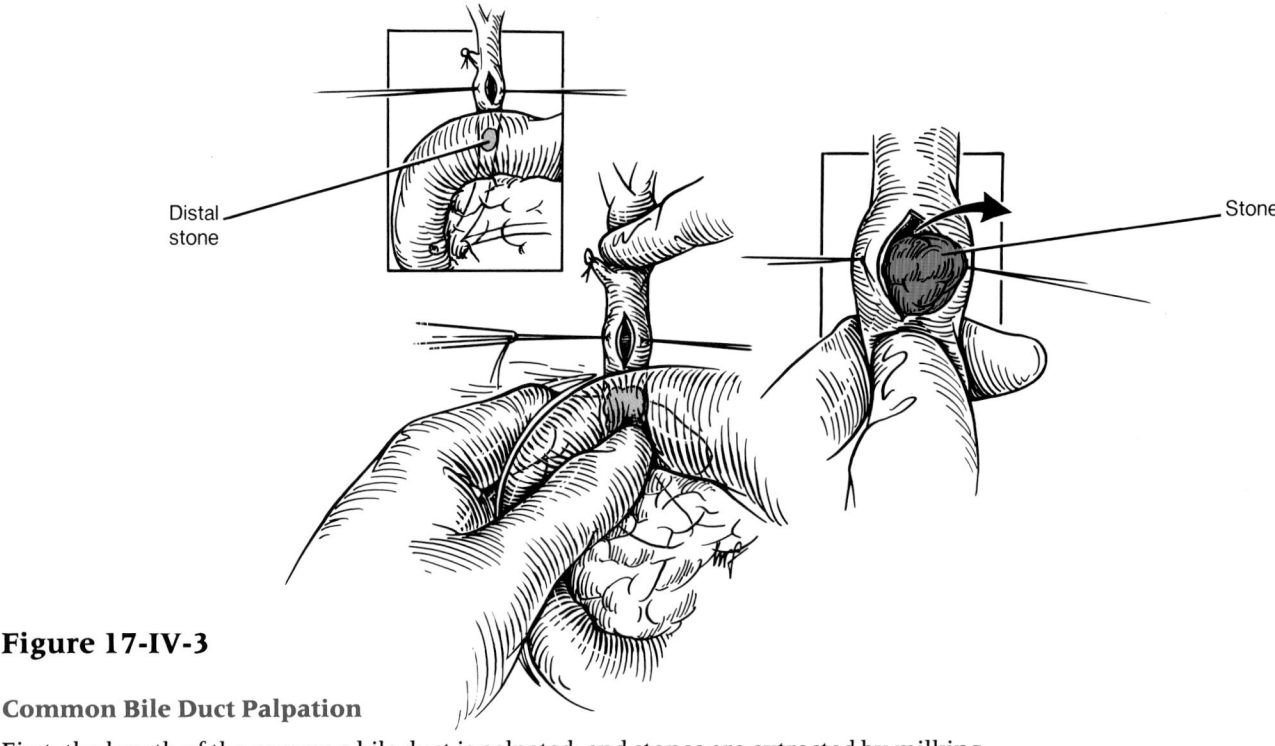

Distal stone

Stone

Figure 17-IV-3

Common Bile Duct Palpation

First, the length of the common bile duct is palpated, and stones are extracted by milking them back through the incision in the common duct. Care is taken so that distal stones are not milked into the proximal duct.

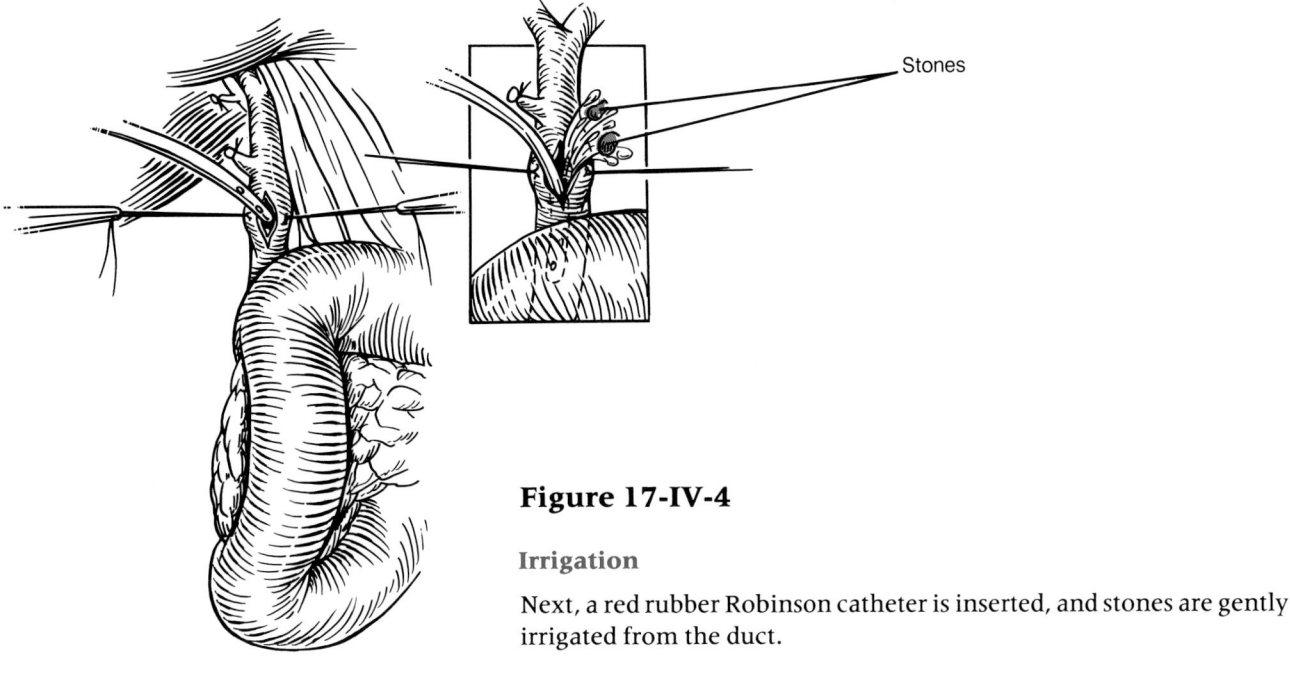

Stones

Figure 17-IV-4

Irrigation

Next, a red rubber Robinson catheter is inserted, and stones are gently irrigated from the duct.

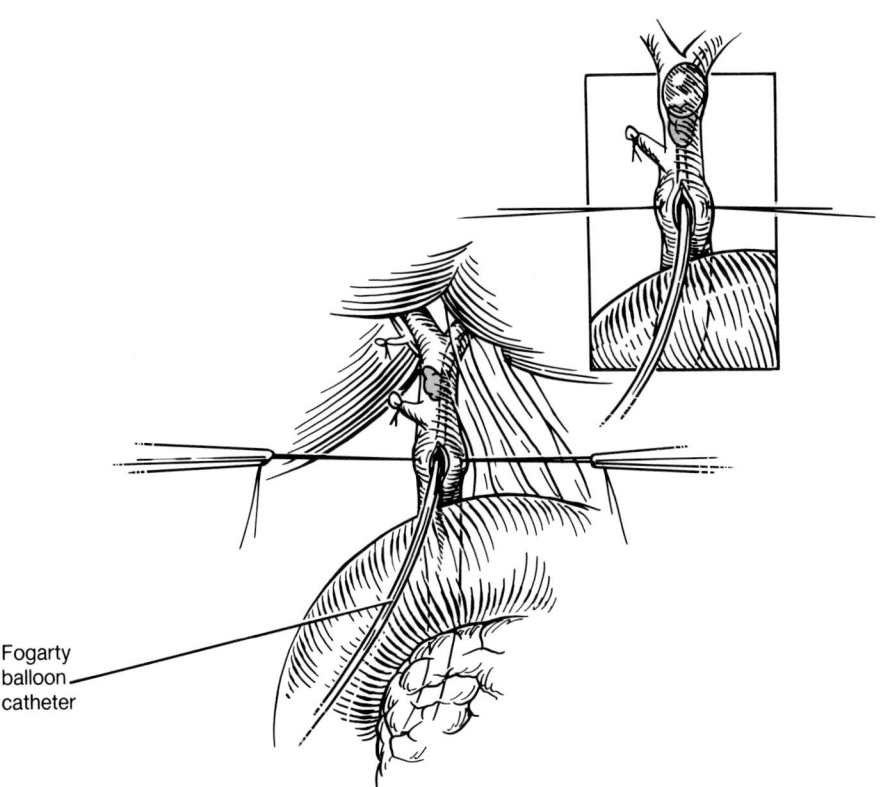

Fogarty balloon catheter

Figure 17-IV-5

Fogarty Balloon Catheterization

Stones not removed by palpation or irrigation are extracted by means of a biliary Fogarty catheter, which is passed beyond the stone before the balloon is inflated.

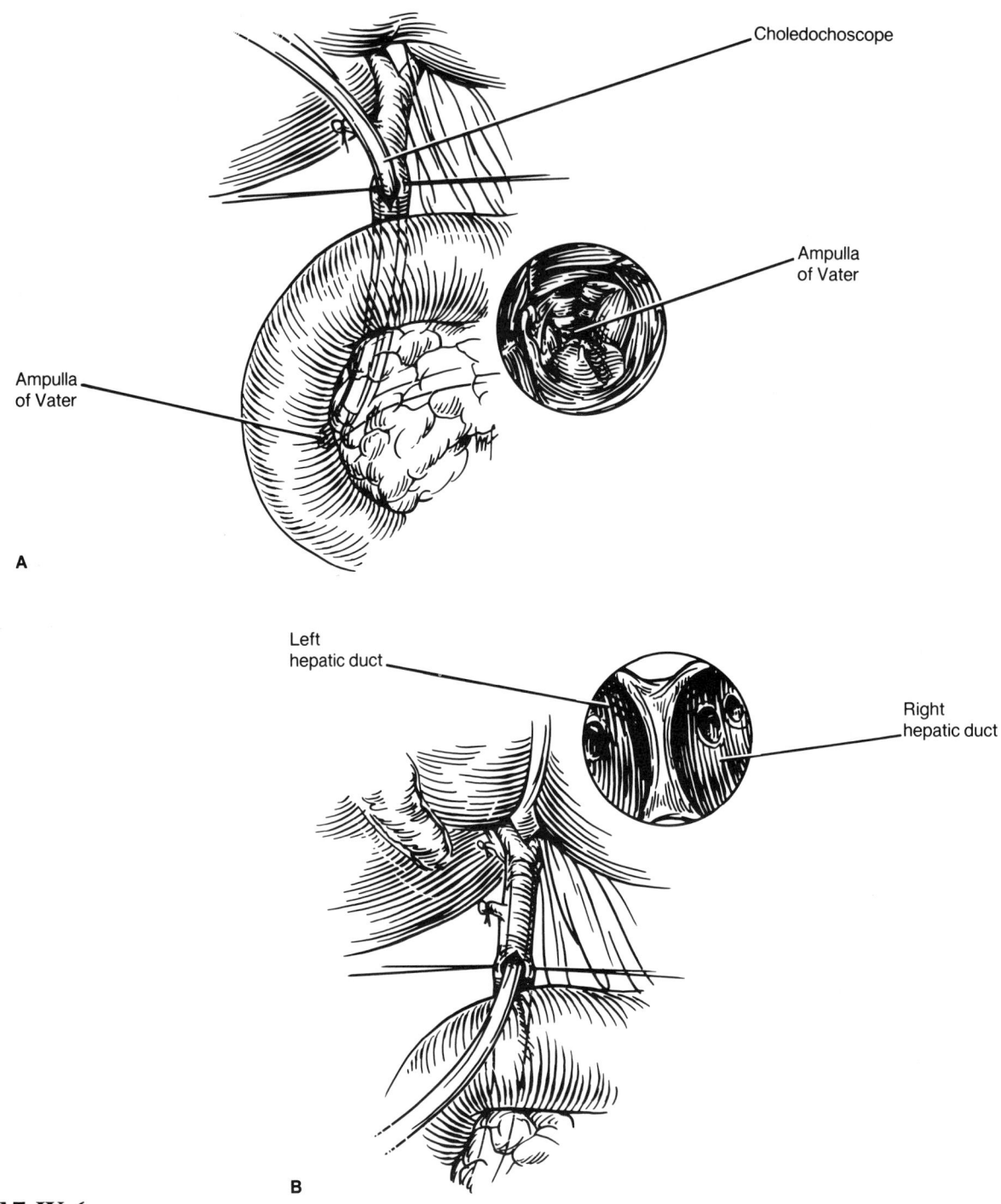

Figure 17-IV-6

Visualization

(**A**) A flexible or rigid choledochoscope is passed through the choledochotomy for thorough visualization of the distal common duct to the ampulla of Vater.

(**B**) The choledochoscope is then passed proximally until secondary biliary radicals are seen in both the right and the left hepatic ducts. The left hepatic duct comes off of the common duct at a more acute and anterior angle than the right hepatic duct.

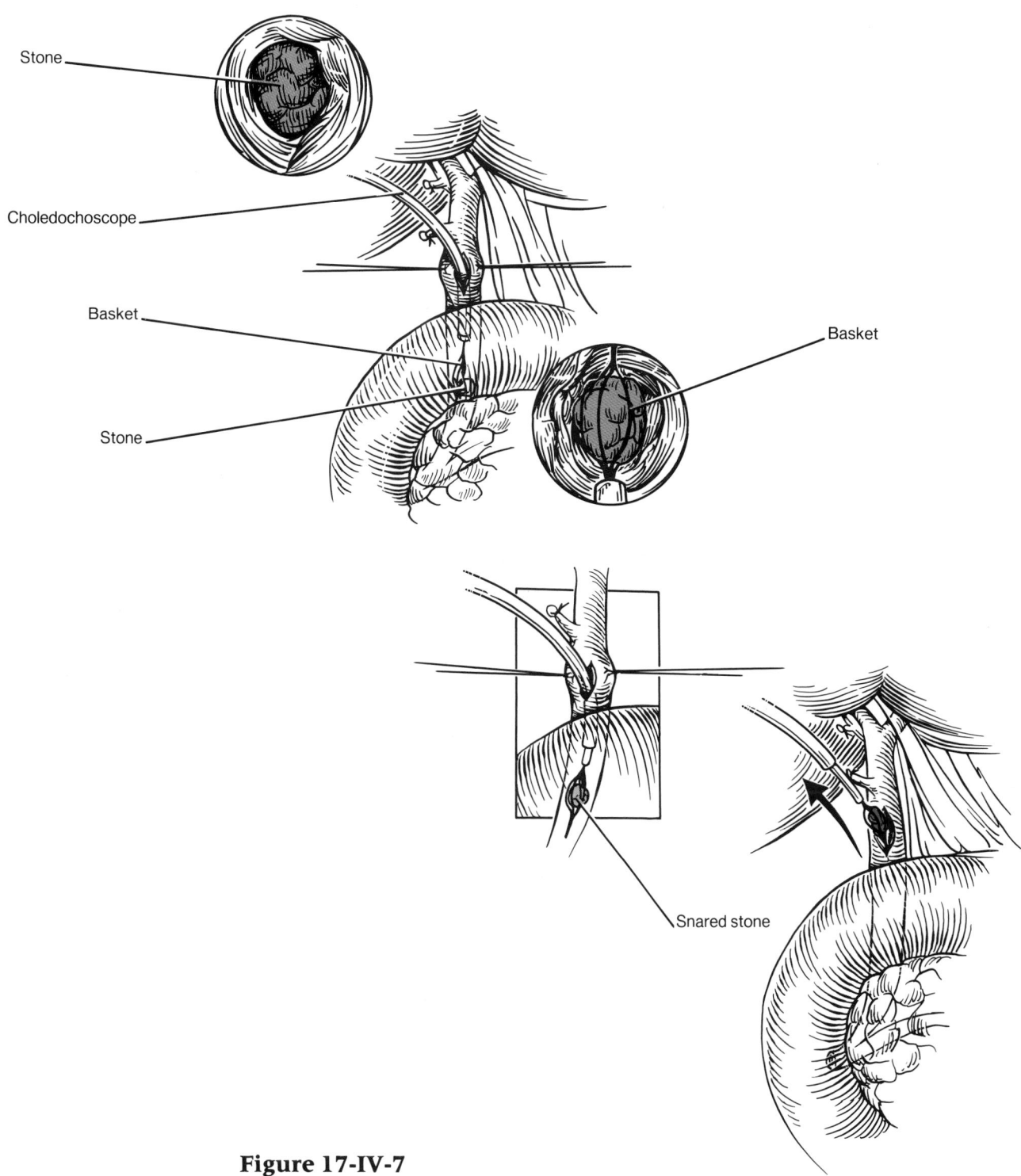

Figure 17-IV-7

Stone Removal

A stone basket or biliary Fogarty catheter can be passed through the instrument port of the choledochoscope and the stone removed under direct visualization. It is important to avoid transferring stones from the distal to proximal ducts, where they are more difficult to extract.

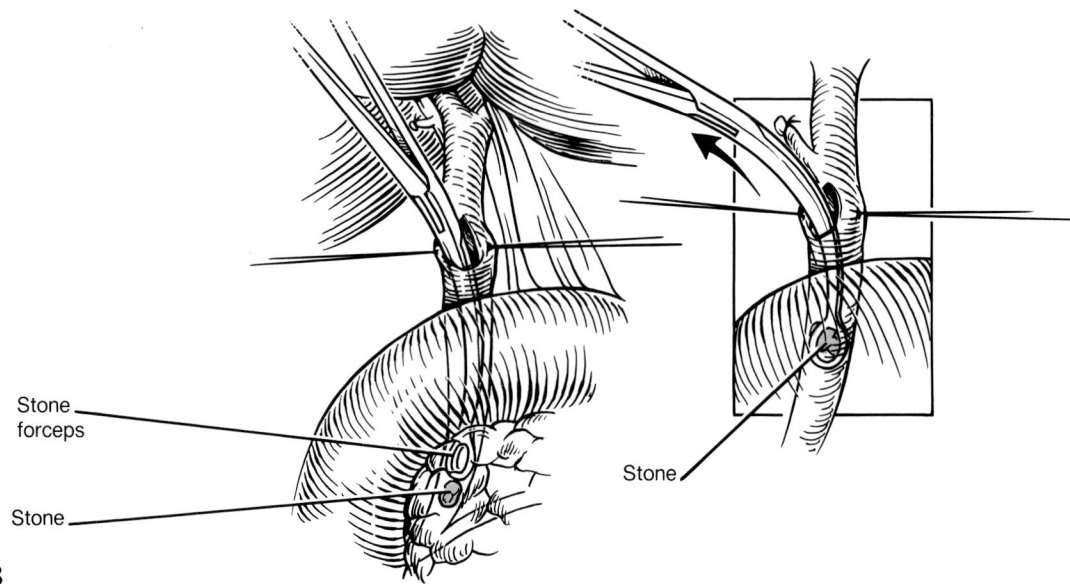

Stone
forceps

Stone

Stone

Figure 17-IV-8

Stone Forceps

If all of these maneuvers fail, a stone forceps can be passed through the choledochotomy for stone extraction. However, this instrument can damage the duct, and it should be used with care. If an impacted stone in the common bile duct persists after complete exploration, extraction from below by means of a transduodenal sphincteroplasty may be necessary.

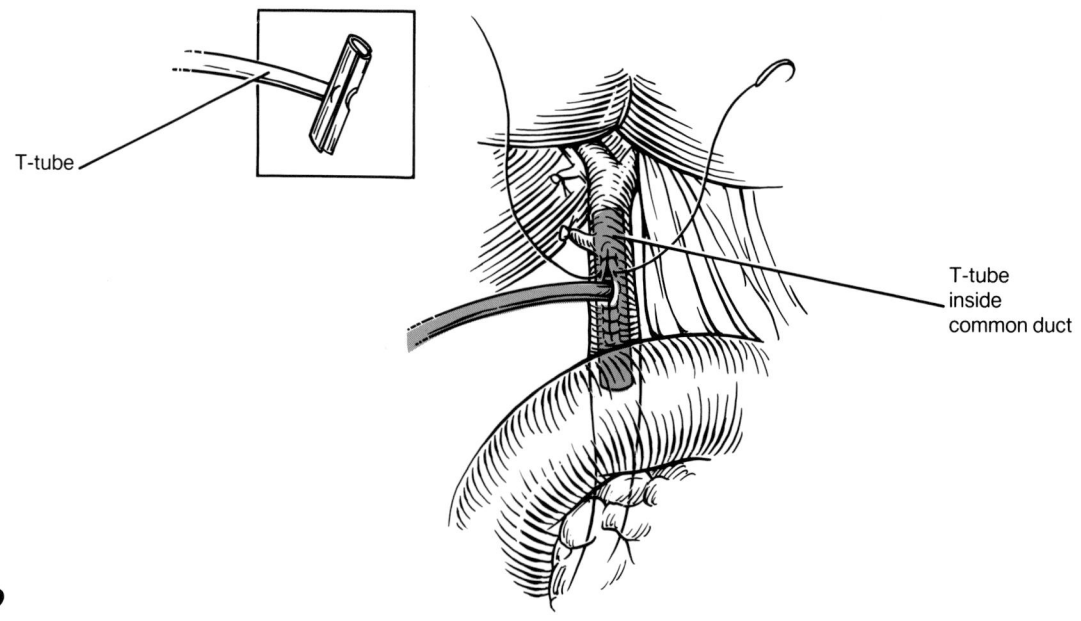

T-tube

T-tube
inside
common duct

Figure 17-IV-9

T-Tube Insertion

After exploration of the common bile duct, a T-tube is inserted. Three or four interrupted sutures are usually necessary to accomplish a watertight longitudinal closure of the duct. The T-tube is fashioned with a hole in its back wall to facilitate removal. A size 14 T-tube is placed so that postoperative extraction of stones through the T-tube tract can be done.

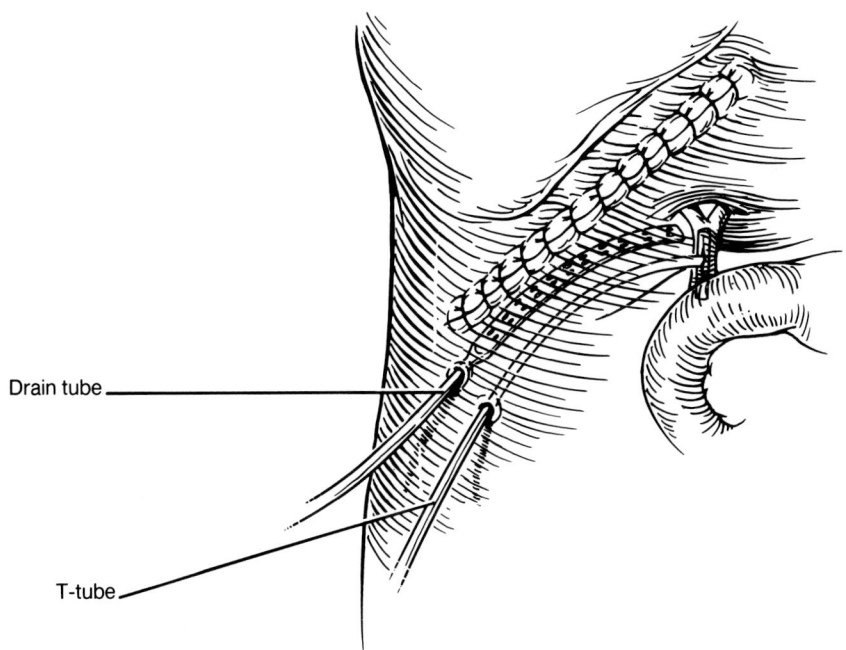

Drain tube

T-tube

Figure 17-IV-10

Wound Closure

The abdomen is closed in two layers with running no. 1 nylon or PDS sutures for the fascia. Small, close-together bites of tissue are important for a secure closure with minimal tension on the suture. The skin is closed with staples or sutures.

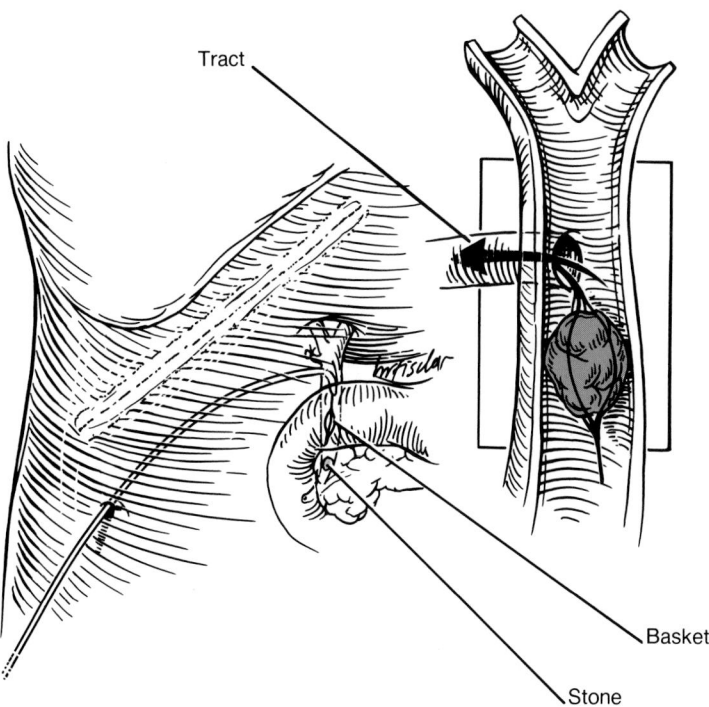

Tract

Basket

Stone

Figure 17-IV-11

Postoperative Stone Extraction

Postoperative extraction of stones through the T-tube tract can be performed as early as 3 weeks after surgery. In the radiologic suite, the T-tube is removed over a guide wire, the tract is dilated, and the stones are removed with a stone basket under fluoroscopic guidance.

SECTION V *Cholecystostomy*

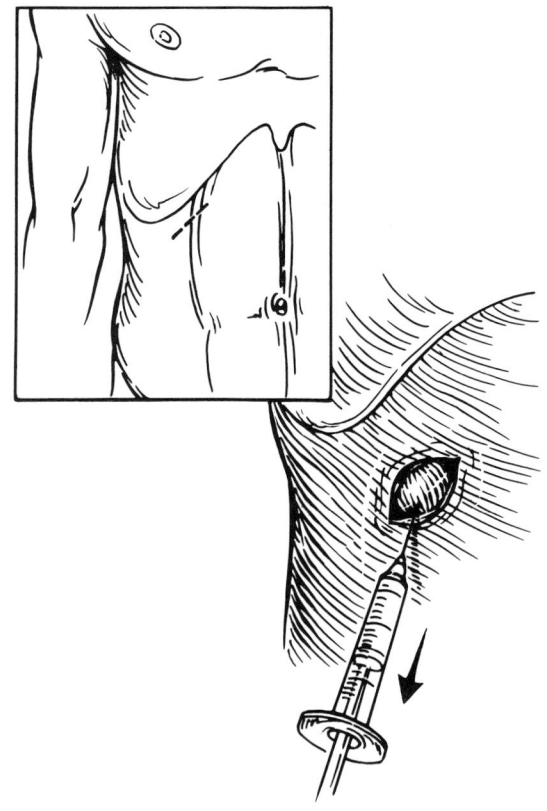

Figure 17-V-1

Bile Aspiration

Open cholecystostomy is now a rarely performed procedure. It is reserved for very ill patients who are unable to undergo general anesthesia and who are not candidates for a radiologic percutaneous approach. Under local anesthesia and sedation, a small incision is made in the subcostal region overlying the position of the gallbladder, which is often palpable. Bile is aspirated with a large-bore needle.

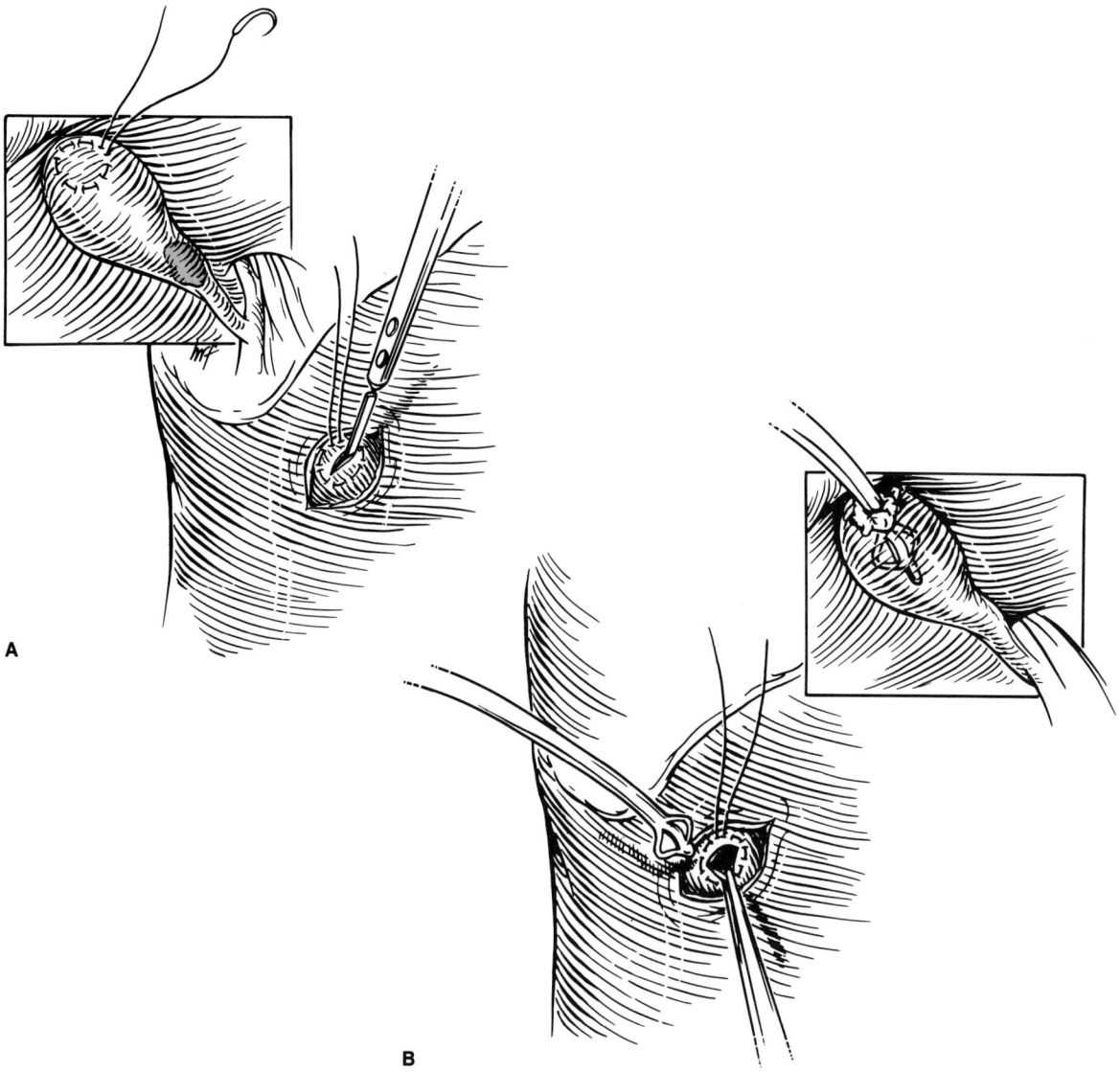

Figure 17-V-2

Indwelling Catheter Insertion

(**A**) A 2-0 silk pursestring suture is placed in the fundus of the gallbladder, and a small puncture is made within the pursestring.

(**B**) A mushroom-tipped catheter or a Foley catheter is inserted into the gallbladder, and the pursestring is secured. A tonsil clamp is used to straighten the mushroom-tipped catheter before it is inserted. Stones can sometimes be evacuated from the gallbladder with a stone clamp before the catheter is inserted.

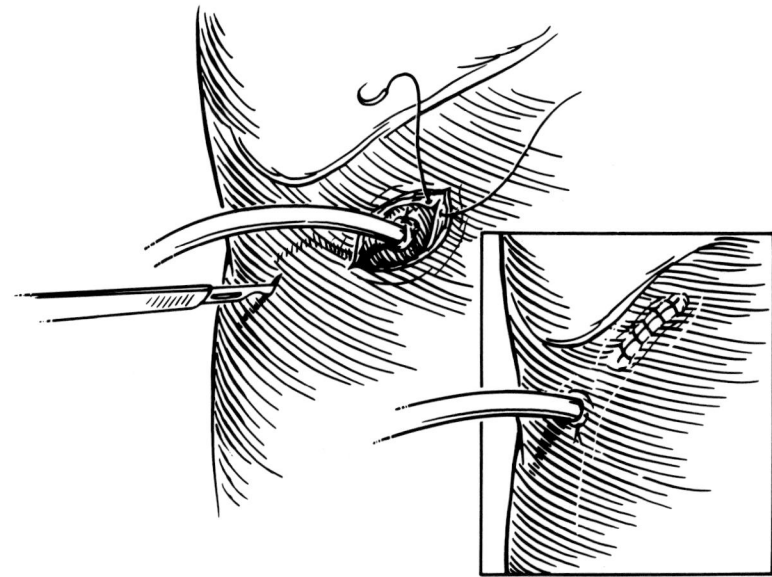

Figure 17-V-3

Drainage Catheter Insertion

The drainage catheter is brought through a separate stab incision and is secured at the skin level. The abdominal incision is closed in two layers with no. 1 Ethilon, and the skin is approximated with staples or sutures.

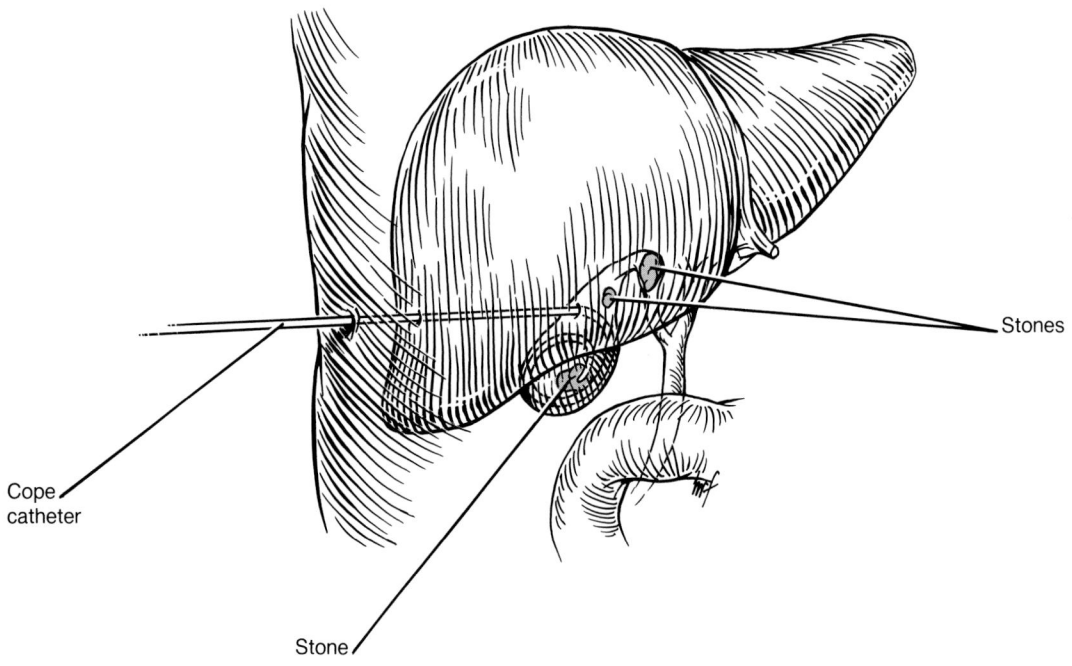

Figure 17-V-4

Percutaneous Drainage

Radiologic percutaneous drainage of the gallbladder is performed under fluoroscopy or ultrasonography. The gallbladder is first entered with a needle, and a guide wire is placed. A transhepatic route is preferred to avoid soiling the peritoneum. A Cope or Ring catheter is inserted into the gallbladder lumen and is secured at the skin.

SECTION VI *Transduodenal Sphincteroplasty*

Indications for sphincteroplasty include an impacted stone in the common bile duct that is not removable by other means; the need for biliary drainage in a patient with a small common duct; ampullary stenosis; as treatment for some patients with the postcholecystectomy syndrome; and after local excision of an ampullary tumor. Sphincterotomy is most commonly accomplished endoscopically, but open sphincteroplasty is preferred when endoscopy has failed or during an open operation (eg, common bile duct exploration).

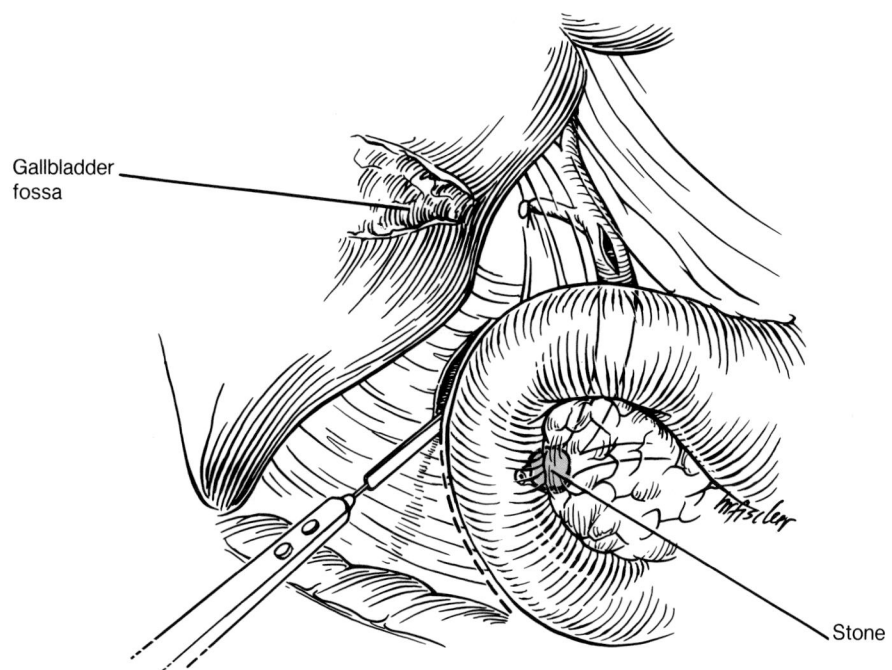

Figure 17-VI-1

Kocher Maneuver

A Kocher maneuver is the initial step. The purposes of duodenal mobilization are both to gain better access to the biliary system and to subsequently achieve a tension-free duodenal closure. A patient with an impacted common duct stone who has undergone an open cholecystectomy and common bile duct exploration is depicted.

Figure 17-VI-2

Duodenotomy

After mobilization of the duodenum, a longitudinal 3- to 4-cm incision is made along the medial aspect of the duodenum. Traction sutures facilitate the duodenal incision.

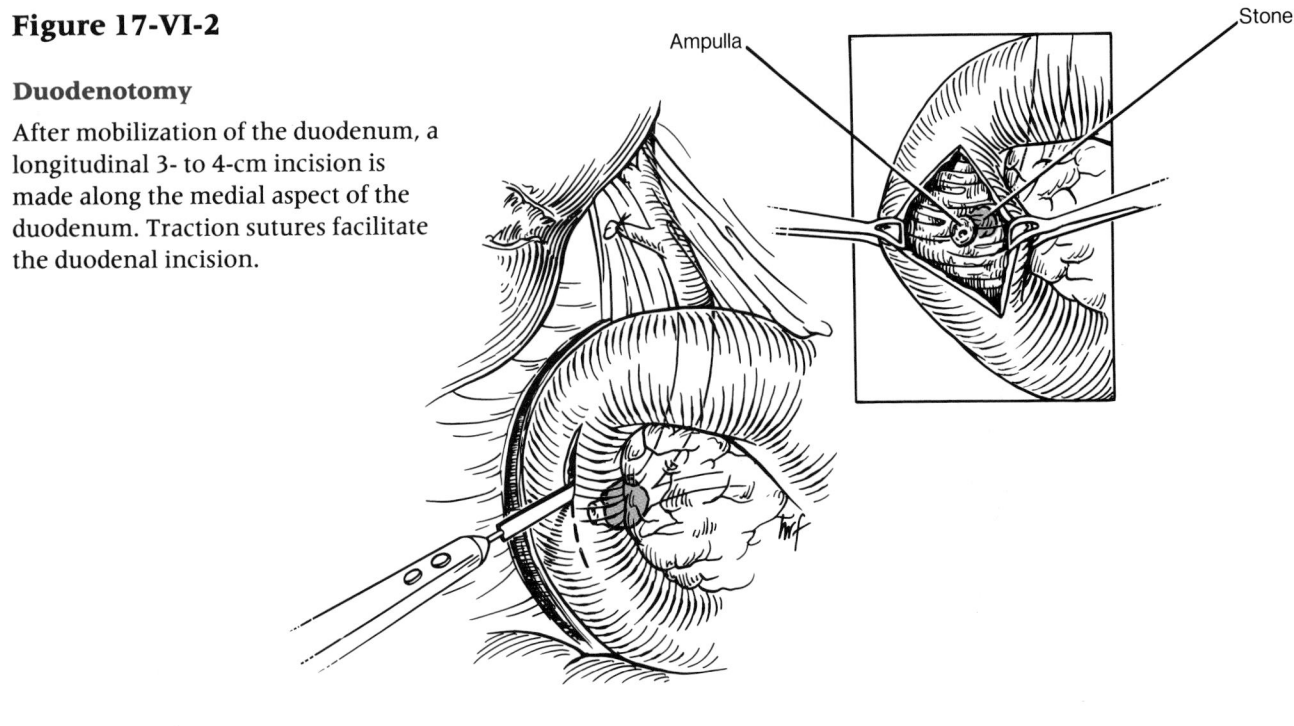

Figure 17-VI-3

Identification of the Ampulla

If the sphincteroplasty is performed in conjunction with common duct exploration, a probe or biliary Fogarty catheter can be inserted through the choledochotomy. The probe exits through the ampulla, making it easily identifiable by a palpating finger. In many cases, however, the sphincteroplasty is performed as a separate operation. The ampulla can usually be identified by palpation at the junction of the third and fourth portions of

(Continued)

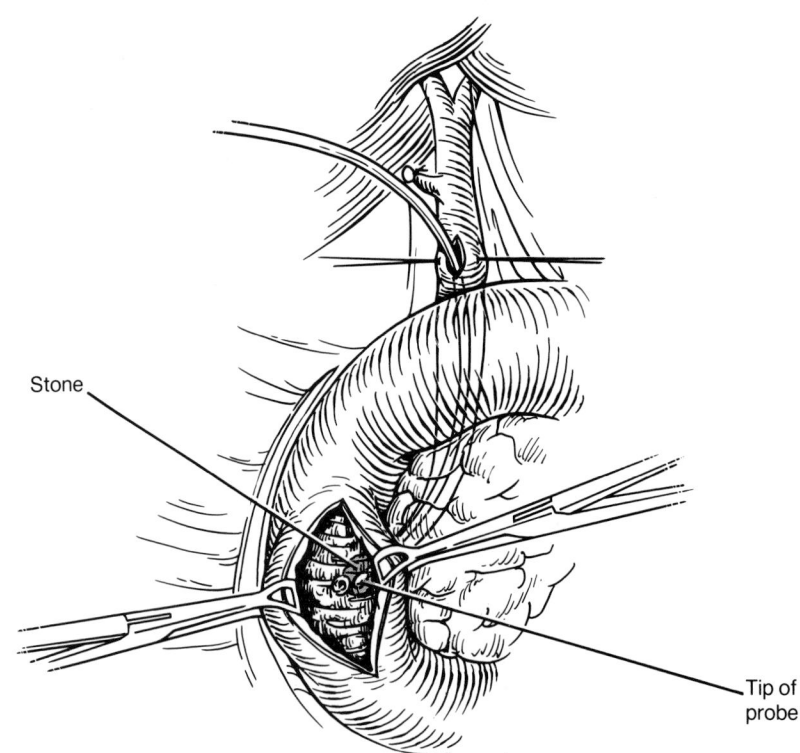

Figure 17-VI-3. *(Continued)*

the duodenum. After the duodenotomy is completed, milking bile from the distal common duct may help identify the ampulla. One needs to be aware of the locations of both pancreatic ducts. The duct of Wirsung is usually located along the inferior edge of the ampulla and slightly to its right side. It may be superficial or deep within the ampulla. The accessory pancreatic duct (duct of Santorini) is usually located 2 to 3 cm proximal and 1 cm medial to the major ampulla.

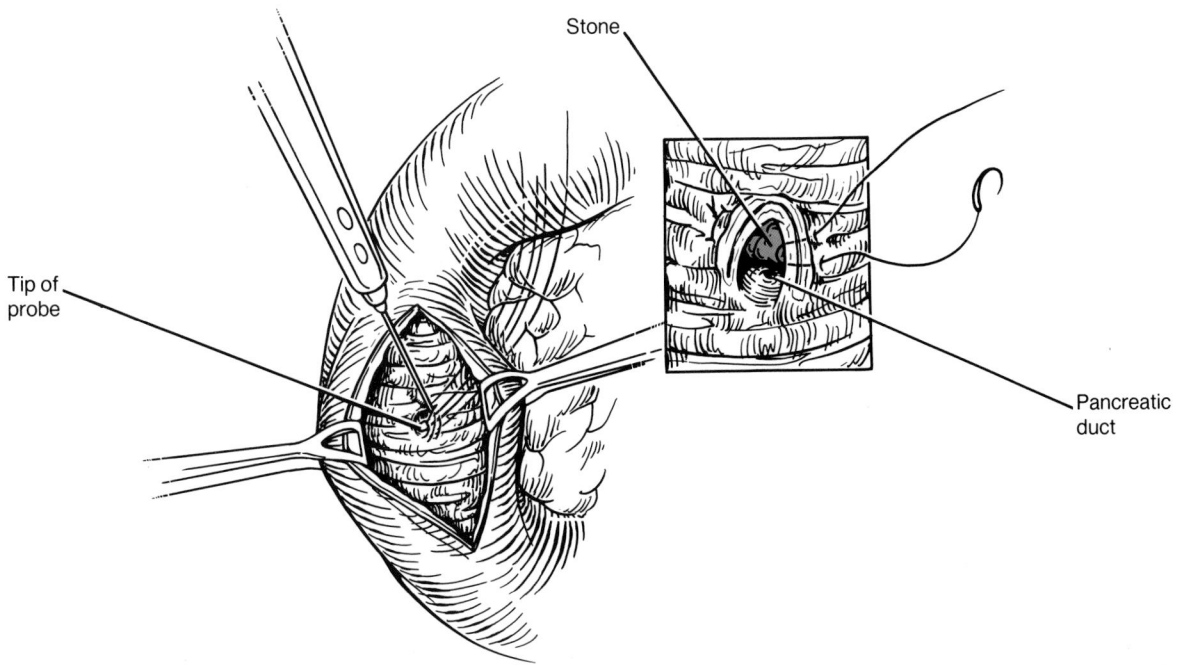

Figure 17-VI-4

Biliary Sphincterotomy

After identification of the major papilla, a probe is inserted into the common bile duct. Using the probe as a guide, the papilla is incised a few millimeters at a time for 2 to 4 cm. The pancreatic duct is almost always identifiable within the first centimeter. As the bile duct is incised, 4-0 or 5-0 interrupted absorbable sutures are placed to approximate the ductal and duodenal mucosa. Care is taken to not occlude the pancreatic duct with a suture.

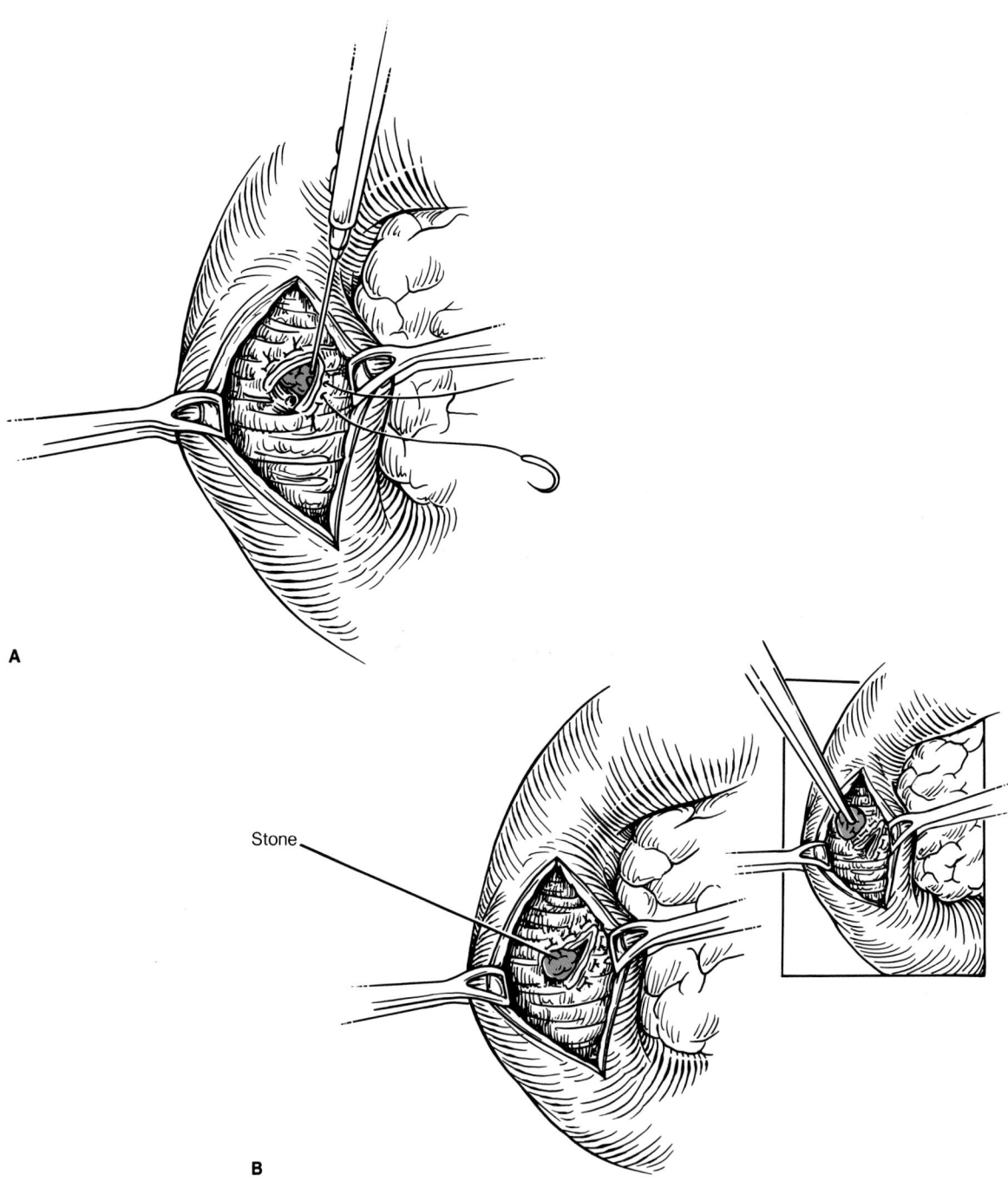

Figure 17-VI-5

Stone Removal

(**A**) The sphincteroplasty is extended, and an apical suture is carefully placed to prevent a duodenal leak.

(**B**) An impacted stone is usually easily removed as the sphincteroplasty is being performed.

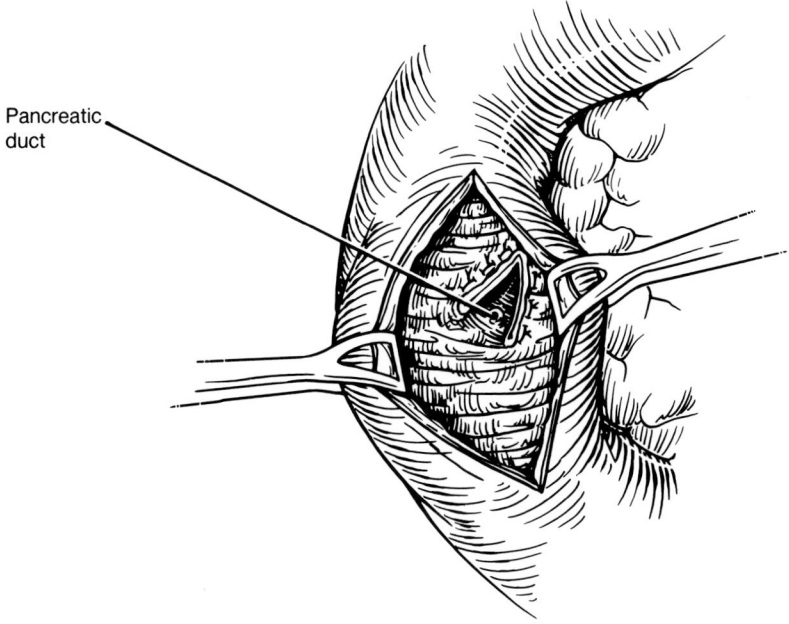

Pancreatic
duct

Figure 17-VI-6

Identification of Pancreatic Duct

After removal of an impacted stone, pancreatic juice can usually be seen flowing from the pancreatic duct orifice. If there is difficulty in identifying the pancreatic duct, secretin, 1 mg/kg, should be administered intravenously to stimulate pancreatic secretion.

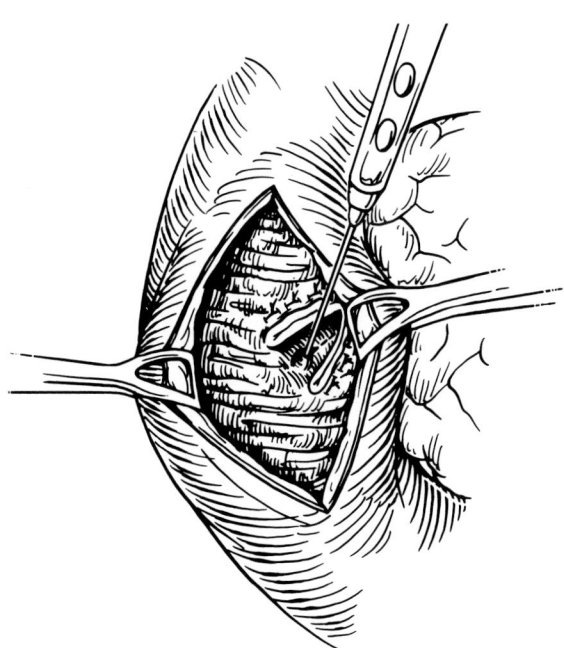

Figure 17-VI-7

Pancreatic Duct Septotomy

If the sphincteroplasty is being done for pancreatic duct stenosis or for postcholecystectomy syndrome, a pancreatic duct septotomy should be added. This is performed using a fine scissors with a probe within the pancreatic duct to indicate its direction. The septum is incised for 0.5 to 1 cm. Sutures are usually not necessary.

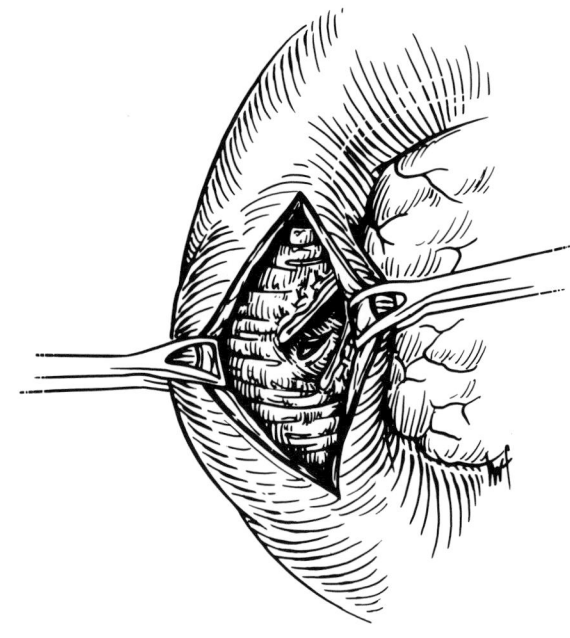

Figure 17-VI-8

Completed Procedure

The completed sphincteroplasty and pancreatic duct septotomy.

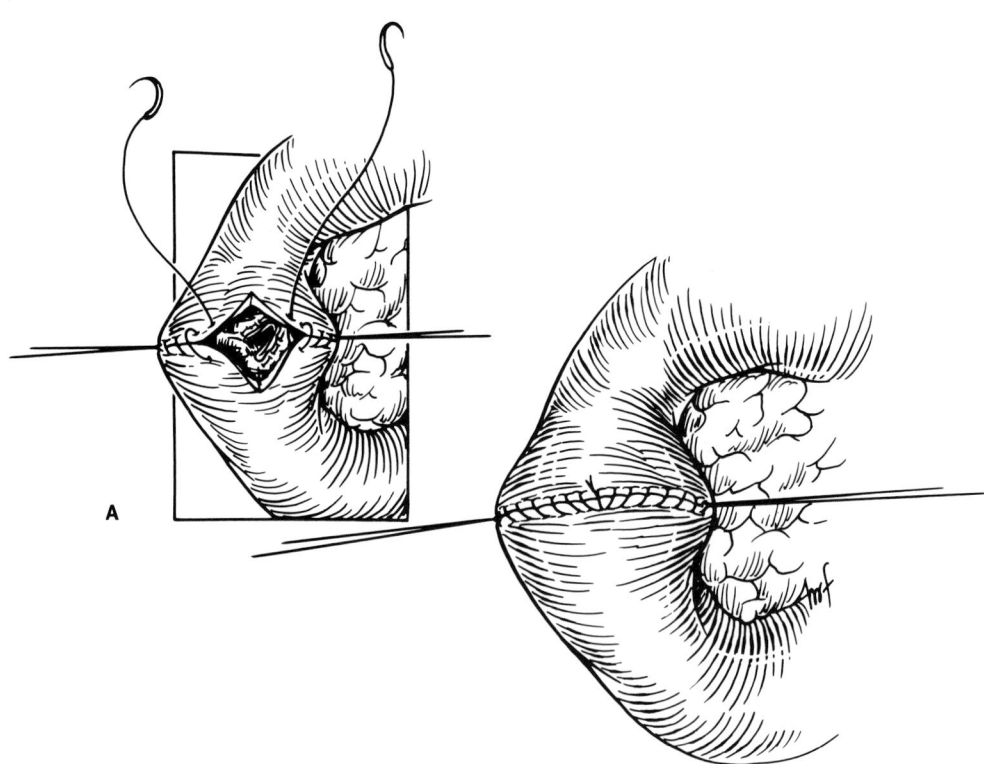

Figure 17-VI-9

Suture Closure of the Duodenum

(**A**) The duodenum is closed transversely in two layers like a Heineke-Mikulicz pyloro-plasty. A running Connell 3-0 chromic suture is used for the inner layer.

(Continued)

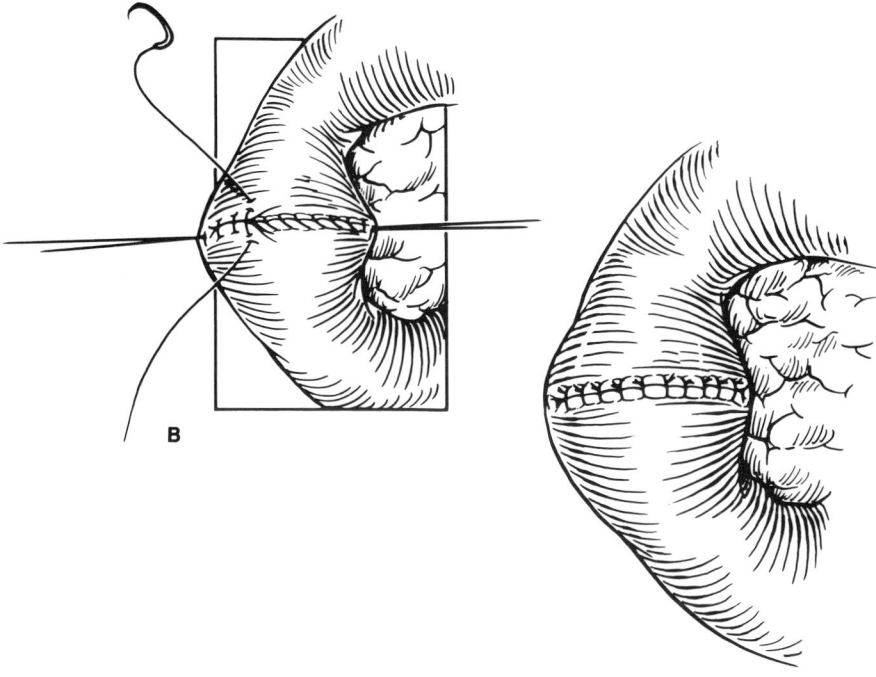

Figure 17-VI-9 *(Continued)*

(B) Interrupted 3-0 silk Lembert sutures are used for the outer layer.

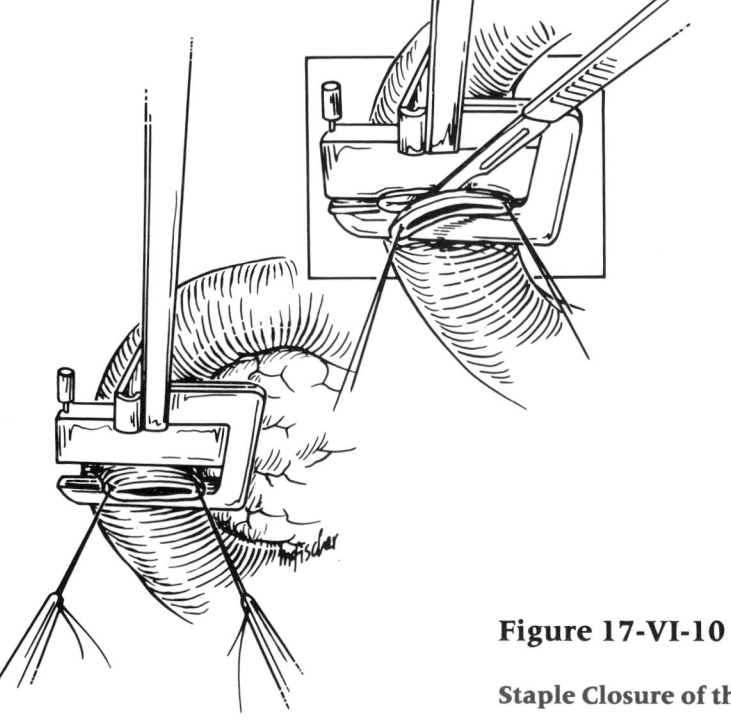

Figure 17-VI-10

Staple Closure of the Duodenum

An alternative to suture closure of the duodenum is stapled closure, using a TA-55 stapler. Although a stapled closure can be accomplished more rapidly, it should be used only when a tension-free closure can be attained.

SECTION VII *Choledochoduodenostomy*

A common indication for choledochoduodenostomy is a benign distal bile duct stricture, which is often secondary to chronic pancreatitis. Retained stones that cannot be removed during common bile duct exploration and the discovery of a large number of stones, which increases the likelihood of a retained stone, are other indications. The presence of primary common bile duct stones, which often form in the duct after cholecystectomy, is another reason to perform a choledochoduodenostomy. Choledochoduodenostomy, like transampullary sphincteroplasty, is performed less commonly since endoscopic sphincterotomy has become available.

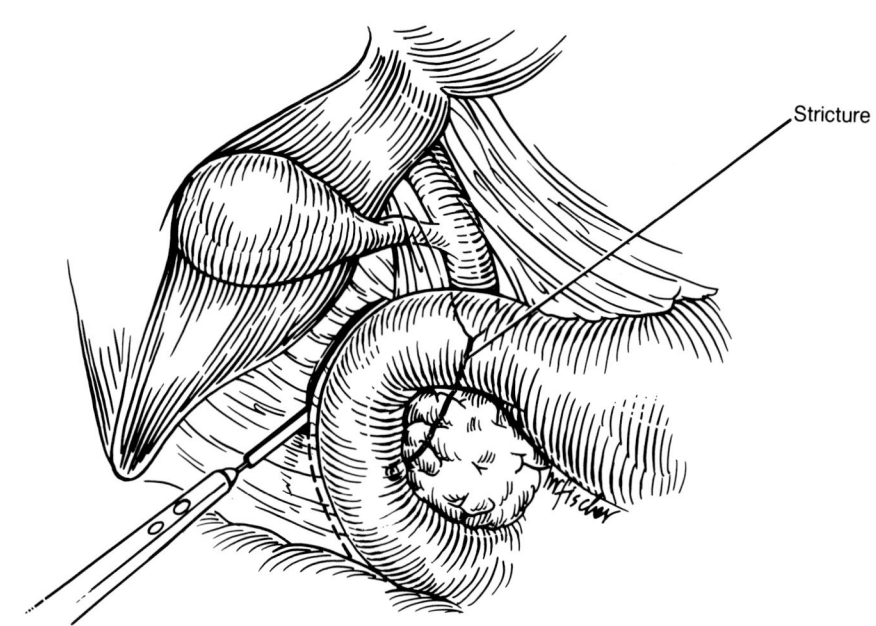

Stricture

Figure 17-VII-1

Initial Steps

If not done previously, cholecystectomy is performed. After the common bile duct is exposed, the duodenum and distal common duct are mobilized (Kocher maneuver).

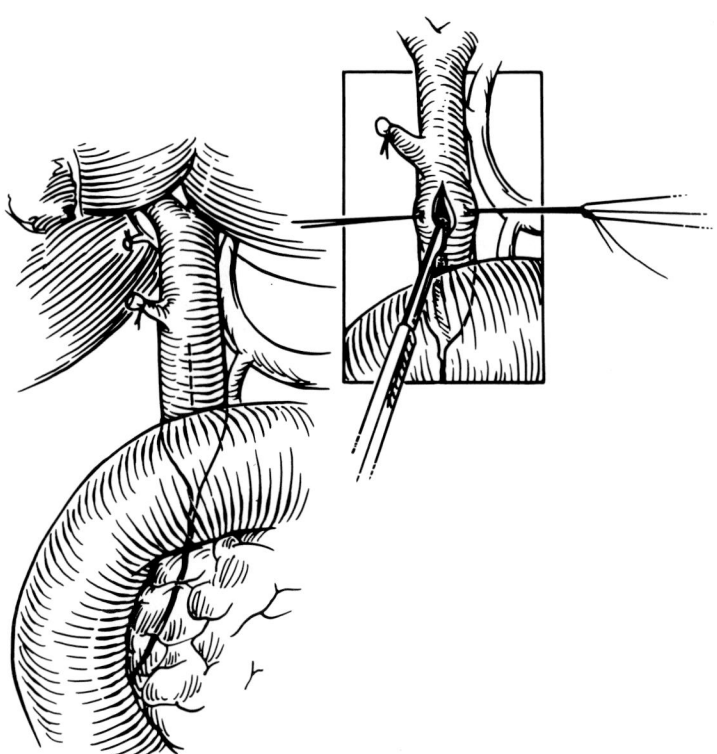

Figure 17-VII-2

Common Bile Duct Incision

A 2- to 3-cm incision is made longitudinally in the common bile duct as for common duct exploration. In fact, the incision for a common duct exploration should be fashioned so it can be used for a choledochoduodenostomy, should one prove necessary. The incision is placed just proximal to where the duodenum crosses over the common bile duct, which optimally should have a diameter of at least 1.5 cm. If the common duct is not dilated and a biliary drainage procedure is necessary, either a transduodenal sphincteroplasty (see Section VI) or a choledochojejunostomy (see Section X) is preferred.

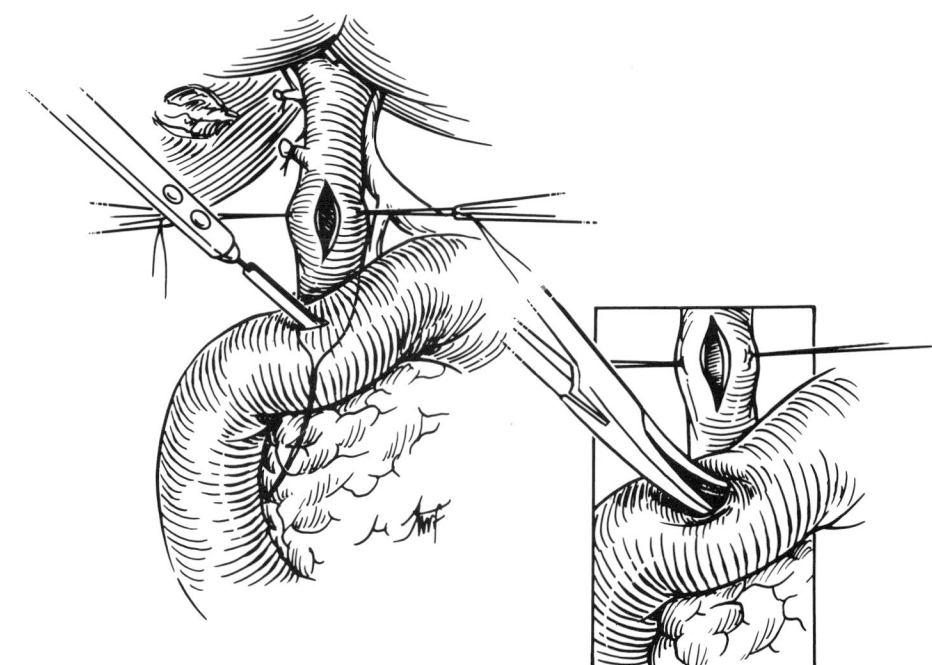

Figure 17-VII-3

Duodenal Incision

A small incision is made in the mobilized duodenum at a site where a tension-free anastomosis can be constructed, generally 7 to 8 cm from the pylorus. A *small* duodenal incision is emphasized because it will stretch to accommodate the bile duct opening, but the reverse does not occur.

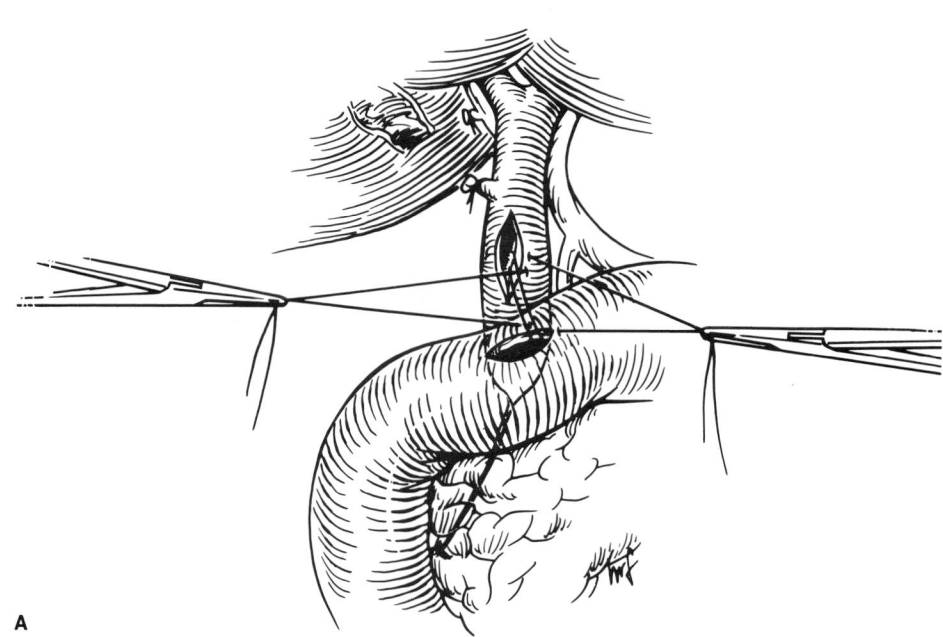

Figure 17-VII-4

Suture Placement

A

(**A**) The anastomosis is accomplished with a single layer of interrupted 4-0 Prolene sutures, all of which are placed so the knots are on the outside. The initial suture is placed at the apex of the duodenal incision and at the midway point on the common duct incision farthest from the operating surgeon, who stands on the patient's right. A second suture is placed adjacent to the first one and posterior to it. These first two sutures serve as apical sutures, and all subsequent sutures of the anterior and posterior rows are placed sequentially from this reference point. Both apical sutures are placed farthest from the surgeon so as not to obscure the placement of subsequent sutures.

(Continued)

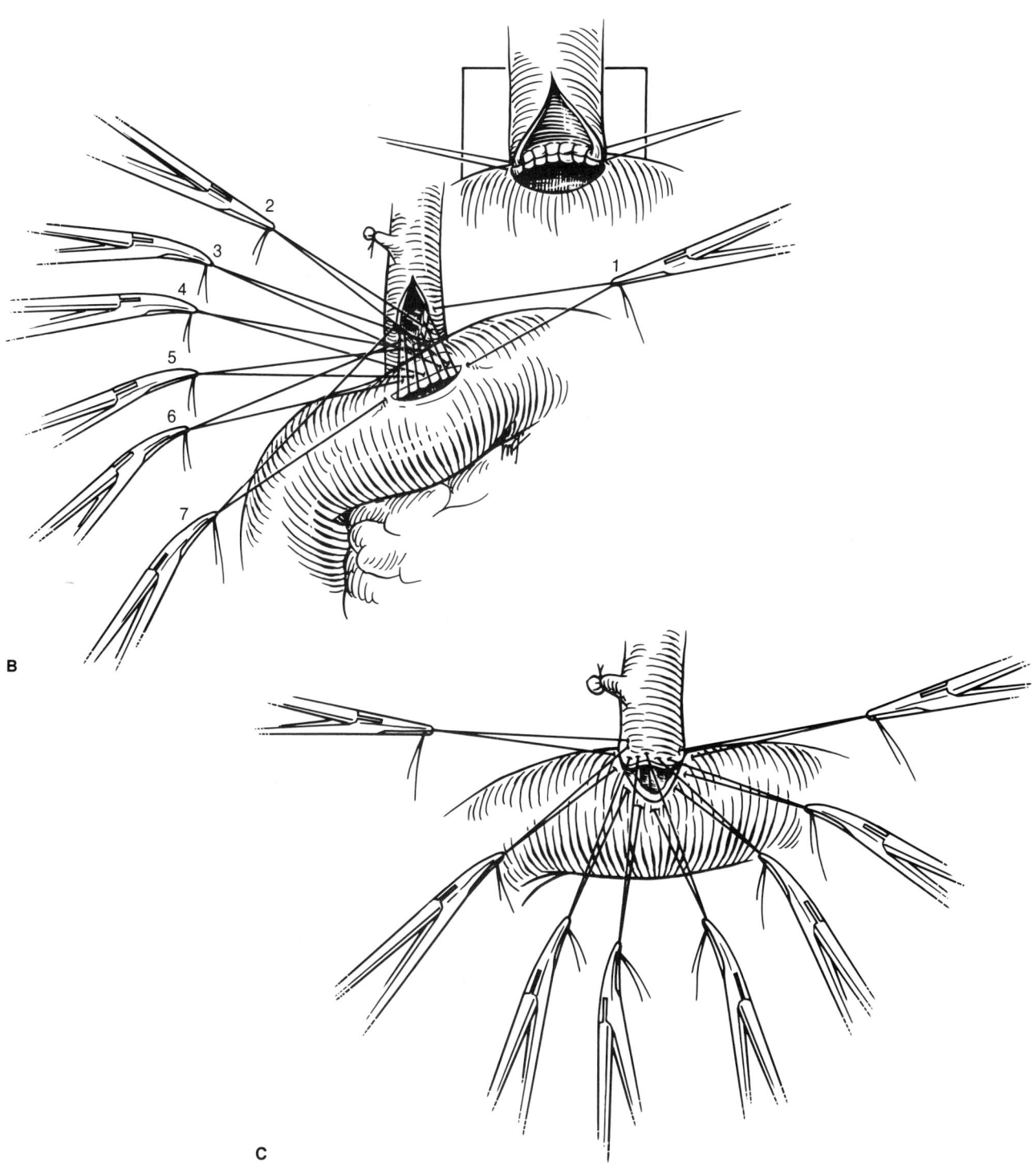

B

C

Figure 17-VII-4 *(Continued)*

(B) Each suture is individually tagged. Halsted clamps distinguish the two end sutures from the others, which are tagged with Crile clamps.

(C) The apical sutures are tied first, after which the remaining sutures are tied in the order in which they were placed.

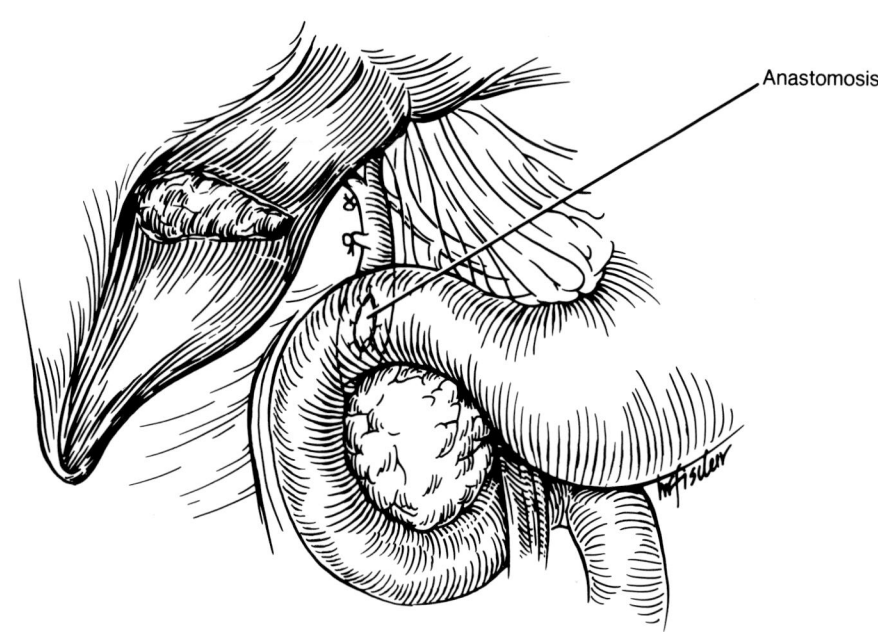

Anastomosis

Figure 17-VII-5

Completed Choledochoduodenostomy

Appearance of the completed anastomosis.

SECTION VIII *Laparoscopic Cholecystojejunostomy*

A laparoscopic cholecystojejunostomy should be selected only for patients in whom the cystic duct–common duct junction is sufficiently far from the site of bile duct obstruction for the gallbladder to serve as an effective long-term conduit.

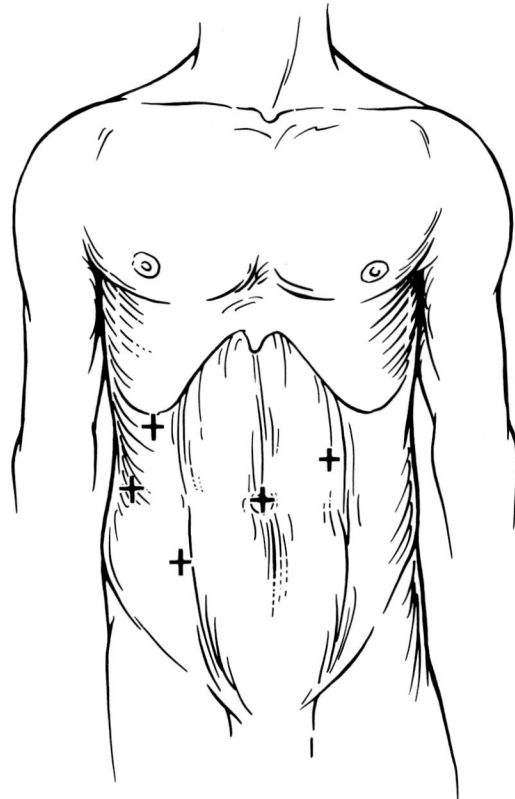

Figure 17-VIII-1

Trocar Ports

Five trocar ports placed at the positions shown are necessary for the operation. Like most other laparoscopic procedures, a 10-mm Hassan trocar is inserted through the umbilicus and is used for the camera.

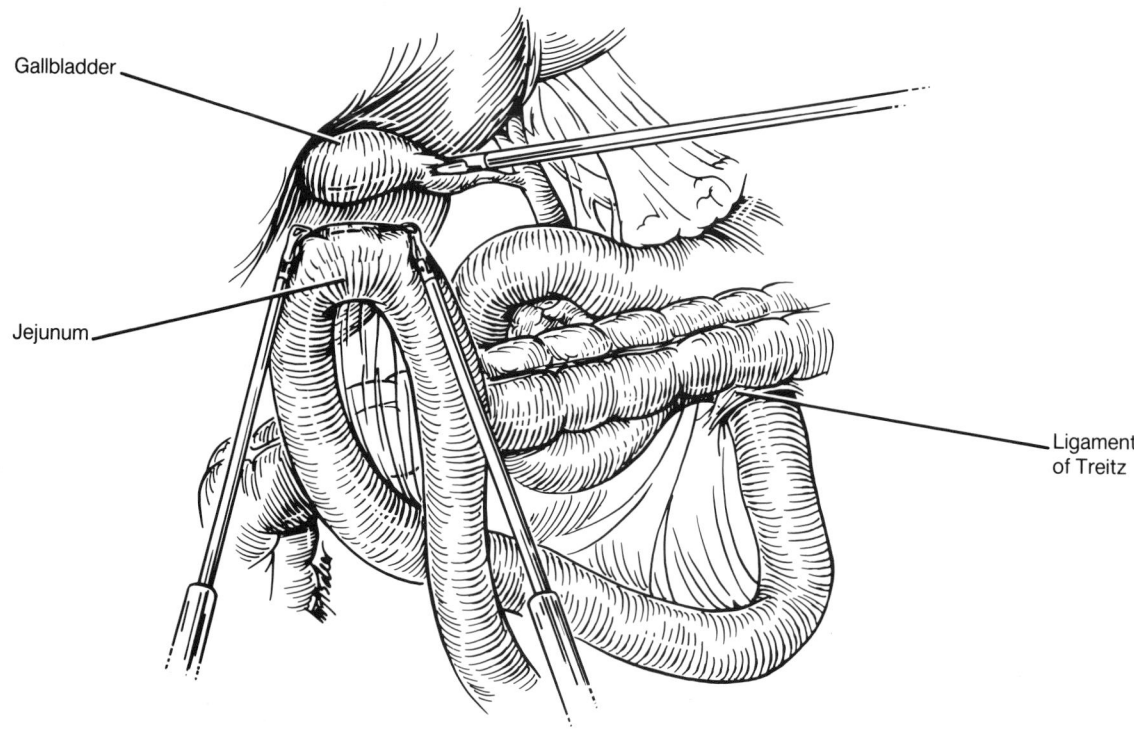

Figure 17-VIII-2

Aligning the Bowel and Gallbladder

After the ligament of Treitz is identified, the proximal jejunum is grasped with a Babcock clamp at a site where it can be approximated to the gallbladder without tension. A 3-0 Ethilon suture is placed to appose the gallbladder and jejunum to facilitate construction of the anastomosis.

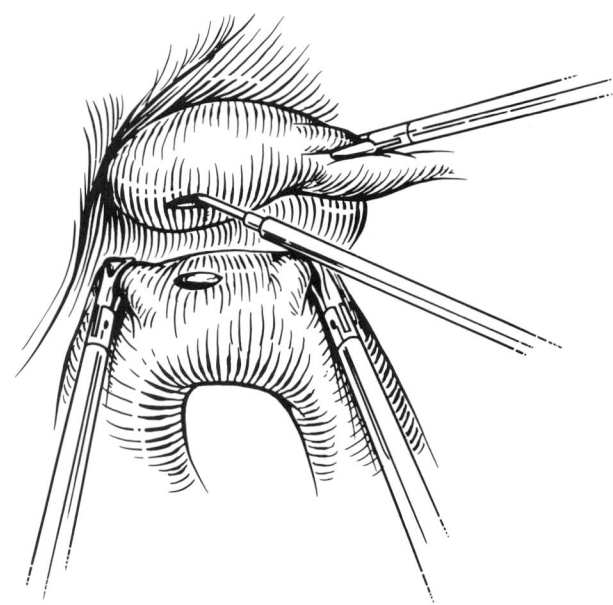

Figure 17-VIII-3

Incisions

Small incisions are made with the cautery in the fundus of the gallbladder and in the antimesenteric border of the jejunum.

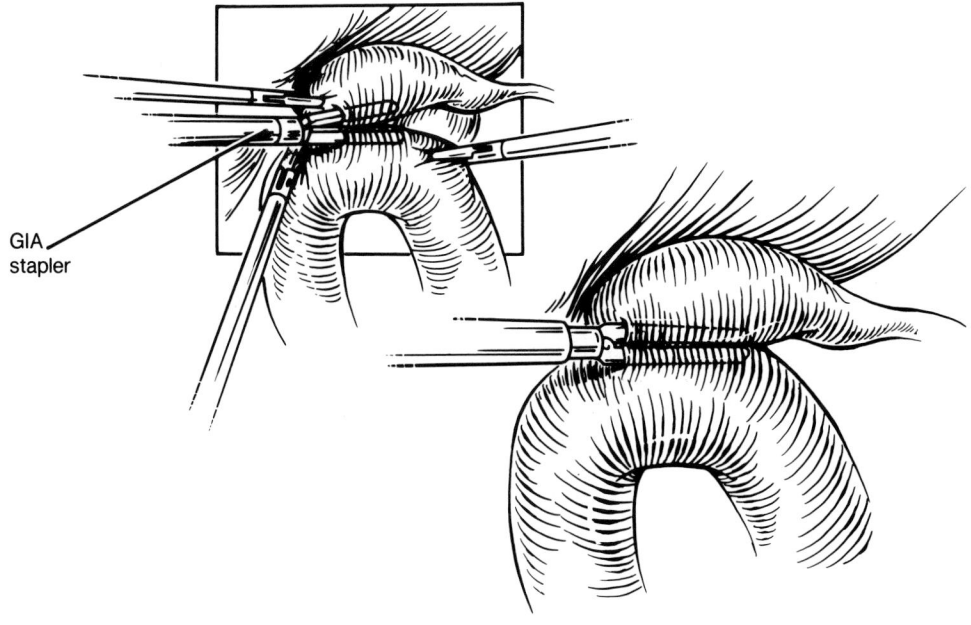

Figure 17-VIII-4

Anastomosis

A GIA stapler is inserted through a 12-mm right lateral trocar site. Generally, only one application of this instrument is necessary to create a sufficient anastomosis.

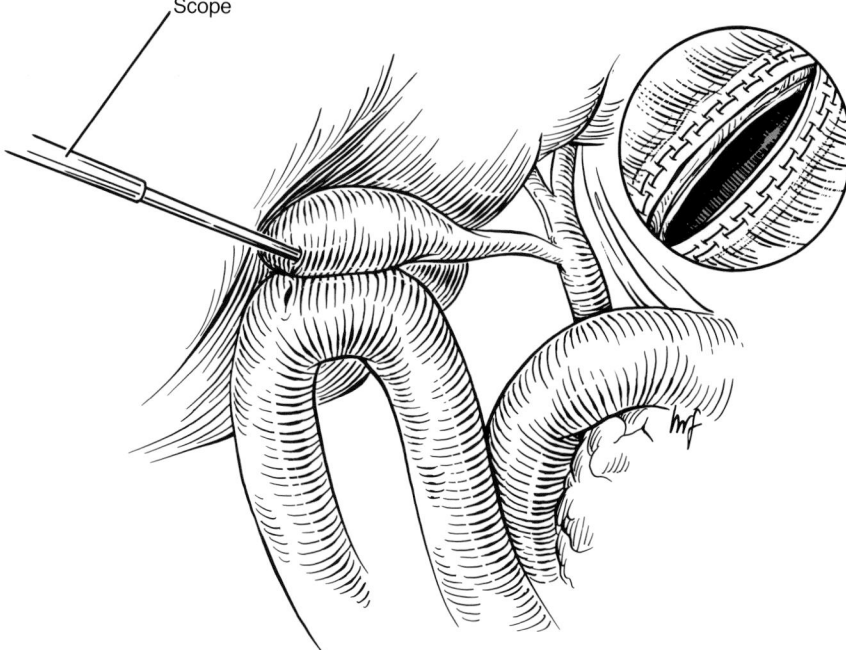

Figure 17-VIII-5

Camera Inspection

Before the anastomosis is closed, the camera is inserted to inspect it for hemostasis and patency.

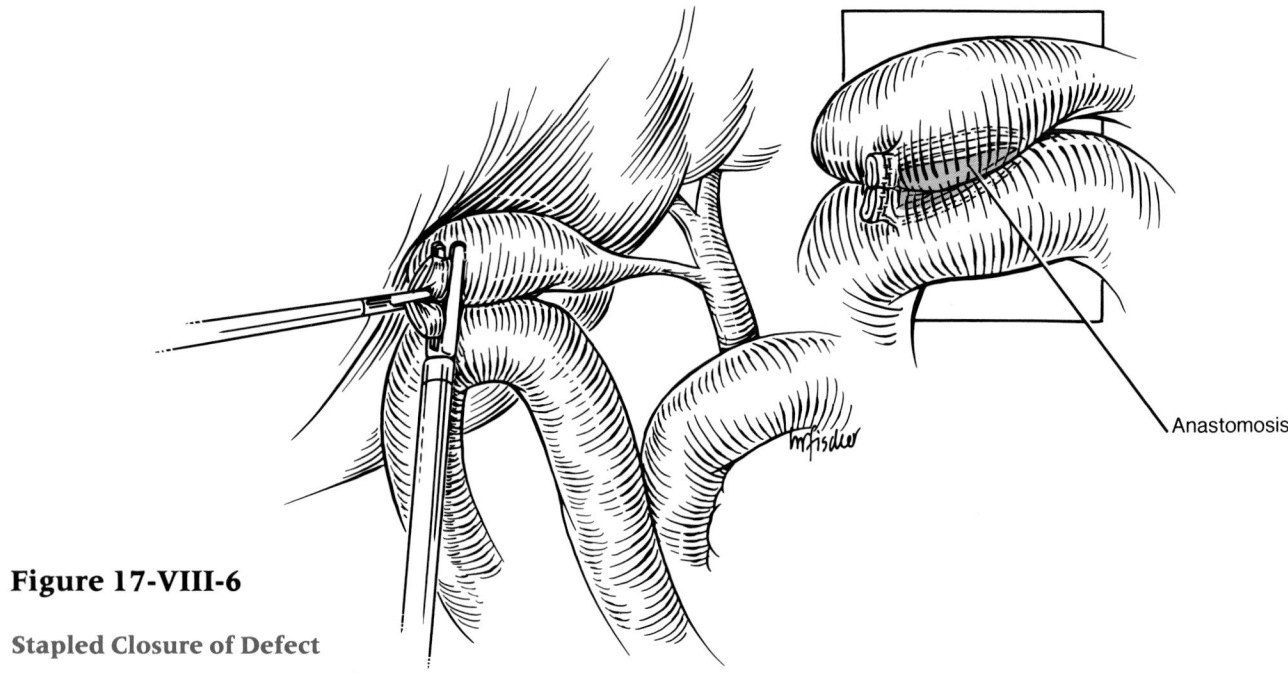

Anastomosis

Figure 17-VIII-6

Stapled Closure of Defect

The remaining gallbladder and jejunal defects are grasped and then closed with another application of the GIA stapler. More than one row of staples is often required to close the defect.

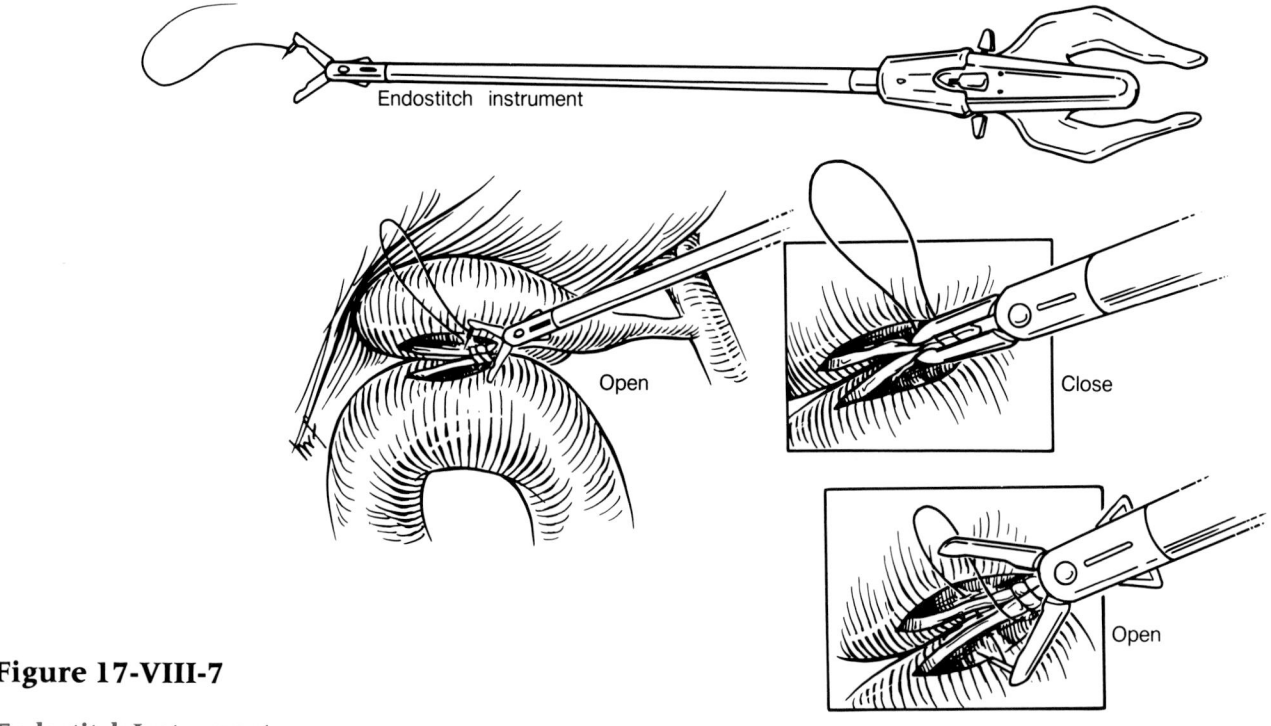

Figure 17-VIII-7

Endostitch Instrument

A laparoscopic cholecystojejunostomy can also be accomplished by a hand suture technique. This can be greatly facilitated by using the Endostitch instrument. The Endostitch instrument self-retrieves and positions the needle after traversing tissue, which reduces operative time. The posterior anastomosis is created with a running 4-0 suture.

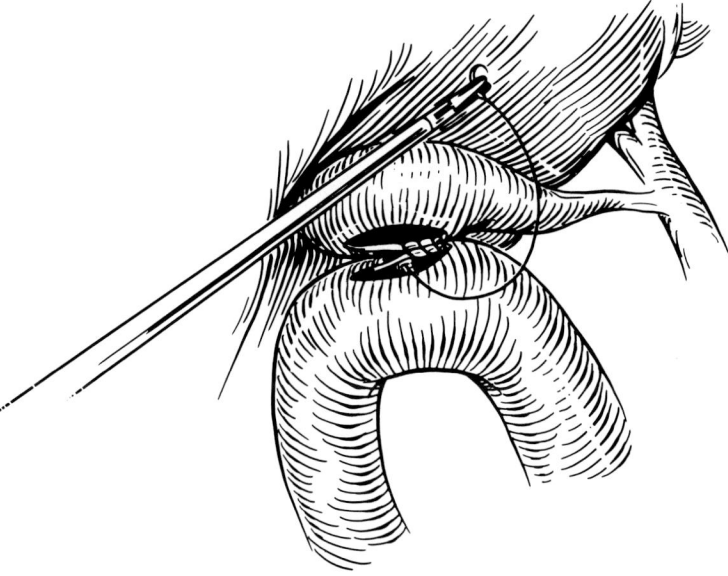

Figure 17-VIII-8

Hand Suturing the Posterior Row

Alternatively, the posterior row can be hand sewn without the Endostitch instrument, but this requires more time.

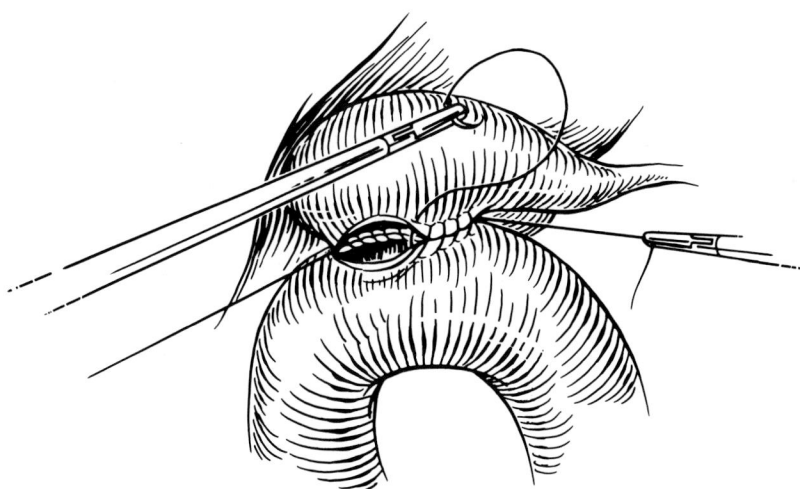

Figure 17-VIII-9

Suturing the Anterior Row

The anterior row is completed with either interrupted sutures or a running suture. Again, this is facilitated with the Endostitch instrument.

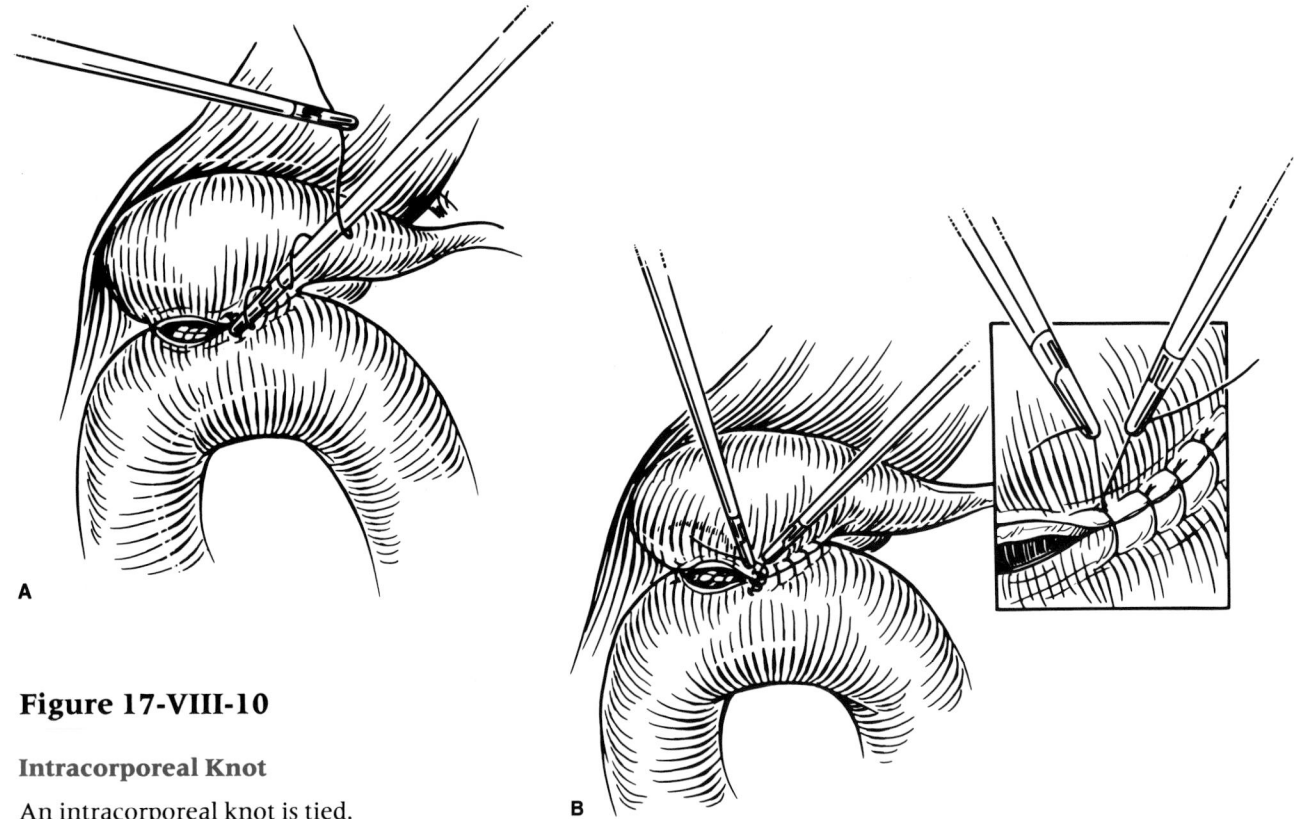

A

B

Figure 17-VIII-10

Intracorporeal Knot

An intracorporeal knot is tied.

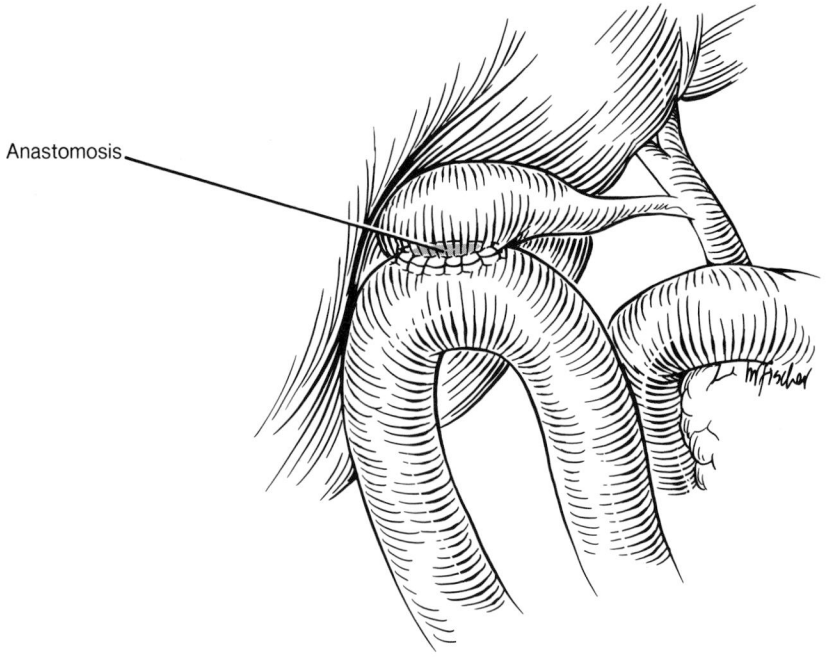

Anastomosis

Figure 17-VIII-11

Completed Cholecystojejunostomy

Although the hand-sewn anastomosis takes more time, it may be more secure.

SECTION IX *Open Cholecystojejunostomy*

A cholecystojejunostomy can be constructed considerably more rapidly than a choledo-chojejunostomy (see Section X). Again, the cystic duct–common duct junction must be proximal to the obstructing lesion (usually an unresectable tumor). Although long-term function of a choledochojejunostomy is probably superior to that of a cholecystojejunos-tomy, the latter is preferred for high-risk patients with limited life expectancies.

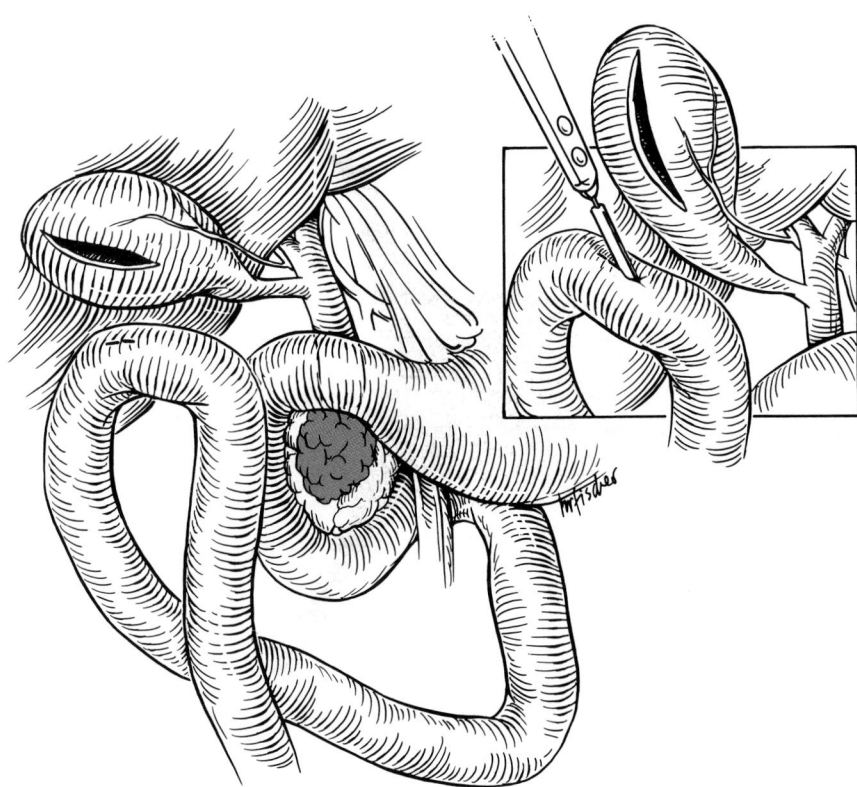

Figure 17-IX-1

Incisions

After identification of the ligament of Treitz, the proximal jejunum is apposed to the gallbladder fundus, and a small incision is made in each.

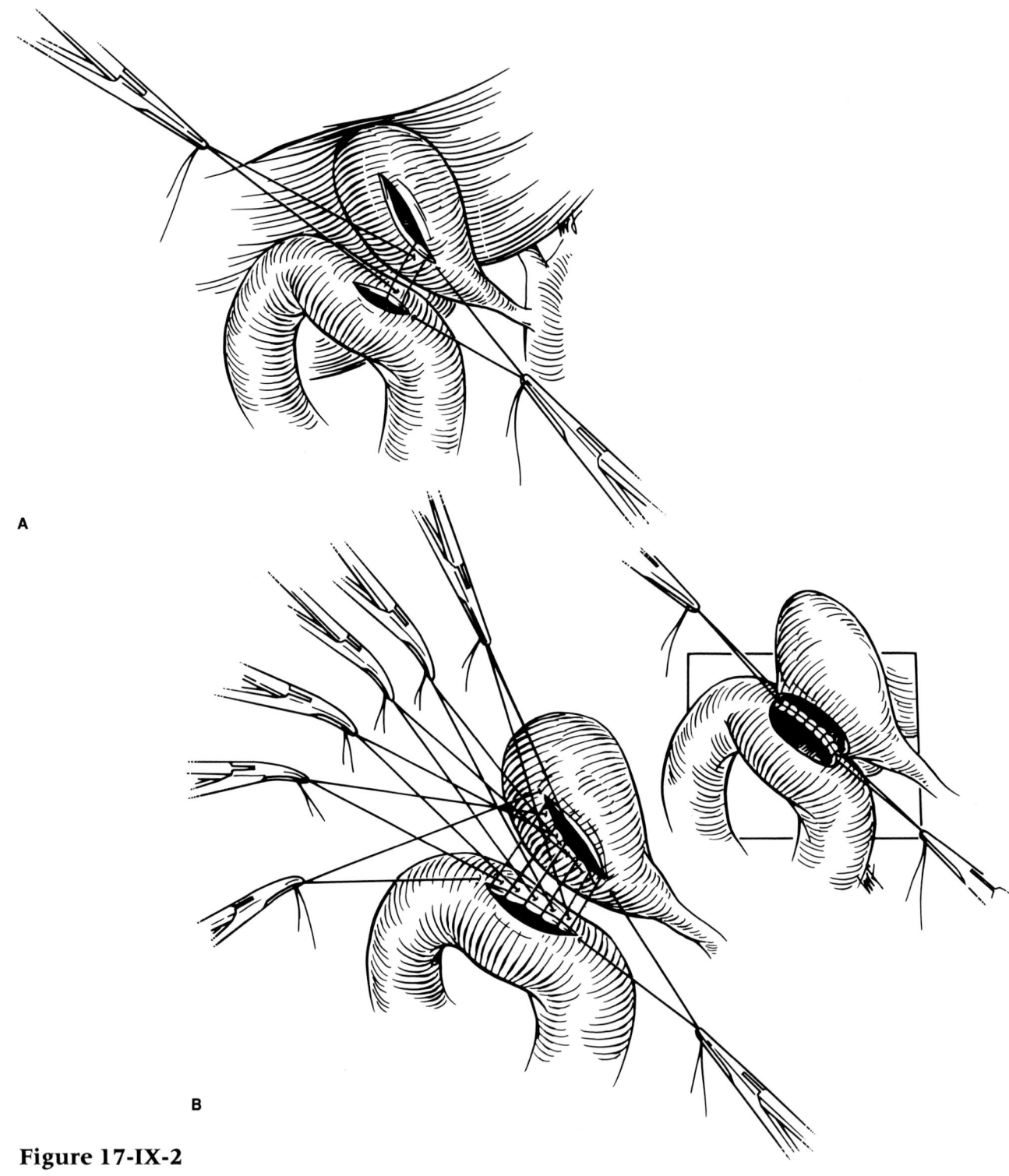

A

B

Figure 17-IX-2

Sutures

(A) Some 4-0 Prolene apex sutures are placed as described for the choledochoduodenostomy (see Fig. 17-VII-4).

(B) The posterior and anterior rows are completed with interrupted 4-0 Prolene sutures.

(Continued)

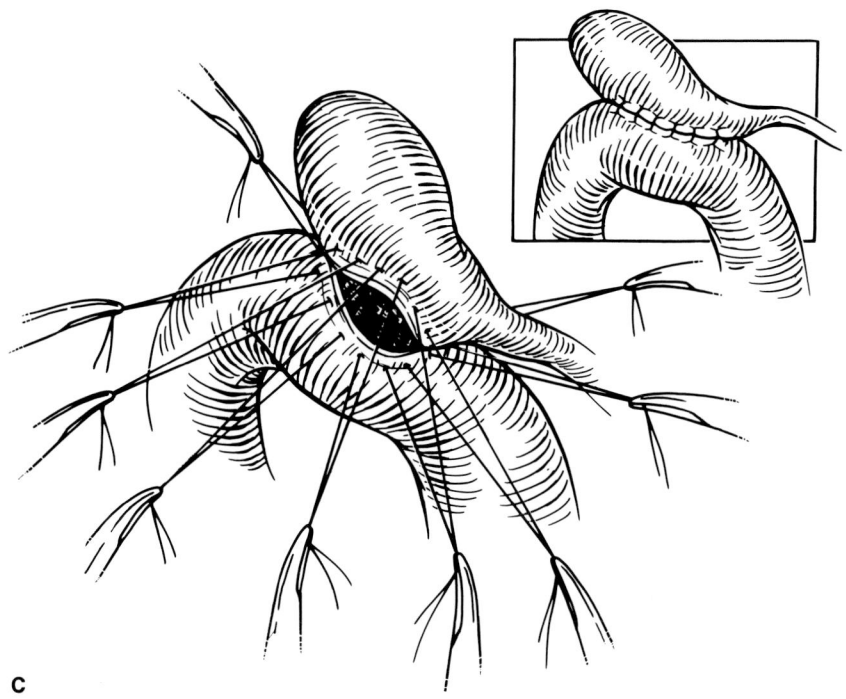

C

Figure 17-IX-2 *(Continued)*

(**C**) These sutures are placed so that the knots lie on the outside.

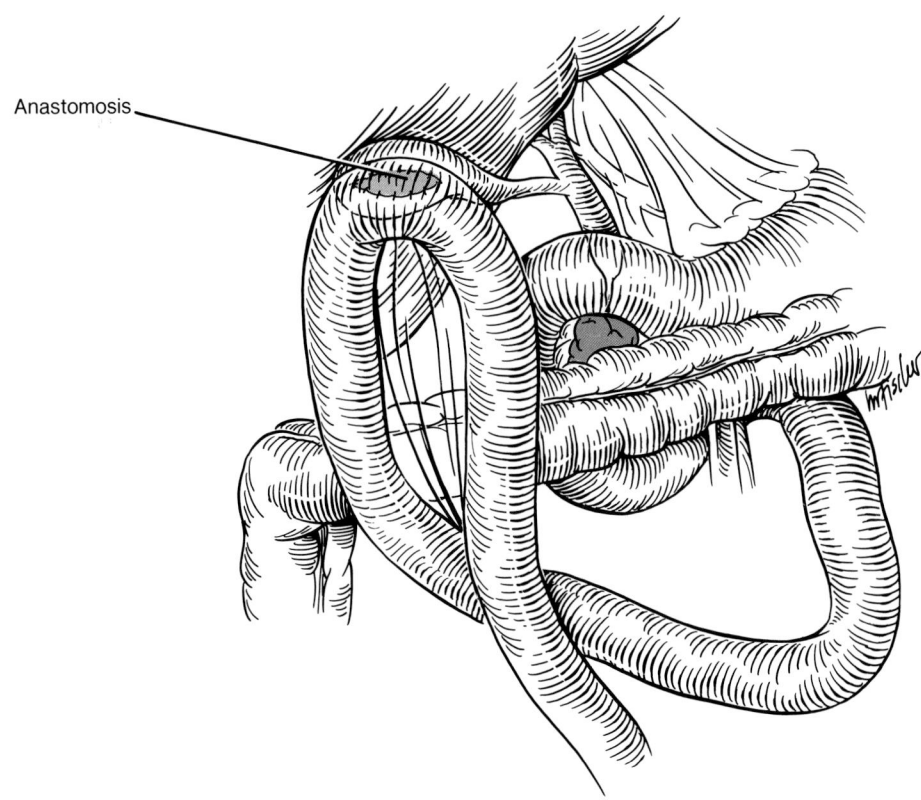

Anastomosis

Figure 17-IX-3

Completed Cholecystojejunostomy

Appearance of the completed anastomosis.

SECTION X *Roux-en-Y Choledochojejunostomy or Hepaticojejunostomy*

The most effective long-term biliary decompression is accomplished by anastomosing a Roux limb of jejunum to the common bile duct or common hepatic duct. With malignant obstruction, an anastomosis to the common hepatic duct is preferred. The duct may be left intact (as depicted here) or divided before it is anastomosed to the jejunum.

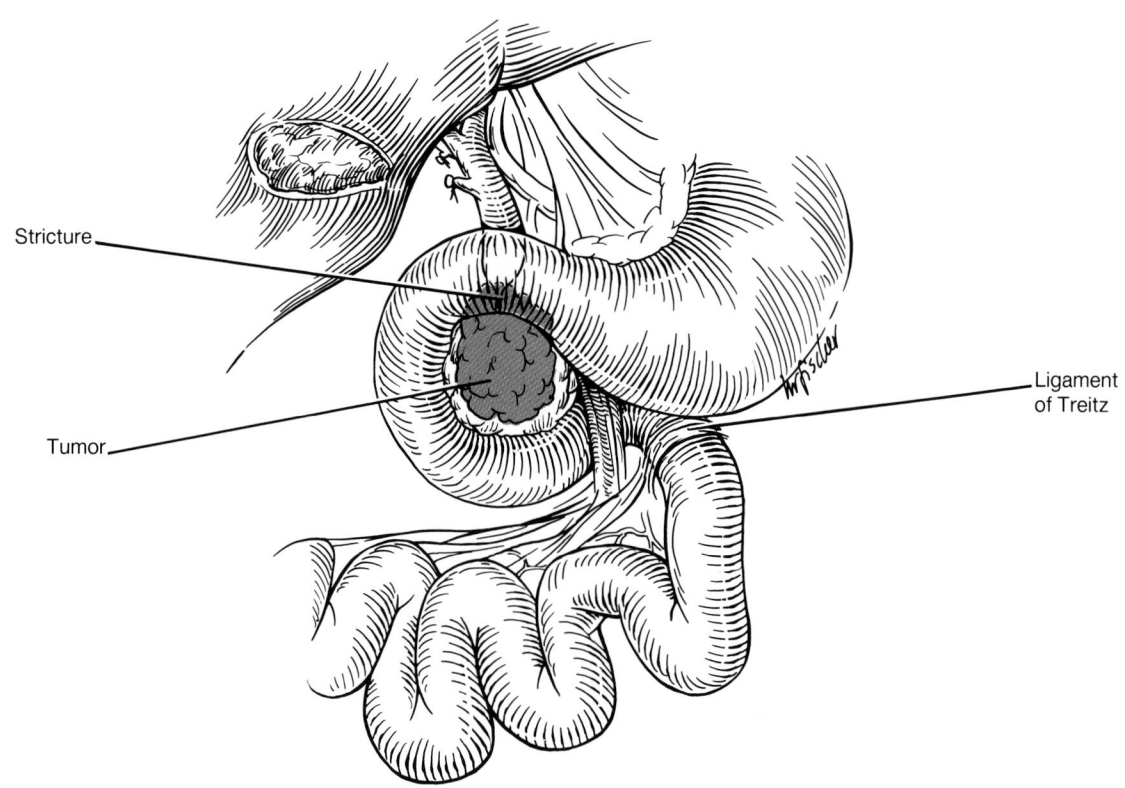

Figure 17-X-1

Duct Obstruction

The distal common bile duct is obstructed by an unresectable tumor. The gallbladder has been removed.

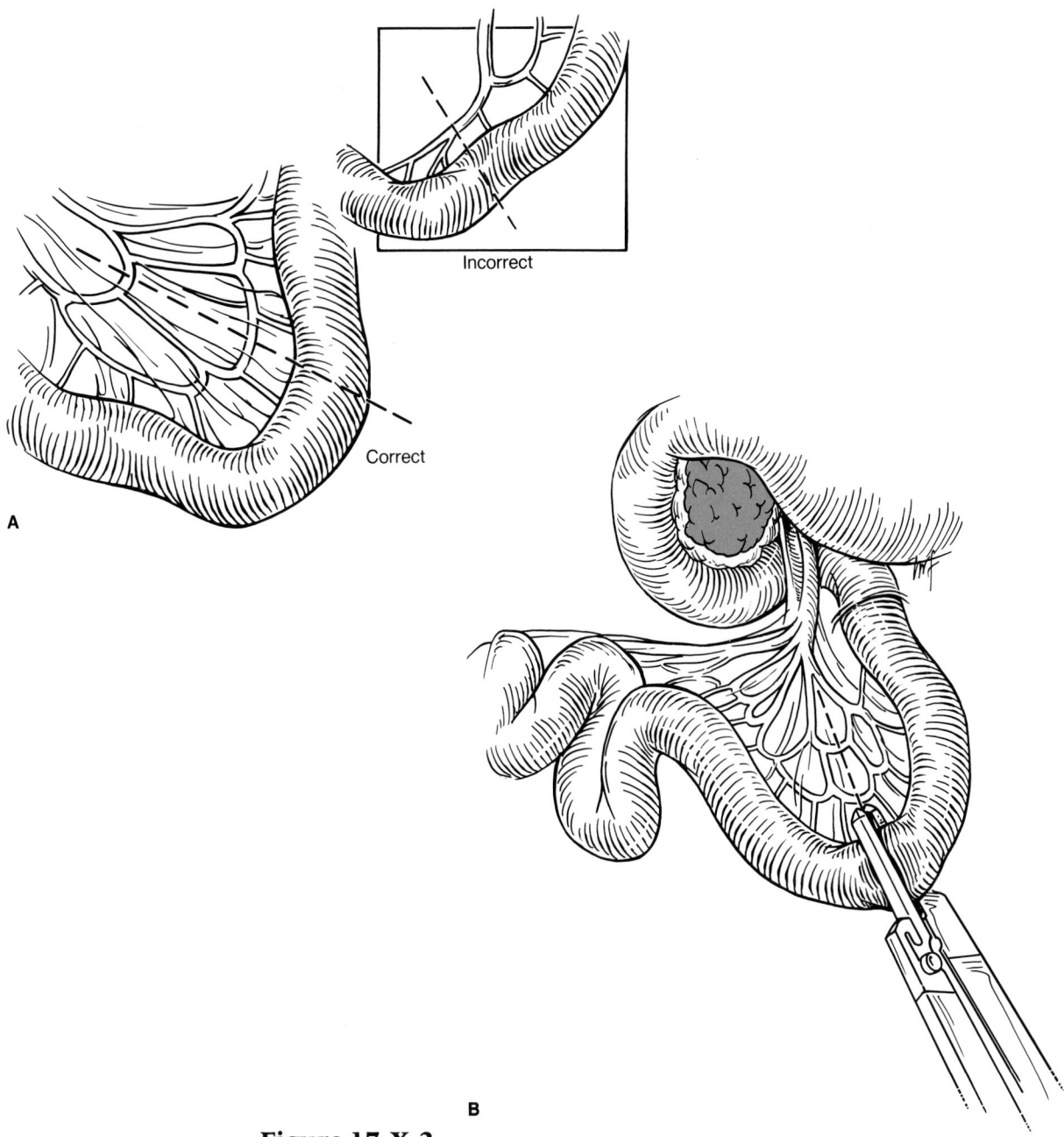

Figure 17-X-2

Division of the Proximal Jejunum and Intestine

(**A**) The site of division of the proximal jejunum and its mesentery is shown. Care is taken to preserve the blood supply of both ends of the jejunum.

(**B**) The GIA stapler is used to divide the intestine.

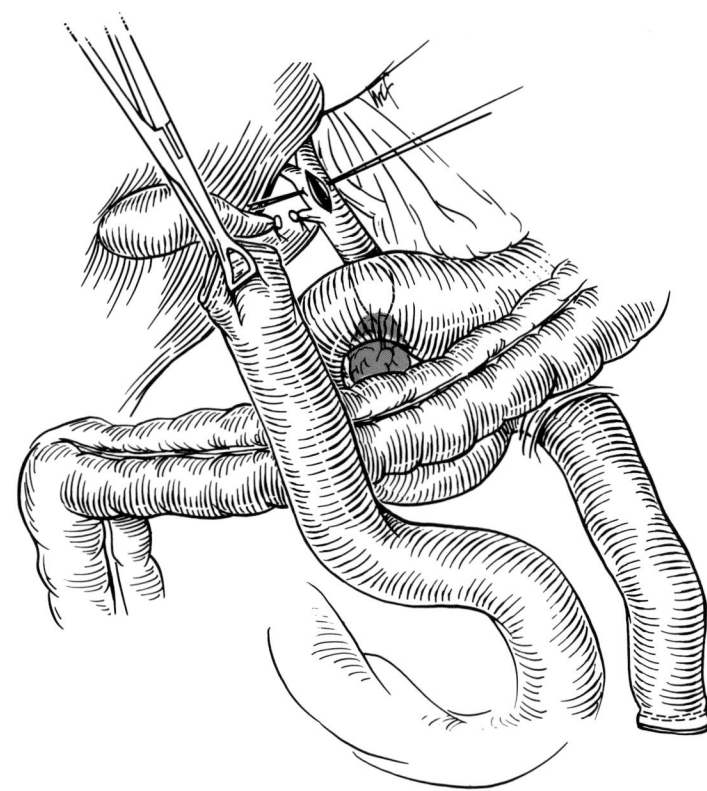

Figure 17-X-3

Antecolic Alignment of Roux Limb

The distal end of jejunum is brought to the incision in the common hepatic duct in an antecolic position to avoid subsequent obstruction by the tumor. A retrocolic position of the jejunum is acceptable when the cause of obstruction is benign. The gallbladder is removed unless infiltrated by tumor.

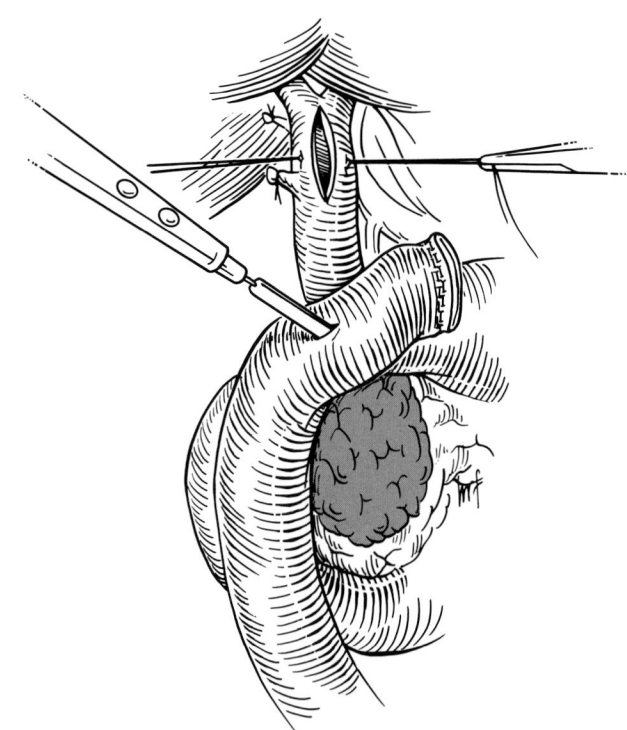

Figure 17-X-4

Incisions

A 2- to 3-cm incision is made longitudinally in the common hepatic duct, and a smaller incision is made in the jejunal limb.

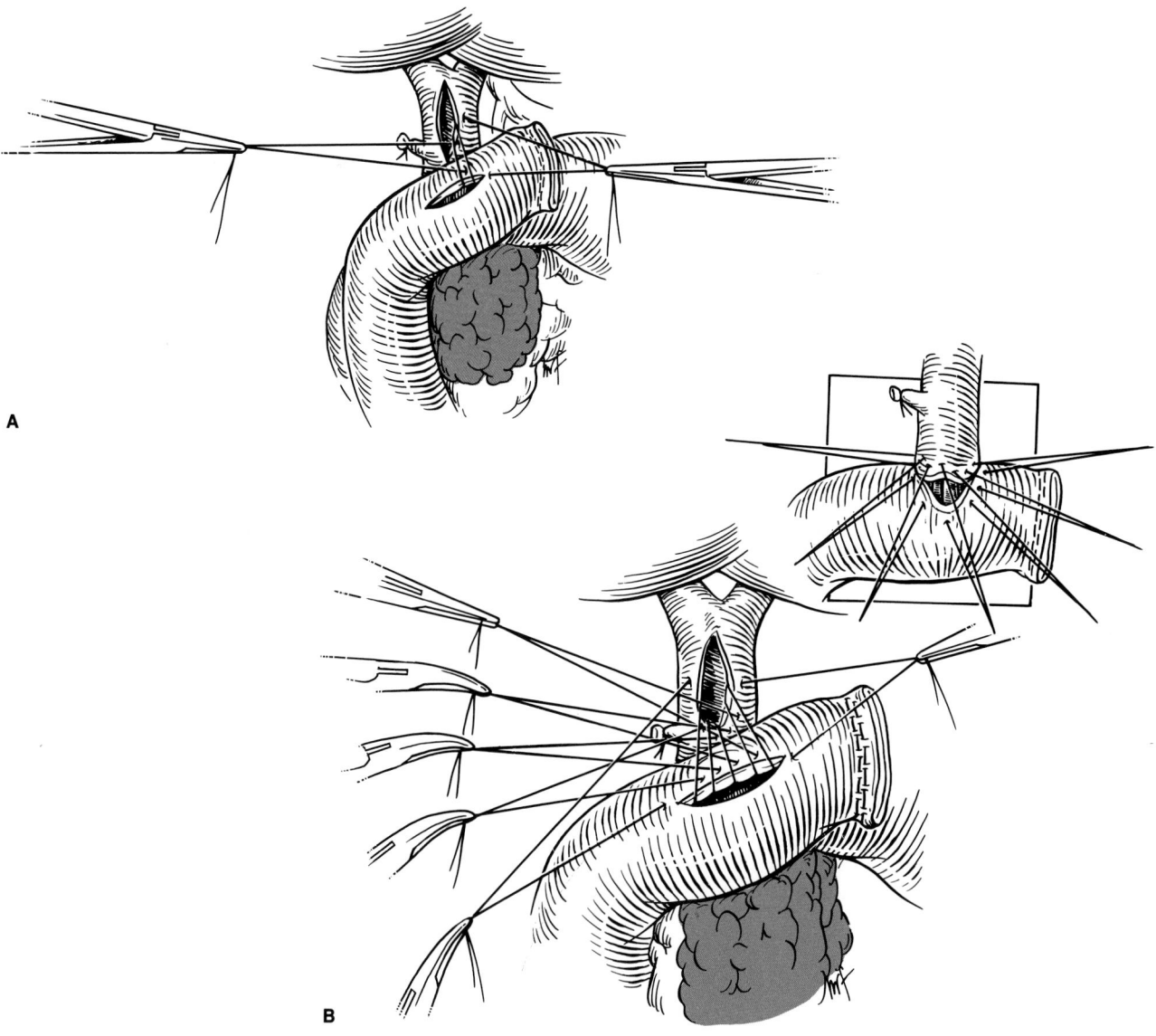

Figure 17-X-5

Suture Placement

(**A**) Interrupted 4-0 Prolene sutures are used for the anastomosis.

(**B**) The sutures are placed so that the knots are on the outside, and all sutures are placed before any are tied. If a mucosa-to-mucosa anastomosis has been accomplished, a stent is not required.

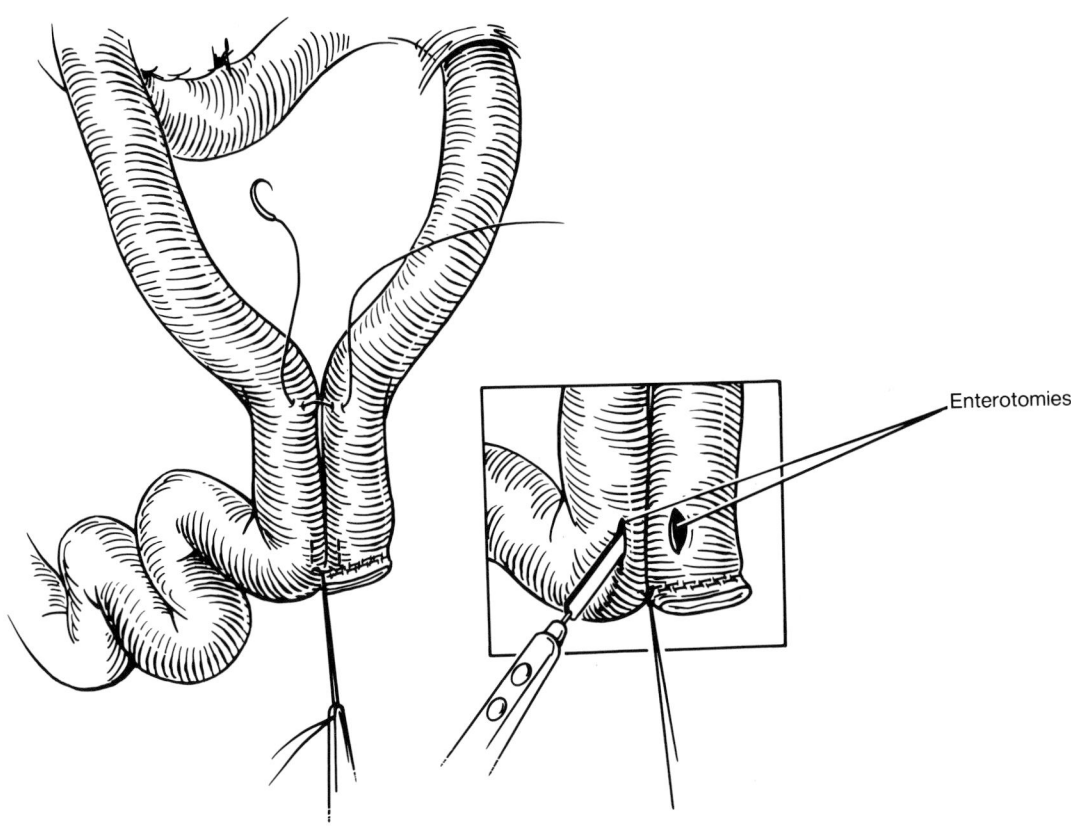

Enterotomies

Figure 17-X-6

Jejunojejunostomy

The jejunojejunostomy is done 18 inches (45 cm) distal to the biliary anastomosis. The jejunal segments are apposed with 3-0 silk sutures, and small enterotomies are made with the cautery.

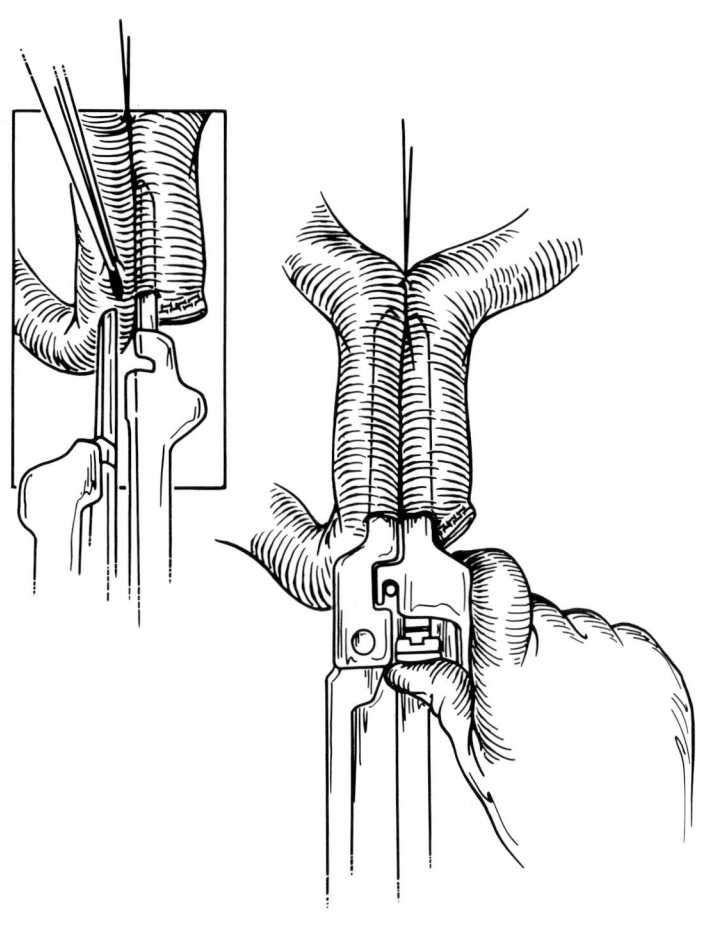

Figure 17-X-7

Creation of the Anastomosis
The anastomosis is created with the GIA stapler.

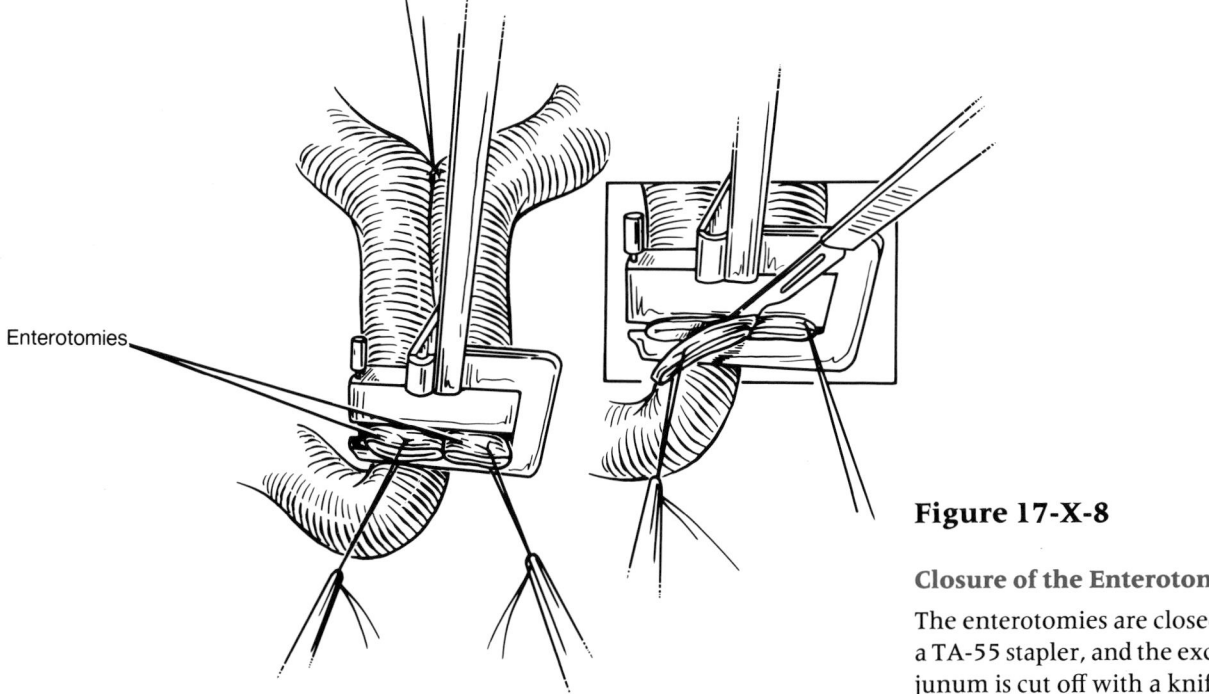

Enterotomies

Figure 17-X-8

Closure of the Enterotomies
The enterotomies are closed with a TA-55 stapler, and the excess jejunum is cut off with a knife.

Anastomosis

45 cm

Anastomosis

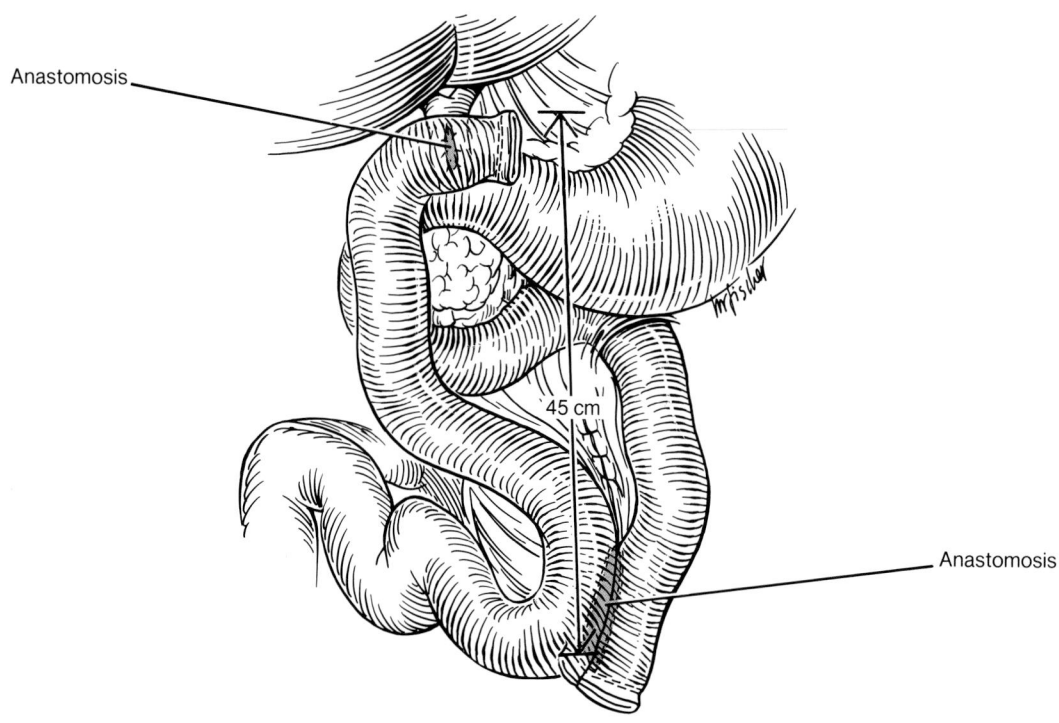

Figure 17-X-9

Completed Hepaticojejunostomy and Jejunojejunostomy

The mesenteric defect is closed with interrupted 3-0 silk sutures.

SECTION XI   *Management of a High Bile Duct Injury From Laparoscopic Cholecystectomy*

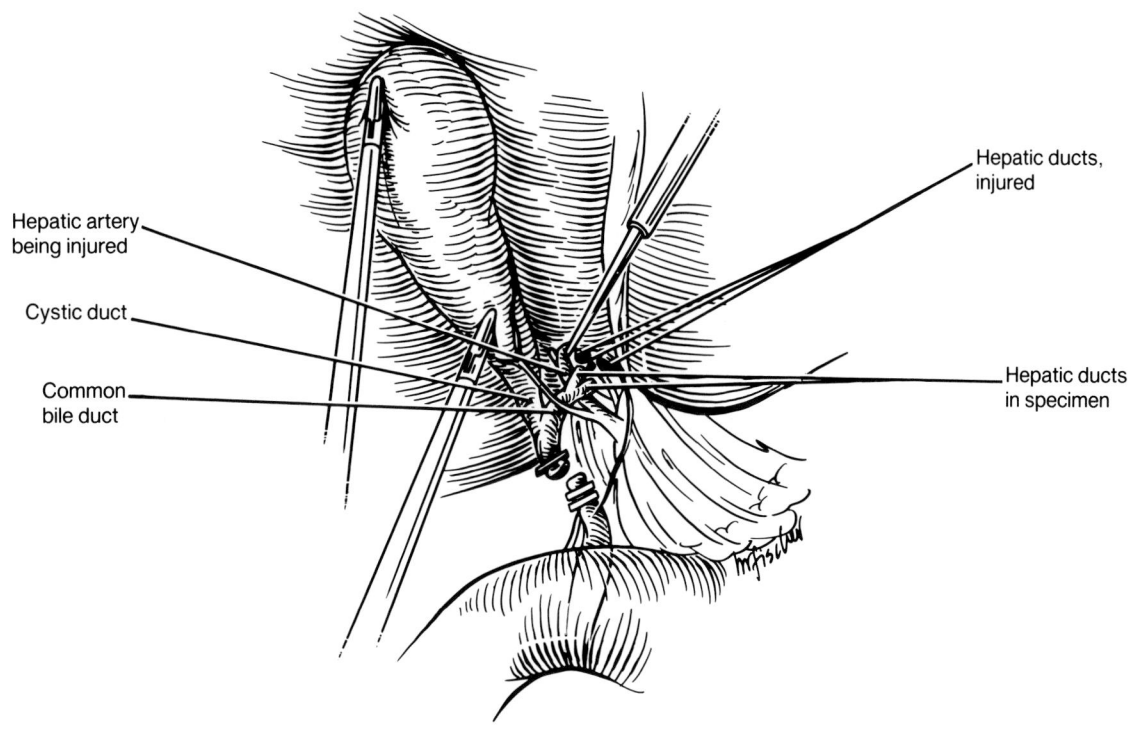

Hepatic ducts, injured

Hepatic artery being injured

Cystic duct

Common bile duct

Hepatic ducts in specimen

Figure 17-XI-1

High Bile Duct Injury

Although a variety of lesser ductal injuries can occur during laparoscopic cholecystectomy, the classic high bile duct injury is depicted. This injury, which invariably has vascular and ductal components, is caused by misidentification of the common bile duct as the cystic duct. The common duct and a small artery supplying it are misidentified as the cystic duct and cystic artery. These structures are doubly clipped and divided. The common duct is dissected into the hilum, where the biliary tract is transected, often above the bifurcation and frequently through secondary hepatic duct radicles, leaving multiple ends of hepatic ducts as shown here. As a result, much of the extrahepatic biliary tree is excised with the gallbladder. The right hepatic artery is often injured as well.

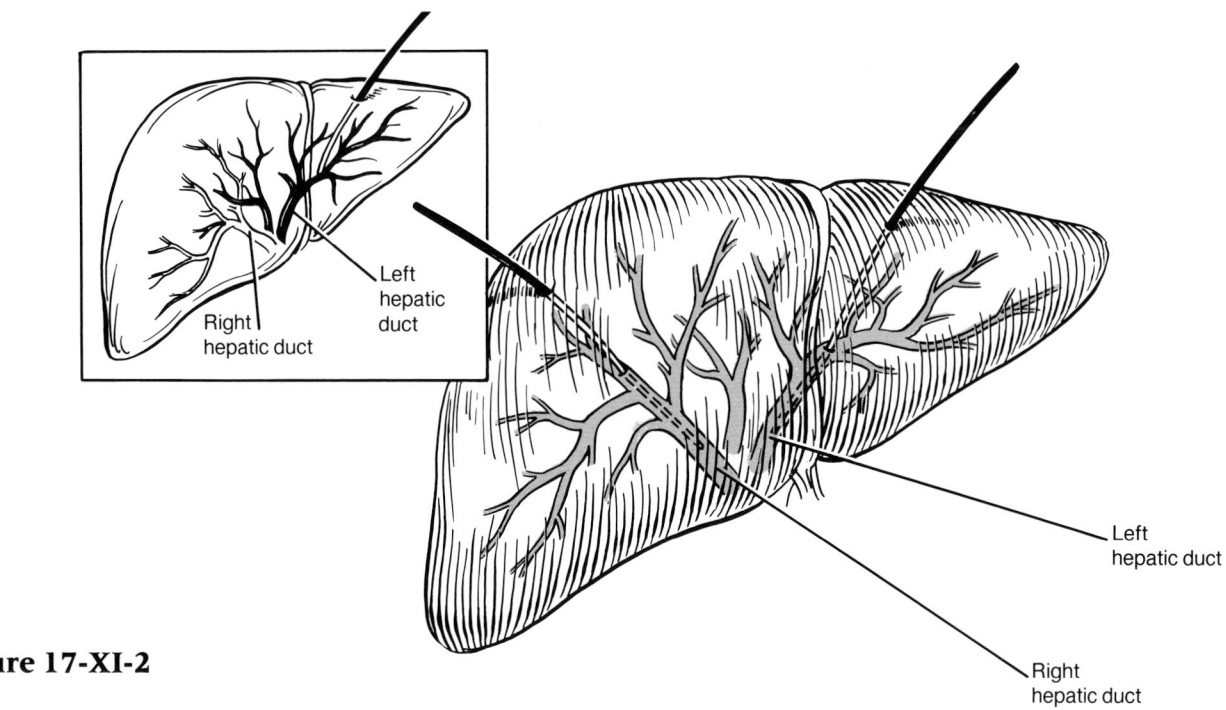

Figure 17-XI-2

Three-Duct Injury

The right hepatic duct has been transected above the junction of the bile duct from segments VII and VIII and the bile duct from segments V and VI. This example illustrates the importance of defining the complete biliary anatomy before repair is begun.

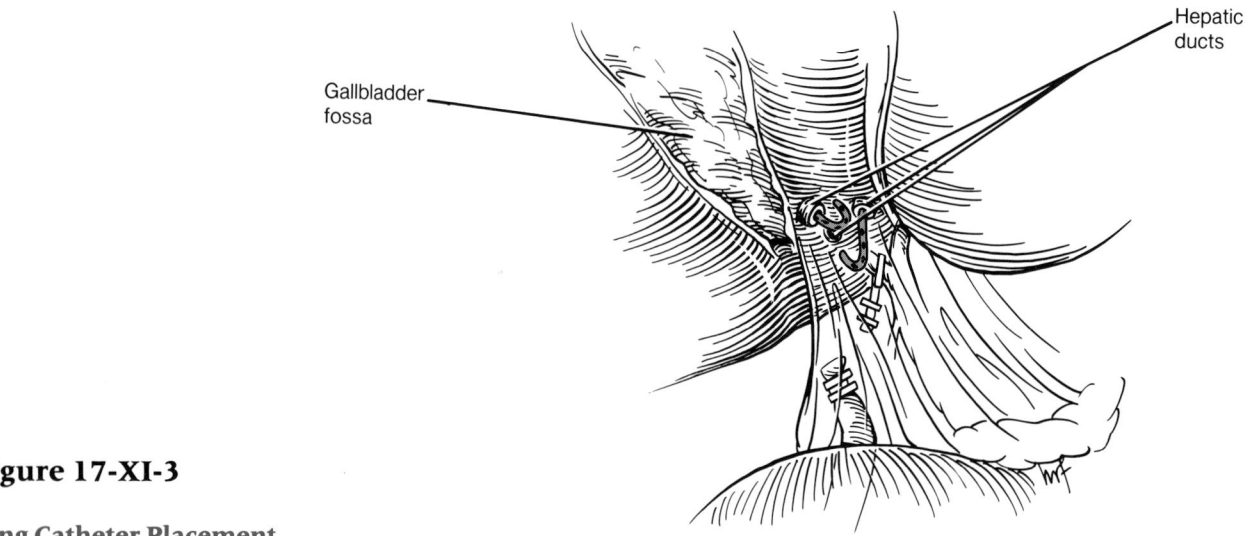

Figure 17-XI-3

Ring Catheter Placement

Bilateral transhepatic Ring catheters are placed before surgery. These catheters assist in identification of the major components of the biliary system at the time of repair. Because part of the biliary tract might be excluded (eg, the duct from segments VII and VIII as shown here), care is taken at the operation to identify all transected ducts. As many as seven separate ducts have been identified after such an injury. The Ring catheters exit through the main right and left hepatic ducts. An additional duct orifice (without a Ring catheter) drains segments VII and VIII.

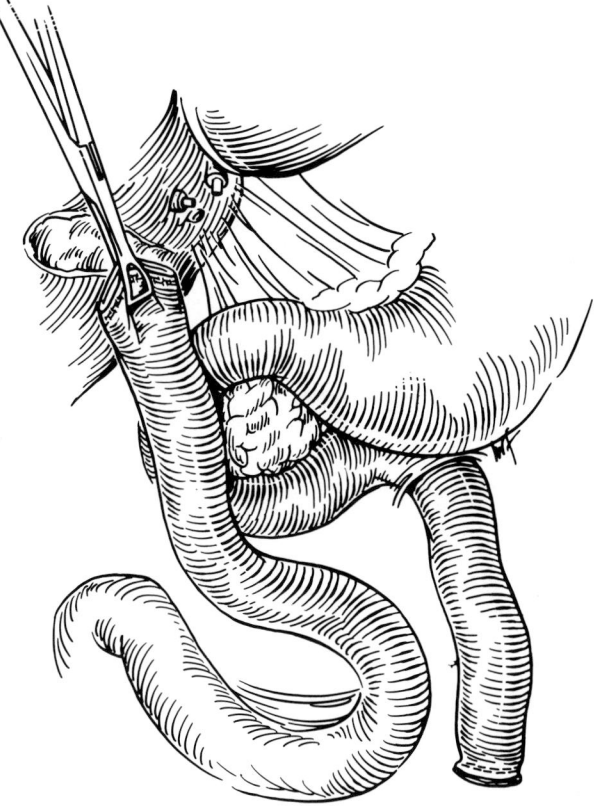

Figure 17-XI-4

Roux-en-Y Reconstruction

After identification of the ducts, a Roux-en-Y limb is constructed as previously described (see Section VII). Either an antecolic or a retrocolic position of the Roux limb is acceptable.

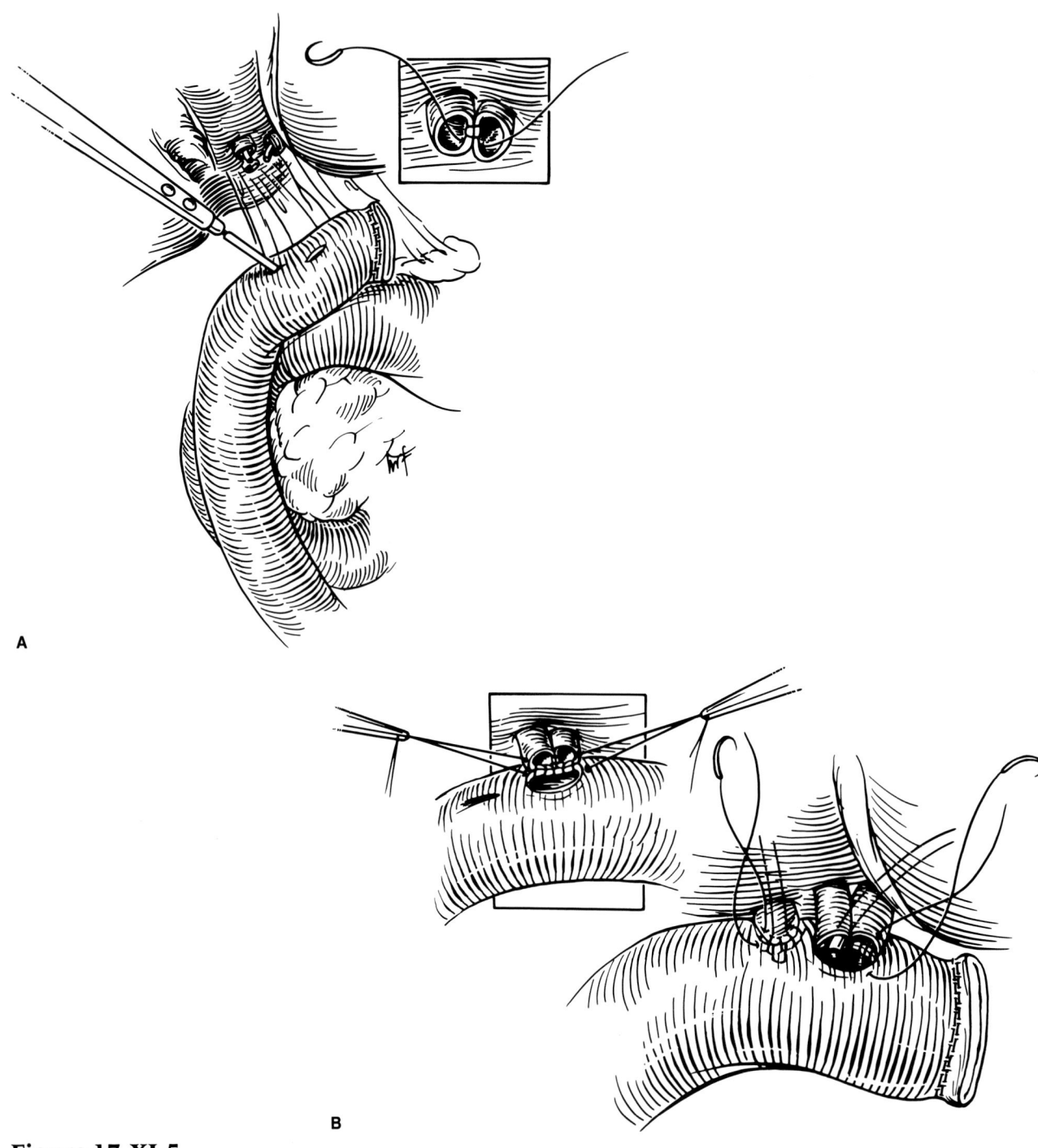

A

B

Figure 17-XI-5

Anastomosis Creation

(**A**) Two of the duct orifices are sewn to each other with fine chromic sutures, creating a bifurcation. Two small enterotomies are made in the Roux limb.

(**B**) The ducts are anastomosed to the Roux limb with interrupted 4-0 or 5-0 Prolene sutures placed so the knots are outside the lumen (see Fig. 17-VII-4).

(Continued)

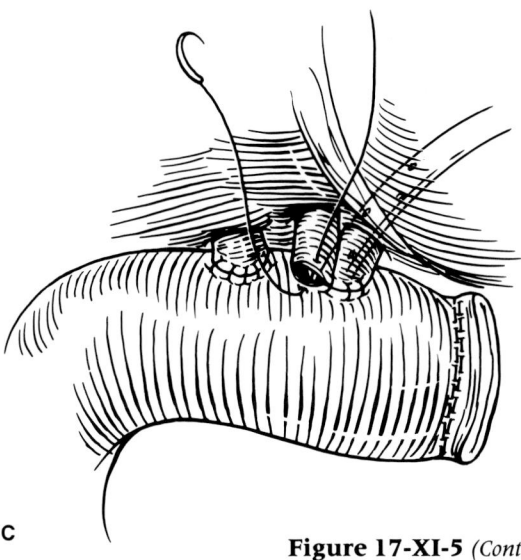

c

Figure 17-XI-5 *(Continued)*

(**C**) The Ring catheters are cut short and left proximal to the anastomoses so that they can be used for postoperative cholangiography. They do not serve as stents and are removed before the patient is discharged from the hospital. The Ring catheter can be used to stent a questionable anastomosis. The anesthesiologist can inject saline through each Ring catheter before abdominal closure to check for anastomotic leaks.

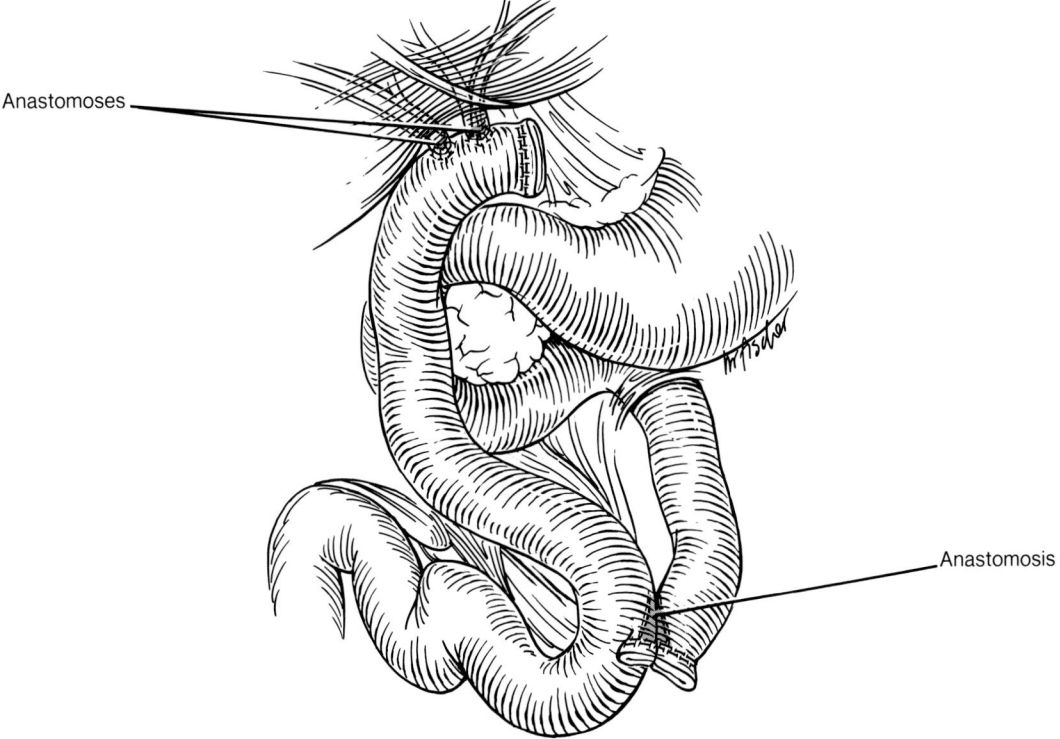

Anastomoses

Anastomosis

Figure 17-XI-6

Jejunojejunostomy Creation

The jejunojejunostomy is constructed with the GIA and TA-55 staplers (see Section VII). The mesenteric defect is closed with interrupted 3-0 silk sutures. The Roux limb should be 45 cm (18 inches) long.

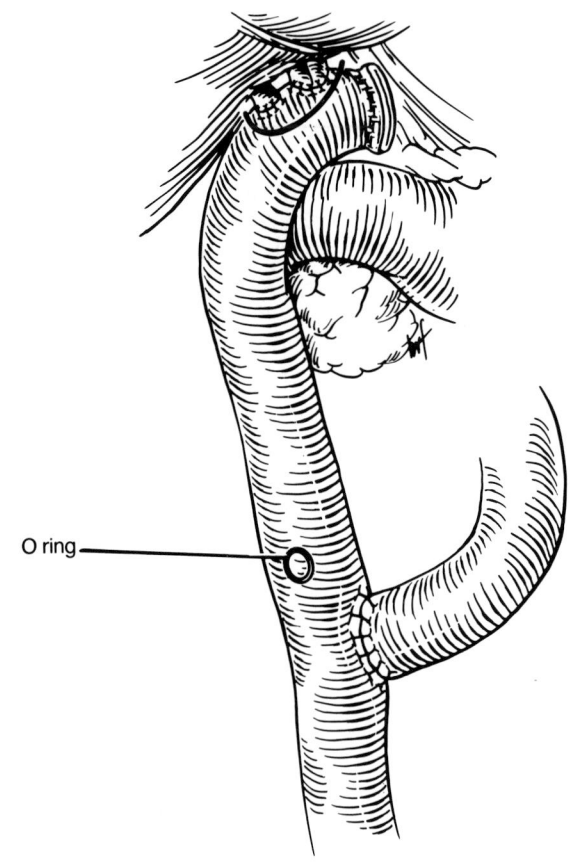

O ring

Figure 17-XI-7

Marking Roux Limb and Anastomosis

After the biliary reconstruction, a metal O ring marker is left on the antimesenteric border of the Roux limb, which is affixed to the anterior abdominal wall. The purpose of the O ring is for potential future radiologic access to the biliary system. A horseshoe-shaped marker is placed at the anastomosis for easy radiologic identification. These markers are particularly useful after biliary reconstruction for sclerosing cholangitis or after resection of a proximal bile duct cancer.

SECTION XII   *Resection of a Mid–Bile Duct Tumor*

The first and second most common locations for bile duct tumors are at the bifurcation of right and left hepatic ducts (a Klatskin tumor) and in the distal common bile duct, respectively.

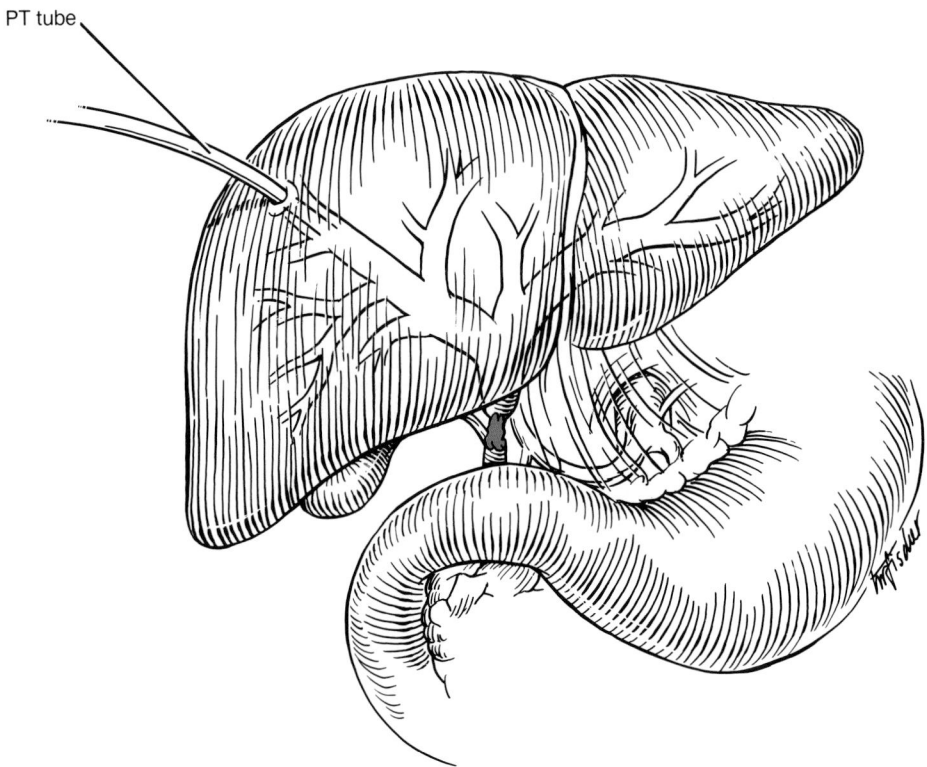

PT tube

Figure 17-XII-1

Tumor Location

Occasionally, a bile duct tumor is found near the junction of cystic and common bile ducts. Resection of a Klatskin tumor is described in the next section, and pancreatoduodenectomy, which is required for a distal tumor, is described in the Atlas Chapter 30.

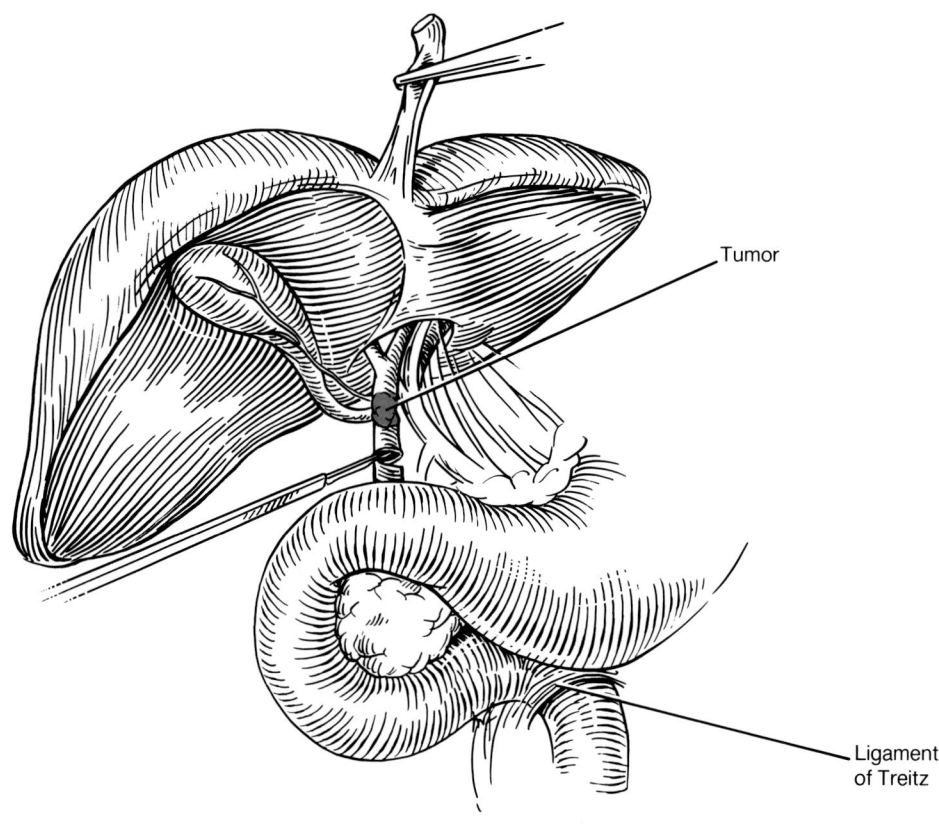

Tumor

Ligament
of Treitz

Figure 17-XII-2

Excision of the Common Bile Duct

A mid–bile duct tumor can be treated by excising the common duct from just above the duodenum to the hepatic duct bifurcation and reconstructing with a Roux-en-Y hepaticojejunostomy. The distal common bile duct is transected after its circumferential dissection.

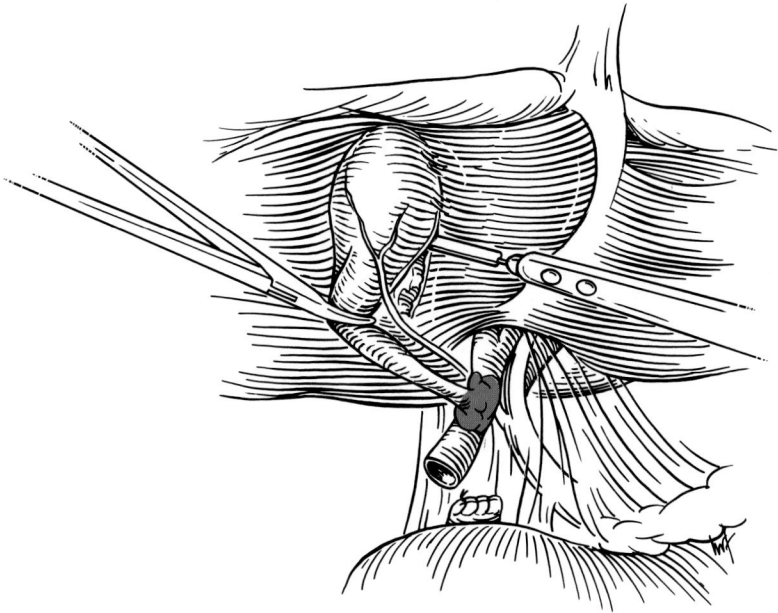

Figure 17-XII-3

En Bloc Resection

The common bile duct and tumor are dissected off of the portal vein. The gallbladder is included in the en bloc resection. The distal bile duct is oversewn.

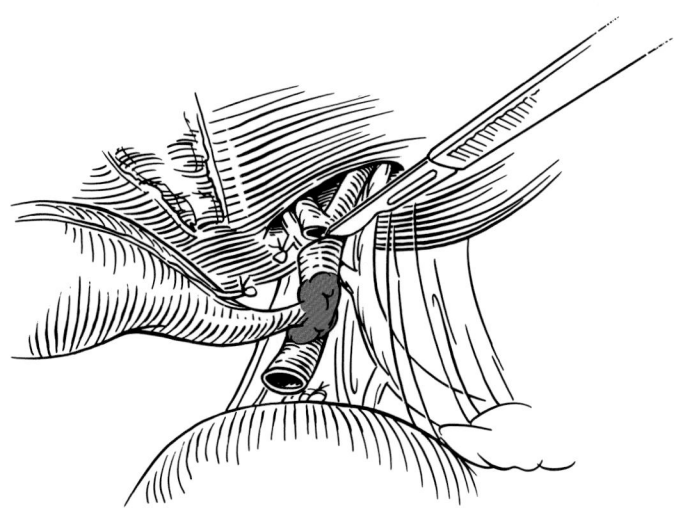

Figure 17-XII-4

Transection of the Common Hepatic Duct

The common hepatic duct is transected just below the bifurcation, and frozen section histologic examination is performed on each end of the excised bile duct.

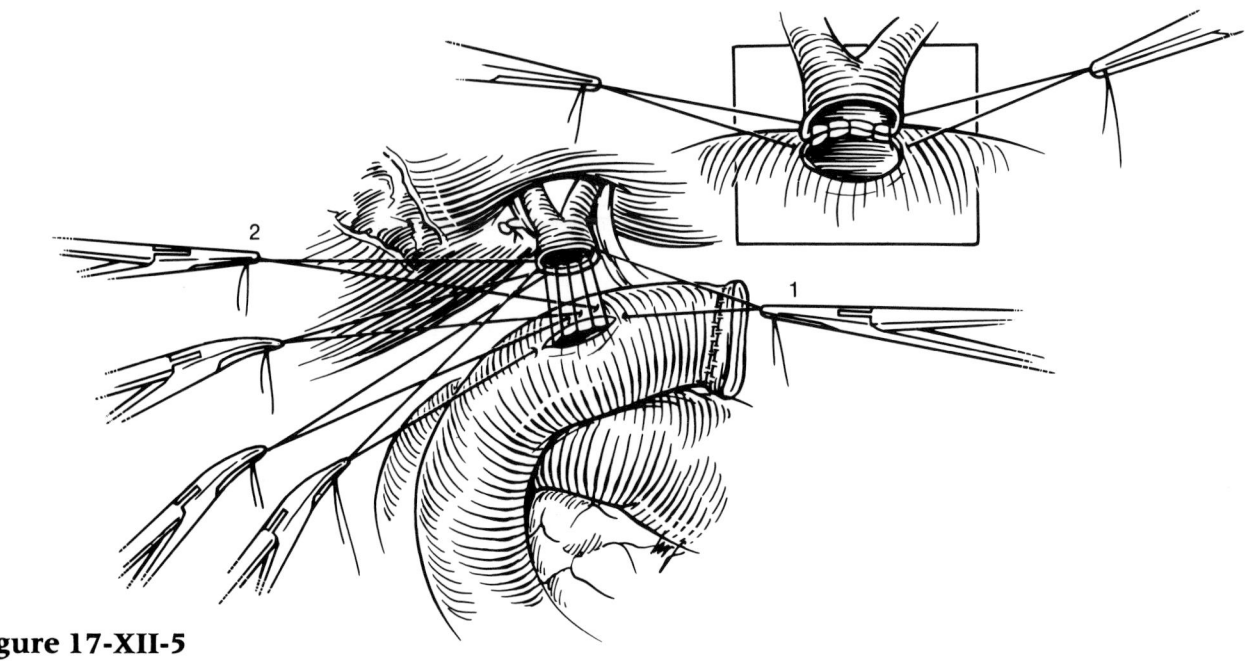

Figure 17-XII-5

Hepaticojejunostomy Creation

An hepaticojejunostomy is constructed as previously described with interrupted 4-0 Prolene sutures (see Fig. 17-VII-4) with the knots tied on the outside.

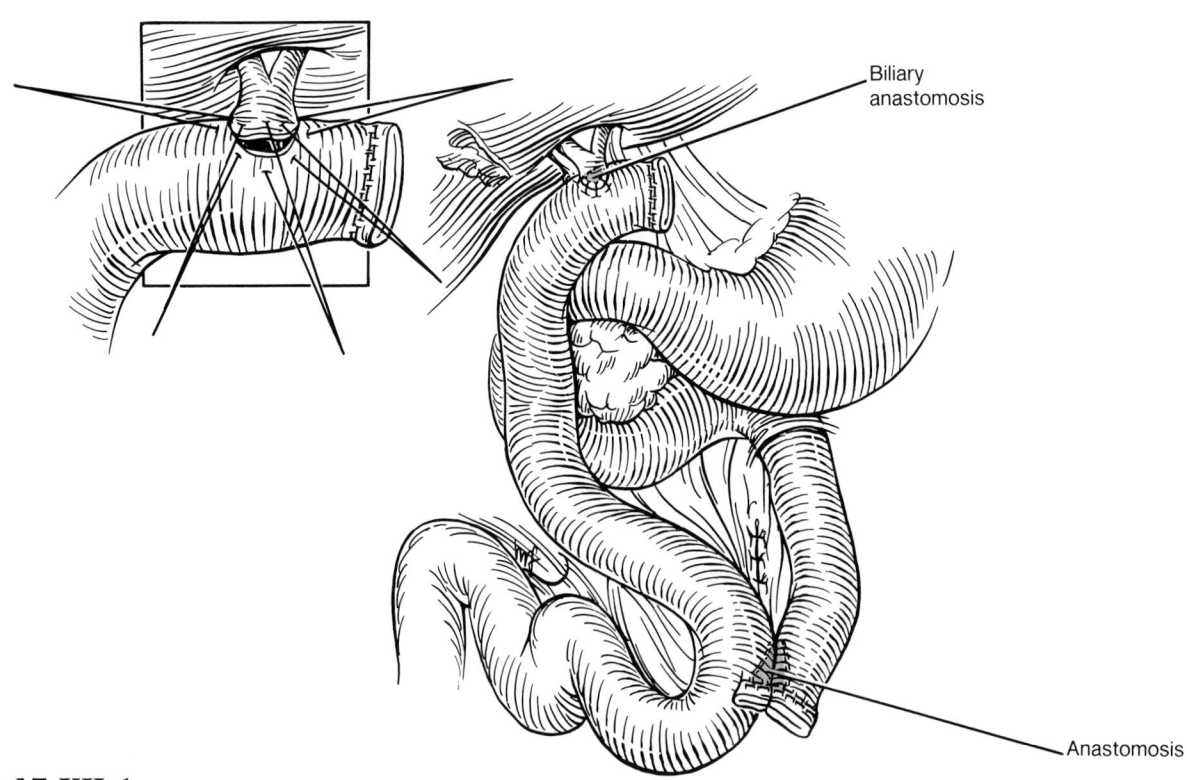

Biliary anastomosis

Anastomosis

Figure 17-XII-6

Completed Procedure

The completed hepaticojejunostomy and jejunojejunostomy (stapled anastomosis; see Section X). The Roux limb should be 45 cm (18 inches) long.

SECTION XIII *Management of a Hilar Bile Duct Tumor (Klatskin Tumor)*

Because of their proximity to portal vein, hepatic artery, and both lobes of the liver, many Klatskin tumors are not resectable. Signs of unresectability include distant metastases, invasion of major vascular structures, and intrahepatic extension to second-order biliary radicles bilaterally. If extension occurs along one hepatic duct, concomitant hepatic lobar resection may be necessary to resect the tumor (see Atlas Chap. 23). Routine resection of the caudate lobe in combination with bile duct resection is controversial.

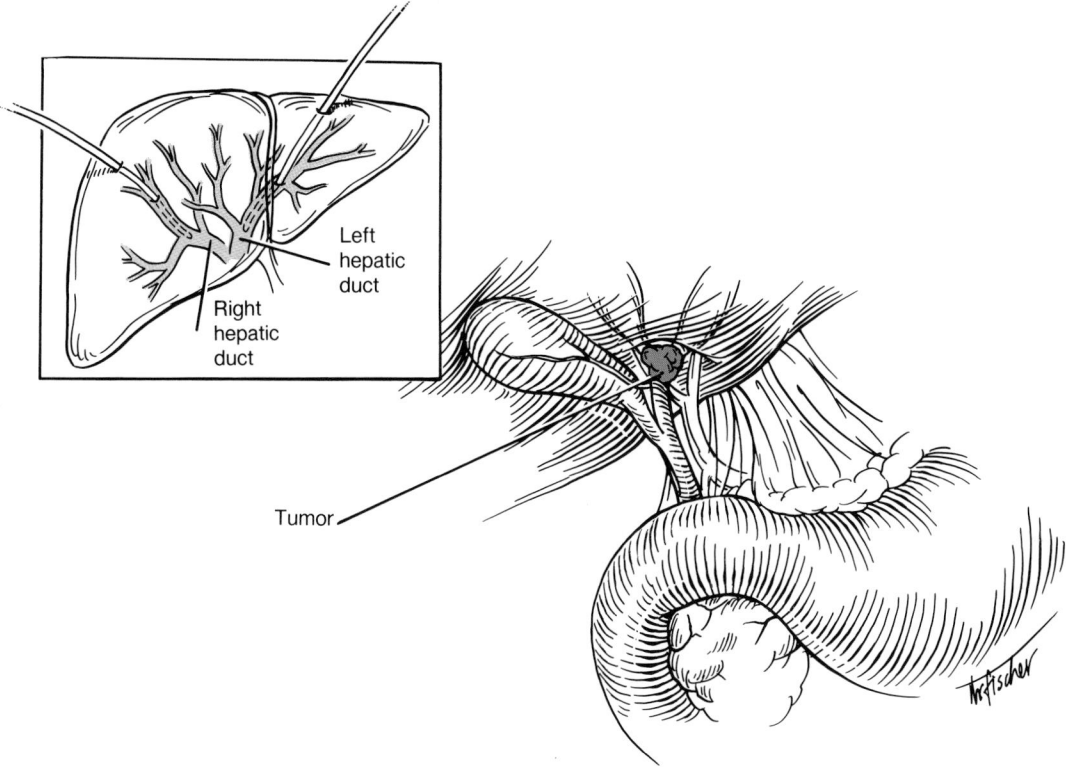

Figure 17-XIII-1

Stent Placement

Bilateral transhepatic stents are placed preoperatively. They traverse the bile duct tumor and are positioned in the duodenum.

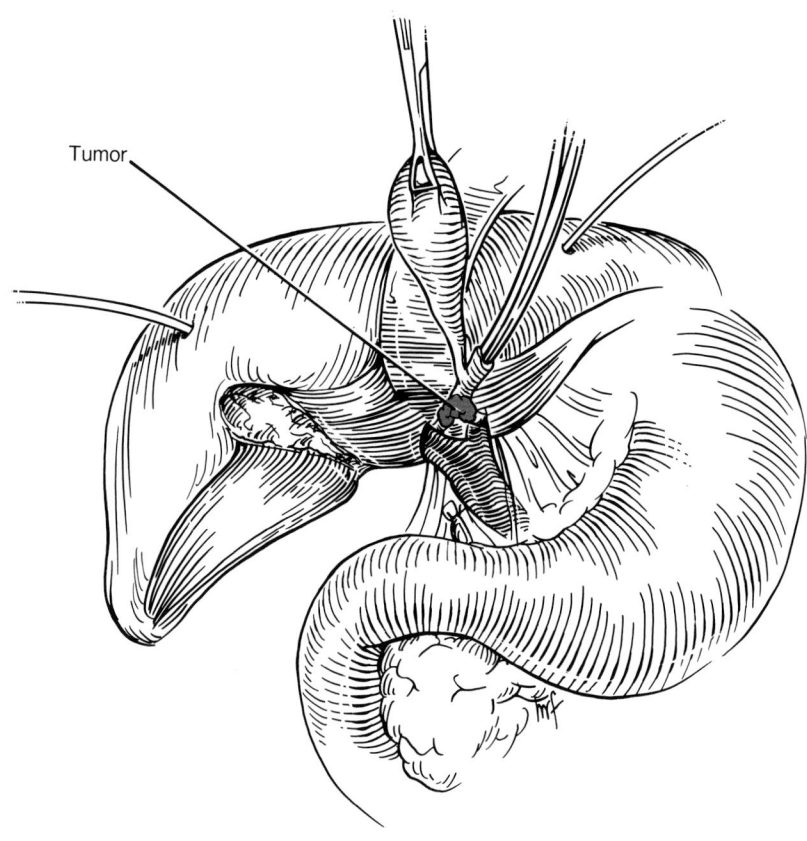

Tumor

Figure 17-XIII-2

Tumor Dissection

If the tumor is deemed resectable, the distal bile duct is divided, and the stents are delivered into the operative field. The distal bile duct is oversewn. The proximal bile duct and the tumor are dissected off of the portal vein into the hilum of the liver. The gallbladder is removed en bloc with the specimen.

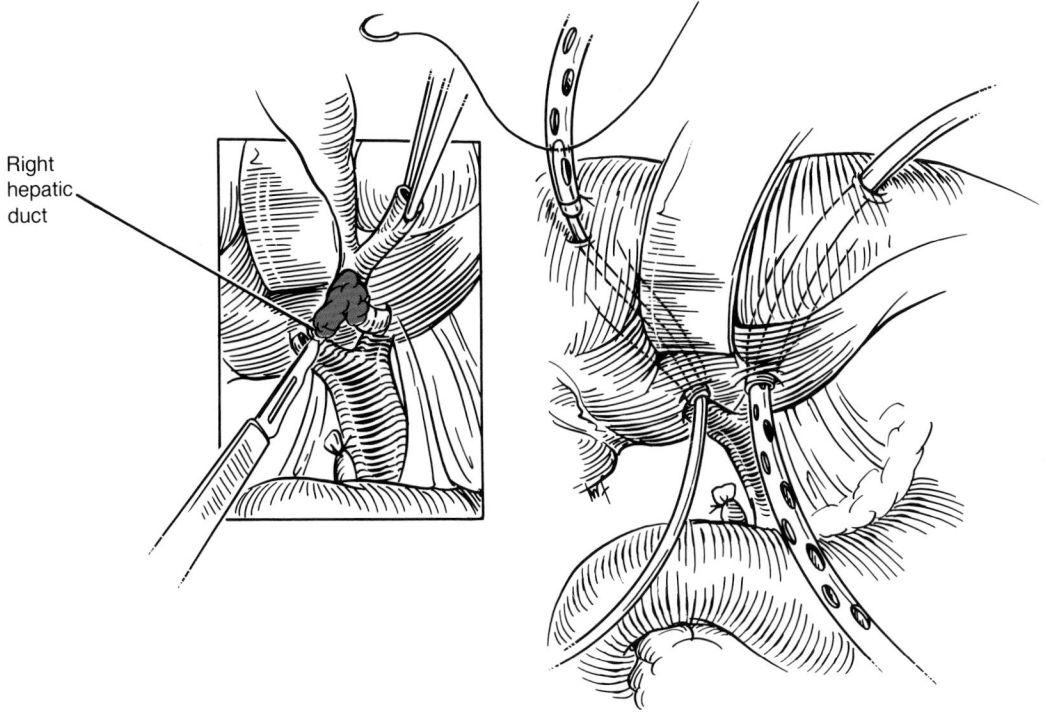

Right
hepatic
duct

Figure 17-XIII-3

Tumor Removal

Both hepatic ducts are dissected proximally until nonfibrotic, normal ducts can be palpated. At this point, the hepatic ducts are divided and the specimen is removed. It is sometimes necessary to resect a portion of central liver parenchyma to reach grossly uninvolved hepatic ducts. Some surgeons routinely resect the caudate lobe, since it is a common site for metastatic disease. The preoperatively placed Ring catheters are used to pull larger Silastic catheters through the liver to stent the anastomoses.

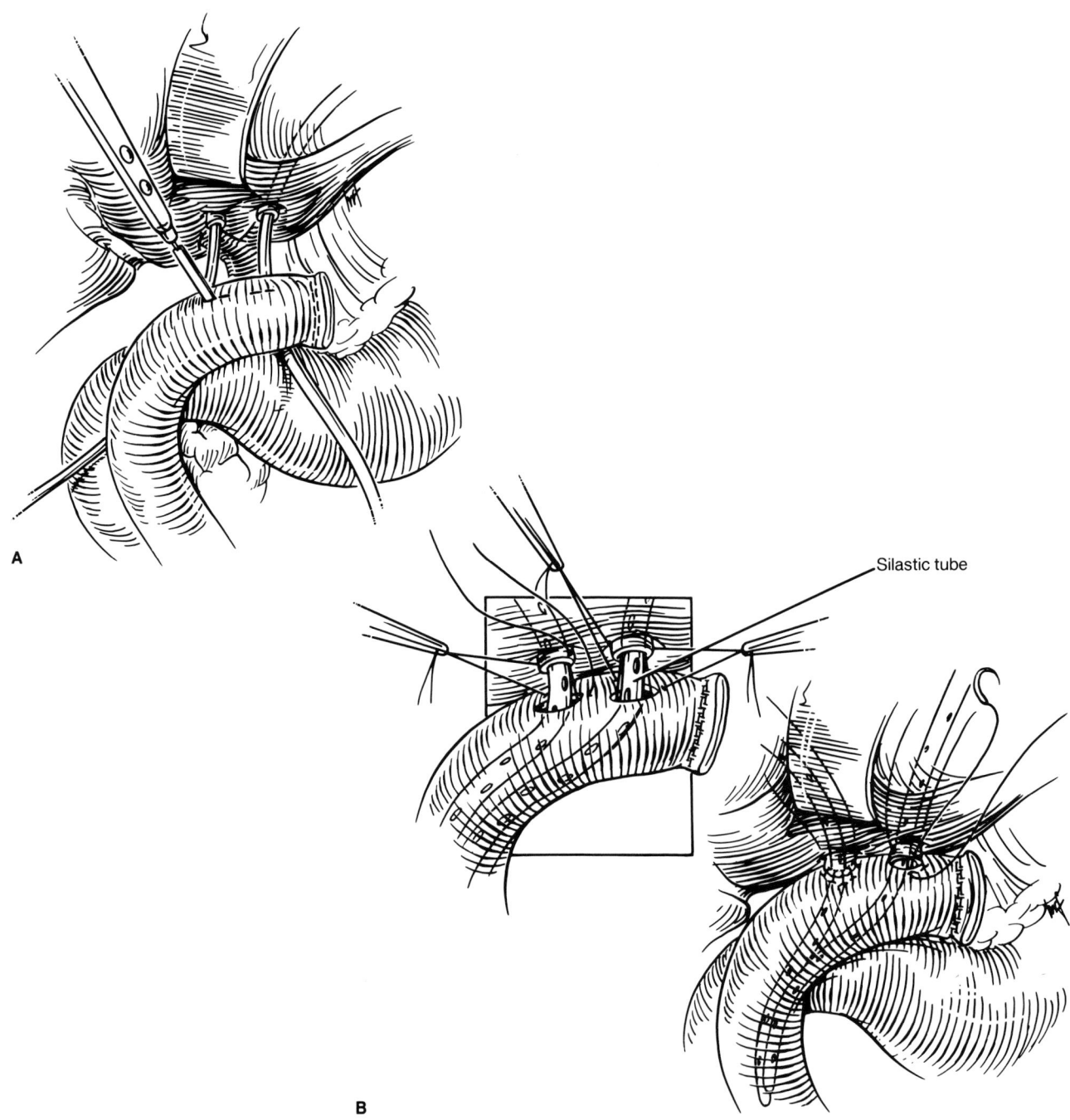

Figure 17-XIII-4

Anastomosis Creation

(**A**) Two small enterotomies are made in a jejunal Roux limb in preparation for the anastomoses.

(**B**) The anastomoses are accomplished with interrupted 4-0 or 5-0 Prolene sutures with the knots on the outside as previously described (see Fig. 17-VII-4).

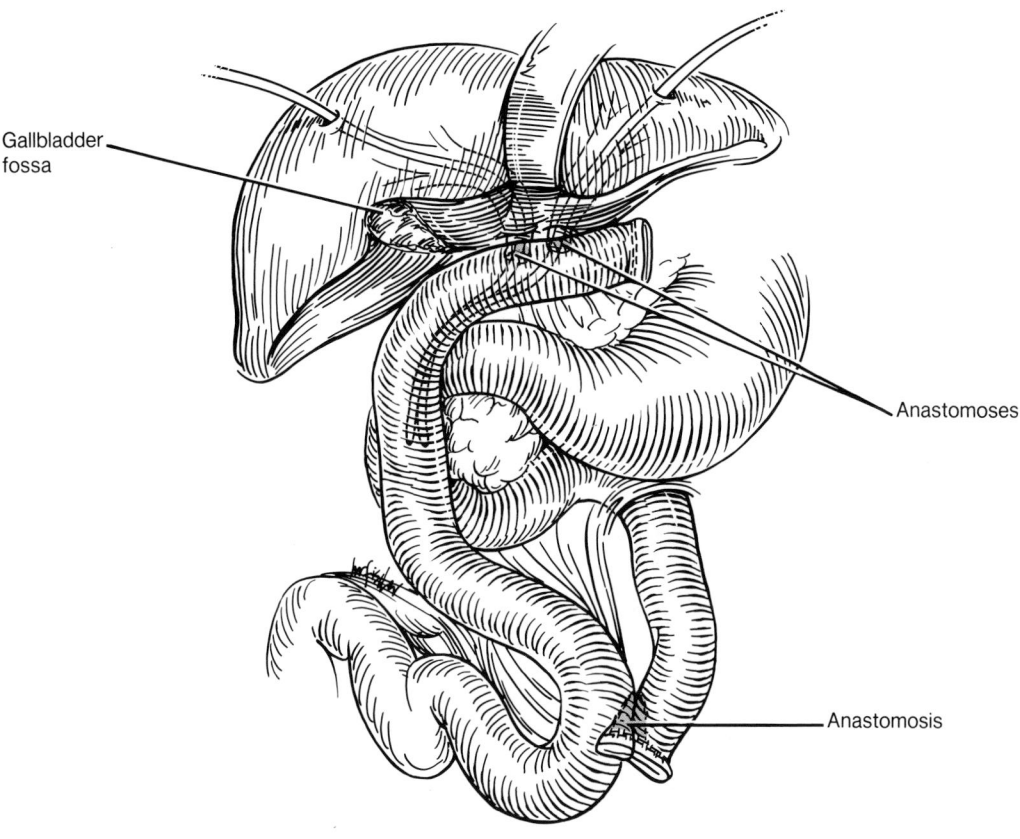

Gallbladder fossa

Anastomoses

Anastomosis

Figure 17-XIII-5

Completed Anastomoses

The Roux limb should be 45 cm (18 inches) long. The stents are left for several months after surgery and can be used for placement of iridium seeds for delivery of postoperative radiation.

SECTION XIV *Local Resection of a Papillary Bile Duct Tumor*

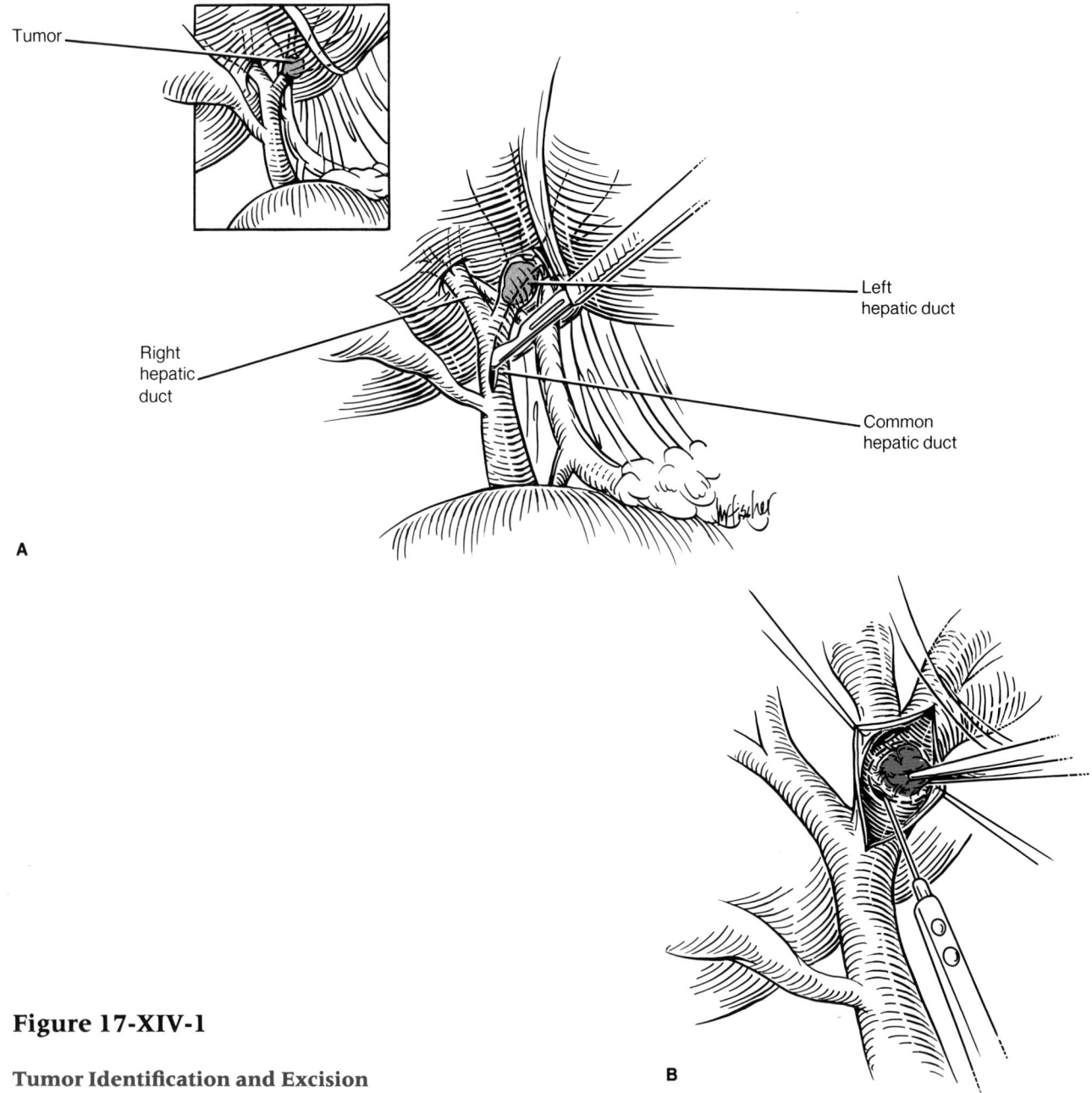

Figure 17-XIV-1

Tumor Identification and Excision

Occasionally, a papillary intrabiliary tumor that can be locally resected is encountered. The tumor depicted here caused intermittent cholangitis.

(A) An incision is made in the common hepatic duct and extended into the left hepatic duct. The obstructing papillary tumor originates from the septum of the secondary hepatic radical to segment IV.

(B) The tumor is identified and excised with cautery.

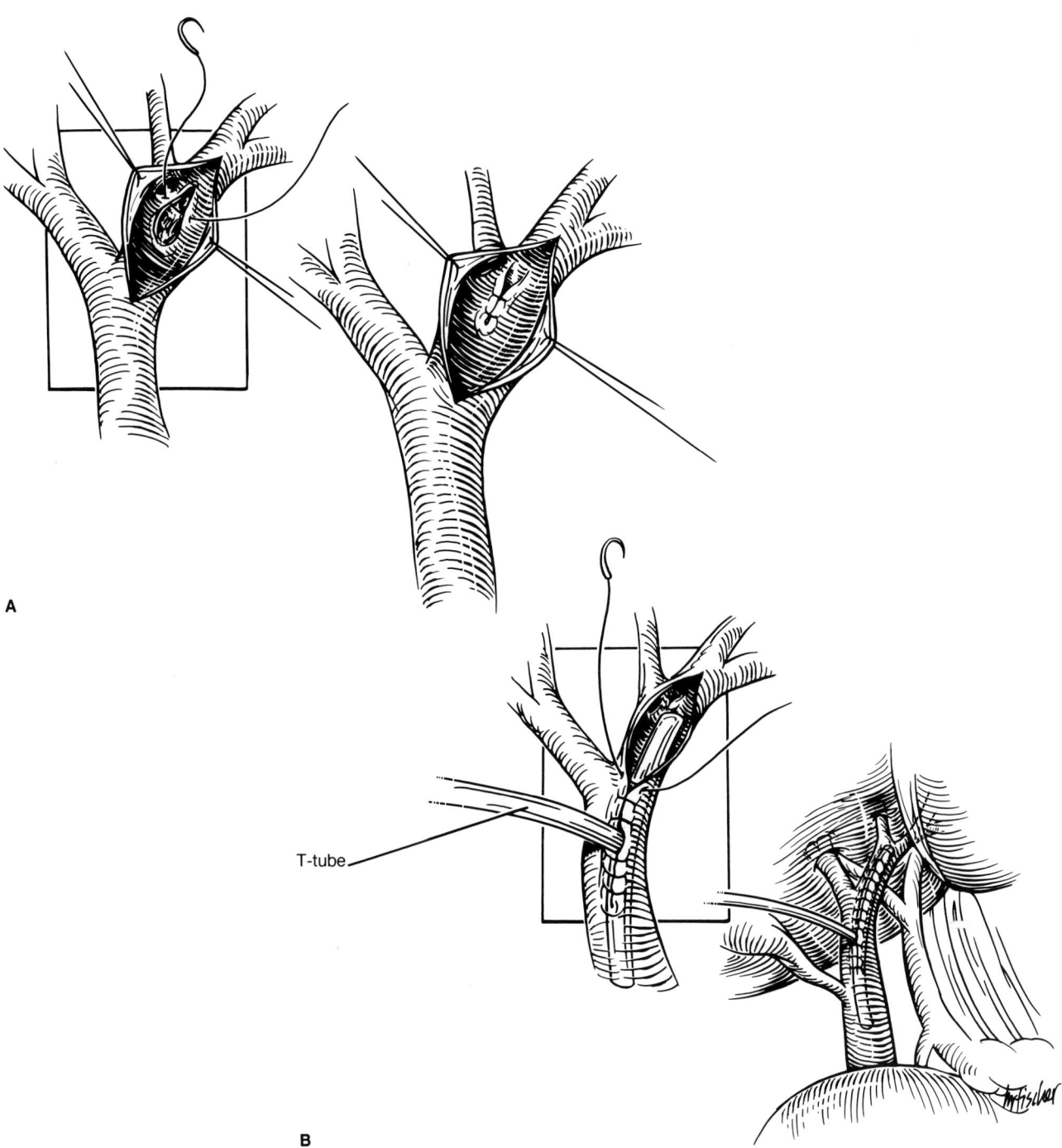

T-tube

A

B

Figure 17-XIV-2

Wound Closure

(**A**) The posterior duct wall is approximated with interrupted absorbable sutures. The upper part of the incision is left open to avoid compromising the secondary biliary radicles.

(**B**) A T-tube is placed with the proximal limb adjacent to the area of excision, and the bile duct is closed with interrupted sutures.

SECTION XV *Biliary Drainage Through the Left Hepatic Duct*

When an unresectable hilar tumor is present, bile drainage from the left lobe can be provided by this approach. This technique is also useful for high benign strictures, especially when previous surgical attempts at repair have obscured the anatomy near the bifurcation.

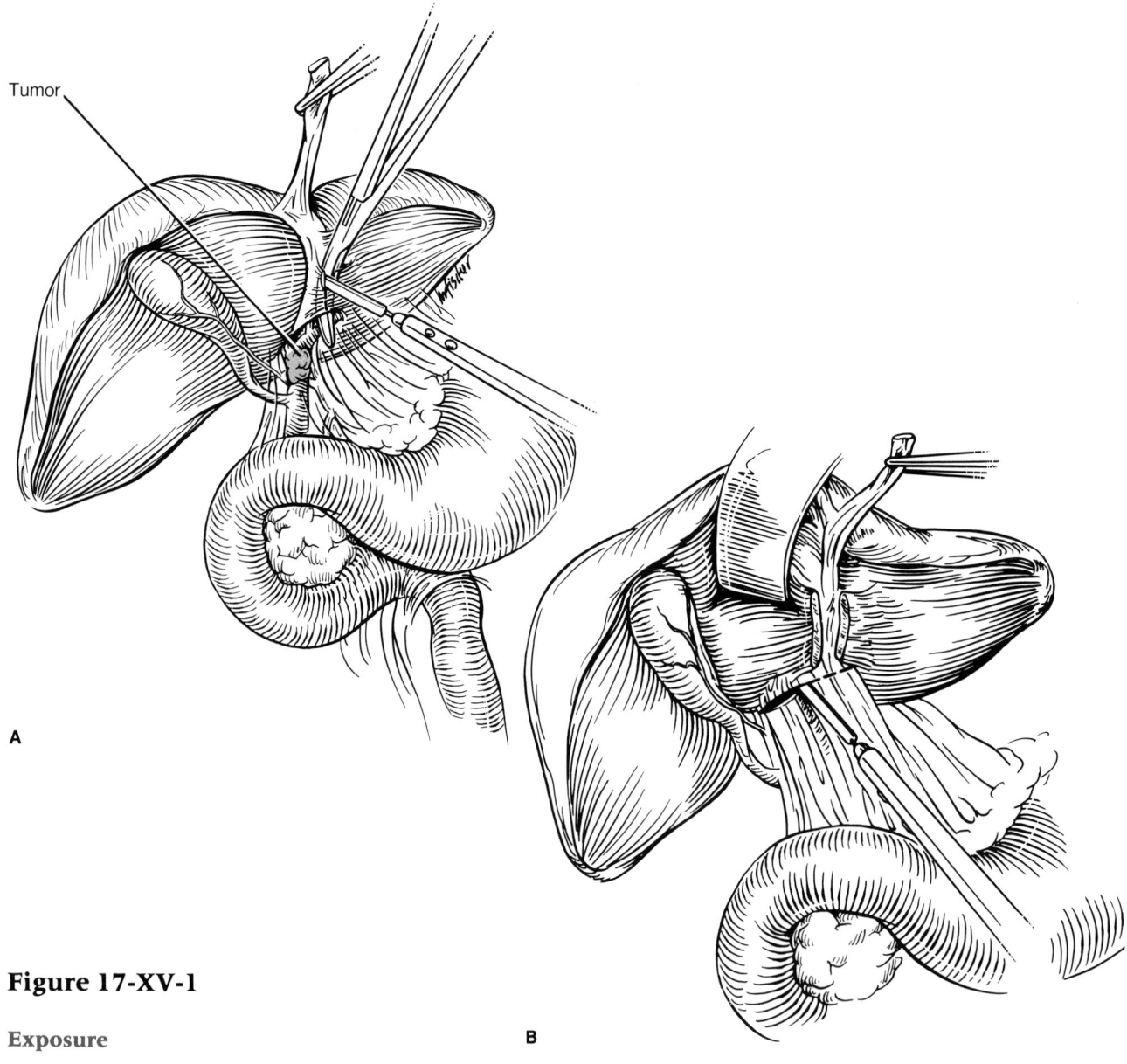

Figure 17-XV-1

Exposure

(**A**) Exposure of the left hepatic duct is gained by incising the bridge of parenchyma.

(**B**) The gastrohepatic ligament is incised along the base of segment IV, which is then elevated to expose the dilated left hepatic duct, which lies over the left main branch of the portal vein.

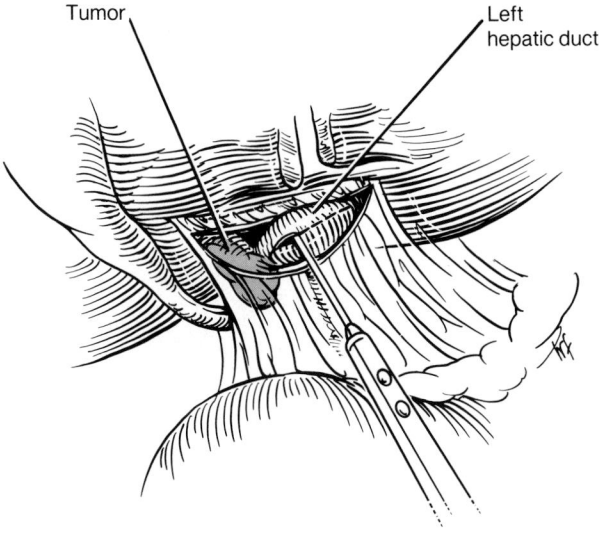

Tumor   Left
               hepatic duct

Figure 17-XV-2

Incising the Left Hepatic Duct

After the left hepatic duct is identified by needle aspiration, it is opened for 2 to 3 cm in preparation for anastomosis to a Roux limb of jejunum.

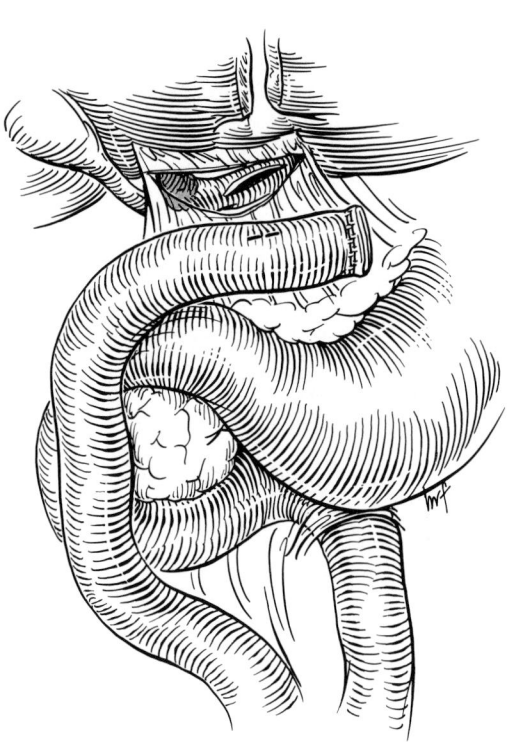

Figure 17-XV-3

Aligning the Bowel

A small incision is made in the jejunum.

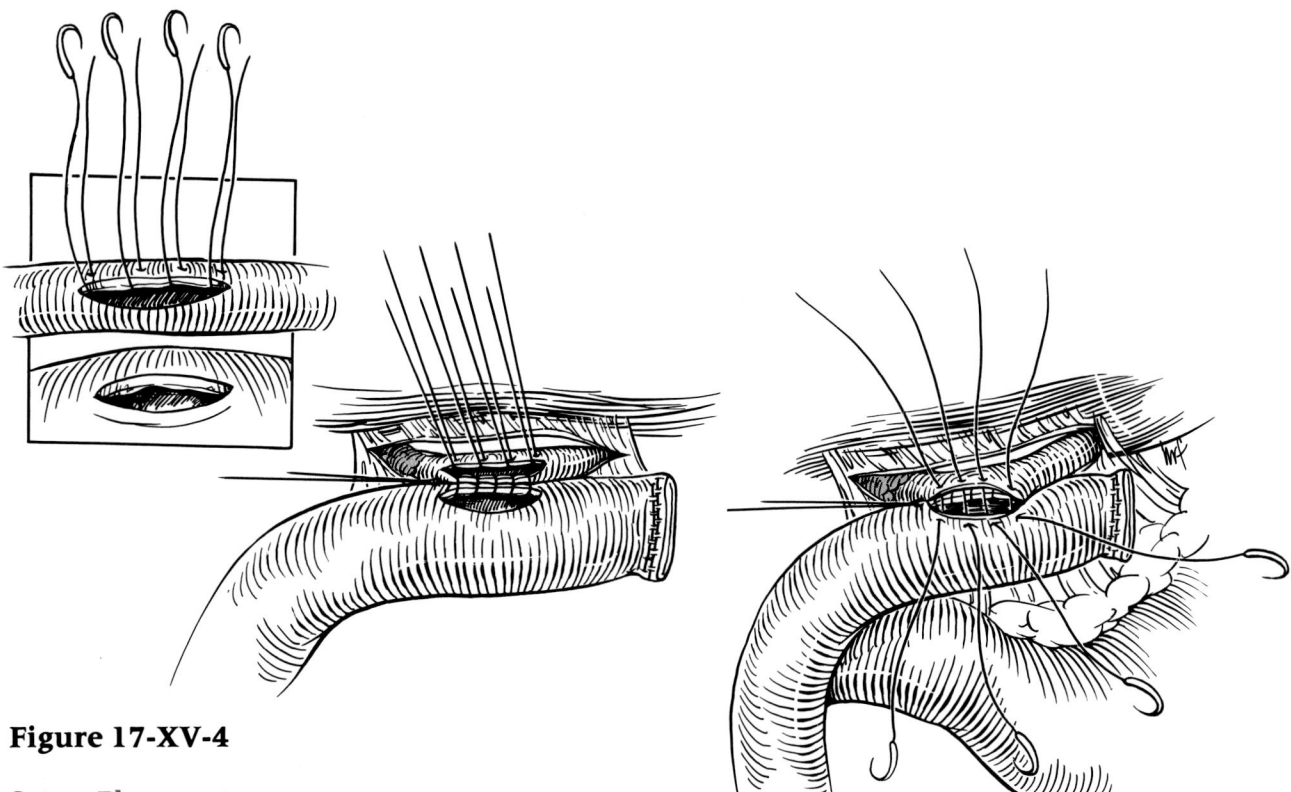

Figure 17-XV-4

Suture Placement

Completion of the anterior anastomosis with the previously placed interrupted sutures. An alternative to the previously described biliojejunal anastomosis is shown. Because the anastomosis is so high in the hepatic hilum, the anterior row of interrupted sutures (4-0 or 5-0) is placed in the bile duct before the posterior anastomosis is created. If the knots cannot be placed on the outside of the posterior row, a slowly absorbable suture material (eg, Maxon) should be used.

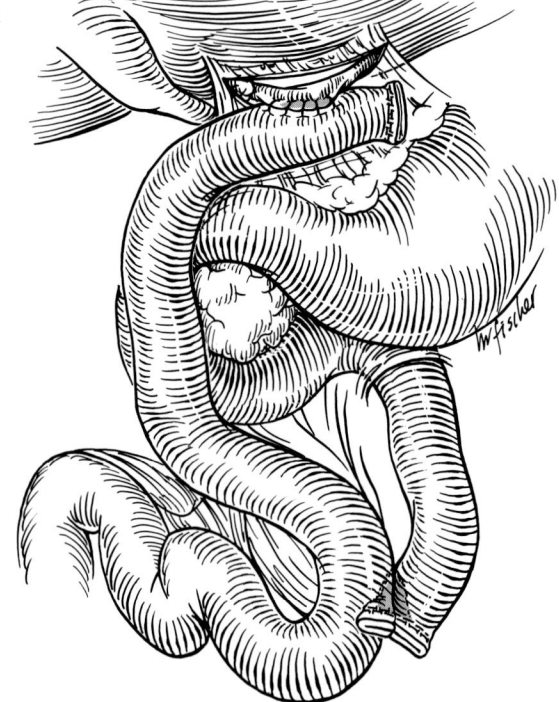

Figure 17-XV-5

Completed Procedure

The completed left hepatic duct–jejunal anastomosis. The jejunal Roux limb is 45 cm (18 inches) long.

586

SECTION XVI *Management of Choledochal Cysts*

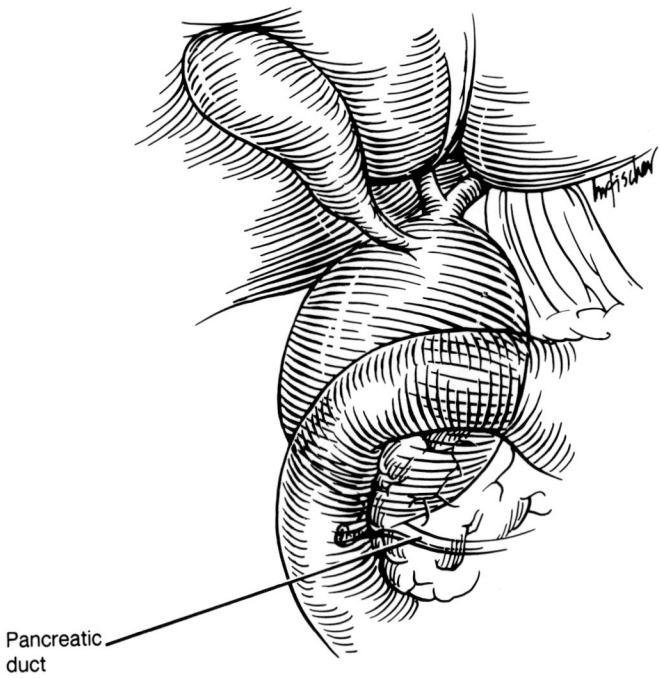

Pancreatic
duct

Figure 17-XVI-1

Type I Choledochal Cyst

A type I choledochal cyst is most common. It is a fusiform dilatation of the bile duct, usually extending from the hepatic duct bifurcation to the pancreas. A relatively consistent finding (70% to 90% of cases) with various types of choledochal cysts is a supraduodenal insertion of the pancreatic duct into the bile duct. This is rarely seen with type III and type V cysts.

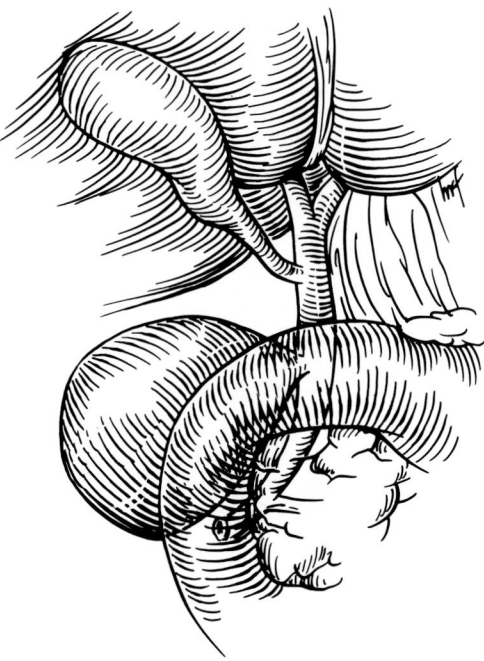

Figure 17-XVI-2

Type II Choledochal Cyst

The much rarer type II cyst is a diverticulum off the common bile duct.

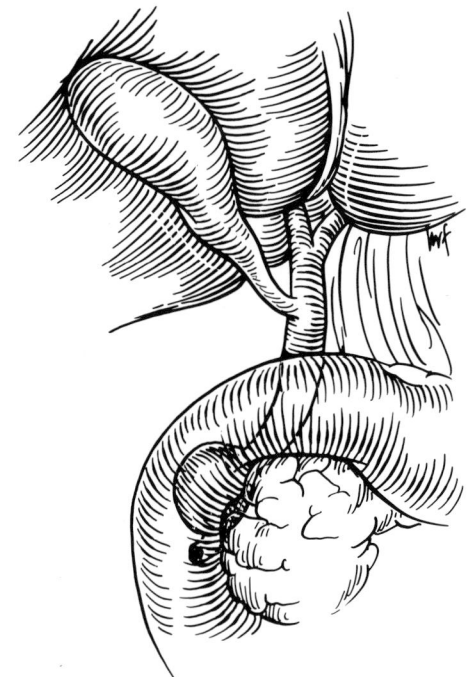

Figure 17-XVI-3

Type III Choledochal Cyst

The type III cyst, or choledochocele, is usually totally within the wall of
the duodenum.

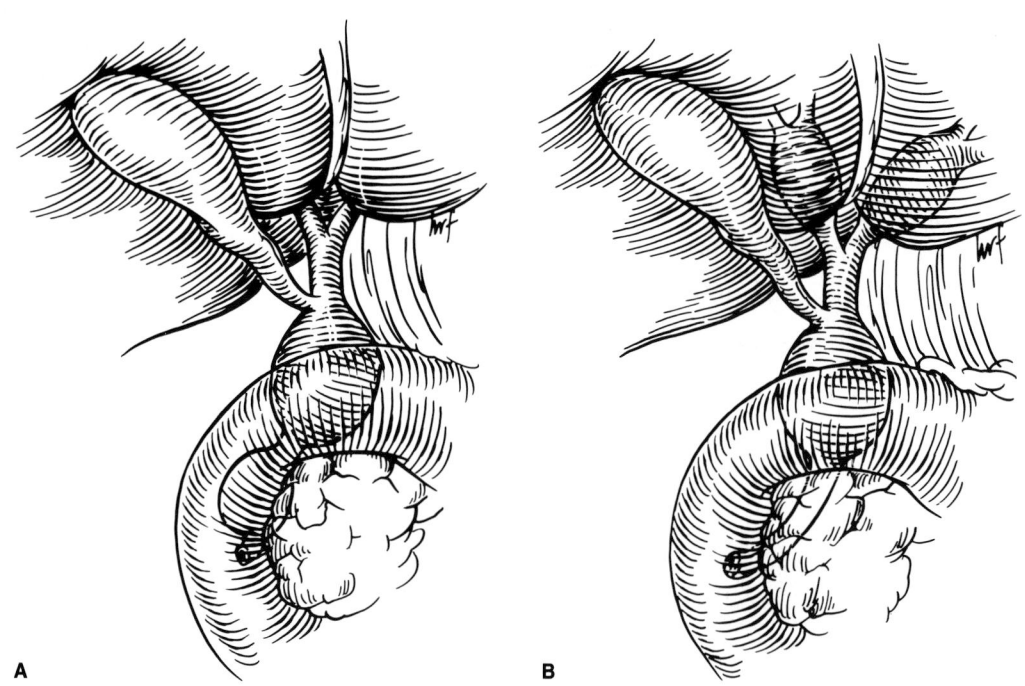

A   B

Figure 17-XVI-4

Type IV Choledochal Cyst

Type IV choledochal cysts are multiple, either entirely extrahepatic (**A**) or extrahepatic
and intrahepatic (**B**).

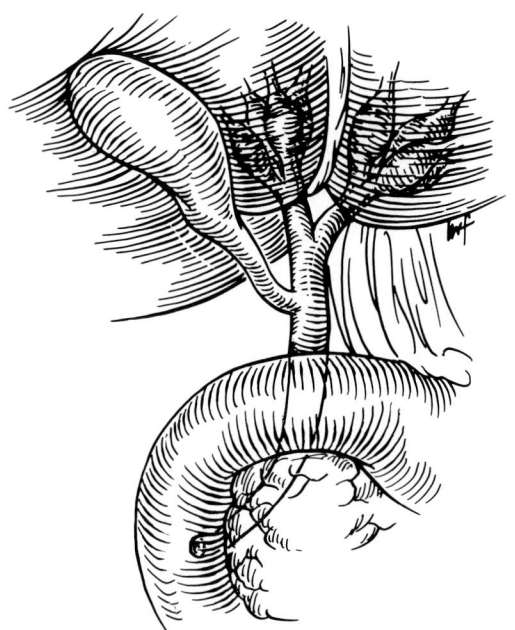

Figure 17-XVI-5

Type V Choledochal Cyst (Caroli's Disease)

Type V choledochal cysts are entirely intrahepatic and multiple. This condition is also referred to as Caroli's disease. Rarely, Caroli's disease is confined to a segment or lobe of the liver, in which case it is treatable by liver resection.

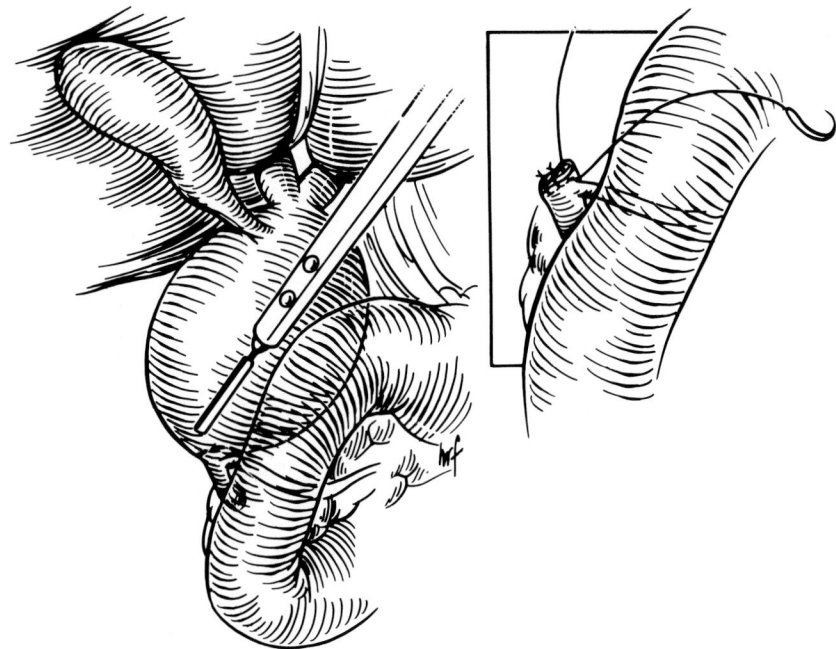

Figure 17-XVI-6

Excision of Type I Cyst

The treatment of choice for type I and II choledochal cysts is complete excision if possible. Simple drainage of the cyst usually leads to persistent biliary stagnation and recurrent cholangitis. In addition, choledochal cysts predispose to development of bile duct carcinoma. The biliary system proximal to the cyst is often significantly dilated, although it is not usually involved in the disease process. The junction between normal duct and cyst can nearly always be appreciated. In the distal dissection of the cyst, the aberrant junction of pancreatic and common bile duct needs to be avoided. If there is a question as to where that junction is, part of the distal cyst is left and oversewn. The cyst may be adherent to the underlying portal vein. If it is difficult to separate these two structures by dissection, a plane can be developed between cyst epithelium and cyst wall, which is left attached to the portal vein.

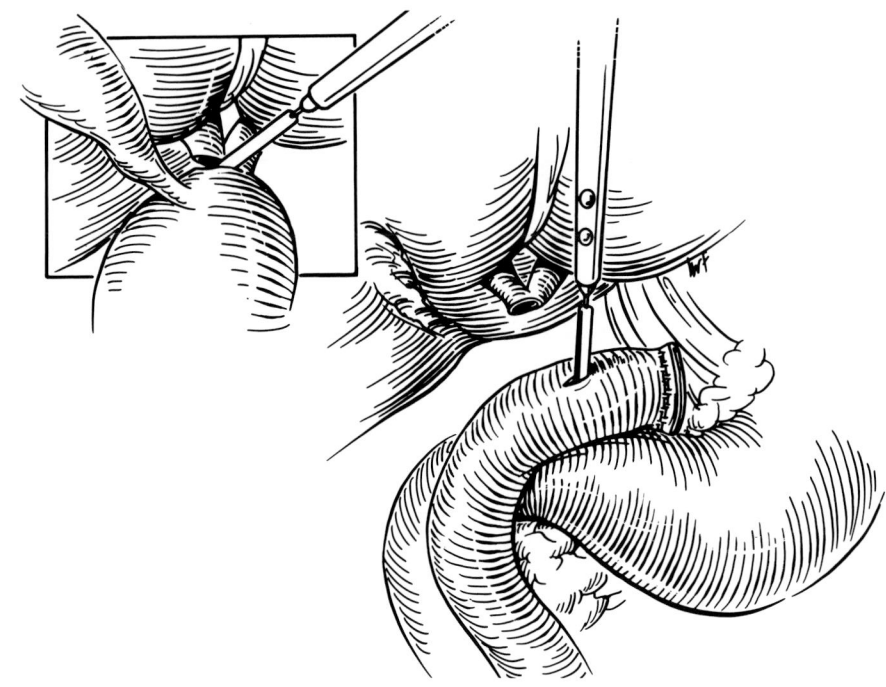

Figure 17-XVI-7

Proximal Dissection and Jejunal Incision

The common hepatic duct is divided just below the bifurcation after full mobilization of the cyst. The specimen consists of choledochal cyst, cystic duct, and gallbladder. An enterotomy is made in a jejunal Roux limb in preparation for a hepaticojejunostomy.

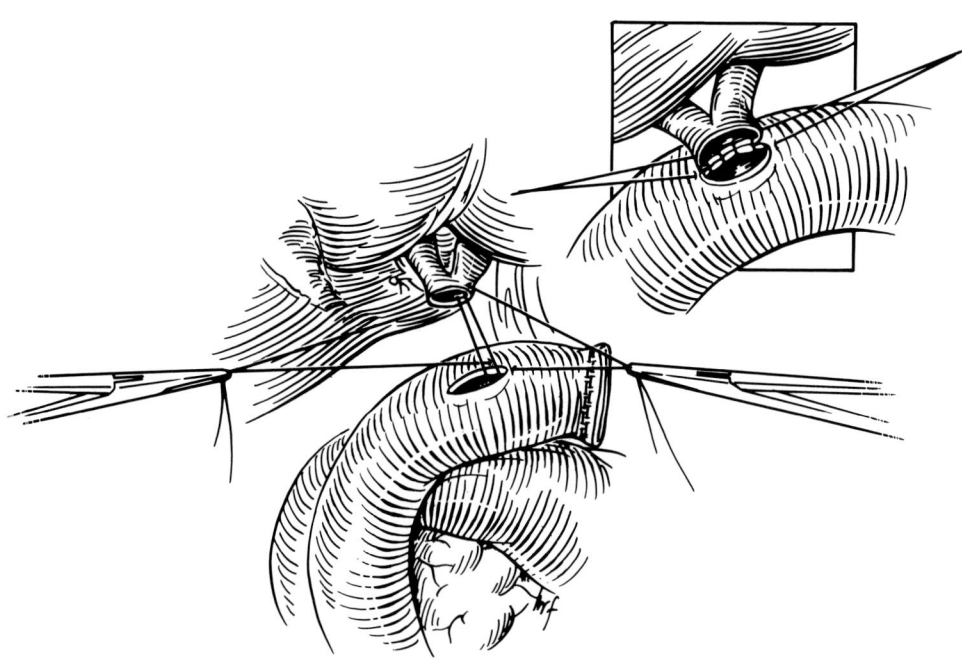

Figure 17-XVI-8

Anastomosis Creation

The bilioenteric anastomosis is constructed with interrupted 4-0 Prolene sutures with the knots on the outside as previously described (see Fig. 17-VII-4). Because of dilation of the proximal bile ducts, this anastomosis usually is not technically challenging.

590

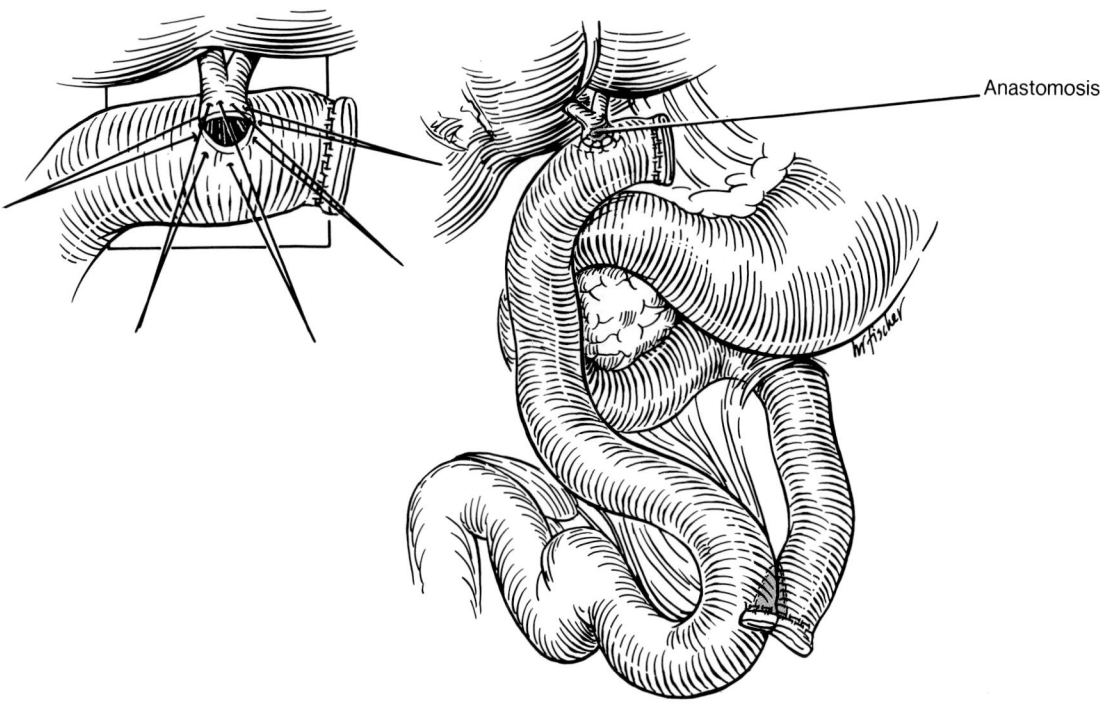

Figure 17-XVI-9

Completed Anastomosis

Completion of the anterior anastomosis. A stent is not necessary.

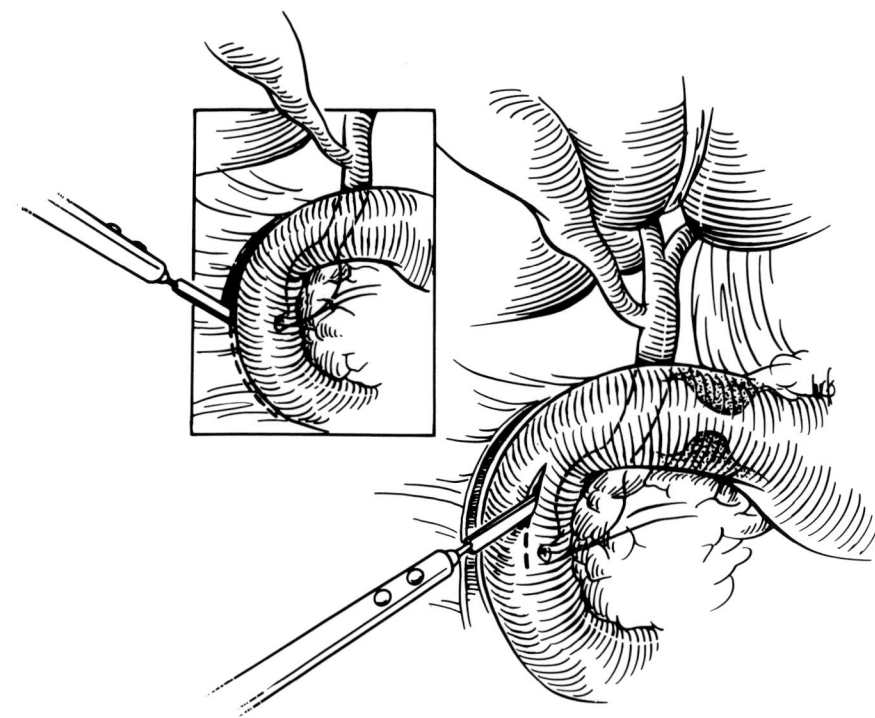

Figure 17-XVI-10

Duodenotomy

The type III cyst (choledochocele) is treated by cystoduodenostomy rather than by excision. The likelihood of carcinoma developing in a type III choledochal cyst is low. The duodenum and cyst are mobilized by the Kocher maneuver, and a duodenotomy is made over the cyst.

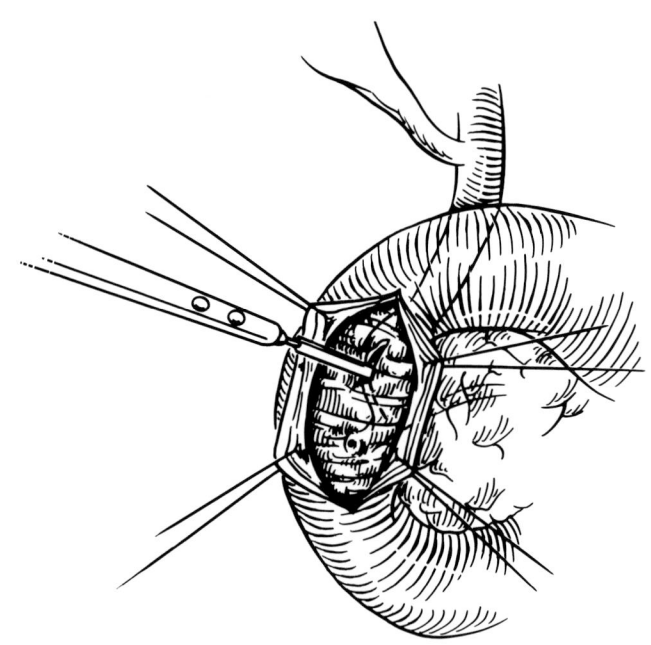

Figure 17-XVI-11

Incision of Duodenum and Cyst

After identification of the cyst by needle aspiration or intraoperative ultrasound, cautery is used to incise the duodenal and cyst walls for a distance of 2 to 3 cm.

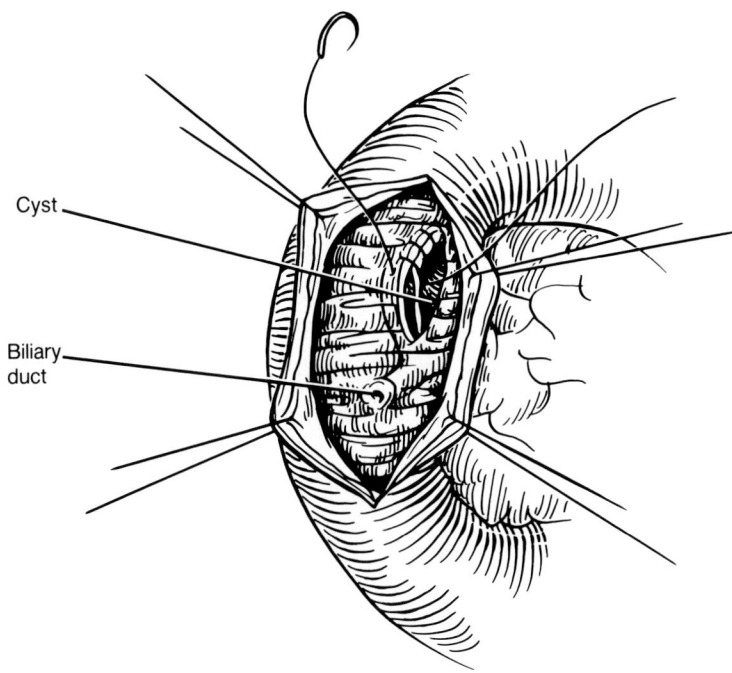

Cyst

Biliary
duct

Figure 17-XVI-12

Suture Placement

The cystoduodenostomy is accomplished intraduodenally with either interrupted or running 4-0 Prolene sutures. Although the ampulla of Vater remains intact, most of the bile drains through the cystoduodenostomy.

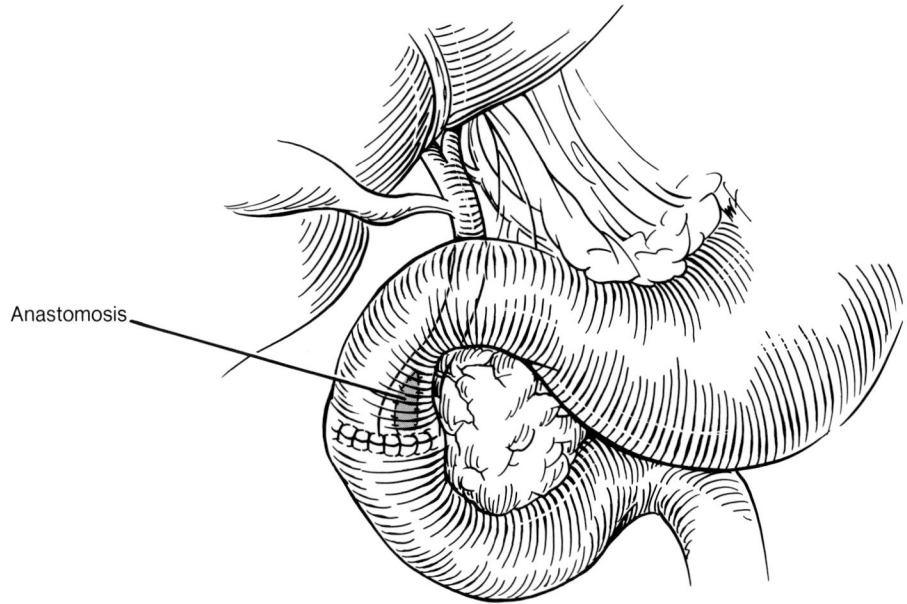

Anastomosis

Figure 17-XVI-13

Closure of Duodenal Incision

The duodenal incision is closed transversely in two layers.

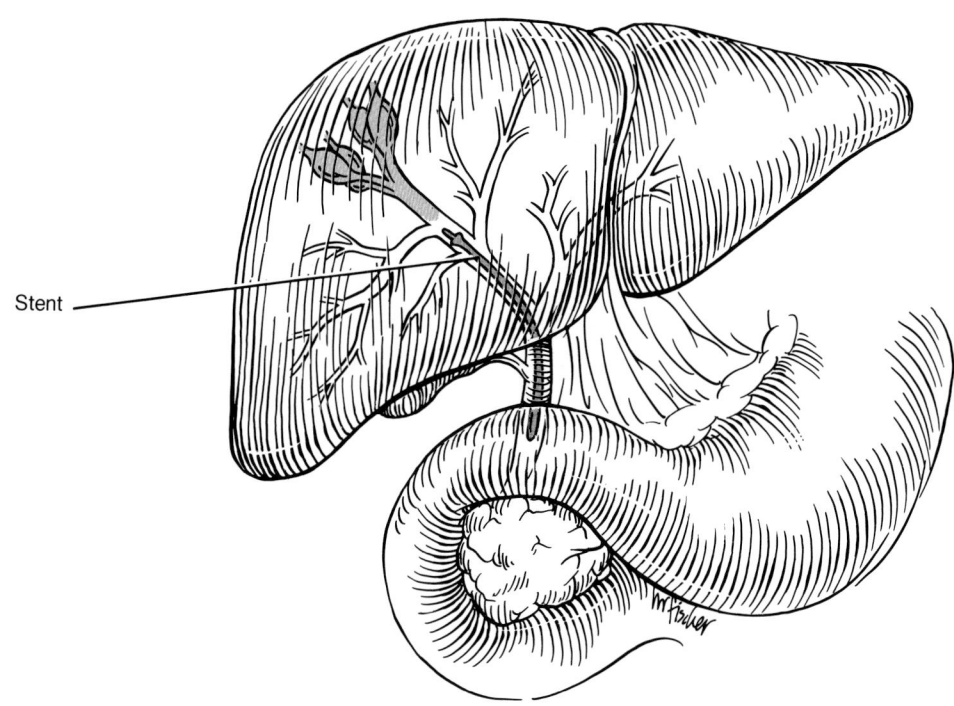

Stent

Figure 17-XVI-14

Stent Placement

Rarely, Caroli's disease (type V choledochal cyst) is segmental, allowing treatment by partial liver resection. A stent is placed endoscopically so that the involved segments can be identified at surgery.

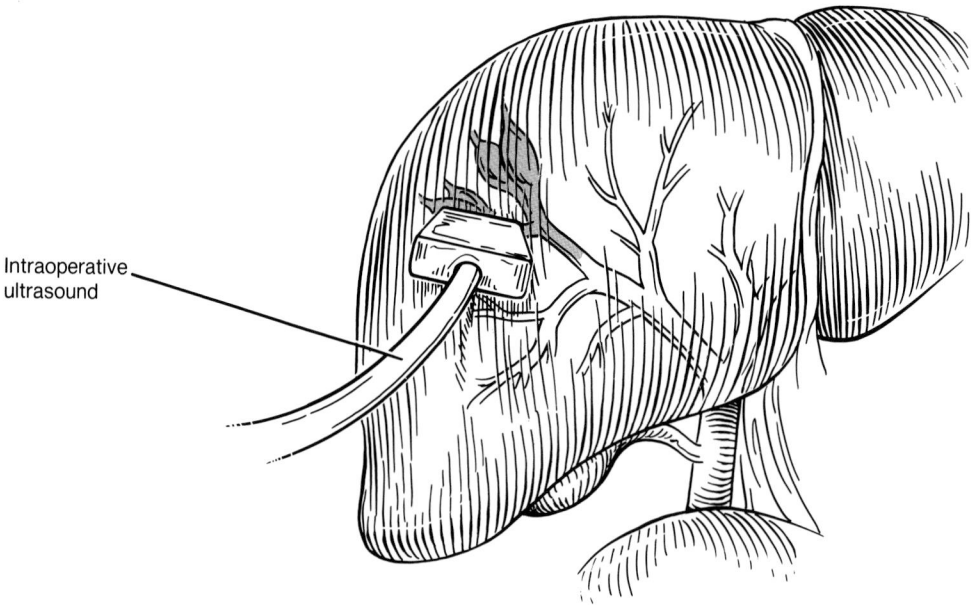

Intraoperative ultrasound

Figure 17-XVI-15

Intraoperative Ultrasound

Intraoperative ultrasound is a useful adjunct to define the part of the biliary system affected by cystic dilation.

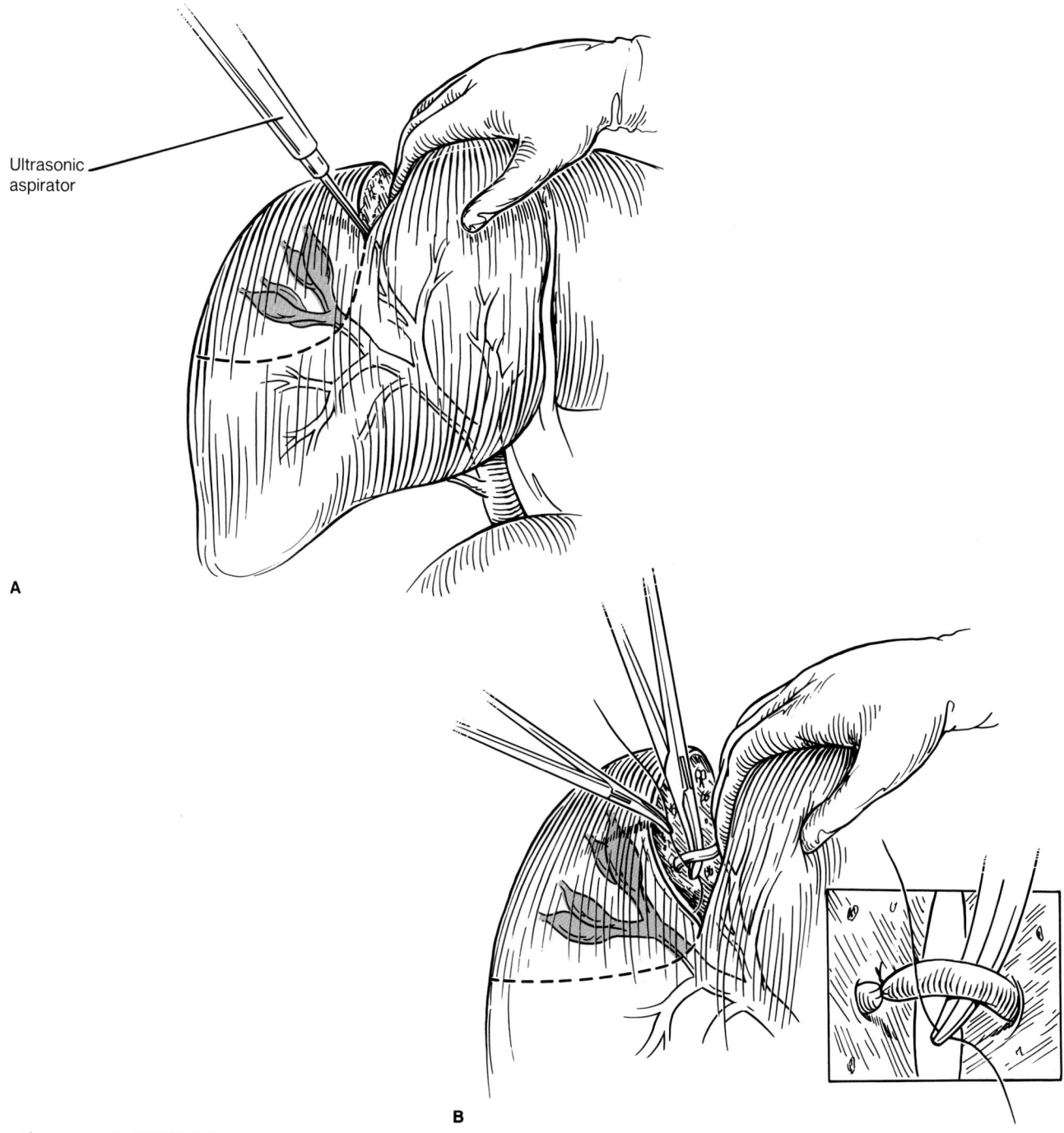

Ultrasonic aspirator

A

B

Figure 17-XVI-16

Ultrasonic Dissection

(**A**) When localized, the dilated ducts are usually confined to one or two hepatic segments. The segments are resected anatomically using the ultrasonic aspirator for parenchymal dissection.

(**B**) The ultrasonic aspirator dissects hepatic parenchyma, leaving major vascular and biliary structures intact. These are then doubly ligated and divided.

(Continued)

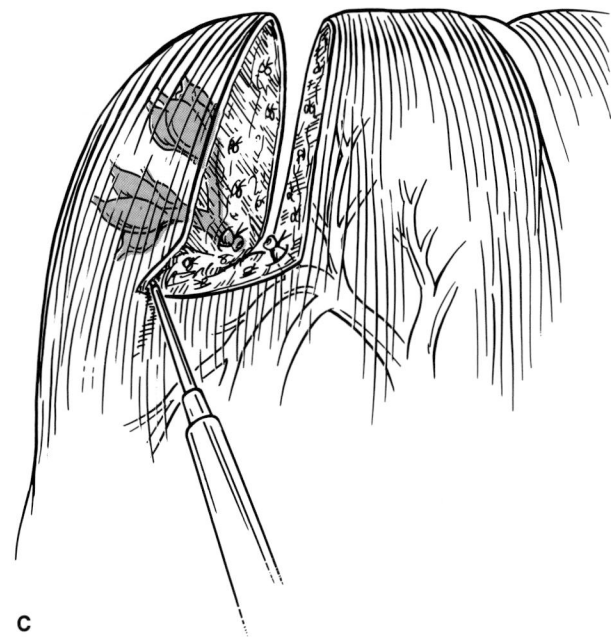

Figure 17-XVI-16 *(Continued)*

(C) Segment VII can be resected with minimal blood loss. C

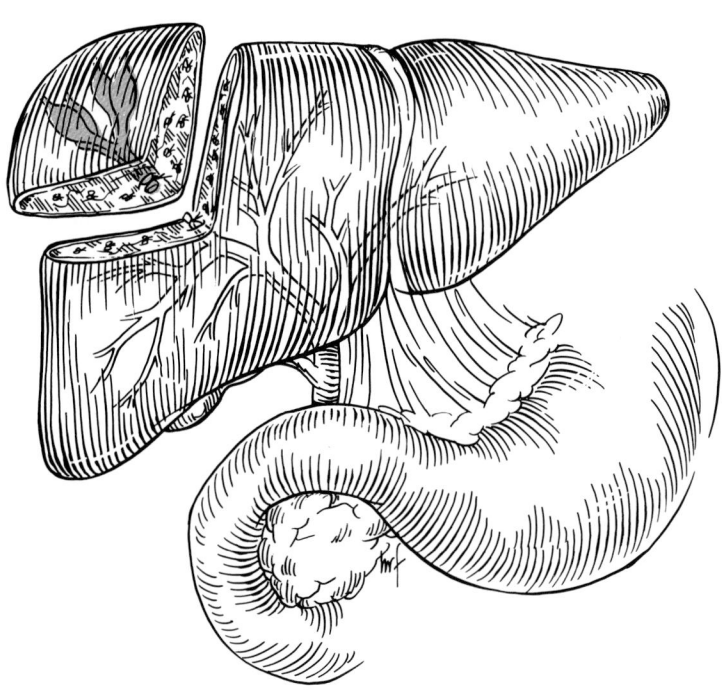

Figure 17-XVI-17

Completed Segmental Resection

Thrombostat spray is applied if bleeding from the parenchymal surface persists. A drain is placed before the abdomen is closed.

SECTION XVII *Management of Gallstone Ileus*

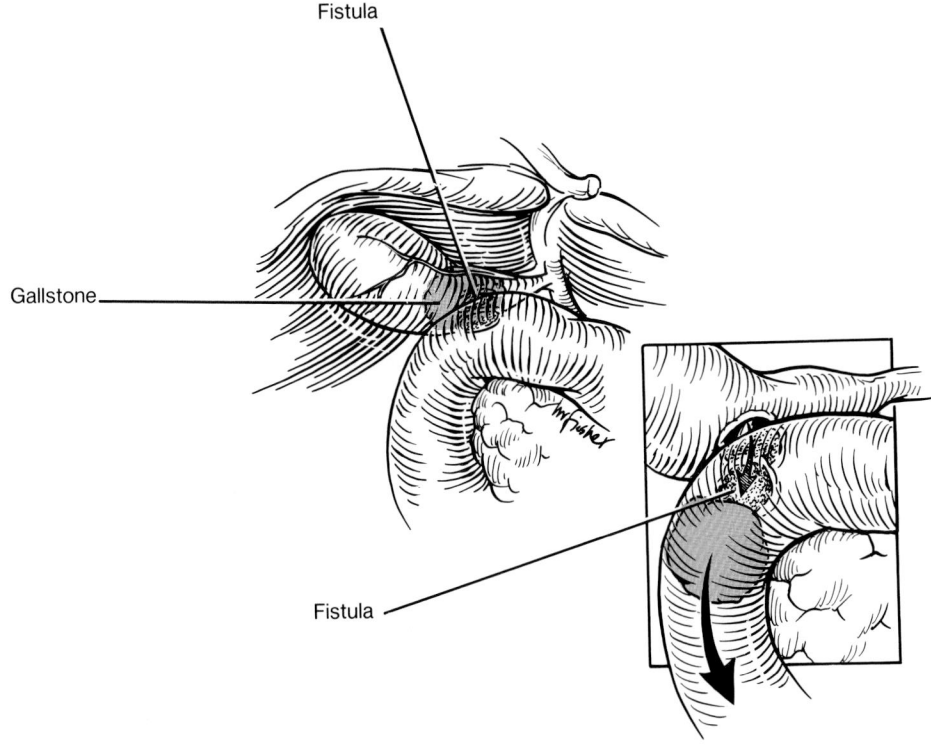

Figure 17-XVII-1

Appearance

Gallstone ileus is caused by erosion of a large gallstone through the gallbladder into the duodenum, resulting in a fistula.

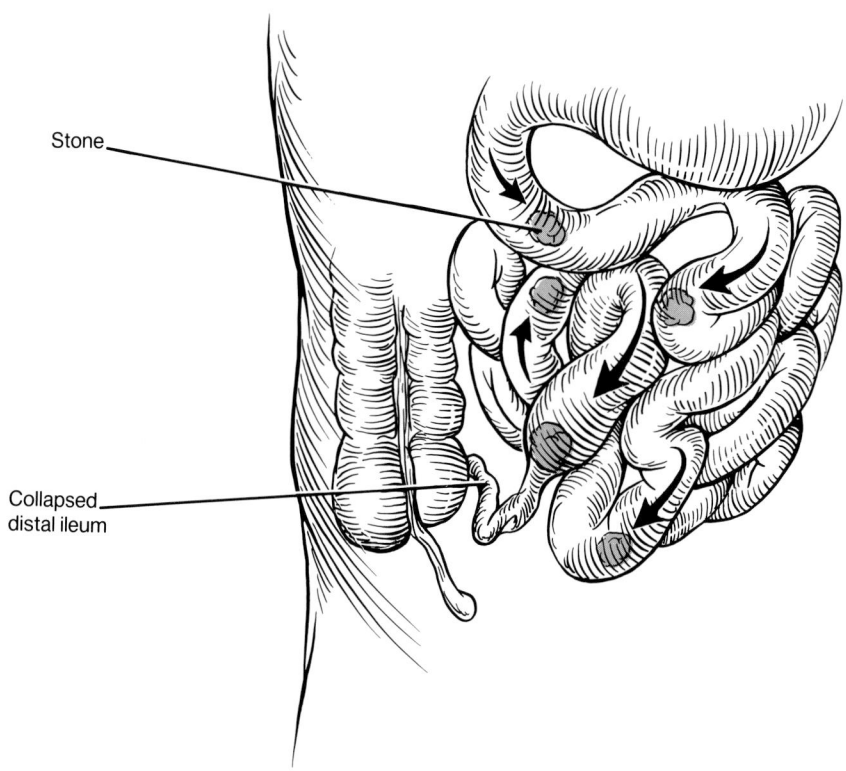

Stone

Collapsed
distal ileum

Figure 17-XVII-2

Multiple Gallstones

The gallstone passes distally in the small intestine, usually lodging in the distal ileum and causing small bowel obstruction. More than one gallstone may pass. Therefore, the full length of small intestine should be examined for stones. Gallstone ileus is usually treated in two stages. First, the small bowel obstruction is relieved by extraction of the gallstone. Cholecystectomy and closure of the duodenal fistula are usually undertaken at a later time, because the right upper quadrant is frequently an inflammatory phlegmon and the patient's condition is often marginal.

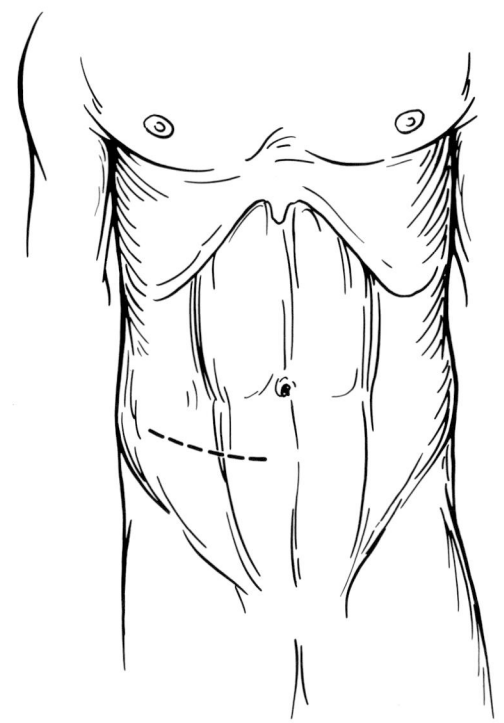

Figure 17-XVII-3

Incision

A transverse incision is made in the right lower abdomen, and the full length of small bowel is examined to identify the point of obstruction at the transition of dilated to collapsed small bowel.

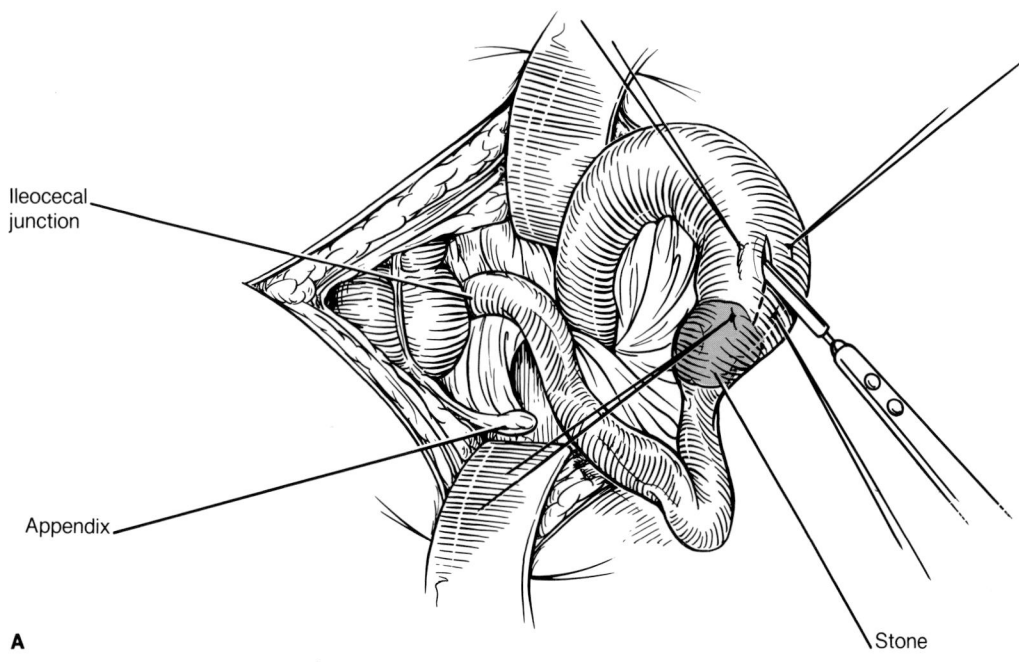

Figure 17-XVII-4

Gallstone Removal

(A) An enterotomy is made proximal to the impacted stone, which is milked back and removed.

(Continued)

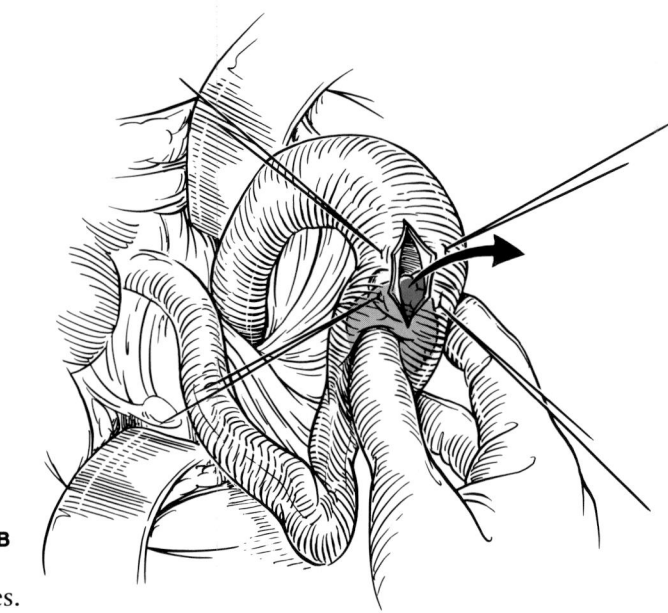

Figure 17-XVII-4 *(Continued)*

(**B**) The entire intestine is inspected for additional stones.

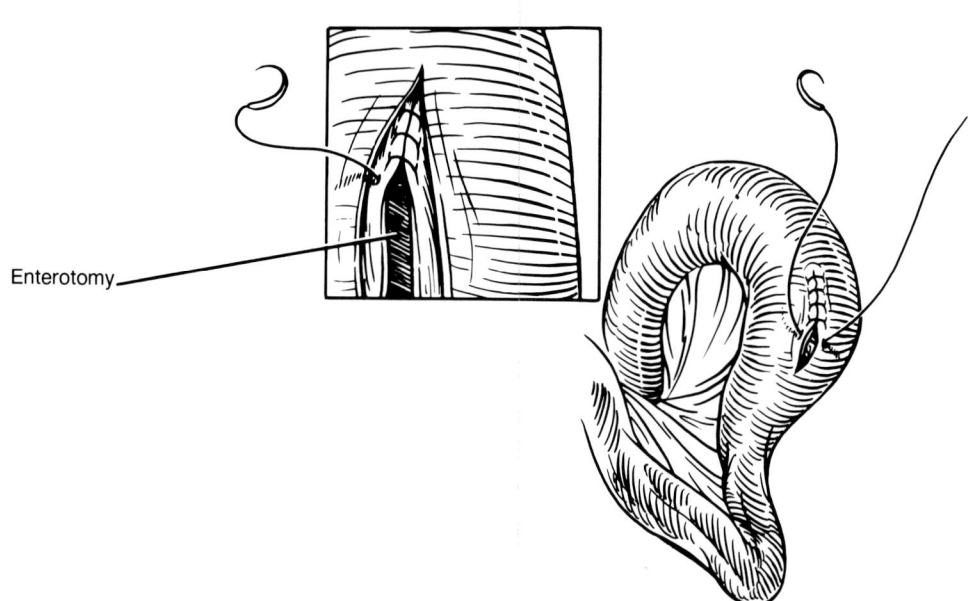

Enterotomy

Figure 17-XVII-5

Enterotomy Closure

The enterotomy is closed in two layers, an inner layer of inverting, running 3-0 chromic suture and an outer layer of interrupted 3-0 silk Lembert sutures. The enterotomy and stone extraction can also be accomplished laparoscopically.

PART IV
Liver

Digestive Tract Surgery: A Text and Atlas, edited by Richard H. Bell,
Layton F. Rikkers, and Michael W. Mulholland.
Lippincott-Raven Publishers, Philadelphia, © 1996.

18

Benign Neoplasms of the Liver

John B. Hanks | *Lynn K. Rosenlof*

Patients with liver masses can have a broad range of nonspecific, nondiagnostic symptoms, such as right upper quadrant pain, fever, bleeding, or jaundice, or they can have no symptoms at all. The differential diagnosis of such masses includes numerous benign liver diseases, such as neoplastic, infectious, cystic, or congenital conditions, and primary and metastatic malignant tumors. A careful history and physical examination often provides important information. Because laboratory tests usually are not helpful, radiologic imaging techniques are used to confirm the diagnosis and develop a surgical plan.

It is important to avoid costly duplication of imaging tests, some of which may be contraindicated or provide little additional information. Advances in surgical techniques (including laparoscopy), interventional radiology, and supportive intraoperative and postoperative care allow surgeons to choose from a wide array of diagnostic and therapeutic modalities. In evaluating and treating patients with liver masses, the following questions should be asked:

1. What is the diagnosis of the mass? What tests are necessary to confirm this diagnosis?
2. Where in the liver is the mass located? Can the lesion be approached surgically?
3. Is surgery required for treatment? Is interventional radiology required for treatment? Is simple observation preferable? Does coexistent cirrhosis alter plans for treatment?

CLINICAL EVALUATION OF PATIENTS WITH LIVER MASSES

Many patients are referred to surgeons for evaluation of liver masses found by chance. Often the patients originally were seen for ill-defined symptoms suggestive of cholelithiasis. During a 5-year period, one group evaluated 64 asymptomatic patients with incidentally found solid hepatic lesions.[1] Thirty-three (51%) lesions were benign hemangiomas and 11 (17%) were malignant. These investigators were unable to define any clinical, biochemical, or imaging process that could differentiate with certainty between benign and malignant lesions. Malignancy was suggested by age greater than 55 years, a palpable mass, or an elevated alkaline phosphatase level.

Important historical points include previous surgical procedures, weight loss, and prior exposure to hepatitis, carcinogens, or oral contraceptives. The physical examination should be directed toward the detection of an abdominal mass, icterus, signs of portal hypertension, or a rectal mass. Appropriate laboratory tests include a complete blood count, serum electrolytes, conventional liver function tests, a hepatitis screen, and tumor markers such as α-fetoprotein and carcinoembryonic antigen. Although a thorough history, physical examination, and laboratory evaluation seldom results in a specific diagnosis, it provides important information to guide the selection of appropriate imaging studies.

RADIOLOGIC EVALUATION OF A LIVER MASS

Methods

Ultrasound

Ultrasound is accurate in detecting localized lesions of the liver but is less useful in diagnosing diffuse liver diseases. The liver parenchyma can be evaluated thoroughly with ultrasound because of its echogenicity. Diffuse disease processes of the liver, such as cirrhosis, obesity, or hepatitis, make the examination more difficult. Normal anatomy, including blood vessels and bile ducts, can be identified reliably with ultrasound. This diagnostic modality is comparable to computed tomography (CT) and is even more sensitive and accurate in some instances, particularly for small lesions. The sensitivity with which a liver mass can be identified or excluded with ultrasound approaches 90%.[2]

Despite its sensitivity in detecting focal masses, ultrasound is less effective in determining the nature of such masses. Purely cystic lesions suggest their diagnosis; solid or complex lesions require further study.

Computed Tomography

Computed tomography is an important imaging modality in the evaluation of liver masses. Many advances have been made in CT scanning as a result of the evolving technology of associated contrast-enhanced imaging. Enhancing techniques include intravenous contrast for imaging the liver parenchyma, direct arterial contrast for delineating the vascular anatomy, and contrast injected by endoscopic retrograde cholangiopancreatography for defining the biliary anatomy. Dynamic CT scanning involves the rapid intravenous infusion of a contrast agent, followed immediately by rapid scans of contiguous images. This technique can elicit differences in the vascularity of various lesions.

Two examples of contrast-enhanced CT scanning are incremental dynamic CT and angiographic CT. Incremental dynamic CT is helpful in differentiating hemangiomas from vascular hepatocellular carcinomas.[3,4] This technique involves rapid sequential scanning 20 seconds after the intravenous bolus injection of a contrast agent. Individual scans are completed rapidly (1 second per scan) while the high-dose contrast agent passes through the hepatic arteries. Additional delayed scans are done 2 or 3 minutes after injection. Certain patterns of contrast enhancement are predictive of benign or malignant masses. In angiographic CT, images are obtained as a contrast agent is injected into the hepatic artery or the superior mesenteric artery. This method has been reported to be particularly effective in diagnosing focal nodular hyperplasia (FNH), in defining hepatic vascular anatomy and its relationship to a mass, and in detecting smaller lesions than is possible with dynamic CT.[4]

Despite the enthusiasm for various contrast-enhanced methods, no specific CT criteria can distinguish benign from malignant liver masses with absolute certainty. However, as experience is gained with bolus injection techniques, characteristic patterns of enhancement may strongly suggest a benign or malignant process.[5–9]

Radionuclide Imaging

Radionuclide imaging assesses regional parenchymal function but does not provide the discrete anatomic information gained from ultrasound and CT. Its advantages include minimal invasiveness and relatively low cost. This imaging technique is sensitive for the detection of focal liver masses, including tumors, cysts, and abscesses; however, like ultrasound and CT, it does not provide a specific diagnosis.[10,11] The sensitivity and specificity of radionuclide imaging vary between 50% and 95%.

The main contrast agent used in radionuclide imaging of the liver is technetium 99m (^{99m}Tc) sulfur colloid, which is extracted efficiently by the phagocytic Kupffer cell.[12] This scan is particularly helpful in distinguishing FNH, which contains Kupffer cells, from hepatic adenoma, which lacks them.

Other radiotracers are used to make specific diagnoses. ^{99m}Tc-labeled red blood cells, in conjunction with early dynamic image sequences of ^{99m}Tc sulfur colloid, determine the vascularity of a lesion. Hemangiomas show a characteristic pattern of uptake. Gallium 67 is differentially concentrated by certain mass lesions, specifically hepatomas and bacterial abscesses, thereby suggesting these diagnoses.[12]

Angiography

Hepatic arteriography can delineate structural relationships of the normal liver to a focal mass, the anatomy of the lesion itself, and the vascularity of the lesion. This invasive procedure can be complicated by thrombosis, bleeding, or segmental hepatic infarction. The availability of ultrasound and CT has reduced the role of angiography from that of a primary diagnostic technique to a complementary diagnostic or therapeutic procedure. Some surgeons use preoperative angiography to define hepatic vascular anatomy, because aberrancies are common. However, experienced surgeons usually can determine the pattern of hepatic arterial blood supply during laparotomy. Angiography helps to differentiate between FNH and adenoma on the basis of anatomic characteristics of the blood supply of these lesions, and it is the gold standard for the diagnosis of hemangioma, although ultrasound and tagged red blood cell scanning are equally effective.[13] Therapeutic uses of angiography include selective hepatic infusion and embolization of malignant lesions.

Magnetic Resonance Imaging

The use of magnetic resonance imaging (MRI) in the evaluation of liver pathology continues to evolve, particularly as new contrast agents are evaluated.[14,15] However, its overall diagnostic accuracy is similar to that of CT. Because it costs considerably more than ultrasound or CT, the use of MRI for liver imaging has been limited.

Intraoperative Imaging

Technologic advances have made it possible to use intraoperative ultrasonography in the evaluation of hepatic masses and anatomy. Intraoperative ultrasound has been embraced enthusiastically by hepatobiliary surgeons because it probably is the most sensitive technique for detecting hepatic masses, and because it aids in hepatic resection by clearly defining intrahepatic vascular anatomy.[16–18] The sensitivity of intraoperative ultrasound in identifying intrahepatic lesions can be as high as 98%, considerably higher than that of preoperative ultrasound or CT. As many as 40% of the lesions seen by intraoperative ultrasound may not be visible or palpable during surgery. This diagnostic technique can reliably define liver masses smaller than 0.5 cm.[17,19] Intraoperative ultrasound has its greatest applicability in patients who are undergoing resection for malignant

primary hepatic tumors or metastatic disease involving the liver. However, it also is useful for defining hepatic anatomy during the resection of benign tumors.

Image-Guided Biopsy

Liver biopsy, which can be performed percutaneously under image guidance by laparoscopy or open laparotomy, can be a valuable part of the diagnostic work-up of a liver mass. Large-bore core tissue biopsy involves the removal of a 1-mm core of tissue, which can be evaluated by either frozen or permanent section. Small-bore fine-needle aspiration followed by cytologic evaluation is gaining increasing acceptance. Conventional large-bore biopsy has a sensitivity of 60% to 82% for diffuse liver disease but is less sensitive for focal lesions.[20,21] The use of ultrasound to guide fine-needle aspiration has been successful in the diagnosis of malignant processes. These biopsy techniques are limited in patients with benign lesions because it can be difficult to differentiate an adenoma or FNH from a malignant lesion. Fine-needle aspiration can be both diagnostic and an important component of the treatment of amebic cysts and pyogenic abscesses. The evaluation of a hypervascular mass by percutaneous biopsy generally is discouraged but may be indicated occasionally.[22,23] When a symptomatic liver mass requires resection regardless of the diagnosis, percutaneous biopsy is not necessary.

Sequence of Imaging Evaluation (Fig. 18-1)

In most cases, ultrasound is a reasonable initial test because it is sensitive, cost-effective, and noninvasive. Although ultrasound may not provide a specific diagnosis,

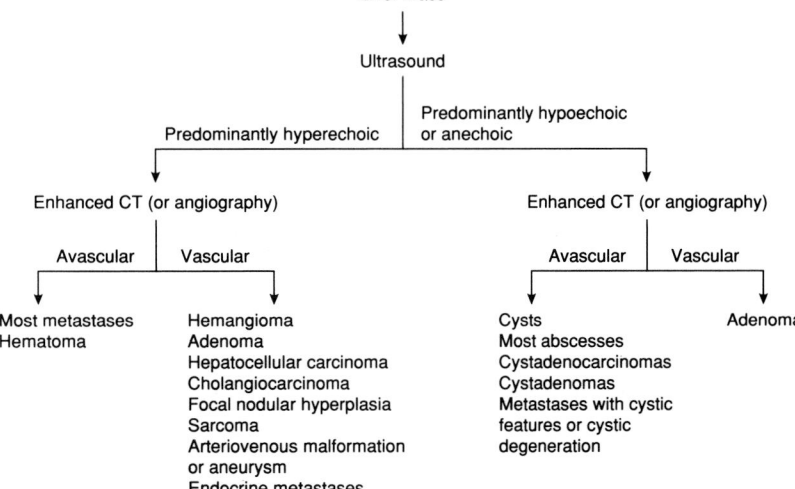

Figure 18-1 An approach to the general characterization of liver masses. The results of carefully selected laboratory tests and the characteristic appearances of masses on CT, ultrasound, and radionuclide imaging usually provide a preoperative diagnosis. Adenomas may be hyperechoic or hypoechoic on ultrasound scans. (Hanks JB, Arnold WS. Hepatic neoplasms. In: Greenfield LJ, Mulholland MW, Oldham KT, Zelenock GB, eds. Surgery: scientific principles and practice. Philadelphia, JB Lippincott, 1992:908)

it is sensitive in detecting coexisting biliary disease, in differentiating cystic from solid masses, and in determining whether there is a solitary mass or multiple masses. If the lesion is solitary and cystic, the likelihood of malignancy is greatly diminished and conservative therapy often can be initiated. When multiple solid lesions are detected, metastatic disease is likely. If resection is not potentially curable, an image-guided biopsy or needle aspiration should be done. Solitary solid lesions must be evaluated cautiously. If the lesion appears to be vascular, needle biopsy is *not* indicated. When ultrasound suggests a hemangioma, the next study should be a tagged red blood cell scan, which usually confirms the diagnosis. For other solid lesions, an enhanced CT scan generally is necessary. The use of this technique in combination with MRI or angiography should be planned thoughtfully in an effort to contain costs. CT angiography or portography is being used more often in many institutions because it more accurately reveals the relationship of the lesion or lesions to vascular structures, and because it is the most sensitive CT technique for detecting additional masses. All the information obtained from imaging studies should be combined and a decision should be made whether to proceed with resection or with a percutaneous image-guided needle biopsy.[24] If the information gained from a biopsy may make surgery unnecessary, the biopsy should be done. However, if surgical treatment of a resectable lesion is indicated regardless of the diagnosis, this step can be omitted.

BENIGN CYSTIC DISEASES

Most cystic lesions of the liver are benign. Although relatively uncommon, cysts are being detected with greater frequency because ultrasound has become the gold standard for the diagnosis of cholelithiasis. In most cases, asymptomatic simple cysts require no treatment.

Congenital (Nonparasitic) Hepatic Cysts

Congenital hepatic cysts can be solitary or multiple and nearly always are benign. The incidence of hepatic cysts is 0.14% to 0.30% in autopsy series.[25] The cause is thought to be a developmental anomaly in which there is interruption of the intralobar ducts during embryologic development. Congenital cysts are lined with cuboidal epithelium and usually do not connect with the biliary tract. An alternative hypothesis is that lymphatic obstruction causes hepatic cysts. They can contain blood or degenerative material. Less common types of hepatic cysts include dermoid cysts, endothelial cysts, retention cysts, and proliferative cysts.

Solitary Congenital Cysts

Solitary cystic lesions usually are discovered in patients with no symptoms as incidental findings at laparotomy or during diagnostic evaluation for other problems. A symptomatic solitary cyst can present with vague right upper quadrant discomfort, a sensation of heaviness, early satiety, or nausea and vomiting. A palpable mass is not commonly found. The fluid within the cyst is under low pressure and is secreted by the endothelial lining. The contents usually are clear, but can be mucoid, bloody, or tinged with bile. There is a female predominance of 3:1.[26]

Evaluation of patients with simple cysts generally reveals normal complete blood counts and liver function test results. The presence of acute abdominal pain suggests intracystic hemorrhage or cyst rupture. Other complications include secondary bacterial infection and obstructive jaundice from compression of the extrahepatic bile duct by the cyst.[26-31] Ultrasound examination reveals an anechoic lesion with smooth borders and occasional septation. CT shows a cystic lesion with low attenuation.

In combination, these studies usually differentiate between a parasitic cyst, an abscess, a simple cyst, and a cystic neoplasm (Fig. 18-2).

An asymptomatic cyst discovered by chance does not require surgical intervention. If the cyst is aspirated, it usually recurs as long as the endothelial lining remains intact.[30] If ultrasound suggests the existence of internal echoes and the possibility of an abscess is raised, the cyst can be aspirated under CT or ultrasound guidance for culture and cytology. In addition, if the cyst is discovered incidentally at laparotomy, aspiration should be performed for Gram stain, culture, and cytology. If this reveals an uninfected cyst, it should be treated conservatively. A symptomatic simple cyst can be resected along with adjacent hepatic parenchyma, or it can be enucleated (Fig. 18-3). Omentum can be placed within the cavity of the excised cyst. If the cyst is infected, external drainage or marsupialization in combination with antibiotic treatment should be performed. If the cyst fluid contains bile, suggesting communication with the biliary tract, construction of a Roux-en-Y limb of jejunum to the cyst should be considered.[27,31]

Adult Fibropolycystic Disease

Adult fibropolycystic disease is uncommon and should be distinguished from childhood fibropolycystic disease (see section on Pediatric Benign Liver Tumors). Adult fibropolycystic disease is inherited as a mendelian dominant trait that does not manifest until adulthood. There is a female predominance. Patients can have con-

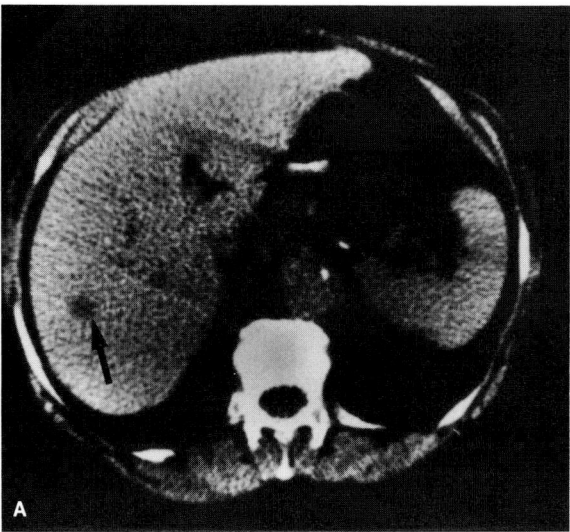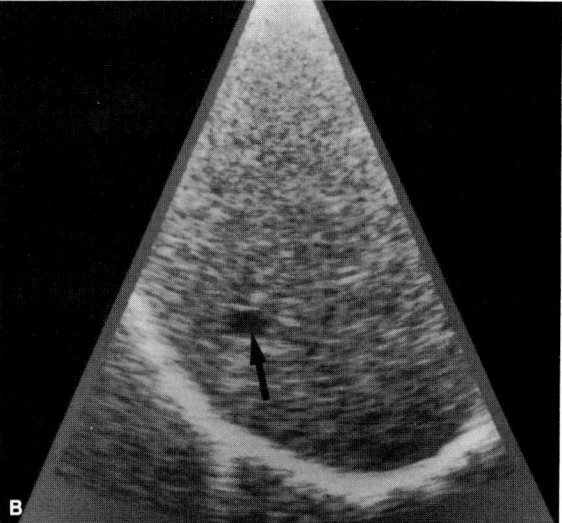

Figure 18-2 Cyst of the right lobe of the liver. A CT scan was performed for evaluation of metastases (**A**). Ultrasound was recommended to assess the lesion further (**B**). These two scans reveal a sharply demarcated wall without internal echoes, which is consistent with the diagnosis of a small hepatic cyst (*arrows*).

comitant cystic involvement of other organs, including the pancreas, the spleen, and, rarely, the lungs. One third of patients have polycystic kidneys. There may be an increased incidence of intracranial vascular aneurysms.[32]

The liver is diffusely involved with multiple cysts, which vary from a few millimeters to more than 20 cm in diameter. These cystic spaces contain a clear fluid secreted under low pressure from a cuboidal epithelial lining. The cystic involvement can be so extensive that nearly all the hepatic parenchyma appears to be re-placed. Microscopic examination reveals normal hepatocytes in the distorted tissue.[32]

Although many patients have no symptoms, some have upper abdominal pain or a gradually enlarging mass.[33] Nearly 75% of patients have a palpable mass. Despite extensive involvement of the hepatic parenchyma, the results of liver function tests are unaltered. Renal function deteriorates before hepatic function in patients with associated polycystic renal disease.

The decision regarding surgical intervention is based on the nature of symptoms and the status of renal

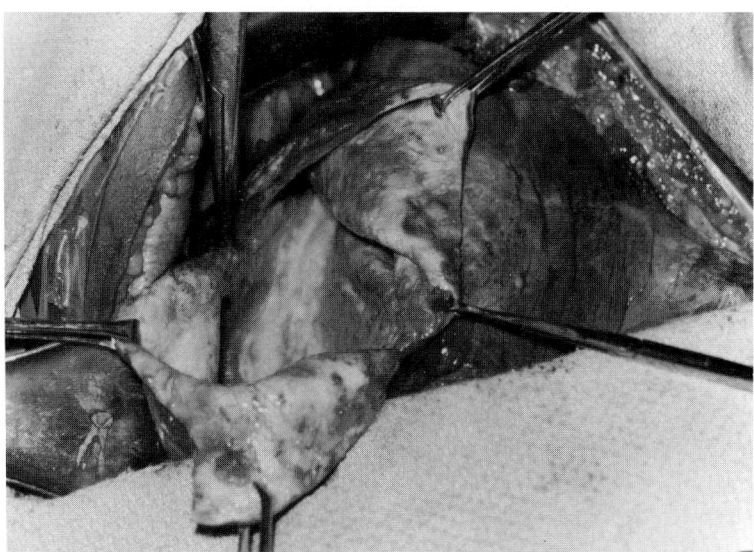

Figure 18-3 Excision of a large unilocular congenital hepatic cyst from the surrounding hepatic parenchyma. (Hanks JB, Jones RS. The liver. In: Fromm P, ed. Gastrointestinal surgery. New York, Churchill Livingstone, 1985:829)

function. If symptoms are minimal, surgical therapy is not necessary. Persistent pain requires consideration of cyst resection, fenestration, or both. Fenestration involves unroofing as many cysts as possible, with digital disruption of the numerous, thin-walled septa separating the cysts.[34] Intraoperative cholangiography should be performed because adjacent bile ducts can be injured. Intraoperative ultrasonography can be helpful in determining cyst location. Resection has been advocated when most of the cysts can be removed while maintaining adequate hepatocellular mass.[35] Hepatic transplantation has been done in selected severe cases.[36]

If renal failure develops, renal transplantation can be considered. However, posttransplant immunosuppressant therapy can cause cyst infection and potentially fatal episodes of hepatic abscess formation.[37]

Hydatid (Parasitic) Cysts

Hydatid disease is the most common cause of hepatic cysts. *Echinococcus granulosis,* a cestode, is the usual cause of unilocular hydatid cyst of the liver. This organism is prevalent in South America, Asia, southern and eastern Europe, and Australia. It is rare in the United States but can be found in Alaska and in the southeastern states.[25,26,38,39] The disease is caused by the larvae of the *Echinococcus* tapeworm, which resides in the gut of its definitive host, the domestic dog. Ova are excreted by the dog and disseminate into groundwater or dwellings, where they are ingested by intermediate hosts (sheep, pigs, and humans). The ova then pass through the intestinal mucosa of the host and are filtered by the liver or lungs. The liver is infected most commonly (nearly 70% of cases). Cysts are found in the right lobe in 60% to 75% of cases, and in both lobes in 20% to 30% of cases. The disease is chronic and affects men and women equally. Hydatid cysts can cause no symptoms, or they can cause right upper quadrant pain or a mass. Most cysts larger than 5 cm are associated with symptoms. The most severe symptoms occur when the cyst ruptures into a bile duct, resulting in abdominal pain, jaundice, and fever.[40] Most cysts are solitary and consist of multiple layers. There is an outside ''host'' capsule composed of compressed liver tissue and fibrous scar. The cyst itself has an outer laminated membrane of proteinaceous material and an intergerminal layer made up of scolices and daughter cysts that float freely in the cystic fluid. This fluid is under high pressure, is slightly alkaline, and is colorless and opalescent. In contrast, alveolar hydatid cysts grow without a capsule and their centers become necrotic as growth progresses.

Diagnosis

It is difficult to diagnose echinococcal cystic liver disease using a single test. Mild abnormalities may be seen in the results of standard liver function tests and eosinophilia may be present. Cyst fluid antibodies develop when the cyst fluid leaks into the peritoneal cavity and is absorbed into the circulation. Immunologic testing consists of an intradermal skin test known as the Casoni test, which produces positive results in 70% of patients with hydatid disease. The results of the complement fixation test are positive in up to 90% of patients with living hydatid cysts. Immunoelectrophoresis is the test of choice and converts to negative results 1 to 2 years after successful surgical treatment of hydatid disease.[26]

Plain films of the abdomen demonstrate a characteristic thin rim of calcification delineating the cyst, strongly suggesting the diagnosis of echinococcal disease. However, ultrasound is a more definitive test for the diagnosis of these cysts. If ultrasound demonstrates daughter cysts, the diagnosis is confirmed. CT has an accuracy of 98% and also is sensitive in demonstrating daughter cysts. It is the best test for differentiating pyogenic and amebic abscesses from hydatid disease. Arteriography plays no role in the diagnosis of echinococcal cysts and adds little to the information obtained by less invasive procedures. If echinococcal cyst is in the differential diagnosis of a hepatic mass, percutaneous needle biopsy or aspiration are contraindicated. Spillage of cyst fluid can result in anaphylaxis and death.

Treatment

No drug is effective for the treatment of living echinococcal cysts. Although there has been enthusiasm for mebendazole and albendazole, long-term results of their use are not available.[40–42] Therefore, the treatment of hydatid disease is primarily surgical, consisting of drainage of the cyst without contamination of surrounding areas or spillage into the peritoneum. Operative management includes careful localization of the cyst followed by aspiration of the contents and irrigation of the cyst with a scolecidal agent. The safest scolecidal agent is 20% hypertonic saline. Although alcohol and formaldehyde have been used, they are associated with greater morbidity. On completion of cyst irrigation, the cyst is opened carefully and evaluated.[43,44] All remaining contents are débrided and the cavity is packed with omentum or simply drained.

Potentially severe complications of hydatid disease include free cyst rupture because of the high internal fluid pressure, and rupture into the biliary tract, which can result in disappearance of the cyst or in biliary obstruction. Cyst rupture into the free peritoneal space can be followed by fatal anaphylaxis. Cysts in the dome of the liver can rupture through the diaphragm into the pleural cavity. Secondary cyst infection can lead to the development of a pyogenic abscess.

Alveolar Hydatid Disease

Alveolar hydatid disease occurs most often in the northern hemisphere, particularly in Alaska and Canada. The causative organism is *Echinococcus multilocularis*, which produces multiple, small, fragile cysts spread diffusely throughout the liver parenchyma. Progressive disease results in liver failure with portal hypertension. Involvement of distant organs includes parasite migration to the brain, lungs, and heart. This disease is associated with a 5-year mortality rate of nearly 50%.

HEPATIC ABSCESSES

Hepatic abscesses first were described in 1836.[45] During the past 150 years, many changes in diagnostic modalities, antimicrobial therapy, and methods of drainage have altered the approach to hepatic abscesses, which are classified as either pyogenic or amebic.

Pyogenic Hepatic Abscesses

Incidence and Etiology

In a 1938 publication, pyogenic hepatic abscesses represented 0.007% of hospital admissions.[46] In that report, about 25% of 186 cases of hepatic abscesses were pyogenic and the remaining 75% were amebic in origin. This experience was updated in 1975, at which time 75% of liver abscesses were found to be pyogenic in origin.[47]

In the era before antibiotics, pyogenic abscesses were caused most frequently by infectious processes in the abdomen, such as suppurative appendicitis complicated by portal thrombophlebitis. In the 1938 report, this accounted for about 35% of cases.[46]

Pyogenic hepatic abscesses now tend to be classified into four etiologic categories: biliary tract disease, cryptogenic, hematogenous spread, or primary hepatic involvement.[47] Biliary tract disease is becoming a more common cause of pyogenic abscesses, accounting for 22% to 51% of these lesions in recent series.[48-51] Hepatic abscesses without an obvious cause are termed idiopathic or cryptogenic. In early series, cryptogenic abscesses accounted for 20% to 45% of pyogenic abscesses. In recent series, cryptogenic abscesses constitute 5% to 21% of liver abscesses.[48,50-52] In a review

of 885 patients collected from the literature, hematogenous spread was responsible for 13% of hepatic abscesses.[52] In another study from a single institution, 14% of liver abscesses were caused by blood-borne infection.[49] The least common cause of hepatic abscesses in most series is primary hepatic involvement, resulting from hepatic trauma, direct extension from intraabdominal infection, or tumor necrosis of primary or secondary intrahepatic tumors.

Causative Agents

Common microbial agents identified in pyogenic hepatic abscesses include streptococci, staphylococci, and colon bacilli.[47] *Escherichia coli* was present on cultureD in 41 of 80 patients in one series.[49] *Klebsiella* and *Staphylococcus aureus* also can be cultured from pyogenic hepatic abscesses. Anaerobic culture techniques have become more sophisticated, particularly in the past 20 years. As a result, organisms are being reported that were not listed in earlier series. Abscesses with foul-smelling pus nearly always contain anaerobic organisms, including *Fusobacterium, Clostridium, Bacteroides fragilis,* and, occasionally, *Actinomyces.* Anaerobic organisms can be cultured from 20% to 45% of liver abscesses.[49]

Diagnosis

Patients with pyogenic hepatic abscesses usually have white blood cell counts of 18,000 to 22,000/μL. Liver function tests generally are not revealing; a nondiagnostic elevation of the alkaline phosphatase level may be the only finding. A chest radiograph or flat plate of the abdomen may suggest a space-occupying lesion or an elevated right diaphragm. Intrahepatic gas and air–fluid levels can be present but are not common.

The diagnostic work-up should begin with ultrasonography, followed by radionuclide scanning, CT, or MRI if necessary (Fig. 18-4). Ultrasonography usually identifies a simple or complex cystic mass within the liver. Neither ultrasound nor radioisotopic scanning is dependable for lesions smaller than 2 cm. CT is the most accurate diagnostic modality for the identification and localization of a hepatic abscess, and it can provide guidance for its percutaneous drainage. Depending on the technique used, CT can demonstrate abscess cavities as small as 1 cm in diameter.

Treatment

The main surgical principle in the treatment of pyogenic hepatic abscess is provision of adequate drainage. Although either surgical or percutaneous drainage can

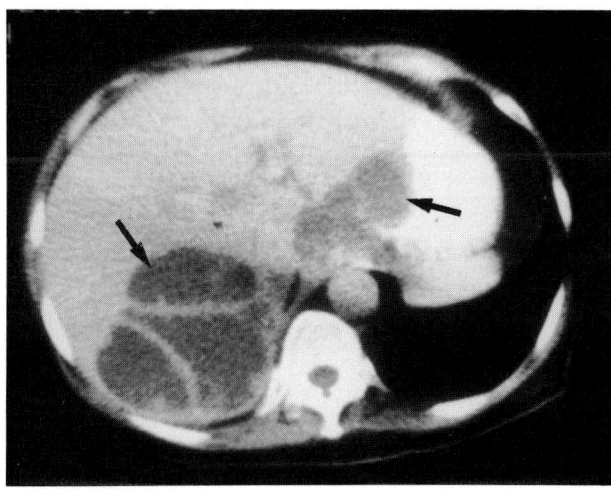

Figure 18-4 CT scan of the liver revealing an extensive pyogenic abscess involving the right and left lobes (*arrows*). Septation is seen, particularly in the extensive right lobe filling defect.

be efficacious for large, solitary lesions, multiple microscopic abscesses, which in the past have been associated with mortality rates approaching 100%, require prolonged antibiotic treatment.[46,49] When biliary tract disease is the cause of the infectious process, it also must be addressed. Open surgical drainage of a hepatic abscess can be accomplished by transabdominal, transpleural, or extraserous routes. These procedures are associated with the risk of contamination of the peritoneal cavity or right hemithorax by abscess contents. An effective alternative to open surgical approaches is percutaneous drainage using radiologic guidance (Fig. 18-5). This was first reported in 1953, when 14 patients underwent direct aspiration of single hepatic abscesses.[53] Another publication reported percutaneous catheter drainage of 58 hepatic abscesses in 51 patients, using either CT or ultrasonography as a localization procedure.[54] Many recent reports have taken an increasingly aggressive posture toward the use of interventional radiologic techniques in the diagnosis and treatment of hepatic abscesses. One institution reviewed 335 image-guided percutaneous catheter abscess drainage procedures in 323 consecutive patients with a 1-year follow-up period.[55] The overall cure rate was 62%. This technique was thought to be particularly valuable in 72 immunocompromised patients, of whom 53% were cured. Overall, this large series had a complication rate of 9.8% and a recurrence rate of 7.1%.

Another report has emphasized the importance of communication of the abscess with the biliary tract.[56] When injection of a contrast agent into the abscess cavity demonstrates biliary tract communication, a longer period of catheter drainage is necessary. Liver abscesses with biliary communication generally do not require alternative interventional techniques or surgical bypass procedures. The overall cure rate in this series was 66%. Although another series of 23 patients had an overall cure rate of 76% with percutaneous drainage, only 3 of 5 patients with secondary complicated abscesses (infected hematoma or necrotic tumor) benefited.[57] Six multilocular or septate abscesses were included in this series; five were cured with the placement of a single catheter.

Whether operations or percutaneous techniques are used, the guiding principles are the same. Patients with hepatic abscesses should be treated initially with intravenous antibiotics, effective drainage, and continued antibiotic therapy until they have recovered clinically and the abscess cavity has disappeared. With the use of sophisticated CT and ultrasound techniques and strict adherence to these principles, improved mortality and morbidity rates are being reported, even with complex abscesses. Segmental or lobar hepatic resection still is necessary on occasion to treat multiple abscesses in complicated clinical situations.[58]

Amebic Abscesses

Amebic abscesses are decreasing in incidence relative to pyogenic abscesses. The infective agent, *Endamoeba histolytica,* occurs in all parts of the United States, although it previously was thought to be confined to tropical or subtropical areas.[42,51]

Diagnosis

In a report describing 181 patients nearly 50 years ago, amebic abscesses most often presented with right upper quadrant abdominal pain (87%) and fever (85%). A history of diarrhea, chills, and nausea was found in about 25% of patients.[59] The white blood cell count can be elevated with amebic abscesses, but when this is associated with fever, a secondary pyogenic infection is suggested. Liver function tests can be abnormal but are not diagnostic. Indirect hemagglutination is a sensitive serologic test when titers exceed 1:128.[26,60]

Treatment

In contrast to pyogenic liver abscesses, the principal therapy for amebic abscesses is medical. Metronidazole is the drug of choice and is effective in most patients. Chloroquine phosphate and emetine hydrochloride were used formerly but are not as effective in combating the amebae residing both within the lumen

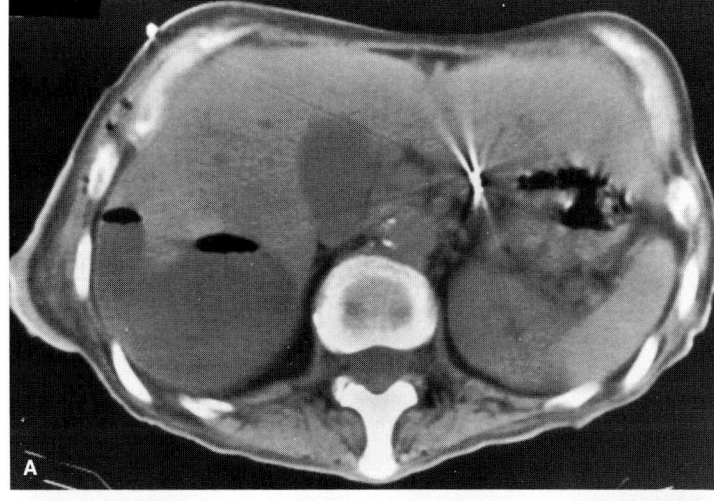

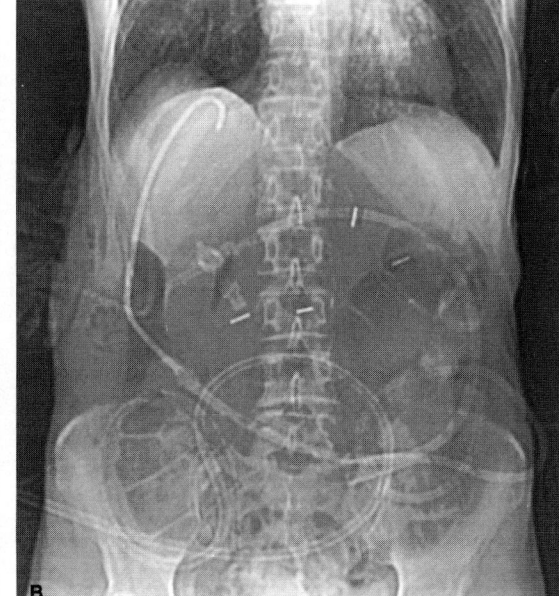

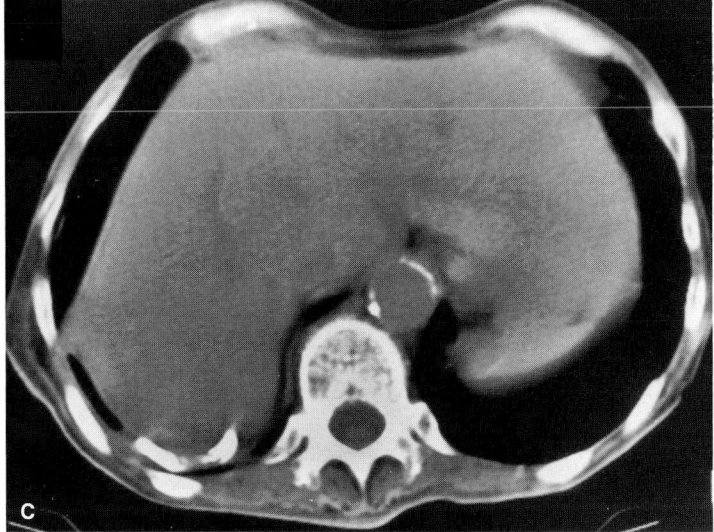

Figure 18-5 A large right lobe hepatic abscess (**A**) is drained percutaneously (**B**), which results in complete resolution of the abscess on a CT scan 2 months later (**C**).

of the abscess and in its periphery. The prompt institution of metronidazole therapy is associated with a cure rate exceeding 90%. Diagnostic modalities include ultrasonographic and CT localization of the abscess (Fig. 18-6). This should be followed by fine-needle aspiration, which demonstrates the classic "anchovy paste" contents of the abscess. The abscess cavity need not be drained completely and is cultured only to exclude secondary infection. Nonhealing abscesses, which are uncommon, can be treated surgically.[51] The most frequent complication of an amebic abscess is secondary infection with conversion to a pyogenic abscess, which must be drained. Other complications include rupture of the abscess cavity into the respiratory system with resultant pulmonary abscesses or empyema, and rupture into the peritoneal cavity with resultant overwhelming sepsis, often resulting in death.[26]

BENIGN NEOPLASMS OF THE LIVER

With the growing use of sophisticated radiologic techniques in the evaluation of abdominal disease, the incidental detection of masses within the liver is increasing. The challenge for clinicians is determining which of these masses require treatment and which can be observed.

Benign Solid Hepatic Neoplasms (Table 18-1)

Hepatocellular Adenomas

Although relatively rare 20 years ago, hepatocellular adenomas have become one of the most common benign hepatic tumors. In a review of 75 cases at the

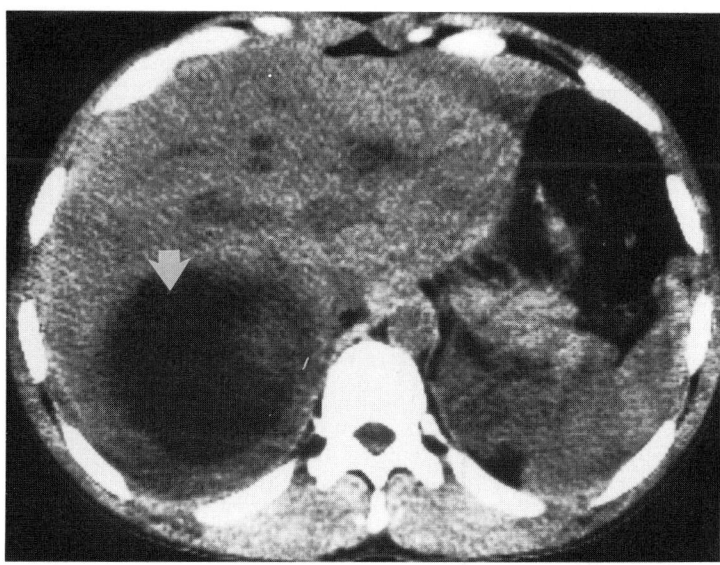

Figure 18-6 CT scan showing an amebic abscess in the posterior aspect of the right lobe of the liver (*arrow*). After documentation of the diagnosis by fine-needle aspiration, the abscess was treated successfully with metronidazole (Flagyl). (Hanks JB, Jones RS. The liver. In: Fromm D, ed. Gastrointestinal surgery. New York, Churchill Livingstone, 1985: 824)

Armed Forces Institute of Pathology, all the patients were women aged 17 to 61 years.[61] Two thirds of them had abdominal masses. Seventeen patients (23%) had circulatory shock due to intraperitoneal rupture of the tumor. In this review, 71% of adenomas were single, and two thirds of these were located in the right lobe. Two thirds of the lesions were 2 to 10 cm in diameter.

The frequency of hepatocellular adenomas has increased over the past 30 to 35 years, primarily as a result of the widespread use of oral contraceptives in Great Britain and the United States. Most hepatic adenomas occur in women of childbearing age who have used contraceptive agents containing estrogen or progesterone.[62–66] The link between initiation of adenoma growth and peripheral levels of estrogen is strengthened further by observations of adenomas in patients receiving conjugated estrogen therapy and in individuals with estrogen-producing tumors.[64] Hepatic adenomas also can be associated with anabolic steroid ingestion in men.[63]

The use of oral contraceptives increases not only the probability of adenoma development but also the

Table 18-1 Characteristics of Common Benign Liver Tumors

Variable	Focal Nodular Hyperplasia	Adenoma	Hemangioma
Age	All ages, mostly third and fourth decades	Third and fourth decades	All ages
Female/male ratio	7:1	7–8:1	Equal
Incidence	Uncommon	Rare	2%–7% of autopsies
Presentation	Largely asymptomatic; one third with abdominal mass or discomfort	25% with bleeding and hypovolemia; 40%–50% with mass associated with oral contraceptives	Usually asymptomatic; oral contraceptives associated with worse symptoms
Malignant potential	None	Minimal	None
Pathology	Stellate, central scar; pseudocapsule, Kupffer cells	Pure hepatocytes, no bile ducts	Fibrous reaction hypervascular, sinusoidal vascularity
Best imaging modality sequence	US, CT, sulfur colloid scan, angiography	US, angiographic CT	US, CT, tagged red blood cell scan
Definitive treatment	Resection, usually because of possible malignant condition	Resection, because of possibility of rupture	Observation if diagnosis is secure for <4 cm; resection for >4 cm or symptoms

US, ultrasound; CT, computed tomography.

risk of serious complications.[67] These tumors are larger than 5 cm in 97% of patients who are taking oral contraceptives compared with 73% of those who are not.[68] In addition, 65% of oral contraceptive users have bleeding or ruptured adenomas compared with 25% of nonusers.

Patients with type IA glycogen storage disease have a high incidence of hepatic adenoma, which always has a tendency to rupture. It is unclear whether dietary therapy is associated with regression of the tumor or amelioration of the symptoms.[67]

Whether hepatic adenomas progress to hepatocellular carcinoma is not clear.[67,69] Despite occasional reports that adenomas are premalignant, it is more likely that well-differentiated malignant lesions are difficult to distinguish from benign adenomas. It is important that the entire resected adenoma be examined diligently for any foci of malignancy, which would change the diagnosis to hepatocellular carcinoma.[67,70]

PATHOLOGY. Hepatic adenomas vary from 1 to 30 cm in size and can be either entirely intrahepatic or pedunculated. Most lesions are in the right lobe of the liver. The gross appearance is of a homogeneous yellow-tan lesion with no obvious capsule. A compressive pseudocapsule can develop from pressure on the adjacent hepatic parenchyma. Intratumor necrosis or hemorrhage may be apparent.

Microscopically, adenoma cells are sharply demarcated from adjacent normal liver by the pseudocapsule. Adenomas consist of cells two or three times the size of hepatocytes and have no bile ducts or bile ductule formation (Fig. 18-7). The cytoplasm of adenoma cells appears clear because of increased glycogen stores, and can contain bile. Nuclei show little variation in size and

no mitotic activity. Occasional areas of hemorrhage and fibrosis may be found throughout the tumor.[61]

DIAGNOSIS. Patients with hepatic adenomas have either no symptoms or nonspecific symptoms. The typical clinical presentation is mild right upper quadrant pain due to expansion, bleeding, or rupture of the tumor (Fig. 18-8). The last circumstance can present as an acute abdomen and shock.[62,67,69] The results of initial routine laboratory tests usually are normal unless bleeding has developed.

No imaging modality is specific for hepatic adenoma. Ultrasound usually demonstrates a solitary mass with nonspecific echogenicity. CT scanning with intravenous contrast often reveals areas of hemorrhage or necrosis within the tumor. Adenomas are hypervascular on both angiography and sulfur colloid scanning.[71-73] These diagnostic tests usually provide only a suggestive diagnosis of adenoma.

TREATMENT. Although some hepatic adenomas regress after oral contraceptive use is discontinued, this is not predictable and the potential for rupture and hemorrhage persists.[65,67]

Surgical resection is the primary therapy for hepatic adenoma. Resection not only eliminates the risk of rupture and bleeding, which occurs in 20% to 25% of patients, it also provides the opportunity to rule out hepatocellular carcinoma. In one recent experience of 14 resections for benign solid liver tumors, 12 were adenomas.[74] Half the patients were treated by wedge resection and four required hepatic lobectomy. Another group reported a 12-year experience of 24 patients with hepatic adenomas.[75] Eighteen patients were women, 16 of whom had been taking oral contraceptives. Fifty percent of the women had bleeding from the tumor.

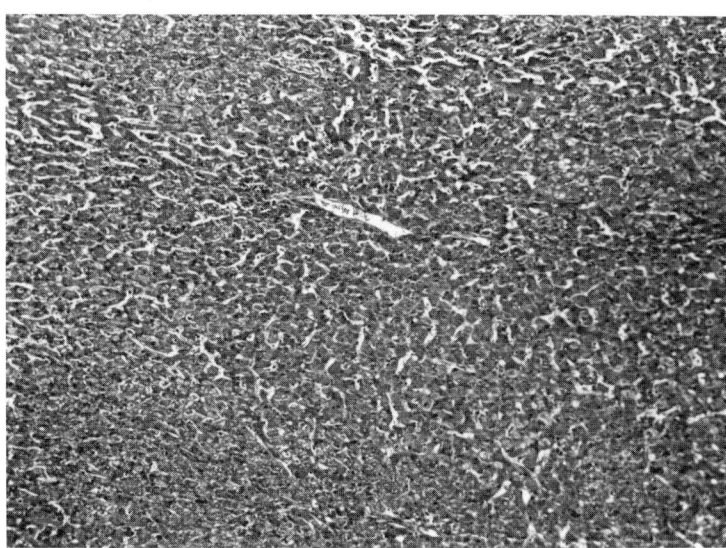

Figure 18-7 Microscopic evaluation of a hepatic adenoma reveals the uniform appearance of normal hepatocytes and the absence of biliary architecture. (See Color Fig. 18-7.) (Hanks JB, Arnold WS. Hepatic neoplasms. In: Greenfield LJ, ed. Surgery: scientific principles and practice. Philadelphia, JB Lippincott, 1992:913)

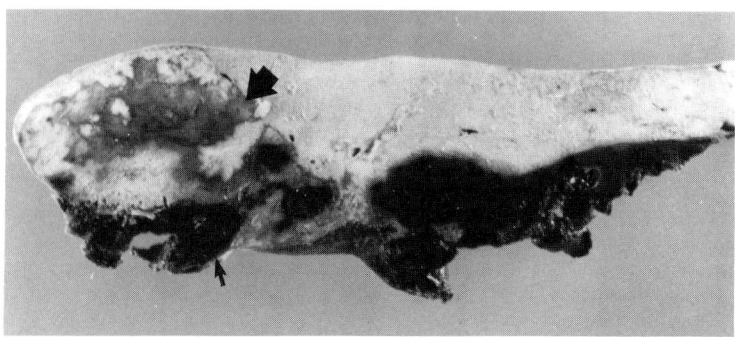

Figure 18-8 Resected left lateral segment showing a hepatic adenoma (*large arrow*) that has hemorrhaged into the inferior aspect of the lobe. A clot (*small arrow*) is visible immediately adjacent to the lesion, which has perforated through the capsule of the liver and dissected extensively.

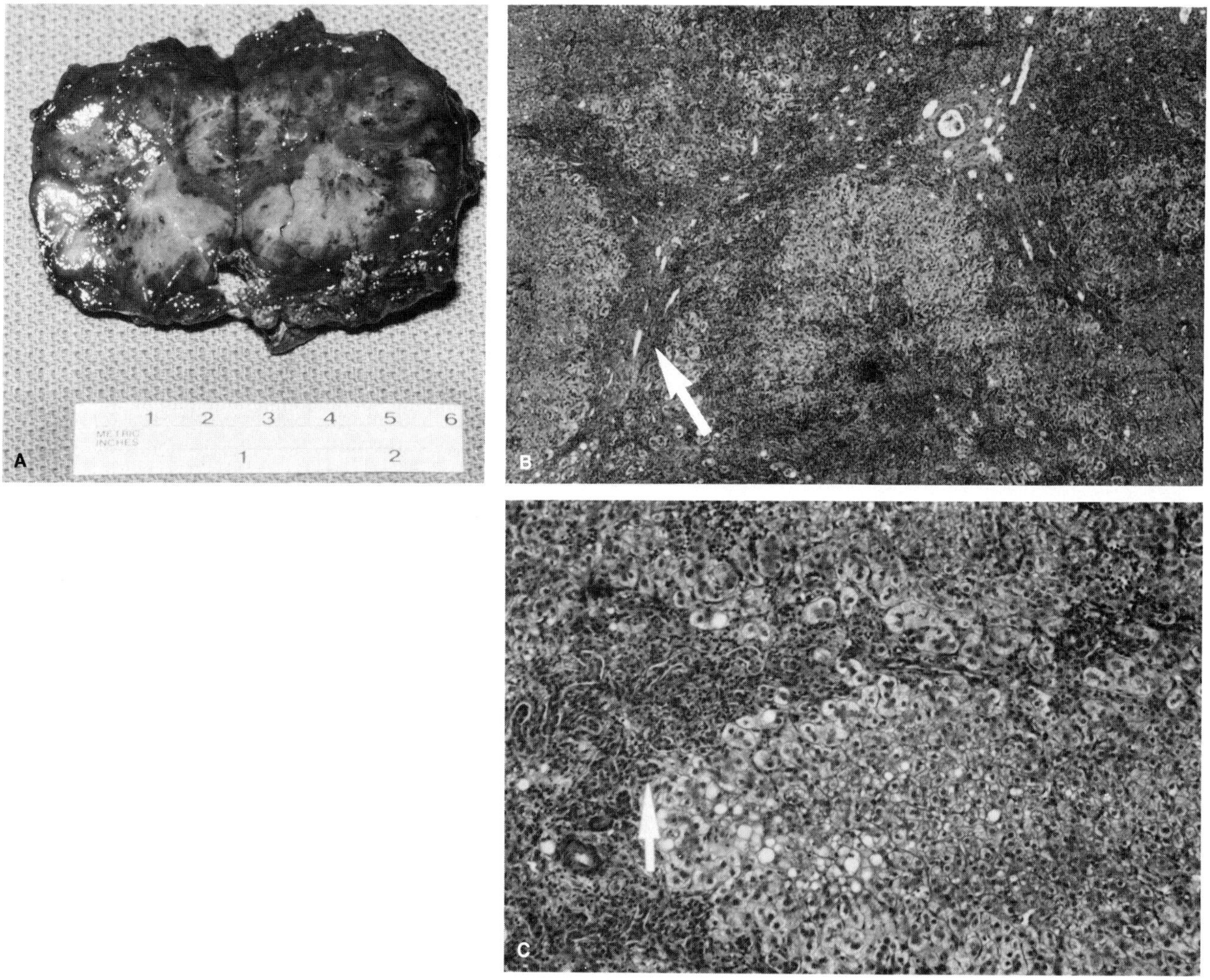

Figure 18-9 Focal nodular hyperplasia. (**A**) The cut specimen has a characteristic internal fibrotic appearance. (**B**) On low-power microscopy, fibrous septa (*arrow*) divide regions of residual hepatic architecture. (**C**) These fibrous septa contain bile ducts (*arrow*).

Seventeen patients underwent successful surgical removal of the lesion, and the remaining patient had preoperative arterial embolization to reduce tumor size before excision. This report also discusses multiple adenomas (or adenomatosis), which is a rare presentation of hepatic adenoma. One patient with adenomatosis underwent transplantation. There was no operative mortality in either of these series.

Focal Nodular Hyperplasia

Although FNH is distinctly different from adenoma, the initial work-up for the two lesions is similar. Many terms have been used for FNH, including *hepatic* *pseudotumor, focal cirrhosis, solitary hyperplastic nodule, benign hepatoma,* and *isolated nodules of regenerative hyperplasia.*

FNH predominantly affects women in the childbearing years; however, it is found more frequently in men and children than are adenomas. There is no correlation between the use of oral contraceptives and the incidence of FNH.[67,69,71] FNH classically presents with few or no symptoms. Most cases are discovered when an imaging study (usually ultrasound) is performed for nonspecific symptoms and demonstrates a solitary mass. Only a few patients have enlarged livers or any other significant signs or symptoms.[62]

In the Armed Forces Institute of Pathology report

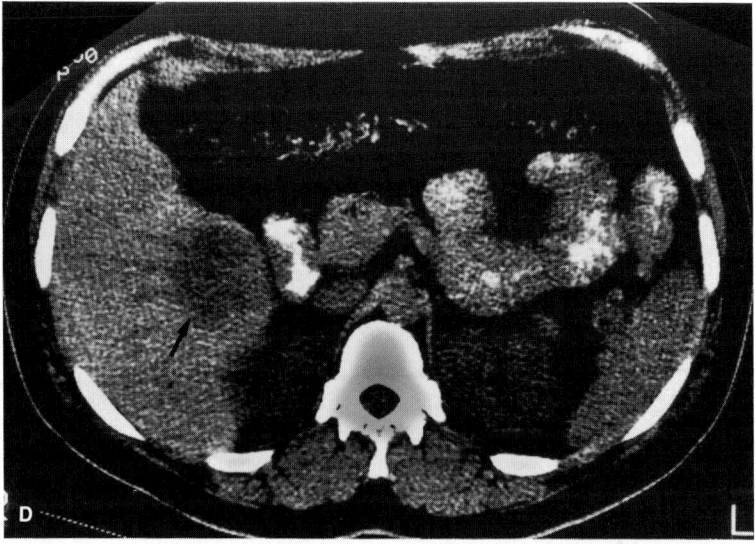

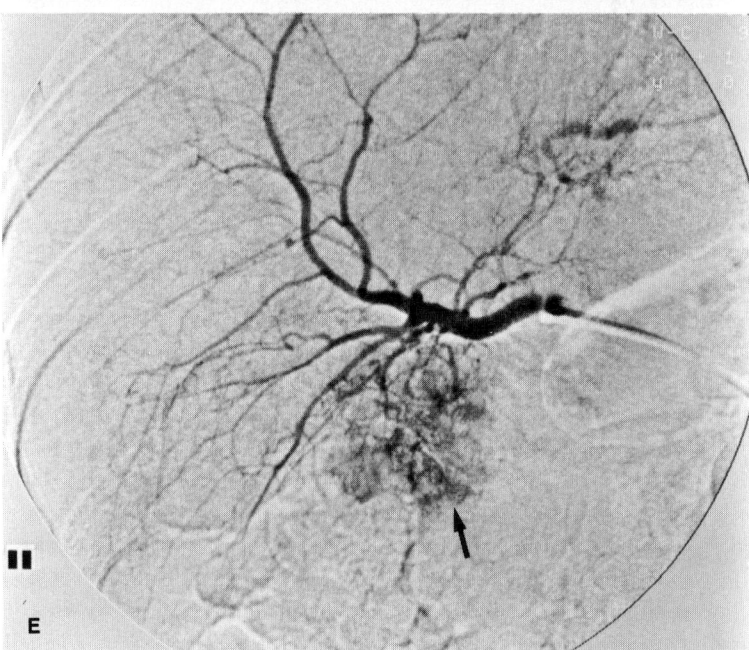

Figure 18-9 *(Continued)* **(D)** CT scan of a 35-year-old woman with minimal symptoms revealed a 5- to 6-cm lesion in the inferior aspect of the right lobe *(arrow)*. **(E)** Preoperative arteriography was performed and delineated a vascular neoplasm with a finely reticular pattern *(arrow)*. The question of malignancy was raised, and the specimen was evaluated during surgery and excised to establish the diagnosis of focal nodular hyperplasia. (See Color Fig. 18-9*A* to *C*.)

of 130 cases of FNH, patients ranged in age from 10 months to 75 years; 96% were between 20 and 40 years of age.[61] The female/male ratio was 2:1 and the lesion was found incidentally at autopsy or surgery in 80% of patients, in contrast to the high rate of symptoms and bleeding seen with adenomas. One hundred two patients (79%) had a single lesion, most of which were in the right lobe. Multiple nodules were found in 9 patients (7%).

Some reports have described an association between FNH and hepatic hemangioma.[76,77] Although coexistence of these lesions was noted in 23% of patients in one report, it was found in only 2% of patients in the Armed Forces Institute of Pathology report.[61,77]

PATHOLOGY. The gross appearance of FNH is globular with a lighter tan color than normal liver. A central stellate scar or, less commonly, areas of hemorrhage may be visible (Fig. 18-9A). Microscopic evaluation shows a central scar with radiation of fibrous tissue to the periphery, which divides the lesion into subunits (see Fig. 18-9B). In contrast to adenomas, the septa between these subunits contain bile ductules and interspersed Kupffer cells (see Fig. 18-9C). Hepatocytes within the subunits generally appear normal, but their cytoplasm contains more glycogen and fat than that of uninvolved hepatocytes in the surrounding liver.[61]

DIAGNOSIS. The results of liver function tests and a complete blood count usually are normal. Ultrasound and CT are sensitive in detecting a mass but are not specific for FNH unless a central scar is seen (see Fig. 18-9D). This finding only suggests the diagnosis. Angiography shows a hypervascular arteriographic appearance, which raises strong suspicion for FNH[71,73] (see Fig. 18-9E). In contrast to adenoma, FNH contains Kupffer cells; therefore, sulfur colloid radionuclide imaging can be useful in conjunction with a nondiagnostic CT or MRI examination. The combined use of ultrasound, CT, and radionuclide scanning usually is successful in diagnosing FNH.[67]

After detection of a mass by ultrasound or CT, radionuclide uptake on a ^{99m}Tc sulfur colloid scan suggests the diagnosis of FNH. If there is little uptake on the scan, angiography should be performed. FNH shows an intense capillary phase on angiography, whereas adenoma classically demonstrates hypovascular areas during the capillary phase.

TREATMENT. Asymptomatic FNH can be treated conservatively if the diagnosis is certain, because these lesions never rupture or bleed. In patients with hepatic masses of unclear origin, image-guided needle biopsy may suggest a diagnosis, particularly if a central scar is demonstrated. Small lesions on the periphery may require excisional biopsy in doubtful cases. Hepatic resection should be performed in patients who have large symptomatic lesions. Resection also is necessary in patients who have few symptoms when the possibility of a malignant process cannot be excluded.

Bile Duct Hamartomas

The terms *bile duct hamartoma* and *bile duct adenoma* often are confused, despite the fact that these are separate entities, both of which are uncommon. These lesions usually are discovered incidentally and can confuse the evaluation of patients with suspected primary or metastatic malignancies.[63]

Benign Vascular Neoplasms

Hemangiomas

The most common benign hepatic tumor is the cavernous hemangioma, found in 2% to 7% of autopsies. Only metastatic disease surpasses hemangioma in frequency.[61,71] Capillary hemangiomas usually are multiple, less than 1 cm in size, and of no clinical significance. Most cavernous hemangiomas found at autopsy are less than 5 cm in diameter. Symptoms correlate with the size of the tumor, which can be as large as 30 cm.[61] Hemangiomas are solitary lesions. Most are intrahepatic, but 15% to 20% are pedunculated, making them easily accessible to local resection.

The pathogenesis of hemangiomas is unknown, although there is debate as to whether oral contraceptives aggravate symptoms. There is no evidence that malignant transformation occurs.

Most patients with cavernous hemangiomas have no symptoms. When symptoms develop, they often include vague right upper quadrant discomfort and a feeling of fullness. Less commonly, patients have fever or a palpable mass.[62] Physical examination may reveal a bruit over the liver. Rarely, jaundice or gastric outlet obstruction is the presenting complaint with large hemangiomas. An unusual condition occasionally associated with cavernous hemangioma is the Kasabach-Merritt syndrome, which consists of a consumptive coagulopathy resulting from platelet trapping within a large hemangioma. Spontaneous rupture and hemorrhage are unusual complications of cavernous hemangiomas.[71,78]

PATHOLOGY. Cavernous hemangiomas appear dark red or brown with a soft, spongy interior (Fig. 18-10C). A dense fibrous pseudocapsule often surrounds the lesions, especially when they are large. Microscopically, vascular spaces of varying size are lined

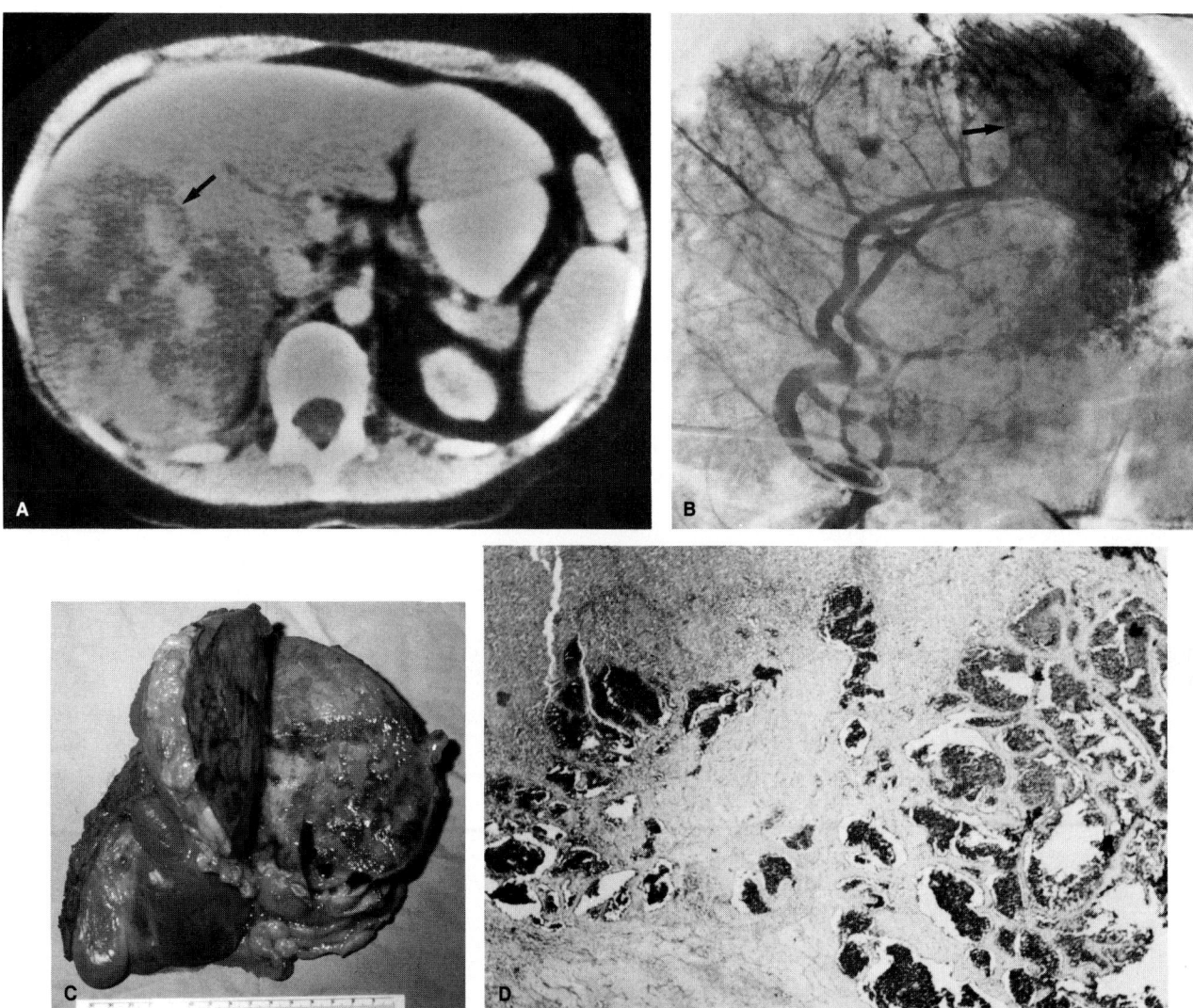

Figure 18-10 Hepatic hemangioma. (**A**) CT scan shows a diffuse mass in the right lobe of the liver (*arrow*). (**B**) Selective arteriography reveals an irregular vascular pattern in the right lobe (*arrow*). Late films demonstrate vascular "lakes" that persist after the contrast disappears from other vascular structures. These two imaging modalities are essentially confirmatory of a hepatic hemangioma. (**C**) Resected specimen shows a brownish lesion contained within an area of dense surrounding fibrous reaction. (**D**) Microscopic evaluation reveals diffuse sinusoids with blood-filled spaces lined by benign-appearing endothelium. (See Color Fig. 18-10*C* and *D*.)

by a single layer of flat, cuboidal cells (see Fig. 18-10*D*). These spaces can be empty, or they can show fresh or old thrombus formation. Surrounding fibrous reaction can be dense, even demonstrating rare stromal calcification.[61]

DIAGNOSIS. Patients with hemangiomas usually have normal results on blood chemistries, complete blood counts, and liver function tests. The work-up can

be initiated with ultrasonography, which detects these lesions with high sensitivity but low specificity. Ultrasound examination usually demonstrates a hyperechoic mass suggestive of hemangioma. CT and radionuclide imaging are useful adjuncts. On CT, hemangiomas show hypoattenuation without contrast, and early peripheral enhancement with progressive enhancement toward the center after contrast injection[73,79] (see Fig. 18-10*A*). Although once considered the gold standard for the diagnosis of hepatic hemangiomas, angiography (see Fig. 18-10*B*) generally has been replaced by the less invasive techniques of CT, ultrasound, and radionuclide imaging (Fig. 18-11). If a lesion has a characteristic CT appearance, the diagnosis often can be confirmed by radionuclide imaging. Although sulfur colloid imaging of the liver can be nonspecific for hemangioma, ^{99m}Tc erythrocyte scanning can add important diagnostic information. In comparing early, or "pool," studies to delayed static studies, hemangiomas, with their increased vascularity, have much higher activity than does the surrounding liver. Because the two scans image different activities, a perfusion-to-blood pool mismatch can be demonstrated that confirms the diagnosis of hepatic hemangioma.[80]

Correct interpretation of radionuclide scans depends on a clear understanding of the anatomy (location and size) and physiology (blood pool mixing) of the lesion. Early phase studies (sulfur colloid) demonstrate the lesion and its location. Late-phase studies suggest the presence of a highly vascular lesion. Thus, accurate diagnosis depends on both choosing appropriate imaging studies and performing them properly, especially the delayed scans.[80]

The T2-weighted MRI is effective for the diagnosis of hemangiomas, especially those smaller than 3 cm.[81] Image-guided needle aspiration or core biopsy usually is contraindicated because of the threat of bleeding, despite reports of its increased use.[22,23]

TREATMENT. Compared with hepatic adenomas, hemangiomas have a low risk of rupture.[67,78] Observation is acceptable treatment in patients who have smaller lesions (less than 4 cm) and few or no symptoms. The only curative therapy is resection, and this should be performed in patients who have larger lesions and significant symptoms. Resection also is indicated in some patients with hemangiomas who are receiving anticoagulant therapy or undergoing dialysis. Although unresectable symptomatic hemangiomas can be treated with radiation or embolization, success rates are lower.[71,82]

Taking advantage of the fibrous pseudocapsule that often accompanies larger hemangiomas, one group reported enucleation of solitary lesions ranging in size from 5 × 7 cm to 25 × 20 cm.[83] This procedure allows preservation of normal hepatic tissue, especially in patients with previous resections or large tumors. There was no operative mortality and one reoperation for bleeding in this series of 10 patients.

Hemangioendotheliomas

Hemangioendothelioma is a vascular lesion, the adult form of which is referred to as epithelioid hemangioendothelioma. In children, the neoplasm is referred

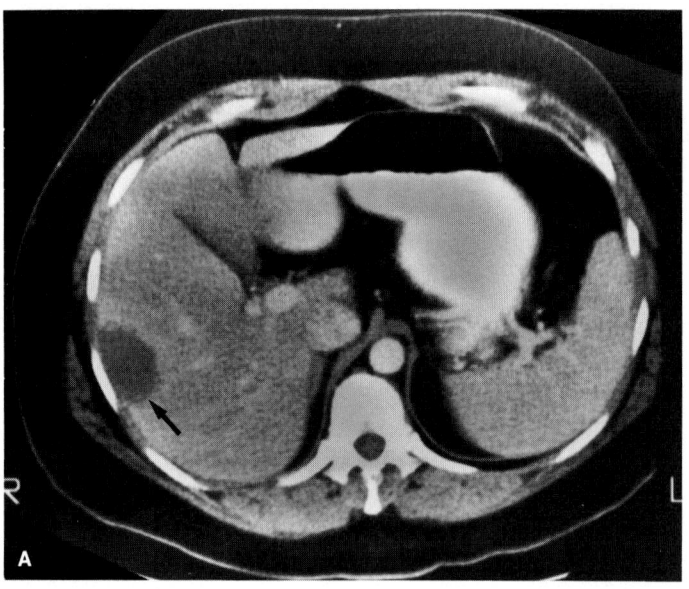
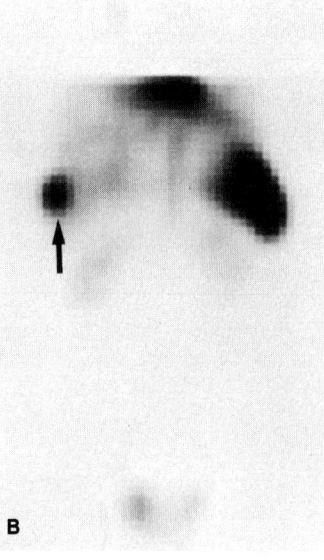

Figure 18-11 (**A**) CT evaluation of a patient with minimal symptoms demonstrates a 3- to 4-cm mass in the lateral aspect of the right lobe of the liver (*arrow*). The peripheral enhancement with contrast study suggests that this is a hemangioma. (**B**) A tagged red blood cell scan demonstrates enhancement of this lesion (*arrow*). The two tests confirm the diagnosis of hemangioma and obviate the need for arteriography. (Hanks JB, Arnold WS. Hepatic neoplasms. In: Greenfield LJ, Mulholland MW, Oldham KT, Zelenock GB, eds. Surgery: scientific principles and practice. Philadelphia, JB Lippincott, 1992:910)

to as infantile hemangioendothelioma and is a benign variant of the adult form. Despite its benign pathology, this tumor can have serious clinical consequences, such as arteriovenous shunting with resultant high-output congestive heart failure, hepatomegaly, and platelet consumption. When these complications develop, resection should be undertaken if possible. In unresectable cases, radiotherapy, selective embolization, or, occasionally, hepatic transplantation may be necessary (Fig. 18-12).

Pediatric Benign Liver Tumors

Primary liver tumors are the third largest category of solid tumors of the abdomen in children. More than half are malignant and carry an unfavorable prognosis. Benign pediatric liver tumors also can be associated with mortality, particularly infantile hemangioendothelioma, which causes high-output cardiac failure.

Hemangiomas

As in adults, hemangiomas are the most common benign liver tumors in children. In one series of 22 benign liver tumors accumulated over 25 years, 16 patients had hemangiomas.[84] Two types of hemangiomas occur in children: cavernous hemangiomas, which are small and usually cause no symptoms, and capillary

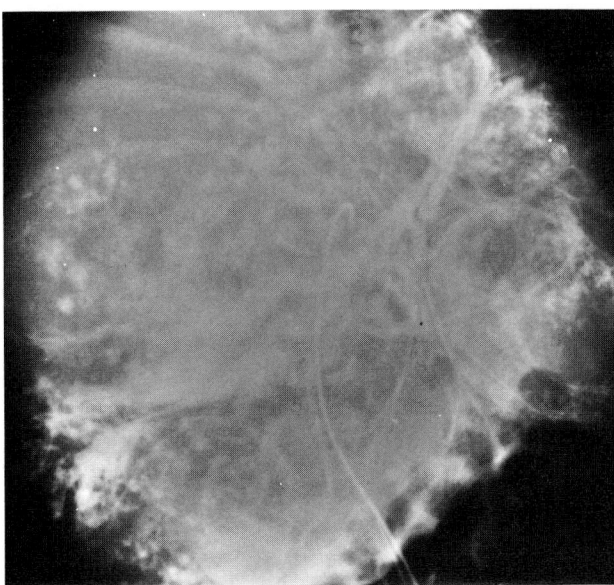

Figure 18-12 Infantile hemangioendothelioma of the liver. Arteriography in this infant demonstrates a highly vascular and extensive lesion. Transcatheter embolization techniques are gaining acceptance as treatment when resection is not possible.

hemangioendotheliomas, which are larger, more cellular, and can have hemodynamic consequences. These lesions can be associated with the triad of hepatomegaly, congestive heart failure, and cutaneous hemangiomas, especially in infants.[84] Platelet trapping within the lesions can result in thrombocytopenia and, rarely, congestive heart failure and consumptive coagulopathy (Kasabach-Merritt syndrome).

The diagnosis of hemangioendothelioma in infants and small children may be suggested by abdominal pain, hepatomegaly, and a right upper quadrant mass. Although arteriography has been the main diagnostic modality, newer imaging techniques include tagged red blood cell scanning and dynamic CT scanning. Doppler ultrasound also is helpful, both for diagnosis and for determination of intrahepatic shunts.

Despite a dramatic presentation, the natural history of infantile hemangioma is involution and disappearance by the age of 5 or 6 years. Rupture, bleeding, and infection are rare, and treatment is reserved for patients with symptoms. Coagulopathy is treated with steroids with or without radiation. Congestive heart failure is treated with diuretics and inotropic agents. If significant clinical symptoms develop, hepatic artery ligation, embolization, radiation, or cyclophosphamide can be considered. If the tumor is confined to a resectable part of the liver and clinical symptoms persist, resection should be performed.[85]

Hamartomas

Hamartomas are the second most common benign liver tumor in children. These lesions often present as large masses that can be either cystic or solid. The cysts contain clear or mucoid material and, in children, the diagnosis usually can be made with ultrasound. Solid hamartomas are difficult to distinguish with certainty from malignant tumors. These lesions can be associated with an increased α-fetoprotein level, further confusing the diagnosis.[84,86] Surgical resection often is necessary for solid lesions, particularly if malignancy is suspected. Large cystic hamartomas should be resected when they cause symptoms.

Childhood Fibropolycystic Disease

Fibropolycystic disease is considerably less common in children than are hemangiomas and hamartomas. Fibropolycystic disease is inherited as an autosomal recessive trait, and is categorized as perinatal, neonatal, or infantile.[87,88] The perinatal and neonatal forms of the condition demonstrate fibrocystic involvement of the liver and kidneys at birth and within the first few months of life, respectively. These patients have progressive renal failure and usually die within the first 12 to 18 months of life. The infantile form usually is detected at 6 to 8 months of age during an evaluation for renal failure. Treatment is directed primarily toward the renal failure. The liver component progresses to hepatic fibrosis with portal hypertension and hepatosplenomegaly by the age of 6 to 10 years, a process termed *congenital hepatic fibrosis.* Histology demonstrates abnormal interlobular bile ducts surrounded by fibrous bands of tissue separated from areas of normal parenchyma.

Renal failure is the predominant problem, and either dialysis or transplantation may be necessary. If portal hypertension and bleeding esophageal varices develop, endoscopic sclerotherapy or portal decompression should be considered. Hepatic transplantation may be required for patients with progressive hepatic failure.[36]

Miscellaneous Tumors

Other benign tumors of the liver are rare. One extensive review of the literature found two hepatic fibromas, four adipose tissue tumors, two leiomyomas, three benign mesotheliomas, three cases of heterotopia, eight benign teratomas, six mesenchymal hamartomas, and a single hepatic myxoma.[61]

REFERENCES

1. Little JM, Richardson A, Tait N. Hepatic dystychoma: a five year experience. HPB Surg 1991;4:291-F.
2. Cottone M, Marcelo MP, Maringhini A, et al. Ultrasound in the diagnosis of hepatocellular carcinoma associated with cirrhosis. Radiology 1993;147:517.
3. Katsuyoshi I, Kazumitsu H, Matsumoto T, et al. Distinction of hemangiomas from hepatic tumors with delayed enhancement by incremental dynamic CT. J Comput Assist Tomogr 1992;16:572.
4. Takayasu K, Muramatsu Y, Moriyama N, et al. Focal nodular hyperplasia of the liver: arterial angio-CT and microangiography. J Comput Assist Tomogr 1992;16:212.
5. Barnett PH, Zerhouni EA, White RI Jr, Siegelman SS. Computed tomography in the diagnosis of cavernous hemangioma of the liver. Am J Radiol 1980;134:439.
6. Itai Y, Araki T, Furui S, Tasaka A. Differential diagnosis of hepatic masses on computed tomography with particular reference to hepatocellular carcinoma. J Comput Assist Tomogr 1981;5:834.
7. Marchal GJ, Baert AL, Wilms GE. CT of non cystic liver lesions: bolus enhancement. Am J Radiol 1980;135:57.
8. Katz DE. Computerized tomography scanning of the normal liver. In: Williams RA, Nunnerly HB, eds. Imaging of the liver, pancreas and spleen. New York, Blackwell Scientific, 1990:25.
9. Karl RC, Morse SS, Halpert RD, Clark RA. Preoperative evaluation of patients for liver resection: appropriate CT imaging. Ann Surg 1993;217:226.
10. Clarke DP, Cosgrove DO, McCready VR. Radionuclide imaging for liver malignancy and its relationship to other hepatic investigation. Clin Oncol (R Coll Radiol) 1986;5:159.
11. Ackery DM, Batty VB. Radionuclide liver imaging. In: Williams RA, Nunnerly HB, eds. Imaging of the liver, pancreas and spleen. New York, Blackwell Scientific, 1990:31.
12. DeLand FH, Wagner HN. Nuclear medicine in hepatic mass lesions. Semin Roentgenol 1993;18:106.
13. Nunnerly HB. Angiography. In: Williams RA, Nunnerly HB, eds. Imaging of the liver, pancreas and spleen. New York, Blackwell Scientific, 1990:39.
14. Smith FW, Mallard JR, Reid A, Hutchison JMS. Nuclear magnetic imaging in liver disease. Lancet 1981;1:963.
15. Bydder GM. Magnetic resonance imaging. In: Williams RA, Nunnerly HB, eds. Imaging of the liver, pancreas and spleen. New York, Blackwell Scientific, 1990:49.
16. Ezacki T, Stansby GP, Hobbs KEF. Intraoperative ultrasonography imaging in liver surgery: a review. HPB Surg 1990;3:1.
17. Makuuchi M, Hasegawa H, Yamazaki S, et al. The use of operative ultrasound as an aid to liver resection in patients with hepatocellular carcinoma. World J Surg 1987;11:615.
18. Bismuth H, Castaing O, Garden OJ. The use of operative ultrasound in surgery of primary liver tumors. World J Surg 1987;11:610.
19. Clark MP, Kane RA, Steele G Jr, et al. Prospective comparison of preoperative imaging and intraoperative ultrasonography in the detection of liver tumors. Surgery 1989;106:849.
20. Sautereau O, Vire O, Cazes PY, et al. Value of sonographically guided fine needle aspiration biopsy in evaluating the liver with sonographic abnormalities. Gastroenterology 1987;93:715.
21. Conn HO. Rational use of liver biopsy in the diagnosis of hepatic cancer. Gastroenterology 1972;62:142.
22. Taavitsainen M, Airaksinen T, Kreula J, Paivansalo M. Fine needle aspiration biopsy of liver hemangioma. Acta Radiol 1990;31:69.
23. Nakaizumi A, Iishi H, Yamamoto R, et al. Diagnosis of hepatic cavernous hemangioma by fine needle aspiration biopsy under ultrasonic guidance. Gastrointest Radiol 1990;15:39.
24. Hanks JB, Arnold WS. Hepatic neoplasms. In: Greenfield LJ, ed. Surgery: scientific principles and practice. Philadelphia, JB Lippincott, 1992:908.
25. Herman RE. Liver cysts. In: Cameron JL, ed. Current surgical therapy. Philadelphia, BC Decker, 1984:156.
26. Hanks JB, Jones RS. Liver. In: Fromm D, ed. Gastrointestinal surgery. New York, Churchill Livingstone, 1985:813.
27. Doty JE, Tompkins RK. Management of cystic diseases of the liver. Surg Clin North Am 1989;69:285.

28. Hudson EK. Obstructive jaundice from solitary hepatic cysts. Am J Gastroenterol 1963;39:161.

29. Sood SC, Watson A. Solitary cyst of the liver presenting as an abdominal emergency. Postgrad Med J 1974;50:48.

30. Saini S, Mueller PR, Ferrucci JT Jr, et al. Percutaneous aspiration of hepatic cysts does not provide definitive therapy. Am J Roentgenol 1983;141:559.

31. Schwartz SI. Liver. In: Schwartz SI, Shires GT, Spencer FS, eds. Principles of surgery, ed 5. New York, McGraw-Hill, 1989.

32. Melnick PJ. Polycystic liver: analysis of 70 cases. Arch Pathol 1955;59:162.

33. Comfort MW, Gray HK, Dahlin DC, Whitesell FB. Polycystic disease of the liver: a study of 24 cases. Gastroenterology 1951;20:60.

34. Wittig JH, Burns R, Longmire WP. Jaundice associated with polycystic liver disease. Am J Surg 1978;136:383.

35. Que FG, Torres VE, Nagorney DM. Surgical resection and polycystic disease. Am J Surg 1993;165:745(A).

36. Madariaga JR, Iwatsuki S, Starzl TE, Todo S, Selby R, Zetti G. Hepatic resection for cystic lesions of the liver. Ann Surg 1993;218:610.

37. Williams JA, Price DE. Liver cysts in end-stage uremia due to polycystic kidney disease. Can Med Assoc J 1970;102:856.

38. Witzelben CL. Cystic disease of the liver. In: Zakim D, Boyer T, eds. Hepatology: a textbook of liver disease. Philadelphia, WB Saunders, 1990:1395.

39. Lewis JW, Koss N, Kerstein MD. A review of echinococcal disease. Ann Surg 1975;181:390.

40. Bartoloni C, Tricerri A, Guidi L, Gambassi G. The efficacy of chemotherapy with mebendazole in human cystic echinococcosis: long-term follow-up of 52 patients. Ann Trop Med Parasitol 1992;86:249.

41. Taylor DH, Morris DL, Richards KS. Perioperative prophylactic chemotherapy of echinococcus granulosus: determination of minimum effective length of albendazole therapy in in vitro proctoscolex culture. HPB Surg 1990;2:159.

42. Brough W, Hennessy O, Rickard MD, Lightowlers MW, Kune GA. Preoperative albendazole therapy for recurrent hydatid disease. Aust NZ J Surg 1989;59:665.

43. Sayek I, Yalin R, Sanac Y. Surgical treatment of hydatid disease of the liver. Arch Surg 1980;115:847.

44. Pitt HA, Korzelius J, Tompkins RK. Management of hepatic echinococcus in Southern California. Am J Surg 1986;152:110.

45. Bright J. Observations on jaundice: more particularly on that form of the disease which accompanies diffused inflammation of the liver. Guys Hosp Rep 1936;1:630.

46. Ochsner A, DeBakey M, Murray S. Pyogenic abscess of the liver. II. An analysis of forty-seven cases with review of the literature. Am J Surg 1938;40:292.

47. DeBakey ME, Jordan GL. Surgery of the liver. In: Schiff L, ed. Diseases of the liver, ed 4. Philadelphia, JB Lippincott, 1975:1103.

48. Kinney TD, Ferrebee JD. Hepatic abscess: factors determining its localization. Arch Pathol Lab Med 1948;45:51.

49. Pitt HA, Zuidema GD. Factors influencing mortality in the treatment of pyogenic hepatic abscess. Surg Gynecol Obstet 1975;140:228.

50. Shapiro M, Rachmilewitz D, Avinoah I, et al. Liver abscess at the Hadassah University Hospital during the years 1967-77. Isr J Med Sci 1980;16:761.

51. Balasegaram M. Management of hepatic abscess. Curr Probl Surg 1981;18:285.

52. McDonald AP, Howard RJ. Pyogenic liver abscess. World J Surg 1980;4:369.

53. McFadzean AJS, Chang KPA, Wong CC. Solitary pyogenic abscess of the liver treated by closed aspiration and antibiotics: a report of 14 consecutive cases with recovery. Br J Surg 1953;41:141.

54. Van Sonnenberg E, Ferrucci JT Jr, Mueller PR, et al. Percutaneous drainage of abscesses and fluid collections: technique, results, and applications. Radiology 1982;142:1.

55. Lambiase RE, Deyoe L, Cronan JJ, Dorfman GS. Percutaneous drainage of 335 consecutive abscesses: results of primary drainage with 1-year follow-up. Radiology 1992;184:167.

56. Do H, Lambiase RE, Deyoe L, Cronan JJ, Dorfman GS. Percutaneous drainage of hepatic abscesses: comparison of results in abscesses with and without intra-hepatic biliary drainage. AJR Am J Roentgenol 1991;157:1209.

57. Johnson RD, Mueller PR, Ferucci JT, et al. Percutaneous drainage of pyogenic liver abscesses. AJR Am J Roentgenol 1985;144:463.

58. Hemming AW, Scudamore CH, Davidson A, Ebb SR. Evaluation of 50 consecutive segmental hepatic resections. Am J Surg 1992;165:621.

59. Ochsner A, DeBakey M. Amebic hepatitis and hepatic abscess: an analysis of 181 cases with review of the literature. Surgery 1943;13:460.

60. Peters RS, Gitlin N, Libke RD. Amebic liver abscess. Annu Rev Med 1981;32:161.

61. Ishak KG, Rabin L. Benign tumors of the liver. Med Clin North Am 1975;59:995.

62. Jones RS. The liver. In: Moody FG, Carey LC, Jones RS, et al, eds. Surgical treatment of digestive disease. Chicago, Year Book, 1986:377.

63. Saul SH. Neoplasms of the liver. In: Sternberg SS, ed. Diagnostic surgical pathology. New York, Raven Press, 1989:1155.

64. Kew MC. Tumors of the liver. In: Zakim D, Boyer TD, eds. Hepatology: a textbook of liver disease. Philadelphia, WB Saunders, 1990:1206.

65. Edmondson HA, Reynolds TB, Henderson B, Benton B. Regression of liver cell adenomas associated with oral contraceptives. Ann Intern Med 1977;86:180.

66. Rooks JB, Ory HW, Ishak KG, et al. Epidemiology of hepatocellular adenoma. JAMA 1979;242:644.

67. Shortell CK, Schwartz SI. Hepatic adenoma and focal nodular hyperplasia. Surg Gynecol Obstet 1991;173:426.

68. Klatskin G. Hepatic tumors. Gastroenterology 1988;73: 386.

69. Kerlin P, Davis GL, McGill DB, et al. Hepatic adenoma and focal nodular hyperplasia: clinical, pathologic, and radiologic features. Gastroenterology 1983;84:994.

70. Cotran RS, Kumar V, Robbins SL. Liver and biliary tract. In: Robbins pathologic basis of disease, ed 4. Philadelphia, WB Saunders, 1989:911.

71. Nichols FC, vanHeerden JA, Weiland LH. Benign liver tumors. Surg Clin North Am 1989;69:297.

72. Welch TJ, Sheedy PJ, Johnson CM, et al. Focal nodular hyperplasia and hepatic adenoma: comparison of angiography, CT, ultrasound, and scintigraphy. Radiology 1985;156:593.

73. Clouse ME. Current diagnostic imaging modalities of the liver. Surg Clin North Am 1989;69:193.

74. Gonzalez F, Marks C. Hepatic tumors and oral contraceptives. J Surg Oncol 1985;29:193.

75. Leese T, Farges O, Bismuth H. Liver cell adenoma: a twelve year surgical experience from a specialist hepatobiliary unit. Ann Surg 1988;208:558.

76. Mathieu D, Bruneton JN, Drouillard J, et al. Hepatic adenoma and focal nodular hyperplasia: dynamic CT study. Radiology 1986;160:53.

77. Mathieu D, Zafrani ES, Anglade M-C, Dhumeaux D. Association of focal nodular hyperplasia and hepatic hemangioma. Gastroenterology 1989;97:154.

78. Trastek VG, van Heerden JA, Sheedy PF, et al. Cavernous hemangioma of the liver: resect or observe? Am J Surg 1983;145:49.

79. Freeny PC, Marks WM. Patterns of contrast enhancement of benign and malignant hepatic neoplasms during bolus dynamic and delayed CT. Radiology 1986;160:613.

80. Front D, Royal HD, Israel O, et al. Scintigraphy of hepatic hemangiomas: the value of TC-99m-labeled red blood cells: concise communication. J Nucl Med 1981;22:684.

81. Nelson RC, Chezmar JL. Diagnostic approach to hepatic hemangiomas. Radiology 1990;176:11.

82. Nishida O, Satoh N, Alam AS, Uchino J. The effect of hepatic artery ligation for unresectable cancerous hemangioma of the liver. Am Surg 1988;54:483.

83. Baer HU, Dennison AR, Mouton W, et al. Enucleation of giant hemangiomas of the liver: technical and pathologic aspects of a neglected procedure. Ann Surg 1992;216:673.

84. Luks FI, Yazbeckk S, Brandt ML, et al. Benign liver tumors in children: a 25 year experience. J Pediatr Surg 1991;26:1326.

85. Stanley P, Geer GD, Miller JH, et al. Infantile hepatic hemangiomas: clinical features, radiologic investigations, and treatment of 20 patients. Cancer 1989;64:936.

86. Ito H, Kiskikawa T, Toda T, et al. Hepatic mesenchymal hamartoma of an infant. J Pediatr Surg 1984;19:315.

87. Sherlock S. Diseases of the liver and biliary system, ed 6. Oxford, Blackwell Scientific, 1981:406.

88. Wright R, Alberti KGMM, Karhan S, Millword-Sapler GH. Liver and biliary disease. London, WB Saunders, 1979:950.

Digestive Tract Surgery: A Text and Atlas, edited by Richard H. Bell, Layton F. Rikkers, and Michael W. Mulholland. Lippincott-Raven Publishers, Philadelphia, © 1996.

19

Malignant Neoplasms of the Liver

Roger L. Jenkins

Malignant tumors of the liver may be categorized as either primary hepatic neoplasms arising from the various structural elements of the liver or secondary metastatic neoplasms arising from other body sites. The type of tumor most commonly seen by the practicing clinician depends in large part on geographic location. Metastatic lesions are more common in Western countries, whereas primary hepatic malignancies, specifically hepatocellular carcinoma (HCC), are more common in the Far East and Africa. The importance of primary liver malignancies is emphasized by the estimate that worldwide, as many as 1 million new cases occur each year.[1] Across the globe, one quarter of a million people die from HCC alone each year. Within the United States, where metastatic liver lesions predominate over primary hepatic malignancies, over 16,000 new primary tumors of the liver and biliary tree are diagnosed annually, accounting for more than 13,000 deaths per year.[2] In comparison, with an estimated 150,000 new cases of colon cancer being diagnosed annually in the United States, about 70,000 patients present with liver metastases annually. Less than 10% of this group with metastases confined to the liver makes up the potential pool of candidates for future surgical resection or ablation.[3]

Primary malignancies of the liver may arise from any cell type within the hepatic parenchyma and supporting tissues. The sheer mass of hepatocytes and biliary structures and the propensity for diseases to affect these two cell types make malignancies arising from hepatocytes and biliary epithelium the most common lesions encountered. Table 19-1 depicts the classification

scheme for the primary hepatic malignancies most commonly seen.

DIAGNOSTIC TECHNIQUES

With few exceptions, most primary liver malignancies have a low resectability rate and a correspondingly poor response to chemotherapy or radiation therapy. Since surgical resection remains the treatment of choice for early primary lesions, diagnosis in the earliest stages of the natural history of the disease becomes an important clinical concern. A carefully obtained history in conjunction with thoughtful attention to physical signs and symptoms form the foundation for any initial clinical evaluation. Combined with astute laboratory testing and logically orchestrated radiologic examination, the clinician should be able to establish the benign or malignant nature of most liver lesions efficiently and to plan an appropriate treatment strategy.

Laboratory Testing

Measurement of a variety of biochemical parameters plays an important role both in the assessment of patients presenting with a liver mass and in the surveillance of patients determined to be at high risk for the development of HCC. A patient with chronic liver disease who manifests sudden aberrations in liver function should be suspected of developing HCC. Similarly, the patient presenting with a recent diagnosis of a liver mass should have standard laboratory measurements of

623

Table 19-1   Classification of Hepatic Malignancies

EPITHELIAL
Biliary cystadenocarcinoma
Cholangiocarcinoma
Hepatoblastoma
Hepatocellular carcinoma

MESENCHYMAL
Angiosarcoma
Embryonal sarcoma
Epithelioid hemangioendothelioma
Fibrosarcoma
Leiomyosarcoma
Lymphoma
Malignant mesenchymoma
Rhabdomyosarcoma

liver function to screen for the presence of underlying parenchymal disease or to measure the degree of hepatic parenchymal compromise by an expanding mass.

Although not true assays of hepatic function, hepatocellular enzyme measurements (aspartate aminotransferase and alanine aminotransferase) should be obtained. Elevations in these enzymes imply ongoing hepatocellular destruction from an ischemic or hepatitic process, whereas an elevated alkaline phosphatase may indicate an element of biliary obstruction. Elevation of the serum bilirubin level in the absence of biliary obstruction suggests impairment of hepatic excretory capacity from an underlying acute or chronic liver disorder. Elevation of the prothrombin time uncorrected by parenteral vitamin K administration is an accurate indicator of hepatic synthetic compromise, whereas depression in the serum albumin level may reflect impaired synthesis, nutritional compromise, or septic stress. Thrombocytopenia and neutropenia may reflect the influence of hypersplenism associated with portal hypertension from cirrhosis or tumor-related portal vein obstruction.

Chromosomal dedifferentiation within tumor cells may be associated with the production of embryonic proteins by tumor cells. α-Fetoprotein (AFP) is a glycoprotein initially produced within fetal yolk sac, liver, and intestine, but its production is almost completely suppressed after birth, with normal values generally falling below 20 ng/mL. Elevation in the AFP level may be observed in patients with chronic hepatitis and cirrhosis, reflecting ongoing liver cell necrosis and regeneration, but the AFP level is rarely elevated above a level of 400 ng/mL in the absence of HCC or certain germ cell tumors.[4–6] There may be considerable fluctuation of the AFP level in patients with hepatitis, indi-

cating the importance of serial measurement. Exponential rises in AFP or absolute levels greater than 400 ng/mL are highly suggestive of the presence of HCC and indicate the need for aggressive radiologic investigation.

Although AFP is elevated greater than 20 ng/mL in 60% to 75% of patients with HCC, it is not specific for this disorder. Serum AFP can also be increased in patients with acute hepatitis as well as in those with chronic active hepatitis. Levels may also be modestly elevated in cirrhosis, in hemochromatosis without cirrhosis, and occasionally in metastatic liver disease of gastric, pancreatic, or lung origin.[7] The availability of AFP as a serologic marker for HCC provides the potential for mass screening of populations at risk in an effort to improve early detection. In combination with ultrasonography, sequential AFP measurements contribute to increased rates of resection and improved survival.[8–13] The positive predictive value of an elevated AFP is greatest in patients with chronic type B hepatitis. In 1986, a National Institutes of Health consensus conference recommended that patients who are hepatitis B surface antigen (HBsAg) positive and have chronic hepatitis or cirrhosis should be screened at 3- to 4-month intervals with AFP determinations and every 4 to 6 months with hepatic ultrasonography.[14] HBsAg carriers without liver disease can be screened less frequently. Such an approach appears to have contributed to a decrease in tumor size at the time of detection and improved resectability and patient survival rate during a 20-year period in China.[15]

Although not yet receiving widespread recognition, the measurement of abnormal prothrombin complexes called des-γ-carboxy prothrombin has been found to be more specific for HCC than AFP. The combination of des-γ-carboxy prothrombin and AFP measurements may further increase the sensitivity and specificity in detection of HCC.[16] Carcinoembryonic antigen (CEA) is another useful serologic marker that may be elevated in a variety of digestive tract malignancies, particularly in colorectal carcinoma. Because CEA is usually not elevated in HCC, an increased level in a patient with a newly discovered liver lesion suggests metastatic malignancy.

Radiologic Techniques

The widespread application of refined techniques of abdominal imaging has contributed to the increased detection of both benign and malignant tumors of the liver that previously went undiscovered or were detected only when associated with clinical symptoms. When employed strategically in conjunction with a knowledge of the pertinent medical history of the patient, radiographic studies of the liver can usually suggest appropriate diagnostic possibilities without requiring percutaneous biopsy techniques. As depicted in Figure 19-1, the diagnostic evaluation of the patient at high risk for HCC because of associated diseases or positive serologic studies can often be abbreviated, with diagnostic studies focused toward assessing for cirrhosis and intrahepatic tumor spread.

Plain films of the abdomen have a minimal role in the radiologic evaluation of most patients with a suspected liver malignancy, although hepatomegaly may be suggested by displacement of surrounding structures. Similarly, diaphragmatic elevation on chest radiography can be seen with large liver tumors. The lack of disease specificity and the restricted resolution of the various radionuclide scanning techniques have limited the utility of these methods of diagnostic imaging. Blood pool scanning with technetium-99m–labeled erythrocytes is the simplest modality for the positive diagnosis of cavernous hemangiomas of the liver.[17]

Ultrasonography

Ultrasonography with Doppler flow imaging is the key diagnostic modality for the hepatobiliary clinician. Its accuracy is dependent on the skills of the technician performing the examination and the radiologist interpreting it. Internal echogenic characteristics of the liver can imply the presence of cirrhosis or fatty change. Changes attributable to portal hypertension, such as splenomegaly, perigastric varices, flow reversal in the portal vein, and ascites, support the presence of chronic liver disease. Estimating the size of a lesion and determining whether it is solid or cystic are important considerations in planning further diagnostic studies. The echogenic properties of a space-occupying lesion can often suggest a particular diagnosis, although both benign and malignant lesions, as well as primary and metastatic malignancies, manifest considerable overlap in transmission characteristics. Although the echo pattern for a particular hepatic tumor varies with tumor histology and the characteristics of the surrounding hepatic parenchyma, small HCCs are initially relatively hypoechoic as compared with metastatic lesions, which tend to be isoechoic or hyperechoic. With continued growth, internal echoes may become more isoechoic or hyperechoic.[8,18] The presence of a fibrous capsule may be detected as a hypoechoic rim, whereas fibrous septa are often displayed as irregular linear structures. The presence of such encapsulation is characteristic of better differentiated, slow-growing, less invasive tumors.[19,20] A carefully performed ultrasound examination has the advantage of being able to detect major portal or hepatic vein tumor involvement. Visualization of the

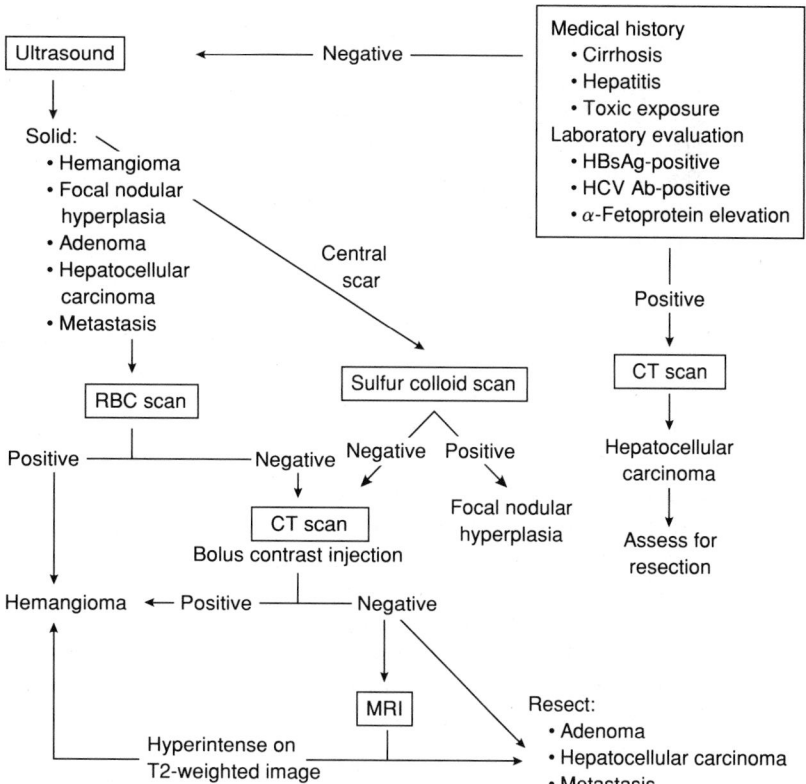

Figure 19-1 Algorithm for the radiologic evaluation of a patient with a suspected liver tumor.

proximity of the lesion to venous outflow structures and hilar inflow structures is vital for the determination of resectability. Portal occlusion by intraluminal tumor extension eventually results in a picture of cavernous transformation as hilar venous collaterals enlarge in a compensatory fashion.[21]

The entire liver should be scanned in an organized fashion to rule out the possibility of multiple lesions. Cavernous hemangioma is the most common solid benign tumor of the liver, occurring in up to 7% of patients in some autopsy series. It represents the most common differential diagnostic entity, usually appearing as a well-circumscribed echogenic mass.[22,23] The presence of multiple lesions within the liver suggests metastatic disease rather than a primary neoplasm. In general, a nodule visualized within a cirrhotic liver represents HCC until proved otherwise. Despite its inability to convey a contiguous pictorial view of hepatic anatomy and pathology, ultrasonography still represents one of the most sensitive radiologic diagnostic modalities.[24]

Intraoperative ultrasonography (IOUS) has been validated as an important tool for the more accurate assessment of disease extent as well as for delineation of precise anatomic resection strategy.[25] Offering a sensitivity greater than that of preoperative ultrasonography, computed tomography (CT), or angiography in the detection of hepatic lesions, IOUS is capable of locating tumor nodules unsuspected during initial staging and provides definition of tumor proximity to major portal and hepatic venous structures.[26] IOUS plays an increasingly important role in the aggressive management of both primary and metastatic liver malignancies. When performed at the time of initial laparotomy, it offers the best available technique for defining resectability. Although recent technical developments have led to the development of ultrasound probes that can be introduced through laparoscopic trocars, accurate scanning of the entire liver has been difficult, and the technique cannot yet be recommended as a reliable alternative to open ultrasonography.

Computed Tomography

Although CT is no more accurate than ultrasonography, it has the advantages of operator independence and reproducibility as well as the ability to portray the relation of the liver and its disease processes to the surrounding anatomic structures. CT scanning usually plays a significant early role in defining operability and in planning surgical strategy based on anatomic structure. CT with and without intravenous contrast is important in the evaluation of solid liver masses because diagnostic clues can be obtained from the timing and volume of contrast uptake by the lesion. Early tumor enhancement after intravenous administration of contrast suggests tumor hypervascularity. Tumors with more fibrous tissue, a large extravascular space, and a scanty blood supply may demonstrate a delayed and prolonged enhancement. Thus, both early and late enhanced scans are important in assessing tumor characteristics. Although cavernous hemangiomas usually exhibit delayed uptake of contrast with irregular pooling and a lobulated appearance, HCCs often exhibit earlier uptake of contrast only to become isodense with surrounding liver in later phases of the study. Rapid bolus intravenous contrast techniques produce an enhancement of well-vascularized tumors as well as the surrounding venous anatomic structures. The presence of portal tumor thrombus is often suggested by the presence of decreased attenuation of an entire hepatic lobe.

Although standard hepatic arterial or portal angiography historically figured prominently in the evaluation of liver tumors, these techniques are rarely essential components in the diagnostic work-up today. The direct infusion of contrast into a catheter selectively placed in the celiac axis or superior mesenteric artery provides good definition of vascular structures but has the associated disadvantages of the need for arterial puncture and selective catheterization. CT arterial portography is considered to be one of the more sensitive preoperative imaging techniques for liver tumors, especially when they are less than 2 cm in diameter.[27] Despite the reported sensitivity of this technique, about 20% of lesions diagnosed at surgery with IOUS are not detected preoperatively with CT arterial portography.[28] False-positive findings attributable to the presence of benign lesions or variations in portal perfusion are not uncommon.[29,30] Thus, high sensitivity of CT arterial portography is accompanied by a lack of specificity. A modification of this technique using the selective infusion of iodized oil (Lipiodol) through a hepatic artery catheter followed by delayed CT scanning may improve sensitivity in the detection of HCCs smaller than 2 cm in high-risk patients.[31] Lipiodol is an iodized oil contrast that is actively taken up by hepatic tumor cells when injected into the hepatic artery. This oily contrast persists for weeks to months within the involved hepatic parenchyma before clearance.[32] With the ability to identify lesions as small as 3 mm, it is possible to visualize up to half of small (5- to 10-mm) tumor nodules not discernible with other radiographic imaging techniques.[33] Thus, Lipiodol CT is perhaps the most sensitive of all imaging modalities for the diagnosis of small HCCs. It may play a particularly useful role in the cirrhotic patient with a rising AFP in the absence of a visible lesion on ultrasound scan. Its limitations are related to the need for invasive arterial catheterization and the degree of vascularity of the lesion. Not unexpectedly, small hemangiomas may enhance with this technique and represent a significant source of false-positive findings.

Magnetic Resonance Imaging

Magnetic resonance imaging (MRI) continues to evolve with respect to its role in the evaluation of hepatic tumors and their anatomic relation to surrounding vascular structures. In terms of diagnostic sensitivity, MRI confers little benefit over CT scanning. HCC usually is of higher intensity than the surrounding parenchyma on T2-weighted images and of a lower intensity on T1-weighted images. The presence of a capsule surrounding HCC can be demonstrated in conventional T1- and T2-weighted images as low-density rings. MRI may be diagnostic of a small cavernous hemangioma when red cell–tagged scan or CT scan are nondiagnostic. Hemangiomas have higher T2-weighted values than HCCs, although a few values overlap.[34] It is useful to add MRI with angiographic sequences to the preoperative evaluation when a lesion is centrally located or resides near hepatic venous outflow structures that must be preserved during a planned resection[35] (Fig. 19-2).

Percutaneous Liver Biopsy

The role of liver biopsy in the evaluation of liver tumors should be limited to situations in which the result would change treatment strategy. The ease with which core or aspiration biopsy can be accomplished probably leads to an overuse of this diagnostic modality. Blind or ultrasound-directed percutaneous biopsy plays its major role in the histologic confirmation of malignancy in a patient in whom nonsurgical therapies are under consideration. Such would be the case in patients with suspected coexisting cirrhosis or in patients with prior history of noncolorectal malignancy when histologic confirmation of metastatic disease would mitigate against the need for surgical resection. Patients who are candidates for resection and who have an anatomically resectable lesion are unlikely to benefit from preoperative biopsy. Less than 10% of patients presenting with liver tumors to our hepatobiliary surgery division undergo biopsy. The diagnostic value of aspiration cytology and core biopsy are limited in the presence of well-differentiated HCC when it may be impossible to accurately distinguish normal hepatocytes from HCC or hepatic adenoma. Reliance on biopsy to determine the need for surgical intervention should be discouraged when HCC is suspected clinically. Although standard core biopsy carries the potential for significant hemorrhage from well-vascularized tumors located on the surface of the liver, the technique of fine-needle aspiration can usually be accomplished with relative safety.[36]

HEPATOCELLULAR CARCINOMA

Epidemiology

Although HCC represents one of the most common malignancies that afflicts the human race, epidemiologic investigations give tantalizing clues to its pathogenesis and suggest prospects for earlier intervention and future prevention. Though regarded as rare in Western

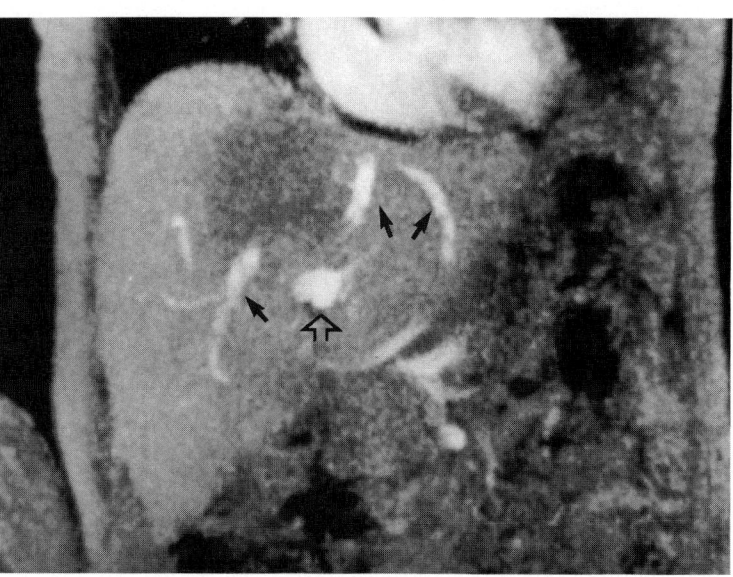

Figure 19-2 T2-weighted MR coronal sectional image demonstrating the relation of the portal vein (*open arrow*) and hepatic veins (*solid arrow*) to a metastatic liver tumor.

medicine, HCC is actually one of the most common tumors in the world, representing the seventh most common cancer in men and the ninth in women.[37] Its incidence varies considerably with geographic regions, presumably because of differences in the major causative factors and their local frequencies. The incidence is low among whites in the United States, Great Britain, and Australia, but the incidence is remarkably high among blacks in Mozambique and sub-Saharan Africa as well as in the Far East. Based on the observed incidence rates, countries may be divided into high-incidence populations (more than 20 cases per 100,000 people per year), intermediate-incidence populations (5 to 20 cases), and low-incidence populations[38] (fewer than 5 cases; Table 19-2). Incidence rates may vary between ethnic groups within the same city or region as a result of differing cultural habits.

Within the United States, the estimated number of new cases of carcinoma of the liver and biliary tract was about 16,000 cases (1.03% of all cancers) for 1994, accounting for almost 13,000 deaths (2% of all cancer deaths).[2] Disappointingly, primary hepatic malignancies are also associated with one of the lowest 5-year survival rates (6% for 1983 through 1989) of any cancer within the United States. Although the 1- to 4-year survival rates have demonstrated improvement since 1973, 5-year survival rates are unchanged from prior decades.[39]

HCC occurs in men five times more often than in women. This ratio is highest in those regions of the world where HCC is more common and considerably lower in regions where the tumor is uncommon. This enhanced susceptibility of men may be related to hormonal factors, genetic predisposition, or carcinogenic environmental exposure.[40] Similarly, in populations with a high incidence of HCC, the tumor tends to occur in younger patients in the third to fifth decade. By contrast, in North America and Europe, the peak incidence tends to be in the fifth and sixth decades. These findings suggest that risk factors for HCC are present at earlier ages or that their carcinogenic effects are more rapid.[41] The observed variations in male to female susceptibility are less evident in younger age groups, in which the frequency of underlying cirrhosis is typically much lower. Although HCC can occur in childhood and adolescence, primary liver cancer in the young is often of the fibrolamellar variant, and children younger than 5 years are more likely to be afflicted with hepatoblastoma.

Most patients with HCC have preexisting cirrhosis. Regardless of cause, cirrhosis appears to be a strong risk factor for the tumor, with 6% to 40% of cirrhotic patients harboring foci of HCC at autopsy.[42,43] Cirrhosis carries a 3-year cumulative HCC risk of 12.5% as compared with 3.8% for chronic hepatitis without cirrhosis. The HBsAg-positive state has been associated with a 7- to 28-fold increased HCC risk as compared with HBsAg negativity.[44–47] A study from Taiwan reported a 1000-fold increase in the annual incidence of HCC in HBsAg-positive patients with cirrhosis as compared with the HBsAg-negative noncirrhotic control group.[48] Hepatitis C is also a risk factor for HCC; anti-HCV positivity carries a four-fold increased HCC risk as compared with anti-HCV negativity.[49] The prevalence of cirrhosis in patients with HCC is about 80% to 90% in most countries. Posthepatitic cirrhosis is more frequently associated with HCC than micronodular cirrhosis secondary

Table 19-2 Correlation Between Prevalence of Primary Liver Cancer (Mortality) and HBsAg Carrier Rate

Country	Primary Liver Cancer Mortality Rate (per 100,000 per Year)	HBsAg Carrier Rate (% of Population)
HIGH-INCIDENCE AREAS		
Mozambique	98.2	14
South Africa (blacks)	22	9
China	17	7.5–14
INTERMEDIATE-INCIDENCE AREAS		
India	—	2.5
Japan	15	2.6
Greece	12	5
LOW-INCIDENCE AREAS		
United States	2.7–4.7	0.2
Scandinavia	2.1–3.5	0.1
Central Europe and United Kingdom	1–7	0.25

(Hadziyannis SJ. Hepatocellular carcinoma and type B hepatitis. Clin Gastroenterol 1980;9:117)

to alcohol. Studies from Japan established that cirrhotic livers with large nodules are more commonly associated with HCC than livers with small nodules.[50,51] The larger nodules may reflect greater regenerative activity with more frequent rearrangements of DNA sequences within the chromosomes. Interestingly, it has been reported that abstinence from alcohol in the presence of established cirrhosis has been associated with an increased risk of HCC.[52] Theoretically, abstinence is associated with an escalation of hepatic regenerative activity, leading to the transformation of small nodules to larger ones, thereby enhancing the potential for malignant change.

Etiology

Hepatocellular carcinoma is associated with a number of clinical disorders and toxic exposures:

CLINICAL DISORDERS
Hepatitis B
Hepatitis C
Alcoholic cirrhosis
Hemochromatosis
α_1-Antitrypsin deficiency
Hereditary tyrosinemia
Budd-Chiari syndrome
Porphyria cutanea tarda
TOXIC EXPOSURES
Aflatoxins
Oral contraceptives
Androgens
Thorotrast

The fact that such a large number of factors have been linked to HCC supports a multifactorial carcinogenic process. The geographic variation in prevalence of HCC correlates with differences in incidence of factors such as hepatitis B virus (HBV), hepatitis C virus (HCV), alcohol intake, and environmental agents. There is a particularly strong correlation between incidence of HCC and prevalence of HBV and HCV. In China and most of Southeast Asia, nearly 100% of adults have serologic evidence of HBV infection, and 10% to 15% are chronic HBsAg carriers.[14]

Hepatitis B Virus

The relation between HBV and the subsequent development of HCC was first noted in 1970.[53] In addition to the epidemiologic evidence linking HBV and HCC, a number of studies have demonstrated that components of the virus can be found within tumor tissue. Hepatitis B viral DNA has been found integrated within the chromosomal DNA of tumor cells, even in patients found to be HBsAg negative with detectable titers of anti-HBsAg.[54-57] The integration of hepatitis B DNA apparently occurs randomly within the genome of the hepatocyte during the course of viral replication. Hepatitis B viral DNA can also be found integrated within the genome of nonneoplastic hepatocytes adjacent to HCC, although the pattern of integration may differ.[58] The integrated HBV DNA may be translated and transcribed along with native DNA, suggesting a carcinogenic role for the virus.[59] As many as one third of HCCs may contain HBsAg detectable by immunohistochemical staining.[60]

Because less than 20% of patients with HCC are candidates for surgical resection, the role for hepatitis B prevention through immunization and the treatment of chronic liver disorders before the development of cirrhosis are critical components of any global treatment plan aimed at reducing mortality figures.

Hepatitis C Virus

In the late 1970s, suspicion of an HCC causative agent other than HBV was supported by the observation in Japan that an increasing number of HBsAg-negative patients who had received blood transfusions developed HCC.[61] It was also observed that the relative proportion of HBsAg-positive cases among all patients with HCC was steadily declining, with increasing numbers of HBV-unrelated cases despite a relatively constant number of HBV-associated cases.[62] Among HBsAg-negative HCC patients, the highest prevalence of HCV antibody positivity is found in Japan, followed by Africa, Italy, France, and China. A lower rate of anti-HCV prevalence is reported for HCC patients from the United States, Switzerland, Austria, and Hong Kong.

Since the hepatitis C virus is an RNA virus, reverse transcription into host DNA would be necessary for an oncogenic potential on the basis of host genome integration. As an etiologic factor in the development of cirrhosis, hepatitis C may promote oncogenesis simply through an associated increase in hepatocyte regeneration and DNA replication. Whatever the mechanism, HCV as a causative factor for HCC appears to be more important than HBV in some countries.[63-66]

Chemical Carcinogens

Vinyl chloride is a halogenated aliphatic hydrocarbon with extensive industrial use that is both hepatotoxic and carcinogenic. Vinyl chloride and related monomers have been most commonly associated with the development of hepatic angiosarcomas but may also be involved in the development of HCC and cholangiocarcinoma.[67]

AFLATOXIN. Aflatoxins are produced by the fungal agents *Aspergillus flavus* and *Aspergillus parasiticus*. The most studied natural carcinogen, aflatoxin B1, is found in a variety of stored grains in hot and humid environments in parts of Africa and China.[68] Aflatoxin contamination of food grains correlates highly with the incidence of HCC in these regions. Aflatoxin may act as a cocarcinogen in concert with HBV or may increase the hepatitis B carrier rate through suppression of the cellular immune response.

STEROIDS. Several studies have shown a relation between the development of hepatic adenomas and the use of oral contraceptives.[69,70] As many as 10% of these lesions are found to be well-differentiated HCCs on histologic examination. The risk of developing hepatic neoplasms secondary to use of androgenic steroids has not been carefully quantified. The magnitude of risk probably relates to the type of anabolic steroid, the dose, and the duration of therapy. These agents may also be associated with other hepatotoxic conditions.

ALCOHOL. The exact etiologic role of ethanol ingestion in the development of HCC remains controversial. Ethanol causes cirrhosis, which is itself a premalignant state. Ethanol is also known to induce the cytochrome P-450–dependent microsomal biotransformation system and interferes with at least one DNA repair mechanism.[71] Other hypotheses regarding the mechanism for ethanol cocarcinogenesis include enhanced solubilization of separately ingested carcinogens, the induction of nutritional deficiencies, and T-cell suppression.[72-74]

Prospective studies suggest that the incidence of HCC in patients with alcoholic cirrhosis is much lower than in HBsAg-positive patients or patients with hemochromatosis and is comparable to that seen in patients with primary biliary cirrhosis.[75] Ethanol abuse may promote the development of cirrhosis and HCC in HBsAg chronic carriers.

An increased prevalence of anti-HCV antibodies has been described in patients with alcoholic cirrhosis and in chronic alcoholics with HCC.[76,77] One study found that 30% to 50% of patients with alcoholic cirrhosis were positive for the anti-C100 antibody, whereas over 70% of drinkers with non–HBsAg-associated HCC were positive for this antibody. In comparison, only 5% of hospitalized alcoholic patients without liver disease were found to be antibody positive.[78,79]

Pathology

The gross appearance of HCC varies considerably depending on the presence or absence of underlying cirrhosis, encapsulation, degree of fibrosis, and pattern of growth. Indeed, HCC may be difficult to differentiate from regenerative nodules in patients with macronodular cirrhosis. Nonneoplastic liver tissue in proximity to HCC may show varying degrees of liver cell dysplasia, especially in hepatitis B carriers. This hepatocytic dysplasia is characterized by nuclear and cellular enlargement, nuclear pleomorphism, multinucleation, and increased nuclear staining. The histology of HCC may have varying trabecular arrangements of hepatocytes and scanty connective tissue stroma (except for the fibrolamellar variant discussed later; Fig. 19-3). Histologic variants of HCC include trabecular, pseudoglandular, multinucleated giant cell, clear cell, scirrhous, sarcomatous, and fibrolamellar forms with varying degrees of cellular differentiation. Well-differentiated forms of HCC may be indistinguishable from normal hepatocytes, and the determination of the hepatocellular origin of a less well-differentiated hepatic tumor may require stains for α_1-antitrypsin or AFP. The variable patterns of growth likely contribute to the differences in the natural history of HCC in various parts of the world and possibly influence the potential for successful surgical resection. Although invasive, nonencapsulated tumors are more common in North American patients, expanding, encapsulated tumors are more frequently reported in Asian and certain European populations.[19,20,80,81] Such territorial variations in tumor growth suggest that resection rates and curability may be influenced by a variety of biologic factors.

Although a multifocal origin of HCC is suggested in patients with underlying cirrhosis, local vascular invasion undoubtedly accounts for many of the cases of diffuse or nodular intrahepatic spread. The tendency of the tumor to spread microscopically along sinusoidal spaces into small hepatic venules is mirrored by its occasional clinical presentation with macroscopic extension into the portal vein or inferior vena cava. Spread may also occur through arteries, lymphatics, and biliary radicals. Lymphatic spread is most commonly to nodes in the hepatic hilum and periaortic and retroperitoneal regions, whereas extrahepatic dissemination is most often to lungs, adrenal gland, and bone.

Clinical Features

Since HCC is usually a slowly growing and asymptomatic tumor in a patient with cirrhosis, initial signs and symptoms are often those related to progression or exacerbation of the underlying liver disease. In recent years, with a more intense focus on screening high-risk patients with ultrasonography and AFP measurements, HCC is being found more often in earlier stages, providing the opportunity for more successful treatment. Most patients, however, continue to present with symp-

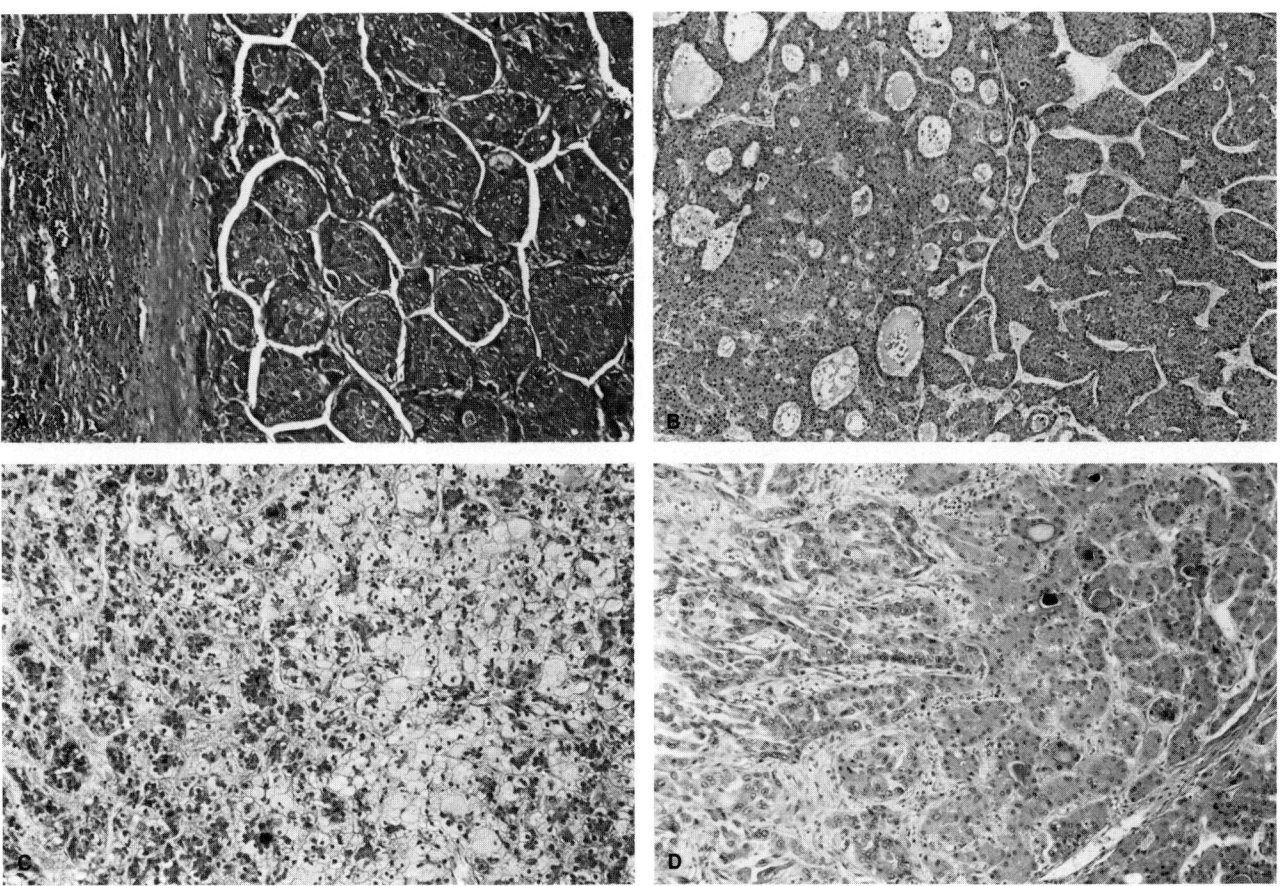

Figure 19-3 Hepatocellular carcinoma. (**A**) Trabecular arrangement with fibrotic capsule. (**B**) Pseudoglandular pattern. (**C**) Clear cell type predominating. (**D**) Infiltration with increased reticular tissue. Cholestasis is evident in neighboring nonneoplastic parenchyma. (See Color Fig. 19-3.)

toms related to hepatic decompensation or direct effects of the enlarging tumor. The duration of symptoms before diagnosis is relatively short and averages 6 weeks in most regions of the world. In reported series, abdominal or shoulder pain represents the most common complaint for 40% to 90% of patients, followed by malaise, abdominal mass or distention, anorexia, weight loss, ascites, fever, nausea or vomiting, and jaundice.[82–88] In countries where HCC is common, presentation as an acute abdominal catastrophe from rupture and hemorrhage may be the first sign of disease and represents the most common cause of nontraumatic hemoperitoneum in men[89] (Fig. 19-4). In up to 30% of cases, the early recognition of the diagnosis is confounded by unusual clinical presentations. Symptoms in these patients may include cholecystitis-like syndromes, progressive hepatic failure, respiratory insufficiency from pulmonary metastases, pathologic fractures from painful bony metastases, fever of unknown origin, or obstructive jaundice. The most common physical sign is hepatomegaly, evident in up to 70% to 90% of patients and frequently

painful. More advanced disease is suggested by the findings of ascites (frequently bloody), splenomegaly, jaundice due to central ductal obstruction or hemobilia, dilated abdominal wall veins, and variceal bleeding. An arterial bruit may be audible over the liver in patients with well-vascularized lesions. The onset of ascites or variceal hemorrhage may reflect either progression of the underlying cirrhosis or tumor invasion of hepatic or portal veins[90,91] (Fig. 19-5).

A variety of paraneoplastic syndromes, including erythrocytosis, hypercalcemia, hypoglycemia, dysfibrinogenemia, porphyria cutanea tarda, and hypertrophic osteoarthropathy, have also been described in association with HCC.[92] The sudden onset of one of these syndromes in a cirrhotic patient should prompt a thorough investigation for HCC.

Detection and Diagnostic Evaluation

Advances in therapy for patients with small HCCs have made early diagnosis important. In China, AFP measurements in endemic regions have led to early detec-

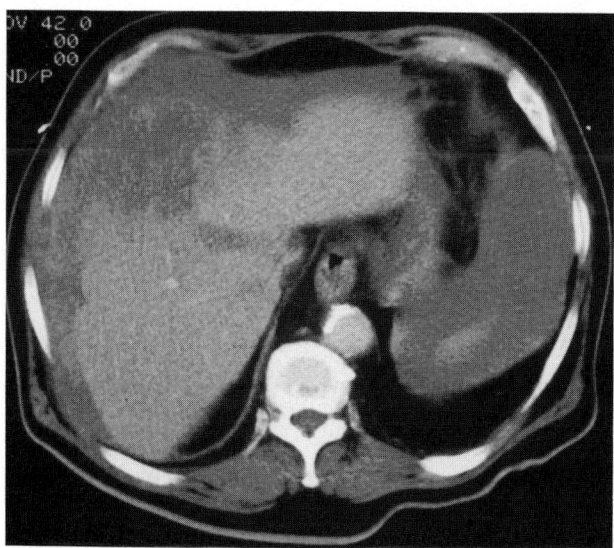

Figure 19-4 CT scan of an 80-year-old man with hemorrhagic rupture of a previously asymptomatic hepatocellular carcinoma who presented with acute abdominal pain and hypotension. Bleeding ceased after palliative hepatic artery embolization.

tion of asymptomatic HCCs, many of which could be successful resected.[15] AFP measurements alone, however, have not significantly increased detection of early, resectable lesions in other regions, probably because most small HCCs are not associated with elevation of AFP.[24,40] Strategies recommended for the surveillance of patients with cirrhosis and advanced chronic hepatitis use abdominal ultrasonography in 3- to 4-month intervals in conjunction with AFP measurements.[93] The recommended interval is based on the observation that HCCs generally require 3 months to increase in size by 1 cm.[8,94]

The work-up of the patient who presents with a liver mass needs to take into account pertinent medical history, the presence of risk factors for a primary hepatic malignancy, and the degree of hepatic reserve remaining. For example, the presence of a breast mass or of guaiac-positive stools or the history of a prior malignancy should focus the clinician on a search for a metastatic disease process. In contrast, a cirrhotic patient with an elevated AFP level should undergo a more focused search for the presence of HCC. A patient with an extensive tumor and signs of advanced liver disease needs an abbreviated evaluation with an emphasis on palliative treatment. Conversely, the patient with an early tumor and excellent functional capacity should be considered a candidate for more precise diagnosis and aggressive surgical intervention.

Treatment

In assessing both the treatment options and the results of treatment of HCC, it is important to take into account the natural history of the disease. The geographic vari-

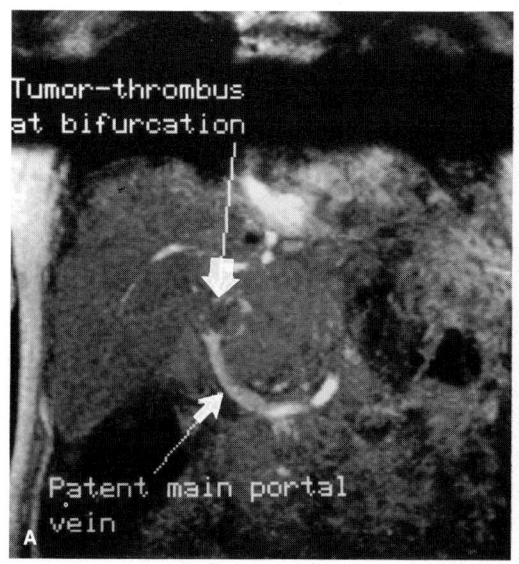
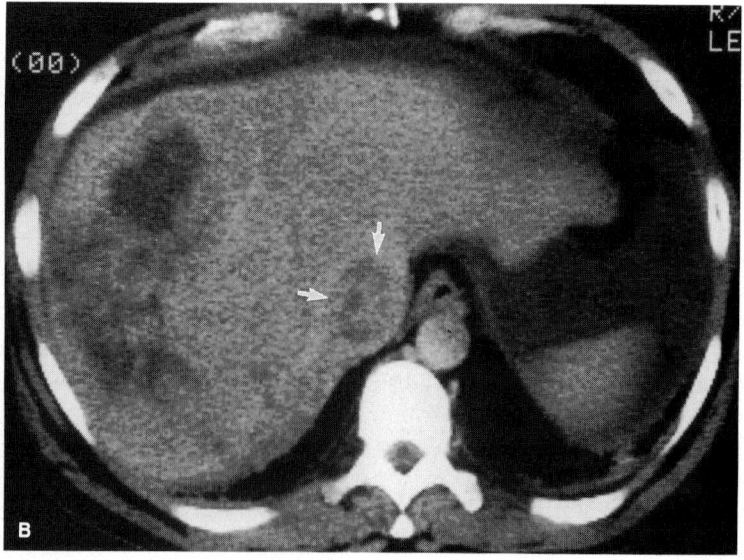

Figure 19-5 (A) MRI demonstrating hepatocellular carcinoma tumor thrombus at portal bifurcation (*large arrow*). Main trunk of portal vein remains patent (*small arrow*). (B) CT scan of a patient who presented with acute Budd-Chiari syndrome. A large hepatocellular carcinoma is present in right lobe of liver with extension through right hepatic vein into vena cava (*arrows*) and atrium.

ations in histologic presentation contribute to considerable heterogeneity in the natural history of HCC. The lower frequency of unifocal, encapsulated, expanding tumors in North American patients in comparison with Asian and southern European patients undoubtedly influences the reported natural history of disease progression and rates of surgical resection. In African patients with HCC, cirrhosis is less common, and tumors generally present at a much larger size with a resultant shortening of the median survival time than is typically seen in Asian populations. HCCs associated with cirrhosis typically have slower growth rates than adenocarcinomas in other sites. Indeed, it has been argued that survival time in cirrhotic patients with HCC is essentially the same with or without resection when similar patient populations are compared. In one investigation,[95] only 12 of 37 asymptomatic Child's class A cirrhotic patients with HCC underwent resection, and 25 patients were not surgically treated because of age or patient refusal. The 2-year survival rate was 39% in the resected group and 50% in the untreated group. Patterns of growth were variable when monitored at 3-month intervals with ultrasonography but generally portrayed significant periods of absent tumor enlargement before or after variable growth spurts. Serial ultrasound examinations performed in patients with established cirrhosis in Taiwan revealed a median doubling time of 4 months, ranging from 1 to 14 months.[96] This suggests that, at least in cirrhotic patients, HCC may be present for several years before becoming detectable or clinically apparent. The diversity in growth rates exhibited by individual tumors is considerable, however, and defines the limits of current surveillance schemes.

Despite the potential for slow tumor growth, most patients with HCC have a poor prognosis, with death resulting from intrahepatic tumor extension or hepatic failure as a result of progressive cirrhosis. The median survival time of patients with symptomatic but untreatable HCC is generally 3 to 4 months. The overall prognosis is dependent on tumor size, tumor growth rate, functional hepatic reserve, and the presence or absence of extrahepatic spread. Staging schemes employed to evaluate disease progression vary and prevent direct comparative studies because of the major influence of coexisting cirrhosis. The influence of underlying liver impairment can be seen when survival of untreated patients with cirrhosis is analyzed by Child's classification. One study reported a median survival of 12 months for 21 patients with Child's class A disease, 6 months for 29 patients with Child's class B disease, and 3 months for 69 patients with Child's class C disease.[97]

In a Japanese series,[98] 850 patients were divided into three stages based on a scoring scheme that included tumor size (assessed as percentage of liver size),

serum albumin level, serum bilirubin level, and the presence or absence of ascites. Surgical exploration was carried out on 157 patients (18.4%). For the untreated patients, median survival rates were 8.3 months for stage I, 2 months for stage II, and 0.7 months for stage III (Fig. 19-6). By comparison, median survival of stage I patients undergoing resection was 25.6 months, whereas those explored but not resected had a median survival of 9.4 months. Stage II patients had a median survival of 12.2 months after resection, but median survival in unresected patients was only 3.5 months. Of note was the observation that 3-year survival was 50% in patients undergoing resection for HCC that was less than 25% of the liver size.

Surgical Resection (Including Transplantation)

Early reports on patient survival after surgical resection of HCC were already influenced by high operative mortality rates secondary to marginal patient selection and technical misadventure. Improvements in preoperative assessment, operative strategy, blood conservation techniques, and postoperative care have greatly improved the rates of successful surgical resection in patients with hepatic tumors. The largest series of patients undergoing treatment for HCC has been compiled by the Liver Cancer Study Group of Japan,[40,99,100] which has periodically analyzed patterns of presentation and treatment results in a high-risk Asian population. In the initial report of 2411 cases managed from 1968 to 1977, 831 patients were treated opera-

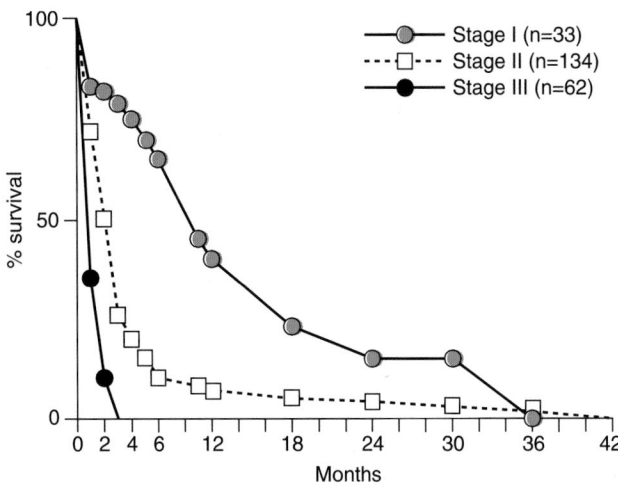

Figure 19-6 Prognosis of patients with untreated hepatocellular carcinoma. (After Okuda K, et al. Natural history of hepatocellular carcinoma and prognosis in relation to treatment: study of 850 patients. Cancer 1985;56:1985)

tively, although only 288 (11.9%) underwent resection, with the remainder receiving vascular ligation or exploratory laparotomy alone. Operative deaths were recorded in 27% of patients, and 1- and 5-year survival rates were 33.3% and 11.8%, respectively. Analysis of the more recent series of 2982 HCC cases revealed an increase in the resectability rate to 20.9%, thought to reflect aggressive use of ultrasonography for earlier detection. The 1-year survival rate had increased to 78%, and the median survival of patients with HCCs smaller than 2 cm approached 80 months. With the introduction of ultrasonography for earlier detection, the tumor size observed at time of resection was considerably reduced. Improvement in survival reflects intervention at an earlier tumor stage, more careful preoperative assessment of hepatic reserve, and the development of ultrasound-guided subsegmental resections in an effort to preserve hepatic mass. Pathologic parameters associated with better prognosis include the presence of a single mass, presence of a fibrous capsule, absence of capsular invasion, and absence of vascular invasion by tumor.

Series from Western countries have rarely achieved as high resectability rates or survival rates as those reported from Japan and Taiwan. The discrepancies in results are generally attributed to more frequent multifocal lesions and a reduced frequency of tumor encapsulation in Western series. A prospective study to evaluate resection for HCC in patients from two major European centers has been published.[101] The diagnosis of HCC was generally made during routine periodic follow-up of 72 asymptomatic cirrhotic patients. Fourteen patients (19%) underwent major hepatic resection, and 58 patients (81%) underwent segmental (48 patients) or nonanatomic (10 patients) resections. Sixty-eight of the 72 patients (94%) had single HCCs. Expanding encapsulated tumors were identified in 53 patients (74%), and infiltrating lesions were seen in the remainder. Sixty percent of tumors were less than 5 cm in largest diameter. Operative mortality was only 6.9%, with death from variceal hemorrhage the most common cause. Recurrence occurred in 16 patients (22%) during follow-up, with more recurrences being noted in the infiltrating HCC group. The 1-, 2-, and 3-year survival rates were 68%, 55%, and 51%, respectively, for all 72 patients. Significantly better survival rates were seen in Child's class A patients and in patients with expanding encapsulated HCC. One- and 3-year survival rates for the 25 Child's class A patients with expanding tumors were both 77%. These results suggest that similar survival rates may be achieved in Western and Asian series when the patient populations are similar.

Most reviews of the Western experience report a reduced incidence of cirrhosis in patients undergoing surgical resection for HCC, with survival rates at 3 years approaching 50% when operative mortality is excluded.[102] Many of the surgeons, however, did not consider cancers growing in cirrhotic livers to be resectable. The results of such studies are difficult to compare because of the small sample size and incompleteness of tumor staging.

The observation that a considerable number of patients with large, unresectable HCCs died of liver failure without gross evidence of extrahepatic spread was strong rational for the initial attempts in the use of total hepatectomy and orthotopic liver transplantation with curative intent. Many such patients were free of the advanced portal hypertension that accompanied chronic cirrhotic states, reducing the technical impediments of recipient hepatectomy. Even as the technical, immunologic, and infectious causes of postoperative death gradually declined, however, death from recurrent disease assumed major significance. Disease recurrence in extrahepatic sites or within the hepatic allograft was common, indicating the influence of systemic tumor dissemination before complete hepatectomy. Exceptions were seen in the case of patients with the fibrolamellar variant of HCC (discussed later) as well as in most patients with small incidental cancers found at the time of transplantation for cirrhotic disease states. The absence of effective alternative therapy for these patients prompted many transplantation programs to continue to offer transplantation as a last resort, with the expectation that survival would gradually improve as better patient selection was established.[103-109] Although the lack of standardized staging information in most of the early transplantation reviews makes comparison of patients and results difficult, the poor prognostic indicators of multifocality, bilobar disease, capsular invasion, and vascular invasion are common threads.

The frustration of rapid disease recurrence and the growing disparity between the number of potential transplantation candidates and donor allografts led to a decline in the use of transplantation for HCC and other tumors. Seminal reports from two centers helped to better define the potential tumor population most likely to benefit from resection or transplantation.[110,111] Both studies retrospectively reviewed data from patients with and without cirrhosis who underwent hepatic resection or liver transplantation, using standardized TNM staging (Table 19-3). One study demonstrated that survival was similar in patients with HCC whether they underwent resection or transplantation, noting the obvious selection biases employed to choose the method of therapy. In the aggregate HCC population, lower TNM stages conferred the best chance of long-term survival in both resection and transplantation groups. When patients with HCC in the presence of underlying

Table 19-3 Staging of Hepatocellular Carcinoma

Stage	Primary Tumor	Nodal Status	Distant Metastases
I	T1	N0	M0
II	T2	N0	M0
III	T1	N1	M0
	T2	N1	M0
	T3	N0, N1	M0
IVA	T4	Any N	M0
IVB	Any T	Any N	M1

Designation	Description
T1	Solitary, ≤2 cm, no vascular invasion
T2	Solitary, ≤2 cm, vascular invasion
	Multiple, one lobe, ≤2 cm, no vascular invasion
	Solitary, >2 cm, no vascular invasion
T3	Solitary, >2 cm, vascular invasion
	Multiple, one lobe, >2 cm, with or without vascular invasion
T4	Multiple, more than one lobe
	Invasion major venous structure
N1	Regional nodal metastases
M1	Distant metastases

cirrhosis were analyzed separately, there appeared to be a long-term survival advantage in the group of patients treated with transplantation. Although TNM stage IV patients fared poorly in both resection and transplantation groups, long-term survival was achieved only in the patients in TNM stage I to III who were treated with transplantation (Fig. 19-7). Death within 4 years invariably occurred in the resection group as a result of recurrent disease or the effects of cirrhosis. This observation lends strength to the argument that transplantation may be the preferred method of treatment in patients with early-stage HCC and underlying cirrhosis. Even with the shortage of donor liver allografts, it appears reasonable to offer transplantation to cirrhotic patients with unifocal HCCs of less than 2 to 3 cm in the absence of extrahepatic disease, but some programs accept a maximal size of 5 cm.

The existence of effective adjuvant or neoadjuvant chemotherapy would theoretically enhance the potential for survival in patients with HCC undergoing transplantation. Although preliminary trials of neoadjuvant therapy have been reported,[112,113] they are hampered by the absence of agents with significant biologic activity against HCC. Any expansion in the use of transplantation for the treatment of unresectable HCC will await the emergence of more effective chemotherapeutic agents.

Chemotherapy and Arterial Infusion

Most of the major classes of cancer chemotherapeutic agents have been tried singly or in combination for the treatment of HCC. The consensus is that no single drug or combination given systemically leads to reproducible response rates of more than 25% or has any substantial effect on survival.[114,115] Given the relative lack of response and the relatively poor tolerance of the cirrhotic patient to systemic drug toxicity, there appears to be little justification for treating patients with single or combination drugs in a systemic fashion outside of clinical trials.

The intraarterial administration of drugs delivered directly into the tumor in high concentrations theoretically increases the local drug delivery while minimizing systemic toxicity. Selective targeting of the tumor seems possible since HCC is almost completely dependent on hepatic arterial inflow, whereas normal liver balances portal venous and hepatic arterial inflow. Moreover, local activity may be increased by using drugs with a high degree of hepatic extraction, high systemic clearance, rapid biotransformation into less toxic metabolites, and evidence of a steep dose–response relation.[116] A number of techniques of arterial catheterization for intermittent or continuous chemoperfusion have been used, ranging from direct operative arterial cannulation to radiologic brachial catheterization. The development of implantable pumps facilitated the controlled delivery of drug into the hepatic artery.[117] Although early trials demonstrated the potential of inducing tumor regression, the small number of patients and the difficulty in assessing tumor response makes the potential role of this approach difficult to evaluate.

Arterial Chemoembolization

Selective arterial embolization with large Gelfoam particles has been widely used throughout Asia and is generally accompanied by necrosis and liquefaction of the central portion of the tumor mass. Eventually rearterialization of the tumor occurs with attendant regrowth. Transarterial chemoembolization (TACE) represents a innovative treatment designed to combine the benefits of intraarterial chemotherapy and segmental hepatic arterial occlusion for the local treatment of HCC. TACE was first reported to be effective for the treatment of unresectable HCC in 1983 and has since been approached by other investigators with variations in chemotherapeutic agent content.[118–122] Tumor response seems to be improved when TACE is followed by segmental arterial occlusion with the infusion of powdered Gelfoam particles. The preferred method has been with the infusion of a mixture of Lipiodol and doxorubicin or cisplatin followed by the injection of fine Gelfoam particles. With the addition of Gelfoam, the response rate of the Lipiodol and chemotherapy mixture is dramatically improved, increasing from 13% to 83% with doxorubicin.[123] Lipiodol is cleared by the nor-

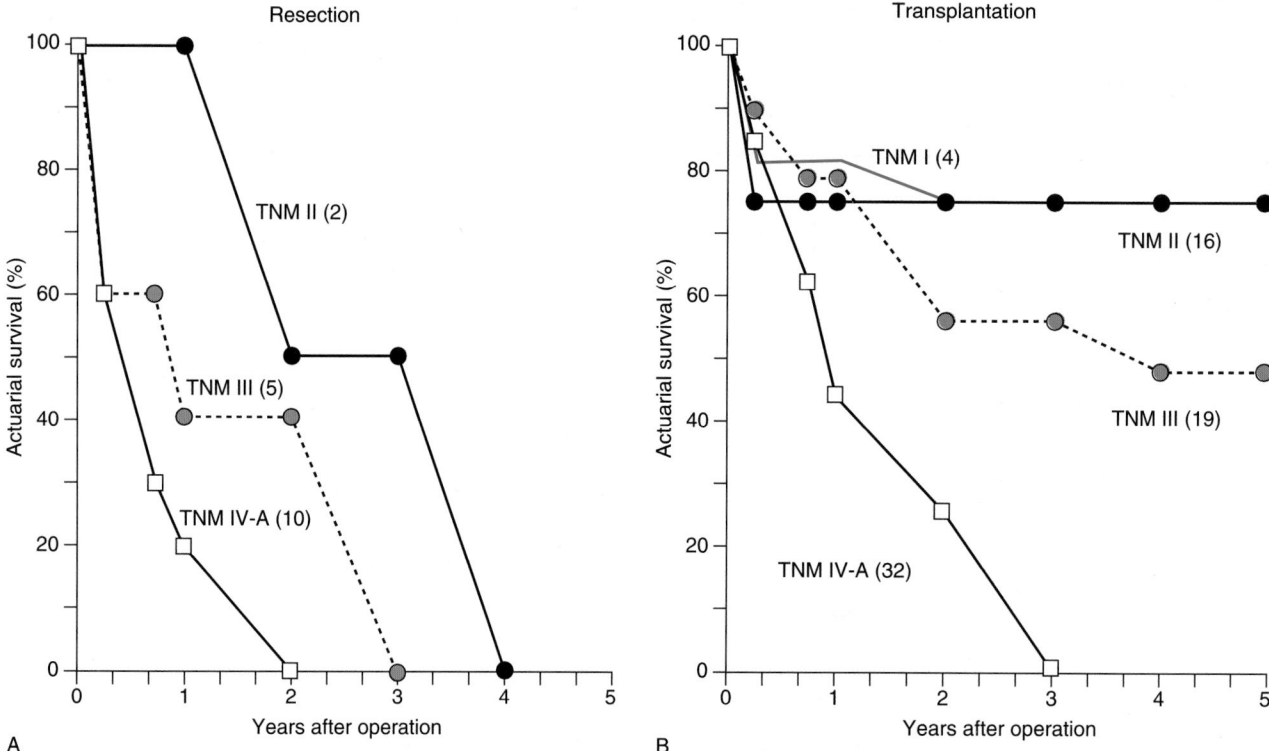

Figure 19-7 Results of hepatic resection (**A**) versus transplantation (**B**) in patients with hepatocellular carcinoma and cirrhosis. Long-term survival was seen only in patients with early-stage disease who underwent transplantation. (After Iwatsuki S, Starzl TE, Sheahan DG, et al. Hepatic resection versus transplantation for hepatocellular carcinoma. Ann Surg 1991;214: 221)

mal hepatic parenchyma in 1 week to 10 days, but it remains visible radiographically within the tumor for weeks to months. The chemotherapy agent becomes trapped within the substance of the tumor, and the segmental hepatic artery occlusion creates relative hypoxia. Necrosis of the tumor with sterile gas formation can be seen within a few days, followed by the gradual involution of the tumor (Fig. 19-8).

Although used as a palliative treatment, TACE has demonstrated improvement in survival rates as compared with systemic chemotherapy or no treatment.[124,125] Not surprisingly, good prognostic factors include encapsulated tumors, unifocal lesions, and tumors less than 5 cm in diameter. To achieve consistent results, chemoembolization needs to be repeated at 4- to 6-month intervals. One institution treated 52 patients considered unresectable because of cirrhosis or multifocal disease with a regimen of doxorubicin, Lipiodol, and Gelfoam powder.[126] Best results were seen in the patient population without portal vein obstruction, in whom median survival rates increased to 24 months. Incomplete TACE, the presence of extrahepatic metas-

tasis, and portal vein thrombosis were all factors associated with poor outcome.

Percutaneous Ethanol Injection

Percutaneous ethanol injection is a technique that uses ultrasound guidance to direct a percutaneously placed needle into an intrahepatic tumor, followed by the direct injection of absolute (99.5%) alcohol.[127] Tissues coming in contact with the alcohol undergo dehydration and denaturation, leading to extensive necrosis. Histopathologic examination of tissues obtained at surgery, autopsy, or biopsy suggest that two thirds of tumors less than 3 cm in diameter become completely necrotic.[128] This technique is commonly applied to patients with HCCs less than 3 to 5 cm in diameter in many Asian and European countries.[129,130] The North Italian Study Group analyzed the results in 207 patients receiving percutaneous ethanol injection and concluded that the efficacy was about the same as that seen with resection.[131] Percutaneous ethanol injection appears to represent a reasonable alternative to surgery in

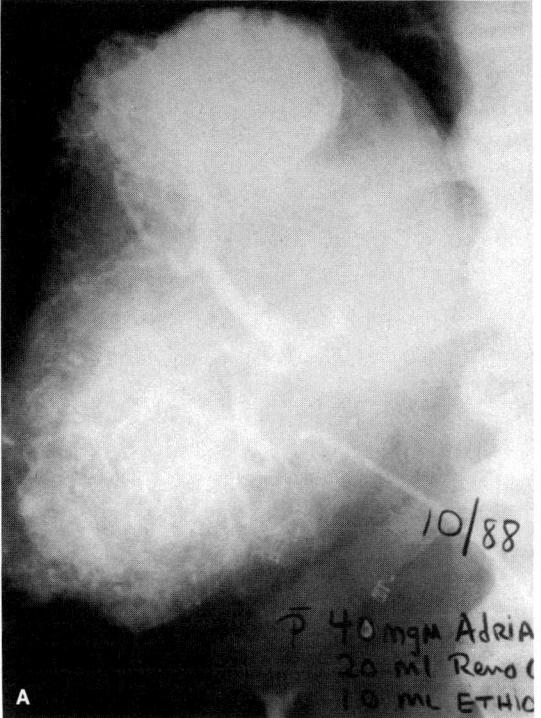
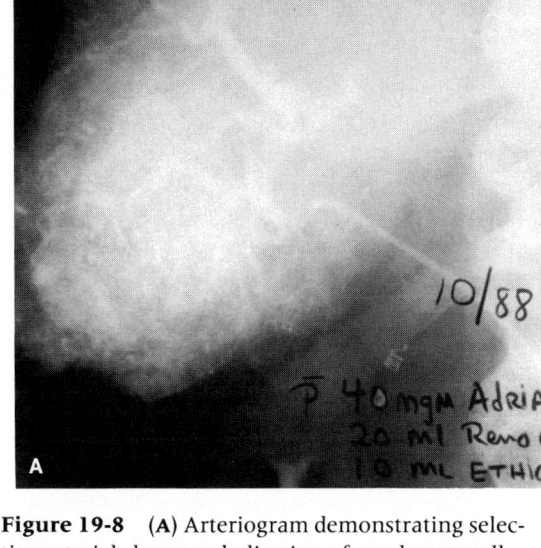

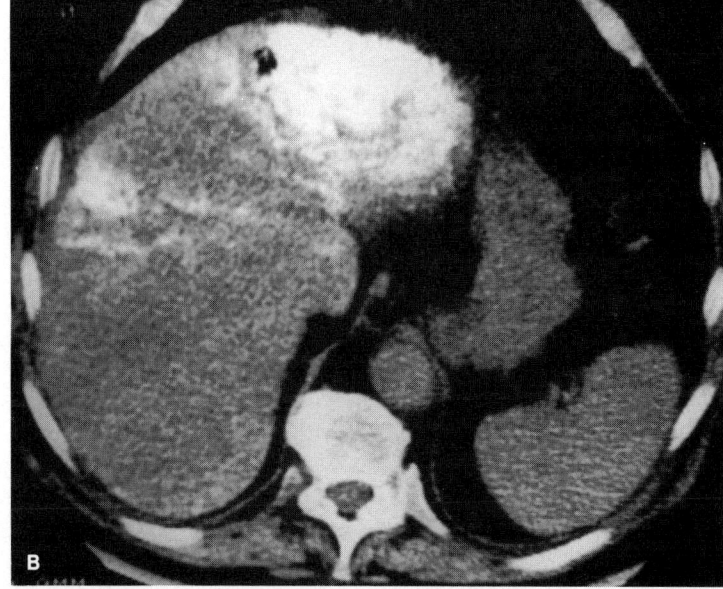
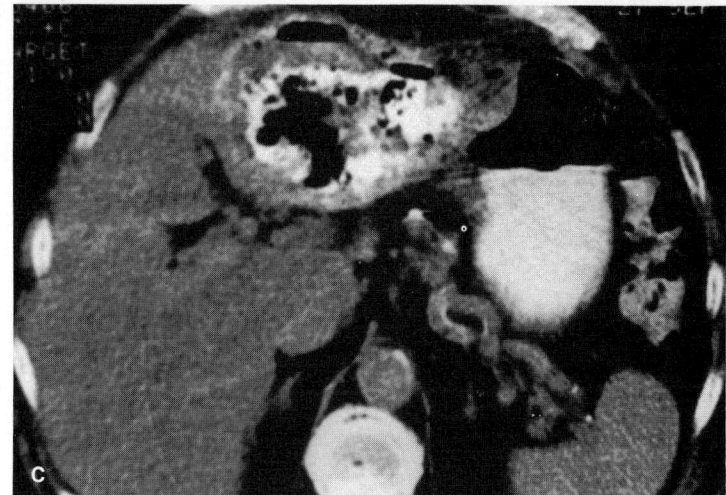

Figure 19-8 (**A**) Arteriogram demonstrating selective arterial chemoembolization of two hepatocellular carcinoma lesions of the right lobe of the liver with doxorubicin (Adriamycin), diatrizoate sodium and diatrizoate meglumine (Renografin), and ethiodized oil (Ethiodol). (**B**) CT scan without intravenous contrast 3 days after arterial chemoembolization of hepatocellular carcinoma in the left lobe of the liver demonstrating persistence of ethiodized oil within tumor parenchyma and early tumor necrosis. (**C**) CT scan of same patient 2 weeks after chemoembolization with extensive necrosis and sterile gas formation within tumor substance.

the management of small HCCs in cirrhotic patients, but prospective controlled trials are needed.

The heterogenous nature of HCC and the influence of coexisting cirrhosis has contributed to the numerous treatment options employed for patient management. Table 19-4 outlines the treatment options as determined by clinical presentation.

FIBROLAMELLAR CARCINOMA

The histologic variant of fibrolamellar hepatocellular carcinoma (FLHC) is often considered separately because of its differing pattern of presentation and clinical behavior. First described in 1956, it was not until 1980 that reports emphasized the occurrence of a fibrolamellar variant of HCC in younger patients with slower

growth rates and a better prognosis than typical HCC.[132] Of the data supporting the distinction between FLHC and HCC, the histologic features of FLHC are the most objective and widely accepted differences. Accounting for only about 1% to 2% of all HCCs, FLHC is predominantly a disease of older children or young adults, without significant sexual predilection.[133] Less than 10% of patients developing this neoplasm are older than 35 years, only 8% have evidence of HBV disease, and only 4% have cirrhosis. Presentation is typically with upper gastrointestinal symptoms, upper abdominal pain, or weight loss. The duration of symptoms is often prolonged, ranging from 4 to 12 months, and the lesion is frequently large enough to be easily palpable.[134–136] Laboratory studies show only mild derangement of liver function, and AFP is elevated in only 11% of cases.

Grossly, the lesions may be single or multiple and

Table 19-4 Treatment Options for Hepatocellular Carcinoma

SURGICAL RESECTION
Noncirrhotic liver
Cirrhotic liver with good function
Anatomically feasible
No extrahepatic disease
Absence of major vascular invasion

ALCOHOL INJECTION
Cirrhotic liver
≤3 cm diameter
Noncirrhotic with medical contraindications
Local recurrence

LIVER TRANSPLANTATION
Cirrhotic liver
≤3 cm diameter
Unifocal
Unresectable fibrolamellar hepatocellular carcinoma

CHEMOEMBOLIZATION
Unifocal or multifocal
Noncirrhotic with medical contraindications
Local recurrence
Patent portal vein

may resemble focal nodular hyperplasia with a central fibrous scar.[137] The histopathologic features of FLHC are characterized by deeply eosinophilic hepatocytes, many of which contain intracytoplasmic hyaline globules and distinct pale bodies.[138] The hepatocytes are well differentiated and well circumscribed within the hepatic parenchyma. The most distinctive and characteristic feature is the separation of the neoplastic hepatocytes by fibrosis arranged in a lamellar fashion (Fig. 19-9).

Imaging characteristics of FLHC are similar to early asymptomatic HCC. Plain films of the abdomen generally show hepatomegaly, occasionally with calcifications overlying the liver shadow. Ultrasound evaluation reveals a moderately echogenic solitary mass with clear demarcation at the periphery.[139] CT generally confirms the ultrasound findings of a discrete, inhomogeneous, low-density single or multicentric lesion (Fig. 19-10).

The surgical resectability rate for FLHC varies from 48% to 75%, in sharp contrast with the less than 20% rate of resectability for nonfibrolamellar HCC.[140] The potential for prolonged survival with resection of FLHC is substantially better than that reported with HCC.[141] Improved results with orthotopic liver transplantation have been reported in patients with otherwise unresectable FLHC, although eventual death from recurrent disease occurs in about half of patients.[142] It is likely the better prognosis generally reported in patients with FLHC could be a result of comparing the particularly

homogeneous FLHC patients with a much more heterogeneous HCC population (coexisting cirrhosis, age, multicentricity). The higher rates of resectability and prolonged survival justify aggressive surgical management, including resection of the primary lesion and regional metastases.

HEPATOBLASTOMA

Principally a tumor of childhood, hepatoblastoma accounts for about 60% of primary malignant tumorsof Western children, affecting about 1 child per 100,000.[143] HCC is far more common than hepatoblastoma in Asian children. Hepatoblastoma is usually diagnosed before the age of 4 years, and 65% to 80% of children with the tumor are younger than 2 years.[144] The lesion has been occasionally reported in adults.

Pathology

Hepatoblastoma usually appears as a large mass lesion in the liver, with its gross appearance depending on the mesenchymal components and the presence of intralesional hemorrhage and necrosis. Cirrhosis is an uncommon association. Histologically, the tumors are classified into epithelial and mixed epithelial–mesenchymal types.[145] An additional anaplastic type has been described that is associated with a poorer prognosis.[146] The epithelial components are made up of fetal and embryonic subtypes. The fetal subtype is characterized by cells that resemble adult hepatocytes and may be associated with varying degrees of extramedullary hematopoiesis. Embryonal cells have poorly defined margins and less cytoplasm. The mixed epithelial–mesenchymal

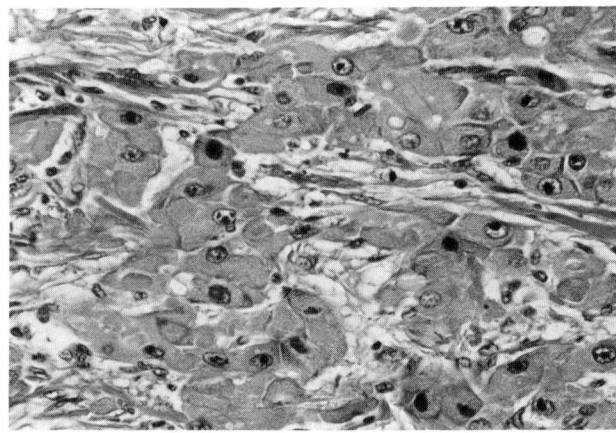

Figure 19-9 Fibrolamellar hepatocellular carcinoma. Deeply eosinophilic tumor cells are separated by fibrous lamellae. (See Color Fig. 19-9.)

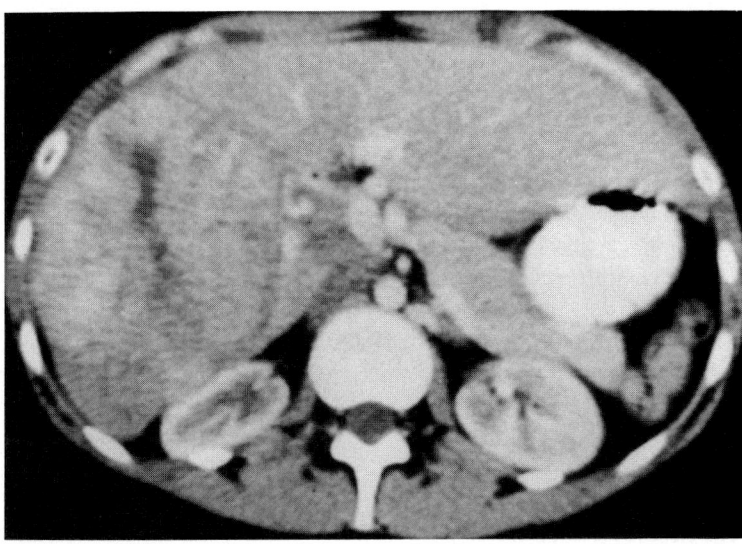

Figure 19-10 CT scan of fibrolamellar hepatocellular carcinoma. A large circumscribed mass with a central scar is seen in the right lobe of the liver.

type has epithelial cells mixed with more primitive spindle-shaped mesenchymal cells. Cartilaginous and osteoid tissue may be present, accounting for the occasional appearance of calcifications on plain abdominal radiography (Fig. 19-11).

Clinical Features

Most patients are brought to the physician because of abdominal swelling accompanied by anorexia, weight loss, nausea and vomiting, or abdominal pain. Physical examination suggests hepatomegaly, and occasionally the tumor is large enough to fill both the upper and lower abdomen. Despite the size of the lesion, jaundice, ascites, and portal hypertension are rarely present. Rupture and intraabdominal hemorrhage may occur, pro-

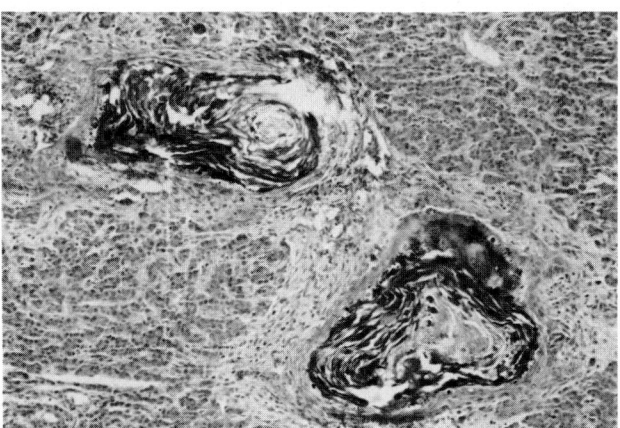

Figure 19-11 Hepatoblastoma. Cords of tumor cells with interspersed stromal tissue and osteoid formation are seen. (See Color Fig. 19-11.)

ducing the picture of an acute abdominal catastrophe. Precocious puberty from tumor-derived hormonal production has been reported in association with hepatoblastoma. As with several childhood malignancies, urinary excretion of cystathionine produced by the tumor is increased in nearly half of patients. Familial occurrence of hepatoblastoma among siblings and identical twins has been described, and an association between this tumor and polyposis of the colon has been found in several families.[147] Congenital anomalies occur in about 5.5% of the reported cases and include cleft palate, macroglossia, earlobe dysplasia, absence of one adrenal, umbilical hernia, and various cardiovascular and renal abnormalities.

Serum AFP is elevated in about 95% of patients with hepatoblastoma and provides a useful tool for assessing disease progression or recurrence. Changes in tests of hepatic function are slight and nonspecific. Plain abdominal radiographs may suggest the diagnosis with the appearance of mottled calcification within the tumor. Pulmonary metastases may be seen on chest radiography. The tumor is echogenic by ultrasonography, with scattered calcifications and regions of necrosis and hemorrhage. On CT, the tumor is generally a lobulated hypodense lesion with minimal contrast enhancement. Adenopathy may be visible in the hilar region.

Hepatoblastoma is a rapidly progressive tumor, with about half of the tumors unresectable at the time of diagnosis because of bilobar disease, extrahepatic spread, or extensive vascular invasion. The complete resection of a hepatoblastoma with purely fetal histology results in a survival rate of 90%, but those with other histologic types have an overall survival rate of only 60%.[148] Long-term survival varies from 15% to 37% and is dependent on resectability and histologic type. Pre-operative chemotherapy or radiation may reduce tumor size and permit subsequent resection. One author concluded that the administration of cisplatin in repeated cycles in conjunction with better staging and surgical techniques is responsible for the improved survival in children with hepatoblastoma.[149] This therapy has been used both in an adjuvant setting and as neoadjuvant treatment to promote tumor shrinkage and allow for surgical resection. Although patients with metastatic disease at diagnosis are potentially curable, most represent a therapeutic challenge.[150]

INTRAHEPATIC CHOLANGIOCARCINOMA

Cholangiocarcinoma is a malignant tumor of biliary epithelial origin arising in peripheral regions of the hepatic parenchyma. Histologically, the lesion represents the intrahepatic counterpart of the extrahepatic or hilar cholangiocarcinoma, commonly referred to as *Klatskin's tumor.*[151] The boundary that differentiates carcinomas of intrahepatic and extrahepatic origin is the point where second-order bile ducts join to become the left and right bile ducts. Overlap may occur when a hilar cholangiocarcinoma extends beyond the boundary, creating confusion in the classification of tumors of hepatic versus biliary origin. True intrahepatic cholangiocarcinomas behave much like HCC in terms of growth rates and spread but are rarely associated with cirrhosis. The average age of patients is about a decade older than that seen with HCC, and the degree of male predominance is only about 2:1. In the United States, cholangiocarcinoma represents 25% of primary liver malignancies and 0.05% of autopsies.[152] In regions where HCC is more common, the tumor represents only 10% of primary liver malignancies. In Thailand and Hong Kong, the ratio of cholangiocarcinoma to HCC is higher and appears to be in association with a high incidence of liver fluke (*Opisthorchis sinensis* or *Opisthorchis viverrini*) infections.[153] These tumors are often found near parasite-infested bile ducts deep within the hepatic parenchyma. Cholangiocarcinoma is also associated withhepaticolithiasis, in which repeated bouts of inflammation of the biliary epithelium may contribute to their development.[154] Of the various hepatic neoplasms reported in association with Thorotrast, cholangiocarcinoma is one of the most frequent malignancies leading to patient death.[155]

Grossly, cholangiocarcinoma has an appearance similar to HCC, white in color and firm in consistency.

The tumors vary in patterns of growth and may appear as well-demarcated nodular lesions or diffusely infiltrative with irregular boundaries and extensive satellitosis. Occasionally, the tumor proliferates along the intrahepatic bile ducts, with adjacent parenchymal infiltration. Large vessel invasion is less common than that associated with HCC. Histologically, most cholangiocarcinomas are well to moderately differentiated mucin-secreting adenocarcinomas with an abundant fibrous stroma (Fig. 19-12). Distinction of cholangiocarcinoma from a metastatic adenocarcinoma of gastrointestinal origin may be difficult. The transition of epithelial cells from normal to neoplastic appearance within ductal structures, free stromal mucin, and nests or isolated tumor cells adrift in the fibrous stroma are distinguishing characteristics of cholangiocarcinoma. Differentiation from a pseudoglandular pattern of HCC is based on the presence of mucin secretion rather than the characteristic bile secretion of HCC. Combined hepatocellular and cholangiocarcinoma tumors are occasionally described and may grow as separate structures or as mixed tumors. Cirrhosis is more frequently associated with this uncommon variant.

Patient presentation is similar to that seen with noncirrhotic HCC, although jaundice is somewhat more common. As many as half of patients are found to have hilar nodal metastases from lymphatic spread at presentation. Elevation of both CEA and CA19-9 levels suggest the diagnosis of cholangiocarcinoma rather than HCC.[40] AFP levels may also be elevated, though usually not to the same level as that seen with HCC.

Cholangiocarcinoma tends to be less vascular than HCC and exhibits only mild contrast enhancement on CT (Fig. 19-13). Bile duct dilation peripheral to the le-

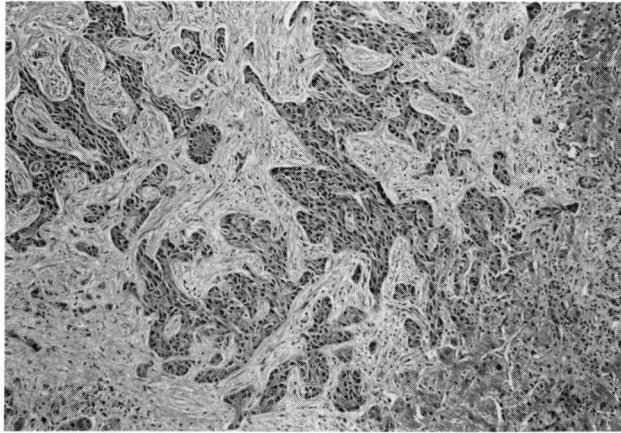

Figure 19-12 Intrahepatic cholangiocarcinoma. Mucin-secreting adenocarcinoma cells with dense fibrous stroma are seen. The absence of bile production helps to differentiate this lesion from hepatocellular carcinoma. (See Color Fig. 19-12.)

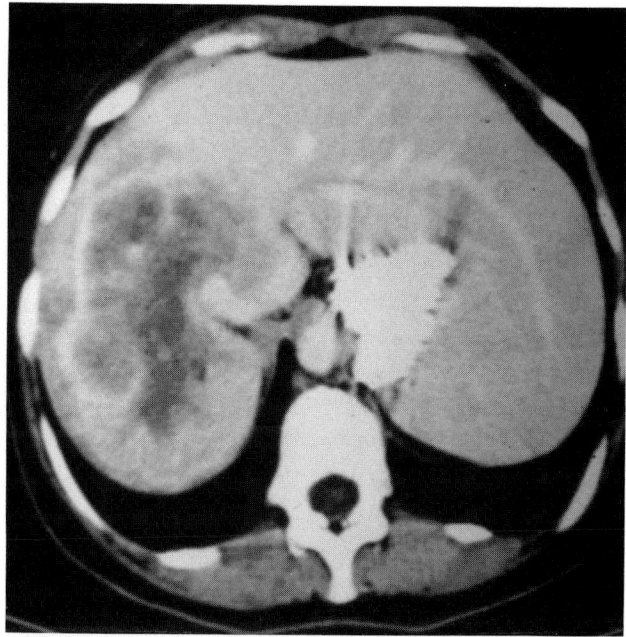

Figure 19-13 CT scan of intrahepatic cholangiocarcinoma. This patient presented with Budd-Chiari syndrome 3 weeks after delivery of her first child and remained well 8 years after total hepatectomy and liver transplantation.

sion is not uncommon, and large celiac nodal metastases are often visualized. The presence of jaundice suggests more proximal tumor extension and should prompt consideration of cholangiography.

Median survival without treatment is only about 6 months. Resection remains the only reliable therapy because the lesion responds poorly to chemotherapy. The fibrous consistency and hypovascular character of cholangiocarcinoma make it less amenable to techniques such as chemoembolization or alcohol injection. Intrahepatic or extrahepatic recurrence, or both, after resection occurs in about half of patients. Survival rates of 40% are attainable in patients resected with curative intent.[40] Thus, aggressive diagnosis and resectional therapy represent the best available management.

BILIARY CYSTADENOCARCINOMA

Biliary cystadenocarcinoma is the malignant counterpart of the more common biliary cystadenoma and represents about 5% of such complex cystic lesions.[156] It is a fluid-filled tumor lined by mucus-secreting columnar epithelium with papillary infoldings. The tumor infiltrates into the septations and occasionally into the hepatic parenchyma, similar to the histologic picture seen with cystadenocarcinomas of the pancreas or ovary.

Distinction between cystadenoma and cystadenocarcinoma can be difficult without evidence of invasion into surrounding parenchyma. The fluid within the loculated spaces may be serous or contain varying proportions of blood, bile, or mucus. Ultrasonography and CT both portray a rounded, fluid-filled structure with internal papillary projections or septations. Evidence of prominent projections or parenchymal infiltration should suggest cystadenocarcinoma rather than cystadenoma (Fig. 19-14).

Presentation is similar to that seen with the benign cystadenoma, with abdominal distention and pain being the most common symptoms. Often confused with simple cysts, they are often instrumented for drainage or biopsy before referral for resection.[157] Because even benign lesions expand and cause biliary or vascular compression, all complex cystic lesions should be resected in operative candidates. Although enucleation may be appropriate for the benign lesion, formal resection should be undertaken for cystadenocarcinoma be-

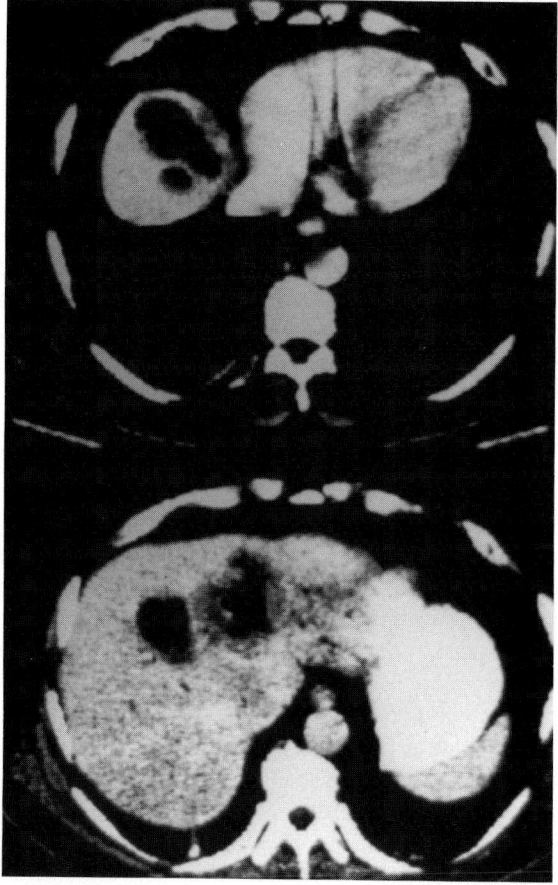

Figure 19-14 CT scan of biliary cystadenocarcinoma demonstrating septated cystic mass with prominent papillary projections along cyst wall.

cause recurrent disease and subsequent metastases are common with inadequate resection.

MALIGNANT MESENCHYMAL TUMORS

Mesenchymal malignancies represent only about 1% to 2% of all primary hepatic malignancies. According to the Registry of Autopsies in Japan,[40] there were only 95 mesenchymal tumors among 17,417 autopsy cases of primary malignant tumors of the liver from 1985 to 1989. Most of these lesions are sarcomas, with prognosis varying by cell type and extent of disease. Although secondary metastasis from an extrahepatic primary tumor is the most common source of hepatic leiomyosarcoma, primary hepatic leiomyosarcoma has been described as arising from the hepatic vasculature, particularly the hepatic veins. Fibrosarcoma resembles that originating from other regions of the body. Undifferentiated sarcomas are primary lesions afflicting children and have been variably referred to as *embryonal sarcoma* or *malignant mesenchymoma*. Such lesions are associated with a poor prognosis except in occasional cases with multimodality therapy that includes radiotherapy, chemotherapy, and surgical resection. Embryonal rhabdomyosarcoma is another rare malignant tumor of childhood, which typically arises from the extrahepatic biliary tree but which can also arise from intrahepatic ductal elements. Primary carcinoids, teratocarcinomas, and primary lymphomas of the liver are occasionally reported. Two of the more common lesions originating from vascular elements, angiosarcoma and epithelioid hemangioendothelioma, are important because of the extraordinary aggressiveness of the former and the slower growing nature of the latter.

Angiosarcoma

Angiosarcoma is an uncommon malignancy of endothelial cells that characteristically grows diffusely along the hepatic sinusoids with often indistinct borders. The lesion is variably associated with exposures to Thorotrast, polyvinylchloride, and arsenic.[158] Despite these associations, most lesions occur in patients without obvious risk factors. There is a slight male predominance, and the lesion characteristically develops in the sixth or seventh decade of life.

Grossly, angiosarcoma presents the appearance of variable-sized nodules spreading throughout vast regions of the liver. Extrahepatic metastases are common at presentation. Histologically, angiosarcoma is characterized by spindle cells and polyhedral cells, often with a multinucleated and pleomorphic appearance (Fig.

19-15). Tumor growth is typically along sinusoids, leaving islands of surviving hepatocytes. Both solid and cavernous areas may be present, with scattered areas of necrosis and hemorrhage. Cirrhosis is rarely present unless the lesion is associated with underlying hemochromatosis. Positive staining of tumor cells for factor VIII–related antigen supports the endothelial origin of angiosarcoma.

The presenting signs and symptoms include abdominal pain, anorexia, nausea, weight loss, fever, tender hepatomegaly, splenomegaly, and ascites. An arterial bruit occasionally is heard over the liver. Tumor rupture may occur in 15% of patients, and hemorrhage after attempted biopsy is common. Progressive tumor infiltration is eventually associated with the development of jaundice and liver failure. Angiosarcoma is characterized by rapid growth, with the duration of symptoms ranging from 1 week to 6 months before deterioration. Ascites is not infrequent and may be bloodstained.

Angiography reveals a characteristic abnormal vascular pattern with diffuse peripheral tumor blushes, and CT reveals scattered areas of contrast enhancement in a diffuse pattern throughout the affected area (Fig. 19-16). Nodal, perihepatic, and splenic metastases are common.

Although resection has been reported, most tumors are too diffuse to consider resection at the time of presentation. Survival beyond 1 year is rare, with most patients succumbing from liver failure or hemorrhagic rupture. Indeed, the diagnosis is made before the patient's death in only about one third of cases. Survival has not been prolonged significantly with any chemotherapeutic regimen to date.

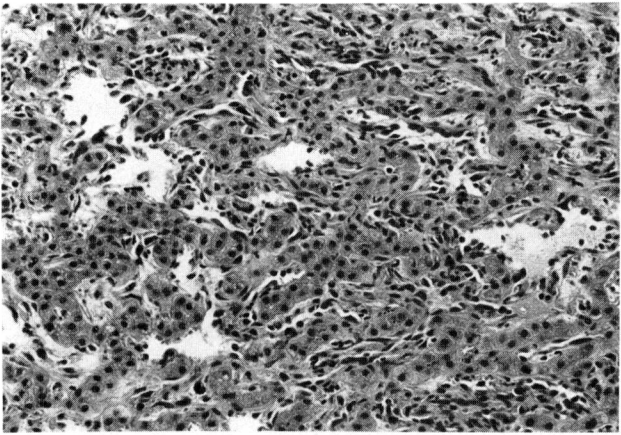

Figure 19-15 Islands of hepatocytes surrounded by elongated tumor cells infiltrating along sinusoids are characteristic of angiosarcoma. (See Color Fig. 19-15.)

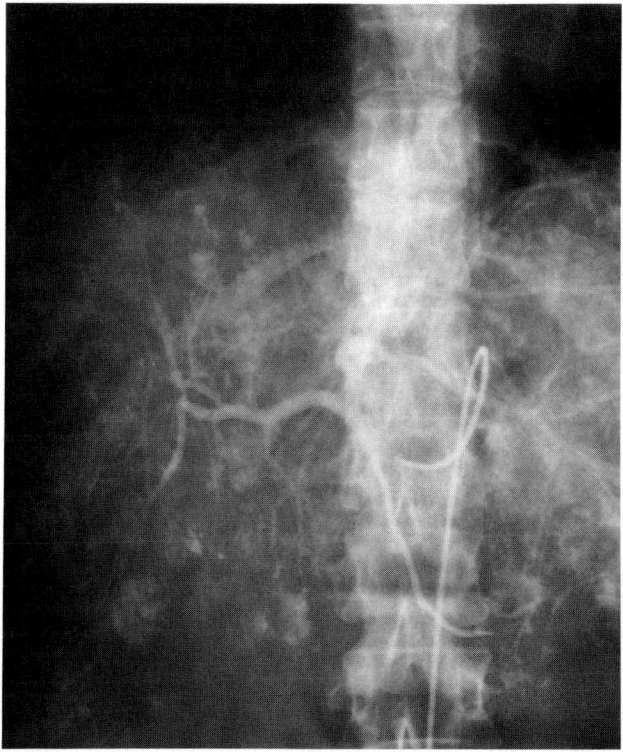

Figure 19-16 Hepatic arteriogram in a patient with diffuse angiosarcoma demonstrating the widespread and hypervascular nature of the tumor.

Epithelioid Hemangioendothelioma

This lesion should not be confused with infantile hemangioendothelioma, which is a tumor of vascular origin typically found in children younger than 6 months, frequently associated with congestive heart failure, and occasionally subject to spontaneous resolution.[159] Epithelioid hemangioendothelioma is a rare, malignant sarcoma of vascular endothelial origin arising in the liver of adults and resembling a similar tumor of the lung (intravascular bronchoalveolar tumor) and soft tissues.[160] The mean age at presentation is 50 years, and about two thirds are found in women. Presenting complaints include right upper quadrant or epigastric pain, weight loss, easy fatigability, fever, and jaundice. The most common laboratory abnormality is elevation of the serum alkaline phosphatase level. Progressive infiltration throughout the liver can lead to death from liver failure. Advanced stages can be associated with hepatic venous outflow occlusion and a Budd-Chiari–type syndrome, and some tumors may bleed with rupture into the peritoneal cavity. Imaging studies usually demonstrate multiple lesions of variable size scattered throughout the liver. CT findings suggest the tumor begins as multiple hepatic nodules that grow and coalesce,

forming large confluent masses preferentially involving the peripheral areas of the liver.[161] At least 40% of patients have extrahepatic tumor at presentation or follow-up. The most common sites of metastases are lung, regional lymph nodes, and peritoneum. Histologically, the tumor consists of combinations of proliferating dendritic or epithelioid cells of endothelial origin scattered singly or in clusters, with a predilection for zone 3 of the liver acini (Fig. 19-17). Progressive vascular occlusion of hepatic venous and portal venous structures is common. Progressive fibrosis and calcification develops within affected areas. The appearance of vacuolated tumor cells embedded within dense fibrous stroma can mimic the appearance of cholangiocarcinoma or mucin-producing adenocarcinoma. The tumor cells may synthesize a factor VIII–related antigen that serves as a useful marker.

The prognosis is variable and unpredictable. Whereas about 20% of the patients die within 2 years, another 20% exhibit prolonged survival, ranging from 5 to 28 years, irrespective of the presence of extrahepatic tumor or the treatment employed. Thus, it is difficult to evaluate the effectiveness of various types of therapy with the available information. The tumor's potential for slow growth and prolonged survival even in the presence of extrahepatic metastases has encouraged aggressive surgical approaches, including metastectomy. One group of researchers reported on 10 patients who had liver transplantations for unresectable epithelioid hemangioendothelioma.[162] Five patients with evidence of at least microscopic metastases were alive at a mean of 40 months (range, 18 to 62 months) after transplantation. Two of the five patients free of metastases at the time of transplantation died of recur-

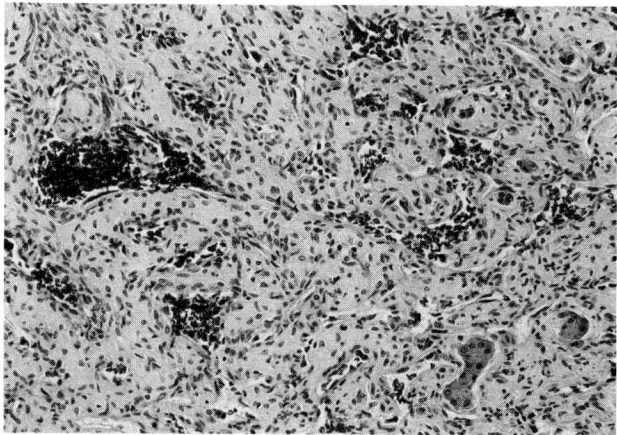

Figure 19-17 Epithelioid hemangioendothelioma consisting of clusters of proliferating endothelial cells trapping scattered islands of normal hepatocytes and forming cavernous vascular channels. (See Color Fig. 19-17.)

rent disease 3 and 16 months after operation. Such favorable biologic behavior supports the continued aggressive use of resection techniques in the management of this rare neoplasm.

METASTATIC HEPATIC NEOPLASMS

Metastatic tumors from extrahepatic origins make up the largest group of malignancies found in the liver. Even in Japan, where HCC is endemic, metastatic malignancies are 2.6 times more common than HCC, with the most common primary sources consisting of bronchogenic, stomach, pancreas, and colon in order of frequency.[40] In comparison, metastatic malignancies were 47 times more common than HCC in a large autopsy series from Los Angeles.[92] As seen in Table 19-5, bronchogenic, colon, pancreas, breast, and stomach were the most common sources in order of frequency. Most patients who present with hepatic metastases have such spread in conjunction with disease in extrahepatic sites. Not uncommonly, the liver tumor is found first during the evaluation of abdominal complaints, leading to a search for the primary site of origin. With the exception of bronchogenic carcinoma, which is characterized by a high frequency of hematogenous spread to multiple sites including the liver, the most common malignancies associated with hepatic metastases are of gastrointestinal origin. The unique vascular arrangement of the liver, with both hepatic arterial and portal venous inflow, contributes to the observed behavior of metastatic spread. Portal inflow from digestive organ sources contributes two thirds of the blood flow to the liver, with the rest attributed to the hepatic artery. Primary lesions developing in the colon, rectum, pancreas, stomach, and small bowel eventually shed viable cells into the adjacent portal circulation, where they are carried to the hepatic sinusoids and trapped by endothelial and Kupffer cells. The cells that are resistant to destruction may become implanted within the hepatic parenchyma and establish an arterial blood supply, which eventually supplants the earlier portal venous source.

Metastatic Colorectal Carcinoma

With the exception of colorectal carcinoma, Wilms tumor, and certain slow-growing neuroendocrine tumors metastatic to the liver, few metastatic diseases lend themselves to effective management by secondary hepatic resection.[163,164] Survival after the development of liver metastases with noncolorectal gastrointestinal malignancies and renal, breast, and gynecologic malignancies is rarely extended by aggressive metastectomy. Of the metastatic diseases afflicting the liver, colorectal carcinoma represents the most important primary site because of behavioral characteristics that allow resection of metastases with curative intent. About half of the annual estimated 147,000 patients with colon or rectal carcinoma are at risk for the development of he-

Table 19-5 Most Common Nonlymphoma Malignant Tumors Metastatic to the Liver

Type of Tumor	No. of Primary Tumors	No. With Hepatic Metastases	Patients With Hepatic Metastases (%)	Patients With Hepatic Metastases Who Were Icteric (%)
Bronchogenic	682	285	41.8	9
Colon	323	181	56.0	34
Pancreas	179	126	70.4	51
Breast	218	116	53.2	30
Stomach	159	70	44.0	60
Unknown primary	102	59	57.0	35
Ovary	97	47	48.0	0
Prostate	333	42	12.6	0
Gallbladder	49	38	77.6	60
Cervix	107	34	31.7	10
Kidney	142	34	23.9	15
Melanoma	50	25	50.0	13
Urinary bladder	66	25	37.9	11
Esophagus	66	20	30.3	29
Testis	45	20	44.4	14
Endometrial	54	17	31.5	20
Thyroid	70	12	17.1	14

(Data obtained at Los Angeles County University of Southern California Medical Center and John Wesley County Hospital. After Edmondson HA, Craig JR. Neoplasms of the liver. In: Schiff L, Schiff ER, eds. Diseases of the liver, ed 6. Philadelphia, JB Lippincott, 1987)

patic metastases during a 5-year period of observation.[3] Only 5000 of these patients have metastases isolated to the liver and are eligible for hepatic resection. The primary stimulus for the application of surgical resection of liver tumors has been the development of technical expertise in an operation historically considered to be fraught with significant morbidity and mortality. Hepatic resection has been espoused as the only treatment option with curative potential in this small subset of patients. Overall, survival appears to hinge on the overall extent of liver involvement with or without resectional attempts.

Natural History

Consideration of the natural history of patients with hepatic metastases from colorectal cancer is crucial to allow proper assessment of the results of resectional therapy. Most reports of results with hepatic resection compare the results of resection with historical controls from earlier periods when referral for resection was uncommon. Comparative interpretation of such studies is marred by the variable extent of liver involvement that determined potential suitability for treatment attempts. Control patients with limited hepatic involvement but no symptoms are probably most comparable to the patients selected as candidates for surgery. It is important to understand the potential for prolonged survival in patients with solitary or limited liver involvement. The fate of 252 patients who had unresected hepatic metastases from 1943 through 1976 at one institution are the basis of one report.[165] Survival rates determined for patients with solitary nodules, multiple unilateral nodules, and widespread hepatic disease were 21%, 6%, and 4%, respectively (Fig. 19-18). Although prolonged survival was possible without treatment, no unresected patient lived 5 years. By contrast, 25% of 116 patients with solitary or multiple metastases confined to the liver were alive 5 years after resection. It was concluded that 2-year survival rates were determined by the biologic activity of the metastatic disease process, whereas long-term survival was determined by successful removal of the tumor. Additional natural history studies and reports of the results of resection have been summarized in one review and serve as the basis for the recommendation for the surgical ablation of limited hepatic disease.[3]

Detection and Staging

Colorectal metastases typically develop within the first 2 years after primary colonic resection in 80% of patients destined to have recurrence, and recurrence develops after 5 years in less than 5%.[166,167] Although

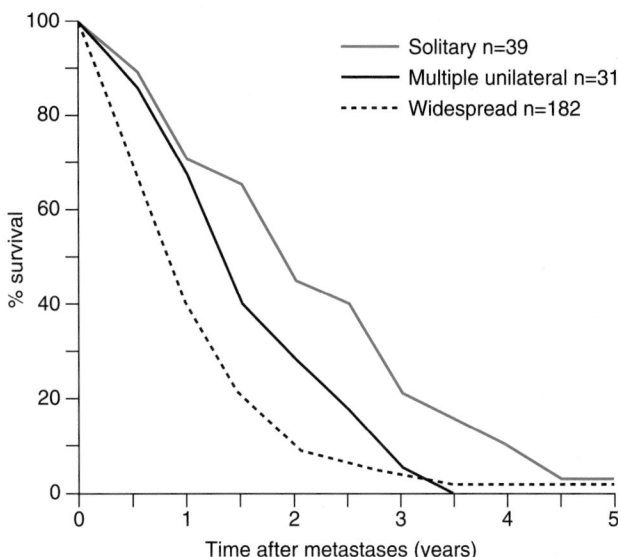

Figure 19-18 Survival rates of untreated patients with metastatic colorectal liver disease as a function of extent of disease at presentation as reported by Wagner and colleagues.[165]

hepatic metastases may present with systemic symptoms of weight loss, pain, fever, and jaundice, such symptoms generally correlate with advanced disease, which is rarely resectable. Most resectable lesions are identified by early detection through routine periodic radiologic surveillance or during the evaluation of abnormal laboratory parameters. Of the standard laboratory parameters obtained as part of liver function testing, elevation of the alkaline phosphatase level correlates best with the presence of hepatic metastases but is generally considered to be inadequate as a routine screening tool. Although elevation of a serum CEA level is not specific for colorectal malignancy, progressive elevation of serial CEA levels after resection of a primary colorectal malignancy indicates recurrent intraabdominal disease in most instances.[168]

Properly performed ultrasound has the capability of detecting lesions as small as 1 cm in diameter that is nearly equivalent to that obtained with CT or MRI but has the added advantages of convenience and reduced cost.[169,170] Ultrasound may be helpful in initiating the differentiation of cystic versus solid lesions and can determine whether the disease is unifocal or multifocal. Even with the most careful preoperative radiographic staging procedures, at least 40% of patients explored are found to have more extensive disease than predicted on the basis of extrahepatic disease or additional small observable liver metastases.[171,172] The application of IOUS with resolution to a level of at least 0.5 cm can further refine the ability to detect additional intrahepatic disease.[3] In our own experience, IOUS leads to modifications in operative planning in at least 30% of instances by identifying additional parenchymal lesions, precluding resection or requiring more extensive resection. IOUS has evolved into a routine diagnostic tool for the intraoperative staging of hepatic colorectal metastases and assumes additional importance in the application of cryosurgical ablation techniques.[173]

Patient Selection

Clearly, only a small subset of patients with colorectal liver metastases actually derive significant benefit from resection of hepatic metastases. Selection of patients for resectional therapy has evolved from the in-depth analysis of large groups of patients undergoing resection with curative intent. The Registry of Hepatic Metastases was created in an attempt to define the importance of various factors in predicting treatment outcome.[174–176] This multiinstitutional retrospective review includes data accumulated on 862 patients undergoing resection for metastatic colorectal carcinoma (Fig. 19-19). The factors associated with prognostic significance include stage of primary tumor, disease-free interval, involvement of hepatic resection margin, number of metastases, and regional lymph node involvement. More advanced Dukes stage of primary tumor with mesenteric nodal involvement confers reduced survival after resection of hepatic recurrence, although the reduction in survival is not significant enough to preclude resection. Patients undergoing resection of metastases within 1 month of colorectal resection achieved a 5-year survival rate of 24% as opposed to those resected more than 1 year after colectomy, in whom a 40% 5-year survival rate was achieved. Although this suggests slower growth rates in biologically less aggressive tumors, a short disease-free interval, including synchronous metastases, should not be a contraindication to resection. The importance of a clean margin of resection is emphasized by a 5-year survival rate of 44% in patients with a margin at least 1 cm as compared with 18% in patients with positive margins. Clearly, the attainment of a resection margin of at least 1 cm should be a major goal of all operative strategies. In general, available evidence suggests that fewer metastatic deposits are associated with better survival. No definitive limit on the number of metastases has been established, but the practical limit is considered to be four lesions if adequate disease-free margins can be obtained. The presence of extrahepatic disease either to regional (portal or celiac) nodes or distant sites is associated with markedly reduced survival as compared with patients resected with isolated hepatic metastases. This observation supports the contention that the surgery should be performed with curative intent rather than as a palliative treatment for prognostic improvement. Of importance are the factors that did not correlate with significant survival differences between groups: age, sex, size of largest metastases, distribution of metastases, or type of resection (anatomic versus wedge).

Surgical Factors

The importance of minimizing blood loss at the time of hepatic resection for metastases is emphasized by the fact that perioperative blood transfusion represents an independent prognostic factor adversely affecting patient survival.[177] Blood transfusion has previously been associated with a reduction in patient survival secondary to recurrent disease, presumably on the basis of transfusion-associated immunosuppression.[178] This suggests that blood conservation techniques, including preoperative autologous donation, intraoperative cell salvage systems, and vascular isolation techniques, may play an important role in eventual outcome after resection of hepatic metastases.

Although delayed resection of synchronous hepatic metastases found at the time of colorectal resection is routine in most centers, simultaneous liver resection may be carried out in selected instances with good results.[179] Such attempts at simultaneous resection should be limited to situations in which the hepatic lesions are accessible through an appropriate incision, situations that require limited resection, and situations with minimal blood loss or bowel contamination. Otherwise, recovery from the colorectal procedure with a period of observation and repeat CT or ultrasound imaging is recommended (Fig. 19-20). The development of additional

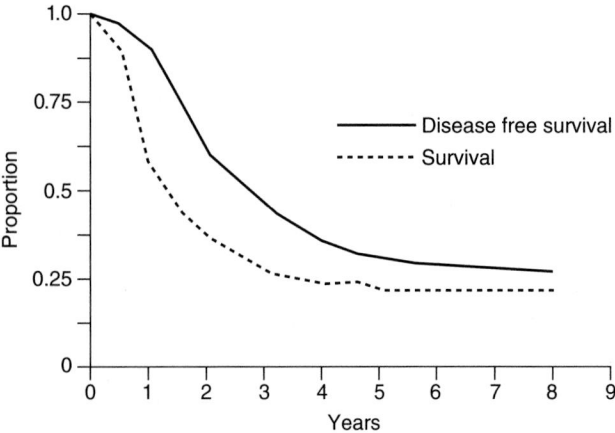

Figure 19-19 Overall survival of 862 patients undergoing resection for colorectal liver metastases as reported to the Registry of Hepatic Metastases.[175]

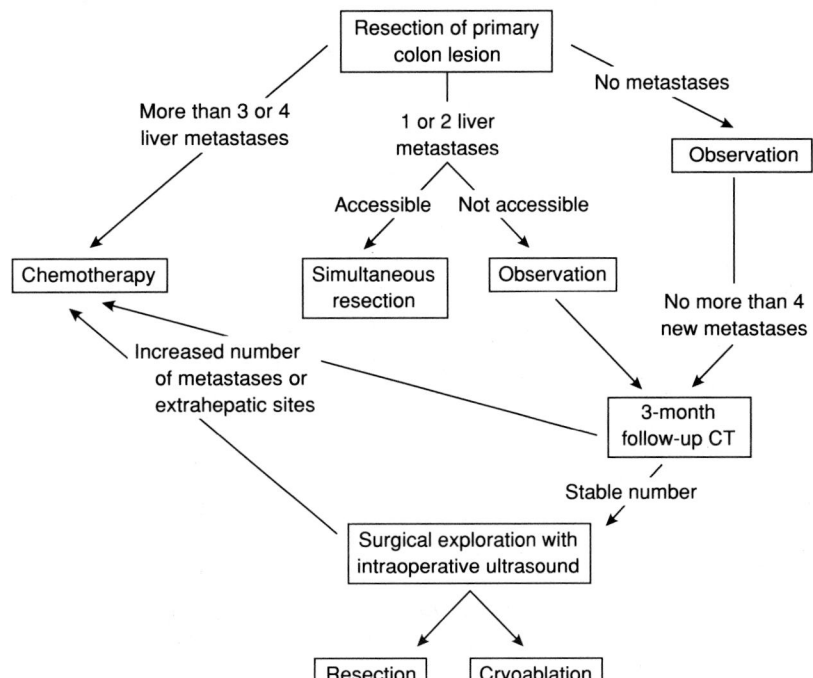

Figure 19-20 Algorithm for the management of hepatic colorectal metastases. IOUS, intraoperative ultrasonography.

intrahepatic or extrahepatic lesions during a 3-month period of observation suggests an aggressive biologic disease less likely to be controlled by resection. For patients presenting with liver metastases at prolonged intervals after the original colorectal resection, colonoscopy is recommended to evaluate for local anastomotic recurrence or the development of a metachronous primary cancer.

Cryosurgical Ablation

The liver is the most common site of recurrence after resection and probably reflects occult tumors not detected at the time of initial hepatic resection.[180] The routine use of IOUS may improve the ability to detect additional small metastases to allow inclusion in a wider resection or to allow more complete extirpation by resection or cryosurgical ablation. Broadly spaced lesions may require separate areas of hepatic resection to effect complete removal with relative preservation of remnant liver mass. Cryosurgical ablation techniques have evolved in an effort to allow the destruction of widely spaced or inconveniently located liver metastases while limiting the amount of normal liver resected or destroyed. It is also an attractive alternative for patients whose underlying medical condition precludes major resection. Cryosurgical ablation uses an ultrasound-guided, operatively placed probe with a core of circulating liquid nitrogen that freezes the lesion in situ, with resultant cell destruction and tissue

absorption. Limitations of the technique include the need for two 10- to 15-minute freeze cycles interspersed with 10-minute thaws, a practical lesion size limitation of 3 to 5 cm, the potential for biliary or vascular injury, and the occasional difficulty of proper probe alignment to encompass the entire lesion. The use of multiple adjacent probes can effect cryoablation of lesions as large as 10 to 12 cm but with reduced assurance of adequate margins. Although reported as a method of treatment for HCC, use of cryosurgical ablation has predominantly been in the management of metastatic liver diseases.[181] When employed as definitive treatment or in combination with resection for hepatic colorectal metastases, cryosurgery appears to demonstrate survival equivalent to that seen with resection alone.[182] Radiologic and serum tumor marker follow-up have shown disappearance of lesions on CT scan and a decrease in the serial serum tumor marker levels.[183,184] Although cryosurgery may be a useful adjunct to allow more complete surgical resection of scattered lesions, the need for complete operative exposure of the liver for probe placement and the time required for the cyclical freezing of multiple lesions limit the utility of the technique. Cryoablation should be considered an adjunctive tool limited to centers fully versed in the conventional methods of major hepatic resection. The development of percutaneous probes placed under ultrasound or laparoscopic guidance is an intriguing concept that may well be in our grasp with improving equipment design.

Infusional and Systemic Chemotherapy

Chemotherapeutic regimens for metastatic colorectal carcinoma are typically centered on the use of 5-fluorouracil alone or in combination with other agents.[185,186] Tumor response rates, however, are generally reported to be no better than 15% to 25%, with little incremental benefit in patient survival. Disappointment with the results of systemic chemotherapy for extensive hepatic metastases led to consideration of the regional delivery techniques to capitalize on the arterial inflow requirements of liver tumors. Design improvements in implantable mechanical delivery systems led to trials with the regional infusion of fluorodeoxyuridine through hepatic artery catheters in an effort to improve the response rate of unresectable colorectal metastases.[187,188] In a randomized trial comparing response rates with systemic versus regional infusion of fluorodeoxyuridine sponsored by the National Institutes of Health, intraarterial therapy had a 62% response rate as compared with 17% for the intravenous systemic group.[189] Nevertheless, 2-year survival rates were not significantly different at 22% and 15%, respectively. The arterial infusions were further associated with significant morbidity from biliary sclerosis, hepatitis, and gastric or duodenal ulceration. The improvement in tumor response with regional infusion was countered by the significant complications from catheter placement or drug toxicity. With little ability to extend life, regional infusion techniques are probably best reserved for patients with symptomatic liver-only disease refractory to systemic therapy. Rekindled enthusiasm for hepatic artery infusion techniques awaits the introduction of new therapeutic agents with demonstrable antitumor effectiveness.

REFERENCES

1. Wands JR, Blum HE. Primary hepatocellular carcinoma. (Editorial) N Engl J Med 1991;325:729.
2. Boring CC, Squires TS, Tong T, Montgomery S. Cancer Statistics, 1994. CA Cancer J Clin 1994;44:7.
3. Steele G, Ravikumar TS. Resection of hepatic metastases from colorectal cancer: biologic perspectives. Ann Surg 1989;210:127.
4. Okuda K. Clinical aspects of hepatocellular carcinoma: analysis of 134 cases. In: Okuda K, Peters RL, eds. Hepatocellular carcinoma. New York, John Wiley & Sons, 1976:387.
5. Liaw YF, Tai DI, Chen TJ, et al. Alpha-fetoprotein changes in the course of chronic hepatitis: relation to bridging hepatic fibrosis and hepatocellular carcinoma. Liver 1986;6:133.
6. Bloomer JR, Waldmann TA, McIntire KR, Klatskin G. Alpha-fetoprotein in non-neoplastic hepatic disorders. JAMA 1975;233:38.
7. Oka H, Kurioka N, Kim K, et al. Prospective study of early detection of hepatocellular carcinoma in patients with cirrhosis. Hepatology 1990;12:680.
8. Ebara M, Ohto M, Shinagawa T, et al. Natural history of minute hepatocellular carcinoma smaller than three centimeters complicating cirrhosis: a study in 22 patients. Gastroenterology 1986;90:289.
9. Wu JC, Lee SD, Hsaio KJ, et al. Mass screening of primary hepatocellular carcinoma by alpha-fetoprotein in a rural area of Taiwan: a dried blood spot method. Liver 1988;8:100.
10. Heyward WL, Lanier AP, McMahon BJ, et al. Early detection of primary hepatocellular carcinoma: screening for primary hepatocellular carcinoma among persons infected with hepatitis B virus. JAMA 1985;254:3052.
11. Cottone M, Turri M, Caltagirone M, et al. Early detection of hepatocellular carcinoma associated with cirrhosis by ultrasound and alpha-fetoprotein: a prospective study. Hepatogastroenterology 1988;35:101.
12. Kobayashi K, Sugimoto T, Makino H, et al. Screening methods for early detection of hepatocellular carcinoma. Hepatology 1985;5:1100.
13. Liaw YF, Tai DI, Chu CM, et al. Early detection of hepatocellular carcinoma in patients with chronic type B hepatitis: a prospective study. Gastroenterology 1986;90:263.
14. Di Bisceglie AM, Rustgi VK, Hoofnagle JH, et al. Hepatocellular carcinoma. NIH conference. Ann Intern Med 1988;108:390.
15. Tang ZY, Yu YQ, Zhou XD, et al. Surgery of small hepatocellular carcinoma: analysis of 144 cases. Cancer 1989;64:536.
16. Okuda H, Obata H, Nakanishi T, et al. Production of abnormal prothrombin (des-γ-carboxy prothrombin) by hepatocellular carcinoma: a clinical and experimental study. J Hepatol 1987;4:357.
17. Birnhaum BA, Weinreb JC, Megibow AJ. Definitive diagnosis of hepatic hemangiomas: MR imagery versus TcPP labelled red blood cell spect. Radiology 1990;176:95.
18. Shinagawa T, Ohto M, Kimura K, et al. Real-time ultrasonographic diagnosis of hepatocellular carcinoma: correlation of echograms and histopathological findings. Jpn J Gastroenterol 1981;78:2404.
19. Nakashima T, Kojiro M, Sakamoto K, Okida K, Shimokawa Y, Kudo Y. Studies of primary liver carcinoma. I. Proposal of new gross anatomical classification of primary liver cell carcinoma. Acta Hepatol Jpn 1974;15:279.
20. Okuda K, Musha H, Nakajima J, et al. Clinicopathologic features of encapsulated hepatocellular carcinoma: a study of 26 cases. Cancer 1977;40:1240.
21. Ohnishi K, Okuda K, Ohtsuki T, et al. Formation of hilar collaterals or cavernous transformation after portal vein obstruction by hepatocellular carcinoma: observation in ten patients. Gastroenterology 1984;87:1150.

22. Ochsner JL, Halpert B. Cavernous hemangiomas of the liver. Surgery 1958;43:577.

23. Bruneton JN, Drouillard J, Feneart D, et al. Ultrasonography of hepatic cavernous hemangiomas. Br J Radiol 1983;56:791.

24. Okuda K. Early recognition of hepatocellular carcinoma. Hepatology 1986;6:729.

25. Makuuchi M, Hasegawa H, Yamazaki S. Ultrasonically guided subsegmentectomy. Surg Gynecol Obstet 1985; 161:346.

26. Traynor O, Castaing D, Bismuth H. Preoperative ultrasonography in surgery of hepatic tumours. Br J Surg 1988;75:197.

27. Heiken JP, Weyman PJ, Lee JKT, et al. Detection of focal hepatic masses: prospective arterial portography and MR imaging. Radiology 1989;171:47.

28. Nelson RC, Chezmar JL, Sugarbaker PH, Bernardino ME. Hepatic tumors: comparison of CT during arterial portography, delayed CT and MR imaging for preoperative evaluation. Radiology 1989;172:27.

29. Peterson MS, Baron RL, Dod GD, et al. Hepatic parenchymal perfusion defects detected with CTAP: imaging-pathologic correlations. Radiology 1992;185:149.

30. Soyer P, Lacheheb D, Levesque M. False positive diagnoses based on CT portography: correlation with pathologic findings. AJR 1992;160:285.

31. Merine D, Takayasu K, Wakao F. Detection of hepatocellular carcinoma: comparison of CT during arterial portography with CT after intraarterial injection of Iodized oil. Radiology 1990;175:707.

32. Shimamura Y, Guven P, Takenaka Y, et al. Combined peripheral and central chemoembolization of liver tumors. Cancer 1988;61:238.

33. Merine D, Takayasu K, Wakao F. Detection of hepatocellular carcinoma: comparison of CT during arterial portography with CT after intraarterial injection of Iodized oil. Radiology 1990;175:707.

34. Ebara M, Ohto M, Watanabe Y, et al. Diagnosis of small hepatocellular carcinoma: correlation of MRI imaging and tumor histologic studies. Radiology 1986;159:371.

35. Finn JP, Longmaid HE, Edelman RR, et al. Portal MR venography: techniques and clinical applications. Dynamic Cardiovascular Imaging 1990;3:96.

36. Smith EH. Complications of percutaneous abdominal fine-needle biopsy. Radiology 1991;178:253.

37. Parkin DM, Stjernsward J, Muir CS. Estimates of the worldwide frequency of twelve major cancers. Bull WHO 1984;62:163.

38. Hadziyannis SJ. Hepatocellular carcinoma and type B hepatitis. Clin Gastroenterol 1980;9:117.

39. Cancer Statistics Review 1973-1986. National Cancer Institute, Bethesda, Maryland. NIH Publication 89-2789. May 1989.

40. Okuda K, Kojiro M, Okuda H. Neoplasms of the liver. In: Schiff L, Schiff ER, eds. Diseases of the liver. Philadelphia, JB Lippincott, 1993:1236.

41. Simonetti RG, Camma C, Fiorello F, et al. Hepatocellular carcinoma: a worldwide problem and the major risk factor. Dig Dis Sci 1991;36:962.

42. Zaman SN, Melia WM, Johnson RD, et al. Risk factors in development of hepatocellular carcinoma in cirrhosis: prospective study of 613 patients. Lancet 1985;1:1357.

43. Hoofnagle JH, Shafritz DA, Popper H. Chronic type B hepatitis and the "healthy" HBs Ag carrier state. Hepatology 1987;7:758.

44. Tsukuma H, Hiyama T, Tanaka S, et al. Risk factors for hepatocellular carcinoma among patients with chronic liver disease. N Engl J Med 1993;328:1797.

45. Trichopoulos D, McMahon B, Sparros L, Merikas G. Smoking and hepatitis B negative primary HCC. JNCI 1980;65:111.

46. Trichopoulos D, Gerety RJ, Sparros L, et al. Hepatitis B and primary HCC in an European population. Lancet 1978;2:1217.

47. Johnson PJ, Krasner N, Portmann B, Eddleston AL, Williams T. Hepatocellular carcinoma in Great Britain: influence of age, sex, HBsAg status and aetiology of underlying cirrhosis. Gut 1978;19:1022.

48. Beasley RP, Hwang LY, Linn CC, Chiens CS. HCC and hepatitis B virus: a prospective study of 22,707 men in Taiwan. Lancet 1981;2:1129.

49. Tsukuma H, Himaya T, Tanaka S, et al. Risk factors for hepatocellular carcinoma among patients with chronic liver disease. N Engl J Med 1993;328:1797.

50. Miyaji T, Imai S. Pathological studies on 639 cases of hepatoma autopsied in Japan during the 10 years from 1946 to 1955 inclusive. Acta Hepatol Jpn 1960;1:100.

51. Shikata T. Primary liver carcinoma and liver cirrhosis. In: Okuda K, Peters RL, eds. Hepatocellular carcinoma. New York, John Wiley & Sons, 1976:53.

52. Lee FI. Cirrhosis and hepatoma in alcoholics. Gut 1966;7:77.

53. Sherlock S, Fox RA, Niazi SP, Scheuer PJ. Chronic liver disease and primary liver-cell cancer with hepatitis-associated (Australia) antigen in serum. Lancet 1970;1:1243.

54. Shafritz DA, Shouval D, Sherman HI, Hadziyannis SJ, Kew MC. Integration of hepatitis B virus DNA into the genome of the liver cells in chronic liver disease and HCC: studies in percutaneous liver biopsies and postmortem tissue specimens. N Engl J Med 1981;305:1067.

55. Fowler MF, Greenfield C, Chu CM, et al. Integration of HBV-DNA may not be a prerequisite for the maintenance of the state of malignant transformation: an analysis of 110 liver biopsies. J Hepatol 1986;2:218.

56. Chen JY, Harrison TJ, Lee CS, Chen DS, Zuckerman AJ. Detection of hepatitis B virus DNA in HCC. Br J Exp Pathol 1986;67:279.

57. Imazeki F, Omata M, Yokosuka O, Okuda K. Integration of hepatitis B virus DNA in HCC. Cancer 1985;58:1055.

58. Kam W, Rall LB, Smuckler EA, et al. Hepatitis B viral DNA in liver and serum of asymptomatic carriers. Proc Natl Acad Sci USA. 1982;79:7522.

59. Yokusuka O, Omata M, Imakezi F, Ito Y, Okuda K. Hep-

atitis B virus RNA transcripts and DNA in chronic liver disease. N Engl J Med 1986;315:1187.

60. Suzuki K, Uchida T, Horiuchi R, Shikata T. Localization of hepatitis B surface and core antigens in human HCC by immunoperoxidase methods: replications of complete virios of carcinoma cells. Cancer 1985;56:321.

61. Okuda H, Obata H, Motoike Y, et al. Hepatocellular carcinoma (HCC) presumably associated with non-B hepatitis virus infection: clinical and pathological observations. Hepatology 1982;2:113.

62. Okuda K, Fujimoto I, Hanai A, et al. Changing incidence of HCC in Japan. Cancer Res 1987;47:4967.

63. Leung NWY, Tam JS, Lai JY, et al. Does hepatitis C virus infection contribute to HCC in Hong Kong? Cancer 1992;70:40.

64. Kew MC, Houghton M, Choo QL, Kuo G. Hepatitis C virus antibodies in Southern African blacks with HCC. Lancet 1990;335:873.

65. Colombo M, De Franchis R, Del Ninno E, et al. HCC in Italian patients with cirrhosis. N Engl J Med 1991;325:675.

66. Hasan F, Jeffers LJ, De Medina M, et al. Hepatitis C-associated HCC. Hepatology 1990;12:589.

67. Gokel JM, Liebezeit E, Eder M. Hemangiosarcoma and HCC of the liver following vinyl chloride exposure. Virchows Arch Path Anat 1976;372:1195.

68. Linsell CA. Environmental carcinogens and liver cancer. In: Lapis K, Johannessen JV, eds. Liver carcinogenesis. Washington DC, Hemisphere 1979.

69. Klatskin G. Hepatic tumors: possible relationship to use of oral contraceptives. Gastroenterology 1977;73:386.

70. Henderson BE, Preston Martin S, Edmondson HA, et al. HCC and oral contraceptives. Br J Cancer 1983;48:437.

71. Naccarato R, Farinati F. HCC, alcohol and cirrhosis: facts and hypothesis. Dig Dis Sci 1991;36:1137.

72. Lieber CS, Garro AJ, Leo MA, et al. Alcohol and cancer. Hepatology 1986;6:1005.

73. Leo MA, Lieber CS. Hepatic vitamin A depletion in alcoholic liver injury in man. N Engl J Med 1982;307:597.

74. Bernstein IM, Webster KE, William RC Jr, Strikland RG. Reduction in circulating T lymphocytes in alcoholic liver disease. Lancet 1974;2:488.

75. Ohnishi K, Lida S, Iwama S, et al. The effect of chronic habitual alcohol intake on the development of liver cirrhosis and hepatocellular carcinoma: relation to hepatitis B surface antigen carriage. Cancer 1982;49:672.

76. Bruix J, Barrera JM, Calvet X, et al. Prevalence of antibodies to hepatitis C virus in Spanish patients with HCC and hepatic cirrhosis. Lancet 1989;2:1004.

77. Pares A, Barrera JM, Caballerian J, et al. Hepatitis C virus antibodies in chronic alcoholic patients: association with severity of liver injury. Hepatology 1990;12:1295.

78. Yamauchi M, Nakahara M, Maezawa Y, et al. Prevalence of hepatocellular carcinoma in patients with alcoholic cirrhosis and prior exposure to hepatitis C. Am J Gastroenterol 1993;88:39.

79. Mendenhall CL, Seef L, Diehl AM, et al. Antibodies to hepatitis B virus and hepatitis C virus in alcoholic hepa-

titis and cirrhosis: their prevalence and clinical relevance. Hepatology 1991;14:581.

80. Scudamore CH, Ragaz J, Kluftinger AM, Owen DA. Hepatocellular carcinoma: a comparison of Oriental and Caucasian patients. Am J Surg 1988;155:659.

81. Franco D, Capussotti L, Smadjac, et al. Resection of hepatocellular carcinoma: results in 72 European patients with cirrhosis. Gastroenterology 1990;98:733.

82. Chlebowski RT, Tong M, Weissman J, et al. Hepatocellular carcinoma: diagnostic and prognostic features in North American patients. Cancer 1984;53:2701.

83. Ihde DC, Sherlock P, Winawer SJ, et al. Clinical manifestations of hepatoma. Am J Med 1974;56:83.

84. Cady B. Natural history of primary and secondary tumors of the liver. Semin Oncol 1983;10:127.

85. Lai CL, Lam KC, Wong KP, et al. Clinical features of hepatocellular carcinoma: review of 211 patients in Hong Kong. Cancer 1981;47:2746.

86. Kew MC, Geddes EW. Hepatocellular carcinoma in rural Southern African blacks. Medicine 1982;61:98.

87. Okuda K. Primary liver cancers in Japan. Cancer 1980;45:2663.

88. Calvet X, Bruix J, Bru C, et al. Natural history of hepatocellular carcinoma in Spain: five years' experience in 249 cases. J Hepatol 1990;10:311.

89. Ong GB, Taw JL. Spontaneous rupture of hepatocellular carcinoma. Br Med J 1972;4:146.

90. Nakashima T. Vascular changes and hemodynamics in hepatocellular carcinoma. In: Okuda K, Peter RL, eds. Hepatocellular carcinoma. New York, John Wiley & Sons, 1976:169.

91. Cooney TG, Bauer DC, Knaver CM. Portal hypertension associated with hepatocellular carcinoma with cirrhosis. Am J Gastroenterol 1980;74:436.

92. Edmondson HA, Craig JR. Neoplasms of the liver. In: Schiff L, Schiff ER, eds. Diseases of the liver, ed 6. Philadelphia, JB Lippincott, 1987:1109.

93. Shinagawa T, Ohto M, Kimura K, et al. Diagnosis and clinical features of small hepatocellular carcinoma with emphasis on the utility of real-time ultrasonography: a study of 51 patients. Gastroenterology 1984;86:495.

94. Sheu JC, Sung JL, Chen DS, et al. Early detection of hepatocellular carcinoma by real-time ultrasonography: a prospective study. Cancer 1985;56:660.

95. Cottone M, Virdone R, Fusco G, et al. Asymptomatic hepatocellular carcinoma in Child's A cirrhosis: a comparison of natural history and surgical treatment. Gastroenterology 1989;96:1566.

96. Sheu JC, Sung JL, Chen DS, et al. Growth rate of asymptomatic hepatocellular carcinoma and its clinical implications. Gastroenterology 1985;89:259.

97. Colombo M. Hepatocellular carcinoma in cirrhotics. Semin Liver Dis 1993;13:374.

98. Okuda K, Ohtsuki T, Obata H, et al. Natural history of hepatocellular carcinoma and prognosis in relation to treatment: study of 850 patients. Cancer 1985;56:1985.

99. Okuda K. Primary liver cancers in Japan. Cancer 1980;45:2663.

100. Liver Cancer Study Group of Japan. Primary liver cancer in Japan: clinicopathologic features and results of surgical treatment. Ann Surg 1990;211:277.

101. Franco D, Capussotti L, Smadjac, et al. Resection of hepatocellular carcinoma: results in 72 European patients with cirrhosis. Gastroenterology 1990;98:733.

102. Adson MA. Primary hepatocellular cancers: Western experience. In: Blumgart LH, ed. Surgery of the liver and biliary tract. London, Churchill Livingstone, 1988:1153.

103. Iwatsuki S, Klintmalm GB, Starzl TE. Total hepatectomy and liver replacement (orthotopic liver transplantation) for primary hepatic malignancy. World J Surg 1982;6:81.

104. Jenkins RL, Pinson CW, Stone MD. Experience with transplantation in the treatment of liver cancer. Cancer Chemother Pharmacol 1989;23(Suppl):S104.

105. Haug CE, Jenkins RL, Rohrer RJ, et al. Liver transplantation for primary hepatic cancer. Transplantation 1992;53:376.

106. OGrady JG, Polson RJ, Rolles K, et al. Liver transplantation for malignant disease: results in 93 consecutive patients. Ann Surg 1988;207:373.

107. Pichlmayr R. Is there a place for liver grafting for malignancy? Transplant Proc 1988;20(Suppl 1):478.

108. Moreno Gonzalez E, Gomez R, Garcia I, et al. Liver transplantation in malignant primary hepatic neoplasms. Am J Surg 1992;163:395.

109. Bismuth H, Chiche L, Adam R, et al. Liver resection versus transplantation for hepatocellular carcinoma in cirrhotic patients. Ann Surg 1993;218:145.

110. Iwatsuki S, Starzl TE, Sheahan DG, et al. Hepatic resection versus transplantation for hepatocellular carcinoma. Ann Surg 1991;214:221.

111. Ringe B, Pichlmayr R, Wittekind C, Tusch G. Surgical treatment of hepatocellular carcinoma: experience with liver resection and transplantation in 198 patients. World J Surg 1991;15:270.

112. Stone MJ, Klintmalm GB, Polter D, et al. Neoadjuvant chemotherapy and liver transplantation for hepatocellular carcinoma: a pilot study in 20 patients. Gastroenterology 1993;104:196.

113. Carr BI, Selby R, Madariaga J, et al. Prolonged survival after liver transplantation and cancer chemotherapy for advanced-stage hepatocellular carcinoma. Transplant Proc 1993;25:1128.

114. Falkson G, Moertel CG, Levin P, et al. Chemotherapy studies in primary liver cancer. Cancer 1978;42:2149.

115. Choi TK, Lee NW, Wong J. Chemotherapy for advanced hepatocellular carcinoma. Cancer 1984;53:401.

116. Ravoet C, Gerard B. Non-surgical treatment of hepatocarcinoma. J Surg Oncol 1993;3(Suppl):104.

117. Daly JM, Kemeny N, Oberman P, et al. Long term hepatic arterial infusion chemotherapy. Anatomic considerations, operative technique, and treatment morbidity. Arch Surg 1984;119:936.

118. Yamada R, Sato M, Kawabata M, et al. Hepatic artery embolization in 120 patients with unresectable hepatoma. Radiology 1983;148:397.

119. Patt YZ, Chuang VP, Wallace S, et al. Hepatic arterial chemotherapy and occlusion for palliation of primary hepatocellular and unknown primary neoplasms in the liver. Cancer 1983;51:1359.

120. Ohnishi K, Tsuchiya S, Nakayama T, et al. Arterial chemoembolization of hepatocellular carcinoma with mitomycin C microcapsules. Radiology 1984;152:51.

121. Shibata J, Fujiyama S, Sato T, et al. Hepatic arterial chemotherapy with cisplatin suspended in an oily lymphographic agent for hepatocellular carcinoma. Cancer 1989;64:1586.

122. Kanematsu T, Furuta T, Takenaka K, et al. A 5-year experience of lipiodolization: selective regional chemotherapy for 200 patients with hepatocellular carcinoma. Hepatology 1989;10:98.

123. Takayasu K, Shima Y, Muramatsu Y, et al. Hepatocellular carcinoma: treatment with intraarterial iodized oil with and without chemotherapeutic agents. Radiology 1987;162:345.

124. Yamada R, Kishi K, Sonomura T, et al. Transcatheter arterial embolization in unresectable hepatocellular carcinoma. Cardiovasc Intervent Radiol 1990;13:135.

125. Hsieh M, Chang W, Wang L, et al. Treatment of hepatocellular carcinoma by transcatheter arterial chemoembolization and analysis of prognostic factors. Cancer Chemother Pharmacol 1992;31(Suppl I):S82.

126. Stuart K, Stokes K, Jenkins R, et al. Treatment of Hepatocellular carcinoma using doxorubicin/ethiodized oil/gelatin powder chemoembolization. Cancer 1993;72:3202.

127. Sugiura N, Takara K, Ohoto M, et al. Percutaneous intratumoral injection of ethanol under ultrasound imaging for treatment of small hepatocellular carcinoma. Acta Hepatol Jpn 1983;24:920.

128. Shiina S, Tagawa K, Unuma T, et al. Percutaneous ethanol injection therapy for hepatocellular carcinoma: a histological study. Cancer 1991;68:1524.

129. Shiina S, Tagawa K, Niwa Y, et al. Percutaneous ethanol injection therapy for hepatocellular carcinoma: results in 146 patients. AJR 1993;160:1023.

130. Okuda K. Intratumoral injection. J Surg Oncol 1993;3(Suppl):97.

131. Livraghi T, Bolondi L, Lazzaroni S, et al. Percutaneous ethanol injection in the treatment of hepatocellular carcinoma in cirrhosis: a study on 207 patients. Cancer 1992;69:925.

132. Edmondson HA. Differential diagnosis of tumors and tumor-like lessions of the liver in infancy and childhood. Am J Dis Child 1956;91:168.

133. Soreide O, Czerniak A, Bradpiece H, et al. Characteristics of fibrolamellar hepatocellular carcinoma: a study of nine cases and a review of the literature. Am J Surg 1986;151:518.

134. Francis IR, Agha FP, Thompson NW, Karen DF. Fibrolamellar hepatocarcinoma: clinical, radiologic and

pathologic features. Gastrointestinal Radiol 1986;11:67.

135. Berman MM, Libbey NP, Foster JH. Hepatocellular carcinoma: polygonal cell type with fibrous stroma—an atypical variant with a favorable prognosis. Cancer 1980;46:1448.

136. Farhi DC, Shikes RH, Murari PJ, Silverg SG. Hepatocellular carcinoma in young people. Cancer 1983;52:1516.

137. Vecchio FM, Fabiano A, Ghirlanda G, et al. Fibrolamellar carcinoma of the liver: the malignant counterpart of focal nodular hyperplasia with oncocytic change. Am J Clin Pathol 1984;81:521.

138. Craig JR, Peters RL, Edmonson HA, Omata M. Fibrolamellar carcinoma of the liver: a tumor of adolescents and young adults with distinctive clinicopathologic features. Cancer 1980;46:372.

139. Adam R, Gibson RN, Soreide O, et al. The radiology of fibrolamellar hepatoma. Clin Radiol 1986;37:355.

140. Nagorney DM, Adson MA, Weiland LH, et al. Fibrolamellar hepatoma. Am J Surg 1985;149:113.

141. Chuong JJ, Livesstone EM, Barwick KW. The histologic and clinical indicators of prognosis in hepatoma. J Clin Gastroenterol 1982;4:547.

142. Penn I. Hepatic transplantation for primary and metastatic cancers of the liver. Surgery 1991;110:726.

143. Weinberg AG, Finegold MJ. Primary hepatic tumors of childhood. Hum Pathol 1983;14:512.

144. Dachman AH, Pakter RL, Ros PR, et al. Hepatoblastoma: radiologic-pathologic correlation in 50 cases. Radiology 1987;164:15.

145. Lack E, Neave C, Vawter GF. Hepatoblastoma: a clinical and pathologic study of 54 cases. Am J Surg Pathol 1982;6:693.

146. Kasai M, Watanabe I. Histologic classification of liver cell carcinoma in infancy and childhood and its clinical evaluation. Cancer 1970;25:551.

147. Stocker JT, Ishak KG. Undifferentiated embryonal sarcoma: report of 31 cases. Cancer 1978;42:365.

148. Haas JE, Muczynski KA, Krailo M, et al. Histopathology and prognosis in childhood hepatoblastoma and hepatocarcinoma. Cancer 1989;64:1082.

149. Douglass EC, Reynolds M, Finegold M, et al. Cisplatin, vincristine and fluorouracil therapy for hepatoblastoma: a Pediatric Oncology Group study. J Clin Oncol 1993;11:96.

150. Feusner JH, Krailo MD, Haas JE, et al. Treatment of pulmonary metastases of initial stage I hepatoblastoma in childhood: report from the Children's Cancer Group. Cancer 1993;71:859.

151. Klatskin G. Adenocarcinoma of the hepatic duct at its bifurcation within the porta hepatis: an unusual tumor with distinctive clinical and pathological features. Am J Med 1965;38:241.

152. Edmundson H, Steiner PE. Primary carcinoma of the liver: a study of 100 cases among 48,900 necropsies. Cancer 1954;7:462.

153. Belamaric J. Intrahepatic bile duct carcinoma and C. sinenesis infection in Hong Kong. Cancer 1973;31:468.

154. Nakanuma Y, Terada T, Tanaka Y, et al. Are hepaticolithiasis and cholangioma aetiologically related? A morphological study of 12 cases of hepaticolithiasis associated with cholangiocarcinoma. Virchows Arch 1985;406:45.

155. Smoron G, Battifora H. Thorotrast-induced hepatoma. Cancer 1972;20:1252.

156. Ishak KG, Willis GW, Cummins SD, et al. Biliary cystadenoma and cystadenocarcinoma: report of 14 cases and review of the literature. Cancer 1977;38:322.

157. Lewis WD, Jenkins RL, Rossi RL, et al. Surgical treatment of biliary cystadenoma: a report of 15 cases. Arch Surg 1988;123:563.

158. Ito Y, Kojiro M, Nakashima T, Takesaburo M. Pathomorphologic characteristic of 102 cases of Thorotrast related hepatocellular carcinoma, cholangiocarcinoma and hepatic angiosarcoma. Cancer 1988;62:1153.

159. Holcomb GW, O'Neill JA, Mahboubi S. Experience with hepatic hemangioendothelioma in infancy and childhood. J Pediatr Surg 1988;23:661.

160. Ishak KG, Sesterhenn IA, Goodman ZD, et al. Epithelioid hemangioendothelioma of the liver: a clinicopathologic and followup study of 32 cases. Hum Pathol 1984;15:839.

161. Radin R, Craig J, Colletti PM, et al. Hepatic epithelioid hemangioendothelioma. Radiology 1988:169:145.

162. Marino IR, Todo A, Tzakis A, et al. Treatment of hepatic epithelioid hemangioendothelioma with liver transplantation. Cancer 1988;62:2079.

163. Wolf RF, Goodnight JE, Krag DE, et al. Results of resection and proposed guidelines for patient selection in instances of noncolorectal hepatic metastases. Surg Gynecol Obstet 1991;173:454.

164. McEntee GP, Nagorney DM, Kvols LK, et al. Cytoreductive surgery for neuroendocrine tumors. Surgery 1990;108:1091.

165. Wagner JS, Adson MA, Van Heerden JA, et al. The natural history of hepatic metastases from colorectal cancer: a comparison with resective treatment. Ann Surg 1984;199:502.

166. Sugarbaker PH, Gianola FJ, Dwyer A, et al. A simplified plan for follow-up of patients with colon and rectal cancer supported by prospective studies of laboratory and radiologic test results. Surgery 1987;102:79.

167. Fantini GA, DeCosse JJ. Surveillance strategies after resection of carcinoma of the colon and rectum. Surg Gynecol Obstet 1990;171:267.

168. Kemeny MM, Sugarbaker PH, Smith TJ, et al. A prospective analysis of laboratory tests and imaging studies to detect hepatic lesions. Ann Surg 1982;195:163.

169. Ward BA, Miller DL, Frank JA, et al. Prospective evaluation of hepatic imaging studies in the detection of colorectal metastases: correlation with surgical findings. Surgery 1989;105:180.

170. Vlachos L, Trakadas S, Gouliamos A, et al. Comparative study between ultrasound, computed tomography, in-

tra-arterial digital subtraction angiography, and magnetic resonance imaging in the differentiation of tumors of the liver. Gastrointest Radiol 1990;15:102.

171. Steele G Jr, Osteen RT, Wilson RE, et al. Patterns of failure after surgical cure of large liver tumors. Am J Surg 1984;147:554.

172. Steele G Jr, Bleday R, Mayer RJ, et al. A prospective evaluation of hepatic resection for colorectal carcinoma metastases to the liver: Gastrointestinal Tumor Study Group protocol 6584. J Clin Oncol 1991;9:1105.

173. Ravikumar TS, Kane R, Cady C, et al. A five year study of cryosurgery in the treatment of liver tumors. Arch Surg 1991;126:1520.

174. Hughes KS, Simon R, Songhorabedi S, et al. Resection of the liver for colorectal carcinoma metastases: a multi-institutional study of patterns of recurrence. Surgery 1986;100:278.

175. Registry of Hepatic Metastases. Resection of the liver for colorectal carcinoma metastases: a multi-institutional study of indications for resection. Surgery 1988;103:278.

176. Hughes KS, Scheele J, Sugarbaker PH. Surgery for colorectal carcinoma metastatic to the liver: optimizing the results of treatment. Surg Clin North Am 1989;69:339.

177. Stephenson KR, Steinberg SM, Hughes KS, et al. Perioperative blood transfusions are associated with decreased time to recurrence and decreased survival after resection of colorectal liver metastases. Ann Surg 1988;208:679.

178. Francis DM, Judson RT. Blood transfusion and recurrence of cancer of the colon and rectum. Br J Surg 1987;74:26.

179. Vogt P, Raab B, Ringe B, et al. Resection of synchronous liver metastases from colorectal cancer. World J Surg 1991;15:62.

180. Stone MD, Cady B, Jenkins RL, et al. Surgical therapy for recurrent liver metastases from colorectal cancer. Arch Surg 1990;125:718.

181. Zhou X, Zhou T, Yu Y, Ma A. Clinical evaluation of cryosurgery in the treatment of primary liver cancer. Cancer 1988;61:1889.

182. Ravikumar TS, Kane R, Cady B, et al. A five year study of cryosurgery in the therapy of liver tumors. Arch Surg 1991;126:1520.

183. Ravikumar TS, Kane R, Cady B, et al. Hepatic cryosurgery with intraoperative ultrasound monitoring for metastatic colon carcinoma. Arch Surg 1987;122:403.

184. Charnley RM, Doran J, Morris DL. Cryotherapy for liver metastases: a new approach. Br J Surg 1989;76:1040.

185. O'Connell MJ. A phase III trial of 5-fluorouracil and leucovorin in the treatment of advanced colorectal cancer. Cancer 1989;63:1026.

186. Valone F, Friedman M, Wittlinger P, et al. Treatment of patients with advanced colorectal carcinoma with fluorouracil alone, high-dose leucovorin plus fluorouracil, or sequential methotrexate, fluorouracil, and leucovorin. J Clin Oncol 1989;7:1427.

187. Sterchi JM. Hepatic artery infusion for metastatic neoplastic disease. Surg Gynecol Obstet 1985;160:477.

188. Kemeny N, Daly J. Intrahepatic or systemic infusion of fluorodeoxyuridine in patients with liver metastases from colorectal carcinoma. Ann Intern Med 1987;107:459.

189. Chang AE, Schneider PD, Sugarbaker PH, et al. Prospective randomized trial of regional versus systemic continuous 5-fluorodeoxyuridine chemotherapy in the treatment of colorectal liver metastases. Ann Surg 1987;206:685.

20

Portal Hypertension

Layton F. Rikkers | *J. Michael Henderson*

Digestive Tract Surgery: A Text and Atlas, edited by Richard H. Bell,
Layton F. Rikkers, and Michael W. Mulholland.
Lippincott-Raven Publishers, Philadelphia, © 1996.

ANATOMY, PATHOPHYSIOLOGY, AND ETIOLOGY

The liver receives its blood supply from dual sources—the portal vein and the hepatic artery. The portal vein is formed beneath the pancreas by the confluence of the superior mesenteric and splenic veins (Fig. 20-1). It courses to the liver as the most dorsal component of the hepatic triad and divides into main right and left branches in the hepatic hilum. Between its confluence and its division into right and left branches, the portal vein is about 6 to 8 cm in length. The left gastric or coronary vein drains the lesser curvature of the stomach and may enter directly the portal vein, the splenic vein, or the confluence of these two vessels. This tributary of the portal venous system assumes particular importance in portal hypertension because it forms the major connection between the portal vein and the esophageal and gastric variceal complex.

The common hepatic artery normally is one of three major branches of the celiac axis, lying in the hepatoduodenal ligament ventral to the portal vein and medial to the common bile duct. Hepatic arterial anatomy can be variable, with the major alterations consisting of origin of the left hepatic artery from the left gastric artery (about 20%) and origin of the right hepatic artery from the superior mesenteric artery (about 20%). The latter variation is of importance to the surgeon because it results in a position of the right hepatic artery lateral rather than medial to the portal vein, potentially interfering with mobilization of the portal vein when it is used in a portosystemic shunt operation.

The portal vein and hepatic artery contribute two thirds and one third, respectively, to the total hepatic blood flow, which approximates 25% of the cardiac output. Portal venous flow is passively controlled; alterations in flow are caused by vasoconstriction or vasodilation of the splanchnic arterial bed, rather than portal venous tributaries. Hepatic arterial flow is regulated primarily through the hepatic artery buffer response to changes in portal venous flow. A decrease in portal venous flow results in an increase in hepatic artery flow, and vice versa. This response is more potent than the direct influence of circulating catecholamines and the sympathetic nervous system, and helps to maintain total hepatic blood flow as near to normal as possible, even in shock, and in the face of intense vasoconstrictive influences.[1]

The relative contributions of portal venous and hepatic arterial components to total hepatic blood flow are of significance because portal venous blood contains hepatotrophic hormones, which are essential to maintaining normal hepatic structure, function, and capacity for liver regeneration.[2] Thus, when an increase in hepatic arterial perfusion compensates for diminished or absent portal venous flow, hepatic atrophy and subsequent failure can develop, even when total hepatic blood flow is maintained at a near-normal level.

Portal hypertension is present when the difference between portal venous pressure and hepatic venous pressure (the portohepatic venous gradient) is greater than 8 mmHg. Although increased resistance to portal venous flow generally is the initiator of portal hypertension, this pathophysiologic state usually is perpetuated and sustained by both the elevated resistance and an increased splanchnic blood flow.[3] The cause of the splanchnic hyperemia in portal hypertension is incompletely understood.

The site of increased resistance to portal venous flow serves as the basis for the classification of portal

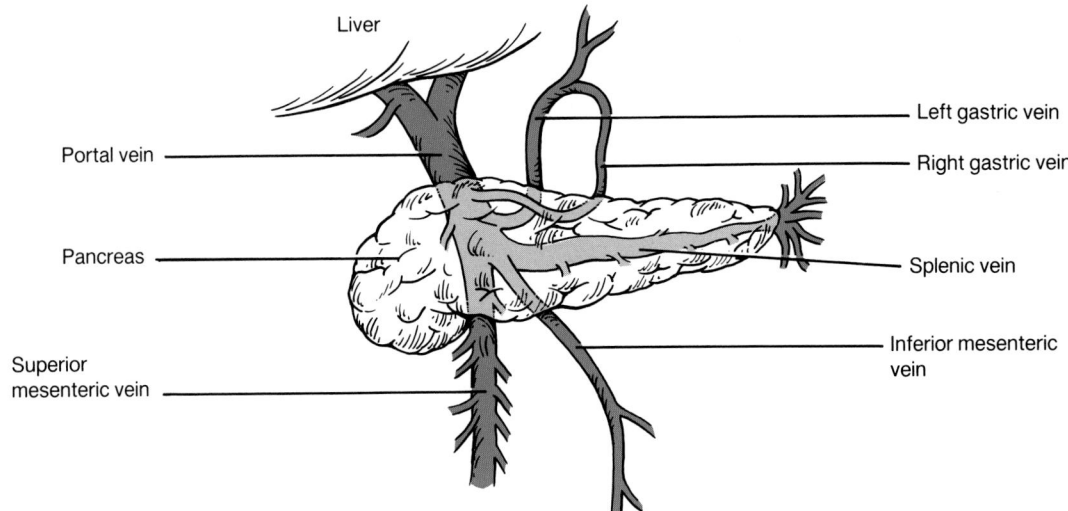

Figure 20-1 The extrahepatic portal venous circulation.

hypertension (Table 20-1). Rarely, elevated portal venous flow is the initiator of portal hypertension, with the development of increased intrahepatic portal venous resistance being a secondary phenomenon. Examples include splanchnic arteriovenous fistulas and "primary" portal hypertension (Banti's syndrome). Increased resistance in the extrahepatic portal venous system (portal vein thrombosis and cavernomatous transformation) accounts for about half of pediatric cases of portal hypertension but is considerably less common in adults. An interesting entity is "left-sided portal hypertension" caused by isolated splenic vein thrombosis.[4] In this situation, the elevated venous pressure is confined to the gastrosplenic venous circulation, and can be eliminated by removal of the spleen. In contrast to most intrahepatic and posthepatic causes of portal hypertension, prehepatic portal hypertension usually is associated with normal hepatic functional reserve; therefore, if bleeding varices can be prevented or controlled, this type of portal hypertension should not compromise long-term survival.

The most common causes of portal hypertension are intrahepatic. Although schistosomiasis is uncommon in North America, it is the most frequent cause of portal hypertension worldwide. Early in the course of most types of nonalcoholic cirrhosis, the major site of increased resistance is presinusoidal, with sinusoidal and postsinusoidal components contributing later in the course of these diseases. The pathophysiology that leads to alcoholic cirrhosis is complex, and results in increased resistance to portal venous flow at the sinusoidal and postsinusoidal levels. This is the most common cause of portal hypertension in the Western world.

All the causes of posthepatic portal hypertension are relatively uncommon.

Whatever the underlying cause, an elevated portal venous pressure is the major stimulus to portosystemic collateralization. Major collateral pathways tend to develop wherever the portal venous and systemic venous circulations are in close apposition (Fig. 20-2). This collateralization results in several of the clinical manifestations of portal hypertension, such as variceal hemorrhage, caput medusae, and hemorrhoids.

DIAGNOSIS AND EVALUATION

Key elements in the assessment of patients with suspected portal hypertension are determination of the cause of portal hypertension, estimation of hepatic functional reserve, evaluation of splanchnic and hepatic hemodynamic status and anatomy, and identification of the site of gastrointestinal hemorrhage, if present.

The first step is a complete history and physical examination. Patients should be interviewed carefully about any history of liver disease, pancreatic disease (splenic vein thrombosis), or gastrointestinal hemorrhage, as well as the presence of other complications of portal hypertension, such as encephalopathy and ascites. The physical examination should be directed at detecting the presence of chronic liver disease or portal hypertension, ascites, and impairment of mental status. Subtle signs of underlying liver disease are spider angiomas (usually on the upper part of the body), palmar erythema, gynecomastia, and testicular atrophy. Visible abdominal wall veins or a palpable spleen are indicative of underlying portal hyperten-

Table 20-1   Causes of Portal Hypertension

Category	Diseases	Frequency	Comments
Prehepatic	Portal vein thrombosis	Uncommon in adults; frequent cause in children	Common causes in adults—malignancy, pancreatitis, and cirrhosis; common causes in children—umbilical vein catheter, umbilical sepsis, and idiopathic (may present as cavernous transformation)
	Splenic vein thrombosis	Uncommon	Pancreatitis most common cause; left-sided portal hypertension only; splenectomy curative
	Splanchnic arteriovenous fistula	Rare	Portal hypertension due to increased portal flow
Intrahepatic			
Presinusoidal	Schistosomiasis	Common	Most common cause of portal hypertension worldwide
	Myeloproliferative diseases	Uncommon	Increased resistance to portal flow caused by hepatic myeloid metaplasia
	Congenital hepatic fibrosis	Rare	Usually present in children
	Nonalcoholic cirrhosis	Common	Increased resistance is presinusoidal in early stages of some types of nonalcoholic cirrhosis (eg, primary biliary cirrhosis)
Sinusoidal	Alcoholic cirrhosis	Common	Most common cause in the United States; may have postsinusoidal component
	Nonalcoholic cirrhosis	Common	Posthepatitic (hepatitis B and C) most common; may be presinusoidal in early stages
Postsinusoidal	Alcoholic cirrhosis	Common	Both sinusoidal and postsinusoidal
	Nonalcoholic cirrhosis	Common	May have increased resistance at all three intrahepatic levels
Posthepatic	Hepatic vein or inferior vena cava thrombosis (Budd-Chiari syndrome)	Uncommon	Common causes are myeloproliferative diseases and malignancy
	Constrictive pericarditis	Rare	
	Right heart failure	Uncommon	Although a common problem, infrequently causes portal hypertension

(Rikkers LF. Portal hypertension. In: Levine BA, ed. Current practice of surgery, vol 3. New York, Churchill Livingstone, 1993:4)

sion. A cirrhotic liver can be large or small, but when palpable, the edge usually is firm and nodular. Although advanced ascites presents with a distended abdomen with a positive fluid wave, lesser degrees of this complication can be detected by careful percussion for shifting dullness. A complete mental status examination and assessment for asterixis (liver flap) are essential. A normal physical examination in a patient with probable portal hypertension (eg, bleeding varices detected on upper gastrointestinal endoscopy) should make the examiner suspicious of a prehepatic or presinusoidal cause of the portal hypertension.

Important laboratory tests in patients with portal hypertension include a complete blood count, platelet count, coagulation profile, tests of liver function, hepatitis serology, serum electrolyte levels, and tests of renal function. Hypersplenism secondary to portal hypertension can be manifested by anemia, leukopenia, or thrombocytopenia. Although one or more of these components frequently are present in patients with portal hypertension, they

rarely are clinically significant. Because many of the coagulation factors are synthesized by the liver, portal hypertension secondary to liver disease often is accompanied by a prolonged prothrombin time. A depressed serum albumin level may be indicative of chronic liver disease, whereas elevation of hepatocellular enzyme, aspartate aminotransferase, or alanine aminotransferase level suggests ongoing liver cell necrosis secondary to hepatitis (viral, alcoholic, or other). Hyperbilirubinemia can be the result of intrahepatic or extrahepatic cholestasis, decreased hepatic functional reserve, or massive blood transfusions. Common serum electrolyte abnormalities in patients with cirrhosis are hyponatremia, hypokalemia, and metabolic alkalosis. An elevated blood urea nitrogen level may indicate blood in the intestinal tract, prerenal azotemia, or the hepatorenal syndrome.

When the diagnosis is in doubt and the clinical situation permits, a percutaneous liver biopsy can be an important part of the evaluation. However, this diagnostic test

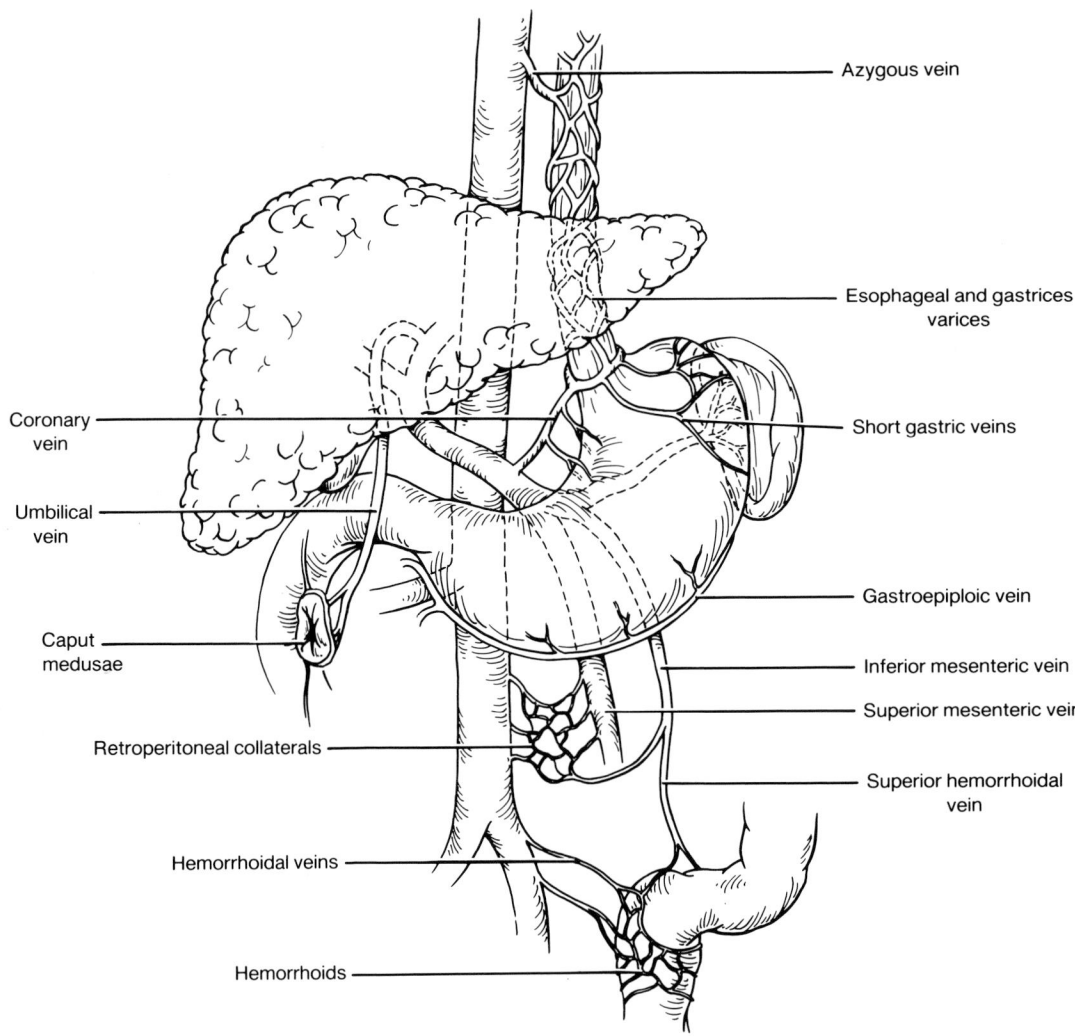

Azygous vein

Esophageal and gastrices varices

Short gastric veins

Gastroepiploic vein

Inferior mesenteric vein

Superior mesenteric vein

Superior hemorrhoidal vein

Coronary vein

Umbilical vein

Caput medusae

Retroperitoneal collaterals

Hemorrhoidal veins

Hemorrhoids

Figure 20-2 Portosystemic collaterals develop wherever the portal and systemic venous systems are in apposition. The coronary vein and short gastric veins link the high-pressure portal venous system with gastric and esophageal varices.

should not be done when moderate ascites or a coagulopathy is present.

In patients with chronic liver disease, estimation of functional hepatic reserve is helpful in determining both the risk of therapeutic intervention for patients with variceal bleeding and the treatment options that should be considered. For example, patients with variceal bleeding who have limited hepatic functional reserve should be considered for hepatic transplantation, whereas those with minimally impaired hepatic reserve may be better served by long-term endoscopic sclerotherapy or shunt surgery. The most common method of assessing hepatic functional reserve is Child's classification or one of its modifications (Table 20-2). Although Child's classification does not directly measure hepatic functional reserve, it is a time-tested method of predicting operative mortality and assessing long-term prognosis. For example, early

mortality rates after shunt surgery are 0% to 5% for patients in Child's class A, 10% to 25% for those in Child's class B, and over 25% for those in Child's class C. In some individuals, Child's class is a dynamic variable and can be improved considerably by conservative medical therapy after recovery from acute variceal hemorrhage or abstinence from alcohol. More direct quantitative measures of hepatocellular function, such as galactose elimination capacity and clearance of a variety of drugs, also are valuable but generally are not available in most institutions. An indirect measure of hepatic reserve is liver size as determined by computed tomography or physical examination.

Portal venous hemodynamic status and anatomy can be assessed by visceral angiography, duplex ultrasonography, and measurement of the hepatic venous pressure gradient. The venous phases of selective superior mesenteric

Table 20-2 Child's Criteria for Hepatic Functional Reserve

Criterion	Class A (Minimal)	Class B (Moderate)	Class C (Advanced)
Serum bilirubin (mg/dL)	<2	2–3	>3
Serum albumin (g/dL)	>3.5	3–3.5	<3
Ascites	None	Easily controlled	Poorly controlled
Neurologic disorder	None	Minimal	Advanced, "coma"
Nutrition	Excellent	Good	Poor, "wasting"

and splenic arteriograms define the anatomy of the portal venous system and provide a qualitative estimate of hepatic portal perfusion. These studies are useful for detecting portal vein or splenic vein thrombosis, and in preparing patients for portosystemic shunt surgery. If a splenorenal shunt is contemplated, the left renal vein also should be cannulated and opacified; 20% of the population have some anomaly that should be defined before surgery. Hepatic portal perfusion is estimated from the venous phase of the superior mesenteric angiogram and is graded from 1 (normal) to 4[5] (nonvisualization of the portal vein; Fig. 20-3). Because the objective of some operations for portal hypertension is preservation of hepatic portal perfusion, it is helpful to know the status of this variable before surgery. Duplex ultrasonography is a noninvasive alternative to angiography, and is being used increasingly for assessing anatomy and flow characteristics of the portal venous system and for determining postoperative shunt patency status.[6,7] However, this technique generally is less accurate than angiography for determining the presence of portal venous thrombi and the patency status of peripheral shunts (eg, distal splenorenal shunts), because large collaterals can mimic the vessels being studied.

Because the portal venous system is interposed between the splanchnic organs and the liver, invasive techniques such as splenic puncture, umbilical vein cannulation, or surgery are required to measure portal pressure directly. However, in patients with sinusoidal and postsinusoidal causes of portal hypertension (eg, alcoholic cirrhosis and many varieties of nonalcoholic cirrhosis), portal pressure can be estimated indirectly by measurement of hepatic venous wedge pressure.[8] Because the magnitude of portal pressure is not predictive of which patients with varices will bleed, the only useful application of this technique is in differentiating between causes of portal hypertension that are presinusoidal and those that are sinusoidal or postsinusoidal.

An essential component of the evaluation of patients

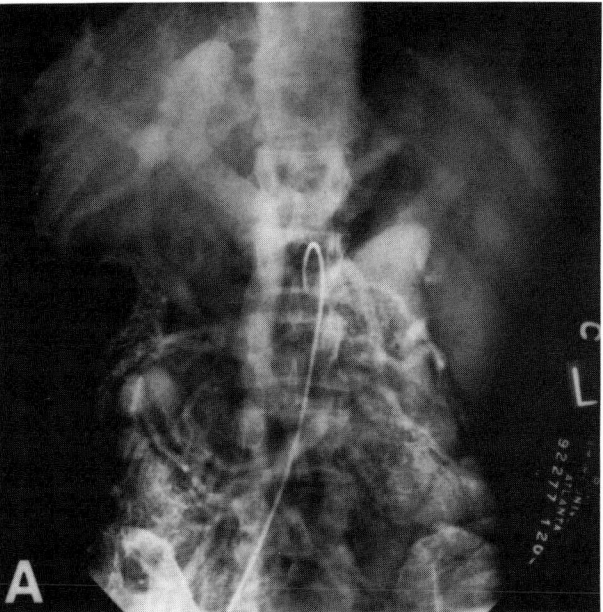
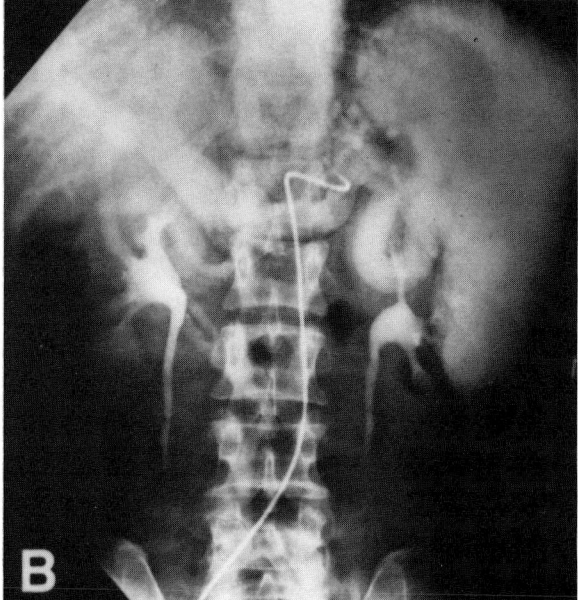

Figure 20-3 The venous phases of superior mesenteric (**A**) and splenic (**B**) angiograms. Superior mesenteric, splenic, and portal veins are opacified. The portal perfusion grade is 2.

with portal hypertension and gastrointestinal bleeding is determination of the site and cause of the bleeding. Variceal hemorrhage may present as hematemesis, hematochezia, or melena. In the absence of hematemesis, a nasogastric tube should be placed to determine whether the bleeding is from the proximal gastrointestinal tract. However, the most important diagnostic procedure is upper gastrointestinal endoscopy, which should be accomplished after patients are hemodynamically stabilized. Even though peptic ulcer disease and Mallory-Weiss tears are more common in patients with cirrhosis than in the general population, upper gastrointestinal bleeding in patients with portal hypertension is secondary to portal hypertension in over 80% of cases.[9] Bleeding is most commonly from esophageal varices, gastric varices, or portal hypertensive gastropathy. Only rarely do varices in other sites in the gastrointestinal tract bleed. Esophageal varices (90%) are more frequently the cause of bleeding than are gastric varices (10%).[10] The endoscopic diagnosis of a bleeding varix can be established by observing the site of bleeding (about 25% of patients), seeing a platelet plug in a recently ruptured varix, or confirming the presence of varices and no other significant lesions in patients who recently have bled from the upper gastrointestinal tract (Figs. 20-4 and 20-5). Portal hypertensive gastropathy is a newly defined entity that mainly involves the fundus and body of the stomach and has the endoscopic appearance of a white reticular network with enclosed erythematous areas[11] (Fig. 20-6). Because some patients with portal hypertension have both varices and portal hypertensive gastropathy, it can be difficult to determine which of these lesions is responsible for bleeding in any individual pa-

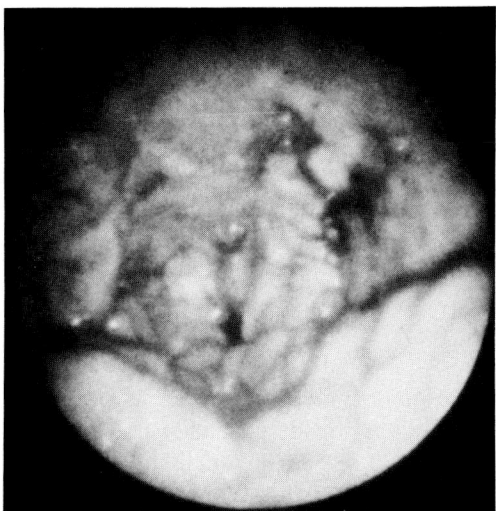

Figure 20-5 Large esophageal varices in a patient who recently bled from the upper gastrointestinal tract. (See Color Fig. 20-5.)

tient. In previously untreated patients, variceal hemorrhage clearly predominates, whereas portal hypertensive gastropathy is a more common cause of bleeding when esophageal varices have been obliterated by long-term sclerotherapy.[12,13]

VARICEAL HEMORRHAGE

Bleeding from esophagogastric varices is a common, dramatic, and life-threatening event in the natural history of patients with portal hypertension. About 25% to

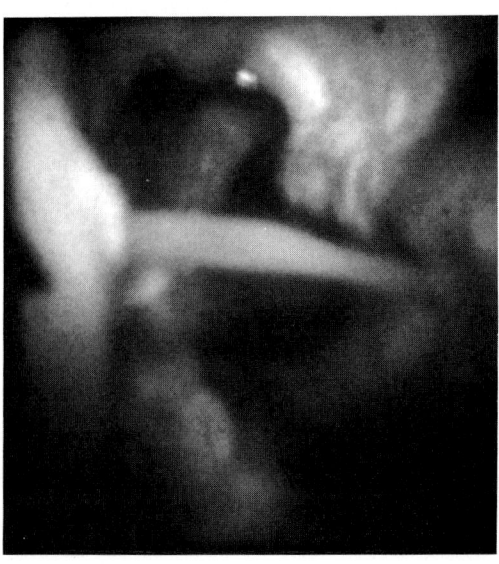

Figure 20-4 Actively bleeding esophageal varix (See Color Fig. 20-4.)

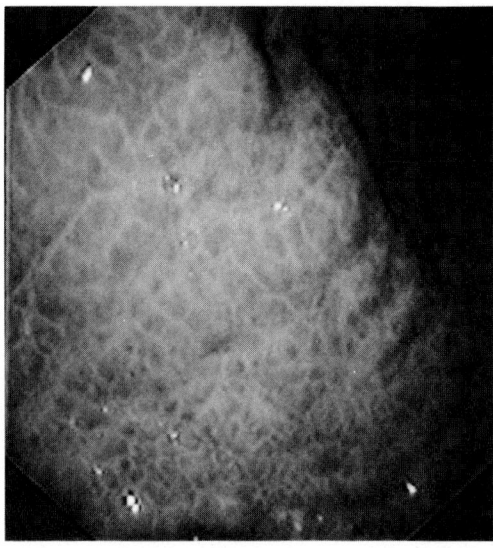

Figure 20-6 Portal hypertensive gastropathy in the fundus of the stomach. A reticular pattern is apparent (See Color Fig. 20-6.)

35% of patients with varices eventually bleed from their varices.[14,15] Variceal hemorrhage is responsible for about one third of all deaths of patients with cirrhosis.[16] Because the risk of death from bleeding in any individual patient is related directly to the hepatic functional reserve, patients with portal hypertension secondary to extrahepatic portal venous obstruction rarely die of bleeding varices, whereas patients with decompensated cirrhosis can have a mortality rate above 50%. The likelihood of dying of variceal bleeding is greatest within the first few days after the onset of hemorrhage, and returns to the prebleeding risk level after 6 weeks.[17]

Although varices can develop at any site throughout the gastrointestinal tract, they are most prone to rupture within 2 cm above or below the esophagogastric junction. The superficial veins in the distal esophagus are in the lamina propria and have relatively little surrounding connective tissue support in comparison to varices at other sites. This allows for dilation, which results in attenuation of the venous wall. Laplace's law states that tension of the variceal wall (T) is related directly to transmural pressure (P) and radius (r) and related inversely to variceal wall thickness (w): $T = P \times r/w$. The minimal portal pressure required for variceal rupture is 12 mmHg.[18] At a constant pressure at or above this level, the likelihood of rupture is greater with large varices than with small varices, and with thin-walled varices than with thicker-walled varices.[18,19] Patients who have large varices with thin epithelial linings, denoted by cherry-red spots and red wale markings seen on endoscopy, are more likely to bleed than are patients with small varices and none of these endoscopic indicators.[20] However, there is considerable overlap between groups, making none of these characteristics reliable predictors of future bleeding.

Patients with varices are treated in three settings: treatment of the acute bleeding episode; definitive therapy to prevent recurrence of bleeding; and prophylactic therapy for varices that have not yet bled. Because patients with acute variceal bleeding often are high operative risks because of decompensated hepatic function, nonoperative therapies usually are preferred. Treatments that are effective and minimally alter hepatic physiology are optimal for definitive treatment to prevent recurrence of bleeding. Most patients with varices never bleed, so prophylactic treatment can be recommended only if it is associated with minimal morbidity and mortality.

Treatment of the Acute Bleeding Episode

In treating acutely bleeding patients, volume resuscitation assumes the highest priority. Fluid resuscitation is achieved through large-bore intravenous catheters with both isotonic fluids and blood. Although these fluids later may contribute to the formation of ascites, immediate concerns take precedence. In patients with chronic liver disease and prolonged prothrombin times, fresh frozen plasma should be a component of the resuscitation volume. Platelet transfusions are necessary only if the platelet count is below 50,000/μL, which is unusual.

After hemodynamic stabilization is achieved, endoscopy should be performed. Although there is controversy regarding the advantages of early endoscopy in upper gastrointestinal bleeding, identification of varices as the cause of the hemorrhage has a major effect on subsequent therapy. Because bleeding varices frequently stop spontaneously, active bleeding may not be observed. However, the presence of medium to large varices and the absence of other lesions confirms varices as the cause of bleeding, especially if an adherent clot on a varix or discoloration of the overlying epithelium is observed. Gastric varices are more subtle than esophageal varices and may be missed by the inexperienced endoscopist. Portal hypertensive gastropathy, which may be the cause of hemorrhage, can be present alone or in combination with varices. It is important to determine whether bleeding is gastric (gastric varices or portal hypertensive gastropathy) or esophageal (esophageal varices) in origin, because this affects subsequent therapy.

The risk of surgery in acutely bleeding cirrhotic patients, who often have associated complications, such as encephalopathy, malnutrition, ascites, or coagulopathy, is frequently high. Therefore, emergency treatment should be nonoperative whenever possible. Endoscopic sclerotherapy or ligation is the mainstay of nonoperative treatment in most centers, but generally is ineffective for bleeding gastric varices and portal hypertensive gastropathy. Patients who are bleeding from these latter lesions may require earlier surgical intervention than patients who are bleeding from esophageal varices. Whenever it becomes evident that nonoperative therapy is unlikely to control hemorrhage, emergency surgery should be performed as soon as possible, and before patients become unsalvageable.[21]

The treatments available for acutely bleeding patients, along with their effectiveness, advantages, and disadvantages, are listed in Table 20-3.

Endoscopic Variceal Sclerosis and Ligation

Although first described in 1939, endoscopic sclerotherapy did not become a common means of treating variceal bleeding until the late 1970s. Endoscopic

Table 20-3 Therapies for Acute Variceal Hemorrhage

Therapy	Effectiveness (%)	Advantages	Disadvantages	Comments
Drugs (vasopressin, vasopressin and nitroglycerin, somatostatin, glypressin)	50–70	Noninvasive; no skill required; widely available	Cardiac complications (vasopressin); early rebleeding common	Only noninvasive therapy for gastric varices and portal hypertensive gastropathy (PHG)
Balloon tamponade	70–85	Immediate control; widely available	Complications frequent; early rebleeding common; not effective for fundal varices or PHG	Use protocol to minimize complications
Endoscopic therapy	80–95	Less invasive than surgery; provides treatment at time of diagnosis; widely available	Late rebleeding common; not effective for gastric varices and PHG; requires skill	More effective than drugs and balloon tamponade for esophageal varices; long-term sclerotherapy may be definitive treatment
Nonoperative shunt (transjugular intrahepatic portosystemic shunt)	75–95	Nonoperative portal decompression	Total portal diversion; frequent shunt stenosis or occlusion; requires skilled personnel	Should be used in acute setting only after other, less invasive therapies have failed
Stapled esophageal transection	70–90	Less operative time than shunt; familiar to most surgeons	High operative mortality; late rebleeding common; not effective for gastric varices and PHG	Coronary vein ligation may be added
Portosystemic shunt	90+	Definitive therapy; maximal effectiveness	High operative mortality; postshunt encephalopathy (nonselective shunts); not familiar to many surgeons	Early consideration for sclerotherapy failures, gastric varices, and PHG

PHG, portal hypertensive gastropathy.
(Modified from Rikkers LF. Portal hypertension. In: Levine BA, ed. Current practice of surgery, vol 13. New York, Churchill Livingstone, 1993:8)

therapy (sclerosis or ligation) now is the most common method of treating acute portal hypertensive bleeding resulting from esophageal varices. Controlled trials have confirmed its effectiveness in controlling acute bleeding.[22–24] However, only one study has demonstrated a survival benefit for patients with acute variceal bleeding treated with sclerotherapy.[24] A significant advantage of endoscopic treatment is that it can be instituted during the initial diagnostic endoscopy. Both intravariceal and paravariceal techniques of sclerosant injection can be used, and often these two methods are combined[25] (Fig. 20-7). Sodium morrhuate and sodium tetradecyl sulfate are the most commonly used sclerosants in the United States. The bleeding varix should be injected first, and if bleeding is reasonably well controlled, all varices should be injected just above the esophagogastric junction and then 5 cm proximal to it. Alternatively,

each varix can be ligated with a rubber band (Fig. 20-8). Studies suggest that rubber-band ligation of varices is associated with fewer complications than sclerosis and may be more effective.[26] Subsequent endoscopic sessions should be planned at intervals of 1 to 2 weeks until all esophageal varices are eradicated.

Endoscopic treatment is effective in 65% to 90% of patients with acute bleeding from esophageal varices and has become the standard therapy.[22–24] Controlled trials show somatostatin to be equally efficacious and reopen the comparative roles of these therapies.[27–29] Pharmacologic therapy and balloon tamponade are useful in patients in whom exsanguinating hemorrhage prevents endoscopic treatment and in those with bleeding from gastric varices or portal hypertensive gastropathy, which is not effectively treated by sclerotherapy.

The most common complication of endoscopic

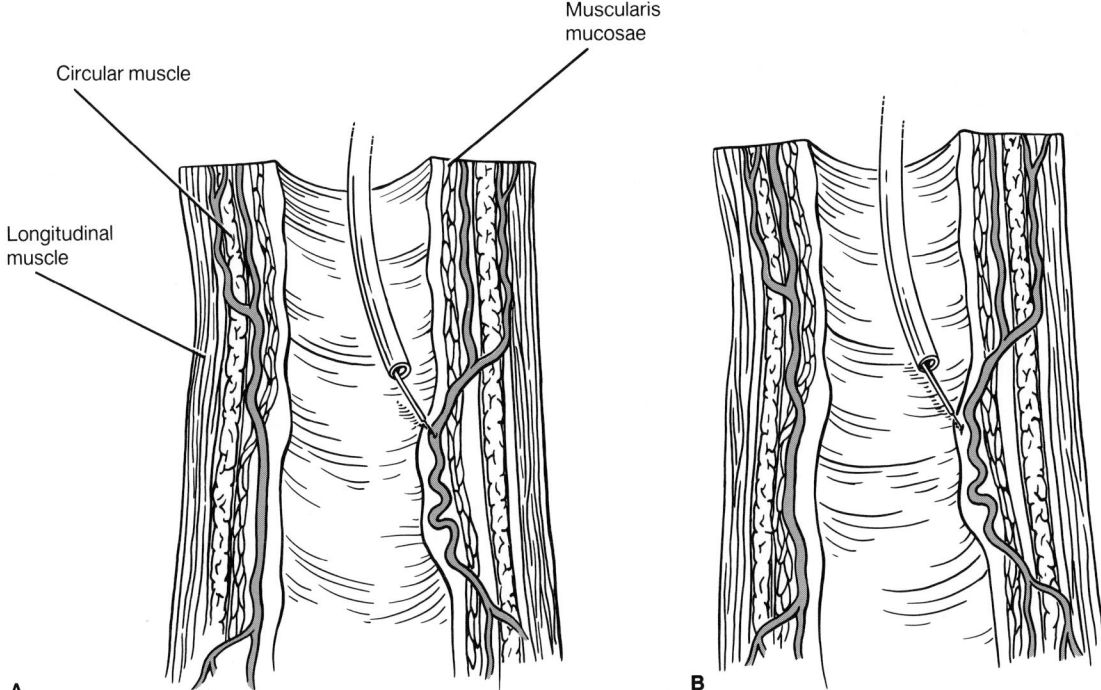

Circular muscle

Longitudinal muscle

Muscularis mucosae

A

B

Figure 20-7 Intravariceal (**A**) and paravariceal (**B**) techniques of endoscopic variceal sclerosis. The former causes variceal thrombosis, and the latter results in a fibrotic thickening of the overlying esophageal epithelium.

treatment is recurrent variceal bleeding, which eventually develops in about half of patients if no other definitive treatment is administered.[30–33] Acute endoscopic treatment failure can be defined as persistent bleeding despite two treatment sessions. Unless urgent surgical therapy or nonoperative shunt (transjugular intrahepatic portosystemic shunt [TIPS]) placement is performed in such patients, the mortality rate exceeds 60%.[31] Other complications of sclerotherapy include esophageal stenosis or perforation, aspiration pneumonitis, esophageal ulceration, and fever.[25]

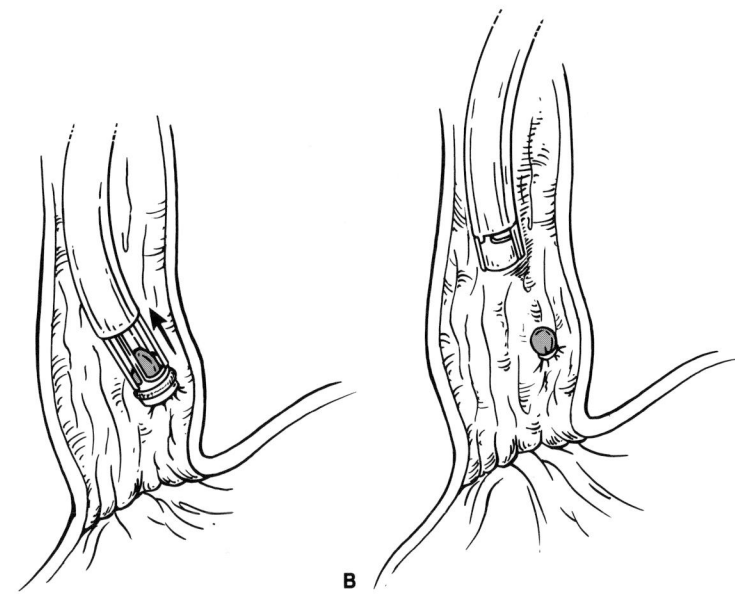

Figure 20-8 Endoscopic band ligation of varices. The varix is brought into the ligating device with suction (**A**) and ligated with an O-ring (**B**).

A

B

Pharmacotherapy

The objective of drug treatment of acute variceal bleeding is to lower the portal pressure, ideally below the critical level of 12 mmHg, which is required for variceal bleeding to occur. Splanchnic vasoconstrictors, which decrease portal venous inflow, have been the most commonly used drugs for acute control of portal hypertensive bleeding. Most experience has been gained with vasopressin, a potent vasoconstrictor, which has been used in this setting for more than 30 years. Because vasopressin also affects other vascular beds, it commonly causes hypertension, bradycardia, decreased cardiac output, and coronary vasoconstriction. Therefore, it should be used only in an intensive care unit setting, where patients can be monitored appropriately. Vasopressin usually is administered as an intravenous bolus dose of 20 U over about 20 minutes, and then as a continuous infusion of 0.2 to 0.8 U/min. To counteract the systemic side effects of vasopressin, nitroglycerin should be given simultaneously, either sublingually (0.6 μg every 30 minutes) or by continuous infusion (40 to 400 μg/min, depending on blood pressure response). This combination therapy not only averts most of the side effects of vasopressin but also is more effective in controlling bleeding, probably because of the dilation of portosystemic collaterals by nitroglycerin.[34,35]

Two splanchnic vasoconstrictors—glypressin,[36] an analogue of vasopressin with a longer duration of action, and somatostatin[37]—also have been used for the treatment of acute variceal hemorrhage. Clinical investigations suggest that both agents are as effective or more effective than vasopressin alone and have fewer adverse effects.

Three randomized trials comparing somatostatin, or its analogue octreotide, with endoscopic sclerotherapy have reopened the question of the role of pharmacologic therapy for acute variceal bleeding.[27–29] Somatostatin is given as a 250-μg intravenous bolus, followed by a continuous infusion of 250 μg/h for 48 to 96 hours.[27] Octreotide is given by continuous infusion of 25 to 50 μg/h for a similar interval.[29] Because pharmacologic therapies and sclerotherapy are equally efficacious in controlling acute bleeding and have similar rates of rebleeding in the first few days, the ease of administration of somatostatin and octreotide may warrant their use. Their cost is high, however, and must be considered in the final decision.

Balloon Tamponade

Balloon tamponade is a temporizing maneuver designed to reduce variceal flow mechanically and to apply pressure directly to acutely bleeding varices.[39] It is particularly applicable to three groups of patients: those with massive hemorrhage preventing effective endoscopic treatment, those with persistent bleeding despite endoscopic treatment, and those being transported from small community hospitals where neither endoscopic treatment nor surgery for portal hypertension is available. The most commonly used device is the Sengstaken-Blakemore tube (Fig. 20-9). The major advantage of balloon tamponade is immediate cessation of bleeding in most patients after balloon inflation. Significant disadvantages include recurrent bleeding in a high proportion of patients after balloon deflation and frequent complications if a strict protocol is not fol-

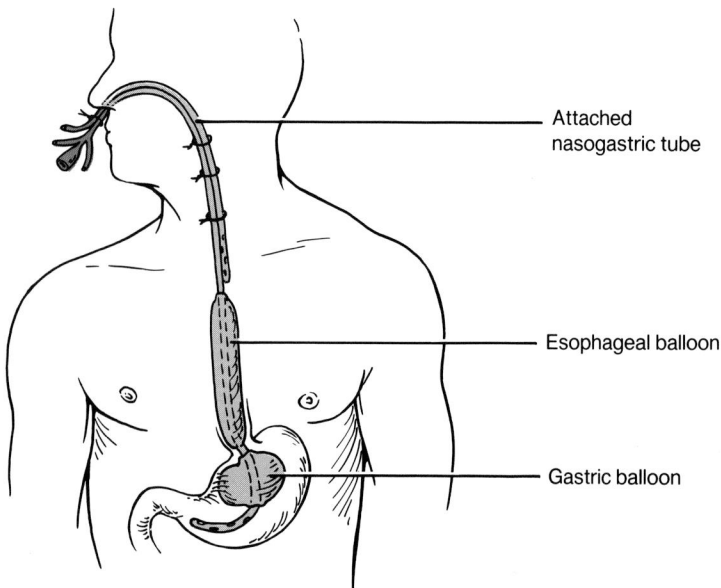

Attached nasogastric tube

Esophageal balloon

Gastric balloon

Figure 20-9 Sengstaken-Blakemore tube with attached nasogastric tube to prevent aspiration. The gastric balloon is pulled up against the esophagogastric junction, and the esophageal balloon is inflated to compress varices directly.

lowed (Table 20-4). The most common complications of balloon tamponade are aspiration and airway compromise. In most patients, nasotracheal intubation should be undertaken if balloon tamponade is to be instituted. Because rebleeding is common after balloon deflation, more definitive treatment (TIPS, surgery, or endoscopic treatment) should be planned for most patients in whom balloon tamponade is used.

Transjugular Intrahepatic Portosystemic Shunt

Insertion of a TIPS is a novel technique for achieving portal decompression without an operation.[40,41] The TIPS procedure is carried out in the interventional radiology suite without anesthesia. Because of the complexity of the technique, a skilled and experienced interventional radiologist is required. An angiography catheter is guided into a large hepatic vein, and a needle is passed from there into the intrahepatic portal vein (Fig. 20-10). The parenchymal tract between the hepatic vein and the portal vein then is dilated with a balloon catheter over a guide wire and a 10-mm expandable metal stent is inserted, creating the shunt.

In experienced hands, the success rate of the TIPS procedure is over 90%.[40,41] Experience with this technique in patients with acute bleeding is limited. When applied in this setting, it has resulted in cessation of active bleeding in about 90% of cases.[40–42] In one report,[43] however, the in-hospital mortality rate for emergency TIPS placement was 56% and bleeding was not controlled in 26% of patients. These authors believe that the TIPS procedure should not be used as a first-line therapy for acute variceal hemorrhage but should be applied only after less invasive treatments, such as endoscopic variceal sclerosis, have failed to control bleeding.

Even though the technique is relatively new, some indications for TIPS insertion are becoming clear. Liver transplant candidates who require transplantation soon and who have failed to respond to sclerotherapy appear to be ideal candidates for the TIPS procedure.[42] The subsequent transplant operation is not compromised, and the intrahepatic shunt is removed when the recipient liver is excised. Patients with advanced hepatic functional decompensation (Child's class C) who are not candidates for transplantation probably also are served better by TIPS placement than by an emergency operation when sclerotherapy fails or cannot be used because of gastric varices or hypertensive gastropathy. The major disadvantages of the TIPS are that it is a nonselective shunt and has been followed by a high frequency of encephalopathy in some series, and that the shunt failure rate (stenosis or occlusion) is high (up to 50% at 1 year in some series).[44,45] TIPS stenosis can be resolved in many patients, however, by further angiographic intervention and shunt dilation.

Table 20-4 Protocol for the Use of the Sengstaken-Blakemore Tube

BEFORE INSERTION
Consider nasotracheal intubation.
Use new tube and inspect balloons for leaks.
Attach no. 18 Salem sump tube above esophageal balloon.
Evacuate blood from stomach with large tube.
Insert through nose using ring forceps if necessary.

AFTER INSERTION
Apply low, intermittent suction to stomach tube.
Apply constant suction to Salem sump.
Inflate gastric balloon with 25-mL increments of air to 100 mL, observing the patient for pain.
Snugly fit gastric balloon to gastroesophageal junction and affix to nose, under slight tension, with soft rubber pad.
Add 150 mL of air to gastric balloon.
Place two clamps (one taped closed) on tube to gastric balloon.
Inflate esophageal balloon to 24 to 45 mmHg, clamp, and assess every hour.
Perform heavily penetrated upper abdomen–lower chest film (portable) to confirm balloon positions.
Determine serial hematocrits every 4 to 6 hours (gastric tube may occlude and fail to detect recurrent hemorrhage).
Tape scissors to head of bed so tube can be transected and rapidly removed if respiratory arrest develops.
Deflate esophageal and gastric balloons after 24 hours.
Remove tube in additional 24 hours if there is no recurrent hemorrhage.

(Modified from Rikkers LF. Portal hypertension. In: Goldsmith H, ed. Practice of surgery. Philadelphia, Harper & Row, 1981:1)

Emergency Surgery

Because most patients with varices have advanced liver disease, which often is made worse by an acute bleeding episode, they are at high risk with emergency surgical intervention. Fortunately, the effectiveness of newer, nonoperative therapies, especially endoscopic treatment and TIPS placement, has made emergency surgery infrequently necessary. Overall, nonoperative methods of controlling bleeding are effective in over 85% of patients, allowing time for improvement of hepatic function, nutritional status, and cerebral function before definitive therapy is undertaken. However, when emergency surgery is required, it should be performed promptly because procrastination usually results in even higher risk. The most common settings in which emergency surgery is required are failure of nonoperative therapies, including endoscopic treat-

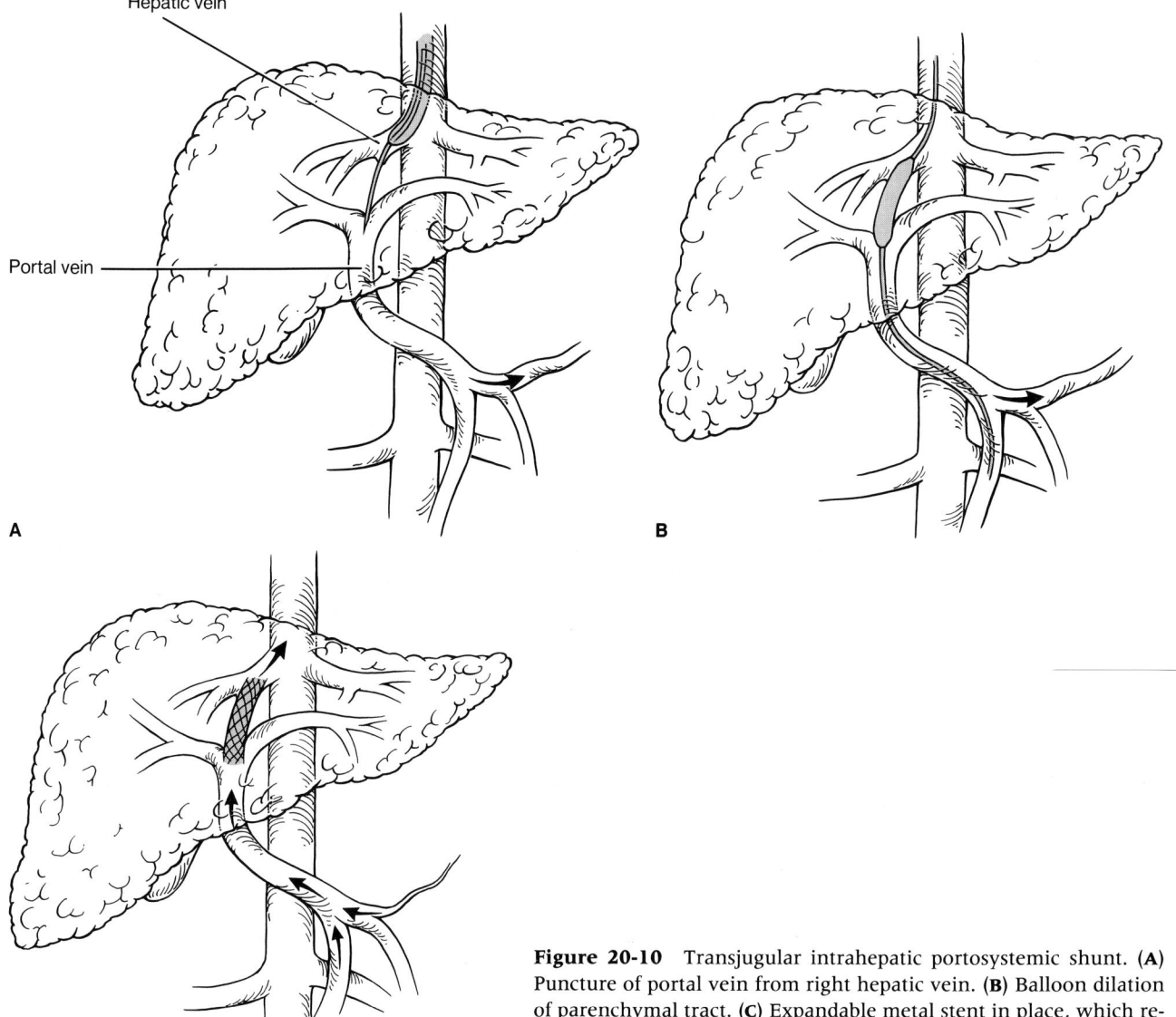

Hepatic vein

Portal vein

A

B

C

Figure 20-10 Transjugular intrahepatic portosystemic shunt. (**A**) Puncture of portal vein from right hepatic vein. (**B**) Balloon dilation of parenchymal tract. (**C**) Expandable metal stent in place, which results in complete diversion of portal flow.

ment, to control acute bleeding; failure of long-term sclerotherapy; and hemorrhage from gastric varices or portal hypertensive gastropathy that is unresponsive to drug treatment.[21]

Although most agree that emergency surgery should be performed when nonoperative therapy fails, there is no consensus about what constitutes nonoperative treatment failure. Although the circumstances of each case must be considered, two frequently used indicators of nonoperative treatment failure are inability to control acute bleeding or recurrence of acute bleeding within 48 hours of admission, and persistent hemorrhage after two endoscopic treatments.[31,46] Continued conservative therapy after either or both of these end points is reached results in mortality rates in excess of 50% in most cases.

There also is no agreement about the best emergency operation. Because it can be performed rapidly and by most surgeons, esophageal transection with a stapling device, sometimes combined with coronary vein ligation, is advocated by many (Fig. 20-11). Controlled trials have shown that early rebleeding rates are lower after esophageal transection than after endoscopic treatment.[47,48] However, late postoperative rebleeding is much more frequent after esophageal transection (over 25%) than after portal decompression (below 10%). In addition, there is little evidence that esophageal transection has a lower operative mortality rate than an emergency shunt if the surgeon is adequately trained to perform both operations.[49] Esophageal transection is clearly a better option for surgeons who have little or no experience with shunt surgery.

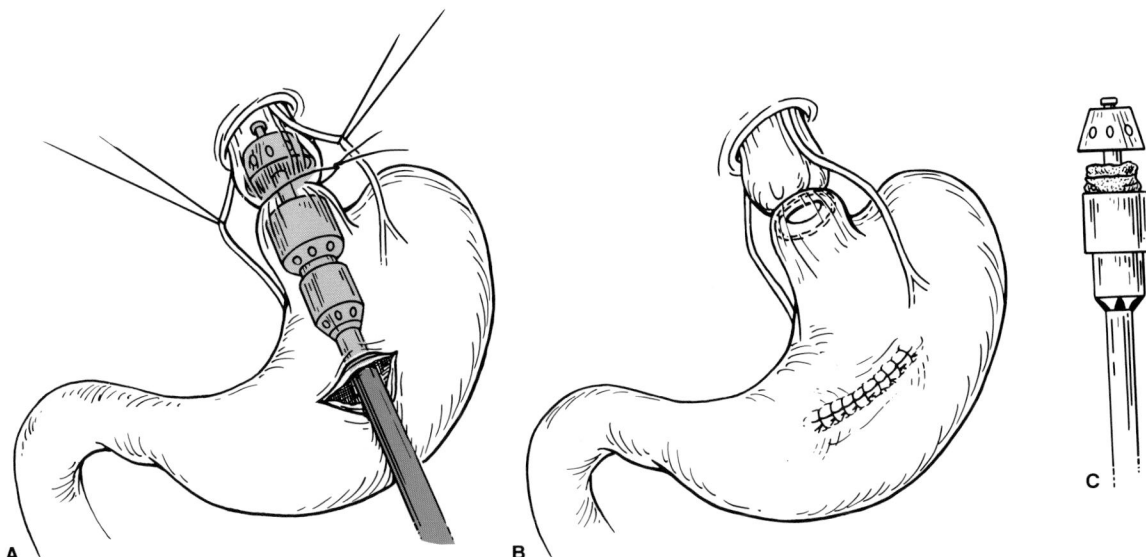

Figure 20-11 Stapled esophageal transection. (**A**) An EEA stapler is inserted in the distal esophagus through a gastrotomy, and the esophagus is tied off while the instrument is in the open position. (**B**) Firing of the stapler results in transection and reanastomosis of the distal esophagus. (**C**) A complete anastomosis is confirmed by obtaining two "doughnuts" of esophageal wall.

Esophageal transection should not be performed if patients are bleeding from gastric varices or portal hypertensive gastropathy.

The most commonly used emergency shunts are the portacaval shunt and the interposition mesocaval shunt. Depending on the Child's class of the patients undergoing surgery, operative mortality rates after emergency nonselective shunt range from 20% to 50%.[21] A selective distal splenorenal shunt also can be considered in the emergency setting if patients otherwise meet the criteria for this operation (appropriate anatomy and absent or medically controllable ascites), and if bleeding can be controlled temporarily by pharmacotherapy or balloon tamponade so that preoperative visceral angiography can be performed. Published operative mortality rates after emergency distal splenorenal shunts have been lower than after emergency nonselective shunts, but patients chosen to undergo emergency selective variceal decompression generally are better operative risks.[21,50]

Acute Treatment Plan

A treatment plan for acute portal hypertensive bleeding is outlined in Figure 20-12. After volume resuscitation, prompt endoscopy should be performed to determine whether patients are bleeding from the esophagus or the stomach. Individuals who are bleeding from esophageal varices should undergo acute sclerotherapy or variceal ligation during the initial endoscopy. Those who are bleeding from gastric varices or portal hypertensive gastropathy should receive initial pharmacotherapy but should be considered for early surgery or TIPS insertion if bleeding persists. The TIPS procedure is the preferred treatment option for poor-risk patients and those who require hepatic transplantation soon. When emergency surgery is necessary, the most important factors in selecting the specific operation are the severity and site of the bleeding and, primarily, the experience of the surgeon.

DEFINITIVE THERAPY FOR PREVENTION OF RECURRENT HEMORRHAGE

Once patients have bled from portal hypertension, the likelihood of a second episode, often within the ensuing 6 weeks, exceeds 70%.[17] Because most patients with portal hypertensive bleeding have chronic liver disease, the goals of long-term therapy are prevention of rebleeding and maintenance of satisfactory hepatic function. The availability of multiple treatment options, each with its own advantages and disadvantages, suggests that none is ideal for all patients in all situations (Table 20-5). Important considerations for the physician or surgeon caring for these patients are optimization of functional hepatic reserve before any surgical therapy, selection of the ap-

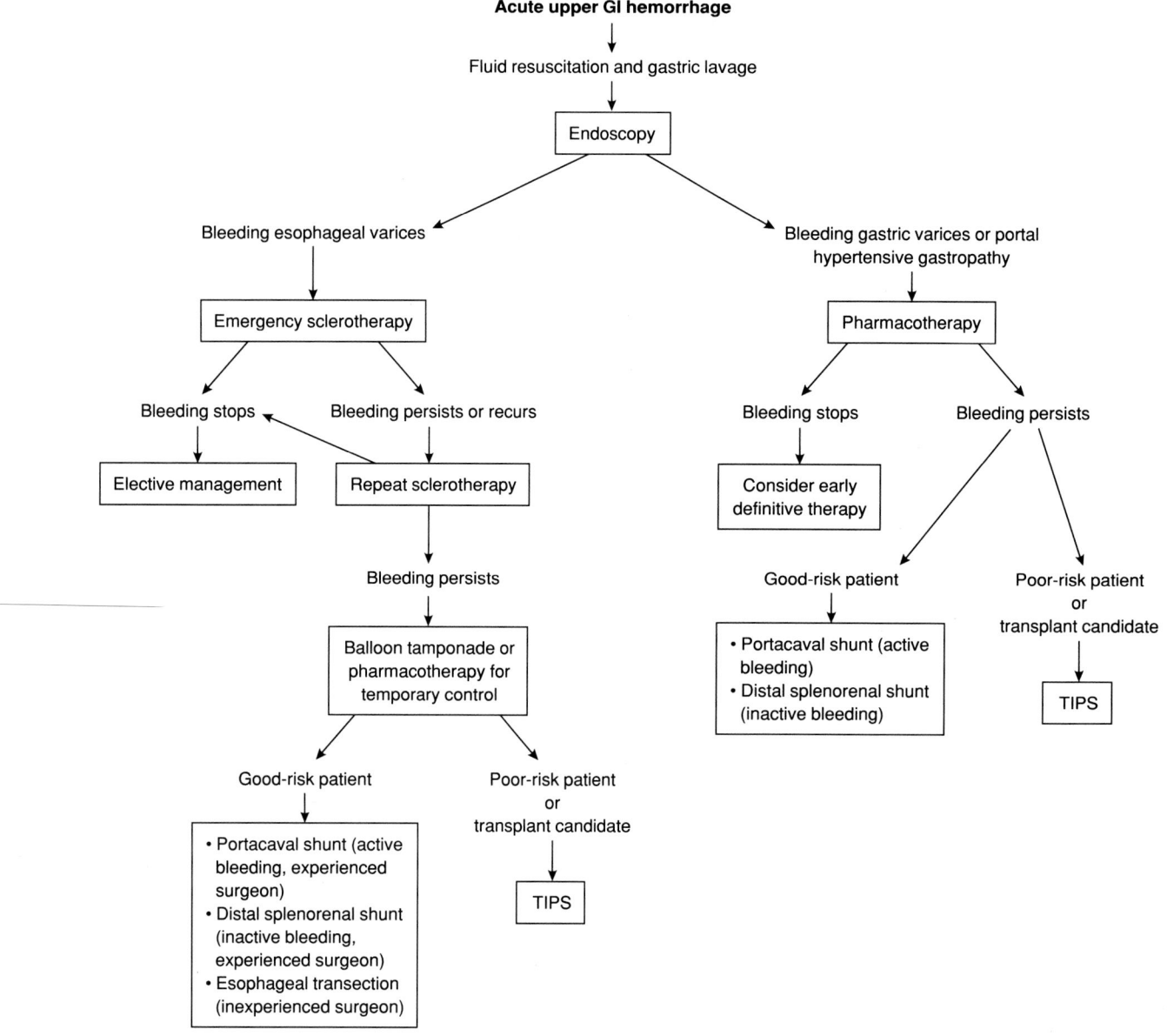

Figure 20-12 Algorithm for the management of acute portal hypertensive bleeding. TIPS, transjugular intrahepatic portosystemic shunt. (After Rikkers LF, Jin G. Surgical management of acute variceal hemorrhage. World J Surg 1994;18:193)

propriate therapy for each clinical setting, and prompt change in the treatment plan when the initial selected therapy fails to control bleeding (eg, endoscopic treatment) or hepatic failure develops (liver transplantation for appropriate candidates).

Pharmacotherapy

The past decade has seen considerable interest in drug therapy for the long-term prevention of recurrent portal hypertensive bleeding. It first was reported in 1981

that a dosage of propranolol sufficient to decrease the heart rate by 25% led to a lower frequency of recurrent hemorrhage and prolongation of survival in good-risk patients with alcoholic cirrhosis.[51] Unfortunately, several subsequent controlled trials using nonselective β-blockers and other agents failed to show a consistent beneficial effect of drugs in the prevention of rebleeding.[52,53] It has been shown that propranolol lowers portal pressure in some patients by decreasing portal venous inflow through a reduction in cardiac output and blockade of β_2-receptors in the splanchnic vasculature,

Table 20-5   Definitive Therapies for Variceal Hemorrhage

Therapy	*Advantages*	*Disadvantages*
Propranolol	Noninvasive; widely available; few side effects	Frequent rebleeding (50%); requires compliance
Endoscopic therapy	Nonoperative; widely available; maintains portal perfusion (95%)	Frequent rebleeding (50%); requires compliance; not applicable to gastric varices
Nonselective shunts	Reliable bleeding control (vein-to-vein, 95%); relatively technically easy; good ascites control (side-to-side)	Loss of portal perfusion; frequent encephalopathy (20%–50%); frequent thrombosis (interposition, 25%)
Selective shunts	Reliable bleeding control (90%); maintains portal perfusion (50%)	May aggravate ascites; not applicable to some patients (advanced ascites); technically difficult
Nonshunting procedures	Maintains portal perfusion (95%); relieves hypersplenism (splenectomy); technically easy (esophageal transection); applicable to splanchnic venous thrombosis	Frequent rebleeding (20%–40%); prevents future selective shunt (splenectomy)
Hepatic transplantation	Reliable bleeding control (95%); restores hepatic function	Limited donor supply; not applicable to many patients; expensive; requires compliance

(Modified from Rikkers LF. Portal hypertension. In: Levine BA, ed. Current practice of surgery, vol 13. New York, Churchill Livingstone, 1993:12)

allowing unopposed α-vasoconstriction. However, this effect is variable from patient to patient, and which patients will respond favorably is not predictable.[54] In addition, no easily measured variable, such as heart rate, has correlated with the portal pressure response in an individual patient.[54]

When a metaanalysis is performed of the many controlled trials of nonselective β-blockade, pharmacotherapy reduces the likelihood of recurrent bleeding by about one third.[55] Surprisingly, propranolol therapy demonstrates more consistent results when it is given prophylactically (ie, to patients who have not previously bled).[56] The use of long-term drug therapy should be limited to compliant patients who are monitored carefully by their physicians. Unfortunately, this noninvasive approach is not yet a practical option for most patients with bleeding varices. The results of ongoing trials of newer drugs and combinations of drugs are awaited with interest.

Long-Term Endoscopic Treatment

Although the efficacy of endoscopic sclerotherapy or ligation as therapy for acute bleeding episodes has been demonstrated, the benefits of long-term endoscopic treatment are less well established. Multiple long-term controlled trials of endoscopic sclerotherapy have shown that 40% to 60% of patients in the treatment group eventually rebleed from portal hypertension.[30–33] There is considerably less experience with rubber-band ligation of varices as definitive treatment, but an initial controlled trial suggests that it is more effec-

tive than sclerotherapy and associated with fewer complications.[26]

Despite its limitations, long-term sclerotherapy has become the most common therapy for the prevention of recurrent variceal hemorrhage during the past 15 years. In most institutions, endoscopic therapy has surpassed shunt surgery as the preferred therapy for esophageal variceal bleeding. There are several reasons for the ascendance of endoscopic treatment:

1. It is less invasive than surgical therapy.
2. There is a general dissatisfaction, especially among gastroenterologists, with shunt surgery.
3. It has no adverse hemodynamic effects.
4. It can be administered by gastroenterologists, to whom most patients initially are referred.
5. Although rebleeding rates are high, most controlled trials have shown that rebleeding is less common among patients treated with sclerotherapy than among untreated patients.[30–33]

Although the technique and timing of repeated endoscopic sessions vary from series to series, esophageal varices are eradicated in about two thirds of patients; these patients then must be monitored by serial endoscopic evaluation because varices can recur. In addition, several trials have shown an increased frequency of bleeding from gastric varices and portal hypertensive gastropathy after esophageal varices have been eradicated.[12,13] Recurrent hemorrhage is most common during the initial year, and the rate decreases to about 15% of patients who experience rebleeding each year thereafter.[57] Rebleeding does not represent sclerotherapy failure because many patients can be treated successfully by further endoscopic therapy. When sclerotherapy failure is defined as either death from rebleeding or the need to perform surgery to salvage patients, failure eventually occurs in 20% to 40% of patients, depending on the length of follow-up in the study.[12,13,58] Because of this relatively high failure rate, individuals undergoing long-term endoscopic treatment should be reliable and live close to centers that provide advanced medical care so that they can undergo subsequent endoscopic treatments or surgery as necessary. Endoscopic sclerotherapy as definitive treatment is associated with a high long-term mortality rate secondary to rebleeding in rural populations.[13]

Transjugular Intrahepatic Portosystemic Shunt

Experience with TIPS placement as a long-term therapy for patients with bleeding from portal hypertension is evolving. The major limitation of this approach is a high incidence (up to 50%) of shunt failure within the first year.[40,41,45] Shunt stenosis, usually secondary to neointimal hyperplasia, is the most common problem and often can be resolved by balloon dilation of the TIPS or insertion of a second shunt. Total shunt occlusion is less common, occurring in 10% to 15% of patients. Both shunt stenosis and shunt occlusion frequently are associated with recurrent portal hypertensive bleeding. In contrast to the TIPS, a surgically created shunt using a vein-to-vein anastomosis rarely fails in the late postoperative interval. Therefore, until TIPS technology improves, the open approach may be preferable for patients who are reasonable operative risks.

Most evidence suggests that the TIPS is a nonselective shunt and completely diverts portal flow away from the sinusoids.[40,41] However, progressive stenosis results in the TIPS functioning as a partial shunt, because there is a progressive rise in portal pressure as stenosis increases and a concomitant restoration of portal flow occurs. Duplex ultrasound and angiographic studies have shown that TIPS placement results in total portal decompression at initial insertion when the shunt is at least 10 mm in diameter. Clinical evidence of the nonselectivity of the TIPS procedure includes its effectiveness in resolving medically intractable ascites and a high frequency of encephalopathy after TIPS insertion in some investigations.[40,41,44,59] All clinical studies are compromised by relatively brief follow-up periods. Because the incidence of encephalopathy after shunt placement tends to be cumulative with time, the full extent of this complication may be considerably greater than reported. A potential answer to the problem of en-

cephalopathy after TIPS insertion may be the development of smaller-diameter stents with reliable long-term patency that cause only partial portal venous diversion.

The major advantage of the TIPS procedure is that it does not involve surgery. Although its indications need to be determined by prospective, controlled trials, it already appears to be the ideal therapy when only short-term portal decompression is required. Liver transplant candidates in whom sclerotherapy fails are well suited for TIPS placement.[40,42] Recurrent bleeding generally is prevented until the transplant operation is performed. The transplant procedure may be made technically easier because portal pressure is reduced, and the shunt presents no problems because it is removed with the recipient liver. Patients with advanced hepatic functional decompensation may not survive long, even when bleeding is controlled. TIPS insertion can be an appropriate therapy for these patients as well.

The TIPS procedure has been used in some centers for the treatment of medically intractable ascites in patients who have not bled.[40,59] Although the TIPS, which functions as a side-to-side portosystemic shunt, has been effective in this setting, it is questionable whether ascites alone is a reasonable indication for its application. The adverse effects of TIPS placement (ie, total portal diversion and encephalopathy) may be more serious problems than ascites. In addition, other reasonably effective therapies for medically intractable ascites are available, such as large-volume paracentesis and peritoneovenous shunting.

Nonselective Shunts

Characteristics common to all nonselective shunts are decompression of the entire portal venous system and complete diversion of portal flow away from the liver. Although nonselective shunts are effective in preventing rebleeding, a major disadvantage of these procedures is that they deprive hepatocytes of portal blood, which contains important nutrients and hepatotrophic hormones.[2] Cerebral toxins, also present in portal blood, bypass the detoxifying mechanisms of the liver and gain direct access to the central nervous system. Thus, adverse consequences of these procedures, such as postshunt encephalopathy, liver atrophy, and accelerated hepatic failure, develop in some patients.

The prototype nonselective shunt is the end-to-side portacaval shunt (Fig. 20-13A). This is the only shunt operation that has been compared extensively with medical therapy in controlled trials. All the investigations were done before the availability of endoscopic treatment or the TIPS procedure. Survival data from the three controlled trials of the therapeutic portacaval shunt (done in patients with prior variceal bleed-

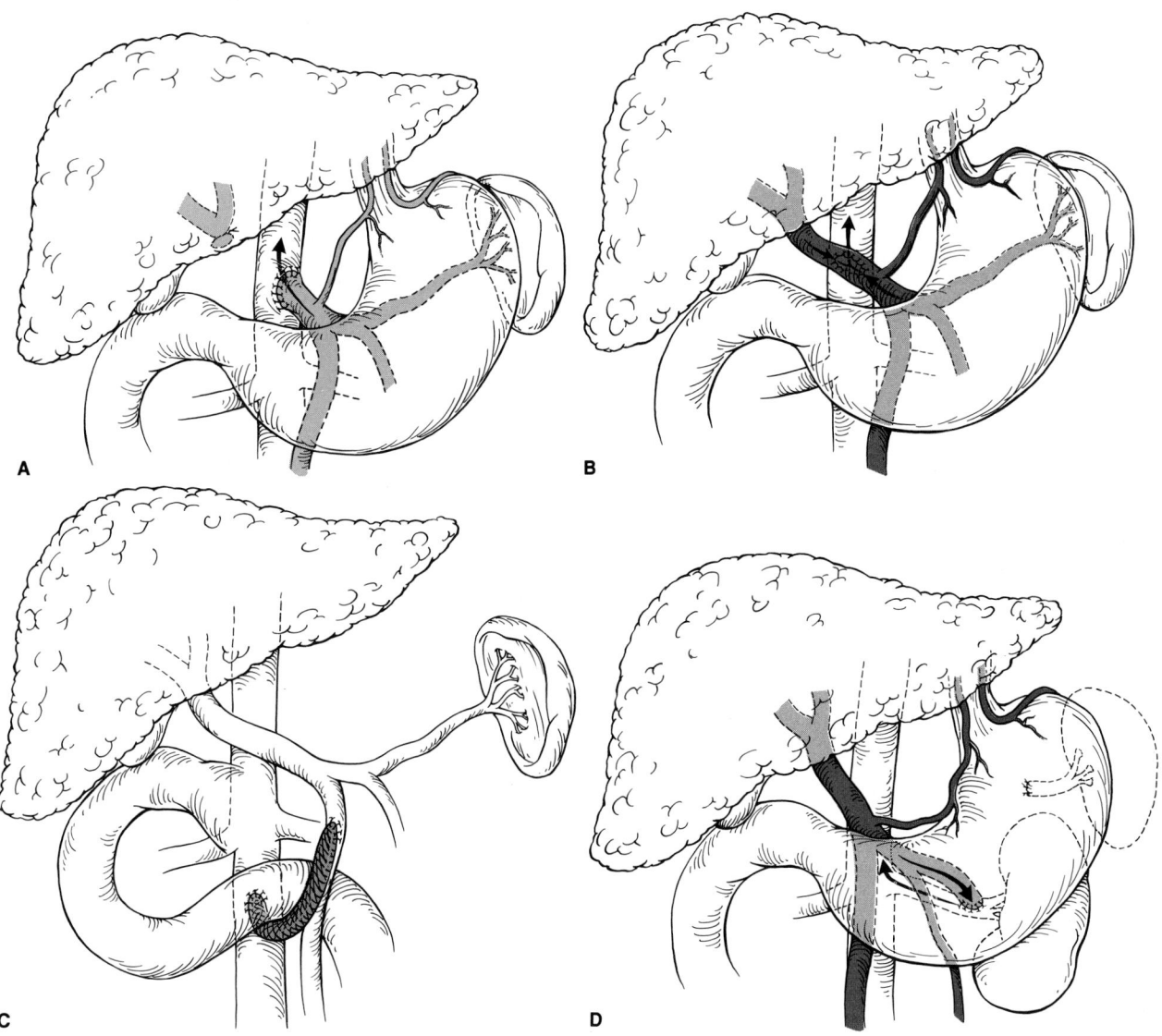

Figure 20-13 Nonselective shunt procedures, which divert all portal flow away from the liver, include the end-to-side portacaval shunt (**A**), the side-to-side portacaval shunt (**B**), the interposition mesocaval shunt (**C**), and the conventional splenorenal shunt with splenectomy (**D**).

ing)[60–62] are combined in the graph shown in Figure 20-14. In all these studies, the most common causes of death in medically treated patients and patients with shunts were variceal rebleeding and hepatic failure, respectively. Neither the individual trials nor the combined data have shown an advantage for either group with respect to long-term survival. However, several surviving control patients eventually received shunts when life-threatening rebleeding developed. Nearly all the patients included in these trials had alcoholic cirrhosis, so the results should not be generalized to patients with other causes of portal hypertension. Although variceal bleeding was controlled effectively in almost all patients who underwent shunt placement,

moderate to severe encephalopathy developed in 20% to 40% of patients, adversely affecting their quality of survival.

All the other shunts in Figure 20-13 are side-to-side portosystemic shunts, which decompress the hepatic sinusoids as well as the splanchnic venous system. Each of these procedures was developed with the hope that it would be partially decompressing, allowing continued portal perfusion of the liver. However, several hemodynamic investigations have shown that all the side-to-side portosystemic shunts, when of a diameter greater than 10 mm, also completely divert portal flow away from the liver.[63–65] Because the liver and splanchnic organs are important contributors to ascites formation,

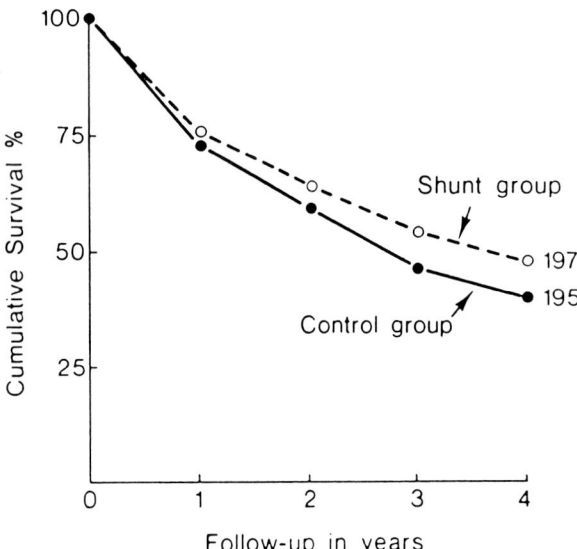

Figure 20-14 Cumulative survival data from four controlled trials of the portacaval shunt versus conventional medical management. (Boyer TD. Portal hypertension and its complications: bleeding esophageal varices, ascites, and spontaneous bacterial peritonitis. In: Zakim D, Boyer TD, eds. Hepatology: a textbook of liver disease. Philadelphia, WB Saunders, 1982:464)

side-to-side shunts are effective in relieving ascites as well as preventing recurrent bleeding. Complete diversion of portal flow by these operations, however, can lead to hepatic failure or encephalopathy in many patients. Controlled and matched controlled comparisons of side-to-side portosystemic shunts with end-to-side portacaval shunts have shown no differences between these procedures, with the exception of better relief of ascites by the side-to-side portosystemic shunts.[60,61]

The direct side-to-side portacaval shunt is somewhat more difficult to construct than the end-to-side portacaval shunt but provides the most reliable patency of any shunt procedure.[66] Shunt occlusion develops in only 2% to 3% of patients. Both the end-to-side and side-to-side portacaval shunts have the disadvantage of dissection in the porta hepatis and use of the portal vein, which may be a detriment with respect to future liver transplantation.

The most commonly performed interposition shunt procedure is the mesocaval variety. This procedure gained popularity because it is technically less challenging than most of the other portosystemic shunt procedures, and because it avoids the hepatic hilum, which is an advantage when future transplantation is a consideration. Although a synthetic graft measuring 14 to 20 mm in diameter generally is used, patency rates are better when an autogenous vein is used. A major disadvantage of prosthetic interposition shunts is a graft throm-

bosis rate that approaches 30% in series with long-term follow-up.[67] A single controlled trial of the interposition mesocaval shunt versus the side-to-side portacaval shunt showed no significant clinical or hemodynamic differences between these two procedures.[68]

In addition to providing a peripheral side-to-side portosystemic shunt, the conventional (central) splenorenal shunt procedure includes splenectomy. A purported advantage of this procedure is effective treatment of hypersplenism, which often accompanies portal hypertension. However, hypersplenism secondary to portal hypertension rarely is clinically significant and generally requires no definitive therapy. Early series of the conventional splenorenal shunt reported a lower frequency of postshunt encephalopathy than with central nonselective shunts. However, further analysis revealed that this resulted from a higher shunt thrombosis rate (about 20% to 25%) with restoration of hepatic portal perfusion after shunt thrombosis had occurred.[66] Matched control studies have shown no significant clinical differences between the conventional splenorenal shunt and other nonselective shunts.[61,69] Because it is technically more demanding and is associated with a higher thrombosis rate than other side-to-side portosystemic shunts, the conventional splenorenal shunt procedure seldom is performed.

In summary, nonselective shunts are the most effective means of controlling variceal bleeding and preventing recurrences. The feature that makes them so effective in controlling bleeding (ie, complete portal decompression) also is responsible for the adverse consequences of postshunt encephalopathy and accelerated hepatic failure, secondary to elimination of hepatic portal perfusion. Despite their associated complications, nonselective shunts remain a reasonable choice in the emergency setting, and when medically intractable ascites is present in patients who are bleeding from portal hypertension. Interposition shunts also can serve as a bridge to liver transplantation when nonoperative therapies fail to control bleeding.

Selective Shunts

Selective portosystemic shunts, which include the distal splenorenal shunt and the left gastric–caval shunt, decompress only a portion of the portal venous system (Fig. 20-15). Objectives of selective shunts are selective decompression of esophagogastric varices, preservation of hepatic portal perfusion, and maintenance of intestinal venous hypertension. The stimulus for the development of these procedures was the high frequency of encephalopathy after use of nonselective shunts. The advantage of a selective shunt is potential preservation of portal flow and continued perfusion of hepatocytes

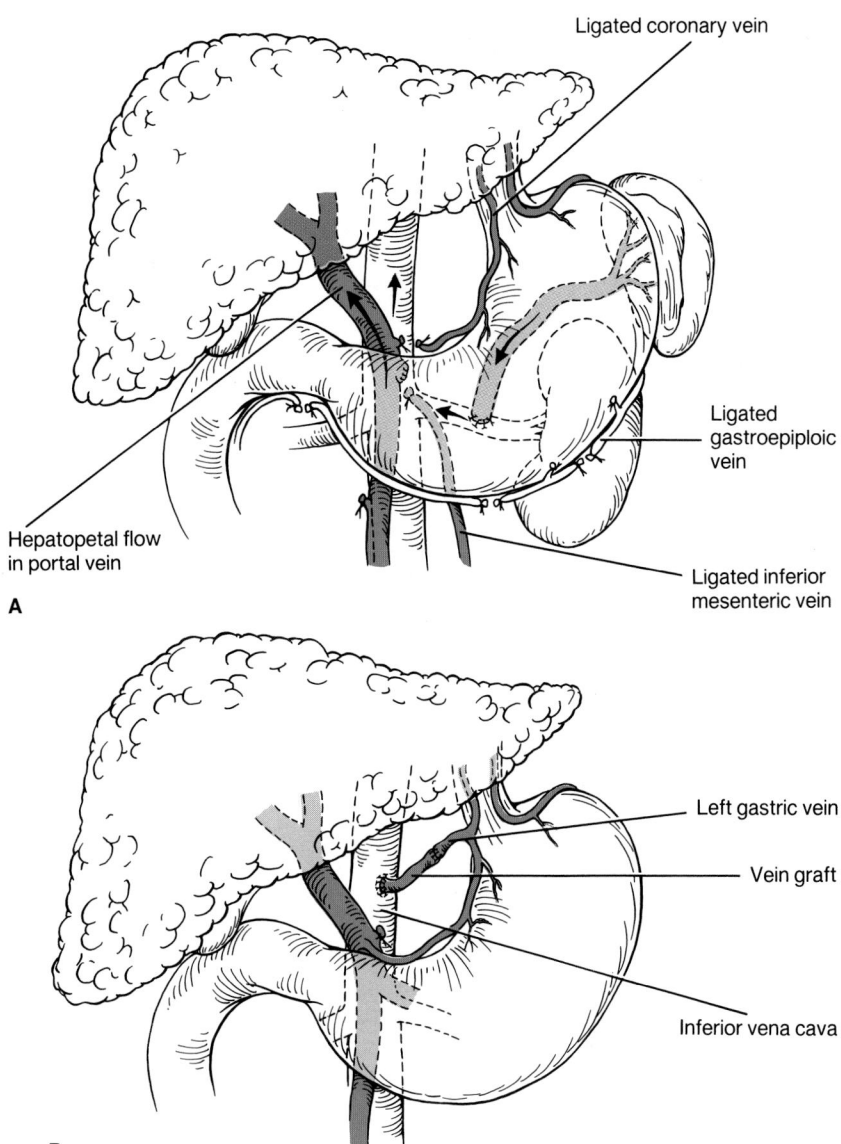

Ligated coronary vein

Ligated gastroepiploic vein

Hepatopetal flow in portal vein

Ligated inferior mesenteric vein

A

Left gastric vein

Vein graft

Inferior vena cava

B

Figure 20-15 Selective shunt procedures, which compartmentalize the portal venous system and preserve hepatic portal perfusion, include the distal splenorenal shunt (**A**) and the left gastric–caval shunt using a vein graft (**B**).

by hepatotrophic hormones that emanate from the portal venous system[2] (Fig. 20-16). A more subtle potential advantage of a selective shunt, even when hepatic portal perfusion is diminished or absent in the late postoperative interval, is maintenance of intestinal venous hypertension, which may inhibit intestinal absorption of purported cerebral toxins, such as ammonia.[70]

The only commonly used selective shunt is the distal splenorenal shunt, which first was described in 1967[71] (see Fig. 20-15). The objectives of the distal splenorenal shunt, namely selective variceal decompression and preservation of hepatic portal perfusion, are achieved by separating the portal venous system into two components—a low-pressure gastrosplenic component and a high-pressure portomesenteric component. The two important technical parts of the proce-

dure are anastomosis of the distal end of the divided splenic vein to the left renal vein and interruption of all collaterals, such as the coronary vein and the right gastroepiploic vein, connecting the two newly formed compartments of the portal venous system.

Although initial clinical experience with the distal splenorenal shunt showed that the objectives of the operation could be attained in a high proportion of patients, it also became apparent that this procedure was not suitable for all patients with portal hypertension. Two main contraindications to the distal splenorenal shunt have evolved—incompatible anatomy and medically intractable ascites. Prior splenectomy precludes construction of a distal splenorenal shunt and a small splenic vein diameter (less than 7 mm) significantly increases the potential for shunt failure. Many patients

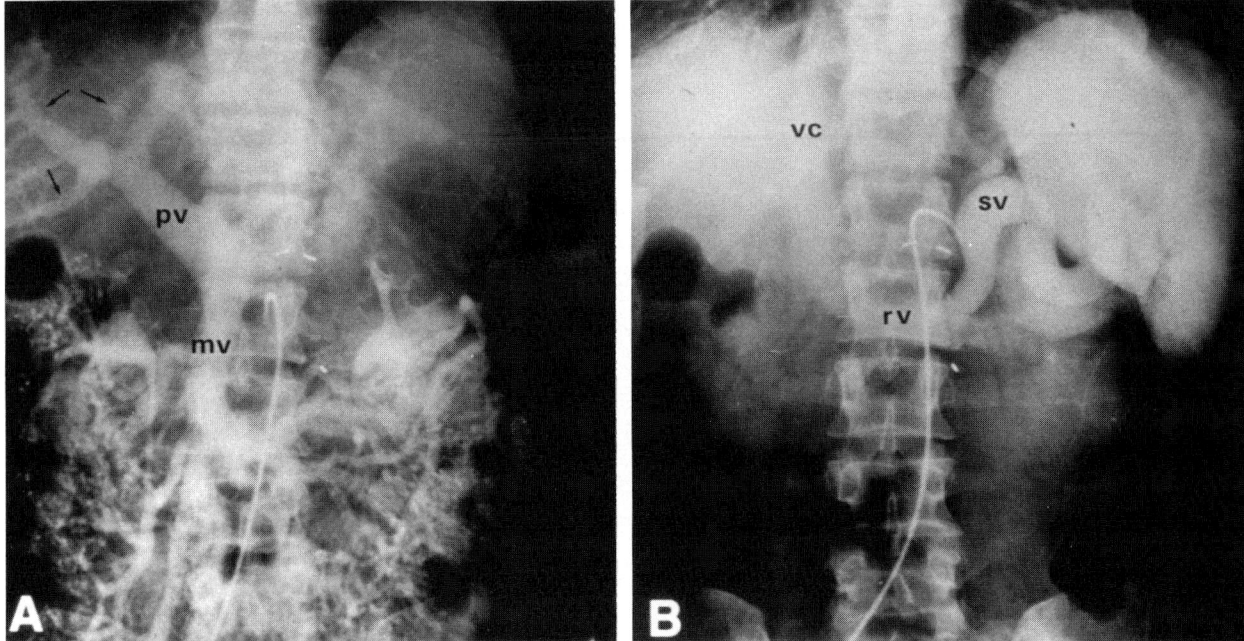

Figure 20-16 Selective superior mesenteric (**A**) and splenic (**B**) angiograms after distal spleno-renal shunting. The former shows continuing portal flow to the liver, and the latter demonstrates a patent shunt. Arrows point to intrahepatic portal venous branches. pv, portal vein; mv, superior mesenteric vein; sv, splenic vein; rv, left renal vein; vc, inferior vena cava.

have or develop mild to moderate ascites when they bleed from varices. As long as their ascites is responsive to medical therapy, they are candidates for the distal splenorenal shunt. However, advanced ascites that is resistant to salt restriction and diuretic therapy is a contraindication to the procedure. Because the distal splenorenal shunt maintains hepatic sinusoidal and intestinal venous hypertension, and because lymphatic pathways are interrupted during shunt construction, this operation can worsen ascites. Preoperative absence of portal flow to the liver is not a contraindication to the procedure because hepatic portal perfusion is restored after collateral ligation in some patients, and maintenance of portomesenteric venous hypertension may lessen the likelihood of postshunt encephalopathy, even when portal perfusion is absent.[70]

Although it is a technically demanding operation, the distal splenorenal shunt operation has been mastered by many surgeons in several countries. During the past quarter century, nearly 4000 patients undergoing distal splenorenal shunt procedures have been described in the surgical literature.[72] In addition, the advantages and disadvantages of selective variceal decompression have been scrutinized by numerous randomized controlled trials comparing the distal splenorenal shunt with a variety of nonselective shunts and to endoscopic sclerotherapy. Despite this extensive expe-

rience, the procedure remains controversial. Still under debate is how effective the distal splenorenal shunt is in the long-term preservation of hepatic portal perfusion and whether the procedure has any significant clinical advantages over the generally easier to perform nonselective shunt procedures and the less invasive long-term endoscopic sclerotherapy.

Although continuing portal flow to the liver can be demonstrated in about 90% of patients soon after the operation by angiographic or ultrasonographic studies, there is gradual attrition of residual portal flow with time because the high-pressure portomesenteric venous compartment gradually undergoes collateralization to the decompressed gastrosplenic compartment.[73,74] Early postoperative loss of hepatic portal perfusion usually is caused by portal vein thrombosis, which develops in 5% to 10% of patients, most likely secondary to stagnant portal flow, which may result from ligation of collaterals.[75] The clinical significance of complete portal vein thrombosis after distal splenorenal shunting ranges from a life-threatening situation to a clinically undetectable event. Long-term hepatic portal perfusion is more likely to be maintained in patients with nonalcoholic causes of portal hypertension than in those with alcoholic cirrhosis.[76] In most investigations, less than 50% of patients with alcoholic cirrhosis have continuing portal flow to the liver 1 year after a distal splenorenal shunt operation. In addition to patients with nonalcoholic cirrhosis, patients with schistosomiasis and those with portal vein thrombosis are likely to maintain portal flow for many years after selective variceal decompression.[77,78] The extent of portal azygous disconnection carried out at the time of the distal splenorenal shunt procedure also is an important determinant of postoperative hepatic portal perfusion. Variations of the distal splenorenal shunt procedure that omit ligation of the coronary vein or other important collaterals are associated with more rapid attrition of hepatic portal perfusion than the originally described operation.[79]

Two groups independently have described better preservation of hepatic portal perfusion after the distal splenorenal shunt procedure, especially in patients with alcoholic cirrhosis, when the devascularization component of the operation is more extensive.[80,81] Splenopancreatic disconnection consists of dissection of the full length of the splenic vein from the body and tail of the pancreas, thereby preventing a "pancreatic siphon" from developing and diverting portal flow to the shunt (Fig. 20-17). One study showed that hepatic portal perfusion was maintained in 84% of alcoholic patients with cirrhosis and in 90% of nonalcoholic patients at 4 years after distal splenorenal shunting combined with splenopancreatic disconnection.[80] However, this extension of the operation has distinct disadvantages, including longer operating time, greater intraoperative blood loss, and a greater likelihood of late postoperative bleeding from gastric varices. Although its

hemodynamic advantages have been established, its clinical benefits have not. Until further studies are done, it seems inappropriate to recommend an even more technically demanding procedure at a time when fewer shunt procedures are performed because of the ready availability of other therapies for portal hypertensive bleeding (endoscopic treatment, TIPS insertion, and liver transplantation).

The most appropriate conclusions to be derived from seven controlled trials of the distal splenorenal shunt versus a variety of nonselective shunts have been argued for several years[82] (Table 20-6). It should be emphasized, however, that the study groups in six of these trials contained almost exclusively patients with alcoholic cirrhosis and that the seventh investigation was applied to a population of patients with schistosomiasis.[64,65,83-87] Although the distal splenorenal shunt frequently is used in patients with nonalcoholic cirrhosis, no investigation has compared selective to nonselective shunts in such patients. To summarize the available data comparing the distal splenorenal shunt to nonselective shunts: none of the trials showed an advantage in survival for either procedure, four demonstrated less frequent encephalopathy after the distal splenorenal shunt,[64,65,86,88] and the remaining three showed no difference in this variable between groups.[83-85] With the exception of one trial in which the portacaval shunt was more effective than the distal splenorenal shunt,[83] nonselective and selective shunts were about equivalent in preventing recurrent portal hypertensive bleeding. Combining the data from all the trials demon-

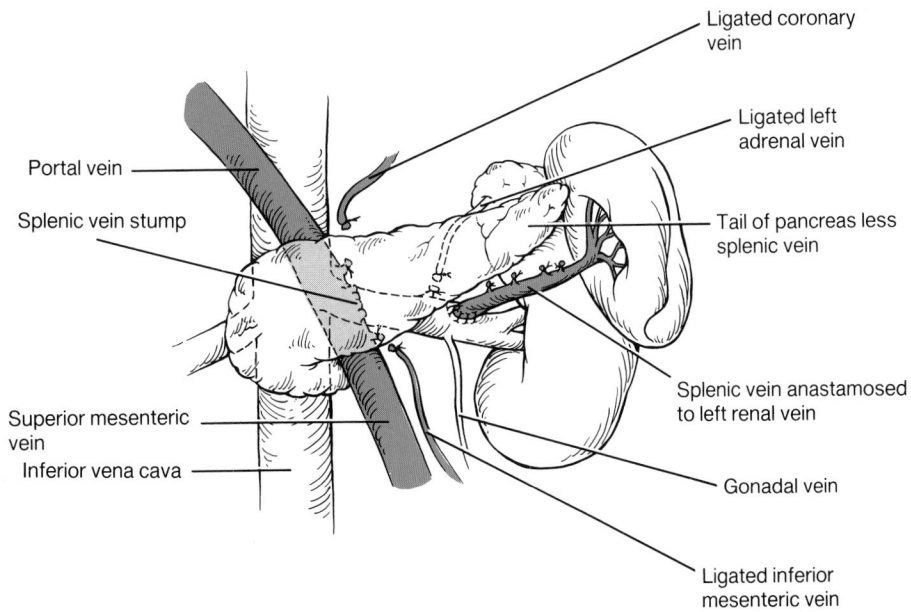

Figure 20-17 Distal splenorenal shunt with splenopancreatic disconnection. The splenic vein is dissected all the way to the splenic hilum, disconnecting it from the tail of the pancreas.

Table 20-6   Randomized, Controlled Trials of Distal Splenorenal Shunt (DSRS) Versus Nonselective Shunts

Trial	Shunt	No.	Alcoholic Cirrhosis (%)	Operative Mortality (%)	PSE (%)	Rebleeding (%)	Survival (%)	Follow-Up (y)
Philadelphia (1979)[72]	DSRS	13	100	8	0.75*†	NA	69	3
	MCS	14	100	7	3.75*†	NA	71	3
Cincinnati (1981)[84]	DSRS	23	96	4	5	13	78	2
	SRS	19	74	0	11	16	100	2
Atlanta (1985)[64]	DSRS	26	69	12	27*	8	42	11
	NSS	29	76	10	76*	14	28	11
Toronto (1985)[86]	DSRS	38	84	13	24*	3	47	5
	PCS	40	80	0	40*	0	53	5
Los Angeles (1986)[83]	DSRS	26	100	12	39	30*	46	5
	PCS	27	100	7	32	4*	33	5
Sao Paolo (1986)[87]	DSRS	30	0	0	7*	7	100	2
	SRS	32	0	0	25*	13	94	2
New Haven/Boston (1988)[85]	DSRS	43	88	9	51	18	53	3.5
	NSS	38	92	13	45	11	32	3.5

PSE, portosystemic encephalopathy; MCS, mesocaval shunt; SRS, conventional splenorenal shunt; NSS, nonselective shunt; PCS, portacaval shunt; NA, not available.
* P < .05.
† Months PSE/months survival.
(Jin G, Rikkers LF. Selective variceal decompression: current status. HPB Surg 1991;5:9)

strates overall incidences of encephalopathy after nonselective and distal splenorenal shunt procedures of 36% and 15%, respectively.[72] A review of the worldwide literature on nonrandomized trials, which comprise some 3700 patients (70% with nonalcoholic cirrhosis), confirms the effectiveness of the distal splenorenal shunt, with rebleeding rates below 10% and overall development of encephalopathy in less than 10% of patients.[72] Two large uncontrolled series also showed higher survival rates after distal splenorenal shunt procedures in patients with nonalcoholic cirrhosis as compared with patients with alcoholic liver disease.[89,90] However, these findings were not duplicated in several other large series.[72,91,92]

The distal splenorenal shunt also has been compared extensively with long-term endoscopic treatment (Table 20-7). The results of four randomized trials should be interpreted only after considering the settings in which they were conducted.[12,13,88,93] All the investigations showed significantly lower rates of recurrent bleeding after distal splenorenal shunting (3% to 17%) than after long-term sclerotherapy (35% to 60%). In the two North American studies,[12,13] sclerotherapy failure, defined as death from bleeding or salvage by shunt surgery, occurred in about one third of patients. Because most sclerotherapy failures could be rescued by surgery in one trial,[12] the sclerotherapy group had a higher survival rate than the distal splenorenal shunt group. However, the survival rate was significantly

higher in the distal splenorenal shunt group in another trial,[13] because salvage of sclerotherapy failures was infrequent. This major difference between these two investigations most likely has to do with the use of an urban population in one study and a predominantly rural population in the other. Three of the controlled trials of sclerotherapy versus the selective shunt operation showed no significant difference between groups with respect to posttreatment encephalopathy.[12,13,88] The fourth trial showed an advantage with respect to this variable in the sclerotherapy group, but this finding may result from the selective shunt technique used in that trial, which omitted ligation of the coronary vein.[93] The two European investigations found no difference in survival between sclerotherapy and selective shunt groups.[88,93] When a metaanalysis is applied to these four investigations, the distal splenorenal shunt is clearly superior to sclerotherapy in preventing rebleeding, and the two treatments are equivalent with respect to survival and posttreatment encephalopathy.[94]

In summary, selective variceal decompression is nearly as effective as nonselective shunts in preventing recurrent hemorrhage. Because portal perfusion is preserved in some patients, and intestinal venous hypertension is maintained, the overall frequency of encephalopathy is lower after distal splenorenal shunting than after the various nonselective shunt procedures. No data have demonstrated an advantage of one type of shunt over another with respect to

Table 20-7 Controlled Trials of Endoscopic Variceal Sclerotherapy (EVS) Versus Distal Splenorenal Shunt (DSRS)

Authors	Treatment	No.	Encephalopathy (%)	Rebleeding (%)	Survival (%)	Follow-Up (y)
Rikkers et al[13]	Shunt	30	25	17*	48*	7
	EVS	30	27	60*	26*	7
Henderson et al[12]	DSRS	35	16	3*	42†	5
	EVS	37	12	59*	65†	5
Teres et al[93]	DSRS	57	24*	14*	71	2
	EVS	55	8*	38*	68	2
Spina et al[88]	DSRS	20	5	5*	95	2
	EVS	20	10	35*	90	2

* $P < .05$.
† $P < .02$.
(Jin G, Rikkers LF. Variceal hemorrhage: surgical therapy. Gastroenterol Clin North Am 1993;22:833)

long-term survival. The distal splenorenal shunt is more effective than long-term endoscopic treatment in preventing recurrent bleeding and is about equivalent to sclerotherapy with respect to survival and postoperative encephalopathy.

The left gastric–caval shunt, which directly decompresses the esophagogastric variceal complex, seldom is used (see Fig. 20-15). Experience with this procedure has been confined almost entirely to Japan, where the results have been good. In one large series,[95] the incidence of recurrent variceal hemorrhage was only 8% and the shunts were patent in 88% of patients who underwent postoperative angiography. In this selected group of patients, the 10-year survival rate was over 50% and postoperative encephalopathy was infrequent. In North America, the left gastric–caval shunt has been used occasionally in patients who are not candidates for the distal splenorenal shunt because of previous splenectomy.[96]

Partial Shunt

Although it is an old concept, partial portal decompression only recently has been achieved consistently using a small-diameter (8- to 10-mm) interposition portacaval shunt[97] (Fig. 20-18). Because the entire portal venous system is partially decompressed, rather than compartmentalized, this is termed a *partial shunt* rather than a selective shunt. The objectives of partial and selective shunts are the same: effective decompression of varices, preservation of hepatic portal perfusion, and maintenance of some residual portal hypertension. Initial attempts at partial shunting consisted of small-diameter vein-to-vein anastomoses (side-to-side portacaval and conventional splenorenal shunts). The general experience with these direct anastomoses has been that they dilate with time and become nonselective shunts.[61]

More recently, a small-diameter interposition portacaval shunt using a ribbed polytetrafluoroethylene graft, combined with ligation of the coronary vein and other collaterals, has been used[97] (see Fig. 20-18). When the shunt diameter is 10 mm or less, hepatic portal perfusion is preserved in most patients, at least during the early postoperative interval. Despite the small diameter, less than 15% of shunts have undergone thrombosis, and most cases of shunt occlusion have been resolved successfully by interventional radiologic techniques. Pilot clinical investigations in two institutions have shown low rates of encephalopathy after partial shunting.[97,98] The results of a prospective, randomized trial of partial (8 mm diameter) and total (16 mm diameter) interposition portacaval shunts have been reported.[99] Survival was similar in both groups, but encephalopathy-free survival was considerably better in the partial shunt group. Most patients with partial shunts maintained portal flow during the early postoperative interval, and no shunts in either group occluded during a follow-up period of slightly less than 2 years. The limitations of this trial are that only 30 patients were randomly assigned and the follow-up has been relatively brief. Further trials need to be done, including a comparison of the small-diameter interposition shunt to the distal splenorenal shunt. If the results of this initial experience are duplicated in subsequent investigations, the partial interposition shunt may be used more often since it is technically easier to perform than the distal splenorenal shunt and could provide longer preservation of

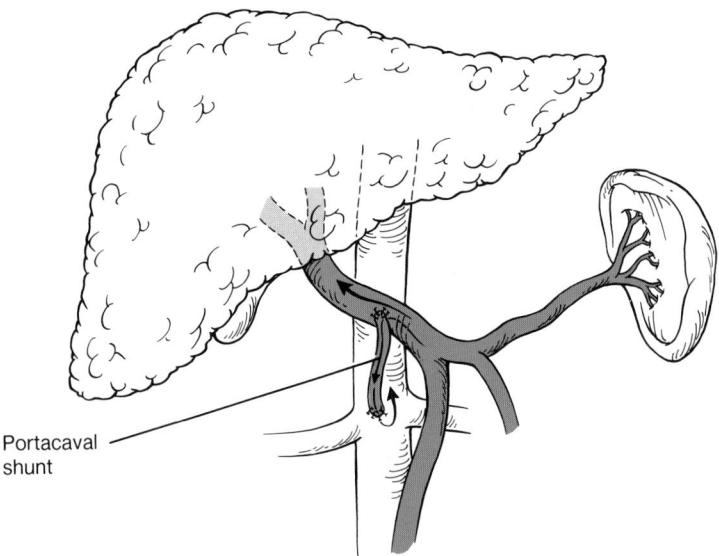

Portacaval shunt

Figure 20-18. A small-diameter (8- to 10-mm) interposition portacaval shunt partially decompresses the portal venous system and may preserve hepatic portal perfusion.

hepatic portal perfusion, because it has a fixed resistance and cannot dilate with time.

Nonshunt Operations

Rather than decompressing varices, the objective of most nonshunt operations is to isolate varices from the hypertensive portal venous circulation. These operations vary from splenectomy alone, which is effective for patients who bleed from varices because of splenic vein thrombosis, to the Sugiura procedure, which consists of extensive devascularization of the esophagus and stomach combined with esophageal transection and splenectomy.

As originally described by its creators, the Sugiura procedure is done in either a single stage or two stages through a laparotomy and a thoracotomy[100] (Fig. 20-19). Through the abdominal incision, the proximal two thirds of the stomach is devascularized and the spleen is removed. Care is taken to preserve the left gastric vein and the paraesophageal collaterals to discourage recurrent formation of varices. A left thoracotomy provides access for devascularization of the esophagus to the inferior pulmonary vein and for esophageal transection and reanastomosis just above the esophagogastric junction. Most North American surgeons have modified the Sugiura procedure so that all its objectives can be accomplished through an abdominal incision. In addition to devascularization of the proximal two thirds of the stomach and removal of the spleen, the esophagus is devascularized proximally for 8 to 10 cm. In Japanese patients with mainly nonalcoholic cirrhosis, the results of the Sugiura procedure have been admirable, with a 66% 5-year survival rate and recurrent variceal hemorrhage in less than 10% of patients.[100] However,

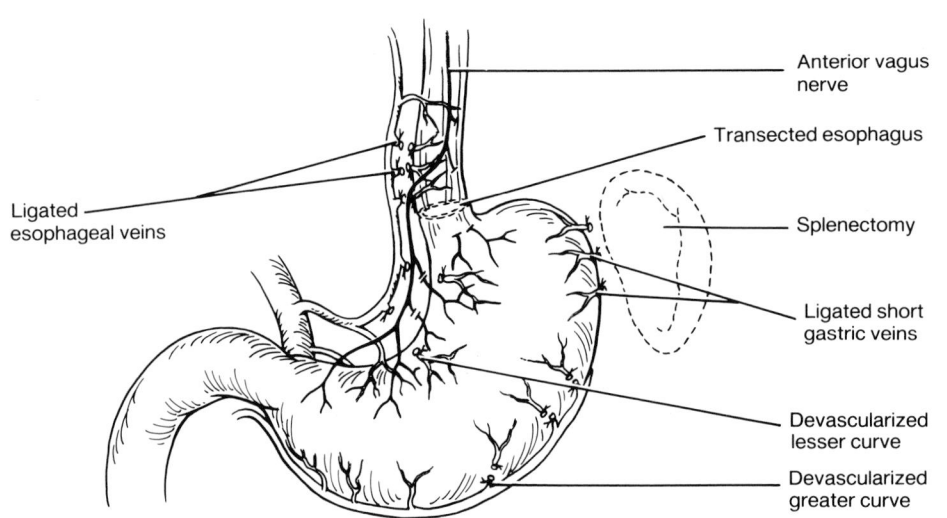

Ligated esophageal veins

Anterior vagus nerve

Transected esophagus

Splenectomy

Ligated short gastric veins

Devascularized lesser curve

Devascularized greater curve

Figure 20-19 The Sugiura operation consists of extensive devascularization of the proximal stomach and distal esophagus, transection of the distal esophagus with an EEA stapler, and removal of the spleen. If the vagal trunks and antral branches are preserved, pyloroplasty is not necessary. The left gastric vein and paraesophageal collaterals are carefully preserved.

the North American experience with this operation in patients with mainly alcoholic cirrhosis has been less successful. Recurrent variceal bleeding has occurred in 10% to 54% of patients, and operative mortality rates have ranged from 10% to 35%.[101]

As discussed earlier, esophageal transection and anastomosis with the EEA stapling device, sometimes combined with left gastric vein ligation, is the most commonly performed nonshunt procedure in the United States and generally is used only in the emergency setting.[47–49] Although it is effective in the emergency control of bleeding from esophageal varices, late rebleeding rates are considerably higher after this procedure than after portal decompressive operations or after the more extensive Sugiura procedure.

In patients with isolated splenic vein thrombosis, splenic venous flow undergoes collateralization through the upper stomach, resulting in the development of gastric varices, which can bleed. If liver disease and portal vein thrombosis are absent, esophageal varices usually do not form. The excess venous flow through the upper stomach can be eliminated by removal of the spleen, which is always curative.[4] This condition most commonly afflicts patients with chronic pancreatitis.

Because their long-term control of bleeding is less complete than that of portal decompressive operations, nonshunt procedures are used infrequently in the elective setting in the United States. Patients in whom sclerotherapy fails and shunts cannot be used because of diffuse splanchnic venous thrombosis are ideal candidates for such operations. A modified Sugiura procedure also is a reasonable option when a distal splenorenal shunt fails, because such patients have a combination of generalized portal hypertension and splenic vein thrombosis.

The advantage of nonshunt operations is that portal flow is preserved indefinitely. Controlled comparisons of the Sugiura procedure or one of its modifications to a variety of shunts, including the distal splenorenal shunt, generally have demonstrated a lower incidence of encephalopathy after the nonshunt operation.[87]

Liver Transplantation

Liver transplantation is not a therapy for variceal bleeding per se but rather is the ultimate therapy for patients with end-stage liver disease, many of whom bleed from portal hypertension. The unique advantage of transplantation over all other approaches to variceal bleeding is that it not only returns portal pressure to normal but also restores hepatic functional reserve. Although hepatic transplantation always should be considered in

the sequence of therapies for patients with cirrhosis who bleed from varices, individual circumstances, economic factors, and a limited supply of donor organs make transplantation a reasonable option for only a small fraction of patients. Common reasons for excluding patients with variceal bleeding from transplant waiting lists include advanced age, active alcoholism or drug abuse, and advanced disease in other organ systems, which make the risk of the transplant operation prohibitive. Individuals with extrahepatic portal hypertension or with schistosomiasis also are not transplant candidates because hepatic functional reserve is retained indefinitely in these disorders.

In addition to determining candidacy for transplantation, another important issue is the timing of transplantation in relation to the variceal bleeding episode. In general, potential transplant candidates with advanced liver disease (Child's class C) should be placed on the waiting list immediately.[102,103] Patients with Child's class A or B liver disease, who have complications of their disease that compromise the quality of their lives, such as advanced ascites, encephalopathy, fatigue, or bone pain, also should be considered for early transplantation.[102,103] Recurrent bleeding can be prevented in most of these patients by endoscopic means until a donor liver becomes available. When endoscopic treatment fails, TIPS placement is an ideal short-term bridge to transplantation.[40,42]

Transplantation usually is not an early consideration for patients with variceal bleeding who have well-preserved hepatic functional reserve and no other significant symptoms of their liver disease.[102,103] Rebleeding generally can be prevented in such individuals by long-term endoscopic treatment, surgical portal decompression, a nonshunt operation, or a sequence of these therapies (eg, long-term endoscopic treatment followed by a selective shunt when sclerotherapy fails). With available technology, TIPS insertion probably is not an effective long-term bridge to transplantation because of its high failure rate after 6 months to 1 year.[40,41,45] All these patients should be followed up carefully and placed on the transplantation list when evidence of hepatic functional decompensation appears.

Overall Plan for Definitive Treatment of Portal Hypertensive Bleeding

Because patients who bleed from portal hypertension form such a heterogeneous group, no single therapy or sequence of therapies is ideal for all. Each individual patient's disease, hepatic hemodynamic alterations, and specific clinical circumstances need to be considered before a definitive treatment plan is formulated. An algorithm for

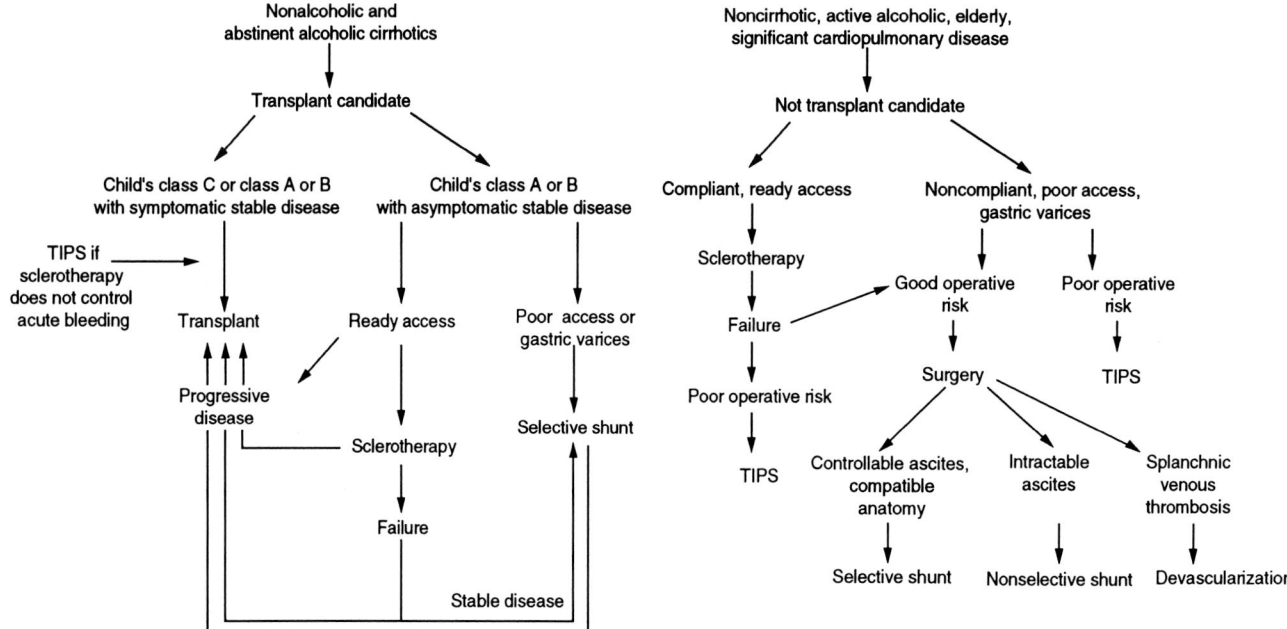

Figure 20-20 Algorithm for definitive treatment of portal hypertensive bleeding. TIPS, transjugular intrahepatic portosystemic shunt. (After Rikkers LF. Portal hypertension. In: Levine BA, ed. Current practice of surgery, vol 3. New York, Churchill Livingstone, 1993:12)

elective treatment of portal hypertensive bleeding is presented in Figure 20-20. Candidacy for hepatic transplantation is assessed first. This decision is based on the cause of portal hypertension, abstinence for patients with alcoholic cirrhosis, the presence or absence of other significant diseases, and the availability of liver transplantation for that individual patient.

If transplantation is not an immediate consideration (Child's class A or B with asymptomatic stable disease), endoscopic treatment is a reasonable initial approach as long as surgery is readily available should sclerotherapy fail to control bleeding. Future transplant candidates who bleed from gastric varices or portal hypertensive gastropathy, or who live in remote geographic locations, are better served by an initial selective shunt as a long-term bridge to transplantation. Because nearly all these patients have less advanced hepatic disease, medically intractable ascites is almost never present, making a nonselective shunt unnecessary.

The definitive treatment plan for patients who will never be transplant candidates is somewhat different. Those who are compliant and who have ready access to medical and surgical care should be treated initially by endoscopic means. Up to one third of these patients eventually fail to respond to sclerotherapy and require another treatment.[12,13] Patients who are reasonable operative risks should undergo surgery. Those who have controllable ascites and compatible anatomy should un-

dergo selective shunting. Patients with medically intractable ascites should receive a nonselective shunt of the side-to-side type; patients with diffuse splanchnic venous thrombosis with or without liver disease should undergo extensive esophagogastric devascularization (modified Sugiura procedure) if endoscopic treatment fails. Patients who have failed to respond to sclerotherapy and who are poor operative risks because of advanced liver disease probably are best served by TIPS insertion. Because the expected survival time for these patients is relatively brief, many of them are likely to die of their advanced liver disease before TIPS malfunction develops. Patients who are noncompliant, have poor access to surgical care, or bleed from gastric varices or portal hypertensive gastropathy are poor candidates for endoscopic treatment. Nonselective β-blockade can be considered for such patients, but the risk of recurrent bleeding remains high with this treatment. Those who are reasonable operative risks should undergo surgery to prevent rebleeding, with the selection of procedure based on clinical and portal hemodynamic circumstances.

Prevention of Initial Variceal Bleeding Episode (Prophylactic Therapy)

Preventing an initial episode of bleeding from portal hypertension is attractive because the mortality rate from this complication is high (15% to 50%). On the other hand, only a few patients with varices eventually bleed (about one third), making prophylactic therapy unnecessary for as much as two thirds of the patient population. To be acceptable, the prophylactic treatment must be associated with lower morbidity and mortality rates than those of the untreated population at risk, only a few of whom will experience an initial bleeding episode. The ideal would be to provide prophylactic treatment only to those patients who are destined to bleed. However, even though endoscopic criteria (eg, size of varices and markings on varices) have been useful in predicting bleeding, considerable overlap between groups make these criteria generally unreliable.[20]

The most commonly used prophylactic treatment is nonselective β-adrenergic blockade with propranolol or nadolol. Nearly all trials of β-blockade as prophylactic therapy have found a reduced incidence of initial variceal hemorrhage in treated patients. A summary of the many available trials has shown a clear benefit of β-blockade, with a reduction of about 40% in the likelihood of initial hemorrhage.[104] Although the frequency of initial bleeding was decreased by β-blockade in most of these studies, survival generally was not prolonged.

In contrast to the consistent results achieved with prophylactic β-blockade, the effects of prophylactic sclerotherapy on the frequency of initial bleeding and survival have been variable. Although a metaanalysis of the many investigations of prophylactic sclerotherapy showed an overall beneficial effect of this treatment, the results were heterogeneous and many of the trials were poorly designed.[105] Two of the studies were terminated because the survival benefit for control patients reached statistical significance.[106,107] This treatment modality cannot be recommended for prophylaxis.

Nearly all controlled investigations of prophylactic surgery to prevent initial variceal bleeding have failed to show any survival benefit. The first such trials in the 1960s compared prophylactic portacaval shunts with conventional medical therapy. Although bleeding developed in few patients with shunts, survival analysis of three American trials showed no advantage, and possibly a disadvantage, for these patients.[108–110] Patients with shunts tended to have an earlier onset of hepatic failure, presumably secondary to complete portal diversion. In addition, encephalopathy developed in many of these patients. A more recent Japanese trial comparing prophylactic surgery (selective shunt [40%] and esophagogastric devascularization [60%]) to medical therapy showed a significant survival advantage for the surgical group.[111] In contrast to the earlier North American trials, most patients included in the Japanese study had nonalcoholic liver disease that was categorized as Child's class A. Although these results are encouraging for this select group of patients, they should not be generalized to all patients with portal hypertension, many of whom in the United States are higher-risk patients with alcoholic cirrhosis.

ASCITES

Ascites also is a common and sometimes life-threatening complication of portal hypertension. Although mild ascites is of little clinical consequence, advanced, tense ascites often precedes the onset of variceal bleeding, can become infected (spontaneous bacterial peritonitis), almost always is present in patients with the hepatorenal syndrome, and compromises normal pulmonary and gastrointestinal function. During the first year after the onset of ascites, 20% to 40% of the afflicted population die.

Although the pathogenesis of ascites is not completely understood, most evidence supports the lymph imbalance theory.[112] According to this concept, the prime factor in the formation of ascites is elevated splanchnic capillary and hepatic sinusoidal pressures, which lead to transudation of fluid into the interstitial space. When the rate of fluid transudation is greater than the capacity for lymph drainage, ascites forms. Because the hepatic sinusoidal lining is more porous than the intestinal capillary endothelium, the liver is a major contributor in most cases. In fact, portal hypertension secondary to extrahepatic portal venous thrombosis almost never is complicated by significant ascites.

As ascites accumulates, a relative circulating volume deficit develops, and a multitude of compensatory mechanisms are set in motion, aggravating the situation. Renal sodium retention is a major factor in this cycle and often can be detected in patients with portal hypertension before the accumulation of ascites and plasma volume depletion.

Because renal sodium retention is a primary mechanism in the initiation and perpetuation of ascites, the condition can be controlled in most patients by the combination of dietary sodium restriction and augmentation of renal sodium excretion by diuretic administration. Because secondary hyperaldosteronism is one of the factors leading to renal sodium retention, spironolactone is the first-line diuretic of choice in these patients. In addition to sodium restriction of 2 to 3 g/d, spironolactone therapy should be initiated at a dosage of 100 to 150 mg/d. If diuresis is not initiated within 2 or 3 days, the dosage can be increased to a maximum of 400 mg/d. Although spironolactone generally is considered a less potent diuretic than furosemide, a controlled trial has shown that it is more efficacious in the treatment of cirrhotic ascites.[113] However, if the desired effect is not achieved with spironolactone alone, hydrochlorothiazide or furosemide can be added to the regimen. Because these diuretics can cause hypokalemia, metabolic alkalosis, azotemia, and the hepatorenal syndrome, renal function and electrolyte balance must be monitored carefully. Daily weight loss secondary to diuresis generally should not exceed 2 lb, because this appears to be the limit at which ascites can be mobilized. More rapid weight loss generally leads to intravascular volume depletion and prerenal azotemia.

The optimal therapy for the 5% to 15% of patients who have diuretic-resistant ascites is controversial. These patients generally have advanced hepatic disease and also are prone to other complications, such as variceal bleeding, encephalopathy, and hepatic functional decompensation. With the exception of those who are candidates for transplantation, the mortality rate for this population of patients is high.

Therapeutic options for patients with diuretic-resistant ascites include intermittent large-volume paracentesis, peritoneovenous shunt placement, TIPS insertion, a nonselective side-to-side portosystemic shunt, and liver transplantation. Intermittent large-volume paracentesis, with or without intravenous administration of colloid, has been resurrected after many years of disuse.[114] In stable patients with ascites, the feared complications of rapid ascites reaccumulation with consequent intravascular volume depletion leading to prerenal azotemia and even shock have not occurred. However, protein loss can be significant and repeated paracentesis can lead to infected ascites, secondary to either bowel puncture or skin organisms.

Because it functions as a megalymphatic, the peritoneovenous shunt appears to be an ideal physiologic therapy for ascites (Fig. 20-21). This device allows transfer of ascitic fluid from the abdomen into the central venous system as long as it is patent and the pressure in the peritoneal cavity exceeds that in the thorax. The peritoneovenous shunt reverses most of the pathophysiologic factors that contribute to the formation of ascites.[115] After shunt insertion, cardiac output and circulating plasma volume are increased, and plasma levels of aldosterone, renin, and antidiuretic hormone are decreased. Both the glomerular infiltration rate and renal plasma flow are increased, with a resultant improvement in urinary volume and salt excretion. In most patients, a brisk diuresis ensues after shunt insertion. However, some degree of renal sodium retention persists even after successful peritoneovenous shunting.

Although the placement of a peritoneovenous shunt is not technically demanding and can be done under local anesthesia, significant morbidity and mor-

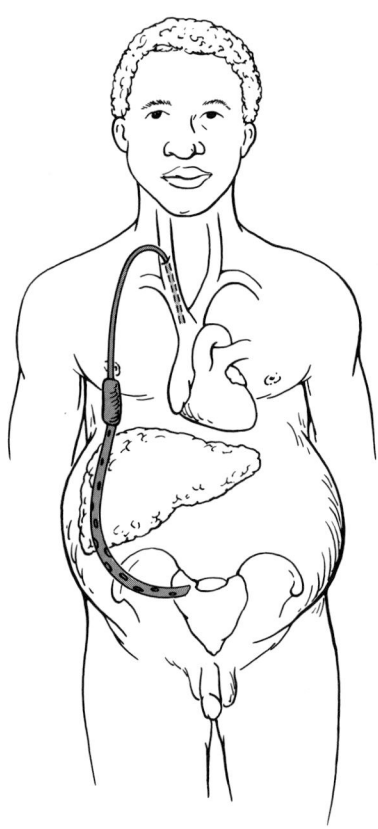

Figure 20-21 As long as intraperitoneal pressure exceeds intrathoracic pressure, the peritoneovenous shunt transfers ascitic fluid from the abdomen to the superior vena cava.

tality may follow this procedure. Complication rates approaching 75% and mortality rates as high as 25% have been reported.[116] The most common complications associated with the peritoneovenous shunt are sepsis, shunt occlusion, and disseminated intravascular coagulation. The last of these complications often is not clinically significant and can be minimized by discarding ascites during the operation and replacing it with saline. The most frequent late complication of a peritoneovenous shunt is shunt occlusion, which eventually occurs in about 30% of patients. After this complication, ascites may reaccumulate.

Use of the peritoneovenous shunt has declined because several controlled trials failed to show any associated survival benefit.[117] In many centers, intermittent large-volume paracentesis or TIPS placement is preferred to the peritoneovenous shunt for patients with diuretic-resistant ascites.

TIPS insertion is being used increasingly for the treatment of medically intractable ascites.[40,59] As long as it remains patent, the TIPS functions as a side-to-side portosystemic shunt, and thereby relieves ascites because of splanchnic venous and hepatic sinusoidal decompression. Although the TIPS is relatively noninvasive and effective, it has a high long-term failure rate and negative effects on portal hemodynamics. To be effective in relieving ascites, the TIPS must divert portal flow completely away from the sinusoids; therefore, in many series,[40,41,44,59] the rate of encephalopathy was high after shunt insertion. Although follow-up is brief in most series, a long-term effect of a patent TIPS would be a more rapid onset of hepatic failure due to the fact that the liver is deprived of the hepatotrophic hormones that are present in portal blood. Because of these adverse consequences, the use of TIPS placement for medically intractable ascites should be limited until controlled trials have demonstrated its overall efficacy.

Because several alternatives are available, and because the morbidity and mortality rates associated with operative shunts are high in patients with advanced ascites, side-to-side portosystemic shunts cannot be justified for the treatment of diuretic-resistant ascites alone. In contrast, these operations are reasonable options for patients with the combination of difficult-to-control ascites and portal hypertensive bleeding.

REFERENCES

1. Lautt WW, Greenway CV. Conceptual review of the hepatic vascular bed. Hepatology 1987;5:952.
2. Starzl TE, Francavilla A, Halgrimson CG, et al. The origin, hormonal nature and action of hepatotrophic substances in portal venous blood. Surg Gynecol Obstet 1973;137:179.
3. Vorobioff J, Bredfeldt JE, Groszmann RJ. Hyperdynamic circulation in portal-hypertensive rat model: a primary factor for maintenance of chronic portal hypertension. Am J Physiol 1983;244:G52.
4. Madsen MS, Peterson TH, Sommer H. Segmental portal hypertension. Ann Surg 1986;204:72.
5. Nordlinger BM, Nordlinger DF, Fulenwider JT, et al. Angiography in portal hypertension: clinical significance in surgery. Am J Surg 1980;139:132.
6. Moriyasu F, Ban N, Nishida O, et al. Clinical application of an ultrasound duplex system in the quantitative measurement of portal blood flow. J Clin Ultrasound 1986;14:579.
7. Ozaki CF, Anderson JC, Rikkers LF. Duplex ultrasound as a noninvasive technique of assessing portal hemodynamics. Am J Surg 1988;155:70.
8. Pomier-Layrarues G, Kusielewicz D, Willems B, et al. Presinusoidal portal hypertension in nonalcoholic cirrhosis. Hepatology 1985;5:415.
9. Dave P, Romeu J, Messer J. Upper gastrointestinal bleeding in patients with portal hypertension: a reappraisal. J Clin Gastroenterol 1983;5:113.
10. Trudeau W, Prindiville T. Endoscopic injection sclerosis in bleeding gastric varices. Gastrointest Endosc 1985;4:264.
11. D'Amico G, Montalbarro L, Traina M, et al. Natural history of congestive gastropathy. Gastroenterology 1990;99:1558.
12. Henderson JM, Kutner MH, Millikan WJ Jr, et al. Endoscopic variceal sclerosis compared with distal splenorenal shunt to prevent recurrent variceal bleeding in cirrhosis: a prospective, randomized trial. Ann Intern Med 1990;112:262.
13. Rikkers LF, Jin G, Burnett DA, et al. Shunt surgery versus endoscopic sclerotherapy for variceal hemorrhage: late results of a randomized trial. Am J Surg 1993;165:27.
14. North Italian Endoscopic Club for the Study and Treatment of Esophageal Varices. Prediction of the first variceal hemorrhage in patients with cirrhosis of the liver and esophageal varices: a prospective multicenter study. N Engl J Med 1988;319:983.
15. Gores GJ, Wiesner RH, Dickson ER, Zinmeister AR, Jorgensen AR, Langworthy A. Prospective evaluation of esophageal varices in primary biliary cirrhosis: development, natural history and influence in survival. Gastroenterology 1989;96:1552.
16. Rigo GP, Merighi A, Chalen NJ, et al. A prospective study of the ability of three endoscopic classifications to predict hemorrhage from esophageal varices. Gastrointest Endosc 1992;38:425.
17. Graham D, Smith JL. The course of patients after variceal hemorrhage. Gastroenterology 1981;80:800.
18. Garcia-Tsao G, Groszmann RJ, Fisher RL, Conn HO, Atterbury CE, Glickmann M. Portal pressure, presence of gastroesophageal varices and variceal bleeding. Hepatology 1985;5:419.
19. Lebrec D, DeFleury P, Rueff B, Nahum H, Benhamou JP. Portal hypertension, size of esophageal varices and risks of gastrointestinal bleeding in alcoholic cirrhosis. Gastroenterology 1980;79:1139.
20. Beppu K, Inokuchi K, Koyanagi N, et al. Prediction of variceal hemorrhage by esophageal endoscopy. Gastrointest Endosc 1981;27:213.
21. Rikkers LF, Jin G. Surgical management of acute variceal hemorrhage. World J Surg 1994;18:193.
22. Larson AW, Cohen H, Zweiban B, et al. Acute esophageal variceal sclerotherapy: results of a prospective randomized controlled trial. JAMA 1986;255:497.
23. Westaby D, Hayes PC, Gimson AES, Polson RS, Williams R. Controlled clinical trial of injection sclerotherapy for active variceal bleeding. Hepatology 1989;9:274.
24. Paquet KJ, Feussner H. Endoscopic sclerosis and esophageal balloon tamponade in acute hemorrhage from esophagogastric varices: a prospective controlled randomized trial. Hepatology 1985;5:580.
25. Schuman BM, Berkmann JW, Tedesco FJ. Complications of endoscopic injection sclerotherapy: a review. Am J Gastroenterol 1987;82:823.
26. Stiegmann GV, Goff JS, Mihaletz-Onody PA, et al. Endoscopic sclerotherapy as compared with endoscopic li-

gation for bleeding esophageal varices. N Engl J Med 1992;326:1527.

27. Planas R, Quer JC, Boix J, et al. A prospective randomized trial comparing somatostatin and sclerotherapy in the treatment of acute variceal bleeding. Hepatology 1994;20:370.

28. Shields R, Jenkins SA, Baxter JN, et al. A prospective randomized controlled trial comparing the efficacy of somatostatin with injection sclerotherapy in the control of bleeding esophageal varices. J Hepatol 1992;16:128.

29. Sung JJY, Chung SCS, Lai CW, et al. Octreotide infusion or emergency sclerotherapy for variceal hemorrhage. Lancet 1993;342:637.

30. Copenhagen Esophageal Varices Sclerotherapy Project. Sclerotherapy after first variceal haemorrhage in cirrhosis. N Engl J Med 1984;311:1584.

31. Terblanche J, Branman PC, Kahn D, et al. Failure of repeated injection sclerotherapy to improve long-term survival after oesophageal variceal bleeding. Lancet 1983;2:1328.

32. Westaby D, MacDougall BRD, Williams R. Improved survival following injection sclerotherapy for oesophageal varices: final analysis of a controlled trial. Hepatology 1985;5:827.

33. Korula J, Balart LA, Radavan G, et al. A prospective, randomised controlled trial of chronic esophageal variceal sclerotherapy. Hepatology 1985;5:564.

34. Gimson AE, Westaby D, Hegarty J, Watson A, Williams R. A randomized trial of vasopressin and vasopressin plus nitroglycerin in the control of acute variceal hemorrhage. Hepatology 1986;6:410.

35. Tsai YT, Lay CS, Lai KH, et al. Controlled trial of vasopressin plus nitroglycerin vs. vasopressin alone in the treatment of bleeding esophageal varices. Hepatology 1986;6:406.

36. Walker S, Stiehl A, Raedsch R, Kommerell B. Terlipressin in bleeding esophageal varices: a placebo-controlled, double-blind study. Hepatology 1986;6:112.

37. Burroughs AK, McCormick PA, Hughes MD, Sprengers D, D'Heygere F, McIntyre N. Randomized, double-blind, placebo-controlled trial of somatostatin for variceal bleeding: emergency control and prevention of early variceal bleeding. Gastroenterology 1990;99:1388.

39. Panes J, Teres J, Bosch J, et al. Efficacy of balloon tamponade in treatment of bleeding gastric and esophageal varices: results in 151 consecutive episodes. Dig Dis Sci 1988;33:454.

40. LaBerge JM, Ring EJ, Gordon RL, et al. Creation of transjugular intrahepatic portosystemic shunts with the Wallstent endoprosthesis: results in 100 patients. Radiology 1993;187:413.

41. Rossle M, Haag K, Ochs A, et al. The transjugular intrahepatic portosystemic stent-shunt procedure for variceal bleeding. N Engl J Med 1994;330:165.

42. Ring EJ, Rade JR, Roberts JP, et al. Using transjugular intrahepatic portosystemic shunt to control variceal bleeding before liver transplantation. Ann Intern Med 1992;116:304.

43. Helton WS, Belshaw A, Althaus S, Park S, Coldwell D, Johansen K. Critical appraisal of the angiographic portacaval shunt (TIPS). Am J Surg 1993;165:566.

44. Martin M, Zajko AB, Orons PD, et al. Transjugular intrahepatic portosystemic shunt in the management of variceal bleeding: indications and clinical results. Surgery 1993;4:719.

45. Dohrenwend M, Saddekni S, Memel DS, Schwartzberg M, Anderson JW, vanLeeuwen DJ. Clinical outcome shunt patency and survival after transjugular intrahepatic portosystemic shunt. Gastroenterology 1994;106:A885.

46. Langer BF, Greig PD, Taylor BR. Emergency surgical treatment of variceal hemorrhage. Surg Clin North Am 1990;70:307.

47. Burroughs AK, Hamilton G, Phillips A, Mezzanotte G, McIntyre N, Hobbs K. A comparison of sclerotherapy with staple transection of the esophagus for the emergency control of bleeding from esophageal varices. N Engl J Med 1989;321:857.

48. Huizinga WKJ, Angorn IB, Baker LW. Esophageal transection versus injection sclerotherapy in the management of bleeding esophageal varices in patients at high risk. Surg Gynecol Obstet 1985;160:539.

49. Teres J, Baroni R, Bordas JM, Visa J, Pera C, Rodes J. Randomized trial of portacaval shunt, stapling transection and endoscopic sclerotherapy in uncontrolled variceal bleeding. J Hepatol 1987;4:159.

50. Potts JR, Henderson JM, Millikan WJ Jr, Warren WD. Emergency distal splenorenal shunts for variceal hemorrhage refractory to nonoperative control. Am J Surg 1984;148:813.

51. Lebrec D, Poynard T, Bernau J, et al. A randomized controlled study of propranolol for prevention of recurrent gastrointestinal bleeding in patients with cirrhosis: a final report. Hepatology 1984;4:355.

52. Burroughs AK, Jenkins WJ, Sherlock S, et al. Controlled trial of propranolol for the prevention of recurrent variceal hemorrhage in patients with cirrhosis. N Engl J Med 1983;309:1539.

53. Villeneuve JP, Pomier-Layragues G, Infante-Riwand C, et al. Propranolol for the prevention of recurrent variceal hemorrhage: a controlled trial. Hepatology 1986;6:1239.

54. Garcia-Tsao G, Grace ND, Groszmann RJ, et al. Short term effects of propranolol on portal venous pressure. Hepatology 1986;6:101.

55. Burroughs AK, McCormick PA. Prevention of variceal rebleeding. Gastroenterol Clin North Am 1992;21:119.

56. Grace ND. Prevention of initial variceal hemorrhage. Gastroenterol Clin North Am 1992;21:149.

57. Snady H. The role of sclerotherapy in the treatment of esophageal varices: personal experience and a review of randomized trials. Am J Gastroenterol 1987;9:813.

58. Burroughs AK. The management of bleeding due to portal hypertension. Part 2. Prevention of variceal rebleeding and prevention of the first bleeding episode in patients with portal hypertension. Q J Med 1988;255:507.

59. Ferral H, Bjarnason H, Wegryn SA, et al. Refractory ascites: early experience in treatment with transjugular intrahepatic portosystemic shunt. Radiology 1993;189:795.

60. Resnick RH, Iber FL, Ishihara AM, et al. A controlled study of the therapeutic portacaval shunt. Gastroenterology 1974;67:843.

61. Bismuth H, Franco D, Hepp J. Portal-systemic shunt in hepatic cirrhosis: does the type of shunt decisively influence the clinical result? Ann Surg 1974;179:209.

62. Reynolds TB, Donovan AJ, Mikkelson WP, et al. Results of a 12-year randomized trial of portacaval shunt in patients with alcoholic liver disease and bleeding varices. Gastroenterology 1981;80:1005.

63. Redeker AG, Kunelis CT, Yamamoto S, et al. Assessment of portal and hepatic hemodynamics after side-to-side portacaval shunt in patients with cirrhosis. J Clin Invest 1964;43:1464.

64. Millikan WJ, Warren WD, Henderson JM, et al. The Emory prospective randomized trial: selective versus nonselective shunt to control variceal bleeding. Ann Surg 1985;201:712.

65. Reichle FA, Fahmy WF, Golsorkhi M. Prospective comparative clinical trial with distal splenorenal and mesocaval shunts. Am J Surg 1979;137:13.

66. Mehigan DG, Zuidema GD, Cameron JL. The incidence of shunt occlusion following portosystemic decompression. Surg Gynecol Obstet 1980;150:661.

67. Smith RB III, Warren WD, Salam AA, et al. Dacron interposition shunts for portal hypertension: an analysis of morbidity correlates. Ann Surg 1980;192:9.

68. Stipa S, Ziparo V, Anza M, et al. A randomized controlled trial of mesentericocaval shunt with autologous jugular vein. Surg Gynecol Obstet 1981;153:353.

69. Malt RA, Abbott WM, Warshaw AL, et al. Randomized trial of emergency mesocaval and portacaval shunts for bleeding esophageal varices. Am J Surg 1978;135:584.

70. Rikkers LF. Portal hemodynamics, intestinal absorption, and postshunt encephalopathy. Surgery 1983;94:126.

71. Warren WD, Zeppa R, Fomon JJ. Selective transsplenic decompression of gastroesophageal varices by distal splenorenal shunt. Ann Surg 1967;166:437.

72. Jin G, Rikkers LF. Selective variceal decompression: current status. HPB Surg 1991;5:1.

73. Belghiti J, Grenier P, Nouel O, et al. Long-term loss of Warren's shunt selectivity: angiographic demonstration. Arch Surg 1981;116:1121.

74. Maillard JN, Flamant YM, Hay JM, et al. Selectivity of the distal splenorenal shunt. Surgery 1979;86:663.

75. Jin G, Rikkers LF. Significance of portal vein thrombosis after distal splenorenal shunt. Arch Surg 1991;126:1011.

76. Henderson JM, Millikan WJ, Wright-Bacon L, et al. Hemodynamic differences between alcoholic and nonalcoholic cirrhotics following distal splenorenal shunt: effect on survival? Ann Surg 1983;198:325.

77. Ezzat FA, Abu-Elmagd K, Sultan A, et al. Schistosomal versus nonschistosomal variceal bleeders: do they respond differently to selective shunt (DSRS)? Ann Surg 1989;209:4.

78. Warren WD, Henderson JM, Millikan WJ, Galambos JT, Bryan FC. Management of variceal bleeding in patients with noncirrhotic portal vein thrombosis. Ann Surg 1988;207:5.

79. Vang J, Simert G, Hansson J, et al. Results of a modified distal splenorenal shunt for portal hypertension. Ann Surg 1977;185:224.

80. Henderson JM, Warren WD, Millikan WJ, et al. Distal splenorenal shunt with splenopancreatic disconnection: a 4-year assessment. Ann Surg 1989;210:332.

81. Inokuchi K, Beppu K, Koyanagi N, et al. Exclusion of nonisolated splenic vein in distal splenorenal shunt for prevention of portal malcirculation. Ann Surg 1984;200:711.

82. Rikkers LF. Is the distal splenorenal shunt better? Hepatology 1988;8:1705.

83. Harley HA, Morgan T, Redeker AG, et al. Results of a randomized trial of end-to-side portacaval shunt and distal splenorenal shunt in alcoholic liver disease and variceal bleeding. Gastroenterology 1986;91:802.

84. Fischer JE, Bower RH, Atamian S, et al. Comparison of distal and proximal splenorenal shunts: a randomized prospective trial. Ann Surg 1981;194:531.

85. Grace DN, Conn HO, Resnick RH, et al. Distal splenorenal vs. portal-systemic shunts after hemorrhage from varices: a randomized controlled trial. Hepatology 1988;8:1475.

86. Langer B, Taylor B, Mackenzie DR, et al. Further report of a prospective randomized trial comparing distal splenorenal shunt. Gastroenterology 1985;88:424.

87. daSilva LC, Strauss E, Gayotto LCC, et al. A randomized trial for the study of elective surgical treatment of portal hypertension in Mansonic schistosomiasis. Ann Surg 1986;204:148.

88. Spina GP, Santambrogio R, Opocher E, et al. Distal splenorenal shunt versus endoscopic sclerotherapy in the prevention of variceal bleeding. Ann Surg 1990;211:178.

89. Warren WD, Millikan WJ Jr, Henderson JM, et al. Ten years' portal hypertensive surgery at Emory. Ann Surg 1982;195:530.

90. Zeppa R, Hutson DG, Levi JU, et al. Factors influencing survival after distal splenorenal shunt. World J Surg 1984;8:733.

91. Rikkers LF, Soper NJ, Cormier RQA. Selective operative approach for variceal hemorrhage. Am J Surg 1984;147:89.

92. Orozco H, Juarez F, Santillan P, et al. Ten years of selective shunts for hemorrhage portal hypertension. Surgery 1988;103:27.

93. Teres J, Bordas JM, Bravo D, et al. Sclerotherapy vs. distal splenorenal shunt in the elective treatment of variceal hemorrhage: a randomized controlled trial. Hepatology 1987;7:430.

94. Spina GP, Henderson JM, Rikkers LF, et al. Distal

spleno-renal shunt versus endoscopic sclerotherapy in the prevention of variceal rebleeding: a meta-analysis of 4 randomized clinical trials. J Hepatol 1992;16:338.

95. Inokuchi K, Sugimachi K. The selective shunt for variceal bleeding: a personal perspective. Am J Surg 1990;160:48.

96. Warren WD, Millikan WJ, Henderson JM, et al. Selective variceal decompression after splenectomy or splenic vein thrombosis. Ann Surg 1984;199:694.

97. Collins JC, Rypins EB, Sarfeh IJ. Narrow-diameter portacaval shunts for management of variceal bleeding. World J Surg 1994;18:211.

98. Rosemurgy AS, McAllister EW, Kearney RE. Prospective study of a prosthetic H-graft portacaval shunt. Am J Surg 1991;161:159.

99. Sarfeh IJ, Rypins EB. Partial versus total portacaval shunt in alcoholic cirrhosis. Ann Surg 1994;219:353.

100. Idezuki Y, Kokudo N, Sanjo K, Sandai Y. Suguira procedure for management of variceal bleeding in Japan. World J Surg 1994;18:216.

101. Wexler MJ, Stein BL. Nonshunting operations for variceal hemorrhage. Surg Clin North Am 1990;70:425.

102. Henderson JM, Gilmore FT, Hooks MA, et al. Selective shunt in the management of variceal bleeding in the era of liver transplantation. Ann Surg 1992;216:248.

103. Wood RP, Shaw BW Jr, Rikkers LF. Liver transplantation for variceal hemorrhage. Surg Clin North Am 1990;70:449.

104. Grace ND. Management of portal hypertension. Gastroenterologist 1993;1:39.

105. Pagliaro L, D'Amico G, Sorensen TIA, et al. Prevention of first bleeding in cirrhosis: a meta-analysis of randomized trials of nonsurgical treatment. Ann Intern Med 1992;117:59.

106. The Veterans Affair Cooperative Variceal Sclerotherapy Group. Prophylactic sclerotherapy for esophageal varices in alcoholic liver disease: a randomized, single-blind, multicenter clinical trial. N Engl J Med 1991;324:1779.

107. The PROVA Study Group. Prophylaxis of first hemorrhage from oesophageal varices by sclerotherapy, propranolol or both in cirrhotic patients: a randomized multicenter trial. Hepatology 1991;14:1016.

108. Conn HO, Lindenmuth WW, May CJ, Ramsby GR. Prophylactic portacaval anastomosis: a tale of two studies. Medicine (Baltimore) 1972;51:27.

109. Resnick RH, Chalmers TC, Ishihara AM, et al. A controlled study of the prophylactic portacaval shunt: a final report. Ann Intern Med 1969;70:675.

110. Jackson FC, Perrin EB, Smith AG, Dagradi AE, Nadal HM. A clinical investigation of the portacaval shunt II: survival analysis of the prophylactic operation. Am J Surg 1968;11:22.

111. Inokuchi K, Sugimachi K, Sato T, et al. Improved survival after prophylactic portal nondecompression surgery for esophageal varices: a randomized clinical trial. Hepatology 1990;1:1.

112. Witte CL, Witte MH, Dumont AE. Lymph imbalance in the genesis and perpetuation of the ascites syndrome in hepatic cirrhosis. Gastroenterology 1980;78:1059.

113. Perez-Ayuso RM, Arroyo V, Planas R, et al. Randomized comparative study of efficacy of furosemide versus spironolactone in nonazotemic cirrhosis with ascites. Gastroenterology 1983;84:961.

114. Gines P, Arroyo V, Vargas V, et al. Paracentesis with intravenous infusion of albumin as compared with peritoneovenous shunting in cirrhosis with refractory ascites. N Engl J Med 1991;325:829.

115. Blendis LM, Greig PD, Langer B, et al. The renal and hemodynamic effects of the peritoneovenous shunt for intractable hepatic ascites. Gastroenterology 1979;77:250.

116. Greig PD, Langer B, Blendis LM, et al. Complications after peritoneovenous shunting for ascites. Am J Surg 1980;139:125.

117. Stanley MM, Ochi S, Lee KK, et al. Peritoneovenous shunting as compared with medical treatment in patients with alcoholic cirrhosis and massive ascites. N Engl J Med 1989;321:632.

Digestive Tract Surgery: A Text and Atlas, edited by Richard H. Bell,
Layton F. Rikkers, and Michael W. Mulholland.
Lippincott-Raven Publishers, Philadelphia, © 1996.

21

Liver Transplantation

Alan N. Langnas | *Byers W. Shaw, Jr.*

Central to any discussion of the management of patients with decompensated chronic liver disease or fulminant hepatic failure is the role of liver transplantation. Liver transplantation has evolved from an onerous surgical exercise attempted at only a handful of institutions to a highly refined operation performed at many medical centers in the United States and throughout the world. At experienced centers, the transplantation procedure has matured to the point at which a 6-hour operation with minimal blood loss has become the rule and innovative advances such as reduced-sized allografts and living-related donation are commonplace. Surgical progress has made liver transplantation possible even in the face of complex technical hurdles. Survival after liver transplantation is not only dependent on the surgeon's ability to perform the operation but is also closely related to the pretransplantation condition of the patient. With the expanding role of liver transplantation in the treatment of patients with liver disease, the dominant factor limiting liver transplantation is an insufficient supply of donor organs.

The major obstacle to long-term patient and allograft survival after liver transplantation is immunologic failure. The myriad of problems related to rejection and infection in the postoperative period highlight the limitations of immunosuppressive regimens. Pharmaceutical advances, combined with a better understanding of the immune response to solid organ transplantation, have prompted the introduction of a variety of novel antirejection agents and strategies. On the horizon are innovative approaches to the induction of donor-specific unresponsiveness. Also in the early clinical stages of development are xenotransplantation and artificial liver support. In this chapter, we expand on the previously mentioned areas in an effort to shed light on

a field that has revolutionized the care of patients with liver disease but that itself is constantly evolving.

INDICATIONS

Epidemiology of Liver Disease

To fully appreciate current and potential needs for liver transplantation, one must understand the scope and magnitude of end-stage liver disease in this country. In the United States, cirrhosis is the cause of about 25,000 deaths annually, or 1.2% of the total 2.1 million deaths.[1] According to a survey sponsored by the American Liver Foundation, with a data base of 5200 nonfederal acute care hospitals, alcohol-related liver diseases affected 215,306 patients at a cost of $1.7 billion in 1992.[2] Nonalcoholic cirrhosis affected 85,490 patients with hospital charges of $1.4 billion. Hospitalizations for 3059 liver transplantation patients amounted to hospital charges of $526 million.[2]

Patient Selection and Timing

Potential liver transplant recipients can be divided into two groups: those with decompensated chronic liver disease and those with acute fulminant liver failure. Decompensated chronic liver disease can be manifested as markedly abnormal liver function tests, refractory ascites, variceal bleeding, portosystemic encephalopathy, or spontaneous bacterial peritonitis. The onset of these complications of chronic liver disease usually portends a poor prognosis and the need for consideration of liver transplantation. As more experience with liver transplantation has been gained, patients with quality-of-life issues, such as incapacitating fatigue, refractory pruritus, and osteogenic bone disease, have been accepted as transplantation candidates even when hepatic functional reserve is well preserved. Considered in the formula for placing a patient on the transplant waiting list is the time it takes to obtain a donor organ. A waiting time of 1 year or longer for small adults or children with certain blood types is common.

Specific Indications

The various liver diseases for which liver transplantation is indicated include the following:

ADULTS
Sclerosing cholangitis
Primary biliary cirrhosis
Postnecrotic cirrhosis
Budd-Chiari syndrome (BCS)
Fulminant hepatic failure
α_1-Antrypsin deficiency
Wilson's disease
Hepatoma
Alcoholic cirrhosis
CHILDREN
Biliary atresia
Neonatal hepatitis
Cirrhosis
BCS
Familial cholestasis
Inborn errors of metabolism
  α_1-Antrypsin deficiency
  Wilson's disease
  Tyrosinemia
  Familial hypercholesterolemia
Hepatic tumors

Primary Biliary Cirrhosis

Primary biliary cirrhosis represents the most common cholestatic liver disease that requires transplantation. The cause of primary biliary cirrhosis is unknown but is suspected to be autoimmune. More than 90% of patients are women, and it is associated with other autoimmune diseases, such as rheumatoid arthritis and scleroderma.[3] Serologic tests for autoantibodies, such as antimitochondrial and antinuclear antibodies, are frequently positive.

Primary biliary cirrhosis is a progressive liver disease with a predictable course. A model for deciding when to consider liver transplantation in patients with primary biliary cirrhosis has been developed.[4] Variables in this model include the histologic stage of the disease and the serum bilirubin level. Indications for transplantation include variceal hemorrhage, encephalopathy,

intractable pruritus, incapacitating fatigue, and hepatic osteodystrophy.

Primary Sclerosing Cholangitis

Primary sclerosing cholangitis is a disorder of unknown cause of the intrahepatic and extrahepatic biliary tree. Although a frequent indication for liver transplantation, this disease is relatively rare. About 70% of patients have inflammatory bowel disease,[5] and about 10% develop cholangiocarcinoma.[6]

The primary indication for transplantation in patients with primary sclerosing cholangitis is decompensated chronic liver disease. Chronic cholangitis or recurrent episodes of acute cholangitis are also reasons to consider transplantation. A predictive survival model similar to the one used for primary biliary cirrhosis incorporates age, serum bilirubin, blood hemoglobin, and liver histology.[7] Many patients with primary sclerosing cholangitis have had previous palliative procedures in an attempt to provide bile drainage. The long-term results of these surgical procedures have been disappointing except for in a select group of patients. Performance of palliative procedures may cause an inappropriate delay in referral for transplantation. Delay in referral may also allow the development of cholangiocarcinoma, which may preclude subsequent transplantation.

Fulminant Liver Failure

Acute fulminant liver failure is characterized by the sudden onset of liver failure associated with encephalopathy and coagulopathy in a previously healthy person. The incidence of fulminant hepatic failure appears to be increasing. Causes include acetaminophen overdose, hepatitis A and B, and tyrosinemia. There is a large group of patients for whom a cause is never found.

Criteria for liver transplantation have been proposed for patients with acetaminophen and nonacetaminophen causes of acute liver failure[8] (Table 21-1). The most frequent cause of death in patients with acute liver failure is cerebral edema with brain-stem herniation. A valuable tool for patient management and for determining prognosis is the intracranial pressure monitor. The decision regarding transplantation in a patient with fulminant liver failure is a dynamic one, often changing within hours. The earliest indicators of irreversible neurologic injury are normally revealed by the intracranial pressure monitor. A cerebral perfusion pressure of less than 40 mmHg for 2 hours or longer is associated with profound neurologic injuries and is a contraindication to transplantation.[9] Alternatively, improved cerebral perfusion and diminishing cerebral hy-

Table 21-1 Criteria for Liver Transplantation in Fulminant Hepatic Failure

ACETAMINOPHEN

pH <7.3 (irrespective of grade of encephalopathy)

or

Prothrombin time >100 s and serum creatinine >300 μmol/L in patients with grade III or IV encephalopathy

NONACETAMINOPHEN

Prothrombin time >100 s (irrespective of grade of encephalopathy)

or

Any three of the following variables (irrespective of grade of encephalopathy):

Age <10 y or >40 y

Etiology—non-A, non-B hepatitis, halothane hepatitis, idiosyncratic drug reactions

Duration of jaundice before onset of encephalopathy >7 d

Prothrombin time >50 s

Serum bilirubin >300 μmol/L

(After O'Grady JG, Alexander GJ, Hayller KM, Williams R. Early indicators of prognosis in fulminant hepatic failure. Gastroenterology 1989;97:439)

pertension may herald hepatic recovery before any other clinical or laboratory variables change.

Hepatitis C

Hepatitis C virus (HCV) has become the most common cause of nonalcoholic cirrhosis to require liver transplantation in the United States. HCV is responsible for nearly all cases of posttransfusion hepatitis. Before routine blood screening for the antibody to HCV, the frequency of transfusion-associated hepatitis was 3% to 4% (150,000 to 300,000 cases annually).[10] Fifty to 70% of sporadic community-acquired non-A, non-B hepatitis cases are also anti-HCV positive.[11] Despite the apparent benign nature of the initial infection, about half of infected patients become chronically infected, and 20% to 40% of these people develop cirrhosis.[12]

The decision to transplant patients with HCV is guided by the degree of hepatic decompensation. There is growing evidence that HCV infection is a precursor to hepatocellular carcinoma (HCC).[13] HCV frequently reinfects the transplanted liver and may be difficult to distinguish from other forms of allograft dysfunction, such as rejection. Studies are investigating the role of antiviral therapy, such as interferon, in preventing or abrogating HCV infections after liver transplantation.

Metabolic Liver Diseases

Metabolic liver diseases that often require liver transplantation include Wilson's disease, hemochromatosis, and α_1-antitrypsin deficiency. Wilson's disease (hepatolenticular degeneration) is characterized by an inborn error of copper metabolism resulting in increased copper stores throughout the body. It is an autosomal recessive disorder located on chromosome 13.[14] The clinical picture of hepatolenticular degeneration is the result of accumulation of toxic levels of copper within the liver and brain. This disease is due to a decreased ability to excrete copper into bile.[15]

Idiopathic hemochromatosis is an autosomal recessive disorder characterized by increased iron stores. The exact cause of this disorder is not known but is suspected to be the result of increased iron absorption by the intestine. These patients are at increased risk for developing HCC. Patients with hemochromatosis are also at increased risk for cardiac disease, particularly conduction abnormalities.[16]

α_1-Antitrypsin deficiency is a genetic disorder that causes cirrhosis in children and adults. Children who are homozygous and present with neonatal cholestasis may be at increased risk for developing cirrhosis.[17] Adults who develop cirrhosis due to α_1-antitrypsin deficiency are at increased risk for developing HCC.[18]

Biliary Atresia and Neonatal Hepatitis

The most common indication for liver transplantation in children is biliary atresia. It is estimated that biliary atresia occurs in about 1 in 15,000 live births.[19] The cause of this disorder is unknown. Despite the liberal use of surgical portoenterostomy (Kasai procedure) for treatment, at least two thirds of these patients require transplantation. One institution reported a 3-year survival rate after portoenterostomy of slightly greater than 50% during the 10-year period from 1973 to 1982.[20] A portoenterostomy often allows a child to grow, increasing the likelihood of obtaining a donor organ. The presence of a previous portoenterostomy does not in itself have a detrimental effect on the outcome of liver transplantation. Numerous revisions of the portoenterostomy, however, may delay timely referral for transplantation. Often, children with a previous Kasai procedure require transplantation because of recurrent cholangitis. Other indications for transplantation include variceal hemorrhage, growth retardation, and nutritional failure. Nutritional support is essential to the pretransplantation preparation of these children. Idiopathic neonatal hepatitis is a waste-basket term for a number of cholangiopathies of infancy and childhood, all histologically characterized by giant cell formation and cirrhosis. Children with neonatal hepatitis should undergo liver transplantation when they demonstrate evidence of decompensated cirrhosis.

Controversial Indications

Alcoholic Liver Disease

The most common cause of chronic liver disease in the United States is alcohol abuse. In 1992, it was estimated that 107,000 hospital admissions were due to complications of alcoholic cirrhosis.[2] To develop alcoholic cirrhosis, it is necessary to consume 120 g (12 beers or 500 mL of whiskey) or more of alcohol per day during an extended period of time.[21] Even with this rate of consumption, less than 20% of people develop cirrhosis.

According to the United Network for Organ Sharing (UNOS) statistics, the most common indication for liver transplantation in the United States is alcoholic liver disease. Studies have demonstrated that patients with alcoholic liver disease have a similar rate of survival to other adults undergoing liver transplantation.[22,23] The best alcohol treatment programs have a 30% to 40% rate of recidivism, and recidivism remains a concern after liver transplantation. The most important factors related to abstinence are family support and patient insight to the fact that alcohol was the cause of the liver disease.[24] The frequency of recurrent alcoholism after transplantation was about 15% in selected groups of patients.[22–24] Essential to the pretransplantation evaluation of these patients are psychiatric and psychological consultation.

The most debatable issue in liver transplantation in 1994 is the role it plays in the treatment of alcoholic liver disease. The controversy revolves around the concept of providing vital and limited resources (ie, donor organs and health care dollars) to patients with self-inflicted disease who may resume their previous behavior and again develop liver disease. Public opinion has begun to influence medical policy. In Oregon, the state Medicaid agency has ruled that it will pay for liver transplantation except in those patients with alcoholic liver disease.

Hepatocellular Carcinoma

Hepatocellular carcinoma is the 10th most common malignancy in the world and the 25th most frequent cancer in the United States.[25] There is a male predominance, with about 75% of patients also having cirrhosis.[26,27] There is a clear relation between hepatitis B and HCC. Reports have also linked HCV to the development of HCC. A variety of carcinogenic substances, including aflatoxin B1, thorium dioxide (Thoratrast), and androgens, have been associated with an increased risk of HCC.[28] α-Fetoprotein levels are elevated in about 70% of cases.[28] Newer diagnostic tests for HCC include computed tomography (CT) portography and iodized oil angiography.[29]

Since most patients with HCC have chronic liver disease, therapy is dictated not only by tumor stage but also by the extent of hepatic reserve. Large series of hepatic resection for HCC have been reported by the Liver Cancer Study Group of Japan.[30] Patients with tumors less than 2 cm in size had a 5-year survival rate of 60%, whereas those with tumors 2 to 5 cm in diameter had a survival rate of only 39%. In a European series, 52 Child's class A patients with small HCCs had a 3-year survival rate of only 57%.[31] Factors influencing survival include histologic grade, encapsulation, vascular invasion, multicentricity, and fibrolamellar variant.[28] Unfortunately, few patients present with tumors that are amenable to resection.

Appealing advantages of transplantation in patients with unresectable HCC or HCC associated with cirrhosis include removing the entire liver, which may harbor other undetected lesions or a preneoplastic environment, and treatment of the cirrhosis. The best results of liver transplantation are in patients with incidental tumors less than 3 cm in diameter.[32–34] When tumor diameter is 5 cm or less, recurrent disease is still relatively infrequent. If tumor diameter is greater than 5 cm or the tumor is multicentric, survival is significantly diminished. When deciding between resection and liver transplantation, important considerations include hepatic reserve, location of the tumor (central versus peripheral), and multicentricity.

Strategies to prevent tumor recurrence after transplantation include the administration in the perioperative period of chemotherapy, radiation therapy, and transcatheter arterial chemoembolization. Most reports of chemoembolization include patients with unresectable HCC not undergoing any form of surgical therapy. These studies have demonstrated the relative safety of the technique as well as the effectiveness of chemoembolization in decreasing the size of the tumor.[35] Several centers have reported preliminary results of patients receiving chemoembolization before liver transplantation.[36,37]

Metastatic Liver Tumors

Liver transplantation has little role in the treatment of metastatic tumors of the liver. When liver transplantation was used to treat metastatic colon and breast cancer, nearly all patients developed recurrent disease. The only group of patients with metastatic disease who may benefit from liver transplantation are those with neuroendocrine tumors.[38]

Hepatitis B

Hepatitis B is an infrequent cause of viral hepatitis in the United States. Less than 1% of the population are chronic carriers of the virus, and less than 10% have evidence of prior exposure. After an infection with hepatitis B, greater than 90% of patients fully recover. The remaining 5% to 10% of patients become chronic carriers, and 5% develop cirrhosis.[39]

Chronic hepatitis B has been a common indication for liver transplantation. In the past, however, the results of transplantation for cirrhosis secondary to hepatitis B have been poor because of reinfection and destruction of the new liver. In a European study, 83% of patients who were positive for hepatitis B DNA reinfected the transplanted liver.[40] In some institutions, patients with hepatitis B are offered liver transplantation only if serum hepatitis B DNA levels are undetectable. Patients with elevated levels of hepatitis B DNA are treated with interferon to stop viral replication so that transplantation may eventually be attempted. The best results with transplantation for hepatitis B have been in France, where patients are treated with intravenous immunoglobulin.[41] Future strategies for the treatment of patients with hepatitis B liver disease may include xenotransplantation from a species (baboon) not susceptible to hepatitis B infection.

Budd-Chiari Syndrome

Budd-Chiari syndrome refers to a group of disorders with obstruction to hepatic venous outflow. Controversy persists regarding appropriate therapy for patients with BCS. With the exception of mild forms of BCS, definitive therapy is necessary to prevent development of hepatic failure. Both portosystemic shunting and liver transplantation have been employed. Advocates of portosystemic shunting emphasize that long-term survival can be achieved and that a shunt prevents the development of cirrhosis. A successful side-to-side portocaval or mesocaval shunt requires favorable anatomy, however, and 20% of BCS patients have portal vein thrombosis, and 30% have inferior vena caval stenosis.[42]

Liver transplantation provides results equal to or better than those obtained with portosystemic shunting. The decision to perform a shunt or transplantation should be based on an estimate of hepatic reserve. When hypoalbuminemia, encephalopathy, or hyperbilirubinemia are present, transplantation is preferred.[43] A portosystemic shunt is reserved for patients who have not yet developed cirrhosis.

CONTRAINDICATIONS

Although previously contraindications, portal vein thrombosis, hepatopulmonary syndrome (HPS), previous right upper quadrant surgery, and age greater than 55 years are no longer barriers to liver transplantation. Absolute and relative contraindications to transplantation include the following:

ABSOLUTE CONTRAINDICATIONS
Active sepsis
Human immunodeficiency virus
Extrahepatic malignancy
Advanced cardiovascular disease
Severe hypoxemia
Active alcoholism
Severe neurologic deficits
RELATIVE CONTRAINDICATIONS
Advanced age
Grade IV coma
Hepatitis B

As experience with the transplant procedure has evolved, surgeons have developed innovative ways to provide splanchnic venous inflow to the new liver in patients with portal vein thrombosis.[44] Techniques include thrombectomy of the portal vein, resection of the phlebosclerotic portal vein with placement of an interposition graft, and extraanatomic bypass with the use of the superior mesenteric vein or a venous collateral for inflow (Fig. 21-1). Avoiding an extensive peripancreatic dissection in search of a suitable vein for inflow

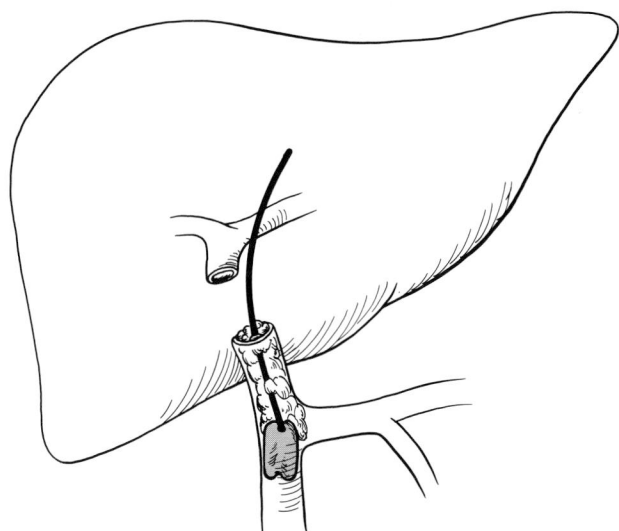

Figure 21-1 Thrombectomy of the portal vein is facilitated by the use of Fogarty catheters. Blood is vented into the peritoneal cavity to ensure that dislodged clots are evacuated. The portal limb of the venous bypass is then inserted.

Table 21-2 Intraoperative and Postoperative Variables of Liver Transplant Recipients With and Without a Prior Portosystemic Shunt (PSS)

	Shunt (N = 17)	*Control (N = 282)*	*P Value*
Operative time (h)	10.4 ± 3.0	8.5 ± 2.6	<.05
Blood loss (U)	25.9 ± 25.6	14.5 ± 15	<.05
Length of hospitalization (d)	26.3 ± 15	35 ± 31	NS
ICU stay (d)	10.2 ± 10.6	15.9 ± 26	NS
Hospital charges ($)	117,575 ± 66,493	139,353 ± 122,746	NS

(After Langnas AN, Marujo WC, Stratta RJ, et al. Influence of a prior portosystemic shunt on outcome following orthotopic liver transplantation. Am J Gastroenterol 1992;87:714)

has been shown to be important in reducing morbidity in these cases. If pretransplantation ultrasonography demonstrates thrombosis of the portal vein, angiography is often helpful in demonstrating potential sources of splanchnic venous inflow for the allograft.

Although a prior portosystemic shunt presents a formidable technical challenge to the transplantation surgeon, most studies have demonstrated no difference in survival between shunted and unshunted patients[45] (Table 21-2). Shunted patients generally experience greater blood loss and require more operative time than unshunted patients. Management of a distal spenorenal shunt at the time of transplantation differs among groups, with some ligating the shunt and performing splenectomy and others leaving it undisturbed.[46,47]

Severe hypoxia (Po_2 less than 60 mmHg) is a contraindication to transplantation if it is the result of an irreversible process such as chronic obstructive disease or pulmonary fibrosis. Some cases of severe hypoxemia, however, are the result of HPS. This syndrome is characterized by severe hypoxemia in patients with liver disease who have morphologically normal-appearing lungs. Arterial blood gases demonstrate hypoxemia (Pao_2 often less than 50 mmHg). The severe pulmonary shunting associated with HPS is potentially reversible and should be considered an indication for transplantation. The work-up to establish the diagnosis of HPS includes pulmonary function tests that include assessment of diffusion capacity, arterial blood gases on room air and while breathing 100% oxygen (shunt study), and contrast echocardiography.[48] In patients suspected of having HPS, a right heart catheterization is required to rule out severe pulmonary hypertension. Patients with HPS demonstrate normal to low pulmonary artery pressures, low pulmonary vascular resistance, and an elevated cardiac output.[48] Severe pulmonary hypertension is a contraindication to transplantation because it often leads to acute right heart failure, an arrhythmia, or sudden death during the posttransplantation in-

terval. Many patients with HPS who have undergone successful liver transplantation are able to discontinue supplemental oxygen within weeks to months.[49-51]

At many centers, liver transplantation is being offered to the elderly. Although acceptable results have been demonstrated with liver transplantation for seniors (older than 60 years), important lessons have been learned.[52,53] For older patients not in the intensive care unit at the time of transplantation, results are similar to those for younger adults; however, morbidity and mortality rates are high for critically ill seniors who undergo liver transplantation. A potential advantage for the elderly patient is a diminished immune system.[54] In a report of renal transplant recipients,[55] those older than 60 years had significantly better graft survival. When considering transplantation for older patients, the evaluation process needs to include a thorough search for concomitant disease (prostate cancer, breast cancer, coronary artery disease) that might preclude transplantation.

DONOR ISSUES

Organ Donation and Distribution

The primary limiting factor to liver transplantation is the availability of suitable donor organs. Although an effort has been made to educate the public as to the need for donor organs, physicians need to improve their skills in identifying potential donors and approaching families regarding organ donation.

The National Organ Transplantation Act mandated the formation of a fair and equitable organ procurement and distribution system. The system is managed under contract to the Department of Health and Human Services by UNOS. All potential transplant recipients must be registered with UNOS to be eligible for a donor organ. The distribution of donor livers follows a local, regional, and national prioritization scheme. UNOS has divided the United States into 11 regions. If a liver cannot be used in the local area, it is then offered to a recipient in the same region. If there are no recipients within the region, the organ is placed into the national pool. Once a satisfactory donor has been identified, it is matched to a potential recipient based on a variety of factors, including size and blood type. The UNOS system stratifies patients into four groups based on medical urgency: status 1, patient at home; status 2, at home but unable to perform normal activities; status 3, hospitalized but not requiring life support; status 4, in the intensive care unit requiring life support. Although both time on the waiting list and medical urgency are included in the formula, medical urgency outweighs waiting time so that sicker patients receive priority.

In 1993, 4824 people donated at least one organ for transplantation, a 7% increase over 1992.[56] There were 3406 cadaveric liver transplantations performed in 1993, a 12% increase over 1992. On January 31, 1994, 3040 patients were waiting for liver transplants in the United States. From 1988 to 1993, the median waiting time for a liver transplant increased from 34 to 163 days. During the same 4-year period, the number of patients awaiting liver transplantation more than doubled. One result of the increased waiting time was an increase in the number of deaths of patients on the waiting list (558 in 1993).

According to UNOS, there were 114 registered liver transplantation programs in the United States in 1994. During 1993, 7 of the 114 programs each performed more than 100 transplantations, accounting for 36% of liver transplantations in the United States, and 32 programs performed fewer than 10 liver transplantations each (UNOS OPTN/Scientific Registry data as of March 18, 1994).

The Organ Donor

Organ donors are people who have sustained an irreversible neurologic injury that results in brain death. Criteria for establishing brain death were first outlined in 1968.[57] The diagnosis of brain death is made by excluding all reversible causes of coma combined with determining the absence of brain stem function. The diagnosis can be confirmed by an electroencephalogram or cerebral blood flow study. Contraindications to organ donation include sepsis and cancer; however, organs from donors with primary central nervous system malignancies are often used. Although this policy is generally accepted, caution should be exercised when the donor does not have an established histologic diagnosis or when a prior ventriculoperitoneal shunt or extensive brain surgery have been performed, all of which increase the risk for metastatic disease.[58] A recent history of active intravenous drug use is another contrain-

dication to organ donation. Organ donors are routinely screened for a number of potentially transmittable diseases, including human immunodeficiency virus, hepatitis B, and hepatitis C. Hemodynamic stability of the donor is preferred but not essential. The use of vasopressors has not been demonstrated to be detrimental to eventual allograft function.[59] In general, all organ donors should be considered potential liver donors.

Prolonged donor starvation (more than 1 week), particularly when combined with other factors believed to be important in predicting poor allograft function, such as hypotension, hypoxemia, and acidosis, may preclude use of the donor liver. The use of older donors (older than 55 years) has become standard practice with many centers using donor livers from patients as old as 70 years.[60] Neonatal donor livers (less than 1 month of age) are infrequently used because of a relatively high rate of primary nonfunction and an increased rate of hepatic artery thrombosis.[61] Even though some neonatal livers function well, obtaining a second liver if the first one fails is so difficult that the risk of using a neonatal liver is prohibitive.

Multiple organ procurement techniques allow for the simultaneous removal of the liver, pancreas, intestine, and kidneys. Principles of the donor operation include a limited surgical dissection and elimination of warm ischemia. In situ perfusion of the abdominal viscera with cold preservation solution allows the donor organs to be flushed and cooled without any warm ischemia. In 1988, the introduction of University of Wisconsin (UW) organ preservation solution (Viaspan, Dupont) revolutionized liver transplantation.[62] Since donor livers can be safely stored for up to 24 hours in UW solution, the logistical constraints imposed by Euro-Collins preservation solution, which had a limit of 6 to 8 hours of safe cold ischemia, have been eliminated. With UW solution, it is no longer necessary for the donor and recipient operations to be performed simultaneously. The extra time afforded allows for increased sharing of livers between distant regions. Local transplantation surgeons can remove the donor liver and send it to the recipient's hospital, often by commercial airlines, thereby eliminating the need for expensive charter jet service.[63] The increased preservation time has also allowed for routine donor liver biopsy, a practice that has been valuable in reducing the incidence of primary nonfunction of the donor liver. The widespread use of reduced-size transplantation, which requires lengthy backtable preparation, would have been impossible without UW solution.

TRANSPLANTATION PROCEDURE

The Standard Operation

The transplantation procedure can be divided into three phases—recipient hepatectomy, the anhepatic phase, and the postrevascularization phase. Although the details of the operation are presented in Atlas Chapter 23, certain basic tenets are reviewed here. As in all surgical procedures, patience, attention to detail, and composure help ensure a favorable outcome.

Formerly, access to the upper abdomen was gained through bilateral subcostal incisions combined with a midline extension. Although the midline extension offers the surgeon excellent exposure, it creates a wound that often heals poorly and may become infected. The exposure that is afforded by the proper application of self-retaining retractors eliminates the need for a midline extension and also reduces the number of assistants required.

The goal of the recipient hepatectomy is to remove the diseased native liver, leaving the blood vessels and common bile duct for anastomosis to the donor organ. The liberal use of electrocautery has been a valuable tool for surgical dissection and hemostasis. When the hepatectomy is difficult, it is tempting to abandon meticulous dissection in favor of blunt dissection and to obtain hemostasis during the anhepatic phase or after revascularization. This approach frequently results in excessive blood loss and increased operative time, and it should be discouraged. The surgeon who takes time to maintain hemostasis during the recipient hepatectomy often is rewarded by decreased bleeding and a shorter operative time, both of which enhance patient outcome.

During the anhepatic phase, the empty right upper quadrant affords easy access to bleeding sites. The surgeon needs to evaluate the cuffs of the suprahepatic and infrahepatic inferior vena cava, the portal vein, and the hepatic artery. If the hepatic artery is unacceptable, a decision needs to be made whether a supraceliac or infrarenal aortic graft is required. Alternatively, the native celiac axis may be dissected and used for arterial inflow to the liver.

Implantation of the donor liver begins with anastomosis of the suprahepatic inferior vena cava, followed by anastomosis of the infrahepatic inferior vena cava. Intima-to-intima approximation between the donor and recipient vessels is essential to prevent thrombosis or bleeding. While finishing the lower caval anastomosis, the liver is flushed with 500 mL of 5% albumin to rinse out the preservation solution and to remove any air trapped in the donor vena cava. If the liver is not flushed, the adenosine and high potassium content of UW solution can cause cardiac arrest after revascularization. The portal vein is reconstructed with a running suture, and a "growth" stitch (see Section IVB in Atlas Chap. 23) is left to avoid narrowing the anastomosis. After the portal vein anastomosis is completed, the inferior vena caval and portal vein clamps are removed. Once hemodynamic stability and hemostasis are obtained, the arterial reconstruction is begun.

The most common method of reestablishing arterial perfusion is anastomosis of the donor celiac axis to the recipient common hepatic artery. Alternatively, a Carel patch of donor aorta may be joined to the juncture of the recipient's right and left hepatic arteries. If the hepatic inflow is not satisfactory, consideration should be given to revising the anastomosis or placing it more proximally on the native common hepatic artery or celiac axis. Occasionally, it is necessary to use an interposition graft of donor iliac artery.

After graft revascularization, the vascular anastomoses are examined, and hemostasis is completed. Continued bleeding is most often related to a coagulopathy, most frequently fibrinolysis and thrombocytopenia. The thromboelastograph and Sonoclot device are helpful in assessing coagulation status.

Finally, biliary reconstruction is performed either as a choledochocholedochostomy over a T-tube or as a Roux-en-Y choledochojejunostomy, the latter being selected when the recipient common bile duct is absent or unacceptable (eg, biliary atresia or sclerosing cholangitis).

Venous Bypass

Venous bypass was introduced to reduce hemorrhage and hemodynamic instability during the anhepatic phase of liver transplantation.[64] The bypass circuit diverts blood from the portal vein and inferior vena cava and returns it to the central circulation (Fig. 21-2). Venous bypass allows for a longer anhepatic phase than would otherwise be possible, an important consideration when placing an aortic graft, in the training of fellows, and in patients with cardiopulmonary disease. The use of percutaneous catheters for the femoral and subclavian veins avoids the complications associated with femoral and axillary cutdowns.[65] The anesthetic management is considerably different when venous bypass is used: intravascular volume support during the anhepatic phase does not need to be nearly as aggressive as when bypass is not used.

Reduced-Size Liver Transplantation

One of the major obstacles to pediatric liver transplantation has been the lack of size-compatible donors. Most pediatric recipients are 2 years of age or less, whereas pediatric donors are more commonly 5 years of age or older. The larger pediatric donor liver often does not fit into the upper abdomen of the younger recipient. In 1987, it was estimated that 25% or more of potential pediatric recipients were dying while awaiting liver transplantation.[66] To provide transplants for

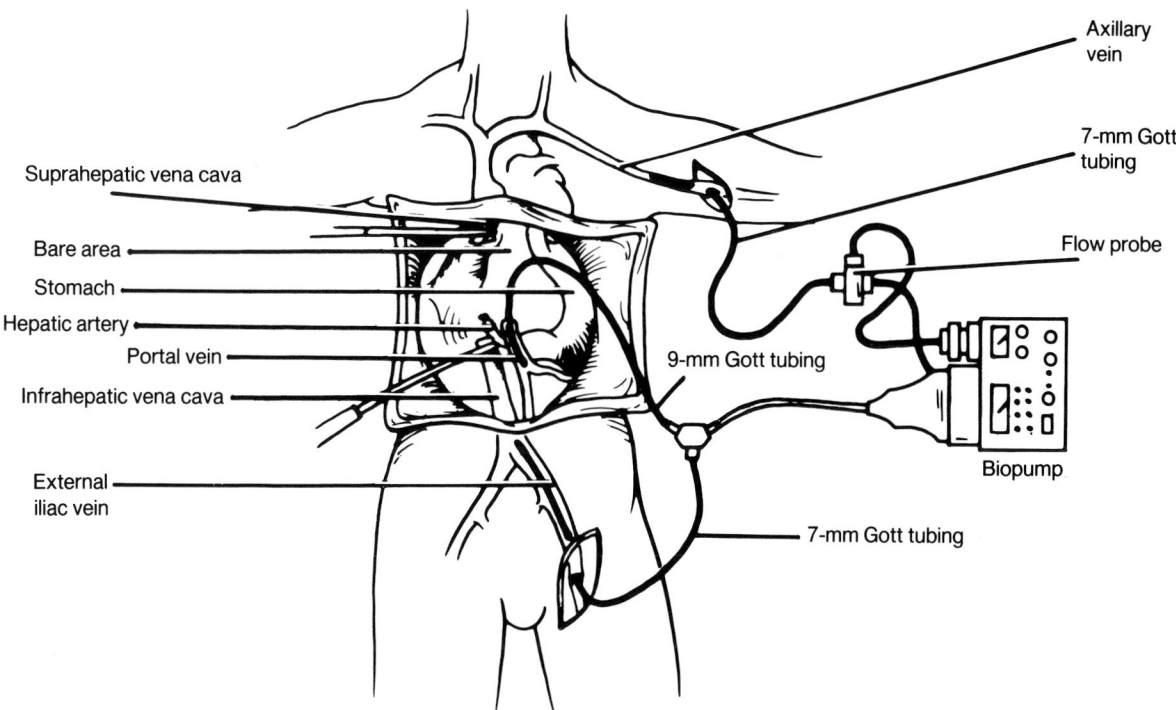

Figure 21-2 The circuit used for venous–venous bypass in liver transplant recipients. The blood is diverted from the splanchnic and infrahepatic systemic venous systems to a pump. It is then returned to the patient through an upper extremity vein. Subclavian and femoral venous access is accomplished percutaneously. Flow can safely be maintained in the range of 2 to 3.5 L/min. When flows are less than 1 L/min, the risk of clot formation within the system increases.

more of these recipients, the size of the large donor liver can be reduced by performing a partial hepatectomy.[67]

The reduced-size allograft typically consists of a left lobe or a left lateral segment of a donor liver, depending on size discrepancy. The caudate lobe is commonly removed from left lobe grafts. An extensive hilar dissection should be avoided to prevent devascularization of the bile duct. The subsequent transplantation procedure is similar to a standard whole-liver graft except that the native vena cava must remain intact. If a left lobe graft is used, it is occasionally necessary to taper the donor vena cava or anastomose the donor hepatic veins to a cloaca of the three native hepatic veins. Concerns regarding adequate function of reduced-size allografts have not been confirmed.[68] Studies have also demonstrated a similar rate of biliary tract complications between whole and reduced-size allografts.[68,69] Some series have suggested that the rate of hepatic artery thrombosis is diminished for recipients of reduced-size allografts.[70] The goal of reducing deaths of patients on the waiting list has been met in most centers.[68]

Split-Liver Transplantations

The technique of split-liver transplantation was first reported in 1988.[71] The enticing feature of this procedure is that it provides two allografts from one donor (Fig.

21-3). The most challenging aspect of split-liver transplantation is the separation of the arterial and biliary systems of the two lobes. Although a transparenchymal approach is preferred for reduced-size grafts, a hilar dissection is required for split-liver grafts. In one se-

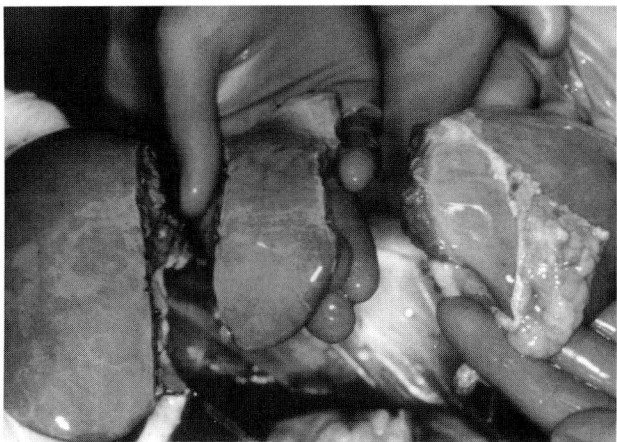

Figure 21-3 Donor liver after backtable preparation. The liver has been divided into two allografts. The right lobe will be transplanted into one recipient, and the left lateral segment into another. The medial segment of the left lobe is discarded.

ries,[68] all five divided livers had different patterns (Fig. 21-4). Overall results of split-liver allografts have been disappointing. Some of the poor results relate to technical complications, and others can be linked to the critical nature of the recipients at the time of transplantation.

Auxiliary Liver Transplantation

Heterotopic

Purported advantages of heterotopic liver transplantation are avoidance of trauma to the native liver, less urgent need for retransplantation if the allograft

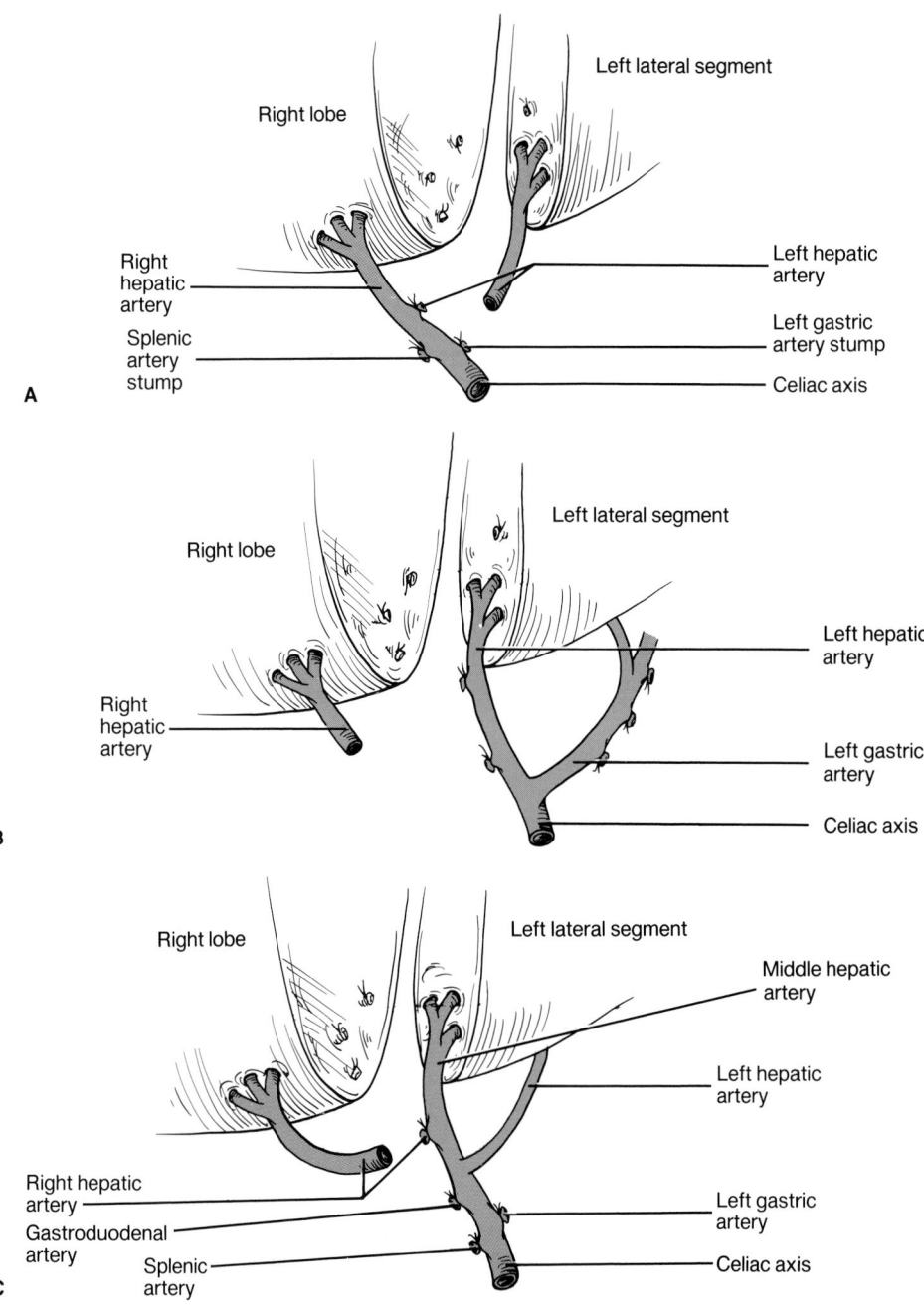

Figure 21-4 Methods of arterial reconstruction used for split-liver transplantation. (**A**) Normal hepatic arterial anatomy. (**B**) Accessory left hepatic artery from left gastric artery. (**C**) Right, middle, and left hepatic arteries. (**D**) Accessory right hepatic artery anastomosed to splenic artery stump. (**E**) Accessory right hepatic artery from superior mesenteric artery.

fails, and less of a requirement to match donor and recipient for size, thereby increasing the potential supply of donors. One important disadvantage of this technique is the competition for splanchnic venous inflow between native and transplanted livers. In addition, by leaving the diseased native liver in situ, the risk for development of a primary hepatic malignancy persists.

The most appealing role for heterotopic liver transplantation is in the treatment of metabolic liver diseases and fulminant liver failure. For patients with a metabolic defect, heterotopic liver transplantation can provide the deficient enzyme without the need for hepatectomy. In patients with fulminant liver failure, if the native liver recovers, immunosuppression can be discontinued, or the heterotopic allograft can be removed.

Orthotopic

The development of auxiliary orthotopic liver transplantation was based on previous experience with reduced-size liver transplantation and the theo-

retic advantages of auxiliary allografts. When performed for correction of a metabolic disorder, the appealing nature of the procedure is that the patient's life is not threatened acutely if the allograft is destroyed either because of immunologic or technical reasons.[72] When done to treat fulminant liver failure, the native liver may recover, allowing for discontinuance of immunosuppression[73] (Fig. 21-5). The technique consists of first doing a left hepatic lobectomy of the native liver and then implanting the donor graft, typically composed of segments 2 and 3, in the newly created space. The donor portal vein is anastomosed to the recipient left portal vein; the donor left hepatic vein is connected to the recipient left hepatic vein; and the hepatic artery of the donor liver is grafted to the recipient's supraceliac aorta (Fig. 21-6). Biliary drainage is provided with a Roux-en-Y choledochojejunostomy to the donor duct or a duct-to-duct anastomosis between the recipient's left hepatic duct and the donor bile duct. Orthotopic auxiliary transplantation has also been achieved by performing a left hepatic triseg-

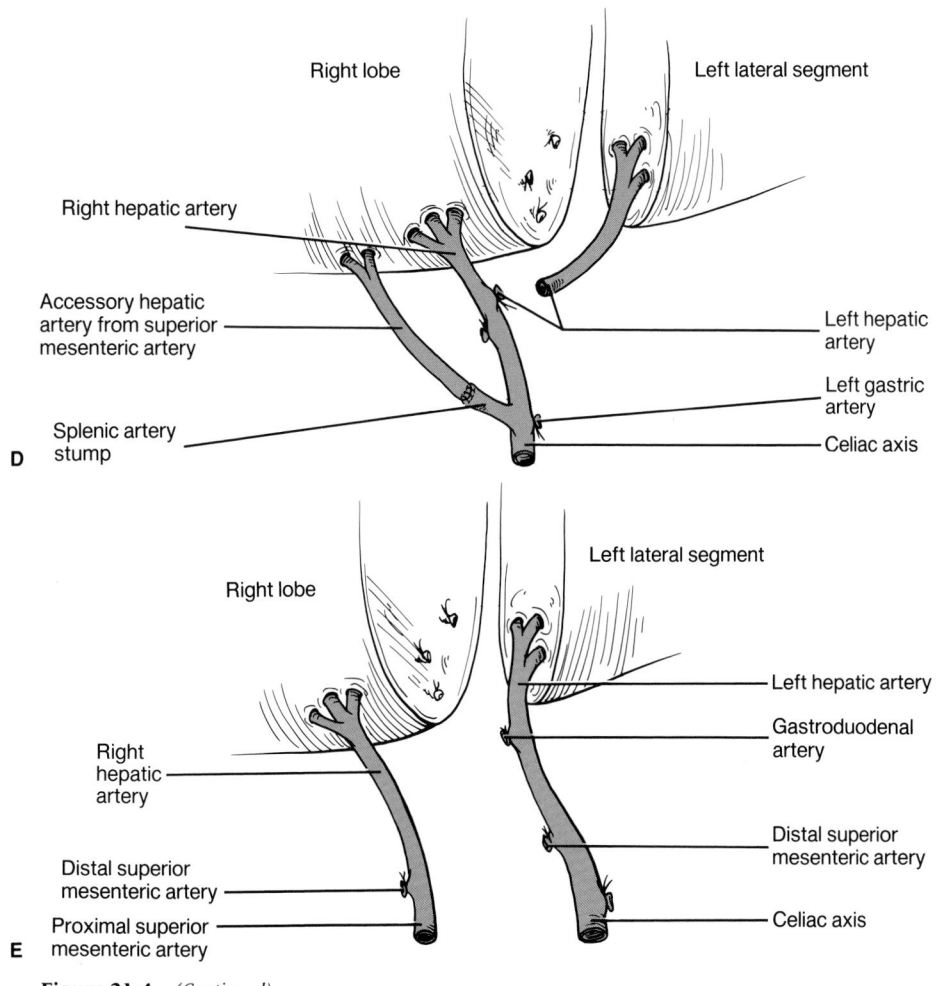

Figure 21-4 *(Continued)*

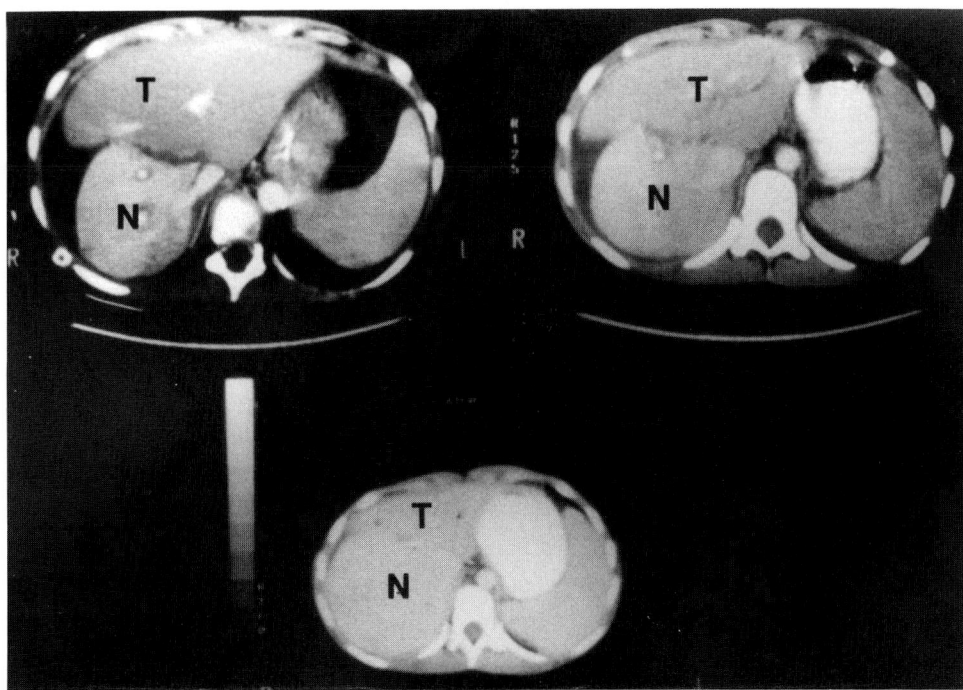

Figure 21-5 CT scans demonstrating the gradual growth of the native liver (N) after transplantation of auxiliary orthotopic liver (T) for fulminant hepatic failure. After adequate recovery of native liver function, immunosuppression was gradually withdrawn.

mentectomy and then placing a relatively small donor liver into the space provided.

Living-Related Transplantation

One of the most exciting new developments in pediatric liver transplantation is living-related donation. Even with the introduction of reduced-size transplant-

ations, there continues to be a shortage of organ donors for pediatric recipients. The number of organ donors has not increased to the same extent as the number of patients on the transplant waiting list.

The concept of living-related transplantation is not new. Living-related kidney transplantation has been used successfully for more than 20 years, with about

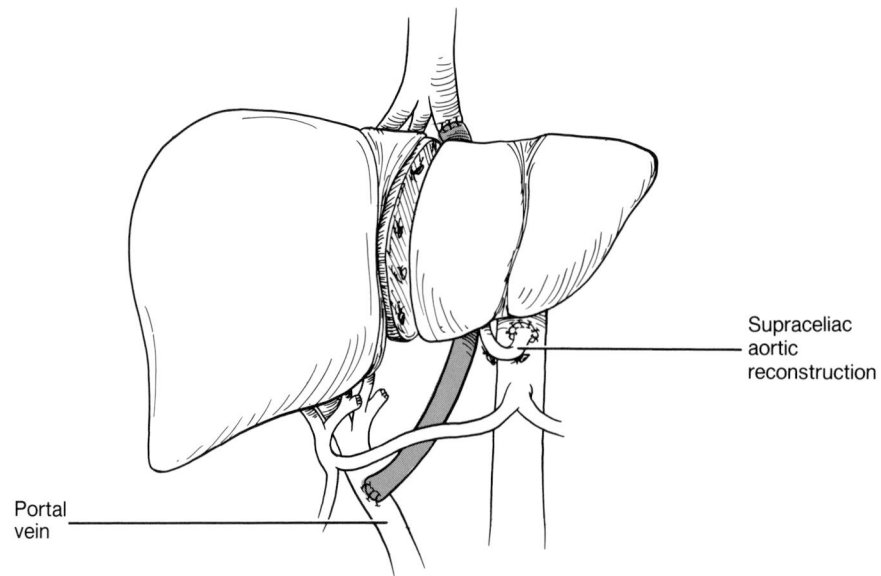

Portal vein

Supraceliac aortic reconstruction

Figure 21-6 Diagram of an auxiliary orthotopic liver transplantation.

2000 procedures performed per year. The major concern with living donation, particularly of the liver, is the risk to the donor. Ethical concerns have also been raised regarding informed consent.[74] Despite these potential obstacles, the first successful living-related liver transplantation was performed in 1989.[75]

The evaluation of a potential donor begins with a thorough history and physical examination. If the patient has no medical or psychiatric contraindications, a variety of blood tests, including blood group typing, are performed. If the recipient and donor are blood type compatible, a volumetric CT scan of the potential donor is performed to ensure a satisfactory volume of liver (10 mL/kg). The final component of the evaluation is arteriography of the potential donor liver to delineate its blood supply. The presence of multiple arteries or small vessels (less than 2 mm) to the donor segment are relative contraindications to donation (Fig. 21-7). The donor operation consists of removing either the entire left hepatic lobe or, more commonly, the left lateral segment.

The recipient operation is similar to a cadaveric reduced-size liver transplantation. The only difference is the frequent need for interposition grafts to the hepatic artery and portal vein. The sources of grafts are usually the saphenous vein from the donor or cryopreserved cadaveric iliac veins.[76] The results of living-related transplantation are similar to those obtained with cadaveric organs.[72] A major advantage of using a living donor is that it allows the transplantation to be performed electively before the child's condition deteriorates. Also, use of living donors increases the availability of cadaveric donors for other pediatric recipients.

A key issue regarding living-related liver transplan-

tation is the risk to the donor. To date, more than 200 donor procedures have been performed. Most donors have had no long-term complications. Unfortunately, there has been at least one donor death secondary to a pulmonary embolism.

COMPLICATIONS

Primary Nonfunction

In the absence of technical or immunologic causes, hepatic allografts that fail to function adequately are classified under the category of *primary nonfunction.* Primary nonfunction of the donor liver may be devastating and usually requires retransplantation to salvage the patient. Fortunately, the incidence of primary nonfunction is low, with most centers reporting rates of less than 10%. Primary nonfunction has been attributed to a number of causes, including hyperacute rejection, donor starvation, cold injury, and reperfusion injury. With the routine application of frozen-section evaluation of donor liver biopsies before transplantation, the rate of primary nonfunction is as low as 1.5% in some series.[77] The primary histologic finding used to exclude donor livers is severe steatosis, defined as greater than 45% macrovesicular steatosis (Fig. 21-8). Some centers have advocated the use of prostaglandins to prevent or reduce the incidence of primary nonfunction.[78]

Biliary Tract Complications

Biliary tract complications occur in 15% to 20% of patients after transplantation.[79,80] Although a frequent source of morbidity, biliary tract complications are an

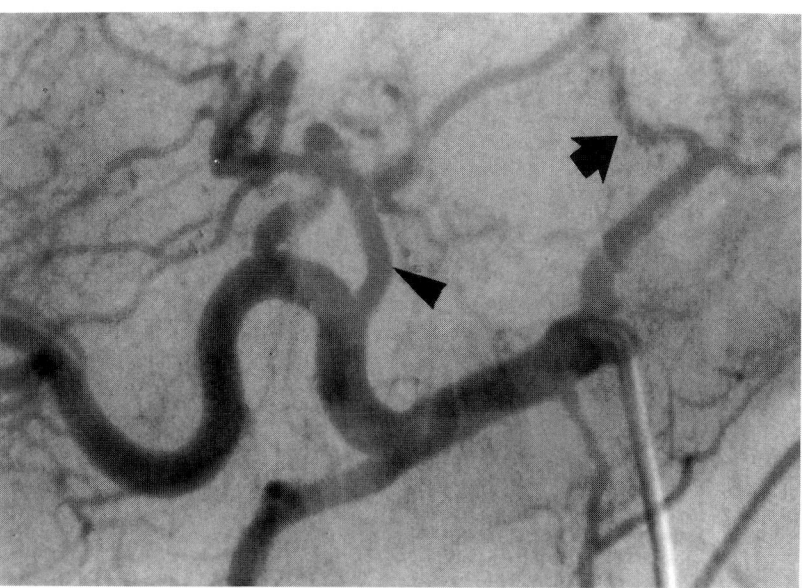

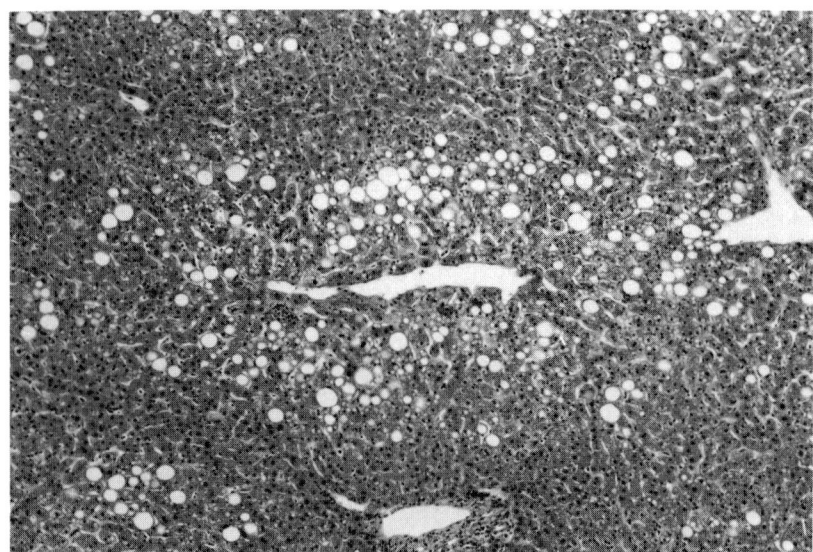

Figure 21-8 Photomicrograph of donor liver showing moderate pericentral steatosis involving about half of the hepatic lobule (hematoxylin–eosin, ×100).

infrequent cause of patient death unless they are associated with hepatic artery thrombosis. Biliary tract complications can be classified as early or late. Early complications (within 4 weeks of the transplantation) include bile leaks and migration or dislodgement of the T-tube. Obstruction of the bile duct is unusual in the early postoperative period, but if present, an expanding mucocele of the cystic duct stump should be considered in the differential diagnosis. Early complications are commonly related to technical errors or ischemia of the distal bile duct. Late biliary tract complications include anastomotic and intrahepatic strictures (Fig. 21-9). Studies have demonstrated an increased risk of intrahepatic biliary strictures when preservation times exceed 15 hours[81] (Fig. 21-10). Late complications can usually be managed nonsurgically with endoscopic and percutaneous techniques. Failure of these approaches necessitates operative repair or, rarely, retransplantation.

Hepatic Artery Thrombosis

Hepatic artery thrombosis is one of the most serious complications of liver transplantation. Dearterialization of the hepatic allograft in the early postoperative period may result in massive hepatic necrosis or uncontrollable biliary sepsis.[82] The incidence of arterial thrombosis differs between adult and pediatric recipients. The rate of arterial thrombosis for adults is about 3%, whereas for children, particularly those less than 10 kg in weight, it is nearly 10%.[83] Risk factors for the development of hepatic artery thrombosis include hypercoagulable states, elevated hematocrit, and weight less than 10 kg.

The cornerstone of therapy for hepatic artery thrombosis has been retransplantation, but this ap-

proach is restricted by a limited donor pool. Even when the damaged liver is replaced, patients with hepatic artery thrombosis often develop infectious and neurologic complications. In an attempt to reduce the morbidity and mortality associated with hepatic artery

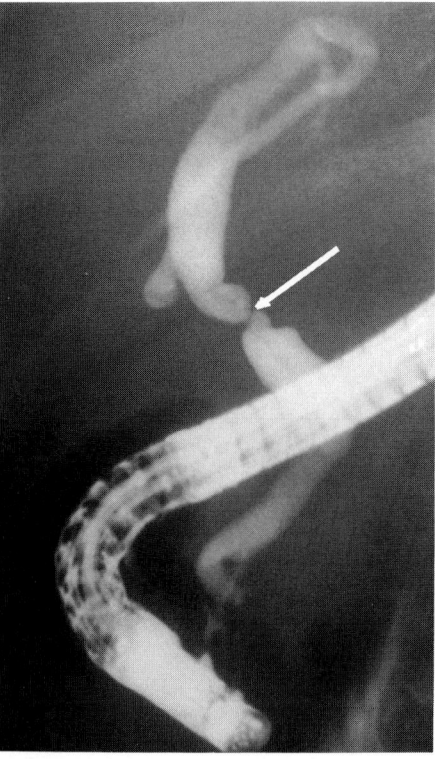

Figure 21-9 Endoscopic retrograde cholangiogram study shows anastomotic stricture (*arrow*) after transplantation. The stricture was successfully dilated by a balloon-tipped catheter and stented by endoscopic techniques.

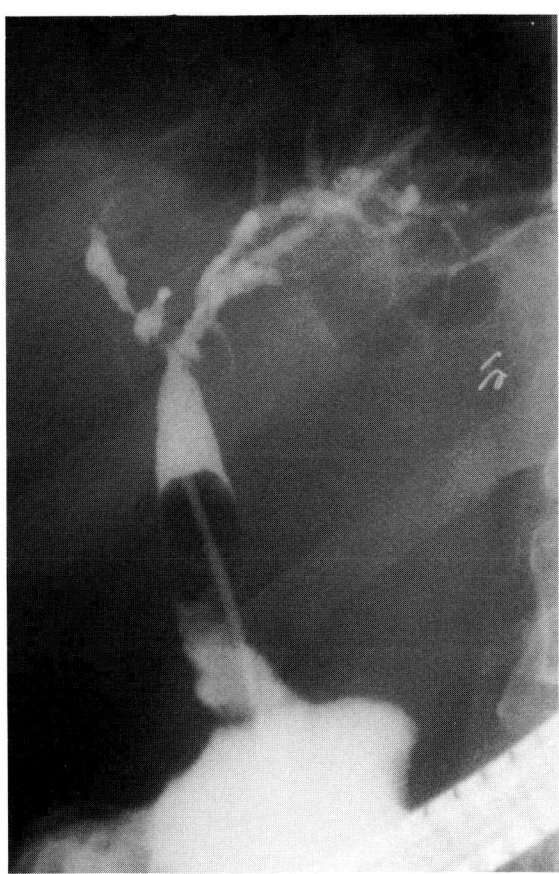

Figure 21-10 Cholangiogram demonstrating multiple intrahepatic strictures. Nonanastomotic strictures, in the absence of hepatic artery thrombosis, are thought to be associated with prolonged cold ischemia. Management of these strictures is mainly by use of percutaneous or endoscopic techniques.

thrombosis, a number of centers have reported success with urgent revascularization of the allograft[84] (Fig. 21-11). The key to successful application of this approach is the early diagnosis of arterial thrombosis. The liberal use of duplex ultrasonography during episodes of allograft dysfunction and as a screening tool on the first postoperative day has enhanced the surgeon's ability to diagnose hepatic artery thrombosis early.

Rejection

Rejection is an inevitable immunologic consequence of human liver transplantation. Rejection can be classified as hyperacute, acute, or chronic. Hyperacute rejection is the result of preformed humoral antibodies reacting against hepatic endothelium. The preformed antibodies bind to class 1 major histocompatability antigens on the endothelium of the hepatic sinusoid, which precipitates

massive hepatic necrosis. Fortunately, hyperacute rejection is rare in liver transplant recipients, and transplantation can be routinely performed despite a positive lymphocytotoxic crossmatch. The resistance of the liver allograft to hyperacute rejection may be related to production of large amounts of soluble class 1 major histocompatibility antigens by the liver that bind and inactivate preformed antibodies.[85] Other explanations for the resistance of the liver allograft to hyperacute rejection include Kupffer cell processing of preformed antibodies and the dual blood supply of the liver.[86] Retransplantation is usually the only alternative for patients who experience hyperacute rejection.

Acute rejection is the most common form of immunologic rejection of liver transplants. Acute rejection has been documented in 60% to 80% of liver transplant recipients, usually occurring within the first 3 postoperative months. According to the National Institutes of Health Liver Transplant Database (NIH-LTDB), nearly half of patients reject within 6 weeks of transplantation.[87] Young adults have more rejection episodes than older recipients, and patients transplanted for acute liver failure have a significantly increased incidence of acute rejection. A positive lymphocytotoxic crossmatch has no influence on the incidence of rejection, whereas an HLA-DR match confers protection. The three centers contributing to the NIH-LTDB all use different immunosuppressive regimens. One group uses quadruple immunosuppression, including induction with an antilymphocyte preparation; the second group uses triple therapy (prednisone, cyclosporine, and azathioprine); and the third group uses cyclosporine and prednisone. There was no difference in the percentage of patients with rejection during the first 6 postoperative weeks among the three centers.[87] The diagnosis of rejection is made by clinical evidence of allograft dysfunction, usually abnormal liver function tests, combined with characteristic pathologic changes on liver biopsy. With cyclosporine-based immunosuppression, the first episode of rejection often occurs after the first week and before the sixth week. The specific therapy employed is directed by the timing and severity of the rejection episode. First episodes of acute rejection are usually managed with steroid boluses. If steroids are ineffective, antilymphocyte therapy (OKT3, Orthoclone, Raritone NJ; ATGAM, Upjohn, Kalamazoo MI) should be administered. Treatment of refractory allograft rejection often requires the use of alternative drug therapy, such as tacrolimus (FK506) or mycophenolate mofetil. For unrelenting rejection episodes, retransplantation is frequently necessary.

Chronic rejection develops in about 10% of patients after transplantation.[88] Chronic rejection is also known as the *vanishing bile duct syndrome* and as *ductopenic rejec-*

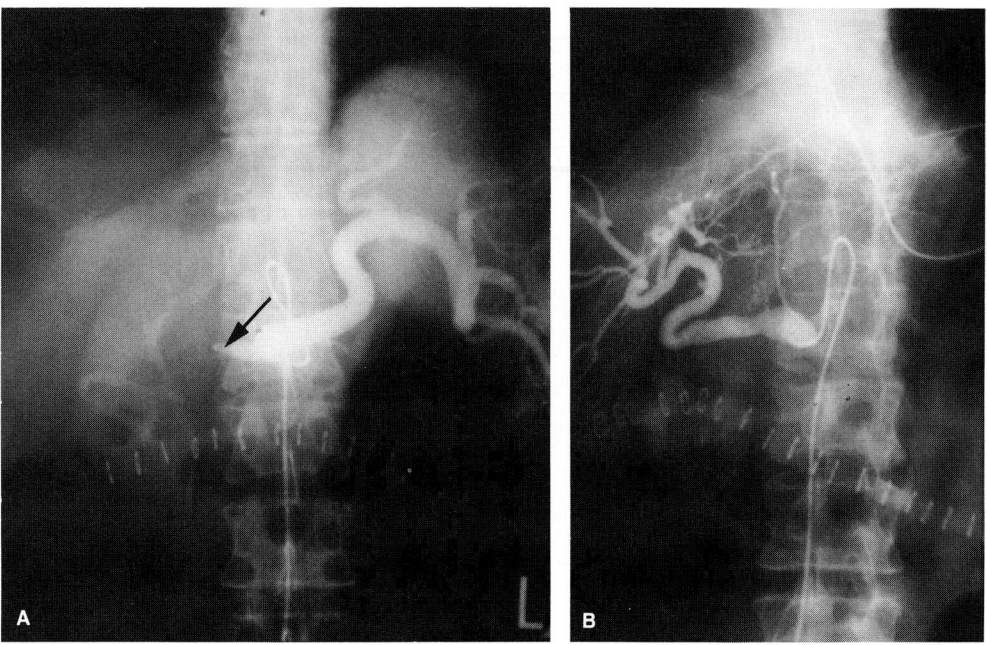

Figure 21-11 (**A**) Arteriogram demonstrating hepatic artery thrombosis (*arrow*) in a patient who recently underwent liver transplantation. (**B**) One day after revascularization of the hepatic allograft, repeat angiography demonstrates patency of the hepatic artery.

tion. The clinical picture of chronic rejection is insidious, with patients often demonstrating no symptoms except the abrupt onset of jaundice. Chronic rejection is usually seen after the first postoperative year but may occur as early as 6 weeks after transplantation. Chronic rejection is characterized histologically by the loss of bile ducts in the portal triads combined with arteriolar thickening or obliteration. The natural history is variable. The only established therapy for advanced chronic

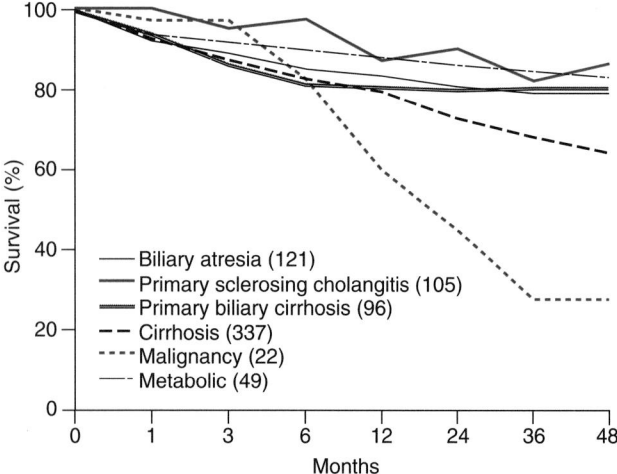

Figure 21-12 Actuarial patient survival after liver transplantation based on preoperative diagnosis.[92]

rejection is retransplantation. Trials are underway to investigate the effectiveness of tacrolimus (FK506) to reverse chronic rejection so that retransplantation can be avoided.

Infections

Infectious complications remain the most common cause of death after liver transplantation. It has been estimated that at least two thirds of patients undergoing liver transplantation develop a postoperative infection. An important principle for the evaluation of fever or suspected infection is that invasive procedures are often required to establish the cause and that specific rather than broad-spectrum antimicrobial therapy should be used. CT, bronchoscopy, and laparotomy are valuable diagnostic tests in establishing the source of an infection. The penalty for frequent use of empiric broad-spectrum antibiotics is the emergence of highly re-sistant organisms, such as vancomycin-resistant *Streptococcus faecium*.[89] Infections after liver transplantation can be categorized into three groups: those directly related to the surgical procedure, those involving the allograft, and those related to immunosuppression.

The most common infection related to the operative procedure is wound infection. Common pathogens include *Staphylococcus* sp, gram-negative aerobes, and *Candida* sp. Although a variety of prophylactic antibiotic strategies have been tried, one of the drawbacks to an aggressive antibiotic regimen is the development of resistant organisms. Common causes of peritonitis are bile leaks and bowel perforations. If a bile leak is identified, hepatic artery thrombosis must be ruled out as a possible cause. An interesting occurrence is the development of multiple small bowel perforations that are unrelated to any obvious cause, including viruses or prior surgical dissection.[90]

A variety of infections may affect the allograft, including hepatitis and abscesses. These infections may manifest as occult fevers, worsening liver function tests, or both. Investigations to determine the source of fever often include abdominal ultrasound, CT, and liver biopsy. A liver abscess may be the result of a biliary stricture, hepatic artery thrombosis, or a prior liver biopsy. Posttransplantation liver abscesses are best managed with percutaneous techniques.

A liver biopsy can usually distinguish between rejection, which requires an increase in doses of immunosuppressive drugs, and an opportunistic infection, which often dictates a decrease in doses of immunosuppressive agents and specific therapy. The liver histology often does not provide conclusive evidence of an opportunistic infection, in which case immunohistologic techniques should be applied.[91] Viral cultures should be routinely performed with each liver biopsy. Effective antiviral therapy is available for cytomegalovirus and other herpes viruses.

Infections unrelated to the operation or the allograft often involve the lungs, central venous catheters, skin, and central nervous system. Nosocomial pneumonia can be caused by common pathogens or opportunistic organisms. A sputum specimen may be helpful, although bronchoscopy is usually required to diagnose the cause of the pneumonia. Community-acquired pneumonia after liver transplantation may be caused by not only common pathogens, such as pneumococcus, but also opportunistic organisms, such as *Legionella* sp, *Pneumocystis* sp, nocardia, and mycobacteria. The differential diagnosis should include posttransplantation lymphoproliferative disorders when pneumonia develops after the first 3 to 6 months.

A common source of infection after transplantation is a central venous catheter. Catheter-related infections are typically manifested by fever and bacteremia, and treatment consists of removing the catheter and administering antibiotics. Occasionally, a central venous catheter infection results in pylephlebitis of one of the central veins or the superior vena cava.

Central nervous system infections are infrequent but can be devastating. The clinical manifestations of a central nervous system infection in the transplantation patient may be subtle, such as a change in visual acuity or atypical neck and shoulder pain due to meningitis. Since a wide variety of organisms can be responsible for such infections, cerebrospinal fluid or tissue cultures should be done. If a CT scan of the head demonstrates a lesion, tissue should be obtained for histology and culture.

Infections of the skin may be a local phenomenon or a manifestation of systemic disease. A rash that does not appear to be related to a specific drug warrants a skin biopsy. Findings of a skin biopsy can include aspergillosis, graft-versus-host disease, and herpes virus.

RESULTS

The results of liver transplantation have improved steadily during the past 10 years. Initial progress was related to better immunosuppressive agents and improved surgical techniques. More recent improvements are related to a better understanding of how the patient's preoperative condition and diagnosis affect posttransplantation survival.

Patient survival at one institution based on diagnosis is depicted in Figure 21-12.[92] Patients with hepatic malignancies and hepatitis B have diminished survival because of recurrent disease. Survival for patients with fulminant liver failure is related to timeliness of referral and capacity to obtain a donor organ. A subgroup of patients with fulminant liver failure develop aplastic anemia, contributing to the relatively high mortality rate in this group.

Patient survival can also be stratified based on the preoperative condition of the patient. A scoring system based on a number of clinical variables has been developed and is referred to as the RISK score[93] (Table 21-3). Important predictors in the RISK scoring system include degree of malnutrition, depth of hepatic coma, prothrombin time, and serum bilirubin. In one report,[94] patients stratified to the high-risk group had markedly diminished survival relative to those in the low-risk group. The survival rate for the high-risk patients was only 44% compared with 85% and 90% for patients in the medium- and low-risk groups, respectively. The high-risk patients (regardless if they lived or died) had considerably higher hospital charges than the low-risk patients who survived.

The NIH-LTDB includes data from patients who received transplants at three transplantation centers.[95] Sixty-seven percent of a total of 668 patients have been followed for at least 1 year. When patients were stratified based on diagnosis, excluding patients with fulminant liver failure, significant differences were noted. The best results were in patients with cholestatic liver disease (92% at 1 year), and the worst results were in

Table 21-3 RISK Score

	Coma	Malnutrition	Ascites
None	0	0	0
Mild/moderate	+1	+1	+1
Severe	+2*	+2	+2
Serum bilirubin >30 mg/dL			+2
Serum bilirubin <10 mg/dL			−1
Prothrombin time <15 s			−1
Patient age >40 y			+1
Subtotal score			
If subtotal >5 and age <25 y			−2
Total preoperative score			
Transfusion requirement >39 units packed red blood cells			+1
Preoperative score >5 and transfusion <10 units			−1
Final postoperative score†			

* Low risk, 0–3 points; medium risk, 4–6 points; high risk, >6 points.

† For stage IV coma, score 6 points. (Shaw BW, Wood RP, Gordon RD, et al. Influence of selected patient variables and operative blood loss on six-month survival following liver transplantation. Semin Liver Dis 1985;5:385)

patients with chronic hepatitis B and in those with a malignancy, whose survival rates at 1 year were 50% and 40%, respectively. Also notable was the role the preoperative condition of the patient had on mortality. When patient survival was analyzed based on UNOS status at the time of transplantation, patients admitted from home had a better chance of 1-year survival than patients hospitalized or those in the intensive care unit.

According to the UNOS Scientific registry, 2-year graft and patient survival rates for liver transplantations performed between 1987 and 1991 were 62% and 69%, respectively. A UNOS investigation assessed the effect transplantation center activity had on patient survival.[96] This analysis demonstrated a 1.5 to 2.5 times increased likelihood of patient death in those liver transplantation programs performing less than 35 to 40 transplantations per year.

IMMUNOSUPPRESSION

An elusive goal of clinical solid-organ transplantation has been the induction of donor-specific unresponsiveness or tolerance. Tolerance can be defined as the suppression of the immune response to donor antigens while retaining the ability to respond to third-party antigens. Unfortunately, with current immunosuppressive regimens, immunologic failure remains the major cause of graft loss after the first postoperative year.

The cornerstone of immunosuppressive therapy is

the combination of cyclosporine and prednisone. Cyclosporine acts by engaging the peptidyl isomerase, cyclophilin.[97] The cyclosporine–cyclophilin complex then binds to calcineurin.[98] This action by cyclosporine prevents the transcription of genes for a number of T-cell activators, including interleukins 2, 3, and 4 and γ-interferon. By blocking the production of these cytokines, activation of cytotoxic and helper T cells is prevented. Cyclosporine may be administered orally or intravenously. The usual starting dose of cyclosporine after liver transplantation is 2 mg/kg twice daily intravenously or 10 mg/kg twice daily orally. The appropriate dose of cyclosporine is determined by blood levels. A problem inherent in the use of cyclosporine is its poor intestinal absorption. The use of liquid vitamin E, taken with oral cyclosporine, increases the bioavailability of cyclosporine.[99] New formulations of cyclosporine (Neoral, Sandoz), with improved absorption profiles, are undergoing clinical trials.[100]

The major side effect of cyclosporine is nephrotoxicity. During the first postoperative year, the glomerular filtration rate often decreases by half.[101] Histologically, interstitial fibrosis and vascular sclerosis can be found on kidney biopsy. Cyclosporine has numerous other side effects, including hypertension, hirsutism, hyperlipidemia, gingival hyperplasia, and neurologic symptoms. Important cyclosporine drug interactions include drugs that affect the cytochrome P-450 system. Cyclosporine OG-37-325, which is purported to have less nephrotoxicity, is undergoing phase II trials in kidney transplant recipients.[102]

Corticosteroids have been an integral part of immunosuppressive regimens since the 1960s. The major action of corticosteroids is to block the transcription of genes for interleukin-1 by macrophages and monocytes. Steroids also indirectly prevent the production of interleukin-2 by lymphocytes, reduce the chemotactic response of monocytes, stabilize lysosomal membranes, and in high doses, produce a cytotoxic effect.[103] Corticosteroids can be used as maintenance immunotherapy and as treatment for rejection. A common adult maintenance dose of prednisone is 20 mg/d, which is then gradually reduced over time. Every-other-day dosing is often used after the first postoperative year, particularly in children. Side effects of corticosteroids include all the typical findings associated with iatrogenic Cushing's syndrome.

Azathioprine is frequently added to cyclosporine- and prednisone-based immunotherapy. Azathioprine is metabolized to 6-mercaptopurine in the liver. Metabolites of azathioprine inhibit purine synthesis through both de novo and salvage pathways. This action of azathioprine on purine synthesis blocks cell replication, in particular clonal expansion of cytotoxic T cells.[103] Azathioprine can be administered orally or intravenously in a daily dose range of 1 to 4 mg/kg. The major side effect of azathioprine is bone marrow suppression, which is dose dependent and self limiting. Other less common side effects include pancreatitis, mucositis, and venoocclusive disease of the liver.

Polyclonal and monoclonal antibodies can be used as either induction therapy or for the treatment of severe or steroid-resistant allograft rejection. Polyclonal antibodies are made by injecting human lymphocytes or thymocytes into a variety of animals (horses, goats, rabbits) and then collecting the antisera. The polyclonal antibodies react against lymphocytes, particularly T lymphocytes. The mechanisms by which the polyclonal antibodies work include complement-mediated destruction and opsonization of lymphocytes with removal by the reticuloendothelial system.[103] ATGAM (Upjohn, Kalamazoo) is the only preparation approved by the Food and Drug Administration. It is given in a dose of 10 to 20 mg/kg/d for 10 to 14 days. Dosing is adjusted based on platelet and white blood cell counts. Side effects include serum sickness, chest pain, and an increased risk for infections, particularly viral.

OKT3 is the only anti-CD3 monoclonal antibody commercially available for clinical use. OKT3 is used as induction therapy or for the treatment of steroid-resistant or severe rejection. OKT3 is a murine-derived antibody to mature T lymphocytes that have the CD3 receptor on the cell surface. The CD3 receptor is essential to the immune function of T lymphocytes, in particular that of allorecognition. The binding of the OKT3 molecule to the CD3 receptor prevents the T cell from recognizing foreign antigen, thereby preventing allograft destruction (ie, rejection).[104] The standard adult regimen is 5 mg/d for 10 to 14 days. The effects of the drug can be monitored by improvement in allograft function, peripheral CD3 counts, and serum OKT3 levels. Use of OKT3 is associated with a number of side effects, particularly with the first two doses. The most severe adverse reactions include pulmonary edema and hypotension. Patients may also develop a viral-like syndrome with fevers, myalgia, and diarrhea. Most of the symptoms related to the use of OKT3 are the result of cytokine release (tumor necrosis factor, interleukin-1, and interferon). OKT3 has been associated with an increased risk of opportunistic infections, particularly viral (cytomegalovirus, herpes simplex).[105,106] When the dose of OKT3 is doubled or a second course is given, an increase in Epstein-Barr virus hepatitis and posttransplantation lymphoproliferative disorders have been reported.[107] A limitation to the use of OKT3 is the development of antimurine antibodies. New monoclonal antibodies in preclinical or phase I clinical trials include humanized anti-CD3, anti-CD4, anti-lL2, and anti-TNF.

A variety of immunosuppressive drugs are undergoing clinical trials. Tacrolimus (FK506, Prograf, Fujisawa) has undergone extensive study in liver transplant recipients and was approved by the Food and Drug Administration. Tacrolimus has a mechanism of action that is similar to cyclosporine, binding to a systolic protein similar to cyclophilin (FK-binding protein). The FK-binding protein–tacrolimus complex blocks the effects of calcineurin, thereby preventing T-cell activation.[98] A multicenter randomized trial comparing cyclosporine based immunosuppression to tacrolimus based therapy demonstrated no differences in patient or graft survival.[108] In the tacrolimus group, there were fewer episodes of steroid-resistant rejection. Tacrolimus has also been used in an attempt to reverse or subdue chronic rejection with variable success. Tacrolimus is water-soluble and is not as dependent on bile production for absorption as is cyclosporine. The toxicity profile for tacrolimus is similar although not identical to cyclosporine and includes nephrotoxicity, neurotoxicity, and glucose intolerance. Blood level monitoring is available.

Other drugs in early clinical trials include mycophenolate mofetil, rapamycin, and deoxyspergualin. Mycophenolate mofetil inhibits de novo purine synthesis.[109] Its actions are similar to azathioprine but are more specific for lymphocytes. Mycophenolate mofetil has been found to be safe and effective for the treatment of refractory rejection in kidney transplant recipients. Rapamycin has a molecular structure (macrolide) that is similar to tacrolimus, although its mechanism of action is different.[110] Rapamycin exerts its immunosuppressive effects by blocking the actions of interleukin-2. Deoxyspergualin is an antitumor agent derived from *Bacillus lactosporus*. Deoxyspergualin appears to suppress antibody formation and delayed-type hypersensitivity reactions.[111] It has been used successfully to treat kidney allograft rejection. Brequinar sodium is an antimetabolite whose mechanism of action is related to the inhibition of de novo synthesis of pyrimidine nucleotides.[112] Brequinar sodium has not yet been tested in a clinical trial. Future therapies include antibodies to intracellular adhesion molecules, such as ICAM-1 and LFA-1.

Total lymphoid irradiation is effective in reducing the requirements for maintenance immunosuppressive drugs when compared with conventional regimens (cyclosporine, azathioprine) in solid-organ recipients. In 25 recipients of cadaveric kidney transplants given total lymphoid irradiation combined with preoperative antilymphocyte globulin, 1-year patient and graft survival were 87% and 76%, respectively.[113] Another group has also demonstrated the effectiveness of total lymphoid irradiation (8 Gy) in prolonging graft survival in human renal allograft recipients.[114] Actuarial 1-year patient and graft survival rates in this series were 94% and 95%, respectively. The mechanism by which total lymphoid irradiation exerts its specific immunologic effect is thought to be by activating suppressor cell populations to create antigen-specific unresponsiveness.

Donor-Specific Bone Marrow

It has been demonstrated that donor bone marrow infusion can induce allograft unresponsiveness in mice treated with antilymphocyte serum but not affect the capacity to respond to other antigens (viral, bacterial, or third-party alloantigens).[115] Two primate studies demonstrated tolerance after donor bone marrow infusion.[116,117] A trial of donor-specific bone marrow infusion in kidney transplant recipients demonstrated the safety of this approach and an improvement in graft survival.[118] Another investigation,[119] using donor-specific bone marrow in liver transplant recipients, did not demonstrate any improvement in outcome.

Chimerism

It has been speculated that prolonged allograft survival after liver transplantation is the result of cell trafficking between donor and recipient.[120] Cells of lymphocyte–macrophage lineage leave the allograft and settle in distant sites, such as recipient skin and the reticuloendothelial system. Simultaneously, recipient-derived dendritic cells enter the allograft. This phenomenon can occur naturally and was first described in Freemartin cattle.[121] Investigations have demonstrated the presence of donor-derived tissues in a variety of organs of patients many years after liver transplantation.[122] In animal studies, donor cells can be found in peripheral blood, skin, lymph nodes, heart, and lungs. The exact mechanism by which microchimerism might induce allograft tolerance is not known.

NOVEL THERAPY

Xenotransplantation

The shortage of human donor organs for transplantation has rekindled interest in the use of xenografts. The first attempts at human xenotransplantation used nonhuman primates as kidney donors.[123] After this limited experience, it became clear that immunologic barriers could not be overcome with conventional immunosuppression (azathioprine and prednisone). Even cyclo-

sporine was not effective in preventing xenograft failure, as demonstrated in one baboon-to-human cardiac transplantation.[124] These failures with human xenotransplantation demonstrated the inability of contemporary immunologic strategies to allow for graft acceptance and stimulated interest in describing the mechanisms of xenograft rejection.

The mechanism by which a xenograft is destroyed is in part determined by the phytogenic similarity between the species. Destruction of xenografts from dissimilar (discordant) species, such as pig-to-human, occurs rapidly (minutes to hours). These discordant transplantations are characterized histologically by antibody and complement deposition, endothelial cell damage, and intravascular coagulation.[125] The damage is the result of natural antibodies in the recipient binding to donor endothelium. A complement-dependent coagulation cascade then ensues through either classic or alternative pathways. Strategies to prevent rejection of discordant xenografts include removal of natural antibodies and complement, plasmapheresis, and extracorporeal organ perfusion.[126] The one pig-to-human liver transplantation was performed heterotopically, as a bridge to human orthotopic transplantation, in a patient with fulminant liver failure.[127] The xenograft functioned initially but underwent coagulative necrosis within 24 hours.

Xenotransplantation between species that do not possess natural antibodies against one another are referred to as *concordant* (eg, baboon to human). In concordant xenotransplantation, rejection is primarily cell mediated.[128] Although a humoral response is probably also involved, it has not been well defined. Xenograft cellular rejection is typically more severe than that seen with allografts. Therapy directed against T-cell and B-cell function has been effective in preventing rejection in concordant animal models. Drugs, such as tacrolimus, brequinar, mycophenolate mofetil, and cyclophosphamide, have been used to promote graft survival in a variety of animal xenograft models.

Experience with human concordant liver xenotransplantation involved transplantation of a baboon liver on two occasions.[129] The first baboon-to-human liver transplantation was performed in a man who had end-stage liver disease secondary to hepatitis B and who was also human immunodeficiency virus–positive. Immunosuppression consisted of tacrolimus, cyclophosphamide, and steroids. The patient had good xenograft function and produced albumin and coagulation factors of baboon phenotype. Unfortunately, the patient died of invasive aspergillosis on postoperative day 70. The second recipient of a baboon liver transplant received an infusion of donor bone marrow at the time of transplantation. The xenograft never functioned properly, and the patient died on the 25th postoperative day.

A practical concern with xenotransplantation is the potential for transmission of infection from animals to humans, often referred to as *zoonoses*.[130] Zoonoses may include organisms that are known to be pathogens in humans and animals, such as *Yersinia* sp and *Salmonella* sp, or organisms whose effects on humans are unknown. Viral infections that may be transmitted from simians include the herpes viruses and retroviruses. In an attempt to prevent the transmission of infections by animals to humans, attempts are being made to raise animals in germ-free or specific pathogen-free environments.

Extracorporeal Liver Support

Before the introduction of liver transplantation, survival of patients with fulminant liver failure after the onset of hepatic coma was 10% to 20%. Because of the limitations of medical therapy, novel approaches to liver support have been undertaken. One of the most successful therapies is extracorporeal liver perfusion (ECLP) with human, baboon, pig, and sheep livers.[131] More than one third of the patients with acute liver failure treated with ECLP regained consciousness. Despite temporary clinical improvement, most patients eventually died of their liver disease. These early clinical attempts with ECLP provided knowledge regarding physiologic and technical requirements needed for the successful application of this technology. In an attempt to either provide a bridge to transplantation or determine whether improved liver function would benefit a patient, ECLP has been attempted at a number of institutions.[132,133] Most cases have made use of human cadaver livers that were otherwise unsuitable for transplantation. The perfusion circuit uses venous access for inflow and outflow, thus avoiding the risks related to arterial cannulation[133] (Fig. 21-13).

A number of other approaches to provide liver support, including plasma exchange, hemodiabsorption, and liver cartridges, are being evaluated. The objective of these approaches is to provide a life-sustaining bridge until a donor liver becomes available or the native liver recovers.

Plasma exchange incorporates the concept that by diluting the patient's blood, toxic substances are removed.[134] Although laboratory parameters, such as coagulation factors and albumin, are normalized, cerebral hypertension is unaffected. Hemodiabsorption makes use of a dialysis membrane surrounded by activated charcoal.[135] Substances speculated to be important in the development of hepatic failure are removed by the hemodiabsorption system. Neurologic and physiologic

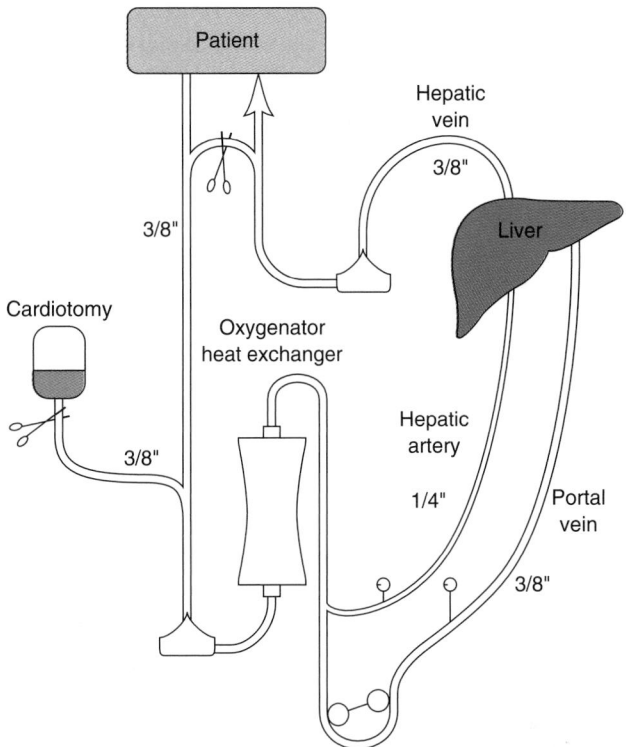

Figure 21-13 Schematic diagram of extracorporeal liver perfusion.

improvement have been demonstrated in the small number of patients treated with this device.

Two bioartificial livers are being tested in humans and animals. The first incorporates a cloned human cell line derived from a hepatoblastoma cultured in a hollow fiber cartridge (Hepatix Inc., Houston).[136] The Hepatix extracorporeal support device has demonstrated efficacy in supporting dogs with acetaminophen-induced hepatic failure. Experience with this liver cartridge in humans is anecdotal. The second extracorporeal liver assist system consists of plasma separation, a charcoal filter, and perfusion through a hollow fiber module seeded with matrix and attached porcine hepatocytes.[137] This bioartificial liver was tested in dogs and reduced serum ammonia and lactate levels. Clinical experience is limited, and human trials are needed to prove its efficacy.

REFERENCES

1. Current trends: mortality patterns—United States, 1991. Mortality and Morbidity Weekly Report 1993;42:891.
2. American Liver Foundation. Progress 1993;14.
3. Sherlock S. Primary biliary cirrhosis and vanishing bile

ducts. In: McIntyre N, Benhamou JP, Bircher J, Rizzetto M, Rodes J, eds. Oxford textbook of clinical hepatology. New York, Oxford University Press, 1991;2:743.

4. Dickson ER, Grambsch PM, Fleming TR, Fisher LD, Langworthy A. Prognosis in primary biliary cirrhosis: model for decision making. Hepatology 1989;10:1.

5. LaRusso NF, Wiesner RH, Ludwig J. Sclerosing cholangitis. In: McIntyre N, Benhamou JP, Bircher J, Rizzetto M, Rodes J, eds. Oxford textbook of clinical hepatology. New York, Oxford University Press, 1991;2:767.

6. Wee A, Ludwig J, Coffey RJ, LaRusso NF, Weisner RH. Hepatobiliary carcinoma associated with primary sclerosing cholangitis and chronic ulcerative colitis. Hum Pathol 1985;16:719.

7. Dickerson ER, Murtaugh P, Wiesner R, et al. Primary sclerosing cholangitis: refinement and validation of survival models. Gastroenterology 1992;102:1893.

8. O'Grady JG, Alexander GJ, Hayllar KM, Williams R. Early indicators of prognosis in fulminant hepatic failure. Gastroenterology 1989;97:439.

9. Schafer DF, Shaw BW Jr. Fulminant hepatic failure and orthotopic liver transplantation. In: Berk PD, Lieber CS, Schaffner F, et al, eds. Seminars in liver disease. New York, Thieme Medical, 1989:189.

10. Donahue JG, Munoz A, Ness PM, et al. The declining risk of post-transfusion hepatitis C virus infection. N Engl J Med 1992;327:369.

11. Alter MJ, Hadler SC, Judson FN, et al. Risk factors for acute non-A, non-B hepatitis in the United States and association with hepatitis C virus infection. JAMA 1990;264:2231.

12. Alter MJ, Margolin HS, Kowczynski, et al. The natural history of community acquired hepatitis C in the United States. N Engl J Med 1992;27:1899.

13. Tsukuma H, Hiyama T, Tanaka S, et al. Risk factors for hepatocellular carcinoma among patients with chronic liver disease. N Engl J Med 1993;328:1797.

14. Frydman M, Bonne-Tamir B, Farrer LA, et al. Assignment of the gene for Wilson's disease to chromosome 13: linkage to the enterase D coccus. Proc Natl Acad Sci USA 1985;82:1819.

15. Gibbsk, Walshe JM. Biliary excretion of copper in Wilson's disease. Lancet 1980;2:538.

16. Bothwell TH, Charlton RW, Cook JD, et al. Iron metabolism in man. Oxford, Blackwell Scientific Publication, 1979.

17. Sveger T. Liver disease in alpha-1-antitrypsin deficiency detected by screening 200,000 infants. N Engl J Med 1976;294:1316.

18. Berg NO, Eriksson S. Liver disease in adults with alpha-1-antitrypsin deficiency. N Engl J Med 1972;287:1264.

19. Danks DM, Campbell PE, Jack I, et al. Studies of aetiology of neonatal hepatitis and biliary atresia. Arch Dis Child 1977;52:360.

20. Karrer FM, Hall RJ, Lilly JR. Biliary atresia and the polysplenia syndrome. J Pediatr Surg 1991;26:524.

21. Lelbach WK. Epidemiology of alcoholic cirrhosis. In: Popper H, Schaffner F, eds. Progress in liver disease, vol 5. New York, Grune & Stratton, 1976:494.

22. Starzl TE, Van Thiel D, Andreas G, et al. Orthotopic liver transplantation for alcoholic cirrhosis. JAMA 1988; 260:2542.

23. Byrd GL, O'Grady JG, Harvey FA, Calne RY, Williams R. Liver transplantation in patients with alcoholic cirrhosis: selection criteria and rates of survival and relapse. Br Med J 1990;301:15.

24. Lucey MR, Merion RM, Henley KS, et al. Selection for and outcome of liver transplantation in alcoholic liver disease. Gastroenterology 1992;102:1736.

25. Parkin DM, Stjernsward J, Muir CS. Estimates of the worldwide frequency of twelve major cancers. Bull WHO 1984;62:163.

26. Colombo M. Hepatocellular carcinoma. J Hepatol 1992;15:225.

27. Kew MC, Popper H. Relationship between hepatocellular carcinoma and cirrhosis. Semin Liver Dis 1984;4: 136.

28. Farmer DG, Rosove MH, Shaked A, Bouttil RW. Current treatment modality for hepatocellular carcinoma. Ann Surg 1994;219:236.

29. Takagaso K, Moriyama N, Muramatso Y. The diagnosis of small hepatocellular carcinoma: efficacy of various imaging procedures in 100 patients. AJR 1990;155:49.

30. Tobe T, Arii S. Improving survival after resection of hepatocellular carcinoma: characteristics and current status of surgical treatment of primary liver cancer in Japan. In: Tobe T, Kaneda H, Okudaira M, et al, eds. Primary liver cancer in Japan. Tokyo, Springer, 1992.

31. Franco D, Capussotti L, Smadja C, et al. Resection of hepatocellular carcinoma: results in 72 European patients with cirrhosis. Gastroenterology 1990;98:733.

32. Iwatsuki S, Starzl TE, Sheahan DG, et al. Hepatic resection versus transplantation for hepatocellular carcinoma. Ann Surg 1991;214:221.

33. O'Grady JG, Polson RJ, Rolles K, Calne RY, Williams R. Liver transplantation for malignant disease: results in 93 consecutive patients. Ann Surg 1988;207:373.

34. Ringe B, Pichlmayr R, Wittekind C, Tusch G. Surgical treatment of hepatocellular carcinoma: experience with liver resection and transplantation in 198 patients. World J Surg 1991;15:270.

35. Yamada R, Kishi K, Sonomura T, Tsuda M, Nomura S, Satoh M. Transcatheter arterial embolization in unresectable hepatocellular carcinoma. Cardiovasc Intervent Radiol 1990;13:135.

36. Bismuth H, Morino M, Sherlock D, et al. A primary treatment of hepatocellular carcinoma by arterial chemoembolization. Am J Surg 1992;163:387.

37. Carr BI, Selby R, Madriaga J, Iwatsuki S, Starzl TE. Prolonged survival after liver transplantation and cancer chemotherapy for advanced-stage hepatocellular carcinoma. Transplant Proc 1993;25:1128.

38. Makowka L, Tzakis AG, Mazzaferro V, et al. Transplantation of the liver for metastatic endocrine tumors of the

intestine and pancreas. Surg Gynecol Obstet 1989;168:107.

39. Dusheiko G, Hoffnagle JH. Hepatitis B. In: McIntyre N, Benhamou JP, Bircher J, Rizzetto M, Rodes J, eds. Oxford textbook of clinical hepatology. New York, Oxford University Press, 1991;1:571.

40. Perrillo RP, Mason AL. Hepatitis B and liver transplantation: problems and promises. (Editorial, comment) N Engl J Med 1993;329:1885.

41. Samuel D, Bismuth A, Mathieu D, et al. Passive immunoprophylaxis after liver transplantation in HBsAg-positive patients. Lancet 1991;337:813.

42. Parker RGF. Occlusion of the hepatic veins in man. Medicine 1959;38:369.

43. Shaked A, Goldstein RM, Klintmalm GB, Drazan K, Husberg B, Busuttil RW. Portosystemic shunt versus orthotopic liver transplantation for the Budd-Chiari syndrome. Surg Gynecol Obstet 1992;171:453.

44. Langnas AN, Marujo WC, Stratta RJ, et al. A selective approach to pre-existing portal vein thrombosis in patients undergoing liver transplantation. Am J Surg 1992;163:132.

45. Langnas AN, Marujo WC, Stratta RJ, et al. Influence of a prior portosystemic shunt on outcome following orthotopic liver transplantation. Am J Gastroenterol 1992;87:714.

46. Brems JJ, Hiatt JR, Kelin AS, et al. Effect of a prior portasystemic shunt on subsequent liver transplantation. Ann Surg 1989;209:51.

47. Mazzaferro V, Todo S, Tzakis AG, et al. Liver transplantation in patients with previous portasystemic shunt. Am J Surg 1990;160:111.

48. Krowka MJ. Management of hepatopulmonary syndrome. Semin Liver Dis 1993;13:414.

49. Hobeika J, Houssin D, Bernard O, Devictor D, Grimon G, Chapuis Y. Orthotopic liver transplantation in children with chronic liver disease and severe hypoxemia. Transplantation 1994;57:224.

50. Starzl TE, Groth CG, Brettschneider, et al. Extended survival in 3 cases of orthotopic homotransplantation of human liver. Surgery 1968;63:549.

51. Stoller JK, Moodie D, Schiavone W. Reduction of intrapulmonary shunt and resolution of digital clubbing associated with primary biliary cirrhosis after liver transplantation. Hepatology 1990;11:54.

52. Stieber AC, Gordon RD, Todo S, et al. Liver transplantation in patients over 60 years of age. Transplantation 1991;51:271.

53. Pirsch JD, Kalayoglu M, D'Allesandro AM, et al. Orthotopic liver transplantation in patients 60 years of age and older. Transplantation 1991;51:431.

54. Fox RA. Immunology of aging. In: Brockelhurst JC, ed. Textbook of geriatric medicine and gerontology. New York, Churchill Livingstone, 1985:82.

55. Tesi RJ, Elkhammas EA, Davies EA, et al. Renal transplantation in older people. Lancet 1994;1:462.

56. UNOS update. 1994;10:372.

57. Report of the Ad Hoc Committee of Harvard Medical School to examine the definition of brain death. Definition of irreversible coma. JAMA 1968;205:337.

58. Morse JH, Turcotte JG, Merion RM, Campbell DA Jr, Burtch GD, Lucey MR. Development of a malignant tumor in a liver transplant graft procured from a donor with a cerebral neoplasm. Transplantation 1990;50875.

59. Makowka L, Gordon RD, Todo S, et al. Analysis of donor criteria for the prediction of outcome in clinical liver transplantation. Transplant Proc 1987;19:2378.

60. Wall WJ, Mimeault R, Grant DR, Bloch M. The use of older donor livers for hepatic transplantation. Transplantation 1990;49:377.

61. Heffron TG, Langnas AN, Fox IJ, et al. Pediatric donors less than one year of age: does donor age affect outcome? Hepatology 1993;18:59A.

62. Kalayoglu M, Solinger HW, Stratta RJ, et al. Extended preservation of the liver for clinical transplantation. Lancet 1988;1:617.

63. Langnas AN, Stratta RJ, Marujo WC, Wood RP, Duckworth RM, Shaw BW Jr. Imported hepatic allografts: use of commercial airlines for transport. Transplant Proc 1991;23:2319.

64. Shaw BW, Martin DJ, Marquez JM, et al. Venous bypass in clinical liver transplantation. Ann Surg 1985;200:524.

65. Ozaki CF, Langnas AN, Bynon JS, et al. A percutaneous method for veno-venous bypass in liver transplantation. Transplantation 1994;57:472.

66. Malatack JJ, Schaid DJ, Urbach AN, et al. Choosing a pediatric recipient for orthotopic liver transplantation. J Pediatr 1987;111:479.

67. Bismuth H, Houssin D. Reduced-size orthotopic liver transplantation in children. Surgery 1984;95:36.

68. Langnas AN, Marujo WC, Inagaki M, Stratta RJ, Wood RP, Shaw BW Jr. The results of reduced-size liver transplantation, including split livers, in patients with end-stage liver disease. Transplantation 1992;53:387.

69. Heffron TG, Emond JC, Whitington PF, et al. Biliary complications in pediatric liver transplantation: a comparison of reduced-size and whole grafts. Transplantation 1992;53:391.

70. Stevens LH, Emond JC, Piper JB, et al. Hepatic allograft thrombosis in infants: a comparison of whole livers, reduced-size grafts and grafts from living related donors. Transplantation 1992;53:396.

71. Pichlmayr R, Ringe B, Gubernatis J, et al. Transplantation einer Spenderleber auf zwei Empfanger (splitting transplant): eine neue Methode in der Weiterentwicklung der Lebersegmenttransplantation. Langenbecks Arch Chir 1988;373:127.

72. Broelsch CE, Emond JC, Whitington PF, Thistlethwaite JR, Baker AL, Lichtor JL. Application of reduced-size liver transplants as split grafts, auxiliary orthotopic grafts and living related segmental transplants. Ann Surg 1990;214:368.

73. Gubernatis G, Pichlmayr R, Kemnitz J, Gratz K. Auxiliary partial orthotopic liver transplantation (APOLT) for

fulminant hepatic failure: first successful case report. World J Surg 1991;15:660.

74. Singer PA, Siegler M, Whitington PF, et al. Ethics of liver transplantation with living donors. N Engl J Med 1989;321:620.

75. Strong RW, Lynch SV, Ong TH, et al. Successful liver transplantation from a living donor to her son. N Engl J Med 1987;322:1507.

76. Heffron TG, Kortz EO, Contis JC, et al. Use of cryopreserved vein allogeneic homografts in liver transplantation. Transplant Proc 1993;2:1091.

77. Markin RS, Wisecarver JL, Radio SJ, et al. Frozen section evaluation of donor livers before transplantation. Transplantation 1993;56:1403.

78. Greig PD, Woolf GM, Sinclair SB, et al. Treatment of primary liver graft nonfunction with prostaglandin E$_1$. Transplantation 1989;48:447.

79. Stratta RJ, Wood RP, Langnas AN, et al. Diagnosis and treatment of biliary tract complications after orthotopic liver transplantation. Surgery 1989;106:675.

80. Lerut J, Gordon RD, Iwatsuki S, et al. Biliary tract complications in human orthotopic liver transplantation. Transplantation 1987;43:47.

81. Li S, Stratta RJ, Langnas AN, Wood RP, Marujo W, Shaw BW Jr. Diffuse biliary tract injury after orthotopic liver transplantation. Am J Surg 1992;164:536.

82. Tzakis AG, Gordon RD, Shaw BW Jr, et al. Clinical presentation of hepatic artery thrombosis after liver transplantation in the cyclosporine era. Transplantation 1985;40:667.

83. Langnas An, Marujo W, Stratta RJ, Wood RP, Shaw BW Jr. Vascular complications following orthotopic liver transplantation. Am J Surg 1991;161:76.

84. Langnas AN, Marujo W, Stratta RJ, Wood RP, Li S, Shaw BW Jr. Hepatic allograft rescue following arterial thrombosis. Transplantation 1991;51:86.

85. Roser BJ, Kamada N, Zimmerman F, Davies HS. Immunosuppressive effect of experimental liver allografts. In: Calne RY, ed. Liver transplantation. New York, Grune & Stratton, 1987.

86. Wardel EN. Kupffer cells and their function. Liver 1987;7:63.

87. National Institutes of Diabetes and Digestive and Kidney Diseases. Incidence of rejection topic. Liver Transplantation Database (database 4/15/90–4/15/93);10-1.

88. Wiesner RH, Ludwig J, Van Hoek B, Krom RAF. Current concepts in cell-mediated hepatic allograft rejection leading to ductopenia and graft failure. Hepatology 1991;14:721.

89. Dominguez EA, David JC, Rupp ME, et al. Vancomycin-resistant Enterococcus faecium (VREF) infections in liver-transplant patients. (Abstract 115) 32nd Annual Meeting of the Infectious Diseases Society of America, Orlando, 1994.

90. Marujo WC, Stratta RJ, Langnas AN, Wood RP, Markin RS, Shaw BW Jr. Syndrome of multiple bowel perforations in liver transplant recipients. Am J Surg 1991;162:594.

91. Markin RS, Langnas AN, Donovan JP, Zetterman RK, Stratta RJ. Opportunistic viral hepatitis in liver transplant recipients. Transplant Proc 1991;23:1520.

92. Langnas AN, Donovan JP, Sorrell MF, et al. Liver transplantation at the University of Nebraska Medical Center from 1985 to 1992. In: Terasaki PI, Cecka JM, eds. Clinical transplants 1992. Los Angeles, UCLA Tissue Typing Laboratory, 1993: Chapter 15.

93. Shaw BW Jr, Wood RP, Gordon RD, Iwatsuki S, Gillquist WP, Starzl TE. Influence of selected patient variables and operative blood loss on six-month survival following liver transplantation. Semin Liver Dis 1985;5:385.

94. Shaw BW Jr, Wood RP, Stratta RJ, et al. Stratifying the causes of death in liver transplant recipients: an approach to improving survival. Arch Surg 1989;124:895.

95. National Institutes of Diabetes and Digestive and Kidney Diseases. Follow-up survival. Liver Transplantation Database (database 4/15/90–4/15/93);3-1.

96. Edwards EB, Hunsicker LG, Guo T, Breen TJ, Daily PO. The impact of liver center volume on the odds of mortality. Presented at the XVth World Congress of the Transplantation Society, Kyoto, Japan, August 1994.

97. Quesniaux VFJ, Schreier MH, Wenger RM, et al. Cyclophilin binds to the region of cyclosporine involved in its immunosuppressive activity. Eur J Immunol 1987;17:1359.

98. Fruman DA, Kiee CB, Bierer BE, Burakoff SJ. Calcineurin phosphatase activity in T lymphocytes is inhibited by FK506 and cyclosporin A. Proc Natl Acad Sci USA 1992;89:3686.

99. Sokol RJ, Johnson KE, Karrer FM, Narkewicz MR, Smith D, Kam I. Improvement of cyclosporin absorption in children after liver transplantation by means of water-soluble vitamin E. Lancet 1991;338:212.

100. Ritschel WA, Adolph S, Ritschel GB, Schroeder T. Improvement of peroral absorption in cyclosporin A microemulsions. Methods Find Exp Clin Pharmacol 1990;12:127.

101. Hay JE, Rorayko MK, Wiesner RH, et al. Withdrawal of cyclosporine from liver transplant recipients is immunologically unsafe and does not improve chronic renal dysfunction. Hepatology 1991;14:53A.

102. Hiestand PC, Traber R, Borel JF. Pharmacological studies with Norvaline^2-cyclosporine (SDZ OG37-325) in comparison with cyclosporine (Sandimmune): a summary. Transplant Proc 1994;26:2999.

103. Lake JR, Roberts JP, Ascher NL. Maintenance immunosuppression after liver transplantation. Semin Liver Dis 1992;12:73.

104. Chatenoud L, Baudrihaye MF, Kreis H, et al. Human in vivo antigenic modulation induced by the anti-T-cell OKT3 monoclonal antibody. Eur J Immunol 1982;12:979.

105. Stratta RJ, Shaeffer MS, Markin RS, et al. Cytomegalovirus infection and disease after liver transplantation: an overview. Dig Dis Sci 1992;37:673.

106. Singh N, Dummer JS, Kusne S, et al. Infections with cytomegalovirus and other herpes viruses in 121 liver

transplant recipients: transmission by donated organ and effect of OKT3 antibodies. J Infect Dis 1988;158: 124.

107. Langnas AN, Castaldo P, Markin RS, Stratta RJ, Wood RP, Shaw BW Jr. The spectrum of Epstein-Barr virus (EBV) infection with hepatitis following liver transplantation. Transplant Proc 1991;23:1513.

108. US Multicenter FK506 Liver Study Group. A comparison of tacrolimus (FK506) and cyclosporine for immunosuppression in liver transplantation. N Engl J Med 1994;331:1110.

109. Mariani R, Fleischmajer R, Schragger AH, et al. Mycophenolic acid in the treatment of psoriasis. Arch Dermatol 1977;113:930.

110. Luo H, Chen H, Daloze P, Chang JY, St-Louis G, Wu J. Inhibition of in vitro immunoglobulin production by rapamycin. Transplantation 1992;53:1071.

111. Groth CG, Ohlman S, Ericson BH, Barholt L, Reinholt FP. Deoxyspergualin for liver graft rejection. Lancet 1990;336:626.

112. Cramer DV, Chapman FA, Jaffee BD, et al. The effect of a new immunosuppressive drug, brequinar sodium, on heart, liver, and kidney allograft rejection in the rat. Transplantation 1992;53:303.

113. Levin B, Collins G, Waer M, et al. Treatment of cadaveric renal transplant recipients with TLI, antithymocyte globulin, and low dose prednisone. Lancet 1985;2: 1321.

114. Myburgh JA, Meyers AM, Thomson PD, et al. Total lymphoid irradiation in kidney transplantation. Transplant Proc 1989;21:3953.

115. Monaco AP, Wood ML, Maki T, Gozzo JJ. Post transplantation donor-specified bone marrow transfusion in polyclonal antilymphocyte serum-treated recipients: the optimal cellular antigen for induction of unresponsiveness to organ allografts. Transplant Proc 1988;20: 1207.

116. Thomas JM, Carver MF, Cunningham PRG, Olson LC, Thomas FT. Kidney allograft tolerance in primates without chronic immunosuppression: the role of veto cells. Transplantation 1991;51:198.

117. Thomas J, Alqaisi M, Cunningham P, et al. The development of a posttransplant TLI treatment strategy that promotes organ allograft acceptance without chronic immunosuppression. Transplantation 1992;53:247.

118. Barber WH, Mankin JA, Laskow DA, et al. Long-term results of a controlled prospective study with transfusion of donor-specific bone marrow in 57 cadaveric renal allograft recipients. Transplantation 1991;51:070.

119. Rolles K, Burroughs AK, Davidson BR, et al. Donor-specific bone marrow infusion after orthotopic liver transplantation. Lancet 1994;343.

120. Starzl TE, Demetris AJ, Murase N, Thomson AW, Trucco M, Ricordi C. Donor cell chimerism permitted by immunosuppressive drugs: a new view of organ transplantation. Immunol Today 1993;14:326.

121. Owen RD. Immunogenetic consequences of vascular anastomosis between bovine twins. Science 1945;102: 400.

122. Starzl TE, Demetris AJ, Trucco M, et al. Chimerism after liver transplantation for type IV glycogen storage disease and type 1 Gaucher's disease. N Engl J Med 1993;328:745.

123. Starzl TE, Marchioro TL, Peters GN, et al. Renal heterotransplantation from baboon to man: experience with six cases. Transplantation 1964;2:752.

124. Jonasson O, Hardy M. The case of baby Fae. JAMA 1985;254:3358.

125. Miyagawa S, Hajime H, Ryota S, et al. The mechanism of discordant xenograft rejection. Transplantation 1988;46:825.

126. Platt JL, Vercellotti GM, Dalmasso AP, et al. Transplantation of discordant xenografts: a review of progress. Immunology 1990;11:450.

127. Makowka L, Cramer DV, Hoffman A, Sher L, Podesta L. Pig liver xenografts as a temporary bridge for human allografting. Xenobiotica 1993;1:27.

128. Moses RD, Auchincloss HJ. Mechanism of cellular xenograft rejection. In: Cooper DKC, Kemp E, Reemtsma K, et al. Xenotransplantation: the transplantation of organs and tissues between species. Berlin, Springer-Verlag, 1991:101.

129. Starzl TE, Fung J, Tzakis A, et al. Baboon-to-human liver transplantation. Lancet 1993;341:65.

130. Michaels MG, Simmons RL. Xenotransplant-associated zoonoses. Transplantation 1994;57:1.

131. Abouna GM, Fisher LM, Porter KA, Andres G. Experience in the treatment of hepatic failure by intermittent liver hemoperfusions. Surgery 1973;137:741.

132. Fox IJ, Langnas AN, Fristoe LW, et al. Successful application of extracorporeal liver perfusion: a technology whose time has come. Am J Gastroenterol 1993;88: 1876.

133. Fristoe LW, Merrill JH, Kangas JA, et al. Extracorporeal support with a donor liver as a bridge to transplantation. J Extracorp Tech 1993;25:133.

134. Agishi T, Nakagawa Y, Teraoka S, Kubo K, Nakazato S, Ota K. Plasma exchange as a rescue strategy for hepatic failure. ASAIO J 1994;40:77.

135. Ash SR. Hemodiabsorption in the treatment of acute hepatic failure. ASAIO J 1994;40:80.

136. Kelly JH, Sussman NL. The hepatic extracorporeal liver assist device in the treatment of fulminant hepatic failure. ASAIO J 1994;40:83.

137. Rozga J, Podesta L, LePage E, et al. A bioartificial liver to treat severe acute liver failure. Ann Surg 1994;219: 538.

Digestive Tract Surgery: A Text and Atlas, edited by Richard H. Bell, Layton F. Rikkers, and Michael W. Mulholland. Lippincott-Raven Publishers, Philadelphia, © 1996.

22

Hepatic Trauma

Jon M. Burch | *Ernest E. Moore*

The liver, because of its expansive mass and central location, is the visceral organ most commonly injured during both blunt and penetrating abdominal trauma.[1] The spectrum of injury severity ranges from trivial (ie, frequently occult and requiring no treatment) to invariably fatal (eg, avulsion of the liver from the vena cava). Numerous techniques are available for the treatment of hepatic injuries, but none is applicable to all lesions. The surgeon's challenge is to assess the nature of the injury rapidly and select the most appropriate initial treatment. The experienced surgeon recognizes when the initial approach is futile and an alternative technique should be used.

PREOPERATIVE EVALUATION AND TREATMENT

General Principles

The surgeon should determine from emergency medical service personnel the circumstances of a patient's injury and the treatment provided in the field. The former information is particularly useful in cases of blunt trauma and may lead the surgeon to suspect liver damage and other associated life-threatening injuries, such as a tear of the thoracic aorta. The probability that an occult injury has occurred is related to the mechanism of injury. If the patient was involved in a motor vehicle accident, emergency personnel should indicate whether the patient was the driver or a passenger; whether the patient was restrained by a seat belt or an air bag; whether the patient was ejected from the vehicle; what the approximate speed of the impact was; what the logistics of the impact (front, rear, or side)

were; and whether any other individuals involved in the accident were dead at the scene. This kind of detailed information generally is not necessary for victims of penetrating wounds because injury is localized to the tracts of these wounds and cannot be assessed in the field.

Treatment priorities in both the field and the emergency department are predicated on the importance of adequate oxygen delivery to the tissues. The basic approach has been outlined succinctly by the American College of Surgeons Committee on Trauma: airway, breathing, and circulation.[2] A secure and patent airway is the highest priority. Patients who are comatose or obtunded, or who cannot otherwise protect their airways should be intubated immediately. Apneic patients must be intubated by the orotracheal route, with care taken after upper torso blunt trauma to immobilize the neck and prevent the exacerbation of a cervical spine injury. Apneic patients with severe maxillofacial or laryngeal trauma that prohibits orotracheal intubation should undergo emergent cricothyroidotomy. Patients who are breathing but require airway control can be intubated by the nasotracheal route. The major advantage of this approach is that neither sedation nor paralysis is needed. In combative patients, rapid-sequence peroral intubation is the safest technique. The availability of oxygen saturation monitoring has made temporary bag-mask ventilation safer, and the risk of aspiration is minimized with cricoid pressure (Sellick maneuver). Caution should be observed in patients with evidence of basilar skull fractures because both nasogastric tubes and nasotracheal tubes can be inserted into the brain parenchyma through the skull fracture. Oxygen supplementation should be provided to all seriously injured patients.

Once the airway has been secured, pulmonary ventilation (breathing) is the next priority. Common causes of poor ventilation include malposition of the endotracheal tube, aspiration of foreign material such as teeth or gastric contents, pneumothorax, hemothorax, and pulmonary contusion. All these possibilities can be confirmed using a combination of physical examination and chest radiography. Endotracheal suctioning and chest tube insertion corrects most ventilatory problems. Patients who have aspirated foreign bodies or gastric particulate contents should undergo bronchoscopy for their removal. Patients with rapidly evolving pulmonary contusions may require mechanical ventilatory support with positive end-expiratory pressure. Chest tubes should be inserted in the fifth intercostal space at the anterior axillary line after digital examination of the pleura. The use of other chest tube insertion sites or failure to palpate the pleura can result in iatrogenic injury to the liver, spleen, or lung.

The treatment of shock (circulation) is the third critical priority. Field treatment of shock in urban environments is controversial because hospital transport times usually are short (10 to 20 minutes). Although some prospective randomized studies of both military antishock trousers and intravenous fluid administration have failed to demonstrate a survival advantage to these treatments,[3,4] others have demonstrated benefit.[5,6] In rural environments, however, where longer transport times are anticipated, the use of antishock trousers and the infusion of crystalloid solutions and blood may be essential to sustain life. In any circumstance, excessive volume loading should be prevented, particularly in the context of active internal bleeding.

In the emergency department, two intravenous catheters (14-gauge or larger) should be inserted for volume resuscitation, and blood should be drawn for typing and hematocrit determination. Additional laboratory studies can be requested (ie, a coagulation profile), but their results are less urgent.

Adult patients with evidence of shock should be given rapidly 2 L of lactated Ringer solution or an equivalent solution. Children should receive an initial fluid challenge of 20 mL/kg. Patients who improve and remain stable have little risk of significant ongoing hemorrhage and can be evaluated systematically. Patients who initially improve but then deteriorate, as well as those who fail to respond, require the administration of O-negative or type-specific blood and urgent operative intervention.

As the resuscitation is being implemented, patients should be examined rapidly but thoroughly. Particular attention should be paid to hidden areas such as the axillae, perineum, and back, because injuries in these regions are easily overlooked. All patients should undergo digital rectal examination, which may reveal blood, perforation, or a high-riding prostate. The last finding or blood at the urethral meatus is suggestive of a urethral laceration. A Foley catheter should be inserted to decompress the bladder and monitor urine output. Patients with evidence of a urethral injury ideally should undergo retrograde urethrography before catheterization. In the case of persistent hypovolemic shock, an initial attempt at Foley catheterization should be made; if this is unsuccessful, a percutaneous suprapubic cystostomy should be done. A nasogastric tube should be inserted to decrease the risk of gastric aspiration and to allow inspection of the contents for blood suggestive of occult gastroduodenal rupture.

Selected radiographs are obtained early in the emergency department evaluation. For patients with severe blunt trauma, lateral cervical spine, anteroposterior chest, and pelvic radiographs should be made as soon as possible. For patients with truncal gunshot wounds, posteroanterior and lateral radiographs of the chest and abdomen are warranted. It also is helpful to mark the entrance and exit sites of penetrating wounds with metallic clips or staples so that the trajectory of the missile can be estimated.

Evaluation and decision making are far more difficult in blunt than in penetrating trauma. In general, more energy is transferred over a wider area during blunt trauma than during gunshot or stab wounds. As a result, blunt trauma is associated with many widely distributed injuries, whereas the damage is localized to the path of the bullet or knife in penetrating wounds. Trauma surgeons often separate patients who have sustained blunt trauma into two broad categories according to their risk for multiple injuries: high energy transfer and low energy transfer. Injuries involving high energy transfer include falls from heights greater than 20 ft, motor vehicle accidents in which the car's change of speed exceeds 20 mph, auto–pedestrian accidents, motorcycle accidents, and motor vehicle accidents in which the patient has been ejected.[2]

Patients who have sustained high-energy trauma have certain patterns of injury related to the mechanism. For example, when unrestrained drivers suffer frontal impacts, their heads strike the windshield, their chests and upper abdomens hit the steering column, and their legs or knees contact the dashboard. The resultant injuries frequently include facial lacerations and fractures, intracranial trauma, laceration of the thoracic aorta, myocardial contusion, injury to the spleen and liver, and fractures of the lower extremities and pelvis. When evaluating such patients, the discovery of one of these injuries should prompt a search for the others.[7]

Low-energy trauma, such as being struck with a club or falling from a bicycle, usually does not result in widely distributed injuries. Potentially lethal lacerations of internal organs, including the liver, still can occur because the net energy transfer to that location can be substantial.

Penetrating injuries are classified according to the wounding agent as stab wounds, gunshot wounds, or shotgun wounds. Gunshot wounds are subdivided further into high- and low-velocity injuries because the speed of the bullet is much more important than its weight in determining kinetic energy transfer. Extensive experience in urban trauma centers has demonstrated that high-velocity gunshot wounds (bullet speed greater than 2000 ft/s) are rare.[7] Shotgun injuries are divided into close-range and long-range wounds. Close-range shotgun wounds are tantamount to high-velocity wounds because the entire energy of the load is delivered to a small area, often with devastating results. Long-range shotgun wounds result in a diffuse pellet pattern in which many pellets miss the victim and those that do strike are widely distributed and of comparatively low energy.

As a rule, little preoperative evaluation is required for firearm injuries that penetrate the peritoneal cavity because the chance of internal injury is over 90% and laparotomy is mandatory.[8,9] Anterior truncal gunshot wounds between the fourth intercostal space and the pubic symphysis are presumed to enter the peritoneal cavity. Gunshot wounds to the back or flank are somewhat more difficult to evaluate because of the greater thickness of tissue between the skin and the abdominal organs. If in doubt, it always is safer to explore the abdomen than to equivocate when the depth of penetration is uncertain.

In contrast to gunshot wounds, stab wounds that penetrate the peritoneal cavity are less likely to injure intraabdominal organs. Anterior and lateral stab wounds to the trunk should be explored under local anesthesia in the emergency department to determine whether the peritoneum has been violated. Injuries that do not penetrate the peritoneal cavity do not require further evaluation. As with gunshot wounds, stab wounds to the flank and back are more difficult to evaluate, and abdominal exploration often is necessary to rule out retroperitoneal injuries. Stab wounds to the lower chest present a unique diagnostic opportunity in the emergency department. After the induction of adequate local anesthesia and extension of the wound as necessary, a finger can be placed into the thoracic cavity to palpate the diaphragm. Confirmation of diaphragm penetration is an indication for laparotomy.

Diagnosis of Intraperitoneal Injury

With few exceptions, it is not necessary to determine which intraabdominal organs are injured, only whether an exploratory laparotomy is necessary. Phys-

ical examination of the abdomen is unreliable in making this determination.[10-13] However, most authorities agree that the presence of abdominal rigidity or gross abdominal distention in a patient with truncal trauma is a reliable indication for mandatory surgical exploration. Patients with evidence of truncal trauma who have persistent hypotension and no other source of blood loss also can be assumed to have significant intraabdominal hemorrhage and should be operated on promptly.

Diagnostic Peritoneal Lavage

Diagnostic peritoneal lavage (DPL) remains the most sensitive test available for determining the presence of intraabdominal injury. For both blunt abdominal trauma and stab wounds to the abdomen, its sensitivity for detecting intraabdominal injury exceeds 95%.[14-16] The results of DPL are considered to be positive if more than 10 mL of blood can be aspirated after insertion of the catheter, or if, after the instillation of 1 L of saline solution, the effluent withdrawn has a red blood cell count greater than $100,000/\mu L$. The detection of bile or of vegetable or fecal material, or the observation of effluent draining through a chest tube, a nasogastric tube, or a Foley catheter also constitutes a positive result. In equivocal cases, measurement of amylase and alkaline phosphatase levels can be helpful in identifying hollow visceral perforation.[17] White blood cell counts of the lavage effluent no longer are considered valid indicators of intraperitoneal injury.[18,19]

Computed Tomography

The use of computed tomography (CT) for the diagnosis of blunt abdominal trauma gained considerable popularity in the early 1980s.[20,21] It was reported that injuries of the liver, spleen, and kidneys could be diagnosed with great precision using this method. However, much of the initial enthusiasm has been tempered by numerous subsequent failures. CT has several limitations[22-26]:

- The need for high-quality radiographs
- The need for radiologists skilled in the interpretation of postinjury CT images
- The need for proper patient preparation
- Inability to identify intestinal injuries reliably
- Relatively poor correlation between splenic and hepatic CT staging and the subsequent risk of bleeding requiring an operation

Despite these limitations, CT remains an important diagnostic tool because of its specificity for hepatic, splenic, and renal injuries.

CT is indicated primarily for hemodynamically stable patients who are candidates for nonoperative therapy, or for those who require further clarification of equivocal DPL findings. Conversely, DPL can be used to clarify equivocal CT findings. CT also is indicated for hemodynamically stable patients who have unreliable results on physical examination and other conditions (ie, intracranial injury) that require CT evaluation. Because of the difficulty in identifying enteric injuries with CT, it may be necessary to supplement this technique with soluble contrast media or barium upper gastrointestinal series.

The results of several studies comparing DPL and CT in patients with blunt trauma indicate that the two techniques have important overlapping roles in the diagnosis of hepatic injuries.[27–29] The best initial test depends on the patient's condition, suspected associated injuries, and the technical capabilities of the radiology service. The newer helical CT scanners may offer better resolution of injury severity; further technologic advances eventually may allow CT to supplant DPL.

Ultrasonography

An ultrasonographic examination performed by a surgeon or an emergency physician in the emergency department has become an alternative to DPL in patients with blunt abdominal trauma.[30,31] Evaluation of the entire abdomen is prohibited by the presence of gas shadows, but ultrasound can be used in specific anatomic regions (eg, Morison's pouch, the left upper quadrant, the pelvis) to identify free intraperitoneal fluid. Although this method is exquisitely sensitive for detecting intraperitoneal fluid collections larger than 500 mL, it is relatively poor for staging solid organ injuries. Insufficient experience with ultrasonography precludes its substitution for DPL in most cases.

Laparoscopy

As laparoscopic cholecystectomy has gained widespread popularity, surgeons have become comfortable with the use of the laparoscope. Because of the excellent view it provides of the liver and anterior diaphragm, laparoscopy seems to be an ideal diagnostic tool for stable patients with possible right upper quadrant anterior abdominal injuries.[32–34] One theoretic concern is carbon dioxide gas embolism through hepatic venous injuries; however, this complication has not been documented in injured patients. Gasless laparoscopy eliminates this potential risk. The precise role of laparoscopy remains to be clarified, but it may expand with the availability of a smaller laparoscope that can be inserted under local anesthesia.

Once the decision has been made to perform a laparotomy, all patients should receive preoperative antibiotics. Numerous prospective randomized studies using single or multiple agents have demonstrated significant reductions in mortality and morbidity rates with appropriate antibiotic therapy. The second-generation cephalosporins and extended-spectrum penicillins have been effective for both blunt and penetrating injuries, and probably are the most cost-effective. Because the tetanus immunization status of most injured patients is not known, all patients with significant blunt or penetrating trauma should receive tetanus prophylaxis.

NONOPERATIVE TREATMENT

The sensitivity of DPL is such that operations have been performed on patients with hepatic injuries that were not bleeding and required no treatment (about 25% of all patients with hepatic injuries). Because of its lack of organ specificity, DPL cannot identify these patients before operation. With the development of whole-body CT and the recognition of its excellent imaging of blunt hepatic injuries, nonoperative treatment has become a reality.

Nonoperative treatment should be used only in patients with blunt trauma who are hemodynamically stable. If the results of physical examination or DPL are equivocal, abdominal CT should be considered. Lesions appear as inhomogeneous hypodense regions that do not enhance with intravenous contrast media (Fig. 22-1). Patients should be placed at bed rest and monitored closely in the surgical intensive care unit (SICU). Transfusions of red blood cells are necessary in 10% to 50% of patients, but should not exceed two units during the first 24 hours of hospitalization. CT should be performed again 5 to 7 days after admission to evaluate the status of the hepatic injury.

The results of nonoperative treatment have been excellent in properly selected patients.[35–39] Mortality related to the hepatic injury is nonexistent. Morbidity, including perihepatic infections, bilomas, and hemobilia, occurs in only 5% to 15% of patients. Delayed hemorrhage requiring operative treatment has been rare. Most bilomas, as well as subcapsular and intrahepatic hematomas, do not require drainage and are reabsorbed over a few months (Fig. 22-2).

There is a marked difference between the success of nonoperative treatment in children and adults. Because of the greater thickness of Glisson's capsule compared with the mass of the liver in children, 60% to 90% of all blunt hepatic injuries in children can be treated without

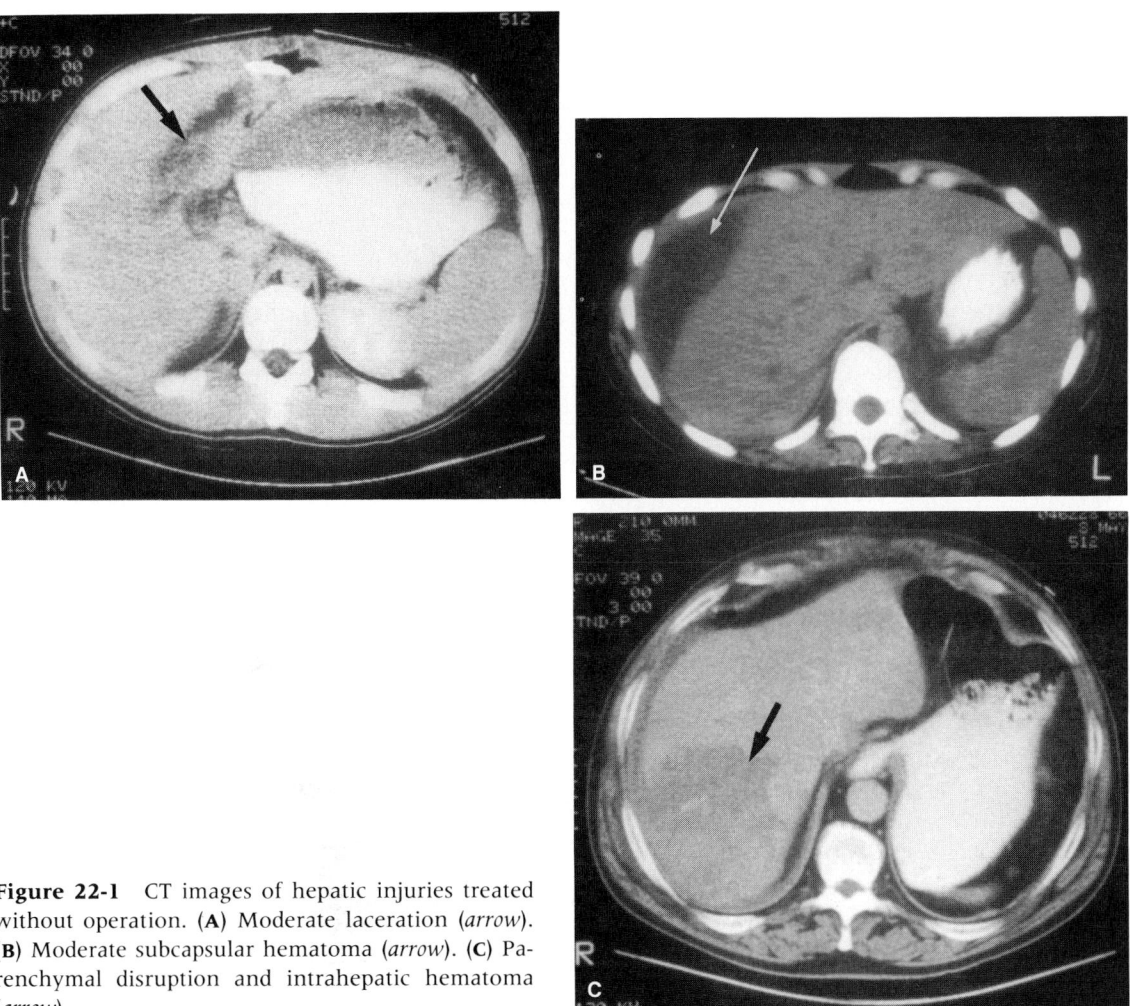

Figure 22-1 CT images of hepatic injuries treated without operation. (**A**) Moderate laceration (*arrow*). (**B**) Moderate subcapsular hematoma (*arrow*). (**C**) Parenchymal disruption and intrahepatic hematoma (*arrow*).

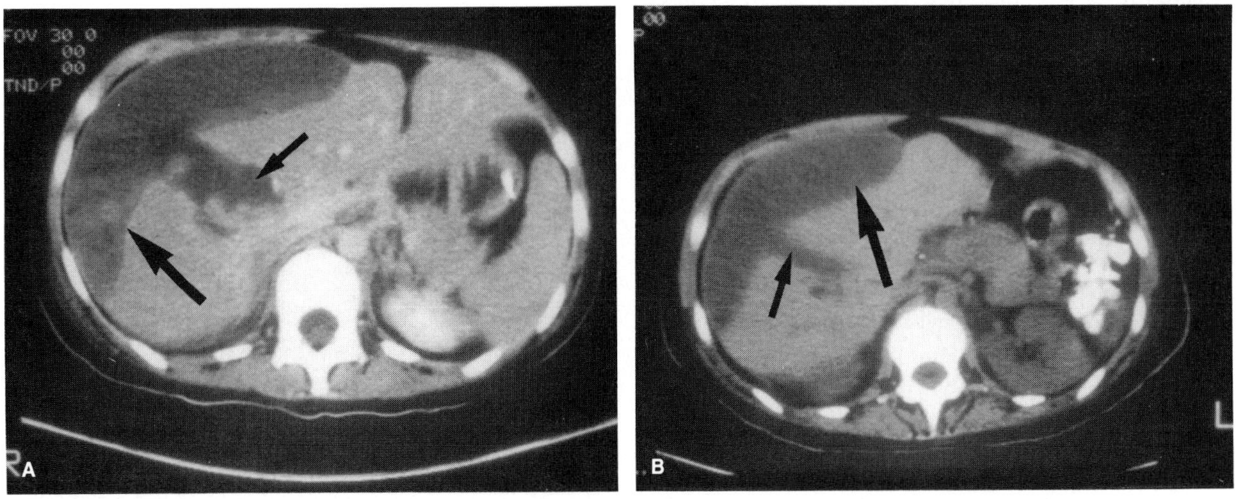

Figure 22-2 (**A**) Initial CT image of a victim of blunt trauma, showing a deep central laceration (*small arrow*) and an extensive subcapsular hematoma (*large arrow*). (**B**) A second CT scan 25 days after injury demonstrates partial resolution of both the hematoma (*large arrow*) and the laceration (*small arrow*).

operation.[40] In contrast, only 20% to 30% of blunt hepatic injuries in adults can be treated in this fashion.

OPERATIVE TREATMENT

General Principles

Patients who sustain minor hepatic injuries without shock can be treated during the perioperative period similar to other emergency surgical patients. However, from the moment seriously injured patients arrive in the emergency department until they can be discharged from the SICU, their physiologic status must be monitored and supported carefully.[41] The three most important physiologic parameters are oxygen transport, core temperature, and coagulation capability. Each of these variables is dependent on the others, and none can be overlooked.

Oxygen transport is a function of cardiac index, hemoglobin saturation, and hemoglobin concentration. In hyperdynamic patients, oxygen delivery should be maintained at greater than 600 mL/min/m^2 to eliminate flow-dependent oxygen consumption.[42] In general, maintaining a cardiac index of greater than 3 L/min/m^2, a hemoglobin concentration of greater than 11 g/dL, and an oxygen saturation over 90% will accomplish this goal. Periodic assessment of oxygen consumption and serum lactate levels is important in severely injured patients.

Cardiac index is determined with the aid of a Swan-Ganz catheter, and critically injured patients should have this device, preferably with oximetric capabilities, inserted as soon as practical. The anesthesiologist can control only a few of the variables that determine cardiac index. The most important of these is left ventricular filling pressure, which should be maintained in the range of 15 to 18 mmHg with crystalloid solutions and blood products. Massively transfused patients develop acidosis and hypothermia, both of which inhibit myocardial contractility. Inotropic agents such as dopamine or dobutamine often are required to maintain adequate cardiac output in the acute setting.

Patients who receive red blood cell transfusions of more than 10 U within 2 hours during an operation require fresh frozen plasma and platelet transfusions to ensure adequate coagulation capability. Although it may appear desirable to measure the prothrombin time, partial thromboplastin time, and platelet count, the time required to perform these tests renders the results invalid during the early phase of emergency surgery because they reflect the patient's condition 30 to 45 minutes previously. Therefore, the transfusion of clotting factors is empiric, usually based on the surgeon's esti-

mation of the patient's ability to form clots. Only through close communication between the surgeon, the anesthesiologist, and blood bank personnel is the correct decision possible.

Hypothermia is an insidious and potentially lethal complication in injured patients undergoing major operations.[43-45] Core hypothermia is a key component of what these authors have termed the *bloody vicious circle* (Fig. 22-3). There are numerous causes of hypothermia, including transfusion of cold blood products and crystalloid solutions at ambient temperature; loss of the shivering reflex because of general anesthesia; evaporative heat loss caused by exposure of the visceral and peritoneal surfaces; conductive heat loss caused by the patient's contact with cold, wet drapes; and inadequate oxygen transport resulting in diminished production of heat by the patient's tissues. As the body's core temperature drops below 34°C, coagulation becomes progressively inadequate, myocardial performance is impaired, and peripheral vasoconstriction inhibits blood flow to skeletal muscle. When the patient's temperature drops below 32°C, the mortality rate rises sharply; few patients survive core temperatures of less than 30°C, because cardiac arrest occurs at this temperature.

Many techniques are used to combat hypothermia. Thermal barrier blankets or warming blankets are placed under the patient's back and wrapped around

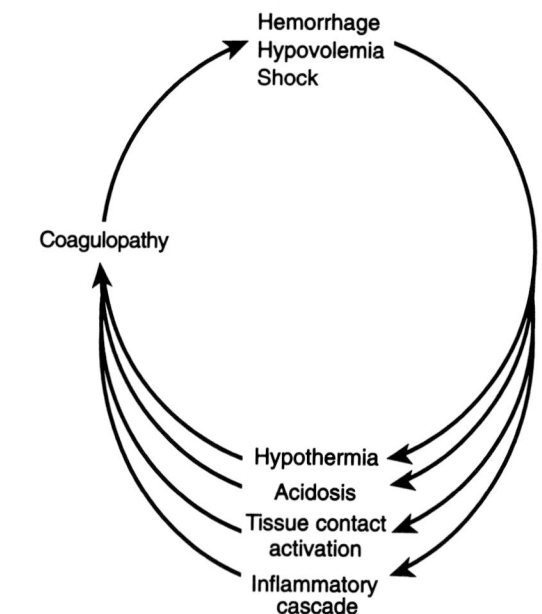

Figure 22-3 The bloody vicious circle. Uncontrolled hemorrhage with attendant hypovolemia and shock induces hypothermia, acidosis, and tissue contact activation of the inflammatory cascade. Each of these factors exacerbates an already existing dilutional coagulopathy, which in turn leads to more hemorrhage.

the extremities and head. Warming humidifiers are used to increase the temperature of inspired anesthetic gases. Crystalloid solutions are stored at body temperature, and blood warmers are used to increase the temperature of transfused blood. Unfortunately, it is difficult to control the heat loss that results from exposure of the patient's peritoneal surfaces and from contact with cold, bloody laparotomy sheets. In cases of recalcitrant hypothermia (temperature less than 32°C), a level I arteriovenous rewarmer is a useful device. However, caution must be exercised to avoid rewarming the patient to a temperature greater than 35°C until oxygen delivery is normalized. If oxygen consumption outstrips oxygen delivery, cellular death can occur.

Assessment of the Hepatic Injury

Anatomic Considerations

The evaluation and treatment of superficial and nonbleeding injuries does not require an exhaustive knowledge of hepatic anatomy. However, in evaluating patients with massive hemorrhage from the liver, knowledge of the hepatic venous system and, to a lesser extent, the arterial supply, is essential. Injuries of the portal vein and its branches can cause severe hemorrhage from the porta hepatis. As the branches of the portal vein penetrate the parenchyma of the liver, they rapidly attenuate and their propensity for severe hemorrhage diminishes. An exception is the left main branch of the portal vein, which travels horizontally until it approaches the falciform ligament. At this point, it turns inferiorly before giving off branches to the left lateral segment. This portion of the portal vein is referred to as the pars umbilicalis (Fig. 22-4). Injuries near

the falciform ligament and the ligamentum teres can result in alarming venous hemorrhage from the pars umbilicalis.

The hepatic veins converge and enter the vena cava within 1 cm of the diaphragm. Injuries in this region can cause catastrophic hemorrhage. A peculiarity of the hepatic venous system is that the right branch of the middle hepatic vein is the only major vessel to cross the anatomic plane between the left and right hepatic lobes (see Fig. 22-4). Rarely, rapid deceleration causes the liver to split through the gallbladder fossa down to the vena cava. Although this wound can appear to be severe, the right branch of the middle hepatic vein may be the only significant vascular injury. It usually can be identified easily and suture ligated.

The retrohepatic vena cava is almost entirely surrounded by the caudate lobe of the liver on both its left and right sides. Severe hemorrhage from behind the right or left lobe or into the lesser sac can be caused by injury to the retrohepatic vena cava. In addition to the major hepatic veins, several other veins enter this segment of the vena cava: the right adrenal vein, the left and right inferior phrenic veins, and the small hepatic veins that drain the caudate lobe and posterior right segment. There can be as many as 18 small veins entering the retrohepatic vena cava.[46] No lumbar or intercostal veins drain into the vena cava above the renal veins.

One of the more common anomalies involving the hepatic arterial supply is origination of the right hepatic artery from the superior mesenteric artery, which occurs in about 20% of patients.[46] As this artery emerges from behind the pancreas, it traverses the hepatic pedicle on the right side of the portal vein and enters the porta hepatis anterior to the right branch of the portal

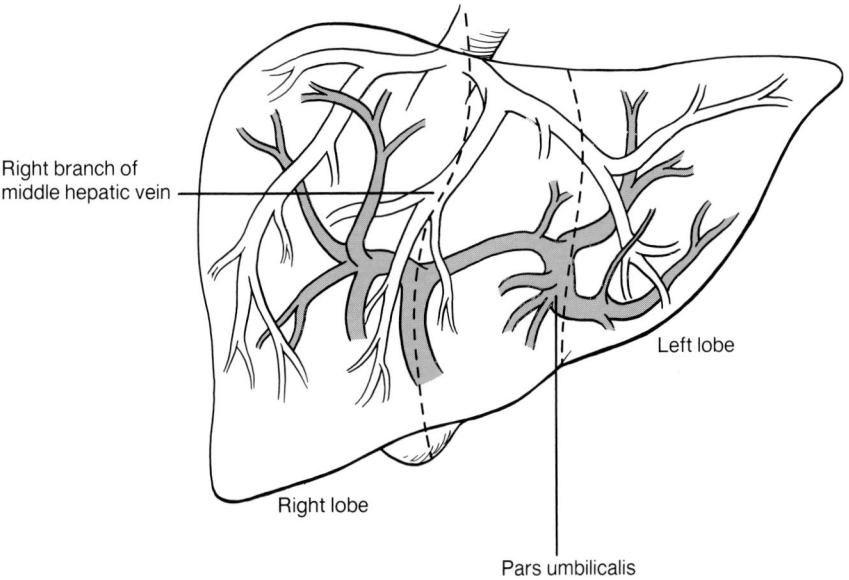

Figure 22-4 Hepatic venous anatomy.

vein. This anomaly can be detected by careful palpation of the hepatic pedicle, which reveals two distinct arterial pulses. An accessory left hepatic artery occurs in 25% to 35% of patients.[46] Either the entire left hepatic artery or one or more accessory left hepatic arteries originates from the left gastric artery. These vessels traverse the gastrohepatic omentum and enter the porta hepatis, either in the usual location or further to the left. Failure to identify these vessels may render clamping of the hepatic pedicle ineffective in controlling arterial hemorrhage from the left lobe.

Exposure of the Liver

Exposure of the liver is hampered by its protected position behind the lower costal margins. Visualization and palpation of the right lobe can be enhanced by elevating the right costal margin with a large Richardson retractor or a fixed retractor (eg, a Bookwalter retractor). Mobilization of the right lobe requires division of the right triangular and coronary ligaments. After division of the right triangular ligament, the surgeon continues medially dividing the superior coronary ligament while taking care not to injure the lateral wall of the right hepatic vein. During division of the inferior coronary ligament, the right adrenal gland can be injured easily because it lies directly beneath the peritoneal reflection. Adjacent to the left border of the right adrenal gland is the retrohepatic vena cava, which also can be injured. After division of the ligaments, the right lobe of the liver can be rotated medially into the surgical incision. This enhances visualization and treatment of posterior, lateral, and superior right lobar injuries. Mobilization of the left lobe poses no unusual problems other than the risk of injury to the left hepatic vein, the left inferior phrenic vein, or the retrohepatic vena cava.

Occasionally, it is necessary to extend the midline abdominal incision into the chest. This is best accomplished with a median sternotomy. The pericardium and diaphragm are divided radially toward the center of the inferior vena cava. This combination of incisions provides excellent exposure of the hepatic veins and the retrohepatic vena cava, and prevents injury to the phrenic nerves.

Grading Hepatic Injuries

The American Association for the Surgery of Trauma Committee on Organ Injury Scaling has developed a useful grading system for classifying hepatic injuries[47] (Table 22-1). Injuries are graded from I, representing superficial lacerations and small subcapsular hematomas, to VI, denoting avulsion of the liver and hepatic veins from the vena cava. Isolated hepatic injuries of grades I to III usually are not life-threatening. In contrast, extensive parenchymal injuries and injuries of the juxtahepatic veins (grades IV to VI) frequently are fatal and require complex maneuvers for successful treatment.

The Pringle Maneuver

One of the most helpful adjuncts in evaluating the extent of hepatic injuries is clamping of the hepatic pedicle, which is known as the Pringle maneuver (Fig. 22-5). Although many authorities prefer to clamp the hepatic pedicle from the right side (see Fig. 22-5A), it usually is preferable to open the lesser omentum manually and place the clamp from the left side while guiding the posterior blade of the clamp through the foramen of Winslow with the aid of the left index finger (see Fig. 22-5B). The advantages of this approach are avoidance of injury to the structures within the hepatic pedicle, assurance that the clamp is properly placed the first time, and inclusion of an aberrant left hepatic artery between the blades of the clamp. In patients with extensive hepatic injuries (grades IV to V), the Pringle

Table 22-1 New Liver Injury Scale

Grade*	Injury	Description†
I	Hematoma	Subcapsular, nonexpanding, <10% surface area
	Laceration	Capsular tear, nonbleeding, with <1 cm deep parenchymal disruption
II	Hematoma	Subcapsular, nonexpanding, hematoma 10%–50%; intraparenchymal, nonexpanding, <2 cm in diameter
	Laceration	<3 cm parenchymal depth, <10 cm in length
III	Hematoma	Subcapsular, >50% of surface area or expanding; ruptured subcapsular hematoma with active bleeding; intraparenchymal hematoma >2 cm
	Laceration	>3 cm parenchymal depth
IV	Hematoma	Ruptured central hematoma
	Laceration	Parenchymal destruction involving 25%–75% of hepatic lobe
V	Laceration	Parenchymal destruction involving >75% of hepatic lobe
	Vascular defect	Juxtahepatic venous injuries (retrohepatic cava or major hepatic veins)
VI	Vascular defect	Hepatic avulsion

* Advance one grade for multiple injuries.
† Based on most accurate assessment at autopsy, laparotomy, or radiologic study.
(Organ Injury Scaling Committee, E. E. Moore, Chair. American Association for the Surgery of Trauma, December, 1988)

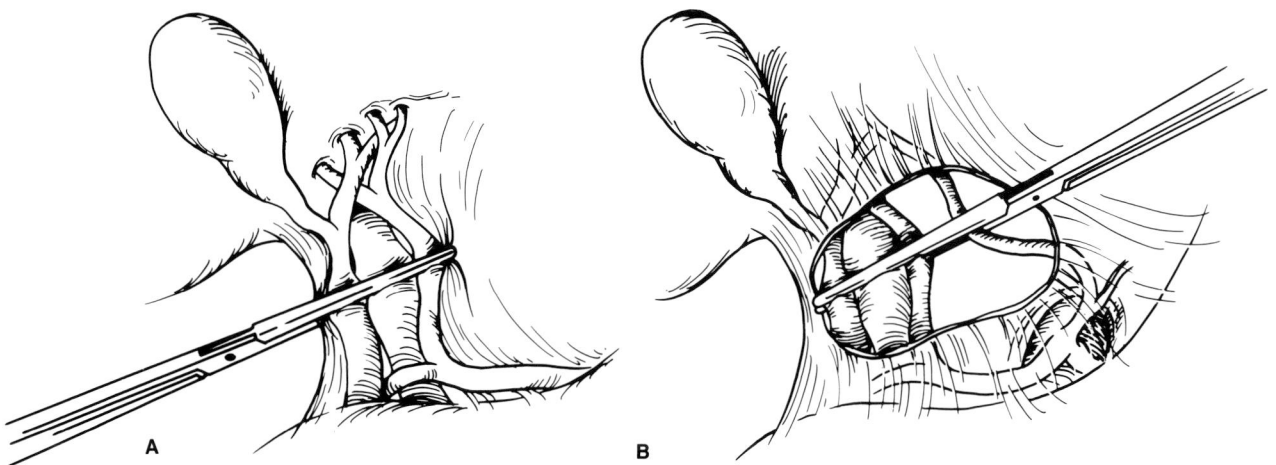

Figure 22-5 The Pringle maneuver. (**A**) The traditional method of clamping the hepatic pedicle. (**B**) Our method increases the likelihood of including an accessory left hepatic artery and lessens the risk of injury to the structures in the hepatic pedicle.

maneuver differentiates between hemorrhage from the hepatic artery and portal vein, which ceases when the clamp is applied, and hemorrhage from the hepatic veins and retrohepatic vena cava, which does not.

Treatment of the Hepatic Injury

The optimal incision for abdominal trauma is a long midline incision. Exposure of upper abdominal injuries can be improved by extending the incision superiorly to the xiphocostal angle. After liquid blood and clots have been evacuated, laparotomy pads are packed into each quadrant of the peritoneal cavity to localize sources of hemorrhage. In the setting of a major liver injury, it is imperative to exclude splenic or mesenteric injuries that may bleed actively as a coagulopathy develops. If the liver appears to be the source of hemorrhage, the pads are removed and the right costal margin is elevated. The surgeon then gently palpates the right and left lobes for traumatic defects. Should additional exposure be necessary, the right or left lobe is mobilized as outlined earlier.

The extent of a hepatic injury can be misjudged during the initial inspection. A minimally bleeding grade III injury can become a grade V injury if a clot occluding a hepatic venous injury is dislodged. The patient's overall condition also can affect the initial evaluation: a quiescent grade II injury may begin to bleed profusely if a coagulopathy develops as a result of blood loss from associated wounds.

Temporary Control of Hepatic Hemorrhage

Temporary control of hemorrhage from the liver is essential for many reasons. During the evaluation and treatment of a major hepatic injury, hemorrhage can

pose an immediate threat to the patient's life. Temporary control is critical to allow the anesthesiologist to restore circulating blood volume before proceeding. Multiple abdominal injuries are common in both blunt and penetrating trauma. Because it is not possible to control simultaneously the hemorrhage from several sites, the surgeon must determine which site constitutes the greatest threat to the patient. If the liver is not the first priority, temporary control will prevent unnecessary blood loss while other injuries are repaired. Of the many temporary techniques available, manual compression, the Pringle maneuver, and perihepatic packing are the most useful.

Manual Compression and Temporary Perihepatic Packing

Periodic manual compression with the aid of laparotomy pads is helpful in the treatment of complex injuries to provide time for necessary resuscitation[1,48,49] (Fig. 22-6). Carefully placed laparotomy pads (perihepatic packing) control hemorrhage from almost all hepatic injuries.[50-54] The pads should remain folded, with two or three stacked together. The right costal margin is elevated, and the pads are placed strategically over and around the bleeding site (Fig. 22-7). Additional pads should be placed between the liver, diaphragm, and anterior chest wall until the bleeding has been controlled. As many as 20 pads may be required to control the hemorrhage from an extensive right lobar injury. The effectiveness of packing can be enhanced by downward pressure on the right costal margin by an assistant. Packing of injuries of the left lobe is not as effective because there is insufficient abdominal and

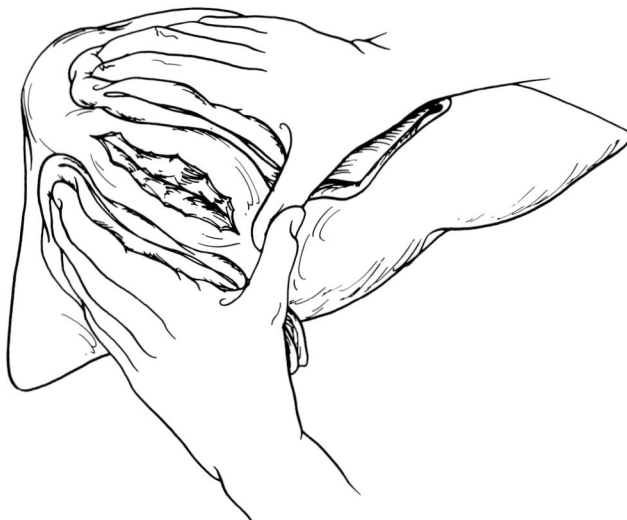

Figure 22-6 Technique for manual compression of a hepatic injury.

thoracic wall anterior to the left lobe to provide adequate compression with the abdomen open. Fortunately, hemorrhage from the left lobe can be controlled by dividing the left triangular and coronary ligaments, and compressing the lobe between the surgeon's hands.

Two complications can occur in packing hepatic injuries. First, tight packing can compress the inferior vena cava and reduce left ventricular filling. The resultant reduction in cardiac output is not tolerated in some patients. Second, the right diaphragm can be forced up-

ward and its motion impaired by perihepatic packing. This causes an increase in airway pressures and a decrease in tidal volume. Depending on the patient's condition, the surgeon must decide whether these potential complications outweigh the risk of additional blood loss.

The Pringle Maneuver

The Pringle maneuver often is used as an adjunct to packing for the temporary control of hemorrhage[48] (see Fig. 22-5). The recommended length of time that a Pringle maneuver can be applied without causing irreversible ischemic damage to the liver has increased over the years. Several authors have documented no hepatic ischemic damage after inflow occlusion for more than 1 hour in patients with complex injuries.[49,55] In dealing with extensive hepatic injuries, the Pringle maneuver should not be released every 20 minutes to allow perfusion of the liver. This not only results in additional uncontrolled blood loss but can contribute to a hepatic reperfusion syndrome and cause more metabolic harm than good.

Consideration can be given to cooling the liver topically with crushed ice.[55] However, this technique has both advantages and disadvantages. Although it allows the liver to tolerate longer ischemic periods, the introduction of ice into the peritoneal cavity lowers the patient's core temperature, impairs cardiac contractility, and aggravates any existing coagulopathy. The use of systemic steroids has been suggested to prolong the liv-

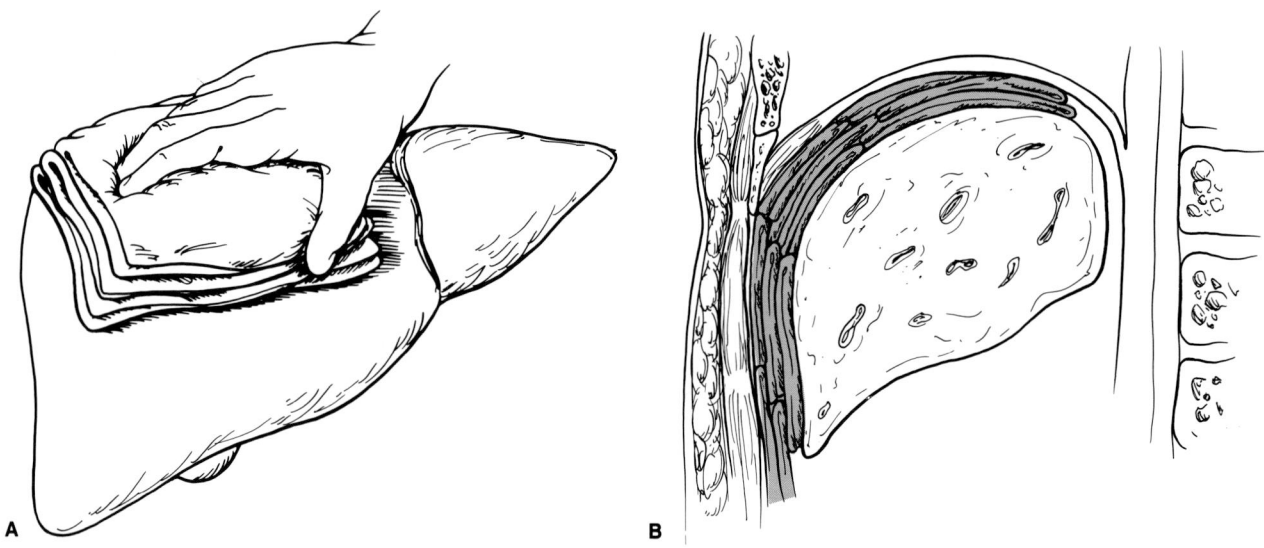

Figure 22-7 Placement of perihepatic packs. **(A)** The initial packs are placed over the injury and between the dome of the liver and the posterior superior aspect of the diaphragm. **(B)** Additional packs are placed between the peritoneal surface of the right lower thorax and the anterior surface of the liver, as shown in the sagittal view.

er's tolerance of portal occlusion, but scientific validation is lacking.[55] The timely administration of antioxidants and other antiinflammatory agents has similar theoretic appeal.

When a life-threatening hepatic injury is encountered on opening the abdomen, the Pringle maneuver should be performed immediately and perihepatic packs placed. This combination of techniques eliminates the forward flow of blood to the liver and controls retrograde venous bleeding.

Lobar Rotation

Rotation of the right or left lobe of the liver can generate sufficient intraparenchymal pressure to control most causes of venous hemorrhage. This technique is used primarily for deep central lacerations of the liver. Extreme rotation of the right lobe twists and partially occludes the retrohepatic vena cava, impairing venous return to the heart.

Hepatic Vascular Isolation

Beyond the simple techniques for temporary control of hepatic hemorrhage are those specifically intended to aid in the treatment of juxtahepatic venous injuries. Among these formidable procedures are hepatic vascular isolation with clamps, the atriocaval shunt, and the Moore-Pilcher balloon. Hepatic vascular isolation is accomplished by applying a Pringle maneuver, clamping the aorta at the diaphragm, and clamping the suprarenal and suprahepatic vena cava.[56] Although this technique has enjoyed considerable success in elective procedures, its use in injured patients has met with mixed results. This presumably is due to the inability of patients in shock to tolerate an acute reduction in left ventricular filling pressure; sudden death has occurred on placement of the venous clamps.[57] If injured patients requiring hepatic vascular isolation have been maintained in a relatively normal physiologic condition, which is rare, it is reasonable to consider this method.

The atriocaval shunt was designed to achieve hepatic vascular isolation and still permit some venous return from below the diaphragm[58] (Fig. 22-8). Trauma surgeons quickly embraced this concept for use in patients with injuries to the hepatic veins or retrohepatic vena cava. After a few early successes, enthusiasm for the atriocaval shunt declined because associated mortality rates were high.[59–63] There are several reasons for these failures.[57] Many trauma surgeons are general surgeons who are unfamiliar or uncomfortable with cannulating the right atrial appendage and guiding a large, stiff tube into the inferior vena cava. Manipulation of the cold, acidotic heart can precipitate a fatal

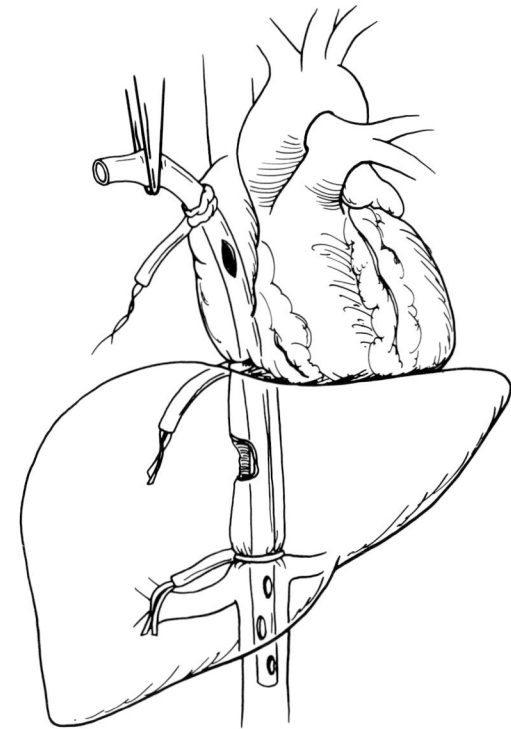

Figure 22-8 The original atriocaval shunt. Using a 36F chest tube, an additional hole is cut about 17 cm from the closest original drainage hole to provide an outlet for blood to enter the right atrium from below the diaphragm. It is wise first to make a visual estimate of the distance: too long a distance is acceptable, too short a distance is a disaster.

arrhythmia. Furthermore, patient selection has a significant effect on results. If the shunt is placed as a desperate maneuver in a patient near death, a fatal outcome is likely. Another factor is the overall complexity of the maneuver. The shunt must be constructed precisely and positioned properly on the first attempt. Patients with juxtahepatic venous injuries tolerate additional blood loss poorly. Finally, iatrogenic injuries to the suprarenal vena cava, the retrohepatic vena cava, and the heart can occur during insertion of the shunt, which also can result in death.

A variation of the original atriocaval shunt involves the substitution of a 9-mm endotracheal tube for the usual large chest tube[64] (Fig. 22-9). The balloon of the endotracheal tube eliminates the need to surround the suprarenal vena cava with an umbilical tape. This minor change eliminated one of the most difficult maneuvers required for the original shunt. Because hemorrhage must be controlled during insertion of the shunt by applying posterior pressure on the liver, access to the suprarenal vena cava is restricted and encircling it with an umbilical tape is difficult.

An alternative to the atriocaval shunt is the Moore-

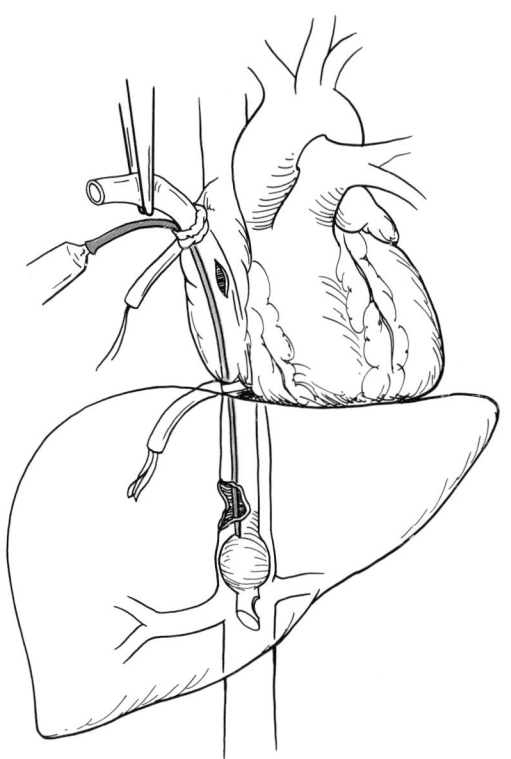

Figure 22-9 An atriocaval shunt using a 9-mm endotracheal tube. The distance between the lateral hole below the balloon (Murphy's eye) and the atrial hole cut by the surgeon should be 15 cm in an adult. When cutting the atrial hole, care is taken not to transect the smaller integral tube used to inflate the balloon.

Pilcher balloon[65] (Fig. 22-10). This device is inserted through the femoral vein and advanced into the retrohepatic vena cava. When the balloon is properly positioned and inflated, it occludes the hepatic veins, thus achieving vascular isolation. The catheter itself is hollow, and appropriately placed holes below the balloon permit blood to flow into the right atrium, similar to the atriocaval shunt. The survival rate of patients with juxtahepatic venous injuries who are treated with this device is similar to that of patients treated with the atriocaval shunt.[62] None of the techniques of hepatic vascular isolation provide complete hemostasis. Drainage from the right adrenal vein, drainage from the inferior phrenic veins, and persistent forward flow from the liver from unrecognized accessory left hepatic arteries contribute to this problem.

A new technique has been developed to expose injuries of the retrohepatic vena cava and hepatic veins.[66] Vascular isolation of the liver is achieved using the clamping technique, and the suprahepatic vena cava is divided between vascular clamps. The liver and suprahepatic vena cava then are rotated anteriorly to provide direct access to the posterior retrohepatic vena cava (Fig. 22-11). Anterior injuries are repaired through an incision in the posterior aspect of the retrohepatic vena cava.

Hepatic Tourniquet

A final technique for temporarily controlling hepatic hemorrhage is the use of a tourniquet.[67] After mobilization of the bleeding lobe, a 1-inch Penrose drain is wrapped around the liver near the anatomic division between the left and right lobes. The drain is stretched until the hemorrhage ceases, and tension is maintained by clamping it. Unfortunately, tourniquets are difficult to use because they tend to slip off or tear through the parenchyma when they are placed over an injured area. An alternative is application of the Lin liver clamp.

Techniques for Definitive Treatment

Topical Measures

Techniques available for the definitive management of hepatic injuries range from manual compression to hepatic transplantation. Minor lacerations of

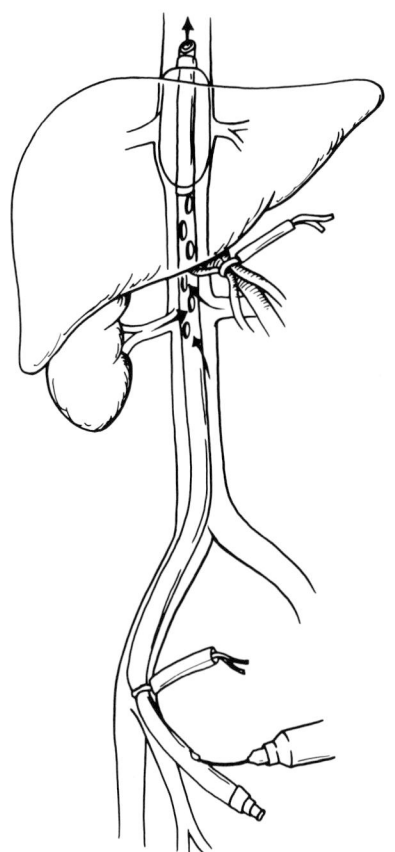

Figure 22-10 The Moore-Pilcher balloon. Similar to the atriocaval shunt, this device offers the advantage of eliminating the need for both a suprarenal caval tourniquet and cannulation of the right atrial appendage.

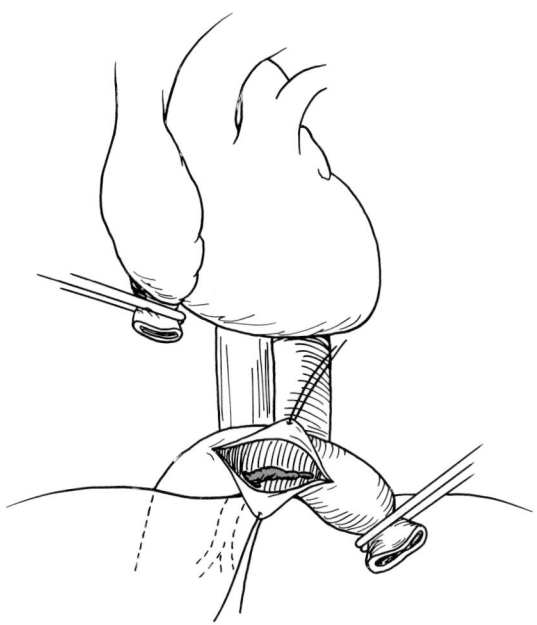

Figure 22-11 An alternative approach to injuries of the retrohepatic vena cava and hepatic veins using the clamping technique to achieve vascular isolation. The suprahepatic vena cava is transected between vascular clamps, and the liver is rotated forward. Injuries to the anterior aspect of the large veins can be approached through a posterior incision in the retrohepatic vena cava.

the hepatic parenchyma of grades I and II can be controlled with manual compression applied directly to the injury site. For similar injuries that do not respond to manual compression, topical hemostatic agents have been used successfully. Small bleeding vessels near the surface of the liver can be controlled with electrocautery, although the power output of the machine may have to be increased. Bleeding from raw surfaces of the liver can be controlled with the argon beam coagulator (Fig. 22-12). This device imparts less heat to the surrounding hepatic tissue than does electrocautery and creates a more consistent eschar, which aids in hemostasis. Microcrystalline collagen in the powdered form can be used in similar situations. The powder is placed on a clean 4 × 4 sponge and applied directly to the oozing surface. Maintaining pressure on the sponge for 5 to 10 minutes often results in cessation of bleeding. Topical thrombin also can be applied to minor bleeding injuries by saturating either a gelatin foam sponge or a microcrystalline collagen pad and applying it to the bleeding site.

Fibrin Glue

Fibrin glue has been used for both superficial and deep lacerations, and appears to be the most effective topical agent. It also can be injected deep into bleeding gunshot and stab wound tracts to prevent extensive dissection and blood loss. Fibrin glue is made by mixing concentrated human fibrinogen (cryoprecipitate) with bovine thrombin and calcium. Because a coagulum forms quickly, the fibrinogen and thrombin–calcium solution are placed in separate syringes joined with a Y connector. The materials are mixed immediately before application. Spray-on applicators also have been used. The use of fibrin glue became popular after the successful management of serious hepatic injuries with this material was reported.[1,68,69] However, enthusiasm has been tempered by recent reports of fatal anaphylactic reactions and the observation of hypotension temporally related to application of the fibrin glue.[70,71] Its role in the treatment of hepatic injuries remains to be defined. Fibrin glue is not approved by the US Food and Drug Administration for general use in hepatic injuries.[72]

Suturing the Hepatic Parenchyma

Some grade II and many grade III and IV lacerations do not respond to topical measures. In these instances, suturing of the hepatic parenchyma can be helpful. Although this technique has been maligned as a cause of hepatic necrosis, it remains the most frequently used hemostatic method.[48,49,55,61,73,74] Hepatic sutures are used most often for persistently bleeding lacerations less than 3 cm in depth. This also is an appropriate technique for deeper lacerations when the urgency of the clinical situation does not allow time for hepatotomy and selective ligation of bleeding vessels. The preferred suture for hepatic parenchyma is 0 or 2-0 chromic attached to a large, blunt-tipped, curved needle. The large diameter of the suture helps prevent it from pulling through Glisson's capsule. If the capsule

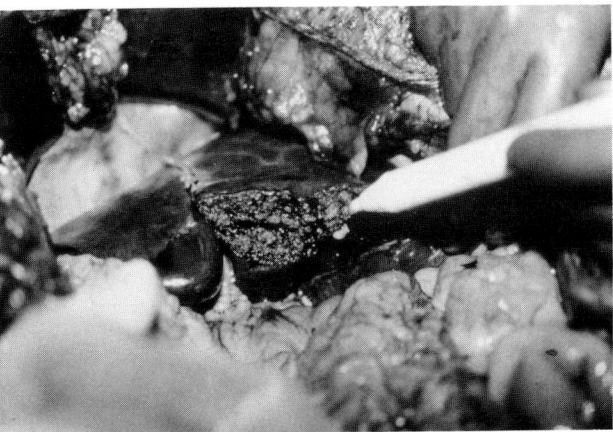

Figure 22-12 The argon beam coagulator can be used to treat diffuse surface hemorrhage from the liver. Eschar forms after its use. (See Color Fig. 22-12.)

of the liver has been stripped away by the injury, suturing of the hepatic parenchyma is less effective. A simple running technique can be used to approximate the edges of a shallow laceration. Deeper lacerations can be managed with interrupted horizontal mattress sutures placed parallel to the edge of the laceration. The knot should be tightened until hemorrhage ceases or the liver blanches around the suture.

Most intrahepatic venous injuries can be managed with parenchymal sutures; however, injuries of larger branches of the hepatic artery may not be controlled. Successful tamponade of injuries of the retrohepatic vena cava and hepatic veins has been achieved by closing the hepatic parenchyma over the bleeding vessel.[57,75] Venous hemor-

rhage from penetrating wounds that traverse the central portion of the liver can be managed by suturing the entrance and exit wounds with horizontal mattress sutures. Although intrahepatic hematomas can form, this may be preferable to an intracaval shunt or deep hepatotomy.

When suturing the hepatic parenchyma fails to control hemorrhage, it is essential that the surgeon remove the sutures to explore the wound and identify the bleeding vessels.

Hepatotomy With Selective Ligation

Hepatotomy with selective ligation of bleeding vessels is an important technique usually reserved for transhepatic penetrating wounds. Many authorities

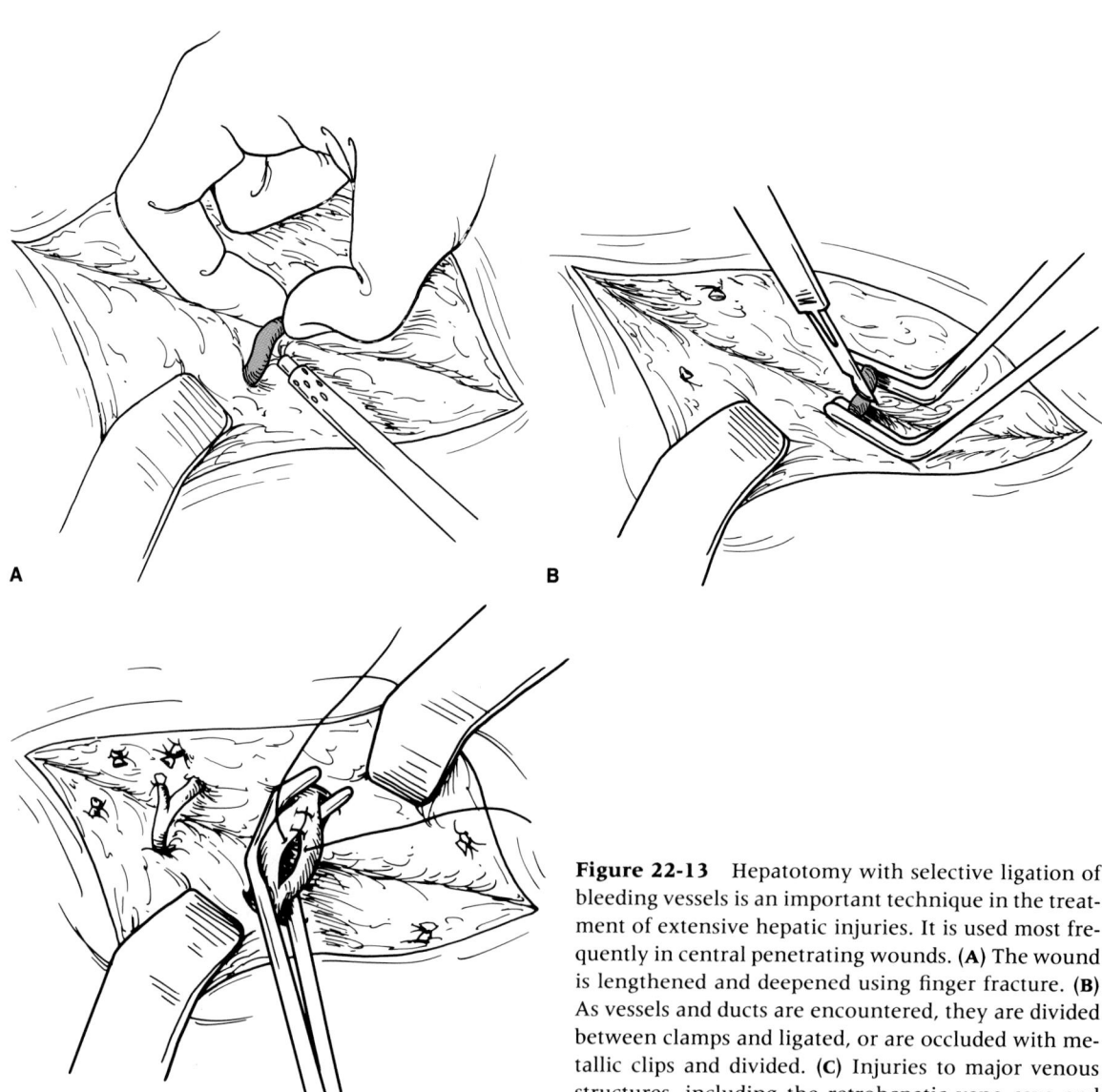

Figure 22-13 Hepatotomy with selective ligation of bleeding vessels is an important technique in the treatment of extensive hepatic injuries. It is used most frequently in central penetrating wounds. (**A**) The wound is lengthened and deepened using finger fracture. (**B**) As vessels and ducts are encountered, they are divided between clamps and ligated, or are occluded with metallic clips and divided. (**C**) Injuries to major venous structures, including the retrohepatic vena cava and the right or left hepatic veins, may be encountered and should be repaired.

prefer this approach to parenchymal sutures.[48,49,55,76,77] Some even favor this technique over an atriocaval shunt for exposing and repairing juxtahepatic venous injuries.[63] The finger fracture technique is used to extend the length and depth of a laceration or missile tract until the bleeding vessels are identified and controlled (Fig. 22-13). Hepatotomy also is indicated if suturing of the hepatic parenchyma has failed to control bleeding. Additional blood loss can be incurred because viable hepatic tissue must be divided to expose the bleeding vessels.

Hepatic Arterial Ligation

Hepatic arterial ligation may be appropriate for patients with recalcitrant arterial hemorrhage from deep within the liver.[78] However, this technique plays a limited role in the treatment of hepatic injuries because hemorrhage from the portal and hepatic venous systems continues.[79] Its primary role is in left or right deep lobar injuries in which application of the Pringle maneuver results in cessation of the arterial hemorrhage. If clamping of the left or right hepatic artery stops the hemorrhage, arterial ligation is a reasonable alternative to deep hepatotomy. Although ligation of the right or left hepatic artery is well tolerated in humans, ligation of the proper hepatic artery (distal to the origin of the gastroduodenal artery) is associated with a significant mortality rate.[80]

Intrahepatic Balloon Tamponade

An alternative to suturing the entrance and exit wounds of a transhepatic injury or performing an extensive hepatotomy is to use an intrahepatic balloon.[81,82] These devices are hand-crafted in the operating room by the surgeon. One method is to tie a 1-inch Penrose drain to a hollow catheter (Fig. 22-14). The balloon then is inserted into the bleeding wound and inflated with soluble contrast media. If the hemorrhage is controlled, a stopcock or clamp is used to occlude the catheter and maintain the inflation. The catheter is left in the abdomen and removed at a subsequent operation 24 to 48 hours later. These devices are particularly useful for deep-seated injuries of the hepatic veins. Recurrent hemorrhage can occur when the balloon is deflated. The balloon catheter may not generate sufficient intraparenchymal pressure to tamponade major arterial hemorrhage.

Resectional Débridement

Resectional débridement is indicated for the removal of peripheral portions of nonviable hepatic parenchyma. The tissue removed rarely should exceed 25% of the liver mass. Because additional blood loss occurs during the removal of nonviable tissue, this technique should be reserved for patients who are in good metabolic condition and can tolerate additional blood loss. Resectional débridement is performed by finger fracture and is appropriate for selected patients with grade III to V lacerations.

Perihepatic Packing

Perihepatic packing has been the most significant development in the treatment of hepatic injuries in the past 15 years. Although packing of hepatic injuries is not new, current concepts and techniques are. In the past, liver lacerations were packed with yards of gauze,

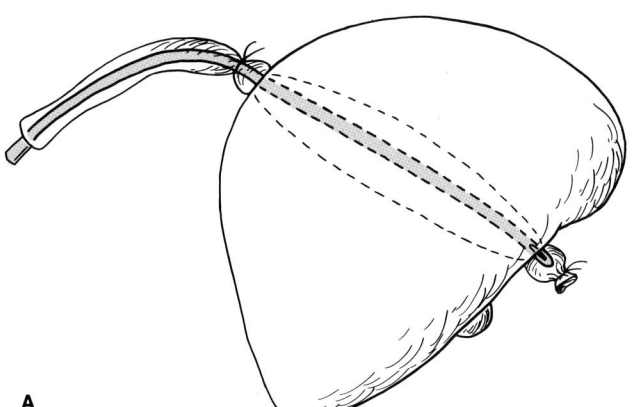
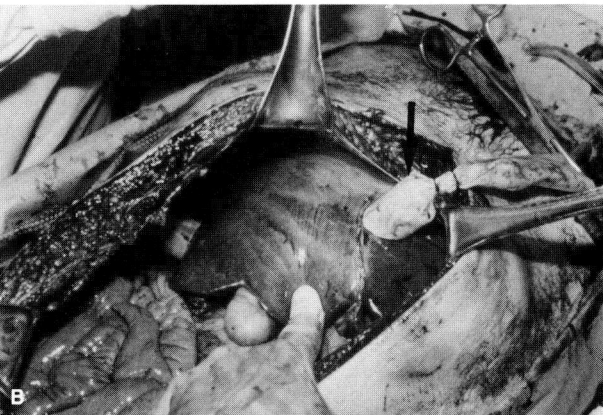

Figure 22-14 (**A**) Schematic representation of an intrahepatic balloon used to treat hemorrhage from a transhepatic penetrating injury. (**B**) Appearance of an intrahepatic balloon in situ (*arrow*).

the end of which was brought out of the abdomen through a separate stab wound.[83] This material then was teased out of the wound over a period of days. Frequent abdominal sepsis and failure to control hemorrhage led to decreasing use of this technique. A newer and preferred method is not to pack the hepatic lacerations themselves but to place the packs over and around the injury to compress the wound by squeezing the liver between the anterior chest wall, the diaphragm, and the retroperitoneum[50–54] (Fig. 22-15). The abdomen then is closed, and the patient is taken to the SICU for resuscitation and correction of metabolic derangements. The patient is returned to the operating room in 24 to 48 hours for removal of the packs. Perihepatic packing is indicated for grade IV and V lacerations, and for less severe injuries in patients with coagulopathies related to associated wounds. The technique is similar to that described earlier (see section on Temporary Control of Hepatic Hemorrhage and Fig. 22-7).

Abbreviated Laparotomy

Most patients with extensive parenchymal damage or juxtahepatic venous injuries have massive blood loss and soon develop the triad of acidosis, hypothermia, and coagulopathy (see Fig. 22-3). As the pH level dips below 7.2, the core temperature drops below 34°C, and coagulation abnormalities develop, the risk of sudden death increases significantly.[84] Red blood cell transfusion requirements in these patients often exceed 10 to 20 units/h, and further attempts to define bleeding areas are futile in the face of the coagulopathy. During the early 1980s, the potentially lethal nature of this condition was recognized and the concept of an abbreviated laparotomy was developed to treat these criti-

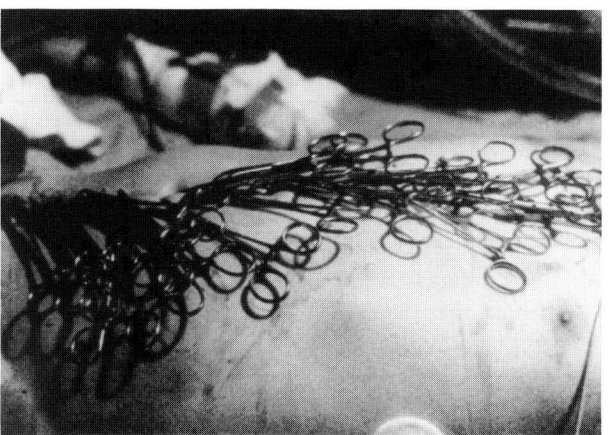

Figure 22-16 Towel clip closure of the abdomen. Towel clips are placed every 1.5 to 2 cm and include only the skin of the abdomen. This approach allows for greater distention of the anterior abdominal wall and lessens the likelihood of an abdominal compartment syndrome. (Burch JM, Ortiz VB, Richardson RJ, Martin RR, Mattox KL, Jordan GL Jr. Abbreviated laparotomy and planned reoperation for critically injured patients. Ann Surg 1992;215:476)

cally ill patients.[84,85] After perihepatic packing is completed, the abdominal incision is closed with towel clips placed 2 cm apart that include only the skin of the abdominal wall (Fig. 22-16). This can be accomplished within 90 seconds. Cold, wet drapes are removed, and the patient is covered from head to toe with layers of warm blankets. If the surgeon believes that a patient's metabolic problems can be corrected in a short time (2 hours or less), the patient can remain in the operating room while additional blood products are administered and rewarming measures are instituted. A patient who is in extremely poor condition and requires several hours for metabolic corrections should be transferred to the SICU. If the patient's condition improves, as evidenced by normalization of coagulation study results, correction of the acid–base balance, and increase of the core temperature to at least 36°C, he or she should be returned to the operating room for removal of the packs and additional treatment of the hepatic injury as necessary.

In addition to the risk of exsanguination, a potentially lethal complication of packing hepatic injuries is the abdominal compartment syndrome.[84,85] After packing, some hemorrhage may continue until the coagulopathy and hypothermia are corrected. During this time, several liters of blood can accumulate in the peritoneal cavity. Added to the space occupied by the packs and the intestinal edema caused by reperfusion injury, this volume of blood can stretch both the diaphragm and the abdominal wall until their loss of compliance

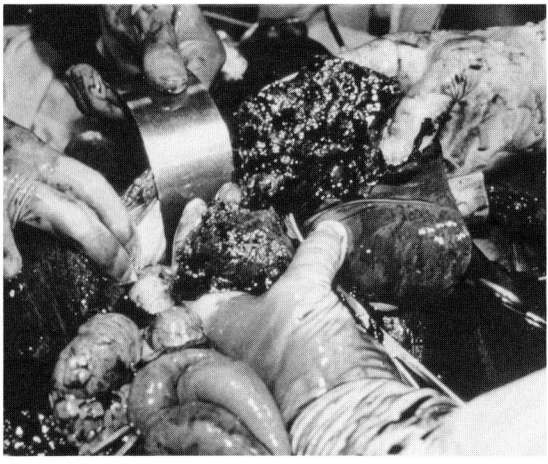

Figure 22-15 Grade V hepatic injury. An injury of this severity is likely to require perihepatic packing.

prevents further distention. The pressure within the abdominal cavity then begins to increase. When the intraabdominal pressure reaches 20 mmHg, blood flow in the inferior vena cava decreases and ventilatory pressures increase. If this condition remains unchecked and the pressure continues to rise, both respiratory failure and renal failure can develop. The only hope for these patients is to return them promptly to the operating room for decompression of the abdomen. If the replacement of blood products has been vigorous, the coagulopathy may have been corrected and further treatment of the hepatic injury may not be necessary. If hemorrhage continues from the liver, it should be packed again, the abdomen should be closed with towel clips, and the patient should be returned to the SICU, where the cycle begins anew. Many patients with seemingly fatal hepatic injuries have been treated successfully in this fashion.

If the abdominal compartment syndrome does not develop, patients are returned to the operating room within 24 to 48 hours. When packing times exceed 48 hours, the risk of intraabdominal sepsis increases. During removal of the packs, care should be taken to prevent additional injury to the liver. Warm saline solution can be used to tease the packs gently off the surface of the liver. Alternatively, a sterile plastic sheet can be placed over the injured liver and the packs applied over it.[50]

Mesh Hepatorrhaphy

If packing fails, the injured portion of the liver can be wrapped with a fine porous material, such as polyglycolic acid mesh, after it has been mobilized (mesh hepatorrhaphy).[86,87] Using a running suture or staples, the surgeon constructs a close-fitting stocking to enclose the injured lobe (Fig. 22-17).

Hepatic Resection

The final alternative for patients with extensive unilobar injuries is anatomic hepatic resection. Although anatomic lobectomy can be performed in elective circumstances with excellent results, the mortality rate for injured patients in most series exceeds 50%.[73,74,76,88–90] Hepatic resection is performed in only a small percentage of patients with liver wounds. Resection has been replaced by perihepatic packing, resectional débridement, and hepatotomy with selective ligation.

There are two circumstances, however, in which anatomic resection may be reasonable. The first is when there are extensive injuries of the lateral segment of the left lobe, which is easier to resect than is an entire right or left lobe. The other indication for anatomic lobectomy is when hemorrhage has been controlled by perihepatic packing and the left or right lobe is nonviable. Because the mass of remaining necrotic liver is large, the risk of subsequent infection is high and resection should be performed as soon as the patient's condition permits.

Hepatic Transplantation

Five injured patients with either devastating hepatic wounds or necrosis of the entire liver have undergone successful hepatic transplantation.[91–94] The

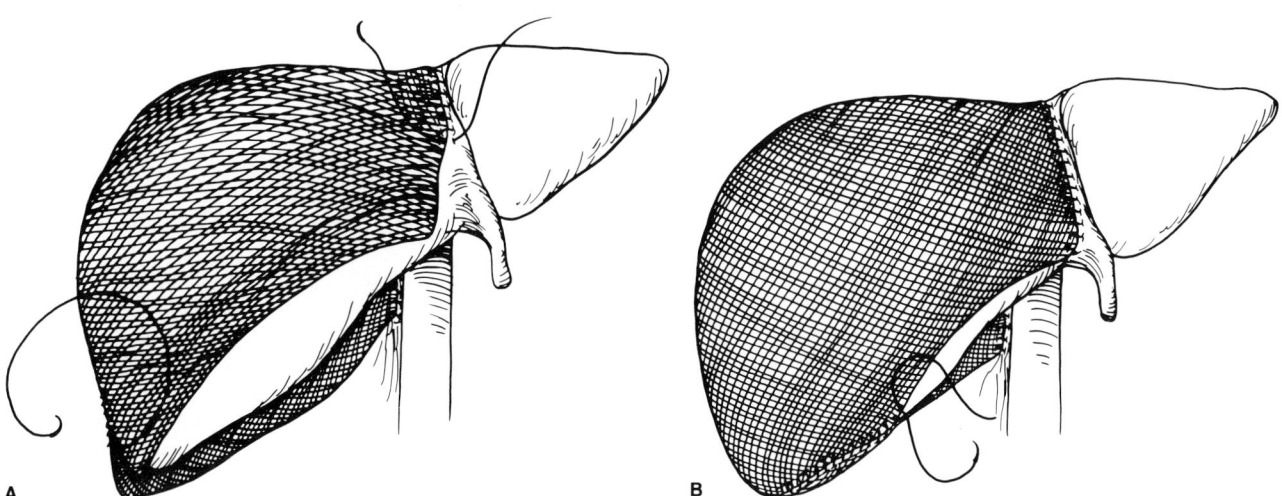

Figure 22-17 (**A**) A fine-mesh absorbable material is wrapped around the right lobe of the liver. The lateral aspect of the mesh is closed with a running suture line or with staples. The posterior leaflet is sutured to the tissues adjacent to the retrohepatic vena cava, and the anterior aspect is sutured to the falciform ligament. (**B**) The remaining inferior leaflets are closely approximated with a suture line or staples.

mean anhepatic period was about 24 hours for these patients. All survived transplantation, although two died of disseminated viral infections within 2 months of the transplant. Two others were alive and well at 16 and 17 months after the procedure. Follow-up of the fifth patient was not stated.

Hepatic transplantation represents the ultimate in aggressive care of the injured patient. All other injuries must be delineated (particularly those of the central nervous system) and the patient should have an excellent chance for survival with the exception of the hepatic injury. Cost and donor organ availability limit this approach, but hepatic transplantation probably will continue to be performed in rare and extraordinary circumstances.

Treatment of Subcapsular Hematomas

Subcapsular hematomas are uncommon but perplexing hepatic injuries. These lesions occur when the parenchyma of the liver is disrupted by blunt trauma but Glisson's capsule remains intact. As noted in the grading system for hepatic injuries, subcapsular hematomas range from minor blisters on the surface of the liver to ruptured central hematomas with severe hemorrhage. These lesions may be recognized either at the time of surgery or before surgery if a CT scan is performed.

Regardless of how these lesions are diagnosed, subsequent decision making often is difficult. Subcapsular hematomas of grades I and II that involve less than half of the hepatic surface, that are not expanding, and that have not ruptured should be left alone when discovered at exploratory laparotomy. Larger hematomas that have not ruptured and are not expanding can be opened and explored, left alone, or packed. If the hematoma is explored, hepatotomy with selective ligation may be required to control bleeding vessels. Even if the hepatotomy is effective, the surgeon still must contend with diffuse hemorrhage from the large denuded surface. Packing also may be required.

Hematomas that are expanding during an operation (grade III) may require exploration. These lesions often result from uncontrolled arterial hemorrhage, and packing alone may not be successful. An alternative strategy is to pack the liver to control venous hemorrhage, close the abdomen, and transport the patient to the angiographic suite for hepatic arteriography and embolization of the bleeding vessel. Ruptured hematomas of grades III and IV require exploration and selective ligation, with or without packing.

Adjuncts in the Treatment of Hepatic Injuries

Drains

For years, all hepatic injuries were drained with Penrose drains brought out laterally or through the bed of the resected 12th rib. More recently, large sump drains and closed suction drains have become popular. The results of several prospective and retrospective studies indicate that the use of Penrose or sump drains is associated with a greater risk of intraabdominal sepsis than is the use of closed suction drains or no drains.[95-98] What is not clear, however, is whether closed suction drains are better or worse than no drains. Experienced trauma surgeons do not agree on the need for drainage, except that it is not necessary for lacerations of grades I, II, and perhaps III. When drains are used, closed suction devices are preferred. A patient who is treated initially with perihepatic packing may require drainage. However, drainage is not indicated at the initial procedure because the patient will be returned to the operating room within 48 hours.

Omental Packing

Another adjunctive treatment involves using the omentum to fill large defects in the liver and to buttress hepatic sutures. The rationale for this approach is that it provides an excellent source for macrophages and fills a potential dead space with viable tissue[99] (Fig. 22-18). The omentum also can provide additional support for parenchymal sutures.

RESULTS

The mortality rate of patients with hepatic injuries is about 10%. The most common cause of death is exsanguination, followed by multiple organ failure and intracranial injury. Other associated injuries are responsible for most of the remaining deaths. Table 22-2 lists mortality and morbidity rates from several large series. A

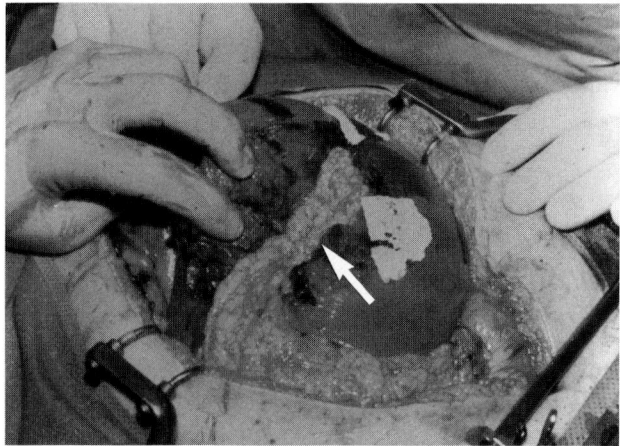

Figure 22-18 Use of a viable omental pedicle to fill a large defect in the liver (*arrow*).

Table 22-2   Results of Treatment of Hepatic Injury in Recent Large Series*

Author	Date	No. of Patients	Mortality Rate	Perihepatic Infections	Hemorrhage	Fistulas	Hemobilia
Pachter[55]	1992	411	7.3	2.8	0.4	2.2	—
Fabian[98]	1991	482	5.6	7.1	—	—	1.5
Feliciano[49]	1986	1000	10.5	3.2	2.5	—	—
Levin[74]	1978	546	10.1	4.6	3.8	1.8	—
TOTAL		2439	8.9	4.2	2.4	2.0	1.5

* All numbers, excluding the number of patients, are percentages. A dash indicates that data were not given.

few generalizations can be made regarding the risk of death and complications with hepatic injuries: (1) both increase proportional to the grade of injury and the complexity of repair; (2) the mortality rate of hepatic injuries is higher with blunt trauma than with penetrating trauma; and (3) infectious complications occur more often with penetrating trauma.

Management of Complications

Postoperative Hemorrhage

Postoperative hemorrhage can be expected in many patients treated with perihepatic packing and abbreviated laparotomy. The cause can be either persistent coagulopathy or a missed vascular injury, usually arterial in nature. In most instances in which postoperative hemorrhage is suspected, patients are best served by reoperation. Arteriography with embolization can be considered in selected cases. If a coagulopathy is the likely cause of postoperative hemorrhage, there is little to be gained by reoperation until the coagulopathy is corrected. An exception is the development of an abdominal compartment syndrome, which must be decompressed in the operating room regardless of the patient's coagulation status.

Perihepatic Infection

Infections within and around the liver occur in about 3% of patients with hepatic injuries. Perihepatic infections develop more often with penetrating trauma than with blunt trauma, presumably because of the greater frequency of enteric contamination in the former. Persistent elevation of the temperature and white blood cell count after the third or fourth postoperative day should prompt a search for intraabdominal infection. In the absence of pneumonia, line sepsis, or urinary tract infection, an abdominal CT scan with intravenous and upper gastrointestinal contrast should be obtained. Many perihepatic infections can be treated with CT-guided drainage. However, infected hematomas and infected necrotic liver cannot be expected to respond to percutaneous drainage. Right 12th rib resection remains an excellent approach for posterior infections and provides superior drainage.

Bilomas, Biliary Ascites, and Biliary Fistulas

Bilomas are loculate collections of bile that can be infected. Infected bilomas are essentially abscesses and should be treated as such. Sterile bilomas eventually will be resorbed. Biliary ascites is caused by disruption of a major bile duct. Reoperation with the establishment of appropriate drainage is the prudent course. Even if the source of bile leakage can be identified, primary repair of the injured duct is unlikely to be successful. It is best to delay definitive repair until a fistulous communication is established with adequate drainage.

Biliary fistulas occur in about 3% of patients with hepatic injuries.[90] They usually are of little consequence and close without specific treatment. Rarely, in patients with associated diaphragmatic injuries, communications develop with intrathoracic structures and result in bronchobiliary or pleurobiliary fistulas. Because of the pressure differential between the biliary tract and the thoracic cavity, most of these fistulas require operative closure.

Hemobilia and Arterial–Portal Venous Fistulas

Hemorrhage from hepatic injuries often is treated without identifying and controlling each individual bleeding vessel. As a result, arterial pseudoaneurysms can develop. As these pseudoaneurysms enlarge, they eventually rupture into the parenchyma of the liver, a bile duct, or an adjacent portal venous branch. Rupture into a bile duct results in hemobilia, which is characterized by intermittent episodes of right upper quadrant pain, upper gastrointestinal hemorrhage, and jaundice.

If the aneurysms rupture into a portal vein, portal hypertension with bleeding varices can develop. These complications are rare and should be treated with hepatic arteriography and embolization.

REFERENCES

1. Feliciano DV, Pachter HL, eds. Heptatic trauma revisited. Curr Probl Surg 1989;26.
2. American College of Surgeons Committee on Trauma. Advanced trauma life support manual. Chicago, American College of Surgeons, 1993.
3. Mattox KL, Bickell W, Pepe PE, Burch J, Feliciano D. Prospective MAST study in 911 patients. J Trauma 1989;29: 1104.
4. Martin RR, Bickell WH, Pepe PE, Burch JM, Mattox KL. Prospective evaluation of preoperative fluid resuscitation in hypotensive patients with penetrating truncal injury: a preliminary report. J Trauma 1992;33:354.
5. Vassar MJ, Perry CA, Holcroft JW. Prehospital resuscitation of hypotensive trauma patients with 7.5% NaCl versus 7.5% NaCl with added dextran: a controlled trial. J Trauma 1993;34:622.
6. Cayten CG, Berendt BM, Dyrne DW, Murphy JG, Moy FH. A study of pneumatic antishock garments in severely hypotensive trauma patients. J Trauma 1993;34:728.
7. Feliciano DV, Wall MJ. Patterns of injury. In: Moore EE, Mattox KL, Feliciano DV, eds. Trauma, ed 2. Norwalk, CT, Appleton & Lange, 1991;81.
8. Lowe RJ, Saletta JD, Read DR, et al. Should laparotomy be mandatory or selective in gunshot wounds of the abdomen? J Trauma 1977;17:903.
9. Moore EE, Moore JB, VanDuzer-Moore S, et al. Mandatory laparotomy for gunshot wounds penetrating the abdomen. Am J Surg 1980;140:847.
10. Olsen WR, Hildreth DH. Abdominal paracentesis and peritoneal lavage in blunt abdominal trauma. J Trauma 1971;11:824.
11. Pacey J, Forward AD, Preto AF. Peritoneal tap and lavage in patients with blunt abdominal trauma: their contribution to surgical decisions. CMA Journal 1971;105:365.
12. Parvin S, Smith DE, Asher M, Virgilio RW. Effectiveness of peritoneal lavage in blunt abdominal trauma. Ann Surg 1975;181:255.
13. Bivins BA, Jona JZ, Belin RP. Diagnostic peritoneal lavage in pediatric trauma. J Trauma 1976;16:739.
14. Root HD, Hauser CW, McKinley CR, LaFave JW, Mendiola RP. Diagnostic peritoneal lavage. Surgery 1965;57: 633.
15. Fisher RP, Beverlin BC, Engrav LH, Benjamin CI, Perry JF. Diagnostic peritoneal lavage. Am J Surg 1978;136: 701.
16. Feliciano DV, Bitondo CG, Steed G, Mattox KL, Burch JM, Jordan GL. Five hundred open taps or lavages in patients with abdominal stab wounds. Am J Surg 1984;148:772.
17. McAnena OJ, Marx JA, Moore EE. Peritoneal lavage enzyme determinations after blunt and penetrating abdominal trauma. J Trauma 1991;31:1161.
18. D'Amelio LF, Rhodes M. A reassessment of the peritoneal lavage leukocyte count in blunt abdominal trauma. J Trauma 1990;30:1291.
19. Soyka JM, Martin M, Sloan EP, Himmelman RG, Batesky D, Barrett JA. Diagnostic peritoneal lavage: is an isolated WBC count $\geq$ 500/mm^3 predictive of intraabdominal injury requiring celiotomy in blunt trauma patients? J Trauma 1990;30:874.
20. Federele MP, Crass RA, Jeffrey BB Jr, et al. Computed tomography in blunt abdominal trauma. Arch Surg 1982;117:645.
21. Meyer AA, Crass RA, Lim RC, Jeffrey RB, Federle MP, Trunkey DD. Selective nonoperative management of blunt liver injury using computed tomography. Arch Surg 1985;120:550.
22. Trunkey D, Federle MP. Computed tomography in perspective. (Editorial) J Trauma 1986;26:660.
23. Meyer DM, Thal ER, Weigelt JA, Redman HC. Evaluation of computed tomography and diagnostic peritoneal lavage in blunt abdominal trauma. J Trauma 1989;29: 1168.
24. Davis JW, Hoyt DB, Mackersie RC, McArdle MS. Complications in evaluating abdominal trauma: diagnostic peritoneal lavage versus computerized axial tomography. J Trauma 1990;30:1506.
25. Marx JA, Moore EE, Jorden RC, Eule J. Limitations of computed tomography in the evaluation of acute abdominal trauma: a prospective comparison with diagnostic peritoneal lavage. J Trauma 1985;25:933.
26. Croce MA, Fabian TC, Kudsk KA, et al. AAST Organ Injury Scale: correlation of CT-graded liver injuries and operative findings. J Trauma 1991;31:806.
27. Peitzman AB, Makaroun MS, Slaksy BS, Ritter P. Prospective study of computed tomography in initial management of blunt abdominal trauma. J Trauma 1986;26: 585.
28. Fabian TC, Mangiante EC, White TJ, Patterson CR, Boldreghini S, Britt LG. A prospective study of 91 patients undergoing both computed tomography and peritoneal lavage after blunt abdominal trauma. J Trauma 1986;26: 602.
29. Sorkey AJ, Farell MB, Williams HJ Jr, Mucha P, Ilstrup DM. The complementary roles of diagnostic peritoneal lavage and computed tomography in the evaluation of blunt abdominal trauma. Surgery 1989;106:794.
30. Gruessner R, Mentges B, Duber C, Ruckert K, Rothmund M. Sonography versus peritoneal lavage in blunt abdominal trauma. J Trauma 1989;29:242.
31. Rozycki GS, Ochsner MG, Jaffin JH, Champion HR. Prospective evaluation of surgeons' use of ultrasound in the evaluation of trauma patients. J Trauma 1993;34:516.
32. Berci G, Dunkelman D, Michel SL, Sanders G, Wahistrom E, Morgenstern L. Emergency minilaparoscopy in abdominal trauma. Am J Surg 1983;146:261.
33. Ivatury RR, Simon RJ, Weksler B, Bayard V, Stahl WM.

Laparoscopy in the evaluation of the intrathoracic abdomen after penetrating injury. J Trauma 1992;33:101.

34. Townsend MC, Flancbaum L, Shoban PS, Cloutier CT. Diagnostic laparoscopy as an adjunct to selective conservative management of solid organ injuries after blunt abdominal trauma. J Trauma 1993;35:647.

35. Federico JA, Horner WR, Clark DE, Isler RJ. Blunt hepatic trauma: nonoperative management in adults. Arch Surg 1990;125:905.

36. Hiatt JR, Harrier HD, Koenig BV, Ransom KJ. Nonoperative management of major blunt liver injury with hemoperitoneum. Arch Surg 1990;125:101.

37. Knudson MM, Lim RC Jr, Oakes DD, Jeffrey RB. Nonoperative management of blunt liver injuries in adults: the need for continued surveillance. J Trauma 1990;30:1494.

38. Burham RM, Buckley J, Keegan M, Fravel S, Shapiro MJ, Mazuski J. Management of blunt hepatic injuries. Am J Surg 1992;164:477.

39. Bynoe RP, Bell RM, Miles WS, Close TP, Ross MA, Fine JG. Complications of nonoperative management of blunt hepatic injuries. J Trauma 1992;32:308.

40. Schiffman MA. Nonoperative management of blunt abdominal trauma in pediatrics. Emerg Med Clin North Am 1989;7:519.

41. Abrams JH, Cerra F, Holcroft JW. Cardiopulmonary monitoring. In: Wilmore DW, Brennan MF, Harken AH, Holcroft JW, Meakins JL, eds. Care of the surgical patient, vol 2. New York, Scientific American, 1994:1

42. Shoemaker WC, Bland RD, Appel PL. Therapy of critically ill postoperative patients based on outcome prediction and prospective clinical trials. Surg Clin North Am 1985;65:811.

43. Luna GK, Maier RV, Pavlin EG, et al. Incidence and effect of hypothermia in seriously injured patients. J Trauma 1987;27:1014.

44. Jurkovich GJ, Greiser WB, Luterman A, Curreri PW. Hypothermia in trauma victims: an ominous predictor of survival. J Trauma 1987;27:1019.

45. Gregory JS, Flancbaum L, Townsend MC, et al. Incidence and timing of hypothermia in trauma patients undergoing operations. J Trauma 1991;31:795.

46. Holinshead WH. Anatomy for surgeons, ed 2, vol 2. New York, Harper & Row, 1971:314.

47. Moore EE, Shackford SR, Pachter HL, et al. Organ injury scaling: spleen, liver, and kidney. J Trauma 1989;29:1664.

48. Moore EE. Critical decisions in the management of hepatic trauma. Am J Surg 1984;148:712.

49. Feliciano DV, Mattox KL, Jordan GL, Burch JM, Bitondo CG, Cruse PA. Management of 1000 consecutive cases of hepatic trauma (1979-1984). Ann Surg 1986;204:438.

50. Feliciano DV, Mattox KL, Burch JM, Bitondo CG, Jordan GL. Packing for control of hepatic hemorrhage. J Trauma 1986;26:738.

51. Ivatury RR, Nallathambi M, Gunduz Y, Constable R, Rohman M, Stahl WM. Liver packing for uncontrolled hemorrhage: a reappraisal. J Trauma 1986;26:744.

52. Carmona RH, Peck DZ, Lim RC. The role of packing and planned reoperation in severe hepatic trauma. J Trauma 1984;24:779.

53. Cue JI, Cryer HG, Miller FB, Richardson JD, Polk HC. Packing and planned reexploration for hepatic and retroperitoneal hemorrhage: critical refinements of a useful technique. J Trauma 1990;30:1007.

54. Beal SL. Fatal hepatic hemorrhage: an unresolved problem in the management of complex liver injuries. J Trauma 1990;30:163.

55. Pachter HL, Spencer FC, Hofstetter SR, et al. Significant trends in the treatment of hepatic trauma: experience with 411 injuries. Ann Surg 1992;215:492.

56. Heaney JP, Stanton WR, Halbert DS, et al. An improved technic for vascular isolation of the liver. Ann Surg 1966;163:237.

57. Burch JB, Feliciano DV, Mattox KL. The atriocaval shunt: facts and fiction. Ann Surg 1988;207:555.

58. Schrock T, Blaisdell TW, Matthewson C. Management of blunt trauma to the liver and hepatic veins. Arch Surg 1968;96:698.

59. Bricker DL, Morton JR, Okies JE, et al. Surgical management of injuries to the vena cava: changing patterns of injury and newer techniques of repair. J Trauma 1971;11:725.

60. Yellin AE, Chaffee CB, Donovan AJ. Vascular isolation in treatment of juxtahepatic venous injuries. Arch Surg 1971;102:566.

61. Walt AJ. The mythology of hepatic trauma: or Babel revisited. Am J Surg 1978;125:12.

62. Millikan JS, Moore EE, Cogbill TH, et al. Inferior vena cava injuries: a continuing challenge. J Trauma 1983;23:207.

63. Pachter HL, Spencer FC, Hofstetter SR, et al. The management of juxtahepatic venous injuries without an atriocaval shunt. Surgery 1986;99:569.

64. Rovito PF. Atrial caval shunting in blunt hepatic vascular injury. Ann Surg 1987;205:318.

65. Pilcher DB, Harman PK, Moore EE. Retrohepatic vena cava balloon shunt introduced via the sapheno-femoral junction. J Trauma 1977;17:837.

66. Buechter KJ, Gomez GA, Zeppa R. A new technique for exposure of injuries at the confluence of the retrohepatic veins and the retrohepatic vena cava. J Trauma 1990;30:328.

67. Murray DH Jr, Borge JD, Pouteau GG. Tourniquet control of liver bleeding. J Trauma 1978;18:771.

68. Kram HB, Reuben BI, Fleming AW. Use of fibrin glue in hepatic trauma. J Trauma 1988;28:1195.

69. Kram HB, Nathan RC, Stafford FJ, et al. Fibrin glue achieves hemostasis in patients with coagulation disorders. Arch Surg 1989;124:385.

70. Berguer R, Staerkel RL, Moore EE, et al. Warning: fatal reaction to the use of fibrin glue in deep hepatic wounds: case reports. J Trauma 1991;31:408.

71. Ochsner MG, Maniscalco-Theberge ME, Champion HR. Fibrin glue as a hemostatic agent in hepatic and splenic trauma. J Trauma 1990;30:884.

72. Feliciano DV. Continuing evolution in the approach to severe liver trauma. (Editorial) Ann Surg 1992;216:521.

73. Trunkey DD, Shires GT, McClelland R. Management of liver trauma in 811 consecutive patients. Ann Surg 1974;179:722.

74. Levin A, Gover P, Nance FC. Surgical restraint in the management of hepatic injury: a review of Charity Hospital experience. J Trauma 1978;18:399.

75. Lucas CE, Ledgerwood AM. Prospective evaluation of hemostatic techniques for liver injuries. J Trauma 1976;16:442.

76. Camona RH, Lim RC Jr, Clark GC. Morbidity and mortality in hepatic trauma: a 5 year study. Am J Surg 1982;144:88.

77. Moore FA, Moore EE, Seagraves A. Nonresectional management of major hepatic trauma: an evolving concept. Am J Surg 1985;150:725.

78. Mays ET. Lobar dearterialization for exsanguinating wounds of the liver. J Trauma 1972;12:397.

79. Flint LM, Polk HC. Selective hepatic artery ligation: limitations and failures. J Trauma 1979;19:319.

80. Lucas CE. Discussion of: Flint LM, Polk HC. Selective hepatic artery ligation: limitations and failures. J Trauma 1979;19:319.

81. Poggetti RS, Moore EE, Moore FA, Mitchel MB, Read RA. Balloon tamponade for bilobar transfixing hepatic gunshot wounds. J Trauma 1992;33:694.

82. Thomas SV, Dulchavsky SA, Diebel LN. Balloon tamponade for liver injuries: case report. J Trauma 1993;34:448.

83. Madding GF, Lawrence KB, Kennedy PA. War wounds of the liver. Tex State J Med 1946;42:267.

84. Burch JM, Ortiz VB, Richardson RJ, Martin RR, Mattox KL, Jordan GL. Abbreviated laparotomy and planned reoperation for critically injured patients. Ann Surg 1992;215:476.

85. Morris JA Jr, Eddy VA, Binman TA, Rutherford EJ, Sharp KW. The staged celiotomy for trauma. Ann Surg 1993;217:576.

86. Reed RL, Merrell RC, Meyers WC, Fischer RP. Continuing evolution in the approach to severe liver trauma. Ann Surg 1992;216:524.

87. Jacobson LE, Kirton OC, Gomez GA. The use of an absorbable mesh wrap in the management of major liver injuries. Surgery 1992;111:455.

88. Lim RC Jr, Knudson J, Steele M. Liver trauma: current method of management. Arch Surg 1972;104:544.

89. Donovan AJ, Michaelian MJ, Yellin AE. Anatomical hepatic lobectomy in trauma to the liver. Surgery 1973;73:833.

90. Defore WW, Mattox KL, Jordan GL, et al. Management of 1590 consecutive cases of liver trauma. Arch Surg 1976;111:493.

91. Esquivel CO, Bernardos A, Makowka L, Iwatsuki S, Gordon RD, Starzl TE. Liver replacement after massive hepatic trauma. J Trauma 1987;27:800.

92. Angstadt J, Jarrell B, Moritz M, et al. Surgical management of severe liver trauma: a role for liver transplantation. J Trauma 1989;29:606.

93. Ringe B, Pichlmayr R, Ziegler H, et al. Management of severe hepatic trauma by two-stage total hepatectomy and subsequent liver transplantation. Surgery 1991;109:792.

94. Jeng LB, Hsu C, Wang C, et al. Emergent liver transplantation to salvage a hepatic avulsion injury with a disrupted suprahepatic vena cava. Arch Surg 1993;128:1075.

95. Fischer RP, O'Farrell KA, Perry JF Jr. The value of peritoneal drains in the treatment of liver injuries. J Trauma 1978;18:393.

96. Gillmore D, McSwain NE, Browder IW. Hepatic trauma: to drain or not to drain? J Trauma 1987;27:898.

97. Noyes LD, Doyle DJ, McSwain NE. Septic complications associated with the use of peritoneal drains in liver trauma. J Trauma 1988;28:337.

98. Fabian TC, Croce MA, Stanford GG, et al. Factors affecting morbidity after hepatic trauma. Ann Surg 1991;213:540.

99. Stone HH, Lamb JM. Use of pedicled omentum as an autogenous pack for control of hemorrhage in major injuries of the liver. Surg Gynecol Obstet 1975;141:92.

Digestive Tract Surgery: A Text and Atlas, edited by Richard H. Bell, Layton F. Rikkers, and Michael W. Mulholland. Lippincott-Raven Publishers, Philadelphia, © 1996.

23

Atlas of Liver Surgery

J. Michael Henderson | *Layton F. Rikkers*

PREOPERATIVE PREPARATION

General factors of preoperative preparation for all procedures in this atlas of liver surgery relate to preparing the patient for a major operation. Cardiac, pulmonary, and renal function must be evaluated and deemed adequate for the extent of procedure planned. This may require appropriate consultation and specialty evaluation. Nutritional status is an important factor in outcome and, although it may not be correctable before surgery, must not be forgotten in the perioperative period. Transfusion of blood and blood products is required for many of these procedures, mandating planning for preoperative preparation or perioperative management. Perioperative and, in the case of liver transplantation, postoperative antibiotics should be given.

Specific factors in preoperative preparation for the different groups of operations are dictated primarily by the status of the liver. Liver resections are done predominantly when the uninvolved part of the liver is normal. Portal hypertension procedures are usually performed on patients with cirrhosis. Liver transplantation is performed for end-stage liver disease. The preoperative status of the liver, or the extent of liver resected, dictates the need for correction of coagulation deficits, determines the details of fluid and electrolyte management, and influences the ability to manage malnutrition.

SECTION I *Surgical Anatomy*

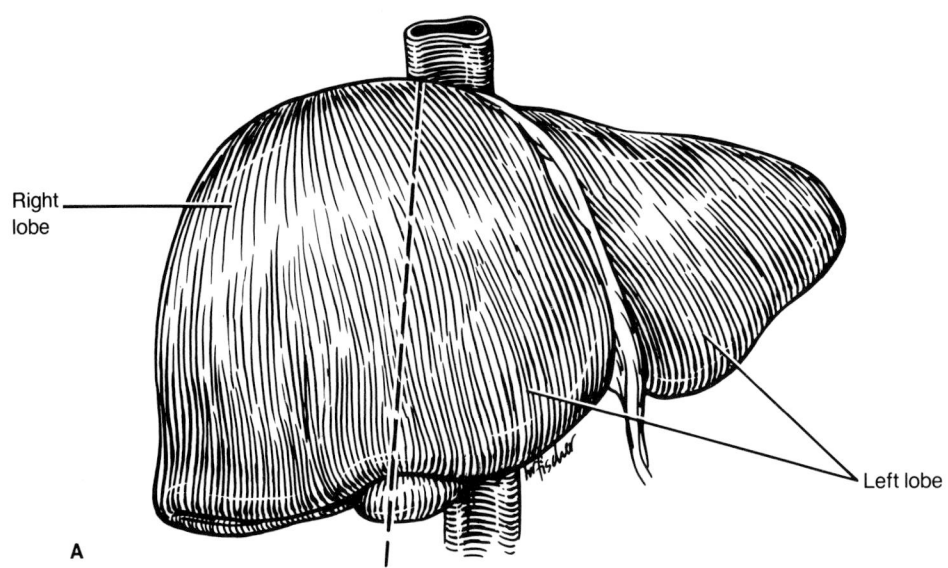

Figure 23-I-1

Anterior and Posterior Surfaces of the Liver

(**A**) The liver sits in the right upper quadrant of the abdomen, protected by the right rib cage, and directly adjacent to the right diaphragm. The left lobe extends across beneath the tendinous portion of the diaphragm toward the spleen in the left upper quadrant.

When viewed from the front, the smooth surfaces of the large right lobe and the wedge projection of the left lobe are clearly visible. The true division of the liver into the right and left lobes is through an imaginary plane from the gallbladder fossa to the suprahepatic inferior vena cava.

(Continued)

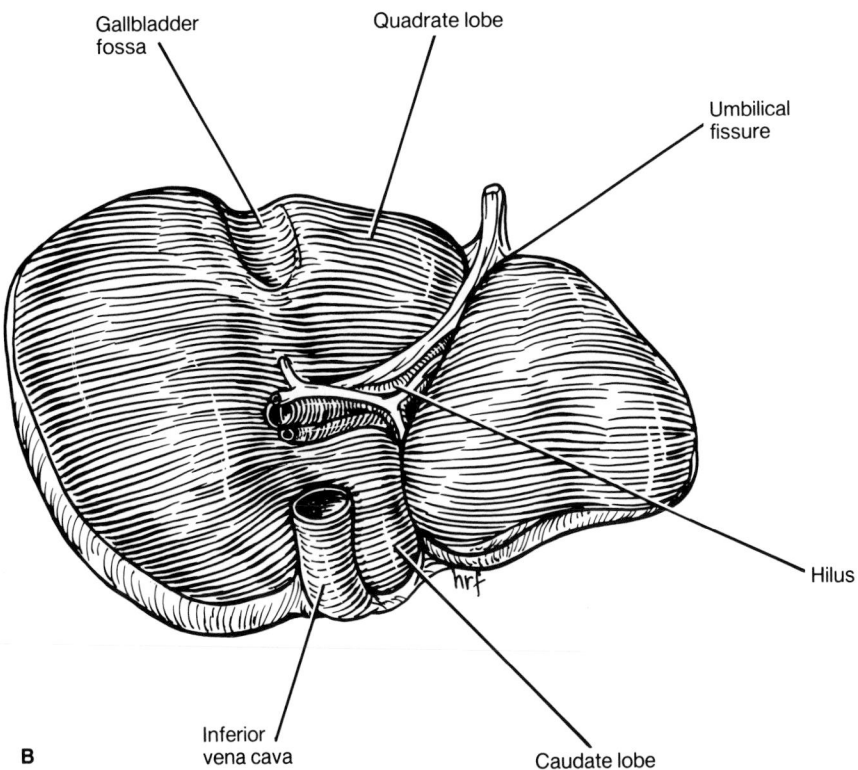

Gallbladder fossa

Quadrate lobe

Umbilical fissure

Hilus

Inferior vena cava

Caudate lobe

B

Figure 23-I-1 *(Continued)*

(B) The posterior surface of the liver. In the explanted liver, as illustrated here, the relations are more complex. Again, the true right and left lobes are delineated by a plane from the gallbladder fossa to the inferior vena cava. The intrahepatic portion of the inferior vena cava has an intimate relation to the caudate lobe. The true left lobe of the liver incorporates not only that segment lateral to the falciform ligament but also the quadrate lobe. The posterior surface of the right lobe of the liver may bear an impression of the right kidney in its inferior portion, while the superior portion is partially delineated by the bare surface of the liver, with the right triangular ligament forming its attachment to the right diaphragm.

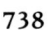

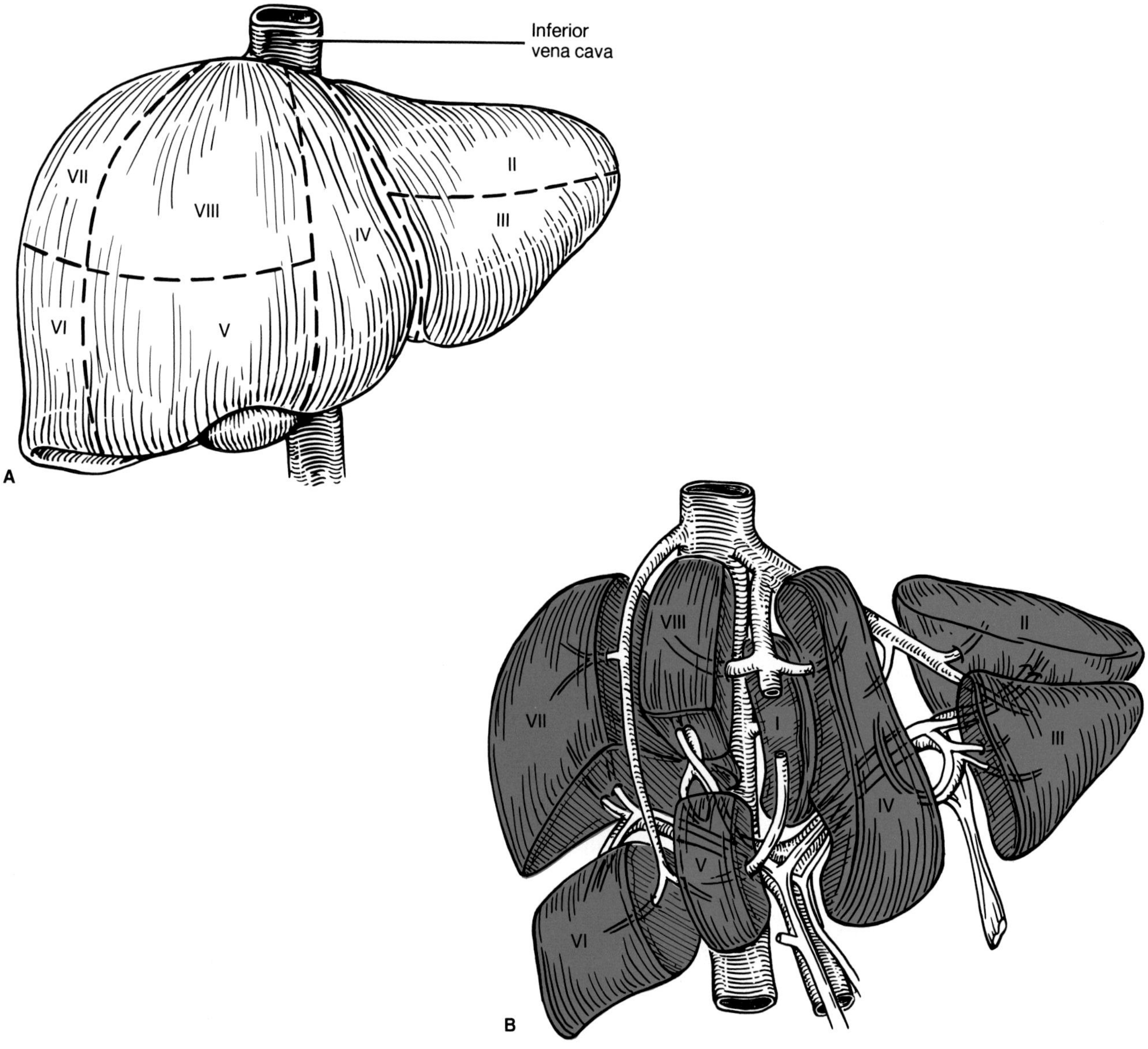

Inferior
vena cava

A

B

Figure 23-I-2

Functional Segments

(**A**) The liver is divided into eight functional segments. Viewed from the anterior surface, segments II through VIII follow a clockwise numbering system from the upper segment of the anatomic left lobe sequentially through to segment VIII on the dome of the right lobe.

(**B**) This exploded illustration of the functional segments of the liver illustrates the vascular inflow and hepatic venous outflow basis for this subdivision. The major hepatic veins lie in the intersegmental planes.

The caudate lobe (segment I) lies posteriorly. The anatomic left lobe consists of segments II, III, and IV: segment IV often is divided into IVa and IVb to represent the inferior and superior halves of this segment. Segments V, VI, VII, and VIII represent the four quadrants of the anatomic right lobe of the liver.

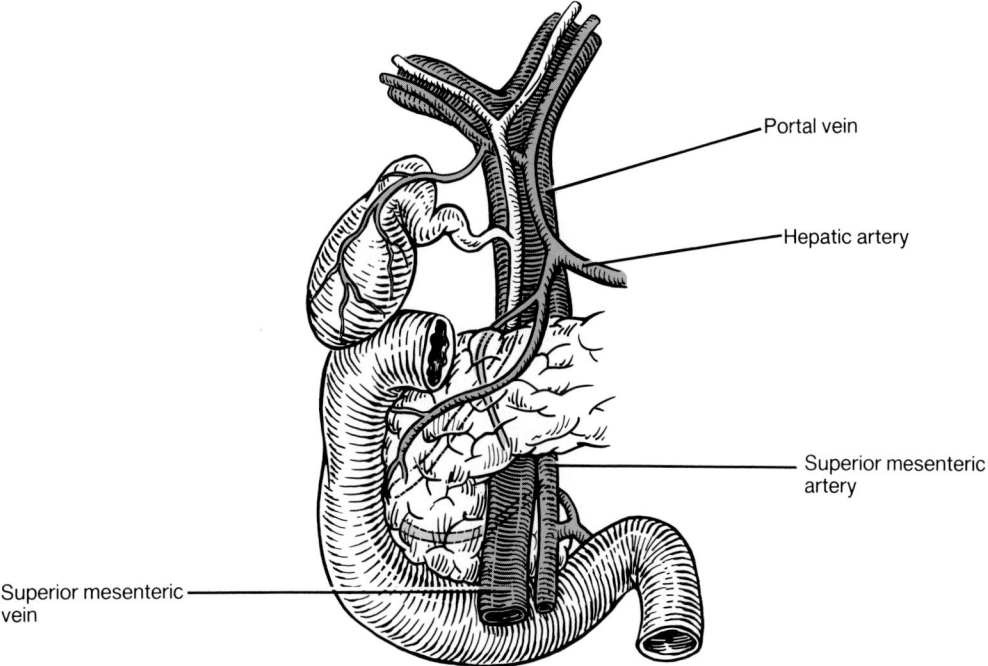

Figure 23-I-3

Normal Relations of Hepatic Artery, Portal Vein, and Bile Duct

The portal vein is formed by the confluence of the superior mesenteric and splenic veins behind the neck of the pancreas. It is the most posterior structure of the hepatoduodenal ligament. It has few tributaries, with the only significant one being the left gastric vein on its left border, usually just above the entrance of the splenic vein. The left gastric vein may also be a tributary of the splenic vein rather than the portal vein.

The common hepatic artery arises from the celiac axis, passes along the superior border of the pancreas, often under the cover of a large lymph node, and then up into the free border of the lesser omentum. The gastroduodenal artery arises from the common hepatic artery. The bifurcation of the hepatic artery proper into its right and left branches is variable, as is the passage of the right hepatic artery in front of or behind the common bile duct.

The common bile duct is anterior and to the right in the free edge of the lesser omentum. It is formed by the union of the right and left hepatic ducts and passes down to the superior border of the pancreas, where it becomes embedded in its posterior surface in its course to the ampulla of Vater. The gallbladder drains into the common bile duct through the cystic duct, which has a variable course.

The cystic artery most commonly arises from the hepatic artery proper or the right hepatic artery to supply the gallbladder.

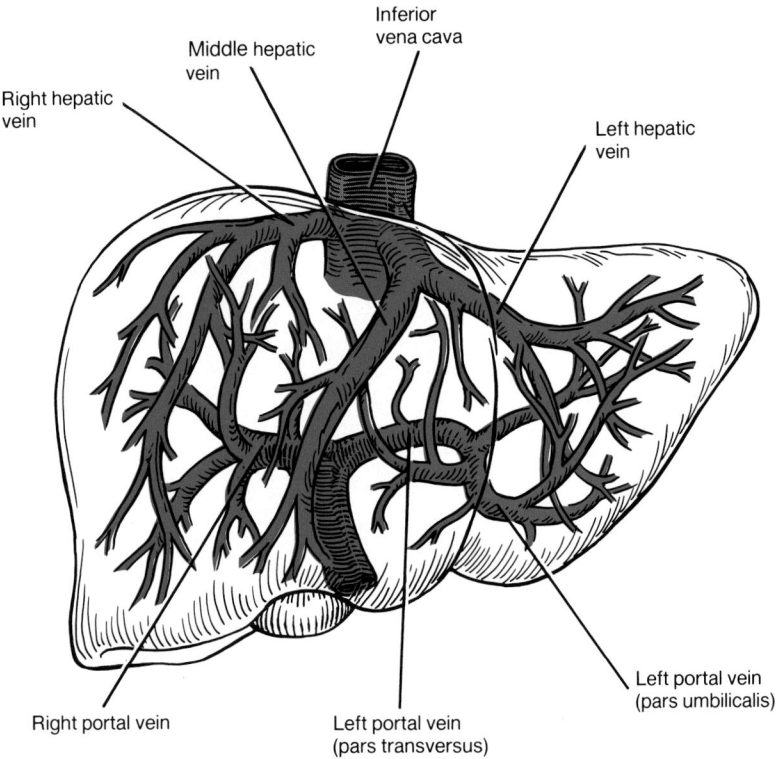

Figure 23-I-4

Venous Anatomy

The portal vein bifurcates into its right and left branches extrahepatically at the hilus. The further main subdivisions of these two branches are the segmental vessels to segments I through VIII. The right portal vein divides early into anterior and posterior divisions. The left vein has a longer course behind the hilar plate of the quadrate lobe (segment IV; see Fig. 23-I-7) but follows the same basic subdivisions to supply segments.

The three major hepatic veins are the right, middle, and left hepatic veins. The middle hepatic vein is a landmark between the right and left anatomic lobes of the liver. The major tributaries to each of the hepatic veins drain the previously described liver segments. The entry of the three main hepatic veins into the suprahepatic vena cava can be identified extrahepatically when the diaphragmatic attachments of the liver are fully dissected down to the suprahepatic inferior vena cava. The left hepatic vein usually joins the middle hepatic vein before the latter's junction with the inferior vena cava.

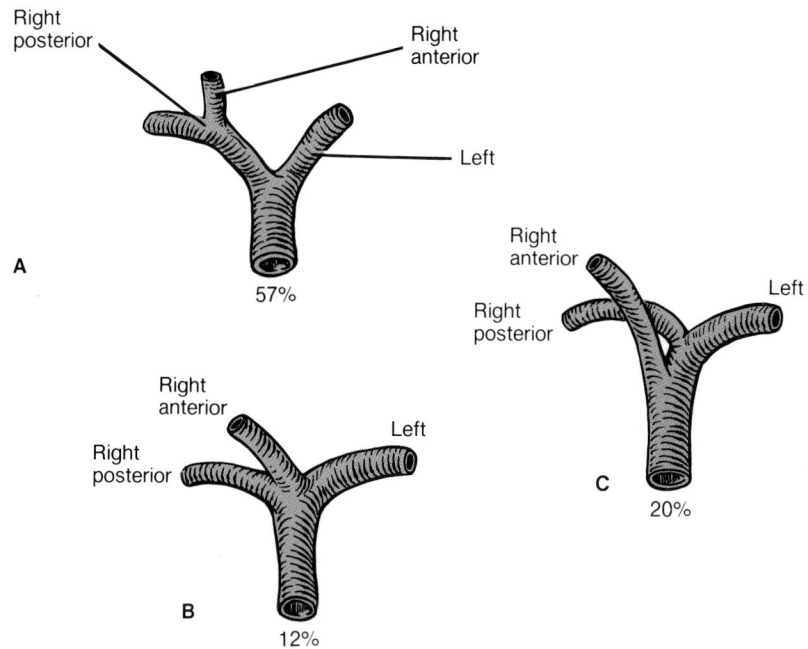

Figure 23-I-5

Anatomy of the Biliary Bifurcation

(**A**) The most common union of the right and left hepatic ducts. The left hepatic duct has a long extraparenchymal course behind the quadrate lobe (segment IV). The right bile duct has a short intraparenchymal course after union of the right anterior and right posterior ducts. Two common variations follow.

(**B**) A trifurcation occurs, as shown in about 12% of the population. In this variation, the right anterior, right posterior, and left hepatic ducts unite at the liver hilus to form the common hepatic duct.

(**C**) In another variation, the right posterior duct drains into the left hepatic duct before the union of the right anterior duct and the left hepatic duct to form the common hepatic duct.

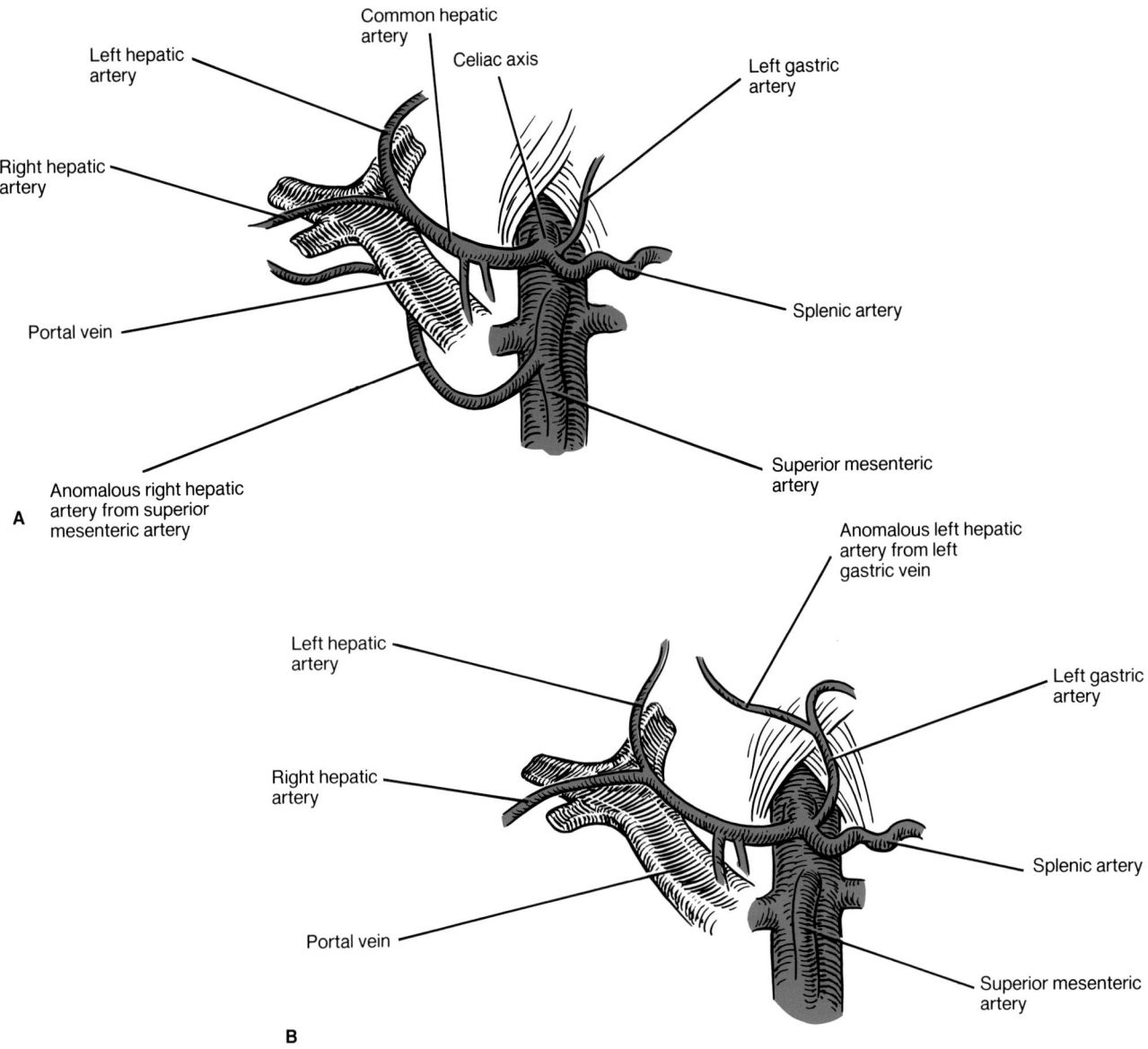

Figure 23-I-6

Abnormal Arterial Anatomy

(**A**) Anomalous right hepatic artery. In about 20% of the population, a right hepatic artery arises from the superior mesenteric artery. This runs beneath the pancreas, then posterior to the bile duct, and on the right side of the portal vein as it passes to the hepatic hilus. This may be a totally replaced right hepatic artery, in which case there is no main branch of the common hepatic artery passing to the right lobe of the liver. Alternatively, it may be an accessory right hepatic artery, in which case there is a significant branch of the hepatic artery proper to the right lobe of the liver.

(**B**) Anomalous left hepatic artery. A replaced, or accessory, left hepatic artery may arise from the left gastric artery. This occurs in about 20% of the population. This arises from the left gastric artery as it reaches the lesser curve of the stomach close to the gastroesophageal junction. It then runs in the gastrohepatic ligament from the gastroesophageal junction to the hepatic hilus.

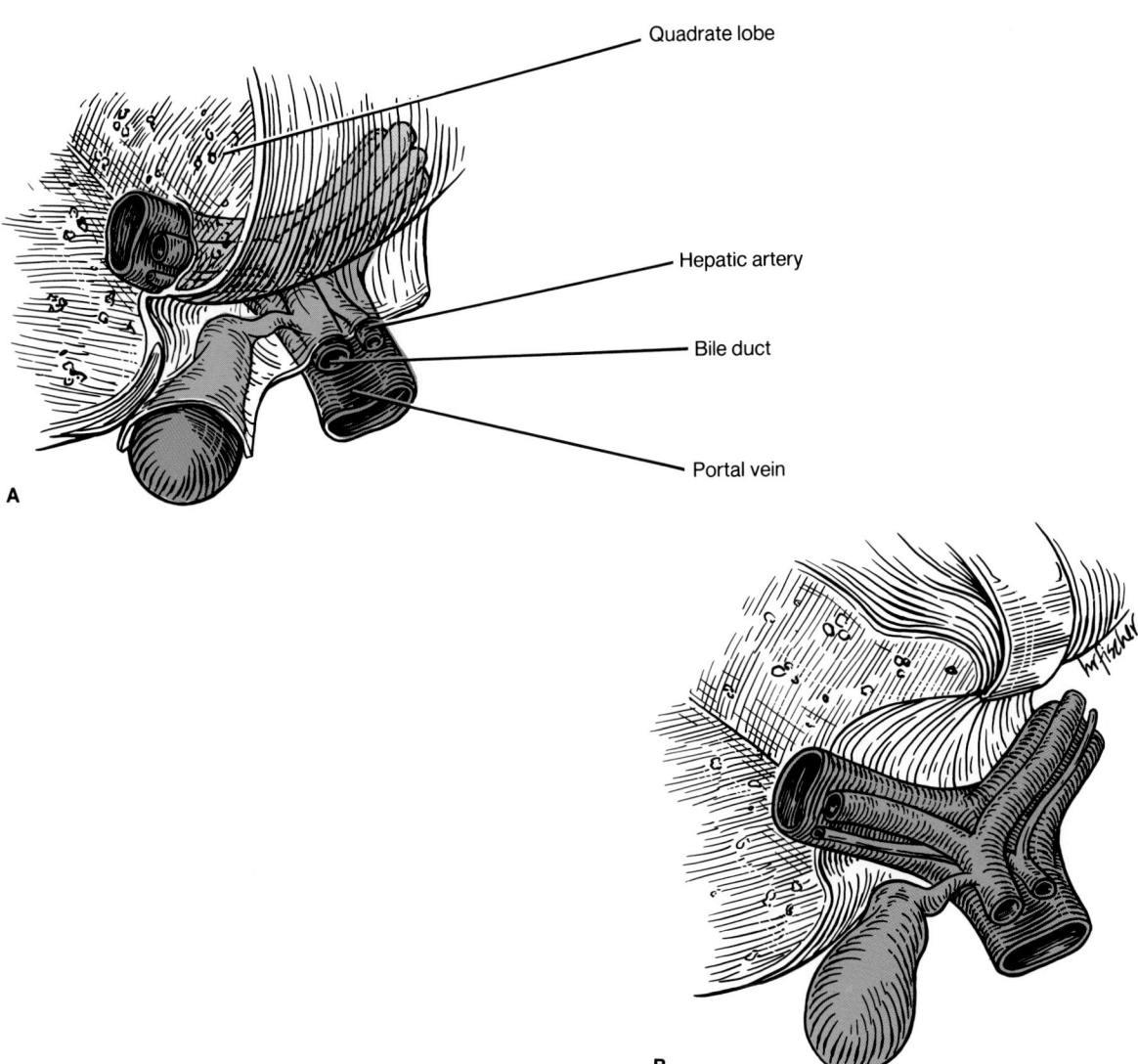

Figure 23-I-7

Hilar Plate

(**A**) The hepatic hilus and the extrahepatic portions of the left hepatic artery, left hepatic duct, and left portal vein are obscured beneath the quadrate lobe (segment IV) of the liver. As illustrated in this figure, the fusion of the liver capsule as it comes together in the hilus contributes to this anatomy.

(**B**) Elevation of the hilar plate. Division of the capsule along the posterior surface of the inferior portion of the quadrate lobe allows elevation of the quadrate lobe and improves exposure of hilar structures.

SECTION II   Liver Resections

A. Major Hepatic Resections

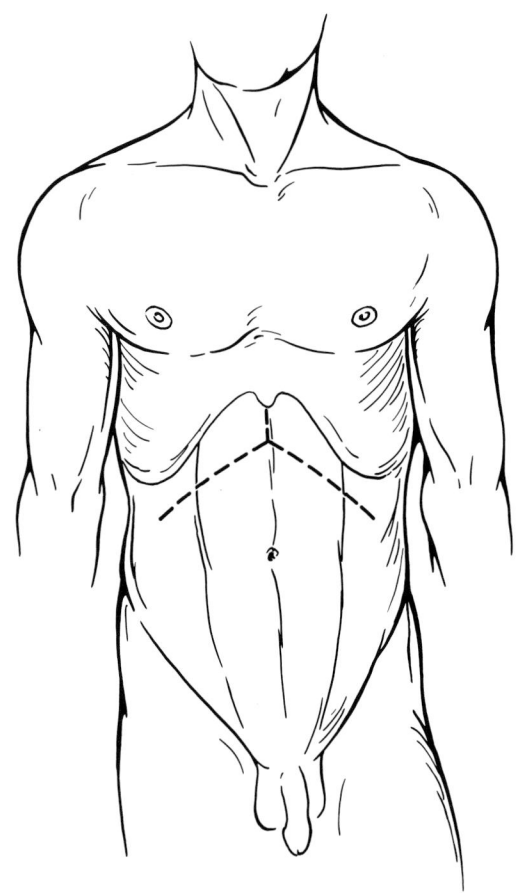

Figure 23-IIA-1

A bilateral subcostal incision, with an upper midline extension, allows access to mobilize fully the whole liver.

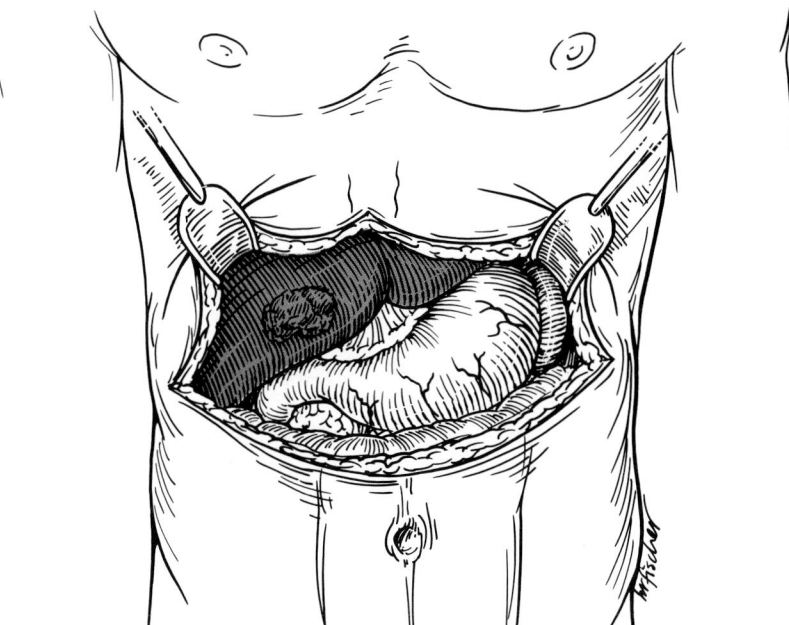

Figure 23-IIA-2

Retraction of Costal Margins

Access for major liver resection is achieved by upward retraction of the costal margins with a "fixed" retractor system. This permits full mobilization of the left and right lobes without having to perform a thoracotomy.

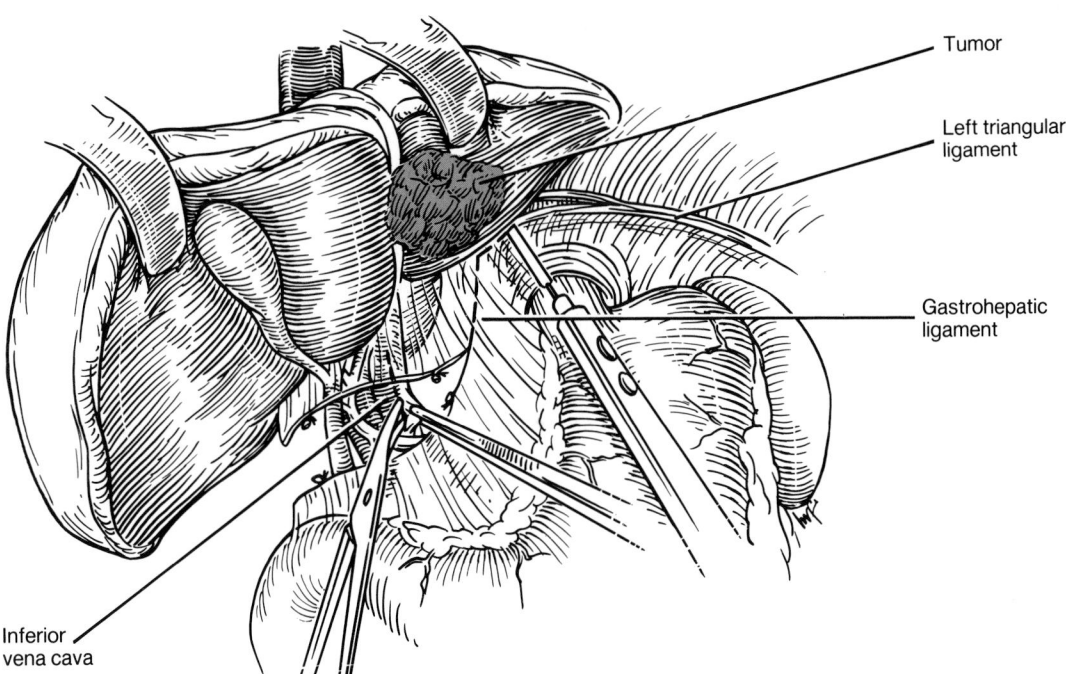

Tumor

Left triangular
ligament

Gastrohepatic
ligament

Inferior
vena cava

Figure 23-IIA-3

Mobilization of Left Lobe

This is achieved by taking down the left triangular ligament, opening the gastrohepatic ligament, and mobilizing the left side of the inferior vena cava. All three of these steps unite superiorly at the vena caval–left hepatic vein junction. The left phrenic vein must be identified and divided.

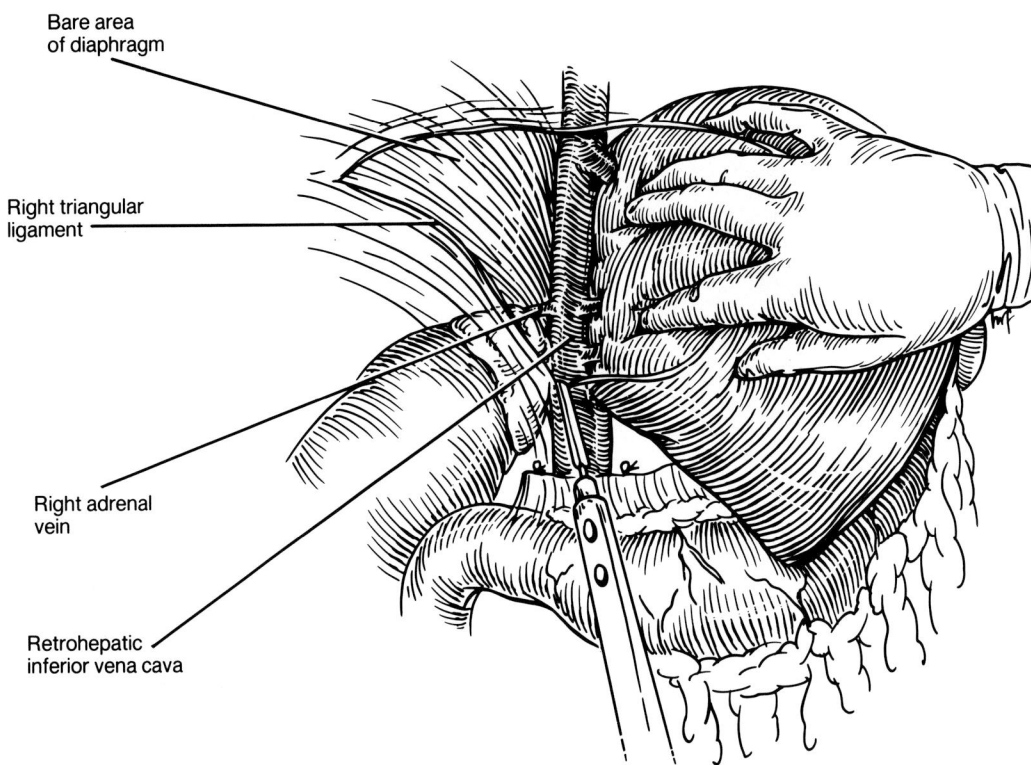

Bare area
of diaphragm

Right triangular
ligament

Right adrenal
vein

Retrohepatic
inferior vena cava

Figure 23-IIA-4

Mobilization of Right Lobe

The right triangular ligament is taken down, and the bare area of the liver is mobilized off the diaphragm. The right lobe is progressively pulled to the left and anteriorly by the assistant on the left of the table. The right side of the vena cava is cleared up to and behind the right hepatic vein. The right adrenal vein is identified.

B. Division of Hepatic Parenchyma During Resection

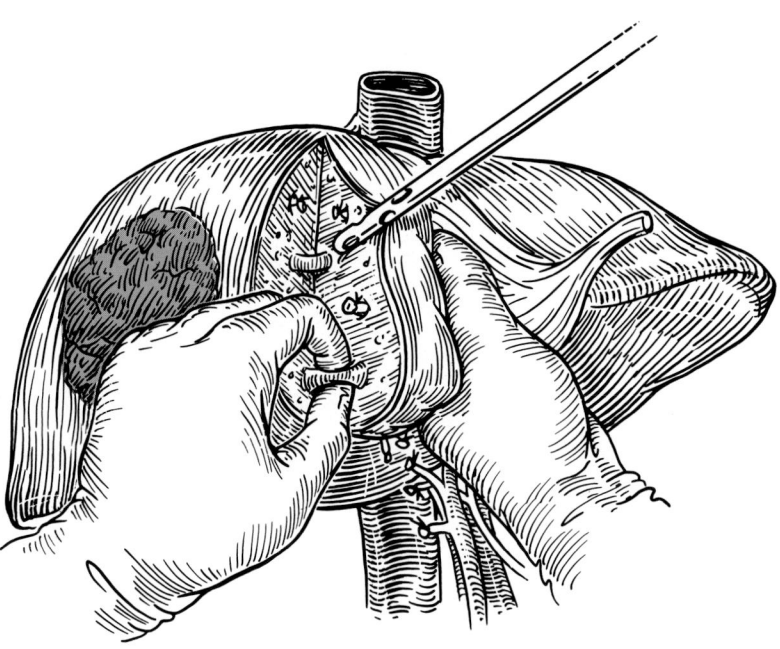

Figure 23-IIB-1

Finger Fracture Technique

Once the capsule of the liver has been incised with the cautery, the hepatic parenchyma can be divided with finger fracture. This allows identification of major structures within the hepatic parenchyma for individual isolation and ligation. The vascularized left lobe of the liver is being compressed by the assistant's left hand.

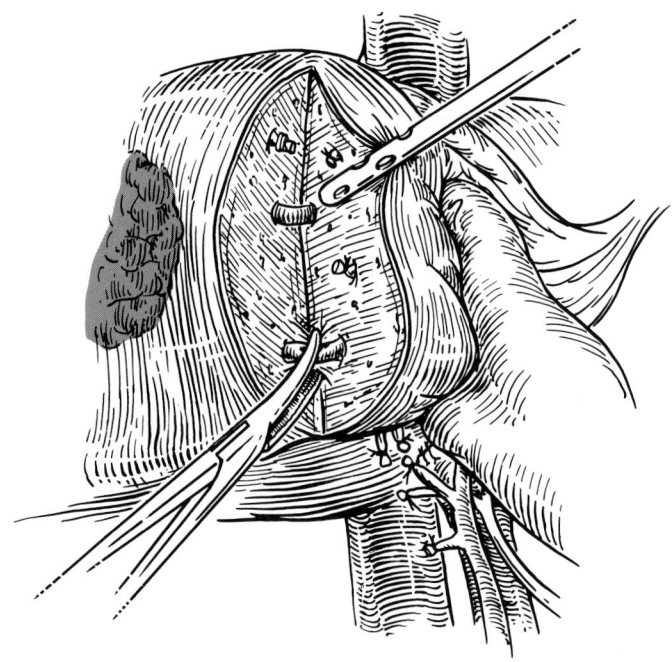

Figure 23-IIB-2

Crush and Clamp Method

In a manner similar to the finger fracture technique, the hepatic parenchyma can be divided by crushing the hepatic parenchyma with a clamp. This allows identification of major vessels and bile ducts in the line of resection. As these are isolated and identified, they are individually ligated.

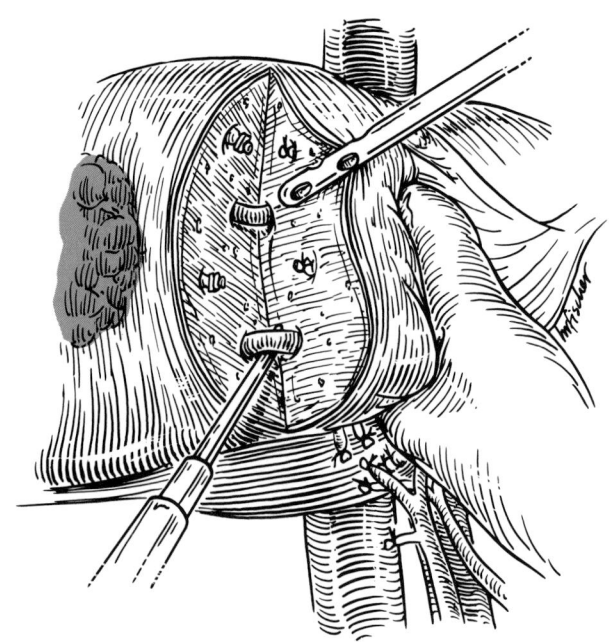

Figure 23-IIB-3

Ultrasonic Dissection

The vibrating tip of an ultrasonic dissector aided with irrigation and suction skeletonizes the hepatic parenchyma, giving clean isolation of structures that need to be individually ligated and divided.

C. Additional Aids in Liver Resection

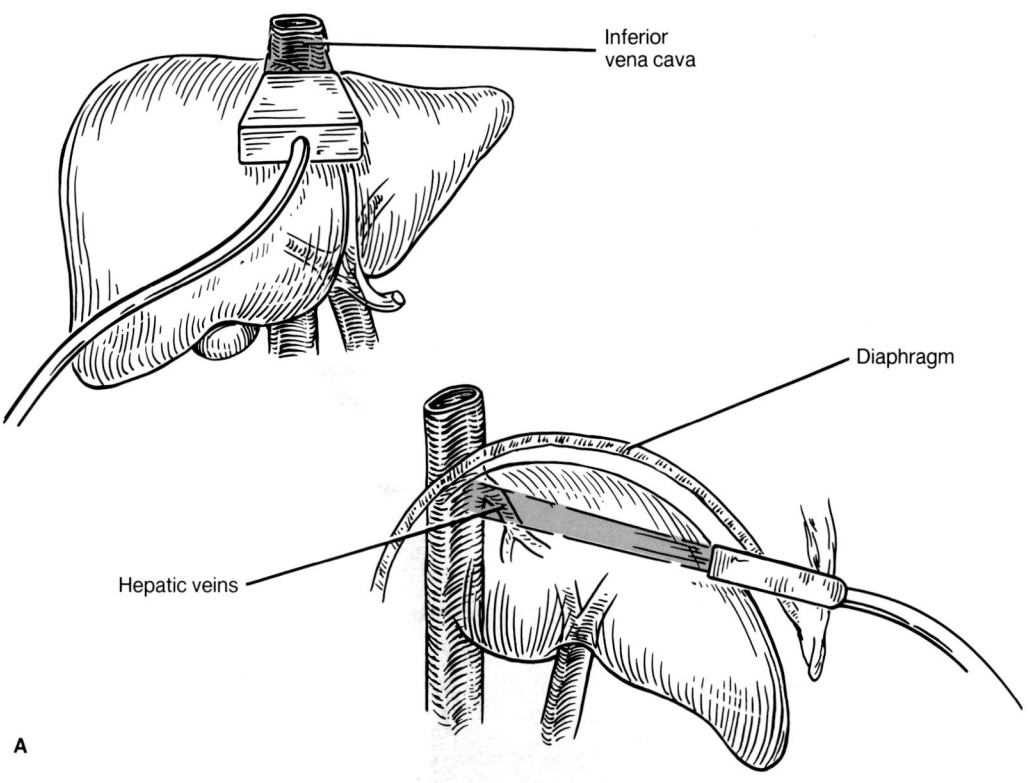

Figure 23-IIC-1

Intraoperative Ultrasound

(**A**) Intraoperative ultrasound has become a useful adjunct in liver resection to identify the tumor and previously unidentified metastases and locate the main vascular structures. The location and configuration of the main hepatic veins and their relation to the tumor are identified superiorly.

(Continued)

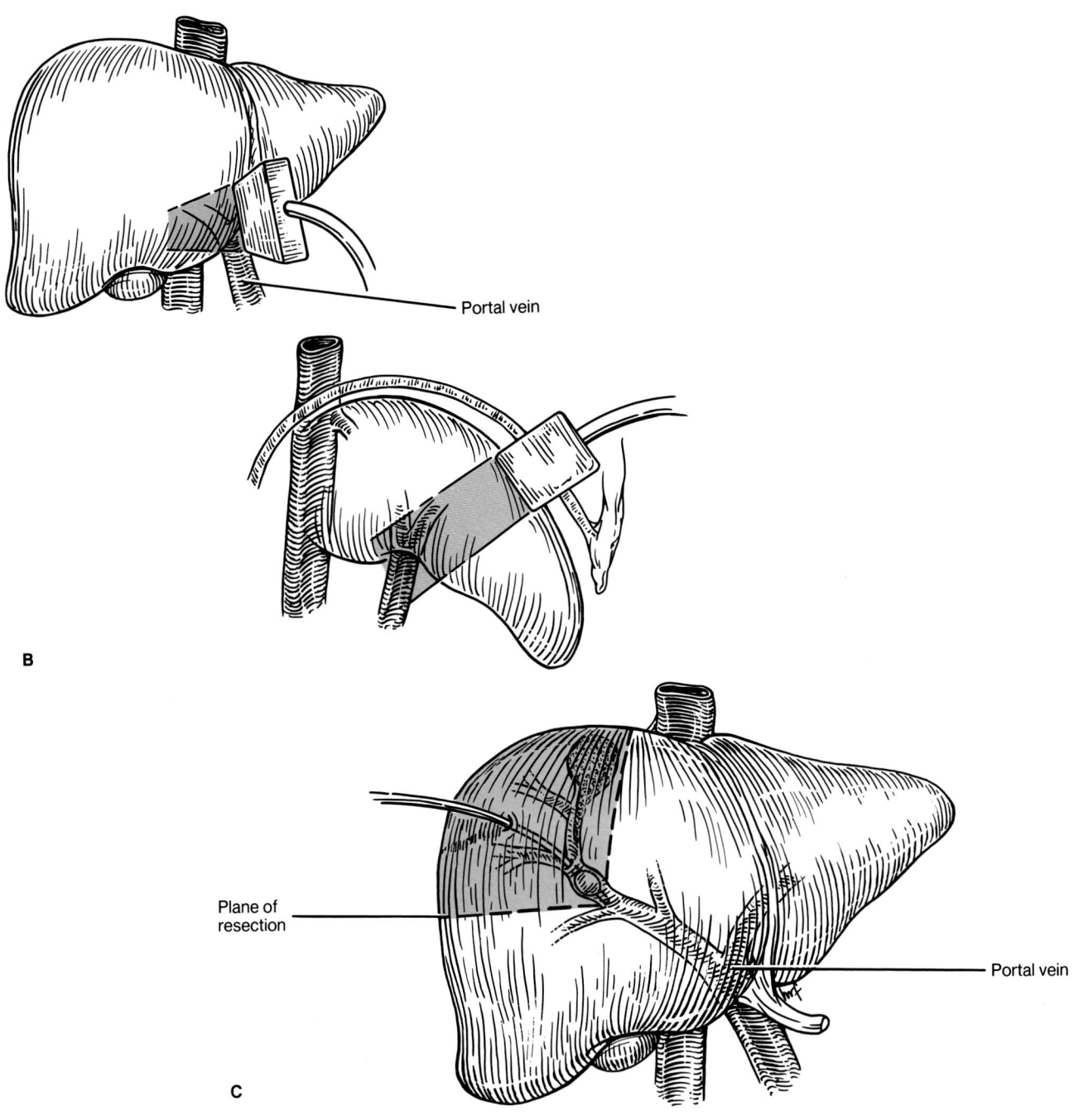

Figure 23-IIC-1 *(Continued)*

(B) Using intraoperative ultrasound, the proximal divisions of the main portal vein can be identified inferiorly, to define their relation to planes of resection and tumor mass.

(C) Isolation of segments for resection. The use of intraoperative ultrasound permits accurate localization of the vessels within the liver. It can also be used to place a transparenchymal balloon occlusion catheter into the main feeding portal vein tributary of any segment planned for resection. This technique is particularly useful in parenchymal sparing resections.

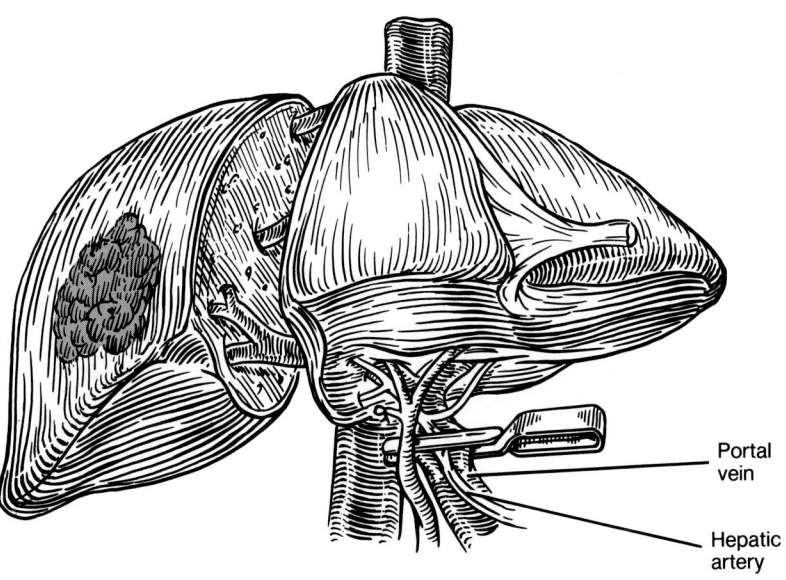

Portal
vein

Hepatic
artery

Figure 23-IIC-2

Inflow Occlusion (Pringle Maneuver)

Cross-clamping of the portal vein and hepatic artery during parenchymal division reduces bleeding from the cut surface, but there will still be significant back-bleeding from the hepatic veins.

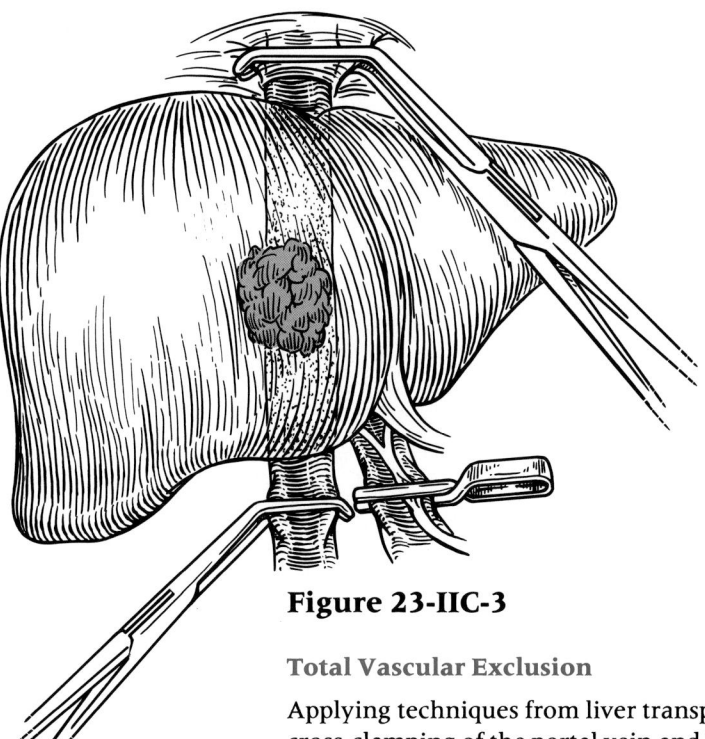

Figure 23-IIC-3

Total Vascular Exclusion

Applying techniques from liver transplantation, the liver can be totally isolated to allow cross-clamping of the portal vein and hepatic arterial inflow and clamping of the inferior vena cava above and below the liver. This permits almost bloodless division of liver substance for major hepatic resections, or isolation of difficult, centrally placed tumors. This is usually tolerated without venovenous bypass after volume expansion by the anesthesiologist. Isolation is achieved as shown by full mobilization as in Figures 23-IIA-3 and 23-IIA-4.

D. Right Hepatic Lobectomy

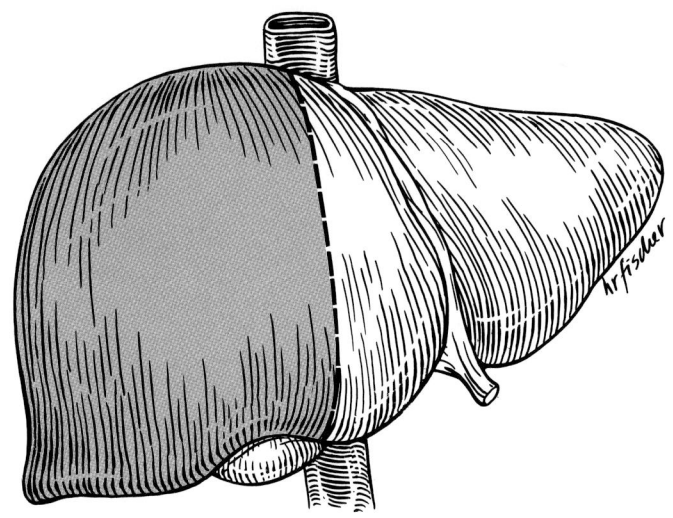

Figure 23-IID-1

Division of the Liver

In right hepatic lobectomy, the colored area is removed.

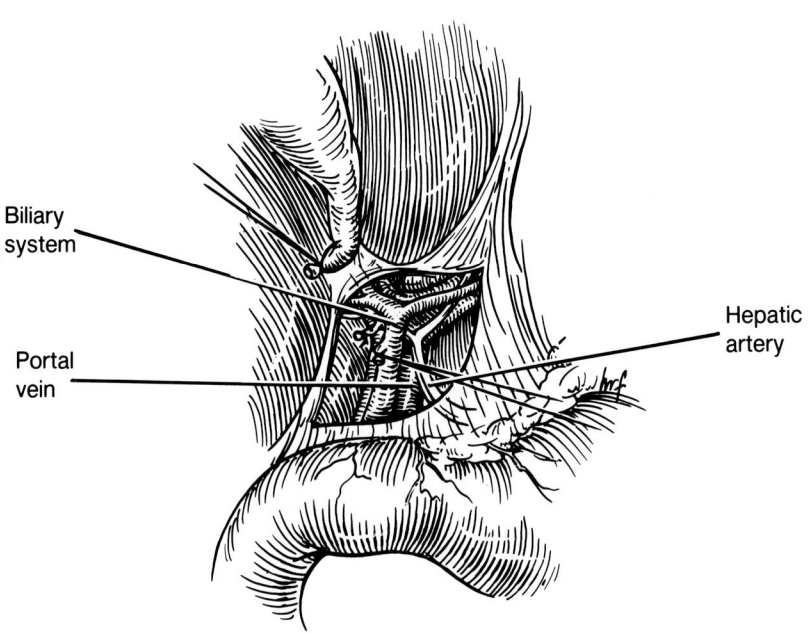

Biliary
system

Portal
vein

Hepatic
artery

Figure 23-IID-2

Hilar Dissection

The hepatic hilus is dissected to identify the common bile duct with its bifurcation, hepatic artery, and portal vein. The cystic duct has been divided to improve exposure for the dissection. The quadrate lobe (segment IV) of the liver has been elevated off the hilus.

Right
hepatic
duct

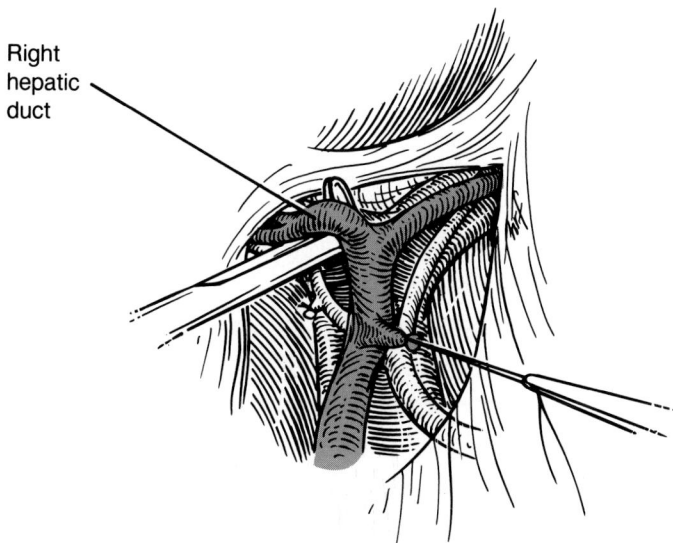

Figure 23-IID-3

Dissection and Division of Hepatic Structures

The right hepatic duct has been isolated and surrounded in preparation for its division. This dissection is difficult when the right posterior hepatic duct arises from or close to the bifurcation.

Right
hepatic
artery

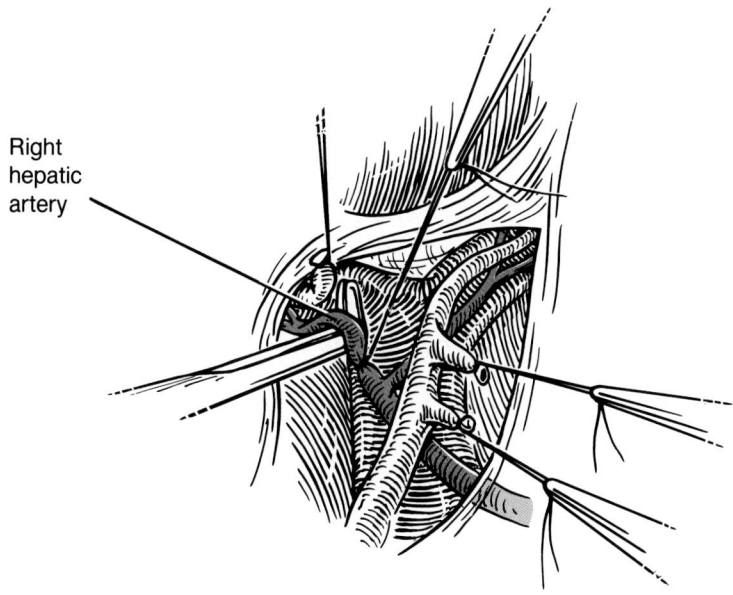

Figure 23-IID-4

Division of Right Hepatic Artery

The right hepatic artery is fully dissected, isolated, and then divided. Both the common bile duct and the bifurcation can be gently retracted to the left.

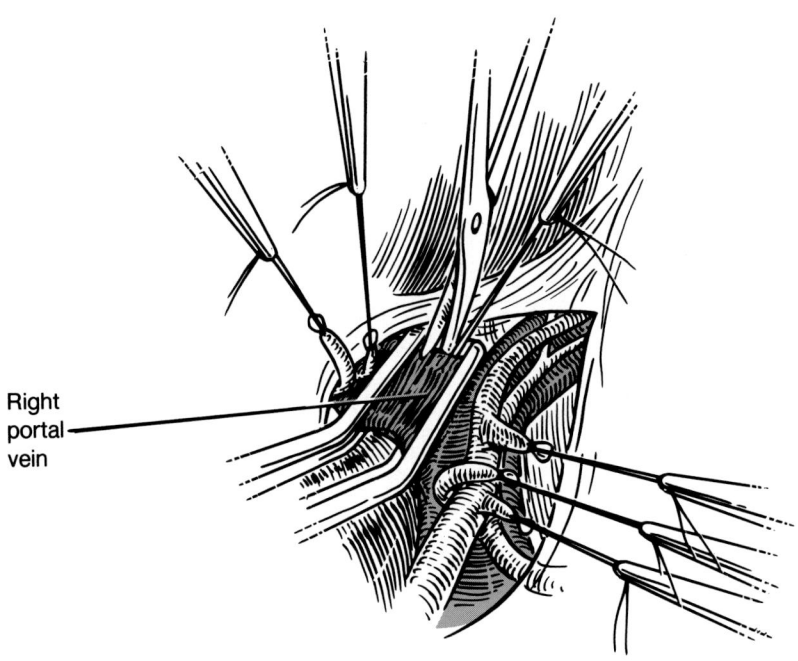

Right
portal —
vein

Figure 23-IID-5

Identification and Division of Right Portal Vein

Clamps are placed on the main right portal vein to obtain better control. Again, both the bile duct and the common hepatic artery can be gently retracted to the left. In isolation of either the main right or left portal vein, it is important to be careful that there is not a major posterior branch of the portal vein coming off the bifurcation.

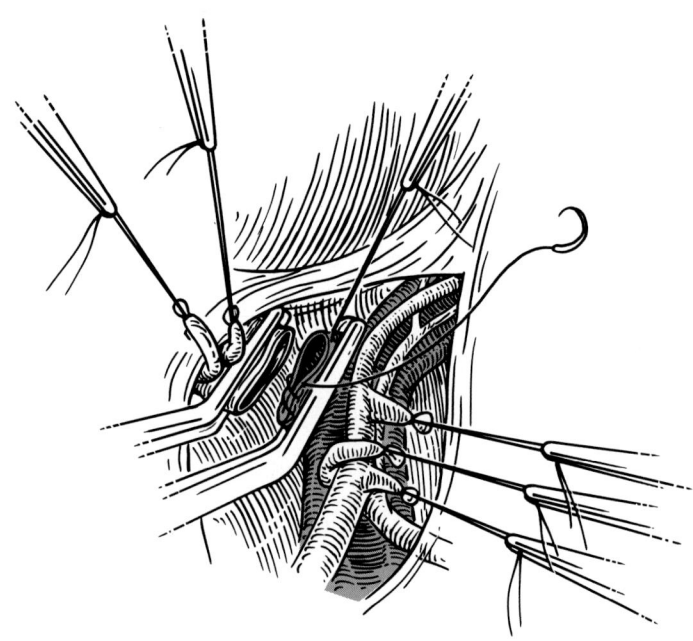

Figure 23-IID-6

Suture Placement

The divided proximal end of the portal vein is oversewn with a 5-0 Prolene suture.

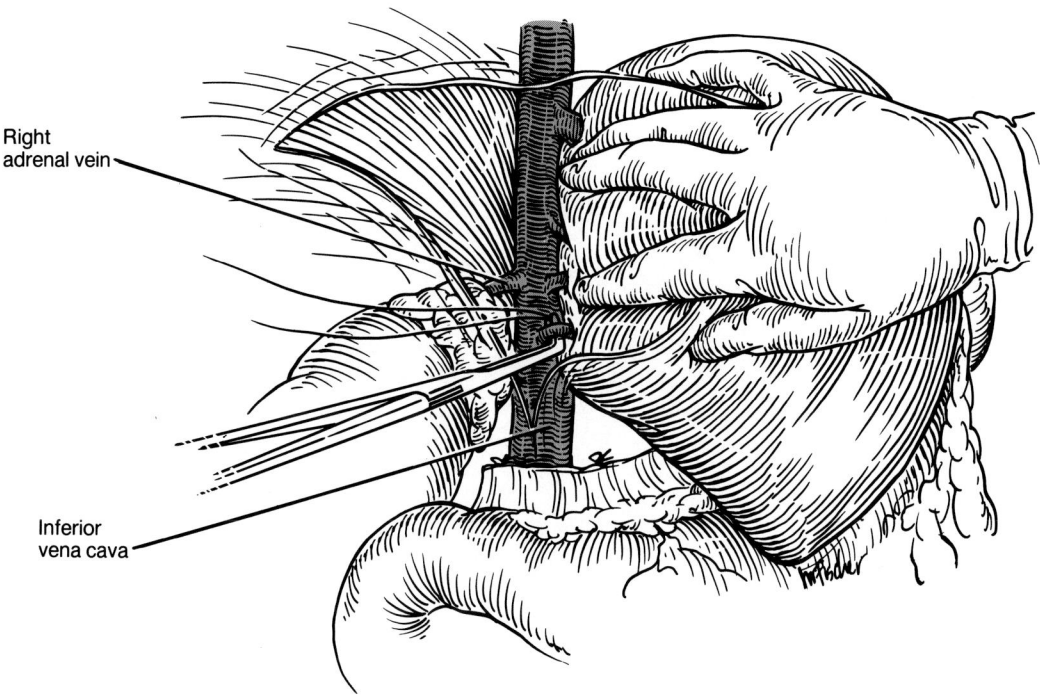

Right adrenal vein

Inferior vena cava

Figure 23-IID-7

Ligation of Retrohepatic Veins

For a major resection, the liver should be mobilized off the vena cava by ligation of retrohepatic veins entering the caudate or right lobes.

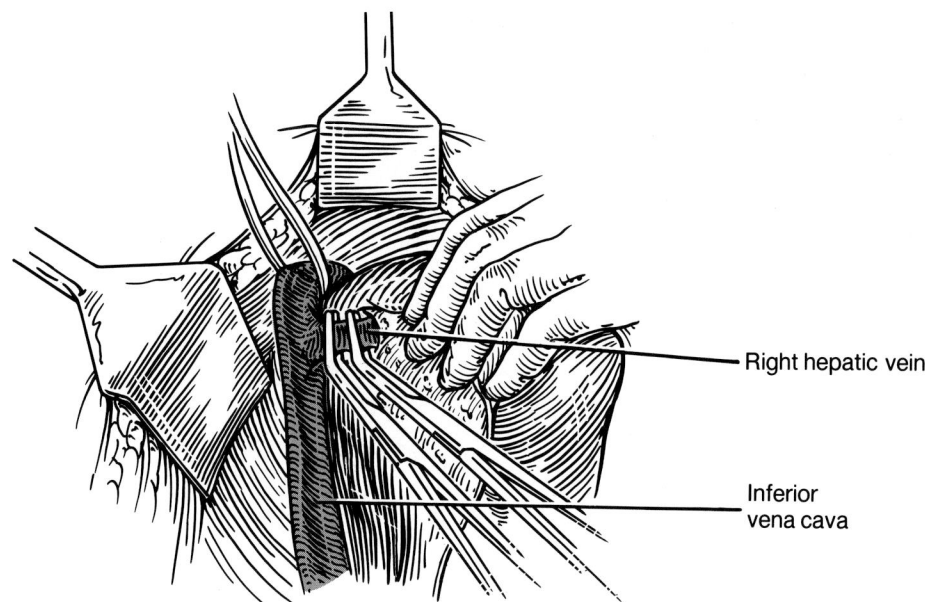

Figure 23-IID-8

Extrahepatic Identification and Ligation of Right Hepatic Vein

After division of the right triangular ligament, the right hepatic vein can be identified extrahepatically as it enters the inferior vena cava. If the right lobe of the liver can be adequately mobilized, and the tumor is not encroaching on the right hepatic vein, it is possible to identify, isolate, and ligate this vein extrahepatically. This maneuver sometimes is limited by the location of tumor or the bulk of the right lobe of the liver. If this is the case, the right hepatic vein should be ligated intrahepatically.

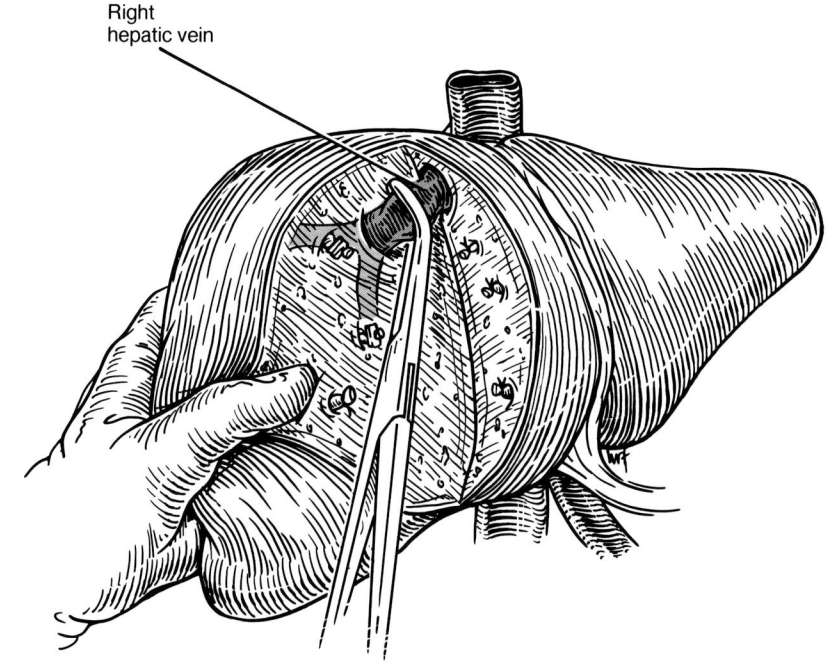

Figure 23-IID-9

Intrahepatic Identification and Ligation of Right Hepatic Vein

Toward the completion of the division of the parenchyma of the right lobe in a formal right hepatic lobectomy, the right hepatic vein will be identified intraparenchymally. With the surrounding parenchyma clear, the vein can be isolated and divided close to the vena cava.

E. Right Trisegmentectomy or Extended Right Hepatic Lobectomy

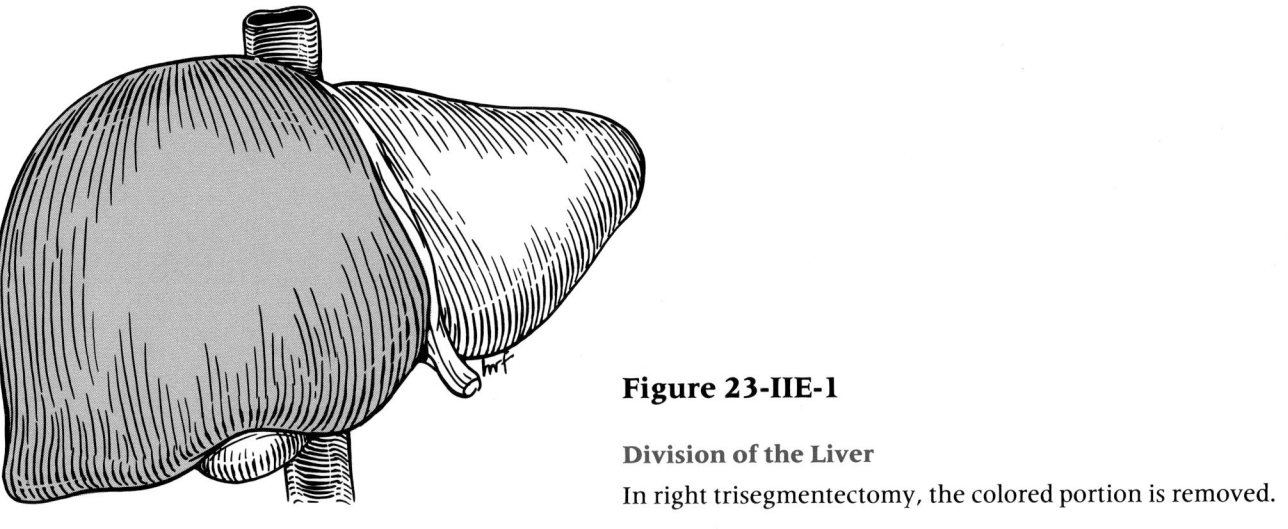

Figure 23-IIE-1

Division of the Liver
In right trisegmentectomy, the colored portion is removed.

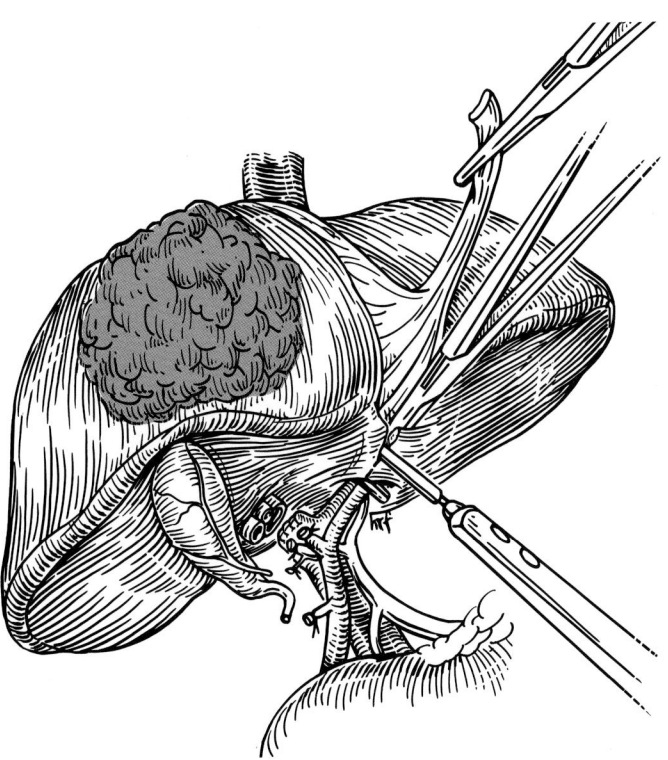

Figure 23-IIE-2

Hilar Dissection
Hilar dissection identifies and divides the main right lobe vessels and bile duct. The left vessels and bile duct must be separated from segment IV. The falciform ligament is pulled anteriorly, and the bridge of liver tissue between segments III and IV is divided to enter the plane of division.

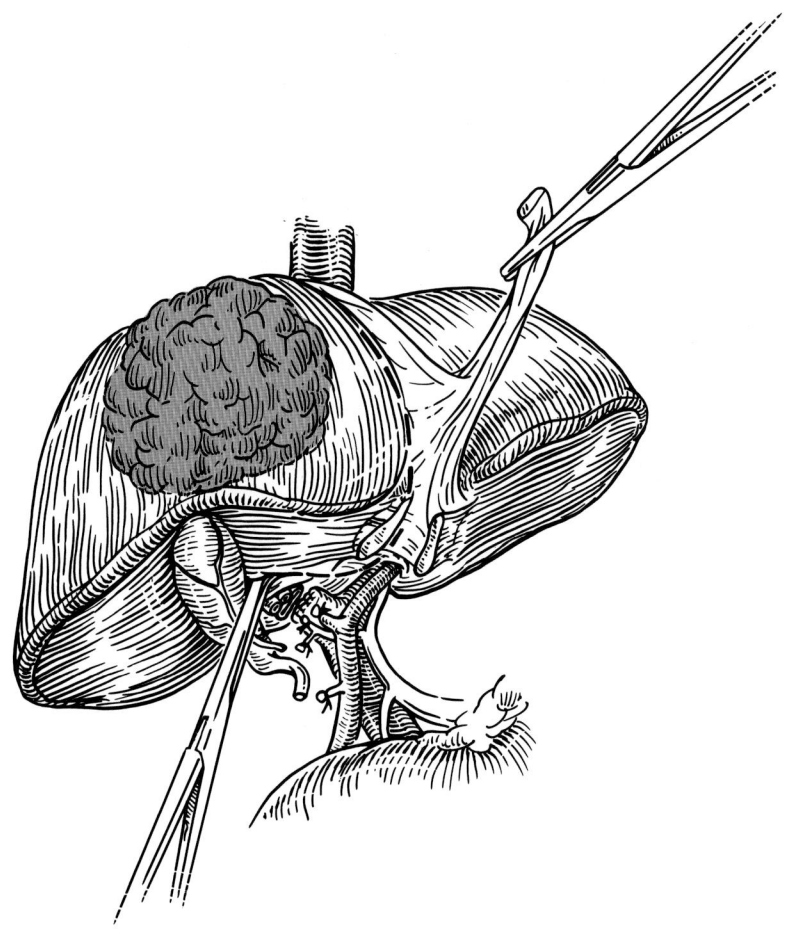

Figure 23-IIE-3

Plane Development

The plane between segment IV and the left vessels and bile duct to segments II and III is developed to protect these structures.

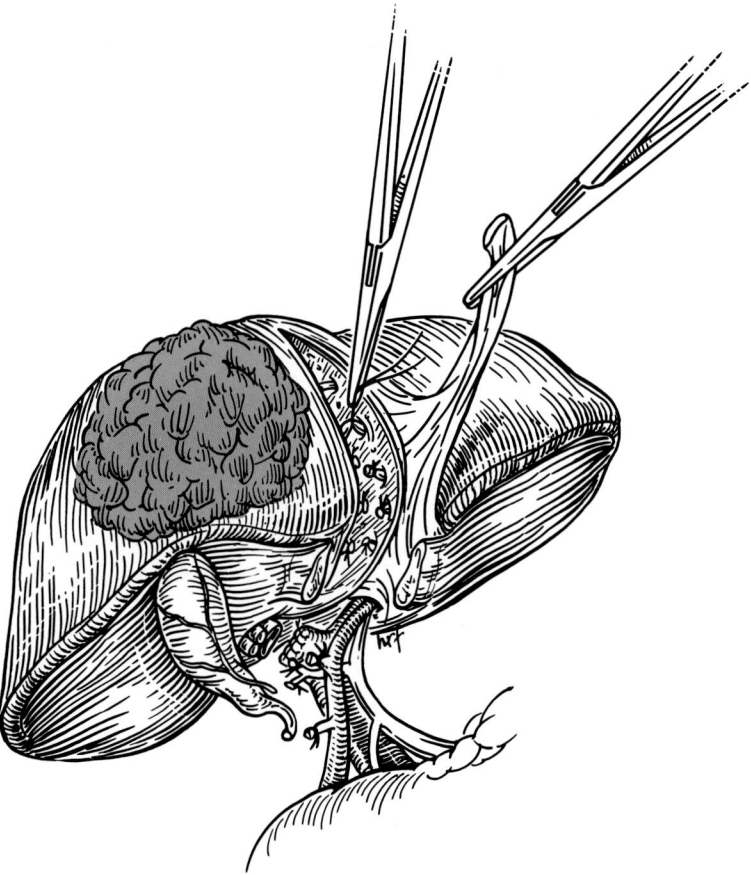

Figure 23-IIE-4

Division of Parenchyma

Parenchymal division is achieved with any of the described methods along the line of the falciform ligament. The right hepatic vein is divided, but the confluence of the middle and left veins must be carefully dissected to ensure preservation of the left hepatic vein for outflow.

F. Left Hepatic Lobectomy

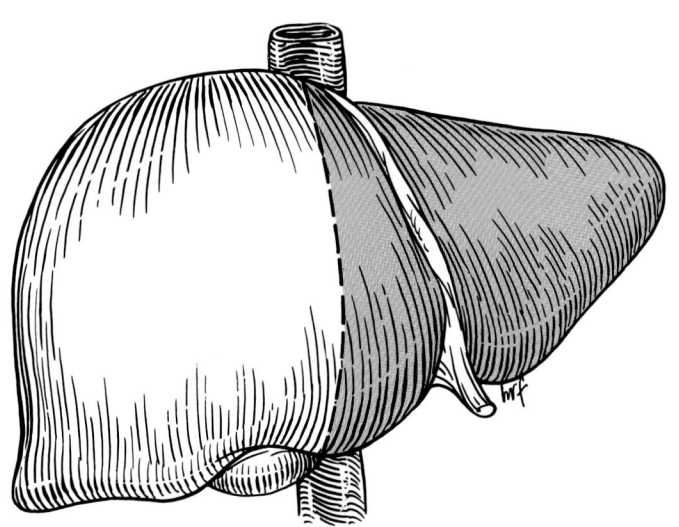

Figure 23-IIF-1

Division of the Liver

In left hepatic lobectomy, the colored portion is removed.

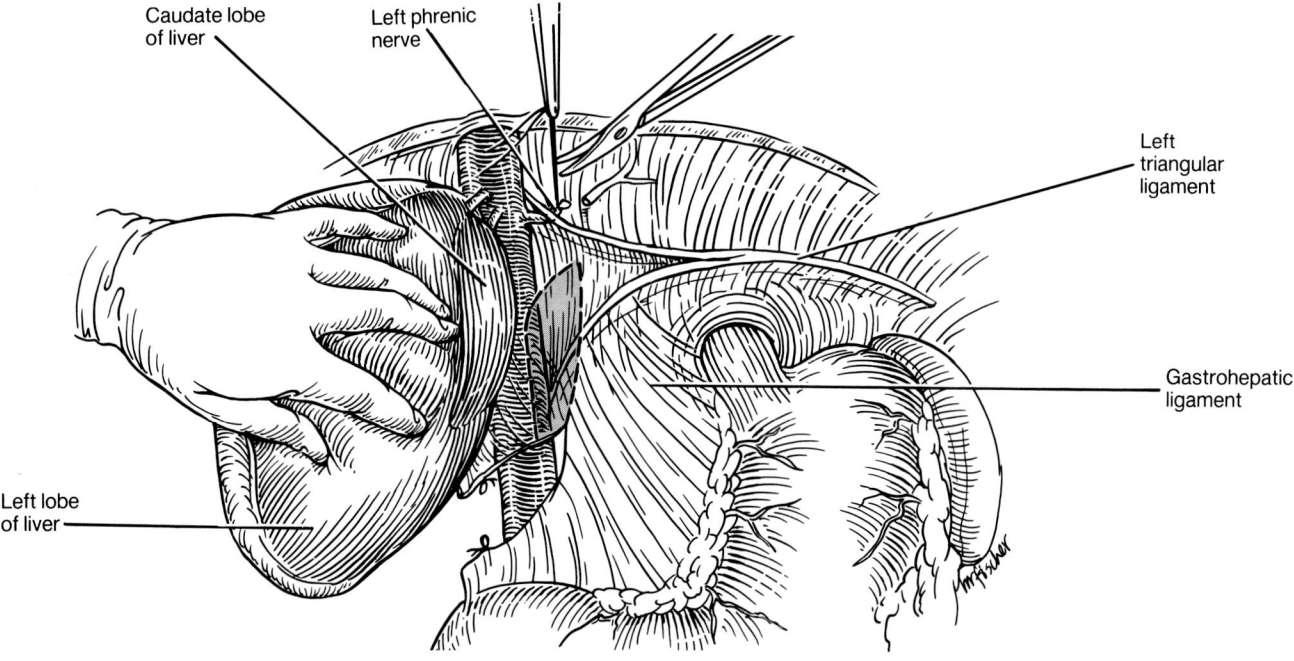

Figure 23-IIF-2

Mobilization of the Liver

The liver is fully mobilized by dividing the left triangular ligament and retracting the left lobe to the right. The gastrohepatic ligament is then opened close to the liver and divided up to the diaphragm; a replaced left hepatic artery arising from the left gastric artery traverses this high up when present. The left side of the vena cava is identified behind the caudate lobe, and its overlying adventitia can be opened to complete this mobilization; this also opens the posterior plane to the suprahepatic vena cava. The left phrenic vein is identified and divided.

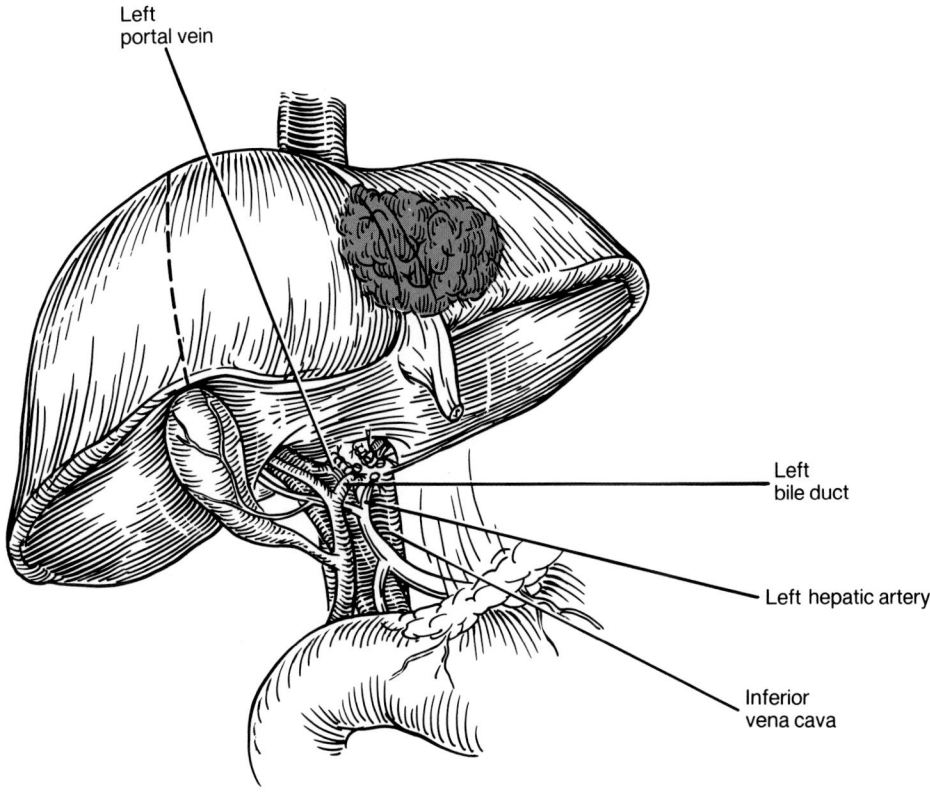

Left
portal vein

Left
bile duct

Left hepatic artery

Inferior
vena cava

Figure 23-IIF-3

Hilar Dissection

Hilar dissection is done by identifying the bifurcations of the hepatic artery, portal vein, and bile duct. For a left lobectomy, the branches of these structures are divided as illustrated.

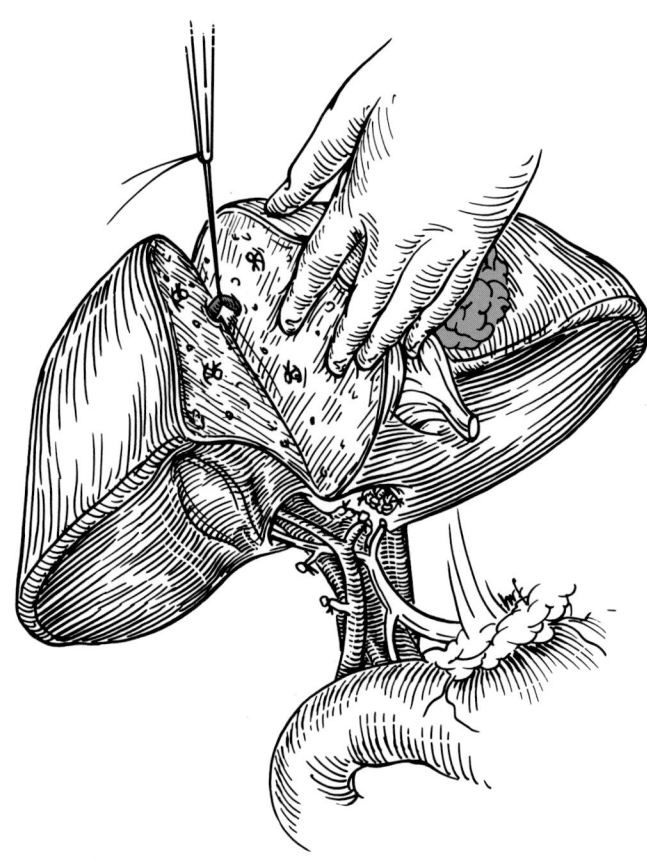

Figure 23-IIF-4

Division of Liver Substance

The liver substance can be divided from the gallbladder fossa along the line of the middle hepatic vein to the vena cava. This can be achieved with any of the methods described.

G. Left Lateral Segmentectomy

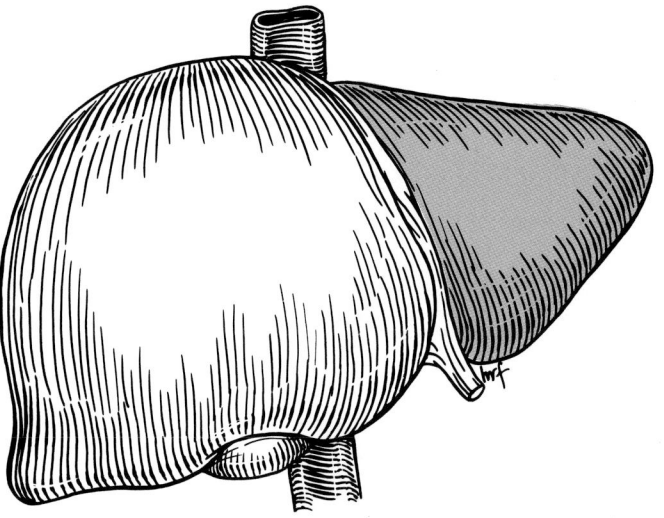

Figure 23-IIG-1

Division of the Liver

This resection entails removal of segments II and III (*colored*) and does not require a formal hilar dissection.

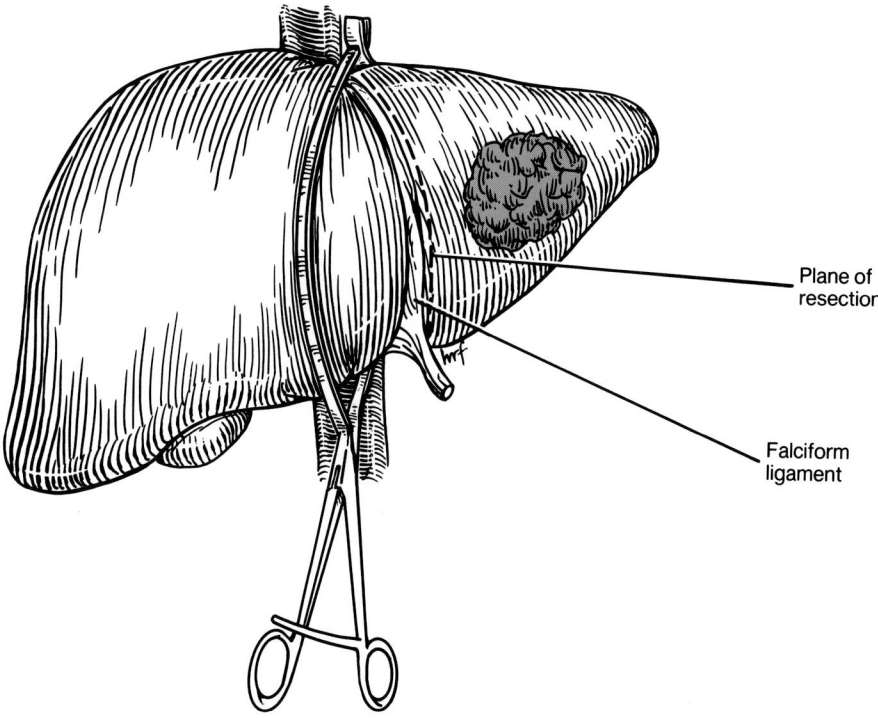

Plane of resection

Falciform ligament

Figure 23-IIG-2

Clamp Placement

The left lobe is fully mobilized as described in Figure 23-IIA-3. This resection can be aided by placement of the large compressing liver clamps just to the right of the falciform ligament.

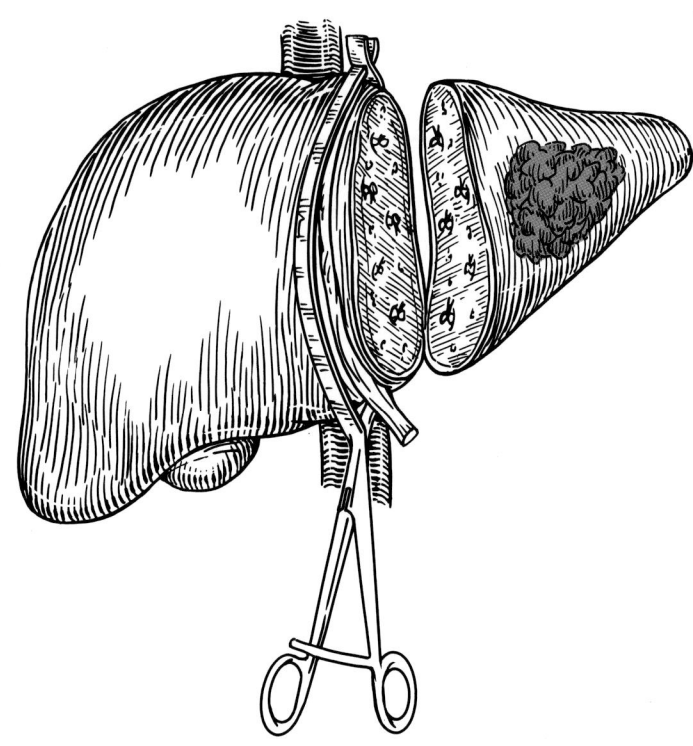

Figure 23-IIG-3

Division of Parenchyma

The parenchyma is then divided along the falciform ligament, vessels are oversewn, and sutures are placed to approximate the divided surface before the clamp is removed.

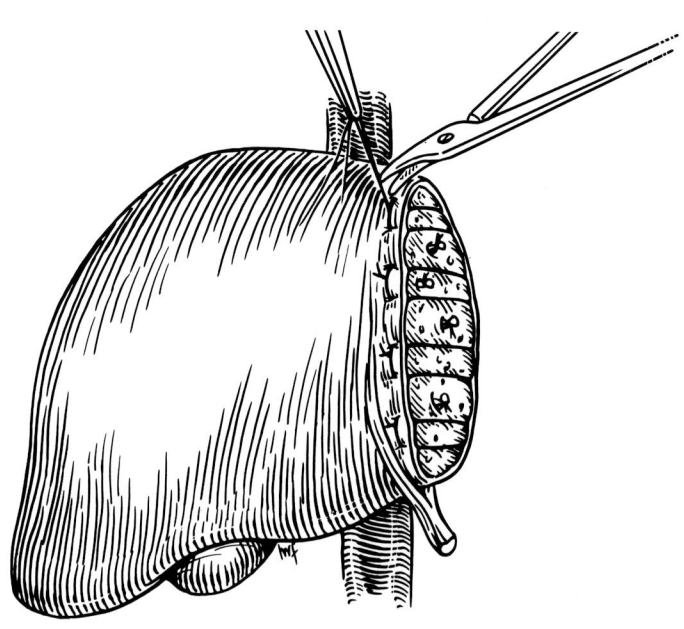

Figure 23-IIG-4

Cut Surface Approximation

The cut surface edges are approximated by through-and-through sutures to compress the divided parenchyma.

H. Other Resections

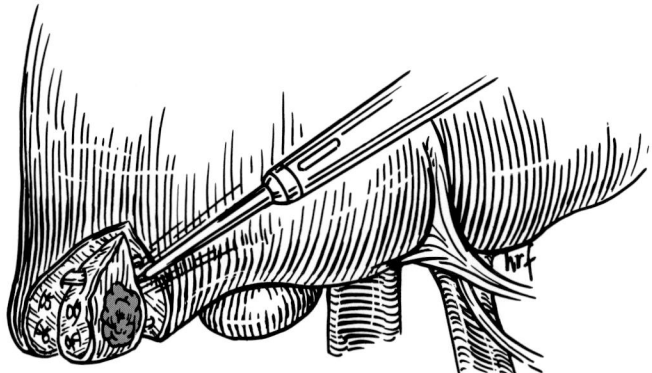

Figure 23-IIH-1

Nonanatomic Resection

Wedge resection of a small lesion can be achieved using any of the parenchymal tissue division methods described previously. In this illustration, the ultrasonic dissector has been used for a small wedge resection. Tumor margins must be 1 cm or greater.

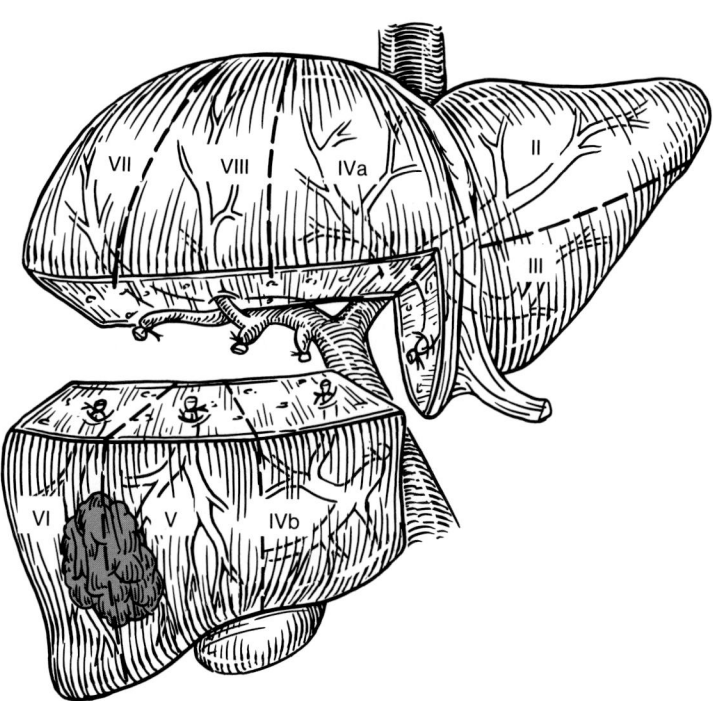

Figure 23-IIH-2

Segmental Resection

Isolated resection of segments V and VI allows preservation of liver parenchyma. By not performing an extended right hepatic lobectomy, the functional parenchyma of segments VII and VIII is preserved. Resections such as this can be accomplished with some of the aids discussed in Figures 23-IIA-3 through 23-IIB-3.

J. Hepatic Cysts

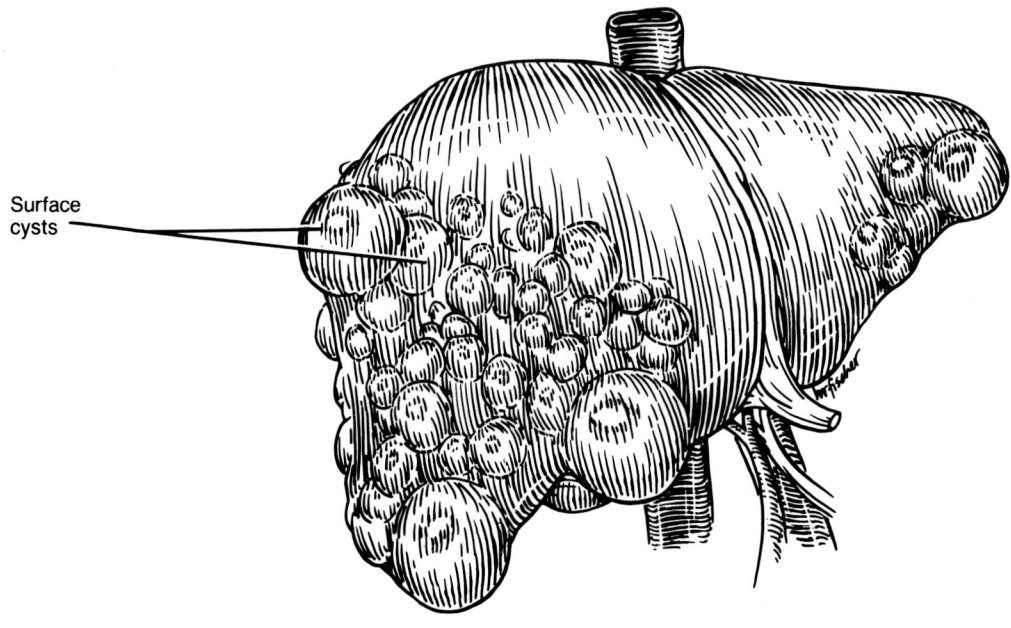

Surface
cysts

Figure 23-IIJ-1

Cyst Appearance

Hepatic cysts may be single or multiple, as illustrated here. They may occur on the surface
of the liver or within the parenchyma.

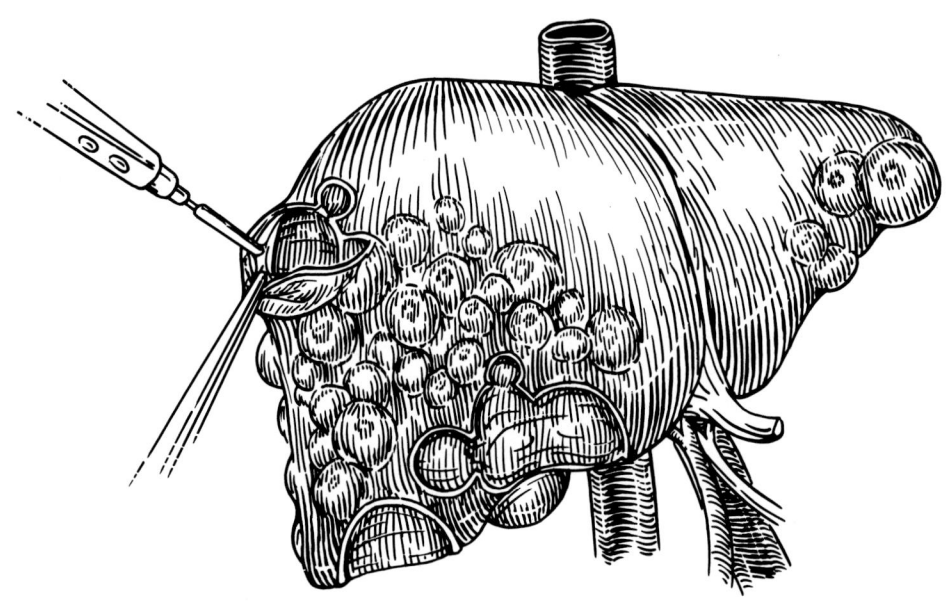

Figure 23-IIJ-2

Unroofing and Fenestration of Hepatic Cysts

Large and symptomatic cysts can be unroofed for decompression. The walls between
cysts can be resected (fenestration) to decompress more of the compressed liver. True
cysts do not communicate with the biliary tree and are left to drain into the free peritoneal cavity. This can also be achieved laparoscopically.

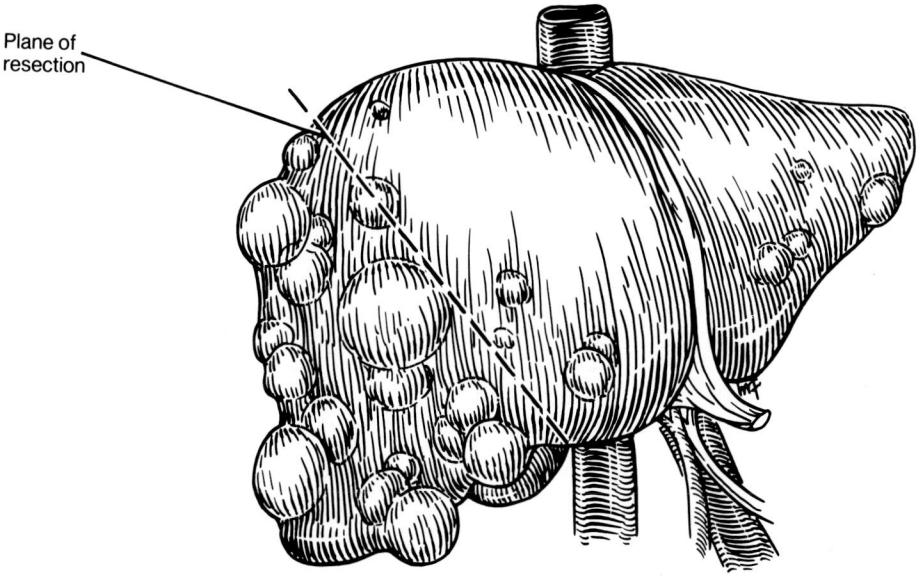

Plane of
resection

Figure 23-IIJ-3

Cyst Resection

In symptomatic patients in whom most cysts are confined to one lobe, resection may be indicated. The rules for parenchymal resections apply.

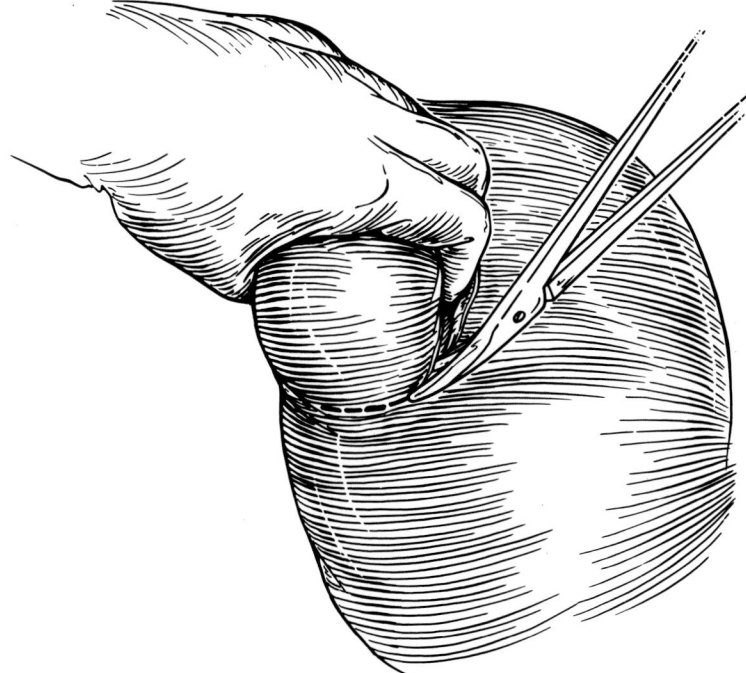

Figure 23-IIJ-4

Cyst Enucleation

Rather than an anatomic resection, many cysts can be enucleated by developing a dissection plane between the cyst and the hepatic parenchyma.

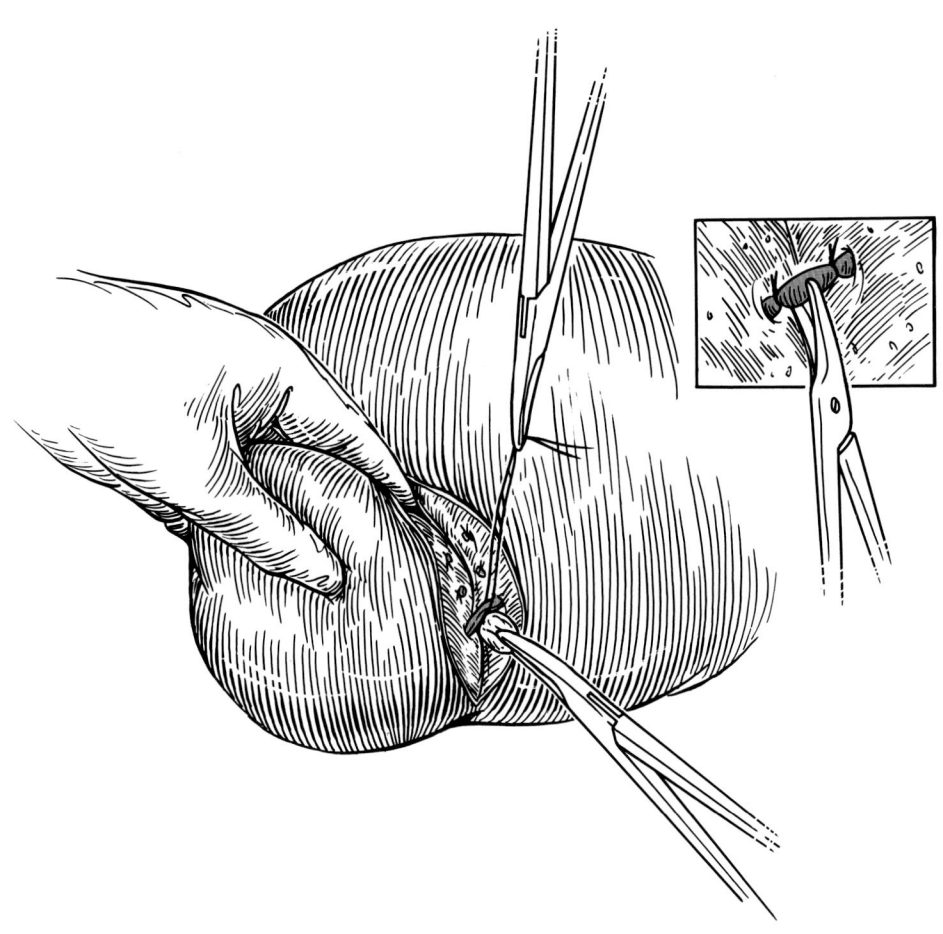

Figure 23-IIJ-5

Ligation and Division of Blood Vessels and Bile Ducts

As blood vessels and bile ducts are encountered during enucleation of a hepatic cyst, they are doubly ligated and divided. Most cysts on the surface can be enucleated with minimal blood loss. Anatomic resection is preferred to enucleation when neoplasia is suspected (eg, biliary cystadenoma or cystadenocarcinoma).

K. Open Drainage of Liver Abscess

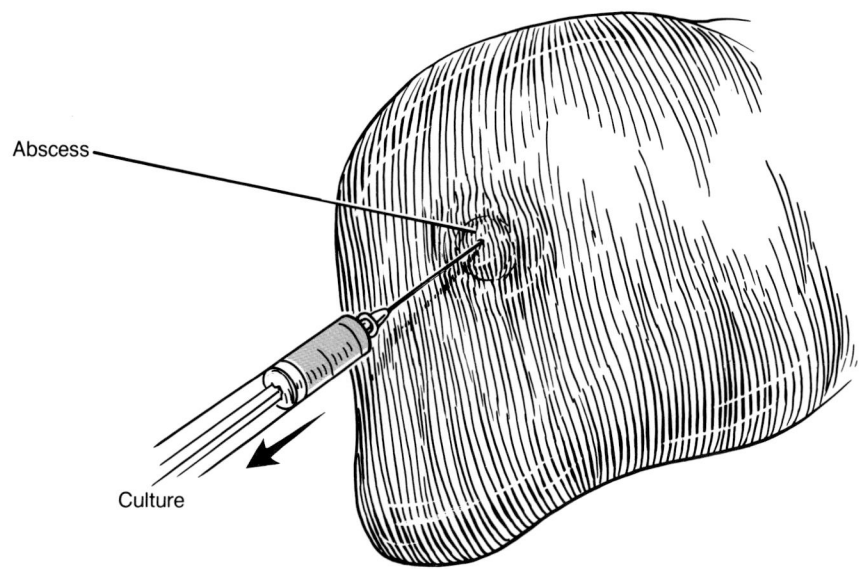

Figure 23-IIK-1

Aspiration

Unilocular liver abscesses generally respond well to percutaneous drainage. Multilocular abscesses often require surgical drainage. After exploration through a right subcostal incision, the abscess in the right lobe of the liver is aspirated, and the syringe contents are sent for aerobic and anaerobic culture.

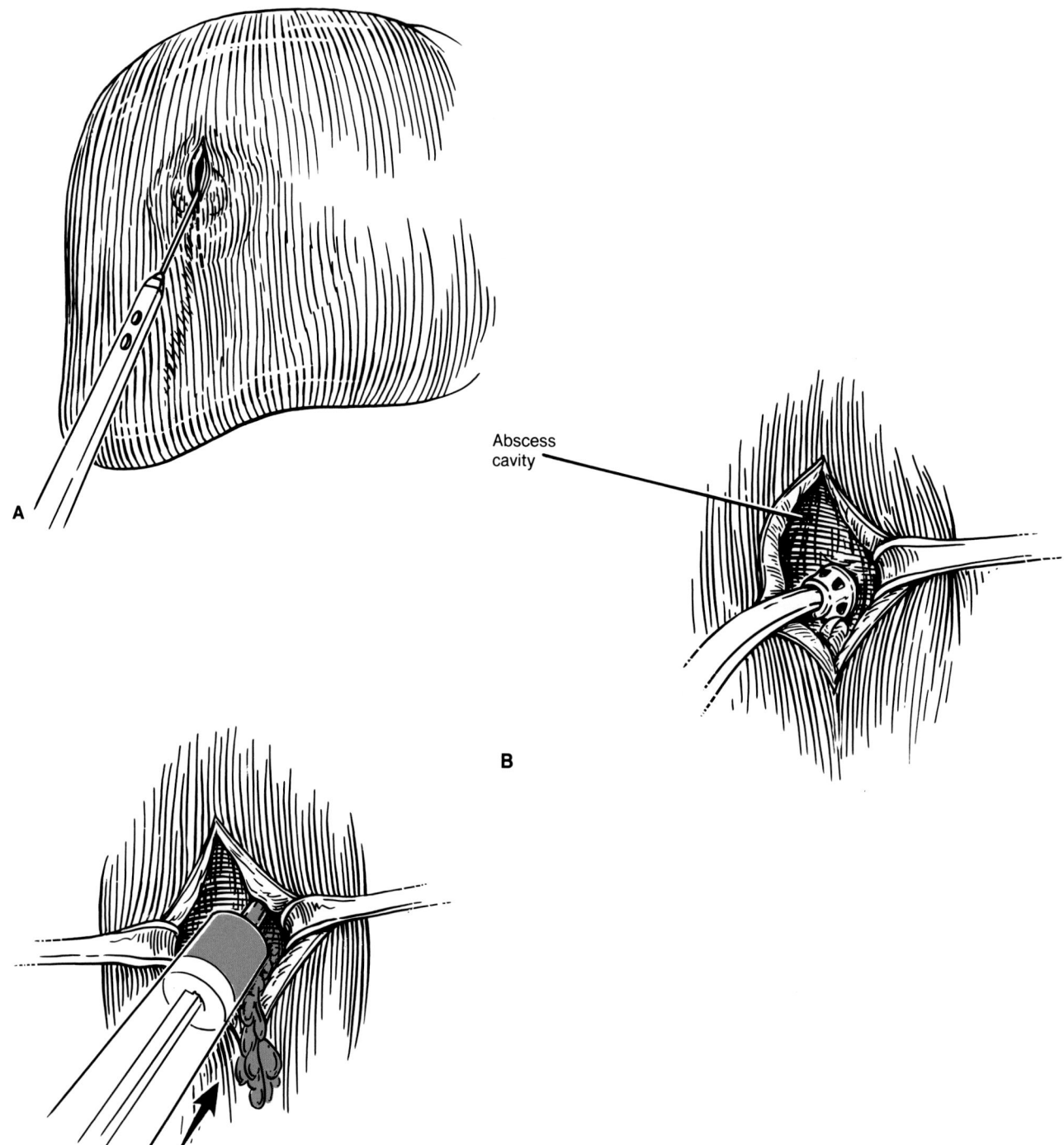

Figure 23-IIK-2

Management of Abscess Cavity

(**A**) The abscess cavity is then opened with cautery.

(**B**) The contents of the abscess cavity are suctioned, and loculations are gently broken down with the palpating finger.

(**C**) The abscess cavity is irrigated thoroughly with saline.

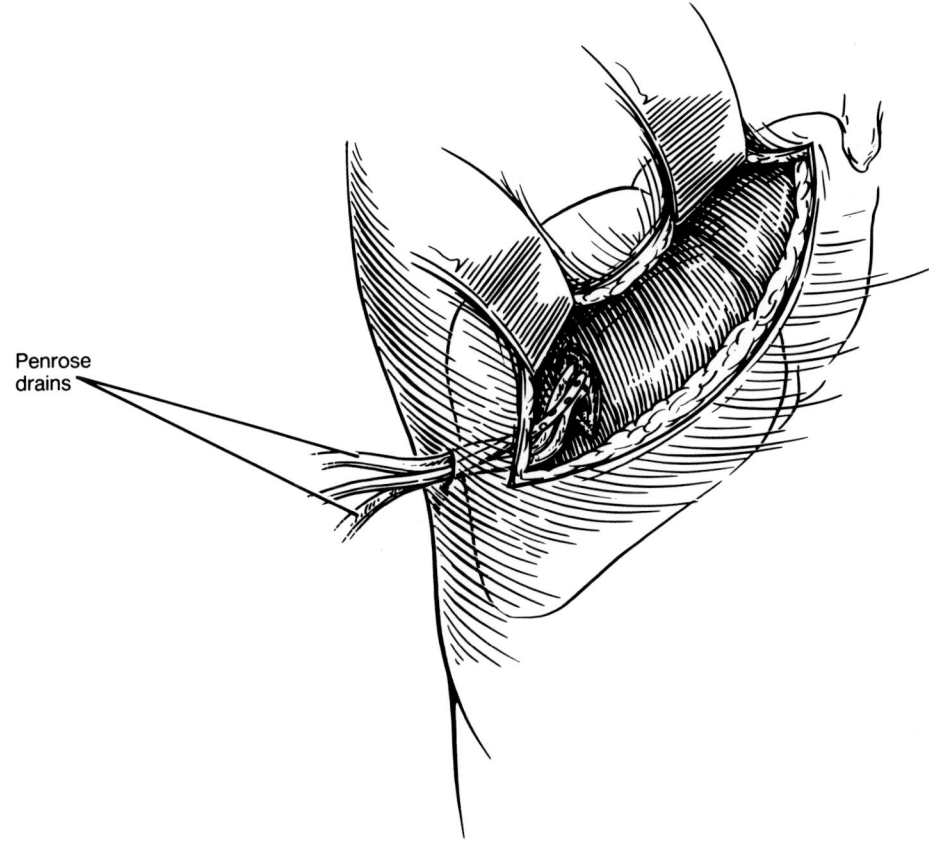

Penrose
drains

Figure 23-IIK-3

Drain Placement

Several Penrose drains and a Jackson-Pratt drain are placed within the abscess cavity and brought through the abdominal wall lateral to the right subcostal incision.

SECTION III   Operations for Portal Hypertension

A. Portacaval Shunt

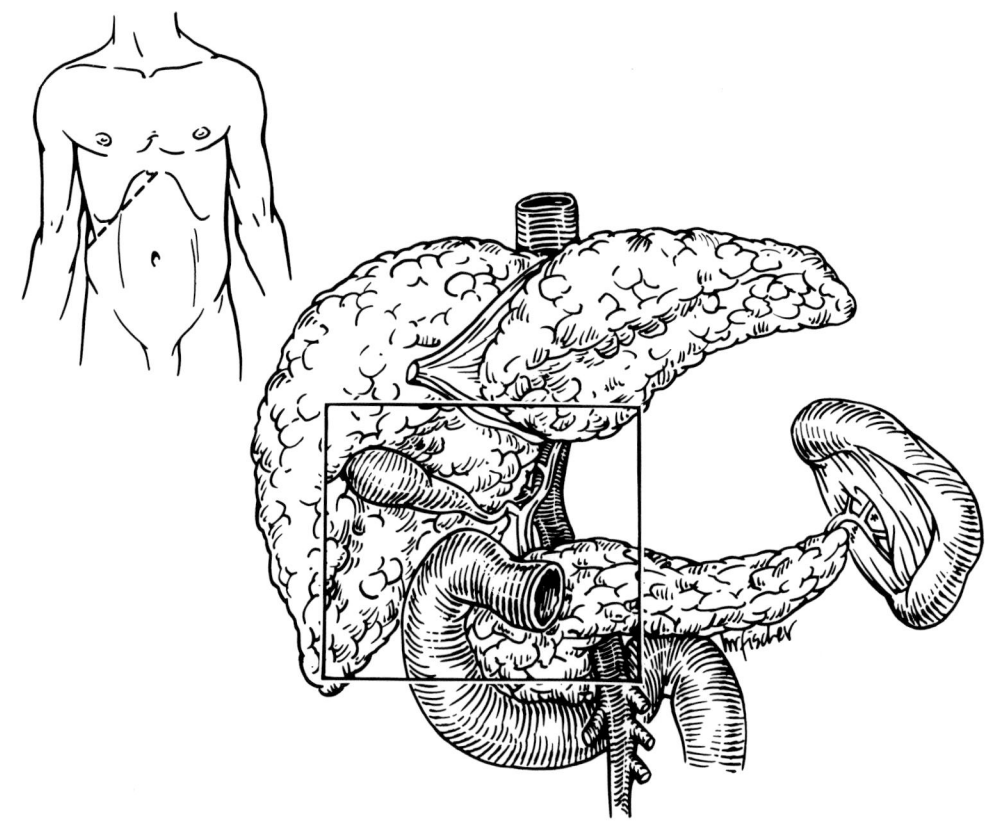

Figure 23-IIIA-1

Incision and Site of Dissection

The incision for portacaval shunt is a right subcostal incision (**inset**). The area of dissection is the hepatic hilus, the right and posterior border of the hepatoduodenal ligament, and the retroperitoneum from behind the duodenum to the caudate lobe of the liver.

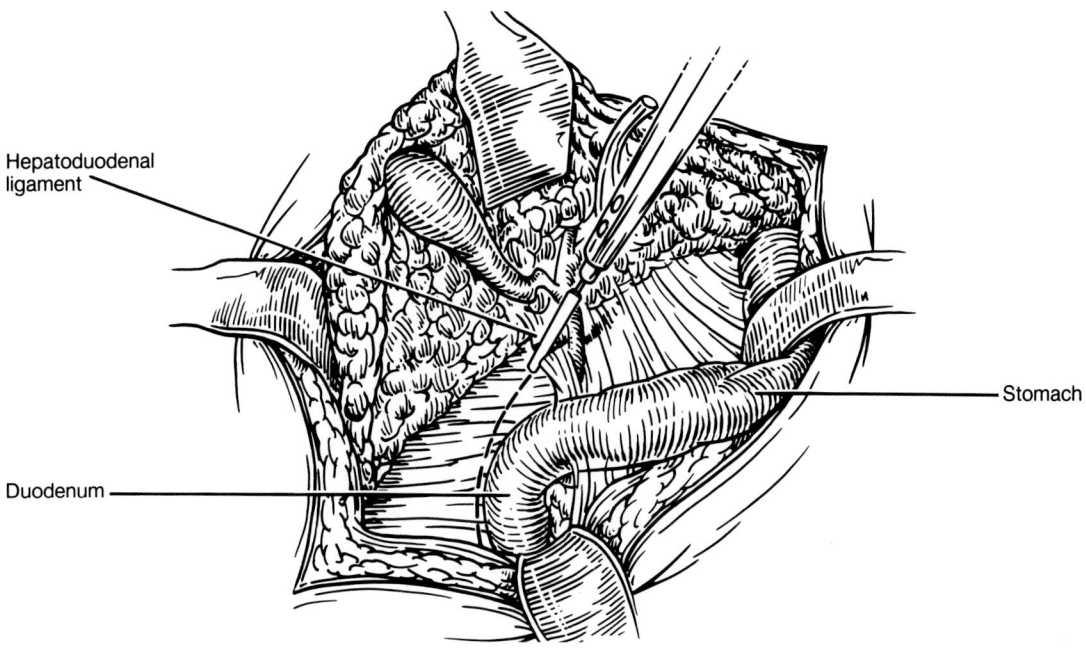

Hepatoduodenal ligament

Stomach

Duodenum

Figure 23-IIIA-2

Exposure

The right costal margin and the liver are retracted superiorly. The peritoneum is incised along the right edge of the hepatoduodenal ligament. The duodenum is "kocherized."

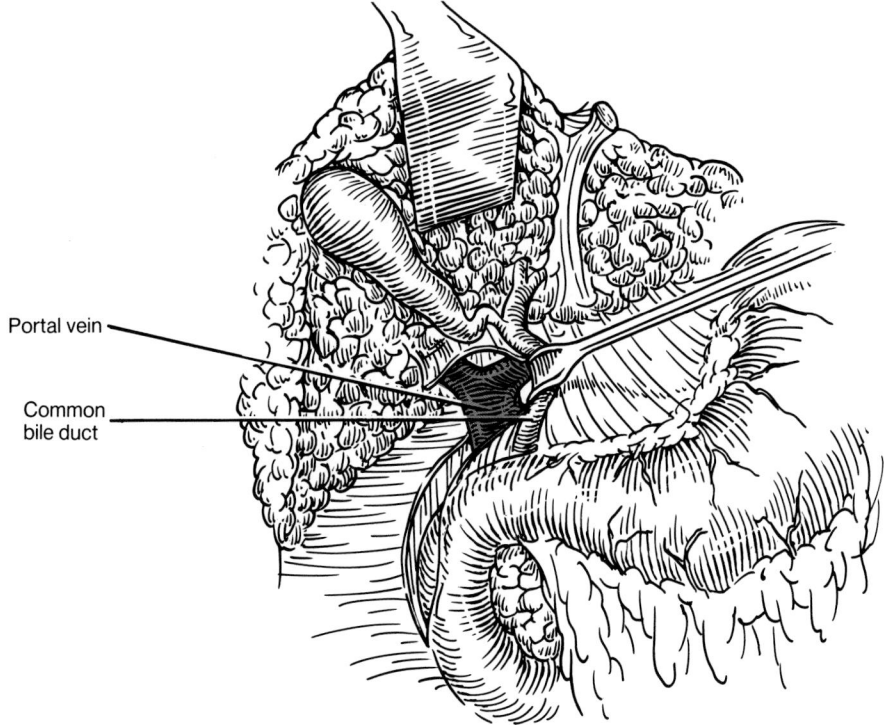

Portal vein

Common bile duct

Figure 23-IIIA-3

Identification of Portal Vein

The portal vein is identified by retracting the common bile duct and hepatic artery to the left and freeing the portal vein over sufficient length between the pancreas and the hepatic hilus.

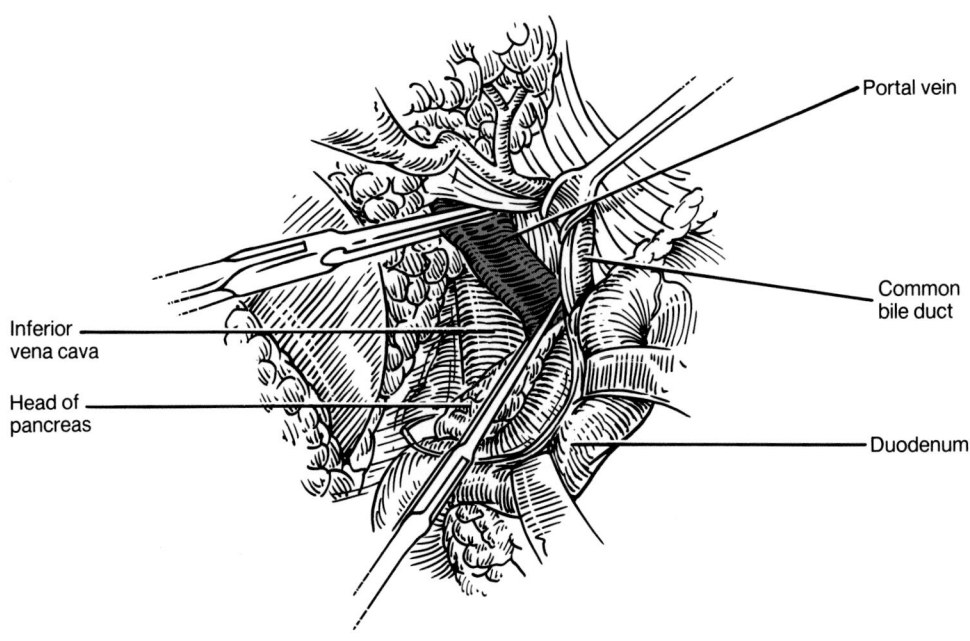

Portal vein

Common
bile duct

Inferior
vena cava

Head of
pancreas

Duodenum

Figure 23-IIIA-4

Identification and Division of Inferior Vena Cava

The inferior vena cava is identified in the retroperitoneum and freed over sufficient
length from the caudate lobe inferiorly so that a partially occluding Satinsky clamp can
be applied. For an end-to-side portacaval shunt, the portal vein is divided at its bifurcation, as illustrated here. It is occluded where it emerges from beneath the pancreas.

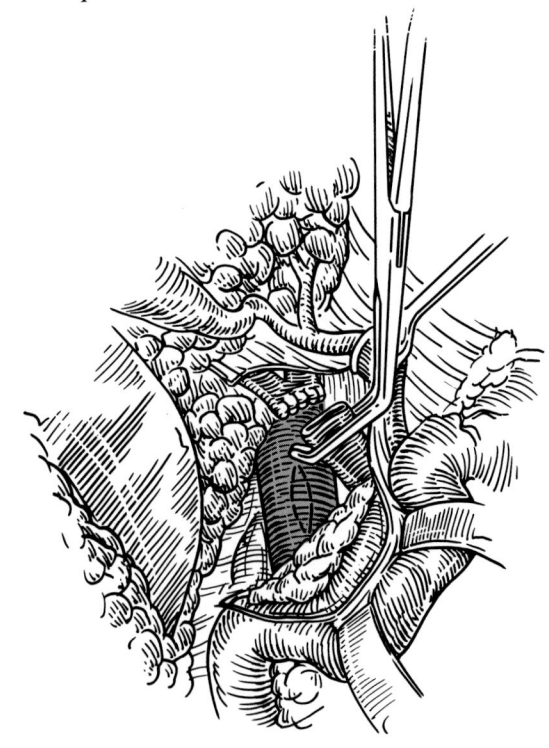

Figure 23-IIIA-5

End-to-Side Portacaval Shunt

The superior end of the portal vein is oversewn. The superior mesenteric end is brought
down for an end-to-side anastomosis to the partially occluded inferior vena cava.

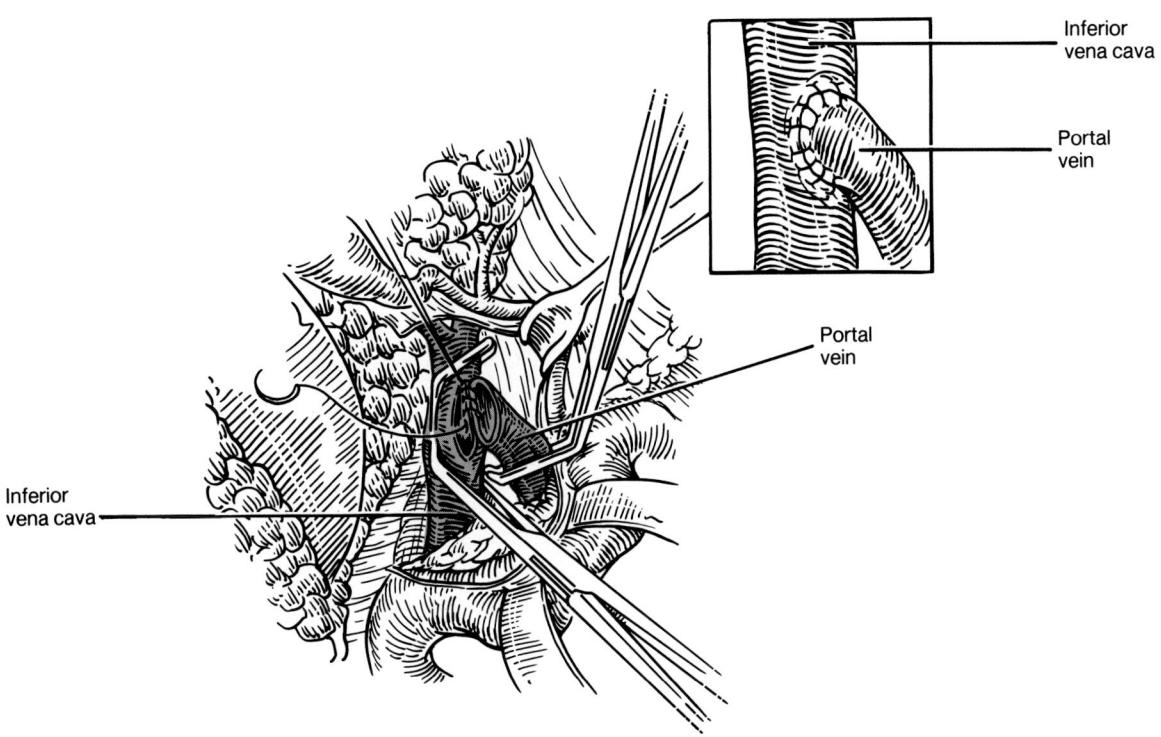

Figure 23-IIIA-6

Anastomosis for an End-to-Side Portacaval Shunt

It is important that sufficient portal vein is isolated and that it is angled correctly to come down to the vena cava without kinking. A button of inferior vena cava, about the diameter of the portal vein, is excised. Two continuous sutures of 4-0 or 5-0 polypropylene are used. The inset shows the completed anastomosis.

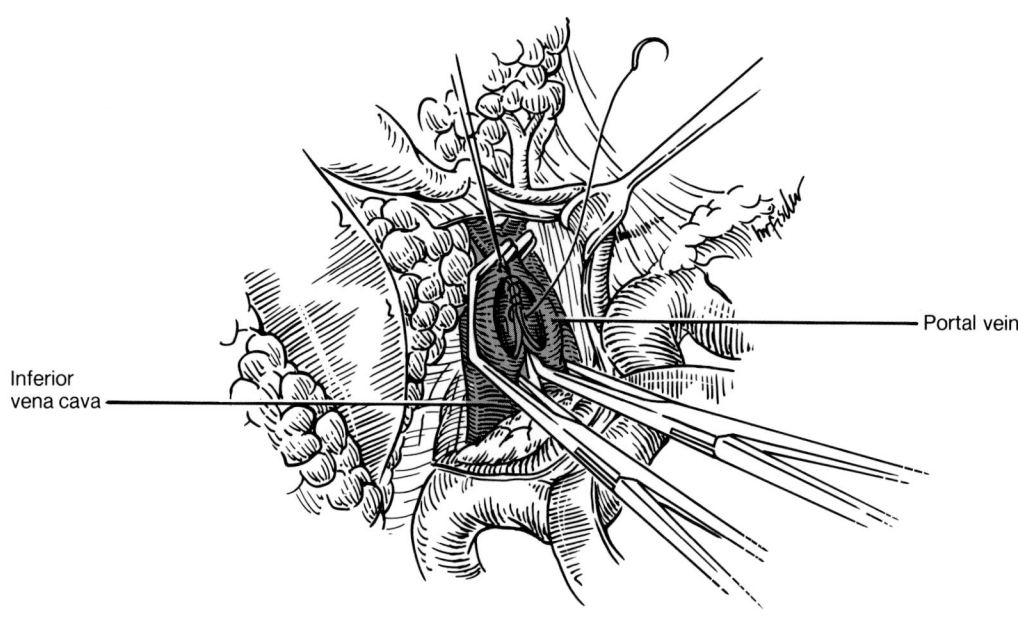

Inferior
vena cava

Portal vein

Figure 23-IIIA-7

Side-to-Side Portacaval Shunt

Following the same dissection as for an end-to-side portacaval shunt, the portal vein is not divided but is anastomosed side to side to the inferior vena cava. More extensive mobilization of the portal vein is required for a side-to-side than for an end-to-side portacaval shunt. When the distance between the portal vein and the vena cava is too great for a vein-to-vein anastomosis, or an enlarged caudate lobe is interposed between these two veins, interposition of a 12- to 16-mm reinforced polytetrafluoroethylene (PTFE; Gore-Tex) graft may be required.

B. Interposition Mesocaval Shunt

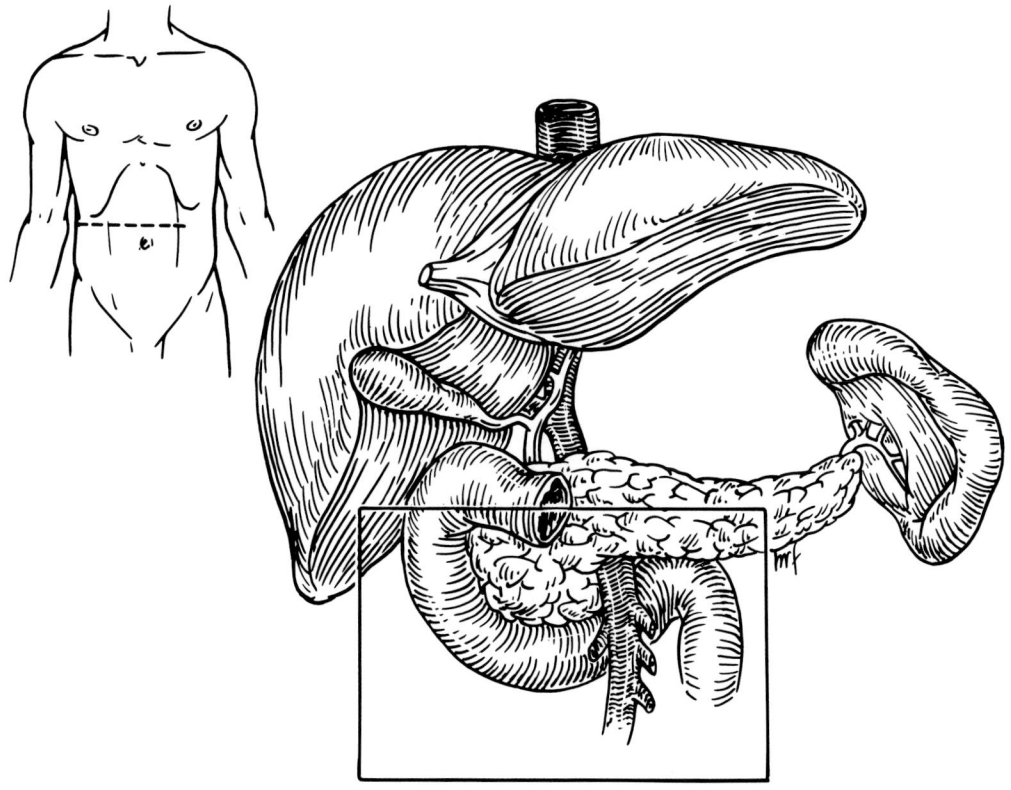

Figure 23-IIIB-1

Site of Dissection

Access for an interposition mesocaval shunt is gained through a right transverse supraumbilical incision (**inset**). The site of dissection is below the transverse mesocolon, approaching the superior mesenteric vein just below the pancreas, and the inferior vena cava behind the third portion of the duodenum.

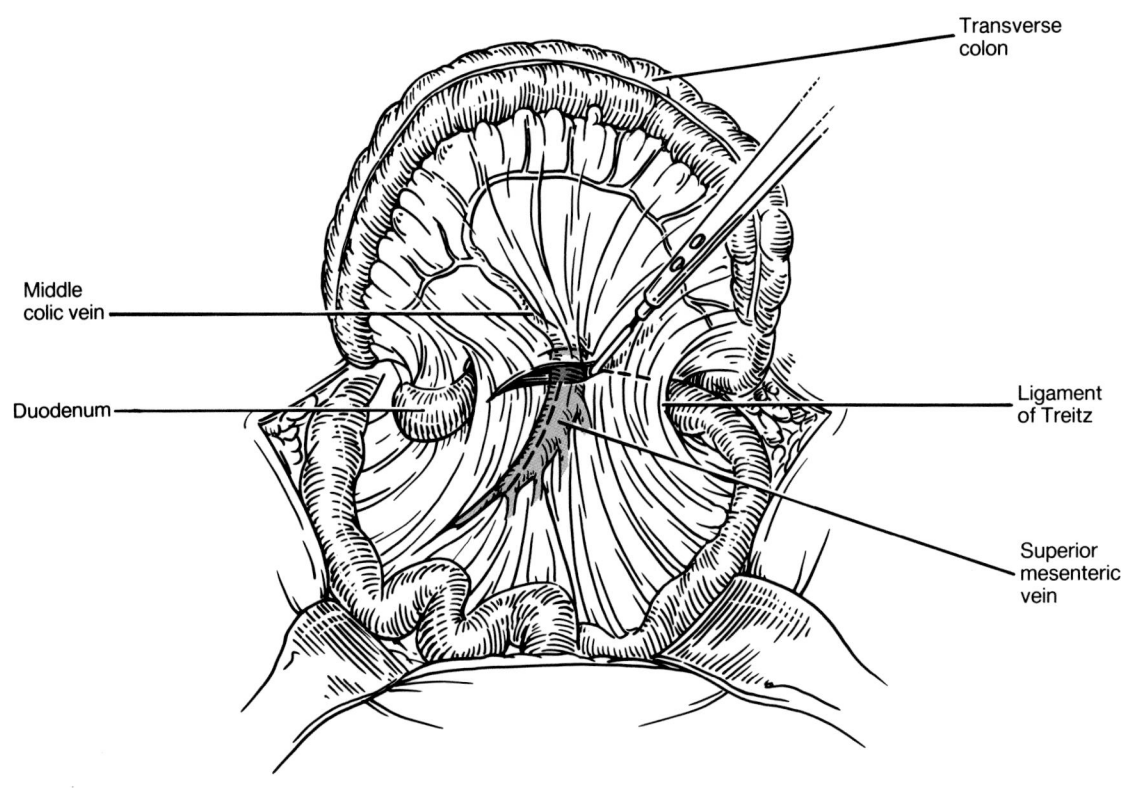

Figure 23-IIIB-2

Identification of Superior Mesenteric Vein

The superior mesenteric vein is identified at the base of the mesocolon. The middle colic vein often acts as a useful guide. Once the vein is identified, it needs to be isolated inferiorly (*dashed line*).

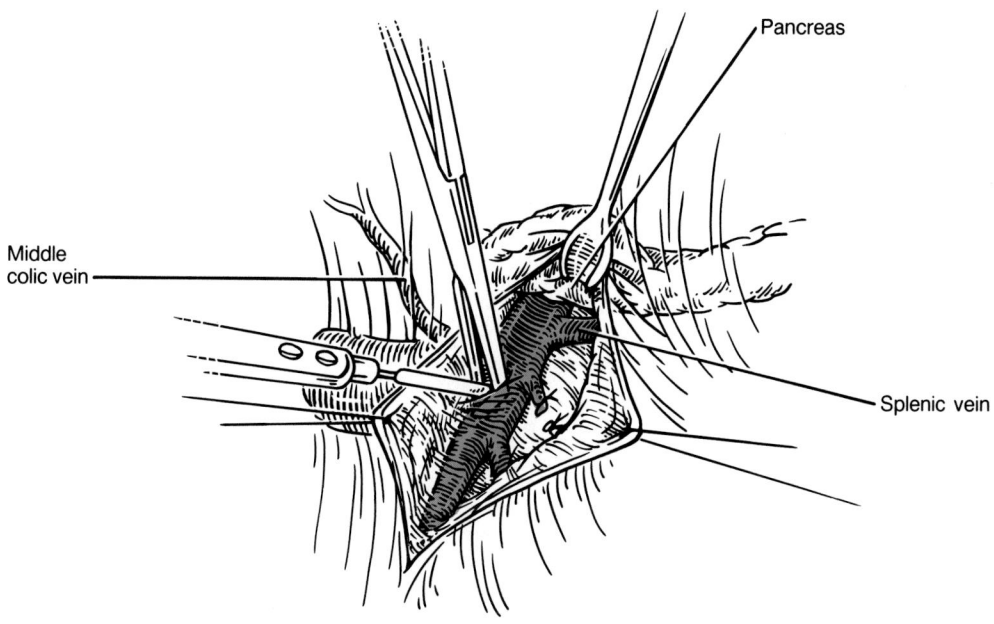

Figure 23-IIIB-3

Isolation of Superior Mesenteric Vein

The middle colic vein is divided, and the superior mesenteric vein is dissected behind the pancreas up to its junction with the splenic vein. The vein is dissected inferiorly over a sufficient length to allow complete isolation for subsequent partial occlusion with a Satinsky clamp. Some tributaries may need to be ligated.

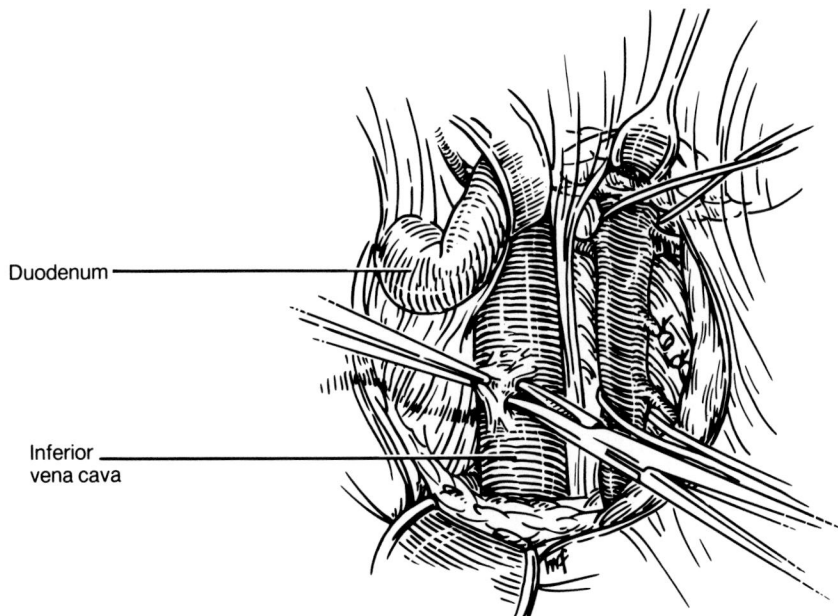

Figure 23-IIIB-4

Identification and Isolation of Inferior Vena Cava

The inferior vena cava is identified by mobilizing the third portion of the duodenum superiorly. Once identified in the retroperitoneum, the inferior vena cava is isolated over sufficient length to allow side clamping with a Satinsky clamp. The more that the duodenum can be mobilized superiorly, the higher the inferior vena cava can be isolated, and the shorter will be the graft between the inferior vena cava and the superior mesenteric vein.

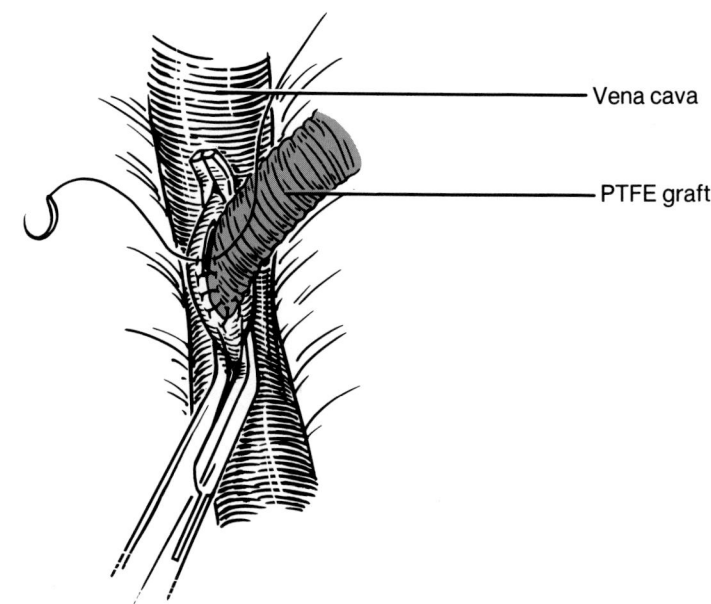

Vena cava

PTFE graft

Figure 23-IIIB-5

Inferior Vena Cava Anastomosis

A reinforced PTFE graft of a size to match the superior mesenteric vein is selected. This is usually 12 to 14 mm in diameter. The initial anastomosis is made to the inferior vena cava with a running 4-0 or 5-0 polypropylene suture. The use of polypropylene allows the graft to be telescoped down onto the inferior vena cava.

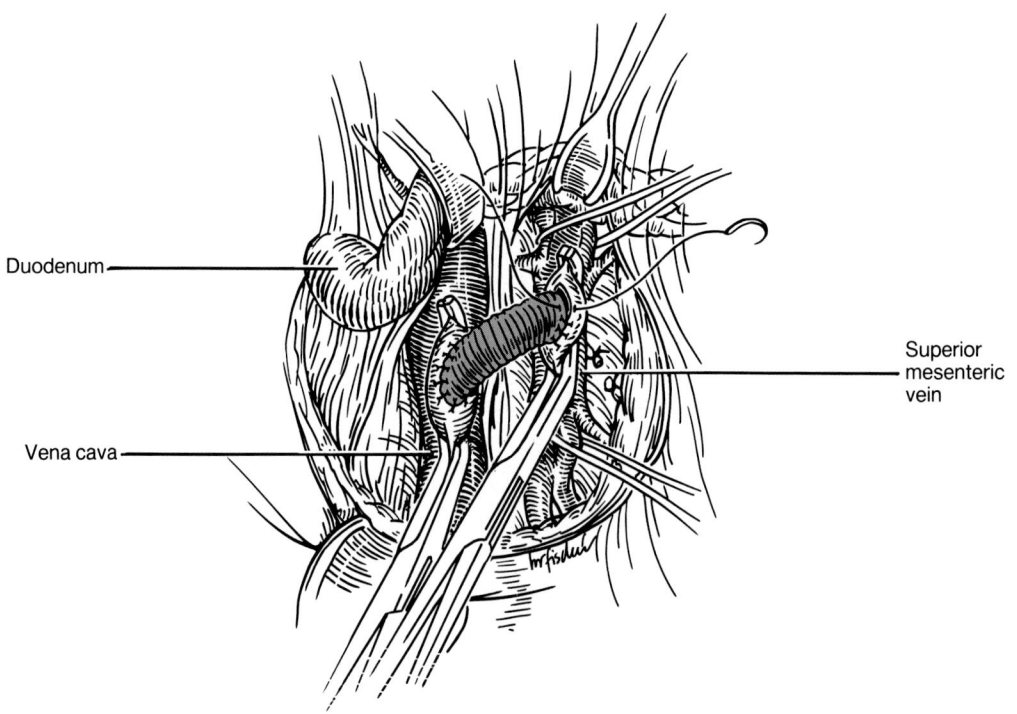

Duodenum

Superior mesenteric vein

Vena cava

Figure 23-IIIB-6

Completion of Mesocaval Shunt

The superior mesenteric vein is anastomosed to the beveled end of the graft with a running 4-0 or 5-0 polypropylene suture. The graft is made as short as possible with a gentle C curve to the inferior vena cava. The anastomosis is made into the right side of the superior mesenteric vein.

C. Distal Splenorenal Shunt

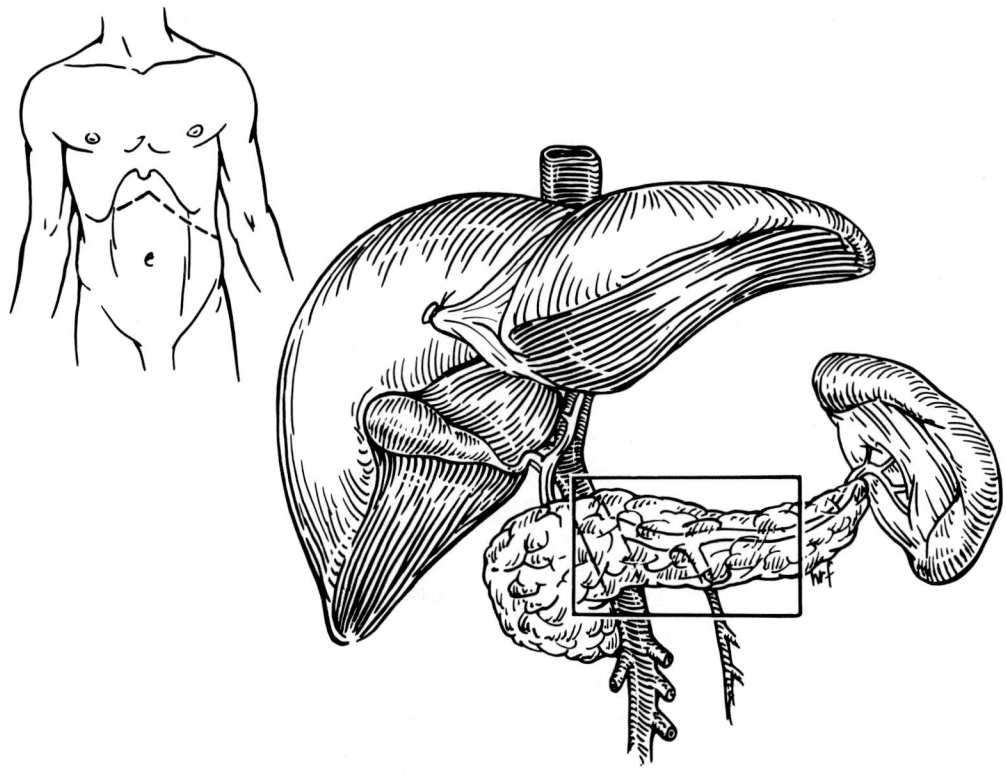

Figure 23-IIIC-1

Incision and Site of Dissection

Access is by a left subcostal incision extended across the midline and right rectus muscle
(**inset**). The falciform ligament is ligated and divided close to the liver to interrupt a
recanalized umbilical vein, if present. The area of dissection for the distal splenorenal
shunt is through the lesser sac by taking down the gastrocolic omentum to identify the
pancreas and then dissecting on its inferior and posterior surface.

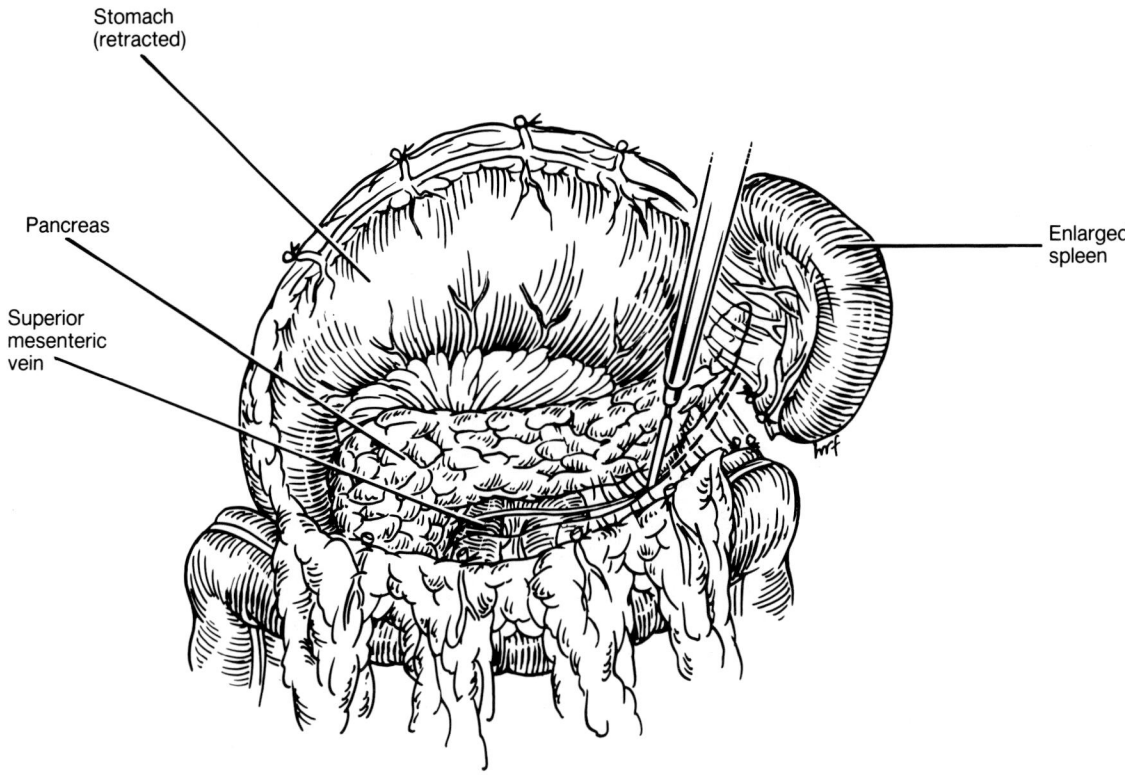

Stomach (retracted)

Pancreas

Superior mesenteric vein

Enlarged spleen

Figure 23-IIIC-2

Exposure of Pancreas

The gastrocolic omentum has been taken down from the pylorus to the short gastric vessels, which must be carefully preserved. In addition, the splenic flexure of the colon is taken down from the spleen to allow access to the tail of the pancreas. The right gastro-epiploic vein is ligated and divided.

   The peritoneum at the inferior border of the pancreas is incised from the superior mesenteric vessels to the splenic hilus. This allows the pancreas to be fully mobilized and turned up on its side.

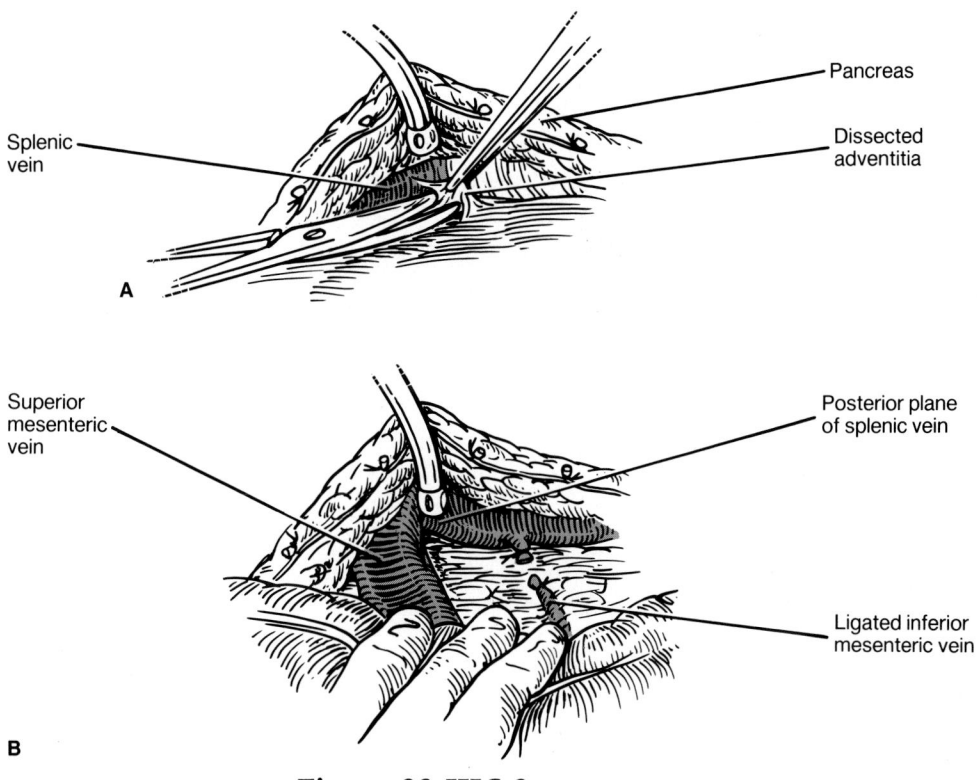

Figure 23-IIIC-3

Dissection of Splenic Vein

(**A**) The splenic vein is identified on the posterior surface of the pancreas. Dissection is carried out directly on the vein by incising the overlying adventitia. The safest initial plane to dissect is the inferior and posterior surface of the splenic vein.

(**B**) The splenic vein is dissected to its junction with the superior mesenteric vein. The inferior mesenteric vein is identified, ligated, and divided. The splenic vein should be fully dissected at its junction with the portal vein where it will be encircled; the initial plane of dissection is the posterior plane.

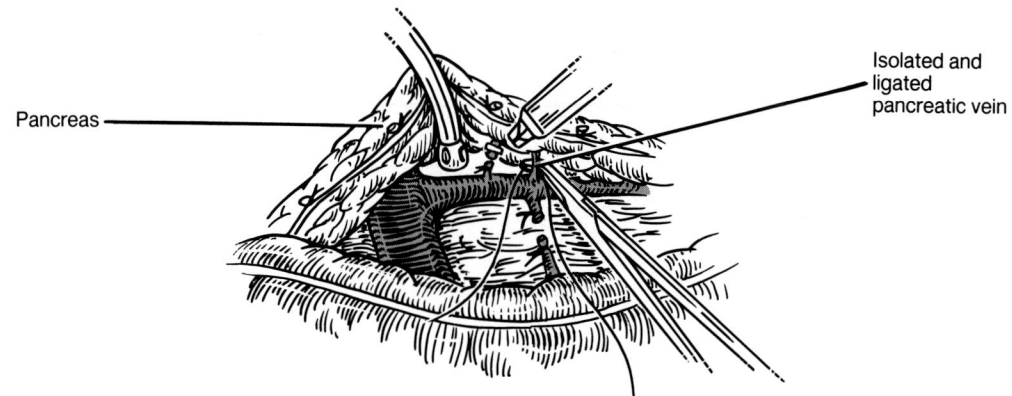

Figure 23-IIIC-4

Dissection of Pancreatic Vein Tributaries

Pancreatic venous tributaries into the splenic vein require delicate dissection. These are isolated from the pancreas by dissecting the tissue at right angles to the splenic vein with a fine-pointed clamp. Once the tributaries are isolated, a 3-0 silk tie is placed on the splenic vein side and a small clip on the pancreatic side.

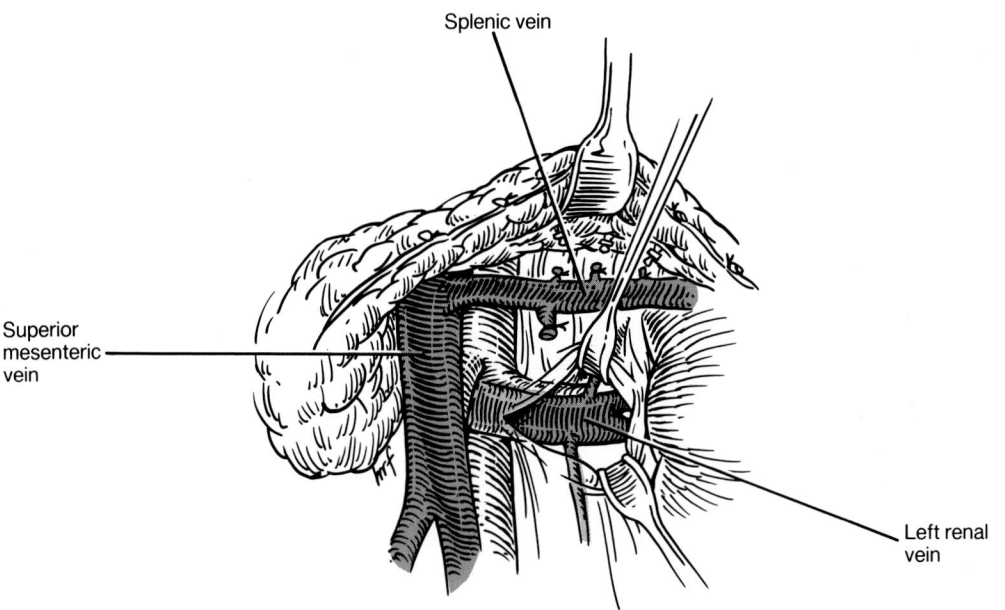

Figure 23-IIIC-5

Identification and Dissection of Left Renal Vein

The left renal vein is identified in the retroperitoneum. This is aided by preoperative left renal venography. This vein is dissected sufficiently to allow its partial occlusion with a Satinsky clamp. The left adrenal vein is ligated and divided. The gonadal vein is left intact.

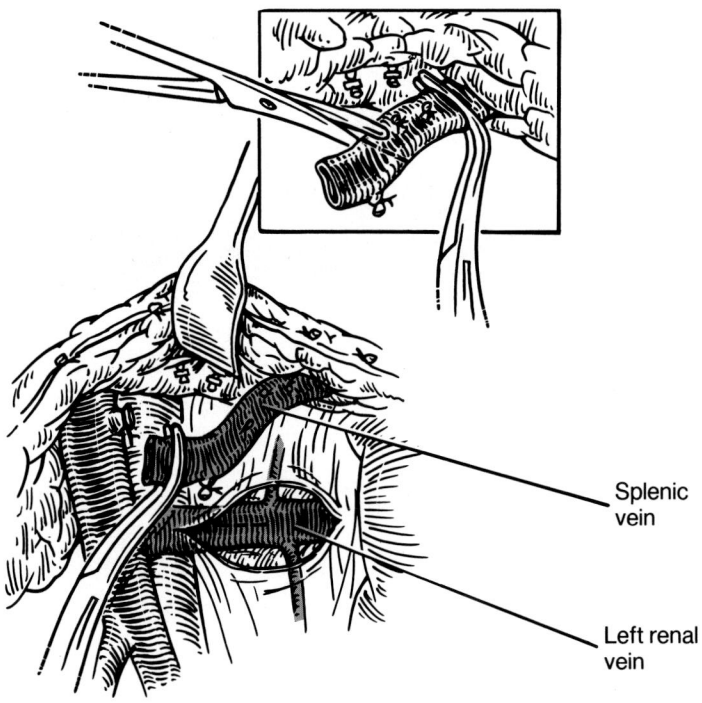

Splenic
vein

Left renal
vein

Figure 23-IIIC-6

Ligation of Splenic Vein

The splenic vein is ligated flush with the portal vein with a single ligature, and a large Ligaclip is placed on the portal vein side of that tie. The length of splenic vein to be used for anastomosis is that which comes down comfortably to the left renal vein without kinking or tension. The splenic vein should be trimmed on an angle to maximize the size of the anastomosis (**inset**).

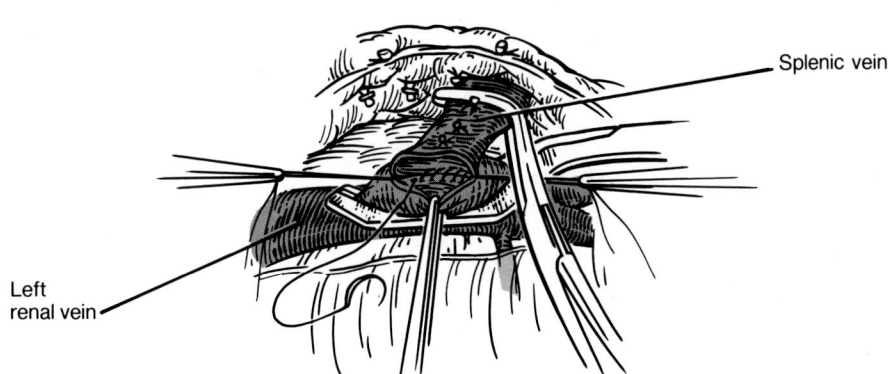

Splenic vein

Left
renal vein

Figure 23-IIIC-7

Left Renal Vein Anastomosis

After a Satinsky clamp is placed on the left renal vein, the vein is opened. The posterior anastomosis is sewn on the inside with stay sutures of 5-0 polypropylene at either end. Knots are placed exteriorly.

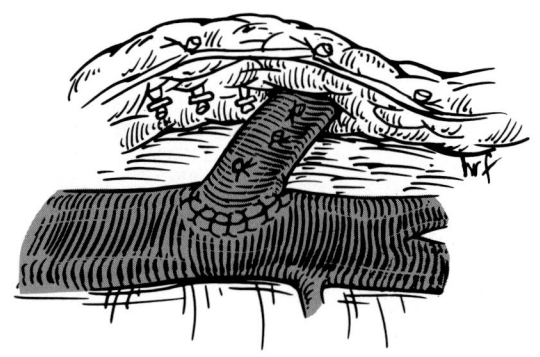

Figure 23-IIIC-8

Suture Placement

The anterior part of the anastomosis is completed with interrupted sutures. When the splenic vein is greater than 10 mm in diameter, a running suture may be used for the anterior anastomosis.

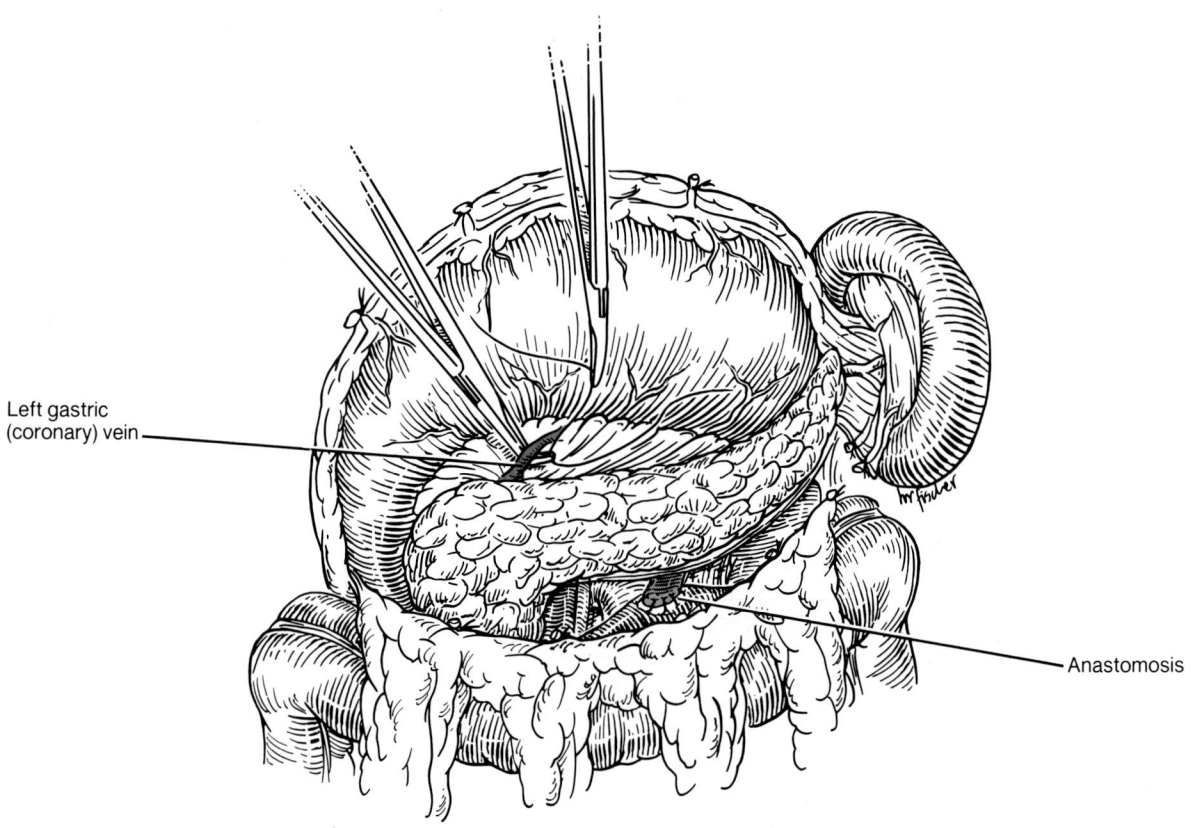

Left gastric (coronary) vein

Anastomosis

Figure 23-IIIC-9

Completion of the Procedure

The operation is completed by dividing the left gastric (coronary) vein above the pancreas as it travels toward the lesser curvature of the stomach. This is a component of the disconnection of portal and splenic systems. When accessible, the coronary vein is also ligated at its entrance into the proximal portal vein or the distal splenic vein.

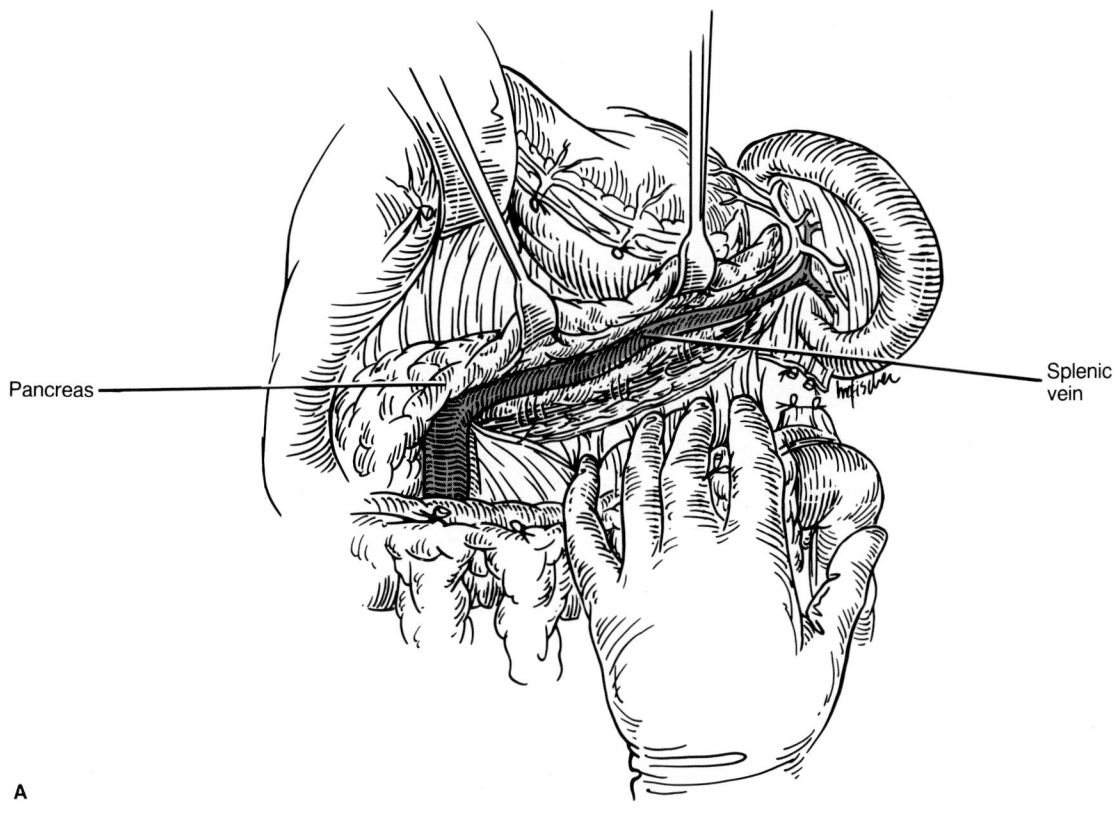

Pancreas

Splenic
vein

A

Figure 23-IIIC-10

Distal Splenorenal Shunt With Entire Splenopancreatic Disconnection

In patients with alcoholic cirrhosis, complete dissection of the splenic vein from the pancreas before its anastomosis to the left renal vein helps prevent the development of portaprival collaterals through the pancreas from the portal vein. The result is a more effective preservation of portal blood flow to the liver.

(**A**) The full extent of dissection of the splenic vein that must be achieved.

(Continued)

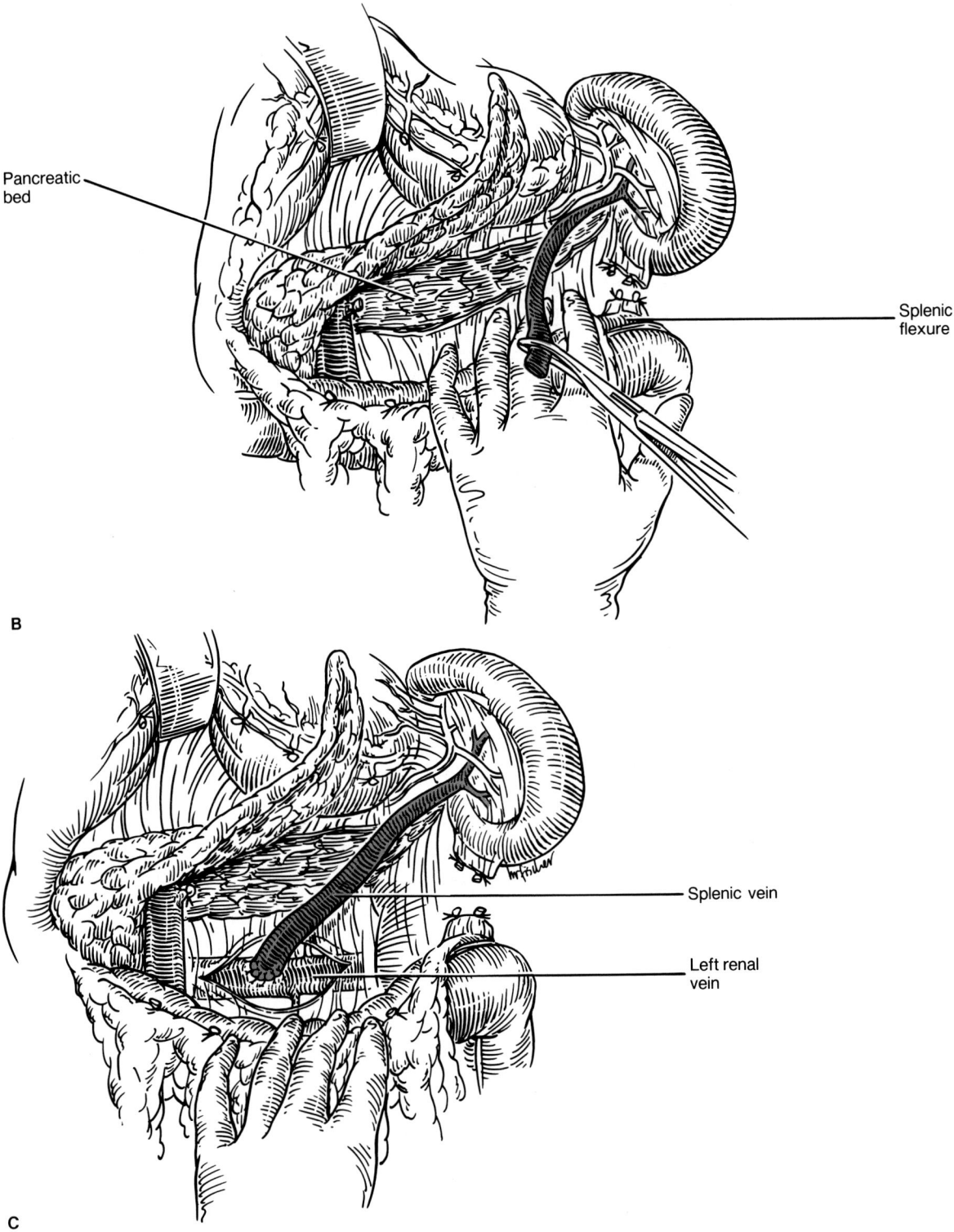

Pancreatic bed

Splenic flexure

B

Splenic vein

Left renal vein

C

Figure 23-IIIC-10 *(Continued)*

(B) The entire splenic vein has been dissociated from the pancreas before the construction of the shunt.

(C) The completed anastomosis for a distal splenorenal shunt with splenopancreatic disconnection.

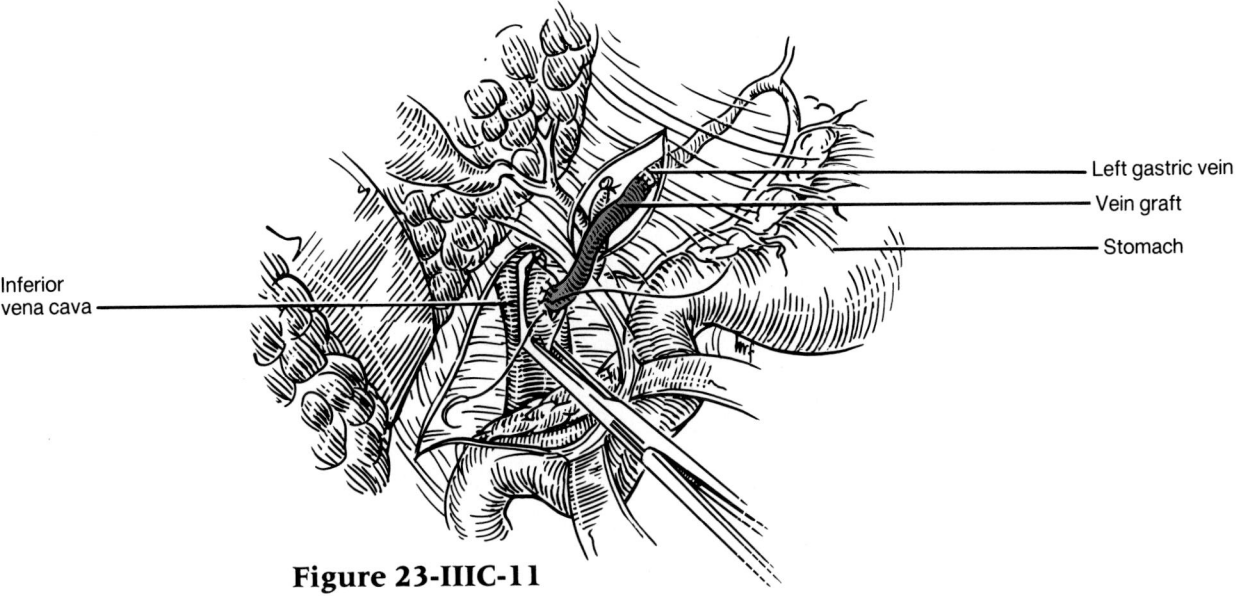

Figure 23-IIIC-11

Coronary Caval Shunt

This selective shunt decompresses gastroesophageal varices through the left gastric vein. A vein graft is interposed between the left gastric vein and the inferior vena cava just below the liver. Saphenous vein can be used for the interposition graft.

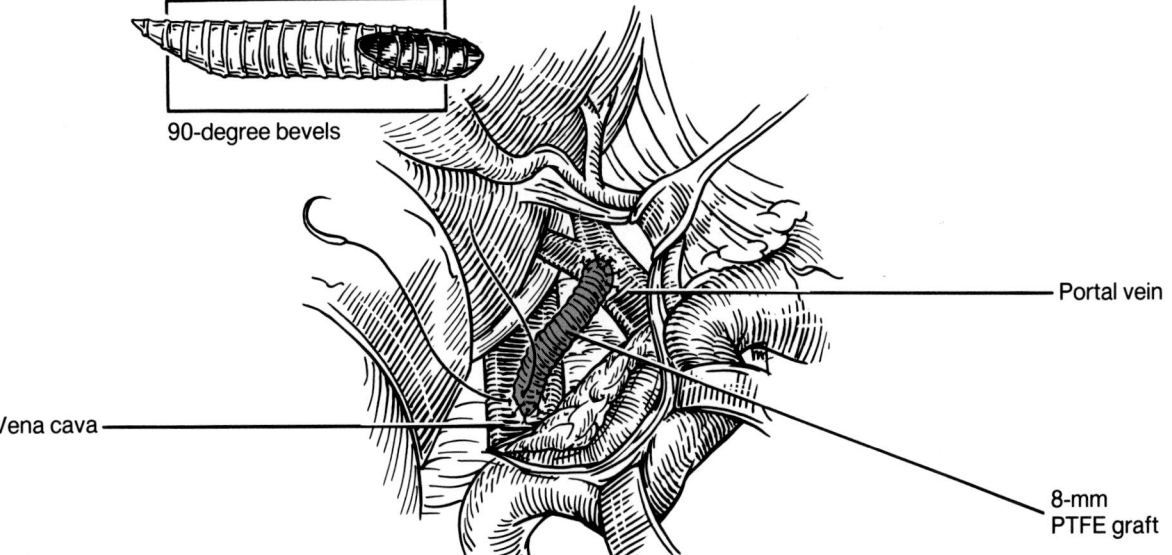

Figure 23-IIIC-12

Small-Bore Interposition H-Graft

When a ribbed polytetrafluoroethylene graft 8 mm in diameter is used for an interposition side-to-side portacaval anastomosis, partial rather than complete portal decompression results. It reduces the portal pressure to about 12 mmHg and maintains some prograde portal flow in 80% of patients. The dissection and exposure for this operation are identical to that described for the portacaval shunt. The graft should be 3 to 5 cm in length, with the end bevels cut at 90 degrees to each other, which conforms to the caval and portal angles of anastomosis (**inset**). To minimize shunt thrombosis, the graft is soaked in a heparin solution before use.

D. Gastroesophageal Devascularization Operation

The following sequence describes an intraabdominal gastroesophageal devascularization operation (modified Sugiura procedure).

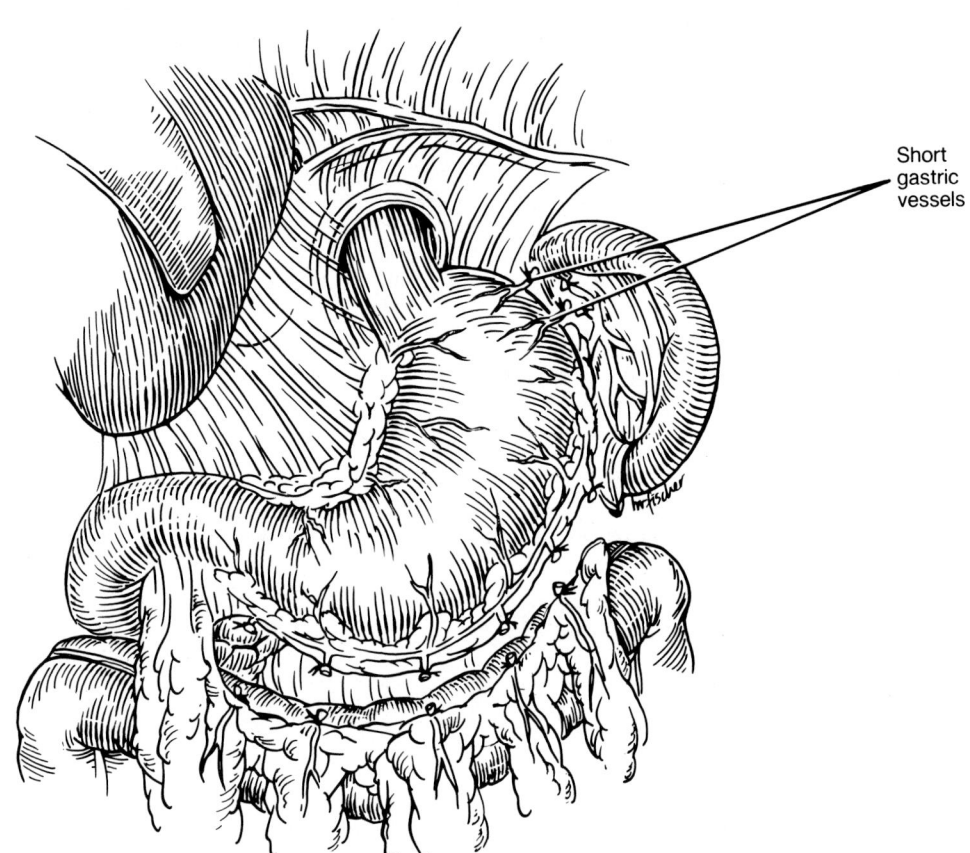

Short gastric vessels

Figure 23-IIID-1

Splenectomy and Devascularization

The spleen is removed, and the proximal two thirds of the greater curve is devascularized.

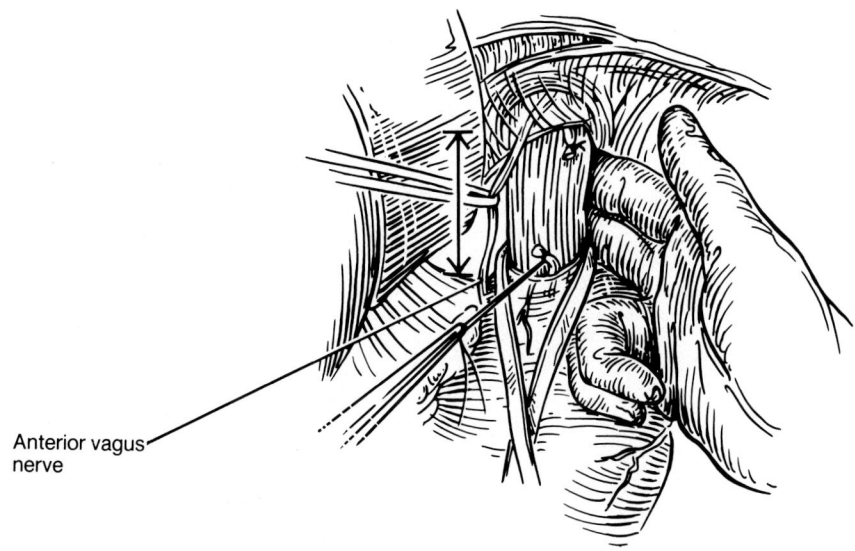

Anterior vagus
nerve

Figure 23-IIID-2

Isolation and Dissection of Esophagus

The esophagus is then isolated. The vagus nerves are identified and retracted to the right. The esophagus should be dissected for 7 cm above the gastroesophageal junction. Particular attention is paid to the posterior surface of the esophagus, where significant penetrating veins may be identified. These should be interrupted.

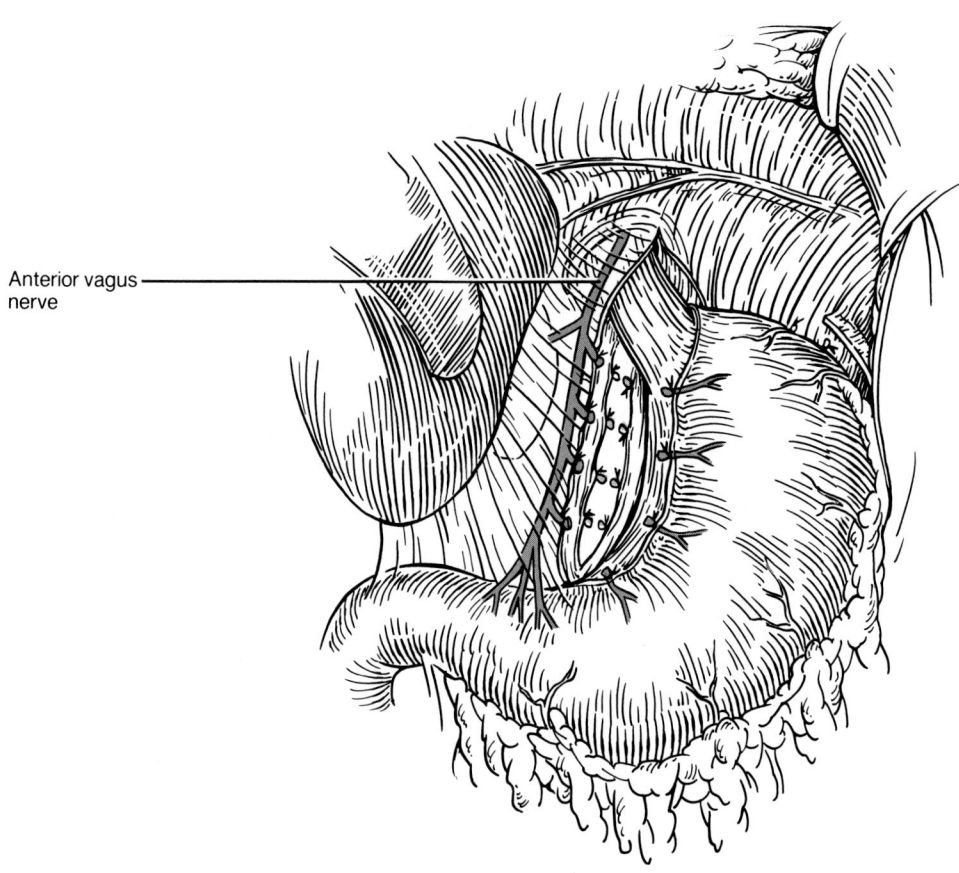

Anterior vagus
nerve

Figure 23-IIID-3

Further Devascularization

With the vagus nerves retracted to the right, the lesser curve is devascularized to 6 cm from the pylorus. This follows the same principles as a highly selective vagotomy, except that the objective is interruption of venous inflow to gastric and esophageal varices. The left gastric vein and paraesophageal collaterals are preserved to maintain portosystemic collateralization and discourage reformation of varices.

Anterior vagus
nerve

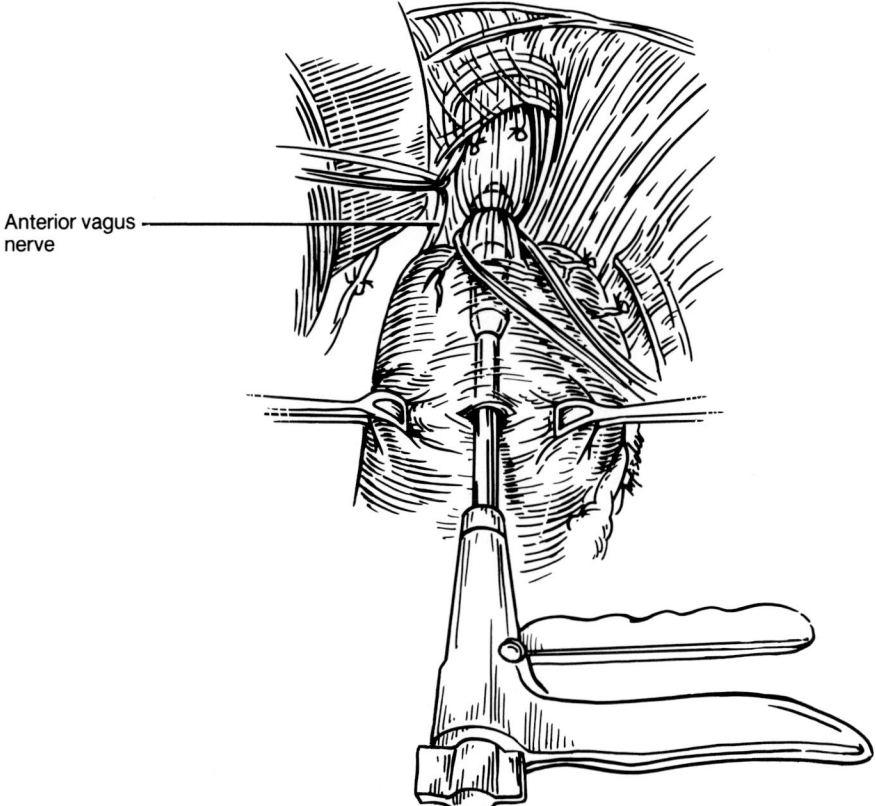

Figure 23-IIID-4

Esophageal Transection

This operation may or may not be combined with esophageal transection. When esophageal transection is a component of the procedure, it can be accomplished with an EEA stapler, which is introduced in the mid-body of the stomach with the anvil placed in the distal 2 cm of the esophagus. The esophagus is tied into the anvil for firing of the stapler, which divides and reanastomoses the esophagus. All intramural varices are interrupted.

In some centers, esophageal transection alone is performed in the management of acute variceal bleeding. In this situation, extensive gastroesophageal devascularization and splenectomy may be omitted, and simple esophageal transection with ligation of the left gastric vein above the pancreas is performed.

SECTION IV   Liver Transplantation

A. Recipient Hepatectomy

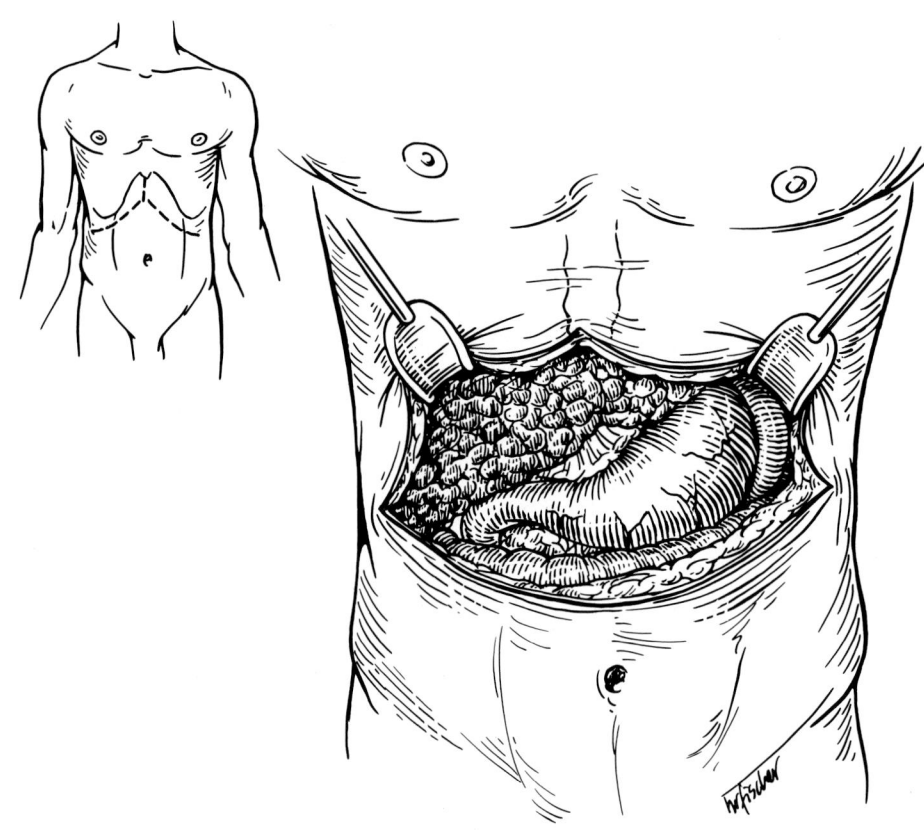

Figure 23-IVA-1

Incision and Exposure

Access is by a bilateral subcostal incision with a midline extension to the xiphoid (**inset**).
Exposure is enhanced by fixed retractors pulling the costal margins upward and outward.

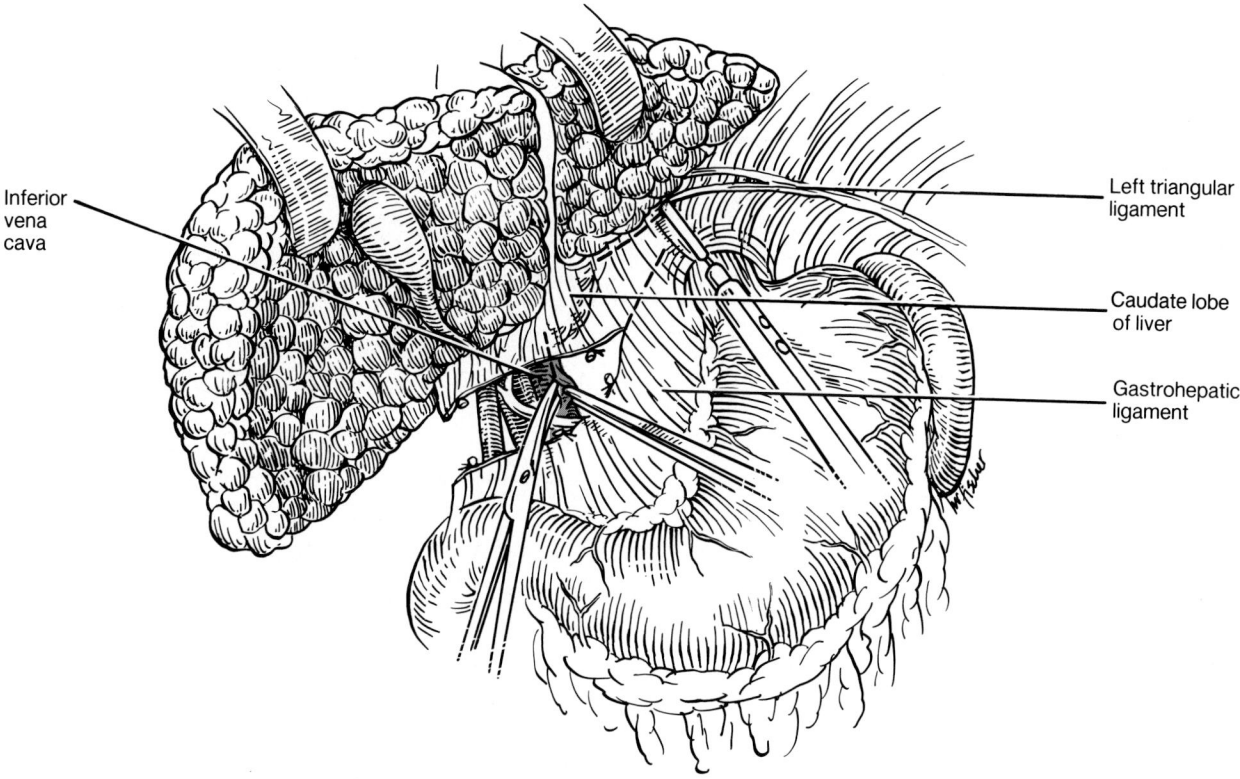

Inferior
vena
cava

Left triangular
ligament

Caudate lobe
of liver

Gastrohepatic
ligament

Figure 23-IVA-2

Mobilization of Left Side of Liver

Mobilization for hepatectomy is achieved by opening the gastrohepatic ligament and dividing it up to the diaphragm. The left triangular ligament is taken down and dissected across to the left hepatic vein and the suprahepatic inferior vena cava.

At this juncture, or later in the dissection, the left side of the inferior vena cava can be identified, the overlying adventitia opened, and the left side of the retrohepatic vena cava dissected up to the diaphragm. This maneuver declares the posterior plane of dissection to the suprahepatic vena cava.

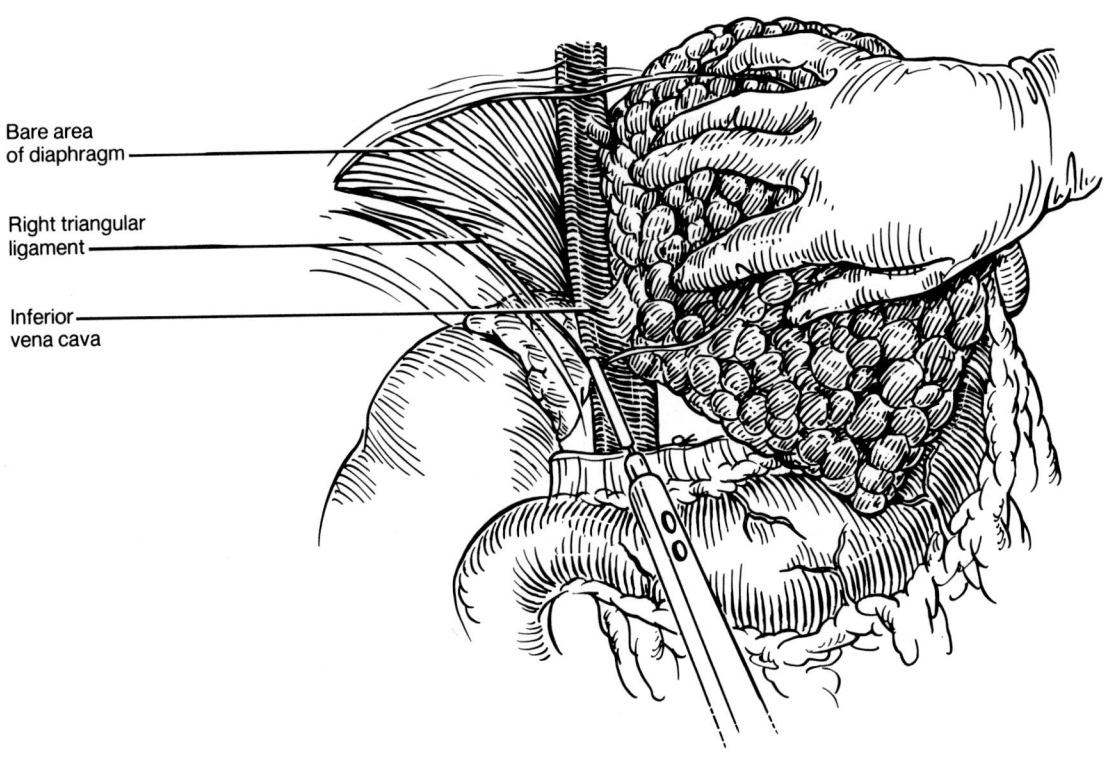

Bare area
of diaphragm

Right triangular
ligament

Inferior
vena cava

Figure 23-IVA-3

Mobilization of Right Side of Liver

Adhesions usually need to be taken down along the inferior border of the right lobe, particularly if there has been a prior cholecystectomy. The right triangular ligament is taken down by dissection along the superior and inferior leaves. The difficulty of this dissection varies depending on its adherence to the diaphragm. Ultimately, the right lobe needs to be fully mobilized to the retrohepatic vena cava. The right adrenal vein should be identified, ligated, and divided.

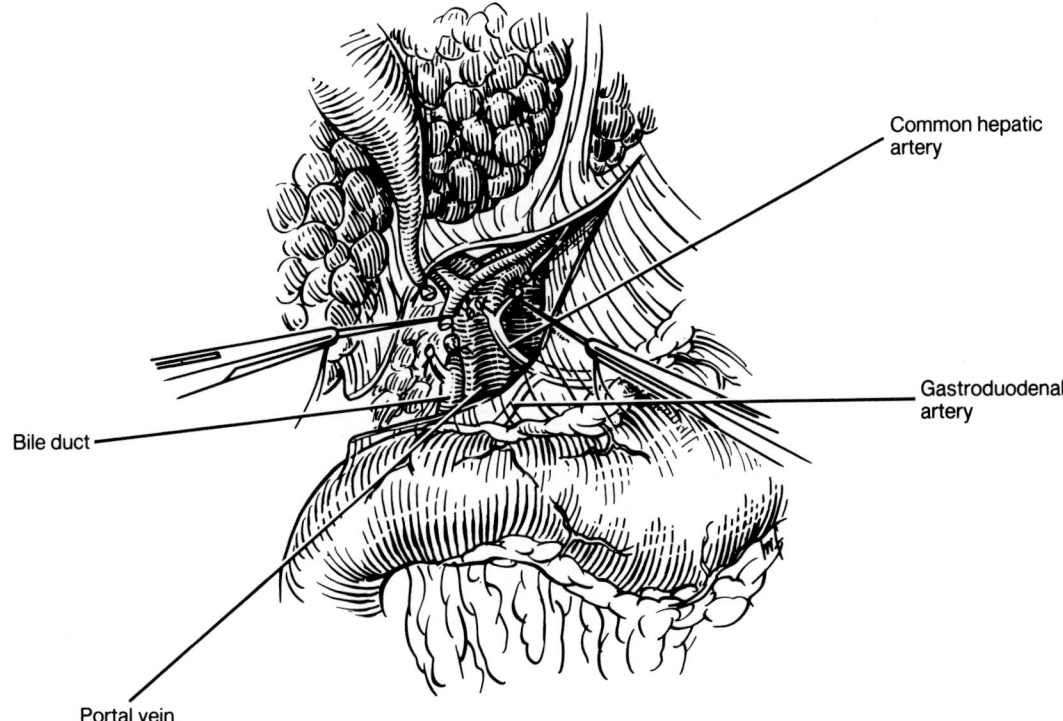

Common hepatic
artery

Gastroduodenal
artery

Bile duct

Portal vein

Figure 23-IVA-4

Hilar Dissection

The essential components of hilar dissection are to identify, isolate, and prepare for subsequent anastomosis a usable portal vein. Other objectives of hilar dissection are to identify, isolate, and prepare a good hepatic arterial inflow and a bile duct suitable for subsequent reconstruction.

The hepatic artery is usually initially identified and dissected high into the hilus, with the right and left branches being divided. Retrograde dissection to identify the common hepatic arterial trunk and the origin of the gastroduodenal artery, which may prove a suitable bifurcation for subsequent anastomosis, should be done.

The portal vein should be dissected to its bifurcation and all overlying adventitia removed from it. The portal vein is left intact until ready for cross-clamping or cannulation for venovenous bypass.

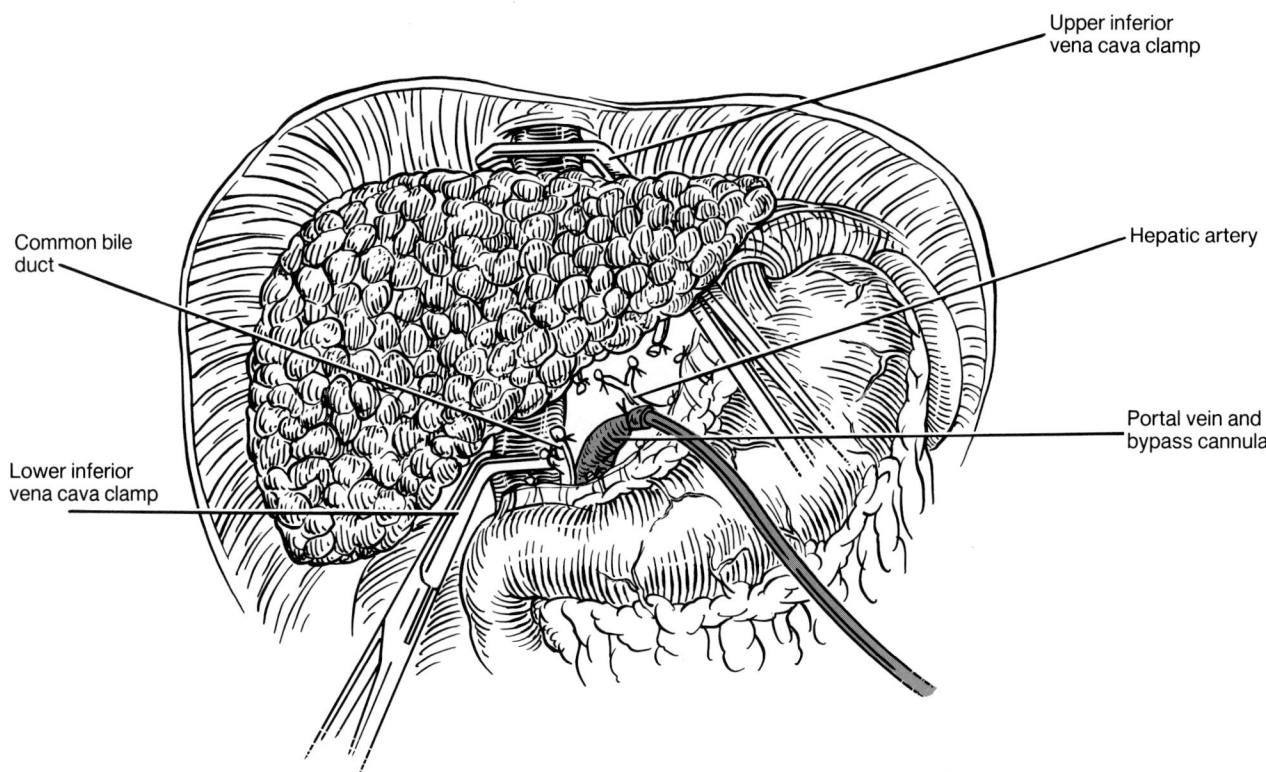

Upper inferior
vena cava clamp

Hepatic artery

Portal vein and
bypass cannula

Common bile
duct

Lower inferior
vena cava clamp

Figure 23-IVA-5

Completion of Hepatectomy

The final steps in preparation for recipient hepatectomy are isolation of the inferior vena cava above and below the liver. This requires accurately identifying and removing overlying adventitia and encircling these structures before cross-clamping. The closer the dissection is on the vena cava, the less bleeding there will be in the retroperitoneum.

If venovenous bypass is being used, a catheter is placed retrograde into the portal vein, as illustrated here. Vena caval drainage is achieved with a catheter placed through the saphenofemoral junction in the groin and advanced to the inferior vena cava. A centrifugal pump with an axillary vein return completes the bypass during the anhepatic phase. Alternatively, some surgeons prefer to proceed to hepatectomy without bypass if the patient is hemodynamically stable.

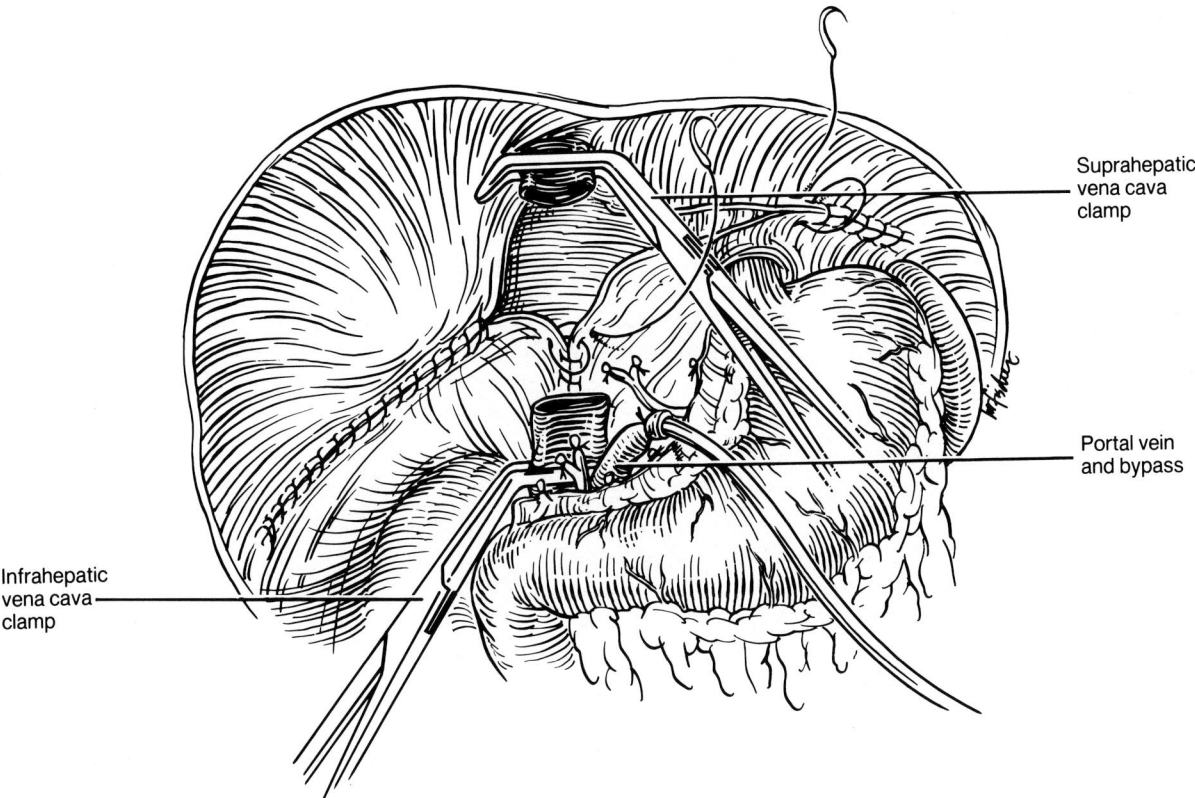

Suprahepatic
vena cava
clamp

Portal vein
and bypass

Infrahepatic
vena cava
clamp

Figure 23-IVA-6

Hemostasis During Anhepatic Phase

After cross-clamping, the liver is dissected off the retrohepatic vena cava. If a piggy-back caval anastomosis is preferred, the vena cava is left intact, and the donor cava is sewn to the hepatic venous orifices. As illustrated here, the retrohepatic vena cava has been excised with the development of appropriate suprahepatic and infrahepatic caval cuffs. The bare area of the diaphragm is electrocoagulated for hemostasis and can be closed with a running suture, as illustrated in this figure. Time spent on hemostasis at this juncture will reap benefits once the new liver has been sewn in and the clamps removed.

B. Implantation of Donor Liver

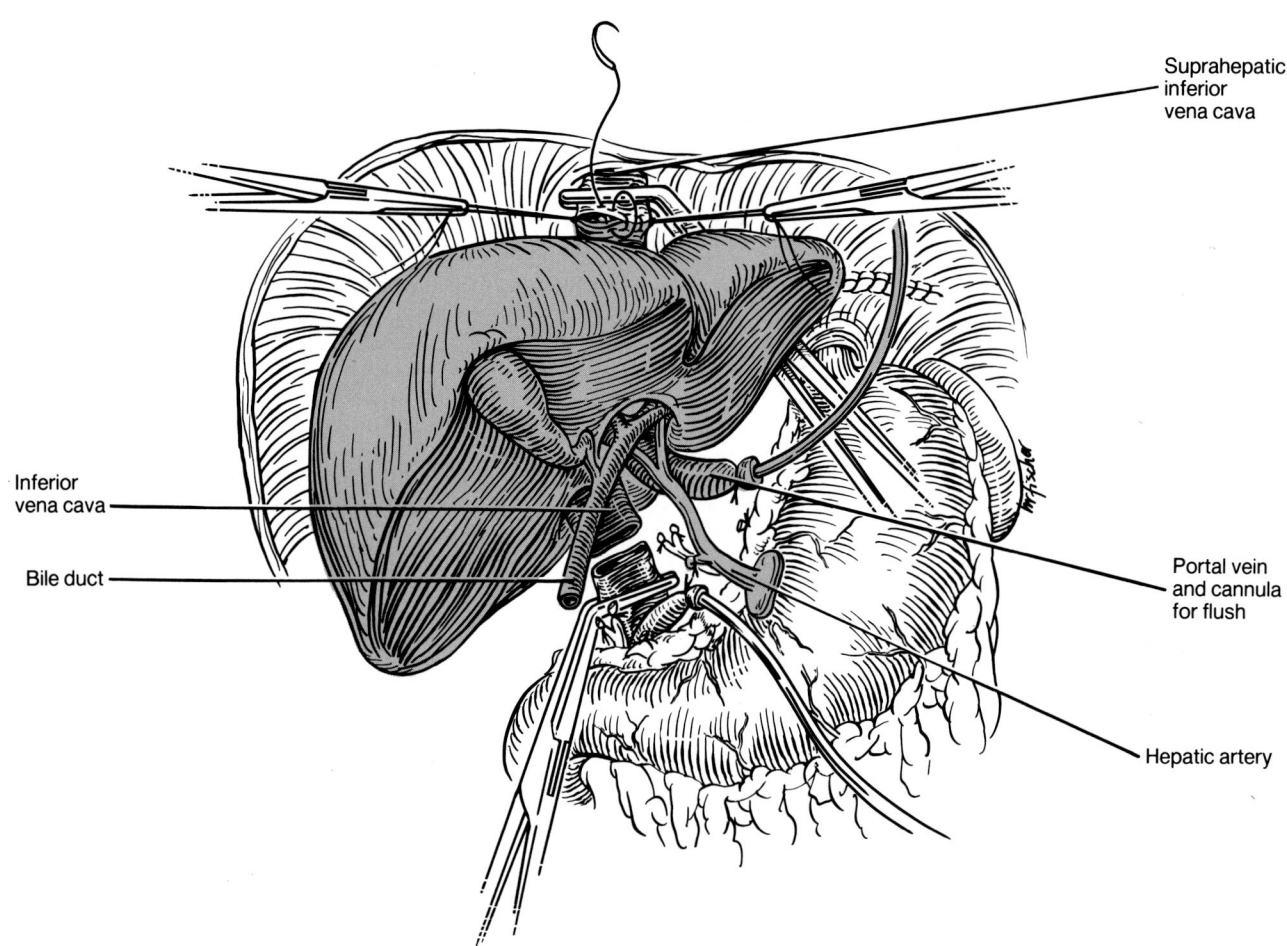

Suprahepatic
inferior
vena cava

Inferior
vena cava

Bile duct

Portal vein
and cannula
for flush

Hepatic artery

Figure 23-IVB-1

Suprahepatic Caval Anastomosis

The initial anastomosis is the suprahepatic caval anastomosis, which is sewn with a running 3–0 polypropylene suture. Access to sew this anastomosis requires downward traction on the donor liver with the assistant's left hand. The alignment of other subsequent anastomoses is shown.

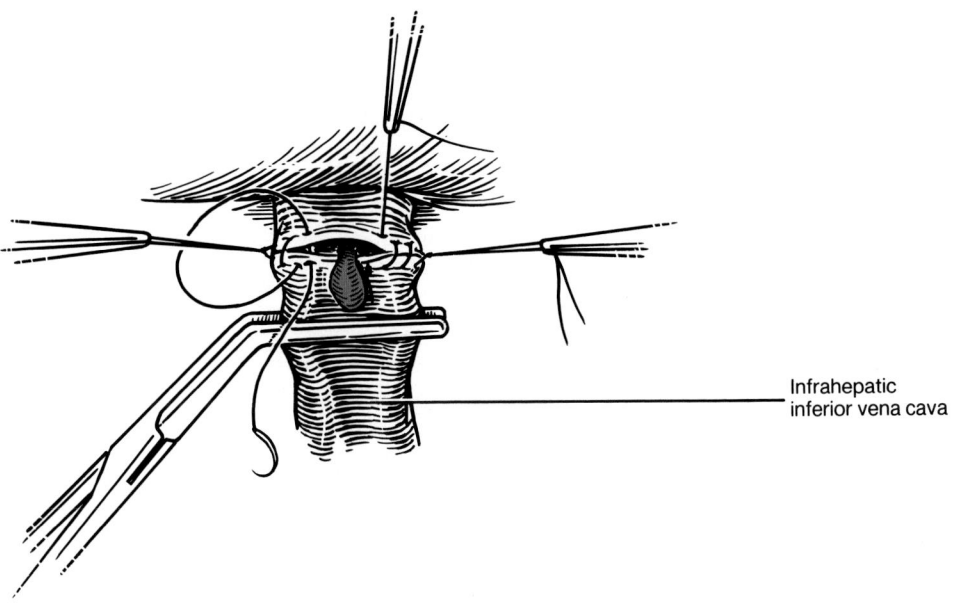

Figure 23-IVB-2

Completion of Infrahepatic Caval Anastomosis

The infrahepatic vena caval anastomosis is fashioned with running 4-0 polypropylene sutures. During this phase of implantation, the donor liver is flushed with a rinse solution to remove the preservative fluids. The drainage of this flush is through the infrahepatic caval anastomosis before its completion. Air from the major vessels is also removed with this flush.

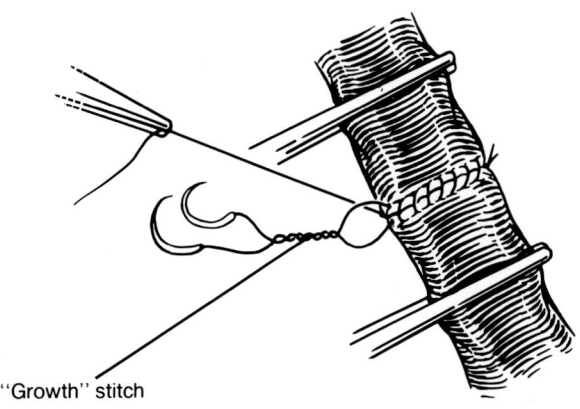

"Growth" stitch

Figure 23-IVB-3

Portal Venous Anastomosis

When venovenous bypass is being used, the portal vein catheter is removed before this anastomosis. Usually, the caval axillary bypass can be maintained at a somewhat reduced total flow. The donor and recipient portal veins are trimmed to an appropriate length before end-to-end anastomosis with a running 5-0 polypropylene suture. As illustrated in this figure, a "growth" stitch of the running polypropylene is left to allow expansion rather than stricture of the anastomosis.

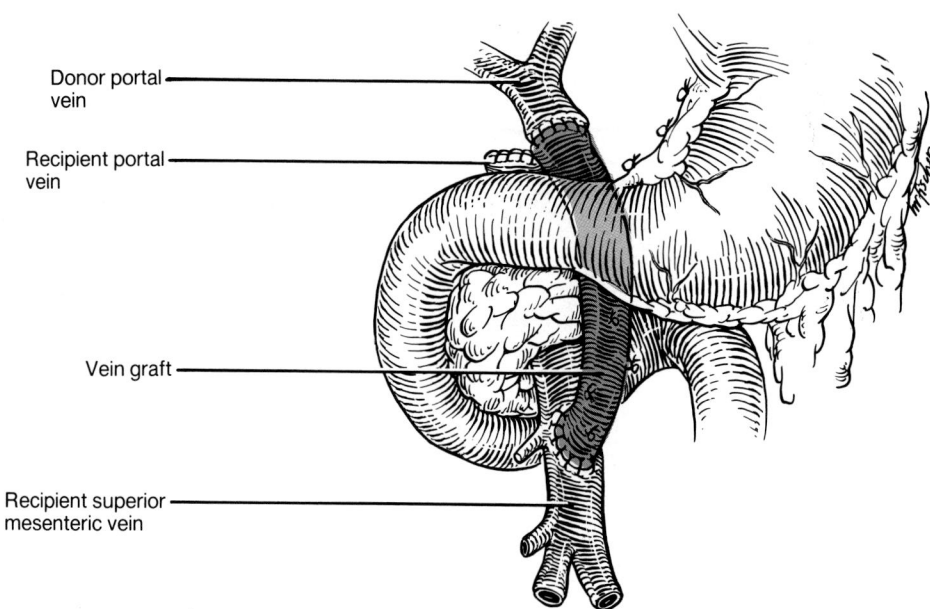

Donor portal vein

Recipient portal vein

Vein graft

Recipient superior mesenteric vein

Figure 23-IVB-4

Portal Venous Reconstruction Requiring a Graft to the Superior Mesenteric Vein

This figure illustrates a method for reconstruction when recipient portal vein thrombosis is present. A venous graft is interposed between the recipient superior mesenteric vein and the donor portal vein, running behind the stomach and anterior to the pancreas.

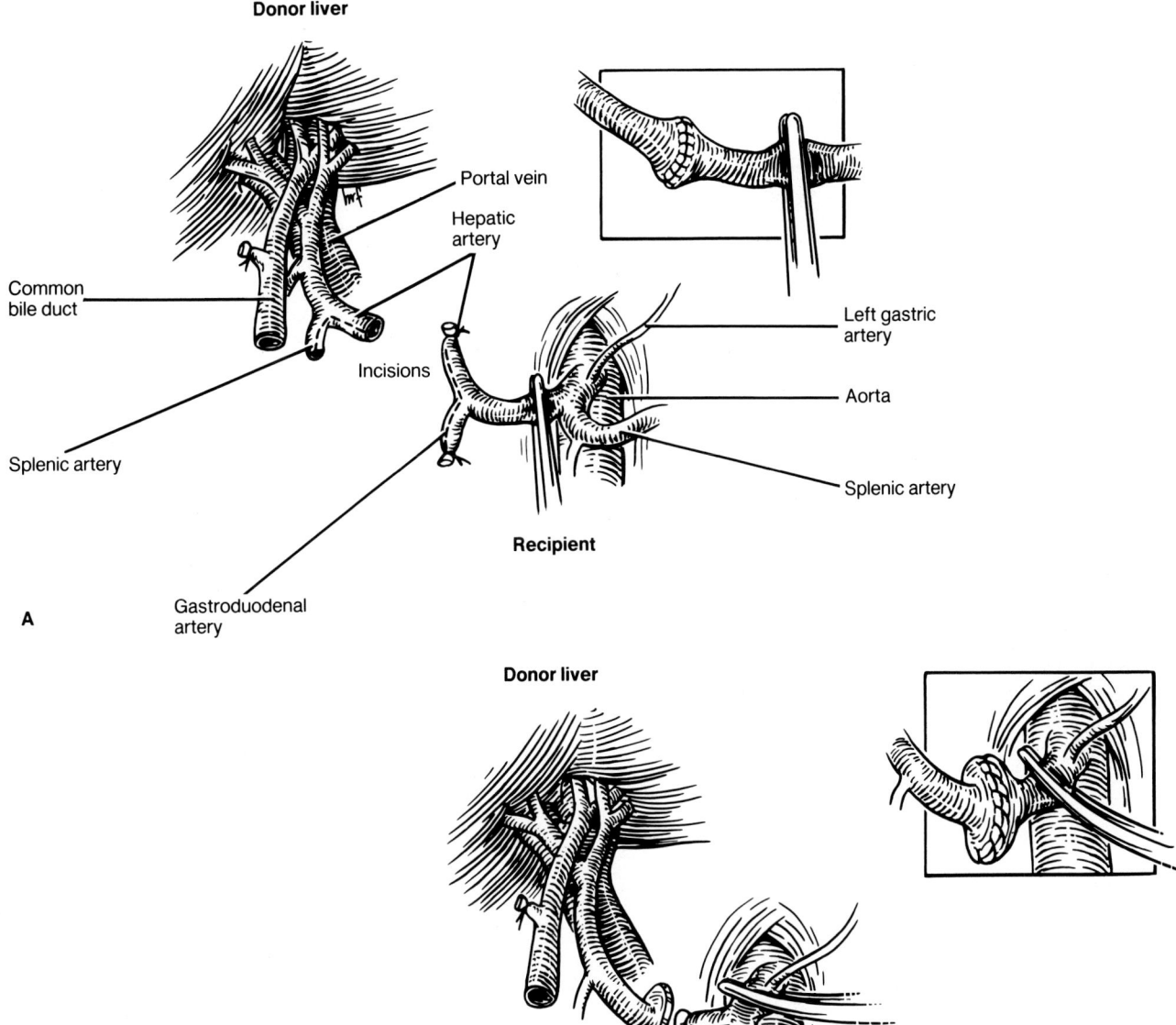

Figure 23-IVB-5

Hepatic Arterial Reconstructions

(**A**) Hepatic artery reconstruction using a Carrel patch of the donor celiac axis and splenic artery orifice to the recipient common hepatogastroduodenal artery bifurcation. The keys to a good arterial anastomosis are provision of an adequate arterial inflow and creation of an adequate-sized anastomosis.

(**B**) The same principle as in **A**, using a Carrel patch of the donor aorta at the celiac axis to the recipient common hepatic artery and splenic artery bifurcation.

(Continued)

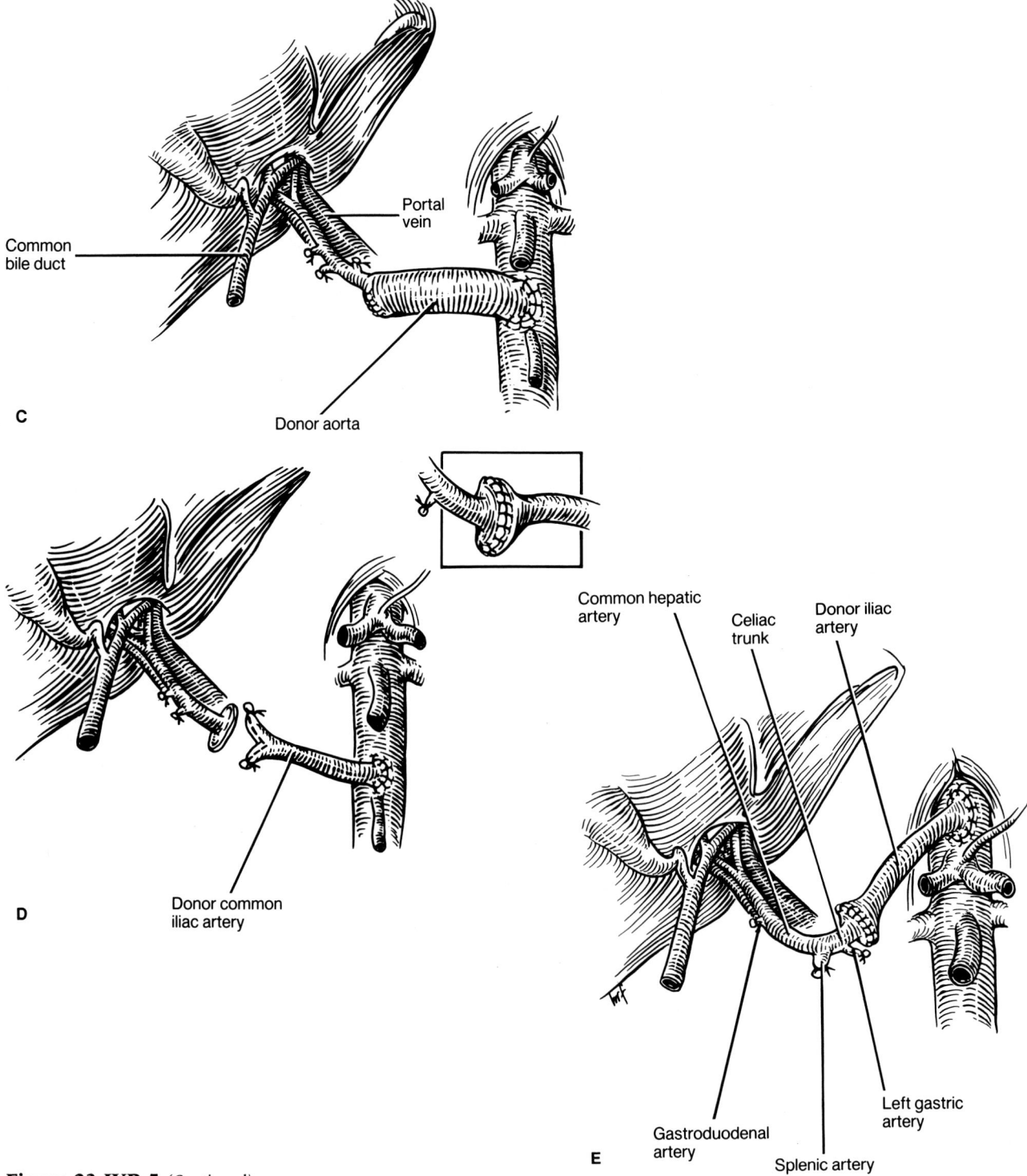

Figure 23-IVB-5 *(Continued)*

(**C**) Arterial reconstruction using donor hepatic artery with attached donor aorta anastomosed to the infrarenal recipient aorta.

(**D**) Arterial reconstruction using the donor common iliac artery graft sewn to the infrarenal aorta of the recipient. Subsequent anastomosis of that graft bifurcation to a celiac axis Carrel patch from the donor aorta completes the arterial reconstruction.

(**E**) The same principle as in the previous figure, with the donor iliac artery graft placed in a supraceliac position. If it is known that an arterial graft to the aorta will be required, it is best to complete the aortic anastomosis during the anhepatic phase.

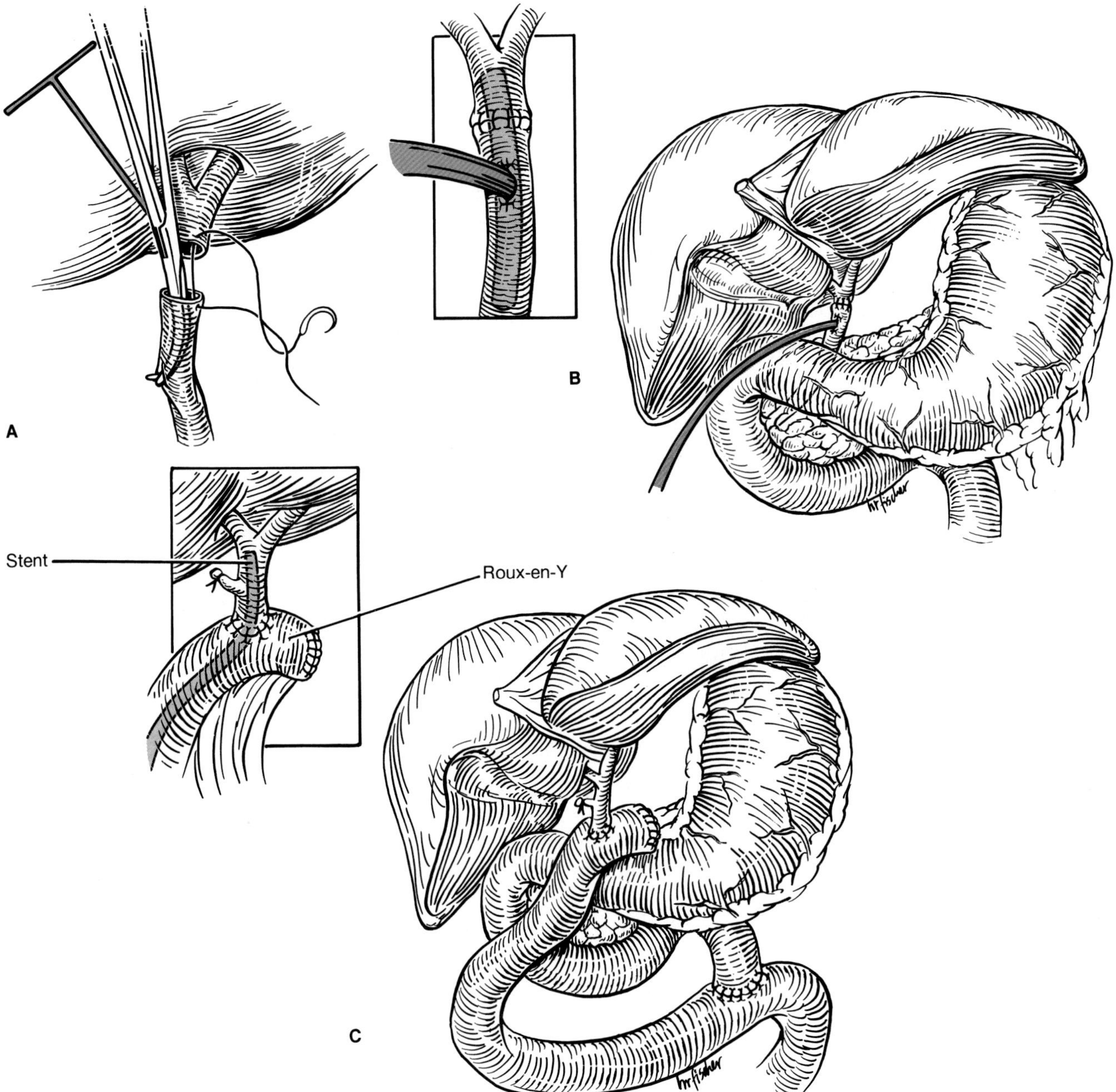

Figure 23-IVB-6

Biliary Reconstructions

(A) Standard choledochocholedochostomy. The T-tube is placed in the recipient common bile duct about 1 to 1.5 cm below the anastomosis. The limb is brought out through a small incision, and the T-limb is then placed into the duct. A longer upper limb is used to stent the anastomosis.

(B) Completion of the stented choledochocholedochostomy. The anastomosis is completed with interrupted sutures. It is also important to close the opening of the T-tube exit to ensure no bile leak at this site.

(C) Roux-en-Y anastomosis for biliary reconstruction. The anastomosis is usually placed over a stent with interrupted sutures from the bile duct to the Roux limb.

C. Donor Hepatectomy

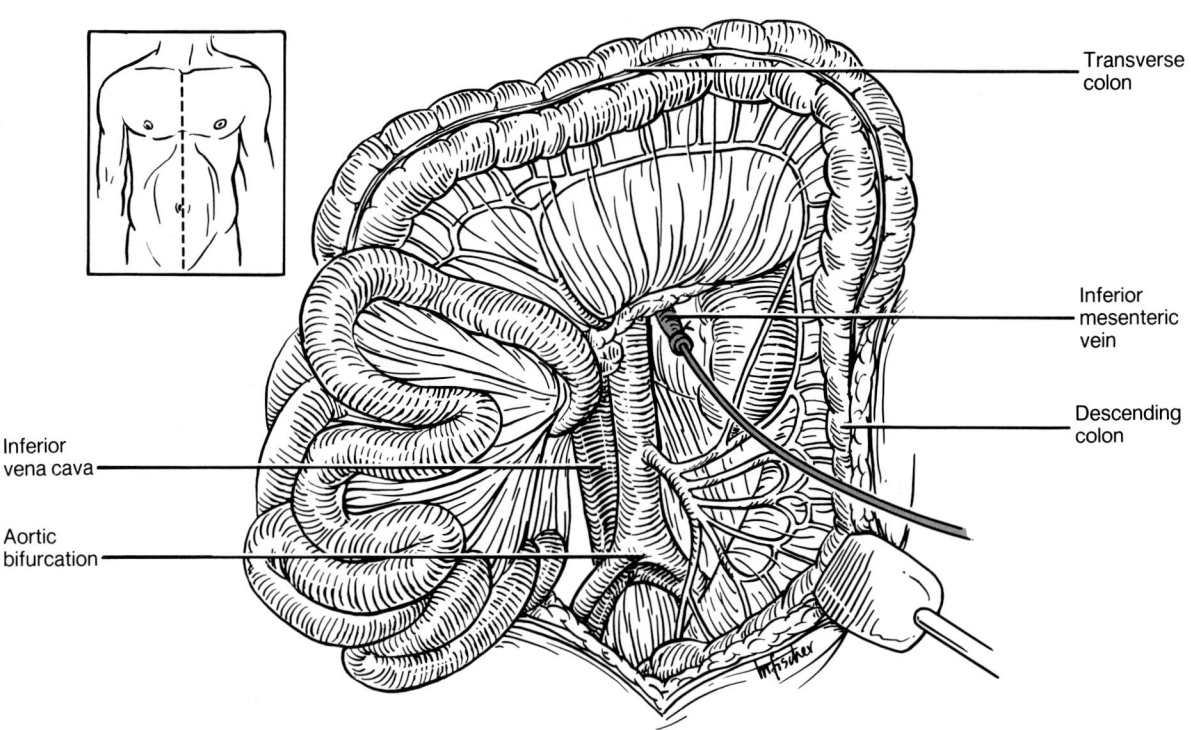

Transverse colon

Inferior mesenteric vein

Descending colon

Inferior vena cava

Aortic bifurcation

Figure 23-IVC-1

Incision and Catheterization

Most organ procurement procedures involve multiorgan harvest. Access is through a midline incision from the suprasternal notch to the symphysis pubis (**inset**). The chest and abdomen should be opened widely.

For liver procurement, the first step is placement of a portal vein catheter, illustrated here as being placed in the inferior mesenteric vein and fed up into the portal vein. Subsequent steps are directed to isolation of the aorta for cannulation for flushing of intraabdominal organs. The degree of hilar dissection depends on the organs being harvested and the preference of the harvesting surgeons.

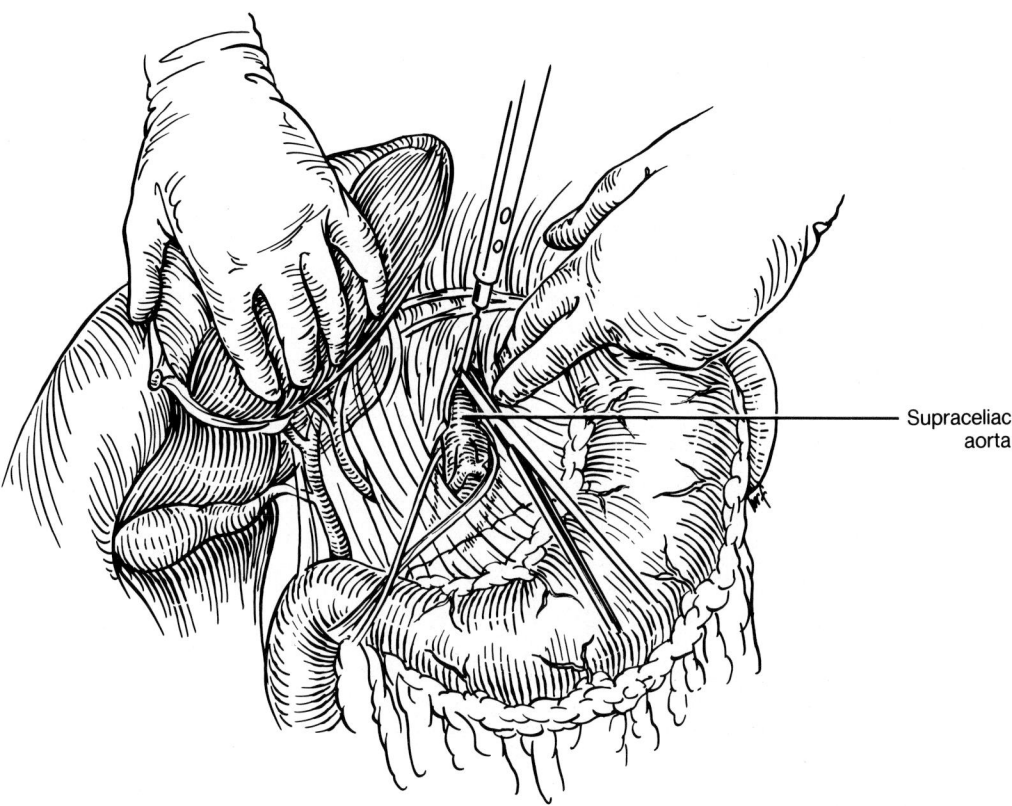

Supraceliac
aorta

Figure 23-IVC-2

Identification and Isolation of Supraceliac Aorta

This is approached through the left crus of the diaphragm after dividing the left triangular ligament and retracting the liver to the right. An abnormal left hepatic artery arising from the left gastric artery must be identified, isolated, and preserved. The aorta is encircled in preparation for subsequent cross-clamping.

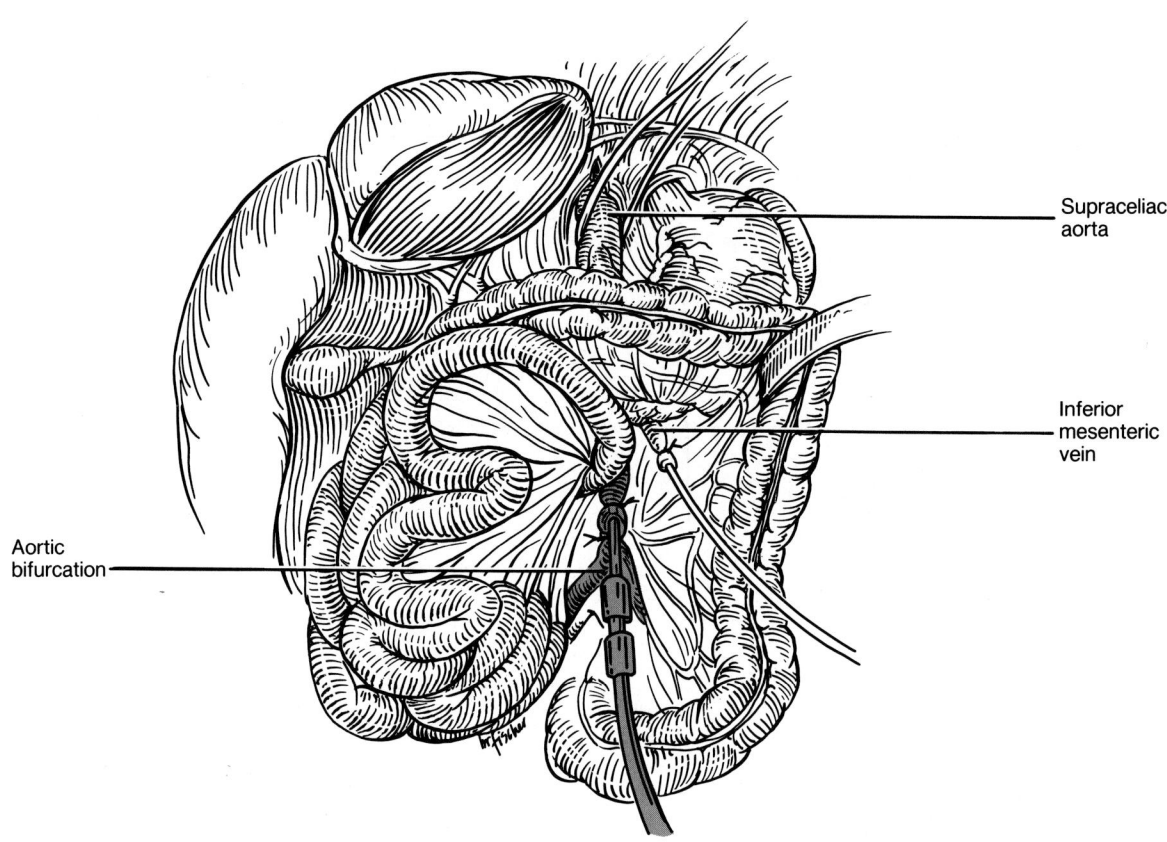

Supraceliac aorta

Inferior mesenteric vein

Aortic bifurcation

Figure 23-IVC-3

Isolation and Cannulation of Distal Aorta

The aorta is isolated at its bifurcation and encircled for control and subsequent cannulation. This cannulation is not performed until all procuring surgeons have done their preliminary dissection and are ready to cross-clamp. All medications, including heparin, should be given before this cannulation.

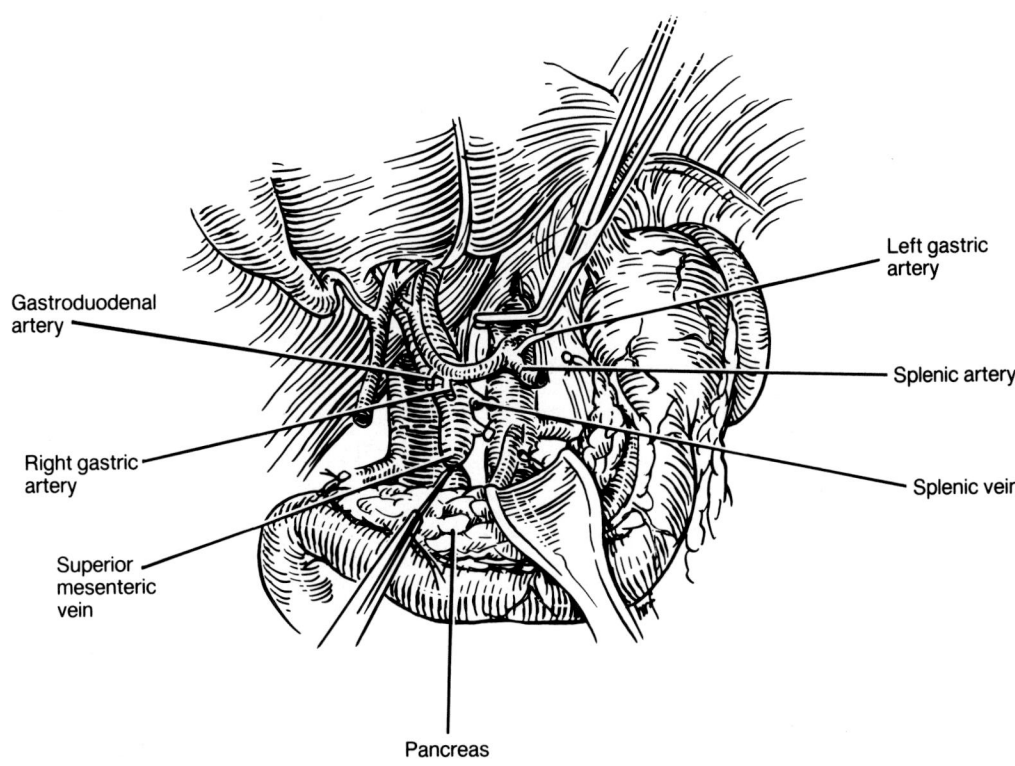

Gastroduodenal
artery

Left gastric
artery

Splenic artery

Right gastric
artery

Splenic vein

Superior
mesenteric
vein

Pancreas

Figure 23-IVC-4

Hilar Dissection

The hilar dissection is performed according to the individual surgeon's preference. The technique used must ensure proper procurement of all organs. From a liver procurement standpoint, the essentials are (1) to acquire an appropriate length of portal vein for subsequent anastomosis, (2) to obtain an adequate length of hepatic artery, at least down to the splenic origin, (3) to identify and preserve aberrant hepatic arteries to the donor liver, and (4) to cleanly divide the bile duct after flushing the gallbladder and biliary system with normal saline.

In this illustration, the pancreas is not being procured. Complete dissections of the portal vein and hepatic artery are illustrated.

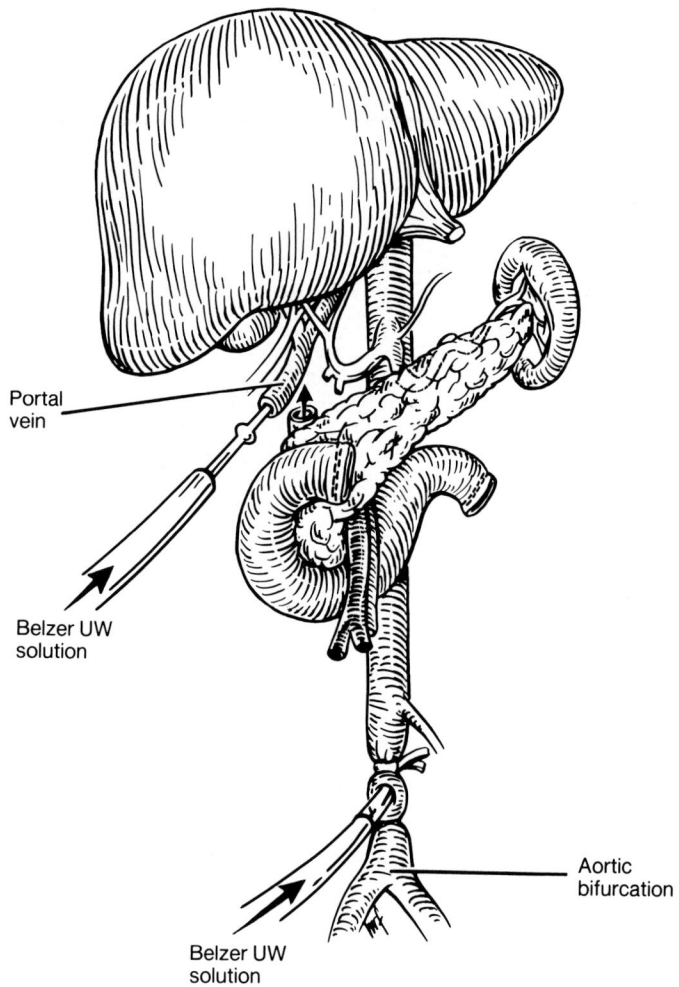

Portal vein

Belzer UW solution

Aortic bifurcation

Belzer UW solution

Figure 23-IVC-5

Combined Liver and Pancreas Procurement

The principles of combined procurement are shown here with the isolation of the pancreas with its duodenal segment. The portal vein is divided above the pancreas, and a catheter is placed to flush the liver. The hepatic artery is dissected down to the splenic artery, making sure there is an adequate splenic stump left for the pancreas graft.

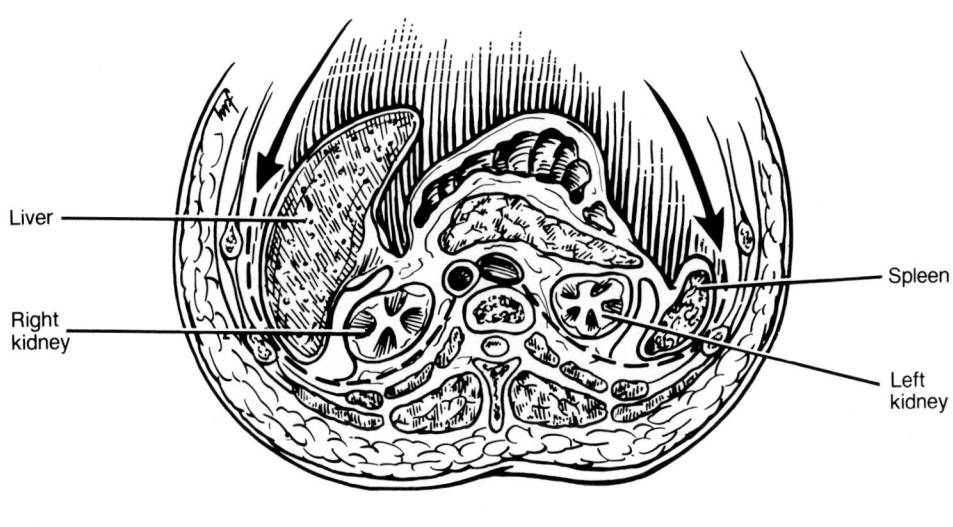

Liver

Right
kidney

Spleen

Left
kidney

A

Posterior

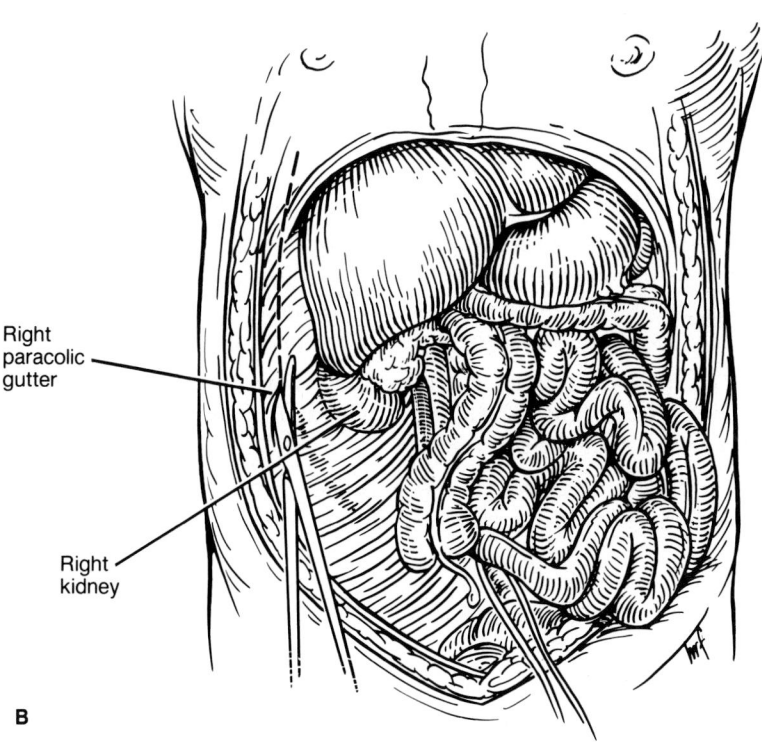

Right
paracolic
gutter

Right
kidney

B

Figure 23-IVC-6

En Bloc Organ Procurement

This method may be used to procure liver, pancreas, and kidneys en bloc. The principle is removal of these organs based on their aortic and vena caval pedicle.

(**A**) Relation of liver, spleen, and kidneys.

(**B**) The infrarenal aorta and inferior vena cava are isolated and cannulated. The organs are flushed and precooled in situ. Dissection for the en bloc removal is done on the right side by full mobilization along the right paracolic gutter, as illustrated here.

(Continued)

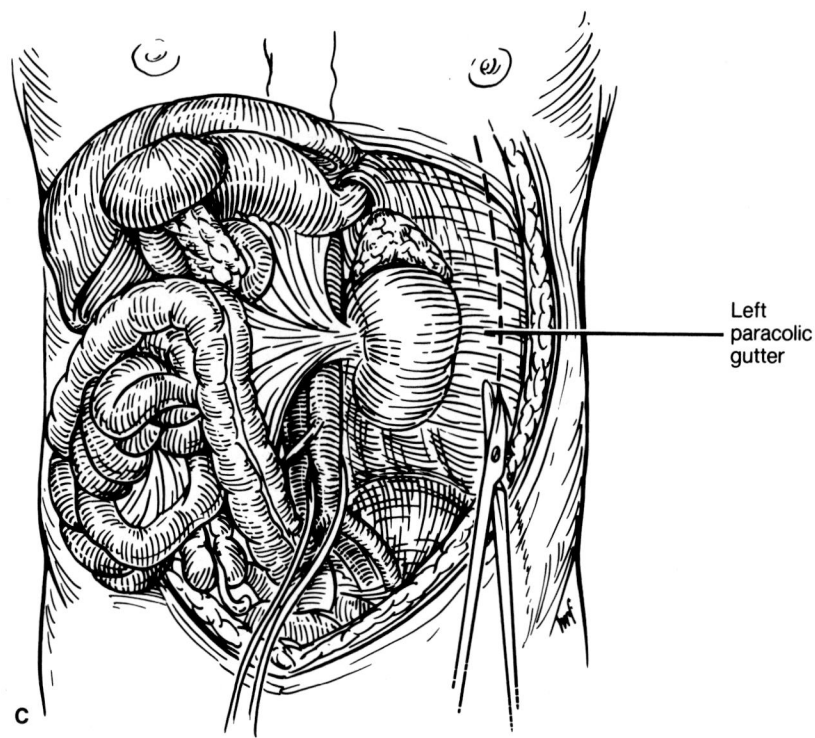

Left paracolic gutter

Figure 23-IVC-6 *(Continued)*

(**C**) The mobilization on the left side is done along the left paracolic gutter and behind the spleen to enter the appropriate retroperitoneal plane along the posterior aspect of the left kidney. The jejunum is transected just distal to the ligament of Treitz. The superior mesenteric pedicle is transected below the pancreas.

(**D**) The en bloc specimen is removed and viewed posteriorly. The aorta is opened to identify vessel origins. The kidneys, with appropriate Carrel patches of the renal arteries, are removed from the specimen.

(**E**) The liver and pancreas are then dissected to retain sufficient lengths of portal vein, hepatic artery, and pancreatic vessels for safe use of these grafts.

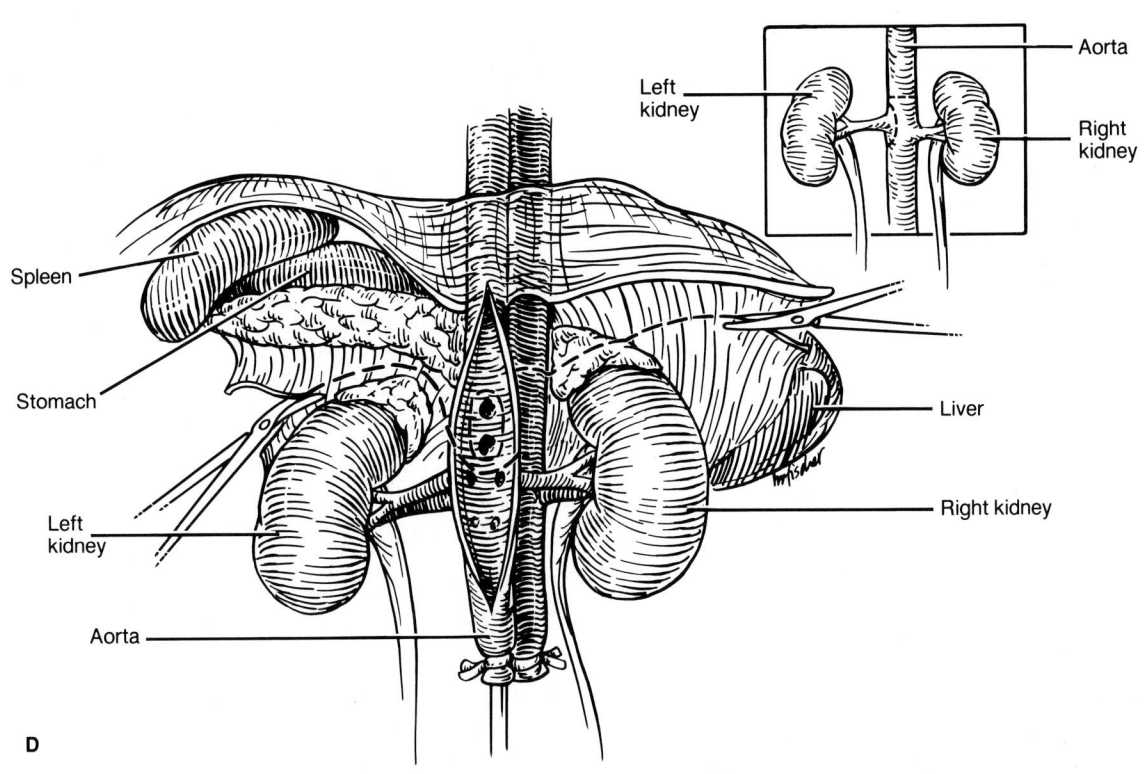

Aorta

Left kidney

Right kidney

Spleen

Stomach

Liver

Left kidney

Right kidney

Aorta

D

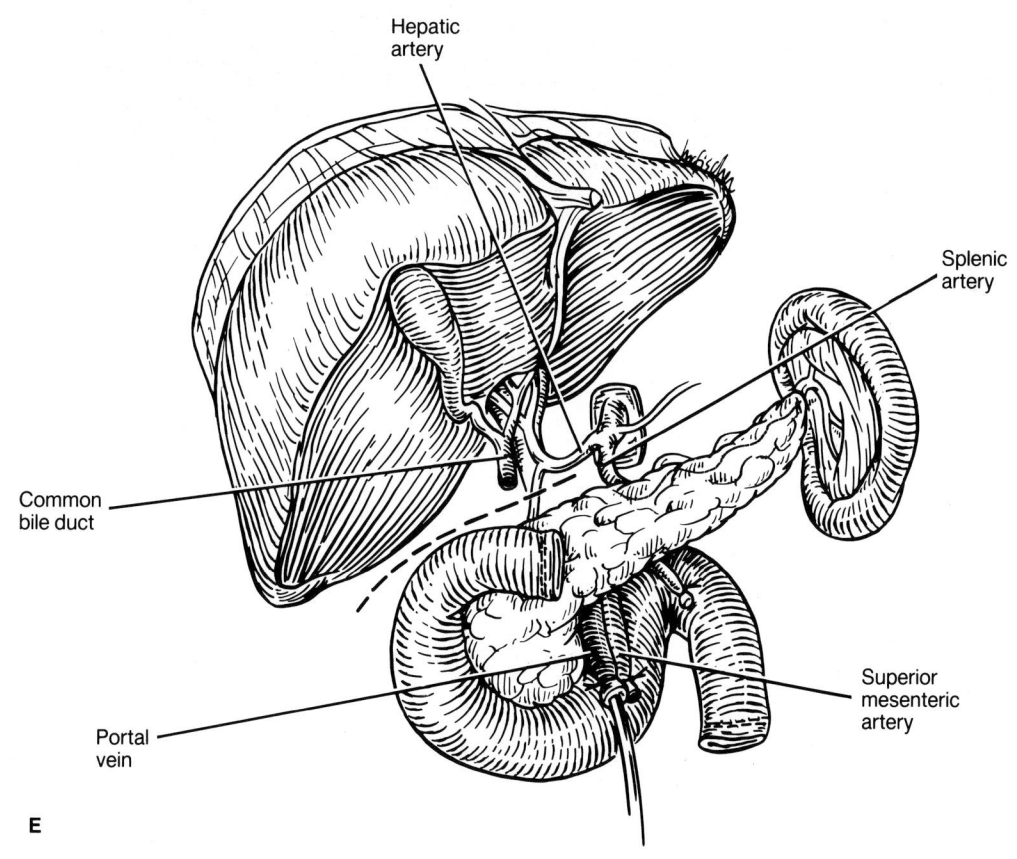

Hepatic artery

Splenic artery

Common bile duct

Portal vein

Superior mesenteric artery

E

PART V
Pancreas

Digestive Tract Surgery: A Text and Atlas, edited by Richard H. Bell, Layton F. Rikkers, and Michael W. Mulholland. Lippincott-Raven Publishers, Philadelphia, © 1996.

24

Acute Pancreatitis

David W. Rattner | *Andrew L. Warshaw*

The corrosive activity of pancreatic digestive enzymes is the driving force that differentiates acute pancreatitis from other abdominal inflammatory conditions. Many etiologic agents trigger acute pancreatitis by a variety of different mechanisms, but they all ultimately result in intraparenchymal enzyme activation, tissue destruction, and ischemic necrosis. Although acute pancreatitis has multiple causes and protean manifestations, the ultimate common denominator is the presence of activated proteolytic enzymes in the pancreatic parenchyma and retroperitoneum.

In mild pancreatitis, the inflammatory response is well controlled. Although there may be edema, usually confined to the pancreas, tissue necrosis is uncommon. In severe pancreatitis, the response is uncontrolled, leading to more widespread tissue injury and the many systemic manifestations of the disease. An inflammatory exudate rich in proteolytic enzymes, kinins, and vasoactive substances escapes from the pancreas into the lesser sac, retroperitoneum, and peritoneal cavity where it can be absorbed into the systemic circulation, leading to shock, respiratory failure, and renal failure. It is the development of necrosis that differentiates mild from severe pancreatitis.

The development of pancreatic necrosis depends on the amount of inappropriate enzyme activation and the degree to which the microcirculation is impaired. The earliest events in the pathogenesis of acute pancreatitis appear to occur intracellularly; they are similar irrespective of the ultimate severity of the ensuing pancreatitis.[1] Thus, events that occur after the intracellular activation of proteases determine the severity of the attack of pancreatitis. Impairment of pancreatic microcirculation occurs as early as 30 minutes after initiation of the disease.[2] In models of edematous pancrea-

titis, microcirculatory perfusion is maintained; but in models of necrotizing pancreatitis, both sluggish capillary flow and reduction in the number of perfused capillaries occur.[3] The use of dextrans in experimental models maintains capillary perfusion, limits the extent of necrosis, reduces the amount of trypsinogen that is activated extracellularly, and improves survival.[2,4] Thus, maintenance of pancreatic microcirculatory perfusion is critical to limiting the extent of necrosis and thus the severity of an attack of pancreatitis.

DIAGNOSIS

No foolproof diagnostic test has been developed for acute pancreatitis. The diagnosis rests on synthesis of clinical and laboratory information. In some cases, the diagnosis is obvious, while in other cases, the protean manifestations of this disease make diagnosis difficult. The typical presentation includes upper abdominal pain, nausea, vomiting, and low-grade fever. Tenderness is generally limited initially to the upper abdomen, although in some severe cases, diffuse peritoneal irritation is present. Laparotomy in cases with severe peritoneal irritation can be the safest means to establish a diagnosis and avoid missing a surgically correctable disease. When acute pancreatitis is found unexpectedly at laparotomy, it should not be a source of embarrassment. Furthermore, it may provide the opportunity to deal with biliary pathology (see later). Rarely, a patient has no pain but presents with distention, ileus, fever, and tachycardia. This form of the disease is more often seen in pancreatic infarction after cardiopulmonary bypass or accidental hypothermia.

The serum amylase level is the single most useful

laboratory test, but there is a significant incidence of false-positive and false-negative results. There is no correlation between the extent of the serum amylase elevation and the prognosis or severity of the disease.[5] The serum amylase level is normal in up to 30% of patients with acute pancreatitis, especially in alcoholics with underlying chronic pancreatitis or patients with hypertriglyceridemia.[6] The development of rapid accurate lipase assays has facilitated measurement of this enzyme as a marker for pancreatitis. Because the pancreas is the only known source of lipase, this may represent a more specific marker for pancreatic disease than total serum amylase. Accurate early discrimination of mild from severe pancreatitis can alter therapy and lead to early intensive care management or early endoscopic retrograde cholangiopancreatography (ERCP). Although amylase and lipase determinations can help establish the diagnosis of acute pancreatitis, they do not reflect or predict the severity of the disease. Therefore, a variety of serum markers and clinical scoring systems have been devised.

Many of the serum markers that have been investigated are nonspecific acute-phase reactants that rise with many acute inflammatory conditions. Polymorphonuclear cell elastase and C-reactive protein are two such markers. Once the diagnosis of acute pancreatitis is established, the peak serum levels of these proteins predict the development of necrosis 80% of the time.[7] Although polymorphonuclear cell elastase reaches peak levels within 1 to 2 days of the onset of illness, C-reactive protein reaches peak levels 3 to 4 days later and remains elevated as long as there is ongoing inflammation.[7] Serum phospholipase A_2 activity correlates with the extent of necrosis and also predicts the likelihood of pulmonary complications but requires a technically difficult assay and thus is employed only for research purposes.

Trypsinogen activation peptides (TAPs) are small peptides cleaved from trypsinogen by enterokinase as the inactive proenzyme is converted to active trypsin. Because this process normally occurs in the gut lumen, trypsinogen activation peptides are normally not present in the blood or urine. In acute pancreatitis, trypsinogen activation occurs extraluminally (ie, in the retroperitoneum), releasing trypsinogen activation peptides into the circulation, where they are rapidly excreted by the kidney. Thus, they are a specific indicator of the extent of extraintestinal trypsinogen activation. Because of its specificity, TAPs may be the most useful biochemical marker for assessing the severity of acute pancreatitis. In one study,[8] trypsinogen activation peptide assay in urine correctly predicted severity of acute pancreatitis in 87% of cases, whereas C-reactive protein predicted 55%. The sensitivity and specificity for tryp-

sinogen activation peptides were 80% and 90%. Mild forms of pancreatitis may have little or no extraintestinal trypsinogen activation, and thus TAP assay is not useful as a general diagnostic tool.

Because most institutions do not yet have the capability to assay the serum markers mentioned earlier, clinical scoring systems are widely used. The most widely used system is Ranson's system (Table 24-1), consisting of 11 easily obtainable clinical parameters at admission and 48 hours later.[9] The presence of up to three signs suggests a favorable outcome, whereas patients with four or more positive signs are likely to have a complicated course. The APACHE II score also has been used to stratify patients with acute pancreatitis.[10–13] Although initially designed for use in critical care,[14] it can provide useful discrimination between mild and severe cases of pancreatitis on admission to the hospital without a 48-hour delay. Furthermore, it can be recalculated daily to reflect continuing disease activity, with rising scores suggesting ongoing and untreated complications.

Dynamic contrast-enhanced computed tomography (CT) scanning has been shown to identify accurately areas of the pancreas that are not perfused and are likely to undergo necrosis subsequently.[15–17] Because the extent of necrosis correlates with severity of illness, early CT scans can predict the likelihood of subsequent complications.[18,19] After obtaining standard CT images of the pancreas, a bolus of intravenous contrast (usually 150 mL) is given at a rate of 2.5 mL/s. Twenty seconds after contrast administration, 5-mm sections at 5-mm intervals are obtained through the previously determined area of the pancreas. Normally perfused pancreas enhances about two thirds as much as the aorta,[15] or by 40 Hounsfield units.[17] Areas that fail to enhance have been shown to be hypoperfused and to undergo

---

Table 24-1   Ranson's Signs of Severe Acute Pancreatitis

AT ADMISSION
Age >55 years
Blood glucose >200 mg/dL
Serum lactate dehydrogenase >300 IU/L
Serum glutamic–oxaloacetic transaminase >250 U
White blood cell count >16,000/μL

48 HOURS AFTER ADMISSION
Hematocrit fall >10%
Blood urea nitrogen rise >5 mg/dL
Serum calcium <8 mg/dL
Arterial P_{O_2} <60 mmHg
Base deficit >4 mEq/L
Estimated fluid sequestration >6 L

necrosis subsequently.[18] The amount of the hypoperfused pancreas has been shown to correlate with the number of positive Ranson's signs,[15] APACHE II score,[17] and severity of illness.[16,19] Thus, early dynamic contrast-enhanced CT pancreatography has the potential to identify areas of necrosis that could be targeted for early débridement as well as to predict which patients are likely to have a complicated episode of acute pancreatitis so that early therapeutic (medical or surgical) intervention can be employed. Similar information, however, can also be discerned from clinical scoring criteria so that these criteria are generally used to select patients who need a contrast-enhanced CT scan.

MEDICAL TREATMENT

Many measures have been tried in an effort to modify the natural history of pancreatitis. Unfortunately, no known agent arrests or reverses the inflammatory process in pancreatitis. Most cases of acute pancreatitis are self-limited and subside spontaneously. In about 90%, endogenous control mechanisms are successful in resolving the inflammation. Existing treatment need only be supportive and reactive to complications that develop. Future attacks can be prevented if a remediable cause is identified. Severe pancreatitis may require intensive medical management for a multitude of associated complications.

Fluid Replacement

The most important requirement in the early treatment of pancreatitis is maintenance of adequate hydration. If the patient becomes hypovolemic and splanchnic circulation is compromised, the pancreas may become ischemic, with the potential to convert uncomplicated into complicated pancreatitis. In cases of severe pancreatitis, in which large fluid shifts occur, measurements of cardiac output and pulmonary capillary wedge pressure with a Swan-Ganz catheter may be necessary, especially if cardiac or renal compromise complicate fluid management. If significant anemia develops, transfusion may be required. When there is hemodynamic instability despite adequate fluid replacement, peritoneal lavage should be considered (see later).

Treatment of Hypoxemia

Hypoxemia is common in acute pancreatitis, with up to 45% of patients in one series having arterial Po_2 of less than 50 mmHg.[20] Four types of pulmonary disease are associated with acute pancreatitis: (1) early hypoxia without radiographic abnormality; (2) respiratory insufficiency with nonspecific radiologic abnormalities (diaphragmatic elevation, atelectasis, pulmonary infiltrates, pleural effusions); (3) pulmonary edema occurring early in illness; and (4) late respiratory failure secondary to systemic sepsis. Respiratory failure is most likely to occur in the sickest patients, and the need for intubation and ventilatory support indicates a high chance of fatal outcome.[21]

Early hypoxemia is usually associated with hypocarbia and is extremely common during the first 48 hours of acute pancreatitis. It occurs during clinically mild as well as severe pancreatitis. The only clues to the presence of hypoxemia may be subtle tachypnea and hyperventilation. The chest radiograph is usually normal. Impaired diffusion capacity, decreased compliance, increased airway resistance, and decreased vital capacity have all been demonstrated during this early phase, although the underlying cause or causes have eluded definitive documentation.[22] Because early hypoxemia is both common and insidious, supplemental oxygen should be part of the routine treatment of older patients with acute pancreatitis.

Of those patients who survive beyond the first 48 hours of illness, 30% to 60% have radiographically demonstrable pulmonary complications.[23] Unlike early occult hypoxemia, these complications correlate directly with the severity of the underlying pancreatitis. They usually occur with continuing pancreatic injury and are associated with increased mortality. Atelectasis, bibasilar infiltrates, and diaphragmatic elevation are nonspecific abnormalities common to any disease that involves subdiaphragmatic inflammation. They are in part the result of splinting of the abdominal wall and restricted excursion of the diaphragm due to pain, localized peritonitis, and ascites. These phenomena usually resolve as the underlying pancreatitis subsides. Pneumonitis, commonly the result of aspiration of vomitus, can complicate recovery, and its prevention remains a reason for using nasogastric suction in patients with acute pancreatitis. Pleural effusions that occur during the acute phase of the illness are sympathetic collections in response to subdiaphragmatic inflammation. They are usually sterile exudates with low amylase content. These effusions are not generally large enough to compromise ventilation significantly and rarely require removal by thoracentesis.

Treatment of these forms of respiratory compromise is supportive and directed primarily at the underlying pancreatitis. Humidification of the airways, supplemental tracheal suctioning, and ventilatory exercise to keep alveoli open are helpful. Antibiotics are not necessary unless radiographic evidence of pneumonia appears and should then be chosen on the basis of sputum Gram stain and culture. If the patient is already being treated with antibiotics for the pancreas, a resistant organism may have been selected in the respiratory tract, and a change of antibiotics is often necessary to treat the pulmonary infection effectively.

Noncardiogenic pulmonary edema occurs in 10% to 30% of patients with acute pancreatitis, usually 2 to 4 days after the onset of the attack.[24] The early circulatory dysfunction phase of pancreatitis is generally over by the time respiratory failure occurs. In fact, all the other clinical features of the attack may be subsiding or may have resolved when respiratory failure first begins to evolve. The chest radiograph shows pulmonary vascular congestion, perihilar fluffy infiltrates, and finally full-blown pulmonary edema. The edema fluid has a high protein content, unlike cardiogenic pulmonary edema, in which the fluid is a transudate. The clinical picture resembles that of the adult respiratory distress syndrome, but it evolves rapidly and without sepsis playing a part.

The treatment of pulmonary edema secondary to pancreatitis is again primarily supportive. Diuresis may be beneficial if filling pressures are high, but overdiuresis should be avoided because of potential renal compromise. If severe pulmonary edema and hypoxia supervene, endotracheal intubation, positive pressure ventilation, and positive end-expiratory pressure are necessary. Ventilatory support may be required for several weeks. Most commonly, however, the alveolar membrane injury heals within 7 to 10 days. It is important to be vigilant for the development of pneumonia in this setting. Daily sputum Gram stains should be obtained, and the development of purulent sputum with a predominant organism should be treated as evidence of bacterial pneumonia.

Minimizing Pancreatic Secretion

''Putting the pancreas at rest'' by fasting the patient has been a traditional part of medical treatment. The availability of somatostatin analogues, which completely inhibit pancreatic secretion, has allowed this hypothesis to be tested. In two large multicenter trials,[25,26] somatostatin treatment had no effect on the course of illness. Experimentally, it is known that pancreatic secretion is shut down during acute pancreatitis, and thus the failure to demonstrate an effect of somatostatin in clinical trials is not surprising.

All patients with pancreatitis are at risk of vomiting and aspirating because of ileus. Therefore, when ileus or significant abdominal distention is present, a nasogastric tube is useful. However, prolonged nasogastric suction is not necessary and can even promote aspiration. Histamine-2 blockers in theory might confer the same benefits as nasogastric suction. However, as with nasogastric tubes, studies have not shown them to have any effect on the course of pancreatitis. Histamine-2 blockers or antacids are still helpful in prophylaxis against hemorrhagic gastritis, to which these patients are susceptible.

Antibiotic Therapy

Antibiotics have never been shown to be effective in preventing the late septic complications of acute pancreatitis, and their use can even promote selection of organisms that are more difficult to treat later on. It seems reasonable to withhold antibiotic therapy in mild to moderate cases of alcoholic pancreatitis. In severe pancreatitis, however, tissue necrosis is likely. Withholding prophylactic antibiotic therapy in these patients is problematic because there is a high risk of subsequent infection. In a large German study,[27] 40% of patients with severe pancreatitis requiring surgery had bacterial infection of the pancreas or peripancreatic tissue. Bacteria can be recovered from the peripancreatic fluid in fulminant cases early in the course of the disease. Therefore, preemptive treatment with broad-spectrum antibiotics can be justified in hope of limiting bacterial invasion in this period of vulnerability. Imipenem and mezlocillin are two antibiotics that have been shown to achieve high concentrations in the pancreas relative to other commonly employed aminoglycosides and cephalosporins.[28] A randomized trial of imipenem in 74 patients with necrotizing pancreatitis demonstrated a significant reduction in pancreatic sepsis (12% versus 30% in patients not receiving antibiotics).[29]

SURGICAL TREATMENT

Surgical approaches to pancreatitis have generally been employed in two clinical settings. In the first, surgery is used in an effort to modify the course of pancreatitis in its earliest stages. In the second and more common setting, surgery is employed when patients deteriorate or fail to improve after appropriate medical management.

Attempts to Modify the Early Course of Pancreatitis

The demonstration that gallstones can be recovered from the stools of most patients with gallstone pancreatitis emphasized the importance of gallstones passing into the common bile duct and then obstructing or traumatizing the pancreatic duct orifice.[30] About two thirds of patients have stones impacted at the ampulla during the first 48 hours of gallstone-induced pancreatitis.[31] This observation has led some to advocate early common duct exploration (within 48 hours) to remove impacted stones, with the intent that the progression from edematous to necrotizing pancreatitis will be aborted.

Proving that early stone removal is beneficial has been problematic. First, many of the patients studied undoubtedly had only chemical hyperamylasemia induced by the obstructing stone, not true pancreatic inflammation. Second, the differentiation of gallstone-induced from other forms of pancreatitis is often difficult. Biochemical criteria are helpful, but direct cholangiography is needed to be sure.[32,33] Although mild jaundice frequently accompanies acute pancreatitis of any etiology (owing to common bile duct compression by inflammation in the head of the gland), a bilirubin of more than 40 μmol/L has a sensitivity and specificity of 80%. Combining this value with a γ-glutamyl transpeptidase of more than 250 IU/L, alkaline phosphatase of more than 225 IU/L, and age of more than 70 years, biochemical tests can correctly predict the presence of common duct stones in 93% of patients. However, the sensitivity is only 44%.[34] These values, which were determined in a retrospective fashion, have yet to be confirmed in a prospective study. In fact, in a carefully controlled study evaluating the efficacy of early endoscopic stone removal,[35] only half of patients with apparent gallstone-induced pancreatitis who underwent ERCP within 72 hours of the onset of pancreatitis had stones demonstrated in the common duct. Third, even when cholangiography demonstrates the presence of common duct stones, less than 5% are impacted at the ampulla.[32,35,36] Nonetheless, 60% of patients who die from gallstone-induced pancreatitis are found at autopsy to have choledocholithiasis. This has led some to propose that nonimpacted stones can intermittently obstruct the pancreatic duct, playing a key role in either preventing resolution of mild pancreatitis or promoting progression from mild to severe pancreatitis.[36]

In an uncontrolled series, removal of the impacted stone during the first 48 hours of the attack by common duct exploration and, if necessary, transduodenal sphincteroplasty appeared to reduce the mortality rate from 16% to 2%.[31] In contrast, others found that operating on 22 patients with gallstone pancreatitis during the first week after the attack led to a 23% mortality rate (three quarters of the patients operated on within 48 hours died), whereas there were no deaths among 58 patients treated nonoperatively until the pancreatitis subsided, with subsequent cholecystectomy and common duct exploration.[37] Similarly, in a study of 172 patients, impacted stones were found in 63% of patients operated on within 72 hours, but a 12% operative mortality rate was observed in these patients.[38] In contrast,

if operation was delayed 5 to 7 days, only 5% still had impacted stones, and the operative mortality rate was nil. Pancreatitis in 15% of patients did not subside but progressed and forced earlier operative treatment.

Transduodenal sphincteroplasty in the presence of acute pancreatitis has an appreciable risk of causing an abscess or a duodenal fistula.[39] Because 95% of cases of gallstone pancreatitis "quiet down" with medical management and without progression to a fulminant form, and 95% of stones pass spontaneously in the first week, surgical intervention to remove the stone within 48 hours does not appear justifiable. Cholecystectomy and, if still necessary, common duct exploration can be safely and effectively delayed until pancreatitis subsides, generally during the same hospital admission.

An alternative to early surgery is ERCP, which can be carried out safely by experienced endoscopists in up to 90% of cases of gallstone pancreatitis.[40–42] Prophylactic antibiotics should be employed, and injections into the pancreatic duct should be avoided. The earlier ERCP is performed, the more frequently common duct stones are found, an observation confirming the surgical studies.[31,38] When an impacted stone is found and endoscopic sphincterotomy (ES) with stone removal is successfully performed, most authors report a rapid improvement in the clinical course. In patients with an impacted stone with complicating cholangitis, a situation that is rare, urgent decompression is beneficial.[42]

Two prospective randomized clinical trials of early ERCP and ES have been published. In the first,[35] overall complications appeared to be less in the patients undergoing early ERCP and ES (17% versus 34%), and the mortality rate appeared to be diminished (2% versus 8%), although the numbers were too small to achieve statistical significance. ES was of no benefit in patients with mild pancreatitis. When the data were analyzed only for those patients with severe pancreatitis, there was a significant decrease in rates of both morbidity (24% versus 61%) and mortality (4% versus 18%). This study has been criticized because the control group was significantly older than the ERCP and ES group and because only 12 patients who underwent urgent ERCP and ES actually had common duct stones. Therefore, the important conclusion was based on a small number of patients. Nonetheless, the implication of this study is that early removal of common duct stones in patients with severe pancreatitis may be beneficial. A larger trial failed to confirm that local and systemic complications of pancreatitis were reduced by early ERCP and ES.[42] Hospital mortality was reduced in those patients undergoing early ERCP and ES, but the difference was not statistically significant. However, this trial conclusively demonstrated that early ERCP and ES resulted in a reduction in biliary sepsis in both mild and severe cases of pancreatitis. In all patients who had unrelenting biliary sepsis, persistent ampullary or common duct stones were identified. These studies indicate that patients with evidence of cholangitis benefit from early ES. Patients who present with indices of severe nonalcoholic pancreatitis (either by clinical scoring system, CT scan, or serum markers) should be considered for early ERCP and ES if biliary sepsis is suspected and a highly skilled endoscopist is available.

Pancreatic Drainage and Defunctionalization

Several years ago, an operation was devised to drain the pancreatic bed and reduce stimulation of the gland by placement of sump drains in the lesser sac, cholecystostomy tube or T-tube, gastrostomy tube, and jejunostomy tube.[43] Review of our own experience with this procedure revealed that only patients who were judged to be dying in shock after 24 to 48 hours of maximal supportive care appeared to benefit.[44] The success of the operation in these patients was believed to be due to the removal of toxic ascites—a result that could also have been achieved with placement of percutaneous peritoneal lavage catheters. Thus, this operation is no longer a viable form of therapy.

Pancreatic Resection

Major distal pancreatic resection can be accomplished in the face of acute pancreatitis with a mortality rate of about 40%, while pancreaticoduodenectomy or total pancreatectomy raises the mortality rate to 60% or more.[45,46] A key question is how to select those patients likely to benefit. The surgeon must decide which part of the pancreas to resect and how much to resect. This decision can be difficult because surface changes may

not represent the degree of central pancreatic injury and because several days are required for the changes of pancreatic devitalization to become visible (Fig. 24-1). In the first few days, there is only massive swelling with or without hemorrhagic staining. Early dynamic contrast-enhanced CT pancreatography can identify areas of necrosis that could be targeted for early débridement. Nonetheless, there are patients with substantial areas of necrosis who remain clinically well, and no reports have demonstrated improved survival in patients with preemptive early resection, compared with those treated by later débridement of clearly demarcated necrotic tissue. In a trial comparing early pancreatic resection versus peritoneal lavage,[47] resection was not found to be superior to intensive conservative management (including peritoneal lavage) and led to a longer intensive care unit and hospital stay. Because the operative mortality rate of early pancreatic resection is high, it seems preferable to delay surgery until areas of necrosis are clearly demarcated and there is proven bacterial infection or clinical deterioration.

Recommended Surgical Responses to Specific Complications of Acute Pancreatitis

Early Phase (First 4 Days): Peritoneal Lavage

Many of the systemic effects of pancreatitis are believed to be mediated by kinins and other vasoactive amines, such as kallikrein and bradykinin, which can be found in the dark brown exudate accompanying fulminant pancreatitis. The effects of these metabolic substances are manifested by capillary leak, low peripheral vascular resistance, and hyperdynamic shock. Peritoneal lavage to remove this toxic ascites frequently leads

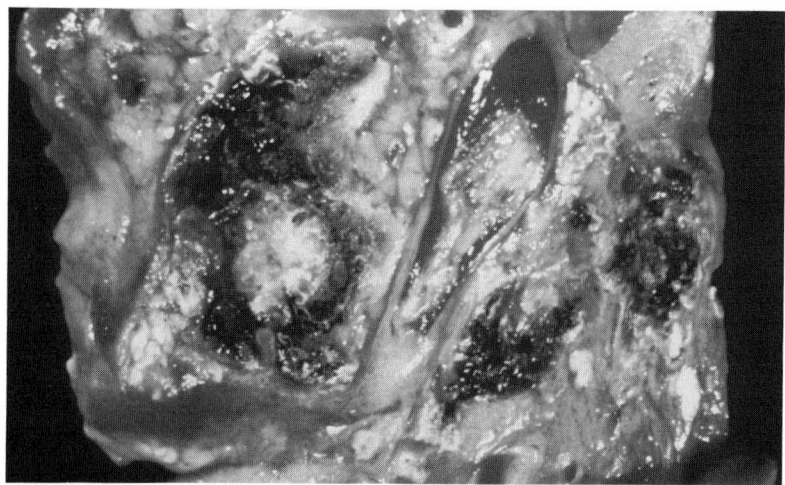

Figure 24-1 Cross section of resected pancreas showing focal areas of necrosis (*dark areas*) surrounded by viable tissue. These foci of necrosis would not be visible if examination were limited to the surface of the pancreas. (See Color Fig. 24-1.)

to a rapid improvement of hemodynamic and respiratory dysfunction, whereas hemodialysis does not.

The precise role of peritoneal lavage is controversial. Peritoneal lavage is not a treatment of pancreatitis but only reverses some of the early-phase systemic effects that are mediated by circulatory toxins. It is therefore of no benefit in mild to moderate degrees of pancreatitis and does not alter the progression of pancreatic injury or prevent the intermediate or late-phase developments of pancreatic necrosis and abscess.[45,48,49] Likewise, there is no benefit in treating the signs and symptoms that develop after the first few days because the cause of late inflammation is more likely to be necrosis, abscess, or pseudocyst.

Attempts have been made to select patients in whom lavage would be helpful. Studies based on Ranson's signs or similar systems,[49,50] which stratify for severity and risk of dying, have demonstrated no benefit in any objective parameter.[33,48] However, Ranson's signs are only statistical predictors of mortality and do not characterize the clinical course of individual patients. No study has yet been performed that addresses the use of peritoneal lavage in the treatment of early-phase shock or even identifies a subset of patients in early-phase shock. These are precisely the patients in whom striking immediate improvement is commonly seen. Therefore, many still believe that peritoneal lavage is beneficial when there is early evidence of major plasma volume loss, hypotension, pulse greater than 140 beats/min, or continued clinical deterioration. Lavage should be instituted within 24 hours of the onset of illness.

Lavage is performed through a percutaneously placed dialysis catheter. One or 2 L of dialysate is used per "run." The lavage fluid need not equilibrate, as for peritoneal dialysis, but can be evacuated immediately. The purpose is to wash out the ascitic fluid and its toxins, and the process need be continued only until the systemic effects are reversed. The response to lavage should be rapid, occurring within several hours. If it is not rapid, the surgeon may be dealing with an error in diagnosis, gallstone pancreatitis complicated by cholangitis, or inaccessible loculation of toxic ascites in the lesser sac. The latter can be reached by percutaneous catheter placed under ultrasound or CT guidance.

In one small but intriguing series,[51] prolonged peritoneal lavage for 7 days reduced the incidence of late pancreatic sepsis and death. In this study, 29 patients with severe pancreatitis collected during a 10-year period were randomized to receive peritoneal dialysis (48 L/d) for either 2 or 7 days. Although little difference in mortality rates was observed in the overall series, when patients with more than five Ranson's signs were evaluated, long peritoneal lavage reduced the incidence of pancreatic sepsis from 57% to 30%. Furthermore, no patient who received long peritoneal lavage died from pancreatic sepsis, compared with a 33% death rate from pancreatic sepsis in patients treated with standard 48-hour peritoneal lavage. All patients in this study received broad-spectrum antibiotics from the outset of their treatment, and the peritoneal dialysate contained ampicillin. Although the number of patients in this study was small, the results are stimulating and await confirmation from other centers.

Middle Phase (4 Days to 2 Weeks)

It is ordinarily only after several days of acute pancreatitis that irreversible tissue destruction becomes recognized. Phlegmon or swelling is apparent on ultrasound and CT in 30% to 50% of patients and palpable in 15% to 20%. This swelling represents edema and inflammation. The combination of tissue ischemia and release of activated enzymes into these areas produces an ongoing necrotizing process. Liquefaction may occur in small, well-defined geographic patches or even in large segments, such as the distal two thirds of the gland, with extension of the necrotizing process into the retroperitoneum, perirenal spaces, and mesentery. This process often includes peripancreatic as well as pancreatic necrosis. A general scheme for the management of patients with acute pancreatitis complicated by necrosis is shown in Figure 24-2.

The greatest benefit of dynamic contrast-enhanced CT scans can be seen in patients who are in the middle or late phase of acute pancreatitis. In these patients, with smoldering symptoms and inflammation, routine CT scans often demonstrate solid-appearing inflammatory masses that do not appear amenable to débridement or drainage. However, dynamic contrast-enhanced CT scans often delineate substantial areas of necrosis (Fig. 24-3). This can direct subsequent intervention to hasten resolution of the process. Contrast-enhanced CT scans may also show the pancreas to be well perfused but in the midst of extensive necrosis of peripancreatic tissue.

When necrosis develops, several factors determine the ultimate outcome—the amount of necrosis, the extent of extrapancreatic necrosis, bacterial contamination of necrosis,[52] and perhaps most important, the overall status of the patient as reflected in the APACHE II score.[10,11] Because the factors affecting outcome are multiple, no single parameter, except the presence of infection, is an absolute indication for débridement. There is virtually universal agreement that infected necrosis must be surgically débrided. Percutaneous radiology–guided drainage is not capable of removing infected solid material.[10,53] Therefore, although percu-

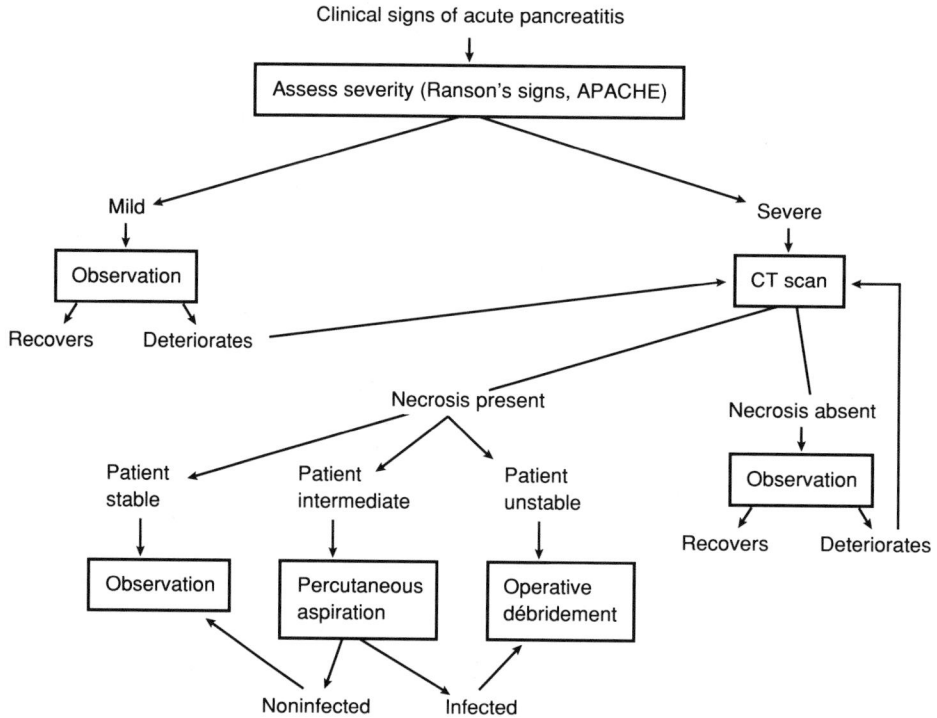

Clinical signs of acute pancreatitis

Assess severity (Ranson's signs, APACHE)

Mild

Severe

Observation

CT scan

Recovers   Deteriorates

Necrosis present

Necrosis absent

Patient
stable

Patient
intermediate

Patient
unstable

Observation

Recovers   Deteriorates

Observation

Percutaneous
aspiration

Operative
débridement

Noninfected   Infected

Figure 24-2 General scheme for the diagnosis and management of pancreatitis complicated by necrosis. However, exploratory laparotomy may well be indicated in patients who are unstable or clinically deteriorating despite negative CT or bacteriologic studies. Occasionally, such exploration reveals a diagnosis other than pancreatitis; on other occasions, deterioration in patients with pancreatitis is due to intraabdominal complications (eg, visceral perforation, ischemia) other than pancreatic necrosis.

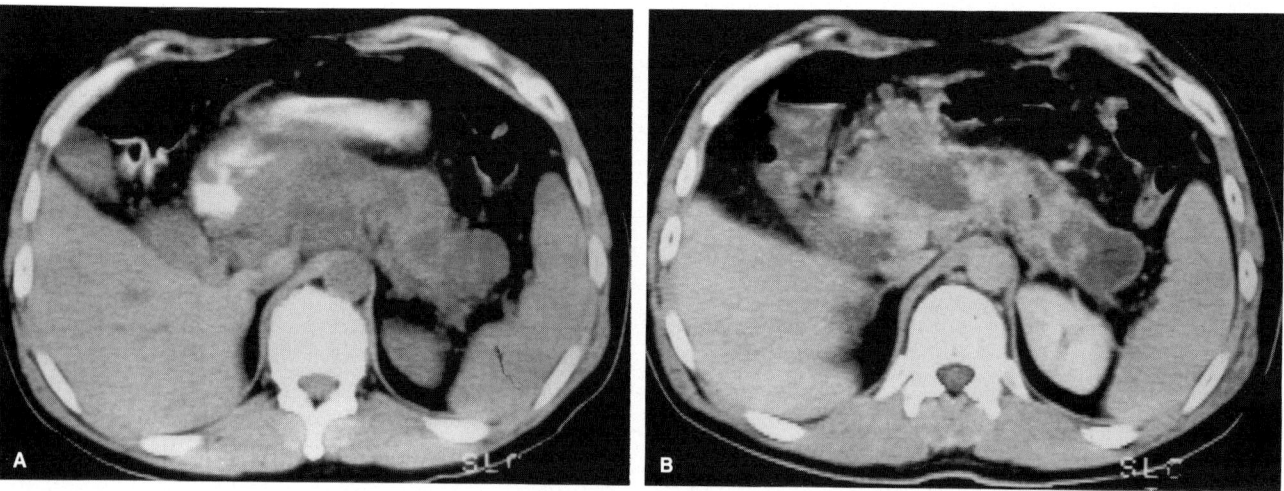

Figure 24-3 (**A**) CT scan of the abdomen showing an amorphous inflammatory mass in the area of the pancreas. (**B**) After administration of intravenous contrast, multiple areas of necrosis are apparent. Subsequent intervention can thus be accurately directed at these nonperfused areas.

taneous radiologic intervention plays a major role in the management of collections that are primarily fluid, it should not be used as an initial therapy for patients with necrosis.

In 40% to 70% of patients, pancreatic necrosis becomes infected.[10,27,52] The incidence of infection is maximum during the third week of the disease process. The appearance of infection, in some series, has been correlated with a higher mortality rate (37.8% versus 8.7% in one experience[51]). In this series, which differentiated between infected necrosis and pancreatic abscess, patients with infected necrosis were operated on earlier and with a higher mortality rate than those with pancreatic abscess. It appears that the combined ill effects of active pancreatitis and the infected necrosis forced early surgical intervention in some of these patients. In contrast, patients whose active phase of pancreatitis was over, leaving them with infected necrotic tissue, had a more indolent process that evolved during a longer period of time. When surgery finally became necessary, the necrotic tissues had become fully liquefied, that is, abscessed. This view is supported by studies in which needle aspiration of pancreatic phlegmon shows unexpectedly high rates of bacterial colonization, often with little or no clinical signs of infection.[54] Thus, it is not necessarily infection alone that creates the toxic state. Furthermore, the hemodynamic consequences of pancreatic necrosis are virtually identical whether infected or sterile.[55] If infected necrosis can be indolent, and if sterile necrosis can produce severe hemodynamic consequences, the difference between the unstable patient with infected necrosis and the stable patient with a pancreatic abscess (and their correspondingly different mortality rates) must be due to another factor, most likely the enzymatic and other biochemical events of ongoing acute pancreatitis.

The management of patients with sterile necrosis is extremely controversial. Several authors have reported high mortality rates in patients with sterile necrosis,[10,11,56] casting further doubt on the primacy of infection as the major determinant of outcome. Minimally invasive therapy (such as diagnostic needle aspiration) or observation alone has been advocated for sterile necrosis.[57,58] Successful nonoperative management of 11 patients with sterile necrosis was reported despite the presence of renal or respiratory failure in 6 patients.[57] Operative mortality is rare in patients with sterile necrosis operated on after the first week. However, postoperative complications (fistula, abscess) are frequent (13% to 24%), leading some to question whether sterile necrosis should be operated on at all.[57,58] There is, however, no controlled series comparing operative and observational therapy for this group of patients. If necrotic areas are small, sterile collections may resolve.

When signs of inflammation are present, percutaneous aspiration should be undertaken to determine if infection is present. When bacteria are found in the aspirate, débridement and drainage are indicated. Larger necrotic areas are problematic because of concern that they will become infected before there is sufficient time to reabsorb and heal. The decision to operate on large collections is often made because of clinical signs of inflammation, and thus the actual bacteriologic status of the necrotic tissue does not necessarily alter the clinical decision. If large collections are truly asymptomatic, they can be managed nonoperatively with the expectation that a small percentage will become infected and require débridement and drainage.

Some sterile collections produce symptoms by mass effect or local inflammation. Patients who are symptomatic (systemically ill, unable to eat, anorexic, febrile, or in pain) should not be denied a laparotomy simply because a necrotic collection is sterile. Some patients suffer low-grade symptoms for up to a year because their physicians are overly committed to avoiding an operation. In some cases, symptoms due to mass effect and local inflammation can be relieved only by débridement and drainage.

There are three main surgical approaches to débridement of necrosis. We have performed aggressive initial débridement of the lesser sac and retroperitoneum, often through a transmesocolic approach (Fig. 24-4). In this technique, it is imperative that the initial operation be thorough, and therefore the results are best in the hands of experienced pancreatic surgeons.[10] At the time of laparotomy, the entire pancreas from head to tail must be explored. Reference to the preoperative CT scan provides a road map to direct the operation. Often, the capsule of the pancreas must be incised to find a necrotic sequestrum (Fig. 24-5). All necrotic tissue must be removed. Simply placing drains adjacent to dead tissue is not adequate therapy.

We prefer to use a midline laparotomy for débridement of pancreatic necrosis (see Section III in Atlas Chap. 30). This allows easy access to the entire abdomen and does not interfere with placement of stomas, which may be required if colonic necrosis is encountered. Once the abdomen is entered, cultures are obtained of any free fluid that is present. The surgeon must make a decision about the easiest way to expose areas of pancreatic necrosis. Access through the transverse mesocolon is the least vascular of all approaches to the lesser sac, and that is why we prefer it. This approach also provides excellent access to the tail of the pancreas. Frequently, collections in the lesser sac "point" just lateral to the ligament of Treitz. This area is bluntly explored with a sucker or finger, and if a soft spot is identified, it is easily opened to allow egress of

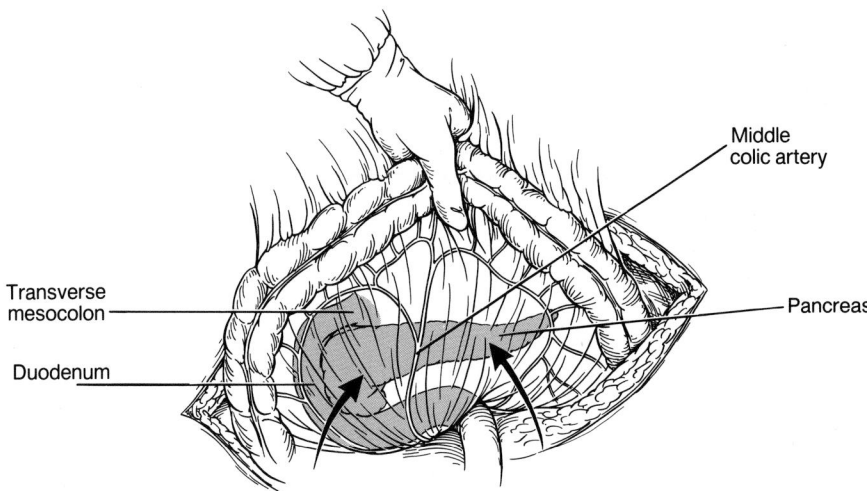

Figure 24-4 Access to the pancreas for débridement can be gained by approaching the lesser sac through the avascular areas of the transverse mesocolon.

fluid and necrotic material. The mesocolon is then opened toward the left side to create a large enough defect to allow a hand to be placed into the lesser sac. Occasionally, branches of the left colic artery are encountered, and these must be ligated if they have not previously thrombosed. Division of these branches does not result in colonic necrosis unless the marginal artery has been occluded from either atherosclerotic disease or concomitant inflammation. Collections to the right of the spine can also be approached through the right transverse mesocolon. These collections often track down into the root of the small bowel mesentery and thus are accessible through the infracolonic approach. If the collections do not appear to point toward the transverse mesocolon, it is necessary to go through the

gastrocolic omentum (see Section III in Atlas Chap. 30). This is usually thick and vascular, and it sometimes is difficult to identify the wall of the transverse colon because of severe inflammatory changes. By placing a hand into the lesser sac through the avascular area of the mesocolon, dissection through the gastrocolic ligament can be guided and injury to the wall of the colon and stomach avoided. Rarely, collections arising cephalad to the pancreas must be approached through the lesser omentum. Once the focus of necrosis is exposed, débridement is carried out bluntly. Both finger dissection and dissection with a sponge stick or suction are appropriate. Often, a necrotic sequestrum is present and attached by a thin strand or thread of tissue. This thread of tissue should be divided between clamps be-

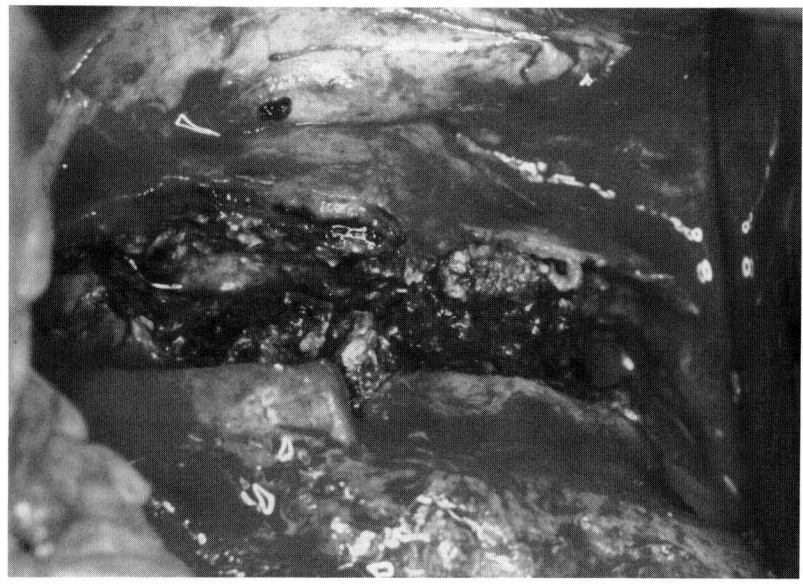

Figure 24-5 Often, the capsule of the pancreas appears viable. It is important, however, to incise the pancreatic capsule to find the necrotic material. Preoperative CT scans showing nonenhancement of the central portion of the pancreas are commonly associated with this finding. (See Color Fig. 24-5.)

cause it usually represents a major vessel, which may bleed after the débridement. Sharp dissection is not usually required. After all loose debris has been removed, the cavities are irrigated forcefully with saline. The cavity is then filled with multiple, large, gauze-filled Penrose drains as well as suction drains.[59] This ensures easy egress of residual necrotic material and also serves to pack the abscess cavity. This packing maneuver often controls minor bleeding.

Because of the pancreas's proximity to splenic and portal veins, major venous bleeding can occur during the course of débridement. The veins are often friable and do not hold sutures. Nonetheless, a preliminary attempt to suture ligate bleeding vessels should be made. If tissue is too friable to hold the sutures, however, the débridement cavity should be packed with laparotomy pads to control bleeding. On rare occasions, it may be necessary to leave the cavity packed for control of bleeding, close the abdomen, and return to the operating room a day or two later to remove the packs. Gastrostomy and jejunostomy tubes are used sparingly. If evidence of bile duct compression is present, a cholecystostomy tube is placed at the time of surgery. It is usually not possible to perform a cholecystectomy in patients with substantial necrosis because of inflammation in the porta hepatis.

It is important to bring all drains out laterally (in the flanks) to provide dependent drainage. Furthermore, this isolates the infected material from the healing midline incision. All drains are left in for a minimum of 7 days. If sump drains are draining a significant amount of fluid, they remain on suction. If no fluid is draining, they are converted to passive drains. One drain is removed every other day until no drains remain. This is akin to removing gauze packing from an abscess cavity and allows the cavity to collapse slowly around the residual drains.

Because the necrotizing process may continue after the initial operation, alternative operative approaches have been proposed. These approaches aim to provide continuing débridement in the lesser sac as more tissue is sloughed. One technique involves necrosectomy and continuous postoperative lavage of the lesser sac.[60] In this technique, the pancreas is approached through the gastrocolic ligament. Necrotic tissue is débrided sharply and bluntly; irrigation and drainage catheters are placed in the lesser sac; the gastrocolic ligament is then reapproximated to create a closed space for the postoperative lavage. Two days after surgery, lavage with isotonic solution begins at a rate of 7 to 48 L/d. The median duration of lavage is 25 days, and the median hospital stay is 60 days.[60] Lavage can be discontinued when the effluent no longer contains particulate debris and the amylase content of the effluent is similar to se-

rum levels. Even with lavage, however, reoperation was required in 31% of patients with infected necrosis and 21% of patients with sterile necrosis. This technique requires substantial nursing care to manage the lavage system. Despite these drawbacks, the reported mortality rate was impressively low (8.1%).

Another popular technique is open packing (see Section III in Atlas Chap. 30). The abdomen is entered through a chevron or transverse incision, and the pancreas is exposed through the gastrocolic ligament. After blunt débridement, the lesser sac is packed with moist gauze, and the abdominal wound is partially closed. The patient is returned to the operating room every 48 hours for further débridement and packing until all necrotic debris is removed and healthy granulation tissue appears. After the first four or five débridements, these reoperations can be performed in the intensive care unit. When healing occurs, the abdomen can be closed over drains, with or without delayed lavage of the cavity.[11,57] Good results have been reported with this technique despite the relatively high rate of development of enteric fistulas (15% to 20%). Mortality rates were as low with sequential débridement as with the previously described methods.[11]

Finally, there are proponents of combined anterior and retroperitoneal approaches for pancreatic débridement.[61] Because the necrotizing process often tracks retroperitoneally behind the colon, this approach allows dependent drainage, packing, and simultaneous access to intraabdominal and retroperitoneal pathology. It is possible, however, to access retrocolic areas by the transabdominal approach if necessary (see Section III in Atlas Chap. 30).

It is difficult to compare the results of these three techniques because published series contain patients with differing severity of illness and indications for surgery. Circumstances in which greater than 100 g of necrotic tissue are removed, in which there is poor delineation of viable from nonviable tissue, or in which there is extensive peripancreatic necrosis with extension into the root of the mesentery, pararenal spaces, and lateral gutters are most likely to require more than one débridement. If there is concern that the initial débridement is likely to be incomplete, greater consideration should be given to open packing or continuous postoperative lavage.

PANCREATIC PSEUDOCYSTS. Pseudocysts are localized collections of pancreatic juice due to disruption of the pancreatic duct by inflammation. These cysts lack a true epithelial lining; rather, their walls are composed of fibrous and granulation tissue derived from peritoneum, retroperitoneal tissue, or the serosal surface of adjacent viscera. Pseudocysts occur in 10% to

20% of cases of acute pancreatitis. Pseudocysts that occur as part of the ongoing necrotizing process are different and more dangerous than pseudocysts associated with chronic pancreatitis.[62]

Since the introduction and widespread use of ultrasonography, it has been appreciated that many acute pseudocysts resolve spontaneously. Although it is difficult early in the course of acute pancreatitis to differentiate a bland peripancreatic fluid collection from a true pseudocyst, 15% to 30% of acute pseudocysts resolve within 6 weeks.[63,64] Size appears to be the best predictor of resolution. Cysts larger than 6 cm that remain 6 weeks after detection are unlikely to resolve spontaneously.[62,65] CT scanning is the preferred initial test for detection of pseudocysts, while ultrasound is more practical for follow-up, is less costly, and does not expose patients to ionizing radiation. Endoscopic retrograde pancreatography adds little to the management of acute pseudocysts unless a percutaneous radiologic approach is planned (see later), and it risks introducing bacteria into a previously sterile collection.

Most patients with acute pseudocysts have epigastric pain, nausea, and vomiting. For symptomatic pseudocysts, decompression is indicated to relieve discomfort and prevent complications. The management of asymptomatic cysts, on the other hand, is controversial. In a series from Johns Hopkins,[66] 36 patients with asymptomatic pseudocysts (both acute and chronic) were managed nonoperatively. Sixty percent of the cysts completely resolved, and the remainder were stable. Most other series, however, have reported about a 10% death rate during expectant management of acute pseudocysts, due primarily to hemorrhage and sepsis. In our experience,[62] 4 of 22 patients with pseudocysts developed these complications while awaiting maturation of the cyst wall. Therefore, the surgeon must balance the desire to allow spontaneous resolution against the risk of complications while waiting.

Ideally, surgical drainage of pancreatic pseudocysts should be performed when the cyst wall is fibrotic enough to allow placement of sutures (mature cyst wall). A rule of thumb is that most cyst walls mature within 6 weeks of the onset of symptoms. "Old amylase" determinations can provide a biochemical marker for cyst wall maturity.[62] In the absence of infection, internal drainage is the preferred mode of decompression because both the complication rate (68% versus 32%) and the mortality rate (11% versus 1%) are lower than with external drainage.[67] The choice of surgical procedure for internal drainage depends on the local topography. Cysts adherent to the posterior wall of the stomach are ideally drained through a cystogastrostomy (see Section III in Atlas Chap. 30). Cysts larger than 15 cm,

however, should not be anastomosed to the stomach because these giant cysts tend to retain material in the dependent portions of the cyst, leading to retroperitoneal sepsis.[68] Most other cysts are best drained into a Roux-en-Y loop of jejunum. Occasionally, cysts in the head of the pancreas impinge on the duodenum, and cystoduodenostomy can be easily performed (see Section III in Atlas Chap. 30). It is important to excise a small portion of the cyst wall at the time of surgery. If epithelium lines the cyst, the surgeon is probably dealing with a neoplastic cyst (or, rarely, a duplication cyst or simple cyst) rather than a pseudocyst. Neoplastic cysts should be resected rather than drained. If the surgeon encounters a pseudocyst containing a large amount of necrotic material, it is preferable to débride the cavity and drain it externally rather than risk disruption of the anastomosis by an ongoing necrotizing process. If at the time of surgery the cyst wall is soft, friable, and will not hold sutures, external drainage must be performed. The higher mortality rate reported for external drainage procedures reflects a greater proportion of patients who are operated on earlier in the course of pancreatitis. External drainage is necessary in about 25% of acute pseudocysts. Postoperatively, up to 20% of externally drained patients develop a pancreatic fistula. More than 90% of these fistulas close within 3 to 4 months.

Resection of pancreatic pseudocysts is rarely necessary. Because the walls of the cyst often include adjacent viscera, it is not practical to excise the pseudocyst in most instances. However, some pseudocysts arising from the tail of the pancreas dissect into the splenic hilum or beneath the splenic capsule. These pseudocysts have a propensity to cause life-threatening hemorrhage from the spleen and are best managed by resection with splenectomy and distal pancreatectomy.

Percutaneous drainage has gradually gained acceptance in the treatment of selected pancreatic pseudocysts. Simple aspiration of acute pancreatic pseudocysts is associated with a recurrence rate of 75% or more. Drainage of pseudocysts with indwelling catheters is more successful and is similar to surgical external drainage without débridement of associated necrotic debris. When there is a complex collection of solid and liquid in an acute pseudocyst, percutaneous drainage is generally not as effective as operative drainage because large amounts of necrotic material cannot be adequately drained through small percutaneous catheters. Infected pseudocysts that do not have a significant solid component can be successfully treated with percutaneous drainage.[69,70] The success rate appears to correlate with the degree of ongoing inflammation, as reflected in the APACHE II score.[70] Repeated catheter manipulation and replacement is often required to achieve a successful outcome.[69,71] Complications are common, although these can often be managed nonoperatively. Nearly half of all patients develop external pancreatic fistulas, occasionally involving the colon, but most of these close with conservative means. When anatomic abnormalities in the proximal pancreatic duct prevent fistula closure, however, subsequent surgery is more difficult than it would have been if an initial internal drainage procedure had been performed. Those factors associated with failure of percutaneous drainage of abdominal abscess[53] also apply to failed percutaneous pseudocyst drainage and include the presence of multiple system organ failure, presence of foreign body or necrotic tissue, and hematoma. It appears that the ideal patients for percutaneous drainage are those who are relatively well and have a discrete fluid collection. If the surgeon plans percutaneous drainage of a pseudocyst, ERCP can be useful to demonstrate communication with the pancreatic duct or to demonstrate a site of proximal duct obstruction, which indicates a higher likelihood of subsequent development of a fistula. Use of somatostatin to diminish pancreatic secretion can be combined with percutaneous drainage when communication with the pancreatic duct is demonstrated. Normal pancreatic ductal anatomy or ERCP is reassuring if percutaneous drainage is planned. Patients with multiple pseudocysts and ongoing inflammation are probably best managed with surgical techniques.

Endoscopic techniques can be used to create cystogastrostomies and cystoduodenostomies.[72,73] In patients with chronic pancreatitis, endoscopic cystoduodenostomy has been shown to be safe and efficacious,[72] but its role in the presence of acute inflammation is less well established. Endoscopic cystogastrostomy carries a significant risk of hemorrhage and does not afford the endoscopist a chance to assess cyst wall maturity.

Therefore, these procedures are best performed only by expert endoscopists. If there is any reason to suspect a neoplastic cyst, endoscopic drainage is contraindicated. The surgeon must resist the temptation to use endoscopic and percutaneous drainage procedures inappropriately just because they are less invasive. All forms of intervention have their unique benefits and risks.

OTHER COMPLICATIONS OF ACUTE PANCREATITIS. Hemorrhage, a highly lethal complication, is caused by erosion of major blood vessels by elastase and other proteases. The initial vascular lesion is a pseudoaneurysm (Fig. 24-6). Infection is almost always present. If rupture occurs, life-threatening hemorrhage into the pseudocyst or retroperitoneum occurs. Angiography should be the initial step in management for this problem. Eight of 12 patients in our experience had bleeding fully controlled with angiographic techniques, and in the others, angiography provided a road map for the surgeon to follow or allowed débridement and vessel ligation to take place under more favorable conditions.[74] When bleeding is from the main hepatic or splenic artery, angiographic control is more difficult to achieve. Although the effects on ultimate survival are difficult to establish without question, reduction in the rate of bleeding or complete cessation of bleeding saves blood, adds time for planning, and can reduce the expenditure of the patient's reserves. Surgery is inevitably required at some point for débridement of the associated regional necrosis and to control sepsis. When the affected area is inadequately drained or débrided, progression of sepsis or recurrence of bleeding usually follows, resulting in the death of the patient.

Vascular thrombosis may involve the colic branches of the superior mesenteric artery, the splenic artery, or the gastroduodenal artery. Arterial occlusion

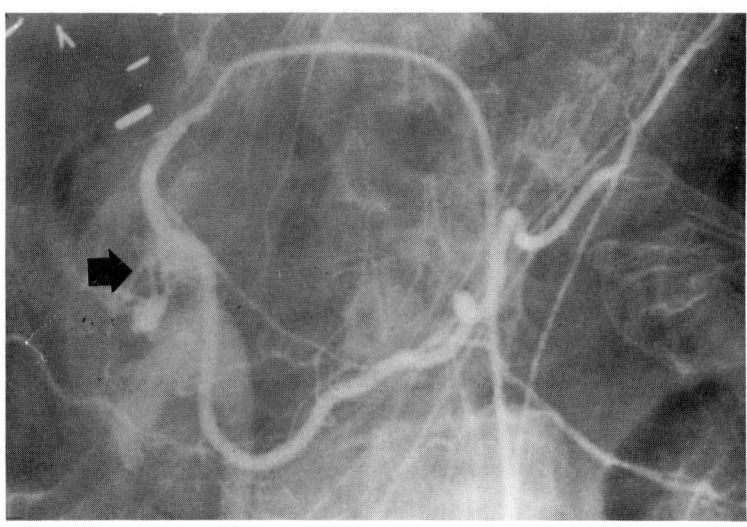

Figure 24-6 Selective arteriogram with injection of contrast into the gastroduodenal artery demonstrating hemorrhage from a pseudoaneurysm (*arrow*).

is manifested as gastrointestinal bleeding from sloughed mucosa, infarction of a viscus with perforation, fistulas, or late stenosis and stricture. If bowel infarction occurs, it is necessary to exteriorize two stomas rather than risk breakdown of an anastomosis. If the duodenum perforates, attempts at local repair with thorough external drainage should be made in preference to pancreaticoduodenectomy. If fistulization occurs, adequate drainage allows some fistulas to close, with healing of the underlying process. Gastric fistulas, on the other hand, usually do not heal (only 33% heal in our experience) and the rate of hemorrhage from those fistula tracts is high.[75] Biliary fistulas, particularly after choledochotomy, have been successfully treated by percutaneous and endoscopic internal stenting.[76]

Failure of gastric emptying may be due to duodenal compression or to localized ileus from the nearby phlegmon. Gastroenterostomy is occasionally necessary because gastric emptying can be impaired for long periods. A gastrostomy tube is helpful as the surgeon awaits resolution of the obstruction.

Partial common bile duct obstruction due to compression of the intrapancreatic portion of the common bile duct is common. The serum bilirubin can rise to 3 or 4 mg/dL. Operative decompression is almost never necessary unless common duct stones and cholangitis are present. An occasional patient requires an endoscopic or percutaneous stent for temporary relief of biliary obstruction (Fig. 24-7). The common duct returns to its normal configuration when the pancreatitis subsides.

Late Phase

Abscesses are the most common cause of death in acute pancreatitis. They occur in about 2.5% of all patients with acute pancreatitis and are related to the severity of the attack.[77] Abscesses are the most likely complication after the second week and arise from secondary infection of necrotic and liquefied pancreas. Abscesses usually contain enteric bacteria, but if broad-spectrum antibiotics have been used, *Candida* sp may become a major pathogen. In two reports,[59,77] 20 of 45 patients and 18 of 27 patients, respectively, had multiple organisms cultured from their pancreatic abscesses. Patients who require peritoneal lavage in the early phase of their disease appear to have an increased incidence of abscess formation. However, it is probable that early lavage is indicative of the severity of the pancreatitis rather than the portal by which infection enters.

The best means for diagnosing a pancreatic abscess is CT scanning (Fig. 24-8). Although it is possible to predict which patients are statistically more likely to form abscesses by the use of early CT scan and clinical severity score,[78,79] patients must be evaluated individually. Early CT of the pancreas is recommended in moderate or severe pancreatitis. Patients with persistent clinical evidence of pancreatic inflammation should have CT evaluation every week to monitor change in the retroperitoneal anatomy. Fever and leukocytosis are not always present with infection and do not reliably differentiate infected from sterile collections. In one report,[59] 13% of patients with pancreatic abscess had no fever or leukocytosis. Unless extraintestinal gas is present, the CT often cannot distinguish sterile from infected collections, and needle aspiration sampling can be helpful. Infection presenting early (first 2 to 3 weeks), especially in the patient who has never become free of inflammatory signs, is likely to be due to ongoing pancreatitis (see earlier). Abscesses manifesting late (3 weeks or longer) in the disease tend to be more well-defined collections of pus and to behave similarly to other types of

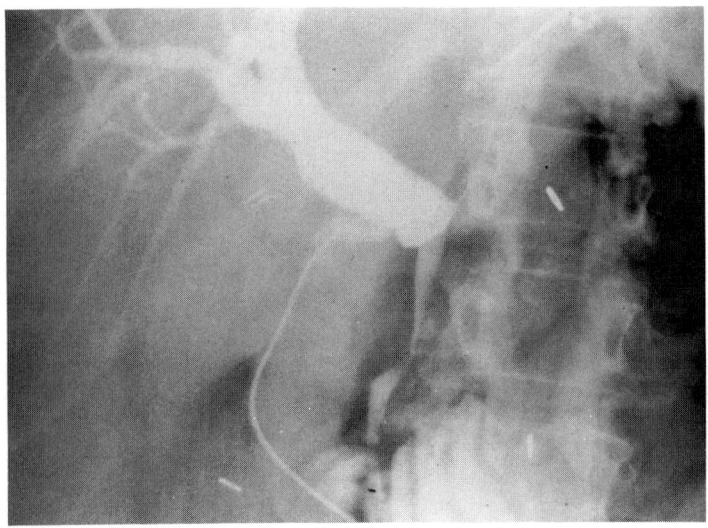

Figure 24-7 Intraoperative cholangiogram demonstrating compression of the distal common bile duct by acute inflammation in the head of the pancreas.

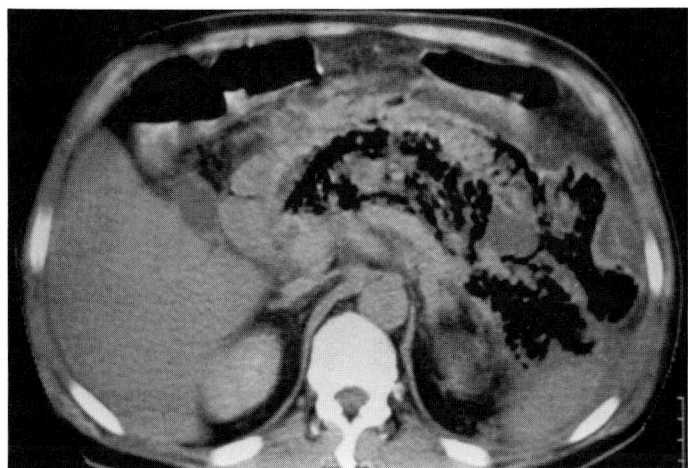

Figure 24-8 Abdominal CT scan showing extensive retroperitoneal inflammation with gas in the retroperitoneum due to a pancreatic abscess. CT findings in most pancreatic abscesses are not as dramatic.

intraabdominal abscesses. Adequate drainage is nonetheless essential; without it, the mortality rate approaches 100%. Antibiotics alone have never cured an abscess, and while limiting bacteremia, they may select for late fungal superinfection.

Guarded enthusiasm has developed for percutaneous drainage of pancreatic abscesses,[53,69] with some authors claiming up to a 70% success rate; others have not been as successful.[80] The major shortcoming of percutaneous drainage is the inability to débride thick necrotic material (Fig. 24-9) and thus to open all the extensions and loculations of what may be a labyrinthine cavity. Abscesses presenting late in the course of pancreatitis and those developing after initial surgical drainage are most appropriate for percutaneous cathe-

ter drainage. These tend to be well-defined collections of pus, perhaps similar to infected pseudocysts. In one report,[81] only 8 of 25 patients had successful treatment of pancreatic abscesses by percutaneous drainage alone. Most required a combination of surgical and radiologic drainage. Although the fluid component of the abscess is often adequately drained percutaneously, surgery is required to remove pieces of necrotic debris. Patients in whom the abscess can be successfully drained percutaneously may require multiple catheter insertions, multiple catheter manipulations, and long-term catheter drainage (averaging 3.5 weeks in this series).

Experience with pancreatic abscesses, emphasizing aggressive débridement of any associated necrosis, has reduced the mortality rate to 5%.[59] Late endocrine and

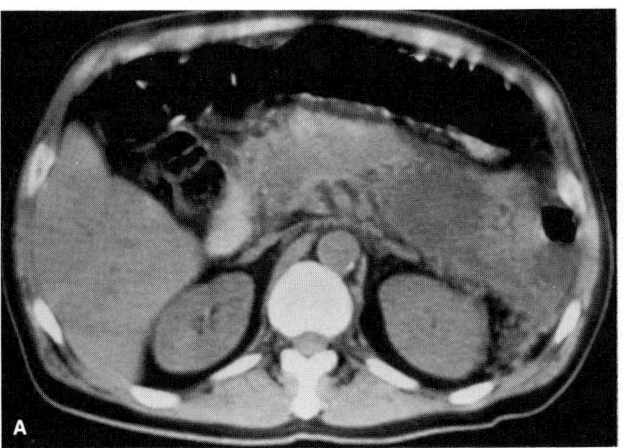
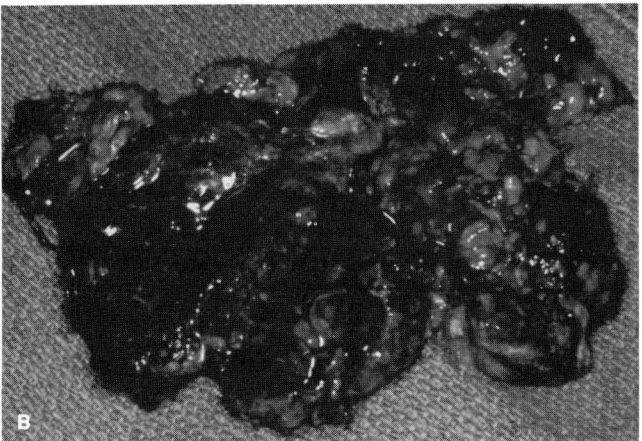

Figure 24-9 (A) Abdominal CT scan from a patient with necrotizing pancreatitis showing a collection in the region of the body of the pancreas. **(B)** Surgical specimen obtained from débridement. The necrotic debris resulting from acute necrotizing pancreatitis has the consistency of mud and is often too thick to drain through a percutaneously placed catheter. (See Color Fig. 24-9*B*.)

exocrine insufficiency is rare, probably because much of the removed tissue is peripancreatic tissue. Reoperation is required in 20% of patients. Complications occur frequently after abscess drainage and include fistulas, new abscesses, hemorrhage, renal failure, and wound infection.

PERSISTING PANCREATITIS

Some patients have lingering symptoms, such as inability to eat, abdominal pain, or even intermittent fever, long after a bout of acute pancreatitis. Often, there is no evidence of infection or other apparent reason for failure to improve. Most of these patients require intravenous nutritional support either at home or in the hospital. At some point (usually 2 to 3 months after the onset of illness), the physician must look for a reversible problem that will alter the course of the illness. When patients fail to progress during this prolonged interval, continued supportive therapy alone is not adequate treatment. For example, patients with sterile necrotic collections have occasionally been maintained on total parenteral nutrition for up to 1 year in the vain hope that surgery could be avoided. However, only débridement of necrotic tissue or removal of an inflammatory mass allows these patients to recover normal gastrointestinal function and return to a normal life-style.

Surgically correctable causes of persisting pancreatitis include undrained collections, irreversible injury to the pancreatic duct, or inflammatory masses pressing on the stomach or duodenum. If a focal collection is seen on CT scan, débridement or drainage is the appropriate intervention. If no explanation for persistent pancreatitis is seen on CT scan, ERCP may identify irreversible injury to the pancreatic duct causing persistent obstructive pancreatitis distal to the ductal injury. Distal pancreatectomy is indicated in such patients.[82]

A few patients continue to have low-grade signs of pancreatic inflammation for weeks or months, without focal collections or areas of necrosis demonstrable by CT scan to target for débridement or drainage. In patients who have persistent swelling or phlegmon in the head of the pancreas, pancreaticoduodenectomy is an appropriate option.[83] Usually, the resected specimen demonstrates microabscesses or unrecognized duodenal wall injury. Resection of the head of the pancreas in this setting is technically demanding and should only be performed by an experienced pancreatic surgeon.

REFERENCES

1. Steer ML. How and where does acute pancreatitis begin? Arch Surg 1992;127:1350.
2. Klar E, Mall G, Messmer K, Rattner DW, Warshaw AL. Improvement of impaired pancreatic microcirculation by isovolemic hemodilution protects pancreatic morphology in acute biliary pancreatitis. Surg Gynecol Obstet 1993;176:144.
3. Knoeffel WT, Kollias N, Warshaw AL, Nishioka N, Waldner H, Rattner DW. Pancreatic microperfusion in experimental pancreatitis of graded severity. Digestion 1991;49:31.
4. Schmidt J, Fernandez-del Castillo C, Rattner DW, Lewandrowski K, Warshaw AL. Ultra-molecular dextran (500,000 d) reduces trypsinogen activation, lowers mortality, and prevents necrosis in acute experimental pancreatitis. Am J Surg 1993;165:40.
5. Abruzzo JL, Homa M, Houck JC, et al. Significance of the serum amylase determination. Ann Surg 1958;147:921.
6. Lesser PB, Warshaw AL. Diagnosis of pancreatitis masked by hyperlipemia. Ann Intern Med 1975;82:795.
7. Uhl W, Buchler M, Malfertheiner P, Martini M, Beger HG. PMN elastase in comparison with CRP, antiproteases, and LDH as indicators of necrosis in human acute pancreatitis. Pancreas 1991;6:253.
8. Gudgeon AM, Heath DI, Hurley P, et al. Trypsinogen activation peptides assay in the early prediction of severity of acute pancreatitis. Lancet 1990;335:4.
9. Ranson JHC, Rifkind KM, Roses DF, et al. Prognostic signs and the role of operative management in acute pancreatitis. Surg Gynecol Obstet 1974;139:69.
10. Rattner DW, Legermate DA, Lee MJ, Mueller PR, Warshaw AL. Early surgical débridement of symptomatic pancreatic necrosis is beneficial irrespective of infection. Am J Surg 1992;163:105.
11. Stanten R, Frey CF. Comprehensive management of acute necrotizing pancreatitis and pancreatic abscess. Arch Surg 1990;125:1269.
12. Wilson C, Heath DI, Imrie CW. Prediction of outcome in acute pancreatitis: a comparative study of APACHE II, clinical assessment, and multiple factor scoring systems. Br J Surg 1990;77:1260.
13. Roumen RM, Schers TJ, deBoer HH, Goris RJ. Scoring systems for predicting outcome in acute hemorrhagic necrotizing pancreatitis. Eur J Surg 1992;158:167.
14. Knaus WA, Draper EA, Wagner DP, Zimmerman JE. APACHE II: a severity of disease classification. Crit Care Med 1985;13:818.
15. Bradley EL, Murphy F, Ferguson C. Prediction of pancreatic necrosis by dynamic pancreatography. Ann Surg 1989;210:495.
16. Puolakkainen PA. Early assessment of acute pancreatitis: a comparative study of computed tomography and laboratory tests. Acta Chir Scand 1989;155:25.
17. Larvin M, Chalmers AG, McMahon MJ. Dynamic contrast enhanced computed tomography: a precise technique for identifying and localizing pancreatic necrosis. Br Med J 1990;300:1425.
18. Nuutinen P. Contrast enhanced computed tomography in acute edematous pancreatitis. Surg Res Comm 1987;27:1035.

19. Block S, Maler W, Bittner R, Buchler M, Malfertheiner P, Beger HG. Identification of pancreas necrosis in severe acute pancreatitis: imaging procedures versus clinical staging. Gut 1986;27:1035.

20. Imrie CW, Whyte AS. A prospective study of acute pancreatitis. Br J Surg 1975;62:490.

21. Jacobs ML, Daggett WM, Civetta JM, et al. Acute pancreatitis: analysis of factors influencing survival. Ann Surg 1977;185:43.

22. DeTroyer A, Naeije R, Yernault JC, Englert M. Impairment of pulmonary function in acute pancreatitis. Chest 1978;73:360.

23. Ranson JHC, Turner JW, Roses DF. Respiratory complications in acute pancreatitis. Ann Surg 1974;179:557.

24. Warshaw AL, Lesser PB, Rie M, et al. The pathogenesis of pulmonary edema in acute pancreatitis. Ann Surg 1975;182:505.

25. Glorup I, Roikjaer O, Andersen B, et al. A double blind multicenter trial of somatostatin in the treatment of acute pancreatitis. Surg Gynecol Obstet 1992;175:397.

26. D'Amico D, Favia G, Biasiato R, et al. The use of somatostatin in acute pancreatitis: results of a multicenter trial. Hepatogastroenterology 1990;37:92.

27. Beger HG, Krautzberger W, Bittner R, et al. Results of surgical treatment of necrotizing pancreatitis. World J Surg 1985;59:972.

28. Bassi C, Fontana R, Vesentini S, et al. Antibacterial and mezlocillin enhancing activity of pure human pancreatic juice. Int J Pancreatol 1991;10:293.

29. Pederzoli P, Bassi C, Vesentini S, Campedelli A. A randomized multicenter clinical trial of antibiotic prophylaxis of septic complications in acute necrotizing pancreatitis with imipenem. Surg Gynecol Obstet 1993;176:480.

30. Acosta JM, Ledersma CL. Gallstone migration as a cause of acute pancreatitis. N Engl J Med 1974;290:484.

31. Acosta JM, Pellegrini CA, Skinner DB. Etiology and pathogenesis of acute biliary pancreatitis. Surgery 1980;88:118.

32. Coppa GF, LeFleur R, Ranson JHC. The role of Chiba needle cholangiography in the diagnosis of possible acute pancreatitis with cholelithiasis. Ann Surg 1981;193:393.

33. Mayer AD, McMahon MJ. Biochemical identification of patients with gallstones associated with acute pancreatitis the day of admission to the hospital. Ann Surg 1984;201:68.

34. Neoptolemos JP, London N, Bailey I, et al. The role of clinical and biochemical criteria and endoscopic cholangiopancreatography in the urgent diagnosis of common bile duct stones in acute pancreatitis. Surgery 1986;100:732.

35. Neoptolemos JP, London N, Slater ND, et al. A prospective study of ERCP and endoscopic sphincterotomy in the diagnosis and treatment of gallstone acute pancreatitis. Arch Surg 1986;121:697.

36. Neoptolemos JP. The theory of persisting common bile duct stones in severe gallstone pancreatitis. Ann R Coll Surg Engl 1989;71:326.

37. Ranson JHC. The timing of biliary surgery in acute pancreatitis. Ann Surg 1979;189:654.

38. Kelley TR. Gallstone pancreatitis: the timing of surgery. Surgery 1980;88:345.

39. Welch JP, White CE. Acute pancreatitis of biliary origin: is urgent operation necessary? Am J Surg 1982;143:120.

40. Rosseland AR, Solhaug JH. Early or delayed endoscopic papillotomy in gallstone pancreatitis. Ann Surg 1984;199:165.

41. Sanfray L, Cotton PB. A preliminary report: urgent duodenoscopic sphincterotomy for acute gallstone pancreatitis. Surgery 1981;89:424.

42. Fan ST, Lai ECS, Mok FPT, Lo CM, Zheng SS, Wong J. Early treatment of acute biliary pancreatitis by endoscopic papillotomy. N Engl J Med 1993;328:228.

43. Lawson DW, Daggett WM, Civetta JM, et al. Surgical treatment of acute necrotizing pancreatitis. Ann Surg 1970;172:605.

44. Warshaw AL, Imbembo AL, Civetta JM, et al. Surgical intervention in acute necrotizing pancreatitis. Ann Surg 1974;179:484.

45. Hollender LF, Meyer C, Marrie A, et al. Role of surgery in the management of acute pancreatitis. World J Surg 1981;5:361.

46. Kivilaakso E, Lempinen M, Makelarnen A, et al. Pancreatic resection versus peritoneal lavation for acute fulminant pancreatitis. Surg Gynecol Obstet 1981;152:493.

47. Schroder T, Sainio V, Kivisaari L, Puolakkainen P, Kivilaakso E, Lempinen M. Pancreatic resection versus peritoneal lavage in acute necrotizing pancreatitis: a prospective randomized trial. Ann Surg 1991;214:663.

48. Ihse I, Evander A, Holmberg JT, Gustafson I. Influence of peritoneal lavage on objective prognostic signs in acute pancreatitis. Ann Surg 1986;204:122.

49. Kauste A, Hookersted EK, Ahonen J, et al. Peritoneal lavage as a primary treatment in acute fulminant pancreatitis. Surg Gynecol Obstet 1983;156:458.

50. Ranson JH, Spencer FC. The role of peritoneal lavage in severe acute pancreatitis. Ann Surg 1978;187:565.

51. Ranson JHC, Berman RS. Long peritoneal lavage decreases pancreatic sepsis in acute pancreatitis. Ann Surg 1990;211:708.

52. Beger HG, Bittner R, Block S, Buchler M. Bacterial contamination of pancreatic necrosis: a prospective clinical study. Gastroenterology 1986;91:433.

53. Gerzof SG, Robbins AH, Johnson WC, et al. Percutaneous catheter drainage of abdominal abscess: a five year experience. N Engl J Med 1981;305:653.

54. Gerzof SG, Banks PA, Robbins AH, et al. Early diagnosis of pancreatic infection by CT-guided aspiration. Gastroenterology 1987;93:1315.

55. Beger HG, Bittner R, Buchler M, et al. Hemodynamic data pattern in patients with acute pancreatitis. Gastroenterology 1986;90:74.

56. Karimgani I, Porter KA, Langevin RE, Banks PA. Prognostic factors in sterile pancreatic necrosis. Gastroenterology 1992;103:1636.

57. Bradley EL, Allen K. A prospective longitudinal study of

observation versus surgical intervention in the management of necrotizing pancreatitis. Am J Surg 1991;161:19.

58. Reber HA. Surgical intervention in necrotizing pancreatitis. Gastroenterology 1986;91:479.

59. Warshaw AL, Jin G. Improved survival in 45 patients with pancreatic abscess. Ann Surg 1985;202:408.

60. Beger HG, Buchler M, Bittner R, Oettinger W, Block S, Nevalaainen T. Necrosectomy and postoperative local lavage in patients with necrotizing pancreatitis: results of a prospective trial. World J Surg 1988;12:255.

61. Villazon A, Villazon O, Terrazas F, Rana R. Retroperitoneal drainage in the management of the septic phase of severe acute pancreatitis. World J Surg 1991;15:103.

62. Warshaw AL, Rattner DW. The timing of surgical drainage for pancreatic pseudocysts: clinical and chemical criteria. Ann Surg 1985;202:720.

63. Crass RA, Way LW. Acute and chronic pancreatic pseudocysts are different. Am J Surg 1981;142:660.

64. Agha FP. Spontaneous resolution of acute pancreatic pseudocysts. Surg Gynecol Obstet 1984;158:22.

65. Bradley EL, Gonzales AC, Clements JL. Acute pancreatic pseudocysts: incidence and implications. Ann Surg 1976;184:734.

66. Yeo CJ, Bastidas JA, Lynch-Nyhan A, Fishman EK, Zinner MD, Cameron JL. The natural history of pancreatic pseudocysts documented by computed tomography. Surg Gynecol Obstet 1990;170:411.

67. Martin EW Jr, Catalano P, Cooperman M, et al. Surgical decision making in the treatment of pancreatic pseudocysts: internal vs. external drainage. Am J Surg 1979;138:821.

68. Johnson LB, Rattner DW, Warshaw AL. The effect of size of giant pancreatic pseudocysts on the outcome of internal drainage procedures. Surg Gynecol Obstet 1991;173:171.

69. Gerzof SG, Johnson WC, Robbins AH, Spechler SJ, Nabseth DC. Percutaneous drainage of infected pancreatic pseudocysts. Arch Surg 1984;119:888.

70. Adams DB, Harvey JS, Anderson MC. Percutaneous drainage of infected pancreatic and peripancreatic fluid collections. Arch Surg 1990;125:1554.

71. Van Sonnenberg E, Wittich GR, Casola G, et al. Complicated pancreatic inflammatory disease: diagnostic and therapeutic role of interventional radiology. Radiology 1985;15:335.

72. Sahel J, Bastiel C, Pellat B, Schurgers P, Sarles H. Endoscopic cystoduodenostomy of cysts of chronic calcifying pancreatitis: a report of 20 cases. Pancreas 1987;2:447.

73. Kozarek RS, Bryako CM, Harlan J, Sanowski RA, Cintora I, Kovac A. Endoscopic drainage of pancreatic pseudocyst. Gastrointest Endosc 1985;31:322.

74. Waltman AC, Luers PR, Athanasoulis CA, Warshaw AL. Massive arterial hemorrhage in patients with pancreatitis: complementary roles of surgery and transcatheter occlusive techniques. Arch Surg 1986;121:439.

75. Warshaw AL, Moncure AC, Rattner DW. Gastrocutaneous fistulas associated with pancreatic abscess: an aggressive entity. Ann Surg 1989;210:603.

76. Smith AC, Shapiro RH, Kelsey PB, Warshaw AL. Successful treatment of non-healing biliary–cutaneous fistulas with biliary stenting. Gastroenterology 1986;90:764.

77. Bradley EL, Fulenwider JT. Operative treatment of pancreatic abscess. Surg Gynecol Obstet 1984;150:509.

78. McMahon MJ, Playforth MJ, Pickford IR. A comparative study of methods for the prediction of severity of attacks of acute pancreatitis. Br J Surg 1980;67:22.

79. Ranson JHC, Balthazar E, Caccavale R, Cooper M. Computed tomography and the predication of pancreatic abscess in acute pancreatitis. Ann Surg 1985;201:656.

80. Rotman N, Mathieu D, Anglade MC, Fagniez PL. Failure of percutaneous drainage of pancreatic abscesses complicating severe acute pancreatitis. Surg Gynecol Obstet 1992;174:141.

81. Steiner E, Mueller PR, Hahn PF, et al. Complicated pancreatic abscesses: problems in interventional management. Radiology 1988;167:443.

82. Warshaw AL, Cambria RP. False pancreas divisum: acquired pancreatic duct obstruction simulating the congenital anomaly. Ann Surg 1984;200:595.

83. Rutledge PL, Warshaw AL. Persistent pancreatitis: a variant treated by pancreatico-duodenectomy. Arch Surg 1988;123:597.

Digestive Tract Surgery: A Text and Atlas, edited by Richard H. Bell, Layton F. Rikkers, and Michael W. Mulholland. Lippincott-Raven Publishers, Philadelphia, © 1996.

25

Chronic Pancreatitis

David W. McFadden | *Howard A. Reber*

Chronic pancreatitis is an inflammatory disease of the pancreas characterized by replacement of its exocrine and endocrine tissue with fibrous scar. In the United States, most cases are attributable to chronic alcoholism, and confirmed alcoholics are 20 to 50 times more likely to have chronic pancreatitis than are members of the general population.[1] The disease process usually is inexorable, even if the patient stops drinking. Chronic pain is the primary reason for surgical therapy in most patients. Other complications of chronic pancreatitis that may require surgery include pseudocysts, biliary and intestinal obstruction, and splenic vein thrombosis.

Gallstone pancreatitis, the second most common cause of acute pancreatitis, rarely leads to chronic pancreatitis. The pancreas is believed to return to normal between attacks. It is this difference in the capability of the pancreas to recover that forms the basis for the classification of pancreatitis into acute and chronic forms (Table 25-1). Nevertheless, patients with chronic pancreatitis may have intermittent episodes of acute pancreatic inflammation.

Surveillance studies of patients with chronic pancreatitis suggest that few die as a direct result of the disease. Prognosis is determined by the adequacy and availability of medical care, the socioeconomic conditions and intellectual capacity of the patient, and the presence of continued alcoholism and narcotic addiction.[2-4] Several large cohort studies have revealed that chronic pancreatitis is the direct cause of death in only 20% of patients, with most patients succumbing to alcohol-induced liver disease, cancer, or postoperative complications.[5-8] Between 25% and 35% of patients operated on for chronic pancreatitis are dead within 5 years.[5,7,9] The mortality rate is higher in patients who continue to drink alcohol (63% versus 25% at 6 years).[10]

ETIOLOGY

Alcohol-Induced Pancreatitis

Alcoholism is the cause of 75% of the cases of chronic pancreatitis in the United States and other developed countries. Several clinical forms of chronic pancreatitis have been described. Episodes of binge drinking may produce attacks typical of acute pancreatitis. These usually occur in patients who have been drinking for years but who have not had any symptoms of pancreatic disease before the first attack. Nevertheless, such patients are thought already to have suffered permanent damage to the pancreas.[10] Another clinical scenario occurs in individuals with chronic abdominal or back pain, often accompanied by steatorrhea and diabetes, the result of exocrine and endocrine insufficiency. These patients may never have had a recognized episode of acute pancreatic inflammation.

Pancreatic calcifications are seen in one third of patients with alcohol-induced chronic pancreatitis,[9] but their presence does not imply a worse clinical prognosis. In fact, freedom from pain was correlated with the presence of calcifications in one prospective review.[5] Significant weight loss is common because eating may aggravate the pain, and patients avoid food. Narcotic addiction also is common. The usual age of onset is in the mid-30s, and men are affected more commonly than women (Table 25-2). Cessation of alcohol use may lessen the continued deterioration in endocrine pancreatic function, but does not stop the progression of the disease.[5,11] Abstinence also may increase the chances of pain relief after surgical intervention.[5]

Symptomatic chronic pancreatitis has been diagnosed as early as 2 years after the beginning of significant alcohol consumption, but most cases involve a de-

Table 25-1 Classification of Pancreatitis

Classification	Description	Clinical Characteristics	Morphologic Characteristics
ACUTE PANCREATITIS	Exocrine and endocrine functions are temporarily impaired. Functional restitution to normal usually occurs. Rarely leads to chronic pancreatitis.	Acute abdominal or back pain. Increased pancreatic enzymes in blood or urine. Usually benign course, but can be severe and fatal. May be a single episode or recurrent.	Gradation of lesions from mild (interstitial edema, periglandular fat necrosis) to severe (peripancreatic and pancreatic necrosis and hemorrhage). Clinical features and morphologic findings may not correlate.
CHRONIC PANCREATITIS	Demonstrates irreversible morphologic changes leading to progressive and permanent deficits in endocrine and exocrine function. In obstructive chronic pancreatitis, improvements are noted after the obstruction is removed.	Persistent and recurrent abdominal pain in most patients, evidence of pancreatic insufficiency (eg, steatorrhea or diabetes).	Irregular sclerosis, with destruction and permanent loss of exocrine parenchyma in focal, segmental, or diffuse patterns. Varying degrees of ductular and ductal dilatation. Cysts, pseudocysts, and intraductal calculi are common, as are edema and focal necrosis. Islets of Langerhans appear relatively well preserved. In obstructive chronic pancreatitis, the ductal system is dilated proximal to the point of occlusion (by tumor or scarring), with diffuse atrophy and fibrosis. Calculi are uncommon.

cade or more of ethanol ingestion. Daily consumption averages 100 to 150 g, and the type of alcoholic beverage consumed is irrelevant. Alcoholics who ingest a diet high in protein and fat may have a greater risk of chronic pancreatitis.[10] An estimated 10% to 15% of alcoholics develop chronic pancreatitis; a similar percentage develop cirrhosis of the liver. The factors that control individual susceptibility remain unknown.

Initial investigations suggested that ethanol produced pancreatitis by evoking spasm of the sphincter of Oddi, creating an outflow obstruction to exocrine pancreatic secretion. However, this does not appear to be a full explanation for the development of pancreatitis. Ethanol also is a cellular metabolic toxin, with detrimental effects on both the synthetic and secretory capacities of pancreatic acinar cells. An increase in pancreatic juice concentrations of enzyme protein has been described, along with precipitation of protein plugs in the ductules. Calcium can complex within the matrix of these plugs, resulting in multiple points of ductal obstruction scattered throughout the pancreas.[10] Further parenchymal damage follows as secretion continues against this multifocal obstruction. Pancreatic ductal permeability also is increased by ethanol, perhaps allowing pancreatic enzymes to leak into and damage the surrounding tissue.

Duct Obstruction

Mechanical obstruction to pancreatic juice secretion is the primary cause of chronic pancreatitis in about 5% of cases. It is important to establish obstruction as the

Table 25-2 Clinical Features of Chronic Pancreatitis

Feature	Incidence	Etiology	Remarks
Pain	85%	Unknown; fibrosis, low blood flow, neural encasement are suggested reasons	Back or abdominal pain postprandial in nature and relieved by postural changes
Weight loss	Common	Fear of eating, because of pain; malabsorption	Typically gradual; if rapid, consider pancreatic cancer
Malabsorption	Subclinical in almost all patients	Exocrine insufficiency	Diarrhea, steatorrhea, and azotorrhea
Diabetes	Glucose intolerance common; frank diabetes in 30%	Endocrine insufficiency	Ketoacidosis and nephropathy are rare. Retinopathy and neuropathy have similar incidences

cause, because reversal of some of the damage to the pancreas may be possible if the obstruction is removed early enough.[12] Ductal obstruction as a cause of chronic pancreatitis occurs in a variety of clinical settings.

Congenital and Acquired Strictures of the Pancreatic Duct

Fusion of the ventral and dorsal pancreatic ducts occurs during fetal development, and narrowing of the duct at this junction occurs normally in 3% of the population.[13] If this finding is seen on endoscopic retrograde cholangiopancreatography (ERCP), it is pathologically significant only if proximal ductal dilation exists. Chronic pancreatitis has been reported in patients with severe strictures. These patients tend to be young adults who have weight loss and abdominal pain.[14] Any part of the pancreatic duct can develop a stricture after scarring from trauma or severe acute pancreatitis. Posttraumatic strictures tend to be in the mid-body of the gland, where the duct is compressed over the underlying vertebral bodies. The resultant chronic pancreatitis affects only the distal pancreas.

Cystic Fibrosis

Cystic fibrosis, transmitted as an autosomal recessive trait, is the most common lethal genetic disease in the United States. Pancreatic insufficiency is present in up to 95% of patients, usually manifesting as steatorrhea and azotorrhea.[15] Recurrent episodes of acute or chronic pancreatitis occasionally develop in older children or adults with this disorder. Pancreatic calcifications, diabetes, and abdominal pain are often described. Surgical therapy is the same for these patients as for those with chronic pancreatitis from other causes, but the chronic pulmonary disease of patients with cystic

fibrosis puts them at higher risk for perioperative complications.[16]

Pancreas Divisum

Pancreas divisum (Fig. 25-1) is a normal variant of the pancreatic ductal system in which most pancreatic secretions enter the duodenum through the minor papilla. Only the secretions from the uncinate process of the gland (the ventral pancreas) empty through the major papilla with the bile. Pancreas divisum occurs in about 7% of the population and usually is not associated with clinical pancreatic disease. Sometimes the opening at the minor papilla is too small for the large amount of pancreatic juice secreted, and the obstruction results in repeated episodes of acute pancreatitis or chronic obstructive pancreatitis.[17] In some patients with this problem who have undergone pancreatic resection, the changes of chronic pancreatitis were confined to the area of the pancreas that drained through the minor papilla.[10] Such patients tend to be young women (mean age 29 years) with no history of significant alcohol abuse.[18] In patients with established chronic pancreatitis and pancreas divisum, efforts to relieve the obstruction at the minor papilla usually are ineffective.[10]

Duct Obstruction by Tumors

Cancer of the head of the pancreas often obstructs the pancreatic duct and produces chronic obstructive pancreatitis. However, clinically significant chronic pancreatitis is unusual in this setting. Rarely, in patients with slow-growing cancers, pain and steatorrhea may be present for some time and may be attributed to chronic pancreatitis. Episodes of acute pancreatic inflammation also may occur. These patients usually are older than those with alcohol-induced chronic pancre-

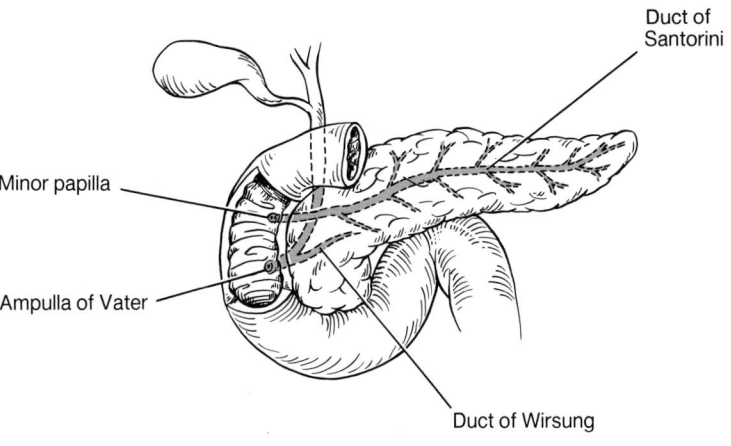

Minor papilla

Ampulla of Vater

Duct of Santorini

Duct of Wirsung

Figure 25-1 Pancreas divisum, a congenital anomaly of the pancreas in which the duct of Santorini (dorsal pancreatic duct) is the predominant duct draining the pancreatic parenchyma.

atitis and often have no apparent cause for the pancreatitis. A high index of clinical suspicion is necessary to make a correct and early diagnosis.

Inflammation of the Papilla of Vater

The papilla of Vater rarely is chronically inflamed, and obstruction of the duct of Wirsung by such a process is even less common.[10] When inflammation is present, it usually is caused by the passage of common bile duct stones through the papilla, although the vigorous use of metal dilators at the time of common bile duct exploration also has been implicated. In some cases, there is no apparent explanation. Clinicians must be extremely cautious in attributing chronic pancreatitis to this entity, and all other possible factors must be eliminated first. As with pancreas divisum, treatment directed toward relief of the obstruction is not effective.[10]

Protein Malnutrition

A specific type of chronic pancreatitis is seen in children with severe protein-calorie malnutrition and kwashiorkor. Adequate dietary replenishment is curative, provided parenchymal fibrosis is minimal. Abdominal pain and pancreatic calcifications are uncommon.[10] Another kind of chronic pancreatitis, possibly related to malnutrition, occurs only in certain tropical areas (eg, Nigeria). Beginning in childhood, it is associated with abdominal pain, pancreatic calcification, steatorrhea, and diabetes. The pancreatic ducts usually are dilated and obstructed. Nutritional repletion does not reverse this process.[19]

Hypercalcemia

Hypercalcemic states, most commonly hyperparathyroidism, can cause both acute and chronic pancreatitis by unclear mechanisms. Hypercalcemia may encourage the intraductal precipitation of calcium stones, which are seen in nearly half these patients. Calcium also influences the activation of certain pancreatic enzymes and acinar cell synthetic and secretory events. Acute hypercalcemia increases pancreatic ductal permeability, which may allow enzymatic leakage into the parenchyma. Hypercalcemia also increases the secretion of protein into the pancreatic juice.[20]

Hereditary Pancreatitis

Hereditary, or familial, pancreatitis is a rare form of progressive chronic pancreatitis associated with a variable clinical course.[19] It is inherited as an autosomal dominant trait with incomplete penetration. Symptoms

begin in early adolescence and are typical of acute pancreatitis. Relentless progression with parenchymal destruction is the rule, and calcifications, diabetes, and steatorrhea are seen in as many as 73% of patients. Most patients have dilated pancreatic ducts; therefore, lateral pancreaticojejunostomy often provides effective pain relief. The incidence of pancreatic carcinoma (9% to 20%) is increased in these patients, mandating close follow-up.[19]

Idiopathic Pancreatitis

No definitive cause of chronic pancreatitis is found in about 10% of patients in the United States, and in as many as 30% to 50% of patients in countries with low ethanol consumption. Patients with idiopathic chronic pancreatitis tend to be older than those with the alcohol-induced variety.[2] ERCP usually documents dilated pancreatic ducts; pancreatic calcifications are less common than in alcohol-induced pancreatitis. Patients with idiopathic chronic pancreatitis usually have less pain; disease progression and complications also occur less frequently.[21] The aging process itself can lead to pathologic changes similar to chronic pancreatitis (4.2% at 70 years; 16.7% at 90 years), although symptoms are unusual.[2] Idiopathic calcifying chronic pancreatitis in Europe has been linked to the ingestion of diets high in fat and protein.[20]

PATHOLOGY

Early in the disease, the pancreas is grossly normal in appearance and ERCP may reveal normal ducts. As the disease progresses, the pancreas may become enlarged, indurated, and edematous. The ducts still may be normal, or slight dilatation may be seen. Later, the pancreas usually is small, with rounded edges and a rubbery or firm consistency.[19] By this time, ERCP usually reveals dilated ducts. Ductal calculi are common, and vary from 1 mm to more than 1 cm in diameter. All pancreatic calcifications are located within the ducts. At surgery, the dilated main pancreatic duct often is palpable as a longitudinal soft depression on the anterior surface of the gland. In the normal pancreas, the main duct is posterior and not palpable. Microscopically, the disease initially is scattered irregularly throughout the gland, and is characterized by sclerosis of the exocrine parenchyma[2,19] (Fig. 25-2). Protein deposits, which later may calcify to form stones, obstruct the ducts. As the disease advances, fibrosis extends through the gland, although normal lobules still may be found. In the most advanced stages, the pancreas is replaced almost completely with fibrous tissue, with cysts seen in

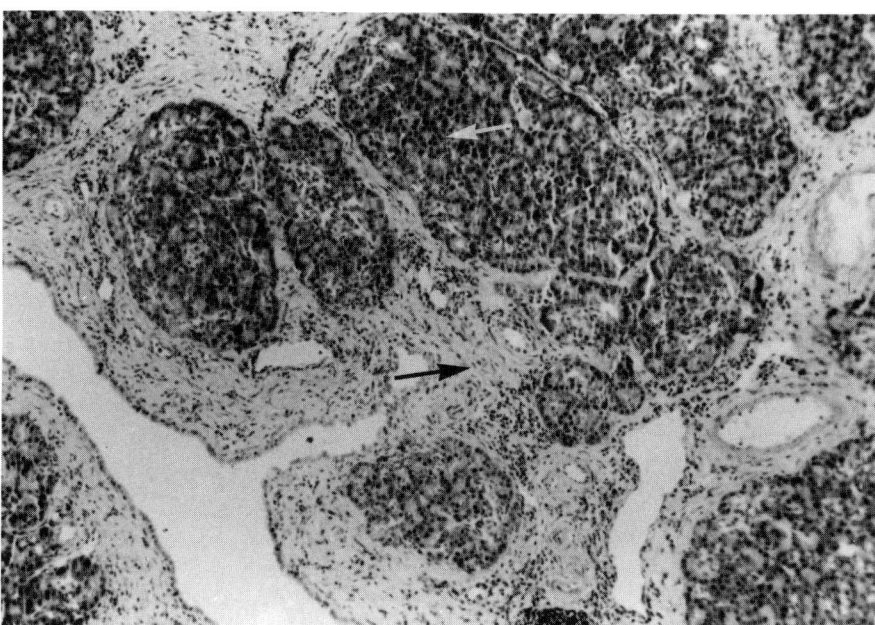

Figure 25-2 Histologic appearance of moderately advanced chronic pancreatitis (×50). Some normal acinar units are present (*white arrow*), but others have been replaced by fibrosis (*black arrow*). Numerous chronic inflammatory cells also are present.

lieu of ductal epithelium. Islets of Langerhans are relatively well preserved and may be histologically hyperplastic, despite functional deficiencies. Intrapancreatic nerves are distributed more densely as a result of parenchymal contraction and fibrosis. The neurilemmal sheaths appear destroyed, possibly allowing noxious substances to contact and irritate them.

In chronic pancreatitis secondary to chronic obstruction of the main duct, the lesions are more diffuse and all the lobules are evenly affected. Only moderate ductal dilatation is seen, and protein plugging and calculi are rare.

DIAGNOSIS

Clinical Manifestations

Abdominal pain is the presenting symptom in up to 95% of patients with chronic pancreatitis. The intensity of the pain can be severe and often is described as boring, dull, cramping, or aching in quality. Usually located in the epigastrium, the pain of chronic pancreatitis is felt in the back in about half of patients.[2] The pain may be partially relieved by sitting with the trunk bent forward or by lying prone. Patients also characteristically lie curled in a fetal position. The pain may be episodic or constant. In most cases, the pain-free intervals shorten and the painful attacks become longer. When the disease is so far advanced that most exocrine function is lost, about one third of patients experience spontaneous pain relief. Another 10% to 20% have tempo-

rary remissions that last 1 to 3 years.[2] The "burnout" theory of pain has led many clinicians to postpone surgical consultation for these patients, in the hope that the pain eventually will subside spontaneously. Unfortunately, there is no way to predict in which patients this will occur.

The aggravation of pain by food is characteristic of chronic pancreatitis as well as carcinoma of the pancreas. It probably is related to meal-induced stimulation of pancreatic secretion, which may acutely reduce blood flow to the gland. Drinking ethanol may worsen the pain, although many patients claim that pain develops or worsens after 12 to 24 hours of abstinence, and they continue to drink.[21] Patients often fear eating, and about 75% lose weight because of decreased intake. Significant weight loss from malabsorption or diabetes is less common, because most of these patients are able to maintain their weight by eating more frequently and in greater amounts. Narcotic addiction is common, and correlates with a worsened surgical prognosis.[4] Painless chronic pancreatitis occurs 5% to 10% of the time, and is more likely to be of the idiopathic variety.[18,22]

The pathogenesis of the pain in chronic pancreatitis remains unclear. Suggested causes include pancreatic inflammation, increased pancreatic parenchymal or intraductal pressure, neural inflammation, and pancreatic ischemia.[9,23] Most likely, the pain of chronic pancreatitis is multifactorial, and different factors may predominate depending on the etiology, structural changes, degree of pancreatic insufficiency, and severity of the disease.[23]

Diarrhea, steatorrhea, and azotorrhea are hallmarks of significant pancreatic exocrine insufficiency but usually do not occur until 90% of the secretory capacity of the pancreas is lost.[23] These symptoms can be the result of either progressive parenchymal destruction or major ductal obstruction. Steatorrhea is an earlier and more significant problem than azotorrhea, because troublesome diarrhea usually accompanies significant fat malabsorption.[2,23] Carbohydrate digestion is unaffected, because salivary amylase production continues normally. Patients complain of bulky, offensive, fatty, or oily stools. Deficiencies in the fat-soluble vitamins are rare.[23]

Almost 70% of patients with chronic pancreatitis have abnormal glucose tolerance, and half of these have frank diabetes mellitus. Some degree of malabsorption also is present in these patients. The diabetes usually is easily controlled with insulin, but hypoglycemia can be a problem in alcoholics with irregular eating habits.[10] Although ketosis and nephropathy are less common, retinopathy and neuropathy occur with the same frequency as in idiopathic diabetes mellitus.[24]

Many patients with chronic pancreatitis have failed to adapt to societal stresses and have inadequate personalities. The burdens of the disease often result in depression and anxiety.[10] These character traits must be recognized and addressed by the treating physician.

Abnormal physical findings are rare in patients with chronic pancreatitis. There may be some epigastric tenderness and evidence of weight loss. Occasionally, jaundice is present. A palpable mass usually is a pancreatic pseudocyst. Painful nodules over the lower extremities, from subcutaneous fat necrosis, and polyarthritis of the small hand joints are seen occasionally.

Laboratory Findings

Routine blood studies are rarely of benefit in the diagnosis of chronic pancreatitis. Leukocytosis, hyperamylasemia, and hyperlipasemia can be seen during acute exacerbations but may not be present later in the course of the disease. Explanations for the often normal serum pancreatic enzyme concentrations noted during acute exacerbations of chronic pancreatitis include previous acinar cell destruction that limits the amount of enzyme available for release, and chronic fibrosis that restricts leakage of enzymes into the circulation during inflammation. About two thirds of patients with alcohol-induced chronic pancreatitis have abnormal results on liver function studies, usually mild elevations of serum levels of bilirubin, alkaline phosphatase, and

aspartate aminotransferase.[23] Mild depression of the serum albumin level also may be present.

Numerous tests of pancreatic function have been evaluated for their ability to provide diagnostic and prognostic information in chronic pancreatitis. These include measurements of serum concentrations of trypsin, elastase, pancreatic isoamylase, and pancreatic polypeptide, as well as tests of pancreatic function such as cholecystokinin–secretin stimulation or test meals (Lundh test).[24] Such tests rarely are indicated in patients with chronic pancreatitis or pancreatic cancer, because they seldom influence therapy or distinguish between the two diseases. They may be of some value in the evaluation of patients with suspected pancreatic disease for which there is no radiologic evidence.

Imaging Studies

The finding of diffuse speckled calcifications within the pancreas on plain abdominal radiographs is diagnostic of chronic pancreatitis, and is seen in 30% to 50% of patients[25] (Fig. 25-3). Accordingly, plain films of the abdomen often are the first imaging procedure performed.[24] Ultrasound is the next simplest and least expensive radiographic method. Dilated pancreatic ducts (more than 4 to 5 mm in diameter), pseudocysts, and calcifications all can be detected with overall sensitivities of 70% and specificities of 90%.[26]

Computed tomographic (CT) scanning is 10% to 20% more sensitive than ultrasound for diagnosing chronic pancreatitis, but has a similar specificity.[26] Although CT is more expensive and requires the use of ionizing radiation, it provides the most reliable overall assessment of the pancreas and peripancreatic area, and should be performed in all patients in whom surgery is contemplated or a complication of chronic pancreatitis is suspected.[10,23] The most common CT findings in chronic pancreatitis include ductal dilatation, calcifications, and cystic lesions in or near the pancreas (Fig. 25-4). Less commonly, enlargement or atrophy of the gland, heterogenous parenchymal density, and splenic vein thrombosis are seen.[27] When the duct is dilated, it usually can be seen traversing the gland. Biliary dilatation, if present, also is evident.

ERCP is the radiologic procedure of choice in the diagnosis of chronic pancreatitis. The accuracy of ERCP in making the diagnosis increases with the duration of disease, reaching 92% in patients who have been affected for more than 5 years.[27] ERCP should be performed in most patients with chronic pancreatitis who are being evaluated for operation. The radiologic appearance of the ductal system may show caliber variations, strictures, obstructions, ductal filling defects consistent with stones, pseudocysts, and areas of dilata-

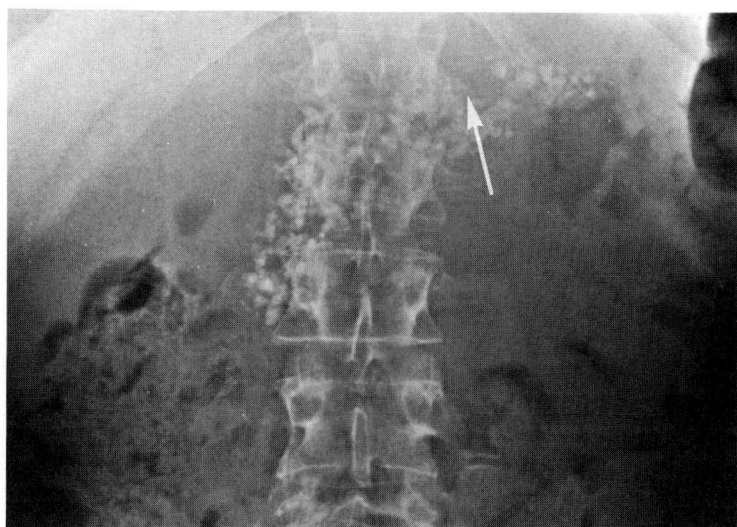

Figure 25-3 Plain abdominal radiograph demonstrating extensive abdominal calcification (*arrow*) in a patient with chronic pancreatitis.

tion.[25] If a preoperative ERCP cannot be obtained, intraoperative pancreatography may be required. This usually is done by needle puncture of the main pancreatic duct through the anterior surface of the gland. Occasionally, duodenotomy and cannulation of the duct through the ampulla are necessary.[28] Intraoperative ultrasound may be useful in cases in which the main pancreatic duct is difficult to localize.

In most patients with advanced chronic pancreatitis, the main pancreatic duct is dilated up to 1 cm in diameter, often with intermittent points of obstruction (chain-of-lakes appearance; Fig. 25-5). The common bile duct usually is opacified during ERCP, which may reveal bile duct compression and influence the therapy (see later).

Differential Diagnosis

Although the diagnosis of chronic pancreatitis usually is straightforward, at times it can be difficult to differentiate from cancer of the pancreas, especially from tumors of the head of the gland. Although CT scans and ERCP images help to distinguish the two, laparotomy and biopsy may be required. Even then, it may not be possible to identify a small cancer situated deeply within an indurated, enlarged, and chronically in-

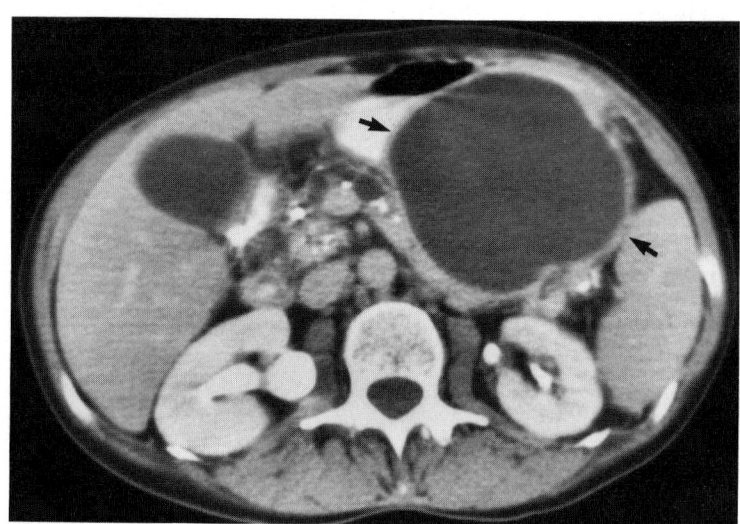

Figure 25-4 CT scan of the abdomen demonstrating a pseudocyst in the region of the pancreatic tail (*arrows*). The main pancreatic duct is dilated, and the gland contains calcifications.

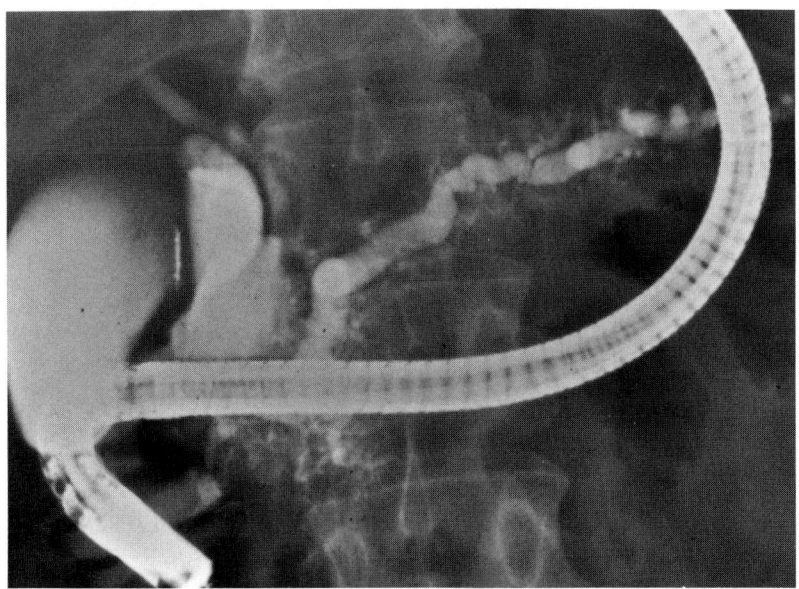

Figure 25-5 Endoscopic retrograde cholangiopancreatography demonstrating alternating areas of stricture formation and dilation (chain-of-lakes sign) in the main pancreatic duct of a patient with chronic pancreatitis. Clubbing of side branches of the pancreatic duct also is present.

flamed head of the pancreas.[8] Then, the decision whether to resect must be based on the surgeon's judgment and on the ability to perform the Whipple operation with an acceptably low mortality rate (less than 5%). Because chronic pancreatitis primarily affecting the head of the pancreas also is treated effectively by the same operation, resection is an acceptable approach in most patients in whom occult carcinoma of the head of the gland is suspected.

TREATMENT

Management of Acute Exacerbation of Pancreatitis

The medical treatment of episodes of acute inflammation in patients with chronic pancreatitis is the same as in patients with acute pancreatitis from other causes (see Chap. 24).

Pancreatic Insufficiency

Fat malabsorption causing steatorrhea and diarrhea is the primary problem requiring treatment in affected patients. Protein digestion is aided by gastric pepsin and small intestinal brush-border enzymes; salivary amylase facilitates carbohydrate digestion. Diarrhea can be eliminated and steatorrhea minimized if about 30,000 IU of lipase is supplied with each meal. This requires the ingestion of multiple tablets, the exact number depending on the amount of lipase present per tablet, which is highly variable in commercial preparations of pancreatic enzymes. If diarrhea persists, a H_2 receptor

antagonist can be added in the hopes of preventing inactivation of lipase by acidic gastric contents. Another approach is to use commercially available enzyme preparations with a pH-sensitive polymer coating, which may improve enzyme delivery in patients with significant levels of gastric acid production.

Diets for patients with chronic pancreatitis should supply 3000 to 6000 kcal/d, emphasizing carbohydrate (40 g or more) and protein (100 to 150 g).[2,23] Fat intake should not exceed 100 g/d, divided among four meals. Fat malabsorption can never be eliminated, but diarrhea should cease and weight gain is possible in most patients.[2,10]

Diabetes Mellitus

Patients with diabetes from chronic pancreatitis are sensitive to exogenous insulin, and hypoglycemia may result even from small doses. The absence of exogenous glucagon probably is a factor in this phenomenon.[10] Conversely, ketoacidosis is rare, even if blood glucose levels are high. Maintenance of fasting glucose levels between 150 and 200 mg/dL is acceptable. Less than 20 to 30 U/d of insulin usually is required. Oral agents rarely are effective.

The risk of developing diabetes after pancreatic resection is related directly to the preoperative glucose tolerance and the amount of pancreas resected. Most patients with abnormal glucose tolerance before operation require insulin after a resection of 50% or more of the pancreas.[2,10,23]

Pain

Up to 75% of patients experience substantial pain relief simply by stopping the intake of alcoholic beverages,[29] but over 50% continue to drink despite chronic pain.[2]

In theory, oral enzyme replacement should reduce pain by suppressing endogenous pancreatic enzyme synthesis and secretion. Although several studies have shown improvement in up to 75% of patients, most responders were middle-aged women with idiopathic chronic pancreatitis.[30–32] Most clinicians have been disappointed when this treatment has been applied to patients with alcohol-induced pancreatitis.

Celiac plexus block by percutaneous alcohol injection, using either ultrasound or CT guidance, has produced inconsistent results in chronic pancreatitis. Analgesic benefits may last only a few months, and repeated injections tend to be less effective.[32]

Analgesics remain the mainstay of nonoperative methods of pain control in patients with chronic pancreatitis. Initially, nonnarcotic agents should be used, and their administration before meals to decrease postprandial pain is suggested. Oral nonsteroidal antiinflammatory drugs are useful, but their tendency to cause gastric upset may require concomitant H_2 receptor antagonist treatment. Later, mild narcotics such as codeine or hydrocodone are used in combination with acetaminophen.[10] In severe cases, potent opiates are required, and addiction is common.[23]

Chronic pain is the most common indication for operation in chronic pancreatitis. All too often, patients are denied surgical treatment until they have become addicted to narcotics and are severely depressed from the constant pain. Operation earlier in the course of the disease (especially in patients with dilated ducts amenable to pancreaticojejunostomy) should be considered for most patients.[10] In patients who would require major pancreatic resections, or who have associated medical conditions that would significantly complicate the use of general anesthesia, continued management with analgesics may be warranted.

Extrapancreatic Involvement

Common Bile Duct Obstruction

Jaundice is seen in as many as one third of patients with chronic calcific pancreatitis sometime during the course of the disease. It most often results from transient obstruction of the intrapancreatic portion of the common bile duct during an episode of acute pancreatic inflammation, and subsides when the acute process resolves. However, some 10% of patients have persistent common duct obstruction from fibrous constriction of the duct in the head of the gland. On radiography, such

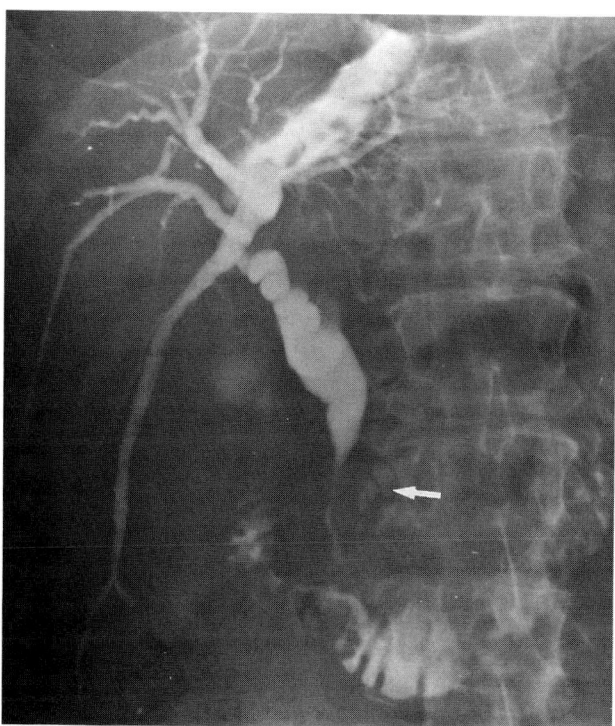

Figure 25-6 Percutaneous transhepatic cholangiogram demonstrating biliary obstruction resulting from tapered distal common bile duct stenosis caused by chronic pancreatitis. Calcification can be seen in the head of the pancreas (*arrow*).

strictures are smoothly tapered, longitudinal, and symmetric (Fig. 25-6). The common duct proximal to the stricture usually is moderately dilated. The gallbladder and cystic duct also may be distended. The obstruction is almost never complete, in contradistinction to pancreatic cancer, in which the stricture is shorter, asymmetric, and complete. When the obstruction is caused by chronic pancreatitis, and the duct is freed surgically from the constricting pancreas, it often expands to relieve the obstruction. Most often, the obstruction is simply bypassed with a choledochoduodenostomy or a choledochojejunostomy.

Duodenal Obstruction

Less than 1% of patients with chronic pancreatitis have persistent duodenal obstruction from inflammation in the adjacent pancreatic head. Duodenoscopy shows marked narrowing of the second or third portion of the duodenum with intact mucosa. The differential diagnosis includes pancreatic cancer, peptic ulcer, and rare conditions such as duodenal diverticulitis and annular pancreas. The correct diagnosis may not be made until the time of operation. Gastrojejunostomy is effective in bypassing the obstruction.

Colonic Obstruction

Occasional patients with chronic pancreatitis have colonic obstruction. In 80% to 90%, the transverse colon, splenic flexure, or both are involved. The hepatic flexure is involved in 15% of cases. In 80% of patients, the obstruction is partial. When colonic obstruction is associated with an episode of acute pancreatitis, the obstruction often resolves with conservative therapy. When obstruction is due to chronic fibrosis, operation is required for relief. Carcinoma of the colon generally can be ruled out by preoperative colonoscopy because benign strictures are associated with an intact mucosa. Colon resection with end-to-end anastomosis is curative.

Splenic Vein Thrombosis

Thrombosis of the splenic vein may result from repeated episodes of pancreatic inflammation, compression of the vein by pancreatic fibrosis, or a combination of both. Splenic vein thrombosis produces left-sided portal hypertension with gastric varices, and may be associated with life-threatening episodes of upper gastrointestinal hemorrhage. Splenectomy is curative and indicated in patients who have symptoms.

Pseudocysts

Pseudocysts are discussed in depth in Chapter 24, and usually occur after an episode of acute pancreatitis. Nevertheless, they complicate as many as 40% of cases of chronic pancreatitis, and can produce similar symptoms and complications in the chronic setting. The pathogenesis of pseudocysts in chronic pancreatitis probably is related to ductal obstruction with continued secretion into the obstructed duct segment. The duct dilates and eventually ruptures into the surrounding tissue, where it enlarges to form a clinically evident cyst. Pseudocysts that develop in patients with chronic pancreatitis usually have a mature wall by the time they are detected, so a preoperative waiting period for cyst maturation is unnecessary.

Surgical Treatment of Chronic Pancreatitis

The goals of surgery in chronic pancreatitis are to relieve intractable pain and to treat complications while preserving as much functioning pancreatic tissue as possible.[8] Several points must be made clear to patients and their families:

1. Surgery is unlikely to affect the relentless dete-

rioration of pancreatic function in most patients.
2. There is no completely satisfactory operation for chronic pancreatitis, and results of surgery are variable.
3. Third, patients with continued narcotic or alcohol use have limited life expectancies and tend to have the worst results from surgery.[4,8]

Most operations for chronic pancreatitis are performed for intractable pain that interferes substantially with the patient's quality of life. Factors that are considered include employability, frequency of hospitalization, psychiatric disturbances (usually depression), weight loss, deterioration of family life, and the need for narcotic analgesics.[10]

Patients being evaluated for surgery should undergo an abdominal CT scan and an ERCP in addition to the standard preoperative assessment for a major abdominal procedure. Arteriography may be considered if resection is entertained. Surgical care of each patient should be individualized, and preoperative psychiatric assessment frequently is beneficial.[10,23]

Historically, there have been three surgical approaches to the management of pain in chronic pancreatitis: ductal drainage, pancreatic resection, and denervation procedures.[33] The choice of operation is dictated by ductal anatomy and comorbid conditions.

Drainage Operations

Puestow and Gillesby[34] introduced a new standard for surgical management of chronic pancreatitis in 1956 with their description of 21 patients who underwent pancreaticoenterostomy. Four of these patients had a side-to-side pancreaticojejunostomy. The modern operation of longitudinal pancreaticojejunostomy was described in 1960 by Partington and Rochelle,[35] who eliminated splenectomy and excision of the tail of the gland (Fig. 25-7; see Section IVA in Atlas Chap. 30).

The normal diameter of the main pancreatic duct is 4 to 5 mm in the head, 3 to 4 mm in the body, and 2 to 3 mm in the tail of the gland.[10] When the diameter in the head and body expands to 7 to 8 mm or more, a pancreaticojejunostomy becomes technically feasible and has a good chance of producing lasting pain relief. Results are poor in glands with smaller ducts, possibly because of anastomotic strictures.

Most series report operative mortality rates of less than 5% from pancreaticojejunostomy, with morbidity rates that range from 7% to 30%.[25,36-41] Diabetes does not result directly from the operation, because little or no pancreatic tissue is removed.[42] Some studies have

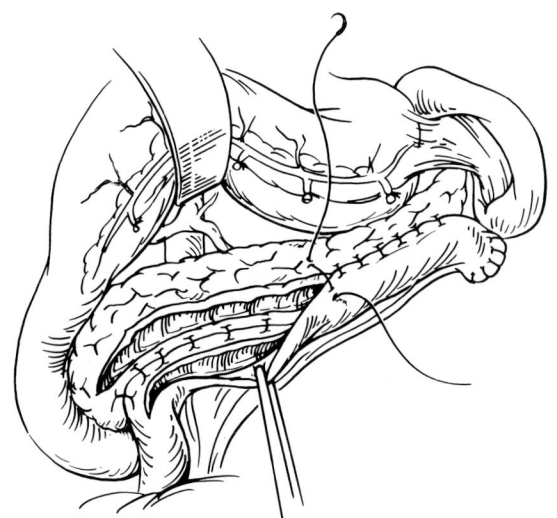

Figure 25-7 Longitudinal pancreaticojejunostomy.

suggested that the operation slows the deterioration of pancreatic function.[12,43]

Postoperative pancreatic fistulas are unusual, probably because the fibrotic pancreas holds sutures well. Closed suction drainage controls the rare leakage that occurs, and spontaneous closure is the rule. Clinical improvement in malabsorption is uncommon, but most patients with pain relief gain weight because they eat more. Pain is relieved completely or substantially in 75% to 85% of patients for the first few years after surgery.[36-41] Unfortunately, pain recurs in as many as half of patients after 5 years.[5,8,10,23] Recurrence of pain is an indication for ERCP. If stenosis of the pancreaticojejunal anastomosis is present, revision is reported to be successful in 71% of patients.[44] If the anastomosis is widely patent, pancreatic resection should be considered.

Pancreatic Resection

Resection is the treatment of choice when operation is indicated in patients whose ducts are normal or narrow in diameter. As a rule, the portion of the pancreas in which the disease is most severe should be resected.[33] Often, the head of the pancreas is significantly involved, making a pancreaticoduodenectomy a reasonable option. The traditional Whipple pancreaticoduodenectomy offers an 85% chance of long-term pain relief.[45-47] The operative mortality rate is less than 5% in the hands of experienced pancreatic surgeons.[48-50] Alternatives to the standard Whipple operation include the pylorus-preserving Whipple operation and the duodenum-preserving resection of the head of the pancreas (see later).[33,50]

Distal resections (50% to 60% of the gland) are in-

dicated less often, when the disease is concentrated in the body or tail of the pancreas. Such may be the case in patients who have chronic pancreatitis caused by a traumatic stricture of the main pancreatic duct in the body of the gland. Subtotal (80% to 95%) or total pancreatectomy can be considered in patients with diffuse disease and small ducts, or if pain persists after more limited resection or drainage. Extensive resections often are complicated by brittle diabetes, and should be done infrequently for that reason. Careful preoperative selection is mandatory if resection is considered.

PANCREATICODUODENECTOMY (WHIPPLE PROCEDURE). Many patients have extensive disease that involves mainly the head of the pancreas, which may be swollen to 5 to 6 cm in diameter or more and contain multiple cysts and calcifications. The bile duct or duodenum also may be obstructed by chronic fibrosis associated with the inflammatory process. In these circumstances, a Whipple resection may be appropriate (see Section V in Atlas Chap. 30). In addition, pancreaticoduodenectomy is indicated if there is clinical suspicion that pancreatic cancer is present.

DUODENUM-SPARING RESECTIONS OF THE HEAD OF THE PANCREAS. Beger and colleagues[51-53] described a duodenum-preserving resection of the head of the pancreas for patients with chronic pancreatitis who have inflammatory masses in the head of the gland (see Section IVB in Atlas Chap. 30). Normally, these patients would have been candidates for Whipple resections. The body and tail of the pancreas, as well as a thin rim of the head of the gland along the duodenum, are preserved.

The operation consists of two major steps. First, the pancreas is transected at the junction of the neck and the body of the gland. A subtotal resection of the head is performed, leaving a small piece of pancreatic tissue between the common bile duct and the duodenal wall. Second, pancreatic secretory flow is reestablished into the proximal jejunum by interposition of a Roux-en-Y jejunal limb, preserving gastroduodenal continuity. The same jejunal limb is anastomosed to the dissected tissue in the concavity of the duodenum. In Beger's experience, excision of the head of the gland resolved concomitant biliary obstruction in 83% of affected patients. The remaining patients required a choledochojejunostomy, again using the same Roux-en-Y limb. In patients with dilated main pancreatic ducts, a longitudinal side-to-side pancreaticojejunostomy was added to the procedure.

In 141 patients thus treated, the reported hospital mortality rate was only 0.7%, and 77% of patients were free of pain (average follow-up of 3.6 years). Glucose metabolism was unchanged or improved in 90% of patients. These results are encouraging, but longer follow-up and confirmation by other investigators are needed.

Another resection procedure for patients with chronic pancreatitis associated with an enlarged pancreatic head and a dilated pancreatic duct has been described by Frey[54] (see Section IVC in Atlas Chap. 30). In this procedure, the head of the pancreas is "cored out" rather than resected. The operation is easier than the one described by Beger because the neck of the pancreas is not divided, and dissection near the mesenteric vessels is avoided. As with the Beger procedure, a 0.5- to 1-cm rim of pancreatic tissue is left in situ next to the duodenum to maintain the duodenal blood supply and viability. The pancreatic duct is opened along its length and drained along with the cored-out head as in the usual side-to-side pancreaticojejunostomy. In both operations, the intrapancreatic segment of the common bile duct can be freed from the surrounding fibrosis, thus frequently avoiding the need for biliary bypass.[55] In these authors' experience with 30 such procedures, there have been no operative deaths. One patient had a leak from the pancreaticojejunostomy, which closed spontaneously. Only short-term follow-up is available (less than 2 years), but all the patients have had significant pain relief.

DISTAL PANCREATIC RESECTION. A 95% distal pancreatectomy entails the removal of all but a thin rim of pancreatic tissue that lies within the C-loop of the duodenum (see Section IVD in Atlas Chap. 30). Usually the spleen also is removed, although it can be preserved either by maintaining the integrity of the short gastric vessels or by performing meticulous ligation of the pancreatic branches of the splenic artery and vein, preserving them as well. This operation rarely is indicated because of the endocrine and exocrine insufficiency that results.[56] Pain relief is afforded to 60% to 80% of patients with 4 to 8 years of follow-up.[46,56]

Total pancreatectomy rarely is performed because it uniformly results in diabetes and exocrine insufficiency,[56] and because pain relief usually can be achieved with a less radical operation. It is used most often when a previous Whipple procedure or distal pancreatectomy has failed to provide pain relief. If possible, the pylorus should be preserved. The results appear to be satisfactory, although only a few series are available for evaluation. Pain relief occurs in 56% to 86% of this select group of patients in whom previous operations have failed.[57–59]

A duodenum-preserving total pancreatectomy has been described.[60] Nine of the 14 patients so treated were reported to be free of analgesic requirements, and only 2 had significant problems with diabetes. In a carefully selected group of young patients (mean age 34 years), this operation may have some utility.

Denervation Procedures

Surgical sympathectomy and celiac ganglionectomy relieved pain effectively in more than 200 patients treated by Mallet-Guy.[61] Because these good results have not been duplicated in other series, the procedure has not gained widespread acceptance.[26,33] Encouraging results were reported in 15 patients treated by left transthoracic splanchnicectomy and bilateral truncal vagotomy.[62] Five patients subsequently required right transthoracic splanchnicectomy. Fourteen patients (93%) had excellent results, albeit with mean follow-up of only 16 months. This procedure can be performed using the thoracoscope.

A denervated splenopancreatic flap procedure for chronic pancreatitis also has been described.[63,64] The operation consists of subtotal resection of the head of the pancreas, division of the gland at the junction of the neck and body, and complete mobilization of the distal pancreas and spleen from the retroperitoneum with division of the splenic artery and vein. The blood supply to the spleen and distal pancreas is maintained retrograde through the short gastric vessels, and the pancreatic remnant is drained into a Roux-en-Y limb of jejunum. Theoretically, this operation severs all neural pathways to the pancreas, excises the scarred pancreatic head, and drains the pancreatic duct. Long-term follow-up has not been reported; the complexity of the procedure makes its widespread application unlikely.

Pancreatic Autotransplantation

To avoid the complication of diabetes, which has limited the applicability of pancreatic resection, autotransplantation of the distal pancreas has been performed.[65] After a 95% pancreatectomy, the duct of the distal 50% to 60% of the pancreas is injected with neoprene and ligated. The pancreatic remnant then is placed in a subcutaneous pocket overlying the vastus lateralis muscle in the thigh. Vascular anastomoses are performed to the distal common femoral vessels. Because the number of patients treated by this approach is small and the length of follow-up is limited, this procedure must be regarded as experimental.

Islet Cell Autotransplantation

A series of 26 patients who underwent total or near-total pancreatectomy with autotransplantation of dispersed islet tissue have been described.[66] Prepared islet cells were injected slowly into a mesenteric vein while portal pressure was measured at intervals. There were no episodes of disseminated intravascular coagulation, significant portal hypertension, or hepatic dysfunction

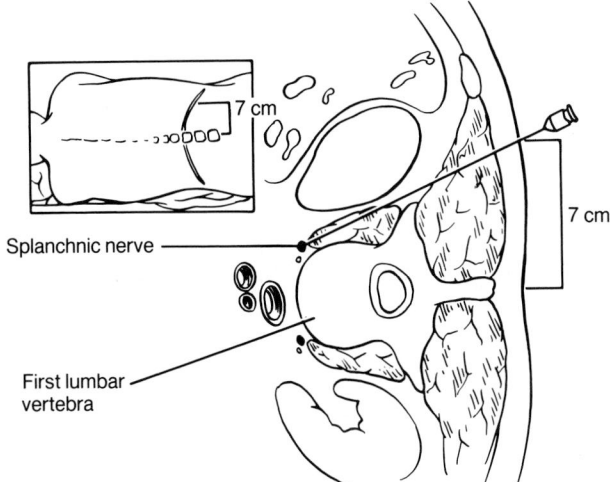

Figure 25-8 Technique of celiac plexus nerve block.

previously associated with the procedure. There was one perioperative death and a 44% operative morbidity rate. Ninety percent of patients experienced partial or complete pain relief, and 20% were insulin-independent at a mean follow-up of 5.7 years. Insulin independence correlated with the number of islets recovered, which was less when pancreatic fibrosis was more severe.[66] Although still experimental, islet autotransplantation may prove to be a useful adjunct to extensive pancreatic resection in this setting.[66,67]

Percutaneous Neurolysis

Percutaneous neurolysis of the celiac ganglia by injection of ethanol or phenol may be valuable in patients with small pancreatic ducts who are not candidates for drainage or resection[33] (Fig. 25-8). Neurolysis is effective in about two thirds of patients, but pain recurs within 1 year in most.[68] Although the procedure can be repeated, it is less likely to be effective.[32]

REFERENCES

1. Sarles H. Alcohol and the pancreas. Adv Exp Med Biol 1977;856:429.
2. Bank S. Chronic pancreatitis: clinical features and medical management. Am J Gastroenterol 1986;81:153.
3. Miyake H, Harada H, Kunichika K. Clinical course and prognosis of chronic pancreatitis. Pancreas 1987;2:378.
4. Little JM. Alcohol abuse and chronic pancreatitis. Surgery 1987;101:357.
5. Lankisch PG, Lohr-Happe A, Otto J, Creutzfeldt W. Natural course in chronic pancreatitis. Digestion 1993;54:148.
6. Levy P, Milan C, Pignon JP. Mortality factors associated with chronic pancreatitis. Gastroenterology 1989;96:1165.
7. Ammann RW, Akovbiantz A, Schueler G. Course and outcome of chronic pancreatitis. Gastroenterology 1984;86:820.
8. Moossa AR. Surgical treatment of chronic pancreatitis: an overview. Br J Surg 1987;74:661.
9. Prinz RA, Greenlee HB. Pancreatic duct drainage in 100 patients with chronic pancreatitis. Ann Surg 1981;194:313.
10. Reber HA. Chronic pancreatitis. In: Schwartz SI, Ellis H, eds. Maingot's abdominal operations, ed 9. Norwalk, CT, Appleton & Lange, 1990:1583.
11. Gullo L, Barbara L, Labo G. Effect of cessation of alcohol use on the course of pancreatic dysfunction in alcoholic pancreatitis. Gastroenterology 1988;95:1063.
12. Nealon WH, Townsend CM, Thompson JC. Operative drainage of the pancreatic duct delays functional impairment in patients with chronic pancreatitis. Ann Surg 1988;208:321.
13. Turner LJ. Chronic pancreatitis and congenital strictures of the pancreatic duct. Am J Surg 1983;145:582.
14. Leese T, Chiche L, Bismuth H. Pancreatitis caused by congenital anomalies of the pancreatic duct. Surgery 1989;105:125.
15. di Sant'Agnese PA, Davis P. Cystic fibrosis in adults. Am J Med 1979;66:121.
16. Fernald GW, Boat TF. Cystic fibrosis: overview. Semin Roentgenol 1987;22:87.
17. Britt LG, Samuels AD, Johnson JW. Pancreas divisum: is it a surgical disease? Ann Surg 1983;197:654.
18. Miller AR, Nagorney DM, Sarr MG. The surgical spectrum of hereditary pancreatitis in adults. Ann Surg 1992;215:39.
19. Agha FP, Williams KD. Pancreas divisum: incidence, detection and clinical significance. Am J Gastroenterol 1987;82:315.
20. Sarles H. Etiopathogenesis and definition of chronic pancreatitis. Dig Dis Sci 1986;31:91S.
21. Ammann RW, Buehler H, Muench R. Differences in the natural history of idiopathic and alcoholic chronic pancreatitis: a comparative long-term study of 287 patients. Pancreas 1987;2:368.
22. Kalthoff L, Layer P, Calin JE. The course of alcoholic and nonalcoholic chronic pancreatitis. Dig Dis Sci 1984;29:953.
23. Owyang C, Levitt M. Chronic pancreatitis. In: Yamada T, Alpers DH, Owyang C, Powell DW, Silverstein FE, eds. Textbook of gastroenterology. Philadelphia, JB Lippin-.cott, 1991;1879.
24. Covet C, Genton P, Pointel JP. Prevalence of retinopathy is similar in diabetes mellitus secondary to chronic pancreatitis with or without pancreatectomy and in idiopathic diabetes mellitus. Diabetes Care 1985;8:323.
25. Rossi RL, Heiss FW, Braasch JW. Surgical management of chronic pancreatitis. Surg Clin North Am 1985;65:79.
26. Hessel SJ, Siegelman SS, McNeil BJ. A prospective evaluation of computed tomography and ultrasound of the pancreas. Radiology 1982;143:129.
27. Karasawa E, Goldberg HI, Moss AA. CT pancreatogram

in carcinoma of the pancreas and chronic pancreatitis. Radiology 1983;148:49.

28. Desa LA, Williamson RCN. On table pancreatography: importance in planning operative strategy. Br J Surg 1990;77:1145.

29. Trapnell JE. Chronic relapsing pancreatitis: a review of 64 cases. Br J Surg 1979;66:471.

30. Slaff J, Jacobson D, Tillman CR. Protease-specific suppression of pancreatic exocrine secretion. Gastroenterology 1984;87:44.

31. Isaksson G, Ihse I. Pain reduction by an oral pancreatic enzyme preparation in chronic pancreatitis. Dig Dis Sci 1983;28:97.

32. White TT. Pain relieving procedures in chronic pancreatitis. Contemp Surg 1983;22:43.

33. Alvarez C, Widdison AL, Reber HA. New perspectives in the surgical management of chronic pancreatitis. Pancreas 1991;6S:76.

34. Puestow CB, Gillesby WJ. Retrograde surgical drainage of pancreas for chronic relapsing pancreatitis. Arch Surg 1956;76:898.

35. Partington PF, Rochelle REL. Modified Puestow procedure for retrograde drainage of the pancreatic duct. Ann Surg 1960;152:1037.

36. Bradley EL. Long-term results of pancreaticojejunostomy in patients with chronic pancreatitis. Am J Surg 1987;153:207.

37. Sarles JC, Nacchiero M, Garani F. Surgical treatment of chronic pancreatitis. Am J Surg 1982;144:317.

38. Mannell A, Adson MA, McIlrath DC. Surgical management of chronic pancreatitis: long-term results in 141 patients. Br J Surg 1988;75:467.

39. Drake DH, Fry WJ. Ductal drainage for chronic pancreatitis. Surgery 1989;105:132.

40. Morel P, Rohner A. Surgery for chronic pancreatitis. Surgery 1987;101:130.

41. Potts JR, Moody FG. Surgical therapy for chronic pancreatitis: selecting the appropriate approach. Am J Surg 1981;142:654.

42. Jalleh RP, Williamson RCN. Pancreatic exocrine and endocrine function after operations for chronic pancreatitis. Ann Surg 1992;216:656.

43. Nealon WH. Progressive loss of pancreatic function in chronic pancreatitis is delayed by main pancreatic duct decompression: a longitudinal prospective analysis of the modified Puestow procedure. Ann Surg 1993;217:458.

44. Prinz RA, Aranha GV, Greenlee HB. Redrainage of the pancreatic duct in chronic pancreatitis. Am J Surg 1986;151:150.

45. Rossi RL, Rothschild J, Braasch JW. Pancreaticoduodenectomy in the management of chronic pancreatitis. Arch Surg 1987;122:416.

46. Keith RG, Saibil FG, Sheppard RH. Treatment of chronic alcoholic pancreatitis by pancreatic resection. Am J Surg 1989;157:156.

47. Howard JM, Zhang Z. Pancreaticoduodenectomy in the treatment of chronic pancreatitis. World J Surg 1990;14:77.

48. Carey LC. Pancreaticoduodenectomy. Am J Surg 1992; 164:154.

49. Cameron JC. Rapid exposure of the portal and superior mesenteric veins. Surg Gynecol Obstet 1993;176:395.

50. Traverso LW, Kozarek RA. The Whipple procedure for severe complications of chronic pancreatitis. Arch Surg 1993;128:1047.

51. Beger HG, Buchler M. Duodenum-preserving resection of the head of the pancreas in chronic pancreatitis with inflammatory mass in the head. World J Surg 1990;14:83.

52. Beger HG, Buchler M, Bittner RR. Duodenum-preserving resection of the head of the pancreas in severe chronic pancreatitis. Ann Surg 1989;209:273.

53. Beger HG, Krautzberger W, Bittner R. Duodenum-preserving resection of the head of the pancreas in patients with severe chronic pancreatitis. Surgery 1985;97:467.

54. Frey CF, Smith GJ. Description and rationale of a new operation for chronic pancreatitis. Pancreas 1987;2:701.

55. Frey CF, Suzuki M, Isaji S. Pancreatic resection for chronic pancreatitis. Surg Clin North Am 1989;69:499.

56. Frey CF, Childs CG, Fry WF. Pancreatectomy for chronic pancreatitis. Ann Surg 1976;184:403.

57. Stone WM, Sarr MG, Nagorney DM. Chronic pancreatitis: results of Whipple's resection and total pancreatectomy. Arch Surg 1988;123:815.

58. Cooper MJ, Williamson RCH, Benjamin IS. Total pancreatectomy for chronic pancreatitis. Br J Surg 1987;74:912.

59. Keith RG, Shepard RH, Saibil FG. Resection for chronic alcoholic pancreatitis. Can J Surg 1981;24:119.

60. Lambert MA, Lincham IP, Russel RC. Duodenum preserving total pancreatectomy for end-stage chronic pancreatitis. Br J Surg 1987;74:987.

61. Mallet-Guy PA. Late and very late results of resections of the nervous system in the treatment of chronic relapsing pancreatitis. Am J Surg 1983;145:234.

62. Stone HH, Chauvin EJ. Pancreatic denervation for pain relief in chronic alcohol associated pancreatitis. Br J Surg 1990;77:303.

63. Warren WD, Millikan WJ, Henderson JM. A denervated pancreatic flap for control of chronic pain in pancreatitis. Surg Gynecol Obstet 1984;159:581.

64. Shires GT, Warren WD, Millikan WJP. Denervated splenopancreatic flap for chronic pancreatitis. Ann Surg 1986;203:568.

65. Rossi RL, Soelder JS, Braasch JW. Long-term results of pancreatic resection and segmental pancreatic autotransplantation for chronic pancreatitis. Am J Surg 1990;151:51.

66. Farney AC, Najarian JS, Nakleh RE. Autotransplantation of dispersed pancreatic islet tissue combined with total or near-total pancreatectomy for treatment of chronic pancreatitis. Surgery 1991;110:427.

67. Morrow CE, Cohen JI, Sutherland DER. Chronic pancreatitis: long-term surgical results of pancreatic duct drainage, pancreatic resection, and near-total pancreatectomy and islet cell autotransplantation. Surgery 1984;96:608.

68. Leung JWC, Bowenwright M, Aveling P. Coeliac plexus block for pain in pancreatic cancer and chronic pancreatitis. Br J Surg 1983;70:730.

Digestive Tract Surgery: A Text and Atlas, edited by Richard H. Bell,
Layton F. Rikkers, and Michael W. Mulholland.
Lippincott-Raven Publishers, Philadelphia, © 1996.

26

Neoplasms of the Exocrine Pancreas

Richard H. Bell, Jr.

DUCTAL ADENOCARCINOMA OF THE EXOCRINE PANCREAS

About 28,000 new cases of adenocarcinoma of the pancreas are diagnosed annually in the United States. These represent about 2% of all malignancies excluding skin cancers. The outlook for patients with carcinoma of the pancreas is poor enough that pancreatic cancer accounts for 5% of yearly cancer deaths and is the fifth most common cause of cancer death in the United States, after carcinoma of the lung, colorectum, breast, and prostate.[1] During the past 30 years, there has been modest improvement in the treatment of patients with carcinoma of the pancreas; the overall 5-year survival increased from 1% in 1960 to 4% in 1990. Nevertheless, it is clear from these figures that most patients with pancreatic cancer are not curable. Surgery plays an important role in the minority of patients who present with early tumors limited to the pancreas. Mortality rates for major pancreatic resections have improved significantly[2,3]; there is no longer much debate, as there was some years ago, about the advisability of surgery for patients with early tumors. Surgery also plays an important role in the palliation of biliary and duodenal obstruction in selected patients with advanced carcinoma of the pancreas.

Further progress in the treatment of pancreatic cancer will depend to a certain extent on the development of more effective adjuvant therapies, which are discussed in some detail later. More important, however, will be the development of methods for earlier diagnosis. Most patients present with tumors that have invaded outside the pancreas into the retroperitoneum or have spread to regional lymph nodes or distant viscera. Until it becomes possible to detect carcinoma of the pancreas at an earlier stage, therapy will be limited by the advanced state of malignancy with which most patients present.

Epidemiology, Etiology, and Risk Factors

The number of cases of pancreatic cancer reported annually began to rise in the early part of this century and rose steadily between 1930 and 1970, when the total incidence began to stabilize at its current level (Fig. 26-1). The reasons for the increased frequency of pancreatic cancer cases during the past decades is not known but probably relates in part to increased cigarette smoking (see later) and in part to better diagnosis and reporting.

A considerable amount of epidemiologic research has been performed in pancreatic cancer. The epidemiology of this neoplasm is important for at least two reasons. First, it may be possible to identify environmental factors leading to pancreatic cancer, the effects of which could be negated by behavioral modification (eg, smoking cessation). Second, it may be possible through epidemiologic research to identify high-risk groups for whom population screening would be appropriate, although this goal has not yet been achieved, with the exception of the identification of a limited number of high-risk families (see later).

In the course of epidemiologic investigation of pancreatic cancer, both host and environmental factors

849

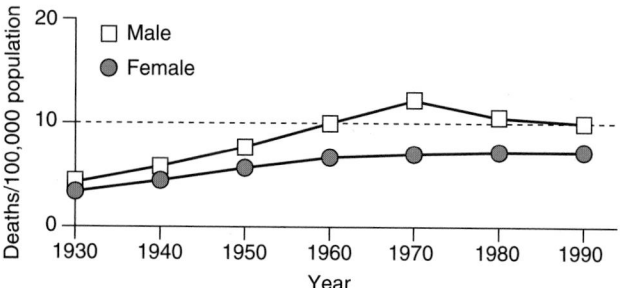

Figure 26-1 Age-adjusted annual rate of deaths from pancreatic cancer in the United States for 1930 through 1990. (After Boring CC, Squires TS, Tong T, Montgomery BA. Cancer statistics, 1994. CA Cancer J Clin 1994;44:7)

have been found to contribute to the likelihood of developing carcinoma of the pancreas. The most predictive host factor is age. The incidence of pancreatic cancer rises steadily with advancing years.[4] About 80% of cases occur in people older than 60 years. The risk of developing pancreatic cancer is about three-fold higher for people in the eighth decade of life than for the general population. Although pancreatic cancer is seen at all ages and even in children, cases in people younger than 40 years are extremely rare.

In addition to age, sex and race are both predictive of the risk of development of pancreatic cancer. Men are slightly more likely to develop carcinoma of the pancreas than women. Blacks born in the United States are at increased risk compared with whites.[5]

There has been increased awareness of familial proclivity to the development of pancreatic cancer. In a case control study,[6] 7.8% of patients with pancreatic cancer had a positive family history for pancreatic cancer compared with 0.6% of control patients. A number of families have been identified and followed in whom multiple cases of pancreatic cancer appear to have been inherited through an autosomal dominant factor.[7] About 3% to 5% of all pancreatic cancer cases have a hereditary origin. It is hoped that study of families prone to pancreatic cancer will yield information about the genetic abnormalities associated with the development and progression of pancreatic cancer in a manner analogous to colon cancer after the discovery of the location of the gene for familial adenomatous polyposis.[8]

Further evidence of a hereditary role in the cause of pancreatic cancer comes from the observation that the risk of pancreatic cancer is increased in several familial disorders. These include hereditary pancreatitis, multiple endocrine adenomatosis type I, Lynch's syndrome type II, von Hippel–Lindau syndrome, ataxia telangiectasia, and the familial atypical multiple mole melanoma syndrome.

Among other host factors suspected to be associ-

ated with the development of pancreatic cancer is diabetes mellitus. If searched for carefully, the incidence of glucose intolerance in patients with newly diagnosed pancreatic cancer is as high as 80%.[9] In several case control studies, there was a higher than expected incidence of frank diabetes in patients with pancreatic cancer compared with controls. It appears, however, that long-standing diabetes is probably not a major risk factor for the development of pancreatic cancer. Rather, the diabetes associated with pancreatic cancer is usually of recent onset and may in fact be a marker for the development of pancreatic cancer. It was proposed that the glucose intolerance associated with pancreatic cancer is caused by increased pancreatic production of the hormone islet amyloid polypeptide and that diabetes may actually improve after tumor resection.[10]

For many years, the role of preexisting pancreatitis as a risk factor for the development of pancreatic cancer was debated. A recent large retrospective cohort study of patients with chronic pancreatitis from six countries,[11] however, revealed a high risk for the development of pancreatic cancer (20 times that of the general population). The risk for development of pancreatic cancer appeared to be independent of the type of pancreatitis, a finding consonant with the fact that most studies have shown little effect of alcohol ingestion per se on the risk for pancreatic carcinoma. The mechanisms involved in carcinogenesis in patients with preexisting pancreatitis are unknown. However, the mutated K-*ras* oncogene, which is present in most cases of pancreatic cancer, has been detected in the ductal epithelium of some patients with chronic pancreatitis.[12]

Among the various environmental factors that have been investigated as possible predisposing agents in the development of pancreatic cancer, the role of cigarette smoking is clearly established. Smoking is associated with a two- to three-fold increased risk of developing carcinoma of the pancreas.[13] Many studies demonstrate a correlation between the number of cigarettes smoked and the risk for pancreatic cancer. About 30% of cases of pancreatic cancer can be directly attributed to cigarette consumption.

The role of dietary habits in the development of pancreatic cancer has been extensively evaluated, with somewhat conflicting results. The incidence of pancreatic cancer in various countries appears to parallel the intake of dietary fat, but results of individual studies relating dietary fat intake and the risk of pancreatic cancer are variable. It may be that only certain types of fats are associated with increased risk. It is well known, however, that dietary fats are tumor promoters in animal models of pancreatic cancer.

Other studies suggest that overeating is associated

with an increased risk of developing pancreatic cancer.[14] On the other hand, certain foods appear to be protective, particularly fruits and vegetables and dietary items high in fiber content.

As noted earlier, there is little evidence that ingestion of alcohol is directly associated with increased risk for pancreatic cancer. Likewise, a number of recent studies suggest little adverse effect of coffee consumption.

In reviewing the available epidemiologic data on pancreatic cancer, it is clear that, with the exception of rare pancreatic cancer families, there are not well-established high-risk groups for whom population screening for pancreatic cancer is practical. Most available serum markers for pancreatic cancer have an appreciable false-positive rate (see section on diagnosis). The ratio of false-positive to true-positive results is high when screening for a disease like pancreatic cancer, which has a relatively low incidence in the population (about 25 cases per 100,000 population). The expense and risk of working up all false-positive results in population screening make such an approach impractical. There is therefore a need both for truly tumor-specific markers and for an improved definition of high-risk people before mass screening for pancreatic cancer will become a reality.

Pathology

It is generally believed that most of exocrine pancreatic carcinomas arise from the cells lining the pancreatic ducts, despite the fact that these cells constitute only a small percentage of the pancreatic mass, which is predominantly made up of acinar cells. The question of whether tumors with a ductal phenotype might actually arise through a process of dedifferentiation of acinar cells has been debated for some time and is still not resolved. There are examples of conversion from acinar to ductal phenotype in animal tumor cell lines.[15] In addition, the targeting of oncogenes to acinar cells in transgenic mice has resulted in the unpredicted development of tumors with a ductal phenotype.[16] Foci of acinar cell dysplasia have been noted in the human pancreas at autopsy, but their significance is uncertain. The prevailing opinion is that most human pancreatic carcinomas arise from pancreatic ducts.

One classification of pancreatic exocrine tumors that takes their biologic behavior into account is shown in Table 26-1.[17] Of the malignant lesions, ductal adenocarcinoma accounts for 80% to 90% of tumors in most large series.[18,19]

Table 26-1   Classification of Pancreatic Exocrine Tumors

BENIGN
Serous cystadenoma
Mature cystic teratoma

UNCERTAIN BIOLOGIC BEHAVIOR
Intraductal tumors
    Intraductal papillary tumor
    Intraductal mucin hypersecreting tumor
Mucinous cystic tumor
Solid and papillary (solid and cystic) tumor

MALIGNANT
Ductal adenocarcinoma
Variants of ductal adenocarcinoma:
    Mucinous noncystic carcinoma
        Well differentiated
        Poorly differentiated with signet-ring cells
    Adenosquamous carcinoma
    Anaplastic carcinoma
Mucinous cystadenocarcinoma
Acinar cell carcinoma
    Acinar cell cystadenocarcinoma
Pancreatoblastoma
Small cell carcinoma
Miscellaneous tumors

(After Kloppel G. Pathology of nonendocrine pancreatic tumors. In: Go VLW, DiMagno EP, Gardner JD, et al, eds. The pancreas: biology, pathobiology, and disease, ed 2. New York, Raven, 1993)

Hyperplastic Changes in the Pancreatic Ducts

To diagnose pancreatic cancer at an earlier stage, it is important to understand as thoroughly as possible lesions in the pancreatic duct that may be precursors of pancreatic carcinoma. This task is unfortunately complicated by difficulty in access to these lesions in comparison, for example, to colonic polyps, for which the study of premalignant lesions has contributed significantly both to our understanding of colon cancer and to the treatment of patients. The task in the pancreas is more formidable, but a better understanding of early pancreatic duct lesions and their significance is emerging.

Three major types of early hyperplastic change in the pancreatic duct have been described—nonpapillary (flat) ductal hyperplasia, ductal papillary hyperplasia, and ductal hyperplasia with atypia. Nonpapillary epithelial hyperplasia is common; foci of nonpapillary hyperplasia are found frequently in patients with no known pancreatic disease and are numerous in patients with chronic pancreatitis. The change consists of replacement of the normal cuboidal ductal epithelium by columnar cells containing mucin. This lesion is not considered premalignant. On the other hand, ductal papillary hyperplasia is considered by some authorities to be a precursor lesion for pancreatic cancer. The incidence of this lesion increases with age and is more common in patients with frank pancreatic cancer elsewhere in the gland. It is not, however, uniformly accepted that ductal papillary hyperplasia is a premalignant lesion; some authorities note that clearcut evidence of transition of these lesions to carcinoma is lacking. Areas of ductal papillary hyperplasia are reported to be negative for the mutated K-*ras* oncogene, which is present in most invasive pancreatic carcinomas.[20] Finally, even the significance of ductal hyperplasia with atypia is controversial. Although the lesions are malignant histologically, there is controversy about whether this lesion is really seen in isolation in otherwise normal pancreatic ducts or whether it is only seen in the pancreas of patients with invasive carcinoma, suggesting that this lesion may represent intraductal extension of invasive carcinoma. Thus, the morphologic classification of ductal hyperplastic changes has been clarified to some extent, but there is still considerable debate concerning the biologic significance and behavior of these lesions.

Invasive Ductal Adenocarcinoma

Invasive ductal adenocarcinoma accounts for 80% to 90% of pancreatic malignancies in most series. Sixty to 70% of these tumors arise in the head of the pancreas; the reason for this predilection for the head of the gland is unknown. As a consequence of the location of these tumors, they obstruct the common bile duct, pan-creatic duct, or both as they enlarge. Bile duct obstruction leads to jaundice, which is the presenting complaint in most patients with carcinoma of the head of the pancreas. Obstruction of the pancreatic duct usually is asymptomatic, but about 5% of cases of carcinoma of the pancreas present with evidence of acute pancreatitis or a pseudocyst. The incidence of occult pancreatitis, determined on histologic examination of the pancreas at autopsy or surgery, is much higher.

The size of the tumor in resected specimens averages about 3 cm, whereas average size at autopsy is 5 to 6 cm. The tumors are hard and irregular; their consistency is typically even firmer than that of chronic pancreatitis. Histologic examination reveals neoplastic glands lined by cuboidal or columnar epithelium embedded in a dense fibrous matrix (Fig. 26-2). In many specimens, the fibrous stroma occupies more area than the tumor cells. The appearance of the glands ranges from well differentiated to markedly anaplastic. The better-differentiated tumors tend to produce mucin within the glands.

Some debate has occurred about the incidence of multicentric tumors within the pancreatic ductal system. Some reports suggested that as many as 40% of resected cases of pancreatic cancer demonstrated multifocal areas of carcinoma within the specimen, and this finding was used as a rationale for the routine performance of total pancreatectomy for adenocarcinoma of the pancreas.[21] Other careful studies,[22] however, reveal that true "skip" lesions are rare. In about 10% of total pancreatectomy specimens, there is direct exten-

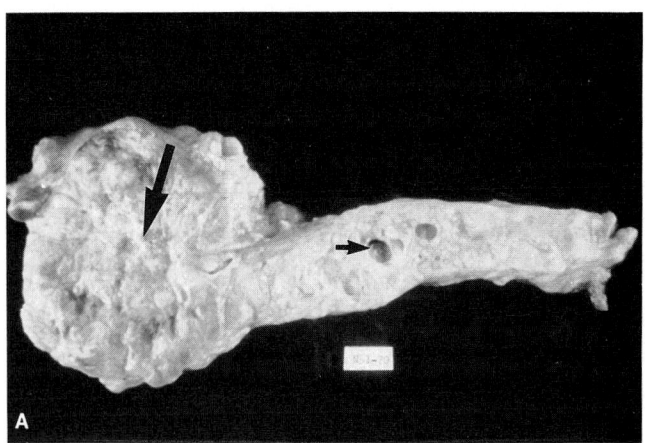 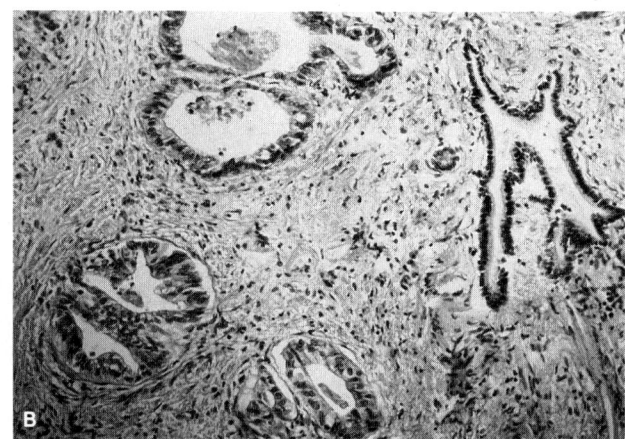

Figure 26-2 Gross and microscopic appearance of ductal adenocarcinoma of the head of the pancreas. (**A**) In the gross specimen, there is a mass and marked scirrhous reaction (*large arrow*) and dilation of the main pancreatic duct in the body of the gland (*small arrow*). (**B**) Microscopic examination reveals anaplastic glands from a well-differentiated adenocarcinoma (*lower left*) embedded in a fibrous matrix. Some normal residual ductal structures remain (*right*). (Bell RH. Neoplasms of the exocrine pancreas. In: Greenfield LJ, Mulholland MW, Oldham KT, Zelenock GB, eds. Surgery: scientific principles and practice. Philadelphia, JB Lippincott, 1993:818)

sion of tumor from the head into the body and tail. This sort of extension can be detected during pancreaticoduodenectomy by frozen section of the margin of division of the pancreas over the portal vein, which should be done routinely. The incidence of true multicentricity in pancreatic cancer is low and does not justify the routine performance of total pancreatectomy.

Extension beyond the confines of the pancreas is present in most resected specimens of carcinoma of the pancreas. The duodenum is the most common site of visceral invasion but is included in the pancreaticoduodenectomy specimen. The stomach, colon, and gallbladder may also be directly invaded; involvement of these organs generally indicates incurability even if the organs can be excised en bloc. Direct extension beyond the pancreas into the retroperitoneum is extremely common in carcinoma of the pancreas. These tumors invade lymphatic channels and perineural spaces early in their course, and tumor cells move along these conduits into the retroperitoneum. Histologic examination of the retroperitoneal margins after pancreaticoduodenectomy reveals tumor involvement in up to half of cases.[23] This high incidence of direct retroperitoneal spread has been used as a rationale for extended en bloc retroperitoneal dissection in the surgical treatment of pancreatic cancer and for adjuvant radiation therapy (see later).

Lymph node metastases are present in 50% to 60% of resected specimens of pancreatic cancer. Even in pancreatic carcinomas smaller than 2 cm, the incidence of lymph node metastases is 30%.[24] Figure 26-3 shows

that the most commonly involved lymph nodes are those in the posterior pancreaticoduodenal and superior pancreatic head regions, followed by those in the inferior head and superior body areas, the anterior pancreaticoduodenal region, and the inferior body region.[25] The lymphatic groups along the superior and inferior borders of the body of the pancreas are not routinely excised during pancreaticoduodenectomy.

Distant metastases are already present at the time of diagnosis of pancreatic cancer in 80% or more of patients. The most commonly involved site is the liver, followed by the lungs, but metastases to a multitude of distant sites have been described. In addition to hematogenous metastases, a significant number of patients have peritoneal carcinomatosis at the time of diagnosis. Although multiple, the individual tumor implants may be too small to be seen by computed tomographic (CT) scan. Peritoneal carcinomatosis can be detected by laparoscopy with peritoneal washings for cytology, which many surgeons perform before pancreaticoduodenectomy in patients who appear to have resectable tumors by CT scan criteria (see Diagnosis).

Staging of Pancreatic Cancer

Table 26-2 shows a staging system for pancreatic cancer oriented toward surgical resectability. Using this system, it was shown in an evaluation of 924 patients that survival in patients with stage I disease was higher (33% at 1 year) than in patients with stages II and III disease (combined survival of 13% at 1 year). Survival

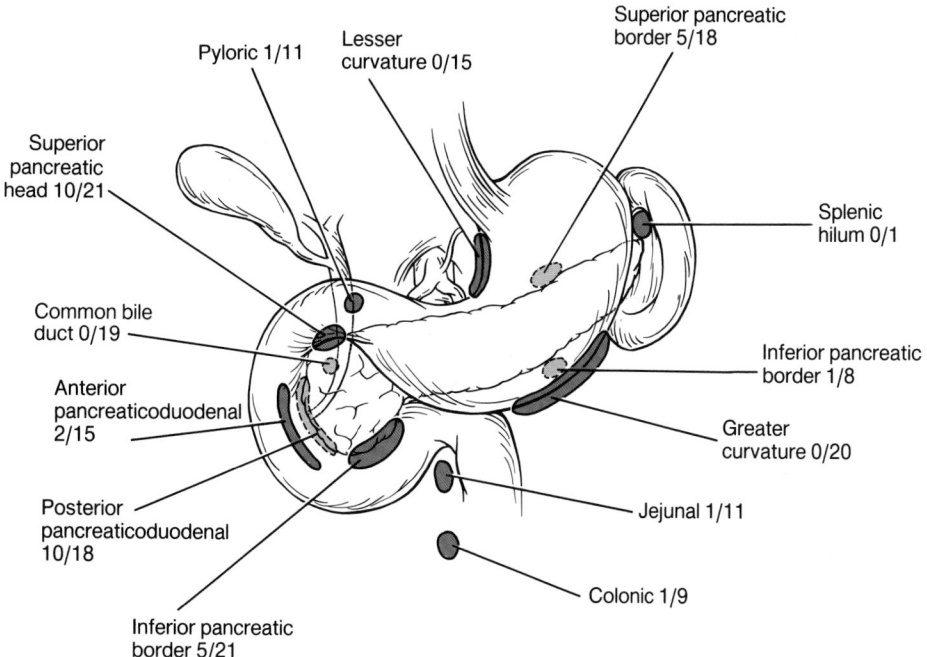

Figure 26-3 Lymph node involvement in 21 patients who underwent apparently curative resection of ductal carcinoma of the head of the pancreas, most of whom were treated by total or regional pancreatectomy. For each nodal group, the denominator indicates the number of patients in whom nodes were found in that area. The numerator indicates the number of patients in whom lymph nodes contained microscopically verified cancer. (After Cubilla AL, Fitzgerald PJ. Surgical pathology aspects of cancer of the ampulla-head-of-pancreas region. In: Fitzgerald PJ, Morrison AB, eds. The pancreas. Baltimore, Williams & Wilkins, 1980:72)

Table 26-2   Staging of Pancreatic Carcinoma

Stage	Primary Tumor	Nodal Status	Distant Metastases	Description
I	T1, T2	N0	M0	No or limited direct extension to adjacent viscera, with no regional node extension and absence of distant metastases (limited direct extension defined as involvement of the organs adjacent to the pancreas that could be removed en bloc with the pancreas if a curative resection were attempted)
II	T3	N0	M0	Further direct extension of tumor into adjacent viscera, with no lymph node involvement and no distant metastases, which precluded surgical resection
III	T1, T2, or T3	N1	M0	Regional node metastases without clinical evidence of distant metastases
IV	T1, T2, or T3	N0, N1	M1	Distant metastatic disease in liver and other sites

Designation	Description
PRIMARY TUMOR	
T1	No direct extension of the tumor beyond the pancreas
T2	Limited direct extension (to duodenum, bile ducts, or stomach), still possibly permitting tumor resection
T3	Further direct extension, incompatible with tumor resection
TX	Tumor extension not assessed or not recorded
REGIONAL LYMPH NODE INVOLVEMENT	
N0	Regional nodes not involved
N1	Regional nodes involved
NX	Regional node involvement not assessed or not recorded
DISTANT METASTASIS	
M0	No distant metastasis
M1	Distant metastatic involvement
MX	Distant metastatic involvement not assessed or not recorded

(After Pollard HM, et al. Staging of cancer of the pancreas. Cancer of the Pancreas Task Force. Cancer 1981;47:1631)

with advanced local extension (stage II, 15%) was similar to cases with lymph node metastases (stage III, 11%). Survival was significantly worse in patients with distant metastases at the time of presentation (stage IV, 5% at 1 year).[26]

In general, a correlation exists between tumor size and stage. Nevertheless, even small tumors of the pancreas may be biologically aggressive. In primary tumors smaller than 2 cm, metastasis to regional lymph nodes has already occurred in 30% to 40% of cases, and extrapancreatic invasion is demonstrable in at least 30%. Overall, less than half of patients with tumors smaller than 2 cm have stage I disease (tumor confined to the pancreas).[27]

Diagnosis

Pancreatic carcinoma is difficult to diagnose in its earliest stages, when there is the most potential for a curative resection. Many patients give a history of abdominal symptoms for several months before diagnosis, but these early symptoms of pancreatic cancer generally consist of vague abdominal pain or dyspepsia, which is often minimized both by patients and physicians. It is usually not until patients develop jaundice or significant weight loss that the correct diagnosis is made. In the past several years, there has been steady improvement in imaging techniques for carcinoma of the pancreas, and these tumors can now be detected in the size range of 1.5 to 2 cm by CT scan. Unfortunately, many patients do not undergo imaging tests until their symptoms and their tumors are advanced. The advent of serum markers, such as CA19-9 (see later), may have some impact on earlier diagnosis in that a physician may be more willing to order a blood test than a CT scan in the face of equivocal symptoms. Unfortunately, CA19-9 and similar serum markers may be normal in patients with small tumors. New imaging tests, such as endoscopic ultrasonography, appear to be pushing the limits of resolution to even lower levels than CT, but such expensive and complex tests are unlikely to be ordered in patients with early symptoms. To improve our ability to diagnose pancreatic cancer earlier, a highly sensitive, specific, low-risk, and inexpensive screening test needs to be developed, and practitioners need to be more alert to the possibility of pancreatic cancer in elderly patients with subtle digestive complaints.

Clinical Signs and Symptoms

The most common presenting symptoms and signs of pancreatic cancer are listed in Tables 26-3 and 26-4. Virtually all patients with pancreatic cancer experience weight loss, and it is usually substantial, averaging 10

Table 26-3 Symptoms of Pancreatic Cancer

Symptom	Patients (%)
HEAD	
Weight loss	92
Jaundice	82
Pain	72
Anorexia	64
Dark urine	63
Light stools	62
Nausea	45
Vomiting	37
Weakness	35
Pruritus	24
Diarrhea	18
Melena	12
Constipation	11
Fever	11
Hematemesis	8
BODY AND TAIL	
Weight loss	100
Pain	87
Weakness	43
Nausea	43
Vomiting	37
Anorexia	33
Constipation	27
Hematemesis	17
Melena	17
Jaundice	7
Fever	7
Diarrhea	3

(After Howard JM, Jordan GL Jr. Cancer of the pancreas. Curr Probl Cancer 1977;2:5)

kg. Initially, weight loss may occur with a seemingly normal appetite, but eventually most patients develop anorexia as well. Documented unexplained weight loss in adult patients should lead to a search for an occult malignancy and is sufficient justification for the performance of an abdominal CT scan.

Jaundice, scleral icterus, dark urine, light stools, or some combination of these symptoms usually is responsible for patients first seeking medical attention. Often, jaundice is noticed by friends or relatives before it is apparent to the patient. The jaundice is progressive. Pruritus due to bile salt deposition in the skin is present in about one fourth of jaundiced patients and may be debilitating.

Although it was often taught in the past that pancreatic cancer presents with painless jaundice (as a distinguishing point from choledocholithiasis), most patients in fact experience pain. In the early stages, pain may be vague or mild, but as the disease progresses, about three fourths of patients experience moderate to severe abdominal pain, often radiating directly through to the back. Occasionally, pain is confined to the back.

Digestive symptoms are common in patients with pancreatic cancer. Nausea and vomiting may be due to duodenal obstruction by tumor. In other cases, no apparent mechanical obstruction is present when contrast studies are performed, but it may be that motility is affected by subtle tumor invasion that is below the limits of radiologic detection. Patients may note a change in bowel habits; both constipation and diarrhea can occur. Steatorrhea occurs in less than 10% of patients.

The most common physical findings in patients with newly diagnosed pancreatic cancer are icterus and hepatomegaly. Enlargement of the liver is often due to congestion as a result of biliary obstruction and does not necessarily imply the presence of metastases. A dilated gallbladder (Courvoisier's sign) is present in about one fourth of patients. In most cases, the tumor is not palpable. Ascites is present in about 15% of patients with pancreatic cancer and implies incurability. Rectal examination may reveal occult blood in the stool as a result of tumor invasion into the duodenum.

Laboratory Findings

Patients with pancreatic cancer may be anemic because of blood loss into the gastrointestinal tract due to tumor invasion. Fasting plasma glucose levels are elevated in about one third of patients with pancreatic cancer, and in some patients, this may be the first evidence of diabetes. In patients with previously diagnosed diabetes, worsening hyperglycemia may be a warning sign of the development of pancreatic cancer. Standard liver

Table 26-4 Signs of Pancreatic Cancer

Sign	Patients (%)
HEAD	
Jaundice	87
Palpable liver	83
Palpable gallbladder	29
Tenderness	26
Ascites	14
Abdominal mass	13
BODY AND TAIL	
Palpable liver	33
Tenderness	27
Abdominal mass	23
Ascites	20
Jaundice	13

(After Howard JM, Jordan GL Jr. Cancer of the pancreas. Curr Probl Cancer 1977;2:5)

function tests usually reveal elevation of the serum bilirubin level and alkaline phosphatase characteristic of extrahepatic biliary obstruction. Transaminase levels may also be elevated, but usually not to the extent of the alkaline phosphatase. The prothrombin time is sometimes elevated as a result of an inability to absorb vitamin K. Mild elevations of the serum amylase occur in about 5% of patients; marked elevations are unusual.

Certain mucins produced by well-differentiated pancreatic cancers are shed into the serum and have been exploited as tumor markers. Mucins are large glycoproteins whose function appears to be protection and lubrication of cells. Mucin epitopes have been isolated from pancreatic cancer cells and monoclonal antibodies raised against these antigens to detect mucins in the serum of patients with suspected pancreatic cancer. CA19-9 is the most widely used antibody test.[28,29] The CA19-9 antigen has been identified as sialosyl-fucosyl-lactotetrose, which is the sialylated form of the Lewis[a] (Le[a]) blood group antigen found on erythrocytes. About 5% of people lack the Lewis gene and are therefore unable to make either the blood group antigen or the tumor marker. CA19-9 is normally present in pancreatic juice and pancreatic duct cells. Because CA19-9 is detected in normal tissues, it is a tumor-associated rather than a tumor-specific antigen. CA19-9 levels in pancreatic juice are not useful in the diagnosis of pancreatic cancer.[30] In normal people, only low levels of CA19-9 are detectable in serum. Elevated serum levels of CA19-9 (more than 37 U/mL) are observed in about 80% of patients with pancreatic cancer.[31,32] The reported specificity of the test for pancreatic cancer varies from 60% to 90%. Elevated levels of CA19-9 in anicteric patients have a high positive predictive value for pancreatic cancer. High serum levels of CA19-9 (more than 1000 U/mL) are also virtually pathognomonic for pancreatic cancer and usually indicate advanced disease. CA19-9 may be elevated in 20% to 70% of other gastrointestinal malignancies and in about 15% of nongastrointestinal malignancies. CA19-9 may also be elevated in cirrhosis of the liver and biliary disease, particularly with cholangitis, and also in a minority of cases of chronic pancreatitis. Serum levels of CA19-9 are unfortunately less likely to be elevated in patients with small pancreatic tumors (about 50% sensitivity for tumors smaller than 3 cm) and may not be elevated at all in patients with poorly differentiated tumors, which presumably have lost the genetic ability to express the antigen. Nevertheless, CA19-9 is a useful test when attempting to differentiate benign from malignant pancreatic disease. A negative CA19-9 test in combination with negative imaging studies has a high negative predictive value. Because both false-positive and false-negative results do occur, it is important not to rely on

the CA19-9 value alone in reaching a diagnostic conclusion. CA 19-9 has been shown, however, to improve sensitivity and specificity in the diagnosis of pancreatic cancer when combined with standard radiologic techniques. Several studies also suggest that combining the measurement of CA19-9 with other tumor markers improves sensitivity and specificity. In one study,[33] a discriminant system based on a combination panel of nine tumor markers was able to distinguish completely between patients with ductal pancreatic adenocarcinoma and those with benign pancreatic disease. Such computer-based diagnostic systems are not generally available.

The era of molecular biology has ushered in new possibilities for the diagnosis of pancreatic cancer. Of particular interest thus far is the observation that about 90% of human ductal pancreatic carcinomas contain a mutated form of the K-ras gene.[34] The ras genes encode the production of proteins that are involved in the control of intracellular signaling and are thought to have an important regulatory role in cellular growth. Mutations in the ras genes appear to result in loss of normal cellular growth regulation and may be an important early step in initiating the change from normal to malignant cell. In pancreatic cancer cells, the most common alteration in the K-ras gene is a single nucleotide substitution in codon 12 of the genetic sequence.[35] In addition to being able to demonstrate K-ras mutations in pancreatic tissue from surgery or autopsy, investigators have been able to detect the mutated gene in fine-needle aspirates of the pancreas, in pancreatic juice, and in stool by taking advantage of molecular biology techniques that amplify minute amounts of the gene by repeatedly copying it until it can be detected. K-ras mutations are more common in pancreatic cancers of cigarette smokers than nonsmokers. In general, no correlation has been found between the presence of K-ras mutation and tumor grade or stage or patient survival. This finding is consonant with the belief that K-ras mutation is an early event in carcinogenesis and that further subsequent genetic changes may be responsible for defining tumor biology. At any rate, the fact that K-ras mutations occur early in pancreatic cancer makes the detection of such mutations an attractive strategy for the early detection of pancreatic cancer. The ability to measure K-ras mutations in serum, which has been suggested in some preliminary studies, is a particularly exciting prospect. In one study,[36] mutant K-ras was detected in the pancreatic juice of six patients with pancreatic cancer and was detected in the serum of two of six additional patients. At this point, there are a number of important questions remaining to be answered about the value of mutated K-ras as a diagnostic tool in pancreatic cancer. It is not clear, for example, whether

K-*ras* mutations are tumor specific. They have been detected by some investigators in ductal tissue in chronic pancreatitis.[12] On the other hand, the increased risk of pancreatic cancer in patients with chronic pancreatitis suggests the possibility that K-*ras* mutations in chronic pancreatitis may be a marker for future malignancy. It is also not clear whether K-*ras* mutation by itself predicts the development of malignancy with sufficient accuracy to justify resection of pancreatic tissue on this basis alone. Nor is it known how long the process of malignant transformation takes once mutated K-*ras* appears. Nevertheless, this is a field of active investigation, and it is likely that these answers will be forthcoming. Finally, K-*ras* is not the only oncogene that has been found in patients with pancreatic cancer. For example, about half of patients with pancreatic cancer demonstrate overexpression of the p53 nuclear transcription factor by tissue immunohistochemistry; in one study,[37] such changes were not seen in chronic pancreatitis. The study of the molecular biology of pancreatic cancer will no doubt accelerate and is likely to provide significant diagnostic advances.

Imaging Studies

The imaging modalities used with some frequency in the diagnosis and staging of pancreatic cancer are transcutaneous ultrasonography, CT scanning, endoscopic retrograde cholangiopancreatography (ERCP), and visceral arteriography. Endoscopic ultrasonography (EUS), a relatively new technique, shows promise in being able to detect small pancreatic masses. Scanning using radiolabeled monoclonal antibodies to tumor antigens is in the development phase.

Ultrasonography is an extremely useful, low-risk, and relatively inexpensive initial test in the evaluation of patients with jaundice. The presence of dilated extrahepatic or intrahepatic bile ducts is essentially diagnostic of mechanical extrahepatic biliary obstruction. This finding directs the further evaluation toward defining the nature of the obstruction, usually by CT or ERCP. Ultrasonography has the additional virtue of being the best imaging modality for the diagnosis of gallstones. If stones are present, choledocholithiasis ordinarily is entertained as part of the differential diagnosis of jaundice in the elderly. If gallbladder stones are not present by ultrasonography, choledocholithiasis is unlikely. The finding of normal caliber bile ducts by ultrasonography makes cancer of the head of the pancreas unlikely and ordinarily directs the evaluation toward hepatocellular disease. Although ultrasonography is said to be as sensitive in detecting a mass in the pancreas as CT scanning, this comparison usually does not take into account the fact that about 20% of ultrasound examinations are technically unsatisfactory in imaging the pancreas because of overlying bowel gas. In addition, ultrasonography is more operator-dependent than CT. Finally, ultrasonography is not as useful as CT in defining local invasion, vascular involvement, or lymph node metastases. For these reasons, ultrasonography is generally used as a screening tool in patients with jaundice; those with evidence of duct obstruction should be further evaluated by CT scan.

One study comparing the effectiveness of transcutaneous ultrasonography and CT in making the diagnosis of pancreatic cancer in jaundiced patients came to the conclusion that ultrasonography and CT had similar specificity: they were both more than 90% effective in ruling out the disease.[38] On the other hand, the sensitivity of CT was superior: a firm diagnosis of pancreatic cancer was made in more than 90% of the cases by CT but in only 60% of cases by transcutaneous ultrasonography.

In a series of 1220 patients consecutively evaluated for suspicion of pancreatic cancer, ultrasonography was an effective initial diagnostic tool when combined with signs, symptoms, and routine laboratory tests.[39] The finding of a focal mass on ultrasound had a sensitivity of 83% and excellent specificity (99%).

CT scanning is by far the most useful single imaging test in the diagnosis of pancreatic cancer (Fig. 26-4). As noted, CT scanning is not only able to detect the pancreatic mass in more than 90% of patients with pancreatic cancer, it also provides important information about the stage of the disease and the likelihood of resectability. Technical modifications of CT, such as spiral scanning and three-dimensional CT arteriographic reconstruction, have further improved the usefulness of the test. Invasion of contiguous organs, involvement of major adjacent vessels such as the portal vein or superior mesenteric artery, the presence of lymphadenopathy, and the presence of ascites, peritoneal implants, or liver metastases are all findings that can be detected by CT scan with varying degrees of accuracy, but when present indicate a low or absent likelihood of resectability or cure. CT scanning is over 90% accurate in predicting unresectability. It is less accurate in predicting resectability; slightly more than half of patients deemed resectable by CT scan are not in fact resectable when explored. CT scanning thus has its primary value in detecting unresectability and sparing some patients unnecessary laparotomy; most patients who are scanned are found to be unresectable by CT criteria. For example, in a series of 213 patients undergoing CT with a suspected diagnosis of pancreatic cancer, 188 (88%) were found to have inoperable tumors by radiologic criteria.[40] CT findings in this series of patients are shown in Table 26-5.

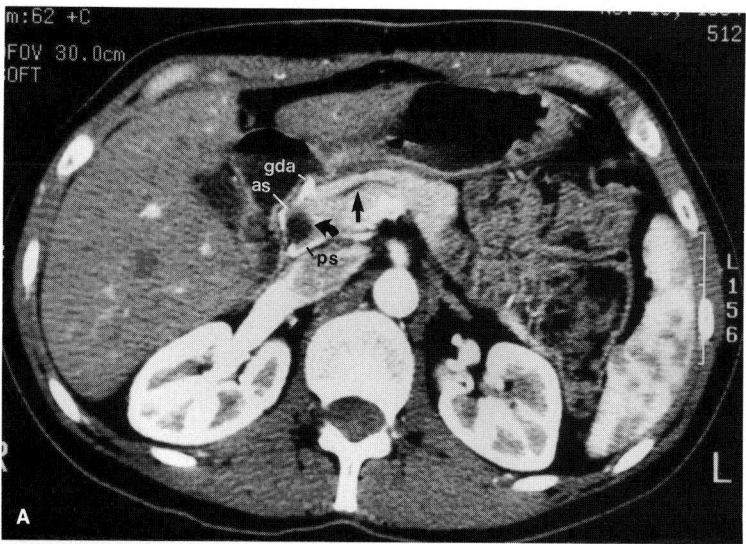

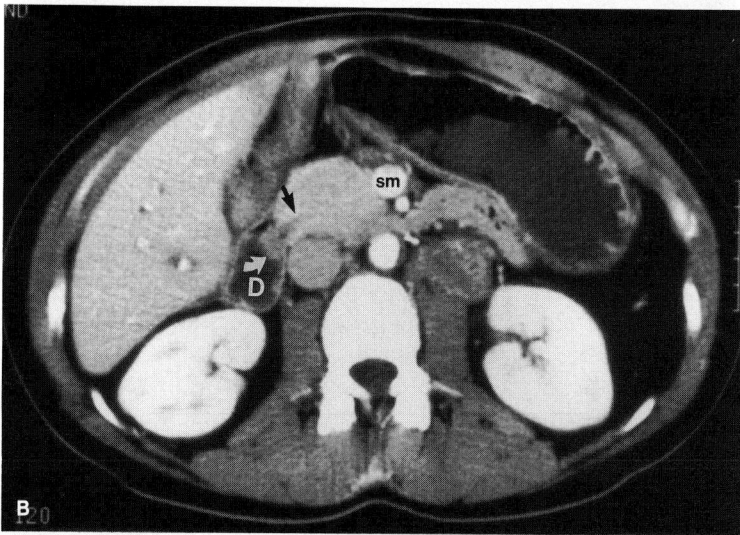

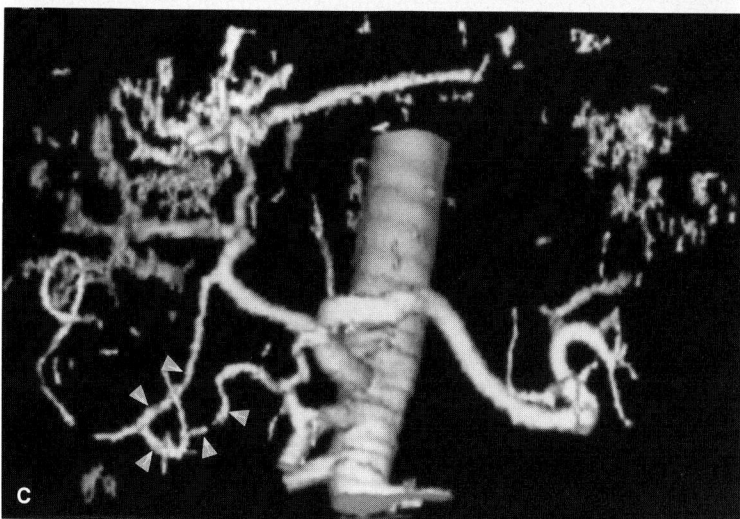

Figure 26-4 CT scan evaluation of the pancreas. (A) Normal double-spiral CT scan at the level of the head of the pancreas during early arterial phase showing intense contrast enhancement of pancreatic parenchyma and positions of common bile duct (*curved arrow*), pancreatic duct (*straight arrow*), and small peripancreatic arteries. gda, gastroduodenal artery; as, anterior superior pancreaticoduodenal artery; ps, posterior superior pancreaticoduodenal artery. (B) Normal double spiral scan during portal phase showing excellent contrast enhancement of the superior mesenteric vein (sm) as well as delineation of the pancreatic duct (*straight arrow*). Water has been used as the oral contrast agent to distend the duodenum (D), allowing visualization of the normal papilla (*curved arrow*). (C) Three-dimensional CT arteriogram obtained from computer processing of axial CT spiral images showing normal vascular anatomy, including pancreaticoduodenal arcade (*arrowheads*). (D) Three-dimensional arteriogram demonstrating a vascular anomaly. The right hepatic artery (H) arises from the superior mesenteric artery (SM). The splenic (S), left gastric (LG), left hepatic (LH), and gastroduodenal (GD) arteries arise from the celiac artery (C). (E) CT scan of resectable pancreatic carcinoma showing a 1.5-cm hypodense mass (*arrows*) in the head of the pancreas. (F) CT scan of unresectable pancreatic carcinoma. Contiguous scans of the pancreas show soft tissue density tumor (*arrowheads*) adjacent to the aorta (a) and celiac artery (c) and encasing the splenic artery (s). (Courtesy of Patrick C. Freeny, MD, Department of Radiology, University of Washington School of Medicine, Seattle)

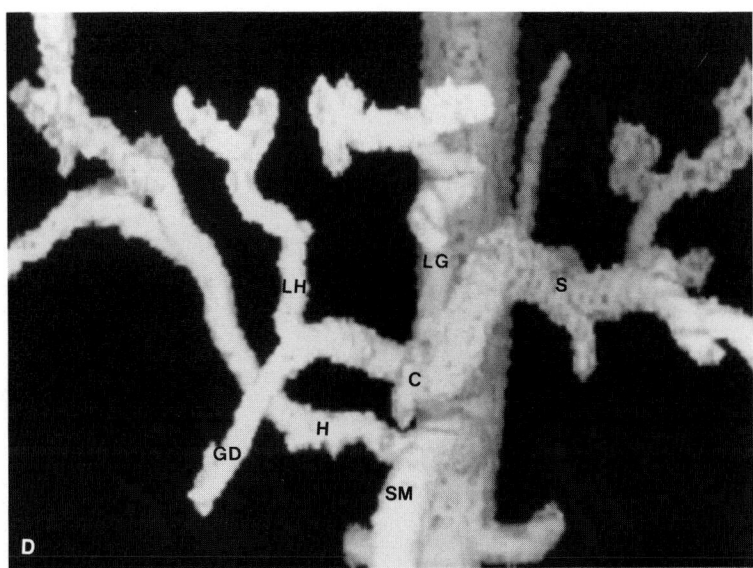

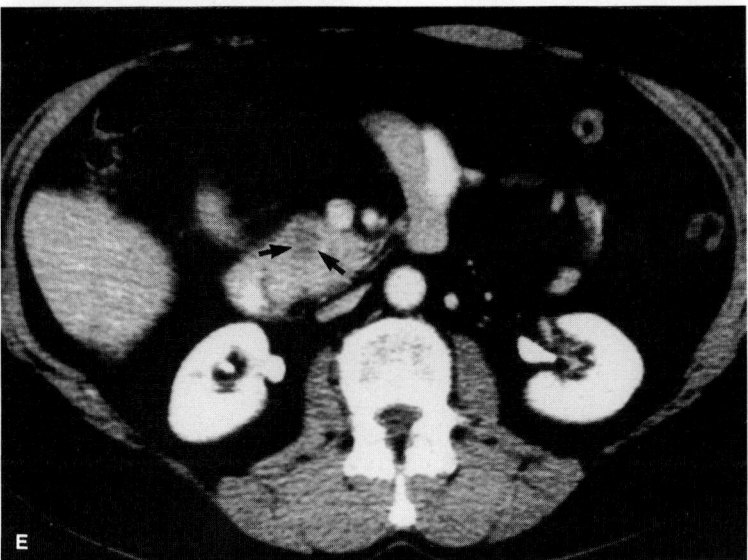

Figure 26-4 *(Continued)*

ERCP is a sensitive test for pancreatic cancer. The cost, complexity, and potential risk of ERCP, however, mandate its judicious and appropriate use in the evaluation of suspected pancreatic cancer. ERCP is primarily useful in two groups of patients. The first consists of those patients in whom CT scanning reveals dilation of the biliary duct, pancreatic duct, or both, but in whom no mass is evident. A subset of this group includes patients who have gallstones and bile duct dilation by ultrasound and no pancreatic mass by CT scan. Not all such patients require ERCP to differentiate choledocholithiasis from malignant obstruction, but ERCP is appropriate in older patients, particularly if there is associated weight loss or other symptoms that may suggest carcinoma. A second group of patients in whom ERCP is indicated are those with a mass in the head of

the pancreas and either clinical or CT signs of chronic pancreatitis. ERCP, particularly when combined with cytologic examination of the pancreatic juice, is probably the best available test to differentiate chronic pancreatitis from carcinoma.

Overall, ERCP has about a 90% sensitivity and specificity for diagnosis of pancreatic cancer.[41] The most common finding is abrupt obstruction of the common bile duct, pancreatic duct, or both (*double-duct sign;* Fig. 26-5). Although bile duct strictures due to pancreatic cancer can be variable in their appearance, they tend to be irregular and abrupt, whereas strictures due to chronic pancreatitis are typically long and smoothly tapered. Small pancreatic carcinomas may cause only focal obstruction of the pancreatic duct. In some cases, this finding has been misinterpreted as pancreas divisum.

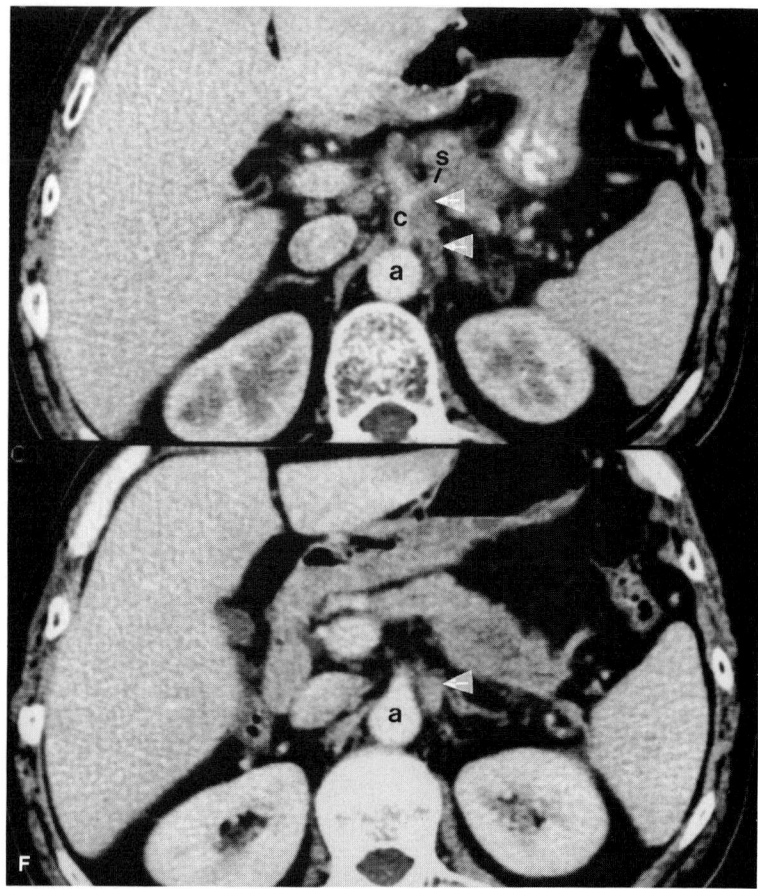

Figure 26-4 *(Continued)*

The selective use of ERCP in the diagnosis of pancreatic cancer was endorsed in a review designed to assess the value of various diagnostic tests in 126 patients with pancreatic cancer.[42] ERCP did not alter management in patients with a mass in the pancreas detected by CT or in patients with metastatic disease detected on noninvasive imaging. On the other hand, ERCP was useful in patients whose clinical course was suggestive of pancreatic cancer but whose CT scans were read as normal or indeterminate.

Cytologic examination of pancreatic juice increases the sensitivity of ERCP in the diagnosis of pancreatic carcinoma, although conventional cytologic examination of secretin-stimulated pancreatic juice by itself is associated with a significant percentage of false-negative examinations. Cytologic examination of the pancreatic juice appears to be more accurate in tumors of the head of the pancreas than in tumors in the body and tail. Direct insertion of a cannula into the pancreatic duct to collect pure juice appears to offer the possibility for increased sensitivity of this test.[43]

Visceral angiography is not an appropriate test to establish the diagnosis of pancreatic cancer. It is, however, used by many surgeons to evaluate vascular invasion in patients who have apparently resectable disease on CT scanning (Fig. 26-6). There is debate, however, as to the value of angiography now that dynamic CT scanning has improved to the point at which vascular

Table 26-5 Computed Tomographic Findings in 213 Patients With Pancreatic Cancer

Finding	Patients
Tumor mass	205 (96%)
MPD/CBD dilation	168 (79%)
Contiguous organ invasion*	91 (43%)
Local peripancreatic extension	154 (72%)
Vascular invasion	175 (82%)
Metastases	106 (50%)
Liver	72 (34%)
Lymph nodes	57 (27%)

MPD, main pancreatic duct; CBD, common bile duct.
* Includes stomach, spleen, duodenum, and small bowel mesentery.
(After Freeny PC, Traverso LW, Ryan JA. Diagnosis and staging of pancreatic carcinoma with dynamic computed tomography. Am J Surg 1993;165:600)

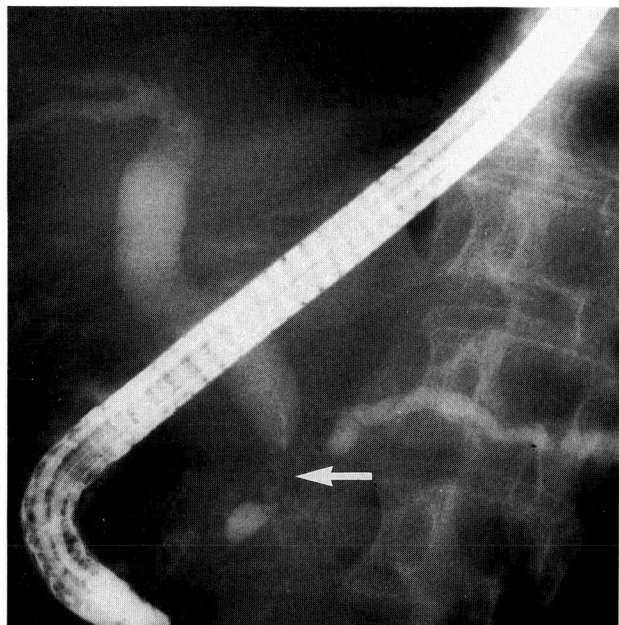

Figure 26-5 Endoscopic retrograde cholangiopancreatographic study in a patient with ductal adenocarcinoma of the pancreas demonstrating circumferential stenosis of both the distal common bile duct and the main pancreatic duct in the head of the pancreas. The location of the tumor is indicated by the arrow. (Bell RH. Neoplasms of the exocrine pancreas. In: Greenfield LJ, Mulholland MW, Oldham KT, Zelenock GB, eds. Surgery: scientific principles and practice. Philadelphia, JB Lippincott, 1993:823)

with high frequency with newer-generation CT scanners and spiral three-dimensional techniques (see Fig. 26-4).

An imaging technique that shows promise in the diagnosis and staging of carcinoma of the pancreas is EUS. The use of mechanically rotating ultrasound probes at the tip of an upper gastrointestinal endoscope produces a 360-degree image. Pancreatic carcinomas appear as hypoechoic masses in the pancreatic substance (Fig. 26-7). EUS appears to be significantly better than transcutaneous ultrasound or CT in the detection of pancreatic tumors smaller than 2.5 cm[48]; the lower limits of detection of pancreatic tumors by EUS may be less than 1 cm. EUS is not capable of distinguishing pancreatic carcinoma from focal areas of pancreatitis (pseudotumors). The place of EUS in the diagnosis of pancreatic cancer is not established, nor is EUS widely available yet. Clearly, it is too expensive and complex for screening. It is probably useful at this point primarily in patients who have clinical symptoms or serum CA19-9 levels suggestive of pancreatic cancer, but negative CT scan and ERCP. In addition to detection of pri-

involvement can be assessed with considerable accuracy by CT alone.[44,45] A retrospective review of 32 patients undergoing both CT and angiography revealed that in 5 patients (16%), CT disclosed contiguous tumor growth around major vessels not detected by angiography.[46] Angiography, on the other hand, appeared to add no valuable information beyond CT concerning major vascular involvement. In another review of 60 patients who had both tests, CT detected vascular invasion missed on angiography in 20% of patients, whereas angiography detected invasion missed on CT in only 5%.[40] In the latter group, other signs of unresectability were present, so angiography was believed to have provided no significant additional information regarding staging. On the other hand, a review of preoperative angiography in 64 patients undergoing pancreaticoduodenectomy revealed findings in 19 patients (30%) that altered treatment strategy.[47] These included examples of celiac axis occlusion requiring revascularization, replaced hepatic arteries requiring preservation, preoperative embolization for pseudoaneurysm or arteriovenous fistula, and splenectomy for splenic vein thrombosis. Such findings, however, may be detected

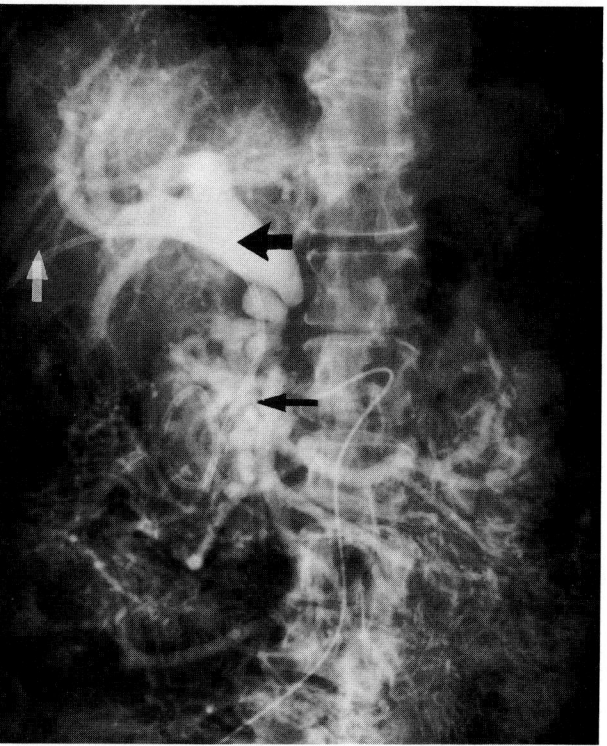

Figure 26-6 Venous phase of a superior mesenteric angiogram in a patient with carcinoma of the head of the pancreas. The junction of the superior mesenteric vein (*small black arrow*) and portal vein (*large black arrow*) is occluded, and multiple collateral vessels have formed in an attempt to bypass the obstruction. A previously placed transhepatic biliary drainage tube is visible (*white arrow*).

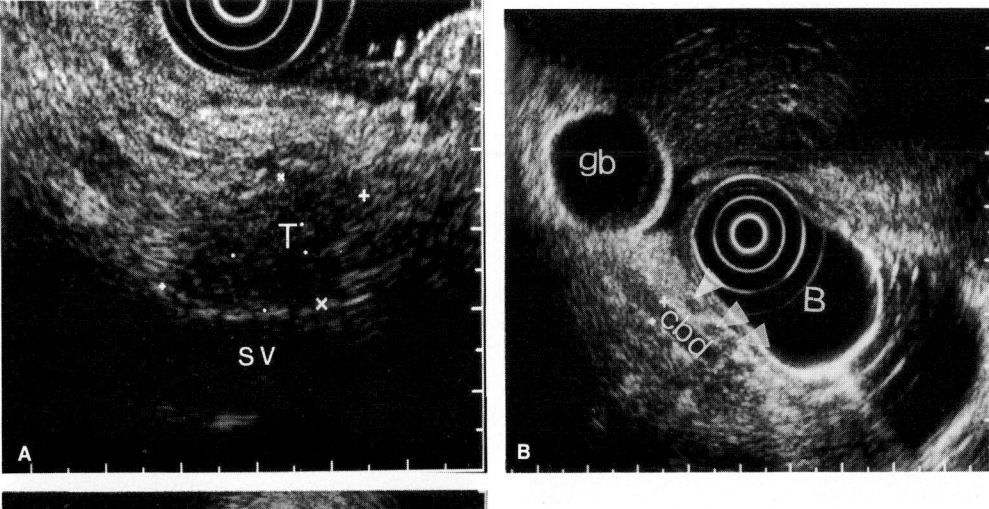

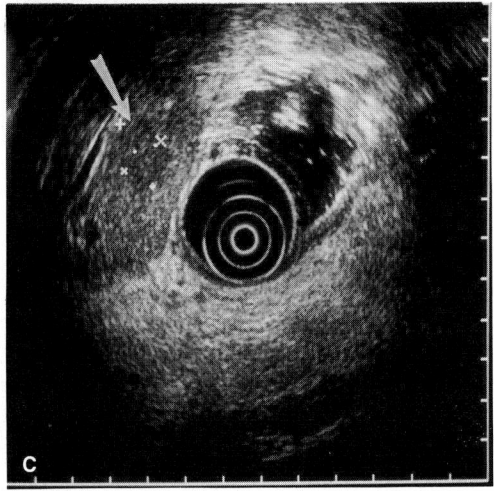

Figure 26-7 Endoscopic ultrasound examination in a patient with carcinoma of the body of the pancreas. (**A**) The ultrasound transducer is in the stomach. The tumor mass (T) and splenic vein (sv) are seen. (**B**) Image taken with the probe in the duodenum demonstrates the gallbladder (gb), a normal 4-mm diameter common bile duct (cbd), and small lymph nodes (*arrowheads*). A water-filled balloon (B) surrounds the transducer. (**C**) Image taken with the transducer in the stomach shows a metastasis (*arrow*) in the left lobe of the liver. (Courtesy of Michael B. Kimmey, MD, Division of Gastroenterology, University of Washington School of Medicine, Seattle)

mary tumors, EUS appears to be an effective tool in staging pancreatic cancer. In one study,[49] EUS was more effective than transcutaneous ultrasound or CT in detecting local invasion and vascular involvement. EUS is better at detecting portal vein invasion than arterial involvement. There are differing reports about the ability of EUS to detect nodal involvement. It appears to be effective in detecting nodal invasion near the pancreas but may lose effectiveness in detecting more distant nodal enlargement.

Two other diagnostic techniques that are under development but that do not yet have a defined clinical role are direct endoscopy of the pancreatic duct using 1- to 3-mm diameter pancreatoscopes and intraductal ultrasound of the pancreatic duct with transpapillary probes.[50,51]

Computed Tomography–Guided Fine-Needle Aspiration

The technique of CT-guided fine-needle aspiration (CT-FNA) of pancreatic cancer (Fig. 26-8) can provide a histologic diagnosis at virtually no risk.[52] The reported sensitivity of the technique varies widely in the literature from 45% to 100%. False-positive aspirations are extremely rare. Some have expressed concern that preoperative CT-FNA in patients with potentially resectable pancreatic tumors may result in dissemination of tumor cells throughout the peritoneal cavity.[53] Others have not confirmed such a risk.[54] At any rate, preoperative CT-FNA is not necessary in patients in whom laparotomy is planned unless they are to undergo preoperative irradiation (see later); CT-FNA may be as easily and accurately performed intraoperatively before resection or bypass.[55,56] CT-FNA is primarily indicated in patients with radiologic evidence of unresectable disease who are not candidates for laparotomy. In such cases, histologic evidence of malignancy allows for an accurate prognosis. Some pancreatic lesions suspected of being ductal carcinoma by CT may in fact be more favorable tumors (lymphoma, islet cell tumors) or may not be malignancies at all (chronic pancreatitis). These occasional cases of mistaken identity justify the use of CT-FNA in virtually all patients with suspected pancreatic cancer in whom operative confirmation of histology is

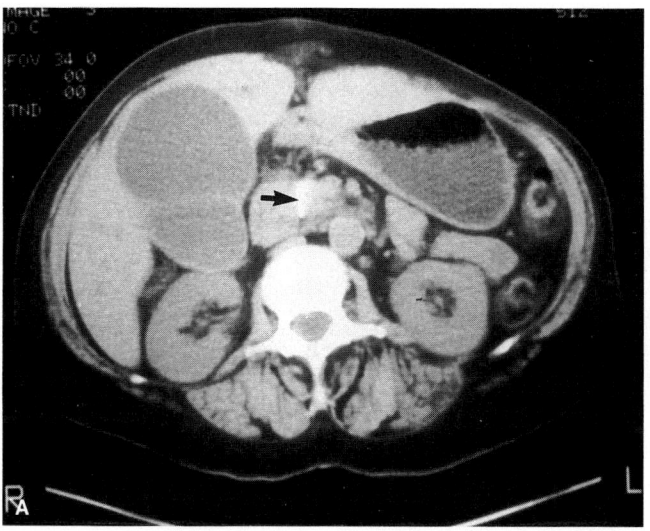
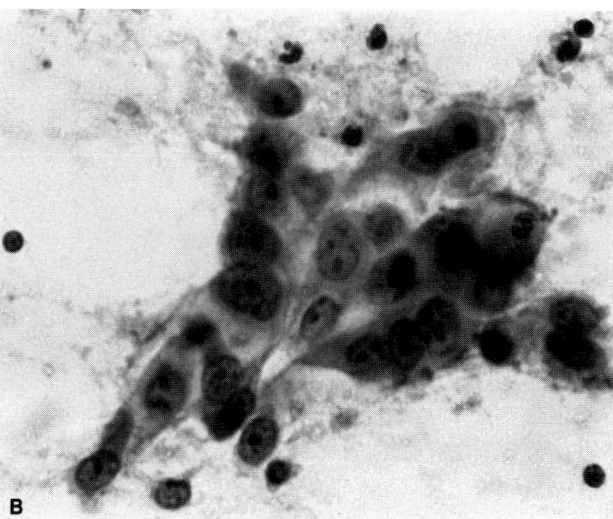

Figure 26-8 Percutaneous CT-guided fine-needle aspiration biopsy of the pancreas. (**A**) A 22-gauge needle is passed into a mass in the head of the pancreas (*arrow*). (**B**) The stained cytologic aspirate is compatible with ductal adenocarcinoma of the pancreas. (Bell RH. Neoplasms of the exocrine pancreas. In: Greenfield LJ, Mulholland MW, Oldham KT, Zelenock GB, eds. Surgery: scientific principles and practice. Philadelphia, JB Lippincott, 1993:823)

not planned.[57] In patients who in fact have pancreatic cancer, CT-FNA also may be required before initiating palliative chemoradiotherapy (see later).

Laparoscopy

Laparoscopy has been used increasingly as part of the diagnostic evaluation of patients with potentially resectable disease. Of those patients who appear to have resectable tumors by standard radiologic techniques, about one fourth are found at the time of laparoscopy to have small tumor implants on the peritoneal surface or omentum or superficial liver metastases indicative of incurability.[58,59] At the time of laparoscopy, saline can be infused into the peritoneal cavity, recovered, and spun down for cytologic examination of the cell block.[53] About 30% of patients who otherwise appear to have disease localized to the pancreas have malignant cells in the peritoneal washings. This finding appears to be associated with a high likelihood of the development of peritoneal carcinomatosis, incurability, and shortened survival. There is not yet sufficient experience with this technique, however, to determine whether a positive peritoneal cytology should be considered a categorical contraindication to resection in patients with otherwise apparently curable disease.

Laparoscopy can be performed immediately before proceeding to pancreaticoduodenectomy. When combined with cytologic examination of the peritoneal cavity, laparoscopy requires an additional anesthetic be-

cause of the time lag in preparing the washings for examination. Laparoscopy and peritoneal washings appear to be of value in avoiding laparotomy in patients who will not benefit from pancreatic resection. The decision about whether to perform laparoscopy also depends on whether the patient will require laparotomy for relief of jaundice or duodenal obstruction (see later). Laparoscopy is most reasonably used only if a positive finding will result in avoidance of laparotomy.

Curative Therapy for Ductal Pancreatic Adenocarcinoma

Surgery

Surgical resection is the only therapy that offers the prospect of permanent cure in ductal carcinoma of the pancreas. Of all patients presenting with pancreatic cancer, 10% to 15% are found to have resectable lesions after a complete preoperative evaluation and operative exploration.[60,61] About 90% of resectable pancreatic adenocarcinomas are located in the head of the gland rather than the body or tail. This may be due both to the fact that carcinoma overall is more common in the head of the gland and to earlier presentation in patients with tumors in the head of the gland because of the development of obstructive jaundice.

CARCINOMA OF THE HEAD OF THE PANCREAS. Resectable carcinomas in the head of the gland are traditionally managed by pancreaticoduodenectomy (Fig. 26-9) or one of its variants (described

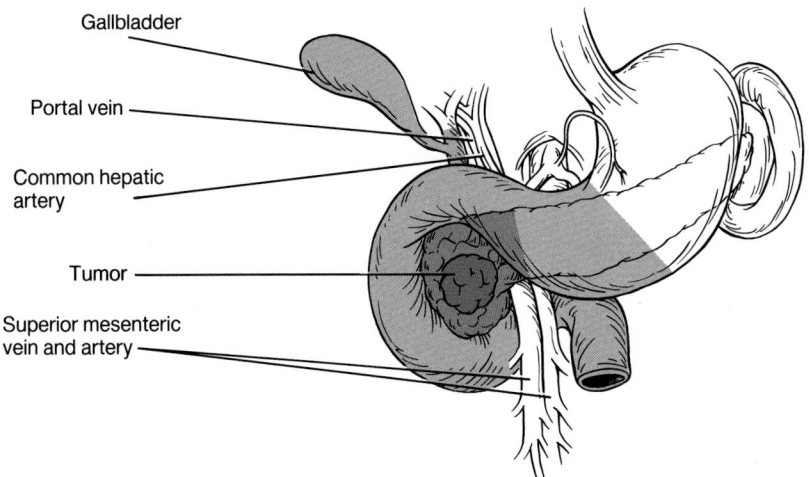

Gallbladder

Portal vein

Common hepatic
artery

Tumor

Superior mesenteric
vein and artery

Figure 26-9 Pancreaticoduodenectomy. The tissues to be resected, including the distal stomach, duodenum, proximal jejunum, head of pancreas, distal common bile duct, and gallbladder, are indicated.

later). The first resection of the head of the pancreas and duodenum for tumor was described by Whipple in 1935[62]; the operation was performed in two stages for a tumor of the ampulla of Vater, but Whipple's name remains associated with the modern version of the operation for pancreatic cancer. Two years later, the performance of a pancreaticoduodenectomy for carcinoma of the pancreas was reported.[63] In the 1940s, the operation was modified, culminating in the report by Child in 1948 of 22 cases of one-stage radical pancreaticoduodenectomy,[64] in which he described the operation as it is performed today.

The indication for pancreaticoduodenectomy is the presence of a potentially resectable mass in the head of the pancreas. Histologic confirmation of the diagnosis is not required preoperatively if the clinical setting makes carcinoma of the pancreas a possibility. For patients to be appropriate candidates for resection, preoperative studies should show no evidence of distant metastases (liver, nodes outside the proposed resection margins), no major arterial invasion, and patency of the superior mesenteric and portal veins. Tumors immediately adjacent to the veins may be amenable to resection, so contiguity to the major veins is not a contraindication to resection if the veins are patent.

Pancreaticoduodenectomy (see Section V in Atlas Chap. 30) is most easily performed through a bilateral subcostal incision. Upon entering the abdomen, a careful inspection of the entire peritoneal cavity should be undertaken in search of metastatic disease, which would render resection unproductive. The most common sites for such previously unsuspected metastases are the liver and the peritoneal surfaces, including the omentum. The lesser omentum should be opened to allow inspection of the lymph node beds around the celiac axis. It is common to find soft 1- to 1.5-cm nodes in this area, and biopsy of such soft and movable nodes is

time-consuming and usually unproductive. If, on the other hand, the nodes are hard, matted, or fixed, biopsy is warranted, and pancreatic resection should not be performed if the nodes harbor carcinoma. The base of the inferior surface of the transverse mesocolon should be examined in the area of the superior mesenteric vessels. This is a relatively common site for direct tumor extension and nodal disease, which, depending on their extent, may render the disease unresectable.

If the general abdominal exploration is negative for metastasis, the hepatic flexure of the colon is mobilized and retracted caudally to expose the head of the pancreas and duodenum. An extensive Kocher maneuver is performed so that the entire duodenum and head of the pancreas can be palpated. Ordinarily, the tumor is detectable by its hardness in contrast to the surrounding tissues. Often, the remainder of the pancreas is firm because of coexisting pancreatitis due to ductal obstruction, but even in these circumstances, the tumor is usually firmer than the rest of the gland. As noted earlier, FNA cytology may be performed at this point with little risk and a 70% to 80% chance of a successful tissue diagnosis. Multiple passes with the needle can be made if necessary. With the fine-needle (22-gauge) technique, it is not necessary to perform biopsies transduodenally, as was recommended in the past when large-bore needles were used. Incisional biopsy of the pancreas is not as accurate as FNA, is considerably riskier, and is therefore rarely if ever indicated. If the results of FNA are negative, the surgeon must decide if the combination of clinical features, radiologic evaluation, and operative findings justify proceeding with pancreaticoduodenectomy. If there is a mass in the head of the pancreas or obstruction of the biliary or pancreatic ducts that cannot be otherwise explained, pancreaticoduodenectomy is generally justifiable even in the absence of tissue confirmation of malignancy. The smallest tumors, which are the most difficult to biopsy, are also the most likely to be cured by extirpation.

Once the decision to proceed with pancreaticoduodenectomy is made, the lesser sac is opened widely through the gastrocolic omentum. If the pylorus-preserving variant of the pancreaticoduodenectomy (PPPD) is planned, the gastroepiploic vessels should be preserved in continuity with the stomach. After opening the lesser sac, the body and tail of the pancreas are examined for evidence of direct tumor extension; lymph nodes above and below the body of the pancreas should also be evaluated since these node groups may be affected in carcinoma of the head of the gland. The finding of positive nodes in this area does not necessarily preclude resection, but it necessitates a more extensive pancreatectomy and node dissection.

The middle colic vein is identified and followed to its junction with the superior mesenteric vein. Cautious dissection is then undertaken between the anterior surface of the superior mesenteric vein and the posterior aspect of the neck of the pancreas to determine if the portal vein is free of direct invasion. If there is any difficulty in this dissection, it should not be forced because injuries to the portal vein behind the neck of the pancreas may be extremely difficult to control. If the tunnel anterior to the vein can only be partially completed, it is best to move above the duodenum, ligate and divide the gastroduodenal artery, identify the portal vein above the pancreas, and continue to try to develop the plane anterior to the portal vein working both from above and below the neck of the pancreas. Although the development of a free plane anterior to the vein is an encouraging sign, it does not preclude the possibility that the vein is invaded laterally or posterolaterally, a finding that may not become apparent until the end of the operation. If such limited invasion is ultimately encountered, it can usually be dealt with by a partial or segmental resection of the portal vein.

If the portal vein appears uninvolved, the operation proceeds by dividing the stomach, removing the gallbladder, and dividing the common hepatic duct as portrayed in Section V in Atlas Chapter 30. The jejunum is divided beyond the ligament of Treitz, and the proximal jejunum and fourth portion of the duodenum are pulled beneath the superior mesenteric vessels to exit on the patient's right side. With both the stomach and the duodenum retracted to the right, the neck of the pancreas is divided over the portal vein. The resection is completed by carefully ligating the branches entering the portal vein from the head of the pancreas and uncinate process and by dividing the retroperitoneal attachments of the pancreas along the superior mesenteric artery beneath the portal vein.

After removing the operative specimen, recon-struction requires three anastomoses (Fig. 26-10). The most common approach is to perform the anastomosis between the cut surface of the pancreas and the free end of the jejunum first (see Section V in Atlas Chap. 30). It is extremely important to drain the area of the pancreaticojejunostomy with closed suction drains. The common hepatic duct is then anastomosed to the side of the jejunum, and finally an end-to-side gastrojejunostomy is performed.

Many surgeons prefer to perform PPPD, which preserves the entire stomach, pylorus, and first few centimeters of the duodenum.[65] In this variant of the operation (Fig. 26-11), the blood supply to the distal stomach and pyloric region is maintained by preserving the right gastric and right gastroepiploic arcades by ligating those vessels close to their origin off the hepatic and gastroduodenal arteries, respectively (see Section V in Atlas Chap. 30). After resection of the operative specimen, gastrointestinal continuity is restored by anastomosing the cut end of the duodenum to the side of the jejunum. In most cases of pancreatic cancer, it is technically possible to preserve the pylorus. On occasion, the proximity of a tumor in the upper head of the pancreas to the pylorus may suggest that a standard resection would be more advisable.

EXTENDED PANCREATICODUODENECTOMY. Pathologic examination of resected specimens after standard pancreaticoduodenectomy often reveals positive retroperitoneal margins. In addition, lymph node metastases from pancreatic cancer may involve nodal groups along the superior or inferior body of the pancreas or along the common hepatic artery and superior mesenteric artery, which are not routinely removed in a standard pancreaticoduodenectomy. For these two reasons, surgeons have proposed that operation for carcinoma of the pancreatic head be expanded to include an wide en bloc dissection of the retroperitoneal soft tissue adjacent to the pancreatic head and a more extensive nodal dissection. To perform the latter, it is generally necessary to extend the pancreatic resection line slightly to the left, allowing better exposure of the celiac axis and the base of the superior mesenteric artery. In practical terms, extended pancreaticoduodenectomy (EPD) requires a revision of the Kocher maneuver to provide for a wider excision of peripancreatic soft tissue and in addition includes skeletonization of the aorta, inferior vena cava, portal vein, and hepatic, proximal splenic, and superior mesenteric arteries (see Section V in Atlas Chap. 30). The results of EPD in comparison to standard resection are discussed later.

TOTAL PANCREATECTOMY. As discussed earlier, the rationale for total pancreatectomy for carcinoma of the head of the pancreas was based on the belief that as up to 30% of patients had multicentric

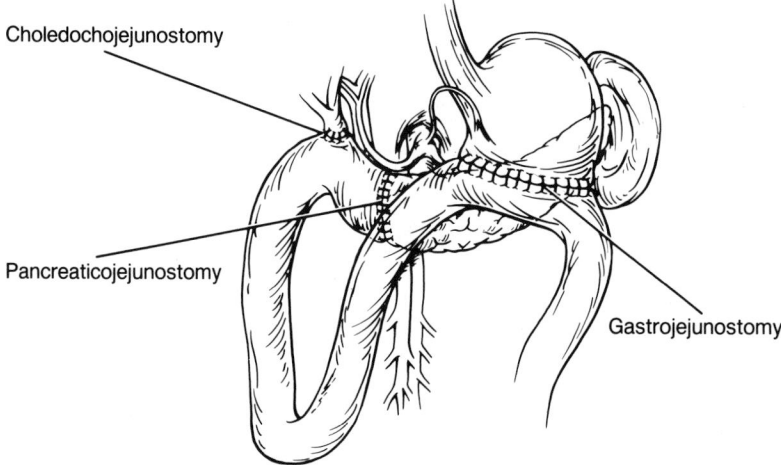

Figure 26-10   Completed reconstruction after standard pancreaticoduodenectomy.

disease within the pancreas, a belief that is probably fallacious for the reasons previously indicated. Total pancreatectomy also has the virtue of avoiding the need for a pancreaticointestinal anastomosis. After total pancreatectomy and duodenectomy, the free end of the jejunum is ordinarily oversewn, and the biliary and gastric are anastomoses performed in the usual end-to-side fashion. The results of total pancreatectomy for carcinoma of the head of the pancreas are discussed later.

POSTOPERATIVE COURSE AFTER PANCREATICODUODENAL RESECTION.   Historically, pancreaticoduodenectomy was associated with a high rate of postoperative mortality, in the range of 20%. In the last

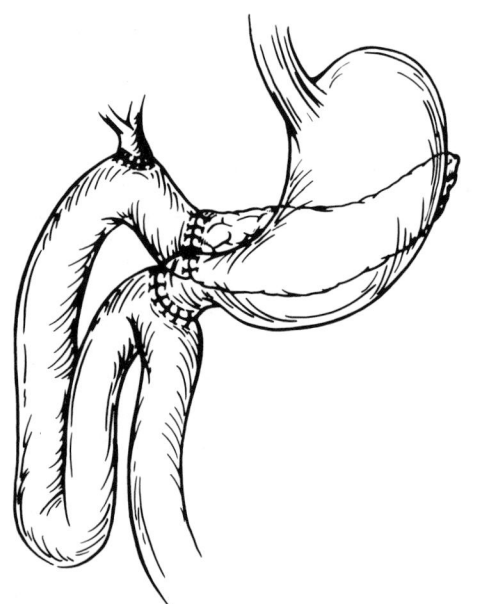

Figure 26-11   Completed reconstruction after pylorus-sparing variant of pancreaticoduodenectomy.

decade, considerable evidence has been published indicating that the operation is being done more safely and that postoperative mortality rates of 5% or less are now the norm in centers with significant experience with the operation.[2,3,66] An analysis of reduction in mortality after pancreaticoduodenectomy suggests that improvement is due in great part to increased concentration of the procedures in the hands of a few experienced surgeons. Better perioperative care, particularly the availability of interventional radiology, has also contributed to the improvement in mortality.[67]

Consonant with the magnitude of the operation, morbidity remains substantial after pancreaticoduodenectomy, with about 20% to 40% of patients experiencing postoperative complications. Of these, the most dreaded is disruption of the pancreaticojejunostomy, which occurs in 10% to 15% of patients. The use of subcutaneous injections of somatostatin analogue in the perioperative period has been shown in one randomized trial to reduce the incidence of pancreatic leaks after pancreatic resection.[68] If the anastomosis is adequately drained, many leaks are controlled, persist for a time as a pancreaticocutaneous fistula, and ultimately close spontaneously with no adverse effect other than prolongation of the hospital stay. If leakage from the pancreaticojejunostomy becomes manifest by drainage of amylase-rich fluid in the first 7 to 10 days after operation, cessation of oral intake is recommended. Such patients should be maintained on total parenteral nutrition or fed by jejunostomy (if available) until the fistula closes or the fistula volume is low (less than 100 mL/d) and stable, at which point oral alimentation can be cautiously reintroduced. Some patients leave the hospital with a persistent low-volume fistula. Most of these close within 2 to 3 months.

In a few patients after pancreaticoduodenectomy,

leakage from the pancreatic anastomosis is a fatal complication. In such patients, leakage leads to invasive retroperitoneal sepsis, which in turn results in erosion of blood vessels and life-threatening hemorrhage. Erosion may occur into the portal vein or its branches or into any of the major arteries around the operative bed. Sometimes, patients experience a small-volume herald bleed through their drains, which is then followed hours or days later by a massive hemorrhage. Significant bleeding from postoperative drains in association with a pancreatic leak usually mandates reoperation. Although bleeding may be temporarily controlled by angiographic embolization, reexploration is required to control sepsis, which is the underlying cause of the bleeding. Often, such sepsis is diffusely invasive in the retroperitoneum and not amenable to percutaneous drainage. Open packing of the operative bed, as used in necrotizing acute pancreatitis, may be life-saving.[69] Completion pancreatectomy is an extremely high-risk undertaking under such circumstances but has been reported to succeed in controlling sepsis and bleeding in isolated cases.[70] In all, postoperative hemorrhage is the most common cause of death after pancreaticoduodenectomy.

Disruption of the choledochojejunostomy with development of a biliary fistula occurs in about 5% of patients after pancreaticoduodenectomy. If adequately drained and not associated with retroperitoneal sepsis, most of these fistulas close spontaneously. Persistence of drainage should prompt a percutaneous transhepatic cholangiogram, which occasionally reveals a technical problem with the anastomosis that requires operative revision.

Generally, patients undergoing pancreaticoduodenectomy receive antiulcer prophylaxis in the perioperative period. Despite this precaution, upper gastrointestinal bleeding occurs in about 5% of patients after pancreatic resection. The gastroenterostomy is the most common site, and bleeding can sometimes be controlled endoscopically. Bleeding can also occur from the gastric or jejunal mucosa. Classic marginal ulceration occurs in 5% to 10% of patients after pancreaticoduodenectomy. In the past, it was common practice to perform a truncal vagotomy as part of the Whipple procedure, but recent studies demonstrated that vagotomy does not prevent postoperative marginal ulceration and has the unwanted side effect of exacerbating delayed gastric emptying,[2] which is common after pancreaticoduodenectomy even when a vagotomy is not performed. For these reasons, vagotomy is not recommended in conjunction with pancreatic resection. Finally, retroperitoneal bleeding due to breakdown of the pancreaticojejunal anastomosis may present as an upper gastrointestinal hemorrhage secondary to the entrance of blood into the disrupted jejunal limb.

As noted earlier, delay in gastric emptying is a common complication of pancreaticoduodenectomy, occurring in 10% to 30% of patients. Some patients may not be able to be weaned from gastric suction for 2 to 3 weeks and require parenteral nutrition or jejunal feeding during this period. Delayed gastric emptying is more common after PPPD than standard pancreaticoduodenectomy. Ordinarily, the gastric outlet obstruction is functional and not anatomic, but occasionally a mechanical obstruction occurs because of technical problems with the anastomosis or scarring around the pancreatic bed. If outlet obstruction persists in the postoperative period, a barium upper gastrointestinal series should be obtained. If contrast enters the small bowel, even sparingly, the likelihood is that function will return with continued expectant management. Complete failure of contrast to enter the intestine usually is indicative of complete mechanical obstruction; the cause of the obstruction may be apparent on endoscopy but in any event is likely to require operative intervention for correction.

RESULTS OF SURGERY FOR CARCINOMA OF THE HEAD OF THE PANCREAS. In a review of the literature published from 1980 to 1989, 42 (5.4%) of 768 patients who underwent standard pancreaticoduodenectomy for carcinoma of the pancreas were actual 5-year survivors.[71] The percentage of patients cured by resection, however, appears to be slowly increasing; 5-year survival rates in the range of 20% have been reported from centers with significant operative experience (Table 26-6). Because of the large number of patients followed, the data from the pancreatic cancer registry of the Japan Pancreas Society is probably the most meaningful. Among 2311 patients who underwent resection for pancreatic cancer between 1981 and 1987, the actual 5-year survival rate was 18%, although survival for ductal carcinoma of the pancreas was probably slightly lower because of the inclusion in this registry of a small number of patients with malig-

Table 26-6 Survival After Surgery for Pancreatic Cancer

Investigation	Patients	Dates of Operations	Actuarial 5-Year Survival Rate (%)
Cameron et al[74]	89	1969–1990	19
Trede et al[66]	133	1972–1989	24
Geer et al[73]	146	1983–1990	24

nant islet cell tumors or cystadenocarcinomas.[72] Reported median survival after pancreaticoduodenectomy remains relatively fixed at about 1 year. Thus, some fortunate patients are cured by resection, but many live only a short time after surgery. Factors that predict a poor outcome after resection include lymph node involvement, poor histologic tumor differentiation, and tumor size greater than 2.5 cm.[73,74] Tumor size less than 2 to 2.5 cm is associated with a lower likelihood of lymph node metastasis and retroperitoneal and vascular invasion. It may be the lower frequency of these findings rather than tumor size per se that is most important in determining survival because occasional patients with larger tumors are long-term survivors if spread outside the pancreas is absent.[75,76] In a review of nearly 500 surgically treated patients with pancreatic cancer,[77] a short history of symptoms, absence of back pain, and a CA19-9 value of less than 400 U/mL were also favorable prognostic signs in addition to small tumor size, well to moderately differentiated histology, and absence of nodal metastases. Age alone does not appear to strongly influence prognosis after pancreaticoduodenectomy,[78,79] but postoperative morbidity is increased in patients older than 70 years in some series, and mortality is influenced adversely if patients older than 70 years have significant comorbid illnesses, such as cardiac disease.[80,81]

The most common site of tumor recurrence after macroscopically ''curative'' resection of pancreatic carcinoma is in the retroperitoneum (80% of cases)—in regional lymph nodes, the retroperitoneal soft tissue, or both. Hepatic metastases are found in 60% to 70% of patients who develop recurrent disease, and peritoneal carcinomatosis is found in 40% to 50%.[82,83]

In attempting to improve survival and quality of life after resection for carcinoma of the head of the pancreas, surgeons have evaluated other operative approaches in addition to traditional pancreaticoduodenectomy. As noted earlier, these include the pylorus-sparing variant of pancreaticoduodenectomy, pancreaticoduodenectomy with extended retroperitoneal and regional node dissection, and total pancreatectomy.

Most evaluations of the safety and efficacy of PPPD indicate that operative morbidity and mortality and long-term survival are equivalent to those after traditional pancreaticoduodenectomy.[84,85] One group of surgeons,[86] however, noted a significantly lower survival rate in pancreatic cancer patients after PPPD compared with traditional pancreaticoduodenectomy, particularly in patients with stage III tumors. The two operations have not been compared in a prospective, randomized fashion.

In terms of quality of life after resection, it was hoped that PPPD would permit improved nutritional and digestive well-being in comparison to traditional pancreaticoduodenectomy. In fact, no such advantage has been documented.[87] Most patients who are tumor free after either method of pancreaticoduodenectomy experience relatively little digestive difficulty, which is rather surprising in view of the considerable disruption of normal upper gastrointestinal physiology that both operations entail.

Total pancreatectomy appears to offer no advantage over traditional pancreaticoduodenectomy in the management of cancer of the head of the pancreas. Although pancreaticoduodenectomy and total pancreatectomy have not been compared in a controlled clinical trial, comparative studies suggest that long-term survival after total pancreatectomy is no better than after pancreaticoduodenectomy and may even be slightly worse.[88,89] Although the rationale for total pancreatectomy was the observation that about one fourth of patients with carcinoma of the head of pancreas have multifocal disease within the gland, the accuracy of that observation is debated (see section on pathology), and the prognosis of patients with multicentric disease is poor even after total pancreatectomy.[90] Finally, patients who have undergone total pancreatectomy experience unstable diabetes with frequent hypoglycemia and other metabolic consequences not observed after traditional pancreaticoduodenectomy.[91]

Considerable interest has been generated in EPD, which includes an aggressive resection of the retroperitoneal soft tissue and lymph nodes surrounding the celiac axis and the superior mesenteric artery in comparison to traditional pancreaticoduodenectomy or PPPD. To provide exposure for the nodal dissection around the celiac trunk, the line of division of the pancreatic parenchyma is slightly more to the patient's left than in traditional pancreaticoduodenectomy. Sometimes, EPD is combined with segmental resection of the portal vein if the tumor is adherent to the vein, but venous resection is not an integral part of EPD. The rationale for EPD is based on the observations that the retroperitoneal soft tissue invasion is present in as many as 80% of patients with resectable pancreatic cancer, that retroperitoneal margins are inadequate in as many as 30% to 40% of patients undergoing traditional pancreaticoduodenectomy, and that nodal involvement is present along the common hepatic and superior mesenteric arteries in a significant number of patients with grossly resectable disease.[23,92] Two initial reports from Japan noted 5-year survival rates of 33% and 29% after EPD compared with historical survival rates after traditional pancreaticoduodenectomy in the same institutions of 0% and 9%.[93,94] Early results of a small prospective trial likewise suggested improvement in survival in patients with pancreatic cancer treated by EPD.[95]

Long-term survival after so-called regional pancreatectomy (which usually includes total pancreatectomy, extensive upper abdominal lymphadenectomy, and en bloc resection of involved major vascular structures) is not better than after traditional pancreaticoduodenectomy, suggesting that expanding the scope of operations for pancreatic cancer is not fruitful beyond a certain point.[96,97] Although it has become relatively common practice to resect a portion of the portal vein involved by tumor, this maneuver probably benefits only patients with limited venous involvement.[90,98] It is appropriate to perform a segmental resection of the portal vein to avoid a positive retroperitoneal margin in an otherwise resectable tumor. Attempts at venous resection in patients with grossly invaded, thrombosed major veins are not warranted. Most authorities no longer advocate segmental resection of the hepatic or superior mesenteric arteries if they are invaded. In general, however, the optimal extent of resection for carcinoma of the head of the pancreas is not yet clearly defined. The reported results with EPD are encouraging and warrant continued investigation.

CARCINOMA OF THE BODY AND TAIL OF THE PANCREAS. Carcinoma of the body and tail of the pancreas is usually advanced at the time of diagnosis, and the resectability rate is 5% to 10%.[99] Splenic vascular involvement does not necessarily preclude resection.[100] In one series of 26 patients who underwent distal pancreatectomy for ductal carcinoma of the pancreas, median survival was 10 months, and the 5-year survival rate was 8%.[101] These figures are not significantly different than those reported after pancreaticoduodenectomy for carcinoma of the head of the pancreas during the same period.

Adjuvant Therapy Combined With Surgical Resection

Because most patients who undergo pancreatic resection for ductal carcinoma of the pancreas ultimately develop recurrent cancer, there has been interest in trying to improve the results of surgery with adjuvant therapy. Because a high percentage of patients develop local recurrence after pancreatic resection, radiation therapy, either external or intraoperative or both, has been added to the treatment regimen in an attempt to improve local control. Most adjuvant therapy programs include 5-fluorouracil (5FU) as a radiation sensitizer. Other chemotherapeutic agents have also been added in an attempt to eradicate presumed micrometastases. Adjuvant therapy has been used in both the postoperative and preoperative settings.

The first firm demonstration of the value of adju-vant therapy after resection for pancreatic carcinoma was provided by a study[102] in which 43 patients who underwent apparently curative pancreatic resection were randomly assigned to receive no further therapy or to a combination of 40 Gy of external radiation therapy and 5FU weekly for 2 years. The adjuvant program was well-tolerated and resulted in a significantly increased median survival (20 months) for the treated group compared with the control group (11 months). The beneficial effect of postoperative 5FU and radiation therapy was confirmed in a second trial of the same regimen.[103] The low toxicity of this regimen and its proven efficacy suggest that it should be instituted in all otherwise suitable patients after resection for ductal carcinoma of the pancreas.

Interest has increased in the use of preoperative chemoradiotherapy in patients who have apparently resectable tumors. In such programs, patients are carefully staged radiologically before beginning preoperative therapy. After the completion of chemoradiotherapy, patients are restaged radiologically (and sometimes laparoscopically) to be sure they still appear to have resectable tumors before proceeding to laparotomy. The ability to palliate jaundice by endoscopic or transhepatic routes (see later) allows sufficient time for a course of preoperative radiation therapy. The rationale for preoperative therapy as opposed to postoperative therapy includes the following considerations:

1. Most patients can proceed promptly to chemoradiotherapy, whereas postoperative therapy is delayed in a significant number of patients because of complications of surgery or because of general debilitation.
2. Preoperative therapy may prevent dissemination of live tumor cells at the time of laparotomy.
3. Tumors may shrink during preoperative therapy, improving the chances for a complete surgical resection.

The first consideration has proved accurate. Nearly all patients who enter preoperative adjuvant protocols are able to complete them and undergo surgery at the scheduled time. The second and third considerations have not been validated yet. Although studies of preoperative therapy show that most resected specimens contain varying amounts of necrotic tumor cells, most tumors do not shrink substantially by radiologic criteria during preoperative therapy; there is conflicting evidence whether tumors are significantly down-staged by preoperative therapy.[54,104,105] The studies available suggest that the risk of operation is not increased by preoperative therapy. Survival in patients undergoing preoperative chemoradiotherapy appears to be about equivalent to that of patients receiving postoperative therapy. Preoperative therapy continues to be modified and evaluated in several centers, however, and further evidence concerning its role in the treatment of pancreatic cancer should be forthcoming soon.

A number of centers have employed intraoperative radiation therapy as part of an adjuvant program for resectable pancreatic cancer. It involves the single application of high-dose (usually 20 Gy) radiation to the bed of the resected pancreas before performing the pancreatic, biliary, and gastric anastomoses. Intraoperative radiation is ordinarily employed in combination with either preoperative or postoperative external-beam radiation therapy. Despite its theoretic appeal, a randomized trial suggested that intraoperative radiation therapy offered no survival advantage in pancreatic cancer when compared with conventional external-beam radiation therapy in the adjuvant setting.[106]

Palliative Therapy for Ductal Pancreatic Adenocarcinoma

Because most patients have unresectable tumors when first diagnosed, palliation of symptoms in those with incurable disease is an important part of the care of patients with pancreatic cancer. The symptoms for which palliation is usually considered are jaundice (with or without pruritus), vomiting due to gastric outlet obstruction, and pain. In addition, chemoradiotherapy may be advised in the hopes of slowing tumor progression (see later). In choosing the best palliation possible for an individual patient, it is useful for a multidisciplinary group of physicians to participate along with the patient in choosing the most appropriate therapy. This group should include a medical oncologist, a radiation therapist, a pain specialist, a gastroenterologist, and a surgeon, since all have something to offer in the palliation of pancreatic cancer. The difficulty comes in choosing the best therapy for an individual patient. The functional status of the patient should be carefully assessed. For patients with advanced disease who are significantly debilitated, it may be appropriate to offer pain control and not perform any invasive procedures for the relief of other symptoms, since the morbidity and mortality of surgical bypass, for example, can be significant in patients with poor performance status. In the past, choledochoenterostomy and gastroenterostomy were associated with an operative mortality of about 20%.[107] Clearly, this is unacceptable for a palliative procedure and underscores the need to tailor the therapy to the patient's performance status and life expectancy.

Treatment of Jaundice

In general, procedures for the relief of jaundice should be entertained in any patient of reasonable functional status who is expected to live more than a few weeks. Relief of jaundice is associated with improved appetite, an enhanced sense of well-being, and disappearance of pruritus, which can be disabling. In choosing the best procedure for the relief of jaundice, the first decision that must be made is whether to use an endoscopic or a traditional surgical technique. Percutaneous transhepatic approaches may also be used,[108] although the endoscopic route is generally less risky and simpler. The decision between endoscopic and surgical therapy depends in part on the presence of symptoms of gastric outlet obstruction; if present, these mandate a surgical approach.

Endoscopic relief of jaundice in patients with pancreatic cancer is accomplished by performing a papillotomy at the sphincter of Oddi and then passing a guide wire up the common bile duct (Fig. 26-12). A 10F or 11.5F plastic catheter is then piggybacked over the wire until it is positioned across the obstruction. If the catheter eventually becomes clogged, it may be replaced by extracting the occluded catheter endoscopically and repeating the same procedure. Surgical relief of jaundice is accomplished by choledochojejunostomy or cholecystojejunostomy as the situation dictates—the latter is simpler and is the operation of choice if the cystic duct is not obstructed by tumor (see Section V in Atlas Chap. 30). The issue of whether to perform concomitant gastroenterostomy is discussed later.

Endoscopic and surgical approaches to the relief of jaundice have been compared in a number of studies.[109–111] In general, endoscopic approaches are associated with less initial morbidity, mortality, and expense than surgical bypass, but surgical bypass is more durable. In one series of 118 patients undergoing biliary bypass, only 2% developed recurrent jaundice.[112] In contrast, 20% to 50% of patients treated with endoscopically placed plastic stents develop recurrent jaundice requiring treatment. These episodes may be associated with cholangitis and cause significant morbidity and mortality. For these reasons, the advantages of endoscopic treatment in comparison to surgery diminish with increasing time. Therefore, surgical bypass has been proposed in patients with an anticipated life expectancy of 6 months or more; endoscopic stenting is preferred in patients with a shorter predicted life expectancy. The presence of distant metastases at the time of presentation is an indication for endoscopic rather than surgical relief of jaundice. Because surgeons have been more selective about recommending surgical bypass, operative mortality for these procedures has fallen from

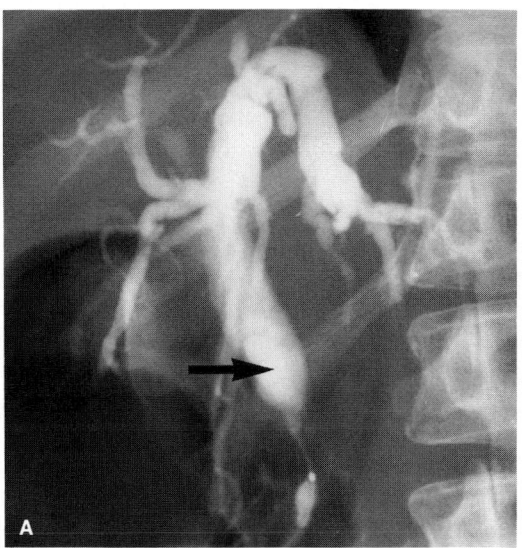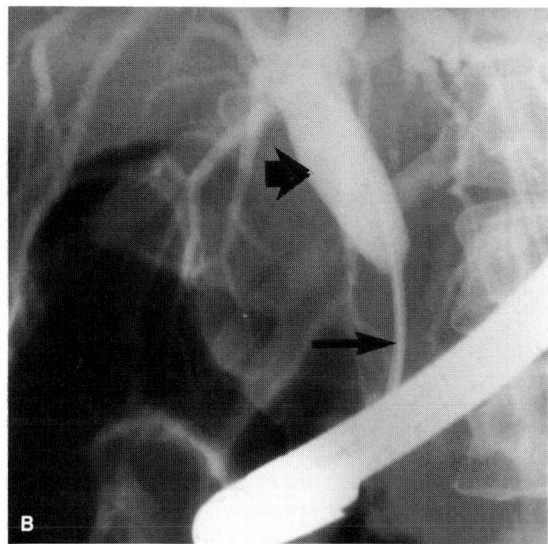

Figure 26-12 Endoscopic relief of jaundice in a patient with unresectable carcinoma of the pancreas. (**A**) A guide wire is passed from the duodenum through the malignant stricture into the dilated proximal bile duct (*arrow*). (**B**) A plastic stent (*thin arrow*) was passed over the guide wire into the dilated bile duct (*thick arrow*). The guide wire is removed after satisfactory placement of the stent.

the traditionally reported 20% to 25% to less than 5%.[112,113]

When surgical relief of jaundice is chosen, the options are cholecystoenterostomy or choledochojejunostomy. If the cystic duct communicates with the common bile duct (which should be confirmed by cholangiography through the gallbladder) and is grossly separated from tumor by 1 cm or more, cholecystoenterostomy is the procedure of choice because of its simplicity.[114]

Treatment of Gastric Outlet Obstruction

Debate has been long-standing about the value of gastroenterostomy in the palliative treatment of patients with pancreatic carcinoma. In patients with symptomatic gastric outlet obstruction, gastrojejunostomy is indicated for the relief of vomiting, but these symptomatic patients have a poor prognosis, any many are never discharged from the hospital.[115] The question of whether to perform a prophylactic gastroenterostomy in asymptomatic patients at the time of biliary bypass continues to be debated. The argument for gastric bypass is based on the observation that 10% to 20% of patients undergoing biliary bypass alone develop gastric outlet obstruction before death.[116] Because it is not possible on clinical grounds to predict which patients will develop gastric outlet obstruction, some have recommended liberal use of prophylactic gastric bypass.[117]

The case against prophylactic gastroenterostomy is based on the argument that patients may develop gastric outlet obstruction even after prophylactic gastroenterostomy[118] and that concomitant gastric bypass adds to the morbidity of biliary bypass.[113,118] The question cannot be resolved definitively on the basis of available studies, but the weight of the evidence is against the performance of prophylactic gastric bypass.

Treatment of Pain

Most patients with carcinoma of the pancreas experience abdominal or back pain before their death, and in most, the pain is described as moderate to severe. Therefore, the relief of pain is one of the most important aspects of the palliative therapy of pancreatic cancer. Chemical splanchnicectomy (celiac plexus block with 50% alcohol) performed at the time of biliary or gastric bypass has been shown to significantly lower mean pain score at 2, 4, and 6 months after operation and at final assessment.[119] This technique is simple, associated with virtually no complications, and should be considered in all patients undergoing bypass, even if they are not experiencing pain before bypass, since celiac block delays or prevents the subsequent onset of pain. In patients who are not candidates for surgical bypass, celiac plexus block can be performed percutaneously and has been shown to provide pain relief equivalent to oral narcotics but with fewer side effects.[120]

Antineoplastic Therapy

In patients with unresectable pancreatic cancer, the combination of 5FU and 40 Gy of external-beam radiation therapy has been shown to increase median survival from 5 to 10 months compared with radiation therapy alone.[121] Occasional patients achieve relatively prolonged survival after chemoradiotherapy, and about 40% are alive after 1 year. These survival figures must be viewed in light of the fact that most treated patients have moderate to good performance status. Nevertheless, the toxicity of this regimen is limited. About 80% of patients are able to complete a full course of treatment. Therefore, combination therapy with 5-FU and radiation should be seriously considered in all patients with unresectable pancreatic cancer who appear to be able to tolerate therapy. More aggressive combinations of chemotherapy and radiation show some promise and are under evaluation.[122]

CYSTADENOMA AND CYSTADENOCARCINOMA OF THE PANCREAS

Two varieties of cystic neoplasms of the pancreas have been described—serous cystadenoma and mucinous cystic neoplasm (mucinous cystadenoma and mucinous cystadenocarcinoma). The distinction between these two forms of cystic neoplasm is clinically significant since the serous tumors appear to be uniformly benign, whereas the mucinous variety has clear malignant potential.

Both serous and mucinous cystic neoplasms usually present when the tumors are already large (average, 10 cm). Serous tumors are slightly more common in women, whereas the mucinous variety occurs six times as often in women as in men. About one fourth of patients, and particularly those with benign neoplasms, are asymptomatic. In asymptomatic patients, tumors are usually discovered during imaging or operation for some other condition. Symptomatic patients ordinarily present with abdominal pain, and many have a palpable abdominal mass. Tumors in the head of the pancreas may cause obstructive jaundice, but this is decidedly less common than in patients with ductal adenocarcinoma of the pancreas. Weight loss suggests that the cystic lesion is malignant.

Serous cystadenomas are classically described as containing multiple small cystic spaces and having the appearance of a honeycomb on cut section. Histologically, the cystic spaces are lined by bland cuboidal epithelial cells containing glycogen. The cyst spaces contain clear fluid, and no mucin is present. Typically,

these tumors contain a stellate central core of fibrosis. CT scanning is the most useful diagnostic test for the detection of serous cystadenoma. About 30% of the tumors contain central calcifications on CT; the cysts themselves are ordinarily too small to detect.

Mucinous cystic neoplasms differ in that they usually contain one or a few large cystic spaces. The spaces are filled with thick mucus. Additional small cysts may be embedded in the fibrous capsule of the tumor. Microscopically, the cysts are lined by columnar epithelium containing mucin. Papillary ingrowths from the cyst lining are frequent and may be detectable on visual inspection of the cyst lining. CT typically demonstrates a large cystic mass with internal septations (Fig. 26-13).

Although cystic tumors are clearly of two types pathologically, it is often difficult to distinguish serous from mucinous lesions before or at surgery. The CT and ERCP findings are not pathognomonic, and inspection and palpation at operation are unreliable.[123,124] Some serous lesions may have large cystic spaces, causing further confusion.[125] Open biopsy of these tumors at the time of laparotomy is subject to misinterpretation and is probably contraindicated because of the possibility of disseminating tumor cells after entering a cyst cavity. An attempt has been made to distinguish benign from malignant cystic neoplasms by sampling the cyst contents before surgery under CT guidance. In one study,[126] the carcinoembryonic antigen content of cysts accurately predicted the presence of mucinous or serous histology, being elevated only in the former. Confirmation of this finding would potentially provide a mechanism for avoiding surgery in patients with asymptomatic serous tumors. The practical reality, however, is that all cystic neoplasms of the pancreas require resection, usually by a distal pancreatectomy and occasionally by pancreaticoduodenectomy for lesions located in the head. Rarely, a total pancreatectomy is required. Simple enucleation of cystic neoplasms has been associated with a high complication rate and is inappropriate from the point of view of surgical margin should the histology prove malignant.

Cystic neoplasms of the pancreas have been mistaken for pancreatic pseudocysts and drained internally with resultant widespread tumor dissemination. Cystic pancreatic masses in patients without a history of pancreatitis should always be viewed as potentially malignant tumors.

Other tumors sometimes confused with cystic neoplasms are the mucinous variety of ductal adenocarcinoma or ductal adenocarcinoma associated with an obstructive pseudocyst. These latter carcinomas have a much poorer prognosis than mucinous cystadenocarcinoma.

After successful resection of a cystic neoplasm of the

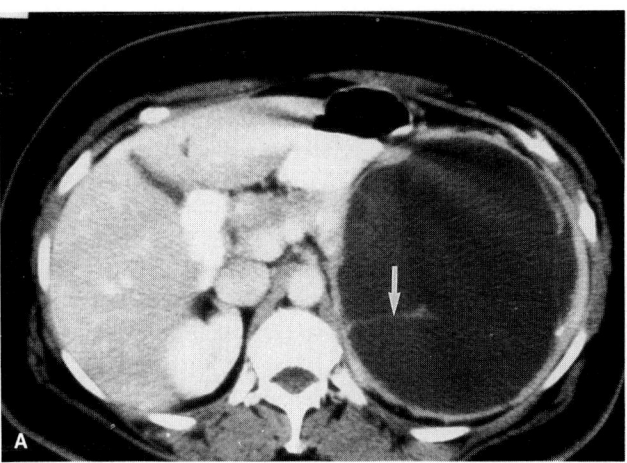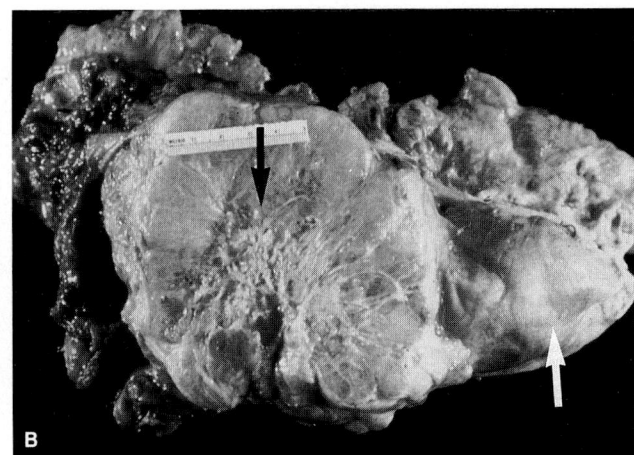

Figure 26-13 (**A**) CT appearance of mucinous cystadenocarcinoma of the pancreas. A large cyst with a single internal septation is visible (*arrow*). (**B**) A mucinous cystadenocarcinoma of the pancreas is seen that contains a large single cyst (*white arrow*) as well as an extensive solid component (*black arrow*). (Bell RH. Neoplasms of the exocrine pancreas. In: Greenfield LJ, Mulholland MW, Oldham KT, Zelenock GB, eds. Surgery: scientific principles and practice. Philadelphia, JB Lippincott, 1993:832)

pancreas, virtually all patients with serous tumors are cured. The 5-year survival for patients with resectable mucinous cystadenocarcinomas is about 60% to 70%.[127]

SOLID AND CYSTIC TUMOR OF THE PANCREAS

Solid and cystic tumor of the pancreas is also referred to as *papillary–cystic neoplasm of the pancreas* or *papillary and solid neoplasm.* About 150 cases of this neoplasm have been reported; it is distinctive because of the age group in which it occurs and its generally good prognosis compared with other pancreatic neoplasms.

Solid and cystic tumor is primarily a disease of young women between the ages of 10 and 35 years. The most frequent presenting symptom is abdominal pain. The tumors are large at the time of presentation (average 10 cm), and many patients have a palpable abdominal mass. CT scanning demonstrates a mass consisting of varying amounts of solid and liquefied material. Some tumors contain peripheral calcifications. Although the CT findings are nonspecific, the finding of a pancreatic mass in a young woman is highly indicative of solid and cystic neoplasm.

Grossly, solid and cystic tumors are rounded, soft, and light brown in color. The center of the tumor contains old blood and cystic spaces filled with necrotic debris. The rim of the tumor is fibrous and may be partially calcified. Histologically, the tumors consist of sheets of uniform cells, often arranged in pseudorosettes around a fibrous stalk. The histogenetic origin of the cells in solid and cystic tu-

mors is uncertain; features of both exocrine and endocrine cell lineage may be found. It is possible that these are tumors of a primordial pancreatic stem cell.

The treatment for solid and cystic neoplasm of the pancreas is formal pancreatic resection with a margin of normal pancreatic tissue. The results of surgery are gratifying: about 90% of patients are permanently cured.[128,129]

PANCREATIC LYMPHOMA

Although lymphoma is not a pancreatic exocrine tumor in the true sense, it may arise in the pancreas and present as a pancreatic mass lesion, which is difficult to distinguish radiologically from pancreatic carcinoma.[130] Although many non-Hodgkin's lymphomas include at least microscopic involvement of the pancreas, the term *pancreatic lymphoma* is reserved for those cases in which the lymphoma appears to arise in the pancreas itself and in which the bulk of the tumor involves the pancreas and peripancreatic tissues. Defined in this way, pancreatic lymphoma accounts for 1% to 2% of pancreatic neoplasms and about 1% of non-Hodgkin's lymphomas.

Pancreatic lymphoma usually has a rapid onset. The tumors grow quickly and are typically 6 to 10 cm at the time of presentation. Abdominal pain, weight loss, and jaundice are the most common presenting symptoms. The findings on abdominal CT scan are not specific for lymphoma, but the presence of a large tumor with extensive peripancreatic lymphadenopathy should suggest the possibility (Fig. 26-14).

When the diagnosis of lymphoma is suspected preop-

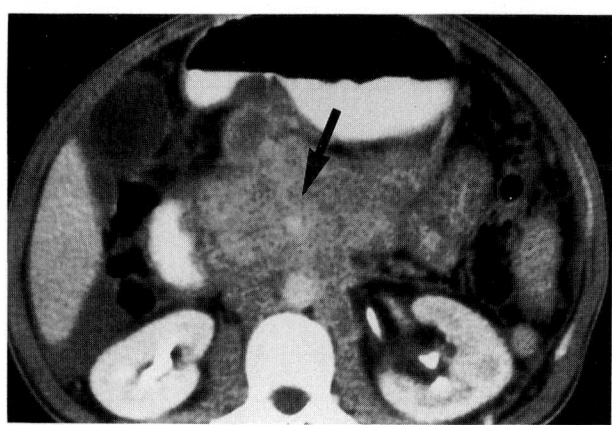

Figure 26-14 CT scan of pancreatic lymphoma demonstrating a large mass virtually replacing the pancreas (*arrow*) and extensive peripancreatic lymphadenopathy. (Bell RH. Neoplasms of the exocrine pancreas. In: Greenfield LJ, Mulholland MW, Oldham KT, Zelenock GB, eds. Surgery: scientific principles and practice. Philadelphia, JB Lippincott, 1993:832)

eratively, guided percutaneous biopsy of the mass should be performed. If the diagnosis of lymphoma can be made, and there is sufficient tissue for typing, laparotomy is usually unnecessary since the tumors are only rarely resectable and since jaundice and other symptoms resolve with chemotherapy, which is the treatment of choice. Surgical exploration is appropriate if the diagnosis cannot be made by needle biopsy. Open biopsy is uniformly successful in such circumstances.[131] Surgical resection of the tumor is indicated in the rare case in which the tumor is relatively small and entirely confined to the pancreas on CT scan. Exploration for the purpose of biliary compression alone is not indicated. Jaundice may be relieved by endoscopic stent placement before the institution of chemotherapy. If the jaundiced patient is explored for a biopsy, a cholecystojejunostomy is appropriate since the improvement in hepatic function allows for rapid institution of multidrug chemotherapy. About half of patients with pancreatic lymphoma undergo a initial remission with chemotherapy alone[131,132]; long-term follow-up suggests, however, that most patients ultimately succumb to recurrent disease.[133]

OTHER PANCREATIC EXOCRINE NEOPLASMS

Because the normal pancreas contains a variety of cell types, a broad spectrum of tumors may arise there. Among these is *acinar cell carcinoma*, which is a rare tumor despite the fact that acinar cells make up about 95% of the bulk of the exocrine pancreas. Acinar cell carcinomas typically present as a large tumor in the el-

derly. The tumors are usually advanced, with both lymphatic and hematogenous metastases present. Some patients develop an accompanying syndrome of metastatic fat necrosis with skin, bone, and joint lesions, fever, and leukocytosis, which is thought to be due to elevated serum lipase levels. The histopathologic diagnosis of acinar cell tumor is made by the demonstration of acinar enzymes immunohistologically or by the demonstration of zymogen granules by electron microscopy. Surgical resection is indicated in the rare patient with disease restricted to the pancreas.[134]

Besides the common scirrhous ductal adenocarcinoma described in detail earlier, there are other variants of ductal cancer of the pancreas. Two described entities are *intraductal papillary carcinoma* and *mucin-producing intraductal carcinoma*, the latter sometimes referred to as *duct-ectatic carcinoma*. The features of these two conditions overlap somewhat since they both occur in dilated, mucin-filled ducts and tend to be multifocal. The duct-ectatic carcinomas occur against a background of *mucin-producing duct ectasia*, a condition characterized by focal or diffuse dilation of the main pancreatic duct and excessive mucin production. At endoscopy, mucin can be seen emanating from the papilla of Vater. Not all patients with mucin-producing duct ectasia have carcinoma, so optimal management has not yet been clearly defined. Intraductal papillary carcinomas and tumors arising in these patients may have a better prognosis than the usual variety of pancreatic carcinomas.[135,136]

Although pancreatic exocrine neoplasms are rare in children,[137] there are isolated reports of a childhood tumor referred to as *pancreatoblastoma*, which contains both epithelial and mesenchymal elements. The tumors tend to be encapsulated, and the prognosis in the few reported cases appears to be good if the tumor can be completely resected.

REFERENCES

1. Boring CC, Squires TS, Tong T Cancer statistics, 1993. CA Cancer J Clin 1993;43:7.
2. Grace PA, Pitt HA, Tompkins RK, DenBesten L, Longmire WP Jr. Decreased morbidity and mortality after pancreaticoduodenectomy. Am J Surg 1986;151:141.
3. Crist DW, Sitzmann JV, Cameron JL. Improved hospital morbidity, mortality, and survival after the Whipple procedure. Ann Surg 1987;206:358.
4. Maruchi N, Brian D, Ludwig J, Elveback LR, Kurland LT. Cancer of the pancreas in Olmsted County, Minnesota, 1935–1974. Mayo Clin Proc 1979;54:245.
5. Fraumeni JF Jr. Cancers of the pancreas and biliary tract: epidemiological considerations. Cancer Res 1975;35:3437.
6. Ghadirian P, Boyle P, Simard A, Baillargeon J, Maisonneuve P, Perret C. Reported family aggregation of pan-

creatic cancer within a population-based case-control study in the Francophone community in Montreal, Canada. Int J Pancreatol 1991;10:183.

7. Lynch HT, Fitzsimmons ML, Smyrk TC, et al. Familial pancreatic cancer: clinicopathologic study of 18 nuclear families. Am J Gastroenterol 1990;85:54.

8. Vogelstein B, Fearon ER, Hamilton SR, et al. Genetic alterations during colorectal tumor development. N Engl J Med 1988;319:525.

9. Schwartz SS, Zeidler A, Moossa AR, Kuku SF, Rubenstein AH. A prospective study of glucose tolerance, insulin, C-peptide, and glucagon responses in patients with pancreatic carcinoma. Am J Dig Dis 1978;23:1107.

10. Permert J, Larsson J, Westermark GT, et al. Islet amyloid polypeptide in patients with pancreatic cancer and diabetes. N Engl J Med 1994;330:313.

11. Lowenfels AB, Maisonneuve P, Cavallini G, et al. Pancreatitis and the risk of pancreatic cancer. N Engl J Med 1993;328:1433.

12. Caldas C, Hahn SA, Hruban RH, Redston MS, Yeo CJ, Kern SE. Detection of K-ras mutations in the stool of patients with pancreatic adenocarcinoma and pancreatic ductal hyperplasia. Cancer Res 1994;54:3568.

13. Whittemore AS, Paffenbarger RS Jr, Anderson K, Halpern J. Early precursors of pancreatic cancer in college men. J Chronic Dis 1983;36:251.

14. Howe GR, Jain M, Miller AB. Dietary factors and risk of pancreatic cancer: results of a Canadian population-based case-control study. Int J Cancer 1990;45:604.

15. Pettengill OS, Faris RA, Bell RH Jr, Kuhlmann ET, Longnecker DS. Derivation of ductlike cell lines from a transplantable acinar cell carcinoma of the rat pancreas. Am J Pathol 1993;143:292.

16. Sandgren EP, Quaife CJ, Paulovich AG, Palmiter RD, Brinster RL. Pancreatic tumor pathogenesis reflects the causative genetic lesion. Proc Natl Acad Sci USA 1991;88:93.

17. Kloppel G. Pathology of nonendocrine pancreatic tumors. In: Go VLW, DiMagno EP, Gardner JD, et al, eds. The pancreas: biology, pathobiology, and disease. New York, Raven Press, 1993:871.

18. Morohoshi T, Held G, Kloppel G. Exocrine pancreatic tumors and their histological classification: a study based on 167 autopsy and 97 surgical cases. Histopathology 1983;7:645.

19. Cubilla AL, Fitzgerald PJ. Morphological patterns of primary nonendocrine human pancreas carcinoma. Cancer Res 1975;35:2234.

20. Lemoine NR, Jain S, Hughes CM, et al. Ki-ras oncogene activation in preinvasive pancreatic cancer. Gastroenterology 1992;102:230.

21. Tryka AF, Brooks JR. Histopathology in the evaluation of total pancreatectomy for ductal carcinoma. Ann Surg 1979;190:373.

22. Kloppel G, Lohse T, Bosslet K, Ruckert K. Ductal adenocarcinoma of the head of the pancreas: incidence of tumor beyond the Whipple resection line. Histological and immunocytochemical analysis of 37 total pancreatectomy specimens. Pancreas 1987;2:170.

23. Willett CG, Lewandrowski K, Warshaw AL, Efird J, Compton CC. Resection margins in carcinoma of the head of the pancreas: implications for radiation therapy. Ann Surg 1993;217:144.

24. Tsuchiya R, Noda T, Harada N, et al. Collective review of small carcinomas of the pancreas. Ann Surg 1986;203:77.

25. Cubilla AL, Fortner J, Fitzgerald PJ. Lymph node involvement in carcinoma of the head of the pancreas area. Cancer 1978;41:880.

26. Pollard HM. Staging of cancer of the pancreas: Cancer of the Pancreas Task Force. Cancer 1981;47:1631.

27. Satake K, Nishikawa H, Yokomatsu H, et al. Surgical curability and prognosis for standard versus extended resection for T1 carcinoma of the pancreas. Surg Gynecol Obstet 1992;175:259.

28. Koprowski H, Herlyn M, Steplewzki Z, Sears HF. Specific antigen in serum of patients with colon carcinoma. Science 1981;212:53.

29. Del Villano BC, Brennan S, Brock P, et al. Radioimmunometric assay for a monoclonal antibody-defined tumor marker, CA19-9. Clin Chem 1983;29:549.

30. Hyoty M, Hyoty H, Aaran RK, Airo I, Nordback I. Tumor antigens CA 195 and CA 19-9 in pancreatic juice and serum for the diagnosis of pancreatic carcinoma. Eur J Surg 1992;158:173.

31. Steinberg W. The clinical utility of the CA19-9 tumor-associated antigen. Am J Gastroenterol 1990;85:350.

32. Malesci A, Montorsi M, Mariani A, et al. Clinical utility of the serum CA19-9 test for diagnosing pancreatic carcinoma in symptomatic patients: a prospective study. Pancreas 1992;7:497.

33. Saito S, Taguchi K, Nishimura N, et al. Clinical usefulness of computer-assisted diagnosis using combination assay of tumor markers for pancreatic carcinoma. Cancer 1993;72:381.

34. Almoguera C, Shibata D, Forrester K, Martin J, Arnheim N, Perucho M. Most human carcinomas of the exocrine pancreas contain mutant c-K-ras genes. Cell 1988;53:549.

35. Hruban RH, van Mansfeld AD, Offerhaus GJ, et al. K-ras oncogene activation in adenocarcinoma of the human pancreas: a study of 82 carcinomas using a combination of mutant-enriched polymerase chain reaction analysis and allele-specific oligonucleotide hybridization. Am J Pathol 1993;143:545.

36. Tada M, Omata M, Kawai S, et al. Detection of ras gene mutation in pancreatic juice and peripheral blood of patients with pancreatic adenocarcinoma. Cancer Res 1993;53:2472.

37. Casey G, Yamanaka Y, Friess H, et al. p53 Mutations are common in pancreatic cancer and are absent in chronic pancreatitis. Cancer Lett 1993;69:151.

38. Pasanen PA, Partanen KP, Pikkarainen PH, Alhava EM, Janatuinen EK, Pirinen AE. A comparison of ultrasound, computed tomography and endoscopic retro-

grade cholangiopancreatography in the differential diagnosis of benign and malignant jaundice and cholestasis. Eur J Surg 1993;159:23.

39. Maringhini A, Ciambra M, Raimondo M, et al. Clinical presentation and ultrasonography in the diagnosis of pancreatic cancer. Pancreas 1993;8:146.

40. Freeny PC, Traverso LW, Ryan JA. Diagnosis and staging of pancreatic adenocarcinoma with dynamic computed tomography. Am J Surg 1993;165:600.

41. DiMagno EP, Malagelada J-R, Taylor WF, Go VLW. A prospective comparison of current diagnostic tests for pancreatic carcinoma. N Engl J Med 1977;297:737.

42. Alvarez C, Livingston EH, Ashley SW, Schwarz M, Reber HA. Cost-benefit analysis of the work-up for pancreatic cancer. Am J Surg 1993;165:53.

43. Nakaizumi A, Tatsuta M, Uehara H, et al. Cytologic examination of pure pancreatic juice in the diagnosis of pancreatic carcinoma: the endoscopic retrograde intraductal catheter aspiration cytologic technique. Cancer 1992;70:2610.

44. Dooley WC, Cameron JL, Pitt HA, Lillemoe KD, Yue NC, Venbrux AC. Is preoperative angiography useful in patients with periampullary tumors? Ann Surg 1990;211:649.

45. Gulliver DJ, Baker ME, Cheng CA, Meyers WC, Pappas TN. Malignant biliary obstruction: efficacy of thin-section dynamic CT in determining resectability. AJR 1992;159:503.

46. Aspestrand F, Kolmannskog F. CT compared to angiography for staging of tumors of the pancreatic head. Acta Radiol 1992;33:556.

47. Biehl TR, Traverso LW, Hauptmann E, Ryan JA Jr. Preoperative visceral angiography alters intraoperative strategy during the Whipple procedure. Am J Surg 1993;165:607.

48. Palazzo L, Roseau G, Gayet B, et al. Endoscopic ultrasonography in the diagnosis and staging of pancreatic adenocarcinoma: results of a prospective study with comparison to ultrasonography and CT scan. Endoscopy 1993;25:143.

49. Yasuda K, Mukai H, Nakajima M, Kawai K. Staging of pancreatic carcinoma by endoscopic ultrasonography. Endoscopy 1993;25:151.

50. Riemann JF, Kohler B. Endoscopy of the pancreatic duct: value of different endoscope types. Gastrointest Endosc 1993;39:367.

51. Yasuda K, Mukai H, Nakajima M, Kawai K. Clinical application of ultrasonic probes in the biliary and pancreatic duct. Endoscopy 1992;24(Suppl 1):370.

52. Kocjan G, Rode J, Lees WR. Percutaneous fine needle aspiration cytology of the pancreas: advantages and pitfalls. J Clin Pathol 1989;42:341.

53. Warshaw AL. Implications of peritoneal cytology for staging of early pancreatic cancer. Am J Surg 1991;161:26.

54. Evans DB, Rich TA, Byrd DR, et al. Preoperative chemoradiation and pancreaticoduodenectomy for adenocarcinoma of the pancreas. Arch Surg 1992;127:1335.

55. Earnhardt RC, McQuone SJ, Minasi JS, Feldman PS, Jones RS, Hanks JB. Intraoperative fine needle aspiration of pancreatic and extrahepatic biliary masses. Surg Gynecol Obstet 1993;177:147.

56. Edoute Y, Lemberg S, Malberger E. Preoperative and intraoperative fine needle aspiration cytology of pancreatic lesions. Am J Gastroenterol 1991;86:1015.

57. Benning TL, Silverman JF, Berns LA, Geisinger KR. Fine needle aspiration of metastatic and hematological malignancies clinically mimicking pancreatic carcinoma. Acta Cytol 1992;36:471.

58. Warshaw AL, Tepper JE, Shipley WU. Laparoscopy in the staging and planning of therapy for pancreatic cancer. Am J Surg 1986;151:76.

59. Warshaw AL, Gu ZY, Wittenberg J, Waltman AC. Preoperative staging and assessment of resectability of pancreatic cancer. Arch Surg 1990;125:230.

60. Michelassi F, Erroi F, Dawson PJ, et al. Experience with 647 consecutive tumors of the duodenum, ampulla, head of pancreas, and distal common bile duct. Ann Surg 1989;210:544.

61. Sener SF, Fremgen A, Imperato JP, Sylvester J, Chmiel JS. Pancreatic cancer in Illinois: a report by 88 hospitals on 2,401 patients diagnosed 1978–84. Am Surg 1991;57:490.

62. Whipple AO, Parsons WB, Mullins CR. Treatment of carcinoma of the ampulla of Vater. Ann Surg 1935;102:763.

63. Brunschwig A. Resection of head of pancreas and duodenum for carcinoma: pancreatoduodenectomy. Surg Gynecol Obstet 1937;65:681.

64. Child CG 3rd. Radical one-stage pancreaticoduodenectomy. Surgery 1948;23:492.

65. Traverso LW, Longmire WP Jr. Preservation of the pylorus in pancreaticoduodenectomy. Surg Gynecol Obstet 1978;146:959.

66. Trede M, Schwall G, Saeger HD. Survival after pancreatoduodenectomy. Ann Surg 1990;211:447.

67. Pellegrini CA, Heck CF, Raper S, Way LW. An analysis of the reduced morbidity and mortality rates after pancreaticoduodenectomy. Arch Surg 1989;124:778.

68. Fiess H, Klempa I, Hermanek P, et al. Prophylaxis of complications after pancreatic surgery: results of a multicenter trial in Germany. Digestion 1994;55(Suppl 1):35.

69. Bradley EL III. Management of infected pancreatic necrosis by open drainage. Ann Surg 1987;206:542.

70. Trede M, Schwall G. The complications of pancreatectomy. Ann Surg 1988;207:39.

71. Bell RH. Exocrine pancreatic neoplasms. In: Greenfield LJ, Mulholland MW, Oldham KT, Zelenock GB, eds. Surgery: scientific principles and practice. Philadelphia, JB Lippincott, 1993;826.

72. Tsuchiya R, Tsunoda T. Tumor size as a predictive factor. Int J Pancreatol 1990;7:117.

73. Geer RJ, Brennan MF. Prognostic indicators for survival after resection of pancreatic adenocarcinoma. Am J Surg 1993;165:68.

74. Cameron JL, Crist DW, Sitzmann JV, et al. Factors influencing survival after pancreaticoduodenectomy for pancreatic cancer. Am J Surg 1991;161:120.

75. Tsuchiya R, Harada N, Tsunoda T, Miyamoto T, Ura K. Long-term survivors after operation on carcinoma of the pancreas. Int J Pancreatol 1988;3:491.

76. Martin FM, Rossi RL, Dorrucci V, Silverman ML, Braasch JW. Clinical and pathologic correlations in patients with periampullary tumors. Arch Surg 1990;125:723.

77. Bottger T, Zech J, Weber W, Sorger K, Junginger T. Relevant factors in the prognosis of ductal pancreatic carcinoma. Acta Chir Scand 1990;156:781.

78. Tannapfel A, Wittekind C, Hunefeld G. Ductal adenocarcinoma of the pancreas: histopathological features and prognosis. Int J Pancreatol 1992;12:145.

79. Kojima Y, Yasukawa H, Katayama K, Note M, Shimada H, Nakagawara G. Postoperative complications and survival after pancreatoduodenectomy in patients aged over 70 years. Surg Today 1992;22:401.

80. Baumel H, Huguier M, Manderscheid JC, Fabre JM, Houry S, Fagot H. Results of resection for cancer of the exocrine pancreas: a study from the French Association of Surgery. Br J Surg 1994;81:102.

81. Bakkevold KE, Kambestad B. Morbidity and mortality after radical and palliative pancreatic cancer surgery: risk factors influencing the short-term results. Ann Surg 1993;217:356.

82. Kayahara M, Nagakawa T, Ueno K, Ohta T, Takeda T, Miyazaki I. An evaluation of radical resection for pancreatic cancer based on the mode of recurrence as determined by autopsy and diagnostic imaging. Cancer 1993;72:2118.

83. Griffin JF, Smalley SR, Jewell W, et al. Patterns of failure after curative resection of pancreatic carcinoma. Cancer 1990;66:56.

84. Klinkenbijl JH, van der Schelling GP, Hop WC, van Pel R, Bruining HA, Jeekel J. The advantages of pylorus-preserving pancreatoduodenectomy in malignant disease of the pancreas and periampullary region. Ann Surg 1992;216:142.

85. Tsao JI, Rossi RL, Lowell JA. Pylorus-preserving pancreatoduodenectomy: is it an adequate cancer operation? Arch Surg 1994;129:405.

86. Roder JD, Stein HJ, Huttl W, Siewert JR. Pylorus-preserving versus standard pancreatico-duodenectomy: an analysis of 110 pancreatic and periampullary carcinomas. Br J Surg 1992;79:152.

87. Fink AS, DeSouza LR, Mayer EA, Hawkins R, Longmire WP Jr. Long-term evaluation of pylorus preservation during pancreaticoduodenectomy. World J Surg 1988;12:663.

88. van Heerden JA, McIlrath DC, Ilstrup DM, Weiland LH. Total pancreatectomy for ductal adenocarcinoma of the pancreas: an update. World J Surg 1988;12:658.

89. Tsuchiya R, Tsunoda T, Yamaguchi T. Operation of choice for resectable carcinoma of the head of the pancreas. Int J Pancreatol 1990;6:295.

90. Launois B, Franci J, Bardaxoglou E, et al. Total pancreatectomy for ductal adenocarcinoma of the pancreas with special reference to resection of the portal vein and multicentric cancer. World J Surg 1993;17:122.

91. Dresler CM, Fortner JG, McDermott K, Bajorunas DR. Metabolic consequences of (regional) total pancreatectomy. Ann Surg 1991;214:131.

92. Kayahara M, Nagakawa T, Kobayashi H, et al. Lymphatic flow in carcinoma of the head of the pancreas. Cancer 1992;70:2061.

93. Ishikawa O, Ohhigashi H, Sasaki Y, et al. Practical usefulness of lymphatic and connective tissue clearance for carcinoma of the pancreas head. Ann Surg 1988;208:215.

94. Manabe T, Ohshio G, Baba N, et al. Radical pancreatectomy for ductal cell carcinoma of the head of the pancreas. Cancer 1989;64:1132.

95. Henne-Bruns D, Kremer B, Meyer-Pannwitt U, Vogel I, Schroder S. Partial duodenopancreatectomy with radical lymphadenectomy in patients with pancreatic and periampullary carcinomas: initial results. Hepatogastroenterology 1993;40:145.

96. Fortner JG. Regional pancreatectomy for cancer of the pancreas, ampulla, and other related sites: tumor staging and results. Ann Surg 1984;199:418.

97. Sindelar WF. Clinical experience with regional pancreatectomy for adenocarcinoma of the pancreas. Arch Surg 1989;124:127.

98. Ishikawa O, Ohigashi H, Imaoka S, et al. Preoperative indications for extended pancreatectomy for locally advanced pancreas cancer involving the portal vein. Ann Surg 1992;215:231.

99. Nordback IH, Hruban RH, Boitnott JK, Pitt HA, Cameron JL. Carcinoma of the body and tail of the pancreas. Am J Surg 1992;164:26.

100. Johnson CD, Schwall G, Flechtenmacher J, Trede M. Resection for adenocarcinoma of the body and tail of the pancreas. Br J Surg 1993;80:1177.

101. Dalton RR, Sarr MG, van Heerden JA, Colby TV. Carcinoma of the body and tail of the pancreas: is curative resection justified? Surgery 1992;111:489.

102. Kalser MH, Ellenberg SS. Pancreatic cancer: adjuvant combined radiation and chemotherapy following curative resection. Arch Surg 1985;120:899.

103. Gastrointestinal Tumor Study Group. Further evidence of effective adjuvant combined radiation and chemotherapy following curative resection of pancreatic cancer. Cancer 1987;59:2006.

104. Ishikawa O, Ohhigashi H, Teshima T, et al. Clinical and histopathological appraisal of preoperative irradiation for adenocarcinoma of the pancreatoduodenal region. J Surg Oncol 1989;40:143.

105. Hoffman JP, Weese JL, Solin LJ, et al. A single institutional experience with preoperative chemoradiotherapy for stage I–III pancreatic adenocarcinoma. Am Surg 1993;59:772.

106. Johnstone PA, Sindelar WF. Patterns of disease recurrence following definitive therapy of adenocarcinoma

of the pancreas using surgery and adjuvant radiotherapy: correlations of a clinical trial. Int J Radiat Oncol Biol Phys 1993;27:831.

107. Pretre R, Huber O, Robert J, Soravia C, Egeli RA, Rohner A. Results of surgical palliation for cancer of the head of the pancreas and periampullary region. Br J Surg 1992;79:795.

108. Glattli A, Stain SC, Baer HU, Schweizer W, Triller J, Blumgart LH. Unresectable malignant biliary obstruction: treatment by self-expandable biliary endoprostheses. HPB Surg 1993;6:175.

109. van den Bosch RP, van der Schelling GP, Klinkenbijl JH, Mulder PG, van Blankenstein M, Jeekel J. Guidelines for the application of surgery and endoprostheses in the palliation of obstructive jaundice in advanced cancer of the pancreas. Ann Surg 1994;219:18.

110. Shepherd HA, Royle G, Ross AP, Diba A, Arthur M, Colin-Jones D. Endoscopic biliary endoprosthesis in the palliation of malignant obstruction of the distal common bile duct: a randomized trial. Br J Surg 1988;75:1166.

111. Andersen JR, Sorensen SM, Kruse A, Rokkjaer M, Matzen P. Randomised trial of endoscopic endoprosthesis versus operative bypass in malignant obstructive jaundice. Gut 1989;30:1132.

112. Lillemoe KD, Sauter PK, Pitt HA, Yeo CJ, Cameron JL. Current status of surgical palliation of periampullary carcinoma. Surg Gynecol Obstet 1993;176:1.

113. de Rooij PD, Rogatko A, Brennan MF. Evaluation of palliative surgical procedures in unresectable pancreatic cancer. Br J Surg 1991;78:1053.

114. Rappaport MD, Villalba M. A comparison of cholecysto- and choledochoenterostomy for obstructing pancreatic cancer. Am Surg 1990;56:433.

115. Weaver DW, Wiencek RG, Bouwman DL, Walt AJ. Gastrojejunostomy: is it helpful for patients with pancreatic cancer? Surgery 1987;102:608.

116. Huguier M, Baumel H, Manderscheid JC, Houry S, Fabre JM. Surgical palliation for unresected cancer of the exocrine pancreas. Eur J Surg Oncol 1993;19:342.

117. Potts JR 3rd, Vogt DP, Broughan T, Hermann RE. Indications for gastric bypass in palliative operations for pancreatic carcinoma. Am Surg 1991;57:24.

118. van der Schilling GP, van den Bosch RP, Klinkenbijl JH, Mulder PG, Jeekel J. Is there a place for gastroenterostomy in patients with advanced cancer of the head of the pancreas? World J Surg 1993;17:128.

119. Lillimoe KD, Cameron JL, Kaufman HS, Yeo CJ, Pitt HA, Sauter PK. Chemical splanchnicectomy in patients with unresectable pancreatic cancer: a prospective, randomized trial. Ann Surg 1993;217:447.

120. Mercadante S. Celiac plexus block versus analgesics in pancreatic cancer pain. Pain 1993;52:187.

121. Moertel CG, Frytak S, Hahn RG, et al. Therapy of locally unresectable pancreatic carcinoma: a randomized comparison of high dose (6000 rads) radiation alone, mod-

erate dose radiation (4000 rads + 5-fluorouracil), and high dose radiation + 5-fluorouracil: The Gastrointestinal Tumor Study Group. Cancer 1981;48:1705.

122. Bruckner HW, Kalnicki S, Dalton J, et al. Combined modality therapy increasing local control of pancreatic cancer. Cancer Invest 1993;11:241.

123. Pyke CM, van Heerden JA, Colby TV, Sarr MG, Weaver AL. The spectrum of serous cystadenoma of the pancreas: clinical, pathologic, and surgical aspects. Ann Surg 1992;215:132.

124. Gazelle GS, Mueller PR, Raafat N, Halpern EF, Cardenosa G, Warshaw AL. Cystic neoplasms of the pancreas: evaluation with endoscopic retrograde pancreatography. Radiology 1993;188:633.

125. Lewandrowski K, Warshaw A, Compton C. Macrocystic serous cystadenoma of the pancreas: a morphologic variant differing from microcystic adenoma. Hum Pathol 1992;23:871.

126. Lewandrowski KB, Southern JF, Pins MR, Compton CC, Warshaw AL. Cyst fluid analysis in the differential diagnosis of pancreatic cysts: a comparison of pseudocysts, serous cystadenomas, mucinous cystic neoplasms, and mucinous cystadenocarcinoma. Ann Surg 1993;217:41.

127. Talamini MA, Pitt HA, Hruban RH, Boitnott JK, Coleman J, Cameron JL. Spectrum of cystic tumors of the pancreas. Am J Surg 1992;163:117.

128. Zinner MJ, Shurbaji MS, Cameron JL. Solid and papillary epithelial neoplasms of the pancreas. Surgery 1990;108:475.

129. Pezzi CM, Schuerch C, Erlandson RA, Deitrick J. Papillary-cystic neoplasm of the pancreas. J Surg Oncol 1988;37:278.

130. Van Beers B, Lalonde L, Soyer P, et al. Dynamic CT in pancreatic lymphoma. J Comput Assist Tomogr 1993;17:94.

131. Tuchek JM, De Jong SA, Pickleman J. Diagnosis, surgical intervention, and prognosis of primary pancreatic lymphoma. Am Surg 1993;59:513.

132. Webb TH, Lillimoe KD, Pitt HA, Jones RJ, Cameron JL. Pancreatic lymphoma: is surgery mandatory for diagnosis or treatment? Ann Surg 1989;209:25.

133. Behrns KE, Sarr MG, Strickler JG. Pancreatic lymphoma: is it a surgical disease? Pancreas 1994;9:662.

134. Klimstra DS, Heffess CS, Oertel JE, Rosai J. Acinar cell carcinoma of the pancreas: a clinicopathologic study of 28 cases. Am J Surg Pathol 1992;16:815.

135. Nishihara K, Fukuda T, Tsuneyoshi M, Kominami T, Maeda S, Saku M. Intraductal papillary neoplasm of the pancreas. Cancer 1993;72:689.

136. Yanagisawa A, Ohashi K, Hori M, et al. Ductectatic-type mucinous cystadenoma and cystadenocarcinoma of the human pancreas: a novel clinicopathological entity. Jpn J Cancer Res 1993;84:474.

137. Grosfeld JL, Vane DW, Rescorla FJ, McGuire W, West KW. Pancreatic tumors in childhood: analysis of 13 cases. J Pediatr Surg 1990;25:1057.

Digestive Tract Surgery: A Text and Atlas, edited by Richard H. Bell,
Layton F. Rikkers, and Michael W. Mulholland.
Lippincott-Raven Publishers, Philadelphia, © 1996.

27

Neoplasms of the Endocrine Pancreas

Jeffrey A. Norton | *Jeffrey F. Moley*

Few patients in surgical practice provoke as much interest as those with functional tumors of the endocrine pancreas. These patients challenge the clinical skill of the surgeon and provide a rare opportunity to view human physiology and pathophysiology at work.

The islets of Langerhans are neural crest–derived tissues that are scattered throughout the pancreas. Histologic, ultrastructural, and immunohistochemical analysis has made possible the classification of several islet cell types. The β cells, which produce insulin, reside in the center of the islets; the α cells, which produce glucagon, are situated on the periphery; and the δ cells, which make somatostatin, are in between. Gastrin-secreting cells are not found in the normal adult pancreas, but normally are found in the antrum of the stomach and with decreasing density distally within the duodenum. Islet cells that secrete pancreatic polypeptide and vasoactive intestinal polypeptide (VIP) also have been described, and other types of islet cells undoubtedly exist.

The existence of pancreatic islet cell tumors was postulated as early as 1902. Shortly after the discovery of insulin, a patient with symptoms of hyperinsulinism was described who was found to have a cystic neoplasm of the pancreas with metastases to the liver and lymph nodes. Extracts of the resected tumor were found to contain insulin. In 1955, Zollinger and Ellison[1] described the presence of islet cell tumors of the pancreas in several patients with atypical extensive peptic ulcer disease. These tumors later were found to produce gastrin, a gut hormone normally secreted by the antral G cells.[2,3] Subsequently, pancreatic functional endocrine tumors were described in association with other characteristic syndromes: the glucagonoma syndrome,[4] the somatostatinoma syndrome,[5] and the watery diarrhea hypokalemic alkalosis vipoma syndrome[6] (also called the Verner-Morrison syndrome; Table 27-1). These syndromes arise from specific islet cell types. Although the clinical picture usually is dominated by a single hormone excess, many of these tumors secrete several substances in addition to the primary hormone, including adrenocorticotropic hormone (ACTH), melanocyte-stimulating hormone, pancreatic polypeptide, VIP, secretin, insulin, gastrin, glucagon, and somatostatin.[7–13]

MULTIPLE ENDOCRINE NEOPLASIA TYPE 1

The first detailed reports of familial disease in multiple endocrine neoplasia type 1 (MEN-1) were made by Wermer in 1954.[14] In MEN-1 patients, tumors develop in the parathyroid glands, pancreatic islet cells, and pituitary gland. Lipomas, carcinoids, and benign tumors of the thyroid and adrenal cortex can also occur. Hyperparathyroidism almost always is present.[15–17] Clinical evidence of pituitary and pancreatic islet cell tumors is found in approximately 25% and 60% of patients, respectively.[18–21] Autopsy studies of patients with MEN-1 reveal neoplasia of the parathyroid glands, pituitary gland, and pancreatic islets, even though patients do not always manifest clinical evidence of hyperfunction from each of these tissues. The diagnosis of MEN-1 depends on the presence of at least three of the following

Table 27-1 Signs and Symptoms, Hormone, Incidence, and Pathology of Islet Cell Tumors

Tumor	Signs and Symptoms	Hormone	Incidence	Percentage of Tumors Identified at Surgery	Location Duodenum (%)	Location Pancreas (%)	Percentage With Metastases	Percentage With MEN-1
Gastrinoma	Ulcer pain, diarrhea, esophagitis	Gastrin	2 per 5 million	52–87	38	62	50	18–24
Insulinoma	Hypoglycemia	Insulin	4 per 5 million	80–100	—	>99	5	5
Vipoma	Watery diarrhea	VIP	Rare	100	15	85	40	Occasional
Glucagonoma	Rash, weight loss, malnutrition	Glucagon	Rare	98–100	—	>99	70	Occasional
Somatostatinoma	Diabetes, cholelithiasis, steatorrhea	Somatostatin	Rare	100	50	50	70	—
ACTH-producing	Cushing's syndrome	ACTH	Rare	100	—	100	100	—
Nonfunctioning tumor	Pain gastrointestinal bleeding, mass	Pancreatic polypeptide, neuron-specific enolase, none	1 per 5 million	100	—	>99	60	High

ACTH, adrenocorticotropic hormone; MEN-1, multiple endocrine neoplasia type 1; VIP, vasoactive intestinal polypeptide.

criteria: primary hyperparathyroidism; pancreatic islet cell tumor (Zollinger-Ellison syndrome [ZES], insulinoma, vipoma); pituitary tumor; and positive family history. Molecular genetic analysis of four families with MEN-1 localized the disease locus to the long arm of chromosome 11 (11q) in tight linkage to the human skeletal muscle glycogen phosphorylase gene.[22] In subsequent collaborative studies, the gene was localized further, first to a 12-centimorgan region,[23] then to an 8-centimorgan region in the vicinity of the MEN-1 locus.[24] The gene for MEN-1 has not been found and characterized. There is no widely available genetic test to identify MEN-1 gene carriers, but one is expected soon.

The mechanism by which these genetic defects lead to tumor formation in affected individuals is not understood. According to one hypothesis, the first step in tumor formation is a germinal level mutation that predisposes the individual to tumor development in certain cells or tissues. The second event is a somatic mutation that eliminates the normal wild-type allele in the susceptible cell population, thereby unmasking a recessive mutation in the germ line and leading to tumor transformation.[25] This mechanism appears to exist for hereditary retinoblastoma (chromosome 13) and Wilms' tumor (chromosome 11).[26,27] It also appears to exist for MEN-1. Analysis of tumor and constitutional tissue genotypes in two brothers with insulinomas who had acquired the gene for MEN-1 from their mother revealed a loss of the normal paternal chromosome 11 allele in the tumor tissues of both individuals, consistent with the above model.[22]

Blood relatives of patients with MEN-1 should be

screened for this disorder starting in their early teenage years. Because hyperparathyroidism almost always is the first detectable abnormality in patients with MEN-1, serum calcium measurements should be performed yearly on asymptomatic kindred members at risk for the disease. If the history or physical examination suggests pituitary or pancreatic tumors, an appropriate diagnostic evaluation, including biochemical testing and radiologic imaging studies, should be initiated.

Pancreatic islet cell tumors occur in about 60% of patients with MEN-1. Although these tumors often secrete more than one type of polypeptide hormone, they rarely produce a mixed clinical picture. Several distinct clinical syndromes have been described. The most common islet cell tumors in patients with MEN-1 are gastrinomas, which produce the clinical picture of ZES. Insulinomas are the second most common functional islet cell tumors in patients with MEN-1. VIP-secreting tumors (vipomas), glucagonomas, and somatostatinomas also are encountered. As opposed to the management of sporadic islet cell tumors, the management of pancreatic tumors in patients with the MEN-1 syndrome is complicated by the fact that the pancreas usually is diffusely involved with islet cell hyperplasia and multifocal tumors.[28] In patients with MEN-1 who have ZES, the duodenum may be similarly involved with solitary or multiple gastrinomas.[29,30] Somatostatinomas in patients with MEN-1 also may be found in the proximal duodenum and peripancreatic areas, and the tumors usually are malignant. The treatment of these tumors must be focused on two goals: relief of symptoms related to excessive hormone production and cure or palliation of the malignant process if possible. Patients with islet cell tumors almost always suffer more from the systemic effects of hormone overproduction than from the local effects of the tumor mass. Before surgical exploration is undertaken for an islet cell tumor, any patient with clinical evidence of hypercortisolism or virilization should be evaluated for the presence of an adrenal tumor by measuring urinary excretion rates of glucocorticoids, mineralocorticoids, or sex hormones. The adrenal glands should be palpated at surgery, even if the results of preoperative studies are normal.

In patients with MEN-1 who have unresectable or metastatic malignant islet cell tumors, the administration of streptozotocin and 5-fluorouracil (5-FU) or doxorubicin (Adriamycin) results in a 40% 3-year response rate.[31-33] In patients who experience disease relapse on that regimen, interferon treatment has produced some responses.[34-36]

Gastrinoma and Multiple Endocrine Neoplasia Type 1

Gastrin increases acid and pepsin output by parietal and chief cells of the gastric fundus. Overproduction of gastrin results in the clinical picture of gastric acid hypersecretion, severe peptic ulcer disease, esophagitis, and watery diarrhea. The diagnosis of gastrinoma in patients with MEN-1 is the same as that in other patients (Table 27-2). It depends on the detection of increased basal acid output (normally less than 4 mEq/h for women and less than 6 mEq/h for men) and concomi-

tant elevated fasting serum gastrin levels (more than 100 pg/mL). H_2 blockers or omeprazole should be discontinued before these parameters are measured. If basal acid output is greater than 15 mEq/h, and fasting serum gastrin levels are higher than 100 pg/mL, the diagnosis of gastrinoma is established. Provocative testing with secretin (2 U/kg intravenously) further increases serum gastrin levels to more than 200 pg/mL in 85% of patients with gastrinomas. Serum calcium levels also should be determined; if these are elevated, serum parathyroid hormone levels should be measured. Most patients with MEN-1 and ZES have primary hyperparathyroidism before they develop gastrinomas. Surgery to correct the primary hyperparathyroidism (either $3\frac{1}{2}$-gland parathyroidectomy or 4-gland parathyroidectomy with autograft) should be performed before surgery to correct the hypergastrinemia, because successful parathyroid surgery markedly alleviates the signs and symptoms of ZES in these patients.

Preoperative anatomic localization of large islet cell tumors can be achieved by computed tomography (CT), magnetic resonance imaging (MRI), or angiography (Table 27-3). Percutaneous transhepatic selective venous sampling may be necessary in some cases. In this technique, blood samples for hormone levels are obtained along the splenic, mesenteric, and portal veins. Some suggest that this study can determine the region of the pancreas containing the gastrinoma.[37-39] Similar information can be obtained with the secretin angiogram.[40,41] Most patients with MEN-1 who have ZES are treated with omeprazole or H_2 antagonists, be-

Table 27-2   Diagnostic Criteria for Islet Cell Tumors

Tumor Type	Test	Results
Gastrinoma	Fasting gastrin	↑Gastrin (>100 pg/mL)
	BAO	↑BAO (>15 mEq/h)
	Secretin test	↑Gastrin (>200 pg/mL)
Insulinoma	72-h fast	Symptoms of hypoglycemia
		↑Insulin (>6 U/mL)
		↓Glucose (<40 mg/dL)
		↑C peptide (>1.7 ng/mL)
		↑Percentage of proinsulin (>30%)
Vipoma	Fasting VIP	↑VIP (>250 pg/mL)
Glucagonoma	Fasting glucagon	↑Glucagon (>500 pg/mL)
Somatostatinoma	Fasting somatostatin	↑Somatostatin (somatostatin-like peptide)
ACTH-producing tumor	Urinary free cortisol	↑Cortisol
	Plasma ACTH	↑ACTH
	Dexamethasone	Failure to suppress
	Corticotropin-releasing hormone	Failure to increase
Nonfunctional tumor	Open biopsy or aspiration	Islet cell tumor

ACTH, adrenocorticotropic hormone; BAO, basal acid output; VIP, vasoactive intestinal polypeptide.

Table 27-3 Preoperative Localization of Islet Cell Tumors

	Number	True-Positives (%)	References
Ultrasound	43	23	48, 77
Octreotide scanning	21	86	125, 129
Computed tomography	60	43	48, 131
Magnetic resonance imaging	35	26	48, 120
Endoscopic ultrasound	38	82	123
Selective angiography	70	56	48, 132
Portal venous sampling	92	76	48, 138, 139
Provocative angiography*	17	65	40, 175

* Secretin (gastrinoma) or calcium (insulinoma) is injected sequentially into arteries that perfuse different areas of the pancreas. Hormone levels are measured in the hepatic vein. When the artery that perfuses the tumor is injected, there is a rapid rise in hormone in the hepatic vein (true-positive).

cause the islet cell neoplasia is not cured by pancreatic resection. Evidence suggests that the gastrinomas in patients with MEN-1 sometimes are located within the duodenum, as in patients with sporadic gastrinomas.[29,30] Occasional patients with MEN-1 who have ZES can be cured by resection of duodenal gastrinomas,[38] but this is not uniformly successful.[19,42] Patients with CT, MRI, or angiographic evidence of apparently resectable islet cell tumors are candidates for surgery; half of these patients have metastases at the time of surgical exploration.[42] In these cases, the tumors generally are located in the body or tail of the pancreas, and patients are treated best by subtotal pancreatectomy and additional resection of any obvious gastrinomas within either the pancreatic head or the duodenum. The presence of lymph node metastases in the peripancreatic tissue does not necessarily imply incurability, and even small, easily resected peripheral liver metastases may be excised with some benefit to the patient. After operation, gastrin levels decrease in most patients in whom gastrinoma tissue has been resected; however, secretin-stimulated gastrin levels may remain high. For this reason, some argue against surgery for grossly localized gastrinomas in patients with MEN-1,[43] but long-term benefits are achieved by surgery in selected patients.

Treatment of patients with unresectable disease should consist of H_2 blockers (ranitidine, famotidine) or proton pump inhibitors (omeprazole) to inhibit gastric acid secretion, or the somatostatin analogue octreotide[44] with or without chemotherapy (streptozotocin with 5-FU or doxorubicin) as antitumor drugs.[45] Total gastrectomy and parietal cell vagotomy have no place in the treatment of acid hypersecretion in patients with ZES, including patients with MEN-1. The condition can be controlled easily with omeprazole. There also is no role for debulking of grossly unresectable disease. Some patients with unresectable malignant gastrinomas develop evidence of hypercortisolism secondary to ectopic

ACTH secretion by the tumor.[11,46,47] These patients are best treated by bilateral adrenalectomy.[47]

Insulinoma and Multiple Endocrine Neoplasia Type 1

Twenty-five to 30% of patients with MEN-1 who have pancreatic islet cell tumors have evidence of hyperinsulinemia and develop the clinical picture of hypoglycemia, including weakness, dizziness, behavioral disorders, seizures, neurologic deficits, palpitations, nausea, vomiting, and diarrhea.[48] The presence of Whipple's triad (symptoms of hypoglycemia brought on by exercise, blood glucose level less than 50 mg/dL, relief of symptoms with ingestion of glucose) often suggests the diagnosis.[49] The most reliable test in establishing the diagnosis of insulinoma is the simultaneous measurement of insulin and glucose levels during a 72-hour fast (see Table 27-2). Determination of the insulin/glucose ratio is helpful.[50] The ratio in unaffected patients is less than 0.4, whereas that in patients with insulinomas often is more than 1.0. Measurements of C peptide (a connecting peptide between proinsulin and insulin) levels in response to insulin infusion also can be helpful in establishing the diagnosis in difficult cases. Unlike in normal subjects, in patients with insulinomas, C peptide secretion is not suppressed in response to the hypoglycemia produced by insulin infusion.[51]

Similar to patients with gastrinomas, patients with insulinomas may have diffuse pancreatic islet cell disease characterized by microadenomatosis, islet cell hyperplasia, and multifocal tumors.[52] However, many patients with insulinomas and MEN-1 have solitary, large islet cell tumors that not only are responsible for the hyperinsulinism, but may be malignant[42] (Fig. 27-1). Anatomic localization of insulinomas in patients with hyperinsulinism and MEN-1 is best achieved by CT, MRI, or angiography (see Table 27-3). Intraoperative

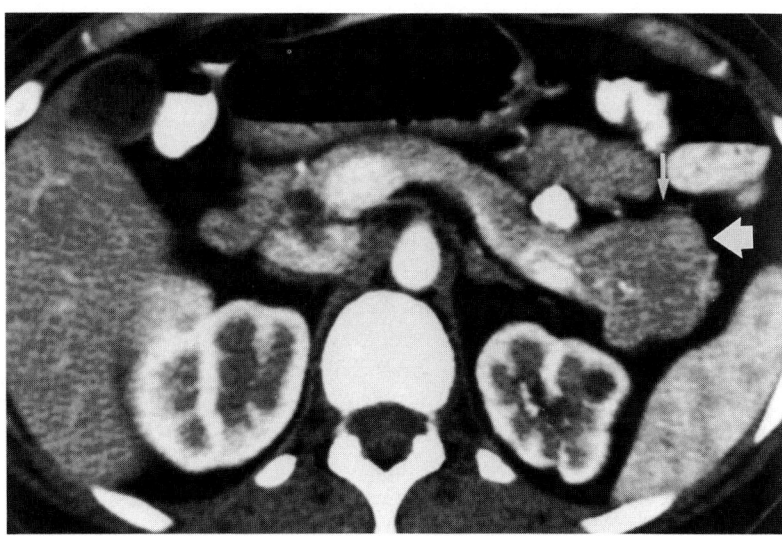

Figure 27-1 A large insulinoma in the pancreatic tail (*arrow*) in a patient with hypoglycemic syndrome and MEN-1. There are small calcifications within the tumor, suggesting that this large islet cell tumor may be malignant.

ultrasound also is helpful in precise operative localization of these tumors. All methods of localization, however, underestimate the true number of tumors found in the pancreas at histologic examination. The dominant tumor usually is located in the body or tail of the pancreas. Distal subtotal pancreatectomy is used for tumors within the body and tail of the pancreas; simple enucleation is advised for tumors of the pancreatic head. After resection, some patients have recurrent hypoglycemia. Diazoxide is an antihypertensive agent that also inhibits insulin secretion from the pancreatic islet cells. Given at a dosage of 100 to 150 mg every 8 hours, it is effective in relieving hypoglycemia in 60% of patients with persistent postoperative hyperinsulinemia. Octreotide also is useful in some patients.[53] If these treatments are unsuccessful, completion pancreatectomy or resection of metastatic disease may be necessary. If tumors are widely metastatic, a debulking procedure may relieve symptoms for some time.[54,55]

Vipoma and Multiple Endocrine Neoplasia Type 1

Vasoactive intestinal polypeptide is found in the nervous tissue as well as in the D_1 cells of the pancreas. Vipomas are extremely rare tumors, even in patients with MEN-1. These tumors cause the watery diarrhea, hypokalemia, achlorhydria syndrome. Patients have profound secretory diarrhea and metabolic abnormalities. The diagnosis is established by the measurement of fasting VIP levels (normal, 0 to 170 pg/mL; see Table 27-2). Preoperative fluid and electrolyte management is greatly facilitated by the use of octreotide.[53,56] Localization is accomplished best by CT, although arteriography has been reported to be helpful in some cases (see Table

27-3). Treatment is surgical in most patients, with removal of the tumor by enucleation or partial pancreatectomy. In patients who are poor surgical risks, or who have widely metastatic malignant disease, octreotide, in combination with chemotherapeutic agents such as streptozotocin and 5-FU, offers effective palliation.[56]

Other Tumors Associated With Multiple Endocrine Neoplasia Type 1

Other functional islet cell tumors occur in patients with MEN-1, including somatostatinomas, pancreatic polypeptidomas, and glucagonomas. Their presentation and management is much the same as that of sporadic tumors, except for the fact that in patients with MEN-1, the pancreas is diffusely involved with islet cell hyperplasia and nesidioblastosis, and the tumors usually are multifocal. Therefore, preoperative localization studies rarely identify all abnormal tissue, and distal subtotal pancreatectomy may be necessary to relieve symptoms and decrease recurrences.

Bronchial and other foregut carcinoids have been described in patients with MEN-1. Their management is the same as that of sporadic carcinoids.

Follow-Up of Patients With Known Multiple Endocrine Neoplasia Type 1

Patients with known MEN-1 should be observed closely for the development of new abnormalities and the recrudescence of endocrinopathies already treated. This should include yearly determinations of plasma calcium, glucose, gastrin, fasting insulin, VIP, prolactin, growth hormone, and β human gonadotropin hormone levels. In addition, a detailed history and physical examination should be directed toward detecting abnormalities in the parathyroid, pituitary, or pancreatic islet cell systems.

The role of provocative test regimens in the evaluation of patients with MEN-1 is not as well defined. Because the most common initial presentation in patients with MEN-1 is primary hyperparathyroidism, affected individuals usually are identified by the detection of an increased serum calcium level. The islet cells of the pancreas are the second most frequent site of neoplasms in patients with MEN-1. These tumors may be benign or malignant and may secrete a variety of peptide hormones, including gastrin, insulin, VIP, pancreatic polypeptide, and glucagon. In patients with symptoms, the diagnosis is confirmed by the demonstration of elevated hormone levels in the blood. However, the rate of discovery of occult tumors that are not detectable by routine hormone screening in these patients would be much higher if a more sensitive screening method were used. Provocative agents (calcium, secretin, insulin) have been helpful in the diagnosis of pancreatic endocrine tumors, but their role in routine screening for pancreatic islet cell disease in patients with MEN-1 has not been determined.

ZOLLINGER-ELLISON SYNDROME

Incidence and Pathology

Gastrinomas of the pancreas and duodenum, the second most common functional islet cell tumors, are rare, with an annual incidence of less than 1 per million population per year.[57,58] Gastrinoma is the most common functional islet cell tumor in patients with MEN-1, and about 20% of patients with ZES have it in the context of MEN-1 (see Table 27-1).[59]

Between 60% and 75% of patients with gastrinomas have either undetectable (by imaging) or localized disease at the time of diagnosis; the remaining 25% to 40% have metastatic disease, usually to the liver.[60-62] Nearly 75% of gastrinomas are malignant, with metastases initially to local lymph nodes and subsequently to the liver and other distant sites.[63,64] Metastases to the brain, lung, heart, and bone have been described.[65-67] Some suggest that gastrinomas originating to the left of the superior mesenteric artery are more malignant than those originating to the right of the artery.[68] It also has been stated that pancreatic gastrinomas are more likely to be malignant than are duodenal gastrinomas.[69] Whether either of these statements is true is not clear, because about 55% of duodenal wall primary gastrinomas have lymph node metastases at the time of surgery.[70] It is clear that duodenal gastrinomas are much

more common than previously expected[62,70-72] and that most primary gastrinomas (80%) occur within the confines of the gastrinoma triangle,[73] an area that is bordered by the superior mesenteric artery, the cystic duct, and the celiac axis, and includes the head of the pancreas and the duodenum. Duodenal tumors are more common within the first or second portion of the duodenum[74] (Fig. 27-2). Extraintestinal, extrapancreatic primary gastrinomas have been described within lymph nodes. The removal of such tumors may result in postoperative normalization of the serum gastrin concentration, suggesting that they are true primary gastrinomas.[75-78] However, many believe that these lymph node gastrinomas are really metastases from occult duodenal primaries.[62,71] Finally, unusual primary sites for gastrinomas include the ovary, the stomach, and the liver.[77,79-82]

In patients with MEN-1, gastrinomas may originate within the pancreas or the duodenum. Most patients with MEN-1 who have ZES have multiple primary islet cell tumors within the pancreas.[28] Studies indicate that these patients also have single or multiple neuroendocrine tumors within the duodenum. Immunoperoxidase staining for gastrin suggests that duodenal wall tumors are more likely to be gastrinomas.[29,30] Although some have suggested that gastrinomas within the context of MEN-1 seldom are malignant,[43] others have reported that about half of tumors identified by CT or arteriography are cancerous, as determined by distant spread.[42] Therefore, because it is unclear which of the multiple tumors really are gastrinomas, and because

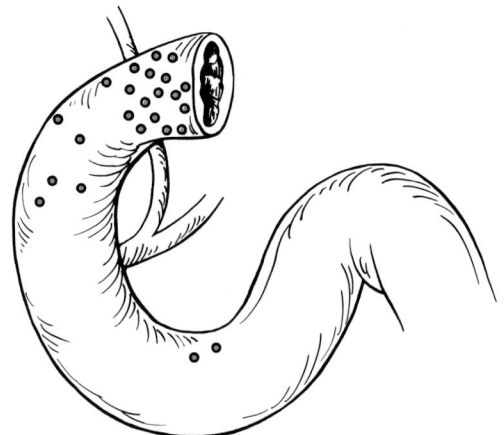

Figure 27-2 Location of 24 duodenal gastrinomas. Each dot represents a gastrinoma in an individual patient. There were 17 in the first portion of the duodenum, 5 in the second, and 2 in the third. Most duodenal gastrinomas are in the first and second portion of the duodenum. (After Thom AK, Norton JA, Axiotis CA, Jensen RT. Location, incidence and malignant potential of duodenal gastrinomas. Surgery 1991;110:1089)

the true malignant potential of these tumors is not well defined, controversy exists about the correct treatment of islet cell tumors in patients with MEN-1. These points were considered earlier in this chapter.

It is impossible by histologic criteria alone for pathologists to determine reliably whether an individual islet cell tumor is a gastrinoma or a malignant growth.[21] Pathologists use immunoperoxidase staining for gastrin to determine whether a removed neuroendocrine tumor is a gastrinoma. This is especially important in patients with MEN-1, who may have multiple tumors removed. However, studies suggest that there is no clear correlation between the proportion of cells that stain positive for gastrin and the true secretory nature of the tumor.[11] For gastrinomas, as for other islet cell tumors, determining malignancy depends on careful surgical exploration and biopsy of tumors at distant extrapancreatic extraintestinal sites, such as the lymph nodes or liver.[21] Thus, the determination of malignancy is made by surgeons at the time of exploration and confirmed by pathologists on examination of biopsy samples.

Signs and Symptoms

Patients with ZES usually are men in the fourth or fifth decade of life. The syndrome occurs less commonly in women. Patients who have ZES as part of the MEN-1 syndrome generally are younger (in their third decade) and are equally likely to be men as women.[42,83]

Patients with gastrinomas classically have severe peptic ulcer disease associated with profound gastric acid hypersecretion.[10,54,79,84] There generally is a long interval (average of 8 years) between the onset of symptoms and diagnosis of the disease. Gnawing epigastric pain is the most common symptom, and about 90% of patients have evidence of duodenal peptic ulcer disease at the time of diagnosis.[62,85–88] Patients may experience recurrent or atypically located ulcers, such as ulcers within the fourth portion of the duodenum or the jejunum. However, some patients with ZES do not have any evidence of peptic ulcer disease. Diarrhea and weight loss are other symptoms associated with ZES.[62,79] In addition, esophagitis, stricture with dysphagia, and endoscopic abnormalities of the distal esophagus are present in 60% of patients.[89–91] Gastrinomas may be more common than previously thought and should be included in the differential diagnosis for patients who have peptic ulcer disease, secretory diarrhea, or esophagitis. ZES should be excluded (see the section on diagnosis for details) in patients who are undergoing planned surgery for peptic ulcer or esophageal reflux disease.

Diagnosis

The diagnosis of ZES depends on two critical components—gastric acid hypersecretion and fasting hypergastrinemia.[73,85,92–95] Therapy with all medications that affect gastric acid secretion, such as histamine receptor antagonists (cimetidine, ranitidine, famotidine) and omeprazole, should be discontinued before gastric acid secretion is measured. A nasogastric tube is passed and acid secretion is collected for a timed interval. The amount of acid secreted, measured in milliequivalents per hour, is equal to the amount of $1N$ sodium hydroxide that must be added to the output to neutralize it. Patients with ZES always have acid secretion greater than 15 mEq/h, unless they have had previous surgery to decrease acid secretion, in which case they have levels above 5 mEq/h.[92,93] Another, simpler method is to measure the pH of the stomach secretions. In patients with ZES, it is always less than 4.0.

Achlorhydria must be excluded carefully during the evaluation, because it causes false-positive elevations in serum gastrin levels. Once the presence of gastric acid hypersecretion has been established, fasting serum gastrin levels should be measured (again, in the absence of all medications that affect acid output). All patients with ZES have increased fasting serum gastrin levels (over 100 pg/mL). The combination of elevated gastric acid output and increased fasting serum gastrin levels provides the unequivocal biochemical diagnosis of ZES[73,85,92–95] (see Table 27-2).

Provocative tests to increase serum gastrin levels further also have been used to aid in the diagnosis of ZES. Three different studies have been advocated in the past: the secretin test,[96,97] the calcium infusion test,[98–100] and the protein meal test.[101,102] The calcium infusion test relies on an infusion of calcium over 4 hours (54 mg/kg/h of calcium gluconate) to increase serum gastrin levels in patients with ZES.[99,100] A positive result is an increment of gastrin greater than 395 pg/mL. However, the calcium infusion test provides true-positive information in only 65% of patients with ZES, so its routine use no longer is recommended. The protein meal test has been advocated by some to exclude antral G cell hyperplasia as a cause of hypergastrinemia.[101,102] A 40-g protein meal causes an increment in serum gastrin levels in patients with antral G cell hyperplasia, but not in patients with ZES. This study no longer is recommended either, because antral G cell hyperplasia does not appear to be an important entity in the differential diagnosis, and many doubt that it has any clinical significance. The only provocative study still used in the evaluation of patients with ZES is the secretin test. In this study, serum gastrin levels are measured before and at 15, 30, 60, and 90 minutes after the intravenous administration of 2 U/kg of secretin. At either the 30-minute or the 60-minute sample, there is a greater than 200 pg/mL increment over the baseline gastrin level in patients with ZES. The results of this study are positive in 85% of patients with ZES.[100]

Control of Acid Hypersecretion

Controlling acid hypersecretion is an important part of the treatment of patients with ZES.[85] The gastric acid hypersecretion of ZES is life-threatening unless it is properly controlled. In 1955, when Zollinger and Ellison[1] described the first two patients with this syndrome, they discussed several important points regarding the management of gastric acid secretion in ZES. These researchers carefully measured the amount of acid output in each patient. The peptic ulcer disease could not be controlled until there was essentially no acid output. To achieve this, they performed total gastrectomy, and this became the procedure of choice for controlling gastric acid output in patients with ZES. In 1980, the H_2 blocker cimetidine was reported to control gastric acid hypersecretion in some patients with ZES.[103] However, this method was found to be cumbersome because patients became refractory to the medication, so most physicians used the drug only to prepare patients for total gastrectomy.[104] More potent H_2 blockers have since become available, and proton pump inhibitors such as omeprazole have been approved for use in patients with ZES, greatly simplifying the medical control of gastric acid hypersecretion.[105–110] As a result, total gastrectomy no longer is necessary to control gastric acid hypersecretion in patients with ZES.

The most important technique in controlling acid secretion in patients with ZES is careful measurement of acid output.[85] Complete relief of symptoms and freedom from all complications of peptic ulcer disease, including diarrhea, can be achieved if gastric acid secretion is reduced to less than 10 mEq/h in previously unoperated patients and to less than 5 mEq/h in patients who have had prior surgery to reduce acid output.[92,93] The medication dosage must be chosen to maintain these levels constantly. Symptoms of pain or diarrhea cannot be used to determine whether the dosage is adequate. Furthermore, the results of medical management cannot be monitored adequately by repeated endoscopy. Patients with ZES may require two to five times the dosage of H_2 receptor antagonist needed to treat idiopathic peptic ulcer disease. Most patients can be given omeprazole, 60 to 120 mg once daily. In patients with severe esophageal disease, it may be necessary to decrease acid output to less than 1 mEq/h to heal strictures and reduce the need for subsequent esophageal dilatation.[111] Finally, medical control of

acid secretion also is important at the time of surgical exploration to resect the gastrinoma. Therapy must be changed to an intravenous drug preparation that keeps the acid output at less than 10 mEq/h.[112] A continuous infusion of intravenous ranitidine at an hourly dosage previously determined to maintain the proper acid control is effective.

The complications associated with the high drug dosages necessary to control acid output have led some to criticize medical management of acid hypersecretion. When cimetidine is used as a primary agent, some patients develop gynecomastia and thrombocytopenia, as well as tachyphylaxis to the acid-reducing effects of the drug.[113] These side effects have not been observed with ranitidine and famotidine, however. Omeprazole has been associated with the development of gastric carcinoid tumors in rodents receiving long-term treatment.[79,114–117] This tumor has not been seen in humans; however, the drug has not been used for long periods in patients with ZES. Long-term follow-up requires heightened awareness and careful examination for the development of these potentially malignant tumors.

Surgery, besides total gastrectomy, can be used to help control gastric acid hypersecretion. Some recommend parietal cell vagotomy at the time of surgery in all patients with ZES.[118] However, this procedure is controversial. Advocates of this approach cite the facts that it reduces acid output in patients with ZES and appears to be safe and well tolerated, with no dumping or other associated symptoms. Furthermore, even if all the tumor is completely removed and patients are apparently cured of ZES, half still have some element of gastric acid hypersecretion secondary to an increased parietal cell mass.[112] Critics suggest that vagotomy alone does not control acid output in patients with ZES. At best, it reduces the amount of medication needed to control acid secretion. With the advent and ease of administration (once or twice daily dosing) of omeprazole, most argue that parietal cell vagotomy is unnecessary.[79,114–117]

Surgery to help control acid output appears to be indicated in patients with MEN-1 who have both ZES and primary hyperparathyroidism. Surgery directed at the primary hyperparathyroidism may help in the management of acid output in these patients. Several patients with both endocrine problems have required less acid-reducing medication after successful parathyroidectomy.[18,119] Some patients no longer have any biochemical evidence of ZES after successful surgical correction of primary hyperparathyroidism.[18] Because these patients always have parathyroid hyperplasia, the appropriate operative procedure is either 3½-gland parathyroidectomy or 4-gland parathyroidectomy with immediate autograft.[16,17]

Radiographic Localization

Despite the availability of sophisticated radiographic imaging studies, about half of patients with sporadic gastrinomas have no tumor identified on complete preoperative examination.[62] Modalities may be categorized as noninvasive and invasive imaging studies, and regionally localizing studies. In general, invasive localizing studies are more effective than are noninvasive studies, but are associated with greater expense and potential for significant complications. Noninvasive studies include ultrasound, CT, MRI, and labeled octreotide scanning. Invasive imaging studies include endoscopic ultrasound, intraoperative ultrasound, and selective angiography. Invasive regional localization studies include transhepatic portal venous sampling for gastrin levels in selected veins, and secretin angiography (see Table 27-3).

Gastrinomas, like all islet cell tumors and most neuroendocrine tumors, appear as sonolucent mass lesions that can be seen in two planes by ultrasound[120–122] (Fig. 27-3). In general, the pancreas and the liver are more echodense than are islet cell tumors, so tumors are more readily visible within these structures. Real-time color-flow imaging can be used to distinguish tumors from other sonolucent structures such as blood vessels and ducts. The basic tenet underlying both endoscopic[123] and intraoperative[122] ultrasound is that greater resolution can be obtained by positioning the transducer closer to the tumor. Enhanced imaging during invasive ultrasound is achieved by the use of near-field higher megahertz transducers that can image objects closer to the transducer with improved resolution. This belief has been supported by studies demonstrating that endoscopic and intraoperative ultrasound have much greater sensitivity and specificity than does standard ultrasound.[122–124] Standard ultrasound reveals only about 20% of gastrinomas and provides essentially no advantage over standard CT, so it cannot be recommended.[120,121] Endoscopic ultrasound has been demonstrated to have a sensitivity of 80% and appears to be a major advance in the imaging of islet cell tumors.[124] Endoscopic ultrasound is performed with a side-viewing endoscope placed within the duodenum. Rarely, a primary gastrinoma within the duodenum can be identified as a submucosal mass on endoscopy. A saline-filled balloon is expanded in the duodenum to distend this area and provide a uniform substance through which to send sound waves. A 7.5-mHz transducer is used that can provide excellent resolution in the region of the pancreatic head.[124] Intraoperative ultrasound has been effective in revealing islet cell tumors within the pancreas but not gastrinomas within the duodenum.[122,123] It is performed with a 10-mHz transducer

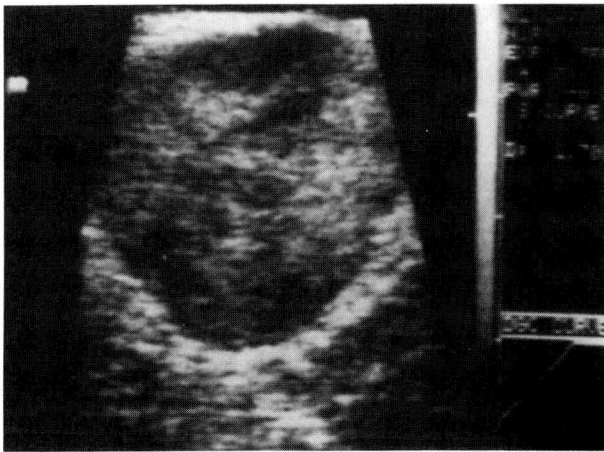

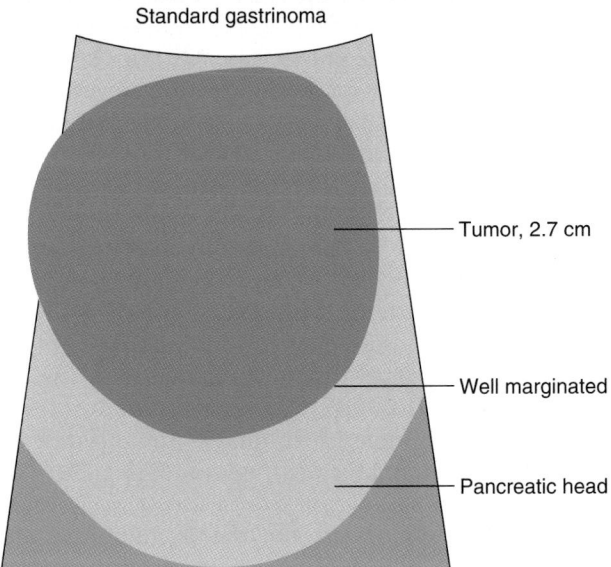

Standard gastrinoma

Tumor, 2.7 cm

Well marginated

Pancreatic head

Figure 27-3 Intraoperative ultrasound of a gastrinoma within the pancreatic head. Operative sonographic appearance of a typical islet cell tumor. The tumor is sonolucent compared with the surrounding pancreas, which is more echogenic. The margin of the tumor and the pancreas is discrete with an echogenic rim around the entire tumor. This appearance is consistent with a benign islet cell neoplasm. (After Norton JA, Cromack DT, Shawker TH, et al. Intraoperative ultrasonographic localization of islet cell tumors. Ann Surg 1988;207:163)

imaging through a pool of saline. Unfortunately, most gastrinomas that are overlooked on preoperative imaging are within the wall of the duodenum, and intraoperative ultrasound has not proven helpful in identifying these small lesions.[74] There is no evidence that endoscopic ultrasound reliably reveals occult duodenal tumors either. The duodenum appears to be a difficult area to examine by ultrasound because it has a heterogeneous background including gas, liquid, and solid.[74,122]

Octreotide scanning uses radioactive iodine-labeled octreotide to image gastrinoma and islet cell tumors based on the density of somatostatin receptors.[125–127] The ability to image tumor correlates with the density of the receptor in in vitro studies and appears to correlate with the clinical response to octreotide therapy in vivo.[127] Octreotide scanning is not widely available in the United States and most of the available information comes from the European experience.[126–130] This study correctly reveals 80% of islet cell tumors, including gastrinomas, and yields few false-positive results. As octreotide scanning becomes available in the United States, it should be useful in determining the exact location of islet cell tumors.

CT is performed with intravenous contrast and gastrinomas are identified based on increased vascularity as bright spots on the scan.[48,131] This study can reliably detect liver metastases with a sensitivity of 85%. CT reveals all primary gastrinomas larger than 3 cm in diameter and about 50% of those 1 to 2 cm in diameter. However, because primary gastrinomas usually are small, CT detects only about 30% to 40% of these tumors.[48,131] The sensitivity of MRI is nearly identical to that of CT.[48,120] The detection of gastrinomas, like other islet cell tumors, is enhanced by the T2-weighted or stir sequence in which islet cell tumors appear as bright spots compared with the surrounding pancreas, liver, or duodenum. Some suggest that imaging of gastrinomas is enhanced by the use of gadolinium. Like CT, the usefulness of MRI appears to be limited by the size of the primary tumor in that small tumors are not readily identifiable by this method. Thus, MRI or CT are used to exclude large tumors within the pancreas or the presence of unexpected liver metastases. Endoscopic ultrasound should be attempted if no tumor is seen on CT or MRI, because it may be able to detect smaller primary gastrinomas.[124]

Selective angiography is the single best overall imaging study because it reveals at least 50% of primary gastrinomas and accurately detects liver metastases[48,132] (see Table 27-3). Gastrinomas are visible because of an increased blood supply and vascular blush. Few false-positive results are obtained and the blush enables accurate localization of the tumor. Of the 50% of patients with gastrinomas who have negative results on angiography, many have duodenal gastrinomas.[70–72,74,133] Islet cell tumors of the pancreatic tail also may be overlooked on angiography, although gastrinomas in this location are rare.[62,134] Regional localization of gastrinomas is possible when selective angiography is combined with selective injections of secretin to different regions of the pancreas.[40,41,135,136] Catheters are placed into three different arteries (gastroduodenal, hepatic, and splenic) and the hepatic vein. Secretin is injected sequentially into each of the vessels and levels of gastrin are measured in the hepatic vein effluent and in one peripheral vein. When the artery that perfuses the gastrinoma is injected with secretin, there is a marked rise in the hepatic vein concentration of gastrin. Secretin angiography enables correct regional localization of gastrinomas in 75% of cases.[40] Elevation of venous gastrin levels after injection of the gastroduodenal artery suggests the presence of a duodenal wall gastrinoma.[133] Some have advocated performing a pancreaticoduodenectomy if there is a gradient in gastrin after injection of the artery that perfuses the area of the pancreatic head, and if there is no evidence of distant metastatic disease at the time of operation.[136] Others have used selective injection of methylene blue into the gastroduodenal artery at the time of surgical exploration to help identify small duodenal wall gastrinomas that are difficult to find.[137]

Gastrinomas also may be localized by transhepatic sampling of the portal vein and its tributaries for gastrin levels.[37,138,139] In this technique, a catheter is passed through the liver into the portal vein and blood is sampled from its major branches and selective tributaries for determination of gastrin concentrations. Twenty to 30 samples are obtained. The closer the selective catheter can be positioned to the tumor (the source of gastrin), the higher the concentration of gastrin and the greater the ratio compared with peripheral levels. This study is able to pinpoint the region of the pancreas containing the gastrinoma in about 80% of cases[37,138,139] (see Table 27-3). It is highly invasive and has been associated with complications, including hemobilia and bleeding in 10% of patients.[139] It also is expensive and tedious, and requires considerable expertise. Because most occult gastrinomas are located within the gastrinoma triangle,[134] regional localization to the pancreatic head obtained by portal venous sampling does not provide much additional information. Secretin angiography provides identical information with less expense and technical difficulty, and also may image the tumor; therefore, it is preferable to portal venous sampling for regional localization of gastrinomas.

In summary, the initial imaging test in patients with gastrinomas should be CT or MRI to identify large malignant tumors within the pancreas or liver. If the tumors are occult and not identified on initial tests, the next appropriate studies are endoscopic ultrasound, octreotide scanning, and secretin angiography. It is possible to identify and remove gastrinomas in most patients in whom all studies are uninformative with the exception of a gastrin increment on the secretin angiogram.[62,74,133]

Preoperative Preparation

Once the surgeon is confident of the diagnosis of gastrinoma based on the results of biochemical studies, acid output has been controlled with drugs, and imaging and regional localizing studies have been performed, the patient is made ready for surgery. Immediate preoperative preparation is similar to that for any major operation except for certain specific issues related to surgery on the pancreas. Because tumors located in the body or tail of the pancreas may be removed by subtotal pancreatectomy with splenectomy, antipneumococcal vaccine generally is administered to further reduce the low likelihood of postsplenectomy sepsis. The use of octreotide before surgery to diminish the risk of pancreatic fistula formation is controversial.[140,141] In the immediate preoperative period, a complete mechanical bowel preparation is recommended. The use of perioperative antibiotics also is indicated. The operative plan is based on the results of localization studies. Consideration should be given to the unexpected finding of metastatic tumor or the failure to identify any gastrinoma.

Exploration for Gastrinoma

On the day of surgery, the patient should receive continuous intravenous ranitidine at a dosage previously determined to maintain acid output at a rate of less than 10 mEq/h. The goal of surgery is to find and remove all gastrinoma for cure of ZES. The surgeon must be aware of the results of preoperative localization studies and have a clear understanding of all potential tumor locations, including the duodenal wall, which is believed to be the site of many occult gastrinomas[70,71,133,142] (see Fig. 27-2). The fact that about 80% of primary gastrinomas are found within the gastrinoma triangle is critical information.[134]

The surgery generally is performed through either a midline or a bilateral subcostal incision (see Section VIA in Atlas Chap. 30). Initially, the entire abdomen is examined carefully. This is important because primary tumors have been located within the kidney, liver, ovary, mesentery, omentum, and other atypical sites.[81] Furthermore, metastatic gastrinoma also can occur within the mesentery and the liver. A clear assessment of the extent of disease is important for prognostic reasons. It also is possible in some patients to remove all metastatic tumor at surgery and induce a complete remission.[143]

Critical to the procedure is complete exposure of the pancreas and duodenum. In the past, it was thought that pancreatic gastrinomas often were occult, so intraoperative ultrasound was used to improve the detection of these tumors (see Fig. 27-3). However, the use of ultrasound during pancreatic exploration for gastrinomas did not improve the detection rate of pancreatic gastrin-producing tumors.[74,122] It became clear that duodenal gastrinomas are more common than previously believed and often had been overlooked.[70,72,144] New techniques to improve the detection of duodenal wall gastrinomas appear to increase the likelihood of surgical cure. These include preoperative catheterization of the gastroduodenal artery followed by intraoperative injection of methylene blue, and intraoperative endoscopy with transillumination, both of which aid in the discrimination of duodenal wall tumors (Fig. 27-4). Extensive duodenotomy with inspection, palpation, and eversion of the duodenal mucosa to detect small duodenal gastrinomas as small nodules within the wall also is appropriate if other measures fail.[72,74] Examination of the duodenal wall that abuts the pancreas may be hazardous, because both the main and accessory papillae can be mistaken for tumors. The surgeon should pass a catheter through the cystic duct into the common bile duct and the duodenum for correct identification of the am-

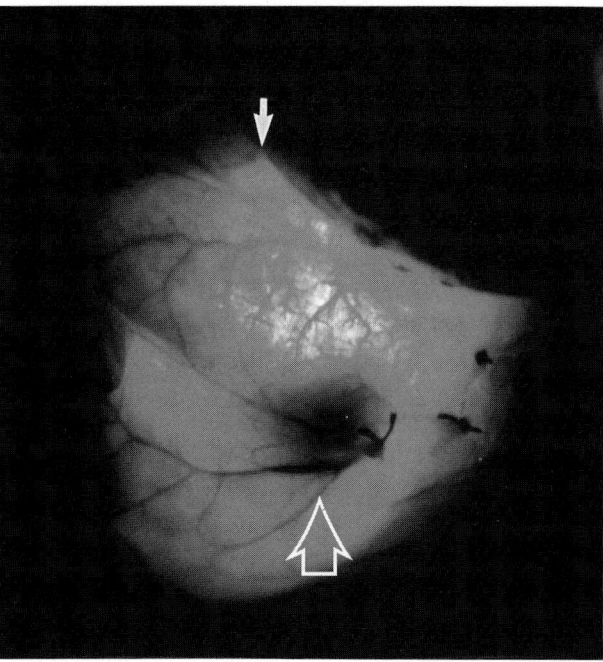

Figure 27-4 Transillumination of duodenal wall gastrinoma. Operating room lights are dimmed. Endoscopy is performed with the scope passed into the duodenum (*small arrow*). The gastrinoma (*large arrow*) is identified as a focal area of opacification to the transmission of light. (See Color Fig. 27-4.)

pulla. Intravenous secretin, 1 U/kg, also can be used during the operation to allow identification of the pancreatic duct, which responds rapidly by emitting clear juice. Direct inspection of the duodenal mucosa can identify tumors on the medial wall of the duodenum that were missed by transillumination. The concentration of gastrinomas is greatest in the first and second portions of the duodenum (see Fig. 27-2). Localized duodenal wall gastrinomas usually are excised with a full-thickness wall of duodenum, with the expectation of excellent long-term survival. Others recommend pancreaticoduodenectomy if a gastrinoma appears to be localized to the region, based on both a clear increment in hepatic vein gastrin levels when the gastroduodenal artery is injected with secretin and the finding that tumor is localized to that region at laparotomy.[136] Pancreaticoduodenectomy may result in an increased cure rate, but also is associated with greater short- and long-term morbidity. Studies are necessary to determine its exact role in patients with ZES. Most experts recommend simple resection of duodenal wall tumors, enucleation of pancreatic head tumors, and resection of pancreatic body and tail tumors. This strategy has been associated with acceptable complication and cure rates[62,145] (Tables 27-4 and 27-5).

Gastrinomas in the pancreatic body and tail appear to be more malignant than those in the pancreatic head and, therefore, usually are removed by subtotal pancreatectomy with splenectomy.[146] Intraoperative ultrasound has facilitated the identification of gastrinomas within the pancreas, and always should be used[122] (see Fig. 27-3). Ultrasound also can help in determining the best way to remove the tumor based on evidence of invasion or proximity to the pancreatic duct. In addition, ultrasound can detect deep liver metastases that may not be apparent from palpation, and can be used to plan the exact method of resection. Isolated liver metastases usually are removed by wedge resection at the same operation.[147] Some authors[143,147] also have resected larger liver metastases by formal lobectomy at the same procedure in selected individuals based on the results of preoperative imaging studies. Gastrinoma in lymph nodes also should be removed.

If a duodenal gastrinoma is removed by simple resection, the duodenum is closed in a transverse direction so as not to constrict the lumen.[74,142] No postoperative drains are placed and the patient is maintained on a continuous infusion of ranitidine.[112] After incision into the pancreas to enucleate a gastrinoma from the pancreatic head, or after subtotal pancreatectomy with splenectomy, large closed suction drains are placed to prevent the pooling of pancreatic exocrine drainage within the operative site.[141] The level of amylase in any drainage should be measured to determine whether it is coming from the pancreas. If the level of amylase in the fluid is markedly elevated compared with the level in plasma, the drains should not be removed until the amount of drainage measures less than 15 mL/d for 2 consecutive days.

Results of Curative Surgery for Gastrinoma

Surgery, as outlined earlier, has resulted in cure for some patients with ZES.[62,142,145] Even patients with liver metastases may experience complete remission after resection of all tumor.[143,147] As gastrinomas are detected in more patients at exploratory laparotomy, the proportion of patients cured of ZES will continue to rise. Of patients who have the sporadic, nonfamilial form of ZES with either imaging evidence of localized gastrinoma or no identifiable gastrinoma, studies suggest that gastrinomas will be found and resected in about 90% and evidence of remission will be seen in about 60%.[61,62,148] Of patients with metastatic gastrinoma, about 40% to 50% have localized metastatic disease and are candidates for curative surgery. Of all those who undergo surgery, about 80% have completely resectable disease, and 40% of those who undergo resection have no biochemical evidence of disease afterward.[62,143,147] However, long-term follow-up studies of patients with localized disease indicate that 50% will have evidence of recurrent disease after 5 years.[62,64] The most efficient and economical way to detect recurrence is to perform secretin stimulation tests at regular intervals after surgery.[149] Increased secretin-stimulated

Table 27-4 Islet Cell Tumor Identification and Cure Rate in Various Series

Tumor	Number	Number With Tumor Identified	Number Cured	References
Insulinoma	502	499 (99%)	499 (99%)	48, 153, 180, 185
Gastrinoma	209	168 (80%)	83 (40%)*	62, 145, 203

* Cure rate means immediate cure rate (ie, no evidence of residual disease).

Table 27-5 Morbidity and Mortality of Islet Cell Tumor Surgery

Location of Tumor	Number	Morbidity	Deaths	References
Pancreas	468	139 (30%)	10 (2%)	48, 141, 185
Duodenum	35	6 (17%)	0 (0%)	74

serum gastrin levels are the earliest sign of recurrence. Long-term follow-up studies of patients who undergo resection of distant metastatic gastrinomas indicate that those with only solitary liver metastases have the best prognosis and survive the longest.[143] However, all patients with metastatic disease at presentation eventually develop evidence of recurrence if they are observed long enough. Recurrence may take many years, suggesting that resection of distant disease still has some benefit. Incomplete resection of metastatic gastrinoma does not appear to be justified; subsequent survival is the same as in patients who do not undergo surgery.[143]

INSULINOMA

Incidence and Pathology

Despite the fact that insulinoma is the most common functional islet cell tumor, with an incidence of about 1 per million population per year,[58,150] it still is a rare lesion. Most physicians and surgeons will treat only one or two patients with insulinoma during their careers.[151] Therefore, a complete understanding of the evaluation and surgical treatment of this tumor is imperative.

Insulinomas generally are solitary, benign, small tumors occurring anywhere within the pancreas.[48,152,153] Typical insulinomas are not identifiable on most imaging studies and must be found during exploratory laparotomy. About 5% of insulinomas are malignant.[55] Malignant insulinomas should be apparent on standard imaging studies as large pancreatic masses, perhaps associated with liver metastases. About 10% of patients with insulinomas have the MEN-1 syndrome[42] (see Table 27-1). Unlike gastrinomas, which frequently occur within the duodenum, insulinomas almost always (over 99%) occur within the pancreas; when present at sites outside the pancreas, these tumors are associated with ectopic pancreas.[154,155] The distribution of insulinomas within the pancreas also is different than that of gastrinomas. Gastrinomas are located most commonly within the pancreatic head (gastrinoma triangle),[134] whereas insulinomas are distributed uniformly throughout the gland.[48,155] Occasionally, nesidioblas-

tosis has been described as a cause of hyperinsulinism in adults with hypoglycemia.[52] However, nesidioblastosis occurs much more commonly in infants with hypoglycemia and is manifested by diffuse enlargement of the islets throughout the pancreas.[156] In such cases, no discrete tumors are present and the appropriate surgical procedure is near-total pancreatectomy. It is unlikely that nesidioblastosis is a true pathologic entity in adults with hypoglycemia.[156] Careful examination of the pancreas in patients with MEN-1, for example, always demonstrates multiple islet cell tumors and diffuse islet cell hyperplasia,[20,30] but most of these tumors produce pancreatic polypeptide and not insulin and, therefore, do not cause symptoms.[157,158] Surgeons should remember that patients with insulinomas generally have solitary islet cell tumors located within the pancreas that usually are small and benign, and can be found and removed to restore normal glucose homeostasis.[48,152,153]

Signs and Symptoms

Patients with insulinomas generally have symptoms of neuroglycopenia.[151–153] These symptoms usually are more apparent during a period of fasting and include altered consciousness, decreased arousal in the morning, tremulousness, and seizures. Most patients subconsciously realize that symptoms are associated with fasting, so they increase food intake to compensate, which in turn results in weight gain.

Insulinoma is more common in women than in men. It usually occurs in the third or fourth decade of life.

Diagnosis

The diagnosis of insulinoma is based on the presence of symptomatic fasting hypoglycemia and hyperinsulinism.[159] The study of choice is the supervised fast with measurement of serum levels of glucose and insulin[151,159] (see Table 27-2). This study requires hospitalization with placement of a peripheral heparin lock for blood drawing and possible administration of glucose when symptoms arise. Patients fast for a maximum of 72 hours and are allowed to ingest only noncaloric beverages. Monitoring is performed at 5- to 15-minute intervals, and serum levels of glucose and insulin are measured before and every 6 hours during the fast. If symptoms of neuroglycopenia consistent with hypoglycemia develop, the fast is terminated and serum levels of glucose, insulin, C peptide, and proinsulin are measured.[48,151,152,159] All patients with insulinomas have symptoms of neuroglycopenia during a 72-hour fast[48]; normal persons do not. Most of these patients have symptoms after fasting for only 24 or 48 hours. At the time symptoms develop, 90% of patients have serum glucose levels below 40 mg/dL and the remainder have levels below 45 mg/dL.[48] All patients with insulinomas have abnormally high levels of insulin for the degree of hypoglycemia (over 5 μU/mL). Most of these patients also have abnormal levels of C peptide (over 1.75), indicating that the high levels of insulin are being produced by the tumor and not being administered from a surreptitious source. Similarly, most patients with insulinomas have elevated proportions of proinsulin, an insulin precursor. Most tumors make a greater proportion of proinsulin than does the normal pancreas (over 25%). Some suggest that malignant islet cell tumors produce chorionic gonadotropin, and that it can be used as an indicator of malignancy.[160]

Stimulation and suppression tests have been used to aid in the diagnosis of insulinoma.[161] Provocative agents include calcium, tolbutamide, glucagon, and leucine. Suppression tests involve the administration of porcine or fish insulin to suppress serum levels of human insulin. Provocative agents cause a further elevation of plasma levels of insulin in patients with insulinomas but not in normal individuals. The administration of fish insulin does not affect plasma levels of C peptide and human insulin in patients with insulinomas, but reduces them in normal individuals.[51] These tests are not recommended for routine use.

The major concern in the differential diagnosis of insulinoma is factitious hypoglycemia.[162] This usually occurs in young women who have some knowledge of the medical profession as health care workers, or who have a relative with diabetes mellitus. Urinary levels of sulfonylureas can be measured by mass spectroscopy and used to rule out the use of oral hypoglycemic drugs. Close observation during the fasting period is necessary to prevent patients from using any medications. Elevated serum levels of C peptide and proinsulin are not present in factitious hypoglycemia. Finally, antiinsulin antibodies are measured. Their presence suggests the administration of exogenous nonhuman insulin. Antibody testing does not detect the administration of commercial recombinant human insulin. Factitious hypoglycemia is a real concern in the differential diagnosis of insulinoma. One series indicates that 80% of patients with factitious hypoglycemia have undergone unnecessary pancreatic surgery. These patients have significant psychiatric problems and the long-term prognosis is poor.[162]

Control of Hypoglycemia

Hypoglycemia can be life-threatening in patients with insulinomas and should be controlled before localization studies and surgery are performed. The ability to control hypoglycemia before surgery affects the intraoperative care of these patients. If hypoglycemia can be well controlled with drugs and diet, it becomes relatively less critical to find and remove the insulinoma at the time of surgery. However, if hypoglycemia is not controlled, the tumor must be found and removed for cure, which may necessitate more aggressive operative procedures. Therefore, the best possible management of hypoglycemia should be attempted before surgery to determine the necessity of successful removal of the insulinoma at the time of operation.[159]

The mainstay in the management of hypoglycemia is careful dietary regulation, which may include the use of cornstarch to slow the absorption of nutrients and awakening patients at night for feedings to prevent morning hypoglycemia. Dietary management requires the intake of excessive calories and results in weight gain. Drugs may help control the hyperinsulinism. Diazoxide has been the drug of choice, but 40% of patients cannot tolerate it because of nausea, vomiting, and hypotension. In a similar proportion of patients, it is ineffective. Diazoxide use must be discontinued 1 week before surgery because it has been associated with life-threatening intraoperative hypotension. Calcium-channel blockers, such as verapamil, also have been used to decrease insulin secretion in patients with insulinomas.[163] However, significant hypotension and poor control of hyperinsulinism limits their efficacy. Finally, octreotide has been used to control hypoglycemia in a few patients with malignant insulinomas; however, it generally has been ineffective in patients with typical sporadic insulinomas.[164-166] In summary, the medical management of hypoglycemia associated with insulinoma is based primarily on dietary manipulation. Drugs are effective in few patients, and most must rely on successful surgical resection of the tumor for control of symptoms.

Preoperative Radiographic Localization

The radiographic localization studies used for insulinoma are the same as those used for gastrinoma. Because insulinomas usually are small, imaging results for these tumors also are similar to those for gastrinomas (ie, tumor is not identified in about half of patients even with invasive localization procedures[48]; see Table 27-3). However, unlike gastrinomas, which typically lie within the confines of the gastrinoma triangle, insulinomas are distributed evenly throughout the pancreas, and correct regional localization may suggest the area of the gland that should be removed if no tumor is identified at laparotomy.[48,167] This is advantageous because it eliminates blind removal of pancreas that may not contain tumor.

Table 27-3 lists the accuracy of various localization procedures for insulinoma. Many insulinomas are smaller than 2 cm in diameter and cannot be detected with noninvasive techniques such as ultrasound,[48,168,169] CT,[138,153,169] or MRI.[48,169] However, one of these studies should be performed to exclude the unlikely possibility of a large malignant insulinoma with liver metastases. Selective celiac angiography, which produces hypervascular blushing of insulinomas, previously was considered the best localization study, and initial reports suggested that it detected 95% of these tumors.[168,170] However, recent reports do not confirm this high accuracy rate and suggest that the true sensitivity is 50%.[48] Portal venous sampling for insulin has a sensitivity of 82% (range, 70% to 95%) independent of tumor size, but it only suggests which part of the pancreas contains the tumor.[167] Although it does not provide precise imaging of the tumor, portal venous sampling has been shown to be the most sensitive test for detecting small insulinomas[48,168,171-174] (Fig. 27-5). Some suggest that the diagnostic ability of portal venous sampling falls considerably when insulinomas are located within the pancreatic tail. Other disadvantages of portal venous sampling include its considerable expense, complication rate of 3%, and mortality rate of 0.4%.[139]

A new technique for localizing insulinomas is calcium angiography.[175,176] It is a modification of the secretin angiography used to localize gastrinomas in which calcium is used as the provocative agent instead of secretin. In this study, pancreatic arteriography is performed in an attempt to image the insulinoma and identify which arteries perfuse different areas of the pancreas. Calcium gluconate then is injected rapidly into each selectively catheterized artery and plasma samples are obtained from the hepatic veins for determination of insulin concentrations. A two-fold elevation of insulin levels is considered to be a positive localization. A published evaluation of this method indicates that it provided insulin gradients in the hepatic vein in nine of nine patients (100%) with insulinomas and unequivocal positive localization of the correct region of the pancreas with tumor in six of nine patients (66%).[176]

Studies describe the advantages of endoscopic ultrasound in localizing pancreatic islet cell tumors.[123] The use of a high-frequency transducer with this technique can distinguish tumors as small as 2 mm. Islet cell tumors appear as homogeneous sonolucent mass lesions with smooth borders. Endoscopic ultrasound was found to have a sensitivity of 80% to 85% and a specificity of 95%. It is especially useful for insulinomas, because these tumors are located within the pancreas and stand out against a uniform, more echodense background.

Scanning with isotope-labeled somatostatin analogues such as iodine- and indium-labeled octreotide has been used to visualize insulinomas.[126,127,129] However, only 60% of insulinomas were visualized with this technique, because octreotide receptors were not present on all tumors. Positive scan results predict those patients who will have positive responses to octreotide therapy.[128]

Exact recommendations for individual studies de-

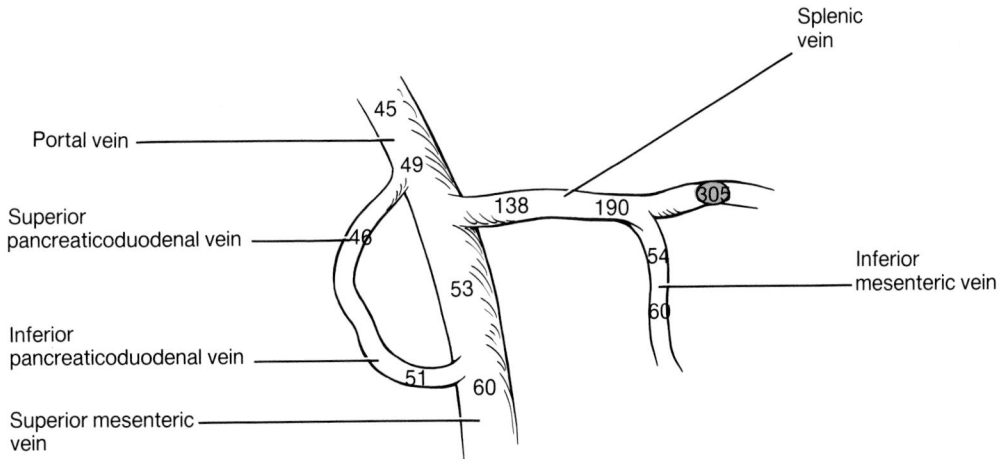

Figure 27-5 Transhepatic selective venous sampling of the portal vein and its tributaries for insulin. Serum insulin levels are markedly elevated in the distal splenic vein, localizing the insulinoma to the tail of the pancreas. All measurements are in microunits per milliliter. Peripheral insulin is 56 µU/mL. (After Norton JA, Shawker TH, Doppman JL, et al. Localization and surgical treatment of occult insulinomas. Ann Surg 1990;212:618)

pend on the availability of the techniques in different institutions and on the experience of the operating surgeon. Some experienced endocrine surgeons believe that localization studies are not necessary for patients with insulinomas because they usually find the tumors regardless of the results.[177] However, individual cases may be difficult, leading others to suggest that invasive localization studies should be performed in all patients.[178,179]

Initially, an imaging study that includes the pancreas and the liver is performed in an attempt to identify the primary tumor and to exclude the presence of a malignant insulinoma with liver metastases. CT with intravenous contrast is preferred because of its excellent images and the fact that the tumor may appear as a vascular blush. Endoscopic ultrasound and labeled octreotide scanning are not widely available and must be considered experimental in the evaluation of patients with insulinoma, although both studies appear promising. If either study is available, it should be used.

The use of invasive localization studies in patients with insulinomas is controversial. These studies are expensive and, at institutions with experience in the treatment of insulinoma, surgery usually is successful even when the test results are negative.[167,177–179] As a result, many believe these studies are not indicated. However, difficulty may arise if no insulinoma is identified during surgical exploration. This situation previously was managed by performing blind subtotal pancreatectomy based on the probability that 66% of insulinomas would be removed in the specimen. However, recent studies indicate that the most common location of nonpalpable insulinomas is in the pancreatic head because the increased thickness makes the tumors more difficult to feel.[167] No study always provides accurate localization, but both portal venous sampling for insulin and calcium arteriography provide correct regional localization in 80% to 100% of patients.[48,167,175,176] Portal venous sampling for insulin (see Fig. 27-5) is an established method, used with excellent results at many institutions. Calcium angiography is a promising new study with comparable sensitivity and specificity. Therefore, unless noninvasive imaging studies provide unequivocal identification, the use of arteriography and portal venous sampling for regional localization and potential arteriographic imaging of insulinomas is recommended.

Immediate Preoperative Preparation and Surgical Plan

The preoperative preparation of patients with insulinomas is similar to that of patients with gastrinomas. The use of a pneumococcal vaccine (Pneumovax), bowel preparation, and perioperative antibiotics is recommended. The results of localization studies and the images themselves should be reviewed extensively. The results of regional localization studies, including either portal venous sampling or calcium angiography, also should be reviewed to determine which portion of the pancreas harbors the insulinoma. This information is especially useful when no tumor is identified because it allows the surgeon to remove the area suspected of containing the tumor. This task is relatively simple if the studies suggest that the insulinoma is within the pancreatic tail. It is more difficult if they indicate that the tumor is within the pancreatic head. In this case, guidance should be obtained from discussions with the patient, the family, and the endocrinologist. Because occult, unidentified insulinomas in the pancreatic head usually are benign, the major factor in determining whether to remove the tumor is the severity of the symptoms and the degree to which they can be controlled. Therefore, the patient's response to medical therapy is a prime consideration in deciding to perform a pancreaticoduodenectomy if no tumor is identified and localization studies suggest that it lies within the pancreatic head. In some patients, it is necessary to remove the head of the pancreas when the results of regional localization studies are definitive and symptoms are poorly controlled. Each step of the operation should be reviewed with the endocrinologist, the patient, and the family so that a reasonable strategy can be designed before surgery is undertaken.

Exploration for Insulinoma

The abdomen is entered through an upper midline or bilateral subcostal incision (see Section VIA in Atlas Chap. 30) and a fixed upper abdominal retractor is used to improve exposure. A general exploration of the entire abdomen is performed. Unlike gastrinomas, which usually are malignant and often are located outside the pancreas, insulinomas rarely are malignant and almost always are found within the pancreas. Therefore, the initial part of the exploration should exclude significant pathology outside the pancreas in organs such as the liver and ovary, but it may be performed expeditiously because disease in these organs resulting from insulinoma is large and easy to identify.

Excellent exposure of the pancreas is essential in patients with insulinomas. This requires complete mobilization of the hepatic and splenic flexures of the colon. Full division of the gastrocolic ligament and wide visualization of the body and tail of the pancreas also are necessary. A complete Kocher maneuver always must be done to reveal the posterior head of the pancreas. Complete dissection and mobilization along the inferior border of the pancreas is necessary to palpate the body and tail of the gland between the thumb and forefinger. Ligation of the short gastric vessels, detachment of the splenic ligaments, and mobilization of the spleen may be required to allow proper examination of the tail of the pancreas. Complete and meticulous mobilization, examination, and careful palpation of the pancreas is an essential component of the operation.

Identification of insulinomas is crucial. Surgeons must use every technique available to accomplish this goal and avoid excessive biopsy of normal pancreas and anatomic variations, which may be associated with complications such as fistula, pseudocyst, and abscess. The first maneuver used to identify insulinomas is visualization. These tumors appear reddish brown against the pale, pinkish yellow pancreas. However, most tumors are not on the anterior surface of the pancreas and are not visible on initial examination of the gland. The second maneuver used to identify insulinomas is palpation. Insulinomas feel firm compared with the surrounding pancreas, because these tumors generally have a small inflammatory reaction of pancreatitis around them. Palpation is a dependable maneuver for identifying most insulinomas. Tumors within the pancreatic head may be overlooked by this technique, however, because the gland is thicker there and small tumors are hard to find deep in the substance of the head.[167] Intraoperative ultrasound is a relatively new method that has significantly improved the operative detection of insulinomas[152,167,180] (Fig. 27-6). It is performed by the operating surgeon in conjunction with an ultrasonographer. The pancreas is scanned with a near-field, high-resolution, real-time transducer, usually either a 7.5- or 10-MHz device. Mass lesions always are scanned in two directions to confirm the presence of a true mass. Insulinomas appear as sonolucent tumors within the more echodense pancreas. Tumors that are not palpable or visible within the pancreatic head have been detected by this technique[152,167,180] (Fig. 27-7). Intraoperative ultrasound also provides useful information about adjacent vital structures, such as the pancreatic duct, superior mesenteric vein, and common bile duct. It can be used to plan the least morbid path of dissection for removal of the insulinoma, or it may suggest that the tumor should be resected by distal pancreatectomy because of its relationship to the pancreatic duct. Intraoperative ultrasound correctly identifies almost all insulinomas and clearly enhances outcome. It should be used in all surgical explorations for insulinomas.

Some authors have described the use of intraoperative glucose monitoring to facilitate localization of insulinomas.[181–184] This is performed either by frequent measurement of circulating glucose levels or by intra-

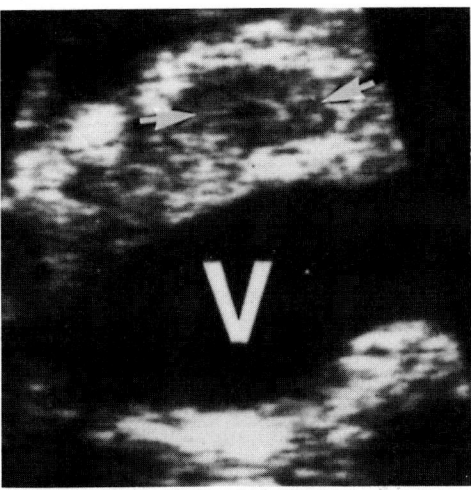

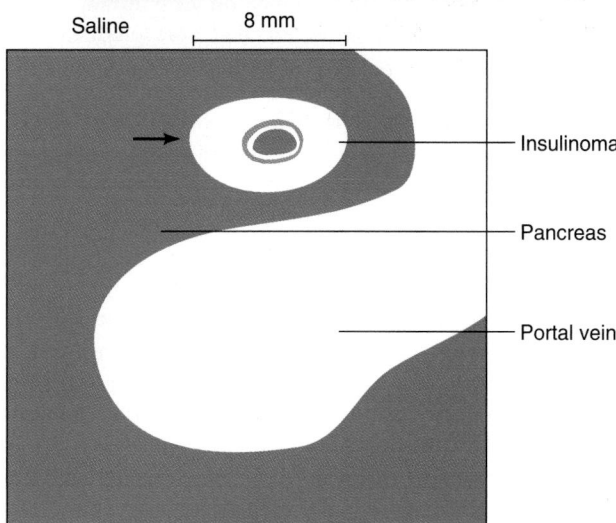

Figure 27-6 A transverse intraoperative ultrasound scan of a small pancreatic insulinoma. The insulinoma (*arrows*) appears sonolucent and is within the head of the pancreas overlying the portal vein (V). The tumor measures 8 mm in length. The tumor has been partially exposed using ultrasound, because it was not palpable within the pancreatic head. (After Norton JA, Shawker TH, Doppman JL, et al. Localization and surgical treatment of occult insulinomas. Ann Surg 1990; 212:617)

operative determination of glucose and insulin levels using a glucose clamp device. The former method depends on an absolutely constant infusion of glucose and has yielded false-positive results. The latter method is reliable, but it is cumbersome, expensive, and unnecessary.

After the insulinoma is identified and removed, the specimen is given to the pathologist, who uses frozen section to determine whether it is an islet cell tumor. Postoperative serum glucose levels usually rise to slightly more than 200 mg/dL. Insulin should not be

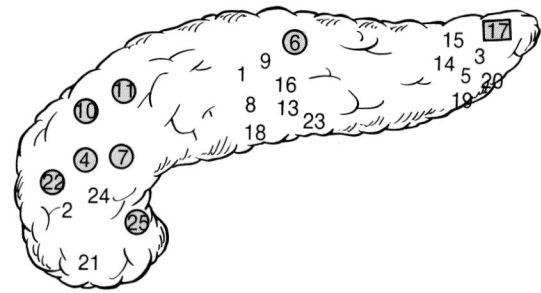

Figure 27-7 The locations of insulinomas in 25 patients with sporadic disease and the methods by which they were identified. Each number represents an insulinoma in a separate patient. The tumors are uniformly distributed throughout the pancreas. Numbers without a circle or square indicate tumors that were identified by palpation or visualization. Circles indicate tumors that were identified only by intraoperative ultrasound. Square indicates tumors that were found after resection based on portal venous sampling gradient. One patient did not have a tumor identified; subsequently, his tumor was removed from the pancreatic tail. (After Doherty GM, Doppman JL, Shawker TH, et al. Results of a prospective strategy to diagnose, localize and resect insulinomas. Surgery 1991;110:993)

used to treat this mild hyperglycemia. After several days, the suppressed normal islets secrete more insulin and serum glucose levels return to normal without treatment. The major postoperative concern is drainage of pancreatic fluid. Large-bore, closed, low-suction drains are placed at the pancreatic incision site to minimize the accumulation of pancreatic enzymes in the abdomen. During the postoperative period, the amylase level of the drainage fluid is analyzed to determine whether the drainage is from the pancreas. If amylase levels are high, the drains should not be removed until the drainage is minimal and the patient is eating a regular diet. As mentioned previously, some believe that octreotide may reduce the amount of drainage from the pancreas and may improve healing and reduce complications after pancreatic surgery.[140] However, no beneficial effect has been seen in patients undergoing insulinoma resection.[141]

Results of Surgery

Surgical treatment of insulinomas produces excellent results (see Table 27-4). In several large series,[48,50,185] the cure rate was about 95%. The complication rate was 10% to 20%, but the mortality rate was less than 2% (see Table 27-5). Furthermore, the use of major pancreatic resection in patients with insulinomas is decreasing, because surgeons realize that these tumors generally are benign and can be enucleated. For instance, pancreat-

icoduodenectomy hardly ever is indicated for benign insulinomas. Favorable surgical results also are associated with the increasing use of intraoperative ultrasound, which allows precise operative detection and localization of islet cell tumors (see Fig. 27-6).

In one series of 25 consecutive patients with insulinomas and no evidence of metastases or MEN-1,[48] 24 patients were cured of the hyperinsulinism by resection of a small islet cell tumor. The remaining patient underwent reoperation and was found to have a small insulinoma within the tail of the pancreas, which was easily resected. There were no operative deaths and no long-term morbidity. Despite the fact that the treatment of insulinomas can be challenging, most patients are cured with few complications.

Metastatic insulinomas are rare, accounting for less than 10% of all insulinomas[54,55] (see Table 27-1). Affected patients generally have tumors identified by CT or other noninvasive imaging studies, and usually have large mass lesions within the pancreas, often measuring 5 to 6 cm. If surgeons can resect all tumor, including lymph node or liver metastases, patients have an excellent chance of being free of hyperinsulinism.[55] Some patients have enjoyed a durable response from such therapy. However, it also has been noted that subtotal resection or debulking of the tumor mass does not appear to improve control of the hypoglycemia.[54,55] In general, aggressive surgery for distant disease should be undertaken only if all visible tumor can be resected.

It is not clear whether resection of metastatic tumors improves survival in these patients. Although some suggest it does,[147] no randomized studies have been performed and patients with metastatic islet cell tumors may have indolent disease for long periods. Among patients with gastrinomas, those who undergo resection of multiple metastatic lesions do not live any longer than those who do not undergo resection.[186] Resection of distant disease is performed to improve control of hypoglycemia, because regulating serum glucose levels in individuals with malignant insulinomas can be difficult. Octreotide has been used with some success, but it only works in 40% of patients.[53,165] Other approaches include the use of chemotherapeutic drugs such as streptozotocin, doxorubicin, 5-FU,[31–33] and interferon-α,[34–36] each of which has had some success in patients with metastatic insulinomas. However, none of these drugs have provided a complete response or prolonged survival. Embolization of metastases within the liver has been used with limited success. The combination of chemotherapy and embolization for liver metastases has resulted in dramatically high response rates within the liver (90%), but this therapy does not appear to affect extrahepatic disease or to improve survival.[187,188]

In summary, most experts recommend resection of metastatic insulinomas if it can be done safely and all tumor can be removed. If it appears unlikely that all tumor can be removed and the disease is not progressive, most experts do not treat until there is clear evidence of disease progression. If there is evidence of progression and the disease is localized to the liver, chemoembolization may be helpful. If there is evidence of progression and the disease is systemic in nature, chemotherapy with doxorubicin, streptozotocin, and 5-FU is appropriate. Control of hypoglycemic symptoms should be accomplished with diet, diazoxide, verapamil, or octreotide. More than one of these agents may be necessary.

UNUSUAL AND NONFUNCTIONING ISLET CELL TUMORS

Incidence

Nonfunctioning islet cell tumors include truly nonfunctional tumors that do not appear to produce known peptides as well as tumors that produce pancreatic polypeptide and tumors that produce other hormones that do not cause a characteristic syndrome. Nonfunctional tumors are about as common as insulinomas and gastrinomas (ie, about 1 per million population). Unusual islet cell tumors include those that produce VIP (vipomas), glucagon (glucagonomas), ACTH, somatostatin (somatostatinomas), and growth hormone–releasing factor. These tumors occur at an approximate rate of less than 0.1 per million people. Each of the unusual functional islet cell tumors produces a characteristic syndrome that distinguishes it from other tumors and aids in its clinical detection (see Table 27-1).

Signs and Symptoms

Nonfunctioning islet cell tumors cause symptoms related to the mass effect or malignant nature of the tumor, with invasion into the stomach, bowel, or splenic vein and associated gastric varices, gastrointestinal hemorrhage, and hypersplenism.[189] These patients have pain, upper or lower gastrointestinal bleeding or fullness, and early satiety (see Table 27-1).

Patients with vipomas have severe secretory diarrhea, often exceeding 5 L/d.[6,190] These patients also have hypochlorhydria, hypokalemia, and, occasionally, hypercalcemia. The secretory diarrhea is so severe that dehydration and weakness are common. Recognition of secretory diarrhea by noting the presence of continued high output of stool despite the absence of oral intake is the clinical key to the diagnosis.

Patients with glucagonomas have a characteristic rash called *necrolytic migratory erythema* that is pathognomonic for the disease.[191,192] The rash is red, raised, scaly, and itchy, and it can come and go for no apparent reason. The rash usually is located in the groin, on the buttocks, or on the distal lower extremities. Patients with glucagonomas almost always scratch the rash incessantly, making it worse. These patients have type II diabetes with mild glucose intolerance. They usually have profound evidence of cancer cachexia, with marked wasting, weight loss, and decreased body fat. Measurements of fasting plasma levels of amino acids indicate that these patients have severe hypoaminoacidemia with decreased circulating levels of nearly every amino acid.[4] Patients with glucagonomas also have an unusually high incidence of deep venous thrombosis; most have symptoms secondary to either venous obstruction or pulmonary embolus.

Patients with ACTH-producing tumors have the signs and symptoms of Cushing's syndrome.[47] These include truncal obesity, weight gain, hypertension, diabetes, striae, abnormal menstrual periods (including amenorrhea), a high incidence of severe infections, easy bruising, personality change with mood swings, atherosclerosis, and coronary artery disease at a young age. Patients with ACTH-producing tumors usually have evidence of hypersecretion of other peptide hormones, such as gastrin.[193]

Patients with somatostatinomas have gallstones, mild type II diabetes mellitus, and steatorrhea.[194] These patients also may have MEN-1. Patients with tumors that produce growth hormone–releasing factor have evidence of acromegaly. These tumors also occur in the presence of MEN-1.

Diagnosis

The diagnosis of nonfunctional islet cell tumors is dependent on biopsy proof of islet cell tumors. Because these patients have symptoms related to tumor size and invasion, imaging studies such as CT almost always reveal the lesions. Surgical resection or CT-guided needle biopsy provides the unequivocal diagnosis (see Table 27-2).

The diagnosis of vipomas depends on the presence of severe secretory diarrhea with concomitant hypokalemia, hypochlorhydria, hypercalcemia, and elevated fasting levels of VIP. The plasma assay for VIP has been relatively imprecise, but good assays are now available. The diagnosis of glucagonomas is dependent on the characteristic symptom complex, especially the rash, the fasting hypoaminoacidemia, and the hyperglucagonemia (greater than 500 pg/mL). The diagnosis of somatostatinomas is dependent on the presence of the symptom complex of gallstones, steatorrhea, and diabetes, as well as elevated circulating levels of somatostatin-like peptide. Biopsy of a tumor within either the pancreas or the duodenum and staining of the sample with immunoperoxidase for somatostatin also may be necessary, because some tumors are able to synthesize but not secrete somatostatin, and the plasma assay is not widely available. The diagnosis of ectopic ACTH-producing tumors is dependent on the presence of hypercortisolism, increased plasma levels of ACTH, failure to suppress cortisol with dexamethasone, failure to increase ACTH with corticotropin-releasing hormone, and the presence of a source for the ectopic production of ACTH. The most common sources in order of prevalence are small cell lung cancer, bronchial carcinoid, thymic carcinoid, and islet cell cancer. Islet cell tumors that secrete excessive amounts of ACTH also secrete other hormones, such as gastrin, and may cause other syndromes. Ectopic ACTH secretion is a sign of an extremely malignant islet cell tumor. Tumors that produce growth hormone–releasing factor are diagnosed by the presence of acromegaly and the detection of large islet cell tumors of the pancreas.

Pathology and Location of Tumors

Unusual and nonfunctional islet cell tumors are considered to be cancerous until proven otherwise. They are much more likely to be malignant than are insulinomas and appear to be malignant more often than are gastrinomas. Nonfunctional islet cell tumors generally originate within the pancreas and spread to distant sites, usually the liver. These tumors frequently are large at the time of diagnosis because the symptoms they produce result primarily from the local effects of tumor. All localized nonfunctional islet cell tumors should be treated as potentially malignant lesions and resected.

Glucagonomas originate within the pancreas and usually are not resectable for cure at the time of diagnosis. All glucagonomas are potentially malignant and should be considered as such. These tumors seldom are found outside the pancreas. Vipomas can be located outside the pancreas, but usually are found within the gland. These tumors have a malignancy rate similar to that of gastrinomas (about 60%) and sometimes can be cured. Somatostatinomas originate with equal frequency in the duodenum and the pancreas. Somatostatinomas almost always are malignant; patients have distant disease at the time of diagnosis and seldom are cured. Some suggest that patients with pancreatic somatostatinomas usually have the somatostatinoma syndrome and patients with duodenal tumors do not. Some duodenal somatostatinomas appear to synthesize but

not secrete somatostatin, and they stain positively for somatostatin using immunoperoxidase methods. Duodenal somatostatinomas have been associated with von Recklinghausen's disease. Pancreatic ACTH-producing tumors usually present as large pancreatic primary tumors with unresectable metastatic disease. Patients with tumors that produce growth hormone–releasing factor are rare, but most have had large pancreatic primary tumors that may have been malignant.

In summary, these less common islet cell tumors usually are cancerous, but are slower growing than standard exocrine cancer of the pancreas. These tumors often are diagnosed in younger patients, who can withstand more aggressive surgical procedures to remove them. Complete resection of all tumor is associated with durable long-term responses.

Control of Symptoms With Medication

Patients with nonfunctional islet cell tumors have symptoms related to the mass of the tumor or the invasion of adjacent structures. These symptoms can be relieved only by resection of the tumor. Patients with glucagonomas have a severe rash and poor nutrition related to excessive plasma levels of glucagon. These symptoms can be controlled using total parenteral nutrition with added insulin.[195] Studies have demonstrated that the rash is related to a nutritional deficiency in plasma levels of either amino acids or zinc. Total parenteral nutrition with added insulin normalizes plasma levels of amino acids and zinc, resulting in rapid improvement in the rash. However, the administration of octreotide at dosages of 450 μg/d normalizes plasma levels of glucagon, improving the rash and nutritional abnormalities in most patients without the use of total parenteral nutrition.[196] The rash associated with glucagonomas is so severe that medical control of this symptom results in a major improvement in the quality of life.

The diarrhea and electrolyte abnormalities associated with vipomas are debilitating and can be life-threatening. Affected patients have numerous stools with a total daily volume of about 10 L. They also have profound hypokalemia, which results in more weakness and difficulty with ambulation. About one third of patients with vipomas also have significant hypercalcemia. In the past, each of these abnormalities was treated by the vigorous administration of intravenous fluids in preparation for surgery. This method of resuscitation required large volumes of fluid and potassium, and corrected the abnormalities only partially (the severe watery diarrhea persisted). Therefore, patients underwent major surgery with contracted plasma volumes. The use of octreotide in dosages similar to those mentioned earlier has greatly simplified and improved the fluid and potassium management of patients with vipomas.[56,196] Octreotide reduces plasma VIP to normal levels and stops the diarrhea promptly, allowing fluids and potassium to restore patients rapidly.

The hypercortisolism associated with ectopic ACTH-producing tumors must be controlled medically before major surgery is undertaken. Ketoconazole and other drugs may be effective for short periods. However, patients with ectopic ACTH syndrome have the most severe form of hypercortisolism, and bilateral adrenalectomy usually is necessary to control their symptoms.[47]

Imaging Studies to Localize Tumors

In patients with unusual islet cell tumors or nonfunctioning islet cell tumors, tumor localization usually is achieved by CT. Most of these patients have large identifiable tumors within either the pancreas or the duodenum. The typical tumor is within the pancreas; however, somatostatinomas and vipomas may be located outside the gland. Because these tumors often are large at presentation, the extent of disease is a major concern. Therefore, CT also must include accurate images of the liver. In determining resectability, the surgeon may need to use other studies, such as selective arteriography or endoscopic ultrasound to exclude vascular invasion. In operated patients, intraoperative ultrasound may assist in accurately determining the extent and resectability of disease.

Surgery

Unusual islet cell tumors and nonfunctional islet cell tumors almost always are malignant, but they tend to grow and spread slower than do most adenocarcinomas. Surgery improves survival if all tumor can be resected, and may prove curative in selected patients with limited resectable metastatic disease. Unlike the situation with insulinomas and gastrinomas, major pancreatic resection to remove these unusual islet cell tumors is worthwhile because of the greater probability of malignancy.

SURGICAL MANAGEMENT OF UNRESECTABLE METASTATIC ISLET CELL TUMORS

The treatment of patients with unresectable or metastatic islet cell tumors poses a difficult challenge. These patients frequently have advanced disease (the resectability rate of malignant islet cell tumors has been reported to be 26% to 65%). Treatment is directed toward two goals—control of symptoms caused by hormone excess and arrest of the progress of the malignancy.

Numerous pharmacologic approaches have been used to treat symptoms of hormone excess in patients with advanced islet cell tumors (eg, omeprazole for gastrinomas; octreotide for insulinomas, glucagonomas, and vipomas).[197] Although these drugs have been successful in controlling symptoms, they do not appear to influence the progress of the malignancy. Radiotherapy, hepatic artery embolization, single- and combined-agent chemotherapy, and the synthetic peptide somatostatin analogue octreotide all have been used to decrease tumor growth, with response rates as high as 50%.[197]

In general, subjecting patients with locally advanced or metastatic cancer to morbid procedures to reduce tumor bulk has not been a widespread practice. However, patients with metastatic disease from islet cell carcinomas may benefit from surgery in which all grossly evident disease can be removed. This is because symptoms are related directly to the volume of tumor present, and tumor growth is more indolent and survival times are longer than in other carcinomas. Success has been reported with reoperation for metastatic deposits in other neuroendocrine tumors.

In 1978, a patient with insulinoma was described who demonstrated a "marked though transient" improvement after distal pancreatectomy and resection of three liver metastases.[198] Since that time, a few additional reports have confirmed the efficacy of an aggressive surgical approach to patients with locally advanced islet cell tumors or liver metastases. For example, five patients with extensive metastatic gastrinomas were treated prospectively with attempted surgical resection of all tumor from the pancreas, regional nodes, and liver.[147] The patients also were treated with streptozotocin, doxorubicin, and 5-FU chemotherapy. All gross disease was removed in four cases, and these patients had a significant reduction in antisecretory medicine requirements and no demonstrable tumor at follow-up. In two patients, fasting and provoked gastrin levels remained normal 32 months after surgery.

Table 27-6 summarizes several publications describing the results of surgery for metastatic or unresectable pancreatic islet cell tumors. Four cases of palliative resection of advanced glucagonoma were reported between 1978 and 1981.[198,199] In each case, pancreatic resection was performed, and in two cases, liver metastases were resected. These patients all had initial improvement in symptoms, rash, and biochemical parameters. Chemotherapy was initiated in three patients after several months, when signs or symptoms of progression developed. It is difficult to evaluate the contri-

Table 27-6   Surgery for Metastatic Islet Cell Tumors

Author, Year	Tumor Type	Number of Patients	Extent of Disease	Treatment	Complete Resection Possible?	Results	Follow-Up
Murray et al, 1978	Glucagonoma	1	Pancreas, spleen, liver	Distal pancreatectomy, removal of 3 liver metastases, streptozotocin	No	Decrease in insulin and glucagon levels, improved symptoms	23 mo
Montenegro et al, 1980	Glucagonoma	1	Pancreas, liver	Distal pancreatectomy, splenectomy	No	Resolution of rash, symptoms	15 mo
Prinz et al, 1981	Glucagonoma	2	Pancreas, liver	Distal pancreatectomy (2), dacarbazine (2), removal of liver metastases (1)	No	Resolution of rash, improvement of symptoms	3 y 5 y
Danforth et al, 1984	Insulinoma	8	Pancreas 8 of 8, liver 4 of 8, lymph nodes 8 of 8	Excision 1/8, pancreatectomy 7/8, liver resection 1/8, chemotherapy 4/8	6 of 8	7.5-y median survival after curative resection	2.8–22 y
Thompson GB et al, 1988	Islet cell tumor	43	Not stated for this subgroup of patients	Not stated for this subgroup of patients	Not stated for this subgroup of patients	51% symptomatic improvement	6 y
Makowka et al, 1989	Glucagonoma (2); gastrinoma (1)	3	Hepatic metastases	Hepatic transplant (3), nodal dissection (3), pancreatectomy (2)	Yes	All 3 patients alive with no evidence of disease	7–34 mo
Norton et al, 1985	Gastrinoma	5	Pancreas (3), nodes (1), liver (3)	Pancreatectomy (3), nodal dissection (1), hepatic resection (3)	4 of 5	Benefit to 4 patients in whom all disease resected; 2 patients have normal biochemical testing after 32 months	14–32 mo
McEntee et al, 1990	Islet cell tumor	13	Liver	Hepatic resection	6 of 13	Effective palliation, complete relief of symptoms, 10 of 13; alive with no evidence of disease, 5 of 13	4–82 mo

bution of chemotherapy to the outcome of these patients. The patient who was not treated with any adjuvant therapy also had complete resolution of rash and other symptoms for more than 15 months. Since these encouraging initial reports, several larger series have been described. In a series of 17 patients with islet cell tumors, 8 underwent resection of insulinomas with lymph node or liver metastases. Five of these patients also received chemotherapy. All patients showed improvement in symptoms and signs of hyperinsulinemia, and a median survival of 7.5 years was reported.[55] In another report of 43 patients with islet cell tumors, 28 patients underwent palliative operations for unresectable or metastatic disease. Of these patients, 51% were reported to have had improvement in symptoms after surgery.[200]

In a series of 37 patients who underwent hepatic resection for metastatic neuroendocrine tumors, 13 had metastatic pancreatic islet cell tumors. Curative resection was possible in 6 patients, and complete relief of symptoms was reported in 10 patients; 5 patients were alive and free of disease after follow-up of 4 to 82 months.[201] Five patients have been described in whom liver transplantation, pancreatectomy, and extensive nodal dissection was performed for unresectable liver metastases from neuroendocrine tumors.[202] Three of these patients had islet cell tumors (two with metastatic glucagonomas and one with a gastrinoma); the other two patients had metastatic carcinoids. The patient with a gastrinoma died of metastatic disease 10 months after surgery. The two patients with glucagonomas were alive and free of disease at 23 and 41 months after surgery, respectively.

The results of these studies indicate that some patients with metastatic islet cell tumors benefit from extensive surgery to resect primary and distant disease. Because these patients also can survive for years with unresected metastatic islet cell tumors, this extensive surgery must be performed with minimal mortality and acceptable morbidity. If this can be done (as suggested by these reports), survival and quality of life may be improved in selected patients with metastatic islet cell tumors.

REFERENCES

1. Zollinger RM, Ellison EH. Primary peptic ulceration of the jejunum associated with islet cell tumors of the pancreas. Ann Surg 1955;142:709.
2. Gregory RA, Grossman MI, Tracy HJ, Bentley PH. Nature of the gastric secretagogue in Zollinger-Ellison tumors. Lancet 1967;2:543.
3. Gregory RA, Tracy JH, Agarwal KL. Amino acid constitution of two gastrins isolated from Zollinger-Ellison tumor tissue. Gut 1969;10:603.
4. Mallinson CN, Bloom SR, Warin AP, et al. A glucagonoma syndrome. Lancet 1974;2:1.
5. Larsson LI, Hirsch MA, Holst J, et al. Pancreatic somatostatinoma: clinical features and physiologic implications. Lancet 1977;1:666.
6. Verner JV, Morrison AB. Islet cell tumor and a syndrome of refractory watery diarrhea and hypokalemia. Am J Med 1958;29:529.
7. Kloppel G, Heitz PU. Pancreatic endocrine tumors. Pathol Res Pract 1988;183:155.
8. Mukai K, Greider MH, Grotting JC, Rosai J. Retrospective study of 77 pancreatic endocrine tumors using the immunoperoxidase method. Am J Surg Pathol 1982;6:387.
9. Creutzfeldt W. Endocrine tumors of the pancreas: clinical and morphological patterns. In: Fitzgerald PS, Morrison AB, eds. The pancreas. Baltimore, Williams & Wilkins, 1980:208.
10. Jensen RT, Gardner JD. Gastrinoma. In: Go VLW, Brooks FA, DiMagno EP, et al, eds. The exocrine pancreas: biology, pathobiology, and disease, ed 2. New York, Raven, 1986:727.
11. Larsson LI, Grimelius L, Hakanson R, et al. Mixed endocrine pancreatic tumors producing several peptide hormones. Am J Pathol 1975;79:271.
12. Chiang HCV, O'Dorisio TM, Huang SC, Maton PN, Gardner JD, Jensen RT. Multiple hormone elevations in Zollinger-Ellison syndrome: prospective study of clinical significance and of the development of a second symptomatic pancreatic endocrine tumor syndrome. Gastroenterology 1990;99:1565.
13. Wynick D, Williams SJ, Bloom SR. Symptomatic secondary hormone syndromes in patients with established malignant pancreatic endocrine tumors. N Engl J Med 1988;319:605.
14. Wermer P. Endocrine adenomatosis: peptic ulcer in a large kindred. Am J Med 1963;35:205.
15. Marx SJ, Attie MF, Levine MA, Spiegel AM, Downs RW Jr, Lasker RD. The hypocalciuric or benign variant of familial hypercalcemia: clinical and biochemical features in fifteen kindreds. Medicine (Baltimore) 1981;60:397.
16. Marx SJ, Spiegel AM, Levine MA, et al. Primary hyperparathyroidism in familial multiple endocrine neoplasia type I: long-term follow-up of serum calcium after parathyroidectomy. Am J Med 1982;307:416.
17. Marx SJ, Menczel J, Campbell G, Aurbach GD, Spiegel AM, Norton JA. Heterogeneous size of the parathyroid glands in familial multiple endocrine neoplasia type 1. Clin Endocrinol (Oxf=+) 1991;35:521.
18. Norton JA, Cornelius MJ, Doppman JL, Maton PN, Gardner JD, Jensen RT. Effect of parathyroidectomy in patients with hyperparathyroidism, Zollinger-Ellison syndrome, and multiple endocrine neoplasia type 1: a prospective study. Surgery 1987;102:958.
19. van Heerden JA, Srnith SL, Miller LJ. Management of

the Zollinger-Ellison syndrome in patients with multiple endocrine neoplasia type I. Surgery 1986;100: 971.

20. Thompson NW, Lloyd RV, Nishiyama RH, et al. MEN I pancreas: a histological and immunohistochemical study. World J Surg 1984;8:561.

21. Norton JA, Doppman JL, Jensen RT. Cancer of the endocrine system. In: DeVita VT, Hellman S, Rosenberg SA, eds. Cancer: principles and practice of oncology, ed 3. Philadelphia, JB Lippincott, 1989:1269.

22. Larsson C, Skogseid B, Oberg K, Nakamura Y, Nordenskjold M. Multiple endocrine neoplasia type 1 gene maps to chromosome 11 and is lost in insulinoma. Nature 1988;332:85.

23. Nakamura Y, Larsson C, Julier C, et al. Localization of the genetic defect in multiple endocrine neoplasia type I within a small region of chromosome II. Am J Hum Genet 1989;44:751.

24. Fujimori M, Wells SA, Nakamura Y. Fine-scale mapping of the gene responsible for multiple endocrine neoplasia type 1 (MEN 1). Am J Hum Genet 1992;50:399.

25. Knudson AG. Mutation and cancer: statistical study of retinoblastoma. Proc Natl Acad Sci USA 1971;68:820.

26. Francke U, Holmes LB, Atkins L, Riccardi VM. Aniridia-Wilms tumor association: evidence for specific deletion of 11p13. Cytogenet Cell Genet 1979;24:185.

27. Hansen MF, Cavenee WK. Retinoblastoma and the progression of tumor genetics. Trends Genet 1988;4:125.

28. Thompson NW, Lloyd RV, Nishiyama RH, et al. MEN-1 pancreas: a histological and immunohistochemical study. World J Surg 1984;8:561.

29. Pipeleers-Marichal M, Somers G, Willems G, et al. Gastrinomas in the duodenums of patients with multiple endocrine neoplasia type 1 and the Zollinger-Ellison syndrome. N Engl J Med 1990;322:723.

30. Pipeleers-Marichal M, Donow C, Heitz PU, Kloppel G. Pathologic aspects of gastrinomas in patients with Zollinger-Ellison syndrome with and without multiple endocrine neoplasia type I. World J Surg 1993;17:481.

31. Moertel CG, Hanley JA, Johnson LA. Streptozotocin alone compared with streptozotocin plus fluorouracil in the treatment of advanced islet-cell carcinoma. N Engl J Med 1980;303:1189.

32. Moertel CG, Hanley JA. Combination chemotherapy trials in metastatic carcinoid and malignant carcinoid syndrome. Cancer Clin Trials 1979;2:327.

33. Moertel CG, Kvols LK, O'Connell MJ, Rubin J. Treatment of neuroendocrine carcinomas with combined etoposide and cisplatin. Cancer 1991;68:227.

34. Oberg K, Ericksson B, Norheim I. Interferon treatment of neuroendocrine gut tumors. J Clin Oncol 1987;6:80.

35. Oberg K, Lindstrom H, Alm G, Lundquist G. Successful treatment of therapy-resistant pancreatic cholera with human leukocyte interferon. Lancet 1985;1:725.

36. Oberg K, Norheim I, Lind E, et al. Treatment of malignant carcinoid tumors with human leukocyte interferon: long term results. Cancer Treat Rev 1986;70: 1297.

37. Glowniak JV, Shapiro B, Vinik AI, Glaser B, Thompson NW, Cho KJ. Percutaneous transhepatic venous sampling of gastrin: value in sporadic and familial islet-cell tumors and G-cell hyperfunction. N Engl J Med 1982;307:293.

38. Thompson NW. Surgical treatment of the endocrine pancreas and Zollinger-Ellison syndrome in the MEN I syndrome. Henry Ford Hosp Med J 1992;40:195.

39. Thompson NW. Surgical considerations in the MEN-1 syndrome. In: Johnston IDA, Thompson NW, eds. Endocrine surgery. London, Butterworths, 1983:144.

40. Doppman JL, Miller DL, Chang R, et al. Gastrinomas: localization by means of selective intraarterial injection of secretin. Radiology 1990;174:25.

41. Imamura M, Takahashi K. Use of selective arterial secretin injection test to guide surgery in patients with Zollinger-Ellison syndrome. World J Surg 1993;17:433.

42. Sheppard BC, Norton JA, Doppman JL, Maton PN, Gardner JD, Jensen RT. Management of islet cell tumors in patients with multiple endocrine neoplasia: a prospective study. Surgery 1989;106:1108.

43. Malagelada JR, Edis AJ, Adson MA, van Heerden JA, Go VLW. Medical and surgical options in the management of patients with gastrinoma. Gastroenterology 1983;84:1524.

44. Arnold R, Benning R, Neuhaus C, Rolwage M, Trautmann B. Gastroenteropancreatic endocrine tumors: effect of sandostatin on tumor growth. The German Sandostatin Study Group. Metabolism 1992;41:116.

45. von Schrenck T, Howard JM, Doppman JL, et al. Prospective study of chemotherapy in patients with metastatic gastrinoma. Gastroenterology 1988;94:1326.

46. Heitz PU, Kasper M, Polak JM, Kloppel G. Pancreatic endocrine tumors. Hum Pathol 1982;13:263.

47. Zeiger MA, Pass HI, Doppman JD, et al. Surgical strategy in the management of non-small cell ectopic adrenocorticotropic hormone syndrome. Surgery 1992;112:994.

48. Doherty GM, Doppman JL, Shawker TH, et al. Results of a prospective strategy to diagnose, localize and resect insulinomas. Surgery 1991;110:989.

49. Whipple AO. Hyperinsulinism in relation to pancreatic tumors. Surgery 1944;16:289.

50. Pasieka JL, McLeod MK, Thompson NW, Burney RE. Surgical approach to insulinomas: assessing the need for preoperative localization. Arch Surg 1992;127:442.

51. Service FJ, O'Brien PC, Kao PC, Young WF. C-peptide suppression test: effects of gender, age, and body mass index: implications for the diagnosis of insulinoma. J Clin Endocrinol Metab 1992;74:204.

52. Harrison TS, Fajans SS, Floyd JC, et al. Prevalence of diffuse pancreatic beta islet cell disease with hyperinsulin problems in recognition and management. World J Surg 1984;8:583.

53. Maton PN. Use of octreotide acetate for control of symptoms in patients with islet cell tumors. World J Surg 1993;17:504.

54. Fraker DL, Norton JA. The role of surgery in the man-

agement of islet cell tumors. Gastroenterol Clin North Am 1989;18:805.

55. Danforth DN, Gorden P, Brennan MF. Metastatic insulin secreting carcinoma of the pancreas: clinical course and the role of surgery. Surgery 1984;96:1027.

56. Maton PN, O'Dorisio TM, Howe BA, et al. Effect of a long-acting somatostatin analogue (SMS 201-995) in a patient with pancreatic cholera. N Engl J Med 1985;312:17.

57. Stadil F, Stage JG. The Zollinger-Ellison syndrome. Clin Endocrinol Metab 1979;9:433.

58. Jensen RT, Norton JA. Pancreatic endocrine tumors. In: Yamada T, Alpers DH, Owyang C, Powell DW, Silvenstein FE, eds. Textbook of gastroenterology. Philadelphia, JB Lippincott, 1991:1912.

59. Norton JA. Neuroendocrine tumors of the pancreas and duodenum. Curr Probl Surg 1994;31:77.

60. Zollinger RM. Gastrinoma: factors influencing prognosis. Surgery 1985;97:49.

61. Ellison EC, Carey LC, Sparks J, et al. Early surgical treatment of gastrinoma. Am J Med 1987;82:17.

62. Norton JA, Doppman JL, Jensen RT. Curative resection in Zollinger-Ellison syndrome: results of a 10 year prospective study. Ann Surg 1992;215:8.

63. Zollinger RM, Martin EW, Carey LC. Observations on the postoperative tumor growth of certain islet cell tumors. Ann Surg 1976;184:525.

64. Zollinger RM, Ellison EC, O'Dorision T, Sparks J. Thirty years' experience with gastrinoma. World J Surg 1984;8:427.

65. Slimak GG, Pisegna J, Metz DL, Gardner JD, Jensen RT, Maton PN. Use of alpha interferon in patients with metastatic gastrinoma. Gastroenterology 1991;100:A299.

66. Tjon Tham RT, Falke TAM, Jensen JB, Lamers CB. CT and MR imaging in advanced Zollinger-Ellison syndrome. J Comput Assist Tomogr 1989;13:821.

67. Barton JC, Hirschowitz BI, Maton PN, Jensen RT. Bone metastases in malignant gastrinoma. Gastroenterology 1986;91:915.

68. Howard TJ, Sawicki MP, Stabile BE, Watt PC, Pasarro E. Biologic behavior of sporadic gastrinoma located to the right and the left of the superior mesenteric artery. Am J Surg 1993;165:101.

69. Kaplan EL, Horvath K, Udekwu A, et al. Gastrinomas: a 42 year experience. World J Surg 1990;14:365.

70. Thom AK, Norton JA, Axiotis CA, Jensen RT. Location, incidence and malignant potential of duodenal gastrinomas. Surgery 1991;110:1086.

71. Thompson NW, Vinik AI, Eckhauser FE. Microgastrinomas of the duodenum. Ann Surg 1989;209:396.

72. Thompson NW, Pasieka J, Fukuuchi A. Duodenal gastrinomas, duodenotomy, and duodenal exploration in the surgical management of Zollinger-Ellison syndrome. World J Surg 1993;17:455.

73. Stabile BE, Morrow DJ, Passaro E. The gastrinoma triangle: operative implications. Am J Surg 1984;147:25.

74. Sugg SL, Norton JA, Fraker DL, et al. A prospective study of intraoperative methods to diagnose and resect duodenal gastrinomas. Ann Surg 1993;218:138.

75. Wolfe MM, Alexander RW, McGuigan JE. Extrapancreatic, extraintestinal gastrinoma: effective treatment by surgery. N Engl J Med 1982;306:1533.

76. Delcore R Jr, Cheung LY, Friesen SR. Outcome of lymph node involvement in patients with Zollinger-Ellison syndrome. Ann Surg 1988;206:291.

77. Norton JA, Doppman JL, Collen MJ, et al. Prospective study of gastrinoma localization and resection in patients with Zollinger-Ellison syndrome. Ann Surg 1986;204:468.

78. Friesen SR. Are "aberrant nodal gastrinomas" pathogenetically similar to "lateral aberrant thyroid" nodules? Surgery 1990;107:236.

79. Jensen RT, Gardner JD. Zollinger-Ellison syndrome: clinical presentation, pathology, diagnosis and treatment. In: Dannenberg A, Zakim D, eds. Peptic ulcer and other acid-related diseases. New York, Academic Research Association, 1991:117.

80. Harmon JW, Norton JA, Collen MJ. Removal of gastrinomas for control of Zollinger-Ellison syndrome. Ann Surg 1984;200:396.

81. Maton PN, Macken SM, Norton JA, Gardner JD, O'Dorisio TM, Jensen RT. Ovarian carcinoma as a cause of Zollinger-Ellison syndrome. Gastroenterology 1989;97:464.

82. Primrose JN, Maloney M, Wells M, Bulgin O, Johnston D. Gastrin-producing ovarian mucinous cystadenomas: a cause of Zollinger-Ellison syndrome. Surgery 1988;104:830.

83. Podevin P, Ruszniewski P, Mignon M, et al. Management of multiple endocrine neoplasia type I (MEN I) in Zollinger-Ellison syndrome. Gastroenterology 1990;98:A230.

84. Andersen DK. Current diagnosis and management of Zollinger-Ellison syndrome. Ann Surg 1989;210:685.

85. Wolfe MM, Jensen RT. Zollinger-Ellison syndrome: current concepts in diagnosis and management. N Engl J Med 1987;317:1200.

86. Friesen SR. Treatment of the Zollinger-Ellison syndrome: a 25 year assessment. Am J Surg 1982;143:331.

87. Thompson JC, Reeder DD, Villar HV, Fender HR. Natural history and experience with diagnosis and treatment of the Zollinger-Ellison syndrome. Surg Gynecol Obstet 1975;140:721.

88. Cameron AJ, Hoffman HN. Zollinger-Ellison syndrome: clinical features and long-term follow-up. Mayo Clin Proc 1974;49:44.

89. Bondeson AG, Bondeson L, Thompson NW. Stricture and perforation of the esophagus: overlooked threats in Zollinger-Ellison syndrome. World J Surg 1990;14:361.

90. Waxsman I, Gardner JD, Jensen RT, Maton PN. Peptic ulcer perforation as the presentation of Zollinger-Ellison syndrome. Dig Dis Sci 1991;36:19.

91. Miller LS, Vinayek R, Frucht H, Gardner JD, Jensen RT, Maton PN. Reflux esophagitis in patients with Zollinger-Ellison syndrome. Gastroenterology 1990;98:341.

92. Maton PN, Gardner JD, Jensen RT. Recent advances in the management of gastric hypersecretion in patients with Zollinger-Ellison syndrome. Med Clin North Am 1989;18:847.

93. Maton PN, Frucht H, Vinayek R, Wank SA, Gardner JD, Jensen RT. Medical management of patients with Zollinger-Ellison syndrome. Gastroenterology 1988;94:294.

94. Bonfils S, Landor SH, Mignon M, et al. Results of surgical management in 92 consecutive patients with Zollinger-Ellison syndrome. Ann Surg 1981;194:692.

95. Deveney CW, Deveney KE, Stark D, Moss A, Stein S, Way LW. Resection of gastrinomas. Ann Surg 1983;198:546.

96. McGuigan JE, Wolfe MM. Secretin injection test in the diagnosis of gastrinoma. Gastroenterology 1980;79:1324.

97. Okunieff P, Zietman A, Kahn J, et al. Lack of efficacy of water-suppressed proton nuclear magnetic resonance spectroscopy of plasma for the detection of malignant tumors. N Engl J Med 1990;322:953.

98. Isenberg JI, Walsh JH, Passaro EJ, Moore EW, Grossman MI. Unusual effect of secretin on serum gastrin, serum calcium, and gastric acid secretion in a patient with suspected Zollinger-Ellison syndrome. Gastroenterology 1972;62:626.

99. Lamers CBH, van Tongeren JHM. Comparative study of the value of calcium, secretin, and meal stimulated increase in serum gastrin in the diagnosis of the Zollinger-Ellison syndrome. Gut 1977;18:128.

100. Frucht H, Howard JM, Slaff JF. Secretin and calcium provocative tests in patients with Zollinger-Ellison syndrome: a prospective study. Ann Intern Med 1989;111:713.

101. Slaff JI, Howard JM, Maton PN, et al. Prospective assessment of provocative gastrin tests in 81 consecutive patients with Zollinger-Ellison syndrome. Gastroenterology 1986;90:1637.

102. Friesen SR, Tomita T. Pseudo–Zollinger-Ellison syndrome: hypergastrinemia, hyperchlorhydria without tumor. Ann Surg 1981;194:481.

103. McCarthy DM. The place of surgery in the Zollinger-Ellison syndrome. N Engl J Med 1980;302:1344.

104. Thompson JC, Lewis BG, Wiener I, Townsend CMJ. The role of surgery in the Zollinger-Ellison syndrome. Ann Surg 1983;197:594.

105. Maton PN, Vinayek R, Frucht H, et al. Long term efficacy and safety of omeprazole in patients with Zollinger-Ellison syndrome: a prospective study. Gastroenterology 1989;97:827.

106. Meijer JL, Jansen JB, Lamers CB. Omeprazole in the treatment of Zollinger-Ellison syndrome and histamine H2-antagonist refractory ulcers. Digestion 1989;44:31.

107. Vinayek R, Amantea MA, Maton PN, Fruchet H, Gardner JD, Jensen RT. Pharmacokinetics of oral and intravenous omeprazole in patients with Zollinger-Ellison syndrome. Gastroenterology 1991;101:138.

108. Vinayek R, Frucht H, London JF, et al. Intravenous omeprazole in patients with Zollinger-Ellison syndrome undergoing surgery. Gastroenterology 1990;99:10.

109. McArthur KE, Collen MJ, Maton PN. Omeprazole: effective convenient therapy for Zollinger-Ellison syndrome. Gastroenterology 1985;88:939.

110. Lamers CDHW, Lind T, Moberg S, Jansen JBMJ, Olbe L. Omeprazole in Zollinger-Ellison syndrome: effects of a single dose and of long term treatment in patients resistant to histamine H2-receptor antagonists. N Engl J Med 1984;310:758.

111. Metz DC, Pisegna JR, Fishbeyn VA, Benya RV, Jensen RT. Control of gastric acid hypersecretion in the management of patients with Zollinger-Ellison syndrome. World J Surg 1993;17:468.

112. Fraker DL, Norton JA, Saeed ZA, Maton PN, Gardner JD, Jensen RT. A prospective study of perioperative and postoperative control of acid hypersecretion in patients with Zollinger-Ellison syndrome undergoing gastrinoma resection. Surgery 1988;104:1054.

113. McCarthy DM, Hyman PE. Effect of isopropamide on response to oral cimetidine in patients with Zollinger-Ellison syndrome. Dig Dis Sci 1982;27:345.

114. Norton JA, Jensen RT. Unresolved surgical issues in the management of patients with Zollinger-Ellison syndrome. World J Surg 1991;15:151.

115. Ekman L, Hansson E, Havu N. Toxicological studies on omeprazole. Scand J Gastroenterol 1985;20(Suppl 108):53.

116. Poynter D, Pick CR, Harcourt RA. Association of long-lasting unsurmountable histamine H2 blockage and gastric carcinoid tumors in the rat. Gut 1985;26:1284.

117. Larsson H, Carlsson E, Mattsson H. Plasma gastrin and gastric enterochromaffin cell activation and proliferation: studies with omeprazole and ranitidine in intact and antrectomized rats. Gastroenterology 1986;90:391.

118. Richardson CT, Peters MN, Feldman M. Treatment of Zollinger-Ellison syndrome with exploratory laparotomy, proximal gastric vagotomy, and H2-receptor antagonists. Gastroenterology 1985;89:357.

119. McCarthy DM, Peikin SR, Lopatin RN. Hyperparathyroidism: a reversible cause of cimetidine-resistant gastric hypersecretion. BMJ 1979;1:765.

120. Frucht H, Doppman JL, Norton JA, et al. MR imaging of gastrinomas: comparison with computed tomography, angiography and ultrasound. Radiology 1989;171:713.

121. London JB, Shawker TH, Doppman HL, et al. Prospective assessment of abdominal ultrasound in patients with Zollinger-Ellison syndrome. Radiology 1991;178:763.

122. Norton JA, Cromack DT, Shawker TH, et al. Intraoperative ultrasonographic localization of islet cell tumors. Ann Surg 1988;207:160.

123. Rosch T, Lightdale CJ, Botet JF, et al. Localization of pancreatic endocrine tumors by endoscopic ultrasonography. N Engl J Med 1992;326:1721.

124. Ruszniewski P, Mouyal PA, Combes R, et al. Endoscopic ultrasonography (EUS) is useful for localization of primary gastrinomas. Gastroenterology 1991;100:A297.

125. VanEyck CHJ, Bruining HA, Reubi JC, et al. Use of iso-tope-labelled somatostatin analogs for visualization of islet cell tumors. World J Surg 1993;17:444.

126. Lamberts SW, Bakker WH, Reubi JC, Krenning EP. So-matostatin receptor imaging in the localization of endo-crine tumors. N Engl J Med 1990;323:1246.

127. Lamberts SW, Hofland LJ, van Koetsveld PM, et al. Par-allel in vivo and in vitro detection of functional somato-statin receptors in human endocrine tumors: conse-quences with regard to diagnosis, localization and therapy. J Clin Endocrinol Metab 1990;31:566.

128. Lamberts SW, Hofland LJ, van Koetsveld PM, et al. Par-allel in vivo and in vitro detection of functional somato-statin receptors in human endocrine pancreatic tumors: consequences with regard to diagnosis, localization and therapy. J Clin Endocrinol Metab 1990;71:566.

129. Lamberts SW, Reubi JC, Krenning EP. Somatostatin re-ceptor imaging in the diagnosis and treatment of neuro-endocrine tumors. J Steroid Biochem Mol Biol 1992;43:185.

130. Lamberts WH, Krenning EP, Breeman WA, et al. So-matostatin receptor imaging: in vivo localization of tu-mors with a radiolabeled somatostatin analog. J Steroid Biochem Mol Biol 1991;37:1079.

131. Wank SA, Doppman HL, Miller DL, et al. Prospective study of the ability of computerized axial tomography to localize gastrinomas in patients with Zollinger-Ellison syndrome. Gastroenterology 1987;92:905.

132. Maton PN, Miller DL, Doppman HL, et al. Role of selec-tive angiography in the management of Zollinger-El-lison syndrome. Gastroenterology 1987;92:913.

133. Thom A, Norton JA, Doppman JL, Miller D, Chang R, Jensen RT. A prospective study of the use of intraarterial secretin injection and portal venous sampling to localize duodenal gastrinomas. Surgery 1992;112:1002.

134. Stabile BE, Morrow DJ, Passaro E. The gastrinoma tri-angle: operative implications. Am J Surg 1984;147:25.

135. Imamura M, Takahaski K, Adachi H, et al. Usefulness of selective arterial secretin injection test for localization of gastrinoma in the Zollinger-Ellison syndrome. Ann Surg 1987;205:230.

136. Imamura M, Takashi MP, Isobe Y, Hattori Y, Satomura K, Tobe T. Curative resection of multiple gastrinomas aided by selective arterial secretin injection and intra-operative secretin test. Ann Surg 1989;210:710.

137. Ko TC, Flisak M, Prinz RA. Selective intra-arterial meth-ylene blue injection: a novel method of localizing gas-trinoma. Gastroenterology 1992;102:1062.

138. Cherner JA, Doppman JL, Norton JA, et al. Prospective assessment of selective venous sampling for gastrin to localize gastrinomas. Ann Intern Med 1986;105:841.

139. Miller DL, Doppman JL, Metz D, Maton PN, Jensen RT. Portal venous sampling in Zollinger-Ellison syndrome: technique, results and complications in 95 procedures. Radiology 1992;182:235.

140. Buchler M, Friess H, Klempa I, et al. Role of octreotide in the prevention of postoperative complications fol-lowing pancreatic resection. Am J Surg 1992;163:125.

141. Lange JR, Steinberg S, Doherty GM, et al. A randomized prospective trial of postoperative somatostatin analogue in patients with neuroendocrine tumors of the pan-creas. Surgery 1992;112:1033.

142. Thompson NW, Vinik AI, Eckhauser FE. Microgastrino-mas of the duodenum: a cause of failed operations for the Zollinger-Ellison syndrome. Ann Surg 1989;209:396.

143. Carty SE, Jensen RT, Norton JA. Prospective study of aggressive resection of metastatic pancreatic endocrine tumors. Surgery 1992;112:1024.

144. Frucht H, Norton JA, London JF, et al. Detection of du-odenal gastrinomas by operative endoscopic transillu-mination: a prospective study. Gastroenterology 1990;99:1622.

145. Howard TJ, Zinner MJ, Stabile BE, Passaro EJ. Gas-trinoma excision for cure. Ann Surg 1990;211:9.

146. Stabile BE, Passaro E. Benign and malignant gas-trinoma. Am J Surg 1984;149:144.

147. Norton JA, Sugarbaker PH, Doppman JL, et al. Aggres-sive resection of metastatic disease in selected patients with malignant gastrinoma. Ann Surg 1986;203:352.

148. McCune CS, Marquis DM. Interleukin 1 as an adjuvant for active specific immunotherapy in a murine tumor model. Cancer Res 1990;50:1212.

149. Fishbeyn VA, Norton JA, Benya RV, et al. Assessment and prediction of long-term cure in patients with Zol-linger-Ellison syndrome: the best approach. Ann Intern Med 1993;119:199.

150. Norton JA, Levin B, Jensen RT. Cancer of the endocrine system. In: DeVita VT Jr, Hellman S, Rosenberg SA, eds. Cancer: principles and practice of oncology, ed 4. Phila-delphia, JB Lippincott, 1993:1333.

151. Norton JA, Whitman ED. Insulinoma. Endocrinologist 1993;3:258.

152. Norton JA, Sigel B, Baker AR, et al. Localization of an occult insulinoma by intraoperative ultrasonography. Surgery 1985;97:381.

153. Pasieka JL, McLeod MK, Thompson NW, Burney RE. Surgical approach to insulinomas assessing the need for localization. Arch Surg 1992;127:442.

154. Stefanini P, Carboni M, Patrassi N. Surgical treatment and prognosis of insulinoma. Clin Gastroenterol 1974;3:697.

155. Stefanini P, Carboni M, Patrassi N, Basoli A. Beta-islet cell tumor of the pancreas: results of a study on 1,067 cases. Surgery 1974;76:597.

156. Stovroff MC, Norton JA. Changing concepts of islet cell dysplasia in neonatal and infantile hyperinsulinism. World J Surg 1988;12:608.

157. Friesen SR. Tumors of the endocrine pancreas. N Engl J Med 1982;306:580.

158. Friesen SR, Tomita T, Kimmel JR. Pancreatic polypep-tide update: its role in detection of the trait for multiple endocrine adenopathy syndrome, type I and pancreatic polypeptide-secreting tumors. Surgery 1983;94:1028.

159. Comi RJ, Gorden P, Doppman HL, Norton JA. Insu-linoma. In: Go VLW, Gardner JD, Brooks FP, et al, eds.

The exocrine pancreas: biology, pathology and diseases. New York, Raven Press, 1986:745.

160. Kahn CR, Rosen SW, Weintraub BD, et al. Ectopic production of chorionic gonadotropin and its subunits by islet cell tumors: a specific marker for malignancy. N Engl J Med 1977;297:565.

161. Service FJ, Dale AJ, Elveback LR, Jiang N. Insulinoma: clinical and diagnostic features of 60 consecutive cases. Mayo Clin Proc 1976;51:417.

162. Grunberger G, Weiner JL, Silverman R, Taylor S, Gorden P. Factitious hypoglycemia due to surreptitious administration of insulin: diagnosis, treatment and long-term follow-up. Ann Intern Med 1988;108:252.

163. Murakami K, Taniguchi H, Kobayshi T, Seki M, Oimomi M, Baba S. Suppression of insulin release by calcium antagonist in human insulinoma in vivo and in vitro: its possible role for clinical use. Kobe J Med Sci 1979;25:237.

164. Stehouwer CD, Lems WF, Fischer HR, Hackeng WH. Malignant insulinoma: is combined treatment with verapamil and the long-acting somatostatin analogue octreotide (SMS 201-995) more effective than single therapy with either drug? Neth J Med 1989;35:86.

165. Maton PN. The use of the long-acting somatostatin analogue, octreotide in patients with islet cell tumors. Gastroenterol Clin North Am 1989;18:897.

166. Kvols LK, Buck M, Moertel CG, et al. Treatment of metastatic islet cell tumors with a somatostatin analogue. Ann Intern Med 1987;107:162.

167. Norton JA, Shawker TH, Doppman JL, et al. Localization and surgical treatment of occult insulinomas. Ann Surg 1990;212:615.

168. Fraker DL, Norton JA. Localization and resection of insulinomas and gastrinomas. JAMA 1988;259:3601.

169. Liessi G, Pasquale C, D'Andrea AA, Scandellari C, Pedrazzoli S. MRI in insulinomas: preliminary findings. Eur J Radiol 1992;14:46.

170. Dunnick NR, Long JA, Krudy A, et al. Localizing insulinomas with combined radiographic methods. AJR Am J Roentgenol 1980;135:747.

171. Doppman JL, Brennan MF, Dunnick NR, Kahn CR, Gorden P. The role of pancreatic venous sampling in the localization of occult insulinoma. Radiology 1981;138:557.

172. Pedrazzoli S, Pasquali C, Miotto D, Feltrin G, Petrin P. Transhepatic portal sampling for preoperative localization of insulinomas. Surg Gynecol Obstet 1987;165:101.

173. Roche A, Raisonnier A, Gillon-Savouret MC. Pancreatic venous sampling and arteriography in localizing insulinomas and gastrinomas: procedure and results in 55 cases. Radiology 1982;145:621.

174. Vinik AI, Delbridge L, Moattari R, Cho K, Thompson N. Transhepatic portal vein catheterization for localization of insulinomas: a ten-year experience. Surgery 1991;109:1.

175. Doppman JL, Miller DL, Chang R, Gorden P, Norton JA. Insulinomas: localization with selective intraarterial injection of calcium. Radiology 1991;178:237.

176. Doppman JL, Miller DL, Chang R, Gorden P, Eastman RC, Norton JA. Intraarterial calcium stimulation test for detection of insulinomas. World J Surg 1993;17:439.

177. van Heerden JA, Grant CS, Czako PF, Service FJ, Charboneau JW. Occult functioning insulinomas: which localizing studies are indicated? Surgery 1992;112:1010.

178. Bottger TC, Junginger T. Is preoperative radiographic localization of islet cell tumors in patients with insulinoma necessary? World J Surg 1993;17:427.

179. Bottger TC, Weber W, Beyer J, Junginger T. Value of tumor localization in patients with insulinoma. World J Surg 1990;14:107.

180. Grant CS, van Heerden J, Charboneau JW, James EM, Reading CC. Insulinoma: the value of intraoperative ultrasonography. Arch Surg 1988;123:843.

181. Kudlow JE, Albisser AM, Angel A, et al. Insulinoma resection facilitated by the artificial endocrine pancreas. Diabetes 1978;27:774.

182. Tutt GO Jr, Edis AJ, Servie FJ, van Heerden JA. Plasma glucose monitoring during operation for insulinoma: a critical reappraisal. Surgery 1980;88:351.

183. Nauck M, Stockman F, Creutzfeldt W. Evaluation of a euglycaemic clamp procedure as a diagnostic test in insulinoma patients. Eur J Clin Invest 1990;20:15.

184. Krentz AD, Hale PJ, Baddeley RM, Williams AC, Natrass M. Intraoperative blood glucose and serum insulin concentrations in the surgical management of insulinoma. Postgrad Med J 1990;66:24.

185. Rothmund M, Angelini L, Brunt LM, et al. Surgery for benign insulinoma: an international review. World J Surg 1990;14:393.

186. Carty S, Jensen RT, Norton JA. Prospective study of aggressive resection of metastatic pancreatic endocrine tumors. Surgery 1992;112:1024.

187. Moertel CG. An odyssey in the land of small tumors. J Clin Oncol 1987;5:1502.

188. Moertel CG, May GR, Martin JK, et al. Sequential hepatic artery occlusion and chemotherapy for metastatic carcinoid tumor and islet cell carcinoma. Proc Am Soc Clin Oncol 1985;4:80.

189. Kent RB, van Heerden JA, Weiland LH. Nonfunctioning islet cell tumors. Ann Surg 1981;193:185.

190. Marks IN, Bank S, Louw JH. Islet cell tumor of the pancreas with reversible watery diarrhea and achlorhydria. Gastroenterology 1967;52:695.

191. Wilkinson DS. Necrolytic migratory erythema with carcinoma of the pancreas. Trans St John's Hosp Dermatol Soc 1973;59:244.

192. Kahan RS, Perez Figaredo MRA, Neimaius A. Necrolytic migratory erythema: distinctive dermatosis of the glucagonoma syndrome. Arch Dermatol 1977;113:792.

193. Maton PN, Gardner JD, Jensen RT. The incidence and etiology of Cushing's syndrome in patients with Zollinger-Ellison syndrome. N Engl J Med 1986;315:1.

194. Vinik AI, Moattari AR. Treatment of endocrine tumors. Endocrinol Clin North Am 1989;18:483.

195. Norton JA, Kahn CR, Schieberger R, et al. Amino acid deficiency and skin rash associated with glucagonoma. Ann Intern Med 1979;91:213.

196. Maton PN, Gardner JD, Jensen RT. The use of the long acting somatostatin analogue 201-995 in patients with pancreatic endocrine tumors. Dig Dis Sci 1989;34:29S.

197. Modlin IM, Lewis JJ, Ahlman G. Management of unresectable malignant endocrine tumors of the pancreas. Surg Gynecol Obstet 1993;176:507.

198. Murray GT, Nakhood AF, Rae L. Remission of hypoglycemia after partial resection of a metastatic islet cell tumor. Am J Surg 1978;135:846.

199. Prinz RA, Badrinth K, Bunerji M. Operative and chemotherapeutic management of malignant glucagon producing tumors. Surgery 1981;90:713.

200. Thompson GB, van Heerden JA, Grant CS, Camey JA, Ilstrup DM. Islet cell carcinomas of the pancreas: a twenty-year experience. Surgery 1988;104:1011.

201. McEntee GP, Nagorney DM, Kvols LK, et al. Cytoreductive hepatic surgery for neuroendocrine tumors. Surgery 1990;108:1091.

202. Makowka L, Tzakis AG, Mazzaferro V, et al. Transplantation of the liver for metastatic endocrine tumors of the intestine and pancreas. Surg Gynecol Obstet 1989;168:107.

203. Mignon M, Ruszniewski P, Haffar S, Rigaud D, Rene E, Bonfils S. Current approach to the management of the tumoral process in patients with gastrinoma. World J Surg 1986;10:702.

204. Montenegro F, Lawrence GD, Macon W, Pass C. Metastatic glucagonoma: improvement after surgical debulking. Am J Surg 1980;139:424.

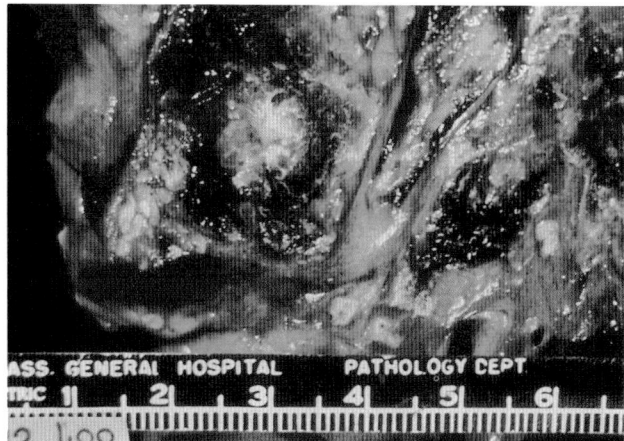

Color Figure 24-1

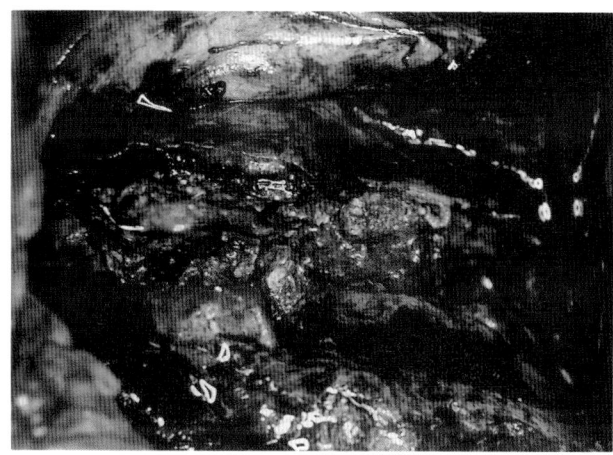

Color Figure 24-5

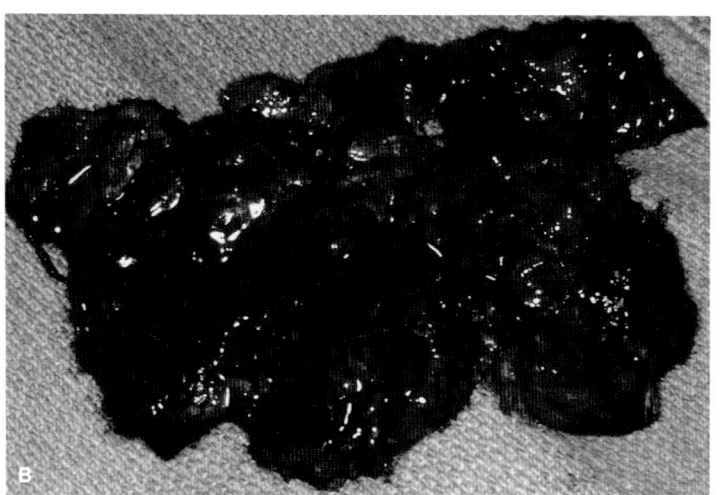

Color Figure 24-9

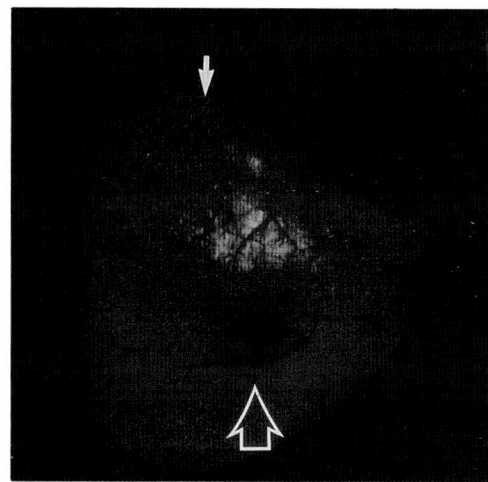

Color Figure 27-4

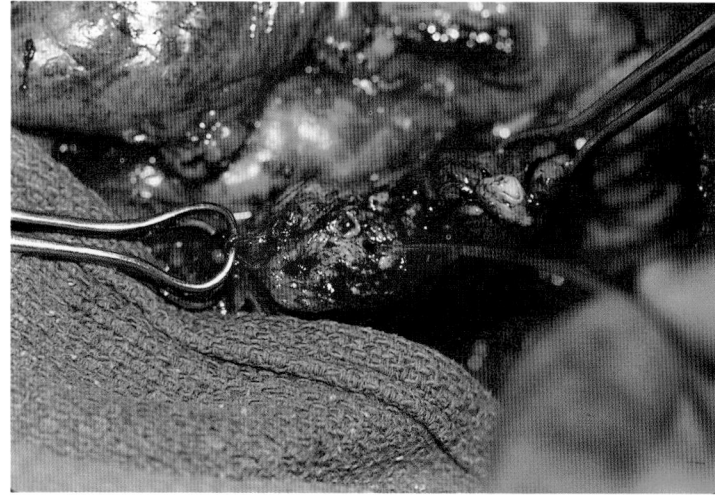

Color Figure 29-8

Digestive Tract Surgery: A Text and Atlas, edited by Richard H. Bell, Layton F. Rikkers, and Michael W. Mulholland. Lippincott-Raven Publishers, Philadelphia, © 1996.

28

Pancreatic Transplantation

Robert J. Stratta | *Rodney J. Taylor*

Diabetes mellitus is a disease of metabolic dysregulation characterized by inappropriate hyperglycemia due to a progressive loss of insulin secretion or action. The syndrome of diabetes mellitus not only is defined by abnormal glucose metabolism but also is associated chronically with specific microvascular and nonspecific macrovascular complications (Fig. 28-1). Diabetes mellitus afflicts about 6% of the population and is the third most common disease and the eighth leading cause of death in the United States.[1] Of the estimated 12 million diabetic patients in the United States, 4 million take insulin, and 1 to 2 million have insulin-dependent diabetes mellitus (IDDM; type I, juvenile onset). Nearly 30,000 new cases of IDDM are diagnosed each year. In most cases of IDDM, progressive β-cell destruction within the pancreatic islets is believed to be due to an autoimmune process resulting in insulin deficiency or absence.[2]

The characteristic long-term complications that are specific to diabetes include retinopathy, nephropathy, and neuropathy.[3] Diabetes mellitus is the leading cause of kidney failure and blindness in adults, the number one disease causing amputations and impotence, and one of the leading chronic diseases of childhood.[1,3,4] In addition, diabetes mellitus is associated with accelerated atherosclerosis, abnormal lipid metabolism, and cardiovascular disease, and it accounts for more than 160,000 deaths per year in the United States.[3]

The discovery of insulin in 1922 changed IDDM from an acute, rapidly fatal disease into a chronic, incurable disease. Although exogenous insulin therapy is effective at preventing acute metabolic decompensation and is life-saving, most patients with IDDM develop one or more end-organ complications during their lifetime (Table 28-1). During the past decade, evidence that the microvascular complications of diabetes mellitus result from hyperglycemia has increased.[3,4] Long-term hyperglycemia may result in excessive glycosylation of circulating and membrane-bound proteins, leading to basement membrane thickening and microangiopathy.[5] Even with tight control, exogenous insulin cannot achieve the glucose metabolism of an endogenous insulin source that responds to moment-to-moment changes in glucose concentration and therefore protects against the development of microvascular complications over time.

Efforts to develop a closed-loop insulin pump coupled to a glucose sensor, mimicking β-cell function in which the secretion of insulin is closely regulated, have not been successful. The transplantation of free grafts of insulin-producing tissue (islet cells) has likewise not become a reliable therapeutic option.[6] The results of the Diabetes Control and Complication Trial[7] clearly indicated that intensive control of glucose can significantly reduce (but not completely protect against) the long-term microvascular complications of diabetes mellitus. The only form of total endocrine replacement therapy that has been successful in the treatment of diabetes mellitus is pancreas transplantation as an immediately vascularized graft.[8]

RATIONALE FOR PANCREAS TRANSPLANTATION

Vascularized pancreas transplantation was first developed to provide an autoregulating endogenous source of insulin responsive to normal feedback controls. Successful pancreas transplantation is the only known therapy that establishes an insulin-independent eugly-

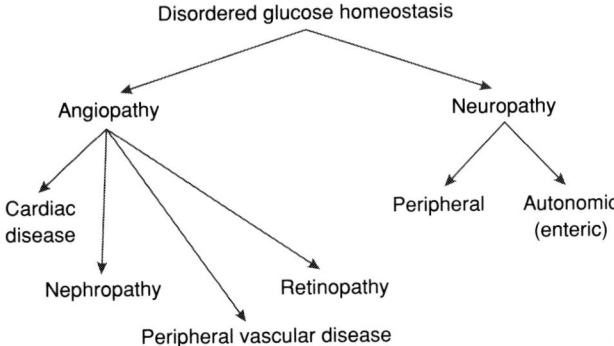

Figure 28-1 Complications of insulin-dependent diabetes mellitus.

cemic state with complete normalization of glycosylated hemoglobin levels.[9,10] The penalties for normal glucose homeostasis are the operative risks of the transplantation procedure and the need for chronic immunosuppression. In some patients, correcting dysmetabolism is the primary goal, and it is clear that a successful pancreas transplantation can result in a markedly improved quality of life.[10,11]

The effects of a functioning pancreas transplantation on the course of established secondary diabetic complications are variable. Although one of the long-range goals of pancreas transplantation is to ameliorate the secondary complications of diabetes, it is difficult to predict who is at risk and what will be the natural history of complications in the individual patient. The morbidity of diabetes is considerable, and it is controversial as to whether the incidence and severity of problems associated with long-term immunosuppression would be less, the same, or more than those associated with long-term diabetes. With improvements in organ retrieval technology, refinements in surgical techniques, and advances in clinical immunosuppression, success rates for vascularized pancreas transplantation have improved dramatically. As a result, pancreas transplantation, (particularly combined pancreas–kidney transplantation) has become an accepted treatment option in appropriately selected patients with IDDM.

BACKGROUND

The first human pancreas transplantation was performed in 1966 at the University of Minnesota.[12] A low level of clinical activity in pancreas transplantation occurred through 1980, with only a few of the earliest attempts being successful.[13,14] These early attempts were fraught with many problems, such as limited graft

and patient survival, difficulties with organ preservation, and management of exocrine secretions. These pioneering efforts demonstrated, however, that the pancreas graft could restore an insulin-independent, euglycemic state to a diabetic patient for a sustained period.

Pancreas Registry

The International Pancreas Transplant Registry (IPTR) was organized in 1980 to provide historical and current data on clinical pancreas transplantation.[15] From December 16, 1966, to August 1, 1994, 6016 pancreas transplantations were performed worldwide and reported to the IPTR.[16] More than three fourths of these cases were performed after September 30, 1987. Since October 1, 1987, all US cases have also been reported to the United Network for Organ Sharing (UNOS) through a subcontract with the IPTR (Fig. 28-2). About 84% of pancreas transplantations have been performed in conjunction with a simultaneous kidney transplantation, whereas the remaining 16% are pancreas transplantation alone, sequential pancreas-after-kidney transplantation, or combined with a single organ other than the kidney or multiple organs (Fig. 28-3).

Registry Results

In the United States, the overall 1-year patient and pancreas graft functional survival (completely insulin-independent) rates are 91% and 72%, respectively (Fig. 28-4). A number of individual centers are reporting even higher graft (more than 90%) and patient (more than 95%) survival rates, particularly with combined pancreas–kidney transplantation[17–19] (Fig. 28-5). Analysis of pancreas transplantation registry data has identified improved results in the following circumstances[16]:

Table 28-1   Morbidity of Diabetes

Complication	Cumulative Prevalence (%)	Relative Risk*
Blindness	16	20
End-stage renal disease	22	25
Amputation	12	40
Myocardial infarction	21	2–5
Stroke	10	2–3

* Relative risk versus nondiabetic population.
(After Nathan DM. Long-term complications of diabetes mellitus. N Engl J Med 1993;328:1676)

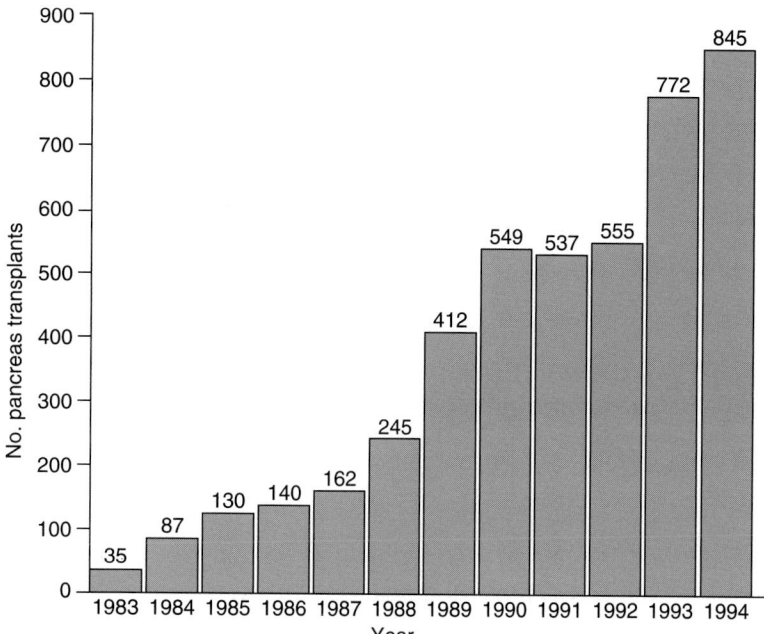

Figure 28-2 Clinical pancreas transplants in the United States from 1983 to 1994 according to the United Network for Organ Sharing registry data.

- In the most recent era
- With better human leukocyte antigen matching
- With pancreas preservation times less than 30 hours
- In patients receiving a combined pancreas–kidney transplant rather than a solitary pancreas transplant
- With bladder drainage of the exocrine secretions
- In patients receiving quadruple immunosuppression
- in recipients younger than 45 years

More than 70 US centers have reported pancreas transplantations to the UNOS registry. Combined pancreas–kidney transplantation in uremic diabetic patients is performed routinely at many transplantation centers. Position statements from the American Diabetes Association and the American Society of Transplant Surgeons have recommended that pancreas transplantation be considered as an acceptable therapeutic alternative to continued insulin therapy in patients with IDDM and end-stage renal disease who either have already had or plan to have a kidney transplantation.

Experience with solitary pancreas transplantation is more limited, with registry results approaching only about 50% 1-year success (Fig. 28-6). For these reasons, recommendations regarding solitary pancreas trans-

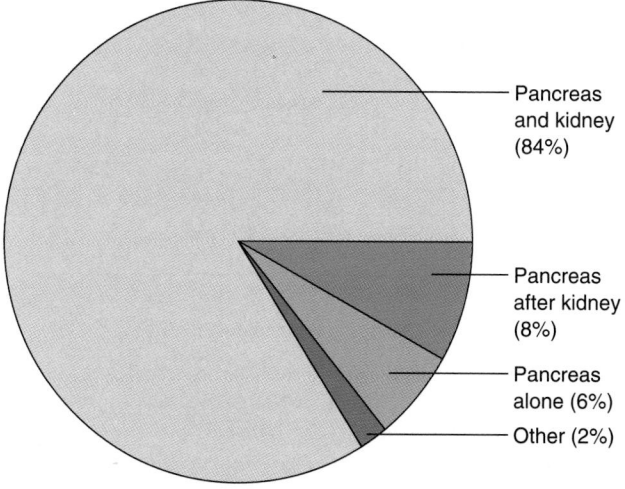

Figure 28-3 Relative numbers of vascularized pancreas transplantations performed according to recipient category.

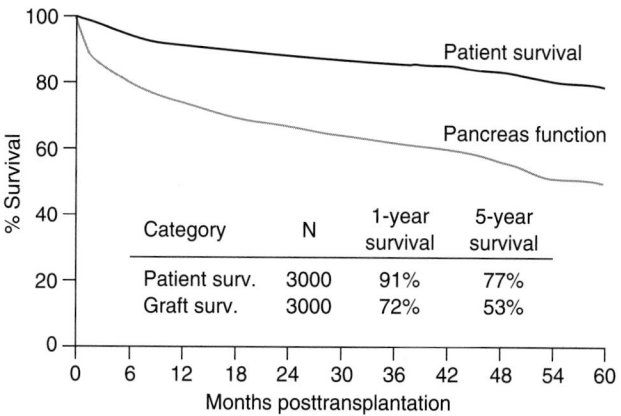

Category	N	1-year survival	5-year survival
Patient surv.	3000	91%	77%
Graft surv.	3000	72%	53%

Figure 28-4 Patient and pancreas functional (insulin-independent) graft survival for all bladder-drained cadaveric pancreas transplantations reported to the United Network for Organ Sharing registry, October 1987 to August 1994.

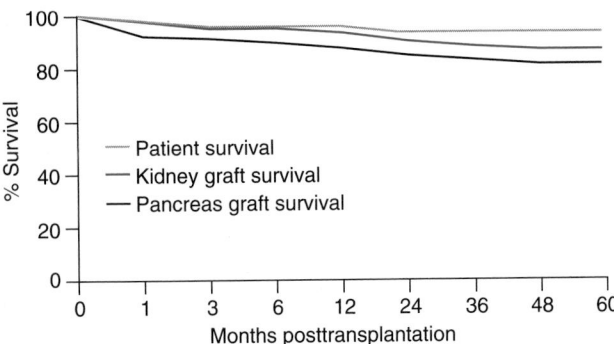

Figure 28-5 Actuarial patient, kidney, and pancreas graft survival for 116 consecutive combined pancreas–kidney transplantations (PKT) performed at the University of Nebraska Medical Center/Clarkson Hospital, April 1989 to January 1995.

plantation are less definite and include patients with IDDM who have failed exogenous insulin therapy.

INDICATIONS

The indications for pancreas transplantation vary among different centers.[20] Nevertheless, certain guidelines have been followed by the leading transplantation centers and have been further modified by clinical experience. Among these are the presence of IDDM, the predicted ability to tolerate the operative procedure, the requisite postoperative immunosuppression, and possible associated complications. In addition, emotional and psychosocial stability to deal with the procedure, possible complications, and sequelae is important. Patients and their families must fully comprehend the nature of the procedure and realize that long-term data are not yet available.

The outcome of pancreas transplantation can be measured in several ways, including patient survival, graft functional survival (insulin independence), normalization of carbohydrate and lipid metabolism, effects on diabetic complications, and impact on quality of life. The assumption that pancreas transplantations are performed primarily to influence the secondary complications of diabetes is not really correct at this time; the overall effect on quality of life is the most important benefit.

PATIENT SELECTION

Typical exclusion, inclusion, and entry criteria for pancreas transplantation are listed in Table 28-2. Combined pancreas–kidney transplantation should be con-

sidered in all type I diabetic patients with significant nephropathy along with the usual options of kidney transplantation alone or dialysis. Patients with significant nephropathy are defined as those who are dialysis dependent or dialysis imminent, with a creatinine clearance of less than 20 mL/min or failure of a prior kidney transplantation. Patients with IDDM and impending or end-stage renal failure who have minimal or limited secondary complications of diabetes (usually between the ages of 20 and 40 years) are considered optimal candidates for combined pancreas–kidney transplantation. However, not all patients with IDDM and renal failure are acceptable candidates. Some centers regard a history of blindness or major amputation as a contraindication to combined pancreas–kidney transplantation.[18] Although these diabetes-related problems are certainly irreversible, a number of patients are well adjusted to these complications and can lead productive lives after dual organ transplantation with facilitated rehabilitation.[11,17]

Pretransplantation Evaluation

Patient selection is aided by a comprehensive multidisciplinary pretransplantation evaluation (Table 28-3). The medical evaluation is tailored to the individual patient based on the investigation of specific signs or symptoms. The work-up confirms the diagnosis of IDDM, determines the patient's ability to withstand the operative procedure, establishes the absence of any ex-

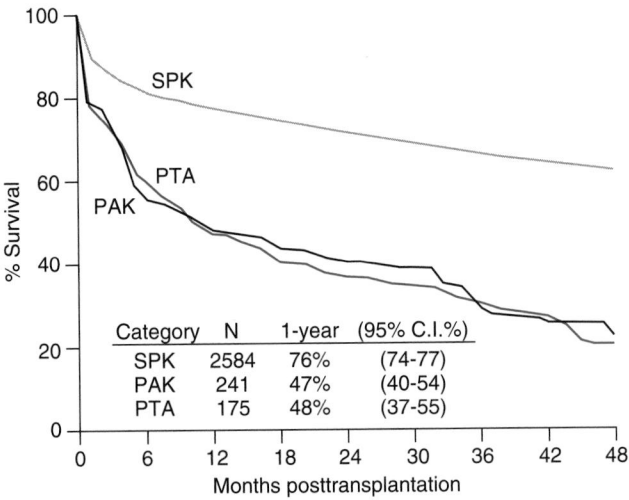

Figure 28-6 Pancreas graft functional survival rates by recipient category for all bladder-drained cadaveric pancreas transplantations reported to the United Network for Organ Sharing registry, October 1987 to August 1994 ($P < .0001$). SPK, simultaneous pancreas–kidney transplantation; PAK, pancreas-after-kidney transplantation; PTA, pancreas transplantation alone.

Table 28-2 Exclusion, Inclusion, and Entry Criteria for Pancreas Transplantation

EXCLUSION CRITERIA

Insufficient cardiovascular reserve (one or more of the following):
  Coronary angiographic evidence of significant noncorrectable coronary artery disease
  Ejection fraction below 50%
  Recent myocardial infarction
Ongoing substance abuse (drug or alcohol)
Major ongoing psychiatric illness
Significant history of noncompliance
Active infection or malignancy
Lack of well-defined diabetic complications
Extreme obesity (>50% ideal body weight)
Inability to understand the therapeutic nature of pancreas transplantation

INCLUSION CRITERIA

Presence of type I diabetes mellitus (documented by metabolic testing when indicated)
Ability to withstand surgery and immunosuppression (as assessed by pretransplantation medical evaluation)
Emotional and sociopsychological suitability
Able to understand investigational nature
Presence of secondary diabetic complications
Financial resources

SPECIFIC ENTRY CRITERIA FOR COMBINED PANCREAS–KIDNEY TRANSPLANTATION

Diabetic nephropathy: creatinine clearance <40 mL/min

SPECIFIC ENTRY CRITERIA FOR PANCREAS TRANSPLANTATION ALONE

The presence of two or more diabetic complications, defined as:
  Proliferative retinopathy
  Early nephropathy with a creatinine clearance >70 mL/min and proteinuria >150 mg/24 h but <3 g/24 h
  The presence of overt peripheral or autonomic neuropathy
  Vasculopathy with accelerated atherosclerosis, *or*
The presence of hyperlabile diabetes as defined by an adverse event scoring system that takes into account the frequency and severity of episodes of ketoacidosis, hypoglycemia, infections, and impairment in quality of life
Creatinine clearance >55 mL/min and serum creatinine <2 mg/dL after cyclosporine challenge test

SPECIFIC ENTRY CRITERIA FOR PANCREAS-AFTER-KIDNEY TRANSPLANTATION

Stable renal allograft function on maintenance immunosuppression with a serum creatinine <2 mg/dL or creatinine clearance >60 mL/min (>40 mL/min if patient on cyclosporine), *and one of the following:*
  Progressive diabetic complications (any one)
  Hyperlabile diabetes with significant impairment in quality of life

(After Stratta RJ, Taylor RJ, Wahl TO, et al. Recipient selection and evaluation for vascularized pancreas transplantation. Transplantation 1993;55:1090)

Table 28-3 Evaluation of the Pancreas Transplantation Candidate

INTERVIEWS AND CONSULTS

History and physical examination by nephrologist, endocrinologist, and transplantation surgeon
Ophthalmology evaluation, including visual acuity, fluorescein angiography, retinal fundus photography with retinopathy score and slit-lamp examination
Transplantation coordinator and medical social worker interview, including completion of quality of life questionnaire
Gynecology consultation for all females (pelvic examination with Pap smear)
Dental evaluation
When indicated, additional evaluations may be required by orthopedic surgery, podiatry, psychology, psychiatry, neurology, or gastroenterology

CARDIOVASCULAR, RESPIRATORY, AND PERIPHERAL VASCULAR EVALUATIONS

Standard testing includes orthostatic vital signs, 12-lead electrocardiogram, chest radiograph, and exercise treadmill or stress thallium study
Additional studies may include arterial blood gases, echocardiography, autonomic and peripheral vasomotor reflexes, Doppler arterial studies, ankle and brachial index, transcutaneous oxygen monitoring, plethysmography, carotid Doppler examination, aortography with run-off, or pulmonary function tests as indicated
Cardiology consultation with or without coronary angiography as indicated

METABOLIC AND ENDOCRINE EVALUATION

Standard testing includes fasting blood glucose, glycohemoglobin, and fasting lipid panel (cholesterol, triglycerides, and high-density lipoprotein-cholesterol)
Fasting and stimulated C-peptide levels are used to assess type of diabetes if needed

GENITOURINARY AND RENAL EVALUATION

Standard testing includes electrolytes, blood urea nitrogen, creatinine, urinalysis with culture, 24-h urine for protein and creatinine clearance, voiding cystourethrogram with postvoid residual, and radiometric glomerular filtration rate
In addition, kidney biopsy or evaluation of erectile dysfunction may be indicated
Cyclosporine challenge test when indicated

SEROLOGY AND IMMUNOLOGY EVALUATION

ABO blood type and human leukocyte antigen tissue type
Cytotoxic antibodies
Viral titers (Epstein-Barr virus, herpes simplex virus, varicella-zoster virus, human immunodeficiency virus, hepatitis B virus, hepatitis C virus, and cytomegalovirus)
VDRL/FTA for syphilis

OTHER LABORATORY TESTS

Complete blood count with differential and platelets, prothrombin time, partial thromboplastin time, chemistry profile, amylase, lipase
Abdominal ultrasound of kidneys and gallbladder
Mammography in women older than 35 y
Hemoccult ($\times$3)
When indicated, nerve conduction studies, gastric emptying scan, electromyography

(After Stratta RJ, Taylor RJ, Wahl TO, et al. Recipient selection and evaluation for vascularized pancreas transplantation. Transplantation 1993;55:1090)

clusion criteria, and documents end-organ complications for future tracking after transplantation. In a suitable candidate, the work-up is also used to determine the type and timing of the pancreas transplantation procedure. The primary determinants for recipient selection are degree of nephropathy and cardiovascular risk. The degree of renal dysfunction (creatinine clearance less than 40 mL/min) may be used to select patients for preemptive combined pancreas–kidney transplantation versus pancreas transplantation alone (creatinine clearance more than 70 mL/min). In patients with intermediate renal function (clearance 40 to 70 mL/min or severe proteinuria), oral cyclosporine challenge testing may be performed to determine renal functional reserve.[20]

Cardiac Evaluation

The cardiovascular evaluation is paramount and used to determine operative risk. Coronary angiography is performed in cases in which the history, physical examination, or noninvasive cardiac studies (especially stress thallium) reveal any abnormality. Characteristics such as age more than 45 years, diabetes for more than 25 years, a positive smoking history, long-standing hypertension, previous major amputation due to peripheral vascular disease, or history of cerebrovascular disease are usual indications for performing cardiac catheterization.[21] A history of previous myocardial infarction, angioplasty, or coronary artery bypass grafting is not necessarily a contraindication to pancreas transplantation. In these cases, stress thallium or echocardiographic imaging (as a functional assessment), in combination with coronary angiography (to provide precise anatomic data), is helpful in defining operative risk.[22] Age more than 60 years, active smoking, and severe obesity (more than 50% ideal body weight) are usually viewed as contraindications to pancreas transplantation. Other contraindications that are applicable to all solid-organ transplantations include the presence of active infection or malignancy, active drug abuse or drug dependence, and a significant history of noncompliance.

Type of Transplantation

Kidney transplantation is the treatment of choice for many patients with advanced diabetic nephropathy.[23] The addition of a pancreas transplantation remains somewhat controversial because of concerns over increased morbidity and mortality.[24–26] A number of groups have reported an actual improvement in graft survival after combined pancreas–kidney transplantation versus cadaver donor kidney transplantation alone in uremic diabetic patients.[26,27] Combined pancreas-kidney transplantation is rapidly becoming accepted as the best treatment option in carefully selected patients with type I diabetes with significant nephropathy. The dual-organ transplantation procedure eliminates the need both for dialysis and exogenous insulin administration, achieves superior metabolic control, and improves quality of life. Despite increased morbidity, the addition of pancreas transplantation to kidney transplantation in appropriately selected patients with IDDM does not appear to jeopardize either the patient or the kidney transplantation and can result in excellent patient and graft survival with greater potential for complete rehabilitation.

Timing of Transplantation

The timing of combined pancreas–kidney transplantation relative to the degree of nephropathy is also a matter of controversy.[17,20] Many diabetic patients with impending renal failure are referred for transplantation before the initiation of dialysis. Combined pancreas-kidney transplantation can be performed safely and effectively in the absence of uremia, thereby facilitating rehabilitation and providing the potential for arresting the progression of diabetic complications before the development of end-stage renal disease.[17] This is not considered preemptive, especially in view of increasing waiting times, the variable progressive nature of diabetic complications, and the diminished survival that diabetic patients have on dialysis.

Solitary Pancreas Transplantation

Specific selection criteria for solitary pancreas transplantation continue to evolve as strategies are designed to minimize the side effects of immunosuppression.[20,28–30] In patients with IDDM and well-functioning kidney transplants, sequential pancreas-after-kidney transplantation has been advocated because these patients are already obligated to chronic immunosuppression.[28] In sequential grafting, the additional risk is primarily that of the surgical procedure. Ideally, solitary pancreas transplantation should be performed before the development of diabetic complications, such as the need for kidney transplantation. No reliable markers exist to predict, before the earliest lesions appear, which diabetic patients will have complications with subsequent progression.[3] The dilemma of patient selection for solitary pancreas transplantation is further compounded by the fact that the probability of success is not as high as with combined pancreas-kidney transplantation.[31]

Therefore, selection criteria for solitary pancreas

transplantation are less clear and are based on the presence of early diabetic complications or exogenous insulin failure.[9,20,28–30] Except for the rare case of extremely hyperlabile diabetes, establishment of insulin independence alone does not justify the need for chronic immunosuppression if an effect on secondary diabetic complications cannot be realized. Solitary pancreas transplantation is restricted by necessity to those patients who have already demonstrated a propensity to early diabetic complications that are (or predictability will be) worse than the potential undesirable side effects of chronic immunosuppression. In these patients, however, the benefit/risk ratio of solitary pancreas transplantation is not clear and will be determined by documentation of the prevention or arrest of secondary diabetic complications and quality-of-life issues. For these reasons, solitary pancreas transplantation is being performed by only a few centers in the United States in highly selected diabetic patients in the setting of strict investigative protocols.

DONOR SELECTION AND MANAGEMENT

Donor Selection

Donor selection and organ procurement are of paramount importance to the success of pancreas transplantation. Most brain-dead donors who maintain a heartbeat and who are appropriate for kidney, heart, lung, and liver donation are also suitable for pancreas donation. Indications and contraindications to pancreas donation are listed in Table 28-4. Although there is some evidence that donor hyperglycemia may have a deleterious effect on initial and long-term allograft function, the presence of hyperglycemia or hyperamylasemia per se are not usual contraindications to pancreas donation.[32,33]

In general, ideal pancreas donors range in age from 10 to 50 years and range in weight from 30 to 100 kg. In donors who weight less than 30 kg, the size of the gland and vessels are such that the risk of vascular thrombosis may be increased. Similarly, in older donors, problems can arise with advanced atherosclerosis extending beyond the origin of the celiac and superior mesenteric arteries and leading to the subsequent risk of thrombosis. In the obese donor, the technical complexity of the multiple-organ procurement, coupled with the potential for latent type II diabetes, places not only the pancreas at risk but other organs removed as well.

Table 28-4   Cadaveric Pancreas Organ Donation

INDICATIONS
Declaration of brain death
Informed consent
Age 6–55 y
Weight 30–100 kg
Hemodynamic stability with adequate perfusion and oxygenation
Normal glycosylated hemoglobin level (in cases of severe hyperglycemia, extreme obesity, or positive family history of diabetes)
Absence of infectious or transmissible diseases (ie, tuberculosis, syphilis, hepatitis, AIDS)
Negative serology (HIV; hepatitis A, B, C; VDRL/RPR for syphilis)
Absence of malignancy (unless skin or low-grade brain cancer)
Absence of pancreatic disease

CONTRAINDICATIONS
History of diabetes mellitus (type I or II)
Previous pancreatic surgery
Pancreatic trauma
Pancreatitis (active acute or chronic)
Intraabdominal contamination
Major (active) infection
Chronic alcohol abuse
Recent history of intravenous drug abuse
Recent history of homosexuality
Prolonged hypotension or hypoxemia with evidence for significant end-organ (kidney, liver) damage
Severe atherosclerosis
Massive transfusions, prior splenectomy, extreme obesity, abnormal anatomy*

* All are relative contraindications.

Donor Management

Management of the multiple-organ donor includes aggressive resuscitation to maintain hemodynamic stability, organ perfusion, and oxygenation. Large-bore intravenous access, central and arterial line pressure monitoring, urinary output measurement, and ventilatory support with 100% oxygen are instituted routinely. Resuscitative efforts usually result in significant hyperglycemia, and there is some evidence to suggest that intensive control with insulin may have a favorable effect on allograft function and survival.[32] Liberal use of intravenous colloid fluids is advocated to minimize pancreatic edema. Judicious administration of vasopressors, such as dopamine, is indicated to maintain the systolic blood pressure higher than 90 mmHg and to promote diuresis.

Living-related pancreas donation is reserved for patients in whom high cytotoxic antibody titers have developed, rendering it difficult if not impossible to find a negative donor crossmatch.[6] A portion of the body and tail of the pancreas can be removed from a living donor, based on a vascular pedicle of the splenic vessels.[34] Although the results of living-related segmental pancreas transplantation have been acceptable, the potential short- and long-term risks to the donor are such that this procedure is reserved for highly selective situations, particularly in the setting of a relative surplus of cadaveric pancreas grafts.

ORGAN PROCUREMENT AND PRESERVATION

Advances in organ retrieval and preservation technology have played an important role in the improving results of pancreas transplantation.[35] Combined liver, kidney, and whole-organ pancreaticoduodenal retrieval can be safely performed in virtually all donors irrespective of vascular anomalies.[35,36] Removal of the whole pancreas is considered the most difficult organ procurement procedure from a technical standpoint, and the success of pancreas transplantation is significantly influenced by the degree of expertise with which the pancreas is retrieved. Until recently, procurement surgeons removed either the liver or the pancreas from the same donor because the combined removal of both organs appeared to compromise their function and survival. In the last several years, a number of experienced groups have reported excellent results with the routine procurement of both the liver and the whole pancreas from the same donor.[35–37]

The pertinent anatomy of pancreas donation is shown in Figure 28-7. Although a number of techniques have been described, most authors advocate combined en bloc hepaticopancreaticoduodenosplenectomy followed by backtable separation of the organs.

Multiple-Organ Retrieval

The operative procedure requires a long midline incision from the sternal notch to the symphysis. The falciform ligament is divided to avoid injury to the liver before median sternotomy. After inspection of the intraabdominal viscera, a nasogastric tube is positioned into the duodenum and is subsequently irrigated with 250 to 500 mL of solution, such as povidone-iodine or amphotericin (50 mg/L amphotericin). The abdominal viscera are then mobilized and retracted cephalad so that the distal aorta and inferior vena cava can be dissected and prepared for cannulation in the event that the donor becomes unstable. The inferior mesenteric artery may be ligated and divided to ensure adequate mobilization of the aorta. The aortic dissection is continued up above the left renal vein, and the proximal superior mesenteric artery is exposed. The dissection then proceeds in the porta hepatis, where the vascular anatomy to the liver is defined and ligamentous attachments are divided. Specific attention is directed to the gastrohepatic ligament to identify an accessory or replaced left hepatic artery. The posterior aspect of the porta hepatis is also carefully inspected, palpated, and dissected to identify a potential accessory or replaced right hepatic artery. The common bile duct is encircled, ligated distally, and transected. A small incision is made in the fundus of the gallbladder to enable saline irrigation of the biliary tract. The gastroduodenal artery is then identified and usually ligated and divided. The common hepatic artery is dissected back to the proximal splenic artery, which is encircled and tagged with a suture. This portion of the dissection usually requires excision of a celiac lymph node. The portal vein is dissected and encircled about 2 cm superior to the pan-

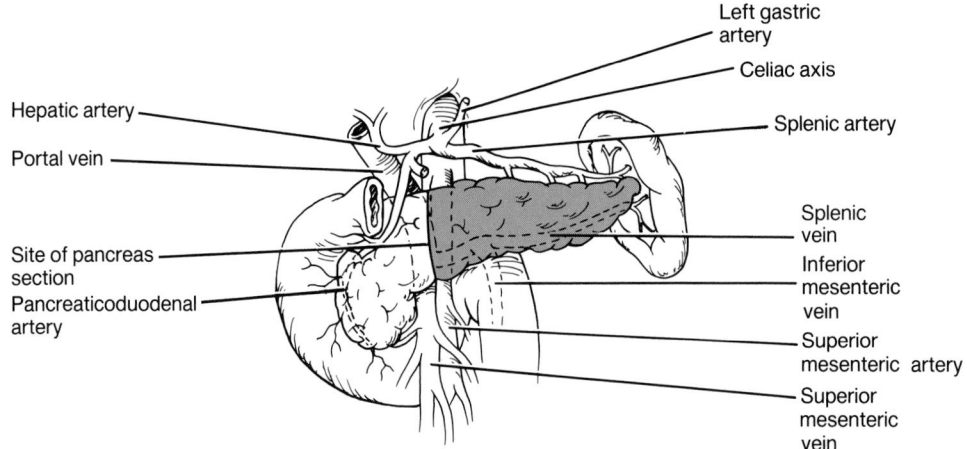

Figure 28-7 Pertinent anatomy for both segmental and whole-organ pancreas donation. Pancreatic transection is performed only in cases of segmental donation.

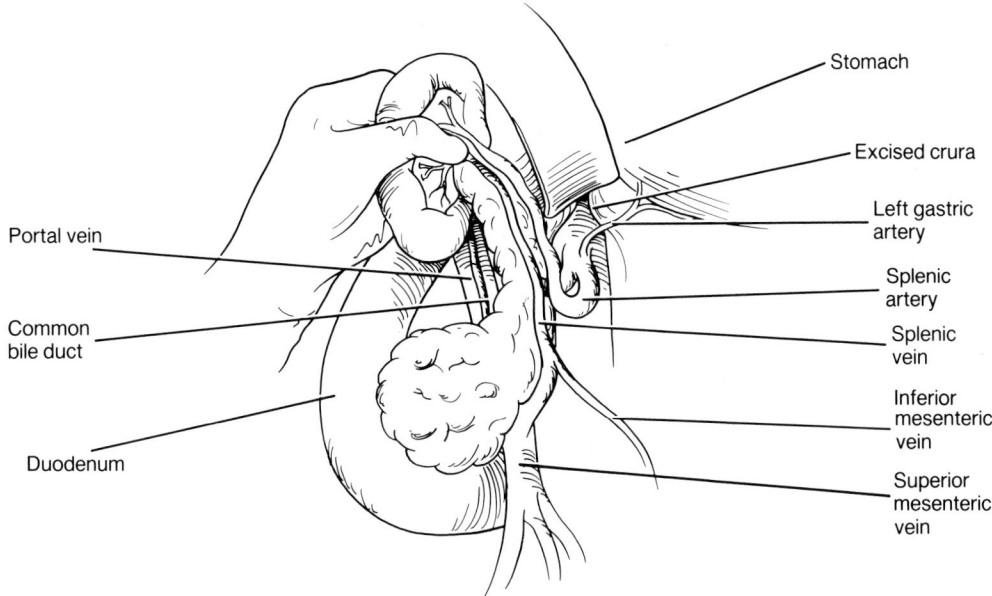

Figure 28-8 Technique of ''no-touch'' donor pancreatectomy using the spleen as a handle.

creas. The diaphragmatic crura are then divided and the supraceliac aorta encircled.

A no-touch pancreatic dissection is then begun with a wide Kocher maneuver to mobilize the duodenum and head of the pancreas. The gastrocolic and gastrosplenic ligaments are divided, including the short gastric vessels, to enable access to the lesser sac and mobilization of the stomach. The left gastric vessels may be ligated and divided depending on the vascular anatomy to the liver. The nasogastric tube is then pulled back into the stomach as the proximal duodenum is transected with a GIA stapling device. The spleen is mobilized and used as a handle to lift the tail and body of the pancreas out of the retroperitoneum (Fig. 28-8). The inferior mesenteric vein is identified and may be used for portal cannulation or ligated and divided. The ligament of Treitz is then taken down and the distal duodenum divided with a GIA stapler. The middle colic vessels are ligated and divided, and the lateral peritoneal attachments to the colon are divided to enable caudad mobilization of the colon. The base of the small bowel mesentery is next isolated.

The donor is then systemically anticoagulated with 20,000 U intravenous heparin. Portal cannulation may be performed through the inferior mesenteric vein, a branch of the superior mesenteric vein, or directly into the portal vein after cardiac arrest with subsequent portal vein transection. In any case, no precooling through the portal vein is necessary. Cannulas are placed in the distal aorta and vena cava. When cardiac arrest is induced, in situ flush with a maximum of 2.5 to 3 L of cold University of Wisconsin (UW) solution (50 mL/kg)

is begun through the aortic cannula, followed by cross-clamping of the supraceliac aorta and base of the small bowel mesentery. Alternatively, the superior mesenteric artery and vein can be separately identified and individually ligated before heparinization or the mesentery can be merely divided after completion of the in situ flush. The vena cava cannula is placed to dependent drainage to ensure adequate decompression. The portal vein is then completely transected 2 cm above the pancreas and cannulated with a hand-held cannula (Fig. 28-9). Alternatively, the portal flush can be performed through the inferior mesenteric vein, superior mesenteric vein, or even on the backtable after organ removal without portal vein transection. In most cases, a maximum 1 to 1.5 L of cold UW solution (25 mL/kg) is flushed through the portal vein simultaneously with the aortic flush.

Liver–Pancreas Separation

Combined en bloc hepaticopancreaticoduodenosplenectomy is performed with the celiac axis and superior mesenteric artery removed on a common aortic segment. Bilateral en bloc nephroureterectomy is then performed by standard techniques. Backtable separation of the liver and pancreas is then begun, with preservation of the celiac axis blood supply to the liver (Fig. 28-10). The splenic artery is usually transected about 1 cm from its origin. Care is taken to preserve an aortic patch with the celiac axis. In cases of an accessory or replaced right hepatic artery off the superior mesenteric artery, the aortic patch should

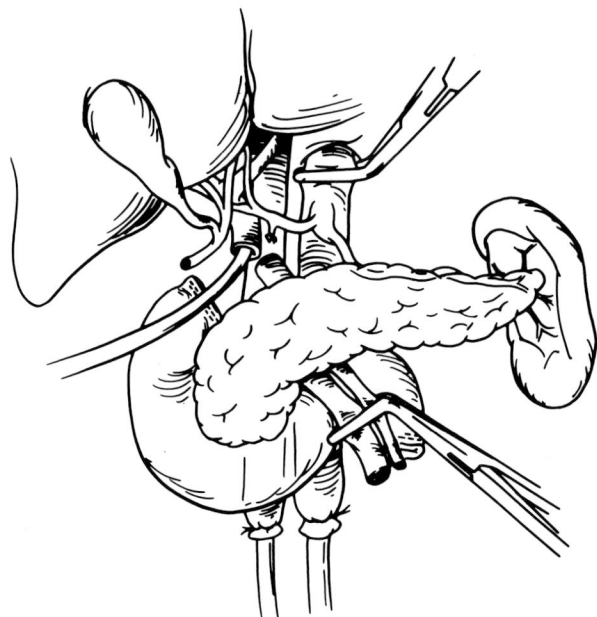

Figure 28-9 Technique of en bloc combined liver–pancreas removal with in situ perfusion of intraabdominal viscera through distal aorta with decompression through distal inferior vena cava, cross-clamping of supraceliac aorta and base of small bowel mesentery, and transection of portal vein 2 cm above pancreas with direct cannulation for portal flush.

include both the celiac axis and the superior mesenteric artery, which is then transected 1 cm distal to the aberrant right hepatic artery to preserve the vascular anatomy to the liver. Ex vivo flush of the liver through the portal vein is performed with an additional 500 mL (10 mL/kg) of cold UW solution. The liver is then immersed and packaged separately in sterile UW solution at about 4°C. The pancreas is then carefully inspected to ensure vascular and parenchymal integrity, and tagging sutures may be placed on the splenic, superior mesenteric, and gastroduodenal arteries. The base of the small bowel mesentery may be trimmed and then oversewn with a running monofilament suture. Alternatively, individual identification and ligation of the superior mesenteric vessels can be performed, or the mesentery may be left long for the recipient surgeon. The duodenum–pancreas–spleen specimen can then be packaged separately in sterile UW solution after splenic fragments are removed for tissue typing. The kidneys are then separated and, likewise, packaged separately in sterile cold UW solution.

Rapid removal of both the liver and pancreas is possible with a minimal dissection technique in an otherwise unstable donor.[38] As previously indicated, the liver and pancreas are removed en bloc, and the organs are separated ex vivo. In highly selected cases, the liver,

pancreas, and kidneys can all be removed as an en bloc specimen with subsequent separation. Whole-organ pancreas retrieval is not compatible with small bowel procurement.

Pancreas Preservation

The introduction of UW solution into clinical transplantation has permitted safe and extended cold storage preservation of the pancreas up to 30 hours without compromise of graft function.[35] Other solutions used include Euro-Collins and Silica Gel Filtered Plasma. The enhanced margin of safety afforded by extended preservation in UW solution has increased the capability for distant organ procurement and sharing, minimized organ wastage, improved the efficiency of organ retrieval, allowed time for crossmatching and adequate preparation of the recipient, and enabled semielective performance of the recipient operation. More important, the quality of preservation has improved, resulting in better initial graft function with fewer complications, such as pancreatitis or vascular thrombosis.

Pancreas Reconstruction

Bilateral donor iliac artery and vein grafts are retrieved at the time of multiple-organ procurement. Before the recipient operation, the pancreas is prepared for transplantation under cold storage conditions in a separate operating suite.[35] Preparation of the pancreas involves several steps that require careful attention to detail to avoid organ injury and facilitate the transplantation. The first step involves mobilization of the portal vein from the pancreatic bed to elongate the vein and allow for a tension-free venous anastomosis in the recipient. If the donor portal vein is shorter than 2 cm, it may be necessary to lengthen the vein with an iliac vein autograft in an end-to-end fashion. The superior mesenteric and splenic arteries are then mobilized and reconstructed with a donor iliac artery bifurcation Y autograft (Fig. 28-11). In general, because of size considerations, the donor internal iliac artery is usually anastomosed end-to-end to the splenic artery and the external iliac artery anastomosed end-to-end to the superior mesenteric artery. The donor common iliac artery can then be trimmed and anastomosed to the recipient iliac artery at the time of transplantation. The splenic hilar vessels are individually ligated in continuity, taking care not to injure the tail of the pancreas. The spleen is left attached to provide a "handle" during the transplantation. The duodenal segment is then prepared by trimming the excess proximal and distal duodenum to leave only 6 to 8 cms of the second portion of the duodenum attached to the pancreas.[39] During this part of the preparation, the common bile

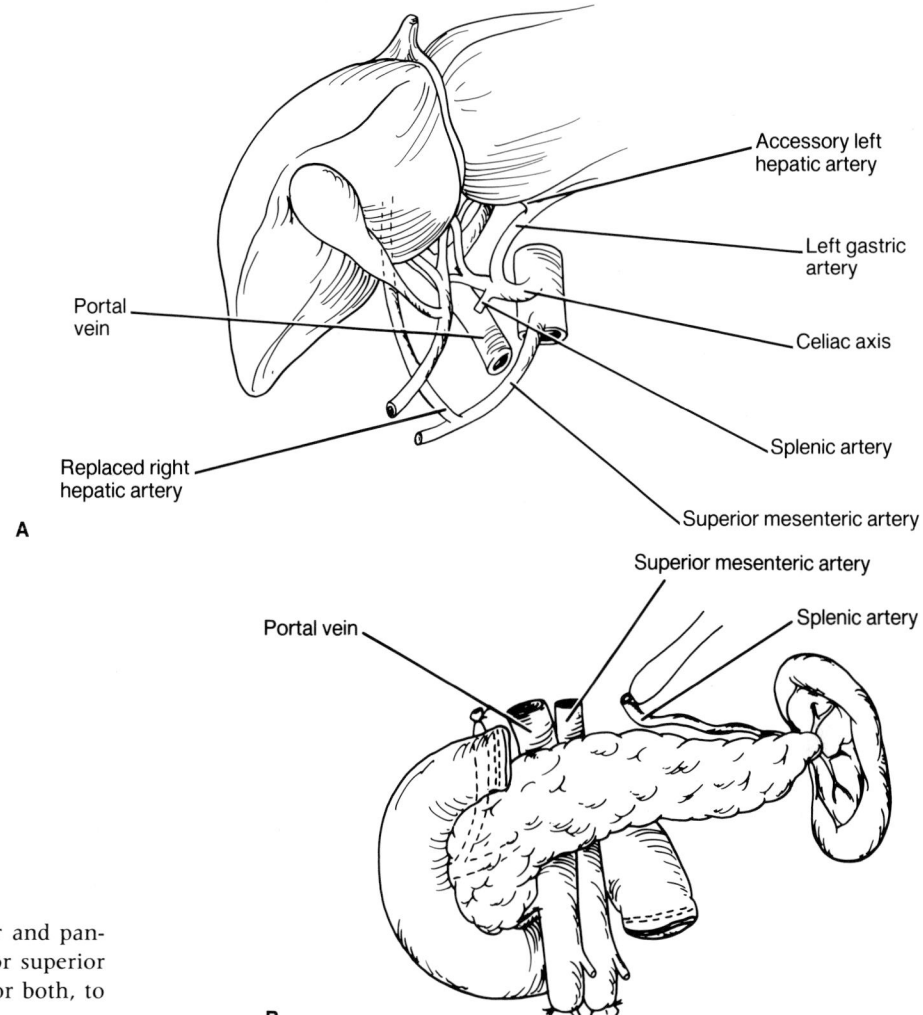

Figure 28-10 Separation of liver and pancreas with preservation of celiac or superior mesenteric arterial blood supply, or both, to the liver.

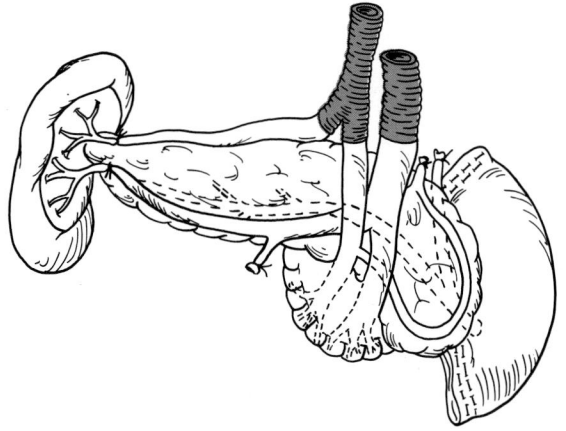

Figure 28-11 Backtable preparation of pancreas with vascular reconstruction, ligation of distal splenic and mesenteric vessels, and trimming of duodenal segment.

duct is cannulated to identify and prevent injury or ligation of the ampulla of Vater. The staple lines on the duodenal ends are inverted with monofilament sutures. The final step involves ligation of the mesenteric bundle near the inferior border of the pancreas with interrupted and running nonabsorbable sutures, particularly if the superior mesenteric vessels have not been specifically identified and ligated. The middle colic vessels, gastroduodenal artery, and common bile duct are also ligated with reinforcement sutures.

SURGICAL TECHNIQUES

Historical Considerations

The history of clinical pancreas transplantation largely revolves around the development and application of various surgical techniques. The first clinical pancreas transplantation, performed by Kelly and Lillehei in December 1966,[12] was a combined kidney–pancreas transplantation, with a segmental pancreas graft transplanted to the iliac fossa and ligation of the pancreatic duct. In their next 13 transplantations between 1966 and 1973, Lillehei and associates[13] used a whole-organ pancreaticoduodenal technique, with either creation of an external ostomy or anastomosis of the graft duodenum to the recipient bowel. In 1973, Gliedman and associates[40] introduced the innovative technique of anastomosis of the duct of a segmental pancreas graft to the recipient ureter in uremic diabetic patients. In the mid-1970s, Groth and colleagues[41] performed segmental pancreas transplantations with anastomosis to a Roux-en-Y limb of recipient bowel (Fig. 28-12).

In 1978, Dubernard and coworkers[42] reported on a new method of segmental pancreas transplantation in which the pancreatic duct was injected with a synthetic polymer to obliterate the exocrine secretions. This technique was adopted by several institutions because it completely avoided bacterial contamination, was safe, and did not require an anastomosis to the exocrine pancreas. Segmental pancreas transplantation by the duct-injection method was the most popular technique until bladder drainage gained prominence in the late 1980s. Also in 1978, the Minnesota group began a series of transplantations using the open duct technique with exocrine drainage into the peritoneal cavity.[14]

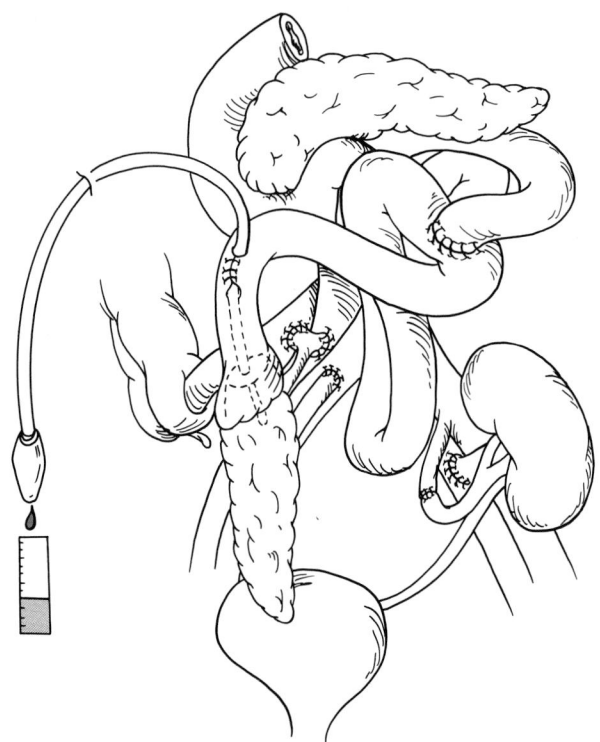

Figure 28-12 Technique of segmental pancreas transplantation with enteric drainage.

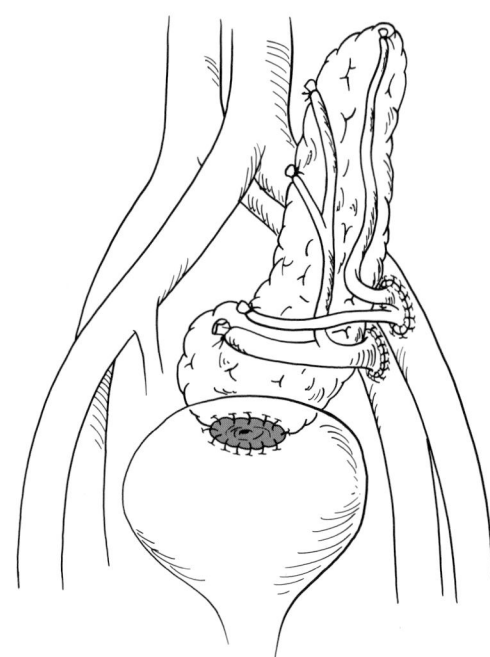

Figure 28-13 Technique of whole-organ pancreas transplantation with bladder drainage by the duodenal button technique.

In 1982, Sollinger's group at the University of Wisconsin described a technique of segmental pancreas transplantation with direct anastomosis of the pancreatic duct to the urinary bladder.[43] Because of a high rate of early vascular thrombosis, this group then switched to whole-organ pancreatic grafting using a duodenal button containing the ampulla for implantation into the urinary bladder[44] (Fig. 28-13). This technique was later modified to incorporate whole-organ pancreaticoduodenal transplantation with anastomosis of a segment of duodenum to the urinary bladder[39] (Fig. 28-14).

Current Techniques

Although a number of different techniques of pancreas transplantation have been described, most North American transplantation centers and an increasing number of European centers have chosen whole-organ pancreas transplantation with the duodenal segment method of bladder drainage as the procedure of choice. Other techniques of pancreas transplantation in use include whole-organ pancreaticoduodenal transplantation with enteric drainage, segmental pancreas transplantation with duct injection, and segmental pancreas transplantation with either enteric or bladder drainage. Advantages of transplanting the whole pancreas include a greater islet cell mass, lower risk of thrombosis

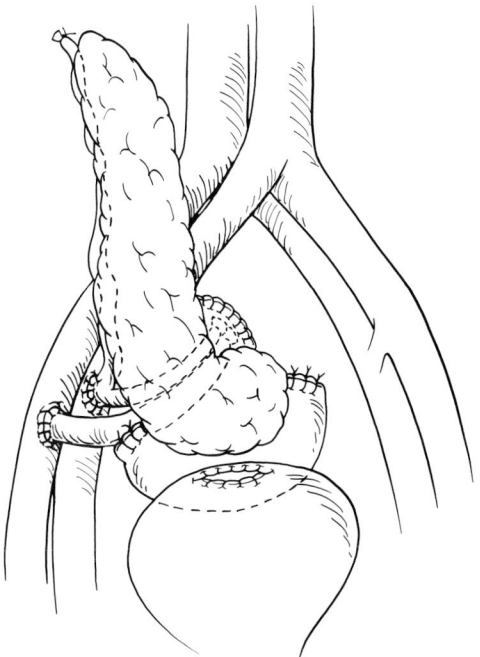

Figure 28-14 Technique of whole-organ pancreas transplantation with bladder drainage by the duodenal segment technique.

because of improved blood flow, and a reduced incidence of pancreatitis or fistulas because the pancreatic parenchyma is not violated. Advantages and disadvantages of the bladder drainage technique are listed in Table 28-5.

In addition to exocrine drainage into the urinary bladder, other nonphysiologic aspects of the procedure include transplantation of a completed denervated organ into an ectopic location with systemic venous drainage of insulin. Most pancreas transplantations are performed in conjunction with a simultaneous kidney transplantation from the same donor (Fig. 28-15). The operation usually lasts 3 to 5 hours, depending on whether the patient is receiving a pancreas alone or combined pancreas–kidney transplantation. During the transplantation procedure, no recipient organs are normally removed, and the patient receives a ''second'' pancreas, a ''third'' kidney, or both.

Operative Approach

Pancreas transplantation can be performed through either a suprainguinal, retroperitoneal approach or through a midline, intraperitoneal incision. With the retroperitoneal approach, it is recommended that the peritoneum be opened after revascularization to facilitate the absorption of peripancreatic secretions.[45] The orientation of the pancreas graft depends on the

method for management of the pancreatic duct and the exocrine secretions. For example, if the bladder drainage technique is used, the graft is oriented so that the pancreatic duct or duodenum projects caudally into the pelvis and bladder. In contrast, with enteric drainage, the pancreatic duct or duodenum can project transversely or cephalad. The same basic techniques for revascularization and management of the exocrine secretions are used for both whole-organ and segmental pancreas transplantation.

Whole-Organ Pancreaticoduodenal Transplantation With Bladder Drainage

For whole-organ pancreas or pancreaticoduodenal transplantation, the graft portal vein (or donor iliac vein extension graft) is anastomosed end-to-side to the recipient iliac vein or vena cava. In most cases, due to liver procurement, a Carrel patch of graft donor aorta encompassing both celiac axis and superior mesenteric artery is not available for direct end-to-side anastomosis to the recipient iliac artery. Therefore, the reconstructed arterial blood supply to the pancreas (donor iliac artery bifurcation graft or end-to-side anastomosis between the donor splenic artery and superior mesenteric artery) is anastomosed end-to-side to the recipient

Table 28-5 Bladder Drainage of Exocrine Secretions

ADVANTAGES
Safety
    Reduced infection rate due to sterility of lower urinary tract
    Control of anastomosis by urethral catheter drainage
Technical considerations
    Anatomic location of bladder favorable
    Bladder mobilization permits tension-free anastomosis
Direct access to exocrine secretions for monitoring pancreas
        allograft function
    Diagnosis of rejection by urinary parameters
    Cystoscopic transduodenal needle biopsy

DISADVANTAGES
Urologic problems
    Hematuria
    Urine leaks
    Cystitis, urethritis, enzyme activation
    Urethral stricture or disruption
    Increased risk of lower urinary tract infections
    Stone formation
Metabolic problems
    Dehydration
    Metabolic acidosis
    Erythrocytosis
Reflux-associated hyperamylasemia or pancreatitis
? Transitional cell (urothelial) dysplasia

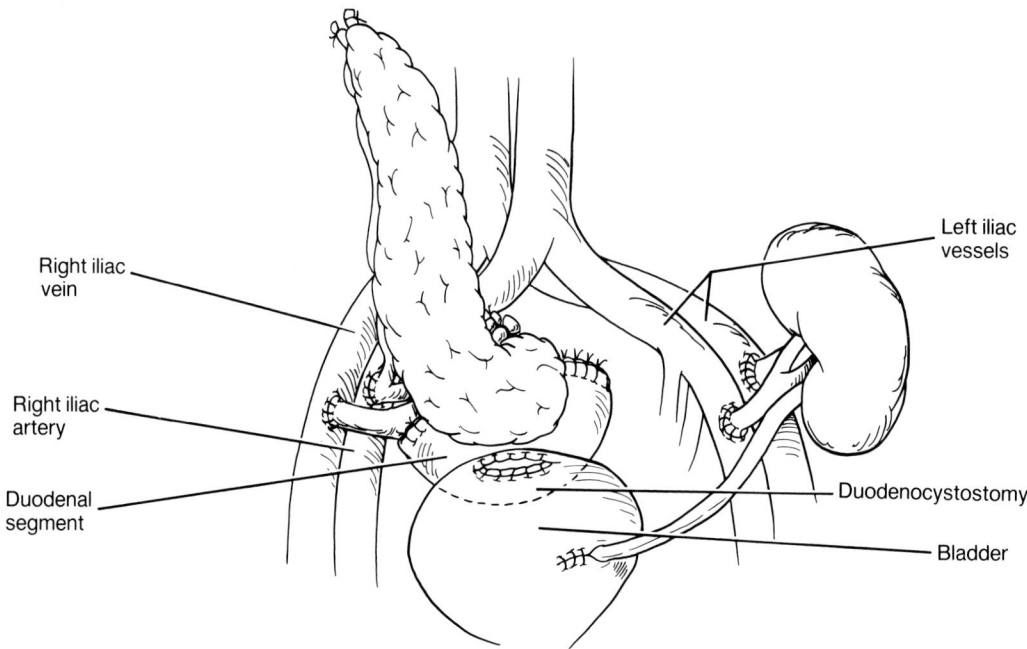

Figure 28-15 Combined pancreas–kidney transplantation with right iliac placement of pancreas after complete mobilization (and lateral displacement) of the iliac vein.

common or external iliac artery. In most cases, the pancreas is anastomosed to the right iliac vessels owing to their favorable anatomic configuration (see Fig. 28-15). If the left iliac vessels are used, particularly with an intraperitoneal approach, the vessels can be isolated in their proximal portion medial to the sigmoid colon, facilitating complete intraperitoneal placement of the graft and avoiding entrapment of peripancreatic secretions within the retroperitoneum lateral and posterior to the sigmoid colon.

A number of studies have reported on the enhanced safety of the midline approach, particularly with regard to infection and performing dual-organ transplantation through a single incision.[45] With the midline approach, the incision extends from the symphysis to the mid-epigastrium (or higher if needed for exposure). The abdomen is explored, and secondary procedures (ie, cholecystectomy, nephrectomy, removal of peritoneal dialysis catheter) are performed as indicated.[46] The bladder is mobilized from its lateral attachments, and the right and left colon are mobilized and reflected into the upper abdomen. The pelvic peritoneum overlying the iliac vessels is incised, and the external iliac artery and vein are exposed. In cases of combined pancreas–kidney transplantation, the kidney transplantation is usually performed to the left iliac vessels with end-to-side vascular anastomoses and an extravesical ureteroneocystostomy. The right iliac artery is then completely mobilized, with preservation of the hypogastric

artery. This enables complete mobilization of the right iliac vein, with ligation and division of the hypogastric vein and any other posterior branches. The iliac vein is placed lateral to the artery to minimize tension on the portal–iliac venous anastomosis, eliminating the need for a vein graft in most cases. The pancreas is then transplanted to the right iliac vessels with end-to-side vascular anastomoses (see Fig. 28-15). In patients undergoing solitary pancreas transplantation, the iliac vessels on the side of the transplantation are completely mobilized as previously described. After release of the vascular clamps, hemostasis is achieved, and the splenic artery and vein are palpated to check for adequate inflow and outflow. A graft splenectomy is then performed.

The duodenal segment is opened along the antimesenteric border for a length of about 3 cm and copiously irrigated with antibacterial and antifungal solutions. An appropriate area on the posterior aspect of the bladder is identified, and a two-layer duodenocystostomy is then performed with a running inner layer and interrupted outer layer of absorbable monofilament suture. Alternatively, techniques of stapling the duodenocystostomy have been described. The duodenocystostomy may lie horizontal or vertical depending on the appropriate orientation of the pancreas in the iliac fossa. The lateral umbilical ligaments are then rolled up around the duodenal segment to help prevent leaks from a potentially ischemic duodenal segment.[47] The pancreas is then placed in the paracolic region, and hemostasis is achieved. Closed-suction drains may be placed medial and lateral to the pancreas and medial to the kidney (if transplanted) to minimize the development of fluid collections. If a simultaneous kidney transplantation is performed, it can then be "retroperitonealized" and the colon tacked over the transplanted kidney to prevent flipping of the intraperitoneal kidney. The peritoneum is closed with absorbable sutures to help keep the fascial closure away from the pancreas. The fascia is then closed with nonabsorbable monofilament sutures.

Whole-Organ Pancreaticoduodenal Transplantation With Enteric Drainage

Another method of whole-organ pancreaticoduodenal transplantation involves enteric drainage of the exocrine pancreas by performing a side-to-side anastomosis of the graft duodenum to the recipient bowel.[48] Alternatively, the graft duodenum can be anastomosed side-to-side to a Roux-en-Y limb of recipient small bowel (Fig. 28-16). A further modification involves placing a small tube or catheter in the pancreatic duct, which is then brought out of the defunctionalized limb and exteriorized. This catheter is usually left in place for several weeks after transplantation in an attempt to avoid an anastomotic fistula, control pancreatic ductal secretions, and enable direct access to pancreatic juice for cytologic or chemical monitoring.[49] Two major drawbacks to enteric drainage techniques include an in-

creased risk of surgical complications (particularly intraabdominal infections) and lack of permanent access to pancreatic ductal secretions as an indicator of allograft function. Despite the complexity of these techniques, they provide a greater range of options for vascular reconstruction, particularly with regard to paratopic pancreas transplantation with portal venous drainage (Fig. 28-17) to prevent systemic hyperinsulinemia.[50]

Segmental Pancreas Transplantation

The pertinent anatomy of a segmental pancreas transplantation is shown in Figure 28-7. The arterial blood supply to the tail and most of the body of the pancreas is derived from the splenic artery, which has its origin in the celiac axis. The dorsal and transverse pancreatic arteries usually ramify with the branches of the superior mesenteric artery through the neck of the pancreas. In certain cases, however, these branches may directly originate from the superior mesenteric artery; lack of recognition of this arrangement can lead to devascularization of the tail of the pancreas during donor hemipancreatectomy. The venous drainage of the tail and most of the body of the pancreas is the splenic vein. Since the narrowest portion of the pancreas is that overlying the portal vein, this is the area of transection of the pancreatic parenchyma during procurement. The splenic artery and vein can be lengthened by vascular grafts in an end-to-end fashion as needed.

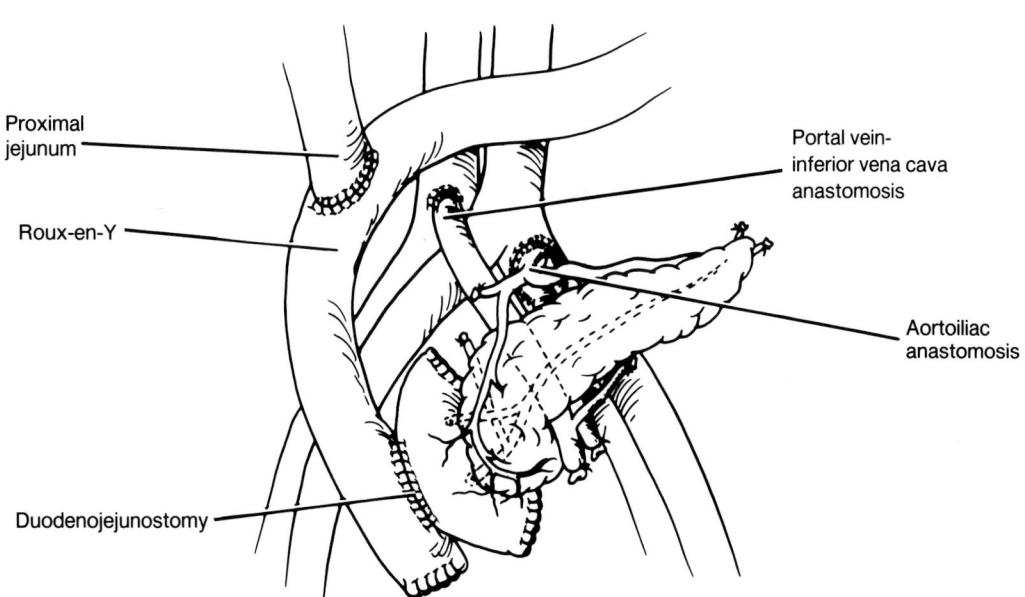

Figure 28-16 Technique of whole-organ pancreaticoduodenal transplantation with enteric drainage.

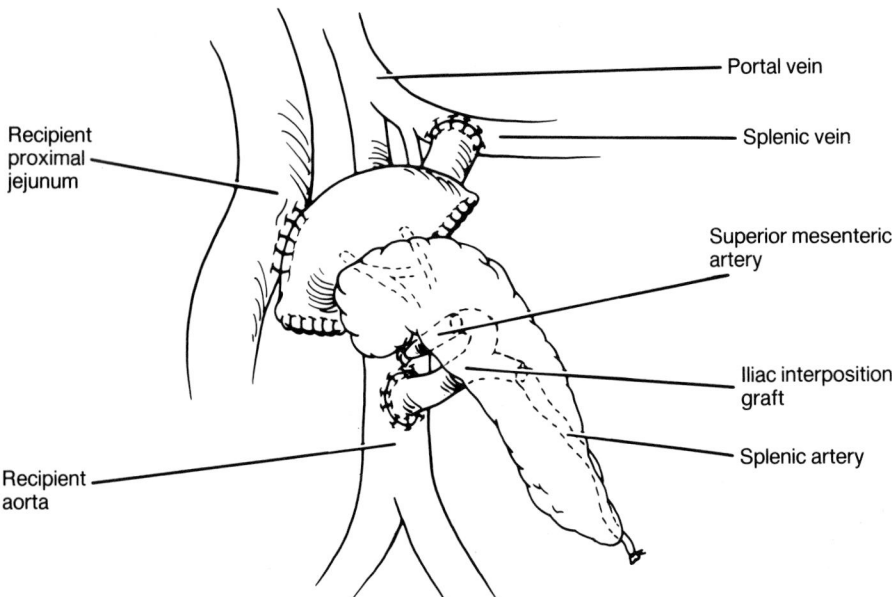

Figure 28-17 Technique of whole-organ pancreaticoduodenal transplantation with portal venous drainage of insulin and enteric drainage of exocrine secretions.

Similar to whole-organ pancreas transplantation, most segmental pancreas transplants are anastomosed to the recipient's iliac vessels in an end-to-side fashion (see Fig. 28-12). In certain cases, the recipient hypogastric artery can be used for an end-to-end anastomosis to a short proximal splenic artery of the graft. Other options for revascularization of segmental pancreas grafts that have been described but not widely used include anastomosis to the recipient's splenic or mesenteric vessels. Although these alternative methods provide portal venous drainage of the segmental graft, a definite metabolic advantage of this technique has not been demonstrated.

Exocrine Drainage Techniques

The three major methods of exocrine drainage after segmental pancreas transplantation include enteric drainage, duct injection, and bladder drainage. Pancreatic duct occlusion by injection of a synthetic polymer gained wide popularity in the early 1980s due to its simplicity and lack of an anastomosis to provide exocrine drainage. A variety of polymers have been used, including neoprene, prolamine, polyisoprene, cyanoacrylate, and silicone rubber. With this technique, several milliliters of synthetic polymer are directly injected into the pancreatic duct, followed by duct ligation to avoid extravasation. The synthetic polymer progressively solidifies after coming in contact with the pancreatic juice. Polymer injection suppresses exocrine function not only by direct toxic effects on the acinar cells but also

by blocking secretions, resulting in acinar atrophy and fibrosis.[51] One potential concern is that duct occlusion may lead to progressive fibrosis, chronic pancreatitis, and eventual islet cell dysfunction. Another problem associated with this technique has been exocrine leakage with the development of pancreatic fistulas and wound complications. In the absence of an anastomosis, however, the infection rate with this technique has remained low.

Exocrine drainage of the segmental pancreas graft into the small intestine is the most physiologic of all ductal management techniques.[48] The transected surface of the segmental pancreas is intussuscepted into the end of a Roux-en-Y limb of small bowel over a ductal stent or catheter (see Fig. 28-12). The pancreatic duct catheter may be exteriorized through the Roux limb, facilitating diversion and allowing external collection of the ductal secretions. The external catheter is usually left in place for 3 to 6 weeks not only to permit anastomotic healing but also for direct monitoring of graft exocrine function.

Segmental pancreas transplantation can also be performed with bladder drainage either by direct mucosal-to-mucosal anastomosis of the graft duct to the bladder over a stent or by intussusception of the transected surface of the pancreas into the bladder as a pancreaticocystostomy.[43,48] Although this technique permits long-term access and control of the exocrine secretions, a potential drawback is an increased risk of leaks with pancreatic fistulas as compared with whole-organ pancreaticoduodenal transplantation with bladder drainage.

PERIOPERATIVE MANAGEMENT

Recipient Selection and Preparation

Preoperative Management

Recipients are selected for transplantation based on ABO blood type compatibility, degree of sensitization, human leukocyte antigen matching, length of time on the waiting list, medical urgency, and a negative T-lymphocytotoxic crossmatch in accordance with UNOS guidelines. With intraperitoneal methods of transplantation, preoperative bowel treatment is helpful and may include mechanical (oral cathartics, cleansing enemas) and antibiotic (selective bowel decontamination) bowel preparation. Preoperative antibiotics and immunosuppression may be administered, intravenous fluid hydration is begun, and serum glucose levels are monitored closely and controlled with sliding-scale insulin therapy. Dialysis, if indicated, is performed preoperatively.

Operative Management

After organ preparation and determination that the final crossmatch is compatible, the recipient is brought to the operating suite. Before the onset of general endotracheal anesthesia, an epidural catheter may be placed for postoperative pain management. After anesthetic induction, a central venous line is inserted, and a radial arterial line may be placed for hemodynamic monitoring during the operative procedure. A nasogastric tube is placed, a 20F to 22F urethral catheter is inserted, and the bladder is irrigated with antibiotic solution.

During the operative procedure, serum glucose levels are monitored frequently and controlled with a continuous insulin infusion. Cautious volume loading is performed with liberal use of colloid, mannitol, and furosemide to promote diuresis and minimize pancreatic edema after reperfusion. Many patients may also benefit from a low-dose dopamine infusion of 3 to 5 $\mu g/kg/$min in an attempt to optimize renal function and hemodynamic support. In patients undergoing solitary pancreas transplantation, consideration may be given to systemic anticoagulation before clamping of the vessels. Pulse oximetry and temperature monitoring are performed, with appropriate interventions to maintain oxygenation and normothermia. Packed red blood cells are transfused to maintain the hematocrit at more than 20%, and fresh frozen plasma may be required in the uremic recipient with excessive oozing. Immunosuppressive and antibiotic medications are administered intraoperatively. Closed-suction drains may be placed around the pancreas after revascularization and exocrine drainage. Dopamine and insulin infusions are continued at the end of the procedure.

Postoperative Management

In the initial postoperative period, because of potential fluid and pulmonary problems, patients are usually observed in the intensive care unit for the initial 2 to 3 days. Once stabilized, they are transferred to the transplantation ward and spend about 2 to 3 weeks in the hospital. Perioperative antibiotics consist of a single preoperative, intraoperative, and three postoperative doses of a first generation cephalosporin. Patients may also receive perioperative vancomycin. Antifungal prophylaxis may consist of fluconazole, ketoconazole, clotrimazole, or nystatin. Antiviral prophylaxis may consist of intravenous ganciclovir, acyclovir, or intravenous immunoglobulin. Pneumocystis prophylaxis consists of trimethoprim sulfamethoxazole or aerosolized pentamidine. Although some centers advocate anticoagulation with heparin or dextran, most centers routinely use antiplatelet agents, such as aspirin or dipyridamole, with or without pentoxifylline.[52,53] Nasogastric suction is continued until the return of intestinal function, which may be assisted by the use of metoclopramide or cisapride. Urethral catheter drainage is maintained for 7 to 10 days, at which time a low-pressure cystogram may be performed to ensure anastomotic integrity before removal of the catheter. Intraabdominal drains are removed over 3 to 5 days depending on the volume and amylase content of drainage. At many centers, however, intraperitoneal suction drains are not routinely used without any apparent adverse sequelae. Patients usually begin ambulation at 48 to 72 hours, and a liquid diet is usually started 3 to 5 days after transplantation.

Postoperative Monitoring

Abdominal ultrasonography and radionuclide scanning are performed on the first postoperative day and whenever clinically indicated to evaluate graft perfusion, anatomy, and fluid collections. Mannitol and albumin supplementation are continued for 24 to 48 hours after transplantation to reduce graft edema and promote diuresis. Urinary output and central venous pressure monitoring are used as guides to fluid replacement. Serum glucose levels are followed closely, and an intravenous insulin infusion is continued to maintain the serum glucose less than 200 mg/dL. Persistent elevation or acute rises in the serum glucose to more than 200 mg/dL require immediate evaluation with duplex ultrasonography or radionuclide scanning to assess graft perfusion and function. Other laboratory determinations include electrolytes, complete blood count with differential and platelet counts, urine and serum amylase, blood urea nitrogen and serum creatinine, urine cytology, and cyclosporine levels. Patients who lose large amounts of bicarbonate through the urinary tract may require bicarbonate supplementation. Patients also receive stress ulcer prophylaxis with a histamine-2 receptor antagonist and antacids. Pneumatic compression boots are applied perioperatively to minimize the risk of venous thrombosis.

Immunosuppression

The introduction of cyclosporine in 1980 was a significant advance in solid-organ transplantation and permitted wider application of pancreas transplantation.[54] Although cyclosporine has become the mainstay of contemporary posttransplantation immunosuppression, immunosuppressive strategies have evolved to achieve effective control of rejection while minimizing injury to the allograft and risks to the patient. Quadruple immunosuppression with antilymphocyte induction in combination with cyclosporine, steroids, and azathioprine is a rational and highly effective protocol that accomplishes these goals. Studies have documented the durability of this protocol in achieving high rates of graft success with low morbidity.[54,55] Despite a diversity of immunosuppressive protocols, most centers employ quadruple immunosuppression with antilymphocyte induction (Fig. 28-18) because the pancreas appears to be a highly immunogenic organ. Controversy exists, however, regarding the type, duration, and dose of antilymphocyte therapy. The antilymphocyte agents most commonly used include the monoclonal antibody OKT3 and polyclonal preparations such as Minnesota antilymphoblast globulin (MALG) or antithymocyte

globulin (ATGAM). From a clinical standpoint, both randomized and nonrandomized trials comparing OKT3 versus polyclonal antilymphocyte induction have yielded mixed results.[54-56] Maintenance immunosuppressive therapy usually consists of cyclosporine, prednisone, or azathioprine or a combination of these. Although IPTR data appear to indicate a trend toward triple or even quadruple immunosuppressive regimens, the diversity of surgical techniques makes it difficult to draw conclusions about which immunosuppressive regimen provides the best patient and graft survival.

OKT3 Induction

With OKT3 induction, the first dose, 2.5 to 5 mg given intravenously, is administered intraoperatively 1 hour after giving 1 g of intravenous methylprednisolone. Postoperatively, OKT3 is administered for 10 to 14 days as a single daily intravenous bolus of 2.5 to 5 mg with dosage adjustments to maintain the absolute peripheral CD3 lymphocyte count less than $10/\mu L$ and the OKT3 level more than 700 ng/mL. Intravenous methylprednisolone is tapered from a daily dose of 3 mg/kg/d (in four divided doses) down to 0.3 mg/kg/d for 5 to 7 days, at which time patients are then switched to a daily oral prednisone dose. Two intravenous methylprednisolone boluses of 500 and 250 mg may be given on consecutive days at the end of OKT3 therapy. Patients also receive intravenous and then oral azathioprine, 1 to 2 mg/kg as a single daily dose, with dosage reductions for a white blood cell count less than $4000/\mu L$ or platelet count less than $100,000/\mu L$. Oral cyclosporine, 5 to 10 mg/kg, may be given preoperatively, and intravenous cyclosporine, 1 mg/kg twice daily, is initiated either on the first postoperative day (quadruple therapy) or after the return of adequate renal func-

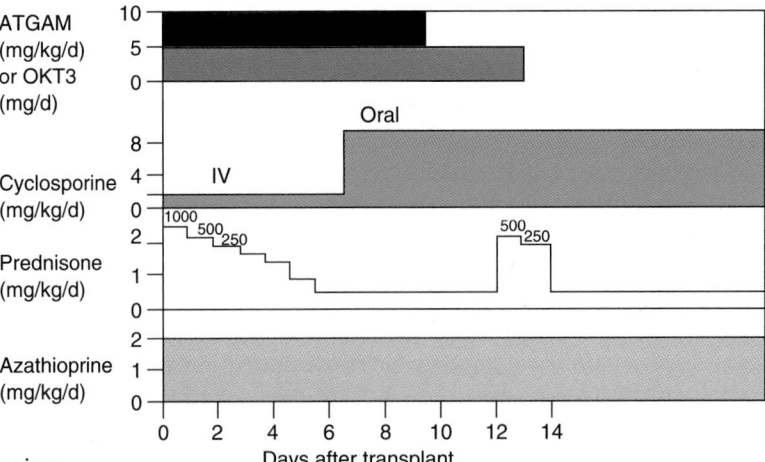

Figure 28-18 Quadruple immunosuppression with either monoclonal or polyclonal antilymphocyte induction.

tion (sequential therapy). When patients begin oral intake, they are converted to oral cyclosporine at a dose of 5 mg/kg twice daily with dosage adjustments to maintain target trough levels in the therapeutic range. Long-term maintenance immunosuppression is triple therapy with cyclosporine, prednisone, and azathioprine, with slow tapering of doses over time.

Antithymocyte Globulin or Minnesota Antilymphoblast Globulin Induction

For patients receiving polyclonal antilymphocyte induction therapy, a similar regimen is followed except that the first dose of antilymphocyte therapy is administered on the first postoperative day. Polyclonal preparations are usually administered for 7 to 10 days (as opposed to 10 to 14 days for OKT3) in a dose of 10 to 20 mg/kg/d as a slow continuous intravenous infusion. Dosage adjustments are made to maintain the white blood cell count more than $4000/\mu L$, the platelet count more than $100,000/\mu L$, and to maintain low peripheral CD3 lymphocyte counts. With the use of any antilymphocyte preparation, dosage adjustments are also made based on adverse effects, and the aggressive use of antiviral prophylaxis is recommended.[57]

Complications of Immunosuppression

Complications of immunosuppressive therapy continue to be the major nonsurgical risk in diabetic recipients of pancreas transplants. Corticosteroids have numerous clinical side effects (see Table 28-6). Glucose intolerance has not been an overwhelming problem despite concerns about the diabetogenic effect of corticosteroids. Steroids induce peripheral insulin resistance but do not have any direct action on insulin-producing capacity. Maintenance immunosuppression with corticosteroids, 0.2 to 0.5 mg/kg/d, does not appear to affect the level of metabolic control achieved by a functioning pancreas allograft, although pulsed steroid therapy may induce hyperglycemia. The effect of corticosteroids alone or in combination with azathioprine on allograft pancreatitis is still unknown.

Polyclonal antilymphocyte preparations and azathioprine have been associated with leukopenia, thrombocytopenia, bone marrow suppression, and increased susceptibility to infection. In the absence of prophylaxis, antilymphocyte induction therapy has been reported to have an unacceptably high risk of viral infections and hematologic malignancies, especially Epstein-Barr virus–associated lymphoma.[57,58] Overimmunosuppression should be avoided because pancreas allograft rejection is not life-threatening, the graft does

Table 28-6 Clinical Effects of Corticosteroids

MODE OF ACTION
Block IL-1 release directly
Reduce capacity of antigen-presenting cells to express class II antigens
Block IL-6 release indirectly
Inhibit gene activation for amplification of IL-1, IL-3, IL-6
Block IL-2 release indirectly
Inhibit activation of T cells
Nonspecific immunosuppressive and antiinflammatory effects
Inhibit migration of immune cells to site of inflammation

SIDE EFFECTS
Increased susceptibility to infection
Impaired wound healing
Growth suppression in children
Myopathy
Osteoporosis, aseptic bone necrosis
Mood swings, psychosis
Cataract formation
Hyperlipidemia
Hyperglycemia, insulin resistance
Sodium retention, edema, hypertension
Cushingoid features, weight gain
Peptic ulcers, gastritis, perforation, pancreatitis, ileus
Acne and other skin changes (striae, easy bruisability)

not usually need to be removed, and exogenous insulin can be resumed.

Cyclosporine has been shown to have direct toxic effects on parenchymal organs, and the pancreas is no exception. Nephrotoxicity remains a major side effect of cyclosporine, but most early cyclosporine-induced changes are transient and dose related. In high doses, cyclosporine causes a deterioration in glucose metabolism, probably by inducing peripheral insulin resistance as well as direct β-cell toxicity.[59] Impaired glucose regulation can be seen particularly in patients receiving cyclosporine and prednisone, but it appears to be a dose-related and reversible phenomenon. Major clinical effects of cyclosporine therapy are listed in Table 28-7.

Undertreatment is another potential hazard of immunosuppressive therapy, with the major problems encountered being either breakthrough rejection or recurrence of diabetes. In identical-twin pancreas allografts managed without immunosuppression, recurrence of disease without evidence of rejection occurs at 6 to 12 weeks.[6,10] Histologic examination of biopsy specimens reveals insulitis, characterized by selective β-cell destruction independent of changes suggestive of rejection. Islet cell antibodies have been implicated in the presumed autoimmune pathogenesis of recurrent diabetes in the allograft. With adequate immunosuppres-

Table 28-7   Clinical Effects of Cyclosporine

MODE OF ACTION
Blocks activation of interleukin-2 gene
Inhibits proliferation of T-helper cells
Prevents γ-interferon release
Prevents release of B-cell activating factors
Hepatotrophic factor
Inhibits peptidyl-prolyl-isomerase system
Spares suppressor cell generation

SIDE EFFECTS
Nephrotoxicity
Hypertension
Hyperkalemia
Hemolytic–uremic syndrome
Hyperuricemia
Neurotoxicity (tremors, seizures, dysesthesia)
Hepatotoxicity
Blocks insulin release
Increased susceptibility to infection
Hyperlipidemia
Gingival hypertrophy
Hirsutism
Breast fibroadenomas
Gastrointestinal (nausea, anorexia)
Increased risk of malignancy

sion, however, recurrence of disease is not inevitable and may be rare.

REJECTION

Pancreas Versus Kidney Rejection

Studies of rejection in recipients of combined pancreas–kidney transplantations from the same donor have provided important clues as to the immunogenicity of the pancreas. In these patients, numerous studies have demonstrated that the manifestations of renal allograft rejection usually precede or parallel those of pancreas rejection.[60] The diagnosis of rejection after combined pancreas–kidney transplantation is usually based on a rise in the serum creatinine level or positive renal allograft biopsy.[61] Although episodes of kidney rejection may occur independently and without concomitant detectable pancreas rejection, isolated pancreas rejection in combined transplantations from the same donor is uncommon. The pancreas allograft may be retained even in the setting of acute irreversible renal allograft rejection. Transplant nephrectomy, however, may subsequently result in vigorous rejection and loss of the pancreas. This finding suggests that a simultaneous kidney transplantation may provide benefit not only from a laboratory monitoring standpoint but also because it

may confer immunologic protection of the pancreas from rejection.

Isolated Pancreas Rejection

With regard to isolated pancreas transplantation (or nonsimultaneous kidney and pancreas transplantation from different donors), the case is different. Isolated pancreas rejection can and does occur in patients with previous kidney transplantations irrespective of renal allograft function. In this setting, the incidence of irreversible pancreas allograft rejection is much higher, leading to a 20% to 30% reduction in overall graft survival.[31] Multiple reports have shown that hyperglycemia is a valid but delayed parameter of pancreas allograft rejection, both experimentally and clinically.[51] Loss of glucose homeostasis occurs late in the sequence of immunologic rejection, with successful reversal of rejection achieved in only 20% to 30% of cases after the onset of hyperglycemia.

Exocrine Versus Endocrine Rejection

The exocrine pancreas is more sensitive to rejection than the endocrine pancreas, with a reduction in exocrine function preceding the onset of hyperglycemia.[52,61–63] Although parallel rejection of the exocrine and endocrine pancreas may occur, histologic studies have noted mononuclear cell infiltration of acinar tissue and vasculitis before any islet cell changes.[51] These observations suggest that early diagnosis of pancreas rejection can be based on exocrine dysfunction. By using ductal drainage techniques that permit easy access and analysis of pancreatic exocrine secretions (pancreaticocystostomy, pancreaticoenterostomy with external stent), one can monitor exocrine function and detect rejection. This approach has revolutionized the technical aspects of pancreas transplantation and may provide further insight into determining the differential susceptibility of the exocrine and endocrine pancreas to rejection.

Diagnosis of Rejection

Pancreas rejection may be subtle and occult, and the development of a noninvasive, reproducible method of detection would certainly enhance allograft survival. A variety of tests are being investigated as potential early markers of rejection (Table 28-8). With regard to clinical presentation, pancreas allograft rejection may be characterized by fever, leukocytosis, ileus, allograft swelling and tenderness, and abdominal pain. Differentiation from pancreatitis is difficult, and none of

Table 28-8   Diagnosis of Pancreas Allograft Rejection

SEROLOGIC PARAMETERS
Endocrine (glucose, insulin, proinsulin, C-peptide, glucagon, pancreatic polypeptide, provocative tests)
Exocrine (amylase, anodal trypsinogen, pancreatic-specific protein, secretory trypsin inhibitor, lipase, bicarbonate, zinc)
Immune (β_2-microglobulin, interleukin-2 (IL-2) receptor, neopterin, soluble human leukocyte antigens (HLA), tumor necrosis factor, thromboxane B_2, prostaglandin E_2, C-reactive protein, platelet-activating factor, IL-1, IL-6, flow cytometry)

PANCREATIC DRAINAGE AND URINARY PARAMETERS
Endocrine (insulin)
Exocrine (amylase, lipase, pH, zinc, trypsinogen)
Immune (β_2-microglobulin, IL-2 receptor, neopterin, HLA, thromboxane B_2, prostaglandin E_2, tumor necrosis factor, interleukins)

CYTOLOGY
Pancreatic juice
Urine (bladder drainage)
Fine-needle aspiration

NONINVASIVE IMAGING
Ultrasonography
Radionuclide perfusion scan
Platelet-labeling scan
Nuclear magnetic resonance
Positron emission tomography

HISTOPATHOLOGY
Open biopsy
Percutaneous needle core biopsy
Percutaneous fine-needle aspiration biopsy
Cystoscopically directed biopsy (bladder drainage)
Endoscopically directed biopsy (enteric drainage)

these features are consistently present or pathognomonic of the rejection process.

Serologic Parameters

Hyperamylasemia is common after pancreas transplantation but is only rarely due to rejection. Hyperamylasemia appears to be a better marker for rejection after solitary pancreas transplantation than combined pancreas–kidney transplantation.[29] Preliminary clinical experience with serum anodal trypsinogen as an early biochemical marker for pancreas rejection has been encouraging.[63] Since hyperglycemia tends to be a terminal event in the rejection process, even minor elevations in the serum glucose must be viewed with suspicion and assumed to be rejection until proved otherwise. Hyperglycemia due to rejection is associated with diminished serum C-peptide levels, but C-peptide and provocative tests are of limited value in the early

diagnosis of rejection. Other serologic parameters of rejection may reflect the immunologic environment of the recipient rather than specific exocrine or endocrine functions of the allograft.

Urinary Parameters

One of the major theoretic advantages of urinary tract diversion of the pancreatic duct is the ability to monitor directly exocrine function by urinary assays. Much experimental and clinical evidence has accumulated to show that reductions in urine amylase levels are an early marker of rejection.[62] A further refinement in urine amylase monitoring involves measuring urine amylase concentration per unit of time (urine amylase activity), which tends to correct for the state of hydration. Elevated urinary insulin levels have been noted during acute rejection and may be due to increased permeability of the islet microvasculature during rejection, with subsequent leakage of insulin into the exocrine secretions. Reductions in the volume of exocrine secretions and the activity and content of enzymes show a clear correlation with cytologic changes and the subsequent development of rejection. These changes revert with successful antirejection therapy.[49] With the development of cytologic monitoring of the pancreatic juice or urine (in patients with bladder drainage), cytologic features of rejection include the appearance of blast cells (lymphoblasts or monoblasts), an increase in the number of eosinophils and mononuclear cells relative to neutrophils, and an increased number of epithelial cells.[64] Positive cytologic signs of rejection appear to precede exocrine dysfunction by 1 to 3 days.

Radiologic Studies

Several attempts have been made at pancreatic imaging. Ultrasonography, computed tomography (CT), and magnetic resonance imaging are excellent at demonstrating anatomy and fluid collections but cannot readily differentiate rejection from pancreatitis or vascular thrombosis. Radionuclide scanning is the best way to evaluate the physiologic status of the pancreas; characteristics of rejection include hypoperfusion, graft swelling, haziness of borders, and diminished visualization, especially in the tail of the pancreas[61] (Fig. 28-19). Perfusion indices can be calculated to further aid in the early detection of rejection based on diminished blood flow. Poor visualization of the pancreas also may occur during radionuclide flow studies despite normal allograft function, so the results must be interpreted in conjunction with clinical findings and other laboratory data.

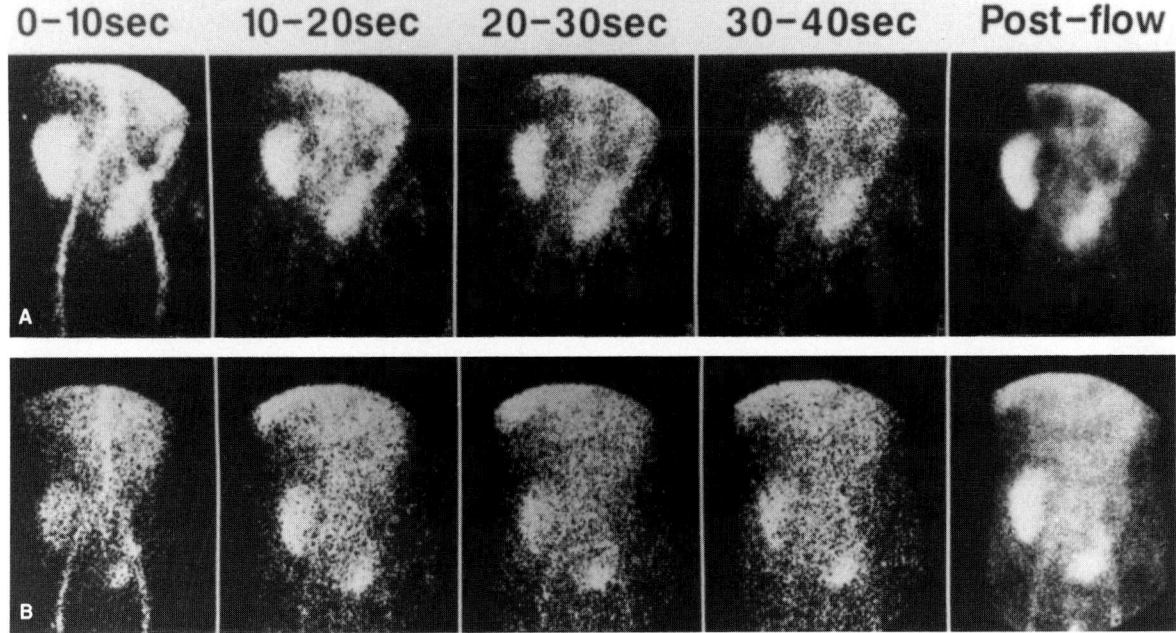

Figure 28-19 (A) Radionuclide perfusion scan performed 1 day after transplantation shows good perfusion and visualization of right iliac kidney and left iliac pancreas grafts. (B) Scan in same patient 6 weeks later shows hypoperfusion of pancreas graft consistent with rejection.

Histopathology

Despite a number of markers for pancreas rejection, histopathologic examination of the pancreas remains the gold standard in the diagnosis of allograft rejection. In contrast to other solid-organ transplantations, however, percutaneous core biopsy of the pancreas allograft is potentially hazardous because of the risks of bleeding, fistula, and pancreatitis.[65] Although safer percutaneous biopsy techniques of the pancreas allograft are being described, most studies of histopathology are based on biopsy findings obtained at laparotomy, which may be attended by serious complications.[51,66] Initial experience with fine-needle aspiration biopsy of the pancreas allograft has met with limited success.[67]

Duodenal Rejection

Techniques of whole-organ pancreas transplantation often involve a portion of the duodenum adjacent to the ampulla, which is employed in the urinary or gastrointestinal anastomosis. Rejection of the duodenum may occur, resulting in mucosal sloughing with subsequent ulceration, perforation, or bleeding.[68] Histologic studies reveal a loss of duodenal mucosal and muscularis layers, with the submucosa densely infiltrated with inflammatory cells. In patients who undergo pancreaticoduodenocystostomy, hematuria may present as an early and ominous sign of impending duodenal rejection that may be a harbinger of subsequent pancreas rejection. With paratopic implantation of the pancreas into the bladder, cystoscopic transduodenal needle biopsy affords an innovative approach to the histopathologic examination of the pancreaticoduodenal allograft.[69] Histologic studies reveal a correlation between duodenal and acinar findings during the rejection process.[68] Although a positive duodenal biopsy is usually indicative of pancreas rejection, pancreas rejection can and does occur independent of duodenal rejection.

Pancreas Allograft Histopathology

Early histologic changes of acute pancreas rejection include a focal interstitial infiltration of transformed lymphocytes into the exocrine pancreas with perivascular cuffing.[51] This progresses to an intense, diffuse mononuclear cell infiltration of the pancreatic parenchyma with increased vascular inflammatory and reactive changes but initial sparing of islet cells (Fig. 28-20). Hyperglycemia is usually not yet apparent at this time. Eventually, coincidental with fibrosis, loss of acinar tissue, pronounced vascular changes, and islet infiltration and destruction occur, resulting in hyperglycemia. Chronic rejection is characterized by dense mononuclear cell infiltrates, nonviable tissue, and subintimal

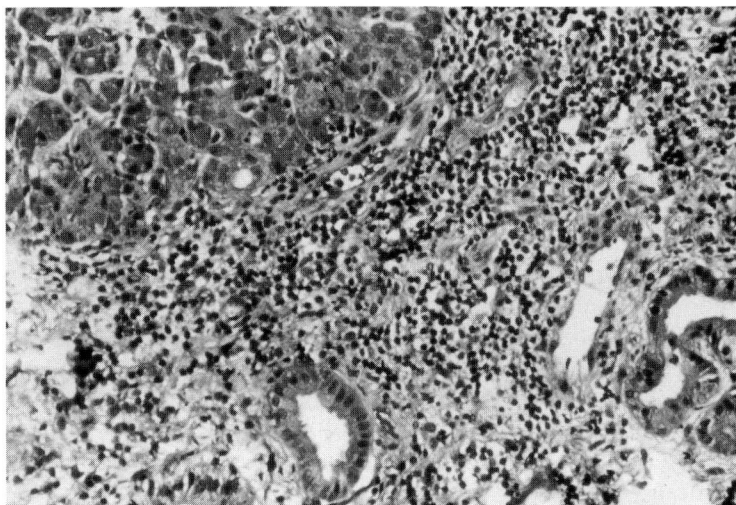

Figure 28-20 Cystoscopically directed core needle biopsy of pancreas allograft showing changes of acute rejection with mononuclear cell infiltration, acinar cell damage, and endotheliitis (hematoxylin–eosin, ×100).

arteriolar hyperplasia with fibromyointimal proliferation and luminal narrowing leading to thrombosis.

Treatment of Rejection

The optimal treatment of rejection is still unknown. The results obtained in renal transplantation in diabetic patients have provided a framework for the development of therapeutic protocols against rejection in pancreas transplantation. The mainstay of antirejection therapy is increased immunosuppression. In combined pancreas–kidney transplantation, aggressive treatment of kidney rejection usually results in functional survival of both organs.[61] Most centers employ pulsed corticosteroids, antilymphocyte preparations, or both as initial therapy for rejection. A paradox of treatment is that bolus steroids, by inducing peripheral insulin resistance, may actually precipitate or aggravate hyperglycemia. Monitoring the efficacy of therapy in this situation can be difficult.

Antilymphocyte therapy alone can reverse pancreas allograft rejection, even in cyclosporine-treated patients, and has no diabetogenic effect.[70] The institution of early treatment of rejection episodes based on decreased urinary amylase levels significantly improves allograft functional survival and is much more effective than treatment started after hyperglycemia.[60–62] For patients receiving antilymphocyte induction therapy, episodes of rejection are initially treated with pulsed steroids. Steroid-resistant rejection or recurrent rejection can be successfully treated with another antilymphocyte preparation or a second course of the induction agent. During courses of antilymphocyte treatment, specific antiviral and antifungal prophylaxis are recommended to prevent infectious complications during and after these periods of heavy immunosuppression.[57] Despite a 20% rate of immunologic graft loss, irreversible allograft rejection results in less than a 10% risk of transplant pancreatectomy.

The best treatment of rejection is prevention. This can be achieved by rendering the graft less immunogenic or by promoting tolerance in the host. Although the degree of immunogenicity of the pancreas is controversial, attempts are being made to alter it with monoclonal antibody technology. Decreasing the immunoreactivity of the recipient by more selective and sophisticated forms of immunosuppression is another form of immunologic conditioning. The ultimate goal of such endeavors is the induction of donor-specific tolerance.

COMPLICATIONS

In addition to rejection, the major causes of graft loss after pancreas transplantation are vascular thrombosis, pancreatitis, and infection. In contrast to other solid organs transplanted, the pancreas is susceptible to a unique set of complications because of its exocrine elements and low blood flow. Furthermore, intraperitoneal placement of a denervated pancreas allograft in a paratopic location with systemic venous drainage of insulin and exocrine drainage into the urinary bladder is associated with a number of unusual problems.

Enteric Conversion

The management of exocrine complications continues to be an area of controversy after pancreas transplantation. For patients with bladder drainage, enteric conversion is recommended for severe problems, such as refractory dehydration and metabolic acidosis, urethral disruption, recurrent urine leaks with severe duodenal pathology, persistent hematuria, refractory cystitis or urethritis, chronic urinary tract infections with foreign-body formation or urosepsis, transitional cell dysplasia, and recurrent reflux pancreatitis.[71,72] Most authors recommend waiting 3 to 6 months before considering an enteric conversion because many of the previously mentioned problems are self-limited and improve with time and nonoperative management. For persistent, refractory, or late cases, however, enteric conversion can be performed with low morbidity and can be effective in treating recurrent urologic or metabolic problems.

The most common technique of enteric conversion involves a side-to-side anastomosis between the allograft duodenal segment and recipient small bowel (Fig. 28-21). After takedown of the duodenocystostomy, the bladder is closed primarily with urethral catheter drainage. In cases of severe duodenal pathology, a Roux-en-Y limb of recipient bowel can be brought down to the duodenal segment with or without pancreatic duct cannulation to protect the bowel anastomosis and promote healing. In extreme cases, the Roux limb can be brought out as an ostomy to provide further control of the exocrine drainage. Despite its physiologic advantage, enteric drainage of the exocrine secretions is not recommended either at the time of transplantation or in the immediate posttransplantation period because of the risk of leakage with subsequent intraabdominal sepsis in the setting of heavy immunosuppression and inadequate bowel preparation. With longer follow-up,

many centers are reporting enteric conversion rates of 10% to 15%.[71,72]

Metabolic Problems

Due to the obligatory loss of sodium and bicarbonate from exocrine drainage into the urinary tract, pancreas transplantation recipients are susceptible to metabolic acidosis and dehydration. Dehydration in the setting of diabetic autonomic neuropathy can result in significant problems with orthostatic hypotension. In the initial postoperative period, the state of hydration is maintained using intravenous normal saline with added sodium bicarbonate (50 to 100 mEq/L). Virtually all patients require supplemental oral sodium bicarbonate once oral intake is resumed, but with time, most patients have a decrease in their requirements.

To further improve fluid status, most patients are strongly encouraged to increase their fluid intake; some patients may in addition require sodium chloride tablets, fludrocortisone, or acetazolamide to help maintain electrolyte balance. The administration of oral pancreatic enzyme supplements appears to have a mild inhibitory effect on pancreatic exocrine output and may be helpful in certain cases.[73] In severe cases of dehydration, patients may present not only with hypotension but also with renal dysfunction and severe constipation. Treatment usually consists of intravenous fluid hydration with salt-containing solutions and added bicarbonate. This metabolic derangement is self-limited and becomes less of a problem after several months. A potential benefit of this condition is that hypertension

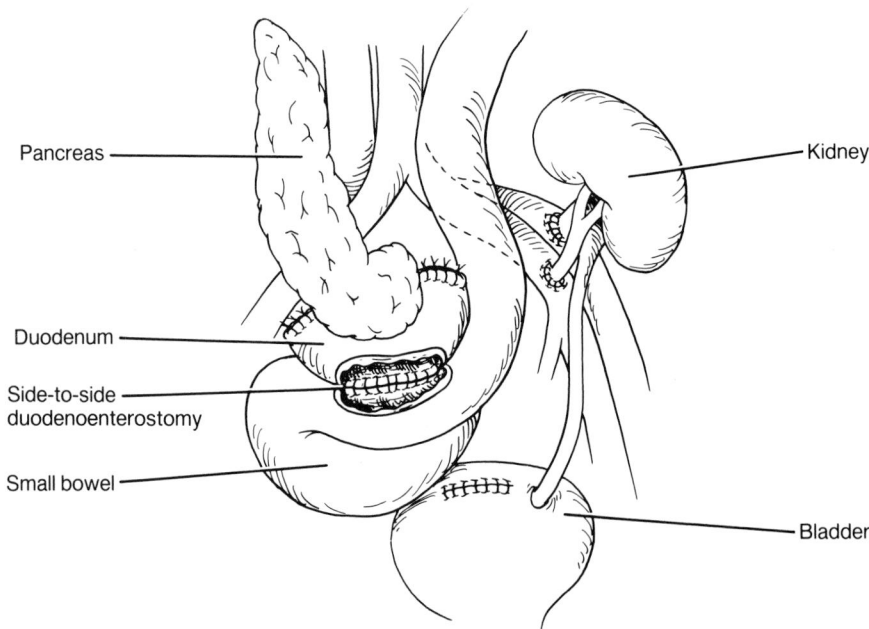

Pancreas

Kidney

Duodenum

Side-to-side duodenoenterostomy

Small bowel

Bladder

Figure 28-21 Technique of exocrine drainage conversion from bladder to enteric drainage.

appears to be less of a problem in pancreas transplant recipients. If patients have continued problems with fluid and electrolyte imbalance, they may be considered candidates for enteric conversion, which is performed for this complication in 5% to 7% of patients.[71,72]

Enzyme Activation

Another complication of urinary drainage of the exocrine pancreas is enzyme activation, leading to "chemical" cystitis, urethritis, or balanitis.[74] This activation exacerbates catheter-induced urethral mucosal injury, leading to persistent urethritis, urethral strictures, or even urethral disruption.[75] These problems are more frequent in men than in women. Although the reported overall incidence is low (3% to 9%), refractory cases may occur that are difficult to treat. Management includes oral or intravenous fluid hydration, alkalinization of the urine, urinary tract analgesics, and treatment of any associated urinary tract infection. Severe cases may require prolonged urethral catheterization for urinary drainage and the administration of oral pancreatic enzymes or somatostatin analogue to decrease exocrine output.[76] Refractory cases may require suprapubic cystostomy or enteric conversion to divert enzymes and allow the healing of the urethral mucosa. For the most part, however, this problem is self-limited and can be managed nonoperatively.

Hyperamylasemia

Hyperamylasemia is another common problem that may or may not signify allograft pancreatitis. In general, the serum amylase is not a reliable parameter of either exocrine function or immune events after pancreas transplantation; peak levels do not correlate with the intensity, duration, or outcome of allograft pancreatitis.[77] The differential diagnosis of hyperamylasemia in the pancreas transplant recipient includes early (ischemic) injury, rejection, reflux pancreatitis, peripancreatic fluid collection (phlegmon, pseudocyst, ascites, abscess), technical problems (leak, fistula), infection (eg, cytomegalovirus), postoperative or postbiopsy injury, and miscellaneous causes related to either the native pancreas or salivary disorders.

Allograft Pancreatitis

Patients with pancreatitis may be asymptomatic or present with fever, lower abdominal pain, allograft swelling or tenderness, ileus, distention, or constipation. The diagnosis of allograft pancreatitis is usually based on clinical presentation; hyperamylasemia; ultrasonographic evidence of pancreatic edema; hyperperfu-

sion with loss of border resolution on radionuclide scanning; CT findings of pancreatic enlargement with edema, peripancreatic fluid, or inflammation (Fig. 28-22); or direct evidence of pancreatitis at laparotomy with edema and saponification. Initial management consists of urethral catheter drainage, urine culture, intravenous fluid hydration, radiologic studies, and blood and urine studies to rule out rejection. Since many patients may have a neurogenic bladder from diabetes, reflux pancreatitis from inadequate bladder emptying is a frequent cause of hyperamylasemia that initially requires catheter drainage and may necessitate short-term intermittent self-catheterization by the patient.

A management algorithm for hyperamylasemia and pancreatitis is presented in Figure 28-23. Urethral catheter drainage is the mainstay of therapy, with somatostatin analogue therapy reserved for persistent hyperamylasemia or pancreatitis. In several uncontrolled nonrandomized clinical studies, somatostatin appears to be safe and effective in reducing the exocrine output of the denervated pancreas allograft, but it also reduces cyclosporine levels.[76]

Allograft pancreatitis may be due to surgical complications, such as leak, fistula, or infection, with development of fluid collections, pseudocysts, or abscesses surrounding the pancreatic graft (Fig. 28-24). The combination of pancreatitis with local tissue breakdown and bacterial contamination can lead to peripancreatic abscess formation that can be difficult to treat. Initial therapy usually consists of percutaneous drainage, but if infection persists, operative exploration is often required.[78] The reported incidence of abscess formation requiring operative drainage ranges from 5% to 22%. The presence of peripancreatic infection portends a poor prognosis, resulting in multiple procedures and eventual allograft pancreatectomy in about 30% to 50% of cases.[46]

Wound Problems

In addition to intraabdominal infections, a high incidence of wound dehiscence and infections has been reported after pancreas transplantation that is not necessarily related to immunosuppression.[45,46] Factors that may be important in preventing wound or intraabdominal infections include intraperitoneal placement of the pancreas through a midline approach, active drainage of the pelvis to prevent fluid collections, selective use of somatostatin, and selective bowel decontamination with appropriate perioperative antibiotic coverage.

Urologic Complications

With the increasing use of bladder drainage, postoperative problems have shifted from intraabdominal to urologic complications.[79–82] A list of the more common urologic

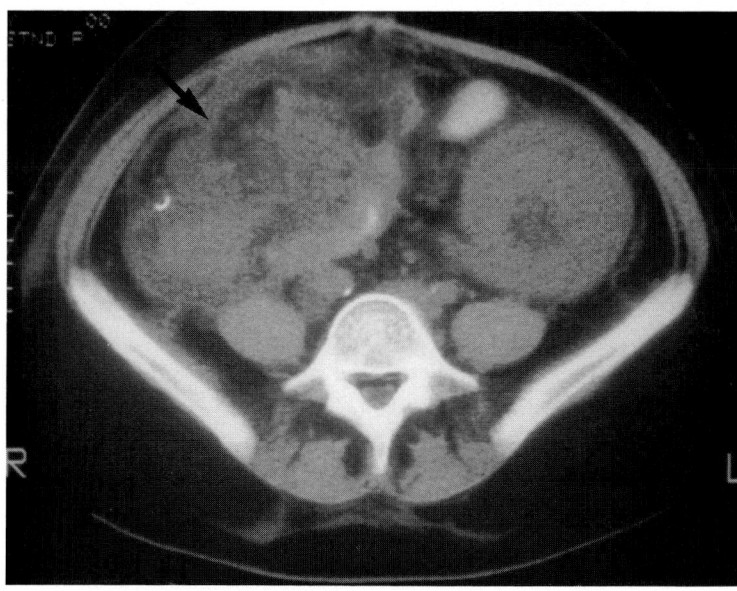

Figure 28-22 CT scan of recipient pelvis showing severe allograft pancreatitis with peripancreatic inflammation and fluid. The transplanted pancreas is on the patient's right, and the transplanted kidney is on the left.

complications and their respective incidence from several of the transplantation centers is shown in Table 28-9.

Urinary tract infections in bladder-drained pancreas transplant recipients are common and multifactorial in nature. The incidence of urosepsis (4%), however, is relatively low. Many of these urinary tract infections are caused by normally nonvirulent organisms that are not commonly associated with urinary tract infections. Among these organisms are *Staphylococcus epidermidis, Citrobacter* sp, and *Enterococcus* sp. The combination of pancreatic enzyme activation, an alka-

line environment, and immunosuppression seems to predispose the bladder to infection by these atypical organisms and makes the eradication of these organisms difficult.[75] Urinary tract infections in bladder-drained pancreas transplant recipients may actually change the pH of the bladder environment and therefore initiate or exacerbate enzyme activation.

With enzyme activation, patients are predisposed to developing urethritis, cystitis, or actual ulceration, which may manifest as hematuria. Gross hematuria is the most frequent major urologic complication, occur-

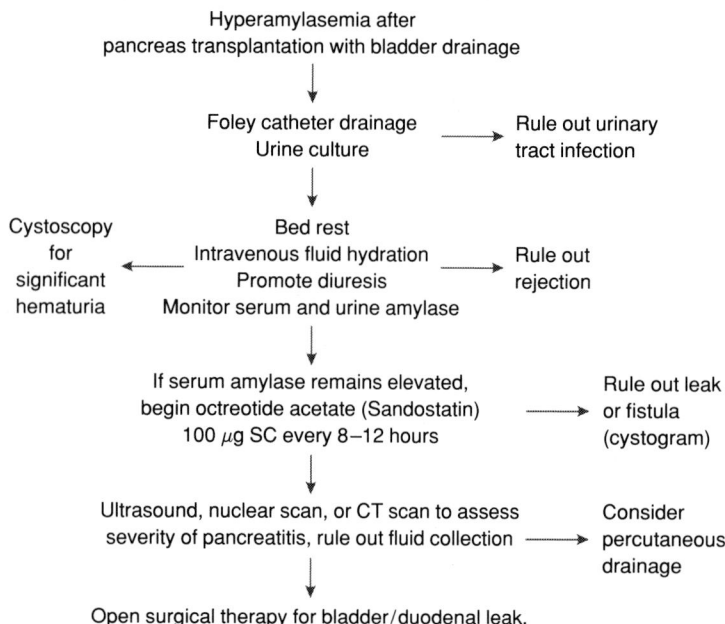

Figure 28-23 Management algorithm for the diagnosis and treatment of hyperamylasemia or allograft pancreatitis after pancreas transplantation.

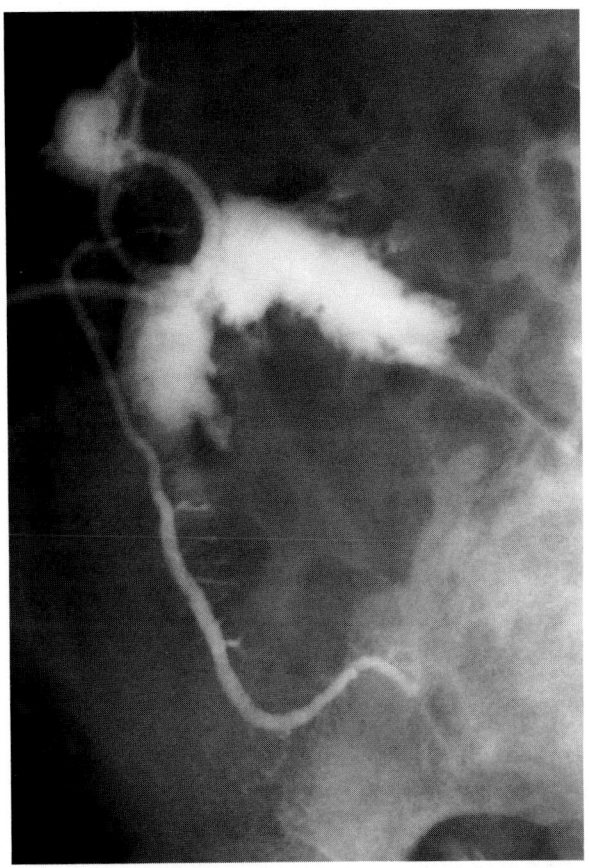

Figure 28-24 Sinogram through percutaneous drainage catheter showing localized cavity adjacent to tail of right iliac pancreas transplant with communication and retrograde filling of the pancreatic duct.

By following a systemic approach, gross hematuria can be successfully treated with minimal morbidity or graft loss and only rarely requires open surgical therapy.[83]

Perforation of the duodenal segment and urinary extravasation occurs nearly as frequently as gross hematuria (4% to 14%) and, if unrecognized, may result in significant morbidity. Most patients present with the sudden onset of lower abdominal pain and hyperamylasemia. A high degree of clinical suspicion is sometimes required because patients may present with only vague abdominal symptoms and fever in the setting of immunosuppression. The most common site of urine leak is the distal staple line of the duodenal segment adjacent to the head of the pancreas. If a standard cystogram does not demonstrate the leak (Fig. 28-25*A*), a CT scan cystogram (see Fig. 28-25*B*) can be helpful in confirming the presence of a perforation. Duodenal segment leaks may occur early or late, with early cases usually due to technical causes or ischemia and late cases due to rejection or infection. Treatment is usually by direct open repair, although some authors advocate nonoperative management with prolonged urethral catheter drainage.[84] Others perform an enteric conversion for duodenal or anastomotic leaks, particularly if recurrent or if associated with significant duodenal segment pathology.[71,72,81]

ring in about 10% of patients with bladder-drained pancreas transplants.[79–82] Early hematuria can be minimized by careful preparation and handling of the duodenal segment to avoid devascularization or mucosal hemorrhage. Urethral catheter drainage is the mainstay of therapy, with most episodes being self-limited.

Vascular Complications

In addition to urologic and exocrine complications, pancreas transplantation is associated with other operative complications inherent to the procedure.[46] Pancreas allografts are prone to vascular problems because of the intrinsically low microcirculatory flow of the organ. Vascular complications include hemorrhage, thrombosis, stenosis, pseudoaneurysm formation, and arteriovenous fistulas.[85] Complications may involve the reconstructed vascular supply to the pancreas, the intrinsic blood supply, or the recipient's native vessels.

Table 28-9   Major Urologic Complications After Pancreas Transplantation With Bladder Drainage

Investigation	Hematuria (%)	Perforation (%)	Urethritis (%)	Urethral Stricture and Disruption (%)	Overall Incidence (%)
Sollinger et al (1993)[81]	15.7	14.2	3.3	2.8	40
Cheung et al (1992)[25]	9.4	4	NA	5.6	24
Smith et al (1991)[80]	9	9	NA	NA	NA
Elkhammas et al (1992)[79]	13	11	9	4	39
Taylor et al (1994)[82]	9	8	8	3	39
AVERAGE	11.2	9.2	6.8	3.9	35.5

NA, Data not available.

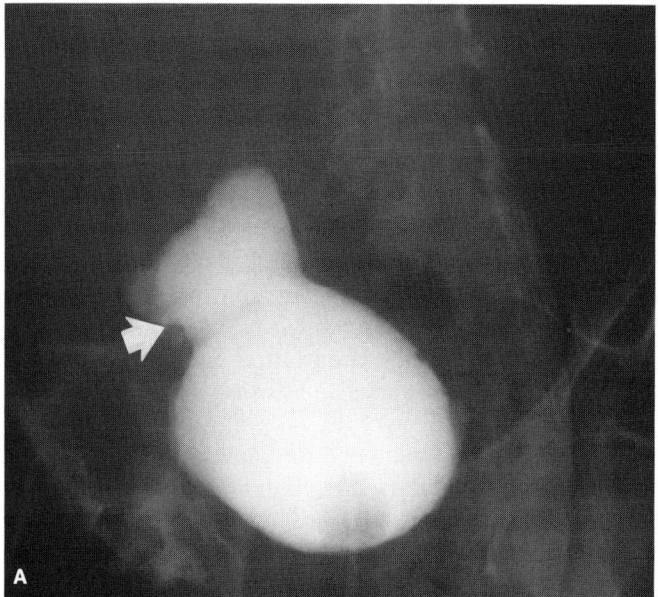

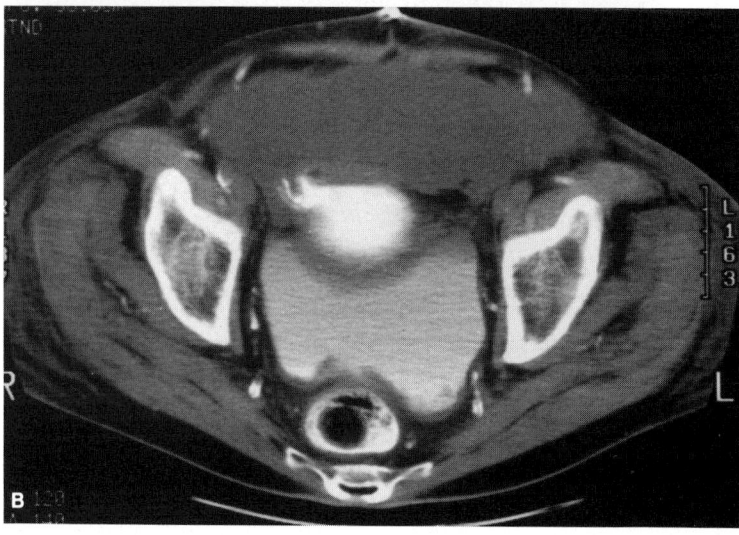

Figure 28-25 (A) Conventional cystogram showing reflux of contrast into duodenal segment with possible extravasation (*arrow*). (B) CT cystogram demonstrating reflux of contrast into duodenal segment with large leak and fluid collection between the bladder and rectum.

Hemorrhage and arteriovenous fistula formation usually involve the transplanted mesenteric bundle (Fig. 28-26). The presence of an arteriovenous fistula may threaten allograft survival and manifest with allograft dysfunction, hematuria, or an asymptomatic bruit or thrill over the allograft. Direct operative repair with individual ligation of the superior mesenteric artery and vein usually results in a successful outcome.

Arterial or venous thrombosis is a dreaded complication after pancreas transplantation because it usually results in allograft pancreatectomy. Whether vascular thrombosis occurs as a manifestation of preservation or immunologic injury or is due to a technical problem may be difficult to determine. Patients usually present with acute hyperglycemia and a dramatic reduction in urine amylase levels. Thrombectomy with attempted graft sal-

vage is potentially dangerous except in the case of isolated splenic artery thrombosis.[86,87] The incidence of vascular thrombosis has decreased because of better preservation, the routine use of an arterial graft, a tension-free portal venous anastomosis (with or without venous extension graft) after complete mobilization of the recipient iliac vein, and antiplatelet (but not full anticoagulation) therapy to reduce the risk of thrombosis without increasing the risk of hemorrhage. Most centers do not routinely employ full anticoagulation therapy with combined pancreas–kidney transplantation. In solitary pancreas transplantation, however, perioperative anticoagulation is indicated because of the higher risk of vascular thrombosis, which may be due to the loss of the "protective" anticoagulant effects of uremia.

Vascular complications are an important source of

morbidity in pancreas transplant recipients, ranging in incidence from 10% to 20%. Clinical presentation is variable but usually includes allograft dysfunction. Physical examination and duplex ultrasonography are usually diagnostic, with angiography reserved for selected cases. Early diagnosis is critical to graft salvage, but prompt surgical intervention may still result in a high rate of graft loss.[85] Although vascular complications are associated with reduced pancreas allograft survival, they are rarely a cause of mortality.

Other Complications

Placement of an intraperitoneal pancreas transplant can also be associated with general surgical complications, such as small bowel obstruction, cholecystitis, and superficial or deep wound infections.[46] Similar to other immunosuppressed transplant recipients, pancreas transplant recipients are at risk not only for bacterial infections but also for opportunistic infections due to viruses (particularly cytomegalovirus), fungi (especially *Candida* sp), and *Pneumocystis* sp.[57] Postoperative management should include regimens of prophylaxis specifically directed against these otherwise unusual infections.

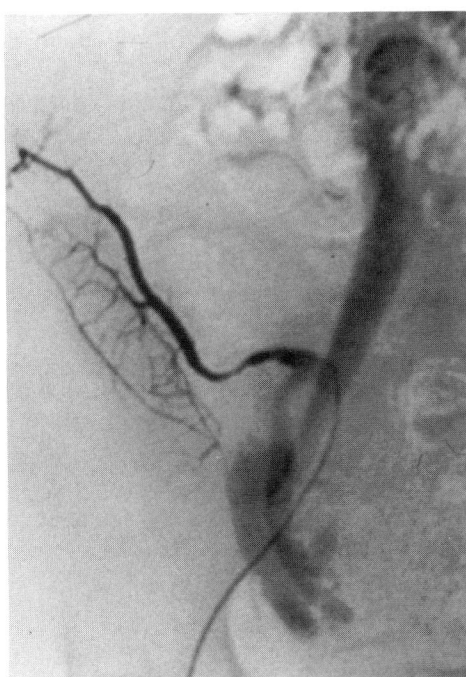

Figure 28-26 Selective arteriography of pancreas allograft revealing patency of the splenic artery and a large superior mesenteric arteriovenous fistula in the head of the pancreas, with early filling of the iliac vein and vena cava.

BENEFITS OF PANCREAS TRANSPLANTATION

Metabolic Effects

From a metabolic standpoint, pancreas transplantation establishes a euglycemic insulin-independent state that is unmatched by any other form of therapy. Carbohydrate metabolism is normalized as documented by 24-hour glucose profiles, stimulation testing, and glycosylated hemoglobin levels.[6,9] Most pancreas transplant recipients receive a pancreas allograft with nonportal venous drainage, which results in fasting and stimulated peripheral hyperinsulinemia.[88] Although concerns have been raised about the possible long-term consequences of hyperinsulinemia, no major sequelae have been identified other than symptomatic hypoglycemia in a minority of patients. Progressive islet cell failure due to insulin resistance has not been well documented in the absence of rejection. In addition, recurrent diabetes (presumably due to autoimmunity) appears to be effectively controlled by the continued immunosuppressive therapy.[6,9,10] There is also evidence that a functioning pancreas transplant may ablate the hyperlipidemic effects of immunosuppression and actually improve lipid metabolism over time.[89]

Effects on Secondary Diabetic Complications

All other existing methods of insulin administration do not provide sufficiently good metabolic control to prevent the progressive diabetic complications of retinopathy, peripheral and autonomic neuropathy, nephropathy, and accelerated atherosclerosis. In addition to correcting dysmetabolism and freeing the patient from exogenous insulin therapy, data on the course of secondary complications after pancreas transplantation are emerging. With regard to nephropathy, preliminary evidence suggests that successful transplantation can induce regression of early but not advanced microscopic lesions of diabetic nephropathy, stabilize renal function, and prevent recurrence of diabetic nephropathy in the kidney transplant.[90] The course of diabetic retinopathy appears to be less favorably influenced by a functioning pancreas transplant.[91] With longer follow-up, however, data are accumulating to suggest that retinopathy may be stabilized. Peripheral and autonomic neuropathy improves or stabilizes in most pancreas transplant recipients, which may actually translate into a survival advantage.[92] Nerve conduction velocities and evoked muscle action potentials increase, and a beneficial effect on microcirculatory blood flow has been demonstrated.[93] These effects may place recipients at a lower overall risk for the development of peripheral ulcers or amputations. Long-term studies are needed, however, to document and characterize the effects of pancreas transplantation on the diabetic condition.

Quality of Life

Pancreas transplantation in patients with hyperlabile diabetes, extreme difficulty with metabolic control, or hypoglycemia unawareness can immediately enhance quality of life simply by inducing insulin independence with improved counterregulation.[10,11] Although the long-term commitment to immunosuppression is the major trade-off of transplantation, most patients find the transition to transplantation easier than continued insulin therapy because of an improved sense of wellbeing with fewer dietary and activity restrictions. A marked improvement in quality of life and rehabilitation potential has been consistently demonstrated after successful pancreas transplantation, particularly in combined pancreas–kidney transplant recipients compared with recipients of kidney transplants alone.[11,94] It is hoped that the changes in carbohydrate and lipid metabolism will also translate into improvements in diabetic end-organ complications and decrease the risk of atherosclerotic vascular disease, although these data are still emerging.

ISLET CELL AND FETAL PANCREAS TRANSPLANTATION

Islet cell and fetal pancreas transplantation represent more sophisticated forms of endocrine replacement therapy for IDDM. As of 1994, about 215 clinical islet cell transplantations had been attempted worldwide, with only a few patients actually achieving complete insulin independence.[6,95] The most popular technique of islet cell transplantation is by intraportal injection, usually through a cutdown on the falciform ligament, with subsequent cannulation of the umbilical vein.[96] Potential advantages of islet transplantation include low morbidity and the possibility of islet immunoalteration or immunoisolation with eventual transplantation without immunosuppression. Problem areas include efficient isolation and purification; safe preservation; identifying the optimal site of transplantation; prevention of rejection, recurrent autoimmune disease, or functional deterioration; and islet cell supply, which will probably need to be from xenograft donors in the future.

Vascularized pancreas transplantation has assumed an increasing role in the treatment of dia-

betes mellitus. Combined pancreas–kidney transplantation should be regarded as the treatment of choice in carefully selected type I diabetic patients with significant nephropathy. Indications for solitary pancreas transplantation are less clearly defined and are based on the presence of early diabetic complications or hyperlability with poor quality of life. The type of transplantation considered has a strong influence on patient (and physician) acceptance. Although transplantation results in euglycemia and complete insulin independence, it is at the expense of hyperinsulinemia and chronic immunosuppression. The net result of these changes on diabetic complications in the long-term remains to be determined. In the short-term, improvement in the quality of life and possible prevention of further morbidity associated with diabetes makes pancreas transplantation an important therapeutic option for selected diabetic patients.

In the future, advances in immunosuppressive strategies and diagnostic technology will only enhance the already good results achieved with pancreas transplantation. Further documentation of the long-term benefits and effects of pancreas transplantation may lead to wider availability and acceptance. Effective control of rejection with earlier diagnosis or better prevention may soon permit solitary pancreas transplantation to become an accepted treatment option in diabetic patients without advanced complications. Although there is significant associated morbidity unique to the pancreas transplantation, this is usually manageable without influencing the outcome. Alternative future strategies, such as islet cell and fetal pancreas transplantations, gene therapy and immunotherapy, more sophisticated insulin pumps, and biohybrid artificial pancreas units, will also play a role in the treatment of IDDM. It will be difficult, however, for these alternative strategies to improve on the metabolic efficiency of the vascularized pancreas transplantation. With the improvement in quality of life and the potential for arresting diabetic complications, pancreas transplantation may become one of the most frequent organ transplantation procedures performed in the future.

REFERENCES

1. Harris M, Hadden WC, Knowles WC, Bennett PH. Prevalence of diabetes and impaired glucose tolerance and

plasma glucose levels in the U.S. population aged 20–74 years. Diabetes 1987;36:523.

2. Eisenbarth GS. Type I diabetes mellitus: a chronic auto-immune disease. N Engl J Med 1986;314:1360.

3. Nathan DM. Long-term complications of diabetes mellitus. N Engl J Med 1993;328:1676.

4. Chase HP, Jackson WE, Hoops SL, Cockerham RS, Archer PG, O'Brien D. Glucose control and the renal and retinal complications of insulin-dependent diabetes. JAMA 1989;261:1155.

5. Brownlee M, Cerami A, Vlassara H. Advanced glycosylation end products in tissue and the biochemical basis of diabetic complications. N Engl J Med 1988;318:1315.

6. Robertson RP. Pancreatic and islet transplantation for diabetes: cures or curiosities? N Engl J Med 1992;327:1861.

7. American Diabetes Association Position Statement. Implications of the Diabetes Control and Complications Trial. Diabetes Spectr 1993;6:225.

8. Sutherland DER. Coming of age for pancreas transplantation. West J Med 1989;150:314.

9. Robertson RP. Pancreas transplantation in humans with diabetes mellitus. Diabetes 1991;40:1085.

10. Sutherland DER. Pancreatic transplantation: an update. Diabetes Rev 1993;1:152.

11. Gross CR, Zehrer CL. Health-related quality of life of outcomes of pancreas transplant recipients. Clin Transplant 1992;6:165.

12. Kelly WD, Lillehei RC, Merkel FK, et al. Allotransplantation of the pancreas and duodenum along with the kidney in diabetic nephropathy. Surgery 1967;61:827.

13. Lillehei RC, Ruiz JO, Acquino C. Transplantation of the pancreas. Acta Endocrinol 1976;83:303.

14. Sutherland DER, Goetz FC, Najarian JS. One-hundred pancreas transplants at a single institution. Ann Surg 1984;200:414.

15. Sutherland DER. Pancreatic transplantation: state of the art. Transplant Proc 1992;24:762.

16. Sutherland DER, Gruessner A, Moudry-Munns K. Analysis of United Network for Organ Sharing (UNOS) United States of America (USA) pancreas transplant registry data according to multiple variables. In: Terasaki PI, Cecka JM, eds. Clinical transplants 1992. Los Angeles, UCLA Tissue Typing Laboratory, 1993:45.

17. Stratta RJ, Taylor RJ, Ozaki CF, et al. A comparative analysis of results and morbidity in type I diabetics undergoing preemptive versus post-dialysis combined pancreas-kidney transplantation. Transplantation 1993;55:1097.

18. Sollinger HW, Knechtle SJ, Reed A, et al. Experience with 100 consecutive simultaneous kidney–pancreas transplants with bladder drainage. Ann Surg 1991;214:703.

19. Schulak JA, Mayes JT, Hricik DE. Combined kidney and pancreas transplantation: a safe and effective treatment for diabetic nephropathy. Arch Surg 1990;125:881.

20. Stratta RJ, Taylor RJ, Wahl TO, et al. Recipient selection and evaluation for vascularized pancreas transplantation. Transplantation 1993;55:1090.

21. Manske CL, Thomas W, Wang Y, Wilson RF. Screening diabetic transplant candidates for coronary artery disease: identification of a low risk subgroup. Kidney Int 1993;44:617.

22. Morrow CE, Schwartz JS, Sutherland DER, et al. Predictive value of thallium stress testing for coronary and cardiovascular events in uremic diabetic patients before renal transplantation. Am J Surg 1983;146:331.

23. Najarian JS, Kaufman DB, Fryd DS, et al. Long-term survival following kidney transplantation in 100 type I diabetic patients. Transplantation 1989;47:106.

24. Gruessner RWG, Dunn DL, Tzardis PJ, et al. Simultaneous pancreas and kidney transplants versus single kidney transplants and previous kidney transplants in uremic patients and single pancreas transplants in non-uremic diabetic patients: comparison of rejection, morbidity, and long-term outcome. Transplant Proc 1990;22:622.

25. Cheung AHS, Sutherland DER, Gillingham KJ, et al. Simultaneous pancreas–kidney transplant versus kidney transplant alone in diabetic patients. Kidney Int 1992;41:924.

26. Stratta RJ, Taylor RJ, Ozaki CF, et al. The analysis of benefit and risk of combined pancreatic and renal transplantation versus renal transplantation alone. Surg Gynecol Obstet 1993;177:163.

27. Schulak JA, Mayes JT, Hricik DE. Kidney transplantation in diabetic patients undergoing combined kidney–pancreas or kidney-only transplantation. Transplantation 1992;53:685.

28. Sutherland DER. Indications for pancreas transplantation: a commentary. Clin Transplant 1990;4:242.

29. Sutherland DER, Kendall DM, Moudry KC, et al. Pancreas transplantation in non-uremic, type I diabetic recipients. Surgery 1988;104:453.

30. University of Michigan Pancreas Transplant Evaluation Committee. Pancreatic transplantation as a treatment of IDDM: proposed candidate evaluation before end-stage diabetic nephropathy. Diabetes Care 1988;11:669.

31. Sutherland DER, Gruessner R, Gillingham K, et al. A single institution's experience with solitary pancreas transplantation: a multi-variate analysis of factors leading to improved outcome. In: Teraski P, ed. Clinical transplants 1991. Los Angeles, UCLA Tissue Typing Laboratory, 1992:141.

32. Gores PF, Gillingham KJ, Dunn DL, Moudry-Munns KC, Najarian JS, Sutherland DER. Donor hyperglycemia as a minor risk factor and immunologic variables as major risk factors for pancreas allograft loss in multi-variate analysis of a single institution's experience. Ann Surg 1992;215:217.

33. Hesse UJ, Sutherland DER. Influence of serum amylase and plasma glucose levels in pancreas cadaver donors on graft function in recipients. Diabetes 1989;38(Suppl 1):1.

34. Sutherland DER, Goetz FC, Najarian JS. Pancreas transplants from related donors. Transplantation 1984;38:625.

35. Sollinger HW, Vernon WB, D'Alessandro AM, Kalayoglu M, Stratta RJ, Belzer FO. Combined liver and pancreas procurement with Belzer-UW solution. Surgery 1989;106:685.

36. Stratta RJ, Taylor RJ, Spees EK, et al. Refinements in cadaveric pancreas-kidney procurement and preservation. Transplant Proc 1991;23:2320.

37. Dunn DL, Morel P, Schlumpf R, et al. Evidence that combined procurement of pancreas and liver grafts does not affect transplant outcome. Transplantation 1991;51:150.

38. Starzl TE, Miller C, Broznick B, Makowka L. An improved technique for multiple organ harvesting. Surg Gynecol Obstet 1987;165:343.

39. Nghiem DD, Corry RJ. Technique of simultaneous renal pancreaticoduodenal transplantation with urinary drainage of pancreatic secretion. Am J Surg 1987;153:405.

40. Gliedman ML, Gold M, Whittaker J, et al. Pancreatic duct to ureter anastomosis for exocrine drainage in pancreas transplantation. Am J Surg 1973;125:245.

41. Groth CG, Lundgren G, Ostman J, et al. Experience with nine segmental pancreatic transplantations in pre-uremic diabetic patients in Stockholm. Transplant Proc 1980;12:68.

42. Dubernard JM, Traegher J, Neyra P, et al. New method of preparation of a segmental pancreatic graft for transplantation: trials in dogs and in man. Surgery 1978;84:634.

43. Cook K, Sollinger HW, Warner T, et al. Pancreaticocystostomy: an alternative method for exocrine drainage of segmental pancreatic allografts. Transplantation 1983;35:634.

44. Sollinger HW, Pirsch JD, D'Alessandro AM, et al. Advantages of bladder drainage in pancreas transplantation. Clin Transplant 1990;4:32.

45. Tesi RJ, Henry ML, Elkhammas EA, Sommer BJ, Ferguson RM. Decreased wound complications of combined kidney–pancreas transplant using intra-abdominal pancreas graft placement. Clin Transplant 1990;4:287.

46. Ozaki CF, Stratta RJ, Taylor RJ, Langnas AN, Bynon JS, Shaw BW Jr. Surgical complications in solitary pancreas and combined pancreas-kidney transplantations. Am J Surg 1992;164:546.

47. Sollinger HW, Knecktle SJ. The current status of combined kidney–pancreas transplantation. In: Sabiston DC Jr, ed. Textbook of surgery, update 6. Philadelphia, WB Saunders, 1990:83.

48. Tyden G, Tibell A, Bolinder J, Ostman J, Groth CG. Pancreatic transplantation with enteric exocrine diversion: experience with 120 cases. Transplant Proc 1992;24:771.

49. Kubota K, Reinholt FP, Tyden G, Bohman SO, Groth CG. Cytologic patterns in juice from human pancreatic transplants: correlation with histologic findings in the graft. Surgery 1991;109:507.

50. Rosenlof LK, Earnhardt R, Pruitt TL, et al. Pancreas transplantation: an initial experience with systemic and portal drainage of pancreatic allografts. Ann Surg 1992;215:586.

51. Sibley RK, Sutherland DER. Pancreas transplantation: immunohistologic and histopathologic examination of 100 grafts. Am J Pathol 1987;128:151.

52. Sutherland DER, Dunn DL, Goetz FC, et al. A ten-year experience with 290 pancreas transplants at a single institution. Ann Surg 1989;210:274.

53. Stratta RJ, Taylor RJ, Zorn BH, et al. Combined pancreas–kidney transplantation: preliminary results and metabolic effects. Am J Gastroenterol 1991;86:697.

54. Sutherland DER. Immunosuppression for clinical pancreas transplantation. Clin Transplant 1991;5:549.

55. Sollinger HW, Stratta RJ, Kalayoglu M, Pirsch JD, Belzer FO. Pancreas transplantation with pancreaticocystostomy and quadruple immunosuppression. Surgery 1987;102:674.

56. Brayman KL, Sutherland DER. Factors leading to improved outcome following pancreas transplantation: the influence of immunosuppression and HLA matching. Transplant Proc 1992;24:91.

57. Stratta RJ, Taylor RJ, Bynon JS, et al. Viral prophylaxis in combined pancreas–kidney transplantation recipients. Transplantation 1994;57:506.

58. Canfield CW, Hudnall SD, Colonna JO, et al. Fulminant Epstein-Barr virus–associated post-transplant lymphoproliferative disorders following OKT3 therapy. Clin Transplant 1992;6:1.

59. Engfeldt P, Tyden G, Gunnarsson R, Ostman J, Groth CG. Impaired glucose tolerance with cyclosporine. Transplant Proc 1986;18:65.

60. Sollinger HW, Stratta RJ, D'Alessandro AM, et al. Experience with simultaneous pancreas-kidney transplantation. Ann Surg 1988;208:475.

61. Stratta RJ, Sollinger HW, Perlman SB, et al. Early diagnosis and treatment of pancreas allograft rejection. Transplant Int 1988;1:6.

62. Prieto M, Sutherland DER, Fernandez-Cruz L, et al. Experimental and clinical experience with urine amylase monitoring for early diagnosis of rejection in pancreas transplantation. Transplant 1987;43:71.

63. Marks WH, Borgstrom A, Sollinger HW, Marks C. Serum immunoreactive anodal trypsinogen and urinary amylase as biochemical markers for rejection of clinical whole-organ pancreas allografts having exocrine drainage into the urinary bladder. Transplantation 1990;49:112.

64. Radio SJ, Stratta RJ, Taylor RJ, Linder J. The utility of urine cytology in the diagnosis of allograft rejection after combined pancreas-kidney transplantation. Transplantation 1993;55:509.

65. Allen RDM, Wilson TG, Grierson JM, et al. Percutaneous biopsy of bladder-drained pancreas transplants. Transplantation 1991;51:1213.

66. Sutherland DER, Casanova D, Sibley RK. Role of pancreas graft biopsies in the diagnosis and treatment of rejection after pancreas transplantation. Transplant Proc 1987;19:2329.

67. Ekberg H, Allen RDM, Greenberg ML, et al. Percutaneous fine needle aspiration biopsy of canine pancreas allo-

graft provides diagnosis of treatable rejection. J Surg Res 1989;47:348.

68. Nakhleh RE, Gruessner RWG, Tzardis PJ, Dunn DL, Sutherland DER. Pathology of transplanted human duodenal tissue: a histologic study, with comparison to pancreatic pathology, in resected pancreaticoduodenal transplants. Clin Transplant 1991;5:241.

69. Perkins JD, Engen DE, Munn SR, Barr D, Marsh CL, Carpenter HA. The value of cystoscopically-directed biopsy in human pancreaticoduodenal transplantation. Clin Transplant 1989;3:306.

70. Stratta RJ, Sollinger HW, D'Alessandro AM, Pirsch JD, Kalayoglu M, Belzer FO. OKT3 rescue therapy in pancreas allograft rejection. Diabetes 1989;38(Suppl 1):74.

71. Sollinger HW, Sasaki TM, D'Alessandro AM, et al. Indications for enteric conversion after pancreas transplantation with bladder drainage. Surgery 1992;112:842.

72. Stephanian E, Gruessner RWG, Brayman KL, et al. Conversion of exocrine secretions from bladder to enteric drainage in recipients of whole pancreaticoduodenal transplants. Ann Surg 1992;216:663.

73. Burton FR, Burton MS, Garvin PJ, Joshi SN. Enteral pancreatic enzyme feedback inhibition of the exocrine secretion of the human transplanted pancreas. Transplantation 1992;54:988.

74. Munda R, Tom WW, First MR, Gartside P, Alexander JW. Pancreatic allograft exocrine urinary tract diversion: pathophysiology. Transplantation 1987;43:95.

75. See WA, Smith JL. Activated proteolytic enzymes in the urine of whole organ pancreas transplantation patients with duodenocystostomy. Transplant Proc 1991;23:1615.

76. Stratta RJ, Taylor RJ, Lowell JA, et al. Selective use of Sandostatin in vascularized pancreas transplantation. Am J Surg 1993;166:598.

77. Stratta RJ, Sollinger HW, Groshek M, et al. Differential diagnosis of hyperamylasemia in pancreas allograft recipients. Transplant Proc 1990;22:675.

78. Hesse UJ, Sutherland DER, Najarian JS, et al. Intra-abdominal infections in pancreas transplant recipients. Ann Surg 1986;203:153.

79. Elkhammas EA, Henry ML, Barone GW, et al. Urological complications in diabetic recipients of combined kidney–pancreas grafts versus kidney grafts alone. Transplant Proc 1992;24:813.

80. Smith JL, See WA, Ames SA, et al. Lower urinary tract complications in patients with duodenocystostomies for exocrine drainage of the transplanted pancreas. Transplant Proc 1991;23:1611.

81. Sollinger HW, Messing EM, Eckhoff DE, et al. Urological complications in 210 consecutive simultaneous pancreas–kidney transplants with bladder drainage. Ann Surg 1993;218:561.

82. Taylor RJ, Bynon JS, Stratta RJ. Kidney–pancreas transplantation: a review of the current status. Urol Clin North Am 1994;21:343.

83. Stratta RJ, Taylor RJ. Prevention and management of hematuria in combined pancreas–kidney transplant recipients with pancreaticoduodenal cystostomy. Transplant Proc 1992;24:788.

84. Elkhammas EA, Henry ML, Tesi RJ, Ferguson RM. Duodenal segment–associated complications following combined kidney/pancreas transplantation. Transplant Proc 1993;25:2230.

85. Bynon JS, Stratta RJ, Taylor RJ, Lowell JA, Cattral M. Vascular reconstruction in 105 consecutive pancreas transplants. Transplant Proc 1994;25:3288.

86. Douzdjian V, Abecassis MM, Cooper JL, Argibay PF, Smith JL, Corry RJ. Pancreas transplant salvage after acute venous thrombosis. Transplantation 1993;56:222.

87. Fernandez-Cruz L, Gilabert R, Sabater L, Saenz A, Astudillo E. Pancreas graft thrombosis: prompt diagnosis and immediate thrombectomy or retransplantation. Clin Transplant 1993;7:230.

88. Diem P, Abid M, Redmon JB, Sutherland DER, Robertson RP. Systemic venous drainage of pancreas allografts as independent cause of hyperinsulinemia in type I diabetic recipients. Diabetes 1990;39:534.

89. Larsen JL, Larson CE, Hirst K, et al. Lipid status after combined pancreas–kidney transplantation and kidney transplantation alone in type I diabetes mellitus. Transplantation 1992;54:992.

90. Bilous RW, Mauer SM, Sutherland DER, Najarian JS, Goetz FC, Steffes MW. The effects of pancreas transplantation on the glomerular structure of renal allografts in patients with insulin-dependent diabetes. N Engl J Med 1989;321:80.

91. Ramsey RC, Goetz FC, Sutherland DER, et al. Progression of diabetic retinopathy after pancreas transplantation for insulin-dependent diabetes mellitus. N Engl J Med 1988;318:208.

92. Navarro X, Kennedy WR, Loewenson RB, Sutherland DER. Influence of pancreas transplantation on cardiorespiratory reflexes, nerve conduction, and mortality in diabetes mellitus. Diabetes 1990;39:802.

93. Abendroth D, Landgraf R, Illner WD, et al. Evidence for reversibility of diabetic microangiopathy following pancreas transplantation. Transplant Proc 1989;21:2850.

94. Nakache R, Tyden G, Groth CG. Quality of life in diabetic patients after combined pancreas–kidney or kidney transplantation. Diabetes 1989;38(Suppl 1):40.

95. Warnock GL, Rajotte RV. Human pancreatic islet transplantation. Transplant Rev 1992;6:195.

96. Scharp DW, Lacy PE, Santiago JV. Results of our first nine intraportal islet allografts into type I (insulin-dependent) diabetic patients. Transplantation 1991;51:76.

Digestive Tract Surgery: A Text and Atlas, edited by Richard H. Bell,
Layton F. Rikkers, and Michael W. Mulholland.
Lippincott-Raven Publishers, Philadelphia, © 1996.

29

Pancreaticoduodenal Trauma

Gregory J. Jurkovich

The unforgiving nature of pancreatic and duodenal injuries is emphasized by dramatic morbidity and mortality statistics. Large series of pancreatic trauma reported during the past decade reveal a mortality rate ranging from 9% to 34%, with a mean rate of 19%.[1] Morbidity rates after pancreatic injury range from 30% to 40%,[2–8] influenced significantly by mechanism of injury (Table 29-1). Reported mortality rates after duodenal injury range from 6% to 25%, and overall morbidity rates range from 30% to 63%, although only about one third of these are directly related to the duodenal injury.[9–11] Major complications of both injuries include fistula, pseudocyst, pancreatitis, anastomotic breakdown, intraabdominal abscess, or pneumonia. These complications account, either directly or indirectly, for the development of septicemia, organ failure, and late mortality. Early mortality rates are largely influenced by the mechanism of injury and are generally due to exsanguination from associated vascular, liver, or spleen injuries.[12–14] A 30-year review of one institution's experience with pancreatic injures emphasizes this point, with a 67% mortality rate due to shotgun wounds, 11% to gunshot wounds, and 6% to stab wounds.[15] One review of 100 consecutive penetrating duodenal injuries[11] documented a 25% mortality rate compared with a 12.5% to 14% mortality rate after blunt duodenal trauma.[10,16] Time from injury to definitive treatment is also an important predictor of mortality. A delay of more than 24 hours in the diagnosis of a duodenal wound increases mortality from 11% to 40%.[17]

Overall mortality in patients with pancreatic trauma is 16% to 20%, depending on the mechanism of injury, the number and type of associated injuries, and the occurrence of complications. Most (50% to 75%) pa-

tients who die with a pancreatic or duodenal injury do so within the first 48 hours of injury, with exsanguination as the primary cause. Infection and subsequent multiple-organ failure account for most of the remaining deaths, with about one third of the patients who survive the first 48 hours developing a complication related to the pancreatic or duodenal injury.[6,9] Fewer than 10% of deaths are primarily attributable to the pancreatic or duodenal injury, and these deaths generally occur 1 to 2 weeks or more after the injury.[6,9,10,18,19]

Fortunately, pancreatic and duodenal wounds are relatively uncommon injuries, primarily because of their protected retroperitoneal location. In Sweden, the annual incidence of pancreatic injury is 0.4 cases per 100,000 population, or 7% of celiotomies for abdominal trauma.[20] In another report,[21] 7.4% of patients undergoing trauma celiotomies were found to have pancreatic injuries. Various other reports estimate that pancreatic injuries occur in only 0.2% to 5% of all abdominal trauma but may occur in up to 10% of severe abdominal trauma.[12–14,22] Reports from urban trauma centers suggest that penetrating pancreatic or duodenal injuries are most common, whereas blunt trauma prevails in other hospitals.

The spectrum of injuries is broad, ranging from simple contusion and hematoma to fracture and laceration or complete disruption. The proximity of the pancreas and duodenum to other vital structures and the high-energy transfer mechanisms involved make isolated injuries distinctly uncommon. For example, the aorta, portal vein, or vena cava are injured in more than 75% of cases of penetrating pancreatic trauma. Injuries to the liver, spleen, or hollow viscus of the gastrointestinal tract are equally common in blunt trauma. In one report,[13] injuries to the liver, colon, and major abdomi-

943

Table 29-1 Pancreatic Trauma: Incidence of Complications According to Mechanism of Injury

Investigation	Total No. of Patients	Stab (%)	Gunshot (%)	Shotgun (%)	Blunt (%)
Jones (1985)[6]	300	7	19	58	18
Werschky & Jordan (1968)[86]	140	10	24	29	18
Wilson & Moorehead (1967)[1]	84	8	45	100	38
Stone, et al (1981)[15]	62	8	20	100	17
TOTAL	486	12	29	57	23

nal vessels accounted for almost half (25 of 55) of all associated injuries. The significance of the associated organ injuries is again illustrated by mortality statistics, which show a 2.5% mortality rate with no or one associated injury, 13.6% with two or three, and 29.6% with four or more associated injuries.[3] Overall, 90% of patients with pancreatic or duodenal injuries have at least one associated injury, with an average of 3.5 to 4.1 associated intraabdominal injuries per patient.[1,5,10,13,15,16,23,24] The single major determinant of outcome after pancreatic injury is the presence or absence of ductal injury. The importance of pancreatic duct injury as a determinant of outcome was probably first recognized and emphasized by Baker and colleagues in 1962 (cited in Laraja and colleagues[25]). Subsequent reviews of experience with pancreatic trauma confirmed and emphasized the importance of determining the status of the pancreatic duct. Resection of distal ductal injures as opposed to drainage alone significantly lowered postoperative morbidity and mortality.[12] In one institution,[8] pancreatic resection distal to site of ductal injury resulted in a decrease in the mortality rate from 19% to 3%. Additional studies documented the importance of intraoperative pancreatography when necessary to determine the status of the pancreatic duct.[26] Aggressive use of intraoperative pancreatography and accurate determination of the status of the pancreatic duct resulted in a decrease in complications from 55% to 15%.

The first priority in managing pancreatic or duodenal trauma should be control of hemorrhage. Limiting bacterial contamination should be the second priority. Duodenal injury is generally apparent intraoperatively, but a diligent search for potential pancreatic injury should follow as the next priority, with an emphasis on determining the status of the pancreatic duct. The presence or absence of pancreatic duct injury is the key determinant of outcome in pancreatic trauma since most postoperative complications can be attributed to inadequate control of major duct disruption.[8,27]

PANCREATIC INJURIES

Anatomy and Physiology

An understanding of pancreatic relational anatomy is essential in planning the surgical approach and understanding the potential for associated injuries (Fig. 29-1). The pancreas lies transversely across the upper part of the posterior abdomen and is about 15 to 20 cm long, 3 cm wide, 1 to 1.5 cm thick, and weighs between 80 and 90 g.[28] Posterior to the pancreas are the inferior vena cava, aorta, left kidney, both renal veins, and the right renal artery. The pancreatic head lies within the concave sweep of the duodenum, with the body crossing the spine and directed obliquely superiorly, with the tail of the pancreas residing in the hilum of the spleen. The splenic artery runs a tortuous route along the upper border of the pancreas, and the splenic vein runs behind the pancreas just superior to its lower edge. The superior mesenteric vein and artery lie just behind the neck of the pancreas and are also enclosed posteriorly by an extension of the pancreatic head known as the *uncinate process*. The uncinate process actually lies between the inferior vena cava and the portal vein. This process can be absent or can almost completely encircle the superior mesenteric artery and vein.

Intraoperative pancreatography is often necessary to determine the status of the pancreatic duct after injury. Knowledge of ductal anatomy assists in obtaining this information. The main pancreatic duct of Wirsung usually traverses the entire length of the gland slightly above a line halfway between the superior and inferior edges (Fig. 29-2) and normally ends by joining the common bile duct and emptying into the duodenum. The accessory duct of Santorini typically branches out from the pancreatic duct in the neck of the pancreas and empties separately into the duodenum about 2.5 cm above the duodenal papilla. A significant number of anatomic variations occur and must be recognized in obtaining intraoperative pancreatograms. In 20% of cases, the accessory duct of Santorini drains into the

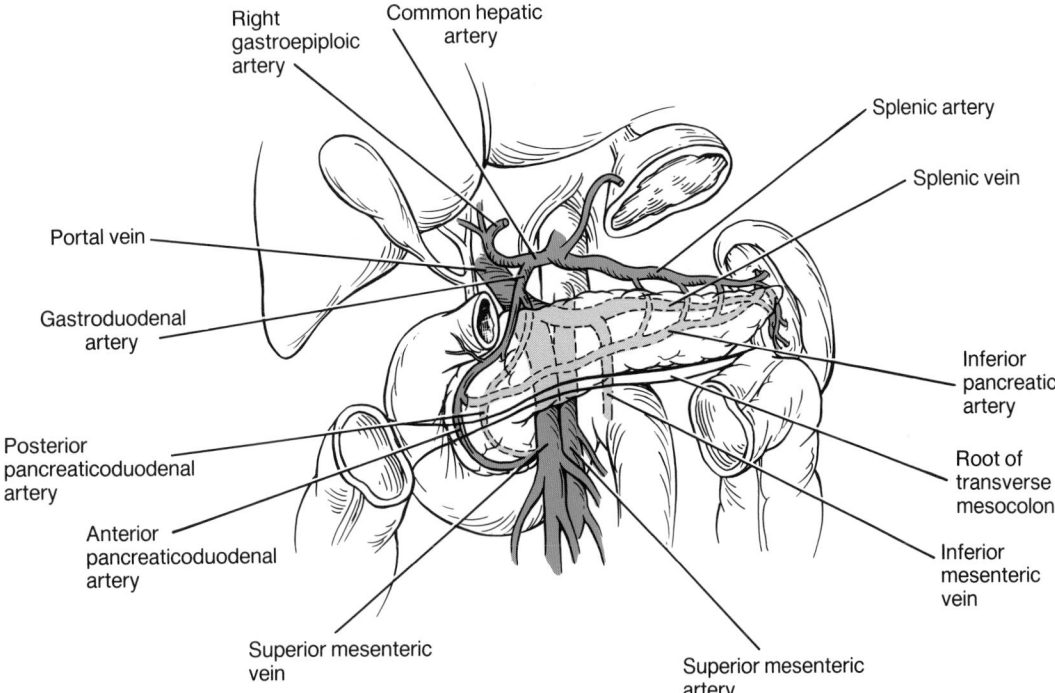

Figure 29-1 Key pancreatic relational anatomy. Note the close association of major vascular structures.

main pancreatic duct, and in 8%, it is the sole duct draining the pancreas.[3] By contrast, absence of the accessory ducts occurs in 10% of cases. Up to half of patients have small additional pancreatic ducts emptying directly from the pancreas into the intrapancreatic portion of the common bile duct. In 2% of patients, the pancreatic and common bile ducts open separately into the duodenum.

The arterial and venous blood supply of the pancreas is relatively constant; however, the frequent anomalous origin of the common hepatic artery (5%) and the right hepatic artery (15% to 20%) from the superior mesenteric artery make these vessels prone to injury during pancreatic surgery. These vessels can pass anterior or posterior to, or directly through, the head of the pancreas, but they subsequently lie posterior to the portal vein.[3,28] Awareness of this relatively common anomaly during dissection of the portal triad should minimize inadvertent injury.

The endocrine cells of the pancreas are histologically separated into nests or islets of cells (islets of Langerhans). The normal pancreas contains 200,000 to 2,000,000 islets distributed throughout its substance. The α-, β-, and δ-islet cells produce glucagon, insulin, and somatostatin, respectively. The secretion of insulin and glucagon is regulated by blood sugar levels: a fall causes glucagon secretion, and a rise triggers insulin secretion. Islet cell concentration in the tail of the pancreas has been shown to be significantly greater than in the body and head,[29] suggesting that resections of the pancreatic tail would be poorly tolerated. Nonetheless, excision of greater than 90% of the pancreas substance is required to produce a state of endocrine deficiency if the pancreas is otherwise normal since partial resection induces hypertrophy or increased physiologic activity of the remaining islets.

Dragstedt initially showed in animals, and others have confirmed in humans, that removal of 80% of pancreatic tissue does not significantly affect carbohydrate or fat metabolism, or digestion and absorption of food, so long as the remaining pancreatic tissue is normal, it remains connected to the duct, and its secretions have free access to the upper intestine.[3,4,30] Other animal studies and human experience with duodenectomy have demonstrated that survival is possible after complete removal of the duodenum, provided there is no obstruction to the flow of bile and pancreatic juice into the upper intestine. Removal of 90% to 95% of the pancreas after trauma produces diabetes, although digestion and absorption of food may be unimpaired. Total pancreaticoduodenectomy, however, results in the need for both hormonal and enzymatic replacement therapy.

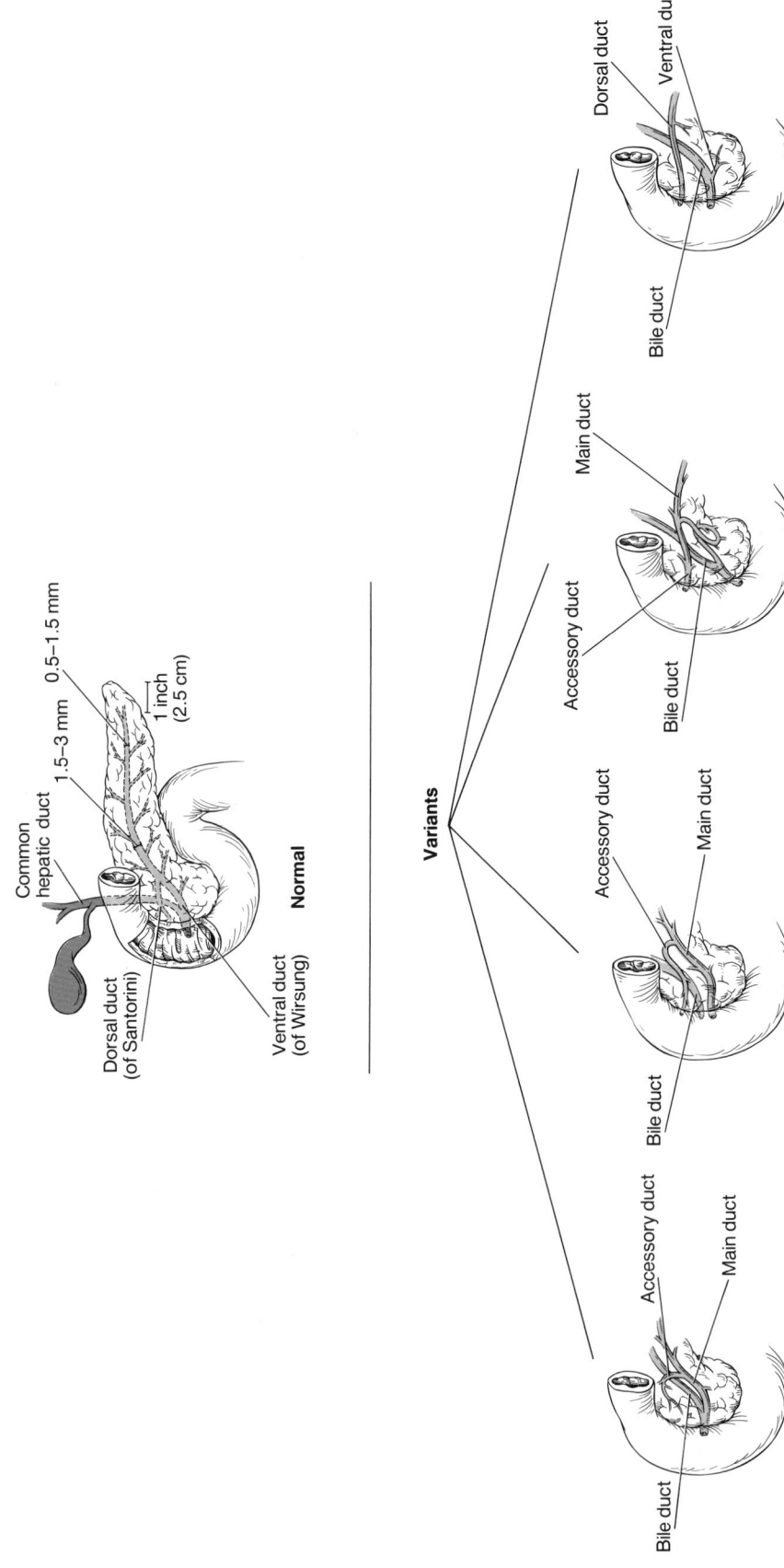

Figure 29-2   Anatomic location and variation of the major and minor pancreatic ducts.

Diagnosis

In evaluating a patient with potential pancreatic injury, it is important to remember that most early morbidity and mortality is due to associated vascular and other intraabdominal organ injury. Therefore, initial priority is given to controlling hemorrhage and containing bacterial contamination. Recognition and precise identification of the pancreatic injury should follow and must not be overlooked. Particular attention must be given to assessing the possibility of major ductal injury. As noted earlier, this single factor has the most direct impact on late morbidity and mortality.

The appropriate procedures and testing involved in the evaluation of a patient with a possible pancreatic injury depend on the mechanism of injury, indications for laparotomy, and time interval after the initial abdominal insult. Patients with clear indications for laparotomy need little or no preoperative evaluation directed at identifying a possible pancreatic injury since the diagnosis of pancreatic injury can be made intraoperatively. Patients without clear indications for laparotomy may require extensive assessment, including efforts to establish the presence of a pancreatic injury. Determining the presence and extent of possible pancreatic injury preoperatively is a challenge, made more difficult by the knowledge that a missed pancreatic injury has dire consequences.[19,31,32]

Preoperative Evaluation

The preoperative evaluation and management of patients with penetrating abdominal wounds is relatively straightforward. Unless injury to the intraperitoneal or retroperitoneal abdominal contents can be definitively ruled out, celiotomy is indicated. The external landmarks that define the abdomen extend from the nipples to the inguinal ligaments anteriorly and from the inferior border of the scapula to the ischial tuberosity posteriorly. At my institution, all patients with gunshot wounds to the abdomen undergo exploratory celiotomy. Stab wound management is more selective, based on location of injury. Anterior abdominal stab wounds that traverse the most superficial investing muscle fascia without obvious peritoneal penetration are evaluated by peritoneal lavage, with more than 1000 red cells per milliliter considered a positive lavage.[33] Posterior and flank stab wounds through muscle fascia, but again with no apparent peritoneal penetration, are assessed by contrast-enhanced computed tomographic (CT) scanning.[34] If celiotomy is indicated, no further diagnostic tests for pancreatic injury are required because thorough intraoperative evaluation will be performed.

The preoperative evaluation of patients with possible blunt pancreatic injury may be more complex and requires a careful evaluation based on location of impact, energy transfer, and associated injuries. The high incidence of associated intraabdominal injuries results in a significant proportion of such patients having clear-cut indications for laparotomy (eg, shock, peritonitis, positive diagnostic peritoneal lavage). As previously stated, these patients require no further preoperative evaluation to identify a possible pancreatic injury because a thorough, direct intraoperative pancreatic examination can be performed.

In contrast, identifying a pancreatic injury in the absence of other indications for laparotomy is challenging. Patients with complete ductal transection have been reported to be asymptomatic for weeks to months after the initial injury.[8,19,31,32] The failure of physical signs and symptoms to develop is likely related to the retroperitoneal location of the pancreas, pancreatic enzymes remaining inactive after an isolated injury, and decreased secretion of pancreatic fluid accompanying parenchymal damage. Early identification of a subtle pancreatic injury therefore requires a high index of suspicion, a carefully planned approach, and close observation.

Blunt pancreatic injuries occur when a high-energy crushing force is applied to the upper abdomen. Most blunt pancreatic injuries result from motor vehicle accidents. The energy of impact is usually directed at the epigastrium or hypochondrium, resulting in a crushing of the retroperitoneal structures. At least 60% of blunt injuries to the pancreas are due to impact with the steering wheel, although any high-energy blow to the epigastric region can damage the pancreatic parenchyma.[18] Soft tissue contusion in the upper abdomen away from bony prominences and disruption of the lower ribs or costal cartilage indicate that a significant force has been dissipated in this area. Epigastric pain out of proportion to the abdominal examination is often a clue to a retroperitoneal injury.

Although the highest concentration of amylase in the human body is in the pancreas, hyperamylasemia is not a reliable indicator of pancreatic trauma. In 1929, Elman first recognized the association between hyperamylasemia and pancreatic disease.[14] It was subsequently suggested (in 1943) that hyperamylasemia was an indicator of pancreatic injury in the blunt abdominal trauma patient.[17] Although initially hailed as a key advance in diagnosing pancreatic trauma, amylase determination has failed to be a reliable indicator. The availability of pancreatic fraction isoamylase (to distinguish salivary from pancreatic amylase) has not improved the sensitivity or specificity of this serum marker of pancreatic injury. In one series,[21] only 8% of blunt abdominal injuries with hyperamylasemia had pancreatic injury. Conversely, as many as 40% of patients with pancreatic injury may have a normal initial serum amylase.[35,36] Table 29-2 highlights the major reports dealing with amylase determination in patients with pancreatic trauma and emphasizes the unreliability of this single test as an indicator of pancreatic trauma. Nonetheless, an elevated serum or peritoneal lavage effluent amylase should intensify concern about a possible pancreatic injury and necessitates further evaluation. Asymptomatic patients with elevated serum pancreatic isoamylase warrant observation and repeat amylase determination. Persistent elevation or the development of abdominal symptoms are grounds for further evaluation, including abdominal CT scan, endoscopic retrograde cholangiopancreatography (ERCP), or surgical exploration.

Patients with hyperamylasemia and abdominal injury who present with a reliable, benign abdominal examination are carefully observed, and serial amylase is remeasured after several hours. If the patient subsequently develops abdominal symptoms or the amylase fails to normalize, consideration must be given to a more careful and directed evaluation of the pancreas. Dual-contrast CT, ERCP, and surgical exploration are all reasonable next-step alternatives. Abdominal CT scans have a reported sensitivity and specificity as high as 80% in diagnosing pancreatic injury, although the accuracy of this examination is largely dependent on interpreter experience, quality of the scanner, and the time from injury.[37,38] The CT signs of pancreatic injury may not yet be apparent if the patient is examined immediately after injury, perhaps contributing to the reports of false-negative CT scans in up to 40% of patients with significant pancreatic injuries.[1] This, however, is not grounds for delaying a CT evaluation but rather is an argument for repeating a CT scan if symptoms persist.

ERCP has no role in the evaluation of the hemody-namically unstable patient but may be helpful in delineating the cause of persistent hyperamylasemia or unexplained abdominal symptoms in a number of other distinct clinical situations involving pancreatic trauma. ERCP is a reasonable method of evaluating the pancreatic duct in the early postinjury period in select hemodynamically stable patients with hyperamylasemia, persistent abdominal pain, or abnormal or questionable abdominal CT findings.[15,39,40] In this circumstance, ERCP must be performed urgently, within 12 hours of injury, because further delays jeopardize subsequent care.[12,41,42] Findings of a disrupted pancreatic duct warrant surgical exploration. Reports of nonoperative management and duct stenting have focused on delayed presentations, not on the acutely traumatized patient.[43] Adequate external drainage and, when possible, resection of the distal gland at the site of injury are the standard of care (see later). Early ERCP that shows intact pancreatic ducts, including the secondary and tertiary radicals, without any extravasation may permit nonoperative therapy if no associated injuries are present.[15,40] The difficulty in this scenario is determining which patients warrant ERCP.[44,45]

The second useful role of ERCP in pancreatic trauma is intraoperative, when the surgeon is faced with the unusual circumstance of being unable to determine pancreatic duct integrity by careful examination alone.[39] In this situation, intraoperative pancreatography is essential and can be obtained by ERCP, duodenotomy, and direct ampullary cannulation or by transection of the tail of the pancreas and distal duct cannulation.[27]

The third use of ERCP in pancreatic trauma is in the evaluation of patients who present with delayed symptoms after abdominal trauma. Several case reports have documented the usefulness of ERCP in diagnosing delayed pancreatic injury and mapping surgical strategy.[44,46,47] Such presentation can be delayed from weeks to years after abdominal trauma; one report de-

Table 29-2 Summary of Reports on Hyperamylasemia and Pancreatic Trauma

Investigation	Mechanism of Injury	Patients With Amylase Measured	Patients With Positive Amylase (%)	Pancreatic Injury	True-Positive Amylase	False-Negative Amylase
Moretz et al (1975)[36]	Blunt	51	23 (45)	5	3	2
Bouwman et al (1984)[85]	Blunt	61	23 (38)	3	2	1
White & Benfield (1972)[21]	Penetrating	33	3 (9)	33	3	30
White & Benfield (1972)[21]	Blunt	25	12 (48)	25	12	13
Olsen (1973)[35]	Blunt	179	36 (20)	4	3	1

scribed 11 patients with pancreatic duct injury who presented 2 weeks to 15 years after abdominal trauma.[10]

Intraoperative Evaluation

Determining the presence and extent of a pancreatic injury intraoperatively requires that the surgeon first recognize the findings that indicate a potential pancreatic injury, then adequately visualize the entire gland, and finally define the integrity of the pancreatic parenchyma and determine the status of the major pancreatic duct when appropriate. This process is often complicated by the extent and severity of associated injuries and occasionally by reluctance to mobilize retroperitoneal structures. Signs suggesting pancreatic injury include the injury mechanisms previously described, the presence of upper abdominal wall contusion or abrasion, and concomitant lower thoracic spine fractures. The presence of a central retroperitoneal hematoma, edema around the pancreatic gland and lesser sac, and retroperitoneal bile staining mandate thorough pancreatic inspection.

Evaluation of the pancreas requires complete exposure of the gland. Exposure of the anterior surface and the superior and inferior borders of the body and tail is obtained by opening the lesser sac through the gastrocolic ligament just outside the gastroepiploic vessels. The transverse colon is retracted downward and the stomach upward and anteriorly. Frequently, a few adhesions between the posterior stomach and the anterior surface of the pancreas need to be incised. Adequate visualization of the pancreatic head and uncinate

process requires mobilization of the duodenum using the Kocher maneuver extended medially to the superior mesenteric vessels. In addition, mobilization of the hepatic flexure of the colon (a frequently overlooked maneuver) greatly facilitates visualization and bimanual examination of the head and neck. Inspection of the tail of the pancreas requires exposure of the splenic hilum. If injury involves the tail of the pancreas, mobilization is achieved first by division of the peritoneal attachments lateral to the spleen and colon. The colon, spleen, and body and tail of the pancreas are then mobilized forward and medially by creating a plane between the kidney and the pancreas with blunt finger dissection. This maneuver permits bimanual palpation of the pancreas and inspection of its posterior surface (Fig. 29-3).

All penetrating wounds of the abdomen should be traced from their entry point through the surrounding musculature to the point of exit or lodging of the missile. Any penetrating wound that goes near the substance of the pancreas requires exposure and careful inspection of the gland in the area. If exploration for penetrating trauma demonstrates no direct penetration or blast effect, further evaluation of the pancreatic duct is unnecessary. If the pancreas has been damaged by a knife or bullet, it is necessary to determine the integrity of the major pancreatic duct. Most penetrating wounds to the margins of the gland can be inspected directly and duct integrity confirmed. Penetrating wounds in the head or neck or central portion of the pancreas gland generally require further evaluation, including pancreatography (see later). Occasionally, intravenous

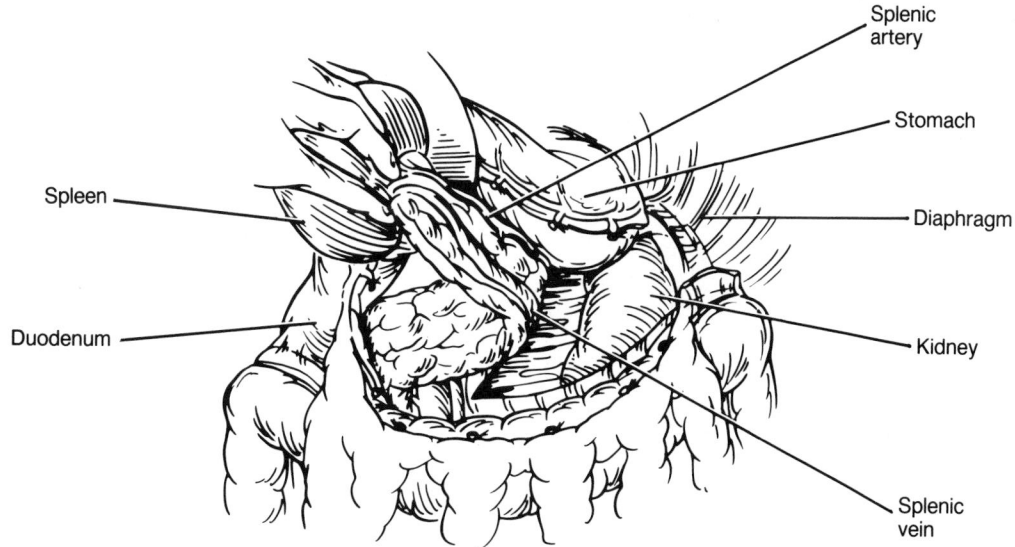

Figure 29-3 Complete mobilization of the tail of the pancreas, allowing for visualization of the dorsal surface.

injection of 1 to 2 μg cholecystokinin (1 to 2 mL sincalide) may stimulate pancreatic secretions enough to localize an otherwise unrecognized major duct injury.

Blunt impact to the pancreas can result in transection of the major duct with or without complete transection of the gland. Minor contusions or lacerations of the pancreatic substance usually do not require further evaluation of the pancreatic duct. An intact pancreatic capsule, however, does not rule out complete division of the pancreatic duct.[8] Establishing the status of the major ductal system under these circumstances is an important step in reducing late morbidity and mortality.

Injuries to the major duct occur in about 15% of cases of pancreatic trauma and are generally the result of penetrating wounds.[5,42] Most of these injuries can be diagnosed by careful inspection after adequate exposure. The remaining few injuries may require the more elaborate investigative techniques noted later to diagnose ductal injury.

The critical influence of ductal injuries on morbidity and late mortality argues for the performance of pancreatography when direct inspection is inadequate to exclude ductal injury. Routine performance of intraoperative pancreatography (see Section VII in Atlas Chapter 30) when proximal duct injury is suspected has decreased the postoperative morbidity rate from 55% to 15% at my institution.[26] A variety of techniques exist for intraoperative pancreatography. The simplest, which should be tried first, is a needle (18-gauge angio-

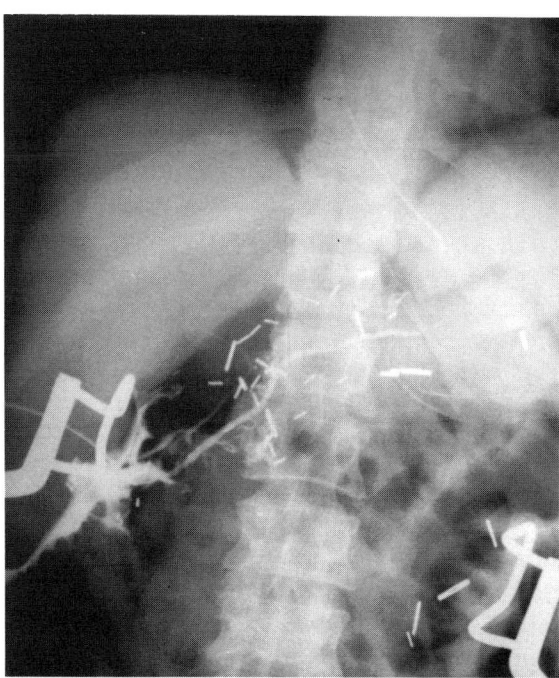

Figure 29-5 Intraoperative pancreatogram obtained by means of direct cannulation of the ampulla of Vater. The main pancreatic duct is normal.

catheter) cholecystocholangiogram (Fig. 29-4). Full-strength or ³/₄-strength water-soluble contrast is injected into the gallbladder under fluoroscopic visualization. About 20 to 30 mL is generally required. Contracture of the sphincter of Oddi with intravenous morphine may enhance the likelihood of pancreatic duct visualization. A cholecystectomy is not necessary after this procedure. Alternatively, duodenotomy and cannulation of the ampulla of Vater can be performed as illustrated in Figures 29-5 and 29-6, or a distal pancreatic resection and distal duct cannulation can be used to obtain pancreatography. Neither of these last two options is particularly attractive in the face of significant concomitant injury. Although perhaps cumbersome and more time-consuming, the performance of intraoperative ERCP by a skilled endoscopist is a reasonable alternative if the surgeon is reluctant to perform a duodenotomy or distal pancreatectomy. Finally, if an open pancreatic duct at the site of injury is visible, pancreatography is advised to evaluate the status of the gland and duct that will remain after resection of the gland distal to the site of injury. Direct cannulation is performed with a small pediatric feeding tube (5F) or cholangiocatheter, and 2 to 5 mL of water-soluble contrast under low pressure (gravity flow) is instilled (Figs. 29-7 and 29-8). The contrast material must not be forcibly injected because of the possibility of duct injury or glan-

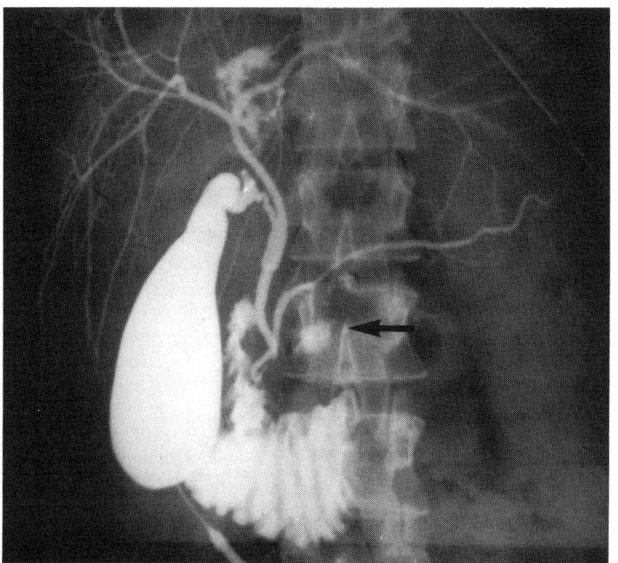

Figure 29-4 Needle cholangiogram performed through the gallbladder with good visualization of the pancreatic duct. Contrast extravasation is visible just over right border of spinal column (*arrow*), indicating proximal duct injury.

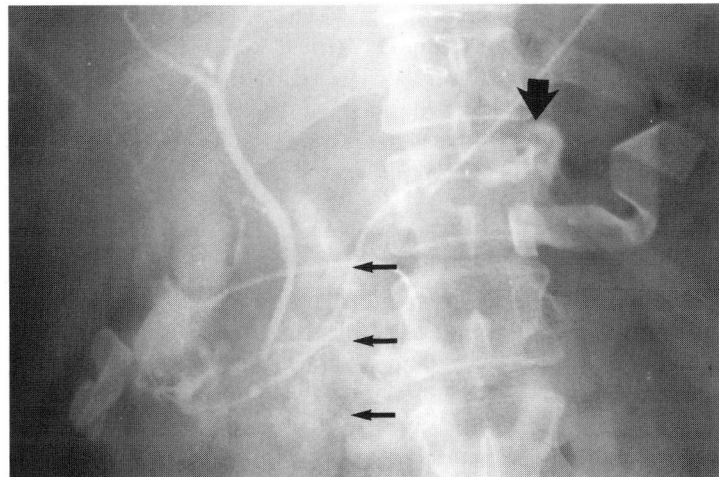

Figure 29-6 Intraoperative pancreatogram obtained by means of direct cannulation of the ampulla of Vater in a patient who had sustained a single stab wound to the back. The injured distal pancreatic duct with contrast extravasation is visible (*large arrow*). Also shown is contrast enhancement of pancreatic head (*small arrows*), indicating excessively forceful injection of contrast.

dular extravasation (see Fig. 29-6), which can cause postoperative pancreatitis.

Classification of Pancreatic Injuries

Although a number of classification systems have been devised to catalogue pancreatic injuries,[24,27,42] the American Association for the Surgery of Trauma has compiled a uniform classification system of all organ injuries, including the pancreas, in an effort to allow comparison of similar injuries between institutions.[48] As is true of any injury classification system, the value of classifying pancreatic injuries is only realized if the system is clinically applicable. To reiterate, the key principles of managing pancreatic injuries are as follows:

1. Control hemorrhage and contain bacterial contamination.
2. Débride devitalized pancreatic tissue.
3. Preserve at least 20% of functional pancreatic tissue whenever possible.
4. Provide adequate drainage of pancreatic injuries or resections.

A management plan based on these principles requires that the surgeon ascertain the presence or absence of associated organ injuries, the degree of pancreatic parenchymal disruption, and the integrity of the main pancreatic duct and ampulla.

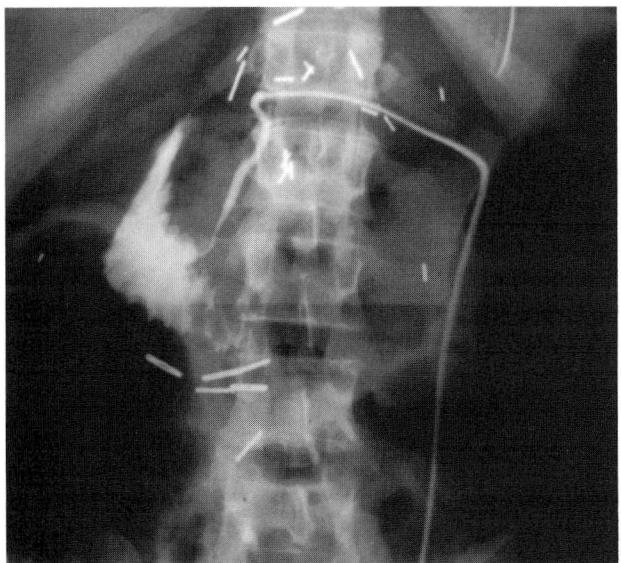

Figure 29-7 Cannulation at the site of mid-pancreatic gland injury, with contrast injected proximally to exclude residual duct injury before distal pancreatic resection and closure of proximal pancreatic stump.

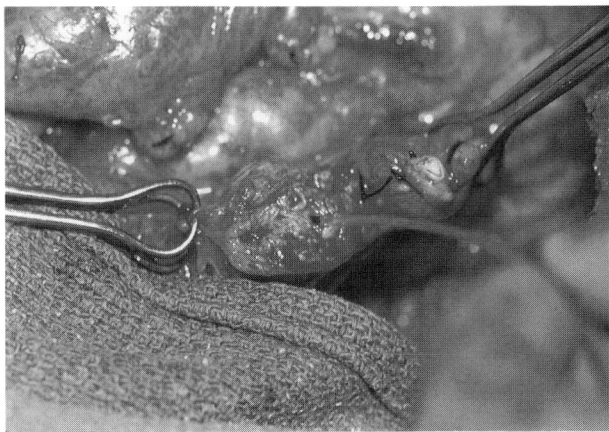

Figure 29-8 Operative photograph of transected pancreatic gland, with cannulation of proximal pancreatic duct to obtain pancreatogram before stump closure. (See Color Fig. 29-8.)

The American Association for the Surgery of Trauma classification system is outlined in Table 29-3. To be consistent with the other organ injury scaling,[48,49] this system has five grades of injury. This system addresses the key issues of treatment of parenchymal disruption and major pancreatic duct status by focusing on the anatomic location of the injury for the more severe (grades III through V) injuries. Proximal duct injuries have different management alternatives than distal duct and parenchymal injuries. Parenchymal contusions or lacerations with minimal or no tissue loss and no ductal injury (grades I and II) need only be externally drained. Combined duodenal and pancreatic head injuries that include the major duct or ampulla require a pancreaticoduodenectomy, although this is only rarely necessary. The difficult decisions in managing pancreatic trauma involve patients with parenchymal disruption and major duct injury. By focusing on the anatomic location of the duct and parenchymal injury (proximal versus distal), this classification provides a useful management guide.

The anatomic distinction between proximal and distal pancreas is generally defined by the superior mesenteric vessels passing behind the pancreas at the junction of the pancreatic head and body. There is no anatomic distinction in the gland itself between head, body, and tail. The anatomic division is useful, however, in estimating residual pancreatic endocrine and exocrine function. Although reports have been made of normal endocrine and exocrine function after 90% pancreatectomy, if possible, every effort should be made to leave at least 20% residual pancreatic tissue to minimize postoperative complications.[50]

Treatment of Pancreatic Injuries

Contusions and Lacerations Without Duct Injury

Minor pancreatic contusions and capsular lacerations account for about 60% of all pancreatic injuries, and lacerations of the pancreatic parenchyma without major ductal disruption account for an additional 20% of pancreatic injuries. These injuries require only hemostasis and adequate external drainage.[23] No attempt should be made to repair capsular lacerations since closure may result in a pancreatic pseudocyst, whereas a controlled pancreatic fistula is usually self-limiting. If the injuries are deep enough to disrupt minor pancreatic ducts, suture repair of the divided parenchymal may reduce the volume of pancreatic drainage, although great care must be taken to avoid injuring the main pancreatic duct. Soft, closed-suction drains are preferred over Penrose drains or sump drains. The rate of intraabdominal abscess formation is less, effluent is more reliably collected, and the excoriation of the skin at the exit site is significantly less with closed-suction drains.[15,18,51]

Table 29-3   Classification System of Pancreatic Injuries: American Association for the Surgery of Trauma Organ Injury Scaling System

Grade*		Injury Description†	ICDM-9‡	AIS-85	AIS-90
I	Hematoma	Minor contusuion without duct injury	863.81–863.84	2	2
	Laceration	Superficial laceration without duct injury		2	2
II	Hematoma	Major contusion without duct injury or tissue loss	863.81–863.84	3	2
	Laceration	Major laceration without duct injury or tissue loss		3	3
III	Laceration	Distal transection or parenchymal injury with duct injury	863.92–863.94	3	3
IV	Laceration	Proximal§ transection or parenchymal injury	863.91	3	4
V	Laceration	Massive disruption of pancreatic head	863.91	5	5

AIS, Abbreviated Injury Score.
* Advance one grade for multiple injuries to the same organ.
† Based on most accurate assessment at autopsy, laparotomy, or radiologic study.
‡ ICDM-9 codes: 863.81 and 863.91, head; 863.92, body; 863.83 and 863.93, tail.
§ Proximal pancreas is to the patient's right of the superior mesenteric vein.
(After Moore EE, Cogbill TH, Jurkovich GJ, et al. Organ injury scaling. III. Chest wall, abdominal vascular, ureter, bladder, and urethra. J Trauma 1992;33:337)

For minor injuries, if the amylase concentration in the drain is equal to or less than that of serum, the drains are removed at 24 to 48 hours. If the effluent amylase concentration persists above that of serum, the drain is left in until there is no evidence of pancreatic leak. Nutrition can be provided through the oral or gastric route as soon as possible, although prolonged gastric ileus and pancreatic complications may preclude standard gastric feeding for long periods in many of the more severely injured patients. In addition, the standard complex protein–carbohydrate–fat diet of most tube feedings increases pancreatic effluent volume and amylase concentration. Because the lower fat and higher pH (4.5) of elemental diets are less stimulating to the pancreas, an elemental formula should be tried before committing the patient to parenteral nutrition.[52,53] Insertion of a needle catheter jejunostomy or small feeding tube jejunostomy at the time of initial celiotomy, particularly in the more complex grade I and all grades II through V pancreatic injuries, allows early postoperative enteral nutrition rather than committing the patient who cannot tolerate oral or gastric feedings to total parenteral nutrition.

Distal Transection and Distal Parenchymal Injury With Duct Disruption

Distal parenchymal transection or injury with duct disruption is best treated by distal pancreatic resection with or without splenectomy. If there is any concern regarding the status of the remaining proximal main pancreatic duct, intraoperative pancreatography should be performed through the open end of the proximal duct (see Figs. 29-7 and 29-8). If the remaining proximal duct is normal, the transected duct should be closed with a direct suture ligature either as a U stitch or a figure-of-eight stitch with nonabsorbable suture.[54] The parenchyma is controlled with mattress sutures placed through the full thickness of the pancreatic gland from anterior to posterior capsule to minimize leakage from the transected parenchyma. Although most surgeons prefer nonabsorbable suture for pancreatic stump closure, one report suggested that a lower complication rate is obtained when nonabsorbable polyglycolic acid suture is used to oversew the pancreatic stump.[41] A small omental patch can be used to buttress the surface, and a drain should be left near the transection line. Stapling devices have been advocated for closure of the pancreatic parenchyma,[54,55] although the duct itself should be individually ligated. The automatic stapling device may also excessively compress and crush the glandular tissue (to about 1.5 mm with a 3.5 mm staple and to 2 mm with a 4.8 mm staple). As with all pancreatic wounds, adequate external drainage

should be established using a closed sump drain. The drain should be monitored and managed as described earlier. In the unusual circumstance in which the proximal remaining duct is abnormal (stricture), distal resection of the injured gland is completed, and the open proximal end is drained internally into a Roux-en-Y jejunal limb.

Concern for the possibility of overwhelming postsplenectomy sepsis may prompt attempted splenic preservation while performing distal pancreatectomy (see Section VII in Atlas Chap. 30). The increased operative time and potential blood loss incurred while performing pancreatectomy without splenectomy must be balanced against the slight risk of postsplenectomy sepsis. The balance would appear to favor splenic salvage only when the patient is completely hemodynamically stable and normothermic and when the pancreatic injury is isolated or present with only minor associated injuries. The technical challenge is in isolating and ligating the splenic vessel branches and in preventing injury to the splenic hilum. This maneuver adds an average of 50 minutes (range, 37 to 80 minutes) to the operative time for distal pancreatectomy,[56] because an average of 22 tributaries of the splenic vein and 7 branches of the splenic artery are encountered.[57] The technique of splenic preservation by ligating and dividing both the splenic artery and vein distal to the tip of the pancreatic tail has been reported in elective distal pancreatectomy.[58] The obvious disadvantage of this technique is the possibility of splenic ischemia because the short gastric vessels remain as the only blood supply to the spleen, and they anastomose to the hilar branching vessels at varying distance from the spleen.[59] It is also unclear whether such a limited blood supply is adequate to prevent future sepsis.

Proximal Transection or Injury With Probable Duct Disruption

Injuries to the pancreatic head present the most challenging management dilemmas. It is essential that the surgeon define the pancreatic duct anatomy in proximal pancreatic injuries. Techniques of intraoperative pancreatography were described earlier and are strongly recommended in this situation (see Figs. 29-4 through 29-8). Some experienced surgeons, however, are hesitant to perform a duodenotomy to perform pancreatography and favor local inspection and exploration of the defect to determine the duct status, if intraoperative ERCP is not an option.[60] If duct injury cannot be excluded by direct inspection, wide external drainage with numerous closed-suction drains and postoperative ERCP is an option. If major duct injury is confirmed, pancreatic duct stenting rather than near-total pancreatectomy may be an option, but there is limited experience with this technique.[43] Intraoperative pancreatography, on the other hand, has proved both safe and extremely accurate, and the advantage of accurate definition at the time of initial exploration outweighs any theoretic disadvantage to pancreatography when there is uncertainty regarding the status of the pancreatic duct.[26,27]

Injuries to the head and neck of the pancreas that spare the major pancreatic duct are best managed by adequate external drainage. Likewise, if the patient is hemodynamically unstable and the status of the pancreatic duct is unclear, wide external drainage (with possible postoperative ERCP) is recommended. If the proximal duct is known to be injured, but the ampulla and duodenum are spared (which is rare), the recommended treatment is distal pancreatectomy that results in subtotal removal of the gland. The proximal residual gland should drain into the duodenum in a normal fashion if the duct is intact. Wide external drainage of the residual pancreatic surface must be provided. Some surgeons add pyloric exclusion or duodenal defunctionalization or diverticulization (Fig. 29-9) to this procedure.[53,60] If there is concern that the residual pancreatic tissue is inadequate to provide endocrine or exocrine function, preservation of the pancreatic tail distal to the injury using a Roux-en-Y pancreaticojejunostomy has been suggested but is rarely used. This requires division of the pancreas at the site of injury, débridement of injured parenchyma, secure closure of the proximal duct and parenchyma, and anastomosis of the open end of the divided distal pancreas to the Roux-en-Y jejunal limb. A review of the three largest reports on pancreatic trauma published since 1990[4,11,41] presents a total of 265 patients, of whom only 2 (0.8%) underwent Roux-en-Y drainage of the distal segment of a transected pancreatic gland. In the two largest published reports of pancreatic trauma, detailing the management of 948 patients (75% penetrating) between 1950 and about 1980,[5,6] a total of 36 (3.8%) patients had Roux-en-Y drainage of the distal gland after resection for injury. The use of this technique is decreasing because of its associated complications and because extensive pancreatectomy is generally safe and well tolerated.[6]

When pancreatic parenchymal transection is incomplete, some surgeons have advocated an anastomosis from the end of the jejunum to the side of the pancreas. This technique is not recommended because of the difficulty in assuring the integrity of the anastomosis and potential for a high-output pancreatic fistula from the posterior pancreatic wound. In 7 patients in whom this technique was used (out of a total of 283 patients), 5 (71%) developed fistulas, and 3 (43%) died.[15]

Provisions should be made for providing early enteral nutritional support in all patients with major pancreatic injury. The surgeon's foresight in placing a jejunal feeding tube at the time of initial celiotomy is rewarded by a simplified and potentially advantageous enteral nutrition regime.[61] Elemental or short-chain polypeptide feeding formulas are particularly useful in this situation, and may be provided through a needle catheter jejunostomy.[52,53]

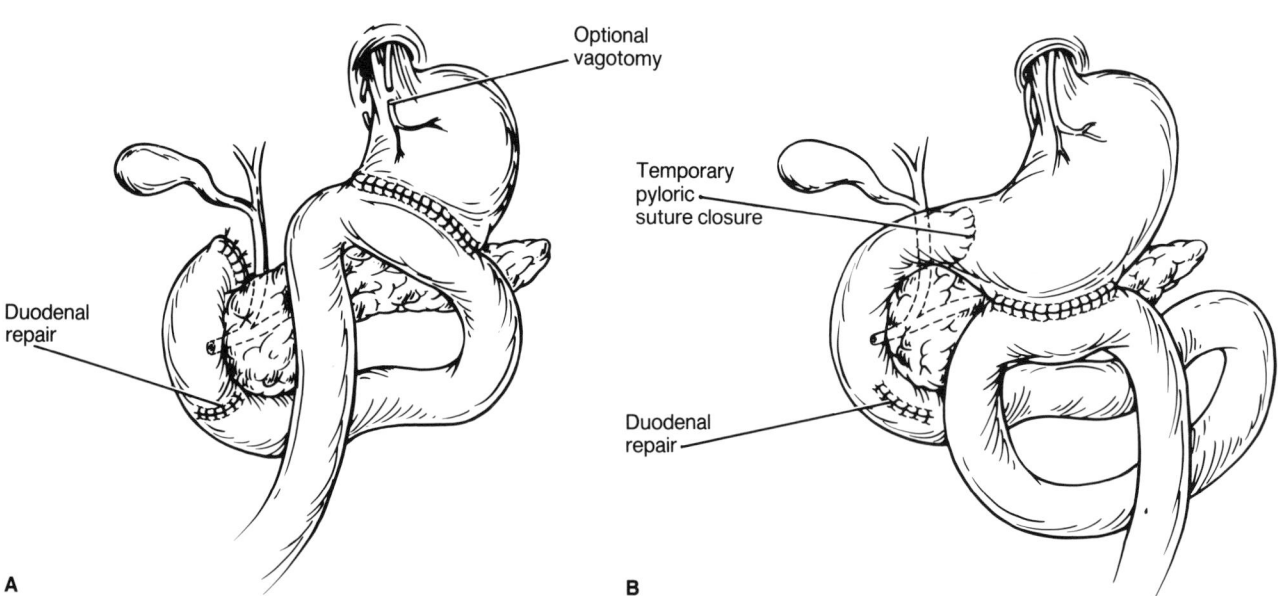

Figure 29-9 Two methods of diversion of gastric contents away from a duodenal repair. (**A**) Duodenal diverticulization. (**B**) Pyloric exclusion.

Combined Pancreatic–Duodenal Injuries

Severe combined pancreatic head and duodenal injuries are rare.[60,62–64] These injuries are most commonly caused by penetrating wounds in patients who routinely have multiple other intraabdominal injuries. Because of the large number of combinations of injuries to the pancreas and duodenum that may occur, no one form of therapy is appropriate for all patients. In a review of 129 cases of combined pancreatic–duodenal injuries, 24% of the patients were treated with simple repair and drainage, 50% underwent repair and pyloric exclusion, and only 10% required a pancreaticoduodenectomy.[60] Selecting the best treatment option is dependent on the integrity of the distal common bile duct and ampulla as well as the severity of the duodenal injury. For that reason, any patient with a combined pancreatic–duodenal injury requires a cholangiogram, a pancreatogram, and evaluation of the ampulla. The cholangiogram can usually be performed through the gallbladder (see Fig. 29-3). If there is unobstructed flow into the duodenum without extravasation, it can be assumed that the common bile duct and ampulla are intact. Occasionally, transduodenal evaluation of the ampulla and pancreatic duct through the injury site can be performed. When the common bile duct and ampulla are intact (as is the situation most cases), the duodenum can be closed primarily and the pancreatic injury treated as previously described. If the status of the pancreatic duct cannot be ascertained intraoperatively, wide external drainage of the pancreatic head with closed-suction drains should be performed rather than a total pancreatectomy. The development of postoperative enterocutaneous fistula, pancreatic fistula, or intraabdominal abscess suggests a major pancreatic duct injury and the need for pancreaticoduodenectomy.[65] If there is concern about the integrity of the duodenal closure, decompression through a side duodenostomy or three-tube system (gastrostomy, retrograde tube jejunostomy for duodenal decompression, and antegrade tube jejunostomy for feeding) may assist by reducing tension at the suture line[66] (see Section VII in Atlas Chap. 30). A retrospective literature review of more than 500 cases of penetrating duodenal trauma and drainage techniques suggests that retrograde drainage is preferable to direct duodenal cannulation[67] (see later).

With severe injury to the duodenum in association with pancreatic head injury, it may be advisable to divert gastric contents away from the duodenal repair. Originally, this was accomplished by duodenal diverticulization.[53,68] A true diverticulization consists of primary closure of the duodenal wound, antrectomy, vagotomy, end-to-side gastrojejunostomy, T-tube common bile duct drainage, and lateral-tube duodenostomy. The concept behind duodenal diverticulization is to completely divert both gastric and biliary contents away from the duodenal injury, provide enteral nutrition through the gastrojejunostomy, and convert a potential uncontrolled lateral duodenal fistula to a controlled fistula (see Fig. 29-9*A*). A less formidable and more popular alternative is the pyloric exclusion, which does not employ antrectomy or biliary diversion (see Fig. 29-9*B* and Section VII in Atlas Chap. 30). This technique has been advocated by several major trauma centers in patients with combined pancreatic and duodenal injuries.[53,60,69,70] The procedure is performed through a gastrotomy and consists of grasping the pylorus with a Babcock clamp, closing the pyloric channel with absorbable size 0 polyglycolic acid sutures, and constructing a loop gastrojejunostomy. Vagotomy is generally not added. This accomplishes temporary diversion of gastric flow away from the duodenum for several weeks while the duodenal and pancreatic injuries heal. The pylorus eventually opens (2 weeks to 2 months), and the gastrojejunostomy functionally closes. Pyloric exclusion has proved useful in managing severe duodenal injuries and combined pancreatic head and duodenal injuries in which a pancreaticoduodenectomy is not required. Few advocate pyloric exclusion for isolated pancreatic injuries.

In massive injuries of the proximal duodenum and head of the pancreas, destruction of the ampulla and proximal pancreatic duct or distal common bile duct may preclude reconstruction. In addition, since the head of the pancreas and the duodenum have a common arterial supply, it is essentially impossible to resect one entirely without making the other ischemic. In this situation, a pancreaticoduodenectomy is required. Although the average mortality for a pancreaticoduodenectomy for trauma has traditionally been reported to be between 30% to 50%,[15,53] more recent experience suggests that with appropriate selection criteria, pancreaticoduodenectomy is a viable option and can be performed for injury with less morbidity and mortality than previously described. During a 6-year period, 10 patients at my center underwent pancreaticoduodenectomy for trauma, out of 117 patients with intraoperatively identified pancreatic injuries. This procedure was performed only in patients with nonreconstructable injury to the ampulla or severe combined pancreaticoduodenal injures. In 8 of 10 patients, the injury was clinically evident. In 2 patients, an injury of this magnitude was suspected, but pancreatography was necessary to prove it. Four of 10 patients developed abdominal abscesses; all these patients had penetrating colon injuries. Two of the patients developed early postoperative pancreatitis that subsequently resolved, and one patient developed a pancreatic fistula. Average follow-up was $2\frac{1}{2}$ years, and half of the patients returned to work or school. Most notably, all patients survived.[62] Two other recent reports also are notable for no deaths and an average hospital stay of 26 days.[65,71]

The major immediate mortality in patients with combined pancreatic–duodenal injuries is attributable to associated major vessel injury in the vicinity of the head of the pancreas (see Fig. 29-1). If immediate control of hemorrhage and resuscitation can be achieved, my experience suggests that the Whipple resection remains the preferred option in that select group of patients with unreconstructable injury to the ampulla or proximal pancreatic duct, or combined massive duodenal and pancreatic head destruction in which pancreaticoduodenectomy in fact represents complete surgical débridement of devitalized tissue.

Complications

Complications related to the pancreatic injury after surgical intervention are seen in 20% to 40% of patients.[7,8,27,31,50] Although most complications related to pancreatic injury are self-limiting or treatable, the overall mortality secondary to the complications ranges from 10% to 20%. In some series, up to half of the postoperative complications could have been avoided with careful inspection of the pancreas and accurate determination of the status of the main pancreatic duct.[31]

Fistula

Fistula is the most common complication after pancreatic injury, with an incidence of 7% to 20%, rising to 26% to 35% after combined pancreaticoduodenal injury.[3,5,6] Most of these are minor (less than 200 mL/d) and spontaneously resolve within 2 weeks of injury if adequate external drainage is provided. In a multicenter review of distal pancreatectomy for trauma, the postoperative fistula rate was 14% (10 of 71), with spontaneous fistula closure in 89% (8 of 9) of survivors in 6 to 54 days.[4] One patient required extirpation of a residual pancreatic sequestrum to facilitate fistula closure. High-output fistulas (greater than 700 mL/d) are rare and generally require longer periods of external drainage or surgical intervention for resolution. If a high-output fistula fails to decrease in volume progressively or persists for more than 10 days, ERCP is indicated and can be most helpful in establishing the cause of the persistent fistula and planning further therapy. Nutritional support must be provided throughout this period. A feeding jejunostomy placed at initial laparotomy may be useful to deliver low-fat, higher pH elemental feeding formulas that cause less pancreatic stimulation than standard enteral formulas. These should be tried before committing the patient to total parenteral nutrition.[52] Somatostatin analogue (octreotide acetate, Sandostatin) has shown promise in treating prolonged, high-output pancreatic fistula, but only after eradicating any infection and in the absence of pancreatic duct obstruction.[72] Treatment typically begins with 50 μg subcutaneously every 12 hours but can increase to up to 1000 μg/d. Alternatively, the dose can be included in total parenteral nutrition solution.[73] Major side effects are unpredictable changes in serum glucose, pain at the injection site, and a variety of nonspecific gastrointestinal complaints.

Abscesses

The incidence of abscess formation after pancreatic trauma ranges from 10% to 25%, depending on the number and type of associated injuries. Early operative or percutaneous drainage is critical, although the mortality rate in this group of patients remains about 25%.[60,74] The intraabdominal abscess is most often subfascial or peripancreatic; a true pancreatic abscesses, resulting from inadequate débridement of dead tissue or inadequate initial drainage, can occur but is unusual.[4–6] Pancreatic abscess associated with necrosis may not be amenable or responsive to percutaneous drainage, and surgical débridement and drainage may be required. Percutaneous decompression may be helpful in distinguishing between abscess and pseudocyst.

Pancreatitis

Transient abdominal pain and elevation of the serum amylase concentration may be anticipated in 8% to 18% of postoperative patients.[4,15,75] This type of pancreatitis is treated with nasogastric decompression, bowel rest, and nutritional support and can be expected to resolve spontaneously. A much more infrequent but deadly complication is hemorrhagic pancreatitis. The first sign of this complication may be bloody pancreatic drainage or a fall in the serum hemoglobin concentration, with the patient rapidly becoming desperately ill. This complication occurs in less than 2% of operative pancreatic trauma patients, but the mortality rate may approach 80%.[5,6]

Secondary Hemorrhage

Postoperative hemorrhage requiring blood transfusion occurs in 5% to 10% of patients with pancreatic trauma, particularly after inadequate external drainage after pancreatic débridement, or when intraabdominal infection has developed.[75,76] These patients generally require reoperation for control, although angiographic embolization may be an effective alternative, providing coexisting sepsis is controlled.

Pseudocysts

Overlooked significant blunt pancreatic injuries often result in the formation of a pseudocyst. One report tabulated the incidence of pseudocyst occurrence in seven studies reported between 1952 and 1983, documenting 22 pseudocysts in 42 blunt pancreatic trauma patients managed nonoperatively.[19] Once again, the major determinant of outcome and indicator of preferred treatment is the status of the pancreatic duct. If the pancreatic duct is intact, percutaneous drainage of the pseudocyst is likely to be effective. Most patients who sustain pancreatic trauma have a normal major pancreatic duct before injury. If the duct is uninjured, percutaneous drainage of a pseudocyst can provide an egress for pancreatic juice and often results in resolution of the pseudocyst. The exception occurs when the pseudocyst is secondary to a major pancreatic ductal disruption that was missed at initial exploration. Percutaneous drainage in this situation does not provide definitive therapy but converts a pseudocyst to a chronic fistula. Endoscopic retrograde pancreatography should therefore precede percutaneous drainage. If pancreatic duct stenosis or injury is demonstrated, treatment options include reexploration and partial gland resection (preferred), distal gland internal Roux-en-Y drainage, and endoscopic transpapillary stenting of the pancreatic duct.[43]

Exocrine and Endocrine Insufficiency

Either problem is unusual after pancreatic trauma. Both animal and human studies suggest that 10% to 20% normal pancreatic tissue is adequate for pancreatic function,[26,77] implying that any resection distal to the mesenteric vessels should leave adequate functioning pancreatic tissue. A multicenter study of 74 cases of distal pancreatic resections documented only one case of endocrine deficiency (diet-controlled hyperglycemia after 80% pancreatectomy) and no instance of exocrine insufficiency.[4] Others have reported no pancreatic insufficiency after up to 90% pancreatic resections.[3]

DUODENAL INJURIES

About three quarters of duodenal injuries are the result of penetrating trauma. Blunt duodenal injuries are the result of a direct blow to the epigastrium—most commonly a steering wheel injury to an unrestrained driver in adults and a direct blow from a bicycle handlebar or similar mechanism in children. The insidious nature of many blunt duodenal injuries makes the initial diagnosis difficult unless a high index of suspension is maintained. In one review of duodenal injury, there was a delay in diagnosis of more than 12 hours in 53% of patients and a delay of greater than 24 hours in 28%.[17] This delay markedly increased morbidity and mortality: mortality was 40% among patients in whom the diagnosis was delayed greater than 24 hours compared with 11% in those operated on within 24 hours. Delays in the diagnosis of duodenal trauma seriously compromise patient outcome.

Diagnosis

In patients with a suspicious mechanism of injury (any direct blow to the epigastrium), a serum amylase should be obtained. Although hyperamylasemia can be diagnostically confusing in both pancreatic and duodenal injuries, a persistently elevated or rising amylase may indicate pancreatic or duodenal injury and mandates further evaluation or operative exploration. The radiologic signs of duodenal injury on the initial plain abdominal or upright chest radiograph are often subtle. They include mild spinal scoliosis or obliteration of the right psoas muscle in addition to retroperitoneal air, which is often difficult to distinguish from the overlying transverse colon. An early suspicion of retroperitoneal duodenal rupture is best confirmed or excluded by either an abdominal CT scan with both oral and intravenous contrast material or an upper gastrointestinal series with water-soluble contrast, followed by barium if the initial results are negative. Diagnostic peritoneal lavage is unreliable in detecting *isolated* duodenal and other retroperitoneal injuries. Nevertheless, it is often helpful, since about 40% of patients with duodenal injuries have associated intraabdominal injuries that result in a positive peritoneal lavage. The findings of amylase or bile in the lavage effluent are more specific indicators of possible duodenal injury. At celiotomy, the presence of retroperitoneal hematoma, bile staining, or air in the central upper abdomen mandates thorough examination of the duodenum.

Treatment

About 80% to 85% of duodenal wounds can safely be primarily repaired. About 15% to 20% are severe injuries that require more complex procedures. Factors that determine whether a duodenal wound can be primarily repaired were examined in a review of 247 patients treated for duodenal trauma.[10] There was an overall duodenal fistula rate of 7% an an mortality rate of 10.5%

in the 228 patients who survived for greater than 72 hours. Five factors (Table 29-4) were most significantly correlated with the severity of duodenal injury and subsequent morbidity and mortality. Patients with mild duodenal trauma had a 0% mortality rate directly attributable to the injury and a 2% duodenal fistula rate, as compared with a 6% mortality rate attributable to the duodenal injury and a 10% fistula rate among those with severe duodenal injuries. Overall morbidity and mortality in both groups are given in Table 29-4. In general, patients with a mild duodenal injury and no pancreatic injury can be primarily repaired. Patients with more severe duodenal injuries and coexistent pancreatic injury may require more complex treatment strategies.

For patients with complete transection of the duodenum, débridement of mucosal edges and primary repair is appropriate in all but those with injury involving the region around the ampulla. An alternative is a Roux-en-Y jejunal limb anastomosis to the proximal duodenal injury and oversewing of the distal injury. Pancreaticoduodenectomy is rarely required for duodenal injuries unless uncontrollable pancreatic hemorrhage or combined duodenal and distal common bile duct or pancreatic duct injury are present. Protection of a tenuous duodenal repair may be accomplished by several techniques, including buttressing the repair with omentum or a serosal patch from a loop of jejunum, although the benefit of such techniques has not been proved.[78,79] Diversion of gastric contents is another option, most commonly accomplished by the pyloric exclusion technique[70] (see Section VII in Atlas Chap. 30), a less disruptive procedure than true duodenal diverticulization.[68,80] Although no prospective randomized trial has shown proven benefit from gastric diversion, several reports suggest that pyloric exclusion and gastrojejunostomy are helpful in severe duodenal injuries.[81,82] Nonetheless, the additional operating time and the extra anastomosis suggest that a good deal of selectivity should be applied to its use. A marginal ulcer at the site of gastrojejunostomy occurred in 4 of 42 patients who underwent postoperative gastrointestinal evaluation in one report,[81] and in 2 of 17 patients in another,[69] prompting some to add truncal vagotomy to the procedure. Vagotomy is not performed by most surgeons since nearly all of the pyloric closures open within a few weeks, regardless of the type of suture material used, and the occasional marginal ulcer can be medically managed in the interim.

An alternative or addition to gastric diversion is duodenal decompression through lateral-tube duodenostomy or retrograde jejunostomy. One group reported a fistula rate of less than 0.5% (1 in 237 patients) in a variety of duodenal injuries treated by retrograde jejunostomy tube drainage,[66] in contrast to a 19.3% incidence of duodenal complications when decompression was not used. Direct drainage with a tube through the suture line gave an even higher dehiscence or fistula rate of 23%. These observations are supported by a review of the literature up to 1984 on penetrating duodenal trauma and tube duodenostomy,[67] which demonstrated an overall mortality of 19.4% and fistula rate of 11.8% without decompression compared with a 9% mortality rate and a 2.3% fistula rate with decompression. This suggested that tube drainage should be performed either through the stomach or by retrograde jejunostomy because these methods resulted in lower fistula and overall mortality rates than lateral-tube duodenostomy. However, there has been no prospective, randomized analysis of the efficacy of various tube duodenal drainage techniques.

Duodenal hematoma is generally considered an injury of childhood play or child abuse but can occur in adults after vehicular accidents. Nearly one third of the patients present with insidious onset of obstruction at least 48 hours after injury, presumably the result of

Table 29-4 Determinants of Duodenal Injury Severity and Outcome

	Mild	*Severe*
DETERMINANTS OF INJURY SEVERITY		
Agent	Stab wound	Blunt or missile wound
Size	<75% wall	>75% wall
Duodenal portion site	3rd, 4th	1st, 2nd
Injury to repair intervals (h)	<24	>24
Adjacent injury	No common bile duct	Common bile duct
OUTCOME		
Overall mortality	6%	16%
Overall morbidity	6%	14%

(After Snyder W, Weigelt J, Watkins W, Bietz DS. The surgical management of duodenal trauma. Surgery 1976;80:523)

fluid shift into the duodenal hematoma. In general, the best results are obtained with conservative or nonsurgical management.[83] The diagnosis can be made either by contrast-enhanced CT scan or upper gastrointestinal study. The initial Gastrografin examination should be followed by barium to provide the greater detail needed to detect the so-called coiled-spring or stacked-coin sign. Although characteristic of intramural duodenal hematoma, this finding is present in only about one fourth of patients with hematoma. Although the initial treatment is nonoperative, associated injuries should be excluded, with particular attention directed toward pancreatic injuries, which occur in 20% of patients.[83] Continuous nasogastric suction should be employed and total parenteral nutrition begun. The patient should be reevaluated with upper gastrointestinal contrast studies at 5- to 7-day intervals if signs of obstruction do not spontaneously abate. Operative exploration and evacuation of the hematoma may be considered after 2 weeks of conservative therapy to rule out contained duodenal perforation or injury to the head of the pancreas as factors that may be contributing to the obstruction.[84]

If a duodenal hematoma is incidentally found at celiotomy for abdominal trauma, a thorough inspection must ensue to exclude perforation. This requires an extended Kocher maneuver, which often successfully drains the subserosal hematoma.

> Pancreatic and duodenal injuries are relatively uncommon and usually accompany injuries to major vessels or other gastrointestinal organs. Because these associated injuries are responsible for much early morbidity and mortality, control of hemorrhage and bacterial contamination takes initial priority over the pancreatic or duodenal injury. The management of specific pancreatic injury depends on the status of the main pancreatic duct, the degree of parenchymal damage, and the anatomic location of the injury. Complete visualization of the gland and accurate determination of duct integrity are the tenets of operative care. Failure to recognize significant duct or parenchymal injury is the major cause of morbidity. Although most pancreatic injuries can be managed by simple drainage, the occasional major transection or pancreatic duct injury necessitates more complex repair. Most duodenal injuries can be managed by débridement and primary repair. The occasional severe duodenal injury, or one with an associated pancreatic injury, may require pyloric exclusion for gastric diversion and retrograde duodenal decompression. Enteral access for nutritional support should be part of the initial operative care of pancreatic or duodenal trauma patients.

REFERENCES

1. Wilson R, Moorehead R. Current management of trauma to the pancreas. Br J Surg 1991;78:1196.
2. Bach RD, Frey DF. Diagnosis and treatment of pancreatic trauma. Am J Surg 1971;121:20.
3. Balasegaram M. Surgical management of pancreatic trauma. Curr Probl Surg 1979;16:1.
4. Cogbill TH, Moore EE, Morris JA, et al. Distal pancreatectomy for trauma: a multicenter experience. J Trauma 1991;31:1600.
5. Graham JM, Mattox KL, Jordan GL. Traumatic injuries of the pancreas. Am J Surg 1978;136:744.
6. Jones RC. Management of pancreatic trauma. Am J Surg 1985;150:698.
7. Sims EH, Mandal AK, Schlater T, Fleming AW, Lou MA. Factors affecting outcome in pancreatic trauma. J Trauma 1984;24:125.
8. Smego D, Richardson J, Flint L. Determinants of outcome in pancreatic trauma. J Trauma 1985;25:771.
9. Shorr R, Greaney G, Donovan A. Injuries of the duodenum. Am J Surg 1987;154:93.
10. Snyder W, Weigelt J, Watkins W, Bietz DS. The surgical management of duodenal trauma. Arch Surg 1980;115:422.
11. Ivatury RR, Nallathambi M, Rao P, Stahl WM. Penetrating pancreatic injuries: analysis of 103 consecutive cases. Am Surg 1990;56:90.
12. Heitsch RC, Knutson CO, Fulton RL, Jones CE. Delineation of critical factors in the treatment of pancreatic trauma. Surgery 1976;80:523.
13. Sukul K, Lont H, Johannes E. Management of pancreatic injuries. Hepatogastroenterology 1992;39:447.
14. Blaisdell F, Trunkey D. Abdominal trauma. In: Trauma management. New York, Thieme-Stratton, 1982.
15. Stone HH, Fabian TC, Satiani B, Turkleson ML. Experiences in the management of pancreatic trauma. J Trauma 1981;21:257.
16. Cuddington G, Rusnak CH, Cameron RDA, Carter J. Management of duodenal injuries. Can J Surg 1990;33:41.
17. Lucas C, Ledgerwood A. Factors influencing outcome after blunt duodenal injury. J Trauma 1975;15:839.
18. Anderson CB, Connors JP, Mejia DC, Wise L. Drainage methods in the treatment of pancreatic injuries. Surg Gynecol Obstet 1974;138:587.
19. Kudsk KA, Temizer D, Ellison EC, Cloutier CT, Buckley DC, Carey LC. Post-traumatic pancreatic sequestrum: recognition and treatment. J Trauma 1986;26:320.
20. Nilsson E, Norrby S, Skullman S, Sjodahl R. Pancreatic trauma in a defined population. Acta Chir Scand 1986;152:647.
21. White P, Benfield J. Amylase in the management of pancreatic trauma. Arch Surg 1972;105:158.
22. Cook DE, Walsh JW, Vick CW, Brewer WH. Upper ab-

dominal trauma: pitfalls in CT diagnosis. Radiology 1986;159:65.

23. Nowak M, Baringer D, Ponsky J. Pancreatic injuries: effectiveness of débridement and drainage for nontransecting injuries. Am Surg 1986;52:599.

24. Sorensen VJ, Obeid FN, Horst HM, Bivins BA. Penetrating pancreatic injuries. Am Surg 1986;52:354.

25. Laraja RD, Lobbato VJ, Cassaro S, Reddy SS. Intraoperative endoscopic retrograde cholangiopancreatography (ERCP) in penetrating trauma of the pancreas. J Trauma 1986;26:1146.

26. Berni G, Bandyk D, Oreskovich M, Carrico CJ. Role of intraoperative pancreatography in patients with injury to the pancreas. Am J Surg 1982;143:602.

27. Jurkovich GJ, Carrico CJ. Pancreatic trauma. Surg Clin North Am 1990;70:575.

28. Quinlan R. Anatomy, embryology, and physiology of the pancreas. In: Shackelford R, Zuidema G, eds. Surgery of the alimentary tract. Philadelphia, WB Saunders, 1983: 3.

29. Wittingen J, Frey C. Islet concentration in the head, body, tail and uncinate process of the pancreas. Ann Surg 1974;179:412.

30. Yellin AE, Vecchione TR, Donovan AJ. Distal pancreatectomy for pancreatic trauma. Am J Surg 1972;124:135.

31. Leppaniemi A, Haapiainen R, Kiviluoto T, Lempinen M. Pancreatic trauma: acute and late manifestations. Br J Surg 1988;75:165.

32. Carr N, Cairns S, Russell R. Late complications of pancreatic trauma. Br J Surg 1989;76:1244.

33. Oreskovich M, Carrico C. Stab wounds of the anterior abdomen: analysis of a management plan using local wound exploration and quantitative peritoneal lavage. Ann Surg 1983;198:411.

34. Feliciano D. Diagnostic modalities in abdominal trauma. Peritoneal lavage, ultrasonography, computed tomography scanning, and arteriography. Surg Clin North Am 1991;71:241.

35. Olsen WR. The serum amylase in blunt abdominal trauma. J Trauma 1973;13:200.

36. Moretz JA, Campbell DP, Parker DE, Williams GR. Significance of serum amylase level in evaluating pancreatic trauma. Am J Surg 1975;130:739.

37. Jeffrey R, Federle M, Creass R. Computed tomography of pancreatic trauma. Radiology 1983;147:491.

38. Peitzman AB, Makaroun MS, Slasky BS, Ritter P. Prospective study of computed tomography in initial management of blunt abdominal trauma. J Trauma 1986;26: 585.

39. Belohlavek D, Merkle P, Probst M. Identification of traumatic rupture of the pancreatic duct by endoscopic retrograde pancreatography. Gastrointest Endosc 1978;24: 255.

40. Whittwell AE, Gomez GA, Byers P, Kreis DJ, Manten H, Casillas VJ. Blunt pancreatic trauma: prospective evaluation of early endoscopic retrograde pancreatography. South Med J 1989;82:586.

41. Wisner D, Wold R, Frey C. Diagnosis and treatment of

pancreatic injuries: an analysis of management principles. Arch Surg 1990;125:1109.

42. Lucas C. Diagnosis and treatment of pancreatic and duodenal injury. Surg Clin North Am 1977;57:49.

43. Kozarek RA, Ball TJ, Patterson DJ, Freeny PC, Ryan JA, Traverso LW. Endoscopic transpapillary therapy for disrupted pancreatic duct and peripancreatic fluid collections. Gastroenterology 1991;100:1362.

44. Gougeon F, Legros G, Archambault A, Bessette G, Bastien E. Pancreatic trauma: a new diagnostic approach. Am J Surg 1976;132:400.

45. Elman R, Arneson N, Graham E. Value of blood amylase estimations in the diagnosis of pancreatic disease. Arch Surg 1929;19:943.

46. Bozymski E, Orlando R, Holt J. Traumatic disruption of the pancreatic duct demonstrated by endoscopic retrograde pancreatography. J Trauma 1981;21:244.

47. Barkin JS, Ferstenberg RM, Panullo W, Manten HD, Davis RC. Endoscopic retrograde cholangiopancreatography in pancreatic trauma. Gastrointest Endosc 1988;34: 102.

48. Moore EE, Cogbill TH, Malangoni MA, et al. Organ injury scaling. II. Pancreas, duodenum, small bowel, colon, and rectum. J Trauma 1990;30:1427.

49. Moore EE, Cogbill TH, Jurkovich GJ, et al. Organ injury scaling. III. Chest wall, abdominal vascular, ureter, bladder, and urethra. J Trauma 1992;33:337.

50. Jones W, Finkelstein J, Barie P. Managing pancreatic trauma. Infect Surg 1990;March:29.

51. Fabian T, Kudsk K, Croce M, et al. Superiority of closed suction drainage for pancreatic trauma: a randomized prospective study. Ann Surg 1990;211:724.

52. Kellum J, Holland G, McNeill P. Traumatic pancreatic cutaneous fistula: comparison of enteral and parenteral feedings. J Trauma 1988;28:700.

53. Cogbill T, Moore E, Kashuk J. Changing trends in the management of pancreatic trauma. Arch Surg 1982;117: 722.

54. Fitzgibbons TJ, Yellin AE, Maruyama MM, Donovan AJ. Management of the transected pancreas following distal pancreatectomy. Surg Gynecol Obstet 1982;154:225.

55. Andersen DK, Bolman RM, Moylan JA. Management of penetrating pancreatic injuries: subtotal pancreatectomy using the auto suture stapler. J Trauma 1980;20:347.

56. Pachter HL, Hofstetter SR, Liang HG, Hoballah J. Traumatic injuries to the pancreas: the role of distal pancreatectomy with splenic preservations. J Trauma 1989;29:1352.

57. Dawson D, Scott-Conner C. Distal pancreatectomy with splenic preservation: the anatomic basis for a meticulous operation. J Trauma 1986;26:1142.

58. Warshaw A. Conservation of the spleen with distal pancreatectomy. Arch Surg 1988;123:550.

59. Schein M, Greinkel W, E'Egidio A. Splenic conservation in distal pancreatic injury: stay away from the hilum. J Trauma 1991;31:431.

60. Feliciano DV, Martin TD, Cruse PA, et al. Management

of combined pancreatoduodenal injuries. Ann Surg 1987;205:673.

61. Kudsk K, Croce M, Fabian T, et al. Enteral versus parenteral feeding: effects on septic morbidity after blunt and penetrating abdominal trauma. Ann Surg 1991;215:503.

62. Oreskovich M, Carrico C. Pancreaticoduodenectomy for trauma: a viable option? Am J Surg 1984;147:618.

63. Graham JM, Mattox KL, Vaughan GD, Jordan GL. Combined pancreatoduodenal injuries. J Trauma 1979;19:340.

64. Lowe R, Saletta J, Moss G. Pancreatoduodenectomy for penetrating pancreatic trauma. J Trauma 1977;17:732.

65. Heimansohn DA, Canal DF, McCarthy MC, Yaw PB, Madura JA, Broadie TA. The role of pancreaticoduodenectomy in the management of traumatic injuries to the pancreas and duodenum. Am J Surg 1990;56:511.

66. Stone H, Fabian T. Management of duodenal wounds. J Trauma 1979;19:334.

67. Hasson J, Stern D, Moss G. Penetrating duodenal trauma. J Trauma 1984;24:471.

68. Berne CJ, Donovan AJ, White EJ, Yellin AE. Duodenal "diverticulization" for duodenal and pancreatic injury. Am J Surg 1974;127:503.

69. Buck JR, Sorensen VJ, Fath JJ, Horst HM, Obeid FN. Severe pancreatico-duodenal injuries: the effectiveness of pyloric exclusion with vagotomy. Am Surg 1992;58:557.

70. Vaughan GD, Grazier OH, Graham DY, Mattox KL, Petmecky FF, Jordan GL. The use of pyloric exclusion in the management of severe duodenal injuries. Am J Surg 1977;134:785.

71. McKone T, Bursch L, Scholten D. Pancreaticoduodenectomy for trauma: a life-saving procedure. Am Surg 1988;54:361.

72. Prinz R, Pickleman J, Hoffman J. Treatment of pancreatic cutaneous fistula with a somatostatin analog. Am J Surg 1988;155:36.

73. Pederzoli P, Bassi C, Falconi M, Albrigo R, Vantini I, Micciolo R. Conservative treatment of external pancreatic fistulas with parenteral nutrition alone or in combination with continuous intravenous infusion of somatostatin, glucagon or calcitonin. Surg Gynecol Obstet 1986;163:428.

74. Wynn M, Hill DM, Miller DR, Waxman K, Eisner ME, Gazzaniga AB. Management of pancreatic and duodenal trauma. Am J Surg 1985;150:327.

75. Moore J, Moore E. Changing trends in the management of combined pancreatoduodenal injuries. World J Surg 1984;8:791.

76. Campbell R, Kennedy T. The management of pancreatic and pancreaticoduodenal injuries. Br J Surg 1980;67:845.

77. Dragstedt L. Some physiologic problems in surgery of the pancreas. Ann Surg 1943;118:576.

78. McInnis W, Aust J, Cruz A, et al. Traumatic injuries of the duodenum: a comparison of primary closure and the jejunal patch. J Trauma 1975;15:847.

79. Ivatury RR, Gaudino J, Ascer E, Nallathambi M, Ramirez-Schon G, Stahl WM. Treatment of penetrating duodenal injuries: primary repair vs. repair with decompressive enterostomy/serosal patch. J Trauma 1985;25:337.

80. Donovan AJ, Hagen WE. Traumatic perforation of the duodenum. Am J Surg 1966;111:341.

81. Martin TD, Feliciano DV, Mattox KL, Jordan GL. Severe duodenal injuries: treatment with pyloric exclusion and gastrojejunostomy. Arch Surg 1983;118:631.

82. Kashuk J, Moore E, Cogbill T. Management of the intermediate severity duodenal injury. Surgery 1982;92:758.

83. Jewett TC, Caldarola V, Karp MP, Allen JE, Cooney DR. Intramural hematoma of the duodenum. Arch Surg 1988;123:54.

84. Touloukian R. Protocol for the nonoperative treatment of obstructing intramural duodenal hematoma. Am J Surg 1983;145:330.

85. Bouwman DL, Weaver DW, Walt AJ. Serum amylase and its isoenzymes: a clarification of their implication in trauma. J Trauma 1984;24:573.

86. Werschky LR, Jordan GL Jr. Surgical management of traumatic injuries to the pancreas. Am J Surg 1968;116:768.

Digestive Tract Surgery: A Text and Atlas, edited by Richard H. Bell, Layton F. Rikkers, and Michael W. Mulholland. Lippincott-Raven Publishers, Philadelphia, © 1996.

30

Atlas of Pancreatic Surgery

Richard H. Bell, Jr.

Preparation of the patient undergoing pancreatic surgery parallels that for other major abdominal operations. Patients who may be volume depleted should receive sufficient intravenous fluid preoperatively to ensure the smooth induction of anesthesia. Patients with pancreatic disease are often malnourished. In those with benign disease, such as chronic pancreatitis, a protracted period of total parenteral nutrition preoperatively may result in improved nutritional parameters and healing. Patients with pancreatic cancer rarely improve nutritionally with prolonged preoperative parenteral nutrition, but it is appropriate to provide intravenous nutrition in the perioperative period since most patients with pancreatic cancer have a prolonged period of impaired nutrition before and after operation. Blood products should be available for all patients undergoing major resections since there is always the possibility of major hemorrhage from the portal or splenic veins or other major vessels in the vicinity of the pancreas. Patients with protracted jaundice in the preoperative period may develop a coagulopathy due to the failure of fat-soluble vitamin absorption; those with elevation of the prothrombin time should be treated with vitamin K to normalize coagulation before surgery. Prophylactic perioperative intravenous antibiotics should be administered. Normal antibiotic bowel preparation is usually reserved for patients with pancreatic cancer because of the possibility that a segment of colon will need to be removed en bloc as a result of tumor invasion of the colonic blood supply in the transverse mesocolon. Patients undergoing a pancreatic resection should receive preoperative and postoperative subcutaneous injections of somatostatin analogue twice daily to reduce the risk of postoperative pancreatic fistula.

It is not clear to what extent patients with preoperative jaundice benefit from relief of jaundice preoperatively. Randomized clinical trials have generally failed to support preoperative measures to relieve jaundice, but endoscopic retrograde cholangiopancreatography and stent placement is probably appropriate in patients with prolonged preoperative jaundice and bilirubin levels greater than 10 mg/dL. The placement of transhepatic stents for the preoperative relief of jaundice is not generally indicated since it is associated with a higher risk of complications (sepsis, bleeding) than stent placement through the ampulla of Vater.

In the operating room, the surgeon should be prepared for the possibility that vascular repairs may have to be performed to the major veins around the pancreas or that partial or segmental resection of vessels, such as the superior mesenteric or portal veins, may have to be performed to allow tumor resection. The operating suite should be fully equipped with vascular instruments that are readily accessible.

As part of most pancreatic procedures, the surgeon should strongly consider the placement of gastrotomy and feeding jejunostomy tubes. With a jejunostomy tube in place in the postoperative period, the patient may be switched from intravenous to enteral alimentation. Since many patients cannot resume oral intake for some time after pancreatic surgery, the presence of a feeding jejunostomy tube simplifies the provision of adequate postoperative nutrition. If it is possible to place one at the time of operation, a gastrostomy tube may provide improved comfort for patients postoperatively since gastric emptying is often delayed after pancreatic surgery, requiring prolonged nasogastric suction if a gastrostomy tube is not available.

SECTION I *Surgical Anatomy*

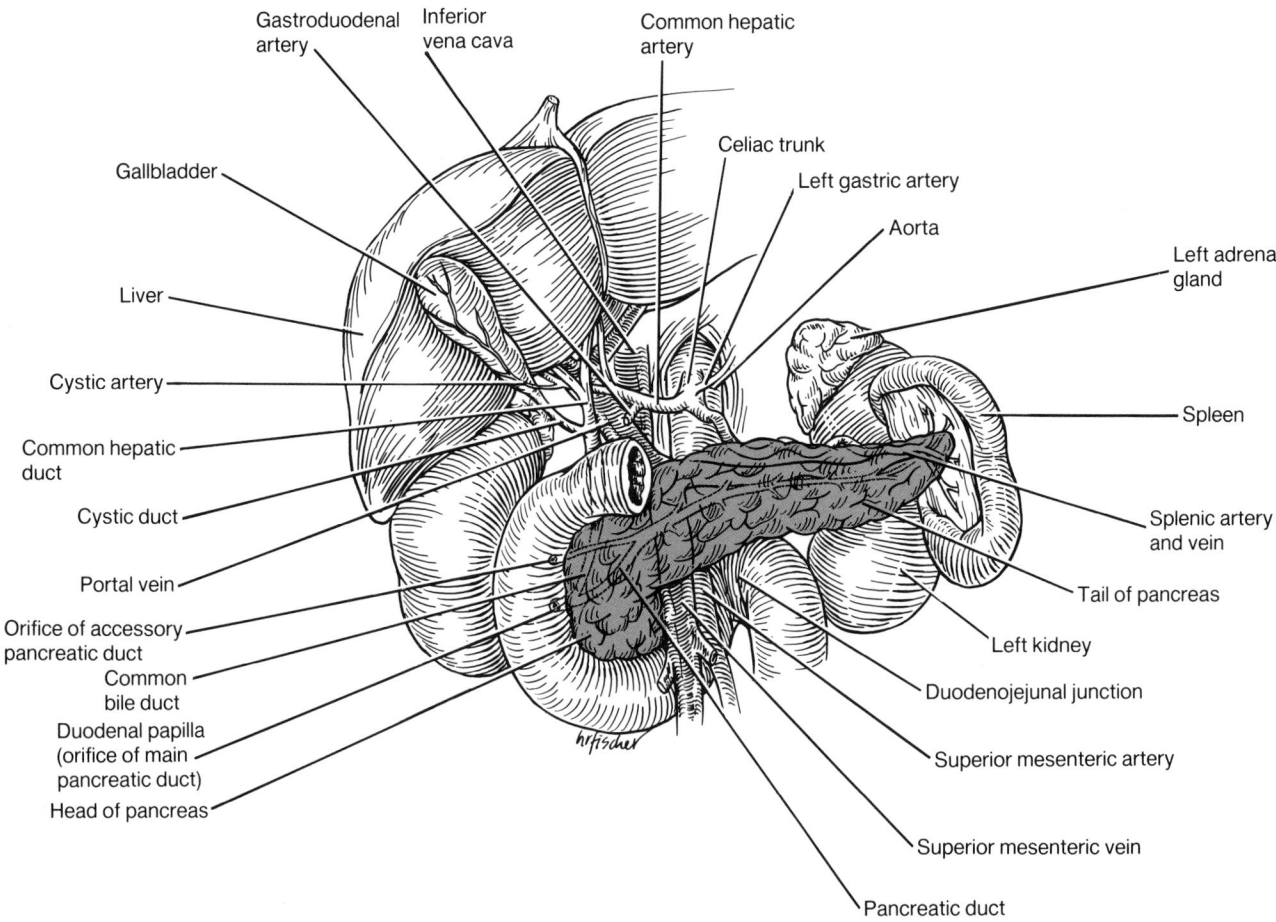

Gastroduodenal artery
Inferior vena cava
Common hepatic artery
Celiac trunk
Left gastric artery
Aorta
Left adrenal gland
Gallbladder
Liver
Spleen
Cystic artery
Common hepatic duct
Cystic duct
Portal vein
Orifice of accessory pancreatic duct
Common bile duct
Duodenal papilla (orifice of main pancreatic duct)
Head of pancreas
Splenic artery and vein
Tail of pancreas
Left kidney
Duodenojejunal junction
Superior mesenteric artery
Superior mesenteric vein
Pancreatic duct

hrfischer

Figure 30-I-1

Anterior View

The superior mesenteric artery and vein pass beneath the neck of the pancreas. The inferior vena cava passes posterior to the duodenum and head of the pancreas. The head of the pancreas can be elevated off the vena cava with a Kocher maneuver (see Section IIA). The common bile duct passes posterior to the duodenum to enter the posterior aspect of the head of the pancreas as it moves toward its junction with the main pancreatic duct. The tail of the pancreas and spleen overlie the left kidney. The body and tail of the pancreas can be elevated by dissection between the pancreas and kidney (see Section IIB).

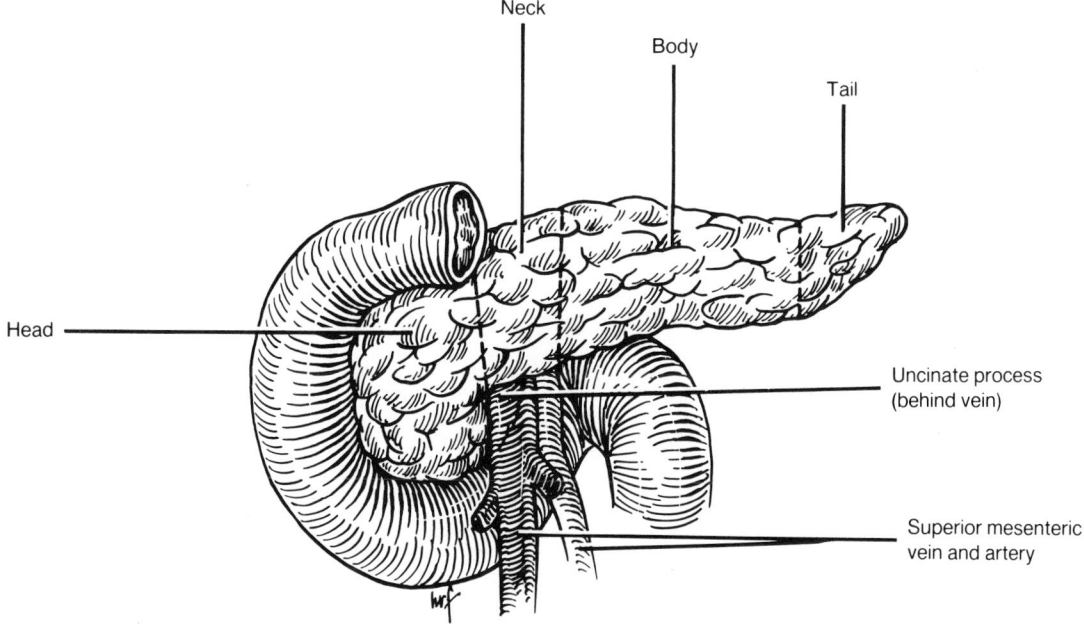

Neck

Body

Tail

Head

Uncinate process
(behind vein)

Superior mesenteric
vein and artery

Figure 30-I-2

Anatomic Regions

The uncinate process of the head of the pancreas extends posteriorly behind the superior mesenteric vein. The neck of the pancreas is that portion immediately overlying the junction of the superior mesenteric and portal veins. The head of the pancreas is intimately associated with the lesser curvature of the duodenal C loop. The head of the pancreas and duodenum share a common blood supply derived from the superior and inferior pancreaticoduodenal arteries. The junction between the body and tail of the pancreas is not delineated by any visible landmark. The tail is that part of the gland which gradually tapers in size, its tip embedded within the splenic hilum. The inferior portion tail of the gland lies in close contact with the splenic flexure of the colon.

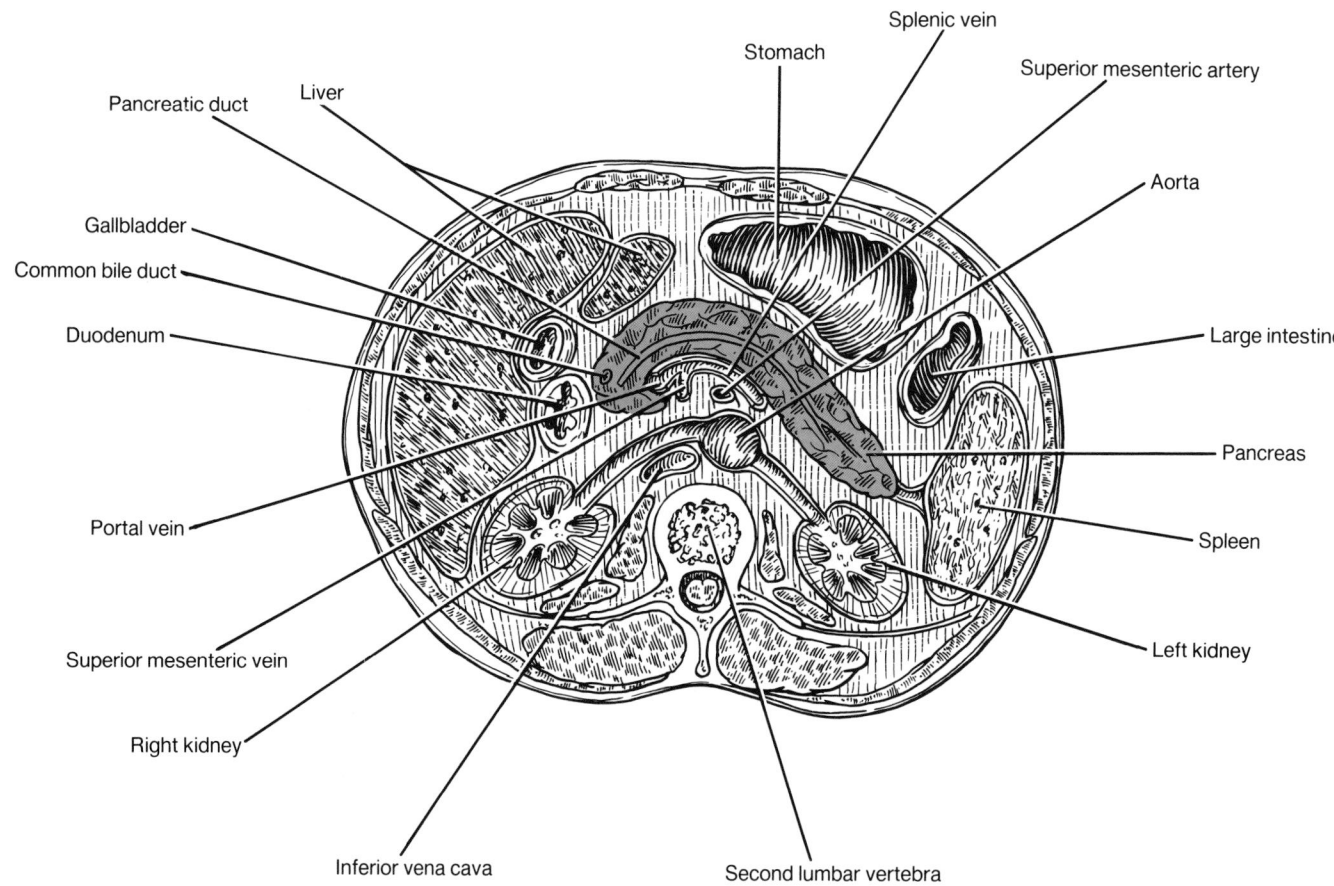

Figure 30-I-3

Cross-Sectional Anatomy

Note the intimate relation of the superior mesenteric and portal veins to the posterior aspect of the neck of the pancreas and the relation of the splenic vein to the posterior aspect of the body and tail of the pancreas. There is a plane of dissection between the posterior aspect of the head of the pancreas and the inferior vena cava. This plane must be entered lateral to the duodenum. It is the area that is opened during a Kocher maneuver and allows the head of the pancreas to be elevated off the vena cava (see Section IIA). Elevation of the head of the pancreas is limited medially by the superior mesenteric artery, which tethers the pancreas to the aorta.

The space seen between the stomach and the anterior surface of the body of the pancreas is the lesser omental sac, which can be opened by dividing the gastrocolic omentum. This is the standard operative approach to the body and tail of the pancreas (see Fig. 30-IIB-1). Finally, there is a plane of dissection between the left kidney and the tail of the pancreas. By elevating the spleen and entering this plane between the spleen and kidney, the body and tail of the pancreas can be mobilized up to the superior mesenteric artery (see Section IIB).

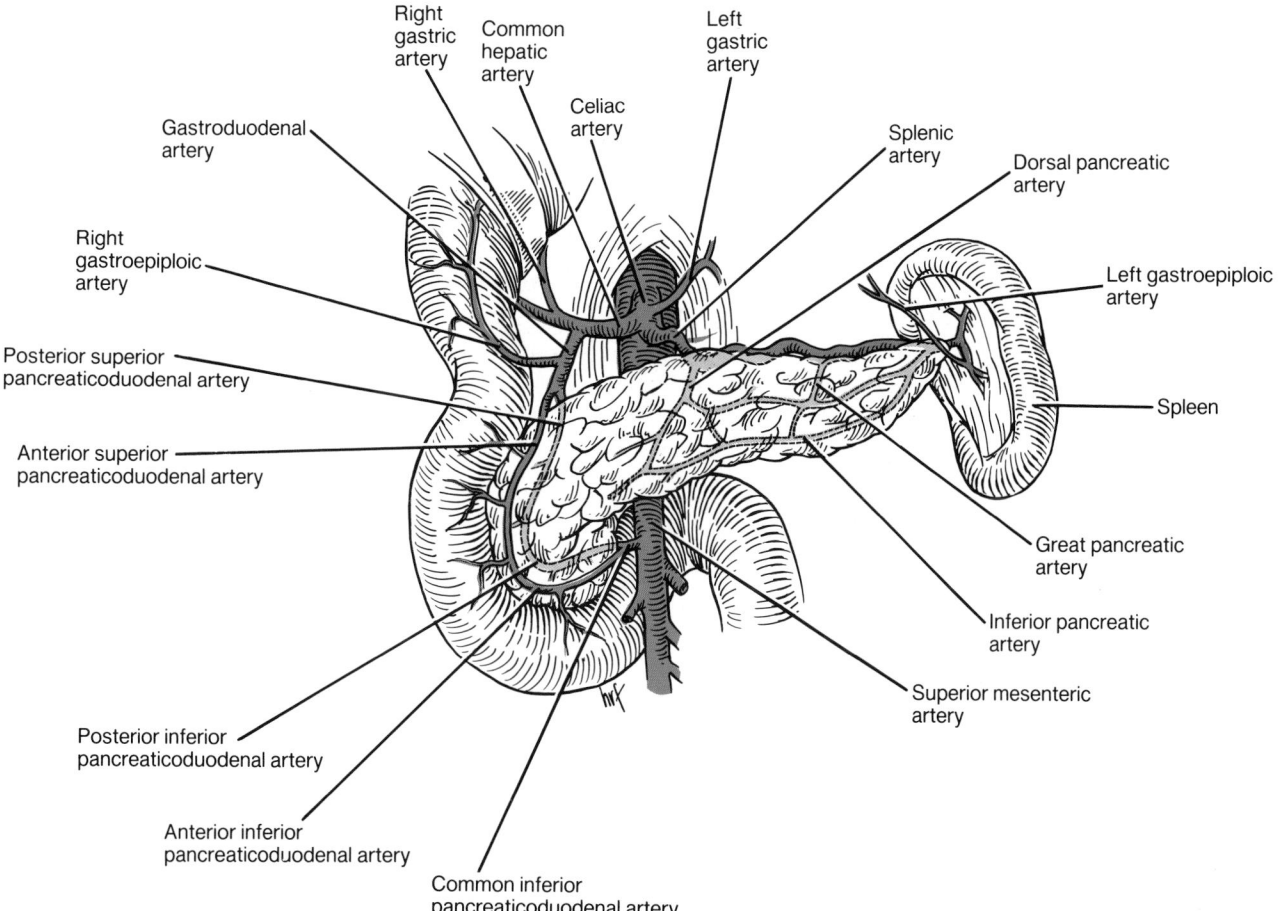

Right
gastric
artery

Common
hepatic
artery

Left
gastric
artery

Celiac
artery

Gastroduodenal
artery

Splenic
artery

Dorsal pancreatic
artery

Right
gastroepiploic
artery

Left gastroepiploic
artery

Posterior superior
pancreaticoduodenal artery

Spleen

Anterior superior
pancreaticoduodenal artery

Great pancreatic
artery

Inferior pancreatic
artery

Posterior inferior
pancreaticoduodenal artery

Superior mesenteric
artery

Anterior inferior
pancreaticoduodenal artery

Common inferior
pancreaticoduodenal artery

Figure 30-I-4

Arterial Supply

The arteries supplying the body and tail of the pancreas are more variable than those supplying the head. The pancreaticoduodenal arcade is formed by branches from both the gastroduodenal artery and the superior mesenteric artery.

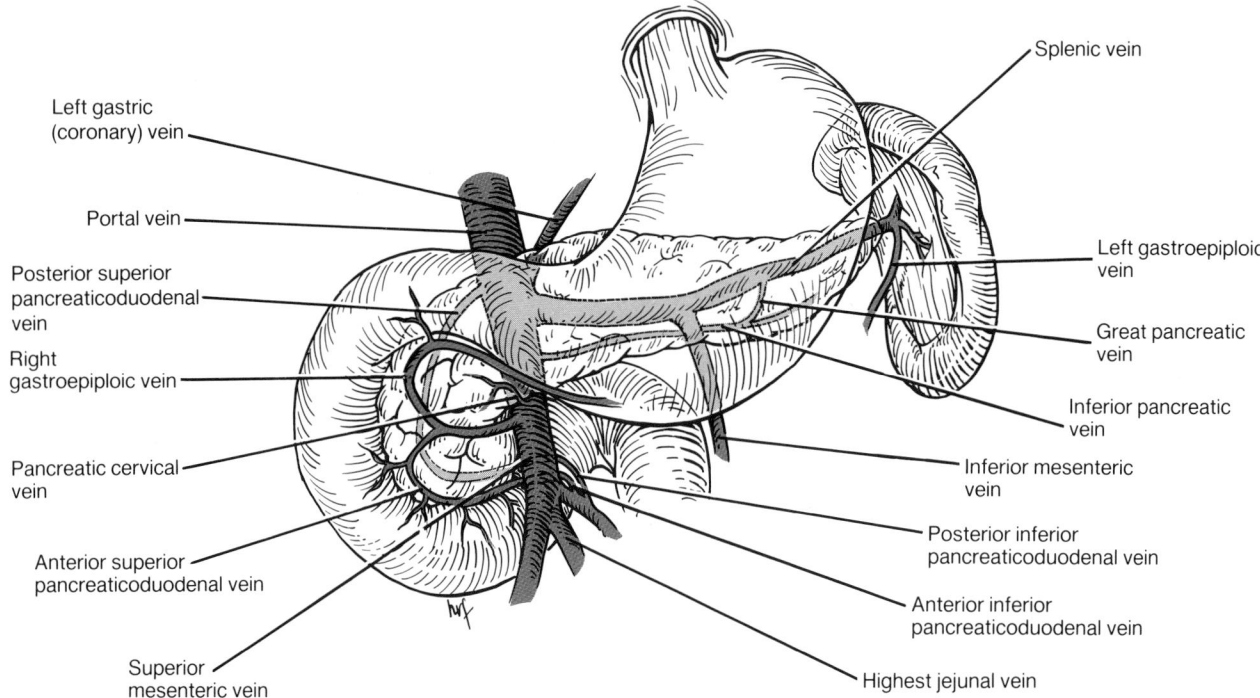

Figure 30-I-5

Venous Drainage

The junction of the superior mesenteric and splenic veins to form the portal vein occurs immediately behind the neck of the pancreas. Ordinarily, there are no venous branches on the anterior aspect of the superior mesenteric–portal vein junction, allowing the development of a surgical plane between the posterior aspect of the neck of the gland and the anterior surface of the veins (see Figs. 30-VA-7 to 30-VA-10).

The entrance of the inferior mesenteric vein into the main portal trunks is variable. The inferior mesenteric vein usually enters the splenic vein as shown and may require formal division during distal pancreatectomy (see Fig. 30-VE-8). On other occasions, the inferior mesenteric vein enters the superior mesenteric vein or the confluence of the superior mesenteric and splenic veins and may not be apparent during distal pancreatectomy.

Unlike the superior mesenteric and portal veins, there is no free plane of dissection between the anterior splenic vein and the posterior aspect of the body and tail of the pancreas. In fact, the splenic vein is often partially embedded within the pancreatic parenchyma. Mobilization of the splenic vein from the pancreas requires division of multiple small branches entering the vein from the posterior aspect of the pancreas.

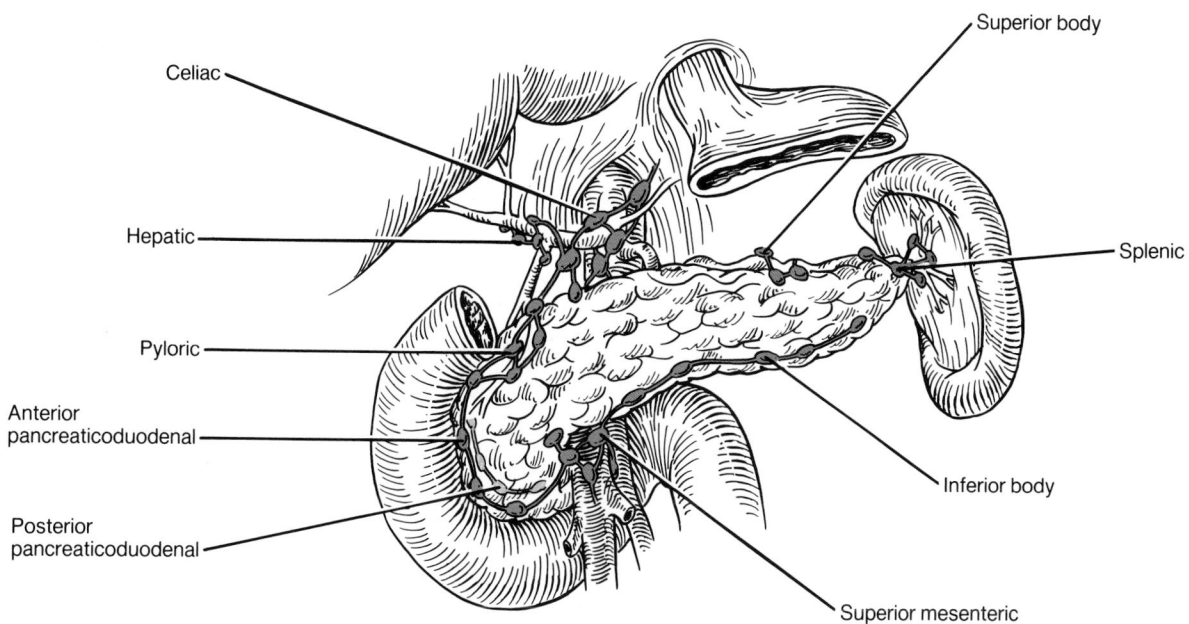

Figure 30-I-6

Lymphatic Supply

For details about the involvement of lymph nodes groups in pancreatic cancer, please refer to Chapter 26 and Figure 26-3.

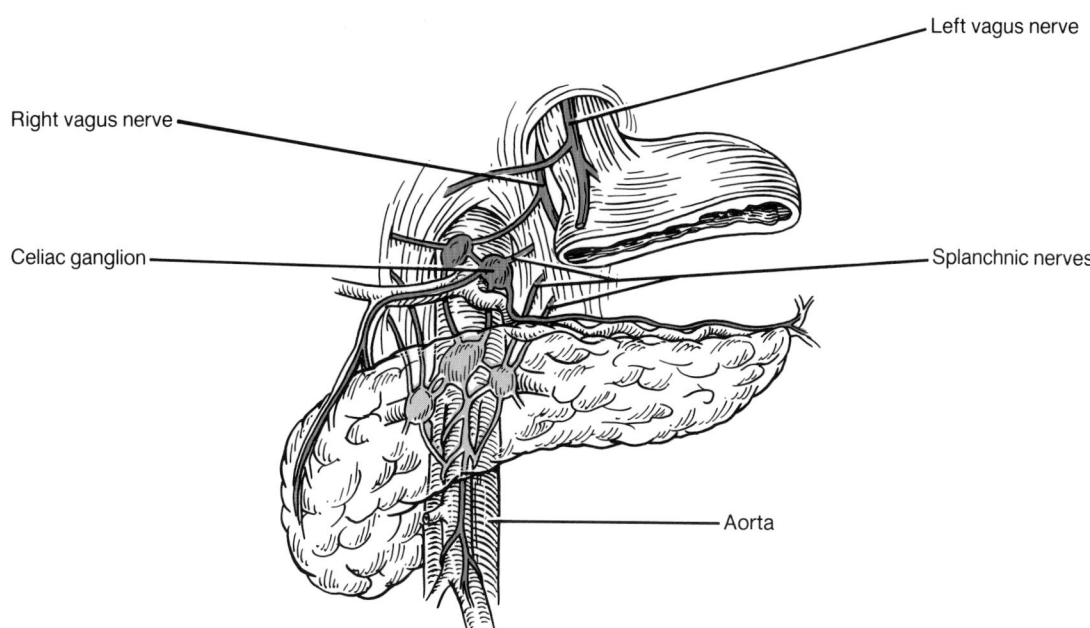

Figure 30-I-7

Innervation

The autonomic supply from the splenic division of the celiac plexus carries both sympathetic postganglionic nerves and parasympathetic preganglionic fibers, the latter forming synapses with ganglion cells within the gland itself. Sensory fibers from the pancreas are mainly carried by the splanchnic nerves. The mass of nervous tissue surrounding the origins of the arteries of the celiac axis can be injected with alcohol percutaneously or at the time of laparotomy for pain control in patients with unresectable pancreatic cancer (see Chap. 26).

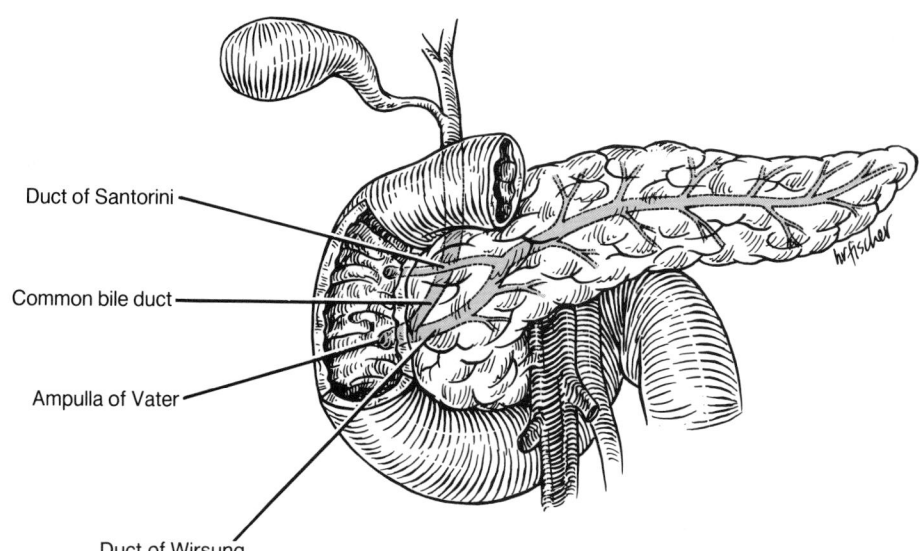

Duct of Santorini

Common bile duct

Ampulla of Vater

Duct of Wirsung

Figure 30-I-8

Ductal System

The most common anatomic arrangement is shown, in which the duct of Wirsung is the dominant duct draining most of the gland and the duct of Santorini is a smaller, accessory duct entering the duodenum through a separate papillary orifice cephalad to the ampulla of Vater. The pancreatic ductal system is subject to considerable variation, including the anomaly referred to as *pancreas divisum,* in which the duct of Wirsung is rudimentary and the duct of Santorini provides the drainage for most of the gland.

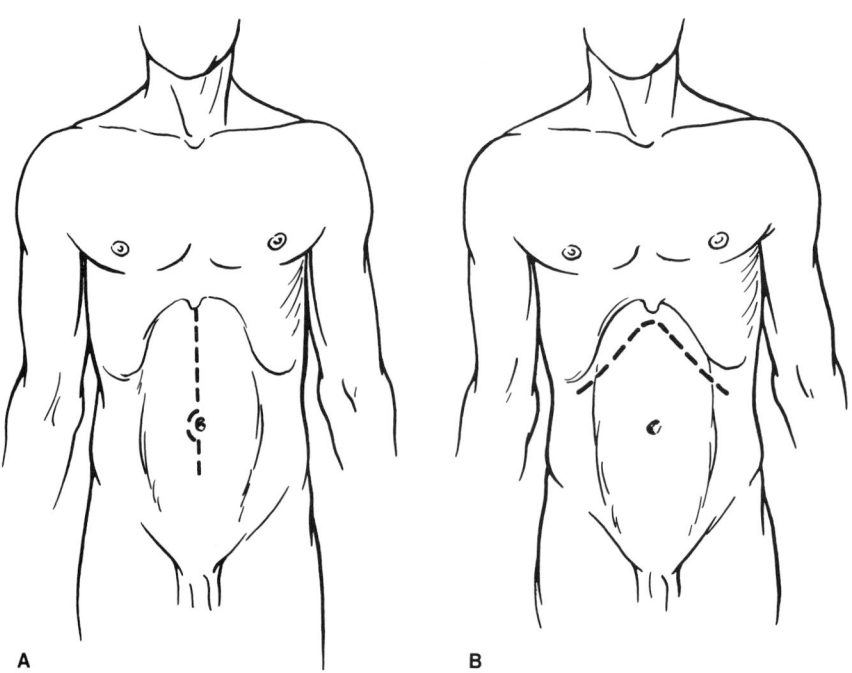

A   B

Figure 30-I-9

Incisions for Pancreatic Surgery

The most useful incisions for pancreatic surgery are the midline laparotomy (**A**) and the bilateral subcostal incision (**B**). Virtually all pancreatic procedures can be performed through either of these incisions.

SECTION II   *Surgical Approaches to the Pancreas*

A. Exposure of the Duodenum and Head of the Pancreas

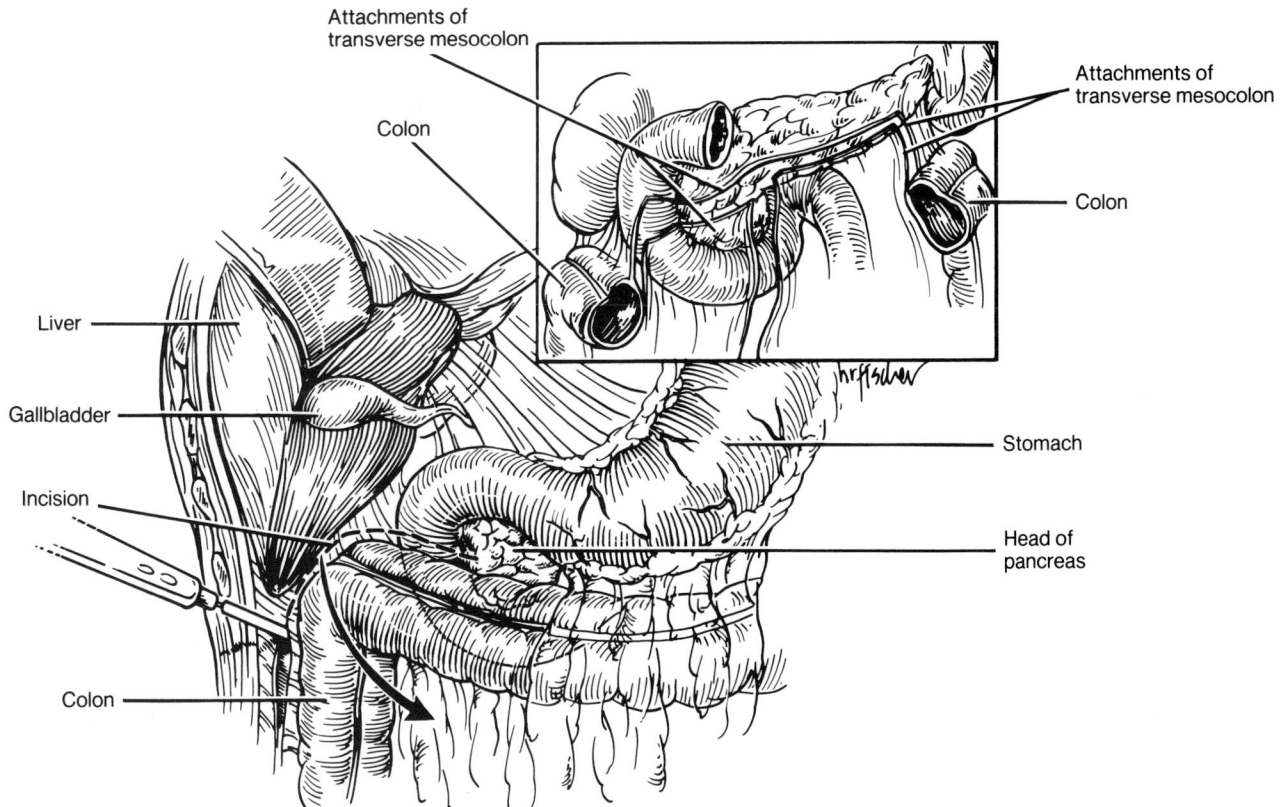

Figure 30-IIA-1

Reflection of Hepatic Flexure

To provide maximal exposure of the head of the pancreas, it is necessary in most patients to mobilize the hepatic flexure of the colon formally and to retract the colon inferiorly. This step should be performed at the outset of any procedure involving the head of the pancreas. The base of the mesocolon crosses the head of the pancreas (**inset**); it is often necessary to mobilize the base of the mesocolon gently off the anterior aspect of the head of the pancreas to gain full exposure of the gland. In doing so, care must be taken not to tear venous branches from the colon entering the superior mesenteric vein.

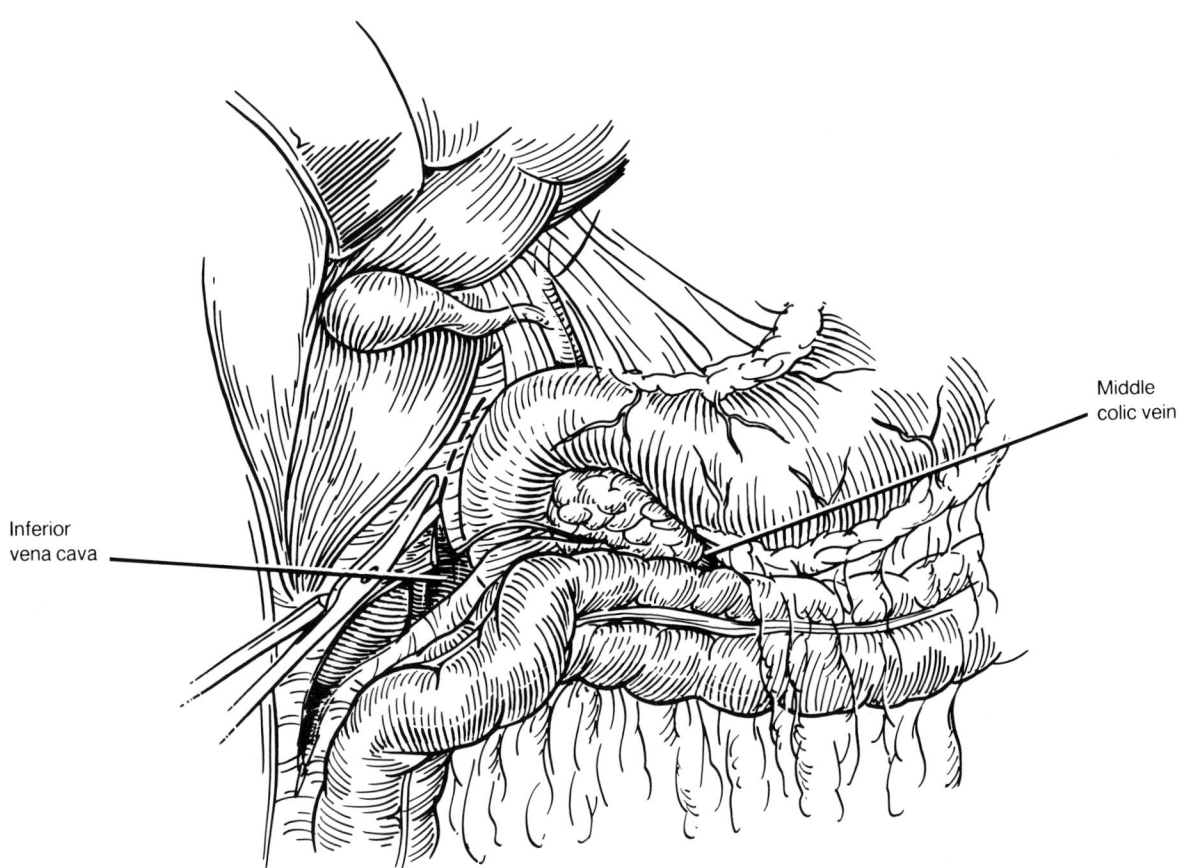

Figure 30-IIA-2

Incision of Lateral Duodenal Peritoneum

After the colon is mobilized inferiorly, the peritoneum lateral to the duodenum is incised. By gentle blunt dissection, the surgeon's hand can then be passed posterior to the duodenum and head of the pancreas and these structures elevated anteriorly off the inferior vena cava (the Kocher maneuver). By a combination of blunt and sharp dissection, the peritoneal attachments on the lateral border of the duodenum should be incised inferiorly to the point at which the duodenum begins to pass beneath the superior mesenteric vessels. The superior limit of the mobilization is the right edge of the hepatoduodenal ligament. The dissection behind the head of the pancreas is limited medially by the superior mesenteric artery, which tethers the pancreas to the aorta. After the head of the pancreas is fully mobilized, it should be possible to visualize the inferior vena cava and to palpate both the aorta and the superior mesenteric artery.

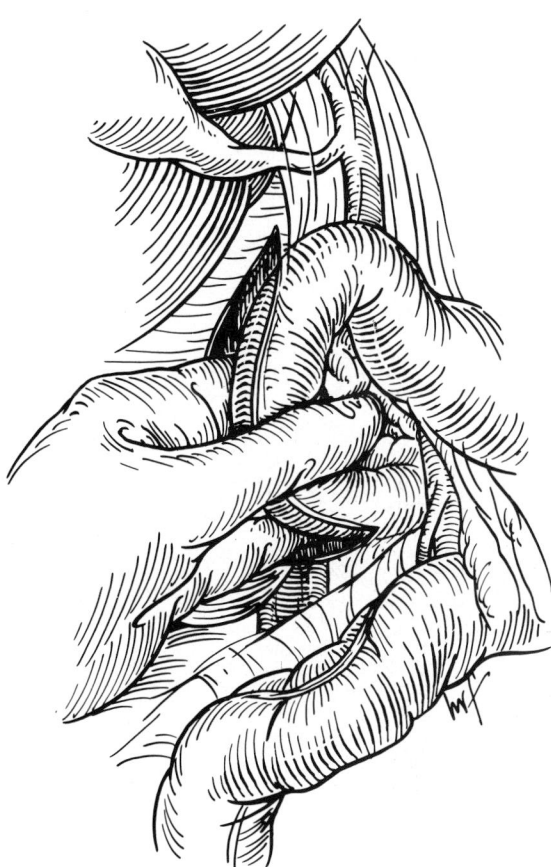

Figure 30-IIA-3

Manual Examination of Pancreatic Head

After the duodenum and the head of the pancreas are fully mobilized, the head and uncinate process of the gland can be palpated between the thumb and fingers. This maneuver is helpful in localizing tumors or identifying areas for biopsy (see Sections V and VI).

B. Exposure of the Body and Tail of the Pancreas

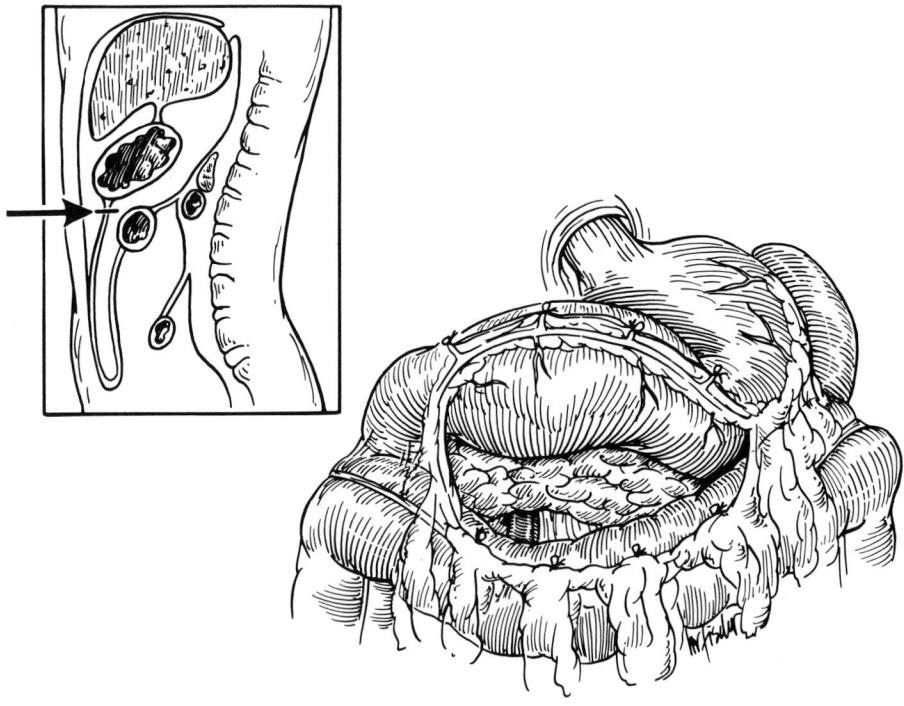

Figure 30-IIB-1

Division of Gastrocolic Omentum

By incising the gastrocolic omentum, the surgeon enters the lesser omental sac (**inset**) and gains access to the anterior surface of the body and tail of the pancreas. Ordinarily, the incision in the gastrocolic omentum is made just below the gastroepiploic vessels to preserve the blood supply to the greater curvature of the stomach. In entering the lesser sac, the stomach is gently retracted superiorly and the transverse colon and mesocolon inferiorly. There are often avascular filmy adhesions between the anterior surface of the body of the pancreas and the posterior wall of the stomach, which can be divided sharply to provide full exposure of the pancreas. The dissection should be kept close to the posterior wall of the stomach to avoid inadvertent entry into the transverse mesocolon and damage to the middle colic vessels.

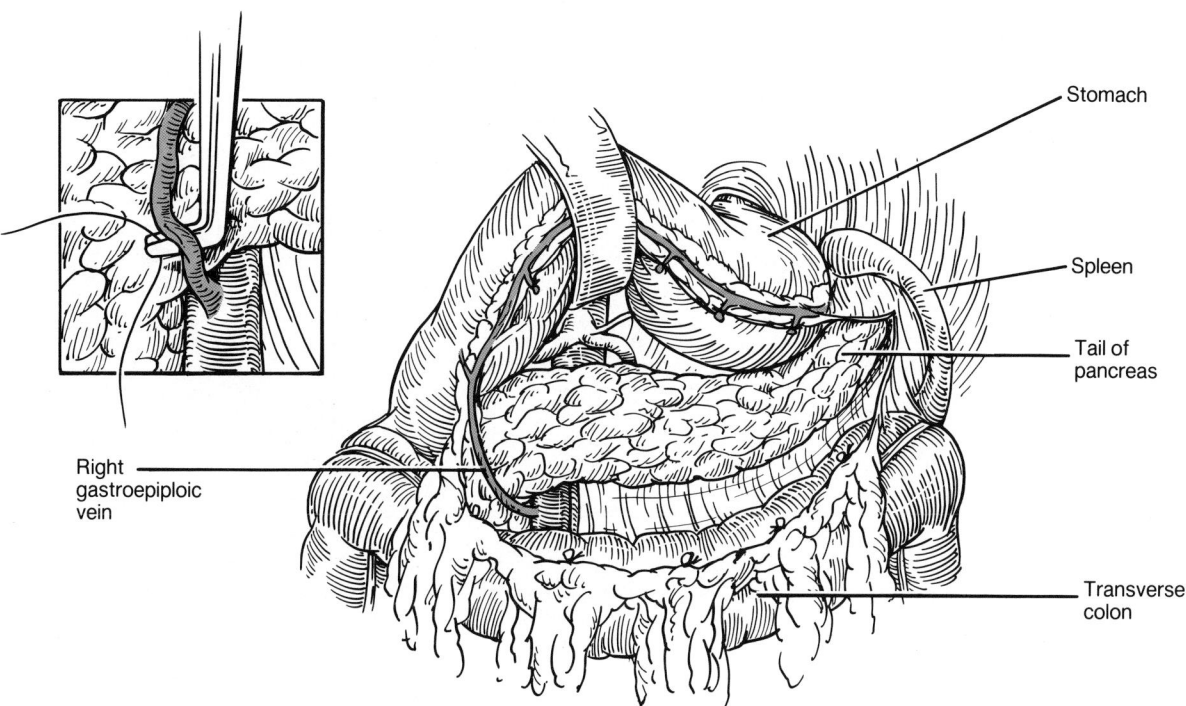

Stomach

Spleen

Tail of
pancreas

Transverse
colon

Right
gastroepiploic
vein

Figure 30-IIB-2

Division of Right Gastroepiploic Vessels

If it is desirable to expose the neck of the pancreas, it is often helpful to divide the right gastroepiploic vein as it crosses the head of the pancreas to enter the superior mesenteric vein. Division of this vein allows the surgeon to expose the entire length of the pancreas, a maneuver which is helpful, for example, during longitudinal pancreaticojejunostomy (see Section IV). Division of the right gastroepiploic vein is not ordinarily necessary for procedures restricted to the body and tail of the pancreas.

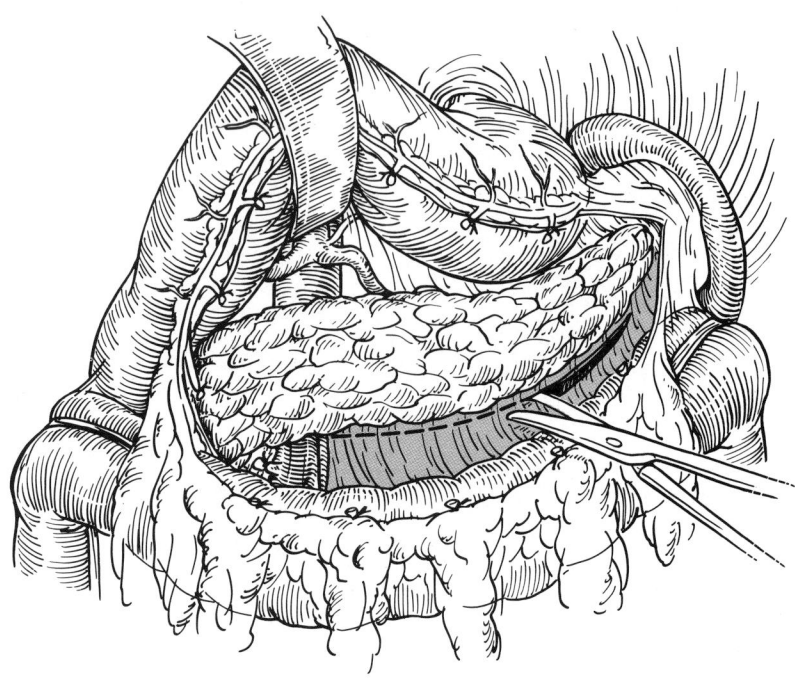

Figure 30-IIB-3

Incision of Peritoneum

Once the body and tail of the pancreas are exposed, an incision is made in the peritoneum along the underside of the gland.

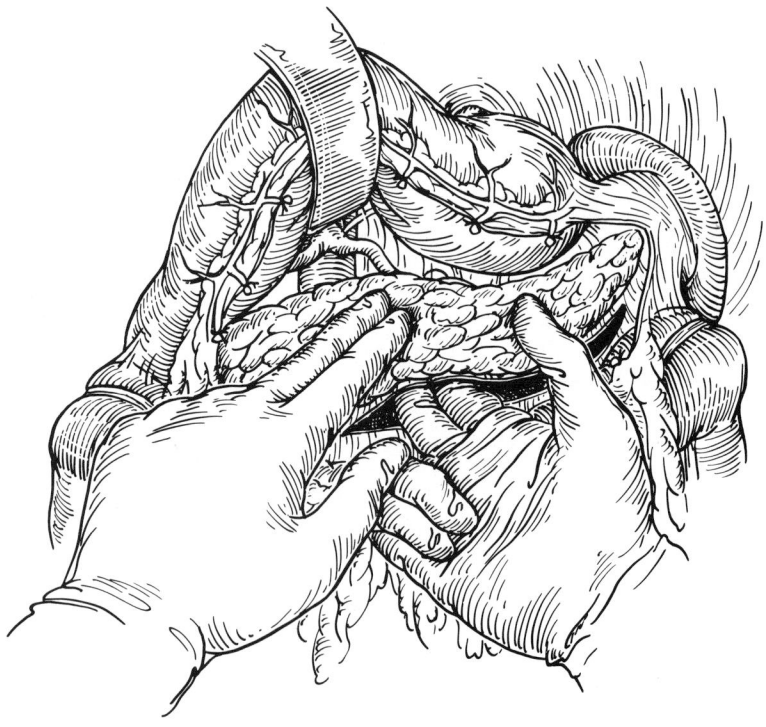

Figure 30-IIB-4

Bimanual Palpation of Pancreatic Tail

By gentle blunt dissection behind the pancreas, the body and tail are mobilized to facilitate bimanual palpation of the gland, which is useful in searching for tumors of the distal pancreas or in palpating the location of the pancreatic duct.

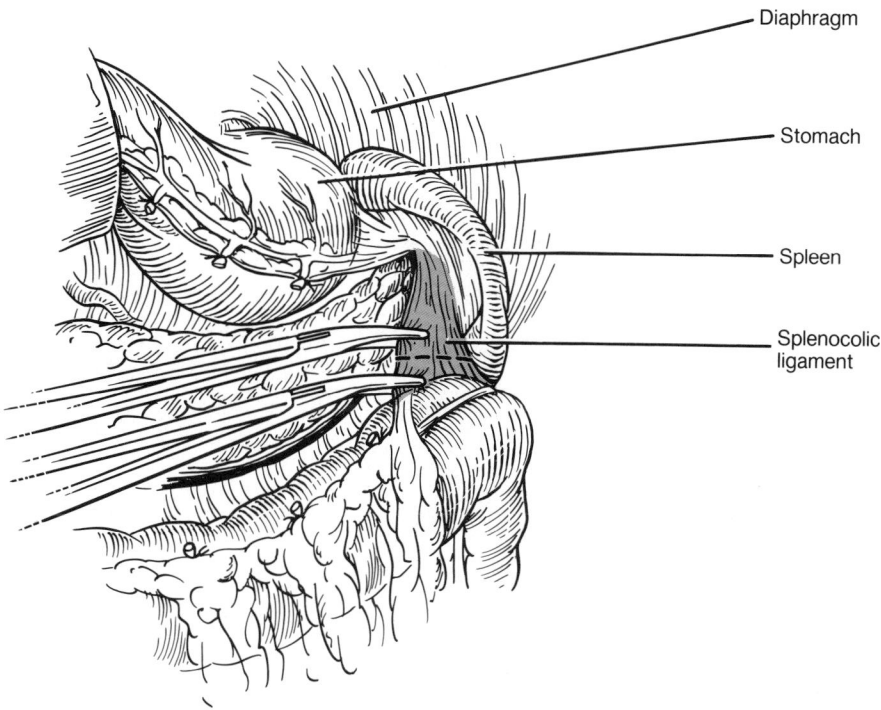

Figure 30-IIB-5

Division of Splenocolic Ligament

To mobilize the body and tail of the pancreas fully, it is necessary to elevate the spleen and distal pancreas off the left kidney and to separate the tail of the pancreas from the left colon. The attachments of the spleen to the splenic flexure of the colon are divided between clamps and ligated.

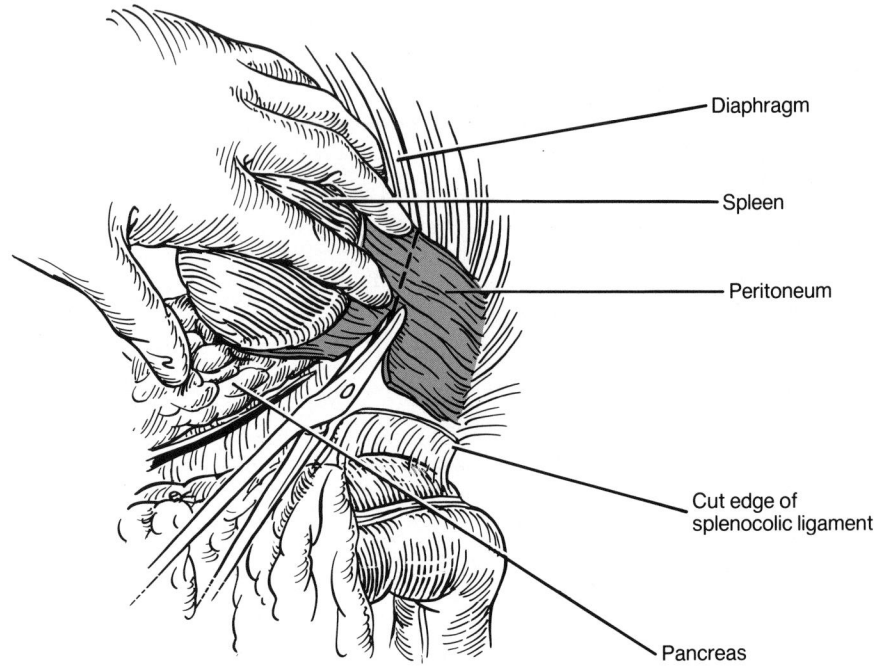

Diaphragm

Spleen

Peritoneum

Cut edge of
splenocolic ligament

Pancreas

Figure 30-IIB-6

Division of Peritoneum

The spleen is gently retracted toward the midline, and the peritoneum lateral to the spleen is fully divided up to the diaphragm to allow the surgeon to pass a hand posterior to the spleen and tail of the pancreas. This maneuver can be performed before the splenocolic ligament is taken down, as shown in Fig. 30-IIB-5. The exact order of these two steps can be varied, depending on the ease of exposure.

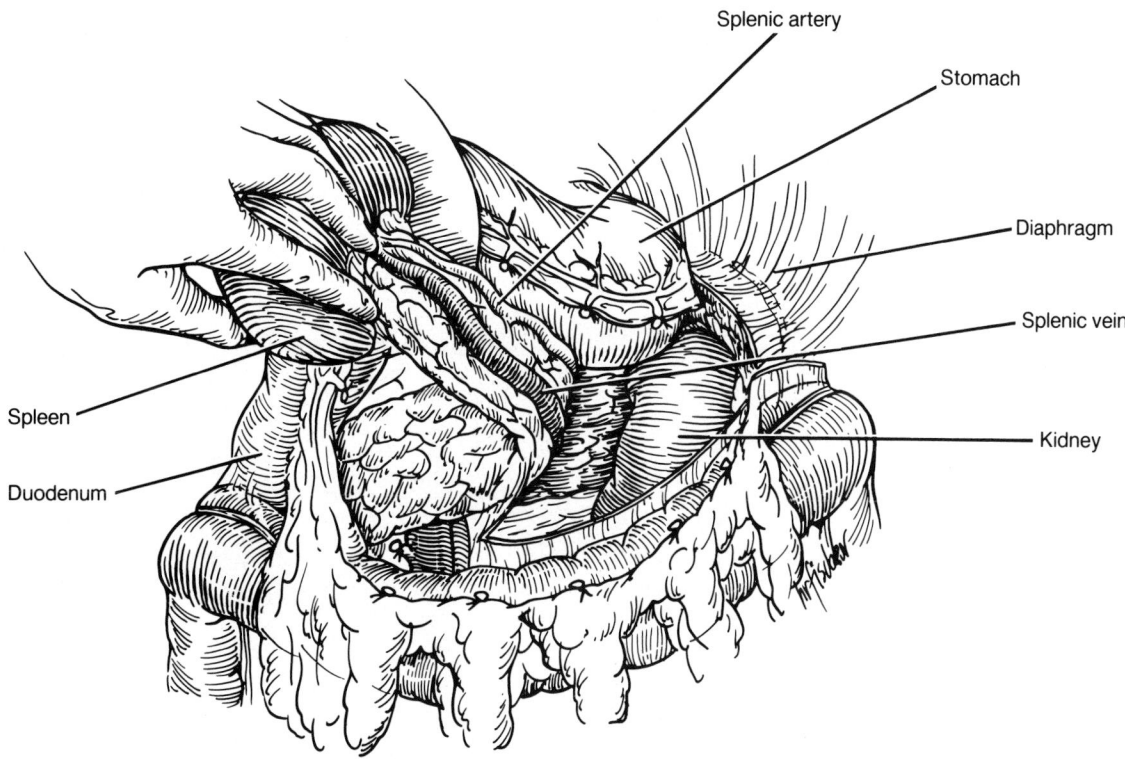

Figure 30-IIB-7

Mobilization of Pancreatic Body and Tail

By passing a hand posterior to the spleen, the tail of the pancreas is gently mobilized off the left kidney and elevated. As the gland is progressively mobilized, the splenic vein becomes apparent coursing along the posterior aspect of the body and tail of the pancreas. In some patients, the inferior mesenteric vein enters the splenic vein from below and requires ligation to elevate the distal pancreas fully (see Fig. 30-VE-8). The mobilization of the distal pancreas ultimately is limited by the superior mesenteric artery, which tethers the gland posteriorly to the aorta.

SECTION III *Operations for Acute Pancreatitis*
A. Débridement of Acute Pancreatic Necrosis

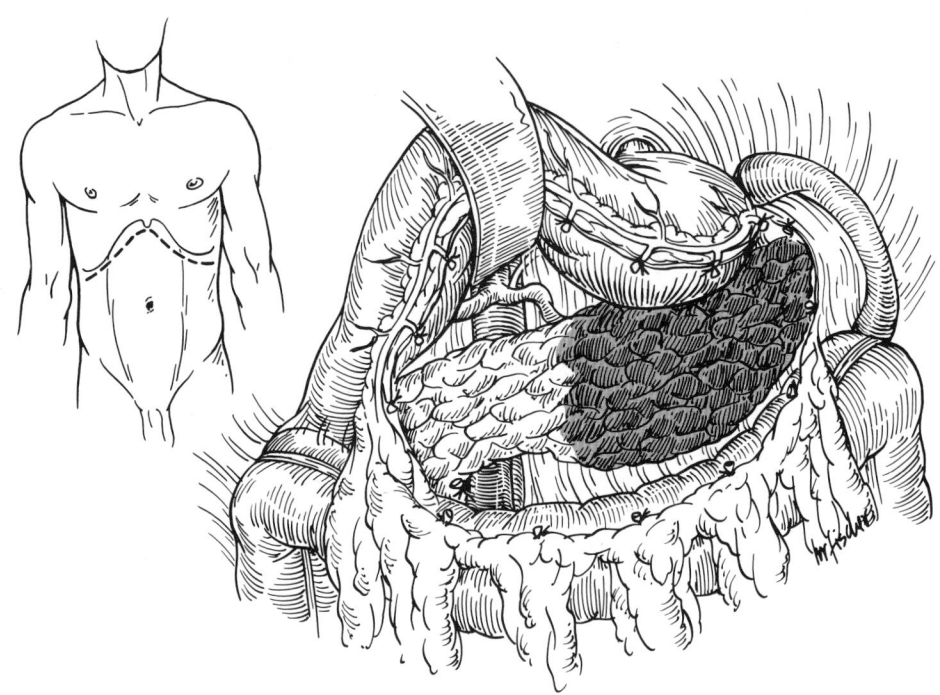

Figure 30-IIIA-1

Approach Through Gastrocolic Omentum

Débridement of acute pancreatic necrosis can be accomplished through a bilateral sub-costal incision (**inset**), which can provide access to the entire gland if necessary. The bilateral subcostal incision has the advantage of paralleling the lesser sac, which facilitates packing the débrided space bounded by the transverse mesocolon below and the posterior wall of the stomach above. After entering the peritoneal cavity, the gastrocolic omentum is opened, providing access to the necrotic body and tail of the pancreas. If possible, the gastrocolic omentum should be entered below the gastroepiploic vessels to preserve blood supply to the greater curvature of the stomach. Entry into the lesser sac, however, may be difficult because of acute inflammation in patients with acute pancreatitis. If entry into the lesser sac is difficult, it is safest to enter the space immediately adjacent to the stomach to avoid injury to the transverse mesocolon and middle colic vessels, or to approach the pancreas through the base of the transverse mesocolon (see Figs. 30-IIIA-6 and 30-IIIA-7).

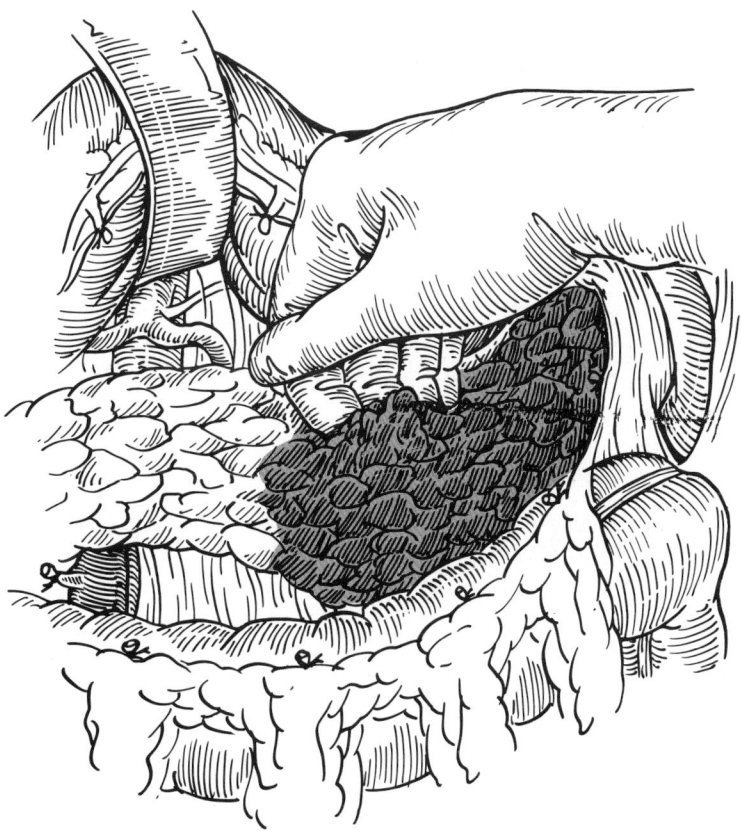

Figure 30-IIIA-2

Débridement

The necrotic portions of the pancreas and peripancreatic tissue can be removed by scooping out the nonviable tissue manually. Tissue that is firmly attached and cannot be easily débrided manually is best left in place. Sharp dissection is potentially dangerous since injuries to major vascular structures can result.

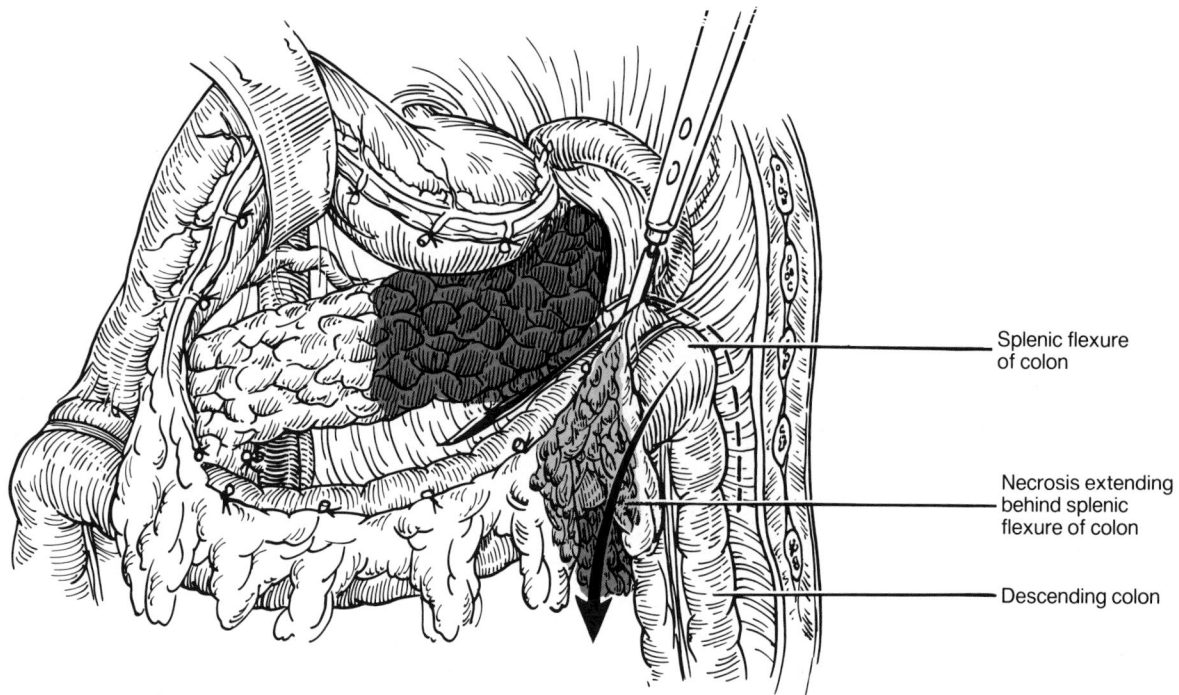

Splenic flexure
of colon

Necrosis extending
behind splenic
flexure of colon

Descending colon

Figure 30-IIIA-3

Division of Splenocolic Ligament and Reflection of Splenic Flexure

Occasionally, peripancreatic necrosis extends behind the splenic flexure of the colon and down into the retroperitoneal space behind the descending colon. In such cases, it is necessary to mobilize the splenic flexure of the colon to allow adequate drainage of retroperitoneal infection. Every effort should be made to "unroof" all areas of peripancreatic necrosis.

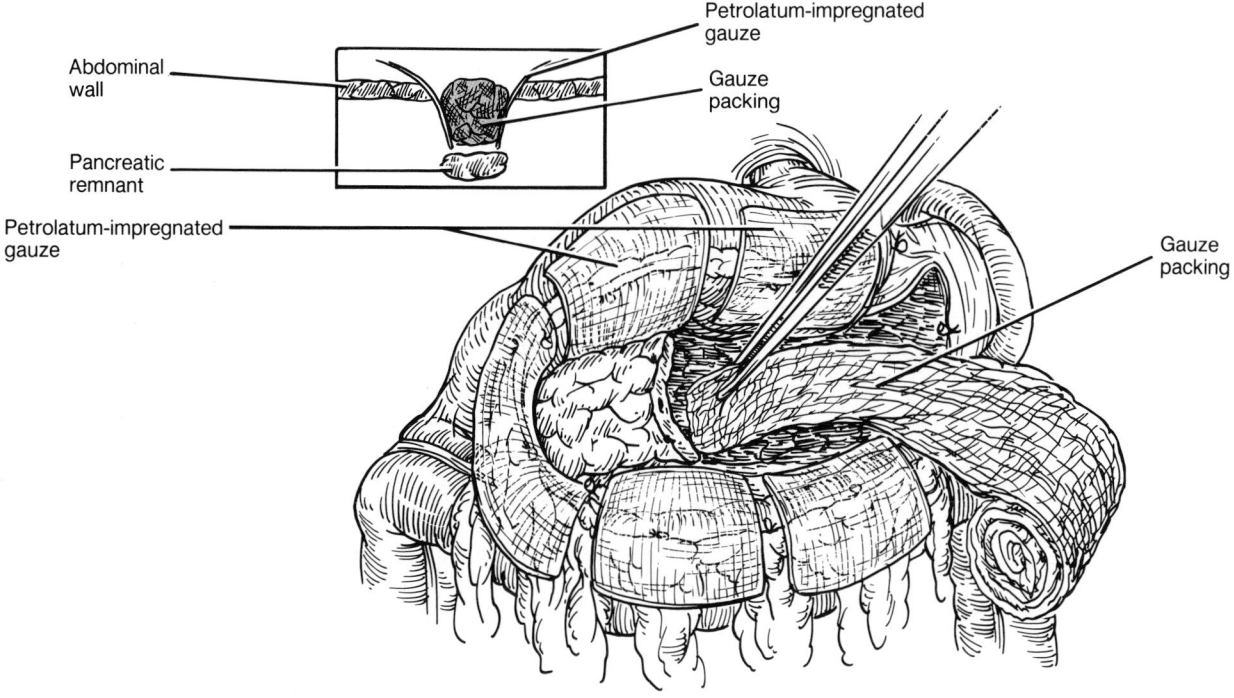

Figure 30-IIIA-4

Gauze Placement

After all areas of necrosis have been débrided, the pancreatic bed, the posterior wall of the stomach, and the transverse mesocolon and colon are covered with nonadherent petrolatum-impregnated (Adaptic) gauze. This prevents packs from sticking to these organs and prevents tearing of these organs when gauze packs are removed on subsequent reexploration. After the surfaces of the viscera are covered with nonadherent gauze, the remainder of the wound cavity is packed with rolled gauze lightly moistened with saline.

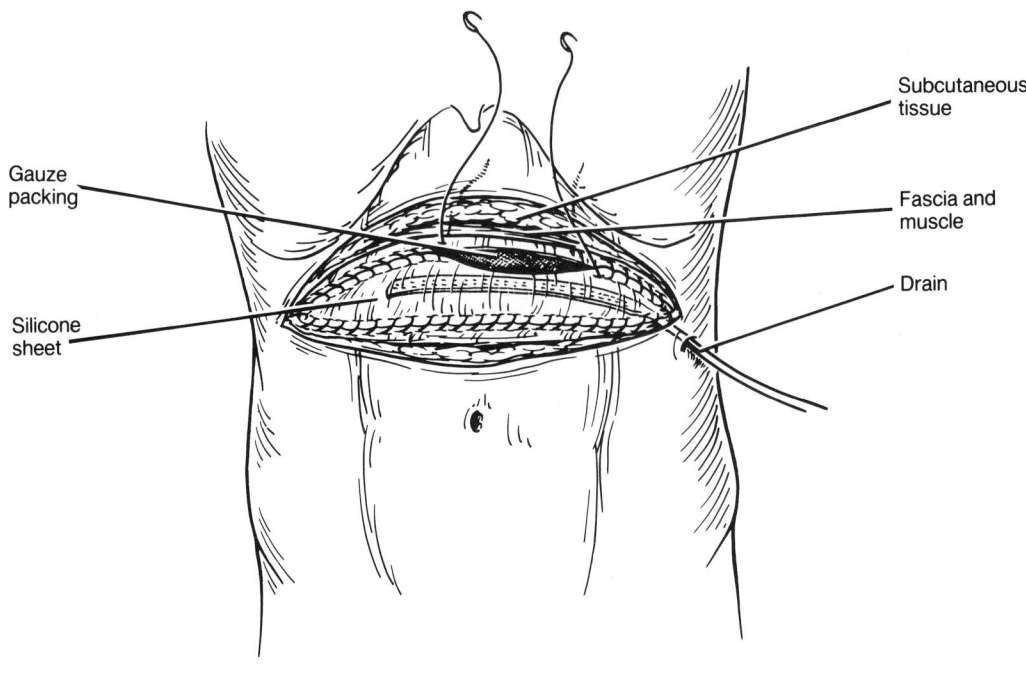

Figure 30-IIIA-5

Placement of Silicone Sheet

Because the treatment of acute pancreatic necrosis usually requires multiple reexplorations for further débridement and dressing changes, the process is greatly facilitated by sewing an elliptical silicone rubber (Silastic) sheet to the fascial edges with a continuous 0 or 2-0 nonabsorbable monofilament suture. In this way, reexplorations can be performed by dividing and then reclosing the silicone sheet, leaving the original fascial closure intact. Closed soft sump drains are placed beneath the silicone sheet to evacuate the fluid that ordinarily accumulates in the packed cavity.

At the time of reexploration, gauze packs are soaked thoroughly with saline before attempting to remove them to avoid tearing the surface of the stomach or colon. The wound is thoroughly explored, further débrided as necessary, and repacked, then the silicone sheet is closed.

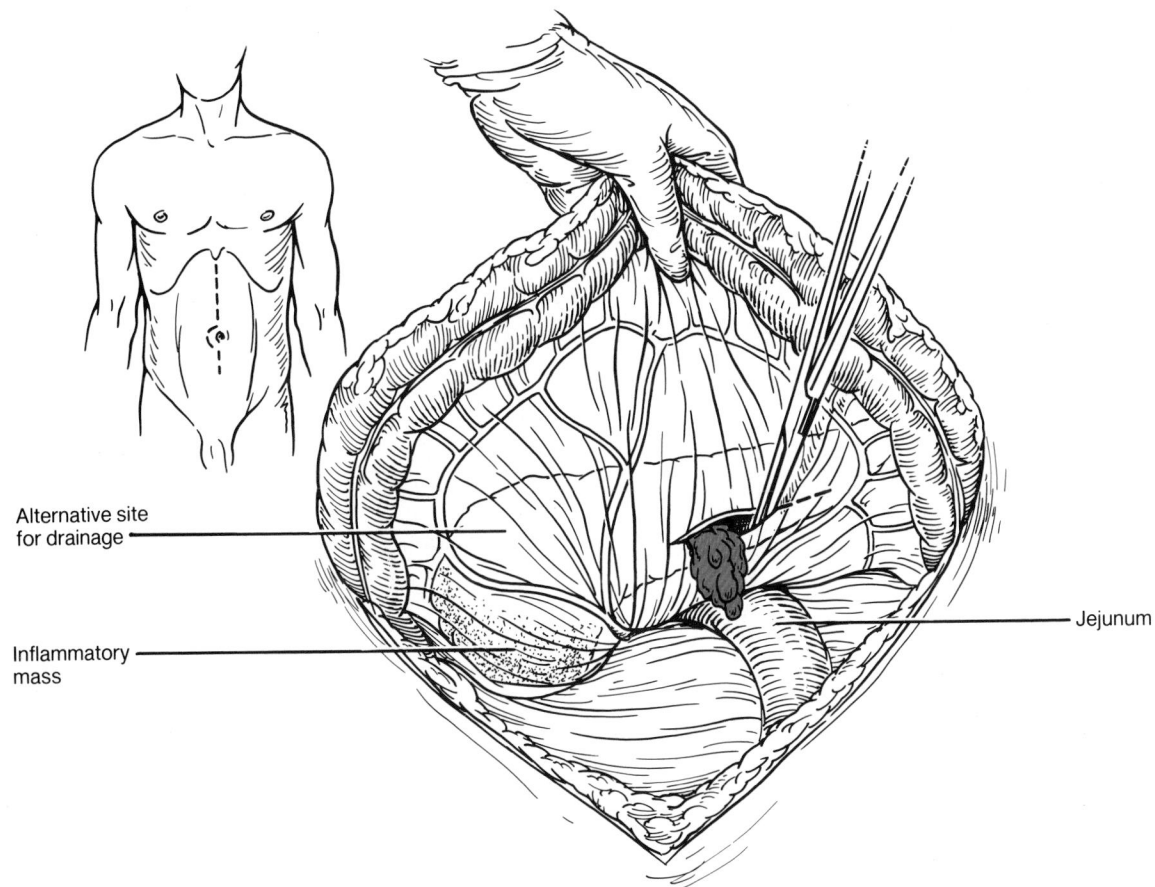

Alternative site
for drainage

Inflammatory
mass

Jejunum

Figure 30-IIIA-6

Approach Through Base of Transverse Mesocolon

An alternative approach to the débridement of pancreatic necrosis is through a midline incision (**inset**) and an incision in the base of the transverse mesocolon. This approach avoids the sometimes difficult entry into the lesser sac through the gastrocolic omentum. On the other hand, exposure of the pancreas itself is somewhat limited. The incision in the transverse mesocolon should be made over areas of fullness or fluctuation. A syringe can be used to aspirate through the mesocolon to identify promising areas for incision. Incisions to the left of the middle colic vessels are used to drain the area of the body and tail of the pancreas. An incision to the right of the middle colic vessels can be used for débridement of the head of the gland and surrounding tissues.

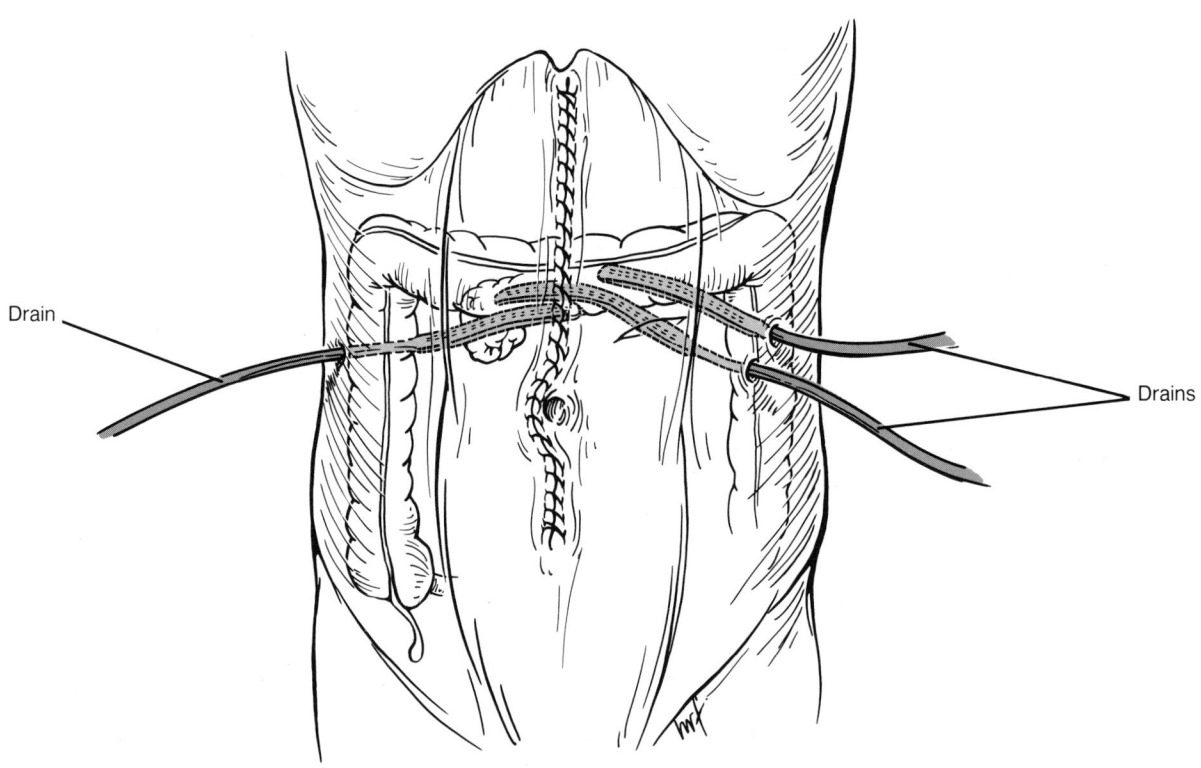

Drain

Drains

Figure 30-IIIA-7

Drain Placement

After débridement, drains are placed through the transverse mesocolon into the peripancreatic space. Numerous drains are advisable. These drains are brought out through stab incisions in the left or right flank. For further details of management of pancreatic necrosis, see Chapter 24.

B. Cystgastrostomy

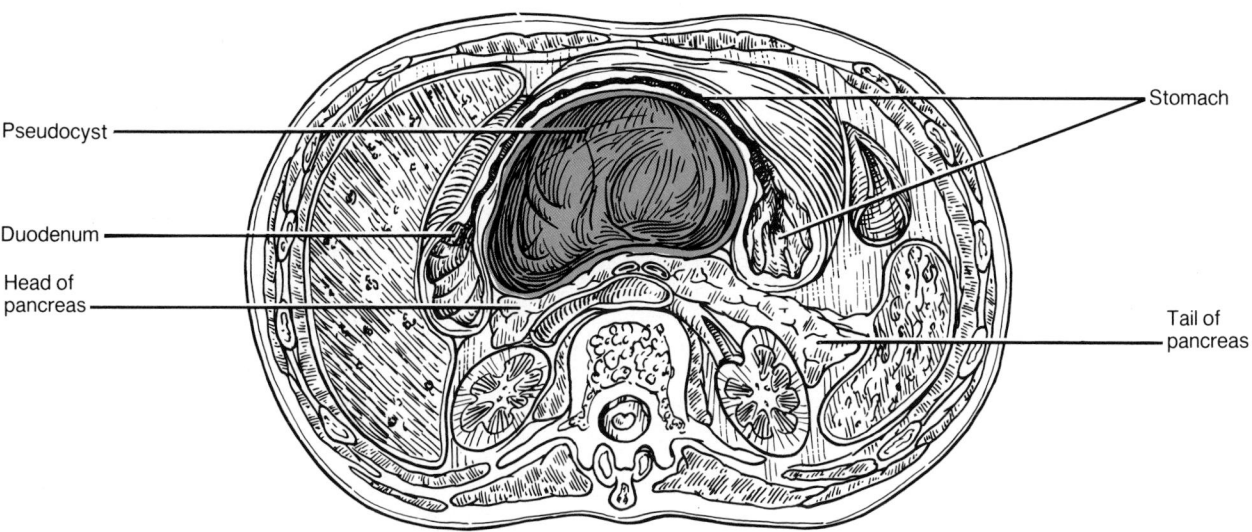

Pseudocyst

Duodenum

Head of
pancreas

Stomach

Tail of
pancreas

Figure 30-IIIB-1

Relation of Stomach and Pancreatic Pseudocyst

Pancreatic pseudocysts are collections of pancreatic juice surrounded by a fibrous capsule. They are ordinarily a complication of an episode of acute pancreatitis, although they may occur in conjunction with chronic pancreatitis. Many pseudocysts associated with acute pancreatitis resolve spontaneously, but persistent pseudocysts require operative drainage. As shown in this cross-sectional view, most pseudocysts lie on the anterior surface of the pancreas in the lesser sac, displacing the posterior wall of the stomach anteriorly.

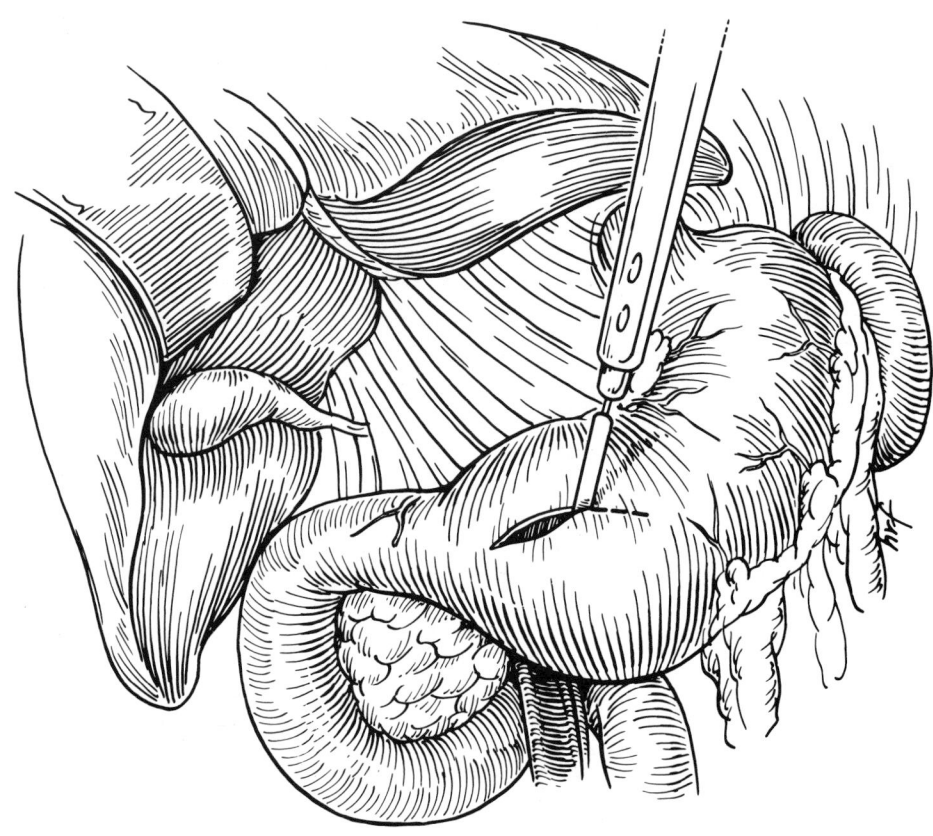

Figure 30-IIIB-2

Anterior Gastrotomy

To drain a pseudocyst internally by the transgastric route, a midline abdominal incision is used. The anterior wall of the stomach is then opened with electrocautery at the point of maximal anterior displacement of the stomach by the pseudocyst.

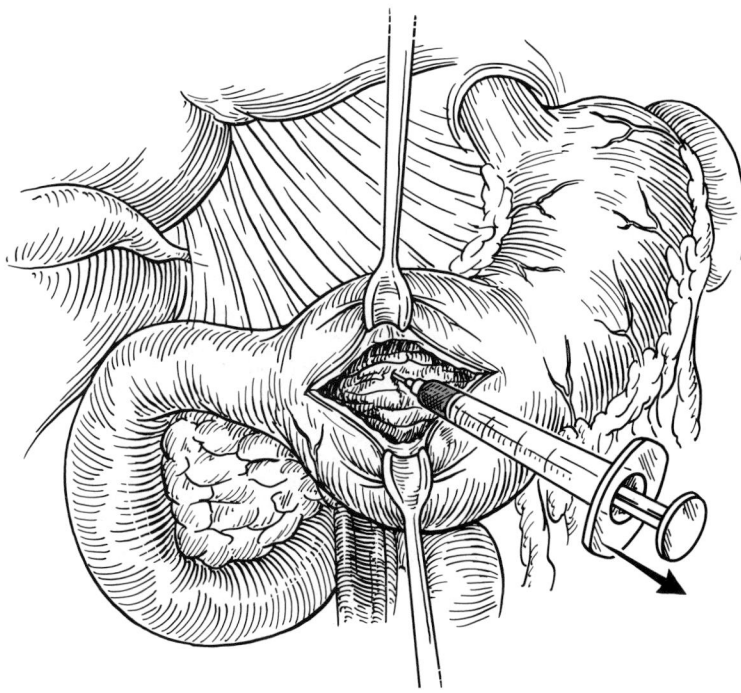

Figure 30-IIIB-3

Confirmation of Cyst Location

A syringe and 18-gauge needle are passed through the posterior wall of the stomach into the mass to confirm the location of the cyst by aspirating fluid.

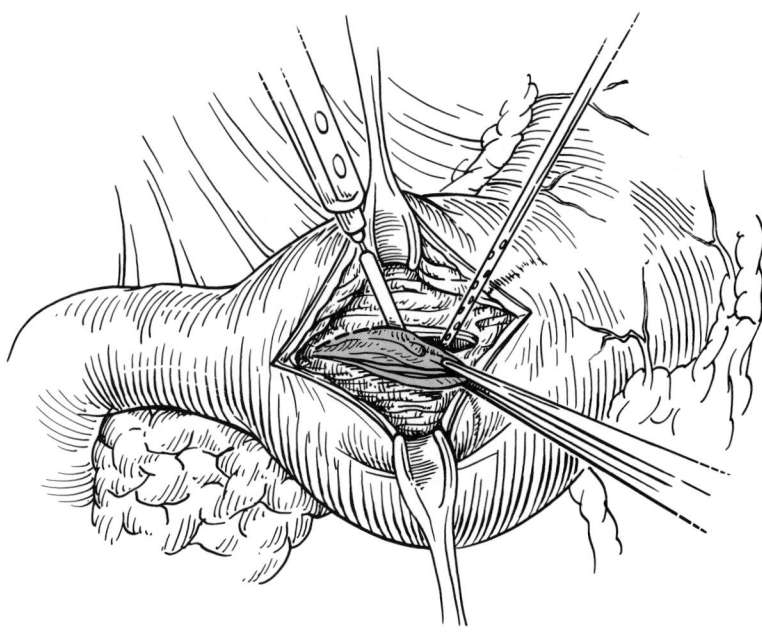

Figure 30-IIIB-4

Opening the Cyst

A full-thickness ellipse of the posterior wall of the stomach measuring 3 to 4 mm in maximal width is excised by cautery at the site of fluid aspiration, making sure that the area chosen for excision appears to be completely adherent to the underlying cyst.

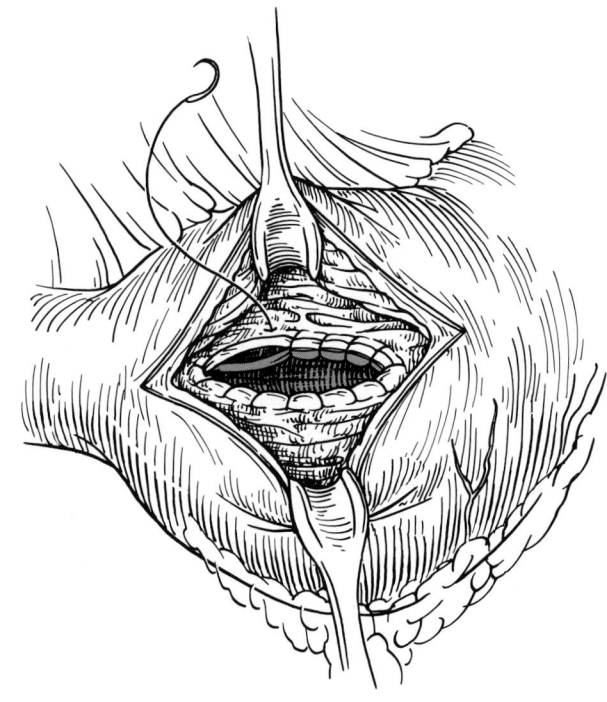

Figure 30-IIIB-5

Oversewing of Cystgastrostomy

The cyst contents are gently aspirated, after which the conjoined posterior gastric wall and cyst wall edges are oversewn with a 2-0 continuous absorbable suture. This step is proposed as a hemostatic maneuver, although its value in preventing postoperative hemorrhage is not established.

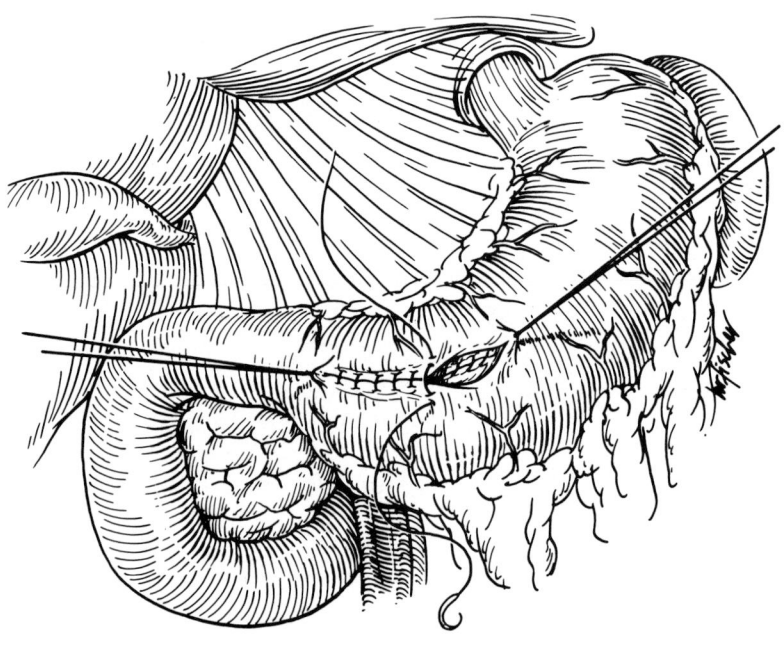

Figure 30-IIIB-6

Closure of Anterior Gastrotomy

The anterior gastrotomy is closed in two layers, with an inner continuous layer of 3-0 absorbable suture and an outer layer of interrupted Lembert sutures of 3-0 silk.

C. Cystduodenostomy

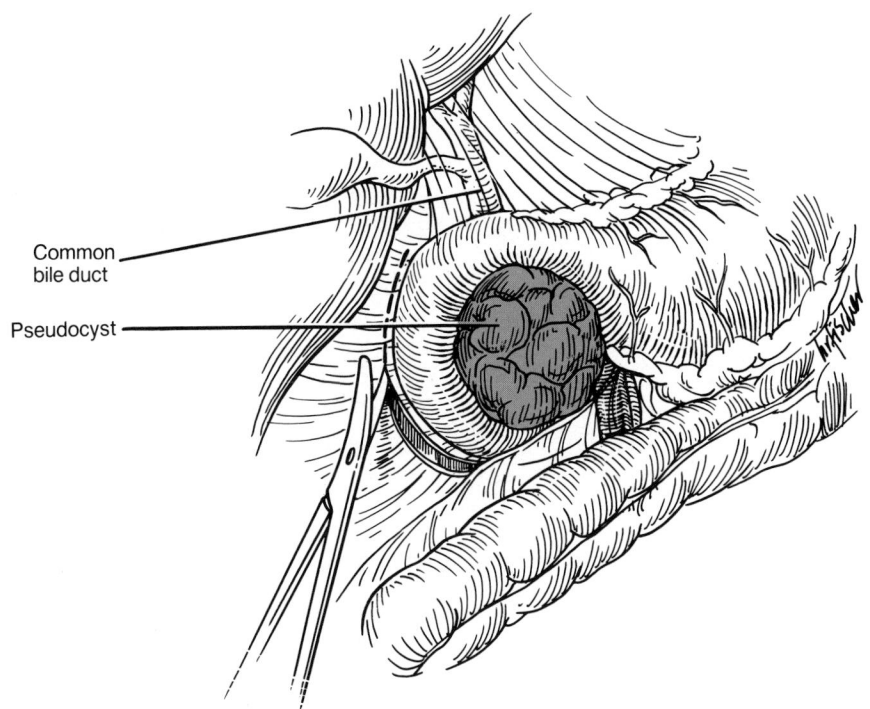

Figure 30-IIIC-1

Relation of Duodenum and Pseudocyst

Pseudocysts located in the head of the pancreas are typically not amenable to cystgastrostomy, but they may abut the medial border of the duodenum, allowing internal drainage by cystduodenostomy. The operation is begun by reflecting the hepatic flexure of the colon inferiorly and then mobilizing the duodenum and head of the pancreas with a Kocher maneuver.

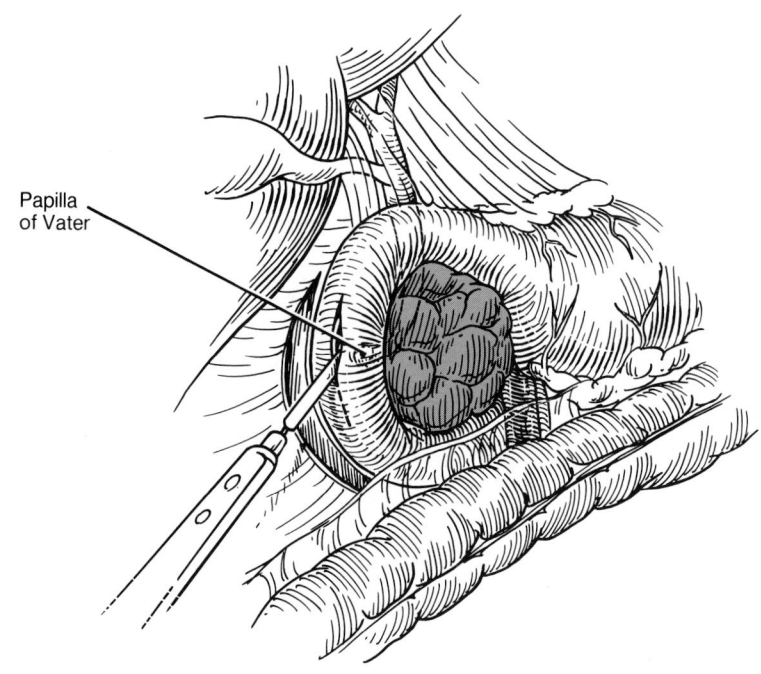

Papilla
of Vater

Figure 30-IIIC-2

Duodenotomy

A full-thickness incision in the antimesenteric border of the duodenum is made opposite the location of the pseudocyst as determined by palpation of the head of the gland or preoperative imaging studies.

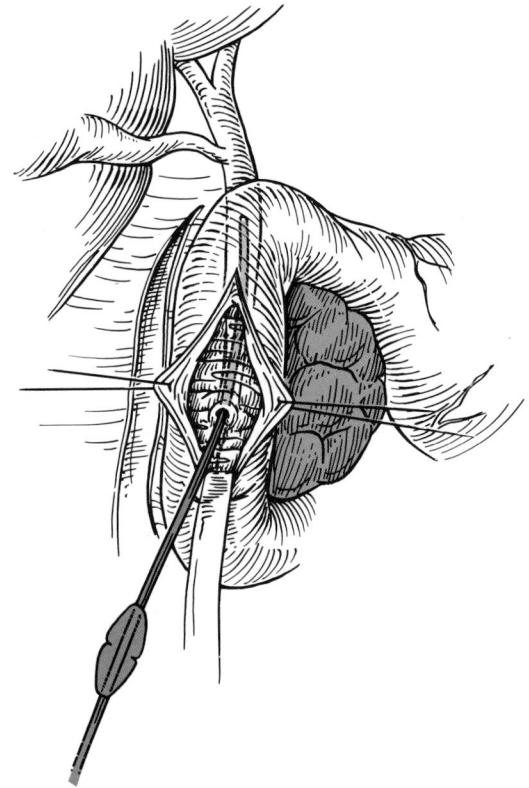

Figure 30-IIIC-3

Identification of Papilla of Vater

The papilla of Vater is located on the medial wall of the duodenum opposite the duodenotomy. It is cannulated with a metal probe to mark its location before incising the medial wall of the duodenum into the pseudocyst.

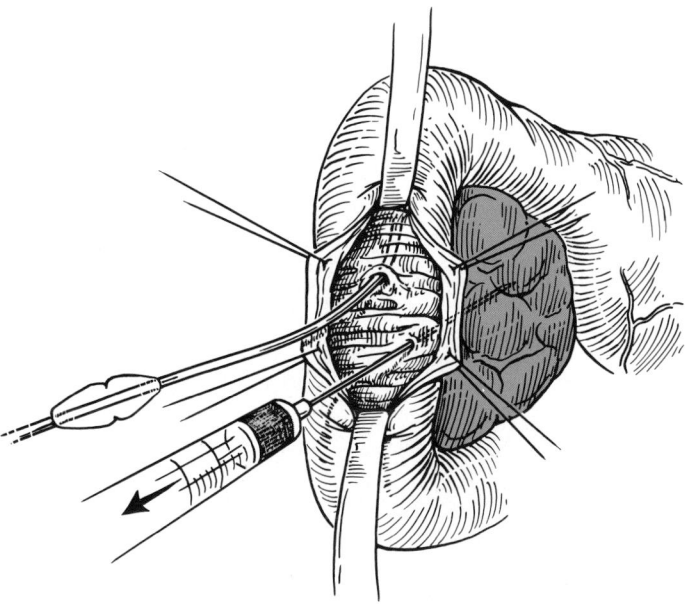

Figure 30-IIIC-4

Confirmation of Cyst Location

The pseudocyst is located by passing an 18-gauge needle attached to a syringe through the medial wall of the duodenum into the suspected location of the pseudocyst in the head of the pancreas. Return of cyst fluid confirms the location of the cyst and guides the location of the medial wall duodenotomy.

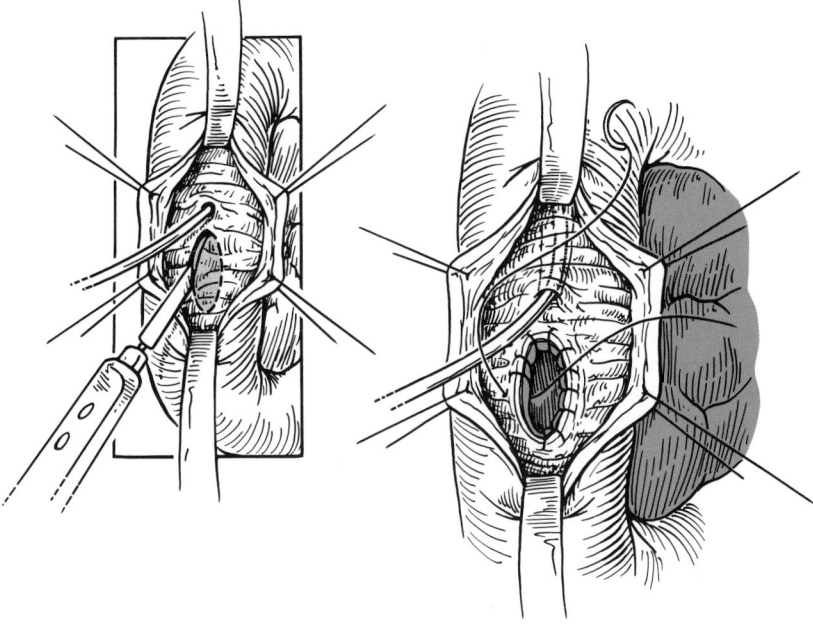

Figure 30-IIIC-5

Creation of Cystduodenostomy

A small full-thickness ellipse of medial duodenal wall is excised over the pseudocyst and the cyst entered, taking care to avoid the papilla of Vater (**inset**). The conjoined edges of the cyst cavity and the medial duodenotomy incision are oversewn with 3-0 absorbable suture. The operation is completed by closing the lateral duodenotomy in two layers, being careful to avoid narrowing of the duodenal lumen.

D. Other Procedures for Pancreatic Pseudocysts

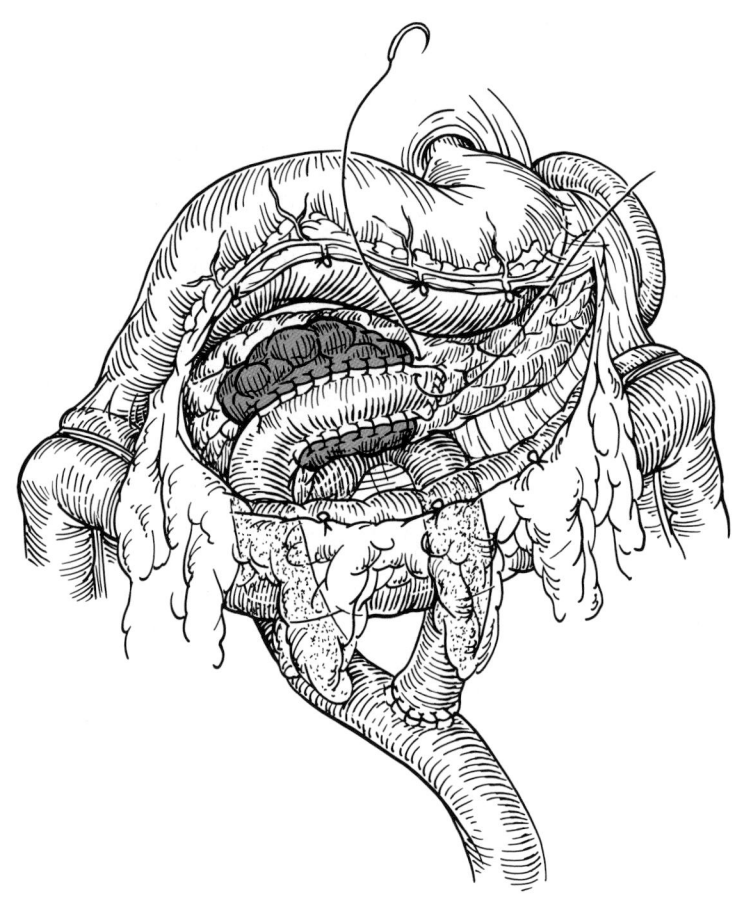

Figure 30-IIID-1

Cystjejunostomy

Some pseudocysts are neither adherent to the stomach nor amenable to cystduodenostomy. In these cases, the pseudocyst can be drained internally into a Roux-en-Y limb of
jejunum. The end of the Roux limb is stapled and oversewn. A longitudinal enterotomy
is made in the jejunal limb, and a single-layer anastomosis is performed between the
opened cyst wall and the small bowel. A soft closed-suction drain (*not shown*) should be
left near the cyst–jejunum anastomosis.

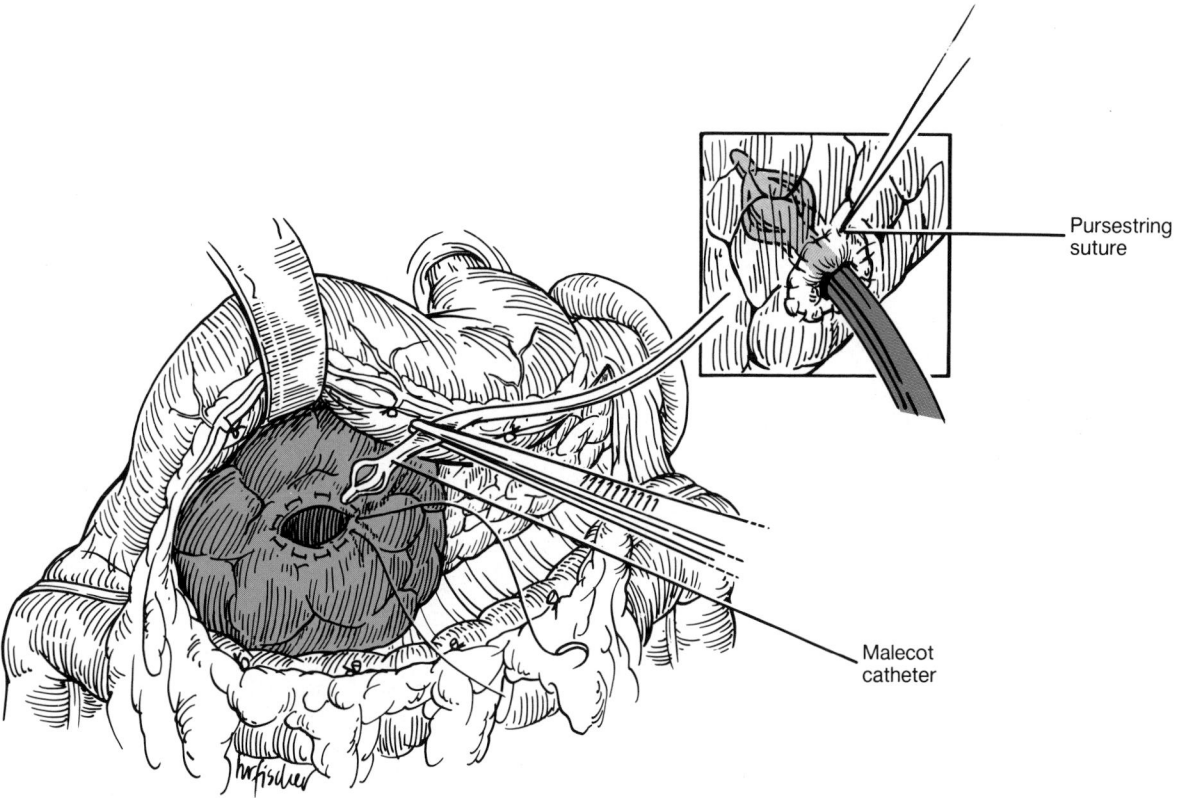

Figure 30-IIID-2

External Drainage

The presence of acute purulent infection in a pseudocyst is a contraindication to internal visceral drainage. Such cysts should be drained externally. This is accomplished by placing a pursestring suture of 2-0 silk in the thickened cyst capsule. A small incision is made into the cyst with electrocautery, allowing the introduction of a 18F to 20F Malecot-style catheter, which is then brought out through a stab incision separate from the abdominal wound. A soft closed-suction drain (*not shown*) should be left in the vicinity of the tube cystotomy.

SECTION IV   Operations for Chronic Pancreatitis

A. Longitudinal Pancreaticojejunostomy

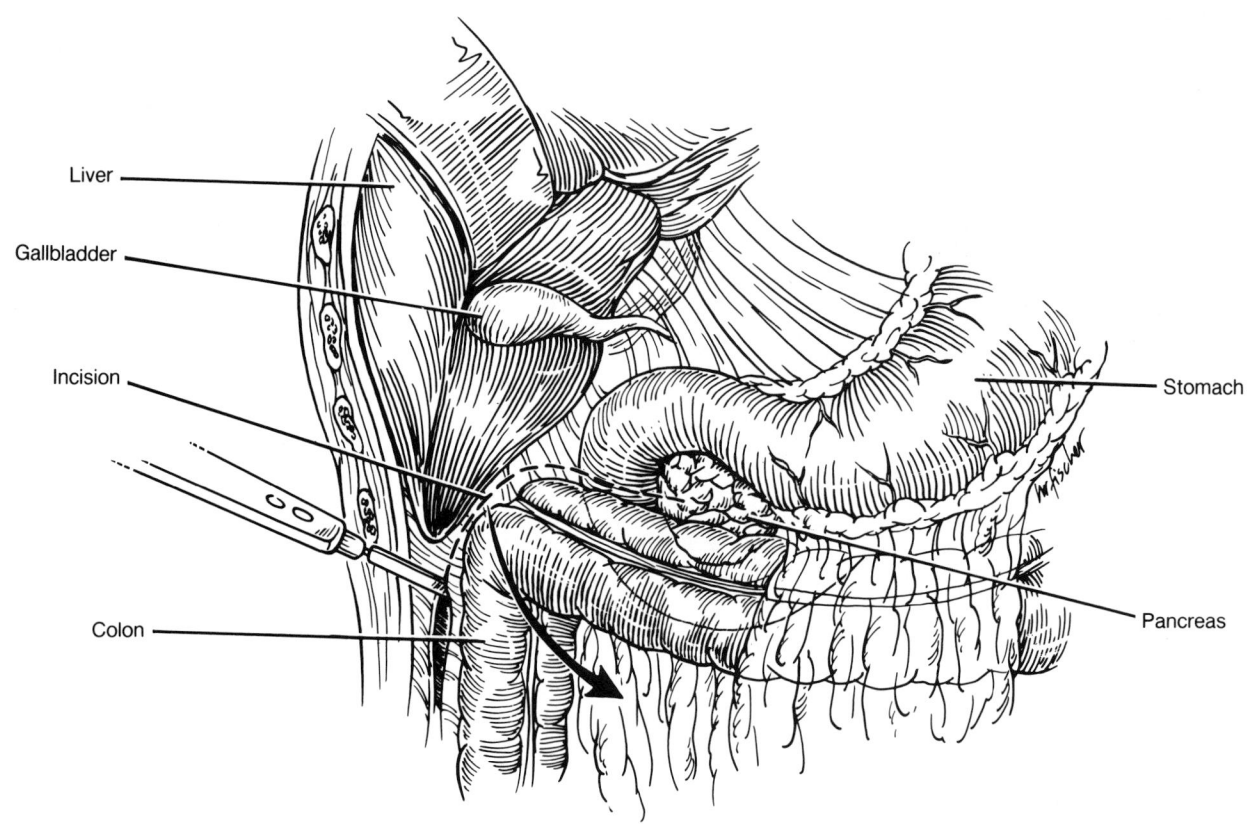

Liver

Gallbladder

Incision

Colon

Stomach

Pancreas

Figure 30-IVA-1

Mobilization of Hepatic Flexure

Longitudinal pancreaticojejunostomy is indicated for the relief of refractory pain in patients with chronic pancreatitis who have a dilated main pancreatic duct. The operation is begun by mobilizing the hepatic flexure of the colon and retracting it inferiorly to expose the head of the pancreas fully.

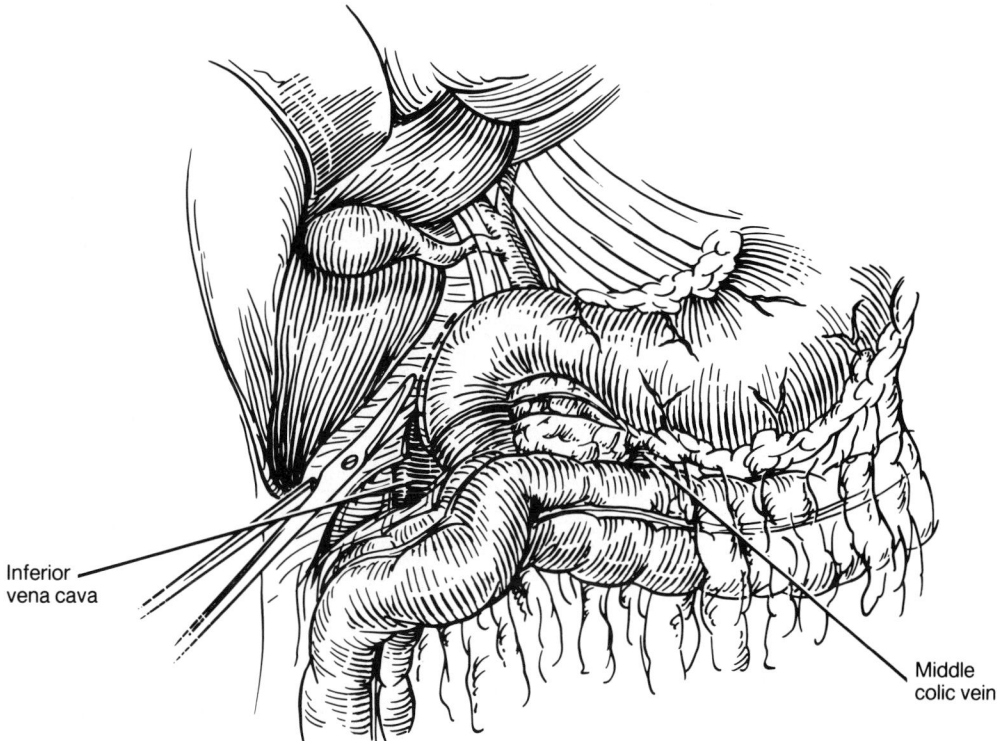

Inferior
vena cava

Middle
colic vein

Figure 30-IVA-2

Mobilization of Head of Pancreas

The peritoneum lateral to the duodenum is fully incised to allow a generous Kocher
maneuver with mobilization and elevation of the entire head of the pancreas.

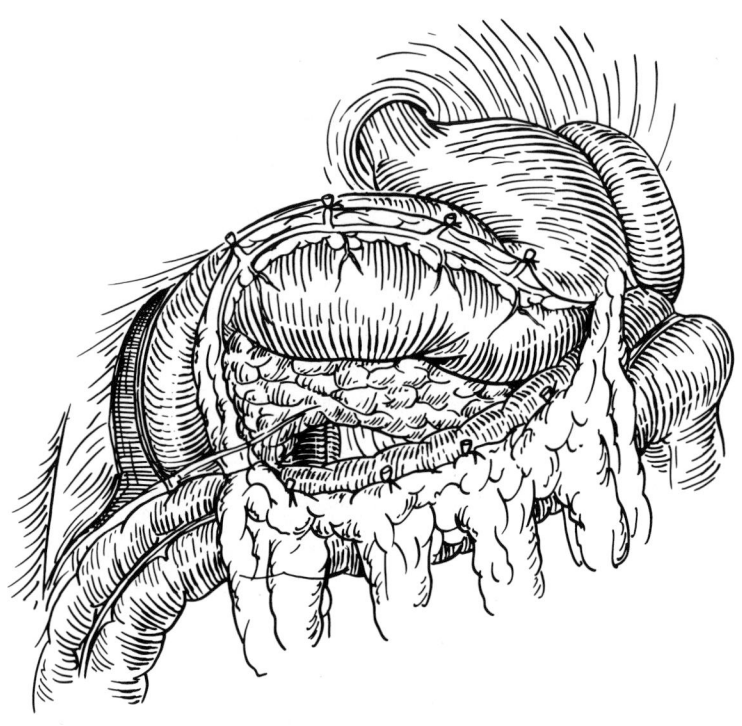

Figure 30-IVA-3

Approach to Pancreas Through Gastrocolic Omentum

The body and tail of the pancreas are exposed by entering the lesser sac through the gastrocolic omentum. The incision in the gastrocolic omentum is usually made outside the gastroepiploic vessels to preserve blood supply to the greater curvature of the stomach. Any adhesions between the posterior wall of the stomach and the pancreas are divided to provide complete exposure of the anterior surface of the body and tail of the pancreas.

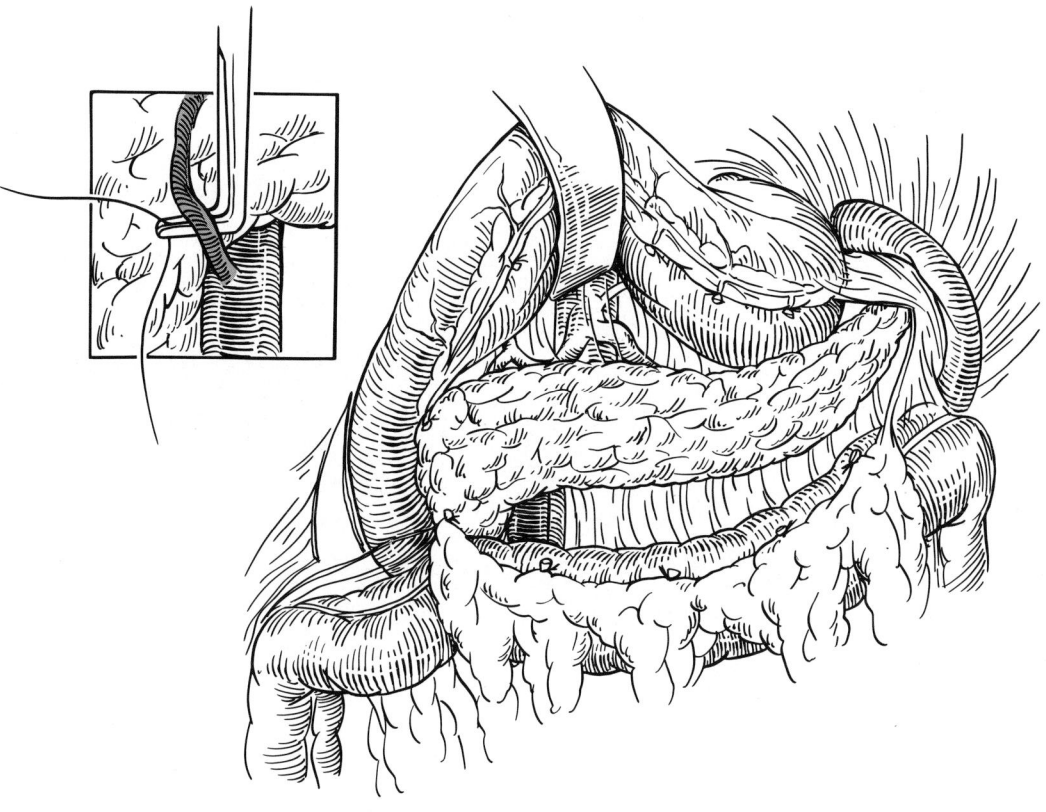

Figure 30-IVA-4

Division of Right Gastroepiploic Vein

The area of the neck of the pancreas is further exposed by ligating the right gastroepiploic vein as it crosses the pancreas to empty into the superior mesenteric vein. Ligation of this vessel allows clearance of adipose tissue from the area of the neck of the pancreas, fully exposing the entire anterior surface of the gland.

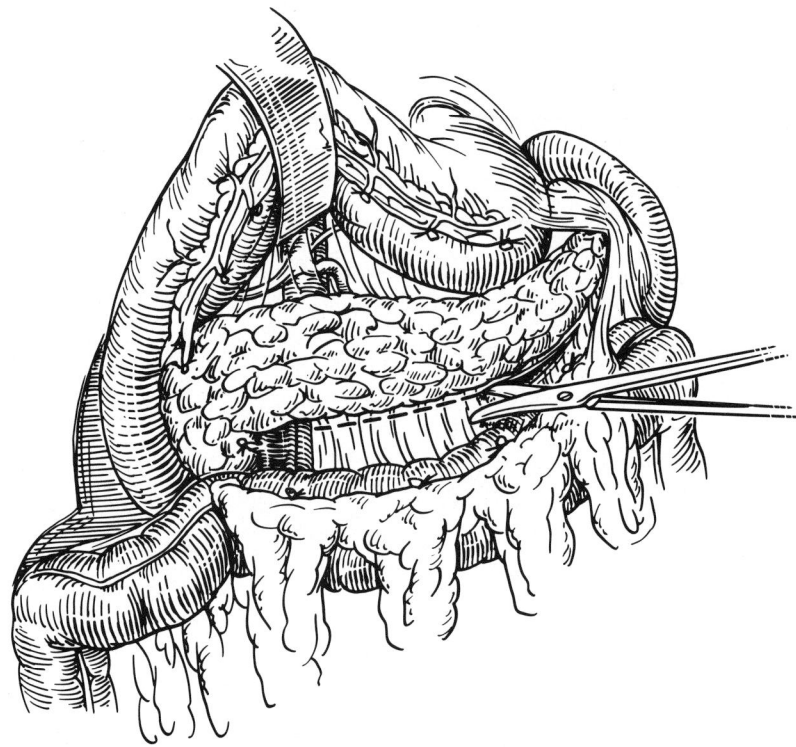

Figure 30-IVA-5

Mobilization of Inferior Border

The peritoneum along the inferior border of the body and tail of the pancreas is incised. Once the peritoneal layer is incised, gentle blunt dissection beneath the lower edge of the gland allows the body and tail to be elevated and mobilized. This step is not absolutely necessary in the performance of pancreaticojejunostomy but is helpful in allowing easier palpation of the pancreas for the location of the pancreatic duct and in providing greater exposed pancreatic surface inferiorly for the placement of subsequent suture lines.

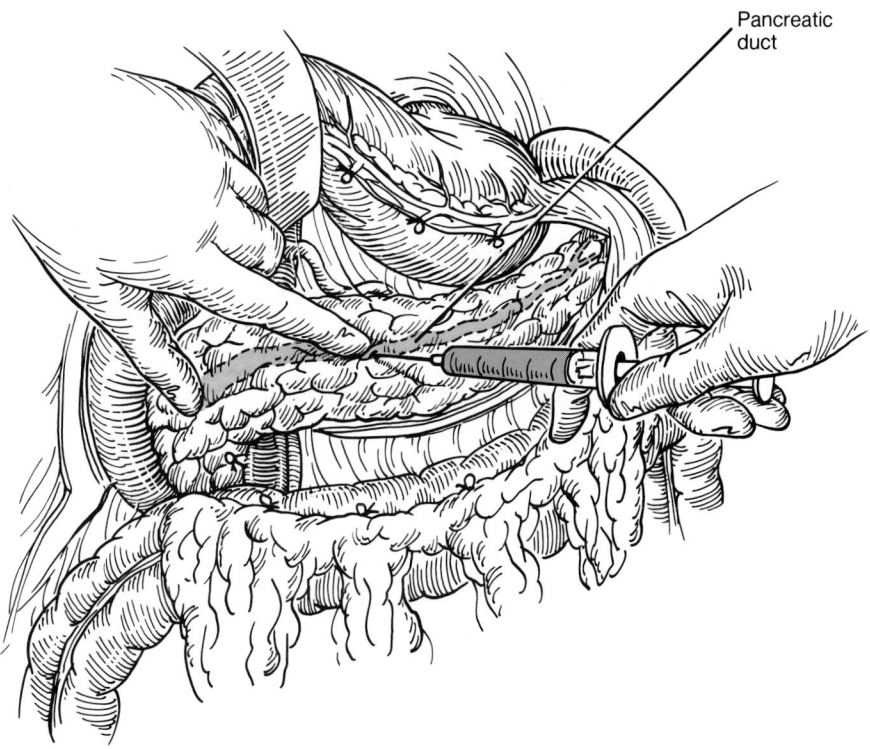

Pancreatic
duct

Figure 30-IVA-6

Palpation and Aspiration

The location of the pancreatic duct is suggested by palpating the body of the gland between the thumb and fingers or bimanually, feeling for a soft tubular structure running longitudinally in the otherwise firm gland. A 20-gauge needle with attached syringe is then passed into the pancreatic duct to confirm its location by the aspiration of clear pancreatic juice. The amount of juice removed should be minimized to avoid collapsing the duct and making incision into it more difficult.

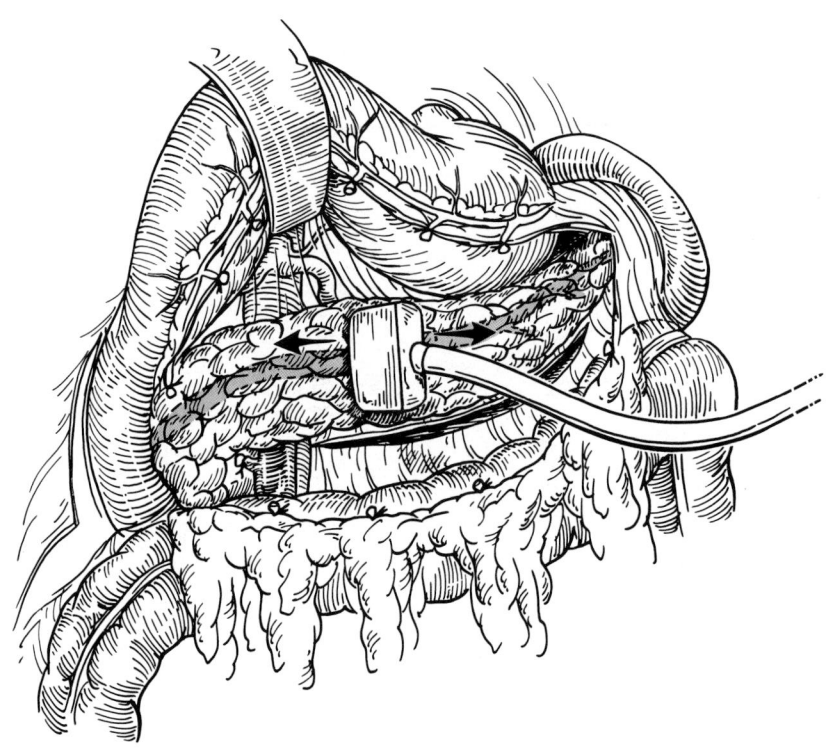

Figure 30-IVA-7

Intraoperative Ultrasonography

Intraoperative ultrasound can be used to determine the location of the pancreatic duct. A needle can be passed into the duct under ultrasound guidance to assist in siting the subsequent incision into the duct.

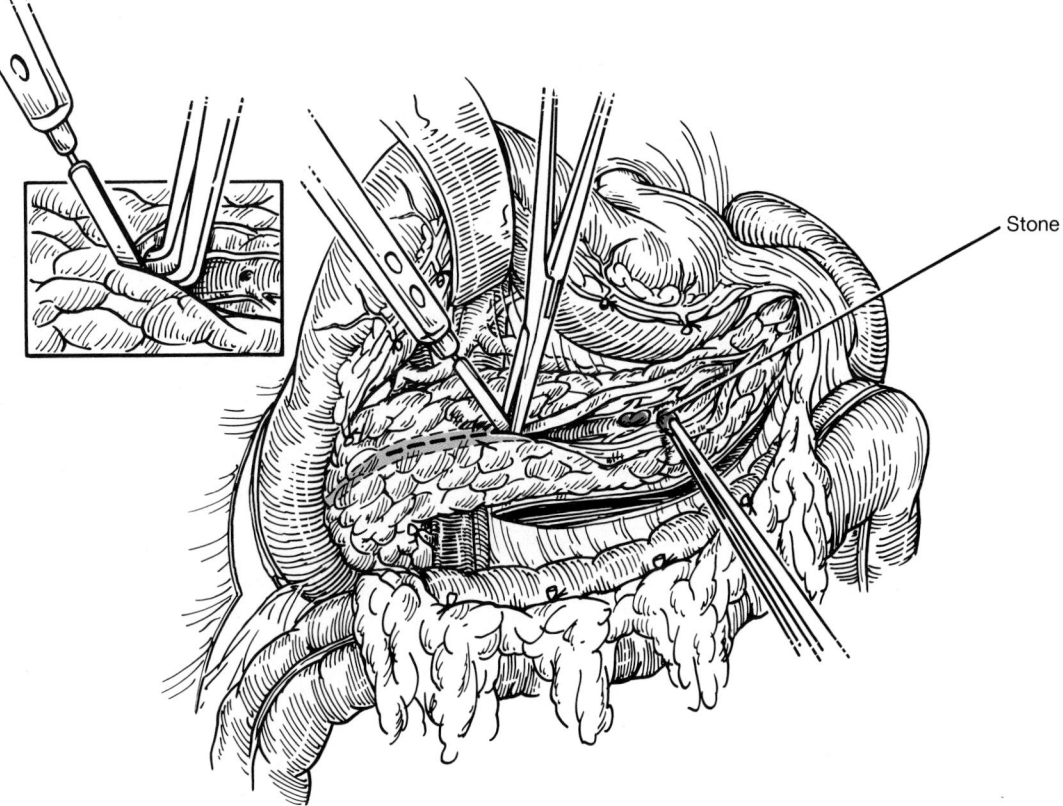

Stone

Figure 30-IVA-8

Incision and Stone Extraction

Once the pancreatic duct has been located by needle aspiration, the pancreatic capsule is incised with electrocautery, and dissection is carried through the pancreatic parenchyma until the duct is entered. A right-angled clamp is placed into the duct and used as a guide to enlarge the ductotomy (**inset**). The duct incision is then progressively extended in both directions using a clamp as a guide to the lumen. Stones in the pancreatic duct, if present, are removed with a forceps.

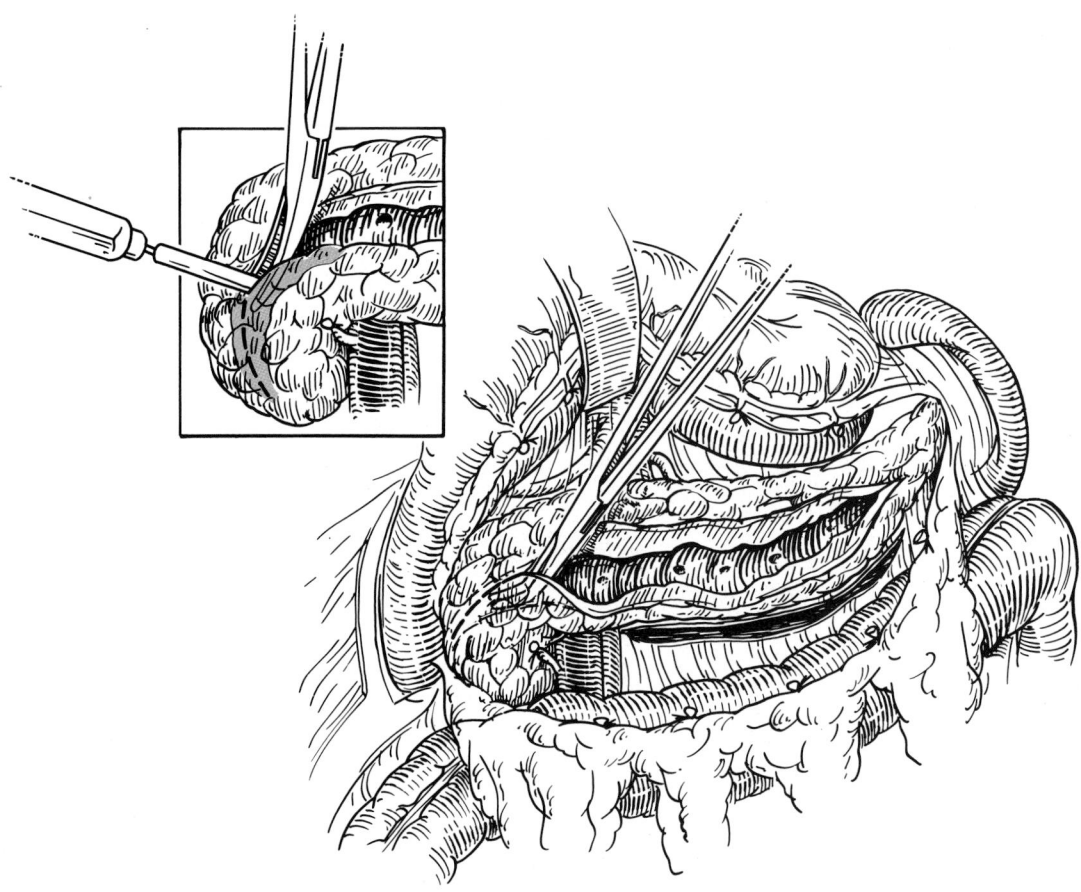

Figure 30-IVA-9

Extension of Operation Into Pancreatic Head

The incision in the pancreatic duct is gradually extended into the head of the gland. As the duct enters the head of the gland, it bends inferiorly and posteriorly (**inset**), and the amount of pancreatic parenchyma overlying the duct increases, making the dissection somewhat more difficult and vascular. Nevertheless, it is important to continue the ductotomy up to within about 1 to 2 cm of the ampulla of Vater. It is critical that no strictures or undrained pockets of the pancreatic duct remain between the right end of the pancreaticojejunostomy and the ampulla.

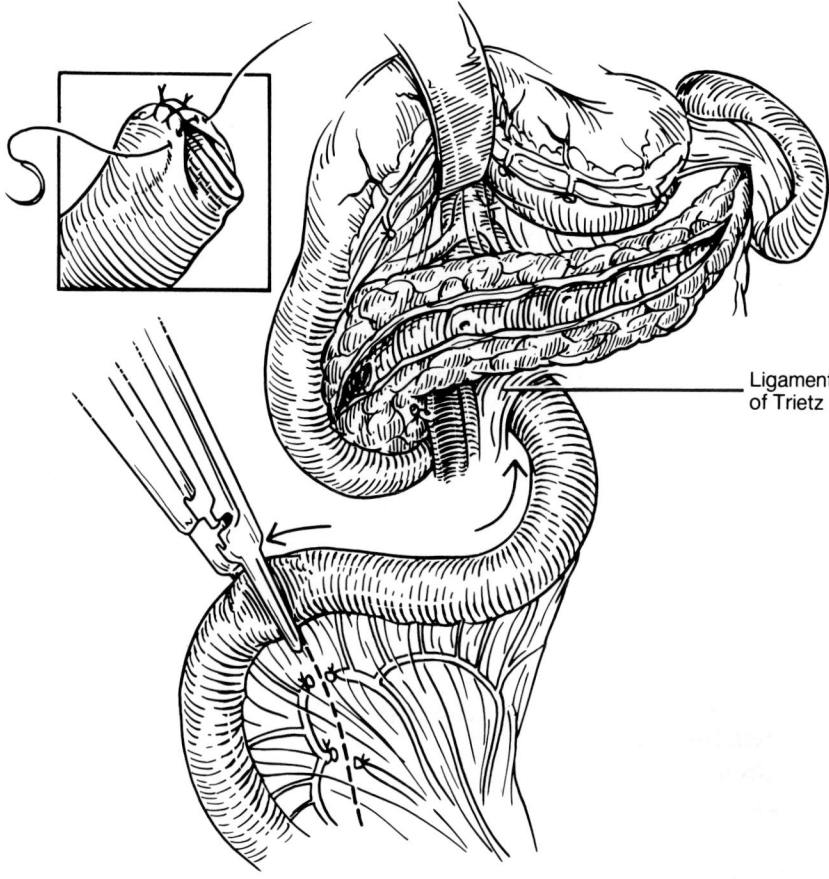

Ligament
of Trietz

Figure 30-IVA-10

Preparation of Roux Limb

After completion of the ductotomy, a Roux-en-Y limb of jejunum is prepared by dividing the jejunum with a gastrointestinal stapler. The distal staple line is oversewn with interrupted sutures of 3-0 silk **(inset)** and brought through the transverse mesocolon so that the jejunal limb overlies the pancreas without tension on the mesentery.

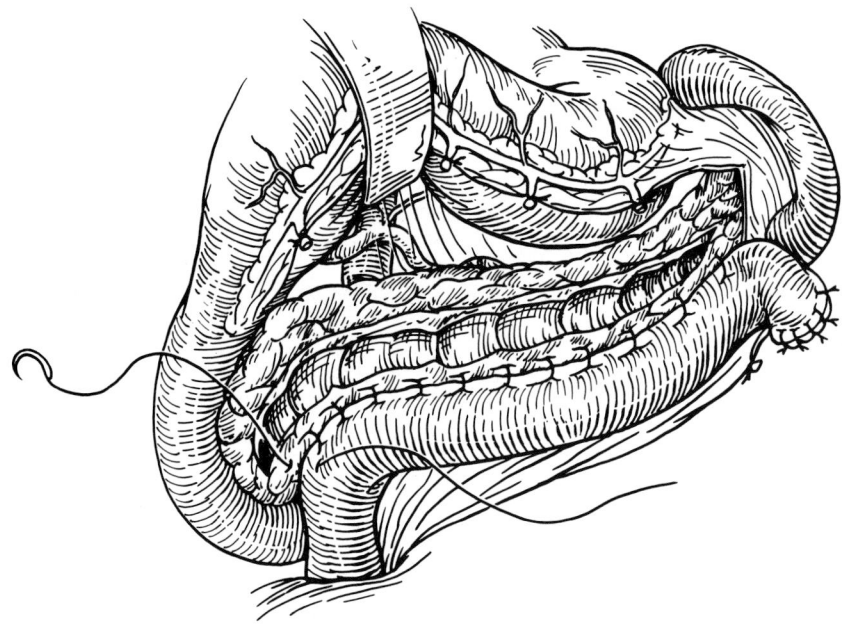

Figure 30-IVA-11

Pancreaticojejunal Suture Line: Posterior Wall

The anastomosis between the pancreas and jejunum can be performed in one or two layers. If a two-layer anastomosis is performed, the outer layer consists of interrupted silk sutures and the inner layer a continuous absorbable suture. A single-layer anastomosis is shown here for clarity. The seromuscular coat of the antimesenteric aspect of the jejunum is sewn to the pancreatic capsule and parenchyma with interrupted nonabsorbable sutures. The sutures in the pancreas are placed away from the edge of the ductotomy. The pancreaticojejunostomy is not a mucosa-to-mucosa anastomosis.

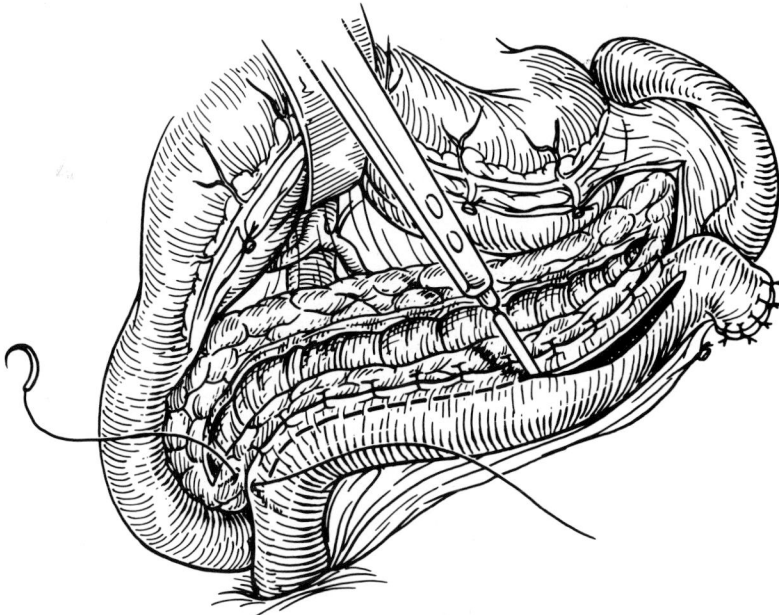

Figure 30-IVA-12

Opening the Roux Limb

The jejunum is opened with electrocautery along a sufficient length to match the length of the pancreatic ductotomy.

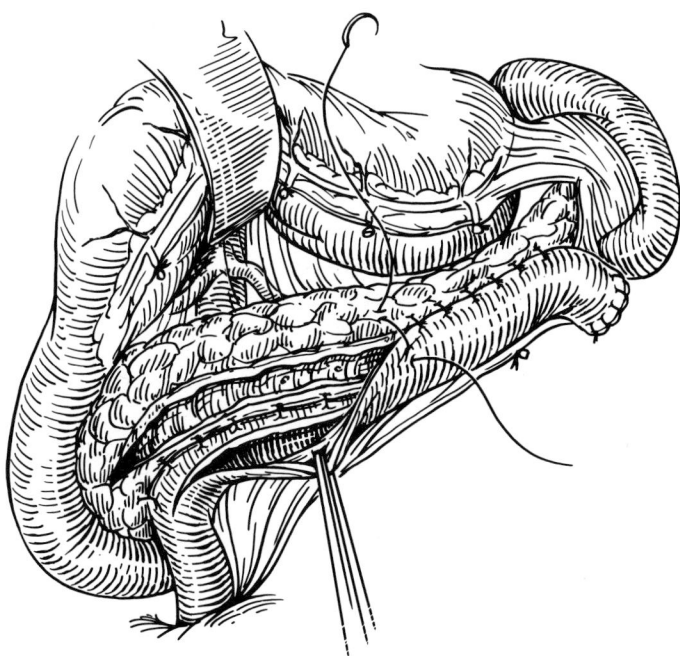

Figure 30-IVA-13

Pancreaticojejunal Suture Line: Anterior Wall

The anastomosis is completed by sewing the anterior jejunal leaflet to the capsule of the pancreas cephalad to the ductotomy.

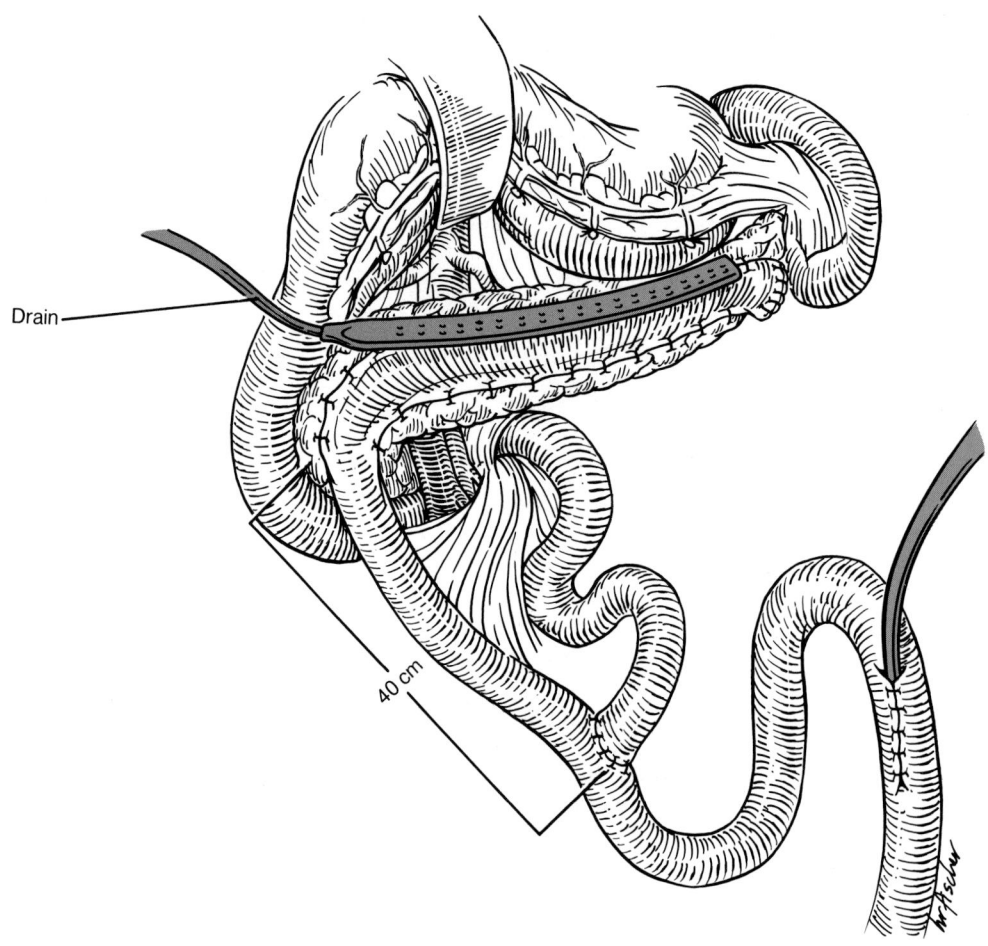

Drain

40 cm

Figure 30-IVA-14

Drain Placement

After completion of the anastomosis, the length of the pancreaticojejunostomy is drained with a soft closed-suction sump drain. Although one drain is shown here for clarity, it is preferable to place a second drain along the inferior aspect of the pancreaticojejunostomy, bringing the latter drain through a stab wound in the left abdominal wall. A feeding jejunostomy completes the operation.

B. Duodenum-Preserving Pancreatic Head Resection: Beger Procedure

The duodenum-preserving resection of the pancreatic head as described by Beger is indicated for patients with intractable pain due to chronic pancreatitis in whom most of the disease is in the pancreatic head. Biliary obstruction due to fibrosis and inflammation can be treated concurrently with this procedure. In this operation, the bulk of the pancreatic head is resected, leaving a rim of pancreas on the medial curvature of the duodenum along with the pancreaticoduodenal blood supply. A portion of the uncinate process can be left behind or completely resected, depending on the technical difficulty involved.

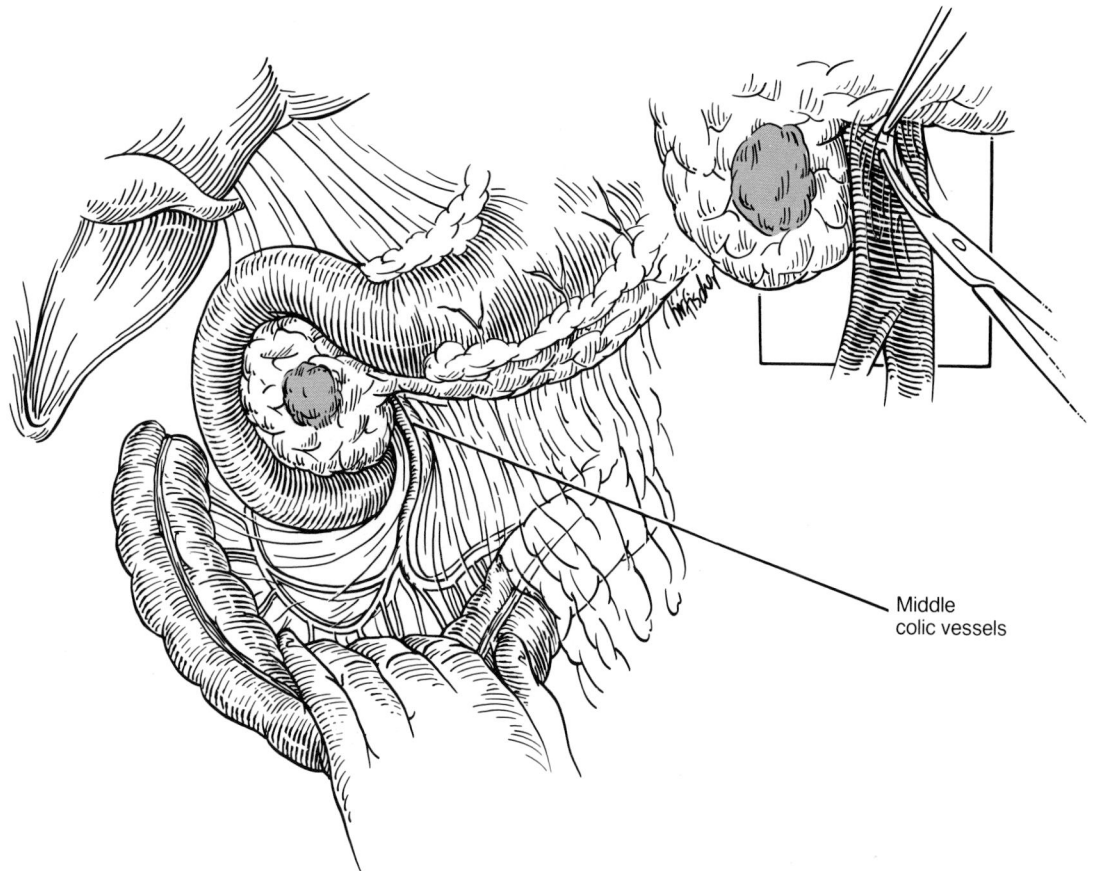

Middle
colic vessels

Figure 30-IVB-1

Identification of the Superior Mesenteric Vein

After full mobilization of the head of the pancreas (for details, see Section IIA) the procedure continues with the identification of the superior mesenteric vein as it passes beneath the neck of the pancreas. The vein is most conveniently located by identifying the middle colic vein and following it down to its entrance into the superior mesenteric vein. To follow the superior mesenteric vein under the neck of the pancreas, periadventitial tissue must be dissected away from the vein (**inset**) so that dissection proceeds immediately along the anterior surface of the vein.

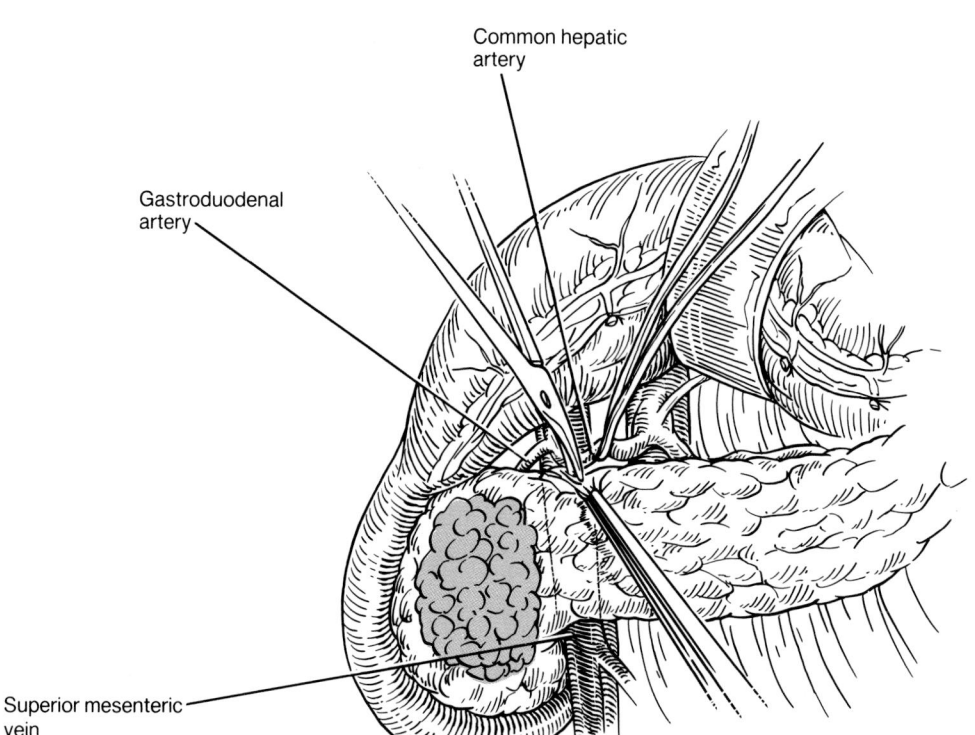

Figure 30-IVB-2

Dissection of Hepatic Artery Away From Pancreatic Head

The common hepatic artery is identified above the neck of the pancreas and carefully dissected away from the edge of the pancreas. The gastroduodenal artery is ordinarily ligated, exposing the anterior surface of the portal vein. Dissection of the tunnel overlying the superior mesenteric and portal veins behind the neck of the pancreas is completed to ensure that the neck of the pancreas can be safely divided over the veins.

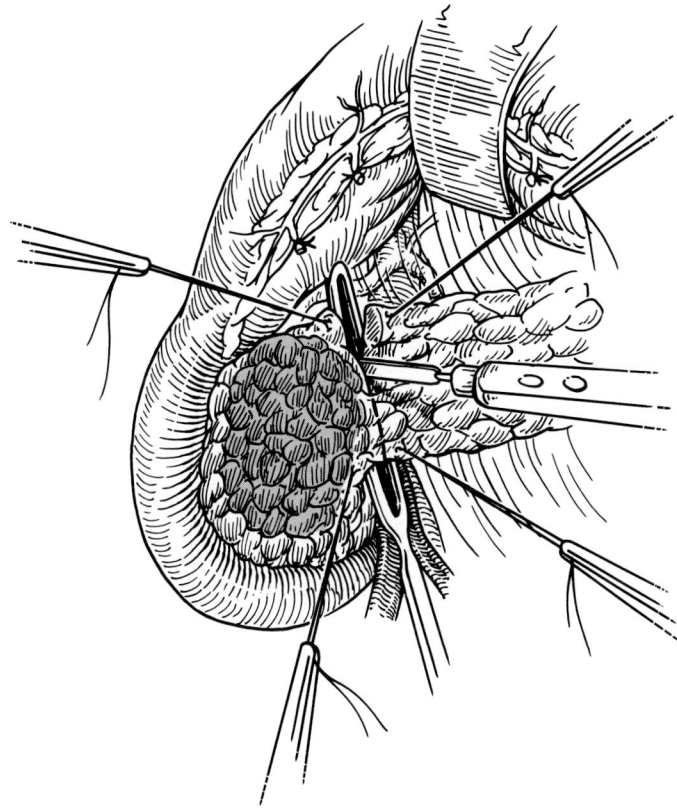

Figure 30-IVB-3

Division of Pancreatic Neck

The neck of the pancreas is divided over the confluence of the superior mesenteric and portal veins. A metal guide is placed beneath the neck of the gland to elevate the pancreas off the veins as it is divided, protecting the veins from inadvertent injury. Before the incision through the neck of the pancreas, hemostatic sutures of 3-0 silk can be placed at the superior and inferior edges of the pancreas in an attempt to decrease bleeding from the marginal arteries running along the upper and lower pancreatic borders.

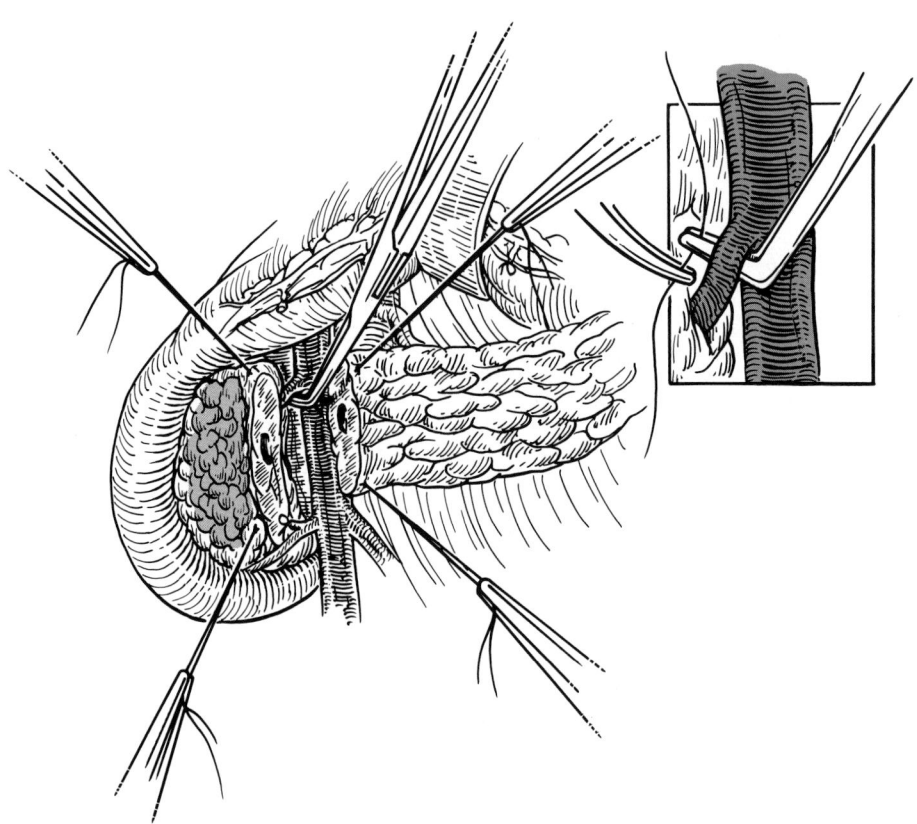

Figure 30-IVB-4

Division of Veins Draining Pancreatic Head

With the head of the pancreas gently retracted to the right, veins draining from the pancreatic head into the portal and superior mesenteric veins are ligated with 4-0 silk ligatures and divided.

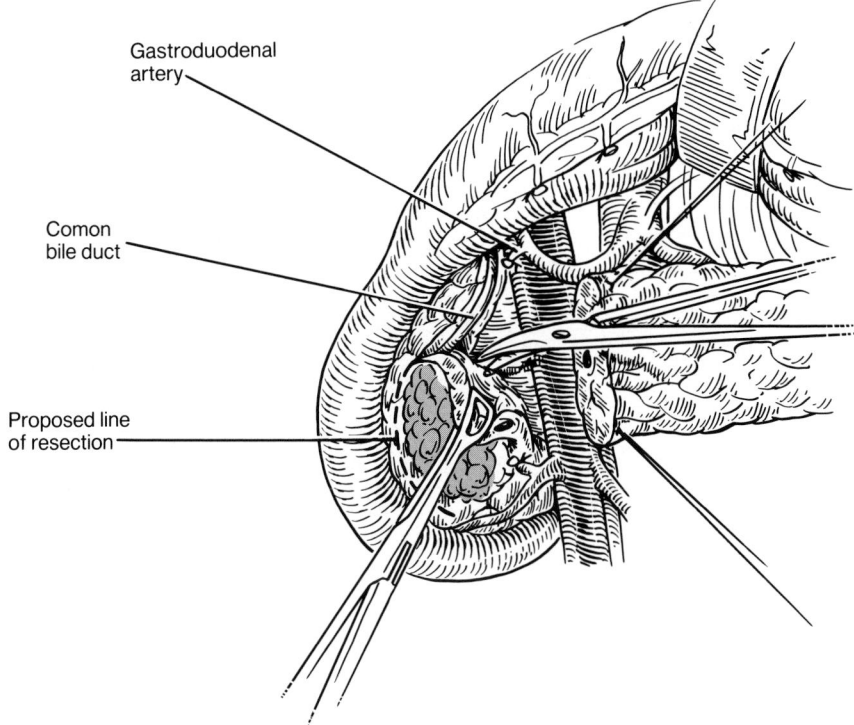

Gastroduodenal artery

Comon bile duct

Proposed line of resection

Figure 30-IVB-5

Separation of Pancreatic Head From Bile Duct

With the bulk of the head of the pancreas free of the portal and superior mesenteric veins, the pancreatic head is trimmed along the margin of the common bile duct, leaving the duct partially embedded in the remaining rim of pancreatic tissue along the medial duodenal wall. If the duct has been obstructed by fibrosis in the pancreatic head, the surgeon should endeavor to free the duct sufficiently that it bulges freely into the space created by the resection of the pancreatic head. The resection of the pancreatic head is continued along the line indicated, making sure to preserve the origin of the inferior pancreaticoduodenal vessels, which, if the gastroduodenal artery has been ligated, provide the blood supply to the pancreatic remnant and duodenum.

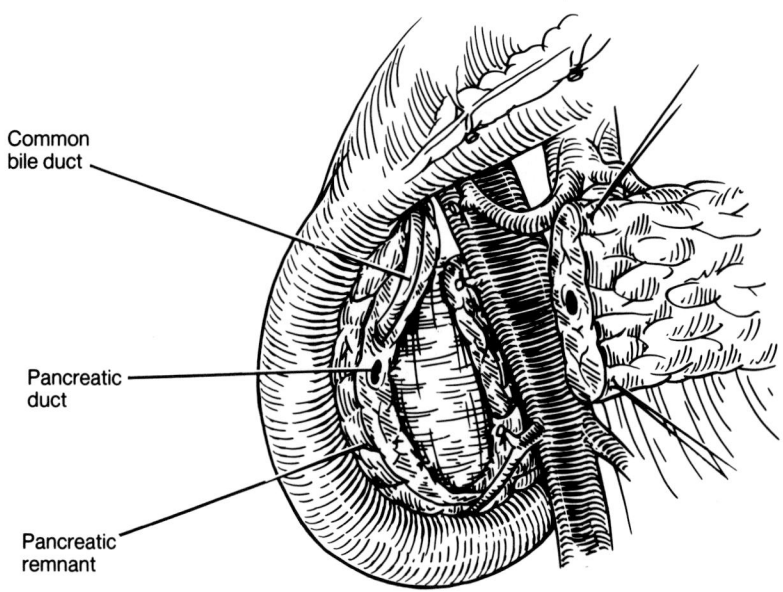

Common bile duct

Pancreatic duct

Pancreatic remnant

Figure 30-IVB-6

Completed Resection

The resection of the pancreatic head has been completed. The common bile duct bulges into the space left by the resection of pancreatic tissue. The inferior pancreaticoduodenal artery and vein have been preserved. In this case, a portion of the uncinate process has been left in place behind the portal and superior mesenteric veins. The pancreatic duct is visible both in the remnant of the pancreatic head and in the remaining body of the pancreas.

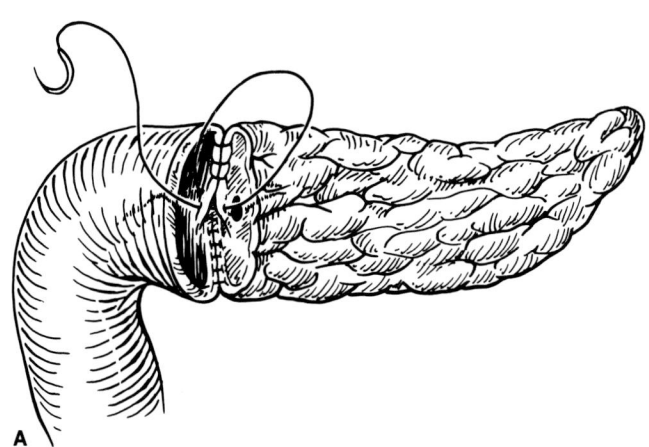

A

Figure 30-IVB-7

Completion of Anastomoses

(**A**) To complete the procedure, a Roux-en-Y loop of jejunum is created. The distal end of jejunum, brought through the transverse mesocolon, is not closed but rather is left open for anastomosis to the remaining body and tail of the pancreas. The anastomosis can be performed in one or two layers. Illustrated here is a two-layer anastomosis with outer interrupted sutures of 3-0 silk and an inner continuous layer of 3-0 absorbable suture.

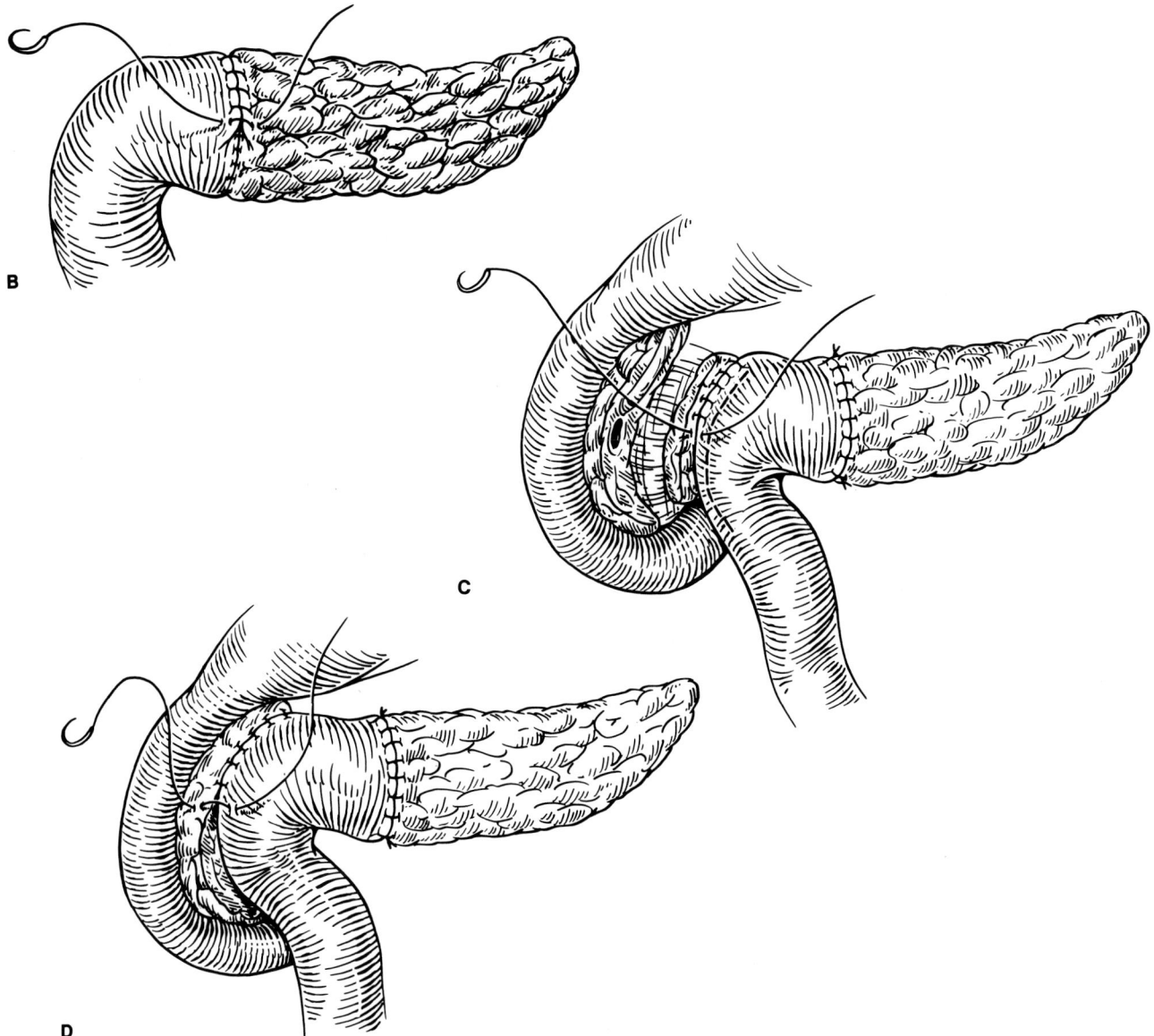

Figure 30-IVB-7 *(Continued)*

(B) The anterior aspect of the anastomosis to the left pancreas is completed with interrupted Lembert sutures of 3-0 silk placed between the seromuscular layer of jejunum and the pancreatic capsule.

(C) After the completion of the anastomosis of the jejunal limb to the left side of the pancreas, the remaining right portion of the pancreas is likewise anastomosed to the jejunal limb. In this case, the portion of the uncinate process left in place must be incorporated into the right anastomosis as well. If common bile duct obstruction has not been satisfactorily relieved by partially freeing the duct from the fibrotic pancreatic head, a lateral choledochotomy can be performed and also incorporated into the right anastomosis to the jejunal limb.

(D) The anastomosis to the right pancreas is completed by placing sutures between the pancreatic remnant along the medial curve of the duodenum and the anterior leaflet of the opened jejunum.

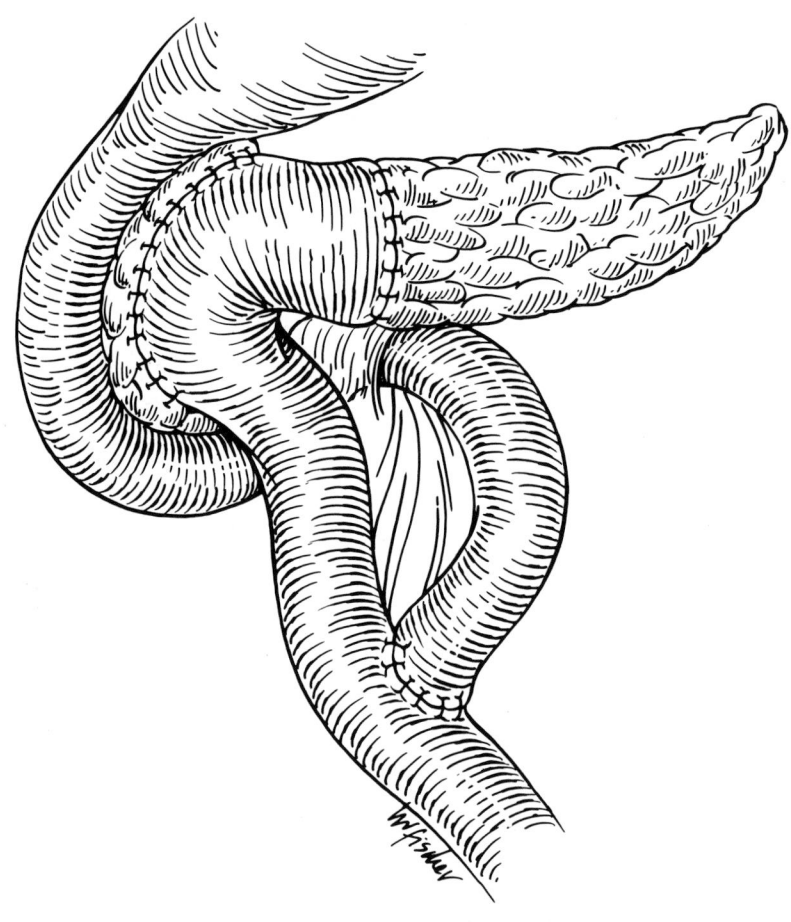

Figure 30-IVB-8

Completed Procedure

The completed operation, showing the dual anastomoses of the right and left pancreatic remnants to the Roux-en-Y jejunal limb. Both anastomoses should be drained with soft closed-suction drains (*not shown*). A feeding jejunostomy and gastrostomy (*not shown*) can be added.

C. Duodenum-Preserving Pancreatic Head Resection: Frey Procedure

The duodenum-preserving resection of the head of the pancreas described by Frey differs from that of Beger in that a central core of the pancreatic head is enucleated, leaving a large central cavity in the head of the pancreas surrounded by a narrow rim of remaining pancreas. The main pancreatic duct is opened longitudinally in communication with the cavity in the head of the pancreas. A large single anastomosis to a Roux-en-Y limb is used to cover the opened pancreatic duct and the cavity in the pancreatic head. The indications for surgery are identical to those described for the Beger procedure.

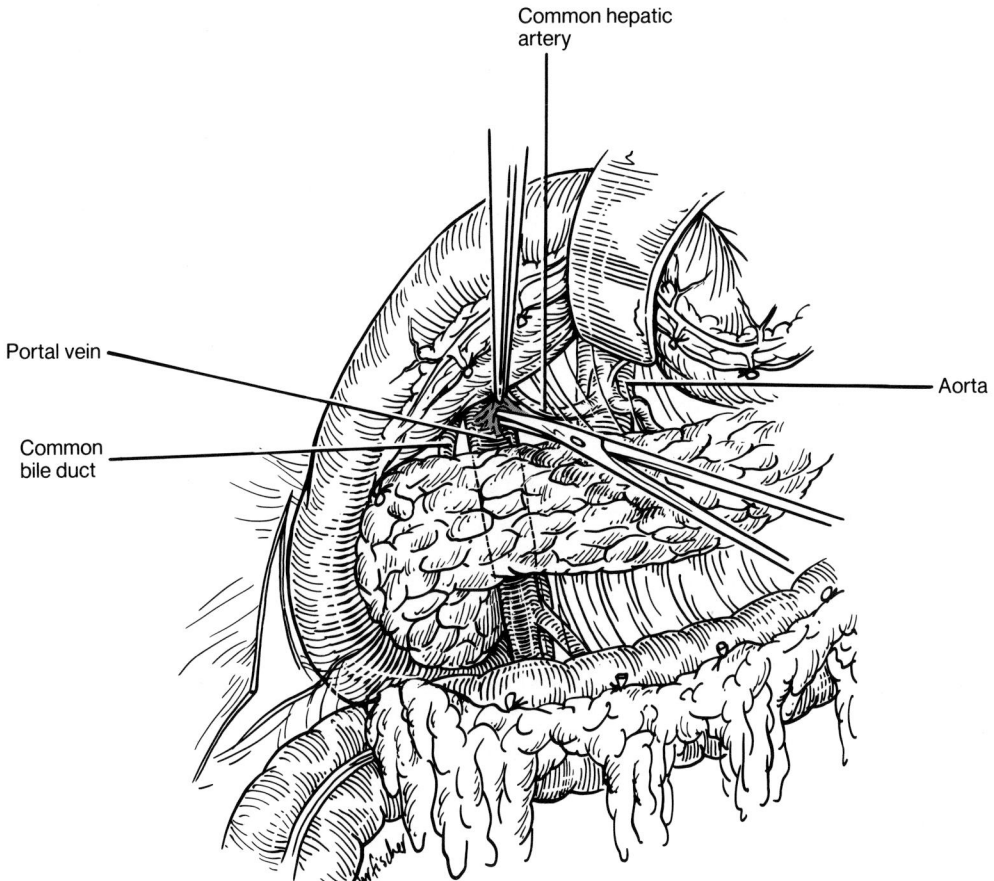

Figure 30-IVC-1

Identification of Superior Mesenteric and Portal Veins

The operation is begun by fully mobilizing the head of the pancreas and by opening the gastrocolic omentum to expose the body and tail of the pancreas. The right gastroepiploic vein is ligated as it crosses the pancreas to allow full exposure of the anterior aspect of the entire gland (see Section II for details of the initial exposure). The superior mesenteric vein is identified below the pancreas and the portal vein above the pancreas. It is not necessary to dissect the tunnel anterior to the veins beneath the neck of the pancreas. The veins serve as landmarks in defining the lateral edge of the pancreatic head resection.

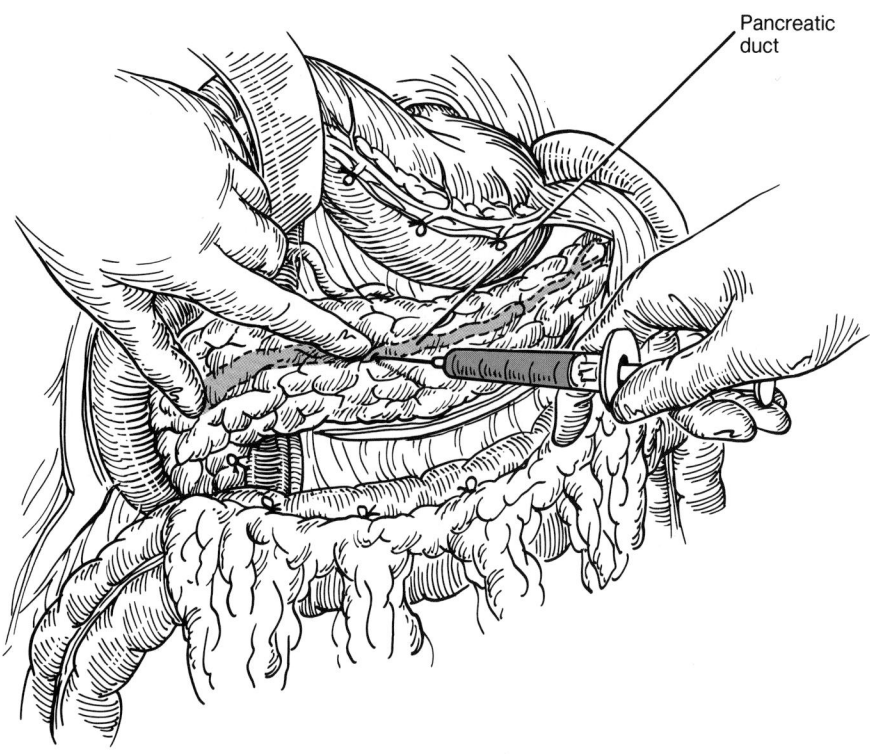

Pancreatic duct

Figure 30-IVC-2

Identification of Pancreatic Duct

The main pancreatic duct, which is typically significantly dilated, is located by aspiration with a 20-gauge needle and syringe, aided by intraoperative ultrasonography if necessary.

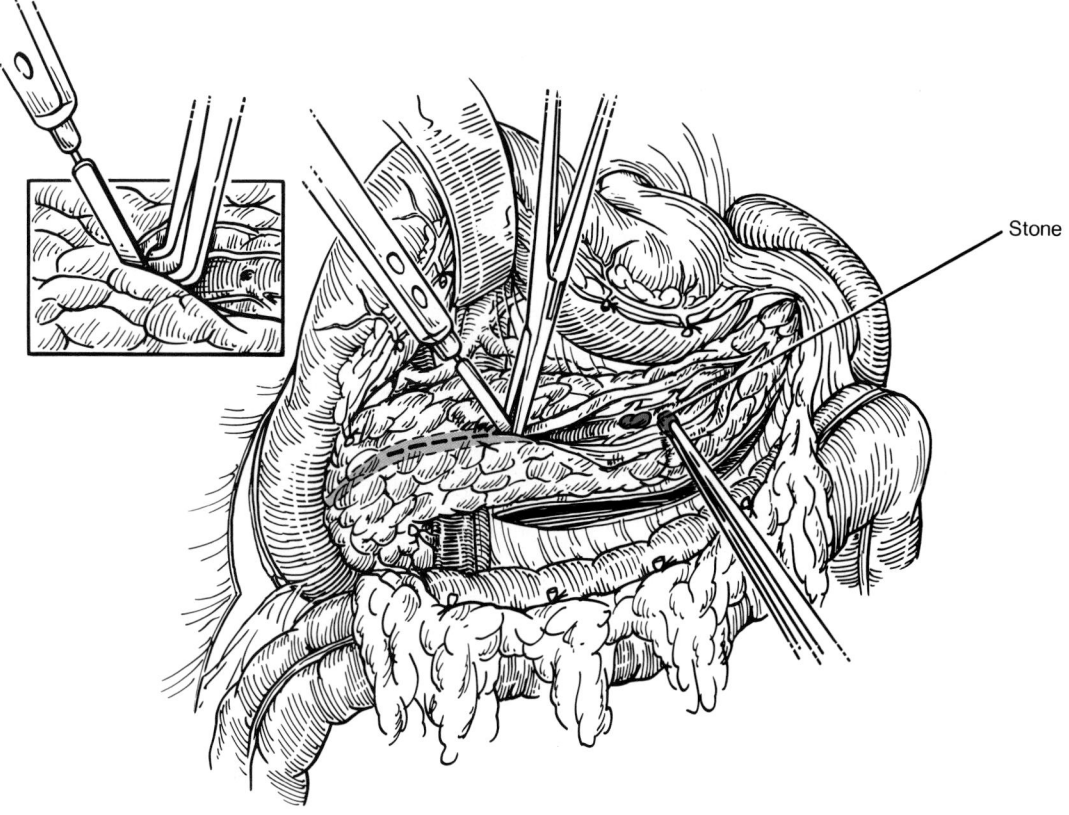

Stone

Figure 30-IVC-3

Duct Incision and Stone Removal

The pancreatic capsule is incised with electrocautery over the location of the pancreatic duct as defined by aspiration. Dissection is carried deeper into the pancreatic parenchyma until the duct is entered. With the aid of a right-angle clamp placed into the duct, the incision into the duct is extended (**inset**). Gradually, the dilated duct is opened throughout the length of the body of the pancreas. Any stones encountered in the pancreatic duct are removed with forceps.

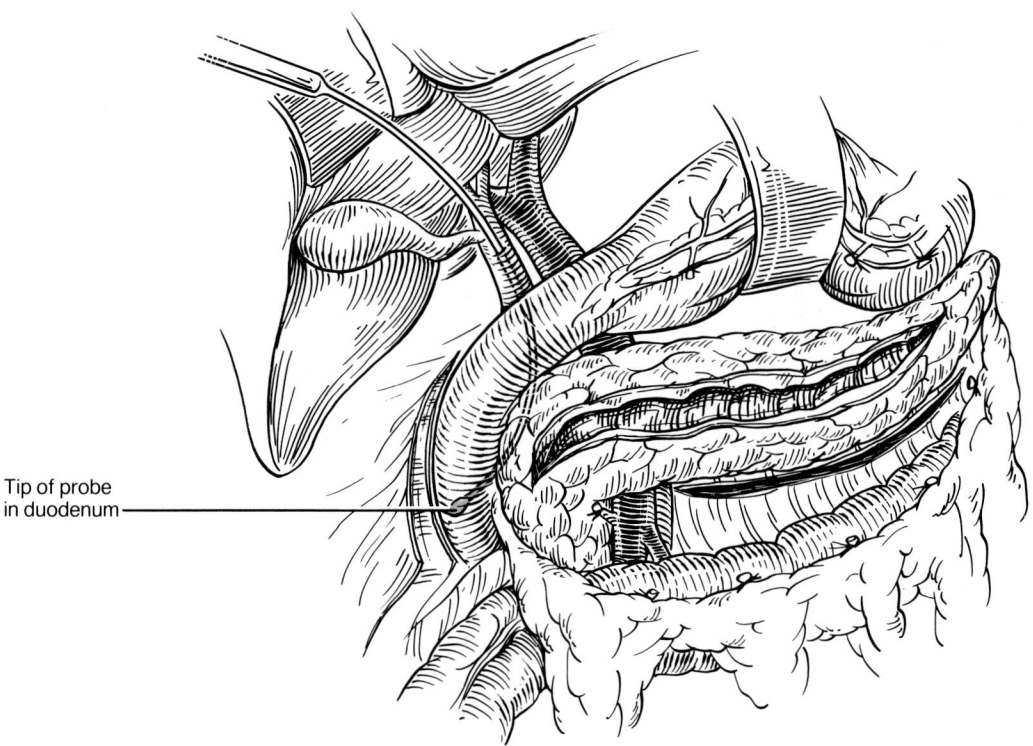

Tip of probe
in duodenum

Figure 30-IVC-4

Placement of Bakes Dilator

The incision in the pancreatic duct is continued into the head of the pancreas. As the duct enters the head of the pancreas, it moves inferiorly and posteriorly, requiring the division of more parenchyma anterior to the duct. The ductotomy should be extended to within 1 to 2 cm of the ampulla of Vater.

A metal probe is placed into the common bile duct through a small choledochotomy. The probe is passed gently into the duodenum and serves as a guide to the location of the common bile duct during the subsequent dissection within the head of the pancreas.

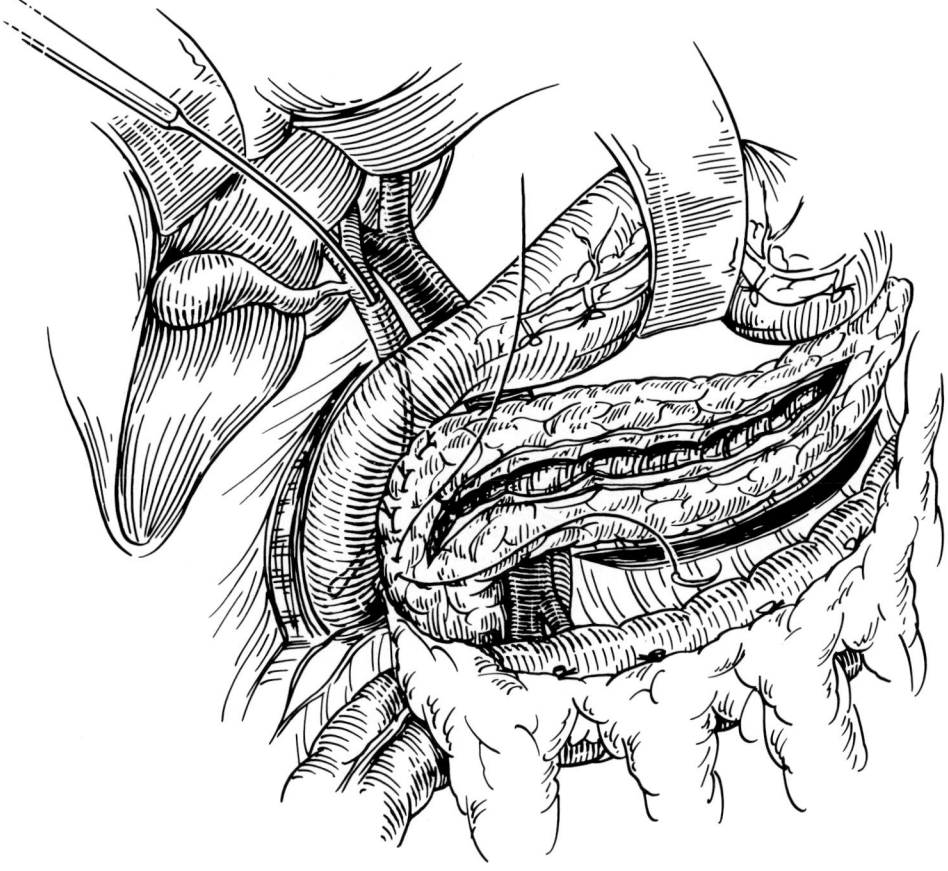

Figure 30-IVC-5

Placement of Hemostatic Sutures

Before commencing the "core-out" of the central portion of the pancreatic head, a series of hemostatic horizontal mattress sutures of 3-0 silk are placed in the portion of the pancreatic head to be preserved along the medial curvature of the duodenum.

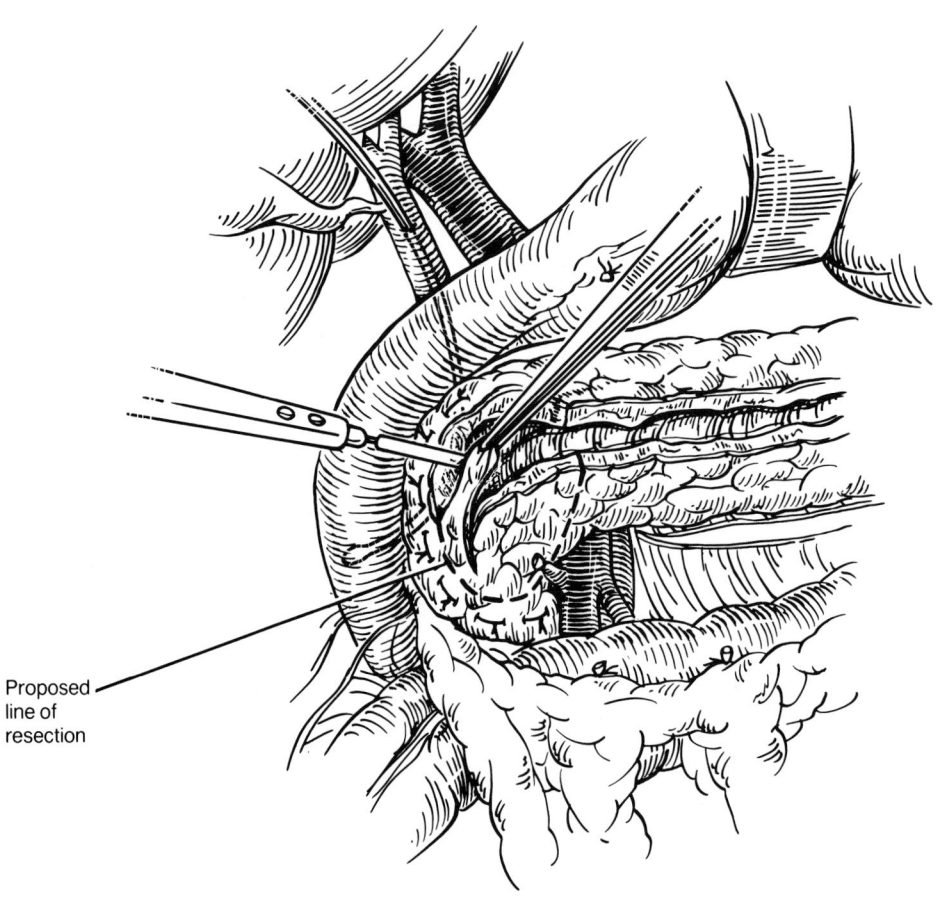

Proposed
line of
resection

Figure 30-IVC-6

Piecemeal Removal of Pancreatic Head

The piecemeal resection of the central core of the enlarged fibrotic pancreatic head is
commenced, working from the opened pancreatic duct outward. The proposed margins
of enucleation are indicated by the dotted line in the diagram. The dissection proceeds
along the edge of the common bile duct, with the location of the duct checked regularly
by palpation of the metal probe within it. The common bile duct is left partially embedded
in the pancreatic head remnant but should be freed medially so that it bulges into the
space left by the central resection of the pancreatic head.

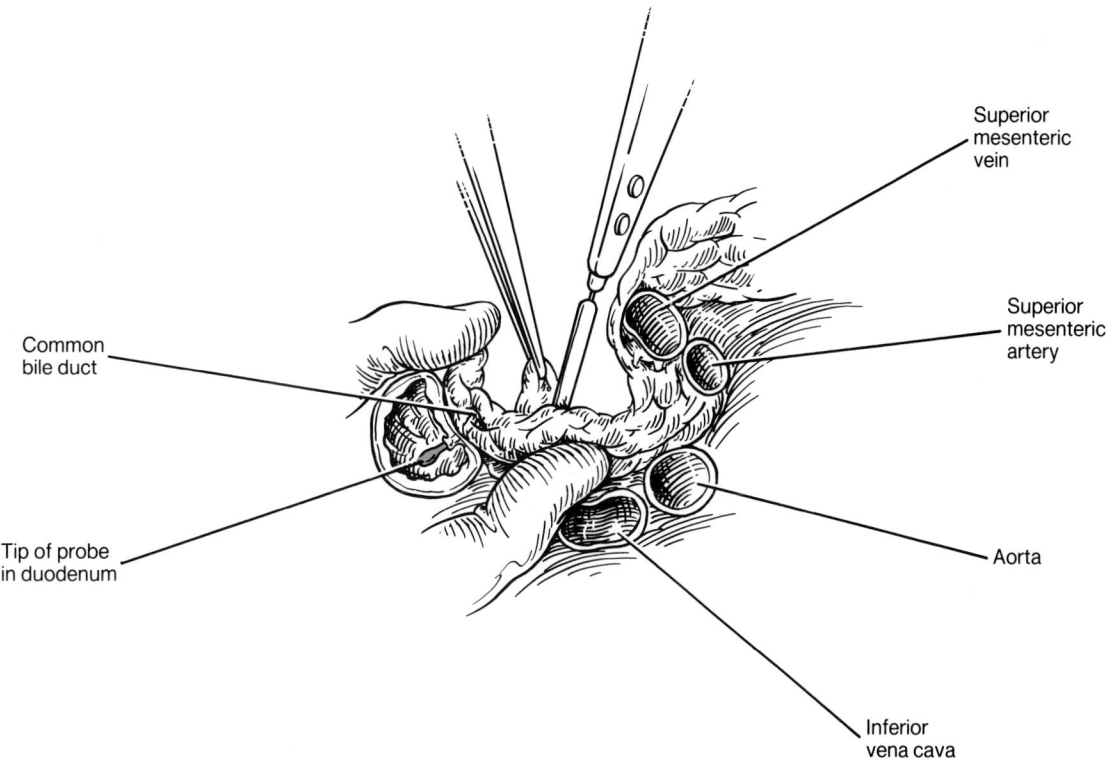

Common
bile duct

Tip of probe
in duodenum

Superior
mesenteric
vein

Superior
mesenteric
artery

Aorta

Inferior
vena cava

Figure 30-IVC-7

Placement of Hand Behind Head of Pancreas to Guide Posterior Dissection

The depth of resection of the pancreatic head is guided by placing the hand behind the mobilized head of the pancreas. A thin margin of pancreatic tissue on the posterior aspect of the head should be left in place as shown. This view also emphasizes the use of the metallic probe in the common duct as a guide to its location and preservation. A thin margin of pancreas is also left on the right lateral aspect of the superior mesenteric and portal veins.

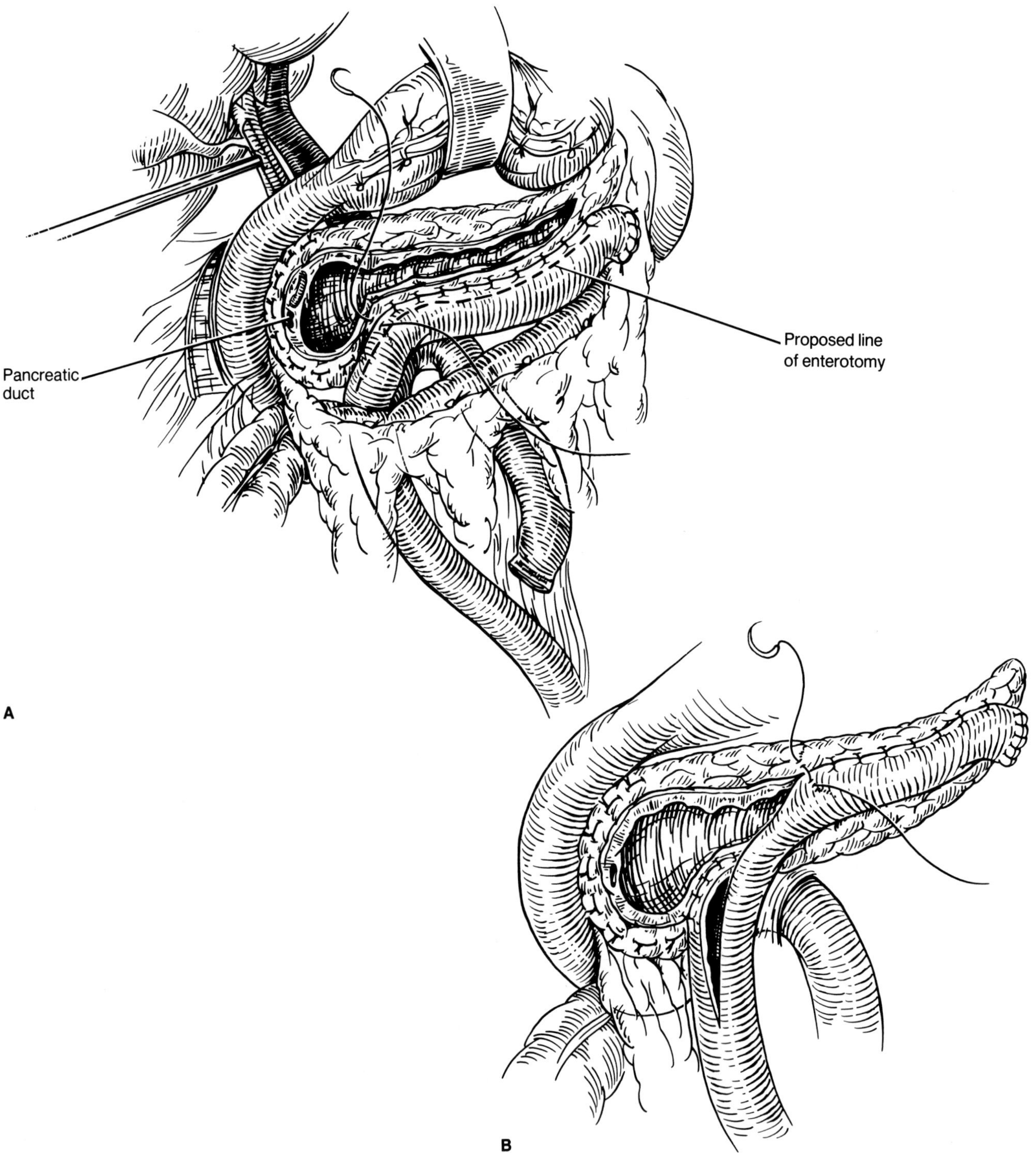

Pancreatic
duct

Proposed line
of enterotomy

A

B

Figure 30-IVC-8

Completion of Anastomosis

(**A**) After the pancreatic head dissection is completed, a Roux-en-Y loop of jejunum is created and passed through the transverse mesocolon so that it overlies the pancreas without tension. The staple line at the end of the jejunum is oversewn with interrupted sutures of 3-0 silk. The anastomosis between the jejunum and the opened pancreas can

Figure 30-IVC-8 *(Continued)*

be performed in one or two layers. If performed in two layers, the outer layer consists of interrupted 3-0 silk sutures between the seromuscular coat of jejunum and the pancreatic capsule. The inner layer is a continuous absorbable 3-0 suture between full thickness of the opened jejunal wall and the pancreatic capsule. In this figure, the anastomosis is shown as a one-layer anastomosis for clarity. Interrupted sutures of 3-0 silk are placed between the seromuscular coat of jejunum and the pancreatic capsule. The proposed line of incision in the antimesenteric border of the jejunum is indicated by the dashed line. Whether a one- or two-layer closure is used, the anastomosis is not intended to provide mucosa-to-mucosa apposition. It is designed to anchor the opened jejunum firmly over the pancreatic defect by suturing the bowel to the fibrotic pancreatic capsule and parenchyma.

(B) The anterior layer of the pancreaticojejunal anastomosis is formed by suturing the seromuscular coat of the jejunum to the fibrotic pancreatic capsule, inverting the bowel mucosa.

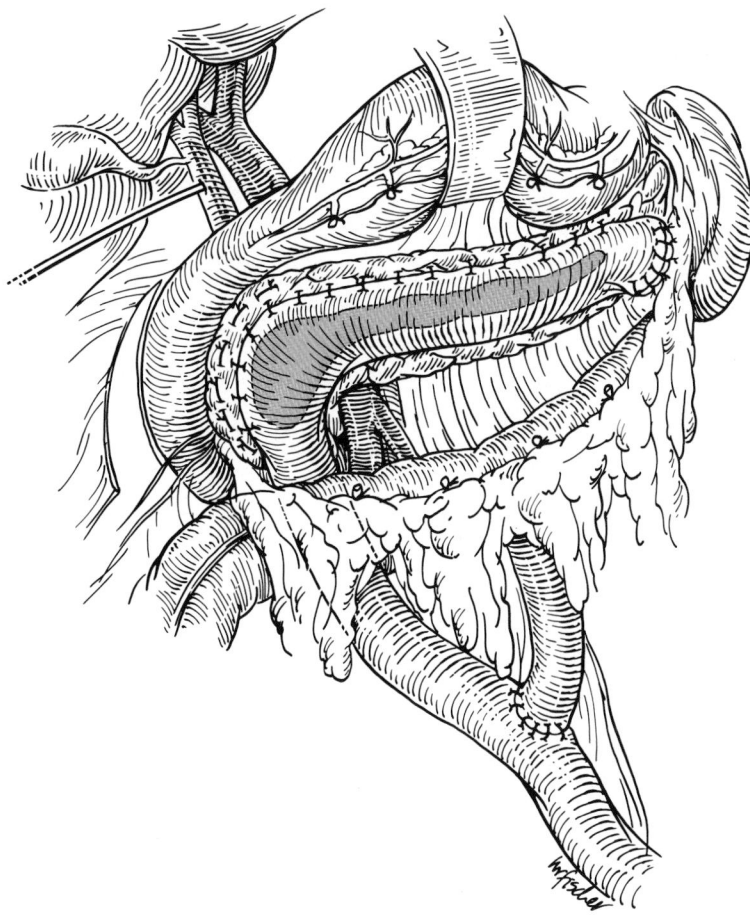

Figure 30-IVC-9

Completed Procedure

Both the upper and lower aspects of the pancreaticojejunal anastomosis should be drained with soft closed-suction drains (*not shown*). A T-tube is customarily left in the common bile duct, and lack of obstruction of the distal common bile duct is confirmed by postoperative cholangiography before removing the T-tube.

D. Subtotal (95%) Pancreatic Resection

Subtotal resection of the pancreas is not as commonly performed as in the past but is occasionally indicated for the treatment of intractable pain due to diffuse chronic pancreatitis when the pancreatic duct is not dilated.

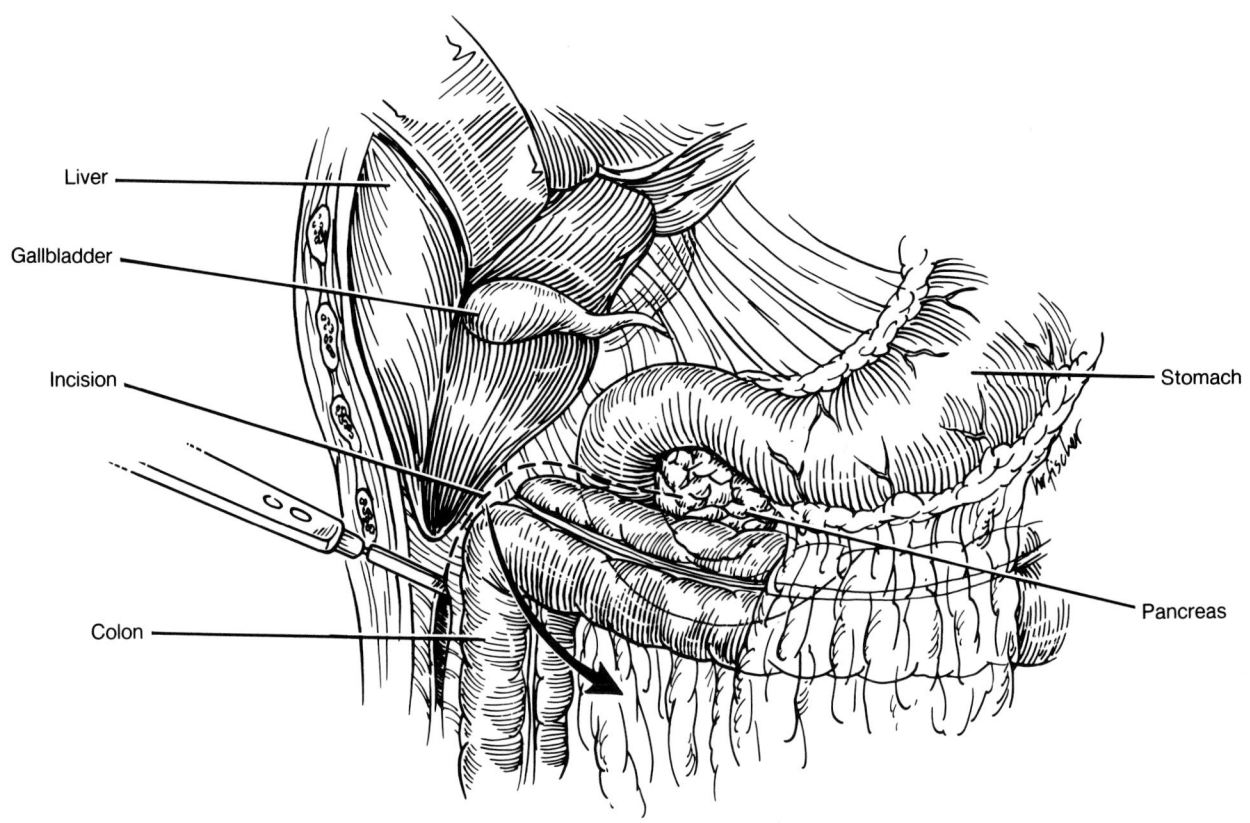

Figure 30-IVD-1

Mobilization of Hepatic Flexure

The operation is begun by fully mobilizing the hepatic flexure of the colon and retracting it inferiorly to expose the head of the pancreas.

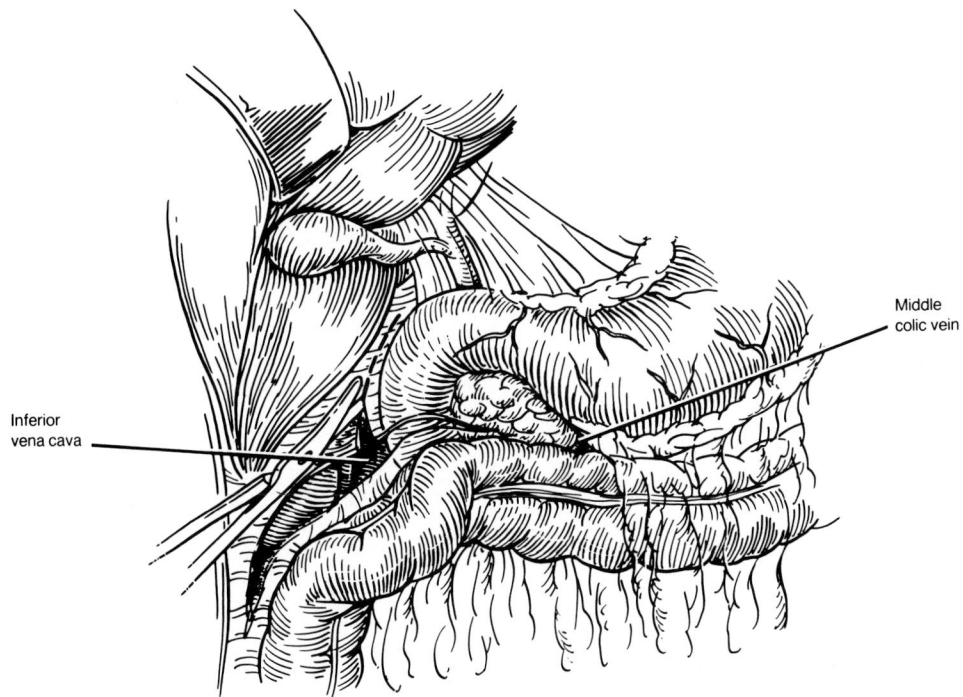

Figure 30-IVD-2

Kocher Maneuver

The peritoneum lateral to the duodenum is excised, and a Kocher maneuver is performed, elevating the duodenum and head of the pancreas.

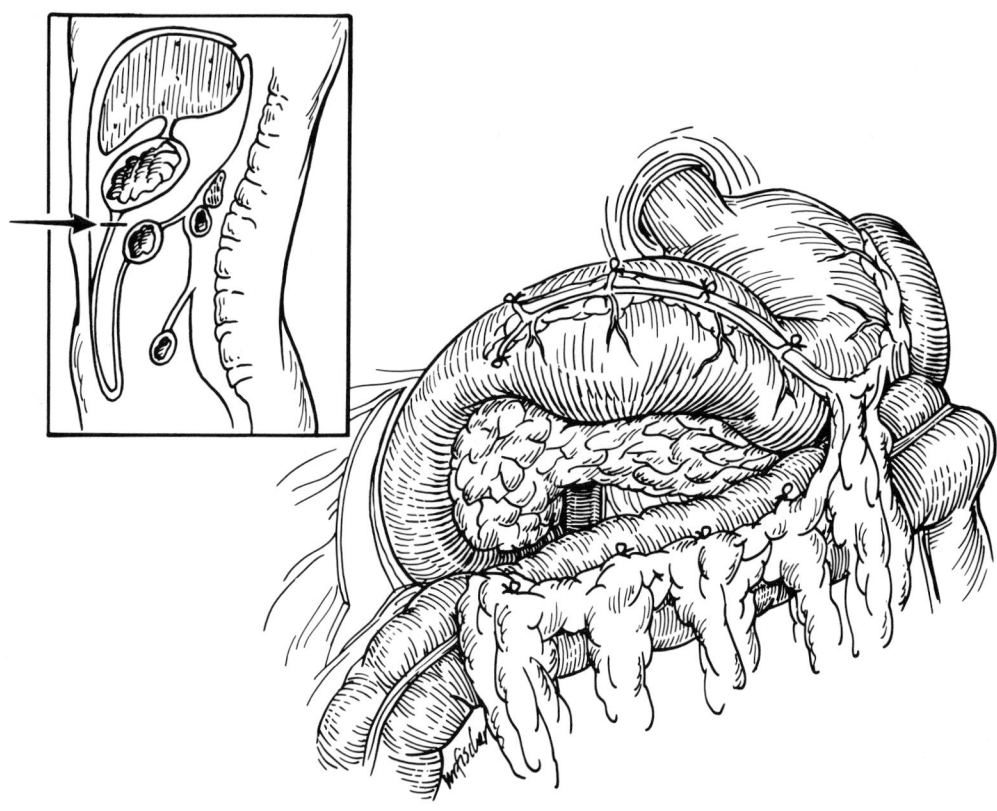

Figure 30-IVD-3

Division of Gastrocolic Omentum

The body and tail of the pancreas are exposed by entering the lesser sac through the gastrocolic omentum (**inset**). Adhesions between the posterior wall of the stomach and the anterior surface of the pancreas are divided sharply to expose the pancreas fully. The right gastroepiploic vein is ligated to provide exposure of the neck of the pancreas and to allow exposure of the anterior surface of the entire gland (see Fig. 30-IIB-2 for details).

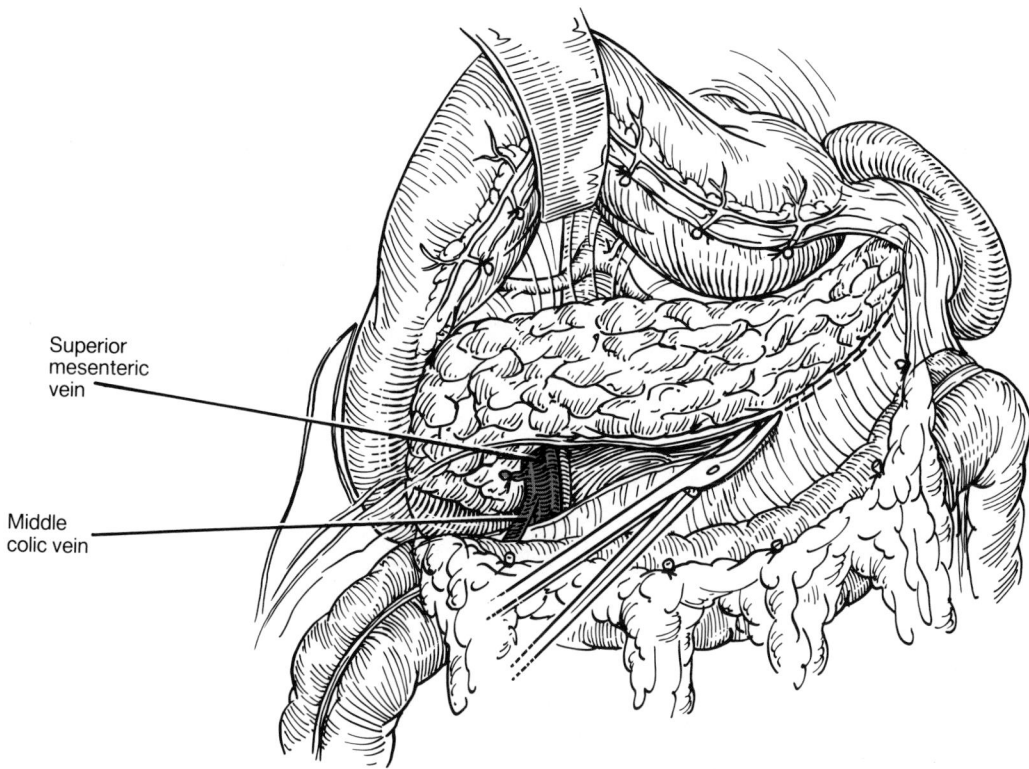

Superior
mesenteric
vein

Middle
colic vein

Figure 30-IVD-4

Opening of Peritoneum

The peritoneum along the inferior border of the pancreas is incised from the superior mesenteric vessels to the tail of the gland. A few small blood vessels may require ligation before the retropancreatic space can be entered. After ligation of these vessels, the body and tail of the pancreas (along with the splenic artery and vein) can be elevated by gentle blunt dissection behind the gland.

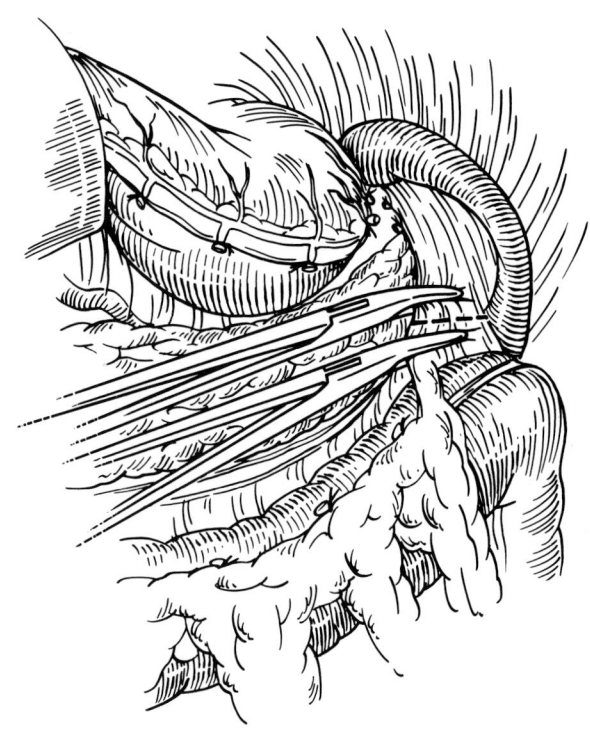

Figure 30-IVD-5

Division of Splenocolic Ligament

To begin the mobilization of the distal pancreas and spleen, the lower short gastric arteries are ligated with 2-0 silk ties and divided. The splenocolic ligament is divided between clamps, and the ends of the cut tissue are ligated with 2-0 silk.

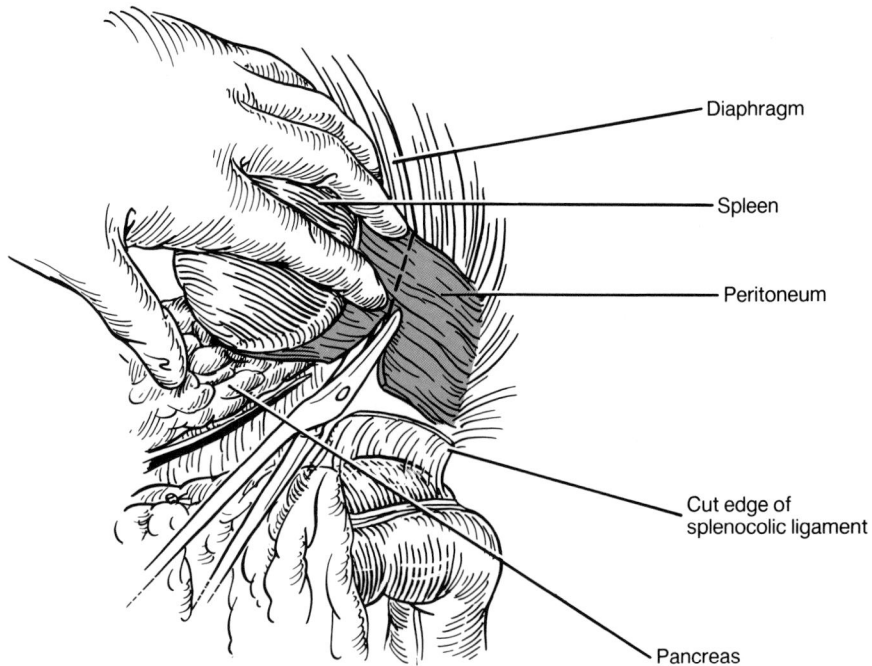

Diaphragm

Spleen

Peritoneum

Cut edge of
splenocolic ligament

Pancreas

Figure 30-IVD-6

Division of Lateral Peritoneal Reflection of Spleen

With the spleen gently retracted to the right, the peritoneum lateral to the spleen is divided from the base of the spleen up to the diaphragm, following a line just outside the curve of the splenic capsule. The order of the steps in Figure 30-IVD-5 and this figure can be reversed, depending on ease of exposure.

1030

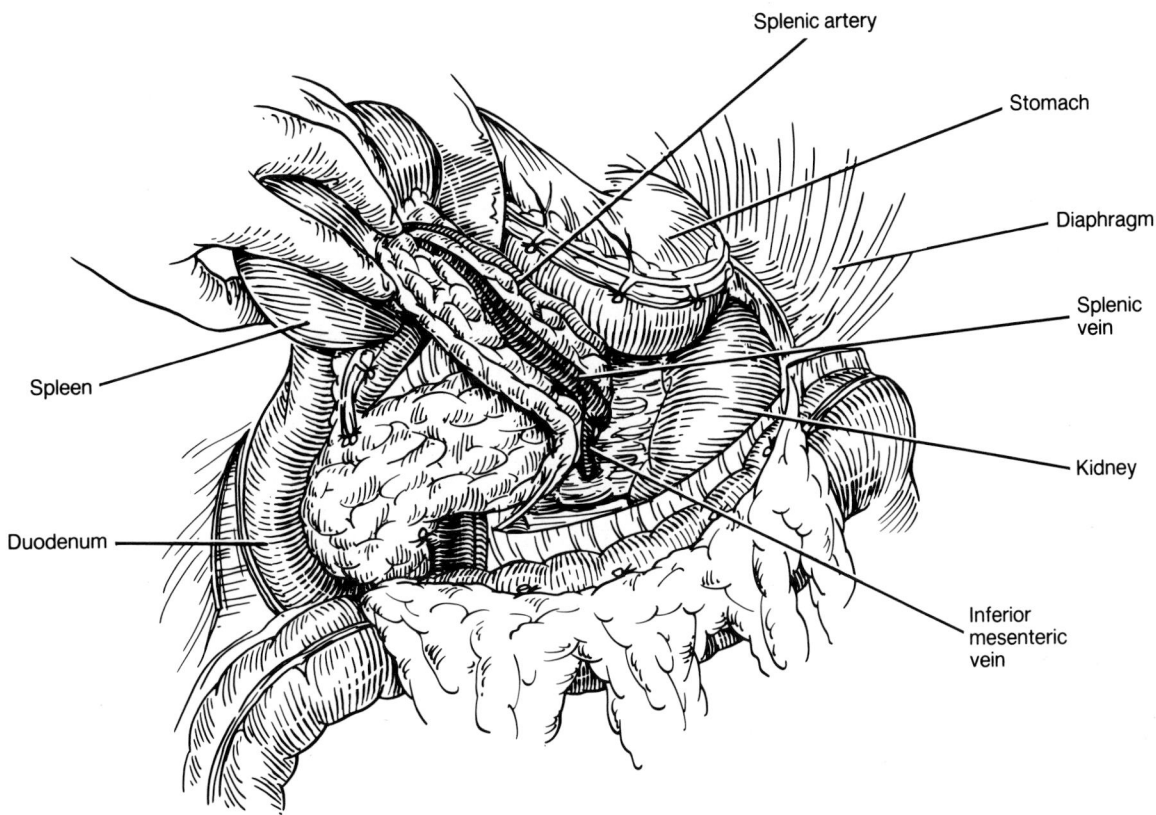

Figure 30-IVD-7

Reflection of Pancreatic Tail and Spleen

The spleen and tail of the pancreas are gently and gradually mobilized anteriorly and to the right. As the spleen is elevated, any remaining short gastric vessels tethering the spleen to the stomach are ligated with 2-0 silk ties and divided. The pancreas and spleen are progressively mobilized off the left kidney. The inferior mesenteric vein may be encountered entering the splenic vein behind the pancreas. If so, it is ligated with 3-0 silk ligatures and divided. The mobilization of the body and tail of the pancreas proceeds until reaching the superior mesenteric artery, which tethers the pancreas to the aorta and is the limit of dissection in this plane.

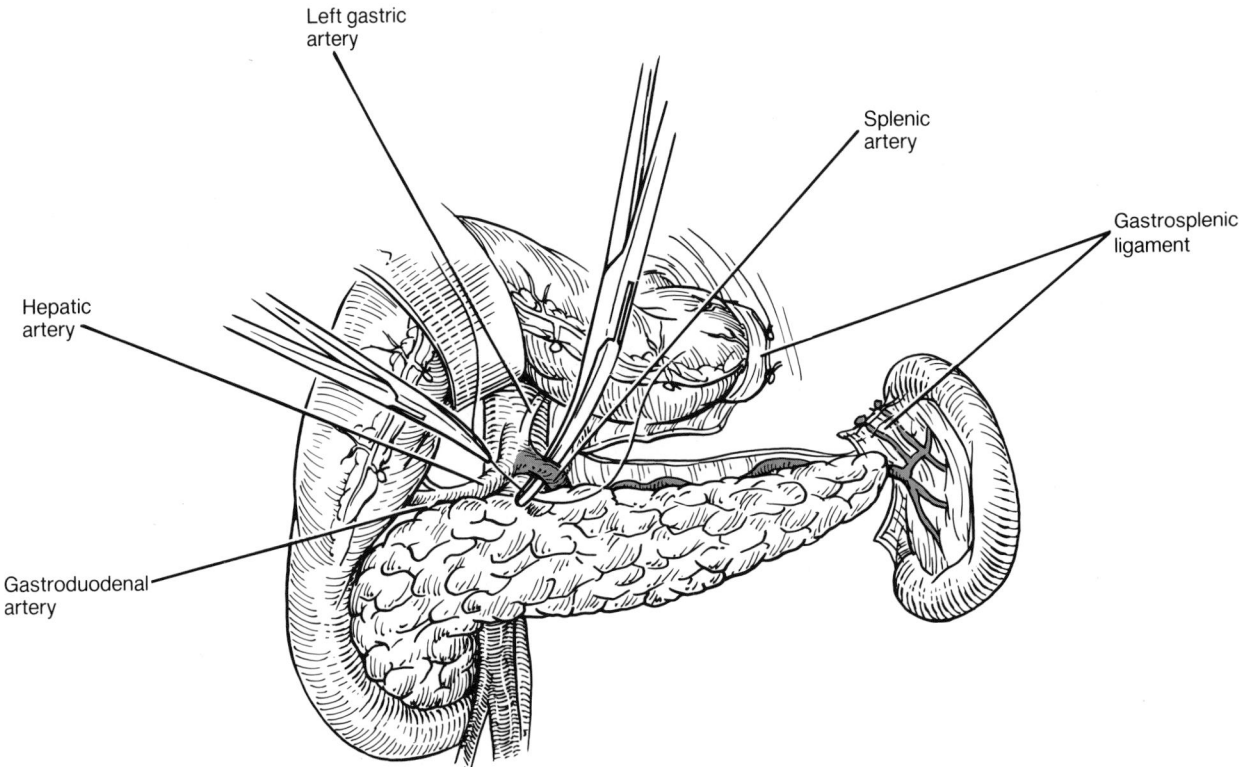

Figure 30-IVD-8

Ligation of Splenic Artery at Origin

The splenic artery is identified at its origin from the celiac axis and is doubly clamped and ligated. A suture ligature of 2-0 silk is placed on the celiac side for security. The splenic end of the artery is tied with a simple ligature of 2-0 silk. If more convenient, the splenic artery can be ligated from the posterior aspect of the gland (see Fig. 30-VE-9*B*).

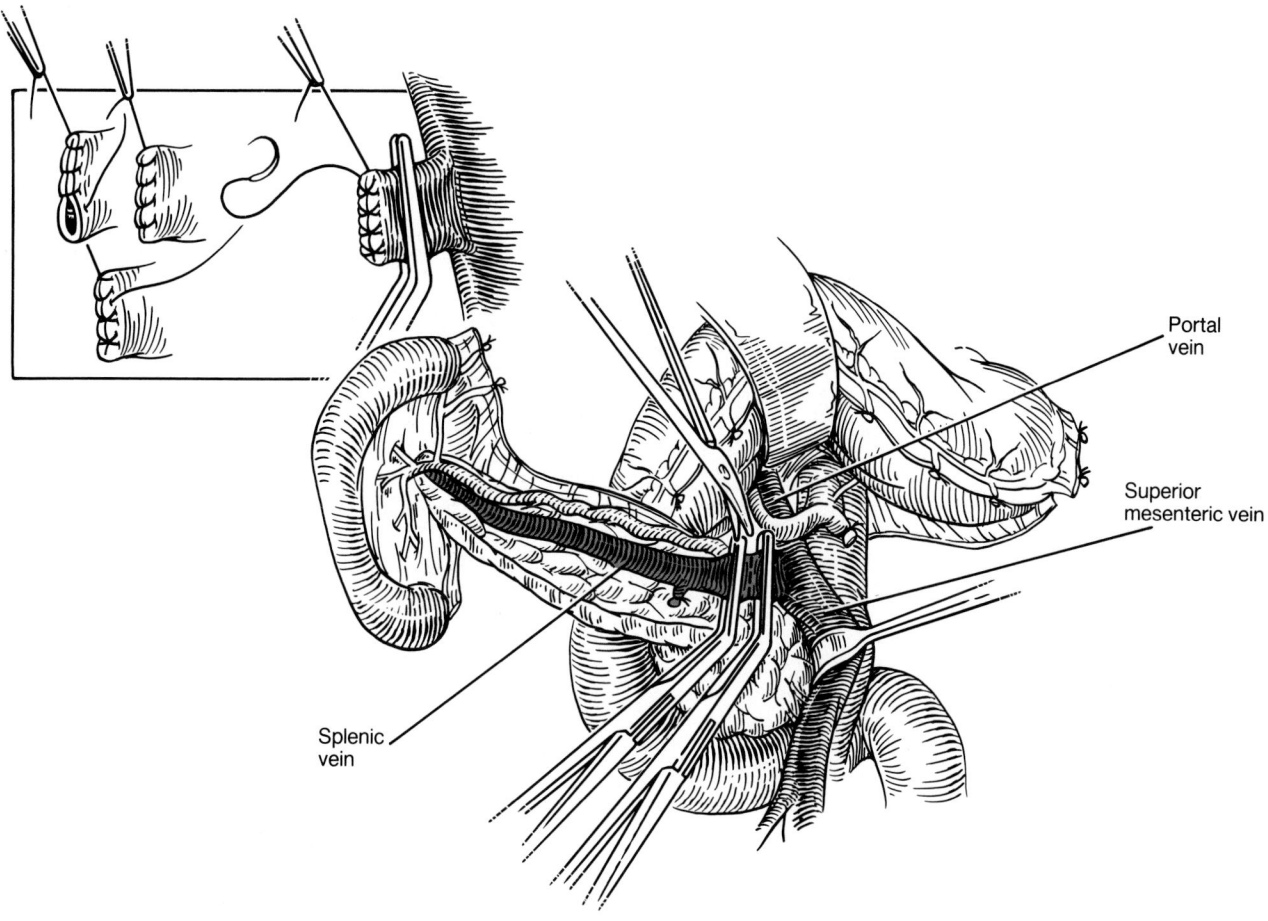

Portal
vein

Superior
mesenteric vein

Splenic
vein

Figure 30-IVD-9

Division of Splenic Vein

The entrance of the splenic vein into the portal vein is slowly and carefully identified on the posterior aspect of the gland. Gentle dissection around the vein at this point, avoiding the small branches of the vein that enter from the pancreas, allows the placement of a pair of fine vascular clamps, between which the splenic vein is divided. Both ends of the vein are oversewn with a running 5-0 monofilament suture (**inset**).

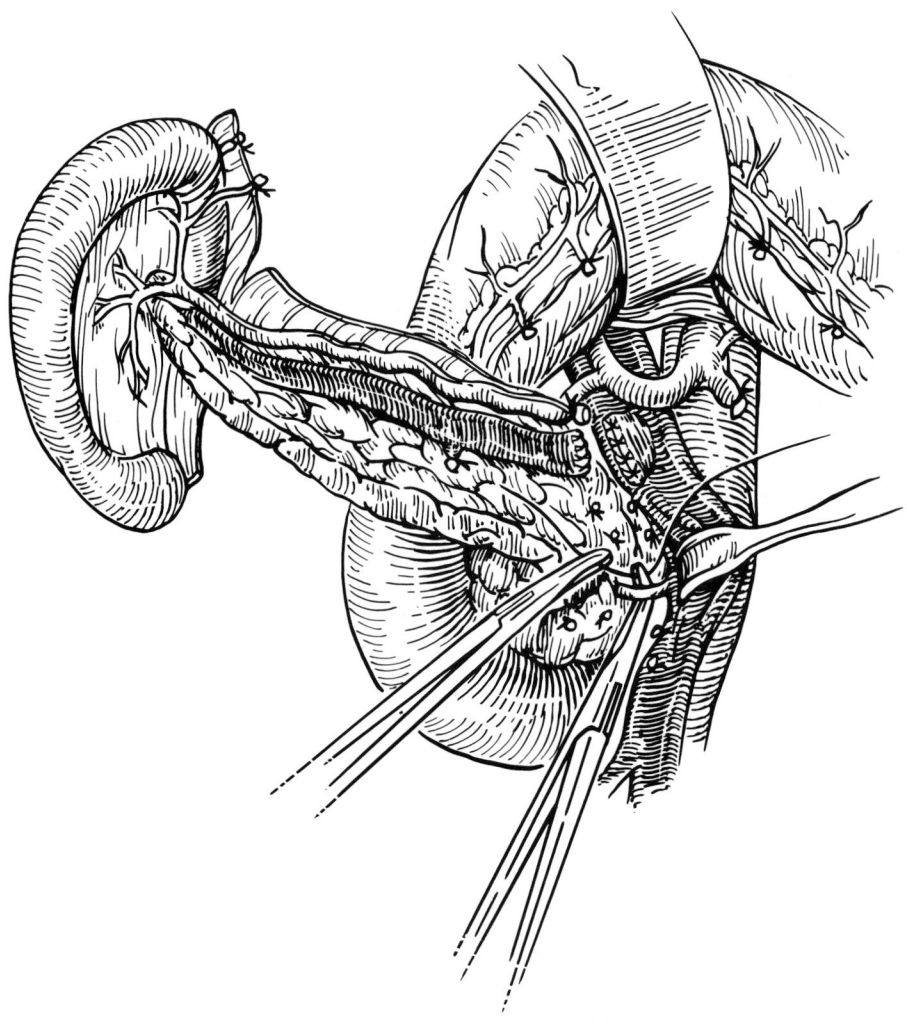

Figure 30-IVD-10

Separation of Uncinate Process

The head of the pancreas must now be separated from the portal and superior mesenteric veins by dividing the veins draining the head of the pancreas into those structures. These veins are delicate and tear easily. The use of very fine clamps for dissection around the veins and fine ligatures (4-0) reduces the risk of hemorrhage.

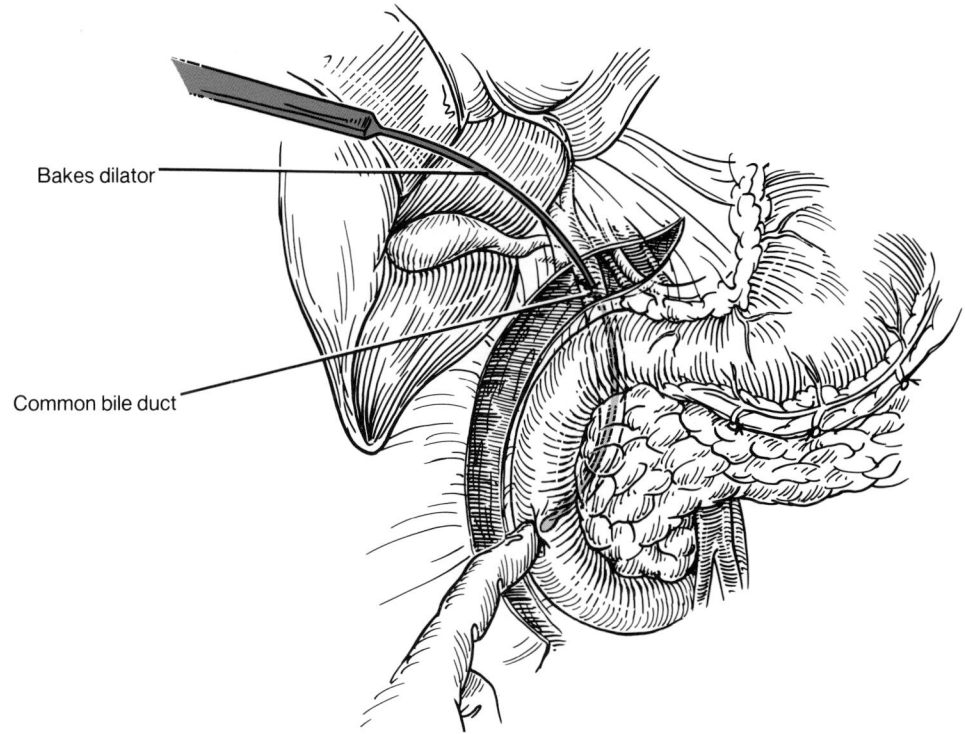

Bakes dilator

Common bile duct

Figure 30-IVD-11

Passage of Bakes Dilator

In preparation for the near-total resection of the pancreas, the common bile duct is cannulated with a metal probe placed through a small choledochotomy. The 5% of pancreas that will not be resected is that portion immediately adjacent to the medial duodenal curve, which contains the distal common bile duct. The dissection through the head of the pancreas proceeds just medial to the common bile duct.

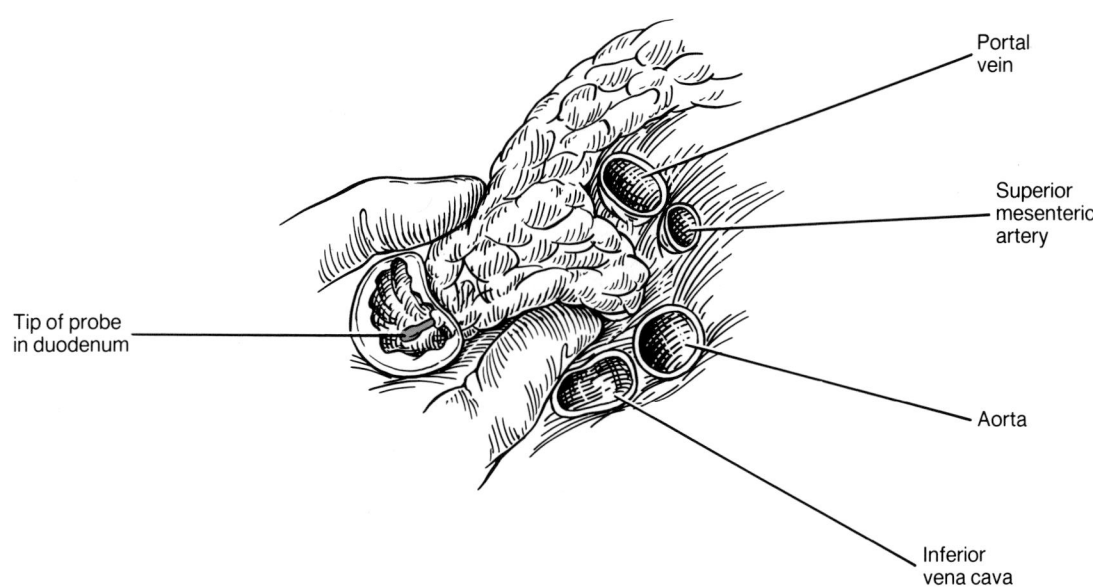

Figure 30-IVD-12

Palpation of Pancreatic Head

This view from below the head of the pancreas shows how the probe in the common bile duct and palpation of the head of the pancreas from the front and back are used to guide the dissection of the pancreatic head. This is done to leave a small remnant of pancreas intact along the medial duodenal curve, containing the intact distal common bile duct.

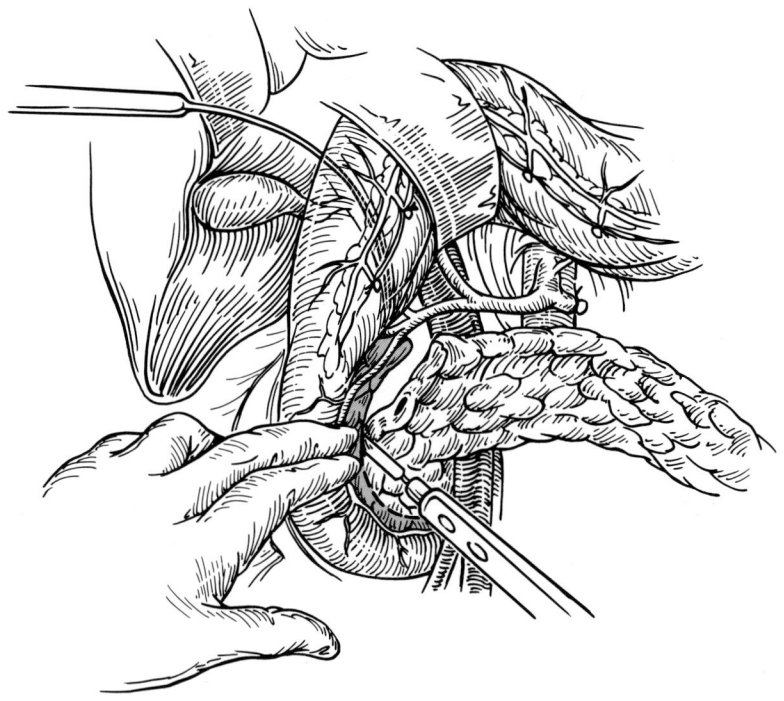

Figure 30-IVD-13

Excision of Pancreatic Head

The curved dissection through the head of the pancreas just medial to the common bile duct follows the dashed line indicated. The pancreaticoduodenal arcade of vessels is preserved to provide blood supply to the duodenum and the remaining pancreatic remnant.

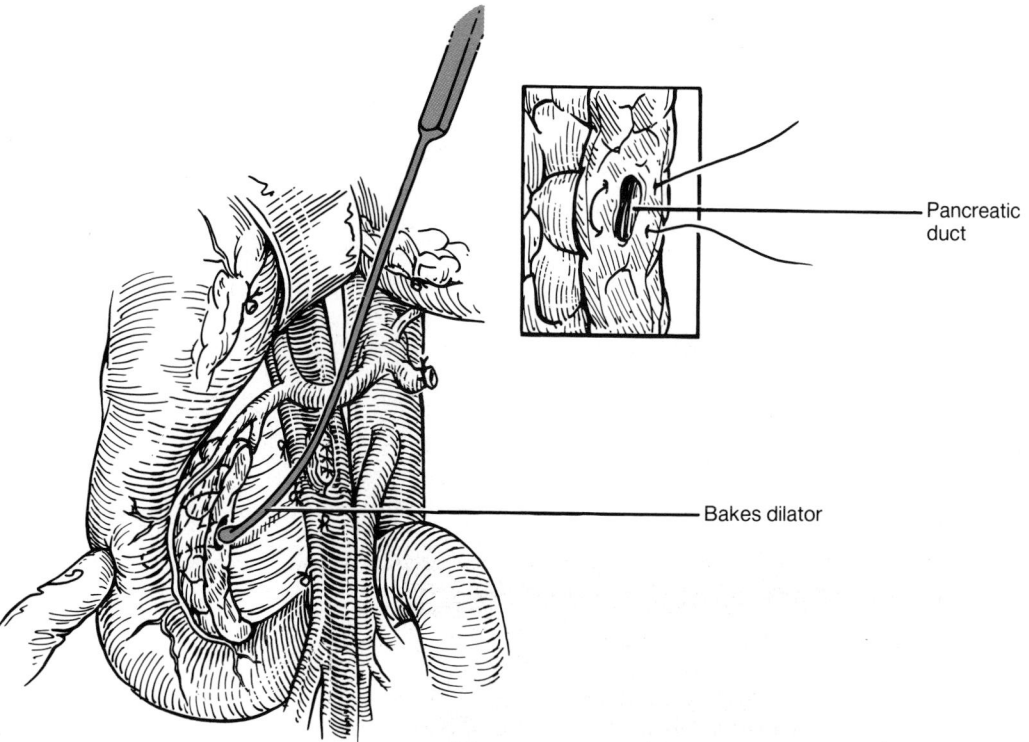

Figure 30-IVD-14

Probing and Ligation of Pancreatic Duct

After removal of the pancreatic specimen, the pancreatic duct is gently probed with a fine Bakes dilator to confirm patency of the ampulla of Vater. The exposed end of the pancreatic duct is then ligated with a horizontal mattress suture of 3-0 silk (**inset**).

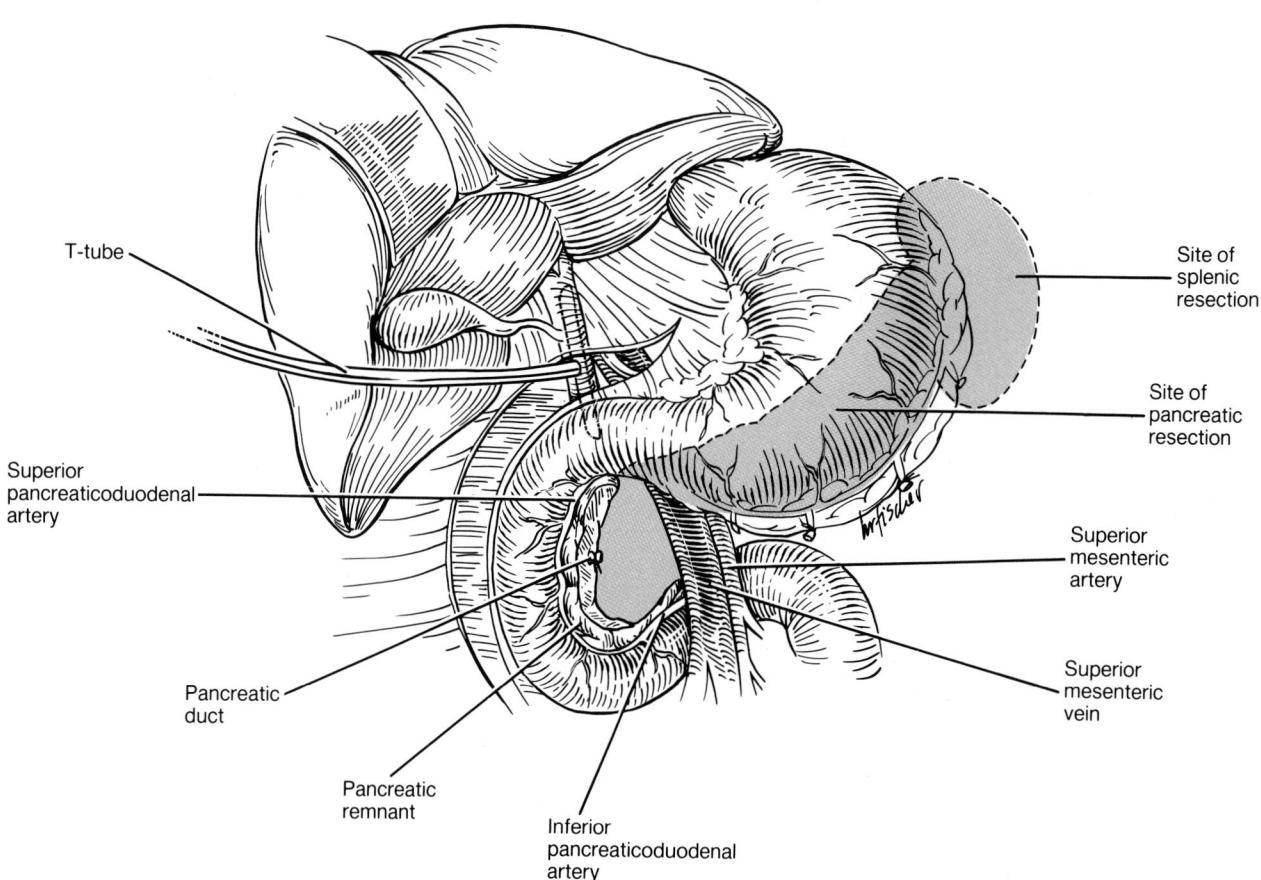

T-tube

Site of splenic resection

Site of pancreatic resection

Superior pancreaticoduodenal artery

Superior mesenteric artery

Superior mesenteric vein

Pancreatic duct

Pancreatic remnant

Inferior pancreaticoduodenal artery

Figure 30-IVD-15

Completed Procedure

A soft closed-suction drain (*not shown*) should be placed immediately adjacent to the cut surface of the pancreatic remnant. Feeding jejunostomy and gastrostomy tubes are advisable (*also not shown*). A T-tube is left in the common bile duct after removal of the metal probe. A postoperative cholangiogram should be performed to confirm patency of the distal common bile duct before removing the T-tube.

SECTION V   *Operations for Pancreatic Exocrine Neoplasms*

A. Pancreaticoduodenectomy for Carcinoma of the Pancreas

Pancreaticoduodenectomy is indicated for resectable carcinomas of the head of the pancreas and for malignant islet cell tumors. The operation described here is the traditional form of the procedure. The pylorus-sparing and extended variants of pancreaticoduodenectomy are described in Sections VB and VC.

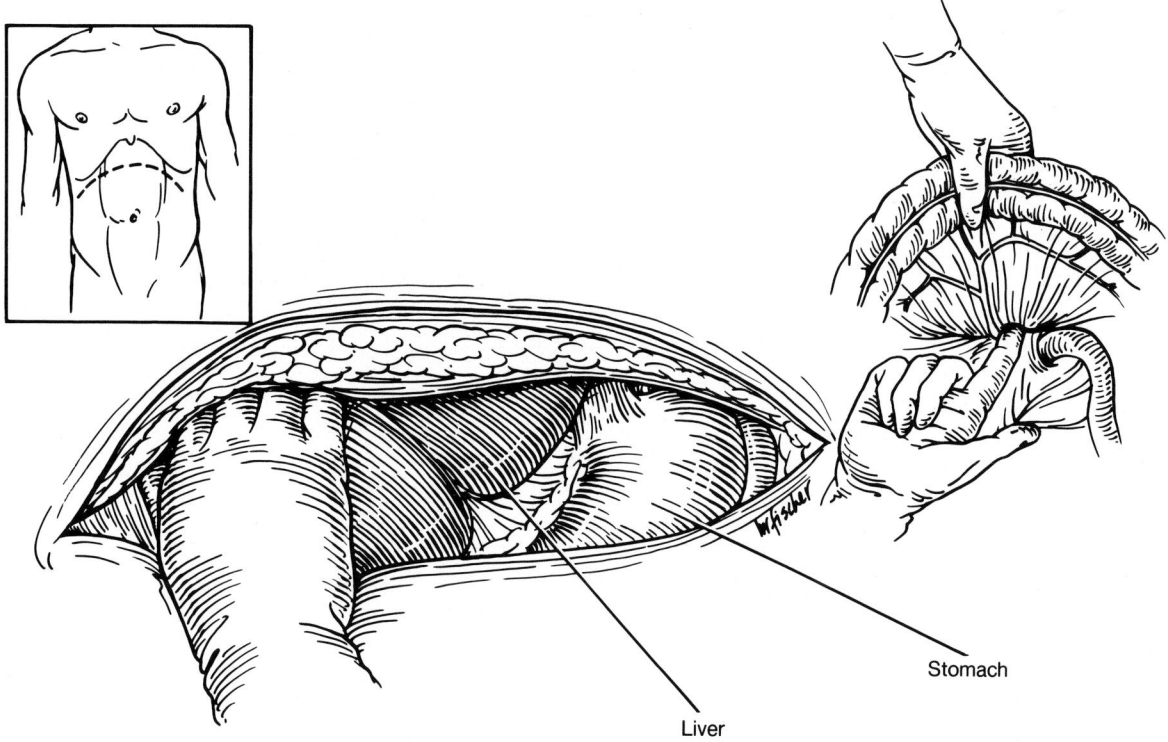

Liver   Stomach

Figure 30-VA-1

Inspection of the Peritoneal Cavity

Pancreaticoduodenectomy can be performed through a bilateral subcostal incision (**inset**) or a midline abdominal incision. Upon entering the abdomen, a thorough inspection of the peritoneal cavity is performed to rule out the presence of metastatic disease that would render the patient incurable by resection. The entire surface of the liver should be palpated as well as the entire peritoneal surface and the omentum. Particular attention should be directed to the area at the base of the transverse mesocolon just medial to the ligament of Treitz (**right**), since direct tumor extension may involve the base of the middle colic vessels. Removing such involvement en bloc may require a partial colonic resection. In addition, lymph node metastases should be sought at the base of the transverse mesocolon along the course of the superior mesenteric artery and vein. Significant direct extension or lymph node involvement in this area is incompatible with surgical cure.

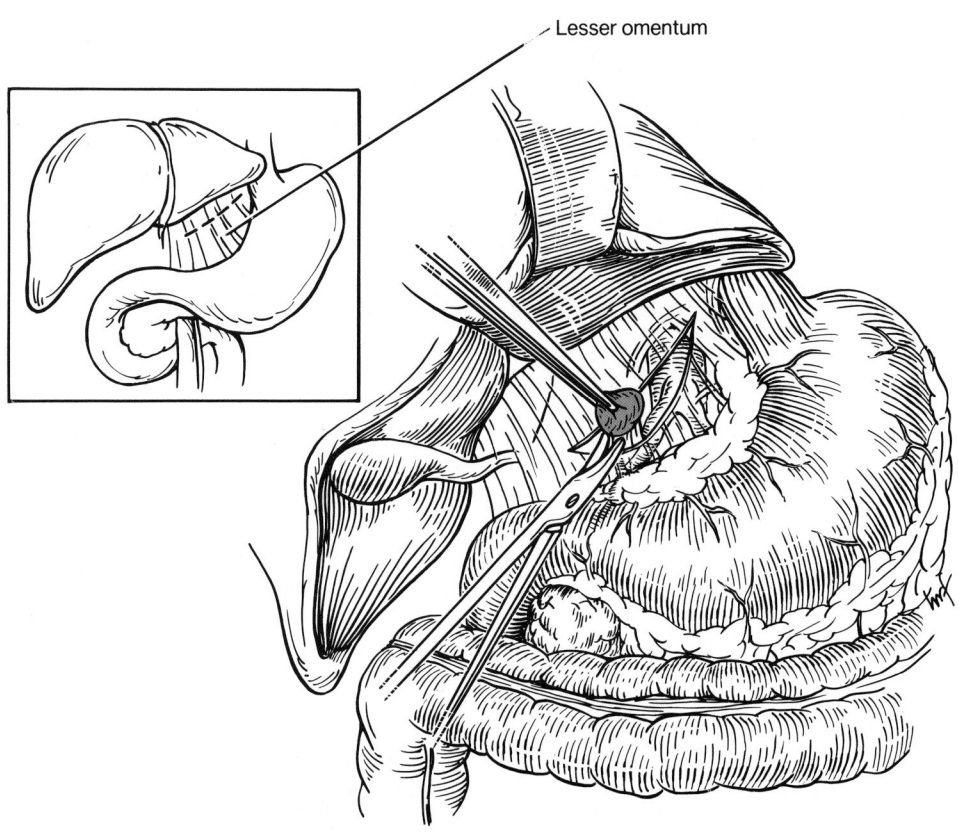

Lesser omentum

Figure 30-VA-2

Biopsy of Celiac Node

As part of the initial examination of the abdomen to determine resectability for cure, the area around the celiac axis should be inspected for lymph node involvement. This region can be easily accessed through the lesser omentum (**inset**). Ordinarily, there are lymph nodes around the celiac axis measuring about 1 cm in diameter. If the nodes are soft and movable, biopsy is not indicated. On the other hand, larger, hard, or matted nodes should undergo biopsy, since metastatic disease at the base of the celiac trunk is generally considered to preclude surgical cure.

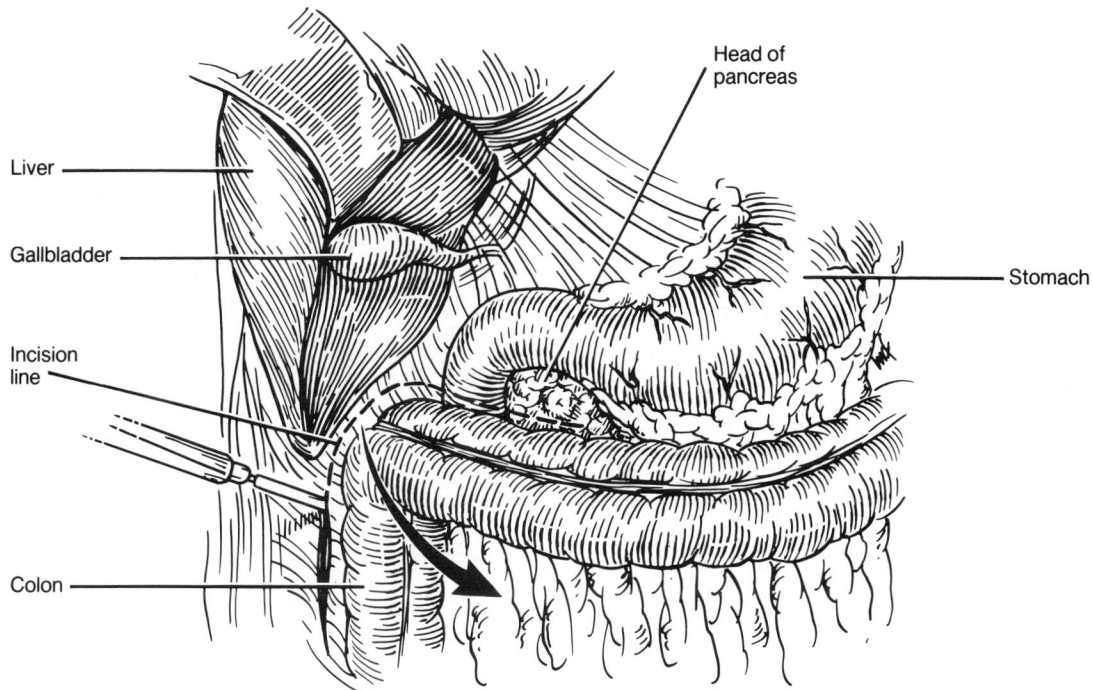

Figure 30-VA-3

Takedown of Hepatic Flexure

If inspection and palpation of the peritoneal cavity indicate that the carcinoma is restricted to the head of the pancreas, the operation is commenced by mobilizing the hepatic flexure of the colon and retracting it inferiorly. The base of the mesocolon crosses the head of the pancreas (see Fig. 30-IIA-1). If it is loosely adherent to the pancreatic head, the mesocolon can be gently swept inferiorly to expose the pancreatic head fully. Occasionally, carcinoma of the head of the pancreas invades the transverse mesocolon as it lies over the anterior surface of the pancreatic head. If the mesocolon is firmly adherent to the pancreatic head, a portion of mesocolon should be left attached to the pancreas as part of the operative specimen. The defect thus created in the mesocolon usually can be closed primarily.

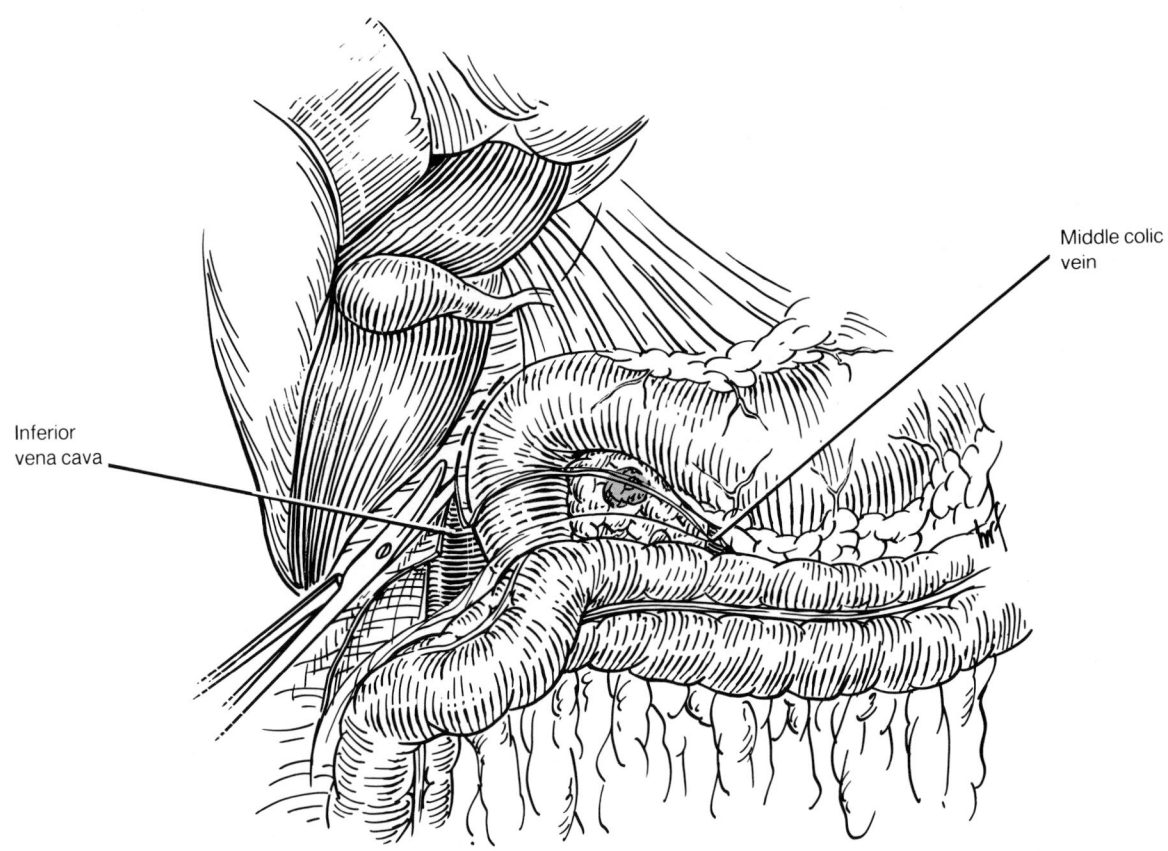

Middle colic
vein

Inferior
vena cava

Figure 30-VA-4

Kocher Maneuver

The peritoneum lateral to the duodenum is incised, and a full Kocher maneuver is performed, mobilizing and elevating the duodenum and head of the pancreas all the way
from the hepatoduodenal ligament to the superior mesenteric vessels. The head of the
pancreas should be completely mobilized off the inferior vena cava and the latter identified. Occasionally, large pancreatic carcinomas invade the anterior aspect of the vena
cava. If this is the case, a Kocher maneuver is impossible, and the tumor is not resectable.

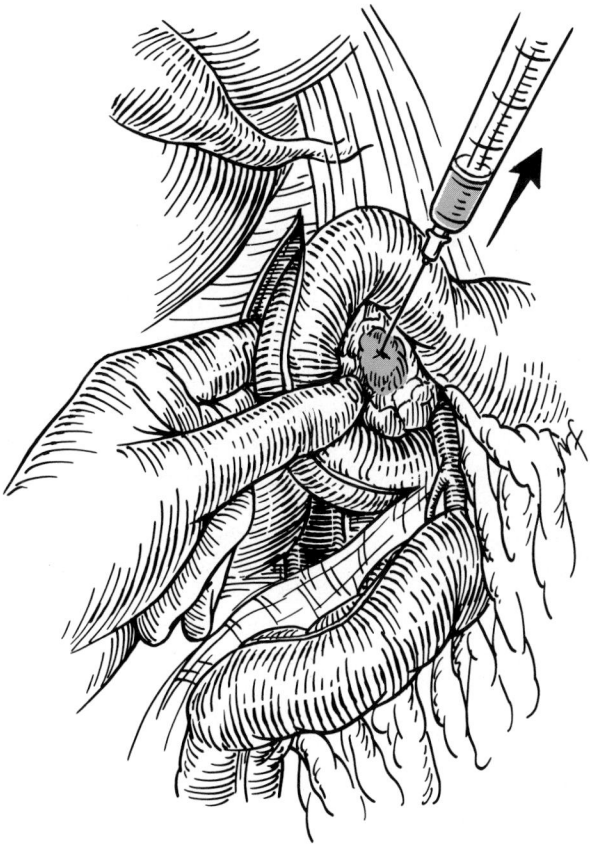

Figure 30-VA-5

Palpation and Aspiration of Tumor

After completion of the Kocher maneuver, the surgeon should carefully palpate the head of the pancreas between the thumb and fingers of the left hand. Tissue confirmation of malignancy can be obtained at this time by fine-needle aspiration of the tumor mass with a 22-gauge needle attached to a dry 10-mL syringe. Multiple needle passes through the tumor increase the likelihood of a positive cytologic diagnosis. If cytologic diagnostic facilities are not available, the tumor biopsy can be performed by traditional core needle biopsy techniques.

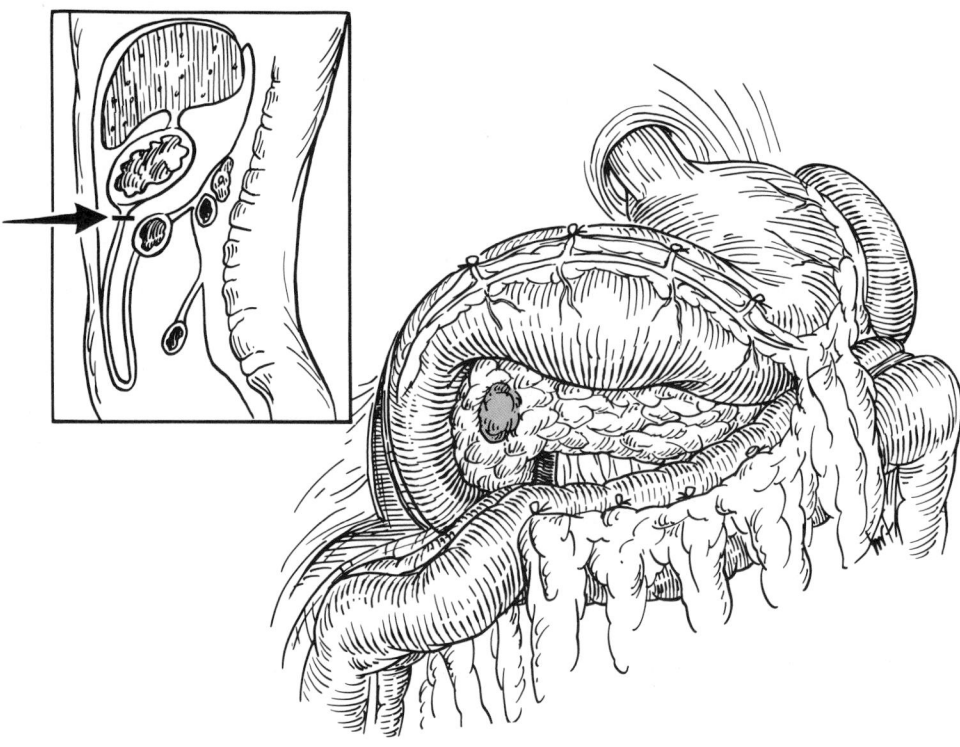

Figure 30-VA-6

Opening Gastrocolic Omentum

The operation continues by dividing a portion of the gastrocolic omentum to expose the anterior surface of the neck and body of the pancreas. The gastrocolic omentum is opened inferior to the gastroepiploic vessels. The right gastroepiploic vein is finally divided as it crosses the neck of the pancreas to provide better exposure of the anterior surface of the gland (see Fig. 30-IIB-2 for details).

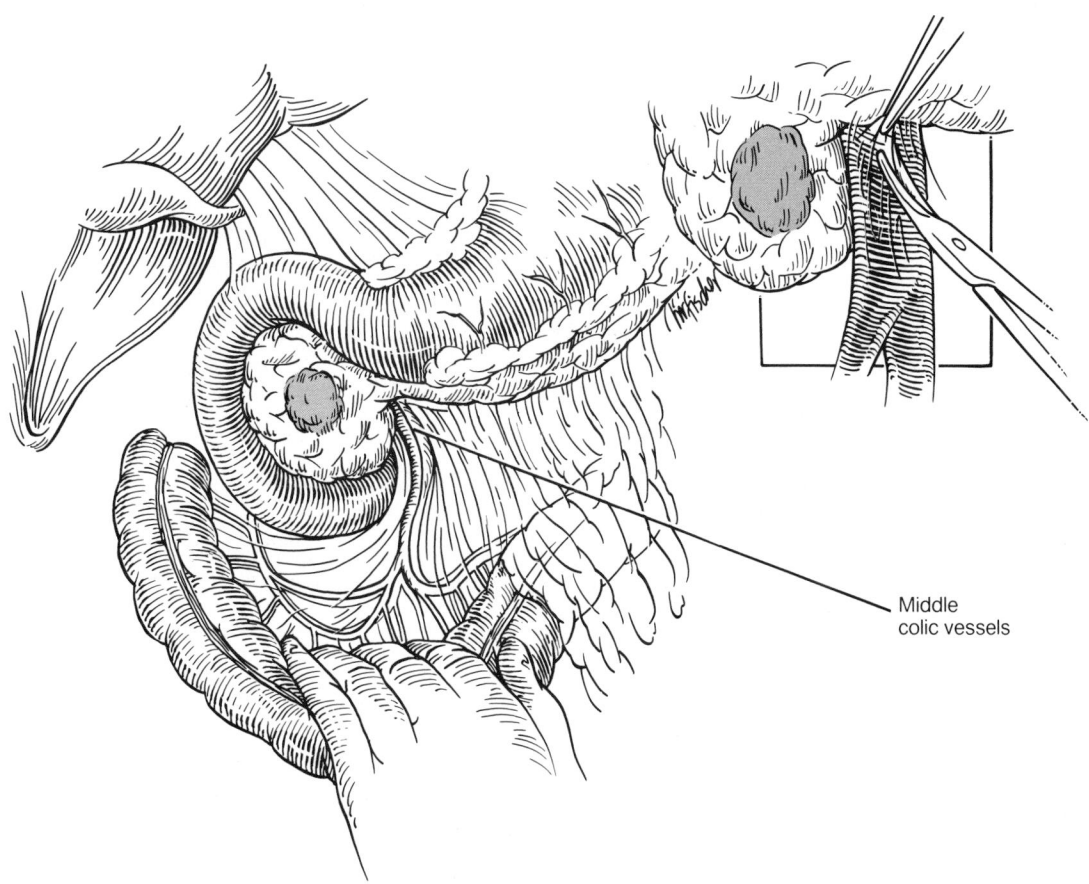

Middle
colic vessels

Figure 30-VA-7

Identification of Superior Mesenteric Vein

In the next stages of the operation, the patency of the space behind the neck of the pancreas anterior to the superior mesenteric and portal veins is determined. To begin this dissection, the middle colic vein is followed downward to its entrance into the superior mesenteric vein. Gentle dissection in this area reveals the superior mesenteric vein beneath a few millimeters of fibroadipose tissue. The periadventitial tissue overlying the anterior surface of the superior mesenteric vein is divided with fine scissors (**inset**) so that further dissection proceeds immediately adjacent to the anterior edge of the vein. Establishment of a plane of dissection directly on the surface of the vein is critical to the success of the following steps in the operation.

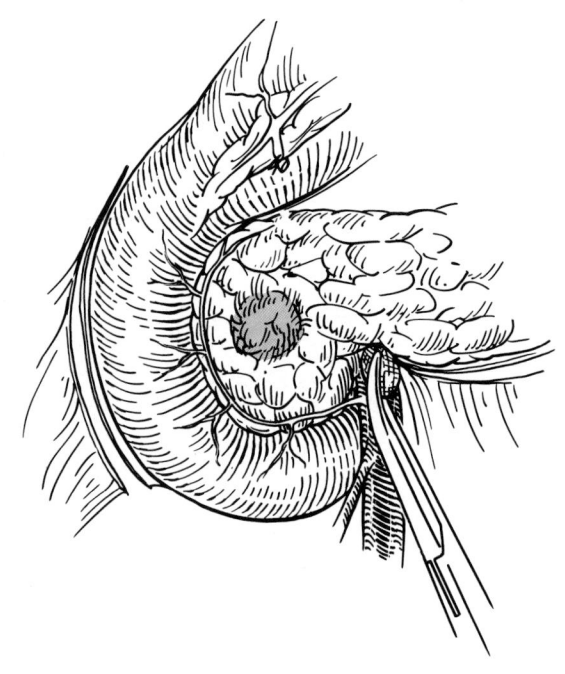

Figure 30-VA-8

Dissection of Superior Mesenteric Vein

The superior mesenteric vein is followed as it disappears under the inferior edge of the neck of the pancreas. Using gentle blunt dissection, a plane is established anterior to the vein and posterior to the back surface of the neck of the pancreas. The dissection must proceed on the anterior surface of the vein; this is an area that is almost always free of branches.

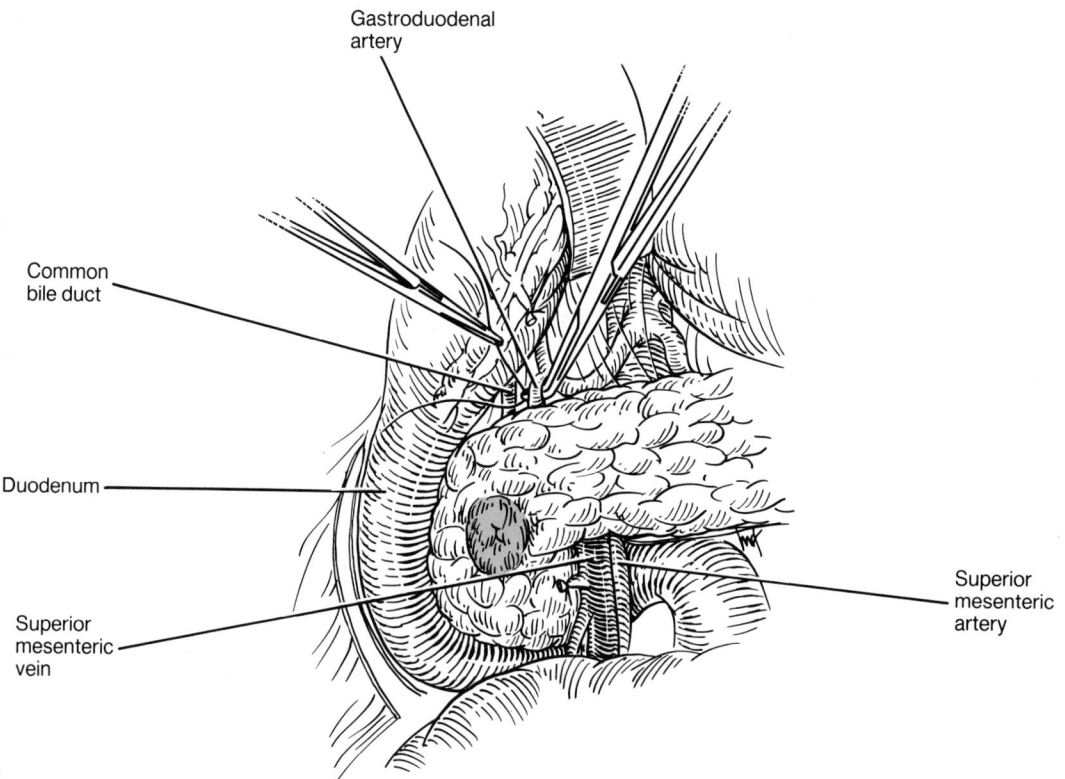

Gastroduodenal artery

Common bile duct

Duodenum

Superior mesenteric vein

Superior mesenteric artery

Figure 30-VA-9

Identification and Ligation of Gastroduodenal Artery

After partial definition of the plane between the neck of the pancreas and the superior mesenteric vein from below the pancreas, it is advantageous to establish the same plane from above the pancreas. To facilitate this, the gastroduodenal artery is ligated with 2-0 silk ties and divided. The closure of the hepatic end of the gastroduodenal artery is reinforced with a 2-0 silk suture ligature. After ligation of the gastroduodenal artery, gentle dissection between the common hepatic artery and the common bile duct reveals the anterior surface of the portal vein.

1046

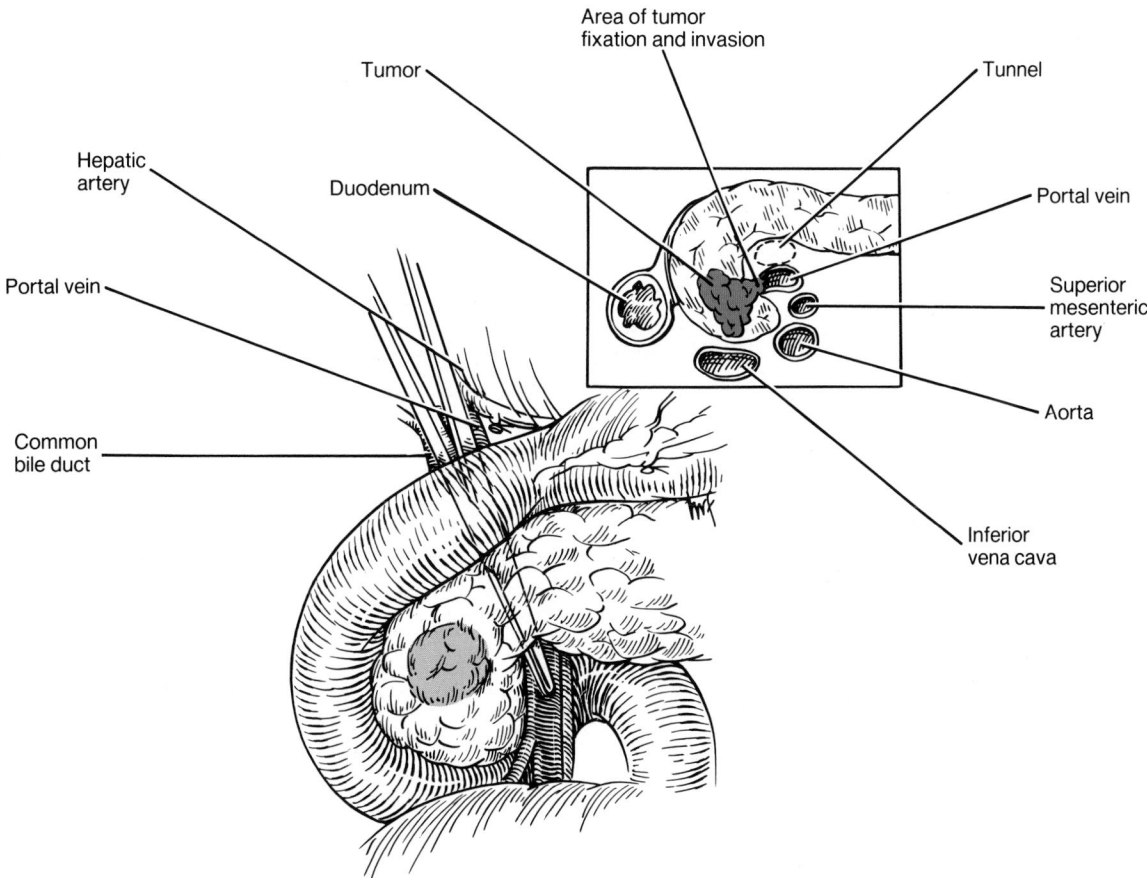

Figure 30-VA-10

Completion of Tunnel Under Pancreas

A plane of dissection is established on the anterior surface of the portal vein and the vein followed inferiorly beneath the neck of the pancreas. By combined gentle probing from above and below the pancreas, a continuous tunnel behind the neck of the pancreas anterior to the portal and superior mesenteric veins is established. If this plane is blocked, the carcinoma is assumed to have invaded the portal vein, and attempts at resection are ordinarily abandoned.

Carcinoma may involve the portal vein posterolaterally even when the tunnel anterior to the veins is patent (**inset**). In this situation, the neck of the pancreas can be safely divided, but in the later stages of the operation, the surgeon becomes aware of the fact that the tumor is adherent to the lateral side of the superior mesenteric or portal vein. In such cases, segmental resection of the veins may be required to avoid a positive tissue margin.

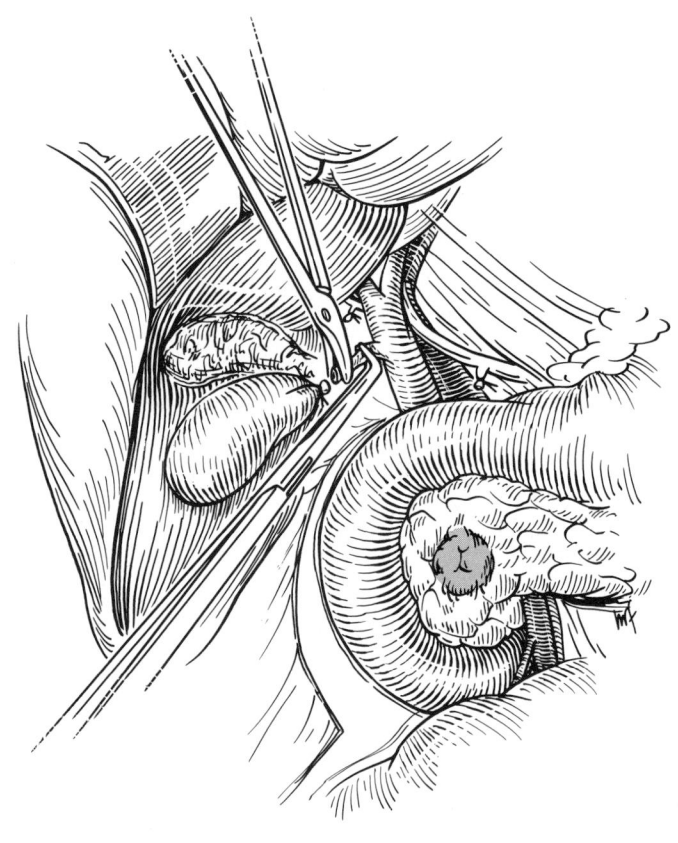

Figure 30-VA-11

Cholecystectomy

At this point in the operation, the surgeon has committed to resection of the tumor, and the extirpating portion of the procedure begins. The cystic duct and cystic artery are ligated with 2-0 silk ties and divided, and the gallbladder is removed.

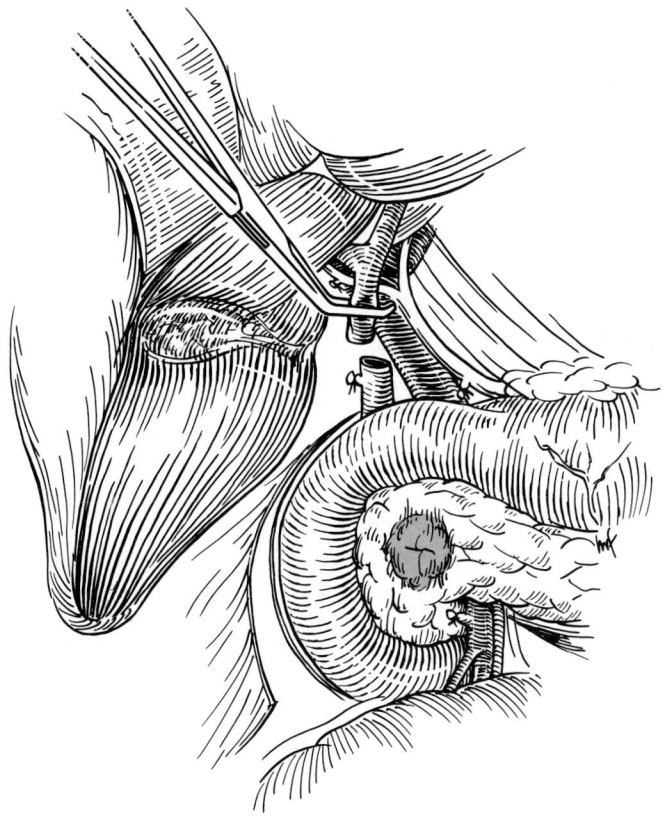

Figure 30-VA-12

Division of Common Hepatic Duct

The common hepatic duct is dissected circumferentially over a short distance just above the entrance of the cystic duct. A fine vascular clamp is placed across the common hepatic duct, and the duct is divided below the clamp.

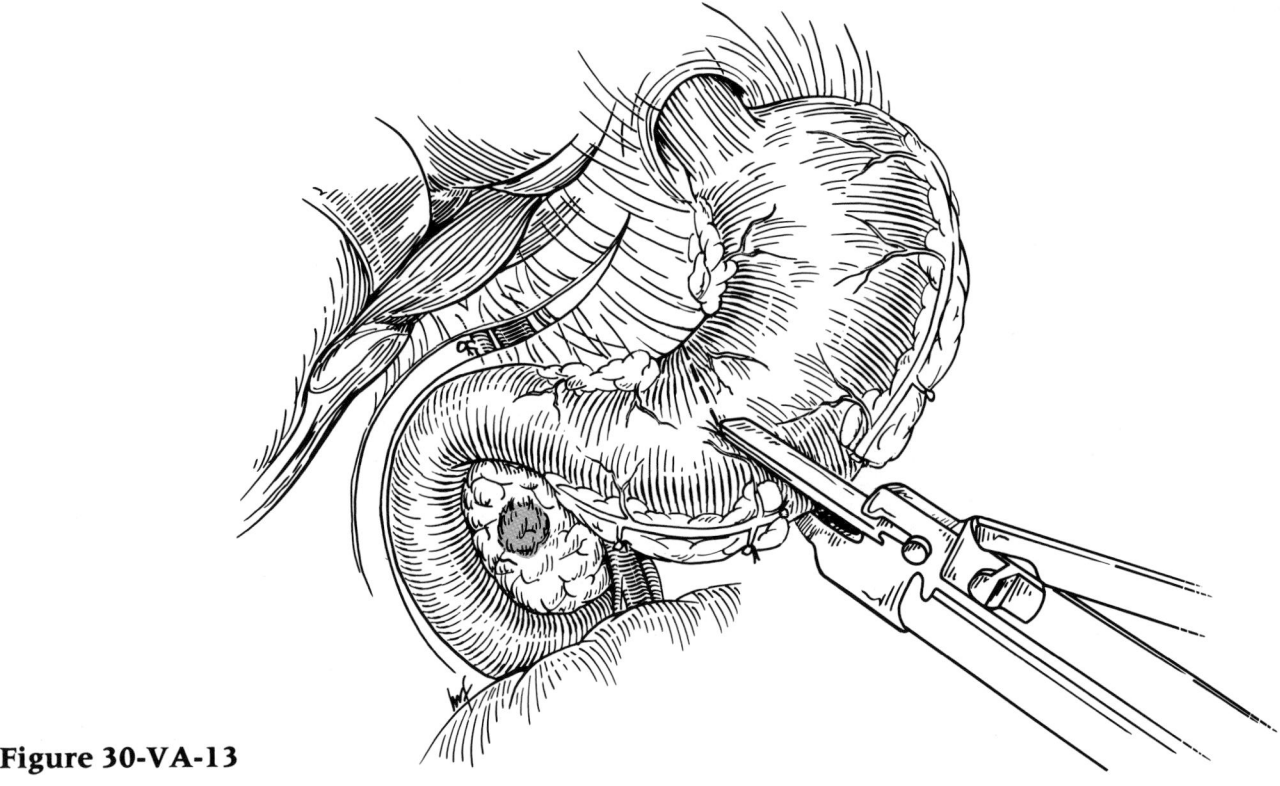

Figure 30-VA-13

Division of Stomach

After cleaning a short segment of the greater and lesser curvature of the stomach for subsequent anastomosis, the stomach is divided with a gastrointestinal stapler. Two fires of the stapler are usually required. The extent of resection is about a 40% distal gastrectomy.

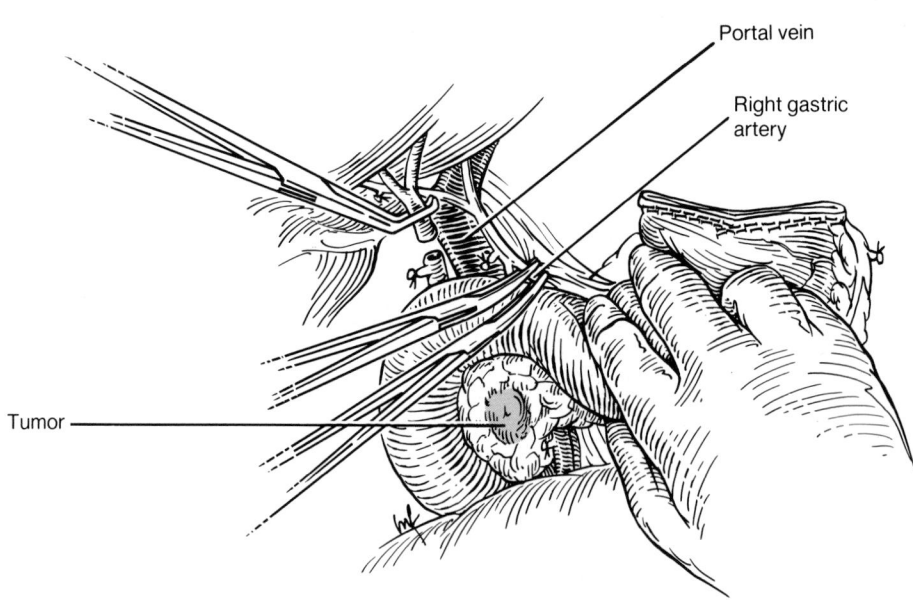

Figure 30-VA-14

Dissection of Distal Stomach

After division of the stomach, the lesser omentum is divided between clamps and ligated with 2-0 silk ties, moving distally along the lesser curvature of the stomach. This dissection is completed by clamping, dividing, and ligating the right gastric artery at its origin from the common hepatic artery.

1050

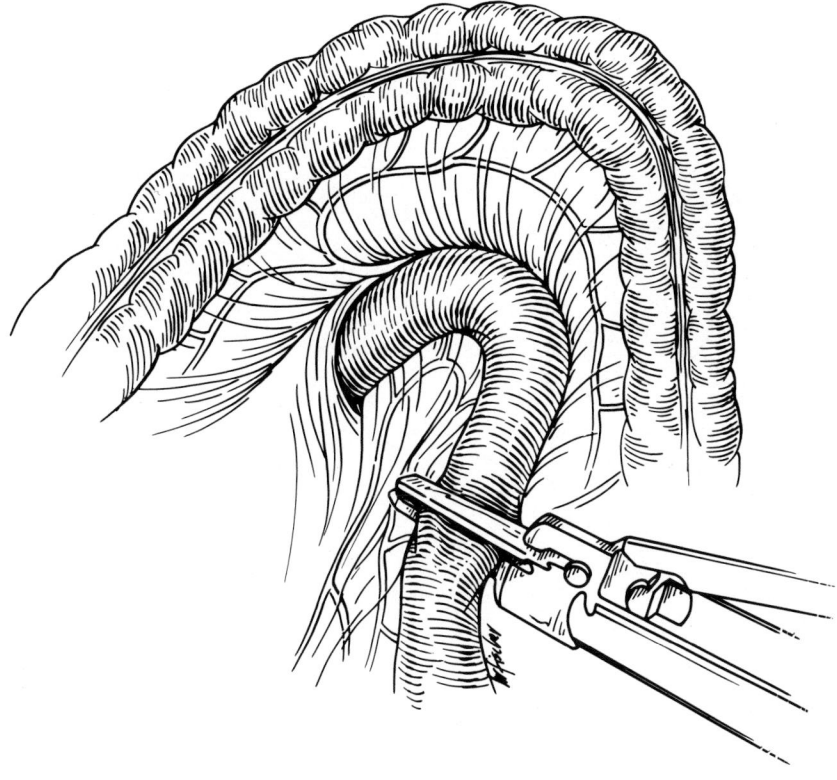

Figure 30-VA-15

Division of Jejunum

Attention is then turned to resection of the distal duodenum and proximal jejunum and preparation of the jejunum for later anastomosis to the pancreas, hepatic duct, and stomach. The transverse colon and mesocolon are retracted upward, and the ligament of Treitz is identified. After clearing the mesentery from a 1- to 1.5-cm segment of proximal jejunum, the small bowel is divided with a gastrointestinal stapler. The site of jejunal transection is usually about 15 cm below the ligament of Treitz, choosing the point where the jejunal mesentery appears to offer the most mobility for bringing the small bowel into the upper abdomen for subsequent anastomosis.

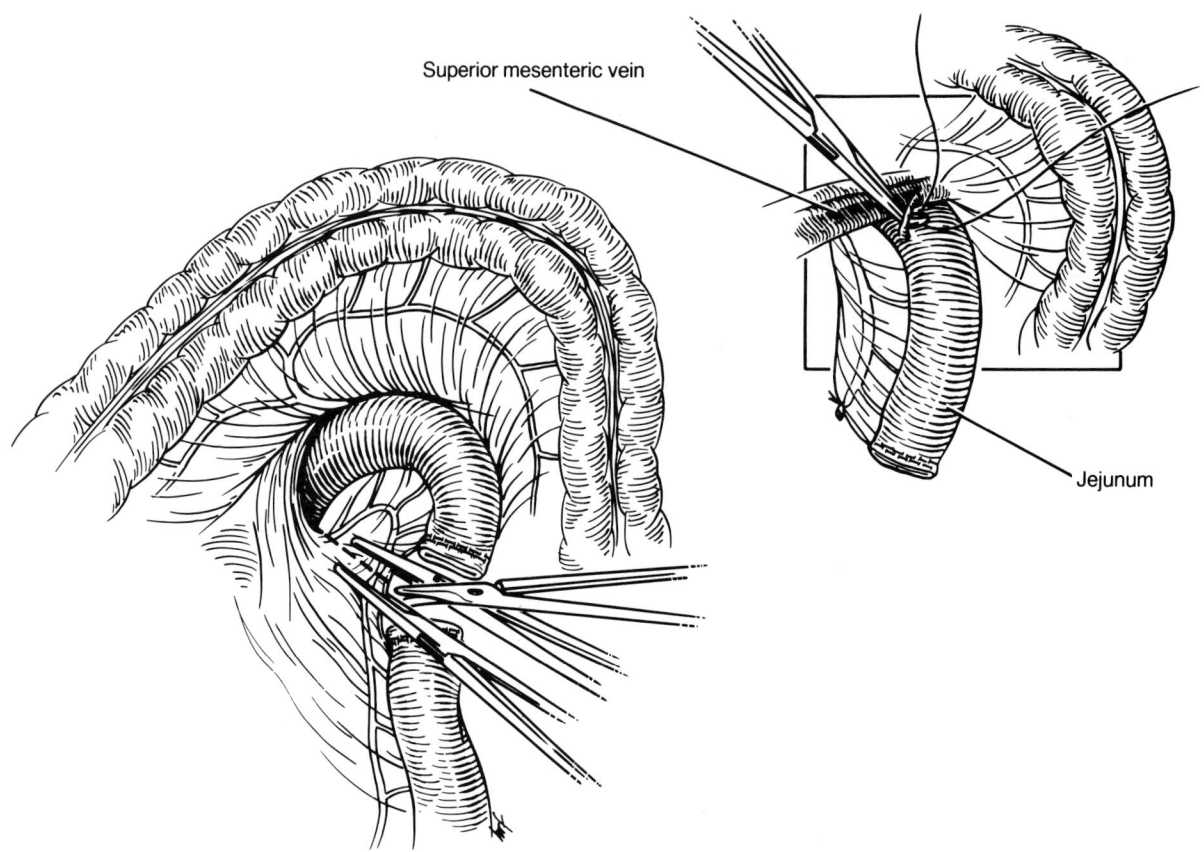

Figure 30-VA-16

Dissection of Jejunal Mesentery

After transection of the jejunum, the mesentery is divided along a line upward toward the superior mesenteric vessels as the vessels pass over the fourth portion of the duodenum. The ligament of Treitz is also completely divided to provide full mobility to the proximal jejunal segment. As the dissection nears completion, small arterial and venous branches from the superior mesenteric vessels to the very proximal jejunum must be ligated with silk ties and divided (**inset**) so that the jejunum can be passed completely beneath the superior mesenteric vessels to emerge on the right side of the vessels.

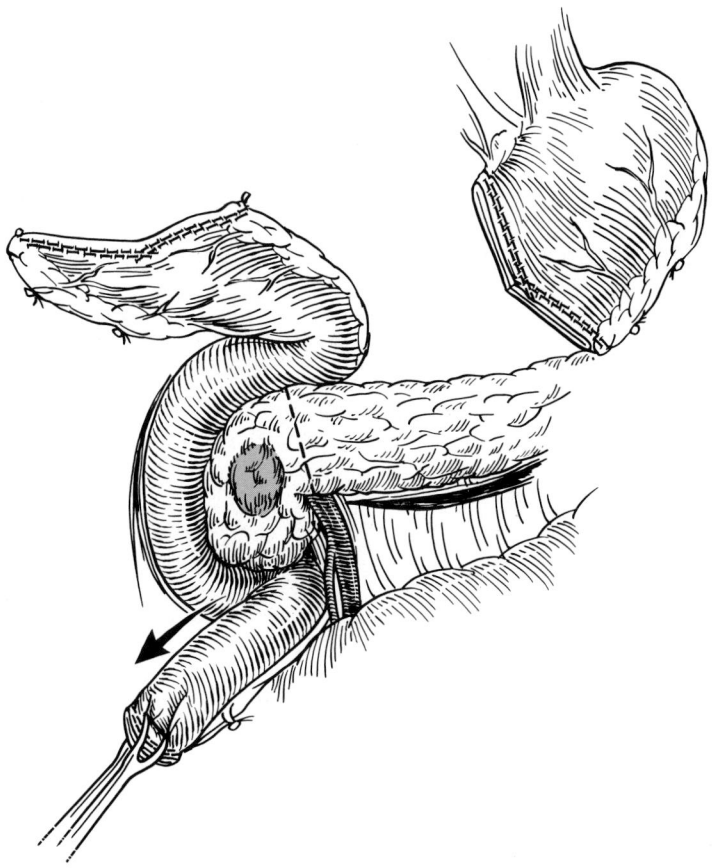

Figure 30-VA-17

Passage of Jejunum Beneath Superior Mesenteric Vessels

The freed jejunum and fourth portion of the duodenum are passed beneath the superior mesenteric vessels to emerge on their right side. If the jejunum cannot be freely passed beneath the vessels, it should be returned to the left side of the abdomen and further dissection of the jejunal mesentery completed before again attempting to pass the bowel beneath the vessels.

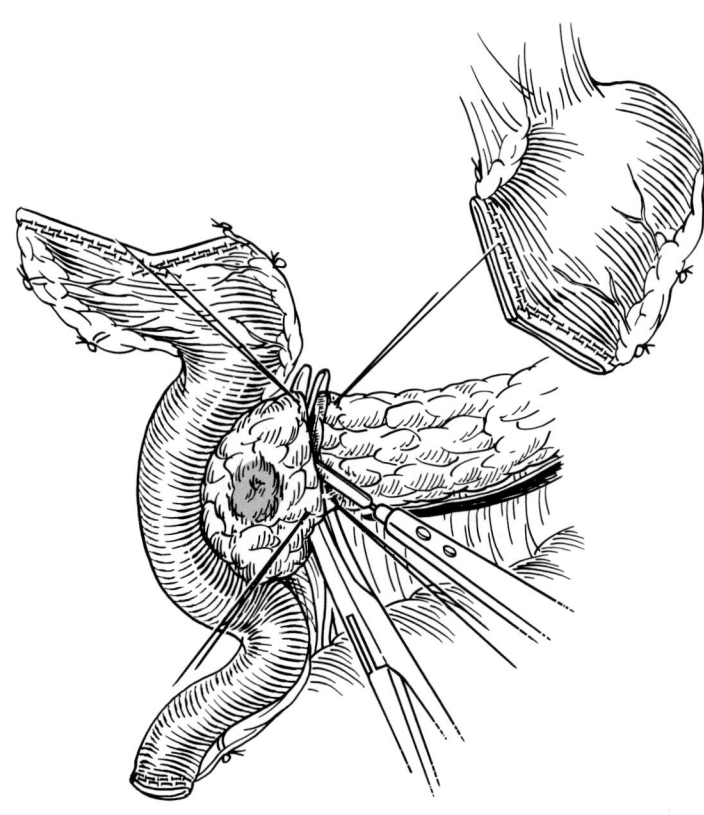

Figure 30-VA-18

Division of Pancreatic Neck

With the stomach and proximal jejunum now retracted to the right, the neck of the pancreas is divided with electrocautery. A large clamp or similar guide is placed beneath the neck of the pancreas anterior to the superior mesenteric and portal veins to prevent inadvertent cautery injury to the veins. Before division of the gland, hemostatic sutures of 3-0 silk are traditionally placed at the upper and lower borders of the pancreas to prevent bleeding from the marginal arteries supplying the neck of the pancreas. If bleeding occurs from the cut pancreatic edges despite this maneuver, it can be easily controlled with suture ligatures of 3-0 silk placed into the pancreatic parenchyma around the responsible vessel, taking care to avoid inadvertent incorporation of the pancreatic duct in the ligature.

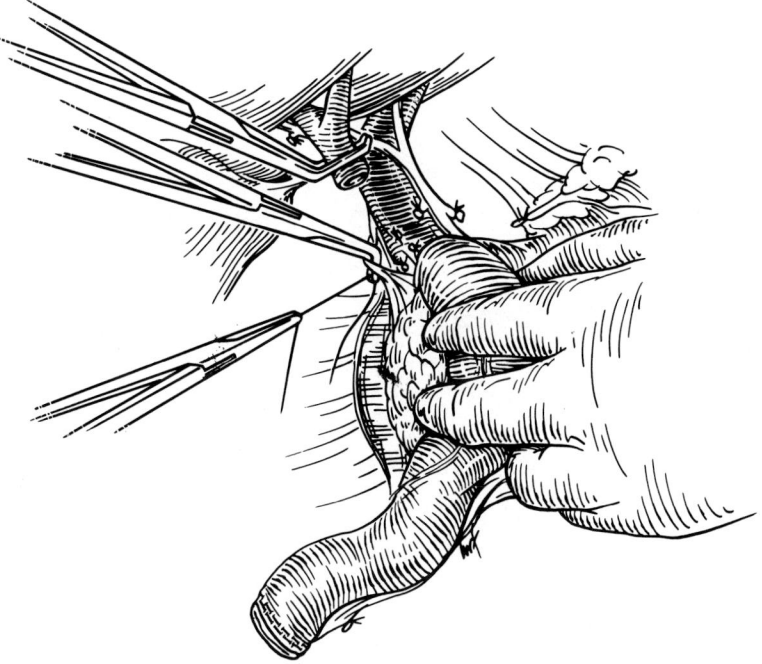

Figure 30-VA-19

Resection of Soft Tissue

Soft tissue on the right lateral aspect of the portal vein is progressively divided between silk ligatures. Ordinarily, lymph nodes are present along the lateral aspect of the lower portal vein. These should be included with the specimen to be resected as the portal vein is skeletonized.

At the lower portion of this dissection, the posterior superior pancreaticoduodenal vein is encountered entering the portal vein posterolaterally from the head of the pancreas. It is a short and fragile vein and easily torn if not carefully dissected. It should be ligated with fine silk ties and divided.

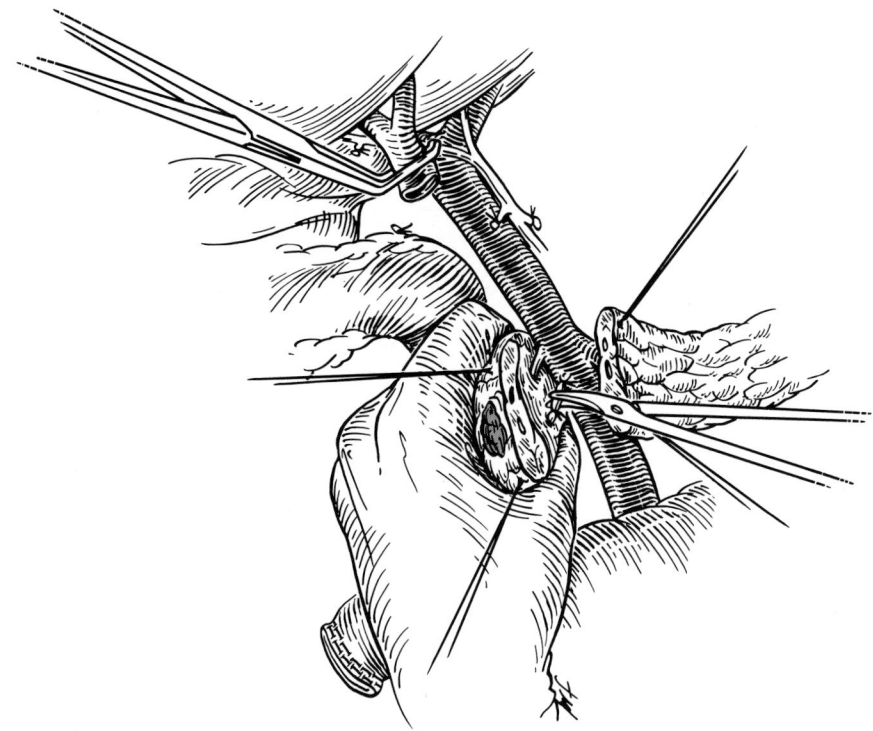

Figure 30-VA-20

Ligation of Branches of Portal Vein to Pancreatic Head

Any remaining veins entering the portal or superior mesenteric veins from the head and uncinate process of the pancreas are carefully ligated with fine silk ties and divided. Retracting the head of the pancreas gently to the right and rolling the portal vein away from the head of the pancreas improves exposure of these short veins.

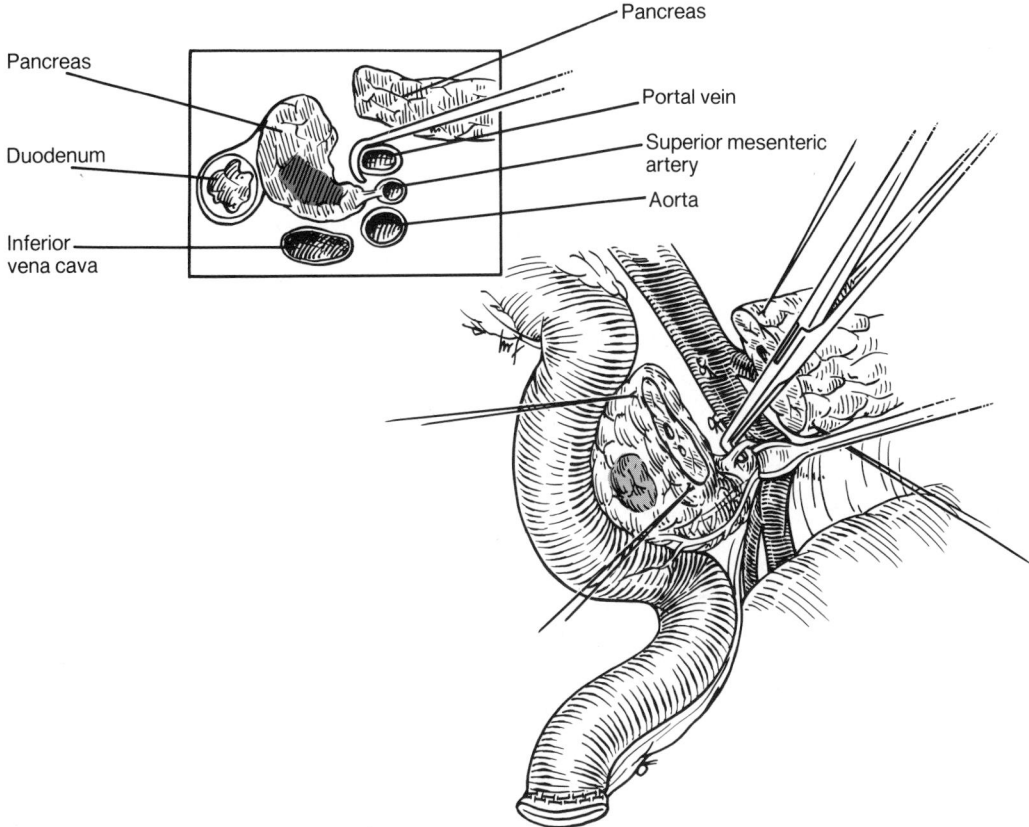

Figure 30-VA-21

Resection of Uncinate Process

As the last step in the resection, the uncinate process of the pancreas is gradually excised by retracting the portal and superior mesenteric veins to the left and dividing the tissue connecting the uncinate process to the superior mesenteric artery (**inset**). This dissection should parallel the artery; in the course of removing the uncinate process, the inferior pancreaticoduodenal artery is divided shortly before removing the specimen.

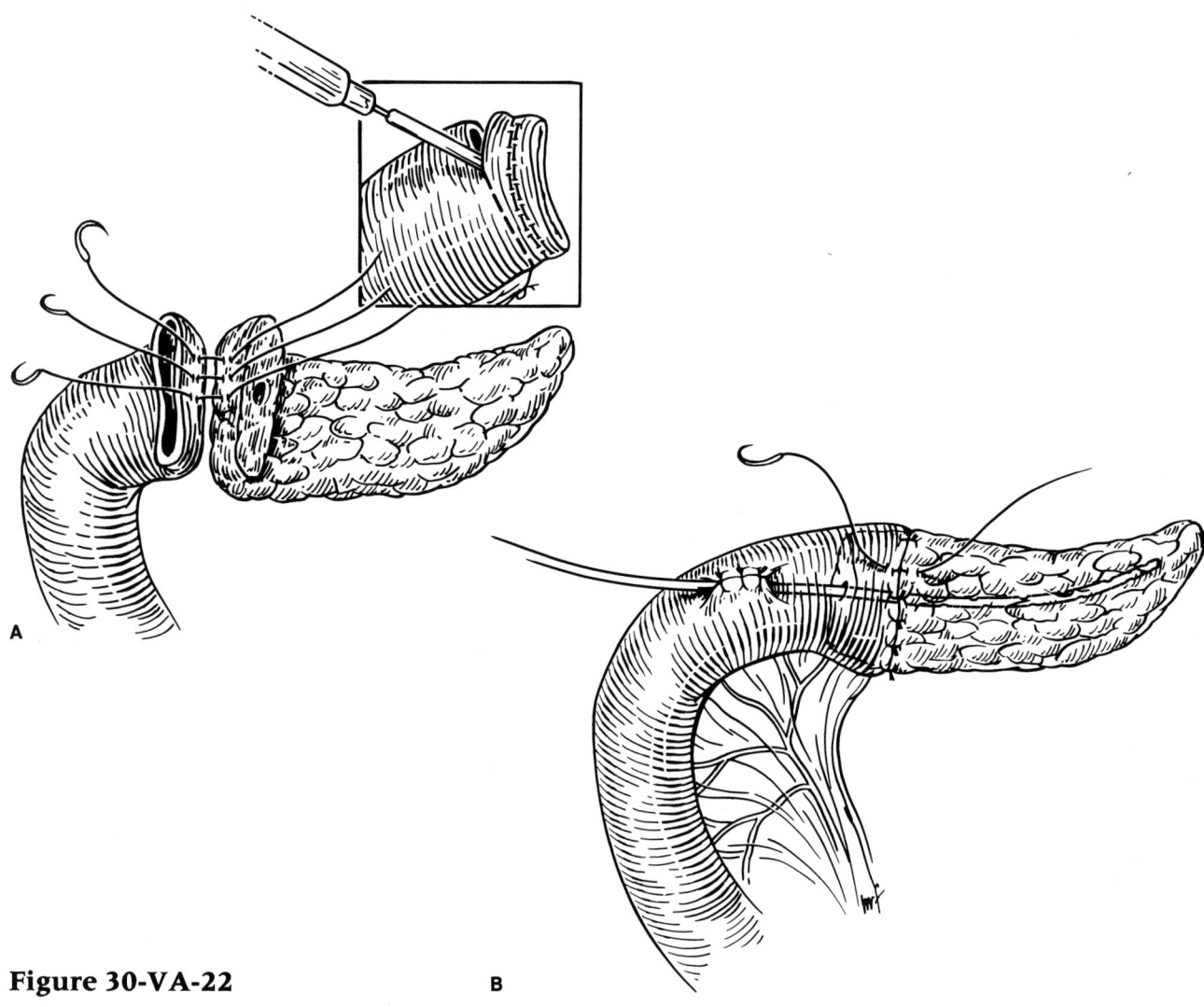

Figure 30-VA-22

B

Pancreatic Anastomosis: Invaginating Technique

After removal of the operative specimen, a retrocolic anastomosis between the pancreas and jejunum is performed. A number of techniques for pancreaticojejunostomy have been described. This figure demonstrates a straightforward end-to-end inversion of the tip of the pancreatic remnant into the jejunum.

(**A**) The staple line at the end of the jejunum is excised (**inset**). A series of 3-0 silk sutures are placed between the seromuscular coat of the posterior jejunum and the posterior aspect of the pancreatic capsule. The sutures in the pancreas should be placed deeply enough to be sure that they do not tear out when tied.

(**B**) Before placing the anterior row of the anastomosis, a 5F feeding tube with multiple end holes is inserted into the jejunal limb and passed into the pancreatic duct as far as possible. The feeding tube is attached to the cut edge of the pancreas with a single 3-0 suture to prevent it from dislodging. The exit site of the tube from the jejunum is covered with a series of interrupted 3-0 silk Lembert sutures.

The anastomosis is completed by sewing the seromuscular coat of the anterior jejunum to the anterior pancreatic capsule. The sutures in the pancreas are placed about 1.5 cm back from the cut edge of pancreas to encourage invagination of the pancreatic remnant into the jejunum when tied.

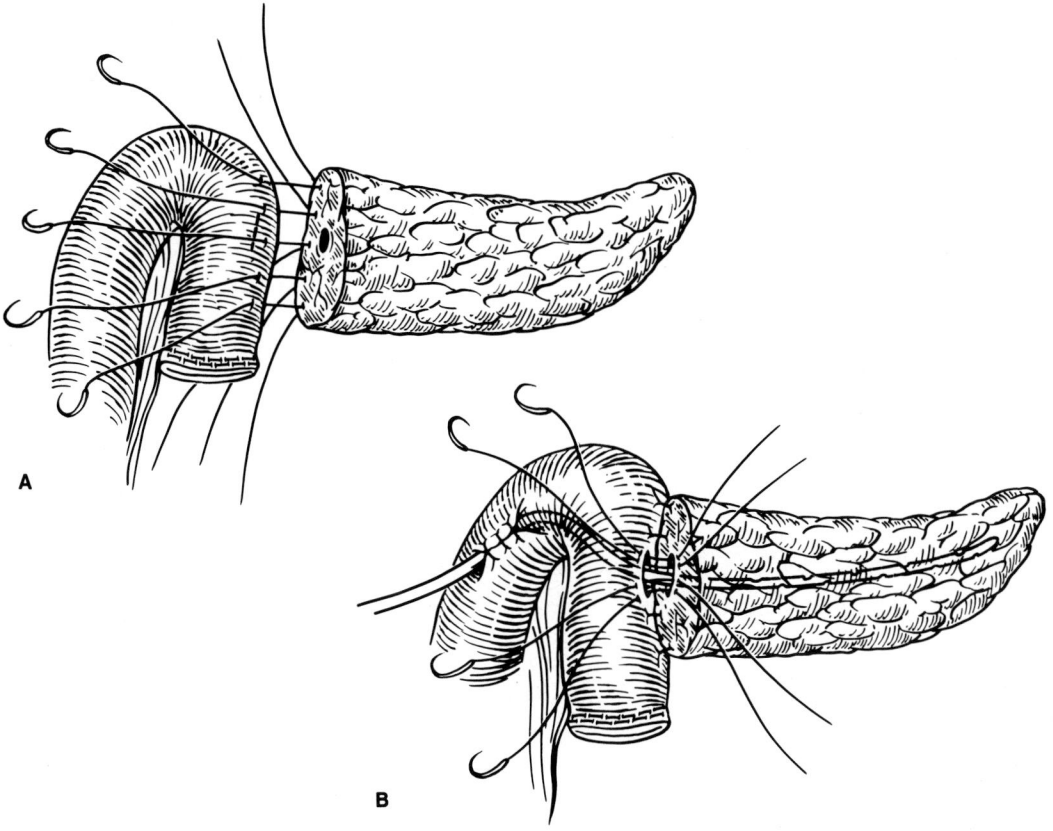

Figure 30-VA-23

Pancreatic Anastomosis: Duct-to-Mucosa Technique

This figure demonstrates an alternative method of pancreaticojejunostomy that includes an end-to-side mucosal anastomosis of the pancreatic duct to the bowel. This method of anastomosis is most appropriate when the pancreatic duct is dilated and the body of the gland is firm.

(**A**) The anastomosis begins by placing a series of Lembert sutures of 3-0 silk from the seromuscular coat of the jejunum to the posterior aspect of the cut edge of the pancreas. Using electrocautery, a small jejunotomy corresponding to the size of the pancreatic duct is created.

(**B**) Interrupted 3-0 absorbable sutures are then placed between the posterior edge of the jejunotomy (full thickness) and the posterior aspect of the pancreatic duct. After completion of the posterior row of the ductal anastomosis, a 5F feeding tube with multiple end-holes is passed into the jejunum and then into the pancreatic duct as far as possible. The exit point of the tube from the jejunum is buried under interrupted 3-0 silk Lembert sutures. After placement of the feeding tube, the anterior row of the ductal anastomosis is completed as shown.

(Continued)

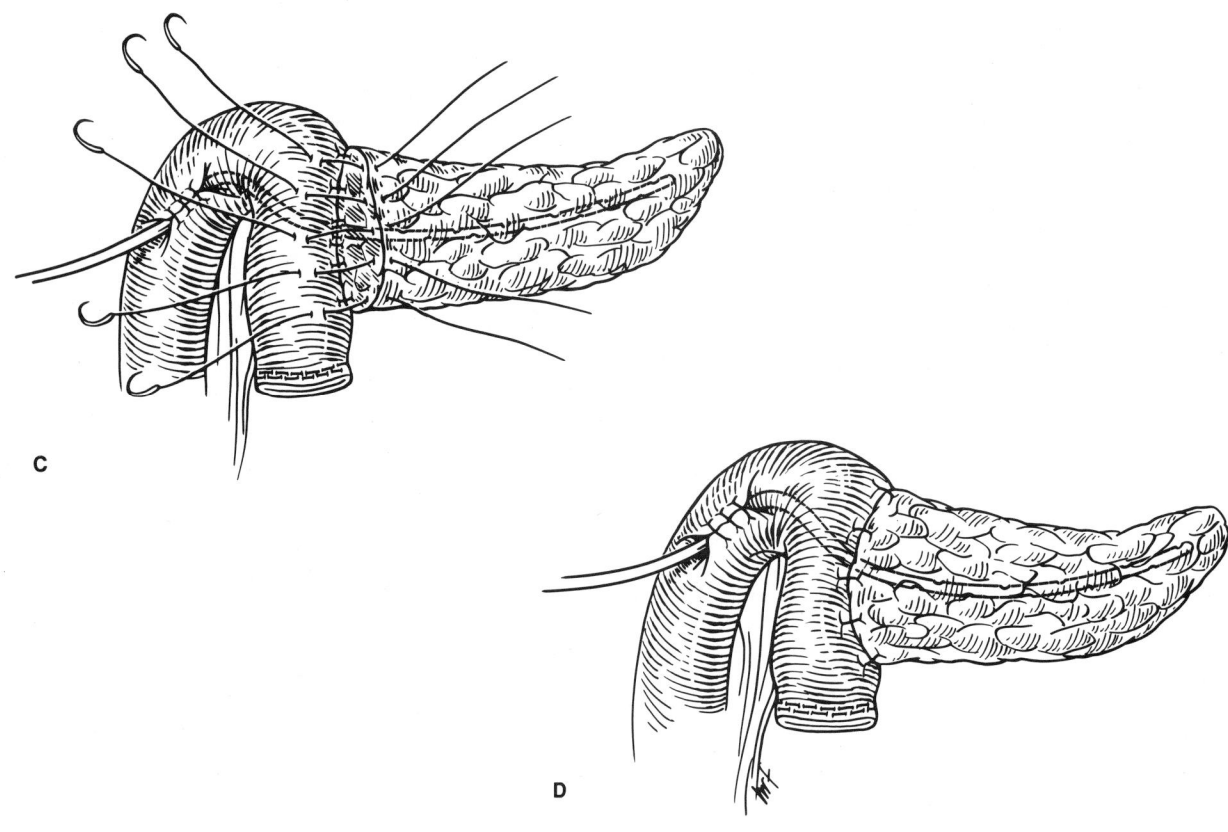

Figure 30-VA-23 *(Continued)*

(**C**) The anterior outer layer of the anastomosis is completed by placing interrupted 3-0 silk sutures between the seromuscular coat of the jejunum and the anterior pancreatic capsule.

(**D**) The completed duct-to-mucosa anastomosis.

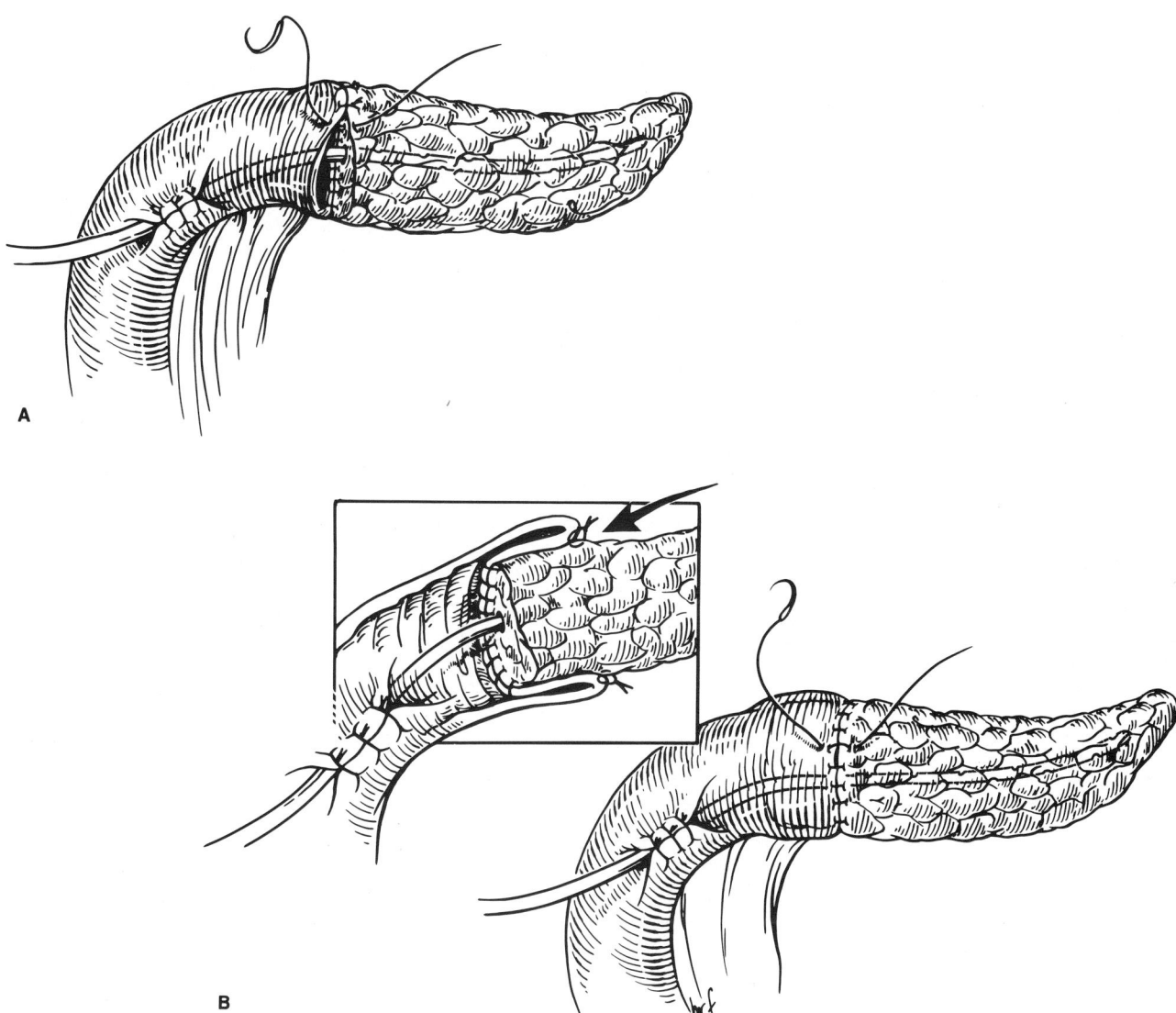

Figure 30-VA-24

Pancreatic Anastomosis: Intussusception Technique

A final method of pancreaticojejunostomy is shown in this figure. This method involves intussuscepting the end of the pancreatic remnant into the open end of jejunum. To provide sufficient pancreatic length for invagination into the jejunum, the pancreatic remnant must be cleared circumferentially for a distance of about 2 cm.

(**A**) The anastomosis is begun by placing interrupted 3-0 silk sutures between the full-thickness end of jejunum and the cut edge of the pancreatic remnant. After completing the posterior portion of this layer of the anastomosis, a 5F feeding tube with multiple end-holes is placed into the pancreatic duct through the jejunum. The anterior portion of this layer of the anastomosis is then completed as shown. The entrance site of the jejunal tube is buried with interrupted 3-0 silk Lembert sutures.

(**B**) The pancreatic remnant is then gently pushed into the jejunal lumen while at the same time rolling the jejunum up over the end of the pancreas to create a intussusception (**inset**). The rounded edge of jejunum that has been advanced over the pancreas is then sutured to the pancreatic capsule with interrupted sutures of 3-0 silk.

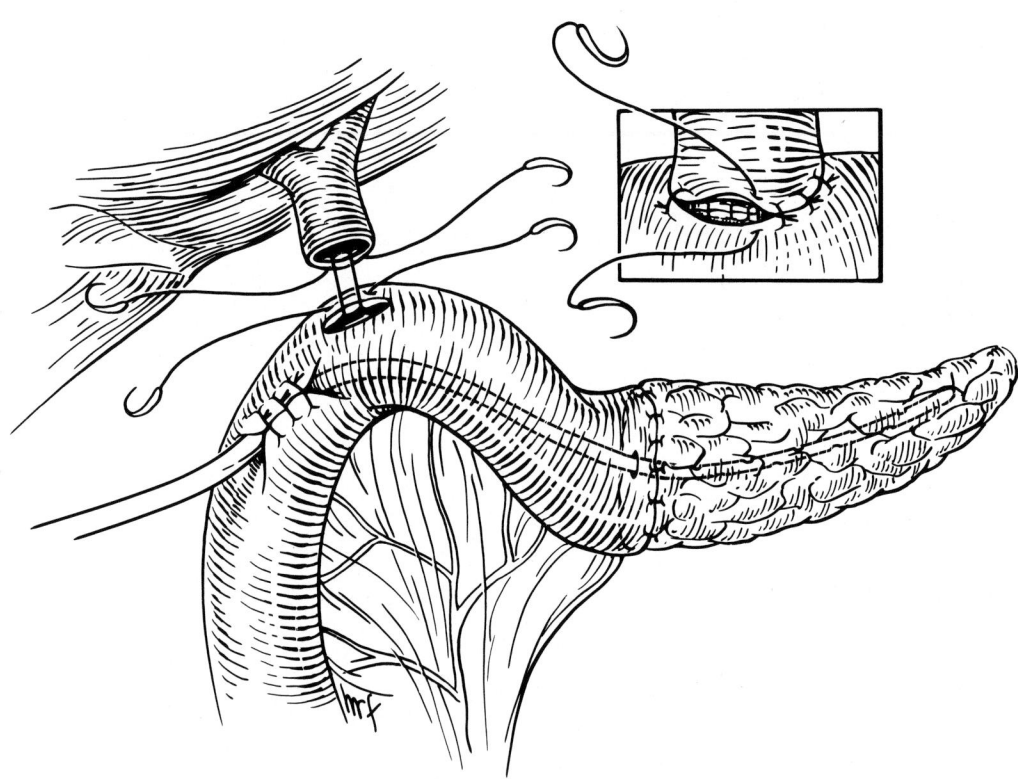

Figure 30-VA-25

Bile Duct Anastomosis

After completion of the pancreaticojejunostomy, the end of the common hepatic duct is sewn to a convenient location on the side of the jejunum. A small enterotomy is made on the antimesenteric side of the jejunum, and the anastomosis is performed with interrupted sutures of 4-0 or 5-0 nonabsorbable monofilament suture, incorporating full-thickness bites of both the bowel and duct, with the knots on the outside of the anastomosis. The anterior wall of the anastomosis is shown in the inset.

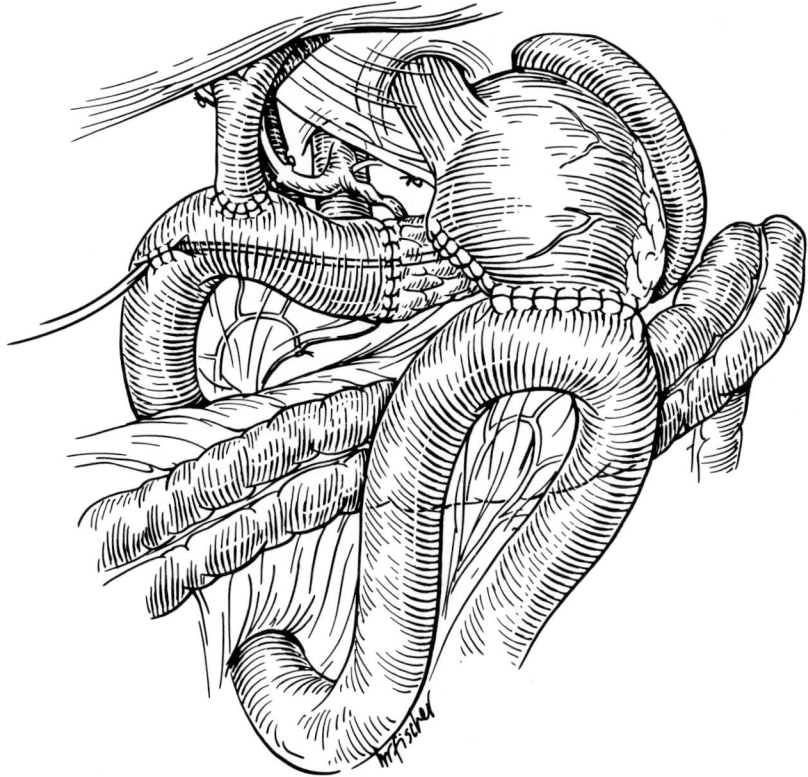

Figure 30-VA-26

Completed Procedure With Gastrojejunostomy

The operation is completed by performing an antecolic gastrojejunostomy. A portion of the gastric staple line extending up the lesser curvature of the stomach is oversewn with interrupted Lembert sutures of 3-0 silk. The remainder of the staple line (about 2.5-cm long) is left exposed in the area chosen for anastomosis to the jejunum.

The anastomosis is begun by placing interrupted sutures of 3-0 silk between the jejunum and the stomach posterior to the staple line. The exposed staple line on the stomach is excised, and a corresponding enterotomy is made on the antimesenteric border of the jejunum. The inner layer of the anastomosis is performed with a running 3-0 absorbable suture. The gastrojejunostomy is completed with an anterior outer row of interrupted 3-0 silk sutures.

A soft closed-suction drain (*not shown*) should be placed immediately adjacent to the pancreaticojejunostomy and brought out through a separate stab incision in the right flank.

B. Pylorus-Preserving Variant of Pancreaticoduodenectomy

In the pylorus-preserving variant of pancreaticoduodenectomy, no gastric resection is performed, the pylorus and first 1 to 2 cm of the duodenum are preserved, and an end-to-side duodenojejunostomy is performed after resection of the pancreatic head and remainder of the duodenum.

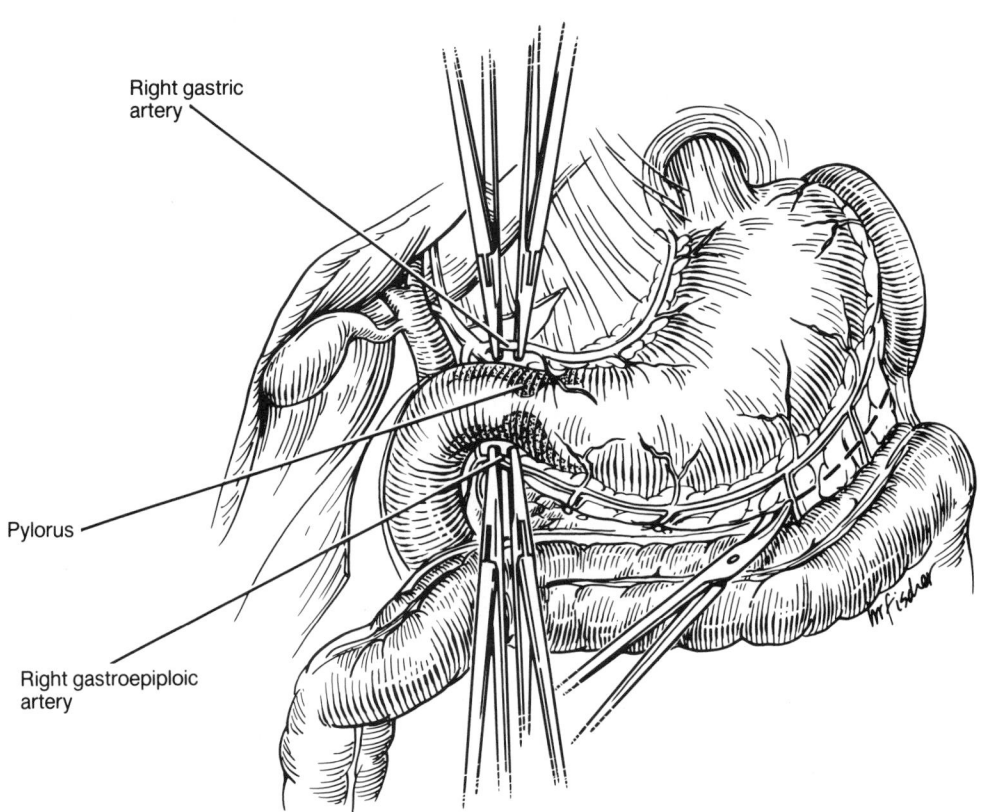

Right gastric artery

Pylorus

Right gastroepiploic artery

Figure 30-VB-1

Ligation of Right Gastric and Gastroepiploic Arteries

In performing a pylorus-preserving pancreaticoduodenectomy, it is critical to maintain the blood supply to the distal stomach and pyloric area. For this reason, the division of the right gastric artery and the right gastroepiploic artery takes place as close to the origin of those arteries as possible.

The incision made in the gastrocolic omentum for exposure of the pancreas must be made outside the right gastroepiploic vessels (*dashed line*).

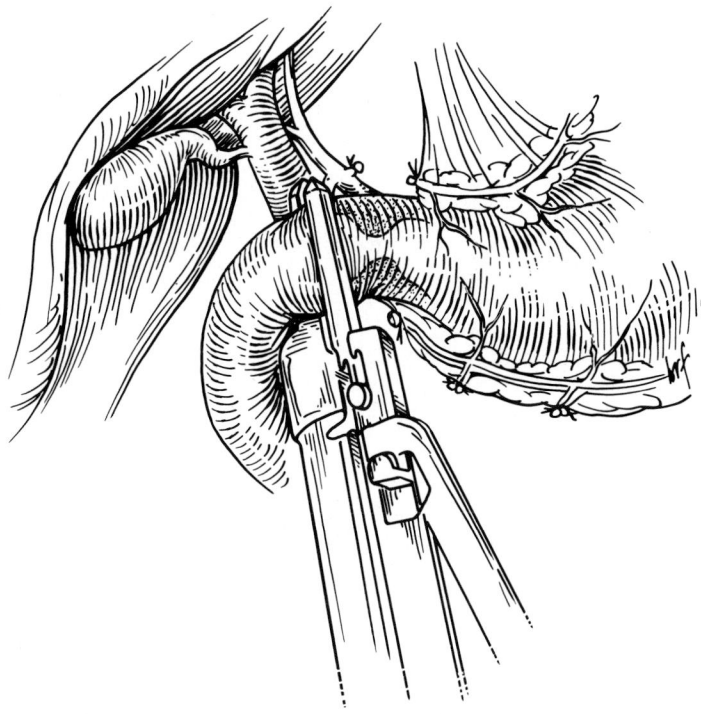

Figure 30-VB-2

Site of Division of Duodenum

The duodenum is divided 1 to 2 cm distal to the pylorus with a gastrointestinal stapler.

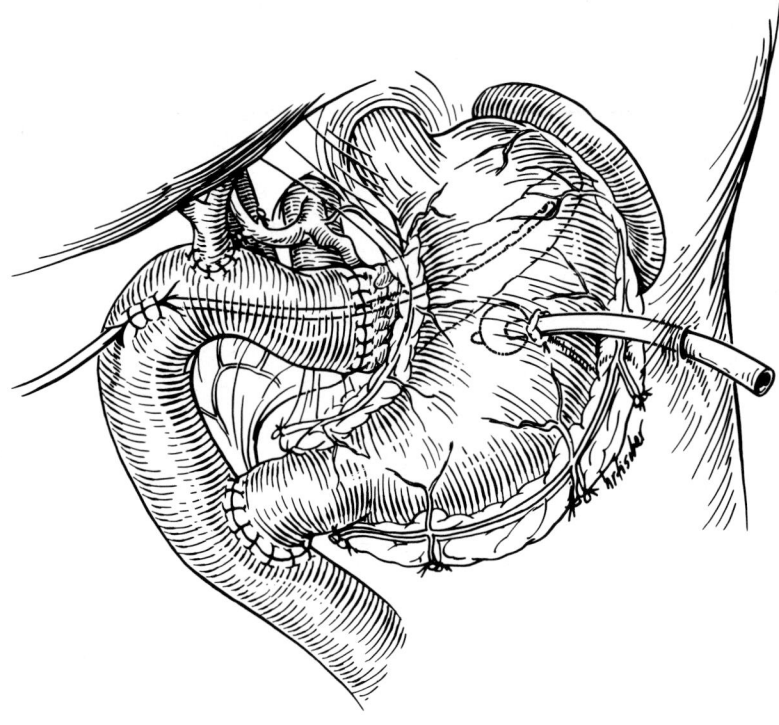

Figure 30-VB-3

Completed Anastomoses

The completed pylorus-preserving variant of pancreaticoduodenectomy. The pancreatic and hepatic duct anastomoses are identical to those in a standard pancreaticoduodenectomy. The anastomosis of the end of the proximal duodenum to the side of the jejunum is performed in two layers, using an outer layer of interrupted 3-0 silk seromuscular sutures and an inner layer of continuous 3-0 absorbable full-thickness sutures.

Because patients undergoing pylorus-sparing pancreaticoduodenectomy frequently experience a prolonged postoperative delay in gastric emptying, the placement of a gastrostomy tube, as shown, can provide enhanced comfort. A feeding jejunostomy tube (*not shown*) should also be strongly considered.

C. Pancreaticoduodenectomy With Radical Lymphadenectomy for Carcinoma of the Head of the Pancreas

Some surgeons advocate an extensive lymphadenectomy and resection of retroperitoneal soft tissue as an integral part of pancreaticoduodenectomy. The value of this extended resection is not clearly established, but it is being practiced with increased frequency.

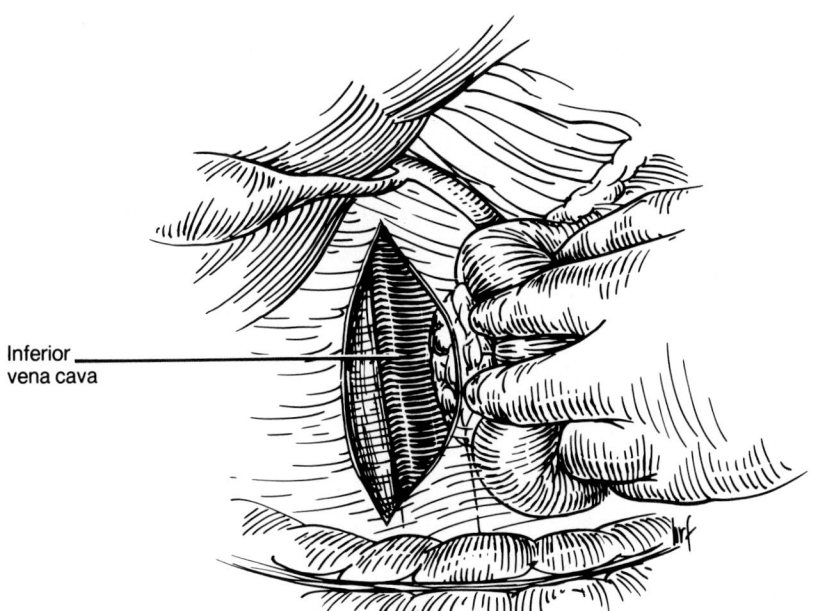

Inferior vena cava

Figure 30-VC-1

Wider Kocher Maneuver

In the initial phases of the procedure, a wider than customary Kocher maneuver is performed by making the peritoneal incision about 2 cm more lateral to the duodenum than is usual. Dissection is carried down immediately to the surface of the inferior vena cava, and the anterior surface of the vena cava is skeletonized, including all soft tissue anterior to the vena cava in the specimen to be resected.

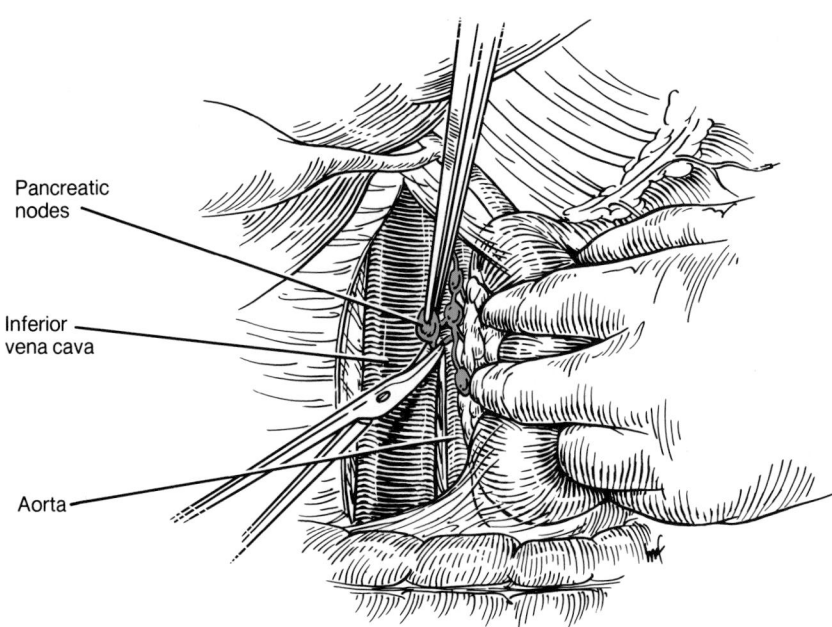

Figure 30-VC-2

Resection of Soft Tissue and Lymph Nodes

As a part of the extended resection of retroperitoneal soft tissue, lymph nodes in the aortocaval groove are dissected in continuity with the pancreatic specimen.

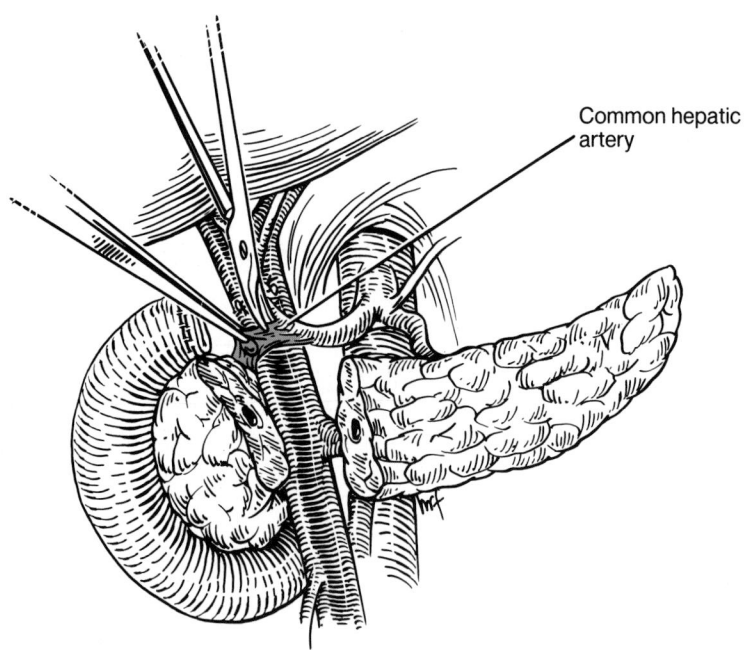

Figure 30-VC-3

Skeletonization of Celiac Axis

An extensive soft tissue clearance is performed around the common hepatic artery. The line of division of the pancreas is moved slightly to the left to expose the area around the origin of the hepatic artery and the remainder of the celiac axis and to allow the removal of additional nodes along the superior and inferior borders of the pancreas. Some surgeons advocate complete clearance of soft tissue around the base of the celiac artery, although this maneuver can increase postoperative complications and is not uniformly practiced.

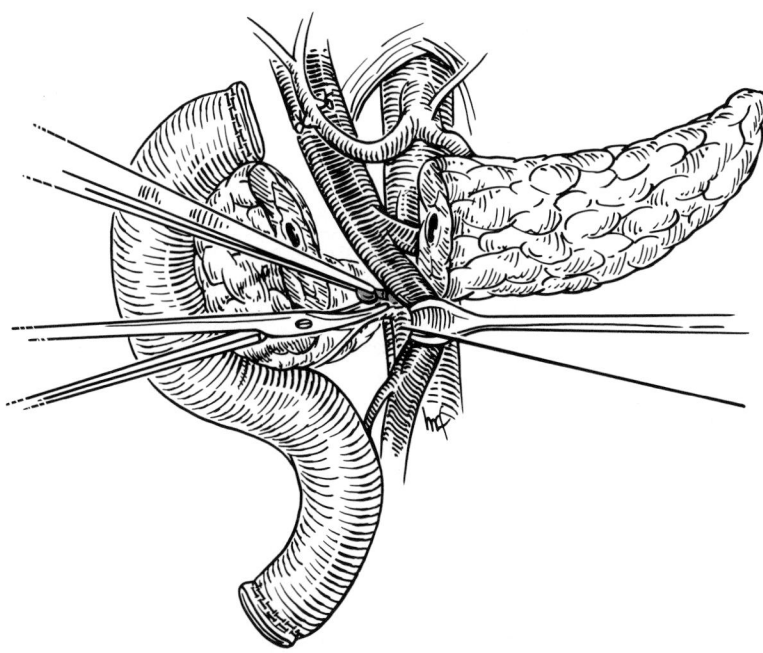

Figure 30-VC-4

Skeletonization of Superior Mesenteric Artery

One of the potentially most important features of extended pancreaticoduodenectomy is the complete skeletonization of the superior mesenteric artery as the uncinate process of the pancreas is removed near the conclusion of the pancreatic resection. This is an area where resection margins positive for carcinoma are relatively common in traditional pancreaticoduodenectomy.

By retracting the portal and superior mesenteric veins up and to the left, the superior mesenteric artery is identified and the plane of dissection continued immediately along the artery, a plane about 1 cm farther to the left than in a traditional pancreaticoduodenectomy. Care must be taken not to injure the superior mesenteric artery in the course of this dissection.

D. Palliative Procedures for Unresectable Carcinoma of the Head of the Pancreas

Traditionally, choledochojejunostomy is recommended for relief of jaundice in patients found to have nonresectable carcinoma of the pancreas at laparotomy. Cholecystojejunostomy is also a satisfactory and simpler alternative if the cystic duct is patent and at least 1 cm removed from the tumor mass, and if the gallbladder is not diseased. If the conditions permitting cholecystojejunostomy are not present, choledochojejunostomy is indicated and can be performed as an end-to-side or side-to-side anastomosis between the common hepatic duct and a Roux-en-Y limb of jejunum. The side-to-side technique is somewhat easier, but an end-to side technique is preferable when the duct is not significantly enlarged, as is often the case when the duct has been stented preoperatively.

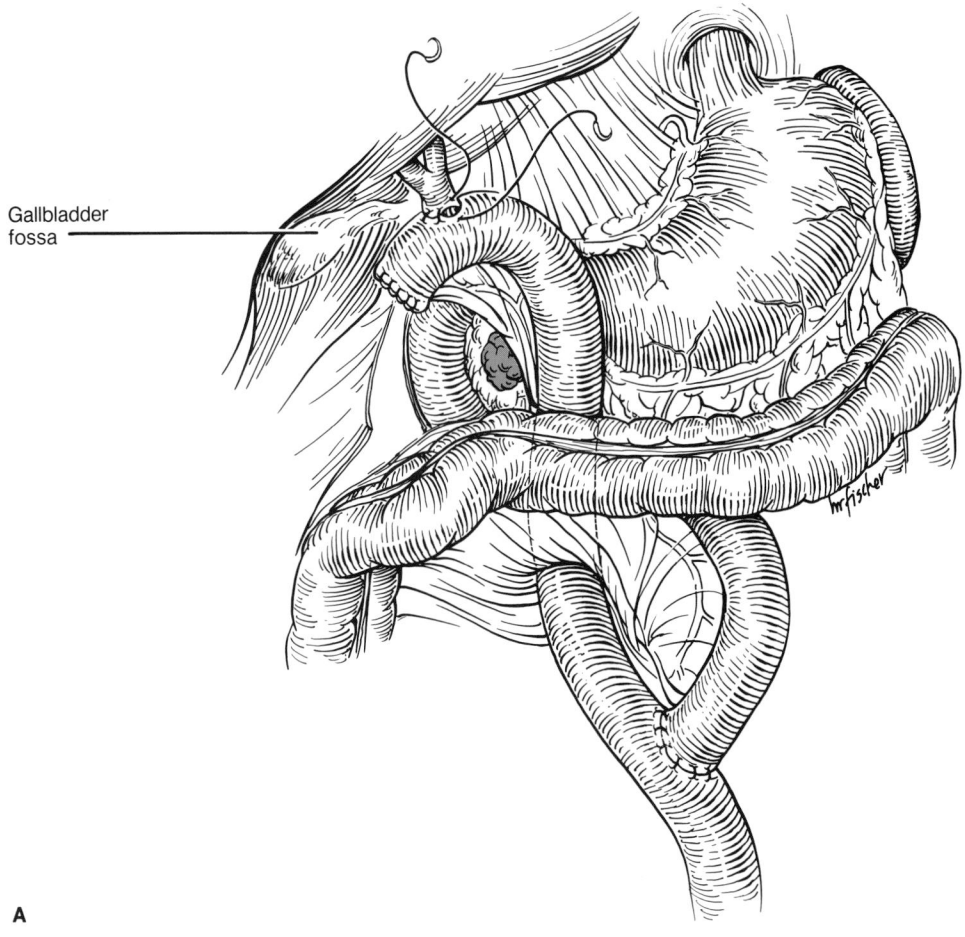

Gallbladder fossa

A

Figure 30-VD-1

Choledochojejunostomy

(**A**) In the end-to-side technique, the gallbladder is removed. The common hepatic duct is divided just above the entrance of the cystic duct, and the distal common duct is oversewn. The proximal duct is anastomosed in a single layer to an equivalent-size enterotomy in the Roux-en-Y limb using interrupted 4-0 or 5-0 monofilament nonabsorbable sutures with the knots tied on the outside of the anastomosis. A soft closed-suction drain (*not shown*) is ordinarily placed adjacent to the anastomosis.

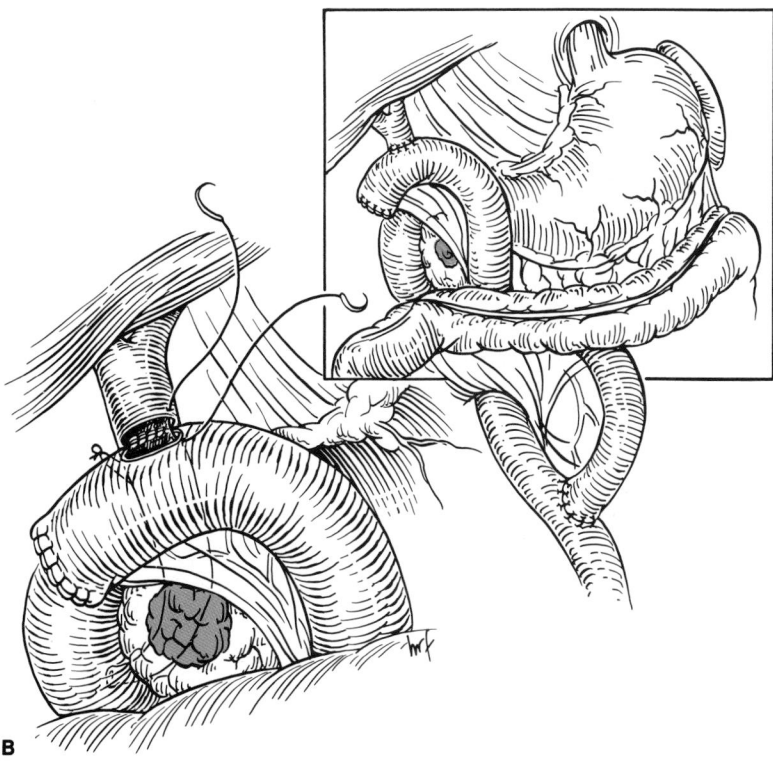

B

Figure 30-VD-1 *(Continued)*

(B) In side-to-side choledochojejunostomy, the gallbladder is removed. A transverse 1-cm incision is made in the common hepatic duct just above the entrance of the cystic duct. The common duct is anastomosed to an equivalent-size enterotomy in a Roux-en-Y limb using 4-0 or 5-0 monofilament nonabsorbable sutures with the knots tied on the outside of the anastomosis. The inset shows the completed retrocolic anastomosis. A soft closed-suction drain (*not shown*) is placed adjacent to the anastomosis.

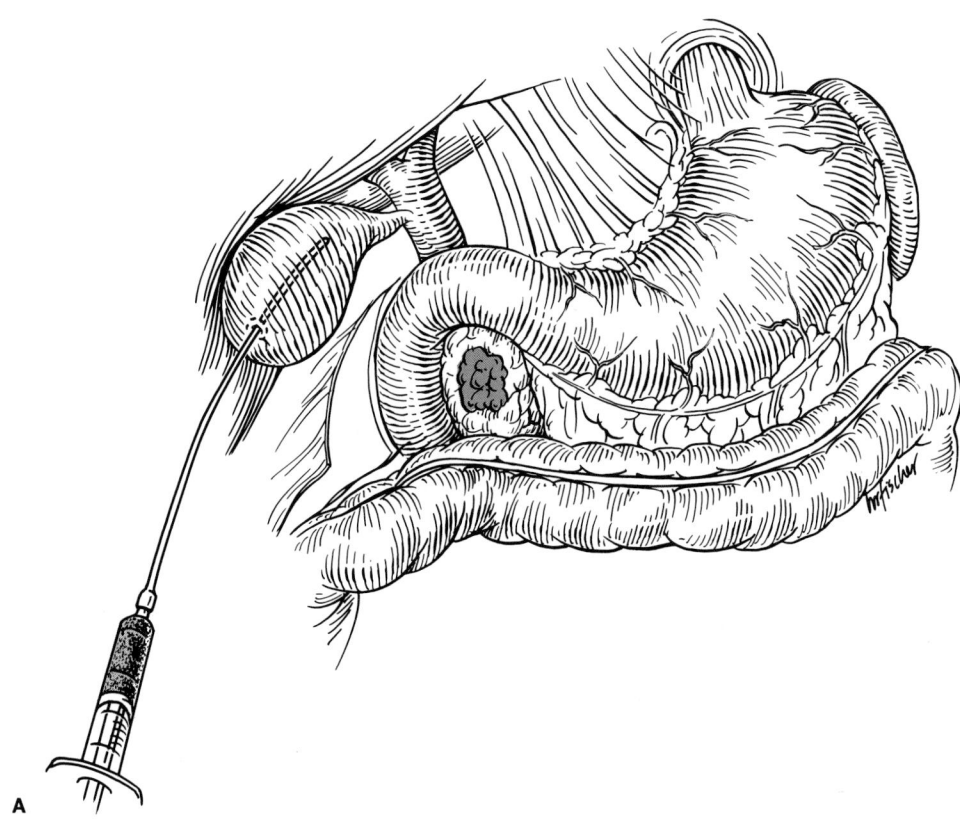

A

Figure 30-VD-2

Cholecystojejunostomy

(**A**) If a cholecystojejunostomy is considered for relief of jaundice in a patient with unresectable pancreatic cancer, a cholangiogram should be performed to demonstrate that the cystic duct is patent and located at least 1 cm away from the pancreatic tumor mass. A 3-0 silk pursestring suture is placed in the dome of the gallbladder, and a small incision is made inside the pursestring into the lumen of the gallbladder. If clear or whitish fluid is present in the gallbladder, it can be assumed that the cystic duct is obstructed and cholecystojejunostomy should be abandoned in favor of choledochojejunostomy. If, on the other hand, there is green fluid in the gallbladder, a cholangiogram should be performed by inserting a short plastic cannula into the gallbladder and injecting 10 to 15 mL of full-strength cholangiography dye. The cholangiogram will give more accurate information about the proximity of the cystic duct and the pancreatic tumor than simple inspection since the cystic duct often travels parallel to and essentially within the wall of the common bile duct for some distance before entering the common duct.

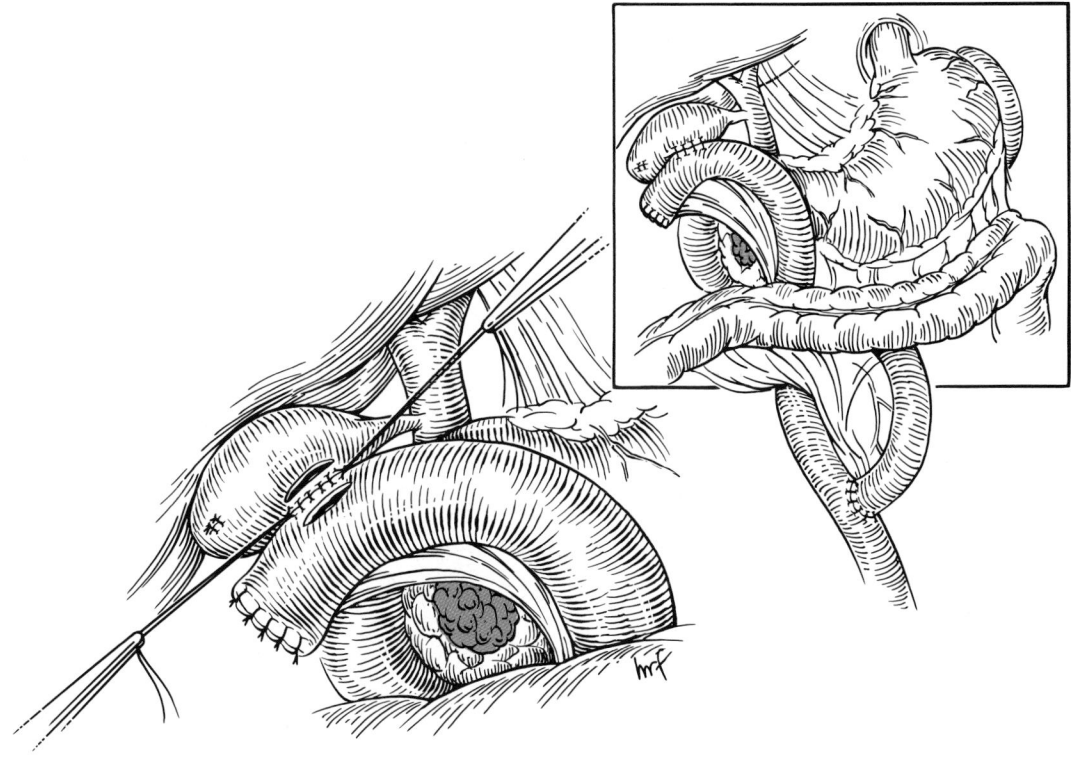

B

Figure 30-VD-2 *(Continued)*

(**B**) In Roux-en-Y cholecystojejunostomy, a posterior layer of 3-0 silk sutures is placed between the seromuscular coats of the jejunum and the gallbladder. Incisions about 2 cm in diameter are made in both organs, and an inner continuous full-thickness layer of 3-0 absorbable suture is added. The anastomosis is completed by an anterior layer of interrupted 3-0 silk sutures. The anastomosis can also be performed in one layer of nonabsorbable full-thickness monofilament suture or with a gastrointestinal stapler passed into small enterotomies in each organ (for stapled and laparoscopic techniques, see Chap. 17). The anastomosis can be performed in either an antecolic or a retrocolic fashion; the latter is shown in the inset.

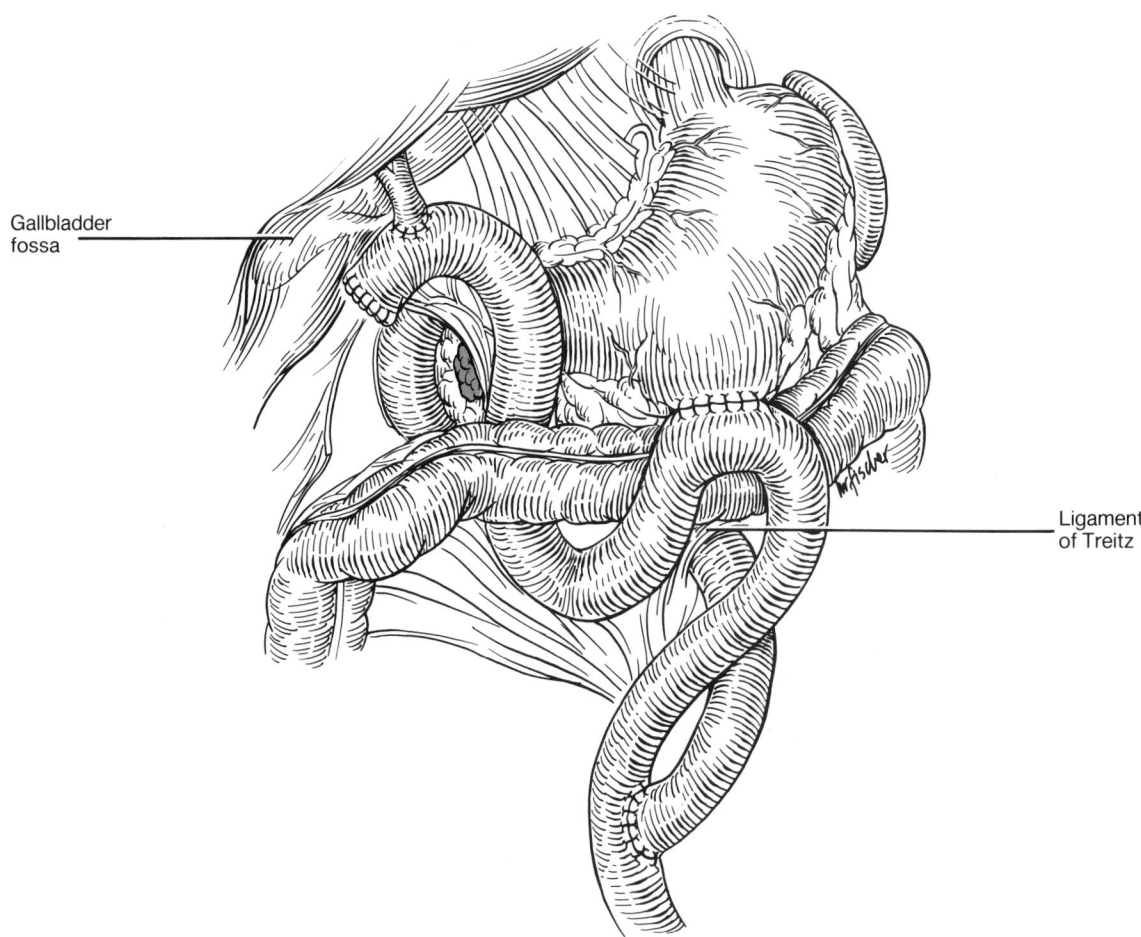

Gallbladder fossa

Ligament of Treitz

Figure 30-VD-3

Combination With Gastrojejunostomy

Gastrojejunostomy is often performed in conjunction with biliary bypass in patients with unresectable pancreatic carcinoma (see Chap. 26). The figure illustrates an antecolic Roux-en-Y gastrojejunostomy coupled with a retrocolic anastomosis to the common hepatic duct. The gastrojejunostomy is performed in two layers, with an outer layer of interrupted 3-0 silk sutures and an inner continuous layer of 3-0 absorbable suture (for details of gastrojejunostomy, see Chap. 11).

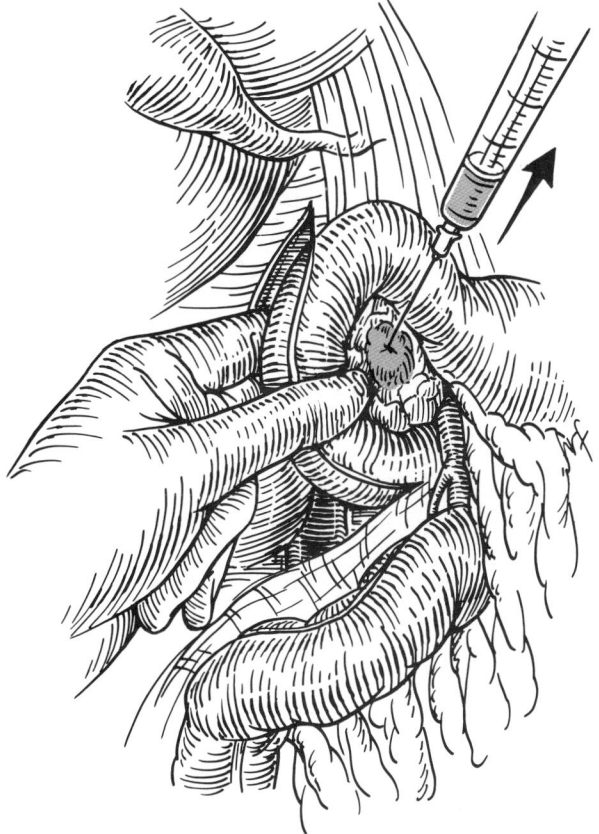

Figure 30-VD-4

Biopsy

When exploration reveals nonresectable carcinoma of the pancreas, it is important to obtain tissue confirmation of malignancy so that the patient can be accurately apprised of the prognosis and in case postoperative chemoradiotherapy is to be offered. After a Kocher maneuver, tissue confirmation of malignancy can be obtained by fine-needle aspiration of the tumor mass with a 22-gauge needle attached to a dry 10-mL syringe. Multiple needle passes through the tumor increase the likelihood of a positive cytologic diagnosis. If cytologic diagnostic facilities are not available, the tumor can undergo biopsy by traditional core needle biopsy techniques. In the case of unresectable pancreatic cancer, it is probably safest to perform the biopsy transduodenally into the tumor mass if a large-bore needle is used.

E. Distal Pancreatectomy and Splenectomy for Carcinoma

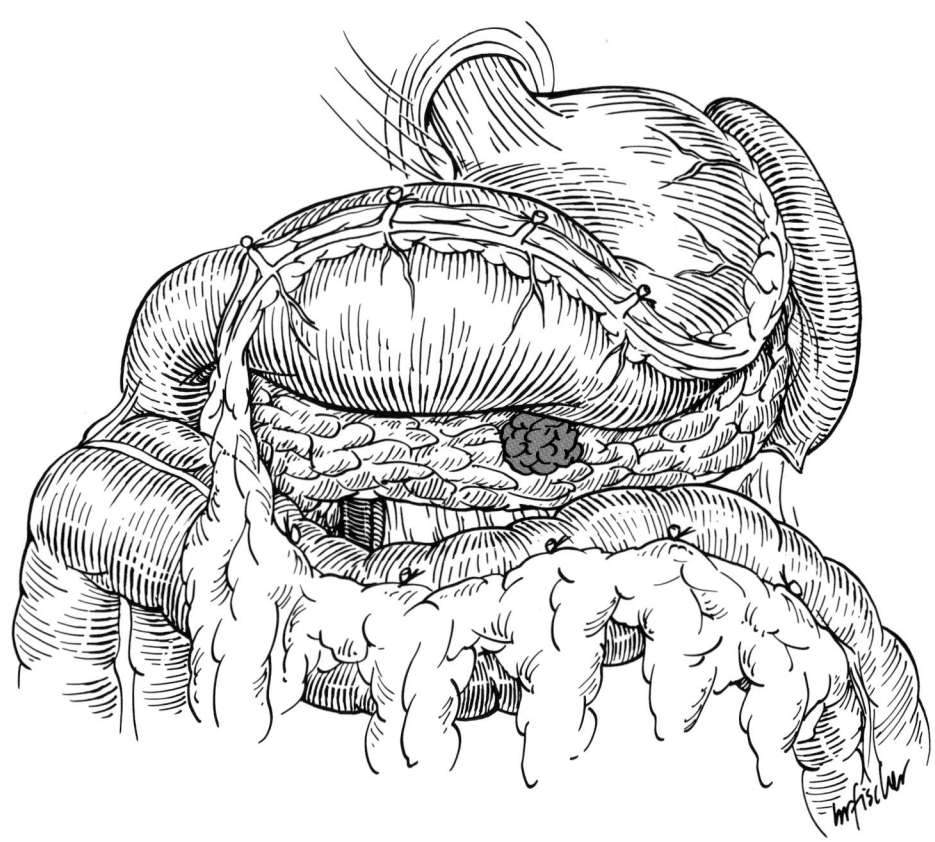

Figure 30-VE-1

Division of Gastrocolic Omentum

Resectable malignant tumors of the body and tail of the pancreas are managed by distal pancreatectomy and splenectomy. Since the line of division of the pancreas is over the superior mesenteric vessels, the tumor should be located such that division of the pancreas at that point yields at least a 1-cm margin free of tumor.

The body and tail of the pancreas are exposed by entering the lesser sac through the gastrocolic omentum. Adhesions between the posterior wall of the stomach and the anterior surface of the pancreas are divided sharply to expose the pancreas fully.

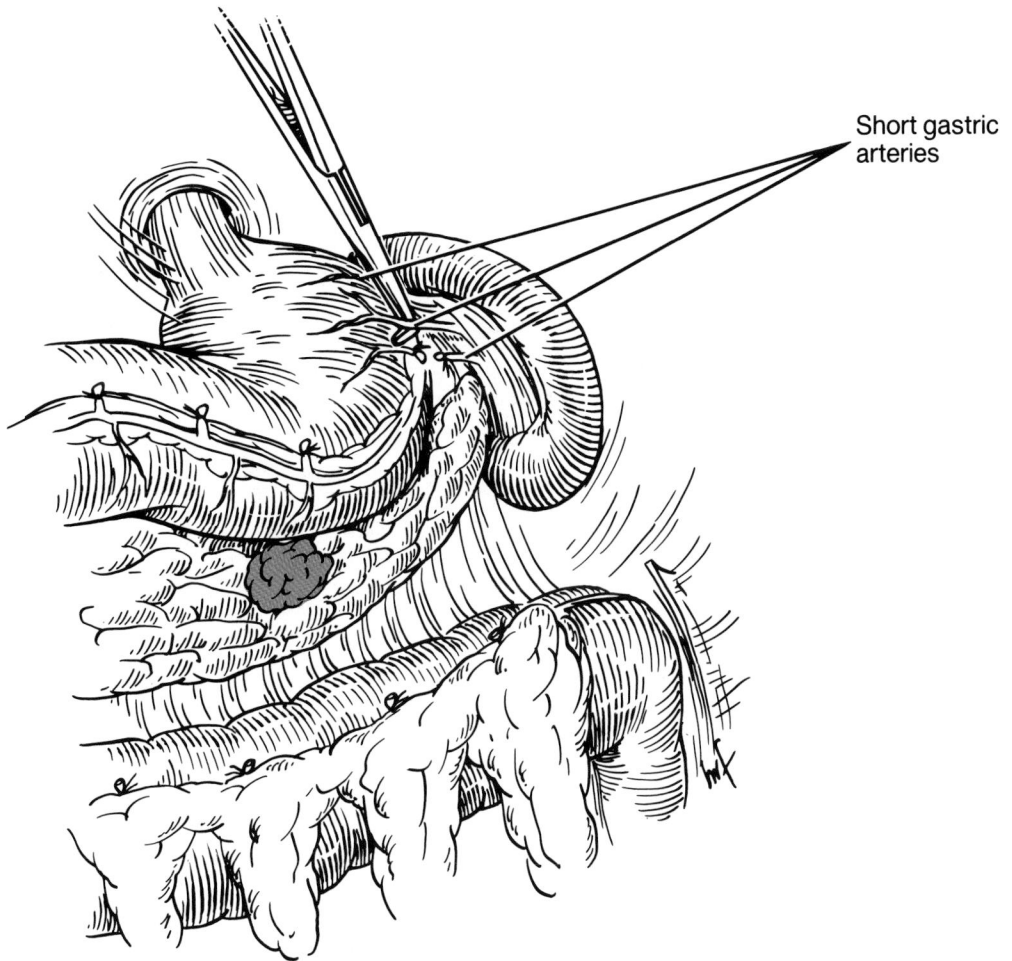

Short gastric
arteries

Figure 30-VE-2

Ligation of Short Gastric Vessels

The process of separating the spleen from the stomach is begun by ligating and dividing the short gastric vessels between the greater curvature of the fundus of the stomach and the splenic hilum. Care must be taken not to retract the stomach too forcibly, tearing these delicate vessels. The highest short gastric vessels near the cardia of the stomach are best ligated after fully mobilizing the spleen (see Fig. 30-VE-6).

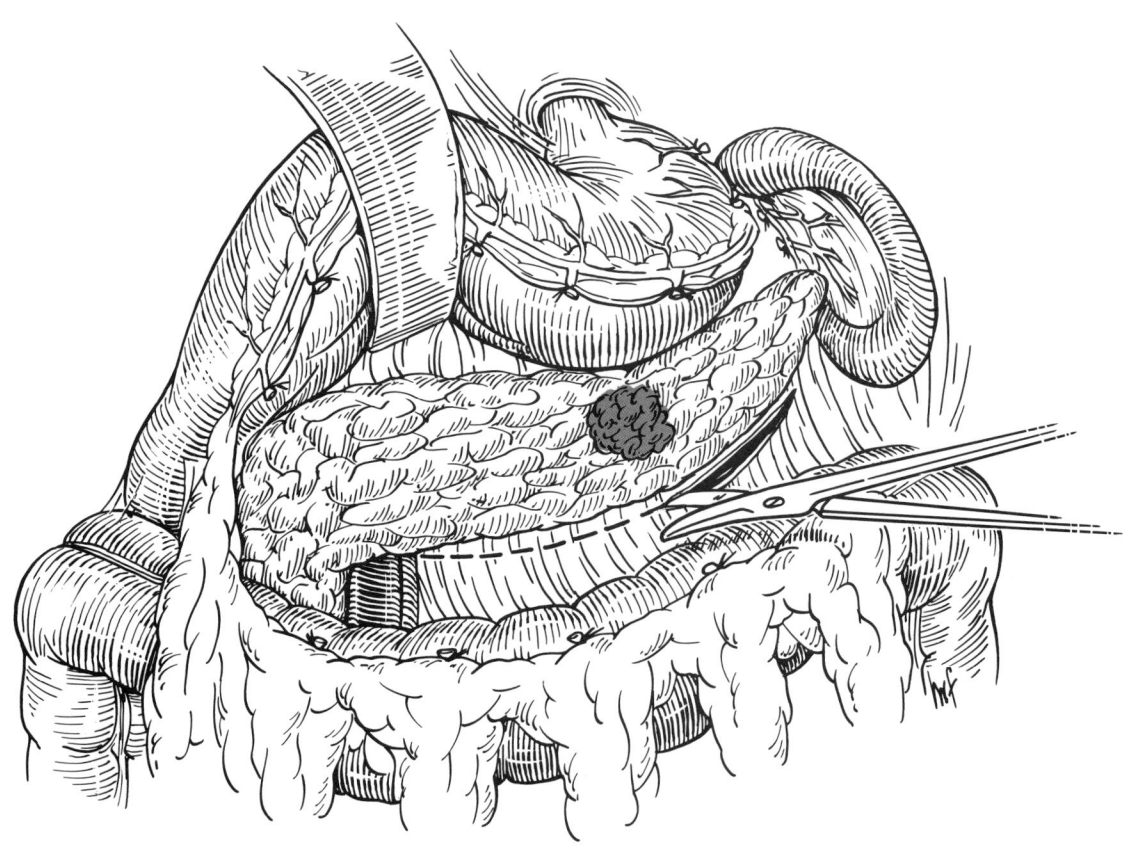

Figure 30-VE-3

Incision of Peritoneum and Identification of Superior Mesenteric Vein

The peritoneum along the inferior border of the pancreas is incised from the superior mesenteric vessels to the tail of the gland. A few small blood vessels may require ligation before the retropancreatic space can be entered. After ligation of these vessels, the body and tail of the pancreas (along with the splenic artery and vein) can be elevated by gentle blunt dissection behind the gland.

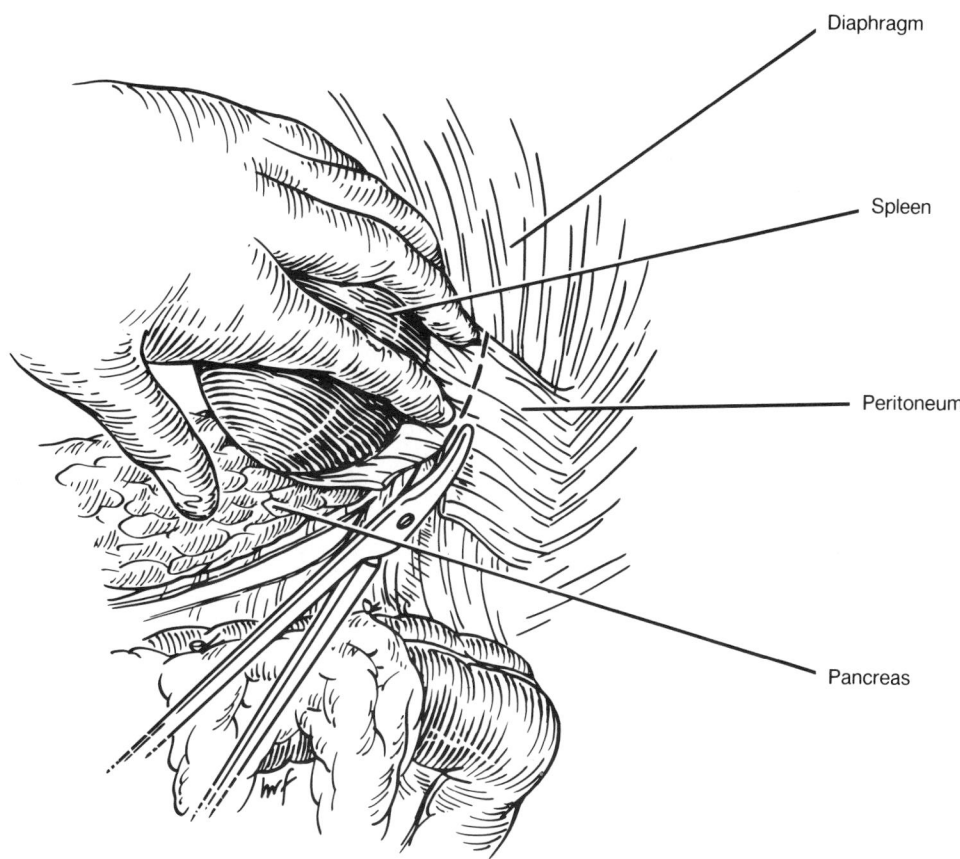

Figure 30-VE-4

Division of Peritoneal Attachments

With the spleen gently retracted to the right, the peritoneum lateral to the spleen is divided from the base of the spleen up to the diaphragm, following a line just outside the curve of the splenic capsule.

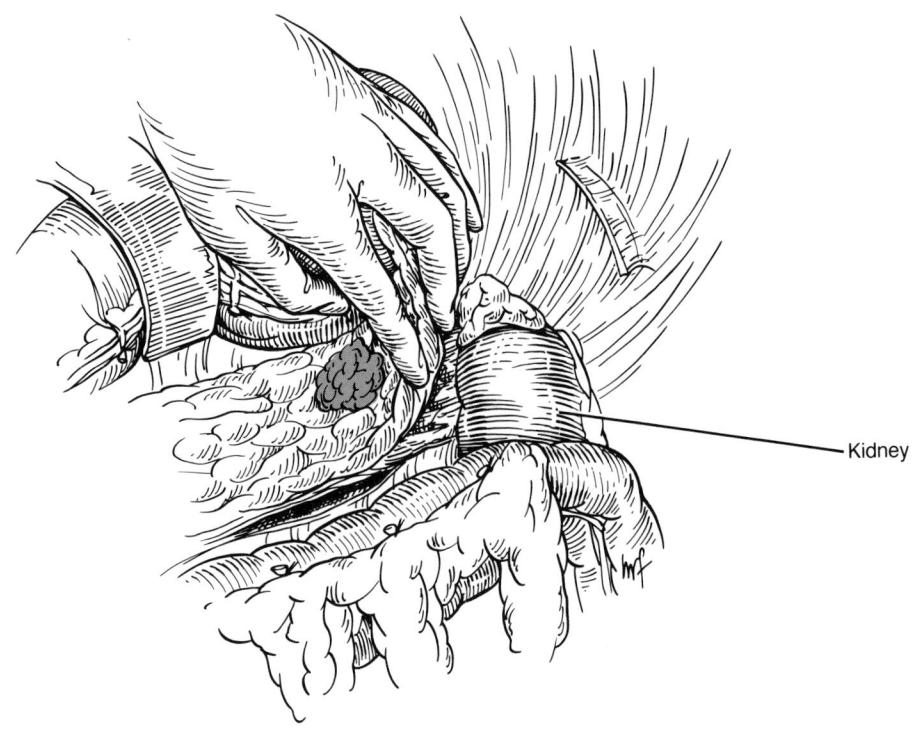

Kidney

Figure 30-VE-5

Mobilization of Spleen and Pancreatic Tail

By gentle manual blunt dissection, the spleen and tail of the pancreas are mobilized anteriorly and to the right, raising them off the left kidney.

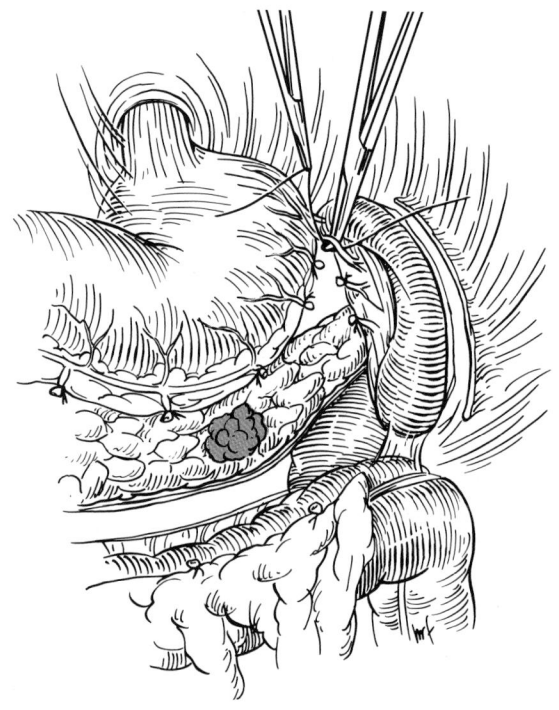

Figure 30-VE-6

Completion of Ligation of Short Gastric Vessels

Once the spleen has been fully mobilized from behind, any short gastric vessels continuing to tether the spleen to the stomach are tied on both sides with silk ligatures and divided. This dissection is continued until the stomach is completely free from the spleen and can be fully retracted to the right.

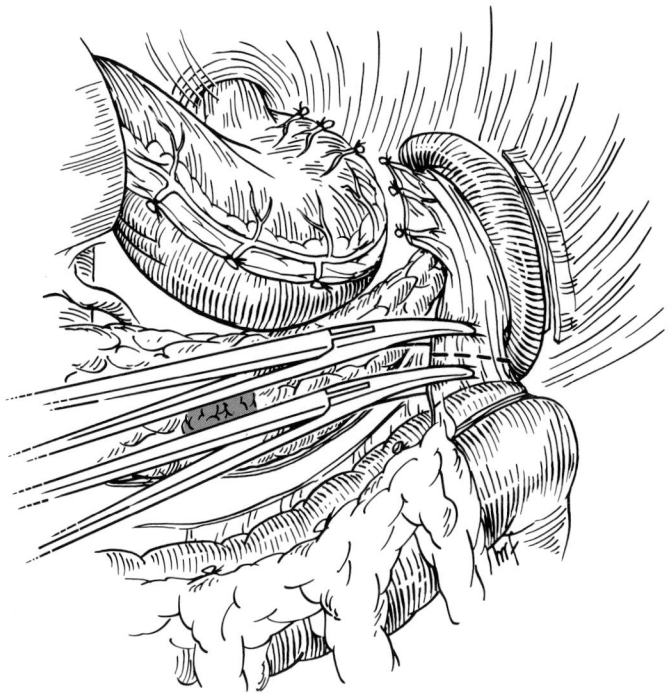

Figure 30-VE-7

Division of Splenocolic Ligament

If not already done, the splenocolic ligament is fully divided between clamps and ligated with 2-0 silk ties, freeing the spleen entirely from the splenic flexure of the colon.

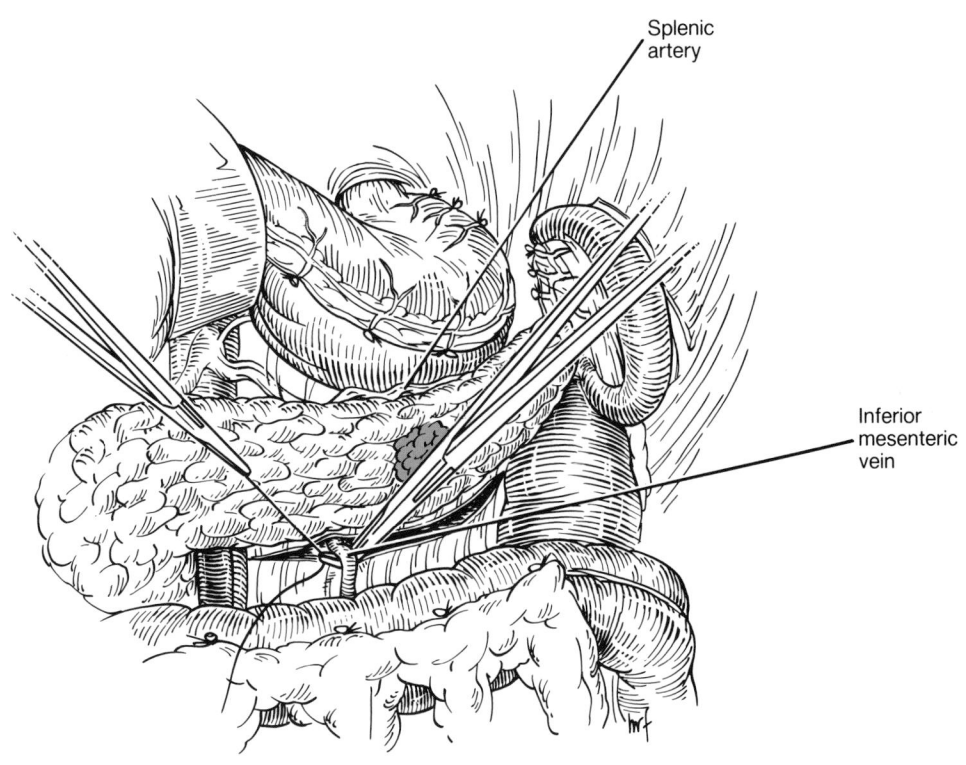

Splenic
artery

Inferior
mesenteric
vein

Figure 30-VE-8

Mobilization of the Pancreatic Tail

The tail of the pancreas and attached spleen and splenic vessels are mobilized by gentle
blunt posterior dissection toward the right. In the course of this dissection, the inferior
mesenteric vein may be encountered as it empties into the splenic vein on the posterior
aspect of the pancreas. If so, the inferior mesenteric vein is ligated with 2-0 silk ligatures
and divided.

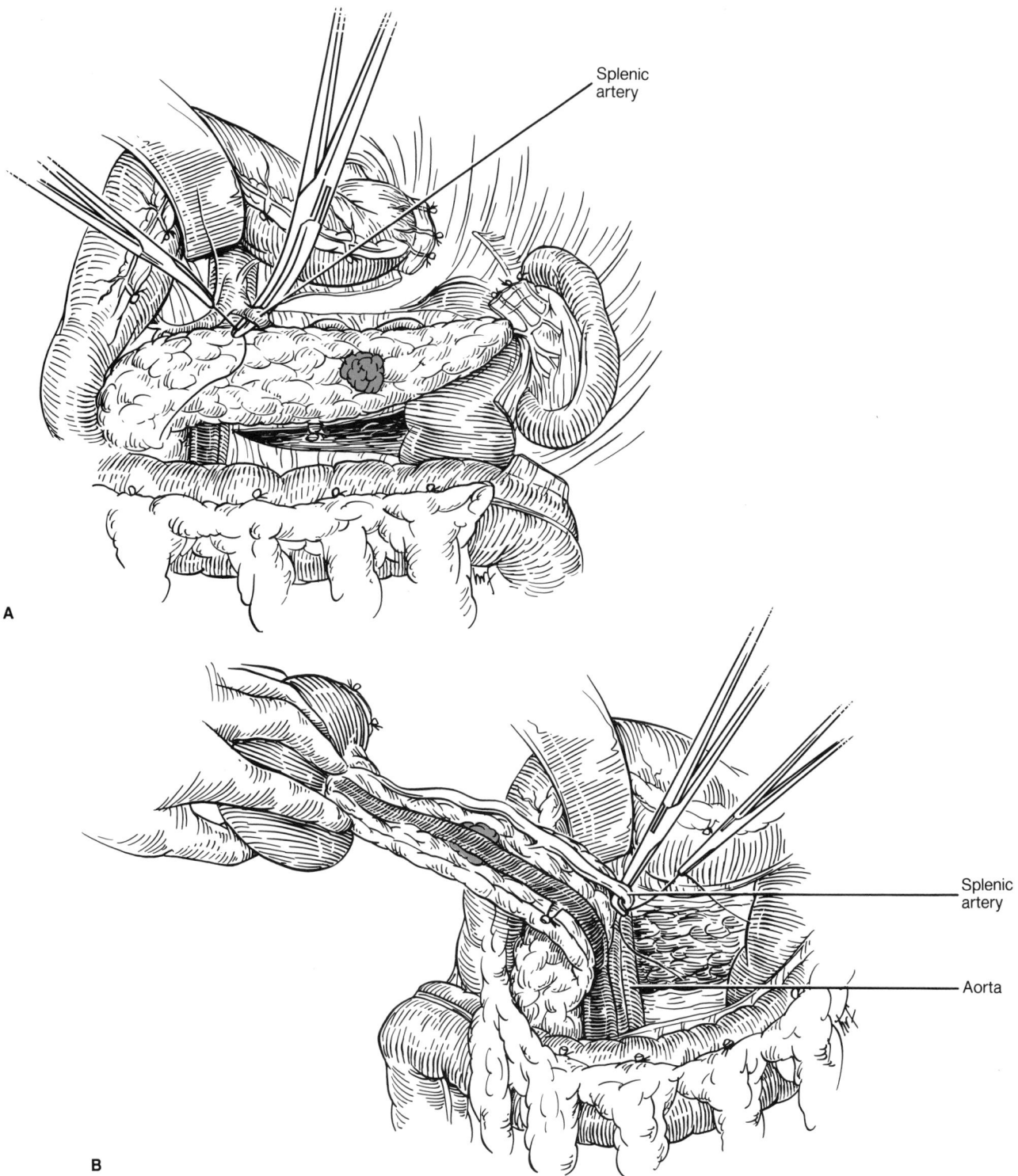

Figure 30-VE-9

Ligation of Splenic Artery

(**A**) The splenic artery is identified at its origin from the celiac axis and is doubly clamped and ligated. A suture ligature of 2-0 silk is placed on the celiac side for security. The splenic end of the artery is tied with a simple ligature of 2-0 silk.

(**B**) If more convenient, the splenic artery can be ligated from the posterior aspect of the gland.

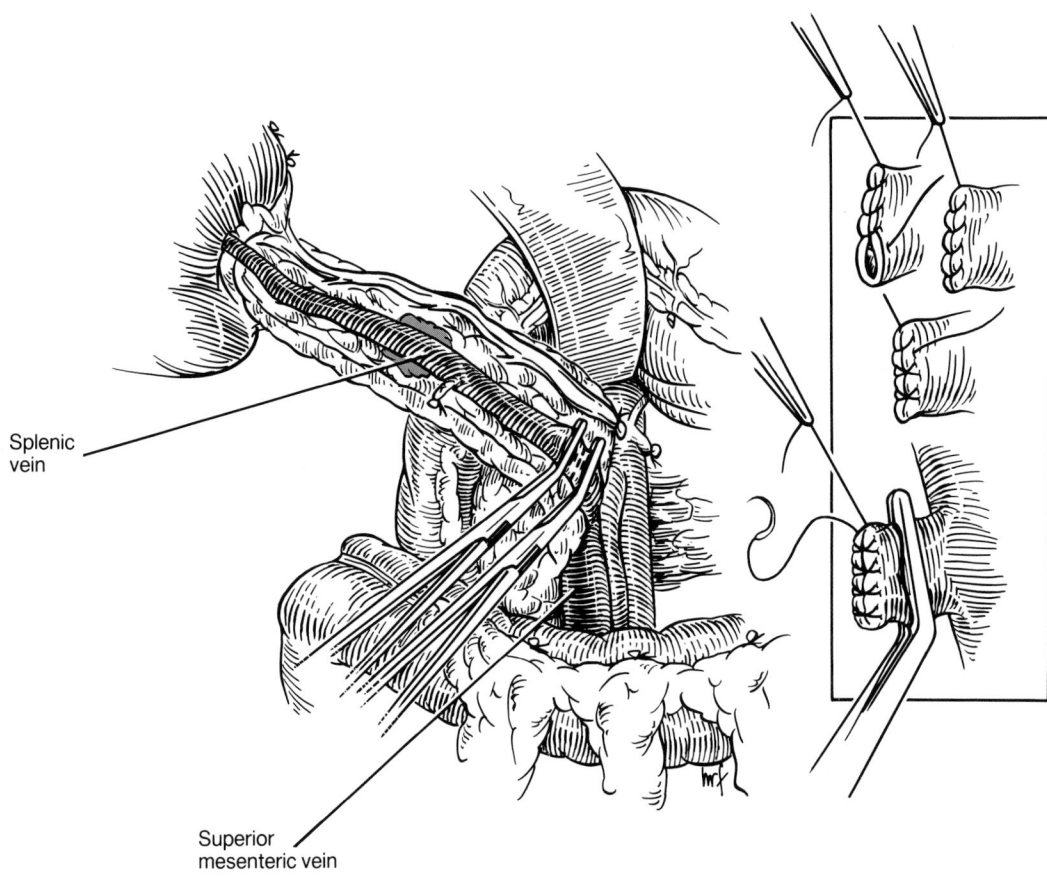

Splenic
vein

Superior
mesenteric vein

Figure 30-VE-10

Division of Splenic Vein

The entrance of the splenic vein into the portal vein is slowly and carefully identified on the posterior aspect of the gland. Gentle dissection around the vein at this point, avoiding the small branches of the vein that enter from the pancreas, allows the placement of a pair of fine vascular clamps, between which the splenic vein is divided. Both ends of the vein are oversewn with a running 5-0 monofilament suture (**inset**).

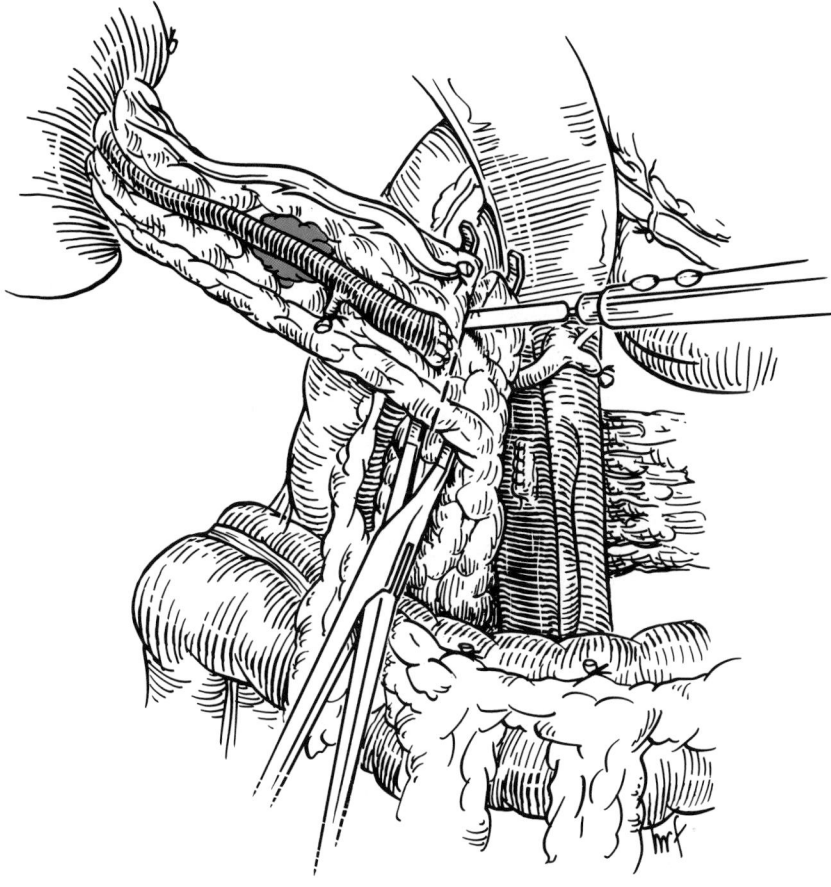

Figure 30-VE-11

Division of Pancreatic Tissue

The pancreatic parenchyma is divided with electrocautery, making sure that there is a margin of at least 1 cm beyond the tumor of the body of the gland.

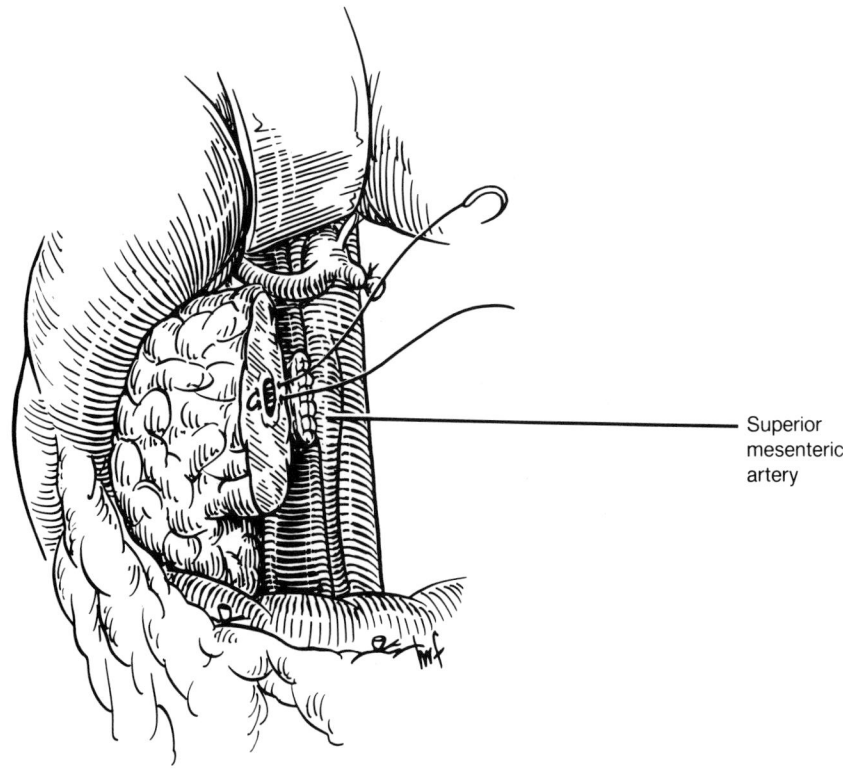

Superior
mesenteric
artery

Figure 30-VE-12

Ligation of Main Pancreatic Duct

The open end of the remaining pancreatic duct is ligated with a horizontal mattress suture of 3-0 silk.

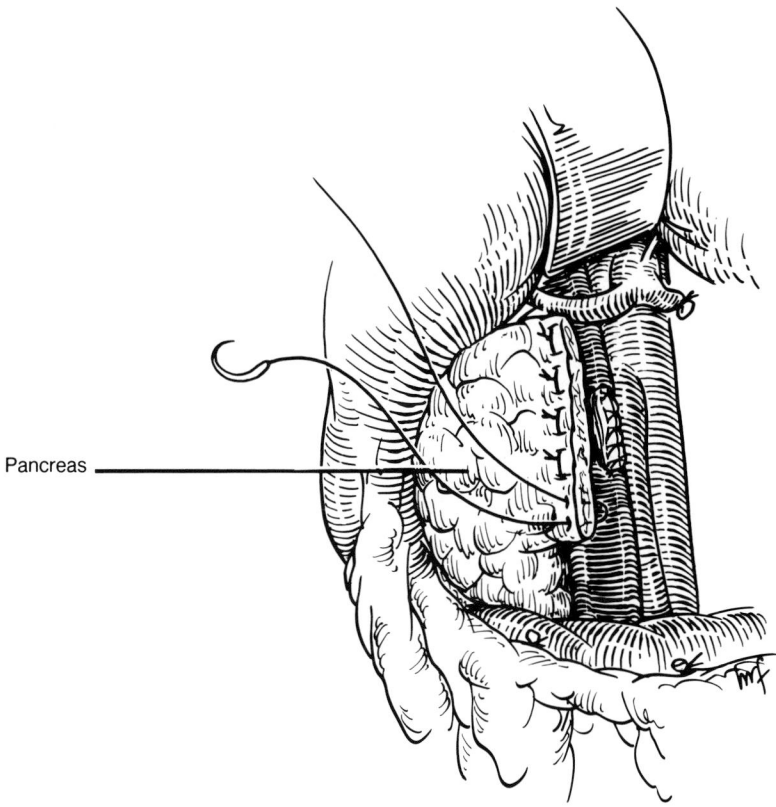

Pancreas

Figure 30-VE-13

Suture Placement

The cut edge of the residual pancreas is gently compressed by a series of interrupted horizontal mattress sutures of 3-0 silk.

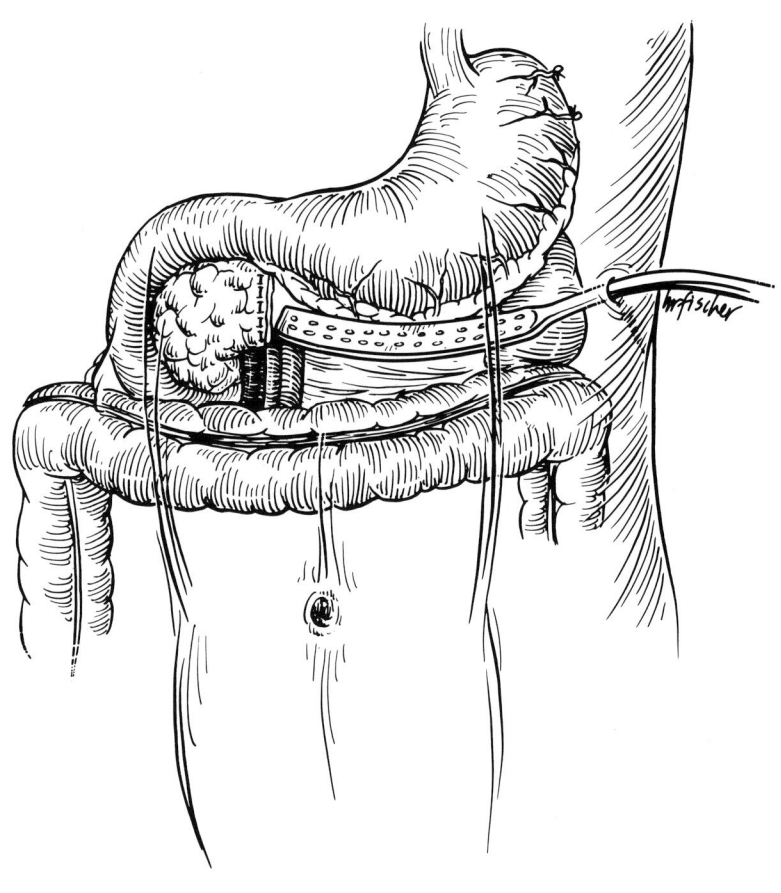

Figure 30-VE-14

Completed Procedure

The completed distal pancreatectomy and splenectomy. A soft closed-suction drain is placed adjacent to the cut edge of the remaining pancreas and brought out through a separate stab incision in the left flank.

F. Transduodenal Excision of Ampullary Tumors

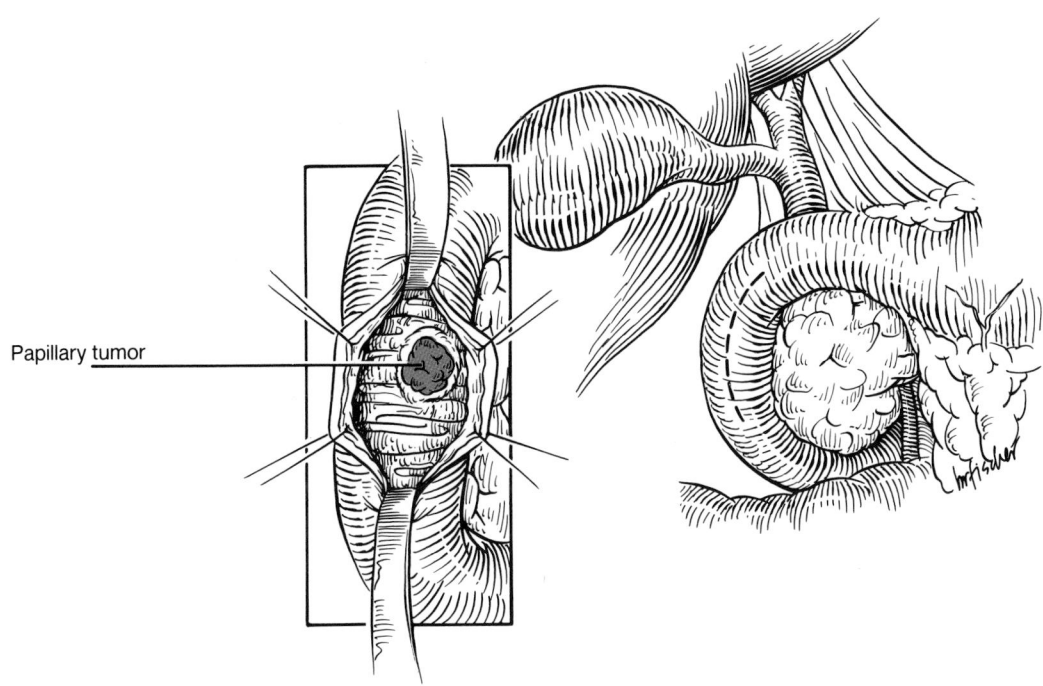

Papillary tumor

Figure 30-VF-1

Longitudinal Duodenal Incision

Benign villous adenomas of the ampullary region can be excised locally. This technique is applicable for small tumors (about 2 cm or less) with no evidence of malignancy by preoperative endoscopic biopsy. The peritoneum lateral to the duodenum is incised, and the duodenum and head of pancreas are elevated (Kocher maneuver), after which a longitudinal duodenotomy is made on the antimesenteric border of the duodenum opposite the tumor (*dashed line*), which often is palpable through the duodenal wall. The edges of the duodenotomy are retracted, revealing a fleshy tumor arising at the ampulla of Vater **(inset)**.

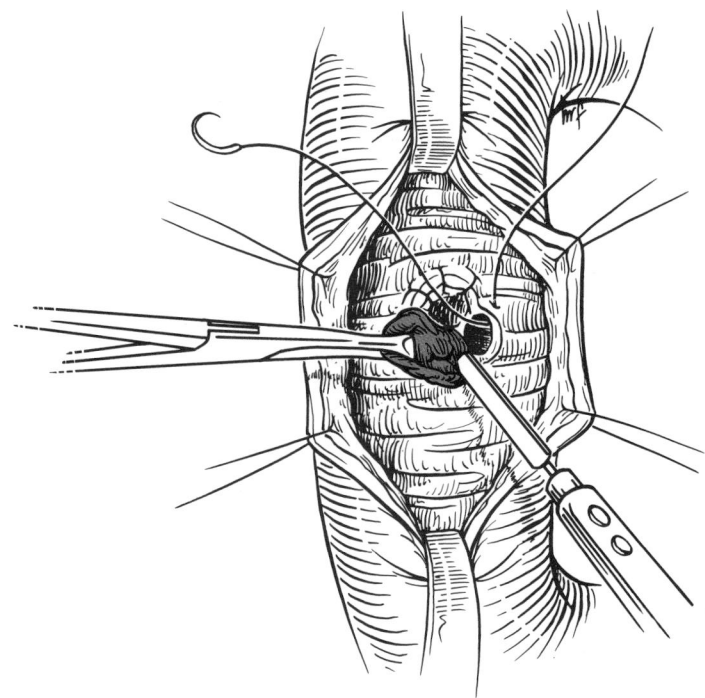

Figure 30-VF-2

Resection of Tumor and Suture Placement

The tumor is gradually excised by electrocautery with a 2- to 3-mm margin of grossly normal duodenal wall around the neoplasm. As the excision exposes the orifices of the common bile duct and pancreatic duct, the edges of these ducts are reapproximated to the normal duodenal wall with interrupted 3-0 absorbable sutures.

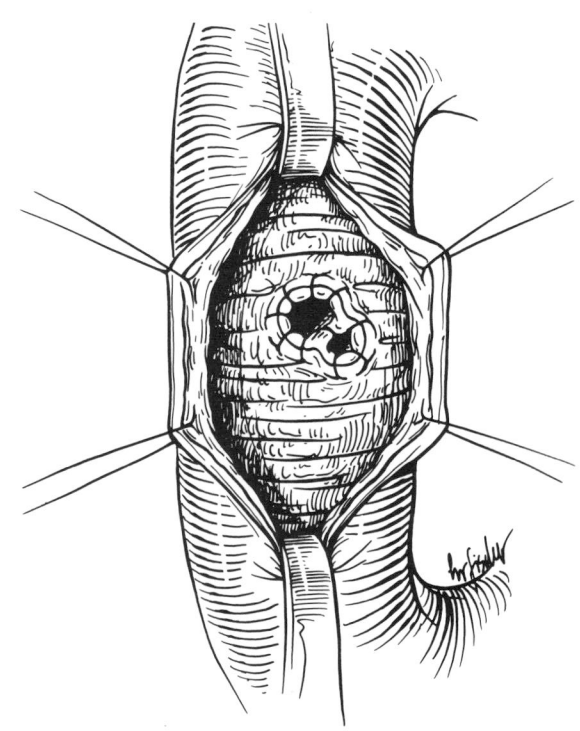

Figure 30-VF-3

Completed Resection

The completed excision of the ampullary tumor showing reapproximation of the edges of the common bile duct and pancreatic duct to the the duodenal wall. The duodenotomy is closed in two layers, taking care not to narrow the duodenal lumen.

SECTION VI *Operations for Pancreatic Endocrine Neoplasms*
A. Gastrinoma

During the past several years, the management of gastrinoma has changed significantly, stressing removal of the primary tumor when possible. In patients with localized gastrinoma identified on preoperative imaging studies or in whom the gastrinoma is not identified on preoperative studies, about 80% are found to have a resectable tumor at laparotomy. This subsection outlines the approach to curative surgery in patients with resectable gastrinoma.

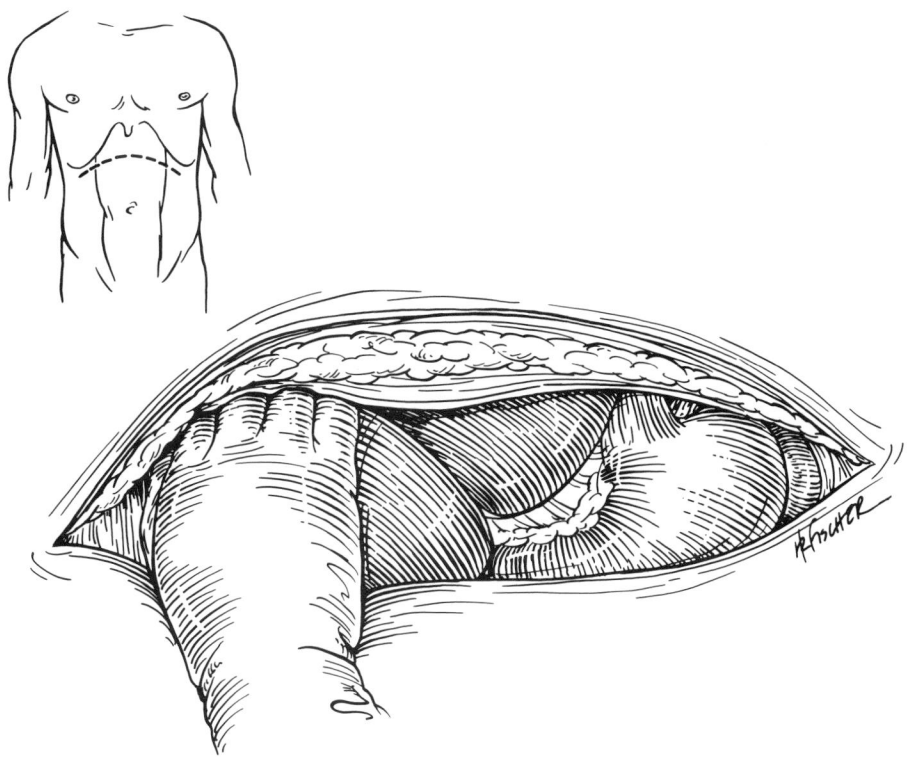

Figure 30-VIA-1

Exploration of Abdomen and Evaluation of Liver

In patients with potentially resectable gastrinoma, the abdomen is explored through a bilateral subcostal incision (**inset**). Upon entering the abdomen, the entire peritoneal cavity should be thoroughly and carefully examined for evidence of nonpancreatic primary tumors or metastatic disease. Any potentially malignant nodules in the liver should be excised for pathologic examination by frozen section.

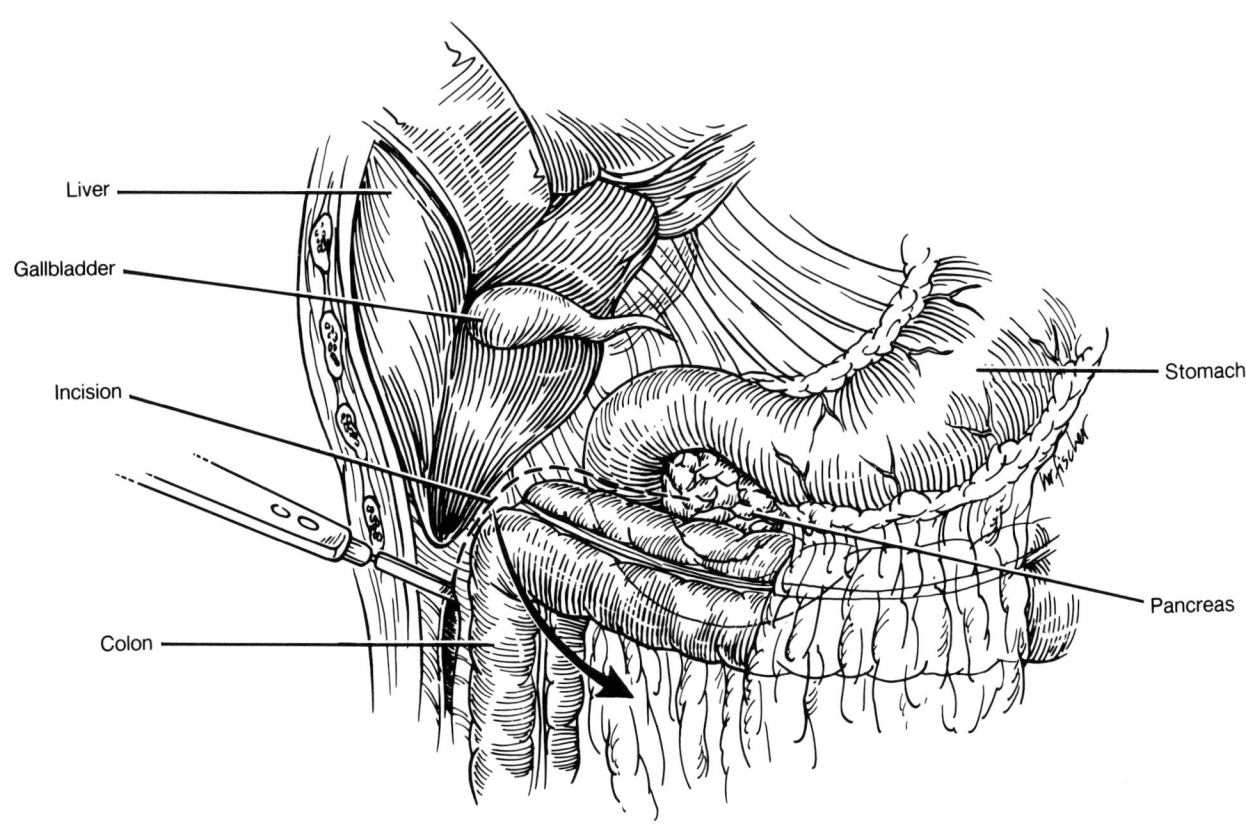

Liver

Gallbladder

Incision

Colon

Stomach

Pancreas

Figure 30-VIA-2

Reflection of Hepatic Flexure

The hepatic flexure of the colon is fully mobilized and retracted inferiorly to expose the head of the pancreas and the duodenum completely. If the transverse mesocolon obscures the head of the pancreas, the base of the mesocolon should be swept down off the pancreas and duodenum to provide optimal exposure.

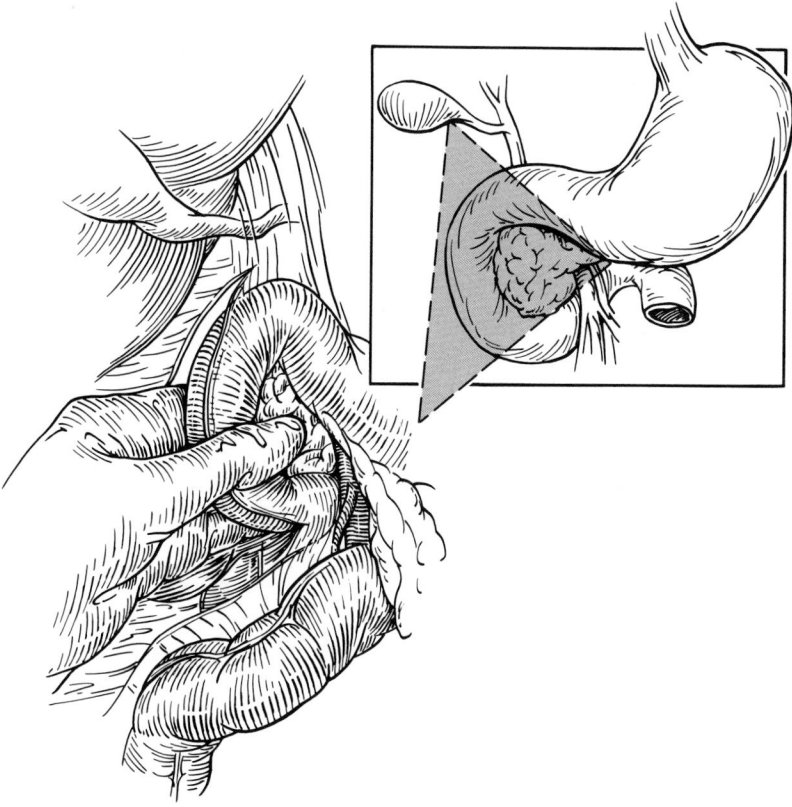

Figure 30-VIA-3

Kocher Maneuver

A complete Kocher maneuver is essential to the success of an exploration for gastrinoma, particularly when the location of the tumor is unknown and must be determined by palpation and inspection. Most gastrinomas are located within the "gastrinoma triangle," an area bounded by the junction of the cystic duct and common bile duct superiorly, the junction of the second and third portions of the duodenum inferiorly, and the junction of the neck and body of the pancreas medially (**inset**). To expose this area fully, a wide Kocher maneuver elevating the duodenum and the head of the pancreas from the hepatoduodenal ligament to the superior mesenteric vessels is performed as shown, and the entire pancreatic head and duodenum are meticulously examined for palpable masses.

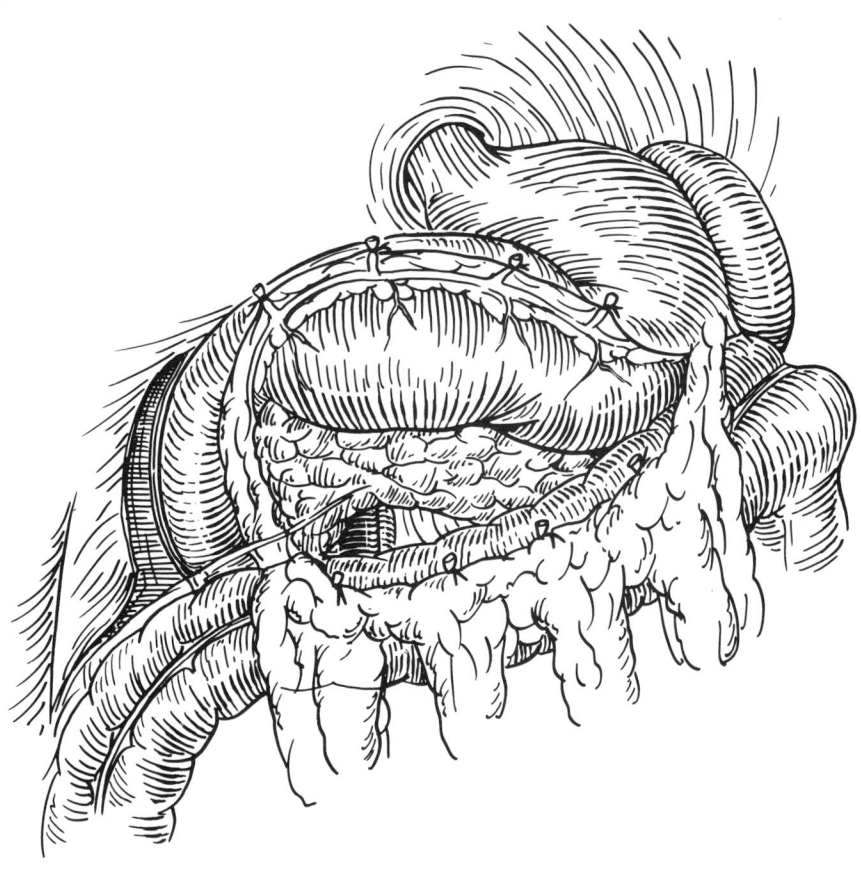

Figure 30-VIA-4

Division of Gastrocolic Omentum

The gastrocolic omentum is divided and the lesser sac entered to expose the body and tail of the pancreas. Any adhesions between the posterior wall of the stomach and the pancreas are divided sharply, and the stomach is retracted cephalad to provide complete exposure of the anterior surface of the pancreas. If the presence of a gastrinoma in the body and tail of the gland is suspected, the peritoneum along the inferior margin of the gland to the left of the superior mesenteric vessels should be incised, allowing entrance into the retropancreatic plane. Elevating the body and tail of the pancreas in this way facilitates bimanual palpation of this portion of the gland (see Figs. 30-IIB-3 and 30-IIB-4).

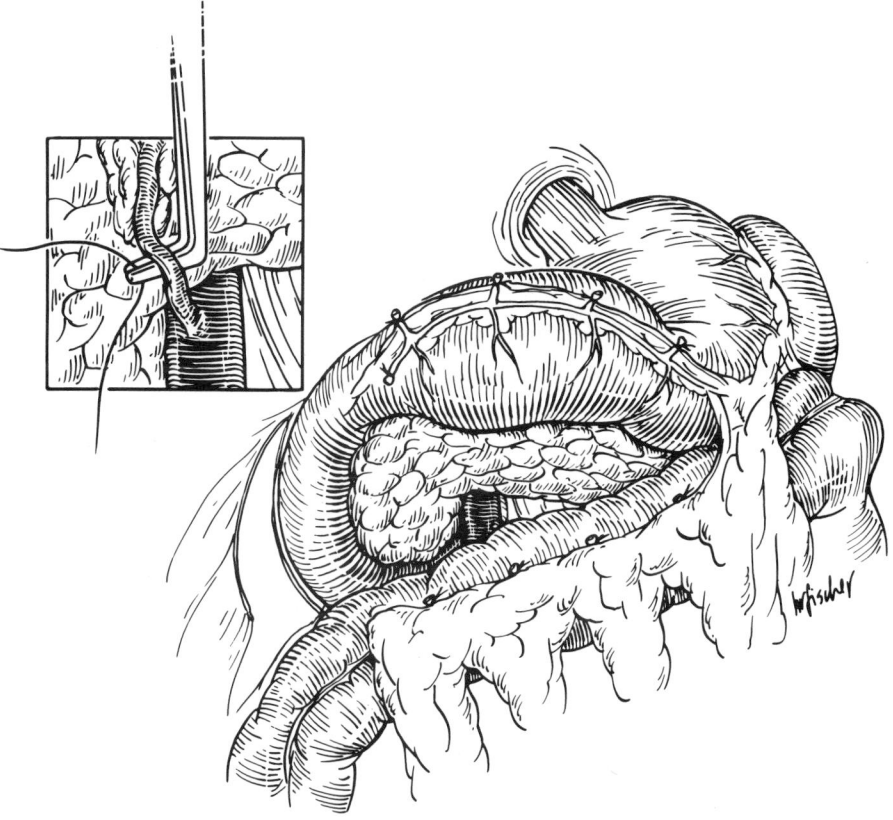

Figure 30-VIA-5

Division of Gastroepiploic Vein

To maximize exposure of the area of the neck of the pancreas, the right gastroepiploic vein is ligated and divided (**inset**). This vein passes from the greater curvature of the stomach across the area of the neck of the pancreas to empty into the superior mesenteric vein. Therefore, the right gastroepiploic vein and fat surrounding it obscure the anterior surface of the head and neck of the pancreas. Dividing this vessel connects the dissection of the head with that of the body and tail and provides complete exposure of the anterior surface of the gland.

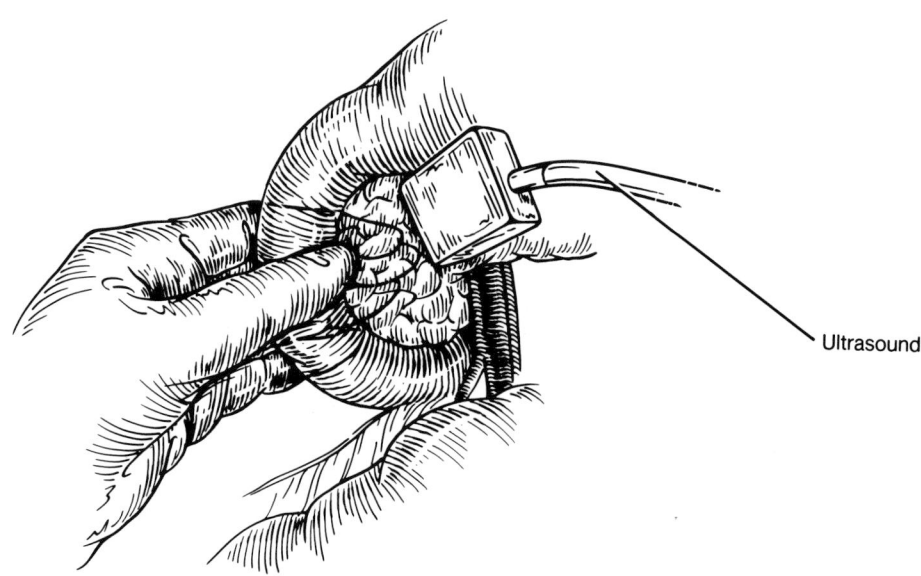

Ultrasound

Figure 30-VIA-6

Ultrasonography of Pancreas

Once exposure of the pancreas is complete, the gland is carefully examined for the presence of tumors by intraoperative ultrasonography (see Chap. 27).

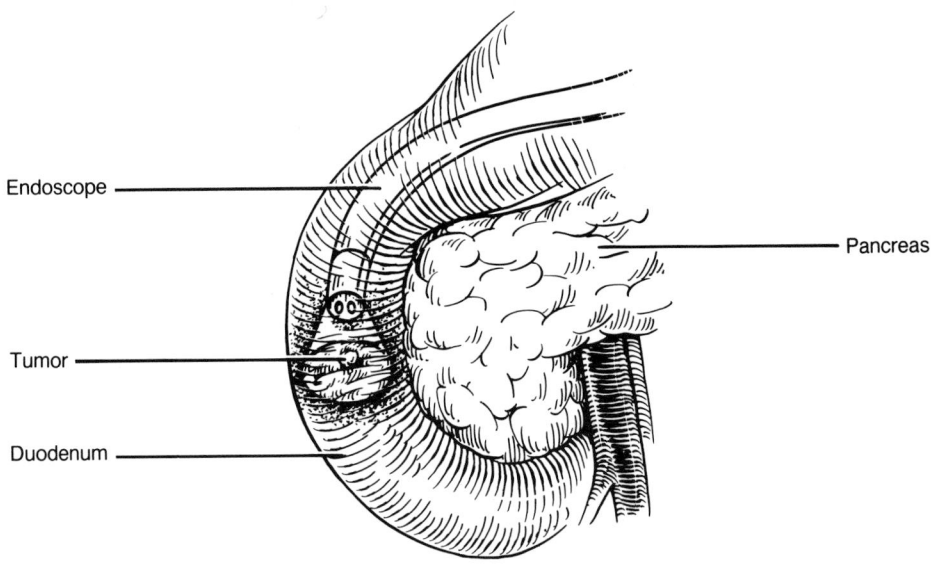

Endoscope

Pancreas

Tumor

Duodenum

Figure 30-VIA-7

Endoscopic Transillumination of Duodenum

About 20% of primary gastrinomas arise in the duodenum. If exploration of the pancreas and external inspection and palpation of the duodenum fail to reveal a gastrinoma, the wall of the duodenum should be transilluminated by the passage of an upper endoscope. Any lesions identified should be excised with a small margin of normal duodenum (see Fig. 30-VIA-8). If transillumination fails to reveal a tumor, the duodenum should be opened through a longitudinal duodenotomy opposite the papilla of Vater to allow direct visual inspection of the duodenal mucosa for tumor. To avoid mistaking the papilla for a tumor or injuring the papilla during biopsy, it is wise to pass a catheter through the papilla into the common duct from below or from the cystic duct into the common duct and through the papilla from above.

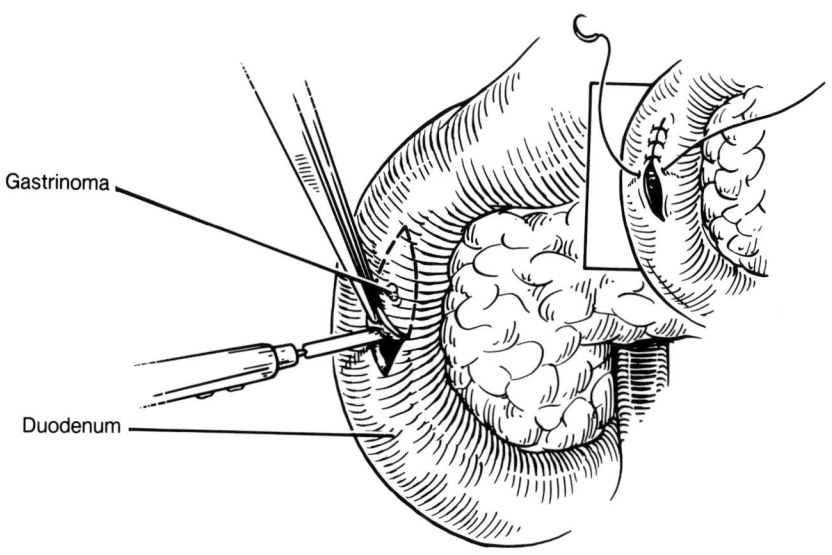

Gastrinoma

Duodenum

Figure 30-VIA-8

Excision of Duodenal Gastrinoma

After being identified by transillumination, the tumor is excised with a small ellipse of normal duodenal wall. Small wounds can be closed with a single layer of 4-0 silk sutures through all layers of the bowel wall. Larger excisions should be closed in two layers with an inner full-thickness layer of continuous 3-0 absorbable suture and an outer layer of interrupted 3-0 silk Lembert sutures.

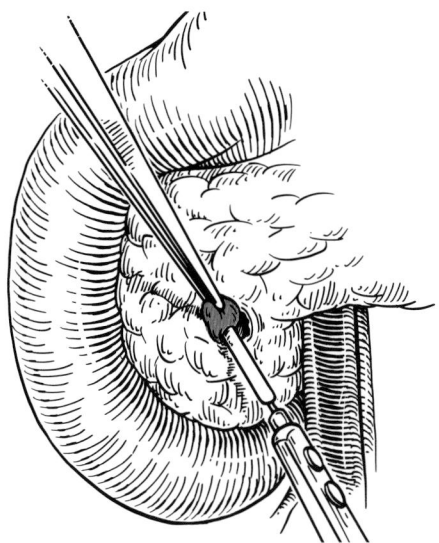

Figure 30-VIA-9

Enucleation of Small Gastrinoma in Pancreatic Head

Lesions in the pancreatic head are managed by enucleation. Intraoperative ultrasound can be used to ascertain the relation of the tumor to the main pancreatic duct and major vessels (see Chap. 27). Only large lesions confined to the head of the pancreas require pancreaticoduodenectomy (see Section VA). Small tumors in the body and tail of the pancreas can be treated by enucleation as well, although distal pancreatectomy should be performed for tumors larger than about 1 cm since the incidence of malignancy in tumors of the body and tail of the gland may be increased. For the technique of distal pancreatectomy, see Section VE.

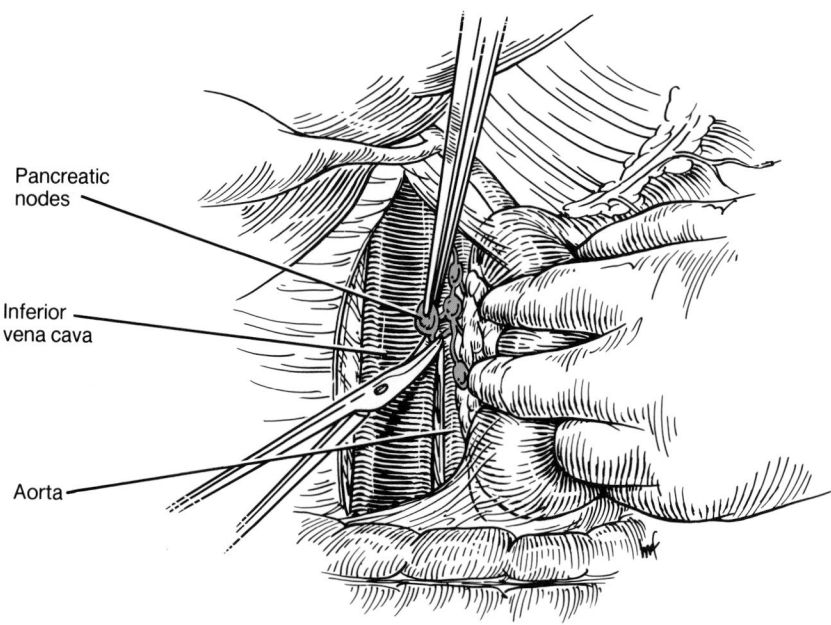

Pancreatic nodes

Inferior vena cava

Aorta

Figure 30-VIA-10

Excision of Peripancreatic Lymph Nodes

As a part of the exploration for gastrinoma, any enlarged lymph nodes in the region of the head of the pancreas should be excised. Occasionally, gastrinoma is found in peripancreatic lymph nodes with no evidence of a pancreatic or duodenal primary. In some patients with isolated lymph node disease, prolonged reduction of serum gastrin levels occurs after node excision. In patients with an identified primary tumor in the pancreas or duodenum, enlarged lymph nodes should also be excised to determine whether metastatic gastrinoma is present.

B. Insulinoma

Insulinomas are usually located in the body and tail of the pancreas. Preoperative localization studies are more likely to be positive with insulinoma than with gastrinoma.

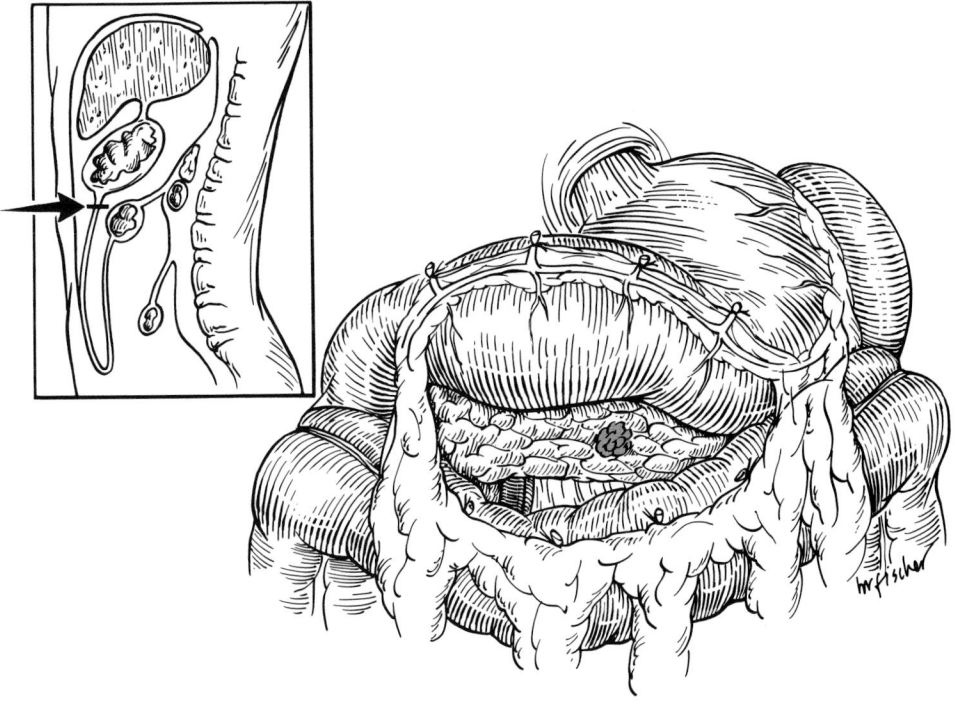

Figure 30-VIB-1

Exposure of Pancreatic Body and Tail

Exploration for insulinoma is begun by entering the lesser sac through the gastrocolic omentum (**inset**). Any adhesions between the posterior wall of the stomach and the anterior surface of the pancreas are sharply divided to provide complete exposure of the anterior surface of the body and tail of the gland.

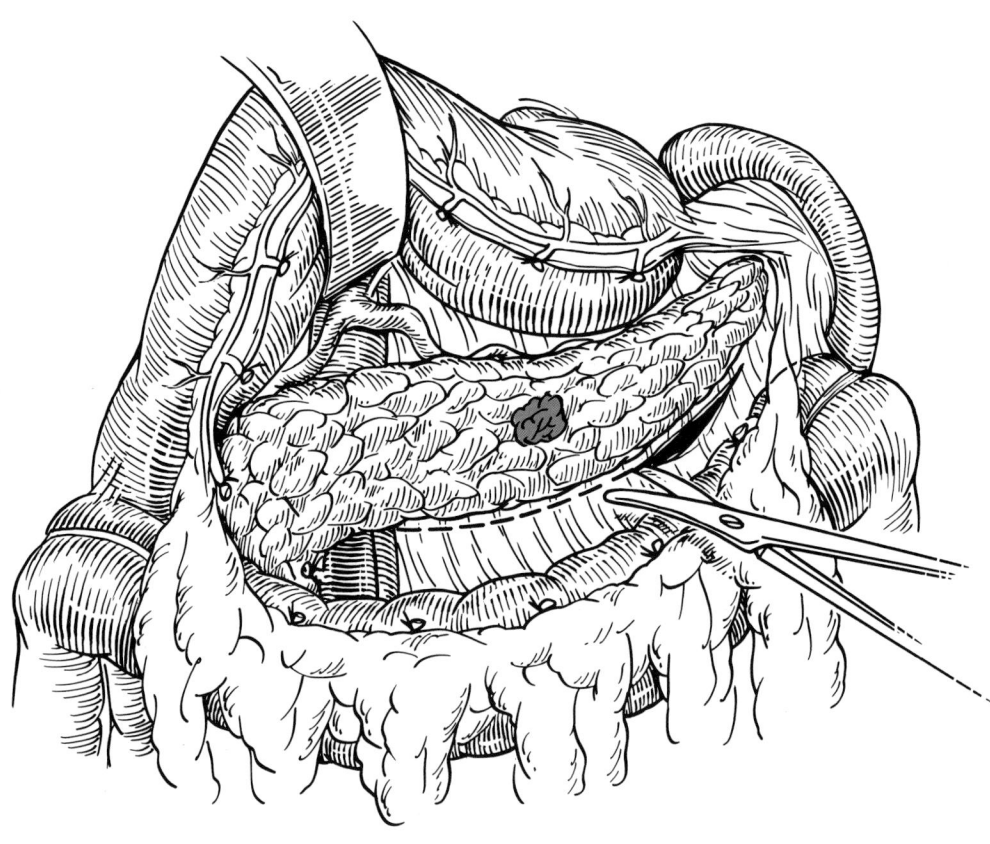

Figure 30-VIB-2

Division of Peritoneum

An incision is made in the peritoneum along the underside of the gland to the left of the superior mesenteric vessels. A few small blood vessels may need to be ligated to enter the retropancreatic plane.

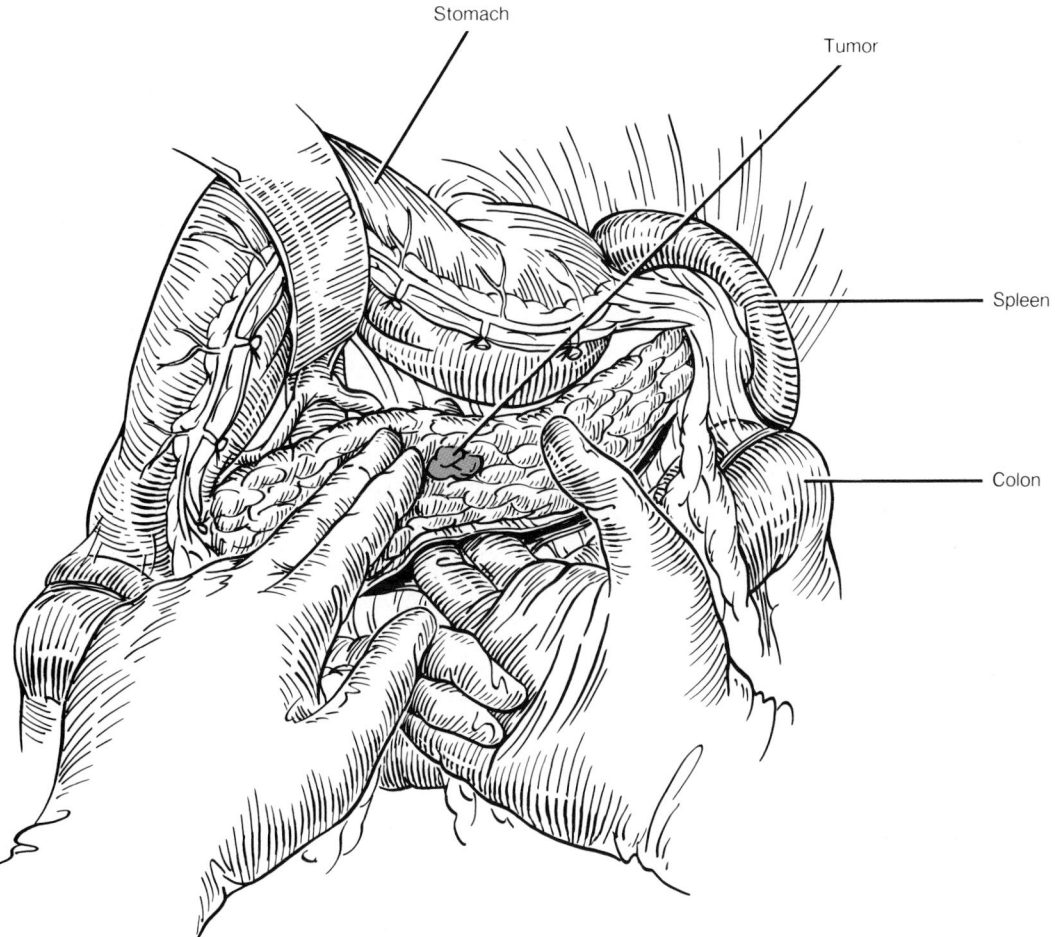

Figure 30-VIB-3

Bimanual Palpation of Pancreatic Tail

By gentle blunt dissection behind the pancreas, the body and tail can be mobilized to facilitate bimanual palpation of the gland, which is useful in searching for insulinomas of the distal pancreas if the exact location of the tumor is not obvious from external inspection of the gland.

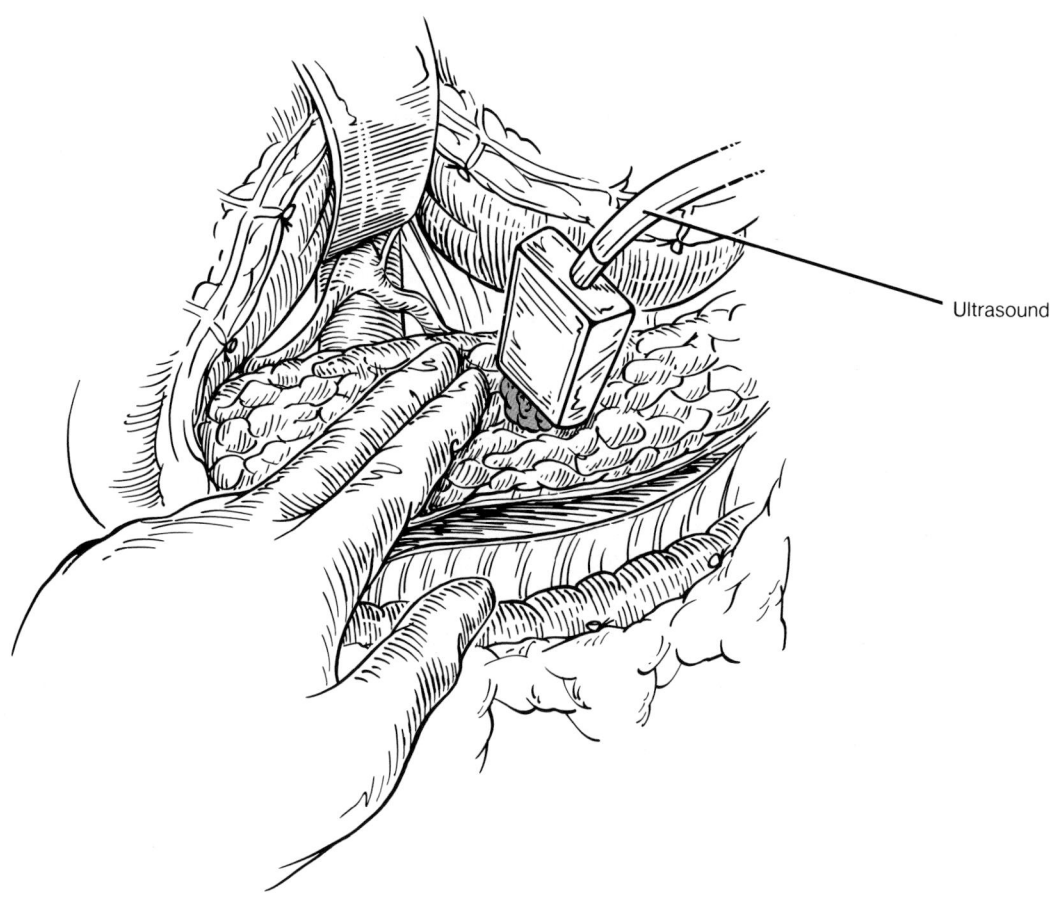

Ultrasound

Figure 30-VIB-4

Ultrasonography of Pancreas

Intraoperative ultrasound is useful for two reasons in the evaluation of insulinoma. First, it can may detect a tumor that is not visible on inspection or palpation of the gland. Second, ultrasound demonstrates the relation of the tumor to the pancreatic duct and to the splenic vein (see Chap. 27). Small tumors of the pancreas (1 cm or less) can be removed by enucleation (see Figs. 30-VIB-5 and 30-VIB-6). Larger tumors and those that abut the pancreatic duct or major vascular structures should be treated with distal pancreatectomy (for technique of distal pancreatectomy, see Section VE).

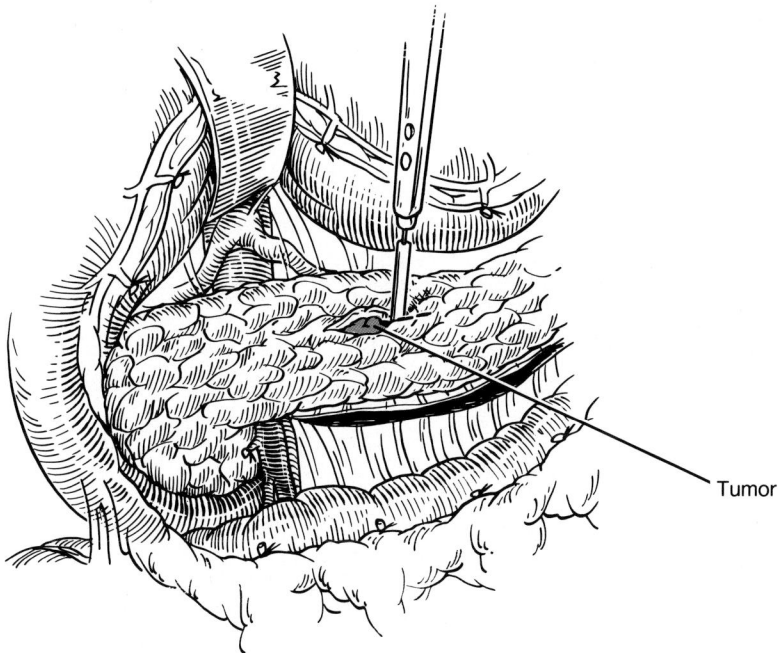

Tumor

Figure 30-VIB-5

Incision for Enucleation

If excision of the tumor will not endanger the pancreatic duct as determined by ultrasonography, the pancreatic parenchyma overlying the tumor is incised with electrocautery.

Tumor

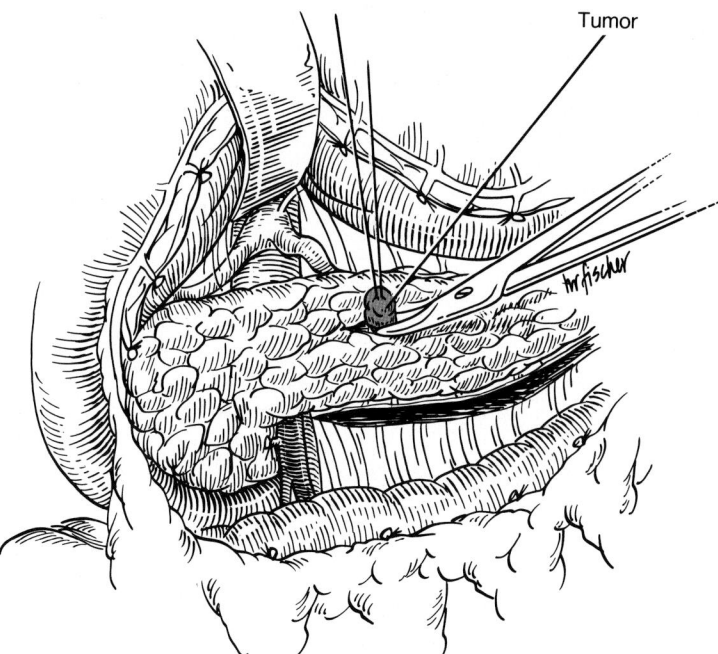

Figure 30-VIB-6

Enucleation of Tumor

A 3-0 silk suture is passed through the tumor as a holder. The tumor is carefully separated from surrounding normal pancreatic parenchyma and excised. The remaining defect in the pancreas is not closed but should be drained with a soft closed-suction drain (*not shown*) brought out through a separate stab incision in the flank.

SECTION VII Operations for Pancreaticoduodenal Trauma
A. Pancreatography

About 15% of cases of trauma to the pancreas result in major ductal disruption, usually from penetrating injuries. If inspection is inadequate to diagnose ductal injury, pancreatography is indicated since recognition of ductal injury at the time of laparotomy for trauma is critical to reducing postoperative morbidity.

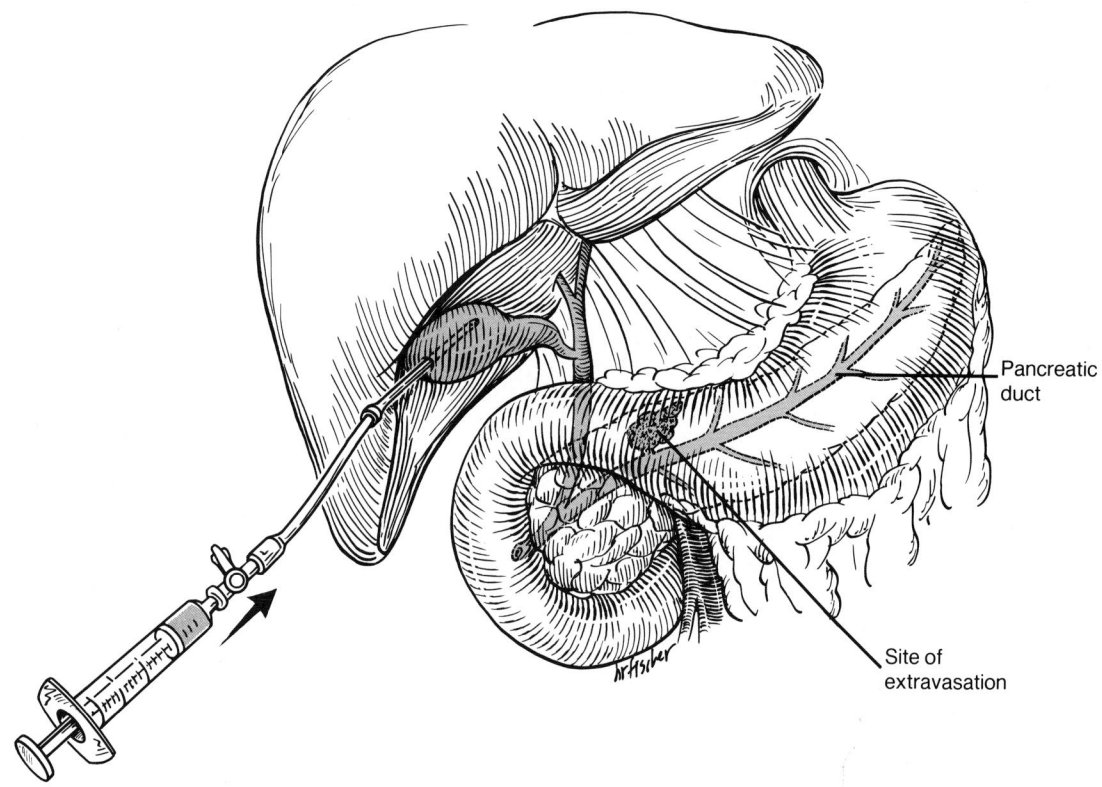

Pancreatic duct

Site of extravasation

Figure 30-VIIA-1

Pancreatography Through Common Bile Duct

Cholecystocholangiopancreatography is performed by inserting an 18-gauge angiocatheter into the gallbladder. Twenty to 30 mL of full-strength water-soluble contrast is injected into the gallbladder under fluoroscopic visualization. The induction of sphincter of Oddi contraction with intravenous morphine can increase the likelihood of refluxing dye into the pancreatic duct. After performance of the cholangiopancreatogram, the catheter is withdrawn and the hole in the gallbladder wall closed with a small pursestring suture of 3-0 silk. Cholecystectomy is not required.

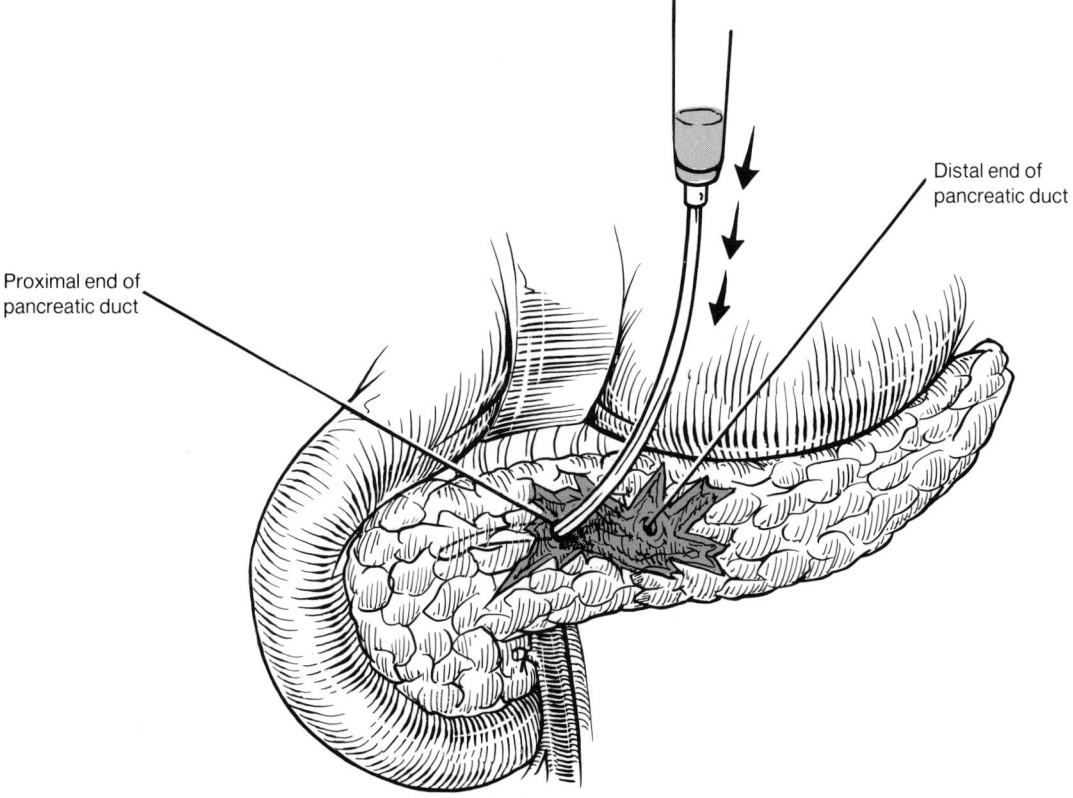

Proximal end of
pancreatic duct

Distal end of
pancreatic duct

Figure 30-VIIA-2

Direct Pancreatography Through Site of Injury

If exploration of a deep parenchymal injury of the pancreas reveals transection of the pancreatic duct, pancreatography is advised to ensure that the duct remaining after a distal pancreatic resection is intact. The proximal pancreatic duct is cannulated with a 5F feeding tube or cholangiogram catheter, and 2 to 5 mL of water-soluble contrast is allowed to flow into the duct by gravity (the plunger is removed from the syringe and the syringe held at the minimal height that allows entrance of contrast into the duct). The contrast medium should not be forcibly injected into the duct because of the possibility of transductal extravasation, which can lead to postoperative pancreatitis.

B. Simple Pancreatic Laceration

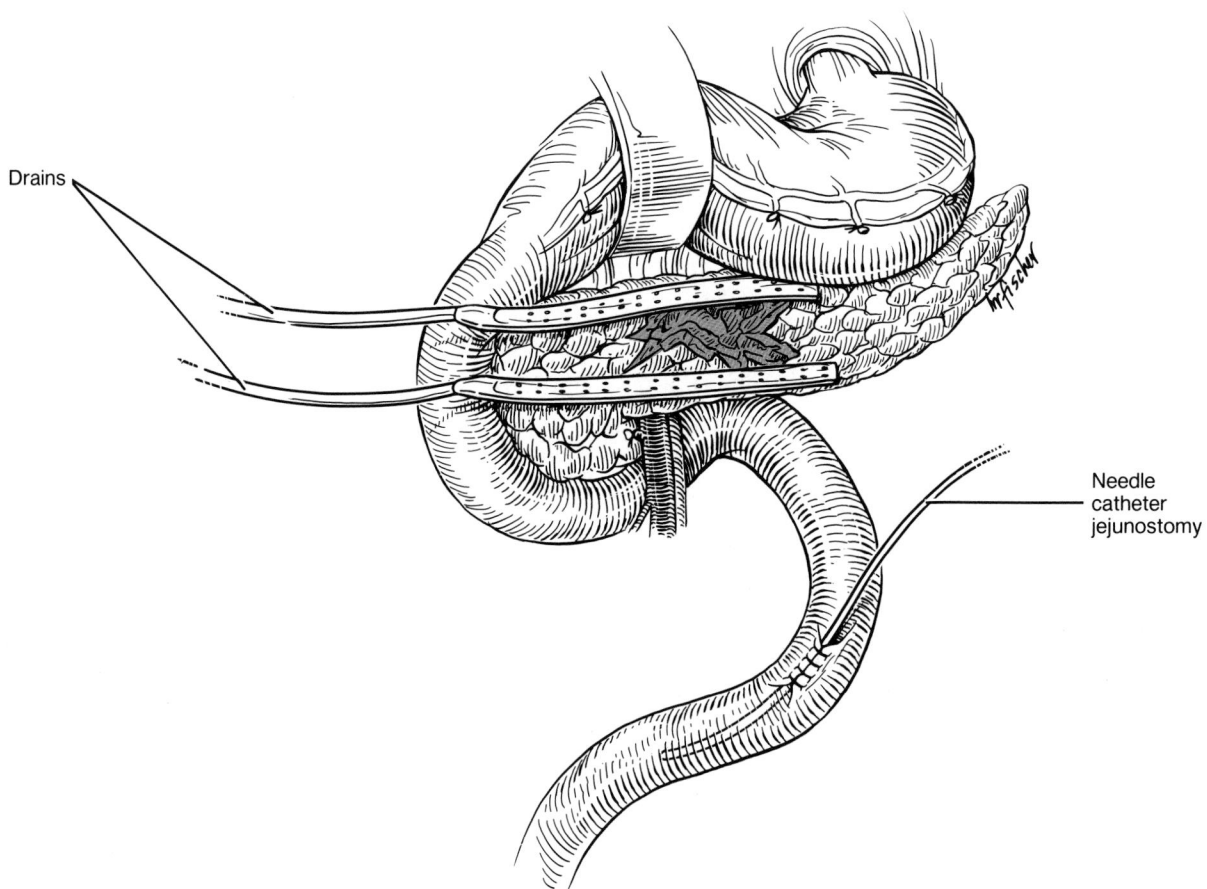

Drains

Needle
catheter
jejunostomy

Figure 30-VIIB-1

Placement of Drains

Superficial injuries to the pancreas that do not cause disruption of the major pancreatic ducts require no therapy other than the placement of drains. As shown, soft closed-suction drains are placed around the site of injury and brought out through separate stab incisions in the flank. A feeding jejunostomy is placed to allow institution of early post-operative nutrition.

C. Distal Pancreatectomy With Splenic Preservation

In rare selected instances of distal pancreatic injury, distal pancreatectomy with splenic preservation should be considered. This procedure is most applicable in children, in whom postsplenectomy sepsis is a more significant concern than in adults. Because distal pancreatectomy with splenic preservation is considerably more difficult and time-consuming than distal pancreatectomy with splenectomy, it should be performed only in patients who are hemodynamically stable and normothermic and who do not have major associated injuries. In all other patients, standard distal pancreatectomy with splenectomy is advised (see Section VE).

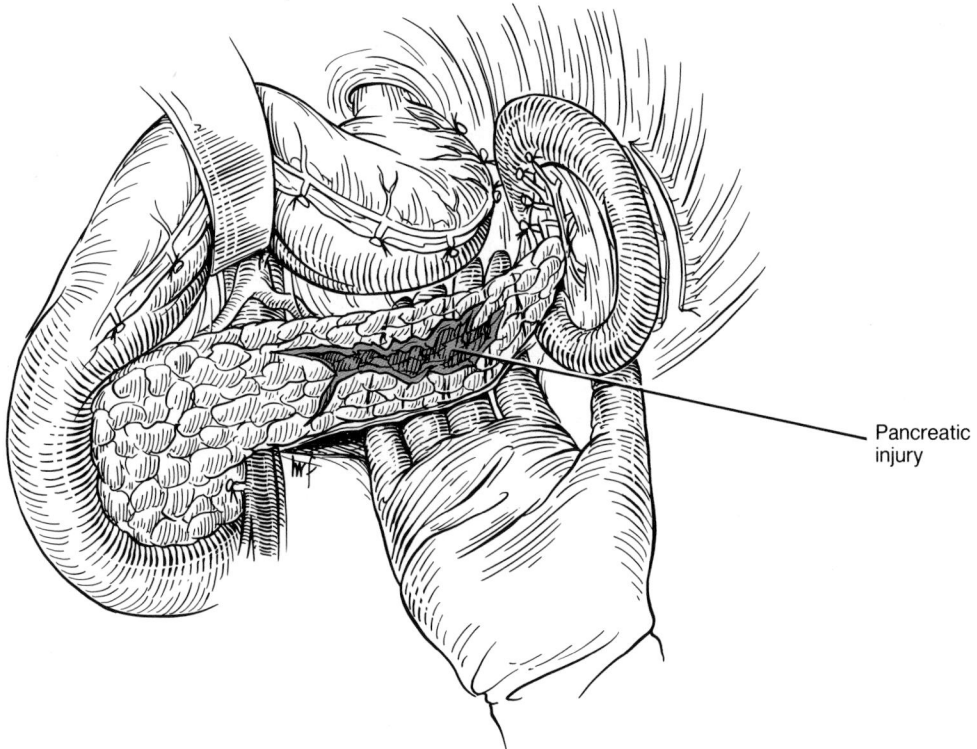

Pancreatic injury

Figure 30-VIIC-1

Mobilization of Pancreas and Spleen

The operation of distal pancreatectomy with splenic preservation is begun by mobilizing the distal pancreas and spleen. The short gastric vessels are divided between the spleen and stomach, and the splenocolic ligament is divided. The peritoneum lateral to the spleen is opened, as is the peritoneum along the inferior surface of the pancreas to the left of the superior mesenteric vessels. By gentle blunt dissection, the spleen and distal pancreas are mobilized anteriorly off the left kidney. For further details of mobilization of the distal pancreas and spleen, see Section IIB.

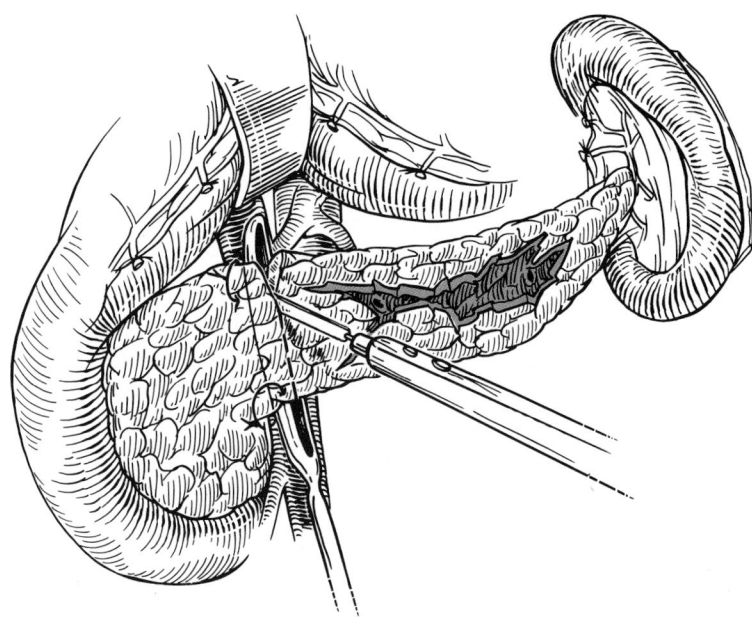

Figure 30-VIIC-2

Division of Neck of Pancreas

The superior mesenteric vein is identified by following the middle colic vein to its entrance into the superior mesenteric vein. The periadventitial tissues overlying the superior mesenteric vein are incised, and a plane of dissection is established on the anterior surface of the vein behind the neck of the pancreas. This dissection is gently continued until an instrument can be passed completely beneath the neck of the pancreas as shown. This dissection can be facilitated by identifying the portal vein within the hepatoduodenal ligament and performing the dissection of the neck of the pancreas from both above and below the gland, taking care to dissect directly on the anterior surface of the veins. Once the neck of the pancreas has been isolated, it is divided with electrocautery.

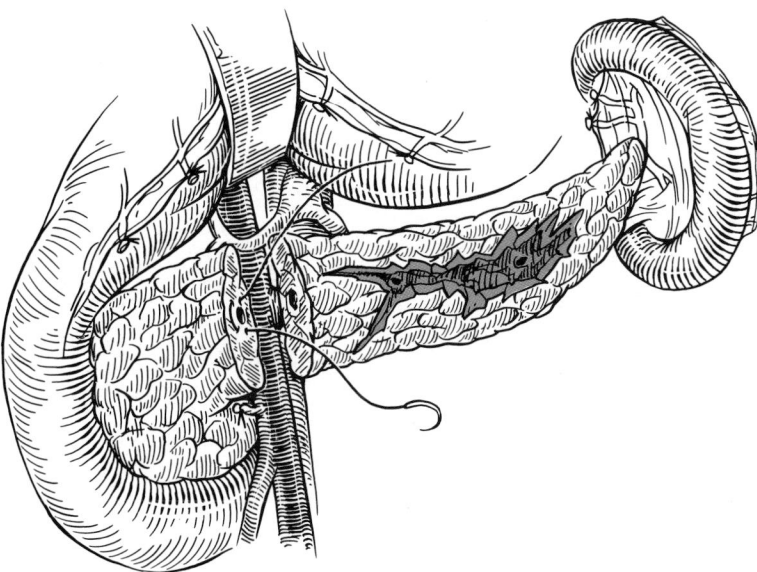

Figure 30-VIIC-3

Closure of Pancreatic Duct

After dividing the neck of the pancreas, the pancreatic duct in the head of the gland is ligated with a horizontal mattress suture of 3-0 silk.

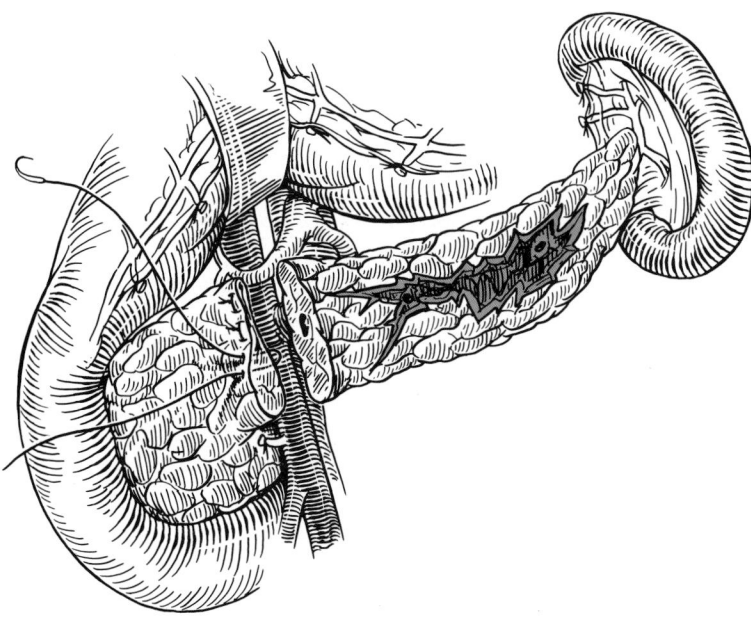

Figure 30-VIIC-4

Closure of Pancreatic Stump

The edges of the cut section of the head of the pancreas are reapproximated by a series of horizontal mattress sutures of 3-0 silk passing through the entire thickness of the gland. These sutures should be tied gently to avoid sawing through the soft pancreatic parenchyma.

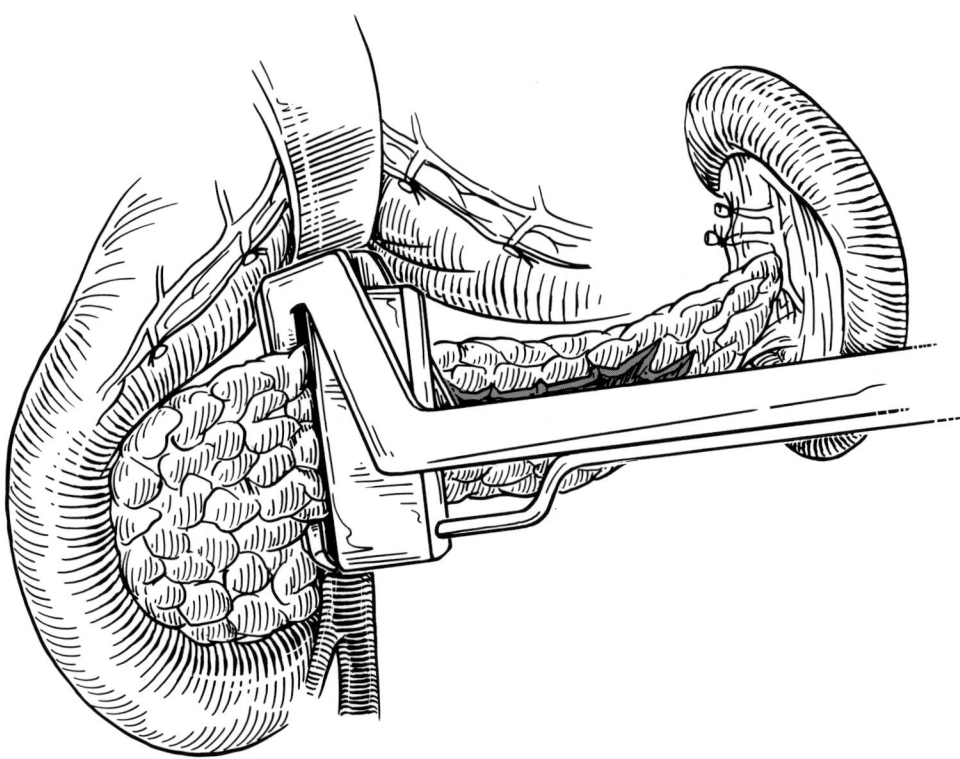

Figure 30-VIIC-5

Alternative Method for Division of the Pancreas

An alternative method for division of the neck of the pancreas and closure of the proximal pancreatic duct remnant. This technique supplants that shown in Figures 30-VIIC-2 through 30-VIIC-4. After completely isolating the neck of the pancreas from the superior mesenteric and portal veins, the lower prong of a thoracic-type stapler is passed behind the neck of the gland anterior to the veins. The stapler is tightened and fired and the pancreas divided with a knife along the guide groove on the distal side of the stapler.

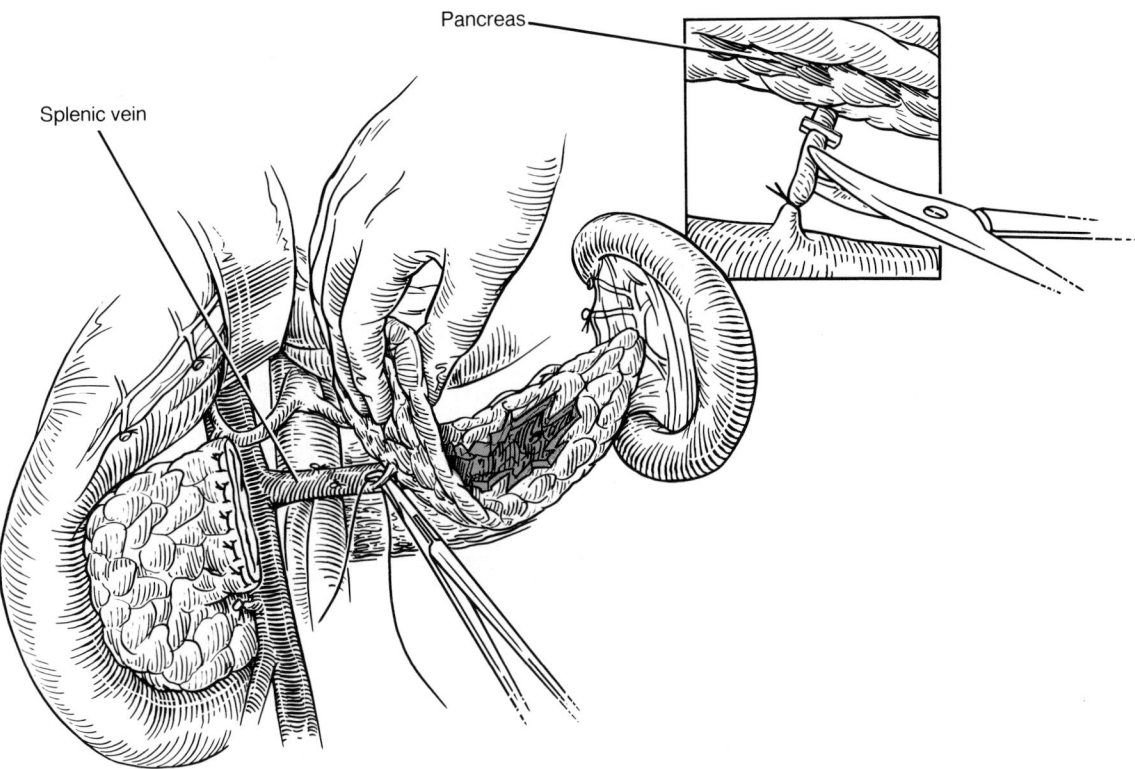

Pancreas

Splenic vein

Figure 30-VIIC-6

Ligation of Branches of Splenic Vein

After division of the neck of the gland as shown previously, the body and tail of the gland must be mobilized off the splenic artery and vein. Whereas separation from the artery is relatively straightforward, the dissection of the splenic vein is difficult because the vein is intimately attached to and sometimes partially obscured within the pancreas and because there are multiple small paired veins entering the anterior surface of the splenic vein from the pancreatic substance. While gently retracting the pancreas anteriorly, these veins are meticulously ligated with 4-0 or 5-0 silk sutures and divided. It is often difficult to place a suture on both ends of these small veins; one solution is to place a tie on the splenic vein side of the branch and a small hemostatic clip on the parenchymal side (**inset**).

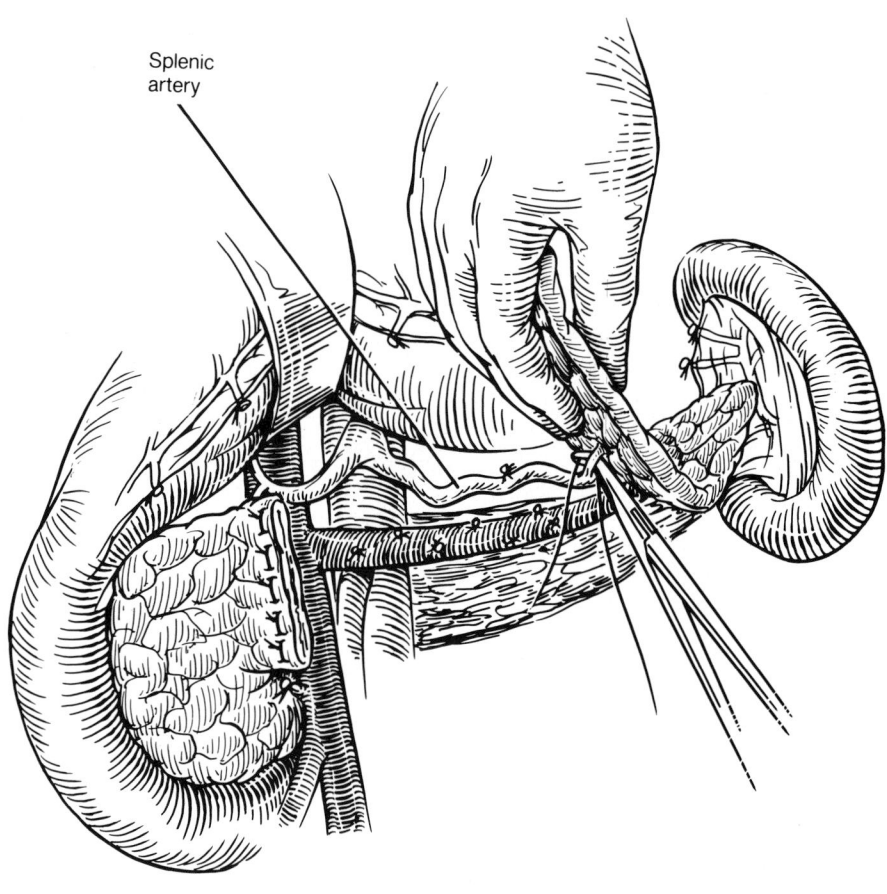

Splenic
artery

Figure 30-VIIC-7

Ligation of Branches of Splenic Artery

As the pancreas is mobilized, branches of the splenic artery entering the pancreatic parenchyma are ligated with 3-0 silk ties, preserving the main artery.

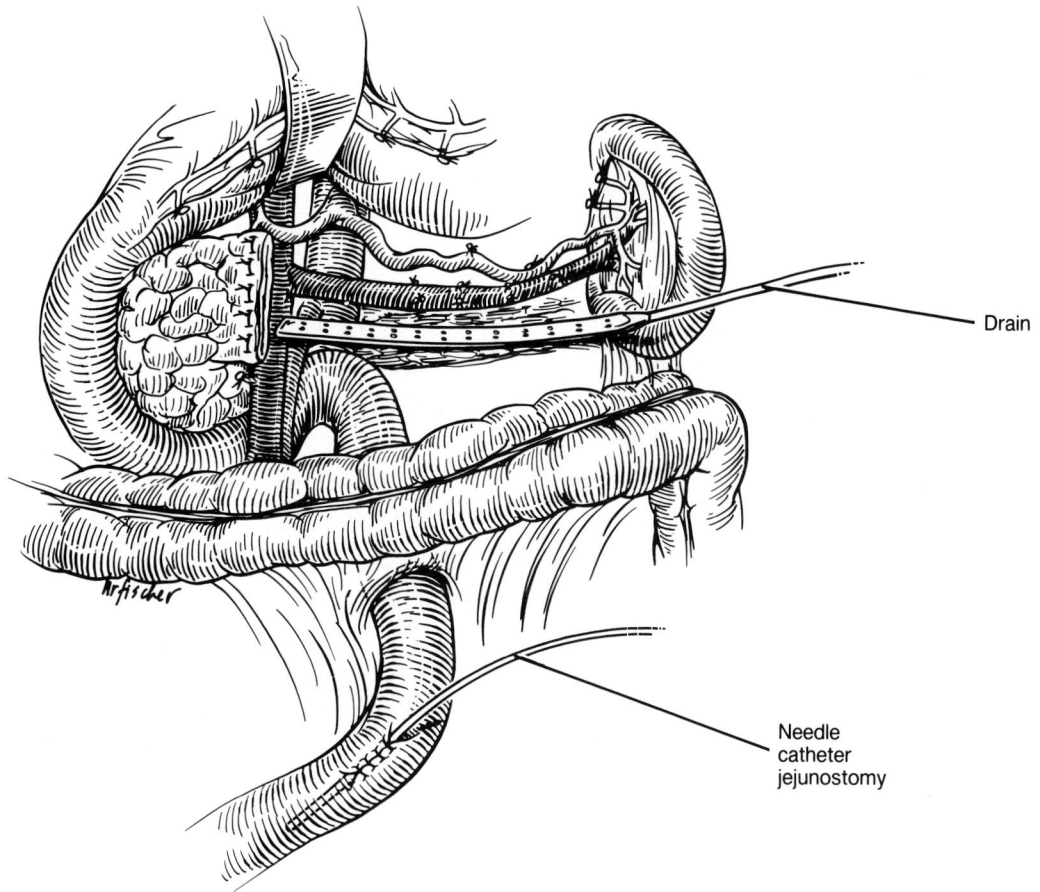

Drain

Needle
catheter
jejunostomy

Figure 30-VIIC-8

Completed Procedure

The completed operation, showing resection of the distal pancreas with preservation of the spleen and the splenic artery and vein. A soft closed-suction drain is placed near the edge of the pancreatic remnant and brought out through a separate stab incision in the flank. A needle catheter or rubber feeding jejunostomy is placed to allow early institution of postoperative nutrition.

D. Duodenal Injuries

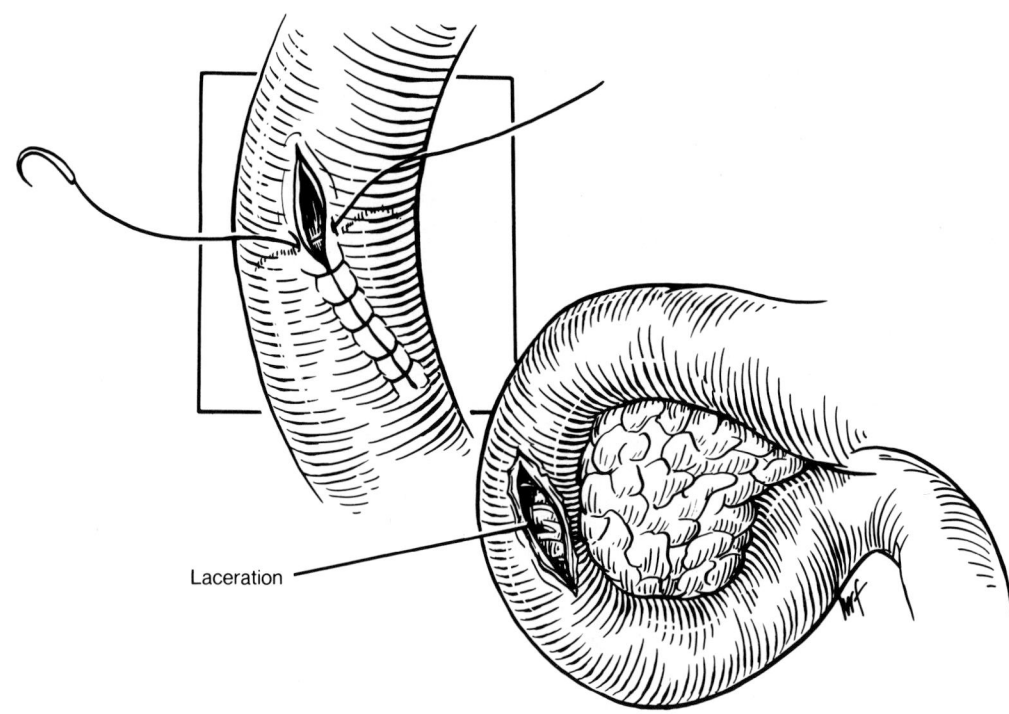

Laceration

Figure 30-VIID-1

Simple Closure of Duodenal Laceration

Simple linear lacerations through otherwise healthy-appearing duodenum can be closed primarily, either with a one-layer closure of interrupted full-thickness 4-0 silk sutures, as shown, or with a two-layer closure (preferable for longer wounds) using an inner continuous closure of 3-0 absorbable suture and an outer layer of interrupted 3-0 silk Lembert sutures.

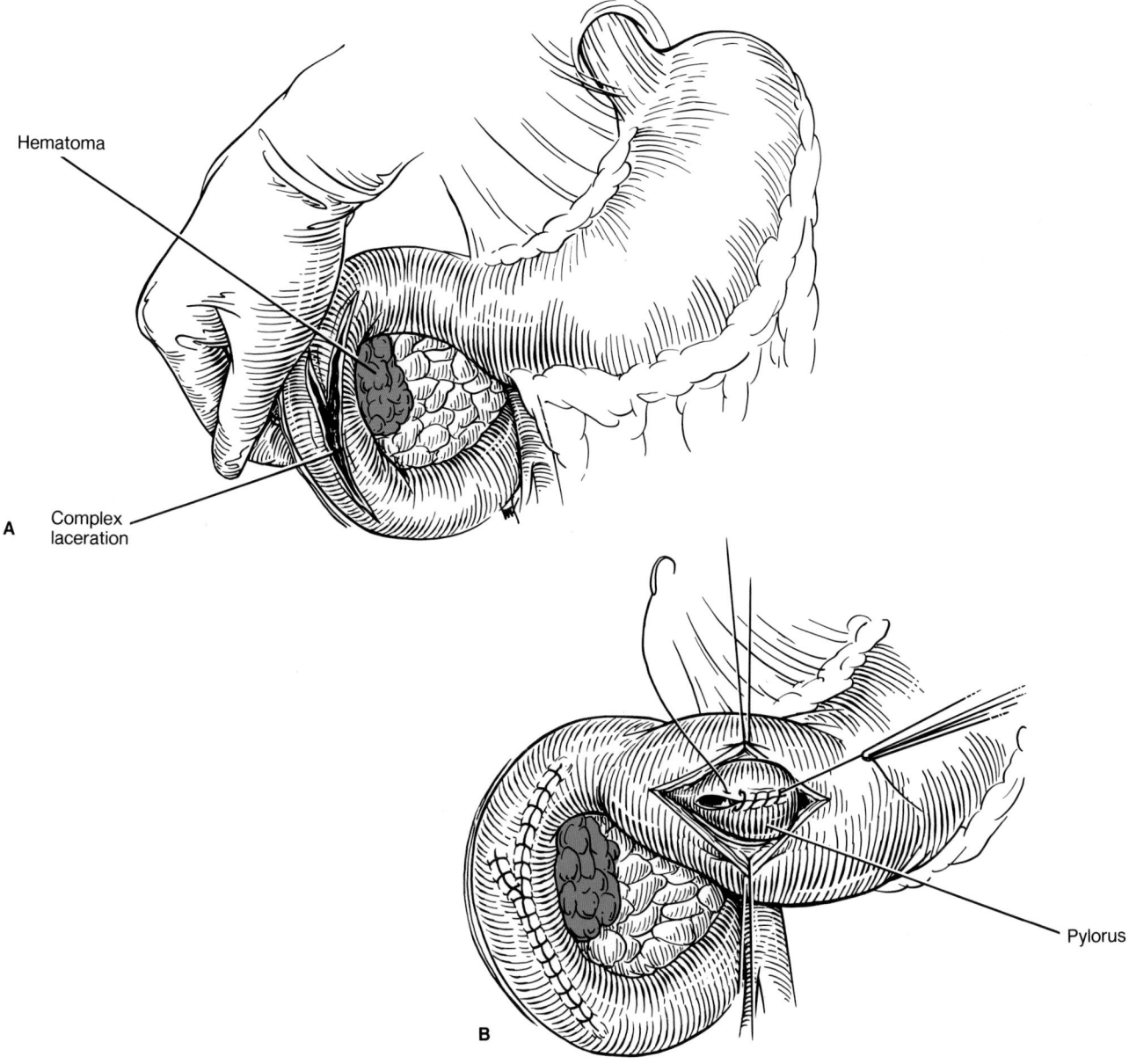

Hematoma

Complex
laceration

A

B

Pylorus

Figure 30-VIID-2

Diverticularization of the Duodenum

In severe and complex lacerations of the duodenum, particularly when associated with injuries of the pancreatic head that do not interrupt the main pancreatic duct, the technique of pyloric exclusion should be considered to temporarily divert gastric contents from the duodenum during the period of healing.

(**A**) The operation is begun by incising the peritoneum lateral to the duodenum and performing a full Kocher maneuver from the hepatoduodenal ligament to the superior mesenteric vessels. This maneuver allows better inspection of the extent of duodenal and pancreatic head injuries and improves the exposure for operative repair.

(**B**) The duodenal injury is closed primarily in one or two layers. A 3- to 4-cm distal gastrotomy is then performed on the anterior and inferior surface of the antrum, and the pylorus is visualized by retracting the edges of the gastrotomy. The pylorus is then closed from within the stomach with a continuous 2-0 absorbable synthetic suture.

(Continued)

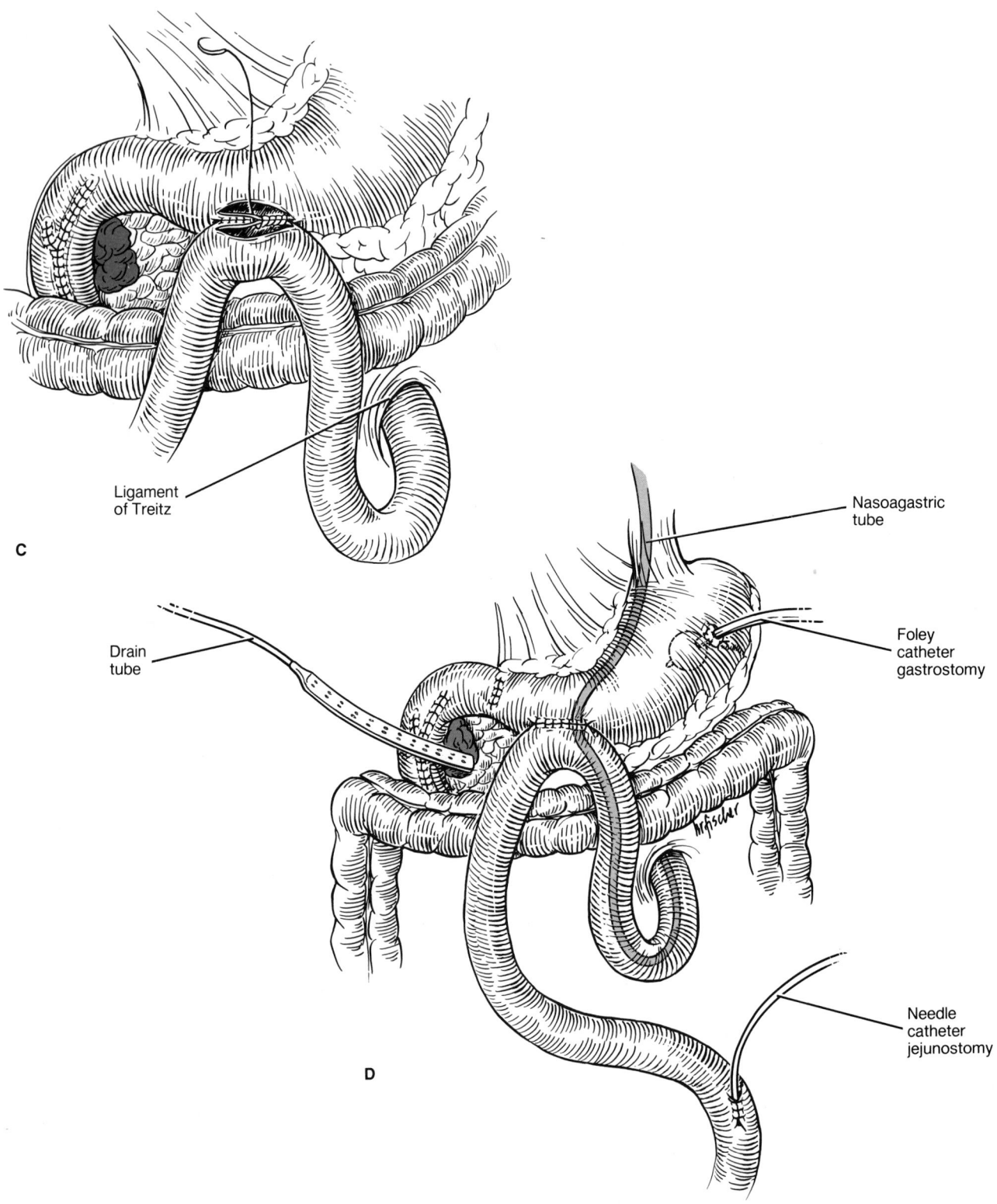

Ligament
of Treitz

C

Drain
tube

Nasoagastric
tube

Foley
catheter
gastrostomy

Needle
catheter
jejunostomy

D

Figure 30-VIID-2 *(Continued)*

(**C**) After closure of the pylorus, a side-to-side gastrojejunostomy is performed in two layers. After placing a posterior row of interrupted 3-0 silk seromuscular sutures to approximate the stomach and jejunum, a longitudinal enterotomy is performed, and an inner continuous layer of 3-0 absorbable full-thickness suture is placed.

(**D**) The gastrojejunostomy is completed with an anterior row of interrupted 3-0 silk seromuscular sutures. A nasogastric tube is guided through the gastrojejunostomy and placed retrograde into the excluded duodenum. A tube gastrostomy and feeding jejunostomy are placed, and a soft closed-suction drain is left adjacent to the duodenal injury and brought out through a separate stab incision in the flank.

PART VI
Small Intestine

31

Intestinal Obstruction, Ileus, and Pseudoobstruction

Jon S. Thompson

Digestive Tract Surgery: A Text and Atlas, edited by Richard H. Bell, Layton F. Rikkers, and Michael W. Mulholland. Lippincott-Raven Publishers, Philadelphia, © 1996.

Intestinal obstruction is a common but challenging diagnostic and therapeutic problem for the surgeon. Intestinal obstruction can be broadly defined as the failure of intestinal contents to continue their orderly progression toward the anus. Mechanical intestinal obstruction occurs when the intestinal lumen is physically constricted or blocked. This condition must be distinguished from ileus, which is an acute derangement in propulsive motility in the absence of luminal obstruction.[1] A third type of obstruction, intestinal pseudoobstruction, is characterized by disordered propulsive motility related to chronic abnormalities of the intestinal muscles and nervous system in the absence of mechanical obstruction. In this chapter, each of these entities is considered in turn, although they have many common diagnostic and therapeutic aspects. Timely operative intervention for mechanical obstruction remains an important management goal, but differentiating between the obstructive conditions has become an increasingly prominent issue. Finally, the surgical management of specific types of obstruction has continued to evolve and also is emphasized in this chapter.

MECHANICAL OBSTRUCTION

Etiology

Mechanical obstruction of the intestinal lumen usually is caused by one of three mechanisms: intraluminal blockade (obturation), intraluminal or intrinsic lesions of the bowel wall, or luminal compression or constriction by lesions extrinsic to the intestine (Table 31-1).

The various conditions that result in intestinal obstruction generally act by a single mechanism, although more than one can be operative (eg, as luminal narrowing occurs, obstruction by a foreign body is more likely). In almost one third of patients, more than one etiologic factor is identified at operation.[2]

The causes of intestinal obstruction vary in frequency according to patient age and site of obstruction. Postoperative adhesions are the most common cause of small intestinal obstruction overall.[2–5] In patients who have not previously undergone operation, inflammatory adhesions, such as those related to gynecologic conditions, must be considered. Adhesions, hernias, and malignant conditions account for 80% of all cases of intestinal obstruction.[2–5] In children, adhesions are the cause of obstruction in less than 10% of cases; intussusception is a more common problem in this age group.[6] Volvulus and intussusception account for about 30% of cases of intestinal obstruction complicating pregnancy and delivery.[7] Cancer should be suspected in elderly patients with intestinal obstruction.[8] Metastatic genitourinary, colonic, pancreatic, and gastric carcinomas cause obstruction more often than do primary small intestinal tumors.[9] Malignancy, diverticular disease, and volvulus are the most common causes of colonic obstruction, with primary colorectal cancer accounting for almost 50% of cases.[10]

Pathophysiology

Small Intestinal Response to Obstruction

Normally, about 2 L of ingested fluids and solids and 8 L of gastric, intestinal, and pancreaticobiliary secretions traverse the intestine daily.[11] Although fluid

Table 31-1   Causes of Mechanical Intestinal Obstruction

INTRALUMINAL OBTURATION	INTRINSIC LESIONS
Foreign bodies	*Congenital*
Iatrogenic	Atresia, stenosis, and webs
Ingested	Duplications
Gallstones	Meckel's diverticulum
Worms	*Inflammatory*
Intussusception	Diverticulitis
Impacted Fluids	Drug-induced
Barium	Infectious diseases
Feces	Ischemic
Meconium	Radiation enteritis
EXTRINSIC LESIONS	Regional enteritis
Adhesions	Ulcerative colitis
Foreign bodies	*Neoplastic*
Hernias	Benign tumors
External	Carcinoma
Internal	Carcinoid
Masses	Lymphoma
Anomalous organs or vessels	Sarcoma
Organomegaly	*Traumatic*
Fluid collections	Intramural hematoma
Neoplasms	
Postoperative	
Volvulus	

fluxes occur in the upper small intestine, most of this fluid is absorbed in the distal small intestine and colon. Intestinal obstruction results in the accumulation of luminal fluid above the level of obstruction because of disruption of the normal intestinal fluid absorptive mechanism proximal to the site of obstruction and failure of luminal contents to reach the avidly absorbing distal intestine.

The progressive accumulation of intraluminal fluid proximal to the site of obstruction occurs within a few hours and is due to several factors. Further ingested fluid and secretions enter the intestinal tract. Intestinal blood flow increases early after the onset of obstruction, particularly proximal to the lesion, which can increase intestinal secretion.[12] This is related, in part, to decreased responsiveness of the splanchnic vessels in the obstructed gut to vasoactive mediators.[13] Rapid infusion of intravenous fluid also increases intraluminal fluid.[14] Net secretion of fluid into the lumen occurs because of impairment of normal absorptive and secretory mechanisms.[15,16] Luminal distention causes venous congestion, intraluminal edema, and, ultimately, ischemia. As intraluminal pressure increases above 20 cm H_2O, fluid flux from lumen to blood is markedly impaired and that from blood to lumen is paradoxically increased.[16] Similar changes occur in sodium and chloride absorption and secretion.[15] However, increased intralu-

minal pressure is not always present and there undoubtedly are other mechanisms for secretory changes. Increased secretion may be mediated by gastrointestinal hormones, such as increased circulating vasoactive intestinal polypeptide, prostaglandins, or endotoxins.[17,18]

Intestinal gas, most of which is ingested, also accumulates during intestinal obstruction.[18,19] Smaller amounts are produced by neutralization of bicarbonate or by bacterial metabolism.[10] Intestinal gas consists predominantly of nitrogen (70%), oxygen (12%), and carbon dioxide (8%), a composition similar to that of air. Thus, only carbon dioxide has a sufficient partial pressure gradient to promote diffusion from the lumen.

The intestine normally tries to overcome a mechanical obstruction by increasing peristalsis. After a period of continuous hyperperistalsis, intermittent quiescent intervals occur, and eventually ileus results.[20,21] The intestine distal to the point of obstruction becomes less active early on. Prolonged mechanical obstruction results in reduced slow-wave frequency and impaired spike activity, but the intestine responds to stimulation.[22] Thus, prolonged ileus can persist after obstruction is relieved. The stagnation of intestinal contents can result in bacterial proliferation. Both aerobic and anaerobic bacteria begin to populate the obstructed intestine.[5,18,23] Bacterial overgrowth can further aggravate absorptive and motor function of the intestine and lead to bacterial translocation and septic complications.[18] The increasing volume of intraluminal contents begins to distend the more proximal intestinal tract, resulting in nausea and vomiting. As the duration of obstruction increases, there is progressive impairment of both absorption and secretion in the more proximal gut. Thus, mechanical obstruction leads to an increasing intravascular fluid deficit related to vomiting, intraluminal fluid accumulation, intramural edema, and intraperitoneal transudation of fluid. Placement of a nasogastric tube further exacerbates the external losses. Hypokalemic hypochloremic metabolic alkalosis commonly complicates high obstruction. Untreated hypovolemia can lead to renal insufficiency, shock, and death.

Strangulation

Strangulation obstruction is the loss of blood supply to an obstructed segment of intestine. This can occur from direct compression of the mesenteric vessels (eg, by a hernia orifice or axial twisting) or as the result of local changes in the intestinal wall. This serious complication is often associated with obstruction from hernia and volvulus, and is found at 15% of operations for small intestinal obstruction.[2-5] The most frequent cause of strangulation obstruction in the colon is volvulus.

Intramural ischemia develops for several reasons. Intraluminal distention and pressure causes venous congestion, capillary leakage, bowel wall edema and hemorrhage, and, ultimately, venous and arterial thrombosis.[24,25] Bacterial overgrowth occurs within a few hours with strangulation obstruction.[23] This results in the production of various intraluminal toxins and can stimulate the release of vasoactive mediators such as prostaglandins.[18,25] The mucosa of the intestine is most susceptible to ischemia, and several factors appear to play a role in this injury, including hypoxia, pancreatic proteases, and oxygen-derived free radicals.[26] The mucosa of the small intestine is more sensitive to ischemia than is the mucosa of the colon.[27] As mucosal necrosis occurs, bacteria and toxins can more readily traverse the intestinal wall into the peritoneal cavity, mesenteric lymph nodes, and circulation.[28] This leads to progressive ischemia, sepsis, frank perforation of the bowel with peritonitis, and, ultimately, death due to septic shock. Gut ischemia and reperfusion also contribute to remote organ failure, such as lung injury.[29]

Closed Loop Obstruction

When a segment of intestine is blocked at two points, a closed loop obstruction occurs. Volvulus is a common cause and can result in twisting of the mesentery as well.[30] Distal obstruction of the large intestine leads to a closed loop obstruction if the ileocecal valve remains competent.[10] As intraluminal pressure increases in the obstructed segment, secretion of fluid into the lumen increases and absorption decreases.[16] The clinical significance of this phenomenon is a high risk of strangulation.[31] A closed loop distends rapidly and often progresses to strangulation before clinical signs of obstruction are obvious.

Partial Intestinal Obstruction

In partial intestinal obstruction, the lumen is not completely occluded. Adhesions are the most common cause and strangulation is unusual.[32] Chronic partial obstruction results in marked thickening of the intestinal wall secondary to muscular hypertrophy. Prolonged simultaneous contractions and an increase in clustered contractions are characteristic manometric findings.[33] These motor abnormalities and the commonly associated bacterial overgrowth can lead to malabsorption, bloating, and secretory diarrhea.[34]

Colonic Obstruction

The pathophysiology of colonic obstruction is different from that of small intestinal obstruction. The colon normally has a limited role in absorption, partic-

ularly distally. Fluid and gas accumulate more slowly in the colon because of its distal position in the gastrointestinal tract and because most fluid is absorbed in the small intestine. This more gradual distention allows the colon to adapt, and decompression can occur through an incompetent ileocecal valve. As mentioned earlier, a competent valve can lead to a closed loop obstruction. Cecal dilation is most marked, and the large diameter and thin wall of the cecum puts it at risk for rupture.[35] Rupture can be related to ischemia of the wall, diastasis of the muscle layers, or bacterial invasion of the wall.[10] With distal obstruction, blood flow is increased to the left colon but decreased to the cecum.[36] Colonic obstruction results in abnormal motility but not hyperperistalsis.[37] Nonperistaltic high-amplitude complexes occur nearly simultaneously throughout the colon, resulting in mass actions that may be the basis for colic and rushing bowel sounds.

Clinical Presentation

Abdominal pain, nausea and vomiting, and failure to pass stool or gas per rectum are the hallmark symptoms of intestinal obstruction. Cramping pain is the initial complaint, which corresponds with hypermotility proximal to the obstructing lesion. The pain is diffuse and poorly localized but generally is felt in the mid-abdomen. As peristalsis becomes intermittent, the colicky pain also becomes intermittent. The onset of constant, generalized pain suggests progression to strangulation and infarction.

Vomiting occurs early secondary to obstruction of the lumen and then becomes more frequent and voluminous as fluid accumulation occurs. The degree of vomiting correlates with the level of obstruction, being a more prominent feature of high obstruction. High obstruction also is characterized by bilious vomiting, whereas low obstruction causes a more malodorous (feculent) vomitus.

Failure to pass gas or stool is an important sign for distinguishing between complete and partial obstruction. Fecal output can continue for hours after a high obstruction due to passage of luminal contents below the obstruction. Episodic diarrhea can be a feature of partial obstruction.

Physical findings can be absent early, but progressive distention will occur, especially with distal obstruction. The patient will begin to show signs of dehydration. Although some guarding may be present on palpation of the abdomen, tenderness is minimal unless complications ensue. A palpable mass should raise concern about malignancy, abscess, or strangulation. Auscultation is useful for dividing patients into three categories: loud, high-pitched bowel sounds with bursts or rushes suggest early mechanical obstruction; absent bowel sounds indicate prolonged mechanical obstruction, paralytic ileus, or intestinal infarction; and normally active or decreased bowel sounds can suggest progressing obstruction but usually are nonspecific findings. With time, dehydration becomes more significant and signs of strangulation can appear. Examination of the groin and incisions for hernias, and rectal examination to evaluate for blood or mass should be performed routinely.

Although the classic findings of strangulation obstruction are constant pain, fever, tachycardia, and tenderness, none of these are present in 10% to 15% of patients with strangulated bowel.[30,38–41] Furthermore, at least one of these findings is present in 90% of patients with simple obstruction. Thus, diagnosis of strangulation obstruction on the basis of clinical findings alone is difficult.

Diagnostic Evaluation

Laboratory Findings

Initial laboratory investigation of the patient with suspected intestinal obstruction should include a complete blood count and serum electrolyte, blood urea nitrogen, serum creatinine, and serum amylase levels. Simple intestinal obstruction does not cause characteristic changes in laboratory results, so these studies rarely are helpful in the diagnosis of intestinal obstruction. Serum electrolyte determinations and renal function tests can detect associated hypokalemia, hypochloremia, and azotemia in 50% of patients.[2] Simple obstruction can be associated with a slight elevation of the leukocyte count and a shift in peripheral leukocyte maturation, but more marked changes are characteristic of strangulation obstruction and other causes of ileus. Although the prevalence of leukocytosis is in-

creased with strangulation, it does not accurately predict this complication.[38,40] Hyperamylasemia can accompany bowel distention and strangulation, making it difficult to exclude acute pancreatitis from the differential diagnosis.[38]

Several tests have been evaluated for their ability to help detect intestinal ischemia due to strangulation obstruction, including serum lactate and phosphate concentrations and various enzyme levels.[38,42–44] Metabolic acidosis is an ominous finding but is not specific for intestinal gangrene. Enzyme levels are not routinely elevated until there is prolonged, extensive ischemia. It is uncertain whether more recently studied mucosal enzymes, such as diamine oxidase and fatty acid binding protein, will prove to be clinically useful.[43,44]

Radiologic Studies

Plain abdominal films are important in the diagnosis and treatment of all patients with obstruction but clearly indicate obstruction in only 50% of patients in whom it is present.[2] A perforation series should be performed initially (upright and supine abdominal views, left lateral decubitus and upright chest films) to evaluate the abdomen for other causes of pain or for complications (eg, pneumoperitoneum from perforated viscus[45]; Fig. 31-1). Upright and supine abdominal films are sufficient after the obstruction has progressed. The presence of gallstones, renal calculi, calcified blood vessels, and radiopaque foreign bodies can suggest other explanations for the patient's complaints.

Small intestinal obstruction is associated with air–fluid levels and dilated intestinal loops (Fig. 31-2). Colonic gas is usually absent.[46–49] Proximal obstruction causes fewer dilated loops and air–fluid levels. If the intestine is primarily fluid filled (eg, closed loop obstruction), the radiographic findings may not suggest

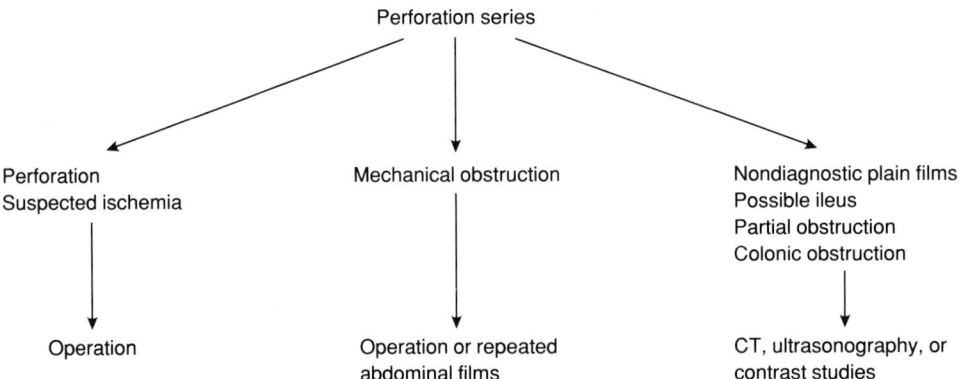

Figure 31-1 Algorithm for radiologic evaluation of patients with suspected intestinal obstruction.

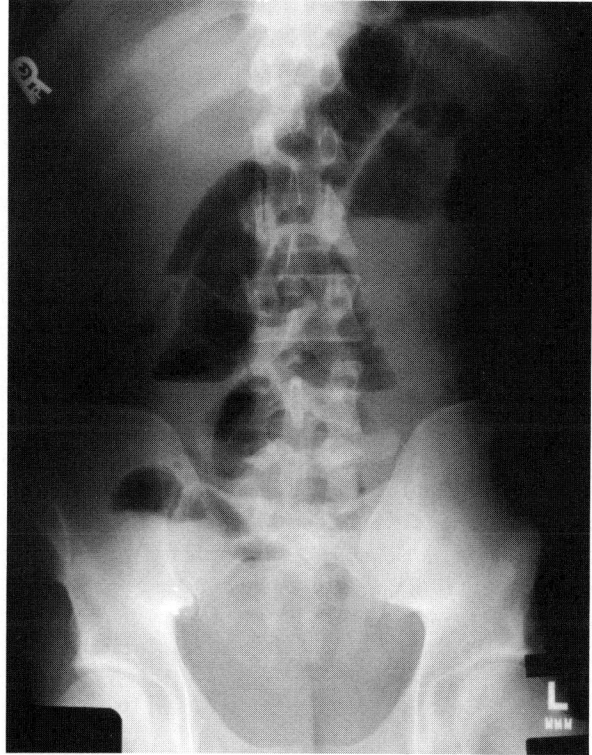

Figure 31-2 Plain abdominal radiograph showing intestinal obstruction. Dilated loops of small intestine are seen in a "stepladder" pattern. Minimal colonic gas is present.

obstruction.[46] Pneumobilia in the absence of a biliary enteric anastomosis suggests gallstone ileus as the cause of obstruction. Several features of plain abdominal films can help in differentiating mechanical obstruction from ileus[46-48] (Table 31-2). However, this distinction can be difficult in 50% of patients.[4,47]

The radiographic appearance of colonic obstruction depends on both the site of obstruction and the competence of the ileocecal valve.[10] The most prominent dilation occurs in the cecum, and a cecal diameter greater than 10 to 12 cm should raise concern about potential rupture. If the ileocecal valve is competent, there may be little associated small bowel distention unless there is a synchronous proximal obstruction or ileus. An incompetent ileocecal valve allows reflux into the small intestine with the radiographic appearance of more generalized dilation. Dilated loops of the large intestine filled with air and fluid, particularly with a bird's beak narrowing, suggest volvulus as the obstructive lesion. A sigmoid volvulus projects into the right upper quadrant with a sausage-like configuration. A cecal volvulus projects into the left upper or mid-abdomen, except for the cecal bascule, where the cecum folds on its transverse axis and, thus, lies on the right side of the abdomen.

Several radiologic findings suggest strangulation obstruction.[46] The bowel wall can be thickened with thumbprinting and loss of mucosal pattern. There can be signs of intraperitoneal fluid. Loop fixation with loss of the valvulae conniventes suggests strangulation. The diaphragm often is elevated but moves normally unless peritonitis develops. Pneumatosis intestinalis and air within the portal venous radicles should raise suspicion of intestinal gangrene.[46,50-52]

Gastrointestinal contrast studies are useful in evaluating partial intestinal obstruction, colonic obstruction, and cases in which the diagnosis is otherwise unclear (eg, loops of bowel with primarily fluid distention and patients who have undergone operation[49,53-55]; Fig. 31-3). These studies yield information on the type and location of the obstruction. They should not be performed if perforation is suspected, because intraperitoneal spillage of barium is a concern.[56] Although water-soluble contrast can be used, it often does not provide good mucosal visualization because of dilution and it poses a risk of potential injury from aspiration.

When ileus is present, the contrast medium slowly advances through the gastrointestinal tract over 4 to 6 hours. Contrast material passes more quickly with partial or complete mechanical obstruction. Enteroclysis, which involves intubation of the duodenum and forceful injection of contrast material, can detect more subtle and distal lesions.[55,57,58] This study generally causes more distention and provides better mucosal detail. If a long intestinal tube is already in place, it can be used for this purpose.

Contrast studies of the colon are particularly valu-

Table 31-2 Radiologic Differentiation of Intestinal Obstruction and Ileus

Radiographic Finding	Mechanical Obstruction	Ileus
Air–fluid levels	Present proximal to obstruction	Prominent throughout
Gas in small intestine	Large bow-shaped loops; "stepladder" pattern	Gas present diffusely; moveable
Gas in colon	Absent or diminished	Increased throughout
Thickened bowel wall	Present if chronic or strangulation	Present with inflammation
Intraabdominal fluid	Rare	Often present
Diaphragm	Slightly elevated; normal motion	Elevated; decreased motion
Gastrointestinal contrast media	Rapid progression to point of obstruction	Slow progression to colon (hours)

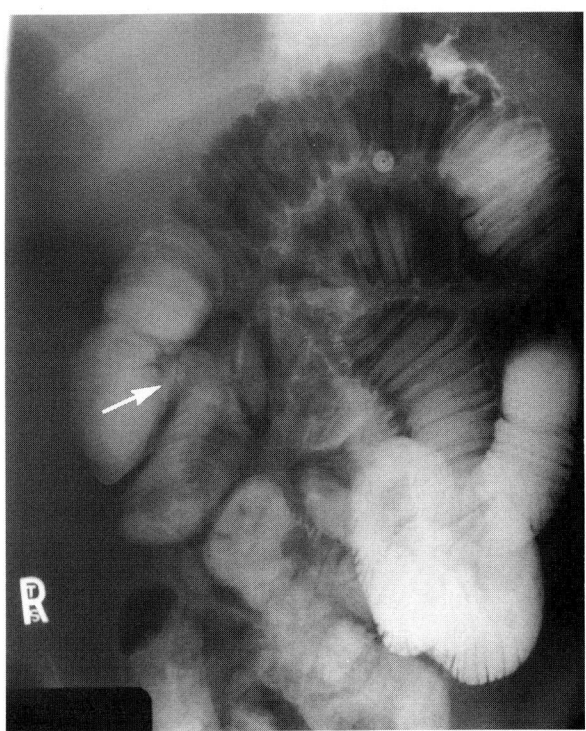

Figure 31-3 Small bowel contrast study showing obstruction. Dilated proximal intestine abruptly changes caliber at a right lower quadrant adhesion (*arrow*).

able in evaluating suspected colonic obstruction.[59,60] Such studies confirm the presence of mechanical obstruction, preventing inappropriate treatment of patients with pseudoobstruction. The point of obstruction and probable etiology can be identified in most cases. Because most patients with large bowel obstruction do not require immediate surgical exploration, contrast studies should be undertaken routinely unless perforation is suspected or marked dilation is present.

Computed tomography and ultrasonography also can suggest mechanical obstruction.[61-64] However, these studies usually are more helpful in evaluating other intraabdominal problems. These imaging techniques can detect bowel wall thickening, luminal stenosis, intramucosal and extraintestinal air, fluid-filled intestine, and other fluid collections. Intussusception has a characteristic appearance of an intraluminal soft tissue mass with an eccentric fatty area of attenuation, corresponding with the intussusception and the intussuscepted mesentery.[63] The coiled-spring sign seen on contrast radiography also can be detected. Computed tomography and ultrasonography should be considered in patients with suspected malignancy, no previous operations, and signs suggesting intraabdominal inflammation.[64]

Treatment

General Considerations

INITIAL THERAPY. The appropriate timing of operative intervention remains a crucial issue in the treatment of intestinal obstruction. The risk of strangulation and the likelihood of resolution with nonoperative treatment are the important factors. Operation should be performed immediately if a closed loop obstruction or strangulation obstruction is suspected. Severe constant pain, rebound tenderness, fever, tachycardia, and leukocytosis suggest the need for emergency surgical intervention. As mentioned earlier, however, clinical findings are not entirely reliable. Early mechanical obstruction can be treated initially without surgery, with about a 25% chance of avoiding operation.[49] Partial intestinal obstruction, early postoperative obstruction, and colonic obstruction are less likely to be complicated by strangulation and thus permit more extended nonoperative therapy. Patients with metastatic cancer, regional enteritis, a history of therapeutic radiation, or multiple recurrent obstruction also should be approached more cautiously.

Although most patients with mechanical obstruction eventually require surgery, preliminary nonoperative therapy for up to 24 hours is appropriate if intestinal ischemia is not a concern (Fig. 31-4). However, persistent pain or tenderness after decompression, leukocytosis, fever, or metabolic acidosis should prompt immediate operation. Patients without histories of previous operations should be explored more expeditiously because volvulus and internal hernia are more likely. Nasogastric suction (with an 18F sump tube) and fluid and electrolyte therapy should be instituted while diagnostic tests are being carried out. Patients who have been vomiting commonly have hypokalemic metabolic alkalosis, necessitating intravenous infusion of normal saline solution with potassium supplementation. Hemodynamic monitoring should be instituted as appropriate. The goals of therapy are to restore the volume deficit, correct electrolyte abnormalities and acid–base imbalance, and detect any other metabolic derangements that need to be addressed.

Prophylactic antibiotics should be administered before operation.[65] Although the small intestine usually harbors few bacteria, obstruction promotes colonization with colonic-type flora, both aerobes and anaerobes.[5,23] Thus, broad-spectrum coverage is indicated. A second- or third-generation cephalosporin or an extended-spectrum penicillin should be adequate. A combination of an aminoglycoside and anaerobic coverage (eg, metronidazole) is a reasonable alternative.

The use of short nasogastric tubes versus long intestinal tubes in the nonoperative management of me-

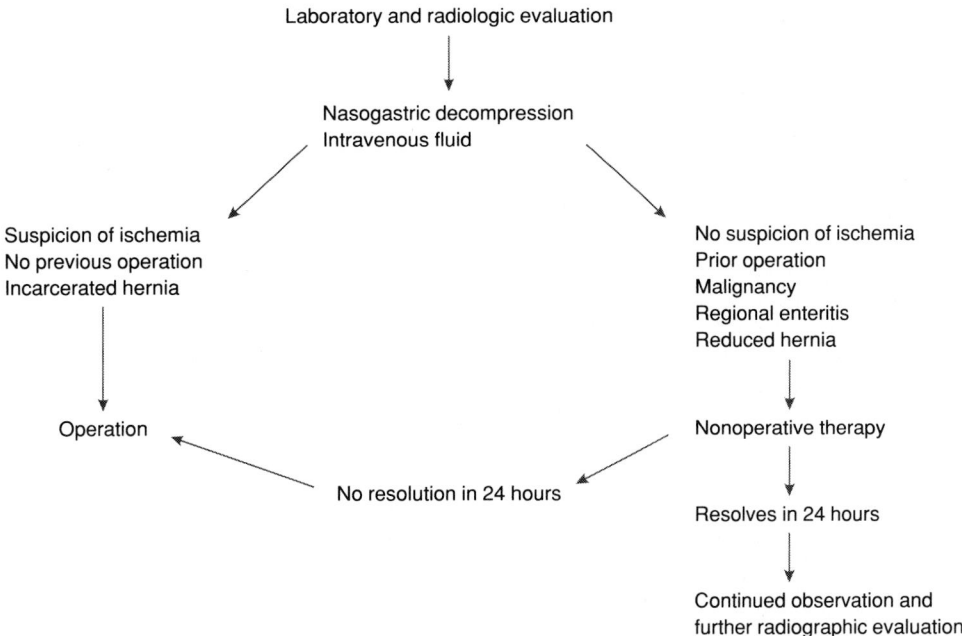

Figure 31-4 Algorithm for evaluation and treatment of patients with suspected complete mechanical bowel obstruction.

chanical obstruction is the subject of ongoing controversy.[49,66-71] Nasogastric suction is more expeditious and removes most of the upper intestinal secretions and swallowed air. Long tubes are more difficult to place and may not adequately decompress the stomach.[67] Their placement can be expedited with endoscopic assistance.[72] The use of long intestinal tubes can lead to unnecessary delay of surgery in patients with complete small bowel obstruction and has been associated with longer hospitalization and greater duration of ileus.[49] Long tubes may have a role in certain situations, including postoperative obstruction, partial intestinal obstruction, recurrent obstruction, inflammatory bowel disease, and carcinomatosis.[61-71] However, there is no convincing evidence that the rate of resolution of obstruction is greater with long intestinal tubes than with nasogastric tubes.[66-71] Complications, including perforation and intussusception, can occur during both insertion and removal of these tubes.[73,74]

SURGICAL STRATEGIES. The abdominal exploration is best carried out through a midline incision so that access is afforded to the entire abdominal cavity. If a previous incision is used, extending it into formerly unoperated territory can permit safer entry into the peritoneal cavity. Laparoscopy can be used as an initial maneuver when the diagnosis of obstruction is uncertain, as well as a means of providing definitive therapy.[75] This technique must be used cautiously, how-

ever, because adhesions and dilated intestine make peritoneal insufflation risky and visualization difficult. If the site of obstruction has been localized at least partially before operation, the appropriate quadrant should be explored first. Identifying the decompressed bowel below the obstruction may assist in finding the point of obstruction. Total evisceration and manipulation of the bowel as the initial maneuver can obscure the cause of obstruction (eg, volvulus) and cause injury because the distended bowel and mesentery tear easily.

Intraoperative decompression of the distended bowel may be necessary to improve exposure, optimize viability, and aid the abdominal closure. Although this can be accomplished by placing a tube through the stomach directly into the intestine or by performing transmural aspiration, it is preferable to milk the intestinal contents backward into a decompressed stomach.[76] This is achieved by a stripping maneuver using the second and third fingers of each hand to occlude the distal lumen and milk the contents in a proximal direction (Fig. 31-5). If this is not possible, passage of a long intestinal tube beyond the pylorus can obviate the need for enterotomy. This is a temporizing maneuver, because the intraluminal fluid will accumulate again in the early postoperative period and there is no evidence that intraoperative decompression improves motility.

Determining the viability of an intestinal segment during operation can be difficult. Improved color, visible mesenteric pulsations, and peristalsis can return im-

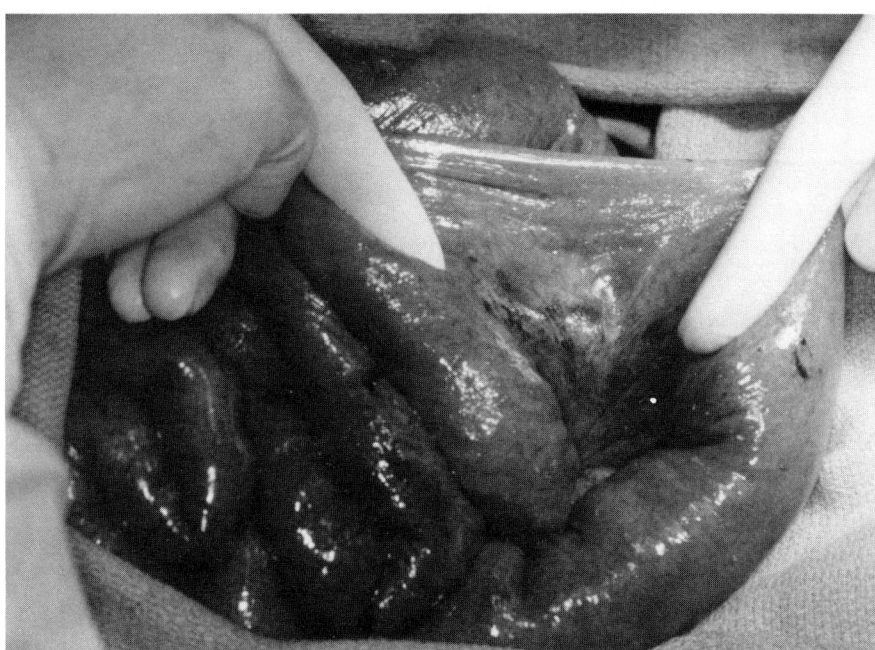

Figure 31-5 Intraoperative decompression of the obstructed bowel. Occlusion of the distal lumen and milking of the contents proximally is accomplished using the fingers of both hands.

mediately after the obstruction is released, but these findings often are questionable. The potentially ischemic bowel should be wrapped in warm packs and left undisturbed for 10 to 15 minutes, and then be reevaluated. The absence of these subjective findings, however, can lead to unnecessary resection.[77] If viability is still questionable, fluorescein staining and Doppler evaluation should be performed.[78-81] The intestines are studied with a Wood lamp after intravenous injection of sodium fluorescein.[78] Patterns of fluorescence include hyperemic, normal, and fine granular patterns indicative of viable intestine, and patchy, perivascular, and nonfluorescent patterns characteristic of nonviable segments.[77] A sterilized Doppler ultrasonic flow probe can be applied lightly to the antimesenteric border of the intestine, as well as to the feeding vessels[78] (Figs. 31-6 and 31-7). Audible flow within 1 cm of the intended anastomosis predicts survival.[79] One study has suggested that fluorescein patterns are more accurate than are Doppler studies and clinical evaluation.[77] These techniques are particularly useful for evaluating the margin of resection of an obviously ischemic segment. Quantitative fluorimetry can improve accuracy.[80]

When ischemia is extensive, the mesenteric vessels should be evaluated for the possibility of restoring circulation. With greater involvement of the small intestine, segments with questionable viability may need to be spared to prevent the short-bowel syndrome. Ongoing evaluation, including a second-look operation, then becomes important.[82] To be effective in reducing mor-

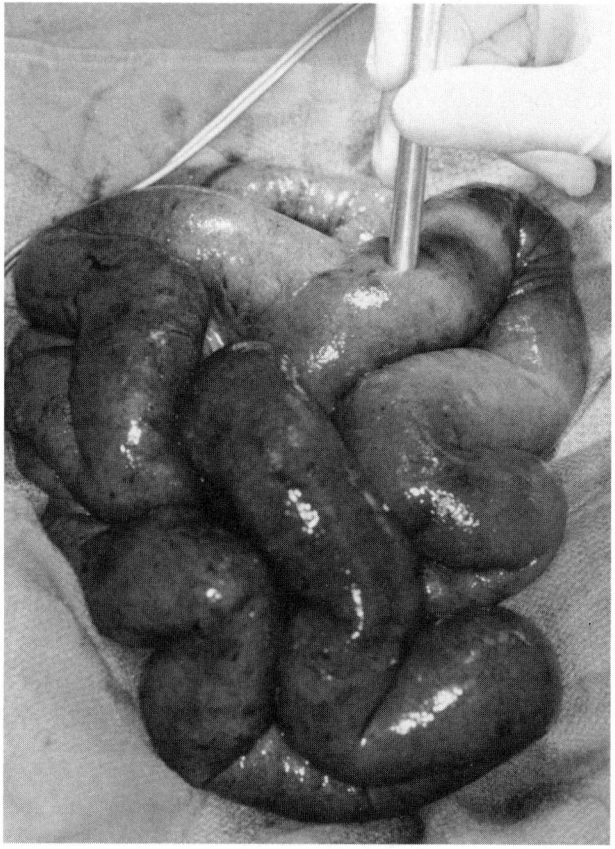

Figure 31-6 Determination of intestinal ischemia. A sterile Doppler probe is placed on the antimesenteric border of the bowel to evaluate perfusion.

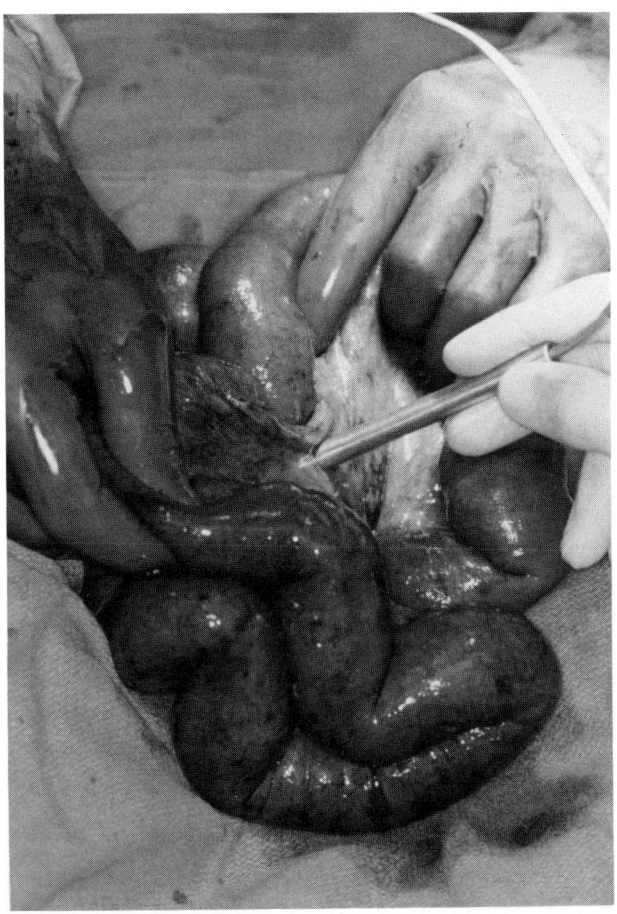

Figure 31-7 A Doppler probe can be used to assess the patency of feeding vessels, which can be difficult to palpate.

bidity and mortality, a second-look procedure must be performed within 24 hours of the initial operation regardless of the patient's condition at the time. Exteriorization of potentially ischemic bowel as a stoma is another consideration and permits endoscopic evaluation.[83] Tissue oximetry, which is expedient and accurate, may prove to be a useful technique for evaluating the viability of extensive segments.[84]

Most obstructions can be resolved by lysis of adhesions. Several techniques, which depend on the nature of the adhesions, can be used for this purpose. Thin, filmy adhesions usually can be distracted and lysed with scissors (Fig. 31-8). Denser adhesions may require sharp dissection with a scalpel. In some situations, vascular adhesions can be divided safely using electrocautery. Enterotomy should be carefully avoided because it increases the risk of postoperative wound infection and is a potential source of obstruction and fistula.[5,75] If enterotomy does occur, it should be repaired immediately or the leakage controlled to prevent further contamination. It is not clear whether serosal injury leads to adhe-

sions, but seromuscular defects with exposed mucosa can lead to perforation, so deep seromuscular injuries generally should be repaired. If large seromuscular deficits occur and mucosal integrity is considered tenuous, buttressing with adjacent bowel wall can be used to avoid resection. Whether all adhesions should be lysed depends on the patient's condition and the difficulty of the operation. Lysis of all adhesions usually is preferable, especially with recurrent obstruction.

The operative maneuvers performed are dictated by the underlying pathology. Enterotomy may be required for removal of a foreign body if it cannot be milked beyond the ileocecal valve. Resection may be required for injury or ischemia. Unresectable obstruction (eg, malignancy or extensive adhesions) may be managed best by enteroenterostomy to bypass the area of obstruction or by construction of a proximal diverting enterostomy. Stricturoplasty also should be considered for benign strictures (see later).

POSTOPERATIVE MANAGEMENT. The postoperative care of patients undergoing surgery for mechanical obstruction is similar to that after laparotomy for other conditions. Fluid and electrolyte management is an important aspect because many patients continue to accumulate intraluminal fluid that requires replacement. The severity and duration of the postoperative ileus depends on the duration of obstruction before operation, on the operation performed, and on patient factors. Most patients have nasogastric tubes in place before surgery. Prolongation of the ileus beyond a few days raises suspicion for underlying problems such as intraabdominal infection, pancreatitis, or intestinal obstruction. The management of ileus is discussed later in this chapter.

Patients who undergo extensive resection have additional problems. Fluid and electrolyte losses are increased. Postoperative gastric hypersecretion must be treated to prevent complications of ulcer disease, improve absorption, and minimize fluid loss. Parenteral nutritional support should be started early to meet caloric needs, but enteral nutrients also are important to stimulate adaptation of the intestinal remnant and maintain the integrity of the mucosal barrier.

Special Considerations

BENIGN STRICTURE. There are several considerations in the management of intestinal strictures. If malignancy is suspected, resection is the appropriate operation. Benign strictures, however, often can be managed by stricturoplasty. Although anastomotic strictures usually are isolated, inflammatory strictures (eg, those related to infection or Crohn's disease), often

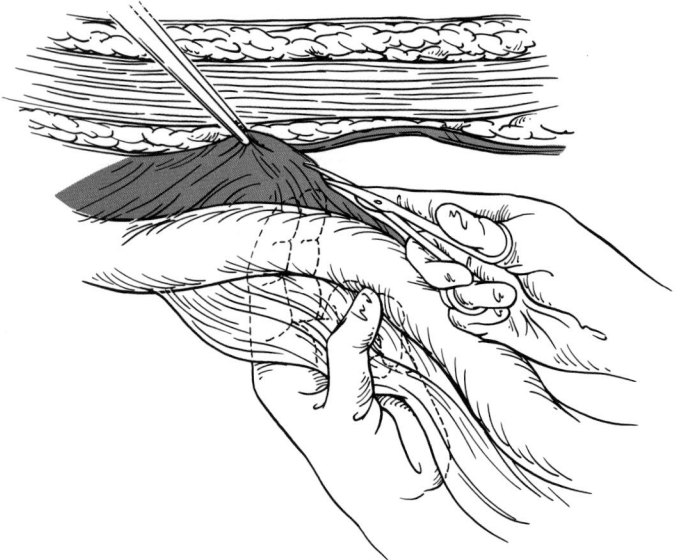

Figure 31-8 The technique for dissection of adhesions depends on their nature. Filmy adhesions often can be distracted easily and divided with scissors.

are multiple. Preoperative contrast studies usually identify these lesions, but it remains important to evaluate the caliber of the lumen further at the time of surgery. A balloon-tipped catheter can be passed from above or through an existing enterotomy to assure an intraluminal diameter of 1.5 to 2 cm. The balloon of a Baker tube filled with 5 mL of water will approximate this size.

Short benign strictures (3 to 4 cm) and most anastomotic strictures can be managed by opening the stricture lengthwise 1 cm beyond its ends and closing it transversely in the manner of a Heineke-Mikulicz pyloroplasty using either a single- or a double-layer closure (Fig. 31-9). Stricturoplasty can be performed, even in the presence of active inflammation, with acceptable morbidity.[85] Longer strictures (up to 12 cm) can be opened by a side-to-side enteroenterostomy using the Finney technique with either sutures or staples. The serosal patch technique is an alternative, but may be more likely to result in recurrent stricture because of contraction of the patched wound. Strictures longer than 15 cm probably are managed best by resection.

With careful attention to detail, stricturoplasty is almost uniformly successful in relieving obstruction. Morbidity rates related to the stricturoplasty (fistula or leak) generally are less than 2%.[85–87] The restenosis rate also is about 2% and, in the case of Crohn's disease, the symptom-free interval is similar to that achieved by resection.[87] However, stricturoplasty for longer strictures can cause problems with intestinal motility and bacterial overgrowth.

INCARCERATED HERNIA. Because incarcerated abdominal wall and groin hernias are a common cause of intestinal obstruction, they always should be looked for at initial examination. Incarceration is most likely when a narrow hernia neck is present, such as the femoral canal, obturator canal, internal inguinal ring, umbilical ring, and area around a stoma. Because strangulation can be difficult to diagnose with certainty, the approach to any incarcerated hernia should include exposure and control of the hernia sac, its contents, and the constricted neck so that the incarcerated segment can be examined. Closed reduction of an incarcerated hernia should be attempted only if strangulation is not suspected (Fig. 31-10). Furthermore, if a hernia is reduced en masse, the constricting neck can continue to cause obstruction.[88]

Incarcerated groin hernias can be approached in several ways.[89] A standard hernia incision above the inguinal ligament is satisfactory in many cases but risks premature reduction and loss of control of a potentially strangulated bowel segment. The preperitoneal approach provides both access and control, and more readily permits intestinal resection. Laparoscopic repair would permit visualization of the segment, but reduction of an incarcerated hernia may prove difficult.[90]

Strangulated incisional hernias also present management problems. Generally, identification, reduction, and resection can be performed by enlarging the hernia defect if necessary. The use of mesh for the repair becomes risky if resection is necessary, and especially in the face of peritonitis. An absorbable mesh can be used as a temporizing maneuver.[89]

A variety of internal hernias can incarcerate and cause intestinal obstruction[91] (Fig. 31-11). These should be considered in patients without histories of laparotomy, but internal hernias also occur through iatrogenic mesenteric defects and around anastomoses and ostomies (Fig. 31-12). Although paraduodenal hernias are the most common, paracecal, foramen of Winslow, transmesen-

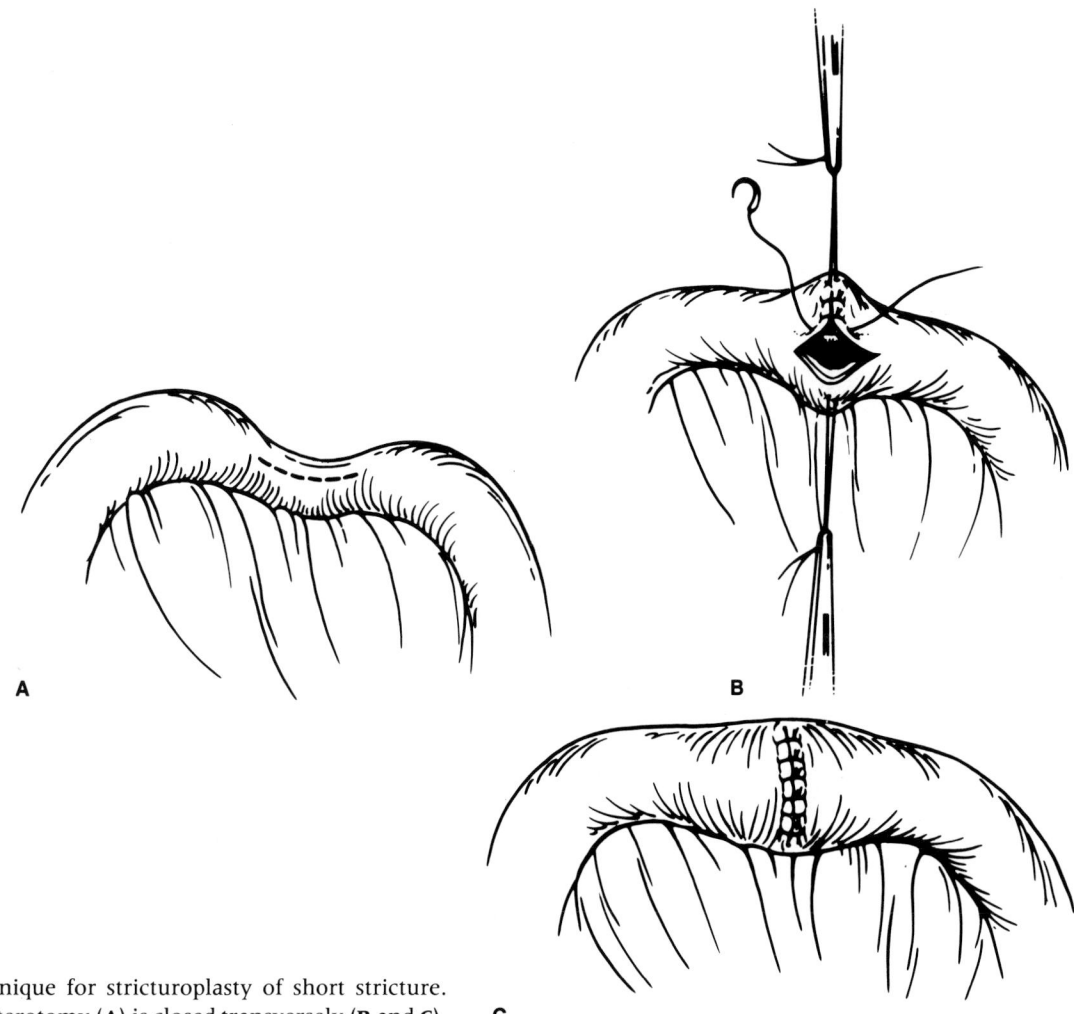

Figure 31-9 Technique for stricturoplasty of short stricture. The longitudinal enterotomy (**A**) is closed transversely (**B** and **C**).

teric, pelvic, and intersigmoid hernias also can occur. Because internal hernias can reduce during early manipulation of the bowel at laparotomy, these sites should be inspected if no obvious obstructive lesion is found.

Reduction of internal hernias can require enlarging the hernial defect, which should be done cautiously to prevent injury to mesenteric vessels. This also can involve mobilization of adjacent intestinal segments (eg, the duodenum) by a Kocher maneuver. After reduction of the hernia, the defect should be either enlarged or closed to prevent recurrent incarceration. Foramen of Winslow hernias are treated adequately by reduction alone. Iatrogenic internal hernias can be minimized by closing defects in the mesentery and omentum, and around anastomoses.

INTUSSUSCEPTION. Intussusception in adults is not as well recognized an entity as it is in children, but it accounts for about 5% of cases overall.[92] About 85% of these cases are associated with a discrete pathologic process, which is malignant half the time.[93] Malignancy is most common with colocolic intussusception (65% versus 30% for enteric intussusception). Because of the high risk of malignancy, operation always should be undertaken for intussusception in adult patients, and resection usually is advisable. Postoperative intussusception, however, is an exception.[94] In these patients, the etiologic factors usually are adhesions, long tubes, suture lines, or other benign conditions, and resection is unnecessary.

All adult patients with intestinal obstruction and suspected intussusception should undergo surgical exploration (Fig. 31-13). If the colon is involved, en bloc resection should be performed without attempted reduction. Sigmoidorectal intussusception should be approached more cautiously to determine whether rectal sparing is feasible. If the risk of malignancy is low, and particularly if the patient has recently undergone surgery, enteroenteric intussusception should be reduced and evaluated before a decision is made regarding resection.

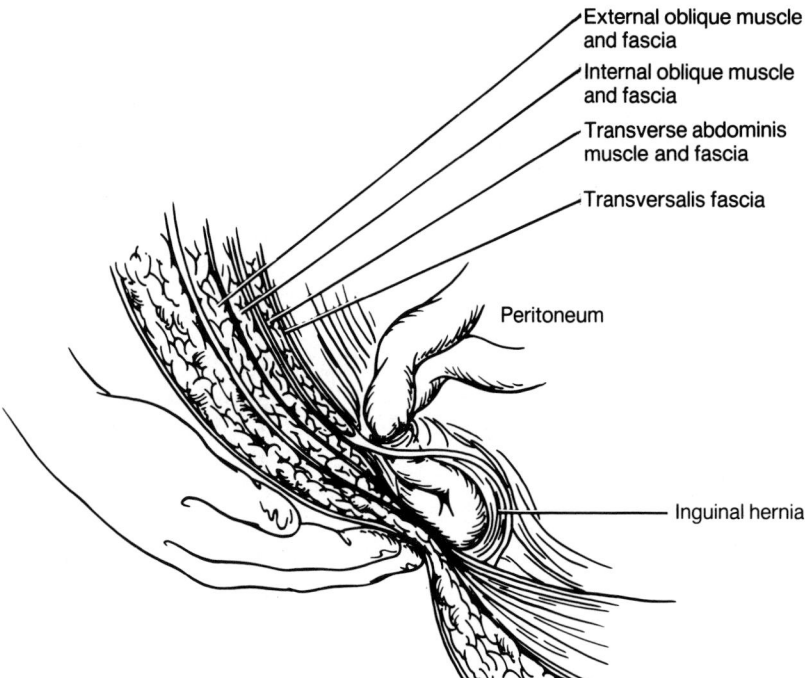

External oblique muscle and fascia

Internal oblique muscle and fascia

Transverse abdominis muscle and fascia

Transversalis fascia

Peritoneum

Inguinal hernia

Figure 31-10 Reduction of incarcerated hernia is undertaken only if strangulation is not suspected. The hernia can be reduced en masse.

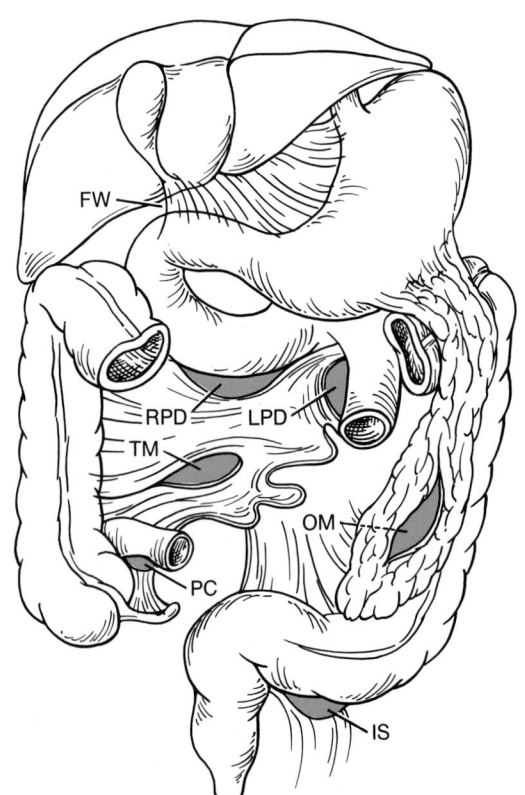

Figure 31-11 Internal hernias. FW, foramen of Winslow; RPD, right paraduodenal; LPD, left paraduodenal; TM, transmesenteric; OM, omental; PC, paracecal; IS, intersigmoid.

MALIGNANT OBSTRUCTION. Obstruction of the small intestine is a common problem in patients who have previously undergone laparotomy for malignancy or have known advanced intraabdominal malignancy. Although there may be a tendency to be reluctant about operating in this setting, an aggressive surgical approach is indicated. Nonoperative management can be successful at first, but recurrent obstruction is common.[9,95] Several studies have emphasized that obstruction in patients with malignancy is due to benign causes, such as adhesions, in at least one third of cases.[9,95–99] Satisfactory palliation of obstruction is achieved with surgery in 60% to 90% of patients with intraabdominal malignancy.[9,95–99] Thus, laparotomy should be undertaken if a patient's overall condition permits. A definitive procedure (eg, resection or bypass)

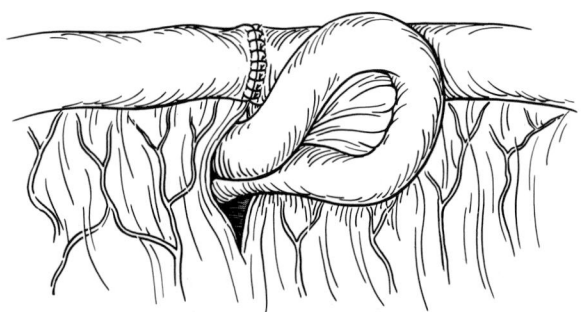

Figure 31-12 Hernia through a mesenteric defect. Such defects should be closed at operation.

should be performed whenever feasible. Tube decompression alone often does not provide successful palliation in these patients.[100] Ovarian cancer has a more dismal prognosis than other malignant tumors because it causes more diffuse obstruction and cannot be palliated as often. However, operation still should be considered in this group of patients.[101,102]

POSTOPERATIVE OBSTRUCTION. Intestinal obstruction occurring within the first 2 weeks after laparotomy is a challenging clinical problem. Postoperative ileus, nasogastric decompression, incisional pain, and analgesic use confound the clinical picture. Bowel sounds are variable and radiologic findings can be difficult to interpret.[103-105] Most cases of mechanical obstruction are due to adhesions and intraabdominal infection.[103-105] Patients undergoing abdominal procedures such as appendectomy, hysterectomy, and colorectal operations appear to be at increased risk.[106] The general debility of these patients and frequent delay in diagnosis result in high morbidity and mortality rates for this condition.[103-107]

Initially, postoperative obstruction should be treated with nasogastric suction. Observation usually is safe for 48 to 72 hours, particularly if there is clinical improvement. The risk of strangulation is low. Observation should be continued for up to 10 to 14 days after the initial operation before reoperation for partial obstruction is considered.[105] Gastrointestinal contrast studies are helpful in differentiating ileus from mechanical obstruction. Long intestinal tubes can be useful in this situation by providing more distal decompression and facilitating radiographic studies.

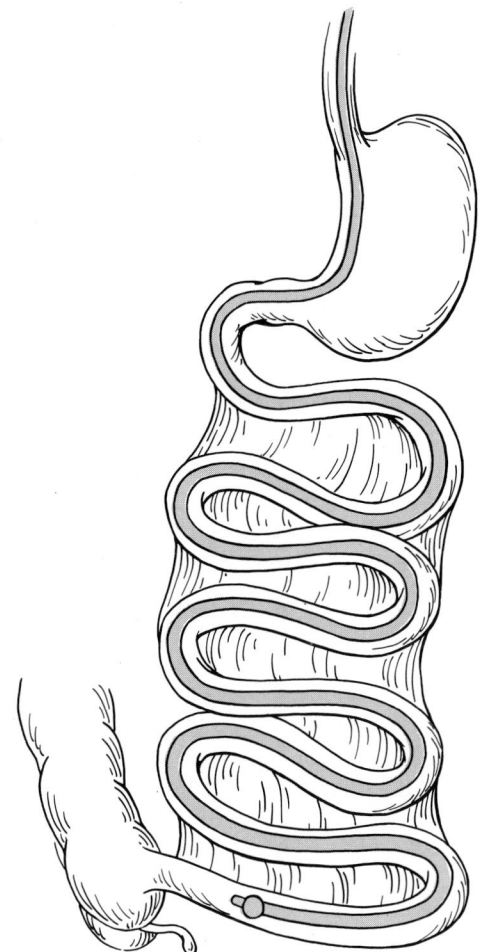

Figure 31-14 Tube plication can be achieved by passing a long intestinal tube and leaving it in place for 10 to 14 days.

RECURRENT OBSTRUCTION. Recurrent intestinal obstruction is a significant problem, especially with adhesive obstruction. Several techniques have been used over the years to prevent this complication.[107-115] The strategy generally has been to fix the intestinal loops into a "nonkinked" configuration so that when adhesions inevitably recur, obstruction does not. The Noble plication consists of performing complete enterolysis and then suturing parallel loops of bowel together, incorporating both mesentery and bowel wall.[108] This procedure has been simplified by using transmesenteric plication.[110] Both these procedures require extensive operating time, have significant complications, and do not eliminate recurrent obstruction.[109,111] Intraluminal support with a long intestinal tube is as effective as the suturing techniques and less morbid[112-115] (Fig. 31-14). The tube usually is left in place for 10 to 14 days. Placing the tube through either the nose or a gastrostomy can prevent the morbidity of transjejunal passage.[74,115] There have been no prospective studies to demonstrate

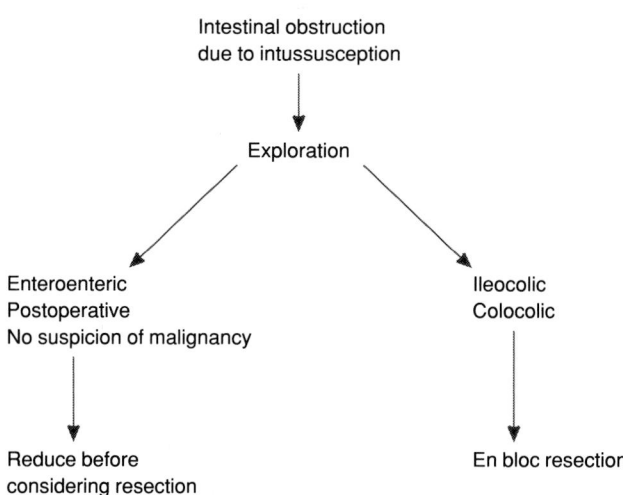

Figure 31-13 Algorithm for management of intussusception in the adult patient.

conclusively that any of these procedures reduce the risk of recurrent obstruction.[107–115]

Because adhesions have become the most common cause of intestinal obstruction, and because recurrent obstruction occurs in 10% to 15% of cases, prevention of adhesions has become a priority. Seventy percent of adhesions are postoperative, 20% are inflammatory, and 10% are congenital.[116,117] Pelvic operations such as hysterectomy, colectomy, and appendectomy are common antecedent procedures.[2] The pathogenesis of adhesions involves an initial serosal injury and subsequent inflammatory response.[118] The inflammatory exudate activates the clotting system, causing the formation of fibrinous adhesions. Enhancement of tissue plasminogen activator results in the resolution of most adhesions. However, reduction of tissue plasminogen activator by various adjuvants results in fibroblast infiltration and vascular ingrowth. Etiologic factors in adhesion formation include ischemic tissue, blood, foreign bodies, peritonitis, thermal injury, and chemical trauma.[117–121] A single adhesive band can pose a greater risk of obstruction and strangulation than more extensive ones.[122] Although many therapies have been used both in scientific trials and in clinical practice to prevent adhesion formation, none has been shown to be efficacious. Agents studied include antihistamines, corticosteroids, dextran 70, heparin, and nonsteroidal antiinflammatory drugs.[117,118,120–128] Preventing exten-

sive dissection and tissue injury remain important surgical principles. Interposing omentum between the wound and intestines also is a valuable maneuver. Laparoscopic procedures can reduce the incidence of adhesions. Antibiotic irrigation actually can increase the formation of adhesions.[121]

COLONIC OBSTRUCTION. The urgency of surgical management of colonic obstruction depends on several factors, including the degree of obstruction, suspicion of strangulation, extent of colonic dilatation, and etiology.[129–133] Most cases of colonic obstruction are caused by cancer or diverticular disease and are partial, so strangulation is unusual. Small bowel dilation is present in 30% of cases and can be due to an incompetent ileocecal valve, synchronous small bowel obstruction, or ileus.[10] Dilation of the colon (usually the cecum) greater than 9 to 12 cm warrants urgent intervention to prevent perforation. About 75% of cases of large bowel obstruction occur in the left colon. Proctoscopy often is advisable to evaluate the rectum before an emergency intraabdominal procedure, because almost 30% of obstructive lesions can be visualized. An overall approach to managing large bowel obstruction is shown in Figure 31-15.

Colonoscopy plays an important role in the management of large bowel obstruction.[134] Initial endoscopic evaluation is useful in establishing the degree of

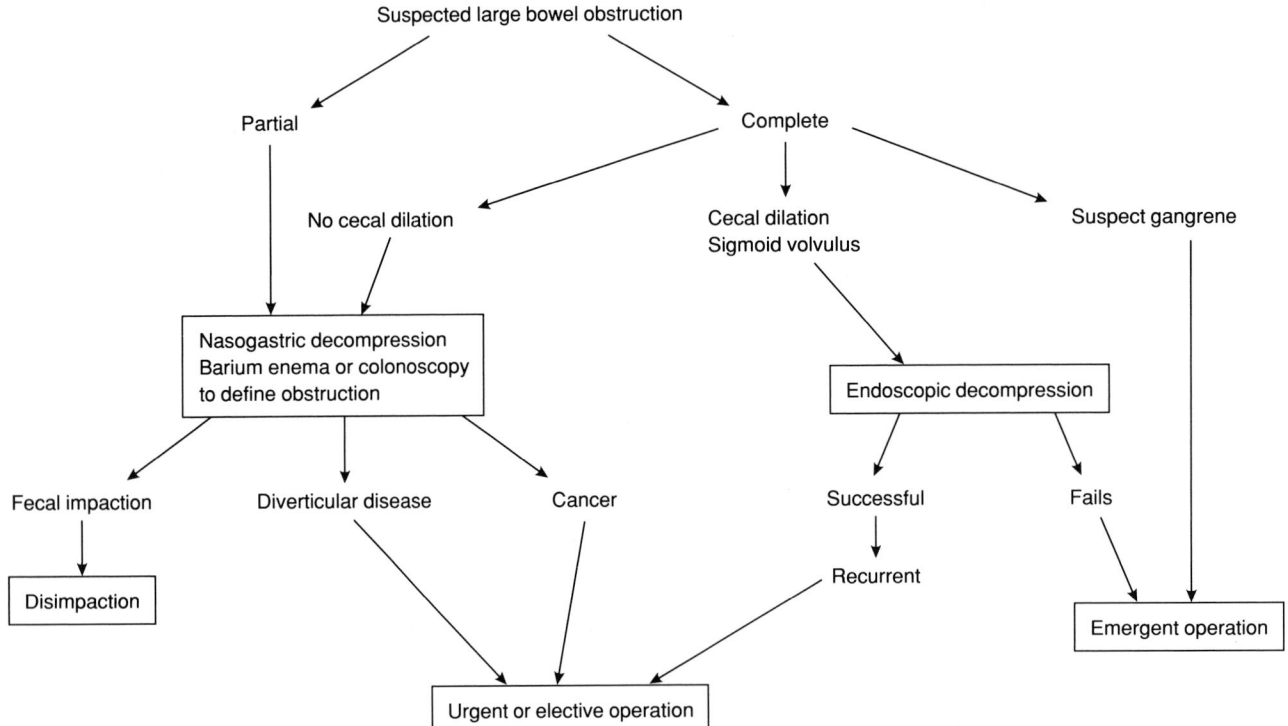

Figure 31-15 Algorithm for management of large bowel obstruction.

obstruction and the cause. If partial obstruction is found, transanal intubation, over a guide wire if necessary, can achieve decompression before surgery and often permit primary resection and anastomosis.[135] An attempt at colonoscopic decompression is valuable in differentiating colonic pseudoobstruction from cecal volvulus.[134,136,137] Colonoscopy can be therapeutic for colonic volvulus. Sigmoid volvulus can be detorsed 80% to 90% of the time but recurs in more than 50% of cases, so definitive operation should be planned.[130,138-140] Successful treatment of cecal volvulus by endoscopy is more sporadic and the incidence of recurrence is less well known. A definitive operation probably is indicated for cecal volvulus as well.[134,137]

Patients often require emergency operation for obstruction from volvulus, especially cecal volvulus, which is treated surgically 80% of the time.[141] Nonviable colon is present in 30% of patients with cecal volvulus and resection is the appropriate treatment.[141,142] Whether intestinal continuity should be reestablished depends on the condition of both the bowel and the patient. When cecal volvulus is not complicated by ischemia, alternatives to resection can be used. Detorsion avoids the morbidity of emergency resection.[136] However, detorsion alone is followed by a recurrence rate as high as 25%.[136,142] The involved cecal segment can be stabilized by cecostomy, cecopexy, or both.[130,141-143] Although there is not a clear difference in recurrence rate between these procedures, cecostomy poses a risk of contamination. Cecopexy can be performed using a peritoneal flap, although there are no convincing studies to support this technique over simple suturing (Fig. 31-16). Insertion of a cecostomy tube decompresses the detorsed bowel, but this goal also can be achieved by an indwelling transrectal tube.[144] If tube cecostomy alone is anticipated, consideration should be given to radiologic placement.[143] Colopexy now is feasible by laparoscopy.[145] These nonoperative approaches generally are reserved for patients who would be at high risk during open operation.

Sigmoid volvulus often is detorsed successfully by sigmoidoscopy, allowing an elective procedure to be performed. Initial tube decompression should be maintained for 48 to 72 hours.[138] Colonoscopy can be more advantageous than rigid sigmoidoscopy because it permits better visualization of the twisted segment and examination of the proximal colon. If emergency operation is required, the options include resection with colostomy and colopexy. Suturing the sigmoid colon to the lateral abdominal wall in a manner similar to cecopexy results in a high recurrence rate.[138] Prosthetic material has been used to secure the colon to the lateral abdominal wall, but this approach has little appeal.[146] Mesosigmoidoplasty is another alternative. The perito-

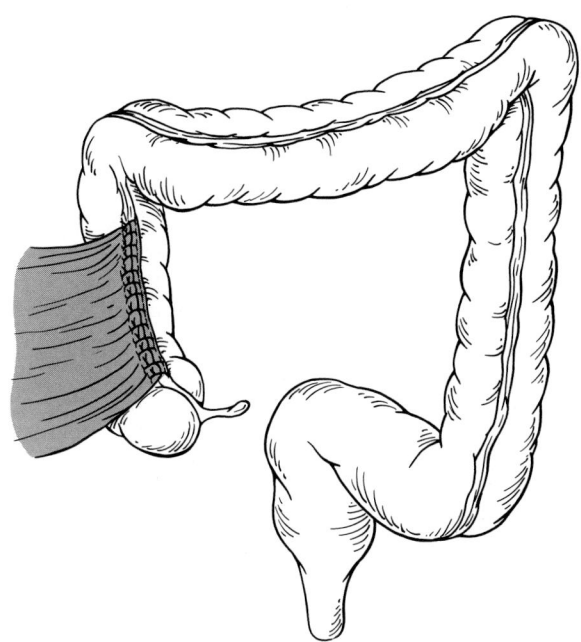

Figure 31-16 Cecopexy is more secure if a peritoneal flap is developed, which increases adhesion to the lateral abdominal wall.

neum of the mesentery is divided from the base of the torsed segment to the mesenteric edge of the bowel and then closed transversely to broaden the mesenteric attachment.[140] Resection is indicated for ischemic twisted colon, which is present in about 10% of cases.[130] The recurrence rate is low when resection is performed after successful detorsion, and this may be the most desirable treatment of sigmoid volvulus. Whereas cecal volvulus involves a mobile, but not necessarily redundant, segment of colon, patients with sigmoid volvulus invariably have redundant sigmoid colon.

When operation is deemed necessary for benign or malignant lesions, there are several possible approaches. If resection of the obstructing lesion is not advisable or required, proximal decompression should be achieved by transverse colostomy or tube cecostomy.[147,148] However, a diverting loop ileostomy also should be considered because it is easy to construct and close and provides satisfactory fecal diversion.[149] Transverse colostomy can be performed either as a loop colostomy or as two stomas after division of the colon. The former is more expeditious and perhaps easier to close, but it has significant morbidity, including prolapse, hernia formation around the colostomy, and retraction and stenosis.[148] Both ends of a divided segment must be matured to decompress the distal obstructed segment. This can be accomplished easily at the stoma site[150] (Fig. 31-17). Because a distal obstructing lesion usually is dealt with at a later time, ease of colostomy closure is not always an issue. Bypass procedures are an alternative to proximal decompression, particularly for widespread cancer.

Resection of the obstructing lesion, and often the entire obstructed segment of bowel, usually is desirable.[151–157] A useful strategy in the management of colonic obstruction is to convert an emergency condition into an elective or urgent situation, thus permitting a one-stage rather than a two-stage operative approach. Certain lesions are amenable to laser recanalization or balloon dilation as either preliminary or definitive maneuvers.[158,159] These approaches are appropriate only for lesions in which the bowel lumen is clearly visible proximal to the point of obstruction so that a guide wire or the colonoscope can be advanced beyond the tumor. The luminal opening created has to be adequate to permit mechanical cleansing and proximal decompres-

sion. Intracolonic stents also have been used for this purpose.[160] These maneuvers then permit a primary resection and anastomosis after bowel preparation. Resection usually is performed within a few days after recanalization. Patients with widespread malignancy and short life expectancy can be treated by repeated recanalization for palliation if the lesion is amenable to this approach. Although some studies have suggested that long-term survival for patients with colon cancer is improved by resection at the initial operation, other studies are less convincing.[156] The patient's general condition, peritoneal contamination, and fecal load are important initial factors in making this decision. Even if anastomosis is not carried out, the colostomy formed in this circumstance generally is more functional than a transverse colostomy.[157] The overall morbidity and mortality of initial resection and anastomosis is similar to the outcome after delayed resection and anastomosis.[129,132,156,157]

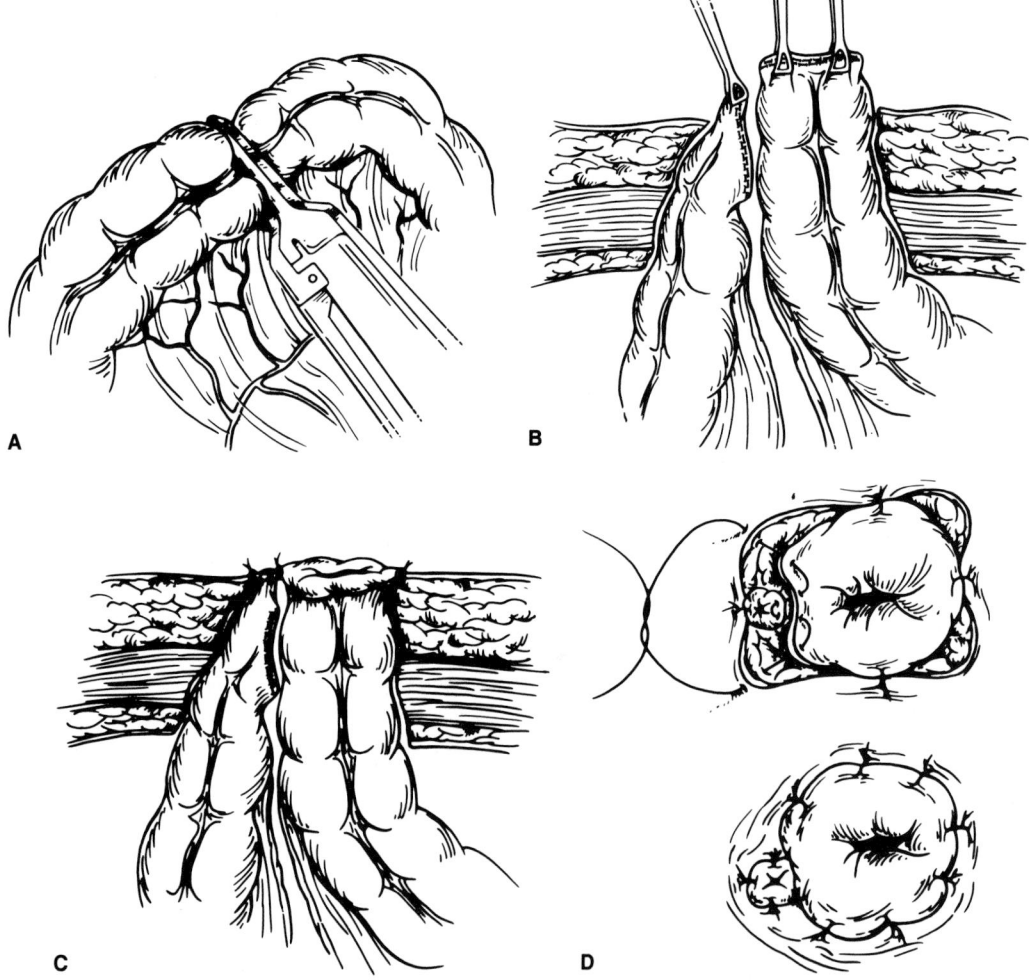

Figure 31-17 When performing a colostomy for obstruction, the distal end needs to be exteriorized. After division of the colon (**A**), both ends can be brought out at a single site (**B** through **D**).

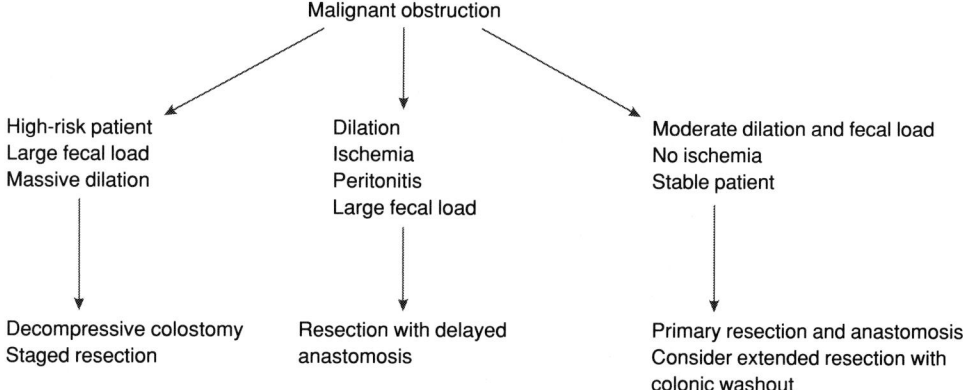

Figure 31-18   Management of malignant obstruction of the left colon.

Resection and anastomosis should be performed only in stable patients, when there is minimal contamination and when the anastomotic ends of the bowel are viable and easily approximated (Fig. 31-18). Patients with complicated obstruction (ie, perforation or ischemia) should undergo delayed anastomosis. Most surgeons are not reluctant to perform a primary anastomosis after an emergency right colectomy, but an anastomosis in the left colon in this setting is more worrisome. A variety of approaches have been used to minimize the potential morbidity of primary resection and anastomosis of the left colon. Both preoperative lavage and intraoperative colonic washout have been advocated[161,162] (Fig. 31-19). Subtotal colectomy with ileorectal anastomosis is thought to be less morbid than seg-

mental resection in terms of anastomotic healing, but it can lead to chronic diarrhea. The use of an intracolonic stent to reduce the risk of anastomotic complications has been reported[163] (Fig. 31-20).

Outcome

About 80% of patients with complete mechanical obstruction require operation compared with 20% of those with partial intestinal obstruction.[49] Strangulation is present in 10% to 15% of cases.[2] Enterolysis alone is performed in 50% of patients, with the rest requiring resection, bypass, or other procedures.[2]

Morbidity rates after operations for intestinal obstruction are 25% to 30% and mortality rates generally

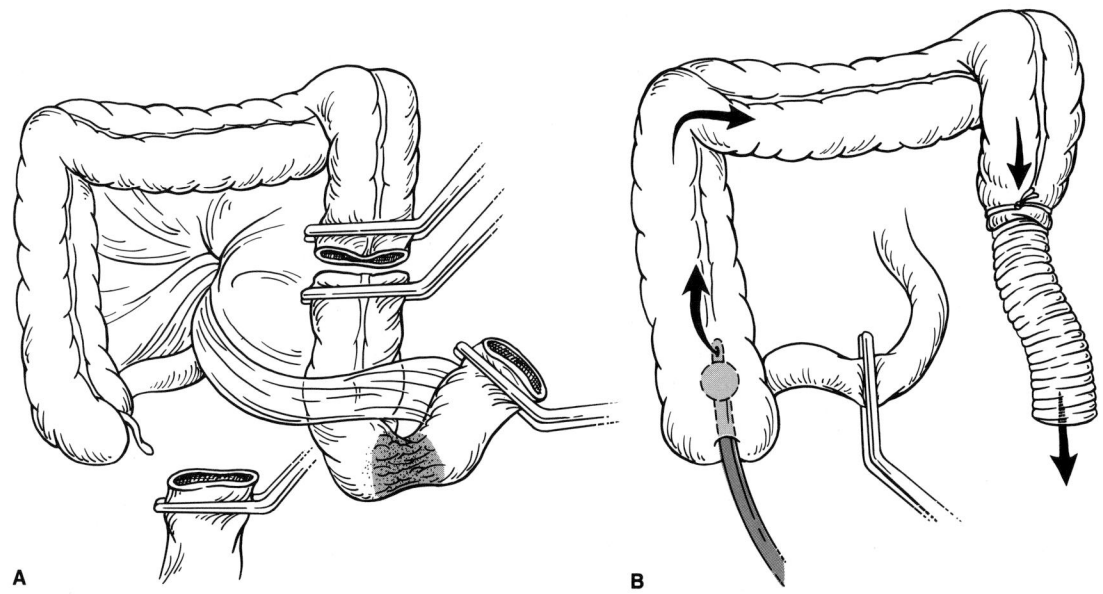

Figure 31-19   On-table lavage can be performed by controlling the distal end of the bowel (**A**) and irrigating through a proximal tube (**B**).

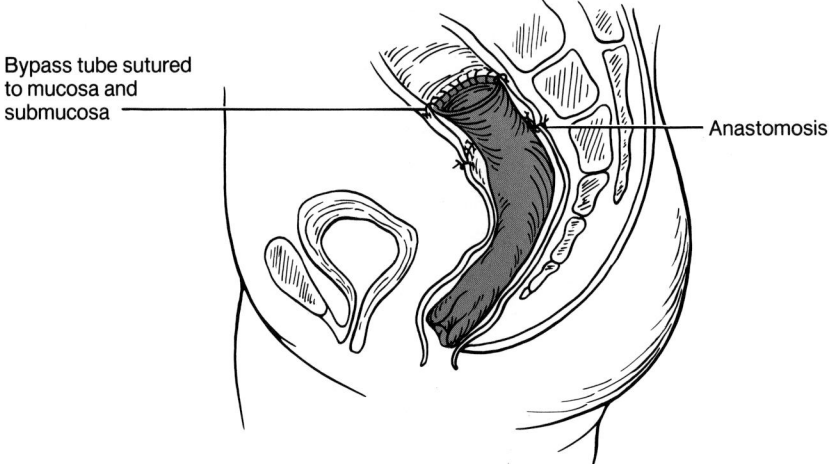

Figure 31-20 Diagram of an intracolonic stent incorporating a proximal cuff, which is sewn to the inner bowel wall, and a soft latex tube for intraluminal diversion of contents.

are less than 10%.[2-5] The incidence of complications is 5 to 10 times greater with strangulation, and death is three times as common.[2-5] These rates also are influenced by patient age, concomitant medical conditions, cause of obstruction, delay in diagnosis and treatment, and site of obstruction.[2-5,9,10] Malignant obstruction has an especially high mortality rate.[9,95-99]

Recurrent obstruction develops in 30% to 40% of patients with episodes of intestinal obstruction.[164] Recurrence is significantly more likely in patients who are treated without operation and in those who have malignant conditions, and it usually occurs within 4 years. Surprisingly, multiple prior episodes of obstruction do not significantly increase the risk of future obstruction.

Acute obstruction complicates 15% of cases of colorectal cancer. The mortality rate of this condition is about 10% but can reach 25% in elderly, high-risk patients.[157] Forty percent of the colostomies that are constructed as part of the initial therapy become permanent.

ILEUS

Etiology

Paralytic ileus has diverse causes[165] (Table 31-3). Intraabdominal and retroperitoneal inflammation and injury are common etiologic factors. Transient ileus occurs after any intraabdominal operation. However, systemic processes such as sepsis, electrolyte abnormalities, endocrine disorders, drugs, and injury also can result in ileus.

Pathophysiology

Ileus usually is the consequence of activating or enhancing the normal inhibitory mechanisms of gastrointestinal motility. In general, parasympathetic vagal fibers are excitatory and sympathetic efferent fibers are inhibitory to motility throughout the gastrointestinal tract. The small intestine has a low level of extrinsic and a high level of intrinsic cholinergic control.[165] Although the enteric nervous system has both α- and β-adrenergic receptors, sympathetic inhibition of intesti-

Table 31-3 Causes of Ileus

DRUG-RELATED
Narcotics
Antidiarrheals
Pro-banthine
Antacids
Warfarin sodium (Coumadin)
Ganglionic blockers
Antidepressants (amitriptyline)
Phenothiazines
Heavy metal poisons

INTRAABDOMINAL INFLAMMATION
Localized (eg, appendicitis)
Peritonitis
Hemorrhage

SYSTEMIC INFECTION
Pneumonia

SYSTEMIC ILLNESS
Acute anemia
Endocrine disorders (myxedema)
Electrolyte abnormalities (Na, Cl, K, Mg)
Hypoosmolality
Myocardial infarction

TRAUMA
Fractured spine
Rib fractures
Hip fracture
Retroperitoneal hematoma

POSTOPERATIVE

nal motility is mediated largely through α-adrenergic receptors. Two types of intestinointestinal inhibitory reflexes have been identified—a low-threshold spinal reflex and a high-threshold peripheral reflex mediated by prevertebral ganglia.[165,166] Ileus can result from inhibition of both spinal and peripheral pathways. The spinal pathways are important in the response to systemic stimuli. Catecholamines have direct effects on muscle but do not appear to play a role in ileus.[165] The intestinal muscle remains potentially receptive to parasympathomimetic agonists.[166] However, the response to these agents can be altered by other factors, such as hypokalemia. Thus, ileus generally is a neurogenic phenomenon secondary to reflex stimulation of adrenergic receptors due to systemic pain or injury or to local responses. The absence of intestinal propulsion results in the accumulation of gas and fluid in the intestine. Impaired absorption further aggravates this problem.[165]

Postoperative ileus is related to many factors, including intestinal sympathetic hyperactivity, hormonal changes, hypokalemia, anesthetic and analgesic drugs, and lack of activity.[167-173] Adrenergic blockade can prevent postoperative ileus.[172] The duration of ileus does not correlate closely with the extent and site of operative dissection.[171] Transit of solids is slowed by suppression of migrating bursts of action potentials and the resultant contractions that normally move intestinal contents abroad.[173-176] This inhibition of bursts occurs for 24 to 48 hours after operations on both the stomach and the small intestine. Myoelectric activity in the colon is decreased for more than 72 hours.

Motility of the colon has less cholinergic drive than that of the small intestine and the sympathetic inhibition is mediated mainly through β-receptors rather than α-receptors.[165,167-169] Acute ileus, or pseudoobstruction, of the colon is thought to occur primarily as a result of diminished parasympathetic stimulation and increased sympathetic inhibition of colonic motor activity.[177,178] The inhibition of sacral parasympathetic pathways may play the predominant role. However, gastrointestinal hormones also regulate colonic motility. Gastrin, cholecystokinin, and motilin stimulate colonic contractions, although peptide YY and secretin inhibit this activity. Elevated prostaglandin levels also may play a role in colonic motility.[179,180] Thus, a variety of systemic and localized inflammatory processes can be implicated in the pathogenesis of colonic ileus. Whatever the mechanism, functional obstruction of the distal colon results in dilation of the proximal colon.

Clinical Presentation

Like mechanical obstruction, ileus usually is accompanied by nausea and vomiting, abdominal distention, and cessation of bowel movements. Whether pain is a significant complaint depends on the underlying cause and degree of distention. Bowel sounds are infrequent and the abdomen is tympanitic with varying degrees of tenderness. Peritonitis results in guarding, direct and rebound tenderness, and, eventually, rigidity.

There are several differences between ileus and intestinal pseudoobstruction. Ileus usually has a sudden onset in a previously well patient. It has a progressive course, as opposed to the intermittent symptoms of pseudoobstruction. Abnormalities of esophageal motility occur with pseudoobstruction, but not with ileus. Ileus should be suspected in the appropriate clinical setting.

Diagnosis

When the diagnosis of ileus is suspected, the most important consideration is identifying and treating the underlying cause. The presence of a recognized cause of ileus helps make the diagnosis. The patient's medications should be reviewed carefully.

Laboratory Studies

No specific laboratory tests are available for the diagnosis of paralytic ileus. Hyperamylasemia can suggest pancreatitis as an underlying cause and anemia should raise suspicion for hemorrhage (eg, retroperitoneal hematoma). Serum electrolyte and magnesium levels should be obtained. Thyroid function test results can suggest a diagnosis of hypothyroidism.

Radiologic Studies

As described in the preceding section, plain radiographs can help differentiate between ileus and mechanical obstruction (see Table 31-2). Gas usually is distributed diffusely throughout the gastrointestinal tract. A water-soluble contrast or barium study demonstrates slow but progressive passage of contrast material through the small intestine into the colon. Barium enema or colonoscopic examination can be important for evaluating suspected colonic ileus, especially to rule out a distal colon obstructing lesion.

Management

Nasogastric suction and intravenous fluid therapy are important aspects of early management. The value of small intestinal drainage tubes is debatable. Hypokalemia should be corrected if present. The important decision to be made early is whether a surgical procedure is required to treat the underlying cause. Prolonged ileus may necessitate parenteral nutritional support.

Prolonged ileus can be managed medically (Table 31-4). However, parasympathomimetic agents such as bethanechol should be used with caution if mechanical obstruction has not been completely ruled out because they are associated with many unwanted side effects.[166,181] Metoclopramide, which is both a cholinergic agonist and a dopamine antagonist, has prokinetic effects throughout the gastrointestinal tract.[182] Metoclopramide has been shown to shorten the duration of ileus.[183,184] Cisapride also is a cholinergic agonist but does not antagonize dopamine. Its prokinetic effects are mediated by serotonin, endorphins, motilin, and pancreatic polypeptide.[185] Cisapride affects all parts of the gastrointestinal tract and also has been shown to shorten postoperative ileus.[186,187] Sympatholytic agents such as chlorpromazine and lidocaine have been used successfully in some cases.[188] Erythromycin is a motilin agonist that stimulates small intestinal motility and can shorten the duration of ileus.[189-191] Octreotide shortens postoperative ileus by inhibiting gastrointestinal hormone release.[192] Prostaglandin inhibition by ketorolac or ibuprofen also can stimulate motor activity.[180,193]

Acute colonic pseudoobstruction also is managed initially without surgery, using nasogastric suction. Such therapy is successful in about 85% of patients.[194,195] However, failure of resolution or dilation of the cecum to greater than 10 cm mandates more aggressive treatment.[194] Colonoscopic decompression is successful in many cases, and this examination can rule out mechanical obstruction.[196-200] Serial colonoscopic procedures may be necessary. Placement of a long intestinal tube at the time of decompression also can be beneficial.[196] In addition, sympathetic blockade with medications or epidural anesthesia has been effective.[195,201,202] Failure of these modalities necessitates surgical approaches such as cecostomy or colectomy.[194-203] Cecostomy can be performed through the skin with radiologic guidance or by laparoscopy using T-fasteners; these are the preferred approaches unless ischemia is suspected.[204,205] Resection should be performed when ischemia or large seromuscular tears are encountered.

Outcome

The outcome of ileus depends primarily on the underlying cause. Although ileus itself usually is a self-limited condition, persistent intestinal dilation can lead to perforation of either the small or large intestine. Nausea and vomiting can result in aspiration of gastric contents.

PSEUDOOBSTRUCTION

Etiology

Chronic intestinal pseudoobstruction is a heterogenous clinical syndrome that has diverse causes and varied clinical presentations[206-209] (Table 31-5). This syndrome is differentiated from ileus by its chronic nature and the underlying disease process involving the intestine. The impaired intestinal motility can be caused by pathologic abnormalities of the intestinal muscle (myopathic) or enteric nervous system (neuropathic). Although some developmental conditions are well recognized (eg, Hirschsprung's disease), most of the causes are acquired. These abnormalities may not be obvious on routine microscopic evaluation. Disease processes can affect both muscle and nerves, and often are diffuse throughout the gastrointestinal tract. Furthermore, the intestinal involvement can be just one component of a more generalized systemic illness.

Pathophysiology

Although the extrinsic nervous system modulates intestinal activity, the musculature and intrinsic enteric nervous system are the predominant factors for normal intestinal motility. Abnormalities of either of these components result in a spectrum of altered motility that includes loss of normal peristalsis and transport, disruption of normal cyclical events such as the migrating motor complex, spontaneous uncoordinated contractile activity, and abnormalities of sphincter activity.[206] In general, myopathic conditions cause low-amplitude pressure activity and hypomotility, whereas neuro-

---

Table 31-4 Pharmacologic Therapy for Prolonged Ileus

HORMONE AGONISTS AND ANTAGONISTS
Erythromycin
Octreotide

OPIATE ANTAGONISTS
Naloxone

PARASYMPATHOMIMETIC AND CHOLINERGIC AGONISTS
Bethanechol
Neostigmine
Metoclopramide
Cisapride

PROSTAGLANDIN INHIBITORS
Indomethacin
Ketorolac

SYMPATHOLYTIC AGENTS
Chlorpromazine

Table 31-5 Causes of Intestinal Pseudoobstruction

DEVELOPMENTAL
Aganglionosis
Hirschsprung's disease

DRUG-INDUCED
Narcotic bowel
Tricyclic antidepressants

ENDOCRINE
Diabetes mellitus
Myxedema

INFECTION
Chagas' disease
Cytomegalovuris

INFILTRATIVE DISEASE
Amyloidosis
Dermatomyositis
Progressive systemic sclerosis
Systemic lupus erythematosus

NEOPLASM
Paraneoplastic syndromes

NEUROLOGIC DISEASE
Brain-stem tumors
Diabetes mellitus
Multiple sclerosis
Muscular dystrophy
Porphyria
Spinal cord injury

FAMILIAL VISCERAL NEUROPATHY AND MYOPATHY
IDIOPATHIC

pathic pseudoobstruction is characterized by excessive and uncoordinated activity. These abnormalities can result from muscle atrophy or infiltration, or from a decreased number of plexuses.

Chronic intestinal pseudoobstruction can be associated with marked dilation of any part of the intestinal tract. This occurs in response to abnormalities of either intestinal muscle or the myenteric plexus and does not always follow a specific pattern. Small intestinal diverticulosis is another potential manifestation of structural abnormalities of muscle or the myenteric plexus.[206]

Clinical Presentation

Intestinal pseudoobstruction occurs in patients of all ages. Recurrent attacks of nausea, vomiting, cramping abdominal pain, and abdominal distention are variable in their frequency, intensity, and duration.[207,208] Constipation and diarrhea can occur but are not constant features. Generally, these recurrent episodes become more persistent until symptoms always are present to some degree.

The clinical presentation can be altered by the extent of involvement of the gastrointestinal tract. Distention can become a permanent feature if bowel dilates in response to the pathologic process. Anorexia and malabsorption often lead to progressive weight loss and malnutrition. Bacterial overgrowth is a common associated problem.

Diagnosis

The nonspecific symptoms and lack of definitive diagnostic tests make accurate diagnosis difficult. Patients with pseudoobstruction often undergo laparotomy for presumed mechanical obstruction. Conversely, mechanical obstruction mistakenly diagnosed as intestinal pseudoobstruction can lead to inappropriate treatment, with disastrous consequences.[210] Intestinal pseudoobstruction should be suspected when there is a long duration of changing symptoms, alternating constipation and diarrhea, and underlying diseases or other factors commonly associated with pseudoobstruction. The surgeon must have an awareness of the syndrome and its presentation, but also must exclude mechanical obstruction through radiologic, manometric, and endoscopic assessment.

Laboratory Studies

No specific laboratory studies aid in the diagnosis of pseudoobstruction. Serum electrolyte determinations and renal function studies can assist in assessing the resultant volume deficit. Other tests, such as thyroid function tests, antinuclear antibodies, serum protein levels, and serologic markers, are useful for evaluating the underlying cause of the pseudoobstruction. Urinary studies and stool analysis also can be helpful in identifying the disease process.

Manometric studies of the upper and lower intestinal tracts should confirm the intestinal dysmotility.[20] Manometric patterns suggesting pseudoobstruction are infrequent low-amplitude contractions characteristic of smooth muscle degeneration and disordered clustered contractions characteristic of nervous degeneration. However, these findings usually are complementary or confirmatory rather than definitive. Biopsy and culture of the small intestine also should be performed. Rectal biopsy should be done if colonic motility is impaired. Endoscopy is important to exclude obstruction and mucosal disease.

Full-thickness biopsy of the small intestine permits definitive histologic study. Histologic sections should be prepared in different orientations to display the var-

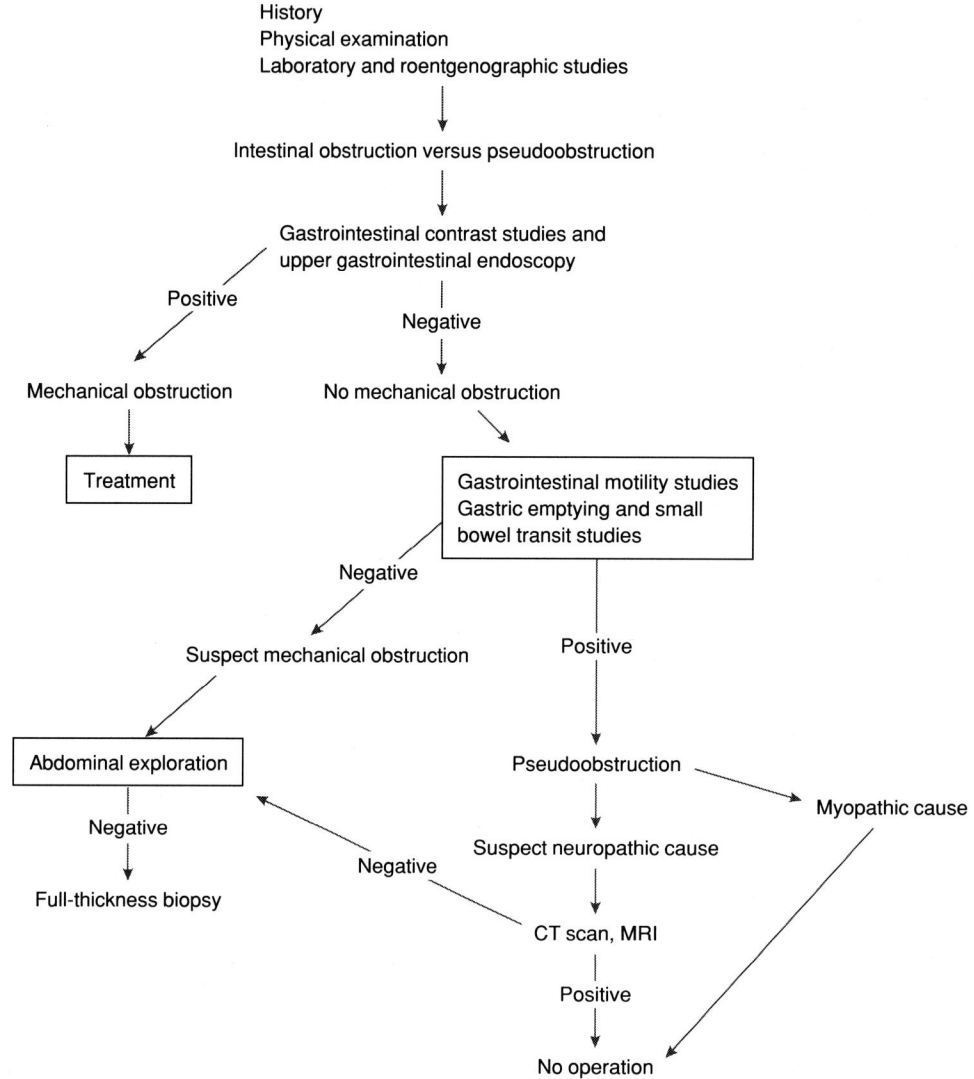

Figure 31-21 Algorithm for evaluation of patients with possible intestinal pseudoobstruction.

ious muscle and nerve components. Silver staining or other techniques for visualizing nerves also should be used.

Radiologic Studies

Radiologic studies are necessary to eliminate the possibility of mechanical obstruction and to localize the disease process. Contrast studies such as enteroclysis can demonstrate changes in bowel caliber, alterations in haustration and valvulae conniventes, and diverticula. There generally is prolonged transit time (4 to 5 hours) of barium from the stomach to the colon. Fluoroscopy can confirm the altered motility. Radionuclide studies (indium-131–fiber and technetium-99–labeled pellets) are useful for evaluating gastric emptying and intestinal transit time.[211] They also can be helpful in assessing the effects of medical therapy on motility.

Management

Therapy for intestinal pseudoobstruction includes identification and treatment of any underlying cause. With primary pseudoobstruction or irreversible gut injury, the options are pharmacologic stimulation of motility, surgical intervention to remove or bypass diseased segments, and prolonged parenteral nutritional support. The agents used to improve motility are similar to those used to hasten the resolution of ileus[212,213] (see Table 31-4). Bacterial overgrowth often is present and antibiotic therapy can transiently improve diarrhea and steatorrhea.

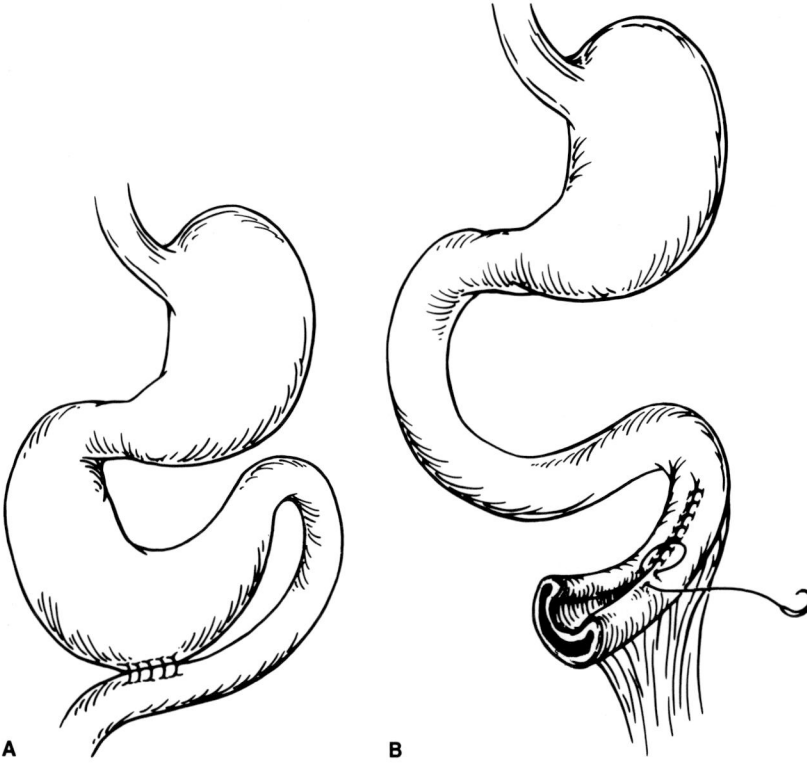

Figure 31-22 Procedures for intestinal pseudoobstruction. (**A**) A side-to-side duodenojejunostomy often is not effective. (**B**) Intestinal tapering can be accomplished by simple imbrication. (After Colemont LS, Camilleri M. Chronic intestinal pseudoobstruction: diagnosis and treatment. Mayo Clin Proc 1989;64:6070)

A   B

Careful preoperative evaluation should decrease the number of unnecessary operations done to rule out mechanical obstruction (Fig. 31-21). If operation is undertaken and no mechanical obstruction is found, a full-thickness biopsy should be performed if pseudoobstruction is a consideration. The sample should measure at least 2 × 2 cm and requires special handling for nerve studies.[214] Operative therapy usually is not effective in the management of intestinal pseudoobstruction because of the diffuse and progressive nature of the underlying disease. However, when the disease is localized, operation can prove beneficial. Although resection or bypass of an apparently localized process is tempting, surrounding areas often are involved and operation can exacerbate the motor dysfunction. This should be considered when patients have well-identified underlying conditions known to be diffuse and progressive, such as diabetes mellitus and scleroderma.

There are several patterns of pseudoobstructive complications, all of which require different surgical approaches. Megaduodenum is a problem in several disorders, and side-to-side duodenojejunostomy often is ineffective[215,216] (Fig. 31-22A). A partial duodenectomy of the anterior wall can improve drainage. The duodenum can be defunctionalized by antrectomy and vagotomy to relieve symptoms as well.[215] Intestinal tapering by either simple imbrication (see Fig. 31-22B) or exci-

sion along the antimesenteric border with a stapler can be used for functional small bowel obstruction.[217] Dysfunctional small intestine can be resected, but symptoms usually recur and creation of the short-bowel syndrome is a concern.[214,215,218] However, as results of intestinal transplantation improve, radical resection and transplantation may become a consideration. Subtotal colectomy with ileorectal anastomosis at the peritoneal reflection has been used with some success for colonic pseudoobstruction.[215] This is successful only in patients in whom colonic dysmotility is confined to the intraperitoneal colon. Preoperative rectal manometry should be performed to demonstrate normal sphincter function, including a preserved rectal inhibitory reflex, when subtotal colectomy is being considered.

A venting enterostomy and long-term parenteral nutritional support have been used for palliation in patients with more diffuse disease.[219] The tube enterostomy can be opened when obstructive symptoms develop, obviating the need for nasogastric tubes in most situations. Additional fluid and nutritional needs can be administered parenterally at home to prevent recurrent hospitalizations.

Outcome

Because most of the underlying causes of pseudoobstruction are not easily remedied, the long-term outcome usually is not satisfactory.[220] The progressive nature of the disorder leads to future obstructive symptoms in most patients. Chronic or recurrent obstruction also can result in a persistent enteropathy in previously normal proximal intestinal segments.[221]

REFERENCES

1. Ballantyne GH. The meaning of ileus. Am J Surg 1984;148:252.
2. Mucha P. Small intestinal obstruction. Surg Clin North Am 1987;67:597.
3. Davis SE, Sperling L. Obstruction of the small intestine. Arch Surg 1969;99:424.
4. Lo AM, Evans WE, Carey LC. Review of small bowel obstruction at Milwaukee County General Hospital. Am J Surg 1966;111:884.
5. Stewardson RH, Bombeck CT, Nyhus LM. Critical operative management of small bowel obstruction. Ann Surg 1978;187:189.
6. Stevenson RJ. Non-neonatal intestinal obstruction in children. Surg Clin North Am 1985;65:1217.
7. Perdue PUS, Johnson HW, Stafford PW. Intestinal obstruction complicating pregnancy. Am J Surg 1992;164:384.
8. Zadeh BJ, Davis JM, Canizaro PC. Small bowel obstruction in the elderly. Ann Surg 1985;51:470.
9. Osteen RT, Guyton S, Steele G, Wilson RE. Malignant intestinal obstruction. Surgery 1980;87:611.
10. Greenlee HB. Acute large bowel obstruction: an update. Surg Annu 1982;14:253.
11. Phillips SF, Wingate DL. Fluid and electrolyte fluxes of the gut. Adv Intern Med 1979;24:429.
12. Papanicolaou G, Nikas D, Ahn Y, Condos S, Fielding LP. Regional blood flow and water content in the obstructed small intestine. Arch Surg 1985;120:920.
13. Neville R, Fielding LP, Cambria RP, Modlin I. Vascular responsiveness in obstructed gut. Dis Colon Rectum 1991;34:229.
14. Sung DTW, Williams LF. Intestinal secretion after intravenous fluid infusion in small bowel obstruction. Am J Surg 1971;121:91.
15. Shields R. The absorption and secretion of fluid and electrolytes by the obstructed bowel. Br J Surg 1965;52:774.
16. Wright HG, O'Brien JJ, Tilson MD. Water absorption in experimental closed segment obstruction of the ileum in man. Am J Surg 1971;121:96.
17. Basson MD, Fielding LP, Bilchik AS, et al. Does vasoactive intestinal polypeptide mediate the pathophysiology of bowel obstruction? Am J Surg 1989;157:109.
18. Roscher R, Oettinger W, Beger HG. Bacterial microflora, endogenous endotoxin and prostaglandins in small bowel obstruction. Am J Surg 1988;155:348.
19. Wangensteen OH, Rea CE. The distention factor in simple intestinal obstruction. An experimental study with exclusion of swallowed air by cervical esophagostomy. Surgery 1939;5:327.
20. Summers RW, Youda R, Prihoda M, Flatt A. Acute intestinal obstruction: an electromyographic study in dogs. Gastroenterology 1983;85:1301.
21. Summers RW, Anuras S, Green J. Jejunal manometry patterns in health, partial intestinal obstruction and pseudoobstruction. Gastroenterology 1983;85:1290.
22. Lausen M, Reichenbacher D, Ruf G, Schoffel V, Pelz K. Myoelectric activity of the small bowel in mechanical obstruction and intraabdominal bacterial contamination. Eur Surg Res 1988;20:304.
23. Cohn I, Bornside GH. Imbalance of the normal microbial flora: influence of strangulation obstruction upon the bacterial ecology of the small intestine. Am J Digest Dis 1965;10:873.
24. Ruf W, Suehiro GT, Suehiro A, Pressler V, McNamara JJ. Intestinal blood flow at various intraluminal pressures in the piglet with closed abdomen. Ann Surg 1980;191:157.
25. Barnett WO. Experimental strangulated intestinal obstruction: a review. Gastroenterology 1960;39:34.
26. Parks DA, Jacobson Ed. Physiology of the splanchnic circulation. Arch Intern Med 1985;145:1278.
27. Leung FW, Su KC, Passaro E, Guth PH. Regional differences in gut blood flow and mucosal damage in response to ischemia and reperfusion. Am J Physiol 1992;263:G301.
28. Deitch EA. Simple intestinal obstruction causes bacterial translocation in man. Arch Surg 1989;124:699.
29. Koike K, Moore FA, Moore EE, Poggetti RS, Tuder RM, Banerjee A. Endotoxin after gut ischemia/reperfusion causes irreversible lung injury. J Surg Res 1992;52:656.
30. Roggo A, Ottinger LW. Acute small bowel volvulus in adults. Ann Surg 1992;216:135.
31. Snyder EN, McCranie D. Closed loop obstruction of the small bowel. Am J Surg 1966;111:398.
32. Brolin RE. Partial small bowel obstruction. Surgery 1984;95:1451.
33. Camilleri M. Jejunal manometry in distal subacute mechanical obstruction: significance of prolonged simultaneous contractions. Gut 1989;30:468.
34. Schwobel M, Hirsig J, Illi O, Battig U. The influence of small bowel contamination on the pathogenesis of bowel obstruction. Prog Pediatr Surg 1989;24:165.
35. Stillwell OK. The law of LaPlace: some clinical applications. Mayo Clin Proc 1973;48:863.
36. Coxon JS, Dickson C, Taylor I. Changes in intestinal blood flow during the development of chronic large bowel obstruction. Br J Surg 1984;71:795.
37. Fraser ID, Condon RE, Schulte WJ, DeCosse JJ, Cowles VE. Intestinal motility changes in experimental large bowel obstruction. Surgery 1980;89:677.
38. Sarr MG, Bulkley GB, Zuidema GD. Preoperative recognition of strangulation obstruction: prospective evaluation of diagnostic capability. Am J Surg 1983;145:176.
39. Silen W, Hein MF, Goldman L. Strangulation obstruction of the small intestine. Arch Surg 1962;85:121.
40. Sosa J, Gardner B. Management of patients diagnosed

as acute intestinal obstruction secondary to adhesions. Am Surg 1993;59:125.

41. Bizer LS, Liebling RW, Delaney HM, Gliedman ML. Small bowel obstruction: the role of nonoperative treatment in simple intestinal obstruction and predictive criteria for strangulation obstruction. Surgery 1981;89:407.

42. Graeber GM, O'Neill JF, Wolf RE, Wukich DK, Cafferty PH, Harmon JW. Elevated levels of peripheral serum creatine phosphokinase with strangulated small bowel obstruction. Arch Surg 1983;118:837.

43. Thompson JS, Bragg LE, West WW. Serum enzyme levels during intestinal ischemia. Ann Surg 1990;221:369.

44. Gollin G, Marks C, Marks WH. Intestinal fatty acid binding protein in serum and urine reflects early ischemic injury to the small bowel. Surgery 1993;113:545.

45. Roh JJ, Thompson JS, Harned RK, Hodgson PE. The value of pneumoperitoneum in the diagnosis of visceral perforation. Am J Surg 1983;146:830.

46. Goldberg HI, Dodds WJ. Roentgen evaluation of small bowel obstruction. Dig Dis Sci 1979;24:245.

47. Dunn JT, Halls JM, Berne TV. Roentgenographic contrast studies in acute small bowel obstruction. Arch Surg 1984;119:1305.

48. Gammill SL, Nice CM. Air fluid levels: their occurrence in normal patients and their role in the analysis of ileus. Surgery 1972;71:771.

49. Brolin RE, Krasna MJ, Mast BA. Use of tubes and radiographs in the management of small bowel obstruction. Ann Surg 1987;206:126.

50. Galandiuk S, Fazio VW. Pneumatosis cystoides intestinalis. Dis Colon Rectum 1986;29:358.

51. Knechtle SJ, Davidoff AM, Rice RP. Pneumatosis intestinalis: surgical management and clinical outcome. Ann Surg 1991;212:160.

52. Liebman PR, Patten MT, Manny J, Benfield JR, Hechtman HB. Hepatic-portal venous gas in adults: etiology, pathophysiology and clinical significance. Ann Surg 1978;187:281.

53. Riveron FA, Obeid FN, Horst HM, Sorensen VJ, Bruins BA. The role of contrast radiography in presumed bowel obstruction. Surgery 1989;106:496.

54. Erickson AS, Krasna MJ, Mast BA, Nosher JC, Brolin RE. Use of gastrointestinal contrast studies in obstruction of the small and large bowel. Dis Colon Rectum 1990;33:56.

55. Maglinte DT, Nolan DJ, Herlinger H. Preoperative diagnosis by enteroclysis of unsuspected closed loop obstruction in medically managed patients. J Clin Gastroenterol 1991;13:308.

56. Dixon JA. Barium sulfate and the obstructed small intestine. Surg Gynecol Obstet 1967;124:838.

57. Maglinte DT, Peterson LA, Vahey TN, Muller RE, Chernish SM. Enteroclysis in partial small bowel obstruction. Am J Surg 1984;147:325.

58. Caroline DF, Herlinger H, Laufer I, Kressel HY, Levine MS. Small bowel enema in the diagnosis of adhesive obstructions. AJR Am J Roentgenol 1984;142:1133.

59. Stewart J, Finan PJ, Courtney DF, Brennan TG. Does a water soluble contrast enema assist in the management of acute large bowel obstruction: a prospective study of 117 cases. Br J Surg 1984;71:799.

60. Chapman AH, McNamara M, Poster G. The acute contrast enema in suspected large bowel obstruction: value and technique. Clin Radiol 1992;46:273.

61. Federle MP, Chun G, Jeffrey RB, Rayor R. Computed tomographic findings in bowel infarction. AJR Am J Roentgenol 1984;142:91.

62. Fleischer AC, Dowling AD, Weinstein L, Jones AE. Sonographic patterns of distended fluid filled bowel. Radiology 1979;133:681.

63. Merine D, Fishman EK, Jones B, Siegelman SS. Enteroenteric intussusception: CT findings in nine patients. AJR Am J Roentgenol 1987;148:1129.

64. Megibow AJ, Balthazar EJ, Cho KC, Medwid SW, Birnbaum BA, Noz ME. Bowel obstruction: evaluation with CT. Radiology 1991;180:313.

65. Myrvold HE, Larsson L, Brandberg A. Systemic prophylaxis with doxycycline in intestinal surgery in patients with high incidence of abnormal fecal flora. Acta Chir Scand 1989;155:277.

66. Wolfson RJ, Bauer JJ, Gelernt IM, Kreel I, Aufses AH. Use of the long tube in the management of patients with small intestinal obstruction due to adhesions. Arch Surg 1985;120:1001.

67. Peetz DJ, Gamelli RL, Pilcher DB. Intestinal intubation in acute, mechanical small bowel obstruction. Arch Surg 1982;117:334.

68. Brightwell NL, Mcfee AS, Aust JB. Bowel obstruction and the long intestinal tube. Arch Surg 1977;112:505.

69. Bizer LS, Liebling RW, Delaney HM, et al. Small bowel obstruction. Surgery 1981;89:407.

70. Helmkamp BF, Kemmel J. Conservative management of small bowel obstruction. Am J Obstet Gynecol 1985;152:677.

71. Snyder CL, Ferrell KL, Goodale RL, Leonard AS. Nonoperative management of small bowel obstruction with endoscopic long intestinal tube placement. Am Surg 1990;56:587.

72. Douglas DD, Morrissey JF. A new technique for rapid endoscope-assisted intubation of the small intestine. Arch Surg 1978;113:196.

73. Nelson RL, Nyhus LM. A new long intestinal tube. Surg Gynecol Obstet 1979;149:581.

74. Chilimindris CP, Stonesifer GL. Complications associated with the Baker tube jejunostomy. Am Surg 1978;44:707.

75. Keating J, Hill A, Schroeder D, Whittle D. Laparoscopy in the diagnosis and treatment of acute small bowel obstruction. J Laparoendosc Surg 1992;2:239.

76. Munro A, Jones PF. Operative intubation in the treatment of complicated small bowel obstruction. Br J Surg 1978;65:123.

77. Bulkley GB, Zuidema GD, Hamilton SR, O'Mara CS, Klacsman PG, Horn SD. Intraoperative determination of

small intestinal viability after ischemic injury. Ann Surg 1981;193:628.

78. Mann A, Fazio VW, Lucas FV. A comparative study of the use of fluorescein and the Doppler device in the determination of intestinal viability. Surg Gynecol Obstet 1982;154:53.

79. Cooperman M, Pace WG, Martin EW, et al. Determination of viability of ischemic intestine by Doppler ultrasound. Surgery 1978;83:705.

80. Carter MS, Fantini GA, Sammartano RJ, Mitsudo S, Silverman DG, Boley SJ. Qualitative and quantitative fluorescein fluorescence in determining intestinal viability. Am J Surg 1984;147:117.

81. O'Donnell JA, Hobson RW. Operative confirmation of Doppler ultrasound in evaluation of intestinal ischemia. Surgery 1980;87:109.

82. Levy PJ, Kraus ZMM, Manny J. The role of second-look procedures in improving survival time for patients with mesenteric venous thrombosis. Surg Gynecol Obstet 1990;170:287.

83. Bellenis IP, Polychronia AB, Papaioannou AN. Preservation of compromised intestine after ischemic injury. Am Surg 1987;53:260.

84. MacDonald PH, Dinda PK, Beck IT, Mercer CD. The use of oximetry in determining intestinal blood flow. Surg Gynecol Obstet 1993;176:451.

85. Fazio VW, Galandiuk S, Jagelman DG, Lavery IC. Stricturoplasty in Crohn's disease. Ann Surg 1989;210:621.

86. Pritchard TJ, Schoetz DJ, Caushaj FP, et al. Stricturoplasty of the small bowel in patients with Crohn's disease. Arch Surg 1990;125:715.

87. Sayfan J, Wilson DA, Allan A, Andrews H, Alexander-Williams J. Recurrence after stricturoplasty or resection for Crohn's disease. Br J Surg 1989;76:335.

88. Kauffman HM, O'Brien DP. Selective reduction of incarcerated inguinal hernia. Am J Surg 1970;119:660.

89. Stoppa RE. The treatment of complicated groin and incisional hernias. World J Surg 1989;13:545.

90. Ger R, Mishnick A, Hurwitz J, Romero C, Oddsen R. Management of groin hernias by laparoscopy. World J Surg 1993;17:46.

91. Ghahremani GG. Internal abdominal hernias. Surg Clin North Am 1984;64:393.

92. Weilbaecher D, Bolin JA, Hearn D, Ogden W. Intussusception in adults. Am J Surg 1971;131:531.

93. Nagorney DM, Sarr MG, McIlrath DC. Surgical management of intussusception in the adult. Ann Surg 1981;193:230.

94. Sarr MG, Nagorney DM, McIlrath DC. Postoperative intussusception in the adult. Arch Surg 1981;116:144.

95. Gallick HL, Weaver DW, Suchs RJ, et al. Intestinal obstruction in cancer patients. Am Surg 1986;8:434.

96. Ellis CN, Boggs HW, Slagle GW, Cole PA. Small bowel obstruction after colon resection for benign and malignant diseases. Dis Colon Rectum 1991;34:367.

97. Walsh HPJ, Schofield PF. Is laparotomy for small bowel obstruction justified in patients with previously treated malignancy? Br J Surg 1984;71:933.

98. Pathak V, Swaminathan AP, Ghuman SS, et al. Intestinal obstruction in carcinomatosis. Am Surg 1980;46:691.

99. Butter SA, Cameron BL, Morrow M, Kahng K, Tom J. Small bowel obstruction in patients with a prior history of cancer. Am J Surg 1991;162:624.

100. Gemlo B, Rayner AA, Lewis B, et al. Home support of patients with end-stage malignant bowel obstruction using hydration and venting gastrostomy. Am J Surg 1986;152:100.

101. Lund B, Hansen M, Lundvall F, Nielsen NC, Sorenson BC, Hansen HH. Intestinal obstruction in patients with advanced carcinoma of the ovaries treated with combination chemotherapy. Surg Gynecol Obstet 1989;169:213.

102. Clarke-Pearson DL, DeLong ER, Chin N, Rice P, Creasman WT. Intestinal obstruction in patients with ovarian cancer. Arch Surg 1988;123:42.

103. Coletti L, Bossard PA. Intestinal obstruction during the early postoperative period. Arch Surg 1964;88:774.

104. Quatromoni JC, Rosoff L, Hauls JM, et al. Early postoperative bowel obstruction. Ann Surg 1980;191:72.

105. Pickleman J, Lee RM. The management of patients with suspected early postoperative small bowel obstruction. Ann Surg 1989;210:216.

106. Stewart RM, Page CP, Brender J, Schwesinger W, Eisenhut D. The incidence and risk of early postoperative small bowel obstruction. Am J Surg 1987;154:643.

107. Baker JW. Stitchless plication for recurring obstruction of the small bowel. Am J Surg 1968;116:316.

108. Noble TB. Plication of small intestine as prophylaxis against adhesions. Am J Surg 1937;35:41.

109. Wilson DO. Complications of the Noble procedure. Am J Surg 1964;108:264.

110. Childs WA, Phillips RB. Experience with intestinal plication and a proposed modification. Ann Surg 1960;152:258.

111. McCarthy JD. Further experience with the Childs-Phillips plication operation. Am J Surg 1975;130:15.

112. Ramsey Stewart G, Shuk A. Nasogastrointestinal intraluminal tube stenting in the prevention of recurrent small bowel obstruction. Aust NZ J Surg 1983;53:7.

113. Brightwell NL, McFee AS, Aust JB. Bowel obstruction and the long tube stent. Arch Surg 1977;112:505.

114. Close MB, Christensen NM. Transmesenteric small bowel plication or intraluminal tube stenting. Am J Surg 1979;136:89.

115. Weigelt JA, Snyder WH, Norman JL. Complications and results of 160 Baker tube plications. Am J Surg 1980;140:810.

116. Raf LE. Causes of abdominal adhesions in cases of intestinal obstruction. Acta Chir Scand 1969;135:73.

117. Ellis H. The cause and prevention of postoperative intraperitoneal adhesions. Surg Gynecol Obstet 1971;133:497.

118. Almdahl SM, Burhol PG. Peritoneal adhesions: causes and prevention. Dig Dis 1990;8:37.

119. Dixon MF, Beck JM. Multiple peritoneal adhesions re-

lated to starch and gauze fragments. J Pediatr Surg 1974;9:531.

120. O'Leary JP, Wickbom G, Cha SO, Wickbom A. The role of feces, necrotic tissue and various blocking agents in the prevention of adhesions. Ann Surg 1988;207:693.

121. Rappaport WD, Holcomb M, Valante J, Chrapil M. Antibiotic irrigation and the formation of intraabdominal adhesions. Am J Surg 1989;158:435.

122. Maetani S, Tobe T, Kashiwara S. Neglected role of torsion and constriction in pathogenesis of simple adhesive bowel obstruction. Br J Surg 1984;71:127.

123. Menzies D, Ellis H. The role of plasminogen activator in adhesion prevention. Surg Gynecol Obstet 1991;172: 362.

124. Fabri PJ, Ellison EC, Anderson ED, Kudsk KA. High molecular weight dextran: effect on adhesion formation and peritonitis in rats. Surgery 1983;94:336.

125. Gazzaniga AB, James JM, Strobe JB, Oppenheim EB. Prevention of peritoneal adhesions in the rat: the effects of dexamethasone, methylprednisolone, promethazine and human fibrolysin. Arch Surg 1975;110:429.

126. Goldberg FCP, Sheets JW, Habal WB. Peritoneal adhesions: prevention with the use of hydrophilic polymer coatings. Arch Surg 1980;115:776.

127. Grosfield JL, Berman JR, Schiller M, Morse TS. Excessive morbidity resulting from the prevention of intestinal adhesions with steroids and antihistamines. J Pediatr Surg 1973;8:221.

128. Gilmore OJA, Reid C. Prevention of intraperitoneal adhesions: a comparison of noxythiolin and a new povidone-iodine/PVP solution. Br J Surg 1979;66:197.

129. Buechter KJ, Boustany C, Caillouette R, Cohn I. Surgical management of the acutely obstructed colon. Am J Surg 1988;156:163.

130. Ballantyne GH, Braudner MD, Beart RW, Ilstrup DM. Volvulus of the colon: incidence and mortality. Ann Surg 1985;202:83.

131. Welch JP, Donaldson GA. Management of severe obstruction of the large bowel due to malignant disease. Am J Surg 1974;127:492.

132. Mackenzie S, Thomson SR, Baker LW. Management options in malignant obstruction of the left colon. Surg Gynecol Obstet 1992;174:337.

133. Leitman IM, Sullivan JD, Brams D, DeCosse JJ. Multivariate analysis of morbidity and mortality from the initial surgical management of obstructing carcinoma of the colon. Surg Gynecol Obstet 1992;174:513.

134. Brothers TE, Strodel WE, Eckhauser FE. Endoscopy in colonic volvulus. Ann Surg 1987;206:1.

135. Lelcuks S, Ratan J, Klausner JM, Skornick Y, Merhav A, Rozin RR. Endoscopic decompression of acute colonic obstruction. Ann Surg 1986;203:292.

136. Andersson A, Bergdahl L, Van De Linden W. Volvulus of the cecum. Ann Surg 1975;181:876.

137. Friedman JO, Odland MD, Bubrick MP. Experience with colonic volvulus. Dis Colon Rectum 1989;32:409.

138. Gibney EJ. Volvulus of the sigmoid colon. Surg Gynecol Obstet 1991;173:243.

139. Peoples JB, McCafferty JC, Scher KS. Operative therapy for sigmoid volvulus. Dis Colon Rectum 1990;33:643.

140. Subrahmanyam M. Mesosigmoplasty as a definitive operation for sigmoid volvulus. Br J Surg 1992;79:683.

141. O'Mara C, Wilson TH, Stonesifer GL, Cameron JL. Cecal volvulus: analysis of 50 patients with long-term follow-up. Ann Surg 1979;189:724.

142. Anderson JR, Welch GH. Acute volvulus of the right colon: analysis of 69 patients. World J Surg 1986;10:336.

143. Patel D, Ansari E, Berman MD. Percutaneous decompression of cecal volvulus. AJR Am J Roentgenol 1987;148:747.

144. Ryan JA, Johnson MG, Baker JW. Operative treatment of cecal volvulus combining cecopexy with intestinal tube decompression. Surg Gynecol Obstet 1985;160:84.

145. Miller R, Roe AM, Eltrigham LOK, Espiner HJ. Laparoscopic fixation of sigmoid volvulus. Br J Surg 1992;79:435.

146. Salim AS. Management of acute volvulus of the sigmoid colon: a new approach by percutaneous deflation and colopexy. World J Surg 1991;15:68.

147. Westdahl PR, Russell T. In support of blind tube cecostomy in acute obstruction of the descending colon: an analysis of 93 emergency cecostomies. Arch Surg 1969;118:577.

148. Winkler MJ, Volpe PA. Loop transverse colostomy: the case against. Dis Colon Rectum 1982;25:321.

149. Fasth S, Hulten L. Loop ileostomy: a superior diverting stoma in colorectal surgery. World J Surg 1984;8:401.

150. Prasad ML, Pearl PK, Abcarian H. End loop colostomy. Surg Gynecol Obstet 1984;158:380.

151. Sjodahl R, Franzen T, Nystrom PO. Primary versus staged resection for acute obstructing colorectal carcinoma. Br J Surg 1992;79:685.

152. Garrison RN, Shively EH, Baker C, Steele M, Trunkey D, Polk HC. Evaluation of the management of the emergent right hemicolectomy. J Trauma 1979;19:734.

153. Hoffmann J, Jensen HE. Tube cecostomy and staged resection for obstructing carcinoma of the left colon. Dis Colon Rectum 1984;27:24.

154. Bat L, Neumann G, Shemesh E. The association of synchronous neoplasms with occluding rectal cancer. Dis Colon Rectum 1985;28:149.

155. Valerio D, Jones PF. Immediate resection in the treatment of large bowel emergencies. Br J Surg 1978;65:712.

156. Carty NJ, Corder AP, Johnson CD. Colostomy is no longer appropriate in the management of uncomplicated large bowel obstruction: true or false? Ann R Coll Surg Engl 1993;75:46.

157. McGregor JR, O'Dwyer PJ. The surgical management of obstruction and perforation of the left colon. Surg Gynecol Obstet 1993;177:203.

158. Daneker GW, Carlson GW, Hohn DC, Lynch P, Roubirn L, Levin B. Endoscopic laser recanalization is effective for prevention and treatment of obstruction in sigmoid and rectal cancer. Arch Surg 1991;126:1348.

159. Stone JM, Bloom RJ. Transendoscopic balloon dilata-

tion of complete colonic obstruction. Dis Colon Rectum 1989;32:429.

160. Keen RR, Orsay CP. Rectosigmoid stent for obstructing colonic neoplasms. Dis Colon Rectum 1992;35:912.

161. Stewart J, Diament RH, Brennan TG. Management of obstructing lesions of the left colon by resection, on table lavage, and primary anastomosis. Surgery 1993; 114:502.

162. Pollock AV, Playforth MJ, Evans M. Preoperative lavage of the obstructed left colon to allow safe primary anastomosis. Dis Colon Rectum 1987;30:171.

163. Rosati C, Smith L, Deitel M, et al. Primary colorectal anastomosis with the intracolonic bypass tube. Surgery 1992;112:618.

164. Landercasper J, Cogbill TH, Merry WH, Stolee RT, Strutt PJ. Long term outcome after hospitalization for small bowel obstruction. Arch Surg 1993;128:765.

165. Nadrowski L. Paralytic ileus: recent advances in pathophysiology and treatment. Curr Surg 1983;40:260.

166. Furness JB, Costa A. Adynamic ileus, its pathogenesis and treatment. Med Biol 1974;52:82.

167. Esser MJ, Mahoney JL, Robinson JC, Cowles RE, Condon RE. Effects of adrenergic agents on colonic motility. Surgery 1987;102:416.

168. Condon RE, Cowles V, Ekbom GA, Schulte WJ, Hess G. Effects of halothane, enflurane, and nitrous oxide in colon motility. Surgery 1987;101:81.

169. Frantzides CT, Cowles V, Salaynzeh B, Tekin E, Condon RE. Morphine effects on human colonic myoelectric activity in the postoperative period. Am J Surg 1992;163:144.

170. Waldhausen JT, Schirmer BD. The effect of ambulation on recovery from postoperative ileus. Ann Surg 1990;212:671.

171. Graber JN, Schulte WJ, Condon RE, Cowles VE. Relationship of duration of postoperative ileus to extent and site of operative dissection. Surgery 1982;92:87.

172. Smith J, Kelly KA, Weinshilboum RM. Pathophysiology of postoperative ileus. Arch Surg 1977;112:203.

173. Condon RE, Frantzides CT, Cowles VE, Mahoney JL, Schulte WOH, Sarna SK. Resolution of postoperative ileus in humans. Ann Surg 1986;203:574.

174. Ducerf C, Duchamp C, Pouyet M. Postoperative electromyographic profile in human jejunum. Ann Surg 1992;215:237.

175. Waldhausen JT, Shaffrey ME, Skenderis BS, Jones RS, Schirmer BD. Gastrointestinal myoelectric and clinical patterns of recovery after laparotomy. Ann Surg 1990;211:777.

176. Schippers E, Holscher AH, Bollschweiler E, Siewert JR. Return of interdigestive motor complex after abdominal surgery: end of postoperative ileus? Dig Dis Sci 1991;36:621.

177. Bachulis BL, Smith PE. Pseudoobstruction of the colon. Am J Surg 1978;136:66.

178. Euphrat EJ. Adynamic ileus of the colon. Arch Surg 1975;110:224.

179. Lauderer JR, Demers LM, Bonnem EM. Elevated prostaglandin E in idiopathic intestinal pseudoobstruction. N Engl J Med 1976;295:21.

180. Thayer ML, Bubrick MP, Jacobs DM, Frykman S. Effects of ibuprofen on postoperative bowel motility and propulsion. Dis Colon Rectum 1988;31:363.

181. Myrhoj T, Olsen O, Wengel B. Neostigmine postoperative intestinal paralysis. Dis Colon Rectum 1988;31:378.

182. James WB, Hume R. Action of metoclopramide on gastric emptying and small bowel transit time. Gut 1968;9:203.

183. Cheape JD, Wexner SD, James K, Jagelman DG. Does metoclopramide reduce the length of ileus after colorectal surgery? Dis Colon Rectum 1991;34:437.

184. Davidson ED, Hersh T, Brinner RA, Barrett SM, Boyle LR. The effects of metoclopramide on postoperative ileus. Ann Surg 1979;190:27.

185. Koop H, Mounikes H, Koop I, Dionysius J, Schwartz C, Arnold R. Effect of the prokinetic drug cisapride on gastrointestinal hormone release. Scand J Gastroenterol 1986;21:907.

186. Boghaert A, Haesert G, Mourisse P, Verlinden M. Placebo controlled trial of cisapride in postoperative ileus. Acta Anaesthesiol Belg 1987;38:195.

187. Tollesson PO, Cassuto J, Rimback G, Faxen A, Bergman L, Mattson E. Treatment of postoperative ileus with cisapride. Scand J Gastroenterol 1991;26:477.

188. Rimback G, Cassuto J, Tollesson PO. Treatment of postoperative paralytic ileus by intravenous lidocaine infusion. Anesth Analg 1990;70:414.

189. Armstrong DN, Ballantyne GH, Modlin IM. Erythromycin stimulates ileal motility by activation of dihydropyridine-sensitive calcium channels. J Surg Res 1992;52:140.

190. Peeters T, Matthijis G, Depoorterc I, Cachet T, Hoogmartens J, Van Trappen G. Erythromycin is a motilin receptor agonist. Am J Physiol 1989;157:G470.

191. Inatomi N, Satoli H, Maki Y, Hashimoto N, Itoh Z, Omura S. An erythromycin derivative, EM-523, induces motilin like gastrointestinal motility in dogs. J Pharmacol Exp Ther 1989;251:707.

192. Cullen JJ, Eagon C, Dozois EJ, Kelly KA. Treatment of acute postoperative ileus with octreotide. Am J Surg 1993;165:113.

193. Kelley MC, Hocking MP, Marchand SD, Sninsky CA. Ketorolac prevents postoperative small intestinal ileus in rats. Am J Surg 1993;165:107.

194. Vanek VW, Al-Salti M. Acute pseudoobstruction of the colon: an analysis of 400 cases. Dis Colon Rectum 1986;29:203.

195. Hutchinson R, Griffiths C. Acute colonic pseudoobstruction: a pharmacological approach. Ann R Coll Surg Engl 1992;74:364.

196. Burke G, Shellito PC. Treatment of recurrent colonic pseudoobstruction by endoscopic placement of a fenestrated overtube. Dis Colon Rectum 1987;30:615.

197. Nano D, Prindiville T, Paulyn M, et al. Colonoscopic

therapy of acute pseudoobstruction of the colon. Am J Gastroenterol 1987;82:145.

198. Strodel WE, Nostraut TT, Eckhauser FE, Dent TL. Therapeutic and diagnostic colonoscopy in non-obstructive colonic dilatation. Ann Surg 1983;197:416.

199. Jetmore AB, Timmcke AE, Gathright JB, et al. Ogilvie's syndrome: colonoscopic decompression and analysis of predisposing factors. Dis Colon Rectum 1992;35:1135.

200. Gosche JR, Sharpe JN, Larson GM. Colonoscopic decompression for pseudoobstruction of the colon. Am Surg 1989;55:111.

201. Lee JT, Taylor BM, Singleton BC. Epidural anesthesia for acute pseudoobstruction of the colon. Dis Colon Rectum 1988;31:686.

202. Sloyer AF, Panella VS, Demas BE, et al. Ogilvie's syndrome: successful management without colonoscopy. Dig Dis Sci 1988;33:1391.

203. Khoo REH, Rothenenberger DA, Wong WD, Buls JG, Najarian JS. Tube decompression of the dilated colon. Am J Surg 1988;56:214.

204. Van Sonnenberg E, Varney RR, Casola G, et al. Percutaneous cecostomy for Ogilvie syndrome: laboratory observations and clinical experiences. Radiology 1990;175:679.

205. Duh OY, Way LW. Diagnostic laparoscopy and laparoscopic cecostomy for colonic pseudoobstruction. Dis Colon Rectum 1993;36:65.

206. Krishnamurthy S, Schuffler MD. Pathology of neuromuscular disorders of the small intestine and colon. Gastroenterology 1987;93:610.

207. Colemont LS, Camilleri M. Chronic intestinal pseudoobstruction: diagnosis and treatment. Mayo Clin Proc 1989;64:6070.

208. Faulk DL, Anuras S, Christensen J. Chronic intestinal pseudoobstruction. Gastroenterology 1970;74:922.

209. Camilleri M. Disorders of gastrointestinal motility in neurologic disease. Mayo Clin Proc 1990;65:825.

210. Richards W, Williams LF. Pseudo-pseudoobstruction: a clinically relevant concept. Am Surg 1989;55:26.

211. Kamm MA. The small intestine and colon: scintigraphic quantitation of motility in health and disease. Eur J Nucl Med 1992;19:902.

212. Camilleri M, Malagelada JR, Abell TL, Brown ML, Hendi V, Zinsmeister AR. Effect of 6 weeks of treatment with cisapride in gastroparesis and intestinal pseudoobstruction. Gastroenterology 1989;96:704.

213. Soudah HC, Haster WL, Gwyang C. Effect of octreotide on intestinal motility and bacterial overgrowth in scleroderma. N Engl J Med 1991;325:1461.

214. Schuffler MD, Leon SH, Krishnamurthy S. Intestinal pseudoobstruction caused by a new form of visceral neuropathy: palliation by radical small bowel resection. Gastroenterology 1985;89:1152.

215. Schuffler MD, Deitsch EA. Chronic idiopathic intestinal pseudoobstruction: a surgical approach. Ann Surg 1980;192:752.

216. Shaw A, Shaffer HA, Anuras S. Familial visceral myopathy: the role of surgery. Am J Surg 1985;150:102.

217. Borgstein ES, Munro A, Youngson GG. Intestinal plication: an alternative to tapered jejunostomy in functional small bowel obstruction. Br J Surg 1991;78:1075.

218. Mughal MM, Irving MH. Treatment of end stage chronic intestinal pseudoobstruction by subtotal enterectomy and home parenteral nutrition. Gut 1988;29:1613.

219. Pitt HA, Mann LL, Berquist WE, Ament ME, Fonkalsrud EW, DenBesten L. Chronic intestinal pseudoobstruction: management with total parenteral nutrition and a venting enterostomy. Arch Surg 1985;120:614.

220. Hanks JB, Meyers WC, Anderson DK, et al. Chronic primary intestinal pseudoobstruction. Ann Surg 1981;89:175.

221. Cezard JP, Aigram Y, Sousino E, et al. Postobstructive enteropathy in infants with transient enterostomy: its consequences in the upper small intestinal functions. J Pediatr Surg 1992;27:1427.

Digestive Tract Surgery: A Text and Atlas, edited by Richard H. Bell,
Layton F. Rikkers, and Michael W. Mulholland.
Lippincott-Raven Publishers, Philadelphia, © 1996.

32

Mesenteric Vascular Diseases

Ronald N. Kaleya | *Scott J. Boley*

Mesenteric vascular diseases are the consequences of insufficient blood flow to all or part of the intestines. The causes of the ischemic insults vary, but the end result for all ischemic intestinal injuries is similar—a spectrum of bowel injury ranging from completely reversible alterations of intestinal function to transmural hemorrhagic necrosis of the intestinal wall. The clinical syndromes associated with mesenteric vascular diseases depend on the severity of the ischemic injury and the site and length of intestine affected. Therefore, the symptoms and signs of the mesenteric vascular diseases vary considerably, obscuring their diagnosis. As awareness of these syndromes and understanding of the pathophysiologic causes and repercussions of intestinal ischemia have increased and diagnostic modalities have improved, an effective approach to the diagnosis and treatment of these diseases has been formulated.

Ischemic disorders of the intestine can be divided into those caused by a transient diminution of blood flow, as in most cases of colonic ischemia, and those caused by a permanent interruption of mesenteric blood flow, as in some forms of acute mesenteric ischemia. Mesenteric vascular diseases also can be broadly classified by site according to whether they affect the midgut or the hindgut. Whereas colonic ischemia affects only the hindgut, acute mesenteric ischemia can affect both the midgut and the hindgut. These diseases can be categorized further as acute or chronic in nature and arterial or venous in origin (Fig. 32-1). Although the viability of the intestine is not compromised in the chronic forms, the blood flow can be insufficient to support the functional demands of the intestine. In contrast, the viability of the intestine is endangered in the acute forms of mesenteric ischemia. Atherosclerotic narrowing and occlusion of the mesenteric arteries,

producing intestinal angina and gradually evolving mesenteric venous thrombosis, are the most common forms of chronic ischemia. The acute form of mesenteric ischemia is more common than the chronic form, and arterial disease is more common than venous disease. The arterial forms of acute mesenteric ischemia include superior mesenteric arterial embolus, nonocclusive mesenteric ischemia, superior mesenteric artery (SMA) thrombosis, and focal segmental ischemia that results from local atherosclerotic emboli or vasculitides. Acute mesenteric venous thrombosis and focal segmental ischemia caused by strangulation obstruction of the small intestine or by localized venous thrombosis comprise the venous forms of acute mesenteric ischemia. Colonic ischemia is almost always the result of acute arterial insufficiency.

ISCHEMIC DISORDERS OF THE COLON

Before 1950, colonic ischemia was considered synonymous with colonic infarction or gangrene. Since that time, it has become recognized as one of the more common disorders of the colon in the elderly and the most common form of ischemic injury of the gastrointestinal tract. Today, the term *colonic ischemia* is used to describe a process that leads to varied clinical outcomes. The spectrum includes reversible ischemic colopathy (submucosal or intramucosal hemorrhage), reversible or transient ischemic colitis, chronic ischemic ulcerative colitis, ischemic colonic stricture, colonic gangrene, and fulminant universal colitis (see Fig. 32-1).

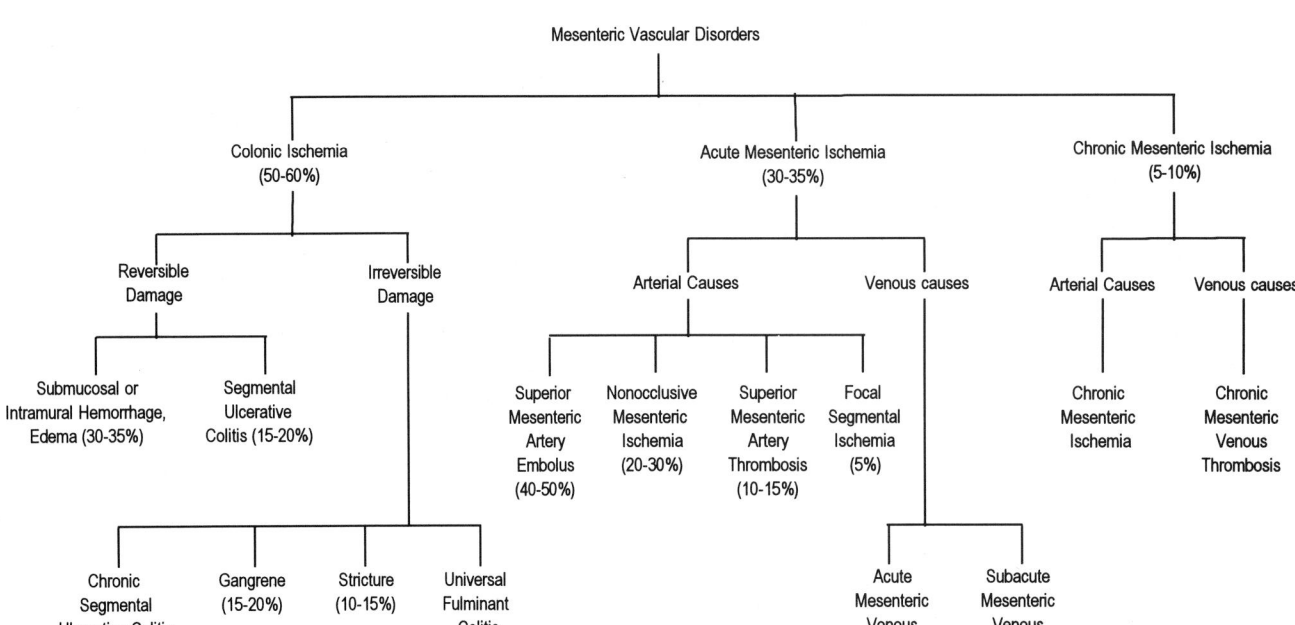

Figure 32-1 Mesenteric vascular disorders.

Colonic Circulation

The colon normally is protected from ischemia by its abundant collateral circulation. Communications between the celiac, superior mesenteric, inferior mesenteric, and iliac arterial beds are numerous. Collateral flow around small arterial branches is made possible by the multiple arcades within the colonic mesentery, and SMA or inferior mesenteric artery (IMA) occlusions are bypassed by the arc of Riolan, the central anastomotic artery, and the marginal artery of Drummond (Fig. 32-2). In addition, within the bowel wall there is a network of communicating submucosal vessels that can maintain viability of short segments of the colon where the extramural arterial supply has been compromised.

The colon has an inherently lower blood flow than the small intestine, making it more sensitive to injury during acute reductions in blood flow. Moreover, experimental studies have shown that functional motor activity of the colon is accompanied by decreased blood flow. In contrast, the blood flow to the small intestine increases markedly during periods of increased peristalsis and digestion. In addition, the pronounced effect of straining on systemic arterial and venous pressure in constipated, as compared with normal, patients provides indirect evidence that constipation can accentuate the adverse circulatory effects of defecation. Geber[1] postulated that "the combination of normally low blood flow and decreased blood flow during functional activity would seem to make the colon (1) rather unique among all areas of the body where increased motor activity is usually accompanied by an increased blood flow and (2) more susceptible to pathology." Other factors that decrease colonic blood flow include changes in the environment, digestion, and emotionally stressful situations. Experiments evaluating hypothalamic influence on gastrointestinal blood flow suggest that the effect of autonomic stimulation is greater on the blood flow of the colon than on any other part of the gastrointestinal tract.[2]

Pathophysiology of Colonic Ischemia

What ultimately triggers an episode of colonic ischemia remains conjectural in most instances. Whether increased demand by colonic tissue is superimposed on an already marginal blood flow or whether the flow itself is acutely diminished has not been determined. However, because colonic ischemia is a disease of the elderly, an association with degenerative changes of the mesenteric vasculature has been postulated. On histologic examination, narrowing of small arteries, arterioles, and veins is evident in colons resected for nonocclusive colonic ischemia. Autopsy studies also have shown abnormal musculature in the wall of the superior rectal artery in the elderly population, confirming an age-related alteration in the mesenteric vasculature.[3] In addition, postmortem angiographic studies have revealed an age-related tortuosity of the longer colonic arteries that can cause increased resistance to colonic blood flow, thus predisposing patients to ischemia.[4]

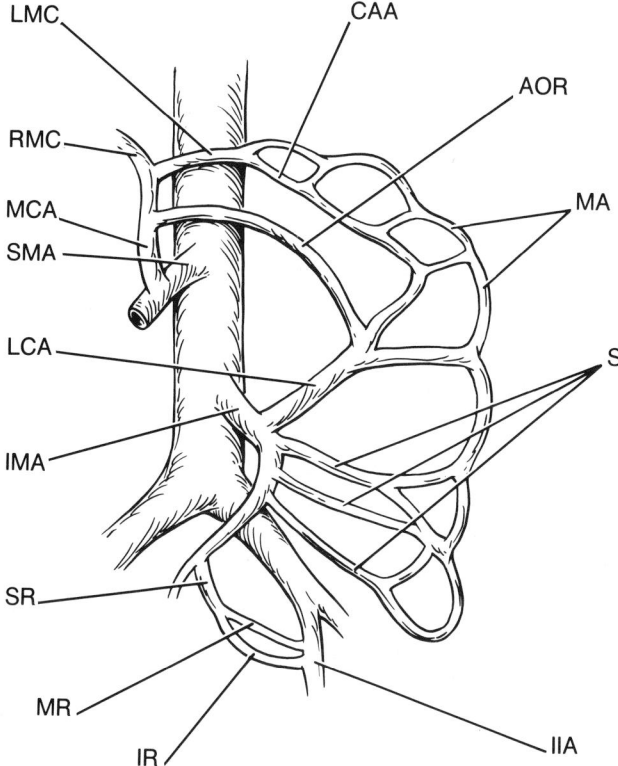

Figure 32-2 Colonic circulation and collateral channels. MCA, middle colic artery; RMC, right branch of the middle colic artery; LMC, left branch of the middle colic artery; CAA, central anastomotic artery; AOR, arc of Riolan (meandering artery); MA, marginal artery of Drummond; SMA, superior mesenteric artery; IMA, inferior mesenteric artery; LCA, left colic artery; S, sigmoid branches; SR, superior rectal artery; MR, middle rectal artery; IR, inferior rectal artery; IIA, internal iliac artery (hypogastric artery).

Despite this suggestive evidence for a vascular or autonomic etiology for colonic ischemia, most cases have no identifiable cause. These spontaneous episodes are thought to be the result of local nonocclusive ischemia in association with small vessel disease. Colonic blood flow can be compromised further by alterations in systemic perfusion accompanying congestive heart failure, digitalis toxicity, or arrhythmia. Many other conditions, spontaneous or iatrogenic, have been associated with colonic ischemia, although a direct cause-and-effect relation has not been established (Table 32-1). Two specific and well-recognized exceptions are the development of colonic ischemia proximal to a potentially obstructing stricture, carcinoma, or diverticulitis and its development after aortic reconstruction.

Demographics

The diagnosis of colonic ischemia often is made after the period of ischemia has passed and blood flow to the affected segment of colon has returned to normal.

Many cases of transient or reversible ischemia probably are missed because the condition resolves before medical attention is sought, or because a barium enema or colonoscopy is not performed early in the course of the disease. In addition, many cases are misdiagnosed as infectious colitis or inflammatory bowel disease. Thus, no study has provided an accurate determination of the true incidence of colonic ischemia.

Table 32-1   Causes of Colonic Ischemia

HEMODYNAMIC CAUSES
Cardiogenic shock
Hemorrhagic shock
Dysrhythmia

OCCLUSIVE CAUSES
Arterial emboli
Cholesterol emboli
Inferior mesenteric artery thrombosis
Volvulus
Strangulated hernia

TRAUMATIC CAUSES
Blunt or penetrating trauma
Ruptured ectopic pregnancy

IATROGENIC CAUSES
Aneurysmectomy
Aortoiliac reconstruction
Gynecologic operations
Colonic bypass procedures
Lumbar aortography
Coronary angiography or angioplasty
Colectomy with high ligation of the inferior mesenteric artery

MEDICATIONS
Estrogens
Danazol
Digitalis
Vasopressin
Gold
Psychotropic drugs
Cocaine

VASCULITIS
Polyarteritis nodosa
Systemic lupus erythematosus
Rheumatoid arthritis and vasculitis
Takayasu's arteritis
Thromboangiitis obliterans

HEMATOLOGIC DISORDERS
Sickle cell anemia
Protein S and C deficiencies
Antithrombin III deficiency
Polycythemia vera

OTHER
Allergy
Long distance running
Parasitic infestation

Several retrospective reviews of older clinical material have revealed many cases of colonic ischemia that were either undiagnosed or misdiagnosed because the various clinical manifestations of this disorder were not recognized. Using the modern clinical, radiologic, and pathologic criteria for the diagnosis of colonic ischemia, two retrospective reviews of 154 patients in whom colitis was identified after the age of 50 years revealed that about 75% of the patients had probable or definite colonic ischemia.[5,6] Inflammatory bowel disease had been diagnosed erroneously in half these patients.

Of the 50 or so cases of gastrointestinal ischemia seen at Montefiore Medical Center each year, 25 to 30 (50% to 60%) are colonic ischemia. Acute mesenteric ischemia accounts for an additional 30% to 40% of cases, and focal segmental ischemia and chronic mesenteric ischemia make up the remainder[7] (see Fig. 32-1).

In our experience with more than 300 cases of colonic ischemia, no significant gender predilection exists. About 90% of patients are older than 60 years and have other evidence of systemic atherosclerotic disease. Colonic ischemia occasionally affects young individuals, however. Causes in the younger population include vasculitis (especially systemic lupus erythematosus)[8]; medications (estrogens,[9,10] danazol,[11] vasopressin,[12] gold,[13] psychotropic drugs[14]); sickle cell anemia[15]; coagulopathies (thrombotic thrombocytopenic purpura,[16] protein C and protein S deficiency,[17] antithrombin III deficiency[18]); competitive long distance running[19]; and cocaine abuse.[20]

Clinical Manifestations

Presentation

Colonic ischemia often presents with the sudden onset of mild, cramping abdominal pain, usually localized to the left lower quadrant. Less commonly, the pain is severe, and in some patients, the description of pain can be elicited only in retrospect, if at all. An urgent desire to defecate frequently accompanies the pain and is followed, within 24 hours, by the passage of either bright red or maroon blood in the stool. The bleeding is not vigorous and blood loss requiring transfusion is so rare that it should suggest an alternative diagnosis. Physical examination can reveal mild to severe abdominal tenderness elicited in the location of the involved segment of bowel.

Distribution of Colonic Ischemia

Any part of the bowel can be affected, but the splenic flexure and descending and sigmoid colon are the most common sites (Fig. 32-3). No prognostic implications can be derived from the distribution of the disease. Nonocclusive ischemic injuries usually involve the "watershed" areas of the colon (ie, the splenic flexure and the junction of the sigmoid and rectum), whereas ligation of the IMA produces changes in the sigmoid colon. Similarly, the length of bowel affected varies with the cause. For example, atheromatous emboli result in short segment changes and nonocclusive injuries usually involve much longer portions of the colon. Depending on the severity and duration of the ischemic insult, fever or leukocytosis can be present. There usually is no acidemia, hypotension, or septic shock. In more severe ischemia, signs of peritonitis can develop.

Natural History of Colonic Ischemia

Despite similarities in the initial presentation of most episodes of colonic ischemia, the outcome cannot be predicted at its onset unless the initial physical findings indicate an unequivocal intraabdominal catastro-

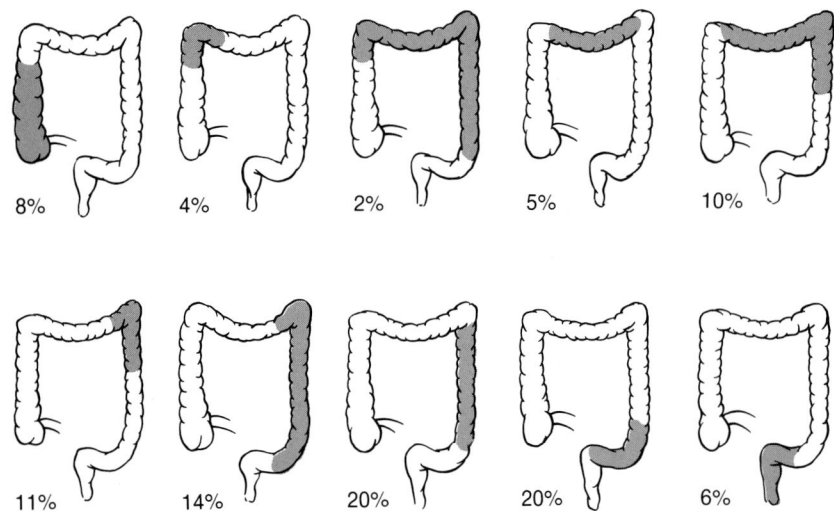

8% 4% 2% 5% 10%

11% 14% 20% 20% 6%

Figure 32-3 Distribution and length of involvement in 300 cases of colonic ischemia. (Brandt LJ, Boley SJ. Colonic ischemia. Surg Clin North Am 1992;72:203)

phe. The ultimate course of an ischemic insult depends on many factors, including the following:

- The cause (ie, occlusive or nonocclusive)
- The caliber of an occluded vessel
- The duration and degree of ischemia
- The rapidity of onset of the ischemia
- The condition of the collateral circulation
- The metabolic requirements of the affected bowel
- The presence and virulence of the bowel flora
- The presence of associated conditions (eg, colonic distention)

Symptoms usually subside within 24 to 48 hours, and clinical, radiologic, and endoscopic evidence of healing is seen within 2 weeks (Fig. 32-4). More severe but still reversible ischemic damage can take 1 to 6 months to resolve. Most patients with reversible disease exhibit only colonic hemorrhage or edema, whereas about one third have transient colitis. At times, with more severe yet reversible ischemia, the entire mucosa can slough as a tube. In one half of patients, the ischemic damage is too severe to heal and irreversible disease ultimately develops. About two thirds of these patients have protracted courses, with either chronic segmental ulcerative colitis or ischemic stricture. The remaining third have signs and symptoms of intraabdominal catastrophe from gangrene with or without perforation, which become obvious within hours of the initial presentation.

Patients who have colonic ischemia as a complication of shock, congestive heart failure, myocardial infarction, or severe dehydration have a particularly poor prognosis. These patients typically are elderly and taking digitalis preparations, which can act as potent splanchnic vasoconstrictors, exacerbating the already compromised colonic perfusion. In one series, such factors were present in one fourth of all patients with colonic ischemia, and 12 of 13 patients who were in shock at the time of presentation died.[21]

Because the outcome of an episode of colonic ischemia usually cannot be predicted, patients must be examined serially for evidence of peritonitis, rising temperature, elevation of the white blood cell count, or worsening symptoms. Patients with diarrhea or bleeding persisting beyond the first 10 to 14 days usually go on to perforation or, less frequently, a protein-wasting enteropathy. Strictures develop over weeks to months and can be asymptomatic or can produce progressive bowel obstruction. Some of the asymptomatic strictures resolve spontaneously over many months.

Diagnosis

Early and accurate diagnosis of colonic ischemia depends on serial radiographic or colonoscopic evaluation of the colon as well as repeated clinical evaluation of the patient. The more severe cases can be difficult to distinguish from acute mesenteric ischemia, whereas the less severe cases can mimic acute or chronic idiopathic ulcerative colitis, Crohn's colitis, infectious colitis, or diverticulitis. A combination of radiographic, colonoscopic, and clinical findings may be necessary to establish the diagnosis of colonic ischemia.

In patients with suspected colonic ischemia, if abdominal radiographs are nonspecific, sigmoidoscopy is unrevealing, and there are no signs of peritonitis, a gentle barium enema or colonoscopy should be performed in the unprepared bowel within 48 hours of the onset of symptoms. The most characteristic finding on barium enema is thumbprinting or pseudotumors (Fig. 32-5), and colonoscopy commonly shows hemorrhagic nodules or bullae. The hemorrhagic nodules seen on colonoscopy are caused by bleeding into the submucosa and are equivalent to the thumbprints seen on barium enema. Segmental distribution of these findings, with or without ulceration, is suggestive of colonic ischemia, but the diagnosis cannot be made conclusively based on a single study. In fact, persistence of the thumbprints suggests a diagnosis other than colonic ischemia (eg, lymphoma or amyloidosis).

Repeated radiographic or endoscopic examinations of the colon together with observation of the clinical course are necessary to make a correct diagnosis. Segmental colitis associated with a tumor or other partially obstructing lesion can behave like ischemic disease. Radiographic findings of universal colonic involvement, loss of haustrations, or pseudopolyposis are typical of chronic idiopathic ulcerative colitis, whereas the presence of skip lesions, linear ulcerations, or fistulas suggests Crohn's colitis.

It is imperative that diagnostic studies be obtained early in the course of the disease because the thumbprinting disappears within days as the submucosal hemorrhages are resorbed or evacuated into the colon when the overlying mucosa ulcerates and sloughs. In colonic ischemia, a second barium enema or colonoscopy performed 1 week after the initial study should reflect evolution of the disease, either by a return to normal or by replacement of the thumbprints with a segmental ulcerative colitis pattern.

If colonoscopy is chosen as the initial study, caution is indicated. Distention of the bowel with air to pressures greater than 30 mmHg diminishes colonic blood flow, shunts blood from the mucosa to the serosa, and causes a progressive decrease in the arteriovenous oxygen difference.[22] Because intraluminal pressure exceeds 30 mmHg during routine endoscopic examination of the colon,[23] colonoscopy can potentially induce or exacerbate colonic ischemia. This risk can be minimized by insufflation with carbon dioxide, which in-

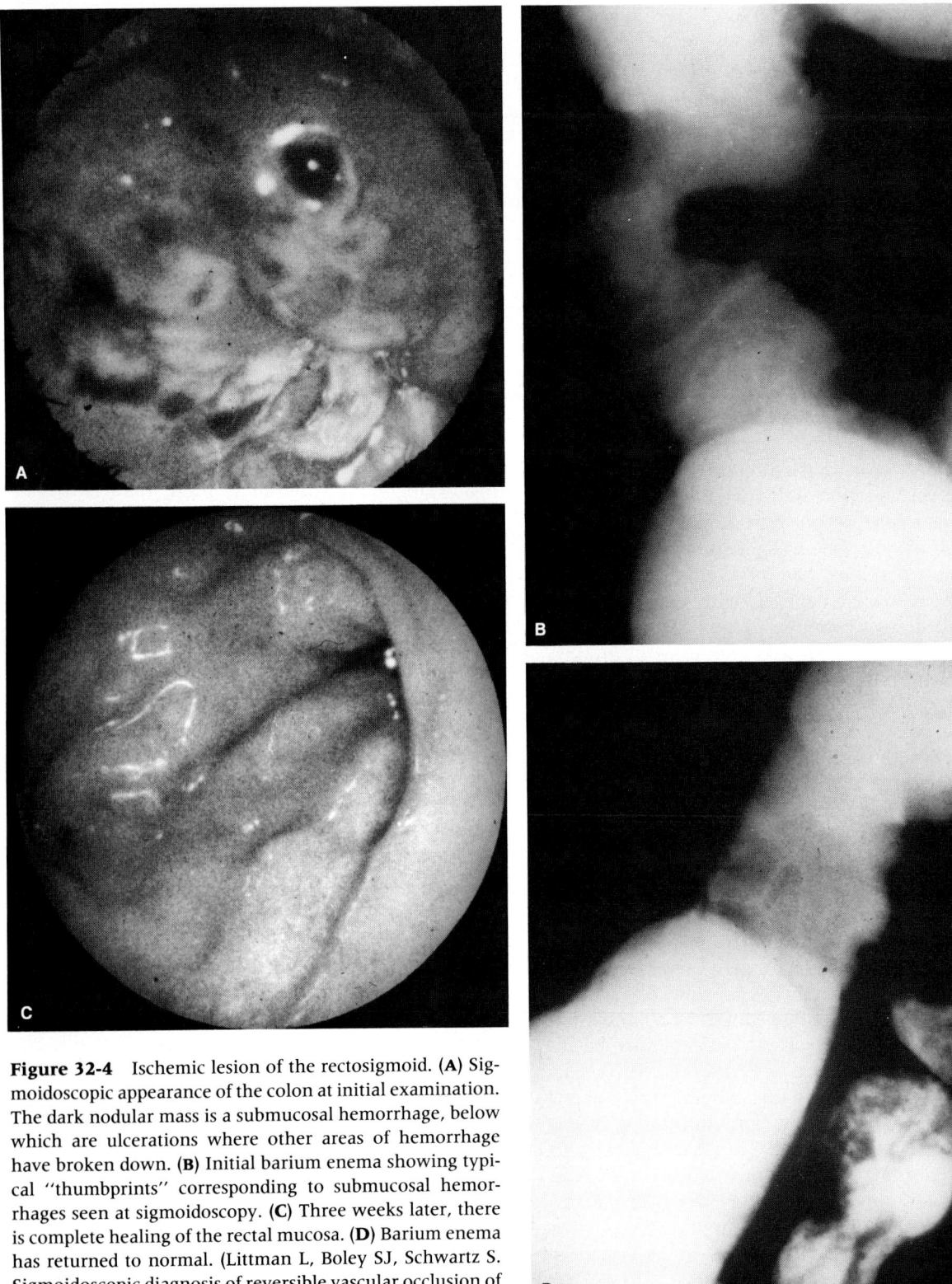

Figure 32-4 Ischemic lesion of the rectosigmoid. **(A)** Sigmoidoscopic appearance of the colon at initial examination. The dark nodular mass is a submucosal hemorrhage, below which are ulcerations where other areas of hemorrhage have broken down. **(B)** Initial barium enema showing typical "thumbprints" corresponding to submucosal hemorrhages seen at sigmoidoscopy. **(C)** Three weeks later, there is complete healing of the rectal mucosa. **(D)** Barium enema has returned to normal. (Littman L, Boley SJ, Schwartz S. Sigmoidoscopic diagnosis of reversible vascular occlusion of the colon. Dis Colon Rectum 1963;6:142)

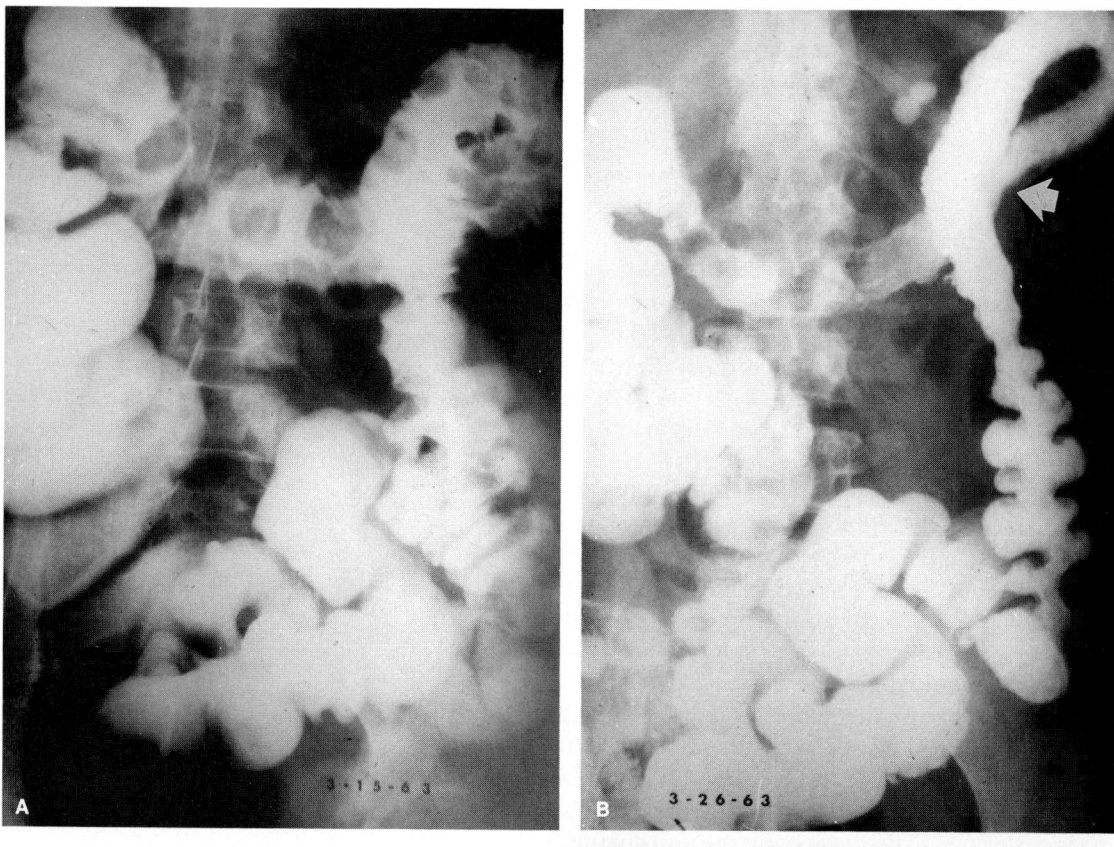

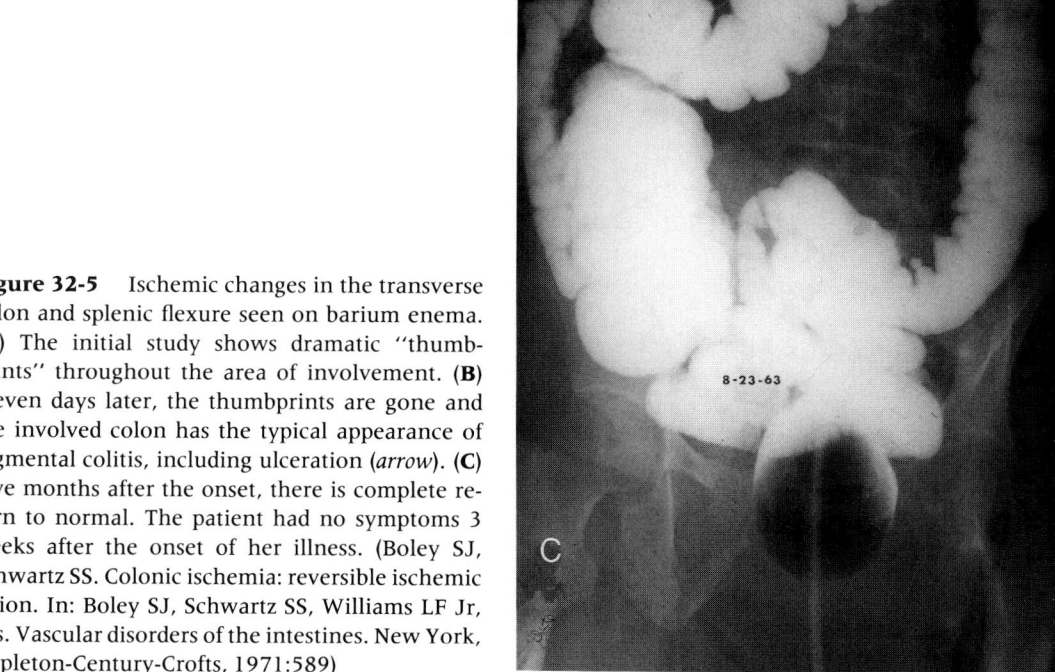

Figure 32-5 Ischemic changes in the transverse colon and splenic flexure seen on barium enema. **(A)** The initial study shows dramatic "thumbprints" throughout the area of involvement. **(B)** Eleven days later, the thumbprints are gone and the involved colon has the typical appearance of segmental colitis, including ulceration (*arrow*). **(C)** Five months after the onset, there is complete return to normal. The patient had no symptoms 3 weeks after the onset of her illness. (Boley SJ, Schwartz SS. Colonic ischemia: reversible ischemic lesion. In: Boley SJ, Schwartz SS, Williams LF Jr, eds. Vascular disorders of the intestines. New York, Appleton-Century-Crofts, 1971:589)

creases colonic blood flow at similar pressures. Furthermore, carbon dioxide is rapidly absorbed from the colon, decreasing the duration of distention and elevation of the intraluminal pressure.[24]

Biopsy samples of nodules or bullae identified by endoscopy early in the course of colonic ischemia reveal submucosal hemorrhage, whereas samples of the surrounding mucosa usually show nonspecific inflammatory changes.[25] Histologic evidence of mucosal infarction, although rare, is pathognomonic for ischemia. Angiography seldom shows significant occlusions or other abnormalities and is not indicated in patients with suspected colonic ischemia. Computed tomography (CT) can show thickening of the bowel wall, but this finding is not specific.

When the clinical presentation does not allow a clear distinction between colonic ischemia and acute mesenteric ischemia, and when plain films of the abdomen do not show the characteristic thumbprinting pattern of colonic ischemia, an "air enema" can be performed by gently insufflating air into the colon under fluoroscopic observation. The submucosal edema and hemorrhages that produce the thumbprinting pattern of colonic ischemia can be accentuated and identified in this manner (Fig. 32-6). Once the provisional diagnosis of colonic ischemia is made, a gentle barium enema is performed to determine the site and distribution of the disease as well as to identify any associated lesion that predisposed to the episode of ischemia (ie, carcinoma, stricture, or diverticulitis). However, if thumbprinting is not observed and the air enema does not suggest the diagnosis of colonic ischemia, a selective mesenteric angiogram is performed immediately to exclude the diagnosis of acute mesenteric ischemia. Because acute mesenteric ischemia progresses rapidly to an irreversible outcome, and because optimal diagnosis and treatment of this condition requires angiography, the diagnosis must be established or excluded before a barium study is performed. Residual barium from a contrast study of the colon obscures the mesenteric vessels, precluding adequate angiographic examination and intervention.

MANAGEMENT OF COLONIC ISCHEMIA

General Principles

Once the diagnosis of colonic ischemia has been established, and if the physical examination does not suggest intestinal gangrene or perforation, patients are treated expectantly. Parenteral fluids are administered and the bowel is placed at rest. Broad-spectrum antibiotics that

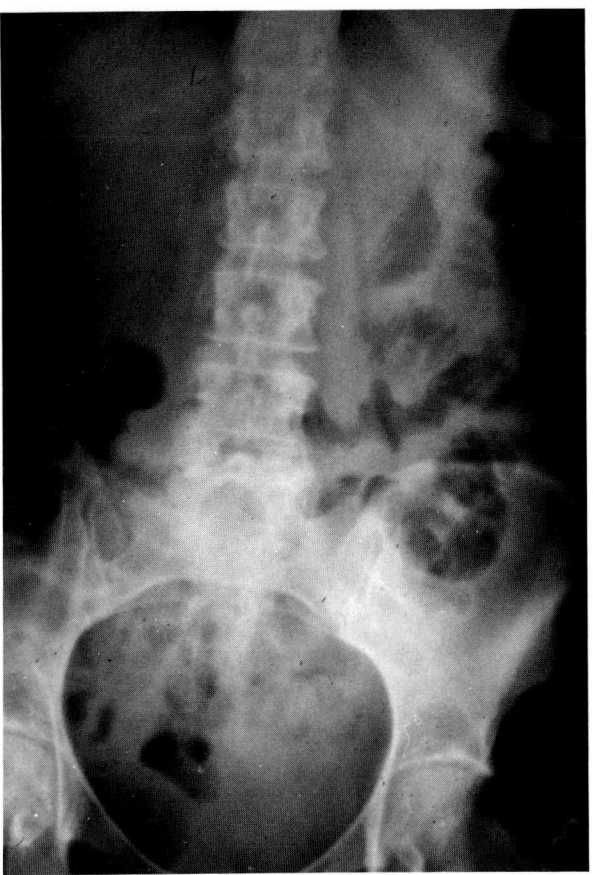

Figure 32-6 Ischemic colitis seen on air enema. (Kaleya RN, Boley SJ. Colonic ischemia. In: Shrock T, ed. Perspectives in colon and rectal surgery. St Louis, Quality Medical, 1990:69)

provide coverage for *Enterococcus* and anaerobic organisms is begun. Antibiotic therapy has been shown to reduce the length of bowel damaged by ischemia, although it does not prevent colonic infarction. Cardiac function is optimized to ensure adequate systemic perfusion. Medications that cause mesenteric vasoconstriction, such as digitalis and vasopressors, should be withdrawn if possible. The urine output is monitored and maintained with parenteral isotonic fluids. If the colon is distended, it can be decompressed with a rectal tube, with or without gentle saline irrigation. Contrary to their efficacy in ulcerative colitis, parenteral corticosteroids are contraindicated because they increase the possibility of perforation and secondary infection.

The white blood cell count, hemoglobin, and hematocrit should be monitored closely during the acute episode. Although they are rarely needed, blood products should be administered according to the patients' requirements. Serum potassium and magnesium must be monitored, because levels of these electrolytes can be disturbed by the associated diarrhea and tissue necrosis. Systemic levels of lactate dehydrogenase, creatine phosphokinase, aspartate aminotransferase, and alanine aminotransferase can reflect the degree of bowel necrosis, but these serum markers are neither sensitive nor specific for colonic ischemia. Patients who have significant diarrhea are begun on parenteral nutrition early. Narcotics should be withheld until it is clear that an intraabdominal catastrophe is not present and that clinical improvement is occurring. Cathartics are contraindicated. No attempt should be made to prepare the bowel for surgery in the acute phase because this can precipitate a perforation.

Increasing abdominal tenderness, guarding, rebound tenderness, rising temperature, and paralytic ileus during the period of observation suggest colonic infarction. These signs, although not absolute indicators of transmural colonic ischemia or infarction, dictate the need for expedient laparotomy for resection of the affected segment of colon. At laparotomy, the serosal appearance of infarcted colon ranges from that of wet tissue paper to mottled, thickened, aperistaltic bowel. The resected specimen should be opened in the operating suite and examined for mucosal injury; if the margins are involved, additional colon should be removed until the margins appear grossly normal.

Management of Reversible Lesions

In the mildest cases of colonic ischemia, in which signs and symptoms of illness disappear within 24 to 48 hours, submucosal and intramural hemorrhages are resorbed, and there is complete clinical and radiographic resolution within 1 to 2 weeks, no further therapy is indicated. More severe ischemic insults result in necrosis of the mucosa with ulceration, inflammation, and the subsequent development of segmental ulcerative colitis. Varying amounts of mucosa can slough that ultimately may heal over several months. Patients with such protracted healing can have no clinical symptoms, even in the presence of persistent radiographic or endoscopic evidence of disease. These patients are placed on high-residue diets and subjected to frequent follow-up evaluations to confirm complete healing or the development of strictures or persistent colitis. Recurrent episodes of sepsis in otherwise symptom-free patients with unhealed areas of segmental colitis usually are caused by the diseased segment of bowel and are an indication for elective resection.

Management of Irreversible Lesions

Patients with persistent diarrhea, rectal bleeding, protein-losing enteropathy, or recurrent sepsis for more than 10 to 14 days usually go on to perforation. Hence,

early resection is indicated to prevent this complication. A polyethylene glycol bowel preparation is administered along with oral and intravenous antibiotics before surgery. Enemas should not be used to prepare the bowel.

Despite a normal serosal appearance, there can be extensive mucosal injury and the extent of resection should be guided by the distribution of disease as seen on the preoperative studies rather than the appearance of the serosal surface of the colon at the time of operation. As in all resections for colonic ischemia, the specimen must be opened at the time of operation to ensure normal mucosa at the margins. If segmental colitis is found to involve the rectum, a mucous fistula or Hartmann procedure with an end colostomy should be performed. The mucous fistula can be fashioned through diseased bowel; in some cases, this segment heals sufficiently to allow subsequent restoration of bowel continuity. Proctocolectomy rarely is indicated except in patients with colonic ischemia after abdominal aortic replacement.

Patients who have had concurrent or recent myocardial infarctions and those who have major medical contraindications to surgery can undergo a trial of prolonged parenteral nutrition with concomitant intravenous antibiotic therapy as an alternative, albeit less optimal, method of management.

Management of the Late Manifestations of Colonic Ischemia

Colonic ischemia may not cause clinical symptoms during the acute insult but still produce chronic segmental ulcerative colitis. This form of colonic ischemia often is misdiagnosed when patients are not seen during the acute episode. Barium enema studies can show a segmental colitis pattern, a stricture simulating a carcinoma, or even an area of pseudopolyposis (Fig. 32-7). The clinical course at this stage of disease often is indistinguishable from other causes of colitis or stenosis. Crypt abscesses and pseudopolyposis usually considered histologically diagnostic of chronic idiopathic ulcerative colitis also can be seen in ischemic colitis. The de novo occurrence of a segmental area of colitis or stricture in an elderly patient should be considered ischemic and treated accordingly. Patients with chronic segmental ischemic colitis initially are treated according to their symptoms. Local corticosteroid enemas can be helpful but parenteral corticosteroids should not be used. In patients whose symptoms cannot be controlled by medication, segmental resection of the diseased bowel should be performed. Resection ordinarily is curative; recurrence is unlikely.

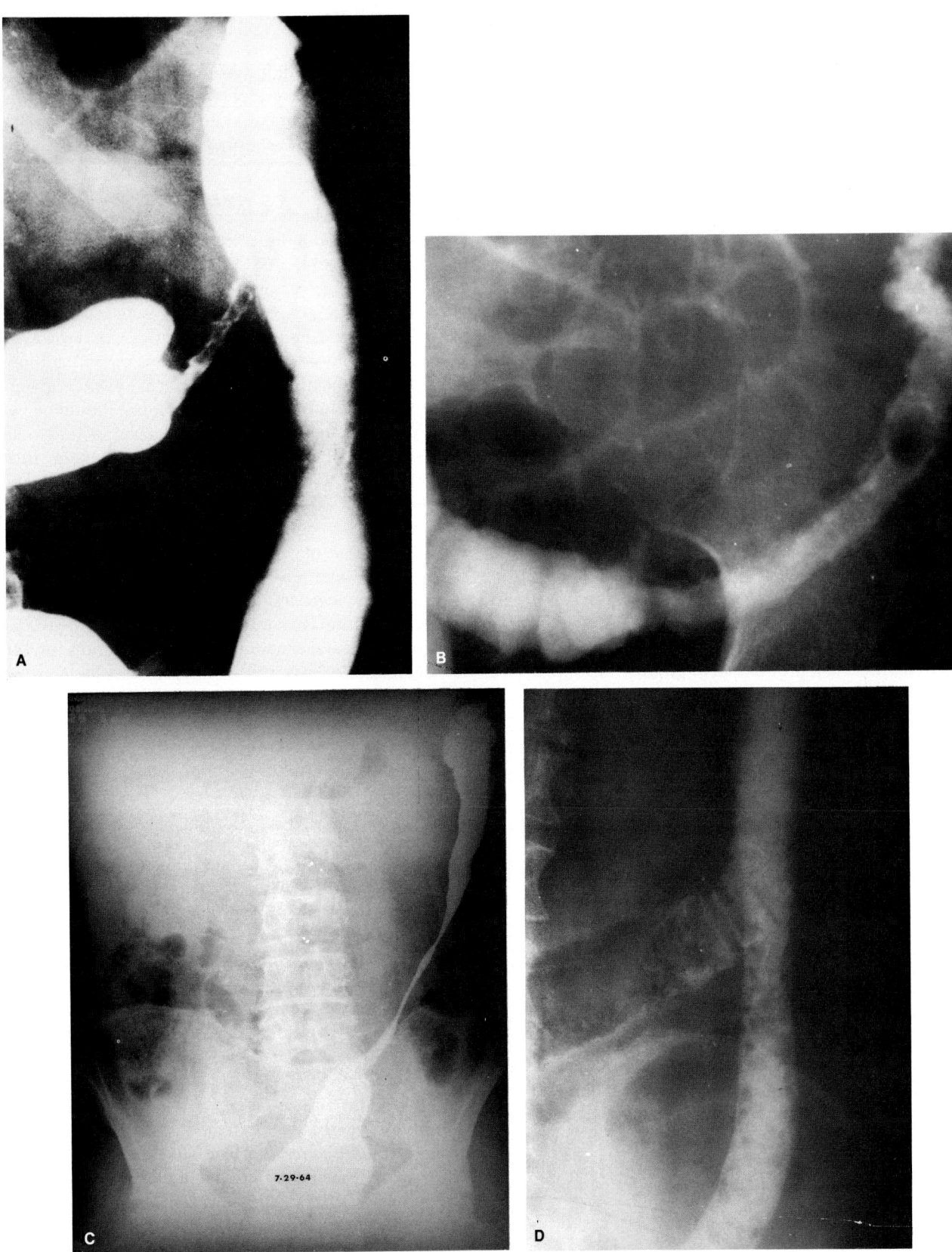

Figure 32-7 Appearance on barium enema of irreversible ischemic lesions of the colon. (**A**) Ischemic stricture with characteristics of carcinoma. (**B**) Chronic segmental ulcerative colitis. (**C**) Stricture. (**D**) Pseudopolyposis. (**A** from Brandt LJ, Katz HJ, Wolf EL, Mitsudo S, Boley SJ. Simulation of colonic carcinoma by ischemia. Gastroenterology 1985;88:1137; **B** through **D** from Boley SJ, Brandt LJ, Veith FJ. Ischemic disorders of the intestines. Curr Probl Surg 1978;15:55)

Management of Ischemic Strictures

Patients with asymptomatic segmental ulcerative colitis can go on to develop stenosis or strictures of the colon. Strictures that produce no symptoms should be observed; some return to normal over 12 to 24 months with no further therapy. If symptoms of obstruction develop, however, a segmental resection is required.

Management of Specific Clinical Problems

Colonic Ischemia Complicating Abdominal Aortic Surgery

Mesenteric vascular reconstruction is not indicated in most cases of colonic ischemia, but it can be required to prevent colonic ischemia during and after aortic reconstruction. After elective aneurysmectomy, 3% to 7% of patients have colonoscopic evidence of ischemia.[26,27] The incidence of ischemia after repair of ruptured aortic aneurysms can be as high as 60%.[28] Although clinical evidence of this complication is found in only 1% to 2% of patients, it is responsible for about 10% of deaths after aortic replacement.[29] Factors that contribute to the occurrence of postoperative colonic ischemia include rupture of the aneurysm, hypotension, operative trauma to the colon, hypoxemia, arrhythmias, prolonged crossclamp time, and improper management of the IMA during aneurysmectomy.

The most important aspect of therapy for the colonic ischemia that can develop after aortic surgery is prevention. Collateral blood flow to the left colon after occlusion of the IMA comes from the SMA through the arc of Riolan (the meandering artery) or the marginal artery of Drummond, and from the internal iliac arteries through the middle and inferior hemorrhoidal arteries. If these collateral pathways are intact, postoperative colonic ischemia can be minimized. Therefore, aortography as well as full mechanical and antibiotic bowel preparation must be performed before aortic reconstruction is undertaken. Aortography is recommended to determine the patency of the celiac axis, SMA, IMA, and internal iliac artery. The presence of a meandering artery, in and of itself, does not allow safe ligation of the IMA, because the blood flow in the meandering artery frequently originates from the IMA and reconstitutes an obstructed SMA. Ligation of the IMA in this circumstance can be catastrophic, with infarction of the small and large bowel (Fig. 32-8A). Ligation of the IMA is safe only when it has been confirmed by angiography that the blood flows into the meandering artery from the SMA to the IMA. Reimplantation of the IMA is required, therefore, in patients in whom the

SMA is occluded or tightly stenosed and the IMA provides inflow to the meandering artery (see Fig. 32-8B).

Occlusion of both hypogastric arteries on the preoperative arteriogram indicates that the rectal blood flow is dependent on collateral flow from the IMA or from the SMA through the meandering artery. In this circumstance, reconstitution of flow to one or both hypogastric arteries is desirable at the time of aneurysmectomy (see Fig. 32-8C).

At operation, crossclamp time should be minimized and hypotension prevented. If a meandering artery is identified, it should be carefully preserved. Because the serosal appearance of the colon is not a reliable indicator of collateral blood flow, several methods have been suggested to determine the need for IMA reimplantation. A stump pressure in the transected IMA greater than 40 mmHg or a ratio of mean IMA stump pressure to mean systemic blood pressure greater than 0.4 indicates adequate collateral circulation and can be used reliably to avoid IMA reimplantation.[30] The presence of Doppler ultrasound flow signals at the base of the mesentery and at the serosal surface of the colon with temporary IMA inflow occlusion also suggests that the IMA can be ligated safely without reimplantation.

Tonometric determination of the intramural pH of the sigmoid colon has been used to identify inadequate colonic blood flow during aneurysmectomy.[31,32] A balloon is passed into the sigmoid colon through the anus before the aorta is crossclamped to evaluate the effect of occlusion and restoration of aortic flow on colonic intramural pH. The intramural pH is a metabolic marker of tissue acidosis and will reflect any clinically significant ischemia, thus indicating the need for revascularization while the abdomen is open. When IMA reimplantation is deemed necessary, the IMA should be excised with a patch of aortic wall (Carrel patch) and sutured into the side of the aortic prosthesis.

If the SMA is occluded, it can be revascularized by reimplanting it into the graft wall or by creating a lateral extension of the prosthesis and performing an end-to-side anastomosis to the SMA. Liberal use of these adjunctive procedures has reduced substantially the incidence of colonic ischemia and eliminated it as a cause of death after aortic surgery.[27]

The difficulty in accurately assessing colonic ischemia after surgery and the significant mortality associated with its occurrence mandates the use of postoperative colonoscopy in high-risk patients. Patients at high risk for the development of postoperative colonic ischemia after aortic reconstruction are those with ruptured abdominal aortic aneurysms, prolonged crossclamping time, patent IMAs on preoperative aortography, nonpulsatile flow in the hypogastric arteries at operation, and postoperative diarrhea. In these cases, colonoscopy

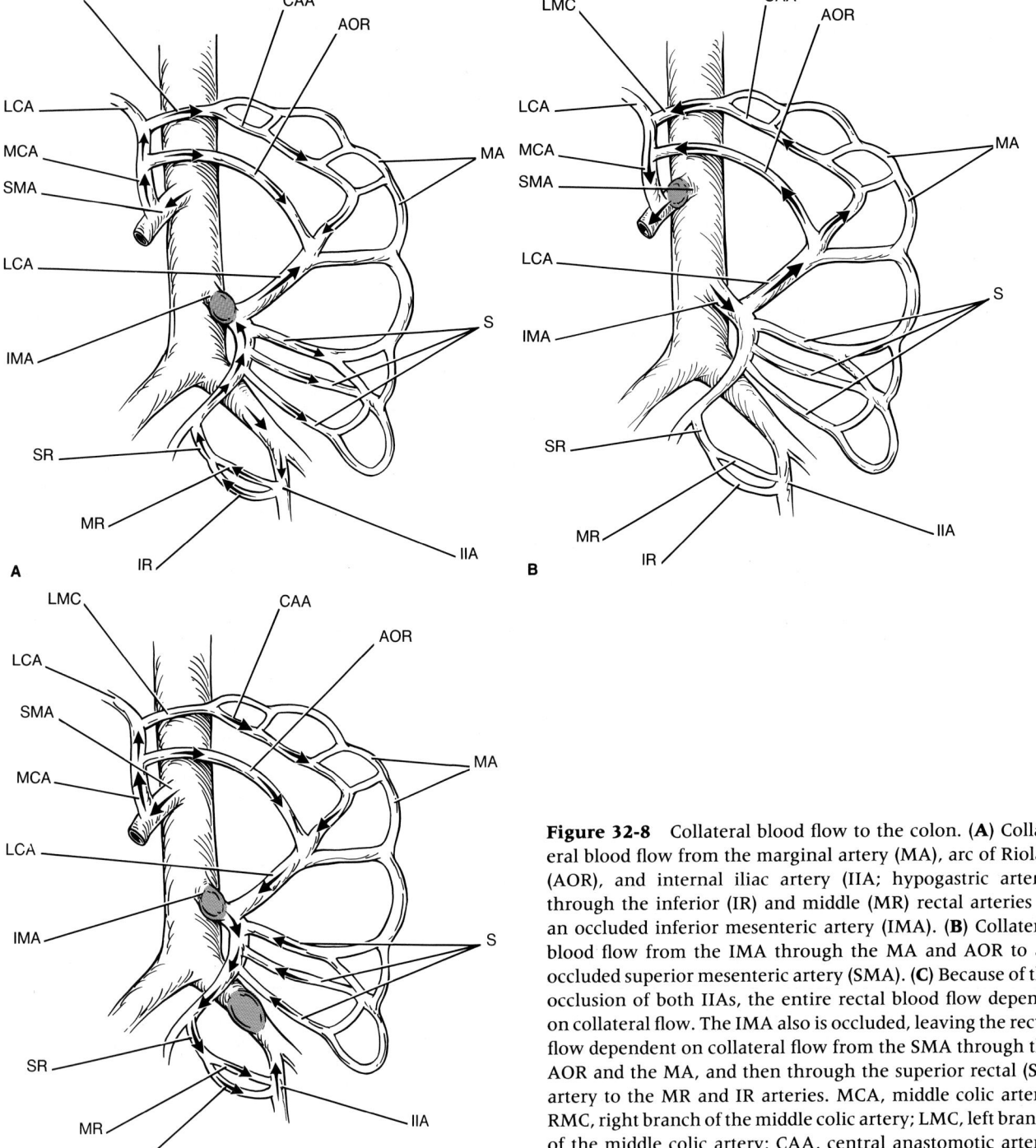

Figure 32-8 Collateral blood flow to the colon. **(A)** Collateral blood flow from the marginal artery (MA), arc of Riolan (AOR), and internal iliac artery (IIA; hypogastric artery) through the inferior (IR) and middle (MR) rectal arteries to an occluded inferior mesenteric artery (IMA). **(B)** Collateral blood flow from the IMA through the MA and AOR to an occluded superior mesenteric artery (SMA). **(C)** Because of the occlusion of both IIAs, the entire rectal blood flow depends on collateral flow. The IMA also is occluded, leaving the rectal flow dependent on collateral flow from the SMA through the AOR and the MA, and then through the superior rectal (SR) artery to the MR and IR arteries. MCA, middle colic artery; RMC, right branch of the middle colic artery; LMC, left branch of the middle colic artery; CAA, central anastomotic artery; LCA, left colic artery; S, sigmoid branches.

is performed routinely within 2 to 3 days of the operation and, if colonic ischemia is identified, therapy is begun before major complications develop. Clinical deterioration indicating progression of the ischemic insult to transmural necrosis necessitates reoperation. These patients should undergo resection and colostomy. Primary anastomosis is contraindicated because of the potential for contamination of the aortic prosthesis in the event of an anastomotic leak. If the rectum is involved, it also must be resected. Every effort should be made protect the aortic graft from contamination by covering it with local tissues or the omentum.

Fulminating Universal Colitis

A fulminating form of colonic ischemia involving most or all of the colon and rectum has been identified in a few patients. It is characterized by the sudden onset of a toxic universal colitis picture. Bleeding, fever, severe diarrhea, and abdominal pain and tenderness, often with signs of peritonitis, are present. The clinical course is rapidly progressive. The management of this condition is similar to that of other forms of fulminating colitis. Total abdominal colectomy with an ileostomy usually is required. A second-stage proctectomy has been necessary in some patients within 1 month of the original surgery. Histologic examination of the resected colon usually reveals ischemic changes, severe ulcerating colitis, and necrosis.

Lesions Mimicking Colon Carcinoma

Late ischemic colitis can present with strictures that mimic colon carcinoma. Colonoscopy may be able to distinguish the malignant lesions from those resulting from ischemic cicatrization, and is advisable when an annular lesion is identified on barium enema. The treatment is local resection with immediate restoration of bowel continuity.

Colitis Associated With Colon Carcinoma

Acute colitis in patients with carcinoma of the colon has been recognized for many years.[33] The colitis usually is proximal to the tumor and occurs with and without clinical obstruction. It is of ischemic origin and has the radiologic and endoscopic appearance of ischemic colitis. Clinically, patients can have symptoms of colonic ischemia or symptoms related to the primary cancer. In many cases, however, the predominant complaints are related to the ischemic episode and include sudden onset of mild to moderate abdominal pain, fever, bloody diarrhea, and abdominal tenderness.

It is important for both radiologists and surgeons to be aware of the association between colonic ischemia and colon cancer. Radiologists must be careful to exclude cancer in every case of colonic ischemia, and surgeons should examine any colon resected for cancer for the presence of an ischemic process in the area of the anastomosis, because involvement can lead to stricture or a leak.

Colonic Ischemia as a Manifestation of Acute Mesenteric Ischemia

Colonic ischemia localized to the right side of the colon can be a manifestation of acute mesenteric ischemia. If radiographs or colonoscopy reveal evidence of colonic ischemia isolated to the right colon, selective mesenteric angiography should be performed before the patient is discharged from the hospital to evaluate the status of the SMA. Demonstration of a partially or completely obstructed SMA in this setting is an indication for revascularization of the artery.

ACUTE MESENTERIC ISCHEMIA

The term *acute mesenteric ischemia* is applied to a wide spectrum of bowel injury within the distribution of the superior mesenteric vessels, ranging from reversible alterations in bowel function to transmural necrosis of the bowel wall. Acute mesenteric ischemia can result from an SMA embolus, nonocclusive mesenteric ischemia, or thrombosis of the SMA or the superior mesenteric vein (SMV; see Fig. 32-1). Depending on the degree and duration of the ischemia, as well as the length of bowel involved, a variety of clinical presentations are observed. Clinical and animal research has led to the development of a multidisciplinary diagnostic and therapeutic approach that has improved the prognosis for patients with suspected acute mesenteric ischemia.

Demographics

Acute mesenteric ischemia has been diagnosed increasingly in the past 25 years, but its exact incidence is difficult to determine. The increased incidence has been attributed to the aging of the population, because acute mesenteric ischemia occurs predominantly in geriatric patients, especially those with significant cardiovascular and systemic disorders. The widespread use of coronary and surgical intensive care units and other extraordinary means of cardiopulmonary support has salvaged patients who previously died rapidly of cardiovascular conditions, only to have them go on to develop acute mesenteric ischemia as a later consequence of their primary disease. At our large metropolitan medical center, acute mesenteric ischemia is responsible for about 0.1% of all admissions.

Together, superior mesenteric arterial emboli and nonocclusive mesenteric ischemia are responsible for 70% to 80% of reported cases of acute mesenteric ischemia. The incidence of nonocclusive ischemia has declined, possibly because of the increasing use of systemic vasodilators, such as calcium channel blockers and nitrates, in coronary intensive care units. These agents may protect the mesenteric vascular beds from vasospasm and decrease the period of profound hypotension associated with acute myocardial events. In addition, the more common use of left ventricular assist devices in the treatment of cardiogenic shock has decreased the period of profound hypotension associated with left ventricular failure and, presumably, attenuated its effect on the mesenteric circulation.

Types of Acute Mesenteric Ischemia

Arterial Causes

SUPERIOR MESENTERIC ARTERY EMBOLUS. Responsible for 40% to 50% of episodes of acute mesenteric ischemia, SMA emboli usually originate from left atrial or ventricular mural thrombi. The thrombi migrate after being dislodged or fragmented during a period of dysrhythmia, or after cardiac catheterization. Many patients with SMA emboli have histories of previous peripheral artery emboli, and about 20% have synchronous emboli in other arteries. Emboli to the SMA tend to lodge at points of normal anatomic narrowing, usually immediately distal to the origin of a major branch (Fig. 32-9). In 10% to 15% of patients, the emboli lodge peripherally in branches of the SMA, or in the SMA itself distal to the origin of the ileocolic artery. The embolus can occlude the arterial lumen completely, but often occludes the vessel only partially.

Experimental studies suggest that initially, the collateral circulation is adequate to maintain intestinal viability after most cases of acute SMA occlusion, but after a period of partial occlusion and diminution of blood

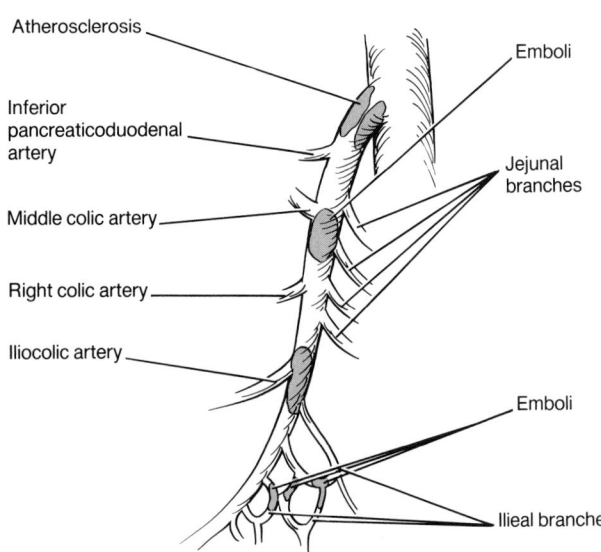

Figure 32-9 Common sites of superior mesenteric artery (SMA) emboli. Emboli distal to the ileocolic branch or in segmental branches are considered minor emboli. All others are major emboli. Thrombosis usually occurs near the origin of the SMA. (Kaleya RN, Boley SJ. Mesenteric ischemic disorders. In: Maingot R, ed. Abdominal operations, ed 9. East Norwalk, CT, Appleton & Lange, 1990:398)

flow distal to the embolus, vasoconstriction develops in arteries both proximal and distal to the embolus. This vasoconstriction can impair the collateral blood flow to the SMA and its branches distal to the embolus sufficiently to cause or exacerbate ischemic injury.

NONOCCLUSIVE MESENTERIC ISCHEMIA. This causes 20% to 30% of episodes of acute mesenteric ischemia and is thought to result from splanchnic vasoconstriction initiated by vasoactive medications or by a period of decreased cardiac output associated with hypotension secondary to dysrhythmias, myocardial depression, or hypovolemia. The vasoconstriction can persist even after the precipitating cause has been eliminated or corrected. Predisposing factors for nonocclusive mesenteric ischemia include acute myocardial infarction, congestive heart failure, aortic insufficiency, hepatic diseases, renal diseases (especially in patients requiring hemodialysis),[34,35] and major cardiac or intraabdominal operations. Frequently, a more immediate precipitating cause such as acute pulmonary edema, cardiac arrhythmia, or shock is present, although the consequent intestinal ischemia may not become manifest until hours or days later.

SUPERIOR MESENTERIC ARTERY THROMBOSIS. This occurs at areas of severe atherosclerotic narrowing, most often at the origin of the SMA (see Fig. 32-9). The acute ischemic episode commonly is superimposed on chronic mesenteric ischemia; hence, about 20% to 50% of these patients have histories of abdominal pain with or without evidence of malabsorption and weight loss during the weeks to months preceding the acute episode. In addition, most patients with SMA thrombosis have severe and diffuse atherosclerosis with a prior history of coronary, cerebrovascular, or peripheral arterial insufficiency.

Venous Causes

Mesenteric venous thrombosis can present as an acute, subacute, or chronic process. About 2 patients per 100,000 admissions to our institution have had mesenteric venous thrombosis confirmed by operative or pathologic means. This represents less than 5% of all cases of acute mesenteric ischemia. This entity is discussed separately.

Pathophysiology of Mesenteric Ischemia

The severity of ischemia-induced intestinal injury is inversely related to blood flow.[36] Ischemic injury to the intestinal mucosa occurs when the tissue is deprived of oxygen and other nutrients necessary to maintain cellular metabolism and integrity. Reduction of blood flow to the intestine can reflect generalized poor systemic perfusion, as in shock or with a failing heart, or it can result from local morphologic or functional changes of the splanchnic vasculature. Narrowing of the major mesenteric vessels, focal atheromatous emboli, vasculitis as a consequence of a systemic disease, or mesenteric vasoconstriction can lead to inadequate circulation at a cellular level.

Several factors contribute to ischemic injury of the bowel, including the state of the general circulation, the extent of collateral blood flow, the response of the mesenteric vasculature to autonomic stimuli, circulating vasoactive substances, local humoral factors, and the normal and abnormal products of cellular metabolism before and after reperfusion of the ischemic segment of intestine. In addition, the functional demands of the bowel as dictated by motor, absorptive, and secretory activities; the intestinal microflora; and the rate of cellular turnover affect the extent and severity of intestinal injury. Because these factors are so diverse and cannot all be controlled in the experimental or clinical setting, investigation of the role of individual factors often does not reflect the full and profound pathophysiologic consequences of intestinal ischemia.

Collateral Circulation

The intestines have an extensive collateral circulation that protects them from ischemic insults. The SMA, IMA, and celiac artery are connected by a vast array of collateral vessels. As a general rule, at least two of the major splanchnic vessels must be compromised to produce symptomatic intestinal ischemia. However, the converse is not true. Occlusion of two of the three vessels occurs frequently without evidence of ischemia, and total occlusion of all three vessels in patients with no symptoms has been observed.

Collateral pathways around occlusions of smaller arterial branches in the mesentery are provided by the primary, secondary, and tertiary arcades in the small bowel, and by the marginal artery of Drummond, the central anastomotic artery, and the arc of Riolan in the colon. The intestine responds to reductions in blood flow by redistributing flow to the various layers. In general, the intramural blood flow in regional ischemia redistributes to favor the mucosa, especially the superficial portion.[37,38]

Collateral pathways open immediately when a major vessel is occluded, in response to the fall in arterial pressure distal to the obstruction. Initially, an acute decrease in perfusion pressure is compensated for by local regulatory mechanisms so that the reduction in flow is

proportionately less than the reduction in perfusion pressure.[39] This physiologic action, termed *autoregulation,* is due to vasodilation of the resistance vessels downstream from the occlusion, largely in response to the release of local metabolites from the ischemic tissue. Some of this vasodilation also is due to relaxation of vascular smooth muscle in direct response to a decreased perfusion pressure.[40] Autoregulation of flow can be maintained only for a brief period. Experimentally, occlusion of the SMA is followed by a transient increase in celiac artery and IMA flow. The increased blood flow through this collateral circulation continues as long as the pressure in the vascular bed distal to the obstruction remains below systemic pressure, and is almost always sufficient to maintain intestinal viability. With prolonged ischemia, vasoconstriction develops in the involved vascular bed, elevating the pressure in the distal bed, causing a reduction in collateral flow, and potentially compromising bowel viability.

The degree of reduction in blood flow that the bowel can tolerate without damage is remarkable. In one study, mesenteric arterial flow was reduced by 75% for 12 hours. No morphologic changes could be identified by light microscopy, and there was normal distribution of Patent Blue V dye (Boley SJ, unpublished data). One reason for these findings is that only one fifth of mesenteric capillaries are open at any time, and uptake of oxygen occurs only in these open vessels. Therefore, normal oxygen consumption can be maintained with only 20% to 25% of normal blood flow. When intestinal blood flow is reduced, oxygen extraction is increased, allowing a fairly constant oxygen consumption over a wide range of blood flow. In addition, the arteriovenous oxygen difference widens as a reflection of the enhanced oxygen extraction. However, below a critical level of blood flow, oxygen consumption falls precipitously because increased oxygen extraction no longer can compensate for the diminished blood flow.[41]

Microcirculation and Collateral Flow

An extensive network of vessels within the bowel wall arises from the vasa recta and vasa brevia on the mesenteric border of the bowel. These vessels give rise sequentially to the external muscular vascular plexus, then penetrate the muscular coat and form a rich submucosal plexus. The submucosal plexus is more extensive in the small bowel than in the colon, and may make the small intestine more resistant to ischemia than is the colon.[42] A central arteriole originates from the submucosal plexus, loses its muscular coat, and branches into an extremely rich subepithelial capillary network within each individual villus.

The flow through this redundant system is controlled by a network of resistance and capillary vessels, which in turn are affected by many functional, humoral, local, and neural influences. There are two primary mechanisms for the control of splanchnic vascular resistance. The first is neural, mediated by the autonomic nervous system. The second is humoral, consisting of a variety of circulating hormones, including catecholamines, vasoactive peptides, and inflammatory mediators such as histamine and the arachidonic acid metabolites. Numerous pharmaceutical agents have either primary or secondary effects on the splanchnic vasculature, and many of these are splanchnic vasoconstrictors. In the clinical setting, use of these agents can cause splanchnic ischemia.

Control of Intestinal Blood Flow

AUTONOMIC FACTORS. The sympathetic nervous system, primarily by activation of the α-adrenergic receptors, is important for the maintenance of resting splanchnic arteriolar tone. Although circulating catecholamines also play a role, the primary mechanism of sympathetic control is neural. Particularly, stimulation of afferent adrenergic fibers releases norepinephrine from the nerve synapses supplying the smooth muscle of the precapillary resistance vessels. However, as seen elsewhere in the body,[43,44] reduction of blood flow is associated with disproportionate vasoconstriction in the postcapillary venous beds that make up the capacitance vasculature.[45] The combined effect of vasoconstriction of the arterial and venous beds cannot be predicted, but in animals, blood flow to the villi is preserved at normal or nearly normal levels, even in instances where overall blood flow is reduced by 50%. Within minutes of initial vasoconstriction, blood flow rises to nearly normal levels (autoregulatory escape). The exact nature of this process has not been elucidated, but it seems to be a generalized process inherent to all vascular smooth muscle. The most appealing explanation is the differential effects of the α- and β-adrenergic stimuli. β-Adrenergic agonists cause vasodilation, whereas α-adrenergic agents cause vasospasm. The net alteration in intestinal blood flow produced by sympathetic stimulation cannot be predicted from experimental studies, because adrenergic stimuli also change bowel motility and wall tension, absorption, and secretion, all of which can have a pronounced effect on the regional and local blood flow.[46]

Circulating catecholamines influence the splanchnic vasculature in a manner similar to norepinephrine released at local sympathetic nerve terminals, as discussed earlier. The major sympathetic response in circulatory shock is mediated by the neural pathway.

HUMORAL FACTORS. The important vasoconstrictor peptides include angiotensin II and vasopressin. Vasopressin selectively affects the splanchnic resistance vasculature, and this response is disproportionately greater than in the systemic circulation.[47] This differential vasoconstriction is exploited in the use of vasopressin for the therapeutic control of gastrointestinal hemorrhage. Vasopressin is released as a result of systemic hypotension; if the hypotension results from mesenteric ischemia, the vasopressin can exacerbate vasoconstriction in the splanchnic vessels. The preferential constriction of ischemic segments of intestine by vasopressin has been demonstrated in a canine model of occlusive mesenteric ischemia.[48]

Similarly, a differential vasoconstriction also is seen in the response of the splanchnic vasculature to angiotensin II. This probably is due to an increased number of angiotensin II receptors in the splanchnic vascular smooth muscle.[49] Clinically, splanchnic hypersensitivity to angiotensin II generated by renin released from the hypotensive kidney during a low-flow state may be a contributory mechanism underlying mesenteric ischemia. In an experimental cardiogenic shock model of nonocclusive mesenteric ischemia, disproportionate mesenteric ischemia was found to be the result of severe splanchnic vasospasm. This response was unaffected by blockade of the sympathetic nervous system, but was abolished by inhibition of the renin–angiotensin axis. These hemodynamic changes correlated closely with plasma renin levels and could be reproduced, in the absence of shock, by the infusion of angiotensin II directly into the mesenteric vessels. In addition, the histologic intestinal damage resembles that seen with nonocclusive mesenteric ischemia.[50]

LOCAL FACTORS. Although many arachidonic acid metabolites cause splanchnic vasodilation, the prostaglandins PGF_{2a}, PGB_2, and PGD_2, the leukotrienes C_4 and D_4, and some thromboxane analogues produce splanchnic vasoconstriction.[51] Blockade of prostaglandin synthesis with aspirin, indomethacin, or meclofenamate decreases the resting level of splanchnic flow, suggesting that one or more of the arachidonic metabolites plays a role in maintaining vasodilator tone.[52]

Local factors that accompany ischemia have potent vasodilative effects on intestinal vessels. Hyperkalemia, hyperosmolarity of the blood, decreased local oxygen tension, adenosine released on breakdown of adenosine triphosphate, and local acidosis dilate resistance vessels and produce local hyperemia. High intraluminal potassium concentrations cause an initial vasodilation followed by severe vasoconstriction leading to local ischemia of the affected bowel segment in dogs.[53] This mechanism is believed to be responsible for small bowel ulcers in patients receiving enteric-coated potassium chloride tablets.[54]

Gastrointestinal hormones, including cholecystokinin, gastric inhibitory peptide, glucagon, neurotensin, and secretin, have been studied for an effect on intestinal blood flow. These hormones administered in physiologic concentrations have no appreciable effect on intestinal blood flow.[55]

EXOGENOUS VASODILATORS. Locally administered vasodilators such as papaverine prevent and reverse the persistent vasoconstriction that follows a decrease in SMA blood flow. This observation suggested that intraarterial papaverine could be used in a clinical setting to treat vasoconstriction associated with the low-flow syndrome. Papaverine is a potent inhibitor of the enzyme, phosphodiesterase, which is the major enzyme in the degradation of cyclic adenosine monophosphate (cAMP). cAMP modulates vascular smooth muscle relaxation.[56] Inhibition of this enzyme system potentiates the vasodilative effect of cAMP by allowing it to accumulate rather than be metabolized by the phosphodiesterase. Other agents, such as prostaglandin E_1 and glucagon, also may act through this pathway by increasing the formation of cAMP.[57]

Mesenteric Vasoconstriction

Despite adequate collateral pathways in most cases, acute interruption or diminution of blood flow in the mesenteric circulation caused by emboli or hypotension can result in intestinal ischemia secondary to persistent vasospasm. A decrease in SMA flow initially produces local mesenteric vascular responses that tend to maintain intestinal blood flow, but if the diminished flow is prolonged, active vasoconstriction develops that can persist even after the primary cause of decreased flow is corrected.

After an acute 50% reduction in SMA blood flow in anesthetized dogs, the mesenteric arterial pressure in the peripheral mesenteric arteries falls to 49% of mean control values.[58] When SMA flow is maintained at 50% of normal, mesenteric arterial pressure returns to control values in 1 to 6 hours, whereas celiac flow, which initially increases, falls to control levels. The greater fall in mesenteric pressure suggests lowered resistance or vasodilation. However, the changes in active resistance cannot be deduced when pressure and flow are changing in the same direction.[59] The increased vascular resistance caused by vasoconstriction ultimately results in decreased collateral perfusion through the celiac system. If SMA occlusion is discontinued as soon as mesenteric arterial pressure rises to control values, flow through the SMA immediately returns to normal. How-

ever, if SMA occlusion is maintained for 30 to 240 minutes after mesenteric arterial pressure returns to control levels, flow in the SMA does not return to normal after release of the occlusion; rather, it remains at 30% to 50% of control values because of persistent arterial vasoconstriction. This decreased flow continues for up to 5 hours of observation. In this manner, mesenteric vasoconstriction plays a significant role in the development of ischemia in both acute occlusive and nonocclusive arterial forms of mesenteric ischemia.

When papaverine is infused during 50% flow restriction, the mesenteric arterial pressure remains low and increased celiac flow persists throughout 4 hours of observation, and the SMA flow returns to normal on release of the obstruction. Based on these observations, the use of intraarterial papaverine infusions is recommended in the management of both the occlusive and nonocclusive forms of acute mesenteric ischemia. Intraarterial papaverine also is recommended for selected patients with acute mesenteric venous thrombosis because venous thrombosis has been shown in experiments to cause arterial spasm.[60]

The presumption that bowel injury occurs during the period of diminished cardiac output or hypotension, and that correction of these problems returns the mesenteric blood flow to normal, does not explain adequately the operative findings of persistent bowel ischemia when no arterial or venous obstruction is found and cardiac function has been optimized. The onset of abdominal signs and symptoms caused by intestinal ischemia actually can begin after correction of the primary systemic problems in patients with nonocclusive mesenteric ischemia. This paradox can be explained by the experimental observations that an episode of low mesenteric flow, as short as 2 hours in duration, can produce mesenteric ischemia as a result of persistent vasoconstriction that continues after correction of the initiating problem. Because vasospasm can persist even after the initial cause of the ischemia is corrected, bowel injury continues unless the vasospasm is relieved. An aggressive radiologic and surgical approach to these diseases targets both the cause and the persistent vasospasm.

Cellular Response

Intestinal ischemia induces a spectrum of injury ranging from subtle changes in capillary permeability to transmural necrosis. The final outcome is dependent on local as well as systemic factors. Two separate processes are responsible for the subsequent damage: tissue hypoxia and reperfusion injury. Hypoxia occurs during the period of ischemia and the reperfusion injury occurs when flow is reestablished. As an episode of intestinal ischemia progresses and homeostatic changes occur, one region can experience hypoxic injury while another undergoes reperfusion-induced damage.

Both metabolic and morphologic changes occur when intestine is deprived of an adequate blood supply. Ultrastructural changes occur within 10 minutes; by 30 minutes, extensive changes, including accumulation of fluid between cells and the basement membranes, are present.[61] The tips of the villi then begin to slough and a membrane of necrotic epithelium, fibrin, inflammatory cells, and bacteria accumulates. Later, edema appears, followed by bleeding into the submucosa. Cellular death progresses from the lumen outward until there is transmural necrosis of bowel wall.[62,63]

A major consequence of bowel ischemia is enhanced transcapillary filtration, interstitial edema, and, ultimately, fluid movement into the lumen of the bowel. Comparison of vascular permeability in control intestinal preparations and preparations subjected to 1 hour of ischemia, with and without subsequent reperfusion, indicated that both ischemia and reperfusion increase vascular permeability.[64]

Several endogenous substances, including oxygen free radicals, platelet-activating factor, arachidonic acid metabolites, and bacterial endotoxins, have been implicated in the pathogenesis of reperfusion injury. These substances are released during small bowel ischemia, and are thought to be major mediators of the intestinal damage. In addition, a rapidly growing body of evidence suggests that oxygen free radicals such as superoxide, hydrogen peroxide, and hydroxyl radical mediate the cellular injury produced by reperfusion of ischemic intestine.

Effect on the Mucosal Barrier

Although the primary function of the small intestinal mucosa is to absorb nutrients, it also functions as an important barrier against luminal bacteria and their toxins. The barrier function of the intestinal mucosa is deranged in experimental animals subjected to ischemia. Changes in mucosal permeability induced by ischemia and reperfusion have been studied by measuring either the clearance of various agents from blood to intestinal lumen or the translocation of luminal bacteria to mesenteric lymph nodes. Complete ischemia followed by reperfusion leads to a marked increase in gut mucosal permeability.[65,66] The increment in mucosal permeability is related directly to the extent and duration of the ischemic insult. However, oxygen uptake must be reduced to less than half of control values for ischemia–reperfusion to increase mucosal permeability.[67]

Clinical Response to Acute Mesenteric Ischemia

The response to reduced intestinal blood flow is complex and the consequences of mesenteric ischemia are only now being fully appreciated. On occlusion of the SMA, there initially is a marked increase in bowel activity. This increase in motor function results in rapid bowel evacuation and increases the oxygen demands of the affected intestine. Shortly thereafter, bowel motility ceases either as a result of the massive sympathetic response to mesenteric ischemia or as a consequence of local factors associated with the ischemia itself. Within hours, the bowel becomes hemorrhagic and edematous as capillary integrity is compromised. Intramural hydrostatic pressure rises with increased edema and hemorrhage. In normal bowel, increased intramural pressure usually is well tolerated, but as perfusion pressure to the edematous bowel decreases, the edema can compromise further an already marginal blood flow. In addition, bacterial utilization of a marginally adequate intestinal oxygen supply and production of toxic metabolites can exacerbate the ischemic injury.

The shift of intravascular volume into the bowel wall causes severe hemoconcentration and hypovolemic shock. Vasoactive mediators and bacterial endotoxins are released from the ischemic bowel into the peritoneal cavity and absorbed into the general circulation, causing a variety of physiologic effects, including cardiac depression, septic shock, and acute renal failure. These effects can contribute to the death of the patient even before there is complete necrosis of the bowel wall.

Diagnosis and Management

Early identification of acute mesenteric ischemia requires a high index of suspicion in patients who have significant risk factors for this disease. It occurs most frequently in patients more than 50 years of age who have chronic heart disease and long-standing congestive heart failure, especially those in whom the cardiac disease is poorly controlled with diuretics or digitalis. Cardiac arrhythmias (commonly atrial fibrillation), recent myocardial infarction, and hypotension due to burns, pancreatitis, or hemorrhage all predispose patients to acute mesenteric ischemia. Previous or synchronous arterial emboli increase the likelihood of an acute SMA embolus. The development of sudden abdominal pain in patients with any of these risk factors should suggest the diagnosis of acute mesenteric ischemia.

Presentation

Acute abdominal pain varying in severity, nature, and location occurs in 75% to 98% of patients with intestinal ischemia. A previous history of abdominal pain in the weeks to months preceding the acute onset of severe abdominal pain is present only in the few patients in whom acute mesenteric ischemia is caused by SMA thrombosis complicating chronic mesenteric ischemia. In early acute mesenteric ischemia, the pain experienced is markedly out of proportion to the physical findings. Therefore, sudden severe abdominal pain accompanied by rapid and often forceful bowel evacuation, especially with minimal or no abdominal signs, strongly suggests an acute arterial occlusion in the mesenteric circulation.

Unexplained abdominal distention or gastrointestinal bleeding can be the only indications of acute intestinal ischemia, especially in nonocclusive disease, because pain is absent in up to 25% of these patients. Patients surviving cardiopulmonary resuscitation who have culture-proven bacteremia and diarrhea without abdominal pain also should be suspected of having nonocclusive mesenteric ischemia.[68] Distention, although absent early in the course of mesenteric ischemia, often is the first sign of impending intestinal infarction. The stool contains occult blood in 75% of patients, and this bleeding can precede all other symptoms of ischemia. Right-sided abdominal pain associated with the passage of maroon or bright red blood in the stool is characteristic of colonic ischemia but also suggests the diagnosis of acute mesenteric ischemia.

Although there are no abdominal findings early in the course of intestinal ischemia, increasing tenderness, rebound tenderness, and muscle guarding reflect the progressive loss of intestinal viability and the presence of transmural gangrene as infarction develops. Significant abdominal findings strongly indicate the presence of infarcted bowel. Nausea, vomiting, hematemesis, massive abdominal distention, back pain, and shock are other late signs often indicating compromise of bowel viability.

Laboratory Signs

Leukocytosis exceeding 15,000 cells/μL occurs in about 75% of patients with acute mesenteric ischemia. About 50% of patients have metabolic acidemia. Elevated levels of amylase and phosphate in the blood and of alkaline phosphatase and inorganic phosphate in the peritoneal fluid have been described, but the sensitivity and specificity of these markers of intestinal ischemia have not been established.[69] Leukocytosis out of proportion to the clinical findings, an elevated hemoglobin and hematocrit indicating hemoconcentration as a result of fluid loss into the bowel and peritoneal cavity, and blood-tinged peritoneal fluid, often with an elevated

amylase content, are not specific for acute mesenteric ischemia, but suggest advanced intestinal necrosis and sepsis.

Radiographic Signs

Before infarction occurs, plain abdominal radiographs usually are normal.[70] As the disease progresses, a pattern of adynamic ileus, a gasless abdomen, or small bowel pseudoobstruction can be noted. Late in the course of the disease, formless loops of small intestine or small intestinal "pinkyprinting" can suggest the diagnosis of acute mesenteric ischemia. Less commonly, isolated thumbprinting of the right colon is the only radiologic abnormality. The finding of ischemia in the right colon can result from disease in the main SMA rather than simply interference with local colonic blood flow (Fig. 32-10). Rare findings that accompany all types of bowel infarction include pneumatosis and gas in the portal venous system.

Upper gastrointestinal series can show dilated loops of

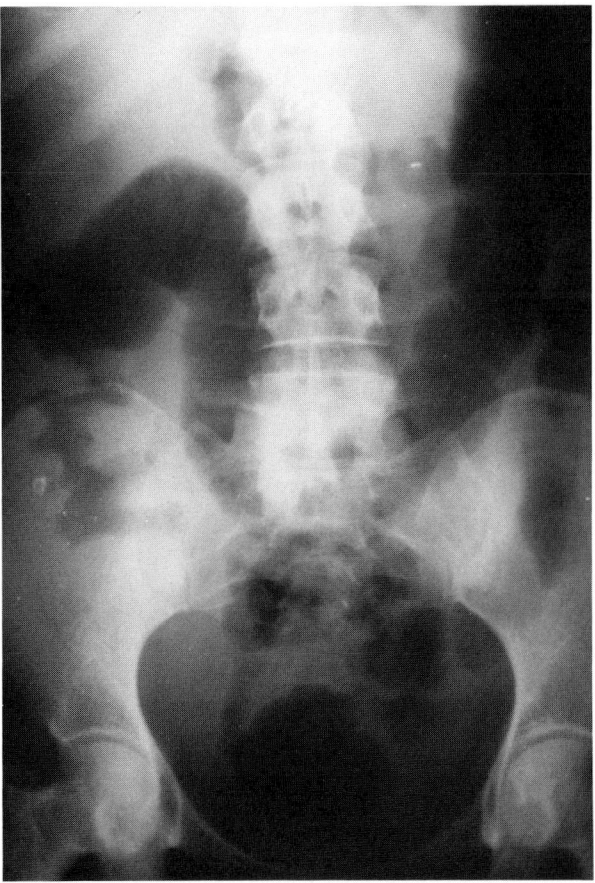

Figure 32-10 Air enema showing isolated right-sided colonic ischemia. (Brandt LJ, Boley SJ. Colonic ischemia. Surg Clin North Am 1992;72:203)

small intestine with thickened folds, mucosal ulceration, or a scalloped bowel border. These findings are more characteristic of focal segmental ischemia. Duplex scanning has been of some value in identifying portal and superior mesenteric venous thrombosis, as well as SMA occlusion in a few patients. CT has been used to identify both arterial and venous thromboses and ischemic bowel, but only in the late stages of the disease. Magnetic resonance imaging (MRI) and positron emission tomography soon may prove helpful in the diagnosis of mesenteric ischemia.

Laparoscopy

Laparoscopy can be useful in patients whose clinical status precludes angiography.[71] However, laparoscopic examination of the bowel is limited to the serosal surface, making it unreliable for diagnosing early mucosal necrosis.

Angiography

Angiography is used to identify major arterial occlusion by embolus or thrombosis. Selective angiography also is the mainstay of diagnosis and initial treatment of nonocclusive forms of acute mesenteric ischemia. Four reliable angiographic criteria for the diagnosis of mesenteric vasoconstriction (Fig. 32-11), the cause of nonocclusive mesenteric ischemia, have been identified[72]:

- Narrowing of the origins of multiple branches of the SMA
- Alternate dilatation and narrowing of the intestinal branches (string-of-sausages sign)
- Spasm of the mesenteric arcades
- Impaired filling of intramural vessels

Mesenteric vasoconstriction occurs commonly in hypotensive patients and in those with pancreatitis, but

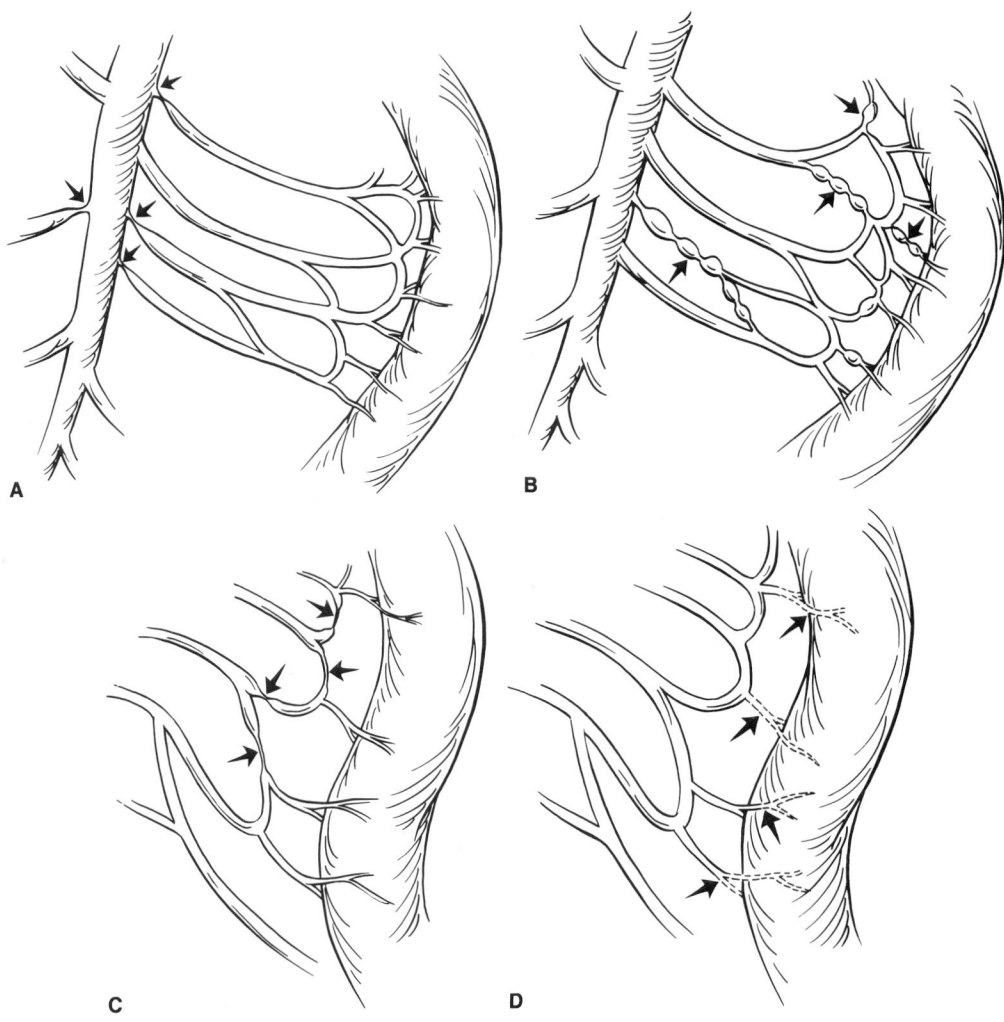

Figure 32-11 Angiographic criteria for acute mesenteric ischemia. (**A**) Narrowing of multiple branches. (**B**) Alternate spasm and dilatation of intestinal branches ("string of sausages" sign). (**C**) Spasm of arcades. (**D**) Impaired filling of intramural vessels. (Kaleya RN, Boley SJ. Mesenteric vascular diseases. In: Maingot R, ed. Abdominal operations, ed 9. East Norwalk, CT, Appleton & Lange, 1990:400)

its presence in patients with suspected intestinal ischemia who are not in shock, do not have pancreatitis, and are not receiving vasopressors is diagnostic of nonocclusive mesenteric ischemia. Therefore, if angiography is performed sufficiently early in the disease, patients with occlusive and nonocclusive acute mesenteric ischemia can be identified before bowel infarction develops.

Aggressive Diagnostic and Therapeutic Approach to Suspected Acute Mesenteric Ischemia

Patients older than 50 years with any of the previously enumerated risk factors for acute mesenteric ischemia who experience the sudden onset of abdominal pain lasting for more than 2 hours should be suspected of having acute mesenteric ischemia. These patients should be treated according to an aggressive radiologic and surgical algorithm (Fig. 32-12). Less absolute indications for inclusion into this protocol include unexplained abdominal distention, colonoscopic evidence of isolated right-sided colonic ischemia, and acidosis without an identifiable cause. Because the presence of diagnostic clinical or nonangiographic radiologic signs usually indicates irreversible intestinal injury, broad selection criteria are essential if early diagnosis and successful treatment are to be achieved. Some negative study results must be accepted to identify and salvage those patients who do have acute mesenteric ischemia.

General Principles of Management

Initial treatment is directed toward correcting the underlying cause of the ischemia. Relief of acute congestive heart failure and correction of hypotension, hypovolemia, and cardiac arrhythmias must precede any diagnostic evaluation. Efforts to improve mesenteric blood flow will be futile if low cardiac output, hypovolemia, or hypotension persists. Patients with acute mesenteric ischemia often have sepsis, with low systemic vascular resistance and sequestration of fluid into the third space. Optimal cardiac performance can be achieved best under these circumstances with the aid of a Swan-Ganz catheter, using serial cardiac profiles to ensure maximal systemic perfusion.

After resuscitation is accomplished, plain films of the abdomen are obtained. These films are taken not to establish the diagnosis of acute mesenteric ischemia, but to exclude other identifiable causes of abdominal pain (eg, a perforated viscus with free intraperitoneal air). Normal results do not exclude acute mesenteric ischemia; ideally, patients should be studied before ra-

diologic signs are present, because such findings indicate the presence of infarcted bowel. If no alternative diagnosis is made on the basis of the plain abdominal films, selective SMA angiography is performed immediately. Based on the angiographic findings and the presence or absence of peritoneal signs that persist for more than 20 minutes after the administration of a bolus dose of intraarterial vasodilator, patients are treated according to the algorithm in Figure 32-12.

Even when the decision to operate has been made based on clinical grounds, a preoperative angiogram must be obtained to manage the patient properly at celiotomy. Relief of mesenteric vasoconstriction is an essential part of the treatment of SMA emboli and thrombi, as well as nonocclusive low-flow states. Intraarterial infusion of papaverine though the angiography catheter into the origin of the SMA is the best method of relieving mesenteric vasoconstriction both before and after operation. The drug is infused at a constant rate of 30 to 60 mg/h in a concentration of 1 mg/mL. The clinical and angiographic responses of patients to vasodilator therapy determine the duration of the papaverine infusion.

Although almost all the papaverine infused into the mesenteric circulation is cleared during its passage through the liver, under some circumstances, this drug can have systemic effects at this dosage. Therefore, systemic arterial pressure and cardiac rate and rhythm must be monitored constantly during the infusion. The most common cause of hypotension with papaverine infusion is dislodgment of the catheter from the orifice of the SMA. Therefore, hypotension during a papaverine infusion should be managed by changing the infusate to saline solution and obtaining a plain abdominal film to confirm proper placement of the arterial catheter.

Management at Laparotomy

Laparotomy is indicated in patients with acute mesenteric ischemia to restore intestinal arterial flow after an embolus or thrombosis, or to resect irreparably damaged bowel. Revascularization should precede evaluation of intestinal viability because bowel that initially appears infarcted can show surprising recovery after the restoration of adequate blood flow.

Tests of Intestinal Viability

After revascularization, intestinal viability can be assessed by several methods. Traditionally, the bowel is placed in warm, saline-soaked laparotomy pads and observed over 10 to 20 minutes for return of normal color, peristalsis, and the presence or absence of pulsa-

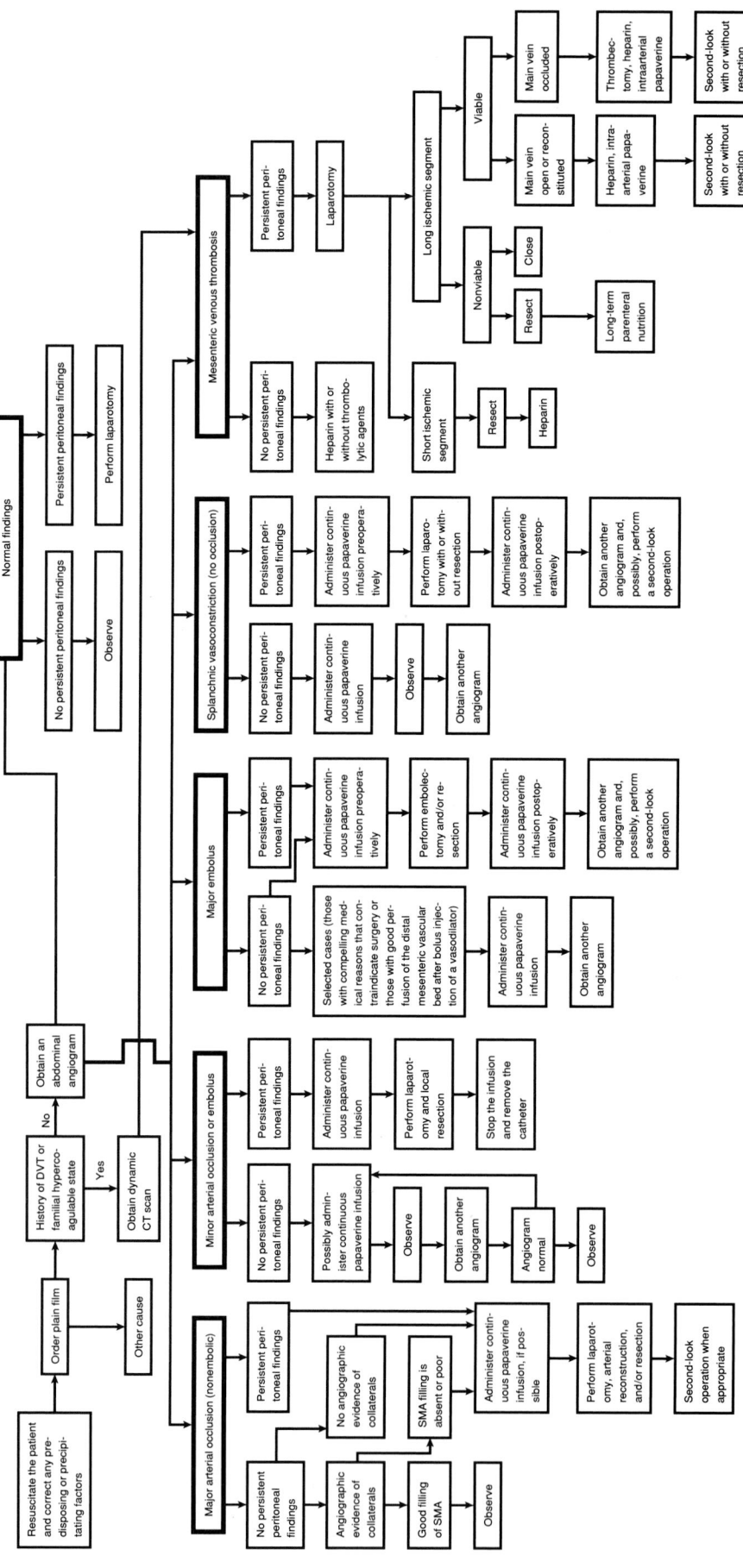

Figure 32-12 Management of acute mesenteric ischemia based on angiographic and CT findings.

1170

tions in the intestinal arteries. This clinical assessment is of limited accuracy, however, and more sensitive and specific evaluation depends on technologic aids. Techniques that have been proposed include surface fluorescence,[73] perfusion fluorometry,[74] Doppler measurements of arterial flow,[75] electromyography,[76] surface temperature, serosal pH, surface oxygen consumption, and radioisotope uptake determinations. Only Doppler pulse determinations, fluorescence using an ultraviolet light after intravenous injection of fluorescein, and perfusion fluorometry have gained wide clinical acceptance. Surface fluorescence increases the accuracy with which viable bowel can be differentiated from nonviable bowel; the equipment is inexpensive and the dye is safe, but the technique remains subjective. Perfusion fluorometry is more objective, allows repeated determinations, and is more accurate than surface fluorescence. The equipment is expensive, however, and only small areas of the bowel can be evaluated at one time. Although Doppler probes are available in most operating rooms, only small areas of the intestine can be examined with this modality. A practical solution is the initial use of surface fluorescence, with either perfusion fluorometry or Doppler examination reserved for evaluation of the equivocal areas.

Decision to Resect Intestine

Short segments of bowel that are nonviable or questionably viable after revascularization are resected. If extensive portions of the bowel are involved, only the clearly necrotic bowel is resected and a planned reexploration (second-look operation) is performed within 12 to 24 hours. The decision to perform a second-look procedure is made during the initial celiotomy if major portions or multiple segments of intestine are of equivocal viability. The purpose of the second-look celiotomy, as proposed by Shaw,[77] is "not just to allow a clear definition between dead and live bowel to take place, but also to allow time for the institution of supportive measures which may render more of the bowel viable." Such measures can include optimization of cardiac output, SMA infusion of papaverine, and institution of antibiotic or anticoagulant therapy. The decision to perform a second-look procedure is a commitment and the operation should be done irrespective of the patient's clinical course. If a second operation is planned, bowel ends can be exteriorized at the first operation and no anastomoses need be made until the time of the reexploration. It has been estimated that only 18% of second-look operations contribute to patient survival.[78]

If, at initial laparotomy, there is obvious infarction of all or most of the small bowel with or without a portion of the right colon, the surgeon must decide whether to do anything further. Resection of all involved bowel inevitably results in short-bowel syndrome and, in these older patients, a commitment to lifelong parenteral nutrition. A frank preoperative discussion of this potential problem with patients and their families is important so that an acceptable decision can be reached if extensive bowel necrosis is encountered at surgery.

Postoperative Care

The use of anticoagulants in the management of acute mesenteric ischemia is controversial. Heparin can cause intestinal, submucosal, or intraperitoneal hemorrhage and, except in the case of mesenteric venous thrombosis, should not be used in the immediate postoperative period. Late thrombosis after embolectomy or arterial reconstruction, however, occurs frequently enough that initiating anticoagulant therapy 48 hours after operation seems advisable.

Both systemic and locally administered antibiotics have been shown to improve the survival of ischemic bowel.[79] In addition, the high incidence of positive blood culture results in patients with acute mesenteric ischemia, as well as the clinical and experimental evidence that ischemic bowel permits translocation of intraluminal bacteria, support the use of broad-spectrum systemic antibiotics as soon as the diagnosis is entertained and throughout the postoperative period, as dictated by the findings at celiotomy.[80]

Management of Specific Types of Acute Mesenteric Ischemia

Superior Mesenteric Artery Embolus

On identification of an SMA embolus at angiography (Fig. 32-13), a papaverine infusion is begun through the catheter placed selectively in the origin of the SMA, proximal to the occlusion. Patients then are treated according to the algorithm in Figure 32-12, based on the site of the embolus, the presence or absence of peritoneal signs, the extent of the collateral blood flow, and the degree of vasospasm in the vascular beds both proximal and distal to the embolus as determined by a second angiogram performed after a selective intraarterial bolus injection of 25 mg of tolazoline.

Minor emboli are those found in the branches of the SMA or in the SMA distal to the origin of the ileocolic artery. Patients with minor emboli whose pain is relieved by vasodilator therapy can be treated expectantly. Patients with major emboli who are selected for nonoperative therapy must have significant contraindications to surgery, no peritoneal signs, and adequate

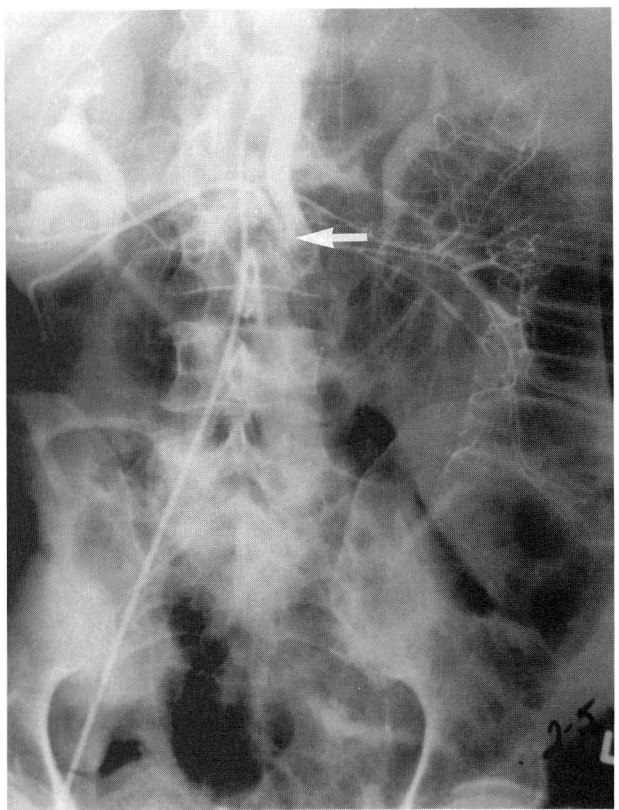

Figure 32-13 Arteriogram showing embolus completely occluding the superior mesenteric artery (*arrow*) with associated vasospasm occluding blood flow. (Brandt LJ, Boley SJ. Ischemic intestinal syndromes. Adv Surg 1981;15:16)

perfusion of the vascular beds distal to the embolus after the initiation of vasodilator therapy. Direct infusion of thrombolytic agents through selectively placed catheters has been used successfully in a few patients, most of whom had partial occlusion of the SMA. However, thrombolytic agents can require up to 36 hours to dissolve the embolus,[81] during which time there can be continued ischemia and ultimate necrosis of the bowel. Furthermore, because the extent of injury to the small intestine cannot be monitored during the infusion of thrombolytic agents, their use for acute mesenteric ischemia is not recommended.

If embolectomy is performed, it should be done before final decisions are made about intestinal viability. The embolus is approached directly or, less optimally, through a proximal arteriotomy (Fig. 32-14). The proximal SMA is exposed by drawing the transverse colon cephalad and forward, as the small intestine is retracted backward. The inferior leaf of the transverse mesocolon is incised and the proximal SMA is dissected free between the pancreas and the fourth portion of the duodenum. The SMA is exposed for 2 to 3 cm proximal and

distal to the origin of the middle colic artery. The SMA is palpated gently to determine the most distal extent of arterial pulsation or is examined directly with a Doppler probe to identify the site of the embolus. Once the site of the embolus is found, proximal and distal control of the SMA and its branches is achieved with vessel loops or gentle vascular clamps. A longitudinal arteriotomy is made over the embolus or just proximal to it, the embolus is removed, and residual clots are flushed out of the artery by briefly releasing the vessel loops. A balloon embolectomy catheter then is passed in proximal and distal directions to remove all remaining clots. The arteriotomy is closed with or without a vein patch, depending on vessel diameter.

After embolectomy, bowel viability is determined. If no second-look operation is planned, infusion of papaverine is continued for an additional 12 to 24 hours. An arteriogram is then obtained to exclude persistent vasospasm before the arterial catheter is removed. If a reoperation is performed, the infusion is continued through the second procedure and until no vasoconstriction is present on a follow-up angiogram.

Nonocclusive Mesenteric Ischemia

Nonocclusive mesenteric ischemia is diagnosed when the angiographic signs of mesenteric vasoconstriction are seen in patients who have the clinical picture of mesenteric ischemia and are neither in shock nor receiving vasopressors. The angiographic findings can range from the previously described local signs to a pruned appearance of the entire mesenteric vasculature. A selective SMA infusion of papaverine is begun in all patients with nonocclusive mesenteric ischemia as soon as the diagnosis is made. In patients with persistent peritoneal signs, the infusion is continued during and after surgical exploration. At operation, manipulation of the SMA is minimized. Overtly necrotic bowel is resected, and a primary anastomosis is performed only if no second-look procedure is planned. It is better to leave bowel of questionable viability than to perform a massive enterectomy, because the bowel frequently improves with supportive measures or is demarcated more clearly by the time of reoperation.

When a papaverine infusion is used as the primary therapy for nonocclusive mesenteric ischemia, it is continued for about 24 hours, then the infusate is changed to normal saline solution for 30 minutes and another angiogram is performed. Based on the clinical course of the patient and the presence or absence of vasoconstriction on the second angiogram, the infusion is either discontinued or maintained for an additional 24 hours. Angiography is performed daily until there is no radiographic evidence of vasoconstriction and the patient's

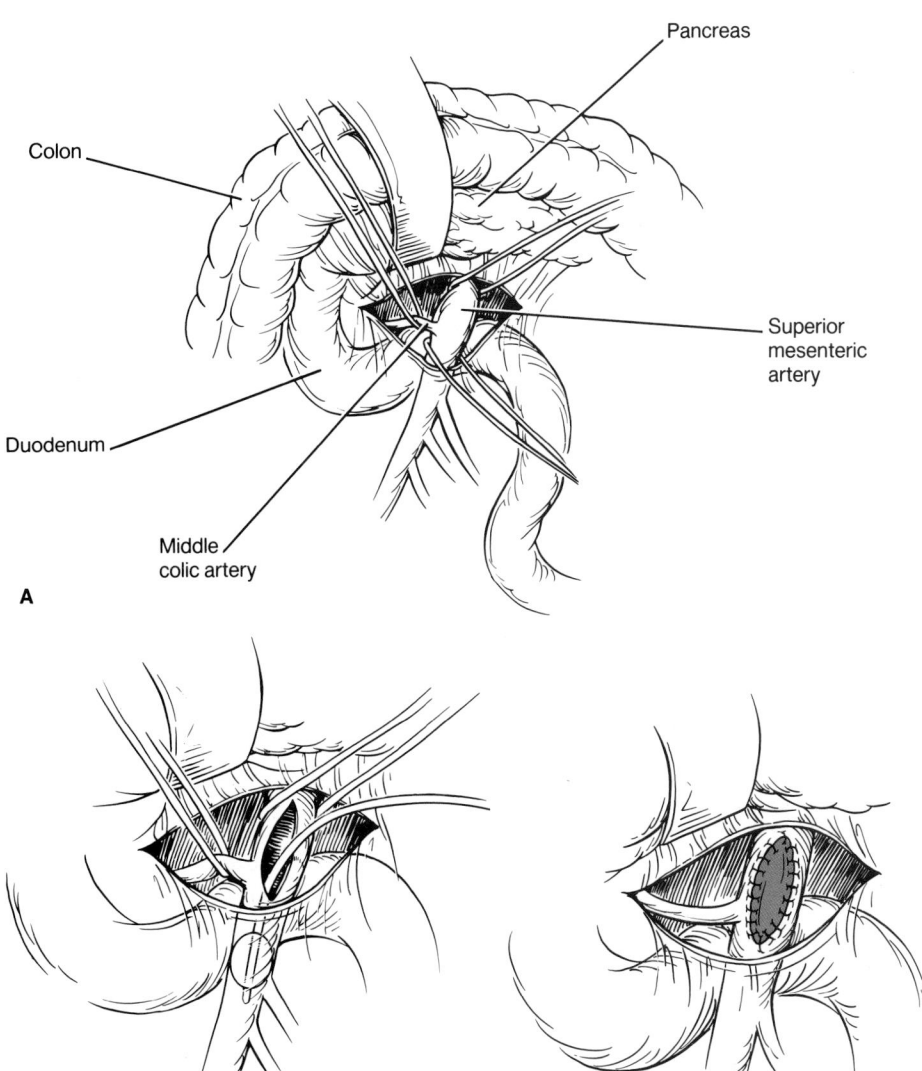

Colon

Duodenum

Middle
colic artery

A

Pancreas

Superior
mesenteric
artery

B

C

Figure 32-14 Technique of superior mesenteric artery embolectomy. **(A)** The artery is isolated at the base of the mesentery over the site of the embolus. **(B)** A longitudinal arteriotomy is made and the vessel is cleared of debris. **(C)** The arteriotomy is closed primarily or with a vein patch (shown). (Boley SJ, Sprayregen S, Veith FJ, et al. An aggressive roentgenologic and surgical approach to acute mesenteric ischemia. In: Nyhus LM, ed. Surgery annual, vol 5. New York, Appleton-Century-Crofts, 1973:375)

clinical symptoms and signs are gone. Infusions usually are discontinued after 24 hours, but have been maintained for as long as 5 days.

When papaverine is used in conjunction with surgery for nonocclusive disease, a second-look operation frequently is necessary. In such cases, the infusion is continued as previously described for second-look operations after embolectomy. The arterial catheter is removed when no angiographic signs of vasoconstriction are seen 30 minutes after cessation of vasodilator therapy.

Acute Superior Mesenteric Artery Thrombosis

Superior mesenteric artery thrombosis is identified most often on a flush aortogram showing complete occlusion of the SMA within 1 to 2 cm of its origin. Some filling of the SMA distal to the obstruction through col-

lateral pathways almost always is present. Branches both proximal and distal to the obstruction can show local spasm or diffuse vasoconstriction. Differentiation between thrombosis and embolus can be difficult; in such cases, patients are treated initially for SMA embolus. A more difficult problem arises in patients with abdominal pain without abdominal signs who demonstrate complete occlusion of the SMA on aortography. In these cases, it is important to differentiate between an acute and a long-standing occlusion, because the latter can be an incidental finding unrelated to the acute illness. Prominent collateral vessels between the superior mesenteric and the celiac or inferior mesenteric circulations are characteristic of chronic SMA occlusion. If large collaterals are present and there is good filling of the SMA on the late films during the angiogram, the occlusion can be considered chronic and the abdominal pain probably is unrelated to mesenteric vascular disease. In the absence of peritoneal signs, such patients are treated expectantly. The absence of collateral vessels, or the presence of collateral vessels with inadequate filling of the SMA, indicates an acute occlusion. Prompt intervention is indicated irrespective of the abdominal findings in these cases.

If possible, an angiographic catheter is placed in the proximal SMA and a papaverine infusion is begun. If the origin of the SMA cannot be identified or cannulated at angiography, a small Silastic catheter should be advanced proximally into the SMA through a jejunal artery at the time of operative revascularization to treat the associated vasospasm. This catheter is brought out through a separate incision in the abdominal wall and is used for postoperative papaverine infusion.

Revascularization procedures for SMA thrombosis are similar to those used for chronic mesenteric ischemia, in which reimplantation, thrombectomy and endarterectomy, or some form of bypass graft to the SMA distal to the obstruction is used. These are discussed in the section on chronic mesenteric ischemia. Percutaneous balloon and laser angioplasty of the SMA also have been reported.[82] Because there is no effective method of monitoring end-organ injury, and because of the danger of recurrent thrombosis with irreparable bowel loss, we do not recommend these techniques for acute SMA occlusion.

Complications of This Aggressive Approach to the Management of Acute Mesenteric Ischemia

Complications caused by angiographic studies and prolonged infusions of vasodilative drugs have not been excessive. Three of our first 50 patients had transient acute tubular necrosis after angiography and treatment of mesenteric ischemia. One patient had arterial occlusion in both lower extremities during a papaverine infusion for an SMA embolus, probably representing synchronous emboli. However, the SMA catheter could not be excluded as an etiologic factor. Several patients had local hematomas at the arterial puncture sites, but no major problems were encountered with blood flow to the lower extremities in these cases.

Problems caused by prolonged papaverine infusions have been minimal. Infusions lasting more than 5 days have been used without significant systemic effects. Fibrin clots on the arterial catheter have been observed commonly, but have not caused any difficulty. Three catheters underwent thrombosis and had to be removed, but this complication subsequently has been prevented by using a continuous infusion pump to deliver the papaverine solution. Catheter dislodgment requiring replacement occurred several times.

Septic complications, including wound infections, pneumonia, intraabdominal abscesses, and hepatic abscesses, are common. Intraoperative and postoperative myocardial infarctions occur frequently in this population with advanced atherosclerotic disease and other predisposing comorbid conditions. Long stays in the intensive care unit are the rule rather than the exception, even after early diagnosis.

Late thrombosis after embolectomy or arterial reconstruction has been minimized by the initiation of anticoagulant therapy 48 hours after surgery. Earlier treatment is not advised because it can precipitate postoperative bleeding or hemorrhage into the ischemic bowel wall.

Results of Therapy for Acute Mesenteric Ischemia

Mortality rates of 70% to 90% have been reported using traditional methods of diagnosis and treatment of acute mesenteric ischemia. The aggressive approach described earlier can significantly reduce these catastrophic figures.[83-94] Of the first 50 patients treated by this approach, 35 (70%) proved to have acute mesenteric ischemia. Of these, 33 had angiographic signs of ischemia. The remaining 2 patients had normal results on angiography. Of 65 patients from two institutions treated according to this protocol, 36 (55%) survived, including 14 of 26 with nonocclusive mesenteric ischemia, 14 of 23 with SMA embolus, 4 of 6 with SMA thrombosis, and 4 of 6 with superior mesenteric venous thrombosis. Most of the survivors lost less than 3 ft of small intestine.

In 47 patients with intestinal ischemia resulting from SMA emboli, a survival rate of 55% was achieved in those treated according to an aggressive protocol compared with only 20% in those treated by traditional methods. Intraarterial papaverine as the primary treatment was successful in 4 patients; 2 of these did not undergo operation, and the other 2 had normal intestine at the time of delayed laparotomy. Of those patients with SMA emboli who were placed in the protocol within 12 hours of reporting their pain to their physicians, and who were treated strictly according to the protocol, two thirds survived.

Using the aggressive approach outlined earlier, at least 50% of patients with acute mesenteric ischemia who were treated according to the algorithm survived, and about 70% to 90% of them lost less than a meter of intestine.[83,84] Ninety percent of patients with acute mesenteric ischemia who underwent angiography before they had signs of peritonitis survived, demonstrating the value of early diagnosis. Ideally, all patients with acute mesenteric ischemia should be studied at a time when plain films of the abdomen are normal and an acute surgical abdomen has not developed. Other published studies that did not use vasodilator therapy have had significantly higher mortality rates (Table 32-2). Therefore, wider use of this aggressive protocol for patients at risk may improve overall results of therapy for acute mesenteric ischemia.

MESENTERIC VENOUS THROMBOSIS

Mesenteric venous thrombosis is an infrequent, but distinct, form of intestinal ischemia. Improvements in diagnostic modalities and therapy have altered our concepts of the disorder, and we now recognize that thrombosis of the SMV can develop slowly with no symptoms, in a more subacute manner with pain but no intestinal infarction, or in an acute fashion with the classic presentation. Other contributions have altered our understanding of the etiology, methods of diagnosis, and management so that much of what has been written about mesenteric venous thrombosis is no longer applicable.

Demographics

Patients with operative or pathologic confirmation of mesenteric venous thrombosis represent 2 per 100,000 hospital admissions and well below 10% of patients with acute mesenteric ischemia seen during this period. About 0.01% of all emergency surgical service admissions to a Dutch hospital were attributable to mesen-

Table 32-2 Mortality Rates for Acute Mesenteric Ischemia With or Without Intraarterial Vasodilator Therapy

Investigators	Patients	Vasodilator Therapy	Survival Rate (%)
Levy et al, 1990[87]	62	No	60
Batellier & Kieny, 1990[88]	65	No	50
Finucane et al, 1989[89]	32	No	34
Georgiev, 1989[90]	175	No	7
Paes et al, 1988[91]	38	No	47
Clavien & Muller, 1986[92]	81	No	29
Koveker et al, 1985[85]	39	No	15
Clark & Gallant, 1984[83]	27	Yes/no	48
Sachs et al, 1982[78]	49	No	35
Rogers et al, 1982[93]	12	No	33
Krausz & Manny, 1978[94]	40	No	22
Boley et al, 1977[84]	35	Yes	55

Table 32-3 Conditions Associated With Mesenteric Venous Thrombosis

HYPERCOAGULABLE STATES
Peripheral deep venous thrombosis
Neoplasms
Protein C deficiency
Protein S deficiency
Antithrombin III deficiency
Oral contraceptive use
Pregnancy
Polycythemia vera
Thrombocytosis

INFLAMMATION
Pancreatitis
Peritonitis (eg, perforated appendicitis or diverticulitis)
Inflammatory bowel disease
Pelvic or intraabdominal abscess

PORTAL HYPERTENSION
Cirrhosis
Congestive splenomegaly
After sclerotherapy for varices

TRAUMA
Postoperative states
After splenectomy
Blunt abdominal trauma

OTHER
Decompression sickness

teric venous thrombosis.[95] Although a review of the literature suggests a male predilection of up to 1.5:1,[96,97] a review of our experience showed no such preference. The mean patient age was 48 years in the literature, but 60 years at our institution.[96] We have attributed these differences to the higher proportion of geriatric patients seen at our medical center as compared with most other institutions.

Etiologic Factors

Many conditions have been associated with mesenteric venous thrombosis (Table 32-3). In older studies, up to 55% of cases were thought to have no etiologic factor. In more recent reports, however, contributing disorders are identified in up to 81% of patients.[97] This discrepancy can be explained by the fact that many of the cases in retrospective reviews occurred before conditions such as antithrombin III, protein S, and protein C deficiencies had been described.[98] Therefore, with increasing knowledge, the number of cases of primary mesenteric venous thrombosis in which no cause can be identified should decrease. Hypercoagulable states are especially important, being found in 14 of 16 patients in one report.[99] Oral contraceptive–related mesenteric venous thrombosis accounted for about 9% of cases seen in the women in our study, but for only 4% of the total series.[100] This finding is corroborated by a literature review that also showed a 5% incidence in the total population; however, there was an 18% incidence among women.[97] The lower incidence of oral contraceptive–related episodes in our series may reflect the large proportion of geriatric patients seen at our institution. In addition, a spate of isolated case reports relating oral contraceptive use to mesenteric venous thrombosis may skew the composition of cases in the literature. Mesenteric venous thrombosis also has been seen as a complication of sclerotherapy for esophageal varices.[101]

Natural History of Mesenteric Venous Thrombosis

The location of the initial thrombosis within the mesenteric venous circulation varies with the etiology. SMV thrombosis secondary to cirrhosis, neoplasm, or operative injury clearly starts at the site of obstruction and extends outward, whereas thrombosis caused by hypercoagulable states tends to start in smaller venous branches and propagate into the major trunks. Infarction of intestine rarely occurs unless the branches of the peripheral arcades and the vasa recta are involved, even when the junction of the portal vein and the SMV is occluded. Inferior mesenteric vein thrombosis leading to infarction has been reported in less than 6% of cases of mesenteric venous thrombosis.

When collateral circulation is inadequate and venous drainage from a segment of bowel is compromised, there is increasing congestion of the involved intestine. The bowel becomes edematous, cyanotic, and thickened with intramural hemorrhages, and similar changes ultimately involve the subjacent mesentery. Serosanguineous peritoneal fluid accompanies early hemorrhagic infarction. Arterial vasoconstriction can be marked, but pulsations persist up to the bowel wall. Late in the process, transmural infarction occurs, and it can become impossible to differentiate venous from arterial occlusion.

Clinical Manifestations

Presentation

Superior mesenteric vein thrombosis can present with a sudden onset, a subacute onset of weeks to months, or a chronic onset in which there usually are no symptoms until late complications occur. Up to 60%

of patients have histories of deep venous thrombosis in the extremities.[102,103]

Acute Superior Mesenteric Venous Thrombosis

The symptoms and signs of acute SMV thrombosis (the form of the disease classically described) are both varied and nonspecific, and the disorder has long been known as the great imitator of other abdominal diseases. In series that predate angiography and imaging studies, a correct preoperative diagnosis was made infrequently. Except for abdominal pain, which was present in over 90% of patients (Table 32-4), no symptoms pointed to the diagnosis of mesenteric venous thrombosis. Moreover, even the duration, nature, severity, and location of the pain varied widely, although it typically was out of proportion to the physical findings. In our review, the mean duration of pain before hospital admission was 5 days, but others found it to range from 2 weeks to more than 1 month.[104,105] Some of the last patients probably would be considered to have the subacute form of SMV thrombosis that we are beginning to recognize today. An initially surprising finding is that survivors had a longer interval (6 days) before admission than did patients with a fatal outcome (4.4 days). This can be explained by assuming that patients with a more indolent course are those who have less extensive bowel infarction and, hence, a better prognosis.

Other prominent symptoms include nausea and vomiting, which occur in more than half the patients. Lower gastrointestinal bleeding or bloody diarrhea, in up to 15% of patients, and hematemesis, in up to 13%, are indications of bowel infarction. The presence of hematemesis as well as bleeding per rectum should alert the physician to the possibility of a mesenteric ischemic catastrophe. Occult blood is present in the stools of more than half the patients.

The initial physical findings in acute SMV thrombosis vary greatly, reflecting both different stages and

Table 32-4 Symptoms Associated With Mesenteric Venous Thrombosis

Symptom	Occurrence (%)
Abdominal pain	90
Vomiting	77
Nausea	54
Diarrhea	36
Constipation	14
Hematemesis	9
Hematochezia	5

degrees of ischemic injury. Although almost all patients have abdominal tenderness (Table 32-5), and most have decreased bowel sounds and abdominal distention, only two thirds manifest clear signs of peritonitis. Guarding and rebound tenderness develop later in the course, however, as bowel infarction evolves. Most patients have temperatures greater than 38°C, but only one fourth have clinical signs of septic shock.

Laboratory studies for the diagnosis of all forms of intestinal ischemia have proved to have low specificity or low sensitivity. In our series of 22 patients, only a white blood cell count above 12,000 cells/μL and an increase in the proportion of polymorphonuclear cells were present in more than two thirds of the patients. These laboratory tests can suggest, but not confirm or exclude, the diagnosis of intestinal ischemia.

Patients with personal or family histories of deep venous thrombosis or other thrombotic episodes who have symptoms compatible with mesenteric ischemia should undergo evaluation for a hypercoagulable state. The work-up should include antithrombin III, protein S, and protein C levels, as well as the routine coagulation profile. Antithrombin III binds to the serine protease portion of thrombin, thereby preventing the conversion of fibrinogen to fibrin. Protein S and C are vitamin K–dependent clotting factors. When activated, protein C and its cofactor protein S inactivate factors V and VIII. In addition, the protein C and protein S complex can stimulate fibrinolysis by activation of plasminogen activator. In deficiency states, patients have a tendency to clot. Because protein C and S are vitamin K dependent, and because antithrombin III deficiency states are heparin resistant, warfarin therapy is used in these patients.[106]

Subacute Superior Mesenteric Venous Thrombosis

The term *subacute SMV thrombosis* is used to describe patients who have abdominal pain for several weeks to months without intestinal infarction. This presentation can be attributable either to extension of the thrombotic process at a rate rapid enough to cause pain but slow enough to allow collaterals to develop before infarction occurs, or to acute thrombosis of only enough venous drainage to produce reversible ischemic injury. Most often, the condition has been an incidental finding on imaging studies done for other suspected diagnoses, and the pain has subsided spontaneously or after the initiation of anticoagulant therapy.

Typically, pain is the only symptom, although some patients have nausea or diarrhea. Physical examination and laboratory test results are normal. The pain is related to meals in a few patients, but usually is nonspecific in site and nature. Some patients whose disease begins with this type of presentation ultimately have intestinal infarction; hence, the distinction between the acute and subacute forms of SMV thrombosis can become blurred. The late occurrence of infarction can be the result of recurrent SMV thrombosis. On histologic examination, new and old thromboses have been found at the time of autopsy in nearly half of pateints with major vein involvement.[107] Moreover, some patients with disease of subacute onset, in which the symptoms subside, later develop the problems seen with chronic SMV thrombosis.

Chronic Mesenteric Venous Thrombosis

The term *chronic mesenteric venous thrombosis* has been applied to patients who have no symptoms during the period when the thrombosis occurs. Some patients never have problems related to the SMV thrombosis, but others have gastrointestinal bleeding from esophageal or intestinal varices.[108] The esophagus is the most common site of varices and always is associated with thrombosis of the portal vein, the splenic vein, or both. The physical findings of chronic mesenteric venous thrombosis are those of portal hypertension if the main portal vein is involved, but there can be no abnormal findings when only the SMV is involved. Laboratory studies in cases of portal or splenic vein involvement often show secondary hypersplenism with thrombocytopenia or pancytopenia.

Diagnosis

Acute Mesenteric Venous Thrombosis

The absence of any reliable specific symptoms, signs, or laboratory studies makes preoperative diagnosis of acute mesenteric venous thrombosis difficult. Moreover, the variability in the course of the disease, with some patients having an indolent course of days to weeks and others having a relatively acute onset and

Table 32-5 Physical Findings on Hospital Admission for Mesenteric Venous Thrombsis

Physical Finding	*Occurrence (%)*
Abdominal tenderness	97
Abdominal distention	80
Decreased bowel sounds	77
Occult blood in stool	54
Guarding or rebound tenderness	53
Temperature >38°C	47
Systolic blood pressure <90 mmHg	23

progressive course, further obscures the diagnosis. The difficulty in diagnosing mesenteric venous thrombosis was graphically described by Anane-Sehaf[109]: ''Perhaps the best overall finding was an uneasy feeling on the part of the examining physician that his patient looks sick but that he could not say why or from what.'' In the past, the correct diagnosis almost always was made at laparotomy. In more recent series in which the newer diagnostic modalities have been used, the diagnosis was made without, or before, operation.

Plain films of the abdomen, if abnormal, almost always reflect the presence of infarcted bowel; when present, these changes rarely permit differentiation of venous and arterial forms of ischemia. In our series, 75% of patients had abnormal plain films, but 50% showed only a nonspecific ileus pattern and only 25% suggested the presence of some form of acute mesenteric ischemia. Gas in the wall of the bowel or in the portal vein, and free air in the peritoneal cavity, all late signs of intestinal infarction, can be seen on plain films.

Barium enemas are of little value because mesenteric venous thrombosis rarely involves the colon. Some authors report small bowel studies to be both specific and sensitive.[110] Characteristic findings include marked thickening of the bowel wall and valvulae conniventes due to congestion and edema, separation of loops due to mesenteric thickening, a long transition zone between involved and uninvolved bowel with progressive narrowing of the lumen by the thickened wall, and thumbprints or pseudotumors.

Selective mesenteric arteriography can establish a definitive diagnosis before bowel infarction occurs, can differentiate venous thrombosis from arterial forms of ischemia, and provides access for the administration of intraarterial vasodilators when relief of the associated arterial vasoconstriction is deemed important. The angiographic findings of mesenteric venous thrombosis have been determined by experimental and clinical means, and include the following:

- Demonstration of a thrombus in the SMV with partial or complete occlusion
- Failure to visualize the SMV or portal vein
- Slow or absent filling of the mesenteric veins
- Arterial spasm
- Failure of arterial arcades to empty
- A prolonged blush in the involved segment

In addition, the angiogram can show reconstitution of venous blood flow above the thrombus, which can be an important factor in planning therapy.

Ultrasonography,[111,112] CT,[113] and MRI[114] all have been used to demonstrate thrombi in the SMV and the portal vein before bowel infarction. Ultrasonography is of less value in pure SMV thrombosis because overlying gas can prevent good visualization of the vein, but it can be used as a screening test (Fig. 32-15). Thickening of the bowel wall and free peritoneal fluid are sonographic findings suggesting intestinal ischemia.

Gastrointestinal CT scanning can establish the diagnosis in over 90% of patients with mesenteric venous thrombosis by demonstrating the thrombus, venous collateral circulation, and involved intestine.[103] Specific findings include thickening and persistent enhancement of the bowel wall, enlargement of the SMV, a central lucency in the lumen of the vein representing a thrombus, a sharply defined vein wall with a rim of increased density, and dilated collateral vessels in a thickened mesentery (Fig. 32-16). These findings may be

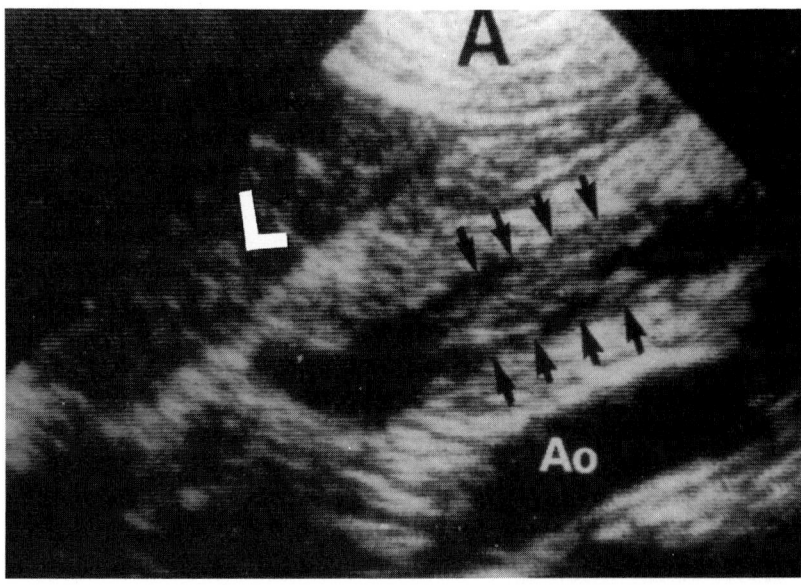

Figure 32-15 Longitudinal ultrasonographic section showing thrombus (*arrows*) in the distended superior mesenteric vein. Ao, aorta; L, liver. (Kidambi H, Herbert R, Kidambi AV. Ultrasonic demonstration of superior mesenteric and splenoportal venous thrombosis. J Clin Ultrasound 1986;14: 199)

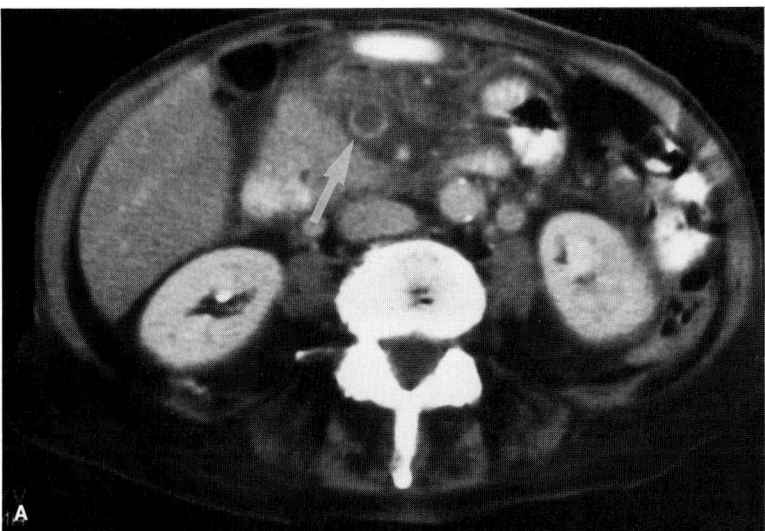

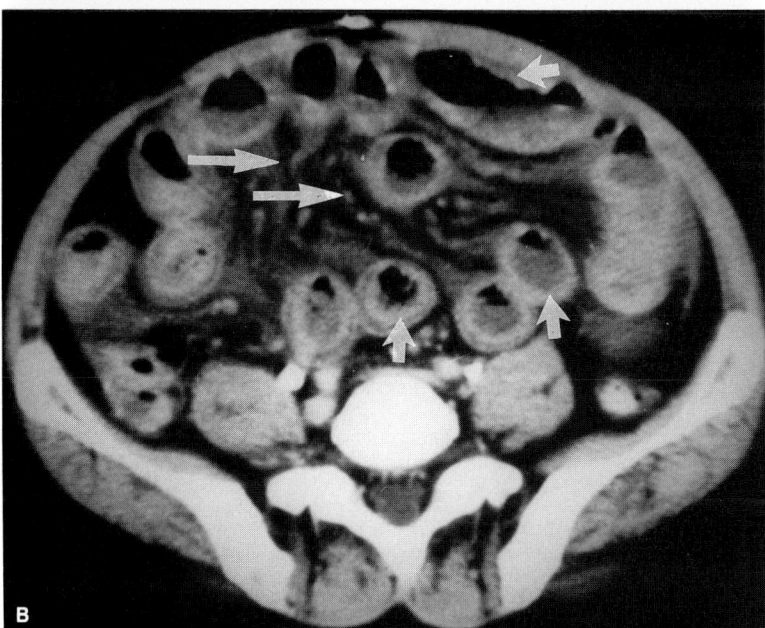

Figure 32-16 (**A**) Abdominal contrast CT demonstrating an enlarged superior mesenteric vein with central lucency in the lumen representing the thrombus. The vein wall is sharply defined, with a rim of increased density surrounding the thrombus (*arrow*). (**B**) Abdominal contrast CT showing thickening and persistent enhancement of the bowel wall (*small arrows*) and dilated collateral vessels within a thickened mesentery (*large arrows*). (**A** courtesy of Dr. Scott Harrison, University of Washington School of Medicine, Seattle; **B** courtesy of Dr. Lawrence Carl)

more indicative of the chronic form of mesenteric venous thrombosis because many patients in whom they have been described underwent CT for another indication and the mesenteric thrombosis was an incidental finding. Some believe that when a diagnosis of mesenteric venous thrombosis is made by CT, little is gained by a subsequent selective mesenteric angiogram. However, the better delineation of thrombosed veins and the access for administration of intraarterial vasodilators make angiography of value in selected patients.

There is no firm information regarding the desirability of performing angiography and CT in patients with acute mesenteric venous thrombosis. A few patients evaluated by imaging techniques who had no ab-

dominal findings have been treated successfully without angiography or operation. MRI also has been used to diagnose mesenteric venous thrombosis in some patients, but its only apparent advantage is that it does not require the use of ionizing radiation.

There have been isolated reports of mesenteric venous thrombosis being diagnosed by various endoscopic methods. Routine gastroduodenoscopy and colonoscopy rarely are of value because the duodenum and colon are infrequently involved, but examination of the proximal jejunum with a long endoscope can suggest the diagnosis if that portion of the bowel is involved. Laparoscopy can be useful in circumstances where the diagnosis is uncertain. Scintiangiography has been diagnostic of mesenteric venous thrombosis; however, it has not been proved clinically reliable.[115]

As previously stated, the correct diagnosis of mesenteric venous thrombosis often is made at laparotomy. The hallmarks of mesenteric venous thrombosis are serosanguineous peritoneal fluid, dark red to blue-black edematous bowel, striking thickening of the mesentery, good arterial pulsations in the involved segment, and thrombus in cut mesenteric veins; at this stage, some degree of intestinal infarction invariably has occurred. Thus, as with the other forms of acute mesenteric ischemia, improved survival will come only from earlier diagnosis. For this reason, during the past 15 years, we have used the same diagnostic protocol for patients suspected of having mesenteric venous thrombosis as for those suspected of having arterial forms of acute mesenteric ischemia. However, the successful nonoperative pharmacologic treatment of several patients in whom mesenteric venous thrombosis was diagnosed by imaging techniques suggests that use of the aggressive protocol is not always necessary.

In patients suspected of having mesenteric venous thrombosis, we first obtain a contrast-enhanced CT. A past history of deep venous thrombosis and a family history of an inherited coagulation defect are examples of factors that warrant the use of CT as the first imaging study. Patients with no factors suggesting venous thrombosis are promptly resuscitated and undergo selective mesenteric angiography.

Chronic Mesenteric Venous Thrombosis

Because chronic mesenteric venous thrombosis causes no symptoms or presents as gastrointestinal bleeding, the evaluation is directed toward determining the source of the hemorrhage. Upper and lower gastrointestinal endoscopy and the same imaging studies used for acute mesenteric venous thrombosis should establish the diagnosis, the extent of the thrombosis, and the site of the bleeding. Transhepatic splenoportography can be used to better define the extent of the thromboses and varices if necessary, but papaverine-enhanced selective SMA angiography is a better choice if the portal vein is occluded.

Management of Mesenteric Venous Thrombosis

Acute Mesenteric Venous Thrombosis

Until recently, a diagnosis of mesenteric venous thrombosis mandated prompt laparotomy. However, with the advent of newer methods of diagnosis, mesenteric venous thrombosis is being identified before bowel infarction occurs, and nonoperative therapy is proving successful in these cases. In the select group of patients in whom there are no physical findings suggestive of intestinal infarction, and in whom the diagnosis of mesenteric venous thrombosis is made by ultrasonography, CT, MRI, or angiography, a trial of anticoagulant or thrombolytic therapy can prove worthwhile. Heparin and streptokinase have been used successfully in the few case reports of this type of therapy[116] (see Fig. 32-12). If signs of intestinal infarction develop, immediate operation is indicated.

All other patients should undergo prompt laparotomy. In the past, therapy consisted of resection of infarcted bowel and immediate institution of anticoagulant therapy. Although the value of anticoagulant therapy has been a matter of debate, recent studies show a clear benefit to the immediate use of heparin. Only 13% of patients who received this therapy had disease recurrence or progression and only 13% died; in contrast, 20% to 25% of patients who did not receive anticoagulants after surgery had recurrence and 50% died.[97,100]

The extent of bowel resection also has been a subject of disagreement. Older articles recommended wide resection beyond the apparently infarcted bowel because the thrombosis often extended past the resected mesentery. More recent experience suggests that it is not necessary to sacrifice viable bowel when heparin and second-look operations are used. We believe that only the nonviable bowel should be excised as determined by clinical evaluation and, if necessary, by administration of fluorescein with examination under a Wood lamp. Although routine second-look operations have been recommended,[117] most surgeons use this procedure only in selected patients.

Other therapeutic options are mesenteric venous thrombectomy[118] and intraarterial papaverine infusions through the SMA angiographic catheter,[119] both of which have been used in only a few patients. The limited experience with these two modalities makes it impossible to define their value.

If a short segment of ischemic bowel is found at operation, local resection should be done and heparin should be administered promptly. Extensively involved bowel that is not all frankly nonviable presents a more difficult problem, and the angiographic findings can be essential to the decision-making process. If the angiogram shows the major vein to be open or reconstituted, indicating that blood is flowing through the vein or around the obstruction, a second-look operation should be performed 12 to 18 hours later and the intervening time should be used to improve circulation with papaverine infused into the SMA. Mesenteric venous thrombosis has been shown in experiments to have associated arterial spasm, which contributes to the ischemia. Relieving the arterial vasoconstriction may improve the blood supply enough to preserve viability.

If a long segment of questionable bowel is found at laparotomy and the angiographic or operative findings indicate complete thrombosis of the SMV at its junction with the portal vein, with or without extension into the portal vein, venous thrombectomy is indicated. A second-look operation should be performed after thrombectomy if the bowel is not clearly viable. Again, heparin therapy is instituted promptly. Intraarterial papaverine can be beneficial if there appears to be arterial vasoconstriction after the thrombectomy.

This surgical approach is predicated on salvaging the maximum length of bowel. Thrombectomy is not indicated when short segments of bowel are involved, and there is no evidence that it is advantageous when venous flow is reconstituted around a thrombus.

Chronic Mesenteric Venous Thrombosis

Treatment of chronic mesenteric venous thrombosis is directed at controlling gastrointestinal bleeding, which usually is from esophageal varices. Sclerotherapy, various portosystemic shunts, devascularization procedures, and resection of bowel (when the bleeding arises from intestinal varices) all have a place in selected patients. No surgical treatment is indicated for asymptomatic chronic mesenteric venous thrombosis when the collateral venous drainage is adequate to prevent bleeding from portal hypertension.

Results of Therapy for Mesenteric Venous Thrombosis

The mortality rate for acute mesenteric venous thrombosis is lower than for the other forms of acute mesenteric ischemia, ranging from 20% to 50%. The overall recurrence rate has been 20% to 25%, but falls to 13% to 15% if heparin therapy is instituted promptly when the diagnosis is made.

In the past, almost all patients with acute mesenteric venous thrombosis had some infarcted bowel. This was true of the patients in our series as well. However, the amount of bowel resected was significantly less than in patients with arterial forms of acute mesenteric ischemia. The mean length of bowel resected in our series was 151 cm, with a range of 43 to 450 cm. There was no correlation between the length of involved bowel and mortality. Ninety-five percent of our patients had segmental involvement of the jejunum, the ileum, or both; 5% had involvement of the terminal ileum and right colon.

The natural history of chronic mesenteric venous thrombosis is not known. It appears that less than half of patients never develop bowel infarction. Many patients have no symptoms. The percentage of patients who have late gastrointestinal bleeding has not been determined but probably is small. As mesenteric venous thrombosis is recognized more frequently, our understanding of the natural history of this disorder should increase.

CHRONIC MESENTERIC ARTERIAL ISCHEMIA

Chronic mesenteric arterial ischemia results from inadequate perfusion of the midgut during periods of increased oxygen demand. The oxygen requirements of the bowel increase significantly in the postprandial period because of rises in motility, secretion, and absorption, all of which are energy-dependent functions. Although experimental studies have shown increases in mesenteric blood flow after meals, vascular resistance also increases during peristalsis, impairing intramural perfusion. In normal individuals, these changes in blood flow are well tolerated and lead to no untoward effects; in patients with impaired mesenteric circulation resulting from atherosclerotic disease, oxygen requirements can exceed oxygen delivery, resulting in cellular hypoxia. This hypoxic injury is manifested by ischemic visceral pain and abnormalities in gastrointestinal absorption or motility. The pain is similar to that which arises in the myocardium with angina pectoris or in the calf with intermittent claudication.

Atherosclerotic involvement of the large mesenteric arteries is almost always the cause of this form of intestinal ischemia; however, small vessel diseases such as thromboangiitis obliterans (Buerger's disease) or polyarteritis nodosa also can produce chronic intestinal ischemia. Although partial or complete occlusion of the celiac artery, the SMA, or the IMA is fairly common in the general population, relatively few patients have chronic intestinal ischemia. Moreover, many patients with occlusion of two or even three of these vessels never have symptoms.

Clinical Features

The one consistent feature of chronic mesenteric ischemia is abdominal pain. Most commonly, this occurs 10 to 15 minutes after meals, gradually increases in severity, finally reaches a plateau, and then slowly dissipates over the course of 1 to 3 hours. The pain pattern is so intimately associated with eating that patients reduce their food intake and experience massive weight loss. Bloating, flatulence, and derangements in motility with constipation or diarrhea also occur.

The physical findings rarely are helpful, although the presence of an abdominal bruit has been reported in up to 75% of patients. Occasionally, patients have occult blood in the stool. Weight loss in the setting of occult fecal blood often leads to an unproductive search for a gastrointestinal malignancy.

Diagnosis

Postprandial abdominal pain associated with weight loss strongly suggests chronic intestinal ischemia. No specific, reliable diagnostic test is available for abdominal angina. The diagnosis must be based on the clinical symptoms, the arteriographic demonstration of occlusion of the splanchnic arteries, and, to a great degree, the exclusion of other gastrointestinal diseases.

Angiographic evaluation includes flush aortography in the frontal and lateral views and selective injection of the SMA, the celiac artery, and the IMA. The degree of occlusion of the three major arteries can be assessed best on the lateral projections and the collateral circulation and patterns of flow are most evident on the frontal views (Fig. 32-17). The presence of prominent collateral vessels not only indicates significant stenosis of a major vessel, but also connotes a chronic process. Stenosis or occlusion of one or more of the major visceral vessels demonstrated on an angiogram does not by itself establish the diagnosis of arterial insufficiency.

In the past, the prevention of acute intestinal infarction was considered a justification for early surgical intervention. However, over 75% of cases of acute mesenteric ischemia are caused by embolus or nonocclusive disease, and in neither condition are prodromal symptoms present, nor has the incidence of intestinal infarction in patients with chronic occlusive disease of the splanchnic vessels been established. The fear of impending intestinal infarction, therefore, is not a sufficient indication for operation. There is one special case in which reconstruction or bypass of obstructed visceral

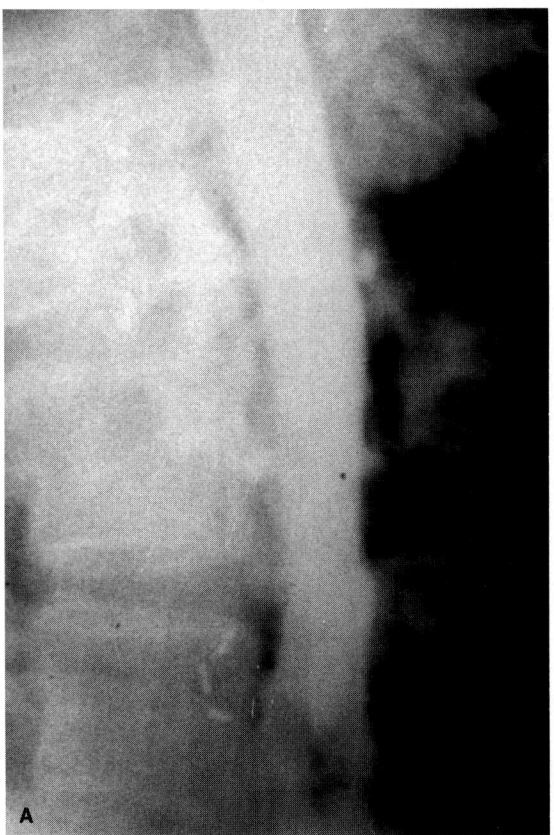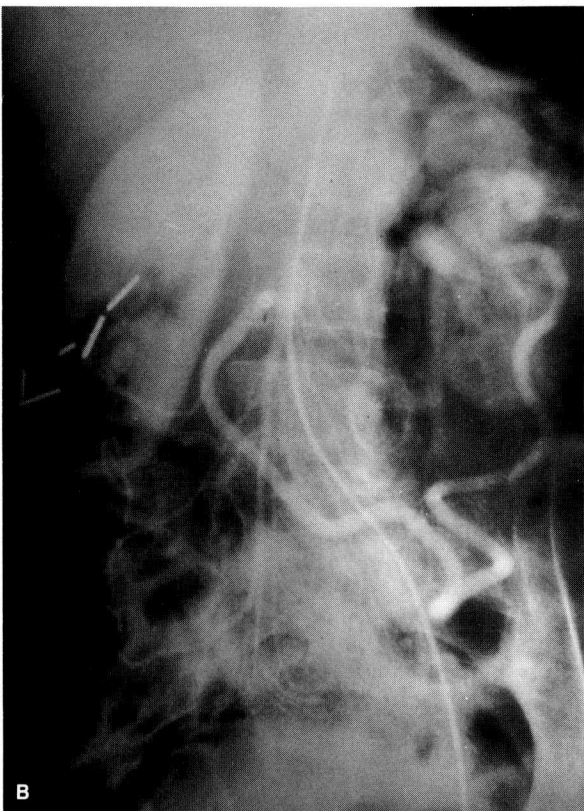

Figure 32-17 Chronic versus acute superior mesenteric artery (SMA) occlusion. **(A)** Lateral projection showing occlusion of major vessels. **(B)** Chronic occlusion with a large meandering artery providing collateral flow to the SMA through the middle colic artery. (Boley SJ, Brandt LJ, Veith FJ. Ischemic disorders of the intestines. Curr Probl Surg 1978;15:55)

arteries is recommended in the absence of chronic abdominal pain. This occurs in patients who are undergoing aortic reconstruction for peripheral vascular disease and in whom aortography demonstrates occlusive disease of the SMA or celiac artery and the presence of a large meandering artery.

Management

The difficulty in establishing an unequivocal diagnosis of chronic mesenteric ischemia, the fragility of these elderly patients, and the risks of a major operation for revascularization of the gut have made the selection of patients for surgery difficult. More recently, limited success with balloon angioplasty, which can be performed with much less morbidity, has made it less critical to establish the diagnosis with absolute certainty before undertaking treatment.

With no available method for measuring intestinal blood flow accurately, precise criteria to define the need for operative arterial reconstruction are lacking. There is agreement that patients with the typical pain of abdominal angina and unexplained weight loss, whose diagnostic evaluations have excluded other gastrointestinal diseases and whose angiograms show occlusive involvement of at least two of the three major mesenteric arteries, should benefit from revascularization. The issue is less clear if only one major vessel is involved or if the clinical presentation is atypical. Lacking a quantitative test, most patients with atypical symptoms are observed. Revascularization is indicated when pain and weight loss do not respond to other treatment and balloon angioplasty is unsuccessful, even if only one vessel is occluded.

Patients with chronic intestinal ischemia often are severely malnourished and generally require a period of parenteral alimentation before revascularization. Albumin levels and prothrombin times should be corrected before intervention is undertaken. Vitamin deficiencies also can be apparent and require supplementation with parenteral folate, vitamin C, vitamin K, thiamine, or vitamin B_{12}.

Several procedures have been advocated for restoring normal flow and pressure distal to an occlusion of the SMA or celiac artery, including reimplantation, endarterectomy, and bypass. The preferred procedure is bypass to the SMA distal to the occlusion, although several surgeons believe that both the SMA and the celiac artery must be revascularized if both are occluded.

Reimplantation

Reimplantation is performed by transecting the artery distal to the occlusion and performing an anastomosis directly to the aorta. This procedure is technically difficult because of the short length of available vessel and the presence of severe aortic atherosclerotic disease in the region of the takeoff of the celiac artery and SMA trunks. Reimplantation should be reserved solely for those situations in which the aorta is being replaced and the revascularization is done as a preventive measure.

Endarterectomy

Endarterectomy has been attempted both through the diseased vessel and through the aorta itself (Fig. 32-18). Both procedures are technically difficult and

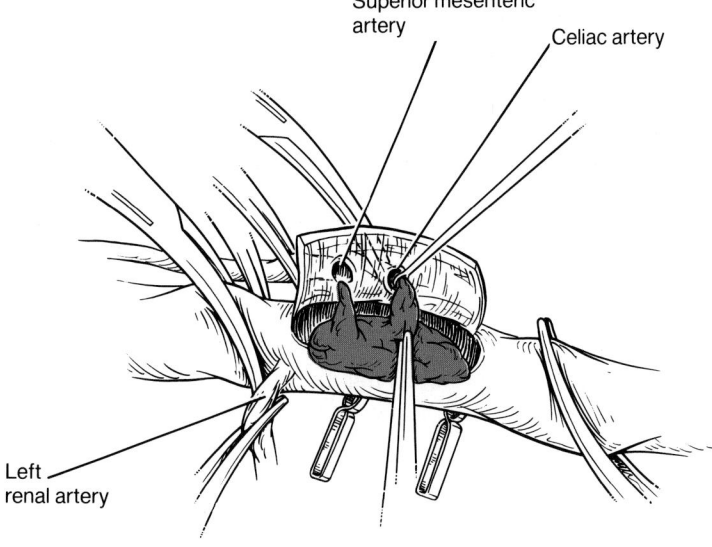

Figure 32-18 Diagrammatic representation of trapdoor aortotomy circumscribing the visceral orifices. Note total proximal and distal aortic occlusion and control of individual intercostal arteries. Trapdoor has been opened and is hinged on the right aortic wall. The endarterectomy is proceeding with removal of the superior mesenteric artery lesion. (Cunningham CG, Reilly LM, Rapp JH, Schneider PA, Stoney RJ. Chronic visceral ischemia: three decades of progress. Ann Surg 1991;214:276)

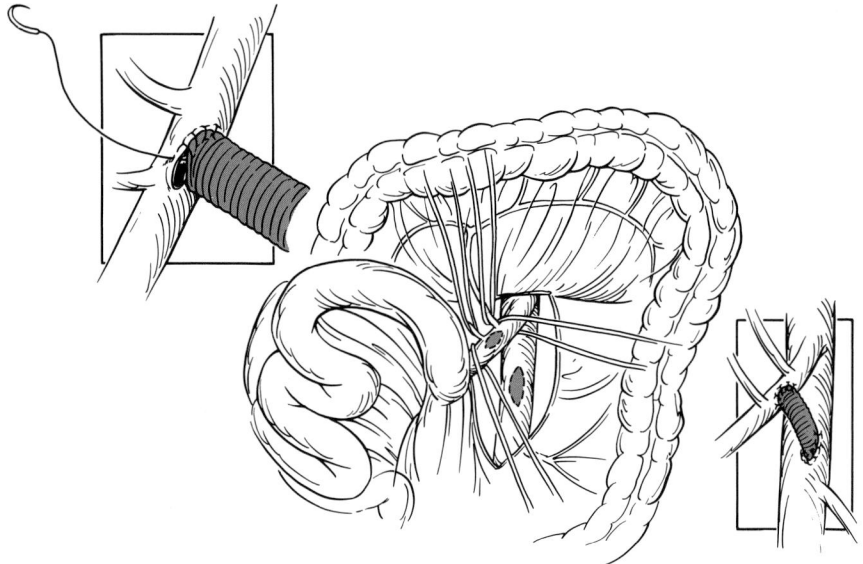

Figure 32-19 Technique of aorta–to–superior mesenteric artery (SMA) bypass. An incision in the retroperitoneum has been made over the aorta and carried superiorly to divide the ligament of Treitz. This provides exposure of the aorta and the SMA in the region of the middle colic artery. Sites of the anastomosis are shown. The left inset shows the fine suture technique of anastomosis. The right inset shows the completed anastomosis. (Boley SJ, Brandt LJ, Veith FJ. Ischemic disorders of the intestines. In: Ravitch MM, ed. Curr Probl Surg 1978;15:55)

can result in embolization of atheromatous fragments into the distal visceral and systemic circulations. The transarterial approach usually is unsuccessful because the most proximal extent of the occlusion is difficult to remove safely. The transaortic trapdoor endarterectomy requires crossclamping the aorta in the supraceliac position, which increases the possibility of ischemic injury to the kidneys and distal circulation. Although this approach is completely autogenous and offers the theoretic advantage of clearing both the visceral and renal vessels, the extensive nature of the operation makes it applicable to few patients.

Bypass

Mesenteric bypass from the aorta or the iliac artery to the side of the SMA distal to the occlusion is the procedure of choice (Fig. 32-19). Reversed autologous saphenous vein is the preferred graft material. Polytetrafluoroethylene or knitted Dacron are suitable substitutes if the saphenous vein is unavailable or smaller than 5 mm in diameter.

The optimal site of origin of the graft has been debated. Because of the mobility of the SMA, grafts originating from the infrarenal aorta can become occluded with movement of the mesentery of the small intestine. In addition, late failure due to progressive atherosclerotic disease of the infrarenal aorta has led some surgeons to use the supraceliac aorta as the inflow for the graft (Fig. 32-20). Occasionally, it is necessary to use the iliac artery as the inflow for the graft when dissection of the supraceliac aorta is difficult and the infrarenal aorta is too diseased.

Results of Therapy for Chronic Mesenteric Ischemia

Patency rates of bypass grafts to the SMA and celiac artery have been generally good, and symptomatic relief in properly selected patients has been excellent. Stoney and associates, however, have reported poor results with retrograde bypass procedures. They attribute this to an unusual and rapidly progressive form of atherosclerosis that involves the subdiaphragmatic aorta and that occurs more commonly in women and in relatively young patients. On the basis of their extensive experience, they advocate either an antegrade prosthetic bypass from the supraceliac aorta by a transabdominal approach or a thoracoabdominal retroperitoneal trapdoor endarterectomy.[120]

FOCAL INTESTINAL ISCHEMIA

Ischemic insults localized to short segments of the small intestine produce a broad spectrum of clinical features without the life-threatening systemic consequences associated with damage to more extensive portions of the gut. The most frequent causes are atheromatous or small thrombotic emboli, strangulated hernias, blunt abdominal trauma, and segmental venous thrombosis. In the late 1960s, enteric-coated thiazide–potassium chloride preparations caused short ulcerating stenoses that proved to be localized venous infarctions. Focal ischemia associated with systemic collagen vascular diseases can occur late in the course of the illness or can be the heralding event of the generalized disorder.

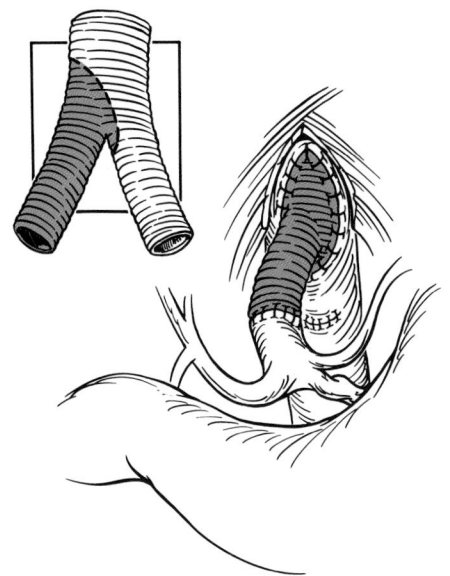

Figure 32-20 Antegrade aortovisceral bypass to the celiac axis. (Wylie EJ, Stoney RJ, Ehrenfeld WK. Manual of vascular surgery, vol 1. New York, Springer-Verlag, 1980:211)

Clinical Features

Pathophysiology

Focal intestinal ischemia usually occurs in the presence of adequate collateral circulation to prevent transmural hemorrhagic infarction. Infected infarcts can occur from partial necrosis of the bowel wall and secondary invasion by intestinal bacterial flora. Limited tissue necrosis can result in complete healing, a chronic enteritis simulating Crohn's disease, or a stricture with partial or complete intestinal obstruction. Transmural necrosis with perforation or localized peritonitis can follow a severe local insult.

Presentation

The presentation of short segment ischemic bowel injury differs according to the severity of the infarct. In the acute presentation, seen with transmural necrosis, there is a sudden onset of abdominal pain that often mimics acute appendicitis. Such patients have clinical signs of peritonitis and sepsis. Another common presentation is that of chronic enteritis, with cramping abdominal pain, diarrhea, fever, and weight loss. This clinical picture is indistinguishable from Crohn's disease of the small intestine. The most common presentation, however, is that of chronic small bowel obstruction, with or without a history of some antecedent episode of trauma, pain, or hernia incarceration. Cramping abdominal pain, distention, and vomiting are the direct results of the obstruction, and bacterial

overgrowth in the dilated loop proximal to the obstruction can lead to the metabolic and clinical derangements associated with the blind loop syndrome (ie, anemia, diarrhea, and steatorrhea). A preoperative diagnosis of focal ischemia is difficult to make. A previous episode of transient pain, trauma, incarcerated hernia, or a known systemic illness can suggest the correct diagnosis.

Diagnosis and Management

The treatment of acute focal intestinal ischemia usually is surgical, but some patients without signs of peritonitis can be treated expectantly. In those instances, the diagnosis is based on the radiologic findings of thumbprinting indicative of acute ischemia. Serial studies should reveal an improving pattern. Both clinical and radiologic findings must resolve or the nonoperative approach is abandoned.

Patients with chronic enteritis or obstruction should undergo surgical exploration after proper preparation. A limited resection is the procedure of choice for both focal enteritis and obstructing lesions.

REFERENCES

1. Geber WF. Quantitative measurements of blood flow in various areas of the small and large bowel. Am J Physiol 1960;198:985.
2. Delaney JP, Leonard AS. Hypothalamic influence on gastrointestinal blood flow in the awake cat. Fed Proc 1970;29:260.
3. Quirke P, Campbell I, Talbot IC. Ischaemic proctitis and adventitial fibromuscular dysplasia of the superior rectal artery. Br J Surg 1984;71:33.
4. Binns JC, Issacson P. Age-related changes in the colonic blood supply: their relevance to ischaemic colitis. Gut 1978;19:384.
5. Brandt L, Boley S, Goldberg L, Mitsudo S, Berman A. Colitis in the elderly: a reappraisal. Am J Gastroenterol 1981;76:239.
6. Wright HG. Ulcerating colitis in the elderly: epidemiological and clinical study of an in-patient hospital population. Submitted as thesis for M.D. degree, Yale University, 1970.
7. Brandt LJ, Boley SJ. Colonic ischemia. Surg Clin North Am 1992;72:203.
8. Ho MS, Teh LB, Goh HS. Ischaemic colitis in systemic lupus erythematosus: report of a case and review of the literature. Ann Acad Med Singapore 1987;16:501.
9. Tedesco FJ, Volpicelli NA, Moore FS. Estrogen and progesterone associated colitis: a disorder with clinical and endoscopic features mimicking Crohn's colitis. Gastrointest Endosc 1982;28:247.

10. Barcewicz PA, Welch JP. Ischemic colitis in young adult patients. Dis Colon Rectum 1980;23:109.

11. Miyata T, Tamechika Y, Torisu M. Ischemic colitis in a 33 year old woman on danazol treatment for endometriosis. Am J Gastroenterol 1988;83:1420.

12. Schmitt W, Wagner-Thiessen E, Lux G. Ischaemic colitis in a patient treated with glypressin for bleeding oesophageal varices. Hepatogastroenterology 1987;34:134.

13. Wright A, Benfield GF, Felix-Davies D. Ischaemic colitis and immune complexes during gold therapy for rheumatoid arthritis. Ann Rheum Dis 1984;43:495.

14. Gollock JM, Thompson JP. Ischaemic colitis associated with psychotropic drugs. Postgrad Med J 1984;26:449.

15. Gage TP, Gagnier JM. Ischemic colitis complicating sickle cell crisis. Gastroenterology 1983;84:171.

16. Dubois A, Lyonnet P, Cohendy R, et al. Ischemic colitis as a manifestation of Moschkowitz's syndrome. Ann Gastroenterol Hepatol (Paris) 1989;25:19.

17. Blanc P, Bories P, Donadio D, et al. Colite ischemique et thromboses veineuses recidivante par deficit familial en proteine S. (Letter) Gastroenterol Clin Biol 1989;13:945.

18. Knot EAR, Ten Cate JW, Bruin T, Iburg AHC, Tytgat GNJ. Antithrombin III metabolism in two colitis patients with acquired antithrombin III deficiency. Gastroenterology 1985;89:421.

19. Heer M, Repond F, Hany A, Sulser H, Kehl O, Jäger K. Acute ischaemic colitis in a female long distance runner. Gut 1987;28:896.

20. Fishel R, Hamamoto G, Barbul A, Jiji V, Efron G. Cocaine colitis: is this a new syndrome? Dis Colon Rectum 1985;28:264.

21. Guttorson NL, Bubrick MP. Mortality from colonic ischemia. Dis Colon Rectum 1989;32:469.

22. Boley SJ, Agrawal GP, Warren AR, et al. Pathophysiologic effects of bowel distention on intestinal blood flow. Am J Surg 1969;117:228.

23. Kozarek RA, Emest DL, Silverman ME. Air pressure induced colon injury during diagnostic colonoscopy. Gastroenterology 1980;78:7.

24. Brandt LJ, Boley SJ, Sammartano RJ. Carbon dioxide and room air insufflation of the colon. Gastrointest Endosc 1986;32:324.

25. Boley SJ, Brandt LJ, Veith FJ. Ischemic disorders of the intestine. Curr Probl Surg 1978;15:1.

26. Ernst CB, Hagihara PF, Daugherty ME, Satchello CR, Griffen WO Jr. Ischemic colitis incidence after abdominal aortic reconstruction: a prospective study. Surgery 1976;80:417.

27. Zelenock GB, Strodel WE, Knol JA, et al. A prospective study of clinically and endoscopically documented colonic ischemia in 100 patients undergoing aortic reconstructive surgery with aggressive colonic and direct pelvic revascularization, compared with historic controls. Surgery 1989;106:771.

28. Hagihara PF, Ernst CB, Griffen WO Jr. Incidence of ischemic colitis after abdominal aortic reconstruction. Surg Gynecol Obstet 1979;149:571.

29. Kim MW, Hundahl SA, Dang CR, McNamara JJ, Straehley CJ, Whelan TJ Jr. Ischemic colitis after aortic aneurysmectomy. Am J Surg 1983;145:392.

30. Ernst CB, Hagihara PF, Daugherty ME, Griffen WO Jr. Inferior mesenteric artery stump pressure: a reliable index for safe IMA ligation during abdominal aortic aneurysmectomy. Ann Surg 1978;187:641.

31. Fiddian-Green RG, Amelin PM, Hermmann JB. Prediction of the development of sigmoid ischemia on the day of aortic surgery. Arch Surg 1986;121:654.

32. Poole JW, Sammartano RJ, Boley SJ, Miller L, Stretch J, Veith FJ. The use of tonometry to detect sigmoid ischemia during aneurysmectomy. Presented at the New York Surgical Society, November, 1987.

33. Teitjen GW, Markowitz AM. Colitis proximal to obstructing colonic carcinoma. Arch Surg 1975;110:1133.

34. Dahlberg PJ, Kisken WA, Newcomer KL, Yutuc WR. Mesenteric ischemia in chronic dialysis patients. Am J Nephrol 1985;5:327.

35. Dumazer P, Dueymes JM, Vernier I, Thierry FX, Conte JJ. Ischemie mesenterique non occlusive chez l'hemodialyse periodique. Presse Med 1989;18:471.

36. Chiu CJ, McArdle AH, Brown R, Scott HJ, Gurd FN. Intestinal mucosal lesion in low-flow states. I. A morphological, hemodynamic, and metabolic reappraisal. Arch Surg 1970;101:478.

37. Redfors S, Hallback DA, Haglund U, et al. Blood flow distribution, villous tissue osmolality and fluid and electrolyte transport in the cat intestine during regional hypotension. Acta Physiol Scand 1963;57:270.

38. Lundgren O, Svanik J. Mucosal hemodynamics in the small intestine of the cat during reduced perfusion pressure. Acta Physiol Scand 1973;88:551.

39. Folkow B. Regional adjustments of intestinal blood flow. Gastroenterology 1967;52:423.

40. Shephard AP, Granger DN. Metabolic regulation of the intestinal circulation. In: Shepherd AP, Granger DN, eds. Physiology of the splanchnic circulation. New York, Raven Press, 1984:38.

41. Poole JW, Sammartano RJ, Boley SJ. The use of tonometry in the early diagnosis of mesenteric ischemia. Curr Surg 1987;44:21.

42. Spjut HJ, Margulis AR, McAlister WH. Microangiographic study of gastrointestinal lesions. AJR 1964;92:1173.

43. Gershon MD, Erde SM. The nervous system of the gut. Gastroenterology 1980;80:1571.

44. Banks RO, Gallavan RH, Zinner MJ, et al. Vasoactive agents in control of the mesenteric circulation. Fed Proc 1985;44:2743.

45. Rothe CF. Reflex control of veins and vascular capacitance. Physiol Rev 1983;63:1281.

46. Jacob H, Brandt LJ, Farkas P, Frishman W. Beta-adrenergic blockade and the gastrointestinal system. Am J Med 1983;74:1042.

47. Said SI. Vasoactive peptides: state of the art review. Hypertension 1983;5(Suppl 1):17.

48. Bulkley GB, Womack WA, Downey JM, Kvietys PR,

Granger DN. Collateral blood flow in segmental intestinal ischemia: effects of vasoactive agents. Surgery 1986;100:157.

49. Gunther S, Gimbrvne MA Jr, Alexander RW. Identification and characterization of the high affinity vascular angiotensin II receptor in rat mesenteric artery. Circ Res 1980;47:278.

50. Bailey RW, Bulkley GB, Hamilton SR, Morris JB, Haglund UH. Protection of the small intestine from nonocclusive mesenteric ischemia injury due to cardiogenic shock. Am J Surg 1987;153:108.

51. Chapnick BM, Feigen LP, Hyman AL, Kadowitz PJ. Differential effects of prostaglandins in the mesenteric vascular bed. Am J Physiol 1978;235:H326.

52. Gerkens JF, Shand DG, Flexner C, Nies AS, Oates JA, Data JL. Effect of indomethacin and aspirin on gastric blood flow and acid secretion. J Pharmacol Exp Ther 1977;203:646.

53. Boley SJ, Schultz L, Krieger H, Schwartz S, Elguezabal A, Allen AC. Experimental evaluation of thiazides and potassium as a cause of small-bowel ulcer. JAMA 1965;192:763.

54. Boley SJ, Allen AC, Schultz L, Schwartz S. Potassium-induced lesions of the small bowel. I. Clinical aspects. JAMA 1965;193:997.

55. Premen AJ, Kvietys PR, Granger DN. Postprandial regulation of intestinal blood flow: role of gastrointestinal hormones. Am J Physiol 1985;249:G250.

56. Kukovetz WR, Poch G. Inhibition of cyclic 3',5'-nucleotide phosphodiesterase as a possible mode of action of papaverine and similarly acting drugs. Naunyn Schmiedebergs Arch Pharmacol 1970;267:189.

57. Boorstein JM, Dacey W, Cronenwett JL. Pharmacologic treatment of occlusive mesenteric ischemia. J Sci Res 1988;44:555.

58. Boley SJ, Regan JA, Tunick PA, Everhard ME, Winslow PR, Veith FJ. Persistent vasoconstriction: a major factor in nonocclusive mesenteric ischemia. Curr Top Surg Res 1971;3:425.

59. Selkurt EE, Scibetta MP, Cull TE. Hemodynamics of intestinal circulation. Circ Res 1958;6:92.

60. Laufman H. Significance of vasospasm in vascular occlusion. Thesis. Chicago, Northwestern University Medical School, 1948.

61. Brown RA, Chiu CJ, Scott HJ, Gurd FN. Ultrastructural changes in the canine ileal mucosal cell after mesenteric arterial occlusion: a sequential study. Arch Surg 1970;101:290.

62. Ahren C, Haglund U. Mucosal lesions in the small intestine of the cat during low flow. Acta Physiol Scand 1973;88:1.

63. Chiu CJ, McArdle C. Intestinal mucosal lesion in low flow states. Arch Surg 1970;101:478.

64. Granger DN, McCord JM, Parks DA, Hollwarth ME. Xanthine oxidase inhibitors attenuate ischemia-induced vascular permeability changes in the cat intestine. Gastroenterology 1986;90:80.

65. Crissinger KD, Granger DN. Mucosal injury induced by ischemia and reperfusion in the piglet intestine: influence of the age and feeding. Gastroenterology 1989;97:920.

66. Parks DA, Grøgaard B, Granger DN. Comparison of partial and complete arterial occlusion models for studying intestinal ischemia. Surgery 1982;92:896.

67. Bulkley GB, Kvietys PR, Parks DA, Perry MA, Granger DN. Relationship of blood flow and oxygen consumption to ischemic injury in the canine small intestine. Gastroenterology 1985;89:852.

68. Gaussorgues P, Gueugniaud PY, Vedrinne JM, Salord F, Mercatello A, Robert D. Bacteremia after cardiac arrest and cardiopulmonary resuscitation. Intens Care Med 1988;14:575.

69. Thompson JS, Bragg LE, West WW. Serum enzyme levels during intestinal ischemia. Ann Surg 1990;211:369.

70. Smerud MJ, Johnson CD, Stephens DH. Diagnosis of bowel infarction: a comparison of plain films and CT scans in 23 cases. AJR 1990;154:99.

71. Serreyn RF, Schoofs PR, Baetens PR, Vandekerckhove D. Laparoscopic diagnosis of mesenteric venous thrombosis. Endoscopy 1986;18:249.

72. Segelman SS, Sprayregen S, Boley SJ. Angiographic diagnosis of mesenteric arterial vasoconstriction. Radiology 1974;122:533.

73. Stolar CJ, Randolph JG. Evaluation of ischemic bowel viability with a fluorescent technique. J Pediatr Surg 1978;3:221.

74. Carter MS, Fantini GA, Sammartano RJ, Mitsudo S, Silverman DG, Boley SJ. Qualitative and quantitative fluorescein fluorescence in determining intestinal viability. Am J Surg 1984;l147:117.

75. Shah S, Andersen C. Prediction of small bowel viability using Doppler ultrasound. Ann Surg 1981;194:97.

76. Brolin RE, Semmlow JL, Koch RA, Reddell MT, Mast BA, Mackenzie JW. Myoelectric assessment of bowel viability. Surgery 1987;102:32.

77. Shaw RS. The "second-look" after superior mesenteric arterial embolectomy or reconstruction for mesenteric infarction. In: Ellison EH, Frieser SR, Mulholland JH, eds. Current surgical management. Philadelphia, WB Saunders, 1965:509.

78. Sachs SM, Morton JH, Schwartz SI. Acute mesenteric ischemia. Surgery 1982;92:646.

79. Cohn I, Floyd CE, Dresden CF, Bornside GH. Strangulation obstruction in germ-free animals. Ann Surg 1962;156:692.

80. Wells CL. Relationship between intestinal microecology and the translocation of intestinal bacteria. Antonie Van Leeuwenhoek 1990;58:87.

81. Vujic I, Stanley J, Gobien RP. Treatment of acute embolus of the superior mesenteric artery by topical infusion of streptokinase. Cardiovasc Intervent Radiol 1984;7:94.

82. Becker GJ, Katzen BT, Dake MD. Noncoronary angioplasty. Radiology 1989;170:921.

83. Clark RA, Gallant TE. Acute mesenteric ischemia: angiographic spectrum. AJR 1984;142:555.

84. Boley SJ, Sprayregan S, Siegelman SS, Veith FJ. Initial results from an aggressive roentgenological and surgical approach to acute mesenteric ischemia. Surgery 1977;82:848.

85. Hibbard JS, Swenson JC, Levin AG. Roentgenology of mesenteric vascular occlusion. Arch Surg 1933;26:20.

86. Koveker G, Reichow W, Becker HD. Ergebnisse der Therapie des akuten Mesenterial gefassverschlusses. Langenbecks Arch Chir 1985;366:536.

87. Levy PJ, Krausz MM, Manny J. Acute mesenteric ischemia: improved results: a retrospective analysis of 92 patients. Surgery 1990;107:373.

88. Batellier J, Kieny R. Superior mesenteric artery embolism: 82 cases. Ann Vasc Surg 1990;4:112.

89. Finucane PM, Arunachalam T, O'Dowd J, Pathy MSJ. Acute mesenteric infarction in elderly patients. J Am Geriatr Soc 1989;37:355.

90. Georgiev G. Acute obstruction of the mesenteric vessels: a diagnostic and therapeutic problem. Chirurgia 1989;42:23.

91. Paes E, Vollmar JF, Hutschenreiter S, Schoenberg MH, Kübel R, Schölzel E. Der mesenterialinfarkt: neue aspekte der diagnostik und therapie. Der Chirurg 1988;59:828.

92. Clavien PA, Muller C. Infarctus mesenterique: etude retrospoective sur 17 ans. Schweiz Med Wochenschr 1986;116:977.

93. Rogers DM, Thompson JE, Garrett WV, Talkington CM, Patman RD. Mesenteric vascular problems: a 26-year experience. Ann Surg 1982;195:554.

94. Krausz MM, Manny J. Acute superior mesenteric arterial occlusion: a plea for early diagnosis. Surgery 1978;l83:482.

95. Hansen HJB, Christofferson JK. Occlusive mesenteric infarction: a retrospective study of 83 cases. Acta Chir Scand 1976;472(Suppl):103.

96. White R, Boley SJ. Mesenteric venous thrombosis (MVT): an unusual cause of acute mesenteric ischemia. Read before the 50th Annual Scientific Meeting of the American College of Gastroenterology, Philadelphia, October 9–11, 1985.

97. Abdu RA, Zakhaur BJ, Dallis DJ. Mesenteric venous thrombosis: 1911 to 1984. Surgery 1987;101:383.

98. Broekmans AW, van Rooyen W, Westerveld BD, Briët E, Bertina RM. Mesenteric vein thrombosis as presenting manifestation of hereditary protein S deficiency. Gastroenterology 1988;92:240.

99. Harward TRS, Green D, Bergan JJ, Rizzo RJ, Yao JST. Mesenteric venous thrombosis. J Vasc Surg 1989;9:328.

100. Kaleya RN, Boley SJ. Mesenteric venous thrombosis. In: Najarian JS, Delaney JP, eds. Progress in gastrointestinal surgery. Chicago, Year Book, 1989:417.

101. Thatcher BS, Sivak MV, Ferguson DR, Petras RE. Mesenteric venous thrombosis as a possible complication of endoscopic sclerotherapy: a report of two cases. Am J Gastroenterol 1986;81:126.

102. Clavien PA, Durig M, Harder F. Venous mesenteric thrombosis: a particular entity. Br J Surg 1988;75:252.

103. Clavien PA, Huber O, Mirescu D, Rohner A. Contrast enhanced CT scan as a diagnostic procedure in mesenteric ischaemia due to mesenteric venous thrombosis. Br J Surg 1989;76:93.

104. Sack J, Aldrete JS. Primary mesenteric venous thrombosis. Surg Gyneçol Obstet 1982;154:205.

105. Matthews J, White RR. Primary mesenteric venous occlusive disease. Am J Surg 1971;122:579.

106. Bertina RM. Hereditary protein S deficiency. Haemostasis 1985;15:241.

107. Johnson CC, Baggenstoss AH. Mesenteric venous occlusion: study of 99 cases of occlusion of veins. Mayo Clin Proc 1949;24:628.

108. Warshaw AL, Gongliang J, Ottinger LW. Recognition and clinical implications of mesenteric and portal vein obstruction in chronic pancreatitis. Arch Surg 1987;122:410.

109. Anane-Sehaf JC, Blair E. Primary mesenteric venous occlusive disease. Surg Gynecol Obstet 1975;41:740.

110. Clemett AR, Chang J. The radiological diagnosis of spontaneous mesenteric venous thrombosis. Am J Gastroenterol 1975;63:209.

111. Kidambi H, Herbert R, Kidami AV. Ultrasonic demonstration of superior mesenteric and splenoportal venous thrombosis. J Clin Ultrasound 1986;14:199.

112. Matos C, Van Gansbeke D, Zalcman M, et al. Mesenteric venous thrombosis: early CT and US diagnosis and conservative management. Gastrointest Radiol 1986;11:322.

113. Rosen A, Korobkin M, Silverman PM, Dunnick NR, Kelvin FM. Mesenteric vein thrombosis: CT identification. AJR 1984;143:83.

114. Al Karawi MA, Quaiz M, Clark D, Hilali A, Mohamed AE, Jawdat M. Mesenteric vein thrombosis: non-invasive diagnosis and follow-up (US + MRI) and non-invasive therapy by streptokinase and anticoagulants. Hepatogastroenterology 1990;37:507.

115. Smith RW, Selby JB. Scintiangiographic diagnosis of acute mesenteric ischemia. AJR 1979;132:67.

116. Verbanck JJ, Rutgeerts LJ, Haerens MH, et al. Partial splenoportal and superior mesenteric venous thrombosis: early sonographic diagnosis and successful conservative management. Gastroenterology 1984;86:949.

117. Khodadadi J, Rosencwajg J, Nacasch N, Schmidt B, Feuchtwanger MM. Mesenteric vein thrombosis: the importance of a second-look operation. Arch Surg 1980;112:315.

118. Bergentz SE, Ericsson B, Hedner U, Leandoer L, Nilsson IM. Thrombosis in the superior mesenteric and portal veins: report of a case treated with thrombectomy. Surgery 1974;76:286.

119. Lanthier P, Lepot M, Mahieu P. Mesenteric venous thrombosis presenting as a neurological problem. Acta Clin Belg 1984;29:92.

120. Cunningham CG, Reilly LM, Stoney R. Chronic visceral ischemia. Surg Clin North Am 1992;72:231.

Digestive Tract Surgery: A Text and Atlas, edited by Richard H. Bell, Layton F. Rikkers, and Michael W. Mulholland. Lippincott-Raven Publishers, Philadelphia, © 1996.

33

Neoplastic Disease of the Small Intestine

Steven E. Raper

Neoplastic disease of the small intestine can be either benign or malignant, with lesions arising from an epithelial or mesenchymal origin. Cancers of the small intestine are rare compared with cancers of the esophagus, stomach, or colon. Predisposing factors for the development of cancer of the small intestine include the familial polyposis syndromes, Crohn's disease, and celiac sprue. In most clinical series, malignant tumors are more common, whereas in autopsy series, benign tumors are more common. This discrepancy has led to the notion that most malignant tumors cause symptoms, whereas a significant proportion of benign tumors are discovered incidentally. Diagnosis requires suspicion and the use of diagnostic studies such as enteroclysis or computed tomography (CT). Surgery is the treatment of choice for benign lesions that cause symptoms. Surgery is the only hope for cure of malignant lesions and can provide significant palliation if cure is not possible.

BENIGN TUMORS

Pathology

Benign tumors of the small intestine can arise from the epithelium, lymphoid tissue, or mesenchymal elements. Adenomas of the small intestine are histologically similar to those of the large bowel, an both tubular and villous features may be present. The periampullary area is the most common site for villous tumors in the duodenum. In one series,[1] 90% of sporadic and familial polyposis villous tumors were seen in the second portion of the duodenum. The association of familial adenomatous polyposis and duodenal tumors is discussed later. Brunner's gland adenomas arise from submucosal duodenal glands but are histologically similar to hamartomas in other locations in the small intestine. Leiomyomas are lobulated and arise from smooth muscle cells of the muscularis propria or blood vessel wall.

Clinical Presentation

Benign tumors rarely present in childhood and usually begin to cause symptoms by the sixth decade. Intermittent pain from partial obstruction or emesis are the most frequent manifestations. Intussusception is a common mechanism of obstruction. Benign tumors are rarely palpable. Guaiac-positive stool is present in up to 25% of cases. Weight loss, massive hemorrhage, and melena are unusual in benign lesions, and these symptoms indicate a malignant process. Benign tumors are biochemically silent, and the diarrhea and flushing observed with carcinoid tumors do not occur.

Therapy

Adenomas

All three types of duodenal adenomas are amenable to endoscopic resection. Tubular and tubulovillous adenomas are pedunculated, have a low malignant potential, and can be excised piecemeal if necessary. Villous adenomas, especially those larger than 3 cm, have a malignant potential similar to that of colonic tumors, and total excision is necessary. Up to 30% of large benign tumors harbor foci of invasive cancer. Pedunculated lesions can be excised endoscopically, but sessile lesions, especially in the region of the ampulla of Vater, should be treated with local operative excision if possible or with pancreaticoduodenectomy if not.

Lipomas and Leiomyomas

Lipomas and leiomyomas have similar radiographic features, usually appearing as ovoid, eccentric, extraluminal masses arising from submucosal adipose tissue or vessel walls. They arise most often in the jejunum and on cut section have either a yellow and fatty (lipoma) or fibrous, firm, and gray-white (leiomyoma) appearance. If an asymptomatic lipoma is diagnosed by CT, observation is recommended. For symptomatic lipomas, leiomyomas, and lesions in which histologic identification is not possible, segmental resection is performed.

Hamartomas

Brunner's gland adenomas usually do not cause symptoms and excision is not often necessary. Hamartomas of the small intestine are part of the inherited Peutz-Jeghers syndrome, an autosomal dominant disease that also includes mucocutaneous pigmentation. The hamartomas of Peutz-Jeghers syndrome cause symptoms most frequently as the leading point for an intussusception and less frequently as blood loss. The lesions are extensive, and resection should be limited to the segment responsible for the symptoms. The need for repeated laparotomy can be decreased by the use of intraoperative endoscopy to excise additional polyps.[2]

MALIGNANT TUMORS

Clinical Presentation

A constellation of clinical symptoms is common to all types of small bowel tumors. Abdominal pain is the most common symptom in patients with both benign and malignant small bowel tumors. Given the frequency of abdominal pain in the population at large and the relative rarity of small bowel tumors, the disease usually is far advanced when diagnosed, or is accompanied by other symptoms such as obstruction or bleeding. Vague symptoms such as anorexia, dyspepsia, and malaise may be overlooked initially but are found frequently when assiduously sought. When diagnostic efforts are reviewed, patients seek help relatively early, whereas misinterpretation of symptoms by clinicians

can be responsible for delays of up to 12 months.[3] Physical examination is usually unrevealing, although large, bulky masses may be palpated in lymphomas and sarcomas.

Partial or complete obstruction occurs in half of cases of small bowel cancer. The tumor causes an annular constriction of the small bowel and encroaches on the lumen. A polypoid tumor may act as the lead point, or intussuscipiens, as a cause of obstruction. An acute angulation or mesenteric fixation can fold the bowel and obstruct the flow of intestinal chyme. Carcinoid tumors can generate an intense desmoplastic reaction involving large portions of the mesentery.

When bleeding is massive, the usual cause is erosion of a small to medium-sized artery in the base of a rapidly growing tumor that has undergone central necrosis. Perforation of small bowel tumors generally occurs with lymphomas or leiomyosarcomas and results from loss of blood supply to a transmurally invasive tumor.

Periampullary carcinomas of the duodenum can cause obstructive jaundice, and biochemical confirmation should be sought. Some small bowel tumors, specifically carcinoid neoplasms, are biochemically active and patients manifest specific clinical syndromes, depending on tumor location.

Diagnostic Studies

Small bowel tumors have no pathognomonic features on plain radiographs. They are rarely calcified and, therefore, are not directly detectable. Occasionally, with large, bulky tumors, a paucity of bowel gas is noted in one quadrant of the abdomen as the tumor mass displaces bowel loops. The most common abnormalities on plain radiographs are findings suggestive of small bowel obstruction.

Barium contrast studies are usually the definitive diagnostic tests for patients with small bowel tumors. The small bowel follow-through is technically the easiest of the contrast procedures to perform and is a natural extension of the barium swallow used to evaluate the stomach and duodenum. Proper interpretation of the small bowel follow-through depends on the use of a standard technique and familiarity with the procedure. An initial dose of 500 mL of barium sulfate is generally administered and the patient is placed in a right lateral decubitus position. A prokinetic agent, such as metoclopramide, is administered with additional barium ingestion. Fluoroscopy and compression radiography are performed until contrast reaches the cecum. Diagnostic yield is increased by the administration of an effervescent solution that forces gas into the bowel to delineate partially obstructive lesions. To evaluate the distal ileum, it occasionally is necessary to insufflate air or CO_2 gas into the rectum.[4]

Enteroclysis is a variant small bowel contrast study that is useful for detecting tumors of the small intestine. In addition to providing information on narrowing of the bowel, enteroclysis can determine distensibility of the small intestine, which may be abnormal in relatively early stage lesions. There are two major differences in technique relative to usual contrast techniques. Methylcellulose is compounded with the barium to allow for better evaluation of mucosal detail, and a tube is passed fluoroscopically to bypass the stomach and duodenum. In general, enteroclysis should be reserved for the diagnosis of intermittent obstruction, or partial obstruction. Enteroclysis can also be useful when the results of other diagnostic studies are negative in cases of chronic intestinal bleeding.[5]

Noninvasive imaging studies such as CT are useful in determining tumor resectability. CT features indicating malignancy in duodenal tumors include the presence of an exophytic or intramural mass, central necrosis, ulceration or excavation, and invasion of the tumor into the bowel wall. In general, polypoid tumors within the lumen are benign. Vascular encasement, invasion of contiguous organs other than the head of the pancreas, distant lymphadenopathy, and metastatic hepatic lesions all can be assessed and are indicative of unresectability.[6]

Arteriography is not usually performed for patients with small bowel tumors but occasionally helps make the diagnosis. Arteriographic identification of a small bowel tumor usually occurs in a patient who is undergoing a work-up for occult gastrointestinal (GI) bleeding. Lesions of the small intestine, including tumors, account for up to 20% of cases of occult GI hemorrhage.[7] The diagnostic yield can be increased by selective celiac or superior mesenteric catheterization. Sarcomas and leiomyomas are hypervascular and often have a circumscribed tumor blush. Adenocarcinomas are frequently hypovascular, with arteries that are encased or occluded.

Endoscopy is assuming an increasing role in the diagnosis of tumors of the small intestine. Enteroscopy can be performed by a variety of techniques. The conventional approach is to use a long endoscope, generally 160 to 170 cm, which is passed orally. A less conventional approach is to pass a string from the mouth to the anus as a guide for the passage of small-diameter tubing, usually the size of a biopsy forceps, which is then passed through the biopsy port of the endoscope. This allows the scope to be passed with a lower likelihood of bowel perforation resulting from looping of the scope within the bowel lumen. The third approach is to use a sonde-type enteroscope. This device has a balloon at the tip that is inflated when the scope has passed into the duodenum. Intestinal peristalsis then advances the enteroscope into the distal ileum. In expert hands, satisfactory evaluation of the mucosa is accomplished in a high proportion of patients.[8] Disadvantages include the length of time required for passage and the ability to evaluate only 50% to 70% of the mucosa.

Endoscopic ultrasound is used primarily for staging of periampullary and duodenal tumors. Evaluation of the duodenum, ampulla, common bile duct, pancreas, portal vein, and regional lymph nodes can be performed. Accurate assessment of the tumor stage and nodal status is possible in a high proportion of cases. In one series,[9] accuracy rates for staging periampullary tumors were 78% for ampullary carcinoma and 81% for common bile duct carcinoma.

Adenocarcinoma

Pathogenesis

Adenomas and carcinomas constitute an important group of neoplasms found in the small bowel. The microscopic features, histogenetic relationships, and clinical significance mimic those of colonic tumors. Recent advances in the molecular biology and genetics of the adenoma–carcinoma sequence in colon cancer appear to apply to duodenal tumors as well. In the familial adenomatous polyposis syndrome, autosomal dominant inheritance of a mutant adenomatous polyposis coli gene results in the growth of hundreds of adenomas in the colon and rectum and lesser numbers in the duodenum. The overall prevalence of duodenal polyps in patients with familial adenomatous polyposis is about 80%, making routine upper endoscopic surveillance of this patient population mandatory.[10] There is an increased relative risk of duodenal carcinoma and ampullary carcinoma in patients with familial adenomatous polyposis compared to the general population.[11]

The adenomatous polyposis coli gene, responsible for familial adenomatous polyposis, has been localized to the long arm of chromosome 5 (5q21). Although the exact nature of the adenomatous polyposis coli gene product is not known, the protein is similar in amino acid sequence to cytoskeletal proteins and appears to be associated with cellular differentiation. Additional gene defects are necessary for the development of invasive cancer in patients with familial adenomatous polyposis who have duodenal adenomas. The development of severe dysplasia in duodenal adenomas associated with familial adenomatous polyposis has been linked to mutations in the K-*ras* gene.[12] Although not yet proved, the progression from dysplastic polyp to invasive cancer may involve another mutation, in the p53 gene (short arm, chromosome 17) or the DCC gene (long arm, chromosome 18).

Epidemiology

In 1993, about 2900 new cases and 950 deaths from malignant small bowel tumors occurred in the United States, for an age-adjusted incidence of about 1 per 100,000.[13] The small intestine accounts for about 1% of digestive malignancies, and the most common primary cancer of the small intestine is adenocarcinoma. The incidence of small bowel cancer is essentially equal in men and women, reaching a peak in the sixth and seventh decades. Malignant tumors are more common in affluent Western countries, and there is a correlation between small bowel and large bowel cancer within a given country.

Treatment

SURGERY. Total excision, by endoscopic polypectomy or surgery, is the only definitive therapy for duodenal and periampullary tumors. Endoscopic polypectomy is an ideal therapy for pedunculated polyps. For small, sessile, benign duodenal adenomas, transduodenal local resection is an acceptable option. In selected cases, local resection has been used as a palliative operation for periampullary cancer in patients too frail to undergo a major resection. However, of six patients treated with local resection at one university medical center, one of three patients with benign pathology and all three patients with cancer had recurrence within 2 years of resection.[14]

Although conceptually simple, periampullary local excision is a procedure requiring expert judgment and technique. Given the high reported incidence of recurrent malignant tumors treated by local resection, it is important to ensure that a locally excised tumor is benign. Endoscopic biopsy is inaccurate for the diagnosis of cancer because biopsy fails to include malignant tissue in up to half of cases.[15] Performed improperly, injury to the common bile duct, pancreatic duct, or both can occur. Reimplantation of the common duct is generally accomplished by a technique similar to transduodenal sphincteroplasty. Another factor in the recurrence of seemingly benign tumors of the duodenum is the observation that a high proportion of tumors of the small intestine are located in a relatively small area surrounding the ampulla.[16] This suggests that a field effect in the remaining duodenum is responsible for the development of new, rather than recurrent, tumors.

Pancreaticoduodenectomy is the standard operation for curative resection of periampullary cancer, as well as for large benign neoplasms of the ampulla and second and third portions of the duodenum. For patients with an otherwise normal duodenum, a pylorus-preserving operation can provide more normal upper GI function. In centers with the necessary patient volume and expertise to perform this operation on a regular basis, the operative mortality rate should be less than 5%, and significant procedure-related morbidity, such as anastomotic leak, should be less than 20%. In patients with distal duodenal adenocarcinoma, segmental resection can be performed with acceptably low perioperative morbidity and recurrence rates.[17]

If adenocarcinomas of the small intestine cannot be resected for cure, excision of the primary tumor occasionally can be worthwhile in an attempt to provide palliation. Tumor resection alleviates problems associated with ulceration and bleeding or obstruction. Radical lymphadenectomy and resection of all midgut-derived tissues have not been shown to improve survival. If resection of the involved bowel is likely to result in short-bowel syndrome in the absence of possible cure, bypass is a good option to decompress a patient with obstruction. Laser therapy can provide palliation in patients with friable ulcerated tumors that can be reached by the endoscope.

ADJUVANT THERAPY. No effective chemotherapeutic agents are available for adjuvant use. 5-Fluorouracil and the nitrosoureas are associated with partial response rates of 10% to 20% and can provide some benefit in individual cases. Because adenocarcinomas are generally resistant to radiotherapy, this approach is not used routinely.

PROGNOSIS. Five-year survival rates for nonselected patients with adenocarcinoma range from 5% to 30%. In one series,[18] a resectability rate of 65% and an overall survival rate of 30% were reported. In patients without lymph node metastases, the 5-year survival rate was 70%; the survival rate was 13% in patients with positive lymph nodes. Another series reported an overall survival rate of 24%.[19]

Carcinoid Tumors

Pathogenesis

Carcinoid tumors arise from pluripotential cells in the crypts of Lieberkühn. The responsible cells are called argentaffin or chromaffin cells (in the past, they were referred to as Kulchitsky cells). The embryologic origin of these cells is still debated, but most authors believe they arise from a common neuroectodermal origin.[20] Carcinoid tumors of the GI tract are classified according to the embryologic region of the tissue in which they arise: foregut, midgut, or hindgut. Carcinoid tumors in each of these three sites tend to produce and secrete different humorally active compounds. On gross appearance of the cut surface, the typical carcinoid tumor is bright yellow. There is often an associated intense infiltration of collagen and other matrix components known as desmoplasia. Carcinoid tumors are differentiated histochemically by an affinity for silver stains (Grimelius, chromaffin) and immunologically by antibodies to a variety of GI peptides or neuronal markers (neuron-specific enolase).

Numerous chemical compounds have been identified in blood, urine, and tumor tissue. Among the biologically active substances are 5-hydroxytryptamine (serotonin), 5-hydroxytryptophan, kallikrein, adrenocorticotropic hormone, histamine, substance P, prostaglandins, catecholamines, gastrin, somatostatin, and insulin.[20] In general, carcinoid tumors of the GI tract are biochemically silent until extraintestinal metastases are present.

Histologically, the tumors are composed of a monotonous population of cells with uniform nuclei and cytoplasm and few mitotic figures. All carcinoid tumors are malignant, but with variable aggressivity. Many look like undifferentiated adenocarcinomas or other anaplastic tumors. Immunohistochemical staining with antibodies directed against a variety of GI peptides, immunocytochemical staining with silver stains, or electron microscopy (to demonstrate secretory granules) allows the correct diagnosis. The somewhat variable appearance of carcinoid tumors has probably led to underdiagnosis of these lesions.

Clinical Presentation

CARCINOID SYNDROME. Small lesions do not cause symptoms and usually are discovered incidentally at laparotomy performed for another reason. Medium to large lesions generally cause symptoms of bowel obstruction, similar to adenocarcinomas. Although carcinoid tumors can secrete numerous substances, as discussed earlier, the ability of the liver to degrade such compounds usually results in the absence of symptoms attributable to biochemically active agents.

Once carcinoid tumors of the small intestine have metastasized to the liver or other sites that do not drain into the portal venous circulation, a spectrum of symptoms develops that is collectively called the carcinoid syndrome. The hallmarks of the syndrome are intermittent flushing and diarrhea. The flushing of midgut, or small intestinal, carcinoid tumors is of a violaceous hue and can last from seconds to minutes. Flushing may be precipitated by many foods, alcohol, physical stress, and anesthetic induction. Less common manifesta-

tions, usually indicative of advanced disease, include bronchospasm, venous suffusion and telangiectasia, and heart failure. Heart failure associated with the carcinoid syndrome is due to endocardial and valvular fibrosis of the right side of the heart, and is thought to be related to the high levels of vasoactive amines passing through the heart on the way to the lungs, although no clear correlation between the onset of symptoms and elevated blood levels of any of the substances known to be produced by carcinoid tumors has been proved.

ASSOCIATED ENDOCRINOPATHIES. Rarely, carcinoid tumors secrete biologically active peptides that mimic other tumors. Gastrin-secreting carcinoid tumors, when metastatic, may be associated with virulent ulcer disease and hypergastrinemia suggestive of primary gastrinomas. Adrenocorticotropic hormone–secreting carcinoid tumors can cause Cushing's syndrome. Insulin-secreting tumors may mimic insulinomas. Histologically, carcinoid tumors often resemble islet cell tumors. The diagnosis often is made only at laparotomy.

Diagnosis

The diagnostic studies used for small carcinoid tumors are similar to those used for other tumors of the small intestine. Biochemical diagnosis of the carcinoid syndrome is aimed at detecting serotonin overproduction. The most consistent finding is an elevation in the concentration of urinary 5-hydroxyindoleacetic acid (5-HIAA). Urinary 5-HIAA levels in excess of 10 mg/dL are highly suggestive of an underlying carcinoid tumor. False-negative results are usually due to inadequate collection, but alternate pathways for serotonin metabolism do exist and occasionally yield misleading results. A more important problem is the false-positive test result. Many common foods (eg, bananas, tomatoes, pineapples) cause increased excretion of 5-HIAA, which falsely elevates the urinary 5-HIAA test result. Phenothiazines and other diuretics can also confound interpretation of the results.

New diagnostic modalities take advantage of the ability of carcinoid tumors to concentrate radioisotope complexed to somatostatin analogues such as indium-111 pentetreotide and iodine-131 MIBG.[21,22]

Treatment

SURGERY. Surgery is the most important aspect of the curative treatment of carcinoid tumors of the small intestine. Surgery also has an important place in the palliation of metastatic disease.

PREOPERATIVE MANAGEMENT. Physical stress, such as anesthetic induction, can precipitate the development of carcinoid crisis, a life-threatening complication of persistent generalized flushing, severe diarrhea, central nervous system effects, and cardiovascular derangements such as tachycardia, arrhythmia, and shock. For patients with known carcinoid tumors who undergo surgery, the anesthesiologist should have available the long-acting somatostatin analogue octreotide. The rapid administration of a single dose of octreotide to a patient with carcinoid crisis can be life-saving.[23] The carcinoid crisis precipitated by anesthetic induction is so severe that some recommend preoperative prophylaxis with octreotide.[24] Patients with manifestations of the carcinoid syndrome must be evaluated for congestive heart failure related to endomyocardial fibrosis. In addition to assignment of New York Heart Association functional class, echocardiography can allow determination of the severity of disease. Judicious use of central pressure monitoring devices is necessary to optimize fluid management.

PRIMARY TUMOR. In planning an operation, carcinoid tumors should be considered malignant. There is a clear correlation between the presence of metastases and the size of the primary tumor. Tumors of less than 1 cm metastasize to the liver infrequently, with nodal metastases occurring in 20% of cases.[20] Resection should include en bloc wedge resection of the mesentery, as well as generous margins. The remaining intestine should be examined for the presence of multicentric disease, which can occur in 20% to 30% of patients.

METASTATIC DISEASE. Even if residual disease is left after primary resection, carcinoid tumors tend to grow slowly and, in the absence of gross hepatic metastatic disease, patients may remain free of symptoms for years. If an operation is being performed to relieve obstruction, but gross total removal would leave the patient an intestinal cripple, bypass of the obstructed segment is an acceptable option. Radical operations, such as gross total intestinal resection for involvement of the mesentery, can result in short-gut syndrome and trouble the patient more than residual metastatic disease.

Several options exist for the patient with hepatic metastases secondary to carcinoid tumors. It is reasonable to resect solitary metastases, if adequate margins can be obtained. In general, hepatic metastases are diffuse and not amenable to resection or debulking. Hepatic artery ligation has been tried, and ischemia and necrosis of the tumor can result in short-lived relief of symptoms.[25] Similarly, hepatic artery chemotherapy infusion through an implantable pump can provide palliation in some patients. Palliation is usually limited in

duration, but repeated treatment can be considered. A final surgical option is hepatic transplantation for metastatic carcinoid tumors, which has been performed successfully in five patients.[26]

If surgery is not possible, numerous drugs can be tried in an attempt to relieve the uncomfortable flushing and diarrhea of the carcinoid syndrome. Octreotide, already discussed with respect to intraoperative carcinoid crisis, is the drug of first choice for metastatic carcinoid syndrome. Octreotide can be given subcutaneously two or three times a day or can be administered intravenously with total parenteral nutrition. The clinical effects last 8 to 12 hours. Octreotide decreases circulating levels of serotonin and urinary 5-HIAA and relieves symptoms. One mode of action is a decrease in splanchnic blood flow.[27] Tachyphylaxis can occur, but a significant proportion of patients (25% to 30%) experience relief for 1 to 2 years. Other useful drugs include cyproheptadine and methysergide, which are serotonin antagonists, and phenoxybenzamine, which prevents kallikrein release.

CHEMOTHERAPY. Radiotherapy has been of no benefit, but chemotherapy can achieve partial response rates in 30% to 40% of these patients. Partial responses have not translated into increased survival, however. Agents most commonly used are combinations of streptozotocin and 5-fluorouracil. More recently, doxorubicin and cisplatin have been used with success.[28] In a phase II study,[29] doxorubicin was administered intraarterially, followed by gelatin sponge embolization, and was associated with an 80% partial response rate. The biologic response modifiers interferon-α and interferon-γ have been used in patients with advanced disease.[30–32]

Prognosis

The overall 5-year survival is relatively good, reflecting the long interval between diagnosis of recurrence and death. In one large series,[33] the 5-year survival rate was 75% in patients who underwent complete resection for cure and 19% in patients with distant metastases. Survival is shorter, stage for stage, in patients with the carcinoid syndrome. Patients with nonmetastatic disease have survival rates similar to those of the general population, whereas the presence of resectable nodal disease is associated with survival times of 10 to 15 years.

Lymphoma

Predisposing Factors

Non-Hodgkin's lymphoma of the small intestine is not as common as primary gastric lymphoma and accounts for about 20% of all GI lymphomas. The ileum is involved more frequently than is the jejunum. The risk of developing small bowel lymphoma is increased in patients with Crohn's disease, celiac sprue, idiopathic steatorrhea, organ transplantation, and the acquired immunodeficiency syndrome (AIDS).

The association between Crohn's disease and lymphoma of the small intestine has been recognized for several decades, but the magnitude of increased risk, time to development, and relationship to severity of the underlying Crohn's disease are not well understood. Delay in diagnosis is common due to similar clinical and radiographic appearances.

Intestinal lymphoma was first reported as a complication of celiac sprue in the 1960s. The typical presentation is a relapse of sprue-like symptoms years after the initial diagnosis, or sudden clinical deterioration (weight loss, abdominal pain, emesis) after a relatively stable, mild course. Many of the tumors are T-cell lymphomas. In one large series,[34] lymphoma developed in 5% of patients with sprue, with the incidence increasing with age. Other malabsorptive states that are associated with the development of intestinal lymphomas include idiopathic steatorrhea and dermatitis herpetiformis.

Another important association is that of small bowel lymphoma and organ transplantation. The frequency of all lymphomas in transplant recipients has been estimated to be 40- to 400-fold greater than that of the normal population. The lymphomas are often extranodal, occurring in the GI tract and the central nervous system. The disease is frequently diffuse by the time of diagnosis, but isolated intestinal disease has been reported. The lymphomas are almost always of B-cell lineage and the patients often have serologic evidence of Epstein-Barr virus infection.[35] There is a correlation between the emergence of these aggressive tumors and the intensity of immunosuppression. A decrease of immunosuppression is one of the mainstays of therapy for this complication.[36]

Congenital immunodeficiency states such as Wiskott-Aldrich syndrome, X-linked agammaglobulinemia, and severe combined immunodeficiency syndrome also are associated with an increased incidence of lymphoma of the small intestine. Autoimmune diseases, including Wegener's granulomatosis, Sjögren's syndrome, systemic lupus erythematosus, and rheumatoid arthritis, also appear to have an increased incidence of lymphomas in intestinal locations.

A variant of primary intestinal lymphoma—rare in Western nations but common in the Middle East, Africa, Southeast Asia, and South America—is immunoproliferative small intestinal disease (IPSID). The involved cells are immunoglobulin A–secreting B cells, with a heavy-chain paraprotein detectable in the urine

of a significant proportion of patients. The tumors arise from a single abnormal clone. Poor standards of hygiene found in endemic areas and the ability to reverse early changes with the administration of tetracycline suggest that microbial colonization may play a role in pathogenesis.[37] Pseudolymphoma is a premalignant lesion histologically similar to true lymphomas of the small intestine, except for the lack of necrosis and mitotic figures. The diagnosis of pseudolymphoma is usually made after intestinal resection. If the diagnosis of pseudolymphoma is made before operation, resection is still indicated because foci of true lymphoma may be present in areas adjacent to the biopsy site.

Pathology

In Western countries such as the United States, primary lymphomas of the small intestine usually are localized to a segment of small bowel. This pattern of involvement is different from that seen in Middle Eastern countries or in patients with IPSID-related lymphomas. Most lymphomas of the small intestine are non-Hodgkin's in type, but the incidence of primary Hodgkin's disease of the small intestine has been increasing, especially in patients with AIDS. A commonly used classification for non-Hodgkin's lymphomas, the Ann Arbor system, has been adapted for staging lymphomas of the small intestine (Table 33-1).

Although lymphomas associated with celiac disease are predominantly T-cell in origin, most intestinal lymphomas are of B-cell origin. Histogenetically, B-cell lymphomas of the intestine share a similarity with tumors at other sites, such as the salivary glands, lung, and thyroid. These tumors are associated with a high rate of chromosomal rearrangements.[38] This tissue has been collectively called mucosa-associated lymphoid

Table 33-1 Staging of Primary Lymphoma of the Small Intestine

Stage	Description
1E	Involvement of a localized segment of bowel without nodal involvement
IIE	Involvement of a localized segment of bowel with regional nodal involvement
IIIE	Involvement of bowel and lymph nodes on both sides of the diaphragm; the spleen may be involved in stage IIIES
IV	Diffuse involvement of more than one extralymphatic organ or tissue, with or without nodal involvement

(Modified from Lance P. Tumors and other neoplastic diseases of the small intestine. In: Yamada T, ed. Textbook of gastroenterology, ed 1. Philadelphia, JB Lippincott, 1990:1491)

tissue, and a characteristic centrocyte-like cell that predominates in these tumors is thought to be derived from the mantle zone of Peyer's patches, not the follicles.[39] Centrocyte-like cells do not demonstrate a bcl-2 gene (t[14:18]) translocation that is often seen in follicular lymphomas of peripheral lymph nodes.[40,41]

Clinical Presentation

The symptoms of lymphoma of the small intestine are similar to those of other neoplasms of the small bowel (ie, abdominal pain, weight loss, intestinal obstruction). Lymphomas most frequently occur before the age of 10 years or after the age of 50 years. Palpable masses are noted in up to 50% of patients. Perforation does occur, is a more common presentation in patients with AIDS, and is associated with a poorer prognosis.[42,43]

Ultrasound has been reported to be of benefit in the radiologic diagnosis of intestinal lymphoma. The diagnostic modality is rapid, inexpensive, and noninvasive, making it a good first choice. Characteristic findings include hypoechoic bowel wall thickening, bulky masses, and nodular extraluminal disease.[44] Contrast studies are also helpful because GI lymphomas have characteristic findings. Double contrast studies can demonstrate the extramucosal origin of a mass. CT examination can determine segmental wall thickness of an involved segment and the relationship of adjacent structures.[45]

Treatment

Although common practice dictates the use of combination radiotherapy and chemotherapy to treat diffuse intestinal lymphoma, localized disease is best treated by surgical resection. Laparotomy may be indicated for symptoms even when curative resection is not possible, as in peritonitis from perforation or debulking for obstruction. Formal staging laparotomy, with splenectomy, is not usually recommended for non-Hodgkin's lymphoma of the small bowel. In the past decade, the development of CT and magnetic resonance imaging, as well as advances in the treatment of lymphoma, have decreased the number of cases in which staging laparotomy is necessary.[46] Splenic involvement can usually be identified by noninvasive imaging studies (ie, CT or magnetic resonance imaging). At the time of surgical resection, liver biopsy and aortic node sampling should be performed because these procedures contribute little to morbidity and can alter staging and management in up to 30% of patients.

Adjuvant chemotherapy with a multiple-drug regimen is usually recommended for resected lesions that involve mesenteric lymph nodes, but the data support-ing this approach are sparse. The role of postoperative radiotherapy is also a matter of debate. One retrospective series[47] has documented a 5-year disease-free survival rate of 50% using adjuvant radiation in stage IE and IIE lymphomas of the small intestine and ileocecum; other data have not been as convincing. For palliation of stage IIIE and IVE disease with or without partial surgical debulking, combination chemotherapy and localized radiation therapy can provide a partial response.

The prognosis of intestinal lymphomas is dependent primarily on the stage of the tumor (see Table 33-1). In contrast to gastric lymphomas, tumors of the small intestine tend to be more diffuse, involving essentially the entire small bowel or its mesentery. Multicentricity is also a significant problem, as are malabsorption and malnutrition. For stage IE and IIE disease, 5-year survival rates are in the 80% range, but for advanced disease, survival beyond 12 months is rare. Variables that favor improved prognosis include lower tumor stage, younger patient age, and resectability.[48]

Sarcoma

Epidemiology

Sarcomas make up 10% to 20% of all malignant tumors of the small intestine. In the adult population, peak incidence occurs between the fourth and sixth decades. Despite the ability to induce sarcomas chemically or virally in various animal models, no geographic, occupational, or ethnic associations are known to exist in humans. Chromosomal abnormalities have been noted, and Carney's syndrome of GI leiomyosarcoma, pulmonary chondroma, and functioning paraganglionoma in young women suggests a genetic predisposition in at least some of these tumors.[49,50]

Pathology

Most sarcomas of the small intestine are leiomyosarcomas. Kaposi's sarcoma has become more common in patients with AIDS but is rarely confined to the small intestine. Fibrosarcomas, liposarcomas, and essentially all other histologic types have been reported to arise primarily in the small intestine. Two independent variables for differentiation between benign leiomyomas and leiomyosarcomas exist: initial tumor size and the number of mitotic figures per high-power microscopic field. Tumors larger than 10 cm behave as if malignant, regardless of the histologic findings, and metastasis can occur even in the absence of mitotic figures.[51] Marked cellular atypia is also an important finding, usually occurring in association with a high mitotic rate. Symptomatic lesions are more likely to be malignant than benign, and a higher relative incidence of sarcomas has been reported in Meckel's diverticula. Sarcomas of the small intestine can grow intraluminally, serosally, or circumferentially. These lesions are extremely vascular, but necrosis is often seen as the tumors rapidly outgrow the available blood supply. The resulting central ulceration is likely to bleed and to manifest as melena. Lymph node metastases are rare. Sarcomas of the small intestine spread hematogenously, as do sarcomas at other sites.

Clinical Presentation

As do other types of small intestinal tumors, sarcomas often present with vague symptoms of abdominal pain or bloating. Sarcomas tend to grow extrinsically and are much further advanced at the time of presentation than are adenocarcinomas or carcinoid tumors. Obstruction is usually due to extrinsic compression rather than circumferential growth. On physical examination, palpable masses are often evident, and peritoneal signs occur in the 10% of patients who have perforation of necrotic bowel. The diagnosis is suggested by the presence of extrinsic compression on small bowel follow-through. A barium-filled cavity indicative of central tumor necrosis suggests sarcoma, as opposed to other cancers of the small intestine. CT can also document an extrinsic mesentery-based mass and a contrast-filled cavity suggestive of sarcoma. In addition, CT can demonstrate intratumoral calcifications and may identify hepatic, intraperitoneal, or pulmonary metastases in up to 30% of cases. Angiography should be performed to help in the assessment of resectability. Angiography usually shows a hypervascular mass, in contrast to adenocarcinoma or carcinoid tumors, which are usually hypovascular.

Treatment

The only curative therapy is surgical resection with en bloc removal of the mesentery and associated lymph nodes. Resection for cure can be accomplished in 50% to 75% of patients.[51] Failure is usually due to locoregional recurrence. Extended lymph node dissection is not necessary because sarcomas tend to spread through the bloodstream. Duodenal sarcomas generally require pancreaticoduodenectomy because the tumors are bulky and not amenable to local resection. Even in the presence of some intraperitoneal disease or hepatic metastases, primary tumor resection may be indicated to prevent the complications of bleeding or obstruction. Successful resection of isolated hepatic or pulmonary metastases has been reported.

Adjuvant chemotherapy and radiotherapy have not been documented to confer any survival benefit. Combination chemotherapy for unresectable disease has been tried with doxorubicin, cyclophosphamide, dacarbazine, and other agents; however, there are data to suggest that GI sarcomas are less responsive than other soft tissue sarcomas.[52] Partial response rates vary between 12% and 43%.[51]

Survival rates depend on the histologic grade of the tumor, the number of mitoses per high-power field, and the size of the primary tumor. For low-grade, completely resected tumors, 5-year survival can be expected in 55% to 80% of patients.[53,54] Patients with high-grade lesions or lesions with a poor prognosis fare worse, with survival rates of 5% to 20%.[53,54] The development of recurrent intraabdominal disease portends a worse outcome, with a median survival of only 7.5 months.[51]

Metastatic Tumors

Many tumors can metastasize to the small intestine, either by direct extension from intraperitoneal disease, such as colon or ovarian carcinoma, or by spread from distant sites, such as skin, breast, or lung. Such metastases can occur either at the time of diagnosis or later. With some tumors (ie, melanoma), bowel obstruction occasionally predates diagnosis of the primary lesion. Although cure is not possible in such cases, significant palliation can be achieved by resection or bypass of the metastases.

Clinical Presentation

Presenting signs and symptoms of small bowel metastatic disease are usually those of intestinal obstruction. Obstruction can be partial or complete and acute or chronic. Patients with malignant obstruction are often malnourished and in chronic pain. The inability to eat and drink without emesis is physiologically and psychologically devastating. Lesions can cause obstruction due to extrinsic compression, volvulus, or intussusception. Abdominal masses can be palpated. The diagnosis is usually confirmed by CT of the abdomen and pelvis. Postoperative elevation of the carcinoembryonic antigen or CA-125 level in a patient with previously normal levels points to recurrent colorectal or ovarian cancer as the cause of obstruction. The major differential diagnosis is adhesive bowel obstruction after prior abdominal surgery. Most bowel obstructions occurring after operation for colon cancer are due to benign adhesions, whereas those occurring after operation for ovarian or gastric cancer usually result from recurrent tumor.[55]

Treatment

In deciding whether to undertake surgical exploration of a patient with metastatic bowel obstruction, a general rule is that one attempt at relief of the obstructed segment (or segments) is worthwhile. Findings can range from a "frozen abdomen," for which nothing can be done, to one simple lesion that is easily removed. Complicating factors such as preoperative radiation, extent of disease, malignant ascites, or type of anastomosis have not been associated with excessive abscess or fistula complications.[56] In one large series of 102 patients with melanoma who underwent exploratory laparotomy for malignant obstruction,[57] no operative mortality was recorded and symptomatic relief was reported in 92% of cases. The mean overall survival time after first exploration for melanoma metastasis is close to 1 year, but this fell to 3.6 months for a second exploration.[58]

For patients whose tumor burden is not amenable to resection, bypass is a good option for restoring intestinal continuity. Disease may be so advanced that only gastrostomy can be performed to at least allow the removal of an uncomfortable nasogastric tube. Nonoperative decompression of the intestinal tract has been achieved with percutaneous gastrostomy.[59] This approach has merit for extensive disease but may miss a subset of patients with obstruction who would benefit from excision of metastases.

REFERENCES

1. Galandiuk S, Hermann RE, Jagelman DG, et al. Villous tumors of the duodenum. Ann Surg 1988;207:234.
2. Spigelman AD, Thomson JPS, Phillips RKS. Towards decreasing the laparotomy rate in the Peutz-Jeghers syndrome: the role of preoperative small bowel endoscopy. Br J Surg 1990;77:301.
3. Maglinte DD, O'Connor K, Bessette J, Chernish SM, Kelvin FM. The role of the physician in the late diagnosis of primary malignant tumors of the small bowel. Am J Gastroenterol 1991;86:304.
4. Maglinte, DD, Lappas JC, Kelvin FM. Small bowel radiography: how, when, why? Radiology 1987;158:553.
5. Rex DK, Lappas JL, Maglinte DD. Enteroclysis in the evaluation of suspected small intestinal bleeding. Gastroenterology 1989;15:265.
6. Kazerooni EA, Quint LE, Francis IR. Duodenal neoplasms: predictive value of CT for determining malignancy and tumor resectability. AJR 1992;159:303.
7. Allison DJ, Hemingway AP, Cunningham DA. Angiography in gastrointestinal bleeding. Lancet 1982;2:30.
8. Lewis BS, Waye JD. Total small bowel enteroscopy. Gastrointest Endosc 1987;33:435.
9. Mukai H, Nakajima M, Yasuda K, Mizuno S, Kawai K. Evaluation of endoscopic ultrasonography in the pre-operative staging of carcinoma of the ampulla of Vater and common bile duct. Gastrointest Endosc 1992;39:676.
10. Church JM, McGannon E, Hull-Boiner S, et al. Gastroduodenal polyps in patients with familial adenomatous polyposis. Dis Colon Rectum 1992;35:1170.
11. Offerhaus GJ, Giardiello FM, Krush AJ, et al. The risk of upper gastrointestinal cancer in familial adenomatous polyposis. Gastroenterology 1992;106:1980.
12. Odze RD, Quinn PS, Terrault NA, et al. Advanced gastroduodenal polyposis with ras mutations in a patient with familial adenomatous polyposis. Hum Pathol 1993;24:442.
13. Silverberg E, Boring CC, Squires TS. Cancer statistics, 1993. CA Cancer J Clin 1993;43:9.
14. Farouk M, Niotis M, Branum GD, Cotton PB, Meyers WC. Indications for and the technique of local resection of tumors of the papilla of Vater. Arch Surg 1991;126:650.
15. Ryan DP, Shapiro RH, Warshaw AL. Villous tumors of the duodenum. Ann Surg 1986;203:301.
16. Ross RK, Hartnett NM, Bernstein L, Henderson BE. Epidemiology of carcinomas of the small intestine: is bile a small bowel carcinogen? Br J Cancer 1991;63:143.
17. Lowell JA, Rossi RL, Munson JL, Braasch JW. Primary adenocarcinoma of the third and fourth portions of the duodenum. Arch Surg 1992;127:557.
18. Ouriel K, Adams JT. Adenocarcinoma of the small intestine. Am J Surg 1984;197:66.
19. Desa LA, Bridger J, Grace PA, Krausz T, Spencer J. Primary jejunoileal tumors: a review of 45 cases. World J Surg 1991;15:81.
20. Thompson GB, van Heerden JA, Martin JK, Schutt AJ, Ilstrup DM, Carney JA. Carcinoid tumors of the gastrointestinal tract: presentation, management and prognosis. Surgery 1985;98:1054.
21. Jodrell DI, Irvine AT, McCready VR, Woodcraft E, Smith IE. The use of 131I-MIBG in the imaging of metastatic carcinoid tumors. Br J Cancer 1988;58:663.
22. Dorr U, Rath U, Sautter-Bihl ML, et al. Improved visualization of carcinoid liver metastases by indium-111 pentreotide scintigraphy following treatment with cold somatostatin analogue. Eur J Nucl Med 1993;20:431.
23. Kvols LK, Moertel CG, O'Connell MJ, et al. Treatment of malignant carcinoid syndrome: evaluation of a long-acting somatostatin analog. N Engl J Med 1986;319:663.
24. Basson MD, Ahlman H, Wangberg B, Modlin IM. Biology and management of the midgut carcinoid. Am J Surg 1993;165:288.
25. Persson BG, Nobin A, Ahren B, Jeppson B, Mannsson B, Bengmark S. Repeated hepatic ischemia as a treatment for carcinoid liver metastases. World J Surg 1989;13:307.
26. Makowka L, Tzakis AG, Mazzaferro V, et al. Transplantation of the liver for metastatic endocrine tumors of the intestine and pancreas. Surg Gynecol Obstet 1989;168:107.
27. Cho KJ, Vinik AI. Effect of somatostatin analogue (octreotide) on blood flow to endocrine tumors metastatic to

the liver: angiographic evaluation. Radiology 1990;177: 549.

28. Porter AT, Ostrowski MJ. Successful treatment of malignant carcinoid tumour with intravenous cis-platinum. Eur J Surg Oncol 1988;14:703.

29. Ruszniewski P, Rougier P, Roche A, et al. Hepatic arterial chemoembolization in patients with liver metastases of endocrine tumors: a prospective phase II study in 24 patients. Cancer 1993;71:2624.

30. Spiegel RJ. Additional indications for interferon therapy: basal cell carcinoma, carcinoid, and chronic active hepatitis. Semin Oncol 1988;15:41.

31. Andersson T, Wilander E, Eriksson B, Lindgren PG, Oberg K. Effects of interferon on tumor tissue content in liver metastases of human carcinoid tumors. Cancer Res 1990;50:3413.

32. Janson ET, Kauppinen HL, Oberg K. Combined alpha- and gamma-interferon therapy for malignant midgut carcinoid tumors: a phase I-II trial. Acta Oncol 1993; 32:231.

33. Godwin DJ. Carcinoid tumors: an analysis of 2,837 cases. Cancer 1975;36:560.

34. Cooper BT, Holmes GKT, Ferguson R, Cooke WT. Celiac disease and malignancy. Medicine 1980;59:249.

35. Haber DA, Mayer RJ. Primary gastrointestinal lymphoma. Semin Oncol 1988;15:154.

36. Cohen JI. Epstein-Barr virus lymphoproliferative disease associated with acquired immunodeficiency. Medicine 1991;70:137.

37. Khojasteh A, Haghshenass M, Haghighi P. Immunoproliferative small intestinal disease: a "Third World lesion." N Engl J Med 1983;308:1401.

38. Wotherspoon AC, Pan LX, Diss TC, Isaacson PG. Cytogenetic study of B-cell lymphoma of mucosa-associated lymphoid tissue. Cancer Genet Cytogenet 1992;58:35.

39. Isaacson PG, Dogan A, Price SK, Spencer J. Immunoproliferative small-intestinal disease. An immunohistochemical study. Am J Surg Pathol 1989;13:1023.

40. Pan L, Diss TC, Cunningham D, Issacson PG. The bcl-2 gene in primary B-cell lymphoma of mucosa associated lymphoid tissue. Am J Pathol 1989;135:7.

41. Shepherd NA, McCarthy KP, Hall PA. 14:18 Translocation in primary intestinal lymphoma: detection by polymerase chain reaction. Histopathology 1991;18:415.

42. Davidson T, Allen-Mersh TG, Miles AJ, et al. Emergency laparotomy in patients with AIDS. Br J Surg 1991;78: 924.

43. Domizio P, Owen RA, Shepherd NA, Talbot IC, Norton AJ. Primary lymphoma of the small intestine: a clinico-pathological study of 119 cases. Am J Surg Pathol 1993;17:429.

44. Goerg C, Schwerk WB, Goerg K. Gastrointestinal lymphoma: sonographic findings in 54 patients. AJR 1990;155:795.

45. Dodd GD. Lymphoma of the hollow abdominal viscera. Radiol Clin North Am 1990;28:771.

46. Marble KR, Deckers PJ, Kern KA. Changing role of splenectomy for hematologic disease. J Surg Oncol 1993;52: 169.

47. Herrmann R, Panahon AM, Barcus MP, et al. Gastrointestinal involvement in non-Hodgkin's lymphoma. Cancer 1980;46:215.

48. Rackner VL, Thirlby RC, Ryan JA. Role of surgery in multimodality therapy for gastrointestinal lymphoma. Am J Surg 1991;161:570.

49. Carney JA. The triad of gastric epithelioid leiomyosarcoma, pulmonary chondroma, and functioning extraadrenal paraganglionoma: a five year review. Medicine 1983;62:159.

50. Sreekantaiah C, Sandberg AA. Ring(13)(p11q34) as the sole abnormality in a leiomyosarcoma of the small bowel. Cancer Genet Cytogenet 1991;54:115.

51. Licht JD, Weissmann LB, Antman K. Gastrointestinal sarcomas. Semin Oncol 1988;15:181.

52. Celik C, Lopez C, Douglass HO. Advanced leiomyosarcoma of the stomach. J Surg Oncol 1984;26:83.

53. Akwari OE, Dozois RR, Weiland LH, et al. Leiomyosarcoma of the small and large bowel. Cancer 1978;42: 1375.

54. Chiotasso PJP, Fazio VW. Prognostic factors of 28 leiomyosarcomas of the small intestine. Surg Gynecol Obstet 1984;155:197.

55. Cox MR, Gunn IF, Eastman MC, Hunt RF, Heinz AW. The operative aetiology and type of adhesions causing small bowel obstruction. Aust NZ J Surg 1993;63:848.

56. Donato D, Angelides A, Irani H, Penalver M, Averette H. Infectious complications after gastrointestinal surgery in patients with ovarian carcinoma and malignant ascites. Gynecol Oncol 1992;44:40.

57. Branum GD, Seigler HF. Role of surgical intervention in the management of intestinal metastases from malignant melanoma. Am J Surg 1991;162:428.

58. Khadra MH, Thompson JF, Milton GW, McCarthy WH. The justification for surgical treatment of metastatic melanoma of the gastrointestinal tract. Surg Gynecol Obstet 1990;171:413.

59. Adelson MD, Kasowitz MH. Percutaneous endoscopic drainage gastrostomy in the treatment of gastrointestinal obstruction from intraperitoneal malignancy. Obstet Gynecol 1993;81:467.

Digestive Tract Surgery: A Text and Atlas, edited by Richard H. Bell,
Layton F. Rikkers, and Michael W. Mulholland.
Lippincott-Raven Publishers, Philadelphia, © 1996.

34

Crohn's Disease

Fabrizio Michelassi

Crohn's disease can involve any segment of the gastrointestinal tract and manifests with varied symptoms and complications. Medical treatment aims at alleviating symptoms and improving the patient's quality of life. Surgical treatment becomes necessary when medical treatment fails or when complications develop. A complete understanding of the indications and the limitations of medical and surgical treatment is essential in the treatment of patients affected by Crohn's disease.

Many patients with Crohn's disease require surgical intervention during their lifetime. One review of an 18-year experience with 639 patients with Crohn's disease reported that two thirds of patients required at least one surgical procedure.[1] Nevertheless, the decision to operate on a patient is rarely an easy one and requires balancing the risks and benefits of continued medical therapy with those of surgery.

To determine an optimal treatment plan for the patient, a team approach is essential, including surgeon and gastroenterologist, helped by the radiologist and pathologist. At some point in the patient's treatment, the benefits of surgery, resulting in medication-free periods, may be greater than the risks. Similarly, Crohn's disease involves disease-free periods along with relapses, and nonclinical factors also play a role in the choice of therapies appropriate for the individual patient.

GENERAL CONSIDERATIONS

Surgical Indications

The three most common indications for surgical treatment in Crohn's disease are septic complications, intestinal obstruction, and failure of medical treatment.

Other less common indications include hemorrhage, neoplastic degeneration, fulminant colitis with or without toxic megacolon, and, in the pediatric population, growth retardation (Table 34-1). In any given patient, several indications may be present.

Septic Complications

Septic complications include fistulas, inflammatory masses, abscesses, and rarely, free perforation or hepatic abscesses.

Fistulas are common; in one series,[2] fistulas were found in 35% of patients at operation. The presence of a fistula by itself, however, is responsible for surgical treatment in a minority of patients. These conditions include enterocutaneous and enterovaginal fistulas, when the enteric drainage becomes a matter of personal and social embarrassment for the patient; enterovesical or colovesical fistulas, when the connection of the intestine to the genitourinary system causes repeated urinary tract infections and eventual renal function impairment; and enteroenteric fistulas that produce functional and anatomic bypass of a major segment of intestine with consequent malabsorption or profuse diarrhea. The clinical presentations of fistulas depend on their location and are described in a different section of this chapter under the heading of the specific location.

Inflammatory masses and abscesses occur less frequently than fistulas. The preoperative diagnosis of an intraabdominal mass may indicate that the patient harbors an intraabdominal abscess and needs surgical treatment. In one series,[3] preoperative diagnosis of an inflammatory mass or an abscess was accomplished by physical examination in 110 of 653 patients (17.2%). In

Table 34-1 Primary Indications for Surgery in Crohn's Disease

SEPTIC COMPLICATIONS
Inflammatory mass or abscess
Fistula, considered an indication for surgery if one of the following is present:
 Drainage is a matter of personal embarrassment (eg, enterocutaneous or enterovaginal fistula)
 Fistula communicates with the genitourinary system (eg, enterovesical or colovesical fistula)
 Fistula produces a functional or anatomic bypass of a major segment of intestine with consequent malabsorption or profuse diarrhea (eg, duodenocolic or enterorectosigmoid fistula)
Free perforation
Hepatic abscess

OCCLUSIVE COMPLICATIONS
Obstipation
Intestinal obstruction (partial or complete)

FAILURE OF MEDICAL TREATMENT
Corticosteroid therapy inadequate to control patient's symptoms
Recurrence of symptoms with tapering from high-dose corticosteroids
Worsening of symptoms or new onset of complications while on maximal medical therapy
Occurrence of steroid-induced complications (cushingoid features, cataracts, glaucoma, systemic hypertension, aseptic necrosis of the head of the femur, myopathy, or vertebral body fractures)

HEMORRHAGE

CARCINOMA

GROWTH RETARDATION

FULMINANT COLITIS WITH OR WITHOUT TOXIC MEGACOLON

half of these patients, an intraabdominal abscess was confirmed at laparotomy; the other half had an inflammatory mass without an abscess component. An additional 3% of patients were found to have masses on radiologic evaluation, all of which were found to be abscesses at operation. Intraabdominal abscesses were found in another 39 patients, in whom the diagnosis was not suspected preoperatively; these patients underwent surgery because of the presence of other surgical indications. In total, 165 of 639 patients (26%) in the series had either an intraabdominal abscess or an inflammatory mass at the time of operation.

Because abscesses are unlikely to respond to medical treatment, the presence of an abscess indicates the need for surgical treatment. Moreover, the physical finding of an inflammatory mass is usually an indication that the disease has reached a degree of severity and complexity that warrants surgical treatment. Most

patients develop symptoms related to worsening of the disease (anorexia, fatigue, and weight loss) or to the development of obstructive complications (abdominal pain and diarrhea). Others have generalized signs of sepsis, such as fever, which, coupled with the presence of a tender abdominal mass, strongly suggest the presence of an abscess. A thorough physical examination can identify most patients with intraabdominal abscesses. Radiographic imaging studies that are useful in diagnosing additional cases include abdominal computed tomography (CT), abdominal ultrasound, and gastrointestinal contrast studies.

The location of the mass or abscess can influence the clinical presentation. For example, limb pain and flexion contracture of the hip suggest a psoas abscess; in the presence of a right lower quadrant inflammatory mass, swelling and pitting edema of the right lower extremity may indicate compromise of venous return due to compression or thrombosis of the right common iliac vein.

Free perforation is a rare complication of Crohn's colitis because transmural disease usually leads to the formation of inflammatory adhesions with neighboring viscera, parietal peritoneum, or omentum that wall-off the perforation. Usually, free perforation results from a secondary rupture of an abscess into the peritoneal cavity and requires prompt surgical intervention with resection of the perforated bowel. Symptoms and findings are consistent with an acute abdomen unless masked by the effects of corticosteroid treatment. The loss of the hepatic dullness on abdominal percussion and the presence of pneumoperitoneum on an upright radiograph of the thorax indirectly demonstrate the presence of free intestinal perforation.

Pyogenic hepatic abscess is a rare complication of Crohn's disease, despite extensive intraabdominal sepsis and frequent portal pyemia. Because of its rarity, pyogenic hepatic abscess represents a difficult diagnostic problem. The presence of sepsis out of proportion to the abdominal findings should alert the physician to the possibility of a liver abscess. Liver ultrasonography and CT are the initial diagnostic studies when a liver abscess is suspected.

Intestinal Obstruction

Often chronic in nature, intestinal obstruction can also be acute. The obstruction may be due to one narrow stricture or to long diseased segments and can be partial, high-grade, or complete. Symptoms differ depending on the location of the disease in the gastrointestinal tract: delayed gastric emptying in gastroduodenal disease; postprandial cramps in ileojejunal disease; abdominal distention, pain, and diarrhea in ileocolic disease. At times, dilated loops of small bowel are identifiable on physical examination of the abdomen.

Failure of Medical Treatment

Although septic complications and intestinal obstruction represent operative indications based on specific findings, medical treatment is judged a failure and surgery is considered (see Table 34-1) when one of the following conditions is present:

1. High-dose corticosteroid therapy proves inadequate.
2. The patient has no symptoms while on high-dose corticosteroid therapy but has recurrence of symptoms with tapering of the steroid dose.
3. The disease progresses with worsening symptoms or a new onset of complications while the patient is receiving maximal medical therapy.
4. Significant treatment-related complications develop, including steroid-induced cushingoid features, cataracts, glaucoma, hypertension, aseptic necrosis of the head of the femur, myopathy, and vertebral body fractures.

The decision to operate on a patient because of failure of medical treatment is not an easy one and needs to be shared with the gastroenterologist and the patient. The surgeon and gastroenterologist need to balance the risks and benefits of continued medical therapy with those of surgery. The number of previous resections, the amount of diseased bowel, and the length of grossly normal intestine remaining are all important considerations. The surgeon and the patient need to consider the risks and benefits of surgery with the changes in the quality of life of the patient, especially if a temporary or permanent stoma is likely to be required.

Hemorrhage

Massive hemorrhage is a rare but potentially lethal complication of Crohn's disease, occurring in about 1% of patients. In a review of seven patients with intestinal hemorrhage,[4] investigators reported that patients experiencing one episode of hemorrhage were likely to have at least one additional episode. Therefore, emergency surgical intervention may be necessary because of unremitting hemorrhage or electively because of the increased likelihood of recurrent bleeding. During active bleeding, a preoperative angiogram showing the exact location of the hemorrhage can assist intraoperative decisions regarding the extent of resection, especially in the presence of multiple segments of gastrointestinal tract involvement.

Carcinoma

The first reports of large intestinal carcinoma and small bowel adenocarcinoma in Crohn's disease were published in 1948[5] and 1956,[6] respectively. By 1991, 100 case reports of small intestinal adenocarcinoma complicating Crohn's disease had appeared in the literature.[7,8] A similar number of case reports have appeared for colorectal adenocarcinoma in Crohn's disease. Although the association between intestinal carcinoma and Crohn's disease has been documented by several authors, the precise calculation of the relative risk has been difficult. Estimates of relative risk have varied from 6 to 320 times that of the normal population, with most figures falling between 40 and 115 for patients with small bowel Crohn's disease and between 6 and 20 for patients with large bowel involvement. Estimates indicate a prevalence of 0.6% for small bowel adenocarcinoma and of 1.4% for large intestinal adenocarcinoma in patients with Crohn's disease.[9]

The development of carcinoma in the presence of Crohn's disease presents a difficult diagnostic problem. Both diseases frequently cause altered bowel habits, symptoms of obstruction, and anemia. The radiographic changes in Crohn's disease complicated by cancer may be similar to those caused by advanced inflammatory disease alone. Preoperative diagnosis of carcinoma is unlikely in the small intestine and difficult to obtain in the large intestine, except when recognized on colonoscopy or proctosigmoidoscopy or palpated on rectal examination. Even at laparotomy, tumors may not be detected. In one review of the literature,[10] half of the carcinomas were not suspected at operation and were diagnosed only on microscopic examination.

Because several reports have stressed the association between small bowel adenocarcinoma and bypassed intestinal segments,[11,12] bypass surgery should not be performed for Crohn's disease of the small bowel. Additionally, the occurrence of carcinoma in defunctionalized rectal stumps[13–15] dictates that rectal stumps should be either restored to their function or excised. Although surveillance of the large bowel is feasible, it is difficult to distinguish neoplastic from inflammatory stricture and to make early diagnosis of adenocarcinoma. The diagnosis of adenocarcinoma is suspected or obtained preoperatively in a minority of patients.

Growth Retardation

Growth retardation occurs in 15% to 30% of children affected by Crohn's disease.[16] If developmental retardation persists in the presence of adequate medical and nutritional therapy, surgical treatment should be elected before puberty, or else longitudinal growth will not occur because of closure of epiphyses.[17]

Fulminant Colitis With or Without Toxic Megacolon

Toxic megacolon occurs in about 6% to 15% of patients with Crohn's colitis.[18] Fulminant colitis with or without toxic megacolon represents a surgical emergency and should be treated by rapid resuscitation and operation. Patients who develop either toxic megacolon or fulminant colitis may require operation during the first flare of the disease and may come to operation before a specific determination of the type of colitis can be made. In these instances, it is important to determine the status of the rectum before commencing operation. If the rectum is free of disease, the patient may be suffering from Crohn's colitis, and the entire rectum that is without disease should be preserved as a mucous fistula or as a long Hartmann's pouch for subsequent anastomosis to the ileum. If the rectum is diseased, the patient may be suffering from ulcerative colitis. As much rectum as possible should be preserved as a Hartmann's pouch to facilitate subsequent completion restorative proctectomy with ileoanal pouch anastomosis. If Crohn's colitis is unequivocally diagnosed (presence of a rectovaginal fistula or perineal sepsis), the rectum should be resected and a short Hartmann's pouch constructed. After the patient has recovered from the first operation, a completion proctectomy can be accomplished with minimal morbidity through a perineal approach.

Preoperative Evaluation and Preparation

When the decision to proceed with surgical treatment is made, the extent of gastrointestinal involvement must be determined. This can be accomplished by a combination of upper gastrointestinal radiographs with small bowel examination, air contrast barium studies or colonoscopy, abdominal CT scan, and intravenous pyelogram. For Crohn's disease of the colon, the surgeon should perform the colonoscopy or at least be present at the time of the examination to evaluate the status of the entire colon. Proctoscopy may ascertain the presence or absence of rectal disease, the extent of perianal disease, and the length of disease-free rectum, if any, suitable for possible anastomosis. The final decision regarding the condition of the bowel is made at operation during inspection of the gut and open examination of any resected bowel.

In preparing a patient with Crohn's disease for operation, the condition of the patient and degree of obstruction dictate the need for nutritional support and an incremental bowel preparation. The debilitated patient can be placed on bowel rest to facilitate mechanical preparation, and nutrition can be delivered parenterally. A combination of total parenteral nutrition with specific vitamin and mineral additives and transfusions of whole blood improves anemia and hypoproteinemia but rarely results in a positive nitrogen balance.

If an anastomosis is contemplated, mechanical preparation must be meticulously obtained, perhaps over the course of several days, by a combination of bowel rest and catharsis with hyperosmolar solutions. In the presence of a small bowel obstruction, a nasogastric or a nasoenteric tube may be needed to decompress the bowel. Enemas should be used sparingly, particularly in patients with perianal disease. Adequate preparation of the rectum can be achieved in the operating room by proctoscopy with aspiration and irrigation of the rectum of the anesthetized patient before commencing the procedure. Oral or systemic antibiotics, or both, should be used as prophylaxis.

If a stoma may be necessary, the site should be marked before the day of operation to ensure proper placement based on body habitus and to avoid compromising the site by the abdominal incision. With the exception of the rare patient who requires operation because of gastroduodenal Crohn's disease, an infraumbilical transverse incision affords excellent exposure to the small bowel, colon, and rectum.

OPERATIVE STRATEGY

The indications for surgical treatment described in the previous section are found with different incidence along the gastrointestinal tract. Also, the operative procedure of choice (bypass, strictureplasty, resection) depends on the location of the disease within the gastrointestinal tract. This section analyzes indications for surgical treatment and operative strategy according to the location of Crohn's disease in the gastrointestinal tract. When resection with removal of all gross disease is indicated, a clear margin of 5 cm should be obtained on either side of the resected specimen. Wider margins, as well as the radical inclusion of the entire lymph nodal basin related to the resected specimen, have not reduced the recurrence rate of Crohn's disease and have inappropriately sacrificed normal small bowel.

Gastroduodenal Disease

Two to 4% patients affected by Crohn's disease present with involvement of the stomach or duodenum, but only 33% of these ever require surgical treatment. Reporting on 1670 patients, investigators described 70 patients (4.2%) with duodenal involvement[19]; of these, only 22 required surgical intervention. The most common indication for surgical treatment is chronic, worsening obstruction (Fig. 34-1). Patients complain of early satiety with prolonged gastric emptying, nausea, and vomiting.

When Crohn's disease is limited to the third or fourth portion of the duodenum, a Roux-en-Y duodenojejunostomy is the preferred procedure. When the disease extends to the first or second portion of the duodenum, a gastrojejunal bypass is the procedure of choice, although considerable debate exists about whether a vagotomy should be added. The debate focuses on the risk of postvagotomy diarrhea versus the risk of marginal ulceration. Because of the high incidence of marginal ulceration after a gastrojejunostomy without vagotomy, a vagotomy is usually performed. Gastroduodenal disease is the only indication for the use of bypass surgery in Crohn's disease. Bypass surgery in other segments of the gastrointestinal tract has been abandoned because of the risk of developing septic, hemorrhagic, and neoplastic complications originating from the unresected diseased segment.

Acute, massive gastroduodenal hemorrhage is a rare complication that requires immediate surgical treatment. Hemostasis by suture ligation or electrocoagulation, vagotomy, and a gastric drainage procedure constitute effective surgical treatment.[20]

Because of its proximity to the terminal ileum and the colon, the duodenum can be the site of ileoduodenal or coloduodenal fistulas. In these cases, the duodenum is usually not primarily involved by Crohn's disease. Instead, the fistula originates from a diseased ileocolic segment and drains into the duodenum. Appropriate surgical management follows the principle of resection of the primary disease with extirpation of the fistula and closure of the duodenum.[21–23]

Acute pancreatitis can develop in the presence of duodenal disease,[24] probably as a result of refluxed duodenal contents into the pancreatic duct. When other, more common causes of pancreatitis have been excluded, a gastrojejunostomy and vagotomy are indicated to prevent recurrent attacks of pancreatitis.[25]

Jejunoileal Disease

Crohn's disease of the jejunum and midgut occurs in 3% to 10% of patients.[26] The two most common complications of severe jejunoileal disease are obstruction and sepsis. Chronic, high-grade small bowel obstruction are due to single or multiple strictures. When multiple tight strictures are present, the small bowel is transformed into a sequence of dilated saccular segments separated by tight, ringlike strictures (Fig. 34-2). The dilated segments, which contain partially digested food particles, vegetable fibers, and seeds, become an environment for bacterial overgrowth. Because of bacterial overgrowth and stagnation, patients report symptoms of nausea, abdominal cramps, and occasional vomiting or diarrhea. Malabsorption and anemia can also occur. This clinical picture is an indication for operation.

Septic complications, such as an inflammatory mass or an abscess, are also considered evidence of medical treatment failure and an indication for surgical treatment. A fistula requires surgery when it produces a bypass of a sizable portion of small bowel with consequent diarrhea and malabsorption. Enterocutaneous or enterovaginal fistulas are almost always indications for surgical treatment because of drainage that may be difficult to contain. Nevertheless, most of the time, fistulas represent a marker of disease severity rather than an absolute indication for surgical treatment. Treatment of fistulas of the jejunum and ileum are discussed with fistulas of the ter-

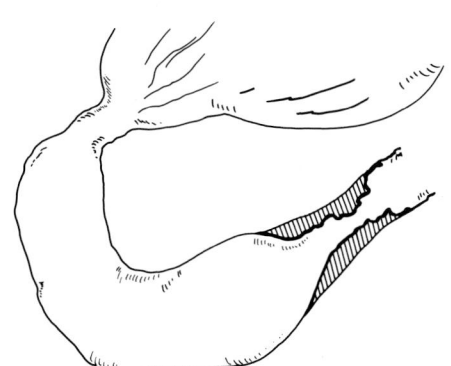 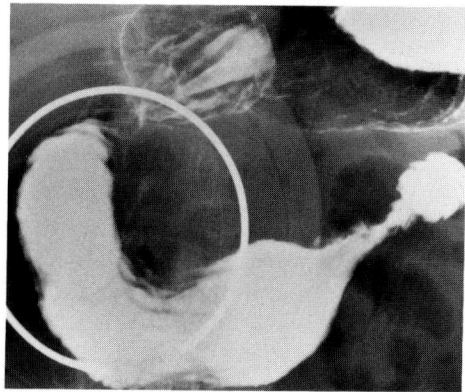

Figure 34-1 Upper gastrointestinal barium study showing Crohn's disease affecting the third portion of the duodenum.

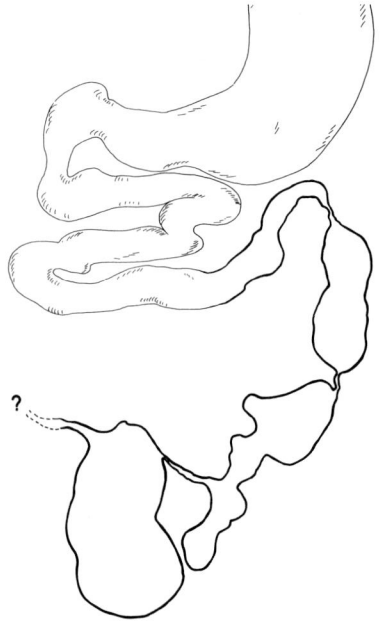

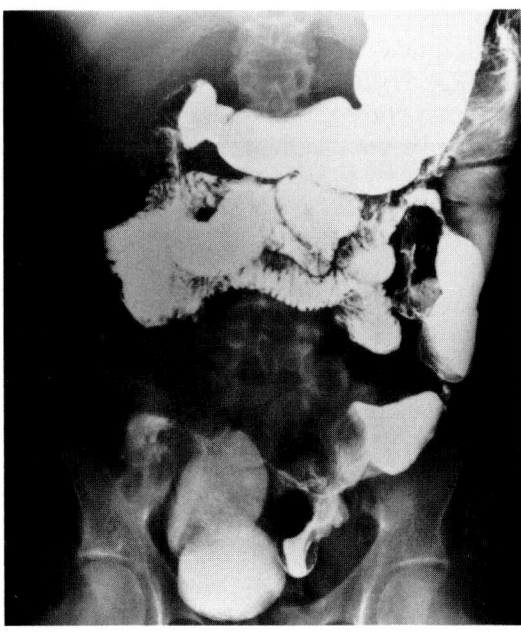

Figure 34-2 Small barium study showing extensive jejunoileal disease with dilated saccular segments separated by tight ringlike strictures. The transit of barium is so impeded that radiographic definition of further distal disease is difficult.

minal ileum because they often produce the same symptoms and physical findings.

When the disease is limited, the operation of choice is small bowel resection with primary anastomosis. When the disease is widespread or when pre-vious resections have greatly decreased the length of the remaining small bowel, the surgeon is confronted with the problem of how to care for the patient's symptoms and complications without risking a chronic short gut syndrome. In this case, stricture-

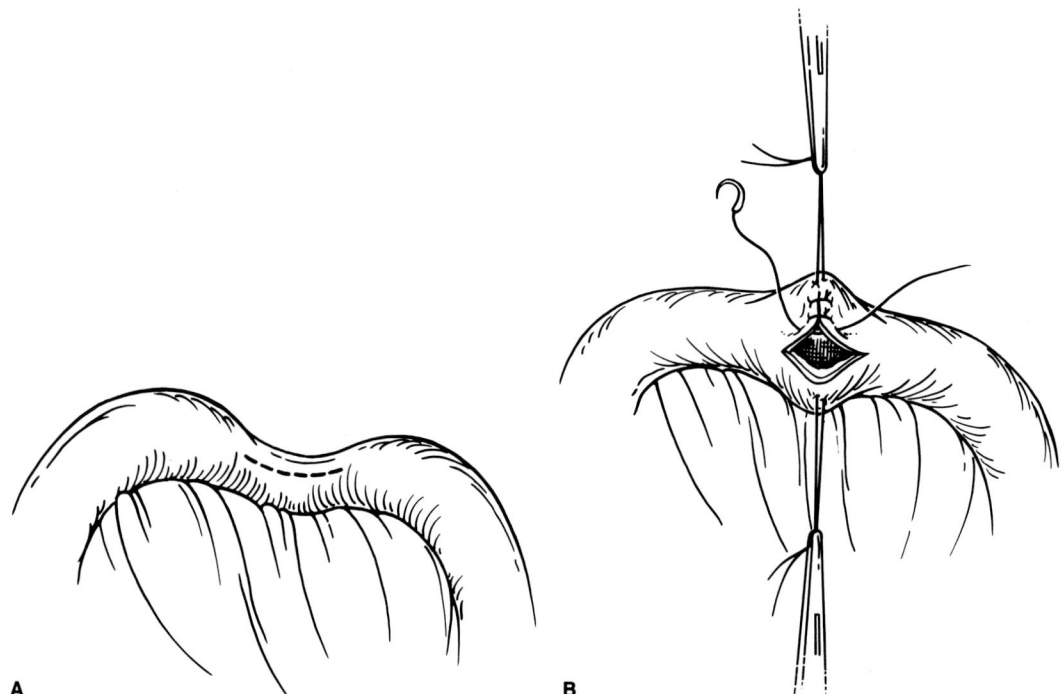

A   B

Figure 34-3 Heineke-Mikulicz strictureplasty for short stenosis (up to 7 cm). (After Fazio VW, Galandiuk S, Jagelman DG, Lavery IC. Strictureplasty in Crohn's disease. Ann Surg 1989; 210:621)

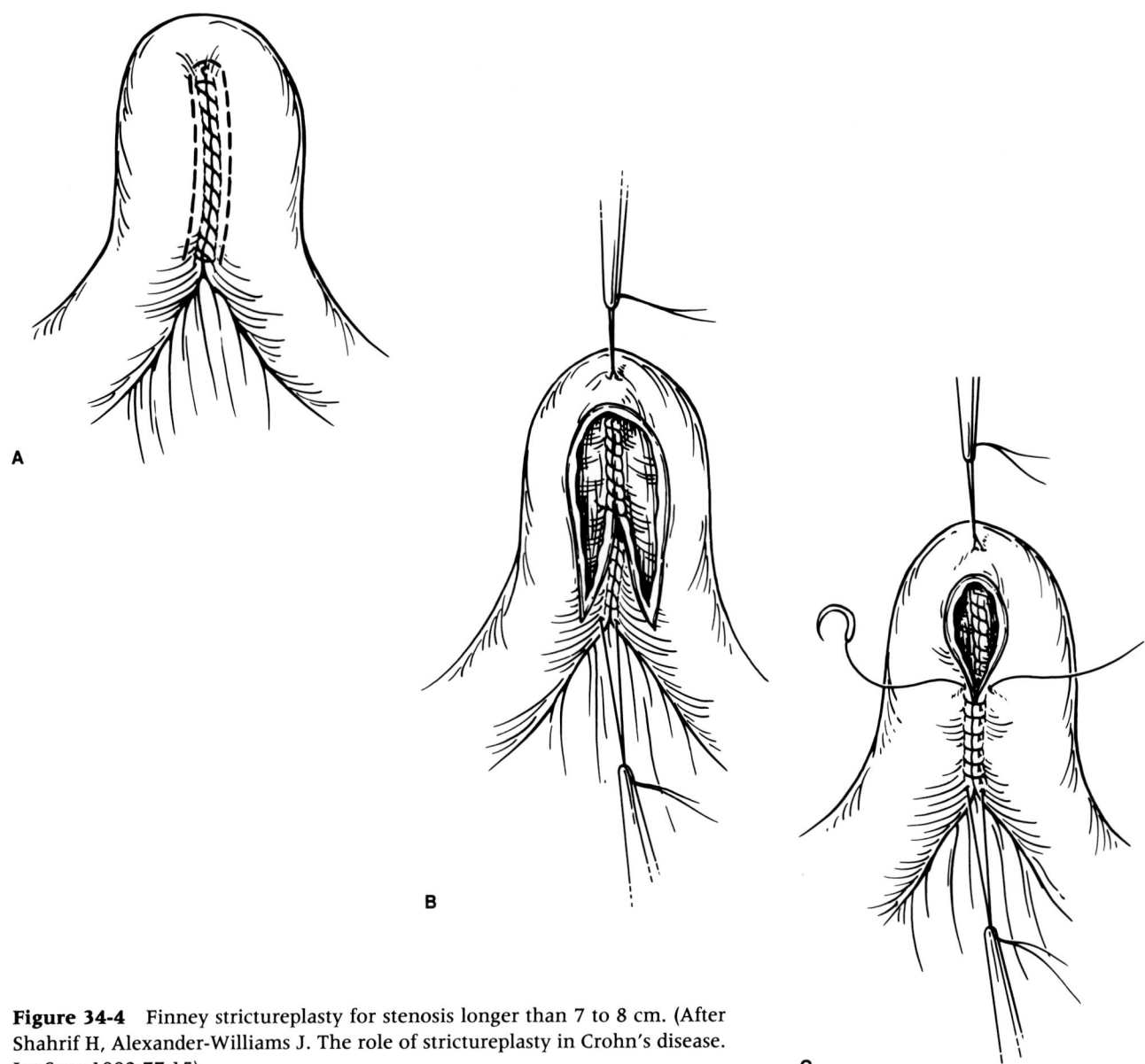

A

B

C

Figure 34-4 Finney strictureplasty for stenosis longer than 7 to 8 cm. (After Shahrif H, Alexander-Williams J. The role of strictureplasty in Crohn's disease. Int Surg 1992;77:15)

plasty alone or in combination with limited resections should be employed in an effort to limit intestinal resection and to overcome the symptomatic obstruction. The choice of the strictureplasty to be employed depends mainly on the length of the segment affected by the stenosis. For stenosis up to 7 cm long, it is preferable to use the Heineke-Mikulicz technique (Fig. 34-3); for stenosis between 7 and 15 cm, a Finney strictureplasty is a better alternative (Fig. 34-4); for stenosis and skip lesions up to 20 cm long, a combination of Heineke-Mikulicz and Finney strictureplasties can be employed (Fig. 34-5); for segments of stenosis and skip lesions up to 30 cm long, a side-to-side isoperistaltic enteroenterostomy can be used (Fig. 34-6). Modifications of the Heineke-Mikulicz strictureplasty have been described in the case of stenosis associated with a proximal dilation (Fig. 34-7) or a chronic fistula (Fig. 34-8).

Disease of the Terminal Ileum

Obstruction

In up to half of patients affected by Crohn's disease, the terminal ileum represents the primary area of involvement (Fig. 34-9). Because the terminal ileum is the narrowest portion of the small bowel, obstructive symptoms are frequently encountered. Unremitting

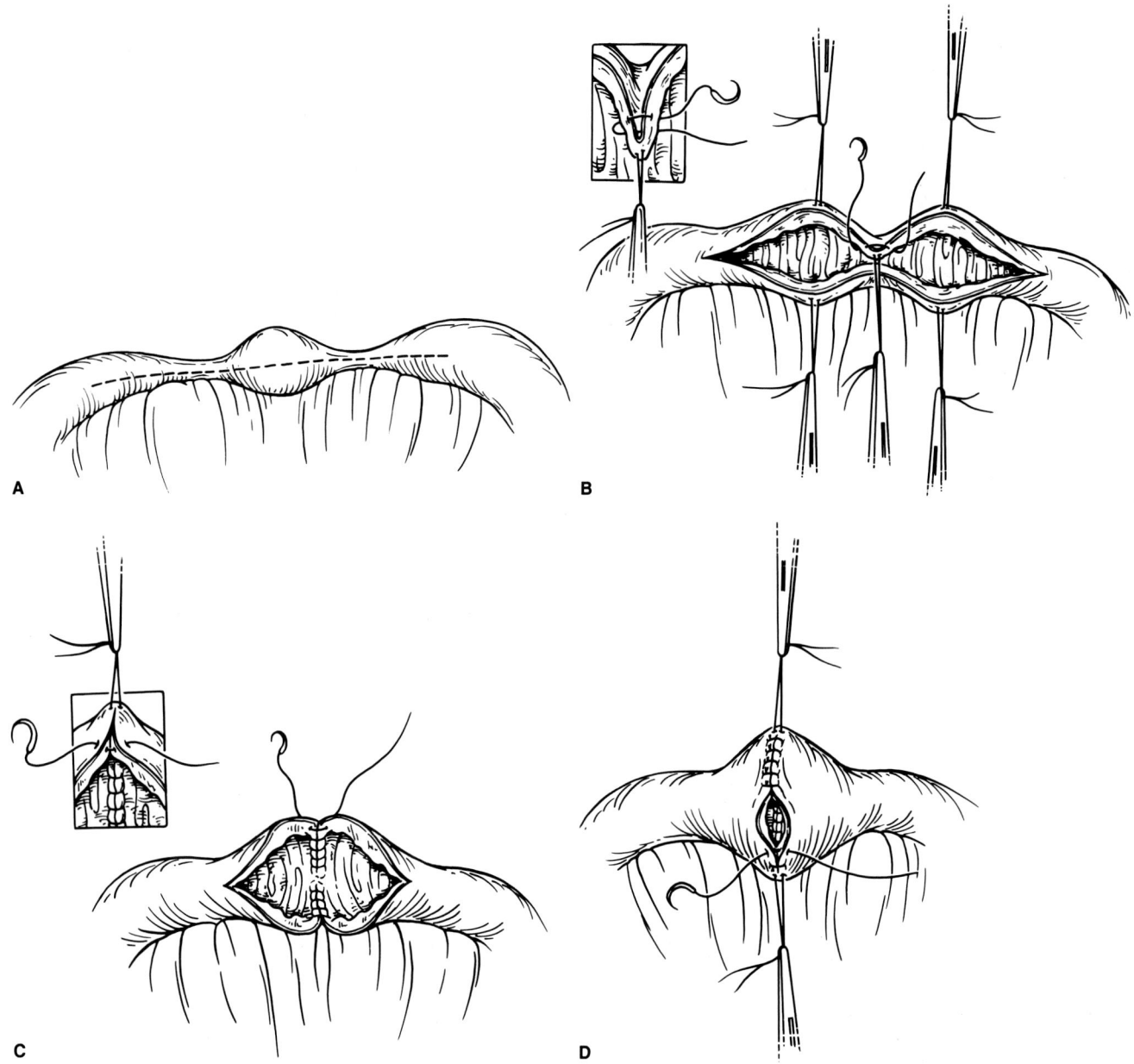

Figure 34-5 Combined Heineke-Mikulicz and Finney strictureplasty for stenosis and skip lesions of up to 20 cm in length. (After Fazio VW, Tjandra JJ. Strictureplasty for Crohn's disease with multiple long strictures. Dis Colon Rectum 1993;36:71)

chronic obstructive symptoms or an episode of high-grade obstruction indicates that the degree of cicatricial stenosis is such that medical treatment is unlikely to be effective and surgical treatment is necessary.

When evaluating a patient with Crohn's disease who has a complete intestinal obstruction, other causes of complete intestinal obstruction, including volvulus, intussusception, incarcerated hernias, and adhesive bands, that require emergent surgical treatment must be ruled out. When the physician is certain that the obstruction is due

to Crohn's disease alone, even in the presence of high-grade or complete obstruction, careful observation and supportive treatment may be instituted. A conservative approach can be adopted because, unlike with volvulus, intussusception, hernias, and adhesive bands, obstruction from Crohn's disease is unlikely to cause vascular insufficiency and ischemic complications. Moreover, the obstruction in Crohn's disease is often the result of undigested food occluding the stenotic, diseased terminal ileum; eventual fermentation and decomposition facilitate

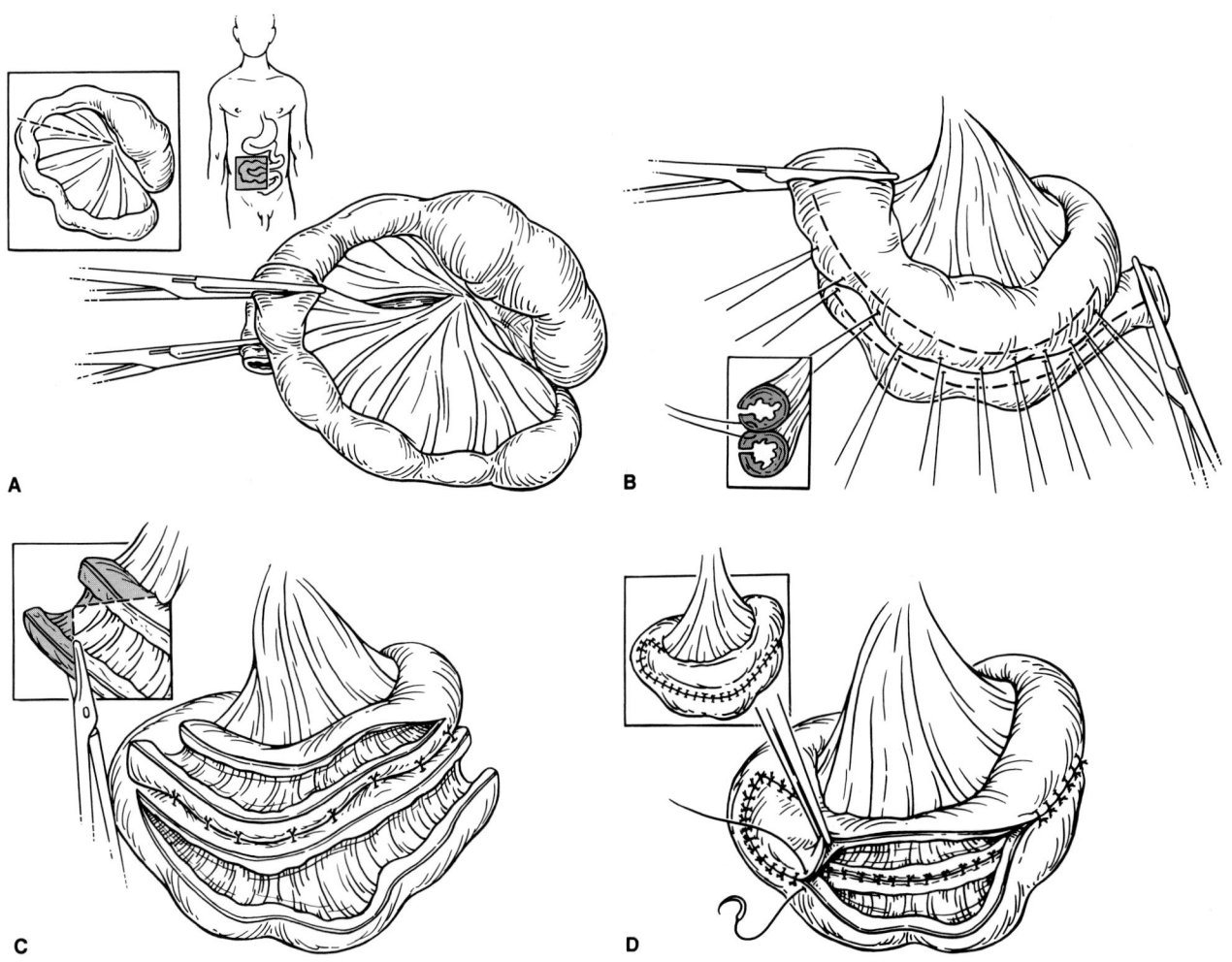

Figure 34-6 Side-to-side isoperistaltic enteroenterostomy for stenosis and skip lesions of combined length of up to 30 cm. (After Michelassi F. Side-to-side isoperistaltic strictureplasty. J Colon Rect Dis [submitted])

passage and restoration of gastrointestinal function. If the obstruction resolves without operation, an elective procedure can be performed during the same hospitalization after mechanical intestinal preparation. Immediate surgical treatment must be instituted if the patient's condition deteriorates.

When a patient presents with partial, chronic intestinal obstruction due to several tight strictures, the small bowel may be dilated (Fig. 34-10A). Placement of a nasoenteric decompressing tube may be necessary to accomplish a thorough preoperative intestinal preparation. Long nasoenteric decompressing tubes facilitate mechanical preparation of the dilated intestine, both as a suction device and as a conduit for slow instillation of hyperosmolar electrolyte-containing solutions (see Fig 34-10B). No matter how prolonged the preoperative decompression, chronically dilated small bowel does not

resume original size before surgical intervention. Fortuitously, persistent intestinal dilation can facilitate end-to-end anastomosis with the ascending colon after ileocecal resection.

Fistulas

Recognized early by Crohn,[25] fistulas are common in Crohn's disease of the terminal ileum; however, they rarely represent the only indication for surgical treatment. In one series of 639 patients undergoing surgery for Crohn's disease,[2] 331 patients had disease in the terminal ileum. Of these, 217 patients (65.6%) were found to harbor 285 intraabdominal fistulas, but in only 6% did fistulas represent the primary indication for surgical treatment.

Fistulas result from full-thickness disease rupturing

(Text continues on page 1212)

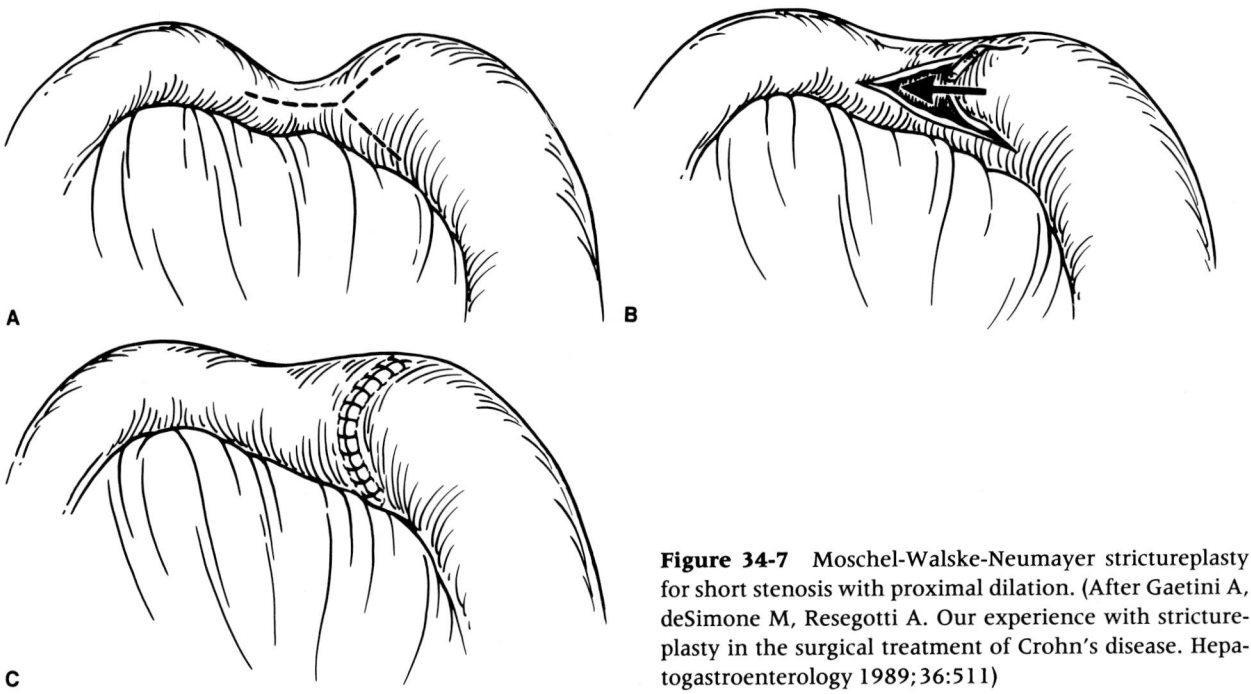

Figure 34-7 Moschel-Walske-Neumayer strictureplasty for short stenosis with proximal dilation. (After Gaetini A, deSimone M, Resegotti A. Our experience with strictureplasty in the surgical treatment of Crohn's disease. Hepatogastroenterology 1989;36:511)

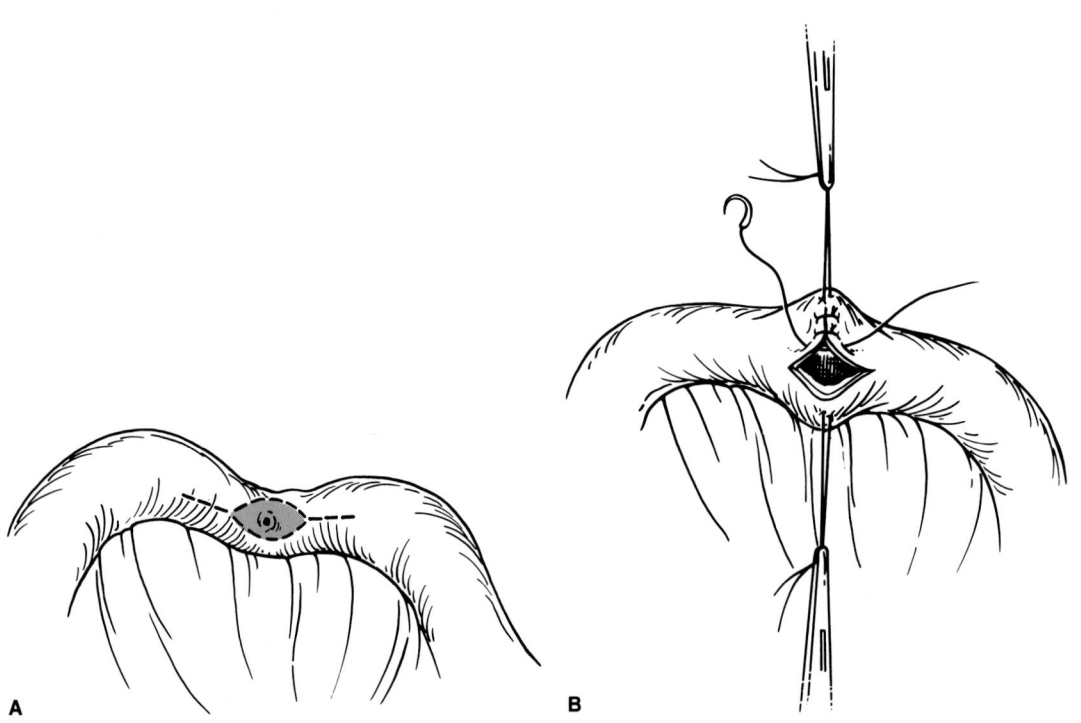

Figure 34-8 Judd strictureplasty for stenosis with a chronic fistula. (After Gaetini A, deSimone M, Resegotti A. Our experience with strictureplasty in the surgical treatment of Crohn's disease. Hepatogastroenterology 1989;36:511)

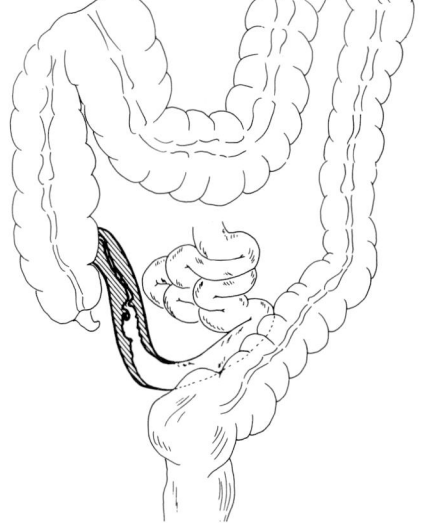

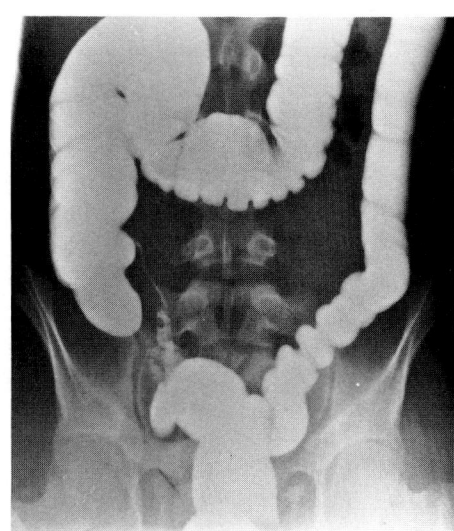

Figure 34-9 Barium enema with reflux in the terminal ileum showing a long stenosis ("string sign") in the intestinal segment just proximal to the ileocecal valve.

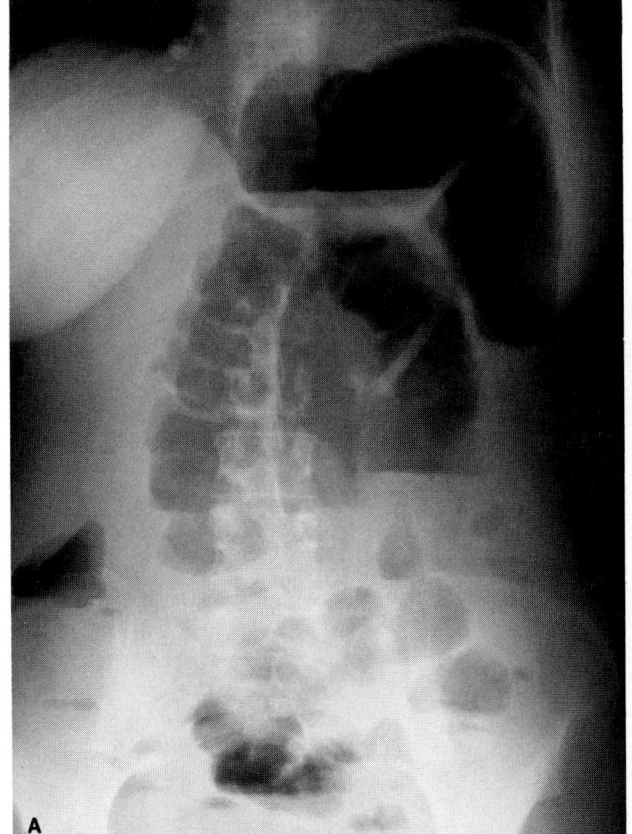

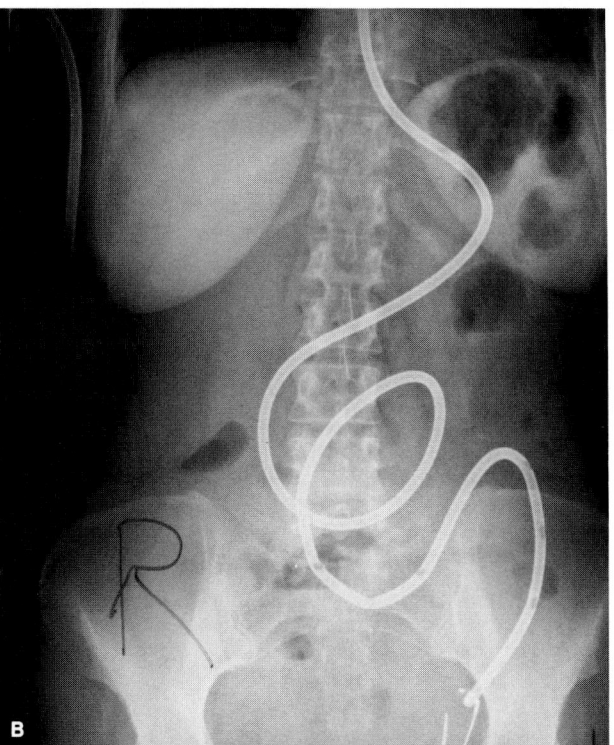

Figure 34-10 (**A**) Abdominal radiograph taken in upright position showing dilated loops of small bowel and air–fluid levels consistent with partial small bowel obstruction in a patient known to have Crohn's disease of the terminal ileum. (**B**) Same patient after passage of a nasoenteric tube for decompression and mechanical preparation of the small bowel before operation.

into an adjacent hollow viscus. At times, an abscess may intervene. In any case, the nearby viscus or organ is usually not affected by Crohn's disease, and Crohn's disease does not spread to it.

Fistulas have been traditionally classified as internal or external. *Internal fistulas* connect a diseased intestinal segment to another portion of the gut, or to extraintestinal hollow viscera, such as genitourinary, biliopancreatic, or bronchopleural structures. *External fistulas* connect diseased intestinal segments with the body surface and include enterocutaneous or colocutaneous fistulas, anal fistulas, and enterovaginal fistulas.

Among internal fistulas, only enterovesical fistulas cause symptoms (pneumaturia, fecaluria) that are so characteristic as to be diagnostic. To diagnose external fistulas, including enterocutaneous and enterovaginal fistulas, only an accurate history and physical examination are needed. In all cases, preoperative radiologic and endoscopic examinations are required to determine the extent of gastrointestinal involvement by Crohn's disease and to delineate the anatomy of the fistula accurately. In some instances, fistulas are discovered at the time of operation or only after a careful examination of the resected specimen.

ENTERODUODENAL FISTULAS. Enteroduodenal fistulas (Fig. 34-11) are rare, with fewer than 100 cases reported in the English literature.[27-31] They occur with equal frequency in primary and recurrent disease: in primary Crohn's disease, fistulas usually originate from a diseased colon; after operation, the fistula originates from disease at the ileocolic anastomosis. In all these cases, the duodenum is not primarily involved by Crohn's disease; in fact, there is only one reported enteroduodenal fistula in the English literature with histologic evidence of duodenal Crohn's disease.[30]

The appropriate surgical management of enteroduodenal fistulas follows the principle of resection of the primary disease with extirpation of the fistula.[21-23] Controversy exists about how the duodenal defect should be managed. Some authors have proposed to protect duodenal repairs routinely by applying a serosal patch to cover the defect.[32] In this technique, the serosa of a jejunal loop is sutured to the healthy duodenal serosa surrounding the duodenal repair. Some also prefer the serosal patch technique for defects that are not suitable for primary closure because of edema or friability of the duodenal wall. In contrast, in the presence of edema or friability of the duodenal wall, other authors advocate incorporating the duodenal defect in a side-to-side or Roux-en-Y duodenojejunostomy.[22] In most patients, a primary closure is feasible; when the duodenal defect is close to the pancreatic border, however, a tedious and meticulous dissection is necessary to mobilize healthy duodenal wall from the pancreas. Although other maneuvers, including omental or peritoneal patch and side-to-side or Roux-en-Y duodenojejunostomy, are not

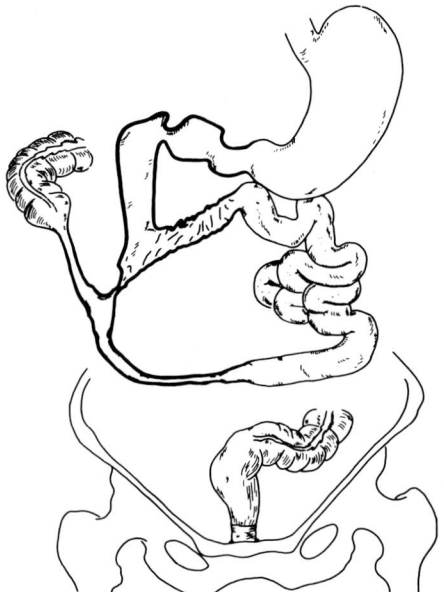
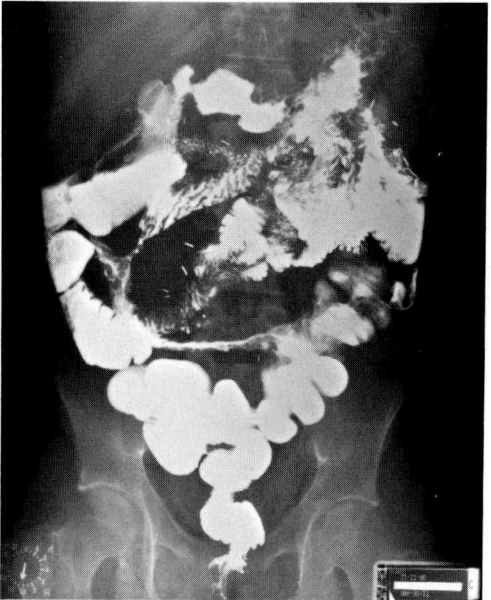

Figure 34-11 Upper gastrointestinal series showing an ileoduodenal fistula in a patient with a recurrence proximal to the ileoascending anastomosis. (Michelassi F, Balestracci T, Chappell R, et al. Primary and recurrent Crohn's disease: experience with 1379 patients. Ann Surg 1991;214:23)

necessary as routine procedures, they should be used to protect a difficult primary closure or to avoid a primary closure when local conditions render it inadvisable. Most authors routinely use a decompressing tube, entering the gastric lumen as a gastrostomy and traversing the pylorus to protect the duodenal closure.

ENTEROENTERIC FISTULAS. Enteroenteric fistulas (Fig. 34-12) are often asymptomatic and are discovered in as many as 46% of cases[31] during abdominal exploration or on careful inspection of the resected specimen. One investigator,[33] reporting on 64 patients with enteroenteric fistulas, concluded that fistulas are not an absolute indication for surgery. This investigator considered surgical intervention only when fistulas were complicated by sepsis or intestinal obstruction or when they caused massive diarrhea because of the bypass of a sizable length of intestine. Enteroenteric fistulas are often treated by en bloc resection with the diseased segment. In cases in which this approach would lead to excessive sacrifice of uninvolved intestine, an attempt to separate the normal-appearing loops adherent to the diseased segment should be made. Care is necessary to contain or minimize contamination of the operative field due to transection of fistulas or to opening of an interloop abscess. The resulting defect in the normal, adjacent intestinal wall is closed with meticulous technique after débriding its edges to healthy tissue.

ILEOCOLIC FISTULAS. Ileocecal and right ileocolic fistulas (Fig. 34-13) are the most common internal fistulas encountered. Although they are usually asymptomatic and rarely represent the only indication for sur-

gical treatment, fistulas usually indicate the presence of severe disease. Ileocecal and right ileocolic fistulas usually lend themselves to en bloc resection with the diseased intestinal segment.

When an ileorectosigmoid fistula (Fig. 34-14) is present, the sigmoid is involved most often because of its proximity but is otherwise not affected by Crohn's disease. Although some authors[34] have advocated resection of both terminal ileum and sigmoid in the treatment of these fistulas, the defect through the sigmoid wall can also be closed primarily after débridement of the edges. Sigmoid resection is necessary when there is evidence of primary Crohn's disease in the sigmoid colon; when the intestinal wall is inflamed, thickened, and rigid; when débridement of the edges of the fistula results in a large defect in the sigmoid wall; and when the opening of the fistula is on the mesenteric side of the sigmoid and primary closure is difficult.

ENTEROCUTANEOUS FISTULAS. Enterocutaneous fistulas usually drain through a previous abdominal scar or through the umbilicus.[35,36] At times, enterocutaneous fistulas result from surgical incision and drainage of a subcutaneous abscess complicating severe intraabdominal disease[37,38] or from percutaneous drainage of an abdominal abscess. The presence of an enterocutaneous fistula does not necessarily dictate immediate surgical intervention. Patients may be reluctant to undergo surgical treatment when the enterocutaneous fistula has a minimal output and the underlying disease is under satisfactory control. Surgical

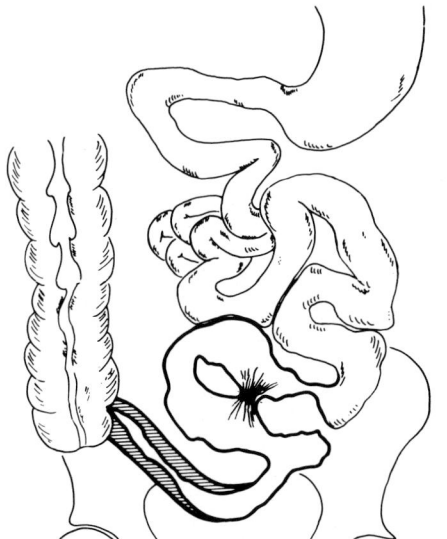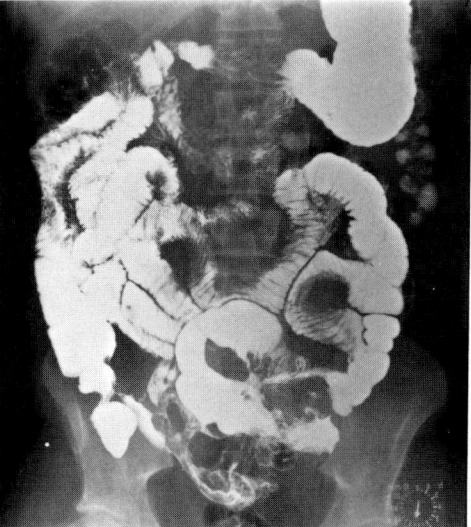

Figure 34-12 Small bowel follow-through series showing an enteroenteric fistula in Crohn's disease of the terminal ileum. (Michelassi F, Balestracci T, Chappell R, et al. Primary and recurrent Crohn's disease: experience with 1379 patients. Ann Surg 1991;214:23)

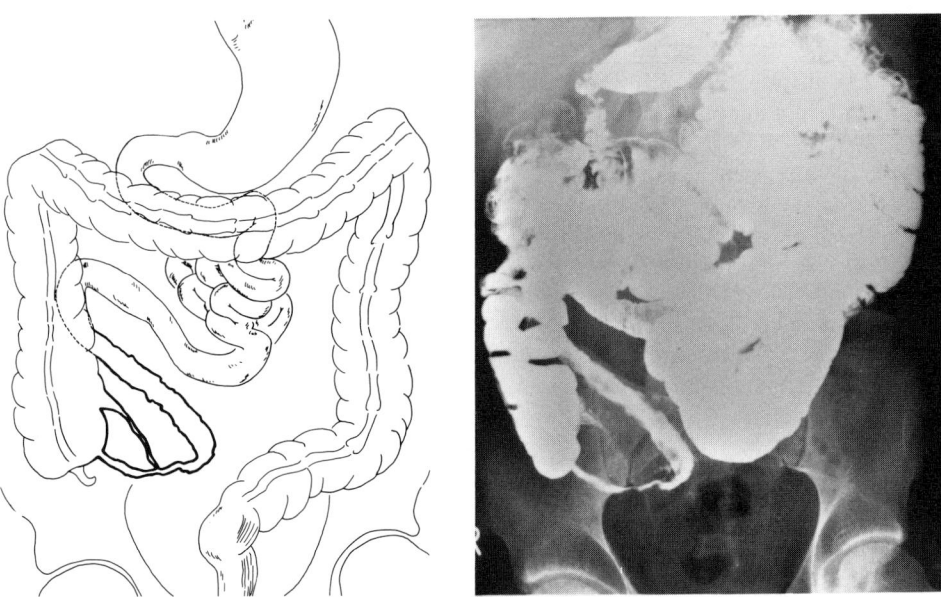

Figure 34-13 Small bowel follow-through series showing an enteric–right colic fistula.

intervention may not be needed when the cutaneous opening of the fistula drains near an intestinal stoma and can be incorporated into the stoma appliance. In most cases, difficulty in maintaining personal hygiene and fear of social embarrassment, bothersome symptoms associated with the diseased segment that led to the formation of the fistula, and skin excoriation that invariably forms around the cutaneous opening of the fistula all become factors indicating the need for surgical treatment. Surgical treatment of an enterocutaneous fistula is based on resection of the diseased intestinal segment, extirpation of the fistula, and débridement of the fistulous tract through the abdominal wall and subcutaneous tissue. This usually requires several subcutaneous fistulotomies, which are left to heal by secondary intention.

ENTEROGENITAL FISTULAS. Enterovaginal fistulas are rare complications of Crohn's disease[39] and most often occur in women who have undergone a hysterectomy. The vaginal discharge is cause for discomfort, social and sexual embarrassment, and difficulty in maintaining personal hygiene. Most of these patients demand treatment of this condition and readily accept a recommendation for an operation. The surgical treatment of an enterovaginal fistula involves resection of the diseased bowel with extirpation or débridement of the fistulous tract and drainage of any intervening abscesses. The opening into the vaginal cuff is usually small. Often located in the center of an area of induration and inflammation, the opening does not need to be sutured and invariably closes by secondary intention. Enterosalpingeal fistulas are rare; one report describes

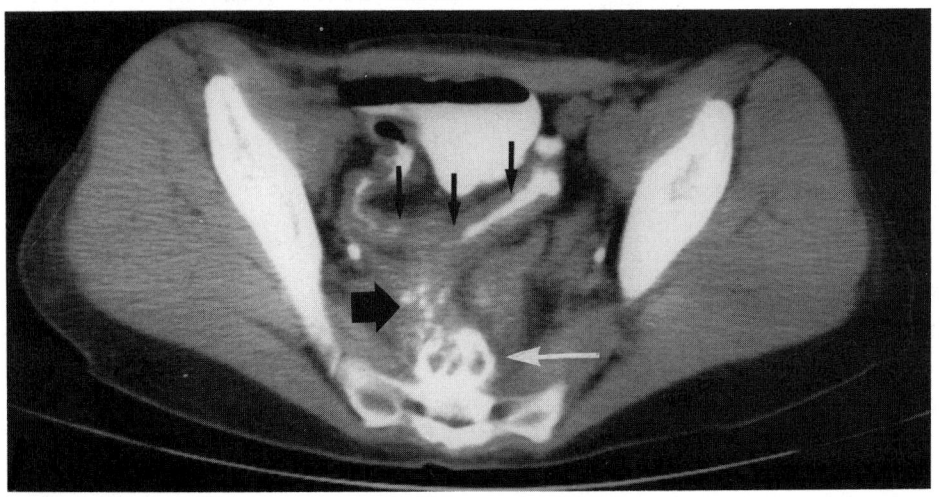

Figure 34-14 CT showing a thickened, diseased terminal ileum (*small arrows*) with extravasation of contrast in the perirectal space (*large arrow*). Contrast is also seen in the rectal lumen (*white arrow*). At exploration, an ileorectal fistula was confirmed. (Michelassi F, Balestracci T, Chappell R, et al. Primary and recurrent Crohn's disease: experience with 1379 patients. Ann Surg 1991; 214:23)

enteric fistula to the right fallopian tube and enteric fistula to the uterus.[40] Another large experience encountered only two enterosalpingeal fistulas during the course of 20 years.[2]

ENTEROVESICAL FISTULAS. Enterovesical fistulas (Fig. 34-15) occur in 2% to 5% of patients with Crohn's disease[41-43] and usually cause pneumaturia. Some patients also experience fecaluria. Because of associated urinary tract infection, most patients also complain of urgency, frequency, dysuria, suprapubic discomfort, strangury, and occasionally passage of blood-tinged urine. The consequences of chronic urinary tract infection on renal function, in addition to the symptoms of the intestinal disease,[42-44] represent an urgent indication for operation. The need for surgery is not mitigated by the ability of antibiotics and urinary antiseptics to control symptoms of urinary infection.[42,44]

Surgical treatment parallels that for other fistulas—resection of the diseased segment of intestine with extirpation of the fistulous tract. The opening in the bladder is usually located at the dome, and débridement and primary closure can be affected without danger to the trigone. After repair, the bladder is drained for several days with an indwelling catheter, which is removed after radiologic confirmation that the bladder repair has healed. A closed suction drain is placed at the time of operation in proximity to the bladder repair to drain urine that may extravasate.

Inflammatory Masses and Abscesses

Inflammatory masses and abscesses often produce the same symptoms and physical findings and can be accurately classified only during an exploratory laparotomy. A *phlegmonous mass* is an expression of severe disease and inflammation that has remained contained in the affected intestinal segment. In contrast, an *abscess* is the result of a walled-off perforation. In either case, the physical finding of an inflammatory mass is an indication that the disease has reached a degree of severity and complexity to warrant surgical treatment. In one series,[3] preoperative diagnosis of an inflammatory mass or an abscess was accomplished by physical examination in 129 patients (20.2%). Thirty-six more patients, in whom preoperative examination had not suggested the presence of an inflammatory mass, were found to have an intraabdominal abscess at laparotomy.

Because the terminal ileum is the intestinal segment most often affected by Crohn's disease, most inflammatory masses are located in the right lower quadrant (Fig. 34-16). In the presence of a right lower quadrant mass, the right ureter may be compressed or encased in retroperitoneal fibrosis near the pelvic brim,

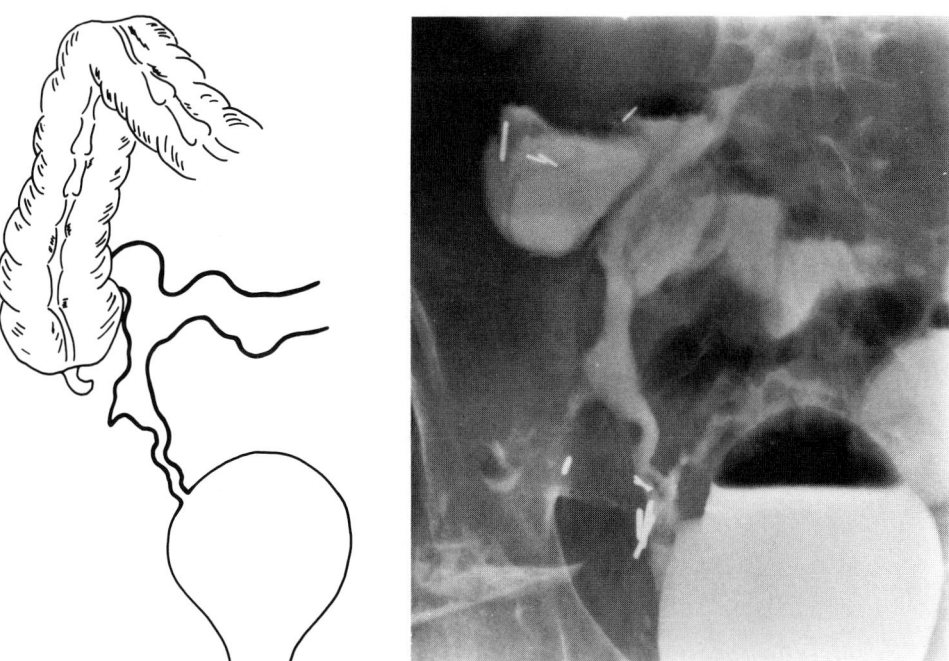

Figure 34-15 Cystogram revealing an ileovesical fistula. (Michelassi F, Balestracci T, Chappell R, et al. Primary and recurrent Crohn's disease: experience with 1379 patients. Ann Surg 1991;214:23)

causing right hydronephrosis. Because obstructive uropathy is usually asymptomatic, a preoperative ultrasound study of the right kidney and ureter should be obtained in patients with a right lower quadrant mass. If hydronephrosis is documented, an intravenous pyelogram should follow to delineate the degree and location of the obstruction. As an alternative approach, if abdominal CT is necessary in the course of the preoperative evaluation, the infusion of intravenous iodine contrast at the time of the study can help the physician to visualize a dilated ureter and renal pelvis.

For most abdominal masses diagnosed preoperatively, an abscess is found at the time of the surgical treatment, either alone or in combination with a phlegmonous mass. In one series,[3] 57% of patients diagnosed preoperatively with an intraabdominal mass had an abscess. Therefore, the preoperative diagnosis of an intraabdominal mass should raise the clinical suspicion that the patient harbors an intraabdominal abscess. Nevertheless, in up to one third of cases, there is no preoperative suspicion of an abdominal abscess. This is common with interloop abscesses and in cases in which the abscess and the surrounding inflammatory reaction is not sizable enough to be appreciated on physical examination. Misdiagnosis also occurs when the usual signs of sepsis, such as fever, chills, and general malaise, are attributed to an exacerbation of the disease or are masked by steroid therapy.

In the absence of peritoneal signs, patients may undergo gentle intestinal mechanical preparation and elective resection. In the presence of localized peritoneal signs, patients can usually be treated safely with intravenous fluids, antibiotic administration, and bowel rest. If close observation indicates progressive improvement, continuation of nonoperative treatment is justified. This approach can transform an emergent situation into a semielective procedure, increasing the chances of performing a resection with primary anastomosis and avoiding a temporary stoma. Peritonitis or failure to improve dictates immediate operation, even if this results in the need for a temporary stoma after resection of the diseased segment.

CLASSIFICATION. Abdominal abscesses defy easy classification,[45-47] and many authors group them all together. Intraabdominal abscesses can be classified as retroperitoneal or intraperitoneal, with subdivision of the latter category into interloop, intramesenteric, and enteroparietal.

RETROPERITONEAL ABSCESSES. The overall incidence of retroperitoneal abscesses in Crohn's disease ranges from 2.7% to 5%.[35,36] The most common symptoms and physical findings are pain referred to the back and to the lower limb, fever, and flexion contracture of the hip. Abdominal pain is present in only 40% and an inflammatory mass in 12.5% of cases. Retroperitoneal abscesses are often psoas abscesses. Although psoas abscesses were initially described as secondary to tubercular spondylitis, investigators have reported that Crohn's disease is the most common cause of retroperitoneal psoas abscesses worldwide and that 80% of these abscesses are located on the right side[48] (Fig 34-17). The right side is more commonly involved because the terminal ileum is the most common location of Crohn's disease.

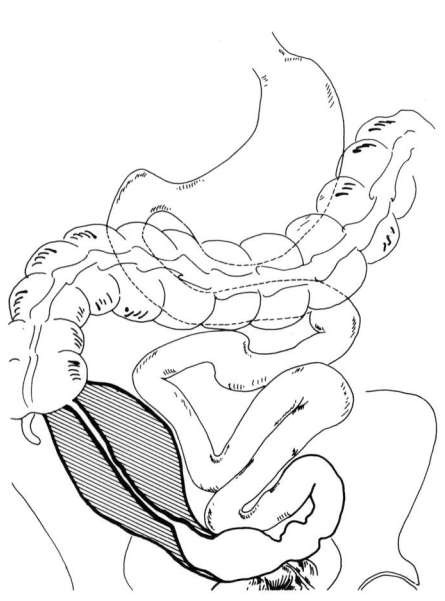

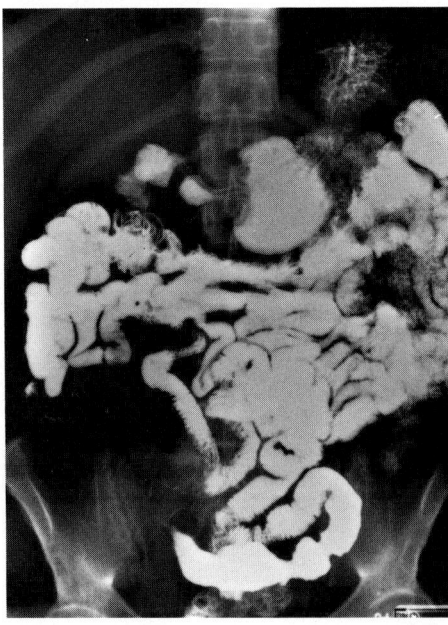

Figure 34-16 Upper gastrointestinal series showing displacement of small intestinal loops by a large right lower quadrant mass in a patient with disease confined to the terminal ileum. (Michelassi F, Balestracci T, Chappell R, et al. Primary and recurrent Crohn's disease: experience with 1379 patients. Ann Surg 1991; 214:23)

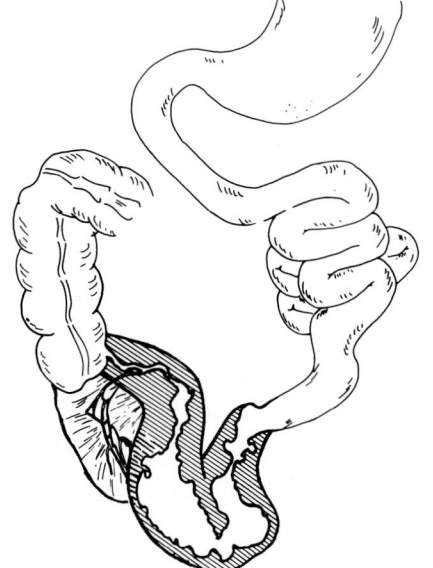

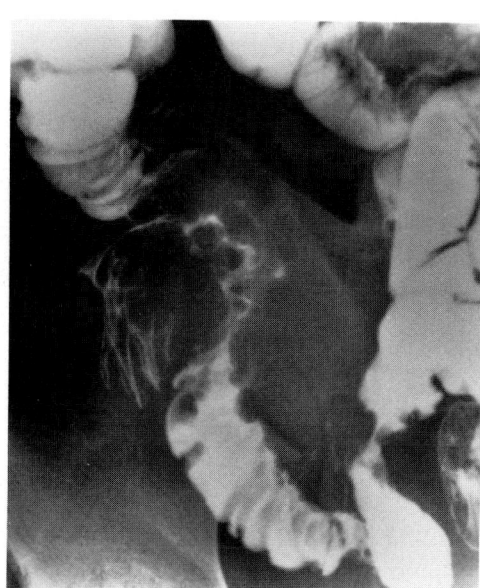

Figure 34-17 Small bowel follow-through series showing a right psoas abscess originating from a walled-off perforation of the terminal ileum.

Usually, retroperitoneal abscesses are drained and the walls débrided during the performance of a laparotomy for resection of the diseased intestinal segment. In advanced cases in which the abscess points to the inguinal region, a limited incision in the groin can be used to obtain drainage preliminary to resection of the diseased intestine.

INTRAPERITONEAL ABSCESSES. The overall incidence of intraperitoneal abscesses in Crohn's disease ranges from 12% to 28%.[37,38,49] Interloop abscesses are usually diagnosed at the time of operation, during the mobilization of macroscopically healthy intestinal loops from the diseased segment. Part of the wall is resected with the specimen; whatever is left adherent on healthy loops must be débrided to minimize the postop-

erative recurrence. The mechanical débridement must be carefully performed to minimize the chance of iatrogenic injuries to normal bowel.

An intramesenteric abscess (Fig. 34-18) develops from perforation of the diseased intestinal segment at its mesenteric border and is totally contained within the leaflets of the mesentery. These abscesses usually contain a minimal amount of pus and should be resected en bloc with the diseased intestinal segment.

Enteroparietal abscesses are located between intestinal loops and the abdominal wall. They are more easily appreciated on preoperative physical examination than interloop, mesenteric, or retroperitoneal abscesses.

Retroperitoneal, interloop, and intramesenteric abscesses do not lend themselves to preoperative percutaneous drainage. Percutaneous drainage is easily accom-

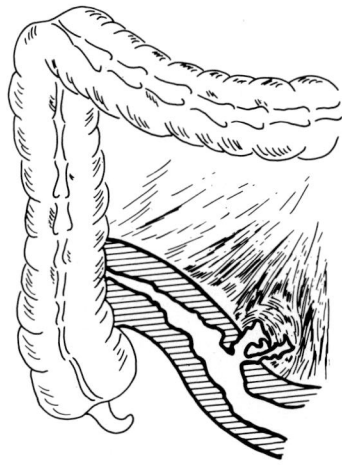

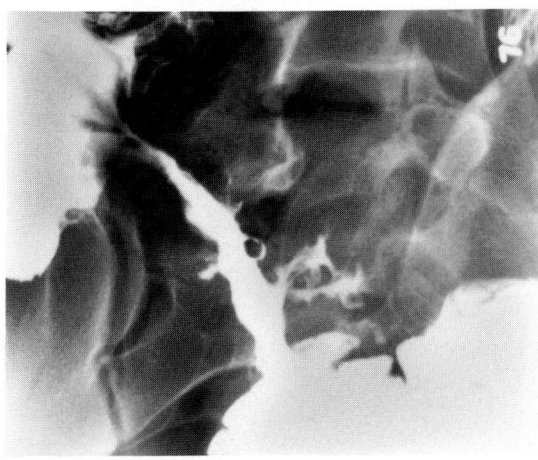

Figure 34-18 Small bowel follow-through series showing an intramesenteric abscess originating from a perforation of the terminal ileum in the mesentery.

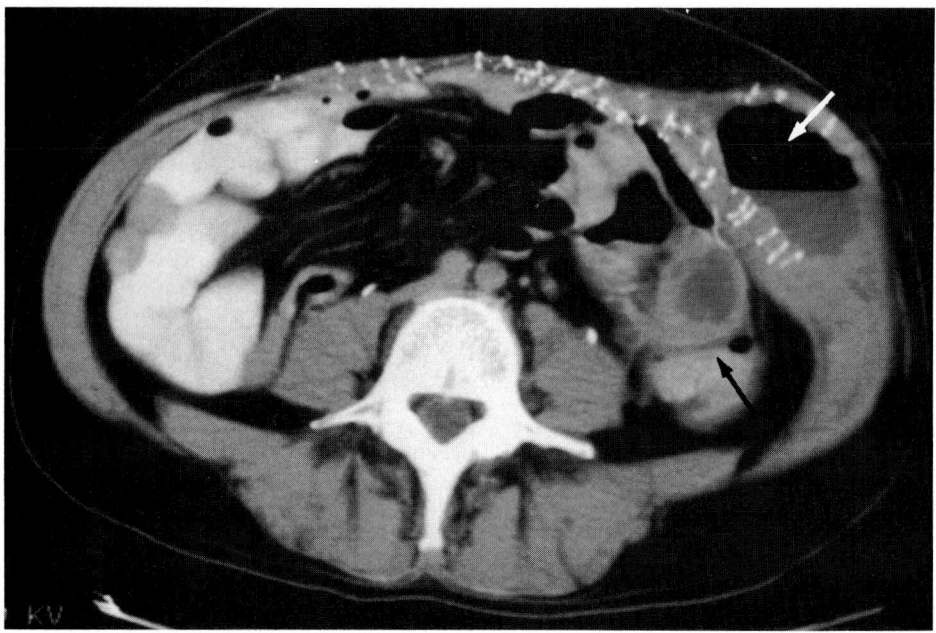

Figure 34-19 CT scan showing a left flank abscess (*black arrow*) originating from Crohn's disease of the descending colon, perforated through the abdominal wall into the subcutaneous planes. An air–fluid level is evident in the subcutaneous extension (*white arrow*). (Michelassi F, Stella M. Intraabdominal septic complications in Crohn's disease. In: Levine B, ed. Perspectives in surgery, vol 3. St Louis, Quality Medical Publishing, 1993: 63)

plished for subcutaneous extensions of intraabdominal abscesses (Fig. 34-19) and for some favorably located enteroparietal abscesses (Fig. 34-20). If percutaneous drainage is elected, CT and ultrasound are excellent techniques to guide catheter insertion.[50,51] This technique can be used advantageously in seriously ill patients as a temporary measure to facilitate subsequent surgical intervention. According to one report,[45] however, external fistulas developed in 21 of 37 patients (56.8%) after surgical incision and drainage of the abscess, and only 6 of 37 (16%) patients required no fur-

ther treatment. The presence of necrotic tissue in the abscess cavity, the persistence of the primary disease, and the development of a fistulous tract are all indications for definitive surgical treatment.

When exploratory laparotomy and surgical drainage are elected, the abscess should be drained completely and its walls débrided if not resected with the specimen. Steps should be taken early in the operative procedure to minimize contamination of the abdominal wound and peritoneal cavity by protecting the edges of the incision with an impermeable wound protector and

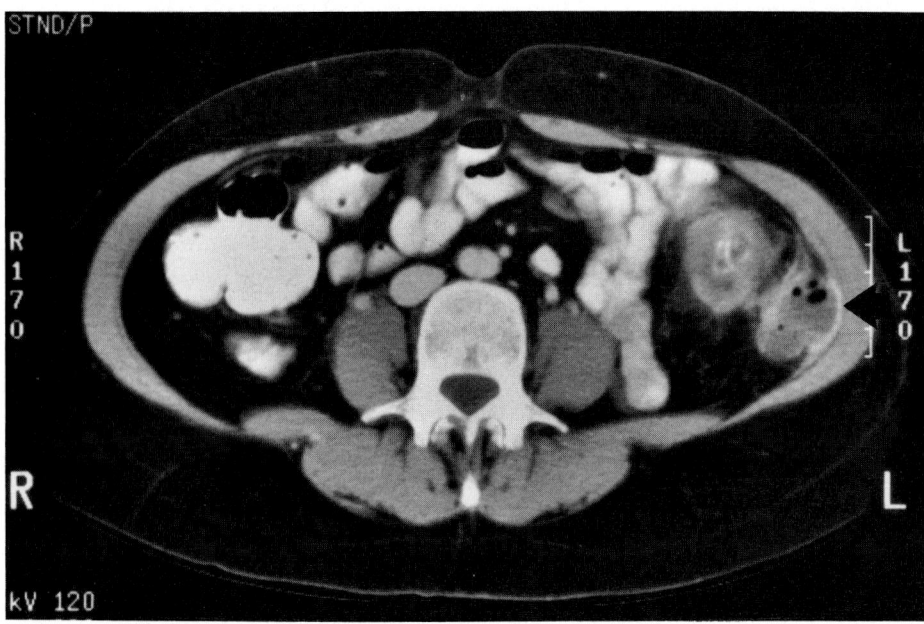

Figure 34-20 CT scan showing a left flank enteroparietal abscess (*arrow*) originating from Crohn's disease of the descending colon. Air is evident in the abscess cavity. This location lends itself to percutaneous drainage.

by walling off the uncontaminated peritoneal cavity with laparotomy pads. An attempt should be made to enter abscesses extraperitoneally or in a nondependent location to allow suctioning of the liquid component before uncontrollable spillage occurs.

Ureteral Obstruction

Ureteral obstruction (Fig. 34-21) is a well-recognized complication of ileal disease and occurs in about 5% of patients.[52,53] Resection of the inflammatory mass usually relieves the compression on the ureter and cures the right hydronephrosis. When the hydronephrosis is caused by retroperitoneal fibrosis secondary to the presence of an inflammatory mass or an abscess, however, constriction of the ureter can be released only by ureterolysis.

Free Perforation

Free perforation is a rare occurrence in Crohn's disease and usually results from secondary rupture of an abscess into the peritoneal cavity. An emergency laparotomy is needed in these cases, with resection of the diseased segment and exteriorization of the proximal bowel as a terminal ileostomy. The distal end can be exteriorized as a mucous fistula or closed as a defunctionalized pouch, depending on the degree of peritoneal contamination.

Hemorrhage

Acute massive intestinal hemorrhage occurs in less than 1.5% of patients with Crohn's disease,[4] but patients experiencing one episode of hemorrhage are likely to have at least one additional episode. Age of the patient, duration and activity of the disease, and use of corticosteroids do not influence the occurrence of bleeding. Because of the increased likelihood of recurrent bleeding, these patients should undergo a resection of the diseased segment.

Disease of the Colon

Patients with Crohn's colitis represent the second largest group of patients affected by Crohn's disease. In a series of 639 patients operated on for Crohn's disease,[1] about one third had Crohn's colitis: 38 had disease confined only to the colon, 27 had pancolitis, and the remainder had disease affecting various segments of the colon, rectum, and small bowel. In another report of 615 patients,[54] 27% had Crohn's colitis, and an additional 3.4% had Crohn's disease primarily involving the rectum and anus.

When colonic Crohn's disease is limited to the right colon, it is usually a manifestation of Crohn's ileocolitis (Fig. 34-22). In these instances, an ileocolic resection is performed with a primary anastomosis of the ileum to the ascending or transverse colon in either an end-to-side or end-to-end fashion. The type of anastomo-

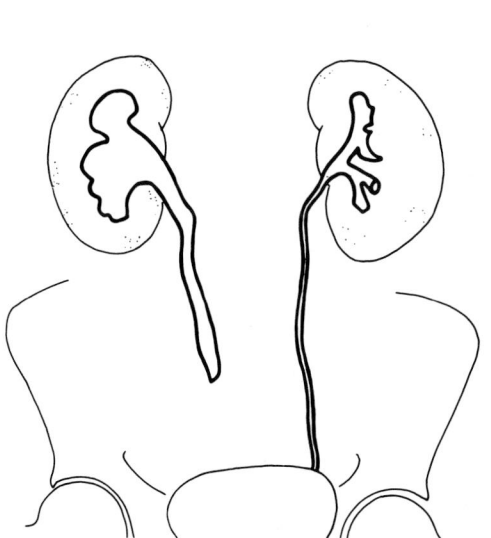
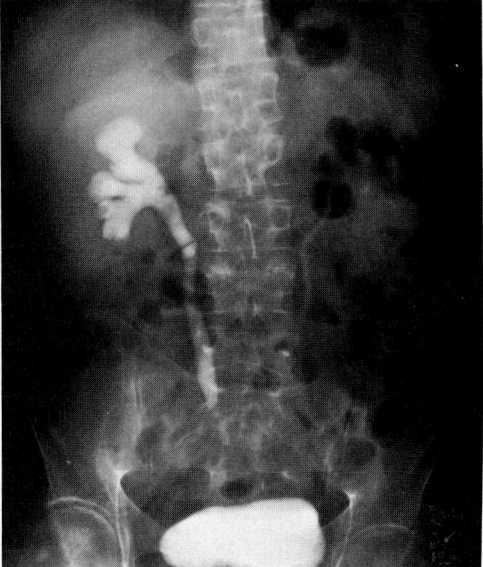

Figure 34-21 Complete right ureteral obstruction with ipsilateral hydronephrosis. (Michelassi F, Stella M. Intra-abdominal septic complications in Crohn's disease. In: Levine B, ed. Perspectives in surgery, vol 3. St Louis, Quality Medical Publishing, 1993:63)

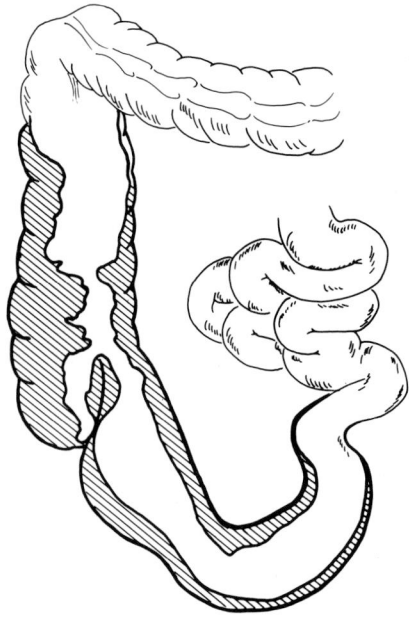
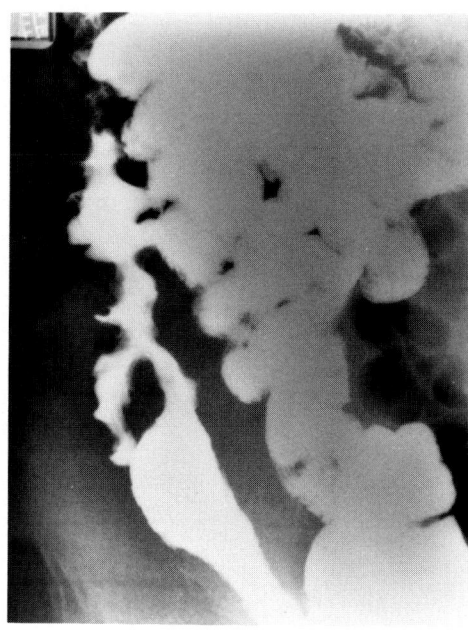

Figure 34-22 Small bowel follow-through series showing Crohn's disease of the terminal ileum and right colon.

sis employed is dictated by convenience and lumen disparity.

Segmental colitis of the transverse colon (Fig. 34-23) and left colon (Fig. 34-24) is rare, and operation is usually indicated because of a localized inflammatory process mimicking diverticulitis with abscess formation, incomplete obstruction, or rarely, hemorrhage. In these instances, local resection with a primary colonic anastomosis is indicated, but recurrence in the remaining colon is frequent and rapid.[55]

Crohn's colitis with rectal sparing (Fig. 34-25) occurs in about 20% of the colitic population.[56] The determination of rectal sparing is made by inspection of the mucosa by rigid proctoscopy. Histologic evaluation by means of biopsy is unnecessary and often confusing. In

the colitic patient whose rectum is spared, abdominal colectomy with an ileoproctostomy is the procedure of choice when there is no severe perineal disease or sphincter dysfunction. For this operation to be worthwhile, 10 to 14 cm of rectum should be free of disease, and ideally, all or most of the terminal ileum should be preserved. If significant ileal resection has been performed or if the rectal segment is too short, the patient may suffer disabling diarrhea.

Although the risk of recurrence of disease after an ileoproctostomy is greater than that after proctocolectomy with endoileostomy, it is the procedure of choice if there is significant rectal sparing.[57] Avoidance of a permanent stoma and maintenance of an intact perineum are important quality-of-life factors. After ileo-

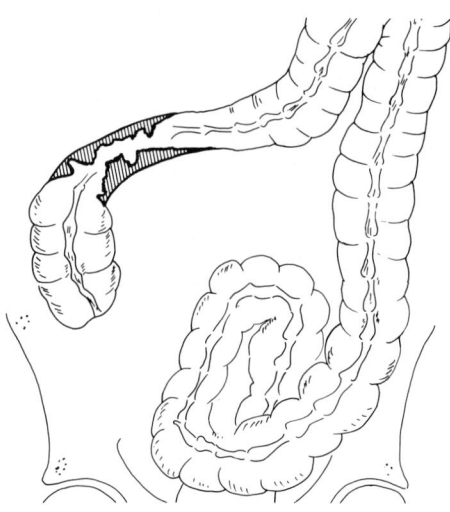
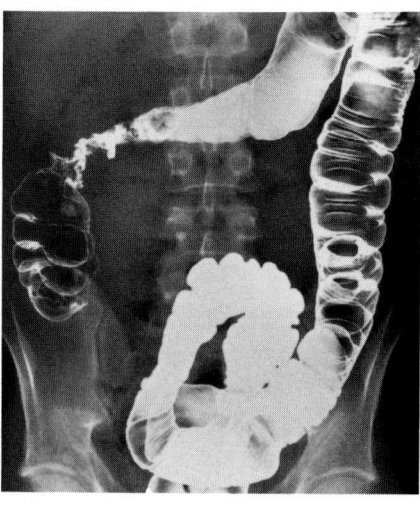

Figure 34-23 Barium enema showing Crohn's colitis limited to the right side of the transverse colon.

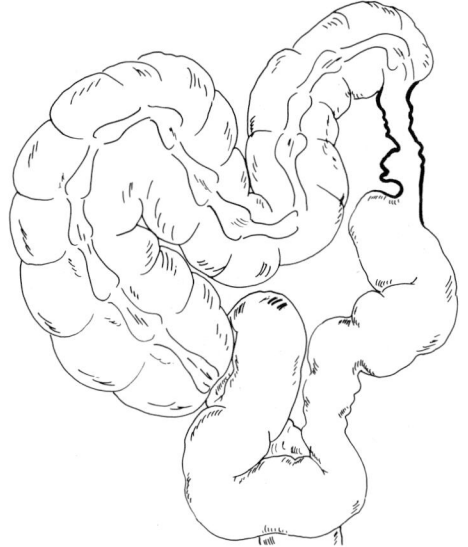
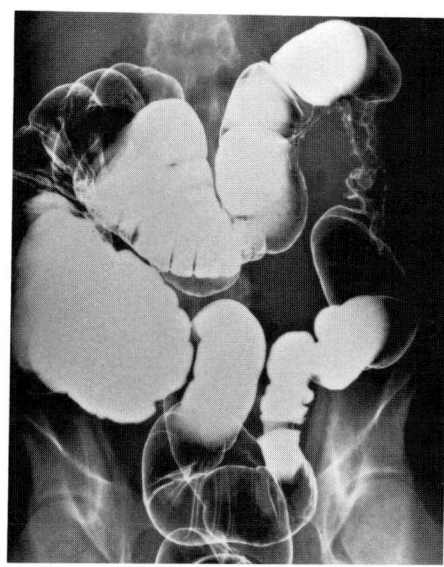

Figure 34-24 Barium enema showing Crohn's colitis limited to the proximal portion of the descending colon.

proctostomy, recurrence appears in about half of patients within 5 years.[58] The recurrence may involve the small bowel, rectum, or both. In many patients, a second resection and anastomosis is possible, although a large number of patients eventually require a proctocolectomy.

In a few patients, Crohn's colitis is confined to the anorectum or rectosigmoid (Fig. 34-26). For these patients, a proctectomy and descending colostomy are satisfactory.

For patients with pancolitis or severe perineal disease, total proctocolectomy and end ileostomy are the procedures of choice. In this operation, as much terminal ileum as possible is preserved. Gross inspection of the mucosa of the terminal ileum determines the amount of ileum to be resected. Resection should en-

compass all gross lesions of Crohn's disease, but in some patients, aphthous ulcers extend throughout the ileum. The presence of aphthous ulcers alone is not an absolute indication for resection.

In some patients with pancolitis, the patient seeks operation because of unbearable perineal sepsis resulting from rectocutaneous fistulas. These patients are best treated by a two-stage operation. At the first operation, the intraabdominal colon and upper and mid-rectum are removed, creating a short (4- to 6-cm) Hartmann's pouch in the hollow of the sacrum. A permanent end ileostomy is established. Before the procedure is terminated, the perineal abscesses are drained, and the fistulas and sinus tracts are opened. After the perineum has healed by secondary intention and the perineal sepsis has cleared, usually a period of 8 to 12

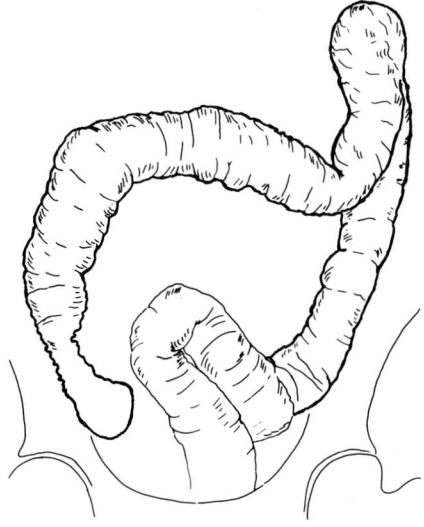
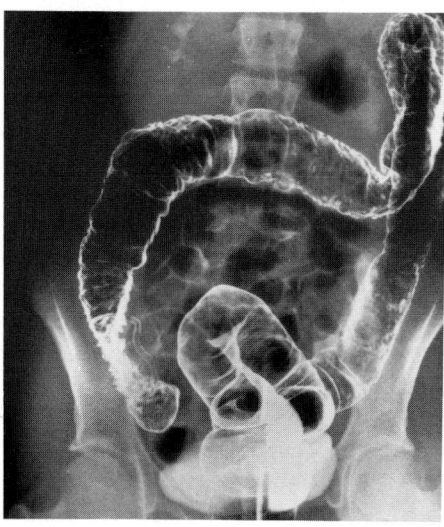

Figure 34-25 Barium enema showing Crohn's colitis with sparing of the rectum and rectosigmoid.

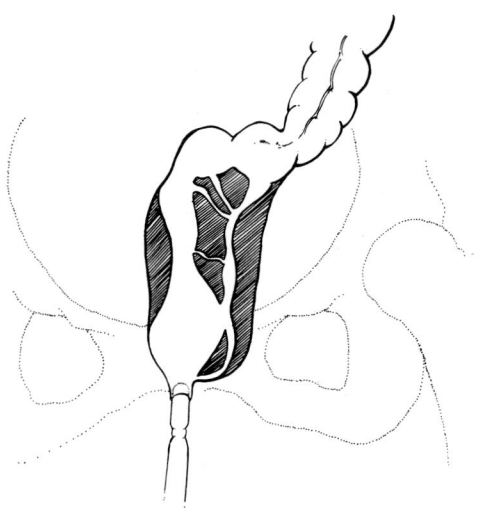
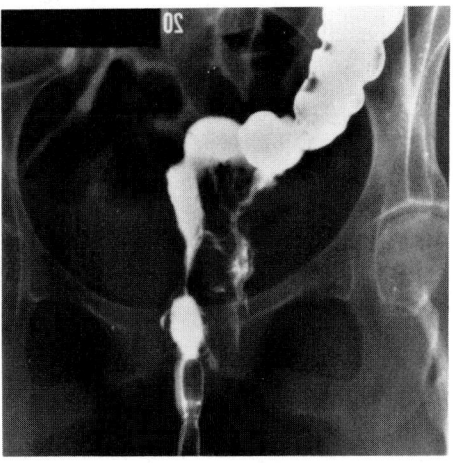

Figure 34-26 Barium enema showing Crohn's proctitis with loss of the rectal ampulla, several rectosigmoid fistulas, and an intervening perirectal abscess.

weeks, the short Hartmann's pouch is removed using a perineal approach. At this second stage, primary closure can usually be accomplished, avoiding persistent perineal wounds.

Because of the importance that the colon and rectum have regarding anal continence, frequency of bowel movements, and stool consistency, emergent operations for acute colitis should be performed in a manner that spares as much as possible of the anorectal region. If the rectum is free of disease, it should be preserved either as a mucous fistula or as a long Hartmann's pouch for subsequent anastomosis to the ileum. If the rectum is severely diseased, a proctocolectomy is accomplished with a short Hartmann's pouch. A perineal proctectomy can then be accomplished after the patient has recovered from the first operation.

The most common indication for operation for Crohn's colitis is failure of medical treatment, followed by sepsis. Hemorrhage, acute colitis with or without toxic megacolon, carcinoma, and obstruction are less frequent indications.

Obstruction

In contrast to the ileocolic variety of Crohn's disease, in which obstruction is the most frequent indication for operation, obstruction of the colon by the granulomatous process is a relatively rare complication, necessitating operation in only 5% of patients with Crohn's colitis who are treated surgically. The symptomatic obstruction is usually partial. The obstructive process can occur anywhere in the abdominal colon, occasionally at the anorectal junction, and rarely in the mid-rectum. Right-sided obstructions are usually associated with ileocolic disease, and most patients can be prepared by decompression for

an elective ileocolic resection with primary anastomosis. Obstructions occurring at the left side of the colon can be treated electively by segmental resection of varying magnitude, but total obstruction requiring emergency operation is best treated by a resection and exteriorization. High-grade, partial obstruction at the anorectal junction can be successfully treated by repeated dilations under anesthesia. Strictureplasty has little or no application in colonic obstruction caused by Crohn's disease.

Fistulas

Investigators[3] have reported that 16% of patients affected by Crohn's colitis have either internal or cutaneous fistulas and that 36% have perineal fistulas. Fistulas arising from Crohn's colitis do not close by nonoperative treatment despite a decrease in output with bowel rest and total parenteral nutrition.[38] Successful and complete closure of colonic fistulas requires resection of the segment of colon that gives rise to the fistula. Fistulas arising from the colon and connecting to the abdominal wall, bladder, vaginal stump, small bowel, or adjacent, nondiseased colon are best treated by division of the fistula, resection of the diseased colon, and repair of the adjacent viscera. The resection of the colon can vary from segmental resection with reanastomosis to total proctocolectomy. Attempts to preserve short segments of the right colon involved in the fistulous process are ill conceived. Involvement of the sigmoid colon by a diseased ileocolic segment is best treated by ileocolic resection and repair of the defect in the sigmoid colon, which is rarely the locus of granulomatous disease.[59]

Fistulous lesions between the small bowel and colon often involve a segment of small bowel that also harbors Crohn's disease. In these instances, great care must be taken to determine the status of the small bowel before attempting repair. If Crohn's disease is found in the small bowel, the bowel should be resected to disease-free margins before attempting an anastomosis or establishing a terminal ileostomy.

Abscesses

Intraabdominal abscess is an infrequent complication of Crohn's colitis. The diagnosis of intraabdominal abscess is suggested by the symptoms of chills and fever with leukocytosis and the presence of a mass. The abscess cavity is localized either by contrast radiographs or by CT scan with contrast. The presence of an abscess is an indication for resection of the diseased segment of colon. This procedure can be preceded by open (extraperitoneal) or closed (percutaneous) drainage. Small abscess cavities adjacent to the bowel are excised without undue spillage and do not preclude primary anastomosis. If intraabdominal contamination prohibits primary anastomosis, proximal ileostomy or end colostomy is established, and the distal segment is brought out as a mucous fistula or closed within the abdominal cavity. Anastomosis may be considered after subsidence of inflammation, usually in 6 to 12 weeks.

Anorectal Disease

About one fourth of patients affected by Crohn's disease undergo some type of operative procedure for treatment of anorectal disease. Because of the obvious importance of the anorectal region for continence, the surgeon should treat perineal complications of Crohn's disease without jeopardizing anal function. The experienced surgeon also should recognize a degree of septic perineal complications that preclude successful repair and help the patient in accepting a resection and permanent stoma.

The most common indications for surgical treatment of anorectal disease are septic (abscess, anal fistula, rectovaginal fistula, extensive perineal sepsis). Occasionally, patients present with an isolated anorectal stricture. Many physicians mistakenly believe that perineal wounds do not heal in patients with Crohn's disease and have adopted a philosophy of therapeutic nihilism. This attitude can result in continued suffering and may lead to the development of new abscesses and fistulas, progression of the process to produce a "watering-pot" perineum, and destruction of the sphincter mechanism, introitus, and vagina.

The treatment of perineal complications of Crohn's disease should be based on a clinical evaluation of anal continence and degree of colorectal disease. In patients with a grossly normal rectal mucosa, anal stenosis can be dilated, ischiorectal abscesses can be drained, fistu-

lotomies can be performed, and repair of low rectovaginal fistulas can be attempted with expectation of successful outcome. In patients with mild to moderate involvement of the rectal mucosa, treatment with topical antiinflammatory agents can occasionally affect dramatic improvement. If improvement persists, surgical repair of complicated defects can result in complete healing and normal function. In patients with severe perineal disease or incontinence, only proctocolectomy with a permanent stoma can be expected to bring relief. Extensive perineal disease is usually associated with destruction of the sphincter mechanism and incontinence. Following this algorithm, only 9% of all patients with complications of Crohn's disease require permanent stomas. All patients with perineal complications of Crohn's disease in whom a sphincter-saving operation is advised should be informed that new fistulas can develop in the future.

Rectovaginal fistulas that occur as a complication of anorectal Crohn's disease require special mention. Most fistulas are at or near the introitus. In about half of patients, discharge through the vagina is so minimal that patients do not require operative treatment. In the remaining patients, the discharge is great enough to cause embarrassment, sexual inhibition, and difficulty maintaining personal hygiene. Several operative techniques are available that differ in anatomic approach, which can be transanal, transvaginal, or perineal. All share the principles of interruption of the fistula with débridement of both openings of the fistula and its tract. In the perineal approach, the levator ani muscle is interposed between the rectum and vagina, and both fistulous openings are excised and closed.[60] In the transanal and transvaginal approaches, a rectal or vaginal mucosal flap is advanced to cover the fistulous tract (Fig. 34-27).

Anal strictures occur in less than 5% of patients with Crohn's disease and may be the only manifestation of gastrointestinal disease. More commonly, anal strictures are associated with colorectal disease. In the absence of diffuse or severe colorectal or perianal disease, the stenosis can be dilated under anesthesia, and a program of self-dilation can be begun by the patient.

Disease of the Ileoanal Pouch

Restorative proctocolectomy with ileoanal pouch anastomosis is contraindicated in patients with verified Crohn's colitis because of the likelihood of recurrent disease in the pouch and the eventual need for pouch excision and a permanent ileostomy. Historical recollection of perineal disease or evidence of perineal disease on physical examination should alert the phys-

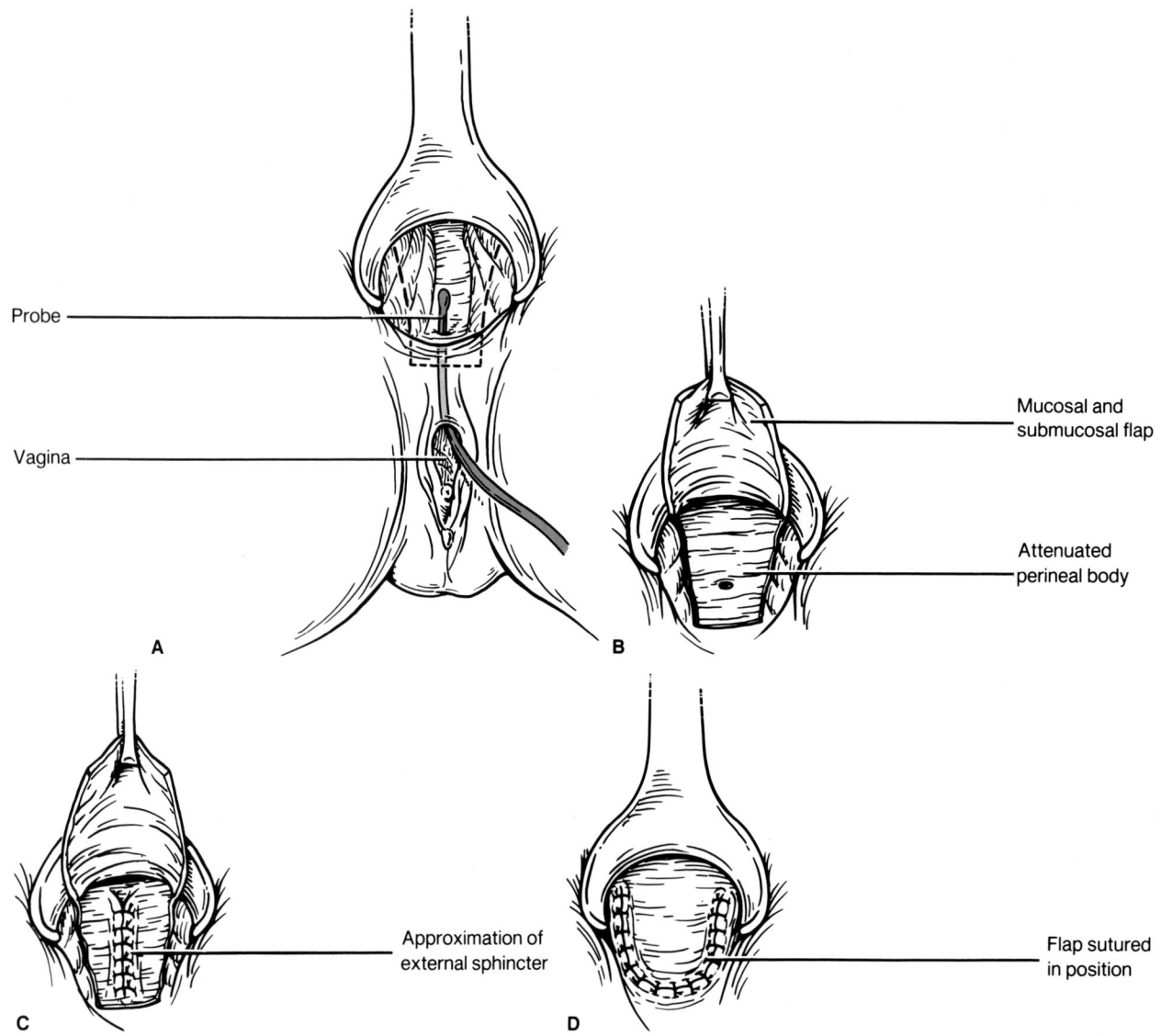

Figure 34-27 Endorectal advancement flap for low rectovaginal fistula. (**A**) The patient is in the jackknife prone position, and the probe identifies the rectovaginal fistula. (**B**) The advancement flap of the rectal mucosa and submucosa is elevated from the rectal wall, starting at the dentate line. (**C**) Plication of the external sphincter with closure of fistula. (**D**) The flap is advanced over the plicated external sphincter; the redundant portion with the fistula opening is excised; the flap is then sutured in position with interrupted sutures.

ician that the patient may be affected by Crohn's colitis rather than ulcerative colitis. Other endoscopic, radiologic, and pathologic characteristics of Crohn's disease should be actively sought before proceeding with an ileoanal pouch anastomosis procedure. Nevertheless, between 2% and 7% of patients who have undergone an ileoanal pouch procedure for ulcerative or indeterminate colitis develop Crohn's disease in the pouch.[61,62] If the patient continues to have a functional pouch and normal continence, there is no indication for any surgical procedure. Crohn's disease in ileoanal pouches may eventually become complicated with pelvic or perineal sepsis, obstructive complications, or poor function unresponsive to medical treatment. Complications such as hemorrhage and carcinoma are rare. When complications occur, the pouch should be excised and a terminal ileostomy fashioned. The procedure is complemented by removal of the internal anal sphincter and primary closure of the perineum. In the presence of perineal sepsis, the pelvic floor is closed primarily, and the skin and subcutaneous tissues of the perineum are débrided and left to heal by secondary intention.

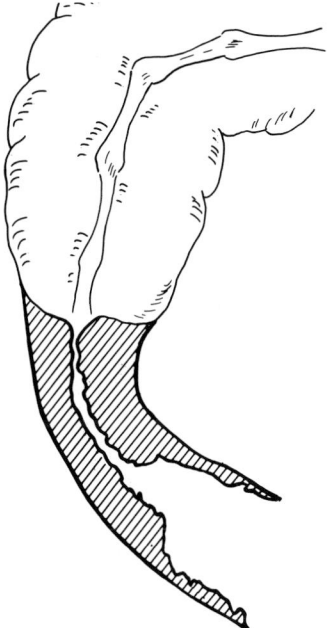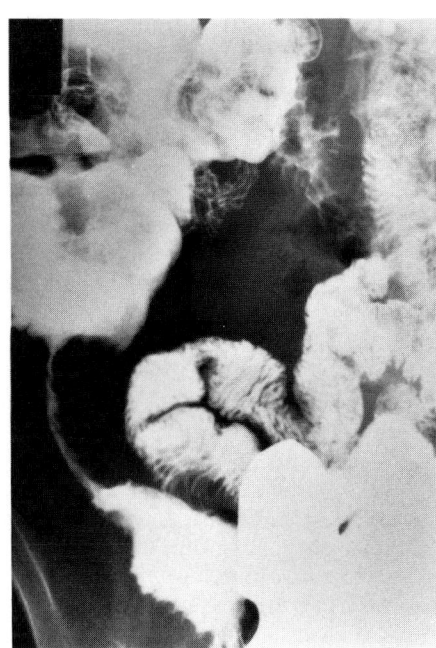

Figure 34-28 Small bowel follow-through series showing recurrent disease at the site of a previous end-to-end ileocolic anastomosis.

RECURRENT DISEASE

Crohn's disease is a panenteric disease that tends to recur after surgical treatment. No definitive therapy reduces Crohn's disease recurrence rates. Although data about the use of mesalamine formulations[63] or immunosuppressive agents to prevent postoperative recurrence are encouraging, further clinical trials are necessary to substantiate the promising results of preliminary trials.[64]

The incidence of recurrent disease varies according to the end point considered. Recurrence is lowest if only patients in need of surgical treatment are considered and highest if endoscopic recurrences are considered. In one experience covering 18 years,[1] the recurrence rate was 20% at 5 years and 34% at 10 years when only disease that required additional surgical treatment was considered. The number of sites involved was the only variable that was significantly associated with recurrence rate. The annualized risk for recurrence was 1.6% for patients with single-site involvement and 4% for those with multiple-site involvement. The risk for reoperation for Crohn's disease is higher when the original disease involves both the small and large bowel than when it is confined to either segment alone.[54,65–67]

When disease involves the terminal ileum (Fig. 34-28) or the abdominal colon, and gastrointestinal continuity is reestablished with an ileocolic anastomosis, the recurrence rate is similar whether the original localization was in the small or large bowel. Patients with small intestinal disease have a recurrence rate similar (44%) to patients with colonic disease (45%) during a follow-up period of more than 10 years.[65] Others reported recurrence rates of 21% and 16% for small and large bowel involvement, respectively.[54] A review of 13 studies showed that the average surgical recurrence rate was 34% for large bowel disease and 29% for small bowel disease.[66]

Recurrence rates are lowest after proctocolectomy with permanent ileostomy.[68–70] Disease in the neoterminal ileum appears in only 5% to 10% of the operated population during a follow-up period of 10 years.[71] When Crohn's disease recurs in the neoterminal ileum and is complicated by stenosis, fistula, or abscess, resection is necessary. Establishment of a secondary ileostomy involves placement of the ileostomy on the left side of the abdomen in a mirrored position to the first stoma. If there are no septic complications involving the external portion of the stoma, the original site can be used.

Patients suffering from Crohn's disease present to the surgeon with an almost unlimited variety of problems. The solution to these clinical problems requires a thorough understanding of the pathogenesis of the disease, appropriate use of nonoperative therapy and knowledge of its limitations, and application of the various surgical algorithms based on conservatism. The operative procedures performed for the patient with Crohn's disease are usually palliative, and in most instances the disease, but not the specific complication, recurs and may well require further operations. Therefore, conservatism both in the decision for operation and in the extent of operation must be the guiding principle for the surgeon.

REFERENCES

1. Michelassi F, Balestracci T, Chappell R, et al. Primary and recurrent Crohn's disease: experience with 1379 patients. Ann Surg 1991;214:230.
2. Michelassi F, Stella M, Balestracci T, Giuliante F, Marogna P, Block GE. Incidence, diagnosis and treatment of enteric and colorectal fistulae in patients with Crohn's disease. Ann Surg 1993;218:660.
3. Michelassi F, Balestracci T, Stella M, Giuliante F, Block GE. Incidence, diagnosis and treatment of abdominal abscesses in Crohn's patients. J Colon Rect Dis (submitted).
4. Homan WP, Tang CK, Thorbjarnason B. Acute massive hemorrhage from intestinal Crohn's disease. Arch Surg 1976;111:901.
5. Warren S, Sommers SC. Cicatrizing enteritis (regional ileitis) as a pathologic entity: an analysis of 120 cases. Am J Pathol 1948;24:475.
6. Ginzburg L, Schneider KM, Dreizin DH, Levinson C. Carcinoma of the jejunum occurring in a case of regional enteritis. Surgery 1956;39:347.
7. Greenstein AJ, Sachar D, Pucillo A, et al. Cancer in Crohn's disease after diversionary surgery: report of seven carcinomas occurring in excluded bowel. Am J Surg 1978;135:86.
8. Riberio MB, Greenstein AJ, Heimann TM, Yamamraki Y, Aufses AJ. Adenocarcinoma of the small intestine in Crohn's disease. Surg Gynecol Obstet 1991;173:343.
9. Michelassi F, Testa G, Pomidor WJ, Lashner BA, Block GE. Adenocarcinoma complicating Crohn's disease. Dis Colon Rectum 1993;36:654.
10. Fleming KA, Pollock AC. A case of Crohn's carcinoma. Gut 1975;16:533.
11. Greenstein AJ, Sachar DB, Smith H, Janowitz HD, Aufses AH Jr. Patterns of neoplasia in Crohn's disease and ulcerative colitis. Cancer 1980;46:403
12. Perzin KH, Peterson M, Castiglione P, et al. Intramucosal carcinoma of the small intestine arising in regional enteritis (Crohn's disease): report of a case studied for carcinoembryonic antigen and review of the literature. Cancer 1984;54:151.
13. Hamilton SR. Colorectal carcinoma in patients with Crohn's disease. Gastroenterology 1985;89:398.
14. Traube J, Simpson S, Riddell RH, Levin B, Kirsner JB. Crohn's disease and adenocarcinoma of the bowel. Dig Dis Sci 1980;25:939.
15. Lavery IC, Jagelman DG. Cancer in the excluded rectum following surgery for inflammatory bowel disease. Dis Colon Rectum 1982;25:522.
16. McCafferty TD, Nasr K, Lawrence AM, Kirsner JB. Severe growth retardation in children with inflammatory bowel disease. Pediatrics 1970;45:386.
17. Homer DR, Grand RJ, Colodny AH. Growth course and prognosis after surgery for Crohn's disease in children and adolescents. Pediatrics 1977;59:717.
18. Buzzard AJ, Baker WNW, Needham PRG, et al. Acute toxic dilatation of the colon in Crohn's colitis. Gut 1974;15:416.
19. Murray JJ, Schoetz DJ Jr, Nugent FW. Surgical management of Crohn's disease involving the duodenum. Am J Surg 1984;147:58.
20. Paget ET, Owens MP, Peniston WO. Massive upper gastrointestinal tract hemorrhage: a manifestation of regional enteritis of the duodenum. Arch Surg 1972;104:397.
21. Goldwasser B, Mazor A, Wiznitzer T. Enteroduodenal fistula in Crohn's disease. Dis Colon Rectum 1981;24:485.
22. Wilk PJ, Fazio V, Turnbull RB Jr. The dilemma of Crohn's disease: ileoduodenal fistula complicating Crohn's disease. Dis Colon Rectum 1977;20:387.
23. Smith TR, Goldin RR. Radiographic and clinical sequelae of the duodenocolic anatomic relationship: two cases of Crohn's disease with fistulization to the duodenum. Dis Colon Rectum 1977;20:257.
24. Legge DA, Hoffman HN II, Carlson HC. Pancreatitis as a complication of regional enteritis of the duodenum. Gastroenterology 1971;61:834.
25. Crohn BB. Regional ileitis. New York, Grune & Stratton, 1949.
26. Cooke WT, Swan CHJ. Diffuse jejunoileitis of Crohn's disease. Q J Med 1974;43:583.
27. Spirt M, Sachar DB, Greenstein AJ. Symptomatic differentiation of duodenal from gastric fistulas in Crohn's disease. Am J Gastroenterol 1990;85:455.
28. Lee KKW, Schraut WH. Diagnosis and treatment of duodenoenteric fistulas complicating Crohn's disease. Arch Surg 1989;124:712.
29. Thompson WM, Cockrill H Jr, Rice RP. Regional enteritis of the duodenum. AJR 1975;123:252.
30. Fitzgibbons TJ, Green G, Silberman H, et al. Management of Crohn's disease involving the duodenum, including duodenal cutaneous fistula. Arch Surg 1980;115:1022.
31. Glass RE, Ritchie JK, Lennard-Jones JE, et al. Internal fistulas in Crohn's disease. Dis Colon Rectum 1985;28:557.
32. Pettit SH, Irving MH. The operative management of fistulous Crohn's disease. Surg Gynecol Obstet 1988;167:223.
33. Broe PH, Bayless TM, Cameron JL. Crohn's disease: are enteroenteral fistulas an indication for surgery? Surgery 1982;91:249.
34. Fazio VW, Wilk P, Turnbull RB Jr, Jagelman DG. The dilemma of Crohn's disease: ileosigmoid fistula complicating Crohn's disease. Dis Colon Rectum 1977;20:381.
35. Jensen JA, McClenathan JH. Umbilical fistulas in Crohn's disease. Surg Gynecol Obstet 1987;164:445.
36. Veloso FT, Bardoso V, Fraga J, Carvalho J, Dias LM. Spontaneous umbilical fistula in Crohn's disease. J Clin Gastroenterol 1989;11:197.

37. Steinberg DM, Cooke WT, Alexander-Williams A. Abscess and fistulae in Crohn's disease. Gut 1973;14:865.

38. Greenstein AJ, Kark AE, Dreiling DA. Crohn's disease of the colon. I. Fistula in Crohn's disease of the colon, classification, presenting features and management in 63 patients. Am J Gastroenterol 1974;63:419.

39. Heyen F, Winslet MC, Andrews J, Alexander-Williams J, Keighley MRB. Vaginal fistulas in Crohn's disease. Dis Colon Rectum 1989;32:379.

40. Fazio VW, Jones IT, Jagleman DG, et al. Recto-urethral fistulas in Crohn's disease. Surg Gynecol Obstet 1987;164:148.

41. Crohn BB, Yarnis H. Regional enteritis, ed 2. New York, Grune & Stratton, 1958.

42. Talamini MA, Broe TJ, Cameron JL. Urinary fistulas in Crohn's disease. Surg Gynecol Obstet 1982;154:553.

43. Kyle J, Murray CM. Ileovesical fistula in Crohn's disease. Surgery 1969;66:497.

44. Greenstein AJ, Sachar DB, Tzakis, et al. Course of enterovesical fistulas in Crohn's disease. Am J Surg 1984;147:788.

45. Ribeiro MB, Greenstein AJ, Yamazaki Y, Aufses AH Jr. Intra-abdominal abscess in regional enteritis. Ann Surg 1991;213:32.

46. Nagler SM, Poticha SM. Intraabdominal abscess in regional enteritis. Am J Surg 1979;137:350.

47. Cybulsky IJ, Tam P. Intra-abdominal abscesses in Crohn's disease. Am Surg 1990;56:678.

48. Ricci MA, Meyer KK. Psoas abscess complicating Crohn's disease. 1985;80:970.

49. Edwards H. Crohn's disease, an inquiry into its nature and consequences. Ann R Coll Surg Engl 1969;44:121.

50. Flancbaum L, Nosher JL, Brolin RE. Percutaneous catheter drainage of abdominal abscesses associated with perforated viscus. Am Surg 1990;56:52.

51. Lambiase RE, Cronan JJ, Dorfman GS, Paolella LP, Haas RA. Percutaneous drainage of abscesses in patients with Crohn disease. AJR 1988;150:1043.

52. Present DH, Rabinowitz JG, Banks PA. Obstructive hydronephrosis: a frequent but seldom recognized complication of granulomatous disease of the bowel. N Engl J Med 1969;280:523.

53. Block GE, Enker WE, Kirsner JB. Significance and treatment of occult obstructive uropathy complicating Crohn's disease. Ann Surg 1973;17:322.

54. Farmer RG, Hawk WA, Turnbull RB Jr. Clinical patterns in Crohn's disease: a statistical study of 615 cases. Gastroenterology 1975;68:627.

55. Alan A, Andrews H, Hiltin CJ, Keighley MR, Alan RN, Alexander-Williams S. Segmental colonic resection as an appropriate operation for short skip lesions due to Crohn's disease of the colon. World J Surg 1989;13:611.

56. Trnka YM, Glotzee DJ, Kasdon EJ. Long term outcome of restorative operation in Crohn's disease: influence of location, prognostic factors in surgical guidelines. Ann Surg 1982;196:345.

57. Fawaz KL. Ulcerative colitis and Crohn's disease of the colon: a comparison of the long term postoperative courses. Gastroenterology 1976;71:372.

58. Watts J, Hughes ESR. Ulcerative colitis and Crohn's disease: results after colectomy and ileorectal anastomosis. Br J Surg 1977;64:77.

59. Block GE, Schraut WH. The operative treatment of Crohn's enteritis complicated by ileosigmoid fistula. Ann Surg 1983;196:356.

60. Buls JG, Rothenberger DA. Anal and rectal vaginal fistulas: repair of the low fistula. In: Kodner IJ, Frey RD, Row JP, eds. Colon, rectal and anal surgery. St Louis, CV Mosby, 1985:63.

61. Deutsch AA, McLeod RS, Cullen J, Cohen A. Results of the pelvic-pouch procedure in patients with Crohn's disease. Dis Colon Rectum 1991;34:475.

62. Hyman NH, Fazio VW, Tuckson WB, Lavery IC. Consequences of ileal pouch–anal anastomosis for Crohn's colitis. Dis Colon Rectum 1991;34:653.

63. Prantera C, Pallone F, Brunetti G, Cottone M, Miglioli M, the Italian IBD Study Group. Oral 5-aminosalicylic acid (Asacol) in the maintenance treatment of Crohn's disease. Gastroenterology 1992;103:363.

64. Tremaine WJ. Maintenance of remission in Crohn's disease: is 5-aminosalicylic acid the answer? Gastroenterology 1992;103:694.

65. Whelan G, Farmer RG, Fazio VW, Goormastic M. Recurrence after surgery in Crohn's disease: relationship to location of disease (clinical pattern) and surgical indication. Gastroenterology 1985;88:1826.

66. Chardavoyne R, Flint GW, Pollack S, Wise L. Factors affecting recurrence following resection for Crohn's disease. Dis Colon Rectum 1986;29:495.

67. Mekhjian HS, Switz DM, Watts HD, et al. National cooperative Crohn's disease study: factors determining recurrence of Crohn's disease after surgery. Gastroenterology 1979;77:807.

68. Crohn BB, Ginsburg S, Oppenheimer GD. Regional ileitis: a pathological and clinical study. JAMA 1932;99:1323.

69. Bargen JA, Weber H. Regional migratory ulcerative colitis. Surg Gynecol Obstet 1930;50:964.

70. Glotzer DJ, Gardner RC, Goldman H, et al. Comparative features and course of ulcerative and granulomatous colitis. N Engl J Med 1960;282:582.

71. DeDombal FT, Burton I, Goligher JC. The early and late results of surgical treatment for Crohn's disease. Br J Surg 1971;58:805.

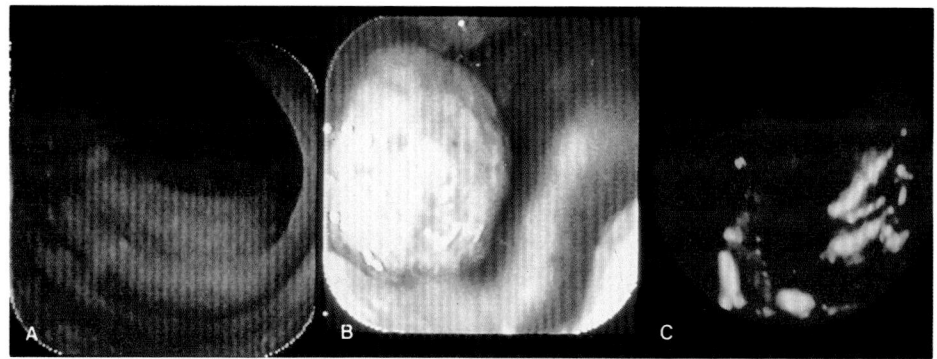

Color Figure 35-15

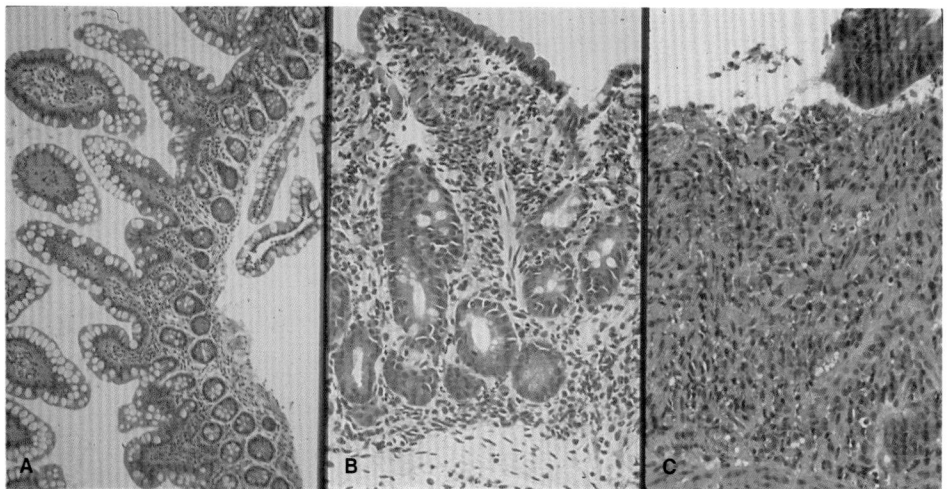

Color Figure 35-16

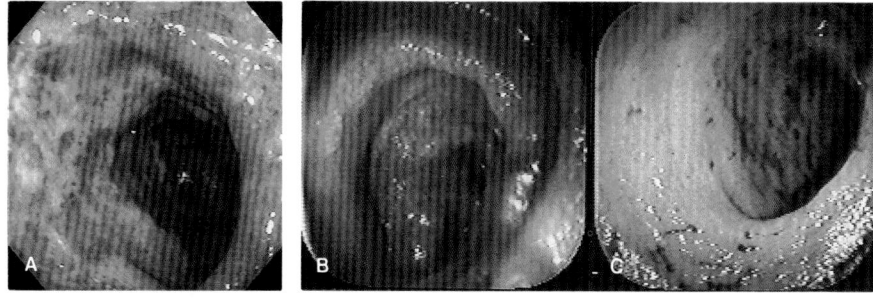

Color Figure 35-17

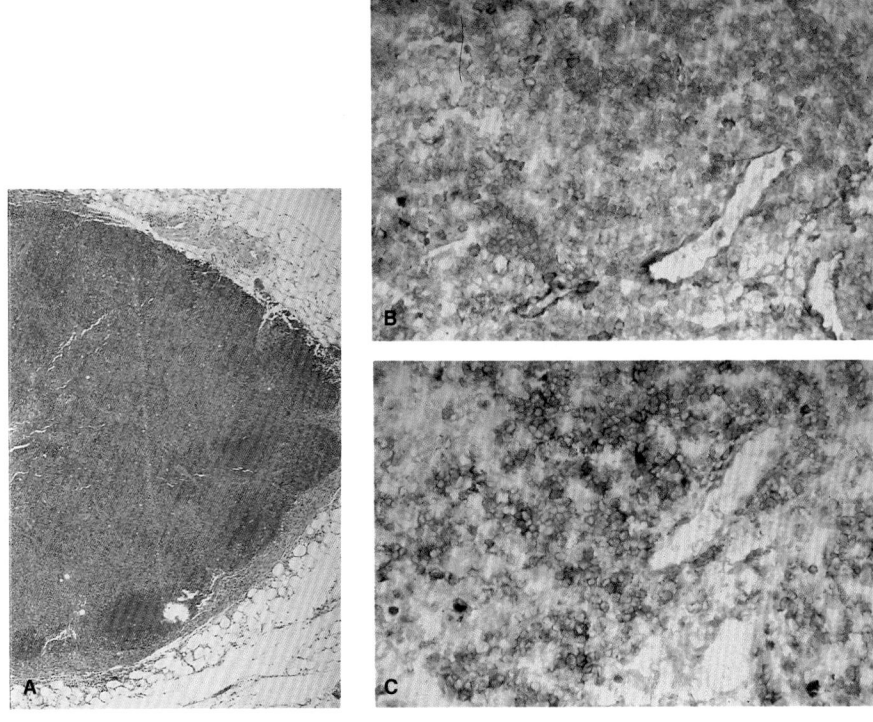

Color Figure 35-23

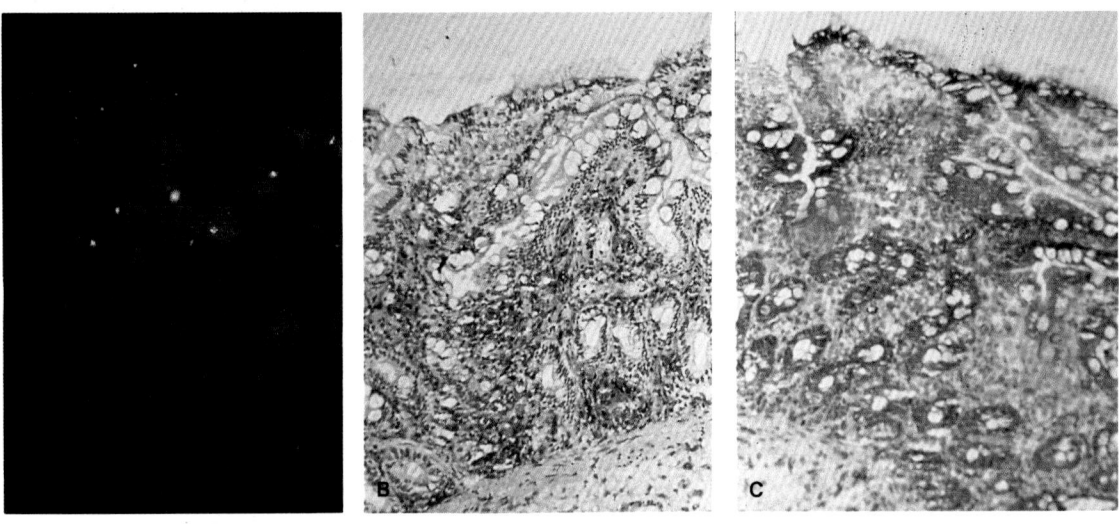

Color Figure 35-24

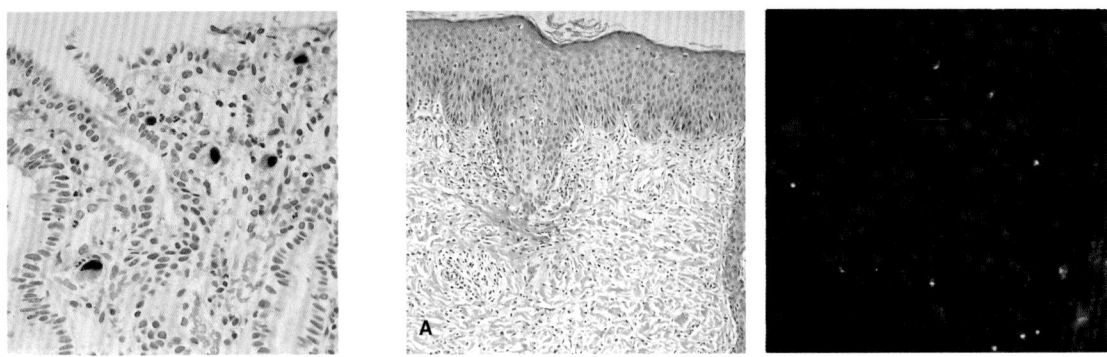

Color Figure 35-26   Color Figure 35-29

Digestive Tract Surgery: A Text and Atlas, edited by Richard H. Bell,
Layton F. Rikkers, and Michael W. Mulholland.
Lippincott-Raven Publishers, Philadelphia, © 1996.

35

Intestinal and Multivisceral Transplantation

John J. Fung | *Kareem Abu-Elmagd* | *Satoru Todo*

After the successful evolution and widespread clinical use of hepatic transplantation in the 1980s, intestinal transplantation remained as the sole elusive achievement for the next era of transplant surgeons. The initial attempts in the 1960s were suspended because of poor graft and patient survival.[1-5] During the 1980s, the successful clinical use of cyclosporine for solid organ transplantation triggered further clinical attempts at intestinal transplantation, but the results were still unsatisfactory.[6-15] During the first half of 1990, FK506, a more potent immunosuppressive drug, ushered in the new era of small bowel and multivisceral transplantation with initially promising results.[16-18]

In the late 1960s, several clinical attempts at intestinal transplantation were conducted at different centers.[1-5] These trials were unsuccessful, even in cases of perfectly HLA-matched transplants from related donors, because of the ineffective immunosuppressive regimen available at that time.[5]

During the 1980s, the use of cyclosporine facilitated the achievement of long-term survival after experimental intestinal transplantation; together with continuous progress in the field of organ transplantation, this justified further clinical attempts at small bowel transplantation.[19,20] The key factors for potential success were the availability of adequate immunosuppressive therapy and effective antimicrobial agents. Nonetheless, worldwide long-term success rates were unsatisfactory.[6-15] Based on data collected for the Small Bowel Transplant Registry, the cumulative survival of small intestinal allografts under cyclosporine was less than 10% (Dr. David Grant, London, Ontario, personal communication). The causes of patient and graft loss were unrelenting rejection, sepsis, and disseminated posttransplantation lymphoproliferative disease (PTLD). In addition to the two isolated intestinal allograft survivors reported from European trials,[12,15] the Canadian group has reported another three survivors among five patients who received combined hepatic and intestinal grafts.[21]

In 1989, the new immunosuppressive agent FK506 was introduced to clinical transplantation.[16,22] The demonstration of its superior therapeutic index for both solid organ transplantation and experimental intestinal and multivisceral transplantation triggered new trials with these procedures at our center.[23-26] FK506 is a macrolide antibiotic that is produced by the soil fungus, *Streptomyces tsukubaensis,* and has a potent immunosuppressive effect.[27-30] Its molecular structure is unrelated to that of cyclosporine, and the two drugs have different cytosolic binding sites.[31,32] Both agents inhibit T-lymphocyte activation, in part by suppressing the synthesis and expression of the cytokine, interleukin-2.[30] Yet there is a practical difference in the utilization of these drugs. FK506 has a greater ability to reverse ongoing or established rejection and its dose adjustability allows the physician to titrate the immunosuppressive baseline to the threshold of rejection, rather than to rely arbitrarily on target drug levels.[33-35] In addition, FK506 has more long-term advantages, including rapid withdrawal or even complete discontinuation of corticosteroid therapy, absence of hirsutism and gingival hyperplasia, and a low incidence of hypertension.[36-38] Of practical interest are the absorption characteristics of

FK506, which make this agent more suitable for visceral transplantation.[39] The intestinal absorption of FK506 does not appear to depend on the presence of bile salts and is less affected by the development of gastrointestinal motility or absorptive dysfunction.[40]

INTESTINAL FAILURE

Maintenance of normal gastrointestinal function involves the integration of numerous complex physiologic interactions. Despite the essential regulatory role of the central nervous system, primary impairment of the digestive, absorptive, neuroendocrine, and motor functions of the gastrointestinal system is the leading cause of gastrointestinal insufficiency. Primary intestinal failure, therefore, is defined as the inability to maintain nutrition or adequate fluid and electrolyte balance without special support due to the loss of absorptive surface or function of the native gut.[41]

Surgical removal and congenital absence of a significant length of the intestine (short-gut syndrome) are common causes of temporary or permanent gastrointestinal insufficiency. Under these circumstances, the residual bowel undergoes adaptive changes to compensate for the lost absorptive surface area by widening its circumference and increasing the villus height. The adaptive process is facilitated by intraluminal nutrients, pancreaticobiliary secretions, hormones, and enterotropic factors. Clinically, the process has three phases: phase I (7 to 10 days), when diarrhea is severe and patients require massive fluid and electrolyte replacement; phase II (1 to 3 months), when diarrhea stabilizes and patients still need total parenteral nutrition (TPN) and other medical treatment; and phase III (3 to 12 months), when diarrhea is controlled enough to allow enteral feeding and weaning from TPN.[42] If TPN cannot be discontinued 12 to 24 months after the initial insult, intestinal failure approaches an irreversible state, necessitating permanent TPN therapy.

The irreversibility of surgical intestinal failure, although difficult to determine at the time of small bowel resection, correlates with the length of remaining native bowel, the site of intestinal resection, and the presence or absence of the ileocecal valve.[43,44] Concomitant loss of the large bowel is another risk factor because the gastrointestinal tract loses the ability to absorb water. In general, resection of over 80% of the small bowel along with the ileocecal valve is associated with failure of the adaptive process and permanent loss of the intestinal absorptive function. In contrast, patients who require resection of the jejunum only have a good chance of successful recovery because the ileum has more adaptive capacity.

Functional failure of the gastrointestinal system results from defects in either enterocyte function or mural neuromuscular activity. Microvillus inclusion disease and radiation enteritis are examples of enterocyte abnormalities, and myopathy and neuropathy of the intestinal wall are examples of motility disorders (pseudoobstruction).

TPN has been the primary life-saving therapy for patients with temporary or irreversible intestinal failure. TPN was first introduced by Dudrick in 1968 and has been used widely during the past two decades. Medicare data indicate that about 19,700 patients, or 80 persons per 1 million population, received home TPN in the United States in 1987; this figure is much higher than the 2 to 4 persons per million population reported in Europe because of the more liberal use of TPN in this country.[41,45] Unfortunately, long-term TPN therapy has many limitations, including metabolic abnormalities, bone disease, cholelithiasis, cholestatic liver failure, impaired quality of life, and substantial cost. Of the 1594 TPN-dependent patients followed up by the OASIS registry since 1984, those with benign intestinal diseases experienced 2.6 complications requiring hospitalization per year.[45] The 3-year survival rate for the entire population ranged from 65% to 80% according to the cause of the intestinal disease, and 6.7% of the deaths were from TPN-related complications. In Europe, sepsis, thrombosis of major vessels, and liver failure contribute to 28% of the deaths that occur during TPN therapy.[46] In the pediatric population, cholestasis with the potential risk of liver failure is more common, occurring in 30% to 40% of children who receive long-term TPN.[47] The same trend was observed among the pediatric patients referred to our center for possible intestinal transplantation either alone or as part of a composite graft. Of 99 children, 25 (25%) died of liver failure and sepsis while waiting for organs.[48]

Because of limited social and personal activities, some patients receiving TPN become overly dependent on their caregivers and experience psychiatric disturbances and drug abuse. The severity of such morbidity correlates significantly with the duration and nature of the primary intestinal disease, the coexistence of extraintestinal disorders, and the degree of family support.

The cost of TPN has increased rapidly over the last decade. In 1980, the cost per patient ranged from $16,506 to $24,939 per year.[49] By 1983, it had increased to $17,000 to $127,000 per year, and it currently is estimated at $75,000 to $150,000 per year.[41]

INDICATIONS FOR TRANSPLANTATION

Intestinal transplantation can be an alternative to TPN for patients with irreversible intestinal failure. However, it is the only treatment option for those in whom simultaneous intestinal replacement is an absolute surgical necessity to technically replace an irreversibly damaged liver with parenchymal or vascular decompensation.

At our center, only patients with irreversible intestinal failure who require permanent TPN are considered for isolated intestinal transplantation. The most common cause is loss of over 70% of the native small bowel (short-gut syndrome). The leading indications for intestinal resection among adults include abdominal trauma, Crohn's disease, surgical adhesions, Gardner's syndrome, desmoid tumor, and occlusion of the superior mesenteric vessels. In the pediatric population, the indications are different and include necrotizing enterocolitis, intestinal atresia, midgut volvulus, and complicated gastroschisis. A less common indication for intestinal transplantation in both adults and children is defective gastrointestinal motility (chronic pseudoobstruction) due to hollow visceral myopathy, neuropathy, or generalized absence of the myenteric plexus (total intestinal aganglionosis). Impairment of the enterocyte absorptive capacity that is significant enough to warrant permanent TPN therapy occurs in patients with microvillus inclusion disease, autoimmune enteropathy, radiation enteritis, extensive inflammatory bowel disease, or massive intestinal polyposis.

Combined hepatic and intestinal transplantation is indicated primarily for patients with combined hepatic and intestinal failure. It also is the only feasible surgical procedure for patients with hepatic failure who have concomitant thrombosis of the entire portomesenteric system. In these patients, enterectomy of the normally functioning native intestine is required. Simultaneous intestinal and hepatic replacement in the absence of liver failure is indicated only in patients with vascular thrombosis due to congenital coagulation defects (protein C, protein S, or antithrombin III deficiency) that can be corrected only by replacing the native liver. In some of these patients, multivisceral transplantation is unavoidable because of concomitant vascular insufficiency of the remaining upper abdominal organs, particularly the stomach and pancreas.

Multivisceral transplantation is indicated for patients with irreversible failure of more than two of the abdominal visceral organs, including the intestine. Common causes of multivisceral failure are extensive thrombosis of the splanchnic vessels, massive gastrointestinal polyposis, and generalized hollow visceral myopathy or neuropathy. Multivisceral transplantation also can be attempted for patients with potentially curable malignant abdominal tumors that require upper abdominal exenteration.

Intestinal transplantation is contraindicated for patients with significant cardiopulmonary insufficiency, the history or presence of aggressive or incurable malignancy, persistent abdominal or systemic infection, or extensive atherosclerosis or severe autoimmune or immunodeficiency syndromes. Isolated intestinal transplantation also should not be performed in patients who tolerate TPN therapy, are older than 60 years, have inactive life-styles, or have failed drug rehabilitation.

PRETRANSPLANTATION EVALUATION

All potential candidates for intestinal transplantation should undergo a thorough evaluation, including a complete history and physical examination, a full nutritional evaluation, and careful hepatic, renal, cardiopulmonary, hematologic, and immunologic assessment. This comprehensive work-up is important to standardize the criteria for patient selection and to explore the potential risk factors in this unique population. Assessment of the etiology, extent, and severity of the primary disease is crucial in every patient. For patients with Crohn's disease, microvillus inclusion disease, polyposis, Hirschsprung's disease, and radiation enteritis, full radiologic, endoscopic, and pathologic examination of the remaining portions of the native gastrointestinal tract is essential for planning a proper surgical strategy. In patients with pseudoobstruction syndrome, motility studies that include both the upper and lower gastrointestinal tracts should be performed. Patients with thrombotic disorders usually need abdominal visceral angiography and special hematologic studies, including protein C, protein S, and antithrombin III measurements. In patients with desmoid lesions, the new imaging techniques should be used to evaluate thoroughly the extent of the tumor, including its relation to adjacent vital structures.

Liver function always should be evaluated. Patients with biochemical evidence of hepatic injury should undergo liver biopsy and other studies that are done routinely for chronic or end-stage liver disease. The extent of the work-up required to assess the cardiopulmonary, renal, hematologic, and immune systems is dictated by the age of the patient, the complexity of the previous medical history, and the nature of the primary disease.

DONOR SELECTION AND TREATMENT

At our center, donor characteristics used for intestinal, hepatic–intestinal, and multivisceral grafts are similar to those used for isolated hepatic allografts. Hemodynamically stable, local donors less than 45 years of age are preferred. All donors are cadaveric, ABO identical to the recipient, and of similar or smaller size and weight. No attempt is made to deplete the donor lymphocyte mass or to match donor and recipient HLA. Donors with positive lymphocytotoxic crossmatch results are not excluded to avoid prolonging the cold ischemia time while waiting for test results. However, transplanting the intestine across a strong positive cytotoxic crossmatch, particularly in the case of an isolated graft, should be avoided.

In the early experience with small bowel transplantation, no attempt was made to match for cytomegalovirus (CMV) status; currently, however, the recommended approach is to use only CMV-seronegative donors for CMV-seronegative patients, particularly those who require isolated intestinal grafts. This strategy has been adopted because of the high morbidity associated with giving CMV-seropositive grafts to CMV-seronegative patients.[50] Recurrent or persistent CMV enteritis has been the most common morbid event in patients with intestinal transplants despite the use of long-term prophylactic or active antiviral therapy with agents such as ganciclovir, foscarnet, and CMV immunoglobulin (Cytogam), given alone or in combination.

Selective bowel decontamination should be attempted in all donors. A combination of amphotericin B, tobramycin/gentamicin, and polymyxin E is given through a nasogastric tube once the donor has been accepted; this procedure is repeated every 6 hours before procurement if time permits. Standard intravenous antibiotic prophylaxis, with cefotaxime and ampicillin, also is administered to all donors.

The intestinal allograft is preserved using University of Wisconsin (UW) solution for both in situ flushing and cold storage. Adult donors usually are flushed with 1 to 2 L and pediatric donors with 50 to 100 mL/kg. Intraluminal flushing with cold lactated Ringer's solution containing amphotericin B, gentamicin, and polymyxin E is performed only when the colon is part of the intestinal graft, and usually is done on the backtable. Until more experience is gained, the cold ischemia time should be kept to a minimum. This can be facilitated by selecting local donors and coordinating the timing of donor and recipient operations. The use of custom-made grafts is important to the success of intestinal transplantation. Because the number of organs that need to be replaced is not always apparent until the time of operation, the intestine should be harvested en bloc with the other abdominal organs (except the kidneys). The decision then can be made during the operation, based on the condition of the recipient's remaining abdominal organs, the status of the residual

splanchnic venous system, the extent of liver damage, and the severity of portal hypertension.

The colon can be harvested and transplanted in continuity with the small bowel to increase the water-absorbing capacity of the graft and to preserve the ileocecal valve. This can reduce the incidence of diarrhea and bacterial overgrowth, which is common among patients who receive intestinal grafts without the colon.[50]

TRANSPLANT PROCEDURES

Donor Operation

As with multiple abdominal organ procurement, the procedure begins with a long midline incision from the pubis to the sternal notch. An abdominal transverse cruciate incision can be added to facilitate dissection and detachment of the abdominal viscera from the peritoneal reflections (Fig. 35-1). The abdominal organs should be examined thoroughly to evaluate their quality and size and to search for vascular anomalies. Because of the segmental vascular supply of the alimentary canal based on the embryonic origin of each part (Fig. 35-2), the details of retrieval of the three different intestinal grafts are described separately.

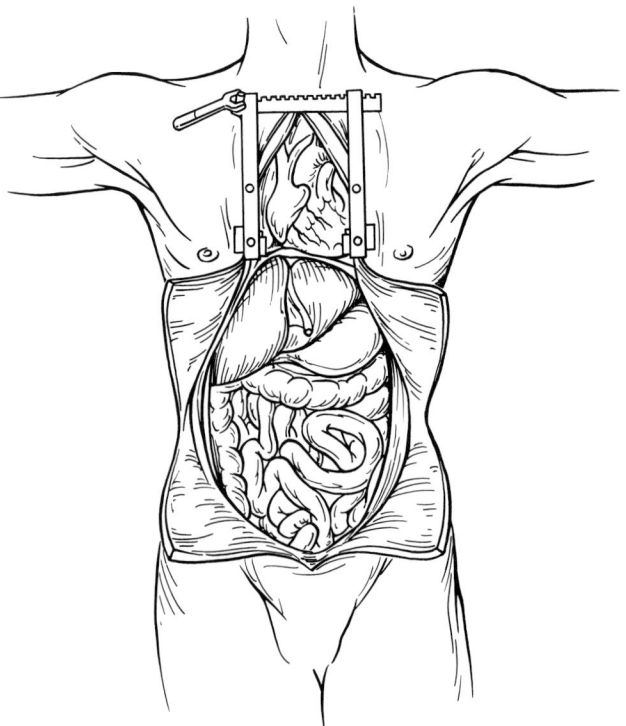

Figure 35-1 Donor operation with an abdominal transverse cruciate incision.

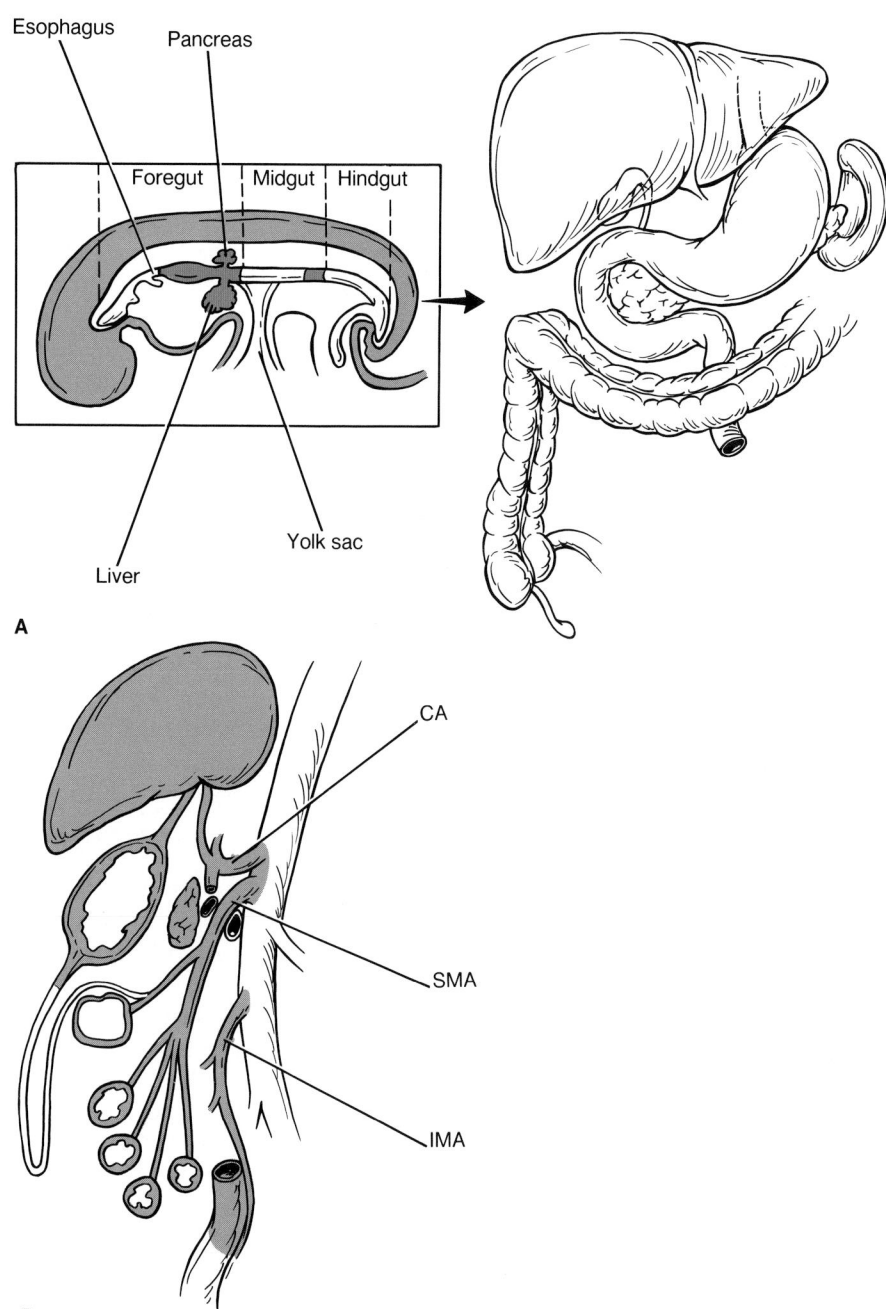

Figure 35-2 (**A**) The embryonic origin of the liver, pancreas, and alimentary canal. (**B**) The segmental blood supply of the different parts of the gastrointestinal tract is shown. CA, celiac axis; SMA, superior mesenteric artery; IMA, inferior mesenteric artery.

Isolated Intestinal Graft

After the initial standard hepatic hilar dissection for liver procurement has been performed, the intestinal procurement procedure begins. The greater omentum is removed from the transverse mesocolon. The peritoneal attachments to the ascending and descending colon are divided. A Kocher maneuver is performed and the duodenum is mobilized until the pedicle of the superior mesenteric vessels is visualized. The root of the mesentery is freed from the retroperitoneal attachments, and the inferior mesenteric artery (IMA) is traced back to its origin and preserved. The mesentery is mobilized further up to the level of the superior mesenteric vessels. Next, the proximal jejunum is transected as close to the ligament of Treitz as possible, using an intestinal stapler (Fig. 35-3). The superior mesenteric vascular pedicle is identified and carefully dissected, and a short length of the superior mesenteric artery (SMA) and superior mesenteric vein (SMV) is

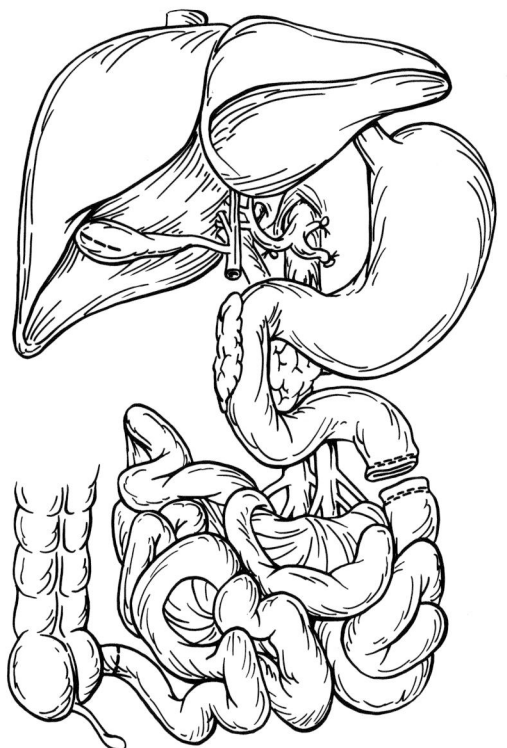

Figure 35-3 Retrieval of the isolated intestinal graft. The initial steps are removal of the greater omentum, mobilization of the duodenum, mobilization of the mesentery, and transection of the proximal jejunum close to the ligament of Treitz.

cleared from the small branches that supply the duodenum and pancreas. If the pancreas is to be used, the SMV and SMA are dissected completely to the level of the inferior border of the pancreas, at or just above the level of the origin of the middle colic vessels. If the pancreas is not to be used, the portal vein and SMV are exposed by transecting the pylorus and the neck of the pancreas that overlies the SMV (Fig. 35-4). Careful dissection of the pancreatic tributaries that enter the SMV completes the lateral mobilization of this vessel (see Fig. 35-4, *inset*). In addition, identification of the confluence of the splenic vein with the portal vein facilitates subsequent cannulation of the splenic vein (Fig. 35-5). Removal of the pancreaticoduodenal segment can be completed either in vivo (see Fig. 35-5, *inset*) or during the backtable dissection. Attention then is directed toward dissection of the SMA at its origin because the presence of an aberrant right hepatic artery would necessitate an alternative approach to division of the SMA. The sigmoid colon is mobilized down to the level of the peritoneal pelvic reflection, where it is divided using an intestinal stapler. The crura of the diaphragm also is divided, and the supraceliac aorta is ex-

posed. Finally, the infrarenal aorta is mobilized just before its bifurcation to the iliac arteries, and systemic heparin is administered. At this point, an aortic cannula and a splenic vein catheter are inserted. UW solution is infused through the aortic and splenic or inferior mesenteric venous cannulas, and the supraceliac aorta is crossclamped (see Fig. 35-5). The venous return is vented into the thorax or through an inferior vena cava cannula. A slush mixture of iced saline is used to achieve topical cooling. After blanching of the intestinal graft, the liver is separated by dividing the portal vein at or preferably above the confluence of the SMV with the splenic vein. The donor hepatectomy is performed using the standard technique and the small bowel graft is removed after the origin of the SMA has been divided with an appropriate Carrel patch (Fig. 35-6). When the colon is retrieved as part of the intestinal graft, the origin of the IMA also is preserved and divided with a patch.

On occasion, with a short SMA or SMV, vascular grafts using donor iliac vessels are attached to one or both vessels during the backtable dissection (see Fig. 35-6, *inset*).

Combined Hepatic–Intestinal Graft

Despite the modifications required to retrieve the liver en bloc with the small bowel, the initial dissection of the liver is similar to that used to harvest the liver alone. The gallbladder is incised, the common bile duct is transected low in the hepatoduodenal ligament, and the bile contents of the gallbladder and biliary tree are flushed with saline. After the arterial anatomy of the liver has been assessed, the gastroduodenal and right gastric arteries are ligated. The splenic and left gastric arteries also are ligated (see Fig. 35-3) and the accessory left gastric artery is preserved if present. Using this technique, the general rule has been to sacrifice the pancreas as a whole-organ allograft because the celiac trunk and SMA are preserved with the en bloc hepatic–intestinal graft (Fig. 35-7). However, segmental harvesting of the pancreas is surgically feasible in these donors and isolation of the islet cells is an alternative approach. The remaining steps of the in situ dissection for the intestinal portion of this composite graft are carried out as described for the intestine alone, except that further dissection and separation of the superior mesenteric vessels from the duodenum and pancreas can be completed on the backtable. After in situ perfusion with UW solution is accomplished through the aortic and splenic cannulas (see Fig. 35-5), a Carrel patch is fashioned around the origins of the celiac trunk and SMA and the combined hepatic–intestinal bloc is removed

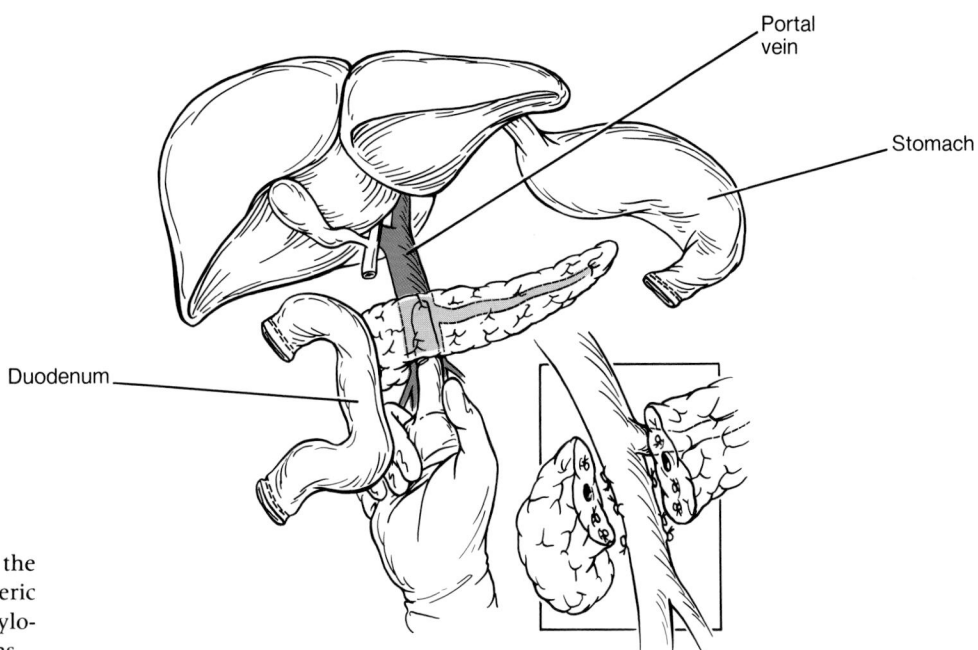

Figure 35-4 Exposure of the portal and superior mesenteric veins by transection of the pylorus and division of the pancreas.

(Fig. 35-8). A Carrel patch around the IMA also is removed if the graft contains the colon.

During the backtable dissection, the vena cava margins are prepared as for an isolated liver allograft. The ganglionic tissue surrounding the celiac trunk and SMA also is cleared. The supportive periportal tissue is preserved in these grafts, in contrast to the practice with isolated liver allografts. An arterial graft always is required to combine the common origin of the ce-

liac trunk and the SMA as a single vascular conduit (Fig. 35-9).

Multivisceral Graft

The retrieval of a multivisceral graft, which usually contains stomach, duodenum, pancreas, intestine, and liver (Fig. 35-10), is an extension of the technique used for multiple abdominal organ procurement.[51-54] A me-

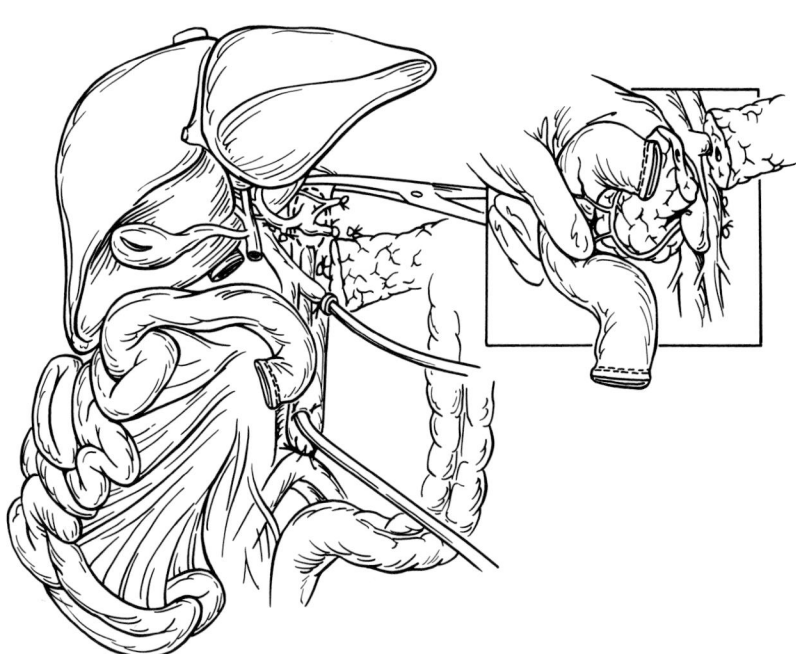

Figure 35-5 Cold perfusion of the in situ specimen. Removal of the pancreaticoduodenal portion (*inset*) can be completed during either the donor or the backtable dissection.

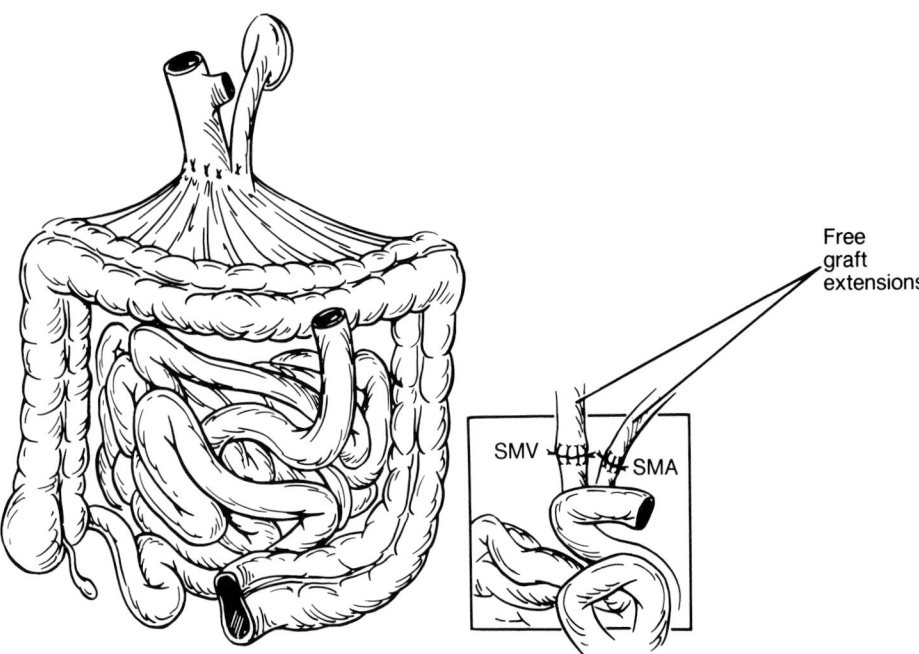

Free graft extensions

Figure 35-6 Isolated intestinal graft containing the colon, with preservation of the ileocecal valve. SMA, superior mesenteric artery; SMV, superior mesenteric vein. (Furukawa H, Abu-Elmagd K, Reyes J, et al. Technical aspects of intestinal transplantation. In: Braverman MH, Tawes RL, eds. Surgical technology international II. 1993:165)

thodical approach to the in situ dissection facilitates proper orientation of the different organs and their vascular pedicles, particularly during backtable dissection and reimplantation.

The technique used for harvesting a combined he-

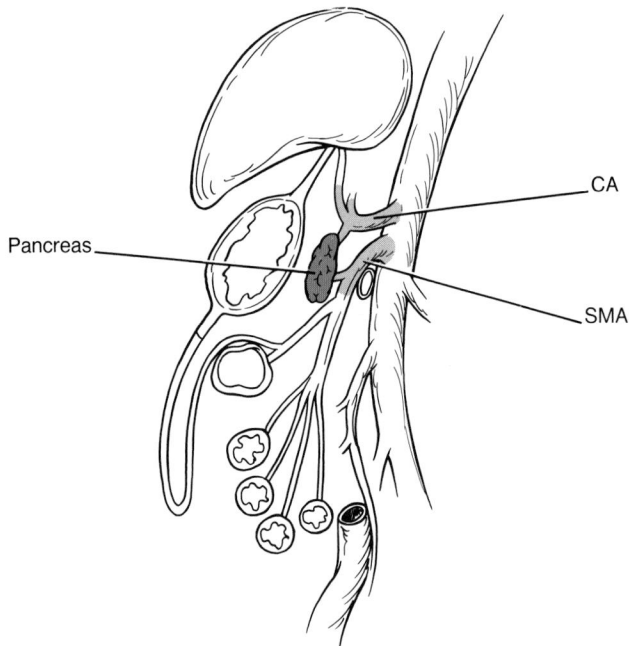

Figure 35-7 The segmental arterial supply of the pancreas from the celiac trunk (CA) and the superior mesenteric artery (SMA), which precludes retrieval of the whole organ from combined liver and intestine donors.

patic–intestinal graft is modified for retrieving a multivisceral graft. The gastrohepatic ligament and its contents are left intact, but the gallbladder is opened and flushed. The stomach is disconnected from the esophagus by transecting the abdominal esophagus with a stapler. This is facilitated by devascularizing the greater curvature of the stomach, including the short gastric vessels, but preserving the gastroepiploic arch. The spleen is removed either in situ or on the backtable. During splenectomy, the splenic vessels should be ligated within the splenic hilus to prevent injury to the tail of the pancreas. The whole graft is infused with the appropriate volume of UW solution only through the aortic cannula. Placement of the arterial graft and pyloroplasty or pyloromyotomy are performed routinely on the backtable.

Recipient Operation

The technical steps of each recipient operation require careful planning based on the frequency and extent of the patient's previous abdominal surgery and the anticipated transplant procedure. Modifications to the described techniques are common, and technical challenges can be formidable.

The recipient operation usually includes a generous midline abdominal incision, with appropriate transverse extensions, particularly in patients with multiple previous abdominal operations, portal hypertension, or marked vascular adhesions. In patients undergoing intestinal transplantation alone, intraabdom-

another technical challenge during closure of the abdominal wall incision in almost every case.

Isolated Intestinal Graft

After dissection of the abdominal adhesions and identification of the remaining portions of the native gut, the surgeon proceeds with identification of the vascular structures required to revascularize the intestinal allograft: (1) the stump of SMV, the splenic vein, the main portal vein, or the inferior vena cava; and (2) the infrarenal aorta. For arterialization of the graft, an area in the anterior aspect of the infrarenal aorta is cleared and the end of the donor SMA is anastomosed to the side of the recipient aorta (Fig. 35-11). Revascularization of the IMA usually can be avoided by limiting the length of the donor colon transplanted. The choice of venous drainage for the intestinal graft depends on the ability to gain access to the remaining recipient mesenteric venous system (see Fig. 35-11, *right inset*). In brief, the donor SMV is anastomosed to either the recipient SMV stump (end to end), the splenic vein (end to side), the main portal vein (end to side),[55] or the infrahepatic vena cava (end to side). Interposition grafts are rarely used in these patients.

Restoration of gastrointestinal continuity usually starts 30 to 60 minutes after reperfusion. During the initial dissection of the recipient organs, the duodenum always is identified and carefully preserved along with the remaining healthy portions of the native small bowel and colon to anatomically reconstruct the alimentary tract. The proximal enteric anastomosis is performed at the most distal accessible level of the recipient gastrointestinal tract (see Fig. 35-11). The proximal end of the graft jejunum is anastomosed to the recipient jejunum, the duodenum, or the stomach. The gastrojejunal anastomosis usually is performed from side to side and the type of duodenojejunal or jejunojejunal anastomosis used is based primarily on anatomic and surgical considerations. The earlier practice of temporarily exteriorizing the proximal end of the donor jejunum has been replaced by simply inserting a jejunostomy tube to prevent excessive loss of gastrointestinal secretions and to facilitate early enteral feeding.

The ability to establish continuity of the distal alimentary tract and the type of enteric anastomosis performed depend on the length of the residual distal native gut and the presence of the colon as part of the intestinal graft. In patients with previous proctocolectomy, a terminal ileostomy or colostomy is performed. In patients with intact colon, the donor transverse colon or ileum is anastomosed to the remaining part of the recipient colon (see Fig. 35-11). In those with intact native terminal ileum, an ileoileal anastomosis can be

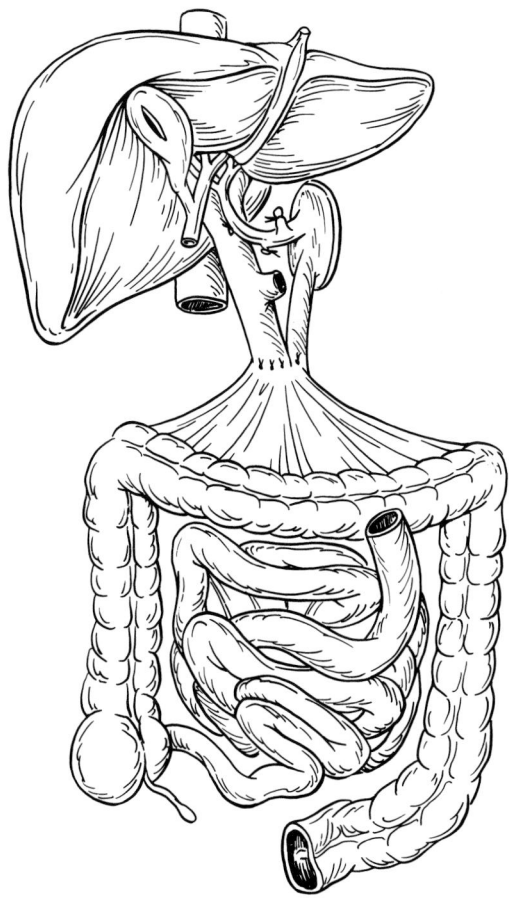

Figure 35-8 Combined hepatic and intestinal graft en bloc, with a common Carrel patch around the origins of the celiac and superior mesenteric arteries. Continuity of the donor portal vein is seen. (Furukawa H, Abu-Elmagd K, Reyes J, et al. Technical aspects of intestinal transplantation. In: Braverman MH, Tawes RL, eds. Surgical technology international II. 1993:165)

inal dissection and identification of the vascular structures required to implant the small bowel are relatively less tedious due to the absence of portal hypertension. In combined hepatic–intestinal transplantation, the operation often is more difficult because of the presence of portal hypertension and abdominal portosystemic collaterals. However, the most challenging procedure is upper abdominal exenteration in patients who require multivisceral transplantation, particularly those with thrombosed splanchnic or systemic abdominal venous systems. In some of these patients, balloon occlusion or embolization of the celiac trunk and SMA reduce the amount of blood loss anticipated during dissection of the native recipient abdominal organs. Contracture of the abdominal cavity in patients with previous multiple enterectomies combined with postperfusion swelling of the implanted intestine presents

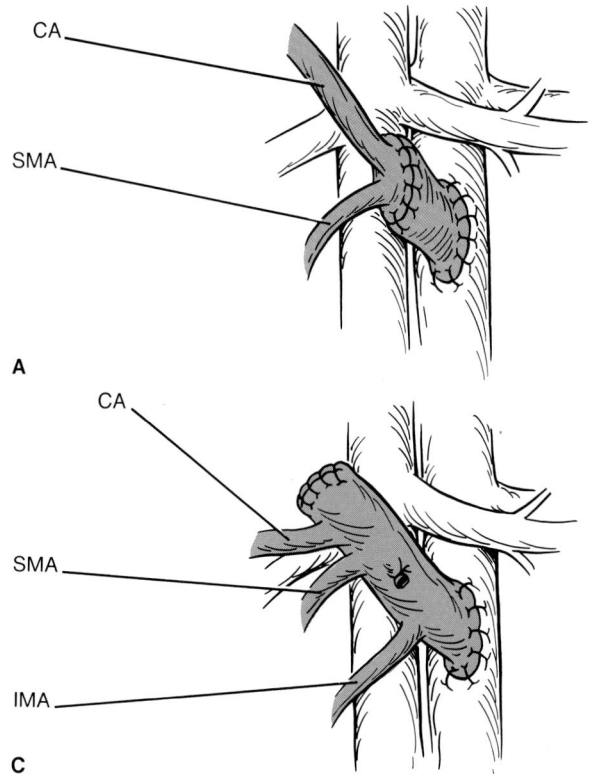

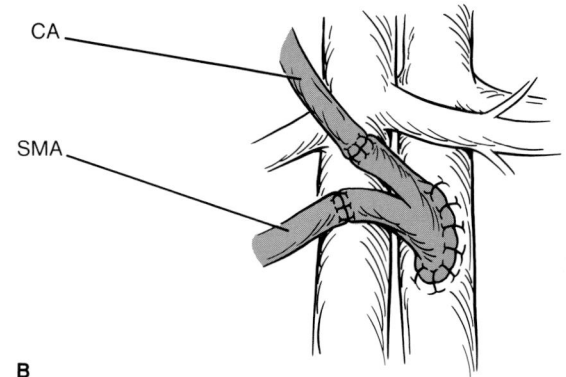

Figure 35-9 Types of arterial grafts used as vascular conduits for combined hepatic–intestinal and multivisceral grafts. The arterial anastomosis shown in **A** is the one most often used. CA, celiac artery; IMA, inferior mesenteric artery; SMA, superior mesenteric artery. (Furukawa H, Abu-Elmagd K, Reyes J, et al. Technical aspects of intestinal transplantation. In: Braverman MH, Tawes RL, eds. Surgical technology international II. 1993:165)

performed with preservation of the native ileocecal valve. A temporary ileostomy always is performed in patients in whom continuity of the distal gastrointestinal tract is achieved. A vent chimney is constructed in small bowel recipients (see Fig. 35-11, *left inset*) and a Bishop-Coop ileostomy is performed in patients who receive small bowel plus colon. These temporary ileostomies help clinicians monitor changes in the graft mucosa and provide easy access for frequent surveillance endoscopy. Surgical closure of these enteric vents is recommended 6 to 12 months after transplantation.

Combined Hepatic–Intestinal Graft

With hepatic–intestinal transplantation, the surgical and anesthetic team must consider the hemodynamic and metabolic changes that occur during the anhepatic phase and after reperfusion. The use of venovenous bypass is compromised in many of these patients by the coexistence of significant stenosis or thrombosis of the superior vena cava system from the long-term use of central intravenous catheters. Therefore, the preferred method of recipient hepatectomy includes preservation of the recipient retrohepatic vena cava (Fig. 35-12). The remaining part of the native splanchnic venous system is drained into the recipient infrahepatic vena cava by creating a portacaval shunt.

In the presence of significant portal hypertension, it is preferable to perform the shunt during the early steps of the operation to minimize blood loss during removal of the native liver and dissection of the residual intestine.

With implantation of the combined hepatic–intestinal graft, the donor suprahepatic vena cava is anastomosed end to side to the recipient vena cava at the level of the hepatic veins[56] (piggyback technique; see Fig. 35-12). Next, the arterial inflow to the entire graft is established by an infrarenal aortic anastomosis with the arterial conduit interposition graft that was connected to the combined celiac trunk–SMA Carrel patch on the backtable.[57] Because both the liver and intestinal grafts are placed in continuity, adequate venous drainage of the remaining native splanchnic organs, such as the stomach, duodenum, pancreas, and spleen, must be achieved. The options are to anastomose the end of the recipient portal vein to the side of the donor main portal vein or to leave the newly fashioned recipient portacaval shunt in place (see Fig. 35-12, *right inset*). The decision is based primarily on the length of the recipient portal vein and the size of the donor portal vein. After the graft is revascularized, about 500 to 1000 mL of blood is vented through the lower infrahepatic vena cava of the donor liver before this vessel is ligated. This is done to minimize the risk and severity of the reperfu-

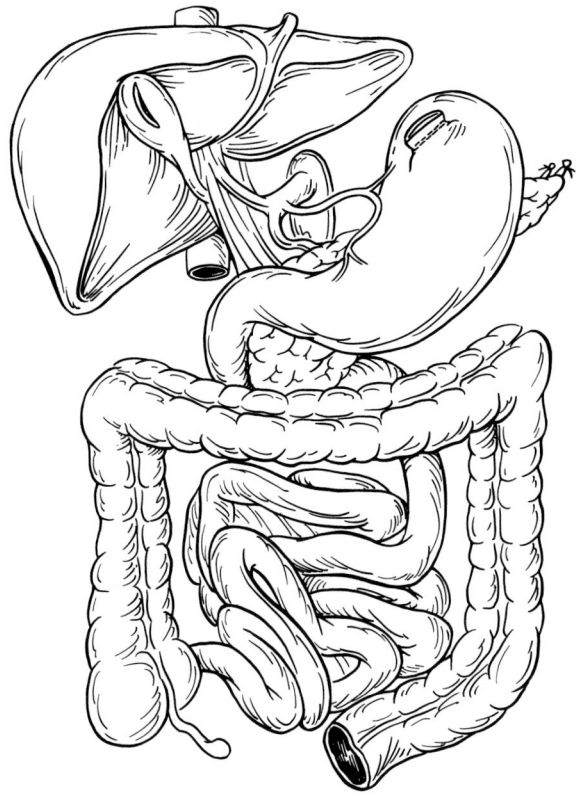

Figure 35-10 Multivisceral graft. Continuity of the visceral, arterial, and portal venous systems is seen. Splenectomy is performed either during the donor operation or on the backtable. (Furukawa H, Abu-Elmagd K, Reyes J, et al. Technical aspects of intestinal transplantation. In: Braverman MH, Tawes RL, eds. Surgical technology international II. 1993:165)

sion syndrome that usually occurs after the stagnant allograft preservation fluid is flushed into the recipient systemic circulation.

Continuity of the gastrointestinal tract is established as in isolated intestinal recipients. Biliary drainage is accomplished by anastomosing the common bile duct to the jejunum of the intestinal graft in a simple loop or Roux-en-Y fashion (see Fig. 35-12).

Multivisceral Graft

With multivisceral transplantation, most of the gastrointestinal organs are replaced en bloc. Arterial inflow and venous outflow of the entire graft are established as in combined hepatic–intestinal transplantation, by using the common arterial conduit and piggyback vena cava drainage (Fig. 35-13). In some of these unique patients, the arterial anastomosis can be performed in the celiac segment of the abdominal aorta

with the advantage of shortening the length of the interposition arterial graft.

Continuity of the proximal gastrointestinal tract is achieved by anastomosing the recipient abdominal esophagus or the remaining portion of the native stomach to the anterior wall of the donor stomach. Continuity of the distal gut is established as in isolated intestinal transplantation. In two pediatric patients with extensive polyposis and Hirschsprung's disease, endorectal pull-through of the transplanted colon was performed without difficulty (Fig. 35-14). Because of inevitable denervation of the stomach, pyloroplasty or pyloromyotomy is performed routinely to prevent gastric outlet obstruction. To minimize the risk of postoperative pancreatitis, bile flow is diverted temporarily by cannulation of the cystic duct[58] (see Fig. 35-13).

POSTOPERATIVE CARE

Immunosuppression

FK506 (Prograf) has been the primary immunosuppressive agent used in intestinal and multivisceral allograft recipients at our center since May 2, 1990. It initially is given intravenously as a constant infusion at a dosage of 0.15 mg/kg/d. Oral administration is begun after the integrity of the gastrointestinal anastomoses is confirmed by radiologic contrast studies, typically at the end of the first postoperative week.[59] Overlap of intravenous and oral FK506 administration is the general rule, with a transition period of about 1 week. The guidelines used for FK506 dosage adjustment are similar to those initially adopted for liver transplantation.[60] The target FK506 plasma level generally is 2 to 3 ng/mL during continuous intravenous therapy. With the oral administration of FK506 and during long-term follow-up, 12-hour trough plasma levels typically are maintained at 1 to 2 ng/mL. The dosage is reduced if there is evidence of nephrotoxicity or neurotoxicity, and is increased if rejection is documented histologically or suspected clinically.[59]

Methylprednisolone is given immediately after reperfusion as a 1-g bolus followed by tapering over 5 days, beginning at 200 mg/d and ending at 20 mg/d, with daily reductions of 40 mg. A maintenance daily dose of 20 mg of methylprednisolone or prednisone is continued and tapered slowly, as tolerated. Corticosteroid doses are scaled down for children.

Prostaglandin E_1 (Prostin) usually is administered immediately after perfusion at a dose of 0.6 μg/kg/h, and is continued if tolerated during the period that intravenous FK506 is given. The role of prostaglandin E_1 in modulating reperfusion injury and rejection and its

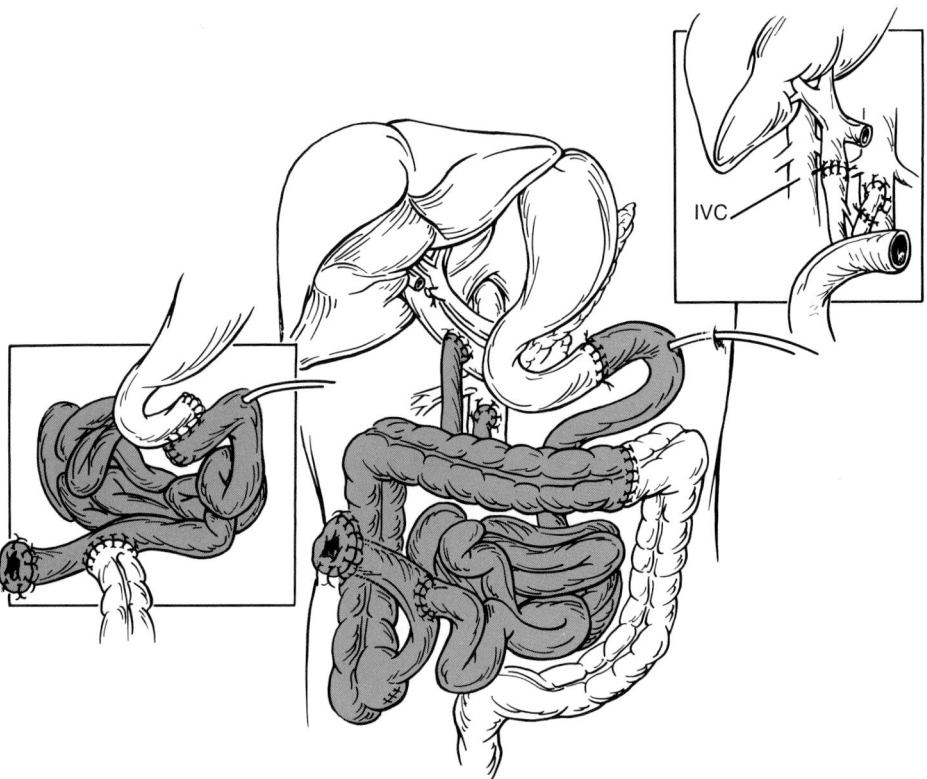

Figure 35-11 Isolated intestinal transplantation including half the colon (*main figure*) or only the small bowel (*left inset*). Graft venous outflow is drained end-to-side (*main figure*) or end-to-end (*right inset*) into the host portal system. IVC, inferior vena cava. (Abu-Elmagd K, Todo S, Tzakis A, et al. Three years clinical experience with intestinal transplantation. J Am Coll Surg 1994;179:385)

renal protective effect have been reported with the transplantation of other organs.[61]

Mild rejection episodes are treated with a single 1-g bolus of methylprednisolone. In addition, a 5-day corticosteroid recycle starting at 200 mg/d and ending at 20 mg/d is administered to patients with moderate rejection. Azathioprine is added for selected cases at dosages of 0.5 to 1 mg/kg/d, and is continued as long as the white blood cell count continues to be above 3000/μL. A 7- to 10-day course of OKT3, 5 to 10 mL/d, is used in patients with corticosteroid-resistant or severe rejection episodes.[62]

Prophylaxis of Infection

Selective decontamination of the native and transplanted gut is continued for 3 to 4 weeks after transplantation. It is reinstituted during severe rejection episodes and in patients with overt symptoms of bacterial overgrowth. A combination of amphotericin B or nystatin, tobramycin or gentamicin, and polymyxin E is given four times a day through the nasogastric or enterostomy tube, or by mouth. Standard intravenous antibiotic prophylaxis with cefotaxime and ampicillin also is administered for 5 to 7 days after transplantation and is continued if necessary, based on the results of blood and body fluid cultures. Quantitative stool cultures are done periodically to monitor changes in the intestinal

flora; simultaneous blood cultures are obtained in patients with active systemic infection to look for evidence of microbial translocation.[59]

Chronic viral and protozoal prophylaxis is accomplished by the administration of acyclovir for CMV and trimethoprim-sulfamethoxazole (Bactrim) for *Pneumocystis carinii.* Because of the high incidence of CMV enteritis in patients who receive CMV-positive grafts, ganciclovir therapy should be initiated early in these high-risk cases and continued for 1 to 3 months after transplantation.

Nutrition

TPN usually is continued during the early postoperative course. After the integrity of the gastrointestinal anastomoses and partial recovery of gut motility are confirmed with the appropriate gastrointestinal contrast studies, enteral feeding through the jejunal tube is commenced with Peptamen. Continuous enteral feeding with gradually increasing volumes is preferred over the bolus method. TPN generally is tapered gradually and discontinued according to the nutritional status of the patient, the enteric caloric intake, and the absorptive capacity of the graft. Peptamen is an isotonic elemental diet that contains peptide-based protein, medium-chain triglycerides, and glutamine. Four to 6 weeks after transplantation in children, the use of Peptamen is con-

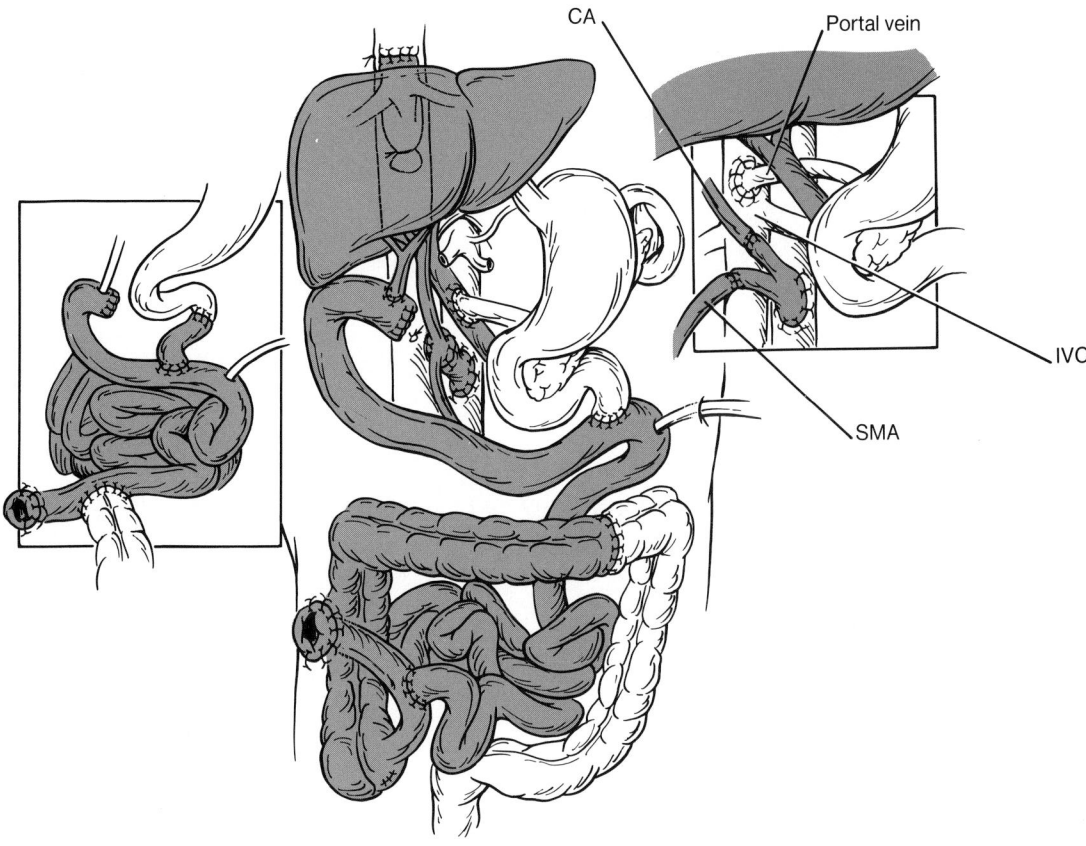

Figure 35-12 Hepatic–intestinal transplantation including part of the colon (*main figure*) or only the small bowel (*left inset*). The host portal vein is drained into the graft portal vein when possible, but in one third of cases this blood is diverted into the vena cava (*right inset*). CA, celiac artery; SMA, superior mesenteric artery; IVC, inferior vena cava. (Abu-Elmagd K, Todo S, Tzakis A, et al. Three years clinical experience with intestinal transplantation. J Am Coll Surg 1994;179:385)

verted to Compleat-B, a lactose- and gluten-free diet that contains dietary fiber to promote normalization of intestinal motility. Enteral tube feedings are decreased gradually as oral intake improves. Weaning from enteral nutritional support is begun by reducing the rate of infusion, then decreasing the daily duration of tube feeding. Opiates, loperamide, and kaolin-pectin mixtures are used in patients who experience high stomal output or diarrhea. Prokinetic agents sometimes are given to patients with gastrointestinal dysmotility. The metabolic advantages of intravenous and enteral use of glutamine in these unique allograft recipients is under investigation.

GRAFT MONITORING

Rejection

Detection of intestinal graft rejection is based primarily on clinical findings, endoscopic observations, and histopathologic examinations of endoscopically guided mucosal biopsies.[62] Surveillance graft endoscopy with random multiple mucosal biopsies should be performed at least weekly for the first 3 months, monthly for the next 3 months, and every 3 to 6 months thereafter and whenever it is clinically indicated. Ileal biopsies are performed using distal ileoscopy or ileocolonoscopy. Jejunal biopsy samples are obtained through a regular upper gastrointestinal endoscope. Given the cumulative histopathologic evidence that the ileal portion of the intestinal allograft is most susceptible to rejection, ileal biopsies are mandatory to confirm or exclude graft rejection.

Acute Rejection

Acute intestinal allograft rejection usually presents with an increase in stomal output, fever, abdominal pain, watery diarrhea, and vomiting. In addition, graft ileus, intestinal bleeding, septic shock, and a clinical picture resembling that of adult respiratory distress syn-

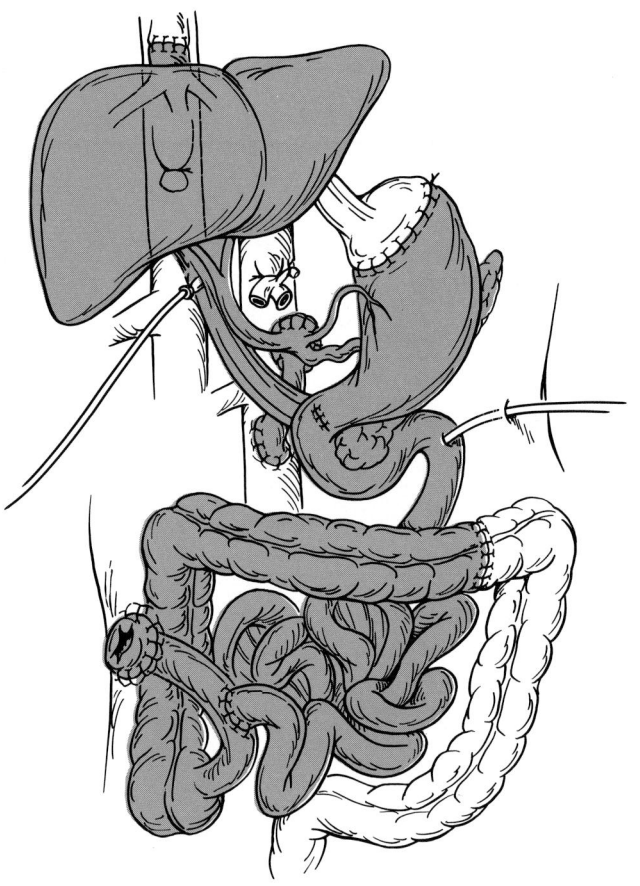

Figure 35-13 Full multivisceral operation including the ascending and right transverse colon. Pyloroplasty or pyloromyotomy was performed, and bile flow was temporarily decompressed in all cases. (Abu-Elmagd K, Todo S, Tzakis A, et al. Three years' clinical experience with intestinal transplantation. J Am Coll Surg 1994;179:385)

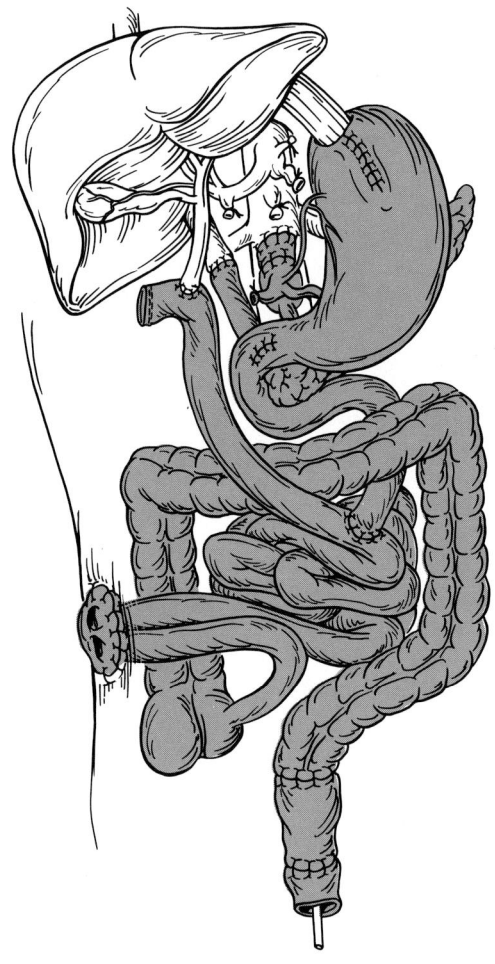

Figure 35-14 The endorectal pull-through operation in a child who received a modified multivisceral graft that combined the stomach, duodenum, pancreas, small bowel, and colon. The native liver was preserved, and the liver allograft was used for another recipient.

drome develop in patients with severe rejection episodes. Endoscopic examination of the intestinal graft usually demonstrates an ischemic or dusky mucosa with focal ulcerations and reduced or absent peristalsis. Grafts with severe rejection show either a nodular mu-

cosa (Fig. 35-15B) or diffuse ulceration with bleeding (see Fig. 35-15C). The histologic criteria for the diagnosis of acute intestinal allograft rejection include a mononuclear cell infiltrate, villus blunting, and cryptitis (Fig. 35-16B). Complete sloughing of the intestinal

A   B   C

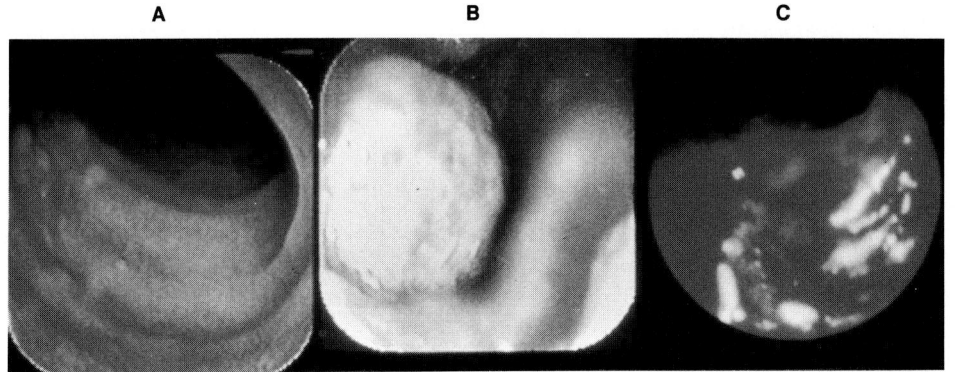

Figure 35-15 The endoscopic appearance of intestinal allograft rejection. (**A**) Normal ileum. (**B**) Moderate rejection with a nodular appearance and small ulcers. (**C**) Severe rejection with diffuse mucosal sloughing and active bleeding. (See Color Fig. 35-15.)

Figure 35-16 The histologic picture of intestinal allograft rejection. **(A)** Normal intestinal mucosa. **(B)** Endoscopic biopsy sample showing widening of the lamina propria, increased mononuclear cells, blunting of the villi, capillary congestion, and significant crypt damage (hematoxylin–eosin, ×140). **(C)** Uncontrolled severe rejection with massive crypt loss and widespread mucosal destruction (hematoxylin–eosin, ×140). (See Color Fig. 35-16.)

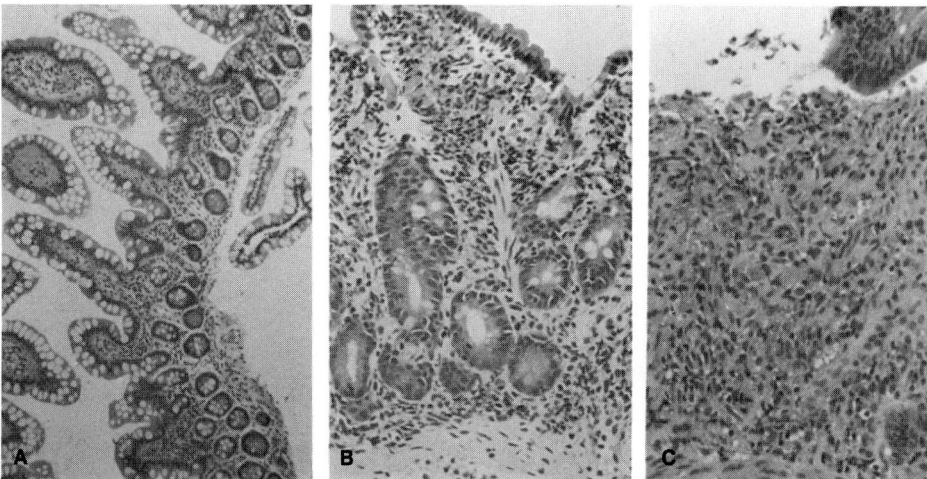

mucosa with crypt destruction is seen in patients with severe rejection episodes (see Fig. 35-16C).

Chronic Rejection

The development of chronic intestinal allograft rejection usually is manifested by intractable diarrhea, abdominal pain, intermittent episodes of sepsis, progressive weight loss, and intermittent intestinal bleeding. Periodic endoscopic examinations reveal pseudomembrane formation, thickened mucosal folds, and finally chronic ulcers in a tubular intestine (Fig. 35-17). Serial radiologic examinations show the development

of dilated intestinal loops with effaced mucosal folds (Fig. 35-18) and thickened walls (Fig. 35-19).

In chronic rejection, intestinal mucosal biopsy samples show apoptosis of crypt cells with a sparse inflammatory cell infiltrate. Angiography sometimes demonstrates segmental narrowing of the mesenteric arterial arcade (Fig. 35-20), which can dictate graft enterectomy. Full-thickness histopathologic examination of the resected grafts in such cases demonstrates mucosal ulceration with intramural abscesses and obliterative arteriopathy (Fig. 35-21).

Grading of intestinal allograft rejection is based on clinical, endoscopic, and histologic criteria (Table 35-1). Immunosuppressive regimens are adjusted ac-

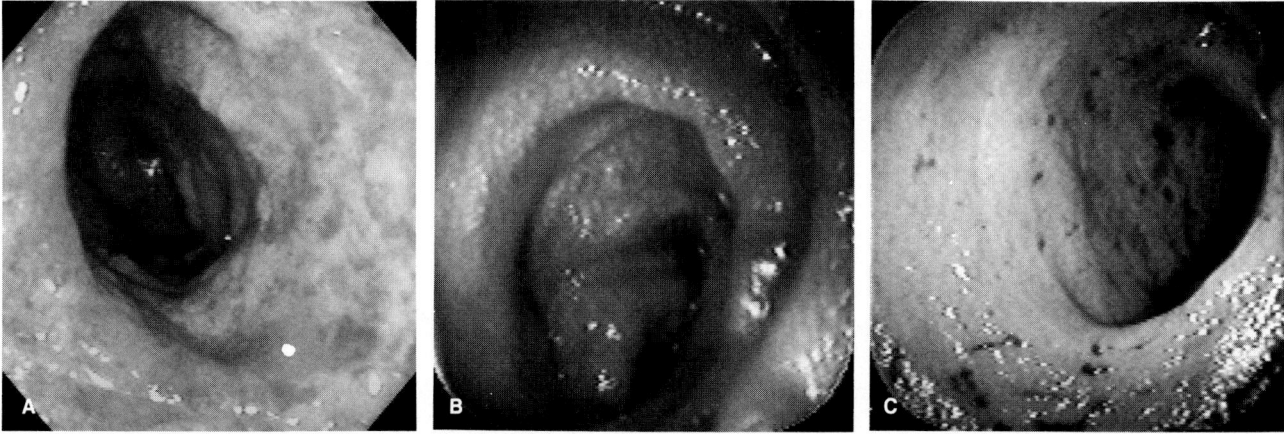

Figure 35-17 The endoscopic appearance of chronic rejection of an intestinal allograft. **(A)** Rejection with pseudomembrane formation. **(B)** Early phase of chronic rejection with granular mucosa and thickened folds. **(C)** Late phase of chronic rejection with tubular intestine and deep ulcers. (See Color Fig. 35-17.)

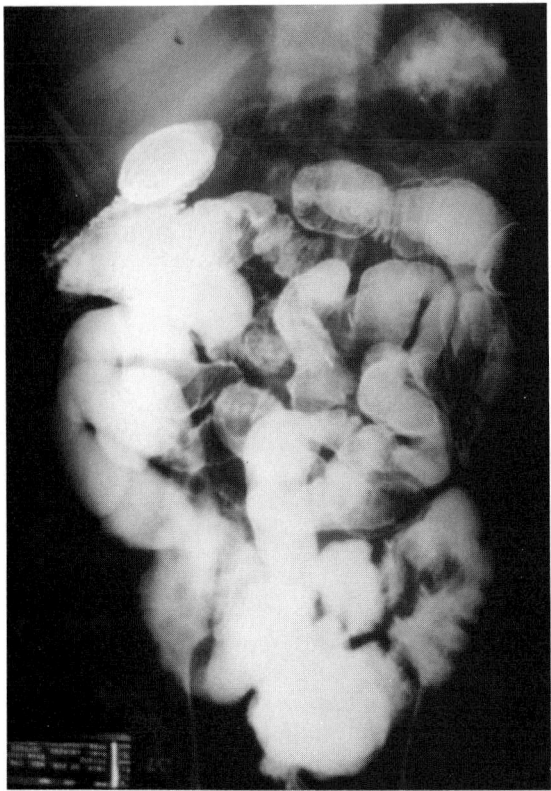

Figure 35-18 Gastrointestinal contrast study showing dilated intestinal loops with loss of the mucosal pattern in a patient with chronic allograft rejection.

cording to the severity of the rejection episodes by administering a corticosteroid bolus and recycle, OKT3, or both.[62] Intractable acute rejection or chronic rejection of isolated intestinal grafts is treated best with early graft enterectomy. Retransplantation in intestinal

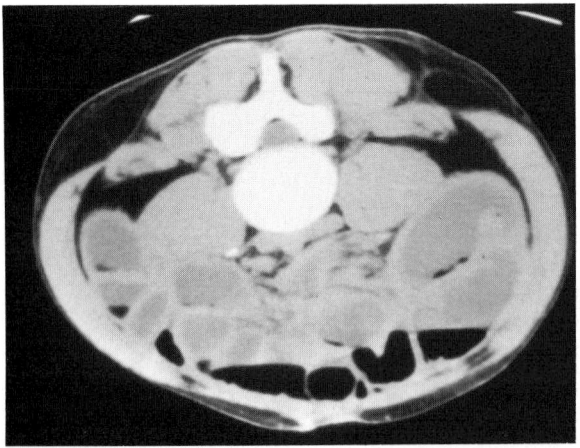

Figure 35-19 Abdominal CT scan showing dilated intestinal loops with thickened walls and radiologic evidence of pneumatosis intestinalis in a patient with chronic rejection of an intestinal allograft.

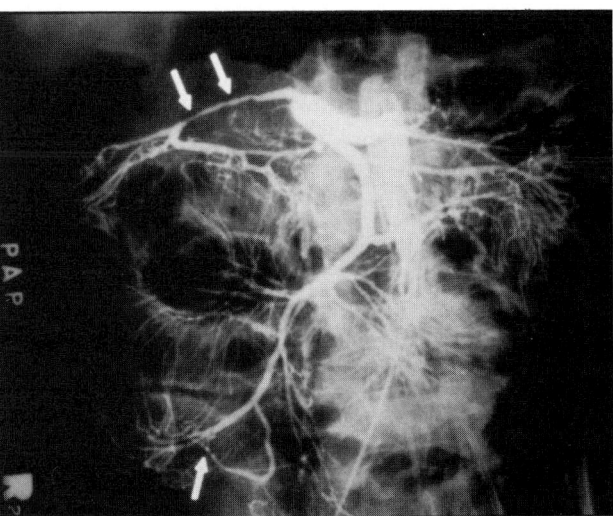

Figure 35-20 Superior mesenteric arteriogram showing segmental narrowing of the jejunal and ileal arterial branches (*arrows*) in a chronically rejected intestinal graft.

allograft recipients carries significant morbidity and mortality.

Function

Graft function is assessed serially and when clinically indicated. The standard biochemical measures of hepatic and pancreatic injury are used to monitor the status of these solid organs. For the transplanted and native parts of the gastrointestinal tract, radiologic contrast studies are performed to determine the duration of gastric emptying, the intestinal transit time, and the pattern of the intestinal mucosa.[63] Serum concentrations of albumin, vitamins, minerals, and trace elements are measured frequently. Oral FK506 kinetic studies are done after the intravenous administration of FK506 has been discontinued. The absorption of d-xylose and fat are helpful tools for monitoring changes in graft function.[64,65] Anthropometric parameters such as body weight and measurements of upper arm fat and muscle also are obtained periodically.

HISTOPATHOLOGY

The intestinal allograft is monitored histologically by frequent endoscopically guided mucosal biopsies. Undirected stomal biopsies have been shown either to miss focal lesions or to document nonspecific changes that can mimic rejection or infection. Histopathologic changes that can be observed in intestinal allografts in-

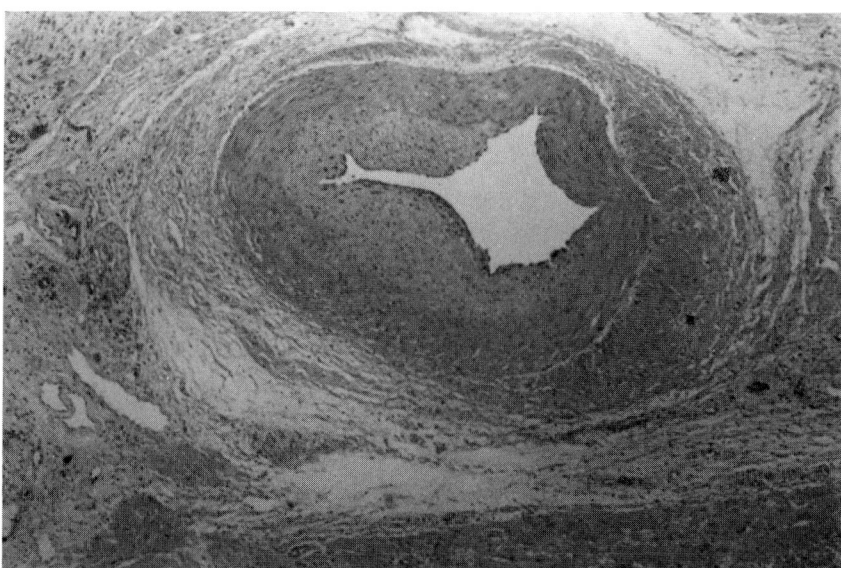

Figure 35-21 The histopathologic picture of a full-thickness intestinal specimen after graft enterectomy. Examination of arteries in the mesenteric root and bowel serosa revealed obliterative arteriopathy, as is typical of chronic rejection in all vascularized organ allografts (hematoxylin–eosin, ×140).

clude preservation injury, immune cell repopulation, graft rejection, and enteric infection.

Preservation Injury

Histologic assessment of preimplantation intestinal biopsy samples usually reveals separation of the villus epithelium from the underlying lamina propria at the level of the basement membrane, or areas of widespread epithelial denudation (Fig. 35-22). Biopsy samples taken after perfusion show variable degrees of epithelial denudation, congestion of the capillaries in the lamina propria, and neutrophilic margination in the submucosal veins. These histopathologic changes are followed by neutrophilic inflammation and the formation of granulation tissue in the lamina propria with a luminal inflammatory pseudomembrane. Epithelial regeneration usually is completed by the second week after transplantation, assuming there is no intervening rejection.

The colon seems to be less susceptible to ischemia than the small bowel. In a canine study, high-energy phosphate levels, electric potential differences, and documented histologic changes suggested that the co-

Table 35-1   Monitoring of Intestinal Allograft Rejection

Rejection	Clinical Findings	Endoscopic Picture	Histopathologic Changes
ACUTE			
Mild to moderate	Fever	Hyperemic friable mucosa	Cell infiltration
	Abdominal distention	Mucosal edema	Villus blunting
	Abdominal pain	Decreased peristalsis	Cryptitis
	Nausea, vomiting	Multiple small ulcers	Mucus and paneth cell depletion
	Increased stomal output		Epithelial cell damage and regeneration
	Diarrhea		
	Ileus		
Severe	Severe bloody diarrhea	Diffuse ulceration	Mucosal sloughing
	Bacteremia	Bleeding	Mural hemorrhage
	Septicemia	Loss of peristalsis	Microabscess
	Adult respiratory distress syndrome		Granulation
CHRONIC	Chronic intractable diarrhea	Loss of mucosal folds	Crypt damage
	Intestinal bleeding	Pseudomembranes	Regenerative epithelium
	Malabsorption	Chronic deep ulcers	Submucosal fibrosis
	Progessive weight loss	Hypoperistalsis	Obliterative arteriopathy
		Loss of mucosal folds	

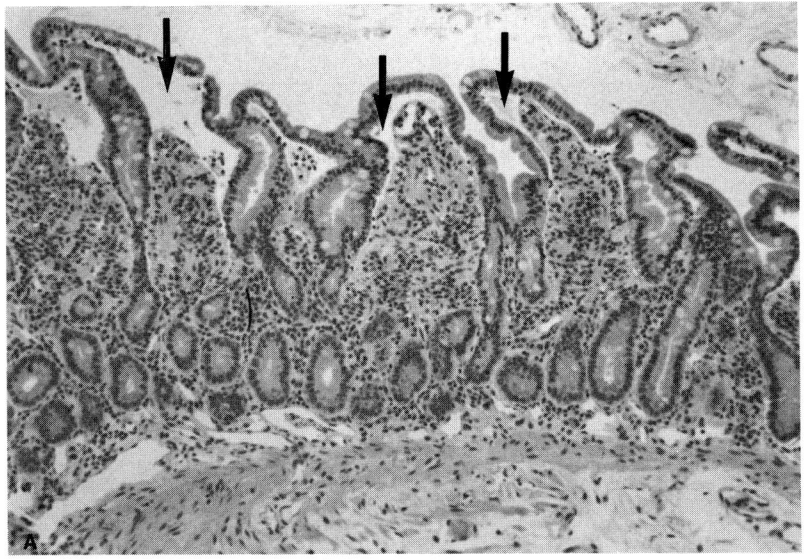

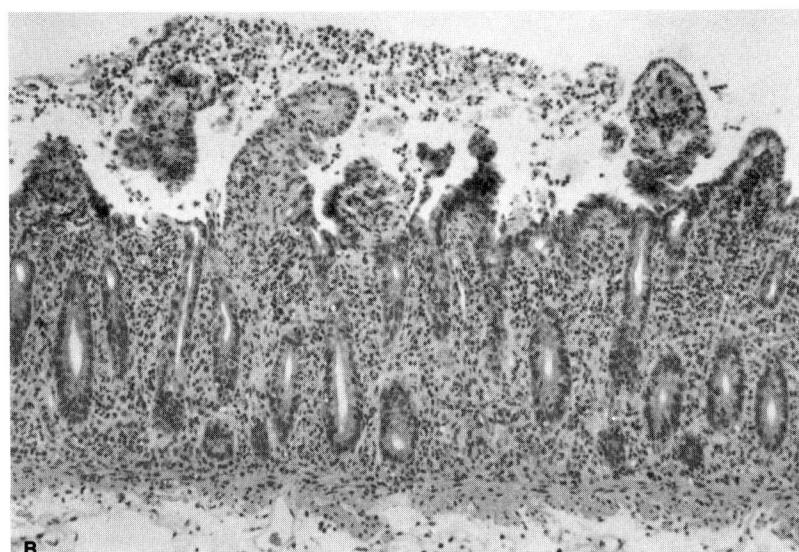

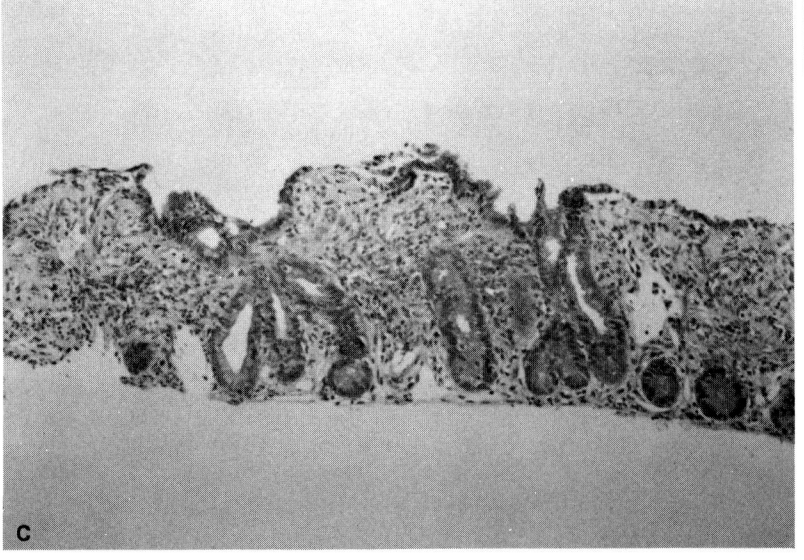

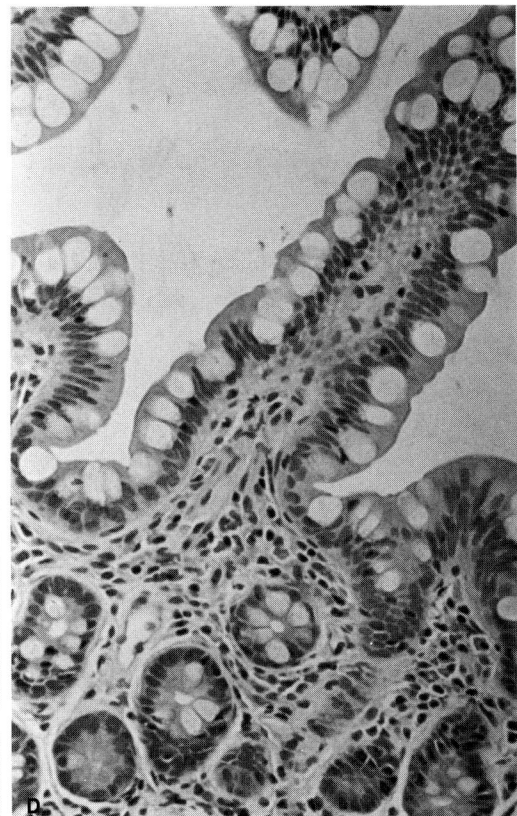

Figure 35-22 Preservation injury of an intestinal allograft. (**A**) Backtable biopsy of the donor small intestine reveals separation of villous epithelium from the underlying stroma (*arrows*; hematoxylin–eosin, ×140). (**B**) Three hours after revascularization, epithelial denudation of the villous tips, a mild inflammatory infiltrate, and regenerative epithelial changes are seen (hematoxylin– eosin, ×140). (**C**) Six to 8 days after transplantation, regeneration begins to restore the normal architecture (hematoxylin–eosin, ×55). (**D**) By 12 days after transplantation, the normal architecture is completely restored (hematoxylin–eosin, ×350).

lon is more resistant to both cold and warm ischemia than is the small intestine.[66] Similar findings are noted in human recipients of large intestine, in whom colonic mucosal preservation changes rarely are seen.

Replacement of Donor Lymphoid Tissue

Within the first 4 weeks after transplantation, the donor mesenteric lymph nodes characteristically show paracortical expansion composed of blastic and prolif-erating lymphocytes, histiocytes, and fewer neutrophils or eosinophils (Fig. 35-23A). At the end of the first week, at least half the lymphocytes are of recipient origin, whereas the remaining lymphocytes and endothelial cells remain of donor origin (see Fig. 35-23B and C). Thereafter, progressively fewer donor cells are found, although the stroma and endothelia remain of donor origin.[67]

Within the intestinal grafts, infiltration of recipient cells occurs irrespective of the diagnosis of rejection. Hybridization studies for the Y chromosome in female-

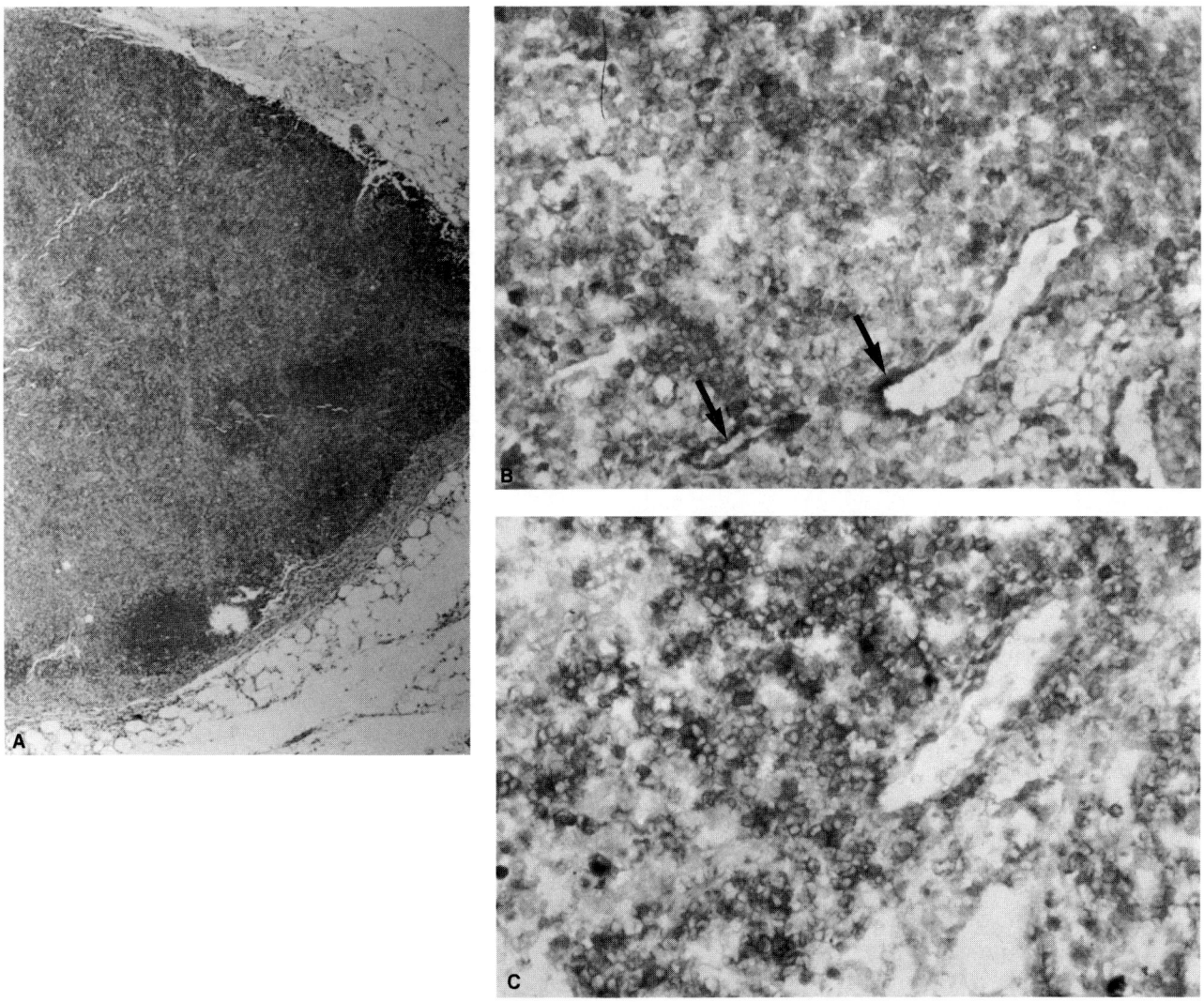

Figure 35-23 Replacement of donor lymphoid tissue in the mesenteric lymph nodes. (**A**) A donor mesenteric lymph node obtained 7 days after transplantation shows a mixture of donor and recipient cells resulting in paracortical expansion and blastogenesis (hematoxylin–eosin, ×55). (**B**) This node was stained with anti-HLA A11, which was present in the donor but not in the recipient (IPEX for anti-HLA A11, ×560). (**C**) A serial section of the same node was stained for anti-HLA A2, which was specific for the recipient (IPEX for anti-HLA A2, ×560). Endothelial staining occurred in **B** (*arrows*) but not in **C**. (See Color Fig. 35-23.)

to-male allografts reveal that recipient hematolymphoid cells infiltrate the lamina propria in the biopsy specimens within the first postoperative week (Fig. 35-24A). Many or most of the cells in the lamina propria are replaced by recipient cells by 70 to 80 days after transplantation (see Fig. 35-24B). In contrast, the epithelial, endothelial, and stromal elements remain of donor origin for up to 2 years after transplantation (see Fig. 35-24C).

Rejection

Acute Rejection

Mild intestinal allograft rejection usually is manifested histopathologically by widening of the lamina propria as a result of edema and by the presence of an increased mononuclear cell infiltrate (see Fig. 35-16B). This infiltrate is composed of blastic lymphocytes, typically cuffed around smaller blood vessels and infiltrating the crypts. Variable numbers of eosinophils and macrophages also can be seen. Peyer's patches can appear enlarged, and as the rejection progresses, superficial mucosal ulcerations appear at these sites. The epithelial cells can show necrosis or reparative changes. An increased nuclear to cytoplasmic ratio can be present in the regenerating glands.

As rejection worsens, the focal mucosal ulceration often is associated with thrombosis of the superficial capillaries of the lamina propria. In cases of severe rejection, extensive mucosal sloughing can occur and is associated with complete loss of the superficial architecture (see Fig. 35-16C). Granulation tissue replaces the mucosa, and the overlying inflammatory pseudomembrane consists of sloughed mucosa, inflammatory cells, and bacteria (Fig. 35-25).

The histopathologic response after successful treatment of acute rejection usually lags behind the clinical response by 5 to 7 days. Microscopic evidence of improvement includes reparative epithelial changes, increased crypt depth with mitosis, decreased edema, and resolution of the mononuclear inflammatory cell infiltrate. However, progression to chronic rejection can be seen in patients with recurrent episodes of rejection that respond partially to augmented immunosuppression.

Chronic Rejection

The transition from acute to chronic rejection is an insidious and slow process. With chronic rejection, histopathologic examination of the full-thickness biopsy specimen demonstrates obliterative vasculopathy of both large and small arteries with fibrosis of the lamina propria and submucosa (see Fig. 35-21). Focal mucosal ulcerations with intramural abscesses, adenomatoid metaplasia, and lymph node fibrosis also can be seen.

Infection

Cytomegalovirus

The histopathologic findings of CMV enteritis vary from a mild mononuclear to a mixed or predominantly neutrophilic infiltrate of the lamina propria that is more localized than that seen in rejection and can occur with or without small mucosal ulcers. Cytoplasmic inclusions also can be detected amidst the focal inflammation in endothelial stromal or, less frequently, epithelial cells (Fig. 35-26). Simultaneously obtained biopsy samples of residual native intestine usually are less severely affected.

In some patients with CMV graft enteritis, serial biopsy samples show a minimal or mild mononuclear cell infiltrate associated with distinct crypt cell apoptosis but without obvious inclusions. In these cases, it is extremely difficult to differentiate between CMV infection and ongoing mild rejection. Examination of multiple levels and use of immunoperoxidase stains for CMV antigens are helpful in distinguishing between the two possibilities. If any histopathologic or immunohistochemical evidence of CMV is detected, the patient is treated primarily for viral infection. However, in some instances, graft rejection and CMV enteritis coexist, and both should be treated promptly.

Epstein-Barr Virus

The histopathologic diagnosis of Epstein-Barr virus infection among intestinal transplant recipients is similar to that described in other allograft recipients.[68] An atypical monomorphic lymphoplasmacytic infiltrate spans the lamina propria and submucosa, but the crypts are relatively spared from damage. The diagnosis usually is confirmed by localization of Epstein-Barr virus DNA in the atypical cells by in situ hybridization.

CLINICAL EXPERIENCE WITH INTESTINAL AND MULTIVISCERAL TRANSPLANTATION

Patient Population

Forty-three patients underwent transplant procedures at the University of Pittsburgh between May 2, 1990, and April 15, 1993. As shown in Table 35-2, 15 patients received isolated intestinal grafts, 21 received hepatic–

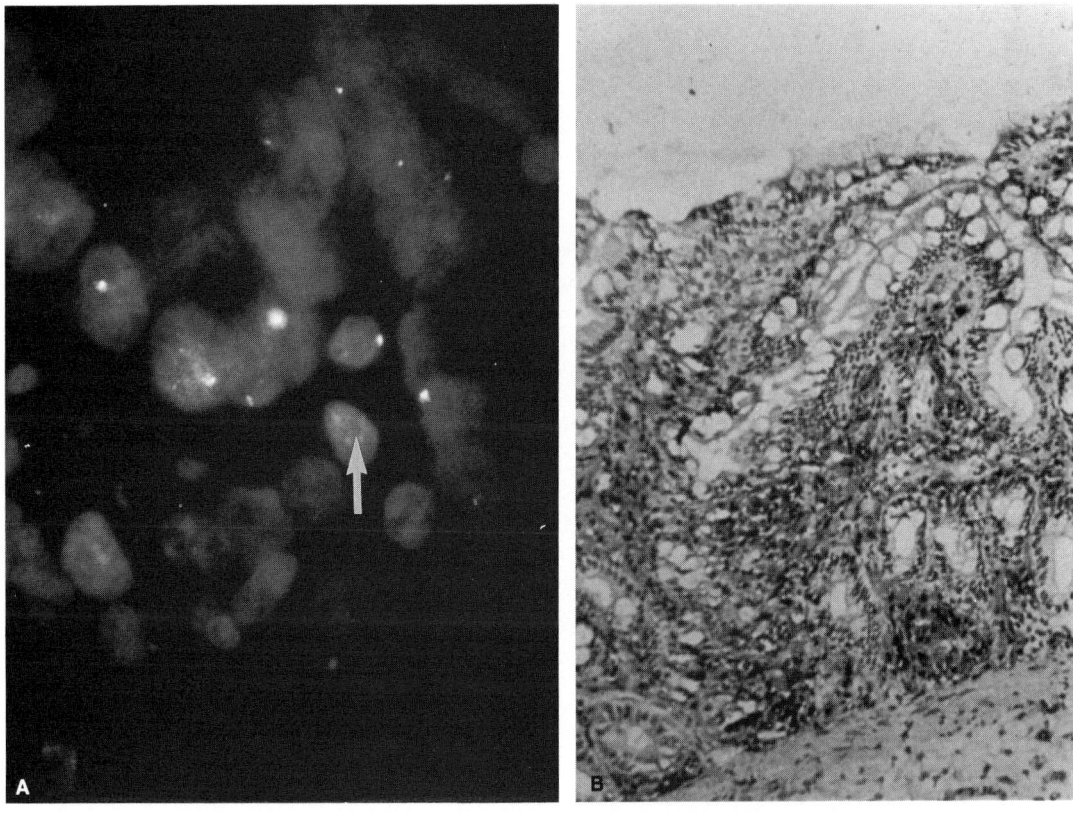

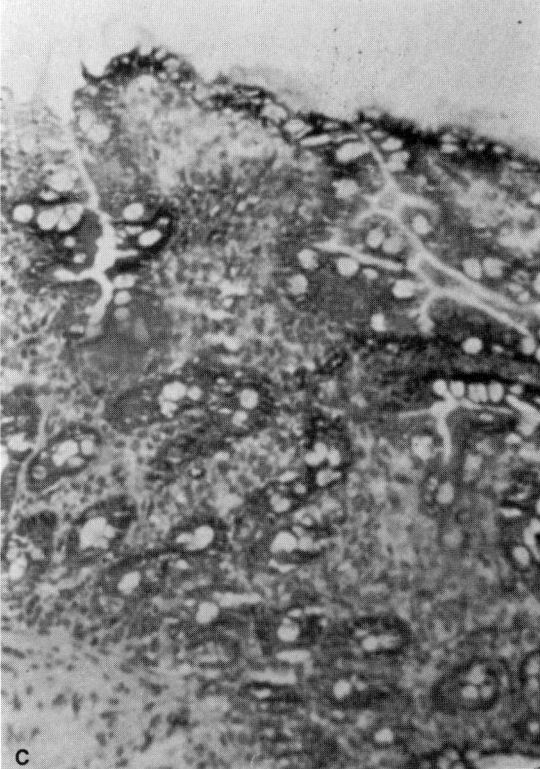

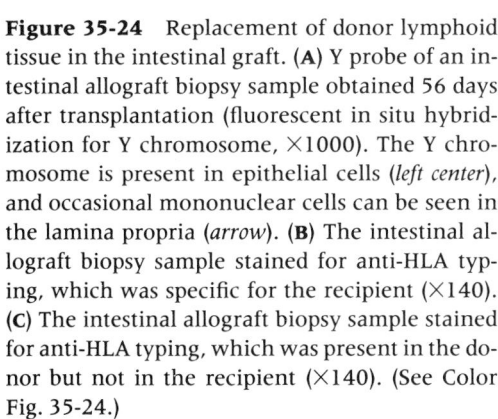

Figure 35-24 Replacement of donor lymphoid tissue in the intestinal graft. (**A**) Y probe of an intestinal allograft biopsy sample obtained 56 days after transplantation (fluorescent in situ hybridization for Y chromosome, ×1000). The Y chromosome is present in epithelial cells (*left center*), and occasional mononuclear cells can be seen in the lamina propria (*arrow*). (**B**) The intestinal allograft biopsy sample stained for anti-HLA typing, which was specific for the recipient (×140). (**C**) The intestinal allograft biopsy sample stained for anti-HLA typing, which was present in the donor but not in the recipient (×140). (See Color Fig. 35-24.)

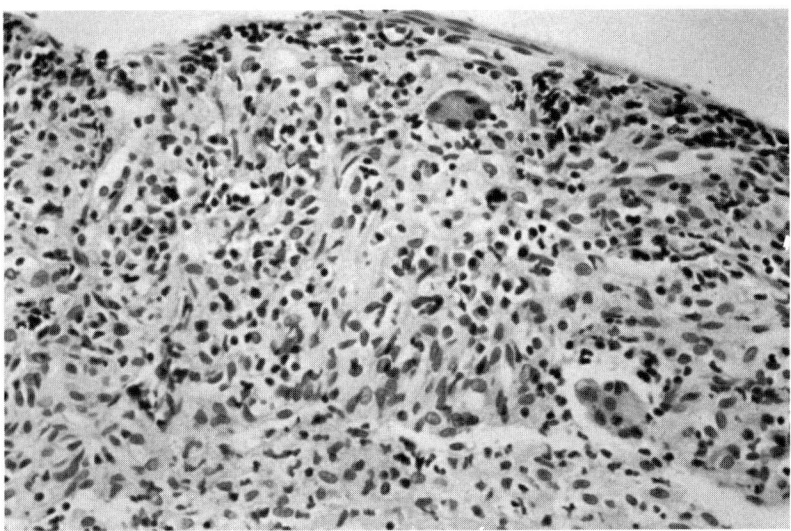

Figure 35-25 Uncontrolled acute rejection eventually results in widespread destruction of the mucosa, which is replaced by granulation tissue. Overlying inflammatory pseudomembrane is visible (*arrow*; hematoxylin-eosin, ×350).

intestinal grafts, and 7 received multivisceral grafts. A total of 45 grafts were used in 43 patients. The 2 extra grafts were given as second grafts to one isolated intestinal graft recipient and one combined hepatic–intestinal graft recipient.

The patients were 22 children and 21 adults, with a preponderance of children requiring hepatic–intestinal transplants and adults receiving isolated intestinal transplants. The mean age was 3.5 ± 3.7 years (range, 0.5 to 15.5 years) for the pediatric population and 33.3 ± 10.2 years (range, 19 to 58 years) for the adult population.

The indications for intestinal transplantation are shown in Table 35-3. Short-gut syndrome due to Crohn's disease was the most common reason for isolated intestinal transplantation, whereas perinatal intestinal complications followed by TPN-induced liver failure was the most common indication for combined hepatic–intestinal transplantation. Mesenteric and celiac vascular occlusion, induced by an inherent hypercoagulopathy, was a common indication for multivisceral transplantation.

Patient and Graft Survival

Thirteen of the 43 intestinal graft recipients died during the study period. The mean length of follow-up for the 30 survivors was 17 ± 9 months (range, 6 to 39 months). The Kaplan-Meier (actuarial) survival curve for the 43 patients is shown in Figure 35-27A. The overall 3-, 6-, 12-, and 24-month patient survival rates were 88%, 84%, 81%, and 74%, respectively. When calculated for each cohort of intestinal allograft recipients (isolated intestinal, hepatic–intestinal, and multivis-

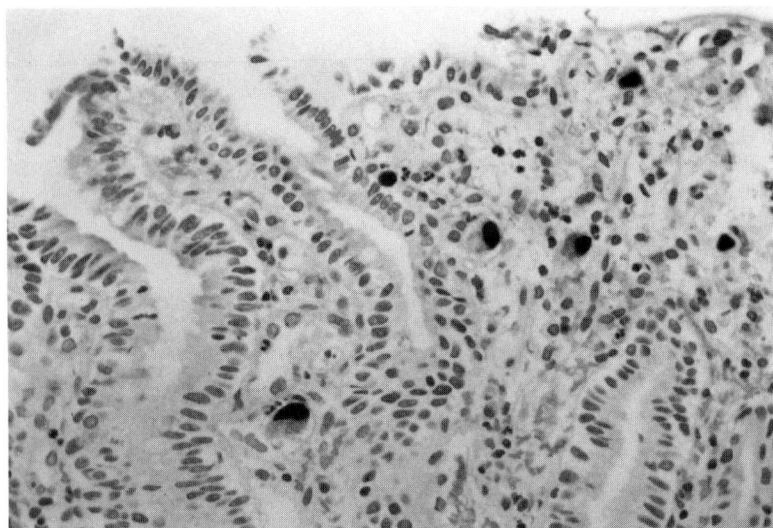

Figure 35-26 Cytomegalovirus enteritis in an intestinal allograft. The diagnosis is confirmed histologically by the presence of characteristic inclusions or staining for viral antigens. Focal neutrophilic inflammation is visible (immunoperoxidase for cytomegalovirus antigens, ×350). (See Color Fig. 35-26.)

Table 35-2 Clinical Characteristics of the Intestinal Transplant Recipients

Clinical Characteristic	Total Population	Isolated Intestine	Intestine + Liver	Multiple Viscera
Patients				
Total	43	15	21	7
Children/adults	22/21	5/10	15/6	2/5
Sex (male/female)	22/21	7/8	11/10	4/3
Duration of TPN (mos)†	37 ± 34	52 ± 47	28 ± 21	26 ± 20
Serum bilirubin (mg/dL)†	11 ± 13	1.0 ± 0.6	19 ± 14	5 ± 9
Graft				
Positive cytotoxic crossmatch	2 (4.7%)	0 (0%)	2 (9.5%)	0 (0%)
Small intestine				
Without colon	30	10	17	3
With colon	13	5	4	4
Follow-up (mos)†	15 ± 10	14 ± 7	16 ± 12	11 ± 8

TPN, total parenteral nutrition.

* Stomach, duodenum, pancreas, intestine, and liver.

† Mean ± SD.

ceral), the 1-year actuarial survival rates were 93%, 71%, and 86%, respectively, and the 2-year survival rates were 83%, 65%, and 86%. Of the 13 deaths, 4 patients had isolated small bowel transplants, 8 had combined hepatic–intestinal transplants, and 1 had a multivisceral transplant. The causes of death were technical complications in 3 patients, opportunistic infections in 2 patients, PTLD in 2 patients, intractable rejection in 2 patients, sepsis after graft removal in 2 patients, and other causes in 2 patients. In one isolated intestinal graft recipient, death resulted from a catheter-related pulmonary embolism that occurred 8 months after removal of the allograft. Details of patient death and graft loss are described elsewhere.[58]

The actuarial survival was estimated for the 45 grafts (43 primary and 2 repeated). The overall graft survival rates were 80%, 78%, 72%, and 59% at 3, 6, 12,

and 24 months, respectively (see Fig. 35-27B). At 18 months, the survival rate was highest for the multivisceral grafts (86%) versus the combined hepatic–intestinal grafts (69%) and the isolated intestinal grafts (64%). Because of the ability to maintain isolated small bowel transplant recipients on TPN after removal of the graft, the discrepancy between patient and graft survival was greatest in this group.

Refractory rejection was the indication for graft enterectomy or replacement in 6 of the 16 lost grafts (5 isolated intestinal grafts in 4 patients and 1 hepatic–intestinal graft; Table 35-4). The remaining 10 grafts were lost because of patient death. Significant reduction in immunosuppression for various reasons preceded intractable rejection of all 6 grafts. Although graft removal with or without retransplantation was technically successful, 5 patients succumbed to sys-

Table 35-3 Indications for Intestinal Transplantation

Adults (n = 21)		Children (n = 22)	
Cause	Patients	Cause	Patients
Crohn's disease	6	Gastroschisis	6
Abdominal trauma	4	Necrotizing enterocolitis	4
Celiac artery occlusion	3*	Volvulus	4
Superior mesenteric artery thrombosis	2	Intestinal atresia	3
Desmoid tumor	2	Microvillus disease	2
Surgical adhesions	2	Pseudoobstruction	2
Metastatic gastrinoma	1	Multiple polyposis	1
Budd-Chiari syndrome	1		

* These patients had short-gut syndrome due to concomitant superior mesenteric artery thrombosis by protein S deficiency, antithrombin III deficiency, or unknown cause (one case each).

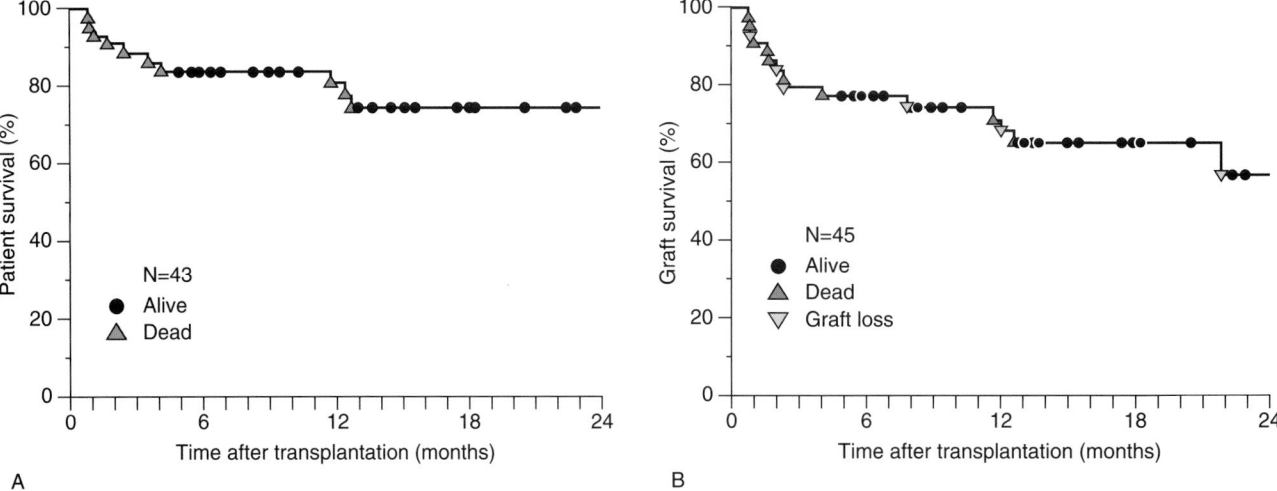

Figure 35-27 Actuarial (Kaplan-Meier) survival of patients (*A*) and grafts (*B*) after intestinal transplantation. (Abu-Elmagd K, Todo S, Tzakis A, et al. Three years' clinical experience with intestinal transplantation. J Am Coll Surg 1994;179:385)

temic sepsis (3 patients), refractory rejection of the second set of organs (1 patient), or late complications of TPN (1 patient). The remaining patient is still alive and receiving TPN.

Loss of part of the composite graft occurred in two transplant recipients because of either severe preservation injury of the pancreas or hepatic artery thrombosis. Pancreaticoduodenectomy was performed in the first case, and liver replacement with salvage of the intestinal graft was accomplished successfully in the second case.

Rejection

The clinical diagnosis of intestinal allograft rejection was made in 95% of the cases but was confirmed by histopathology in only 72% (31 patients). Only 2 patients (both with combined hepatic–intestinal grafts) showed no clinical or histopathologic evidence of intestinal graft rejection at any time after surgery. Most of the episodes of rejection were mild to moderate in severity and the number of episodes per graft was 4.1. Fifty percent of the total population required augmented corticosteroid therapy, and 18% required OKT3. The diagnostic limitation of intestinal mucosal biopsies was underscored in some cases by the discovery of rejection in the whole graft after its removal or at autopsy, despite previous inconclusive biopsy reports.[69]

Beyond 3 months after transplantation, about half of the patients in each transplant group experienced rejection of the intestinal graft. This often was associated with attempts to reduce immunosuppressive therapy because of CMV enteritis, PTLD, or other opportunistic infections.

Although FK506 dosages, FK506 plasma trough levels, and prednisone dosages were similar in the three groups of allograft recipients (Fig. 35-28), the incidence of pathologically confirmed rejection was higher

Table 35-4 Graft Removal or Replacement Due to Refractory Rejection

No.	Graft	Time (days)	Type	Procedure	Fate
1	Intestine	27	Acute*	Enterectomy	Alive, on total parenteral nutrition
2	Intestine	239	Acute*	Enterectomy	Death (pulmonary embolism)
3	Intestine	366	Acute*	Enterectomy	Death (sepsis)
4†	Intestine	667	Chronic*	Enterectomy	Retransplant
5†	Intestine	71	Acute*	Enterectomy	Death (sepsis)
6	Intestine + liver	47	Acute	Retransplantation	Death (rejection)

* Reduction or withdrawal of immunosuppression-precipitated rejection.
† Same recipient.

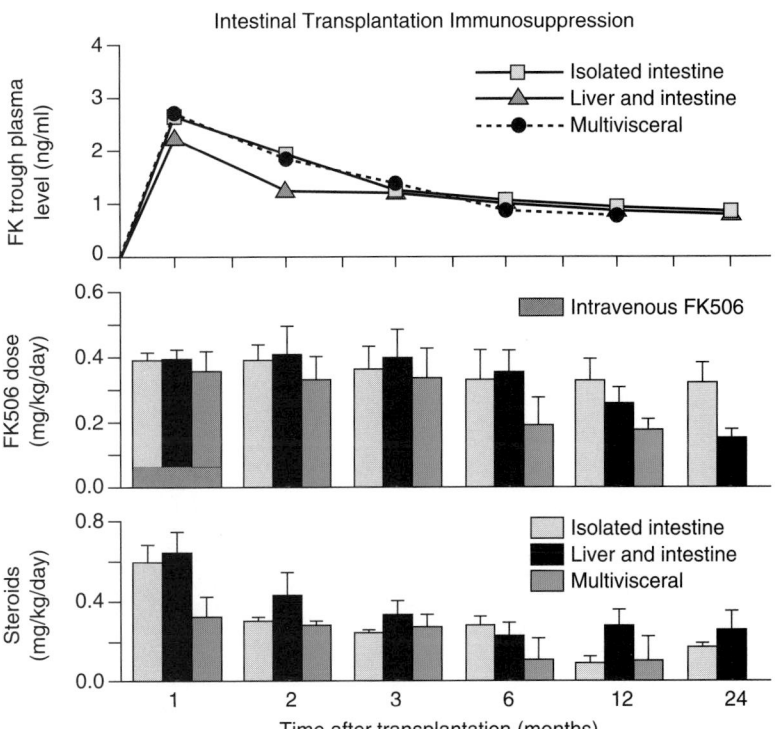

Figure 35-28 FK 506 and prednisone doses in the three cohorts of intestinal allograft recipients and FK 506 plasma trough levels. Values are mean ± SE. (Abu-Elmagd K, Todo S, Tzakis A, et al. Three years' clinical experience with intestinal transplantation. J Am Coll Surg 1994;179:385)

among those with isolated intestinal grafts (93%) than among those with hepatic–intestinal (62%) or multivisceral (57%) grafts. The mean interval between the transplant procedure and the first episode of rejection was 18.8 days (range, 3 to 138 days). However, this mean onset was delayed among patients who received combined hepatic–intestinal grafts (22 days) compared with those who received either isolated intestinal grafts (11 days) or multivisceral grafts (16 days).

The severity of rejection also was greater in the isolated intestinal transplant group than in the combined hepatic–intestinal transplant group, as graded by the need to use OKT3 (31% versus 5%). In addition, augmented corticosteroid therapy was required more often for the isolated intestinal grafts (63%) than for the combined hepatic–intestinal grafts (45%).

Five (36%) of the bowel grafts that included colon showed histologic evidence of colonic rejection at some time. None of the multivisceral grafts had histopathologically proven gastric rejection, but one patient had two episodes of pancreatitis that responded to augmented corticosteroid therapy. Twelve (43%) of the composite visceral grafts that contained liver had histologically diagnosed and clinically treated liver allograft rejection. The number of episodes of rejection per liver allograft was 0.6.

Of the 88 occasions on which both liver and small bowel biopsy samples were taken simultaneously or closely together, 47 (53%) of the dual specimens showed no signs of rejection in either organ, 12 (14%) showed rejection in both organs, 15 (17%) showed rejection only in the liver, and 14 (16%) showed rejection only in the intestine.[58]

Histopathologic examination of full-thickness sections of the 6 resected grafts showed chronic rejection in 2 of the isolated intestinal grafts. In addition, 1 combined hepatic–intestinal graft recipient with a strong positive crossmatch had chronic rejection of both organs. This patient died of hepatorenal failure with the graft in place.

Graft-Versus-Host Disease

Using standard histologic and in situ hybridization techniques, graft-versus-host disease was diagnosed unequivocally in only one case, a child with a combined hepatic–intestinal graft (Fig. 35-29). Limited immunosuppressive therapy was attempted early in the postoperative course because of *P carinii* pneumonia and an intestinal anastomotic leak. The skin lesions appeared 10 days after the transplant procedure. The overall clinical picture simulated life-threatening sepsis. The immunosuppressive regimen was significantly reduced, and 13 days later the patient succumbed to multiple organ failure.[58]

Graft Function

One of the most important parameters in evaluating graft function is the ability to achieve adequate enteral intake and maintain body weight despite discontinua-

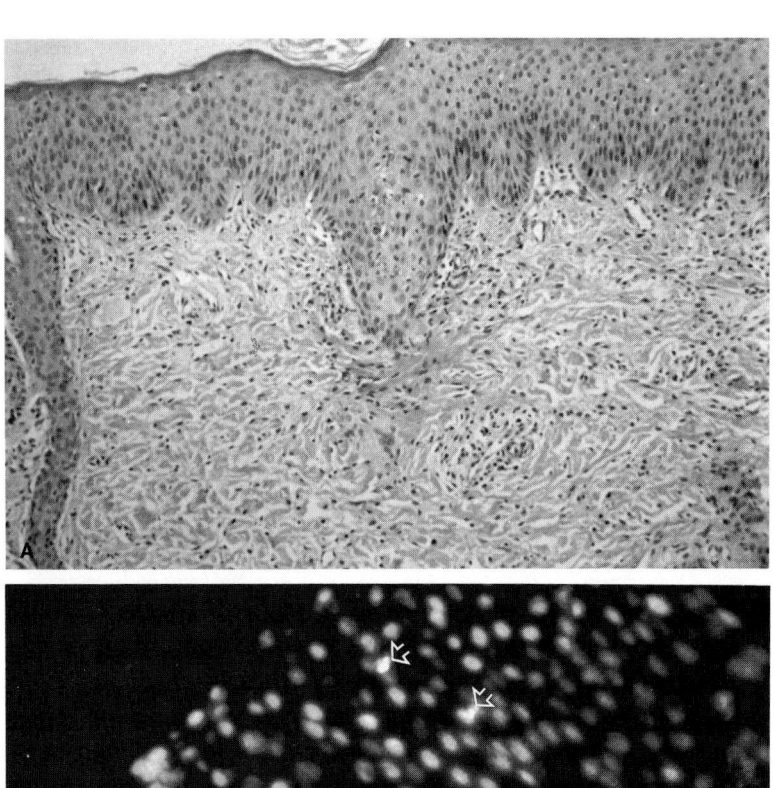

Figure 35-29 (**A**) Graft-versus-host disease. A skin biopsy on day 21 in a female pediatric recipient revealed male donor lymphocytic inflammation at the dermal–epidermal junction (hematoxylin–eosin, ×140). (**B**) The diagnosis of GVHD was confirmed by localizing the Y chromosome in male donor cells (*arrows*) to the areas of damage (fluorescent in situ hybridization for the Y chromosome on paraffin-embedded tissues with propidium iodide counterstain, 450×). (See Color Fig. 35-29.)

tion of TPN. Tube feeding was begun in all intestinal graft recipients at 3 to 54 days (mean: 16 days) after transplantation, and TPN was discontinued after 18 to 210 days (mean: 59 days). Comparing the three different types of graft recipients, enteral feeding was initiated and TPN was discontinued earlier in patients who received intestine alone (Table 35-5). Of the 29 surviving patients with grafts in place, 25 (86%) are free of TPN and enjoy unrestricted oral diets. The remaining patients required reinstitution of partial intravenous nutrition because of the development of gastrointestinal dysmotility (3 patients) or viral enteritis (1 patients). All the children gained weight and had an increase in height. Seven of the adults lost 3% to 27% of their pretransplantation body weight. The current values, however, are within the calculated ideal body weight for each patient.

The absorptive capacity of the intestinal graft was satisfactory in most recipients. Oral administration of the standard FK506 dose (0.3 mg/kg/d) maintained the desired therapeutic plasma trough level of the drug for all patients by the end of the fourth postoperative week. D-Xylose was adequately absorbed by the intestinal graft in most of the 37 studied patients, particularly in the absence of significant preservation injury or graft rejection. The amount of total fecal lipid tended to be high in the early postoperative period, and fat absorption remained abnormal in some patients who were studied 1 year after transplantation.[58]

Motility of the native and transplanted parts of the gastrointestinal tract was evaluated by conventional radiologic contrast and manometric studies.[63,70] Gastric emptying in the early postoperative period was delayed from 2 to 24 hours in 17 (85%) of the 20 adult graft recipients studied. Gastric hypoperistalsis was commonly associated with the use of narcotic analgesics im-

Table 35-5   Nutritional Course

Type of Transplant	Postoperative Time (days)		Current Status		
				TPN	
	Tube Feeding Started	TPN Stopped	Survivors	Free	Partial
Isolated intestine	8 ± 4	43 ± 28	10	9 (90%)	1 (10%)
Intestine + liver	20 ± 9	76 ± 64	13	12 (92%)	1 (8%)
Multiple viscera	24 ± 18	54 ± 21	6	4 (67%)	2 (33%)
Total	16 ± 10	59 ± 49	29	25 (86%)	4 (14%)

TPN, total parenteral nutrition.

mediately after surgery. Recovery of gastric motility was spontaneous and complete in all patients who were studied 4 to 6 months after transplantation. The mean intestinal transit time for the 21 patients who underwent radiologic evaluation was 4.1 hours (range, 0.3 to 24 hours). Thirteen (62%) of these patients had abnormal intestinal transit times, which were markedly accelerated (less than 1 hour) in 6 cases and prolonged (more than 3 hours) in the other 7 cases. When the patients were studied again later, these abnormalities had improved significantly. The myoelectric activity of the native and transplanted gut was characterized by measuring the migrating motor complex. Antral motility was abnormal in all 9 of the studied patients, as evidenced by decreased amplitude or frequency of contraction. Transmission of contraction waves from native to transplanted intestine occurred, although it was not always coordinated.

Bacterial Overgrowth

Quantitative microbial cultures of the terminal ileal contents showed bacterial counts above 10^9 colony-forming units (CFU)/mL on at least one occasion in all but four patients, for an overall incidence of 87%. Of 532 total cultures (17 per patient), 34% showed a bacterial count above 10^9 CFU/mL. The identified microorganisms were either gram negative (6%), gram positive (28%), or both (58%). The remaining 8% were fungal organisms. The composition and concentration of the bacterial colonies were similar among the three types of intestinal transplant recipients.[71]

The ecology of the small bowel graft flora was influenced by gut decontamination, episodes of rejection, and CMV enteritis.[71] During the first 30 postoperative days, the bacterial count exceeded 10^9 CFU/mL in 19% of the 113 cultures, and the populations consisted of 67% gram-positive organisms and 33% gram-negative organisms. With discontinuation of gut decontamina-

tion during the remaining study period, the percentage of bacterial counts above 10^9 CFU/mL gradually increased to 38%. Meanwhile, the concentration of gram-positive organisms decreased and that of gram-negative organisms increased. During significant episodes of rejection and CMV enteritis, total counts of both gram-positive and gram-negative bacteria increased.

Infections

Systemic and local infections were common morbid events after intestinal transplantation.[72] Most patients (90%) experienced at least one episode of clinically significant infection, with a mean of 3.1 episodes per patient. The high incidence of infectious complications in intestinal allograft recipients can be attributed to the loss of the protective intestinal mucosal barrier during rejection or preservation injury, the need for strong immunosuppressive therapy to prevent or control rejection, and the development of bacterial overgrowth. The prolonged need for central venous access in some of these patients is another risk factor that significantly increases the incidence of bacteremia and fungemia.

Translocation of intestinal flora was seen in some patients with moderate to severe episodes of rejection.[71] The diagnosis was made by isolating the same microorganisms in the intestinal lumen and the blood simultaneously, with a quantitative stool culture count above 1×10^9 CFU/mL. Thirteen episodes of translocation occurred in 11 patients, 4 of whom received isolated intestinal grafts and 7 of whom received combined hepatic–intestinal grafts. Ten (77%) of these episodes were associated with rejection. Bacterial and fungal translocation were managed by reversing the underlying immunologic process and effectively controlling infection by selective gut decontamination and specific intravenous antimicrobial therapy.

Similar to lung and kidney transplant recipients,[73,74] the most common viral infection among patients with intestinal allografts was CMV. The incidence of CMV disease in our study was about 40%. The mean onset of the first CMV infectious episode was 48 ± 23 days after transplantation. Despite long-term specific therapy with ganciclovir, foscarnet, or both, over 50% of these patients had recurrent episodes of CMV disease. The placement of CMV-seropositive grafts in CMV-seronegative recipients and the repeated administration of corticosteroid boluses to treat rejection are the two major risk factors that precipitate CMV disease.[75]

The incidence of PTLD among our intestinal allograft recipients was 9.3%. Most of the morbid cases occurred in children who received combined hepatic–intestinal or multivisceral grafts. Another two patients had acute Epstein-Barr viral infection that responded to antiviral therapy. The full clinical picture and histopathology of PTLD has been described elsewhere.[76] The disease affected both the native and transplanted organs. Epstein-Barr virus RNA was found in most of the PTLD lesions by the in situ hybridization technique. Treatment included reduction of immunosuppressive therapy, if possible, and combination antiviral therapy (acyclovir, α-interferon, and ganciclovir or foscarnet).

Disease Recurrence

With follow-up ranging from 8 to 22 months, none of the 13 transplant recipients who had chronic primary disease of their native gut, including Crohn's disease (6 patients), showed any clinical or histopathologic evidence of disease recurrence in the visceral graft.[58]

Postoperative Course

The early convalescence of most patients was prolonged and complicated. The median intensive care unit stay after transplantation was 11 days (range, 2 to 300 days) and the median hospital stay was 11 weeks (range, 3 to 45 weeks). During the study period, the median number of readmissions for all patients was 3 (range, 0 to 14). The primary causes of prolonged hospitalization and frequent readmission were postoperative pulmonary insufficiency, rejection, CMV enteritis, dehydration, Epstein-Barr viral infection, and PTLD. Full details of the postoperative course of the 43 patients have been described elsewhere.[58]

CONTROVERSIES

Our clinical experience, along with the cumulative results of experimental studies of intestinal transplantation done around the world, has brought into question previously accepted assumptions about this procedure.[77-85] Two of these are important technical concerns that need to be addressed individually: the method of venous drainage used for isolated intestinal grafts, and the role of simultaneous liver replacement in intestinal grafting.

Portal Drainage

The venous effluent drained from an isolated intestinal graft can be directed either into the systemic circulation with a mesocaval shunt or through the liver by an anastomosis to the native portomesenteric system. Several experimental studies have indicated that delivery of the venous outflow from the graft into the portal circulation, with consequent perfusion of the host liver, is superior for metabolic and immunologic reasons.[86]

Metabolic changes caused by systemic shunting of allograft intestinal venous outflow are similar to those seen after Eck's fistula, but are less pronounced because of the partial portal diversion.[87,88] Functional and structural abnormalities of the liver have been observed in animals and humans and are attributed to the diversion of so-called hepatotropic factors from the hepatocytes.[89]

Because of its location between the gastrointestinal tract and the systemic circulation, the liver serves as a filter to eliminate bacteria, endotoxins, carcinogens, and toxic substances absorbed into the portal system. This filtration also has been postulated to modulate transplantation antigens to offer immunologic protection to a variety of homografts.[90-98] The specific details and overall results of small and large animal experiments are described elsewhere.[86-108]

In the clinical series described herein, we tried to drain the isolated intestinal grafts physiologically through the host portal veins. The predicted technical difficulties were minimized by using the mesenteric piggyback technique.[55] Inferior vena cava drainage was used in one case of retransplantation with no clinical evidence of undesirable metabolic sequelae. Further clinical trials are needed to determine the long-term metabolic and immunologic effects of systemic drainage of allograft venous outflow in isolated intestinal transplant recipients.[50]

Hepatic Replacement

Numerous experiments have demonstrated the immunologic protection, or tolerance, induced by a concomitantly transplanted liver to other organ allografts procured from the same donor.[86] Evidence of hepatic tolerogenicity was first noted in our original canine multivisceral experiments.[81] The concept was fully de-

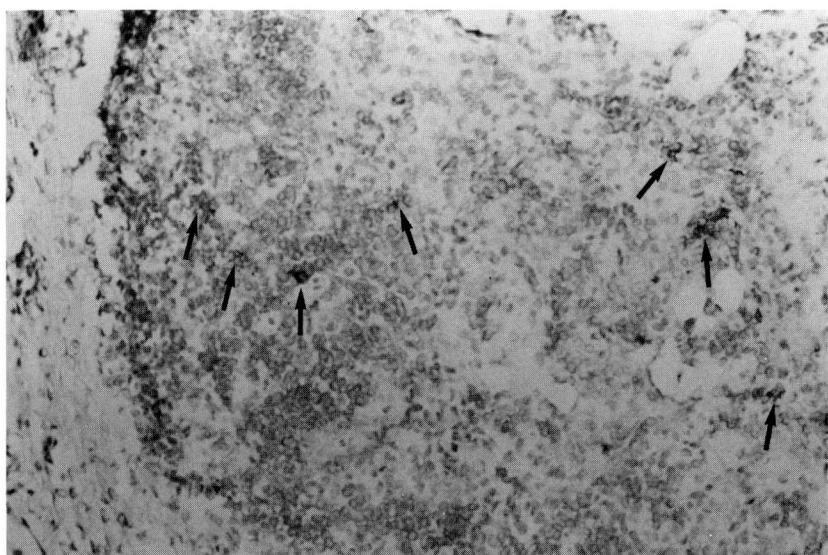

Figure 35-30 Biopsy samples of an inguinal lymph node 29 years after kidney transplantation (×200) stained for HLA-B7 50, an antigen present in the donor but not in the recipient. Donor cells (*arrows*) are visible in the lymph node. (Starzl TE, Demetris AH, Trucco M, et al. Cell migration and chimerism after whole organ transplantation: the basis of graft acceptance. Hepatology 1993;17:1127)

veloped by Calne in 1969, who showed indefinite prolongation of kidney and skin graft survival in pigs receiving concomitant liver transplantation.[109] This finding was confirmed later by others, using rat liver transplantation with various strain combinations.[110–114] The mechanism of hepatic tolerogenicity is unclear, although many explanations have been proposed, including clonal deletion of cytotoxic T cells, production of antibody to class II MHC, antigen inactivation by liver enzymes, antigen alteration by Kupffer cells, inhibition of immune stimulation, and production of soluble donor class I antigen. However, the recent demonstration that migratory tissue leukocytes from the liver allograft create a state of microchimerism in the host (Fig. 35-30) has provided an alternative and more likely explanation.[111–118]

Because of the experimentally proven tolerogenic effect of the liver and the high risk of intestinal allograft loss due to refractory rejection, some have transplanted the liver along with the small bowel in patients with short-gut syndrome, even in the presence of normal liver function.[21] We have chosen to perform hepatic–intestinal transplantation only for patients with irreversible failure of both organs. Nonetheless, the long-term effects and clinical significance of hepatic tolerogenicity on intestinal allograft survival remain to be determined.

Before the introduction of FK506, the small bowel was considered a forbidden organ in transplantation.[119] Recent studies show that intestinal allografts with and without hepatic allografts are vulnerable to rejection and, compared with isolated hepatic allografts, continue to be at high risk long after transplantation.[69]

Because intestinal allograft recipients require strong immunosuppressive therapy, even beyond the first 6 months after transplantation, a new strategy is needed to modulate host and graft immune interactions.[58] One possibility is to amplify the naturally occurring microchimerism through combined bone marrow and intestinal transplantation from the same donor.[58,120] Augmenting chimerism may reduce or eliminate the long-term recipient immunologic response to donor antigens. If this can be accomplished, long-term graft and patient survival, as well as quality of life after intestinal transplantation, will improve significantly because of the low risk of graft rejection and the diminished requirement for strong long-term immunosuppressive therapy.

Research shows that intestinal transplantation still has important limitations. In addition to rejection, recurrent infections, graft dysmotility, dehydration, and bacterial overgrowth are significant morbid events in this unique transplant population. Therefore, we believe that TPN remains the primary treatment option for patients with irreversible intestinal failure. Hepatic–intestinal or multivisceral transplantation, however, is the only available therapy for patients with combined hepatic and intestinal failure.

Our experience has demonstrated the clinical feasibility of intestinal transplantation under improved immunosuppression with FK506. Although many patients achieved a nearly normal quality of life, the intensity of care required during the first year and often thereafter is too great to justify the widespread use of this approach. Until further modifications improve the practicality of isolated intestinal transplantation, this procedure should be offered only to patients with exhausted central venous access and impending hepatic dysfunction. Although hepatic tolerogenicity is a well-established concept, hepatic–intestinal transplantation should be done only in patients with combined hepatic and intestinal failure, thrombosed portomesenteric systems, or inborn hepatic disorders. Multivisceral transplantation should be reserved for special indications. The long-term survival and therapeutic advantages of these surgical procedures have not been determined.

REFERENCES

1. Lillehei RC, Idezuki Y, Feemster JA, et al. Transplantation of stomach, intestine and pancreas: experimental and clinical observations. Surgery 1967;62:721.

2. Okumura M, Fujimura I, Ferrari AA, et al. Transplante de intestino delgaso: apresentacao de um caso. Rev Hosp Clin Fac Med Sao Paulo 1969;2D:39.

3. Olivier CL, Rettori R, Olivier CH, Bauer O, Roux J. Homotransplantation orthotopique de l'intestin grele et des colons droit et transverse chex l'homme. J Chir (Paris) 1969;98:323.

4. Alican F, Hardy JD, Cayirli M, et al. Intestinal transplantation: laboratory experience and report of a clinical case. Am J Surg 1971;121:105.

5. Fortner JG, Sichuk G, Litwin SD, Beattie EJ Jr. Immunological responses to an intestinal allograft with HLA-identical donor-recipient. Transplantation 1972;14:531.

6. Cohen Z, Silverman RE, Wassef R, et al. Small intestinal transplantation using cyclosporine: report of a case. Transplantation 1986;42:613.

7. Starzl TE, Rowe M, Todo S. Transplantation of multiple abdominal viscera. JAMA 1989;26:1449.

8. D'Alessandro M, Kalayoglu M, Sollinger HW, Pirsch JD, Belzer FO. Liver-intestinal transplantation: report of a case. Transplant Proc 1992;24:1228.

9. Tattersall C, Gebel H, Haklin M, Hartsell W, Williams J. Lymphocyte responsiveness after irradiation in canine and human intestinal allografts. Curr Surg 1989;46:16.

10. Revillon Y, Jan D, Goulet O, Ricour C. Small bowel transplantation in seven children: preservation technique. Transplant Proc 1991;23:2350.

11. Hansmann ML, Deltz E, Gundlach M, Schroeder P, Radzun HJ. Small bowel transplantation in a child. Am J Clin Pathol 1989;920:686.

12. Deltz E, Schroeder P, Gebhardt H, et al. Successful clinical small bowel transplantation: report of a case. Clin Transpl 1989;3:89.

13. Grant D, Sommerauer J, Mimeault R, et al. Treatment with continuous high dose intravenous cyclosporine following intestinal transplantation: a case report. Transplantation 1989;48:151.

14. Wallander J, Ewald U, Lackgren G, Tufveson G, Wahlberg J, Meurling S. Extreme short bowel syndrome in neonates: an indication for small bowel transplantation. Transplant Proc 1992;24:1230.

15. Goulet O, Revillon Y, Brousse N, et al. Successful small bowel transplantation in an infant. Transplantation 1992;53:940.

16. Starzl TE, Todo S, Fung J, Demetris AJ, Venkataramanan R, Jain A. FK506 for human liver, kidney and pancreas transplantation. Lancet 1989;2:1000.

17. Todo S, Fung JJ, Starzl TE, et al. Liver, kidney and thoracic organ transplantation under FK506. Ann Surg 1990;212:295.

18. Todo S, Tzakis AG, Abu-Elmagd K, et al. Cadaveric small bowel and small bowel-liver transplantation in humans. Transplantation 1992;53:369.

19. Diliz-Perez HS, McClure J, Bedetti C, et al. Successful small bowel allotransplantation in dogs with cyclosporine and prednisone. Transplantation 1984;37:126.

20. Starzl TE, Demetris AJ. Development of the replacement operation. In: Liver transplantation. Chicago, Year Book, 1989:3.

21. Grant D, Wall W, Mimeault R, et al. Successful small bowel/liver transplantation. Lancet 1990;335:181.

22. Fung J, Todo S, Jain A, et al. Conversion from cyclosporine to FK506 in liver allograft recipients with cyclosporine-related complications. Transplant Proc 1990;22:6.

23. Murase N, Kim D, Todo S, et al. Induction of liver, heart, and multivisceral graft acceptance with a short course of FK506. Transplant Proc 1990;22:74.

24. Murase N, Demetris A, Matsuzaki T, et al. Long survival in rats after multivisceral versus isolated small bowel allotransplantation under FK506. Surgery 1991;110:87.

25. Hoffman AL, Makowka L, Banner B, et al. The use of FK506 for small intestine allotransplantation: inhibition of acute rejection and prevention of fatal graft versus host disease. Transplantation 1990;149:483.

26. Lee K, Stangl MJ, Todo S, et al. Successful orthotopic small bowel transplantation with short term FK506 immunosuppressive therapy. Transplant Proc 1990;22:78.

27. Kino T, Hatanaka H, Miyata S, et al. FK506, a novel immunosuppressant isolated from a streptomyces. II. Immunosuppressive effect of FK in vitro. J Antibiot (Tokyo) 1987;40:1256.

28. Sawada S, Suzuki G, Kawasey Y, et al. Novel immunosuppressive agent, FK506: in vitro effects on the cloned T cell activation. J Immunol 1987;139:1797.

29. Thomson AW. FK506: how much potential? Immunol Today 1989;10:6.

30. Tocci MJ, Matkovich DA, Copllier KA, et al. The immunosuppressant FK selectively inhibits expression of early T cell activation genes. J Immunol 1989;143:718.

31. Siekierka JJ, Hung SHY, Pie M, Lin CS, Sigal NH. A cy-

tosolic binding protein for the immunosuppressant FK506 has peptidyl-prolyl isomerase activity but is distinct from cyclophillin. Nature 1989;341:755.

32. Harding MW, Galat A, Uehling DE, Schreiber SL. A receptor for the immunosuppressant FK506 is cis-trans peptidyl-prolyl isomerase. Nature 1989;341:758.

33. Starzl TE, Abu-Elmagd K, Tzakis A, et al. Selected topics on FK506 with special references to rescue of extrahepatic whole organ grafts, transplantation of forbidden organs, side-effects, mechanisms and practical pharmacokinetics. Transplant Proc 1991;23:914.

34. Fung J, Todo S, Tzakis A, et al. Conversion of liver allograft recipients from cyclosporine to FK506-based immunosuppression: benefits and pitfalls. Transplant Proc 1991;23:14.

35. Jain AB, Fung J, Venkataramanan R, et al. FK506 dosage in human organ transplantation. Transplant Proc 1990;22:23.

36. Todo S, Fung J, Tzakis A, et al. One hundred ten consecutive primary orthotopic liver transplants under FK506 in adults. Transplant Proc 1991;23:1397.

37. Shapiro R, Fung JJ, Jain AB, et al. The side-effects of FK506 in humans. Transplant Proc 1990;22:35.

38. Alessiani M, Cillo U, Fung J, et al. Adverse effects of FK506 overdosage after liver transplantation. Transplant Proc 1993;25:628.

39. Venkataramanan R, Jain A, Warty VW, et al. Pharmacokinetics of FK506 following oral administration: a comparison of FK506 and cyclosporine. Transplant Proc 1991;23:931.

40. Furukawa H, Imventarza O, Venkataramanan R, et al. The effect of bile duct ligation and bile diversion on FK506 pharmacokinetics in dogs. Transplantation 1992;53:722.

41. Mughal M, Irving M. Home parenteral nutrition in the United Kingdom and Ireland. Lancet 1986;2:383.

42. Dowling RH. Small bowel adaptation and its regulation. Scand J Gastroenterol 1982;17(Suppl 74):53.

43. Willmore DW. Factors correlating with a successful outcome following extensive intestinal resection in newborn infants. J Pediatr 1972;80:88.

44. Postuma R, Morez S, Friesen F. Extreme short bowel syndrome in an infant. J Pediatr Surg 1983;18:264.

45. Howard L, Heaphey L, Fleming CR, Lininger L, Steiger E. Four years of North American Registry home parenteral nutrition outcome data and their implications for patient management. JPEN 1991;15:384.

46. Stokes MA, Irving MH. Mortality in patients on home parenteral nutrition. JPEN 1989;13:172.

47. Grosfeld JL, Rescoria FJ, West KW. Short bowel syndrome in infancy and childhood: analysis of survival in 60 patients. Am J Surg 1986;151:41.

48. Todo S, Tzakis A, Abu-Elmagd K, Reyes J, Starzl TE. Current status of intestinal transplantation. Adv Surg 1994;27:295.

49. Wolfe BM, Beer WH, Hayashi JT, Halsted CH, Cannon RA, Cox KL. Experience with home parenteral nutrition. Am J Surg 1983;146:7.

50. Todo S, Tzakis A, Reyes J, Abu-Elmagd K, Furukawa H, Nour B. Small intestinal transplantation in humans with or without colon. Transplantation 1994;57:840.

51. Starzl TE, Todo S, Tzakis A, et al. The many faces of multivisceral transplantation. Surg Gynecol Obstet 1991;172:335.

52. Starzl TE, Hakala TR, Shaw BW, et al. A flexible procedure for multiple cadaveric organ procurement. Surg Gynecol Obstet 1984;158:223.

53. Starzl TE, Miller C, Broznik B, Makowka L. An improved technique for multiple organ harvesting. Surg Gynecol Obstet 1987;165:343.

54. Casavilla A, Selby R, Abu-Elmagd K, et al. Logistics and technique for combined hepatic–intestinal retrieval. Ann Surg 1992;216:85.

55. Tzakis A, Todo S, Reyes J, et al. Piggyback orthotopic intestinal transplantation. Surg Gynecol Obstet 1993;176:297.

56. Tzakis A, Todo S, Starzl TE. Orthotopic liver transplantation with preservation of the inferior vena cava. Ann Surg 1989;210:649.

57. Todo S, Tzakis A, Abu-Elmagd K, et al. Intestinal transplantation in composite visceral grafts or alone. Ann Surg 1992;216:223.

58. Abu-Elmagd K, Todo S, Tzakis A, et al. Three years clinical experience with intestinal transplantation. J Am Coll Surg 1994;179:385.

59. Abu-Elmagd K, Fung JJ, Reyes J, et al. Management of intestinal transplantation in humans. Transplant Proc 1992;24:1243.

60. Abu-Elmagd K, Fung J, Alessiani M, et al. The effect of graft function on FK506 plasma levels, dosages and renal function, with particular reference to the liver. Transplantation 1991;52:71.

61. Takaya S, Iwaki Y, Starzl TE. Liver transplantation in cytotoxic crossmatch cases using FK506, high dose steroids, and prostaglandin E$_1$. Transplantation 1992;54:927.

62. Abu-Elmagd K, Tzakis A, Todo S, et al. Monitoring and treatment of intestinal allograft rejection in humans. Transplant Proc 1993;25:1202.

63. Campbell WL, Abu-Elmagd K, Federal MP, et al. Contrast examination of the small bowel in patients with small-bowel transplants: findings in 16 patients. AJR Am J Roentgenol 1993;161:297.

64. Breiter HC, Craig RM, Levee G, Atkinson AJ. Use of kinetic methods to evaluate d-xylose malabsorption in patients. J Lab Clin Med 1988;112:533.

65. Amenta JS. Lipodol absorption and urinary iodide excretion as a screening test for steatorrhea. Clin Chem 1969;15:295.

66. Takeyoshi I, Kokudo Y, Zhang S, et al. Susceptibility to ischemia: the large bowel versus the small bowel. Transplant Proc 1994;26:1491.

67. Iwaki Y, Starzl TE, Yagihashi A, et al. Replacement of donor lymphoid tissue in human small bowel transplants under FK506 immunosuppression. Lancet 1991;337:818.

68. Starzl TE, Nalesnik MA, Porter KA, et al. Reversibility of lymphomas and lymphoproliferative lesions developing under cyclosporine-steroid therapy. Lancet 1984; 1:583.

69. Abu-Elmagd K, Todo S, Tzakis A, et al. Rejection of human intestinal allografts: alone or in combination with the liver. Transplant Proc 1994; 26:1430.

70. Hutson WR, Putnam PE, Todo S, Abu-Elmagd K, Reynolds J, Rosas F. The effects of small intestinal and multivisceral transplantation on gastric and small bowel motility in humans. Transplant Proc (in press).

71. Abu-Elmagd K, Todo S, Tzakis A, et al. Intestinal transplantation and bacterial overgrowth in humans. Transplant Proc 1994; 26:1684.

72. Kusne S, Manez R, Bonet H, et al. Infectious complications after small bowel transplantation in adults. Transplant Proc 1994; 26:1682.

73. Hutter JA, Scott JA, Wreghitt T, et al. The importance of cytomegalovirus in heart-lung transplant recipients. Chest 1989; 95:627.

74. Nicol D, McDonald AS, Belitsky P, et al. Reduction by combination prophylactic therapy with CMV hyperimmue globulin and acyclovir of the risk of primary CMV disease in renal transplant recipients. Transplantation 1993; 55:841.

75. Manez R, Kusne S, Abu-Elmagd K, et al. Factors associated with recurrent cytomegalovirus disease after small bowel transplantation. Transplant Proc 1994; 26:1422.

76. Reyes J, Bonet H, Green M, et al. Lymphoproliferative disease after combined liver and small bowel transplantation. Transplant Proc (in press).

77. Carrell A. La technique operatoire des anatomoses vasculaires et al transplantation des visceres. Lyon MEO 1902; 98:859.

78. Lillehei RC, Goott B, Miller FA. The physiological response of the small bowel of the dog to ischemia including prolonged in vitro preservation of the bowel with successful replacement and survival. Ann Surg 1959; 150:543.

79. Lillehei Goot B, Miller FA. Homografts of the small bowel. Surg Forum 1960; 10:197.

80. Starzl TE, Kaupp HA Jr. Mass homotransplantation of abdominal organs in dogs. Surg Forum 1960; 11:28.

81. Starzl TE, Kaupp HA Jr, Brock DR, et al. Homotransplantation of multiple visceral organs. Am J Surg 1962; 103:219.

82. Monchik GJ, Russell PS. Transplantation of small bowel in the rat: technical and immunological considerations. Surgery 1971; 70:693.

83. Yoshimi F, Nakamura K, Zhu Y, et al. Canine total orthotopic small bowel transplantation under FK506. Transplant Proc 1991; 23:3240.

84. Grant D, Duff J, Stiller C, et al. Intestinal transplantation in pigs using cyclosporine. Transplantation 1988; 45:279.

85. Grant D. Intestinal transplantation: current status. Transplant Proc 1989; 21:2869.

86. Todo S, Murase N, Tzakis A, Starzl TE. Role of the liver and the portal circulation in intestinal grafting. In: Grant DR, Wood RFM, eds. Small bowel transplantation. Boston, Little, Brown, 1994:101.

87. Starzl TE, Porter KA, Francavilla A. The Eck fistula in animals and humans. Curr Probl Surg 1983; 20:692.

88. Francavilla A, Starzl TE, Porter K, et al. Screening for candidate hepatic growth factors by selective portal infusion after canine Eck fistula. Hepatology 1991; 14:665.

89. Starzl TE, Porter KA, Watanabe K, et al. The effects of insulin, glucagon and insulin/glucagon infusions upon liver morphology and cell division after complete portacaval shunt in dogs. Lancet 1976; 1:821.

90. Mandel MA, Monaco AP, Russel PS. Destruction of splenic transplantation antigens by a factor present in the liver. J Immunol 1965; 95:673.

91. Holman JM Jr, Todd R. Enhanced survival of heterotopic rat heart allografts with portal venous drainage. Transplantation 1990; 40:229.

92. Mazzoni G, DeMartino C, Demofonti A, et al. A comparison of portal and systemic venous drainage in porcine renal allografts. Br J Surg 1972; 59:541.

93. Pfefferman R, Sakai A, Kountz SL. The liver as a privileged site for parathyroid alloimplantation in the rat. Surgery 1976; 79:182.

94. Eloy R, Kedinger M, Garaud K, et al. Isogenic and allogenic transplantation of isolated Langerhans islets into the liver. Langenbecks Arch Chir 1975; 109(Suppl 1):109.

95. Sakai A. Role of the liver in kidney allograft rejection in the rat. Transplantation 1970; 9:333.

96. Boeckx W, Sobis H, Laquet A, et al. Prolongation of allogenic heart graft survival in the rat after implantation on portal vein. Transplantation 1975; 19:145.

97. Mazzoni G, Benichou J, Porter KA, et al. Renal homotransplantation with venous outflow or infusion of antigen into the portal vein of dogs or pigs. Transplantation 1977; 24:268.

98. Gorczynski RM, Cohen Z, Levy G, Koh L. Comparison of functional activity in host and graft mesenteric lymphoid tissue of rats receiving syngeneic heterotopic small bowel allografts with portal or systemic drainage. Transplant Proc 1992; 24:1133.

99. Marchioro TL, Porter KA, Brown BI, et al. The effect of partial portacaval transposition on the canine liver. Surgery 1967; 61:723.

100. Schraut WH, Abraham VS, Lee KW. Portal versus caval venous drainage of small bowel allografts: technical and metabolic consequences. Surgery 1986; 99:193.

101. Koltun WA, Kirkman RL. Nutritional and metabolic aspects of total small bowel transplantation in inbred rats. Transplant Proc 1987; 19:1102.

102. Shaffer D, Diflo T, Love W, et al. Immunologic and metabolic effects of caval versus portal venous drainage in small-bowel transplantation. Surgery 1988; 104:518.

103. Schraut WH, Rosemurgy AS, Riddle RM. Prolongation of intestinal allograft survival without immunosuppressive drug therapy: transplantation of small bowel allografts. J Surg Res 1983; 34:597.

104. Rosemurgy AS, Schraut WH. Small bowel allografts: sequence of histologic changes in acute and chronic rejection. Am J Surg 1986;151:470.

105. Schraut WH, Abraham VS, Lee KW. Portal versus systemic venous drainage for small bowel allografts. Surgery 1985;98:579.

106. Murase N, Demetris AJ, Furuya T, Todo S, Fung JJ, Starzl TE. Comparison of the small intestine after multivisceral transplantation with the small intestine transplanted with portal or caval drainage. Transplant Proc 1992;24:1143.

107. Raju S, Fujiwara H, Grogan JB, Achord JL. Long-term nutritional function of orthotopic small bowel autotransplants. J Surg Res 1989;46:142.

108. Kaneko H, Fischman MA, Buckley TM, Schweizer RT. A comparison of portal versus systemic venous drainage in the pig small-bowel allograft recipient. Surgery 1991;109:663.

109. Calne RY, Sells RA, Pena JR, et al. Induction of immunological tolerance by porcine liver allografts. Nature 1969;223:472.

110. Kamada N, Davies HS, Wright D, Culank L, Roser B. Liver transplantation in the rat: biochemical and histological evidence of complete tolerance induction in non-rejector strains. Transplantation 1983;35:304.

111. Zhong G, Gang H, Sakai Y, et al. Combined small bowel and liver transplantation in the rat: possible role of the liver in preventing intestinal allograft rejection. Transplantation 1991;52:550.

112. Zhong R, He G, Sakai Y, et al. The effect of donor-recipient strain combinations in combined liver/intestine transplantation in the rat. Transplant Proc 1992;24:1208.

113. Sarnacki S, Revillon Y, Cerf-Bensussan N, Calise D, Goulet O, Brousse N. Long-term small-bowel survival induced by a spontaneously tolerated liver allograft in inbred rat strains. Transplantation 1992;54:383.

114. Murase N, Demetris AJ, Kim DG, Todo S, Fung JJ, Starzl TE. Rejection of the multivisceral allografts in rats: a sequential analysis with comparison to isolated orthotopic small bowel and liver grafts. Surgery 1990;108:880.

115. Starzl TE, Demetris AJ, Murase N, Ildstad S, Ricordi C, Trucco M. Cell migration, chimerism, and graft acceptance. Lancet 1992;339:1579.

116. Starzl TE, Demetris AJ, Trucco M, et al. Cell migration and chimerism after whole organ transplantation: the basis of graft acceptance. Hepatology 1993;17:1127.

117. Starzl TE, Demetris AJ, Murase N, Thomson AW, Trucco M, Ricordi C. Donor cell chimerism permitted by immunosuppressive drugs: a new view of organ transplantation. Immunol Today 1993;14:326.

118. Reyes J, Zeevi A, Ramos H, et al. The frequent achievement of a drug free state after orthotopic liver transplantation. Transplant Proc 1993;25:3315.

119. Kirkman RT. Small bowel transplantation. Transplantation 1984;37:429.

120. Fontes P, Rao AS, Demetris AJ, et al. Bone marrow augmentation of donor-cell chimerism in kidney, liver, heart, and pancreas islet transplantation. Lancet 1994;344:151.

36

Atlas of Small Intestinal Surgery

Michael W. Mulholland | *Gerald B. Zelenock* | *Fabrizio Michelassi*

Digestive Tract Surgery: A Text and Atlas, edited by Richard H. Bell, Layton F. Rikkers, and Michael W. Mulholland. Lippincott-Raven Publishers, Philadelphia, © 1996.

PATIENT PREPARATION

The presence of mechanical small bowel obstruction is associated with significant intravascular volume deficits. The small intestine is converted from an organ of net absorption to one of net secretion. Fluid is lost in the form of vomitus, mural intestinal edema, and ascites. Hemoconcentration and azotemia reflect these losses, which must be corrected preoperatively by intravenous repletion. Mechanical obstruction also allows proliferation of luminal bacteria. Luminal flora in obstructed small intestine resemble colonic flora, both qualitatively and quantitatively. Perioperative antibiotics with broad enteric coverage should be selected in the settings of suspected small intestinal obstruction, strangulation or perforation. In elective operations on the small intestine, cathartic preparation to remove particulate residue and oral antibiotic therapy are routinely used, although they are not as well established as for colonic operations.

SECTION I   Small Bowel Resection

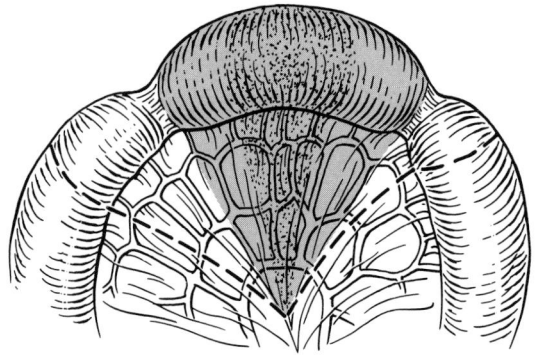

Figure 36-I-1

Exposure

In most instances, a small bowel abnormality is best approached through a vertical mid-line incision. The small intestine, after mobilization from the peritoneal cavity, should be protected with moistened gauze pads.

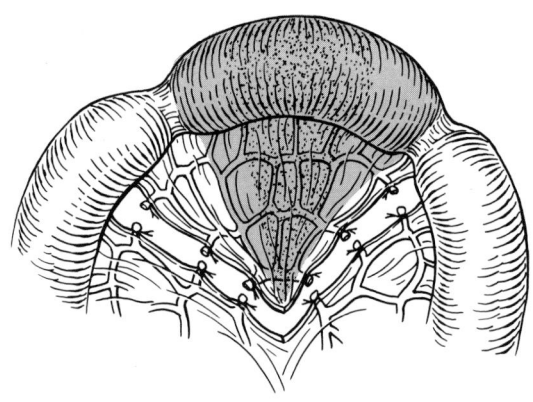

Figure 36-I-2

Division of Mesentery

The mesentery of the diseased segment is divided between hemostats. The mesenteric surface of the intestine should be cleared for a distance sufficient for later anastomosis.

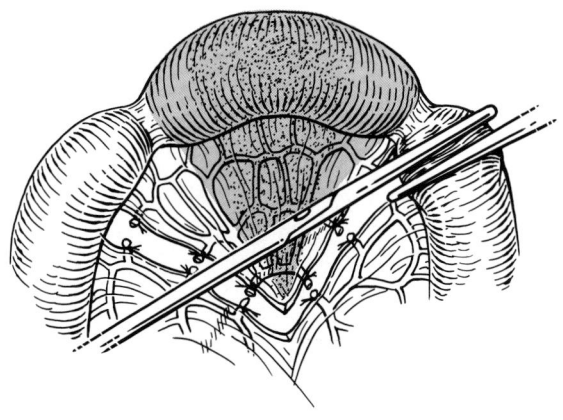

Figure 36-I-3

Resection

Straight atraumatic clamps are placed at the site chosen for transection. A Kocher clamp is used to occlude the bowel on the specimen side of transection to prevent spillage of enteric contents.

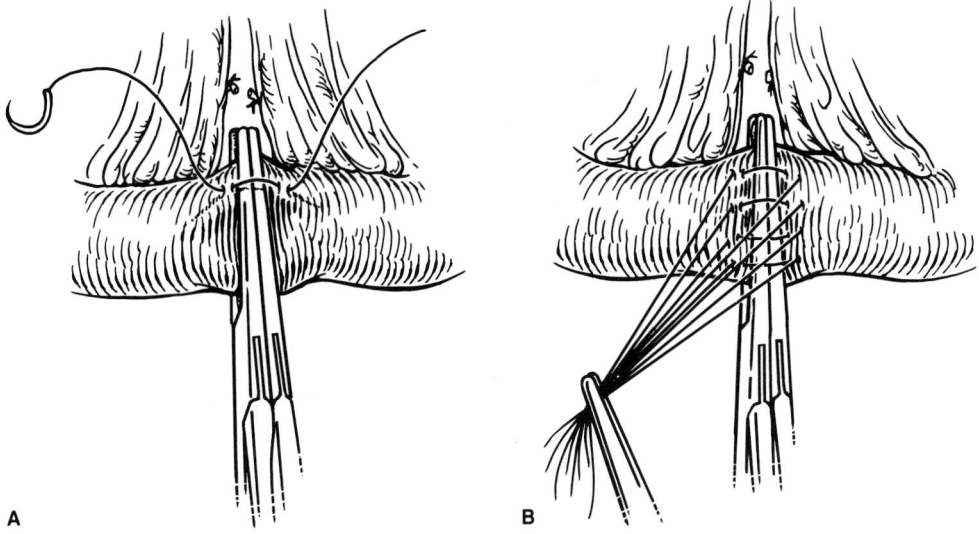

A   B

Figure 36-I-4

Single-Layer Technique

(**A**) The straight clamps are aligned parallel to each other. Interrupted seromuscular sutures are placed adjacent to each clamp. During suturing, care must be taken not to place the needle too deeply and thereby include the opposite wall.

(**B**) All sutures from one side are gathered and held with a hemostat.

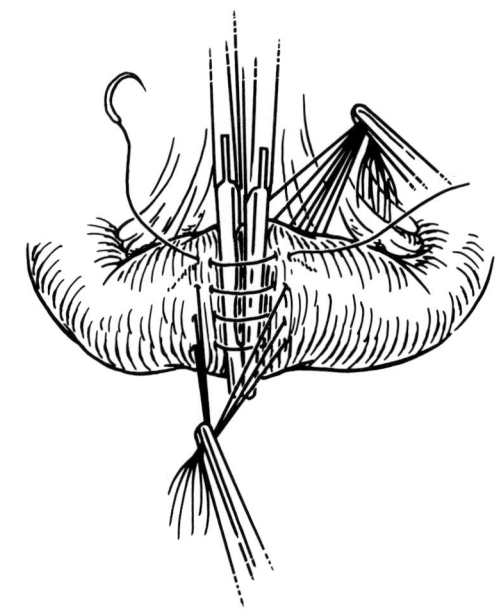

Figure 36-I-5

Posterior Wall

The straight bowel clamps are rotated 180 degrees, exposing the posterior aspect of the anastomosis. A similar set of sutures is placed in the posterior wall.

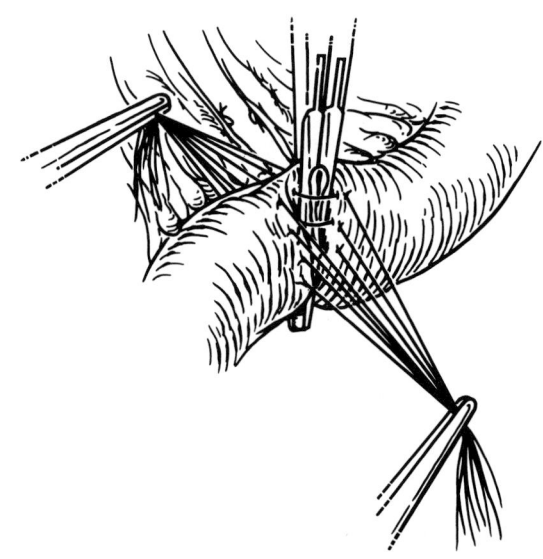

Figure 36-I-6

Removal of Clamps

The tagged sutures are retracted laterally, and the bowel clamps are removed in turn. With sufficient tension on the tagged sutures, the anastomosis remains inverted and no leakage of enteric contents occurs.

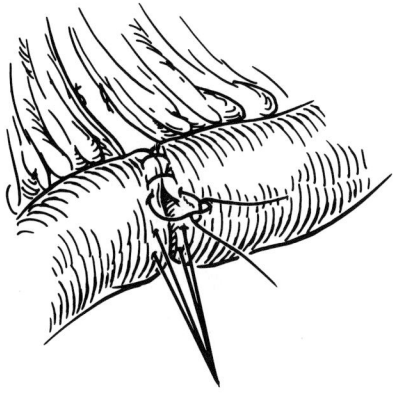

Figure 36-I-7

Completion of Anastomosis

The circumference of the small bowel is gradually rotated as the sutures are tied sequentially. Additional sutures are added during this process, as needed.

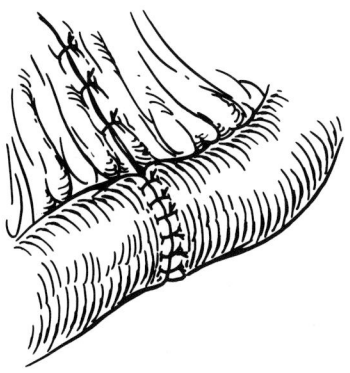

Figure 36-I-8

Mesenteric Defect

The mesenteric defect is closed with interrupted sutures.

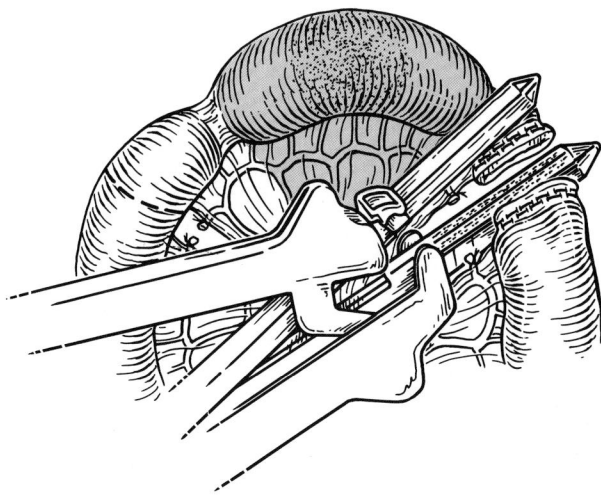

Figure 36-I-9

Double-Layer Technique

The bowel can also be divided using a GIA-type stapler to provide convenience and secure closure.

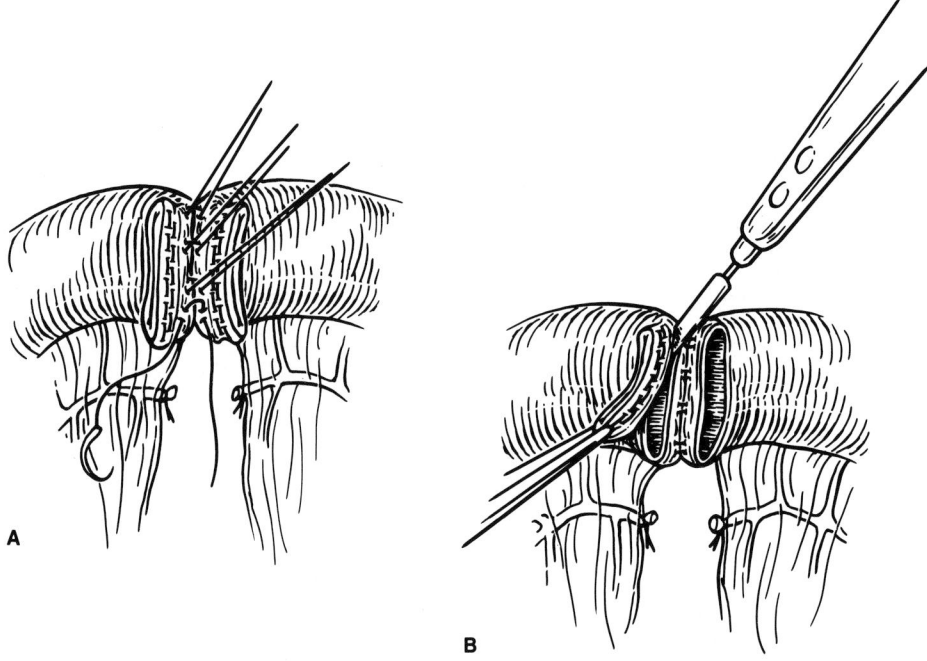

Figure 36-I-10

Posterior Layer

(**A**) Seromuscular sutures of 3-0 nonabsorbable are placed in an interrupted fashion for the posterior layer.

(**B**) Stapled closures are removed with electrocautery.

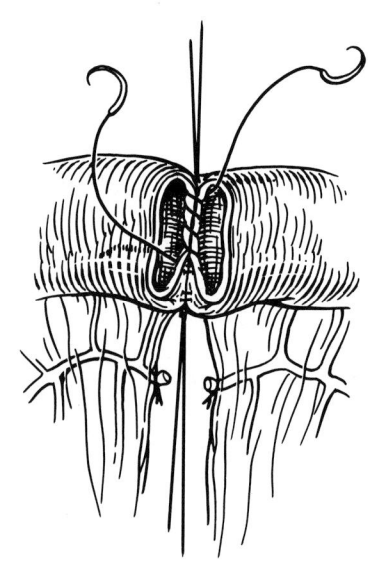

Figure 36-I-11

Posterior Mucosal Suture

A double-armed suture of absorbable material is used for closure of the mucosa. All layers of small intestinal wall should be included in the closure.

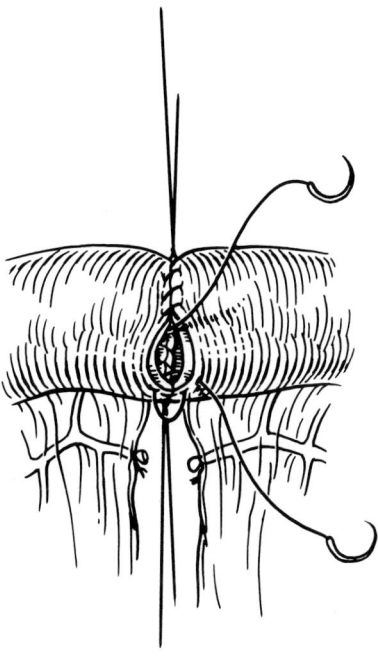

Figure 36-I-12

Anterior Mucosal Suture
The mucosal suture is continued anteriorly.

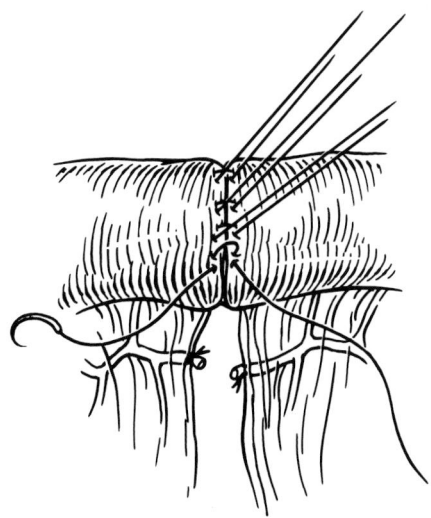

Figure 36-I-13

Anterior Serosal Suture
Anterior seromuscular interrupted nonabsorbable sutures complete the anastomosis.

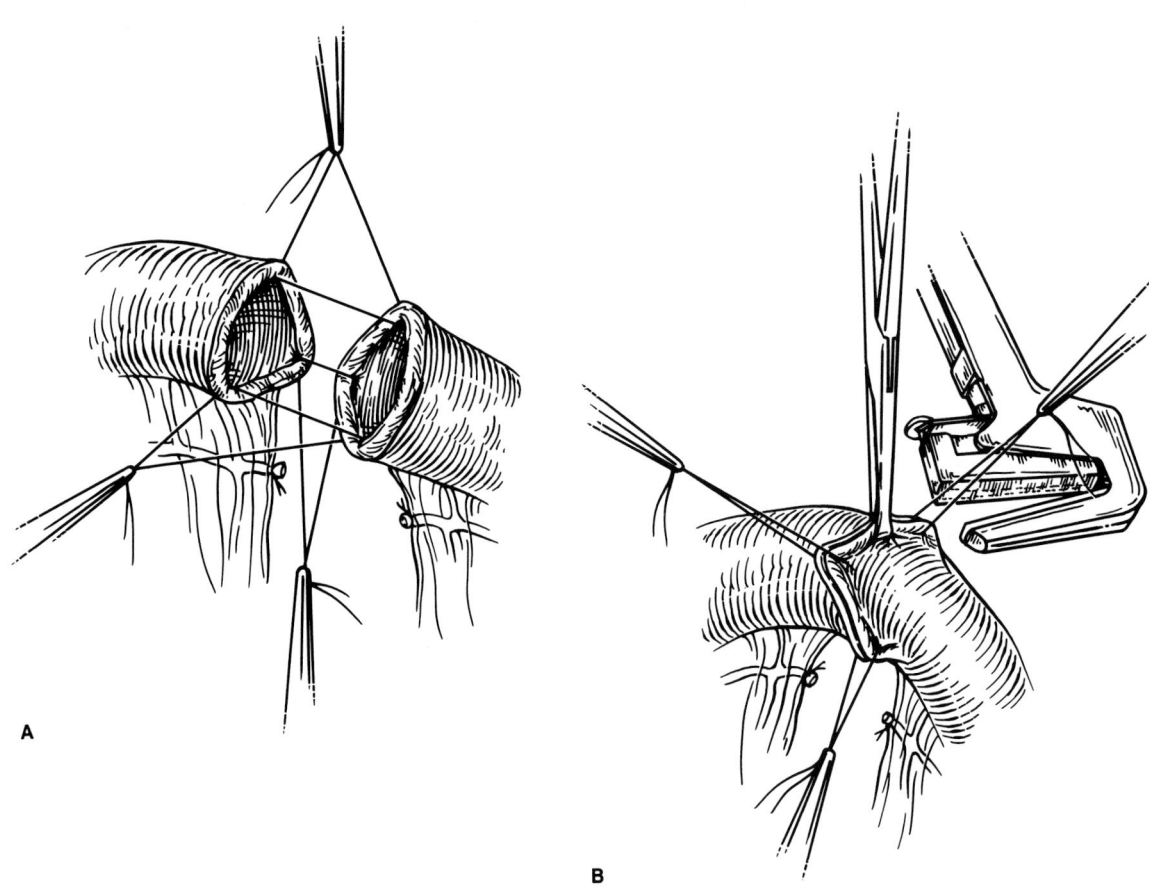

A

B

Figure 36-I-14

End-to-End Stapled Technique

(A) The open ends of the segments to be anastomosed are triangulated by full-thickness sutures placed at 120-degree angles to one another.

(B) Gentle tension on the stay sutures approximates the bowel segments, and forceps or clamps are used to facilitate application of a TA stapling device beneath the elevated segment.

(C) The TA stapler is fired and excess tissue removed before the stapler is released. The stapler is used as a guide for the scalpel tip.

(D) The stay sutures are rotated 120 degrees, and the stapler is applied again.

(E) The staple lines overlap at each corner.

(F) The completed anastomosis with closure of mesenteric defect.

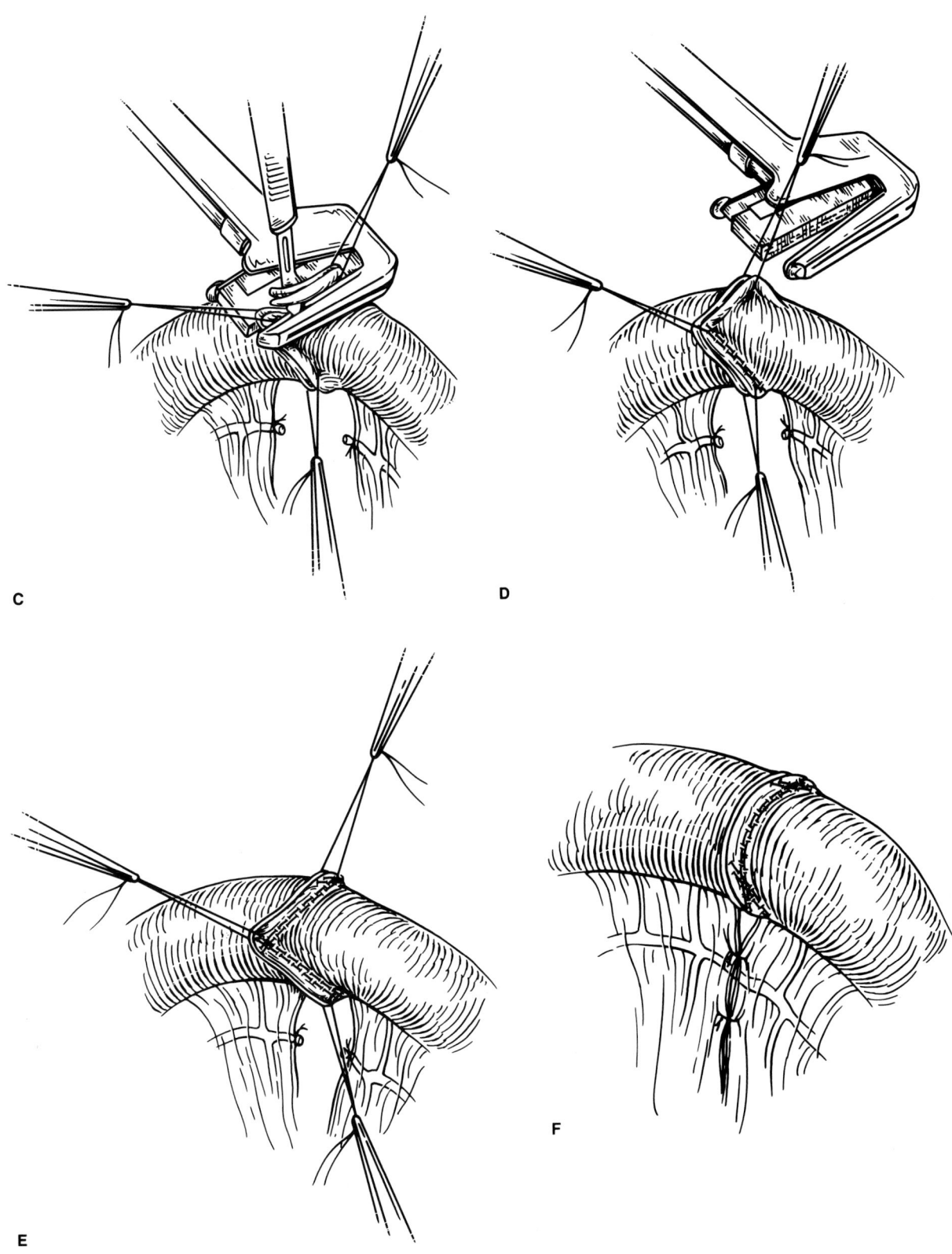

C

D

E

F

Figure 36-I-14 *(Continued)*

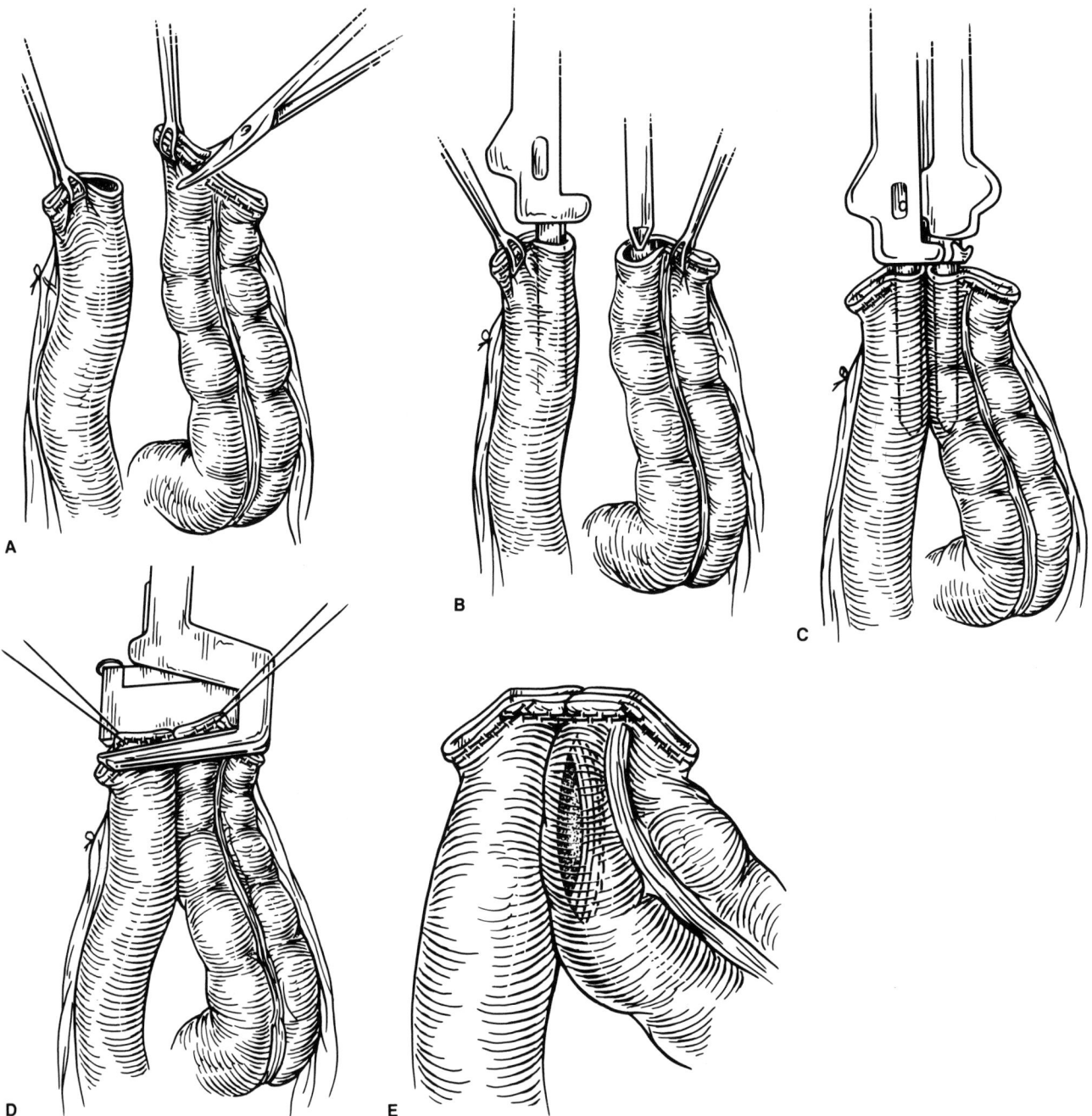

Figure 36-I-15

Side-to-Side Stapled Technique

(**A**) A side-to-side enterocolostomy is illustrated. Both bowel segments have been divided with GIA stapling devices. Bowel segments are aligned with antimesenteric surfaces in apposition. A segment of staple closure large enough to accommodate the fork of a GIA stapler is excised from each segment.

(**B**) One fork of a GIA stapler is inserted into each bowel limb.

(**C**) The stapler is fired, creating an anastomosis. The instrument is removed and the staple lines are inspected for hemostasis.

(**D**) The site of insertion of the GIA stapler is closed by application of a TA stapler.

(**E**) The completed side-to-side enterocolostomy.

SECTION II   *End Ileostomy*

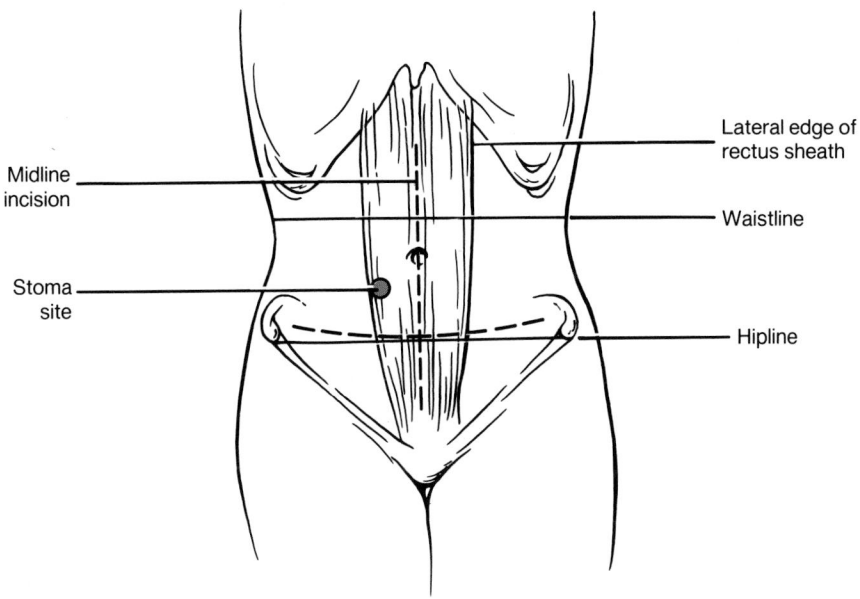

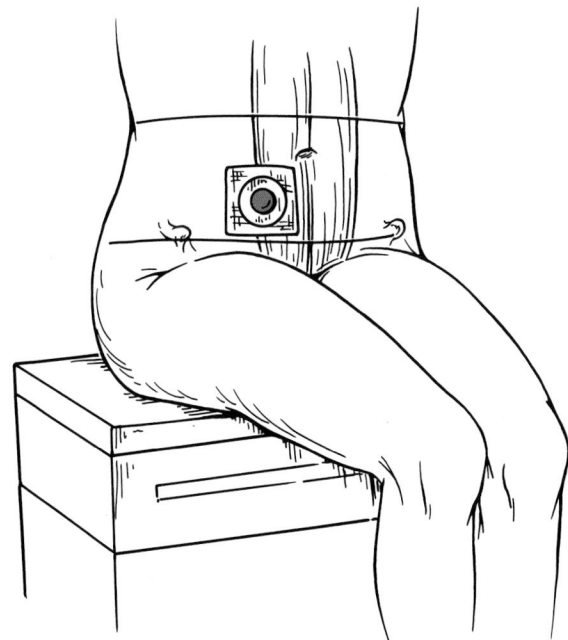

Figure 36-II-1

Ostomy Position

For elective operations, the site of the ostomy should be selected preoperatively, with the patient examined in both standing and sitting positions. The ostomy should be on a flat area of skin away from bony structures, skin folds, scars, or incisions. It should ideally be positioned within the lateral edge of the rectus sheath.

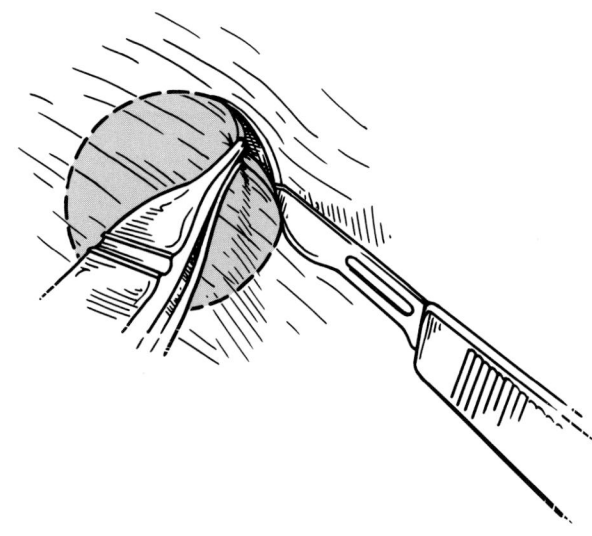

Figure 36-II-2

Ostomy Aperture

A disk of skin approximately 2.5 cm in diameter should be excised. A cylinder of subcutaneous tissue is removed with electrocautery to expose the anterior rectus sheath.

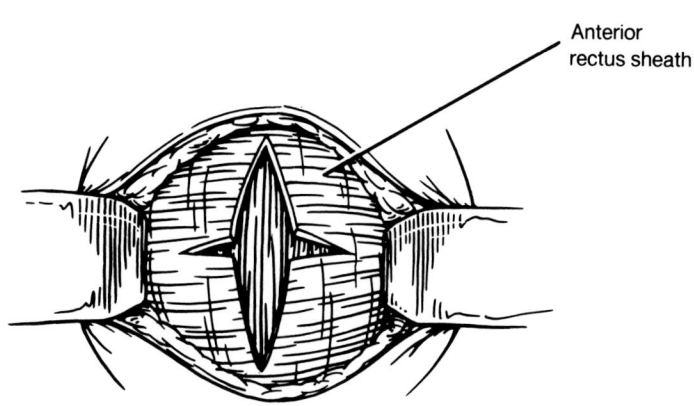

Anterior rectus sheath

Figure 36-II-3

Anterior Rectus Sheath

A cruciate incision is made in the anterior rectus sheath.

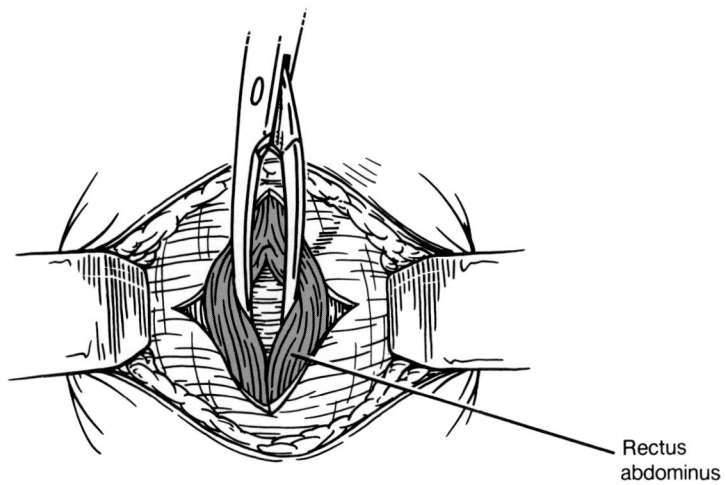

Rectus
abdominus

Figure 36-II-4

Rectus Abdominus Muscle

The rectus abdominus muscle is separated along the direction of the fibers.

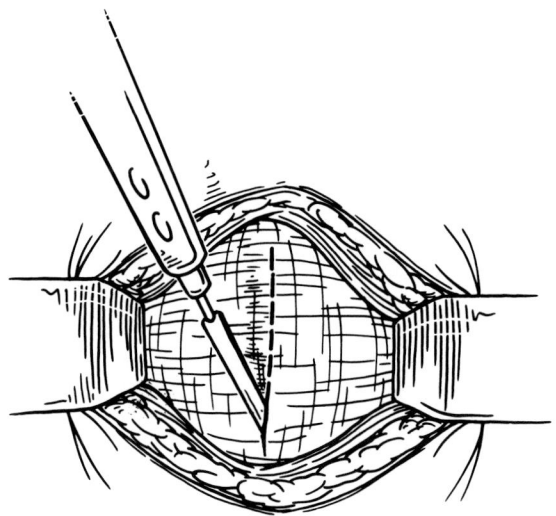

Figure 36-II-5

Posterior Rectus Sheath

The posterior rectus sheath is incised. Underlying abdominal contents should be shielded from injury.

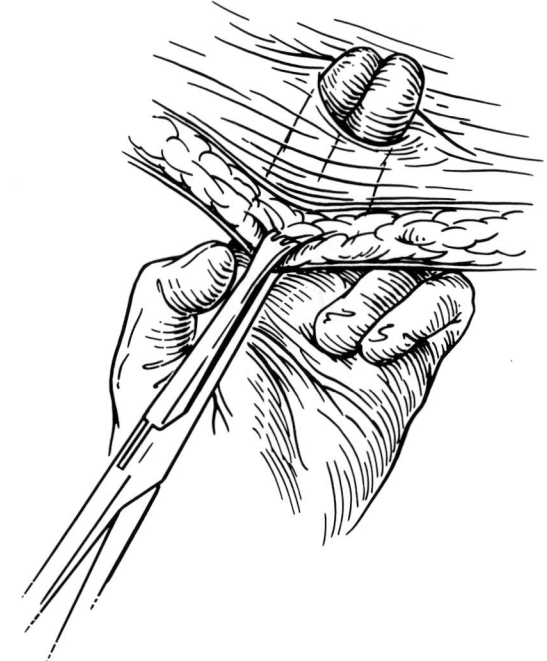

Figure 36-II-6

Ostomy Size

The surgeon must ensure that the ostomy tunnel will not be constrictive for the ileostomy. This condition is generally met if two fingers are accommodated without difficulty.

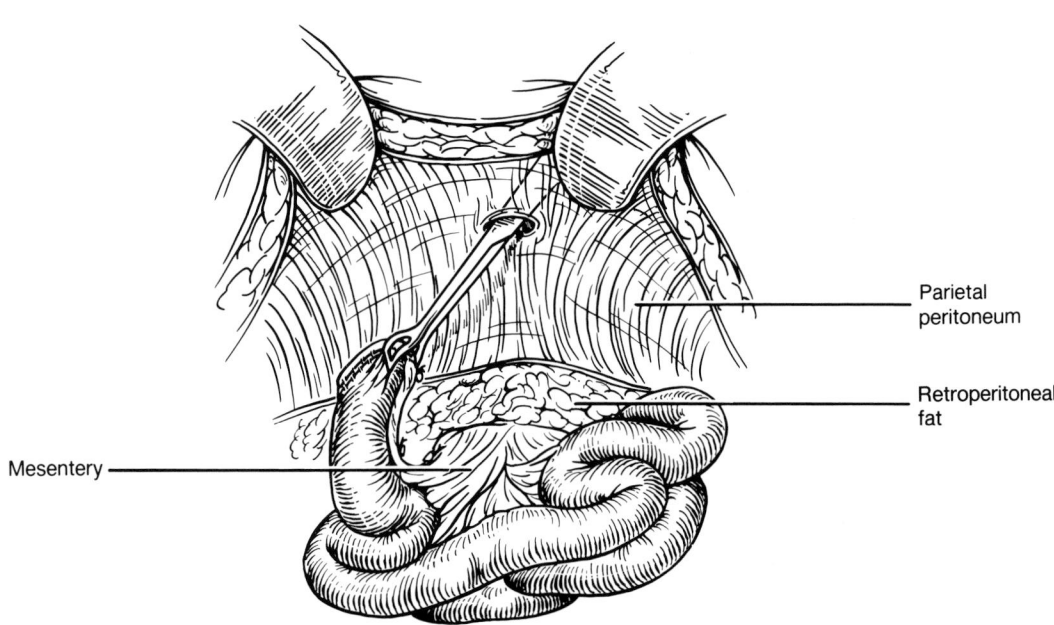

Parietal peritoneum

Retroperitoneal fat

Mesentery

Figure 36-II-7

Delivery of Bowel

A Babcock clamp is passed through the ostomy incision, and the end of the bowel is grasped. As the small intestine is delivered through the ostomy tunnel, the mesentery is observed to prevent twists or constriction.

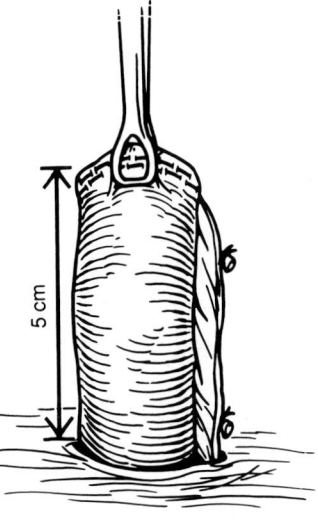

Figure 36-II-8

Ostomy Protrusion

The finished ileostomy should extend 2.5 cm above the level of the skin to provide proper appliance fit. To ensure this, the small intestine must protrude 5 cm above the skin without tension. It is necessary to skeletonize a length of ileum of adherent mesenteric fat to ensure that tension-free eversion of the bowel can subsequently be performed.

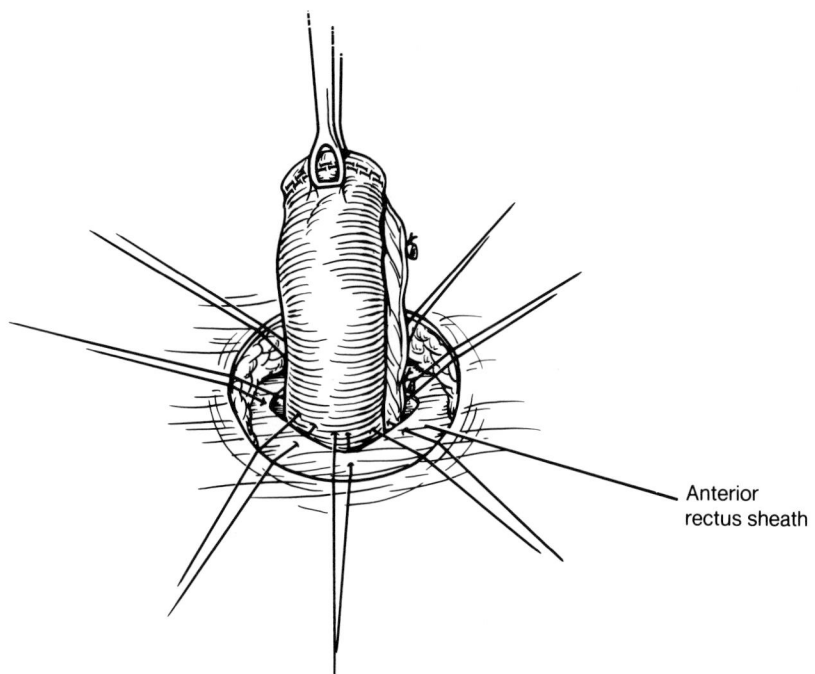

Anterior
rectus sheath

Figure 36-II-9

Fascial Sutures

Interrupted sutures are passed through the rectus sheath and the seromuscular layer of the bowel at the level of the fascia to preclude retraction of the bowel during midline wound closure and to prevent later paraileostomy hernia.

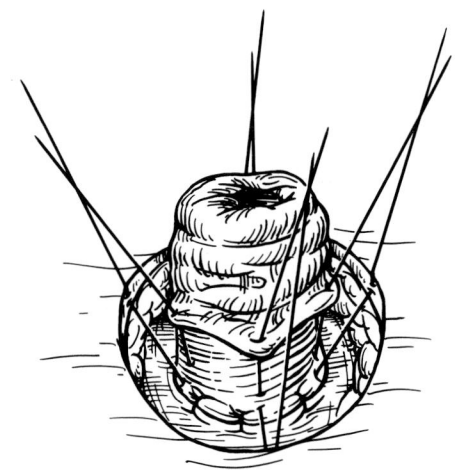

Figure 36-II-10

Four Quadrant Sutures

The ostomy is divided into four quadrants by sutures used to produce eversion. The sutures have three portions—full thickness at the cut end of the bowel, seromuscular at the level of the anterior rectus fascia, and subcuticular at the skin edge.

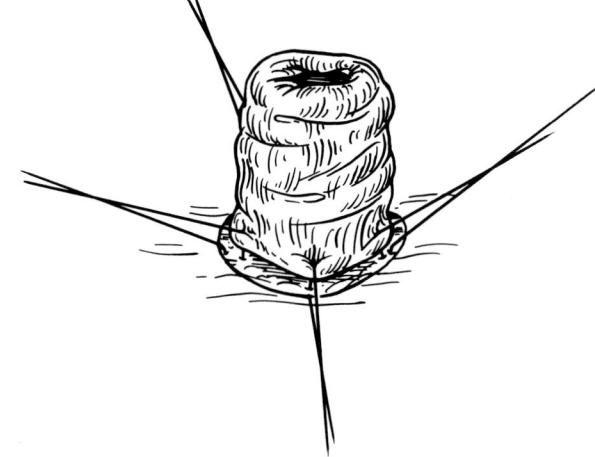

Figure 36-II-11

Ostomy Eversion

As the sutures are tied, the ostomy becomes everted.

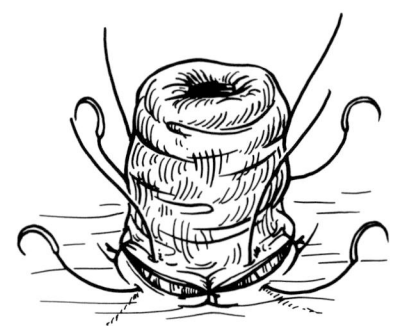

Figure 36-II-12

Completed Ostomy

Simple sutures from the edge of the bowel to the skin complete the anastomosis.

SECTION III *Loop Ileostomy*

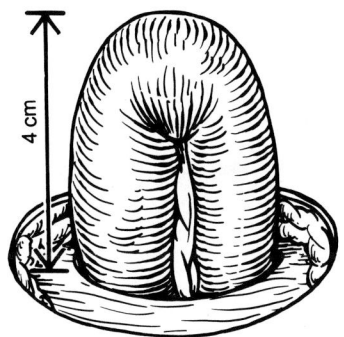

Figure 36-III-1

Loop Protrusion

For a loop ileostomy, the small intestinal loop should protrude 4 cm above the level of the skin.

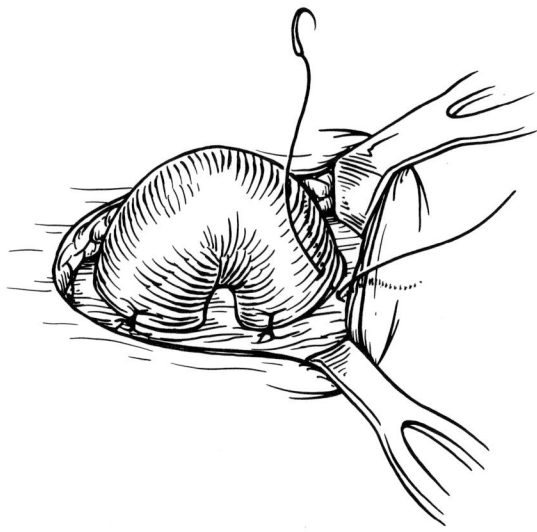

Figure 36-III-2

Fascial Sutures

Interrupted seromuscular sutures are used to secure the intestinal loop to the anterior rectus sheath circumferentially.

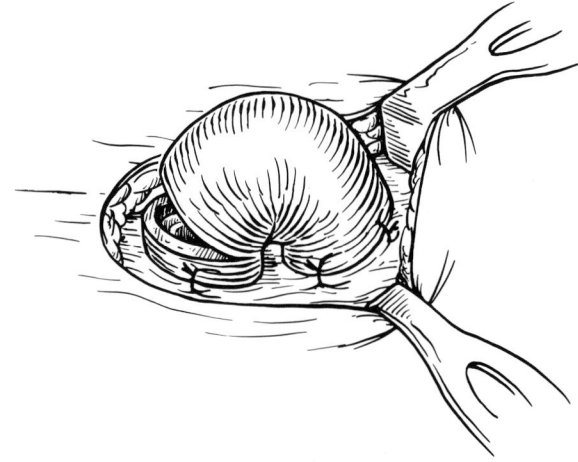

Figure 36-III-3

Incision in Distal Limb

An incision is made in the distal limb that encompasses 80% of its circumference.

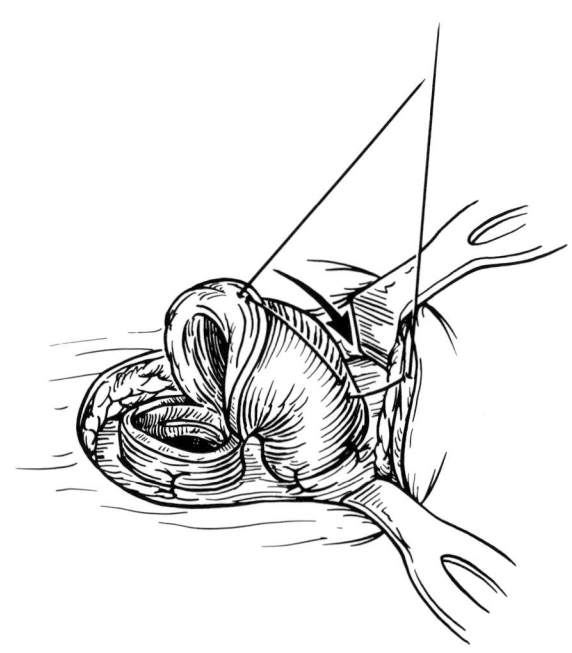

Figure 36-III-4

Eversion of the Proximal Limb

Sutures used to evert the proximal limb have three components—full thickness at the proximal edge of the incision, seromuscular at the level of the anterior rectus sheath, and subcuticular. Usually three or four sutures placed in this manner are necessary to affect eversion. As these sutures are tied, the proximal bowel is everted as a spout; simultaneously, the distal bowel assumes a semiclosed crescent shape.

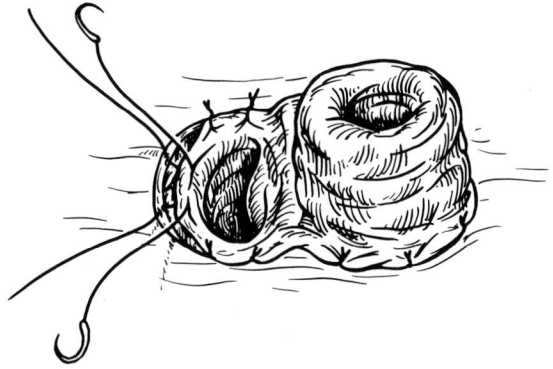

Figure 36-III-5

Completion of Ostomy

Additional sutures are placed circumferentially to produce a secure seal.

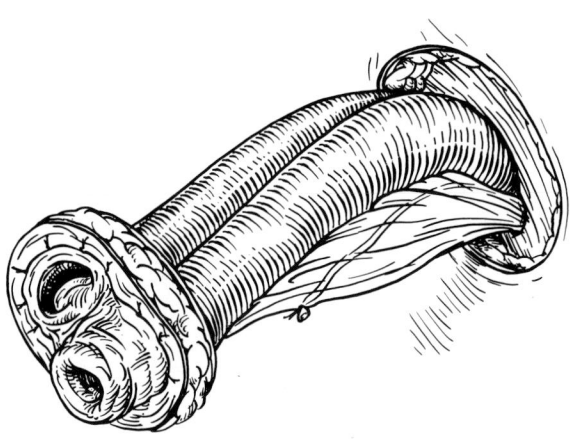

Figure 36-III-6

Ileostomy Takedown

A loop ileostomy can usually be reversed using a paraileostomy incision. An ellipse of skin and subcutaneous tissue surrounding the ostomy is excised, and fascial sutures are divided. A length of bowel, proximal and distal to the ostomy, is delivered externally.

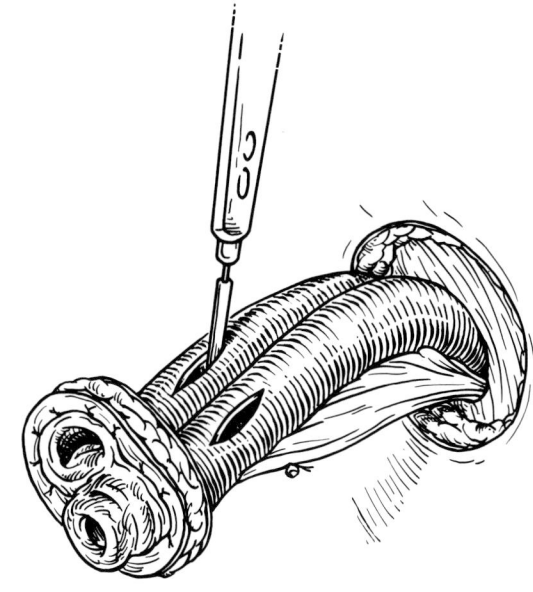

Figure 36-III-7

Alignment of Small Intestine

Proximal and distal bowel loops are aligned with antimesenteric borders facing each other. A small incision is made in each limb using electrocautery.

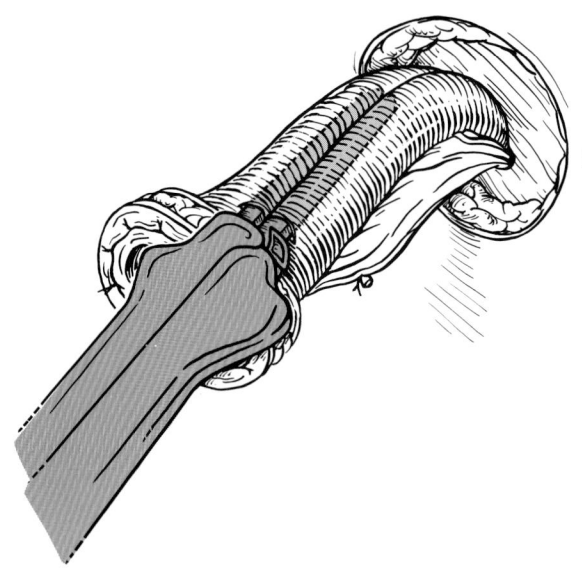

Figure 36-III-8

Insertion of GIA Stapler

A GIA-type stapling device is inserted, one fork in each limb of bowel. The stapler is fired, creating a common lumen. After it is withdrawn, the anastomosis is inspected for hemostasis.

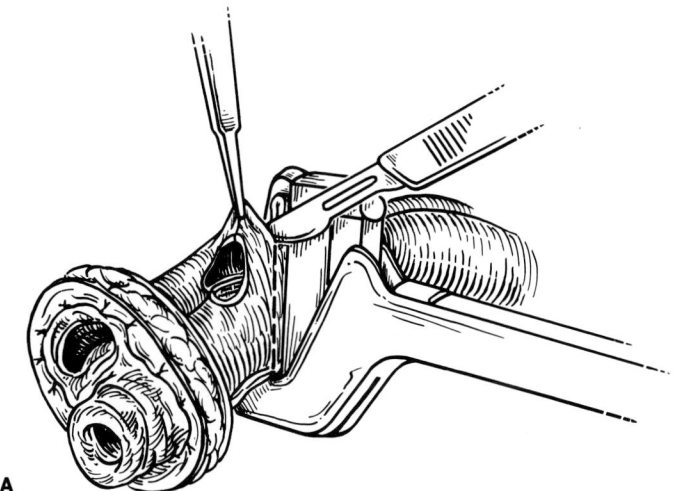

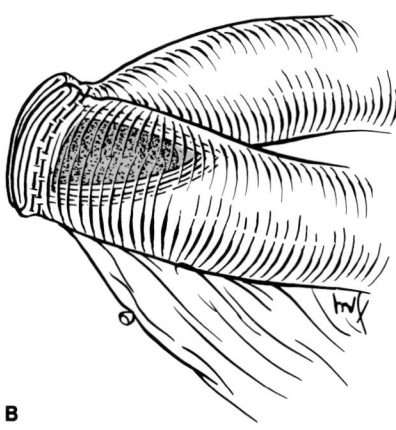

Figure 36-III-9

Completion of Anastomosis

(**A**) A TA stapler is applied distal to the holes used for introduction of the GIA stapler and fired. The ileostomy is resected distal to the TA stapler.

(**B**) The completed anastomosis.

SECTION IV Tube Jejunostomy

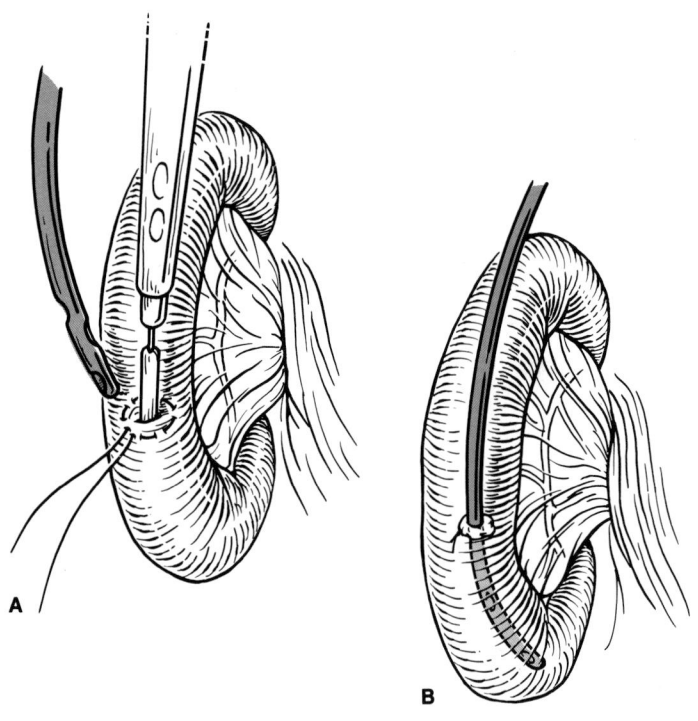

Figure 36-IV-1

Insertion Site

(**A**) Through a short midline incision, a loop of proximal jejunum is delivered. A 3-0 nonabsorbable pursestring suture is placed along the antimesenteric border, and cautery is used to create a small enterotomy. A soft rubber catheter of appropriate size is inserted.

(**B**) The pursestring suture is tied after the catheter has been advanced distally.

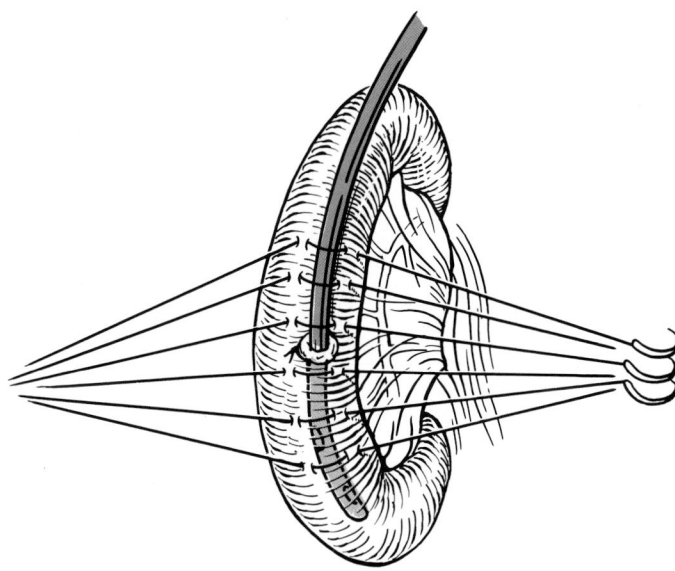

Figure 36-IV-2

Suture Placement

Seromuscular sutures are placed on either side of the tube proximal and distal to the insertion site so that a tunnel of intestinal wall can be created. The needle is left attached to every second suture.

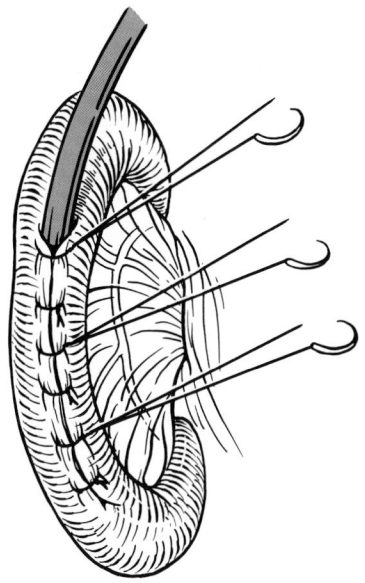

Figure 36-IV-3

Tunnel Creation

Sutures are tied, folding intestinal wall over the insertion site and forming a tunnel-valve to prevent leakage of intestinal contents if the tube is removed. Care must be taken not to include an excessive amount of bowel wall and thereby narrow the bowel lumen beneath the jejunostomy tube.

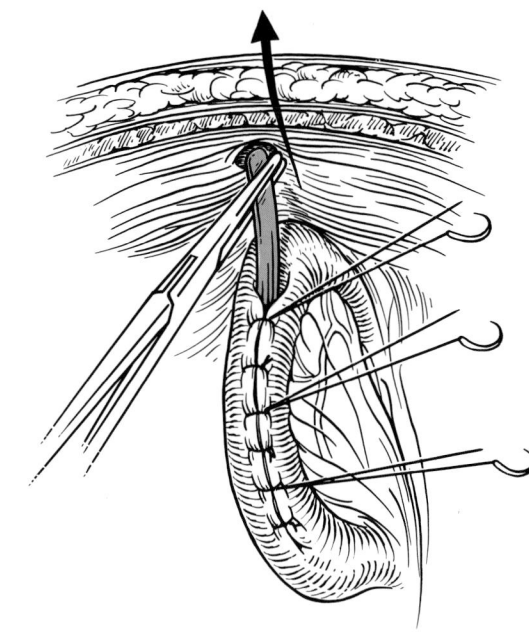

Figure 36-IV-4

Tube Exit Site

The jejunostomy tube exits lateral to the incision in an area away from scars, ostomies, and costal margins.

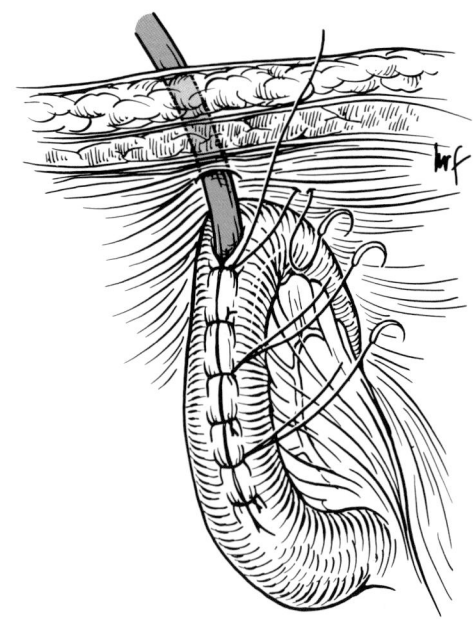

Figure 36-IV-5

Peritoneal Attachment

The needles are used to attach the loop of intestine to the undersurface of the abdominal wall. Additional sutures can be used to ensure a watertight seal at the site of jejunostomy exit.

SECTION V *Laparoscopic Tube Jejunostomy*

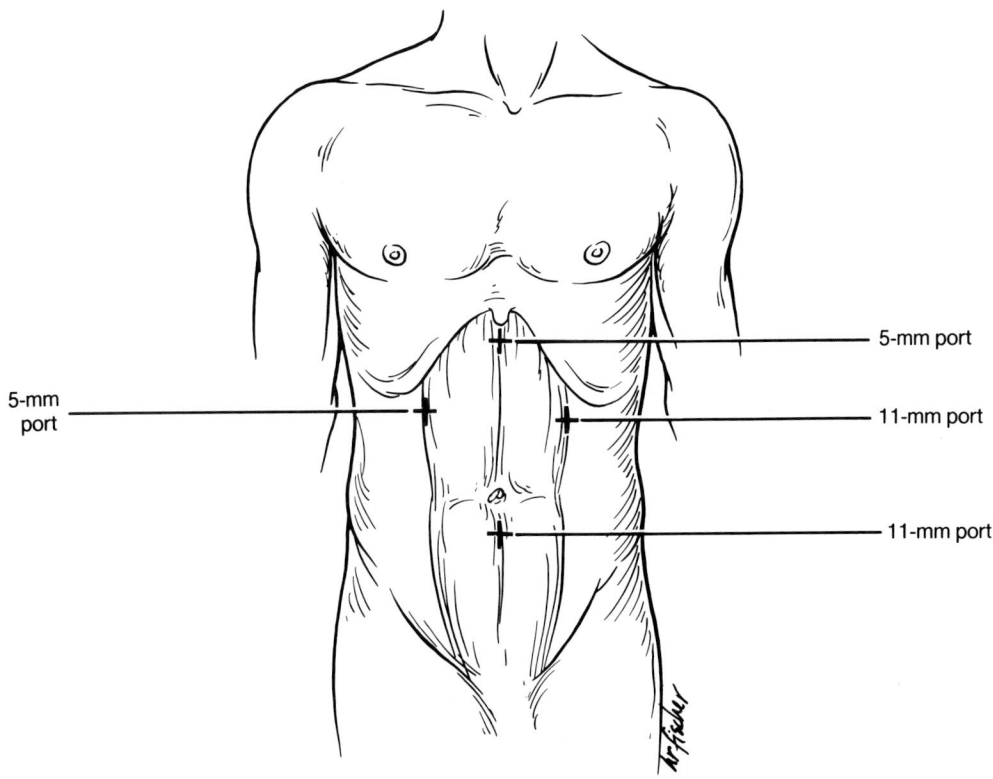

5-mm port

5-mm port

11-mm port

11-mm port

Figure 36-V-1

Port Positioning

After abdominal insufflation, an 11-mm port is introduced through an infraumbilical incision. The laparoscope is placed through this port initially. An 11-mm accessory trochar is placed, under direct vision, in the upper left abdomen. Additional 5-mm ports are placed in the upper midline and right upper quadrant. The laparoscope is moved to the upper left 11-mm port.

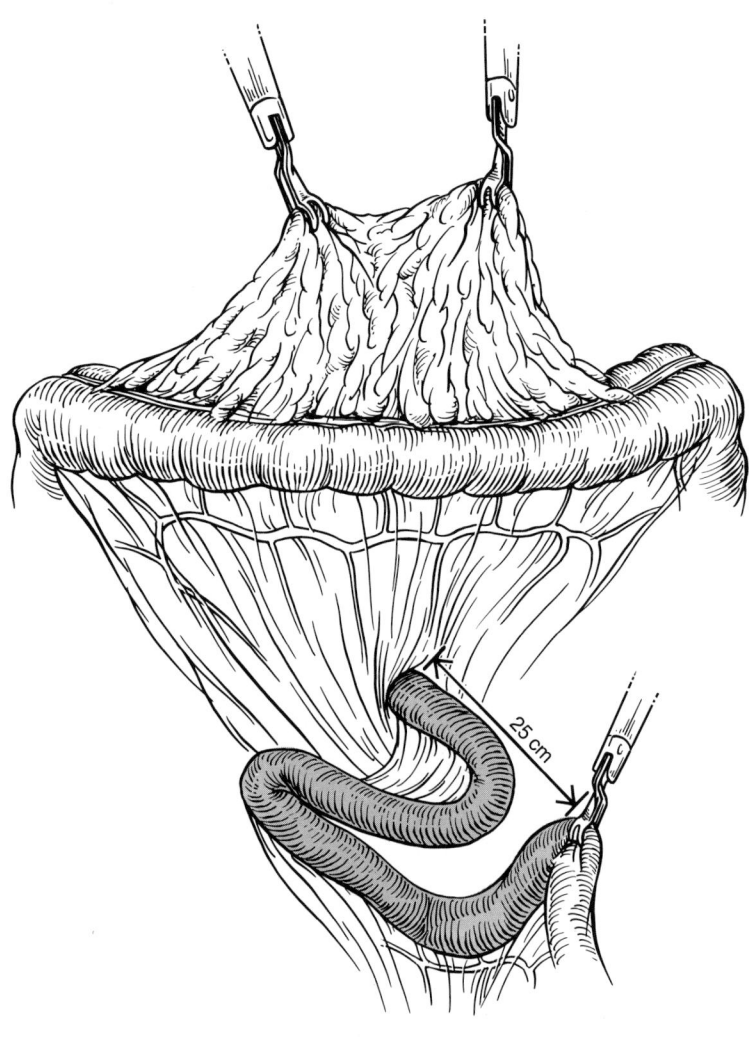

Figure 36-V-2

Identification of Ligament of Treitz

Babcock-type clamps are placed through the 5-mm ports, and the greater omentum and transverse colon are grasped and retracted cephalad. The ligament of Treitz is identified. A segment of jejunum 25 cm distal to the ligament of Treitz is selected.

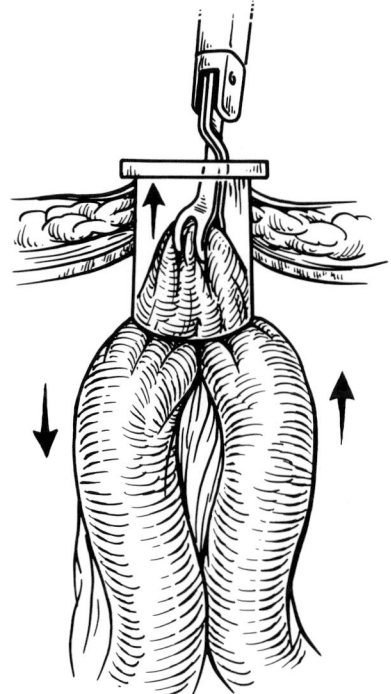

Figure 36-V-3

Laparoscopic Cannula Change

The infraumbilical port is replaced with a 20-mm laparoscopic cannula, using a sleeve converter to allow passage of instruments. The appropriate segment of bowel is grasped and delivered through the 20-mm port. The camera is moved to the left upper abdominal port.

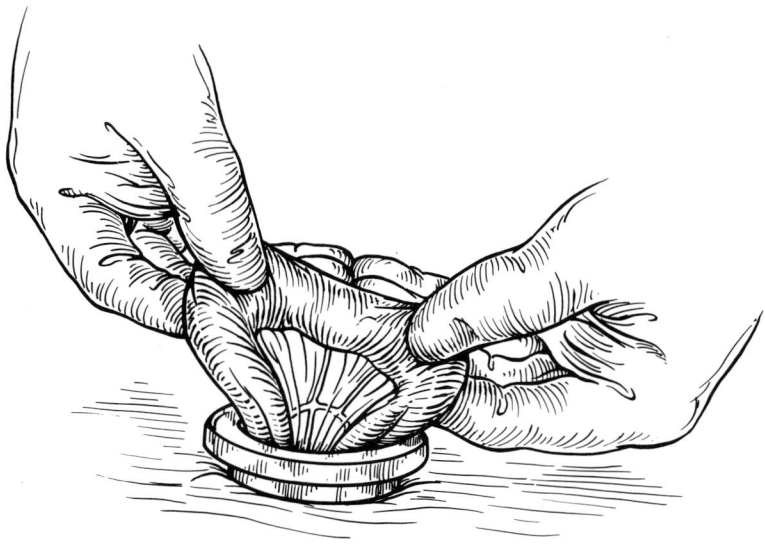

Figure 36-V-4

Bowel Exteriorization

Insufflation is released so that the loop of jejunum can be eviscerated without tension. A Witzel-type tube jejunostomy is constructed. As shown in Figure 36-IV-3, three 3-0 non-absorbable sutures are left with needles attached and the jejunum is returned to the peritoneal cavity. Pneumoperitoneum is reestablished.

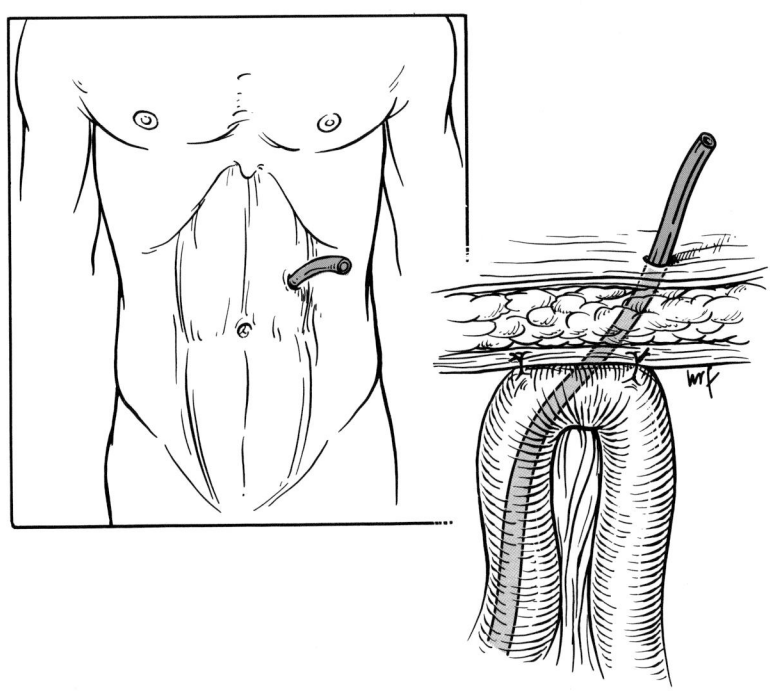

Figure 36-V-5

Tube Exit

The laparoscope is moved to the infraumbilical port. The jejunostomy tube is pulled through the left upper port to externalize it. A laparoscopic suture holder is inserted through the upper midline port to secure the bowel to the anterior peritoneum using the previously placed sutures. Cannulas are removed, and the umbilical incision is closed with interrupted sutures.

SECTION VI *Visceral Revascularization Using Prosthetic Graft*

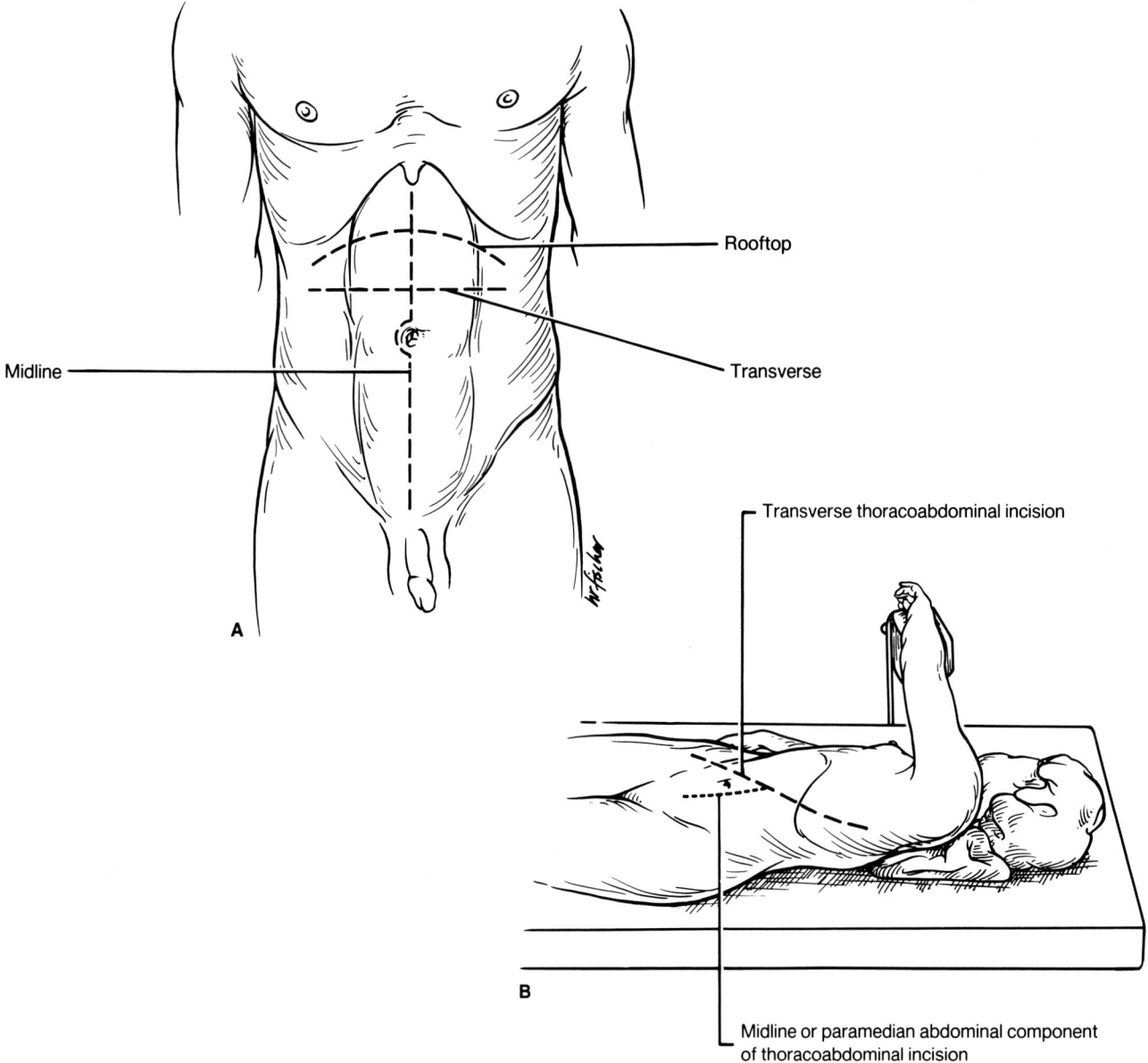

Figure 36-VI-1

Incisions

(**A**) Standard abdominal incisions such as the supraumbilical transverse incision, the chevron (rooftop) incision, and the midline abdominal incision are appropriate for visceral revascularization.

(**B**) For more extensive exposure of the entire mid-abdominal aorta, a transverse thoracoabdominal incision or a thoracoabdominal incision incorporating a midline or paramedian abdominal component provides wide access.

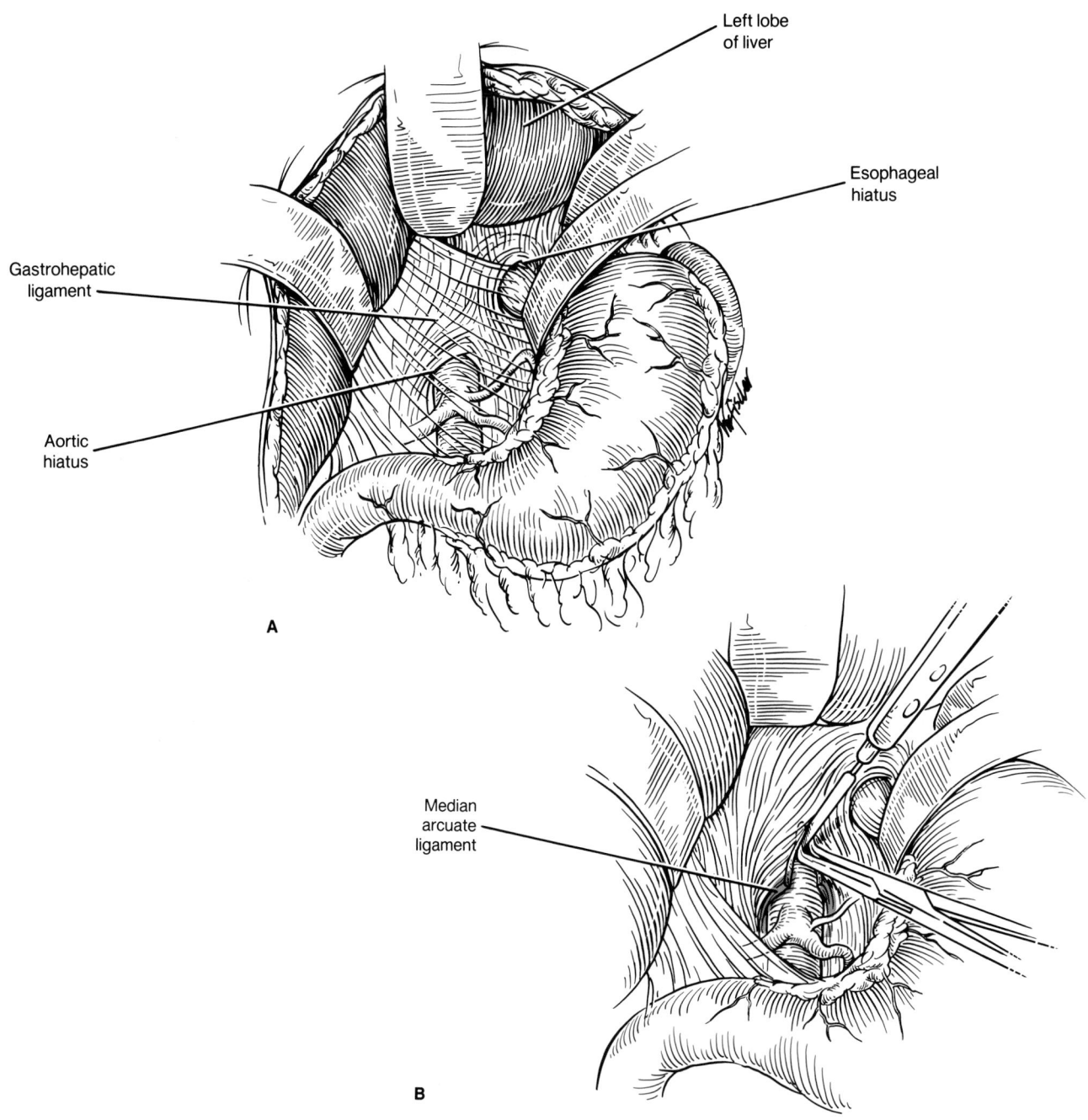

Figure 36-VI-2

Aortic Exposure

(**A**) Cephalad retraction of the left lobe of the liver and left lateral displacement of the stomach tenses the gastrohepatic ligament, which can be divided with Bovie cautery to expose the aortic hiatus. Care must be taken to avoid a replaced left hepatic artery, which courses within the gastrohepatic ligament.

(**B**) Palpation of the aorta and division of the overlying median arcuate ligament and muscular fibers of the aortic hiatus allow exposure of at least 7 cm of supraceliac aorta.

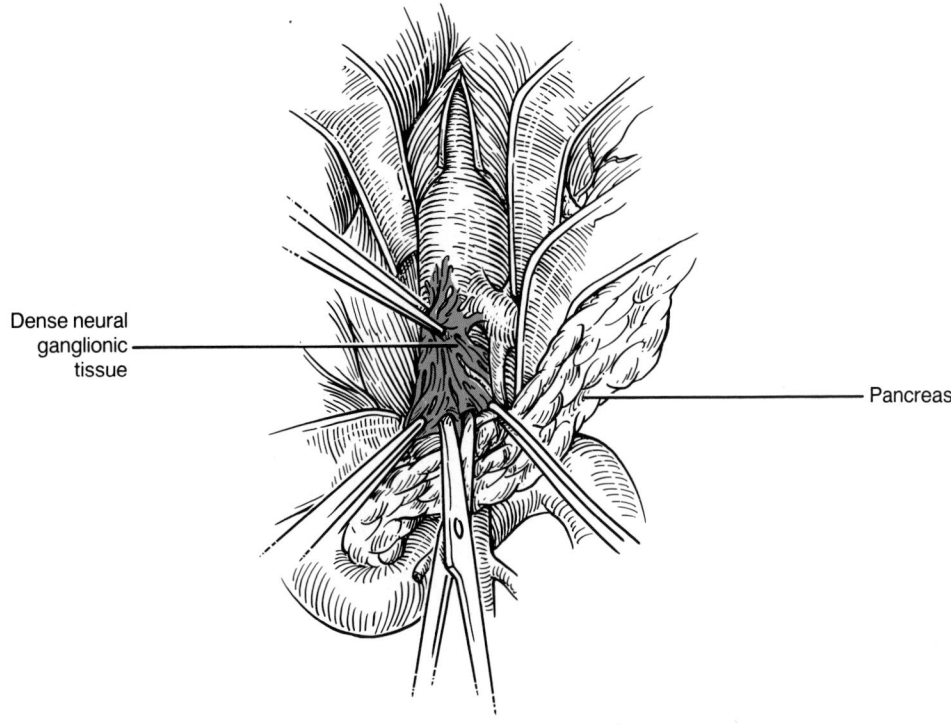

Dense neural ganglionic tissue

Pancreas

Figure 36-VI-3

Dissection of Periaortic Tissue

The supraceliac aorta is typically fully mobilized and then attention is turned to the paraceliac aorta. A dense area of ganglionic tissue is encountered and must be sharply dissected for 1 to 2 cm to expose the proximal celiac axis and its main arterial branches.

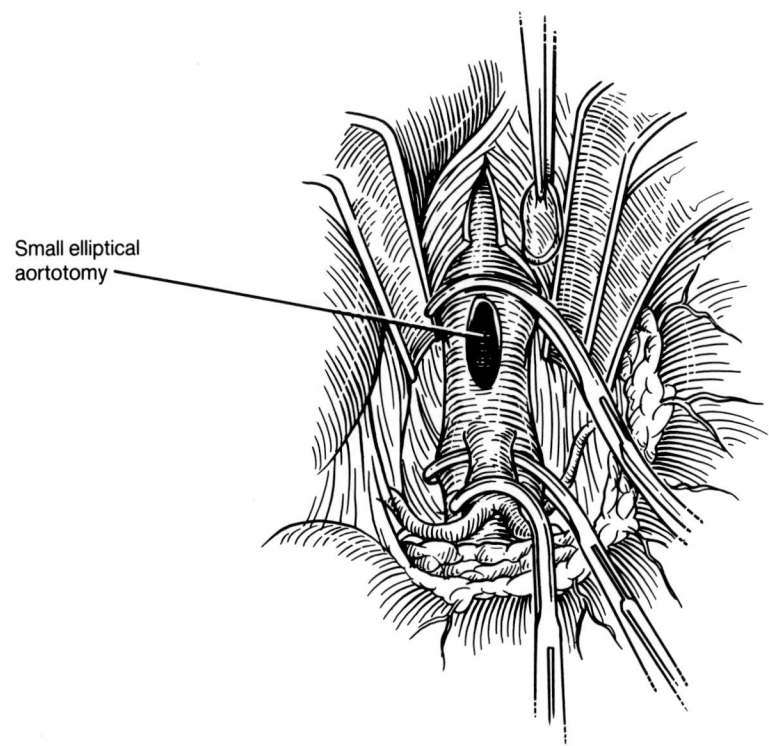

Small elliptical aortotomy

Figure 36-VI-4

Aortic Incision

Proximal and distal control of the supraceliac aorta and clamping of the celiac axis allows a small elliptical aortotomy to be fashioned for the proximal anastomosis. Occasionally, intercostal or lumbar arteries arise at this level. These should be preserved either by external application of a Heifitz clip or by intraluminal tamponade.

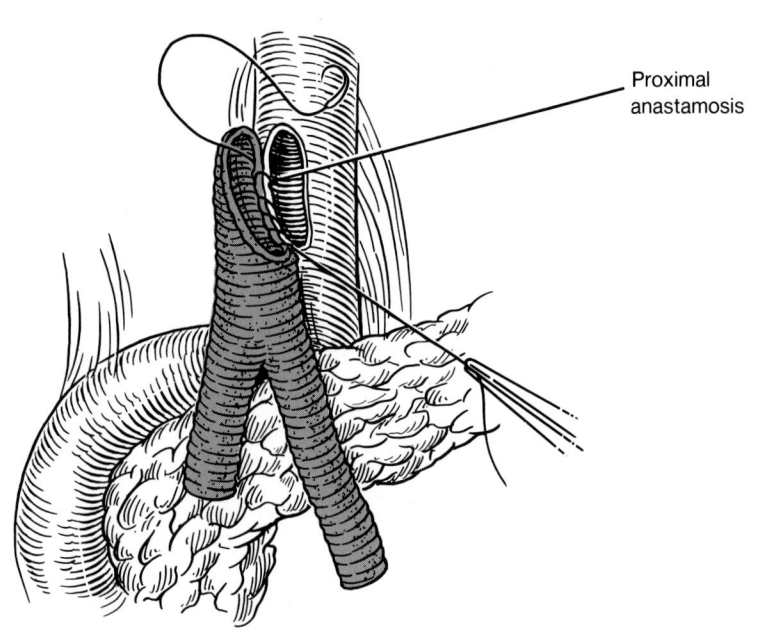

Proximal anastamosis

Figure 36-VI-5

Proximal Anastomosis

The proximal aortic anastomosis begins with an anchoring stitch at the heel of the prosthesis that anastomoses the diagonally cut prosthesis to the elliptical aortotomy. The anastomosis uses a continuous suture technique that proceeds in both directions from the heel and that is completed and tied on the lateral wall of the aortotomy.

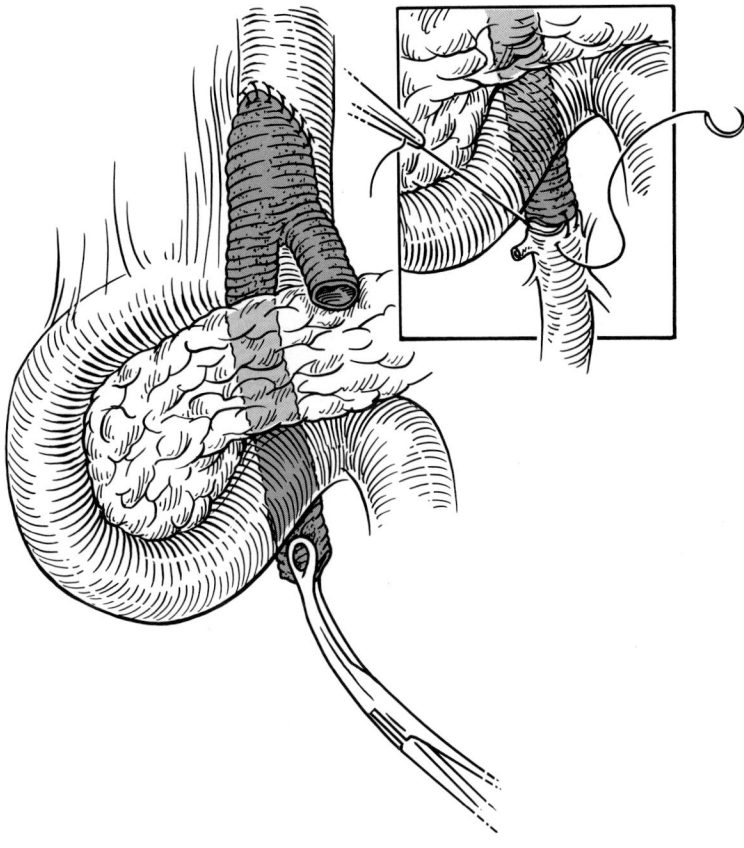

Figure 36-VI-6

Positioning of Graft

The right limb of the prosthesis is passed through a tunnel beneath the pancreas and duodenum with the distal anastomosis to the superior mesenteric artery performed below the duodenum (**inset**).

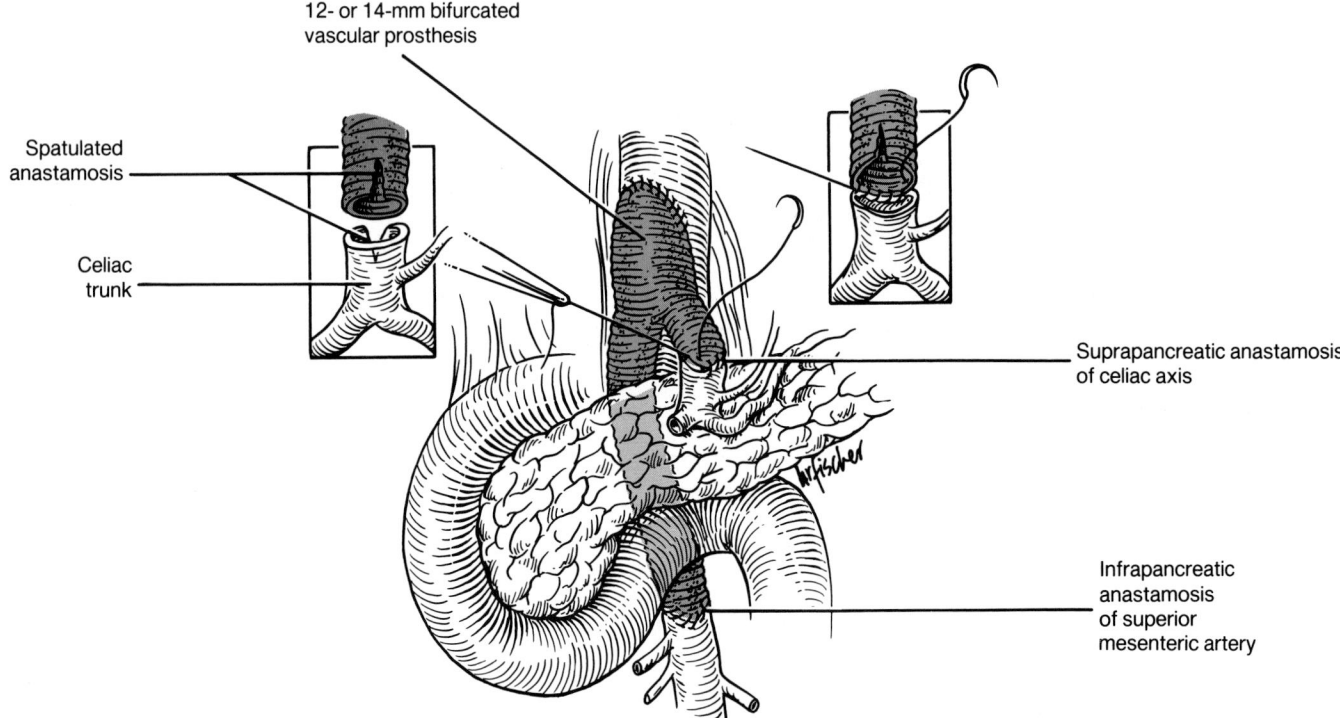

Figure 36-VI-7

Distal Anastomoses

The left limb of the bifurcated vascular prostheses is anastomosed to the superpancreatic portion of the celiac axis. For both the celiac anastomosis and the superior mesenteric artery anastomosis, a spatulated suture technique is used to avoid anastomotic narrowing **(insets)**.

SECTION VII *Visceral Revascularization Through Endarterectomy*

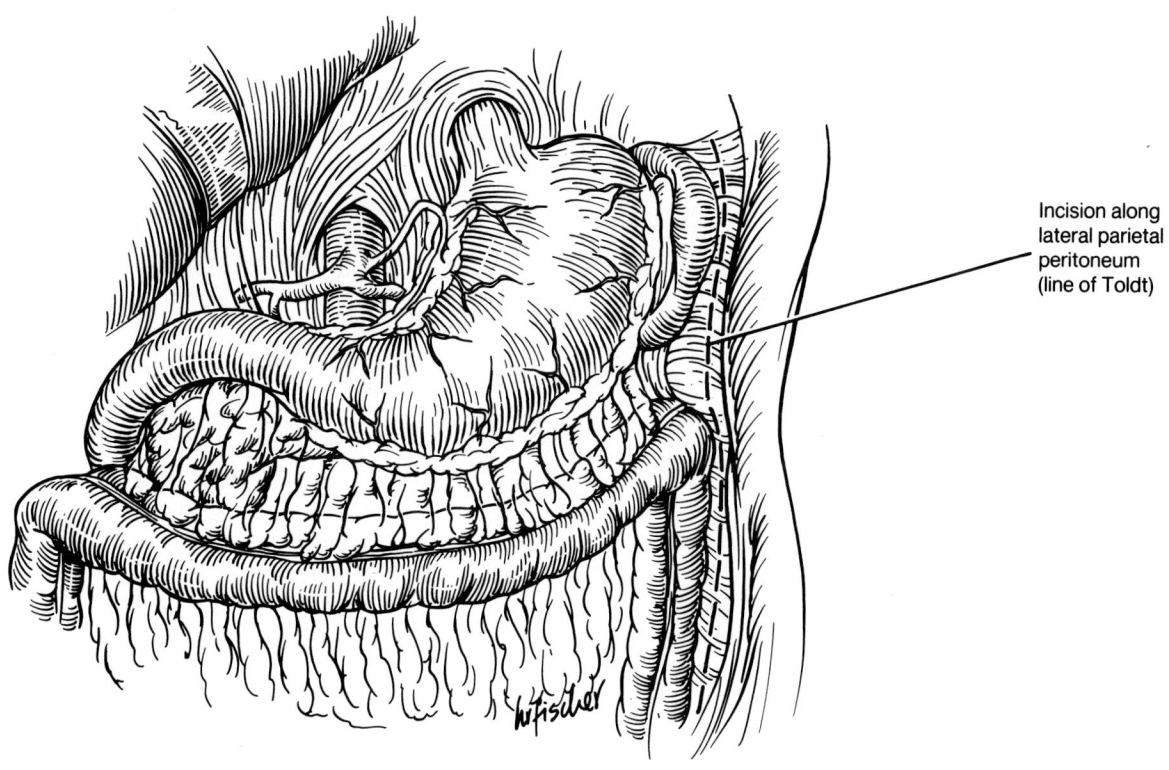

Incision along
lateral parietal
peritoneum
(line of Toldt)

Figure 36-VII-1

Aortic Exposure

Medial visceral rotation allows extensive exposure of the entire visceral aorta. This exposure involves incisions along the left lateral peritoneal reflection (line of Toldt) and mobilization of the left colon, spleen, pancreas, and stomach toward the patient's right.

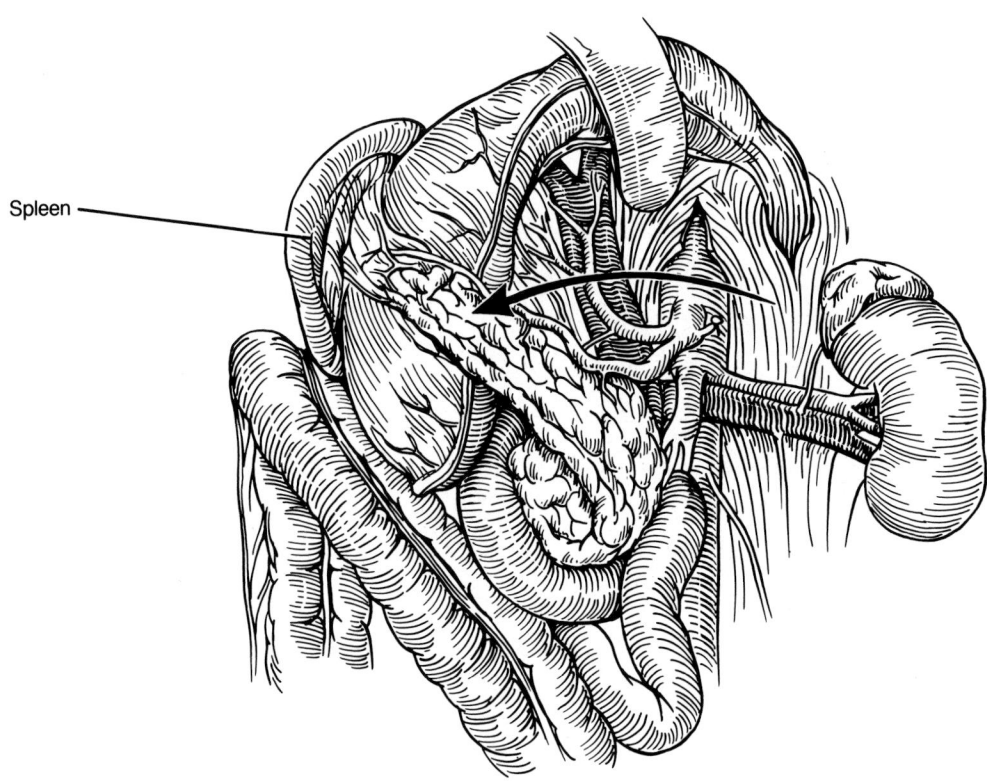

Spleen

Figure 36-VII-2

Visceral Rotation

The dissection can proceed anterior to the left kidney and renal vasculature and provides extensive exposure of the celiac axis and superior mesenteric artery. Wider access to the aorta can be gained by mobilizing the kidney in the same direction.

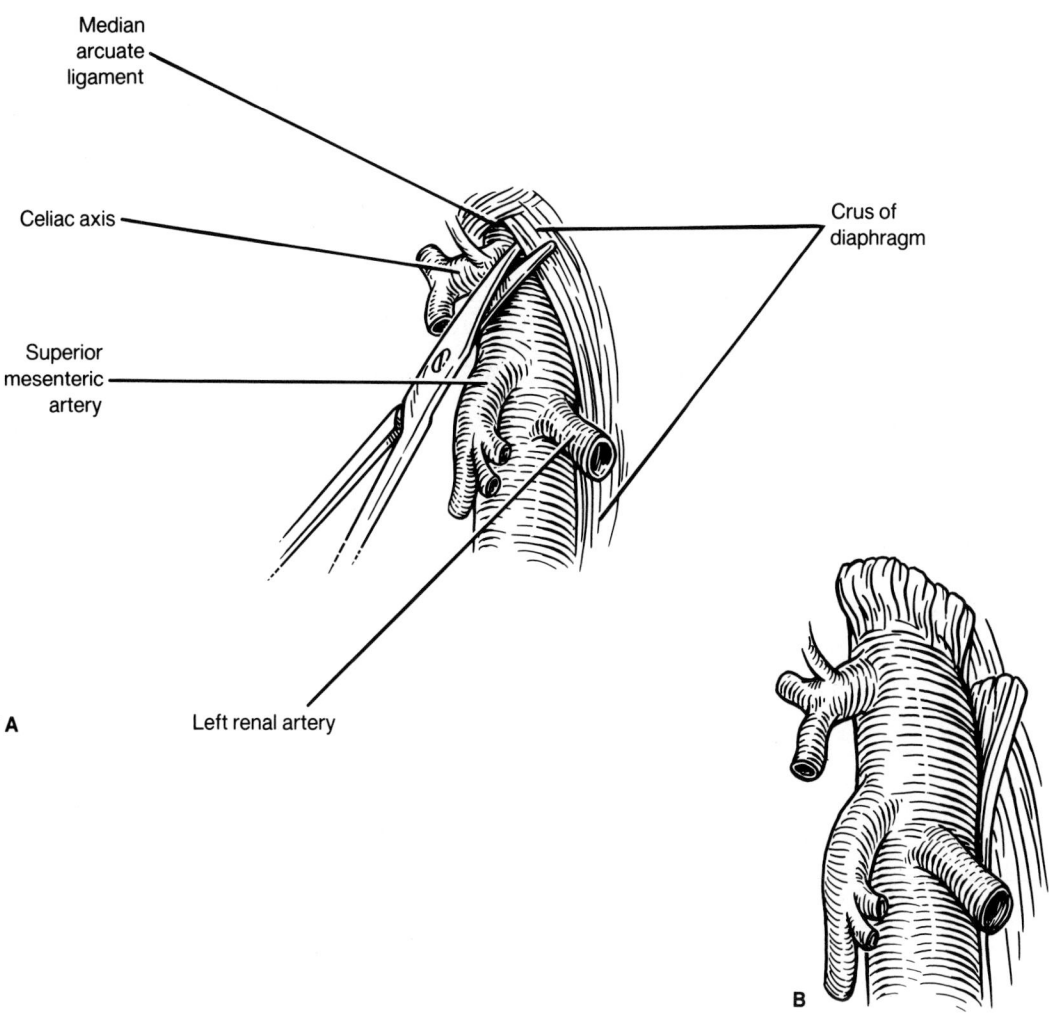

Figure 36-VII-3

Division of Diaphragmatic Crus

(**A**) The crus of the diagram is a more substantial structure and extends further caudally than generally appreciated. Proper mobilization of the visceral aorta requires that the crus be incised with special care taken to avoid the occasional phrenic artery that courses within its substance.

(**B**) The fully mobilized visceral aorta.

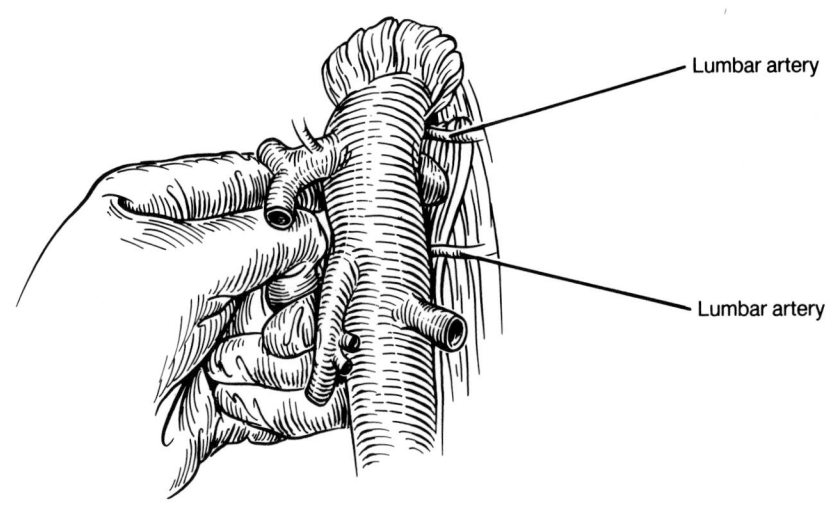

Figure 36-VII-4

Control of Intercostal Arteries

Finger dissection behind the aorta allows recognition of distal intercostal or lumbar arteries; they must be individually clamped to avoid back-bleeding.

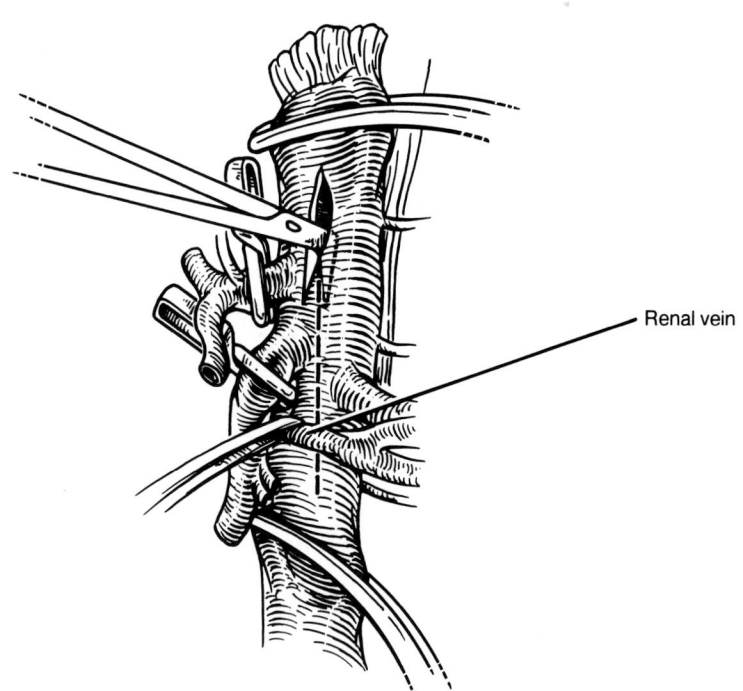

Figure 36-VII-5

Aortotomy

An aortotomy on the left lateral wall of the aorta is made and continues between the superior mesenteric artery orifice and the left renal artery, with care taken to provide an adequate margin for closure.

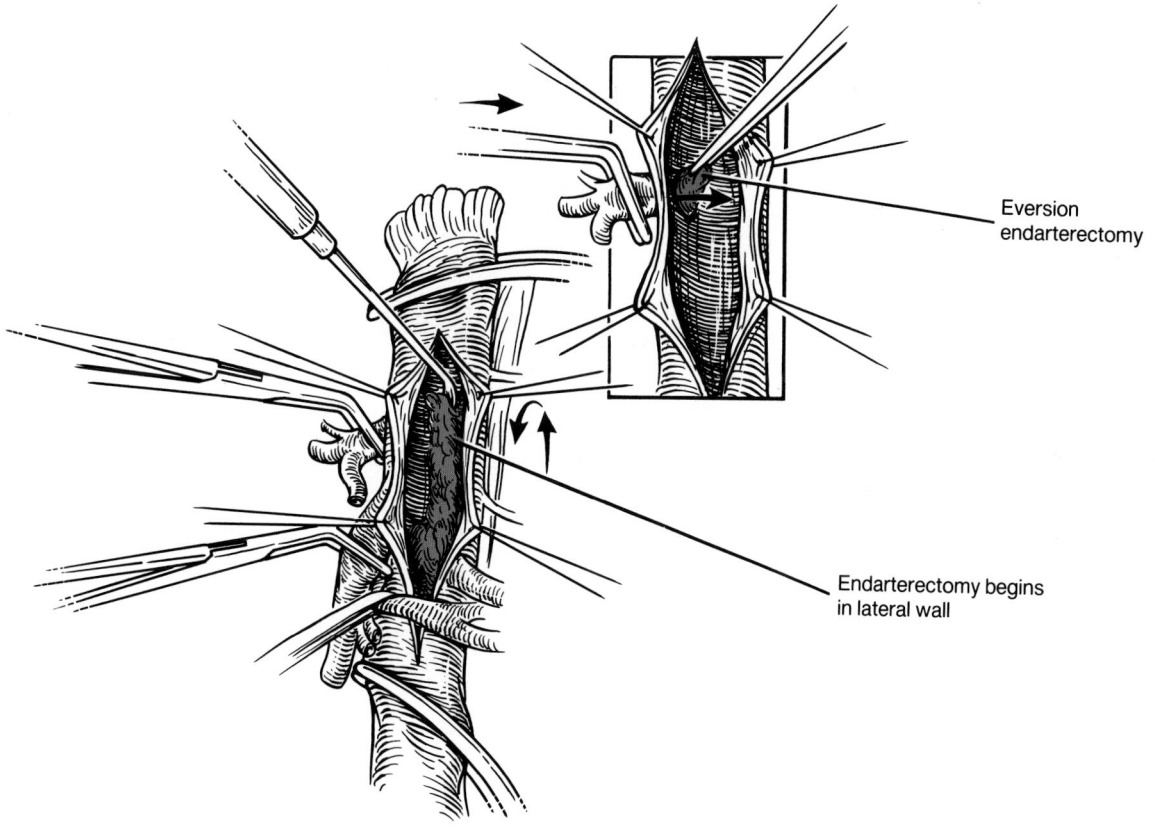

Eversion
endarterectomy

Endarterectomy begins
in lateral wall

Figure 36-VII-6

Endarterectomy

Endarterectomy begins on the left lateral wall of the aorta and proceeds cephalad around the orifices of the visceral vessels. Obtaining the proper plane is key, and gentle traction on the plaque that extends into the visceral vessels combined with intussusception of the luminal contents by a gentle pressure on the visceral artery clamp helps with the eversion endarterectomy (**inset**).

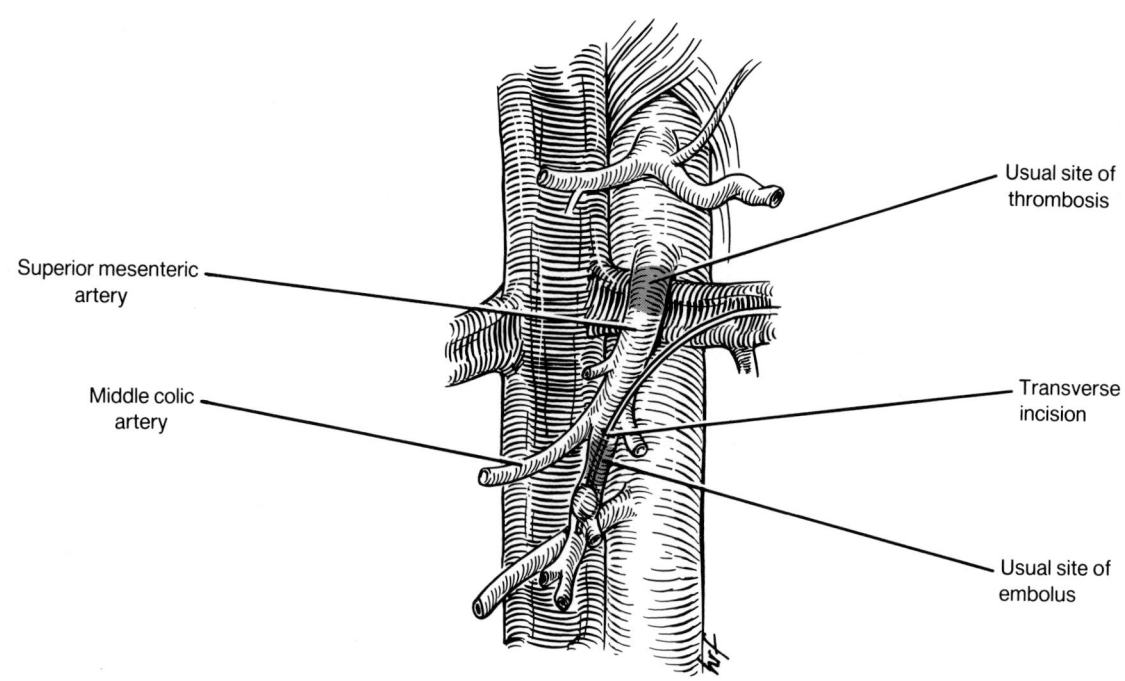

Superior mesenteric artery

Middle colic artery

Usual site of thrombosis

Transverse incision

Usual site of embolus

Figure 36-VII-7

Embolectomy

A superior mesenteric artery embolus usually lodges distal to the origin of the superior mesenteric artery in the region of the middle colic artery, whereas a superior mesenteric artery thrombosis occurs more proximally, at the origin of the vessel.

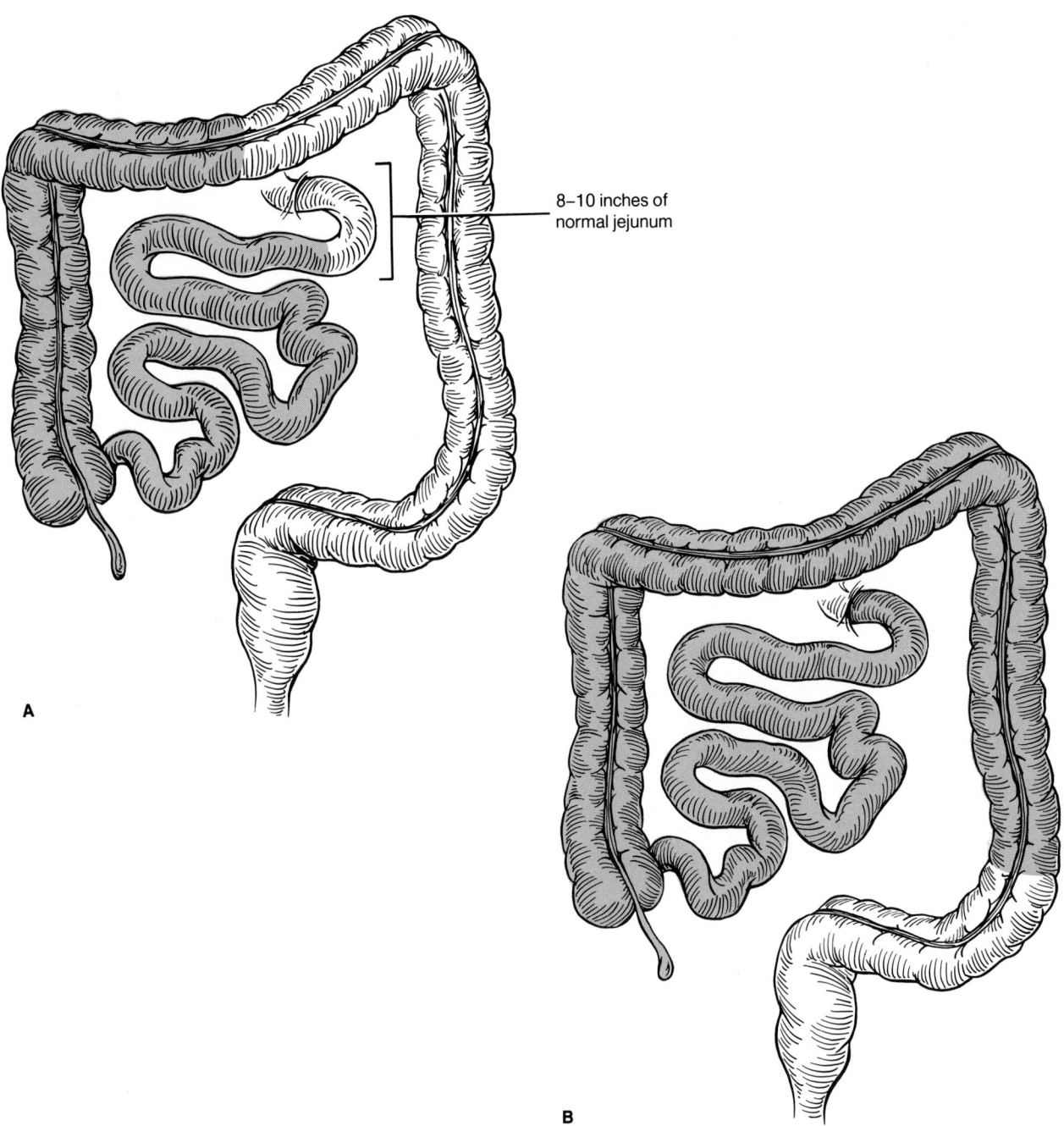

8–10 inches of
normal jejunum

A

B

Figure 36-VII-8

Ischemic Distribution

(**A**) A superior mesenteric artery embolus typically spares the first 8 to 10 inches of jejunum and the colon distal to the mid-colic distribution, including the left half of the transverse colon and the descending colon.

(**B**) A superior mesenteric artery thrombosis results in a more widespread compromise of the intestinal circulation. Virtually all of the small bowel is affected, and more diffuse colonic ischemia occurs.

SECTION VIII *Strictureplasty for Crohn's Disease*

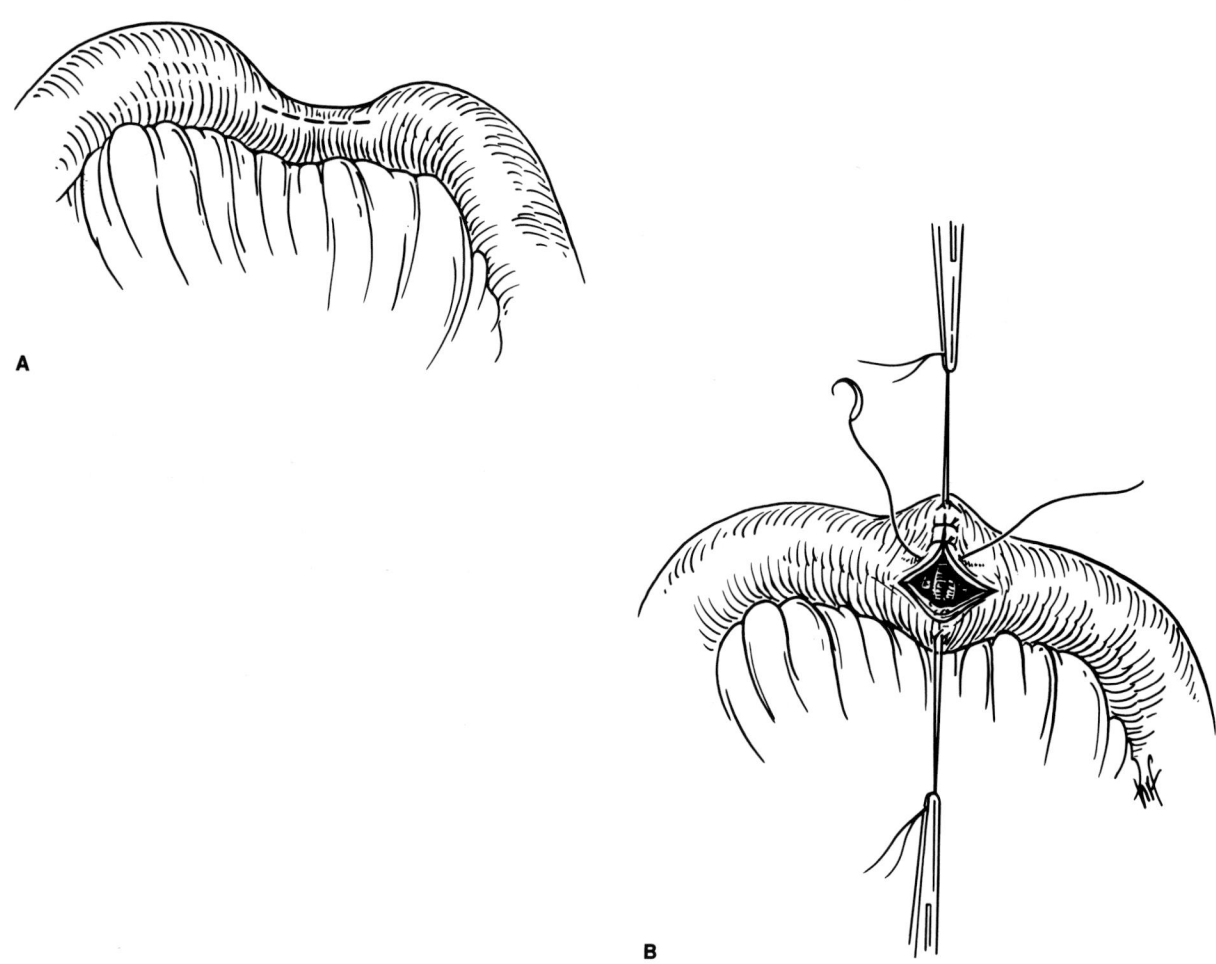

Figure 36-VIII-1

Heineke-Mikulicz Strictureplasty

The Heineke-Mikulicz strictureplasty is appropriate for short stenoses associated with Crohn's disease (up to 7 cm).

(A) A longitudinal incision is created crossing the stricture.

(B) Traction sutures, placed at the midpoints of the incision, are used to transform the longitudinal incision into a transverse incision. Full-thickness nonabsorbable sutures are used to close the incision.

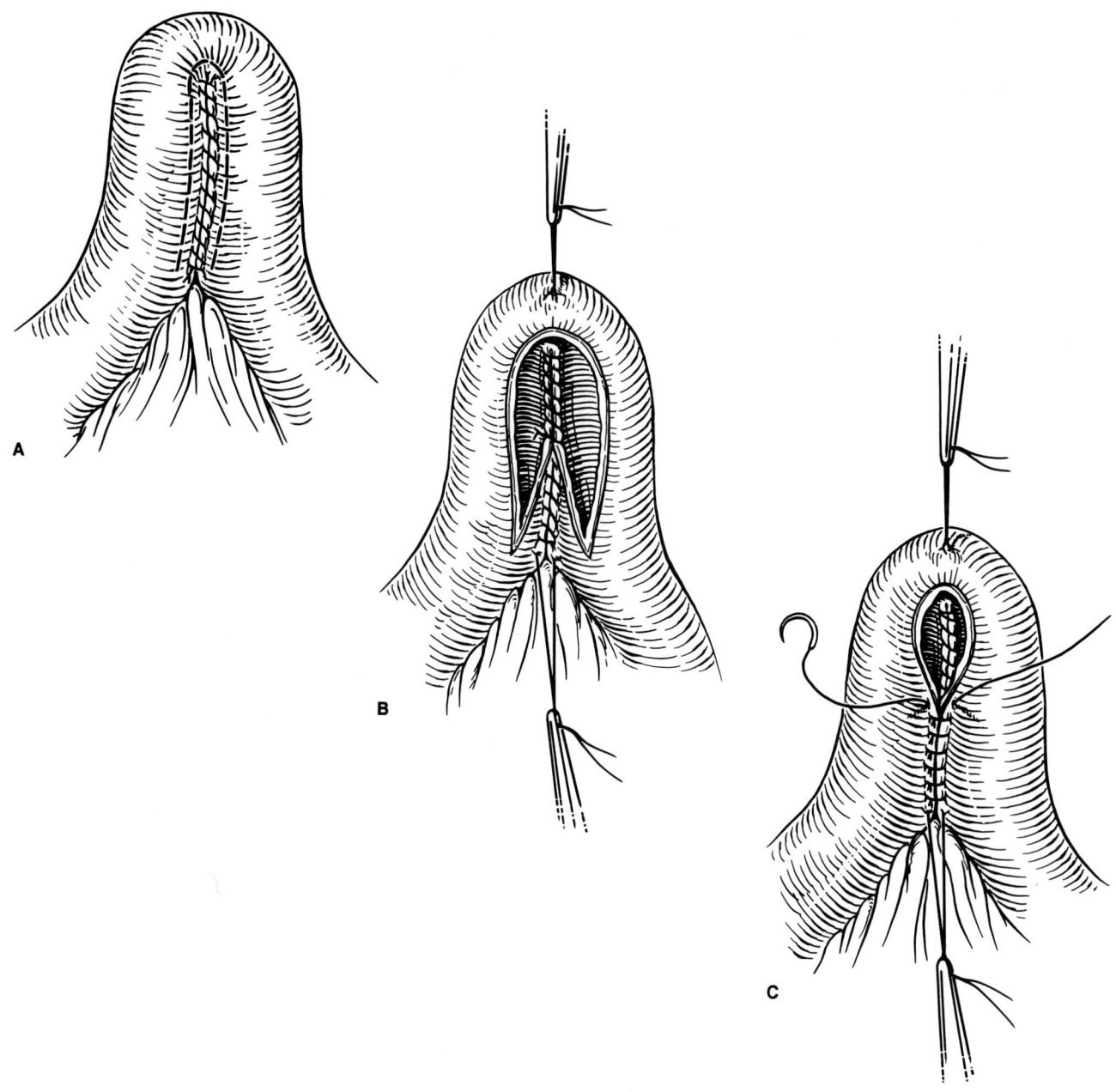

Figure 36-VIII-2

Finney Strictureplasty

For stenoses 7 to 15 cm long, a Finney strictureplasty is preferred.

(**A**) An outer layer of seromuscular nonabsorbable sutures is used to appose bowel proximal and distal to the stricture.

(**B**) An incision is made that traverses the area of narrowing. An inner layer of full-thickness sutures is placed to appose the mucosal edges.

(**C**) The inner suture line is continued anteriorly, and the anastomosis is completed by finishing the outer layer of seromuscular nonabsorbable sutures.

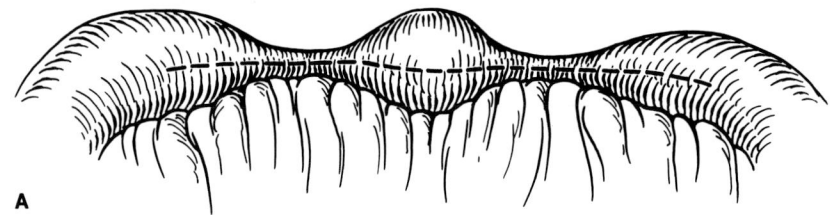

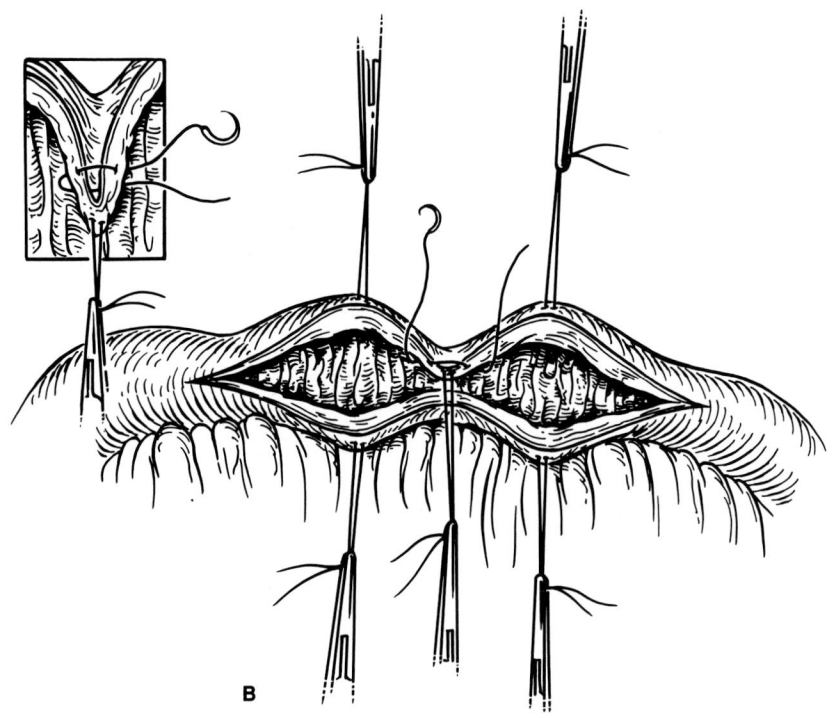

Figure 36-VIII-3

Combined Heineke-Mikulicz and Finney Strictureplasty

A combined Heineke-Mikulicz and Finney strictureplasty can be fashioned for stenoses and skip lesions up to 20 cm long.

(**A**) A longitudinal incision crossing the involved area is created.

(**B**) Sutures are placed at the midpoint of two consecutive strictures, and traction is applied laterally. Subsequently, full-thickness sutures are placed at the midpoint of the saccular dilated segment so that the adjacent narrowed segments are affected.

(**C**) Full-thickness sutures are continued circumferentially, placed so that the knot will lie on the mucosal surface.

(**D**) This placement continues to approximate adjacent segments of bowel while eliminating luminal narrowing.

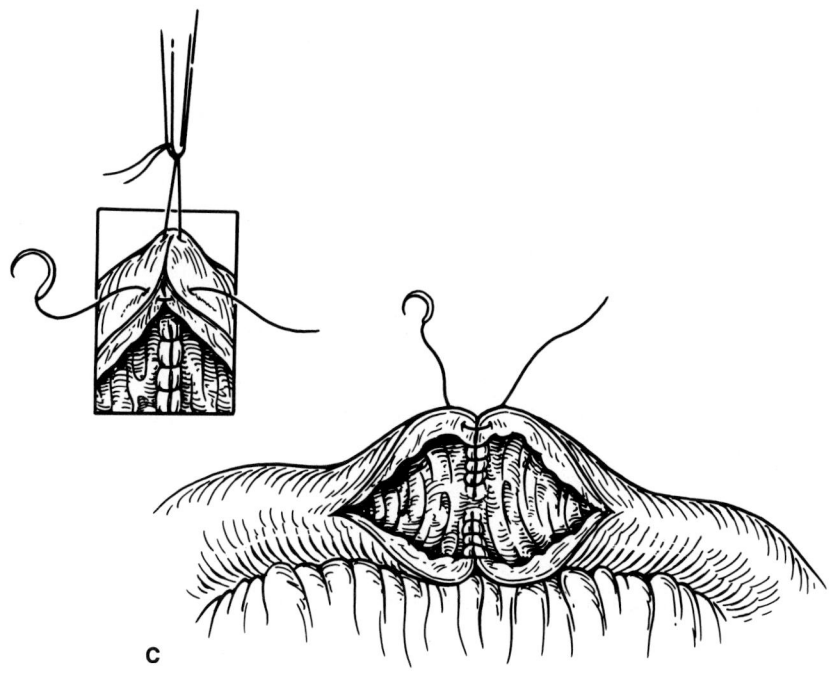

C

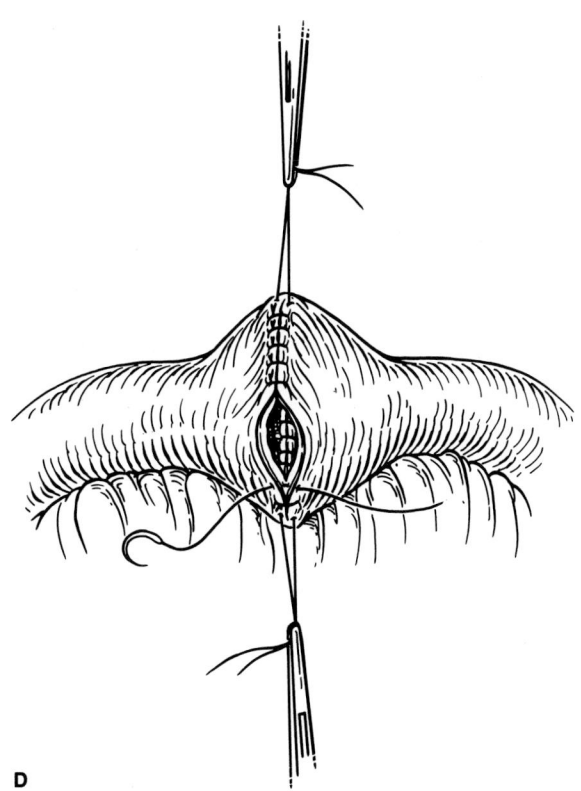

D

Figure 36-VIII-3 *(Continued)*

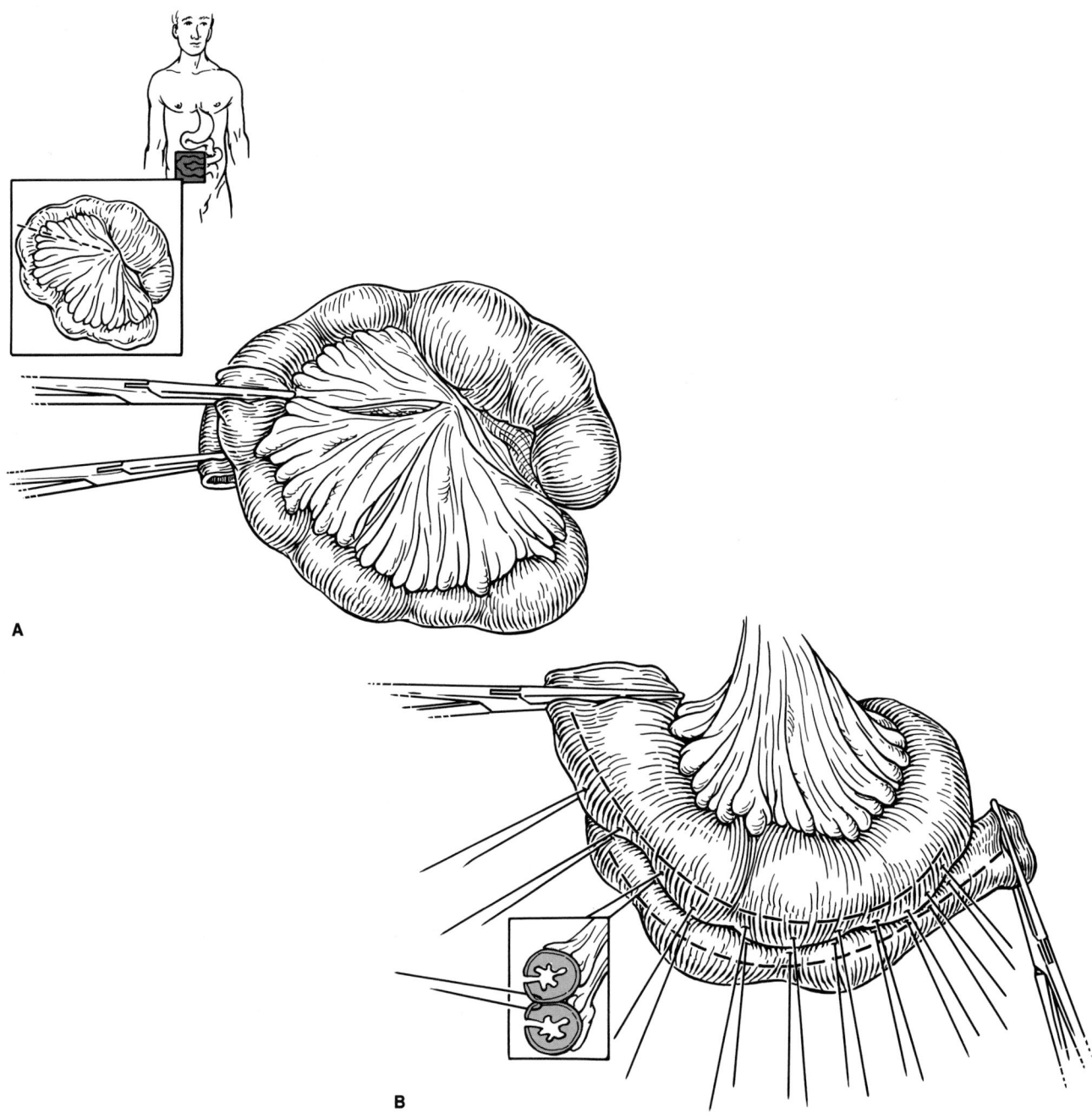

Figure 36-VIII-4

Side-to-Side Isoperistaltic Strictureplasty

Side-to-side isoperistaltic strictureplasty can be used for longer segments affected by stenoses and skip lesions with a combined length of more than 30 cm.

(**A**) The bowel and the mesentery are divided in the middle of the affected segment.

(**B**) The bowel is positioned side-by-side in an isoperistaltic fashion. Nonabsorbable seromuscular sutures are placed from one segment to the other. Parallel longitudinal enterotomies are created along the antimesenteric borders of both segments (**inset**). An inner layer of full-thickness absorbable sutures is used to approximate the mucosal edges.

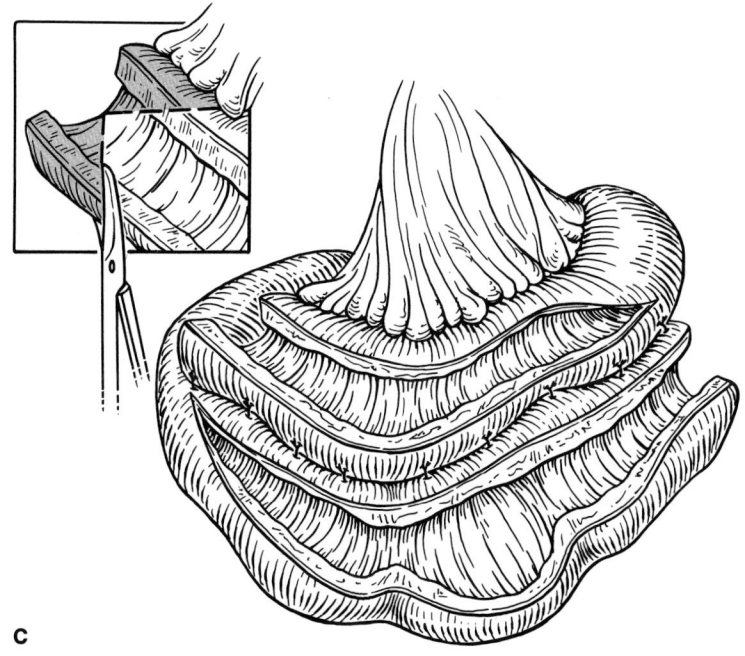

C

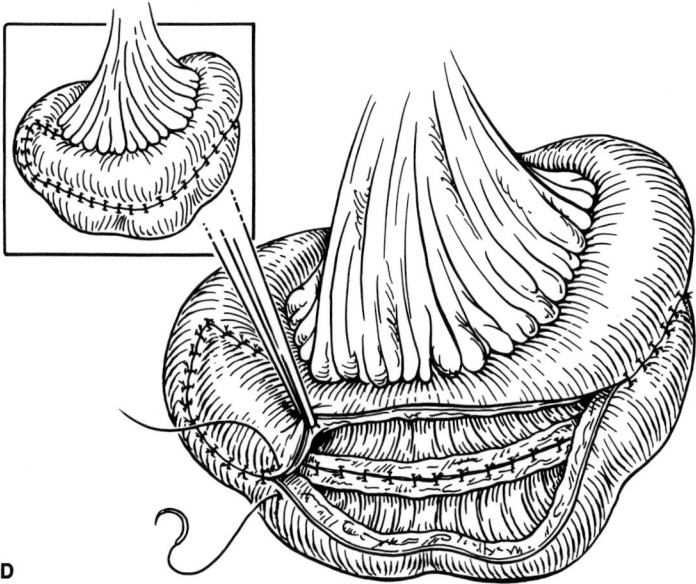

D

Figure 36-VIII-4 *(Continued)*

(C) A wedge-shaped end is created at each point of division of bowel to match the enterotomy performed on the opposite limb of bowel.

(D) The inner layer of full-thickness absorbable sutures and the outer layer of nonabsorbable seromuscular sutures are used to complete the anastomosis.

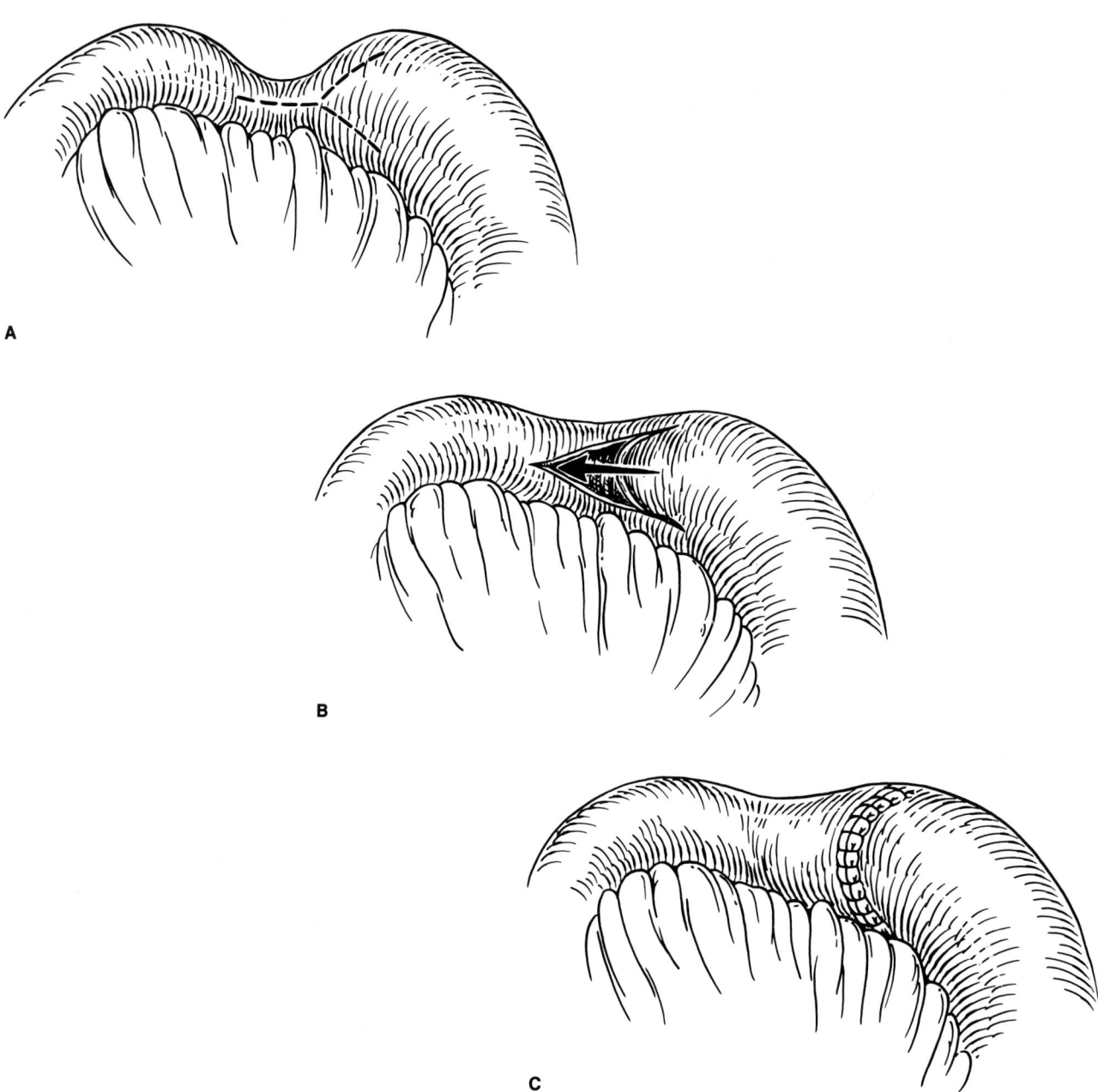

Figure 36-VIII-5

Stenosis and Proximal Dilation

A modification of the Heineke-Mikulicz strictureplasty can be used for lesions that involve stenosis and proximal dilation. A Y-shaped incision (**A**) creates a full-thickness advancement flap (**B**), which is closed with interrupted nonabsorbable sutures (**C**).

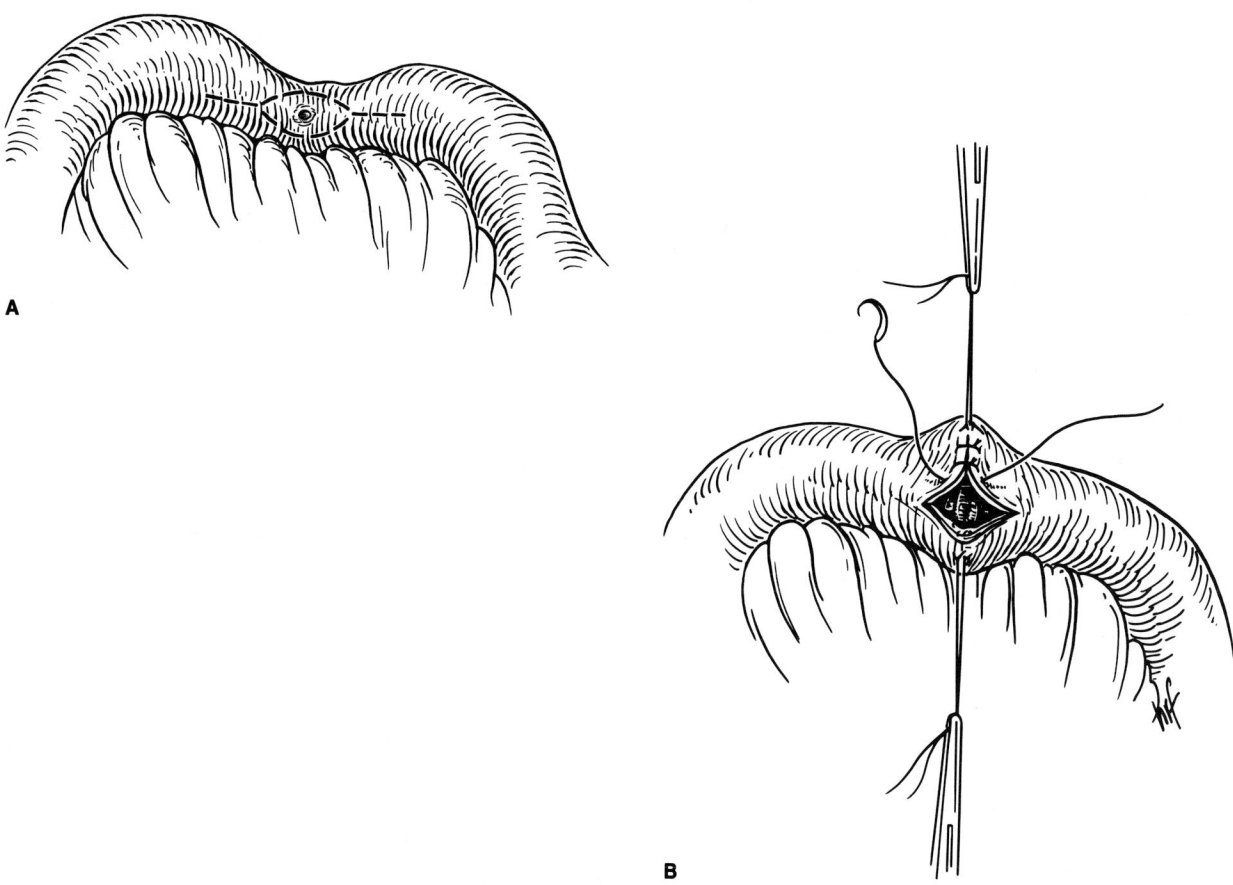

Figure 36-VIII-6

Stenosis and Chronic Fistula

A Judd strictureplasty can be used in the presence of a stenosis with a chronic fistula.

(**A**) The fistulous opening is removed and the edges are débrided.

(**B**) The longitudinal enterostomy is closed in a transverse manner with full-thickness nonabsorbable interrupted sutures.

PART VII

Colon, Rectum, and Anus

Digestive Tract Surgery: A Text and Atlas, edited by Richard H. Bell,
Layton F. Rikkers, and Michael W. Mulholland.
Lippincott-Raven Publishers, Philadelphia, © 1996.

37

Diseases of the Appendix

Michael S. Nussbaum

ACUTE APPENDICITIS

Appendicitis is one of the most common causes of acute
abdominal pain and remains a diagnostic challenge despite advances in laboratory and imaging modalities.
Although appendicitis has been noted since antiquity,
the modern era in the diagnosis and treatment of this
entity began in 1886.[1,2] At that time, the mortality rate
for perforated appendicitis was about 30%. Subsequently, the development of safe operative techniques
for removal of the appendix and the advent of broad-
spectrum antibiotic therapy have reduced the mortality
rate for this disease to less than 1%.[1,3] Successful management of appendicitis depends on prompt diagnosis
and early intervention.

Pathogenesis

Appendicitis is most prevalent in young adults between
the ages of 15 and 25 years; it is less common in infants
and the elderly. However, most deaths resulting from
appendicitis occur at the extremes of age. The pathogenesis of appendicitis is poorly understood, although
several hypotheses have been proposed. The disease is
most common in Western countries and has increased
in prevalence since the late 19th and early 20th centuries. This increase has been attributed to low-fiber diets
that lead to slower fecal transit times, alterations in gut
bacterial flora, and increased intracolonic pressures.[4]
Other factors that may play a role in the development
of appendicitis include familial influences, seasonal factors, enteric viral illnesses, and stressful life events.[1,5]

Luminal obstruction of the appendix appears to be
a key initiating factor in this process. Lymphoid hyperplasia is common in children, teenagers, and young

adults, and is the most frequent cause of luminal obstruction in these age groups. With advancing age, fecaliths, calculi, and luminal fibrosis have a more prominent role. Appendiceal fecaliths and calculi are
associated with an increased risk of complicated appendicitis (eg, perforation, abscess, gangrene).[6] Foreign
bodies, neoplasms, and parasites are less common (5%
to 6%) sources of obstruction.

Once the lumen becomes obstructed, secreted mucus accumulates, leading to an increase in luminal pressure with distention and occlusion of capillaries, venules, and lymphatics (Fig. 37-1). In the presence of
stasis and vascular compromise, luminal bacteria invade the wall of the appendix. Necrosis occurs and progresses to abscess formation or perforation if the process continues unchecked.

Bacterial organisms of colonic origin, such as *Escherichia coli, Staphylococcus epidermidis, Clostridium perfringens,* and other anaerobic species, play a central role
in the inflammatory process.[7,8] Studies have demonstrated increased colonization of the appendix and ileum with anaerobic species (primarily *Bacteroides* and
Fusobacterium sp) in patients with appendicitis as compared with patients undergoing incidental appendectomy.[9] Furthermore, the diversity of bacterial species
cultured from the appendix in patients with complicated disease is much greater than that seen in cultures
of specimens from patients with uncomplicated acute
appendicitis.[10]

Symptoms

Although clinical findings in acute appendicitis can be
variable, certain cardinal symptoms are helpful in making a prompt and accurate diagnosis. A careful history

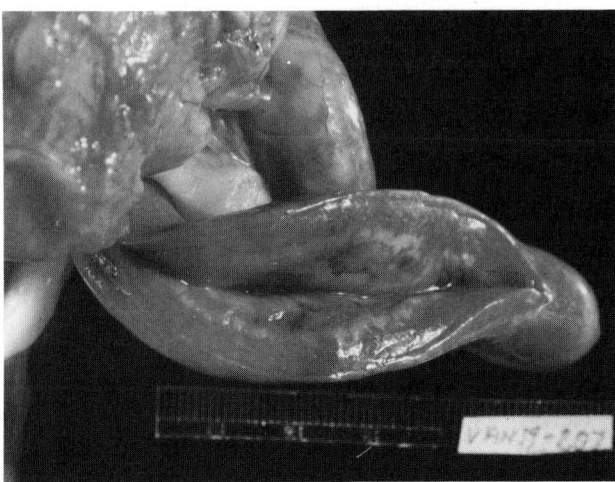

Figure 37-1 Acute nonperforated appendicitis with vascular congestion of the wall and near obliteration of the lumen. (See Color Fig. 37-1.)

and physical examination combined with several laboratory tests should allow the correct diagnosis of appendicitis in over 90% of patients. Appendicitis usually begins with a vague cramping, periumbilical pain that is visceral in nature and thought to be caused by luminal obstruction of the appendix. This early pain can be associated either with constipation accompanied by an urge to defecate or with diarrhea. Diarrhea early in the course is especially common in children with appendicitis. Passage of stool or flatus does not relieve the abdominal discomfort. Anorexia and nausea with or without vomiting generally follow the onset of pain by several hours. If the pain is preceded by anorexia, nausea, and vomiting, appendicitis is unlikely and other diagnoses must be considered.

As the inflammatory response progresses, a localized parietal peritonitis develops, and abdominal pain becomes persistent in the right lower quadrant. Associated with persistent pain is localized muscle spasm (guarding) on palpation of the right lower quadrant. Because the location of the appendix is highly variable, an atypical location (eg, retrocecal, pelvic) may lead to minimal or absent right lower quadrant physical findings. In such patients, additional physical and diagnostic tests may be necessary to diagnose appendicitis accurately.

Diagnostic Evaluation

Physical Findings

Early recognition of the signs and symptoms of appendicitis before the development of peritonitis, gangrene, or perforation is possible in most cases. Despite

advances in imaging modalities and the development of various scoring systems and computer analysis techniques, the key components in diagnosis have remained constant. As described earlier, a history of migratory pain beginning in the umbilical region and settling in the right lower quadrant (McBurney's point) with physical findings of localized muscle spasm and rebound are pathognomonic. Additional findings that support the diagnosis include referred pain in the right lower quadrant on palpation of the left lower quadrant (Rovsing's sign), a heightened sensation to touch and pinprick (cutaneous hyperesthesia) overlying the region of the appendix, and localized distention with tympany in the right lower quadrant. The patient may have mild temperature elevation later in the progression of symptoms, usually after the pain has settled in the right lower abdomen. The temperature rarely rises above 38°C in the presence of uncomplicated appendicitis, and higher temperatures should raise the suspicion of perforation or gangrene. Rectal or pelvic examination may reveal tenderness or a pelvic mass that cannot be appreciated on abdominal examination.

In cases in which the appendix is in an atypical position, further physical maneuvers can aid in the diagnosis. If the appendix is lying behind the cecum or loops of ileum, local signs of inflammation in the right lower quadrant can be markedly diminished. In this position, the inflamed organ is often contiguous with the psoas muscle, and the patient may lie with the right hip flexed to relieve related discomfort. Inflammation in the region of the psoas muscle can be demonstrated by positioning the patient on the left side and extending the hip fully, thus stretching the muscle. An increased sensation of pain is called the iliopsoas sign. When the appendix is situated within the true pelvis, early symptoms are similar to those produced by the appendix in the iliac fossa. Right lower abdominal muscular guarding and localized pain are often absent. The pain is bilateral or suprapubic in nature, and maximal pain is elicited only by performing a rectal examination or by manipulating the internal obturator muscle (obturator sign). If the inflamed appendix is contiguous with the internal obturator muscle, passively flexing the hip (to relax the psoas muscle) and internally rotating the thigh will cause increased pain.

Laboratory Findings

Laboratory studies are of limited value in the early diagnosis of appendicitis. The most valuable laboratory finding, when present, is a leukocytosis of greater than 12,000 cells/μL with a pronounced increase in polymorphonuclear neutrophils. Although as many as 30% of patients with appendicitis have a normal leukocyte count, over 95% have an abnormal differential with an increase in immature forms. In one series of 97 patients,[11] total leukocyte count was not predictive of a diagnosis of appendicitis, whereas an increased number of metamyelocytes in the peripheral blood smear was predictive. An elevated leukocyte count (greater than 20,000 cells/μL) is usually indicative of appendiceal rupture. Other laboratory tests are helpful primarily for identifying alternative causes of the patient's symptoms rather than for confirming the diagnosis of appendicitis. Although a urinalysis is important to rule out urinary tract pathology that may mimic acute appendicitis, abnormal results with microscopic pyuria or hematuria are seen in 20% to 30% of patients with acute appendicitis. These abnormalities are probably caused by a local inflammatory reaction in the ureter or bladder in proximity to the inflamed appendix, especially when the appendix is ruptured or is in the retrocecal or pelvic position.[12,13]

Roentgenologic Findings

In straightforward cases of acute appendicitis, the use of abdominal radiographs is of little additional diagnostic value. When patients have questionable clinical findings, plain abdominal films and more sophisticated imaging studies can be helpful in differentiating appendicitis and excluding other abdominal conditions. The most helpful radiologic finding in patients with appendicitis is an appendiceal fecalith or calculus (Fig. 37-2). Fecaliths are much more common in patients with acute appendicitis than in the general population.[6] These concretions are more frequently associated with perforated appendicitis or abscess formation. Therefore, the presence of a radiopaque appendicolith on radiographs in a patient with equivocal right lower abdominal findings should influence the decision toward earlier surgical exploration. Additional radiologic findings associated with acute appendicitis may be subtle. These include gas in the appendix (rare), localized right lower quadrant ileus, absent bowel gas patterns in the right lower abdomen, right lower quadrant soft tissue density, deformity of the cecal outline, loss of the right properitoneal fat strip, separation of the cecal contents from the right properitoneal fat, gas in a right lower quadrant abscess, and loss of the right psoas muscle shadow. Taken individually, any one of these findings has little significance, but in the presence of multiple signs, the likelihood of appendicitis is greatly increased. Abnormal findings on abdominal radiographs depend on the extent of inflammation in the appendix and adjacent tissues, and plain abdominal radiographs are of little value in the diagnosis of early acute appendicitis.[14]

Barium enema is of limited usefulness in the rou-

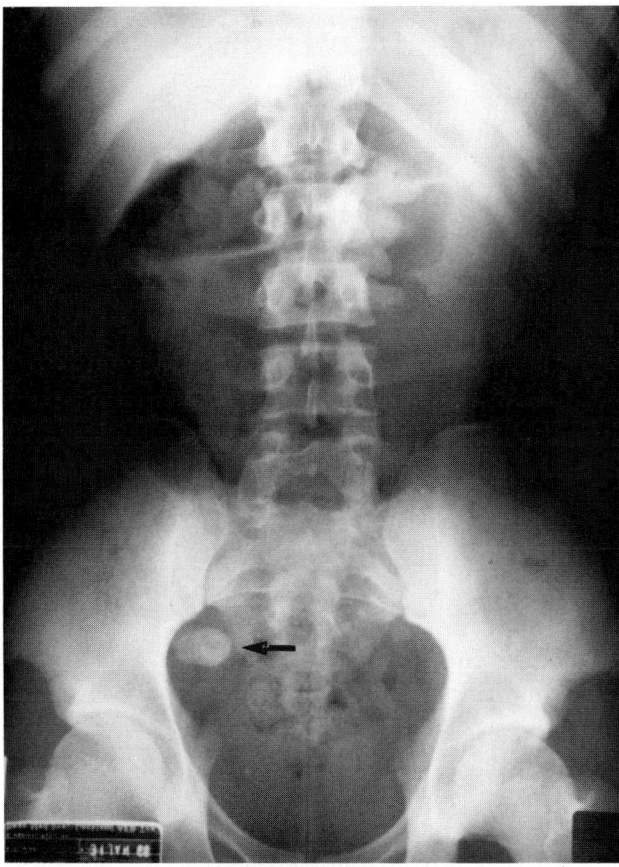

Figure 37-2 Plain abdominal radiograph demonstrating a large appendicolith in the right lower quadrant (*arrow*).

tine diagnosis of appendicitis but can be helpful as an adjunctive test in atypical or equivocal cases. Barium enema examination can be performed as a single contrast technique, without bowel preparation, with no increased risk to patients with appendicitis. Cecal deformity or flattening in combination with nonfilling of the appendix and irritability or spasm of the cecum or terminal ileum are characteristic findings on barium enema (Fig. 37-3). In a recent prospective analysis,[15] barium enema was found to have a negative predictive value of 95% and a positive predictive value of 88%; in the presence of equivocal clinical data, the rate of negative exploration was reduced to 7.2%.

Ultrasonography is a readily available, inexpensive, noninvasive test that, in experienced hands, can be accurate in diagnosing appendicitis (Fig. 37-4). As with barium enema, this modality is most useful as a means of improving decision making in patients with ambiguous clinical findings. Sonography is particularly helpful in women for identifying pelvic and adnexal abnormalities that can mimic the symptoms of appendicitis. In recent years, graded compression ultrasonography of the cecum and

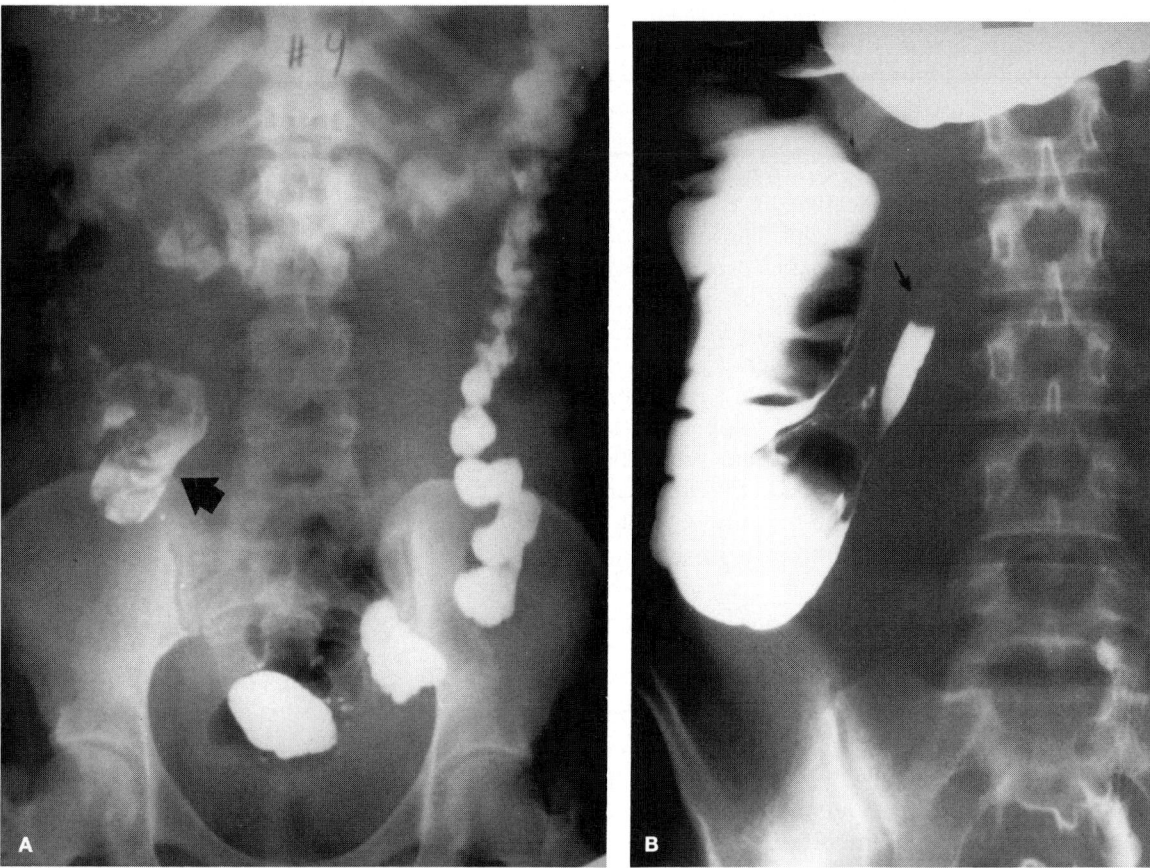

Figure 37-3 Findings on barium enema in patients with appendicitis. (**A**) A cecal deformity (*arrow*) is seen in combination with nonfilling of the appendix. (**B**) Partial filling of the appendix is seen with a fecalith in the tip of the appendix (*arrow*).

appendix has been used in the evaluation of equivocal cases. The most frequent findings in acute appendicitis are noncompressibility of the appendix with a wall diameter greater than 6 mm.[16] By applying these criteria, ultrasonography has been shown to be accurate in evaluation of the appendix, with a reported sensitivity of 75% to 93%, a specificity of 71% to 100%, a positive predictive value of 70% to 80%, and a negative predictive value of nearly 100%.[17–20] Ultrasound appears to permit earlier diagnosis while minimizing the rate of appendectomy in patients with normal appendices.

Another roentgenologic modality for evaluating patients with ambiguous clinical findings is computed tomography (CT). With a reported accuracy rate of 93%, a sensitivity of 98%, a specificity of 83%, and predictive values over 90%, CT is superior to barium enema and compares favorably with ultrasound.[21] Whereas ultrasound can be restricted by excessive obesity or overlying gas-filled loops of small bowel, CT has no such limitations (Fig. 37-5). CT can visualize an appendicolith or an abnormal appendix on cross section or longitudinal section. The

inflamed appendix usually appears as a fluid-filled tubular structure with an enhanced, thickened outer wall. Fluid-filled loops of terminal ileum may be misinterpreted as distended inflamed appendices, and it is important to allow for adequate filling of the terminal ileum and cecum with contrast material to avoid this pitfall. The most common CT finding suggestive of appendicitis is pericecal inflammation, which appears as increased density of pericolic fat. Extensive pericecal inflammation with streaky opacities may represent phlegmons, whereas poorly defined fluid collections constitute abscesses in more advanced cases. The finding of inflammatory changes adjacent to the cecum without visualization of an appendicolith or abnormal appendix is suggestive, but not diagnostic, of appendicitis.[21] In addition to its diagnostic accuracy, CT is of great value in determining the nature and extent of the disease process. If an abscess is identified, CT-guided drainage can be used as a therapeutic modality. CT can also identify other intraabdominal processes unrelated to appendicitis that may explain the patient's symptoms.

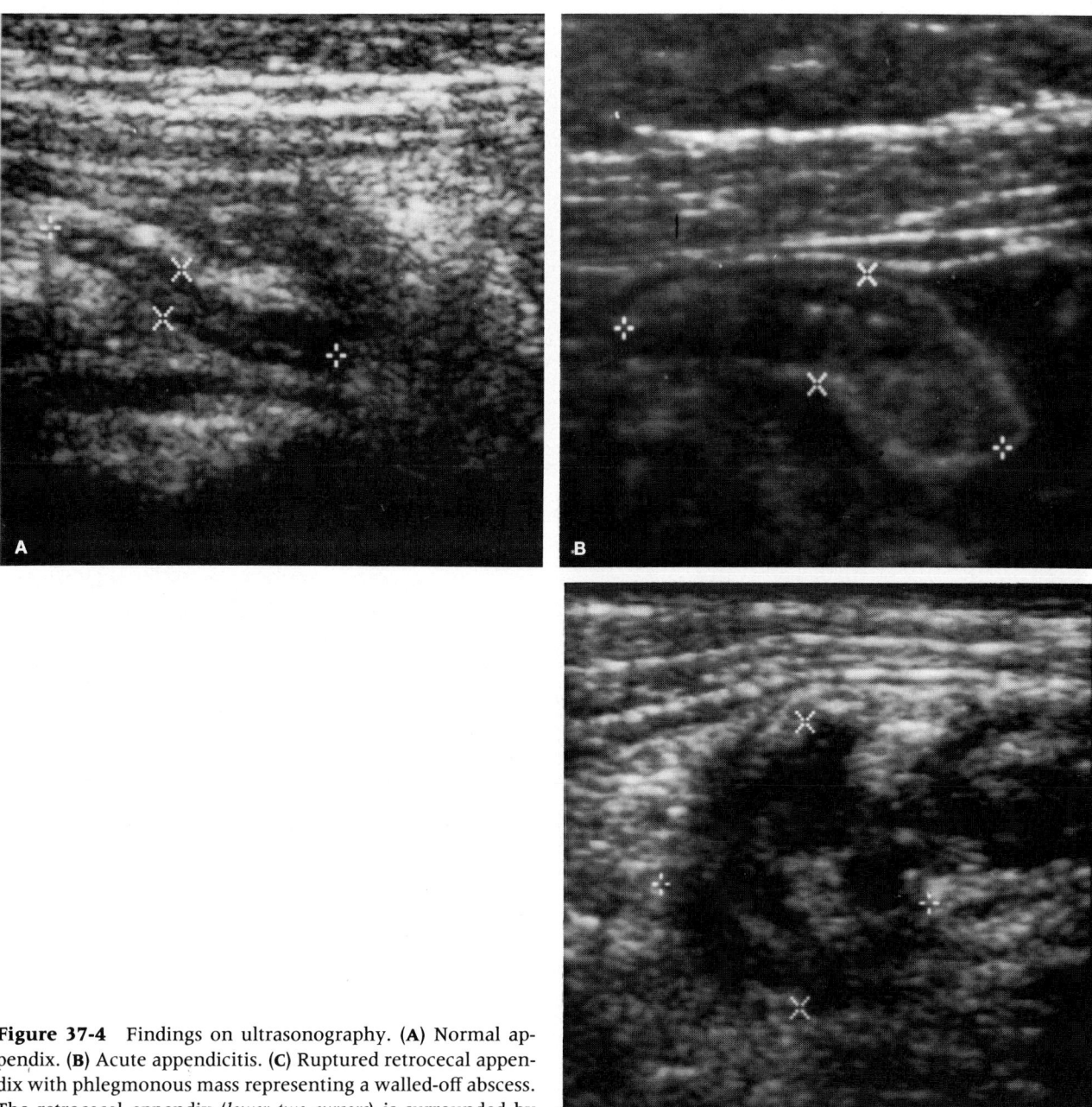

Figure 37-4 Findings on ultrasonography. (**A**) Normal appendix. (**B**) Acute appendicitis. (**C**) Ruptured retrocecal appendix with phlegmonous mass representing a walled-off abscess. The retrocecal appendix (*lower two cursors*) is surrounded by echogenic amorphous material, representing the phlegmon.

Special Circumstances

Infants and Young Children

Appendicitis in childhood remains a serious surgical disorder with reported complication rates as high as 40%. Increased morbidity results from numerous interrelated factors. The initial presentation can mimic gastroenteritis (eg, cramping pain, diarrhea), and children may be unable to communicate effectively the nature of the symptoms. The appendix in children has thinner walls, allowing for more rapid penetration of the infection and earlier perforation. The reported incidence of perforation in children ranges from 30% to 59%, depending on the age range studied.[22–27] Because of the immature omentum in young children, generalized peritonitis is more common in this age group than are well walled-off phlegmons or abscesses. Greater elevation of the temperature and leukocyte count is strongly

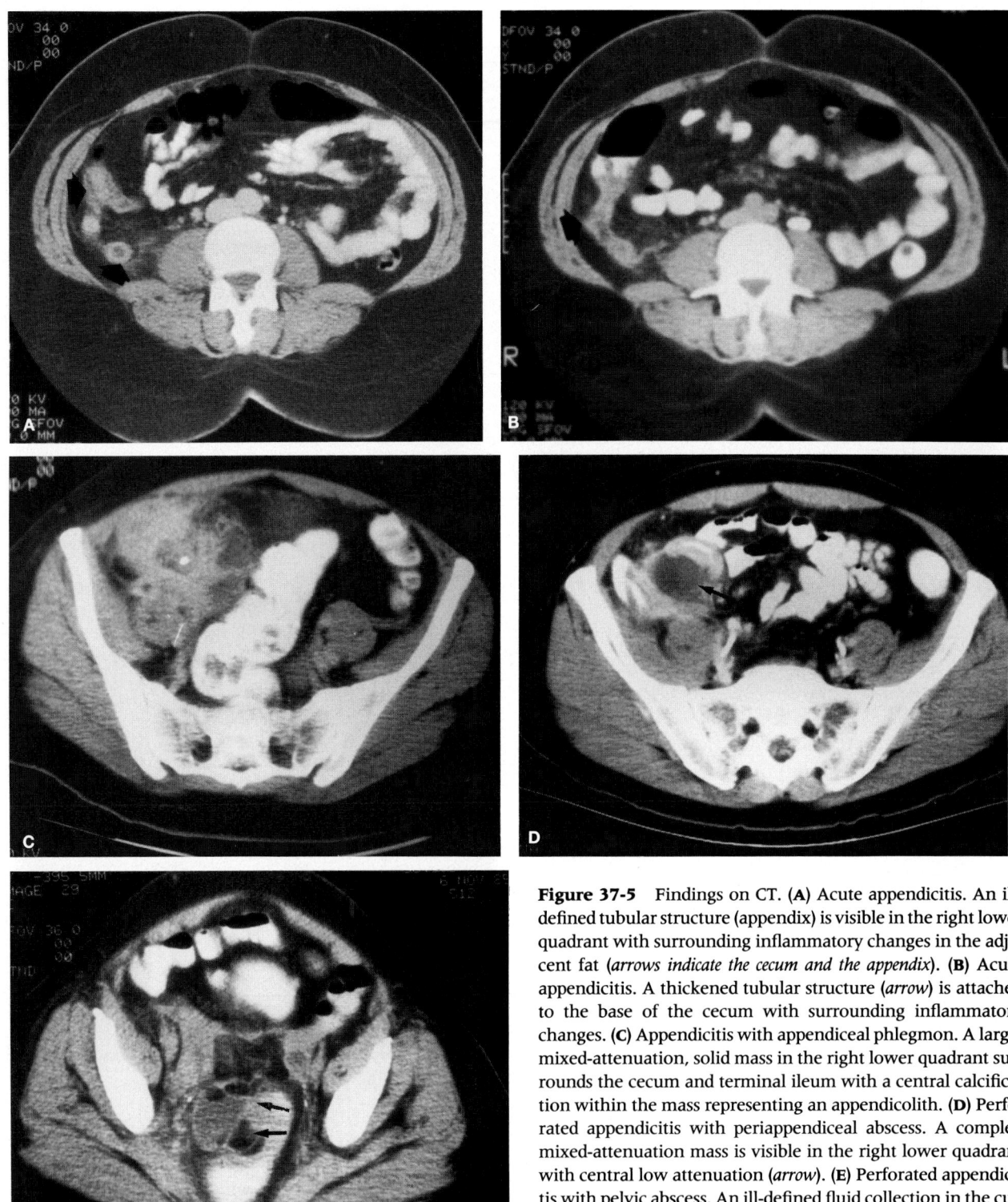

Figure 37-5 Findings on CT. (**A**) Acute appendicitis. An ill-defined tubular structure (appendix) is visible in the right lower quadrant with surrounding inflammatory changes in the adjacent fat (*arrows indicate the cecum and the appendix*). (**B**) Acute appendicitis. A thickened tubular structure (*arrow*) is attached to the base of the cecum with surrounding inflammatory changes. (**C**) Appendicitis with appendiceal phlegmon. A large, mixed-attenuation, solid mass in the right lower quadrant surrounds the cecum and terminal ileum with a central calcification within the mass representing an appendicolith. (**D**) Perforated appendicitis with periappendiceal abscess. A complex mixed-attenuation mass is visible in the right lower quadrant with central low attenuation (*arrow*). (**E**) Perforated appendicitis with pelvic abscess. An ill-defined fluid collection in the cul-de-sac with associated rectal wall thickening, stranding of the pelvic fat, and infiltration of the mesenteric and retroperitoneal fat extending along the right psoas muscle into the retrocecal tissues (*arrows*).

suggestive of perforation in children.[27] Careful attention to physical findings, especially localized right lower quadrant tenderness, is key to the prompt recognition and treatment of appendicitis in children.

Elderly Patients

Acute appendicitis affects about 7% of the population. Its peak incidence occurs between the ages of 15 and 24 years.[28] The risk of appendicitis decreases to about 2% after the age of 50 years and falls to 1.2% to 2.1% after the age of 80 years.[29–31] The mortality rate for appendicitis is between 0.8% and 1.6% in the general population,[30] but over 20% among persons older than 80 years.[31,32] Mortality and morbidity are related primarily to infectious complications resulting from perforation of the appendix.

Elderly patients tend to have less typical symptoms than their younger counterparts, complaining of a more diffuse abdominal pain that is poorly localized or localizes to the mid-abdomen. Careful attention to the physical examination usually reveals right lower abdominal tenderness in most patients. Abdominal distention with an ileus pattern on radiography occurs more frequently in older patients. Because of the atypical presentation, diagnosis and surgical intervention may be delayed. In addition, aging leads to changes in the morphology of the appendix that make the organ structurally weak, with decreased vascularity. These changes include thinning of the mucosa, decreased lymphoid tissue, obliteration of the lumen, fibrosis of the wall, and atherosclerotic changes within the appendiceal artery. Less intraluminal pressure is required to rupture the appendix and the pathologic evolution of the disease is more rapid, often without any prodromal phase.

Delayed diagnosis and the morphologic changes associated with aging make perforation a more common event in older patients (32% to 92%).[31,33] The increased incidence of perforation combined with the diminished physiologic reserve of older patients and their decreased ability to handle infectious complications explain the increased mortality and morbidity described in this population. Conversely, the complication rate for surgery performed for a false-positive diagnosis of appendicitis is low in this group of patients. Therefore, as in the very young, a low threshold for proceeding with surgery is warranted in patients older than 50 years.

Pregnant Patients

Appendicitis is the most common acute abdominal condition requiring operation during pregnancy, with a reported incidence of 1 case per 1500 to 6600 pregnancies.[34] When it is associated with perforation and peritonitis, there is considerable maternal morbidity and mortality, as well as significant fetal loss. Pregnant women are at no greater risk for the development of appendicitis than are members of the general population.[34] The occurrence of appendicitis is equally distributed throughout pregnancy and the natural history of appendicitis is not affected by the stage of pregnancy.[35,36]

The clinical presentation of appendicitis during pregnancy is variable. The early signs of nausea and vomiting may be overlooked and confused with preexisting complaints related to the pregnancy. Early in gestation, the appendix is in its normal position and symptoms are typical, with the development of visceral pain, followed by nausea and vomiting, progressing to right lower quadrant pain and muscle spasm. As the pregnancy progresses, signs and symptoms become less typical. With progressive enlargement of the uterus, the appendix is displaced upward and the tip is rotated counterclockwise into the right upper quadrant.[37] With this displacement, pain becomes less characteristic and may be located on the right side, flank, or upper quadrant. Simultaneously, the abdominal wall is lifted away from the appendix and muscular laxity occurs, obscuring typical guarding and rebound tenderness. Persistent abdominal pain remains the most important symptom in these patients and should never be ignored. A useful test to discern whether the pain is adnexal or uterine in origin is to turn the patient on her left side; if the point of maximal tenderness shifts, the source of the pain is more likely adnexal or uterine.

Leukocytosis is common in pregnancy, and leukocyte counts can be as high as 12,000 to 15,000 cells/μL normally. However, a rising count on serial studies or a shift toward immature forms is indicative of an infectious process. Pyuria and bacteriuria are common in pregnant women and can be misleading in this situation. Roentgenologic studies are rarely helpful in the evaluation of pregnant patients with suspected appendicitis and should not be used during the first trimester. Ultrasonography can be useful in evaluating the appendix using the graded compression technique. In addition, the status of the fetus, placenta, uterus, adnexa, and pelvic cavity can be evaluated for other causes of the patient's symptoms.

Many abnormalities can mimic appendicitis during pregnancy, the most common being pyelonephritis. Pyelonephritis is more common in pregnancy due to the mechanical effect of the gravid uterus on the ureter. However, pyuria and hematuria can also result from extraluminal irritation of the ureter or collecting system by an inflamed appendix. Thus, interpretation of abnormal results on urinalysis in the face of right flank pain during pregnancy is often misleading. Other diagnoses include nephrolithiasis, torsion of an ovary or ovarian cyst, ectopic pregnancy, salpingitis, round ligament pain, ovarian vein thrombosis, cholecystitis, and inflammatory bowel disease.

The risks to the mother and fetus when appendectomy is performed for nonperforated appendicitis or for a normal appendix are minimal.[34] Routine appendectomy does cause a slight increase in premature labor within the first week after operation, decreased mean birth weight, and increased early infant mortality. However, these risks are overshadowed by the markedly increased maternal morbidity and infant mortality that occur with delayed diagnosis and perforated appendicitis.[34,38] When the appendix is located high in the peritoneal cavity, localization appears to be hampered and the large uterus markedly reduces the ability of the omentum to isolate the appendix. Therefore, perforation in pregnancy often leads to generalized peritonitis and the increased virulence associated with this complication. Pregnancy should never be a reason to delay operation. If there is a reasonable suspicion that a patient has appendicitis, early surgical intervention is indicated.

Immunosuppressed or Immunodeficient Patients

The signs and symptoms of acute inflammation that are associated with appendicitis can be blunted or entirely absent in patients who are immunocompromised. Patients who are receiving immunosuppressive therapy—as well as those with leukemia, aplastic anemia, acquired immunodeficiency syndrome, and diabetes—must be considered in this category. In this setting, right lower quadrant symptoms can result from many causes, including appendicitis, diverticulitis, pelvic abscess, pseudomembranous colitis, intestinal hemorrhage, and typhlitis.[39] Because all these entities have similar presentations, distinguishing between them is often difficult. In addition, the usual signs and symptoms may be masked because of the immunosuppressed condition. Physical examination may not be revealing in these situations, and additional diagnostic modalities such as barium enema, graded compression sonography, or CT can play an important role in the evaluation and differential diagnosis.

Differential Diagnosis

Because the signs and symptoms of acute appendicitis can mimic those of nearly any intraabdominal process, the ability to diagnose acute appendicitis requires clear knowledge of acute abdominal pain.[40] In differentiat-

ing the potential causes for a patient's complaints, it is helpful to categorize the possible diagnoses according to age and gender.

Young Children

Gastroenteritis is a frequent disorder that can mimic the symptoms of acute appendicitis, with abdominal pain, diarrhea, nausea, and vomiting. Pain is usually generalized, rather than localized in the right lower quadrant. Vomiting generally precedes the development of abdominal pain in gastroenteritis. Other nonabdominal complaints, such as headache, myalgia, and upper respiratory tract symptoms, may precede or accompany the symptoms of gastroenteritis. Alternative diagnoses to consider in young children include mesenteric adenitis, Meckel's diverticulitis, intussusception, enteric duplication, Henoch-Schönlein purpura, diaphragmatic pleurisy secondary to a posterobasilar pneumonia, and unsuspected abdominal trauma or child abuse. The diagnosis can usually be differentiated by a few simple laboratory tests.

Teenagers and Young Adults

Gastroenteritis and mesenteric adenitis are prominent causes of abdominal complaints that mimic appendicitis in teenagers and young adults. The peak age of onset of regional enteritis occurs in the second and third decades of life. The most common segment of the intestine involved with regional enteritis is the terminal ileum and right colon. Thus, the acute development of an inflammatory mass in the right iliac fossa may be indistinguishable from appendicitis, and it is not unusual to make the initial diagnosis of regional enteritis at the time of exploration for presumed acute appendicitis. Other entities that are common in this age group include infectious mononucleosis, hepatitis, posterobasilar pneumonia, renal or ureteral calculus, and urinary tract infection. Occult trauma or abuse is common in this population, and evidence of abnormal bruising on physical examination should raise this suspicion.

The acute onset of diabetes with diabetic ketoacidosis can cause severe abdominal pain and muscular rigidity. Abdominal symptoms should resolve rapidly with treatment of the ketoacidosis. Testicular abnormalities such as torsion or epididymitis can cause referred pain to the right lower abdomen. Women in this age group may have a variety of gynecologic abnormalities that closely simulate appendicitis, including mittelschmerz, pelvic inflammatory disease (PID), ectopic or normal pregnancy, endometriosis, ruptured ovarian cyst, and ovarian torsion. A complete gynecologic evaluation, including speculum and bimanual pelvic examination, cervical culture, pregnancy testing, and pelvic ultrasonography, is essential in the evaluation of most young women who have symptoms suggestive of appendicitis.

Older Adults

All the entities listed for teenagers and young adults are also common causes of appendicitis-like symptoms in older adults. With aging, many inflammatory and neoplastic abnormalities arise that can be confused with acute appendicitis. One of the most frequent causes of acute peritoneal inflammation in older patients is diverticulitis. The pathogenesis of diverticulitis and appendicitis is identical—obstruction of a diverticulum of the colon. Thus, the sequence of symptoms observed in diverticulitis may be identical to that of appendicitis, but subtle differences can help distinguish the two. Because the sigmoid colon is a hindgut structure, the early visceral pain of diverticulitis is more likely to be hypogastric or suprapubic in nature. Anorexia, nausea, and vomiting are less prominent than with appendicitis. The shift of pain and tenderness associated with parietal peritoneal irritation is usually to an area above the pubis or to the left lower abdomen. Fever and leukocytosis tend to be more pronounced in diverticulitis. Other inflammatory disorders that can be confused with appendicitis include acute cholecystitis, perforated gastric or duodenal ulcer, pancreatitis, torsion or infarction of omentum or epiploic appendix, and prostatitis.

Intestinal obstruction–ileus can develop in conjunction with complicated appendicitis with either perforation or abscess, but it can also result from unrelated causes such as adhesions, hernia, or neoplasm. Carcinoma of the cecum can cause pain in the right iliac region, with a palpable mass that may be indistinguishable from an appendiceal abscess. A history of previous subacute pain in this region, weight loss, and the finding of anemia favor a diagnosis of carcinoma of the colon. Similarly, gynecologic neoplasms in women may also present as a painful right lower abdominal or suprapubic mass that must be differentiated from appendicitis. In patients with peripheral vascular disease or embolic disorders, mesenteric vascular accidents and ruptured abdominal aortoiliac aneurysms can be confused with acute appendicitis in the early phases of these disorders. Pain out of proportion to physical findings should raise the suspicion of mesenteric ischemia, whereas a painful pulsatile mass associated with back or flank pain is characteristic of aneurysmal disease.

The differential diagnosis of appendicitis is relatively straightforward, despite the extensive list of abnormalities that can be confused with this disease. The conditions that account for one third of the errors in diagnosis in women and for two thirds of the errors in men are mesenteric adenitis, gastroenteritis, and abdominal pain of unknown etiology. The historic features, physical findings, and laboratory studies of these disorders are similar. However, certain features distinguish them from appendicitis. Tenderness on palpation is less likely to be well localized in the right lower quadrant, and rebound tenderness is less frequent. In addition, the leukocyte count tends to be lower in these conditions. The other major alternative diagnosis that accounts for most errors in diagnosis in women is PID. PID has a longer duration and gastrointestinal symptoms are less common. Nausea and vomiting occur only half as frequently as in appendicitis. Anorexia is almost always present in appendicitis, whereas patients with PID may be hungry. A history of the last menstrual period beginning within 7 days of presentation is a helpful feature in PID, as is the presence of fever with rigors. The physical finding of bilateral lower abdominal pain and cervical motion tenderness is also more characteristic in PID.[29]

Complications

Left untreated, an acute attack of appendicitis is likely to progress to perforation, resulting in a localized abscess or generalized peritonitis. Perforation occurs in 19% to 32% of patients, and the morbidity and mortality rates in appendicitis are directly related to the presence or absence of perforation. Overall, the mortality rate of appendicitis is about 1%. In nonperforated appendicitis, the complication rate is only 3.1% and the mortality rate ranges from 0.2% to 0.3%; with perforation, the morbidity rate rises to 20% to 50% and the mortality rate is about 8.5%.[41] Little progress has been made in lowering these figures, even with the advent of newer antibiotics and more sophisticated imaging modalities.[42] The single most important factor leading to perforation is patient delay in seeking medical attention,[43] and the most important factor in reducing mortality and morbidity is earlier diagnosis. Suspicion for perforation should increase when the duration of symptoms exceeds 24 hours, the temperature is above 38°C, the leukocyte count is higher than 15,000 cells/μL, and right lower quadrant symptoms progress to generalized signs of diffuse peritonitis.[41]

Additional factors associated with an increased incidence of perforation include patients at the extremes of age and those with concomitant serious medical diseases such as diabetes, cancer, coronary artery disease, hypertension, chronic pulmonary disease, and obesity. Perforation is least common in the group with the highest frequency of appendicitis (age 15 to 25 years), and most common in patients younger than 10 years or older than 80 years. These differences may be related to the structural and morphologic differences in the appendix in these patients (see earlier), which predispose them to more rapid progression to perforation. In addition, delay in treatment is more common at the extremes of age. Young children or infants may be unable to communicate effectively the nature of their symptoms until they have progressed to peritonitis or abscess formation. Similarly, elderly patients tend to wait nearly twice as long to seek medical attention as do younger patients.[43] Associated medical illness contributes significantly to postoperative mortality.

Appendiceal abscess rather than diffuse peritonitis results when the perforated appendix is walled off by adjacent omentum and viscera. In general, abscess formation is rare, seen in less than 5% of cases of acute appendicitis. This entity should be suspected in patients with histories of symptoms lasting longer than 24 hours associated with fever, leukocytosis, and a palpable right lower quadrant mass. Ultrasonography and CT are helpful in evaluating patients with suspected abscess. The perforated pelvic appendix is one of the most easily overlooked, and therefore one of the most dangerous, conditions that can occur in association with appendicitis. When the inflamed pelvic appendix is unruptured, pain due to distention, peristaltic contraction, and localized inflammation may be poorly localized and felt in the epigastrium or periumbilical area. If rupture ensues, abdominal pain diminishes and local pelvic peritonitis results. This usually is not accompanied by muscular rigidity, and patients may actually feel better initially. With progression, the process either tracks upward into the general peritoneal cavity with the development of diffuse peritonitis, or a large pelvic abscess becomes apparent.

Depending on its location, the inflamed appendix may undergo fistulization to contiguous structures such as the small or large bowel, ureter, bladder, uterus, fallopian tube, or retroperitoneal space. These patients may have a variety of symptoms, including urosepsis or ureteral obstruction, and lumbar, psoas, perinephric, tuboovarian, pleural, thigh, or flank abscess.[44–49]

Acute appendicitis may present as a primary small bowel obstruction or paralytic ileus. The inflammatory mass of acute appendicitis or appendiceal abscess may adhere to the small intestine and produce obstruction. Generalized peritonitis resulting from free perforation may precipitate a generalized paralytic ileus.

Portal pyelophlebitis with or without hepatic abscess is an extremely serious, but fortunately uncommon, complication of appendicitis. This entity results from infected thrombi that spread from the inflamed or ruptured appendix through the mesenteric and portal

venous system to lodge in the liver. Before the advent of modern antimicrobial therapy, appendicitis was the most common cause of this complication. Patients had high temperature, jaundice, septic shock, and multiple intrahepatic abscesses, and death was almost inevitable. Since the introduction of modern antibiotic therapy, patients usually have a solitary hepatic abscess. Primary biliary tract disease has replaced appendicitis as the most common cause of portal pyelophlebitis. However, whenever a patient is seen with an intrahepatic abscess of unknown etiology, a spontaneously resolved episode of acute appendicitis or appendiceal abscess should be considered in the differential diagnosis.

The clinical presentation includes right upper quadrant pain, fever, chills, weight loss, anorexia, and hepatic tenderness. Jaundice may or may not be present, and the alkaline phosphatase level and leukocyte count are frequently elevated. CT is the most useful diagnostic modality in evaluating these patients. Treatment consists of intravenous antibiotics and drainage of the abscess, usually by the percutaneous method unless numerous abscesses are inaccessible by this approach.

Recurrent and chronic appendicitis are infrequent but known diseases of the appendix. The former occurs in about 10% to 20% of patients who have acute appendicitis and is pathologically indistinguishable from acute appendicitis except that patients give histories of similar, recurrent attacks of right lower quadrant pain. Chronic appendicitis presents with a history of right lower quadrant pain for more than 2 weeks. Operative and pathologic findings reveal chronic inflammation, and the symptoms are relieved by appendectomy. Chronic appendicitis occurs in only 1% to 2% of appendectomies and should be considered only after an appropriate work-up has eliminated other, more common causes of chronic right lower quadrant pain.[50,51]

Treatment

Preoperative Preparation

Before operation, expeditious preparation of the patient is mandatory. Intravenous fluid is administered until a satisfactory urine output is demonstrated, followed by intravenous infusion of a broad-spectrum antibiotic. To provide effective prophylaxis against wound infection, antimicrobial therapy must be directed against both aerobic and anaerobic gram-negative bacilli. It is not necessary to select anti-*Pseudomonas* antibiotics in uncomplicated appendicitis because infection with *Pseudomonas* is rare in this setting.[9] In nonperforated appendicitis, a single preoperative dose of a second-generation cephalosporin or a combination of a first-generation cephalosporin or ampicillin plus metronidazole or clindamycin is effective prophylaxis against wound infection.[9,52] If perforated appendicitis is suspected before operation, antibiotic coverage should be broadened with the addition of an anti-*Pseudomonas* agent such as an aminoglycoside, a third-generation cephalosporin, or a monobactam.[9,53,54]

Operative Approach

The standard surgical approach has changed over the years since McArthur and McBurney separately and almost simultaneously described the lateral muscle-splitting or gridiron incision.[55,56] Classically, the skin incision is placed lateral to the rectus sheath, in an oblique fashion, parallel to the fibers of the external oblique muscle. The incision should be centered over the point of maximum tenderness because there is considerable individual variation in the location of the appendix. The underlying muscle layers (external oblique, internal oblique, and transverse abdominal) are divided in the direction of their fibers and the peritoneum is identified, stretched tightly in the depths of the wound. The peritoneum can usually be freed of its attachments by passing a finger around the entire circumference of the wound in the plane between the transverse abdominal muscle and the peritoneum. Once mobilized in this fashion, the peritoneum usually bulges upward into the wound and can be incised easily. Most surgeons today prefer to use a transverse skin incision rather than the originally described oblique approach.[55,57,58] This incision is more versatile because it can readily be extended across the lateral portion of the rectus sheath when further exposure is required or when a more extensive exploration is indicated in the face of a normal appendix.[59-61] When the diagnosis is not clear, particularly in elderly patients, a lower midline incision is advantageous because the pathology may reside at a distance from the right lower quadrant. More recently, laparoscopy has become a useful diagnostic and therapeutic approach in patients with equivocal findings rather than committing to a particular incision.

Once the peritoneal cavity is entered, abnormal peritoneal fluid should be aspirated in a syringe and sent for aerobic and anaerobic culture. The appendix should be identified visually or by palpation and mobilized into the incision. It is often necessary to grasp the cecum and gently rock it back and forth into the wound, following the three taeniae to their confluence, until the appendix can be completely exposed. Once exposed, the appendix can be held by placing a Babcock clamp around it. Clamps should not be placed across the appendix and excessive handling should be avoided because the wall of the inflamed appendix is usually edematous and prone to injury. Before proceeding, the wound should be protected with laparotomy pads or towels.

Routine appendectomy entails division of the mesentery of the appendix followed by amputation of the structure. The mesoappendix is isolated, divided between clamps, and ligated. Once the entire mesoappendix is divided, the base of the appendix is crushed with a clamp and an absorbable tie is placed around the base within the crushed groove and tied securely. A clamp is then placed across the appendix distal to the ligature and the appendix is amputated between the ligature and clamp. Most surgeons "sterilize" the stump of the appendix with either phenol or electrocautery, although this step is unnecessary.[62] A commonly debated technical point regards management of the appendiceal stump. The choice is between simple ligation or ligation and inversion. Inversion entails placing a pursestring suture in the cecum around the base of the appendix before ligation and amputation of the structure. Once ligated, the stump is invaginated and the pursestring secured. Many studies have shown that inversion does not provide any advantage over ligation alone,[63] and some studies have demonstrated a slight increase in the risk of infectious complications with inversion of the stump.[64,65] On rare occasions, the entire base of the appendix may be necrotic and secure ligation of the stump is not possible, thus necessitating inversion of the stump with a pursestring suture. Conversely, when the wall of the cecum surrounding the base of the appendix is indurated, inversion may be difficult and should not be attempted.

In certain situations, the appendix and cecum cannot be entirely mobilized into the field. This occurs most commonly in the setting of a retrocecal appendicitis. Forceful attempts to mobilize the appendix in this setting can result in injury to the appendix with contamination of the operative field. Under such circumstances, it is appropriate to ligate and divide the appendiceal base first and then to take down the mesoappendix in a retrograde fashion.

Once the appendix is removed, the field can be irrigated with either normal saline or antibiotic-containing saline, and the wound should be closed in layers, irrigating between each one. The parietal peritoneum is closed with a running absorbable suture. The muscle layers in the gridiron incision tend to fall together as the retractors are removed. Each muscle layer generally requires the placement of a few interrupted absorbable sutures to help approximate the muscle fibers and to aid in hemostasis. The subcutaneous tissue and skin can be safely closed in the setting of nonperforated appendicitis.

Laparoscopic removal of a normal appendix was first described in 1983.[66] In 1987, the first reported series of laparoscopy for acute appendicitis was published.[67] Subsequently, as general surgeons have developed skills in laparoscopic techniques, the use of laparoscopic appendectomy has increased markedly and large experiences with this technique have been reported. The value of laparoscopy in evaluating patients with equivocal or atypical presentations has been well documented.[68,69] This technique is particularly useful in women of childbearing age, in whom the rate of diagnostic error approximates 40%.[69] In pregnant women during the first and second trimesters, laparoscopy has been shown to be as safe and effective as standard laparotomy.[70] Laparoscopic surgery is not feasible in the later stages of pregnancy once the uterus is no longer confined within the pelvis and lower abdomen.

During laparoscopic evaluation, the surgeon is able to visualize the appendix as well as the entire abdomen and pelvis for confirmation or correction of the preoperative diagnosis. Laparoscopic appendectomy is a safe alternative to conventional appendectomy and produces results that are at least equivalent to those of open appendectomy without significant overall cost differences.[71-75] Along with diagnostic advantages, the laparoscopic approach provides superior cosmetic results, less discomfort, fewer abdominal adhesions, and a lower incidence of wound infection; it also allows a more rapid return to normal activity.[76-78] If the preoperative diagnosis of appendicitis is fairly certain, particularly in young men, there is little advantage to the laparoscopic approach and a standard open laparotomy is indicated. However, laparoscopy may be preferable in situations in which the diagnosis is equivocal, particularly in women of childbearing age, in the first two trimesters of pregnancy, and in older patients.

The principles of laparoscopic appendectomy are the same as those of the open approach once access to the abdominal cavity has been gained. After carbon dioxide insufflation of the abdomen with a needle or port through an umbilical incision, a 10-mm port is placed in the umbilical position and two or three additional ports are placed under direct visualization. The placement of these additional ports varies with the position of the appendix and the preference of the surgeon (Fig. 37-6). In general, two 5-mm ports are used for retraction and dissection, with one placed above the pubis in the midline and the other placed directly over the appendix, in the midline 2 cm below the umbilicus, or in the right upper quadrant just lateral to the rectus sheath. A fourth port placed in the left lower or right upper abdomen is occasionally re-

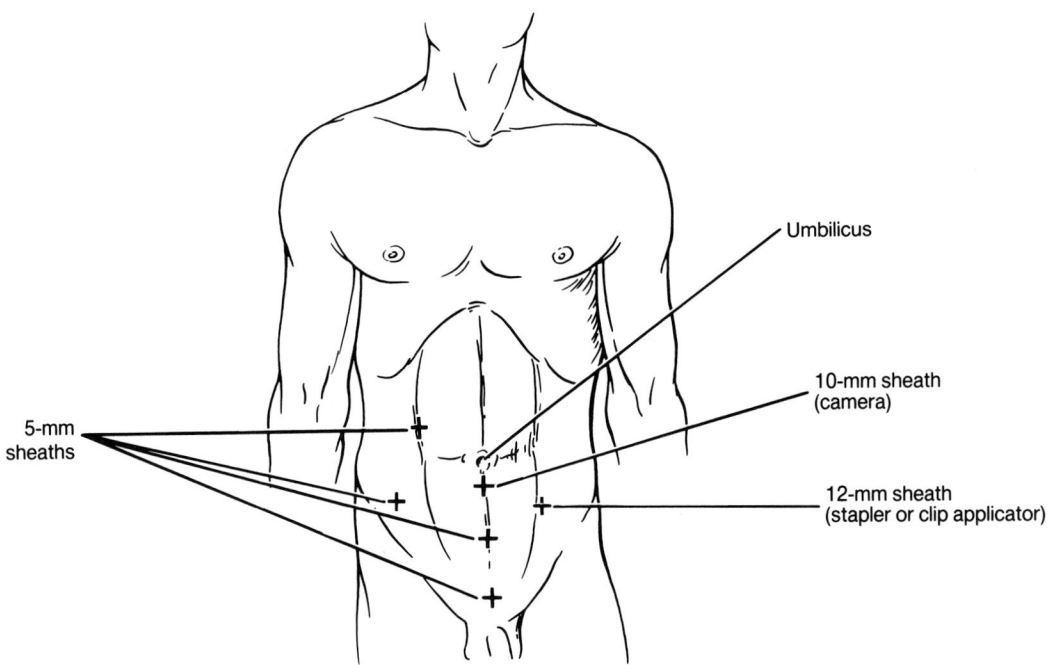

Figure 37-6 Placement of ports for laparoscopic appendectomy. Port positioning is variable and is dependent on the position of the appendix and the method used for securing the mesentery and dividing the appendix. The 10-mm umbilical port is constant and is used for camera access. An additional two or three ports are usually required and should be placed under direct vision once the specific anatomy, pathology, and approach are determined.

quired and can be 5, 10, or 12 mm, depending on the technique used for securing the mesentery and appendiceal stump.

After general laparoscopic evaluation of the abdomen and pelvis, the appendix is identified and mobilized using dissecting forceps or scissors introduced from the right-sided port and atraumatic forceps introduced from the suprapubic port (see Fig. 37-6). Periappendiceal adhesions are divided using electrocautery and the tip of the appendix is grasped with atraumatic forceps. If the tip is too edematous or inflamed to grasp safely with forceps, a pretied loop ligature can be placed around the tip for traction. When the appendix is retrocecal in position, the cecum should be thoroughly mobilized before an attempt is made to grasp the appendix. On occasion, the appendix and cecum may be severely inflamed, making laparoscopic removal hazardous, with an increased risk of rupture and peritoneal contamination. In this situ-

ation, conversion to an open procedure is warranted. In general, however, laparoscopy affords a safer approach to the adherent, difficult to mobilize, retrocecal appendix than does blunt finger dissection in the setting of open appendectomy.

Once the appendix is mobilized and traction is applied to the tip, the mesoappendix is divided and ligated using either sequentially placed endoscopic titanium clips, pretied loop ligatures, or a linear stapler that applies a triple row of hemostatic staples on each side and cuts between the staple lines (Fig. 37-7). The appendix is divided at its base using either the linear stapler or a double ligature of Roeder loops proximal and a single loop distal to the point of amputation. The appendiceal stump and mesentery are inspected for hemostasis. The stump can be invaginated with a laparoscopically placed pursestring suture. However, as discussed earlier, this is probably not necessary and most large laparoscopic appendectomy series have used simple ligation

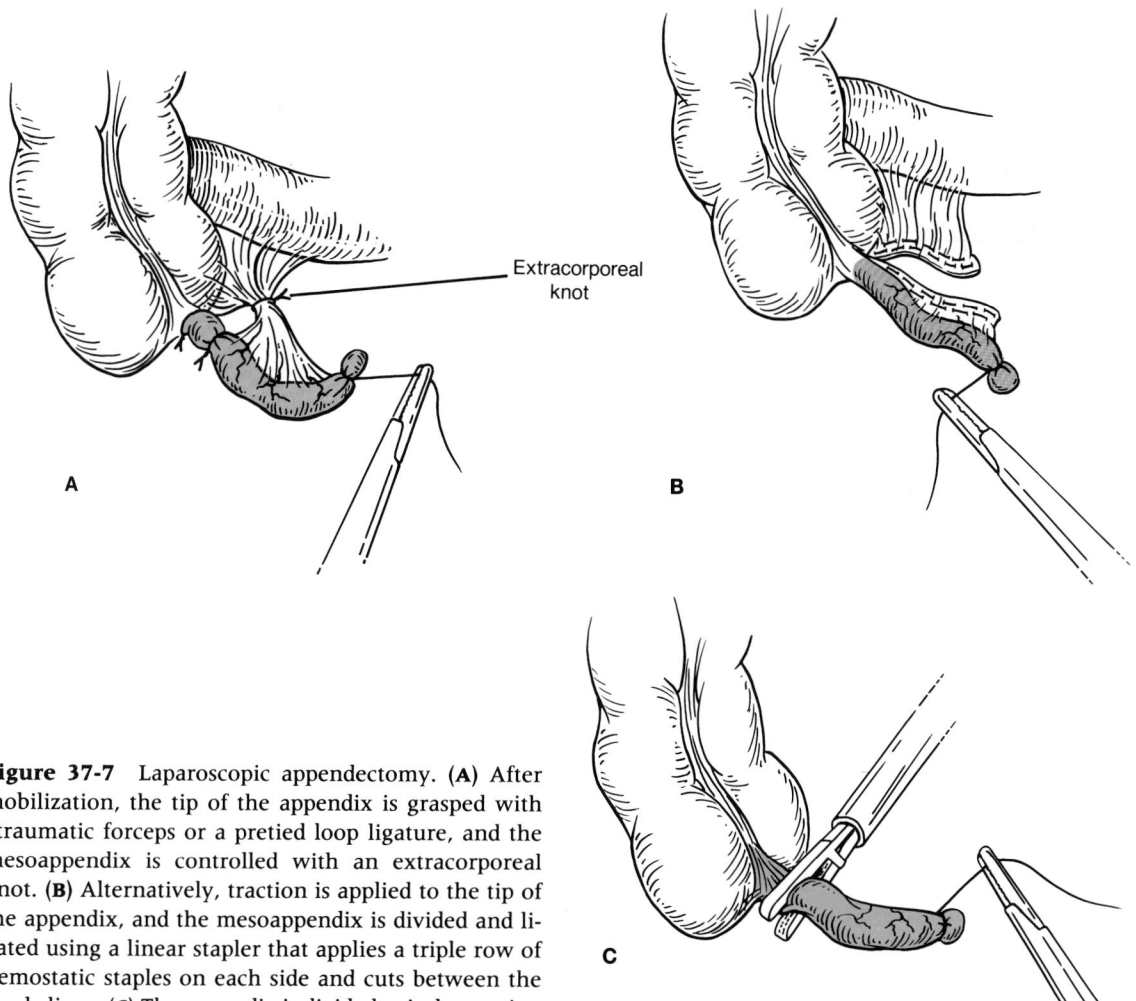

Figure 37-7 Laparoscopic appendectomy. (**A**) After mobilization, the tip of the appendix is grasped with atraumatic forceps or a pretied loop ligature, and the mesoappendix is controlled with an extracorporeal knot. (**B**) Alternatively, traction is applied to the tip of the appendix, and the mesoappendix is divided and ligated using a linear stapler that applies a triple row of hemostatic staples on each side and cuts between the staple lines. (**C**) The appendix is divided at its base using the linear stapler.

and division with no apparent difficulties. The appendix should be extracted by placing it within the 10- or 12-mm port to protect the wound from contamination during removal. If the appendix is larger than the largest port, it should be placed in an endoscopic bag before extraction to eliminate the possibility of contamination of the abdominal wall.

Perforated Appendicitis

In patients with a ruptured appendix and diffuse peritonitis, the appendix should be removed whenever possible. The peritoneal cavity should be irrigated and aspirated, paying particular attention to clearing the gross purulent fluid from the pelvis, right gutter, and abdominal cavity. Drainage is not necessary in the treatment of perforated appendicitis with diffuse peritonitis.[79] Drains are rapidly walled off within the peritoneal cavity and act as a portal of entry for external microorganisms.[42] On the rare occasions when the appendix cannot be identified, a drain can be placed adjacent to the area because of the increased risk of fecal fistula development. The muscular and fascial layers should be approximated, and the skin and subcutaneous tissue packed open or loosely approximated. A delayed primary closure can usually be accomplished within 3 to 5 days once the wound begins to granulate. When a perforated appendix is suspected before operation or encountered at operation, the antibiotic coverage should be broadened to cover *Pseudomonas* as well as the other commonly encountered enteric and *Bacteroides* species.[9,53,54] Antibiotic therapy should be continued after operation until the temperature and leukocyte count have returned to normal.

Appendiceal Abscess

About 2% to 3% of patients with appendicitis have a palpable mass. Therapy for an appendiceal mass or abscess can involve either a conservative, nonoperative approach or early operative drainage with appendectomy. Advocates of conservative therapy point to a complication rate of 15% to 50% with early operation.[80–82] Those who favor early operative intervention note that the abscess can progress to diffuse peritonitis with a 10% treatment failure rate during conservative management.[82,83] No prospective, randomized trials have been performed to evaluate these two approaches, and much controversy exists in the literature.

Before the routine availability of ultrasonography and CT, the entity of appendiceal mass–abscess was a clinical diagnosis. Patients who had symptoms for more than 24 hours associated with fever, leukocytosis, and a right lower quadrant mass were placed in this category.

Conservative management generally includes a period of bowel rest, intravenous hydration, and intravenous antibiotic therapy until the mass and symptoms have resolved. Interval appendectomy in 4 to 6 months is recommended by most authors.[81–83] During the course of conservative therapy, operative intervention is indicated if there is an increase in symptoms or the size of the mass, rupture of the abscess into the peritoneal cavity, persistence of the mass, or development of systemic or localized complications such as pyelophlebitis or small bowel obstruction. About half of all patients with masses have appendiceal phlegmons rather than frank abscesses,[80,81,84] and successful conservative treatment is more likely in these cases.[80]

Any patient with appendicitis and a palpable mass should be evaluated by either ultrasound or CT. If a phlegmon is detected, a nonoperative approach is appropriate with careful observation and repeated imaging to exclude progression and abscess formation. If an abscess is demonstrated, most patients can be treated with percutaneous drainage in combination with intravenous antibiotics.[82,83] Percutaneous catheter drainage has few complications and can achieve more rapid patient response. CT combined with diagnostic needle aspiration is 97% sensitive and 91% specific. About 85% of all intraabdominal abscesses are amenable to percutaneous drainage.[83] With this approach, the need for open operative intervention should be infrequent.

Interval appendectomy after resolution of an appendiceal phlegmon or abscess can be performed with minimal risk. Interval appendectomy is performed to prevent recurrent appendicitis and to identify malignant and premalignant lesions. In an analysis of combined series,[82,83] the mortality rate of interval appendectomy was 0.2% and the morbidity rate was 1.2%, whereas the risk of recurrent appendicitis was about 10%. No clinical features identify patients in whom recurrent appendicitis will develop. Therefore, although the therapeutic gain may be small, elective interval appendectomy after about 4 to 6 months is recommended in most cases.

Normal Appendix at Exploration

If a patient undergoes laparotomy or laparoscopy for suspected appendicitis and the appendix is found to be normal, a careful search should be made for the cause of the patient's symptoms. The distal small bowel, pelvic organs, colon, and upper abdomen should be inspected carefully. An extension of the incision may be required to evaluate these structures adequately during open exploration. The laparoscopic approach allows more complete evaluation of the abdominal and pelvic cavities without increasing the complexity of the operation. In a woman undergoing laparoscopy for suspected appendicitis, a uterine sound or cervical tenaculum should be placed and the patient positioned so that the uterus can be manipulated during the procedure to allow adequate inspection of the pelvic organs.

The appendix should be removed to prevent future appendicitis and to avoid the potential for confusing acute appendicitis with a recurrent attack of a chronic disorder at a later date. The incidence of acute appendicitis is maximal at the age of 15 to 19 years, and the probability of developing acute appendicitis during the rest of the lifetime is as high as 15%.[85,86] Efficacy is far more likely in men who are younger than 50 years and women who are younger than 40 years.[85] As patients age, the risk of developing appendicitis decreases, but the mortality rate from the disorder increases. In several studies of incidental appendectomy,[87–89] there was no increase in complications or length of hospital stay, whereas between 20% and 25% of the "normal" appendices removed were histologically abnormal. Conversely, a large retrospective series of more than 300 incidental appendectomies demonstrated a higher wound infection rate in patients older than 50 years.[90]

A normal appendix should be removed in this situation as long as the procedure can be performed with minimal risk of contamination. This should be done in young patients when there is a preoperative roentgenographic abnormality (eg, appendicolith, abnormal filling or emptying on barium enema) or findings that may lead to recurrent right lower quadrant symptoms in the future. Whether exploration is being performed by the open or laparoscopic method should not influence the decision to perform an incidental appendectomy. Incidental appendectomy generally should not be performed if the cecum is diseased at the base of the appendix (regional enteritis) because of the increased risk of fistula formation.

An alternative approach to conventional appendectomy is inversion-ligation appendectomy. This technique avoids cutting the appendix and thus eliminates the risk associated with exposure of the wound to bacterial contamination from the appendiceal lumen. Inversion-ligation appendectomy involves skeletonization of the appendix by division of the mesoappendix flush with the serosa of the appendix, intussusception of the appendix into the cecal lumen until a 5- to 10-mm nubbin of appendix is left at the base, ligation of the base at the junction with the cecum, and inversion of the ligated nubbin with a cecal pursestring suture. Ligation of the appendix is important to ensure strangulation of the appendix with complete sloughing of the structure into the cecal lumen within 1 week. Without this maneuver, the inverted appendix can serve as a lead point for cecal intussusception. This technique is indicated only for a normal appendix. In cases of acute or chronic appendicitis and those in which the appendiceal lumen has been obliterated by fibrosis or an appendicolith, a standard appendectomy should be performed.[91]

Postoperative Care

In cases of uncomplicated appendicitis, food intake can be advanced once the patient has fully recovered from the anesthetic and the appetite has returned. No postoperative antibiotics are required if there are no complications. The patient should walk early and usually can be discharged from the hospital within 36 to 48 hours of operation.

The postoperative care of patients with appendicitis complicated by perforation with localized or diffuse peritonitis or abscess formation varies with the degree of illness as well as the premorbid condition and other complicating factors. In general, paralytic ileus plays a more prominent role in the early postoperative period and usually requires a period of nasogastric suction until peristaltic action and bowel function return. Parenteral analgesics and antiemetics should be administered as needed. Antibiotics should be continued after operation until the temperature and leukocyte count have returned to normal. When the drain output is scant (less than 10 mL per shift), the drain should be removed. The wound should be left open and delayed primary closure achieved once adequate granulation occurs. Patients should walk as early as tolerated, usually within the first 24 hours after operation. These patients require close observation for the development of complications associated with perforated appendicitis, such as wound infection, intraabdominal abscess, ileus, and bowel obstruction.

Postoperative Complications

The most common complications after surgery for appendicitis are infectious in nature. The development of wound infections and intraabdominal abscesses is directly related to the presence or absence of perforation, doubling the complication rate in these patients.[29,42] The use of preoperative prophylactic antibiotics decreases the incidence of wound infection.[42] If antibiotics are first given during the operation or later, they have no noticeable effect on local wound sepsis.[29] Because of the high incidence of wound complications after perforation, many surgeons leave the wound open and perform delayed primary closure, or allow the wound to heal by secondary intent. When wound infection develops, with signs of localized pain, induration, and erythema, the wound should be opened completely, packed with saline-moistened gauze, and allowed to heal secondarily.

Intraabdominal abscess should be suspected after appendectomy if the patient has fever, abdominal pain, leukocytosis, and diarrhea. The placement of peritoneal drains after perforation, except to drain a specific abscess cavity, is of no use in preventing this complication. Most abscesses arise within the pelvis. Pelvic abscess after appendectomy in the presence of perforation occurs in 1.4% to 18% of patients.[40] The abscess usually becomes manifest 5 to 10 days after surgery. Typical symptoms include fever, abdominal discomfort, dysuria, diarrhea, and painful defecation. On rectal examination, a tender, fluctuant mass can be palpated anteriorly in the cul-de-sac. Because of the frequent occurrence of this complication, baseline rectal examination should be performed immediately after operation for appendicitis. Rectal examination should also be performed on all patients before hospital discharge, especially if they have any of the clinical signs of pelvic abscess. If a pelvic abscess is palpable on rectal or vaginal examination, the preferred route of drainage is through the rectum or vagina. Drainage should be performed only after the abscess has matured and the fluctuant portion has become fixed to the rectum or vagina. Ultrasonography and CT are useful in evaluating the condition and effecting percutaneous drainage in the patient with a postoperative intraabdominal abscess.

Other postoperative complications associated with appendicitis include ileus, early bowel obstruction, and fecal fistula. Prolonged postoperative ileus and early postoperative bowel obstruction after perforated appendicitis often can be treated conservatively with nasogastric decompression. Exploration should be considered if signs of ileus or obstruction do not resolve, if symptoms progress, or if there is evidence of compromised bowel. Fecal fistula is usually a complication of the difficult appendiceal stump. In the presence of perforation and an inflamed or gangrenous stump, a drain should be placed in the vicinity if the surgeon is concerned about the integrity of the closure. If a fistula develops, it is usually low output and should be managed conservatively by placing suction drainage, optimizing the nutritional status of the patient, and addressing any other associated complications (ie, adjacent abscess). This treatment regimen results in spontaneous closure of most fistulas.

Late morbidity from appendicitis is also more common after perforation and peritonitis. The most common late complication is intestinal obstruction secondary to adhesions. The risk of tubal infertility is three to five times higher in women after ruptured appendicitis as compared with a control population or to women with uncomplicated appendicitis.[92]

Rare complications during the early and late postoperative periods include stump appendicitis, intussusception of the appendiceal stump, hemorrhage, and inguinal hernia. Abscess formation due to rupture of the appendiceal stump can occur in the early postoperative period secondary to failure of the appendiceal ligature or pursestring suture, or it can develop years later as a result of an excessively long appendiceal stump.[93] The appendiceal stump may become intussuscepted when inverted and can cause abdominal pain, vomiting, and rectal bleeding. An abdominal mass is evident in half these cases and a barium enema is usually diagnostic, demonstrating cecocolic intussusception. Operative intervention is indicated, with manual reduction and cecopexy or right hemicolectomy. Hemorrhage after appendectomy is rare but can occur within the peritoneum or into the cecum from the appendiceal stump. Intraperitoneal hemorrhage results from inadequate ligation of the appendiceal artery in the mesoappendix and usually requires reoperation to control the source of bleeding. Intraluminal blood results from bleeding from the inverted appendiceal stump and can be controlled by endoscopic means or by reexploration with direct inspection and repeated ligation of the stump. The incidence of right inguinal hernia is about three times greater in patients who have previously undergone appendectomy.[94] Perhaps damage to the iliohypogastric nerve leads to weakening of the transverse muscle of the abdomen. This muscle, along with the transverse fascia and the internal oblique muscle, forms a "shutter mechanism" that closes the internal ring when intraabdominal pressure rises. Placement of the appendectomy incision above the anterior superior iliac spine should avoid this nerve.[94]

NEOPLASIA OF THE APPENDIX

Malignant tumors of the appendix are rare, accounting for less than 0.4% of all intestinal neoplasms. Appendiceal neoplasms are categorized on the basis of their morphology as carcinoid tumors, mucoceles, adenocarcinomas of the colonic type, adenocarcinoid tumors, or other rare lesions.[95,96] Concomitant second malignancies, most often in the gastrointestinal tract, occur with greater than expected frequency in patients with appendiceal tumors.[95]

Carcinoid Tumors

Carcinoid tumors are the most common appendiceal neoplasms, accounting for 50% to 77% of appendiceal tumors and for 66% of appendiceal malignancies. The appendix is the most frequent site for gastrointestinal carcinoid tumors, with an incidence of about 3 to 7 per 1000 appendectomies. Most (70% to 90%) are discovered as an incidental finding at the time of surgery for other indications. There is a slight female-to-male preponderance of 2:1 to 4:1, even allowing for the greater likelihood of incidental appendectomy in women undergoing cholecystectomy or pelvic surgery. As many as 70% of tumors are found at the tip of the appendix, and only 10% result in acute appendicitis. Between 70% and 95% are smaller than 1 cm in diameter without evidence of metastases, and only 2% are larger than 2 cm in diameter. Appendiceal carcinoid tumors rarely present with symptoms and signs of disseminated disease or the malignant carcinoid syndrome; they do so only when distant metastases are present. Multifocal carcinoid tumors within the gastrointestinal tract occur in 4% of cases. Between 8% and 13% of patients with appendiceal carcinoid tumors have a second primary cancer, and the appendiceal carcinoid tumor usually is an incidental finding at the time of laparotomy for the other tumor.[95-99]

On gross examination, carcinoid tumors appear as firm, discrete nodules within the appendix or, less commonly, as areas of diffuse wall thickening. Their microscopic characteristics are similar to those of carcinoid tumors of other origins. The cells are small and uniform, and they contain a central nucleus with punctate chromatin, few mitoses, and a finely granular and usually acidophilic cytoplasm. Virtually all appendiceal carcinoid tumors invade the muscle layer and have lymphatic involvement. Microscopic involvement of the peritoneal surface is common and mesoappendix involvement is observed in 18% of cases.[95]

Despite these histologic findings, few patients have regional or distant dissemination of disease. Carcinoid tumors of the appendix that are less than 1 cm in diameter have a risk of metastatic disease approaching zero. Tumors that are between 1 and 2 cm in diameter rarely metastasize (less than 5% of cases), but the risk of metastasis increases to 30% to 60% in tumors measuring greater than 2 cm. Almost all appendiceal carcinoid tumor metastases are restricted to regional lymph nodes and are found at the time of initial presentation.[98,99] The overall 5-year survival rate is between 90% and 100%.[96] All reported recurrences, distant metastases, and deaths have occurred in patients whose tumors were more than 2 cm in diameter at initial presentation.[98,99]

During any abdominal operation, the discovery of a nodular mass in the appendix should arouse suspicion for carcinoid tumor. Simple appendectomy is adequate therapy for all patients with tumors less than 1 cm in diameter and for most patients with tumors 1 to 2 cm in diameter. Radical right hemicolectomy is appropriate for all tumors larger than 2 cm except in extremely elderly patients or those at high operative risk. In patients who have tumors between 1 and 2 cm combined with positive lymph nodes, vascular invasion, or evidence of involvement of the mesoappendix or the base of the appendix, right hemicolectomy should be considered.[95,96]

Mucoceles

Appendiceal mucoceles are characterized by gross enlargement of the appendix due to hypersecretion and the accumulation of a mucoid substance within the lumen (Fig. 37-8). Mucoceles are rare tumors, with a reported incidence of 0.2% to 0.3% of appendectomy specimens, second only to carcinoid tumors in frequency.[100,101] As in carcinoid tumors, there is a female: male predominance of about 3:1. The average age at the time of diagnosis is 54 years for benign disease and 64 years for malignant disease.[101] Mucoceles of the appendix are classified into four histologic subtypes: retention cysts, mucosal hyperplasia, cystadenomas, and cystadenocarcinomas. Retention cysts have an atrophic, degenerative epithelium, whereas mucosal hyperplasia is characterized by a diffuse mucosal hyperplasia without atypia, similar to hyperplastic colonic polyps. Mucinous cystadenoma is the most common type (52% of all mucoceles) and is characterized by mucosal hyperplasia with some epithelial atypia, similar to colonic villous and adenomatous polyps. Mucinous cystadenocarcinoma is similar to cystadenoma, with the additional finding of glandular invasion into the stroma.[100-102] About 6% of cases of mucinous cystadenoma and cystadenocarcinoma are associated with pseudomyxoma peritonei in which there is diffuse involvement of the peritoneal cavity with gelatinous ascites containing epithelial cells.[101] Pseudomyxoma peritonei may occur, with rupture of mucinous cystadenomas and cystadenocarcinomas originating from

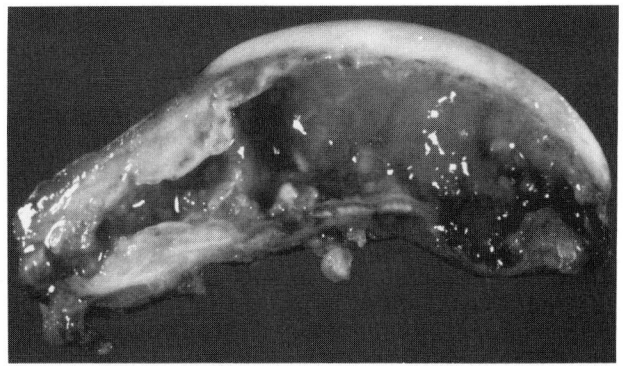

Figure 37-8 Appendiceal mucocele. (See Color Fig. 37-8.)

many different sites, including the ovary (most common) and appendix. The implantation of mucin-producing tumor cells on the peritoneal lining can lead to an inflammatory response, with stimulation of mesothelial cells to produce more mucus and subsequent obstructive and fistulous complications.[95]

About 25% of mucoceles cause no symptoms and are discovered incidentally at surgery or during barium enema.[101] Symptoms are vague, making early diagnosis the exception. Calcium deposition in the wall may appear as a rimlike calcification on plain roentgenograms. Barium enema may reveal a well-circumscribed, smooth-surfaced submucosal or extrinsic mass indenting the cecum. Ultrasonography shows a cystic mass with variable sonographic echogenicity due to anechoic fluid and echogenic mucin. CT demonstrates a low-density mass indenting the cecum, with attenuation values near water density. Both ultrasonography and CT can verify the presence of calcium in the wall of the mass.[95] Pseudomyxoma peritonei appears on sonography as septate ascites with numerous "suspended" echoes that do not move as the patient changes position, whereas CT reveals anterior, septate ascites and scalloping of the liver and spleen margins.[102,103]

If an appendiceal mucocele is identified before operation or incidentally at exploration, it should be removed because of the malignant potential as well as the risk of rupture with development of pseudomyxoma peritonei. Appendectomy alone always cures retention cysts, mucosal hyperplasia, and cystadenomas. If the involved appendiceal wall is contiguous with the cecum or terminal ileum, a right hemicolectomy is indicated. Careful exploration of the entire abdominal cavity is essential because these lesions are associated with synchronous adenomatous tumors of the intestine, ovary, kidney, and breast. Adenocarcinoma of the colon occurs concurrently in about 20% of patients, whereas cystadenocarcinoma of the ovary is found in 18% of patients with an appendiceal cystadenocarcinoma and pseudomyxoma peritonei. If pseudomyxoma peritonei is found, an aggressive approach is recommended and can be associated with extended survival. This includes resection of the mucocele, complete removal of all the peritoneally implanted mucous cysts, omentectomy, and bilateral oophorectomy when ovarian involvement is present. Some surgeons advocate a second-look celiotomy at 6 months with further debulking if necessary.[100,102] The 5-year survival rate of patients with appendiceal cystadenocarcinoma complicated by pseudomyxoma peritonei is significantly decreased (25%). Adjuvant therapy for pseudomyxoma peritonei with radiotherapy or intravenous or intraperitoneal chemotherapy has not proven useful.

Adenocarcinoma

Primary adenocarcinoma of the appendix is rare, with an incidence of 0.01% to 0.08%. Only 250 cases have been reported in the literature. Adenocarcinoma is most common in men during the sixth decade of life and is associated with other solid neoplasms in 11% of cases.[104] Second malignancies most commonly are of gastrointestinal tract origin. These tumors usually originate at the base of the appendix and, because even a small growth can occlude the lumen, most patients have symptoms and findings consistent with acute appendicitis. The diagnosis of appendiceal adenocarcinoma is unlikely to be made before operation, and even during operation, the correct diagnosis is suspected on clinical grounds in less than 40% of cases.[95]

The recommended therapy for most appendiceal adenocarcinomas is right hemicolectomy with lymph node resection. This frequently entails a staged approach because the adenocarcinoma is usually an incidental finding recognized after histologic examination of the appendectomy specimen. Appendectomy alone is sufficient for Duke's A lesions with uninvolved margins.[104] However, if any degree of invasion is demonstrated, hemicolectomy should be performed. Because the muscular layers of the appendix are commonly incomplete or absent, extension to adjacent structures, perforation, and peritoneal seeding is common with this tumor. Because essentially all cases involve the submucosa, appendiceal carcinoma that is truly confined to the mucosa at presentation is uncommon. The prognosis for these lesions after resection is similar, stage for stage, to that of adenocarcinoma of the colon.

Adenocarcinoid Tumors

Adenocarcinoid tumor is an unusual variant of appendiceal carcinoid tumor (also known as goblet cell carcinoid tumor, composite tumor, mucinous carcinoid tumor, crypt cell carcinoma, and microgranular cancer) that has histologic features of both adenocarcinoma and carcinoid tumor. Typical microscopic findings include abundant mucin, neoplastic cells concentrated about the crypts of Lieberkühn, no evidence of malignant transformation of the mucosa, positive staining for argentaffin and argyrophil granules in most cases, and, commonly, vascular, perineural, and serosal invasion.[105] The histogenesis of these tumors is subject to debate. They present most often as acute appendicitis and rarely as an incidental finding. On gross examination, the appendix may appear to have diffuse wall thickening rather than a distinct mass. Intraabdominal spread is a known feature and the tumors have a propensity to metastasize to one or both ovaries. The malignant carcinoid syndrome has not been described in any of these patients.[95]

The appropriate therapy for this entity has not been prospectively evaluated and is not well established. Some authors[105] advocate simple appendectomy for localized lesions, which are histologically low grade without foci of atypia. Other authors[106] treat adenocarcinoid tumors aggressively, with hemicolectomy and resection of ovarian, intraabdominal, and pelvic foci. The 5-year survival rate for appendiceal adenocarcinoid tumors is reported to be 73%, with 10- and 15-year actuarial estimates of 66%.[105]

Miscellaneous Appendiceal Neoplasms

Benign epithelial neoplasms of the appendix have histologic characteristics similar to those of colonic epithelial polyps and should be classified as such. The lesions are categorized as adenomatous, hyperplastic, or mixed hyperplastic–adenomatous. There is a slight female-to-male predominance. These epithelial neoplasms are associated with synchronous carcinoma of the colon in 12% to 21% of cases, and the prognostic significance of the lesions is similar to that of adenomas found elsewhere in the colon.[107]

Other rare malignancies of the appendix include metastatic adenocarcinoma originating in distant abdominal and pelvic sites, lymphoma, granular cell tumor, and paraganglioma of the mesoappendix.[95] These neoplasms require an individualized approach depending on the nature, extent, and concomitant factors associated with the lesion.

MISCELLANEOUS DISORDERS OF THE APPENDIX

Diverticula

Diverticula of the appendix are classified as congenital or true diverticula, which involve all layers of the appendix, and acquired or false diverticula, which do not contain any muscle. The acquired lesions are 10 times more common than the congenital diverticula and are presumed to be caused by excessive muscular activity and luminal obstruction of the appendix. These present as four distinct morphologic and clinical varieties—acute diverticulitis, acute appendicitis with acute diverticulitis, acute appendicitis with diverticulum, and appendix with diverticulum. Relative to acute appendicitis, appendiceal diverticula have a later age of onset, a longer interval of disease, fewer or absent gastrointestinal symptoms, failure of typical abdominal pain progression, delay in surgical treatment, and a high inci-

dence of perforation. Appendiceal diverticulitis is seen most frequently after the third decade of life. A history of previous similar attacks is common. Patients typically have histories of right lower quadrant abdominal pain, leukocytosis, and low-grade fever. The classic progression of periumbilical pain to the right lower quadrant, nausea and vomiting, and anorexia are uncommon features of appendiceal diverticulitis. Appendiceal diverticula are rarely diagnosed on roentgenologic examination. Because of the atypical presentation and longer duration of symptoms, there is a four-fold greater incidence of perforation as compared to acute appendicitis.[108]

Intussusception

Intussusception of the appendix is rare, with a reported prevalence of 0.01%. This disorder usually presents with vague abdominal symptoms and may mimic other, more common causes of acute and chronic abdominal pain. Patients may have symptoms suggestive of acute appendicitis, intussusception, chronic episodic abdominal pain that is poorly localized, painless rectal bleeding, or chronic blood loss. The diagnosis is rarely made before operation. Most cases have been reported in the pediatric and adolescent age groups, with the average patient age being 16 years. The sex distribution is about equal.

Causes of intussusception can be divided into two groups—anatomic and pathophysiologic. Anatomic intussusception is related to a fetal type of cecum with the appendix arising from its tip in a funnel configuration and the proximal lumen having a greater diameter than the tip. The mesoappendix is thin, with a narrow base, and the appendicular wall is particularly mobile, being free of fixation by congenital peritoneal folds or inflammatory adhesions. Pathophysiologic intussusception (Fig. 37-9) is characterized by either intraluminal abnormalities (ie, fecaliths, foreign bodies, parasites) or lesions involving the appendiceal wall (ie, hypertrophic lymphoid follicles, neoplasms, endometriosis, tuberculous granulomas).

Radiologically, these lesions have several distinctive characteristics. On barium enema, there may be a cecal filling defect in association with the absence of appendiceal filling. Double-contrast barium enema may reveal a coiled-spring appearance in the region of the appendiceal lumen. Ultrasonography may demonstrate a target-like abnormality or a concentric ring sign. Endoscopically, an intussuscepted appendix may mimic a colonic polyp and, if endoscopically removed, can result in peritonitis. At operation, an intussuscepted appendix may appear as a cecal mass. If a benign cause for the intussusception can be determined at the

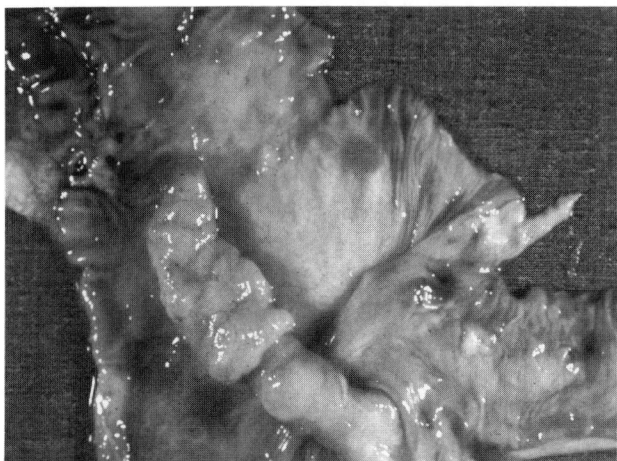

Figure 37-9 Intussusception of the appendix with a villous adenoma as the lead point. (See Color Fig. 37-9.)

time of surgery, an appendectomy is all that is required.[109]

Endometriosis

Ectopic implants of endometrial tissue separate from the uterus (endometriosis) usually involve the pelvic structures and peritoneum. However, other, nonpelvic ectopic sites have been reported, with appendiceal endometriosis occurring in less than 1% of all cases of pelvic endometriosis. The most frequent location of endometrial involvement of the appendix is in the subserosa, with no case of mucosal involvement ever described. The diagnosis of endometriosis of the appendix is usually made incidentally at operation or after histologic examination of the surgical specimen. As mentioned in the previous section, endometriosis is a rare cause of appendiceal intussusception, with 18 such cases reported in the world literature.[110]

Foreign Bodies

Any foreign body ingested can lodge in the appendix and lead to symptoms requiring surgical intervention. Many items found within the appendix have been reported, including pins, lead shot, bones, seeds, glass, teeth, and nails. Pins are the most common foreign body found (37% of cases) and the most likely to cause symptoms (93% of cases). Patients usually have histories of prolonged, intermittent episodes of recurring abdominal pain. Pointed objects are more likely to lead to symptoms. Most patients have no recollection of swallowing a foreign body. The incidence of appendiceal foreign body has decreased during the past 30 to 40

years. The reason for this is unclear but may be related to greater safety awareness in children or less dependence on wild game as a staple in diets. When a foreign body results in symptoms, the appropriate therapy is appendectomy.[111]

Acknowledgments
The assistance of Drs. Diane Babcock, Jonathan Moulton, Amy Nofziger, and Harold Spitz, as well as Beverly Smith, in obtaining the illustrative original radiographs and photomicrographs reproduced in this chapter is greatly appreciated. Roger West provided excellent assistance in photographing all the original items.

REFERENCES

1. Goldman M. Appendicitis: a historical survey. Hosp Med 1966;1:42.
2. Fitz RH. Perforating inflammation of the vermiform appendix with special reference to its early diagnosis and treatment. Am J Med Sci 1886;92:321.
3. McBurney C. Experience with early operative interference in cases of diseases of the vermiform appendix. NY Med J 1889;50:676.
4. Burkitt DP. The aetiology of appendicitis. Br J Surg 1971;58:695.
5. Williams RS. Appendicitis: historical milestones and current challenges. Med J Aust 1992;157:784.
6. Nitecki S, Karmeli R, Sarr MG. Appendiceal calculi and fecaliths as indications for appendectomy. Surgery 1990;171:185.
7. Altemeier WA. The bacterial flora of acute perforated appendicitis with peritonitis. Ann Surg 1938;107:517.
8. Lau WY, Teoh-Chan CH, Fan ST, et al. The bacteriology and septic complications of patients with appendicitis. Ann Surg 1984;200:576.
9. Thadepalli H, Mandal AK, Chuah SK, Lou MA. Bacteriology of the appendix and the ileum in health and in appendicitis. Am Surg 1991;57:317.
10. Baron EJ, Bennion R, Thompson J, et al. A microbiological comparison between acute and complicated appendicitis. Clin Infect Dis 1992;14:227.
11. Nauta RJ, Magnant C. Observation versus operation for abdominal pain in the right lower quadrant. Am J Surg 1986;151:746.
12. Scott JH III, Amin M, Harty JI. Abnormal urinalysis in appendicitis. J Urol 1983;129:1015.
13. Jones WG, Barie PS. Urological manifestations of acute appendicitis. J Urol 1988;139:1325.
14. Janus C. Diagnosis of acute appendicitis: how useful is the abdominal x-ray? Dig Surg 1986;3:27.
15. Ferzli GE, Ozuner G, Davidson PG, Isenberg JS, Redmond P, Worth MW Jr. Barium enema in the diagnosis of acute appendicitis. Surg Gynecol Obstet 1990;171:40.

16. Jeffrey RB Jr, Laing FC, Townsend RR. Acute appendicitis: sonographic criteria based on 250 cases. Radiology 1988;167:327.

17. Puylaert JBCM, Rutgers PH, Lalisang RI, et al. A prospective study of ultrasonography in the diagnosis of appendicitis. N Engl J Med 1987;317:666.

18. Fa EM, Cronan JJ. Compression as an aid in the differential diagnosis of appendicitis. Surg Gynecol Obstet 1989;169:290.

19. Larson JM, Peirce JC, Ellinger DM, et al. The validity and utility of sonography in the diagnosis of appendicitis in the community setting. AJR 1989;153:687.

20. Rioux M. Sonographic detection of the normal and abnormal appendix. AJR 1992;158:773.

21. Balthazar EJ, Megibow AJ, Siegel SE, Birnbaum BA. Appendicitis: prospective evaluation with high-resolution CT. Radiology 1991;180:21.

22. Stone HH, Sanders SL, Martin JD Jr. Perforated appendicitis in children. Surgery 1971;69:673.

23. Marchildon MB, Dudgeon DL. Perforated appendicitis: current experience in a children's hospital. Ann Surg 1977;185:84.

24. Harrison MW, Linder DJ, Campbell JR, Campbell TJ. Acute appendicitis in children: factors affecting morbidity. Am J Surg 1984;147:605.

25. Bennion RS, Thompson JE Jr. Early appendectomy for perforated appendicitis should not be abandoned. Surg Gynecol Obstet 1987;165:95.

26. Putnam TC, Gagliano N, Emmens RW. Appendicitis in children. Surg Gynecol Obstet 1990;170:527.

27. Gamal R, Moore TC. Appendicitis in children aged 13 years and younger. Am J Surg 1990;159:589.

28. Soreide O. Appendicitis: a study of incidence, death rates and consumption of hospital resources. Postgrad Med J 1984;60:341.

29. Lewis FR, Holcroft JW, Boey J, Dunphy JE. Appendicitis: a critical review of diagnosis and treatment in 1,000 cases. Arch Surg 1975;110:677.

30. Mittelpunkt A, Nora PF. Current features in the treatment of acute appendicitis: an analysis of 1,000 consecutive cases. Surgery 1966;60:971.

31. Smithy WB, Wexner SD, Dailey TH. The diagnosis and treatment of acute appendicitis in the aged. Dis Colon Rectum 1986;29:170.

32. Owens BJ III, Hamit HF. Appendicitis in the elderly. Ann Surg 1978;187:392.

33. Burns RP, Cochran JL, Russell WL, Bard RM. Appendicitis in mature patients. Ann Surg 1985;201:695.

34. Horowitz MD, Gomez GA, Santiesteban R, Burkett G. Acute appendicitis during pregnancy. Arch Surg 1985;120:1362.

35. Babaknia A, Parsa H, Woodruff JD. Appendicitis during pregnancy. Obstet Gynecol 1977;50:40.

36. Black WP. Acute appendicitis in pregnancy. BMJ 1960;1:1938.

37. Baer JL, Reis RA, Arens RA. Appendicitis in pregnancy with changes in position and axis of normal appendix in pregnancy. JAMA 1932;98:1359.

38. Mazze RI, Kallen B. Appendectomy during pregnancy: a Swedish registry study of 778 cases. Obstet Gynecol 1991;77:835.

39. Merine DS, Fishman EK, Jones B, Nussbaum AR, Simmons T. Right lower quadrant pain in the immunocompromised patient: CT findings in 10 cases. AJR 1987;149:1177.

40. Silen W. Cope's early diagnosis of the acute abdomen, ed 17. New York, Oxford University Press, 1987:84.

41. Cooperman M. Complications of appendectomy. Surg Clin North Am 1983;63:1233.

42. Berry J Jr, Malt RA. Appendicitis near its centenary. Ann Surg 1984;200:567.

43. Koepsell TD, Inui TS, Farewell VT. Factors affecting perforation in acute appendicitis. Surg Gynecol Ostet 1981;153:508.

44. Sandermann J, Hansen LS. Bilateral ureteral obstruction as a complication to a perforated appendix. Report of a case. Acta Chir Scand 1983;149:535.

45. Turner G, Daniell SJ. Lumbar abscess resulting from appendicitis. J R Soc Med 1984;77:884.

46. Haas GP, Shumaler BP, Haas PA. Appendicovesical fistula. Urology 1984;24:604.

47. Edwards JD, Eckhauser FE. Retroperitoneal perforation of the appendix presenting as subcutaneous emphysema of the thigh. Dis Colon Rectum 1986;29:456.

48. Corder AP. Renal abscess with gas formation secondary to acute appendicitis. Br J Urol 1987;59:90.

49. Ashley S, Corlett SK, Windle R, Cookson JB. Colobronchial fistula: a late complication of appendicitis. Thorax 1988;43:420.

50. Crabbe MM, Norwood SH, Robertson HD, Silva JS. Recurrent and chronic appendicitis. Surg Gynecol Obstet 1986;163:11.

51. Rothman DL, Schwartz SI, Adams JT. Diagnostic laparotomy for fever or abdominal pain of unknown origin. Am J Surg 1977;133:273.

52. Bauer T, Vennits B, Holm B, et al. Antibiotic prophylaxis in acute nonperforated appendicitis: the Danish multicenter study group 111. Ann Surg 1989;209:307.

53. Berne TV, Yellin AE, Appleman MD, Gill MA, Chenella FC, Heseltine PNR. Surgically treated gangrenous or perforated appendicitis: a comparison of aztreonam and clindamycin versus gentamicin and clindamycin. Ann Surg 1987;205:133.

54. Dougherty SH, Saltzstein EC, Peacock JB, Mercer LC, Cano P. Perforated or gangrenous appendicitis treated with aminoglycosides: how do bacterial cultures influence management? Arch Surg 1989;124:1280.

55. Strohl EL, Diffenbaugh WG. The historical background of the gridiron or muscle-splitting incision for appendectomy. Ill Med J 1969;135:287.

56. McBurney C. The incision made in the abdominal wall in cases of appendicitis, with a description of a new method of operating. Ann Surg 1894;20:38.

57. Rockey AE. Transverse incision in abdominal operations. Med Rec 1905;68:779.

58. Davis GG. A transverse incision for the removal of the appendix. Ann Surg 1906;43:104.

59. Fowler GR. A treatise on appendicitis. Philadelphia, JB Lippincott, 1894:153.

60. Harrington FB. Hernia following appendicitis. Boston Med Surg J 1899;141:105.

61. Weir RF. An improved operation for acute appendicitis or for quiescent cases with complications. Med News 1900;76:241.

62. Getzen LC. Appendectomy: ligation of appendiceal stump without cauterization. Surgery 1968;64:514.

63. Watters DAK, Walker MA, Abernethy BC. The appendiceal stump: should it be invaginated? Ann R Coll Surg Engl 1984;66:92.

64. Street D, Bodai BI, Owens LJ, et al. Simple ligation vs stump inversion in appendectomy. Arch Surg 1988;123:668.

65. Sinha AP. Appendicectomy: an assessment of the advisability of stump invagination. Br J Surg 1977;64:499.

66. Semm K. Endoscopic appendectomy. Endoscopy 1983;15:59.

67. Schrieber J. Early experience with laparoscopic appendectomy in women. Surg Endosc 1987;1:211.

68. Leape LL, Ramenofsy MI. Laparoscopy for questionable appendicitis. Ann Surg 1980;191:410.

69. Whitworth CM, Whitworth PW, Sanfillipo J, Polk HC. Value of diagnostic laparoscopy in young women with possible appendicitis. Surg Gynecol Obstet 1988;167:187.

70. Tamir IL, Bongard FS, Klein SR. Acute appendicitis in the pregnant patient. Am J Surg 1990;160:571.

71. Gangal HT, Gangal MH. Laparoscopic appendicectomy. Endoscopy 1987;19:127.

72. Gotz F, Pier A, Bacher C. Modified laparoscopic appendectomy in surgery: a report on 388 operations. Surg Endosc 1990;4:6.

73. Apelgren KN, Molnar RG, Kisala JM. Is laparoscopic better than open appendectomy? Surg Endosc 1992;6:298.

74. Fritts LL, Orlando R III. Laparoscopic appendectomy: a safety and cost analysis. Arch Surg 1993;128:521.

75. Schirmer BD, Schmieg RE Jr, Dix J, Edge SB, Hanks JB. Laparoscopic versus traditional appendectomy for suspected appendicitis. Am J Surg 1993;165:670.

76. Saye WB, Rives DA, Cochran EB. Laparoscopic appendectomy: three years' experience. Surg Laparosc Endosc 1991;1:109.

77. Nowzaradan Y, Westmoreland J, McCarver CT, Harris RJ. Laparoscopic appendectomy for acute appendicitis: indications and current use. J Laparoendosc Surg 1991;1:247.

78. Pier A, Gotz F, Bacher C. Laparoscopic appendectomy in 625 cases: from innovation to routine. Surg Laparosc Endosc 1991;1:8.

79. Greenall MJ, Evans M, Pollock AV. Should you drain a perforated appendix? Br J Surg 1978;65:880.

80. Jordan JS, Kovalcik PJ, Schwab CW. Appendicitis with a palpable mass. Ann Surg 1981;193:227.

81. Skoubo-Christensen E, Hvid I. The appendiceal mass: results of conservative management. Ann Surg 1982;196:584.

82. Bagi P, Dueholm S. Nonoperative management of the ultrasonically evaluated appendiceal mass. Surgery 1987;101:602.

83. Johnson WC, Gerzof SG. Appendiceal abscess: operative drainage or percutaneous drainage? Infect Surg 1985;4:367.

84. Vakili C. Operative treatment of the appendix mass. Am J Surg 1976;131:312.

85. Welch NT, Hinder RA, Fitzgibbons RJ. Laparoscopic incidental appendectomy. Surg Laparosc Endosc 1991;1:116.

86. Ludbrook J, Spears GFS. The risk of developing appendicitis. Br J Surg 1965;52:856.

87. Donaldson DR, Jones K, Aubrey DA. Appendicectomy at cholecystectomy: an appraisal. Br J Clin Pract 1989;43:15.

88. Voitk AJ, Lowry JB. Is incidental appendectomy a safe practice? Can J Surg 1988;31:448.

89. Parsons AK, Sauer MV, Parsons MT, et al. Appendectomy at caesarian section: a prospective study. Obstet Gynecol 1986;68:479.

90. Andrew MH, Roty AR Jr. Incidental appendectomy with cholecystectomy: is the increased risk justified? Ann Surg 1987;53:553.

91. Voeller GR, Fabian TC. Inversion–ligation appendectomy for incidental appendectomy. Am J Surg 1991;161:483.

92. Mueller BA, Daling JR, Moore DE, et al. Appendectomy and the risk of tubal infertility. N Engl J Med 1986;315:1506.

93. Harris CR. Appendiceal stump abscess ten years after appendectomy. Am J Emerg Med 1989;25:238.

94. Arnbjornsson E. Development of right inguinal hernia after appendectomy. Am J Surg 1982;143:174.

95. Lyss AP. Appendiceal malignancies. Semin Oncol 1988;15:129.

96. Roggo A, Wood WC, Ottinger LW. Carcinoid tumors of the appendix. Ann Surg 1993;217:385.

97. Goodwin JD. Carcinoid tumors: an analysis of 2837 cases. Cancer 1975;36:560.

98. Moertel CG, Weiland LH, Nagorney DM, Dockerty MB. Carcinoid tumor of the appendix: treatment and prognosis. N Engl J Med 1987;317:1699.

99. Thirlby R, Kasper C, Jones R. Metastatic carcinoid tumor of the appendix: report of a case and review of the literature. Dis Colon Rectum 1984;27:42.

100. Higa E, Rosai J, Pizzimbono C, et al. Mucosal hyperplasia, mucinous cystadenoma, and mucinous cystadenocarcinoma of the appendix: a re-evaluation of appendiceal "mucocele." Cancer 1973;32:1525.

101. Aho A, Heinonen R, Lauren P. Benign and malignant

mucocele of the appendix: histologic types and prognosis. Acta Chir Scand 1973;139:392.

102. Landen S, Bertrand C, Maddern GJ, et al. Appendiceal mucoceles and pseudomyxoma peritonei. Surg Gynecol Obstet 1992;175:401.

103. Yeh H, Shafir MK, Slater G, et al. Ultrasonography and computed tomography in pseudomyxoma peritonei. Radiology 1984;153:507.

104. Ferro M, Anthony P. Adenocarcinoma of the appendix. Dis Colon Rectum 1985;28:457.

105. Warkel R, Cooper P, Helwig E. Adenocarcinoid, a mucin-producing carcinoid tumor of the appendix: a study of 39 cases. Cancer 1978;42:2781.

106. Edmons P, Merino J, LiVolsi V, et al. Adenocarcinoid (mucinous carcinoid) of the appendix. Gastroenterology 1984;86:302.

107. Williams GR, Du Boulay CEH, Roche WR. Benign epithelial neoplasms of the appendix: classification and clinical associations. Histopathology 1992;21: 447.

108. Lipton S, Estrin J, Lasser I. Diverticular disease of the appendix. Surg Gynecol Obstet 1989;168:13.

109. Jevon GP, Daya D, Qizilbash AH. Intussusception of the appendix: a report of four cases and review of the literature. Arch Pathol Lab Med 1992;116:960.

110. Kaveggia FF, Schaldach FA, Jensen DP, Virata RL. Endometriosis and intussusception of the appendix. Contemp Surg 1992;41:57.

111. Balch CM, Silver D. Foreign bodies in the appendix. Arch Surg 1971;102:14.

Digestive Tract Surgery: A Text and Atlas, edited by Richard H Bell,
Layton F. Rikkers, and Michael W. Mulholland.
Lippincott-Raven Publishers, Philadelphia, © 1996.

38

Ulcerative Colitis

Robert D. Madoff

Ulcerative colitis is a diffuse inflammatory disease of the mucosa and submucosa of the large bowel; its course can range from acute and fulminant to chronic and relapsing. Some patients enter a phase of quiescent colitis that can last for years or decades. Although a variety of medical therapies are available for ulcerative colitis, they are not universally successful and surgery is often necessary. Surgery is also indicated to prevent or treat carcinoma of the large bowel, the risk of which increases markedly over many years of disease. Because ulcerative colitis is limited to the large intestine, total proctocolectomy is curative.

EPIDEMIOLOGY
AND PATHOGENESIS

Ulcerative colitis has a widely variable geographic distribution. The disease is relatively more common in developed countries in North America and Northern Europe, with reported incidences of 4 to 11 per 100,000 people.[1] In contrast, there is a low incidence of ulcerative colitis in developing countries in Africa, Asia, and South America. The disease is rare in Japan, occurring in about 0.4 per 100,000 population. Disease incidence also varies markedly within populations. For example, European- and American-born Israelis develop ulcerative colitis twice as often as do African-, Asian-, or Israeli-born Israelis, and in New Zealand, whites are 10 times as prone to the disease as Polynesians.[1]

Ulcerative colitis can occur at any age, but the disease is most common in the young. The peak incidence in the United States is in the third decade in men and in the fourth decade in women. A second incidence peak occurs later in life during the eighth decade.[2] The sexes are equally affected. The disease clusters in families, with first-degree relatives of patients having 15 times the prevalence of the normal population.[1]

Studies of monozygotic twins demonstrate alterations in colonic mucin in both affected and unaffected siblings, suggesting a genetic predisposition to the disease.[3] Additional support for a genetic predisposition arises from the fact that colitis-associated neutrophil autoantibodies are seen about five times as frequently in unaffected family members of patients with colitis as in unrelated environmental control subjects.[4] On the other hand, the presence of abnormal colonic mucin and neutrophil autoantibodies in unaffected relatives of patients with ulcerative colitis suggests that genetic predisposition alone is not sufficient for the development of the disease.

The etiology of ulcerative colitis remains unknown. Infectious agents and dietary factors have been proposed in large numbers over the years, but a convincing case for any factor remains to be made. Several uncontrolled studies suggest a psychogenic etiology, but careful scrutiny of available data does not support a causal relationship.[5]

One environmental factor of note in the pathogenesis of ulcerative colitis is cigarette smoking. Patients with ulcerative colitis, in contrast to those with Crohn's disease, tend to be nonsmokers. The risk of the disease increases significantly in nonsmoking populations such as Mormons, and cessation of smoking by patients with ulcerative colitis is often associated with relapse of the disease.[1]

The detection of antibodies and lymphocytes cytotoxic to colonic epithelial cells in patients with ulcerative colitis has suggested that ulcerative colitis is an autoimmune disease. Although there is little doubt that the immune system does mediate tissue damage in ulcerative colitis, evidence that the disease is caused by an immunologic reaction against a specific autoantigen is lacking.[6] It is more likely that ulcerative colitis is caused by an "innocent bystander" mechanism, whereby normal colon is injured in the setting of non-autoimmune mucosal T-cell activation.[6] Regardless of the initiating factor, there is ample documentation of the escalating cascade of immune mediators (eg, cytokines, prostaglandins, interleukins, leukotrienes) that characterize the chronic inflammation of ulcerative colitis.[7,8]

Another clue to the pathogenesis of ulcerative colitis comes from patients who have undergone proctocolectomy with creation of an ileoanal reservoir. These patients have a tendency to develop pouchitis, an inflammatory condition of the reservoir that clinically and histologically mimics ulcerative colitis. Although the pathogenesis of this condition remains uncertain, it is intriguing to note that pouchitis is rare to nonexistent in patients who have undergone restorative proctocolectomy for familial adenomatous polyposis. Pouchitis may be related to ulcerative colitis, and elucidation of its pathogenesis may shed light on that of ulcerative colitis.

PATHOLOGY

Ulcerative colitis is limited to the mucosa and submucosa of the large bowel. The disease is invariably present in the rectum and extends proximally in a continuous fashion for variable distances. Skip areas of normal intervening mucosa are not seen. Associated distal ileal inflammation, termed *backwash ileitis,* is seen in about 10% of patients with pancolonic disease.

The histologic hallmark of ulcerative colitis is the crypt abscess, a collection of neutrophils filling a crypt of Lieberkühn (Fig. 38-1). Crypt abscesses expand and coalesce to form mucosal ulcers, whose margins become undermined laterally, forming characteristic collar button–like ulcers seen in profile on barium enema. Confluence of mucosal ulceration can lead to extensive denuding of the colonic surface; residual islands of inflamed mucosa and granulation tissue are termed *pseudopolyps* (Fig. 38-2). Goblet cells lining the crypts are depleted of mucin. An inflammatory infiltrate consisting of neutrophils, lymphocytes, plasma cells, and mast cells is present in the lamina propria, and submucosal edema and hemorrhage are present. Mucosal regeneration is seen during quiescent phases of the disease, characterized grossly by an atrophic mucosal appearance and microscopically by dilated and atypical glands.

CLINICAL FEATURES

The clinical presentation of ulcerative colitis varies with the extent of disease and classically includes passage of bloody diarrhea and mucus. Abdominal pain and tenesmus are variably present. The severity of disease can range from mild rectal bleeding with no increase in stool frequency to fulminant colitis with 20 or more bloody bowel movements per day. Patients with subacute presentations may have associated weight loss and malnutrition. *Toxic megacolon* is characterized by paralytic ileus, dilatation of the colon, and signs of sys-

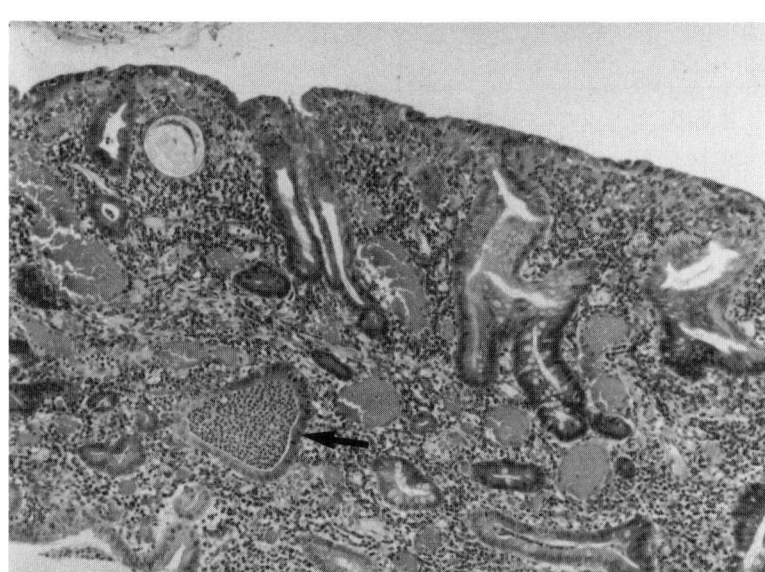

Figure 38-1 Crypt abscess (*arrow*). This crypt of Lieberkühn is filled with polymorphonucleocytes. (See Color Fig. 38-1.)

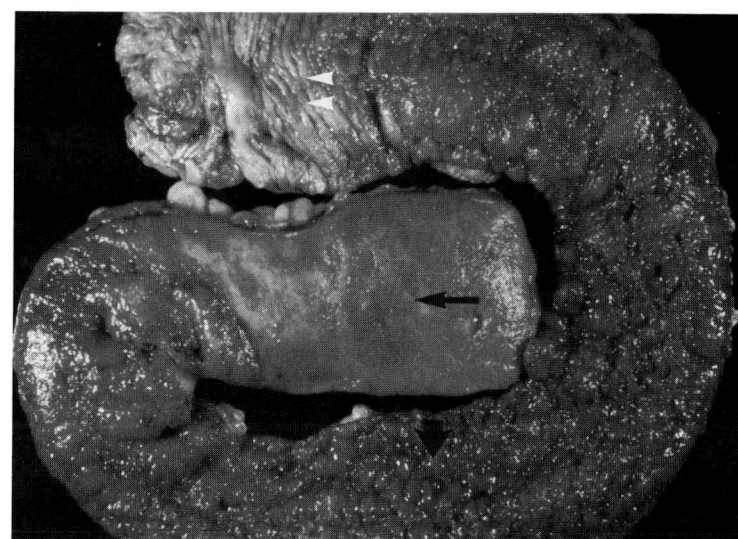

Figure 38-2 Ulcerative colitis. Denudation of rectal mucosa (*black arrowhead*), pseudopolyps (*large black arrow*), and preservation of the normal cecal mucosa (*white arrowheads*) can be seen. (See Color Fig. 38-2.)

temic toxicity (fever, tachycardia, hypotension, and mental status changes).

Ulcerative colitis is a chronic relapsing condition, and it is rare for unoperated patients observed over many years to have only a single attack.[9] Most patients have periods of remission punctuated by episodic recurrences, with frequency and severity varying considerably.[7,8] Smaller groups of patients require surgery for their first attack or fail to obtain full remission and follow a chronic continuous course.[10]

The need for colectomy varies with the extent of disease: at 3 years after diagnosis, about 30% of patients with pancolitis, 10% of patients with limited colitis, and 2% of patients with a distal proctocolitis alone require surgery.[7,8] Subsequently, the annual colectomy rate becomes similar for all three groups. Patients with longstanding ulcerative colitis harbor an increased risk of developing colorectal cancer.

DIFFERENTIAL DIAGNOSIS

Ulcerative colitis must be differentiated from other types of inflammatory bowel disease (Crohn's disease, collagenous colitis, microscopic colitis); radiation colitis; ischemic colitis; and various forms of infectious colitis.

Differentiation of ulcerative colitis from Crohn's disease has important clinical implications. Features suggestive of ulcerative colitis include total colonic involvement with a distal predominance and continuity to the rectum, broad-based ulcers, pseudopolyps, and an absence of skip areas. A diagnosis of Crohn's disease is suggested by a cobblestone mucosal appearance caused by linear ulcers with transverse fissuring. Other features suggestive of Crohn's disease include rectal sparing, skip lesions, transmural inflammation, the presence of microscopic granulomas, and associated small bowel and perianal disease. In about 15% of cases, differentiation between the two disorders is not possible, and the disease is termed *indeterminate colitis.*

Collagenous colitis presents with watery rather than bloody diarrhea and usually occurs in older women. The endoscopic appearance is generally normal and diagnosis of this disorder is made by biopsy. Collagenous colitis is diagnosed by the presence of a characteristic subepithelial collagen layer. Ischemic colitis causes bloody diarrhea, usually in patients with histories of atherosclerotic cardiovascular disease.[11] Abdominal pain is frequently present. The disease usually occurs at the splenic flexure watershed between the superior and inferior mesenteric artery distributions. The rectum is almost always spared due to collateral blood flow from the middle and inferior rectal arteries. Radiation colitis is suggested by a previous history of pelvic radiotherapy, usually for gynecologic malignancy in women and prostatic cancer in men. This disease, usually limited to the rectum and sigmoid, is characterized by rectal bleeding and diarrhea.

Infectious colitis can be caused by a host of organisms, and must be excluded by appropriate stool cultures, direct stool examination for ova and parasites, and, occasionally, colonic biopsies or serologic studies. Important pathogens include species of *Salmonella, Shigella, Campylobacter,* and *Yersinia.* Pseudomembranous colitis caused by *Clostridium difficile* should be considered in patients with histories of recent antibiotic use, and amebiasis (*Entamoeba histolytica*) must be excluded, particularly in patients with histories of travel to endemic areas. Enteroinvasive *Escherichia coli* (serotype 0157)

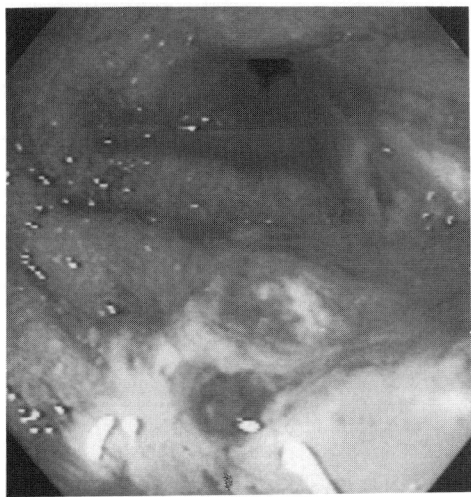

Figure 38-3 Endoscopic appearance of severe ulcerative colitis. (See Color Fig. 38-3.)

produces an acute *Shigella*-like syndrome of abdominal pain and bloody diarrhea.

Immunosuppressed patients are at risk for colitis due to cytomegalovirus, herpes simplex, and *Mycobacterium avium-intracellulare,* as well as neutropenic colitis in those with depressed neutrophil counts. Gonococcal proctitis should be considered in patients with histories of anoreceptive intercourse or other sexually transmitted diseases.

CLINICAL EVALUATION

Endoscopic evaluation of the colon is the cornerstone of diagnosis. The extent of examination is dictated by the disease severity: acutely ill patients can be evaluated unprepared with proctoscopic or flexible sigmoidoscopic examination, whereas patients with subacute or chronic colitis can undergo full colonoscopy after mechanical bowel preparation. The earliest endoscopic changes of colitis are loss of the normal vascular pattern of the colon, followed by mucosal granularity and friability, and finally progressing to ulceration and pseudopolyp formation (Figs. 38-3 and 38-4).

Radiographic evaluation of patients with acute colitis should include plain and upright views of the abdomen without contrast media. This examination allows the diagnosis of pneumoperitoneum and colonic dilatation; the presence of either contraindicates further contrast study (Fig. 38-5). The distal extent of the column of stool in the colon generally corresponds to the proximal extent of inflammation.[12]

Air contrast barium enema demonstrates the mucosal changes of ulcerative colitis, which range from fine granularity to collar button–like ulcers to pseudopolyps (Figs. 38-6 and 38-7). The colonic contour becomes shortened, with depression of the flexures and loss of the normal haustrations in the transverse and ascending colon. (Absence of haustral markings can be a normal finding in the left colon[12] [Fig. 38-8].) Colonic strictures, although often benign, must be considered malignant until proven otherwise, particularly if they are eccentric or do not have a smoothly tapered contour.

An upper gastrointestinal series with small bowel follow-through is useful to exclude the presence of small bowel involvement when Crohn's disease is suspected. Indium-111–labeled leukocyte scans have been used to assess the location and extent of colonic inflammation.[13] Computed tomography is useful in selected circumstances (Fig. 38-9).

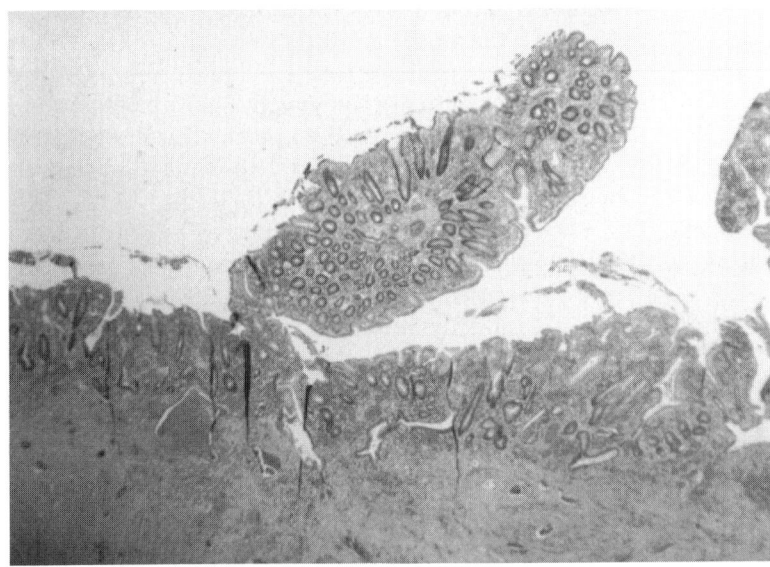

Figure 38-4 Colonic pseudopolyp due to ulcerative colitis. (See Color Fig. 38-4.)

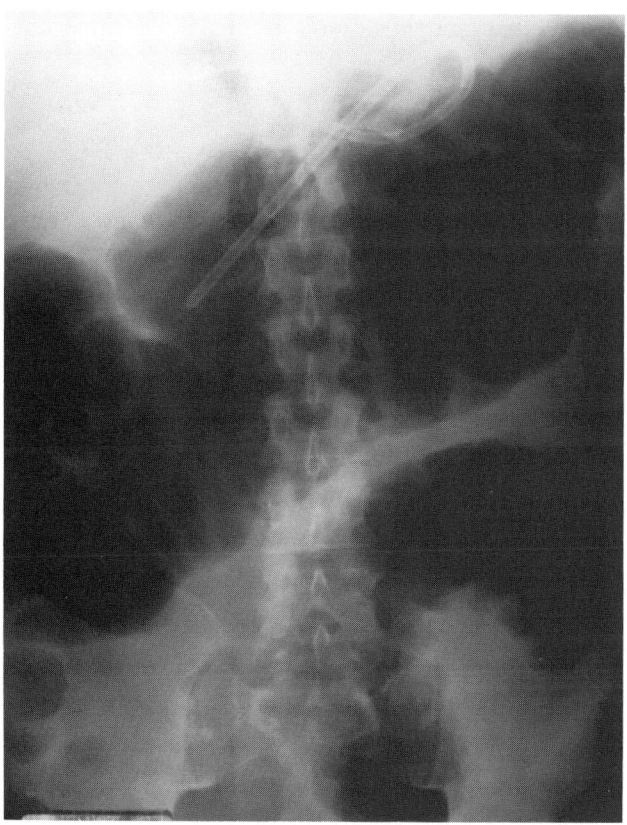

Figure 38-5 Massive colonic dilatation due to ulcerative colitis. This radiologic appearance, combined with clinical toxicity, represents toxic megacolon.

Extraintestinal Manifestations

Extraintestinal manifestations occur in about 25% of patients with ulcerative colitis.[14,15] Sites of involvement include the skin, eyes, joints, and biliary system. Extraintestinal manifestations are seen almost exclusively in patients with colitis extending proximal to the splenic flexure.

Skin

Erythema nodosum consists of nonulcerating nodular lesions that most commonly occur in the pretibial skin (Fig. 38-10). The lesions are seen in about 5% of patients with ulcerative colitis and often correlate with disease activity. *Pyoderma gangrenosum* is a painful, ulcerating skin lesion with overhanging edges and surrounding reddish purple discoloration (Fig. 38-11). Lesions most commonly occur in the lower extremities, and they can occur in more than one site. About half of patients with *pyoderma gangrenosum* have active colitis at the time of diagnosis. Most cases resolve with medical therapy directed at colitis alone. Response to colon surgery is variable, but some cases do resolve after resection of the diseased bowel.[16]

Eyes

Numerous ocular disorders are associated with ulcerative colitis, including episcleritis, anterior uveitis, iritis, and conjunctivitis. Manifestations usually parallel disease activity and remit with treatment of the acute colitis.

Joints

Joint manifestations of ulcerative colitis include acute arthritis, sacroiliitis, and ankylosing spondylitis. Acute monoarticular or polyarticular arthritis, generally affecting large joints, is the most common joint manifestation. Sacroiliitis may cause low back pain or may merely represent an incidental finding on radiologic examination. Most cases do not progress to anky-

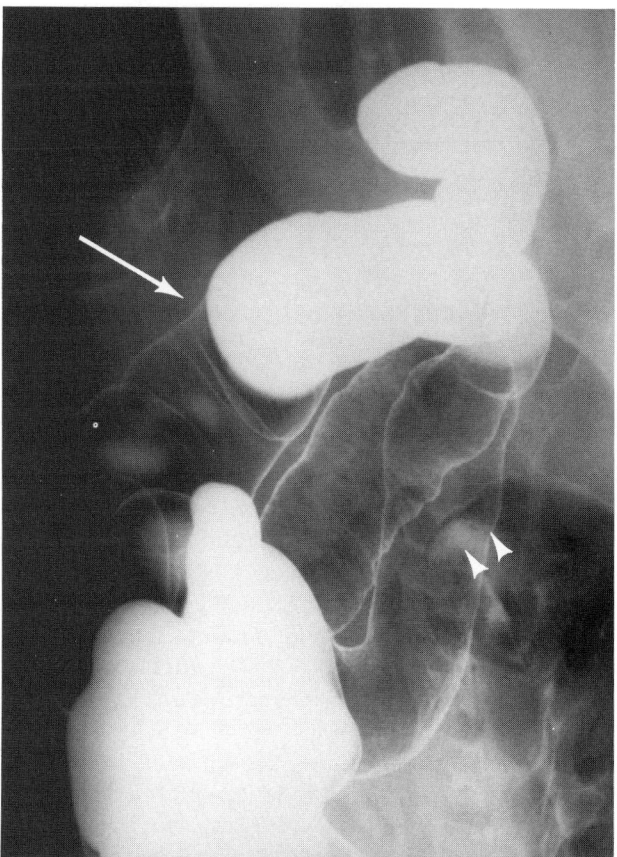

Figure 38-6 Air contrast barium enema showing granularity and fine ulceration of the rectosigmoid (*arrowheads*). The proximal sigmoid is normal (*arrow*).

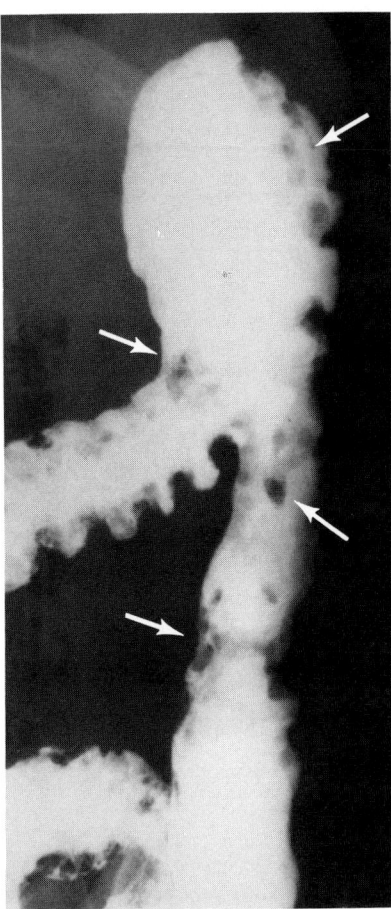

Figure 38-7 Pseudopolyps in the transverse and descending colon (*arrows*).

losing spondylitis, which usually is seen in HLA-B27–positive patients.

Liver

Sclerosing cholangitis is a chronic, progressive, obliterative disorder characterized by fibrosis and inflammation of the intrahepatic and extrahepatic bile ducts (Fig. 38-12). *Pericholangitis* of the intrahepatic ducts is now believed to be part of the spectrum of sclerosing cholangitis. Population studies in Sweden suggest a disease prevalence of 5.5% in patients with colitis extending beyond the splenic flexure.[17] Men are affected twice as frequently as women. Sclerosing cholangitis is an independent risk factor for colonic dysplasia and neoplasia,[18,19] and patients with sclerosing cholangitis harbor an increased risk for developing cholangiocarcinoma. There is no effective medical therapy for sclerosing cholangitis, and proctocolectomy does not influence the course of the disease.[20] Patients with advanced sclerosing cholangitis may de-

velop biliary cirrhosis and ultimately require liver transplantation.

MEDICAL MANAGEMENT

The modern era of ulcerative colitis treatment began in 1942 with the serendipitous observation that sulfasalazine, being used experimentally to treat arthritis in a patient with colitis, led to remission of colitis.[21] The method of action was unknown, and it was not until 1977 that 5-aminosalicylic acid (5-ASA) was shown to be the active moiety of the drug.[22] Corticosteroid therapy was introduced in the early 1950s and efficacy was proved by placebo-controlled trial in 1955.[23] Forty years later, 5-ASA compounds and steroid preparations remain the cornerstones of ulcerative colitis therapy. Advances in the medical management of ulcerative colitis have included a better understanding of the relative roles of these drugs, the development of topical steroid preparations for distal colitis, improved 5-ASA delivery systems, and the use of immunosuppressive agents such as azathioprine, 6-mercaptopurine, and cyclosporine for refractory disease.

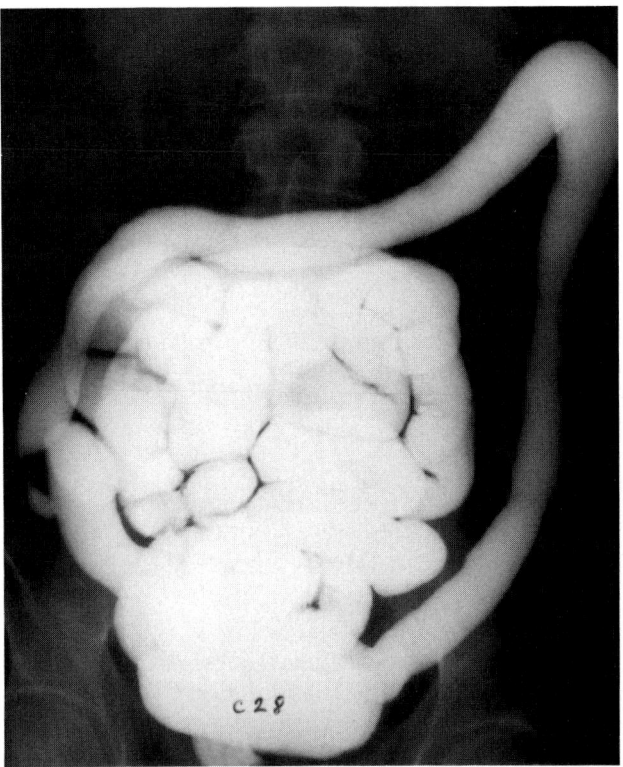

Figure 38-8 Chronic ulcerative colitis. There is a lack of haustration, shortening of the colon, and depression of the hepatic and splenic flexures.

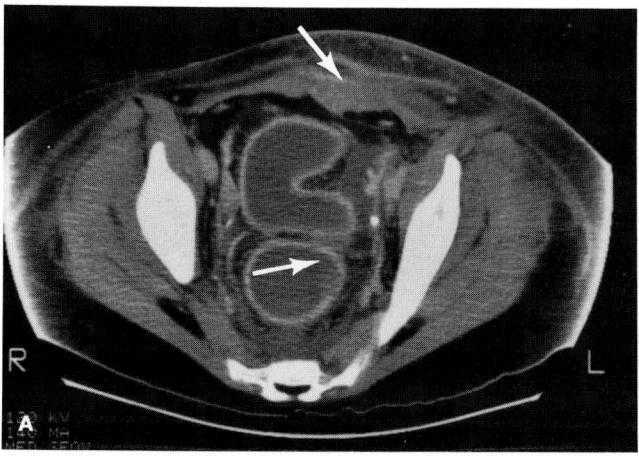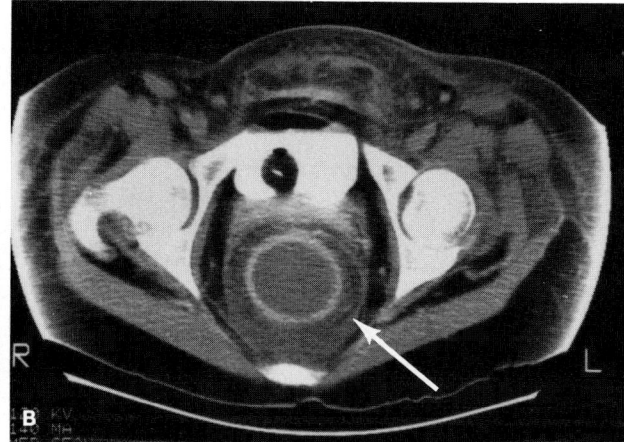

Figure 38-9 (**A**) Severe ulcerative colitis. Rectal and sigmoid walls are markedly thickened (*arrows*). (**B**) Same patient. Edema of perirectal fat is visible (*arrow*).

It is worth reemphasizing that ulcerative colitis is a chronic relapsing disease, rarely cured by medical therapy alone. Accordingly, the goals of drug therapy are to achieve a complete remission, to maintain the remission as long as possible, and to prevent side effects of the medications being used. Conversely, medical therapy can be deemed a failure if it is unable to abort an acute flare of colitis, if only a partial response to therapy is obtained, or if remission can be maintained only at the cost of unacceptable drug side effects.

Drugs

Salicylates

Sulfasalazine consists of 5-ASA bonded to sulfapyridine, with the sulfapyridine acting as a carrier molecule that is cleaved by bacteria in the colon to liberate the therapeutically active 5-ASA. Unbound 5-ASA is absorbed in the small bowel and, thus, cannot be used in its pure form to treat inflamed colonic mucosa. The common side effects of sulfasalazine are largely attributable to the sulfapyridine moiety. These include headache and gastrointestinal upset, which are dose-related, and skin rashes and reversible male infertility, which are not. About 15% of patients are unable to tolerate sulfasalazine because of its side effects.[24]

A variety of 5-ASA compounds have been developed that use alternative delivery systems to prevent premature absorption of the drug by the small bowel. Because these drugs share the same active agent, they are commonly referred to by their proprietary rather than generic names. These new agents include 5-ASA coated in pH-sensitive resin (eg, Asacol, Rowasa); 5-

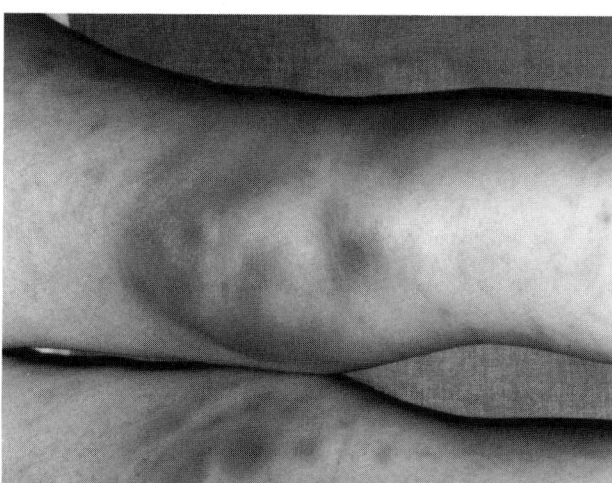

Figure 38-10 Erythema nodosum. (See Color Fig. 38-10.) (Courtesy of William E. Cornatzer, MD)

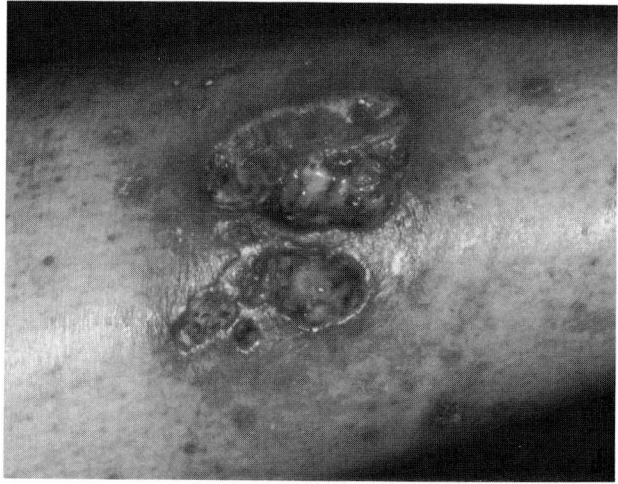

Figure 38-11 Pyoderma gangrenosum. (See Color Fig. 38-11.) (Courtesy of William E. Cornatzer, MD)

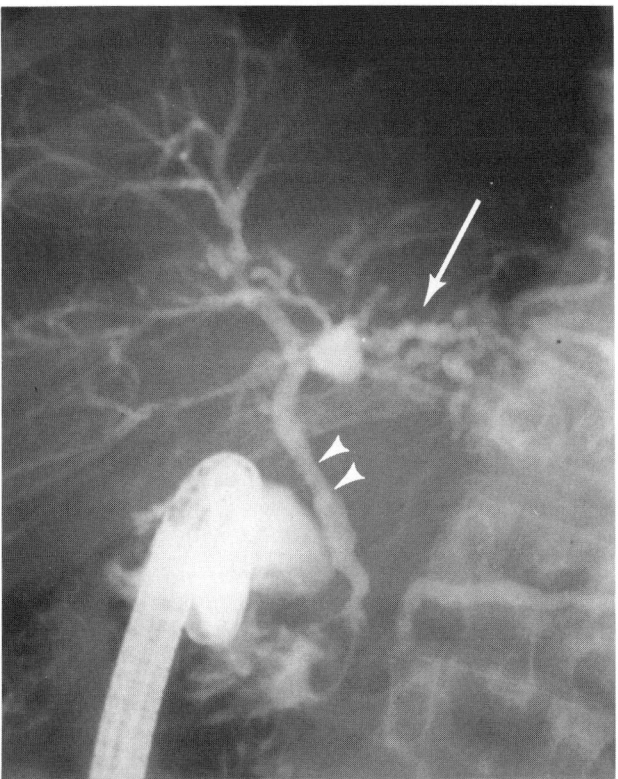

Figure 38-12 Sclerosing cholangitis. There are multiple areas of stenosis with saccular dilatation of the intrahepatic bile ducts, especially in the left lobe (*arrow*). The contour of the common bile duct is irregular (*arrowheads*).

ASA in slow-release microspheres (Pentasa); and 5-ASA linked to itself in an azo bond (osalazine [Dipentum]). 5-ASA compounds are available in oral, suppository, and enema forms. A metaanalysis comparing the various new 5-ASA preparations to sulfasalazine has demonstrated no therapeutic advantage for the new drugs.[25] Accordingly, because the new agents are considerably more expensive, their use should be reserved for patients who are intolerant of sulfasalazine.

Although they are useful in the treatment of acute colitis, 5-ASA compounds have an even more important role in the maintenance of disease remission. Relapse rates at 1 year decrease from about 70% to 20% with the use of sulfasalazine.[24] Prophylactic treatment should be continued for 1 to 2 years after cessation of symptoms.

Corticosteroids

Corticosteroids are powerful antiinflammatory agents that are highly effective in the treatment of ulcerative colitis. Because of the strong mineralocorticoid effect of hydrocortisone, synthetic variants such as

prednisone are generally preferred for therapy. Corticosteroids are available in a variety of preparations, including suppositories, enemas, topical foam, and oral and intravenous forms. Adrenocorticotropic hormone, which stimulates endogenous cortisol production, has no proven benefit over direct administration of the steroids themselves and is rarely used.

The adverse effects of long-term steroid treatment are well known to all clinicians. These include immunosuppression, weight gain, moon facies, acne, hypertension, hyperglycemia, mental depression, osteoporosis, aseptic hip necrosis, premature cataracts, adrenal suppression, and growth retardation in children. These side effects preclude the long-term use of corticosteroids for ulcerative colitis. Accordingly, the inability to wean patients from a steroid-dependent state represents a therapeutic failure and is an important indication for surgery. Furthermore, prophylactic steroid therapy has no role in the management of quiescent ulcerative colitis because it does not decrease the relapse rate without the development of unacceptable side effects.[26]

Attempts are underway to develop new corticosteroid preparations that minimize side effects either by decreasing systemic absorption or by increasing the first-pass hepatic metabolism of the drug.[26] These agents are not yet commercially available and their eventual role awaits definition.

Immunosuppressants

Azathioprine is converted to 6-mercaptopurine in the liver, and both antimetabolites have been used in the treatment of ulcerative colitis. Although this form of therapy has been considered controversial, both therapeutic and steroid-sparing effects have been documented in patients with refractory disease.[27,28] Beneficial effects can take 3 to 6 months or even longer to become apparent. Serious side effects include reversible bone marrow depression and pancreatitis, reported in 2% and 3%, respectively, of patients undergoing treatment with 6-mercaptopurine.[29] Infectious complications were seen in 7.4% of patients in the same series. One fourth of these infections were considered severe.

Cyclosporine is an immunosuppressant that is commonly used for organ transplantation. There are anecdotal reports of the successful use of cyclosporine for refractory colitis, and intravenous cyclosporine has been successfully used in a small series of patients with severe acute colitis that failed to respond to initial steroid therapy.[30]

Other Drugs

Antibiotics should be reserved for specific indications, such as suspected bacterial infection or toxic megacolon. Anticholinergics and antidiarrheals such as loperamide or diphenoxylate with atropine (Lomotil) should not be used in acute colitis, though judicious use in chronic smoldering disease is acceptable.

A miscellany of alternative drugs have had preliminary clinical evaluation in ulcerative colitis.[31] Lipoxygenase inhibitors have been used in an effort to decrease the effects of inflammatory mediators such as leukotriene B_4 and prostaglandin E_2. Examples include ω-3 fatty acids (found in fish oils) and the experimental drug Zileuton. Methotrexate, an antifolate antimetabolite being evaluated as an alternative to azathioprine and 6-mercaptopurine, appears to have a more rapid onset of action than the last two drugs. Uncontrolled studies using the antimalarial chloroquine and the related compound hydroxychloroquine have shown effectiveness in patients with ulcerative colitis. The mechanism of action may be due to interference of antigen processing by colonic epithelial cells.

Because of the protective effects of smoking on ulcerative colitis, nicotine administered as gum or by transdermal patch is undergoing evaluation. New topical treatments for ulcerative colitis include the use of short-chain fatty acid enemas, which provide nutritional substrate for the colonocytes, and lidocaine gel.

Therapeutic Strategy

The choice of treatment for ulcerative colitis depends on the extent and severity of disease. Mild left-sided colitis can be treated either topically or orally with 5-ASA preparations, or topically with steroids. Suppository or foam preparations are useful in patients whose disease is limited to the rectosigmoid, whereas retention enemas can be used for disease extending to the splenic flexure. Patients in whom this regimen fails or those with more severe distal disease usually require a course of oral steroid therapy.

Mild pancolitis requires oral therapy, either with a 5-ASA compound or with oral corticosteroids. Severe colitis, characterized by high stool frequencies (6 to 10 bowel movements per day), marked rectal bleeding, fever, and tachycardia mandates hospital admission. Oral intake is prohibited and fluid and electrolyte deficits are corrected intravenously. Nasogastric suction is appropriate in the presence of ileus with vomiting or colonic dilatation. Intravenous corticosteroids at a dose equivalent to 300 mg/d of hydrocortisone are indicated. Profound anemia is corrected by transfusion, and total parenteral nutrition is administered when nutritional deficits are present. Empiric broad-spectrum antibiotic therapy, including aerobic and anaerobic coverage, is appropriate in the presence of elevated temperature or abdominal tenderness. Patients hospitalized for severe colitis require close clinical follow-up with serial physical examinations and abdominal radiographs.

Indications for Surgery

Acute indications for surgery in ulcerative colitis include known or suspected perforation, fulminant colitis, toxic megacolon, and massive hemorrhage. Subacute or elective indications include intractability, cancer prophylaxis, cancer treatment, and certain refractory extraintestinal manifestations.

The goal of surgery for acute complications of colitis is to remove most of the affected large bowel, to prevent the development of complications, and to correct any complications that have already occurred. In most cases, the correct choice of operation under these circumstances is subtotal colectomy with preservation of the rectal remnant. This approach offers several advantages. First, the acute problem is addressed in an expeditious and effective manner, and all options for definitive surgery remain open. Subsequent surgery can be performed on an elective basis on a patient who is no longer severely ill, who has had an opportunity to regain his or her nutritional balance, and who has been weaned from corticosteroids. Under these circumstances, careful and deliberate rectal dissection can be performed to minimize the risk of pelvic nerve injury, and the infectious morbidity of proctectomy will be lessened. The colon will have been examined pathologically, markedly decreasing the likelihood of an unsuspected diagnosis of Crohn's disease. Finally, the patient will have gained firsthand knowledge of life with an ileostomy. This experience provides a useful perspective as the patient considers the various definitive surgical alternatives available.

The rectal remnant can be managed by several methods after subtotal colectomy. Most surgeons simply close the proximal end of the rectum and return it to the pelvis as a Hartmann pouch. Concerns with this approach include the integrity of the stump closure and technical difficulties that can arise in establishing the proper plane of dissection at the time of subsequent proctectomy. Other surgeons prefer to leave a longer stump and create a mucous fistula. A third option is to place the closed rectal stump outside the fascia in the subcutaneous position. This technique has the advantage of exteriorizing any potential stump blow-outs, and it prevents mucous fistula creation in two thirds of patients (about one third of exteriorized closed rectal stumps spontaneously open to create mucous fistulas).[32]

Perforation

Perforation is the most dreaded acute complication of ulcerative colitis. Although perforation is most commonly seen as a complication of toxic megacolon, it occasionally occurs as a complication of acute colitis without megacolon.[33] Because perforation markedly increases the morbidity and mortality of ulcerative colitis, prevention of this complication is one of the main concerns in the initial management of fulminant or toxic colitis. In one series,[33] perforation occurred in 33% of patients with and 1.3% of patients without toxic dilatation. The mortality rates in these groups were 44% and 57%, respectively. At another center, concern over perforation led to the adoption of a policy of early surgery for acute colitis, which corresponded to decreased rates of perforation (from 32.5% to 11.6%) and operative mortality (from 20% to 7%).[34]

In many cases, the diagnosis of colonic perforation is obvious, based on acute clinical deterioration, new development of a surgical abdomen, marked leukocytosis (or new leukopenia) with left shift, high fever, or pneumoperitoneum on abdominal radiographs. Other times, particularly when the perforation is localized or walled off, definitive diagnosis can be difficult. High-dose corticosteroid therapy can mask the findings of even gross peritonitis, so a "benign" physical examination cannot be relied on to exclude the diagnosis. In general, a clinical suspicion of perforation, even in the absence of a firm diagnosis, is grounds for surgery.

As detailed earlier, subtotal colectomy with ileostomy and a Hartmann pouch or mucous fistula is the appropriate operation in the setting of perforated colitis. There is no role for performing a rectal excision, and even less for a complex reconstructive operation such as an ileoanal pouch.

Fulminant Colitis

Acute severe colitis (characterized by more than six bloody bowel movements per day, fever, and tachycardia) requires aggressive medical therapy and close clinical monitoring. Remission rates of 40% to 55% have been reported.[35,36] Surgery is indicated if the patient fails to improve within 5 days, and urgent surgery is necessary if clinical deterioration occurs at any time.

Toxic Megacolon

Toxic megacolon describes the clinical occurrence of colonic dilatation with systemic toxicity. Dilatation is frequently most prominent in the transverse colon, where a diameter of greater than 6 cm is considered abnormal. Signs of toxicity include fever, tachycardia, hypotension, and altered sensorium. Abdominal examination usually demonstrates distention, tenderness, and hypoactive bowel sounds.

Toxic megacolon can occur either during the initial attack of ulcerative colitis or after disease relapse and can occasionally arise in patients with limited disease rather than pancolitis. The condition is seen in 10% of hospitalized patients with ulcerative colitis[33] and can be precipitated by barium enema or inappropriate use of antidiarrheal or anticholinergic medication in the setting of acute colitis. The presence of toxic megacolon implies severe colitis with marked inflammation, edema, and friability of the colon.

Mortality from toxic megacolon is mainly related to perforation. In one series,[33] perforation occurred in one third of all patients with toxic megacolon and caused a 44% mortality rate. The prognosis was equally bad for sealed or free perforations. In contrast, only 2% of patients with nonperforated toxic megacolon died. Other factors associated with increased mortality rates in this series included age greater than 40 years (30% versus 5%) and need for early (within 5 days after admission) or delayed (more than 1 month after admission) surgery. Eight of 14 patients (57%) in this series who underwent successful medical treatment of their toxic megacolon subsequently required surgery. Similar findings were reported in another study,[37] in which 18 of 38 patients (47%) who had undergone successful medical treatment of toxic megacolon were found to require subsequent surgery, almost always on an urgent basis.

Hemorrhage

Uncontrollable hemorrhage is a relatively uncommon indication for operation in ulcerative colitis. In a series of patients undergoing urgent ulcerative colitis surgery, hemorrhage was the indication in only 6 of 132 cases (4.5%).[38] There were no deaths in this group. In general, colectomy should be considered in the face of ongoing bleeding after a six- to eight-unit transfusion requirement. Subtotal colectomy remains the procedure of choice in the acute situation, although a few patients require early proctectomy for uncontrollable rectal hemorrhage.

Intractability

Some patients with ulcerative colitis are either unable to be weaned completely off steroid therapy or require frequent reinstitution of such therapy. A trial of immunosuppressive drug therapy may prove beneficial for some of these patients. Patients who remain steroid-dependent, or who develop complications from medical therapy, should be considered for surgery. This indication is particularly important in children, in whom growth retardation secondary to chronic disease and prolonged steroid use is an important issue.

Cancer Prophylaxis

Although early estimates of the long-term cancer risk of ulcerative colitis now appear to have been overstated (60% at 30 years), there is no question that patients with long-standing colitis harbor a significant risk of developing colorectal cancer. This risk is greatest in patients with pancolitis but is also present in patients with more limited disease.[7,8] The risk of cancer is not diminished by clinical quiescence.

Biases responsible for the overestimation of cancer risk included generalization of data from referral center populations, inclusion of patients with cancer at the time of referral, inability to identify a true common denominator for patients at risk for malignancy, and limited number of patients followed over the long term. Current estimates of cancer risk vary widely based on geographic location, type of study, definition of population, and method of statistical analysis. One report estimated the cancer risk in a group of New York private practice patients to range from 11.6% to 19.7%, depending on the statistical technique used.[39] The magnitude of cancer risk in other studies following up 20 years of disease ranges from 2% to 25%.[40]

Cancer arising in ulcerative colitis may be difficult to diagnose and tends to present at an advanced stage. For this reason, the concept of prophylactic colectomy after 15 to 20 years of pancolitis was once accepted as surgical dogma. However, a policy of mandatory colectomy carries the inherent disadvantage of removing many colons that never were destined to develop cancer. The clinical problem is identifying which colons these are.

A refinement in the selection of patients for colectomy became available in 1967 with the observation that the development of colorectal cancer in patients with colitis is associated with local or distant dysplastic changes in the colonic mucosa[41] (Fig. 38-13). This observation has led to the development of colonoscopic dysplasia screening programs. Patients participating in these programs undergo annual colonoscopy, beginning in most centers after 8 to 10 years of pancolitis, and multiple biopsy samples are obtained throughout the colon to identify dysplastic foci. Biopsy samples are also obtained of any mass lesions. Identification of high-grade dysplasia or of a dysplasia-associated lesion or mass is an indication for colectomy.

Though widely practiced, the strategy of dysplasia screening has come under considerable criticism.[40]

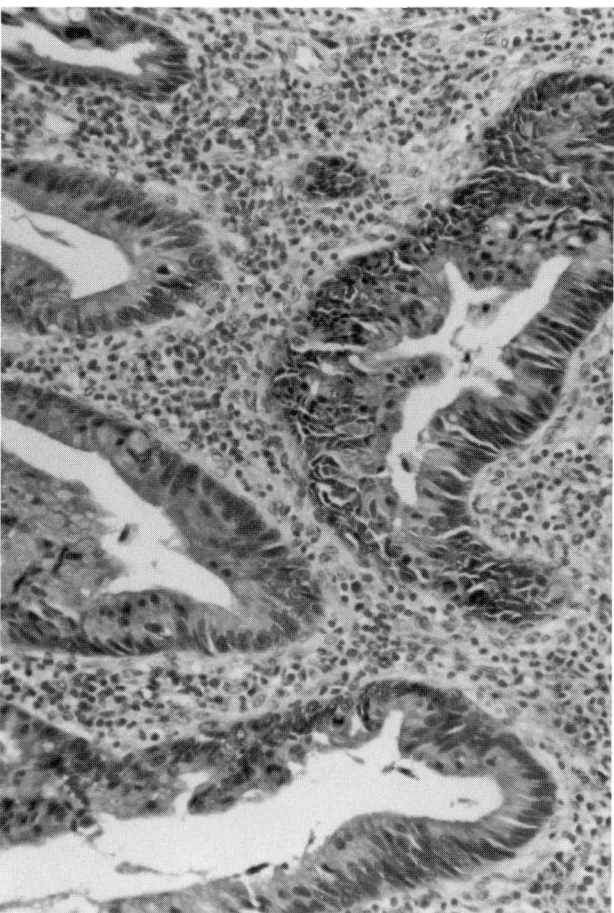

Figure 38-13 Severe dysplasia arising in chronic ulcerative colitis. Marked epithelial crowding, nuclear pseudostratification and hyperchromasia, and scattered mitoses are visible. (See Color Fig. 38-13.)

First, the approach requires lifelong patient compliance with an invasive procedure that is inconvenient, uncomfortable, and costly. Although the risks of colonoscopic complications are small, they become significant in the context of population screening. The histologic diagnosis of dysplasia is imperfect, particularly in the setting of acute inflammation, and the significance of low-grade dysplasia is uncertain.

Dysplasia screening is an imperfectly sensitive tool, and even rigorous dysplasia screening does not guarantee that advanced malignancy will not develop. In blinded studies, high-grade dysplasia was found in only half of colitic colons harboring cancer,[42] and up to 20% of cancers developing in patients undergoing routine dysplasia screening are diagnosed in the absence of dysplasia.[40] Furthermore, if early cancer detection is indeed the mechanism of improved survival in screened populations, it is disturbing that about one third of cancers diagnosed by dysplasia screening in collected series are advanced (Dukes stage C or D).[40]

Despite its many imperfections, dysplasia screening remains the best available approach to colorectal cancer prophylaxis in patients with long-standing ulcerative colitis. There is hope that improved dysplasia markers such as c-k-*ras* mutations[43] and abnormal p53 expression[44] will improve the sensitivity and specificity of the technique. In the meantime, there remains a legitimate role for prophylactic colectomy in the absence of dysplasia after many years of colitis. The decision for surgery under these circumstances must be individualized, and the magnitude of the cancer risk must be balanced with the morbidity and functional results of proctocolectomy with or without reconstruction.

Colorectal Cancer

The development of colorectal cancer is an obvious indication for surgery in ulcerative colitis, and in general the entire large bowel should be resected. Lesser operations can be considered in patients with quiescent colitis who have advanced or metastatic disease at the time of diagnosis. Again, the risk of developing new cancer must be balanced with the likelihood of surviving the initial cancer and with the anticipated functional results of definitive surgery.

Extraintestinal Manifestations

Severe refractory extraintestinal manifestations of ulcerative colitis occasionally require surgical intervention, although the response to surgery is variable. Ankylosing spondylitis and primary sclerosing cholangitis do not improve after colectomy and, therefore, are not indications for surgery.

SURGICAL THERAPY

There are four definitive operations for ulcerative colitis: total proctocolectomy with Brooke ileostomy, total proctocolectomy with continent ileal reservoir (Kock pouch), subtotal colectomy with ileorectal anastomosis, and total proctocolectomy with pelvic pouch and anal anastomosis (restorative proctocolectomy). The functional results of each of these operations are different, and each procedure has distinct advantages and disadvantages (Table 38-1).

Selection of the best operation for an individual patient requires a collaborative effort by the patient and surgeon. The benefits *and* disadvantages of each approach must be candidly discussed because the establishment of unrealistic expectations inevitably leads to

patient dissatisfaction. Optimal patient education is achieved with a combination of written material, enterostomal therapist referral, and contact with patients who have previously undergone the various surgical procedures under consideration.

Preoperative patient preparation depends on the clinical situation. Whenever possible, preoperative mechanical antibiotic bowel preparation should be performed. Perioperative antibiotics can be given orally, intravenously, or both orally and intravenously. Most patients require preoperative steroid coverage because of the adrenal suppression of long-term steroid therapy. Deep venous thrombosis prophylaxis should be used in all patients in whom pelvic dissection is anticipated. One preference is for pneumatic compression stockings.

Preoperative assessment of the patient should be performed by the enterostomal therapist for all patients in whom a temporary or permanent stoma is anticipated. This is important not only for patient education but also for accurate marking of the optimal site for a stoma. The ideal site for a conventional ileostomy is visible and accessible to the patient (not under the panniculus), traverses the rectus abdominis, and avoids previous scars and deformities. It is a truism that the major source of dissatisfaction in patients with ostomies relates to a poorly functioning stoma, and improper positioning of the stoma virtually guarantees a suboptimal result.

Several factors facilitate the technical conduct of ulcerative colitis surgery. Patients are best positioned in the modified lithotomy position with the knees and hips slightly flexed and the legs abducted. This position permits placement of a second assistant surgeon between the patient's legs, where he or she is perfectly located to visualize the splenic flexure during mobilization and to retract during the pelvic dissection. This position also provides exposure for a perineal operator should a synchronous operation be performed. Alternatively, the perineal dissection can be performed with the patient in the prone jackknife position, either before (mucosectomy in restorative proctocolectomy) or after (distal proctectomy) the abdominal portion of the case. Despite the added operative time related to repositioning the patient, exposure of the perineum is vastly improved with the patient prone.

Proctectomy performed for a benign disease such as ulcerative colitis is a different operation from proctectomy performed for malignancy. In the latter case, the widest possible dissection is desired; in the former case, care must be taken to preserve pelvic nerves and, thereby, sexual and urinary function. Although some authors report good results performing the posterior dissection in the anatomic plane immediately posterior to the mesorectal en-

Table 38-1 Surgical Options for Ulcerative Colitis

Procedure	Features	Advantages	Disadvantages
Total proctocolectomy with permanent Brooke ileostomy	Removal of entire colon, rectum, and anus Permanent Brooke ileostomy	Eliminates risk of colorectal cancer Curative for chronic ulcerative colitis Routine procedure for the surgeon Usually one operation Known complications Known long-term results	Permanent ileostomy Requires pouching system Possible sexual and bladder dysfunction Perineal wound Further restorative surgery unlikely
Total colectomy with ileorectal anastomosis	Removal of entire colon Ileum joined to rectum	No ileostomy No external pouching system Best approximates normal bowel function Routine procedure for the surgeon Usually one operation Further restorative surgery feasible	Not curative Risk of cancer in retained rectum Frequent stools (3–8/d) Requires regular follow-up with proctoscopy Further surgery often necessary
Kock pouch (continent ileostomy)	Removal of entire colon, rectum, and anus Permanent ileostomy with nipple valve Internal abdominal ileal reservoir	Eliminates risk of colorectal cancer Curative for chronic ulcerative colitis No external pouching system Continence good when procedure works well Usually one operation Ileostomy may be located lower on the abdomen	Permanent ileostomy Patient must intubate and carry supplies to empty pouch Continence variable Requires specialized surgical expertise Operative revision may be needed Possible sexual and bladder dysfunction Perineal wound Pouchitis Further restorative surgery unlikely
Restorative ileoanal reservoir	Removal of entire colon and upper rectum Lining of lower rectum may be removed (rectal mucosectomy) Internal pelvic ileal reservoir Ileal reservoir joined to the anus Temporary ileostomy usually performed	With complete mucosectomy, risk of colorectal cancer is slight and disease usually is cured No permanent ileostomy No external pouching system Continence usually good	Temporary ileostomy usually necessary Bowel function variable Requires specialized surgical expertise More than one operation usually necessary Increased surgical complications Pouchitis Long-term results unknown (nutritional effects, cancer risk)

(Pena JP, Gemlo BT, Rothenberger DA. Ileal pouch–anal anastomosis: state of the art. Baillieres Clin Gastroenterol 1992;6:113)

velope, preserving the pelvic nerves posteriorly,[37] others prefer a perimuscular dissection. The plane of this dissection is anterior to the superior rectal artery posteriorly and immediately adjacent to the rectal wall anteriorly and laterally (Fig. 38-14). Regardless of surgical technique, patient age has a strong effect on postoperative impotence rates. In one study,[34] sexual dysfunction was reported in none of 8 patients younger than 30 years, in 5 of 25 patients aged 30 to 50 years, and in 6 of 8 patients older than 50 years. Pelvic nerve preservation and perineal wound healing are also optimized by use of the technique of intersphincteric proctectomy (Fig. 38-15). This dissection is

performed in the anatomic plane between the internal and external anal sphincters. The technique leaves behind a small wound surrounded by a cuff of healthy muscle tissue that permits successful primary closure.

Total Proctocolectomy and Brooke Ileostomy

Despite the development of novel procedures for the definitive treatment of ulcerative colitis, total proctocolectomy with Brooke ileostomy remains the time-tested standard operation. Unique benefits derive from the di-

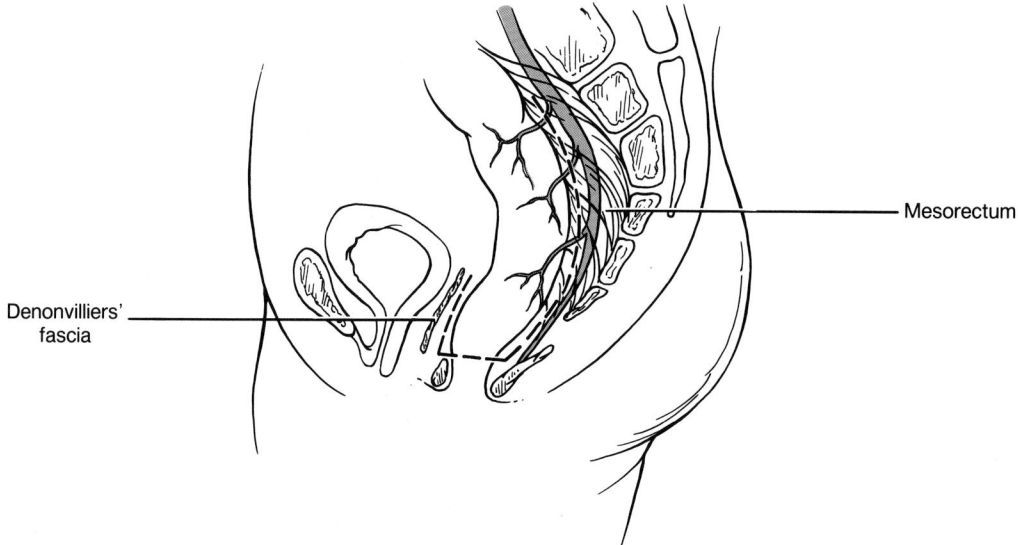

Figure 38-14 Perimuscular rectal dissection. Dissection is performed anterior to the superior rectal artery.

rectness of this approach: it removes all diseased tissue in a single and familiar operation that is curative and eliminates the long-term cancer risk. Its main drawback lies in the need for a permanent stoma that requires an external pouching appliance. Total proctocolectomy also involves pelvic dissection, with possible attendant pelvic nerve injury, and creation of a perineal wound that can heal slowly and sometimes incompletely.

Total proctocolectomy is an option for virtually all patients who require surgery for ulcerative colitis. Total proctocolectomy is the procedure of choice for patients who place a premium on having a single curative operation and for those who are willing to sacrifice the possibility of "normal" bowel function for the more predictable functional outcome of a conventional ileostomy. Total proctocolectomy is also the procedure of choice for patients who are poor candidates for restorative proctocolectomy because of advanced age, compromised sphincter function, and clinical features suggestive of Crohn's disease.

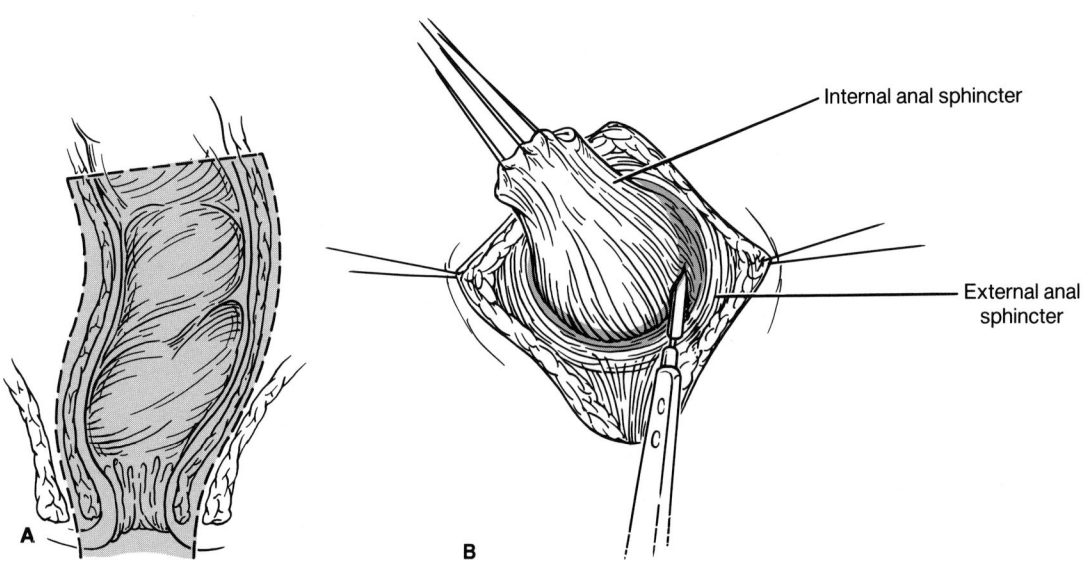

Figure 38-15 Intersphincteric proctectomy. The plane of dissection is between the internal and external sphincters.

Modern series report the incidence of male sexual dysfunction to range from 0%[38] to 17%.[45] Female sexual dysfunction occurs in about 20% of patients.[46] Dyspareunia appears to be related in part to the loss of soft tissue structures in the posterior pelvis.[46]

The incidence of unhealed perineal wounds has markedly decreased since the practice of perineal packing was abandoned in favor of primary perineal closure. At present, open packing of the perineal wound is reserved for patients with uncontrollable hemorrhage. Modern series using intersphincteric proctectomy report early perineal wound healing rates of 75% to 96%.[47,48]

Despite the largely successful results of total proctocolectomy, persisting dissatisfaction with the procedure has stemmed from the need for a permanent stoma. Subsequent developments in ulcerative colitis surgery have all represented attempts to eliminate or modify the conventional Brooke ileostomy.

Abdominal Colectomy With Ileorectal Anastomosis

The first sphincter-saving alternative to total proctocolectomy was abdominal colectomy with ileorectal anastomosis.[49] Like total proctocolectomy, this operation coupled several significant advantages with one major drawback: in this case, retention of a diseased rectum with its potential for continued symptoms and malignant transformation. On the other hand, the procedure does offer technical simplicity, complete avoidance of pelvic dissection, and, in successful cases, avoidance of a permanent stoma. Most modern series limit temporary ileostomy diversion to patients who are severely ill, malnourished, or receiving high-dose steroid therapy, or who have severe rectal disease. Selective use of temporary diversion is associated with anastomotic leak rates as low as 2%.[50]

Although successful results from ileorectal anastomosis can be seen in patients with severe rectal inflammation,[47] the operation is best reserved for patients with only mild to moderate rectal disease. The procedure is particularly useful in young patients, who are rapidly able to return to a normal life-style and avoid all risks of pelvic dissection, and in older patients who are poor candidates for ileoanal anastomosis. Contraindications to ileorectal anastomosis include a fibrotic or strictured rectum, poor anal sphincter function, and preexisting large bowel carcinoma or dysplasia. In one series,[51] rectal cancer or dysplasia occurred in five of seven patients who underwent ileorectal anastomosis with preexisting colon cancer or dysplasia, and a 40% actuarial risk of rectal cancer development has been reported 9 years after the development of moderate to severe dysplasia in the rectal remnant.[52]

Functional results after ileorectal anastomosis are generally good to excellent (Table 38-2). Most patients have four or five bowel movements per 24 hours, with variable rates of nocturnal evacuation.[50,54] Incontinence or seepage is rarely a problem. Conversion to ileostomy, usually with associated proctectomy, is necessary for persisting or recurrent proctitis, poor functional results, or development of rectal dysplasia or cancer. Recent series document failure rates of 11% to 57%, depending on the length of follow-up[56] (Table 38-3).

The risk of developing rectal cancer after ileorectal anastomosis has been estimated to be 0% after 10 years of disease, 2.1% after 15 years, 5% after 20 years, and 12.9% after 25 years.[51] Because these cancers frequently present at an advanced stage, close endoscopic follow-up with biopsies for dysplasia is mandatory in patients with a retained rectum, particularly after 10 years of disease. Fortunately, such follow-up is comparatively simple and can be performed in the office or clinic setting with proctoscopy or flexible sigmoidoscopy.

Table 38-2 Functional Results of Ileorectal Anastomosis for Ulcerative Colitis: Selected Series

Author	Mean Bowel Movements per Day	Excessive Daily Bowel Movements	Nocturnal Evacuations	Incontinence
Newton, 1975[53]	4.5	18% >6	70% sometimes 4% always	17%*
Oakley, 1985[50]	4.3	NA	5.4%	0
Parc, 1985[54]	4.5	17% >6	35%	1% nocturnal seepage 0.5% incontinent
Khubchandani, 1989[55]	1.4	1% >8	NA	0

(Madoff RD, Goldberg SM. Operative approaches to patients with inflammatory bowel disease. In: Cohen AM, Winawer SJ, eds. Cancer of the colon, rectum, and anus. New York, McGraw-Hill, 1995)

Table 38-3 Ileorectal Anastomosis Failures

Author	No.	Follow-Up (y)	Rectal Cancer	Ileostomy/Proctectomy
Baker, 1970[57]	41	2–17	0	18 (44%)
Hughes, 1975[58]	37	Minimum 15	2	12 (32%)
Baker, 1978[59]*	374	2–23	22	47 (13%)
Farnell, 1980[60]	63†	5–17	0	15 (24%)
Oakley, 1985[50]	136	3–25	5	37 (27%)
Johnson, 1986[61]	147	5–36	11‡	22 (15%)
Khubchandani, 1989[55]	53	1–28	2	6 (11%)
Leijonmarck, 1990[62]	51	6–35	0	29 (37%)
Löfberg, 1991[63]	46	12–36	0	25 (54%)

* Aylett's series.
† Patients with ulcerative colitis.
‡ Of 286 subtotal colectomies (147 with ileorectal anastomosis).
(Madoff RD, Goldberg SM. Operative approaches to patients with inflammatory bowel disease. In: Cohen AM, Winawer SJ, eds. Cancer of the colon, rectum, and anus. New York, McGraw-Hill, 1995)

Total Proctocolectomy With Continent Ileostomy

Another approach to the elimination of an external stool-collecting appliance, if not the stoma itself, is the continent ileostomy, described by Kock in 1969[64] (Fig. 38-16). The principle of this technique is to create an internal ileal reservoir with an intussuscepted one-way nipple valve that prevents spontaneous emptying. Pouch evacuation is accomplished by intermittent catheterization. Because ileal effluent is not in contact with the skin, there is no need for stomal eversion, and a small, flush stoma can be created that is less conspicuous than a conventional ileostomy.

The Kock pouch plays a relatively limited role in current surgical practice because of the development and popularization of the ileoanal pouch. Still, there remain specific indications for the continent ileostomy.[65] The procedure can be offered to patients with colitis who have underlying sphincter dysfunction and to those who have undergone previous total proctocolectomy. Rare patients do not have adequate mesenteric length to complete an ileoanal anastomosis, and occasional patients simply prefer the notion of intermittent self-catheterization on a scheduled basis to the risk of excessive stool frequency or possible fecal incontinence after restorative proctocolectomy. On occasion, a failed pelvic pouch can be converted to a continent ileostomy.[66]

Any patient being considered for a Kock pouch must understand the complexity of the operation and the potential for complications. Poorly motivated patients are not good candidates for this procedure and are better served by a conventional ileostomy. Crohn's disease is a strict contraindication to a Kock pouch because of high rates of poor healing, recurrent disease, pouch fistulization, and pouch failure.

Creation of a Kock pouch is a technically challenging operation that is associated with a significant learning curve. Malnourished and acutely ill patients should undergo initial colectomy with ileostomy and be converted to a continent ileostomy on an elective basis. All pouches should have continuous catheter drainage for 2 weeks after surgery, and surgeons inexperienced with the technique should consider the use of a proximal diverting stoma.

The most common technical failure of the Kock pouch is slippage of the nipple valve, which is heralded by difficulty intubating the pouch and loss of pouch continence. Although this complication occurred in up to 50% of patients in early series, experienced surgeons

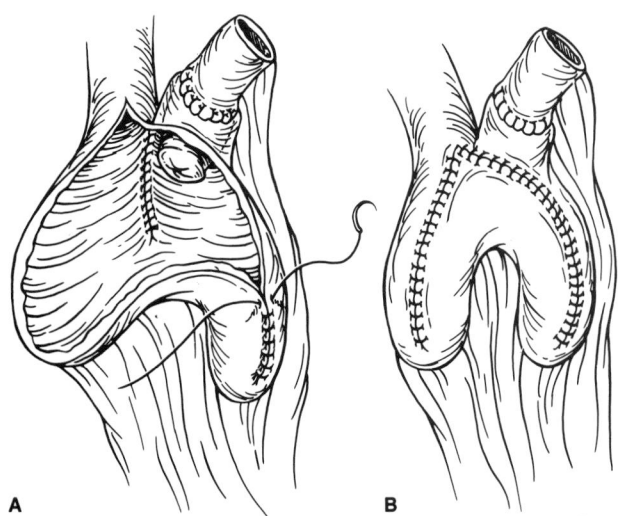

A   B

Figure 38-16 Kock pouch formation.

using improved fixation techniques report about a 10% incidence of nipple valve slippage.[67] Surgical revision is necessary to restore pouch function.

Inflammation of the ileal reservoir, termed *pouchitis*, is reported in 15% to 30% of patients with Kock pouches.[65] An identical syndrome occurs in a similar percentage of patients with pelvic ileal reservoirs.[68] Clinically, patients experience abdominal cramping and increased reservoir output with or without bleeding. Endoscopic evaluation demonstrates inflammatory changes in the pouch mucosa.

The etiology of pouchitis remains uncertain. The fact that the condition, so similar to ulcerative colitis, is rare in patients undergoing ileal reservoir procedures for other indications has already been mentioned and suggests a common pathogenesis. A second clue to the cause of pouchitis lies in its frequent response to the antibiotic metronidazole. Although this observation suggests a bacterial origin, comparative studies have shown no difference in the profile of organisms inhabiting reservoirs with and without pouchitis.[69]

First-line therapy for pouchitis is oral metronidazole. Continuous catheter drainage of Kock pouches can also be helpful. Refractory pouchitis can be treated with topical or oral steroids or 5-ASA preparations. Inability to treat pouchitis successfully occasionally necessitates pouch excision.

Restorative Proctocolectomy

Proctocolectomy without ileostomy was devised to permit complete excision of the entire diseased large bowel while maintaining normal anal continence.[104] The prototype of this operation had been described more than 30 years previously but clinical use in adults was abandoned because of excessive stool frequency and conse-quent perineal excoriation.[70] Interest in anal ileostomy was revived with the parallel development of two seemingly unrelated procedures—the Soave pull-through for Hirschsprung's disease[71] and the Kock continent ileal reservoir. These operations demonstrated the ability of the anal sphincter to function after excision of the proximal rectum and distal rectal mucosa, and the ability of a small bowel pouch to serve as a reservoir capable of holding ileal effluent for prolonged periods between evacuations. Combining these concepts, an operation was devised that included proctocolectomy with anorectal mucosectomy, leaving in place the anal sphincter mechanism, and creation of a three-limbed, S-shaped pouch with sutured anastomosis to the dentate line. Since the introduction of the pouch, its popularity has gained steadily. Problem areas have included the operation's technical complexity, complication rate, need for a temporary diverting ileostomy, and functional results. Technical modifications, some involving compromise of the initial goals of surgery, remain areas of heated debate.

All other things being equal, no patient given the choice between ileostomy and no ileostomy would prefer the latter option. It is important to stress that bowel function after restorative proctocolectomy is not normal. Mean evacuation frequency is four to six bowel movements per 24 hours, often with at least one bowel movement during the night (Table 38-4). Continence, although generally excellent, may be imperfect, with minor nocturnal seepage being a particularly common problem. Patients unwilling to accept this type of result, or patients without ready access to bathroom facilities, may find conventional ileostomy a preferable alternative. Similarly, patients with compromised sphincter function (ie, after childbirth injury or anorectal surgery) are likely to have poor results. Because sphincter

Table 38-4 Functional Results of Ileal Pouch–Anal Anastomosis

Author	No.	Type	Daytime Evacuations	Nocturnal Evacuations	24-Hour Evacuations
de Silva, 1991[72]	88	J/S/W	4.4	0	4.4
Becker, 1985[73]	40	J	5.9	0.5	6.4
Chaussade, 1989[74]	18	J	4.2	1.1	5.3
Everett, 1989[75]	60	W			3.8
Nicholls, 1987[76]	64	W			3.3
Harms, 1992[77]	89*	W	4.6	0.3	4.9
Pemberton, 1987[78]	390	J	6.0	1.0	7.0
Morgan, 1987[79]	72	Straight			8.3
Wexner, 1989[80]	114	S	5.4	1.5	6.9

* Patients with ulcerative colitis; results at 1 year.
(Madoff RD, Goldberg SM. Operative approaches to patients with inflammatory bowel disease. In: Cohen AM, Winawer SJ, eds. Cancer of the colon, rectum, and anus. New York, McGraw-Hill, 1995)

strength decreases with age, patients older than 50 to 60 years should also consider alternative surgical procedures. If there is any question about the adequacy of sphincter function, it should be evaluated before surgery with anal manometry, endoanal ultrasonography, and electromyographic pudendal nerve conduction studies.

As with the Kock pouch, the preoperative diagnosis of Crohn's disease is an absolute contraindication to restorative proctocolectomy. However, patients with indeterminate colitis or Crohn's colitis on final pathology who lack clinical features of Crohn's disease before operation have outcomes similar to those of patients with ulcerative colitis.[81,82]

A variety of pouch configurations are in use (Fig. 38-17). As noted, straight ileal pull-throughs are associated with excessive stool frequency in adults but still see occasional use in children.[83] Two-limbed pouches include the J-shaped pouch[84] and the lateral isoperistaltic reservoir.[85] J-shaped pouches have the advantages of simplicity of construction, adaptability to stapling techniques, and ease of emptying. A potential disadvantage is their small volume compared to three- or four-limbed pouches, but a consistent difference in clinical outcome has yet to be proven. The three-limbed, S-shaped pouch, which is larger than the J-shaped pouch, affords an easier reach to the pelvis because the distal-most ileum is swung downward after division of the ileocolic artery. The pouch is not amenable to stapling techniques and must be hand sutured. Early series reported a high incidence of evacuation disturbances in patients with S-shaped pouches; affected patients required pouch catheterization to permit emptying. The problem of poor emptying has now been solved by lim-

iting the length of the efferent spout to 1 to 2 cm. The four-limbed, W-shaped pouch has the largest volume of current pouch designs. This pouch is formed as adjoining J-shaped pouches that are partially offset to better fit the pelvic outlet.

The functional results after restorative proctocolectomy with various pouch designs are depicted in Table 38-4. Prospective randomized comparisons of different pouch designs are rare, and retrospective comparisons between different groups fail to make a compelling case for the superiority of any single pouch design.

Anal dilatation, necessary to perform mucosectomy, has been shown to decrease resting anal pressure, presumably on the basis of internal anal sphincter injury.[86] This effect is believed to be the cause of the compromised sphincter control that can complicate restorative proctocolectomy. This problem led to development of the double-stapled ileoanal anastomosis, in which mucosectomy is entirely avoided and the anastomosis is completed 1 to 2 cm above the dentate line (Fig. 38-18). Proponents of this approach claim better maintenance of sphincter function and improved clinical results.[87,88] However, randomized comparisons of mucosectomy versus nonmucosectomy techniques have not been performed.

Omission of mucosectomy violates one of the original principles of restorative proctocolectomy in that a strip of diseased tissue remains after operation. The remaining colonic mucosa has not proved to be a clinical problem unless an inappropriately long rectal remnant of greater than 2 cm is left behind. On the other hand, there remains a real concern that the rectal remnant poses a long-term risk for the development of cancer. The magnitude of this risk is entirely unknown, and

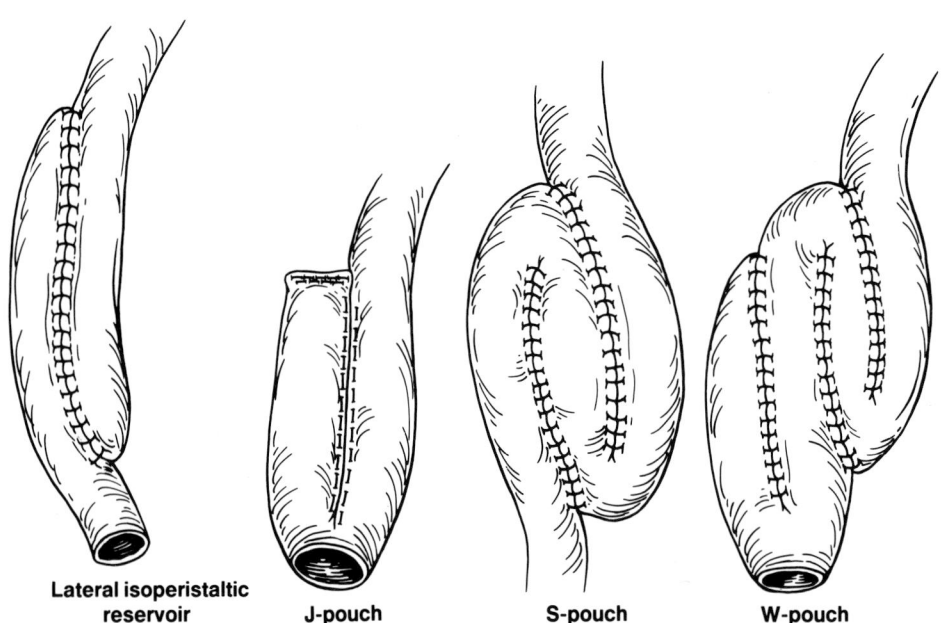

Lateral isoperistaltic reservoir   **J-pouch**   **S-pouch**   **W-pouch**

Figure 38-17 Ileal pouch configurations.

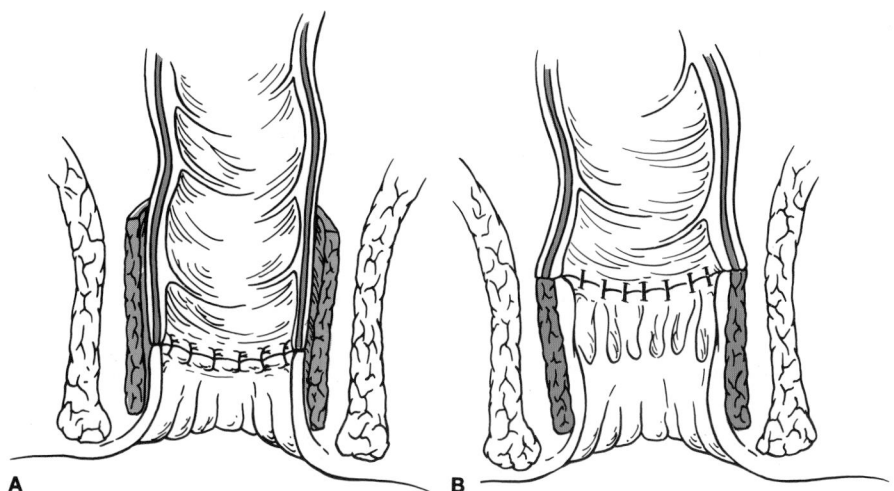

Figure 38-18 Ileal pouch–anal anastomosis. (**A**) Sutured anastomosis at dentate line after mucosectomy. (**B**) Double-stapled anastomosis. There is a residual 1- to 2-cm cuff of rectal mucosa.

even estimates of the incidence of anal dysplasia range widely from 0%[89] to 25%.[90] Proponents of the double-stapled technique point out that mucosectomy is an incomplete solution to a long-term cancer risk because viable rectal mucosa persists in the muscular cuff after mucosectomy[91] and several carcinomas have arisen after restorative proctocolectomy with mucosectomy.[92,93]

Complications of restorative proctocolectomy include small bowel obstruction, infection, and pouchitis. Small bowel obstruction has been reported in 17%[94] to 28%[95] of patients and is frequently related to the temporary ileostomy. Septic complications include perianal, pelvic, and peristomal infections.[95] Pelvic sepsis can result in ileoperineal and ileovaginal fistulas and is often associated with poor subsequent functional results.

Pouch failure, defined as the need for pouch excision or permanent proximal diversion, occurs in many patients. In one series,[96] 25 of 253 patients (10%) had pouch failure. The most common reason was poor functional results (7 patients). Other causes included Crohn's disease (6 patients), pelvic sepsis (5 patients), and refractory pouchitis (4 patients). Forty percent of patients with unsuspected Crohn's disease and 80% of patients who required abdominal exploration for pelvic sepsis had pouch failure. Forty-four percent of failures occurred in the first year after operation.

Early experience with restorative proctocolectomy suggested an unacceptable incidence of pelvic sepsis if the diverting ileostomy was omitted.[97] As familiarity with the operation has grown, a trend toward omission of diversion has developed. This change has been fueled by an increased recognition of ileostomy-associated complications, the desire to avoid the second hospitalization and operation that is necessary even in the absence of complications, and the notion that a double-stapled anastomosis is more secure than that accom-

plished after mucosectomy and hand suture. Retrospective reviews have demonstrated the feasibility and advantages of this approach,[98,99] but case selection appears to be a critical element. In the one available prospective trial,[100] diversion had no effect on pelvic sepsis, and nondiverted patients had fewer complications and markedly decreased hospital stays. Patients receiving systemic corticosteroids and those with unsatisfactory anastomoses were excluded from randomization and all underwent diversion. Omission of diversion can be considered by experienced surgeons after a technically satisfactory operation in patients who are not receiving steroids and are not acutely ill. Should pelvic infection supervene, successful treatment without operation has been reported with the use of percutaneous abscess drainage, intravenous antibiotics, and continuous pouch drainage.[99]

Choice of Operation

Patient satisfaction is high after surgery for ulcerative colitis, predominantly because good health is restored after removal of the diseased large bowel. Physical well-being is the major determinant of quality of life, patients self-select the procedure they prefer, and most patients are capable of adapting to their postoperative status regardless of the operation performed.[101] Nonetheless, helping patients select the operation that is best for them is an important part of surgical care. Conversely, poorly chosen or poorly executed operations almost guarantee bad results and unhappy patients.

Although it is the least glamorous operation, total proctocolectomy with conventional Brooke ileostomy is the time-tested standard that warrants consideration by every patient. It is a particularly attractive option for older patients, patients with abnormal sphincter function, and patients who desire the simplest possible definitive operation with the least likelihood of complications.

Restorative proctocolectomy has gained widespread acceptance since its introduction 15 years ago. It remains the operation of choice for patients who desire a sphincter-saving alternative to conventional ileostomy. Nevertheless, patients choosing this option deserve a candid discussion of the operation's risk and likely functional outcomes. Patients who go into surgery expecting that their neorectum will behave like their native rectum before the onset of colitis invariably face disappointment. Still, even given variable functional results, patient satisfaction after restorative proctocolectomy remains extremely high.[101–105]

The Kock pouch and ileorectal anastomosis have smaller roles to play in the current management of ulcerative colitis. The Kock pouch is mostly used for patients with impaired or previously excised anal sphincters, who are strongly motivated, despite the risk of complications and reoperation, to avoid an external appliance. Ileorectal anastomosis is best reserved for the rare patient with relative rectal sparing, who accepts the long-term risks of developing cancer and understands the likelihood of requiring rectal excision, either prophylactically or therapeutically, later in life.

> Despite continued uncertainty regarding the etiology of ulcerative colitis, recent years have witnessed significant advances in both the medical and surgical treatment of the disease. New drugs and more aggressive use of immunosuppressants are helping some patients to avoid surgery, and new surgical techniques are making conventional ileostomy only one of several options for patients with ulcerative colitis. Because of the enlarged spectrum of therapeutic alternatives, the surgeon's role in the management of patients with ulcerative colitis has broadened considerably. Given the responsibility for both the timing and choice of operation, it is critical that the surgeon be familiar with the full range of therapeutic options and anticipated outcomes. Sound surgical judgment, associated with careful patient education, are the keys to successful results in the long-term management of ulcerative colitis.

REFERENCES

1. Mayberry JF. Recent epidemiology of ulcerative colitis and Crohn's disease. Int J Colorectal Dis 1989;4:59.
2. Garland CF, Lilienfeld AM, Mendeloff AI, Markowitz JA, Terrell KB, Garland FG. Incidence rates of ulcerative colitis and Crohn's disease in fifteen areas of the United States. Gastroenterology 1981;81:1115.
3. Tysk C, Riedesel H, Lindberg E, Panzini B, Podolsky D, Järnerot G. Colonic glycoproteins in monozygotic twins with inflammatory bowel disease. Gastroenterology 1991;100:419.
4. Shanahan F, Duerr RH, Rotter JI, et al. Neutrophil autoantibodies in ulcerative colitis: familial aggregation and genetic heterogeneity. Gastroenterology 1992;103:456.
5. North CS, Alpers DH, Helzer JE, Spitznagel EL, Clouse RE. Do life events or depression exacerbate inflammatory bowel disease? Ann Intern Med 1991;114:381.
6. Shanahan F. Pathogenesis of ulcerative colitis. Lancet 1993;342:407.
7. Podolsky DK. Inflammatory bowel disease. Part I. N Engl J Med
8. Podolsky DK. Inflammatory bowel disease. Part II. N Engl J Med 1991;325:1008.
9. Hendrikson C, Kreimer S, Binder V. Long term prognosis in ulcerative colitis based on results from a regional patient group from the county of Copenhagen. Gut 1985;26:158.
10. Edwards FC, Truelove SC. The course and prognosis of ulcerative colitis. Gut 1963;4:299.
11. Bynum TE, Jacobson ED. Vascular disorders of the large bowel. In: Kirsner JB, Shorter RG, eds. Diseases of the colon, rectum and anus. Baltimore, Williams & Wilkins, 1988:537.
12. Perme CM, Lichtenstein JE. Inflammatory bowel disease. Semin Colon Rectal Surg 1993;4:112.
13. Nelson RL, Subramanian K, Gasparaitis A, Abcarian H, Pavel DG. Indium 111-labeled granulocyte scan in the diagnosis and management of acute inflammatory bowel disease. Dis Colon Rectum 1990;33:451.
14. Monsén U, Sorstad J, Hellers G, Johansson C. Extracolonic diagnoses in ulcerative colitis: an epidemiological study. Am J Gastroenterol 1990;85:711.
15. Danzi JT. Extraintestinal manifestations of idiopathic inflammatory bowel disease. Arch Intern Med 1988;148:297.
16. Levitt MD, Ritchie JK, Lennard-Jones JE, Phillips RKS. Pyoderma gangrenosum in inflammatory bowel disease. Br J Surg 1991;78:676.
17. Olsson R, Danielsson A, Järnerot G, et al. Prevalence of primary sclerosing cholangitis in patients with ulcerative colitis. Gastroenterology 1991;100:1319.
18. Broome U, Lindberg G, Lofberg R. Primary sclerosing cholangitis and ulcerative colitis: a risk factor for the development of dysplasia and DNA aneuploidy? Gastroenterology 1992;102:1877.
19. D'Haens GR, Lashner BA, Hanauer SB. Pericholangitis and sclerosing cholangitis are risk factors for dysplasia and cancer in ulcerative colitis. Am J Gastroenterol 1993;88:1174.
20. Cangemi JR, Wiesner RH, Beaver SJ, et al. Effect of proctocolectomy for chronic ulcerative colitis on the

natural history of primary sclerosing cholangitis. Gastroenterology 1989;96:790.

21. Korelitz BI. Where do we stand on drug treatment for ulcerative colitis? Ann Intern Med 1992;116:692.

22. Azad Khan AK, Piris J, Truelove SC. An experiment to determine the active therapeutic moiety of sulphasalazine. Lancet 1977;2:892.

23. Truelove SC, Witts LJ. Cortisone in ulcerative colitis. Final report on a therapeutic trial. BMJ 1955;4947:1041.

24. Kamm MA, Senapati A. Drug management of ulcerative colitis. BMJ 1992;305:35.

25. Sutherland LR, May GR, Shaffer EA. Sulfasalazine revisited: a meta-analysis of 5-aminosalicylic acid in the treatment of ulcerative colitis. Ann Intern Med 1993;118:540.

26. Hanauer SB. Medical therapy of ulcerative colitis. Lancet 1993;342:412.

27. Hawthorne AB, Logan RFA, Hawkey CJ, et al. Randomised controlled trial of azathioprine withdrawal in ulcerative colitis. BMJ 1992;305:20.

28. Adler DJ, Korelitz BI. The therapeutic efficacy of 6-mercaptopurine in refractory ulcerative colitis. Am J Gastroenterol 1990;85:717.

29. Present DH, Meltzer SJ, Krumholz MP, Wolke A, Korelitz BI. 6-MP in management of inflammatory bowel disease. Short and long term toxicity. Ann Intern Med 1989;111:641.

30. Lichtiger S, Present DH. Preliminary report: cyclosporin in treatment of severe active ulcerative colitis. Lancet 1990;336:16.

31. Linn FV, Peppercorn MA. Drug therapy for inflammatory bowel disease: part II. Am J Surg 1992;164:178.

32. Carter FM, McLeod RS, Cohen Z. Subtotal colectomy for ulcerative colitis: complications related to the rectal remnant. Dis Colon Rectum 1991;34:1005.

33. Greenstein AJ, Sachar DB, Gibas A, et al. Outcome of toxic dilatation in ulcerative and Crohn's colitis. J Clin Gastroenterol 1985;7:137.

34. Goligher JC, Hoffman DC, DeDombal FT. Surgical treatment of severe attacks of ulcerative colitis, with special reference to the advantages of early operation. BMJ 1970;4:703.

35. Meyers S, Janowitz HD. The place of steroids in the therapy of toxic megacolon. Gastroenterology 1978;75:729.

36. Järnerot G, Rolny P, Sandberg-Gertzén H. Intensive intravenous treatment of ulcerative colitis. Gastroenterology 1985;89:1005.

37. Grant CS, Dozois RR. Toxic megacolon: ultimate fate of patients after successful medical management. Am J Surg 1984;147:106.

38. Albrechtsen D, Bergan A, Nygaard K, Gjone E, Flatmark A. Urgent surgery for ulcerative colitis: early colectomy in 132 patients. World J Surg 1981;5:607.

39. Katzka I, Brody R, Morris E, et al. Assessment of colorectal cancer risk in patients with ulcerative colitis. Experience from a private practice. Gastroenterology 1983;85:22.

40. Collins RH, Feldman M, Fordtran JS. Colon cancer, dysplasia, and surveillance in patients with ulcerative colitis. A critical review. N Engl J Med 1987;316:1654.

41. Morson BC, Pang LSC. Rectal biopsy as an aid to cancer control in ulcerative colitis. Gut 1967;8:423.

42. Ransohoff DF, Riddell RH, Levin B. Ulcerative colitis in colonic cancer. Problems in assessing the diagnostic usefulness of mucosal dysplasia. Dis Colon Rectum 1985;28:383.

43. Chen J, Compton C, Cheng E, Fromowitz F, Viola MV. c-Ki-*ras* mutations in dysplastic fields and cancers in ulcerative colitis. Gastroenterology 1992;102:1983.

44. Yin J, Harpaz N, Yong Y, et al. p53 Point mutations in dysplastic and cancerous ulcerative colitis lesions. Gastroenterology 1993;104:1633.

45. Leicester RJ, Ritchie JK, Wadsworth J, Thomson JPS, Hawley PR. Sexual function and perineal wound healing after intersphincteric excision of the rectum for inflammatory bowel disease. Dis Colon Rectum 1984;27:244.

46. Metcalf AM, Dozois RR, Kelly KA. Sexual function in women after proctocolectomy. Ann Surg 1986;204:624.

47. Berry AR, Campos RDE, Lee ECG. Perineal and pelvic morbidity following perimuscular excision of the rectum for inflammatory bowel disease. Br J Surg 1986;73:675.

48. Tompkins RG, Warshaw AL. Improved management of the perineal wound after proctectomy. Ann Surg 1985;202:760.

49. Aylett SO. Three hundred cases of diffuse ulcerative colitis treated by total colectomy and ileo-rectal anastomosis. BMJ 1966;5494:1001.

50. Oakley JR, Jagelman DG, Fazio VW, et al. Complications and quality of life after ileorectal anastomosis for ulcerative colitis. Am J Surg 1985;149:23.

51. Grundfest SF, Fazio V, Weiss RA, et al. The risk of cancer following colectomy and ileorectal anastomosis for extensive mucosal ulcerative colitis. Ann Surg 1981;193:9.

52. Johnson WR, McDermott FT, Pihl E, Hughes ESR. Mucosal dysplasia. A major predictor of cancer following ileorectal anastomosis. Dis Colon Rectum 1983;26:697.

53. Newton CR, Baker WNW. Comparison of bowel function after ileorectal anastomosis for ulcerative colitis and colonic polyposis. Gut 1975;16:785.

54. Parc R, Levy E, Frileux P, Loygue J. Current results: ileorectal anastomosis after total abdominal colectomy for ulcerative colitis. In: Dozois RR, ed. Alternatives to conventional ileostomy. Chicago, Year Book Medical Publishers, 1985:81.

55. Khubchandani IT, Sandfort MR, Rosen L, Sheets JA, Stasik JJ, Riether RD. Current status of ileorectal anastomosis for inflammatory bowel disease. Dis Colon Rectum 1989;32:400.

56. Madoff RD, Goldberg SM. Operative approaches to patients with inflammatory bowel disease. In: Cohen AM,

Winawer SJ, eds. Cancer of the colon, rectum, and anus. New York, McGraw-Hill, 1995.

57. Baker WNNW. The results of ileorectal anastomosis at St. Mark's Hospital from 1953 to 1968. Gut 1970;11:235.

58. Hughes ESR, McDermott FT, Masterton JP. Ileorectal anastomosis for inflammatory bowel disease: 15-year follow-up. Dis Colon Rectum 1979;22:399.

59. Baker WNW, Glass RE, Ritchie JK, Aylett SO. Cancer of the rectum following colectomy and ileorectal anastomosis for ulcerative colitis. Br J Surg 1978;65:862.

60. Farnell MB, Van Heerden JA, Beart RW, Weiland LH. Rectal preservation in non-specific inflammatory disease of the colon. Ann Surg 1980;192:249.

61. Johnson WR, Hughes ESR, McDermott FT, Katrivessis H. The outcome of patients with ulcerative colitis managed by subtotal colectomy. Surg Gynecol Obstet 1986;162:421.

62. Leijonmarck C-E, Löfberg R, Öst Å, Hellers G. Long-term results of ileorectal anastomosis in ulcerative colitis in Stockholm County. Dis Colon Rectum 1990;33:195.

63. Löfberg R, Leijonmarck C-E, Hellers G, Broström O, Tribukait B, Öst Å. Mucosal dysplasia and DNA content in ulcerative colitis patients with ileorectal anastomosis. Follow-up study in a defined patient group. Dis Colon Rectum 1991;34:566.

64. Kock NG. Intra-abdominal "reservoir" in patients with permanent ileostomy: preliminary observations on a procedure resulting in fecal "continence" in five ileostomy patients. Arch Surg 1969;99:223.

65. Vernava III AM, Goldberg SM. Is the Kock pouch still a viable option? Int J Colorectal Dis 1988;3:135.

66. Hulten L. The continent ileostomy (Kock's pouch) versus the restorative proctocolectomy (pelvic pouch). World J Surg 1985;9:952.

67. Kock NG, Brevinge H, Ojerskog B. Continent ileostomy. Perspect Colon Rectal Surg 1989;2:71.

68. Tytgat GN, van Deventer SJ. Pouchitis. Int J Colorectal Dis 1988;3:226.

69. Luukonen P, Valtonen V, Sivonen A, Sipponen P, Jarvinen H. Fecal bacteriology and reservoir ileitis in patients operated on for ulcerative colitis. Dis Colon Rectum 1988;31:864.

70. Ravitch MM, Sabiston DC Jr. Anal ileostomy with preservation of the anal sphincter: a proposed operation in patients requiring total colectomy for benign lesions. Surg Gynecol Obstet 1947;84:1095.

71. Soave F. A new surgical technique for treatment of Hirschsprung's disease. Surgery 1964;56:1007.

72. de Silva HJ, de Angelis CP, Soper N, Kettlewell MGW, Mortensen NJMcC, Jewell DP. Clinical and functional outcome after restorative proctocolectomy. Br J Surg 1991;78:1039.

73. Becker JM, Hillard AE, Mann FA, Kestenberg A, Nelson JA. Functional assessment after colectomy, mucosal proctectomy, and endorectal ileoanal pull-through. World J Surg 1985;9:598.

74. Chaussade S, Verduron A, Hautefeuille M, et al. Proctocolectomy and ileoanal pouch anastomosis without conservation of a rectal muscular cuff. Br J Surg 1989;76:273.

75. Everett WG. Experience of restorative proctocolectomy with ileal reservoir. Br J Surg 1989;76:77.

76. Nicholls RJ, Lubowski DZ. Restorative proctocolectomy: the four loop (W) reservoir. Br J Surg 1987;74:564.

77. Harms BA, Andersen AB, Starling JR. The W ileal reservoir: long-term assessment after proctocolectomy for ulcerative colitis and familial polyposis. Surgery 1992;112:638.

78. Pemberton JH, Kelly KA, Beart Jr RW, Dozois RR, Wolff BG, Ilstrup DM. Ileal pouch–anal anastomosis for chronic ulcerative colitis. Ann Surg 1987;206:504.

79. Morgan RA, Manning PB, Coran AG. Experience with straight endorectal pull-through for the management of ulcerative colitis and familial polyposis in children and adults. Ann Surg 1987;206:595.

80. Wexner SD, Jensen L, Rothenberger DA, Wong WD, Goldberg SM. Long-term functional analysis of the ileoanal reservoir. Dis Colon Rectum 1989;32:275.

81. Hyman NH, Fazio VW, Tuckson WB, Lavery IC. Consequences of ileal pouch–anal anastomosis for Crohn's colitis. Dis Colon Rectum 1991;34:653.

82. Pezim ME, Pemberton JH, Beart RW Jr, et al. Outcome of "indeterminant" colitis following ileal pouch–anal anastomosis. Dis Colon Rectum 1989;32:653.

83. Morgan RA, Manning PB, Coran AG. Experience with straight ileoanal pull-through for the management of ulcerative colitis and familial polyposis in children and adults. Ann Surg 1987;206:595.

84. Utsunomiya J, Iwama T, Imajo M, et al. Total colectomy, mucosal proctectomy, and ileoanal anastomosis. Dis Colon Rectum 1980;23:459.

85. Fonkalsrud EW. Update on clinical experience with different surgical techniques of endorectal pull-through operation for colitis and polyposis. Surg Gynecol Obstet 1987;165:309.

86. Keighley MRB. Abdominal mucosectomy reduces the incidence of soiling and sphincter damage after restorative proctocolectomy and "J" pouch. Dis Colon Rectum 1987;30:386.

87. Nasmyth DG, Johnston D, Godwin PGR, Dixon MF, Smith A, Williams NS. Factors influencing bowel function after ileal pouch–anal anastomosis. Br J Surg 1986;73:469.

88. Holdsworth PJ, Johnston D. Anal sensation after restorative proctocolectomy for ulcerative colitis. Br J Surg 1988;75:993.

89. Schmitt SL, Wexner SD, Lucas FV, James K, Nogueras JJ, Jagelman DG. Retained mucosa after double-stapled ileal reservoir and ileoanal anastomosis. Dis Colon Rectum 1992;35:1051.

90. King DW, Lubowski DZ, Cook TA. Anal canal mucosa in restorative proctocolectomy for ulcerative colitis. Br J Surg 1989;76:970.

91. O'Connell PR, Pemberton JH, Weiland LH, et al. Does rectal mucosa regenerate after ileoanal anastomosis? Dis Colon Rectum 1987;30:1.

92. Stern H, Walfisch S, Mullen B, McLeod R, Cohen Z. Cancer in an ileoanal reservoir: a new late complication? Gut 1990;31:473.

93. Puthu D, Rajan N, Rao R, Rao L, Venugopal P. Carcinoma of the rectal pouch following restorative procto-colectomy: report of a case. Dis Colon Rectum 1992;35:257.

94. Francois Y, Dozois RR, Kelly KA, et al. Small intestinal obstruction complicating ileal pouch–anal anastomosis. Ann Surg 1989;209:46.

95. Wexner SD, Wong WD, Rothenberger DA, Goldberg SM. The ileoanal reservoir. Am J Surg 1990;159:178.

96. Gemlo BT, Wong WD, Rothenberger DA, Goldberg SM. Ileal pouch–anal anastomosis. Patterns of failure. Arch Surg 1992;127:784.

97. Rothenberger DA, Vermeulen FD, Christenson CE, et al. Restorative proctocolectomy with ileal reservoir and ileoanal anastomosis. Am J Surg 1983;145:82.

98. Sagar PM, Lewis W, Holdsworth PJ, Johnston D. One-stage restorative proctocolectomy without temporary defunctioning ileostomy. Dis Colon Rectum 1992;35:582.

99. Cohen Z, McLeod RS, Stephen W, Stern HS, O'Connor B, Reznick R. Continuing evolution of the pelvic pouch procedure. Ann Surg 1992;16:506.

100. Grobler SP, Hosie KB, Keighley MRB. Randomized trial of loop ileostomy in restorative proctocolectomy. Br J Surg 1992;79:903.

101. McLeod RS, Churchill DN, Lock AM, Vandenburg HS, Cohen Z. Quality of life of patients with ulcerative colitis preoperatively and postoperatively. Gastroenterology 1991;101:1307.

102. Köhler LW, Pemberton JH, Zinsmeister AR, Kelly KA. Quality of life after proctocolectomy. A comparison of Brooke ileostomy, Kock pouch, and ileal pouch–anal anastomosis. Gastroenterology 1991;101:679.

103. Keighley MRB, Kmiot W. Surgical options in ulcerative colitis: role of ileo-anal anastomosis. Aust NZ J Surg 1990;60:835.

104. Parks AG, Nicholls RJ. Proctocolectomy without ileostomy for ulcerative colitis. BMJ 1978;2:85.

105. Pena JL, Gemlo BT, Rothenberger DA. Ileal pouch–anal anastomosis: state of the art. Baillieres Clin Gastroenterol 1992;6:113.

Digestive Tract Surgery: A Text and Atlas, edited by Richard H. Bell,
Layton F. Rikkers, and Michael W. Mulholland.
Lippincott-Raven Publishers, Philadelphia, © 1996.

39

Colonic Diverticular Disease

James A. Knol

COLONIC DIVERTICULOSIS

Diverticulosis coli, the presence of colonic diverticula, is a prevalent condition in Western and westernized societies. Diverticular disease is not merely the presence of colonic diverticula, but the conglomerate of complications associated with diverticula. These complications are listed in Table 39-1. Diverticular disease has been categorized into five types: prediverticulosis, multiple diverticulosis, solitary diverticulosis, diverticulitis, and generalized diverticulosis of the small and large intestine.[1] Although most persons in whom diverticulosis occurs never have associated disease, the frequency of diverticulosis is such that diverticular disease is one of the common conditions requiring colon surgery. Despite the frequency with which surgeons encounter diverticular disease, controversy remains in regard to the preferred therapy for several of its manifestations.

The age of occurrence of diverticulosis coli in North American and European populations is skewed toward the elderly. The incidence of colonic diverticulosis is estimated to be 2% to 5% of the population younger than 40 years,[2] 5% to 10% of the population older than 40 years, and 60% to 70% of the population older than 85 years.[3] The true incidence is uncertain. Data acquired from barium enema examinations tend to overestimate the incidence because many patients are studied due to symptoms. Autopsy data are likely to underestimate the incidence because diverticula may be small and not obvious on routine inspection. The gender predilection ratio is 1.5:1 female to male.[2] Diverticulosis is much more prevalent in westernized populations than in Asian or African populations, and the frequency apparently has increased markedly in westernized countries in the 20th century.

The distribution of diverticulosis of the colon differs among world populations. In Western societies, diverticula are distributed predominantly in the sigmoid colon (Fig. 39-1). Diverticulosis occurs most commonly in the right colon in Asian populations, and has been reported chiefly in the descending colon in black South Africans.[4] Inflammatory complications of diverticulosis tend to follow the dominant site for the population.[5] The differing locations in the colon among these populations have cast uncertainty on the etiology of colonic diverticula.

A distinction frequently is made between *true diverticula* and *pseudodiverticula.* Diverticula that occur in the sigmoid colon in Western populations are almost exclusively pseudodiverticula, in which the wall consists of mucosa, minimal submucosa, and no muscularis propria. These histologic features are characteristic for acquired diverticula. The presence of all layers of the bowel wall is the mark of true diverticula and is typical for congenital diverticula. True diverticula are found more commonly in the right colon.[6] However, diverticulitis of the right colon, although occasionally associated with true diverticula, most often occurs in pseudodiverticula.[5]

The etiology of pseudodiverticula is thought to be related to acquired weakness of the colon wall. Diverticula occur at the site of blood vessel penetration of the muscular layer. Some investigators have proposed that two types of acquired diverticular disease can be identified that have differing symptoms, clinical patterns, anatomic distributions, ages of onset, and histologic findings.[7] Under a version of this theory, one group of patients have left-sided diverticula, with associated pain

Table 39-1 Complications Associated With Colonic Diverticula That Constitute Diverticular Disease

DIVERTICULITIS
Phlegmon
Abscess
    Pelvic abscess
    Mesenteric abscess
Perforation into the peritoneal cavity
    Feculent peritonitis
    Purulent peritonitis
Fistula
    Colovesical
    Colovaginal
    Coloenteric
    Colouterine
    Colocutaneous
    Coloureteral, colosalpingal, colocolic, other
Colon stricture with partial or complete obstruction
Ureteral obstruction
Pylephlebitis
Liver abscess

BLEEDING DIVERTICULOSIS

GIANT DIVERTICULA

and bowel symptoms, and histologic evidence of diverticular inflammation. The other group of patients infrequently have bowel symptoms, have a higher density of diverticula in the sigmoid, are older, and are more likely to manifest lower gastrointestinal bleeding.[7] Another version of the theory is that one type of diverticulosis is principally left-sided, associated with muscular hypertrophy, and accompanied more often by inflammation. The other type is not associated with muscular hypertrophy, is more frequently pancolonic in distribution, and is accompanied more often by bleeding complications.[8]

Multiple factors are likely to play a part in the weakness of the colon wall leading to the formation of diverticula.[1] Decreased amounts of elastic and collagen fibers in the colon wall and changes in their character have been described. According to one hypothesis, herniation of the mucosa results from muscular hypertrophy of the circular muscle and the development of high intracolonic pressures with segmentation.[9] Altered physiologic responses associated with the muscular hypertrophy include excessive colonic motility responses to eating and to cholinergic drugs. Similar patterns, including elevated basal motility, were reported in Japanese research subjects with right-sided diverticula.[1] However, some investigators have found no correlation between asymptomatic diverticulosis and colonic motility or pressure measurements. Moreover, pandiver-

ticulosis of the colon often is not associated with muscular hypertrophy.

Inadequate dietary fiber ingestion has been implicated in formation of colonic diverticula. Correlations between low fiber intake and the presence of diverticulosis in a population, and the inverse, have been made.[9] It has been postulated that the increased intraluminal pressure needed to propel stool in the sigmoid colon in the presence of low stool fiber is the impetus for the muscular hypertrophy in the sigmoid colon. Experimental studies in rats have demonstrated an association between high fiber intake and lack of formation of diverticula.[10] Studies in humans also have revealed a consistent correlation between total daily fiber intake and the acquisition of diverticula in populations.[1] Lack of weight gain after the age of 25 years in rural African, rural Indian, Japanese, and Chinese populations also correlates well with decreased tendency to form colonic diverticula.[1]

Complications

Most colonic diverticulosis is asymptomatic, based on autopsy studies relating findings of colonic diverticula and the presence of symptoms in retrospective reviews of subjects' histories.[11] Autopsy studies are likely to underestimate the prevalence of symptoms, and so in-

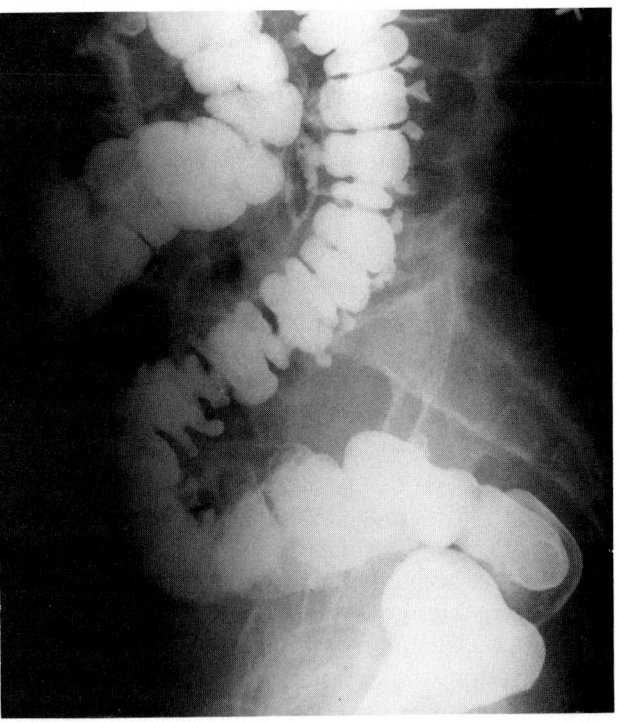

Figure 39-1 Barium contrast radiograph of diverticulosis, principally of the sigmoid and left colon.

crease the percentage of diverticulosis that is asymptomatic. Studies in which the subjects are identified as having diverticula on the basis of barium enema examination are biased toward a high incidence of associated symptoms, because the presence of some symptoms generally is the indication for the contrast study. Nevertheless, irrespective of the type of study done, most persons with diverticulosis have no symptoms.

Among patients who have symptoms, there are a proportion who do not have diverticulitis but who have pain that is attributed to diverticulosis. This condition has been designated *symptomatic or painful diverticular disease.*[12] The pain typically is in the left lower quadrant, occurs in attacks, and may be colicky or steady. Meals often exacerbate or provoke symptoms, and relief may occur after passage of flatus or stool. Constipation, less commonly diarrhea, or both alternating, occur in about half of patients. The physical examination usually exhibits no abdominal findings. Occasionally, there is mild tenderness or a palpable sigmoid colon in the left lower quadrant. Fever, leukocytosis, or peritoneal signs are absent. Whether this syndrome is caused by diverticula or is due to some other coexisting functional syndrome is unclear. Recent onset of symptoms and signs consistent with the syndrome should initiate studies excluding more serious disease, particularly colon cancer. A long history of such episodes suggests irritable bowel syndrome.

COLONIC DIVERTICULITIS

Diverticulitis is the presence of inflammation in the peridiverticular tissue of one or more diverticula. Diverticulitis is the most common complication of colonic diverticulosis.

Epidemiology

Colonic diverticulitis is principally a disease of Western or westernized populations. In these populations, the predominant site of diverticulitis is the sigmoid colon, although diverticula are distributed more widely in 30% of patients.[2] The occurrence of diverticulitis follows the predominant site of diverticulosis, such that in Asian populations, diverticulitis is much more often right-sided.[5]

Sigmoid diverticulitis occurs slightly more frequently in women than in men, at a ratio of about 3:2.[2] The median age of incidence is the seventh decade. In older series, only 2% to 3% of patients with diverticulitis were younger than 40 years at onset[2]; more recent series have found that 20% to 30% of patients with diverticulitis in the United States are 40 years or younger, and in this age group, men predominate.[13,14] Seventy-

five percent of patients with diverticulitis have had symptoms referable to the colon for less than 1 year.[2]

Right colonic and cecal diverticulitis occurs at a younger age than does left colonic diverticulitis, with the median age in the fifth decade and an average age of 40 to 43 years.[15,16] There is a male predominance in right-sided diverticulitis, ranging from a ratio of 3:2 to 5:1 male to female.[15,16]

The prevalence of sigmoid diverticulitis in Western populations is uncertain. Many patients treated as outpatients for an episode of diverticulitis actually may have pain associated with diverticulosis or with some other condition. Conversely, diverticulitis sometimes does occur without any accompanying symptoms. It has been estimated that 10% to 25% of persons with diverticulosis have an episode of diverticulitis.[17] The longer those with diverticulosis are followed up, the more likely is the occurrence of an episode of diverticulitis. The risk that diverticulitis will develop in a person with diverticulosis is about 10% at 5 years of follow-up, 25% at 10 years, and nearly 40% at 20 years.[17]

Etiology

The cause of inflammation in diverticulitis is still a matter of speculation. Obstruction of the neck of a diverticulum with a fecalith or a seed or nut often is postulated as the initiating event, leading to progressively increasing pressure within the diverticulum due to mucus and fluid secretion. The next step is microperforation caused by mucosal ischemia or excessive intraluminal pressure, followed by leakage of fluid into the peridiverticular tissues, with resultant infection and inflammation.[18] Another hypothesis states that high pressure, which develops segmentally between constricting muscle segments, causes perforation of the unsupported mucosa of the diverticulum. Localized pressures within the colonic lumen can reach 90 mmHg.[19] By whatever mechanism microperforation occurs, bacteria and colonic contents gain access to the adjacent tissues or the peritoneal cavity. The etiology of right colonic and cecal diverticulitis is unknown, but is postulated to occur through obstruction of the neck of the diverticulum, with ensuing events as outlined earlier.

Pathology

Perforation occurs almost uniformly at the tip or side wall of the diverticulum, outside the confines of the muscular wall of the colon. There seldom is pathologic evidence of inflammation of the diverticulum neck. The pathologic mechanisms that follow the initiating event depend on the anatomic location of the perforation and the local tissue response. In most cases, microperforation occurs into the mesentery of the sigmoid colon or into the retroperitoneum in the left lower quadrant, and occasionally into an epiploic appendage. Leakage is followed by a local nonsuppurating inflammatory response, with phlegmon formation. The phlegmon may be self-limited, may resolve with antibiotic treatment, or may progress to one of the inflammatory complications of diverticulitis. Resolution of the phlegmon may leave no histologic traces of inflammation but often results in some degree of fibrotic residua. Scarring may result in clinically relevant complications, most commonly luminal stenosis of the sigmoid colon and partial or complete obstruction of the left ureter.

Progression of peridiverticular inflammation, if the diverticulum is in the mesentery or retroperitoneum, results in abscess formation. Uncommonly, adjacent diverticula become involved. More frequently, structures adjacent to the abscess, such as the left ureter or pelvic organs, are involved by the inflammation. Abscesses rarely resolve without treatment, except when they spontaneously decompress into an adjacent hollow viscus.

Colovesical, colovaginal, coloenteric, colouterine, or other fistulas may result if a diverticular perforation or an abscess erodes into adjacent or adherent organs. Fistulas may close spontaneously, with resolution of the associated phlegmon or abscess, or may persist because of the pressure differential between the colonic lumen and the lumen of the involved organ.

Free perforation into the peritoneal cavity may occur under two circumstances. The first is when the diverticulum with microperforation directly abuts the peritoneal cavity and progresses to macroperforation without the initial inflammation becoming adherent to and walled off by omentum or another intraperitoneal organ. If there is a relatively slow leak from the bowel into the peritoneal cavity, purulent peritonitis develops; a larger opening into the peritoneal cavity or a more rapid leak results in fecal peritonitis. The second situation leading to peritonitis is perforation of an abscess into the peritoneal cavity. This is more likely to lead to purulent peritonitis, but may produce fecal peritonitis if there is communication between the colonic lumen and the abscess.

Rarely, distant infections and manifestations of sepsis result from complicated diverticulitis. Distant complications include liver abscess, infected thrombosis of the portal vein, pylephlebitis, and systemic signs of infection. These processes sometimes become clinically evident before the discovery of diverticulitis.

Clinical Manifestations

Uncomplicated Diverticulitis

SIGMOID AND LEFT COLONIC DIVERTICULITIS. Uncomplicated diverticulitis is associated with phlegmon formation and occurs in 63% to 70% of patients

who require hospitalization for a first episode of diverticulitis.[2,20] Only rarely do patients with phlegmon alone require operative therapy. The pathologic process is inferred mainly from the clinical situation, findings on radiologic studies, and results of treatment.

Most patients with diverticulitis have symptoms associated with the inflammatory process, such as cramping or intermittent pain in the lower abdomen, constipation, diarrhea, alternating constipation and diarrhea, dysuria or cramping with micturition, pneumaturia, nausea and vomiting, abdominal distention, vaginal discharge, hematochezia, chills, or rigors. The most common symptom is abdominal pain, although in 20% of patients with evidence of diverticulitis, pain is absent.[20] Pain occurs most frequently in the lower abdomen, on both the right and left sides, and less commonly in the left lower quadrant only.[20] Right-sided pain alone occurs in less than 5% of patients with diverticulitis. The pain is described as cramping or as an intermittent ache, and much less often as continuous.

Alteration in bowel movements occurs in 60% of patients with diverticulitis.[20] A single pattern does not predominate; constant constipation, intermittent constipation, and intermittent diarrhea occur with equal frequency, and alternating diarrhea and constipation are noted less often. Nausea and vomiting are experienced by 20% of patients with diverticulitis. The presence of nausea and vomiting has been associated with more severe diverticulitis, or with its complications.[20] Urinary urgency and frequency occur in 6% of patients, probably because of inflammation adjacent to the bladder.[20] Bleeding per rectum also may occur, although major hemorrhage associated with diverticulitis is unusual.[20]

Fever is often present, and left lower quadrant or suprapubic tenderness usually is noted. Abdominal distention is found in 14% of patients with diverticulitis and also portends more severe disease.[20] In 20% of patients with diverticulitis, a left lower quadrant mass is palpable on the initial abdominal or rectal examination; about half the patients with a palpable mass have complicated diverticulitis.[20]

The most consistent laboratory abnormality is leukocytosis, which is present in 66% of patients with diverticulitis.[21] Microscopic hematuria occurs in as many as 55% of patients.[21]

CECAL AND RIGHT COLONIC DIVERTICULITIS. Most right colonic diverticulitis is misdiagnosed as acute appendicitis, and the correct diagnosis is established in the operating room. Patients almost always experience right lower quadrant pain and tenderness. Other symptoms and signs are variable. Diarrhea occurs in 15% of patients, nausea and vomiting in 7% to 23%, and anorexia in 34%.[22,23] Fever is found in 42% to 59% of patients, a palpable right lower quadrant mass is noted in 7% to 11%, and leukocytosis is detected in 63% to 80%.

Complicated Diverticulitis

Complicated diverticulitis is denoted by the presence of pathology caused by extension of inflammation and infection (see Table 39-1). Fifty to 60% of patients with complicated diverticulitis have no antecedent history of diverticular disease.[20,24] Complicated diverticulitis can be treated with nonoperative therapy only infrequently.

DIVERTICULAR ABSCESS. Diverticular abscess occurs in 14% to 19% of patients hospitalized with diverticulitis.[20,25] The symptoms and signs associated with diverticular abscess are individually indistinguishable from those of uncomplicated diverticulitis, but as a group may be quantitatively more severe. Ileus with associated nausea, vomiting, and abdominal distention is more likely to be present. Fever and leukocytosis are more marked. However, symptoms, signs, and leukocytosis are unreliable in determining the presence or absence of abscess in individual patients.

PERFORATION WITH PERITONITIS. Colonic perforation with purulent or fecal peritonitis occurs in 5% to 10% of patients hospitalized with diverticulitis.[20,26] The distribution between purulent and fecal peritonitis is 86% and 14% of cases, respectively.[27] Abdominal pain is uniformly present. Eighty percent of patients with peritonitis have acute localized left lower quadrant abdominal pain or hypogastric pain with progression to more generalized pain.[27] The remaining 20% of patients have generalized abdominal pain. Other symptoms include obstipation in 50% of patients, vomiting in 30%, diarrhea in 25%, rigors in 20%, and hematochezia in 8%.[27] Physical examination discloses fever in 84% to 90% of patients, hypotension in 15%, and abdominal distention in 50%.[27] Abdominal tenderness is found in all patients with perforation and peritonitis, with the point of maximal tenderness located most frequently in the left lower quadrant. Eighty percent of patients have rebound or percussion tenderness.[28] Leukocytosis occurs in about 90%. Free air on abdominal films is identified in 20% to 44% of patients.[27,28]

FISTULAS. Fistulas between the colon and another hollow organ or the skin occur in 1% to 2% of patients with diverticulitis.[20] Colovesical fistulas occur most frequently, accounting for 65% to 85% of fistulas caused by diverticulitis.[29] Other fistulas associated with diverticulitis, as a fraction of all internal fistulas occurring with diverticulitis, include colovaginal fistulas, 13% to 25%; coloenteric fistulas, 6% to 38%; and colouterine fistulas, 3%.[29] Colocolonic, colosalpingal, and coloureteral fistulas also have been reported. The symptoms of diverticulitis frequently precede or accompany the onset of symptoms from the fistula, although in some cases, the symptoms from the fistula predominate, with few other symptoms pointing to diverticulitis.

Two thirds of colovesical fistulas occur in men. These fistulas are associated with a variety of symptoms that are predictable because the movement of substances is from the colon to the bladder due to the higher pressure in the colon. Urine per rectum is uncommon, occurring in 5% to 10% of patients with colovesical fistulas.[29,30] Pneumaturia, occurring in 60% to 75% of patients, is the most recognizable symptom other than severe urinary tract infection.[29] Other findings include cystitis or dysuria in 70% to 80% of patients, fecaluria in 40% to 70%, abdominal pain in 30% to 90%, fever and sweats in 33%, hematuria in 17%, and diarrhea in 17%. Signs often are absent. Less than 30% of patients exhibit an abdominal or pelvic mass.[29] The natural history of untreated colovesical fistulas from diverticulitis is unclear. Although a colovesical fistula may resolve spontaneously with antibiotic treatment, the usual course is either constant or recurring leak of colonic contents into the bladder, with consequent symptoms.

Colovaginal fistulas are much more likely to occur in women who have undergone hysterectomy.[29] Patients have fecal vaginal discharge as the most prominent symptom. Vaginal symptoms vary from a small amount of brownish discharge to the passage of obviously feculent material and severe vaginitis. Abdominal pain occurs in 50% of patients. On pelvic examination, a vaginal vault opening is seen in 75% to 87% of patients.

Coloenteric fistulas may occur alone, or exist with another fistula. Patients with coloenteric fistulas sometimes have no symptoms but commonly have diarrhea, presumably from fecal contamination of the middle to proximal small intestine.[29] Abdominal pain, fever, and malaise also are experienced by patients with coloenteric fistulas. On physical examination, an abdominal mass, localized peritoneal signs, and abdominal distention are found in one third to one half of patients.

Colouterine fistulas are a rare complication of diverticulitis. Symptoms include feculent, purulent, or hemorrhagic vaginal discharge and also may include constitutional symptoms such as weight loss, fever, malaise, and lethargy.[31] Often, no episode of diverticulitis is identified. On physical examination, there may be a left lower quadrant or pelvic mass, but the results of abdominal and pelvic examinations generally are normal.

Colocutaneous fistulas occur almost exclusively as postoperative complications, usually after operation on the colon (95%), but infrequently after another operation (2%) or after drainage of an intraabdominal abscess involving the abdominal wall (3%).[32] Signs and symptoms include fever and rigors, abdominal mass, abdominal distention, rectal bleeding, and, infrequently, peritoneal irritation. Performance of a colosigmoid anastomosis rather than a colorectal anastomosis is associated with an increased incidence of colocutaneous fistulas.[32] Crohn's disease and cancer should be excluded.[32]

PYLEPHLEBITIS AND LIVER ABSCESS. Pylephlebitis and pyogenic liver abscess associated with diverticulitis are rare complications. Pylephlebitis and pyogenic liver abscess can exist alone or in combination. Pylephlebitis usually results in one or more accompanying liver abscesses. Liver abscess is a more common complication. In patients older than 60 years, diverticulitis is the second most common cause of liver abscess, after cholelithiasis.[33] Diverticulitis is the leading cause of pylephlebitis.[34] Ninety percent of patients with these complications are older than 50 years.[34] Males exceed females by a 3:1 ratio.[34] A subphrenic abscess sometimes accompanies the liver abscess.[34]

Symptoms of liver abscess without pylephlebitis include epigastric pain (53%), nausea and vomiting (47%), weight loss (35%), shortness of breath (29%), malaise (23%), rigors (12%), and diarrhea (12%).[33] Signs include an enlarged liver (55%), tenderness in the epigastrium (41%), jaundice (29%), and fever (23%).[33] Left lower quadrant pain is unusual (9%).[35] Although fever and rigors are almost always present with pylephlebitis, the presence of jaundice is more variable.[34,35] Elevation of the serum bilirubin level may be a reflection of hepatic decompensation more than the presence of pylephlebitis. The results of blood cultures commonly are positive with pylephlebitis. *Escherichia coli* is the most frequently cultured organism from the blood and abscesses, and streptococcal species are the next most common from the liver abscesses.[34,35] Anaerobes, including *Bacteroides fragilis*, and *Clostridium* sp also have been cultured from the blood in patients with pylephlebitis.[35,36]

Diagnostic Methods

Sigmoid and Left Colonic Diverticulitis

When patients have symptoms and signs compatible with acute diverticulitis or one of its complications, the interview and examination should establish that these are congruent with diverticulitis and, if possible, exclude other diseases in the differential diagnosis, which include the following: cancer, Crohn's disease, mesenteric infarction, ischemic colitis, radiation colitis, tuboovarian abscess, stercoral colonic perforation, foreign body perforation, ureteral stone or cancer, and left iliac artery aneurysm. An upright chest radiograph, to evaluate for free intraperitoneal air, and flat and upright abdominal radiographs, to assess for mechanical or paralytic ileus, should be obtained. Initial laboratory studies should include a complete blood count, to assess for leukocytosis and anemia; blood urea nitrogen and serum creatinine levels, to evaluate renal status and guide selection and dosing of antibiotics; serum transaminase, alkaline phosphatase, and bilirubin levels, to survey for liver complications of diverticulitis; and urinalysis, to determine the presence of urinary tract infection and fecaluria. Bladder catheterization should be avoided to prevent introduction of air into the bladder, thereby confounding determination of pneumaturia. Patients with diffuse peritonitis or signs of sepsis should undergo the additional studies required for urgent or emergency operation.

In patients with acute diverticulitis but no initial evidence of complications, additional diagnostic studies are reserved for those who do not respond to medical therapy (see later). Routine use of contrast enema or computed tomography (CT) in the initial evaluation of patients with diverticulitis is discouraged. Twenty-five percent or fewer patients have complicated diverticulitis. It is principally patients with abscesses (14% to 19% of the total) in whom findings on CT are likely to alter markedly the direction of treatment. In the absence of clinical indicators that the disease is progressing, a delay of 2 to 3 days to evaluate for response to medical therapy rarely makes any difference in the outcome of patients with abscesses.

When there is doubt about the diagnosis of diverticulitis, when there are signs of systemic sepsis, or when there is progression of signs or inadequate clinical response to medical therapy, additional diagnostic studies are indicated. Abdominal and pelvic CT are the radiologic studies of choice despite the lower cost and greater availability of contrast enema. The sensitivity of CT for complications of diverticulitis, particularly abscess, is much greater than that of contrast enema.[25] Overall, CT is at least as sensitive as contrast enema in diagnosing diverticulitis, and is more likely to identify other pathology misdiagnosed as diverticulitis.[37,38] Depending on the methods used to visualize the sigmoid colon, the risk of CT for opening a sealed perforation is less than or equal to that of contrast enema. Moreover, CT can be used to guide percutaneous drainage catheter placement in the management of diverticulitis-associated abscesses.[38]

Findings on CT consistent with diverticulitis include local wall thickening (more than 5 mm with at least partial distention of the bowel), inflammation of pericolic fat, and associated diverticula[25,37] (Fig. 39-2). Findings of paracolic fluid collection, with or without extraluminal gas, are highly sensitive and specific for paracolic abscess[25,37] (Fig. 39-3). Thickening of the colon wall adjacent to locally thickened bladder, associated diverticula, and air, or contrast in the bladder, if no intravenous contrast has been administered, are consistent with colovesical fistula.[25]

Isolated from the clinical setting, however, these CT findings are not diagnostic. Thickening of the colon wall occurs in several other conditions, including inflammatory bowel disease, ischemic colitis, pseudomembranous colitis, lymphoma, and colonic adenocarcinoma. Inflammation of pericolic fat also is seen in Crohn's disease and perforated colon cancer. Moreover, in some patients, inflammation of the pericolic fat is minimal or absent on CT, but there is wall thickening, suggesting a process other than diverticulitis. If the CT scan is done in association with clinical findings, confusion based on the similarity of CT findings of diverticulitis to these other conditions is minimized. When uncertainty persists, flexible sigmoidoscopy and contrast enema can be used to differentiate between most of the other pathologic entities.[39]

Certain techniques used by the radiologist performing the CT, particularly in demonstrating the sigmoid

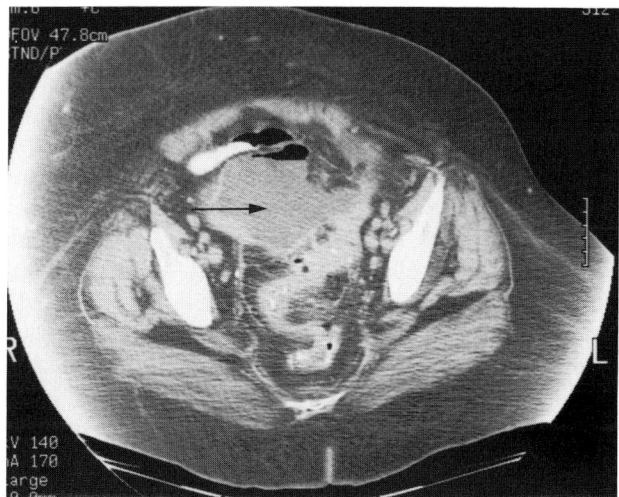

Figure 39-3 CT of a paracolic abscess (*arrow*) complicating diverticulitis.

colon, are of concern to the surgeon. Enteric contrast should be administered by mouth or gastric tube several hours before the examination. Whenever possible, a gentle rectal enema of 150 to 200 mL of water-soluble contrast material should be administered immediately before the CT to improve delineation of the sigmoid colon.[25] Alternatively, air insufflation of the rectum also can display the rectum and sigmoid colon effectively.[38] A scan without intravenous contrast is preferable because, in that context, detection of contrast in the bladder implies either colovesical or enterovesical fistula, or bowel perforation with absorbance of contrast from the peritoneal cavity.[25] Avoidance of bladder instrumentation permits any air seen in the bladder by CT to be attributed to a bowel–bladder fistula.

Cecal and Right Colonic Diverticulitis

Although three fourths of patients with right-sided diverticulitis are operated on with a preoperative diagnosis of acute appendicitis, when the diagnosis of right colonic or cecal diverticulitis is securely made, most patients can be treated successfully by antibiotics without operation. In patients who have had previous appendectomy, the possibility of right colonic or cecal diverticulitis may be more apparent, but the diagnosis also should be considered in Asian patients with right lower quadrant pain and tenderness.

Radiologic studies that may assist in the diagnosis include barium enema, CT, and ultrasonography. Barium enema reveals isolated paracecal or right colonic collections of contrast. Demonstration of diverticula in the right colon suggests the possibility of diverticulitis.

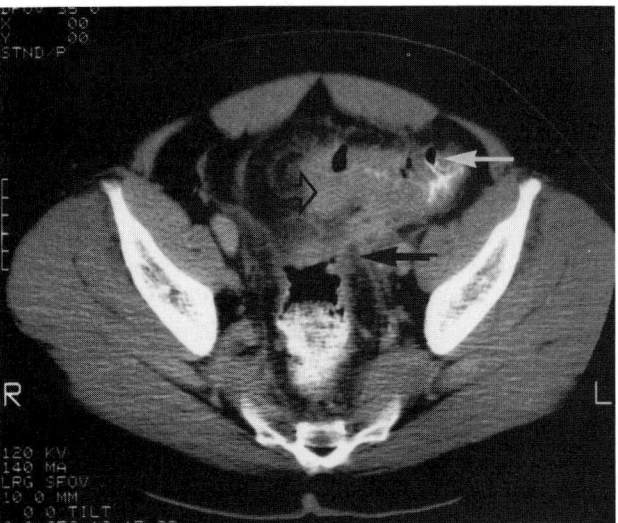

Figure 39-2 CT scan demonstrating the findings of diverticulitis, including local colon wall thickening (*open arrow*), inflammation of pericolic fat (stranding in fat; *black arrow*), and presence of diverticula (*white arrow*).

Demonstration of the entire lumen of the appendix excludes appendicitis. Lack of visualization of a diverticulum in the right colon does not exclude the diagnosis of cecal or right colonic diverticulitis, because diverticulitis often occurs in a solitary right-sided diverticulum. The inflamed diverticulum may not be visualized because of an obstructed ostium.

Inflammatory processes in the cecal area are not easily differentiated from diverticulitis.[40] Ultrasonography may be useful in diagnosing right-sided diverticulitis and distinguishing it from acute appendicitis.[41] The finding in uncomplicated right-sided diverticulitis is a round or oval hypoechoic focus protruding from a segmentally thickened colon wall. Reinforcing the diagnosis is the absence of an enlarged appendix. Extraluminal gas is sometimes present. The existence of an abscess suggests complicated diverticulitis.

Fistulas

Demonstration of a fistula is undertaken in most cases because the portion of the gastrointestinal tract containing the fistula and the nature of the disease process resulting in the fistula are not evident. Less than half of patients with fistulas arising as a complication of diverticulitis have symptoms or signs at presentation indicating diverticulitis as the etiology.[29] For colovesical fistulas, gross inspection of the urine for fecal material, urinalysis, and urine culture confirming infection with fecal organisms are the initial steps. CT and cystoscopy have the highest yield in demonstrating these fistulas (Table 39-2). When barium enema is performed but does not demonstrate the fistula, the presence of barium in the spun urine of the first void confirms communication of the urinary tract with the colon. Despite

Table 39-2 Diagnostic Studies in the Investigation of Colovesical Fistula and the Frequency With Which They Demonstrate the Fistula

Study	Percentage Demonstrated	References
Barium enema	32–42	29, 30
Cystography	22–56	29, 30
Computed tomography		
Demonstrates fistula	11–25	25, 30
Highly suggests fistula	67–92	25, 30
Cystoscopy		
Reveals fistula orifice	30–46	29, 30
Bullous edema, erythema, ulcer	88–92	—
Sigmoidoscopy, colonoscopy	6	30
Intravenous urography	0–8	29, 30

these studies, the origin of these fistulas frequently must be inferred based on an abnormality in the bladder on cystoscopy, the presence of diverticula in the colon adjacent to the bladder, the character of the urine, and the clinical picture.

Colovaginal fistulas can be visualized in 43% to 87% of patients on speculum examination (see Table 39-2). The fistulas usually occur at the apex of the vaginal cuff. Vaginography performed with a balloon catheter inflated in the vagina demonstrates colovaginal fistulas in most cases and is easily performed.[42] Barium enema demonstrates the fistulas in only 34% to 48% of patients.[29]

Treatment

Uncomplicated Diverticulitis

SIGMOID AND LEFT COLONIC DIVERTICULITIS. Uncomplicated diverticulitis is defined by the criterion that it can be treated without operation, whereas complicated diverticulitis almost always requires an operation at some point in treatment. The elements of the initial treatment of diverticulitis are antibiotics and prohibition of oral intake. In patients with mild pain, minimal tenderness, low-grade fever, and insignificant leukocytosis, outpatient therapy with a clear liquid diet and oral antibiotics frequently is successful. In patients with more severe manifestations of inflammation, altered immune status, or additional serious medical problems, and in those in whom 24 to 48 hours of outpatient treatment is unsuccessful, hospitalization, bowel rest, intravenous fluids, and intravenous broad-spectrum antibiotics are indicated. Nasogastric tubes are useful only when there is vomiting or evidence of bowel obstruction. Monitoring of symptoms, vital signs, physical examination, and the white blood cell count must be performed regularly to assess the response to medical treatment, with the initial 72 hours of hospitalization being particularly critical for decision making. Resumption of oral intake should await resolution of signs of inflammation, including normalization of the white blood cell count and temperature, and disappearance of left lower quadrant tenderness. Antibiotic therapy should be continued until signs of inflammation have disappeared. In uncomplicated diverticulitis, it is uncommon for signs of inflammation to persist more than 7 days.

Worsening signs of inflammation, or lack of improvement within 72 hours of initiation of treatment, indicates that the diverticulitis is most likely complicated and that additional intervention is required. Further investigation, usually with CT, is the next step in such patients.

For patients in whom an intraabdominal or pelvic abscess is detected, CT-guided percutaneous drainage, when feasible, is the initial treatment of choice (Fig. 39-4). Advantages of CT-guided percutaneous abscess drainage include rapid resolution of systemic septic manifestations, substitution of elective operation for urgent surgical intervention,[38] and more frequent primary resection and anastomosis. CT-guided percutaneous drainage is successful in 75% of patients. Failure often is associated with grossly feculent discharge.[43] Patients are treated concomitantly with broad-spectrum antibiotics against aerobic coliform bacteria and *B fragilis* until signs of inflammation resolve. Sinograms are obtained at 4- to 7-day intervals to assess for develop-

ment of a fistula to the colon and to monitor collapse of the abscess cavity. Surgery generally is performed after a period of 10 to 14 days after disappearance of the abscess cavity. Patients who respond to percutaneous drainage and antibiotics usually can resume a low-residual diet and be discharged home with the drain in place, followed up at intervals by sinograms until the abscess cavity has resolved. The drain generally is left in place until operation. Patients with persistent signs of inflammation should be restudied with CT to assess for undrained abscess cavities. In the absence of additional collections that are amenable to drainage, patients with persistent sepsis should undergo urgent operation.

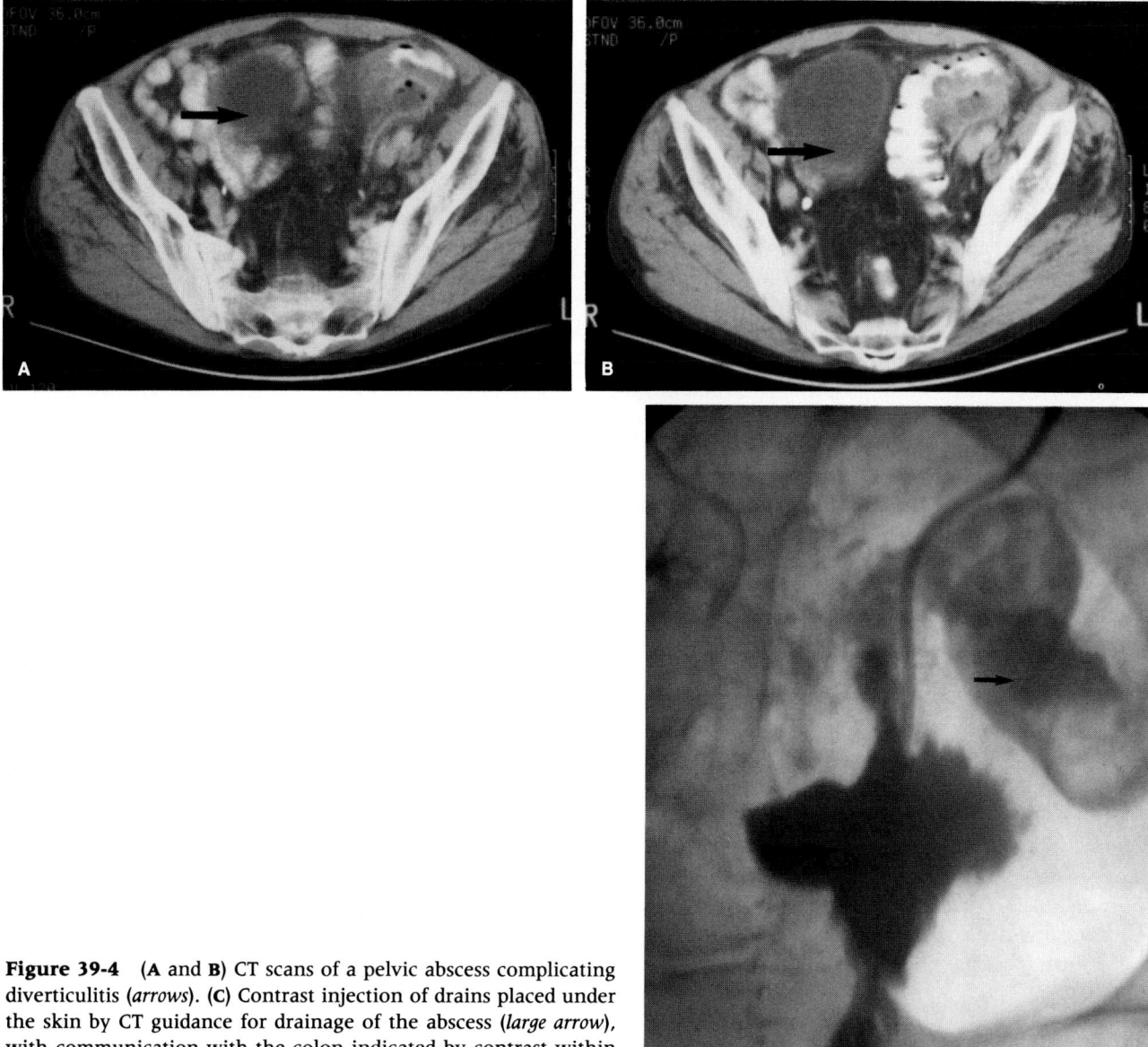

Figure 39-4 (**A** and **B**) CT scans of a pelvic abscess complicating diverticulitis (*arrows*). (**C**) Contrast injection of drains placed under the skin by CT guidance for drainage of the abscess (*large arrow*), with communication with the colon indicated by contrast within the colon lumen (*small arrow*).

Patients with uncomplicated diverticulitis who have had an appropriate response to medical treatment can be discharged from the hospital, usually eating a regular diet. In many of these patients, no diagnostic studies are needed immediately to document diverticulitis or to exclude other disease processes. Performance of such studies can and should wait until 4 to 6 weeks after resolution of the episode of acute inflammation. After that interval, sigmoidoscopy to exclude cancer or inflammatory bowel disease and barium enema to demonstrate diverticulosis can be performed more safely. On documentation of diverticulosis, a high-fiber diet may be initiated.

Symptoms of diverticular disease recur in about one third of patients who have received successful medical therapy for a first attack of diverticulitis, and are severe in 5%.[2] Of those who have a first episode of uncomplicated diverticulitis, 25% are hospitalized a second time, 4% a third time, and 2% a fourth time for recurrent attacks of diverticulitis.[2] Three fourths of those hospitalized a second time have symptoms during the interval, although these usually are mild.[2] Nearly half of second hospitalizations for diverticulitis occur within 1 year of the initial hospitalization, and 91% occur within 5 years.[2] For patients hospitalized a third time, 92% have symptoms during the interval and 42% have severe symptoms.[2] The mortality at the second admission is 7.6%, almost double that of a first attack (4.8%).[2] Twenty-five percent of those hospitalized a second time for diverticulitis require an operation for their diverticular disease, similar to the 18% to 30% who require operation during a first hospitalization.[2,44]

Although the addition of 20 to 25 g of fiber to the daily diet of patients who have experienced an episode of diverticulitis has become standard, the efficacy of a high-fiber diet in preventing future episodes of diverticulitis is unproven. Symptoms and colonic motility after initiation of a high-fiber diet improve compared with a normal-fiber diet. However, there are no long-term prospective studies of the effect of a high-fiber diet on the recurrence of diverticulitis or its complications.

CECAL AND RIGHT COLONIC DIVERTICULITIS. Right colonic diverticulitis is rare in Western populations, but more common in persons of Asian descent. Most cases of right colonic diverticulitis are diagnosed at operation. When a nonoperative diagnosis is made, the principles of nonoperative treatment outlined for left-sided diverticulitis apply. Indications for CT to evaluate for complications are similar to those for left-sided diverticulitis.

The natural history of uncomplicated cecal or right colonic diverticulitis has not been well delineated. Among patients with right colonic or cecal diverticulitis

discovered at operation, without gross perforation or abscess, and treated with appendectomy and postoperative antibiotics, 3% to 14% had recurrent pain and 3% to 7% had more than one episode of recurrent pain, but only 3% required operation for pain or bleeding.[22,23]

As with left-sided diverticulitis, localized abscesses identified by CT can be drained through the skin. Drainage is continued until the abscess cavity has disappeared. After the exclusion of right colonic or cecal cancer and other disease processes, such as Crohn's disease, the drain can be gradually extracted. A fecal fistula present on removal of the drain usually resolves. After resolution of the abscess and any subsequent fecal fistula, there are insufficient data to indicate whether right colectomy or any other operative intervention is advisable.

Operative Treatment of Colonic Diverticulitis and Its Complications

INDICATIONS FOR OPERATION. Operation is necessary in 14% to 30% of patients with diverticulitis.[2,24,44,45] The usual indications for operation during or after diverticulitis are listed in Table 39-3.

The clearest indication for emergent operation is generalized peritonitis with or without evidence of free perforation. Purulent and feculent peritonitis associated with diverticulitis have mortality rates of 8% to 13% and 35% to 50%, respectively.[27,46] There is no role for nonoperative management of these conditions. Urgent or emergency operation also is indicated for pro-

---

Table 39-3 Indications for Operation for Colonic Diverticulitis*

ABSOLUTE
Free perforation
Peritonitis
Acute abdomen with inability to exclude other disease processes
Obstruction
Abscess
Fistula
Inability to exclude carcinoma
Symptomatic stricture
One atack in an immunocompromised patient

RELATIVE
Two or more attacks of diverticulitis
Persistent mass
Persisting urinary symptoms associated with diverticulitis

EQUIVOCAL
One attack of diverticulitis in a patient younger than 40

---

* The timing of the operation differs with the indication.

gressive deterioration due to sepsis and for complete bowel obstruction. For most of the other indications, operation can be delayed for directed evaluation of the extent and site of inflammation, and often can be performed electively or semielectively.

Undrained intraabdominal or pelvic abscesses are associated with persistent sepsis, and urgent operation is indicated. Patients with pelvic abscesses that resolve after percutaneous drainage should undergo resection of the sigmoid colon. Treatment without colectomy in patients with pelvic or intraabdominal abscesses is successful in only 16% to 28% of cases when followed up for 2 years.[47,48] In addition, CT evidence of severe inflammation, including abscess, extraluminal air, and extraluminal contrast, is associated with persistent diverticulitis, colonic stenosis, abscess, or fistula in almost half of patients, and is another indication for resection.[49] In contrast to pelvic and intraabdominal abscesses, isolated mesocolic abscesses associated with diverticulitis resolve with antibiotics and nonoperative treatment in 70% of cases.[48]

Recommendations have been made for resection of the colon in any patient aged 50 years or less who has experienced an attack of diverticulitis.[44] These recommendations remain controversial. Several reports[14,50,51] have indicated a virulent course for diverticulitis in patients younger than 40 years compared with older patients. There is a 2% to 23% incidence of free perforation in younger patients hospitalized for diverticulitis. Between 11% and 85% of patients aged 40 years or less require operation at initial presentation, based on indications other than age.[13,14,50–52] In contrast, limited outcome data on younger patients who have had successful medical treatment of an episode of diverticulitis do not clearly indicate that these patients have a high risk of recurrent disease or subsequent complications. In a group of patients aged 40 years or less who were hospitalized with diverticular disease and treated with medical therapy,[53] investigators reported no operations and absence of symptoms after the index episode in 47% of patients followed up for a few months to 4 years. In another series,[54] 26 patients aged 40 years or less were hospitalized for inflammatory diverticular disease and treated with medical therapy; during a mean follow-up of 52 months, 8% underwent operation for chronic abdominal pain, 38% were readmitted once for recurrent disease, and 4% were readmitted a second time. A less benign course was experienced by 7 of 14 patients in this age group who were treated with medical therapy for diverticulitis at the initial hospitalization and were followed up for 2 to 14 years.[55] Four patients (28%) required emergency operation within 3 years of the index hospitalization, 1 had a colonic obstruction from inflammation, and 2 underwent surgery for repeated episodes of diverticulitis. The other 7 patients, who were followed up for 2 to 10 years, had infrequent and mild symptoms. In another report of 67 patients aged 40 years or less who were treated with medical therapy for diverticulitis and were followed up for an average of 27 months,[50] 45% required no additional hospitalization. The other 37 patients required 54 readmissions for diverticulitis, with the interval to first readmission averaging 22 months. Sixteen patients (24%) required urgent operation after initial medical management, 1 for free perforation, 10 for abscess, 3 for obstruction, and 2 for fistulas. Comparisons with rates of operation and rehospitalization for all age groups do not suggest a markedly higher rate of operation for complications from attacks subsequent to the index episode.[2,47] Available data suggest that patients aged 40 years or less who are treated with medical therapy at the initial hospitalization for diverticulitis have a somewhat more morbid subsequent course, but not enough so to mandate colon resection.

The course of diverticulitis in immunosuppressed patients can be disastrous. In retrospective studies,[56] diverticulitis-associated perforation, sepsis, and peritonitis occur at markedly higher rates than in the absence of immunosuppression. Successful medical treatment of diverticulitis is distinctly unusual in immunosuppressed patients.[56] In general, urgent to emergency operation is necessary at the initial admission for diverticulitis.[57] Attempts at medical treatment should not be prolonged; time should be used to prepare patients for operation.

Patients who have had a recurrent episode of diverticulitis should be considered strongly for elective resection.[18,44,58] Of those who are treated successfully with medical therapy during a second hospitalization for diverticulitis, 20% are admitted a third time for recurrence and 42% have severe symptoms between the second and third hospitalizations.[2] Of those who are treated with medical therapy during a third hospital stay, 42% require a fourth admission for treatment of diverticulitis.[2] A complication rate of 58% for obstruction, abscess, or fistula is associated with multiple attacks.[59]

OPERATIONS FOR SIGMOID AND LEFT CO-LONIC DIVERTICULITIS. The immediate and primary goal of operation for complications of diverticulitis is to reverse the systemic and regional effects of the inflammatory process. Concomitant goals are to prevent injury to important structures in the area and to alter normal functioning of patients as little as possible. The final goal is to restore patients to a normal functional state.

Operations for complications of diverticulitis can

be divided into one-, two-, and three-stage procedures for resection of the involved colon and reestablishment of the integrity of the fecal stream. Because the existence of a rectal diverticulum below the peritoneal reflection is extremely rare, anastomosis of the bowel to restore rectal function almost always is possible and is the ultimate goal of most operations. Although there has been a significant trend toward use of the single-stage procedure, in which resection and reanastomosis are done at the same operation, controversy remains over whether this approach minimizes overall morbidity and mortality. The morbidity and mortality question must be asked about the entirety of the course of treatment, from initial medical treatment to the restoration of anatomic and physiologic function. Focusing on only a segment of the treatment course has led to erroneous conclusions. In addition, the course of treatment must be evaluated with respect to the condition for which the treatment is applied.

Three-stage resection of the colon for the treatment of complications of diverticulitis first was advocated in 1942[60] (Fig. 39-5). The first stage is aimed at facilitating resolution of the inflammatory process and reversing systemic sepsis. It consists of proximal diversion of the fecal stream, usually with a transverse colostomy, with the intention of preventing leakage through a perforation or additional soiling in the inflamed peridiverticular area. Once inflammation has significantly resolved, the second stage is carried out, consisting of resection of the involved colon and any pericolonic inflammation. Finally, when the patient has recovered from the second-stage operation and from any residual inflammation, the third stage is performed by takedown of the ostomy and restoration of bowel continuity. The three-stage approach is used infrequently in current practice because of unacceptable morbidity associated with leaving perforated bowel in place at the first stage. It has been shown by many groups that initial resection of the inflamed colon, although difficult and sometimes tedious, can be performed safely and results in much quicker reversal of sepsis. Cumulative mortality and morbidity associated with the three operations and hospitalizations for the three-stage approach are at least as great as those associated with two-stage resections.

Two-stage resection of left-sided diverticulitis consists of resection of the inflamed or perforated segment of colon and formation of a diverting colostomy at the initial operation, with reestablishment of colon continuity at the second operation. Two approaches have been used (Fig. 39-6). The more common approach to the first stage is the Hartmann procedure, which involves resection of the inflamed colon, formation of a colostomy using the divided end of the remaining proximal bowel, and formation of a rectal pouch. The second stage then involves colostomy closure to the Hartmann pouch. A second approach to the two-stage operation is resection of the involved colon, anastomosis, and formation of a proximal, usually loop, transverse colostomy for diversion of the fecal stream to protect the anastomosis. The advantages of the Hartmann procedure are that the operation is quicker because no time is required for the anastomosis and that an anastomosis is not performed in the presence of unprepared bowel.

The single-stage resection, as the name implies, involves resection and reanastomosis at the same operation (Fig. 39-7). Primary anastomosis in the left colon is accomplished safely only with colon preparation, which cannot be carried out by oral or enema cleansing in most patients with perforation or pelvic abscess. On-table colonic lavage can be accomplished for mechanical bowel preparation to permit safe primary anastomosis.[61]

Several factors must be considered in deciding which operation for complicated diverticulitis is best for a particular patient, including type of complication, associated medical disease, intraoperative hemodynamic status, nutritional status, presence of immunosuppression, extent of bowel preparation, blood supply to the bowel, and degree of edema in the bowel at the margins of resection. The knowledge and experience of the surgeon and other members of the operating team also must be considered.

For patients with feculent or purulent peritonitis caused by sigmoid or left colonic perforation, the two-stage procedure with resection of the inflamed or perforated portion of colon at the initial operation has been the most widely recommended approach. This recommendation is based on retrospective reports from several centers[26,27,62,63] indicating lower mortality and morbidity after primary resection when compared with diverting colostomy as the initial operation. However, recommendation for resection at the initial operation has not been uniform. Similar mortality for primary diversion versus primary resection was noted in one recent retrospective review.[64] Moreover, in a prospective randomized trial,[46] the mortality rate for primary resection versus primary diversion for fecal peritonitis was not significantly different. Surprisingly, there was a significantly worse mortality rate for acute resection in the presence of purulent peritonitis than for diverting colostomy with suture of the perforation and coverage with an omental patch. In this study, complication rates after the first operation were similar for diversion and resection, and a slightly higher percentage of patients in the acute resection group were left with a permanent colostomy. There is agreement in all studies, however,

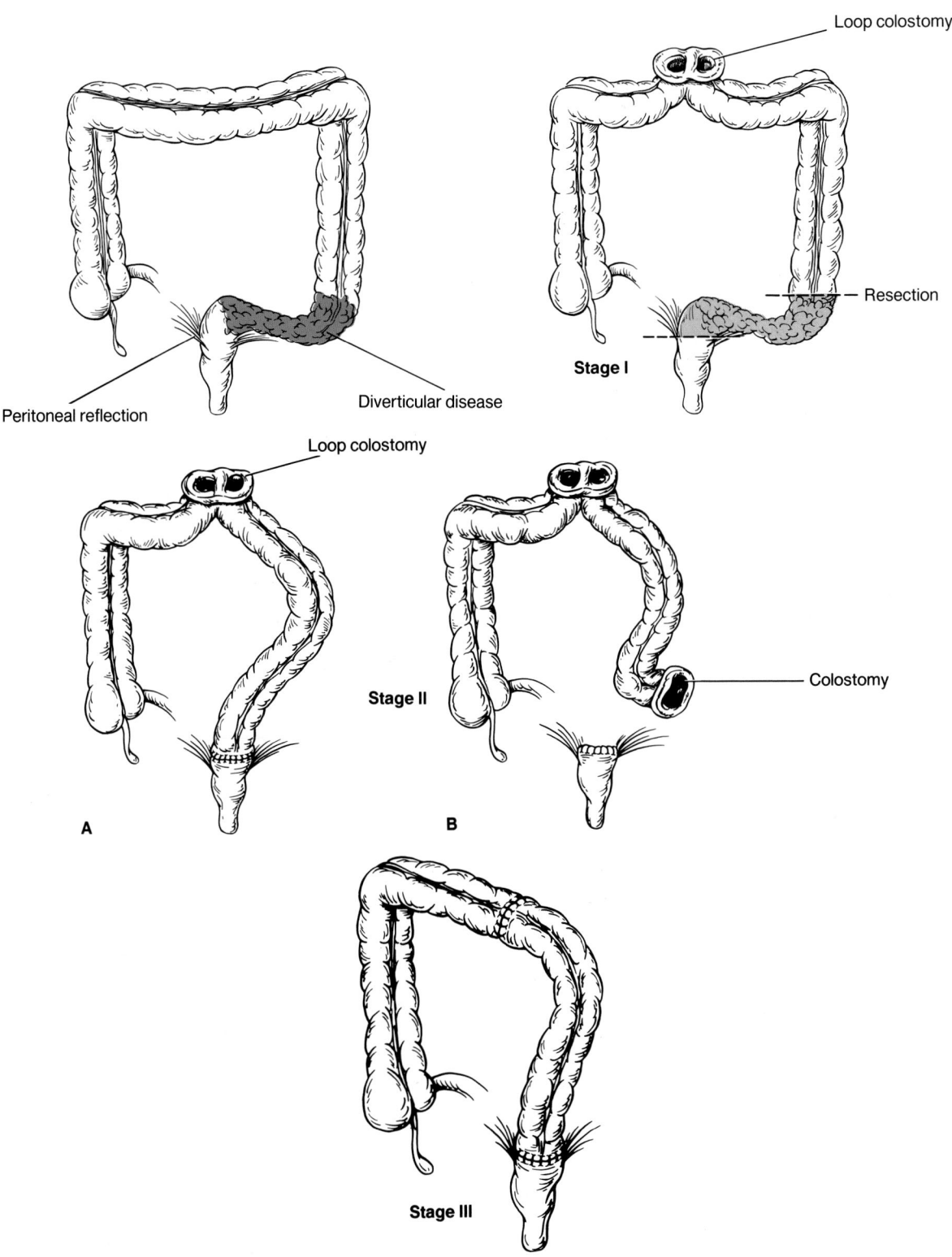

Figure 39-5 Three-stage operation for complicated colon diverticulitis. Stage I: proximal diversion, usually with transverse colostomy, either loop or double-barrel. Stage II: resection of diseased sigmoid colon with anastomosis (**A**), most commonly, or without anastomosis (**B**). (Heavy lines in the stage I diagram indicate lines for resection.) Stage III: restoration of colon continuity.

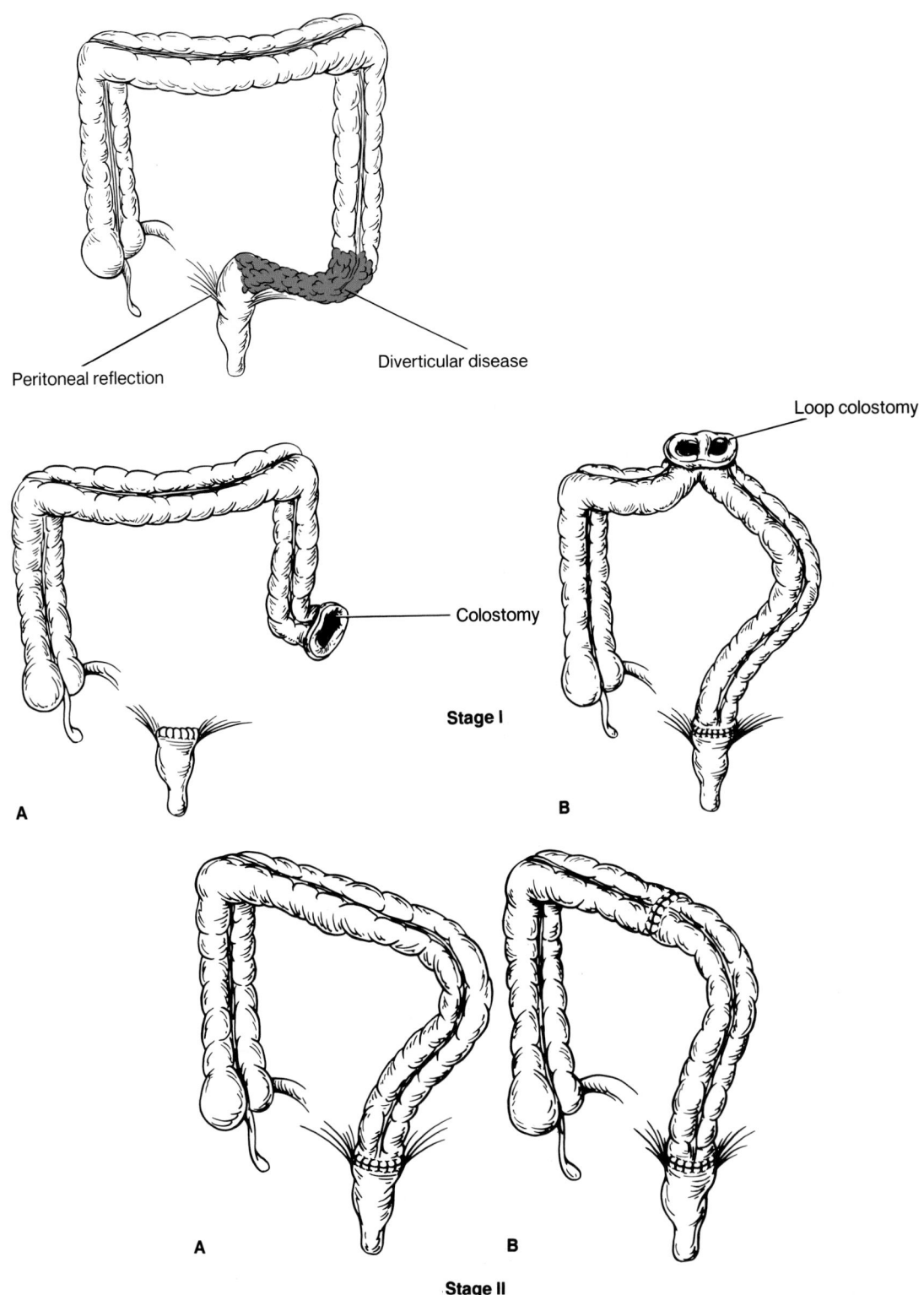

Figure 39-6 Two-stage operation for complicated colon diverticulitis. Stage I: resection of diseased sigmoid colon with descending colostomy and rectal pouch (Hartmann operation; **A**), or descending colorectal anastomosis and proximal diverting colostomy (**B**). Stage II: restoration of colon continuity for the respective procedures.

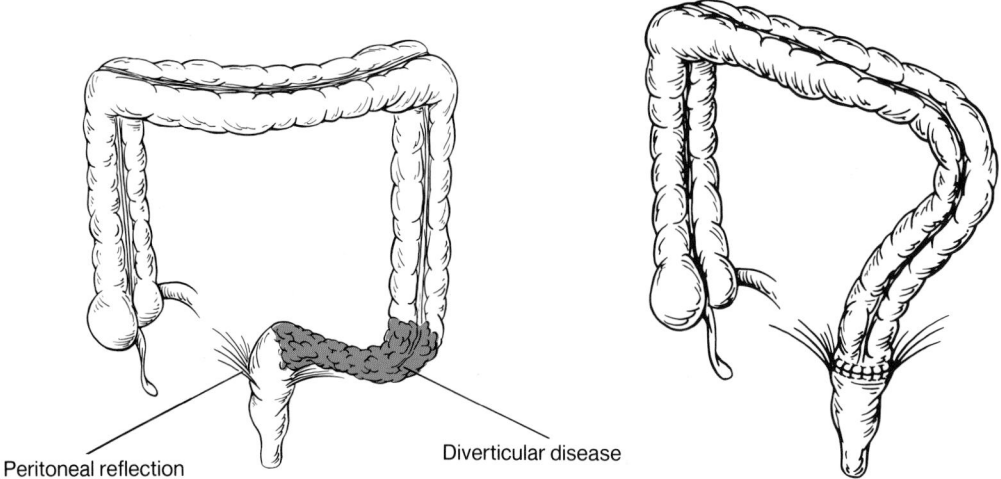

Peritoneal reflection   Diverticular disease

Figure 39-7 Single-stage operation for complicated colon diverticulitis. Resection of diseased sigmoid colon and restoration of colon continuity is accomplished in a single operation.

that patients who undergo acute resection spend fewer days in the hospital.[65]

For patients with walled-off pelvic abscesses without generalized peritonitis, the trend has been toward percutaneous drainage at first, followed by one-stage resection and primary anastomosis of a prepared colon after resolution of the inflammation. For patients requiring urgent operation for abscess, there also has been a trend away from the three-stage approach toward the one- or two-stage approach.[24,44] Retrospective mortality data are not consistent, but in all series in which the variable is examined, there is more prolonged hospitalization with similar or greater morbidity when diverting colostomy is the initial treatment, lending impetus to initial resection as the treatment of choice.

In the presence of an undrained pelvic abscess, the usual operative approach is a two-stage resection using the Hartmann procedure as the initial stage. A two-stage resection with the first stage consisting of resection, anastomosis, and protecting colostomy, if adequate preoperative or intraoperative colon cleansing can be achieved, has similar or lower morbidity and mortality relative to the Hartmann procedure. The colostomy usually is easily closed and infrequently remains permanent.[45]

Patients with small pericolic or mesenteric abscesses almost always can be treated with single-stage procedures. Because of the limited inflammatory process, preoperative bowel preparation is possible, and the abscess can be included within the resected specimen so that no residual inflammation remains.[44]

Similarly, the treatment of patients who have fistulas as a complication of diverticulitis usually involves single-stage resection.[29] Because most fistulas are direct communications between a perforated diverticulum and the secondary organ, or are the site of decompression of an abscess, there typically is no residual associated abscess cavity. Resection of the colon is requisite in the treatment of these fistulas, but treatment of the secondarily involved organ varies. If there is an identifiable bladder opening after dissection of the sigmoid in patients with colovesical fistulas, the opening is closed in two layers.[30] Only nonviable bladder wall is resected, because the disease is not in the bladder. If no identifiable leak can be identified, filling the bladder with 0.5% iodine solution through the urethral catheter may identify a leak. If no leak is readily identified, further search is not indicated. In all cases, the bladder should be decompressed for 7 days using a urethral catheter. A cystogram is performed before removal of the decompressing catheter to exclude residual leak.

For colovaginal fistulas, closure of the vaginal opening after resection of the sigmoid is unnecessary.[29] With enterocolic fistulas, resection of a small segment of bowel encompassing the fistula is recommended. Most patients with colouterine fistulas from diverticulitis have been treated with concomitant hysterectomy and sigmoid colon resection, although the number of reported cases is too small to confirm the necessity of hysterectomy.[29,31]

Resection as a single-stage procedure generally is possible in the treatment of chronic stricture from diverticulitis. Strictures uncommonly cause complete obstruction, so that mechanical bowel preparation usually can be accomplished. Likewise, single-stage resection with anastomosis is the norm for elective resection for diverticulitis. The dissection under such circumstances may be straightforward, or it may be difficult because of extensive fibrosis.

OPERATIONS FOR CECAL AND RIGHT CO-LONIC DIVERTICULITIS. Because right colonic diverticulitis is rare in Western populations, uncertainty and controversy surround the best operative approach to the disease. Randomized trials of differing treatment methods have not been performed. The spectrum of described approaches includes performing right colectomy; leaving the inflamed diverticulum in situ with or without drainage; performing appendectomy; and treating with postoperative antibiotics, cecectomy, diverticulectomy, and diverticular invagination. Based on results of large series of patients treated with surgery, a consistent operative approach can be recommended.

The initial dilemma with right colonic and cecal diverticulitis is that the mass associated with the inflammation must be differentiated from cancer. Other conditions causing inflammation in the right colon include tuberculosis, actinomycosis, amebic colitis, carcinoid, and Crohn's disease. Differentiation of these conditions usually is possible. Experienced surgeons are unable to exclude right colon cancer in only 4% to 8% of patients with right colonic or cecal diverticulitis.[22,23] Findings that identify a diverticulum as the source of the mass include visualization of the inflamed diverticulum, palpation of the ostium of the diverticulum through the colon wall opposite the mass, and inference from the presence of other diverticula in the cecum or right colon.

Free perforation of right colonic diverticulitis occurs only rarely, with no cases reported among 206 patients from several series.[16,23,66–68] There is no literature specifically directed at the management of this complication. Although right colectomy has been recommended for free perforation, if healthy colon wall surrounding the perforation can be exposed, by analogy to perforated appendicitis, closure of the perforation may be wholly satisfactory. In one report,[22] 25 patients with perforated right colonic diverticula were treated by appendectomy and diverticulectomy with no mortality and wound infection as the only complication.

In as many as 40% of patients operated on for right colonic diverticulitis, an abscess with or without communication with the bowel lumen is found.[22] Abscesses can be treated by drainage and resection of the diverticulum through adjacent healthy colon wall, and primary closure.[22] Ileocecectomy is required in a few cases because of proximity of the diverticulum to the ileocecal valve and inability to resect the diverticulum without distortion of the valve. A large associated abscess with thick peel may simulate appendiceal abscess and can be treated initially with drainage; eventual diverticular or colonic resection may be necessary.[66] Appendectomy always should be performed to reduce confusion about recurring symptoms.

Most cases of right colonic and cecal diverticulitis are represented by a mass of the colon caused by peridiverticular inflammation. In a few patients, differentiation from cancer is not possible and right colectomy should be performed. Although right colectomy was the most commonly performed operative procedure (38%) in a review encompassing 635 patients with diverticulitis of the right colon and cecum,[15] it was associated with a 2.5% mortality rate. By contrast, the mortality rate for diverticulectomy (29% of operations) was 0.5%. Reports have emphasized that the optimal therapy for diverticular phlegmon is appendectomy followed by the administration of antibiotics.[16,22] Of 94 patients so treated among three recent series, there were no deaths and only 4 patients had complications (4%). There was agreement among the authors of the reports advocating appendectomy and postoperative antibiotics that colon resection should be avoided whenever possible for right-sided diverticulitis.[16,22]

RESECTION OF SIGMOID DIVERTICULITIS: TECHNICAL ASPECTS. The major considerations in performing resection for sigmoid diverticulitis are preventing injury to adjacent structures, removing or adequately draining purulence, preventing additional fecal contamination, and maintaining viability of the remaining bowel. Although laparoscopic or minimally invasive surgery can be used satisfactorily in selected cases for elective sigmoid resection after resolution of inflammation, laparoscopic resection can be formidable even in that circumstance because of scarring and difficulty in identifying the ureter. The open surgical approach is the only satisfactory approach for urgent or emergency operation and for complications of left-sided diverticulitis.

To allow for mobilization of the splenic flexure of the colon, patients should be prepared for general anesthesia, although epidural anesthesia alone is satisfactory in some cases if expertly administered. A urethral catheter should be placed for drainage of the bladder and for instillation of fluid to define any leaks or fistulas. Placement of ureteral stents for identification of the ureters can assist dissection through dense scar and inflammation. Patients are placed in the lithotomy position with leg holders to permit access to the rectum for irrigation and placement of a stapler for anastomosis.

In general, a midline incision provides the best exposure. The sigmoid colon should be evaluated for free perforation if there is evidence of purulence or fecal material in the abdomen. The structures to which the sigmoid colon is adherent should be noted early in the case; the most frequent structure is the bladder. Often, there are adhesions to the small intestine or cecum.

An early step in mobilization of the sigmoid involves freeing it from the bladder anteriorly. In most cases, the deep pelvis anterior to the upper rectum is relatively uninvolved with inflammation but cannot be accessed until the sigmoid colon is freed from the posterior surface of the bladder. Adhesions of the sigmoid to the bladder usually occur over an area between the dome and the mid–posterior wall, rarely involving the area of the trigone. Particularly dense adhesions to the bladder often are indicative of a colovesical fistula. If the opening of a colovesical fistula is noted, closure is performed in two layers.

Adhesions of the small bowel and cecum to the sigmoid are taken down and any fistulous tracts are controlled for later resection or repair. In women, if a hysterectomy has been performed, there may be dense adhesions between the vaginal cuff and the sigmoid colon, even if no colovaginal fistula has occurred. Dissection of these adhesions usually is easier after posterior and lateral dissection of the upper rectum has been accomplished.

Rather than using a lateral approach to mobilize the sigmoid colon from the left pelvic wall and right posterior rim of the sacrum, the superior to inferior approach facilitates freeing the sigmoid colon while affording better protection to the ureters, iliac vessels, and gonadal vessels. The lateral attachments of the descending colon are divided and the descending colon is mobilized from the retroperitoneum at the level of the inferior pole of the left kidney. The gonadal vessels and the left ureter are identified easily at this level, particularly if there is a stent in the ureter. The distal descending colon then is mobilized from superior to inferior, from lateral attachments to the left aspect of the aorta and anterior to the ureter and gonadal vessels. The site of division of the distal descending colon or proximal sigmoid colon is chosen as the distalmost site where both the bowel wall and its corresponding blood supply are free from the inflammatory or scirrhous process. The colon is divided with a linear-cutting stapler. The presence of diverticula at or near the site of division is of minimal concern, because the presence of diverticula in the remaining proximal bowel does not pose a high risk of recurrence.[69] Furthermore, resection of all diverticula-containing bowel often requires resection of the entire descending colon or more.

The dissection is carried further inferiorly, with attention paid always to the left ureter, but also to the right ureter, and to the iliac vessels. The dissection usually is performed relatively easily by blunt separation of planes. Near the aortic bifurcation, the density of tissue often requires sharp dissection. Although the difficulty of dissection may make it tempting to dissect the plane posterior to the proximal rectum distal to the inflammation, and to begin from inferior to superior along

the left and left-posterior pelvis, that approach almost never should be used because protection of the ureter and iliac vessels is much more difficult. If the inferior approach is used, the ureter and both internal and external iliac vessels must be located and dissection carried anteriorly at all times.

The distal sigmoid or proximal rectum is mobilized below the inflammatory process, usually first posteriorly and to the right, with dissection carried around the circumference. At this point, attachments of the sigmoid to the vaginal cuff can be divided more clearly without risk to the posteriorly lying rectum. The bowel usually is divided between a distal linear stapler and an occluding bowel clamp, and the specimen is removed. The ureter is evaluated for injury, including evidence of devascularization.

If little devitalized inflammatory tissue remains in the pelvis and left gutter, if the patient is not immunocompromised and is tolerating the operative procedure satisfactorily, and if the bowel ends are well vascularized and not excessively edematous, primary anastomosis should be considered. If the bowel is inadequately prepared, on-table preparation can be performed.[70] The proximal bowel is cleansed by insertion of a length of sterile, disposable, corrugated anesthesia respiratory circuit tubing into the end of the proximal colon, tying a length of umbilical tape to hold it in place and running the other end of the circuit tubing down to the floor to a sealed plastic bag. A needle vent is made at the bowel–tubing interface to prevent collapse of the bowel by siphon effect.[71] Warmed saline solution is run through a soft rubber catheter placed into the cecum through an appendicostomy or a pursestring enterotomy in the terminal ileum with the catheter tip in the cecum. The distal ileum is clamped with a noncrushing bowel clamp to prevent retrograde flow of fluid. After the effluent is clear, the bowel can be flushed with 0.5% povidone-iodine solution. The proximal tube is removed, the appendectomy is completed or the ileotomy repaired, and the distal bowel containing the end of the circuit tubing is resected after expressing as much of the residual fluid as possible from the proximal colon. The rectum is irrigated clean using a proctoscope.

The distal anastomosis should be performed in the proximal rectum below all diverticula. The incidence of recurrent diverticulitis is 12% when the anastomosis is performed to the distal sigmoid compared with 7% when it is performed to the proximal rectum.[72] In addition, the risk that a colocutaneous fistula will develop from the anastomosis is increased when it is performed in the distal sigmoid rather than the rectum.[32] Whether the lower recurrence rate for the rectal anastomosis results from the fact that no distal diverticula remain or that the hypertrophic musculature associated with the formation of diverticulosis is removed is not known; both may be important factors.

BLEEDING FROM COLONIC DIVERTICULA

Bleeding from colonic diverticula is one of two common sources of massive lower gastrointestinal bleeding, the other being angiodysplasia. Although diverticular inflammation and bleeding overlap in a small percentage of patients, bleeding from colonic diverticula is an entirely separate complication of diverticulosis. Diverticular bleeding has been reported in 5% to 41% of patients with diverticulosis, about one third of whom bleed massively.[73,74] Investigation of suspected diverticular bleeding by angiography has indicated a significant error rate for diagnosis by exclusion, in which bleeding is attributed to diverticulosis if diverticula can be demonstrated and no other source can be found.[74] Some of the traditional dicta regarding clinical manifestations of diverticular bleeding must be reexamined with respect to current characterization of the sources and natural history of colonic bleeding.

Epidemiology, Anatomy, and Pathogenesis

Bleeding from colonic diverticula is principally a disease of the elderly. Bleeding typically occurs in the seventh to eighth decade, and rarely occurs in patients younger than 50 years.[75-77] The incidence is nearly equal between the sexes.[77]

Although diverticula are found much more commonly in the sigmoid colon in Western populations, careful studies have implicated a diverticulum in the colon proximal to the splenic flexure in 50% to 92% of patients with bleeding diverticulosis.[76,78,79] Diverticular bleeding occurs from the right colon in 41% to 69% of cases, from the transverse colon or splenic flexure in 15% to 25%, and from the descending and sigmoid colon in 8% to 21%.[44,76,80] There are no gross characteristics of the diverticula, the bleeding pattern, or the patients who bleed from diverticula that predict the part of the colon in which the bleeding diverticulum may lie.

Investigation of the pathogenesis of bleeding diverticula has demonstrated a characteristic lesion. There is rupture of the vas rectum, an arteriole, into the lumen of the diverticulum at the dome of the diverticulum or, less frequently, at the antimesenteric margin of the diverticulum.[78] A vas rectum normally runs over the dome of each diverticulum and penetrates the colon wall along the antimesenteric border of the diverticulum. The ruptured vas rectum usually demonstrates fibromuscular intimal thickening, duplicated or focally thickened internal elastic lamina, and thinning of the media. The changes are not associated with acute or chronic diverticulitis. There are no findings that explain the predilection for bleeding from right-sided diverticula.

Clinical Manifestations

The clinical presentation of patients with colonic diverticular bleeding is fecal urgency accompanied by a grossly bloody stool, with dark or bright red blood. Colic sometimes is present, but other accompanying gastrointestinal symptoms are rare.

The hemorrhage stops spontaneously in 90% of patients, even after significant bleeding.[81] Forty-four percent of patients have a single bleeding episode.[82,83] If bleeding stops, 14% to 50% of those patients experience diverticular rebleeding,[75,77,82,83] although the bleeding may be from another diverticular site. About 40% of patients with diverticular bleeding, and as many as 60% of patients older than 65 years, have major bleeding (more than two units of blood replacement, a decrease in the hematocrit of 5% or more, or a systolic blood pressure of 90 mmHg or less on hospital admission).[82] In 45% of patients, bleeding is massive (at least five units of blood replacement required).[84]

Diagnosis

In a series of patients with severe hematochezia,[85] 17% were bleeding from a diverticulum, although 60% had diverticulosis. Of those with diverticulosis, only 27% were bleeding from a diverticulum. Eleven percent of patients were bleeding from an upper gastrointestinal source, and 9% were bleeding from the small bowel. Colonic sources included angiomas, polyps, cancer, colitis, colonic ulcer, and rectal lesions.

The initial steps in diagnosis are exclusion of upper gastrointestinal and anorectal bleeding. For patients in whom the bleeding has ceased, elective or semielective colonoscopy and upper gastrointestinal endoscopy are the initial studies, followed by barium enema to demonstrate diverticula, and then small bowel contrast study to exclude small bowel pathology.

For patients with massive hemorrhage and ongoing bleeding from the rectum, upper gastrointestinal bleeding can be excluded reliably by nasogastric aspiration of clear bile-containing fluid.[85] If bile is not obtained on nasogastric aspiration, upper gastrointestinal endoscopy is indicated. Anoscopy and rigid or flexible sigmoidoscopy should be performed as the next step to exclude anorectal sources of bleeding. Rigid instruments may miss low rectal lesions, which are seen well only with retroversion of a flexible scope.

Controversy exists regarding the best study for evaluating the more proximal colon and bowel. Angiography has been advocated by many if bleeding is ongoing. For angiomas and diverticula, the bleeding lesion is characteristic, and vasoconstrictive or embolic therapy can be used immediately. In many patients, however, bleeding is intermittent and will have slowed or stopped, rendering the angiogram nondiagnostic.[85] In a few patients, visualization of the left colon is poor because of inferior mesenteric artery occlusion. In addition, the contrast material represents a substantial risk for renal injury in elderly or hypovolemic patients. Although the rate of hemorrhage needed to visualize a bleeding point by angiography was 0.5 mL/min in animal studies, in practice, more active bleeding usually is necessary for diagnosis. With active bleeding, detection of a bleeding site can be expected in 50% to 75% of patients.[79,80,86,87] Angiography should be performed as soon as possible after patients arrive at the hospital; a delay of 6 hours or more markedly decreases the chances of successfully identifying a bleeding site.[87] Major complications of angiography occur in 7% of patients, and minor complications in about 17%.[81]

Colonoscopy after purge also can effectively identify the source of diverticular bleeding, although reports of success rates have varied from zero to 85%.[85,87] For experienced endoscopists after purge, despite ongoing bleeding, colonoscopy is a useful diagnostic modality for diverticular and other lower gastrointestinal bleeding. In addition, under some circumstances, endoscopic treatment can be successful for control of lower gastrointestinal bleeding, including diverticular bleeding.[88]

Radionuclide bleeding scans are performed using labeled red blood cells or ^{99m}Tc-labeled sulfur colloid. The sulfur colloid scan is sensitive for active bleeding and able to identify bleeding at a rate of 0.1 mL/min,[89] but it is not useful for bleeding in the region of the liver because of uptake of the sulfur colloid by the reticuloendothelial system. Radionuclide scan diagnosis has major weaknesses, including inability to locate the bleeding site, lack of discrimination between overlying organs, and inability to indicate the nature of the bleeding lesion. Sulfur colloid scans can have utility in documenting active bleeding while mobilizing for angiography.

Intraoperative diagnosis and localization is notoriously inaccurate for lower gastrointestinal bleeding. There is nothing externally visible that indicates that a diverticulum or angioma is the source of bleeding, or that bleeding is from the colon and not from the small bowel. Intraoperative examination using an entero-

scope or colonoscope passed through the mouth can be useful in excluding small intestinal bleeding in many cases, but intraoperative colonoscopy in a blood-containing colon is unlikely to be revealing. Multiple colotomies and transcolotomy examination of the colon are inadvisable because of the gross contamination and usual failure to identify the bleeding locus. All reasonable attempts to define the bleeding site should be made before surgery; the operation cannot be relied on to localize a site or etiology.

Treatment

Initial treatment includes resuscitation and supportive measures. Because many patients with diverticular bleeding have spontaneous cessation, with less than three units of blood replacement, support and observation are appropriate. In elderly patients, however, prolonged waiting and excessive transfusion lead to excess mortality, usually from cardiovascular causes. In a series of 24 patients with presumed diverticular bleeding who were allowed to bleed five units of blood or more,[84] there were 9 deaths. Five deaths were due to myocardial infarction and cardiac failure.

Intraarterial infusion of vasopressin effectively induces cessation of bleeding in 85% to 92% of patients with identified diverticular bleeding sites.[79,87] The effectiveness is postulated to result from thrombosis of the bleeding arteriole induced by the effects of the vasoconstriction. Permanent suspension of bleeding occurs in 42% to 70% of patients.[79,87] Even in patients in whom bleeding recurs, the temporary break allows improvement of the patient's status, converting what would be emergency surgery to urgent surgery.[87] Although embolization of the bleeding colon is a possibility when the bleeding site is identified, embolization should be avoided because of the risk of infarction of a segment of colon wall.[90] There is a case report of epinephrine 1:10,000 injection of the neck of a bleeding diverticulum resulting in successful control of bleeding.[88]

With failure of vasopressin infusion, operation is necessary. Bleeding requiring more than five units of blood replacement is an indication for operation. If the bleeding point can be defined, segmental colectomy is the operation of choice. The mortality rate under those conditions ranges from 0% to 7%, the morbidity rate is about 15%, and the rebleeding rate varies from 0% to 14%.[82,86] If the bleeding point cannot be defined, subtotal colectomy should be performed. The mortality rate for subtotal colectomy is 30% to 50%, the morbidity rate is about 40%, and the rebleeding rate is 0%.[82,86] Despite the high mortality and morbidity for subtotal colectomy for undefined lower gastrointestinal bleeding, patients who have segmental colectomy without identification of a bleeding site have a mortality rate of 57%, a morbidity rate of 83%, and a recurrent bleeding rate of 42%.[86] Under conditions of unlocalized lower gastrointestinal bleeding requiring operation, subtotal colectomy appears to be a better choice than undirected segmental colectomy. After colectomy for massive bleeding, anastomosis usually can be performed without expectations of morbidity.[86]

GIANT DIVERTICULA OF THE COLON

Giant diverticulum of the colon is a rare complication of diverticulosis. Giant colonic diverticula are found most commonly in the sigmoid colon, although they have been reported at other sites.[91] There have been several reports of more than one giant diverticulum in a single patient. The average age at diagnosis is 64 years, with a range from 20 to 89 years, and there is a slight male predominance.[92] The average reported diameter is about 13 cm, with a range from 6 to 27 cm.[92]

Grossly, giant diverticula usually originate on the antimesenteric border of the colon.[93] Inflammatory adhesions to surrounding structures are common.[92] Three patterns are seen under the microscope.[93] In one pattern, designated *giant pseudodiverticulum*, muscularis propria is not found in the wall of the diverticulum but ends at the diverticular neck. Scattered intact mucosa is interspersed with acute and chronic ulcers with granu-

lation. A second pattern, the most common, has been called *giant inflammatory diverticulum*. The wall of this type is fibrous with chronic inflammatory tissue and foreign body giant cell reaction; none of the normal bowel wall elements are present. The least common pattern has been termed *true giant diverticulum*, in which all layers of the bowel wall are present in the diverticular wall. In this last type, there is variable chronic ulceration of the mucosa and evidence of wall injury.

The etiology of giant colonic diverticula is speculative. Although similar elements probably lead to the great size achieved by each type of diverticulum, they likely start from different pathologic entities. Giant pseudodiverticula usually are found in conjunction with other, normal size diverticula. The massive enlargement of the giant diverticulum is thought to be caused by a ball-valve effect at the neck of the diverticulum that allows contents, particularly gas, to enter but not to leave, with gradual enlargement resulting from the increased intraluminal pressure. Giant inflammatory diverticula are considered chronic abscess cavities maintaining some communication with the colonic lumen, but maintained in size or enlarged by a similar ball-valve effect at the neck. True giant diverticula are thought to represent both true diverticula and communicating partial duplications. The mechanism of enlargement is thought to be the ball-valve mechanism.

Symptoms at clinical presentation are principally abdominal pain and complaints related to an abdominal mass, which are present in 85% and 70% of patients,

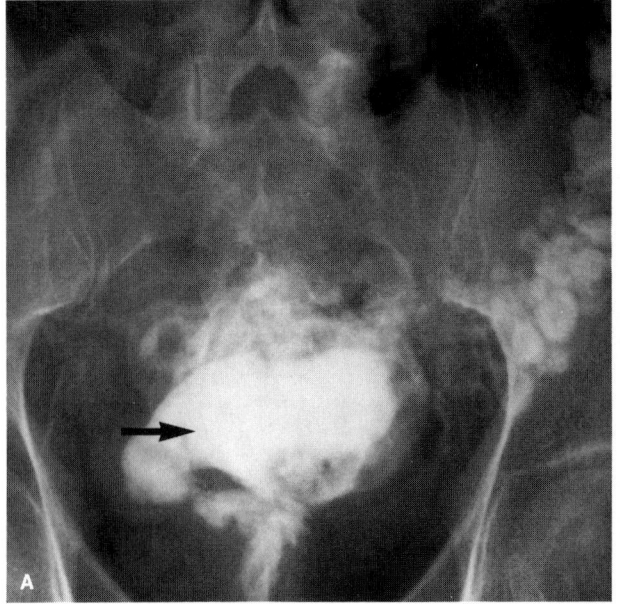
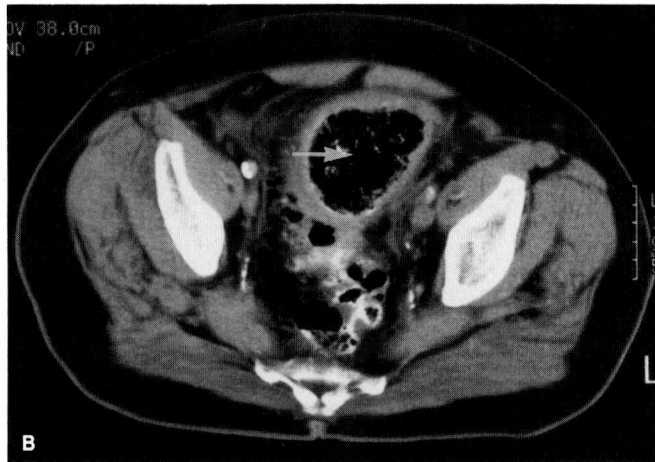

Figure 39-8 (**A**) Barium contrast radiograph of a giant diverticulum of the sigmoid colon (*arrow*). (**B**) CT scan of the giant diverticulum (*arrow*) in the same patient.

respectively.[92] Other symptoms are more sporadic and include melena, hematochezia, nausea and vomiting, abdominal distention, and fever. On physical examination, 70% of patients have a palpable abdominal mass, which sometimes is tender.[94] General abdominal hyperresonance may be present.[92] Infrequently, perforation of the diverticulum occurs and patients may have peritoneal signs.[94] Torsion and partial infarction of giant diverticula also have been described.[92]

The results of plain abdominal radiographs frequently are abnormal, showing a smooth-edged radiolucency in the lower to mid-abdomen, usually anteriorly on a lateral film, containing an air–fluid level in one fourth of all cases[93] (Fig. 39-8). Barium enema fills the giant diverticulum in about 60% of cases, and usually shows a smooth internal wall.[93] Adjacent normal size diverticula generally are seen. There may be compression of the segment of colon adjacent to the giant diverticulum.

The recommended therapy for giant colonic diverticulum is removal by segmental colon resection. Except in the infrequent case of peritonitis associated with perforated diverticulum, colon preparation is possible and primary reanastomosis is usual. Resection of only the diverticulum with closure of the colon has been described, but is not recommended because of the large defect in the colon wall after resection of the diverticulum and possible inflammatory changes in the margins of that opening. Deflation of the diverticulum by manual compression can facilitate the dissection. Dense scar and inflammatory adhesions sometimes are encountered.

REFERENCES

1. Mendeloff AI. Thoughts on the epidemiology of diverticular disease. Clin Gastroenterol 1986;15:855.
2. Parks TG. Natural history of diverticular disease of the colon: a review of 521 cases. BMJ 1969;4:639.
3. Welch CE, Allen AW, Donaldson GA. An appraisal of resection of the colon for diverticulitis of the sigmoid. Ann Surg 1953;138:332.
4. Segal I, Leibowitz B. The distributional pattern of diverticular disease. Dis Colon Rectum 1989;32:227.
5. Markham NI, Li AKC. Diverticulitis of the right colon: experience from Hong Kong. Gut 1992;33:547.
6. Wagner DE, Zollinger RW. Diverticulitis of the cecum and ascending colon. Arch Surg 1961;83:436.
7. Ryan P. Two kinds of diverticular disease. Ann R Coll Surg Engl 1991;73:73.
8. Almy TP, Howell DA. Diverticular disease of the colon. N Engl J Med 1980;302:324.
9. Painter NS, Truelove SC. The intraluminal pressure patterns in diverticulosis of the colon. Gut 1964;5:201.
10. Fisher N, Berry CS, Fearn T, Gregory JA, Hardy J. Cereal dietary fiber consumption and diverticular disease: a lifespan study in rats. Am J Clin Nutr 1985;42:788.
11. Hughes LE. Postmortem survey of diverticular disease of the colon. Gut 1969;10:336.
12. Cheskin LJ, Bohlman M, Schuster MM. Diverticular disease in the elderly. Gastroenterol Clin North Am 1990;19:391.
13. Acosta JA, Grebenc ML, Doberneck RC, McCarthy JD, Fry DE. Colonic diverticular disease in patients 40 years old or younger. Am Surg 1992;58:605.
14. Freischlag J, Bennion RS, Thompson JE Jr. Complications of diverticular disease of the colon in young people. Dis Colon Rectum 1986;29:639.
15. Sardi A, Gokli A, Singer JA. Diverticular disease of the cecum and ascending colon: a review of 881 cases. Am Surg 1987;53:41.
16. Sugihara K, Muto T, Moriaoka Y, Asano A, Yamamoto T. Diverticular disease of the colon in Japan: a review of 615 cases. Dis Colon Rectum 1984;27:531.
17. Parks TG. Natural history of diverticular disease of the colon. Clin Gastroenterol 1975;4:53.
18. Schoetz DJ Jr. Uncomplicated diverticulitis: indications for surgery and surgical management. Surg Clin North Am 1993;73:965.
19. Painter NS. The cause of diverticular disease of the colon, its symptoms and its complications: review and hypothesis. J R Coll Surg Edinb 1985;30:118.
20. Parks TG. Reappraisal of clinical features of diverticular disease of the colon. BMJ 1969;4:642.
21. Morris J, Stellato TA, Haaga JR, Lieberman J. The utility of computed tomography in colonic diverticulitis. Ann Surg 1986;204:128.
22. Ngoi SS, Chia J, Goh MY, Sim E, Rauff A. Surgical management of right colon diverticulitis. Dis Colon Rectum 1992;35:799.
23. Harada RN, Whelan TJ Jr. Surgical management of cecal diverticulitis. Am J Surg 1993;166:666.
24. Alexander J, Karl RC, Skinner DB. Results of changing trends in the surgical management of complications of diverticular disease. Surgery 1983;94:683.
25. Labs JD, Sarr MG, Fishman EK, Siegelman SS, Cameron JL. Complications of acute diverticulitis of the colon: improved early diagnosis with computerized tomography. Am J Surg 1988;155:331.
26. Finlay IG, Carter DC. A comparison of emergency resection and staged management in perforated diverticular disease. Dis Colon Rectum 1987;30:929.
27. Nagorney DM, Adson MA, Pemberton JH. Sigmoid diverticulitis with perforation and generalized peritonitis. Dis Colon Rectum 1985;28:71.
28. Nahrwold DL, DeMuth WE. Diverticulitis with perforation into the peritoneal cavity. Ann Surg 1977;185:80.
29. Woods FJ, Lavery IC, Fazio VW, Jagelman DG, Weakley FL. Internal fistulas in diverticular disease. Dis Colon Rectum 1988;31:591.
30. Kirsh GM, Hampel N, Shuck JM, Resnick MI. Diagnosis and management of vesicoenteric fistulas. Surg Gynecol Obstet 1991;173:91.

31. Huettner PC, Finkler NJ, Welch WR. Colouterine fistula complicating diverticulitis: charcoal challenge test aids in diagnosis. Obstet Gynecol 1992;80:550.

32. Fazio VW, Church JM, Jagelman DG, et al. Colocutaneous fistulas complicating diverticulitis. Dis Colon Rectum 1987;30:89.

33. Sridharan GV, Wilkinson SP, Primrose WR. Pyogenic liver abscess in the elderly. Age Ageing 1990;19:199.

34. Lin C. Suppurative pylephlebitis and liver abscess complicating colonic diverticulitis: report of two cases and review of literature. Mt Sinai J Med 1973;40:48.

35. Perez-Cruet MJ, Grable E, Drapkin MS, Jablons DM, Cano G. Pylephlebitis associated with diverticulitis. South Med J 1993;86:578.

36. Rodning CB, Williams L. Suppurative pylephlebitis due to pseudodiverticulosis coli. South Med J 1984;77:1165.

37. Cho KC, Morehouse HT, Alterman DD, Thornhill BA. Sigmoid diverticulitis: diagnostic role of CT: comparison with barium enema studies. Radiology 1990;176:111.

38. Hachigian MP, Honickman S, Eisenstat TE, Rubin RJ, Salvati EP. Computed tomography in the initial management of acute left-sided diverticulitis. Dis Colon Rectum 1992;35:1123.

39. Balthazar EJ, Megibow A, Schinella RA, Gordon R. Limitations in the CT diagnosis of acute diverticulitis: comparison of CT, contrast enema, and pathologic findings in 16 patients. AJR Am J Roentgenol 1990;154:281.

40. Crist DW, Fishman EK, Scatarige JC, Cameron JL. Acute diverticulitis of the cecum and ascending colon diagnosed by computed tomography. Surg Gynecol Obstet 1988;166:99.

41. Wada M, Kikuchi Y, Doy M. Uncomplicated acute diverticulitis of the cecum and ascending colon: sonographic findings in 18 patients. AJR 1990;155:283.

42. Grissom R, Snyder TE. Colovaginal fistula secondary to diverticular disease. Dis Colon Rectum 1991;34:1043.

43. Stabile BE, Puccio E, vanSonnenberg E, Neff CC. Preoperative percutaneous drainage of diverticular abscesses. Am J Surg 1990;159:99.

44. Rodkey GV, Welch CE. Changing patterns in the surgical treatment of diverticular disease. Ann Surg 1984;200:466.

45. Hackford AW, Schoetz DJ Jr, Coller JA, Veidenheimer MC. Surgical management of complicated diverticulitis: the Lahey Clinic experience, 1967 to 1982. Dis Colon Rectum 1985;28:317.

46. Kronborg O. Treatment of perforated sigmoid diverticulitis: a prospective randomized trial. Br J Surg 1993;80:505.

47. Detry R, Jamez J, Kartheuser A, et al. Acute localized diverticulitis: optimum management requires accurate staging. Int J Colorectal Dis 1992;7:38.

48. Ambrosetti P, Robert J, Witzig JA, et al. Incidence, outcome, and proposed management of isolated abscesses complicating acute left-sided colonic diverticulitis: a prospective study of 140 patients. Dis Colon Rectum 1992;35:1072.

49. Ambrosetti P, Robert J, Witzig JA, et al. Prognostic factors from computed tomography in acute left colonic diverticulitis. Br J Surg 1992;79:117.

50. Ouriel K, Schwartz SI. Diverticular disease in the young patient. Surg Gynecol Obstet 1983;156:1.

51. Hannan CE, Knightly JJ, Coffey RJ. Diverticular disease of the colon in the younger age group. Dis Colon Rectum 1961;4:419.

52. Schauer PR, Ramos R, Ghiatas AA, Sirinek KR. Virulent diverticular disease in young obese men. Am J Surg 1992;164:443.

53. Eusebio EB, Eisenberg MM. Natural history of diverticular disease of the colon in young patients. Am J Surg 1973;125:308.

54. Simonowitz D, Paloyan D. Diverticular disease of the colon in patients under 40 years of age. Am J Gastroenterol 1977;67:69.

55. Chodak GW, Rangel DM, Passaro E Jr. Colonic diverticulitis in patients under age 40: need for earlier diagnosis. Am J Surg 1981;141:699.

56. Perkins JD, Shield CF III, Chang FC, Farha GJ. Acute diverticulitis: comparison of treatment in immunocompromised and nonimmunocompromised patients. Am J Surg 1984;148:745.

57. Misra MK, Pinkus GS, Birtch AG, Wilson RE. Major colonic diseases complicating renal transplantation. Surgery 1973;73:942.

58. Hughes LE. Complications of diverticular disease: inflammation, obstruction and bleeding. Clin Gastroenterol 1975;4:147.

59. Marshall SF. Earlier resection in one stage for diverticulitis of the colon. Am Surg 1963;29:337.

60. Smithwick RH. Experiences with the surgical management of diverticulitis of the sigmoid. Ann Surg 1942;115:969.

61. Allen-Mersh TG. Should primary anastomosis and on-table colonic lavage be standard treatment for left colon emergencies? Ann R Coll Surg Engl 1993;75:195.

62. Himal HS, Ashby DB, Duignan JP, Richardson DM, Miller JL, MacLean LD. Management of perforating diverticulitis of the colon. Surg Gynecol Obstet 1977;144:225.

63. Krukowski ZH, Matheson NA. Emergency surgery for diverticular disease complicated by generalized and faecal peritonitis: a review. Br J Surg 1984;71:921.

64. Peoples JB, Vilk DR, Maguire JP, Elliott DW. Reassessment of primary resection of the perforated segment for severe colonic diverticulitis. Am J Surg 1990;159:291.

65. Greif JM, Fried G, McSherry CK. Surgical treatment of perforated diverticulitis of the sigmoid colon. Dis Colon Rectum 1980;23:483.

66. Arrington P, Judd CS Jr. Cecal diverticulitis. Am J Surg 1981;142:56.

67. Fischer MG, Farkas AM. Diverticulitis of the cecum and ascending colon. Dis Colon Rectum 1984;27:454.

68. Schuler JG, Bayley J. Diverticulitis of the cecum. Surg Gynecol Obstet 1983;156:743.

69. Wolff BG, Ready RL, MacCarty RL, Dozois RR, Beart RW Jr. Influence of sigmoid resection on progression of diverticular disease of the colon. Dis Colon Rectum 1984;27:645.

70. Dudley HAF, Radcliffe AG, McGeehan D. Intraoperative irrigation of the colon to permit primary anastomosis. Br J Surg 1980;67:80.

71. Rothenberger DA, Wiltz O. Surgery for complicated diverticulitis. Surg Clin North Am 1993;73:975.

72. Benn PL, Wolff BG, Ilstrup DM. Level of anastomosis and recurrent colonic diverticulitis. Am J Surg 1986;151:269.

73. Rigg BM, Ewing MR. Current attitudes on diverticulitis with particular reference to colonic bleeding. Arch Surg 1966;92:321.

74. Eisenberg H, Laufer I, Skillman JJ. Arteriographic diagnosis and management of suspected colonic diverticular hemorrhage. Gastroenterology 1973;64:1091.

75. Gostout CJ, Wang KK, Ahlquist DA, et al. Acute gastrointestinal bleeding: experience of a specialized management team. J Clin Gastroenterol 1992;14:260.

76. Athanasoulis CA, Baum S, Rosch J, et al. Mesenteric arterial infusions of vasopressin for hemorrhage from colonic diverticulosis. Am J Surg 1975;129:212.

77. Ramanath HK, Hinshaw JR. Management and mismanagement of bleeding colonic diverticula. Arch Surg 1971;103:311.

78. Meyers MA, Alonso DR, Gray GF, Baer JW. Pathogenesis of bleeding colonic diverticulosis. Gastroenterology 1976;71:577.

79. Welch CE, Athanasoulis CA, Galdabini JJ. Hemorrhage from the large bowel with special reference to angiodysplasia and diverticular disease. World J Surg 1978;2:73.

80. Casarella WJ, Kanter IE, Seaman WB. Right-sided colonic diverticula as a cause of acute rectal hemorrhage. N Engl J Med 1972;286:450.

81. Potter GD, Sellin JH. Lower gastrointestinal bleeding. Gastroenterol Clin North Am 1988;17:341.

82. Boley SJ, DiBiase A, Brandt LJ, Sammartano RJ. Lower intestinal bleeding in the elderly. Am J Surg 1979;137:57.

83. McGuire HH Jr, Haynes BW Jr. Massive hemorrhage from diverticulosis of the colon: guidelines for therapy based on bleeding patterns observed in fifty cases. Ann Surg 1972;175:847.

84. Taylor FW, Epstein LI. Treatment of massive diverticular hemorrhage. Arch Surg 1969;98:505.

85. Jensen DM, Machicado GA. Diagnosis and treatment of severe hematochezia: the role of urgent colonoscopy after purge. Gastroenterology 1988;95:1569.

86. Parkes BM, Obeid FN, Sorensen VJ, Horst HM, Fath JJ. The management of massive lower gastrointestinal bleeding. Am Surg 1993;59:676.

87. Browder W, Cerise EJ, Litwin MS. Impact of emergency angiography in massive lower gastrointestinal bleeding. Ann Surg 1986;204:530.

88. Kim Y, Marcon NE. Injection therapy for colonic diverticular bleeding: a case study. J Clin Gastroenterol 1993;17:46.

89. Alavi A, Ring EJ. Localization of gastrointestinal bleeding: superiority of ^{99m}Tc sulfur colloid compared with angiography. AJR 1981;137:741.

90. Rosenkrantz H, Bookstein JJ, Rosen RJ, Goff WB II, Healy JF. Postembolic colonic infarction. Radiology 1982;142:47.

91. McNutt R, Schmitt D, Schulte W. Giant colonic diverticula: three distinct entities: report of a case. Dis Colon Rectum 1988;31:624.

92. Gallagher JJ, Welch JP. Giant diverticula of the sigmoid colon: a review of differential diagnosis and operative management. Arch Surg 1979;114:1079.

93. Casas DJ, Tenesa M, Alastrue A, Hidalgo F, Barranco LC, Olazabal A. Case report: uncommon radiological and pathological features of giant colonic diverticula. Clin Radiol 1991;44:125.

94. Sutorius DJ, Bossert JE. Giant sigmoid diverticulum with perforation. Am J Surg 1974;127:745.

Digestive Tract Surgery: A Text and Atlas, edited by Richard H. Bell,
Layton F. Rikkers, and Michael W. Mulholland.
Lippincott-Raven Publishers, Philadelphia, © 1996.

40

Neoplasms of the Colon and Rectum

D. Scott Lind | *Wiley W. Souba*

ADENOCARCINOMA

Colorectal neoplasms represent a monumental health problem, with data from the Surveillance, Epidemiology, and End Results program estimating 152,000 new cases and 57,000 deaths due to colorectal cancer in this country in 1993.[1] Excluding basal cell and squamous cell skin cancers, colorectal cancer represents the third most common malignancy among men and the second most frequent among women.[2] It is estimated that 5% of the US population will develop colorectal cancer before the age of 75 years. Unfortunately, the death rate for these tumors has changed little in the past half century.[1]

Despite these discouraging statistics, recent efforts have provided a ripple of optimism. Perhaps the most exciting work involves the molecular and genetic events necessary for colorectal tumorigenesis and progression to metastases. With regard to primary prevention, experimental evidence suggests that modification of dietary factors can reduce the risk of colorectal cancer. Although secondary prevention can be of benefit in high-risk groups, mass screening demands a more sensitive method of detection than the currently available techniques. Molecular and proliferative markers such as oncogenes and flow cytometric DNA analysis provide important prognostic indicators for patients with colorectal cancer. Sophisticated imaging techniques such as endorectal ultrasound and monoclonal antibody immunoscintigraphy may allow more accurate staging.

From a therapeutic standpoint, surgery remains the primary treatment modality for colorectal cancer. It is unlikely that future surgical efforts will have any major effect on overall survival, although refinements in surgical technique may lessen operative morbidity. In addition, sphincter-sparing procedures for low rectal cancer make permanent colostomy unnecessary and prevent impotence and urologic dysfunction.

The contemporary management of colorectal cancer is becoming increasingly multimodal. Many well-designed trials have demonstrated that adjuvant radiotherapy can reduce the local recurrence rate for rectal cancer, and refinements in its use are likely to produce even greater returns. For decades, studies failed to demonstrate any benefit from adjuvant chemotherapy; recent well-designed trials have shown that chemotherapy can prolong survival in subgroups of patients with colorectal cancer. New drug development and the discovery of agents that potentiate existing chemotherapy will further improve the survival of these patients. The optimal integration of all the therapeutic modalities requires definition. Future efforts toward understanding the biology of colorectal cancer will undoubtedly have enormous diagnostic, prognostic, and therapeutic implications.

Etiology

Although the etiology of colorectal cancer remains unknown, it is likely to be the result of a complex interplay of both genetic and environmental factors. Whereas data from both epidemiologic studies and animal experiments suggest a role for diet in the etiology of colorectal cancer,[3] a cause-and-effect relationship between any dietary constituent and colorectal cancer is not proved.

There is substantial evidence to support an association between high intake of fat and colorectal cancer.[4] Possible mechanisms by which a high-fat diet promotes colorectal cancer include changes in carcinogenic fecal bile acids and stimulation of tumor-promoting prostaglandins. There is a correlation between total energy intake and colorectal cancer, and this must be considered when discriminating between the effects of total intake and individual components of the diet.[4]

Investigators have popularized the theory that the high incidence of colorectal cancer in Western societies is the result of a low-fiber diet.[5] Fiber may reduce colorectal cancer risk by increasing intestinal transit and thereby decreasing the time of exposure of the intestinal mucosa to potential carcinogens. Alternative mechanisms include altering the colonic flora and reducing fecal bile acid concentrations.[6] Although the evidence is inconclusive, dietary constituents that may be protective include vitamins A, C, and E; β-carotene; and calcium.[7] Based on the evidence suggesting a relationship between diet and colorectal cancer, the National Cancer Institute recommended the following dietary guidelines to reduce cancer risk[8]:

1. Reduce fat intake to 30% or less of calories.
2. Increase fiber intake to 20 to 30 g/d.
3. Include fruits and vegetables in the daily diet.
4. Drink alcohol in moderation.
5. Minimize consumption of salt-cured, pickled, or smoked foods.

Predisposing Diseases and Factors

Polyposis Syndromes

Several inherited polyposis syndromes are characterized by the development of numerous adenomatous polyps throughout the colon and rectum (Fig. 40-1).

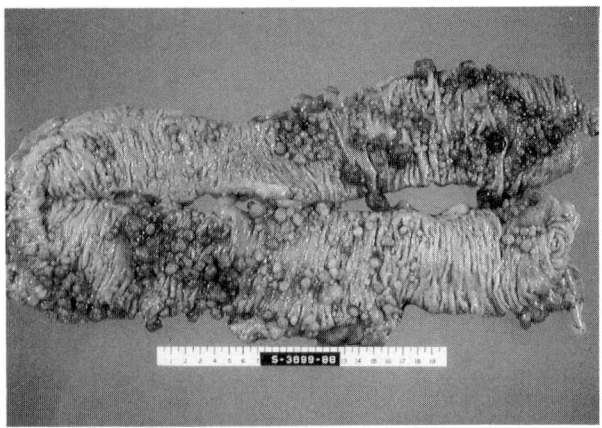

Figure 40-1 Pathologic specimen showing colonic polyposis. (See Color Fig. 40-1.)

Polyps usually appear in the second decade of life and the lifetime risk of colon cancer is virtually 100%, with the average onset of colon cancer occurring between the ages of 35 and 40 years.[9] Because of the high risk of cancer, prophylactic proctocolectomy is recommended. An increased risk of extracolonic cancers, including those of the thyroid, stomach, duodenum, and ampulla of Vater, has been identified in these patients.[10] The gene for familial adenomatous polyposis has been localized to the long arm of chromosome 5.[11]

Inflammatory Bowel Disease

Patients with inflammatory bowel disease are at increased risk for bowel cancer. The risk is greater for patients with ulcerative colitis than for those with Crohn's disease. For patients with ulcerative colitis, the risk depends on the extent and duration of disease.[12] Although cancer incidence rates vary among studies, the risk rises after the first decade of disease activity, and periodic endoscopic surveillance with multiple biopsies throughout the colon is recommended to detect dysplasia.[13] This approach must be viewed with caution because dysplasia does not precede or accompany all cancer associated with inflammatory bowel disease, and controversy exists as to whether periodic endoscopic surveillance reduces mortality from cancer. In addition, even with random biopsies, foci of dysplasia can be missed, and there is interpathologist variation in interpretation of dysplasia. Additional markers of cancer risk such as aneuploidy and loss of an allele for the p53 tumor suppressor gene may improve diagnostic capability.[14] With recent advances in surgical technique, total proctocolectomy and ileoanal anastomosis has gained popularity for the treatment of ulcerative colitis. This operation eliminates the disease and potential for neoplastic change without requiring a permanent stoma. The decision to perform proctocolectomy requires an in-depth assessment of the individual patient, with the discussion involving the patient, the gastroenterologist, and the surgeon.

Cancer Family Syndromes

In certain families, colorectal cancer is inherited in an autosomal dominant fashion.[15] These hereditary nonpolyposis colorectal cancer syndromes may include adenocarcinomas of the breast, ovary, and endometrium. Unlike familial adenomatous polyposis, the gene responsible for these syndromes has not been identified. The average age of detection of colon cancer in these families is 45 years, and family members should undergo aggressive screening beginning in the third decade of life.

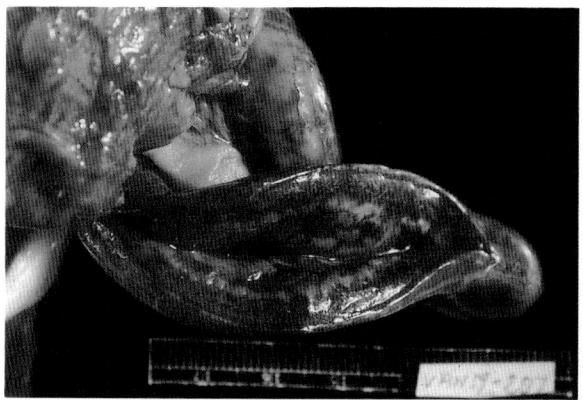

Color Figure 37-1

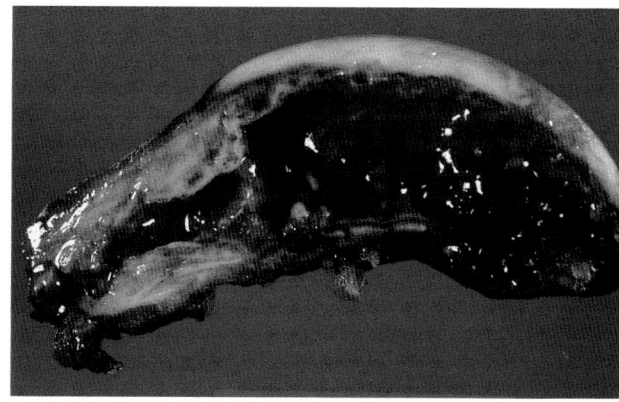

Color Figure 37-8

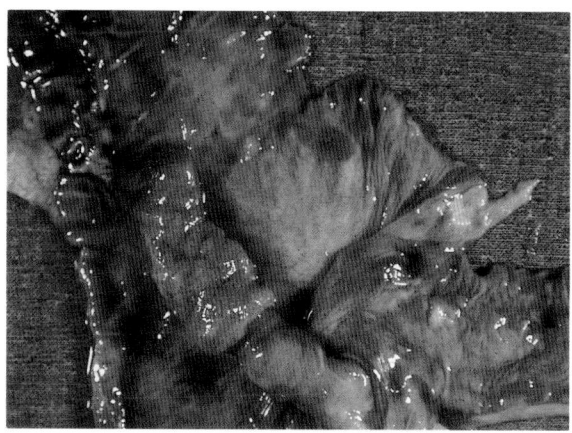

Color Figure 37-9

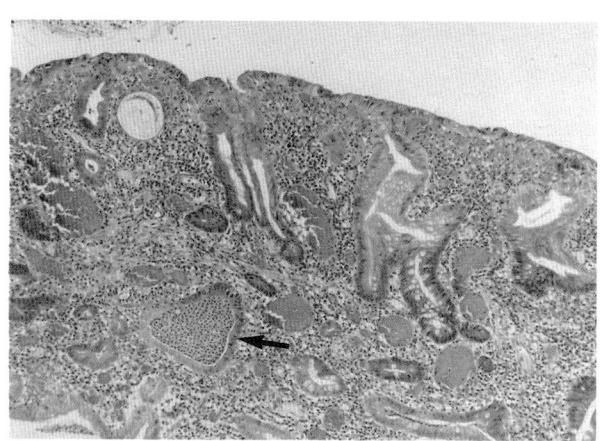

Color Figure 38-1

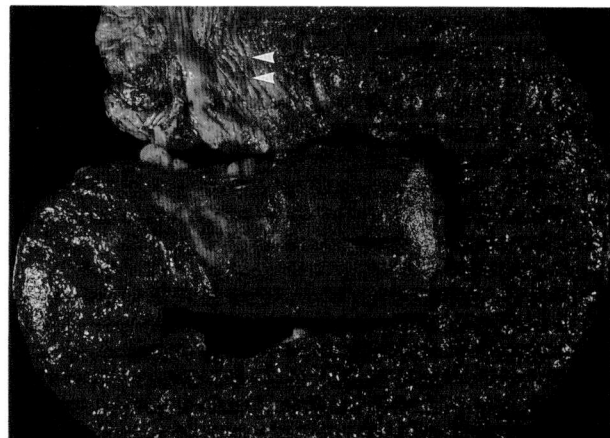

Color Figure 38-2

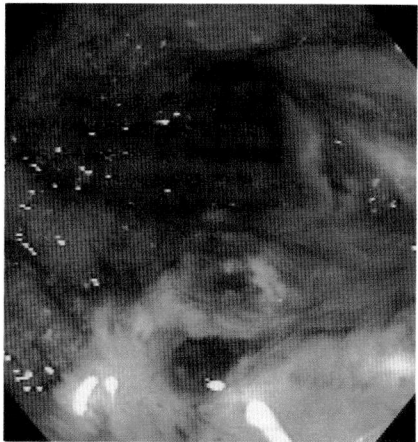

Color Figure 38-3

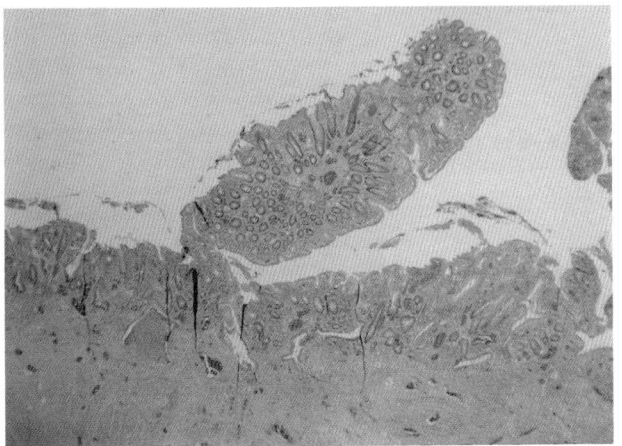

Color Figure 38-4

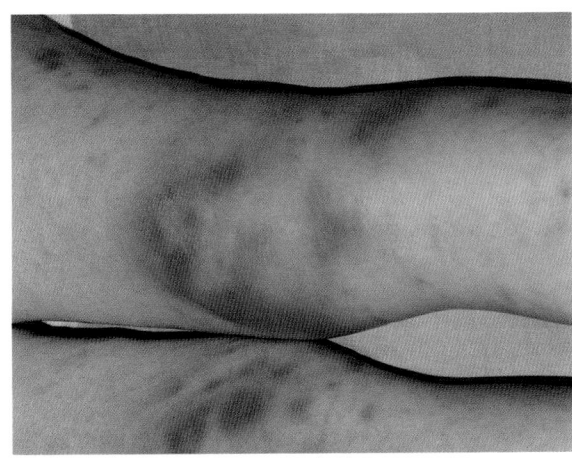

Color Figure 38-10

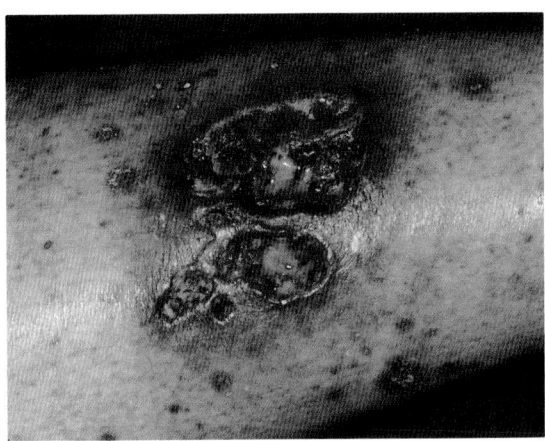

Color Figure 38-11

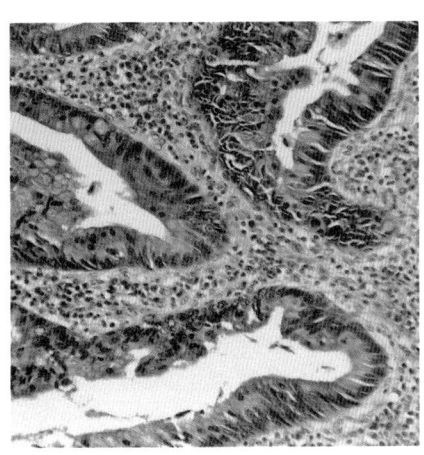

Color Figure 38-13

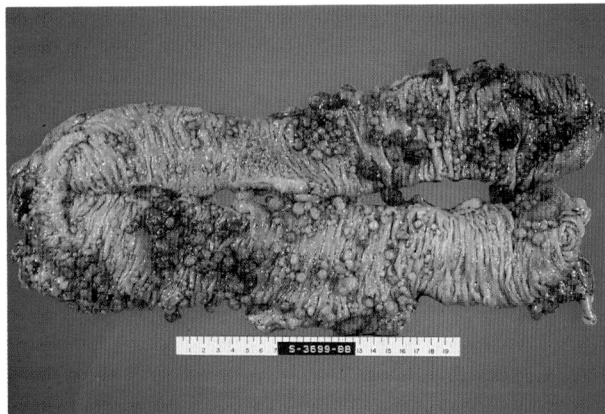

Color Figure 40-1

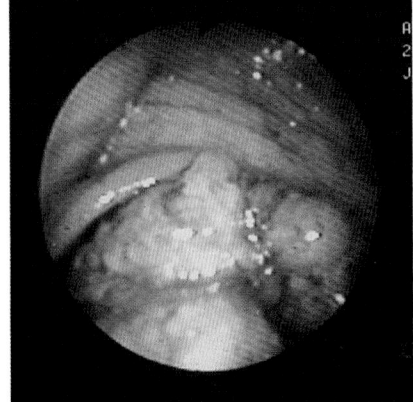

Color Figure 40-2

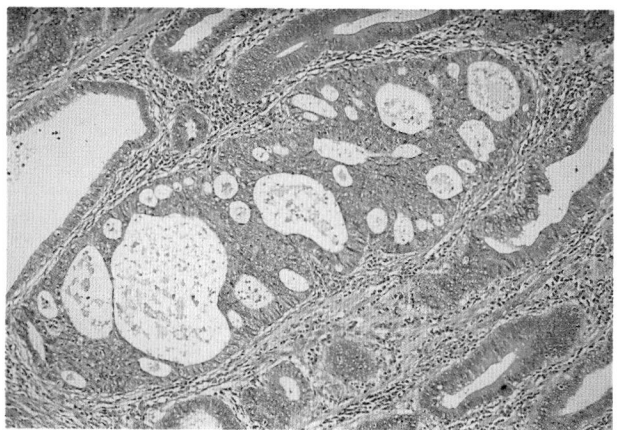

Color Figure 40-6

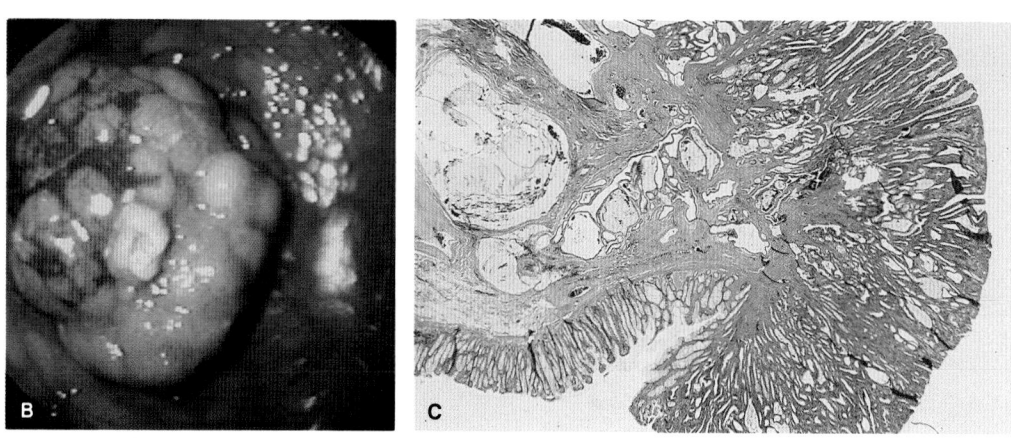

Color Figure 40-12

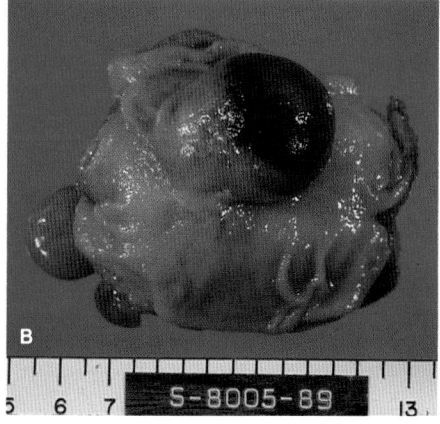

Color Figure 40-13

Molecular Biology

Because of its frequency and clinical accessibility at various stages of development (adenoma–carcinoma sequence), much progress has been made regarding the molecular genetics of colorectal carcinoma. Colorectal oncogenesis appears to be a multistep process, involving abnormal DNA methylation together with the accumulation of both allelic loss or deletion of tumor suppressor genes and dominant oncogene activation[16] (Table 40-1). The progression to metastatic disease is also a complex multistep process with multiple genes involved at each step. Future clinical application of the molecular markers of colorectal neoplasia includes use in identification of high-risk groups, as prognosticators in predicting response to therapy, and as markers to detect recurrence. Using the polymerase chain reaction to amplify minute amounts of RNA and DNA, mutations of the K-*ras* oncogene were detected in the stool of patients known to have colon cancer.[17] Although it is not cost-effective, the potential specificity of such a molecular screening test affords advantages over screening methods that rely on the detection of fecal occult blood.

Screening

Despite their frequency, most colorectal cancers are diagnosed at an advanced stage. Controversy exists over whether current screening techniques, which are designed to detect early disease, improve survival. Some high-risk groups, such as patients with the polyposis syndromes, cancer family syndromes, inflammatory bowel disease, or histories of colorectal cancer and adenomatous polyps, merit special surveillance. Recommendations of the American Cancer Society and the National Cancer Institute for screening the general population appear in Table 40-2. Recent molecular advances may lead to a screening test that is more sensitive and specific than the stool guaiac test. The current climate for controlling health care expenditures demands a cost-effective method of mass screening asymptomatic persons.

Table 40-1   Genetic Alterations in Colorectal Neoplasia

Alteration	Location
DOMINANT TUMOR ONCOGENES	
K-*ras*	Chromosome 12
N-*ras*	Chromosome 1
SUPPRESSOR TUMOR ONCOGENES	
DCC (*deleted in colorectal carcinoma*)	Chromosome 18
APC (*adenomatous polyposis coli*)	Chromosome 5
p53	Chromosome 17

Table 40-2   Screening Recommendations for Colorectal Cancer

Age (y)	Test	Frequency
40+	Digital rectal examination	Yearly
50+	Fecal occult blood test	Yearly
	Sigmoidoscopy	Every 3–5 y

(Modified from American Cancer Society. Guidelines for the cancer-related checkup. CA Cancer J Clin 1980; 30:208)

Clinical Presentation

Most colorectal cancers do not produce symptoms until relatively late in the natural history of the disease. The most common symptoms occur because of an alteration in bowel habits. Signs include persistent diarrhea or constipation, blood per rectum, and a change in the caliber of stools. Other symptoms that can signify more advanced disease include abdominal pain, weight loss, nausea, vomiting, and jaundice. Rectal lesions may produce tenesmus or a sense of incomplete evacuation. Patients with advanced rectal cancers may complain of low back or sacral pain that radiates down the legs, implying tumor involvement of the sacral nerves. Variation in the intraluminal diameter of the right and left colon explains some of the presentations of colon cancer. Cecal lesions characteristically produce bleeding, and patients may have stools that test positive for occult blood, as well as anemia. Alternatively, sigmoid cancers may cause obstructive symptoms. Colon cancers can also cause perforation, either localized or freely intraperitoneal. A diagnosis of cancer may not be considered before operation, and patients may be treated with a presumptive diagnosis of perforated appendicitis or diverticulitis.

Preoperative Evaluation

The preoperative evaluation of patients with colorectal neoplasia can be summarized as follows:

- Thorough history and physical examination
- Chest radiography and routine laboratory work
- Barium enema or colonoscopy
- Computed tomography (CT; optional)
- Endorectal ultrasound (optional for rectal cancer)
- Carcinoembryonic antigen (CEA) level

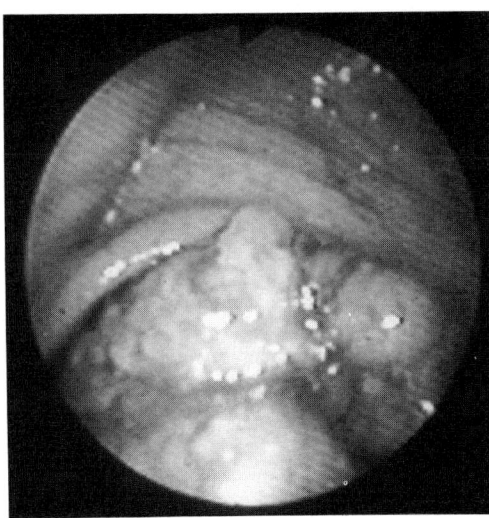

Figure 40-2 Colonoscopic view of adenocarcinoma of the cecum. (See Color Fig. 40-2.)

The history should focus on weight loss, change in bowel habits, and the presence of associated comorbid disease. Depending on body habitus and tumor size, colon cancers occasionally can be palpated on abdominal examination. The abdomen should be examined for hepatomegaly and the presence of ascites. The rectal examination should be thorough; if a mass is palpated, it should be described in terms of morphology (sessile, polypoid, ulcerated); size (proximal and distal extent and degree of circumferential involvement); location (distance from anal verge–dentate line–anorectal sling, anterior–posterior–lateral wall); mobility (fixed to pelvic side walls, sacrum, prostate); and palpable pararectal adenopathy.

Diagnosis and Staging

Once the histologic diagnosis of colorectal cancer has been made, preoperative tests include flexible colonoscopy (Fig. 40-2) and air contrast barium enema (Fig. 40-3) to identify synchronous malignancies (5%) and associated adenomatous polyps (30% to 50%).[18] Colonoscopy has the advantage of allowing biopsy of synchronous lesions or endoscopic removal of polyps outside the area of planned resection. Routine preoperative abdominal CT is not mandatory for carcinoma of the colon because it rarely changes the course of treatment. Even in the presence of widely metastatic disease, palliative resection to obviate obstruction and bleeding is appropriate. In addition, CT is inaccurate for the detection of peritoneal seeding, which can be diagnosed at laparotomy.

CT and magnetic resonance imaging (MRI) are valuable in staging rectal cancers. CT can aid in determining adjacent organ–structure involvement, especially invasion of the bladder, the prostate, or bony pelvic structures. MRI provides no additional information relative to CT for the preoperative evaluation of primary rectal cancer but is more sensitive in differentiating postoperative fibrosis from recurrent rectal cancer. Endorectal ultrasonography has been shown to be more accurate than CT in predicting depth of wall invasion and nodal status in patients with rectal cancer.[19] Although ultrasound appears to be more sensitive than CT in detecting lymph node involvement, neither can distinguish between lymph nodes that are enlarged because of inflammation and those that are enlarged because of tumor. Ultrasound-directed needle biopsy of enlarged pararectal lymph nodes can distinguish histologically involved and reactive lymph nodes. This imaging modality is most valuable in identifying patients with advanced disease who are likely to benefit most from preoperative radiotherapy and in identifying early tumors that are amenable to local therapy. Endoscopic ultrasound provides accurate preoperative staging of tumors in patients who enter randomized clinical trials.

In addition to the routine preoperative laboratory

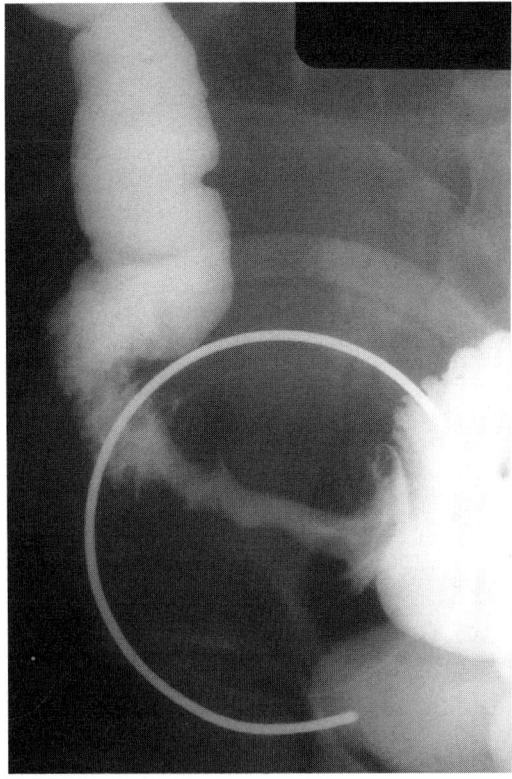

Figure 40-3 Barium enema showing classic apple-core lesion.

work, patients with colorectal cancer should have a CEA level determined to provide prognostic information and serve as a baseline for postoperative follow-up. Preliminary investigative efforts have demonstrated that CEA is concentrated in gallbladder bile compared with serum levels,[20] and in the future, assay of bile for CEA levels may aid in the detection of clinically occult colorectal liver metastases.

Staging Systems

For decades, the Dukes classification or some modification of this staging system, based on depth of penetration of the tumor and lymph node involvement, was the standard method for staging colorectal cancer (Table 40-3). To ensure unanimity and to compare treatment results accurately, the trend is now toward use of the American Joint Committee on Cancer tumor, node, metastases (TNM) classification.[21] Attempts to define the biology of individual colorectal tumors have involved the use of numerous prognostic variables, including CEA level, percentage of positive nodes, histologic grade, presence of lymphatic–vascular invasion, ploidy, and S-phase fraction, as well as specific gene products. In the future, some of these prognostic factors may be incorporated into a staging system that more accurately predicts prognosis and the need for adjuvant therapy. On the other hand, many argue that such sophisticated staging systems lack the simplicity of the original Dukes classification.

Therapy

Contemporary management of colorectal carcinoma demands a multimodal approach involving the primary care physician, gastroenterologist, surgeon, medical oncologist, radiation oncologist, pathologist, enterostomal therapist, nurse, dietitian, and others. Current therapeutic modalities include surgery, radiotherapy, and chemotherapy. The techniques of each modality con-

tinually advance and the optimal sequence of each modality in the course of treatment remains unsettled.

Surgery

Anatomy

Surgery remains the primary therapy for colorectal cancer and the type of resection performed is largely based on the site of the tumor. All surgeons treating colorectal neoplasms must have a complete knowledge of pertinent colorectal anatomy (Fig. 40-4). The cecum, ascending colon, and proximal transverse colon are derived from embryonic midgut and the blood supply is through the superior mesenteric artery and its branches, the ileocolic, right, and middle colic arteries. The remainder of the colon and the rectum are hindgut derivatives and are supplied by the inferior mesenteric artery and its branches, the left colic, sigmoid, and superior rectal arteries. The distal rectum is also supplied by the middle and inferior rectal arteries, which are branches of the hypogastric and pudendal arteries, respectively. The collateral circulation connecting the superior and inferior mesenteric vasculature is through the marginal artery of Drummond. The venous drainage accompanies the respective arteries; thus, the superior and inferior mesenteric veins drain into the portal circulation, whereas the middle and inferior rectal veins drain into the internal iliac vein and the systemic circulation. The lymphatic drainage of the colon and rectum also parallels the vascular anatomy and is conventionally divided into four nodal groups—the epicolic, paracolic, intermediate, and principal lymph nodes. After drainage into the principal nodes, the direction of lymphatic flow is cephalad along the periaortic chain into the cisterna chyli.

The relationship of adjacent organs to the colon and rectum is important with respect to preventing intraoperative injury and contiguous spread with potential multivisceral resection. The mobile parts of the colon can involve the anterior abdominal wall, and curative resection may require wide excision en bloc with the tumor. Reconstruction of the defect is dictated by its size and may require the insertion of prosthetic material. Because of its mobility, the small bowel may be involved by colorectal cancer. Adherent loops of small intestine should never be dissected free from a tumor but resected in continuity. Tumors arising from the cecum and ascending colon on the right and from the descending colon and sigmoid on the left may involve the ureter or kidney. Mobilization of the sigmoid colon demands identification of the ureters to prevent intraoperative injury. In addition, posterior extension of cecal and sigmoid tumors can involve the psoas mus-

Table 40-3 Dukes Staging of Colorectal Cancer

Stage	Description
A	Limited to mucosa
B1	Limited to muscularis propria, nodes negative
B2	Through muscularis propria, nodes negative
B3	Adjacent organ involvement, nodes negative
C1	Limited to muscularis propria, nodes positive
C2	Through muscularis propria, nodes positive
C3	Adjacent organ involvement, nodes positive
D	Distant disease

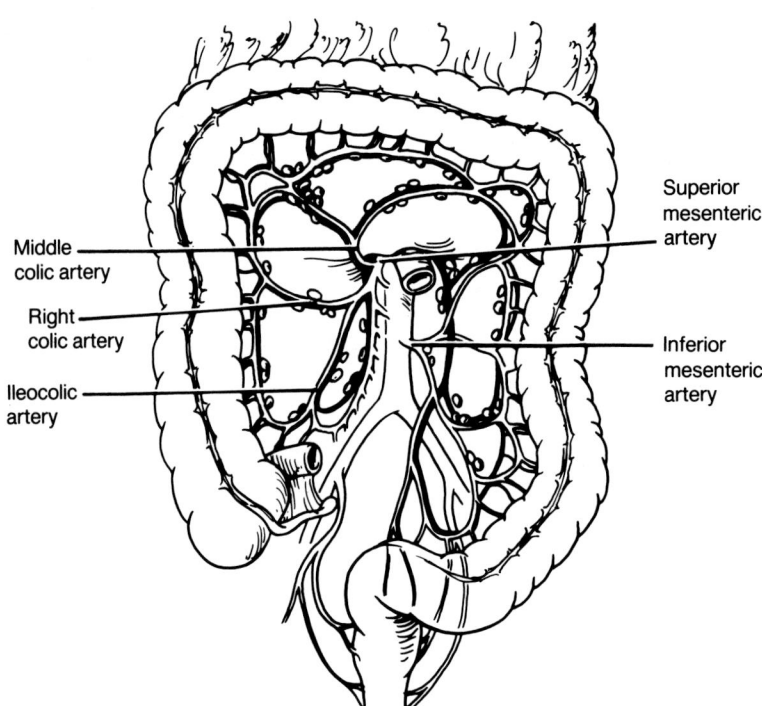

Figure 40-4 Surgically relevant colorectal anatomy.

cle. Neoplasms involving the ascending colon or hepatic flexure may involve the second portion of the duodenum, whereas tumors of the splenic flexure may invade the spleen.

The anatomic constraints of the pelvis place tumors of the rectum in proximity to many organs. In men, rectal tumors may involve the bladder, prostate, and seminal vesicles, whereas in women, the vagina and uterus are adjacent to the rectum.

Oncologic Principles

The goal of surgery for colorectal cancer is to maximize the opportunity for cure while minimizing morbidity and mortality. Laparotomy begins with a thorough evaluation of the entire abdominal cavity. Meticulous bimanual palpation of the liver should be performed, together with palpation and inspection of all serosal surfaces and adjacent and distant nodes. The remaining colon should be palpated carefully for additional lesions that were missed by preoperative studies. Colon resections follow classic oncologic principles, with resection of the tumor-bearing segment of the colon together with the draining lymphovascular pedicle (Fig. 40-5). Segmental or sleeve colon resections are rarely indicated because they compromise oncologic principles and provide no improvement in morbidity over oncologic resections. The advent of stapling devices has allowed the rapid construction of anasto-

moses that are comparable to traditional hand-sewn techniques.

Cancers of the cecum and ascending colon require a right hemicolectomy. Tumors of the hepatic flexure and proximal transverse colon are adequately treated with an extended right hemicolectomy. Ligation of the ileocolic artery for right and extended right hemicolectomy requires resection of the distal part of the terminal ileum because this part of the small bowel derives its blood supply from this vessel. Lesions of the descending colon are treated with left hemicolectomy, whereas lesions of the distal transverse colon and splenic flexure are treated with extended left hemicolectomy. Ligation of the inferior mesenteric artery flush with the aorta provides no improvement in survival because involvement of these nodes denotes distant spread and a poor prognosis, and high inferior mesenteric artery ligation can impair anastomotic blood supply.[22] Therefore, ligation at the level of the takeoff of the left colic artery is usually recommended for left hemicolectomy.

Lesions of the sigmoid colon are frequently treated with a limited segmental resection. An oncologically appropriate resection for a sigmoid cancer requires division of the proximal branches of the left colic artery and wide mesenteric resection with mobilization of the splenic flexure if necessary to construct a tension-free anastomosis. Care must be taken to identify both ureters and prevent injury to these structures.

To prevent dissemination of tumor cells at the time

of surgery, some have advocated early ligation of the lymphovascular pedicle and tape or staple closure of the colon proximal and distal to the tumor before manipulation of the tumor. The benefit of no-touch techniques over conventional methods of colon resection has not been proved.[23] Intraluminal instillation of cytocidal agents has been advocated to reduce tumor cell implantation and anastomotic recurrence but has not been routinely adopted.

Special Considerations

Synchronous Malignancies or Polyps

Patients with synchronous malignancies should be considered for subtotal colectomy depending on the distance between the lesions. Patients with colon cancer accompanied by multiple adenomatous polyps or synchronous cancers are also candidates for subtotal colectomy to reduce the risk of a metachronous lesion and to facilitate surveillance of the remaining colon. Factors that influence the decision to perform prophylactic subtotal colectomy include the number, location, and size of the accompanying polyps, as well as the age and compliance of the patient.

Cancer in a Polyp

Because most colorectal cancers arise from preexisting polyps, the surgeon frequently must determine how to manage cancer arising in a polyp. Complete endoscopic removal of a polyp that contains carcinoma in situ requires no further therapy. When invasive carcinoma is present in a polyp, the surgeon must ensure that endoscopic polypectomy was complete and that the entire polyp was submitted with proper orientation for histologic examination (Fig. 40-6). In the absence of medical problems that would prohibit surgery, carcinoma at the margin of resection is best treated by formal resection. A polyp removed in toto with clear margins requires thorough pathologic review and identification of adverse histologic features (poor differentiation, lymphatic or venous invasion). Invasion into the stalk of the polyp requires formal resection if the patient is an acceptable operative risk. When colectomy is required, it is often difficult to locate the previous polypectomy site during the operation. Even when the polyp has not been removed, it may be soft and difficult to palpate through the colon wall. In addition, endoscopic distance of the lesion from the anal verge or dentate line is often misleading. Therefore, when the surgeon has not performed the endoscopy, the site should be videotaped for later review and the polypec-

tomy site marked with vital dye that can be seen serosally at the time of surgery.

Obstructing Cancers

Ten percent of patients with colorectal cancer have obstructive symptoms.[24] Patients with partial obstruction can be treated with a "gentle" bowel preparation over several days and can then undergo elective resection. This line of therapy must be approached with caution because it can be difficult to distinguish which patients can be prepared safely. Totally obstructing right-sided colon cancers can be treated with right hemicolectomy and immediate ileocolostomy. For the more common obstructing cancers of the left colon, the options include the following, in order of preference:

1. Endoscopic decompression accomplished using a laser or by advancing a tube over a wire passed beyond the obstructed segment. This maneuver allows mechanical preparation and elective resection. Both these endoscopic options require that the narrowed lumen be traversed by the endoscope. They are not appropriate when the obstruction is complete or critical.
2. Primary resection of the cancer and immediate anastomosis with on-table colonic washout with or without proximal colostomy
3. Primary resection of the cancer with immediate colostomy formation and anastomosis at a second stage
4. Subtotal colectomy and primary anastomosis
5. Decompressive colostomy followed by a formal cancer operation later to remove the tumor. If the initial colostomy is a left transverse loop, it can be incorporated into the definitive resection at the second stage.

The decision-making process involves consideration of the physiologic status of the patient, the location of the lesion and duration of the obstruction, the presence of a concomitant perforation or metastatic disease, and the skill and experience of the surgeon.

Adjacent Organ Involvement

Ten percent of patients with colorectal cancer have adjacent organ involvement at the time of exploration,[25] and these patients are often deemed incurable and an inappropriate operation is performed. Locally advanced tumors do not necessarily portend a dismal prognosis and are potentially curable with multiorgan resection.[26] There appears to be a nonmetastasizing variant of colon cancer that grows to a large size without spreading to the regional nodes. Separation of ad-

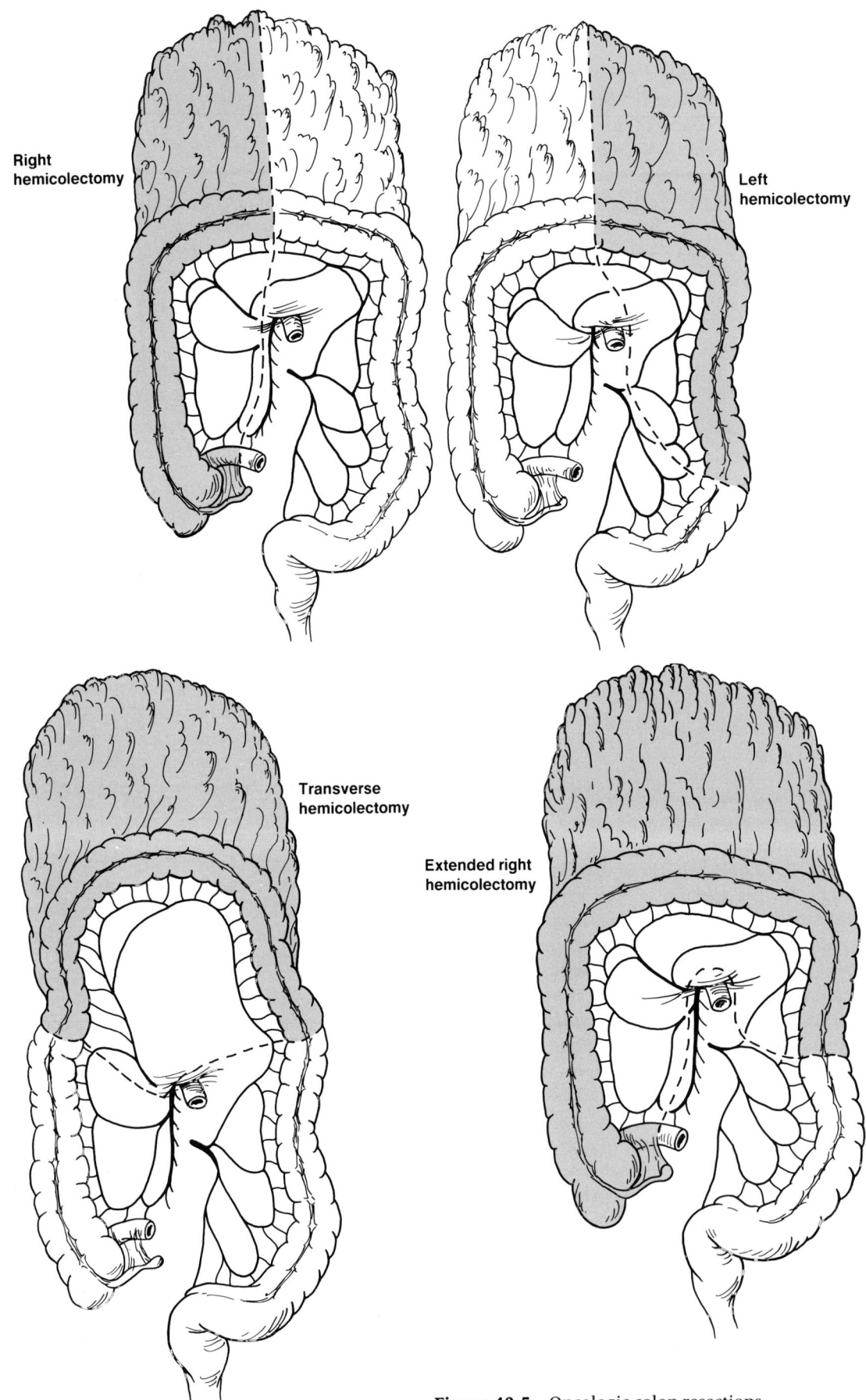

Right hemicolectomy

Left hemicolectomy

Transverse hemicolectomy

Extended right hemicolectomy

Figure 40-5 Oncologic colon resections.

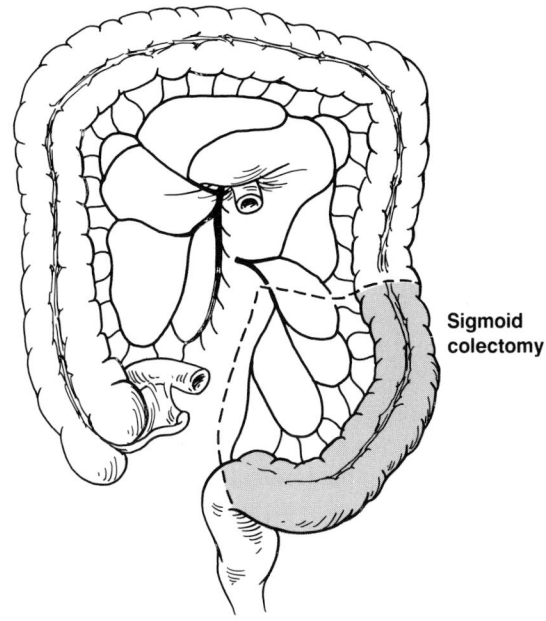

Figure 40-5 *(Continued)*

hesions adjacent to the malignancy can lead to dissemination of tumor cells. En bloc resection of these tumors, depending on their location, can lead to 5-year disease-free survival rates approaching 70%.[26]

Another 10% of patients have metastatic disease in the liver at the time of exploration.[27] Solitary hepatic metastases that can be removed with clear margins by a wedge resection should be removed concomitant with the bowel surgery. Liver metastases that require a formal hepatic resection (ie, right hepatic lobectomy) should be deferred to a later date because of the magnitude of the operative procedure. In addition, the use of intraoperative ultrasound can aid in more accurate staging of hepatic metastases.[28]

Oophorectomy

Oophorectomy is indicated for ovarian metastases or direct extension of the primary tumor to the ovary. The incidence of occult ovarian metastases at the time of colon resection is about 7%.[29] Although there is little evidence to suggest that prophylactic oophorectomy improves survival in patients with colorectal cancer,[30] it may obviate a second palliative operation in women who have large symptomatic ovarian metastases (Krukenberg's tumors); it also has the added benefit of preventing primary ovarian carcinoma. A reasonable approach is to resect overt ovarian metastases, to perform oophorectomy for direct ovarian involvement, and to offer prophylactic oophorectomy to postmenopausal women at the time of colorectal surgery.

Laparoscopic Colectomy

The recent revolution in laparoscopic and minimally invasive surgical techniques has been extended to include colon surgery (Fig. 40-7). Laparoscopic colectomy results in decreased postoperative pain, ileus, and length of hospital stay.[31] Controversy exists regarding the adequacy of margins, nodal dissection, and complication rates. A randomized prospective trial may be required to compare laparoscopic techniques to standard colectomy. Undoubtedly, as technology improves, the number of laparoscopic resections for colorectal cancer will multiply.

Oncologic Principles: Rectum

Abdominoperineal Resection

In 1908, Miles[32] established the oncologic principles of abdominoperineal resection with attention to the "zone of upward spread." This operation remains

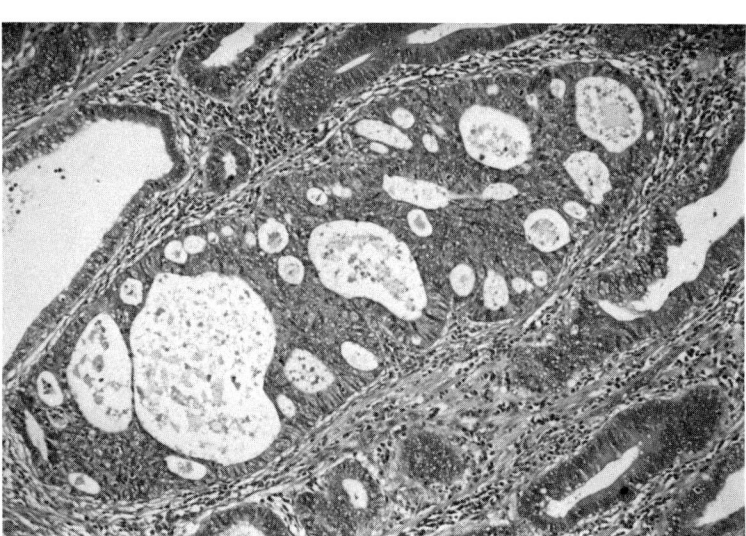

Figure 40-6 Histologic appearance of carcinoma in situ in a polyp. (See Color Fig. 40-6.)

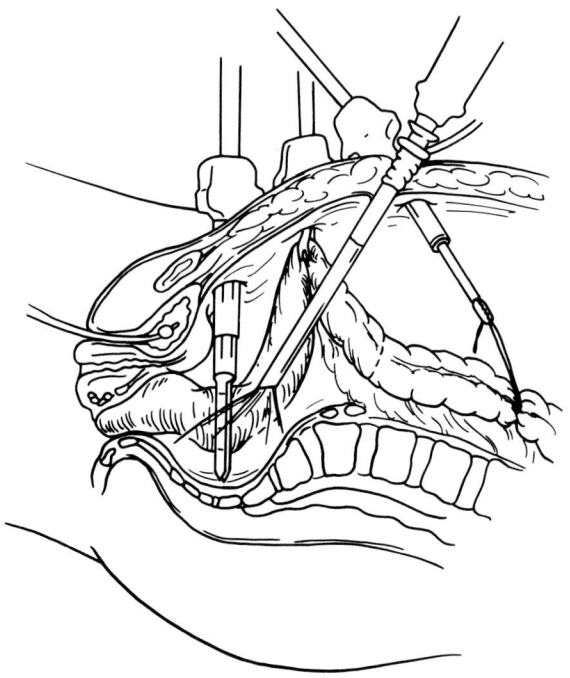

Figure 40-7 Laparoscopically guided dissection preparatory to low anterior resection.

the standard for rectal cancer (Fig. 40-8). Unfortunately, it necessitates a permanent colostomy and is associated with a significant incidence of bladder and sexual dysfunction.[33] Recently, options for the surgical treatment of rectal cancer have expanded to include a variety of sphincter-saving alternatives to abdominoperineal resection. Regardless of the operation performed, sound oncologic principles must be followed so that local control is not compromised.

Low Anterior Resection

Arbitrarily, the rectum is divided into thirds. Most cancers of the proximal and middle thirds can be managed with low anterior resection (resection of the tumor and anastomosis to nonserosalized distal rectum). The use of stapling devices has greatly facilitated the construction of an anastomosis within the confines of the pelvis (Fig. 40-9). Mobilization of the rectum for a low anterior resection is identical to the abdominal dissection for the abdominoperineal resection. Many patients with lower middle third and distal third lesions who were previously treated with the classic abdominoperineal resection are now candidates for a variety of sphincter-saving procedures (see Table 40-2). The "5-cm distal margin rule" has proved false because spread of the tumor is rarely greater than 2 cm.[34] The tangential or radial margin is probably of more importance in minimizing local recurrence than is the length of the distal margin.

Coloanal Anastomosis

For patients with distal, invasive rectal cancers, increasing success with coloanal anastomoses is being reported, and the creation of a J-shaped reservoir can improve continence[35] (Fig. 40-10). The coloanal anastomosis can also be valuable when the surgeon is attempting a low anterior resection and the distal seg-

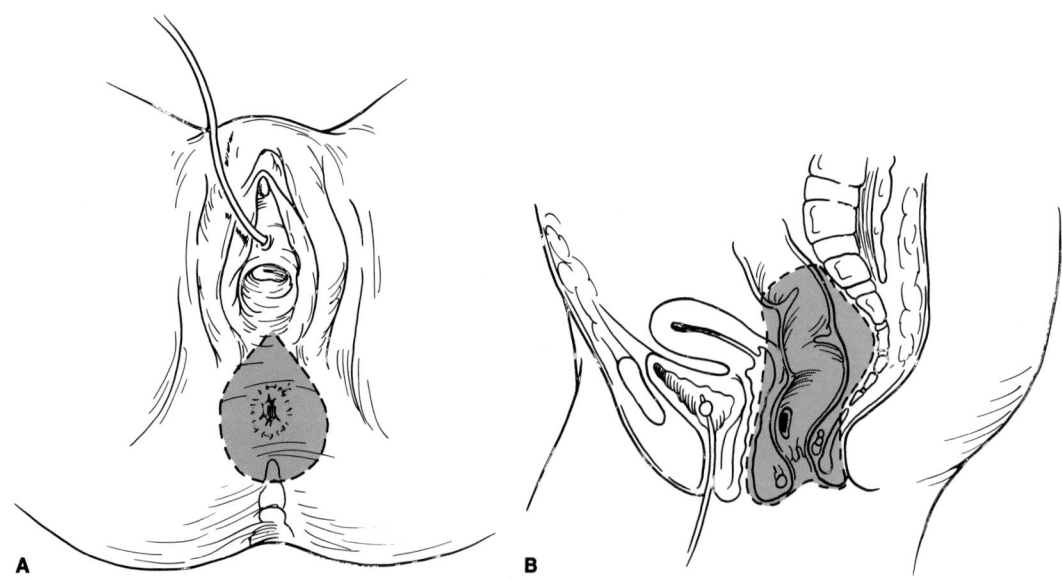

A   **B**

Figure 40-8 Diagrammatic representation of abdominoperineal resection.

of a full-thickness disk of rectum with a 1- to 2-cm margin of normal rectal tissue beyond the tumor (Fig. 40-11). Anterior wall lesions are excised with the patient in the prone or jackknife position, whereas tumors on the posterior wall are excised with the patient in the lithotomy position. The advantage of local excision over destructive techniques (ie, electrocautery, endocavitary radiation) is that the complete specimen is available for histologic analysis. Proposed selection criteria for lesions amenable to local excision are as follows[36]:

- Distance less than 8 cm from anal verge
- Size less than 3 to 4 cm
- Mobile, nonulcerated, noncircumferential
- Well to moderately well differentiated
- T1 or T2 lesion by endorectal ultrasound
- Diploid by flow cytometry

The use of preoperative endorectal ultrasound can aid in determining which lesions are best treated by local excision.

Special Considerations

Complete Excision of the Mesorectum

Some surgeons have advocated total mesorectal excision during low anterior resection as a means of reducing local recurrence.[37] Although pelvic recurrences appear to be less frequent with this technique, complications include increased transfusion requirements and a high anastomotic leak rate requiring routine protective colostomy. The possibility of patient selection bias suggests that a controlled study of total mesorectal excision may be required.

Radical Pelvic Lymphadenectomy

Radical pelvic lymphadenectomy does not result in survival benefit over standard dissections and is associated with an increased incidence of genitourinary com-

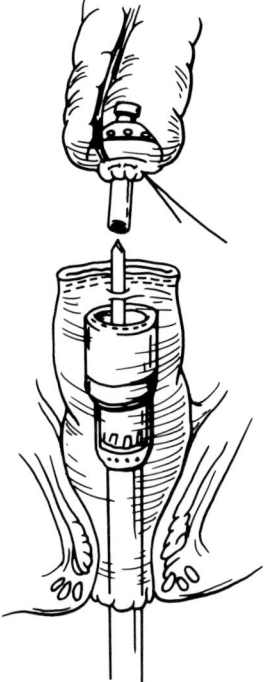

Figure 40-9 Low anterior resection with double-staple technique.

ment retracts or is injured. The coloanal anastomosis is frequently protected with temporary diversion.

Local Excision

Local excision of rectal tumors can be achieved transanally or by the transsphincteric or transsacral route. The principles of local excision involve removal

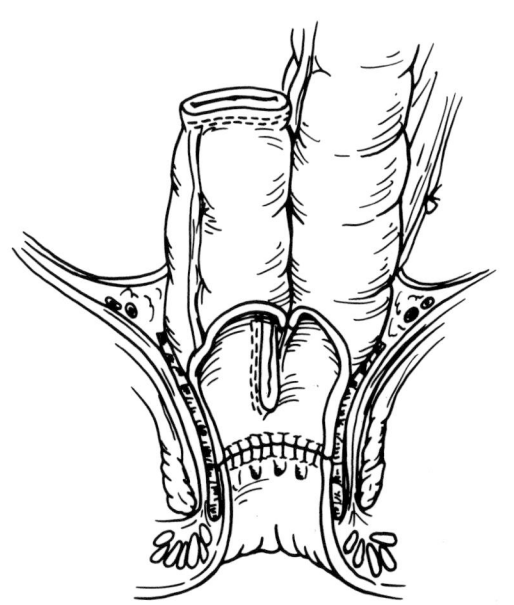

Figure 40-10 Coloanal anastomosis with J-shaped reservoir.

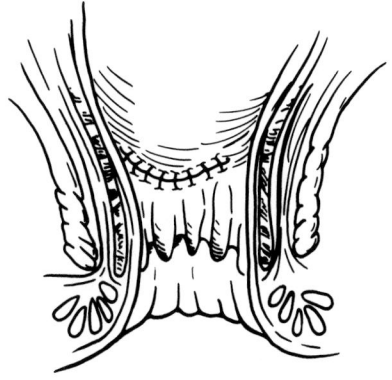

Figure 40-11 Transanal local excision.

plications.[38] Some surgeons perform a posterior vaginectomy in women with anterior lesions because of shared lymphatics between the anterior rectum and posterior vagina, but this has not been shown to reduce local recurrence or to improve survival.[39] If there is any question of direct vaginal tumor involvement, the surgeon should not hesitate to perform partial vaginectomy.

Inadvertent Rectal Perforation

Intraoperatively, the rectum may be perforated during mobilization or during the proctectomy portion of abdominoperineal resection. Because iatrogenic perforation predisposes to local recurrence, perforation warrants adjuvant radiotherapy.

Treatment of Pelvic Dead Space and Perineum

Treatment of the pelvic space that is produced after proctectomy has varied. Although many surgeons reperitonealize the pelvic floor, this maneuver creates a potential site for small bowel obstruction if gaps are left in the closure. If the omentum is of adequate size, an omental sling can be fashioned to fill the space, keeping the small bowel out of the pelvis after operation and reducing enteritis should the patient require postoperative radiotherapy. In the absence of adequate omentum, prosthetic slings have been used to retain the small bowel above the pelvic brim.[40] Prosthetic slings have significant disadvantages, including introduction of foreign material and the need for a second procedure for later removal. Treatment of the perineal wound after proctectomy has also included open packing and healing by secondary intention. The disadvantage of open packing includes the morbidity associated with prolonged healing of the perineal wound. Primary closure prevents this problem, although there is a risk of perineal wound infection if gross contamination occurs during proctectomy.[41] In most circumstances, primary closure is the preferred method of care for the posterior space after proctectomy.

Large Villous Adenoma

Most villous adenomas are found in the rectum, where they are often large and cauliflower-like in appearance, and soft and velvety to palpation (Fig. 40-12). The malignant potential of these tumors increases with their size, and only total histologic examination can ensure that invasive cancer is not present. Management is dependent on size, location, and the presence of invasive cancer.

Extended Resections

Locally advanced rectal cancer may involve the uterus, adnexa, and posterior vaginal wall in women or the seminal vesicles and prostate in men; the bladder may be involved in both sexes. In the absence of distant or extrapelvic disease, an aggressive approach is indicated. Depending on the organs involved, total pelvic exenteration with urinary diversion may be required to obtain tumor-free margins. Posterior rectal tumors fixed to the sacrum can be treated with abdominoperineal resection and sacrectomy in selected patients.[42] Large perineal wounds that result may require muscle flap closure.

Radiotherapy

Despite potentially curative surgery, colorectal cancer frequently recurs locally. Radiotherapy, like surgery, is a local modality and can be used in an adjuvant fashion to destroy tumor cells not removed by surgery. Radiotherapy is not a substitute for an adequate operation. Radiotherapy can be delivered before surgery, after surgery, in a combined fashion ("sandwich technique"), or even during surgery at facilities that possess this capability.

Colon

Although the experience with adjuvant radiotherapy for colon cancer is not as extensive as it is for rectal cancer, radiotherapy is indicated when tumors extend through the wall posteriorly or laterally, particularly in fixed colonic segments.[43]

Rectum

Pelvic recurrence of rectal cancer is a catastrophic event that is often refractory to further surgery and can produce intractable pain. Therapy that can reduce local recurrence of rectal cancer is worthwhile, and evidence strongly suggests that radiotherapy reduces local recurrence. Preoperative radiotherapy is theoretically superior because radiation is more effective in well-oxygenated tissue, whereas surgery renders tissues hypoxic. In addition, the complications of radiotherapy delivered before operation are reduced because of the smaller treatment volumes used. Radiation enteritis is decreased when the small bowel is not fixed by postoperative adhesions.[44] Preoperative radiotherapy can convert marginally resectable lesions to resectability and permit sphincter-sparing surgery for tumors that would have required abdominoperineal resec-

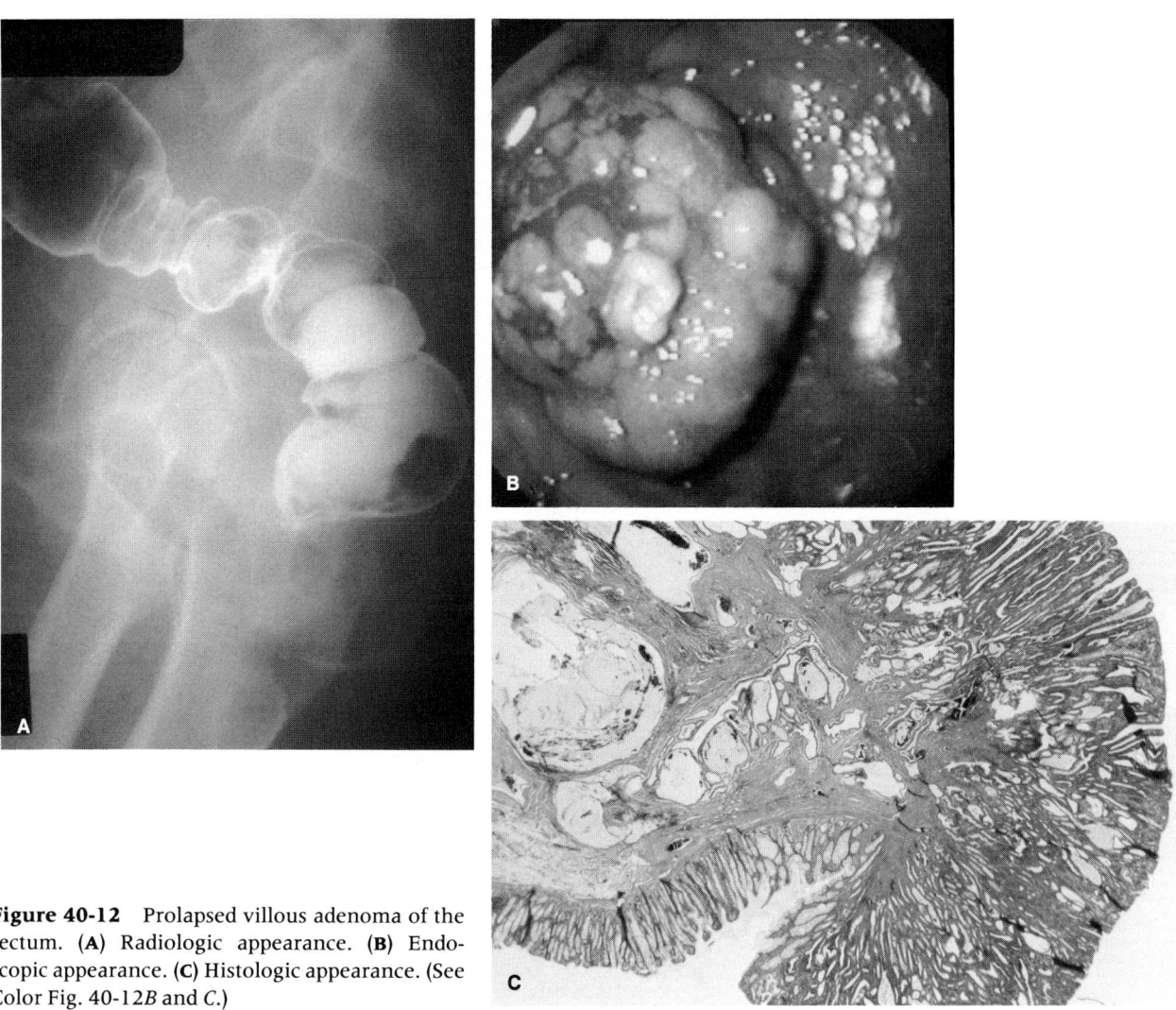

Figure 40-12 Prolapsed villous adenoma of the rectum. **(A)** Radiologic appearance. **(B)** Endoscopic appearance. **(C)** Histologic appearance. (See Color Fig. 40-12*B* and *C.*)

tion. Disadvantages of radiotherapy delivered before operation include the unnecessary treatment of patients at low risk for recurrence and a potentially increased complication rate after resection. An increased incidence of postoperative complications has not been seen in most trials,[45] particularly if proximal bowel outside the irradiated field is used for anastomosis. Improved methods of preoperative staging should allow more appropriate patient selection for preoperative radiotherapy.

Postoperative adjuvant radiotherapy has been used more frequently. For stage B2 and B3 rectal cancers, local recurrences can be reduced from 30% to 35% to 5% with adjuvant radiotherapy. For stage C2 and C3 rectal cancers, reductions in local recurrence from 40% to 60% to 10% to 15% can be achieved. Unfortunately, improved local control does not translate into prolonged survival.

Chemotherapy

Systemic relapse is a major problem after apparently curative surgery for colorectal cancer, with half of patients dying of systemic disease. Early trials of chemotherapy for colorectal cancer, flawed in design, conduct, and statistical analysis, failed to demonstrate any significant benefit for adjuvant chemotherapy.[46] Recent data from well-designed clinical trials demonstrate that adjuvant chemotherapy does prolong disease-free and overall survival when administered to certain subsets of patients with colorectal cancer.[47,48] Patients with stage C colorectal cancer should be offered adjuvant chemotherapy based on a survival advantage demonstrated for treated patients (using 5-fluorouracil–based regimens) relative to untreated control subjects. Efficacy for stage B cancers of the colon and rectum is also likely, although not consistent in all trials of adjuvant therapy.

Regional chemotherapy trials (portal vein or hepatic artery infusion) have been less impressive.[49] Ongoing clinical trials will help define the best drugs and optimal integration of all modalities. Whenever possible, participation in a clinical trial is strongly encouraged because ongoing and future protocols are needed to answer many unresolved issues.

Postoperative Surveillance

The postoperative follow-up of patients with colorectal cancer requires a thorough knowledge of the risk, timing, and patterns of recurrence of the disease. Patients at greatest risk for recurrence are those in whom the primary tumor extends through the bowel wall or involves regional lymph nodes. Most recurrences occur in the first 3 years after operation, and this should be the period of closest follow-up. Local–regional recurrence is more common for rectal tumors. Anastomotic recurrence often represents an extraluminal recurrence that grows into the mucosal surface rather than an isolated suture or staple line recurrence. The most common site of distant relapse is in the liver. Other organs of spread include the peritoneal cavity, lungs, bone, and brain.

As with any cancer, most recurrences after surgery can be detected with a complete history and physical examination. Colonoscopy should be done periodically, not only to detect local recurrence but to discover metachronous polyps and cancers. The frequency of endoscopic follow-up depends on the circumstances and pathologic findings of the initial resection. Patients who undergo resection for perforated or obstructing lesions require postoperative colonoscopy soon after resection to examine the remaining colon. Patients with multiple polyps in the surgical specimen or patients who continue to have polyps detected in postoperative follow-up examinations require more frequent surveillance. Outside the context of an investigational protocol, the use of expensive imaging studies (ie, CT, MRI, bone scanning) for routine follow-up is not cost-effective. The most effective laboratory test for the detection of recurrent disease is a CEA level (if the original tumor was CEA-producing).[50] A persistent rise in the CEA level should prompt a thorough search for recurrent disease. In the absence of any localizing imaging study, the value of a second-look operation is questionable.[51] The use of immunoscintigraphy can aid in detecting occult recurrences, particularly extrahepatic intraabdominal disease.[52]

Treatment of Recurrence

The treatment of recurrent colorectal cancer depends on the location and extent of recurrent disease and the previous therapy. Although hepatic recurrence is not uniformly fatal, most patients die within a year of diagnosis of liver metastases. A select subgroup of patients with hepatic colorectal liver metastases are candidates for hepatic resection because this remains the only potentially curative treatment.[53] Selected patients with isolated hepatic recurrence after liver resection of colorectal metastases can also benefit from repeated resection.[54] Ablative procedures such as alcohol injection and cryotherapy for unresectable hepatic metastases can increase the number of patients with liver metastases who benefit from therapy, but improvement in overall survival has not been shown.[55] Regional intra-arterial chemotherapy, with the advantage of greater drug delivery with minimal systemic toxicity, has an improved response rate over systemic chemotherapy for liver metastases, but this has not translated into improved survival and is associated with significant hepatobiliary toxicity.[56] Patients with solitary lung metastases can benefit from pulmonary resection.[57] Local–regional therapies for liver and lung metastases fail to address the problem of extrahepatic progression of disease, and only the development of more effective systemic therapy will correct this deficiency.

Local–regional recurrence of colon cancer is less frequent than local recurrence of rectal cancer and is often an indicator of systemic failure. Some patients with recurrence after local excision of rectal cancer can be saved with a low anterior resection, coloanal resection, or abdominoperineal resection. However, pelvic recurrence of rectal cancer after a low anterior resection, coloanal resection, or abdominoperineal resection can be a difficult problem, resulting in intractable pelvic pain with limited therapeutic alternatives. In the absence of extrapelvic disease, a few patients are candidates for exenteration or sacral resection.[58] More often, patients are treated with palliative colostomy and radiotherapy. The fecal stream can be maintained in some patients with intraluminal rectal recurrence using the laser or fulguration with electrocautery.

RARE NEOPLASMS

Benign

Endometriomas

Endometrial tissue can implant on the large bowel and produce abdominal or pelvic pain, intestinal obstruction, and bleeding. Treatment is usually medical, but surgery may be required for lesions refractory to medical management, for obstructing lesions, and for distinguishing an endometrioma from a malignant lesion.[59]

Lipomas

Lipomas can arise in the colorectum and may be submucosal or subserosal. Most lipomas are found in the proximal colon (Fig. 40-13). Symptoms are related to tumor size, and ulceration of the overlying mucosa may manifest as gastrointestinal bleeding. Other benign colorectal neoplasms include leiomyomas, fibromas, and neurogenic tumors. Often an operation is required to distinguish these lesions from carcinomas.

Malignant

Squamous Cell Carcinoma

Primary pure squamous cell carcinoma of the colon is rare. Adenosquamous carcinoma is more common and is associated with a less favorable prognosis than is adenocarcinoma. There appears to be an increased incidence of squamous cell carcinoma of the colon in patients with ulcerative colitis.[60]

Lymphoma

The large bowel may be involved secondarily by a generalized lymphoma or a primary gastrointestinal lymphoma. The cecum is the most common location and the diagnosis can be difficult to obtain by colonoscopic biopsy because of the submucosal nature of the lesion.[61] There is an increased incidence of non-Hodgkin's lymphomas of the B-cell type involving the colon in patients with acquired immunodeficiency syndrome.[62]

Carcinoid Tumors

The most common location of a carcinoid tumor of the gastrointestinal tract is the appendix, where they are often discovered incidentally at appendectomy. The next most common location is the small bowel, followed by the rectum, stomach, and colon. In the colorectum, carcinoid tumors appear endoscopically as yellowish, submucosal nodules. Right hemicolectomy is indicated for large appendiceal carcinoid tumors (more than 2 cm) or those with invasion of the mesoappendix. Small rectal carcinoid tumors can be treated by transanal excision.[63]

Sarcomas

Malignant stromal tumors can occur anywhere in the gastrointestinal tract, but are rare in the colon and rectum. Resection following oncologic principles is the treatment of choice. Like sarcomas elsewhere, tumor grade is an important prognosticator.[64] The frequency of Kaposi's sarcoma is greatly increased in patients with acquired immunodeficiency syndrome, and this tumor frequently involves the colorectum. Patients often have accompanying skin lesions. Medical treatment includes α-interferon and cytotoxic chemotherapy, with resection being a last resort.[65]

Metastatic Tumors

Tumors arising from adjacent organs may invade the colorectum. Tumors of the lung, breast, kidney, and skin can metastasize to the large bowel. Frequently, resection or diversion is required for palliation.

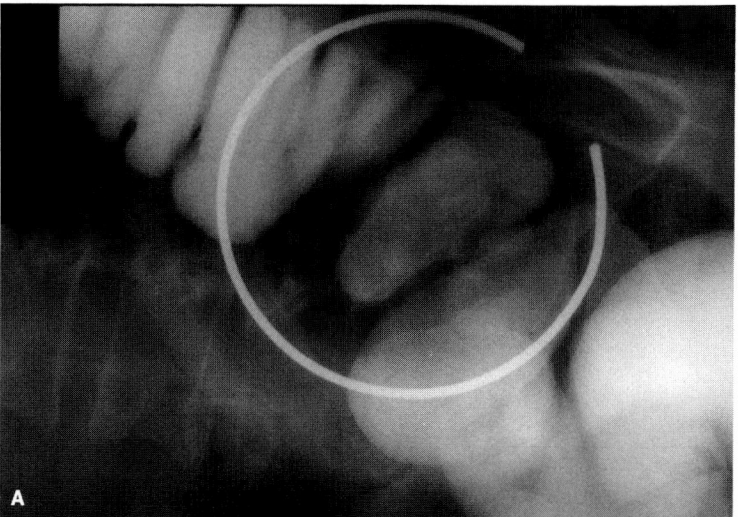
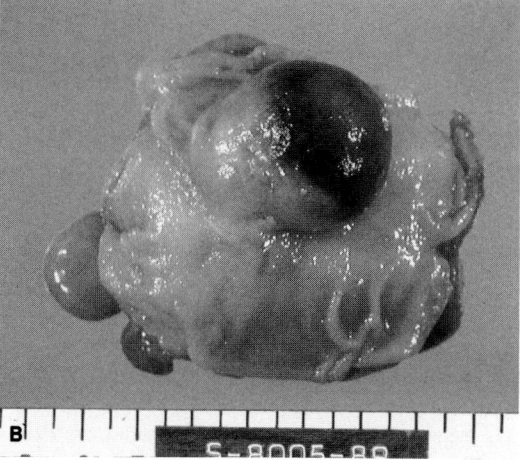

Figure 40-13 Colonic lipoma. **(A)** Radiologic appearance. **(B)** Gross pathologic appearance. (See Color Fig. 40-13*B*.) (Gordon RT, Beal JM. Lipoma of the colon. Arch Surg 1978;113:897)

REFERENCES

1. Boring CC, Squires TS, Tong T. Cancer statistics, 1993. CA Cancer J Clin 1993;43:7.

2. Wynder EL, Shigematsu T. Environmental factors of cancer of the colon and rectum. Cancer 1967;20:152.

3. Armstrong B, Doll R. Environmental factors and cancer incidence and mortality in different countries, with reference to dietary practices. Int J Cancer 1975;15:617.

4. Willett W. The search for causes of breast and colon cancer. Nature 1989;338:389.

5. Burkitt DP, Walker ARP, Painter NS. Dietary fiber and disease. JAMA 1974;229:1068.

6. Kritchevsky D. Fibre and cancer. Med Oncol Tumor Pharmacother 1990;7:137.

7. Burnstein MJ. Dietary factors related to colorectal neoplasms. Surg Clin North Am 1993;73:13.

8. Smigel K. Experts review NCI's dietary guidelines. J Natl Cancer Inst 1990;82:344.

9. Burt RW, Bishop DT, Cannon-Albright L, et al. Hereditary aspects of colorectal adenomas. Cancer 1992;70:1296.

10. Iwama T, Mishims Y, Utsunomiya J. The impact of familial adenomatous polyposis on the tumorigenesis and mortality at the several organs. Ann Surg 1993;217:101.

11. Kinzler KW, Nilbert MC, Su LK, et al. Identification of FAP locus genes from chromosome 5q21. Science 1991;253:661.

12. Ekbom A, Helmick C, Zach M, Adami H-O. Ulcerative colitis and colorectal cancer. N Engl J Med 1990;323:1228.

13. Levin B, Lennard-Jones J, Riddell RH. Surveillance of patients with chronic ulcerative colitis. Bull World Health Organ 1991;64:121.

14. Burmer GC, Rabinovitch PS, Haggitt RC, et al. Neoplastic progression in ulcerative colitis: histology, DNA content and loss of p53 allele. Gastroenterology 1992;103:1602.

15. Fitzgibbons RJ Jr, Lynch HT, Stanislav GV, Watson PA, Lanspa SJ, Marcus JN. Recognition and treatment of patients with hereditary nonpolyposis colon cancer (Lynch syndromes I and II). Ann Surg 1987;206:289.

16. Hamilton SR. Molecular genetics of colorectal carcinoma. Cancer 1992;70:1216.

17. Sidransky D, Tokino T, Hamilton S, et al. Identification of *ras* oncogene mutations in the stool of patients with curable colorectal tumors. Science 1992;256:102.

18. Isler JJ, Brown PC, Lewis FR. The role of preoperative colonoscopy in colorectal cancer. Dis Colon Rectum 1987;30:435.

19. Dershaw DD, Enker WE, Cohen AM, Sigurdson ER. Transrectal ultrasonography of rectal carcinoma. Cancer 1990;66:2336.

20. Yeatman TJ, Kimura AK, Copeland EM, Bland KI. Rapid analysis of carcinoembryonic antigen levels in gallbladder bile. Ann Surg 1991;213:113.

21. Beahrs OH, Myers MH. American Joint Committee on Cancer Manual for Staging of Cancer, ed 3. Philadelphia, JB Lippincott, 1992.

22. Pezim ME, Nichols RJ. Survival after high or low ligation of the inferior mesenteric artery and vein. Dis Colon Rectum 1991;34:1138.

23. Wiggers Y, Jeekel J, Arends JW, et al. No-touch isolation technique in colon cancer: a controlled prospective trial. Br J Surg 1988;75:409.

24. Kelley WE Jr, Brown PW, Lawrence W Jr, Terz JJ. Penetrating, obstructing and perforating carcinomas of the colon and rectum. Arch Surg 1981;116:381.

25. Lopez MJ, Monafo WW. Role of extended resection in the initial treatment of locally advanced colorectal carcinoma. Surgery 1993;113:365.

26. Eisenberg SB, Kraybill WG, Lopez MJ. Long term results of surgical resection of locally advanced colorectal carcinoma. Surgery 1990;108:779.

27. Asbun HJ, Hughes KS. Management of recurrent and metastatic colorectal carcinoma. Surg Clin North Am 1993;73:145.

28. Parker GA, Lawrence W Jr, Horsley JS, et al. Intraoperative ultrasound of the liver affects operative decision making. Ann Surg 1989;209:569.

29. Barr SS, Valentine MA, Bacon HE. Rationale for bilateral oophorectomy concomitant with resection for carcinoma of the rectum and colon. Dis Colon Rectum 1962;5:450.

30. Cutait R, Lesser ML, Enker WE. Prophylactic oophorectomy in surgery for large-bowel cancer. Dis Colon Rectum 1983;26:6.

31. Phillips EH, Franklin M, Carroll BJ, Fallas MJ, Ramos R, Rosenthal D. Laparoscopic colectomy. 1992;216:703.

32. Miles WE. A method of performing abdominoperineal excision for carcinoma of the rectum and of the terminal portion of the pelvic colon. Lancet 1908;2:1812.

33. Kinn A-C, Ohman U. Bladder and sexual dysfunction after surgery for rectal cancer. Dis Colon Rectum 1986;29:43.

34. Pollett WG, Nicholls RJ. The relationship between the extent of distal clearance and survival and local recurrence rates after curative anterior resection for carcinoma of the rectum. Ann Surg 1983;198:159.

35. Drake DB, Pemberton JH, Beart RW Jr, et al. Coloanal anastomosis in the management of benign and malignant rectal disease. Ann Surg 1987;206:600.

36. Graham RA, Garnsey L, Jessup JM. Local excision of rectal carcinoma. Am J Surg 1990;160:306.

37. MacFarlane JK, Ryall RDH, Heald RJ. Mesorectal excision for rectal cancer. Lancet 1993;341:457.

38. Moriya Y, Hojo K, Sawada T, et al. Significance of lateral node dissection for advanced rectal carcinoma at or below the peritoneal reflection. Dis Colon Rectum 1989;32:307.

39. Dozois RR, Perry RE. Rectal cancer: current management. Curr Probl Surg 1990;5:246.

40. Dasmahapatra KS, Swaminathan AP. The use of a biodegradable mesh to prevent radiation-associated small-bowel injury. Arch Surg 1991;126:366.

41. Mazier WP, Surrell JA, Senagore AJ. The bottom end: handling the perineal wound after abdominoperineal resection. Am Surg 1991;57:454.

42. Wanebo HJ, Koness RJ, Turk PS, Cohen SI. Composite resection of posterior pelvic malignancy. Ann Surg 1992;215:685.
43. Sugarbaker PH, Gunderson LL, Wittes RE. Colorectal cancer. In: DeVita VT, Hellman S, Rosenberg SA, eds. Cancer: principles and practice of oncology, ed 2. Philadelphia, JB Lippincott, 1985:842.
44. Cummings BJ. Adjuvant radiation therapy for colorectal cancer. Cancer 1992;70:1372.
45. Mendenhall WM, Bland KI, Copeland EM, et al. Does preoperative radiation therapy enhance the probability of local control and survival in high-risk distal rectal cancer? Ann Surg 1992;215:696.
46. Buyse M, Zeleniuch-Jacquotte A, Chalmers TC. Adjuvant therapy of colorectal cancer: why we still don't know. JAMA 1988;259:1571.
47. Moertel CG, Fleming TR, Macdonald JS, et al. Effective surgical adjuvant therapy of colon carcinoma: an intergroup study. N Engl J Med 1990;322:352.
48. Krook JE, Moertel CG, Gunderson LL, et al. Effective surgical adjuvant therapy for high-risk rectal carcinoma. N Engl J Med 1991;324:709.
49. Wolmark N, Rockette H, Wickerham DL, et al. Adjuvant therapy of Dukes A, B and C adenocarcinoma of the colon with portal vein fluorouracil hepatic infusion: preliminary results of the NSABP protocol C-02. J Clin Oncol 1990;8:1466.
50. Steele G, Ellenberg S, Ramming K, et al. CEA monitoring among patients in multi-institutional adjuvant gastrointestinal therapy trials. Ann Surg 1982;196:162.
51. Steele G Jr. Standard postoperative monitoring of patients after primary resection of colon and rectum cancer. Cancer 1993;71:4225.
52. Sardi A, Workman M, Mojzisik C, Hinkle G, Nieroda C, Martin EW Jr. Intra-abdominal recurrence of colorectal cancer detected by radioimmunoguided surgery (RIGS system). Arch Surg 1989;124:55.
53. Lind DS, Parker GA, Horsley JS, et al. Formal hepatic resection of colorectal liver metastases: ploidy and prognosis. Ann Surg 1992;215:677.
54. Griffith KD, Sugarbaker PH, Chang AE. Repeat hepatic resections for colorectal liver metastases. Surgery 1990;107:101.
55. Ravikumar TS, Steele G Jr, Kane R, King V. Experimental and clinical observations on hepatic cryosurgery for colorectal metastases. Cancer Res 1991;51:6323.
56. Kemeny N, Daly J, Reichman B, et al. Intrahepatic or systemic infusion of fluorodeoxyuridine in patients with liver metastases from colorectal cancer. Ann Intern Med 1987;107:459.
57. Murray KD. Excision of pulmonary metastases of colorectal cancer. Semin Surg Oncol 1991;7:157.
58. Hafner GH, Herrera L, Petrelli NJ. Morbidity and mortality after pelvic exenteration for colorectal adenocarcinoma. Ann Surg 1992;215:63.
59. Goligher JC. Surgery of the anus, rectum and colon, ed 5. London, Bailliere Tindall, 1984:797.
60. Michelassi F, Montag AG, Block GE. Adenosquamous cell carcinoma in ulcerative colitis. Dis Colon Rectum 1988;31:323.
61. Sherlock P, Winawere SJ, Goldstein MJ, et al. Malignant lymphoma of the gastrointestinal tract. In: Glass GB, ed. Progress in gastroenterology, vol 2. New York, Grune & Stratton, 1970:367.
62. Safai B, Diaz B, Schwartz J. Malignant neoplasms associated with human immunodeficiency virus infection. CA Cancer J Clin 1992;42:74.
63. Shakelford PT, Zuidema GD. Surgery of the alimentary tract, ed 2. Philadelphia, WB Saunders, 1982:186.
64. Dougherty MJ, Compton C, Talbert M, Wood W. Sarcomas of the gastrointestinal tract. Ann Surg 1991;214:569.
65. Weber JN, Carmichael DJ, Boylston A, et al. Kaposi's sarcoma of the bowel presenting as apparent ulcerative colitis. Gut 1985;26:295.

Digestive Tract Surgery: A Text and Atlas, edited by Richard H. Bell, Layton F. Rikkers, and Michael W. Mulholland. Lippincott-Raven Publishers, Philadelphia, © 1996.

41

Colorectal Trauma

R. Lawrence Reed II

HISTORY

Intestinal injury has been a part of human experience throughout history, although its recognition and treatment is a relatively recent advance.[1] Most of the improvements in the treatment of colonic trauma have been obtained during the past century. As with many traumatic conditions, much of current practice is based on wartime experiences. Before World War I, most penetrating abdominal wounds were managed nonoperatively. During the Civil War, 3690 recorded nonoperatively managed abdominal wounds had a 90% mortality rate.[2] Operative management of these wounds began during World War I, when a mortality rate of 54% was reported for 1200 British soldiers treated operatively for penetrating abdominal wounds.[2-4] Of the 252 patients who received colonic wounds, primary suture of the wound was used in two thirds, with a mortality rate of 50%, while colostomy exteriorization was employed in the remainder, with a mortality rate of 73%. The predominant approach to colonic wounds for several years was suture repair, with little employment of colostomy.[5-7] During World War II, a change in attitude occurred with regard to colostomy,[8,9] with a resultant reduction in mortality rate to 35%.[10] Initial enthusiasm for colostomy was tempered by investigators who noted that colostomy rates had increased from 33% to 80%, with an increased mortality and morbidity noted in the patients who underwent colostomy.[11-15] Despite these reports, colostomy has become the standard approach for many colonic injuries.

ETIOLOGY AND NATURAL HISTORY

The colon is at risk for injury in multiple abdominal areas because of its course through the abdomen. While the transverse and sigmoid colon are located intraab-dominally, the ascending and descending colon are retroperitoneal structures. The rectum, of course, is a pelvic organ. Thus, the colon is prone to injury in anterior, posterior (flank), superior, and inferior abdominal injuries.

The proportion of colon injuries that are due to blunt or penetrating trauma at any given institution varies as a function of the type of trauma seen by that institution. In inner-city county hospitals with a large volume of penetrating trauma, most colon injuries result from gunshot wounds and stabbing incidents.[16] In rural and suburban institutions, a larger proportion of colon injuries result from blunt vehicular trauma. Some authors have noted a predilection of blunt or penetrating trauma to one side of the colon or the other,[17] but large series have found an equal distribution of injuries throughout the segments of the colon.[16] Rectal injuries account for roughly 20% of colorectal trauma.[11,18-21]

Aside from guns and knives, modern society provides other mechanisms for penetrating injury to the colon and rectum. The increasing use of proctoscopic and colonoscopic techniques and the frequent performance of diagnostic peritoneal lavage (DPL) and peritoneocentesis have produced iatrogenic methods for colonic injury.[22,23] Other mechanisms for rectal injury include anal intercourse and the use of various sexual devices and enema administration kits. Spontaneous perforation of the colon is a rare but reported phenomenon that appears to be most common in immunocompromised patients. In this patient group, spontaneous perforation has a mortality rate of 40% to 100%.[24] The pathogenesis is unclear, but predisposing factors include immunosuppressive medications, uremia, colon ulcerations, and fecal impaction.

Blunt mechanisms of injury to the abdomen often

spare the colon. The transverse and sigmoid portions of the colon can be injured through blunt mechanisms by being compressed against the spine or the sacral promontory, respectively. Avulsion injuries of the colon are unusual. Rectal injuries can occur in the context of severe pelvic fractures, and evidence of such injury should be aggressively sought in these cases.

Blunt abdominal injuries can lead to delayed colonic perforations.[25,26] Patients with preexisting inflammatory bowel conditions, such as Crohn's disease, may be at increased risk of perforation of the intestine from apparently mild trauma.[27] Blunt injuries to the abdomen can also produce an obstructive process in the colon, most likely from intramural hemorrhage and edema. It has been reported that nonoperative management of these injuries can result in complete resolution.[28] The course of resolution may be prolonged, and the overall costs of hospitalization and parenteral nutrition may still be significant.

DIAGNOSTIC AND RESUSCITATIVE MANEUVERS

Penetrating Trauma

Patients with penetrating injuries of the abdomen are managed differently from patients with blunt abdominal trauma (Fig. 41-1). The incidence of internal organ injury approximates 85% for gunshot wounds to the ab-

domen, mandating laparotomy. Only one third of abdominal stab wound victims have suffered significant organ damage requiring operative repair. Routine laparotomy is unnecessary in most patients with stab wounds and must be seen as financially unsound.[29] For lateral flank injuries that are highly suspicious for colonic injury, some have advocated the use of a contrast-enhanced computed tomographic (CT) enema in which multiple images are obtained throughout the tract of the penetration to determine proximity to internal organs.[30] In many trauma centers, such a technique may be unavailable or logistically difficult in an emergency setting. Additionally, the costs associated with finding an injury requiring operative intervention with this technique have been estimated to be high because of the low yield of positive findings.[31] On the other hand, the costs of routine laparotomy for such wounds would certainly be much greater. For stab wounds that are suspicious for colonic injury, such as those involving the lateral abdominal wall, close observation and repeated examinations are necessary. In situations in which a reliable physical examination is not possible, a contrast-enhanced CT enema may be beneficial.

Stab wounds of the anterior abdominal wall do not mandate an exploration unless other conditions exist. In many cases, and in contrast to most patients with blunt abdominal injury, serial abdominal examinations can be relied on to indicate the need for celiotomy. Anterior abdominal stab wound patients who show signs

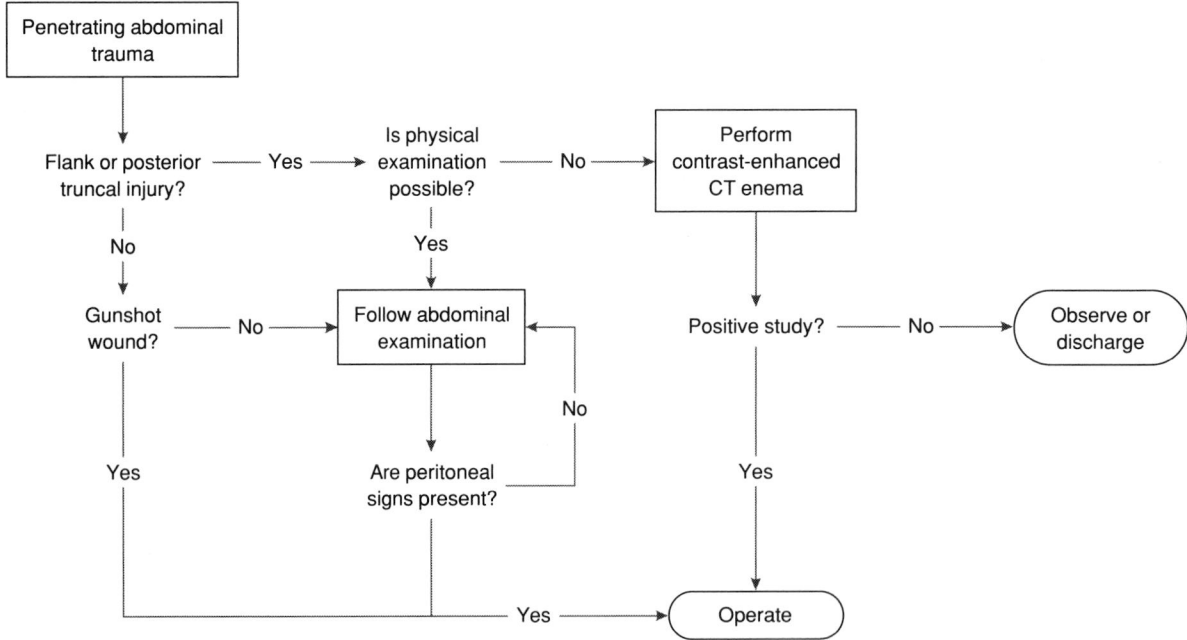

Figure 41-1 Algorithm for the evaluation and management of penetrating abdominal trauma.

of ongoing hemorrhage need exploration. Similarly, those who have signs of peritonitis on abdominal examination warrant laparotomy. Even patients who are initially intoxicated from ethanol ingestion can often be followed in this manner; they manifest signs of guarding or rebound tenderness as their level of intoxication declines.

If physical examination is not reliable, evidence for significant intraabdominal injury should be actively sought. Although DPL is considered a standard in the evaluation of blunt abdominal trauma,[32] no consensus opinion has developed in the case of penetrating abdominal trauma. For example, the red blood cell count criteria for the DPL evaluation of penetrating trauma ranges from 1000[33] to 100,000[34] red cells per milliliter. CT scanning may fail to reveal a small area of intestinal perforation, especially if there is no fluid or air leakage. Laparoscopy may offer a potential diagnostic and therapeutic advantage in cases of penetrating abdominal trauma in which the physical examination is uncertain. With the laparoscope, it is possible to determine if abdominal penetration has occurred. Furthermore, it is possible to assess the intestinal tract in its entirety, visually inspecting for injury. Finally, some perforations may be repaired laparoscopically, especially if there has been minimal enteric spillage. Even with the previously described diagnostic measures, the trauma surgeon should be prepared to undertake a formal laparotomy if he or she cannot be convinced that a colonic injury does not exist.

Potential rectal injuries may be suspected in cases of penetrating trauma because of the path of the wound tract. A rectal examination may reveal local tenderness or blood. If the potential for rectal injury is strong, the patient should undergo proctoscopy in the emergency room. One series showed that gluteal wounds associated with gross blood on rectal examination or in the urine were 100% predictive of an injury warranting exploration with no false-negative results, whereas proctosigmoidoscopy had a false-negative rate of 25%.[35]

Blunt Trauma

Patients with blunt abdominal trauma often have associated injuries or head injuries that make interpretation of abdominal examination difficult (Fig. 41-2). CT scanning can detect hollow viscus injuries, although it is not as sensitive in this regard as is DPL. In one prospective series,[36] CT was diagnostic in only 59% of intestinal injuries, and it was either suggestive or diagnostic in 88% of those with operatively confirmed injuries. CT findings considered *diagnostic* of bowel perforation are pneumoperitoneum (without prior peritoneal lavage); mesenteric, intramural, or retroperitoneal air; and direct visualization of discontinuity of the bowel wall or extravasation of luminal contents. CT findings considered *suggestive* of bowel rupture include intraperitoneal fluid of unknown source, thickened (more than 4 to 5 mm) bowel wall, gross anterior pararenal fluid without a recognized source, and bowel wall hematoma. Thus, even though the patient is hemodynamically stable, the opportunity to prevent significant peritoneal infection at an early stage may be lost.[37,38] DPL, although less likely to miss hollow viscus injuries than CT examina-

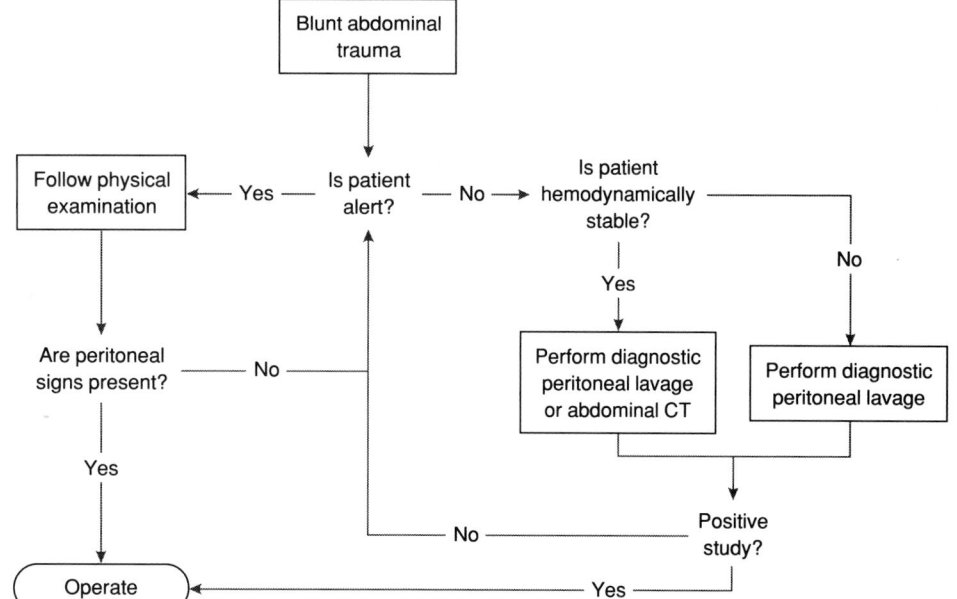

Figure 41-2 Algorithm for the evaluation and management of blunt abdominal trauma.

tion, suffers from its extreme sensitivity, requiring only about 20 mL of intraperitoneal blood to produce a positive result. DPL frequently leads to a nontherapeutic laparotomy, even though the intraoperative findings confirm that the test was truly positive for injury.

PREOPERATIVE PREPARATION

Before laparotomy for suspected colon injury, resuscitation should be initiated as dictated by the patient's vital signs. The basics of this resuscitation involve adherence to the ABC priorities of assessment and management: *a*irway, *b*reathing, and *c*irculation. Oxygen delivery to the tissues is optimized through this approach, and the patient's ability to tolerate the added stress of emergency surgery is improved. Supplemental oxygen should be provided, preparations for anesthetic induction and endotracheal intubation should be made, and at least two large-bore intravenous catheters should be inserted. Foley catheterization is useful for monitoring the renal response to circulatory resuscitation. Nasogastric intubation is used to decompress the stomach before laparotomy, minimizing the risk of aspiration on anesthetic induction and facilitating abdominal exploration.

As a matter of routine for abdominal explorations involving the potential for colon injury, prophylactic systemic antibiotics should be administered. Contamination from colonic injuries imposes a significant risk for subsequent infections because of the bacterial flora that reside in the human colon. The bacterial concentration in the colon is roughly 10^{11} to 10^{12} colony-forming units per milliliter.[39] As much as 60% of the stool's dry weight is bacteria. Anaerobes outnumber aerobic and facultative bacteria by a ratio of 300:1 to 1000:1.[39]

Because of the high bacterial numbers in the colon, any injury or operation that exposes colonic luminal contents to normal tissues creates the potential for infection. Patients undergoing elective colon surgery without the administration of prophylactic antibiotics have an infection rate of roughly 40%.[40,41] Antibiotic prophylaxis for surgical wound infection has emerged as an established and effective practice for elective clean-contaminated and contaminated surgical wounds.[42–46] Standard prophylactic techniques for elective colonic surgery typically involve a mechanical bowel preparation to reduce the fecal mass in combination with prophylactic oral or intravenous antibiotics.[47–49]

Prophylactic use of antibiotics in trauma patients is difficult because antibiotics cannot be administered before injury. Yet, timing of antibiotic administration is still crucial.[50] One study evaluated patients with penetrating abdominal trauma who received prophylactic antibiotics preoperatively, intraoperatively, or postoperatively. The groups were comparable, although the patients who received antibiotics preoperatively actually had more organs injured per patient and a higher incidence of shock than the other groups. Despite this apparent disadvantage, the infection rate in the patients who received antibiotics preoperatively was markedly reduced compared with those who received antibiotics intraoperatively or postoperatively. The potential benefit of prophylactic antibiotics in trauma was also suggested by a study that assessed antianaerobic agents in patients with abdominal trauma.[51] In this study, 100 patients were prospectively randomized to receive either cephalothin plus kanamycin or clindamycin plus kanamycin. The antibiotic coverage differed in that the cephalothin plus kanamycin combination failed to cover anaerobes, whereas clindamycin plus kanamycin did provide coverage. A reduced infection rate was seen in the patients receiving the antianaerobic combination (clindamycin plus kanamycin). Moreover, the infections that did occur were primarily anaerobic, supporting the utility of this form of prophylaxis in abdominal trauma.

Although there is evidence that prophylactic antibiotics are beneficial in trauma, infection rates remain high in severely injured patients. Conditions such as hypovolemic shock, vasoconstriction, and immune suppression increase the severity of infection produced by bacterial contamination; they are considered adjuvants for the development of an infectious process. The effective use of prophylactic antibiotics requires that adequate levels of drugs are present in the contaminated tissues within a time interval of roughly 4 hours. The adjuvant effects for infection just noted are also influenced by the same 4-hour interval after initial bacterial contamination. If adjuvant conditions occur at the time of contamination, the potential for infection is enhanced.[52–54]

A series of studies has shown that the presence of hemorrhagic shock can eliminate the benefit provided by prophylactic antibiotic administration.[55] The benefit of prophylactic antibiotics may be reestablished despite the presence of hemorrhagic shock if an antibiotic dose much larger than the standard dose (a megadose) is given.[55] Clinical evidence shows that larger doses of prophylactic antibiotics in trauma patients can reduce subsequent infection rates.[56] In part, this effect appears to be related to the altered pharmacokinetics seen in trauma patients as a result of massive fluid resuscitation and the hyperdynamic postinjury metabolic state.[57] In reviewing prophylactic antibiotic trials involving patients with colon trauma, it appears that infection rates

(Table 41-1) remain close to the rates observed in patients who received no prophylaxis before elective colon surgery.[40,41] This is especially concerning if one considers the other improvements in patient care (improved resuscitation, nutrition, and newer antibiotic spectra and activities) that have contributed to reducing surgical infection rates during the intervening decades.

A potential explanation for these observations may be an *inoculum effect*,[58] wherein the apparent sensitivity of bacteria toward an antibiotic is reduced as a result of increased bacterial concentrations. If so, then larger doses of antibiotics may be necessary to achieve an effective prophylactic result in colonic trauma, although this hypothesis has not yet been tested. Some have advocated intraoperative lavage, performed by introducing a balloon catheter into the distal ileum and irrigating the colon with several liters of saline, as a method of reducing bacterial load.[59]

Despite disappointing results with antibiotic prophylaxis in colorectal trauma, it is still considered an essential component of patient management. Some have continued antibiotic prophylaxis beyond a 24-hour period, reasoning that because of the heavy bacterial load, treatment for a full 5- to 7-day course rather than prophylaxis is necessary. Unfortunately, prolonged antibiotic treatment in the absence of signs of infection (fever, leukocytosis, local inflammatory changes) does not improve outcome and must be seen as financially unsound (see Table 41-1). Antibiotic prophylaxis should be continued only for a period of 12 to 24 hours.

To be effective, antibiotic prophylaxis in colon injuries must be broad-spectrum, covering facultative gram-negative bacteria, gram-positive aerobes (including *Enterococcus* sp[60]), and anaerobes.[51] In the past, physicians attempted to provide this broad coverage by using regimens such as doxycycline plus penicillin or triple antibiotics (a combination of ampicillin, an aminoglycoside, and clindamycin or metronidazole). Bacterial resistance patterns have since emerged that make doxycycline plus penicillin relatively ineffective against a large proportion of isolates. The concerns over potential drug toxicities and the difficulty with effective dosing given the altered pharmacokinetics make the use of aminoglycosides also unattractive.[57] Triple antibiotic therapy can still be used by substituting the aminoglycoside moiety with effective nontoxic agents targeted against gram-negative organisms, such as aztreonam and third-generation cephalosporins. These should be combined with a drug that has antianaerobic activity, such as metronidazole. In the case of aztreonam, the agent should also be combined with an agent that has activity against gram-positive organisms or that has antienterococcal activity, such as ampicillin or vancomycin. Single-agent prophylaxis for colonic trauma can be provided in the form of broad-spectrum cephalosporins with antianaerobic activity, such as cefoxitin or cefotetan. The lack of enterococcal coverage using cephalosporins makes alternatives such as piperacillin, ampicillin plus sulbactam, and ticarcillin (Timentin) plus clavulanic acid more attractive.[60] Extremely broad-spectrum, single-agent coverage is also available in the form of imipenem plus cilastatin.

OPERATIVE MANAGEMENT

Colon Injuries

The management options for colonic injuries include resection, primary repair, exteriorization, and diversion (Fig. 41-3). Resections can be accompanied by pri-

Table 41-1 Clinical Trials of Prophylactic Antibiotics in Colon Trauma

Investigator	Antibiotics	Duration (h)	Incidence of Infections (%)
Fabian et al (1982)[79]	Cefotaxime with or without cefazolin	8–24	37
Moore et al (1983)[80]	Amikacin, clindamycin, ampicillin	120	27
	Doxycycline and penicillin	120	33
	Carbenicillin	120	33
Nallathambi et al (1984)[81]	Gentamicin, clindamycin, and ampicillin	>120	24
Gentry et al (1984)[82]	Cefamandole	48	23
	Cefoxitin	48	10
	Ticarcillin and tobramycin	48	19
Dellinger et al (1986)[83]	Doxycycline and penicillin	12	17
		120	36
	Cefoxitin	12	27
		120	21
Weigelt et al (1993)[60]	Cefoxitin	24	19
	Ampicillin and sulbactam	24	2

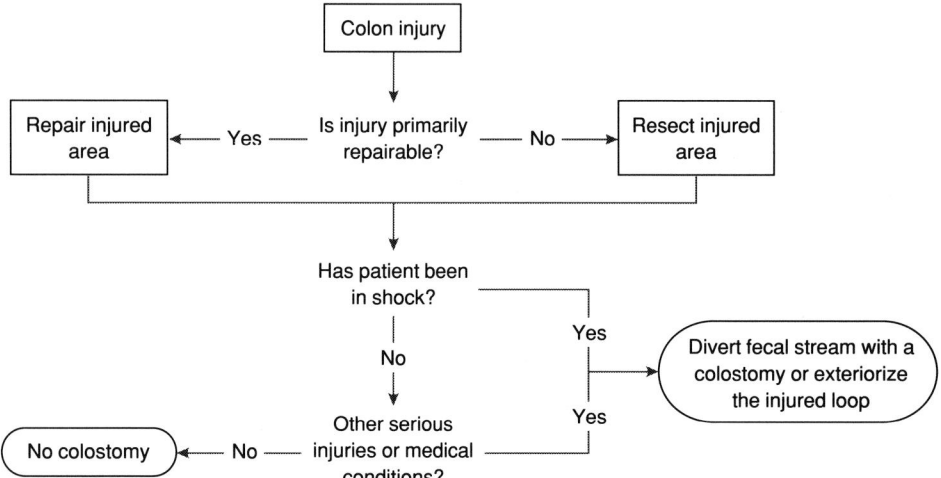

Figure 41-3 Algorithm for the management of colon injuries.

mary anastomosis or by ostomy formation from the proximal severed end of the bowel. In the case of stoma formation, the distal end can be brought out as a mucous fistula or closed as a Hartmann's procedure. In general, these procedures are similar to those undertaken in elective colonic surgery. Stoma maturation may be delayed in some cases pending management of other injuries in a multiple-injury patient.

Resection

Resection should be undertaken when the injured colon is severely damaged and not likely to survive a repair without leakage. Blunt injuries more commonly produce severe contusions of this nature. Gunshot and shotgun injuries can provide a sufficient blast impact to the bowel to make viability questionable. Gross spillage of fecal contents from perforations is often cited as a reason for colon resection, although there is no scientific evidence that such an approach is warranted. If the bowel surrounding the traumatic perforation is otherwise viable, there is no clear rationale for resection. Under such conditions, a repair may be feasible if the following conditions are absent[25]:

- Preoperative shock (blood pressure less than 80/60 mmHg)
- Severe hemorrhage (intraperitoneal blood loss greater than 1000 mL)
- More than two intraabdominal organ systems injured
- Significant fecal contamination of the peritoneum
- Operative start time more than 8 hours after injury
- Severely destructive colon wounds requiring resection

- Major loss of the abdominal wall requiring mesh replacement

The abdomen should be thoroughly irrigated to remove all particulate matter. Many clinicians use an irrigating solution containing antibiotics to aid in the elimination of infective organisms, although the advantage of this method of delivery over intravenously administered antibiotics is controversial.[61,62]

The injured areas should be completely resected, leaving only grossly normal bowel. The mesenteric transection should be performed close to the edge of the bowel wall. There is no need for a wide resection in the trauma setting, and staying close to the edge of the resected bowel helps to prevent inadvertent injury to the nutrient blood supply of the remaining intestine. Suture ligatures are usually preferred on the major vascular structures to prevent later slippage and hemorrhage. A stapling device is preferred to accomplish intestinal transection. The stapler provides a secure closure of the intestinal lumen simultaneously to performance of the transection. The luminal contents are thus controlled until either a stoma or an anastomosis can be constructed.

PRIMARY ANASTOMOSIS. After resection, the surgeon may elect either to perform a primary anastomosis or create a stoma to exteriorize the fecal stream. The issues relevant to this decision are similar to those for primary repair. If a primary anastomosis is chosen, the most expedient method in the injured patient is usually a stapled technique (Fig. 41-4). This is performed by placing one limb of the stapler into the lumen of the proximal bowel and the other limb of the device into the distal bowel. The stapler is fired, joining the two ends of intestine with a side-to-side opening. The opening that remains after removal of the stapler can be

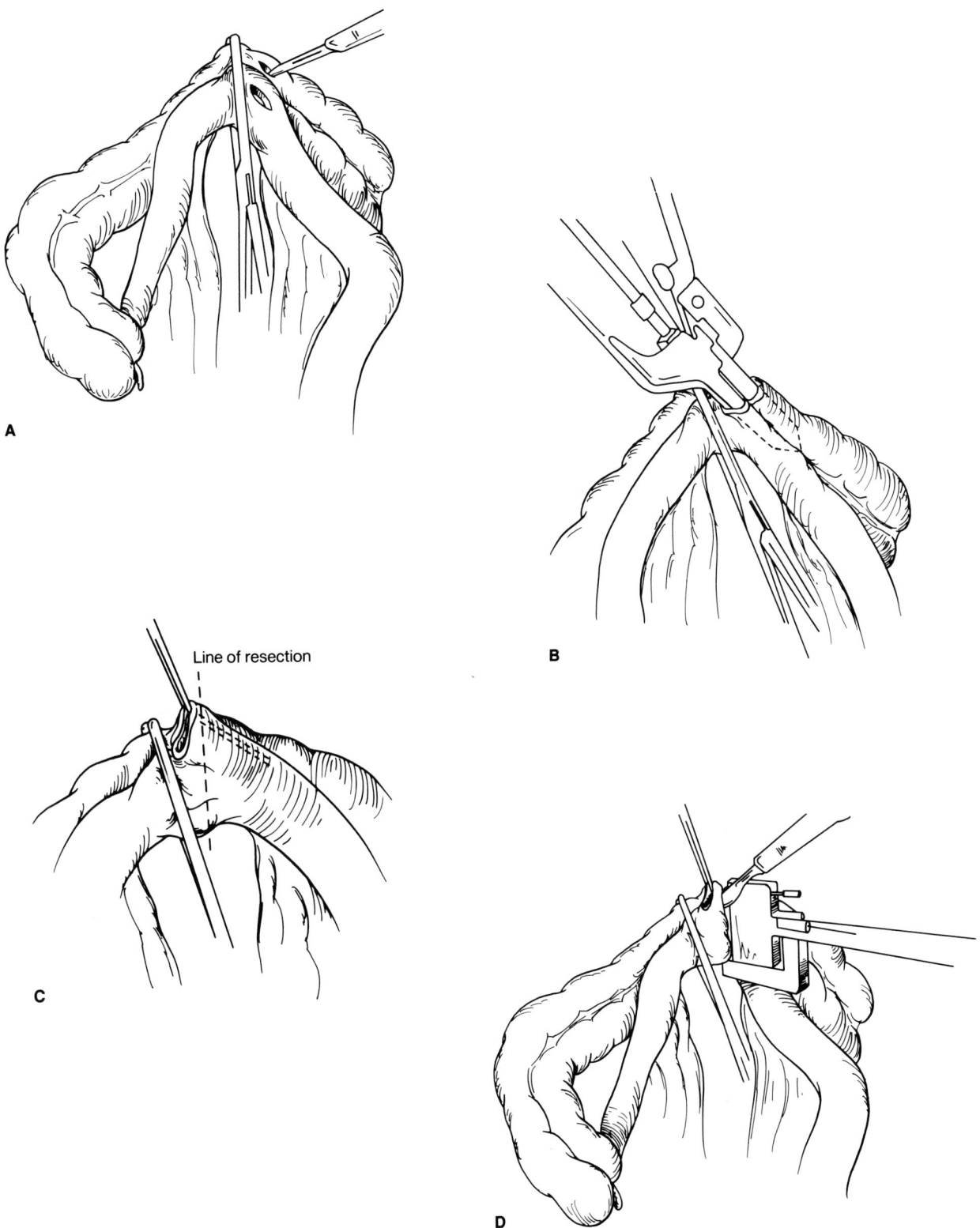

Figure 41-4. Technique for rapid resection of injured colon using stapling devices. **(A)** Right colon is fully mobilized after its blood supply is controlled, and two small enterotomies are made on the antimesenteric side of the bowel to be anasotomosed. **(B)** Insertion and firing of stapler into proximal and distal limbs. **(C)** Completed anastomosis before resection. **(D)** Simultaneous closure of enterotomy, completion of anastomosis, and resection of injured bowel.

closed with a second stapling instrument. The mesenteric defect is closed with a continuous absorbable suture, taking care to place the sutures only in the peritoneal membrane to avoid damage to nutrient mesenteric vessels.

A manually sutured anastomosis can also be constructed, although this usually requires more time. A two-layered intestinal anastomotic technique is preferred, using a continuous absorbable suture for the inner mucosal–submucosal layer and interrupted sutures for the outer serosal layer. The anastomosis is ordinarily constructed in an end-to-end manner, although an end-to-side or even a side-to-side anastomosis may be more easily fashioned. The mesenteric defect should be closed as described for the stapled anastomosis.

STOMA FORMATION. In some cases, it is advisable to create an intestinal stoma to divert the fecal stream and thereby avoid the potential for postoperative intraabdominal fecal spillage. It is generally considered safer in the acute setting to divert the fecal stream whenever there is any concern that the intestinal anastomosis will fail to heal. Circumstances such as circulatory shock, extensive contamination, or other significant medical conditions or injuries may impair the normal healing processes (see list in Resection). Although the complications of colostomy closure can be significant, it is often more prudent in the acute setting to divert the fecal stream if such circumstances exist. The ostomy can be constructed as an end-colostomy or as a loop colostomy.

END-COLOSTOMY. For an end-colostomy, the proximal end of the colon that will drain the fecal stream externally is closed securely, usually with a stapler. An appropriate area for colostomy exit is chosen on the anterior abdominal wall lateral to the midline. The location should be as far lateral as possible to avoid the possibility that the ostomy bag will communicate with the midline laparotomy incision. An effort should be made to locate the stoma away from the patient's belt line. The skin is grasped with a clamp in the center of the desired exit site, and the skin is lifted from the patient. With the scalpel, the surgeon cleanly excises a 1- to 2-inch diameter button of skin by slicing the blade in a head-to-toe direction tangential to the abdominal wall. By using a head-to-toe orientation for this cut, a circle usually results because of the horizontal tension provided by the abdominal wall tissues. The opening is deepened through the abdominal wall, making a cruciate incision in the anterior rectus sheath. The rectus muscle and the posterior rectus sheath or peritoneum are divided longitudinally. Two to three fingers should easily pass through the opening in the abdominal wall.

The closed proximal end of the colon is gently brought through the abdominal wall opening. It is secured in place on the undersurface of the abdominal wall with interrupted sutures placed circumferentially, approximating the serosa of the colon to the posterior rectus sheath and parietal peritoneum. Anteriorly, the serosa of the colon is similarly sutured in interrupted fashion to the anterior rectus sheath with absorbable sutures.

Maturation of the stoma can be performed immediately or in a delayed manner. Delayed maturation is useful as a means of expediting the conclusion of the operation to allow for completion of resuscitation or to devote attention to other life- or limb-threatening conditions. Immediate stoma maturation is ideal in the patient who is hemodynamically stable and who requires no other emergent procedures. It is always advisable to complete the intraabdominal portion of the operation and close the abdominal incision before stoma maturation. If there has been gross contamination or shock, the skin of the abdominal wound should remain open with a temporary hemostatic pack left in place. If the skin is closed, the likelihood of a wound infection is high.

Stoma maturation begins by opening the end of the closed-off colon. The mucosa is everted in a Brooke fashion by using a three-point suture that approximates the skin edge, the serosa of the colon just distal to its exit from the anterior rectus sheath, and the cut mucosal edge of the colonic opening. These sutures are continued circumferentially until the entire ostomy is adequately approximated to the skin surface. A temporary ostomy bag can be applied immediately.

The decision as to whether a mucous fistula or a Hartmann's procedure should be performed is usually based on the nature of the injury. In cases in which the distal end of the bowel consists of the distal sigmoid and rectum, it may be impossible to create a mucous fistula. When the distal end is too low to attach to the skin, a Hartmann's procedure is the only solution possible. The distal end is securely oversewn with nonabsorbable sutures or closed with a stapling device. The rectal stump should be marked with a colored nonabsorbable suture, such as polypropylene, to aid in its identification at the time of reanastomosis. Performing a Hartmann's procedure is usually a fairly rapid process, making this ideal in circumstances in which operative expediency is desired because of the patient's acutely critical condition. On the other hand, a Hartmann's procedure creates an intestinal closure line within the abdomen during the patient's early recovery period, albeit protected by virtue of the proximal colostomy. Should the circulation to the wall of the Hartmann's pouch be poor and healing thereby compromised, leakage of the residual Hartmann's pouch contents could result, producing intraab-dominal sepsis. Most important, the later dissection of the Hartmann's pouch for reanastomosis may be difficult because of the enveloping fibrotic reaction; this may be especially difficult when dissecting for the remnant of the splenic flexure in the left subphrenic space. Alternatively, when a mucous fistula is created, its location is obvious, greatly facilitating dissection during reanastomosis.

Construction of a mucous fistula is accomplished in a manner virtually identical to that of the proximal stoma. It is not necessary or desirable, however, to evert the mucosa using the Brooke technique for the mucous fistula. Furthermore, no ostomy bag is necessary over the mucous fistula; a gauze dressing is usually adequate to absorb any drainage.

LOOP COLOSTOMY. A loop colostomy can effectively divert the fecal stream from a distal injury, is easily created through a single opening in the anterior abdominal wall, and can usually be closed at a later date through a local procedure that avoids formal laparotomy (Fig. 41-5). A segment of colon proximal to the injured area is selected that is mobile or can be easily mobilized by dividing the peritoneal reflection. The mesenteric stalk should allow the colon to pass easily through the anterior abdominal wall without tension and without excessive stretch on the vascular supply. Usually, the transverse colon and sigmoid colon are the most mobile regions, and for this reason, they are commonly used in loop colostomy formation. The distal end of the loop may be closed with a stapler to ensure a complete diversion. By using this method, effective proximal diversion may be accomplished more quickly than with end-colostomy and mucous fistula formation, yet the advantages of a Hartmann's procedure are preserved: complete diversion with an absence of internal staple lines, which could leak, and ease of subsequent identification of the distal bowel.

The skin opening through the abdominal wall usually needs to be larger than for a single-barreled ostomy because two lumens need to pass. The selected loop is brought through the skin opening, and an avascular area in the mesentery is identified. A supporting rod of glass or a plastic bridge is placed through this avascular region and secured to the anterior abdominal wall skin with permanent sutures. The peritoneum and fascia are approximated to the bowel wall in a manner similar to that described for end-colostomy. If complete diversion is desired, a stapler can be placed across the distal end of the loop just proximal to its reentry into the abdomen.[63] Care should be taken to ensure that the proximal and distal ends of the loop are clearly identified and are not twisted in passage through the abdominal wall.

Once the loop is brought out and the abdominal cavity is closed, the loop ostomy can be matured. If the patient is hemodynamically unstable, maturation can be delayed, providing the opportunity to deal with more immediately life-threatening conditions. Maturation is performed by incising the loop transversely along the antimesenteric surface of the bowel and approximating the mucosa to the skin with interrupted sutures. Making the transverse incision over the distal part of the intestinal loop results in a greater tendency for eversion of the mucosa around the proximal end of the stoma with less eversion around the mucous fistula end. This can help the ostomy appliance maintain effective diversion of effluent away from the skin.

Primary Repair

Primary repair of colonic injuries was condemned for a number of years owing to the high rate of complications that appeared to result from its use. During the past two decades, there has been a growing trend toward use of primary repair.[64,65] In 1979, investigators published a prospective, randomized clinical trial of primary repair versus colostomy in 286 patients with perforated colon trauma.[66] Patients were excluded from consideration for primary repair and underwent mandatory colostomy if they met one of the criteria previously presented in the list under Resection. All other patients were randomized, with primary closure being performed in 67 and colostomy performed in 72 patients. This study also included the complications that occurred as a result of colostomy closure. Higher wound and abdominal infection rates were noted in the patients randomized to colostomy than in those who underwent primary repair. Furthermore, hospital stay was 6 days longer in patients who underwent colostomy, exclusive of the stay required for subsequent colostomy closure.

A subsequent report indicated that 64% of 137 patients with colon injuries were managed with primary repair, with an 18% complication rate. The presence of shock, transfusion of four or more units of blood, significant contamination, and associated injuries appeared to contribute more to the development of complications than did the method of management. Significantly, there were no disruptions of the suture line in the patients managed by primary closure.[67]

Given the greater severity of tissue trauma necessary to injure the colon through blunt mechanisms, it is not surprising that primary repair of these injuries is accomplished less frequently than with penetrating trauma.[17] Blunt injuries often are associated with significant contusion of the colonic wall and damage to the nutrient mesentery, making primary repair techni-

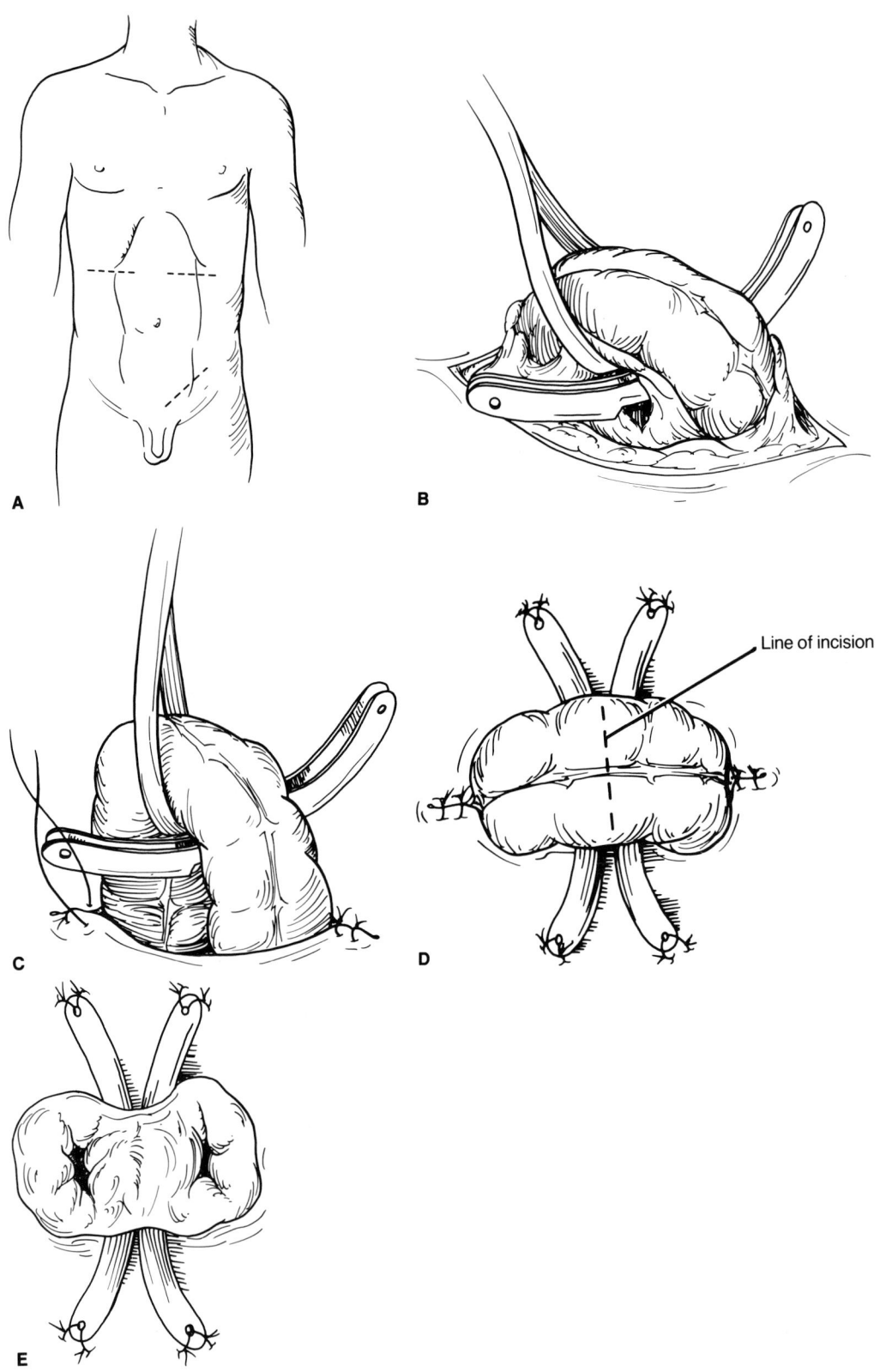

Figure 41-5 Technique for creation of loop colostomy. (**A**) Sites of placement, corresponding to transverse and sigmoid areas of colon. (**B**) Passage of loop of colon through abdominal wall. (**C**) Closure of skin margins. (**D**) Securing plastic bridge to anterior abdominal wall skin. (**E**) Completed colostomy.

cally unsatisfactory. Furthermore, multiple injuries are more commonly associated with blunt trauma.

Exteriorization of the Injured Colon

A technique that is relatively unique to colonic trauma is the exteriorized repair. In this technique, the area of colonic injury is initially repaired in a standard fashion, usually a two-layered intestinal closure or anastomosis; sometimes, this can be accomplished with a stapling device (Fig. 41-6). Because of concerns about the ability of the patient to heal the suture line, either because of the appearance of local tissue or because of the patient's overall critical condition, the repaired segment is exteriorized on the abdominal wall and secured in place over a glass or plastic rod to prevent premature retraction into the abdomen. The exteriorized bowel is kept clean and constantly moist with saline dressings.

If poor healing leads to leakage, the intestinal wound can be converted to a loop colostomy. The leaking area is opened to allow spontaneous mucosal eversion over the exposed bowel wall. Sutured approximation of the mucosal edges to the edges of the skin defect is not usually necessary. Additionally, if complete (non-loop) diversion is desired, the distal end of the exposed bowel can be occluded with an intestinal stapler passed through the exteriorized mesenteric defect. A colostomy bag can then be secured to the converted stoma to collect the fecal stream. The colonic epithelium will ultimately grow to confluence with the skin epithelium, making the final appearance similar to that of an operatively constructed end-colostomy.

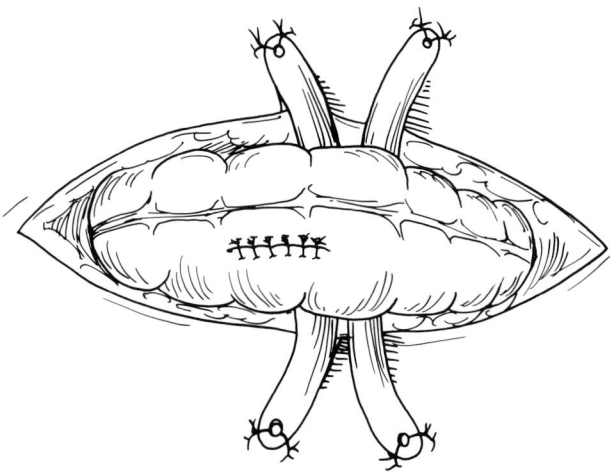

Figure 41-6 Technique for exteriorized repair. The same procedure is followed as described for loop colostomy except that the lumen is not opened. Instead, the repaired area of colon is made visible so that the quality of healing can be assessed.

If leakage has not occurred after 5 to 10 days and if the area shows clear signs of healing, the exteriorized loop can be safely placed back into the abdomen and the fascial defect closed. Reviews of colonic trauma indicate that this method of management is not as commonly employed as colostomy or primary closure, ranging from 9% to 15% of cases.[65,67,68] Complication rates have been reported as high as 40%.[67] A wide range of success rates in terms of colostomy avoidance have been reported, ranging from 22% to 77%. Most authors report success for two thirds to three quarters of patients so treated.[16,65,67,69–72]

Rectal Injuries

Rectal injuries require proximal diversion of the fecal stream with a colostomy (Fig. 41-7). Depending on location, the rectal injury itself may be reparable. Rectal injuries above the peritoneal reflection should be repaired, with proximal diversion. Injuries below the peritoneal reflection are often difficult to repair, especially if associated with a pelvic fracture and hematoma. In such cases, it may be unwise to release the hematoma to repair the injury. Presacral drainage is usually considered key in such circumstances, with the drains exiting the perineum. Although Penrose drains were used for this purpose for a number of years, most believe that closed suction drainage is preferable.[73]

Many trauma surgeons believe it is important to irrigate the distal rectal lumen to clear fecal contents. Potential contamination of the pelvis through the rectal wound could be minimized if the bacterial load is reduced through this maneuver. During the Vietnam conflict, investigators were able to demonstrate a reduction in morbidity of military rectal wounds from 72% to 10% and a drop in mortality from 22% to 0% by using distal washout.[74] Others showed significant benefit using rectal washout in civilian rectal injuries.[75] If a loop colostomy has been created, the distal washout can easily be performed by inserting a Foley catheter into the bowel lumen distal to the staple line (Fig. 41-8).

WOUND MANAGEMENT

Although prophylactic antibiotics are effective in reducing the incidence of wound infections in clean-contaminated cases, they appear to have little effect in colon trauma. Therefore, leaving the operative wound open for delayed primary closure or healing by secondary intention is appropriate, especially in cases of severe contamination. Such an approach is especially fitting for the patient in whom a temporary colostomy

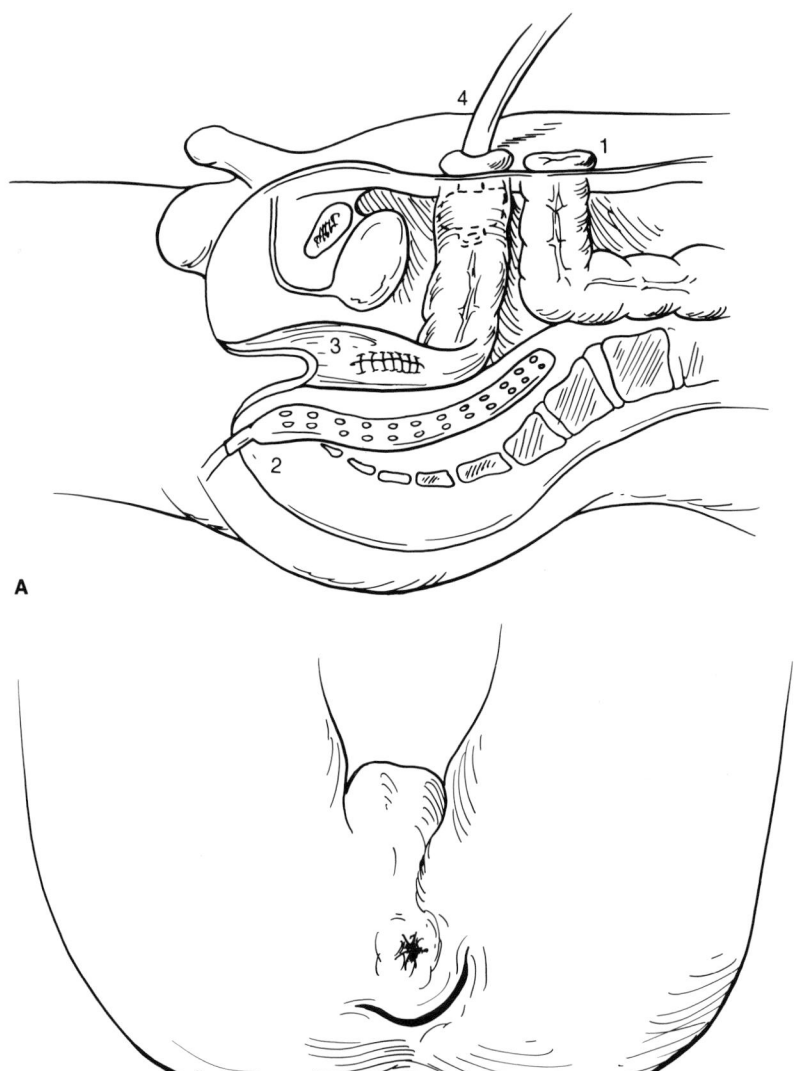

A

B

Figure 41-7 The steps required for effective management of rectal trauma below the peritoneal reflection. (**A**) 1. The fecal stream is diverted with a proximal colostomy. 2. Presacral drainage with closed suction drains is established by way of a blunt presacral dissection and perianal incisions. 3. The rectal injury is repaired. 4. A distal washout of the rectal contents is performed using a Foley catheter temporarily placed in the mucous fistula. (**B**) Site of perianal incisions used for presacral drains.

was created because the midline wound can be revised and closed at the time of elective colostomy closure.

POSTOPERATIVE MANAGEMENT

Postoperatively, the patient recovering from colorectal trauma should be carefully observed for early signs of wound, intraabdominal, or intrapelvic infection. Although some recommend prolonged courses of antibiotics in patients who have heavy contamination, there are no convincing scientific data to indicate that such an approach is effective. Prolonged courses of ineffective prophylaxis are likely to promote the development of infections resistant to the antibiotics in use. If the patient who has undergone primary closure begins to show signs of infection, the wound should be in-

spected. When the wound does not appear to be responsible for the infectious condition, a CT scan of the abdomen should be performed to look for a septic source. Any fluid collections should be drained. If percutaneous CT-guided drainage is not possible or effective, operative drainage should be performed. Enteral nutrition can usually be provided at an early postoperative date, with results equal to or better than parenteral nutrition.[76]

The patient who has sustained colorectal trauma is at high risk for development of a fecal fistula. This complication usually occurs within the first several weeks after primary repair and occasionally occurs after colostomy closure. When a fecal fistula develops, stool drains from the midline abdominal incision or other abdominal wall opening, such as a bullet wound or a prior ostomy site. The fistula exit site should be cared for by

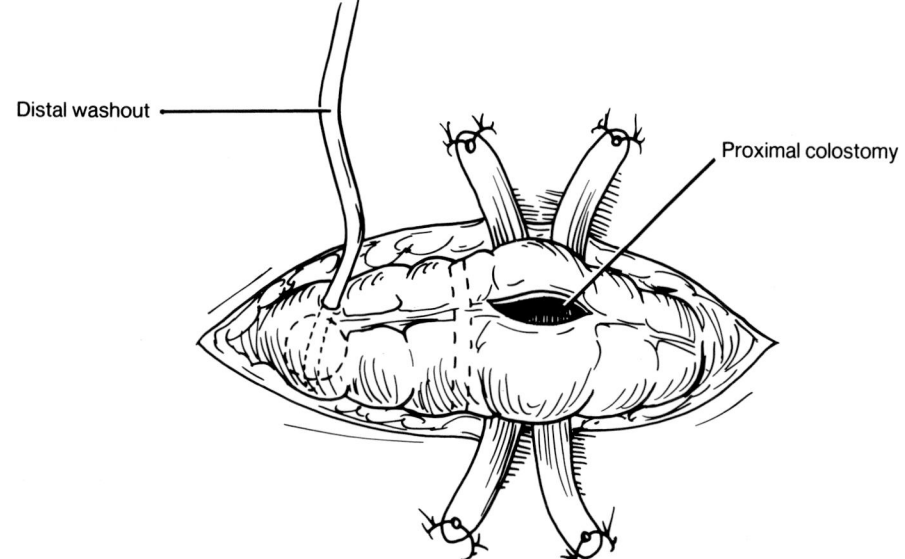

Distal washout

Proximal colostomy

Figure 41-8 Performance of a distal washout for rectal trauma using a loop colostomy for fecal diversion. The bowel lumen is closed with the stapling device. A Foley catheter is placed into the lumen distal to the staple line for irrigation, and the colostomy is fashioned proximal to the staple line for diversion.

ensuring that the fecal effluent is collected in a way that protects the skin. An ostomy bag is usually effective, but in the case of a large raw wound, frequent cleansing is necessary to keep the level of surface contamination at a minimum. With proper care and nutrition, most fecal fistulas heal without surgical therapy. Failure to heal is indicative of tract epithelialization, distal obstruction, or retained foreign body.

COLOSTOMY COMPLICATIONS AND CLOSURE

Although it is clear that mandatory colostomy for all forms of colon trauma is no longer a valid concept, it is also apparent that the risks of colostomy closure may not be as severe as previously thought.[66,77] In one experience, there was no mortality and a 4.9% incidence of major morbidity among 121 patients who underwent closure of a colostomy that had been created for trauma.

Investigators reported on an experience with extremely early colostomy closure.[78] Twenty-nine patients with rectal injuries underwent contrast enema between 5 and 10 days after injury. Only eight patients demonstrated persistent leakage from the rectal injury. Sixteen patients with normal contrast enemas underwent colostomy closures during the same admission, 9 to 19 days after injury. Two of these patients developed a fecal fistula; both underwent a simple closure of the stoma. The authors believe that the patients who underwent a stoma resection with end-to-end anastomosis avoided the complication of a fecal fistula

because the closure involved healthier, uninflamed tissue. The costs of performing a simpler operation versus a resection and anastomosis must be weighed in any comparison of the two techniques. If a slightly more extensive operation is required to provide colostomy closure at an earlier date, overall health care costs, in terms of days of hospitalization and stoma supplies and accessories, may actually be reduced.

REFERENCES

1. Prakash UBS. Shushruta of ancient India. Surg Gynecol Obstet 1978;146:263.
2. Elfin DC, Ward WE. Gunshot wounds of the abdomen: a survey of 238 cases. Ann Surg 1943;118:780.
3. Oberhelman HA, Le Count ER. Peace time bullet wounds of the abdomen. Arch Surg 1936;32:373.
4. Wallace C. A study of 1,200 cases of gunshot wounds of the abdomen. Br J Surg 1917;4:679.
5. Gordon-Taylor G. The abdominal injuries of warfare. Bristol, UK, John Wright & Sons, 1939:24.
6. Jolly DW. Field surgery in total war. New York, Paul B. Hoeber, 1941:186.
7. Division of Medical Sciences of the National Research Council. Abdominal and genito-urinary injuries. Philadelphia, WB Saunders, 1943:78.
8. Ogilvie WH. Abdominal wounds in the western desert. Surg Gynecol Obstet 1944;78:224.
9. Office of the Surgeon General. Circular Letter No. 178, October 28, 1943.
10. Nance FC. Injuries to the colon and rectum. In: Matton KL, Moore EE, Feliciano DV, eds. Trauma. Norwalk, CT, Appleton & Lange, 1988:496.

11. Woodhall JP, Ochsner A. The management of perforating injuries of the colon and rectum in civilian practice. Surgery 1951;29:305.

12. Isaacson JE Jr, Buck RL, Kable HR. Changing concepts of treatment of traumatic injuries of the colon. Dis Colon Rectum 1961;4:168.

13. Axelrod AJ, Hanley PH. Treatment of perforating wounds of the colon and rectum: a re-evaluation. South Med J 1967;60:811.

14. Grablowsky OM, Gage JO, Ray JE, et al. Traumatic colonic and rectal injuries. Dis Colon Rectum 1973;16:296.

15. LoCicero J, Tajima T, Drapanas T. A half century of experience in the management of colon injuries: changing concepts. J Trauma 1975;15:575.

16. Burch JM, Brock JC, Gevirtzman L, et al. The injured colon. Ann Surg 1986;203:701.

17. Bugis SP, Blair NP, Letwin ER. Management of blunt and penetrating colon injuries. Am J Surg 1992;163:547.

18. Bartizal JF, Boyd DR, Folk FA, et al. A critical review of management of 392 colonic and rectal injuries. Dis Colon Rectum 1974;17:313.

19. Ganchow MI, Lavenson GS, McNamara JJ. Surgical management of traumatic injuries of the colon and rectum. Arch Surg 1970;100:515.

20. Strate RG, Grieco JG. Blunt injury to the colon and rectum. J Trauma 1983;23:384.

21. Vannix RS, Carter R, Hinshaw DN, et al. Surgical management of colon trauma in civilian practice. Am J Surg 1963;106:364.

22. Kavin H, Sinicrope F, Esker AH. Management of perforation of the colon at colonoscopy. Am J Gastroenterol 1992;87:161.

23. Martin RR, Burch JM, Richardson R, Mattox KL. Outcome for delayed operation of penetrating colon injuries. J Trauma 1991;31:1591.

24. Alexander P, Schuman E, Vetto RM. Perforation of the colon in the immunocompromised patient. Am J Surg 1986;151:557.

25. Abizeid G, Lepoutre B, Ampe J. Delayed perforation of the sigmoid colon following closed abdominal trauma: apropos of a case report. Acta Chir Belg 1992;92:172.

26. Grandic L, Kukoc M, Vidak V, Saric D, Kostiov D, Aras N. Perforation of the small intestine as a sequela of blunt injuries of the abdomen during a 12-year period. Acta Chir Iugosl 1989;36(Suppl 2)724.

27. Johnson GA, Baker J. Colonic perforation following mild trauma in a patient with Crohn's disease. Am J Emerg Med 1990;8:340.

28. Usui Y, Sasaki S, Hirai R, Kishi A. Sigmoid colon obstruction due to blunt abdominal trauma: a case report. Acta Med Okayama 1991;45:61.

29. Sirinek KR, Page CP, Root HD, Levine BA. Is exploratory celiotomy necessary for all patients with truncal stab wounds? Arch Surg 1990;125:844.

30. Phillips T, Sclafani SJ, Goldstein A, Scalea T, Panetta T, Shaftan G. Use of the contrast-enhanced CT enema in the management of penetrating trauma to the flank and back. J Trauma 1986;26:593.

31. McAllister E, Perez M, Olson SM, et al. Is triple contrast CT scanning useful in the selective management of stab wounds to the back? 24th Annual Meeting of the Western Trauma Association, Crested Butte, CO, March 3, 1994.

32. Fischer RP, Beverlin BC, Engrav LH, Benjamin CI, Perry JF Jr. Diagnostic peritoneal lavage: fourteen years and 2,586 patients later. Am J Surg 1978;136:701.

33. Oreskovich MP, Carrico CJ. Stab wounds of the anterior abdomen: analysis of a management plan using local wound exploration and quantitative peritoneal lavage. Ann Surg 1983;198:411.

34. Thal ER. Evaluation of peritoneal lavage and local exploration in lower chest and abdominal stab wounds. J Trauma 1977;17:642.

35. DiGiacomo JC, Schwab CW, Rotondo MFR, Kauder D, Angood PA, McGonigal M. Who warrants exploration for a gluteal gunshot wound? 24th Annual Meeting of the Western Trauma Association, Crested Butte, CO, February 28, 1994.

36. Mirvis SE, Gens DR, Shanmuganathan K. Rupture of the bowel after blunt abdominal trauma: diagnosis with CT. AJR 1992;159:1217.

37. Rehm CG, Sherman R, Hinz TW. The role of CT scan in evaluation for laparotomy patients with stab wounds of the abdomen. J Trauma 1989;29:446.

38. Fischer RP, Miller-Crotchett P, Reed RL. Gastrointestinal disruption: the hazard of nonoperative management in adults with blunt abdominal injury. J Trauma 1988;28:1445.

39. Sommers HM. Indigenous microbiota in the human. In: Howard BJ, Simmons RL, eds. Surgical infectious diseases, ed 2. Norwalk, CT, Appleton & Lange, 1988:15.

40. Dübgen R. Prophylaxis of infections with antibiotics in colorectal and gastroduodenal operations and appendectomies: a validation of clinical trials. Dissertation, Hamburg University Medical School, Hamburg, Germany, 1988.

41. Condon RE, Wittman DH. The use of antibiotics in general surgery. Curr Prob Surg 1991;28:803.

42. Burke JF. Effective period of preventive antibiotic action in experimental incisions and dermal lesions. Surgery 1961;50:161.

43. Polk HC, Lopez-Mayor JR. Postoperative and wound infection: a prospective study of determinant factors and prevention. Surgery 1969;66:97.

44. Stone HN, Haney BB, Kolb LD, et al. Prophylactic and preventive antibiotic therapy: timing, duration, and economics. Ann Surg 1978;189:691.

45. Bernard HR, Cole WH. The prophylaxis of surgical infection: the effect of prophylactic antimicrobial drugs on the incidence of infection following potentially contaminated operations. Surgery 1964;56:151.

46. Stone HH, Hooper CA, Kolb LD, et al. Antibiotic prophylaxis in gastric, biliary and colonic surgery. Ann Surg 1976;184:443.

47. Nichols RL, Condon RE, Gorbach SL, et al. Efficacy of pre-

operative antimicrobial preparation of the bowel. Ann Surg 1972;176:227.

48. Goldring J, McNaught W, Scott A, et al. Prophylactic oral antibiotic agents in elective colon surgery: a controlled trial. Lancet 1975;2:7943.

49. Matheson DM, Arabi Y, Baxter-Smith D, et al. Randomised multicentre trial of oral bowel preparation and antimicrobials for elective colorectal operations. Br J Surg 1978;65:597.

50. Fullen WD, Hunt J, Altemeier WA. Prophylactic antibiotics in penetrating wounds of the abdomen. J Trauma 1972;12:282.

51. Thadepalli J, Gorbach SL, Broido PW, et al. Abdominal trauma, anaerobes, and antibiotics. Surg Gynecol Obstet 1973;173:270.

52. Burke JF. Fundamentals of wound management: infection. East Norwalk, CT, Appleton-Century-Crofts, 1977.

53. Miles AA, Miles BM, Burke JF. The value and duration of defense reactions of the skin to primary lodgement of bacteria. Br J Exp Pathol 1957;38:79.

54. Miles AA. Natural resistance to infection. Ann NY Acad Sci 1956;66:356.

55. Livingston DH, Shumate CR, Polk HC Jr, et al. More is better: antibiotic management after hemorrhagic shock. Ann Surg 1988;208:451.

56. Ericsson CD, Fischer RP, Rowlands BJ, et al. Prophylactic antibiotics in trauma: the hazards of underdosing. J Trauma 1989;29:1356.

57. Reed RL, Ericsson CD, Wu A, et al. The pharmacokinetics of prophylactic antibiotics in trauma. J Trauma 1992;32:21.

58. Brook I. Inoculum effect. Rev Infect Dis 1989;11:361.

59. Nichols RL. Bowel preparation. In: American College of Surgeons. Care of the surgical patient, vol 2. Elective care. New York, Scientific American, 1988–1993:6.

60. Weigelt JA, Easley SM, Thal ER, Palmer LD, Newman VS. Abdominal surgical wound infection is lowered with improved perioperative Enterococcus and Bacteroides therapy. J Trauma 1993;34:579.

61. Mehigan D, Zuidema GD, Cameron JL. The role of systemic antibiotics in operations on the colon. Surg Gynecol Obstet 1981;153:573.

62. Juul P, Merrild U, Kronborg O. Topical ampicillin in addition to systemic antibiotics prophylaxis in elective colorectal surgery. Dis Colon Rectum 1986;29:165.

63. Maull KI, Sachatello CR, Ernst CB. The deep perineal laceration—an injury frequently associated with open pelvic fractures: a need for aggressive surgical management. J Trauma 1977;17:685.

64. Wiener I, Rojas P, Wolma FJ. Traumatic colonic perforation: review of 16 years' experience. Am J Surg 1981;142:717.

65. Nallathambi MN, Ivatury RR, Shah PM, Rao PM, Rohman M, Stahl WM. Penetrating right colon trauma: the

ever diminishing role for colostomy. Am Surg 1987;53:209.

66. Stone HH, Fabian TC. Management of perforating colon trauma: randomization between primary closure and exteriorization. Ann Surg 1979;190:430.

67. George SM Jr, Fabian TC, Mangiante EC. Colon trauma: further support for primary repair. Am J Surg 1988;156:16.

68. Ivatury RR, Gaudino J, Nallathambi MN, Simon RJ, Kazigo ZJ, Stahl WM. Definitive treatment of colon injuries: a prospective study. Am Surg 1993;59:43.

69. Flint LM, Vitale GC, Richardson JD, Polk HC Jr. The injured colon: relationships of management to complications. Ann Surg 1981;193:619.

70. Dang CV, Peter ET, Parks SN, Ellyson JH. Trauma of the colon: early drop-back of exteriorized repair. Arch Surg 1982;117:652.

71. Lou MA, Johnson AP, Atik M, Mandal AK, Alexander JL, Schlater TL. Exteriorized repair in the management of colon injuries. Arch Surg 1981;116:926.

72. Baker LW, Thomson SR, Chadwick SJ. Colon wound management and prograde colonic lavage in large bowel trauma. Br J Surg 1990;77:872.

73. Vitale GC, Richardson JD, Flint LM. Successful management of injuries to the extraperitoneal rectum. Am J Surg 1983;49:159.

74. Lavenson GS, Cohen A. Management of rectal injuries. Am J Surg 1971;122:225.

75. Shannon FL, Moore EE, Moore FA, McCroskey BL. Value of distal colon washout in civilian rectal trauma: reducing gut bacterial translocation. J Trauma 1988;28:989.

76. Moore EE, Jones TN. Benefits of immediate jejunostomy feeding after major abdominal trauma. J Trauma 1986;26:874.

77. Livingston DH, Miller FB, Richardson JD. Are the risks after colostomy closure exaggerated? Am J Surg 1989;158:17.

78. Renz BM, Feliciano DV, Sherman R. Same admission colostomy closure (SACC), a new approach to rectal wounds: a prospective study. Ann Surg 1993;218:279.

79. Fabian TC, Hoefling SJ, Strom PR, et al. Use of antibiotic prophylaxis in penetrating abdominal trauma. Clin Ther 1982;5(Suppl A):38.

80. Moore FA, Moore EE, Mill MR. Preoperative antibiotics for abdominal gunshot wounds. Am J Surg 1983;146:762.

81. Nallathambi MN, Ivatury RR, Shah PM, et al. Aggressive definitive management of penetrating colon injuries: one hundred thirty-six cases with 3.7% mortality. J Trauma 1984;4:500.

82. Gentry LO, Feliciano DV, Lea AS, et al. Perioperative antibiotic therapy for penetrating injuries of the abdomen. Ann Surg 1984;200:561.

83. Dellinger EP, Wertz MJ, Lennard ES, Oreskovich MR. Efficacy of short-course antibiotic prophylaxis after penetrating intestinal injury. Arch Surg 1986;121:23.

Digestive Tract Surgery: A Text and Atlas, edited by Richard H. Bell,
Layton F. Rikkers, and Michael W. Mulholland.
Lippincott-Raven Publishers, Philadelphia, © 1996.

42

Anorectal Disease

Anthony M. Vernava III | *Robert D. Madoff*

ANATOMY

The dentate line is the most important anatomic land-mark in the anorectum (Fig. 42-1). This crenated, circumferential line in the anal canal represents the junction of the well-innervated squamous epithelium of the anoderm and the relatively insensitive rectal mucosa. It is the reference point from which all lesions in the anorectum should be described. Lesions located cephalad to the dentate line tend to be painless, whereas lesions located caudad to the dentate line are painful. There is a transition zone above the dentate line where sensory fibers can extend for up to 2 cm, so some lesions just at or slightly above the dentate line present with pain.

In the submucosa of the anal canal are three prominent cushions from which most symptomatic hemorrhoids arise. These cushions are in the left lateral, right anterior, and right posterior positions. The anal cushions contain arterioles and venules within a connective tissue matrix; they are not varices. The connective tissue enables adherence of the redundant mucosa and submucosa to the deeper internal anal sphincter.

The anal canal is the termination of the alimentary tract and is responsible for fecal continence. The internal sphincter (Fig. 42-2) is a continuation of the circular muscle of the rectum and is responsible for most resting anal tone (involuntary). Lateral to the internal sphincter is the complex of striated, voluntary muscles known collectively as the external anal sphincter. This muscle complex extends cephalad from the perianal skin to the puborectalis muscle, a U-shaped skeletal muscle that originates at the pubis and loops behind the anorectal junction (Fig. 42-3). The puborectalis can be easily appreciated posteriorly on digital rectal examination as the anorectal ring. This muscle contracts anteriorly and superiorly when the patient is asked to squeeze the sphincter muscle. The functional anal canal measures between 2.5 and 4.5 cm in length.

EVALUATION OF THE ANORECTUM

A comprehensive evaluation of anorectal disorders has four components: history, physical examination, endoscopic assessment, and roentgenographic tests. The examination consists of inspection, palpation, anoscopy, and endoscopy.

Examination of the anorectum can be done with the patient in either the left lateral decubitus or the prone jackknife position; the latter is preferable because it allows a more thorough and complete examination. The left lateral decubitus position is acceptable for a patient who is unable to tolerate the prone position. Inspection reveals skin tags, dermatitis, and external and prolapsed internal hemorrhoids. Anal fissures, typically located just inside the anal verge, are diagnosed by everting the anus with opposing traction on the buttocks. If a painful condition such as fissure or abscess is present, digital examination and endoscopy are deferred until the problem is treated. Internal examination rarely is helpful under these circumstances and never should be performed when it causes acute pain. Affected patients should undergo examination under anesthesia. Gentle digital examination with a well-lubricated index finger notes sphincter tone, mucosal integrity, and the presence or absence of any masses, tenderness, or fluctuation. Anoscopy is a mandatory component of the anorectal examination that allows optimal visualization of the entire anal canal. Rigid or (preferably) flexible proctosigmoidoscopy then should be

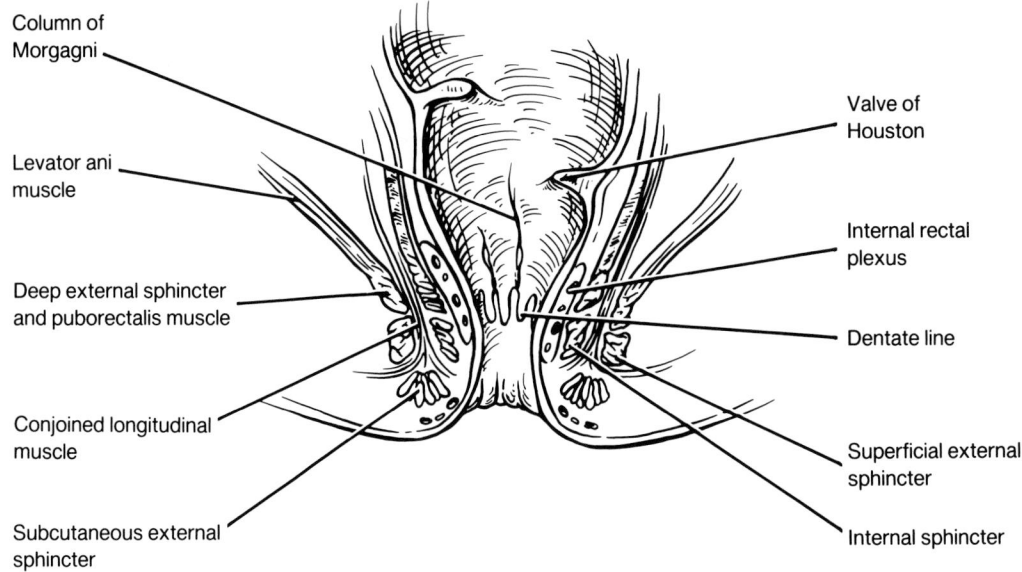

Column of
Morgagni

Levator ani
muscle

Deep external sphincter
and puborectalis muscle

Conjoined longitudinal
muscle

Subcutaneous external
sphincter

Valve of
Houston

Internal rectal
plexus

Dentate line

Superficial external
sphincter

Internal sphincter

Figure 42-1   Anatomy of the anal sphincters.

performed after preparation with one or two mild saline or Phospho-Soda enemas.

ANESTHESIA

Good anesthesia is an essential component of anorectal surgery. Local anesthesia with or without intravenous sedation; regional anesthesia, including caudal, epidural, and spinal blockade; and general anesthesia all can be used for anorectal operations. The selection of the particular anesthetic technique depends on the patient's condition, the specific operation planned, the patient's frame of mind, and the planned positioning of the patient.

Local anesthesia with intravenous sedation is ide-

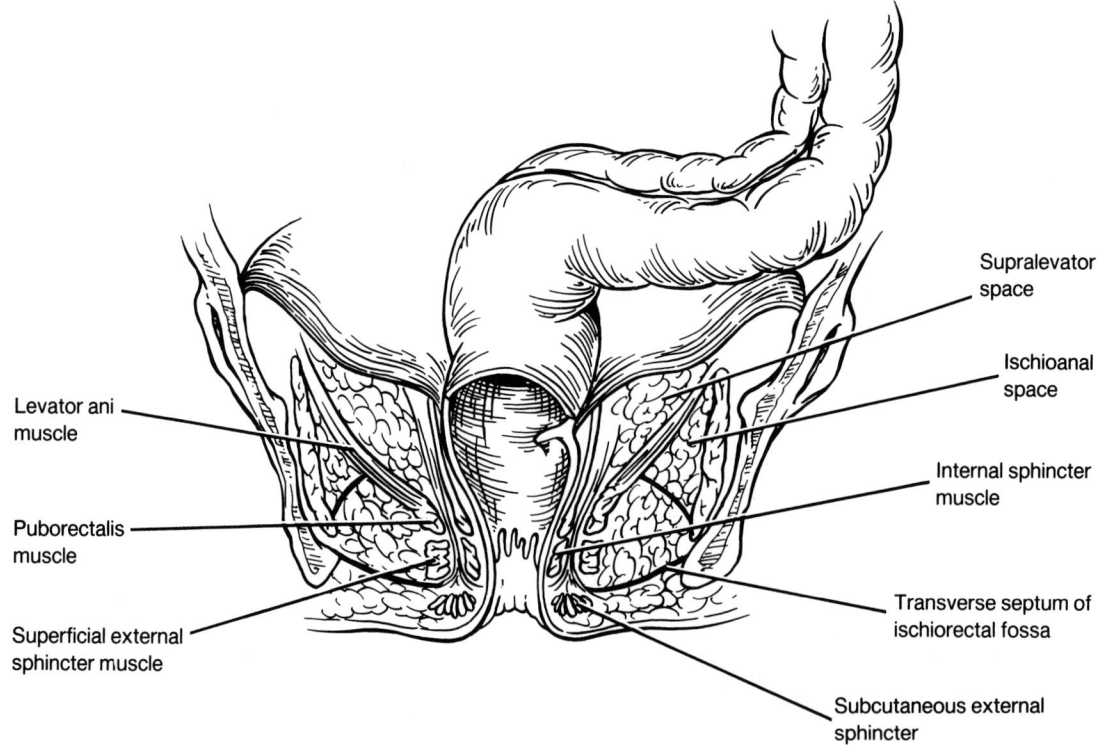

Levator ani
muscle

Puborectalis
muscle

Superficial external
sphincter muscle

Supralevator
space

Ischioanal
space

Internal sphincter
muscle

Transverse septum of
ischiorectal fossa

Subcutaneous external
sphincter

Figure 42-2   Anal canal with perianal spaces.

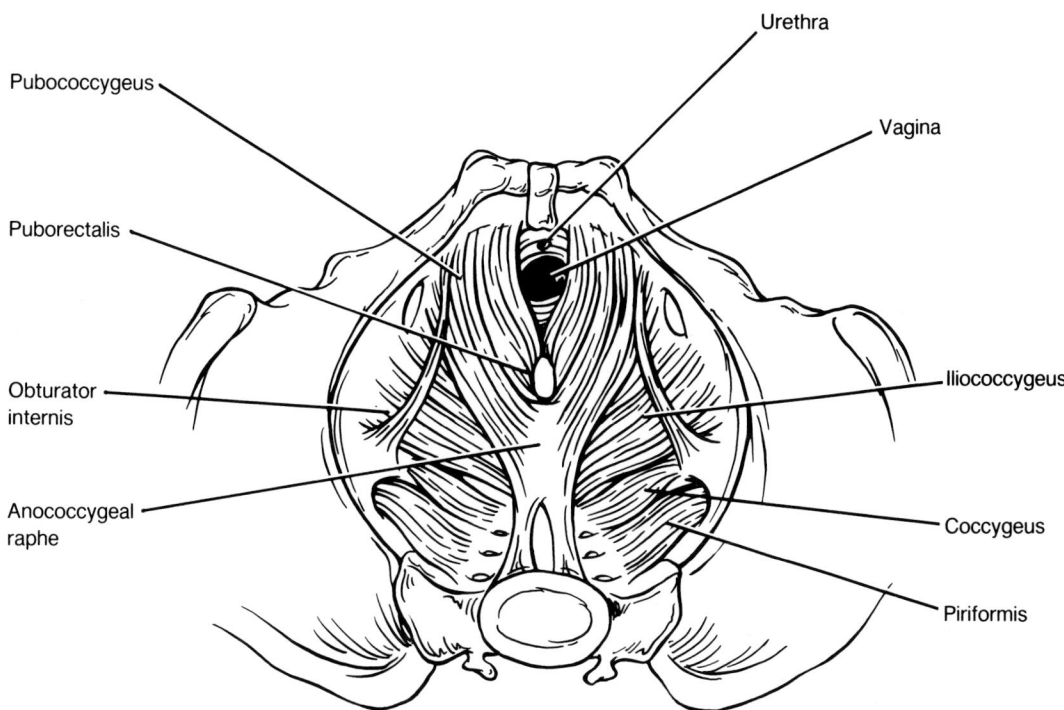

Figure 42-3 Muscular components of the pelvic floor.

ally suited to the performance of many anorectal operations. Benign anorectal conditions, including thrombosed external hemorrhoids, internal hemorrhoids, anal fissure, fistula in ano, and small abscesses, can be managed in this way. The anesthetic agents of choice are lidocaine and bupivacaine. Both are amide compounds that undergo hepatic degradation. Lidocaine is metabolized rapidly and, therefore, is effective for shorter periods, whereas bupivacaine is metabolized more slowly. The addition of epinephrine to the anesthetic prolongs efficacy, delaying absorption by constriction of capillaries.

Because injection of the anesthetic agent into the perianal tissues is painful, intravenous sedation with short-acting agents such as midazolam, fentanyl, or propofol frequently is used. Injection is accomplished using a 25- or 27-gauge needle with a small syringe. The injection should proceed slowly to minimize discomfort.

Caudal anesthesia is well suited for anorectal surgery as a "low" epidural anesthetic placed into the sacral or caudal canal. It is preferred over epidural anesthesia because of the decreased risk of perforation of the dura and spinal headache. Because caudal anesthetics can be placed with the patient in the prone position, repositioning is not necessary. Caudal anesthesia is associated with failure rates as high as 10% and can have a variable level of anesthetic effect. It also carries an increased risk of toxicity compared to epidural and spinal anesthesia because of the high rate of systemic absorption of the anesthetic.

Epidural anesthesia, the injection of an anesthetic into the epidural space, is used frequently for lower abdominal operations but less often for anorectal operations than is caudal anesthesia. The length of effective anesthesia depends on the specific anesthetic used. The primary advantage of epidural anesthesia over spinal anesthesia is the ability to leave a catheter in place so that repeated dosing is possible during the operation. The catheter also can be left in position after the operation for postoperative pain relief.

Spinal anesthesia is achieved by the injection of a local anesthetic into the subarachnoid space. Muscle relaxation and pain relief are excellent with this technique. The major disadvantage of spinal anesthesia is the 3% to 5% risk of postoperative headache caused by cerebrospinal fluid leakage from the needle placed through the dura. The risk of postoperative headache decreases with decreasing size of the needle.

HEMORRHOIDS

Hemorrhoids are diseased variants of highly specialized vascular cushions in the anal canal that are composed of arterioles and venules wrapped in a thickened submucosa and connective tissue.[1,2] The anal cushions are part of the normal anatomy and are located in the left lateral, right posterior, and right anterior positions. Their presumed function is to aid in fecal continence. About 5% of the US population complains of symptoms related to hemorrhoids.[3] All age groups are affected, although the condition occurs most commonly in middle age (45 to 65 years); it is unusual in those younger than 20 years and declines in incidence in those older than 65 years.[3] There is no sex predilection. Blacks are affected less frequently than are whites.[3] The frequency of symptomatic hemorrhoids increases with higher socioeconomic status.[3]

Despite extensive investigation, the etiology of hemorrhoids remains unknown. Suggested theories include varicose vein formation,[4] vascular hyperplasia, portal hypertension,[5] increased anal canal pressure due to internal sphincter abnormality,[6] and chronic straining.[1] The most widely accepted theory is based on gradual downward sliding of the anal cushions.[1] Downward sliding results from weakening of the connective tissue securing the anal cushions due to chronic straining.

The classic association of symptomatic hemorrhoids with chronic constipation has been called into question; the two conditions are not necessarily related.[3,7] Pregnancy is associated with the development and exacerbation of hemorrhoids due to increased abdominopelvic pressure resulting in a relative obstruction of venous return. Portal hypertension is responsible for the development of rectal varices and rectal bleeding, but does not increase the risk of symptomatic hemorrhoids.[8]

Hemorrhoids are classified by their location relative to the dentate line. External hemorrhoids arise from the inferior venous plexus below the dentate line. Internal hemorrhoids arise from the superior hemorrhoidal plexus above the dentate line. External hemorrhoids are covered with innervated squamous epithelium, whereas internal hemorrhoids are lined with insensitive mucosa. Coexisting internal and external hemorrhoids are referred to as mixed hemorrhoids. Further classification of internal hemorrhoids is based on their degree of mucosal prolapse. First-degree hemorrhoids bulge into the lumen of the anal canal; they can bleed but do not prolapse, and are diagnosed best by anoscopy. Second-degree hemorrhoids prolapse outside the anal canal during defecation but spontaneously reduce. Third-degree hemorrhoids are larger still, prolapse outside the anal canal spontaneously, and require manual reduction. Fourth-degree hemorrhoids are chronically prolapsed outside the anal canal and cannot be reduced.

Thrombosed External Hemorrhoids

A thrombosed external hemorrhoid is a common clinical condition resulting from thrombosis of the inferior venous plexus in the anoderm distal to the dentate line. The disorder presents as a tender, palpable mass at the anal verge, with the degree of pain depending on the size of the underlying thrombosis. The natural history of a thrombosed external hemorrhoid is an abrupt onset of an anal mass with exquisite pain that peaks during the initial 2 days. The mass resolves over the ensuing 6 to 10 days. Most patients have resolution of pain by the fourth day after the onset of symptoms.

Treatment of a thrombosed external hemorrhoid is based on the duration of symptoms. If the thrombosis is acute and the pain is disabling, immediate excision under local anesthesia is necessary. The perianal region is anesthetized with 1% lidocaine or 0.5% bupivacaine with epinephrine at a ratio of 1:200,000. An elliptic incision is made around the hematoma, and the entire external hemorrhoidal plexus is excised. Hemostasis is achieved by electrocoagulation and the wound heals by secondary intention. Relief of pain in most patients is prompt and dramatic. Simple incision of the hemorrhoid with extraction of the clot is discouraged because pain relief is not uniform and recurrent thrombosis is common. A thrombosed external hemorrhoid of several days' duration, already symptomatically improved, is treated best without operation using analgesics, warm sitz baths, and an increase in dietary fiber.

Internal Hemorrhoids

Symptoms of internal hemorrhoids are related to the size of the lesions and the degree of mucosal prolapse. Pain is infrequent unless incarceration, thrombosis, or ulceration is present. Bleeding is the most common symptom; it usually is slight and occurs during or after defecation. In some cases, hemorrhage is significant enough to produce anemia. Blood dripping into the toilet after defecation and bloodstains on the toilet tissue are common complaints. Mucus discharge with soiling of the underwear and pruritus are complaints related to mucosal prolapse of third- and fourth-degree hemorrhoids.

The management of hemorrhoidal disease is directed at relieving symptoms; asymptomatic hemorrhoids do not require treatment. Therapeutic options include conservative dietary management[9,10] and office fixation techniques (rubber band ligation,[11-15] infrared coagulation,[10] sclerotherapy,[16-18] and operative hemorrhoidectomy[19-24]).

The medical management of symptomatic hemorrhoids is directed at reducing straining during defecation by increasing fiber intake and using stool bulking supplements.[9,10] Patients initially are given a daily dietary fiber supplement of psyllium or methylcellulose and are encouraged to increase their daily fluid intake to 8 to 10 8-oz glasses of water. The dosage and frequency of the fiber supplement are adjusted to achieve the desired stool frequency and consistency. Minor abdominal cramping and bloating and increased flatulence can occur during the first few weeks of fiber therapy but gradually resolve over time. Patients also are instructed to improve anal hygiene and to use daily sitz baths for comfort. This conservative approach is ideally suited for patients with grade 1 and small grade 2 internal hemorrhoids.

Rubber Band Ligation

Patients with symptomatic grade 2 internal hemorrhoids usually require some other form of therapy in addition to dietary management. Several office techniques are available that fix the redundant, prolapsing hemorrhoidal tissue in the anal canal, thereby relieving symptoms. Rubber band ligation is the most commonly used procedure in the United States. Injection sclerotherapy and infrared coagulation are other options.[25-28]

Rubber band ligation can be performed in the office without anesthesia and has replaced operative hemorrhoidectomy as the treatment of choice for patients with symptomatic grade 2 and small grade 3 internal hemorrhoids.[11] Coexistent fissure, fistula, anal Crohn's disease, and infection with the human immunodeficiency virus are contraindications to the procedure.[29] Patients with synchronous external thrombosed hemorrhoids, hypertrophic papillae, and troublesome skin tags also should be excluded from rubber band ligation in favor of operative hemorrhoidectomy.

The patient is placed in the prone position and digital examination and anoscopy are performed. An anoscope is positioned and the most prominent hemorrhoid is treated first. An alligator forceps is passed through the hollow drum of the ligator and the redundant mucosa is grasped well above the dentate line (Fig. 42-4). The tissue is drawn into the drum of the ligator until it is taut. The trigger of the instrument is fired, releasing two bands around the apex of the redundant hemorrhoidal tissue. It is not critical to include the entire hemorrhoid in the band for ligation to be successful. In fact, this should be avoided to reduce the risk of full-thickness rectal wall banding with subsequent full-thickness necrosis.

Multiple quadrant banding can be performed safely with minimal patient discomfort.[13,30,31] In the past, some authors recommended banding only a single quadrant on the premise that it was safer and better tolerated than multiple banding. Other authors have reported the banding of as many as three quadrants at a single office visit. The complication rates in the latter reports were no different than for single quadrant ligation. Patients are sent home with instructions to take warm sitz baths and dietary fiber supplements, and to return for an office visit in two or three weeks.

Occasionally, patients experience significant pain after banding, necessitating removal of the band.[32] Usually, severe pain indicates that the band has been placed too low in the anal canal and includes anoderm. When this happens, the band should be removed promptly. A local anesthetic is required and should be injected into

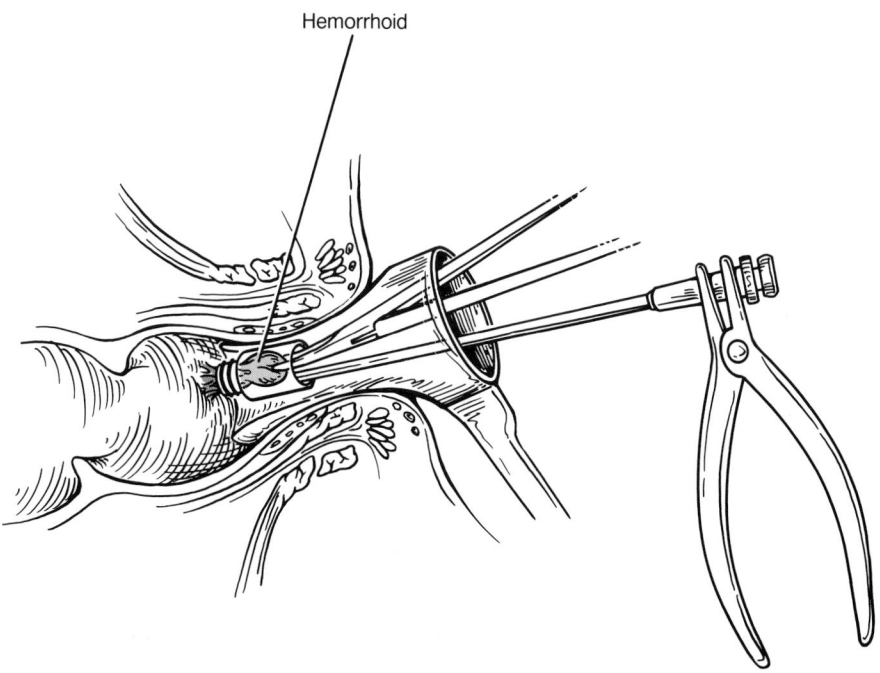

Figure 42-4 Rubber band ligation of internal hemorrhoid. The ligator is passed through the anoscope, and the hemorrhoid is grasped with forceps. The ligator is advanced to the base of the hemorrhoid and fired, placing two bands on the hemorrhoid.

the tissue around the rubber band. The band then can be divided using either scissors or a scalpel.

Minor spotting of blood can occur immediately after banding and continue for several days. Minor bleeding requires no specific therapy. Late hemorrhage occurs in about 1% of patients 7 to 10 days after placement of the band due to sloughing of the hemorrhoidal pedicle. This complication requires reoperation for suture ligation of the bleeding site. Occasionally, the site of bleeding cannot be identified precisely, in which case all three hemorrhoidal excision sites should be oversewn.

Reported complications of rubber band ligation of hemorrhoids also include external hemorrhoidal thrombosis, rubber band slippage, and, rarely, perineal sepsis. External hemorrhoidal thrombosis is seen in about 2% to 3% of patients and should be treated as for spontaneous thrombosis with sitz baths, analgesics, stool softeners, and, occasionally, local excision. The rubber bands themselves can slip off the hemorrhoidal tissues. Slippage usually occurs with the first bowel movement after banding and results from incorrect band placement or defective bands. Repeated banding is required for adequate treatment of symptomatic hemorrhoids.

Necrotizing perineal sepsis also has been reported after rubber band ligation.[33-36] This complication, although rare, is extremely serious and can be fatal. Young men appear to be at greatest risk for necrotizing perineal sepsis. Prodromal symptoms include severe perineal pain, urinary retention, fever, and scrotal edema. Such complaints mandate immediate anorectal examination. If the examination reveals a profoundly tender and boggy anal canal, aggressive surgical therapy is indicated. Broad-spectrum intravenous antibiotics should be administered. Débridement of the area around the band should be performed and the band removed. Fecal diversion with a colostomy can be lifesaving.

The best results with rubber band ligation are achieved in patients with grade 1 and 2 internal hemorrhoids.[12,15,37] Patients with larger hemorrhoids generally require operative hemorrhoidectomy to achieve satisfactory relief of symptoms, although a trial of rubber band ligation may be indicated and can be therapeutic. Failure to achieve remission of symptoms after three banding sessions usually is an indication for operative hemorrhoidectomy.

Injection Sclerotherapy

Symptomatic grade 1 and 2 internal hemorrhoids also can be managed by injection sclerotherapy.[10,16-18] This technique causes fixation of the redundant anorectal mucosa to the underlying tissue by inciting an inflammatory reaction. Injection of the hemorrhoidal pedicle in the submucosal plane is accomplished through an anoscope. No anesthetic is required. If pain is elicited during the procedure, the sclerosant is being injected too low in the anal canal; the injection should be stopped and redirected further cephalad. Effective sclerosing agents include phenol in arachis oil and sodium morrhuate. Complications of sclerotherapy are unusual but include thrombosis, ulceration, and abscess formation. An 8% incidence of bacteremia has been reported with sclerotherapy.[38] The technique is not as effective in eliminating symptoms compared with other treatment options, including rubber band ligation[18] and photocoagulation.[26]

Infrared Coagulation

Infrared coagulation also can be used to treat symptomatic grade 1 and 2 internal hemorrhoids.[25-28] The technique is technically quick and easy to perform; it produces minimal discomfort but requires the use of a special coagulator. The tip of the coagulator is passed through an anoscope and applied to the apex of the hemorrhoid. A trigger device fires the instrument for 1 second. The coagulator "burns" the tissue in the precise location, inciting an inflammatory response that subsequently fixes the tissue. In each hemorrhoidal quadrant, the device must be applied in 4 to 6 different locations around the apex of each hemorrhoid. All three hemorrhoidal quadrants can be treated safely and effectively in a single session. Randomized controlled trials have demonstrated that, for grade 1 and 2 internal hemorrhoids, infrared coagulation has about the same efficacy as rubber band ligation[28] and is better than sclerotherapy.[26]

Cryotherapy

Cryotherapy is mentioned only to caution against its use because of a high rate of complications, including anal stenosis and incontinence, and variable results.[39] It is associated with significant and indiscriminate tissue destruction and a profuse, foul-smelling drainage that can persist for several weeks.

Operative Hemorrhoidectomy

Operative hemorrhoidectomy is reserved for individuals with symptomatic grade 2, 3, and 4 hemorrhoids that fail to improve sufficiently with nonoperative measures.[19-24] About 5% of patients with symptoms attributed to hemorrhoidal disease require operative hemorrhoidectomy.

Most patients undergoing operative hemorrhoidectomy can be treated successfully using local anesthesia with intravenous sedation as described earlier. Local anesthesia without intravenous sedation generally is not used because of pain associated with injection of the local anesthetic. A caudal anesthetic also can be used. General anesthesia is reserved for individuals who refuse local or regional anesthesia. The prone position is preferable and the hips and chest should be well padded.

After local anesthetic has been injected around the anus, attention is directed to the largest hemorrhoidal quadrant. An operating anoscope (usually a Fansler anoscope) is positioned (Fig. 42-5). The hemorrhoid is lifted off the underlying internal sphincter with forceps and excised up to 1 to 2 cm above the dentate line using Metzenbaum scissors. Care is taken to avoid excising too much anal mucosa laterally to prevent tension on the suture lines and postoperative anal stenosis. The mucosa adjacent to the excision site is mobilized using

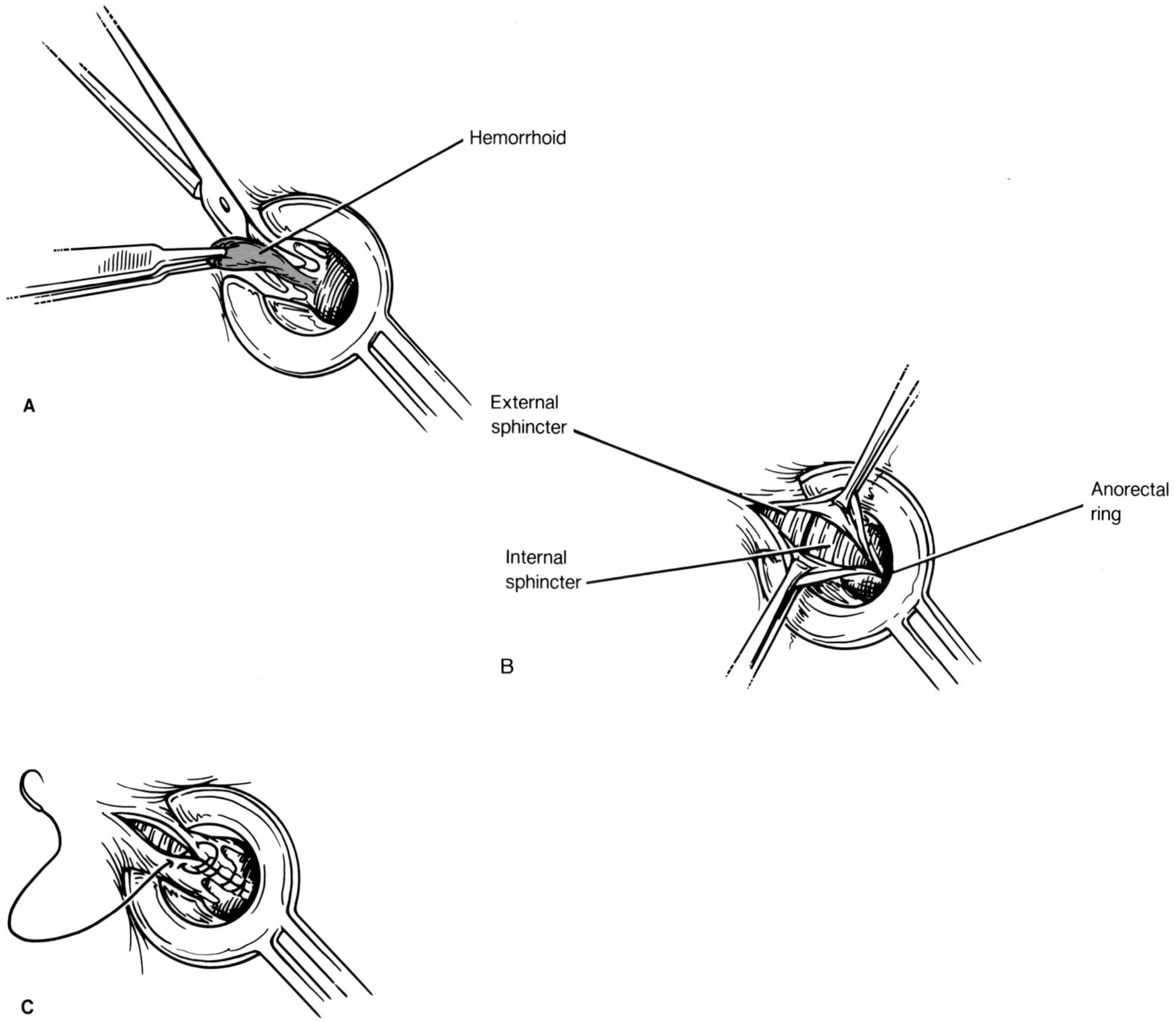

Hemorrhoid

A

External
sphincter

Internal
sphincter

Anorectal
ring

B

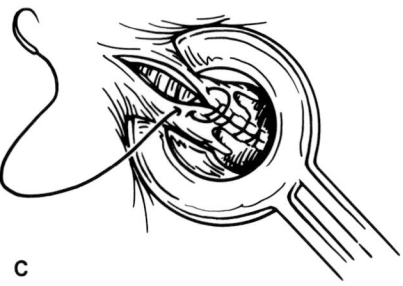

C

Figure 42-5 Operative hemorrhoidectomy. (**A**) With an operating anoscope in place, the largest hemorrhoidal quadrant is excised first. The hemorrhoid is excised beginning in the perianal skin and extending up to 1 to 2 cm above the dentate line. All hemorrhoidal tissue is excised, exposing but not injuring the underlying internal anal sphincter. (**B**) The lateral mucosal edges are gently mobilized to facilitate wound closure. (**C**) The wound is closed with a running absorbable suture. There should be no tension on the wound.

the tip of the scissors to facilitate closure. The operative excision is closed using a running 3-0 absorbable suture, beginning at the hemorrhoidal pedicle and progressing caudad to the perianal skin. All three hemorrhoidal quadrants (right posterior, right anterior, and left lateral) are managed in the same fashion. All external hemorrhoids and skin tags should be treated at the same time. Before the operation is completed, meticulous hemostasis is assured. Bacitracin ointment is placed over the suture lines. The rectum is not packed.

Most patients are discharged from the ambulatory care unit on the day of surgery. Postoperative care includes daily sitz baths, a dietary fiber supplement, and mild analgesics. Constipation must be avoided assiduously because it can lead to fecal impaction. Residual anal tags and mucosal prolapse result from incomplete removal of redundant anoderm and mucosa at operation. Treatment of these anal tags is by local excision in the office. Postoperative mucosal prolapse can be managed by rubber band ligation.

Significant complications after operative hemorrhoidectomy include urinary retention requiring catheterization (3.5% to 15%),[40] constipation, fecal impaction, delayed hemorrhage (1%), mucosal ectropion, anal stricture, and fecal incontinence. Urinary retention can be prevented by minimizing the amount of fluid given during the operation.[40] Constipation and fecal impaction can be prevented by prescribing a dietary fiber supplement, using an analgesic that does not cause constipation, and judiciously administering a gentle laxative if a bowel movement has not occurred by the third postoperative day. Ensuring that the mucosa distal to the dentate line is not sutured can help prevent mucosal ectropion, and preserving anoderm during excision can reduce the incidence of anal stricture. Postoperative delayed hemorrhage is caused by sepsis and ulceration at the ligated hemorrhoidal pedicle. Prevention of this problem depends on meticulous operative technique.

Management of strangulated fourth-degree hemorrhoids is by urgent, closed, three-quadrant hemorrhoidectomy performed in the same manner as described earlier. The operation is safe and produces acceptable results.[41,42] Antibiotics usually are unnecessary.

During pregnancy, hemorrhoidectomy is indicated for irreducible, prolapsed, and thrombosed hemorrhoids. The operation can be performed safely under local anesthesia with the patient in the lateral decubitus or anterolateral position.[43] When fourth-degree hemorrhoids occur during labor or delivery, a hemorrhoidectomy can be performed safely in the immediate postpartum period.[44]

ANAL FISSURE

An anal fissure is a linear tear in the squamous epithelium of the anal canal that can extend from the anoderm to the dentate line. The usual location is in the posterior anal commissure, but fissures also can occur in the anterior midline.[45] Fissures in lateral locations are unusual and mandate biopsy to exclude neoplasm, Crohn's disease, or other inflammatory lesions of the anorectum (eg, syphilis, tuberculosis). Anal fissure is a common disorder that occurs in both sexes at all ages and is the most frequent cause of rectal bleeding in infants. A fissure can be acute or chronic.

Anal fissures typically result from injury to the anal canal during the passage of hard, inspissated stools, but occasionally are caused by diarrheal stools. Anal fissures are associated with "overshoot" contraction of the sphincter mechanism after defecation. This persisting abnormally high pressure results in local ischemia, which leads to persistence of the anal fissure.[46-51]

Pain and bleeding are the most common symptoms of acute anal fissure. The pain, which can be severe, usually begins with defecation and can linger for hours thereafter. Bleeding is minimal and typically limited to spotting. A chronic anal fissure produces less severe pain and bleeding, mucus discharge, and pruritus.

The pain related to an acute fissure is out of proportion to the physical findings. A large "sentinel" tag can be present in chronic fissure. With the patient in the prone position, gentle retraction of the buttocks is performed, revealing the presence of a tear in the lining of the anal canal. In a chronic anal fissure, the fibers of the internal sphincter are visible in the base of the ulcer. Once the diagnosis of fissure is made by inspection, further examination of the anorectum should be deferred.

Anal fissure often is associated with a hypertrophied anal papilla. This can be seen at surgery or on anoscopic examination after the fissure has resolved. Proctosigmoidoscopy should be performed to rule out ulcerative proctitis or Crohn's proctitis. When an anal fissure extends above the dentate line, inflammatory bowel disease is suspected and a complete gastrointestinal evaluation, including colonoscopy and an upper gastrointestinal tract series with small bowel follow-through, should be done before definitive surgical therapy is undertaken.

Treatment

Most anal fissures heal with conservative, nonoperative treatment. The foundation of nonoperative therapy is avoidance of constipation using a high-fiber diet, dietary fiber supplements, and stool softeners. Comfort measures include sitz baths, which provide pain relief by eliminating spasm of the internal sphincter.[52] Occasionally, topical anesthetic creams offer some relief. Medicated suppositories are painful to insert in the presence of an anal fissure and have no therapeutic effect.

Despite the many topical agents and suppositories available for the treatment of fissures, it appears that warm sitz baths and a high-dose daily dietary fiber supplement constitute the most effective treatment protocol. A regimen of warm sitz baths and unprocessed bran resulted in healing of 87% of fissures after 3 weeks of therapy in one prospective study.[53] High-fiber supplements must be taken indefinitely, because recurrence of anal fissures is higher in individuals who discontinue fiber supplementation (68%) compared with those who continue to ingest more than 5 g of unprocessed bran per day (16%) 1 year after successful management of the initial anal fissure.[54]

The indication for operation on an anal fissure is medical intractability. Persistent pain and bleeding after an adequate trial of medical management, usually 3 to 4 weeks, warrants operation. Chronic fissures with a sentinel tag, a hypertrophied anal papilla, or a deep ulcer with exposed internal anal sphincter are more likely to require operation than are acute fissures.[55] Operative management of anal fissures is directed at relieving pain by eliminating internal sphincter spasm and resolving anal stenosis.

Numerous surgical procedures have been used to treat anal fissures, including anal dilatation,[56] excision of the fissure,[57] V-Y anoplasty,[58] and internal anal sphincterotomy.[59] Excision of the fissure is an extensive procedure associated with a large operative wound and incontinence. It is not recommended in the routine surgical management of anal fissure. Excision and V-Y anoplasty closure is better tolerated and has a shorter healing time than excision alone, but requires a more extensive operation. It should be used only in patients who have anal fissures associated with anal stenosis. Anal dilatation is performed in the operating room under general anesthesia. This procedure involves forcefully stretching the sphincter using both hands and tearing the internal anal sphincter muscle. A success rate of 95% has been reported, but 20% of patients are left with some degree of fecal incontinence.[56] Anal dilatation is an uncontrolled method of tearing the muscle and cannot be recommended; more reliable therapies are available. Lateral internal sphincterotomy is the operative treatment of choice for anal fissure. Internal sphincterotomy originally was performed in the posterior midline.[60] It was effective in eliminating symptoms and healing the fissure, but resulted in a keyhole deformity of the anal canal and varying degrees of fecal incontinence. For that reason, more recent authors have advocated division of the internal anal sphincter in the lateral position.[61,62] This modification of the surgical technique retains therapeutic efficacy

and eliminates the keyhole deformity. A subsequent modification of the open, lateral internal sphincterotomy is described later in this chapter.[63]

Internal sphincterotomy is performed in the lateral position of the anal canal (right or left) to prevent a keyhole deformity. Lateral internal sphincterotomy is best performed in an ambulatory surgical unit under monitored local anesthesia. Some surgeons prefer to perform the procedure in the office or emergency department under simple local anesthesia. Local anesthesia with intravenous sedation also can be used for patient comfort. A caudal anesthetic is another alternative. The lateral portion of the operative site and the fissure are infiltrated with a local anesthetic (1% lidocaine plus 0.5% bupivacaine with epinephrine at a ratio of 1:200,000). The operation can be performed using either an open or a closed technique.

In the closed technique, a partial lateral internal sphincterotomy is performed through a small lateral stab wound incision. The sphincterotomy can be performed by inserting the blade into the intersphincteric groove and cutting medially, or by inserting the blade under the mucosa and dividing the internal sphincter laterally (Fig. 42-6). Care must be taken during the latter maneuver to prevent division of the external sphincter muscle. Residual muscle fibers are divided using pressure from the index finger. Hemostasis is achieved with digital pressure.

In the open technique, a radial incision is made in the anoderm at the intersphincteric groove (Fig. 42-7). The internal sphincter is identified, separated from surrounding tissue, and divided with Metzenbaum scissors. The extent to which the internal sphincter is divided varies according to the surgeon's preference and the patient's preexisting fecal continence. For example, a complete internal sphincterotomy would extend cephalad from the intersphincteric groove to the dentate line. Meticulous hemostasis is achieved to prevent a postoperative hematoma and subsequent abscess. The small wound then is closed with an absorbable suture.

After internal sphincterotomy, either open or closed, relief of pain and healing of the fissure usually are prompt. Postoperative care includes sitz baths and mild analgesics.

Complications after internal sphincterotomy are rare and usually can be prevented by familiarity with anorectal anatomy and meticulous surgical technique. Hemorrhage and perianal abscess are unusual. Postoperative hemorrhage occurs in 0.5% of patients, perianal abscess in 1%, thrombosed hemorrhoids in 0.3%, fistula in ano in 0.6%, and hematoma formation in 2.4%. Keyhole deformity is associated with posterior sphincterotomy, which should not be used. Gross fecal incontinence after internal sphincterotomy is rare unless the external anal sphincter is inadvertently divided. There can be a minor change in continence for mucus and

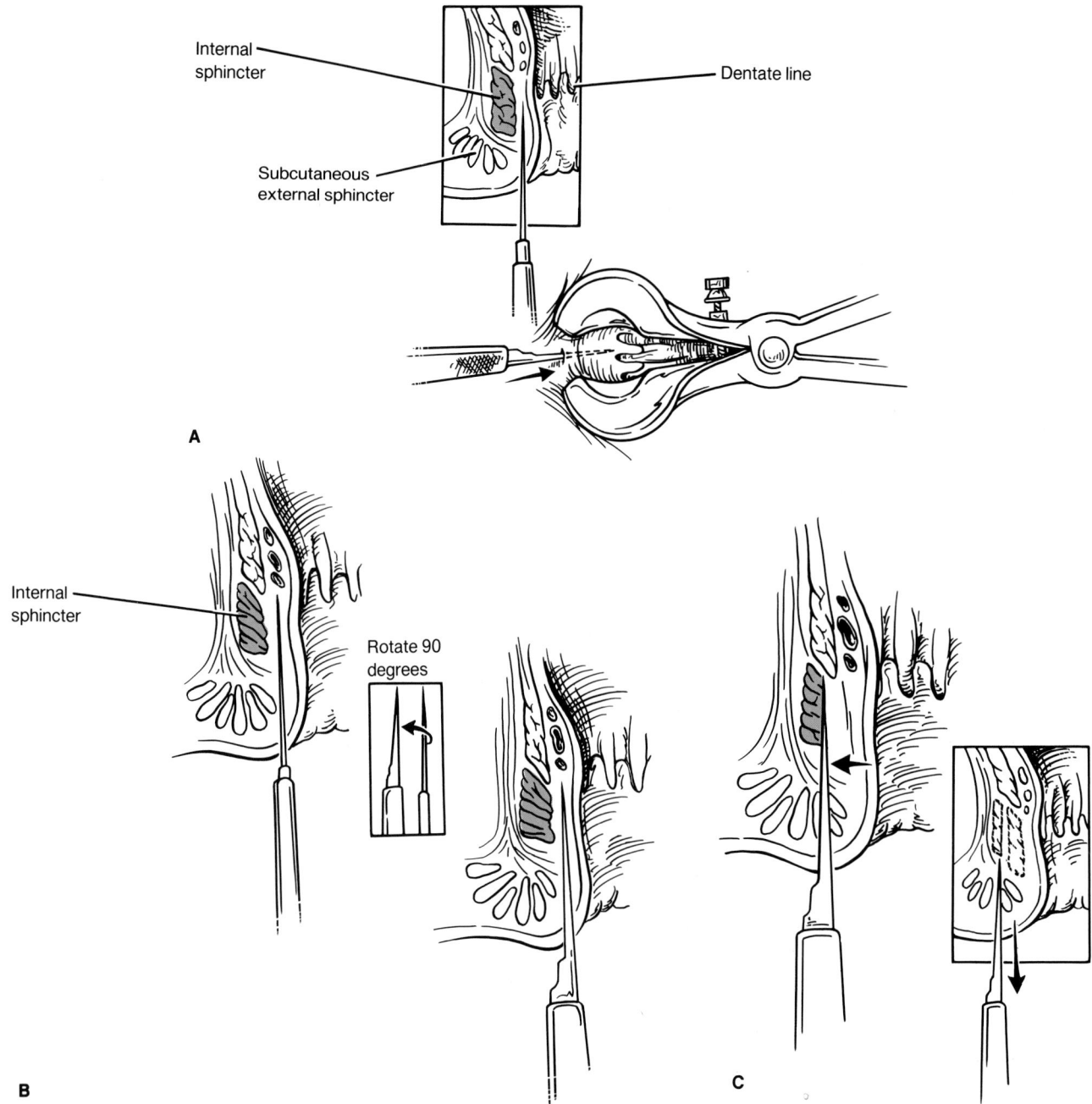

Figure 42-6 Closed lateral internal sphincterotomy. (**A**) With an operative anoscope in place, the intersphincteric groove is palpated. A knife blade is inserted through a small incision into the submucosal plane. (**B**) The knife blade is rotated 90 degrees so that the cutting edge faces the internal anal sphincter. (**C**) Gentle lateral pressure is applied to divide the internal anal sphincter, and the blade is withdrawn. Digital pressure is used to achieve hemostasis.

flatus after sphincterotomy, and patients should be advised of this possibility before operation.[64,65] Recurrence of an anal fissure after lateral internal sphincterotomy occurs in about 2% to 4% of patients.[63,66,67] Conservative therapy is indicated at first, and sphinc-

terotomy is performed again if the fissure fails to heal. Failure to heal or worsening of the fissure after a second lateral internal sphincterotomy is an indication for a complete gastrointestinal evaluation for Crohn's disease as well as a work-up for sexually transmitted dis-

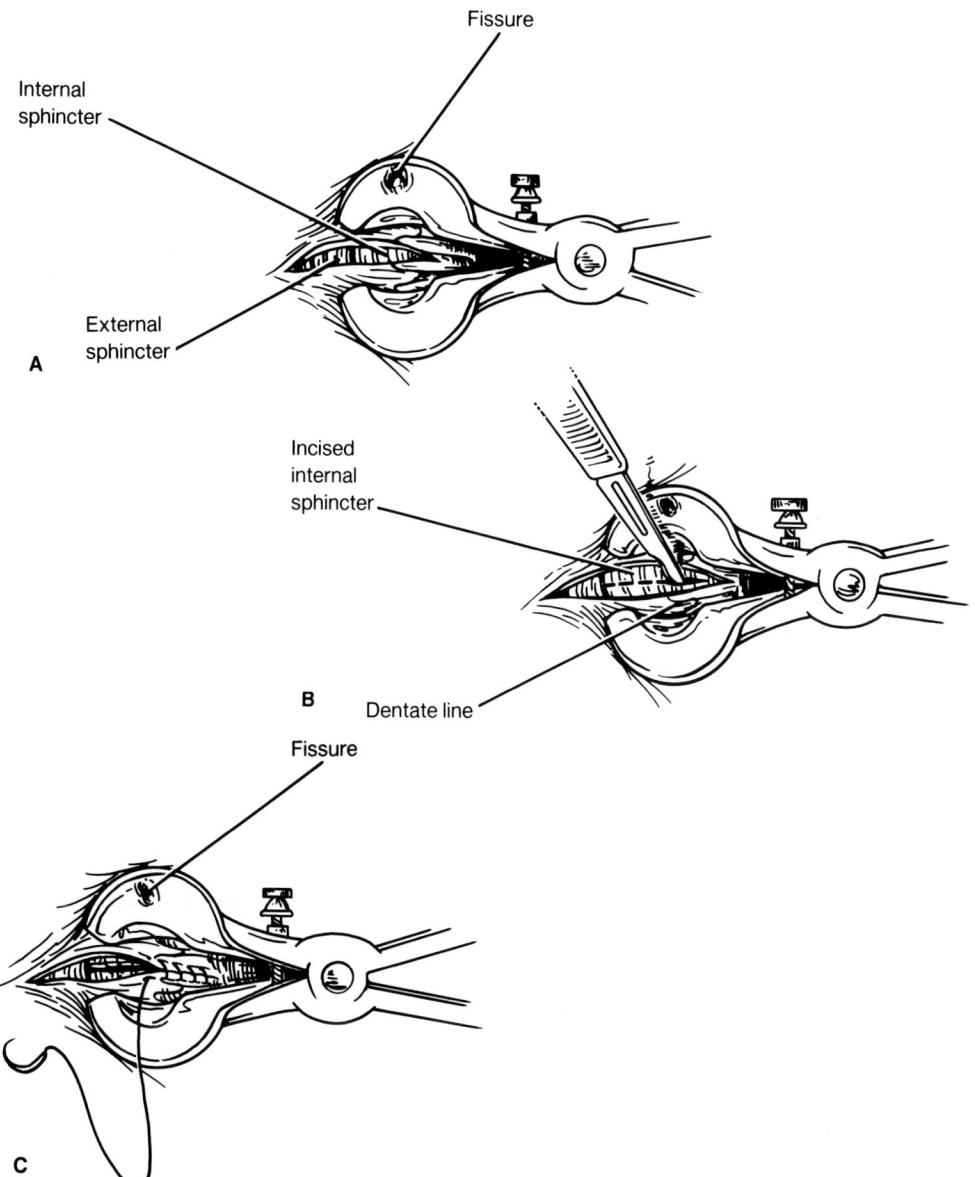

Internal
sphincter

Fissure

External
sphincter

A

Incised
internal
sphincter

B   Dentate line

Fissure

C

Figure 42-7 Open lateral internal sphincterotomy. (**A**) With an operating anoscope in place, an incision is made in the mucosa and anoderm over the intersphincteric groove. (**B**) The internal sphincter is divided from the intersphincteric groove up to the dentate line (a complete sphincterotomy). (**C**) The wound is closed by reapproximating only the mucosa with an absorbable suture.

eases. If no systemic disorders are found, excision of the fissure with V-Y anoplasty should be considered.[58]

PERIANAL SUPPURATIVE DISEASE

Perirectal Abscess

Perirectal abscesses usually present with a painful swelling on the perianal or perineal skin with or without drainage. Most are caused by obstruction and subsequent in-

fection of the anal glands located in the crypts of the anal canal.[68–71] The infection becomes a small abscess, which can localize in a variety of locations (Fig. 42-8). Most crypts are located in the anterior and posterior aspects of the anus, so most perianal abscesses have an anterior or a posterior origin. A partial list of other causes of anorectal infection includes trauma, prior anorectal operation, inflammatory bowel disease (particularly Crohn's disease), neoplasia, and pelvic abscess necessitating in the perineum.

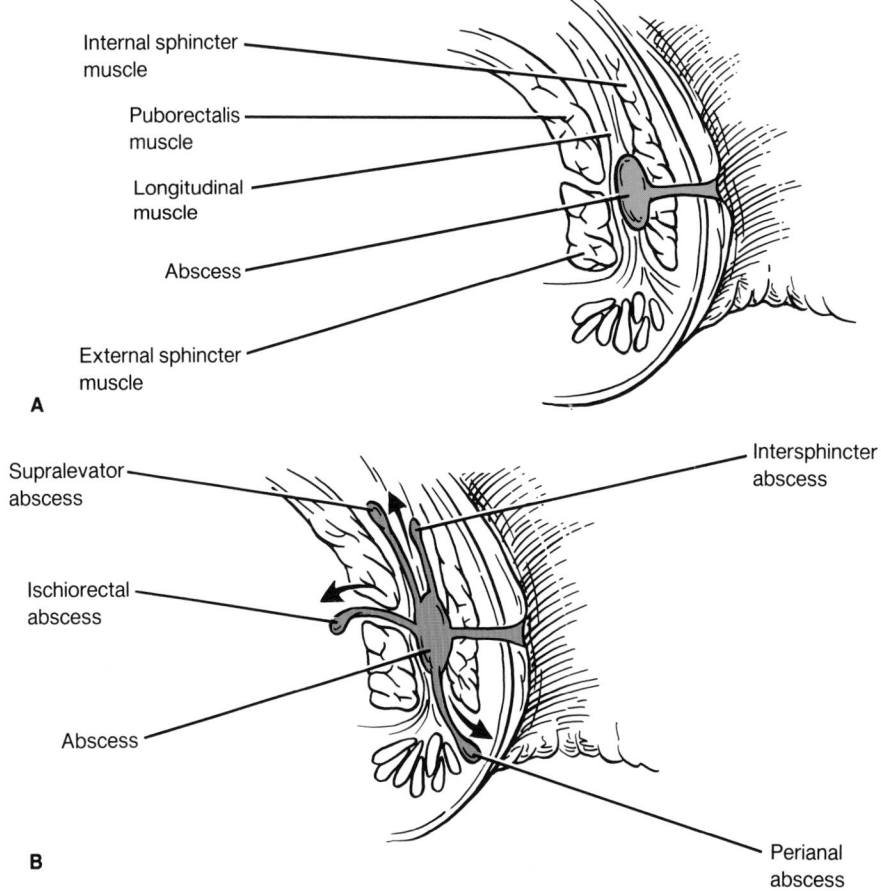

Figure 42-8 Development of perianal abscesses. (**A**) Most perirectal abscesses begin as a result of infection in an anal gland. (**B**) The direction of spread of infection from the initial locus determines the form of abscess.

The most common presenting symptom of acute anorectal infection is pain.[68] Other symptoms include swelling, bleeding, purulent drainage, fever, and change in bowel habits. Pain associated with an abscess is exacerbated with defecation and can be distinguished from pain associated with a fissure in that it never abates. Visual inspection of the perineum can reveal the abscess. The skin can be swollen and erythematous, and even spontaneously draining. Swelling or cellulitis need not be present. The perineum can appear normal without classic signs of acute infection. Digital rectal examination should be performed to identify areas of fluctuation, tenderness, and internal fistulous openings. If the patient is unable to tolerate an examination while awake, one should be performed under general anesthesia. Anoscopy and proctosigmoidoscopy also should be done.

Incision and drainage is the treatment of choice. For small abscesses, drainage can be accomplished in the office or clinic under local anesthesia. The acidic environment of the abscess can make it difficult to achieve anesthesia with a local agent. Patients who cannot be anesthetized adequately in the office are taken to the operating room for regional or general anesthesia.

The prone position is preferred. A perianal abscess is drained through a cruciate skin incision (Fig. 42-9). The skin edges between the cruciate incision should be trimmed so that the wound edges do not close prematurely and result in recurrence. The incision should be made as close to the anal canal as possible to minimize the length of any subsequent fistula in ano. No muscle should be divided, and primary fistulotomy is not advocated at the time of the drainage procedure. An internal opening of the fistula is discovered in one third of patients.[72] When drainage of the abscess is performed without fistulotomy, only 11% of patients subsequently have a fistula and 37% have a recurrent abscess.[68]

In some patients, drainage of a perianal abscess can be accomplished through a small incision with placement of a mushroom catheter.[73] This technique obviates a large incision and accomplishes excellent drainage. Under a local anesthetic, a small incision is made

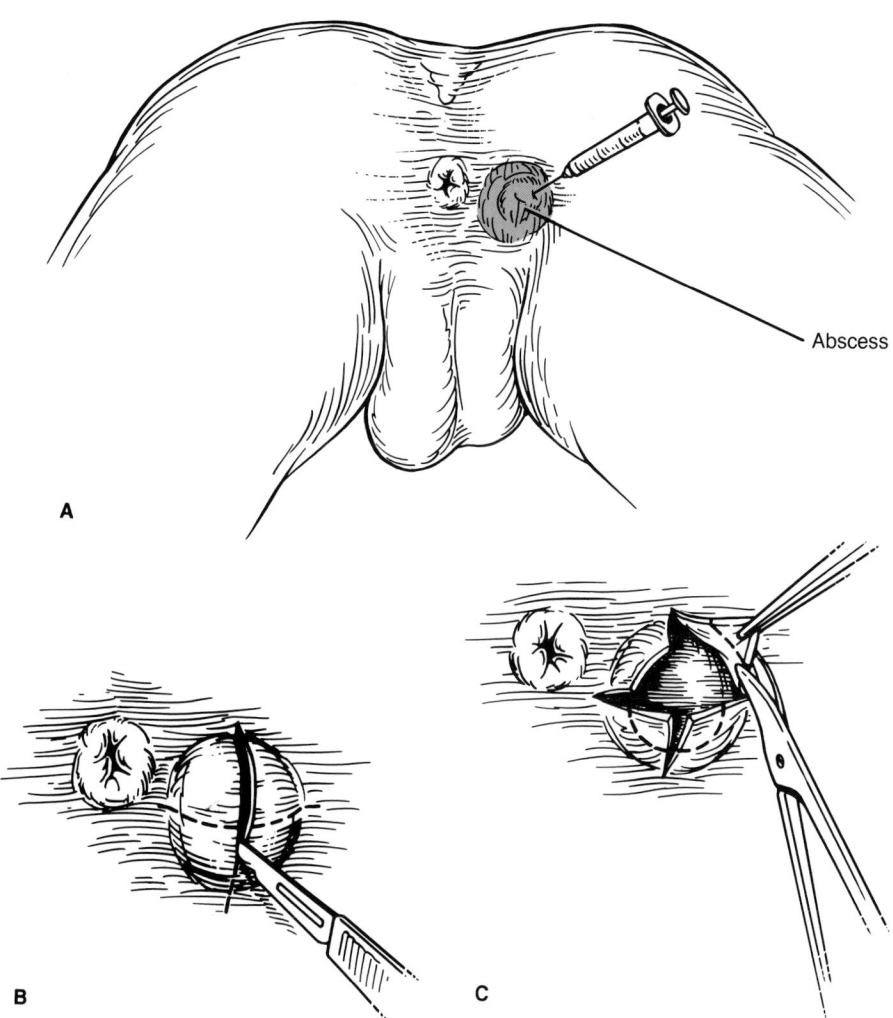

Abscess

Figure 42-9 Drainage of a simple perianal abscess. **(A)** The abscess is anesthetized with a local technique. **(B)** A cruciate incision is made over the abscess. **(C)** The skin edges are trimmed to prevent premature closure of the skin.

over the point of maximal fluctuation. A 10F to 16F mushroom catheter is placed in the abscess cavity, and a dressing is placed over the wound. The patient is instructed to take sitz baths three or four times a day and to return to the office in 1 week. On return, the drain is removed if the cavity has healed.

Antibiotics usually are not necessary for normal individuals after drainage of a perirectal abscess, and are inappropriate as primary treatment. Patients receiving immunosuppressant therapy, such as those with transplanted organs, acquired immunodeficiency syndrome, diabetes mellitus, or cardiac prostheses, are treated with broad-spectrum antibiotics.

Ischiorectal Abscess

Most ischiorectal abscesses can be drained in the same fashion as perianal abscesses, through either a catheter or a cruciate skin incision over the area of fluctuation.

A horseshoe abscess is an ischiorectal abscess that

originates in the deep postanal space and extends into both ischiorectal fossae.[74,75] The deep postanal space is entered and drained by performing an internal sphincterotomy in the posterior midline. Counterdrainage incisions are made over the lateral extensions of the abscess in each ischiorectal fossa. To facilitate evacuation, drains can be placed.

Supralevator Abscess

Suprasphincteric abscesses result from infection that has migrated from elsewhere, either a pelvic abscess caused by diverticulitis or Crohn's disease, or cephalad extension of an intersphincteric or ischiorectal abscess. The precise etiology of the abscess should be determined because it indicates the best site for drainage.

The key to draining a supralevator abscess correctly is to identify its cause. Care must be taken to avoid creating an extrasphincteric fistula. When the supralevator abscess originates from an upward extension of an intersphincteric abscess, it should be drained into the rectum and not through the ischiorectal fossa (Fig. 42-10). When the supralevator abscess originates from a pelvic source, drainage should be either into the rectum or through the ischiorectal fossa, depending on its point of maximum fluctuation. Transabdominal drainage guided by computed tomography (CT) also can be performed. Ultimate resolution of a suprasphincteric abscess caused by intestinal disease requires resection of the diseased intestine. Because of the underlying etiology of the fistula, many patients need antibiotic therapy.

Recurrent Rectal Abscess

Anorectal abscesses recur as the result of inadequate initial drainage, an undiagnosed or untreated fistula in ano, misdiagnosis of a caudal extension of a pilonidal abscess, or hidradenitis suppurativa.[76] Recurrent abscesses can be difficult to diagnose and treat effectively. A thorough evaluation under anesthesia is necessary, and a diligent but gentle search for fistulous tracts should be performed. Any identified fistulas should be treated appropriately. Diagnostic imaging, including CT scanning, may be necessary to determine whether a suprasphincteric abscess is present, and whether there is an associated pelvic abscess.

FISTULA IN ANO

A fistula in ano is an epithelialized tract between the anal canal and perineal skin. It is a direct consequence of anorectal infection in the anal glands or crypts. The intestinal (primary) opening is in the anal canal; the external (secondary) opening is on the perineum. Apart from anorectal infection, etiologic factors include anal or rectal cancer, inflammatory bowel disease, granulomatous disease, foreign body, radiation, and trauma.

Fistulas are classified based on their relationship to the internal and external anal sphincters.[77–79] There are four types of fistulas (Fig. 42-11).

Intersphincteric Fistula

Intersphincteric fistulas are the most common type and account for about 70% of all fistulas in ano. These fistulas originate in the anal canal, traverse the intersphincteric plane, and exit the perineal skin. Simple fistulotomy is the treatment of choice.

Transsphincteric Fistula

Transsphincteric fistulas make up 25% of all fistulas in ano. These fistulas originate in the anal canal, traverse the internal and external anal sphincters, and penetrate the ischiorectal fossa exiting the perineal skin. Operative management of transsphincteric fistulas depends on the amount of external sphincter they involve. If less than 20% of the muscle is involved in the fistulous tract, a simple fistulotomy is appropriate. If over 20% of the external anal sphincter would be divided by a fistulotomy, seton placement with or without fistulotomy should be performed. Another operative approach is to perform an endorectal advancement flap to close the internal fistula opening.[80]

Suprasphincteric Fistula

Suprasphincteric fistulas constitute 5% of all fistulas. They originate at the dentate line, travel superiorly in the intersphincteric groove above the puborectalis muscle, and descend into the ischiorectal fossa. An associated high blind tract can extend above the levator musculature. Treatment involves division of the internal anal sphincter, with seton management of the involved external anal sphincter and adequate drainage of any high blind tract or abscess.

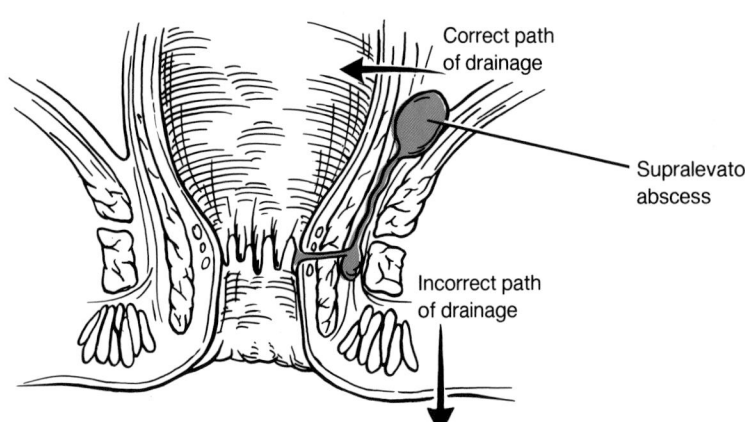

Figure 42-10 Correct operative management of a suprasphincteric abscess. The key to correct management is to avoid creation of an extrasphincteric fistula.

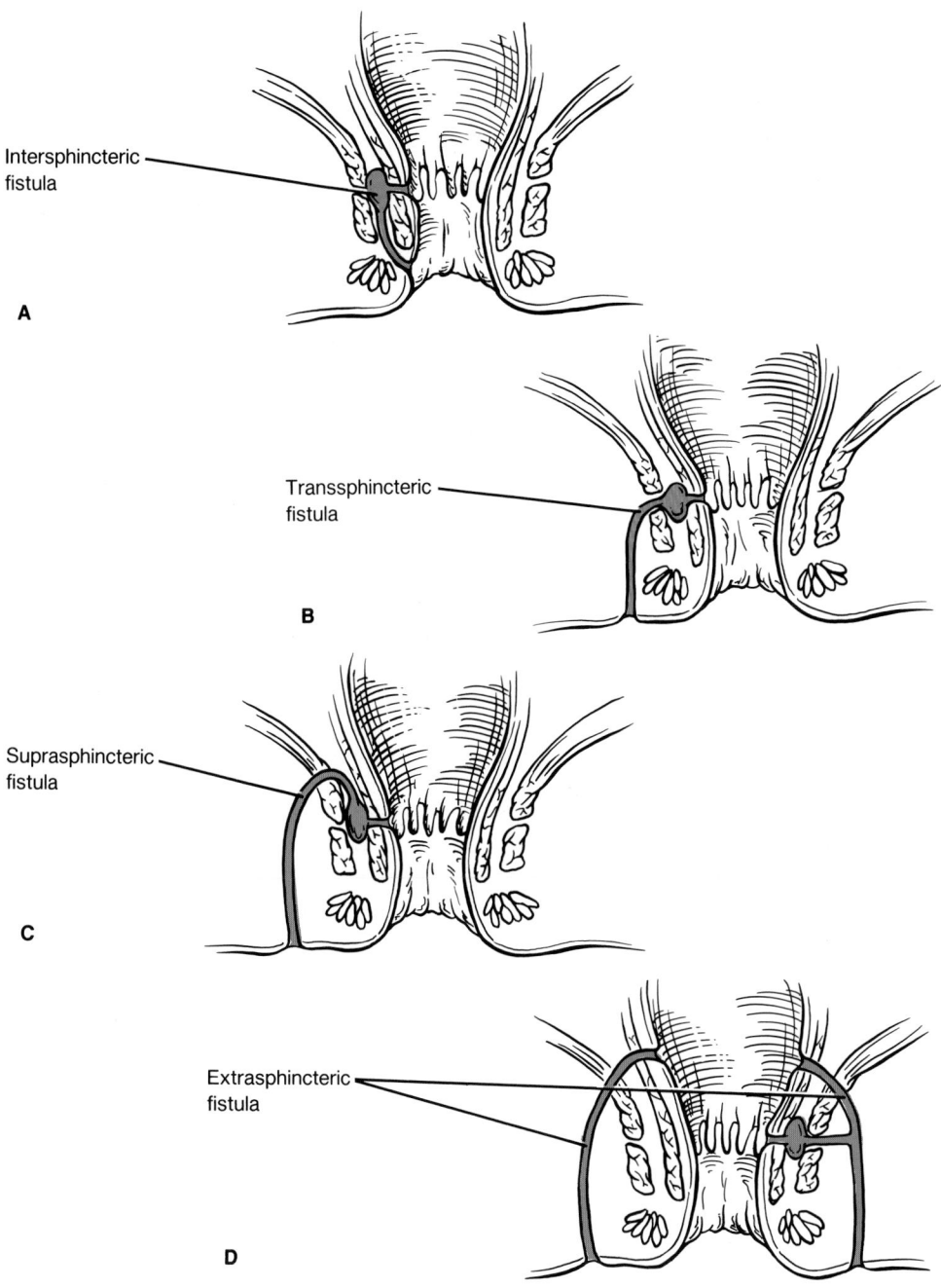

Figure 42-11 Types of fistulas in ano. (**A**) Intersphincteric fistula. (**B**) Transsphincteric fistula. (**C**) Suprasphincteric fistula. (**D**) Extrasphincteric fistulae.

Extrasphincteric Fistula

Extrasphincteric fistulas are rare and account for less than 1% of all fistulas in ano. These fistulas originate high in the rectum, penetrate the levator ani, remain lateral to all the muscles of continence, and exit the skin through the ischiorectal fossa. Extrasphincteric fistulas are the result of pelvic sepsis that has migrated through the perineum. Conditions associated with the development of extrasphincteric fistulas include diverticulitis and perforated Crohn's disease. Successful management of these fistulas depends on adequate treatment of the pelvic sepsis. Resection of the diseased segment of intestine almost always is required, and fecal diversion may be necessary.

Goodsall's Rule

Goodsall's rule predicts the course of an anorectal fistula based on the location of its external opening (Fig. 42-12). The rule states that whenever the external opening of a fistula is anterior to an imaginary transverse plane bisecting the anus, the fistulous tract travels to the anal canal in a straight line. Whenever the external opening lies posterior to this plane, the tract takes a curvilinear course to enter the anal canal in the posterior midline. Bilateral symmetric external openings indicate a horseshoe fistula, and occasionally there are two fistulas present. The use of Goodsall's rule helps in planning definitive operative therapy and preventing division of the external sphincter.

Acute fistulas can present like abscesses with pain, erythema, warmth, and drainage. Chronic fistulas are less dramatic and can present as fibrous cords with minimal inflammation, purulent discharge, and pruritus. Patients frequently complain of constant soiling of their undergarments.

Inspection of the perineum, digital examination, anoscopy, and proctosigmoidoscopy are required. Inspection reveals an external opening, erythema, and discharge. Subcutaneous fibrosis can be noted on digital examination and is an important clue to the course of the fistula. Fluctuation and tenderness in the anal canal reveal the site of a primary abscess. Anoscopy can demonstrate purulent discharge from the internal opening. Identification of the fistula can be aided further by passage of a probe through the external site to the internal

opening. It is important that the probe be maneuvered gently so that a false tract is not created.[78,81,82] Complex and recurrent fistulas in ano are difficult management problems that require careful preoperative evaluation. Fistulography performed with barium sulfate in the radiology suite sometimes can define the course of the fistula. A CT scan of the pelvis and perineum identifies associated deep pelvic sepsis. Intrarectal and intraanal ultrasound has been used to delineate the course of complex fistulas.

Treatment

Fistulotomy is the preferred operative approach to intersphincteric and some transsphincteric fistulas, but it invariably leads to an alteration in continence. Patients should be informed before operation that their ability to control flatus, mucus, and liquid stool can be adversely affected by fistulotomy. True fecal incontinence is unusual after fistulotomy for an intersphincteric fistula. Rates of incontinence after fistula surgery range between 0.001% and 39%, depending on the report and the type of fistula treated.[83-90]

The patient is placed in the prone position and local anesthetic is administered. A small probe is placed through the external opening of the fistula with an anoscope already in place in the anal canal (Fig. 42-13). The probe is advanced gently to avoid creating false passages and then is guided through the internal opening into the anal canal. The tissue overlying the fistula is

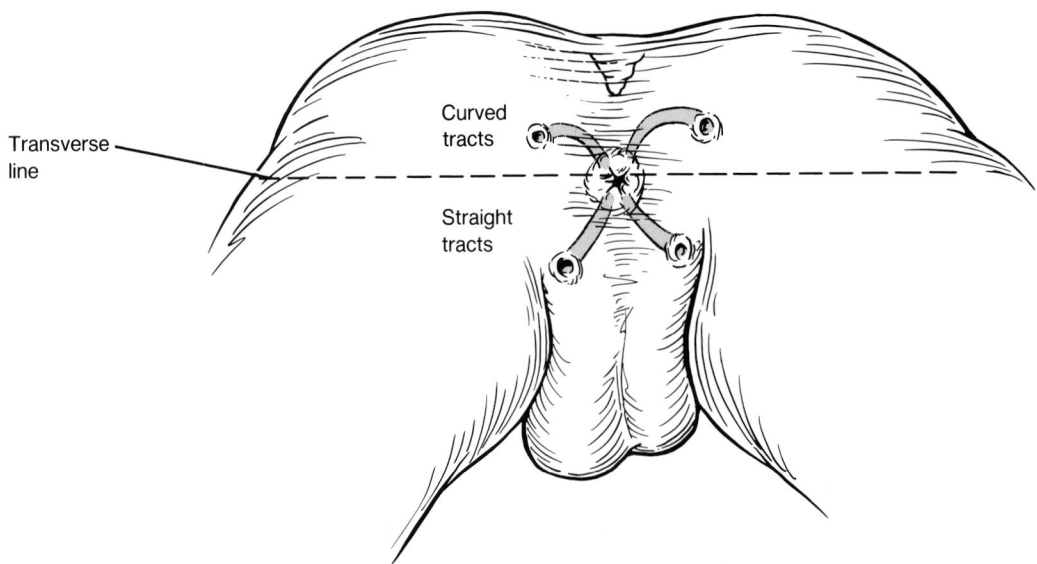

Figure 42-12 Goodsall's rule. When the external opening of a fistula is in the posterior perineum, its course to the rectum is generally curvilinear. When the external opening of a fistula is in the anterior perineum, its course is generally a straight line.

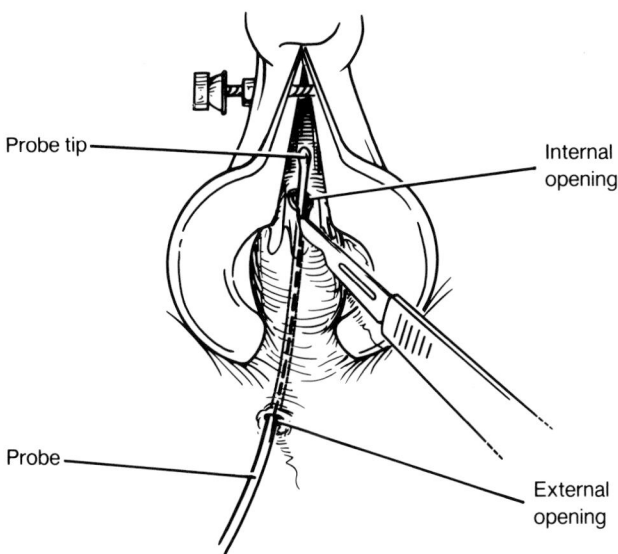

Probe tip

Internal opening

Probe

External opening

Figure 42-13 Primary fistulotomy. With an anoscope in place, a probe is gently passed through the external fistulous opening to discover the internal opening. Great care should be taken to avoid the creation of any false passages. The skin, mucosa, and internal anal sphincter overlying the fistula are divided using a scalpel or electrocautery. The edges of the wound are sutured to the base of the fistula using an absorbable suture.

divided, either sharply or with electrocautery. The technique results in the performance of an internal sphincterotomy. Granulation tissue present in the tract is débrided with a curette. The fistulotomy site can be left completely open or the skin edges can be sutured to the cut edge of the fistula tract. Fistulectomy is not advocated because of the large wound created and because of the risk of injury to the external anal sphincter.

Management of transsphincteric fistulas requires a modification of primary fistulotomy to avoid immediate division of over 10% to 15% of the external anal sphincter. The patient is placed in the prone position and local anesthetic is injected around the fistula. An anoscope is placed in the anal canal and a probe is guided gently into the external opening, through the fistula, and out the internal opening. The external skin, mucosa, and internal sphincter overlying the tract are divided with electrocautery, but the external anal sphincter is left intact (Fig. 42-14). A nonabsorbable suture is passed through the external sphincter component of the transsphincteric fistula and tied loosely around the muscle. The tie should not strangulate the muscle. A rubber band also can be used as a seton. Postoperative care involves sitz baths, dietary fiber supplements, and mild analgesia. Classic seton management involves division of the encircled muscle after about 6 weeks have elapsed to permit fibrosis to occur and to

prevent retraction of the divided muscle ends. Unfortunately, functional results of this approach are suboptimal. An alternative technique involves simple removal of the seton after 4 to 6 weeks. Many fistulas heal spontaneously with this approach, and no loss of muscle function occurs. If a rubber band is used as a seton, it can be tightened in the office to cut through the involved sphincter muscle gradually without significant discomfort to the patient.

An alternative to primary fistulotomy or fistulotomy with seton placement is an endorectal mucosal advancement flap[80] (Fig. 42-15). This technique is particularly useful for patients with suprasphincteric fistulas or with transsphincteric fistulas that involve a large portion of the external anal sphincter. The internal opening is débrided and closed with an absorbable suture. A rectangular flap of mucosa with some internal sphincter is mobilized from the area just cephalad to the internal opening, advanced over the internal opening, and sutured in place using interrupted sutures. The external opening is débrided and widened, and the intervening tract is curetted. A small mushroom-shaped drain can be placed in the tract through the external opening. With this technique, no muscle is divided and there is minimal distortion of the anal canal and minimal risk of incontinence. There is virtually no external wound, so patients have much less discomfort.

The operative management of an extrasphincteric fistula varies according to its cause. If the fistula results from cephalad extension of a transsphincteric anal fistula, the lower half of the fistula should be managed by laying open the fistulous tract with division of the mucosa and internal sphincter. The upper opening can be managed with a seton or an endorectal advancement flap. In difficult cases, a diverting colostomy may be required. An extrasphincteric fistula resulting from caudad extension of a pelvic abscess requires drainage of the pelvic abscess and treatment of the primary pathology.

Fistulas Associated With Crohn's Disease

The incidence of anal disorders in patients with Crohn's disease is 28% to 30%.[91,92] With the exception of external anal tags, anorectal fistulas are the most common type of anorectal disease and are responsible for symptoms of leakage, soiling, pruritus, and chronic sepsis. Management of anorectal fistulas in patients with Crohn's disease can be difficult because of concurrent rectal and proximal intestinal inflammation. This inflammation and the poor healing present in these patients increases the risk of fecal incontinence and nonhealing wounds after operative management.

Some fistulas in Crohn's disease begin as typical

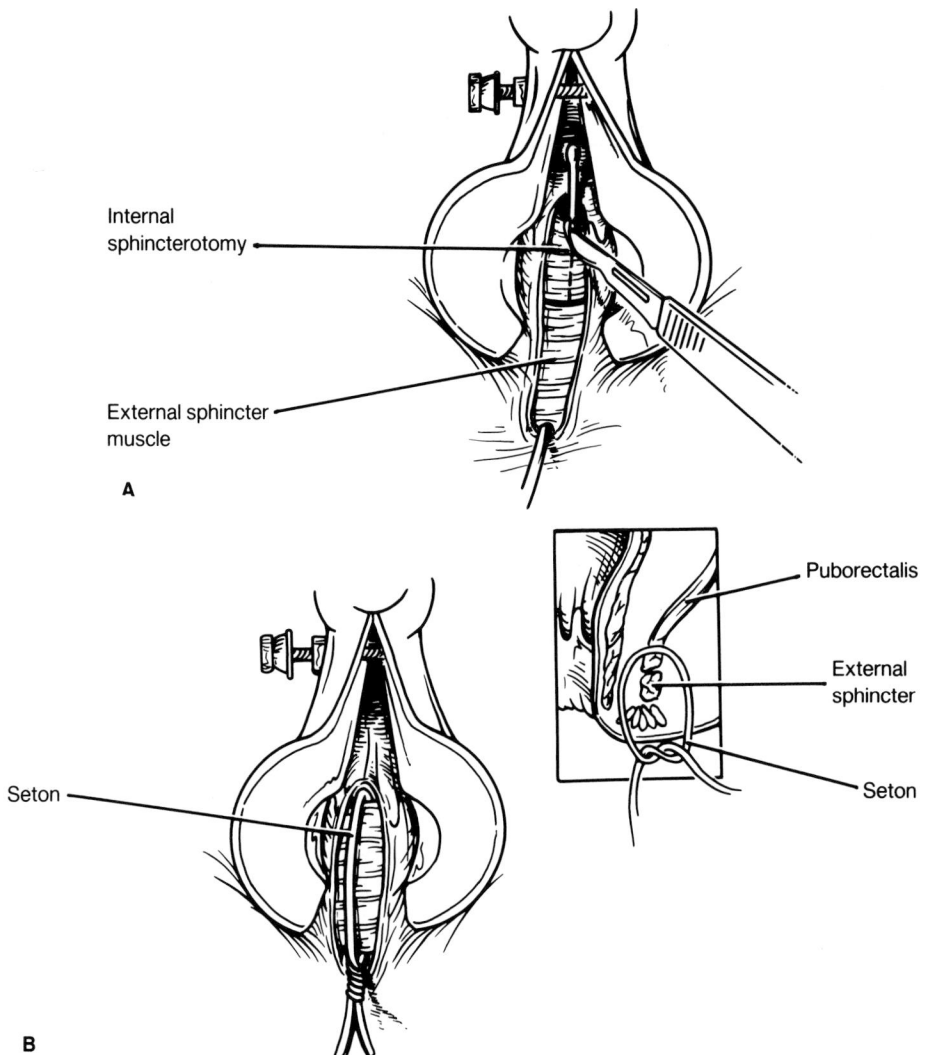

Internal
sphincterotomy

External sphincter
muscle

A

Seton

Puborectalis

External
sphincter

Seton

B

Figure 42-14 Staged fistulotomy with a seton. (**A**) The skin, mucosa, and internal anal sphincter overlying the fistula are divided using a scalpel or electrocautery. The portion of the fistulous tract involving the external anal sphincter or puborectalis muscle is identified. (**B**) A large-caliber, nonabsorbable suture or a rubber band is passed through the fistulous tract using the probe as a guide. The suture is then tied around the muscle—snugly for a cutting seton, loosely for a noncutting seton.

anorectal abscesses of cryptoglandular origin. Others occur as the result of transmural rectal inflammation with ulceration.[93–95] Because of this, unusual and complex perianal fistulas can result, with internal openings in the high, middle, and low rectum. There can be multiple internal openings. An important consideration in the management of perianal fistulous disease is the condition of the rectal mucosa. Active rectal inflammation mandates surgical conservatism because of the associated disturbance in healing and continence. Therapy should be directed at medical treatment of the inflammation of the rectal mucosa with topical and sys-

temic agents such as 5-ASA, corticosteroid enemas, sulfasalazine (Azulfidine), and prednisone.

Although a thorough office evaluation can identify the character of some fistulas, a complete evaluation usually requires an examination under anesthesia. The course of a fistulous tract should be identified using probes gently placed in the tract. Some patients require intraoperative fistulography. Saline with or without hydrogen peroxide injected through the external fistulous opening can be used. Methylene blue should not be used because it rapidly stains adjacent tissue. Extremely complex fistulas may require even more extensive eval-

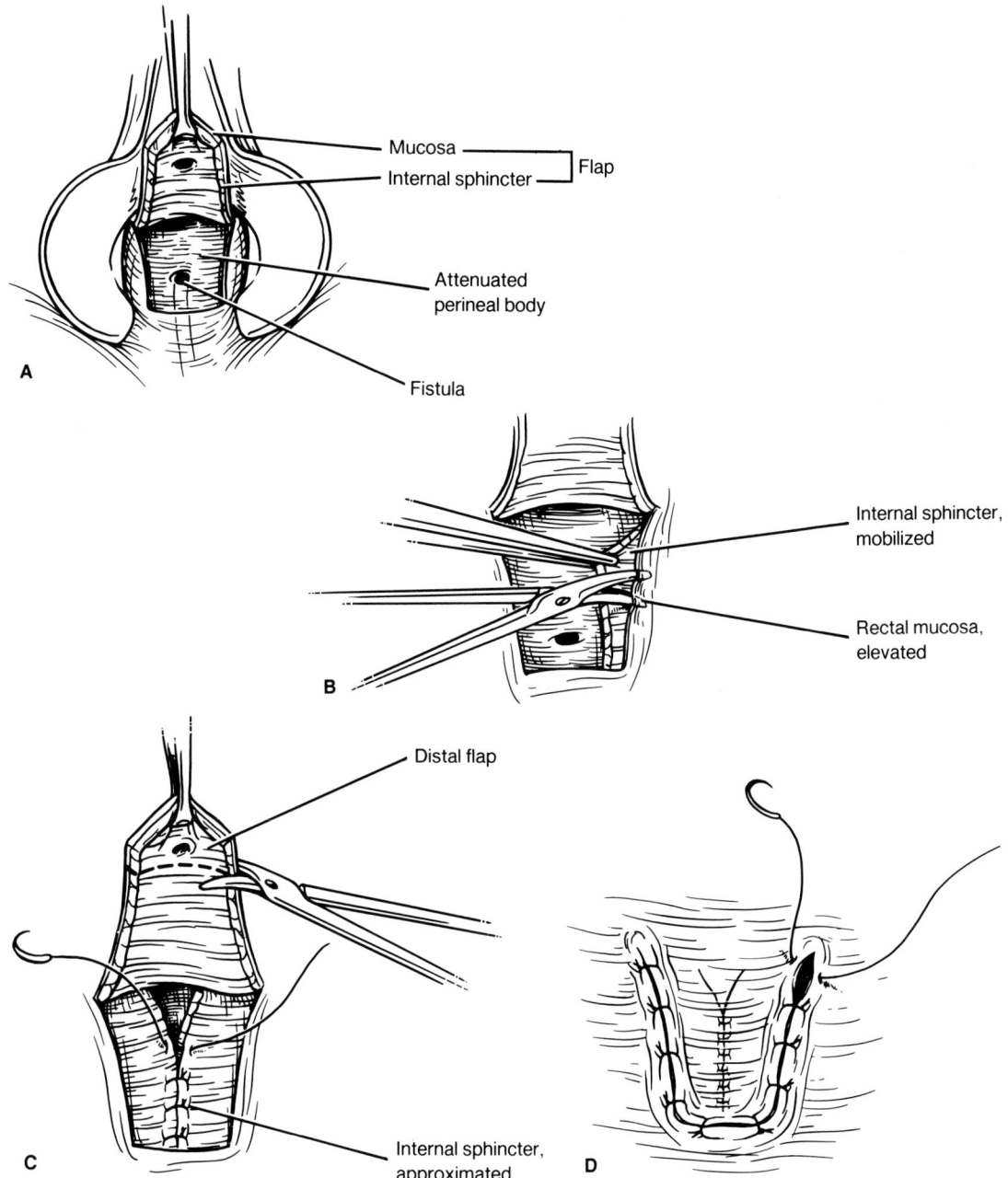

Figure 42-15 Endoanal advancement flap for complex anal fistulas (**A**) Local anesthesia containing epinephrine is infiltrated submucosally to facilitate dissection and hemostasis. A rectangular flap containing mucosa and some internal anal sphincter is fashioned cephalad to the internal fistula opening. (**B**) The flap is mobilized, and the internal anal sphincter is freed from any scar tissue. (**C**) The fistulous opening in the mucosa is excised, and the fistula in the muscle is closed with an absorbable suture. (**D**) The flap is then advanced down over the fistula and sutured in place using 3-0 absorbable suture.

uation using fistulography,[96] CT scanning,[97] magnetic resonance imaging,[98] and intrarectal ultrasound.[99]

Successful management of fistulas in ano in patients with Crohn's disease requires that initial therapy be directed at resolving any inflammation in the rectum and draining sites of active inflammation. Medical therapy using oral metronidazole or ciprofloxacin can be effective in patients without abscesses.[100,101] Surgical management of fistulas in the presence of active rectal disease is associated with poor results.[102-104] When active inflammation is present, the goals of initial therapy should include adequate drainage of pus and control of the fistula with a seton. A fistulotomy that includes division of any muscle should not be performed. Proximal intestinal disease should be managed appropriately as symptoms mandate. Improved control of diarrhea due to proximal disease will help ameliorate the symptoms caused by anorectal fistulas. Fecal diversion may be required.

Surgical management of perianal fistulas in the absence of rectal mucosal inflammation should be performed in the same manner as indicated in patients without Crohn's disease. Primary fistulotomy,[102,103] staged fistulotomy,[104] endoanal mucosal advancement flaps,[104] muscle transfer flaps,[105] fecal diversion,[106] and proctectomy[102,103] all can be used, when appropriate, to manage the spectrum of fistulous disease. Low intersphincteric fistulas can be treated by fistulotomy. Staged fistulotomy with seton management should be used for transphincteric fistulas. Complex fistulas may require staged fistulotomy, endoanal advancement flaps, muscle transfer procedures, or fecal diversion. Transvaginal repair of rectovaginal fistulas also can be used.[107]

Selected operative treatment is the key to success in patients with Crohn's disease who have fistula in ano.[102,108,109] Appropriate operative management of low (superficial) fistulas by fistulotomy results in primary healing after operation in 71% to 91% of cases.[108,109] Most wounds heal within 3 to 6 months. Complications of operation include incontinence and anal stenosis. The incidence of incontinence is variable and it is unclear whether postoperative incontinence after management of complex fistulas is due to the procedure or to the disease. Between 5% and 18% of patients ultimately require proctectomy for resolution of disease.[102,107,108]

PILONIDAL DISEASE

The term *pilonidal* is defined as "containing hair nested in a cyst."[110] Although pilonidal disease can occur at any age, teenagers and young adults are affected most frequently. There is a 3:1 male to female predominance. The prototypic patient is a hirsute young man.

The precise etiology of pilonidal disease is unknown. The most commonly accepted theory attributes pilonidal abscess to a chronic foreign-body reaction resulting from penetration of the subcutaneous tissue by hair shafts.[111–113] Another theory attributes pilonidal disease to infection of the fused caudal end of the medullary canal. According to a third theory, pilonidal disease is acquired as the result of upright posture and the force of gravity. According to this theory, skin between the bottom of the natal cleft and the angle of the sacrum is stretched. Stretching causes skin to break at the thinnest point at the bottom of the follicle. This break in dermal integrity results in acute and chronic follicular infection.

There can be one or more midline pits or external sinus tract openings in the sacrococcygeal area. Each of the pits is lined by squamous epithelium and contains a single hair follicle. Usually, loose hair is present in the tract and the sinus is lined by granulation tissue or squamous epithelium. When inflammation occurs, it proceeds in a cephalad and lateral direction. Secondary pits and sinus tracts then are opened. Chronic inflammation results in the formation of epithelium-lined cavities. Rarely, squamous cell carcinoma occurs within these cavities.[114] The bacteriology of pilonidal infection usually is mixed skin and enteric flora.

Twenty percent of patients have acute inflammation, including localized pain, swelling, and purulent discharge. Fever and leukocytosis are uncommon. Most patients have chronic disease, which is characterized by a persistent painful sensation over the coccyx. There can be intermittent drainage and bleeding.

On physical examination, an acute abscess manifests as cellulitis with induration, erythema, tenderness, and fluctuation. Chronic disease can be innocuous, with only one or more noninflamed midline pits present over the sacrococcygeal area. Hair can protrude through the midline orifice. The differential diagnosis includes anorectal abscess, anorectal fistula, complex abscess due to inflammatory bowel disease, hidradenitis suppurativa, and actinomycosis.

For treatment, the prone position is preferred. The buttocks are taped apart and the skin is carefully shaved. To improve exposure and lighting, a headlight can be used.

Pilonidal Abscesses

Pilonidal abscesses are managed by immediate incision and drainage. The procedure can be accomplished in the office under a local anesthetic. Patients with extremely large abscesses and severe tenderness may require a general anesthetic. The wound is packed and left open. Sixty percent of patients have successful results from simple incision and drainage.[115]

Pilonidal Sinuses

Pilonidal sinuses should not be excised and packed because of prolonged morbidity. Healing can take as long as 6 months with this technique, and multiple operations may be required for delayed healing.

Incision and Marsupialization

In incision and marsupialization, the cyst is laid completely open and all granulation tissue is débrided with a curette.[116] The skin edge then is marsupialized to the cut edge of the sinus wall, which is packed open. Marsupialization decreases the wound size and allows for faster healing. Meticulous perianal hygiene is required for acceptable wound healing and includes skin shaving around the wound and daily cleansing and débridement of the wound.

Excision and Primary Closure

Excision and primary closure, when successful, results in more rapid wound healing and minimal disability.[117] Unfortunately, wounds reopen prematurely and disease recurs in a high percentage of patients treated by this technique. The disadvantages of excision and primary closure are that fascial retention sutures are required for about 14 days and the rate of recurrence is high (20% to 25%).

Some authors advocate excision and primary skin flap closure, including Z-plasty[118] or an advancing flap.[119] The reported results with both these techniques are excellent and the rates of recurrence are low. The significant disadvantage is that these approaches require extensive dissection and postoperative hospitalization is necessary.

Recurrent pilonidal disease and an unhealed wound can be extremely difficult to manage. Initial treatment should involve débridement of granulation tissue and improved wound care. If this is inadequate, excision and primary wound closure with or without a skin flap should be used. Wide excision of recurrent disease with skin grafting also has been recommended.[120] Large or complex recurrences also can be managed using a myocutaneous flap[121] or a cleft closure technique.[122]

HIDRADENITIS SUPPURATIVA

Hidradenitis suppurativa is a dermatologic condition characterized by chronic infection of apocrine glands. The term is derived from the Greek words *hydros,* meaning sweat, and *aden,* meaning gland.[123] The condition is most common in areas with the highest concentration of apocrine glands, such as the axilla, groin, and perineum. Patients usually are 16 to 44 years of age, and men are affected more often than women by a ratio of 2:1.[124,125] The etiology of hidradenitis suppurativa is proposed to be obstruction of apocrine ducts resulting in rupture and secondary bacterial infection. Staphylo-

cocci and streptococci are the most frequently cultured organisms, but enteric organisms also can be present. Patients can have acute abscesses that require drainage or chronic disease that manifests as fibrotic perineal skin with multiple, painful, draining sinus tracts and nodules. Cellulitis can be present. The differential diagnosis of hidradenitis includes pilonidal disease and perianal abscess with multiple fistulas.

Treatment

The treatment of early acute hidradenitis consists of drainage of acute abscesses and administration of oral antibiotics such as tetracycline. Histopathologic examination of the involved skin demonstrates apocrine gland involvement and confirms the diagnosis. After the acute infection has resolved, the diseased skin should be excised completely and the wound closed primarily. Chronic disease is unlikely to respond to nonoperative medical management.[126,127] Any acute infection is drained. After acute infection has resolved, wide local excision of the affected skin is performed to cure the hidradenitis. Management of the wound is tailored to its size. Split-thickness skin grafts or skin flaps can effectively cover the wound and result in rapid healing.[128] However, simply leaving the wound open to heal by secondary intention is a legitimate option and usually results in acceptable cosmesis.[124,129] Fecal diversion generally is not required.[128]

FECAL INCONTINENCE

Fecal incontinence is an embarrassing, distressing, and socially devastating condition. Studies have demonstrated a community prevalence of 2.3%[130] and a nursing home prevalence of 34%.[131] The costs of incontinence, including medical care, adult diapers and stoma supplies, institutionalization, and loss of productivity, are unknown but probably substantial.

Although adequate anal sphincter function is critical for normal continence, several other important factors also are involved.[132] Mental function must be adequate to care about continence, and neurologic pathways must be intact from the brain to the anorectum. Excessive stool volume, liquid stool consistency, and accelerated colonic transit, all characteristic of severe diarrheal states, can lead to incontinence despite an entirely normal sphincter mechanism. Rectal and anal sensation must be intact and normal anorectal reflexes must be present. A stiff rectum that is unable to accommodate a fecal load also predisposes to fecal incontinence.

The causes of fecal incontinence are listed in Table

42-1.[132] These can be subdivided into two groups based on whether or not the pelvic floor is normal. As noted, severe diarrhea occasionally is a primary cause of incontinence. More importantly, any degree of loose stool or enhanced transit can cause decompensation of a partially impaired sphincter mechanism. Overflow incontinence results from functional or anatomic obstruction of the rectum. In the case of fecal impaction, loose stool seeps around the obstructing fecal bolus and out the relaxed anal sphincter.[133] Fecal impaction is believed to be the leading cause of incontinence in institutionalized elderly patients.

A wide variety of neurologic disorders can cause or exacerbate incontinence. Of particular note is the autonomic neuropathy of diabetes mellitus, which leads to incontinence in up to 20% of diabetic patients.[134] Pudendal neuropathy is caused by traction injury of the pudendal nerves.[135] This results from perineal descent

Table 42-1 Causes of Fecal Incontinence

CONGENITAL ANORECTAL ABNORMALITIES
Spina bifida or myelomeningocele
Anorectal malformations

OVERFLOW
Impaction
Encopresis
Rectal neoplasms
Drugs that cause constipation

NORMAL PELVIC FLOOR
Diarrheal States
Infectious diarrhea
Inflammatory bowel disease
Short-gut syndrome
Laxative abuse
Radiation enteritis

Neurologic Conditions
Multiple sclerosis
Dementia, strokes, or tabes dorsalis
Neuropathies (eg, diabetes)
Neoplasms of brain, spinal cord, or cauda equina
Injuries of brain, spinal cord, or cauda equina

INCONTINENCE WITH ABNORMAL PELVIC FLOOR
Trauma
Accidental injuries (impalement, pelvic fractures)
Anorectal surgery
Obstetric injury
Aging
Pelvic Floor Denervation (Idiopathic Neurogenic Incontinence)
Vaginal childbirth
Chronic straining at stool
Rectal prolapse
Descending perineum syndrome

(Madoff RD, Williams JG, Caushaj PF. Fecal incontinence. N Engl J Med 1992;326:1002)

associated with straining at stool or vaginal childbirth; the nerves are stretched between their fixed point of exit at Alcock's canal and the mobile pelvic soft tissue. Pudendal neuropathy, in conjunction with physical dilatation of the anal sphincter, is responsible for the fecal incontinence that frequently complicates rectal prolapse. The term *descending perineum syndrome* refers to the vicious cycle that occurs when excessive straining leads to pudendal nerve injury, consequent pelvic floor weakness, and progressive nerve traction.

Abnormalities of the pelvic floor that lead to incontinence include congenital anorectal malformations and traumatic sphincter injuries. Congenital anorectal anomalies occur in 1 in 5000 liveborn infants.[136] They range in severity from an imperforate anal membrane to total rectal agenesis. The prognosis for continence after surgical correction depends on the adequacy of development of the pelvic floor musculature and its anatomic relationship to the rectum and anus.

Sphincter injury due to trauma occurs in both accidental and iatrogenic settings. Accidental trauma frequently is caused by impalement injuries and pelvic fractures. Iatrogenic sphincter injuries are seen most often after vaginal childbirth. Although studies using endoanal ultrasound have demonstrated anatomic sphincter defects in one third of women after vaginal delivery, only a few have clinically evident sphincter lacerations.[137] As noted earlier, anatomic sphincter injuries after childbirth often are associated with pudendal nerve injuries; risk factors for these injuries include a high-birthweight infant, a prolonged second stage of labor, and use of obstetric forceps.[138]

Partial sphincter division is performed as therapy in surgery for anal fissure and fistula. Alterations in continence, usually minor, are seen in 10% to 30% of patients after these procedures.[139] The extent of impairment correlates with the amount of sphincter muscle divided.[140] Impaired sphincter function also has been documented after vigorous anal retraction, as was frequently performed to permit rectal mucosectomy during the early experience with restorative proctocolectomy.

The evaluation of an incontinent patient begins with a detailed medical history and careful physical examination. The nature and severity of the problem should be assessed and true incontinence differentiated from such conditions as inadequate hygiene, mucus leakage (as from prolapsing internal hemorrhoids or rectal villous tumors), drainage of pus (as from anal fistulas), and fecal urgency without incontinence (as associated with proctitis, irritable bowel syndrome, pelvic irradiation, or low rectal anastomosis). Passage of stool through the vagina due to colonic or rectal fistulas also can be confused with leakage of stool through the anus.

The severity of incontinence is characterized by the frequency of incontinent episodes and the nature of the material being passed. Because gas is the most difficult substance to control, incontinence to gas alone is considered the least severe type of incontinence. Conversely, loss of solid stool, generally the most controllable of bowel contents, bespeaks severe incontinence. The ability to control liquid stool lies somewhere in between. Incontinence occurring during the day is more severe than that occurring at night, when conscious reactions to impending loss of control are suppressed.

A thorough physical examination of the anorectum provides critical diagnostic information: perianal skin breakdown frequently accompanies severe incontinence; scarring and external fistula openings can be identified; and exuberant skin tags are suggestive of Crohn's disease. The anal orifice normally is a slit-like opening with an anteroposterior orientation; deformity can be due to trauma or previous surgical intervention such as fistulotomy. Anal gaping with traction on the buttocks is suggestive of rectal prolapse. Thinning or absence of the perineal body usually is caused by obstetric injury. Digital rectal examination should reveal the presence of a fecal impaction or low-lying rectal cancer, and a qualitative assessment of resting and squeeze anal pressures should be obtained. Particular attention should be paid to the adequacy of puborectalis contraction. This muscle is easily palpable at the posterior anorectal junction, which should be pushed forward when the patient is instructed to squeeze.

Endoscopic inspection of at least the distal large bowel is mandatory in evaluating the incontinent patient. Endoscopic or radiologic investigation of the entire colon and small bowel is indicated when proximal pathology is suspected (ie, in a patient with chronic diarrhea).

Specialized tests for evaluating incontinence include endoanal ultrasound, anal manometry, electromyography, and cinedefecography. Although not always mandatory, these tests are useful to relieve diagnostic uncertainty, confirm a clinical impression, or provide objective data and medicolegal documentation.

Endoanal ultrasound provides an accurate anatomic depiction of the sphincter mechanism. Gaps in the internal and external sphincters, as well as associated pathology such as anal fistulas, are easily identified and localized. Anal manometry measures resting and maximum voluntary contraction pressures, typically using four or eight channels at each level of the anal canal to permit reconstruction of a complete pressure profile.[141] Cinedefecography is a radiologic assessment of rectal emptying in which the patient is instructed to evacuate barium paste under fluoroscopy.[141] This test is useful in diagnosing occult rectal prolapse, abnormal perineal descent, rectocele, and enterocele. Electromyography is most useful for assessing pudendal nerve function; conduction time between the proximal nerve and the sphincter is measured using a glove-mounted electrode.[141] Needle electromyography also is used occasionally to map the external sphincter and to document evidence of denervation injury due to pudendal neuropathy. However, because needle electromyography is painful, this test has been relegated largely to the research setting.

The treatment of fecal incontinence includes conservative medical therapy, surgery, and biofeedback. Underlying causative or aggravating conditions such as inflammatory bowel disease, rectal cancer, fecal impaction, and rectal prolapse should be treated before specific therapy is initiated for the incontinence itself.

Mild disorders of continence often can be treated successfully with simple conservative measures. Adequate dietary fiber intake must be maintained to ensure passage of formed stools, which are most easy to control. Antidiarrheal agents such as loperamide or diphenoxylate with atropine often are beneficial in patients with chronic loose stools or rectal irritability. A program of daily enemas or rectal irrigation after bowel movements frequently is successful in establishing a state of pseudocontinence, whereby fecal leakage is precluded by maintaining an empty rectum.

Anatomic disruption of the anal sphincter is treated best by direct surgical repair. Acute sphincter injuries, including obstetric injuries, generally should undergo immediate primary repair. Proximal diverting colostomy usually is unnecessary. Unstable patients, patients with extensive perineal trauma, and patients with marked fecal contamination should be treated with proximal diversion and delayed repair after 3 months. Other reasons for delayed primary sphincter repair include unrecognized injuries, late loss of function remote in time from the inciting injury, and failed initial sphincter repair.

Overlapping sphincteroplasty is the operation of choice for the late repair of anal sphincter injuries.[142,143] Principles of the operation include wide mobilization of the sphincter mechanism (avoiding branches of the pudendal nerve, which enter the muscle from a posterolateral direction); division of the remaining sphincter at the site of the defect (with preservation of all scar tissue to prevent suture pull-through); and creation of a snug overlapping plication. The levator ani muscles frequently are folded forward to form the superior aspect of the repair. Colostomy is not performed routinely. Good to excellent results are reported in 70% to 80% of patients who undergo the procedure,[142,143] although patients with associated pudendal neuropathy most often have unsatisfactory results[143,144] (Fig. 42-16).

Parks postanal repair was designed to treat patients with anatomically intact sphincters and poor function resulting from pudendal neuropathy.[145] The pelvic floor musculature and external anal sphincter are approached through the intersphincteric plane and plicated posteriorly. Although some patients benefit from the procedure, the ultimate quality of continence often is poor and results tend to deteriorate with time.[146] This operation remains popular in some centers in Great Britain but is performed infrequently in the United States.

Biofeedback therapy is useful for fecal incontinence.[147,148] External anal sphincter function is measured (most commonly by an anal plug electrode) and displayed visually to patients, who use the information to learn to maximize effective sphincter contraction. Patients also undergo sensory training and learn to perceive progressively decreasing volumes of air instilled into a rectal balloon. The mechanism of biofeedback's effect remains uncertain, because manometric studies have failed to demonstrate consistent improvement in anal pressures after training.[149] However, irrespective of its mode of action, biofeedback is successful in alleviating incontinence in more than two thirds of treated patients. The technique is well suited to patients without anatomic sphincter disruptions, patients with combined anatomic and neuropathic lesions, and patients in whom prior sphincter repair has failed.

A variety of anal encirclement operations have been advocated as salvage procedures for patients in whom standard surgical and biofeedback therapy fails. Thiersch originally described the use of silver wire cerclage,[150] and more recent authors have recommended the use of softer and more pliable materials such as Dacron-impregnated Silastic.[151] Although these procedures are simple and easy to perform under local anesthesia, the functional results are poor and the local complication rates (fecal impaction, wound infection, breakage, and erosion of the encircling material) are excessive.[152]

A variation of the Thiersch wire procedure is encirclement of the anal canal with skeletal muscle, usually either the gracilis[153] or a portion of the gluteus maximus.[154] Although this technique avoids many of the local complications of cerclage with foreign material, functional results remain poor because of the patient's inability to maintain continuous voluntary contraction of the muscle and the muscle's tendency to tire. These problems have been obviated by the addition of an implanted nerve stimulator that can be programmed externally.[155] Graded electrical stimulation is used to convert the muscle from fast twitch fibers to slow twitch fibers that are fatigue resistant. The pulse generator then maintains tonic contraction of the muscle until it is deactivated by the patient using a hand-held magnet. Early results using this technique are promising, with success rates of about 65% reported in patients who were not candidates for or failed to respond to standard therapy.[155,156]

If surgery or biofeedback fails to alleviate incontinence, strong consideration should be given to a colostomy. Although many patients initially express reluc-

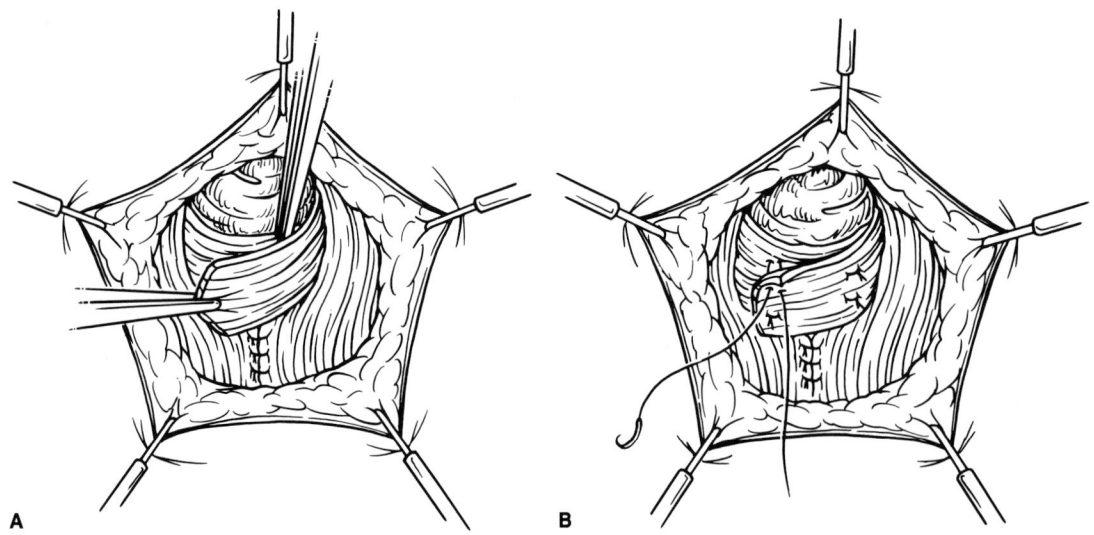

Figure 42-16 Overlapping sphincteroplasty for repair of anal sphincter injury. (**A**) The sphincter is widely mobilized, preserving scar tissue for suture placement. A levatoroplasty is performed. (**B**) Mattress sutures are used to maintain a snug sphincteric overlap.

tance to accept this procedure, they should understand that it essentially converts an unmanageable perineal stoma into a manageable abdominal one. Referral to an enterostomal therapist for preoperative education is essential for alleviating patient fears and concerns. The stoma site should be marked by the therapist before surgery, in a location that is visible to the patient, off the belt line, and away from abdominal scars and deformities. Because patient satisfaction hinges critically on the quality of the stoma itself, the surgeon must exert the effort to create a well-vascularized, tension-free, and technically perfect stoma.

RECTAL PROLAPSE

Complete rectal prolapse, or procidentia, is a full-thickness rectal intussusception that protrudes externally beyond the anal sphincters. Occult or hidden prolapse is an internal rectorectal intussusception that does not protrude beyond the anal verge.

The most common symptom of rectal prolapse is anal protrusion, which initially is caused by straining but eventually can occur spontaneously. Local related symptoms include mucous soiling, perianal excoriation, and mucosal bleeding. Many patients have bowel habit irregularities that range from total incontinence to constipation and incomplete evacuation. Complete rectal prolapse occasionally becomes incarcerated; this situation can lead to vascular compromise and strangulation.

Rectal prolapse in children usually occurs before the age of 4 years. The sex distribution in this group of patients is equal.[157] The condition is associated with functional bowel abnormalities such as constipation or diarrhea. Associated congenital abnormalities include myelomeningocele, spina bifida, and exstrophy of the bladder.[158] There is an increased incidence of pediatric rectal prolapse after repair of imperforate anus.[159] In third-world countries, the condition is associated with parasitic infections that lead to diarrhea.[160] Cystic fibrosis can present with rectal prolapse, and screening for this condition is indicated in young children with unexplained prolapse.[161]

Most adults with rectal prolapse are women. There is an excessive incidence of rectal prolapse in institutionalized patients. The disorder can occur at any age, but the peak incidence is in the fifth to sixth decades. Its incidence and prevalence are unknown.

Anatomic correlates of rectal prolapse include diastasis of the levator ani muscles, a deep cul-de-sac, redundant sigmoid colon, loss of posterior rectal attachments, loss of the horizontal portion of the rectum, and

a patulous anal canal.[162] These abnormalities are most likely a result rather than the cause of prolapse.

Incontinence of varying degrees is reported in 40% to 70% of patients with rectal prolapse.[163] This problem is due in part to direct dilatation of the anal sphincter mechanism and in part to traction injuries of the pudendal nerves. Electromyographic studies have documented normal pelvic nerve function in continent patients with rectal prolapse and pelvic floor denervation in incontinent patients.[164]

The diagnosis of complete rectal prolapse usually is obvious on clinical grounds. Full-thickness prolapse can range from the size of a walnut to that of a melon and is documented best by instructing patients to strain while seated on a commode. Rectal prolapse is difficult to demonstrate when patients are being examined in the prone jackknife position. It is imperative that full-thickness rectal prolapse be distinguished from rectal mucosal prolapse, which is associated with advanced hemorrhoidal disease. The most important factor differentiating these disorders is that full-thickness prolapse is characterized by concentric tissue folds, whereas mucosal prolapse is characterized by radial folds (Fig. 42-17). Other distinguishing features of full-thickness prolapse include the ability to palpate a double thickness of rectal wall by digital examination, the presence of a palpable sulcus between the anal verge, and the fact that mucosal prolapse rarely exceeds 5 cm in diameter.[165]

Rectal prolapse in children usually is a self-limited condition that is treated best with restoration of a normal bowel habit. Surgical therapy, when necessary, is accomplished most often with pararectal injection of sclerosing agents or linear cauterization of the rectal mucosa.[166,167]

Complete rectal prolapse in adults is treated by surgery. This therapy has two goals: to anatomically repair the prolapse itself and to correct the associated functional abnormalities. Dozens of operations directed toward these goals have been described over the years, and the lack of universal acceptance of any single procedure underlies the fact that no perfect operative solution to the problem of rectal prolapse exists.

Operations for rectal prolapse are classified into two groups based on anatomic approach: transabdominal repairs and perineal repairs. Transabdominal repairs involve rectal fixation, bowel resection, or a combination of fixation and resection. Proponents of transabdominal repairs argue that these operations have the lowest reported recurrence rates and are most likely to restore normal continence in incontinent patients. The disadvantage of these approaches is that they entail major pelvic dissection and, thus, impose

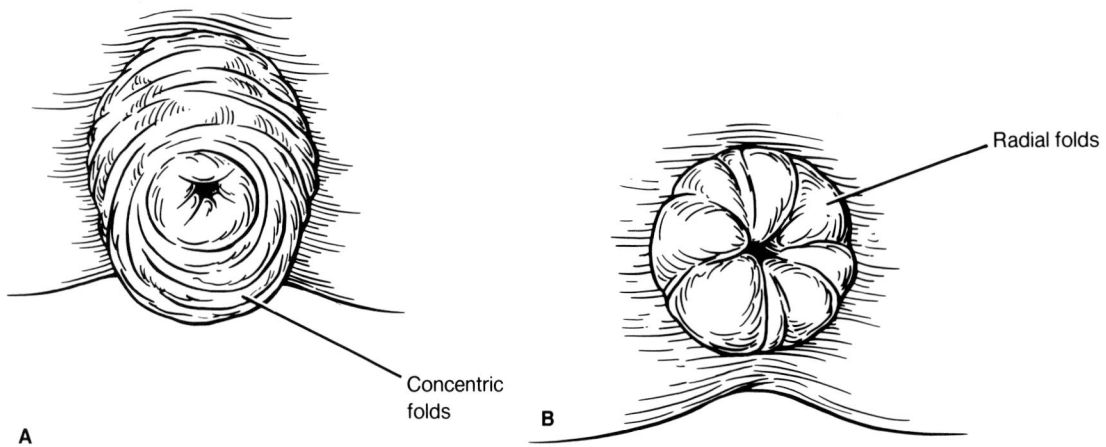

Figure 42-17 (**A**) Full-thickness rectal prolapse is characterized by concentric mucosal folds. (**B**) Rectal mucosal prolapse is associated with radial folds.

significant surgical risk in elderly patients, particularly those with associated medical problems.

Probably the most commonly practiced operation for rectal prolapse in the United States is the anterior sling repair or Ripstein procedure.[168] This operation involves suspension of the mobilized rectum from the sacrum using a completely encircling synthetic sling (Fig. 42-18). The anterior sling repair has been criticized for causing an excessive rate of obstructive complications, but actual sling stricture requiring reoperation has been documented in only a small percentage of patients.[169]

An alternative to the Ripstein procedure was devel-

oped in 1959.[170] The original operation used a piece of Ivalon sponge that was sutured to the sacrum and wrapped around the lateral aspects of the mobilized rectum (Fig. 42-19). Because Ivalon is difficult to remove should infection occur, and because it is associated with sarcoma formation in experimental animals, a variety of alternative sling materials have been used in its place. Proponents of the posterior sling believe that it is associated with fewer postoperative evacuation problems than is the anterior sling, but this contention is poorly documented. The need for any sling is questionable, because excellent results, comparable to those achieved with sling procedures, are reported with direct fixation of the lateral ligaments of the rectum to the sacrum using sutures.[171,172]

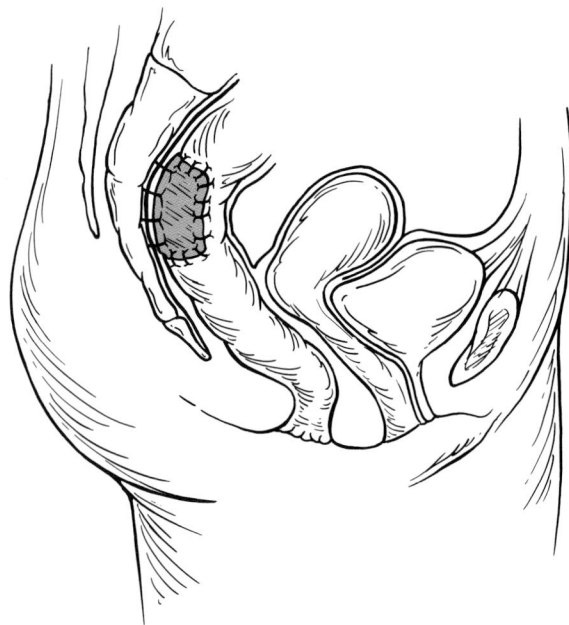

Figure 42-18 Ripstein repair for rectal prolapse.

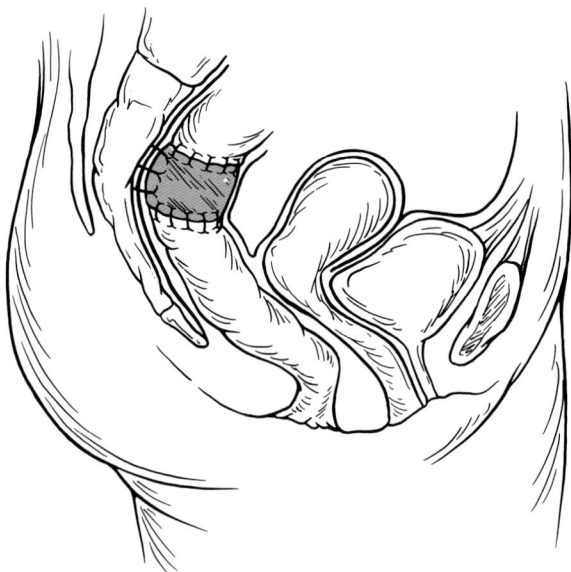

Figure 42-19 Ivalon sponge repair of rectal prolapse.

The use of rectal resection for prolapse repair is based on the notion that the mobilized rectum will scar to the presacral tissue without the need for fixation.[173] Advocates of this approach recommend high (to peritonealized rectum) versus low anterior resection to prevent excessive morbidity, because recurrence rates for the procedures are similar but complications are greatly increased when a low anastomosis is performed.[174]

Resection rectopexy involves complete rectal mobilization, suture fixation of the lateral ligaments to the sacrum, and resection of the redundant sigmoid colon.[175] Although the procedure can help prevent recurrent prolapse by suspending the left colon from the splenic flexure, the significance of resection with rectopexy lies more in its tendency to prevent postoperative constipation. In patients with rectal prolapse and documented slow transit colonic constipation, subtotal colectomy with ileosigmoid or ileorectal anastomosis and rectopexy should be strongly considered.[176]

Perineal prolapse repairs initially were described and popularized before the modern era of safe and routine abdominal and pelvic surgery. Because mixed results were reported at first, their popularity waned in favor of abdominal repairs. However, more recent series have reported excellent results using the perineal approach, particularly when simultaneous pelvic floor repair is carried out. Accordingly, whereas perineal repairs once were reserved exclusively for elderly patients with multiple associated medical problems, many surgeons are now using these repairs as their first line of therapy for all patients of any risk category.

Perineal rectosigmoidectomy first was described in 1889[177] and subsequently was popularized in the United States.[178] The operation, most easily performed with the patient in the prone jackknife position, consists of division of the outer ring of prolapsed rectum, sequential division of the mesenteric vessels until no additional rectum or sigmoid can be mobilized, amputation of the prolapsed segment, and sutured or stapled coloanal anastomosis (Fig. 42-20). Levator repair can be performed before the anastomosis anteriorly, posteriorly, or both, at the surgeon's discretion.

An alternate approach to perineal prolapse repair is the Delorme operation, which entails a long rectal mucosectomy, plication of the denuded rectal muscular wall around the circumference, excision of the redundant mucosa, and mucosal anastomosis at the dentate line[179] (Fig. 42-21). This procedure forms a muscular pessary at the level of the anal sphincter because of the rectal plication. Simultaneous pelvic floor repair can be performed, but this requires a separate posterior incision.

Some surgeons prefer to use anal encirclement procedures for high-risk patients with rectal prolapse. Al-

though these procedures are admittedly simple and can be performed under local anesthesia, they have high recurrence rates and a significant incidence of local complications such as fecal impaction, infection, and breakage and extrusion of the foreign material. Because the other perineal approaches are so well tolerated, even in the presence of multiple associated medical disorders, they are preferred over anal encirclement procedures.

Treatment of internal intussusception is controversial. Although this finding has been associated with symptoms of obstructed defecation and solitary rectal ulcer syndrome,[180,181] it also has been noted in up to 50% of normal volunteers.[182] In the absence of complete rectal prolapse, the results of rectopexy for solitary rectal ulcer syndrome are poor.[183] Better results have been reported using anteroposterior Marlex rectopexy,[184] but these findings await confirmation by other groups.

RECTOVAGINAL FISTULA

Rectovaginal fistulas are epithelialized communications between the rectum and vagina. Patients most commonly complain of passage of flatus or liquid stool through the vagina; passage of solid stool generally indicates an extremely large fistula. Secondary vaginitis frequently is present and often recurs after treatment; recurrent urinary tract infections also can be encountered. Symptoms of fecal incontinence often predominate when associated sphincter injuries are present, and bowel symptoms such as diarrhea, hematochezia, mucous discharge, and tenesmus can be prominent when rectal pathology is present.

The etiology of rectovaginal fistula is depicted here[185]:

Congenital disorders
Acquired disorders
Trauma
    Operative
    Obstetric
    Violent
Infection
Inflammatory bowel disease
Radiation
Carcinoma

The relative frequency of these causes varies widely between series, reflecting individual and institutional referral patterns.

Congenital rectovaginal fistula usually is seen in association with a congenital anorectal malformation, such as a "high" imperforate anus. Obstetric injury is

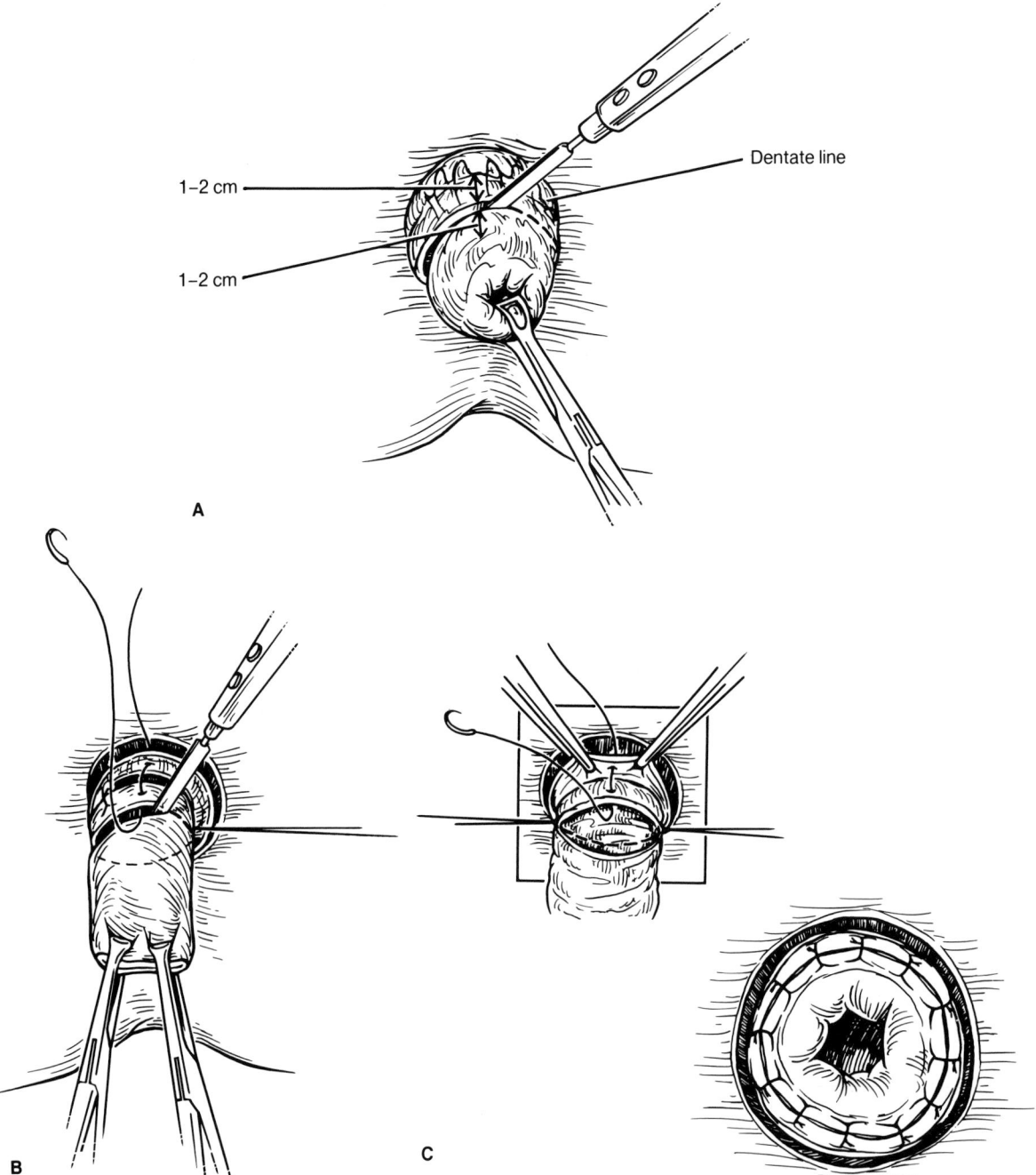

Figure 42-20 Steps in perineal repair of rectal prolapse. (**A**) The prolapsed rectum is grasped and delivered externally. A full-thickness incision of both rectal walls is performed with electrocautery. (**B**) As the incision proceeds, the rectal walls are anastomosed with full-thickness sutures. (**C**) Completion of the perineal anastomosis.

the most common cause of traumatic rectovaginal fistula. The fistula can occur after unrecognized injury, inadequately repaired injury, or late breakdown after repair due to infection or hematoma formation. Postoperative fistula can occur after hysterectomy or low an-

terior resection of the rectum. Cryptoglandular anorectal infection, normally the cause of fistula in ano, occasionally leads to rectovaginal fistula. The fistula also can be associated with inflammatory bowel disease, especially Crohn's disease. Rectovaginal fistula

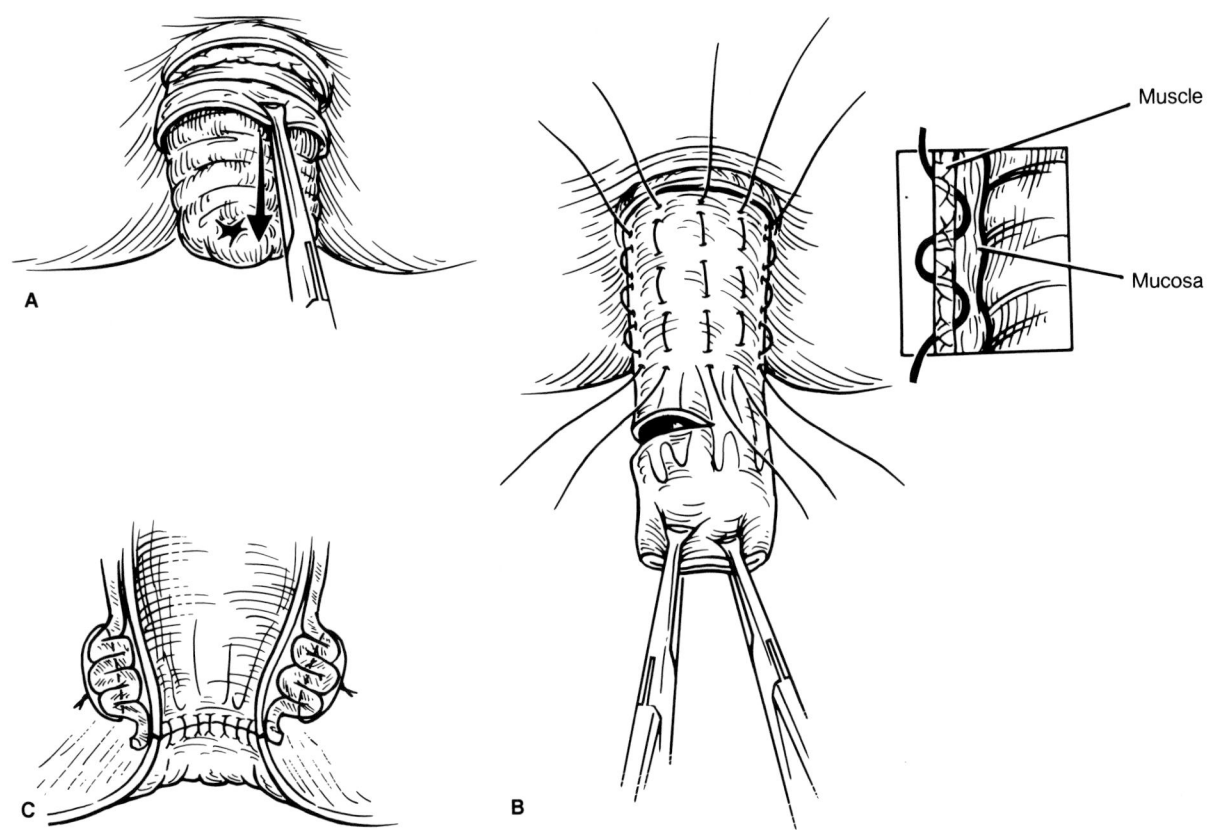

Muscle

Mucosa

A

C

B

Figure 42-21 Delorme operation for rectal prolapse. **(A)** The initial steps involve a long, peri-
neally performed rectal mucosectomy. **(B)** The denuded rectal muscular wall is plicated circumferentially. **(C)** After excision of the redundant mucosa, an anastomosis is performed at the
dentate line. This procedure forms a muscular pessary at the level of the anal sphincter as a
result of the rectal plication. Simultaneous pelvic floor repair can be performed through a separate posterior incision.

can occur as a complication of pelvic radiotherapy for
malignancies, usually gynecologic in origin. Advanced
pelvic malignancy, including primary and recurrent gynecologic and rectal cancer, can cause rectovaginal fistula by direct extension and tumor necrosis.

The diagnosis of rectovaginal fistula generally is
made by history alone and usually can be confirmed
by careful pelvic, rectal, and bidigital examination. The
fistula frequently is surprisingly small and can have the
appearance of a small pit or depression in the rectal or
vaginal mucosa. Communication between the two mucosal surfaces sometimes can be confirmed with gentle
and judicious use of a small fistula probe, but this maneuver usually is too painful to perform in the office
setting. Endoscopic inspection of the rectosigmoid is
mandatory to evaluate and exclude primary large bowel
disorders such as Crohn's disease, cancer, or radiation
proctitis. Details of fecal incontinence should be elicited, and patients with abnormal sphincter function
should undergo anorectal physiologic assessment before surgical repair of the fistula is planned.

Occasionally, it is difficult to confirm the presence
of a rectovaginal fistula that is suspected on clinical
grounds. Contrast enema and vaginography sometimes
are of benefit but often fail to visualize small fistulas.
Endorectal or endovaginal ultrasound, when performed by an experienced examiner, can document the
fistula. Many authors advocate the use of methylene
blue retention enemas with a vaginal tampon in place;
staining of the tampon confirms the presence, if not the
location, of the fistula. An alternate approach is to perform proctoscopy with the patient in the lithotomy position and the vagina filled with warm water; vaginal
air bubbles confirm the presence of a fistula.[186] If a rectovaginal fistula is not identified in the presence of suggestive symptoms, evaluation for a more proximal gastrointestinal source of the fistula should be undertaken.
Common sources include the sigmoid colon from diverticular disease and the small bowel from Crohn's
disease.

It is useful when planning treatment to classify rectovaginal fistulas as either simple or complex.[187] Simple

fistulas are less than 2.5 cm in diameter, occur in the low to middle rectovaginal septum, and are caused by trauma (including iatrogenic and obstetric) or infection. Complex fistulas are greater than 2.5 cm in diameter, occur high in the rectovaginal septum, and are caused by inflammatory bowel disease, radiotherapy, neoplasm, or failed repair of a previous simple fistula. It also is helpful to classify rectovaginal fistulas based on their relationship to the anal sphincter,[188] using the classification systems described by Parks for fistula in ano.[189]

Fistula repair should not be undertaken until the patient and the local tissues are in the best possible condition to obtain a successful outcome. Posttraumatic fistulas should be given at least 6 months to allow maximum spontaneous healing and subsidence of the local inflammatory response. Local sepsis should be treated where appropriate with abscess drainage and antibiotics. Medical treatment of inflammatory bowel disease should be optimized.

Repairs of simple rectovaginal fistulas usually are performed using the perineal approach and do not require fecal diversion. Rectal, vaginal, and combined (conversion of perineal laceration with layer closure) repairs all have been described with excellent success. Simple fistulotomy should not be performed because of the high likelihood of postoperative incontinence.

When anal sphincter function is normal, either endorectal or vaginal repair can be performed. Whereas gynecologists tend to prefer the vaginal approach, most colorectal surgeons opt for the endorectal sliding advancement flap repair. This technique offers the practical advantage of familiar anatomy and the theoretic advantage of closing the high-pressure side of the fistula's opening. The operation is performed after complete bowel preparation with the patient in the prone jackknife position. An endorectal flap that includes the mucosa, submucosa, and circular smooth muscles is elevated beginning just distal to the fistula and progressing proximally about 3 to 5 cm. The cephalad base of the flap is designed to be roughly twice the width of the caudad apex to ensure adequate submucosal blood supply to the flap. The fistula tract is curetted and the divided lateral circular muscle fibers are reapproximated with absorbable sutures. The flap then is advanced without tension over the closure and is secured in place with absorbable suture. The rectal mucosa involved by the fistula is excised and discarded before closure. The vaginal defect is left open to permit drainage.

The success of the endorectal flap advancement closure depends on the number of prior attempts at repair. Failure is likely in patients who have had at least two previous failed attempts at local repair, probably because local tissue is inadequate to sustain healing.[187]

Under these circumstances, a muscle intraposition procedure using the bulbocavernosus or gracilis should be considered.

When rectovaginal fistula is associated with sphincter injury (a common scenario after childbirth injury), conversion to a complete perineal laceration with overlapping layered closure as discussed earlier for fecal incontinence has a high rate of success in correcting both problems.

A detailed discussion of the many surgical approaches to complex rectovaginal fistulas is beyond the scope of this chapter. Perineal approaches to such fistulas require the interposition of healthy muscle tissue such as the bulbocavernosus, gracilis, or sartorius. Abdominal approaches include simple diversion, resection, and restorative resection. Radiation-associated rectovaginal fistulas are treated best with rectal resection and coloanal sleeve anastomosis. Coloanal anastomosis, particularly in the setting of previous radiotherapy, generally should be performed in conjunction with a covering proximal stoma.

Investigators have described an alternate approach to the treatment of radiation-induced rectovaginal fistula using an onlay patch anastomosis.[185,190] In this technique, the sigmoid colon is divided and a proximal end-sigmoid colostomy is created, and the distal rectosigmoid is folded down and anastomosed to the débrided rectal fistula. After complete healing has been documented, the sigmoid colon is anastomosed to the apex of the rectosigmoid loop. This technique has the disadvantage of leaving behind the diseased bowel.

Rectovaginal fistula associated with Crohn's disease often is considered an indication for proctectomy. However, there has been a trend toward attempting local repair in such patients, especially when the rectum is relatively uninvolved. Good results have been reported using this approach in carefully selected patients. Medical and surgical control of any proximal inflammatory bowel disease is important for optimal maintenance of continence.

REFERENCES

1. Thomson WHF. The nature of hemorrhoids. Br J Surg 1975;62:542.
2. Bernstein WC. What are hemorrhoids and what is their relationship to the portal venous system? Dis Colon Rectum 1983;26:829.
3. Johanson JF, Sonnenberg A. Prevalence of hemorrhoids and chronic constipation: an epidemiologic study. Gastroenterology 1990;98:380.
4. Burkitt DP, Graham-Stewart CW. Haemorrhoids: postulated pathogenesis and proposed prevention. Postgrad Med J 1975;51:631.

5. Hosking SW, Smart HL, Johnson AG, Triger DR. Anorectal varices, haemorrhoids, and portal hypertension. Lancet 1989;1:349.

6. Waldron DJ, Kumar D, Hallan RI, Williams NS. Prolonged ambulant assessment of anorectal function in patients with prolapsing hemorrhoids. Dis Colon Rectum 1989;32:968.

7. Gibbons CP, Bannister JJ, Read NW. Role of constipation and anal hypertonia in the pathogenesis of hemorrhoids. Br J Surg 1988;75:656.

8. Goenka M, Kochhar R, Nagi B, Mehta SK. Rectosigmoid varices and other mucosal changes in patients with portal hypertension. Am J Gastroenterol 1991;86:1185.

9. Moesgaard F, Nielsen ML, Hansen JB, Knudsen JT. High fiber diet reduces bleeding and pain in patients with hemorrhoids. Dis Colon Rectum 1982;25:454.

10. Senapati A, Nicholls RJ. Randomized trial to compare the results of injection sclerotherapy with a bulk laxative alone in the treatment of bleeding hemorrhoids. Int J Colorectal Dis 1988;3:124.

11. Barron J. Office ligation treatment of hemorrhoids. Dis Colon Rectum 1963;6:109.

12. Wroblewski DE, Corman ML, Veidenheimer MC, Coller JA. Long-term evaluation of rubber ring ligation in hemorrhoidal disease. Dis Colon Rectum 1980;23:478.

13. Lau WY, Chow HP, Poon GP, Wong SH. Rubber band ligation of three primary hemorrhoids in a single session: a safe and effective procedure. Dis Colon Rectum 1982;25:336.

14. Marshman D, Huber PJ Jr, Timmerman W, Simontaon CT, Odomn FC, Kaplan ER. Hemorrhoid ligation: a review of efficacy. Dis Colon Rectum 1989;32:369.

15. Steinberg DM, Liegois H, Alexander-Williams J. Long term review of the results of rubber band ligation of haemorrhoids. Br J Surg 1975;62:144.

16. Edwards FS. The treatment of piles by injection. BMJ 1888;2:815.

17. Kelsey CB. How to treat haemorrhoids by injections of carbolic acid. NY Med J 1885;42:545.

18. Gartell PC, Sheridan RJ, McGinn FP. Outpatient treatment of haemorrhoids: a randomized clinical trial to compare rubber band ligation with phenol injection. Br J Surg 1985;72:478.

19. Ferguson JA, Heaton JR. Closed hemorrhoidectomy. Dis Colon Rectum 1959;2:176.

20. Fansler WA. Hemorrhoidectomy: an anatomic method. Lancet 1931;51:529.

21. Milligan ETC, Morgan CN, Jones LE, Officer R. Surgical anatomy of the anal canal and the operative treatment of hemorrhoids. Lancet 1937;2:1119.

22. Whitehead W. The surgical treatment of hemorrhoids. BMJ 1882;1:148.

23. Bonello JC. Who's afraid of the dentate line: the Whitehead hemorrhoidectomy. Am J Surg 1988;156:182.

24. Wolff BG, Culp CE. The Whitehead hemorrhoidectomy: an unjustly maligned procedure. Dis Colon Rectum 1988;31:587.

25. Leicester RJ, Nicholls RJ, Mann CV. Infrared coagulation: a new treatment for hemorrhoids. Dis Colon Rectum 1981;24:602.

26. Ambrose NS, Morris D, Alexander-Williams J, Keighley MRB. A randomized trial of photocoagulation or injection sclerotherapy for the treatment of first and second-degree hemorrhoids. Dis Colon Rectum 1985;28:238.

27. Templeton JL, Spence RAJ, Kennedy TL, MacKenzie G, Hanna WA. Comparison of infrared coagulation and rubber band ligation for first and second degree hemorrhoids: a randomized prospective clinical trial. BMJ 1983;286:1387.

28. Ambrose NS, Harres MM, Alexander-Williams J, Keighley MRB. Prospective randomised comparison of photocoagulation and rubber band ligation in treatment of haemorrhoids. BMJ 1983;286:1389.

29. Buchmann P, Seefeld H. Rubber band ligation for piles can be disastrous in HIV-positive patients. Int J Colorectal Dis 1989;4:57.

30. Khubchandani IT. A randomized comparison of single and multiple rubber band ligations. Dis Colon Rectum 1983;26:705.

31. Poon GP, Chu KW, Lau WY, et al. Conventional vs. triple rubber band ligation for hemorrhoids: a prospective, randomized trial. Dis Colon Rectum 1986;29:846.

32. Bartizal J, Slosberg P. An alternative to hemorrhoidectomy. Arch Surg 1977;12:534.

33. O'Hara VS. Fatal clostridial infection after hemorrhoidal banding. Dis Colon Rectum 1980;23:570.

34. Russell TR, Donohue JH. Hemorrhoidal banding: a warning. Dis Colon Rectum 1985;28:291.

35. Shemesh EI, Kodner IJ, Fry RD, Neufeld DM. Severe complications of rubber band ligation of internal hemorrhoids. Dis Colon Rectum 1987;30:199.

36. Scarpa FJ, Hillis W, Sabetta JR. Pelvic cellulitis: a life-threatening complication of hemorrhoidal banding. Surgery 1988;103:383.

37. Gehamy RA, Weakley FL. Internal hemorrhoidectomy by elastic ligation. Dis Colon Rectum 1974;17:347.

38. Adami B, Eckardt VF, Suermann RB, Karbach U, Ewe K. Bacteremia after proctoscopy and hemorrhoid injection sclerotherapy. Dis Colon Rectum 1981;24:373.

39. Smith LE, Goodreau JJ, Fouty WJ. Operative hemorrhoidectomy versus cryodestruction. Dis Colon Rectum 1979;22:10.

40. Bailey HR, Ferguson JA. Prevention of urinary retention by fluid restriction after anorectal operations. Dis Colon Rectum 1976;19:250.

41. Wang CH. Urgent hemorrhoidectomy for hemorrhoidal crisis. Dis Colon Rectum 1982;25:122.

42. Sacco S, Mortilla MG, Tonielli E, Morganti I, Cola B. Emergency hemorrhoidectomy for complicated hemorrhoids. Coloproctology 1987;9:210.

43. Saleeby RG Jr, Rosen L, Stasik JJ, et al. Hemorrhoidectomy during pregnancy: risk or relief? Dis Colon Rectum 1991;34:260.

44. Schottler JL, Balcos EG, Goldberg SM. Postpartum hemorrhoidectomy. Dis Colon Rectum 1973;16:395.

45. Lockhart-Mummery P. Diseases of the rectum and anus. New York, William Wood, 1914:169.

46. Klosterhalfen B, Vogel P, Rixen H, Mittermayer C. Topography of the inferior rectal artery: a possible cause of chronic, primary anal fissure. Dis Colon Rectum 1989;32:43.

47. Hancock BD. The internal sphincter and anal fissure. Br J Surg 1977;64:92.

48. Abcarian H, Lakshmanan S, Read DR, Roccaforte P. The role of internal sphincter in chronic anal fissures. Dis Colon Rectum 1982;25:525.

49. Chowcat NL, Araujo JGC, Boulos PB. Internal sphincterotomy for chronic anal fissure: long-term effects of anal pressure. Br J Surg 1986;73:915.

50. Nothman BJ, Schuster MM. Internal anal sphincter derangement with anal fissures. Gastroenterology 1974;67:216.

51. Arabi Y, Alexander-Williams J, Keighley MRB. Anal pressures in hemorrhoids and anal fissure. Am J Surg 1977;134:608.

52. Dodi G, Bogoni F, Infantino A, Pianon P, Mortellaro LM, Lise M. Hot or cold in anal pain?: a study of the changes in internal anal sphincter pressure profiles. Dis Colon Rectum 1986;29:248.

53. Jensen SL. Treatment of first episodes of acute anal fissure: prospective randomized study of lignocaine ointment versus hydrocortisone ointment or warm sitz baths plus bran. BMJ 1986;292:1167.

54. Jensen SL. Maintenance therapy with unprocessed bran in the prevention of acute anal fissure recurrence. J R Soc Med 1987;80:296.

55. Lock MR, Thomson JPS. Fissure-in-ano: the initial management and prognosis. Br J Surg 1977;65:355.

56. Goligher JC. An evaluation of internal sphincterotomy and simple sphincter stretching in the treatment of fissure-in-ano. Surg Clin North Am 1965;42:1299.

57. Gabriel WB. Principles and practice of rectal surgery, ed 5. Springfield, IL, Charles C Thomas, 1963:250.

58. Samson RB, Stewart WRC. Sliding skin grafts in the treatment of anal fissure. Dis Colon Rectum 1970;13:372.

59. Eisenhammer S. The surgical correction of chronic anal (sphincteric) contracture. S Afr Med J 1951;25:486.

60. Bennett RC, Goligher JC. Results of internal sphincterotomy for anal fissure. BMJ 1962;2:1500.

61. Eisenhammer S. The evaluation of internal anal sphincterotomy operation with special reference to anal fissure. Surg Gynecol Obstet 1959;109:583.

62. Parks AG. The management of fissure-in-ano. Hosp Med 1967;1:737.

63. Notaras MJ. The treatment of anal fissure by lateral subcutaneous internal sphincterotomy: a technique and results. Br J Surg 1971;58:96.

64. Gordon PH. Fissure-in-ano. In: Gordon PH, Nivatvongs S, eds. Principles and practice of surgery for the colon, rectum and anus. St Louis, Quality Medical Publishing, 1992:199.

65. Walker WA, Rothenberger DA, Goldberg SM. Morbidity of internal sphincterotomy for anal fissure and stenosis. Dis Colon Rectum 1985;28:832.

66. Abcarian H. Surgical correction of chronic anal fissure: results of lateral anal internal sphincterotomy vs fissurectomy-midline sphincterotomy. Dis Colon Rectum 1980;23:31.

67. Lewis TH, Corman ML, Prager ED, Robertson WG. Long-term results of open and closed sphincterotomy for anal fissure. Dis Colon Rectum 1988;31:368.

68. Vasilevsky CA, Gordon PH. The incidence of recurrent abscess or fistula-in-ano after anorectal suppuration. Dis Colon Rectum 1984;27:126.

69. Eisenhammer S. The internal anal sphincter and the anorectal abscess. Surg Gynecol Obstet 1956;103:501.

70. Parks AG. Pathogenesis and treatment of fistula-in-ano. BMJ 1961;1:463.

71. Goligher JC, Ellis M, Pissidis AG. A critique of anal glandular infection in the etiology and treatment of idiopathic anorectal abscesses and fistulas. Br J Surg 1967;54:977.

72. Read DR, Abcarian H. A prospective survey of 474 patients with anorectal abscess. Dis Colon Rectum 1979;22:566.

73. Beck DE, Fazio VW, Lavery IC, Jagelman DG, Weakley FL. Catheter drainage of ischiorectal abscesses. South Med J 1988;81:444.

74. Hanley PH. Conservative surgical correction of horseshoe abscess and fistula. Dis Colon Rectum 1965;8:364.

75. McElwain JW, MacLean MD, Alexander RM, Hoexter B, Guthrie JF. Experience with primary fistulectomy for anorectal abscess: a report of 1000 cases. Dis Colon Rectum 1975;18:646.

76. Chrabot CM, Prasad ML, Abcarian H. Recurrent anorectal abscesses. Dis Colon Rectum 1983;26:105.

77. Stelzner F. Die anorektalen Fisteln. Berlin, Springer-Verlag, 1959.

78. Lilius HG. Fistula-in-ano: an investigation of human fetal anal ducts and intramuscular glands and a clinical study of 150 patients. Acta Chir Scand Suppl 1968;383:1.

79. Parks AG, Gordon PH, Hardcastle JE. A classification of fistula-in-ano. Br J Surg 1976;63:1.

80. Lewis P, Bartolo DCCC. Treatment of trans-sphincteric fistulae by full thickness anorectal advancement flaps. Br J Surg 1990;77:1187.

81. Bennett RC. A review of orthodox treatment for anal fistula. Proc R Soc Med 1962;55:756.

82. Hill JR. Fistulas and fistulous abscesses in the anorectal region: personal experience in management. Dis Colon Rectum 1967;10:421.

83. Marks CG, Ritchie JK. Anal fistulas at St. Mark's Hospital. Br J Surg 1977;64:84.

84. Ewerth S, Ahlberg J, Collste G, Holmstrom B. Fistula-in-ano: a six year follow up study of 143 operated patients. Acta Chir Scand 1978;482(Suppl):53.

85. Adams D, Kovalcik PJ. Fistula-in-ano. Surg Gynecol Obstet 1981;153:731.

86. Vasilevsky CA, Gordon PH. Results of treatment of fistula-in-ano. Dis Colon Rectum 1985;28:225.

87. Kuijpers JH. Diagnosis and treatment of fistula-in-ano. Neth J Surg 1982;34:147.

88. Fucini C. One stage treatment of anal abscesses and fistulas: a clinical appraisal on the basis of two different classifications. Int J Colorectal Dis 1991;6:12.

89. Hanley PH, Ray JE, Pennington EE, Grablowsky OIM. A ten-year follow-up study of horseshoe abscess fistula-in-ano. Dis Colon Rectum 1976;19:507.

90. Ani AN, Solanke TF. Anal fistula: a review of 82 cases. Dis Colon Rectum 1976;19:5.

91. Homan WP, Tang CK, Thorbjarnarson B. Anal lesions complicating Crohn's disease. Arch Surg 1976;111:1333.

92. Keighley MRB, Allan RN. Current status and influence of operation on perianal Crohn's disease. Int J Colorectal Dis 1986;1:104.

93. Abcarian H. Perianal Crohn's disease. In: Dozois RR, ed. Management of Crohn's disease. Seminars in colon and rectal surgery, vol 5. Philadelphia, WB Saunders, 1994:210.

94. Hughes LE. Clinical classification of perianal Crohn's disease. Dis Colon Rectum 1992;35:928.

95. Francois Y, Vignal J, Descos L. Outcome of perianal fistulae in Crohn's disease: value of Highes' pathogenic classification. Int J Colorectal Dis 1993;8:39.

96. Weisman RI, Orsay CP, Pearl RK, Abcarian H. The role of fistulography in fistula-in-ano: report of five cases. Dis Colon Rectum 1991;34:181.

97. Sunratter Sehn AV, Lochs H, Vogelsang H, et al. Endoscopic ultrasound versus computed tomography in the differential diagnosis of perianorectal complications in Crohn's disease. Endoscopy 1993;25:582.

98. Lunniss PJ, Barker PG, Sultan AH, et al. Magnetic resonance imaging of fistula-in-ano. Dis Colon Rectum 1994;37:708.

99. Deen KI, Williams JG, Hutchinson R, Keighley M, Kumar D. Fistulas in ano: endoanal ultrasonographic assessment assists decision making for surgery. Gut 1994;35:391.

100. Bernstein LH, Frank MS, Brandt LJ, Boley SJ. Healing of perineal Crohn's disease with metronidazole. Gastroenterology 1980;79:357.

101. Brandt LJ, Bernstein LH, Boley SJ, Frank MS. Metronidazole therapy for perineal Crohn's diease: a follow up study. Gastroenterology 1982;83:383.

102. Morrison JG, Gathright JB Jr, Ray JE, et al. Surgical management of anorectal fistulas in Crohn's disease. Dis Colon Rectum 1989;32:492.

103. Fry RD, Shemesh EI, Kodner IJ, Timmcke A. Techniques and results in the management of anal and perianal Crohn's disease. Surg Gynecol Obstet 1989;168:42.

104. White RA, Eisenstat TE, Rubin RJ, Salvati EP. Seton management of complex anorectal fistulas in patients with Crohn's disease. Dis Colon Rectum 1990;33:587.

105. Brough WA, Schofield PF. The value of the rectus abdominis myocutaneous flap in the treatment of complex perineal fistula. Dis Colon Rectum 1991;34:148.

106. Grant DR, Cohen Z, McLeod RS. Loop ileostomy for anorectal Crohn's disease. Can J Surg 1986;29:32.

107. Sher ME, Bauer JJ, Gelernt I. Surgical repair of rectovaginal fistulas in patients with Crohn's disease: transvaginal approach. Dis Colon Rectum 1991;34:641.

108. Bayer I, Gordon PH. Selected operative management of fistula-in-ano in Crohn's disease. Dis Colon Rectum 1994;37:760.

109. Williams JG, Rothenberger DA, Nemer FD, Goldberg SM. Fistula-in-ano in Crohn's disease: results of aggressive surgical treatment. Dis Colon Rectum 1991;34:378.

110. Kooistra HP. Pilonidal sinuses: review of the literature and report of three hundred fifty cases. Am J Surg 1942;55:3.

111. Patey DH, Scarff RW. Pathology of postanal pilonidal sinus: its bearing on treatment. Lancet 1946;25:484.

112. Patey DH, Scarff RW. The hair of the pilonidal sinus. Lancet 1955;268:772.

113. Bascom J. Pilonidal disease: origin from follicles of hairs and results of follicle removal as treatment. Surgery 1980;87:567.

114. Pilipshen SJ, Gray G, Goldsmith E, Dinem P. Carcinoma arising in pilonidal sinuses. Ann Surg 1981;193:506.

115. Jensen SL, Harling H. Prognosis after simple incision and drainage for a first-episode acute pilonidal abscess. Br J Surg 1988;75:60.

116. Dichateau J, De Mol J, Bostoen H, Allegaert W. Pilonidal sinus: excision-marsupialization-phenolization? Acta Chir Belg 1985;85:325.

117. Kronborg O, Christensen K, Zimmermann-Nielsen C. Chronic pilonidal disease: a randomized trial with a complete three-year follow-up. Br J Surg 1985;72:303.

118. Toubanakis G. Treatment of pilonidal sinus disease with the Z-plasty procedure (modified). Am Surg 1986;52:611.

119. Karydakis GE. New approach to the problem of pilonidal sinus. Lancet 1973;2:1414.

120. Guyuron B, Dinner MI, Dowden RV. Excision and grafting in treatment of recurrent pilonidal sinus disease. Surg Gynecol Obstet 1983;156:201.

121. Perez-Gurri JA, Temple-Walley J, Ketcham AS. Gluteus maximus myocutaneous flap for the treatment of recalcitrant pilonidal disease. Dis Colon Rectum 1984;27:262.

122. Bascom JU. Repeat pilonidal operations. Am J Surg 1987;154:118.

123. Conway H, Strark RB, Climo S, et al. The surgical treatment of chronic hidradenitis suppurativa. Surg Gynecol Obstet 1952;95:455.

124. Thornton JP, Abcarian H. Surgical treatment of perianal and perineal hidradenitis suppurativa. Dis Colon Rectum 1978;21:573.

125. Culp CE. Chronic hidradenitis suppurativa of the anal canal: a surgical skin disease. Dis Colon Rectum 1983;26:669.

126. Broadwater JR, Bryant RL, Petrino RA, et al. Advanced

hidradenitis suppurativa: review of surgical treatment in 23 patients. Am J Surg 1982;144:668.

127. Rosenfeld N, Babar A. Hidradenitis suppurativa of the perianal and gluteal regions, treated by excision and skin grafting. Plast Reconstr Surg 1976;58:98.

128. Masson JK. Surgical treatment for hidradenitis suppurativa. Surg Clin North Am 1969;49:1043.

129. Shaughnessy DM, Greminger RR, Margolis JB. Hidradenitis suppurativa: a plea for early operative treatment. JAMA 1972;222:320.

130. Nelson R, Norton N, Cautley E. Prevalence of fecal incontinence in Wisconsin households. Dis Colon Rectum 1994;37:9.

131. Garrard J, Madoff R, Maldonado G, et al. Prevalence and impact of fecal incontinence (FI) of elderly people in the community and nursing home. (Submitted for publication).

132. Madoff RD, Williams JG, Caushaj PF. Fecal incontinence. N Engl J Med 1992;326:1002.

133. Wrenn K. Fecal impaction. N Engl J Med 1989;321: 658.

134. Schiller LR, Schmulen AC, Hendler RS, Harford WV, Fordtran JS. Pathogenesis of fecal incontinence in diabetes mellitus: evidence for internal-anal-sphincter dysfunction. N Engl J Med 1982;307:1666.

135. Parks AG, Swash M, Urich H. Sphincter denervation in anorectal incontinence and rectal prolapse. Gut 1977;18:656.

136. Pena A. Pediatric surgical problems. In: Corman ML, ed. Colon and rectal surgery, ed 2. Philadelphia, JB Lippincott, 1989:249.

137. Sultan AH, Kamm MA, Hudson CN, Chir M, Thomas JM, Bartram CI. Anal-sphincter disruption during vaginal delivery. N Engl J Med 1993;329:1905.

138. Snooks SJ, Wash M, Henry MM, Setchell M. Risk factors in childbirth causing damage to the pelvic floor innervation. Br J Surg 1985;72(Suppl):S15.

139. Garcia-Aguilar J, Belmonte C, Wong WD, Goldberg SM, Madoff RD. Surgical treatment of fistula-in-ano: factors associated with recurrence and incontinence. Dis Colon Rectum 1994;37:8.

140. Garcia-Aguilar J, Belmonte C, Wong WD, Lowry AC, Madoff RD. Open vs. closed sphincterotomy for chronic anal fissure: long-term results. Dis Colon Rectum 1994;37:9.

141. Smith LE, ed. Practical guide to anorectal testing. New York, Igaku-Shoin, 1990.

142. Fang DT, Nivatvongs S, Vermeulen FD, Herman FN, Goldberg SM, Rothenberger DA. Overlapping sphincteroplasty for acquired anal incontinence. Dis Colon Rectum 1984;27:720.

143. Browning GGP, Motson RW. Anal sphincter injury: management and results of Parks sphincter repair. Ann Surg 1984;199:351.

144. Yoshioka K, Keighley MRB. Sphincter repair for fecal incontinence. Dis Colon Rectum 1989;32:39.

145. Parks AG. Post anal pelvic floor repair (and the treatment of faecal incontinence). In: Todd IP, ed. Operative surgery, ed 3. London, Butterworths, 1977:249.

146. Yoshioka K, Keighley MRB. Critical assessment of the quality of continence after postanal repair for faecal incontinence. Br J Surg 1989;78:1054. (Erratum, Br J Surg 1990;77:356)

147. MacLeod JH. Management of anal incontinence by biofeedback. Gastroenterology 1987;93:291.

148. Jensen LL, Lowry AC. Biofeedback: a viable treatment option for anal incontinence. (Abstract) Dis Colon Rectum 1991;34(Suppl):6.

149. Wald A. Biofeedback for neurogenic fecal incontinence: rectal sensation is a determinant of outcome. J Pediatr Gastroenterol Nutr 1983;2:302.

150. Goldmann J. Concerning prolapse of the rectum with special emphasis on the operation by Theirsch. Dis Colon Rectum 1988;31:154.

151. Labow S, Rubin RJ, Hoexter B, Salvati EP. Perineal repair of rectal procidentia with an elastic fabric sling. Dis Colon Rectum 1980;23:467.

152. Vongsangnak V, Varma JS, Smith AN. Reappraisal of Theirsch's operation for complete rectal prolapse. J R Coll Surg Edinb 1985;30:185.

153. Corman ML. Gracilis muscle transposition for anal incontinence: late results. Br J Surg 1985;72(Suppl):S21.

154. Hentz VR. Construction of a rectal sphincter using the origin of the gluteus maximus muscle. Plast Reconstr Surg 1982;70:82.

155. Konsten J, Baeten CG, Spaans F, Havenith MG, Soeters PB. Follow-up of anal dynamic graciloplasty for fecal continence. World J Surg 1993;17:404.

156. Williams NS, Patel J, George BD, Hallan RI, Watkins ES. Development of an electrically stimulated neoanal sphincter. Lancet 1991;338:1166.

157. Corman ML. Rectal prolapse in children. Dis Colon Rectum 1985;28:535.

158. Freeman NV. Rectal prolapse in children. J R Soc Med 1984;77(Suppl):9.

159. Bhandari B, Ameta DK. Etiology of prolapsed rectum in children with special reference to amoebiasis. Indian Pediatr 1977;14:635.

160. Kulczycki LL, Shwachman H. Studies in cystic fibrosis of the pancreas: occurrence of rectal prolapse. N Engl J Med 1958;259:409.

161. Stern RC, Izant RJ Jr, Boat TF, et al. Treatment and prognosis of rectal prolapse in cystic fibrosis. Gastroenterology 1982;82:707.

162. Goldberg SM, Gordon PH, Nivatvongs S. Essentials of anorectal surgery. Philadelphia, JB Lippincott, 1980.

163. Madoff RD. Rectal prolapse and intussusception. In: Beck DE, Wexner SD, eds. Fundamentals of anorectal surgery. New York, McGraw-Hill, 1992:89.

164. Pemberton JH, Kelly KA. Achieving enteric continence: principles and applications. Mayo Clin Proc 1986;61: 586.

165. Carter HG. Treatment of procidentia of the rectum. South Med J 1971;64:1238.

166. Wyllie GG. The injection treatment of rectal prolapse. J Pediatr Surg 1979;14:62.

167. Hight DW, Hertzler JH, Phillippart AI, et al. Linear cauterization for the treatment of rectal prolapse in infants and children. Surg Gynecol Obstet 1982;154:400.

168. Morgan CN, Porter NH, Klugman DJ. Ivalon (polyvinyl alcohol) sponge in the repair of complete rectal prolapse. Br J Surg 1972;59:841.

169. Gordon PH, Hoexter B. Complications of the Ripstein procedure. Dis Colon Rectum 1978;21:277.

170. Wells C. New operation for rectal prolapse. Proc R Soc Med 1959;52:602.

171. Goligher JC. Surgery of the anus, rectum and colon, ed 4. New York, Macmillan. 1984:246.

172. Blatchford GJ, Perry RE, Thorson AG, Christensen MA. Rectopexy without resection for rectal prolapse. Am J Surg 1989;158:574.

173. Muir EG. A suspension operation for prolapse of the rectum. Ann Surg 1947;126:833.

174. Schlinkert RT, Beart RW Jr, Wolff BG, Pemberton JH. Anterior resection for complete rectal prolapse. Dis Colon Rectum 1985;28:409.

175. Watts JD, Rothenberger DA, Buls JG, Goldberg SM, Nivatvongs S. The management of procidentia: thirty years experience. Dis Colon Rectum 1985;28:96.

176. Madoff RD, Williams JG, Wong WD, Rothenberger DA, Goldberg SM. Long-term functional results of colon resection and rectopexy for overt rectal prolapse. Am J Gastroenterol 1992;87:101.

177. Mikulicz J. Zur operativen Behandlung des prolapsus recti et coli invaginati. Arch Klin Chir 1889;38:74.

178. Altemeier WA, Culbertson WR, Schowengerdt C, Hunt J. Nineteen years experience with the 1-stage perineal repair of rectal prolapse. Am Surg 1971;173:993.

179. Delorme E. On the treatment of total prolapse of the rectum by excision of the rectal mucus membranes or recto-colic. Dis Colon Rectum 1985;28:544.

180. Kuijpers HC, Schreve RH, Ten Cate Hoedemakers H. Diagnosis of functional disorders of defecation causing the solitary rectal ulcer syndrome. Dis Colon Rectum 1986;29:126.

181. Mahieu PHG. Barium enema and defaecography in the diagnosis and evaluation of the solitary rectal ulcer syndrome. Int J Colorectal Dis 1986;1:85.

182. Shorvon PJ, McHugh S, Diamant NE, Somers S, Stevenson GW. Defecography in normal volunteers: results and implications. Gut 1989;30:1737.

183. Keighley MRB, Shouler P. Clinical and manometric features of the solitary rectal ulcer syndrome. Dis Colon Rectum 1984;27:507.

184. Nicholls RJ. Internal intussusception: the solitary rectal ulcer syndrome. Seminars in Colon and Rectal Surgery 1991;2:227.

185. Lowry AC. Rectovaginal fistulas. In: Beck DE, Wexner SC, eds. Fundamentals of anorectal surgery. New York, McGraw-Hill, 1992:145.

186. Corman ML. Colon and rectal surgery, ed 3. Philadelphia, JB Lippincott, 1993:171.

187. Lowry AC, Thorson AG, Rothenberger DA, Goldberg SM. Repair of simple rectovaginal fistulas: influence of previous repairs. Dis Colon Rectum 1988;31:676.

188. Radcliffe AG, Ritchie JK, Hawley PR, Lennard-Jones JE, Northover JMA. Anovaginal and rectovaginal fistulas in Crohn's disease. Dis Colon Rectum 1988;31:94.

189. Parks AG, Gordon PH, Hardcastle JD. A classification of fistula-in-ano. Br J Surg 1976;63:1.

190. Bricker EM, Johnston WD. Repair of postirradiation rectovaginal fistula and stricture. Surg Gynecol Obstet 1979;148:499.

43

Atlas of Colon and Anorectal Surgery

David A. Rothenberger

Digestive Tract Surgery: A Text and Atlas, edited by Richard H. Bell, Layton F. Rikkers, and Michael W. Mulholland. Lippincott-Raven Publishers, Philadelphia, © 1996.

PREOPERATIVE PREPARATION

Preoperative preparation for elective colorectal surgery includes considerations similar to those for other major laparotomies. Cardiovascular stability and pulmonary toilet must be ensured; chronic diseases such as diabetes mellitus and hypertension must be in good control. To ensure postoperative healing, the patient's nutritional status should be adequate. Preoperatively obtained radiographs, both cross-sectional and contrast, are frequently used for preoperative colonic diagnosis and must be reviewed.

The high number of potentially virulent organisms within feces poses special problems for colorectal surgery. The fecal flora can be reduced by mechanical cleaning of the bowel. Mechanical preparation can be further augmented by oral antibiotics, such as erythromycin base and neomycin. Prophylactic intravenous antibiotics should be used routinely. To be effective, prophylactic antibiotics must be administered before the incision is made and should be continued for 24 hours after the operation.

Emergency colorectal surgery does not permit the same sort of measures to reduce fecal bacterial content. When colon perforation exists, fecal peritonitis is frequently associated with septic shock. Adequate hemodynamic monitoring and preoperative fluid resuscitation are essential in this circumstance. Empiric antibiotics, selected to broadly cover aerobic gram-negative and anaerobic organisms, should be modified by intraoperatively obtained bacterial cultures. For both elective and emergent colorectal surgery, the sites for potential ostomies should be indicated preoperatively. Ostomy sites should be marked so that skin folds, creases, incisions, and previous scars are avoided.

SECTION I   Anatomy of the Colon and Rectum

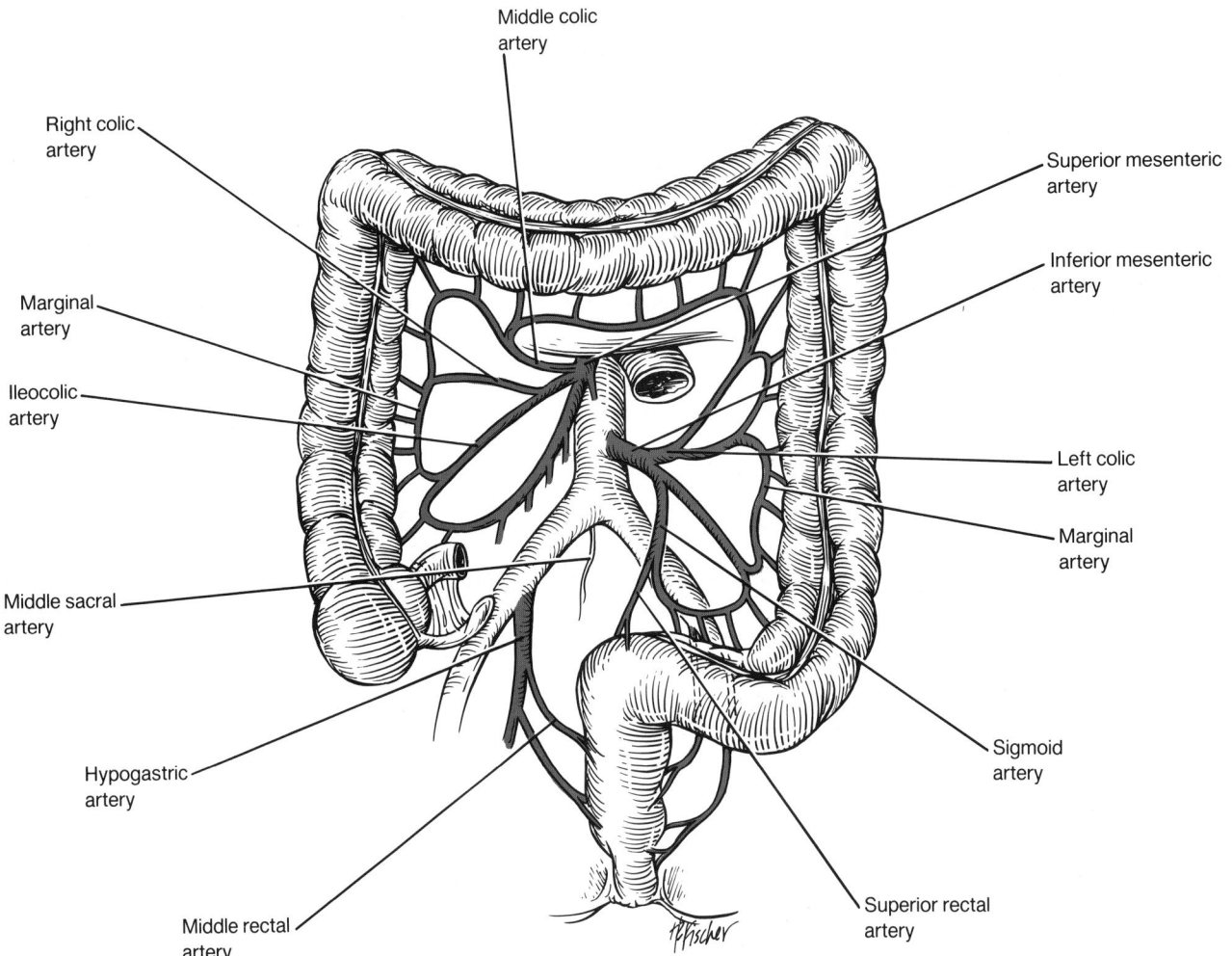

Figure 43-I-1

Arterial Blood Supply to the Colon

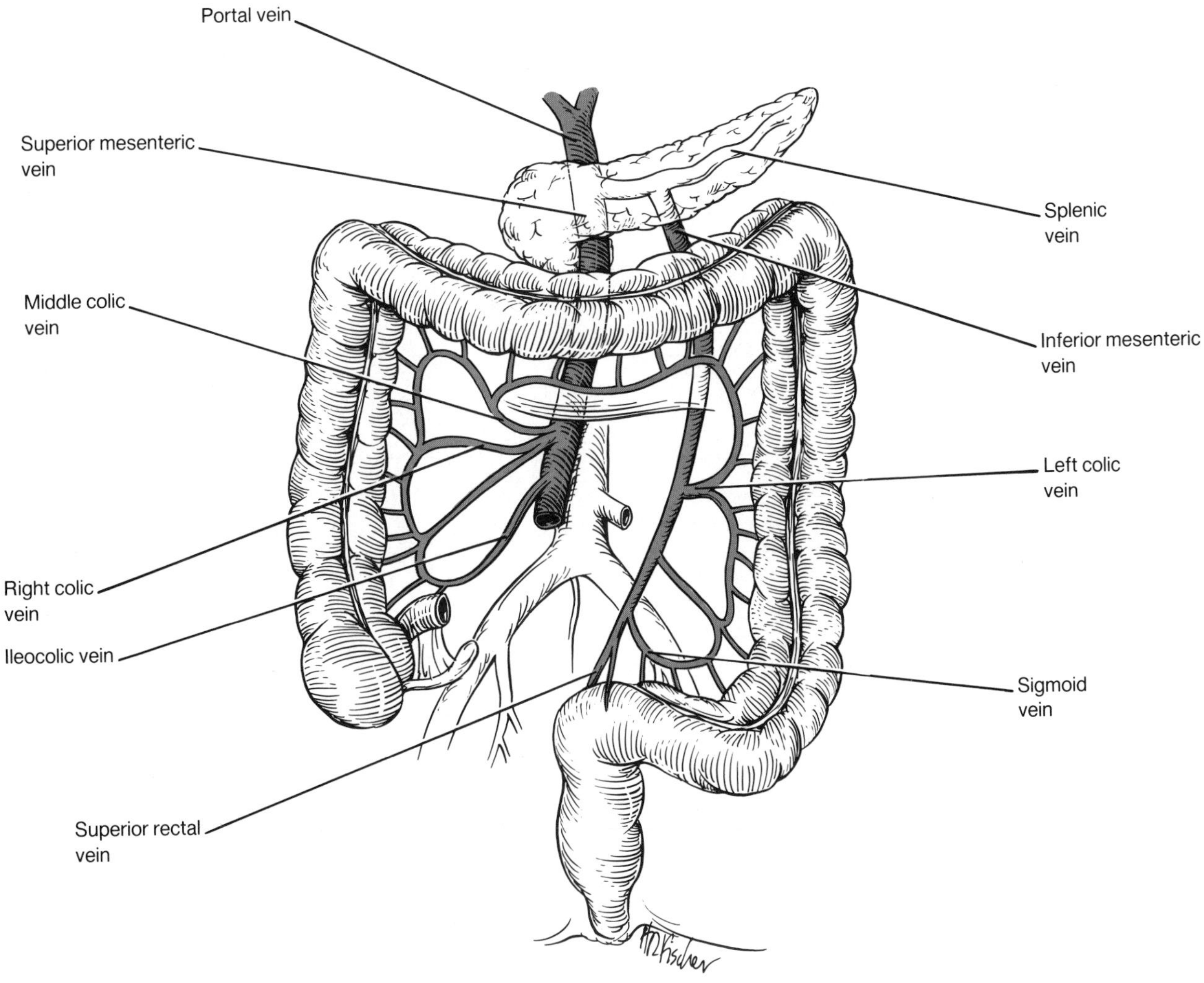

Portal vein

Superior mesenteric
vein

Splenic
vein

Middle colic
vein

Inferior mesenteric
vein

Left colic
vein

Right colic
vein

Ileocolic vein

Sigmoid
vein

Superior rectal
vein

Figure 43-I-2

Venous Drainage of the Colon

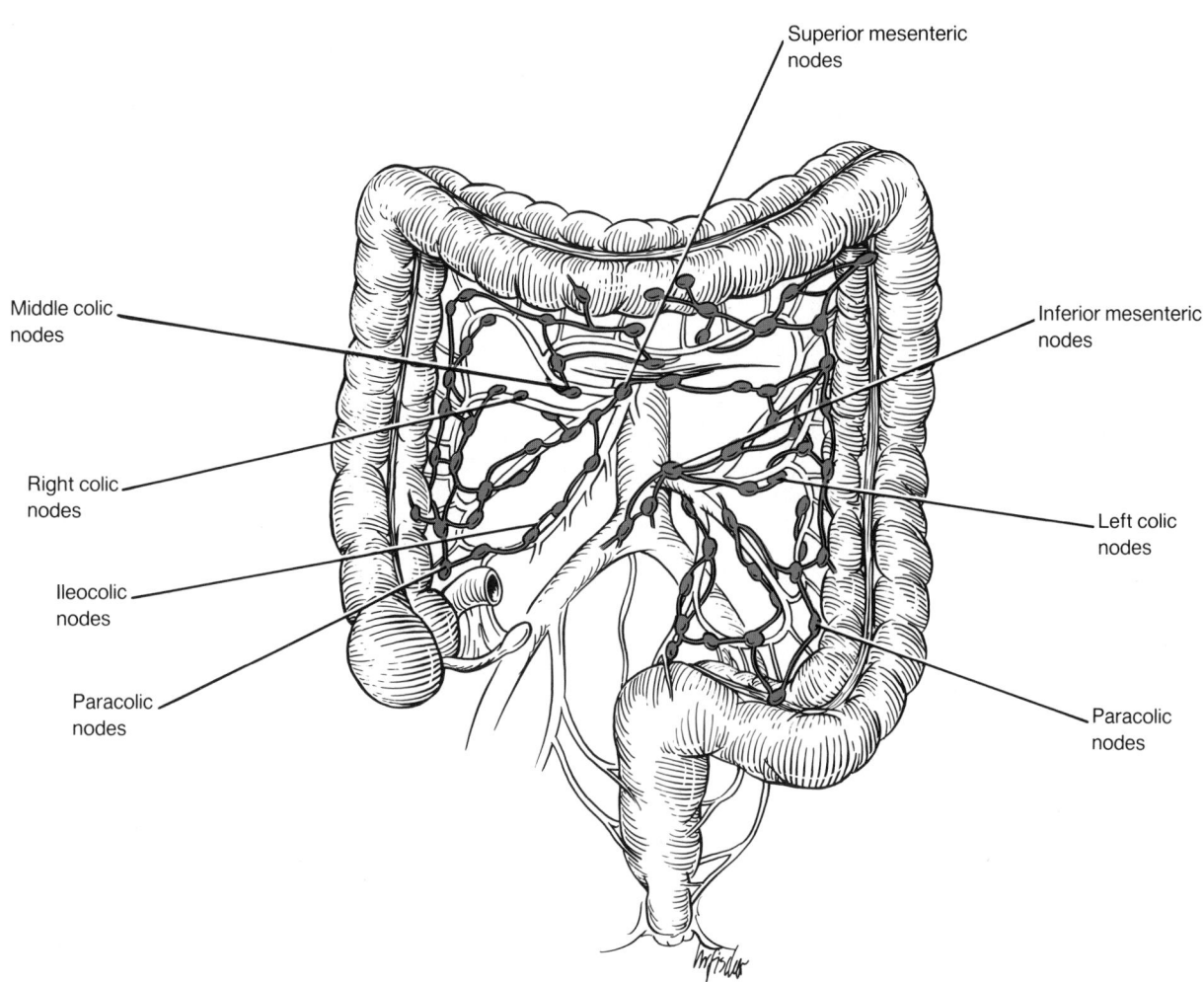

Figure 43-I-3

Lymphatic Drainage of the Colon

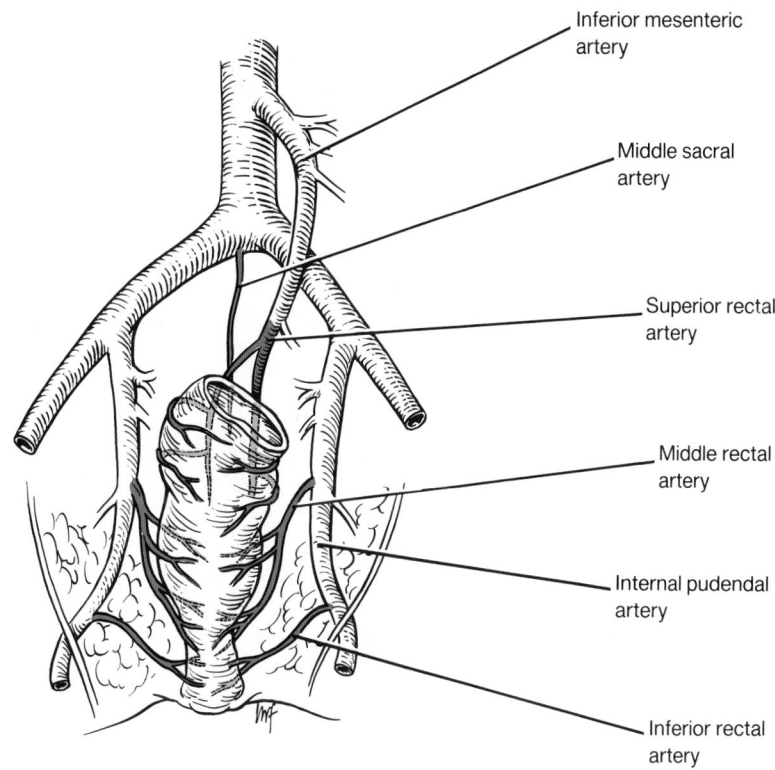

Figure 43-I-4

Arterial Supply to the Rectum

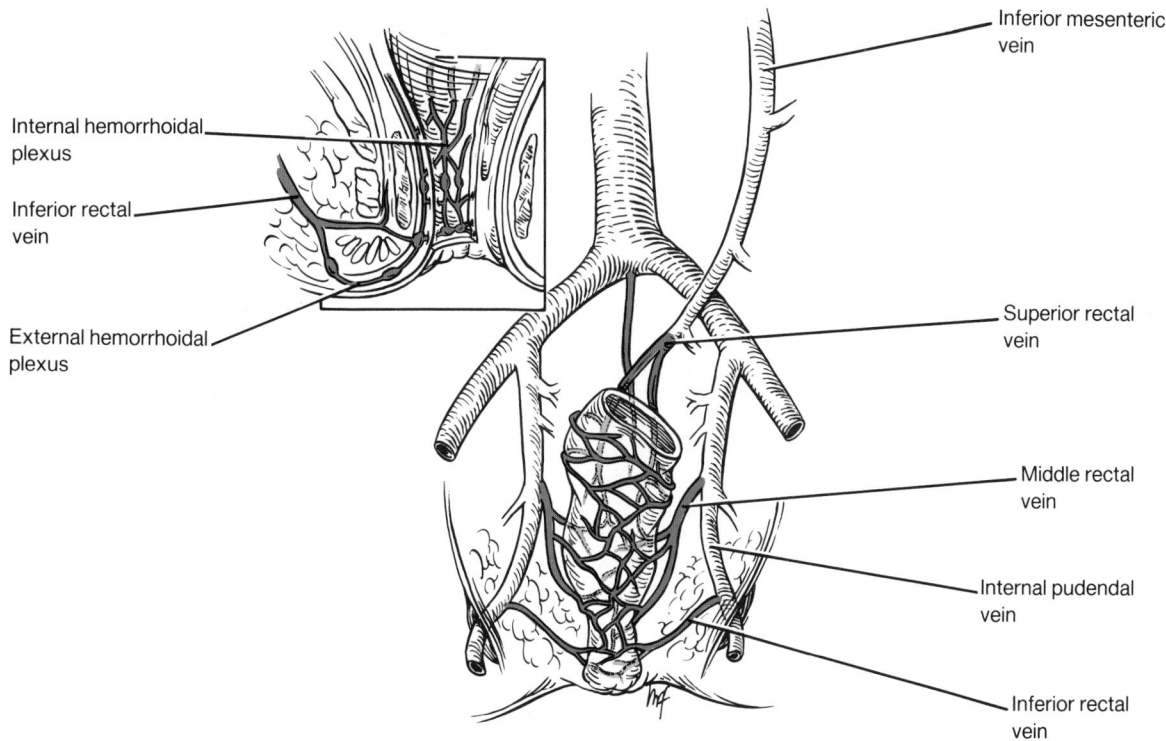

Figure 43-I-5

Venous Drainage of the Rectum and Anal Canal

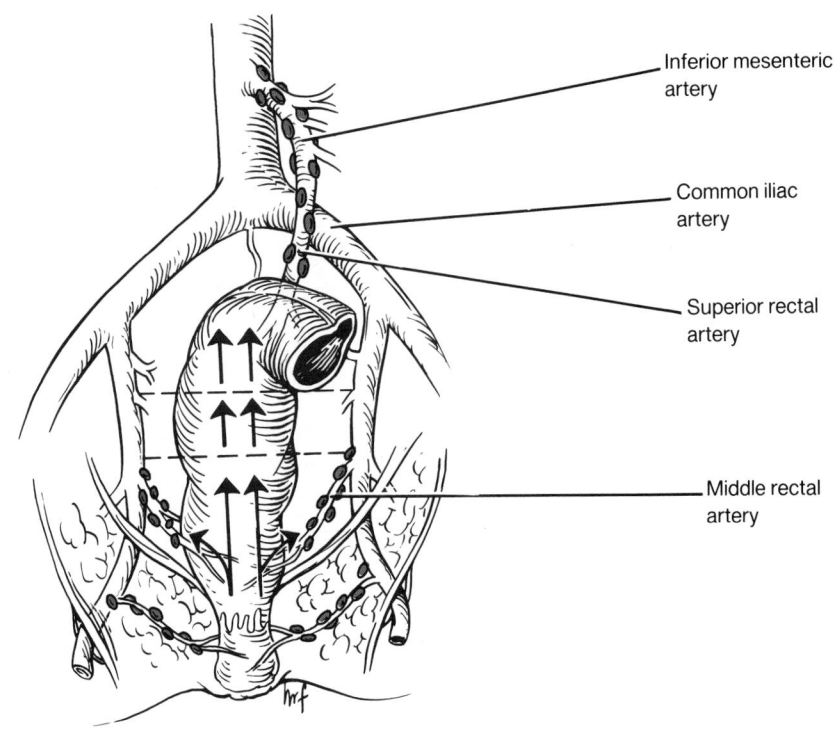

Inferior mesenteric
artery

Common iliac
artery

Superior rectal
artery

Middle rectal
artery

Figure 43-I-6

Lymphatic Drainage of the Rectum

Most rectal lymphatic drainage is through lymph nodes along the superior rectal and inferior mesenteric vessels.

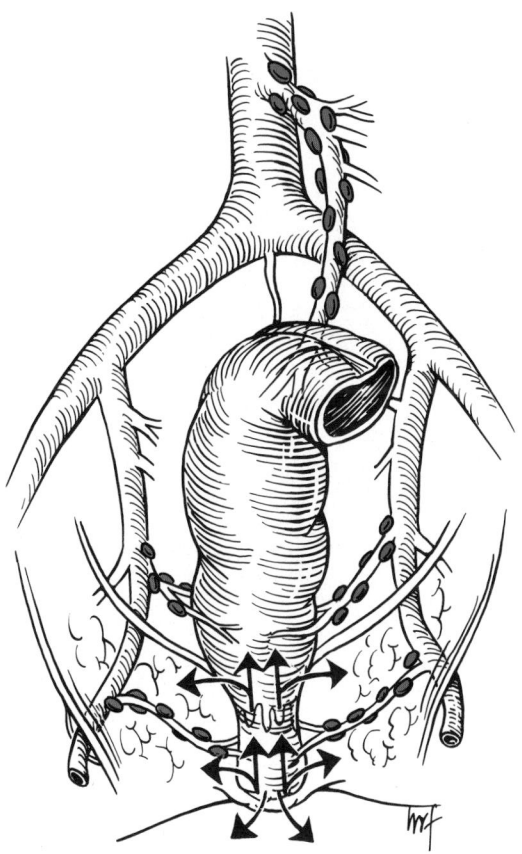

Figure 43-I-7

Lymphatic Drainage of the Distal Rectum and Anal Canal

The main drainage of the distal rectum and anal canal is through superior rectal vessels. Lateral pelvic side wall drainage is possible parallel to the middle rectal artery and its branches. Anal canal drainage may occur as lymphatics traverse the levator ani muscle and follow the inferior rectal artery. Both pathways lead to internal iliac nodes, common iliac nodes, and the lumbar trunks. Lymphatic drainage from the anal canal inferior to the dentate line does not parallel blood vessels, but instead flows anteriorly and superiorly in the perineum to the superior inguinal lymph nodes, and from there to the lumbar trunks through the external iliac nodes.

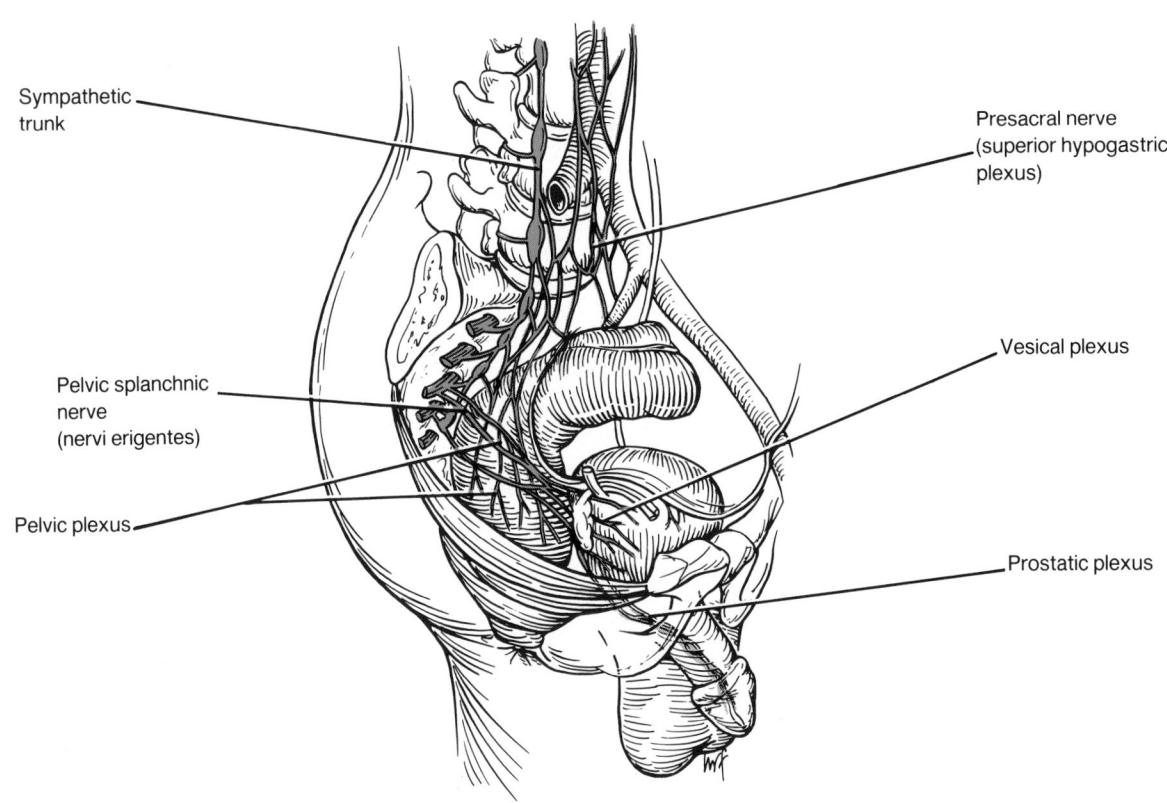

Figure 43-I-8

Autonomic Nerves of the Distal Pelvis: Lateral View

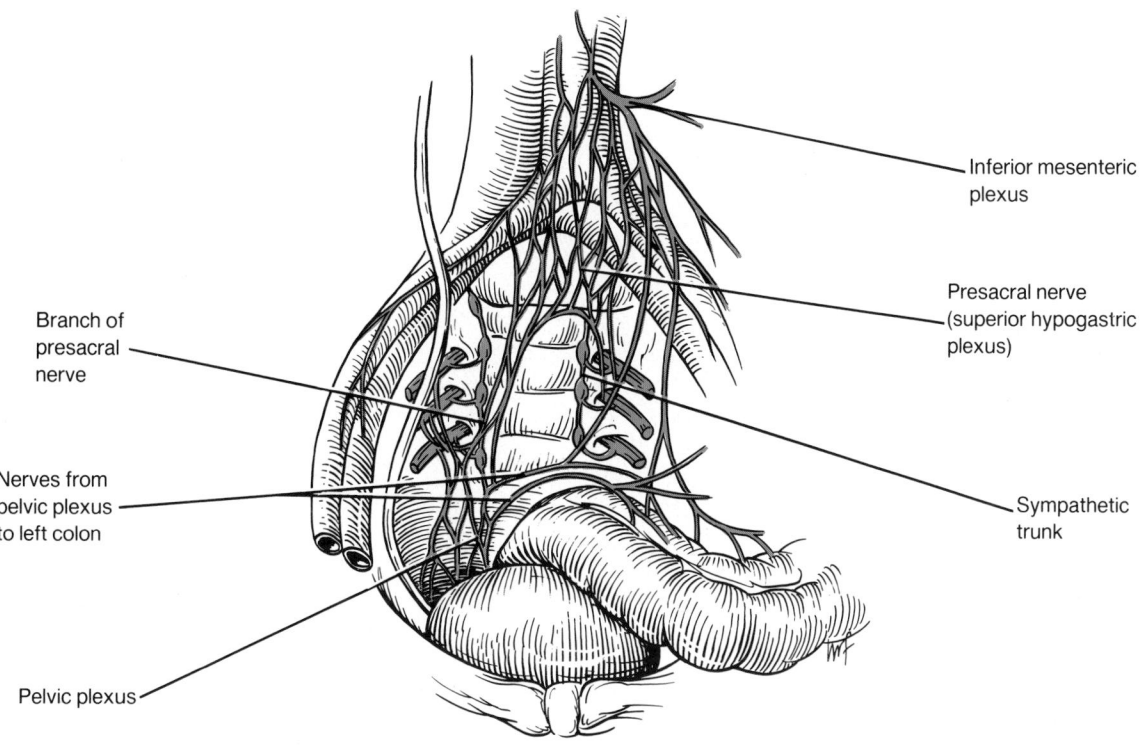

Inferior mesenteric plexus

Presacral nerve (superior hypogastric plexus)

Branch of presacral nerve

Nerves from pelvic plexus to left colon

Sympathetic trunk

Pelvic plexus

Figure 43-I-9

Autonomic Nerves of the Distal Pelvis: Anteroposterior View

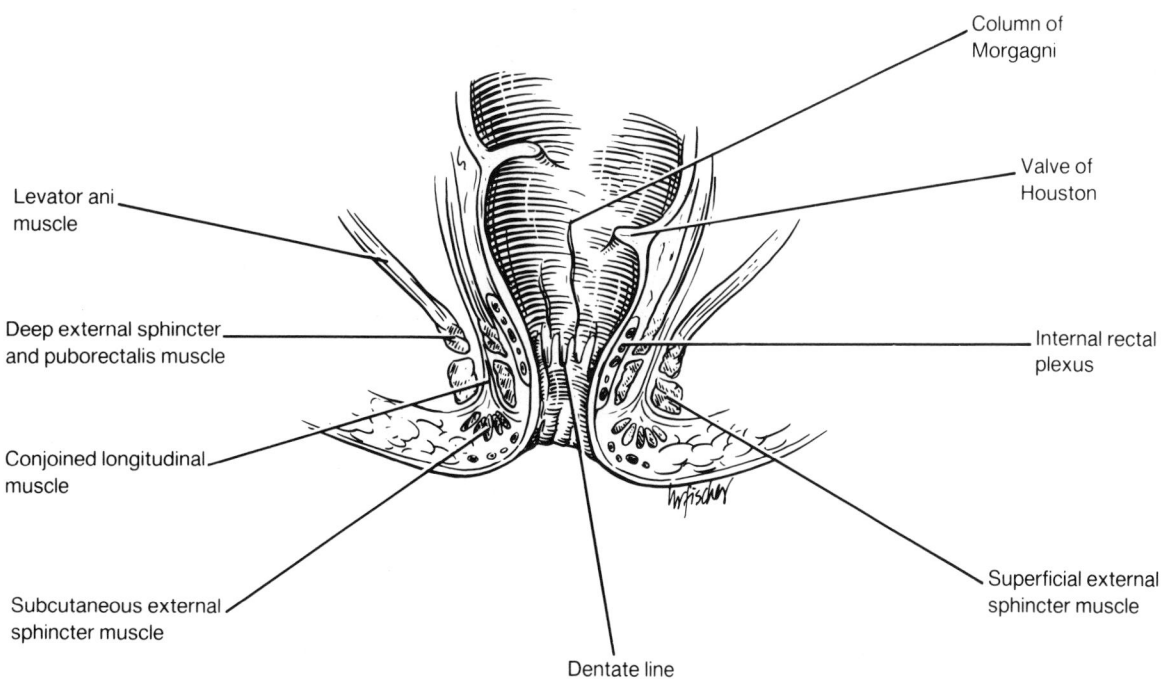

Column of Morgagni

Valve of Houston

Levator ani muscle

Deep external sphincter and puborectalis muscle

Internal rectal plexus

Conjoined longitudinal muscle

Subcutaneous external sphincter muscle

Superficial external sphincter muscle

Dentate line

Figure 43-I-10

Anatomy of the Anal Canal and Sphincter Muscles

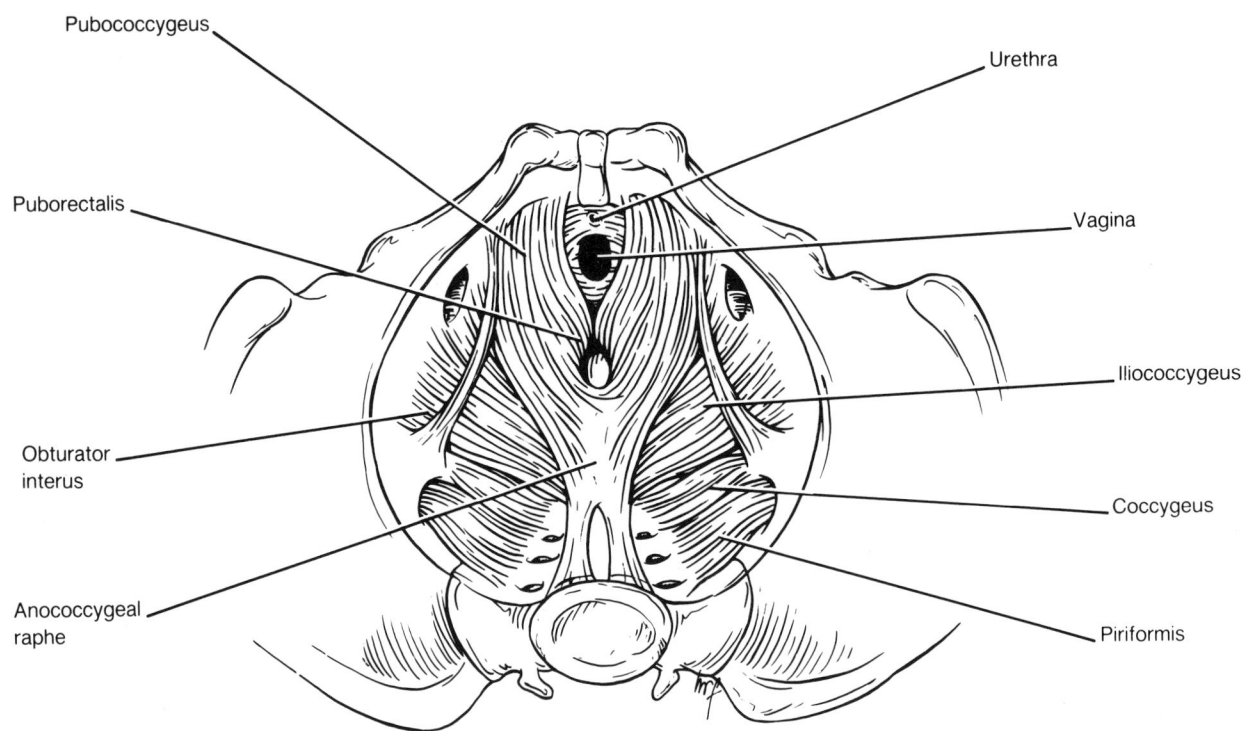

Figure 43-I-11

Pelvic Floor Musculature: Caudal View in Female

Pubococcygeus

Urethra

Puborectalis

Vagina

Obturator interus

Iliococcygeus

Anococcygeal raphe

Coccygeus

Piriformis

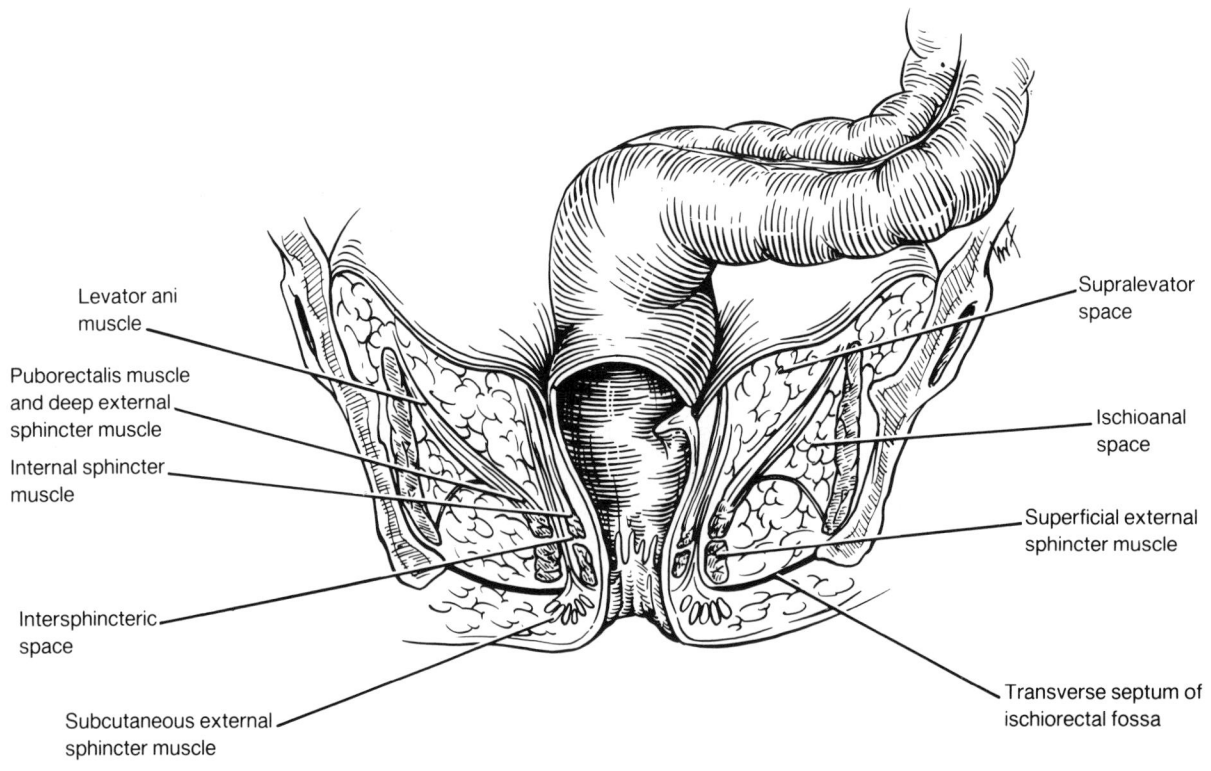

Figure 43-I-12

Lateral Spaces of the Perineum and Deep Pelvis

Levator ani muscle

Puborectalis muscle and deep external sphincter muscle

Internal sphincter muscle

Intersphincteric space

Subcutaneous external sphincter muscle

Supralevator space

Ischioanal space

Superficial external sphincter muscle

Transverse septum of ischiorectal fossa

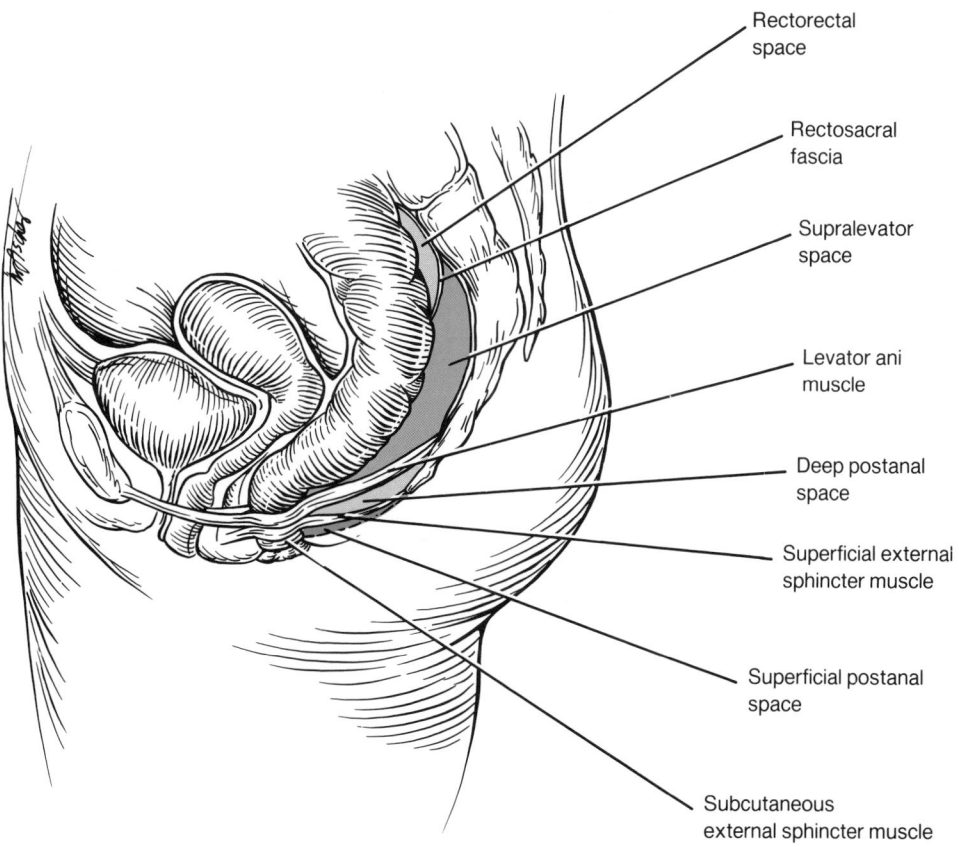

Rectorectal
space

Rectosacral
fascia

Supralevator
space

Levator ani
muscle

Deep postanal
space

Superficial external
sphincter muscle

Superficial postanal
space

Subcutaneous
external sphincter muscle

Figure 43-I-13

Posterior Spaces of the Deep Pelvis and Perineum

These spaces enable the lateral spaces to communicate around the anorectum in a horse-shoe manner.

SECTION II   Colonic Resection

A. Right Hemicolectomy

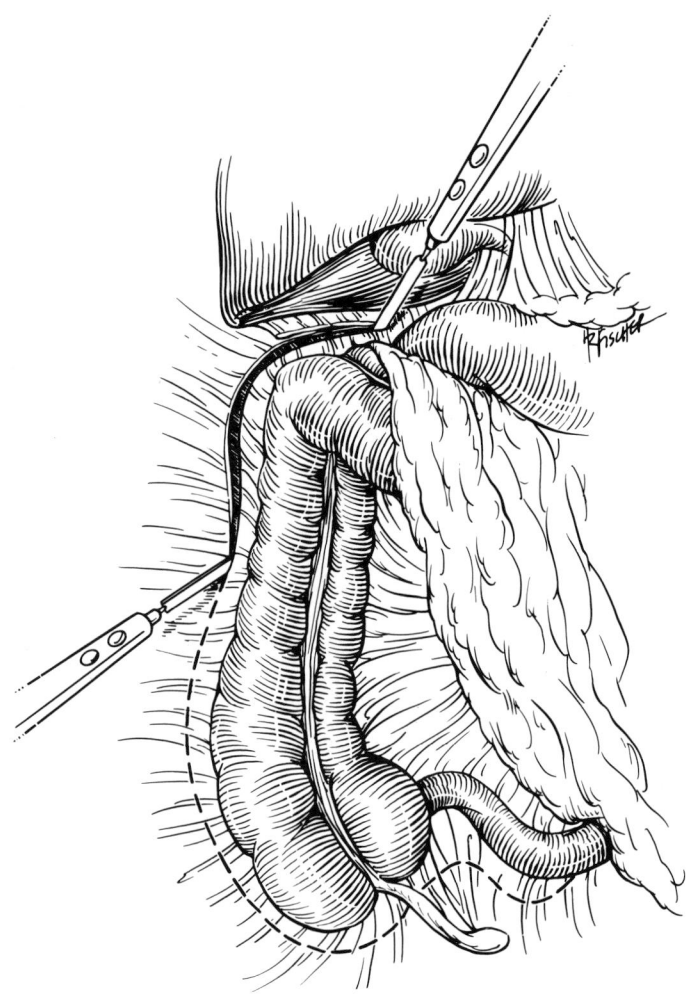

Figure 43-IIA-1

Incision

The extent of peritoneal incision is indicated. Sharp dissection with scissors or electro-cautery, as shown, is used.

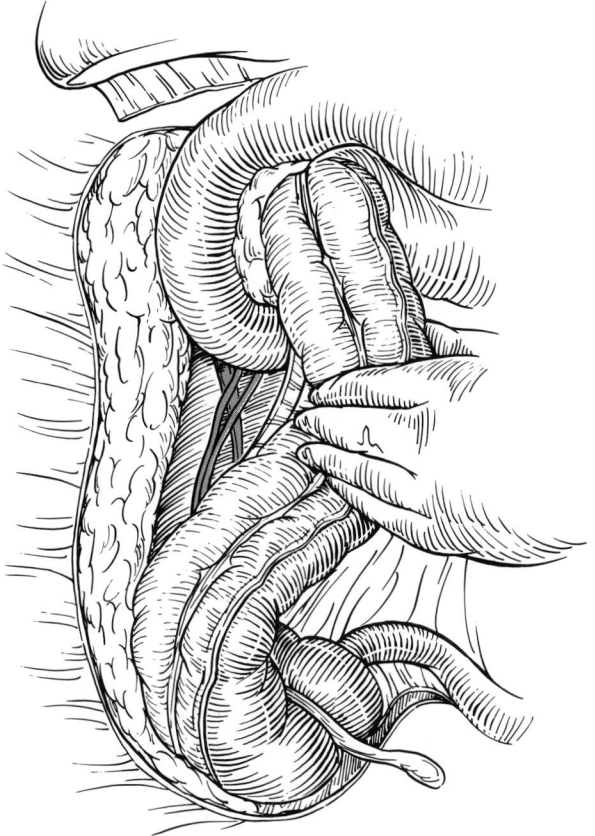

Figure 43-IIA-2

Exposure

The right colon is completely mobilized and reflected medially to expose and avoid injury to the retrocolic structures. The duodenum is easily seen. In thin patients, the right gonadal vessels lying anterior to the right ureter can be seen.

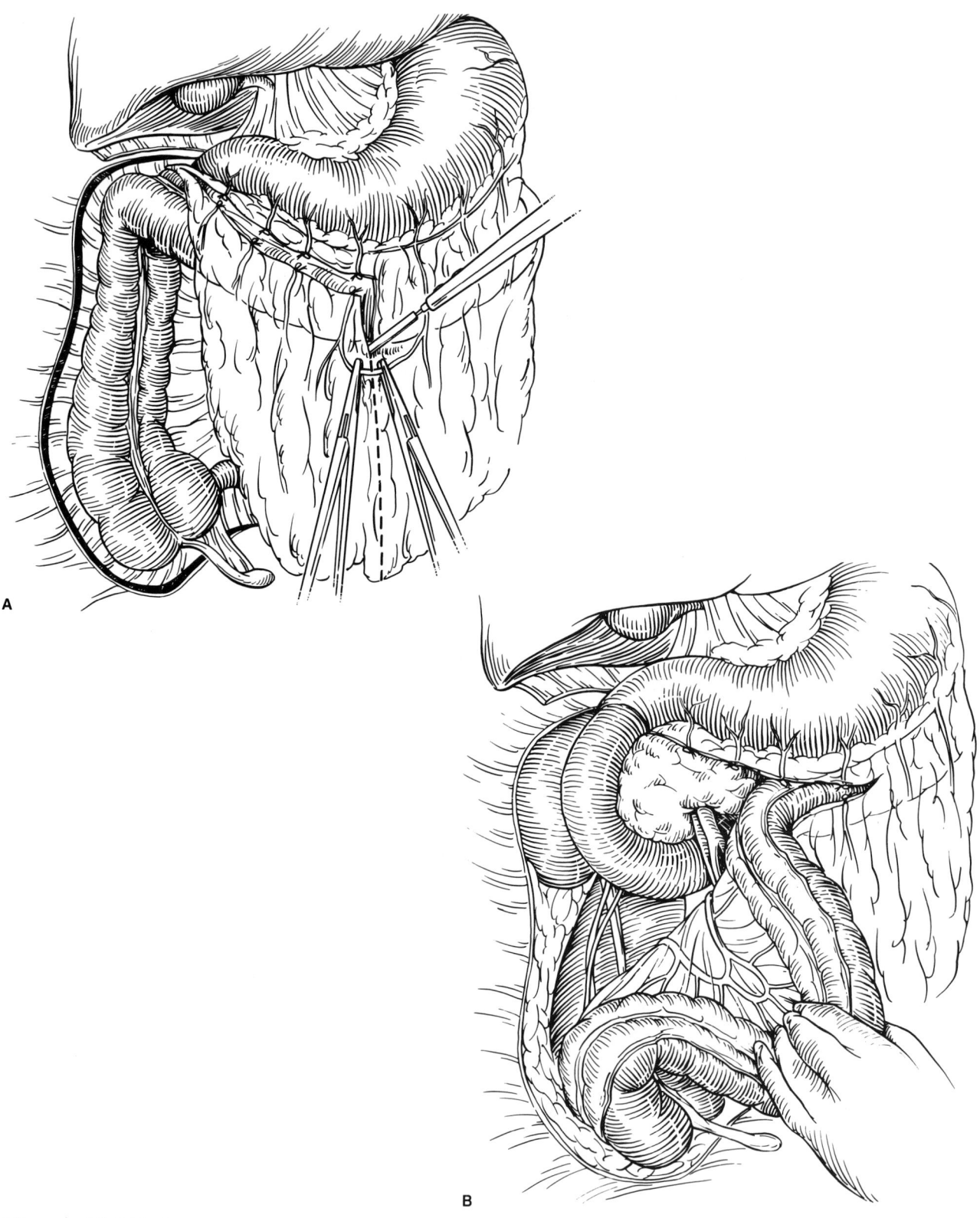

A

B

Figure 43-IIA-3

Division of Omentum

(**A**) The greater omentum is divided inferior to the gastroepiploic vessels, using clamps and ligature. The omentum is split to allow en bloc removal with the right colon.

(**B**) The completely mobilized right colon is ready for resection.

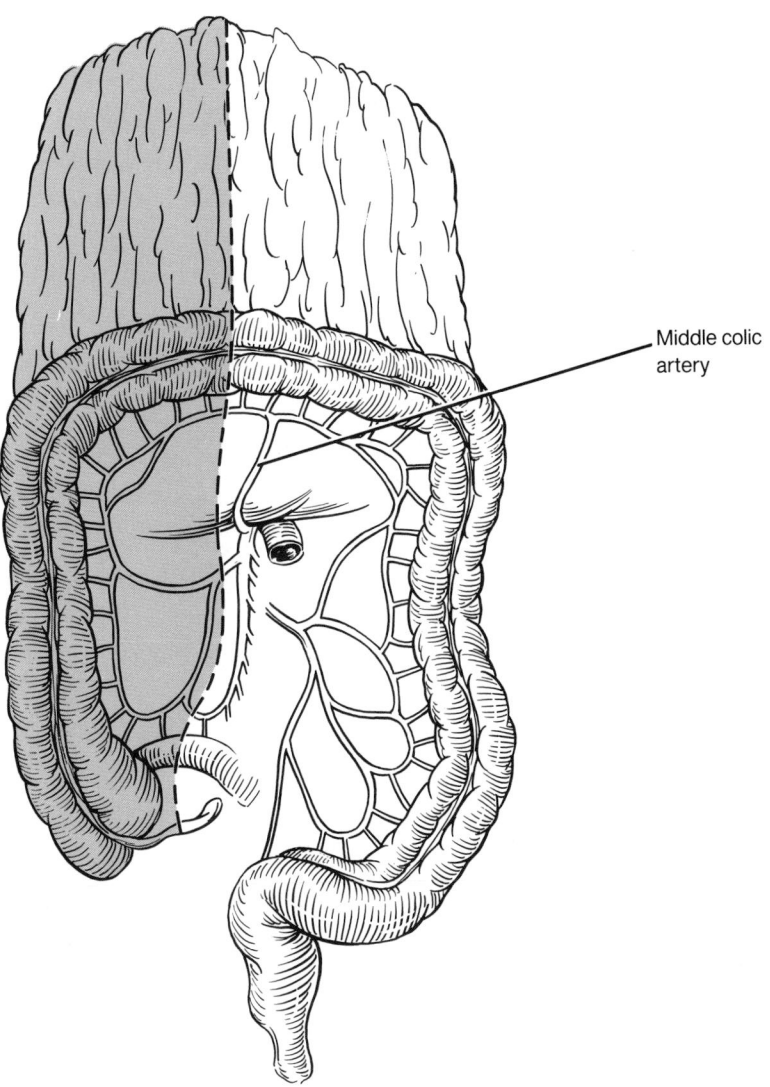

Middle colic
artery

Figure 43-IIA-4

Extent of Colectomy, Mesenteric Excision, and Omentectomy

The right colic artery and the marginal branch of the middle colic artery are ligated. The middle colic artery trunk is preserved.

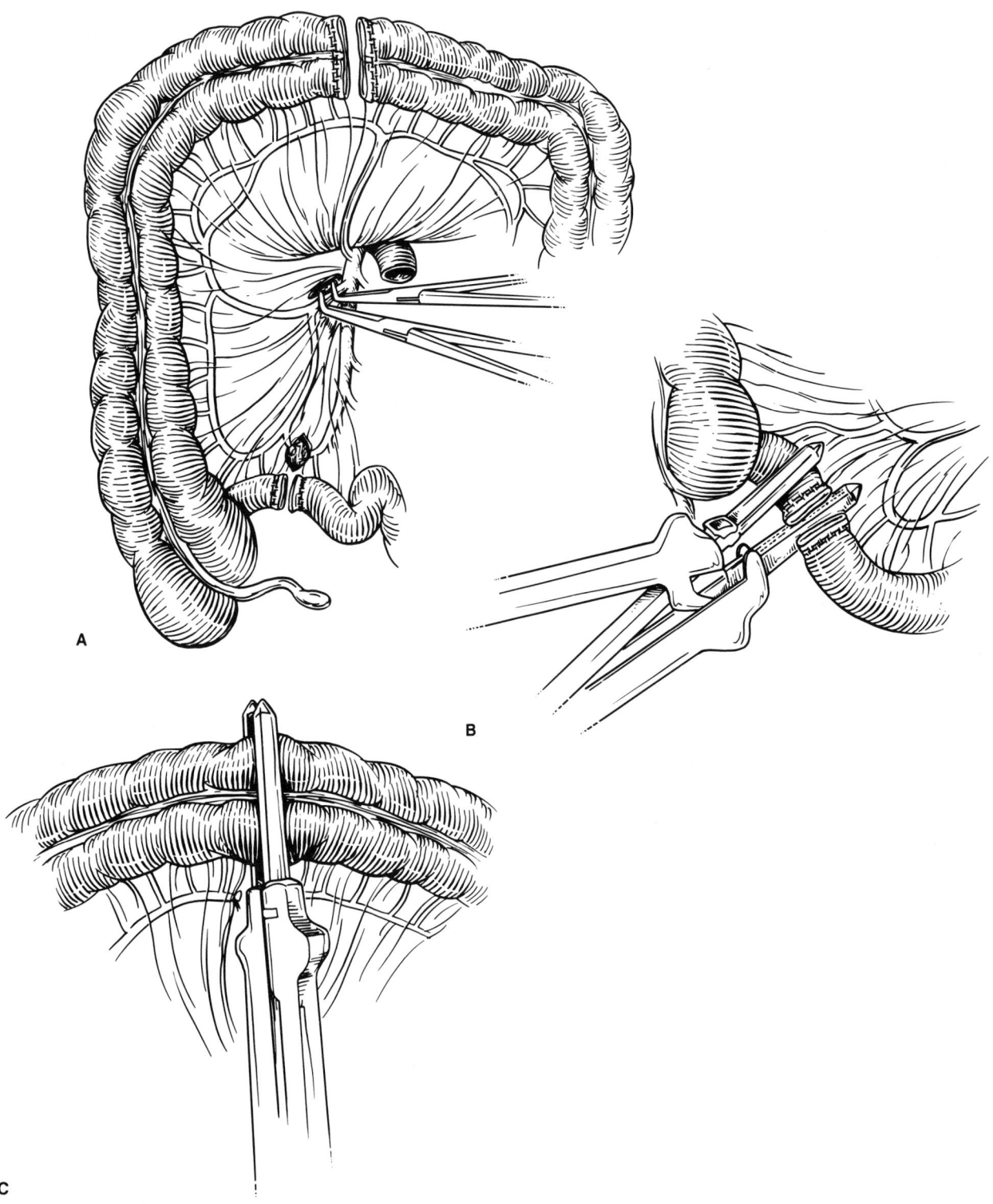

A

B

C

Figure 43-IIA-5

Ligation of Right Colic Artery

(A) The ileocolic and right colic vessels are ligated at the root of the mesentery. The middle colic vessels are preserved.

(B) The distal ileum is divided using a linear cutter-stapler.

(C) The right transverse colon is divided using a linear cutter-stapler.

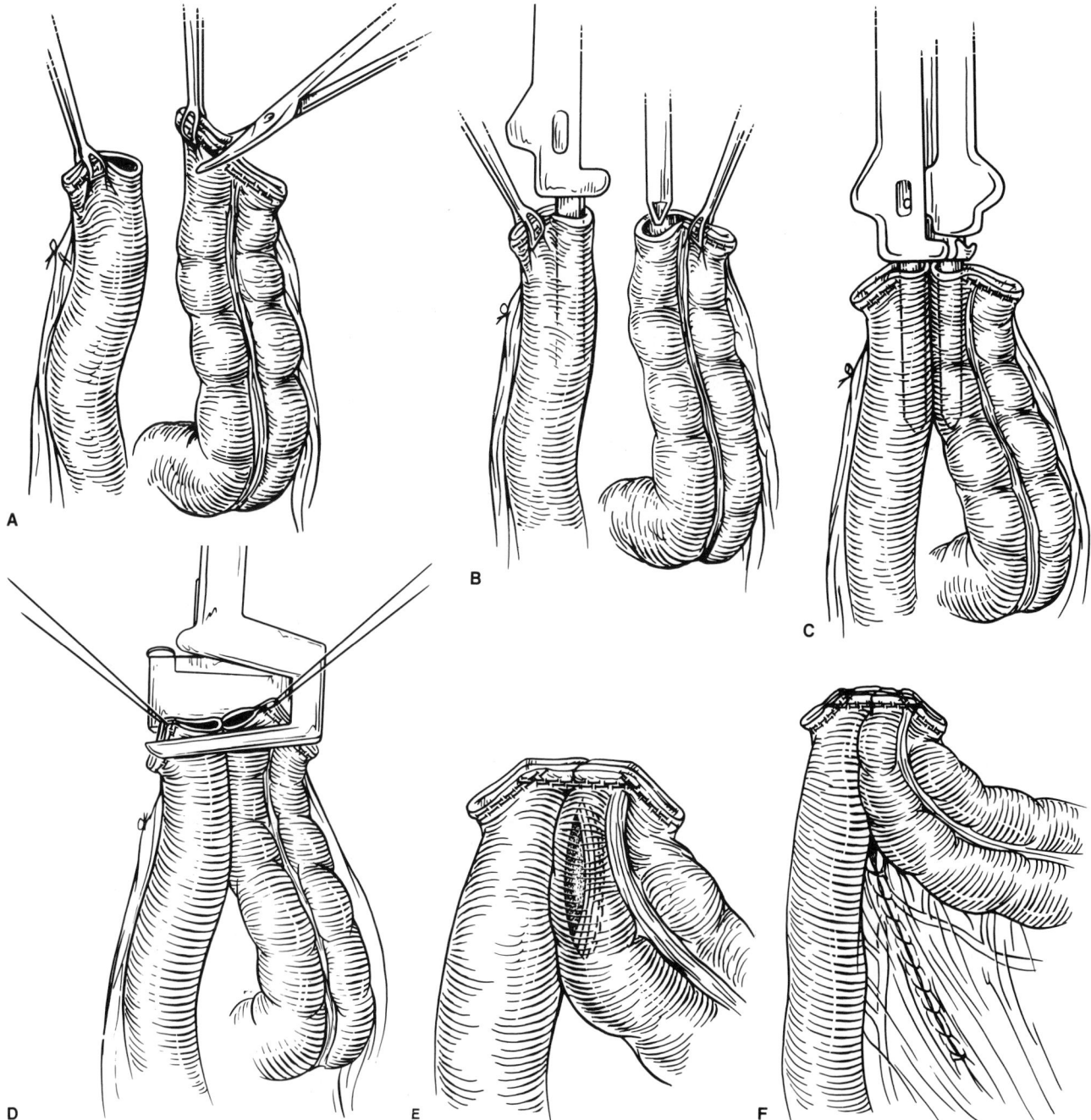

Figure 43-IIA-6

Stapled Side-to-Side Functional End-to-End Ileocolic Anastomosis

(**A**) The antimesenteric corners of both transverse staple lines are amputated with scissors.

(**B**) The linear cutter-stapler is placed into both ends of bowel.

(**C**) The two limbs of bowel are aligned along their antimesenteric borders. The linear cutter-stapler is closed and fired to complete the anastomosis.

(**D**) After removing the linear cutter-stapler, the staple line is inspected for hemostasis and integrity. The enterotomies are closed with a straight stapler.

(**E**) The anatomic result. Some surgeons prefer to suture-reinforce intersecting staple lines and the apex of the anastomosis.

(**F**) The mesenteric defect is closed with a running 3-0 absorbable suture.

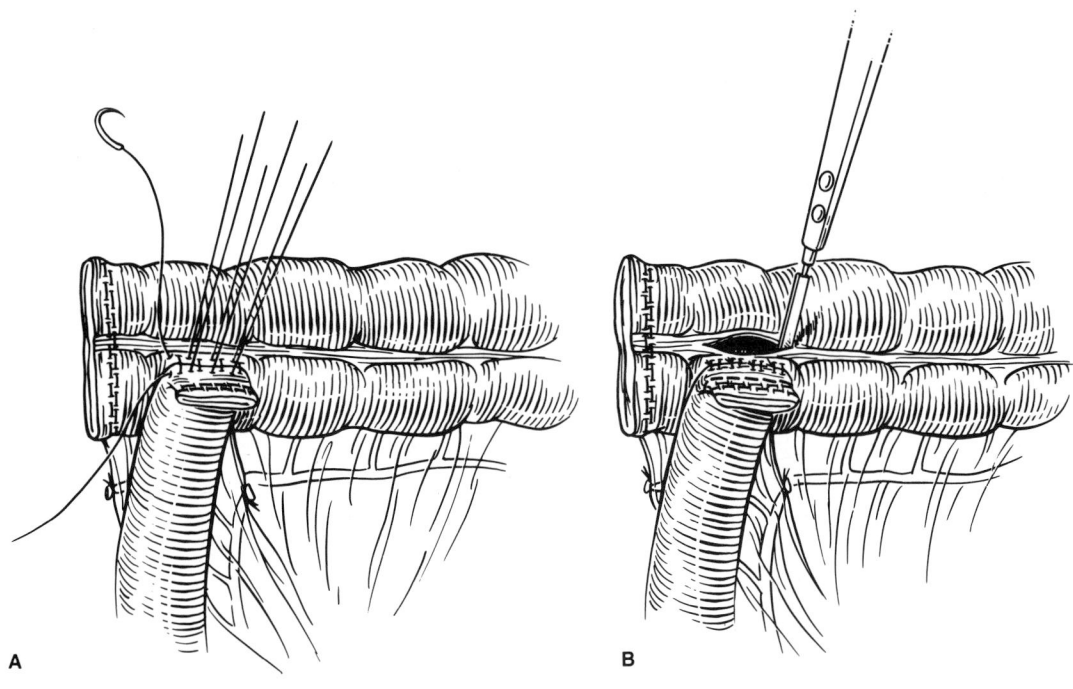

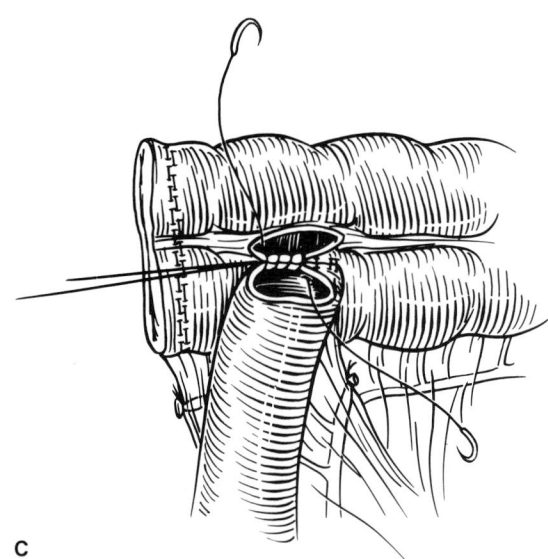

C

Figure 43-IIA-7

Sutured End-to-Side Ileocolic Anastomosis

(A) The right colon has been resected. Both ends of bowel were divided and stapled with a linear cutter-stapler. An outer layer of interrupted 4-0 seromuscular sutures is placed posteriorly between the distal ileum and colon.

(B) A colotomy is made parallel to the suture line. The staple line on the distal ileum is amputated.

(C) An inner continuous full-thickness 3-0 or 4-0 suture is used to approximate the ileum and colon in an end-to-side fashion.

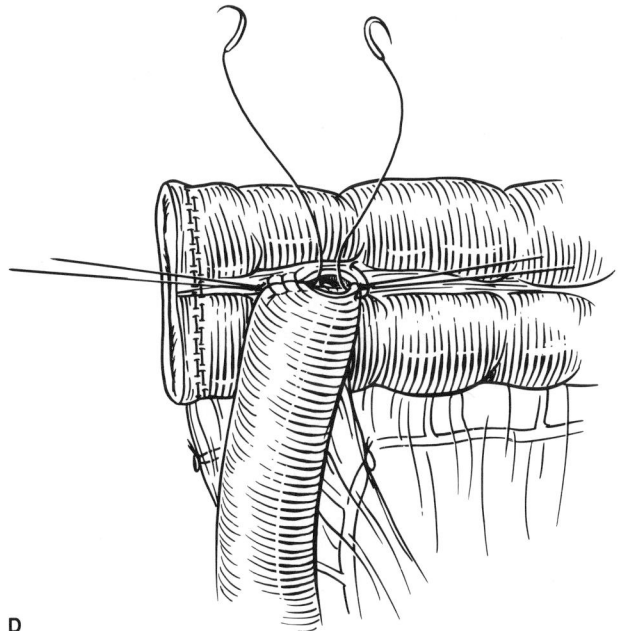

D

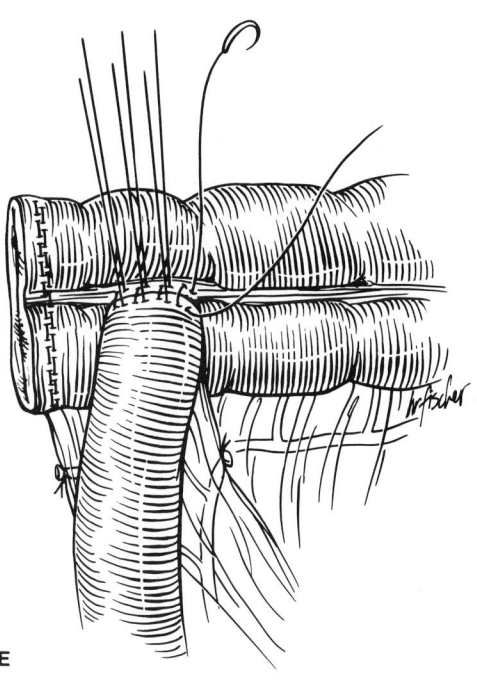

E

Figure 43-IIA-7 *(Continued)*

(D) The continuous full-thickness suture is completed anteriorly.

(E) The anterior row of interrupted 4-0 seromuscular sutures is placed to complete the anastomosis.

B. Left Hemicolectomy

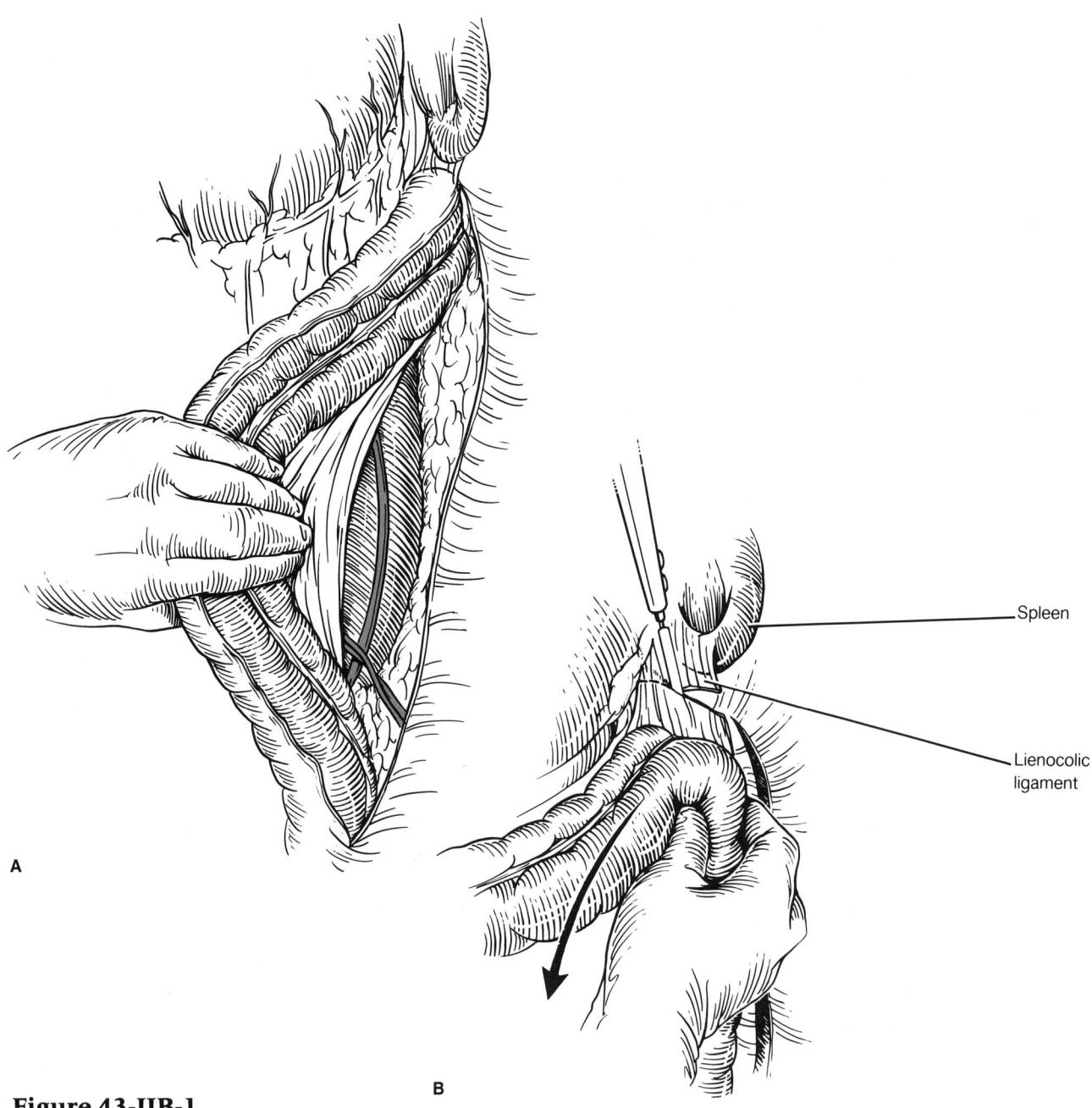

Spleen

Lienocolic
ligament

A

B

Figure 43-IIB-1

Exposure

(A) The sigmoid colon and descending colon are mobilized and reflected by incising the left lateral peritoneal attachments. The retroperitoneal structures—gonadal vessels and left ureter—are identified and pushed posteriorly.

(B) The splenic flexure is mobilized by gentle traction and sharp division of peritoneal attachments to the spleen (lienocolic ligament) and to the diaphragm (phrenocolic ligament).

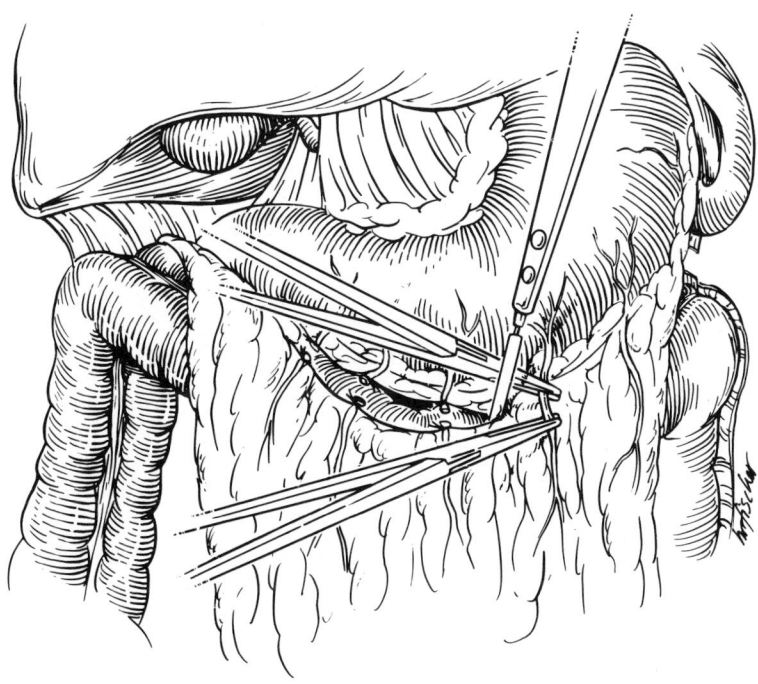

Figure 43-IIB-2

Division of Omentum

The greater omentum is divided inferior to the gastroepiploic vessels using clamps and ligature. The omentum is split to allow its en bloc removal along with the left colon.

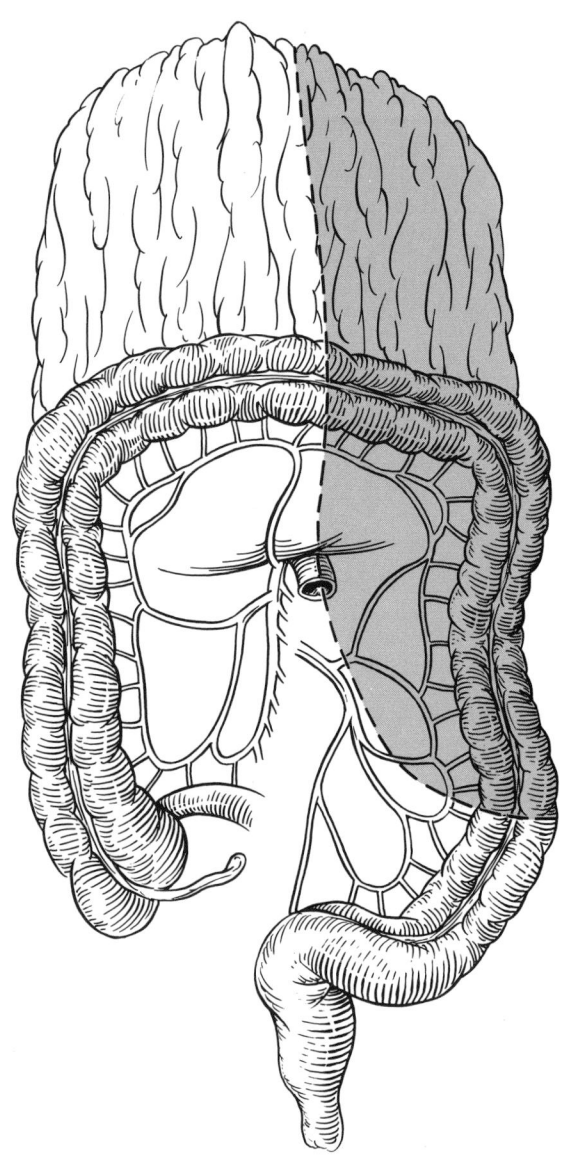

Figure 43-IIB-3

Extent of Colectomy, Mesenteric Excision, and Omentectomy

The left colic, proximal sigmoid, and left branches of the middle colic vessels are ligated.
The main trunk of the middle colic vessel is preserved.

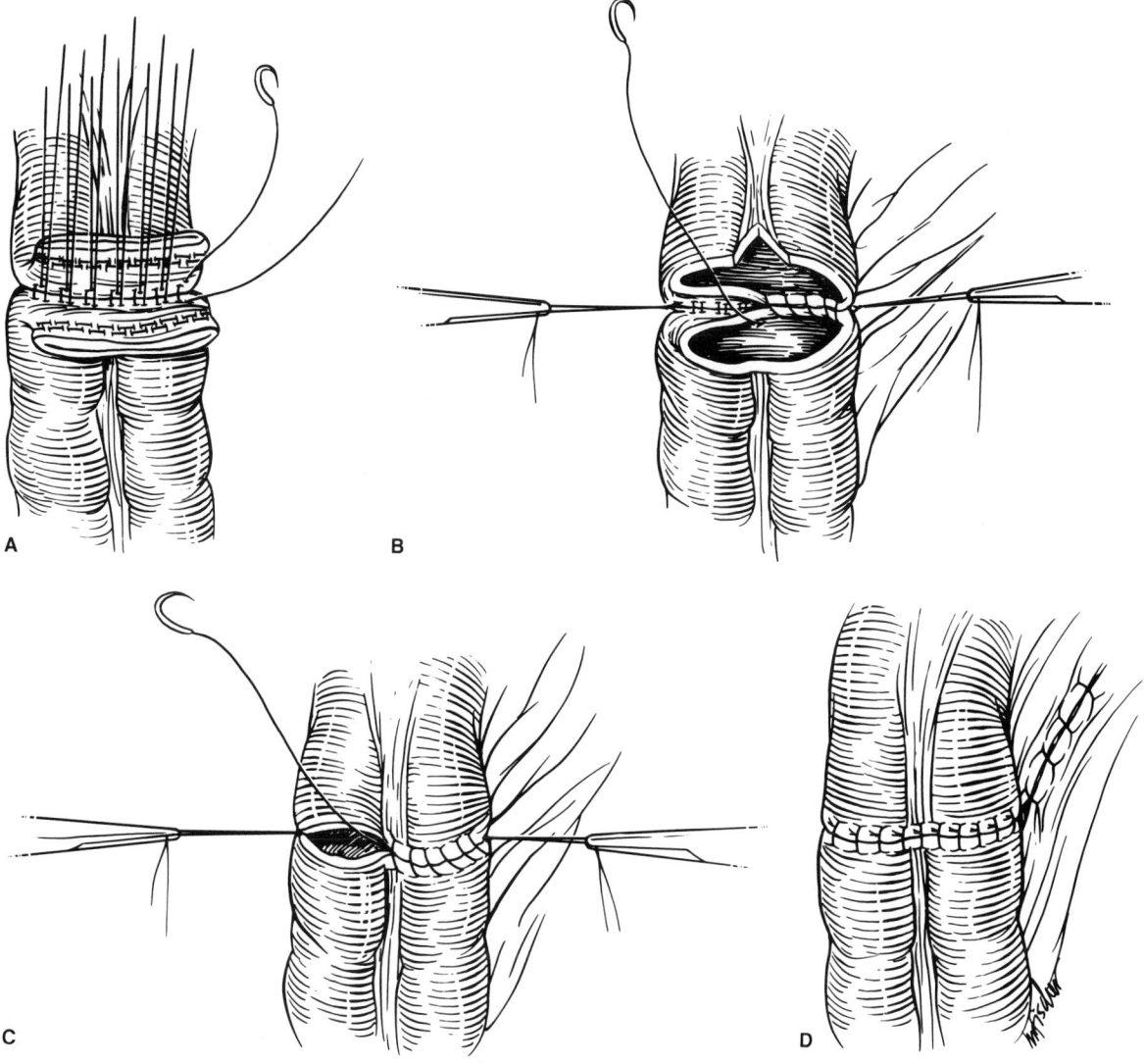

Figure 43-IIB-4

Sutured End-to-End Colocolic Two-Layer Anastomosis

(**A**) The bowel has been resected using a linear cutter-stapler. A posterior layer of interrupted seromuscular 4-0 sutures is placed and tied.

(**B**) Both bowel ends have been opened by excising the staple lines. An inner continuous full-thickness suture is placed. If necessary, the antimesenteric border can be slit, as shown, to increase luminal diameter.

(**C**) The inner continuous suture is completed anteriorly.

(**D**) The anastomosis is completed by placing interrupted 4-0 seromuscular sutures. The mesenteric defect is closed.

C. Sigmoid Colectomy

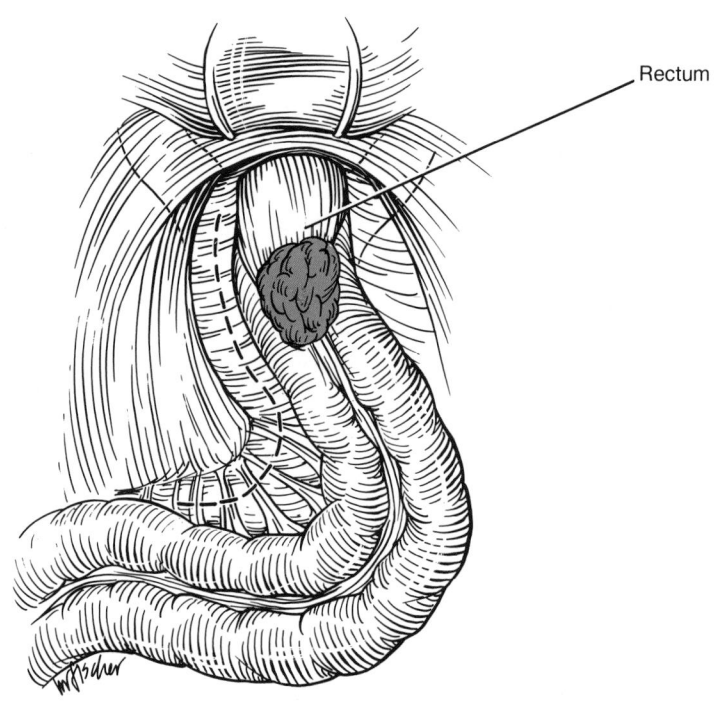

Rectum

Figure 43-IIC-1

Incision

The peritoneum on the left side of the sigmoid colon is incised along the Toldt white line. This incision extends distally into the pelvis along the mesorectum into the cul-de-sac and proximally along the descending colon as far as necessary to achieve mobilization for a tension-free anastomosis.

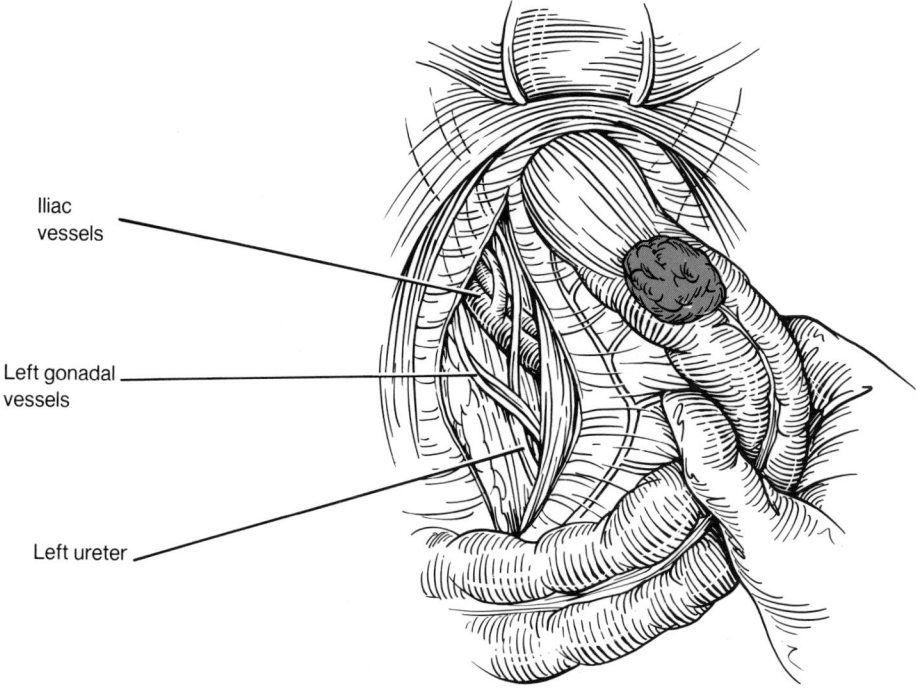

Iliac vessels

Left gonadal vessels

Left ureter

Figure 43-IIC-2

Exposure

The sigmoid and rectosigmoid are reflected to expose the left gonadal vessels crossing anterior to the left ureter as it enters the pelvis anterior to the iliac vessels.

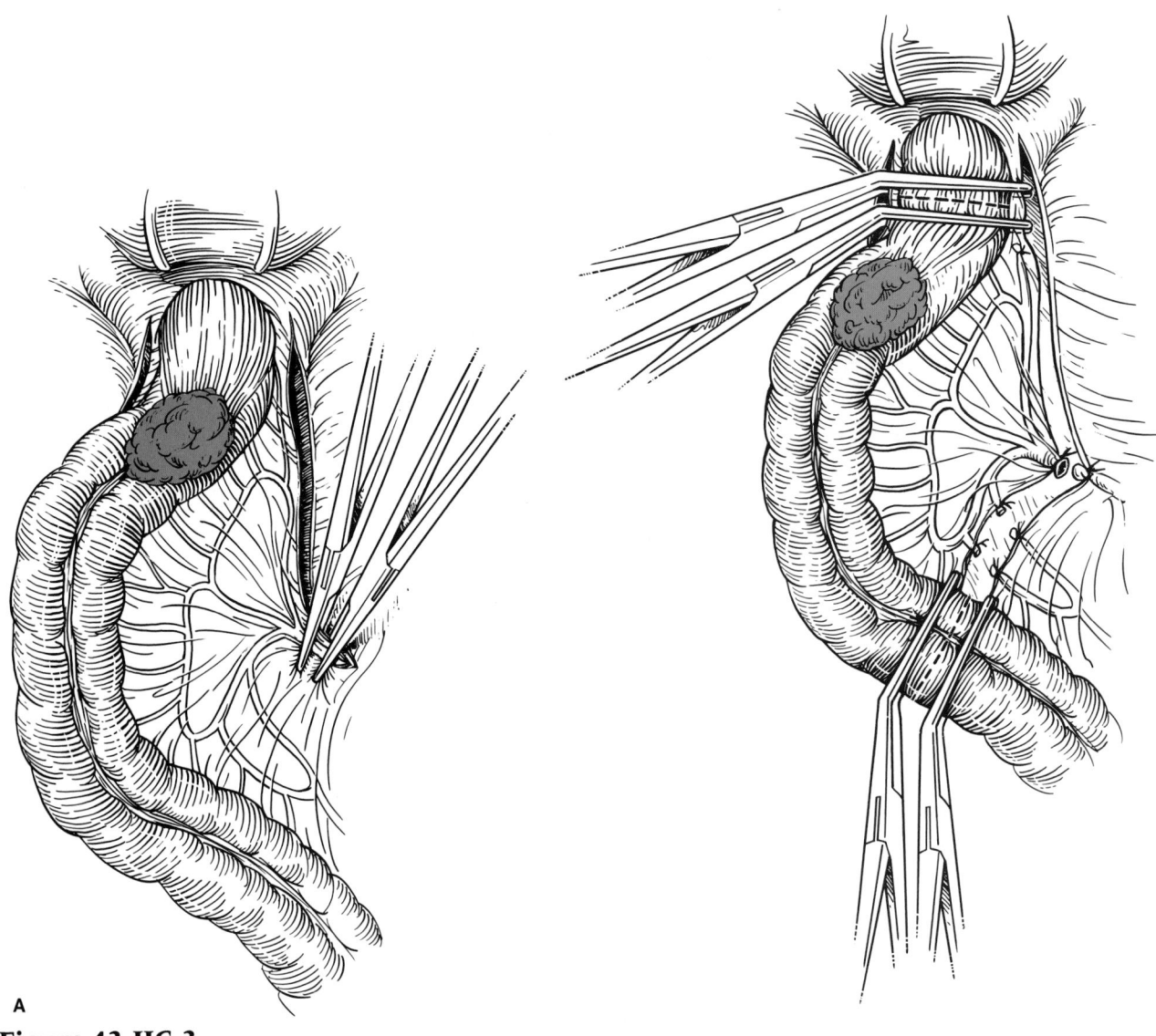

A

Figure 43-IIC-3

Division of Mesentery and Bowel

(A) The peritoneum overlying the sigmoid mesentery has been incised. The sigmoid colon has been completely mobilized. The inferior mesenteric vessels are clamped, divided, and ligated proximally.

(B) The mesentery has been divided up to the sites of proposed resection. Proximally, this is at the sigmoid–descending colon junction where the bowel is being divided between two angled clamps. Distally, two angled clamps are placed in parallel at the recto-sigmoid junction or as dictated by the location of the lesion being resected. The bowel is divided between the two clamps.

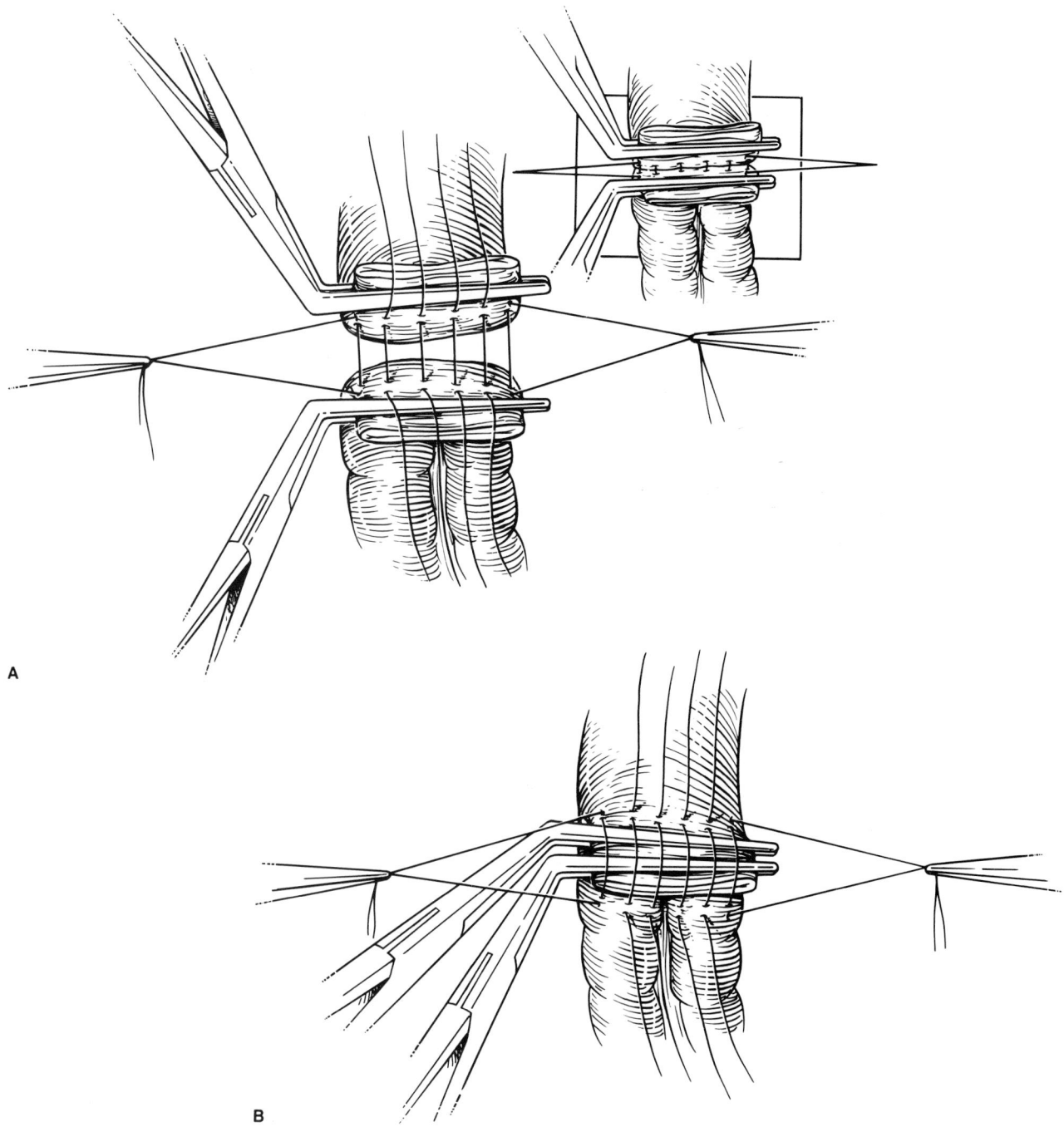

Figure 43-IIC-4

Sutured Single-Layer End-to-End Colorectal Anastomosis

(A) The bowel clamps on the proximal rectum and distal descending colon are aligned in parallel and rotated 90 degrees to expose the posterior walls of the bowel. A posterior row of 4-0 permanent sutures is placed. **(Inset)** Appearance after the posterior row of sutures is tied.

(B) The bowel clamps are rotated to expose the anterior surfaces of the descending colon and rectum. An anterior row of 4-0 permanent sutures is placed.

(Continued)

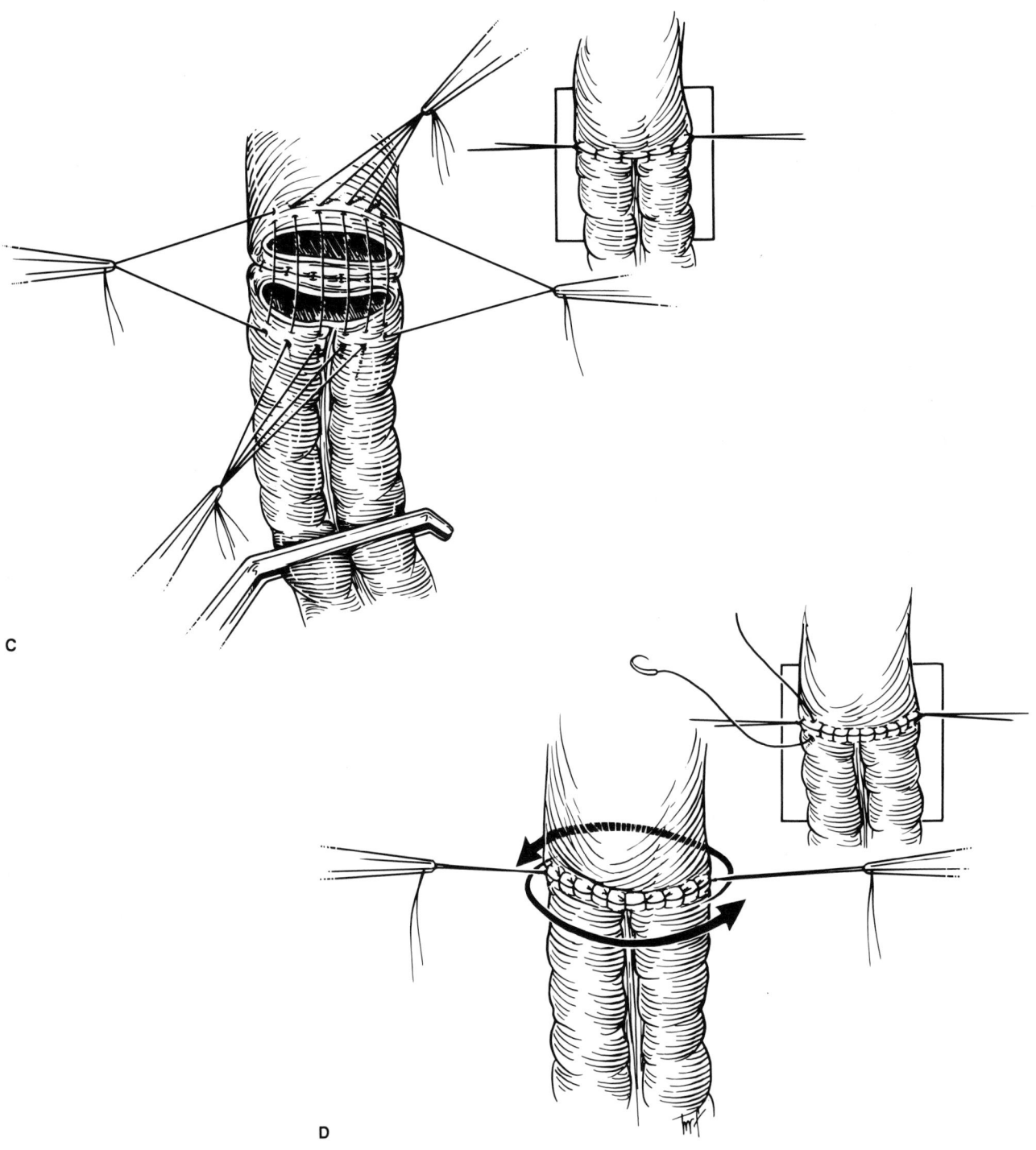

C

D

Figure 43-IIC-4 *(Continued)*

(C) After irrigating the rectum clean through a proctoscope and placing a noncrushing shod clamp proximally, the two bowel clamps are removed while an assistant holds the anterior row of sutures to allow inspection of the anastomosis. This allows the surgeon the opportunity to check to be certain that no suture inadvertently caught the opposite wall and that no major bleeding is present at the anastomosis. **(Inset)** Appearance after the anterior row and corner sutures are tied.

(D) Additional 4-0 sutures are placed between each of the previously placed stitches on the anterior row. The corner sutures tagged with mosquito clamps are then rotated 180 degrees to expose the posterior row of previously placed sutures. **(Inset)** The posterior row is reinforced by additional 4-0 sutures.

1484

D. Rectal Resection

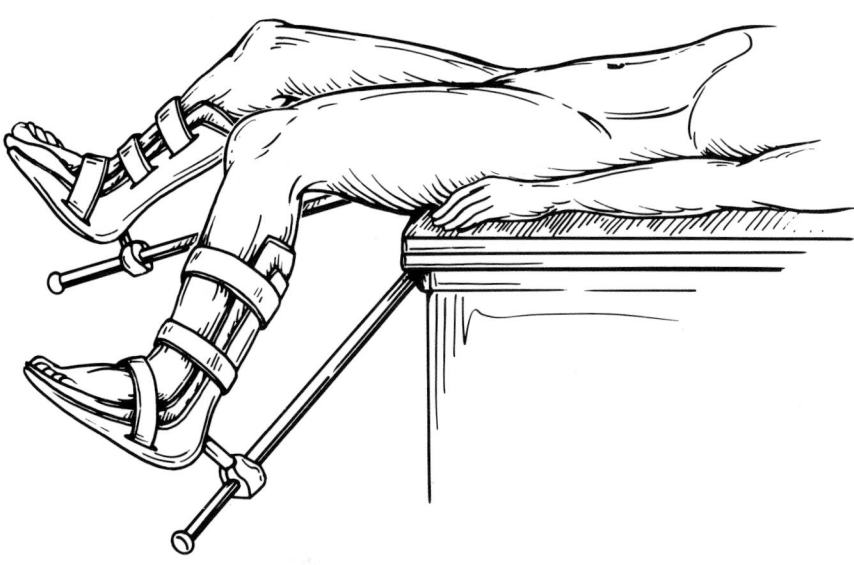

Figure 43-IID-1

Patient Positioning

Proper positioning of the patient before laparotomy facilitates rectal mobilization and resection. The patient is in a modified lithotomy position with the anus at the edge of the table. The legs are placed in padded, adjustable stirrups with the knees flexed such that any pressure is on the heels and not the legs. The hips are minimally flexed and abducted to ensure perineal exposure and access.

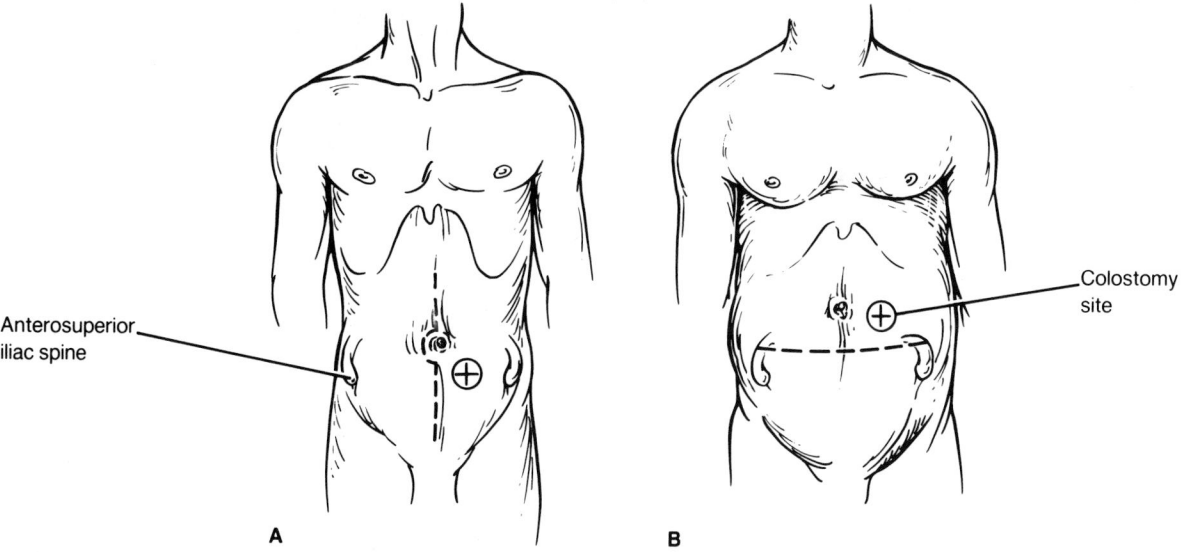

Anterosuperior iliac spine

Colostomy site

A   B

Figure 43-IID-2

Incision

Two possible incisions for rectal resection are presented: midline (**A**), curved to the right of the umbilicus; and transverse (**B**), infraumbilical from iliac crest to iliac crest. In both cases, the site of a potential colostomy is preserved.

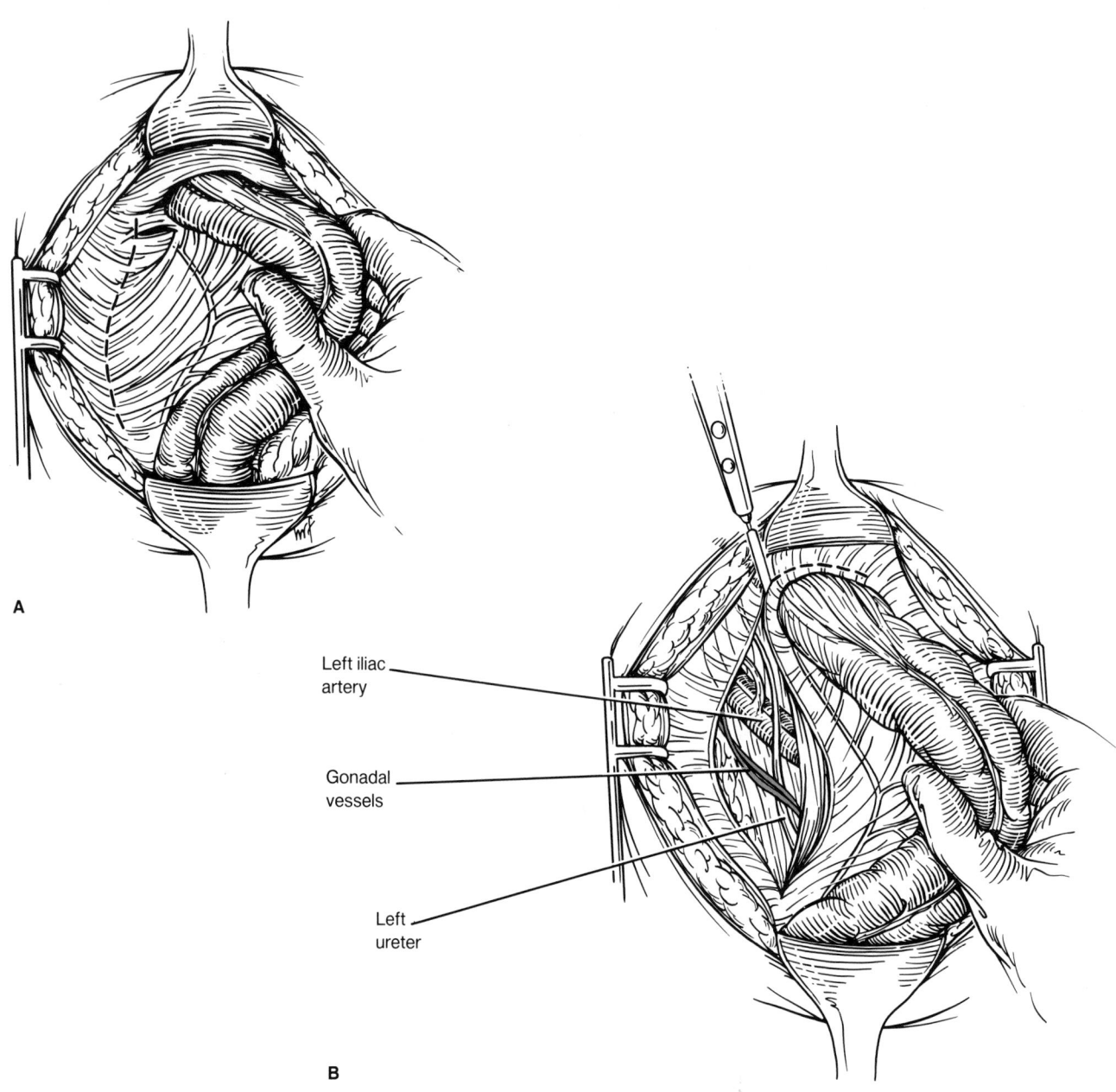

A

Left iliac
artery

Gonadal
vessels

Left
ureter

B

Figure 43-IID-3

Exposure and Dissection

(A) The peritoneum on the left side of the mesorectum is incised. Proximally, this is extended as necessary to ensure mobilization to achieve a tension-free anastomosis or end colostomy.

(B) The rectosigmoid is reflected to expose the left gonadal vessels crossing anterior to the left ureter as it enters the pelvis anterior to the iliac vessels. Distally, the peritoneal incision is extended to open the cul-de-sac anteriorly.

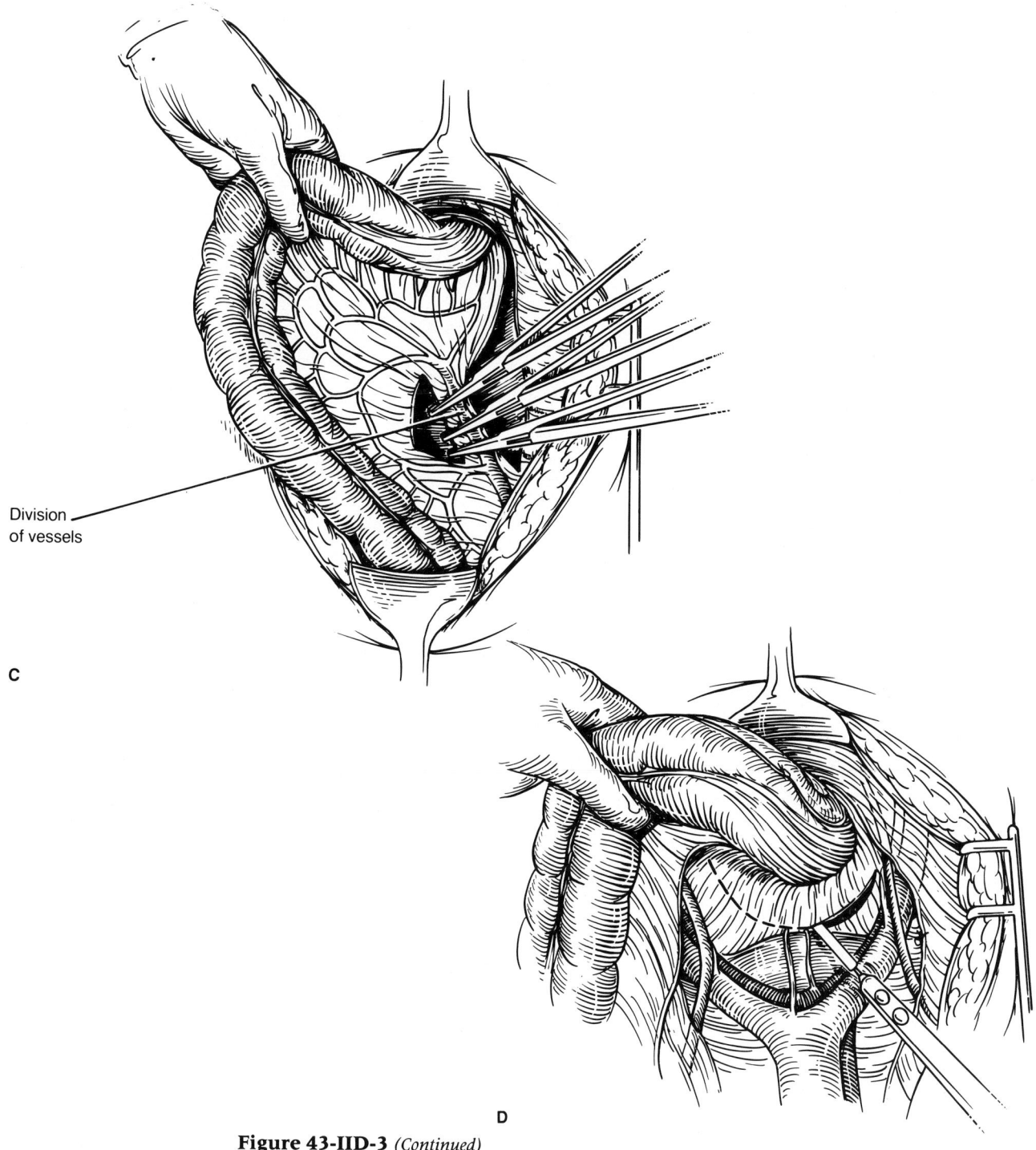

Division
of vessels

C

D

Figure 43-IID-3 *(Continued)*

(C) The peritoneum overlying the rectosigmoid mesentery has been incised and the cul-de-sac completely opened anteriorly. The rectosigmoid has been mobilized to expose the inferior mesenteric vessels, which are triply clamped, divided, and doubly ligated at the pelvic brim, preserving the left colic artery. If a high ligation is preferred, the inferior mesenteric vessels are divided at their origin from the aorta.

(D) The rectum is reflected anteriorly to reveal the endopelvic fascia, which is the anatomic plane to be followed as the rectum is mobilized distally. The thin, fibroareolar tissue posterior to the mesorectum is sharply incised, thus avoiding injury to the presacral nerves and vessels. This dissection is carried distally into the pelvis to the level of the rectosacral (Waldeyer) fascia, which is divided sharply.

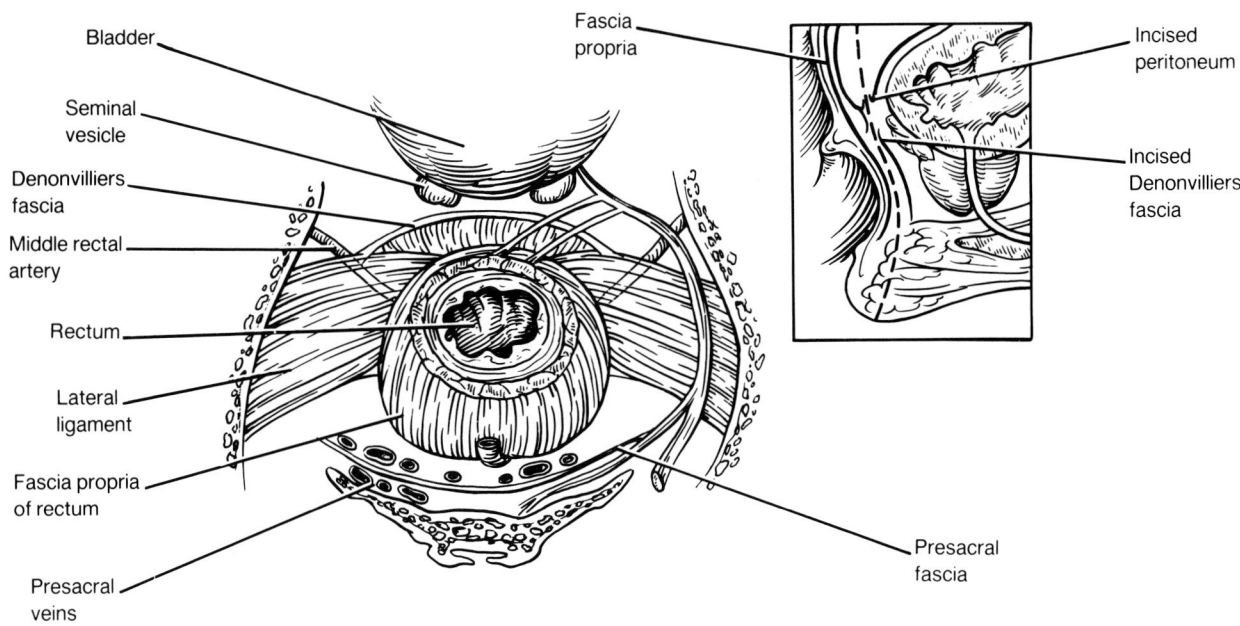

Figure 43-IID-4

Anatomy

The anatomic layers of the distal rectum are shown schematically as viewed looking into the pelvis from above. **(Inset)** Lateral depiction of the anterior plane of dissection used during resection of the rectum. The peritoneum of the cul-de-sac is incised anterior to the rectum, as is the Denonvilliers fascia. Distal dissection is completed in the plane posterior to the Denonvilliers fascia.

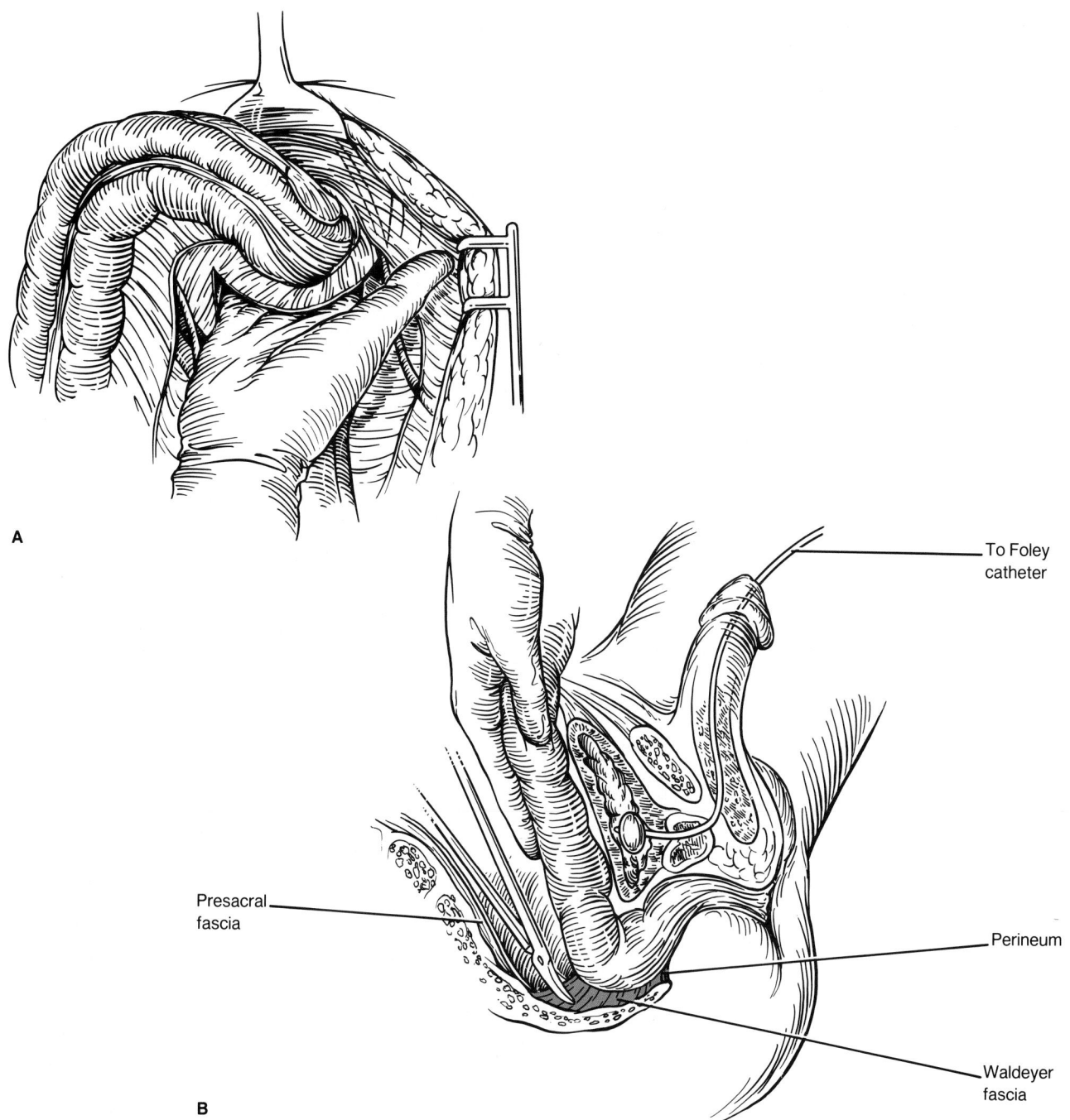

A

To Foley
catheter

Presacral
fascia

Perineum

B

Waldeyer
fascia

Figure 43-IID-5

Manual Manipulation of Posterior Rectum

(A) Some surgeons use a blunt technique for posterior dissection and mobilization of the rectum. The flat of the hand is used to break down the filmy fibroareolar tissue posterior to the mesorectum. By sweeping the slightly cupped hand gently from side to side, the ureters are displaced laterally and a bloodless blunt dissection can be achieved distally to the rectosacral (Waldeyer) fascia posteriorly.

(B) The rectum has been mobilized either sharply or bluntly distally to the rectosacral (Waldeyer) fascia, which is exposed by anterior distraction of the rectum, as shown in this lateral view. The rectosacral fascia is divided sharply to enter the supralevator space and complete the posterior mobilization of the rectum to the tip of the coccyx and levator floor.

(Continued)

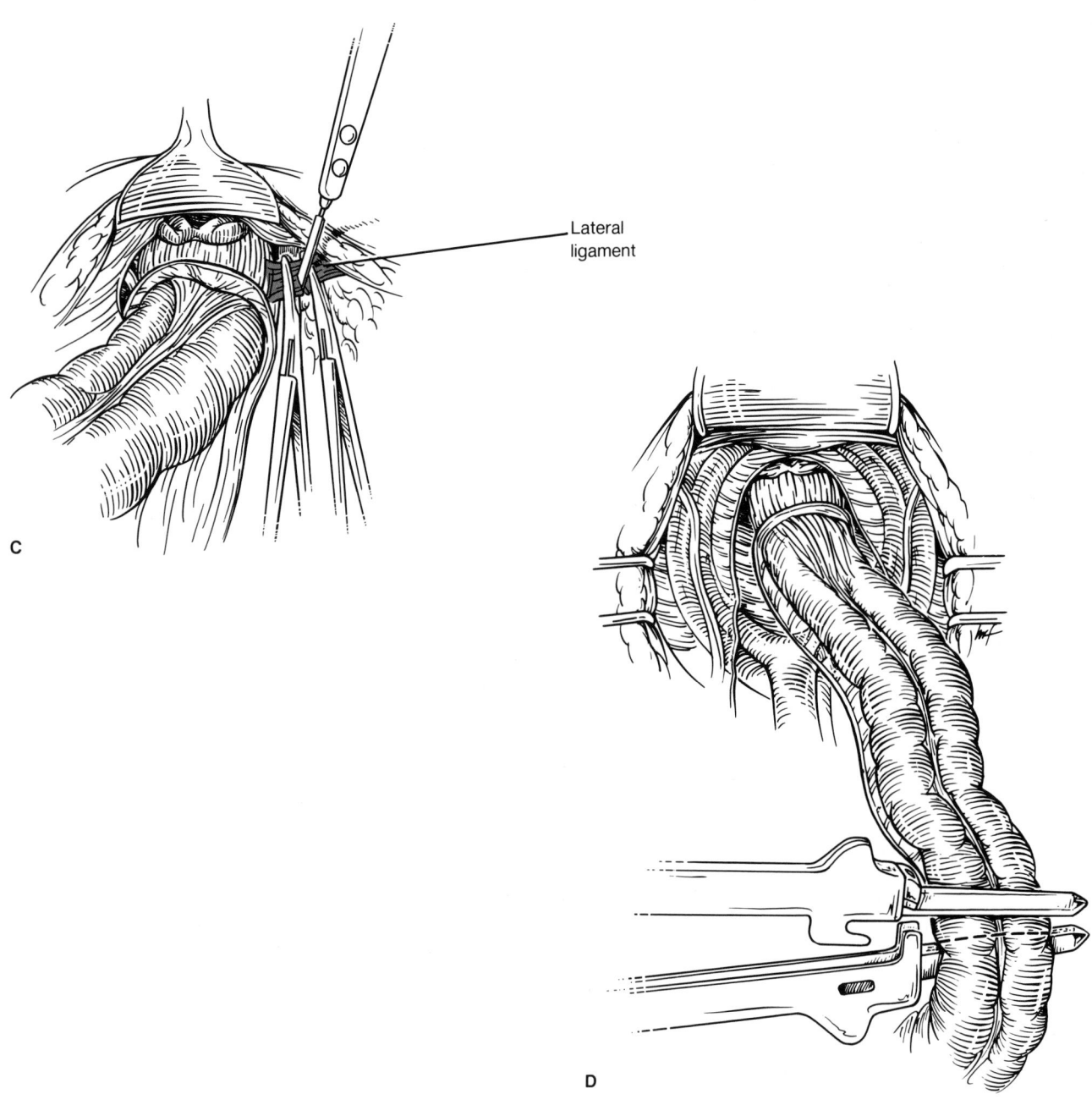

Lateral
ligament

C

D

Figure 43-IID-5 *(Continued)*

(C) The lateral ligaments of the rectum are divided. Often, this is accomplished without need of clamps.

(D) The mobilized proximal colon is transected with a linear cutter-stapler at the junction of the sigmoid colon and the descending colon.

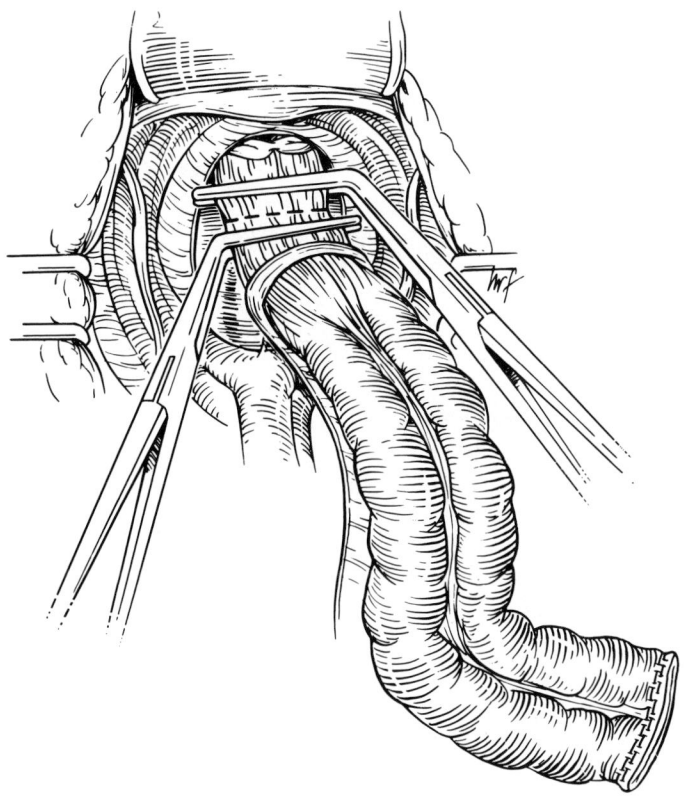

Figure 43-IID-6

Low Anterior Resection of the Rectum

After complete posterior mobilization of the rectum to the coccyx, anterior mobilization to the level of the symphysis pubis, and lateral mobilization by division of the lateral stalks, the surgeon determines whether an anterior resection and colorectal or coloanal anastomosis are feasible. Here, two angled clamps are placed at the level of the distal rectal transection. After dividing the rectum, an assistant can irrigate the distal rectal stump through a proctoscope to minimize risk of pelvic contamination when the clamp is removed.

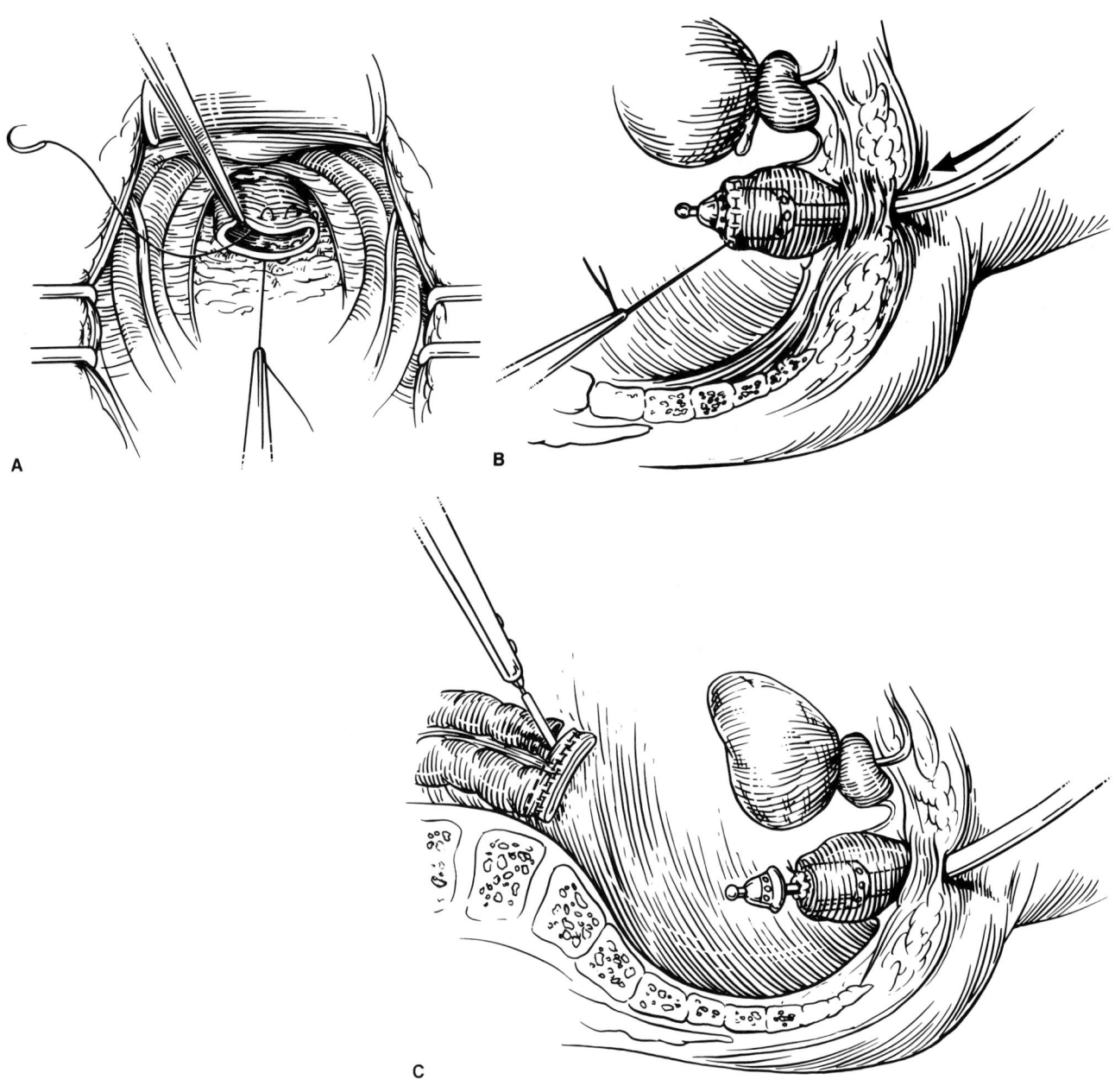

A

B

C

Figure 43-IID-7

Stapled Colorectal Anastomosis

(**A**) The cut end of the distal rectal stump is exposed to allow placement of a pursestring suture before use of a circular stapler.

(**B**) An assistant passes a circular stapler through the anus.

(**C**) The circular stapler has been opened, and the rectal pursestring has been tied around the central rod. The staple line on the proximal bowel is excised to allow placement of a pursestring suture.

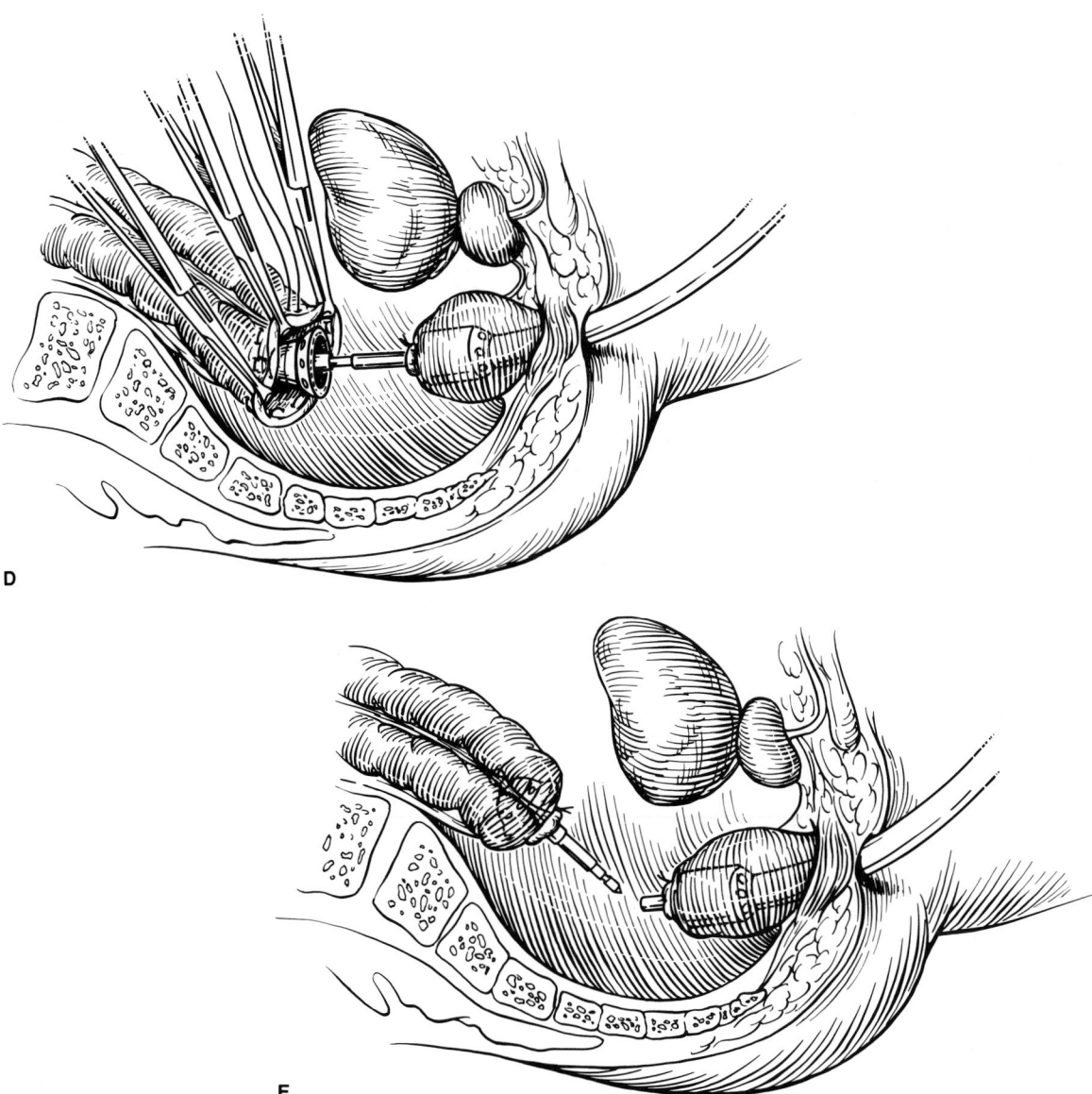

Figure 43-IID-7 *(Continued)*

(D) A pursestring suture has been placed in the cut end of the proximal colon, which is placed over the anvil of the circular stapler.

(E) The proximal pursestring is tied around the central rod. The anvil has been detached from the stapler to allow easier insertion into the proximal bowel.

(Continued)

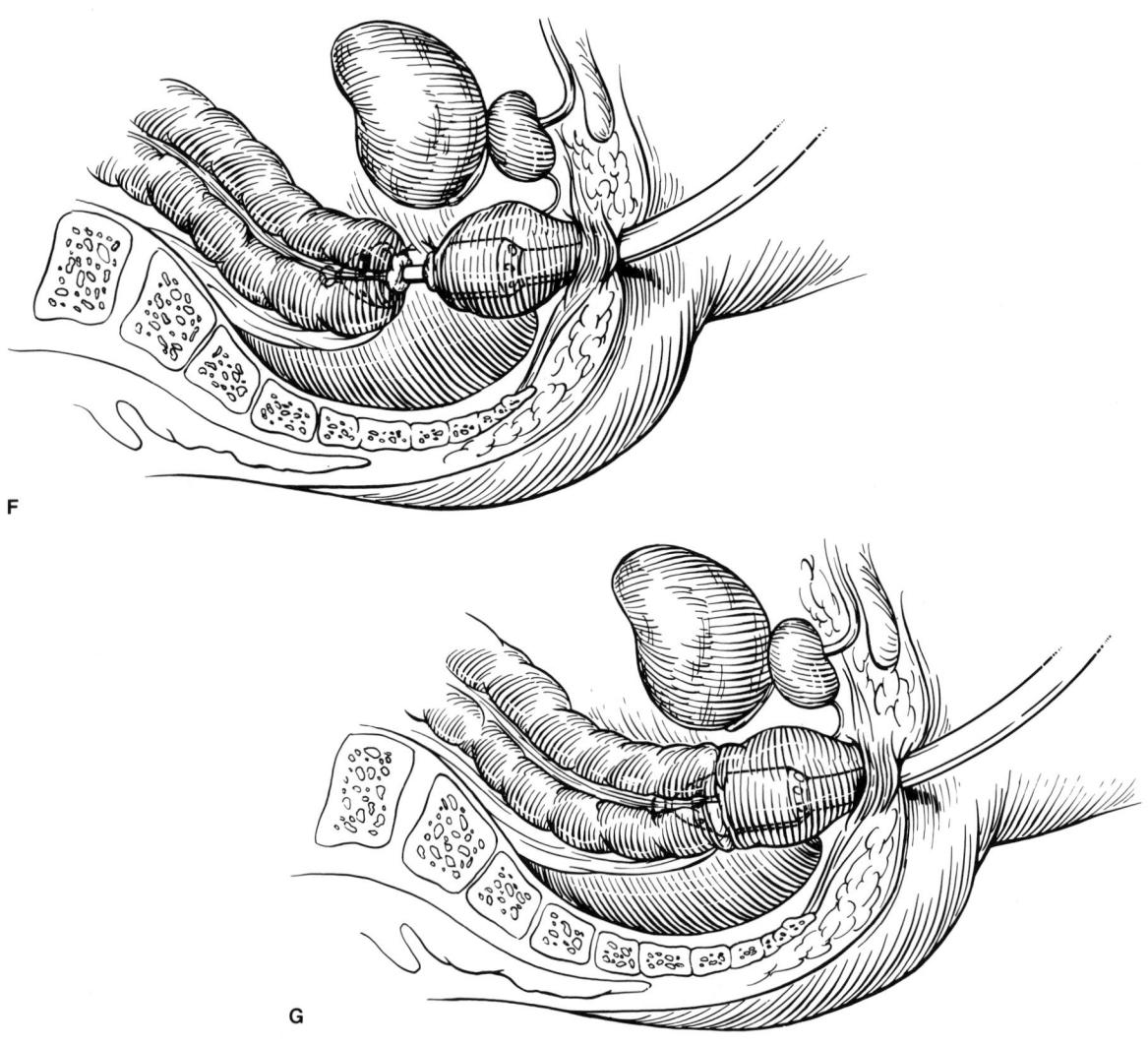

F

G

Figure 43-IID-7 *(Continued)*

(F) The circular stapler is closed.

(G) Once in proper firing range, the circular stapler is fired to create an end-to-end colo-rectal stapled anastomosis.

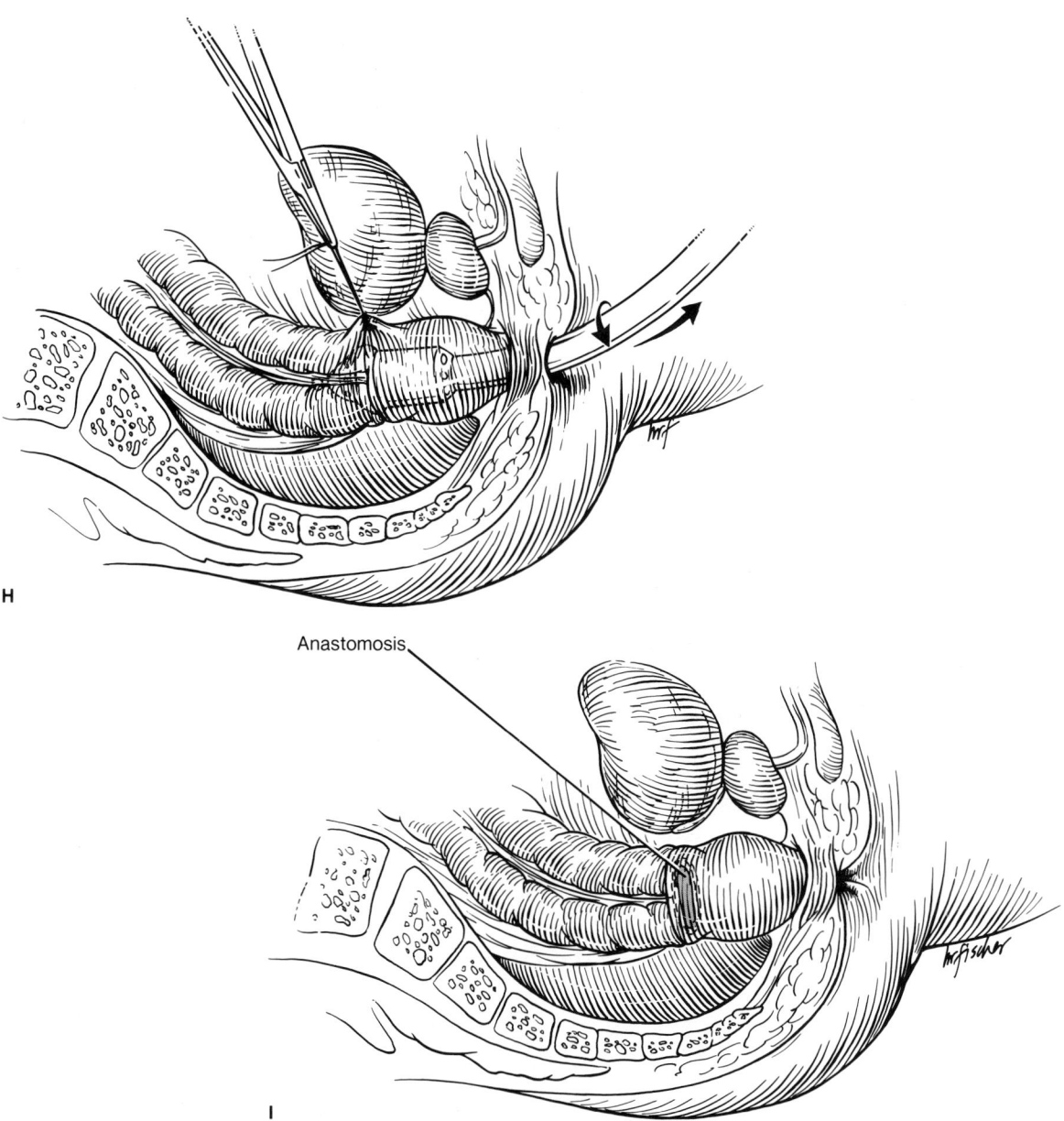

Anastomosis

H

I

Figure 43-IID-7 *(Continued)*

(H) The stapler is opened slightly and removed gently from the completed end-to-end anastomosis. A suture may be used to stabilize the anastomosis while the stapler is withdrawn from the anus.

(I) The completed, inverted, stapled end-to-end colorectal anastomosis is shown.

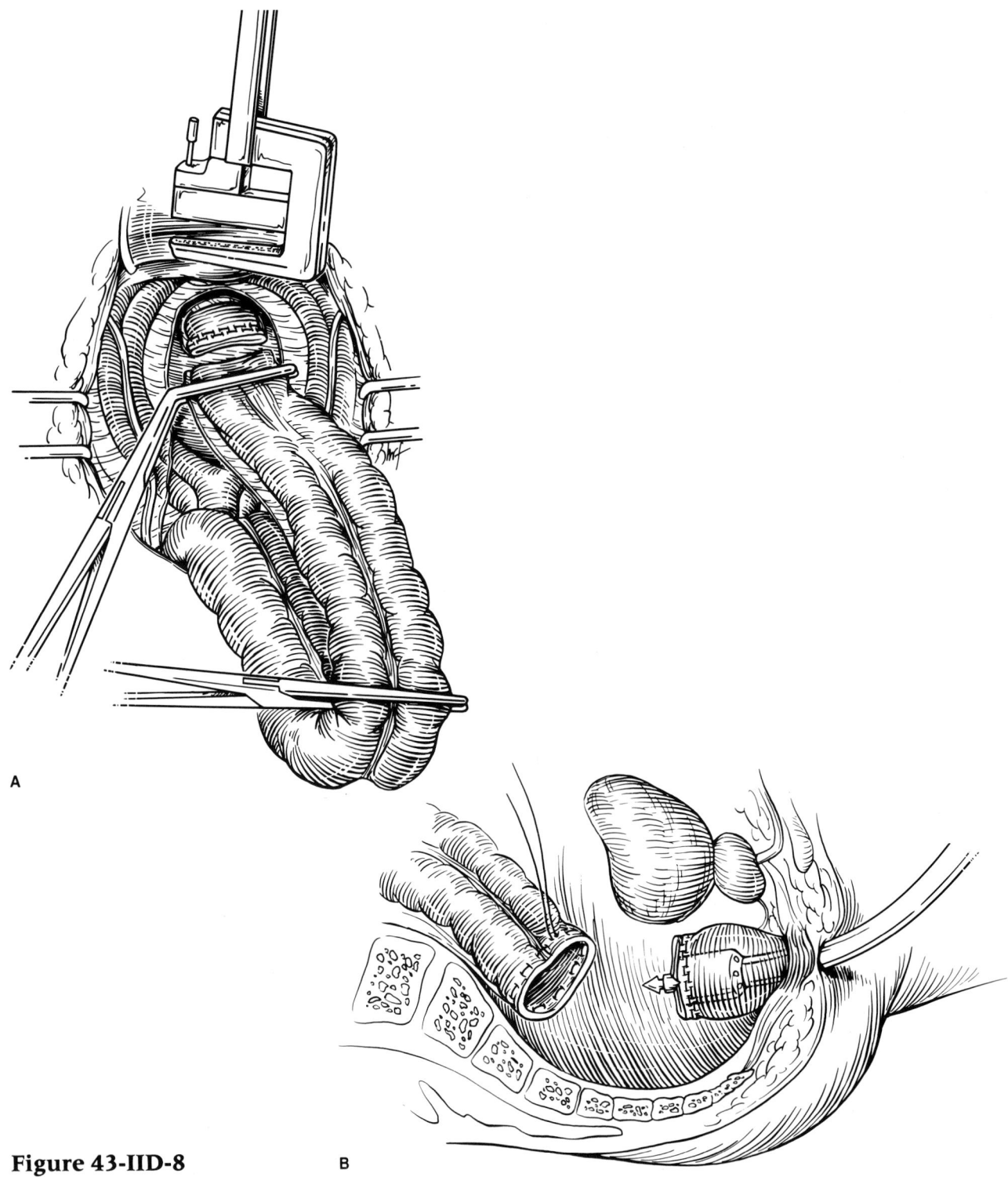

Figure 43-IID-8

Double-Stapled Colorectal Anastomosis

(A) The distal rectum has been closed with a straight stapler and then transected over an angled bowel clamp.

(B) A pursestring suture is placed in the end of the proximal colon. A circular stapler without an anvil but with a disposable trocar within the cartridge is placed into the anus and passed proximally. The trocar is used to pierce the previously placed transverse staple line.

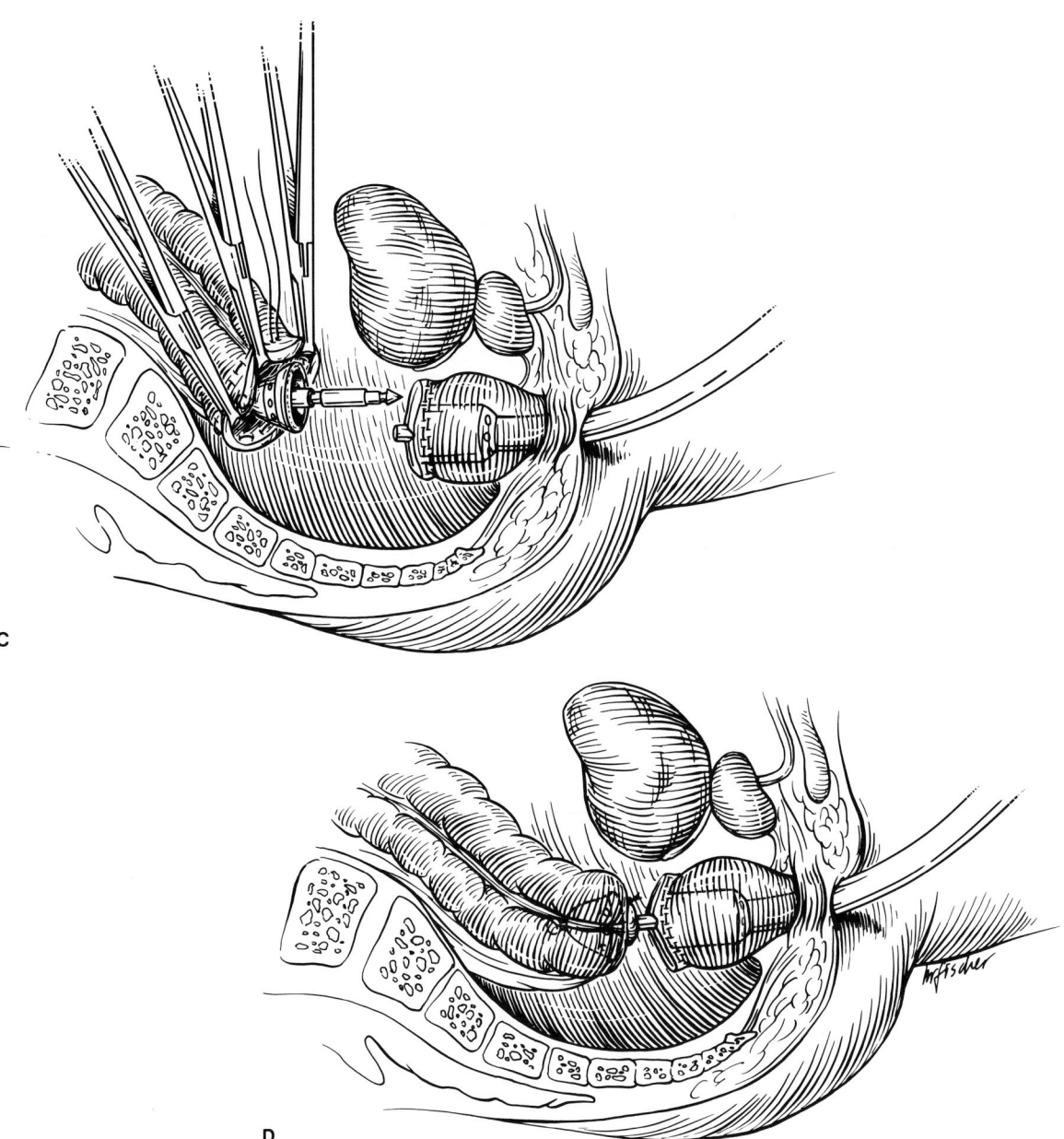

Figure 43-IID-8 *(Continued)*

(C) The disposable trocar has been removed. The anvil for the circular stapler is placed into the proximal bowel, and the pursestring suture is tied.

(D) The circular stapler is closed, fired, and removed in the standard fashion.

(Continued)

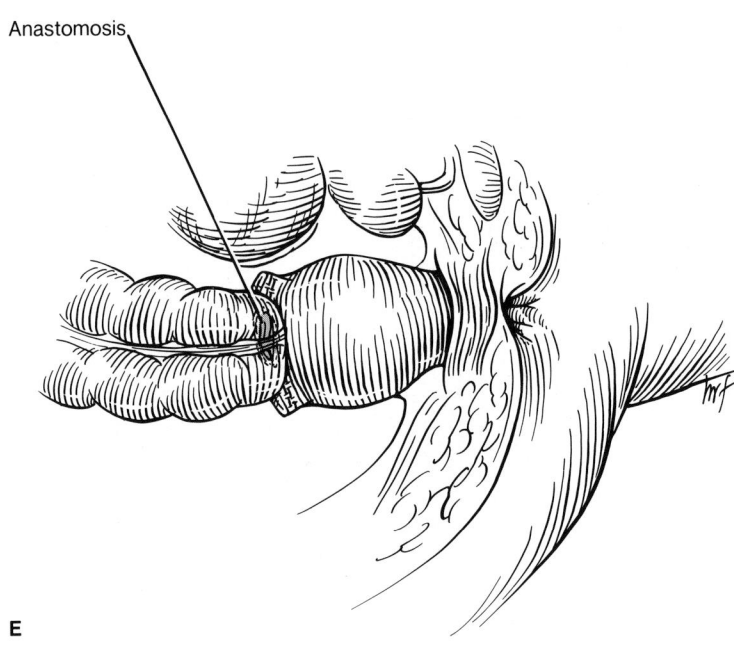

Anastomosis

E

Figure 43-IID-8 *(Continued)*

(E) The completed end-to-end double-stapled colorectal anastomosis is shown.

E. Perineal Dissection

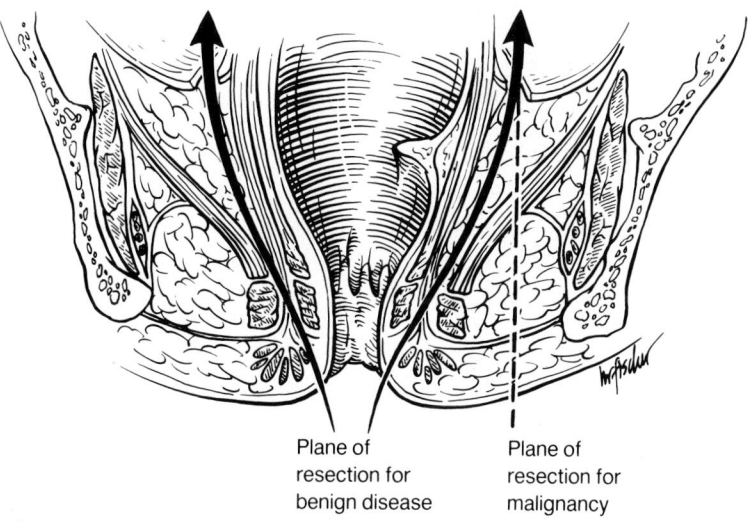

Plane of
resection for
benign disease

Plane of
resection for
malignancy

Figure 43-IIE-1

Perineal Dissection Planes for Benign and Malignant Disease

For benign disease, an intersphincteric dissection plane is used. The external sphincter
and levator ani remain intact. For malignant disease, an extrasphincteric plane is used.
The external sphincter is removed and the levator ani divided.

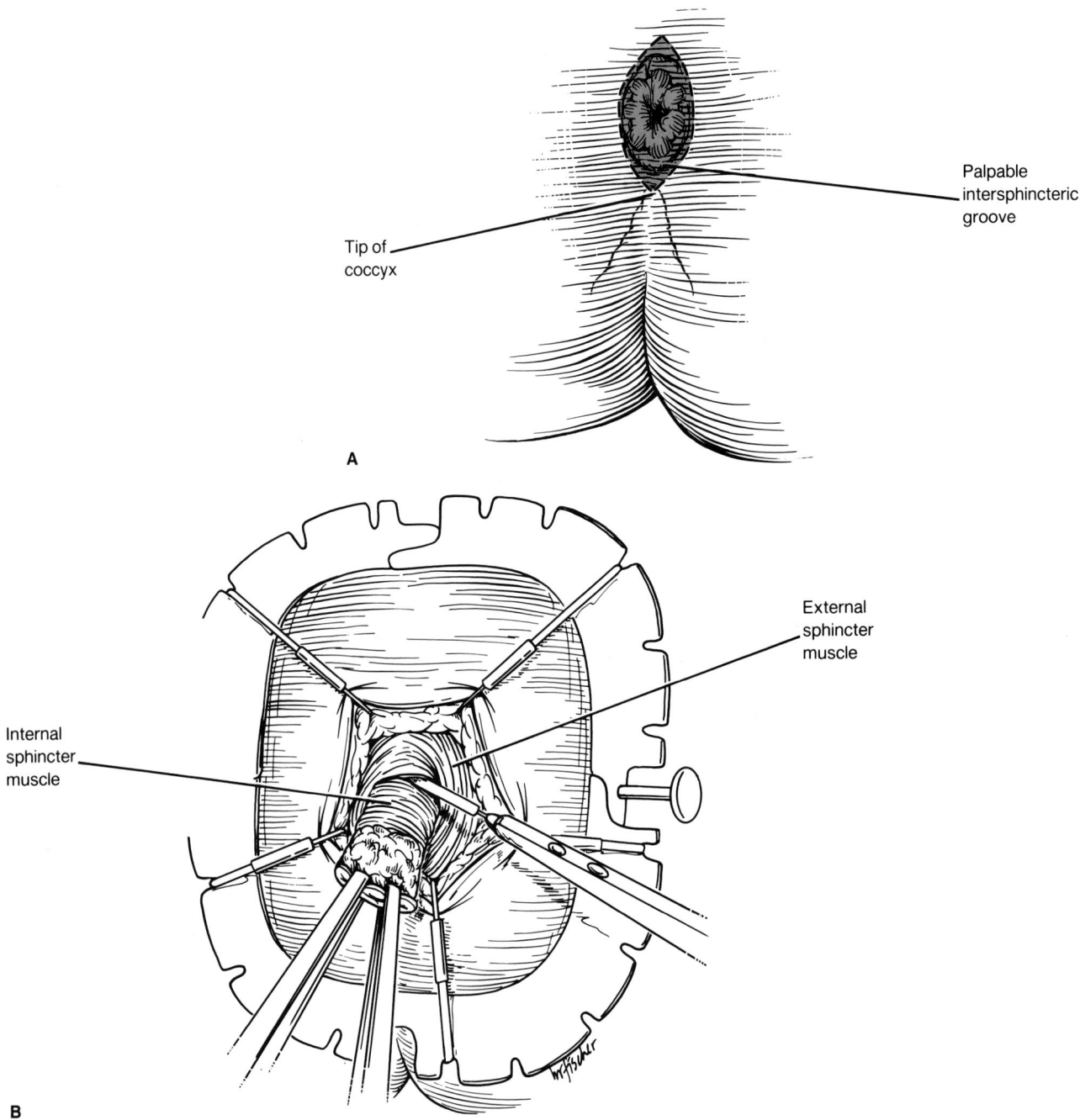

Palpable intersphincteric groove

Tip of coccyx

A

External sphincter muscle

Internal sphincter muscle

B

Figure 43-IIE-2

Dissection for Benign Disease

(**A**) With the patient in a modified lithotomy position, perineal exposure is achieved. The anus is closed with a pursestring suture to prevent fecal spillage during dissection. An incision is made at the level of the intersphincteric groove.

(**B**) Intersphincteric dissection is commenced and continued in the plane between the internal and external sphincters. This is avascular. A multihooked self-retaining retractor (Lone Star) facilitates the exposure.

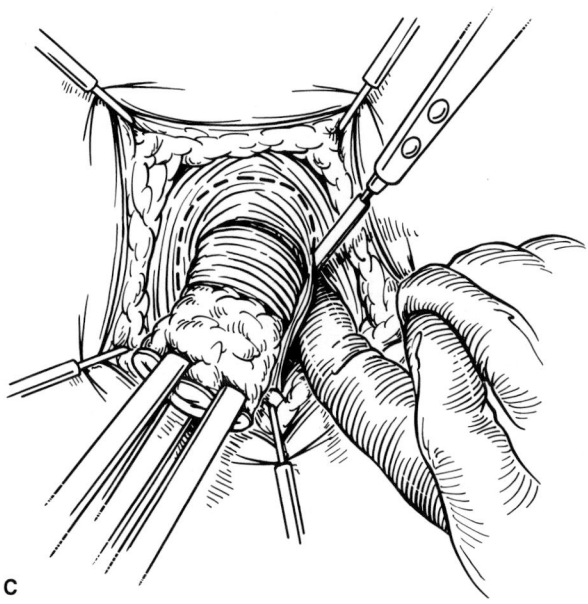

C

Figure 43-IIE-2 *(Continued)*

(C) Posteriorly, the anococcygeal raphe is divided. The dissection proceeds in a cephalad direction to meet the prior pelvic dissection in the posterior midline. The perineal surgeon then inserts a digit into the posterior midline dissection plane and exposes and divides the remaining lateral attachments to the proximal anorectum. Finally, the proctectomy is completed by dissecting anteriorly along the anorectal wall. The resultant defect is small and easily closed with interrupted absorbable sutures in two or three layers.

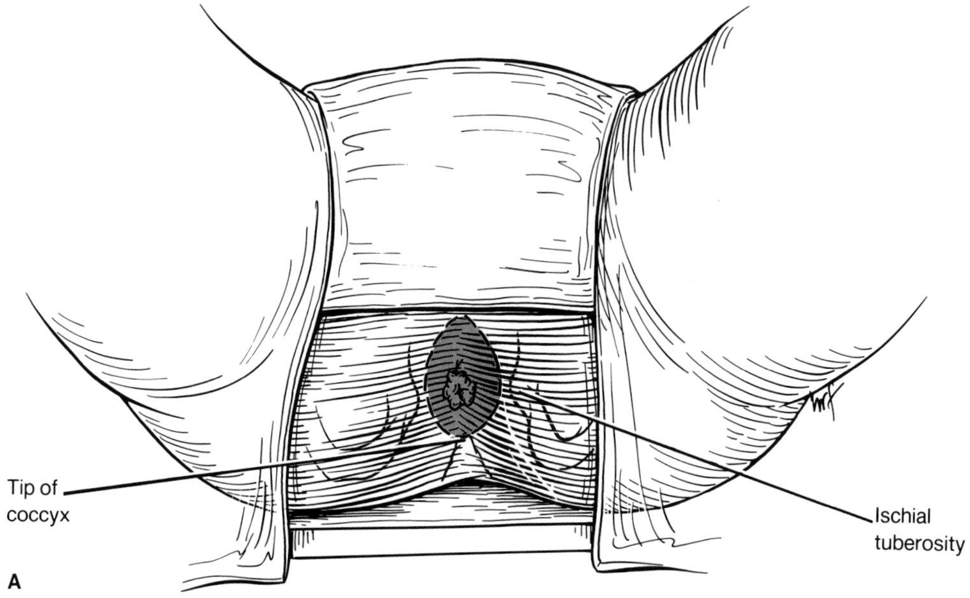

Tip of
coccyx

Ischial
tuberosity

A

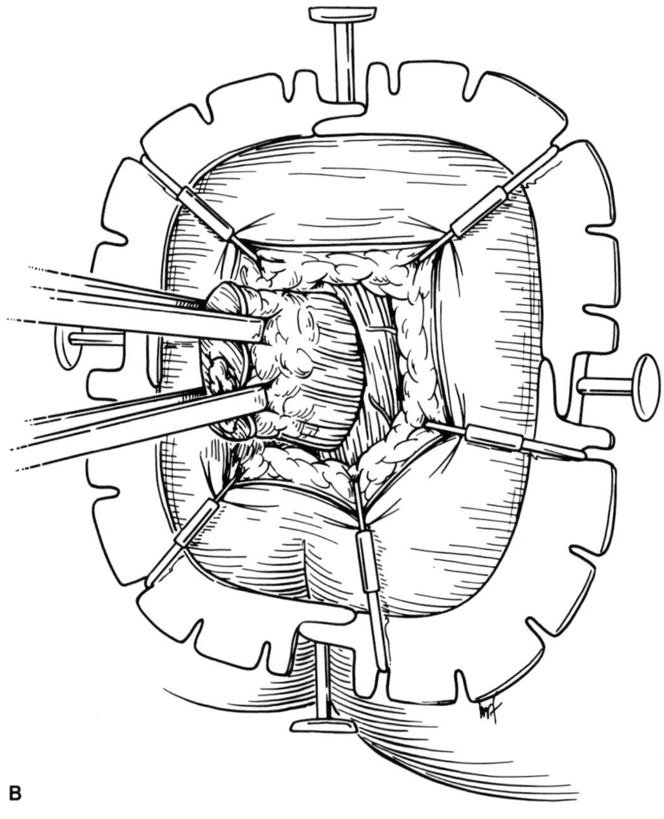

B

Figure 43-IIE-3

Dissection for Malignant Disease

(A) The patient is in a modified lithotomy position. The anus is closed with a pursestring suture to prevent contamination of the wound during proctectomy. An elliptical skin incision is placed over the ischiorectal fossa and meets posteriorly at the tip of the coccyx.

(B) The dissection plane extends proximally through the ischiorectal fat. A multihooked self-retaining retractor (Lone Star) facilitates exposure.

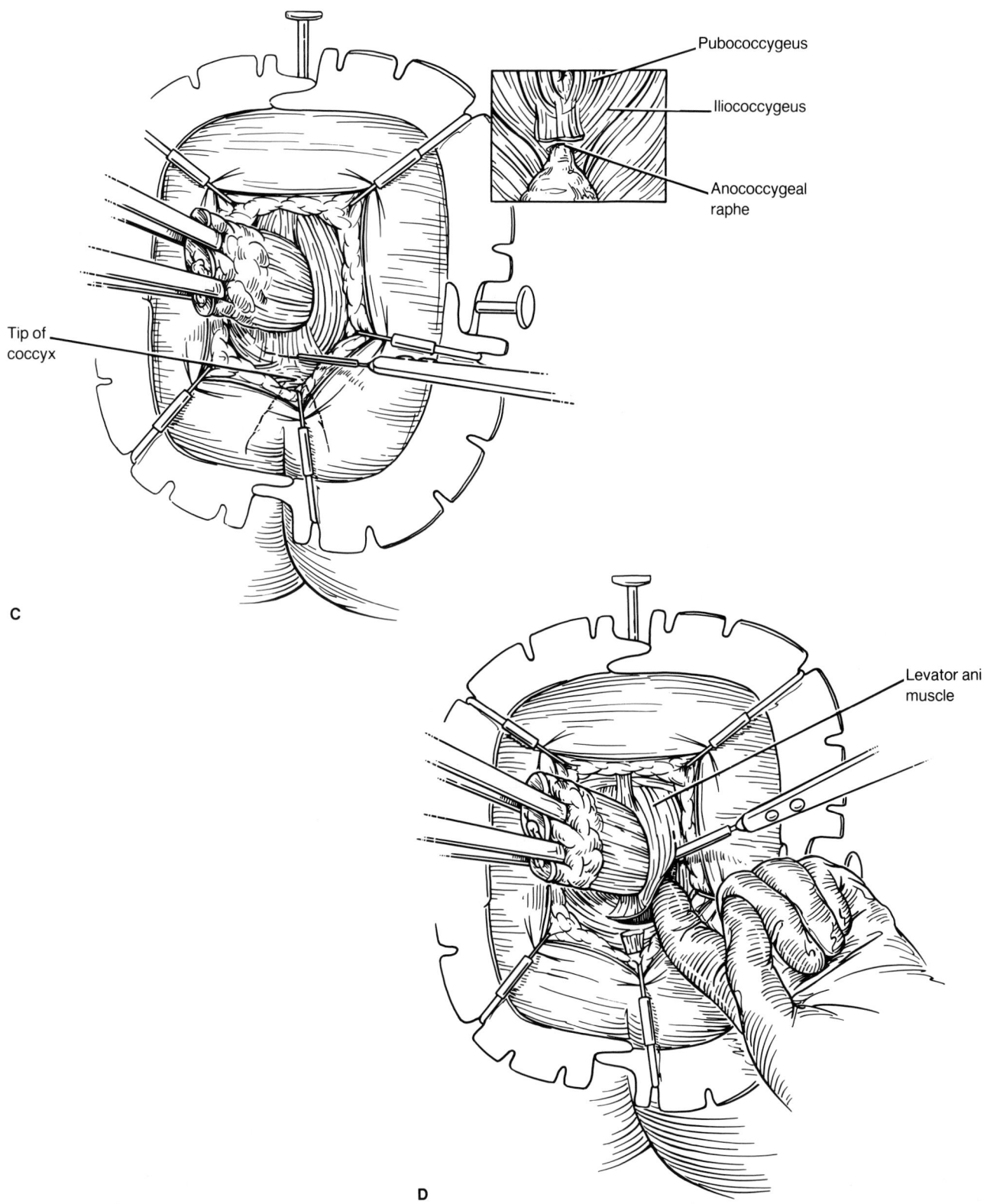

Figure 43-IIE-3 *(Continued)*

(C) Posteriorly, the anococcygeal raphe is divided at the tip of the coccyx. This allows entry into the supralevator space.

(D) After division of the anococcygeal raphe, the levator ani muscles can be hooked with the finger and divided with electrocautery.

(Continued)

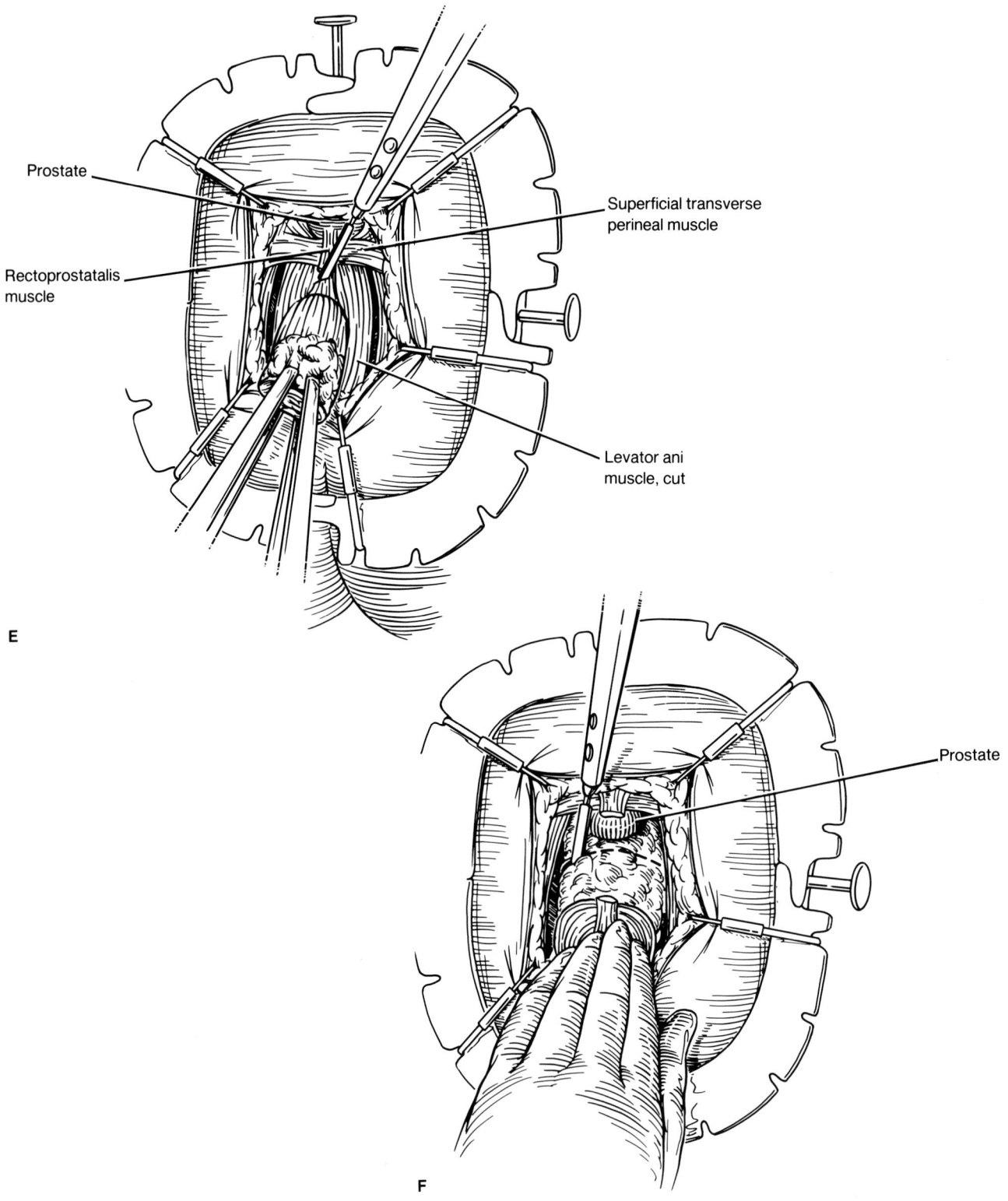

Prostate

**Rectoprostatalis
muscle**

**Superficial transverse
perineal muscle**

**Levator ani
muscle, cut**

E

Prostate

F

Figure 43-IIE-3 *(Continued)*

(E) Anteriorly, the superficial transverse perineal muscles are exposed. In the male, the rectoprostatalis muscles and fascia are divided. This allows dissection of the anterior wall of the rectum in a plane posterior to the Denonvilliers fascia.

(F) After division of the rectoprostatalis, the urethra and prostate are separated from the front of the rectum.

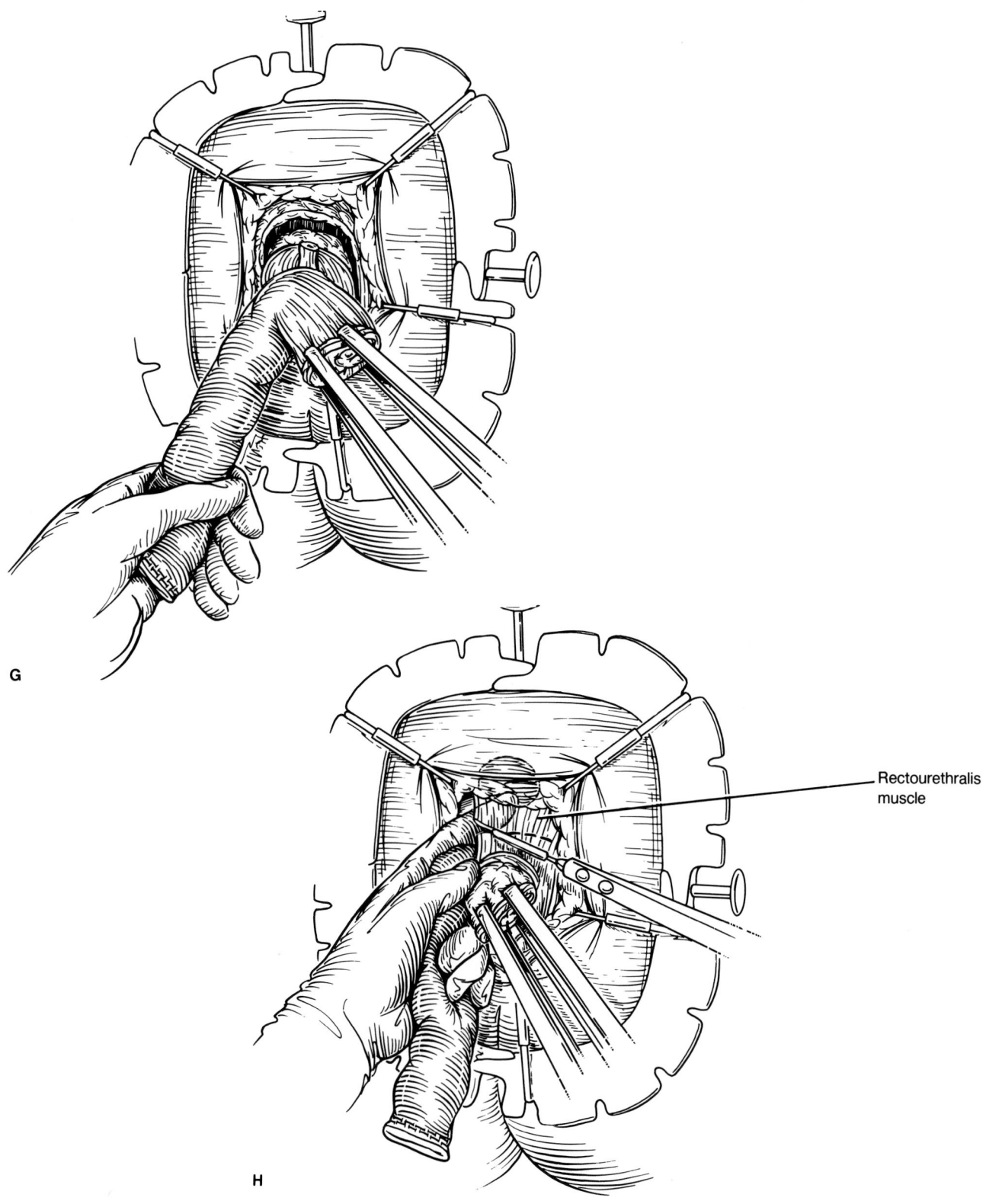

G

H

Rectourethralis
muscle

Figure 43-IIE-3 *(Continued)*

(G) The previously mobilized and divided rectosigmoid can now be protruded through the perineum to allow completion of the dissection.

(H) The remaining attachments of the levator ani muscles and the puborectalis muscles are divided anteriorly. The proctectomy is now completed.

(Continued)

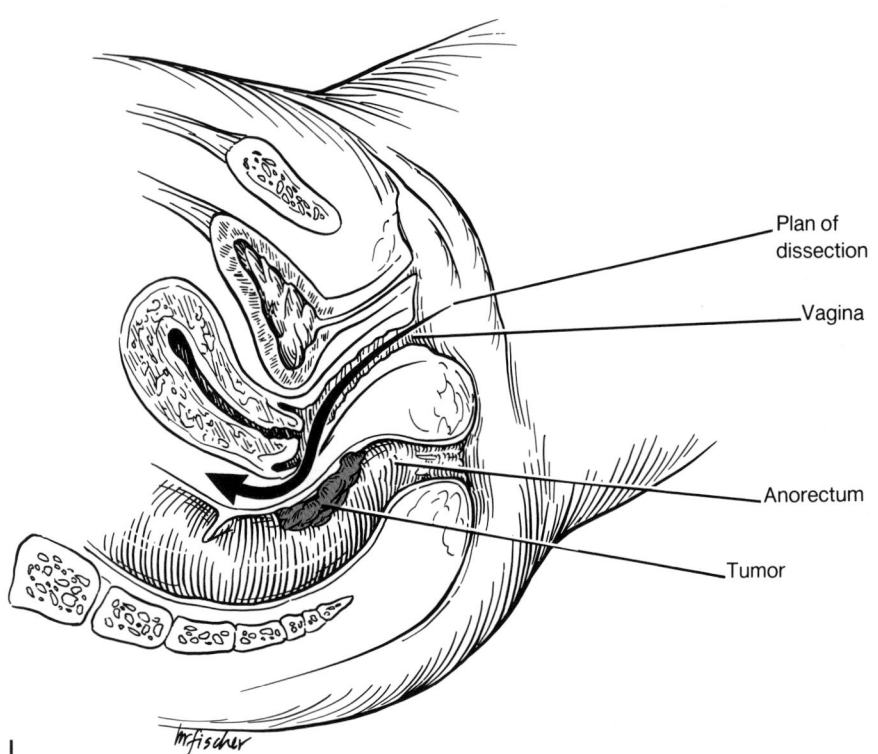

I

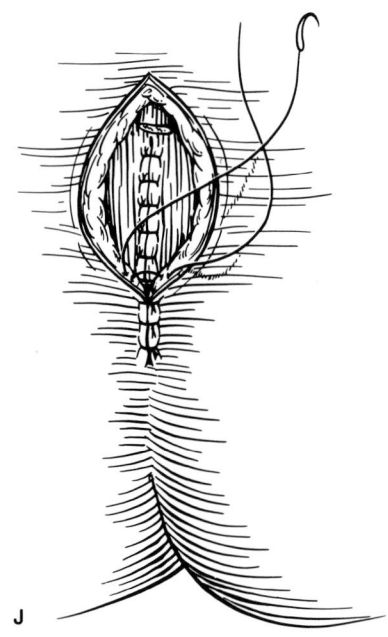

J

Figure 43-IIE-3 *(Continued)*

(I) Anterior rectal cancers in the female may require en bloc excision of the posterior wall of the vagina.

(J) The perineum is closed in layers.

F. Total Colectomy for Benign Disease

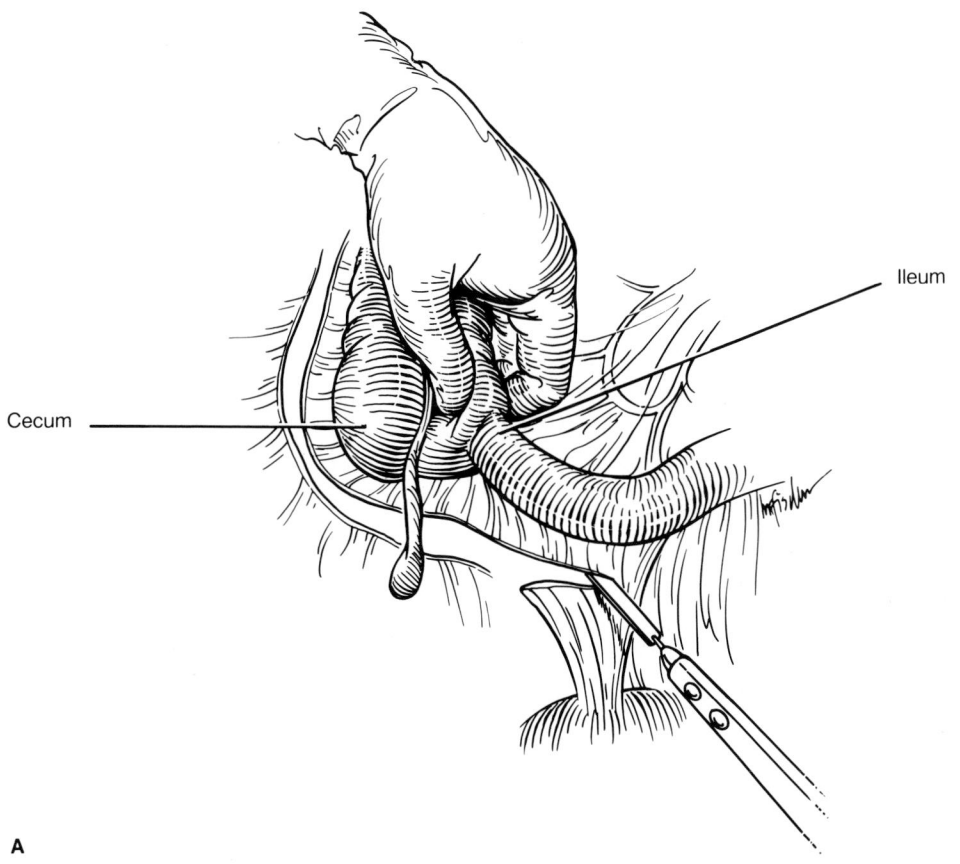

A

Figure 43-IIF-1

Mobilization of the Colon

(**A**) With the patient in a modified lithotomy position, exploration of the abdomen is performed. A total colectomy is commenced by incising the peritoneal attachments of the right colon and terminal ileum with electrocautery. This is facilitated by medial traction on the cecum and terminal ileum.

(Continued)

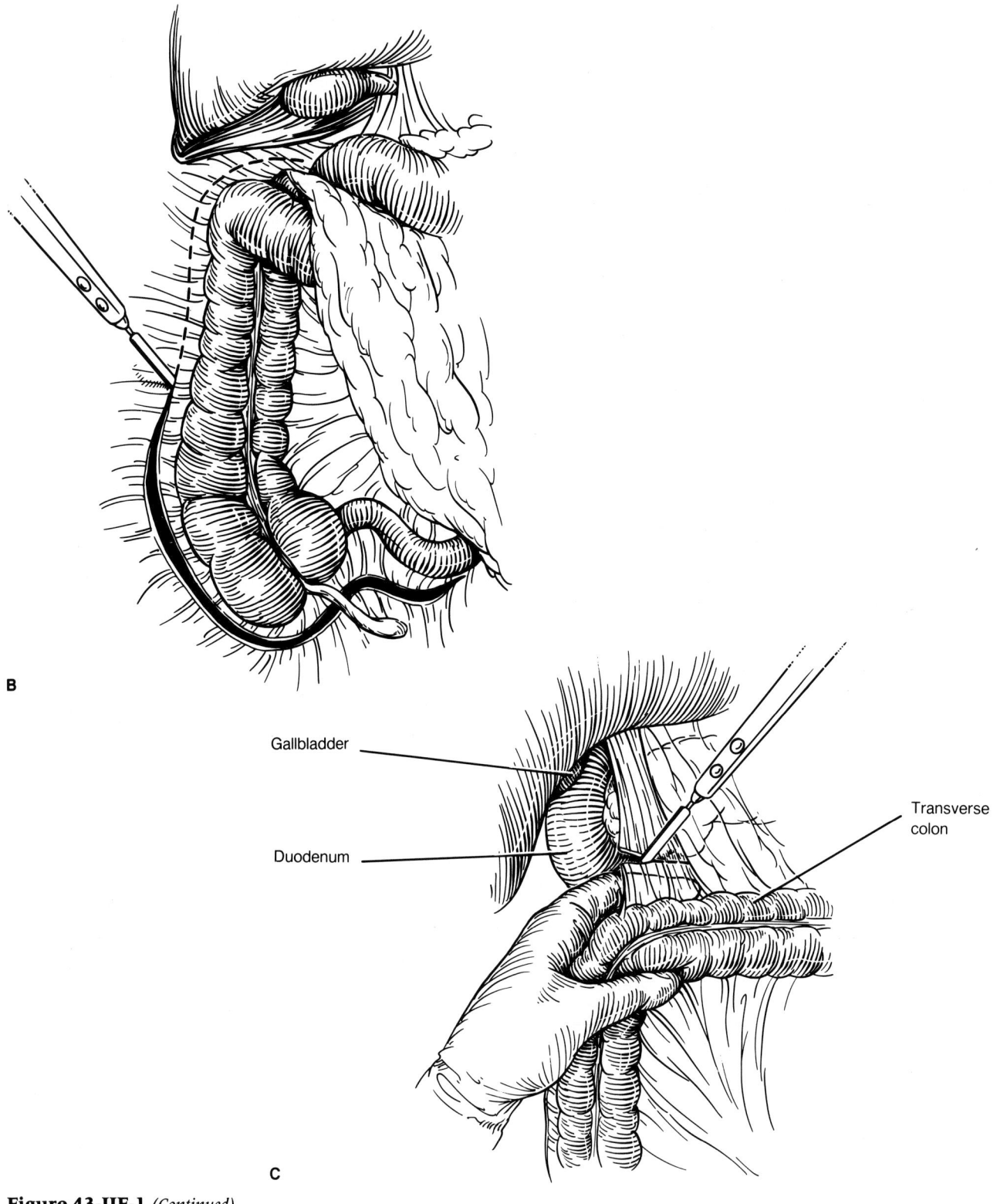

B

Gallbladder

Duodenum

Transverse colon

C

Figure 43-IIF-1 *(Continued)*

(B) The remaining lateral peritoneal attachments are incised up to the hepatocolic ligament.

(C) The hepatic flexure of the colon is mobilized by incising the peritoneal attachments. If the hepatocolic ligament is thick, division between clamps is necessary. The mobilized right colon is reflected medially to expose and avoid injury to the duodenum.

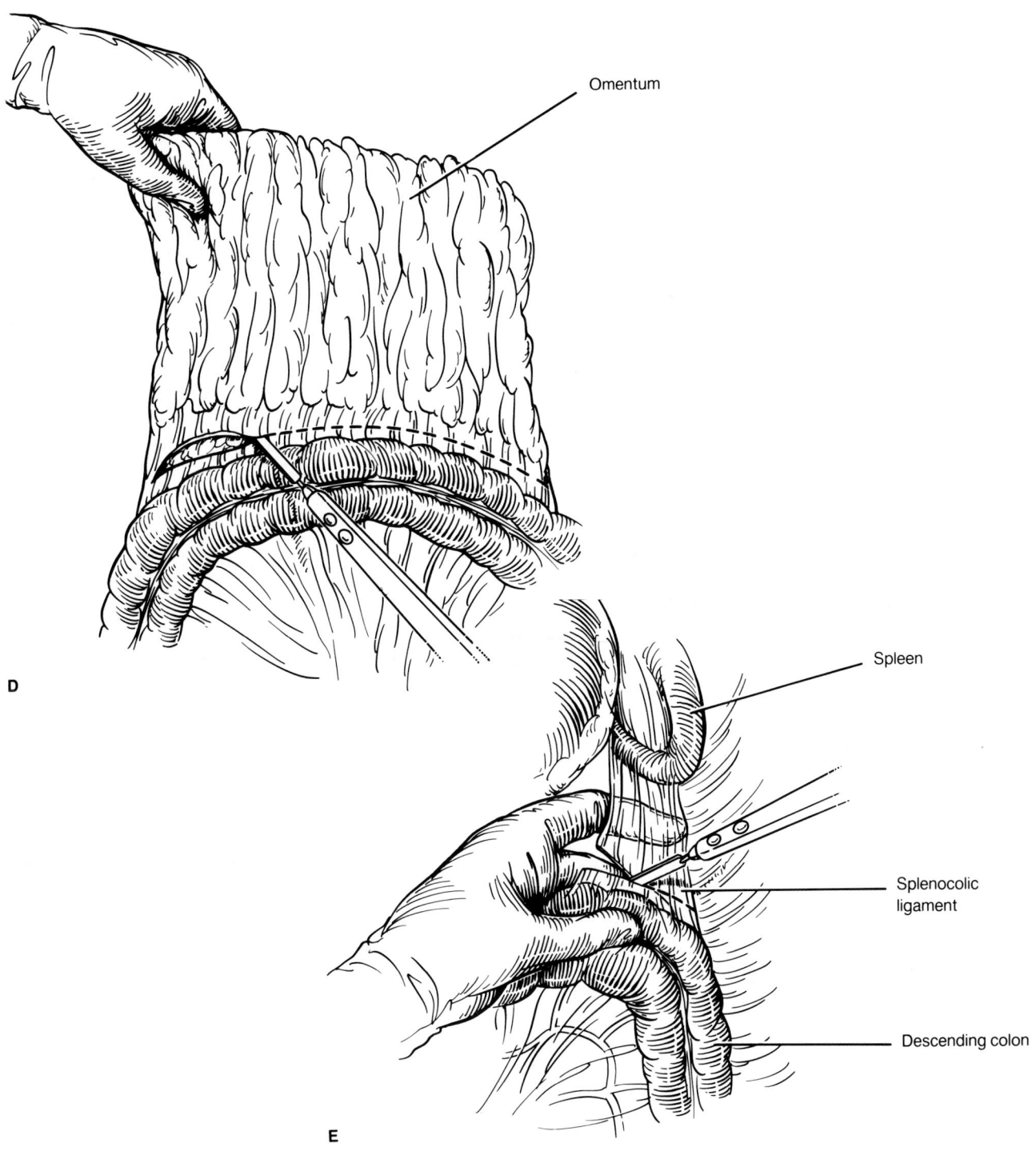

Figure 43-IIF-1 *(Continued)*

(D) The omentum is detached from the transverse colon.

(E) The transverse colon has been mobilized by separating the omentum from the colon from within the lesser sac. The mobilization is continued toward the splenic flexure. The peritoneal attachments are divided with electrocautery. If the splenocolic ligament is thick, it is divided between clamps and ligated. Care is taken not to exert inferior traction on the spleen, or troublesome capsular tears result.

(Continued)

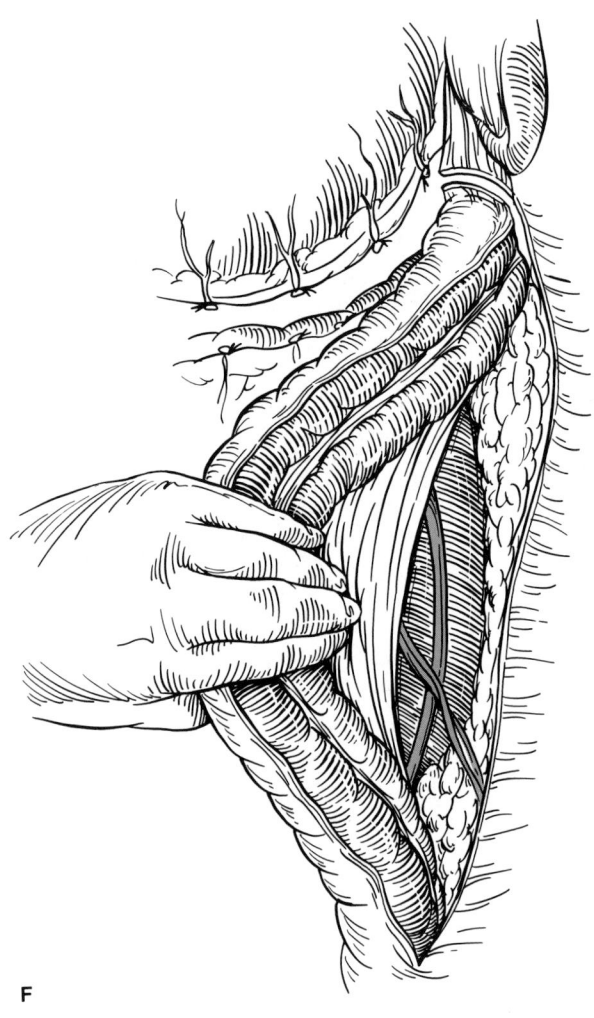

F

Figure 43-IIF-1 *(Continued)*

(F) The peritoneal attachments of the descending colon are incised to complete mobilization of the splenic flexure of the colon. The peritoneal incision is extended inferiorly lateral to the sigmoid colon to the level of the sacral promontory. As medial traction is applied to the mobilized left colon, the ureter and gonadal vessels are identified and gently pushed posteriorly so they are not injured during colectomy.

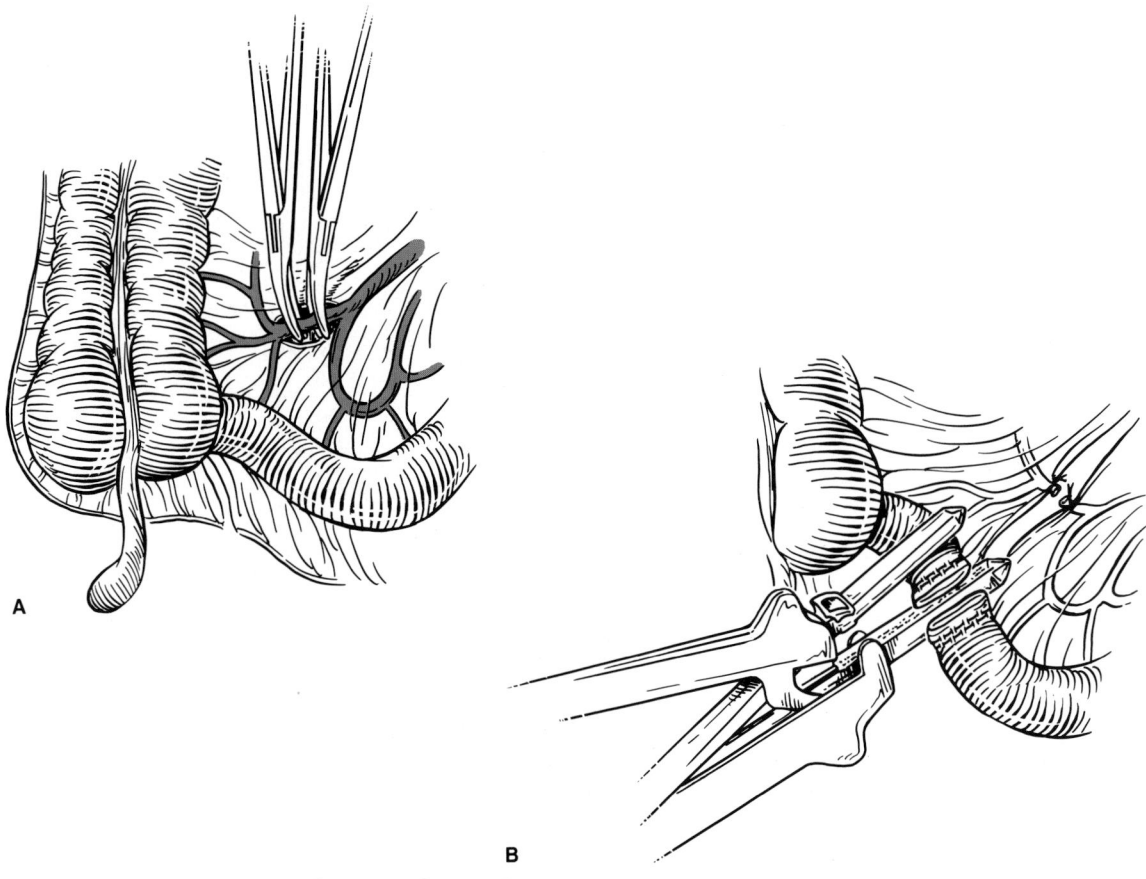

Figure 43-IIF-2

Mesenteric Division

(A) After complete mobilization of the abdominal colon, the major mesenteric vessels are clamped, divided, and ligated. Because the disease process is benign, mesenteric lymphadenectomy is not necessary, and the entire distal ileum can be preserved. Thus, the vascular ligation of the ileocolic vessels can be performed distally, as shown.

(B) The distal ileum is transected with the linear cutter-stapler.

(Continued)

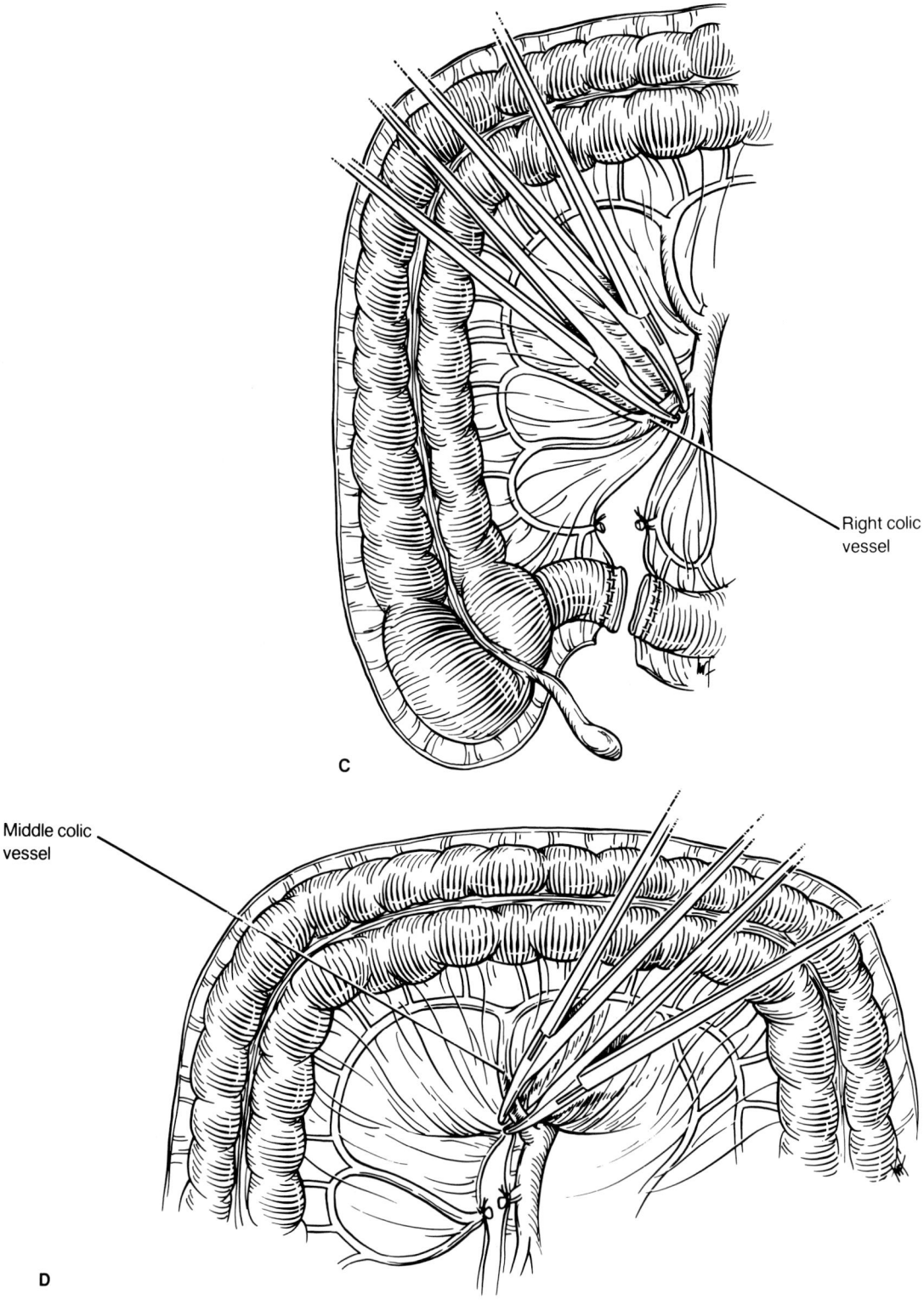

C

Right colic
vessel

Middle colic
vessel

D

Figure 43-IIF-2 *(Continued)*

(C) The right colic vessels are clamped, divided, and ligated.

(D) Mesenteric division continues by clamping, dividing, and ligating the middle colic
vessels.

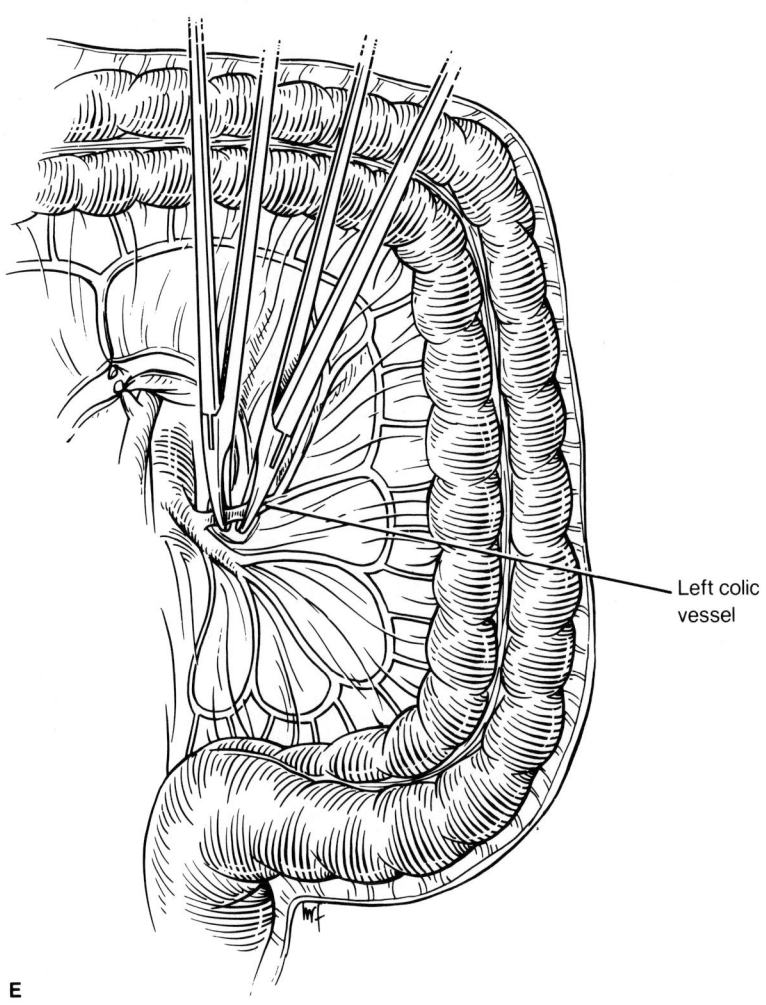

Left colic
vessel

E

Figure 43-IIF-2 *(Continued)*

(E) The left colic vessels are clamped, divided, and ligated after being certain the ureter and gonadal vessels are safely positioned in the retroperitoneum.

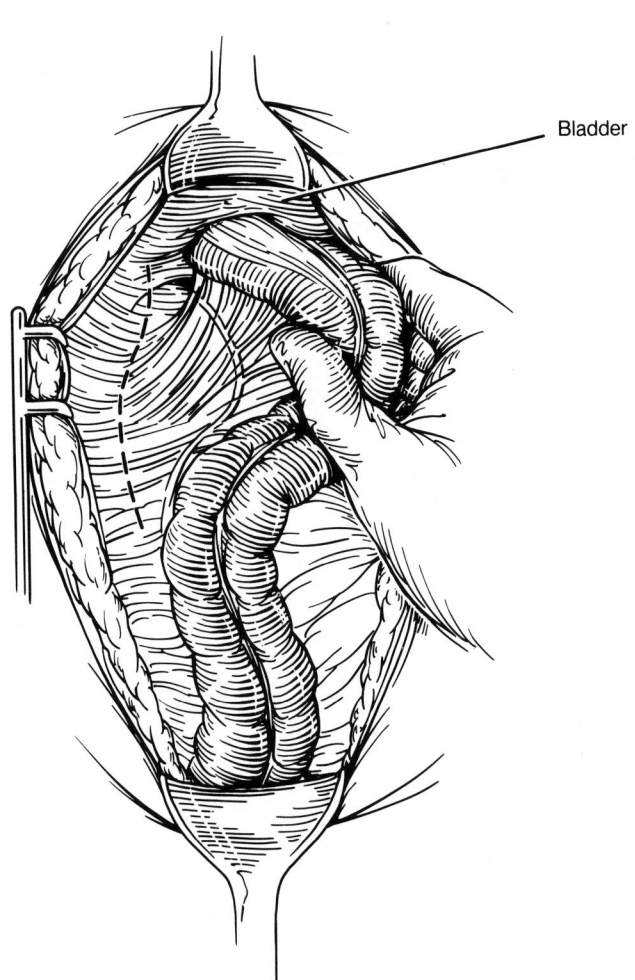

Bladder

A

Figure 43-IIF-3

Mobilization of Rectosigmoid Colon

(A) After the abdominal colon has been mobilized and its mesentery divided to the level of the sigmoidal vessels, the patient is placed in the Trendelenburg position, and the pelvis is exposed by packing the small bowel in the upper abdomen. The peritoneum lateral to the sigmoid colon is incised inferiorly to the level of the cul-de-sac.

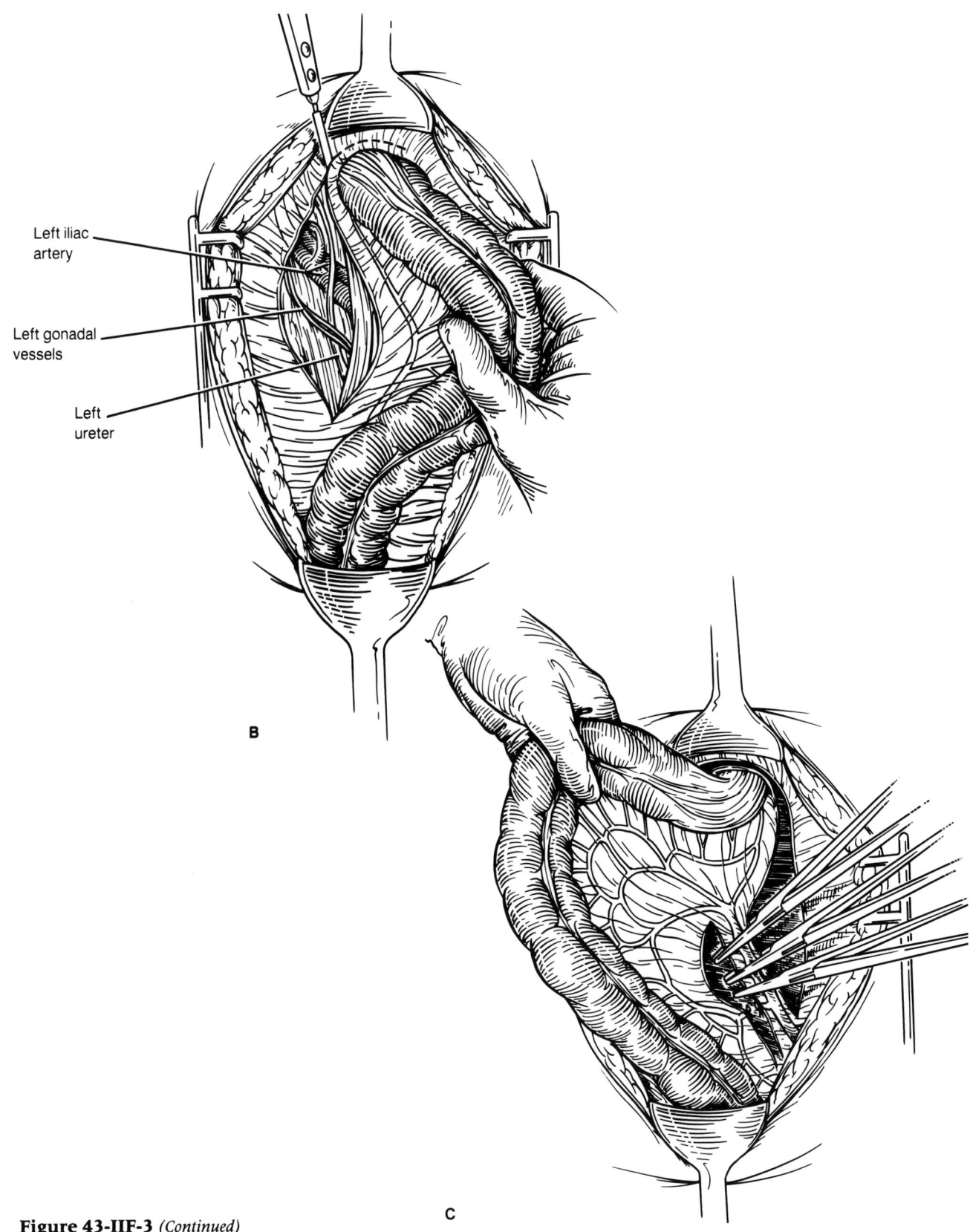

Left iliac artery

Left gonadal vessels

Left ureter

B

C

Figure 43-IIF-3 *(Continued)*

(B) As the sigmoid colon is mobilized, the left ureter, gonadal vessels, and iliac vessels are identified in the underlying retroperitoneum. The anterior cul-de-sac is incised.

(C) Lateral and anterior traction on the mobilized rectosigmoid exposes the sigmoidal vessels, which are triply clamped, divided, and ligated. The peritoneum overlying the right side of the rectosigmoid is incised distally to meet the incision from the left side.

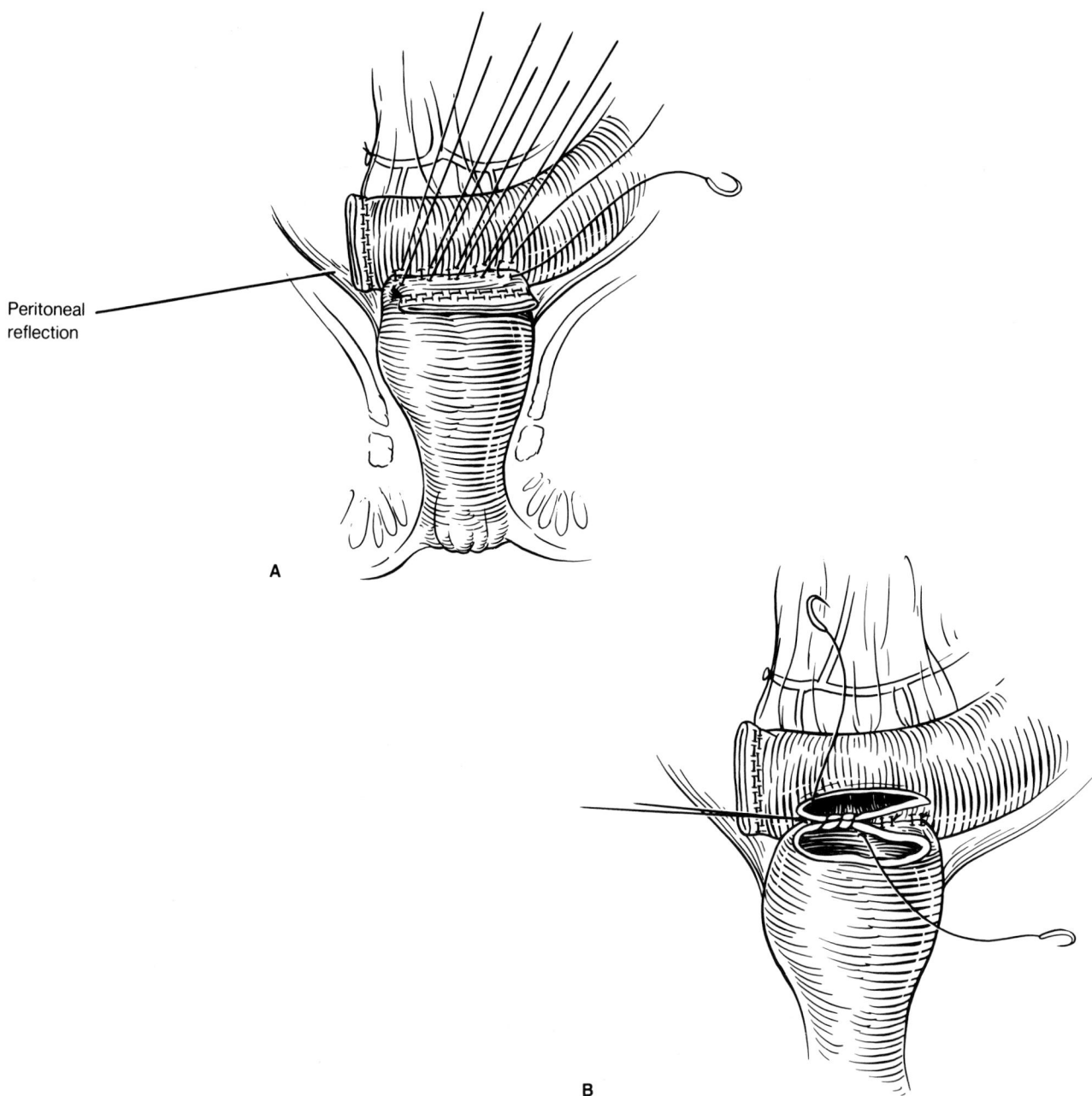

Peritoneal
reflection

A

B

Figure 43-IIF-4

Sutured Side-to-Side Ileorectal Anastomosis

(A) The entire colon has been resected by transecting the rectum with a linear stapler. The terminal ileum is aligned with 4-0 seromuscular interrupted sutures.

(B) After the rectum has been irrigated clean through proctoscopy, the staple line on the rectum is excised, and an enterotomy is made in the terminal ileum, as shown. A running 3-0 or 4-0 absorbable suture is placed on the posterior row.

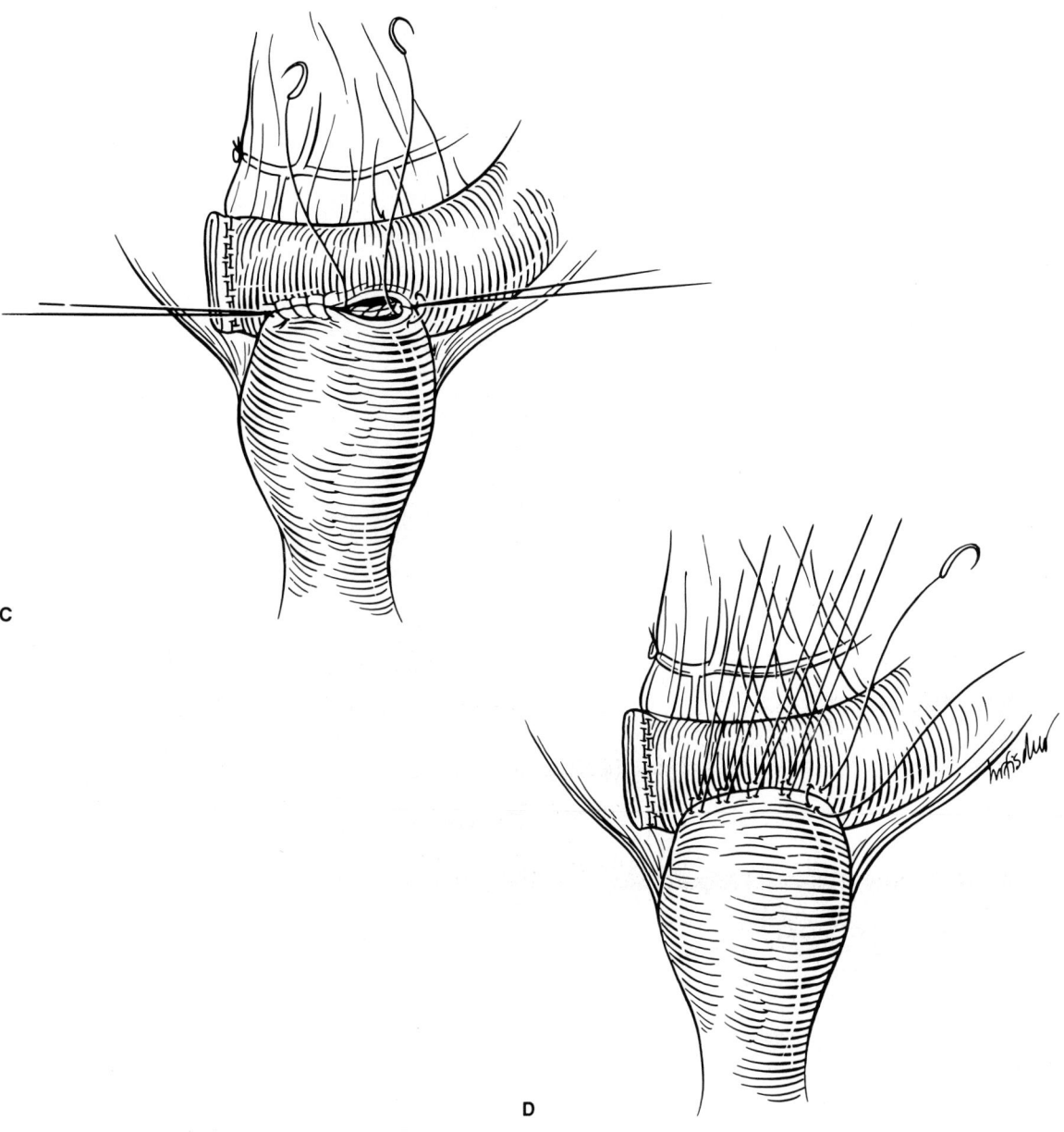

C

D

Figure 43-IIF-4 *(Continued)*

(C) The running suture is continued anteriorly to close the ileorectal defect.

(D) Seromuscular 4-0 interrupted sutures are placed anteriorly to complete the anastomosis.

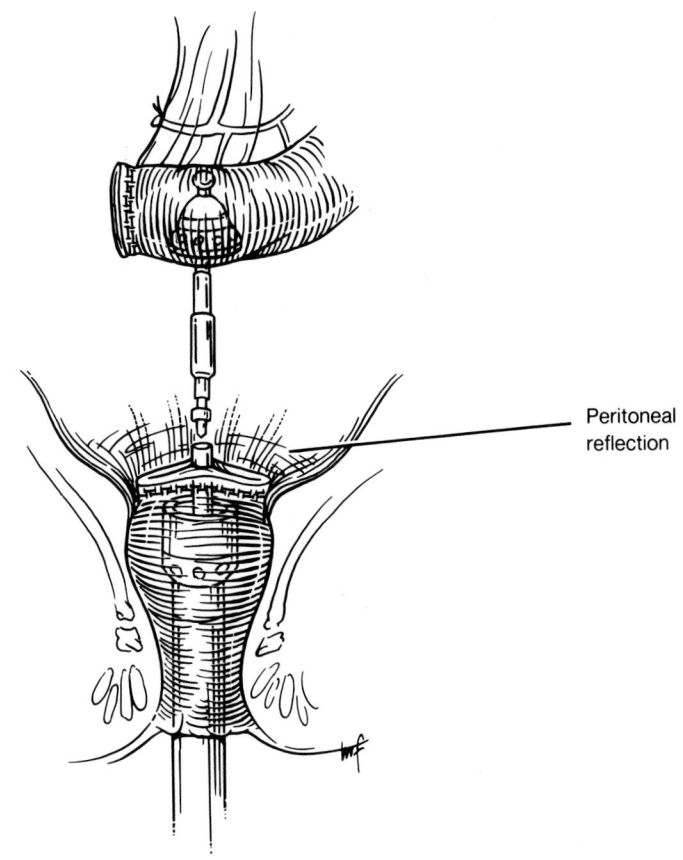

Peritoneal
reflection

Figure 43-IIF-5

Double-Stapled Side-to-End Ileorectal Anastomosis

The entire colon has been resected and the rectum transected with a linear stapler. The rectum has been irrigated clean through proctoscopy, and the integrity of the transverse staple line has been tested by insufflating air into the rectum while the staple line was submerged in saline. After establishing the integrity of the staple line, a circular stapler without anvil but with a retracted trocar was placed into the anus up to the proximal rectum. The trocar was used to penetrate the transverse staple line and has now been removed. An enterotomy was made in the side, which is secured in place by a pursestring suture. The stapler is reassembled, closed, and fired to create a double-stapled side-to-end ileorectal anastomosis.

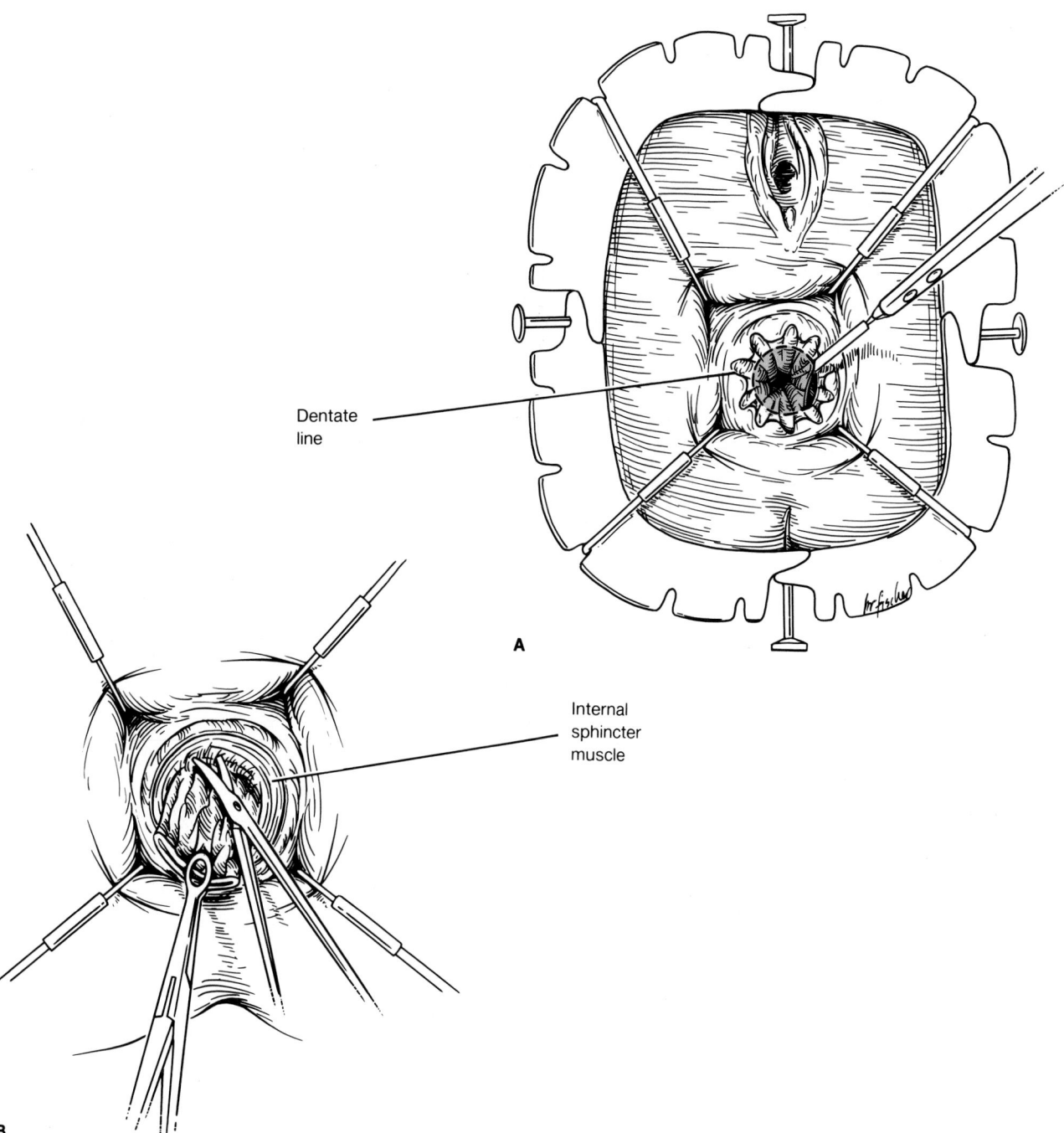

Dentate line

Internal sphincter muscle

A

B

Figure 43-IIF-6

Endoanal Mucosectomy

(A) With the patient in a modified lithotomy position, perineal exposure is achieved by use of a self-retaining ring retractor, which uses skin hooks to efface the anus. A circumferential incision through the mucosa and submucosa to the level of the internal sphincter muscle is made at or just proximal to the dentate line.

(B) A circumferential sleeve of mucosa and submucosa is dissected and mobilized from the underlying internal sphincter muscle.

(Continued)

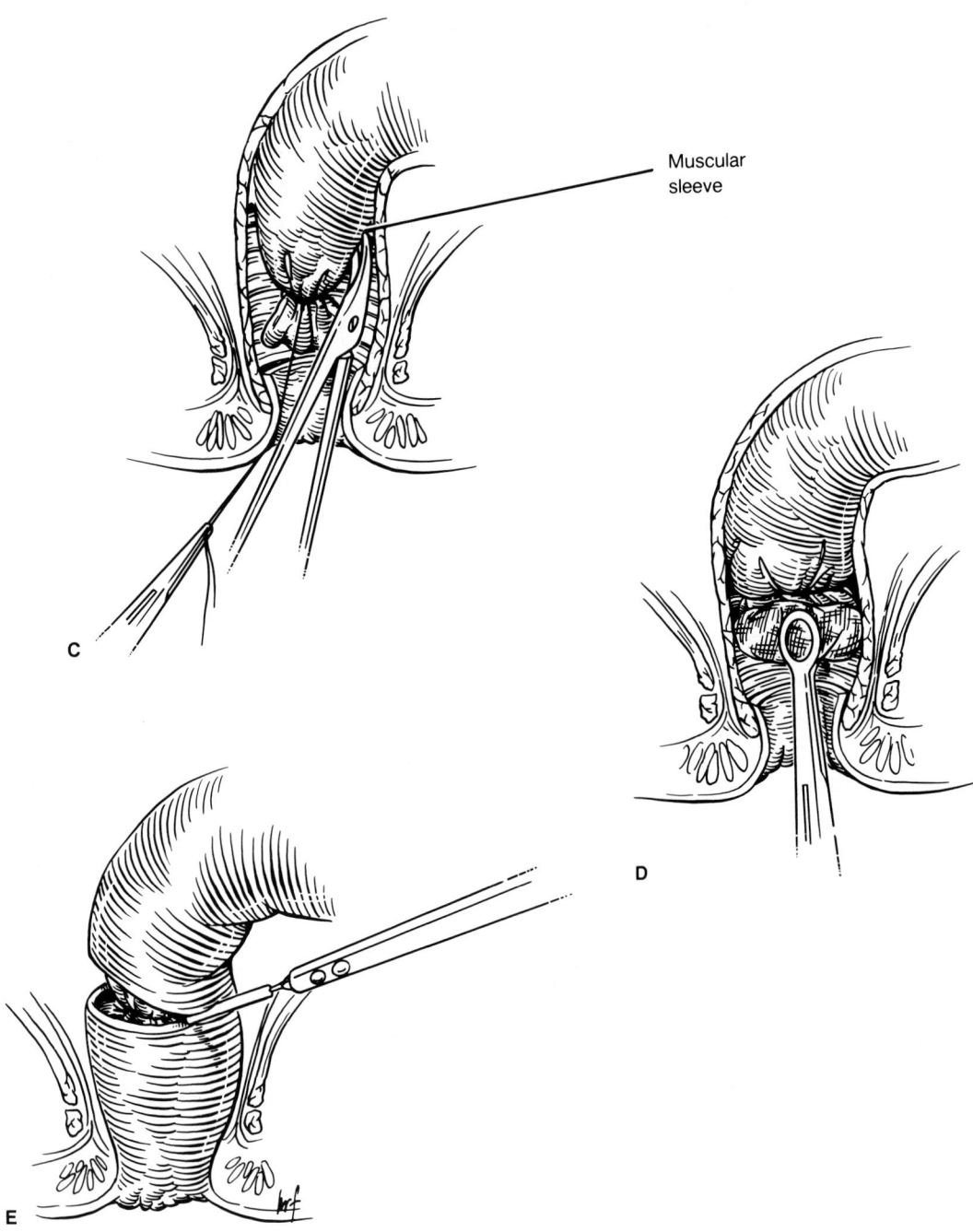

Figure 43-IIF-6 *(Continued)*

(C) A pursestring suture can be placed to gather the distal mucosal sleeve together. Traction on the pursestring can provide additional proximal exposure to complete the mucosectomy up to the top of the anal canal.

(D) After completion of the endoanal dissection, a stick sponge can be used to push the sutured end of the mucosal tube proximally into the rectum. This facilitates the abdominal surgeon's identification of the proximal level of mucosectomy.

(E) A cautery can be used to transect the muscle sleeve of the rectum distal to the mucosectomy, thus ensuring that all of the mucosal sleeve is resected with the proximal colon.

G. Ileal Pouch

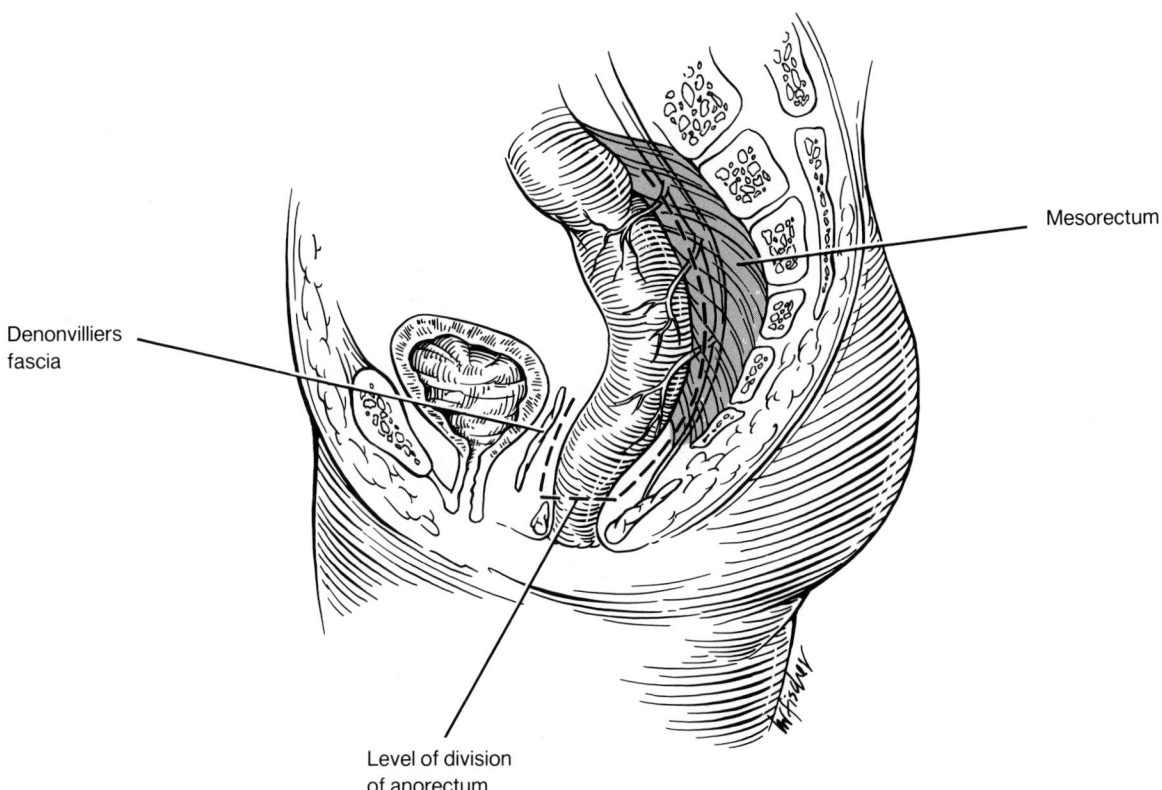

Mesorectum

Denonvilliers
fascia

Level of division
of anorectum

Figure 43-IIG-1

Conservative Pelvic Dissection

The dashed line indicates the conservative plane of dissection sometimes used for benign diseases of the rectum, such as chronic ulcerative colitis or familial adenomatous polyposis. Posteriorly, the dissection is performed anterior to the superior rectal artery within the mesorectum. Anteriorly, the dissection is directly on the rectum and anal canal within the levator muscles and posterior to the Denonvilliers fascia. Technically, this is a more time-consuming and difficult dissection, often with more blood loss than the alternative endopelvic fascial dissection. Whether the more conservative dissection results in less disruption of pelvic nerves and produces less sexual or bladder dysfunction is debated.

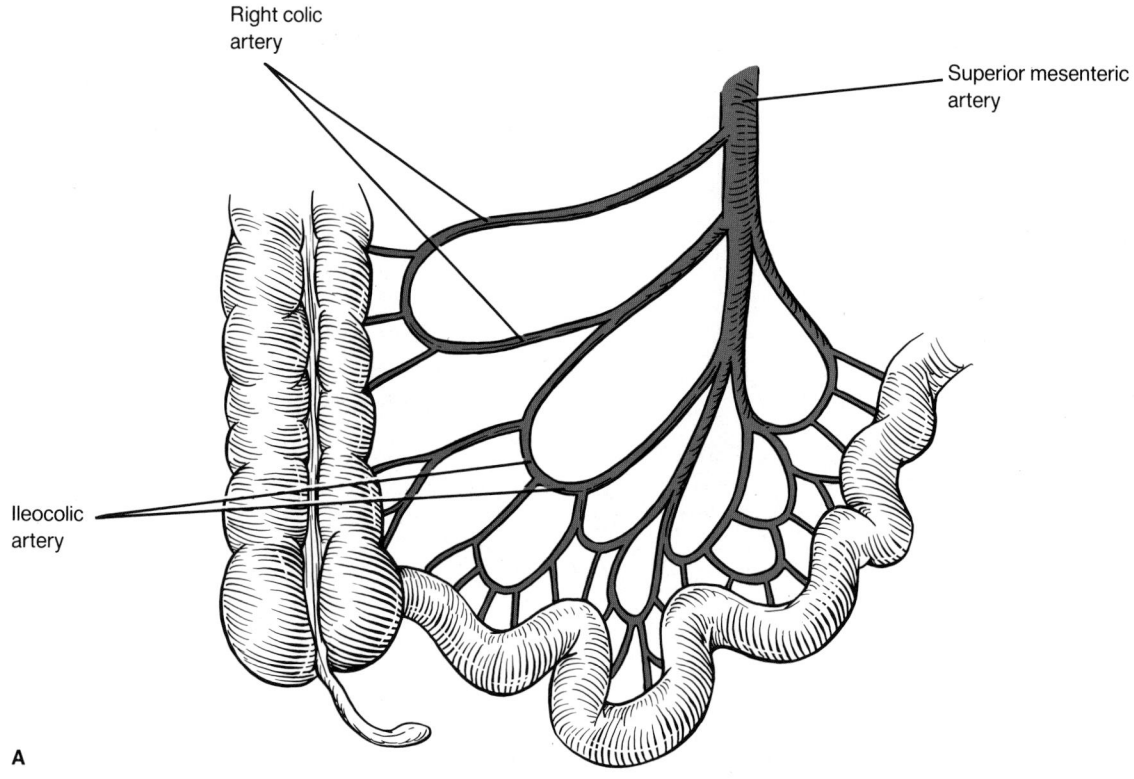

A

Figure 43-IIG-2

Blood Supply

(A) Ileal reservoirs for anastomosis to the anal canal are constructed from the distal 20 to 40 cm of terminal ileum. A variety of pouch configurations can be used, but success is contingent on achieving a tension-free anastomosis and maintaining excellent blood flow to the terminal ileum. The normal anatomy with the blood supply to the terminal ileum, cecum, and right colon is demonstrated here.

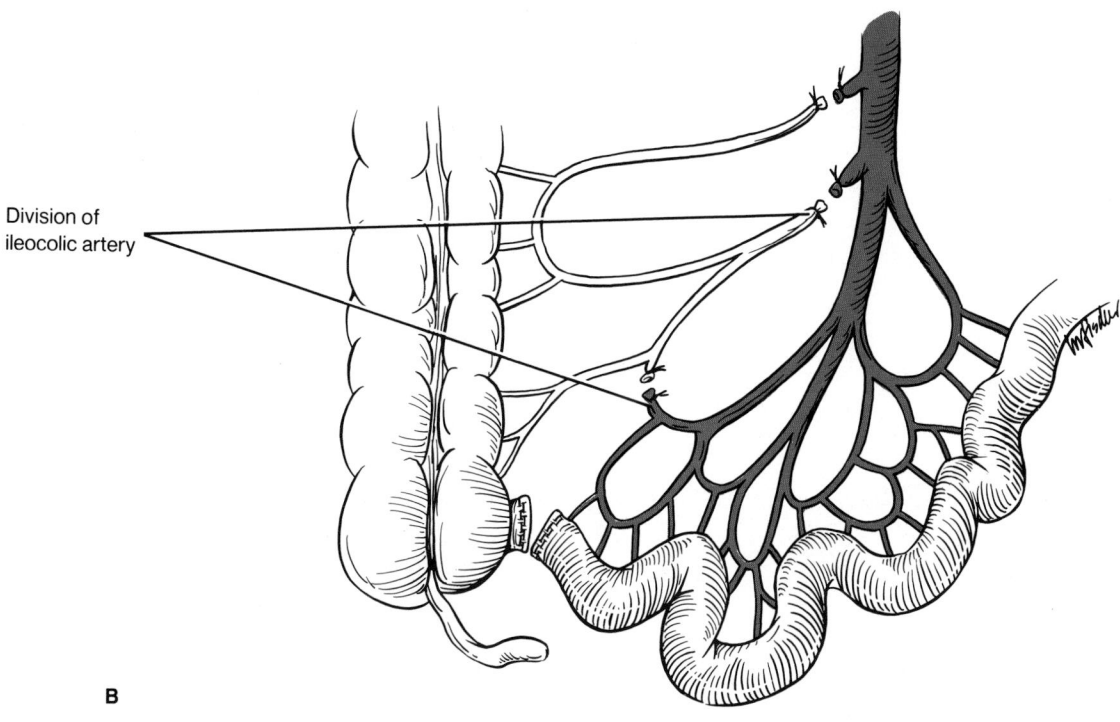

Division of
ileocolic artery

B

Figure 43-IIG-2 *(Continued)*

(B) Regardless of configuration of ileal pouch to be constructed, the ileocolic artery is divided without compromising the blood supply to the terminal ileum, which is divided adjacent to the cecum with a linear stapler. After a standard total colectomy is performed, the terminal ileal peritoneal attachments along the base of the mesentery are divided up to the level of the pancreas, duodenum, and origin of the superior mesenteric artery. The surgeon can then determine which configuration of ileal reservoir is optimal. Most often, a J, S, or W pouch is constructed.

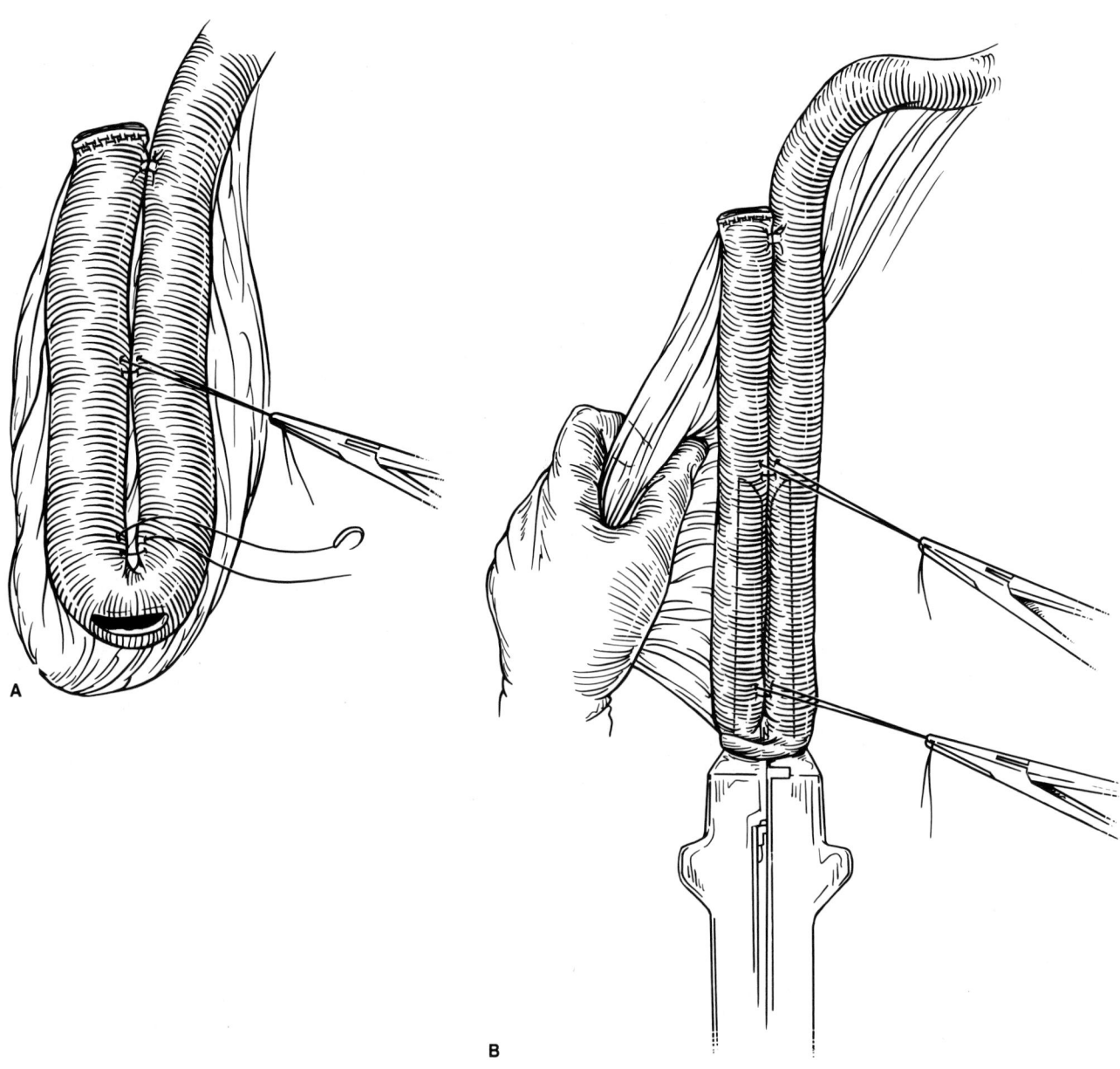

Figure 43-IIG-3

Ileal J Pouch

(A) The most common type of ileal reservoir is the J pouch, consisting of about 20 to 30 cm of ileum. Two limbs of bowel are aligned with temporary 3-0 stay sutures. If the apex of the pouch reaches beyond the symphysis pubis, sufficient length to achieve a tension-free ileoanal anastomosis is usually available. The apex of the pouch is opened on its antimesenteric surface.

(B) Two limbs of a linear stapler are inserted through the apex of the J pouch, aligned, and closed. The surgeon must be sure that the antimesenteric surfaces of the two limbs of bowel are approximated and that their mesentery is retracted as shown. The stapler containing a knife blade is fired to create a side-to-side anastomosis. The stapler is removed and reloaded.

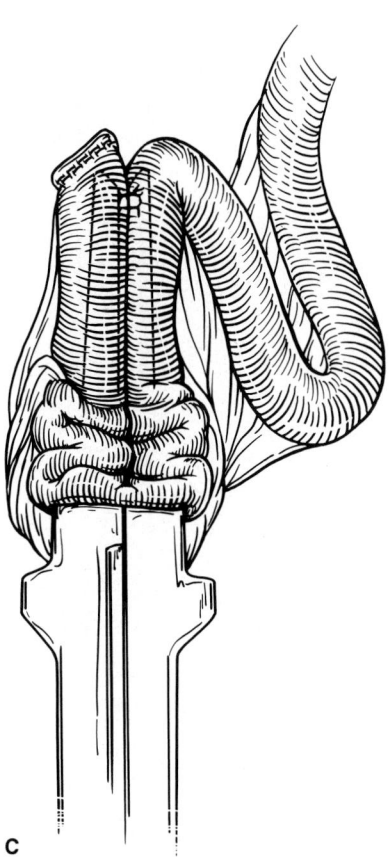

C

Figure 43-IIG-3 *(Continued)*

(C) A second and sometimes third firing of the linear stapler is necessary to complete the J-pouch construction. The already stapled portion of the pouch is gently folded over the linear stapler in an accordion manner.

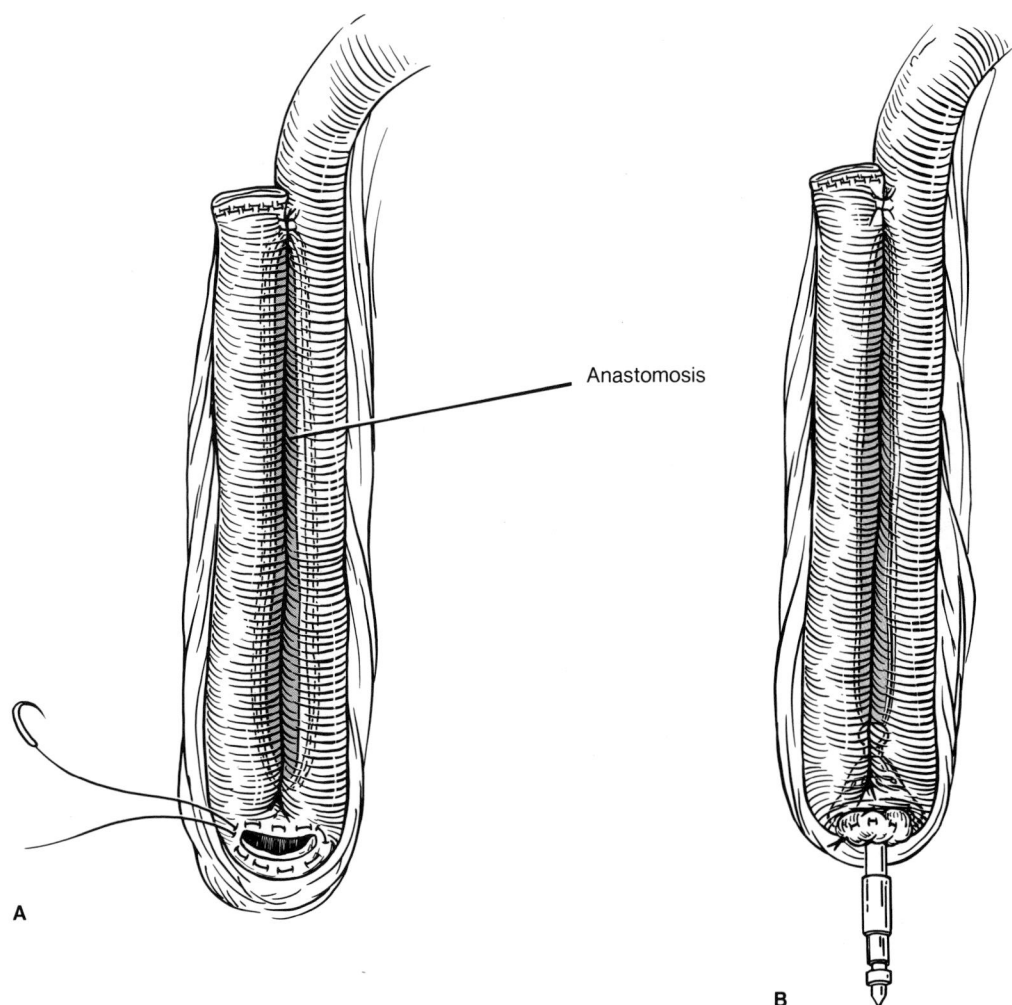

Anastomosis

A

B

Figure 43-IIG-4

Double-Stapled Ileal J-Pouch Anal Anastomosis

(A) After completing the side-to-side anastomosis along the length of the J pouch, a 2-0 polypropylene pursestring suture is placed around the apical enterotomy.

(B) The anvil of a mid-sized circular stapling instrument is tied into the apex of the J pouch.

(C) After completion of the pelvic dissection, the anorectum is divided with a right-angle stapler placed by the abdominal surgeon as close to the dentate line as possible. Care must be taken that extraneous tissues such as the bladder or vagina are not inadvertently closed within the instrument. After closure of the stapler and checking for proper alignment and location, the stapler is fired. The anorectum is divided deep in the pelvis within the levator muscles. In some patients, the anatomy prevents proper distal placement of the stapler, and alternatives such as mucosectomy and hand-sutured ileoanal anastomosis must be undertaken. This is preferable to leaving a long cuff of anorectum.

(D) Before proceeding with the double-stapled anastomosis, the integrity of the transverse staple line is tested by covering the anal stump with saline while an assistant insufflates air through an anoscope. The absence of air leak implies an intact staple line. The assistant next inserts the midsized circular stapler with a trocar in the retracted position within the cartridge. The abdominal operator guides the assistant to position the circular stapler cartridge properly against the anorectal stump and to open the instrument, thus advancing the trocar through the transverse staple line.

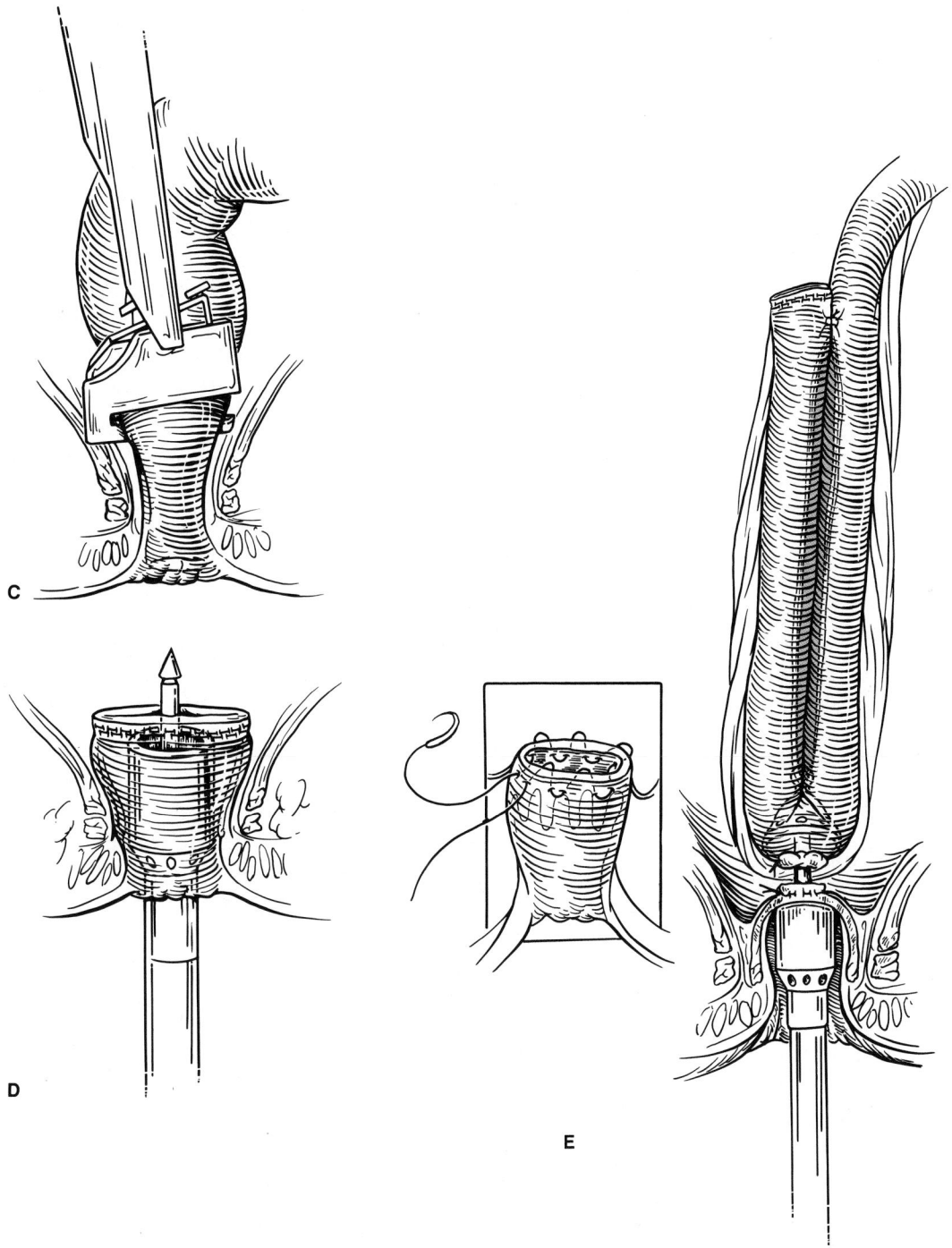

C

D

E

Figure 43-IIG-4 *(Continued)*

(E) The trocar is removed by the abdominal operator, who next inserts the anvil mechanism previously sutured into the apex of the J pouch into the receptacle of the cartridge. The assistant closes the stapler as the abdominal surgeon prevents extraneous tissues from being trapped within the stapling device. When properly aligned, the perineal operator fires the stapler, creating an end-to-end double-stapled ileal J-pouch anal anastomosis. **(Inset)** The alternative involves using a hand-sewn pursestring suture on the anorectal stump in place of the transverse staple line.

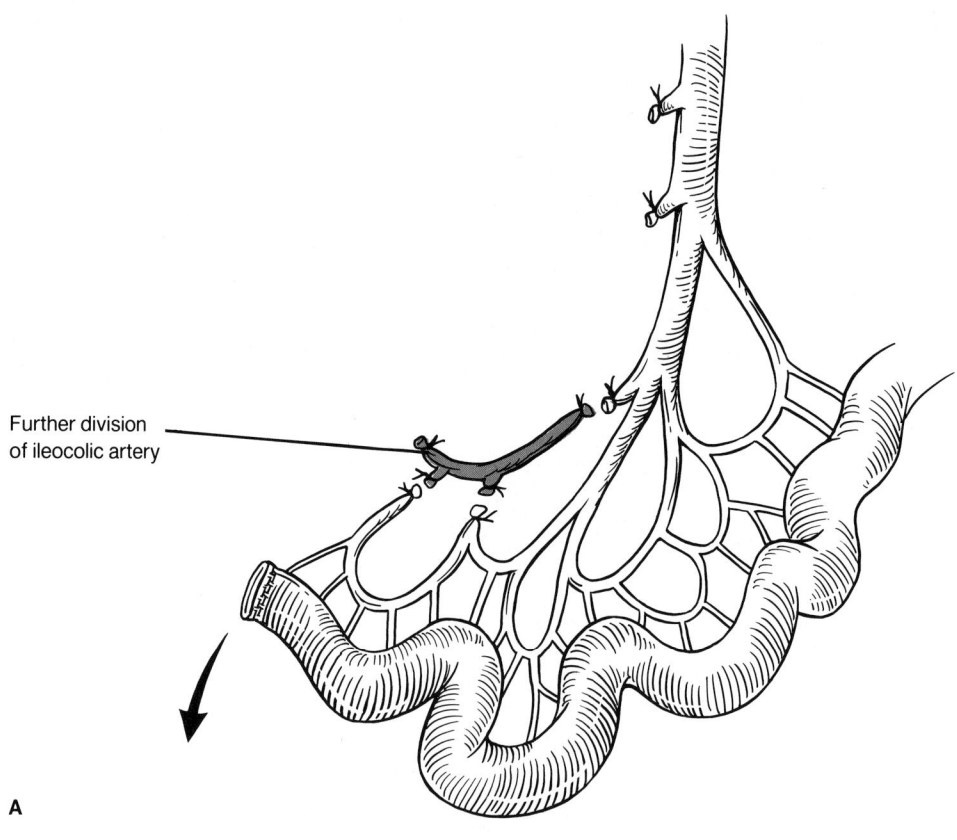

Further division
of ileocolic artery

A

Figure 43-IIG-5

Ileal S Pouch

(A) If the J-pouch configuration does not allow the apex of the reservoir to reach the anal canal without tension, an S-pouch configuration can be performed. Further division of branches of the ileocolic artery, as shown, allows the terminal ileum to be straightened, as depicted by the arrow. Care must be taken to be sure the ileal arcade continues to provide a pulsatile flow of blood to the terminal ileum.

(B) The distal ileum is aligned in an S configuration with three 10-cm limbs and a 1- to 2-cm efferent spout. Temporary stay sutures hold the bowel in this configuration while the pouch is placed into the pelvis to determine whether sufficient length is available to construct a tension-free ileoanal anastomosis.

(C) The antimesenteric borders of the three limbs are incised with electrocautery. Slight tension on the stay sutures maintains the S-pouch alignment.

(D) The antimesenteric borders of the three limbs of bowel are anastomosed side-to-side with running, locked full-thickness 3-0 polyglycolic acid suture lines. The sutures are placed from within the lumen of the open bowel, and the end result is an inverting suture line.

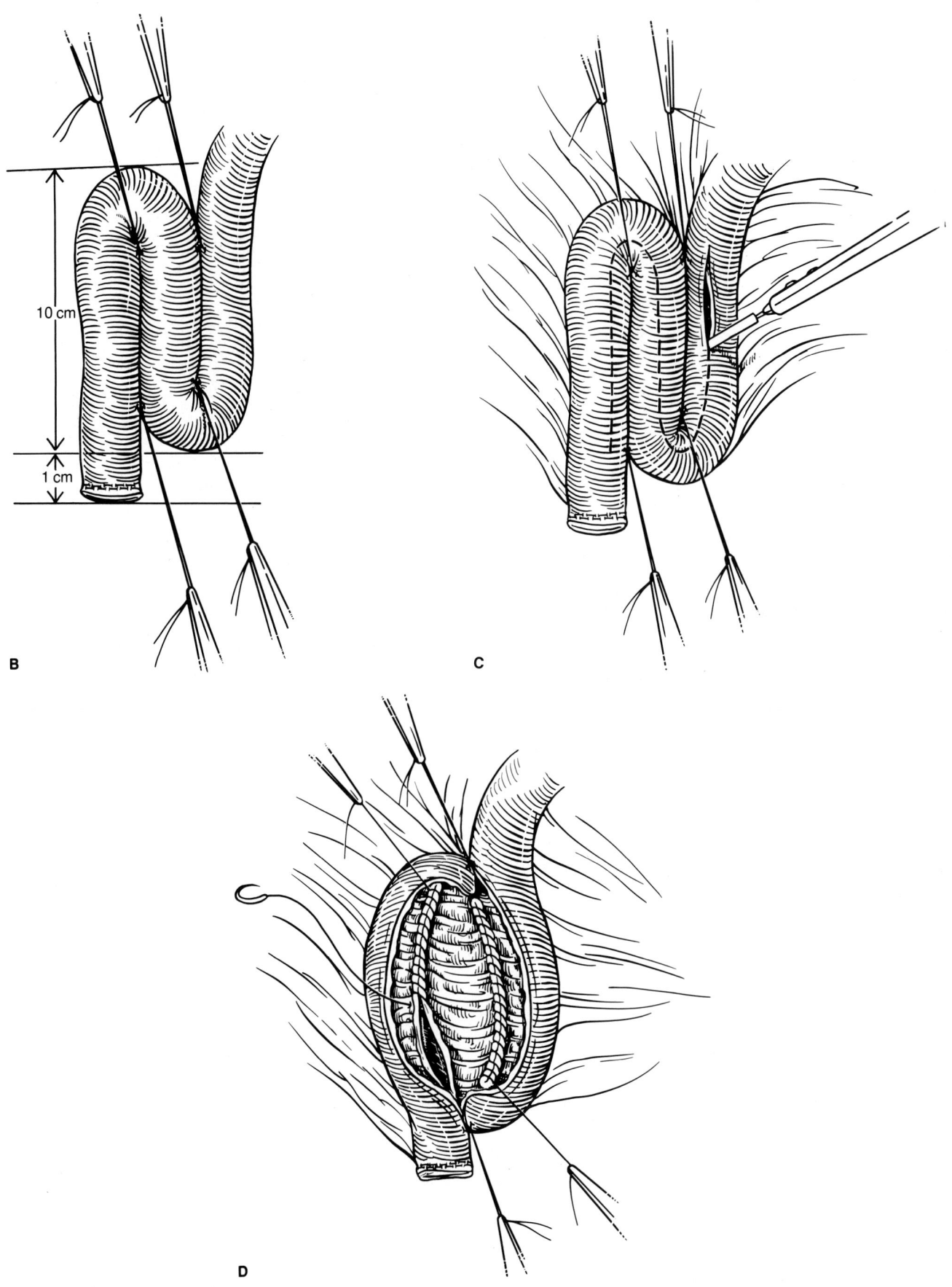

Figure 43-IIG-5 *(Continued)*

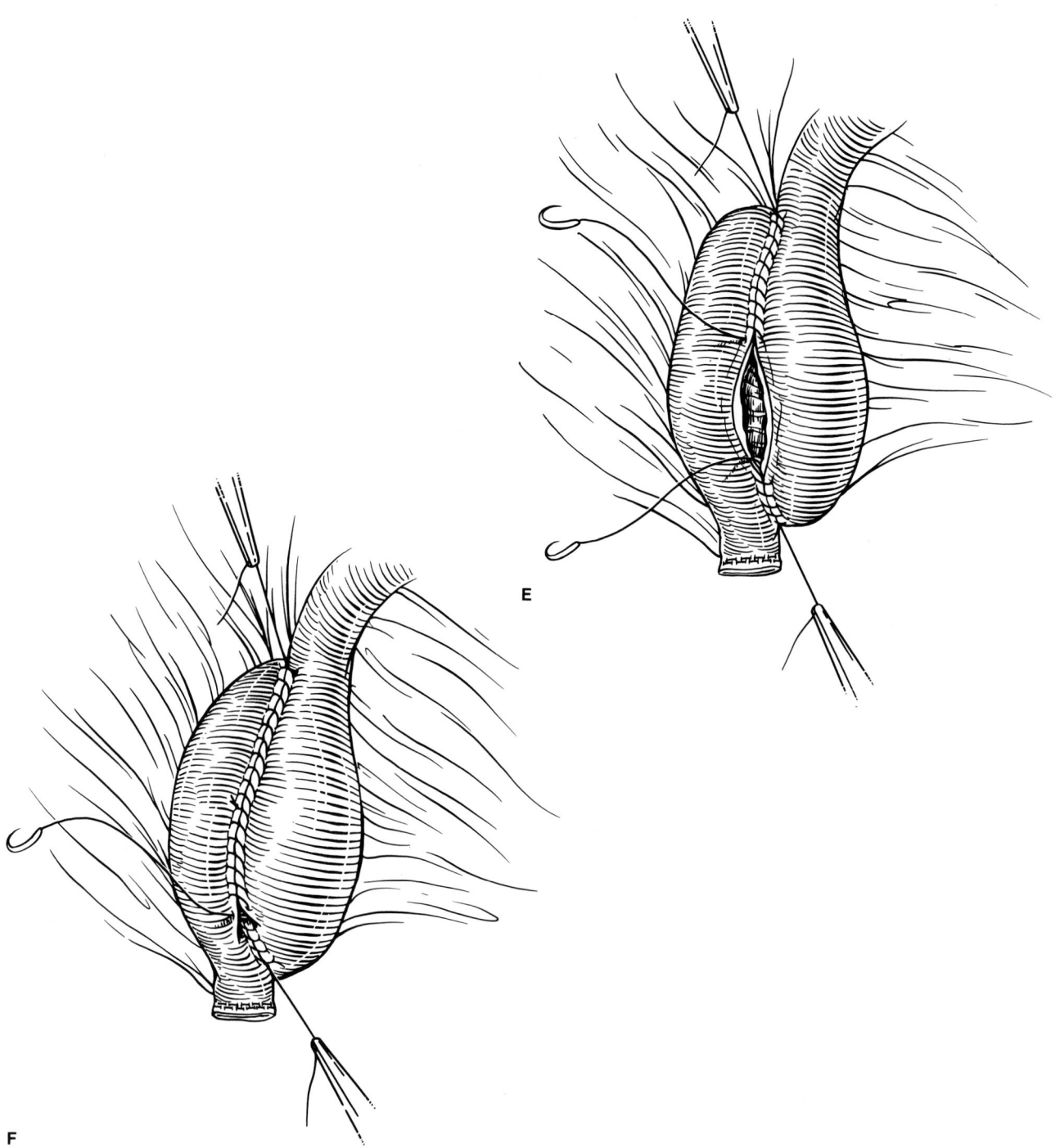

Figure 43-IIG-5 *(Continued)*

(E) The anterior suture line is completed in an identical manner using a running, locked full-thickness suture technique until only a 3- to 4-cm gap remains open.

(F) The final gap in the anterior suture line is closed with a running polyglycolic acid 3-0 suture placed as Connell stitches to achieve inversion of the entire suture line. If a double-stapled technique is used, the distal ileal staple line is excised from the efferent limb, the midsized circular stapler anvil is secured within the efferent limb with a pursestring suture, and a double-stapled anal anastomosis is constructed (see Fig. 43-IIG-4).

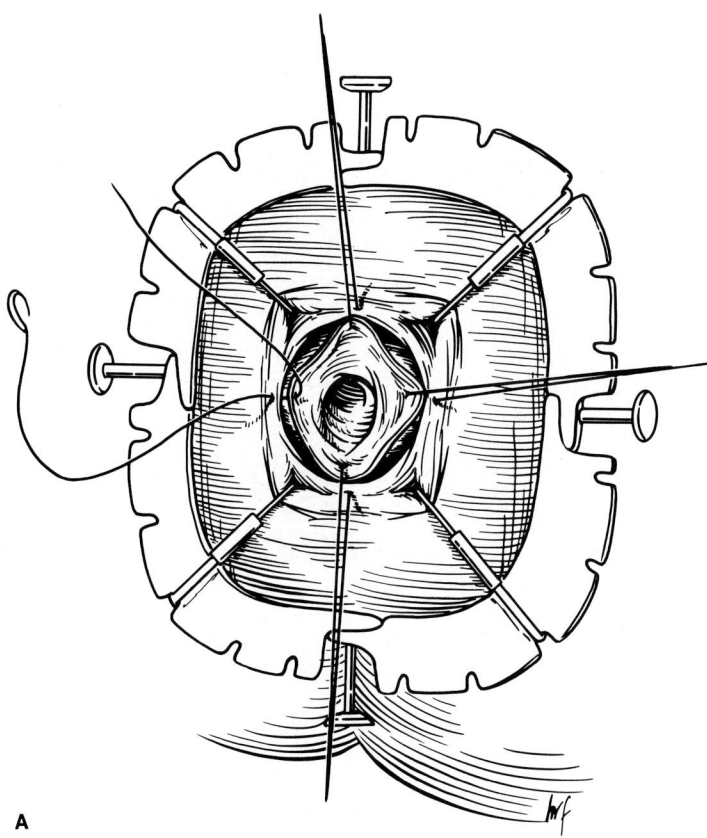

A

Figure 43-IIG-6

Ileal S-Pouch Anal Handsewn Anastomosis

(**A**) If a handsewn end-to-end ileoanal anastomosis is used, as is common after rectal mucosectomy, the S pouch is placed into the pelvis and the efferent limb is gently pulled through the anal canal by the perineal surgeon. A retractor that effaces the anus but does not stretch the anal sphincter facilitates this step. The distal ileal staple line is excised, and four 3-0 polyglycolic acid sutures are placed at right angles to anchor the efferent limb within the anal canal. These sutures incorporate the full thickness of the terminal ileum and a generous bite of internal sphincter muscle at the dentate line.

(Continued)

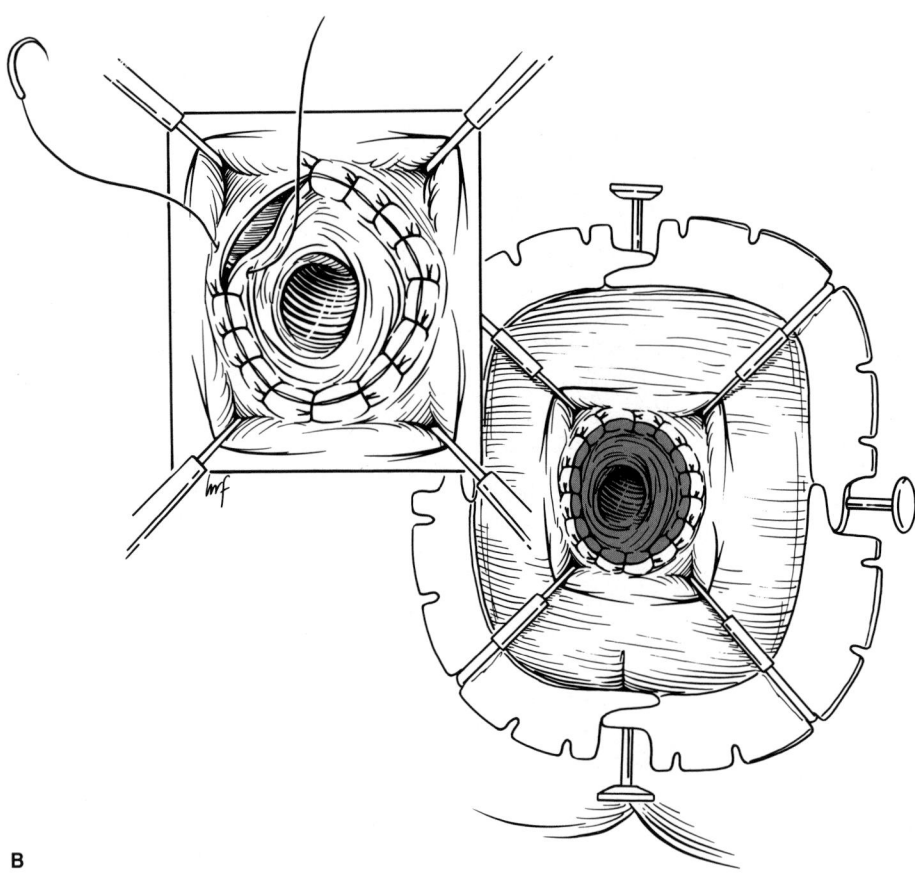

B

Figure 43-IIG-6 *(Continued)*

(B) The ileoanal handsewn anastomosis is completed by placing two or three 3-0 poly-glycolic acid sutures between each anchoring suture. When the retractor is removed, the suture line withdraws inside the anal canal, further lessening any tension on the suture line.

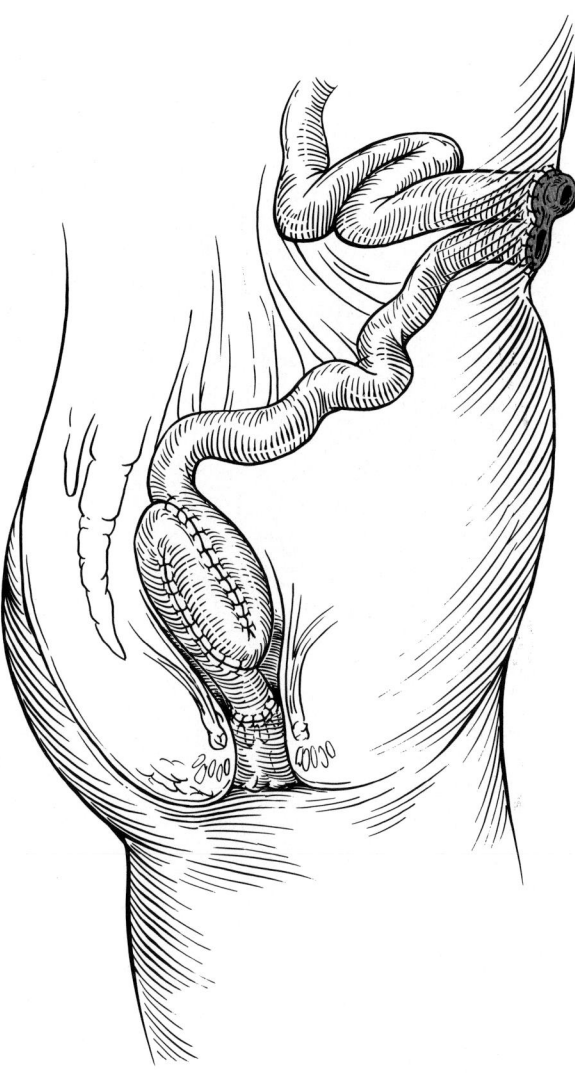

Figure 43-IIG-7

Ileal S-Pouch Anal Anastomosis and Temporary Ileostomy

The completed ileal S-pouch anal anastomosis is shown. A proximal loop ileostomy has been constructed to divert feces temporarily while healing of all suture lines occurs. More ileoanal anastomosis procedures are being performed without a temporary ileostomy. The surgeon must weight the pros and cons of temporary diversion.

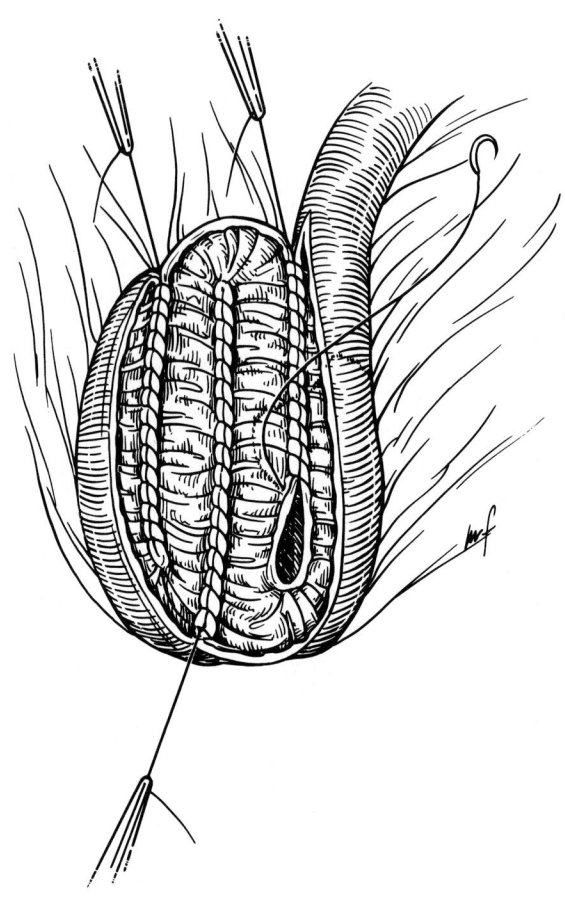

Figure 43-IIG-8

Ileal W Pouch

A third alternative ileal pouch configuration is that of the four-limbed W pouch. Its construction is similar to that of the S pouch.

H. Appendectomy

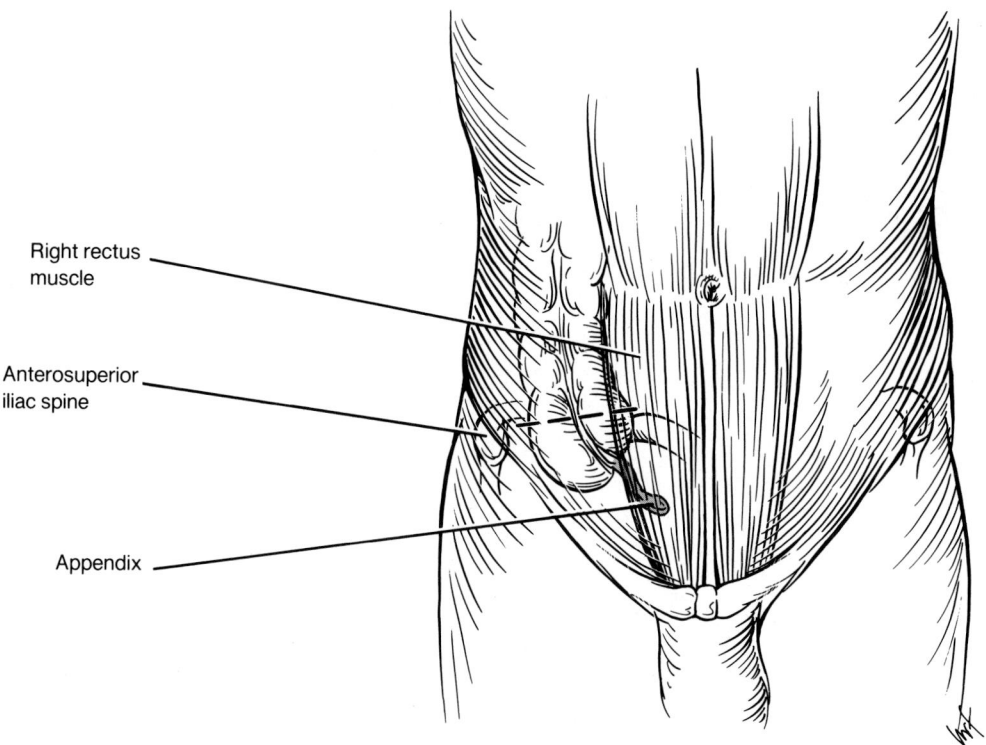

Right rectus
muscle

Anterosuperior
iliac spine

Appendix

Figure 43-IIH-1

Incision

The patient is positioned supine. After the patient is anesthetized, the abdomen is carefully palpated for a mass so the incision can be placed directly over it. If no mass is present, the incision is centered over the McBurney point, defined as the junction of the middle and outer one third of the line that joins the umbilicus to the anterior superior iliac spine. Usually, the incision is oriented transversely in line with the skin creases to produce the most cosmetically acceptable wound.

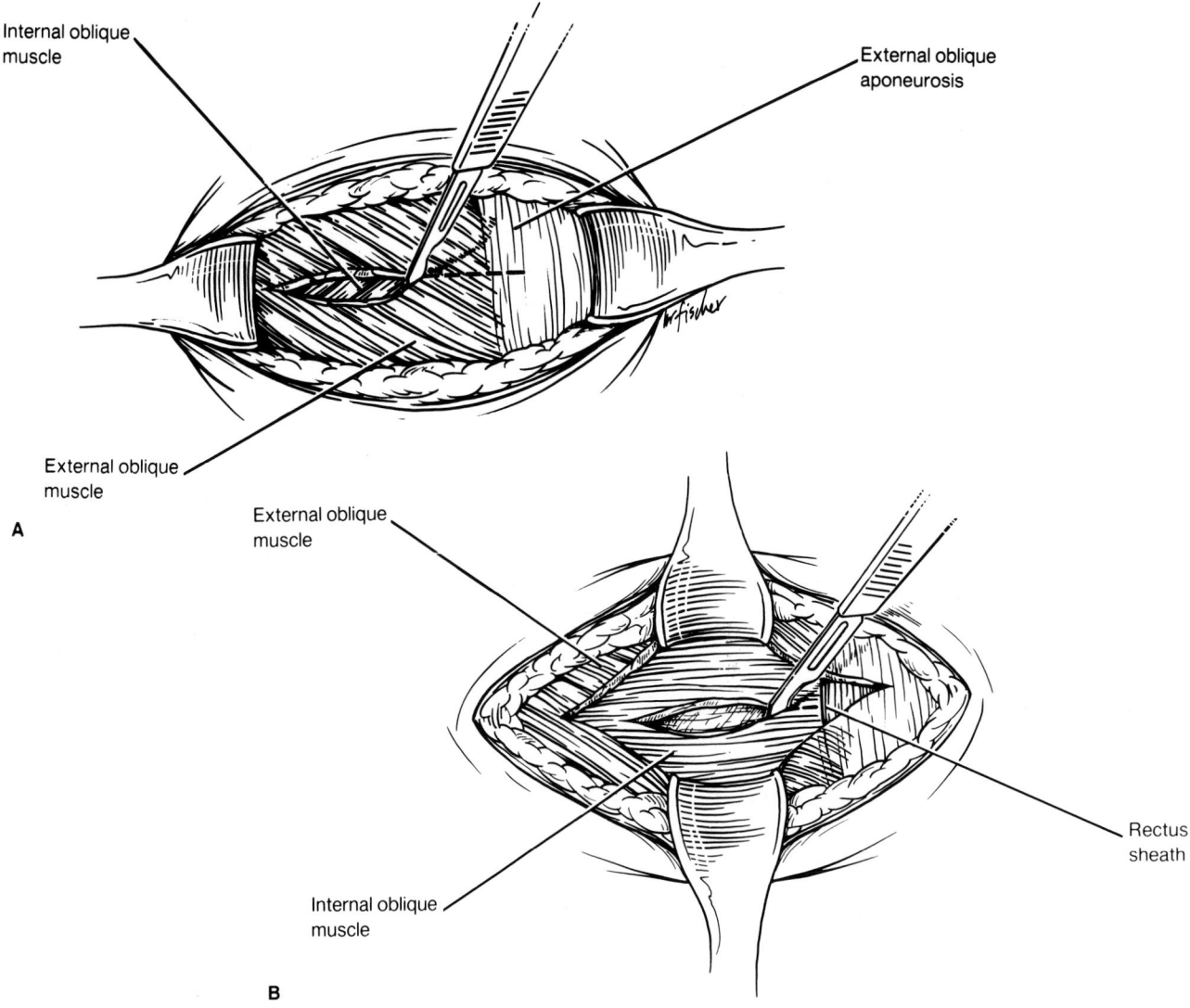

Figure 43-IIH-2

Exposure

(A) The incision is deepened through the external oblique aponeurosis and external oblique muscle to expose the internal oblique muscle. The right rectus abdominis muscle is exposed but usually not divided unless the patient is obese or other circumstances demand greater exposure, in which case the transverse incision is extended medially through the rectus abdominis muscle.

(B) The internal oblique muscle fibers are divided.

(C) Abdominal wall retractors are inserted more deeply to expose the transversalis fascia.

(D) The transversalis fascia is divided transversely to expose the peritoneum.

(E) The peritoneum is grasped with two forceps, tented up, and opened.

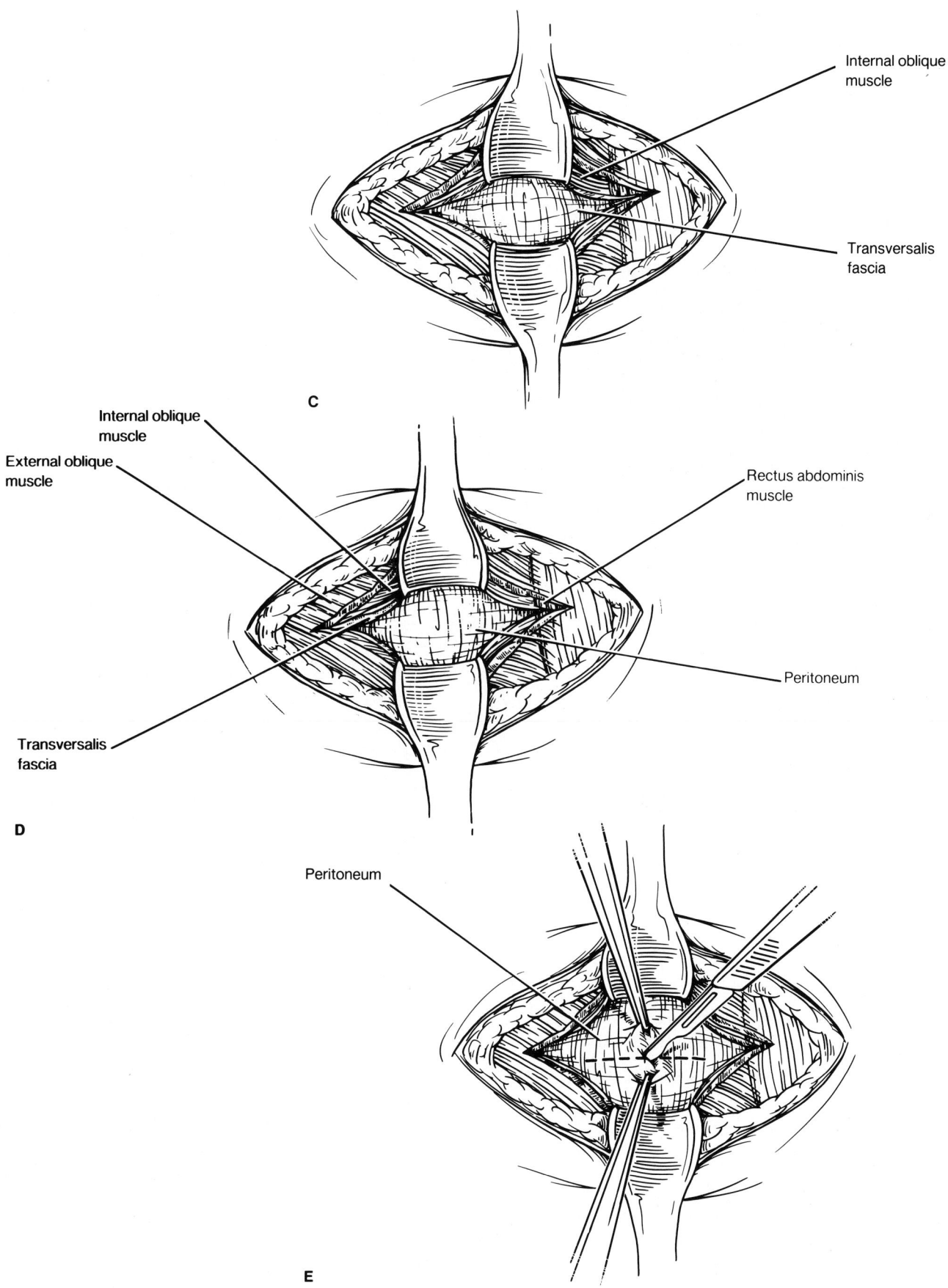

Internal oblique
muscle

Transversalis
fascia

C

Internal oblique
muscle

External oblique
muscle

Rectus abdominis
muscle

Peritoneum

Transversalis
fascia

D

Peritoneum

E

Figure 43-IIH-2 *(Continued)*

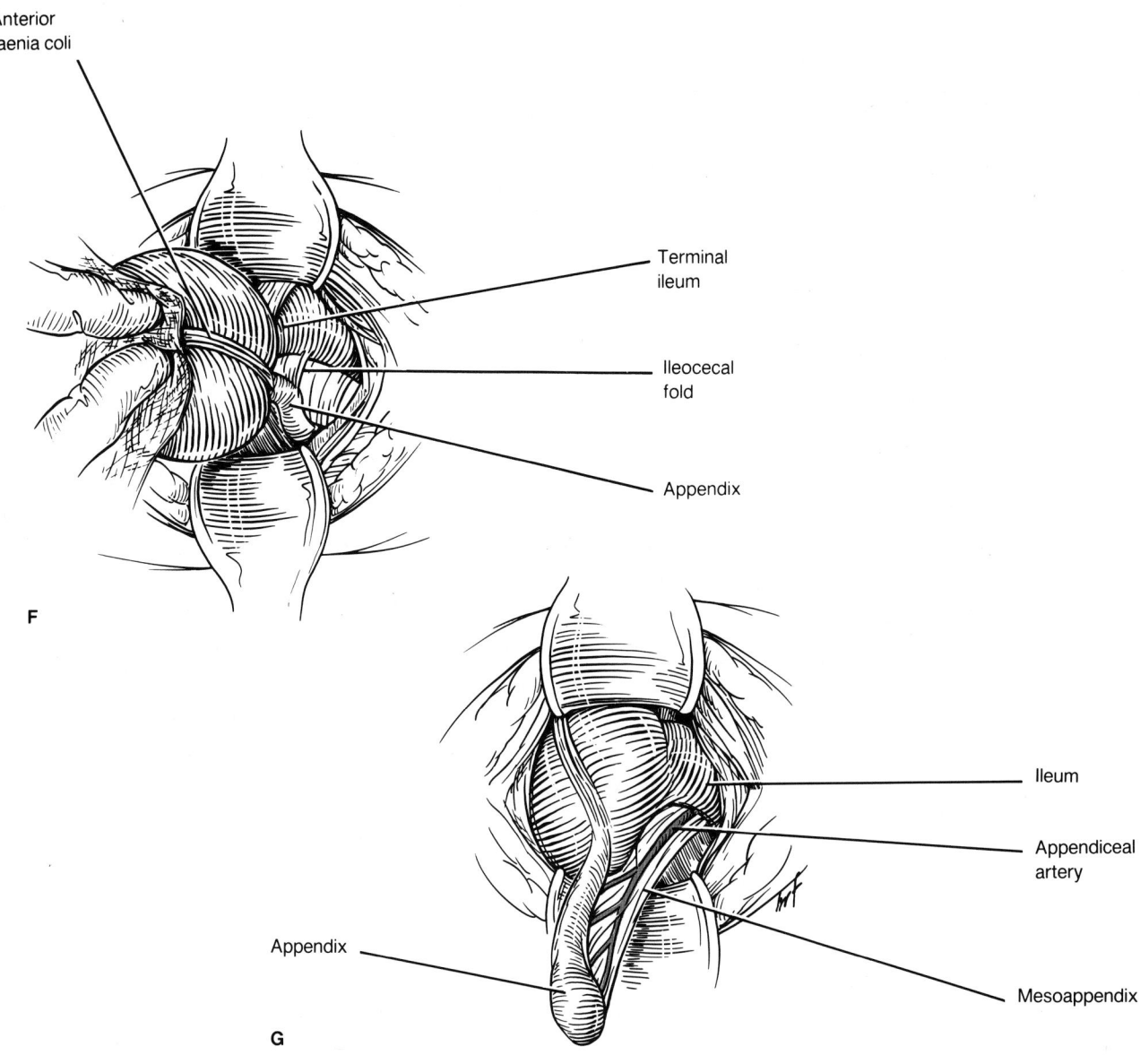

Figure 43-IIH-2 *(Continued)*

(F) The cecum is grasped with a moistened gauze pad and mobilized to expose the appendix at the base of the anterior taenia coli.

(G) Exposure of the base of the cecum, ileocecal junction, and mesoappendix containing the appendicular artery is achieved.

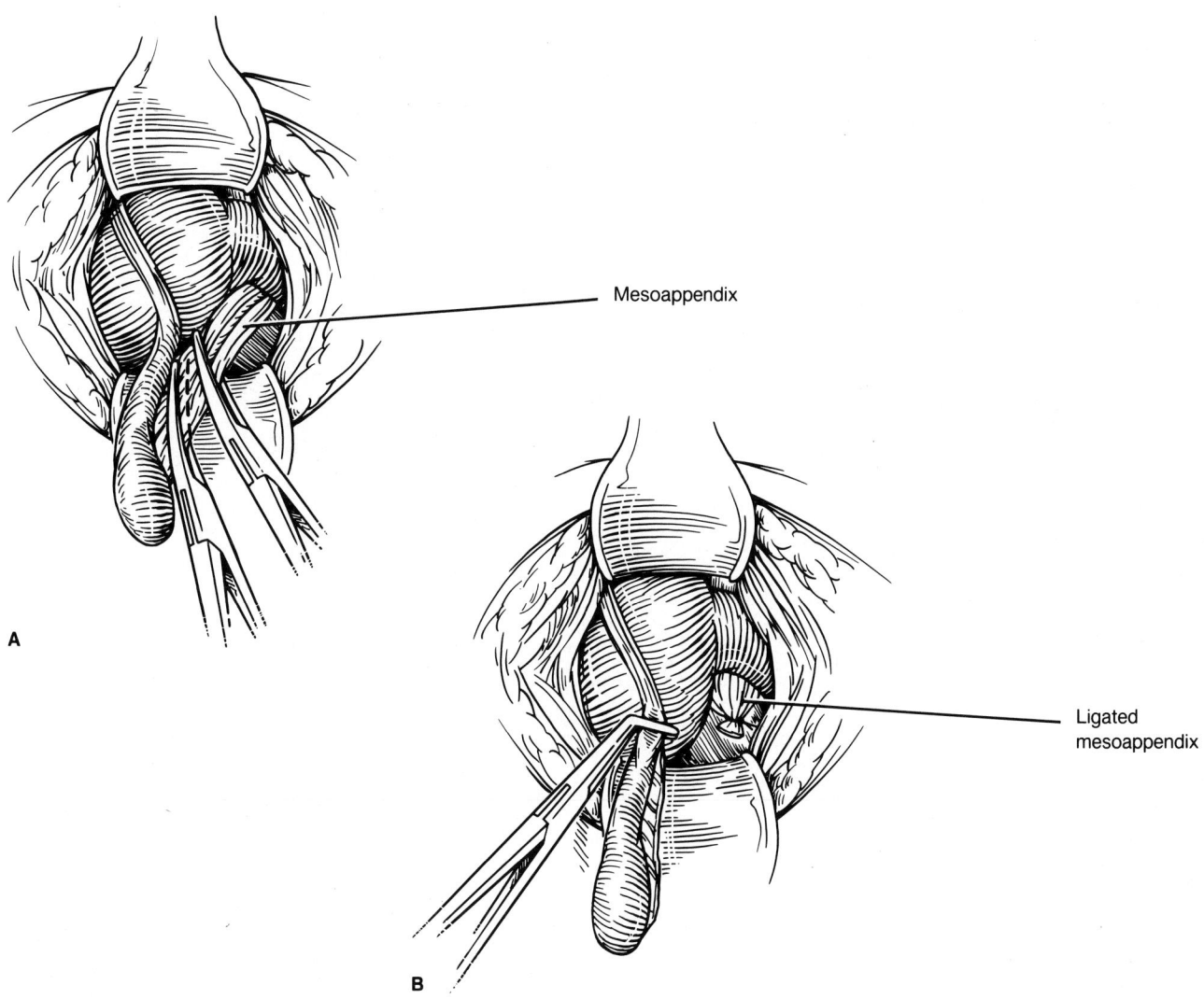

Mesoappendix

Ligated
mesoappendix

A

B

Figure 43-IIH-3

Resection of Appendix

(A) The mesoappendix with the appendicular artery in its free margin is divided between clamps and ligated at its base.

(B) A right-angle clamp is placed just distal to the base of the appendix.

(Continued)

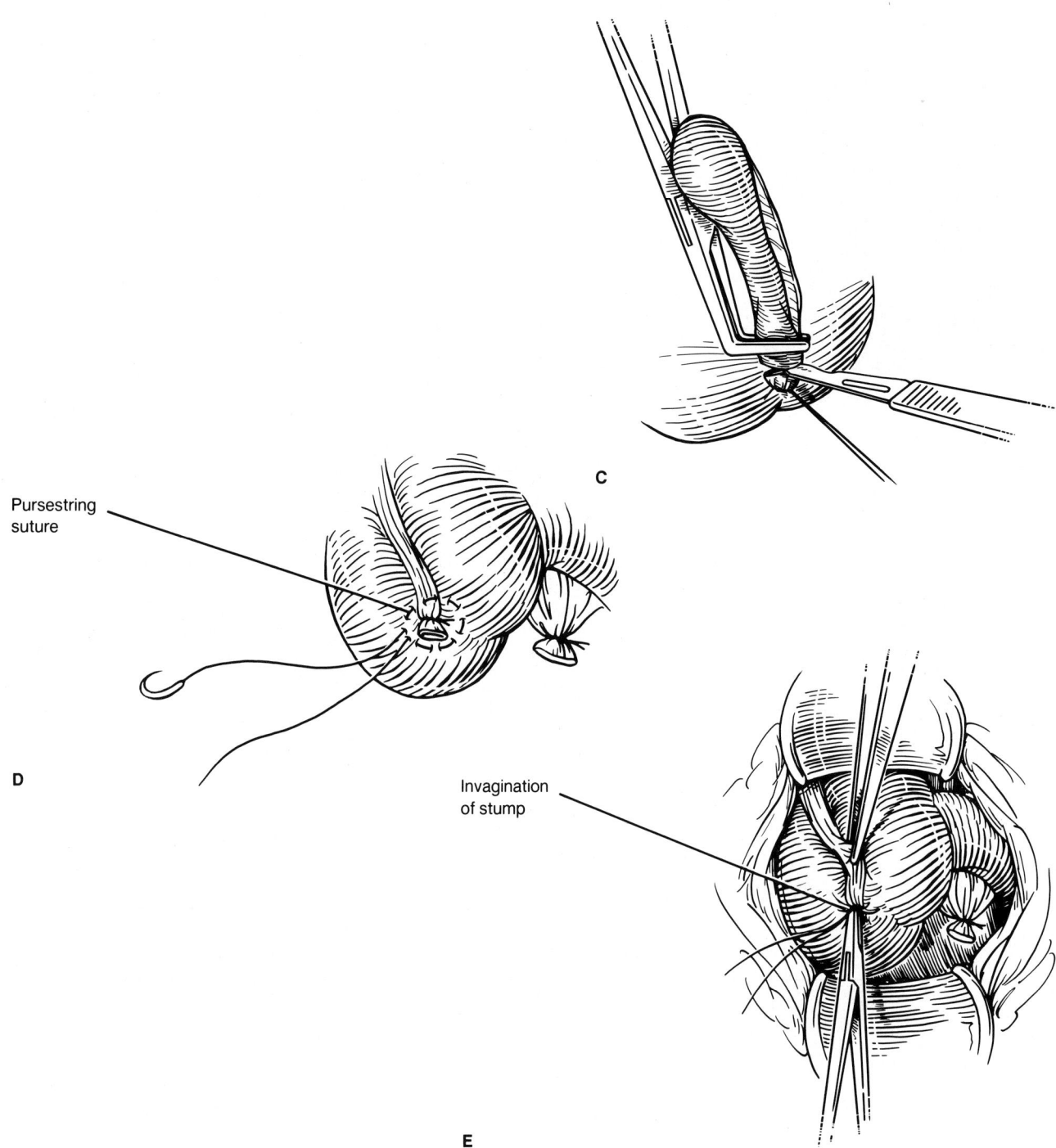

C

Pursestring
suture

D

Invagination
of stump

E

Figure 43-IIH-3 *(Continued)*

(C) The base of the appendix is tied with a 2-0 or 3-0 absorbable suture, and the appendix is divided.

(D) A 2-0 or 3-0 pursestring suture is placed around the appendiceal stump.

(E) The appendiceal stump is inverted and the pursestring tied to complete the appendectomy.

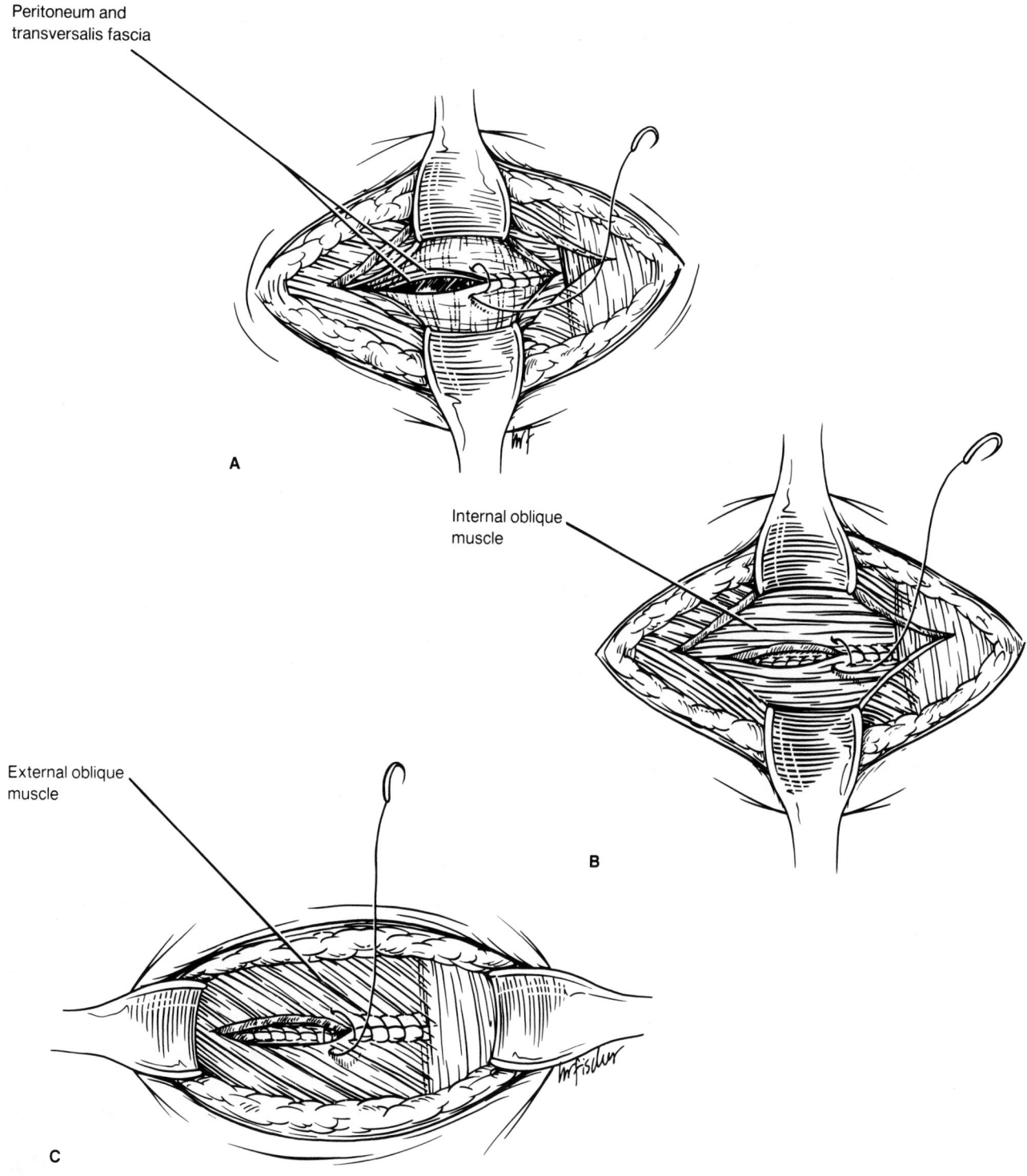

Figure 43-IIH-4

Wound Closure

(A) After wound irrigation, primary wound closure is begun by first closing the peritoneum and transversalis fascia with a running absorbable suture.

(B) The internal oblique muscle is closed with a running 2-0 or 3-0 absorbable suture.

(C) The external oblique muscle is closed with absorbable suture. The subcutaneous tissue is irrigated and the skin closed with sutures or staples unless gross fecal or purulent contamination dictates open packing of the wound.

SECTION III   *Colostomies*

A. End Colostomy

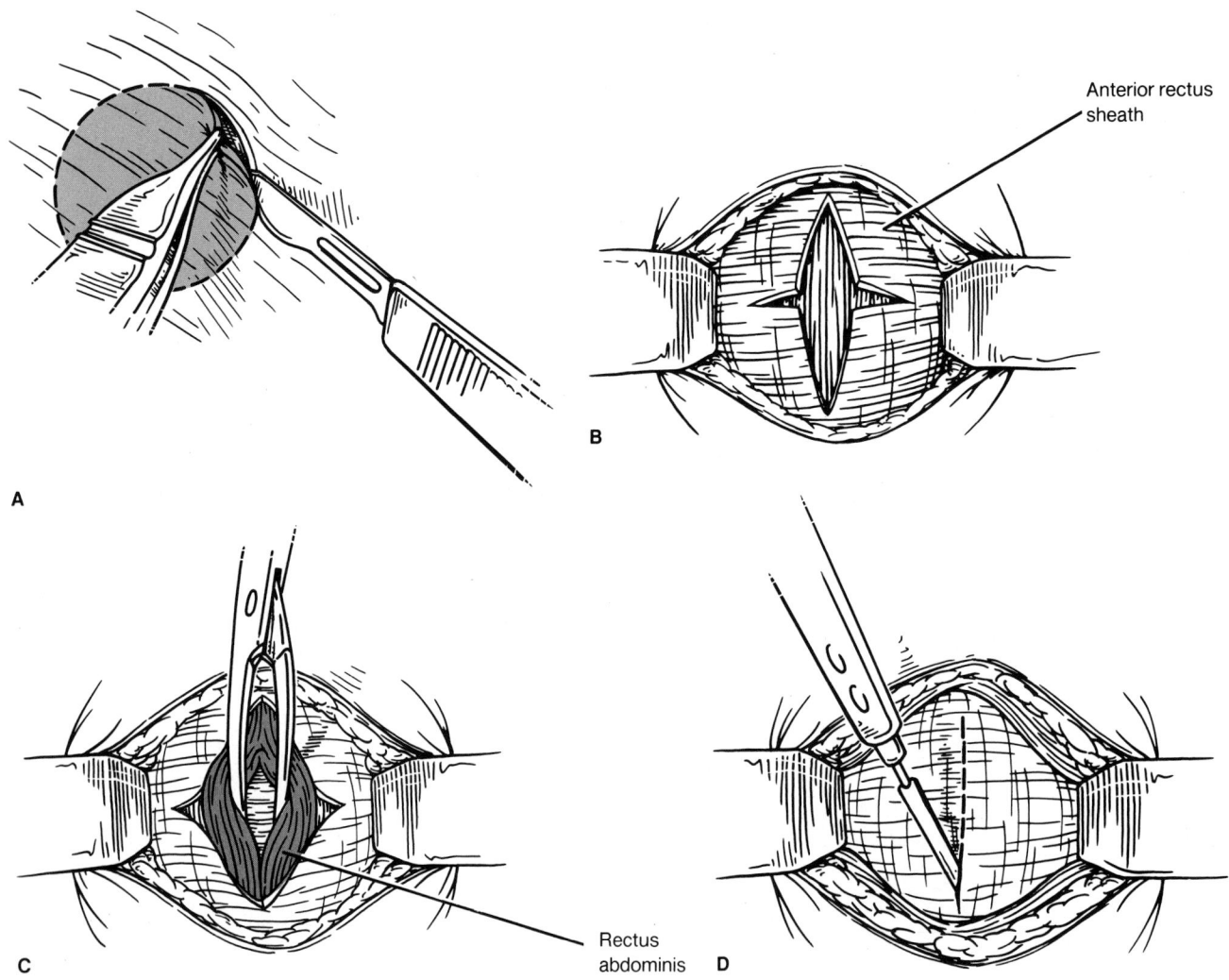

Figure 43-IIIA-1

Incision and Exposure

(**A**) A full-thickness circular skin incision is made at the preselected stoma site located anterior to the rectus abdominis muscle away from the umbilicus, scars, or other irregularities in abdominal wall contour.

(**B**) After excising the skin and subcutaneous tissue, a cruciate incision is made in the anterior fascia of the rectus abdominis muscle.

(**C**) The rectus abdominis muscle fibers are spread apart to expose the posterior fascia and peritoneum.

(**D**) Right-angle retractors are inserted to expose the posterior fascia of the rectus abdominis muscle. The fascia and peritoneum are incised to accommodate the stoma.

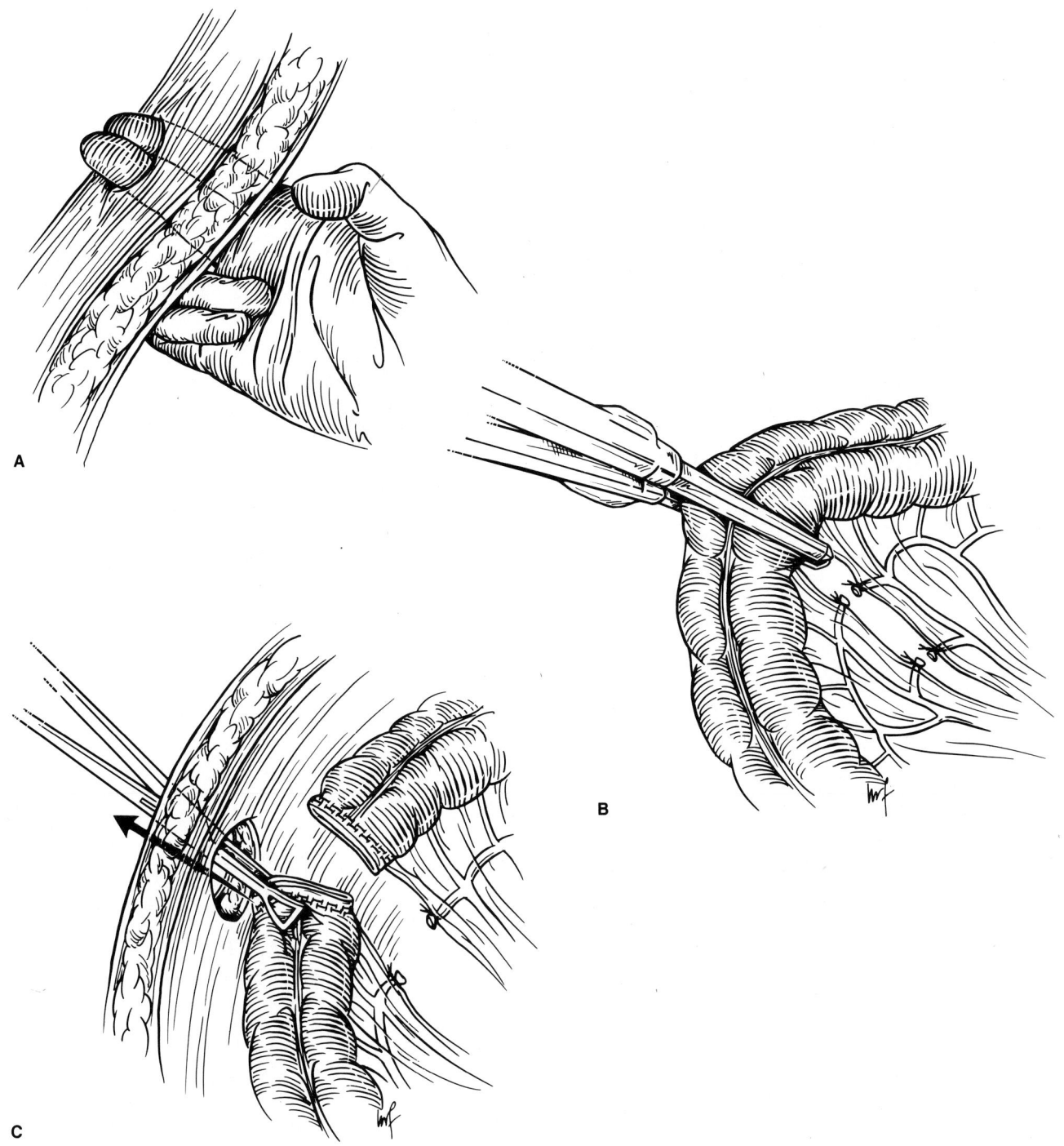

Figure 43-IIIA-2

Construction

(A) The adequacy of the abdominal wall defect created for the colostomy should snugly accommodate passage of two fingers.

(B) The colon is divided with a linear cutter-stapler after dividing and ligating the mesentery.

(C) A clamp is inserted through the abdominal wall defect, and the mobilized colon is delivered to protrude 2 to 3 cm above the skin level. There should be no tension, and the vascularity to the cut end of bowel must be well preserved.

(Continued)

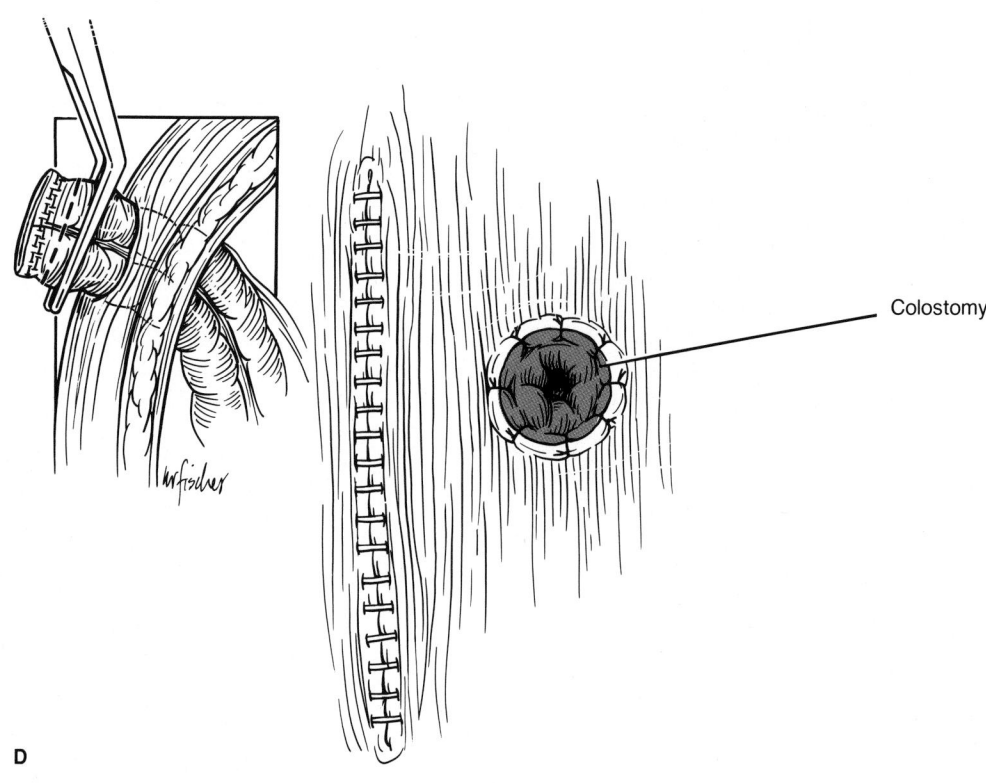

D

Figure 43-IIIA-2 *(Continued)*

(D) The midline incision is closed in the usual fashion. The staple line is then resected and the colostomy matured by suture of the cut edges to the skin with multiple interrupted 3-0 absorbable sutures. The colostomy should protrude at least 1 to 2 cm above the skin level, and vascularity must be preserved.

B. Transverse Loop Colostomy

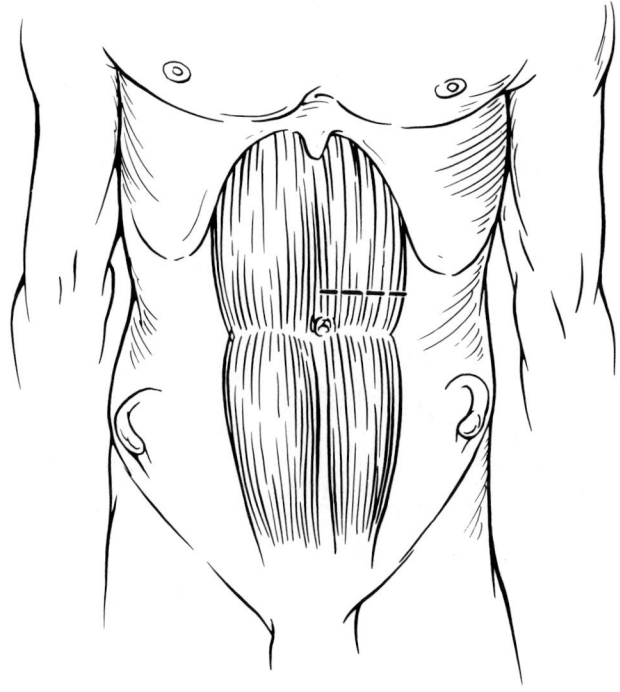

Figure 43-IIIB-1

Incision

If a transverse loop colostomy is indicated without thorough abdominal exploration (as for a patient with carcinomatosis obstructing the left colon), a transverse incision is made over the dilated transverse colon and deepened through the skin, subcutaneous tissue, and anterior rectus fascia.

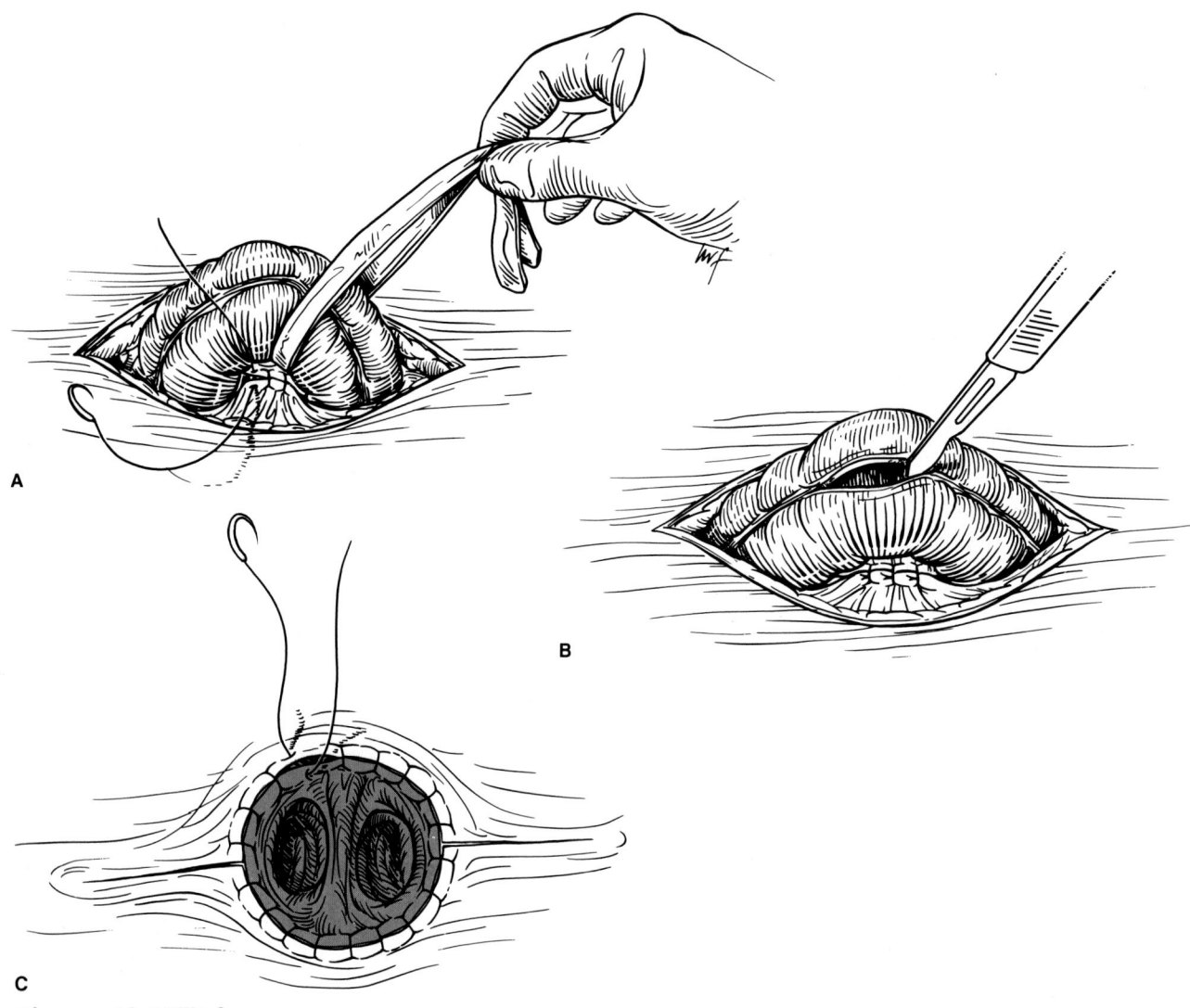

Figure 43-IIIB-2

Construction

(A) The rectus muscle is split to expose the posterior fascia and peritoneum, which is incised transversely for a distance long enough to accommodate careful mobilization of the dilated transverse colon. A small mesenteric window is created beneath the loop of dilated colon, and the cut edges of the anterior rectus fascia are approximated with sutures to close the abdominal wall defect, creating a fascial bridge that supports the loop of colon at the desired height above the level of the skin.

(B) The transverse skin incision is converted from a linear incision to a circular defect by excising a semilunar portion of skin from either side of the incision. If a lateral or medial portion of the skin incision remains linear, it is closed by a subcuticular suture up to the colon wall. The apex of the loop of the mobilized colon is opened with a scalpel to allow immediate decompression of the proximal colon.

(C) The stoma is matured with a running 3-0 absorbable suture to the skin edge. The fascial bridge ensures proper elevation of the stoma above the level of the skin. The resultant stoma should be circular because all stoma appliances are designed for such a stoma. Elliptical stomas create unnecessary difficulties for patients who must alter commercially available appliances to fit their asymmetric stomas.

C. Continent Ileostomy

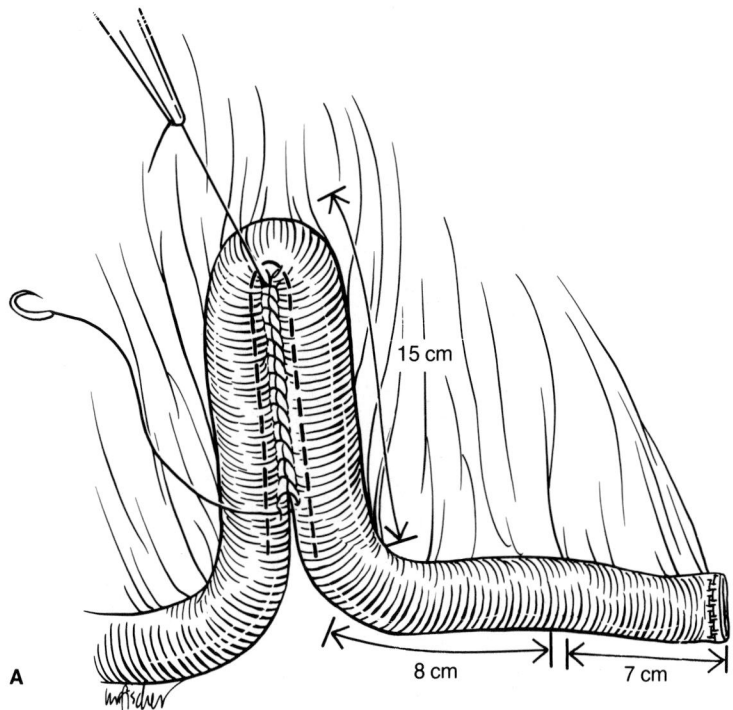

A

Figure 43-IIIC-1

Reservoir and Valve Construction

(**A**) The continent ileostomy involves a reservoir, valve, and stoma, all constructed from the terminal 45 cm of ileum. The apex of the reservoir is 30 cm from the distal ileum. The reservoir is created by folding the loop on itself, suturing the antimesenteric borders together with a 2-0 or 3-0 polyglycolic acid suture over a distance of 15 cm, and then opening the bowel along the dashed line.

(Continued)

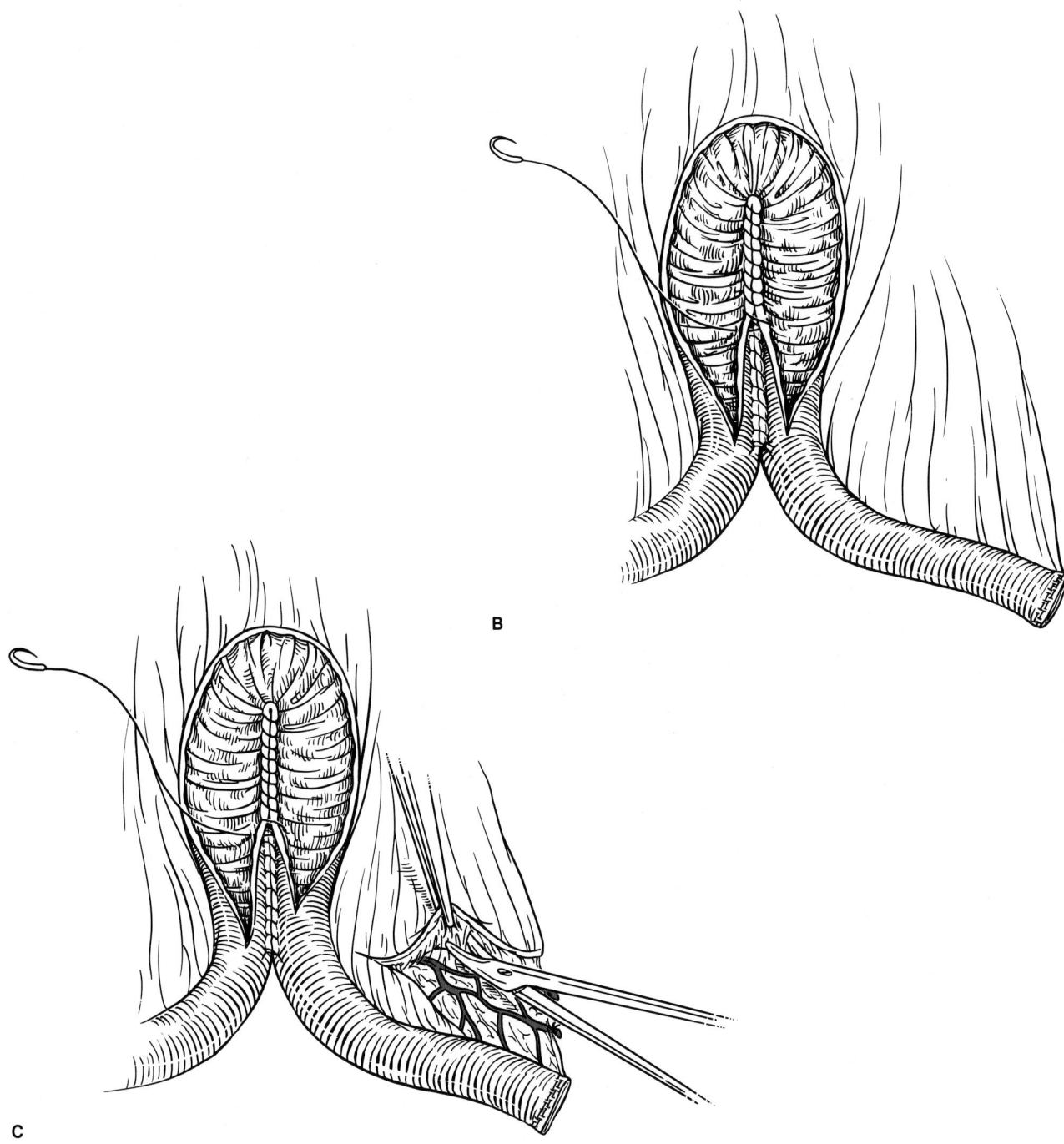

Figure 43-IIIC-1 *(Continued)*

(B) After the enterotomy, a second layer of 2-0 or 3-0 polyglycolic acid suture is placed in a running manner along the cut edges to create the posterior wall of the reservoir.

(C) The ileal segment is prepared for intussusception to create the continent valve by excising the fat between the blood vessels to reduce its mesenteric bulk. The blood supply to the ileum must be preserved. Some surgeons denude the ileum of its peritoneum and score the muscularis with electrocautery or inject tetracycline solution to promote adhesions between the opposing surfaces, or both.

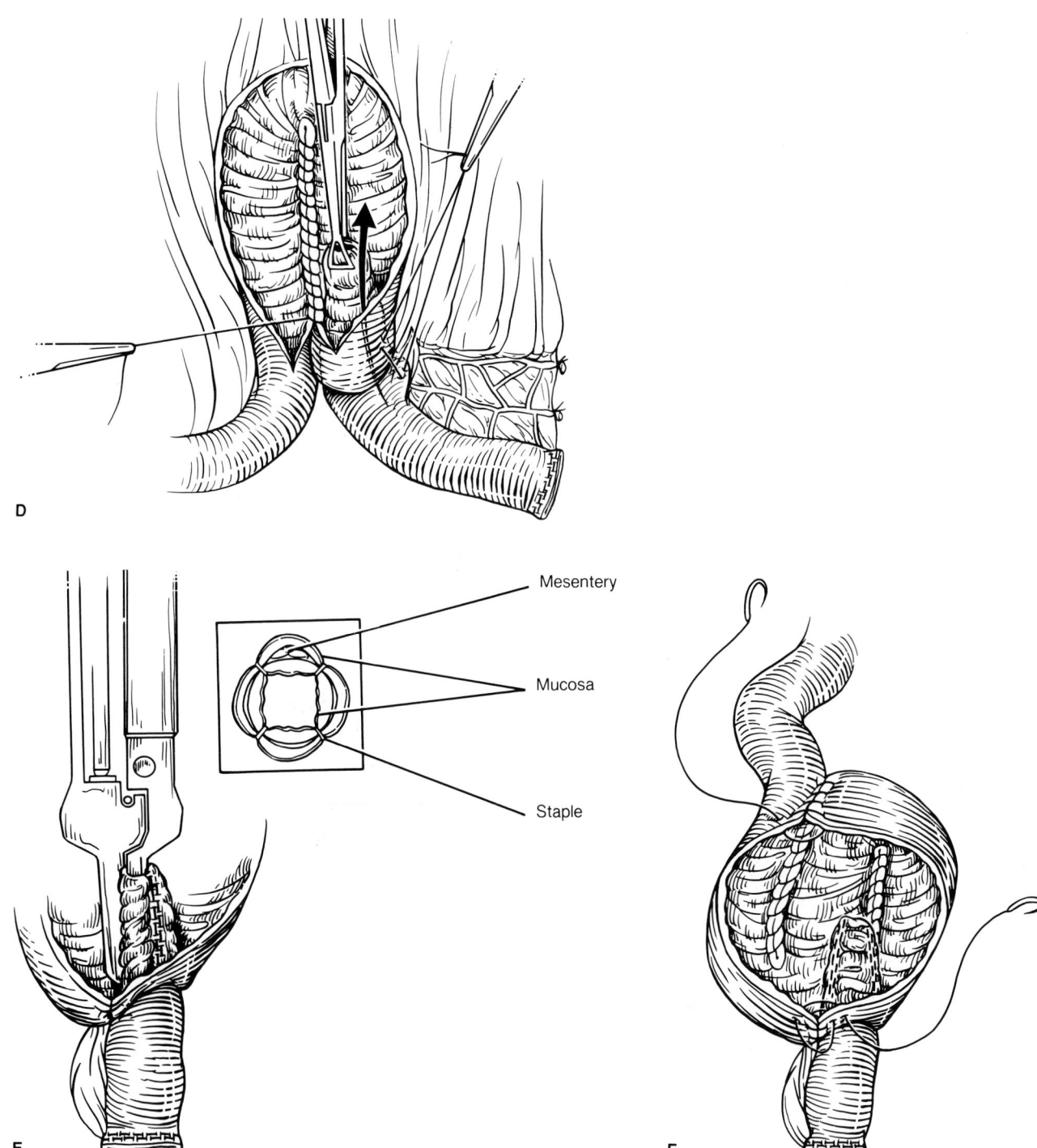

D

Mesentery

Mucosa

Staple

E

F

Figure 43-IIIC-1 *(Continued)*

(D) Three 3-0 silk sutures are placed on both sides of the nipple mesentery proximally and distally to help maintain the intussusception after they are tied. A Babcock clamp is placed from within the pouch into the distal ileal segment, which is grasped at its midpoint. Gentle traction applied in the direction of the pouch lumen, as shown, produces intussusception of the ileum. The previously placed fixation sutures are tied sequentially as the segment is intussuscepted.

(E) The intussuscepted valve is further stabilized by four rows of staples placed on either side of the mesentery and on the antimesenteric border. The surgeon must be sure the linear stapler cartridge has staples only and no knife blade.

(F) The pouch is then closed on its anterior surface by a running 3-0 absorbable suture.

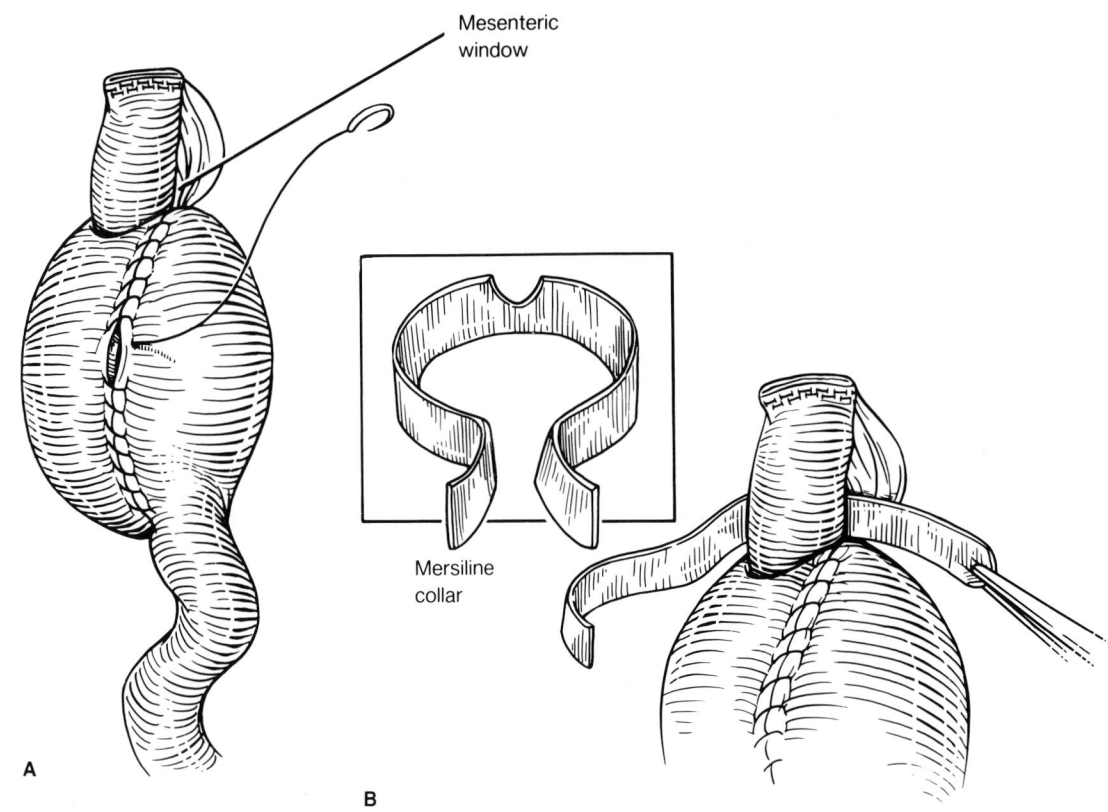

Mesenteric window

Mersiline collar

A

B

Figure 43-IIIC-2

Stoma Construction

(**A**) After the reservoir is completely closed with a running suture, a small mesenteric window is created at the base of the valve.

(**B**) A Mersilene collar is trimmed to accommodate the mesentery and fit around the base of the valve.

(**C**) The free ends of the Mersilene strip are sutured with a permanent stitch at the point where they cross each other.

(**D**) The valve and the pouch are anchored to the collar with multiple interrupted non-absorbable sutures.

(**E**) The reservoir is placed in the pelvis, and the stoma is positioned low in the right lower abdomen near the pubic hair line. The outflow tract traverses the mid-portion of the right rectus abdominis muscle without angulation or redundancy. A 2-cm disc of skin is excised, the subcutaneous fat is retracted, and the rectus fascia is opened in a cruciate incision. The rectus fibers are split, and the posterior fascia and peritoneum are incised to allow insertion of two fingers. Four 2-0 or 3-0 silk anchoring sutures placed at right angles to each other are passed from the pouch to the posterior fascia and peritoneum.

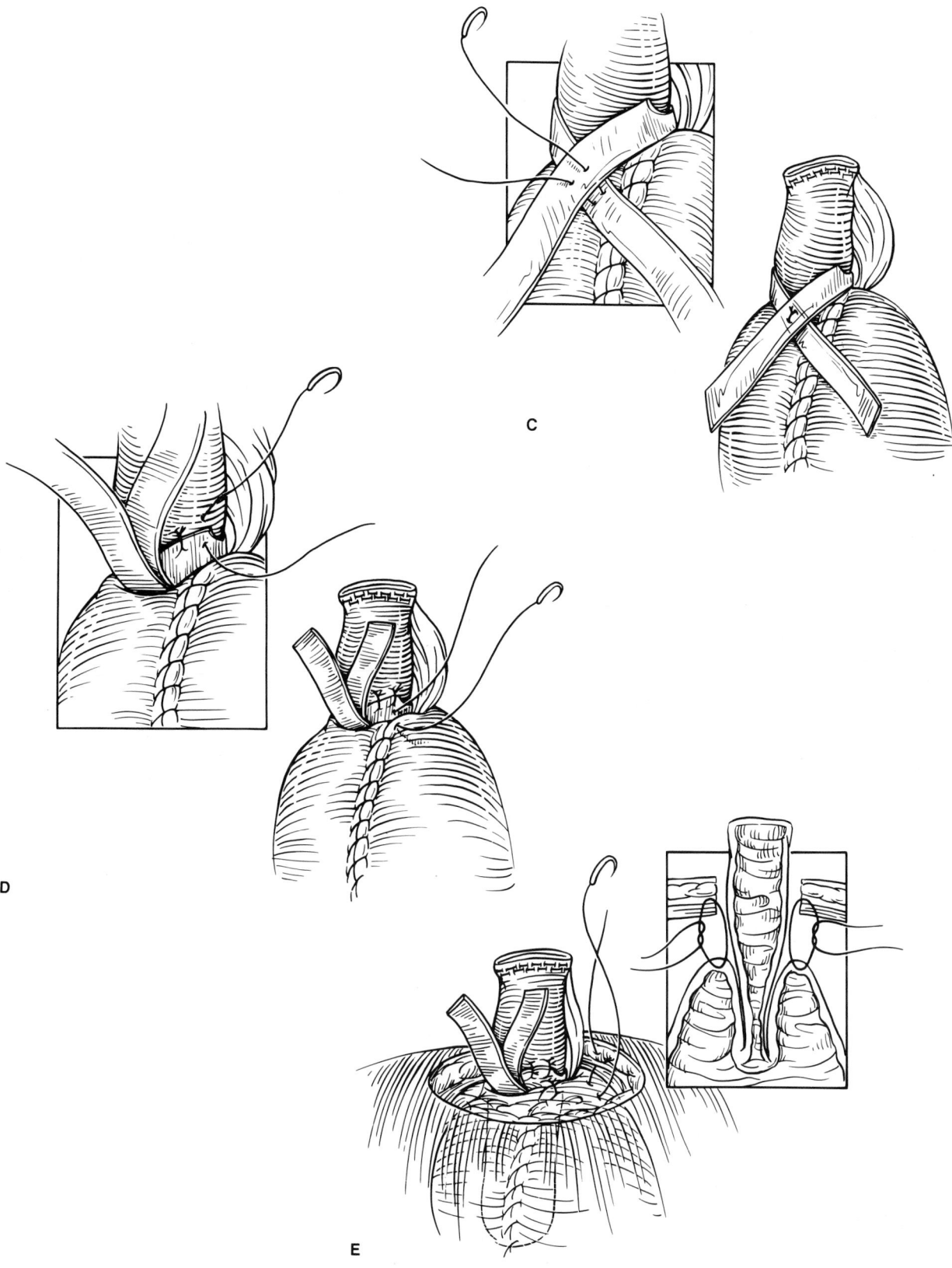

C

D

E

Figure 43-IIIC-2 *(Continued)*

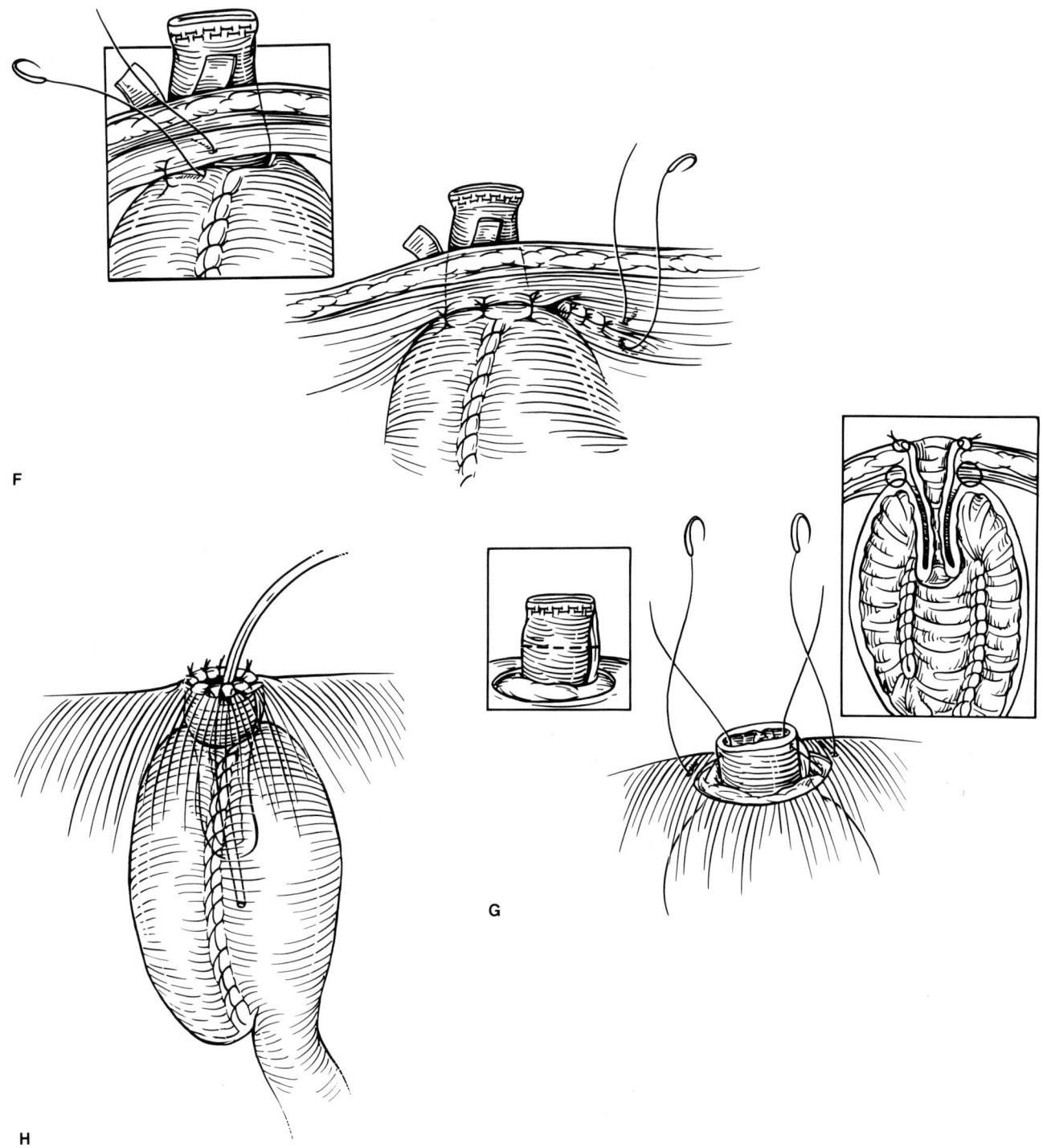

F

G

H

Figure 43-IIIC-2 *(Continued)*

(F) After the outflow tract is passed through the abdominal wall defect, the anchoring sutures are tied. Additional sutures anchor the pouch to the posterior fascia.

(G) The stoma is matured before the abdominal wound is closed by first trimming the exterior ileum so it is flush with the skin. The cut edge of ileum is sewn to the peristomal skin with interrupted 3-0 absorbable suture.

(H) An ileostomy catheter is placed through the stoma into the reservoir. Its position within the reservoir is ascertained by palpation, and it is anchored in place externally. The abdominal wound is closed. The catheter is connected to continuous gravity drainage.

D. Takedown of Loop Stoma With Resection

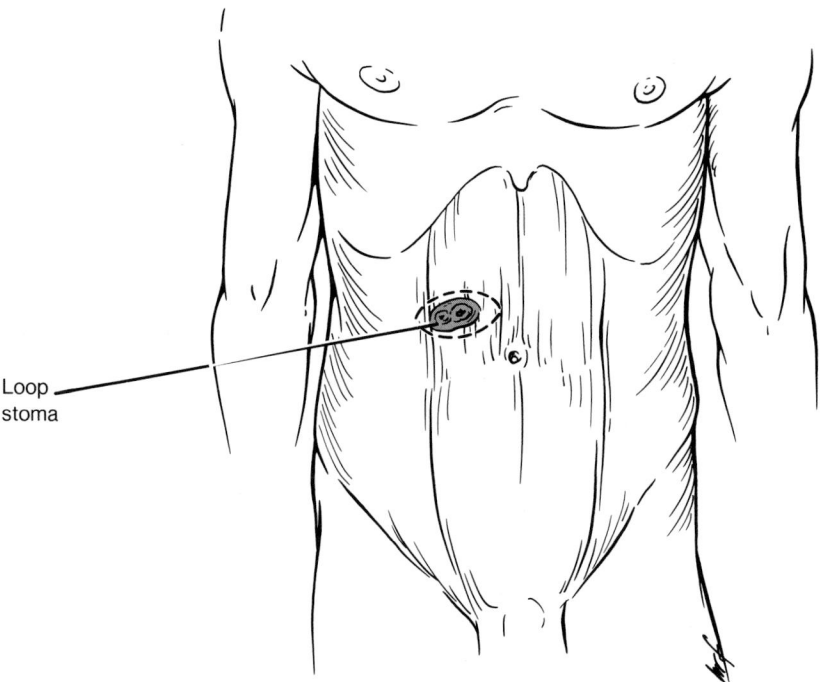

Figure 43-IIID-1

Incision

A transverse elliptical incision through the skin, subcutaneous tissue, and abdominal wall is made around the loop stoma, which has been closed with a suture to prevent intraoperative contamination.

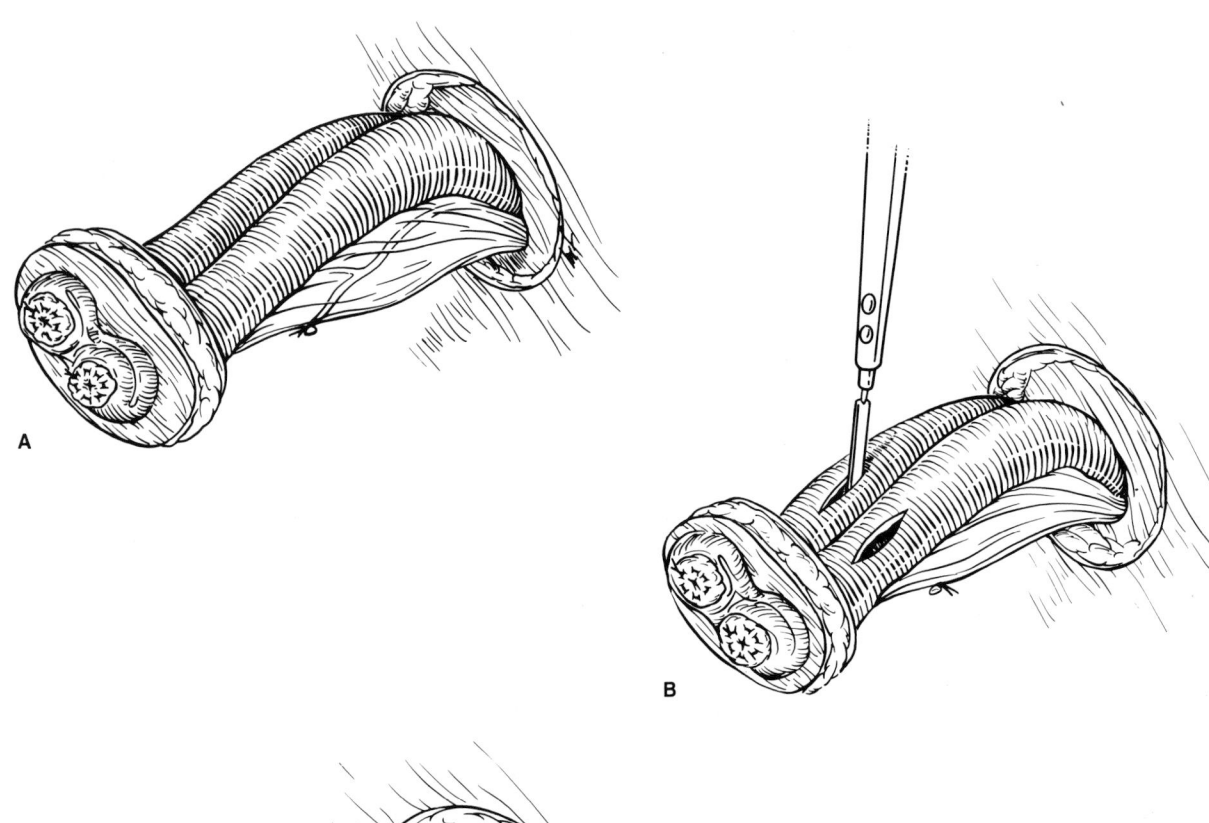

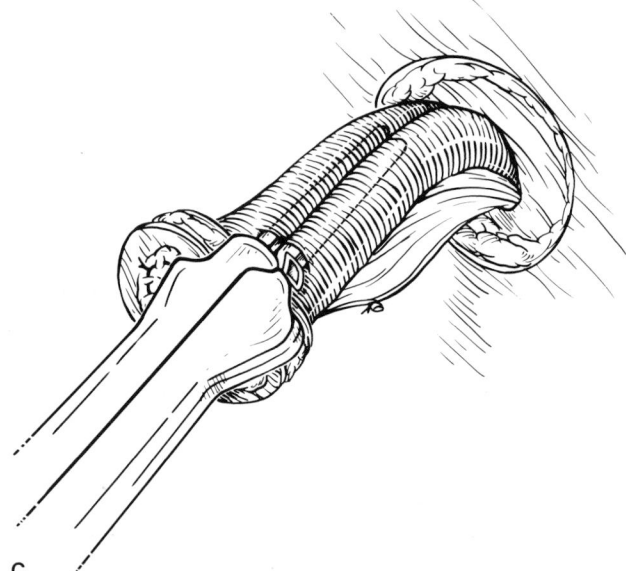

Figure 43-IIID-2

Procedure

(A) The two limbs of bowel used to create the loop stoma are mobilized from the abdomen, and the mesentery is divided at the level of the proposed anastomosis.

(B) Enterotomies are made on the antimesenteric surfaces of the proximal and distal limbs of the loop stoma.

(C) A linear cutter-stapler is inserted through the enterostomies, closed, and fired when properly aligned, thus creating a side-to-side anastomosis.

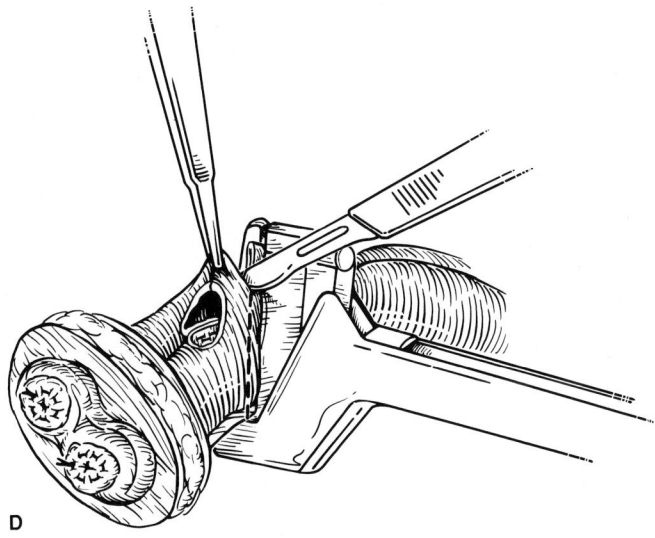

D

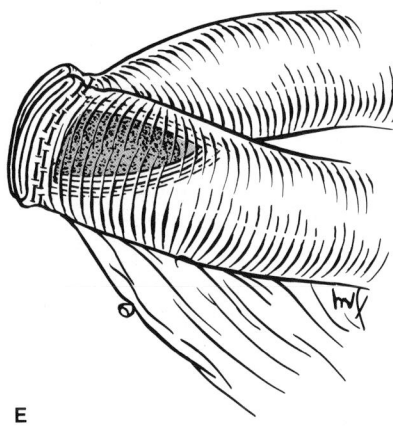

E

Figure 43-IIID-2 *(Continued)*

(D) A transverse stapler is used to close the defect resulting from transection of the portion of bowel involved in the enterotomies and the loop stoma.

(E) The resultant anastomosis is carefully inspected to ensure its vascularity, lack of tension, and accurate approximation of tissues. The apex of the side-to-side anastomosis and the points of crossing staple lines can be reinforced with inverting 3-0 absorbable sutures. The bowel is replaced within the abdomen, and the transverse elliptical incision is closed in layers.

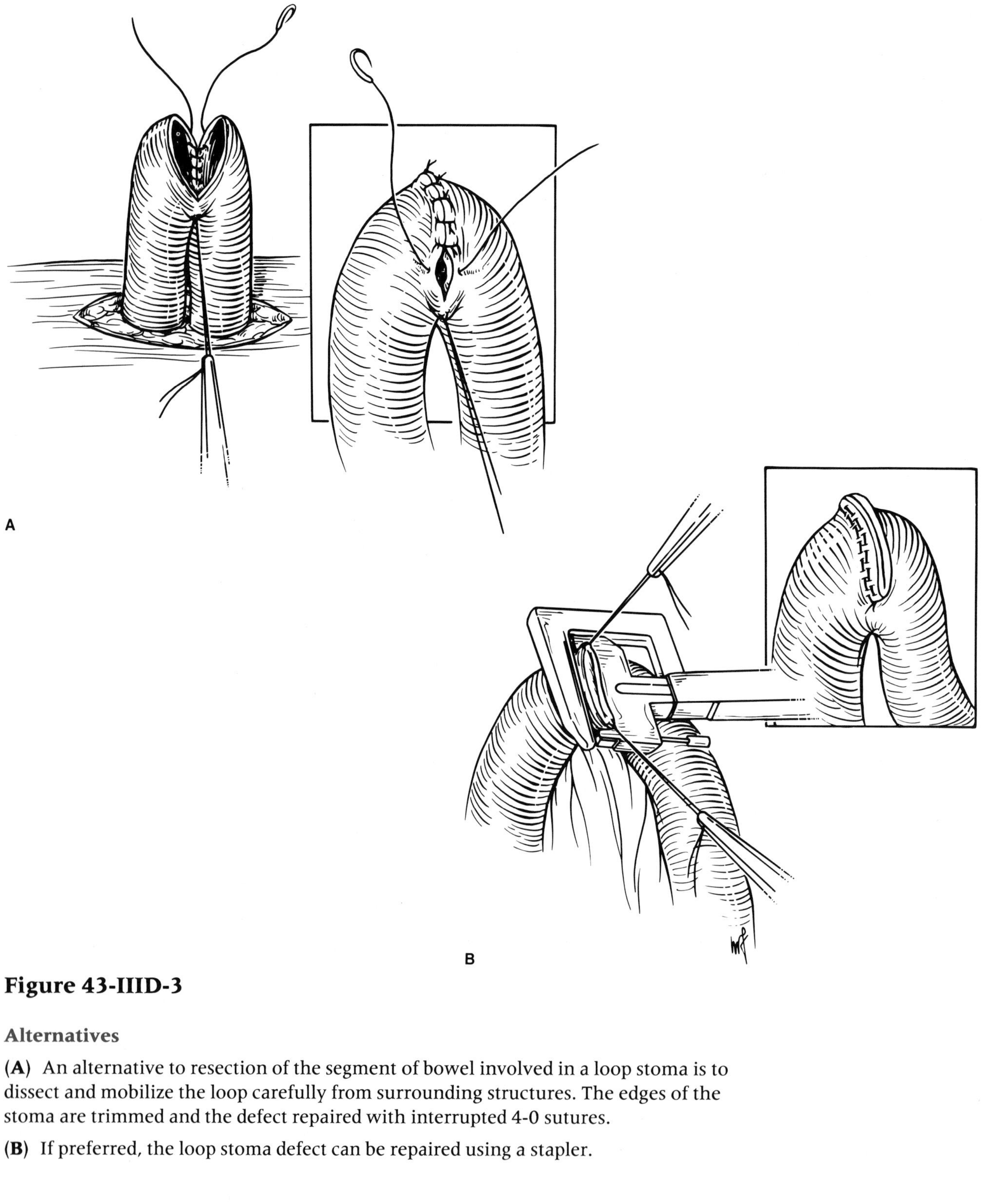

A

B

Figure 43-IIID-3

Alternatives

(A) An alternative to resection of the segment of bowel involved in a loop stoma is to dissect and mobilize the loop carefully from surrounding structures. The edges of the stoma are trimmed and the defect repaired with interrupted 4-0 sutures.

(B) If preferred, the loop stoma defect can be repaired using a stapler.

E. Takedown of End Stoma

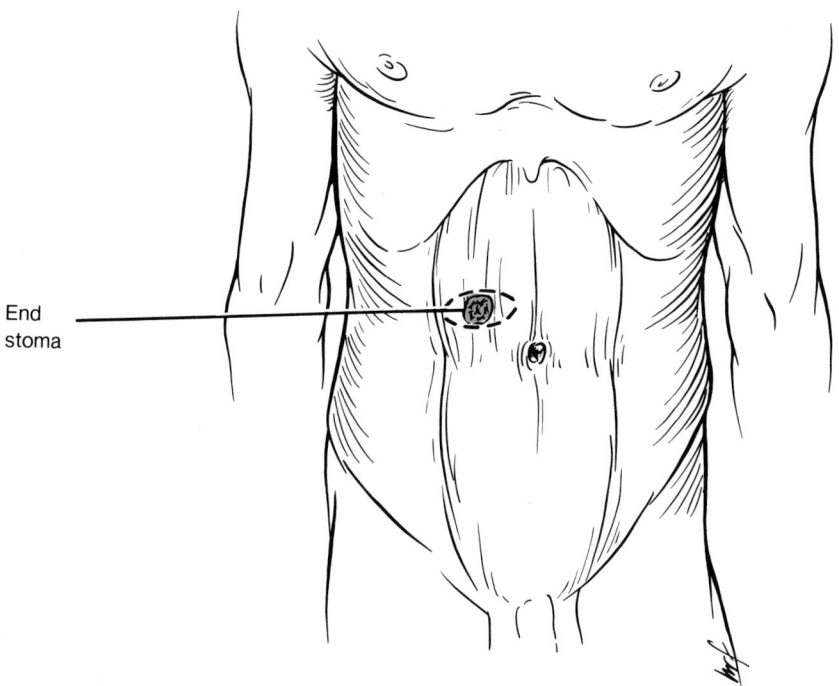

End stoma

Figure 43-IIIE-1

Incision

A transverse elliptical incision is made around the end stoma, which has been closed with a pursestring suture to prevent intraoperative contamination.

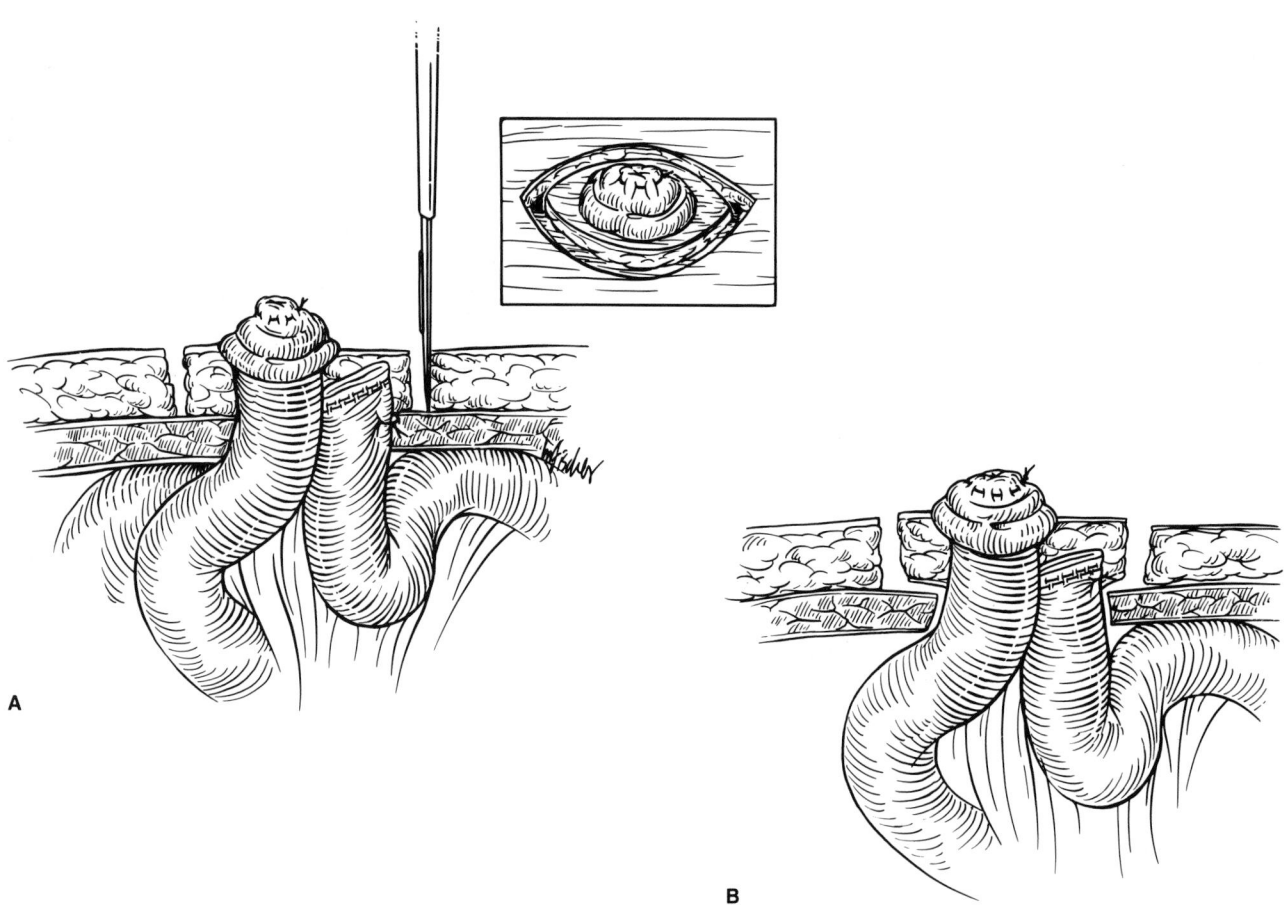

Figure 43-IIIE-2

Mobilization of Colostomy

(**A**) The incision is deepened to the level of the anterior rectus fascia.

(**B**) The proximal and distal limbs of bowel are dissected free from the anterior and posterior rectus fascia and the peritoneum.

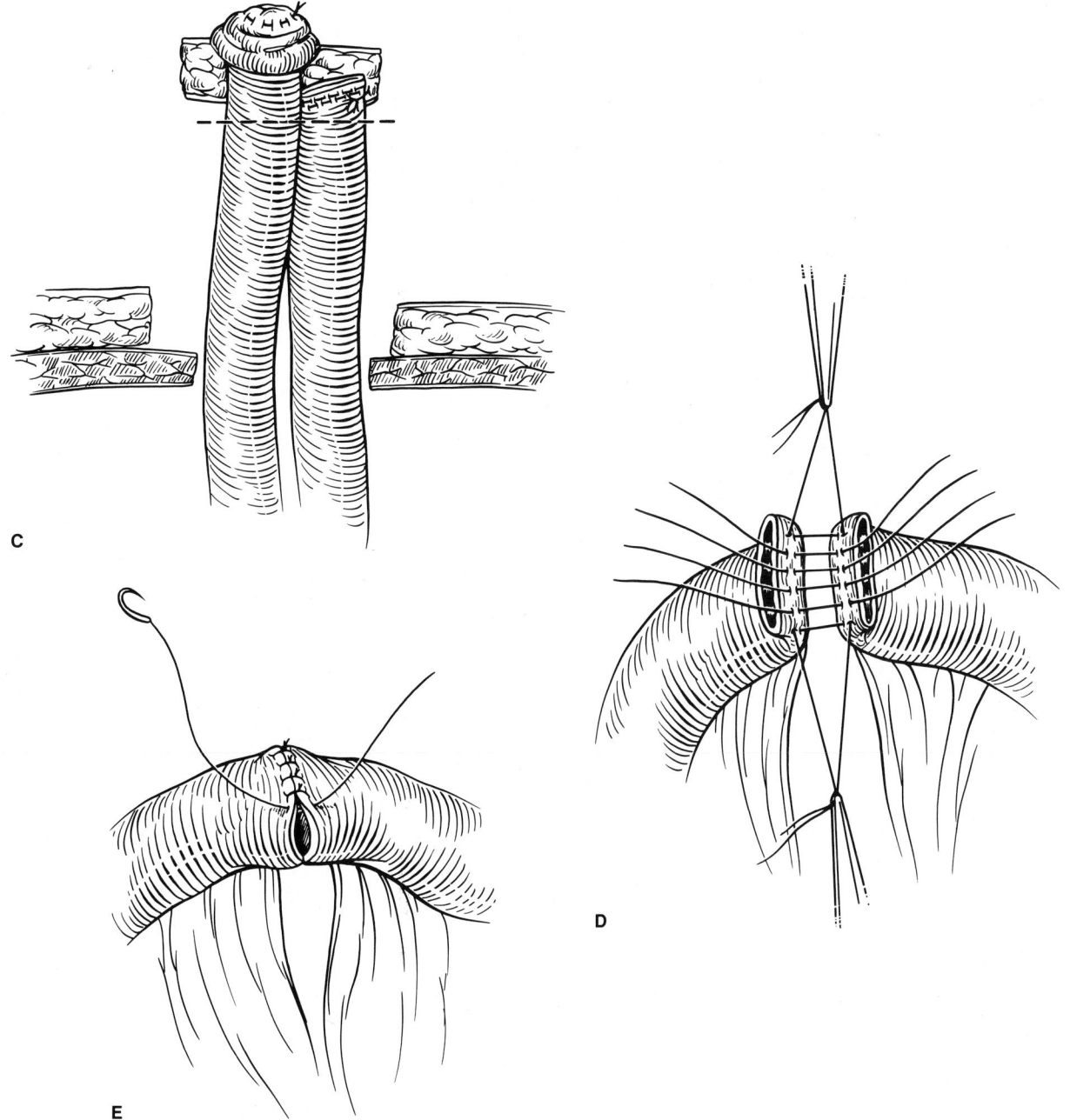

C

D

E

Figure 43-IIIE-2 *(Continued)*

(C) The two adjacent limbs of bowel are mobilized and prepared for anastomosis by resecting the ends and adjacent mesentery.

(D) An end-to-end handsewn enteroenterostomy is performed using 4-0 sutures in a single-layer technique.

(E) The anastomosis is completed with 4-0 interrupted Lembert sutures.

(Continued)

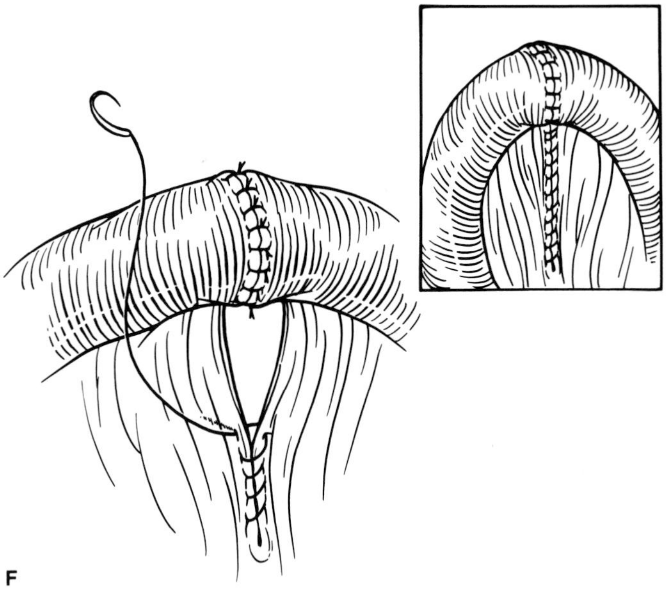

F

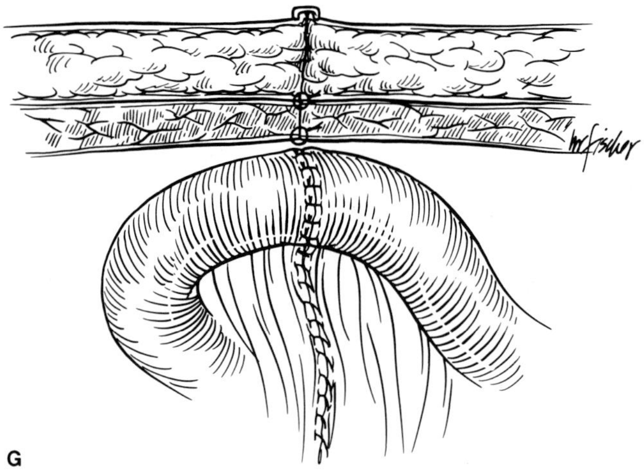

G

Figure 43-IIIE-2 *(Continued)*

(F) The mesenteric defect is closed with a running 3-0 absorbable suture.

(G) After completion of the small bowel anastomosis, the intestine is replaced within the peritoneal cavity, and the wound is closed by a layered technique.

SECTION IV *Laparoscopic Colonic Procedures*

A. Laparoscopic Appendectomy

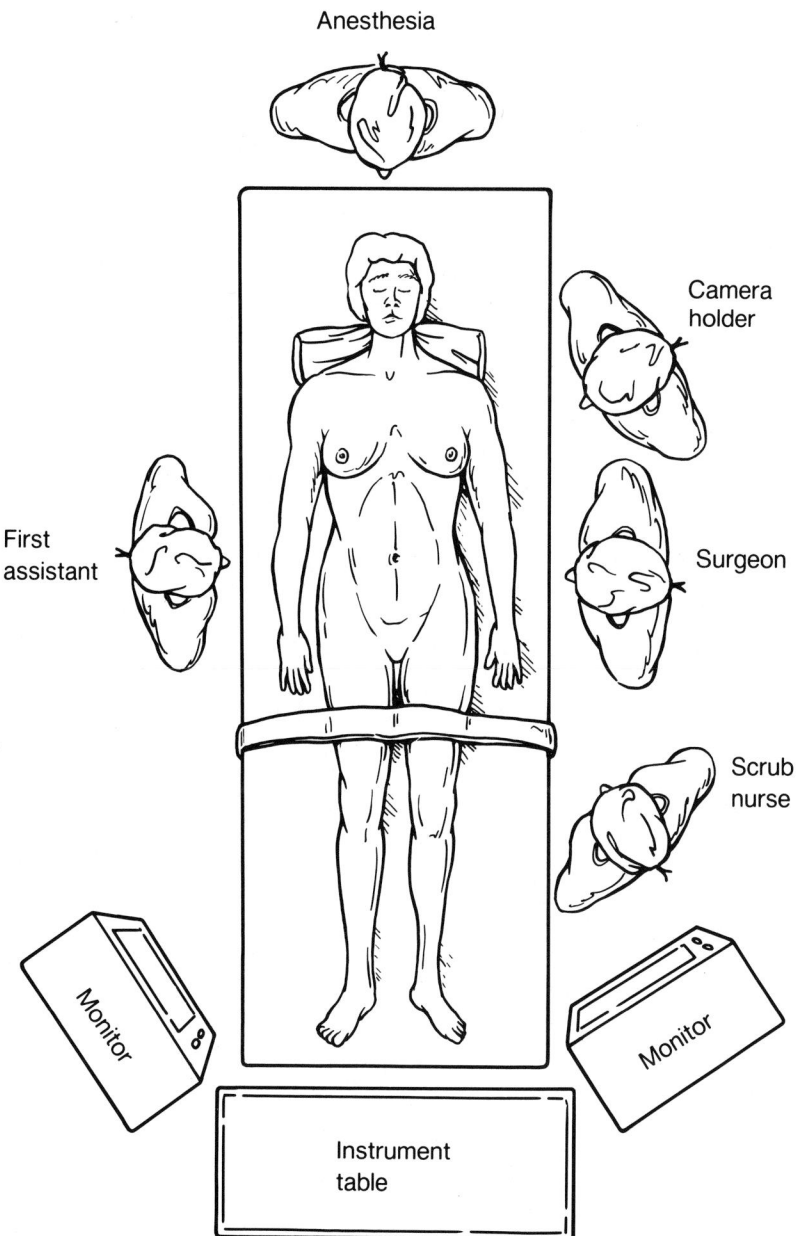

Figure 43-IVA-1

Operating Room Set-Up

A diagrammatic representation demonstrates positioning of equipment and operating room personnel. The patient is positioned supine with the arms tucked in at each side and is secured to the table with shoulder rests and a thigh belt. The camera holder may need to move to an alternate position if the surgeon's functions are inhibited. A catheter is necessary to keep the bladder empty.

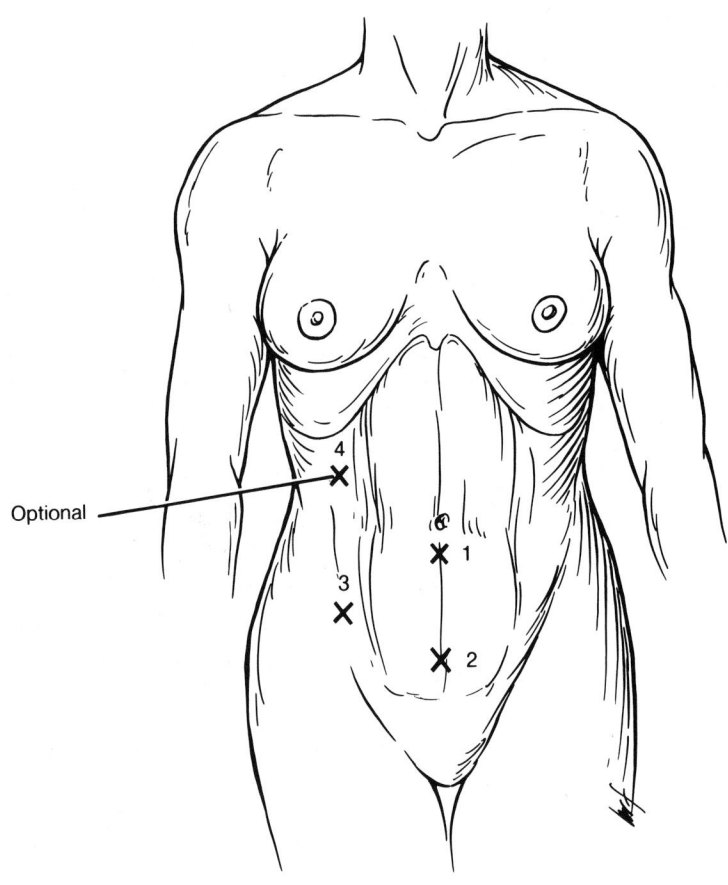

Figure 43-IVA-2

Port Sites

Recommended port sites and functions: (1) infraumbilical port—10/12-mm port for camera; (2) suprapubic port—10/12-mm port for instrumentation; (3) McBurney port—10/12-mm port for instrumentation located over the normal appendectomy incision site so that conversion can be easily made to an open appendectomy if necessary; (4) optional port—10/12-mm port (may be necessary in difficult cases).

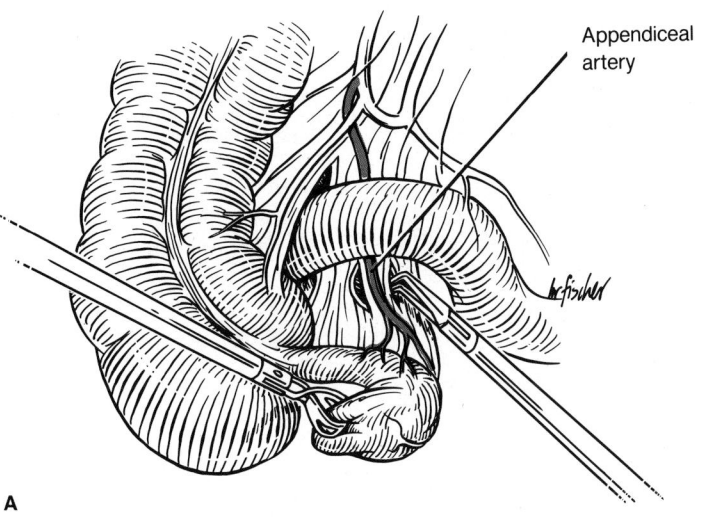

Appendiceal
artery

A

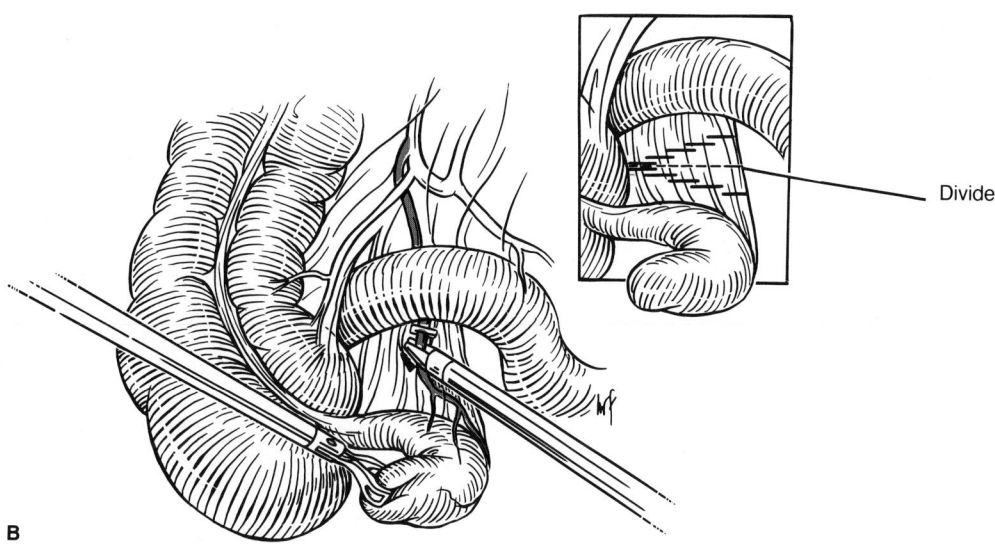

Divide

B

Figure 43-IVA-3

Procedure

(A) The operating table is positioned so that the cecum is easily visualized. Generally, this requires tilting to the left in an almost left lateral decubitus position. The appendix is mobilized by first placing a Babcock clamp or endoloop at the distal end of the appendix. Traction then allows the mesentery to be visualized. The appendiceal artery can thus be identified and isolated.

(B) If the appendiceal artery can be visualized, it is divided using an endoclip applier. Two clips are placed proximally and one distally. The artery is then divided under direct view. **(Inset)** Alternative approach of "stair stepping." Multiple clips are placed, and the mesentery is divided until the cecal wall is identified.

(Continued)

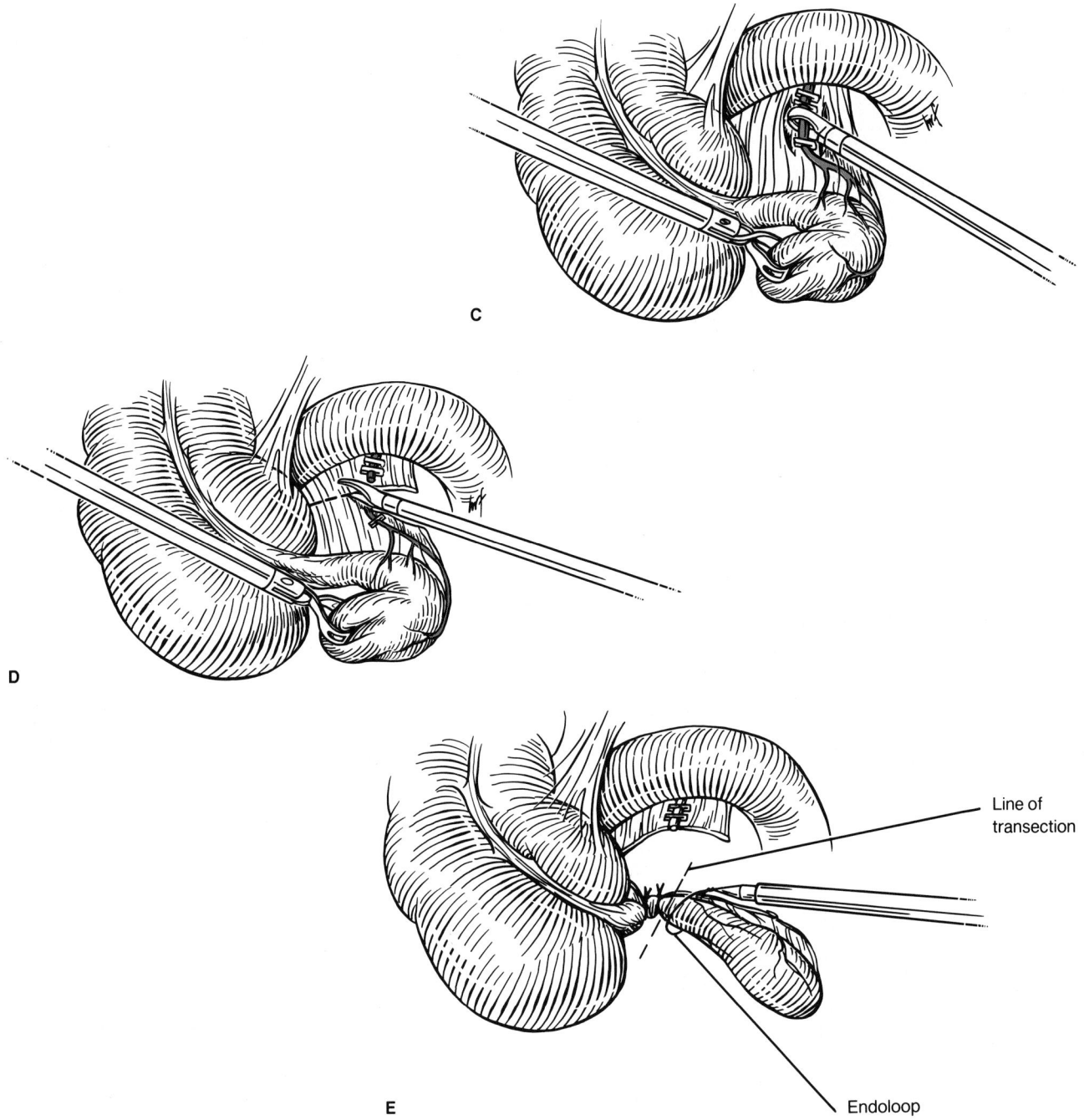

C

D

Line of
transection

Endoloop

E

Figure 43-IVA-3 *(Continued)*

(C) The appendiceal artery has been clipped in two areas, and a second proximal clip has been applied. The artery is being divided with curved scissors.

(D) As traction is placed on the appendix to keep the mesentery under slight tension, an electrocautery scissors is used to divide the clipped artery and adjacent mesoappendix.

(E) One of two approaches to ligating the appendiceal stump is shown. Two endoloops are placed proximally, and one is placed distally. The appendix is then transected.

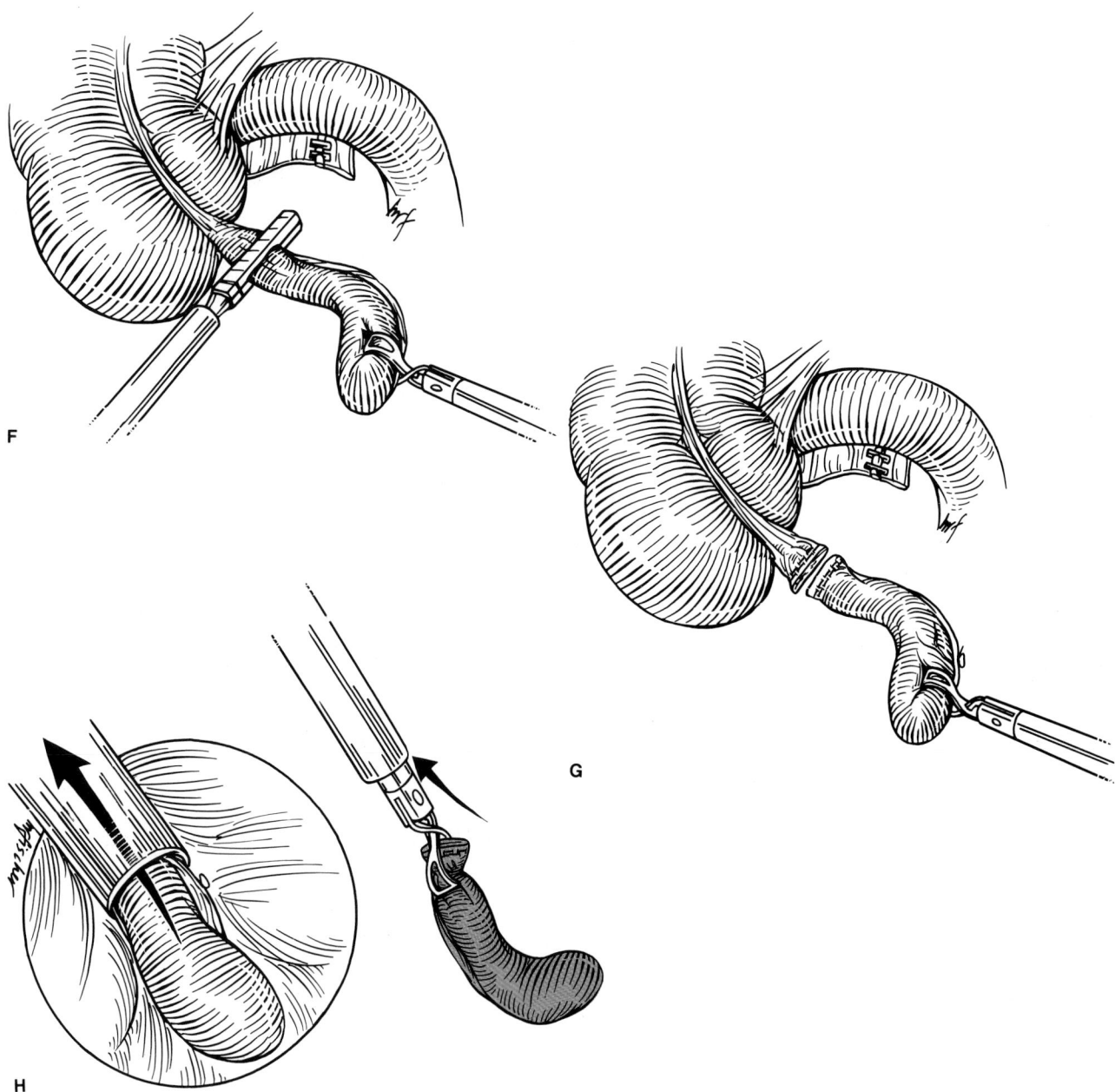

Figure 43-IVA-3 *(Continued)*

(F) An alternative approach to ligating the appendiceal stump is shown. The endolinear cutter stapling device is placed across the appendix adjacent to the cecum. When properly aligned, closed, and fired, this provides a secure closure of the cecum. This has some potential advantages over the endoloop technique because it may be difficult to place two proximal endoloops close to the appendiceal junction with the cecum and because a single endoloop may slip off.

(G) The appendix has been completely mobilized and resected and is ready for extraction.

(H) The appendix can be removed through a 10/12-mm port site, or if large and gangrenous, a sterile condom can be used as a specimen bag. The appendix is placed within the condom, which is then extracted, thus minimizing the chance of wound contamination.

B. Laparoscopic Right Hemicolectomy

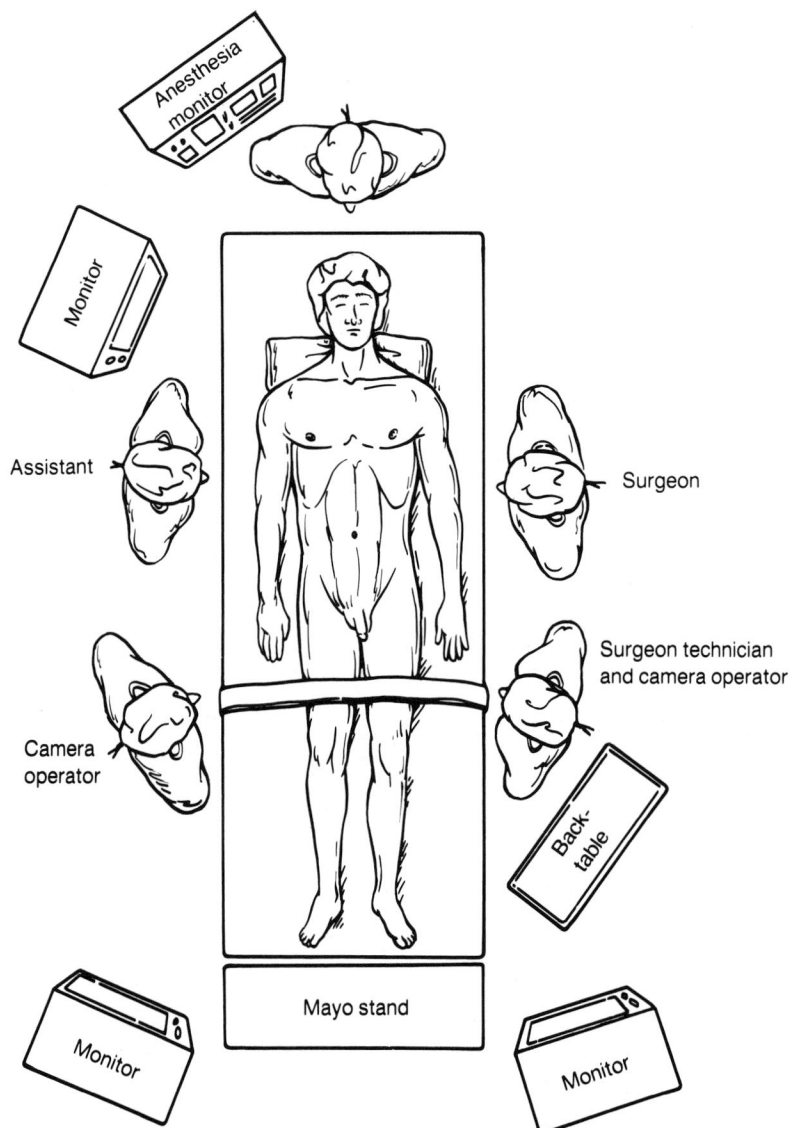

Figure 43-IVB-1

Operating Room Set-Up

Diagrammatic representation of positioning of equipment and operating room personnel. The patient is positioned with a small roll placed under the right flank and is secured to the table with shoulder rests and a thigh belt. The table is moved to the Trendelenburg position and rotated so that the patient is in a left lateral decubitus position. All members of the operating room team must be able to operate the camera and assist the surgeon.

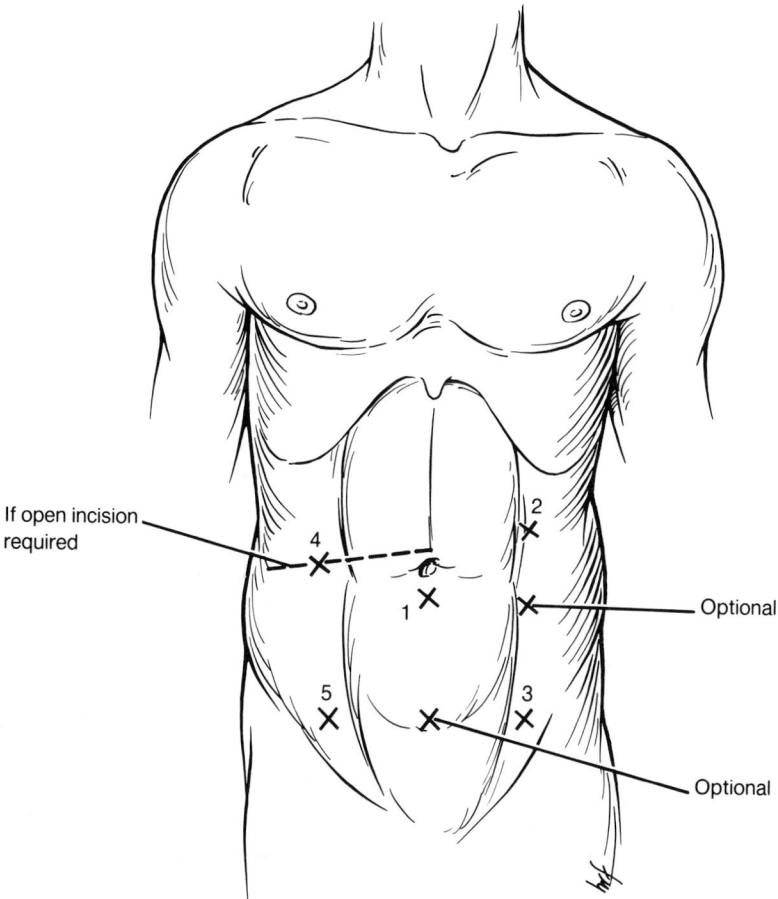

Figure 43-IVB-2

Port Sites

Recommended port sites and functions: (1) infraumbilical port site—10/12-mm port for camera; (2 and 3) left abdominal port sites—10/12-mm ports for instrumentation are placed lateral to the rectus abdominis muscle to avoid epigastric artery injury; (4 and 5) right abdominal port sites—10/12-mm ports for instrumentation are placed lateral to the rectus abdominis muscle to avoid epigastric artery injury. Site 4 is positioned so that if an open laparotomy is required, it can be incorporated into the incision. Two optional port sites are noted and may be used depending on the particular anatomy and difficulties encountered in a specific case.

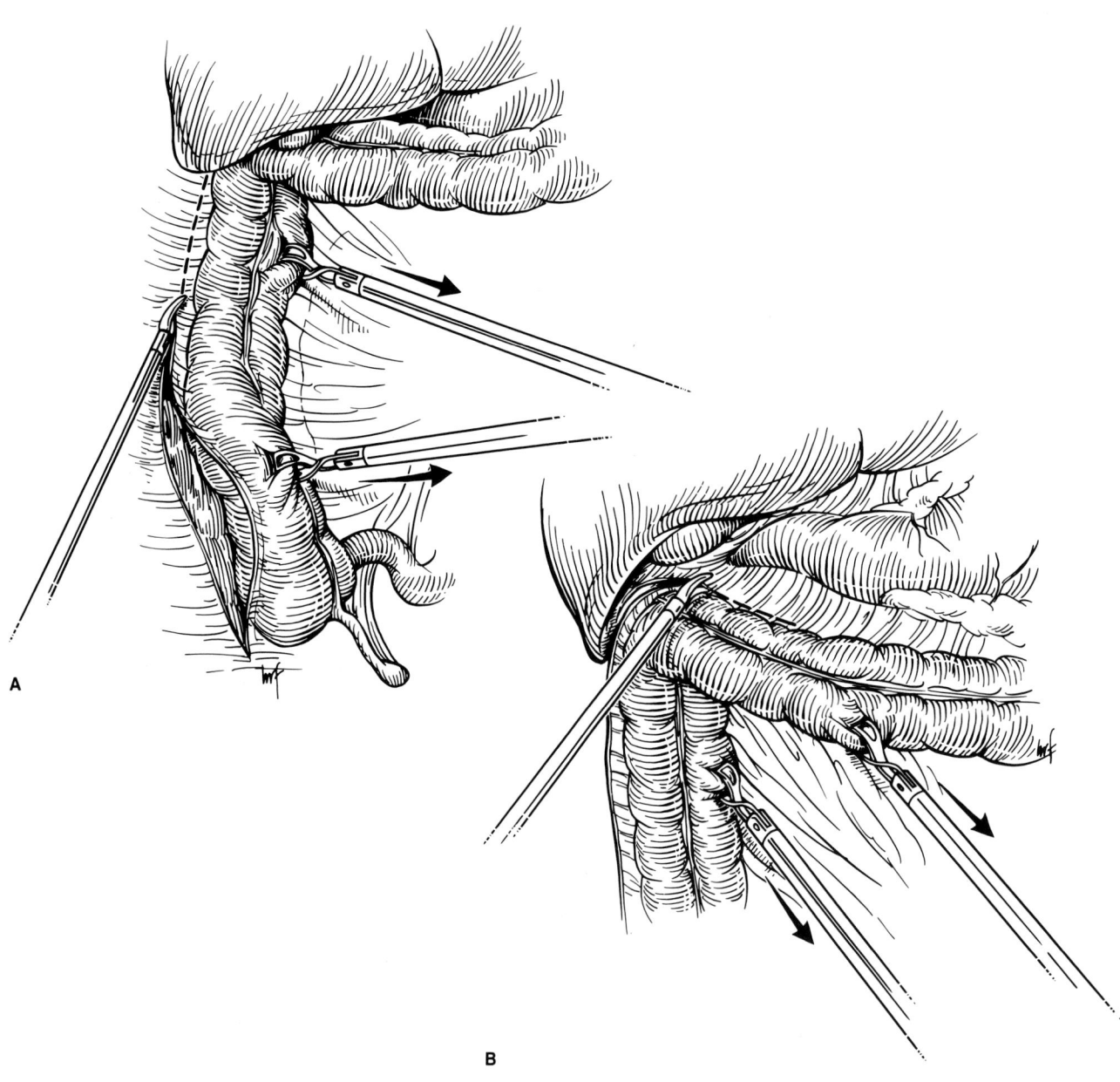

Figure 43-IVB-3

Procedure

(**A**) The ascending colon is mobilized in a manner similar to that used for open right hemicolectomy. Atraumatic Babcock clamps are applied, as shown, to provide counter-traction as the peritoneum is incised with an electrocautery scissors. It is important that only the peritoneum be incised to avoid mesenteric vessel injury and that the duodenum be identified to avoid injury. Blunt dissection can be useful as the peritoneum is being divided. Babcock clamps should only be placed on bowel that ultimately is resected because clamp trauma can sometimes result in late perforations.

(**B**) The hepatic flexure is taken down using Babcock clamps to apply countertraction. If the hepatocolic ligament is thick, clips may be required before the ligament can be divided. The duodenum and gallbladder must be visualized to avoid injury.

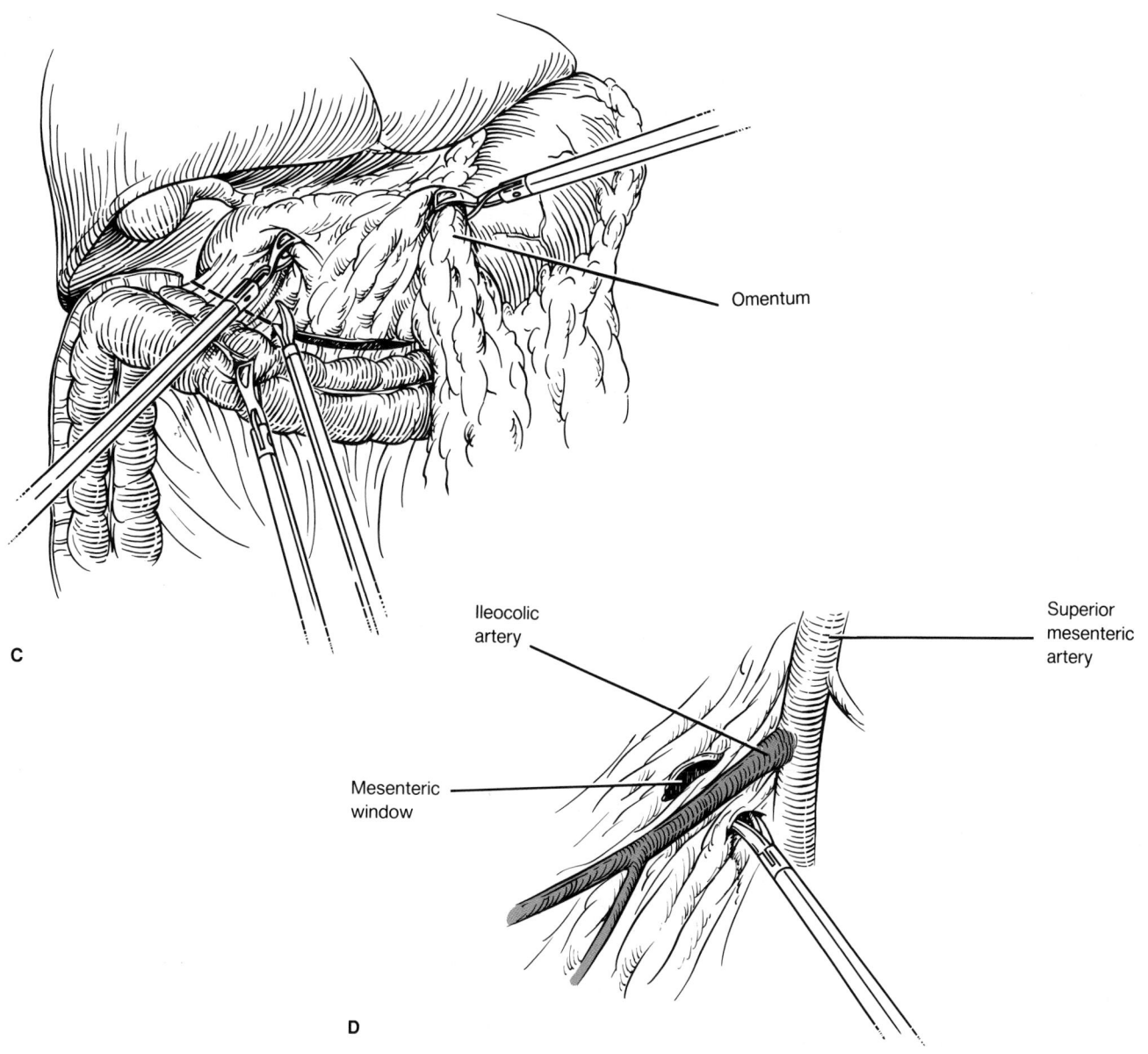

Figure 43-IVB-3 *(Continued)*

(C) The omentum is dissected from the transverse colon. This maneuver is often difficult. Gentle traction with Babcock clamps on the omentum itself is essential. The surgeon must dissect in the plane just adjacent to the transverse colon to minimize bleeding. Electrocautery is generally used, but if larger vessels are encountered, clips must be applied. It is critically important to avoid getting into the mesentery at this point because that causes hemorrhage and distort the plane of dissection. If a malignant lesion is being resected, the omentum is removed en bloc with the specimen.

(D) After the right colon is completely mobilized, the ileocolic artery is identified and isolated proximally as it comes off of the superior mesenteric artery. Gentle traction on the mesentery and careful dissection allow isolation of the vessel.

(Continued)

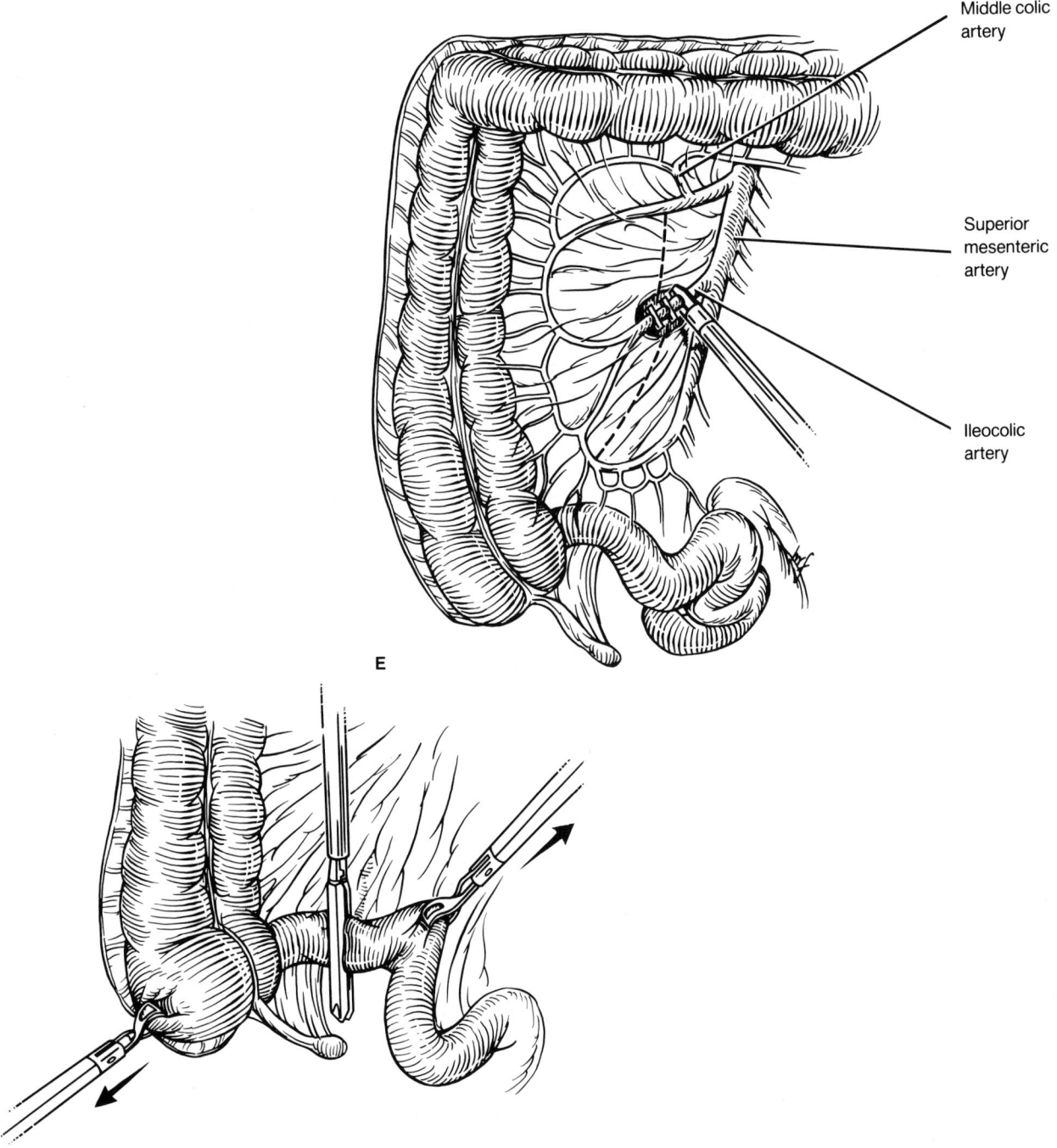

Middle colic
artery

Superior
mesenteric
artery

Ileocolic
artery

E

F

Figure 43-IVB-3 *(Continued)*

(E) The ileocolic artery is clipped twice proximally and once distally, after which it is divided under direct view. The mesentery is then incised with electrocautery up to the points of proposed resection. Additional vessels are encountered near the terminal ileum or transverse colon and must be ligated with clips.

(F) After dividing the mesentery up to the terminal ileum, the endostapling device is inserted and placed across the terminal ileum as shown. When properly aligned, it is fired, thus cutting and stapling simultaneously.

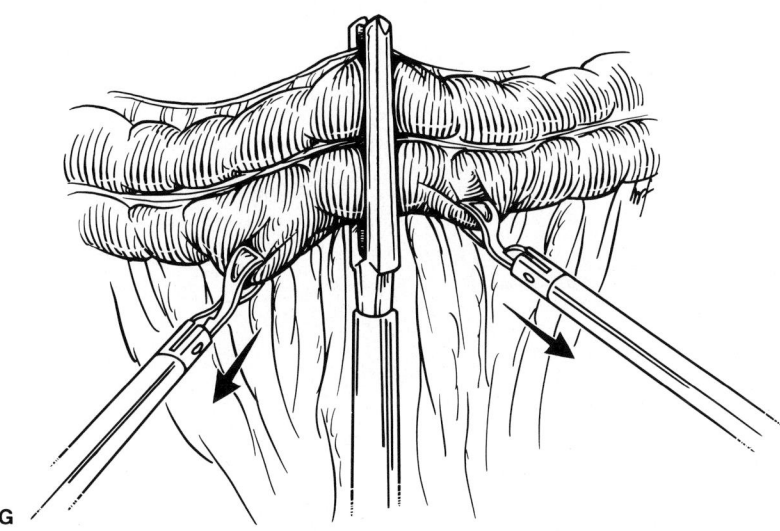

G

Figure 43-IVB-3 *(Continued)*

(G) The transverse colon is similarly transected using an endolinear cutter-stapler. The mesentery leading up to the transverse colon must be divided, including separate division of the right colic artery. The middle colic vessel is generally preserved with a right hemicolectomy, and the endostapler is placed just to the right side of the middle colic vessels. Once properly aligned, it can be closed and fired. The right colon specimen can be removed immediately or placed temporarily in the pelvis for extraction at the completion of the procedure.

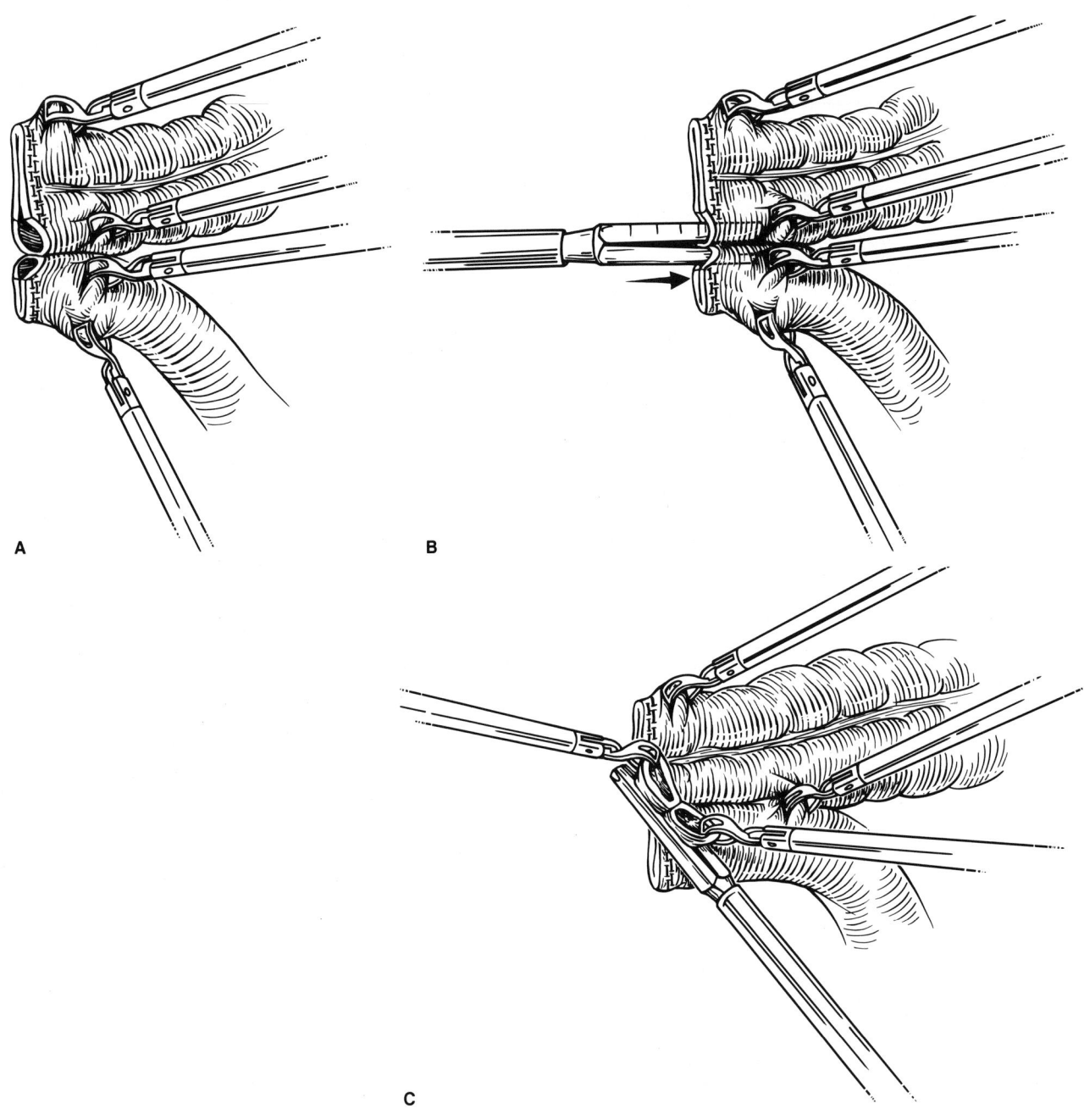

A

B

C

Figure 43-IVB-4

Intracorporeal Stapled Side-to-Side Ileocolic Anastomosis

(**A**) The transverse colon and ileum are aligned along their antimesenteric borders. Enterotomies are made along the antimesenteric edges.

(**B**) The endolinear cutter-stapler is inserted into the enterotomies, closed, and fired, thus creating a side-to-side stapled anastomosis.

(**C**) After removal of the initial stapler, a new endostapler is inserted. Babcock clamps are used to tent up the sites of the enterotomies, which are then resected using the linear cutter-stapler. As in the case of an open anastomosis, it is critical that both enterotomy sites are resected in their entirety.

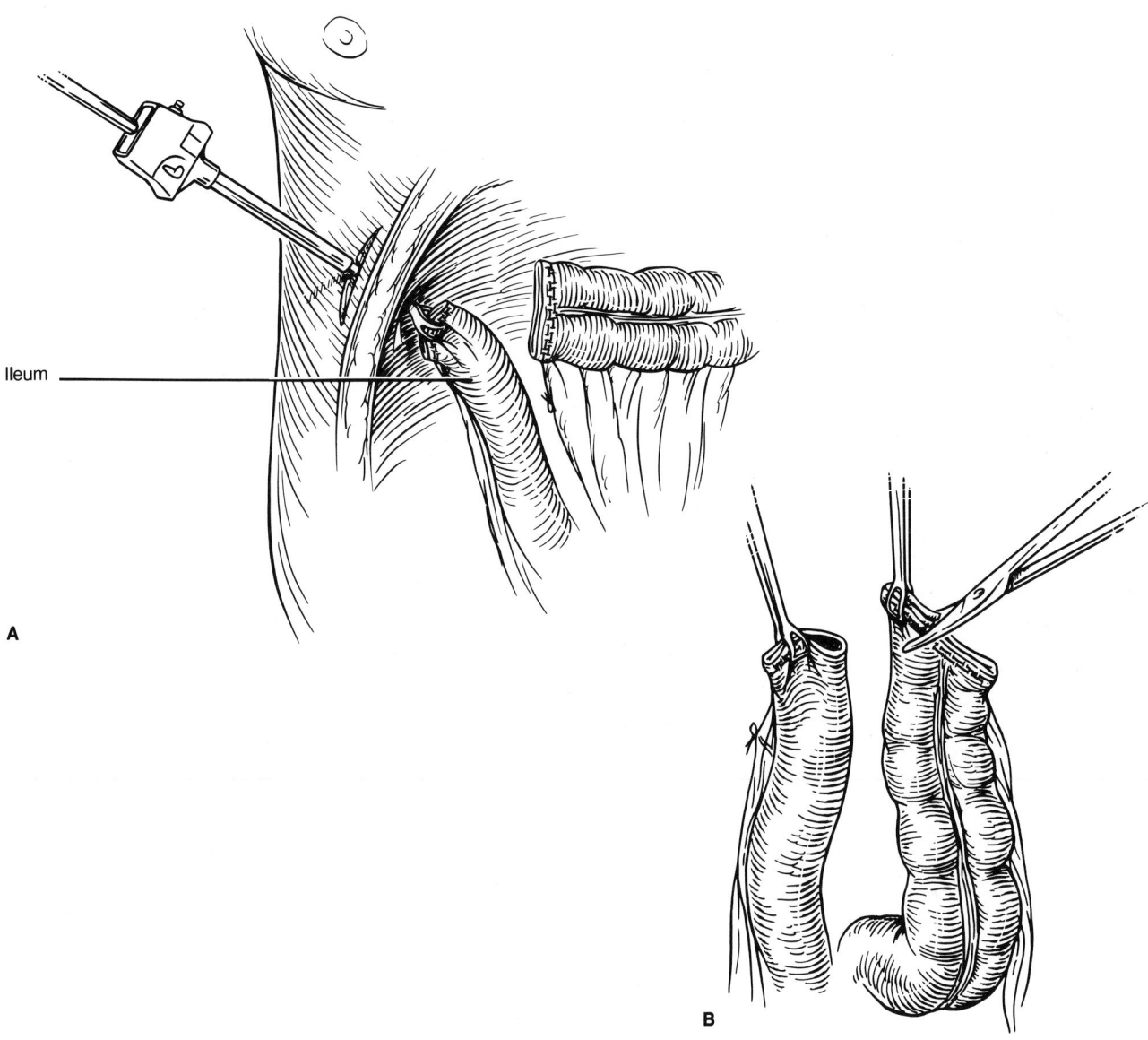

Figure 43-IVB-5

Extracorporeal Stapled Side-to-Side Ileocolic Anastomosis

(**A**) An alternative to the intracorporeal anastomotic technique is to conduct an extra-corporeal anastomosis. To accomplish this, the ileum and the transverse colon are mobi-lized and extracted through a small abdominal incision, which can also be used to extract the specimen. Care must be taken not to tear any of the mesenteric vessels.

(**B**) The ileum and transverse colon are prepared for stapled side-to-side anastomosis by excising a corner of the previous staple line along the antimesenteric borders.

(Continued)

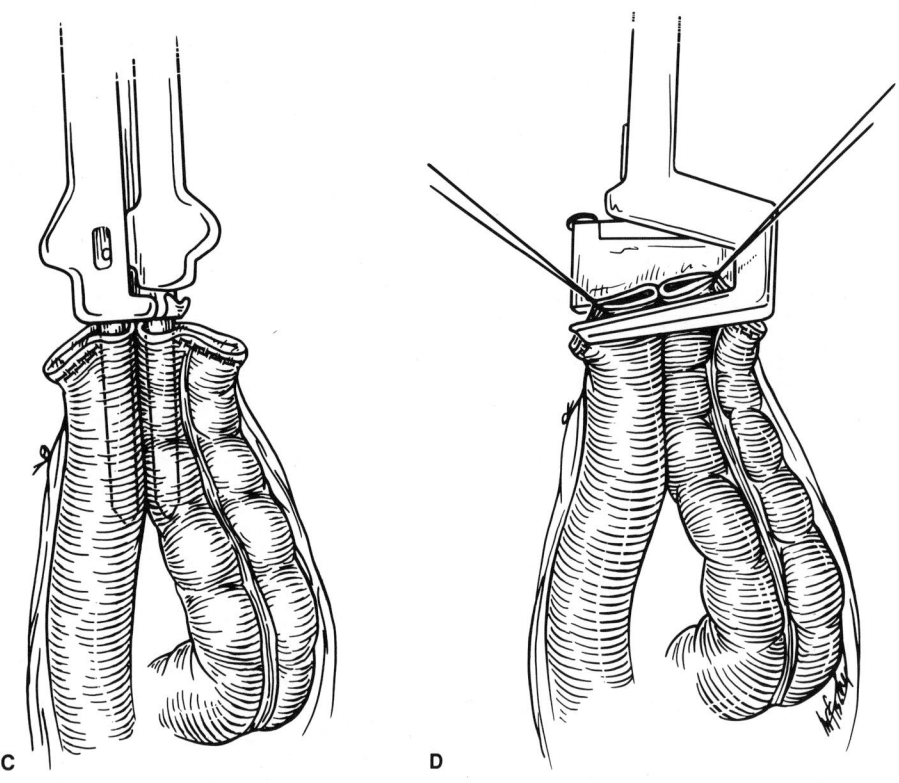

C   D

Figure 43-IVB-5 *(Continued)*

(C) A linear cutter-stapler is inserted through the enterotomies after alignment of the two limbs of bowel on their antimesenteric borders. Once in proper alignment, the stapler is fired, thus creating a side-to-side anastomosis.

(D) After removal of the linear cutter-stapler, the enterotomy defects are repaired either by hand suture technique or with a linear stapler, as shown.

C. Laparoscopic Hartmann Pouch Takedown

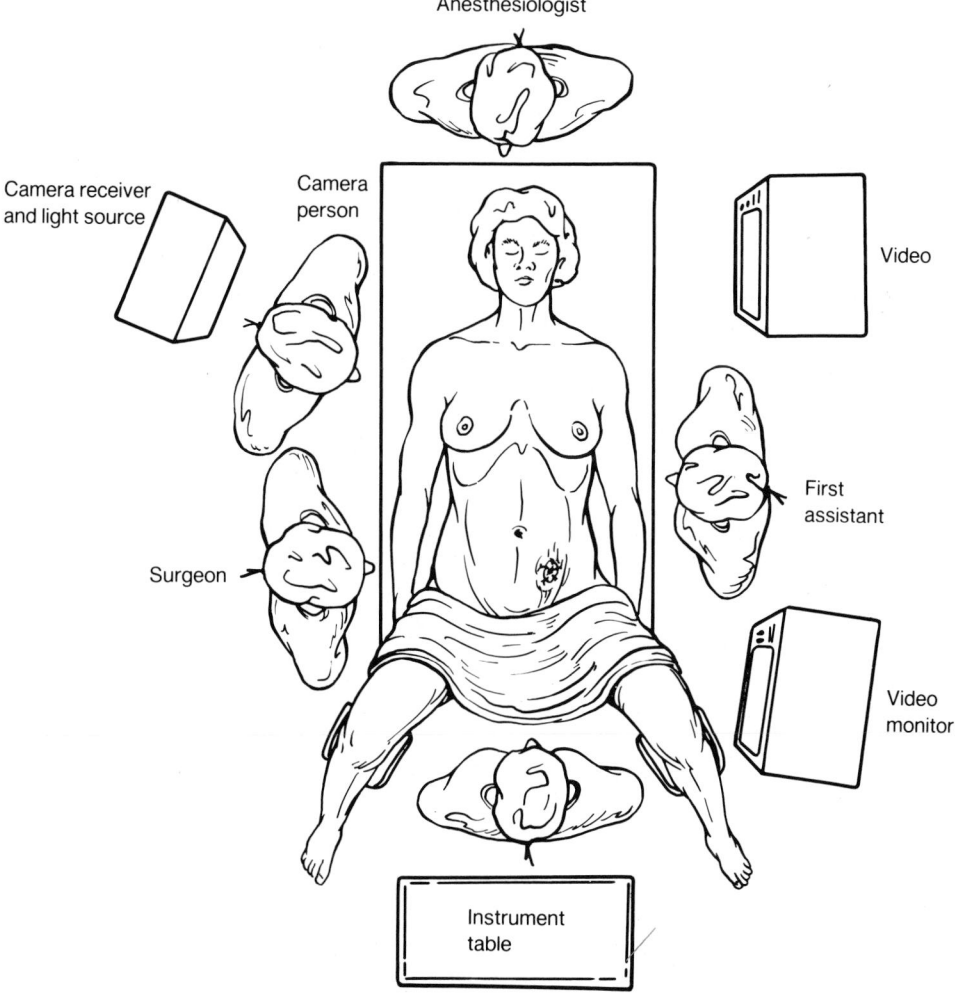

Figure 43-IVC-1

Operating Room Set-Up

A diagrammatic representation demonstrates positioning of equipment and operating personnel. The patient is placed in a modified lithotomy position with the legs in support stirrups that allow the thighs to be in the same plane as the abdomen. A roll is placed under the left flank, and the table is placed in the right lateral decubitus position.

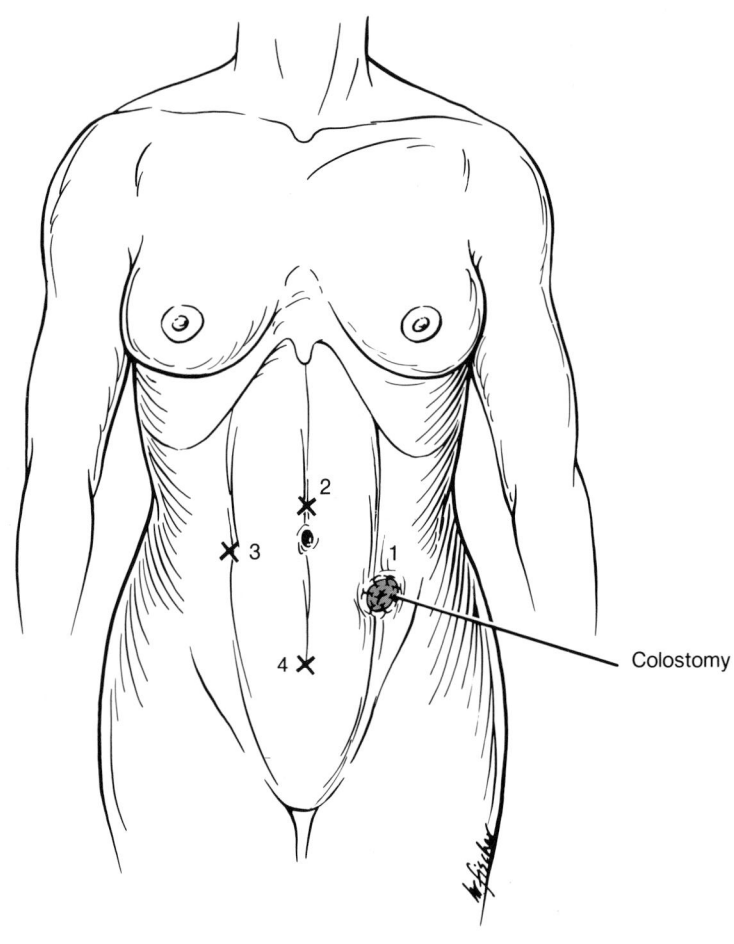

Figure 43-IVC-2

Port Sites

Recommended port sites and functions: (1) Colostomy takedown site. The colostomy is taken down first, thus allowing the surgeon to enter the intraabdominal cavity under direct vision. All subsequent ports can then be placed under direct vision. The colostomy site accommodates the camera. (2) Supraumbilical port site—10/12-mm port for instrumentation. (3) Right abdominal port site—10/12-mm port for instrumentation. (4) Suprapubic port site—10/12-mm port for instrumentation.

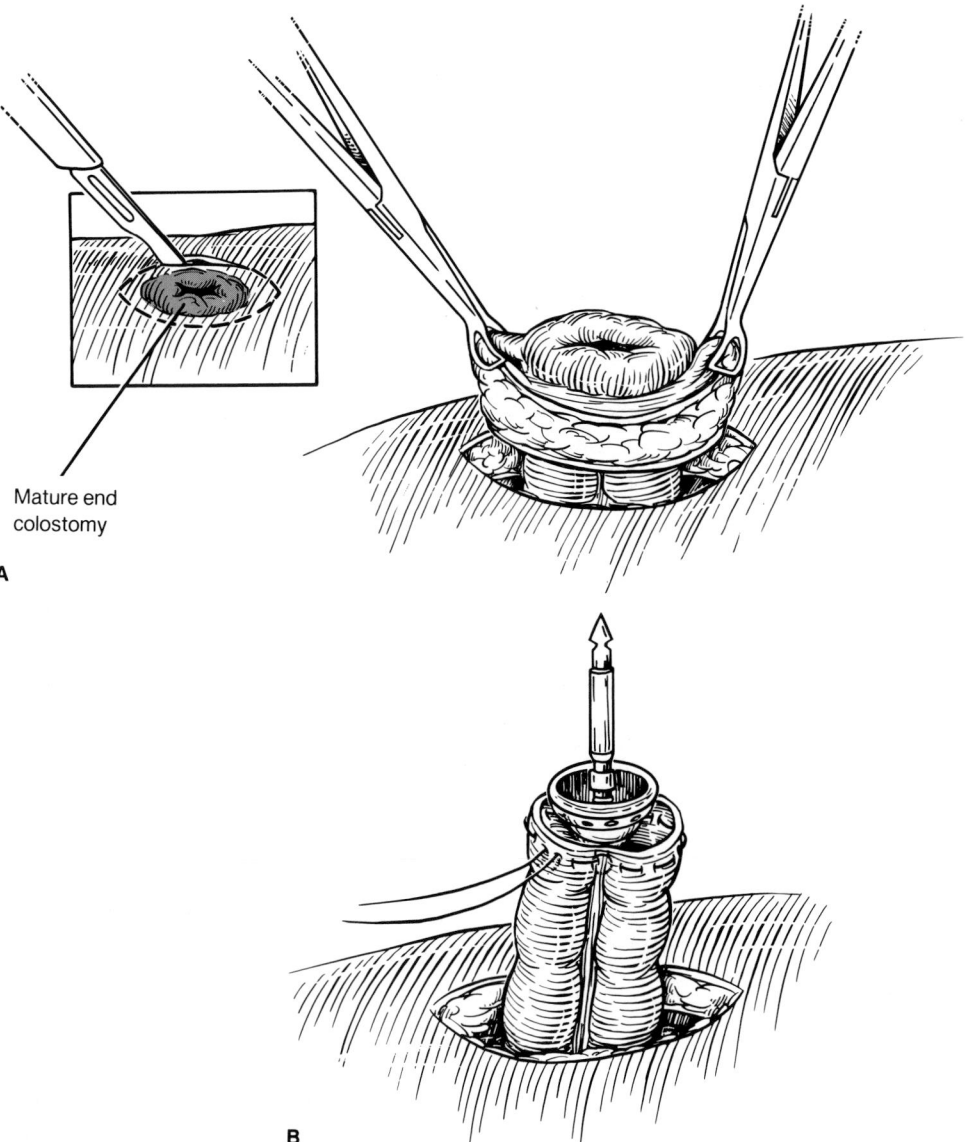

Mature end
colostomy

A

B

Figure 43-IVC-3

Procedure

(A) Colostomy takedown is commenced by making an elliptical skin incision around the stoma. The incision is carried down to the level of the anterior rectus fascia. The colon is then mobilized from the abdominal wall, taking care to avoid any injury to colon itself. Once this is accomplished, the subcutaneous tissue and skin are carefully excised from the end stoma, thus preserving its entire length. The stoma maturation site is unfolded or resected and a pursestring suture placed in the end of the colon.

(B) The anvil mechanism from the circular stapler is placed into the mobilized colon with the pursestring suture in place. The pursestring is tied, securing the anvil.

(Continued)

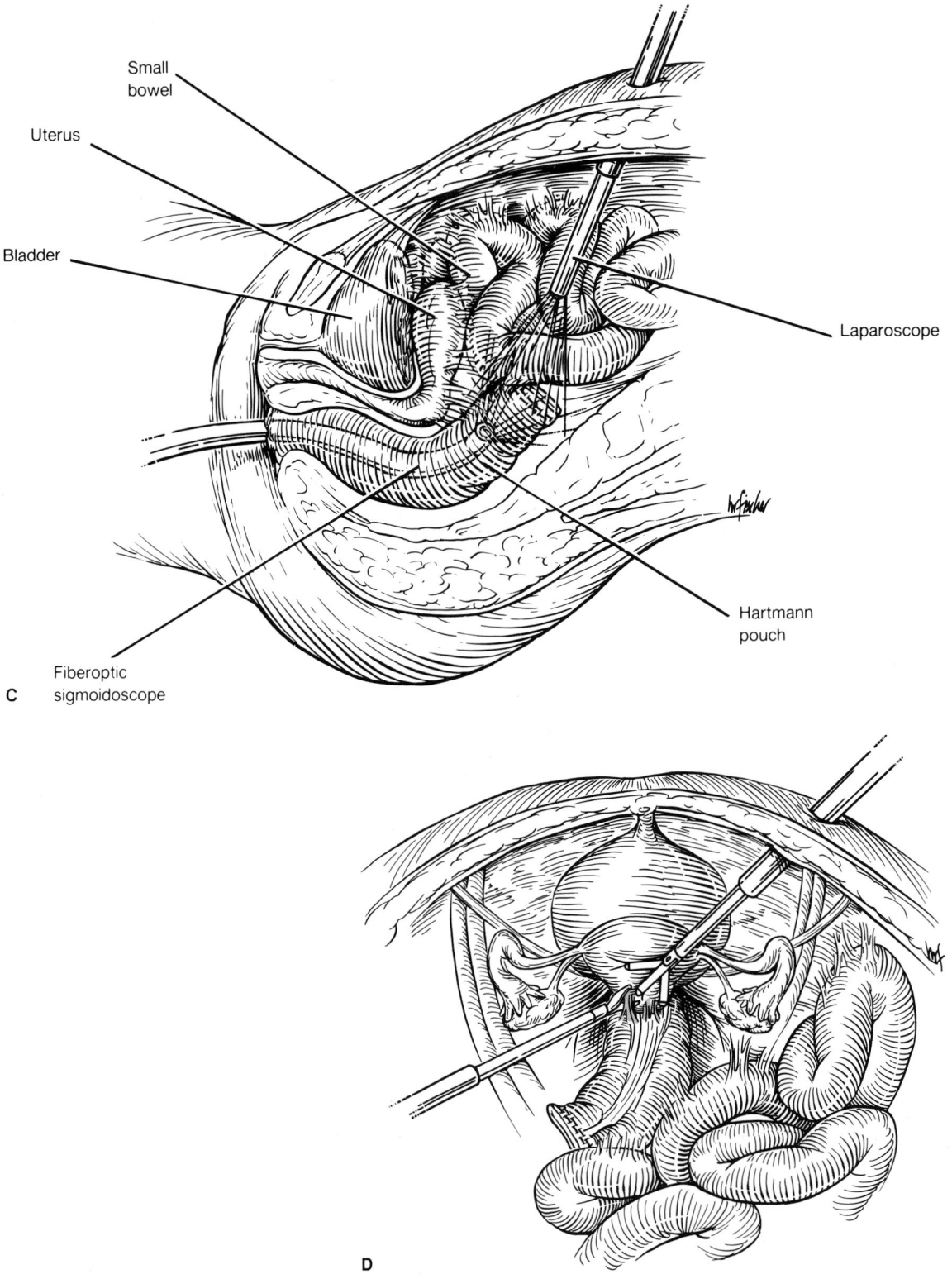

Small
bowel

Uterus

Bladder

Laparoscope

Hartmann
pouch

Fiberoptic
sigmoidoscope

C

D

Figure 43-IVC-3 *(Continued)*

(C) The laparoscope is introduced through the prior colostomy site. Exploration of the abdomen, followed by port placement as depicted earlier, is performed. Rigid proctoscopy or fiberoptic sigmoidoscopy may help identify the proximal Hartmann pouch.

(D) The apex of the Hartmann pouch is mobilized using a combination of sharp and blunt dissection.

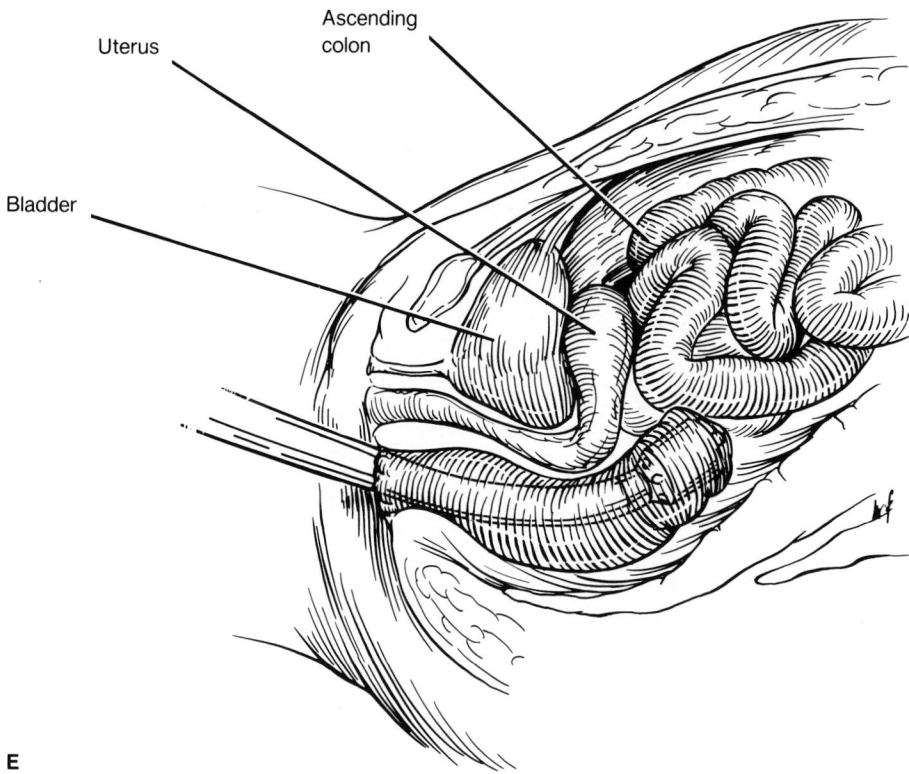

Uterus

Ascending
colon

Bladder

E

Figure 43-IVC-3 *(Continued)*

(E) A circular stapling device without the anvil but with a trocar within the cartridge is gently placed through the anus and passed to the apex of the mobilized Hartmann pouch. This process should be observed carefully by the laparoscopist to ensure no injury to the rectal stump.

(Continued)

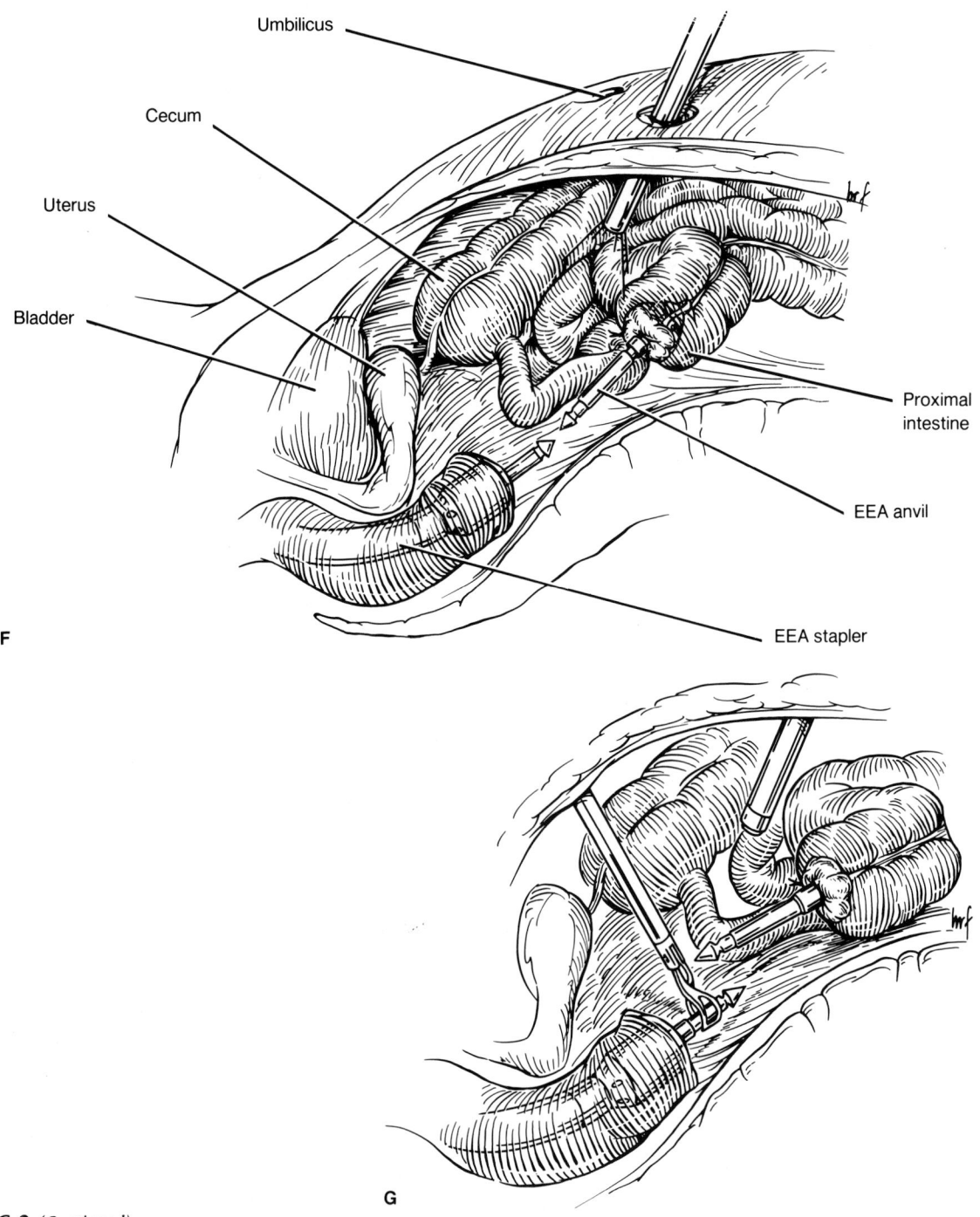

Umbilicus

Cecum

Uterus

Bladder

Proximal intestine

EEA anvil

EEA stapler

F

G

Figure 43-IVC-3 *(Continued)*

(F) Attention is next directed to the descending colon, which already has the anvil mechanism secured to its distal end. The surgeon must be certain that sufficient mobilization is present to allow a tension-free anastomosis to the apex of the Hartmann pouch. If there is any concern, additional mobilization of the splenic flexure must be achieved using electrocautery or clips as necessary. The circular stapling device is opened, thus advancing the trocar through the apex of the Hartmann pouch.

(G) The trocar is removed from the circular stapler cartridge mechanism. The anvil mechanism is inserted into the female receptacle on the cartridge of the circular stapler.

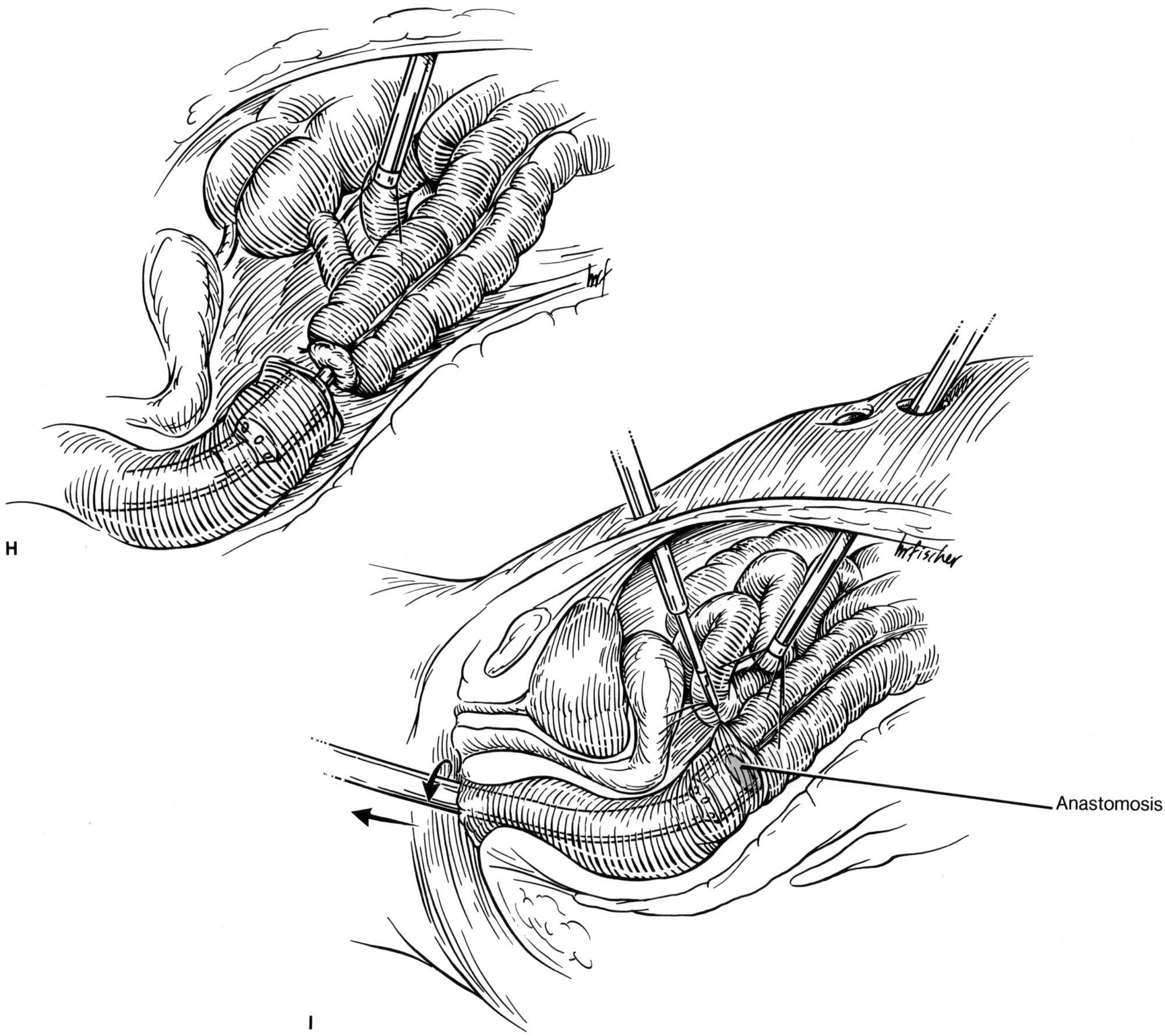

Anastomosis

I

Figure 43-IVC-3 *(Continued)*

(H) The stapling device is closed under laparoscopic visualization. This may require moving the laparoscope from its normal position to a side port.

(I) After firing the circular stapler and creating an end-to-end colorectal anastomosis to the top of the Hartmann pouch, the circular stapler is removed in the standard fashion. A proctoscope can then be inserted into the rectum and the integrity of the anastomosis assessed by insufflating air while the anastomosis is covered with saline. If there is no air leak, if the vascularity is sufficient, if the approximation appears accurate, if there is no tension, and if no extraneous tissue or other organs have been incorporated into the anastomosis, the anastomosis is secure.

D. Laparoscopic Colostomy

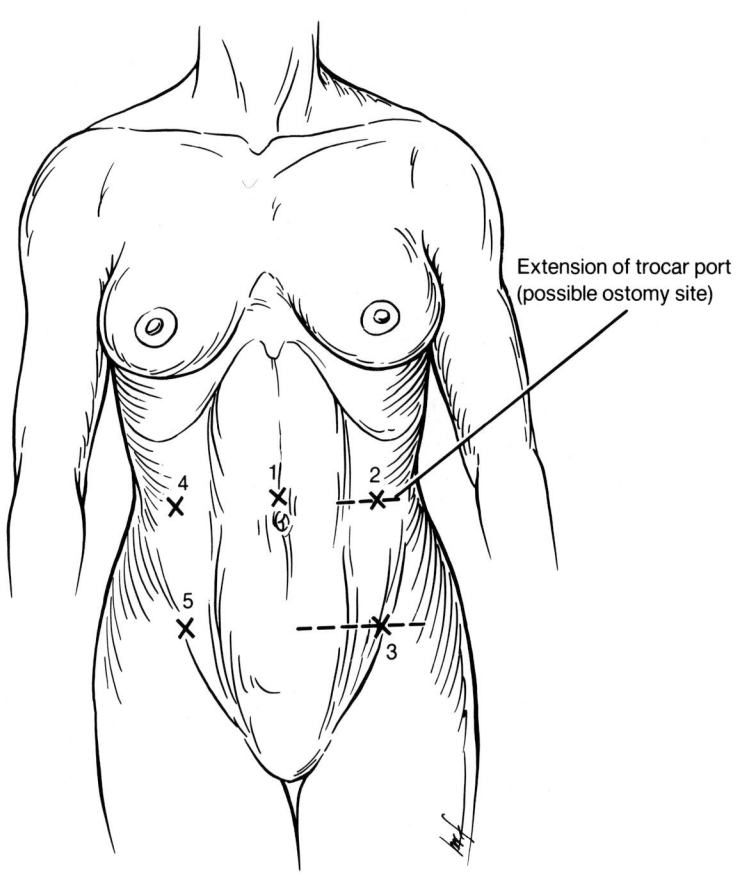

Extension of trocar port
(possible ostomy site)

Figure 43-IVD-1

Port Sites

Recommended port sites and functions: (1) 10/12 mm-port camera site; (2 and 3) 10/12-mm ports—possible sites of colostomy; (4 and 5) 10/12-mm ports—possible sites of ileostomy. The patient's abdominal wall should be carefully assessed in the sitting, standing, and lying positions before surgery to select optimal ostomy sites. Ostomy sites are best placed within the rectus abdominis muscle. The port sites should be adjusted accordingly. Laparoscopic ileostomy can be done in a similar manner as the technique shown here for laparoscopic colostomy.

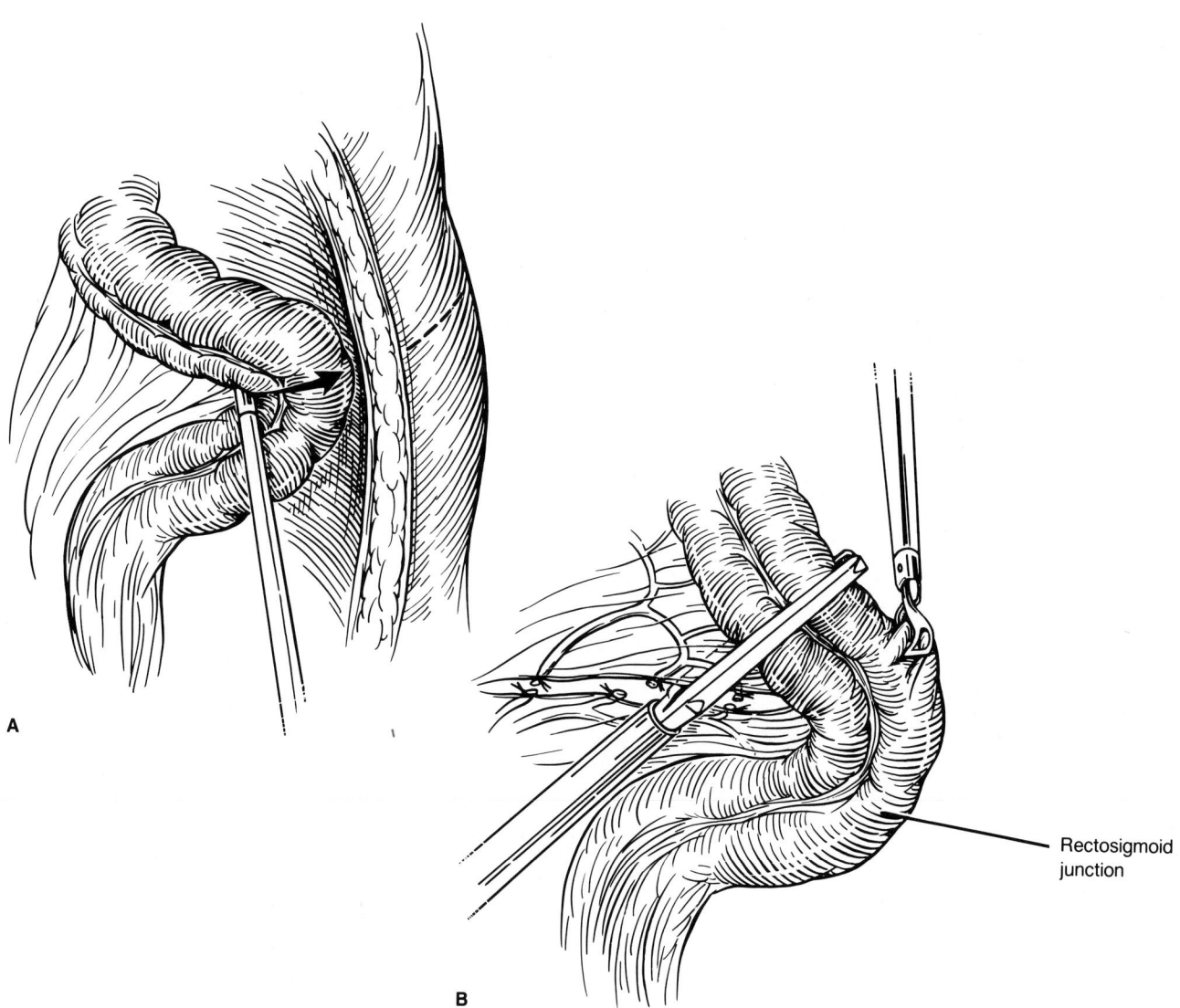

A

B

Rectosigmoid
junction

Figure 43-IVD-2

Procedure

(A) The sigmoid colon is mobilized by incising the lateral peritoneal attachments with electrocautery. Blunt dissection can be used. The left ureter and gonadal vessels should be identified and pushed posteriorly out of the field of dissection.

(B) A mesenteric window is created, and if necessary, several small mesenteric vessels may be clipped and divided. This should be done in manner that preserves blood supply proximally and distally. An endolinear cutter-stapler is placed through the mesenteric window to transect the colon, as shown. Once properly aligned, the stapler is fired, thus cutting and stapling both ends of bowel.

(Continued)

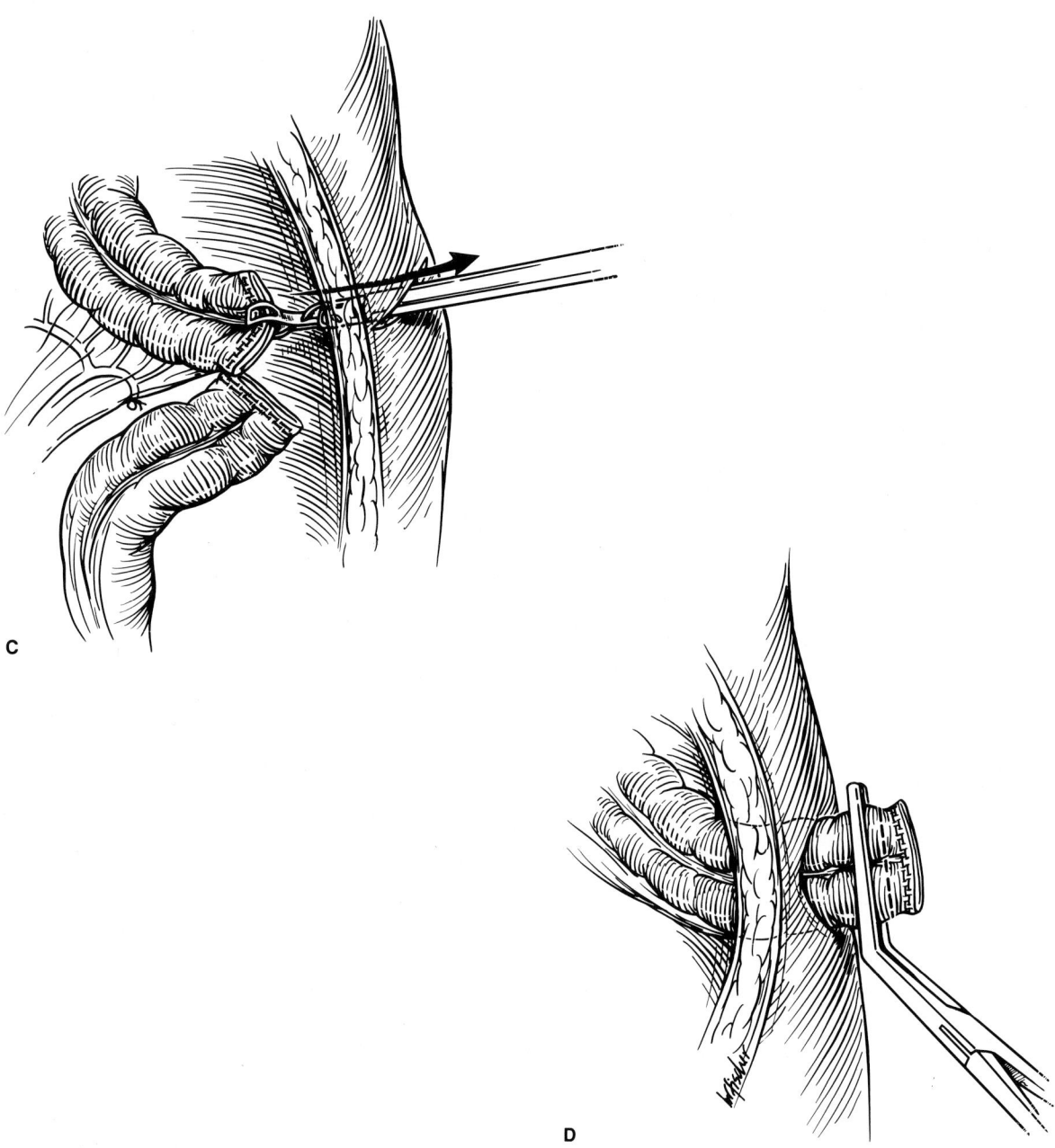

Figure 43-IVD-2 *(Continued)*

(C) The distal staple line is inspected carefully. This can be tested for integrity by insufflating air into the rectum through proctoscopy while the staple line is submerged under saline. Once the surgeon is sure that the staple line is intact distally, the proximal colon, which has been mobilized, is delivered transabdominally through the preselected stoma site in the standard fashion.

(D) The colostomy is matured once it has been delivered to the abdominal wall.

SECTION V Anorectal Surgery

A. Hemorrhoidectomy

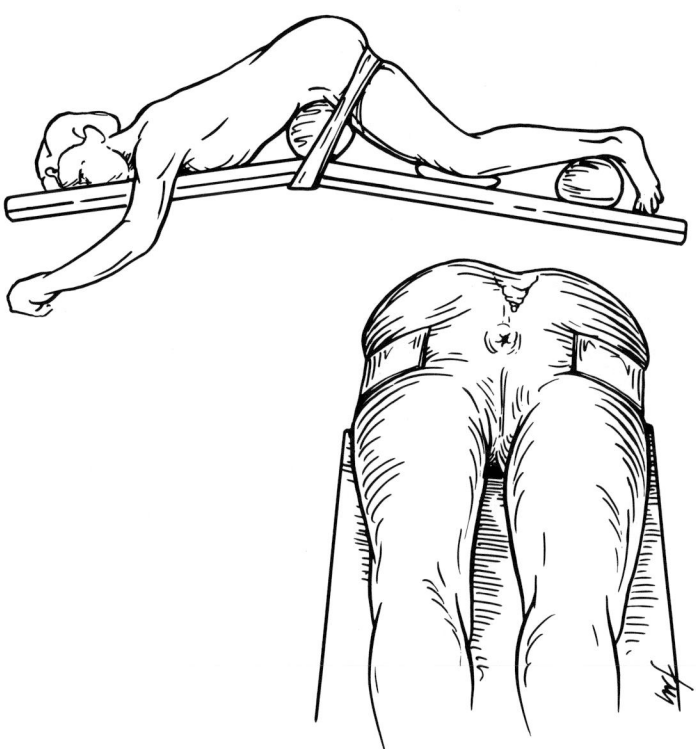

Figure 43-VA-1

Patient Positioning

The patient is placed in a prone position for most anal rectal operations. The table is slightly jackknifed, rolls are placed under the hips and ankles, and pads are placed under the knees. The buttocks are taped apart. No shave is necessary.

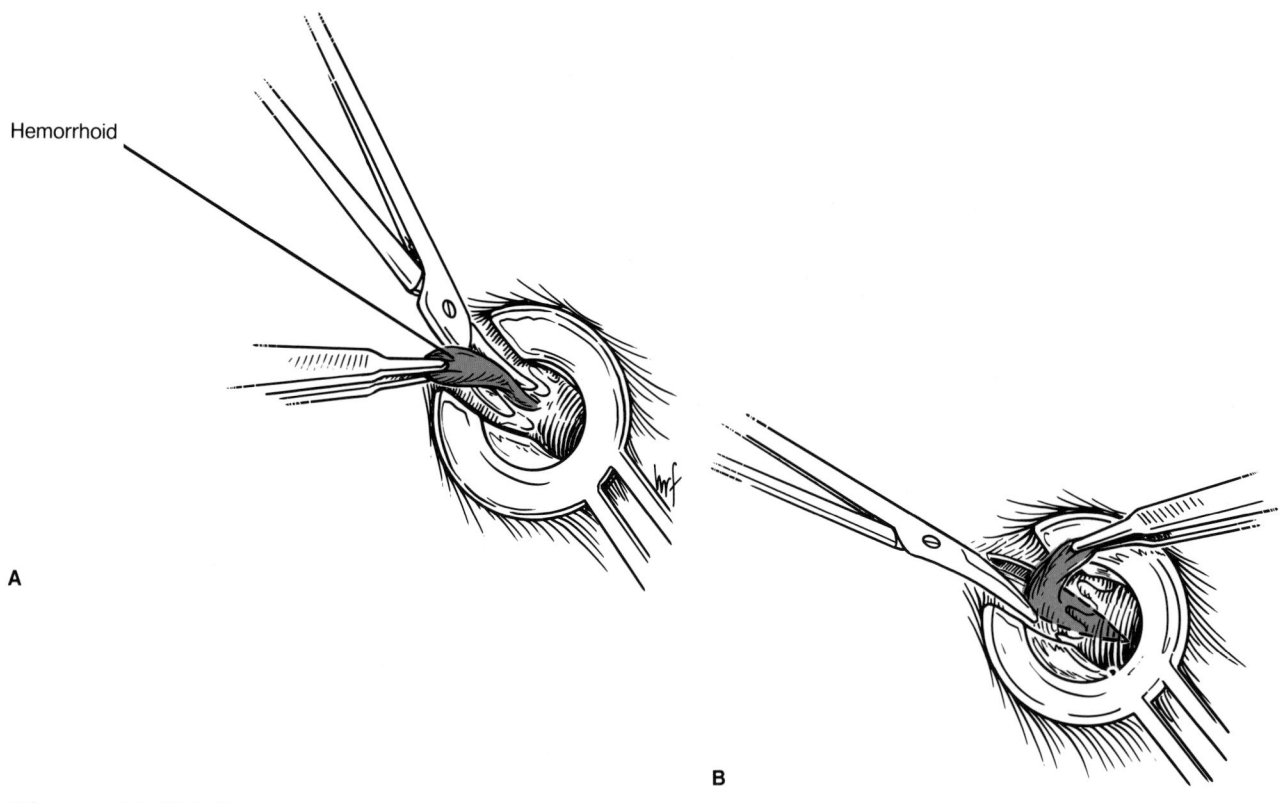

Figure 43-VA-2

Procedure

(A) A Fansler anoscope is inserted into the anal canal to achieve optimal exposure. An elliptical excision of a narrow strip of perianal skin, anoderm, is begun.

(B) The elliptical excision is continued proximally, excising external hemorrhoids, internal hemorrhoids, and redundant rectal mucosa in continuity up to the anorectal ring.

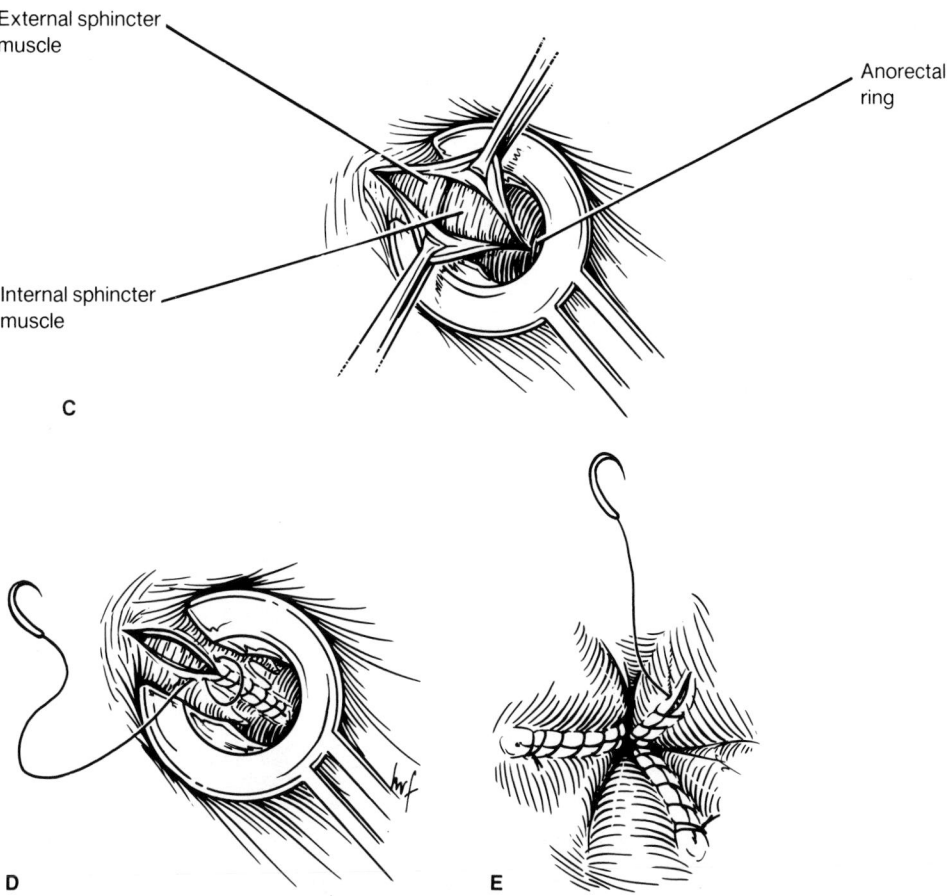

Figure 43-VA-2 *(Continued)*

(C) The resulting elliptical wound exposes the subcutaneous external and internal sphincter muscles. Flaps are elevated on either side of the excision to enable secondary hemorrhoids to be excised submucosally and subcutaneously and to allow the wound to be closed without tension.

(D) Closure of the wound is achieved using a continuous suture of 3-0 chromic cat gut.

(E) Excision and closure are completed in as many areas as necessary. Usually, left lateral, right posterior, and right anterior hemorrhoids are excised.

B. Sphincterotomy for Anal Fissure

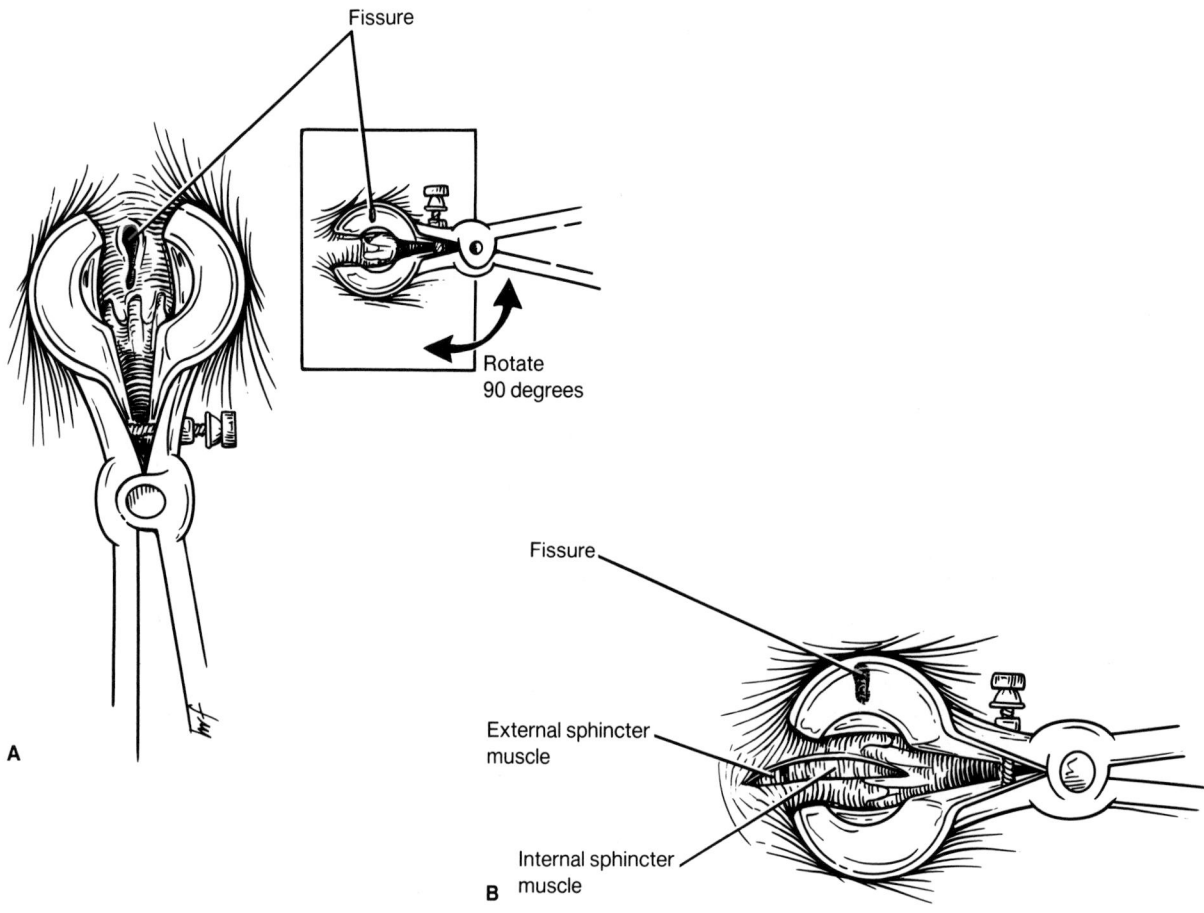

Figure 43-VB-1

Open Internal Sphincterotomy

(**A**) With the patient in a prone jackknife position, a bivalve operating anal speculum is used to identify the fissure in the posterior midline. The speculum is then rotated to expose the left lateral quadrant.

(**B**) A radial incision is made in the anoderm, extending from the dentate line distally to a point beyond the intersphincteric groove. The distal half of the internal sphincter muscle is exposed.

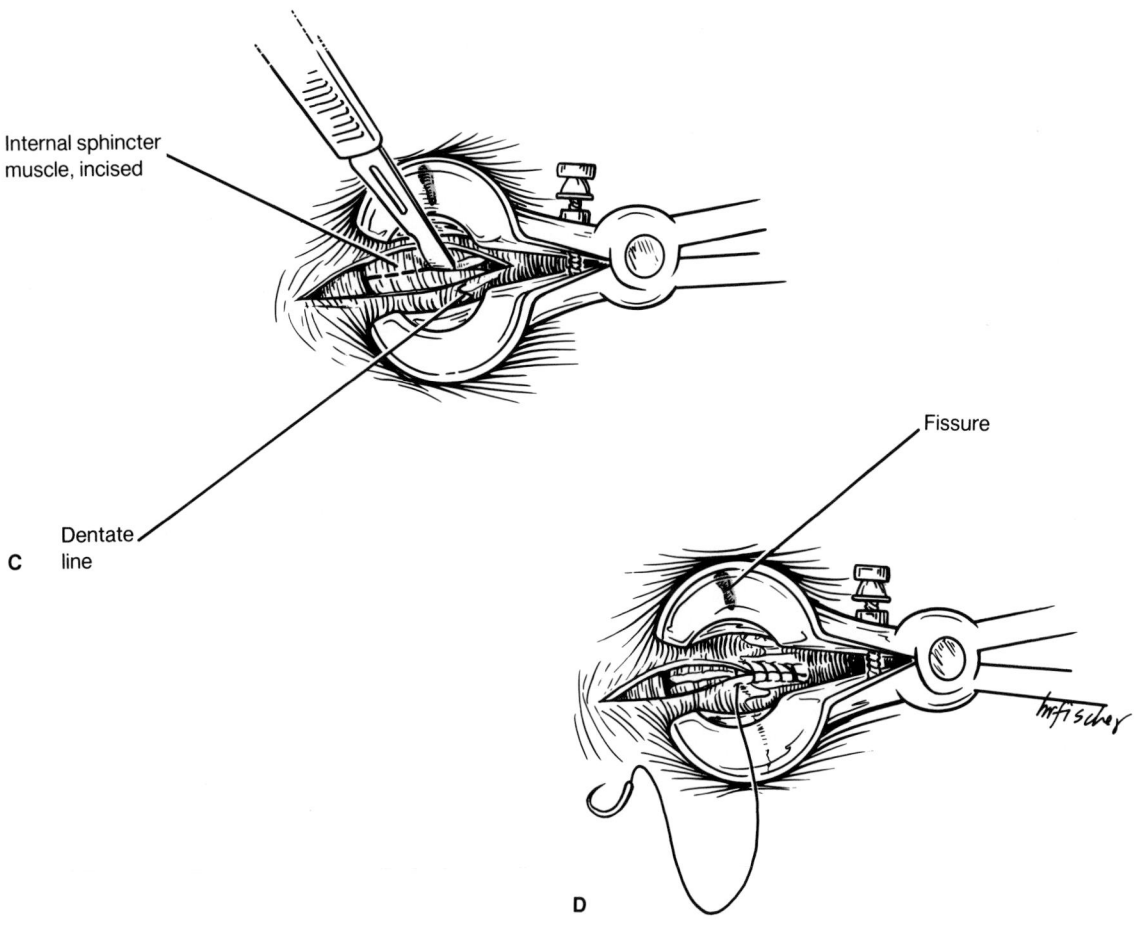

Figure 43-VB-1 *(Continued)*

(C) The distal half of the internal sphincter muscle is divided in its full thickness, extending from the level of the dentate line to its visible lower edge at the intersphincteric groove.

(D) After achieving hemostasis with electrocautery, the radial incision is closed with a continuous 3-0 chromic cat gut suture.

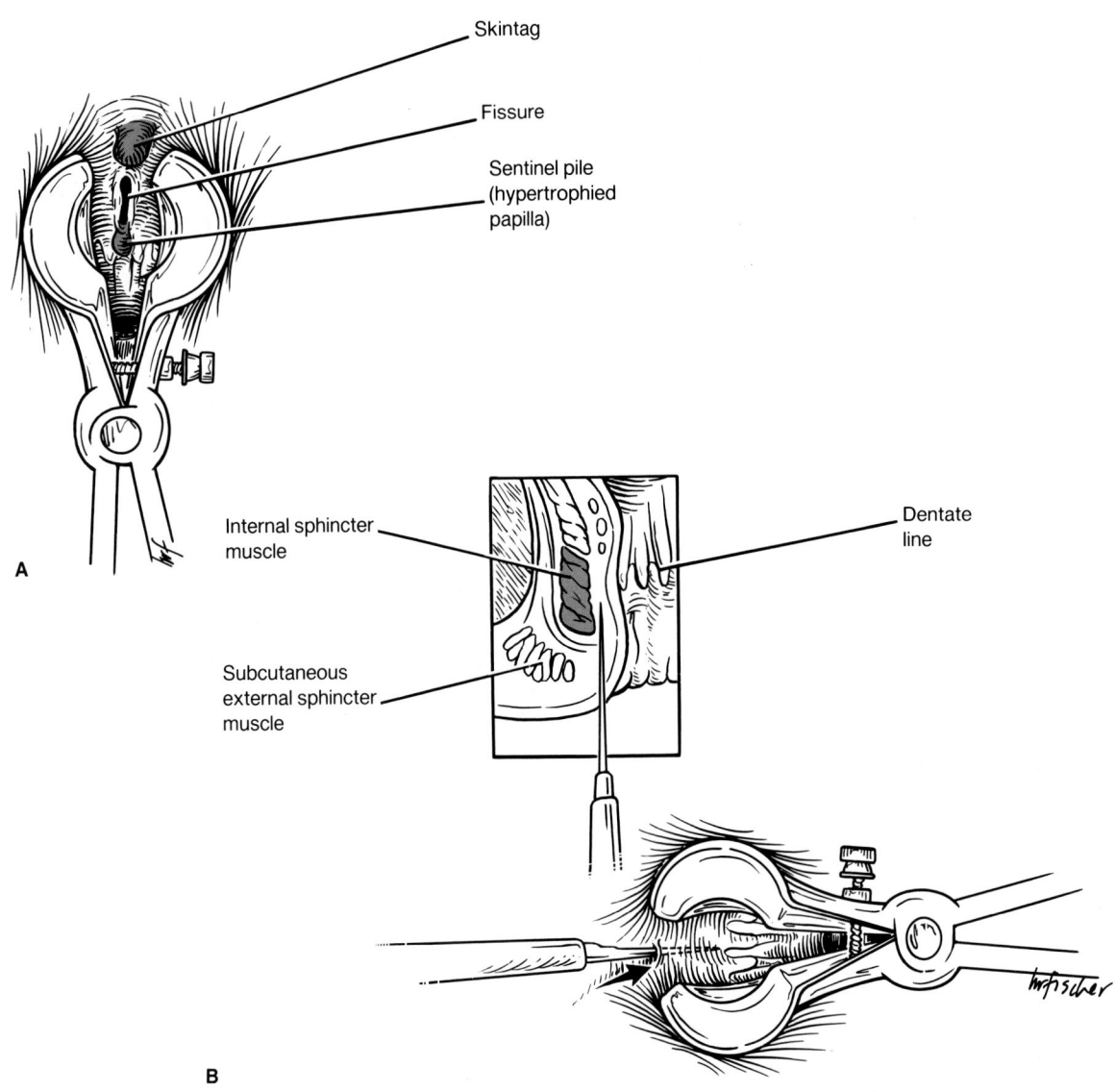

Figure 43-VB-2

Closed Internal Sphincterotomy

(**A**) With the patient in the prone jackknife position, a bivalve operating anal speculum is used to identify the fissure in the posterior midline.

(**B**) The anal speculum is rotated to expose the left lateral quadrant. The intersphincteric groove is easily identified by palpation by spreading the anal speculum. Using a pointed, narrow cataract blade, a stab is made into the anoderm at the intersphincteric groove. The blade is passed under the anoderm to the level of the dentate line at the base of the anal papilla.

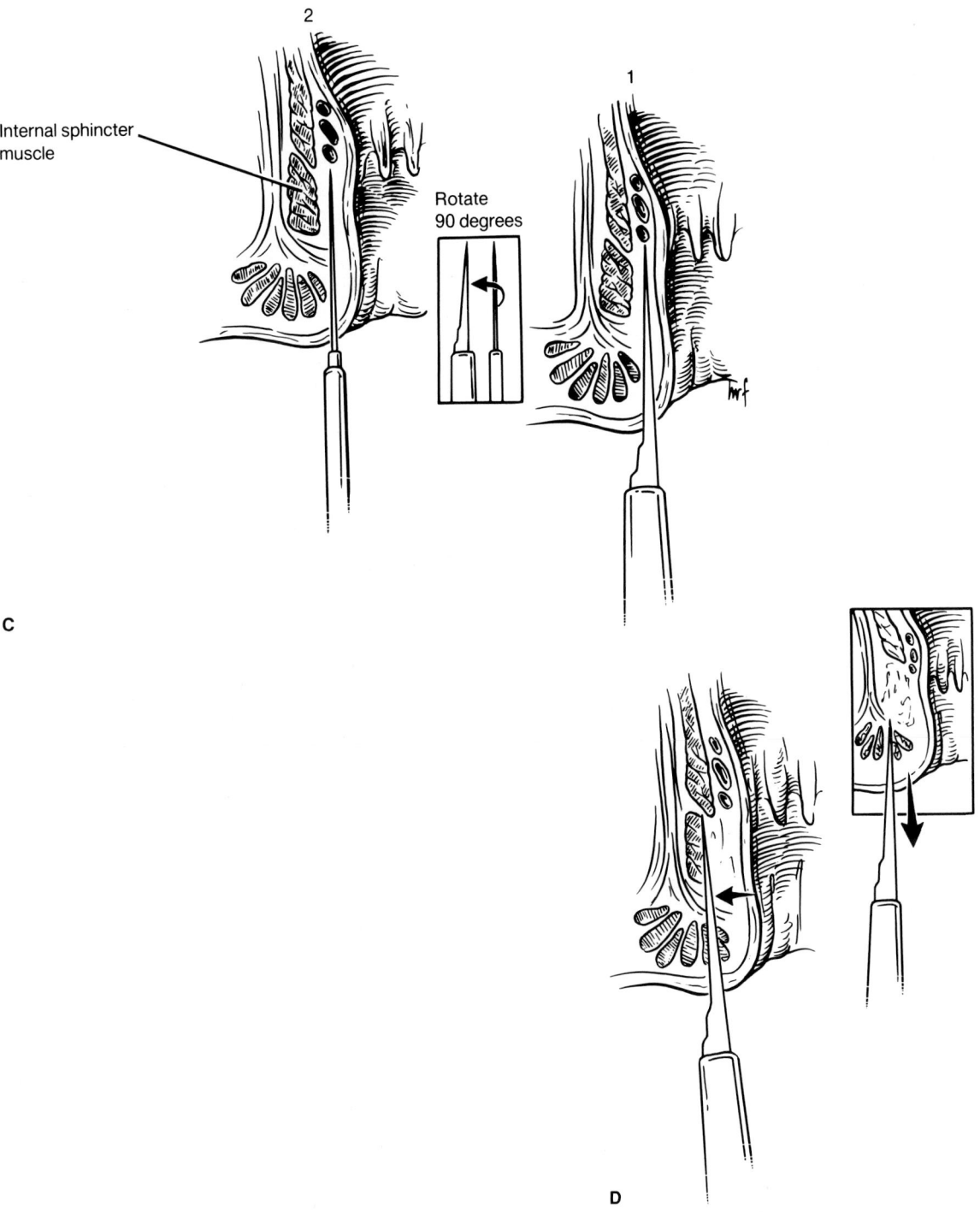

Figure 43-VB-2 *(Continued)*

(C) The blade is rotated 90 degrees so the cutting edge faces externally.

(D) The cutting edge of the blade is passed through the full thickness of the distal half of the internal sphincter muscle and withdrawn. Often, some fibers of the subcutaneous external sphincter muscle are divided as well. The blade is withdrawn from the original stab incision. Complete division of the internal sphincter muscle is confirmed by digital palpation. Hemostasis is achieved by pressure.

C. Anoplasty for Anal Stricture

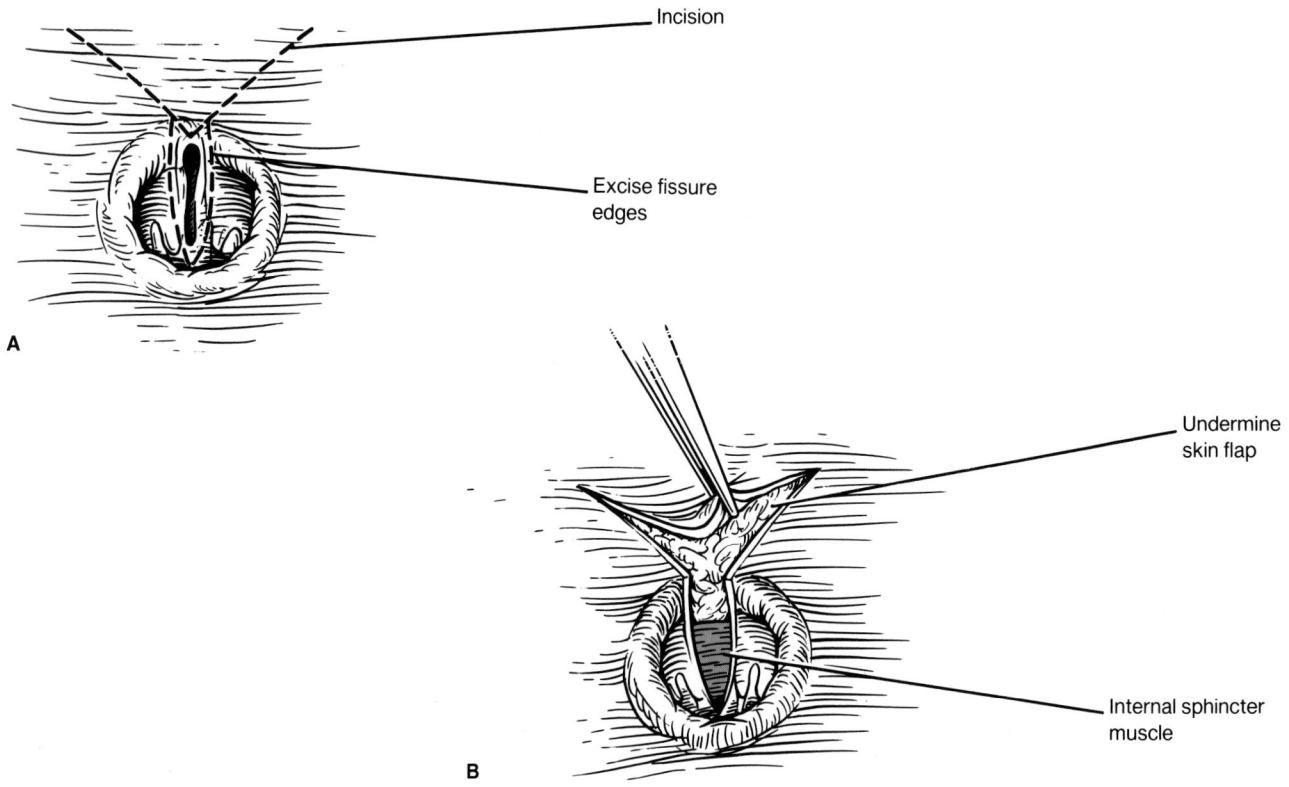

Figure 43-VC-1

Y-V Anoplasty

(**A**) With the patient in the prone jackknife position, the posterior aspect of the anal canal is exposed to exhibit an anal fissure that has resulted in an anal stricture. Often, a speculum cannot be inserted into the anal canal because of the degree of stricture. The anal fissure with the stenotic anoderm is excised. A broadly based posterior V flap of perianal skin is outlined and incised. It is critical that each limb of this flap be at least 4 or 5 cm long.

(**B**) The V flap is undercut and elevated. Lateral skin flaps are undermined. This results in a Y-shaped wound with exposure of the internal sphincter muscle along the stem of the Y.

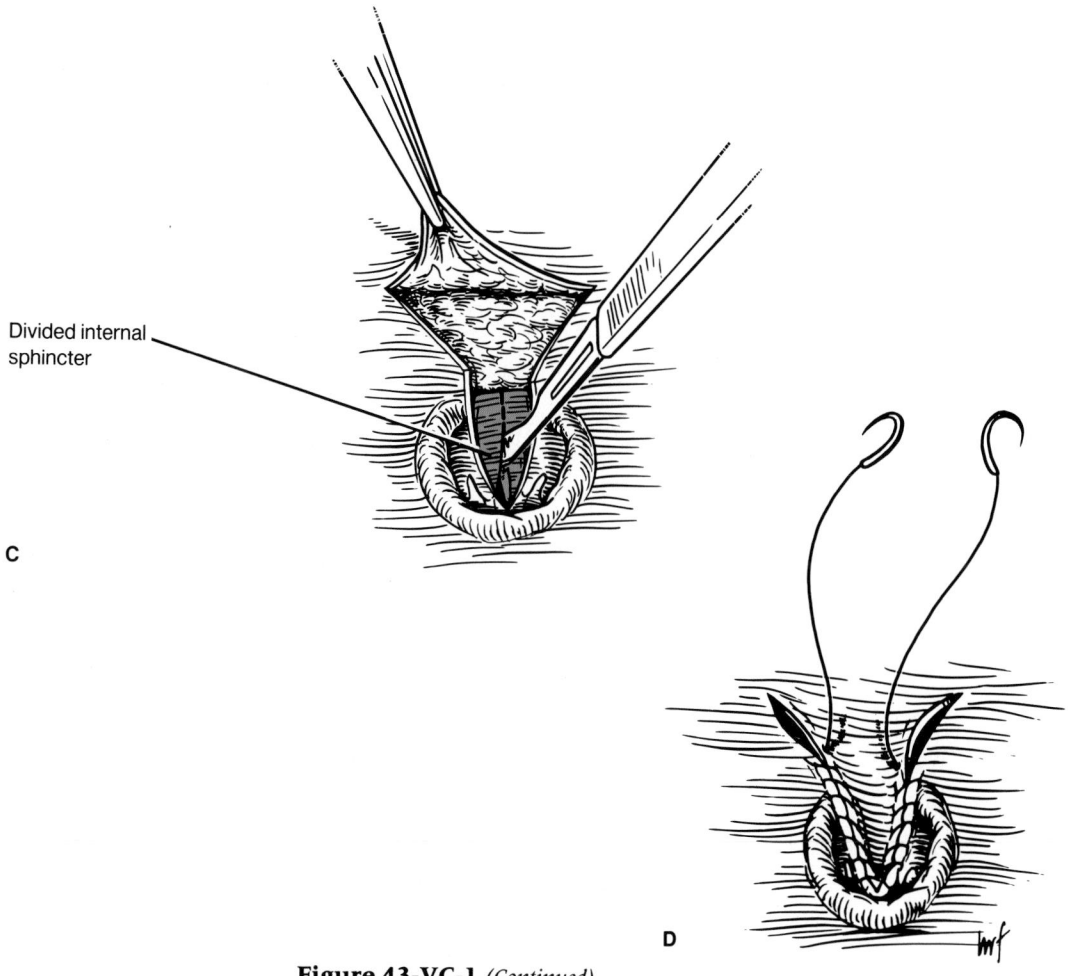

Divided internal
sphincter

C

D

Figure 43-VC-1 *(Continued)*

(C) An open internal sphincterotomy is performed to complete correction of the anal stricture.

(D) The mobilized V flap is advanced into the anal canal. The apex of the flap is sutured to the sphincter muscle at the level of the dentate line, using two or three 2-0 or 3-0 polyglycolic acid sutures. The now V-shaped wound is completely closed with a running polyglycolic acid suture.

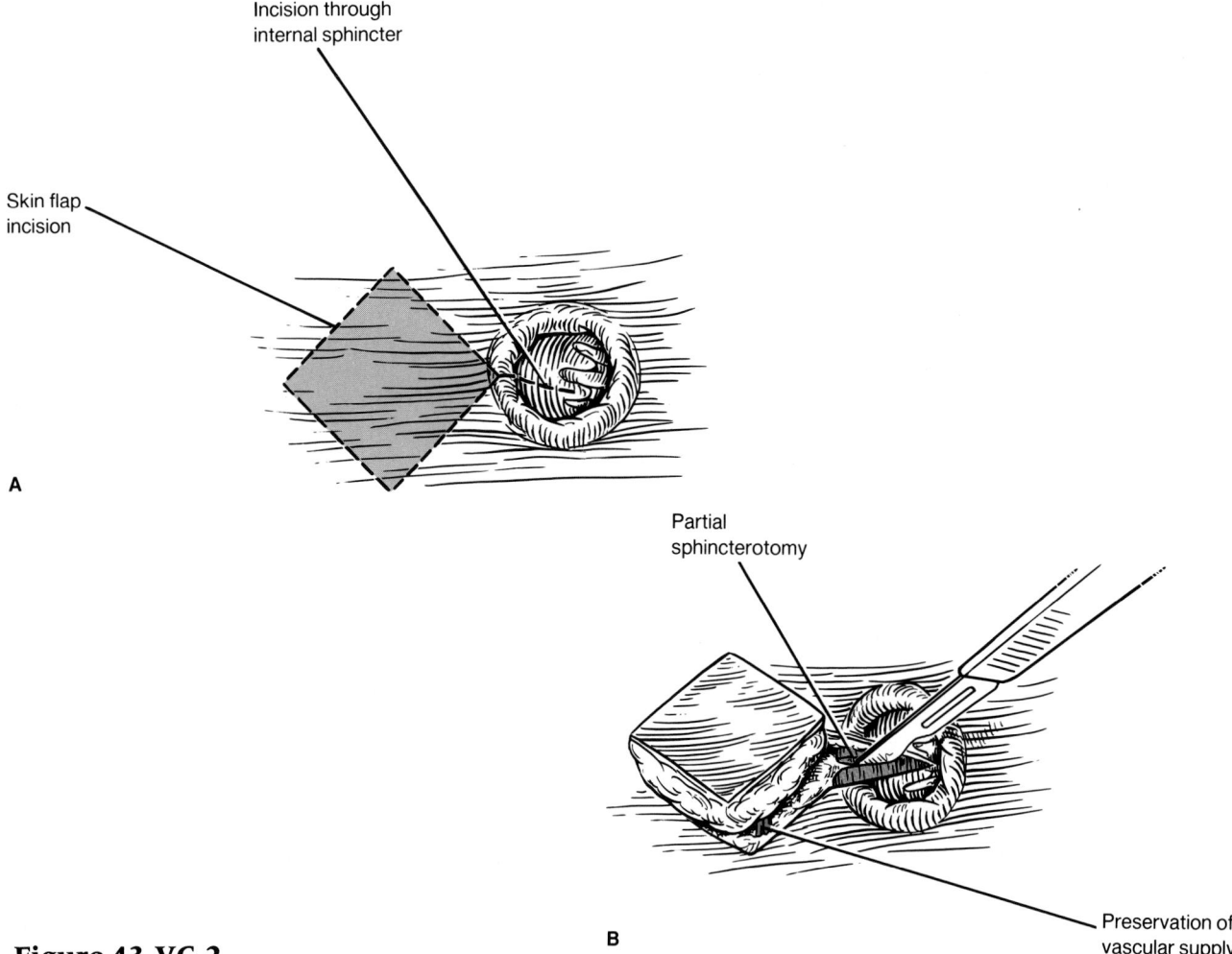

Figure 43-VC-2

Diamond-Flap Anoplasty

(A) With the patient in the prone jackknife position, the left lateral quadrant is exposed and a diamond-shaped skin incision outlined on the perianal skin. The anal stricture is incised radially to enable a partial open internal sphincterotomy to be performed.

(B) The diamond-shaped flap is mobilized by a deep incision into the subcutaneous fat, taking care not to undermine the blood supply to the isolated skin island. A partial internal sphincterotomy is completed.

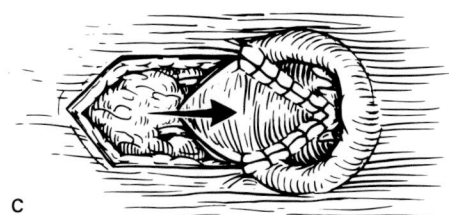

C

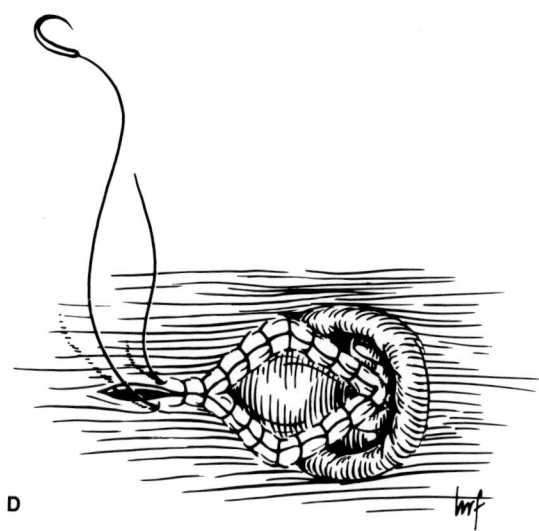

D

Figure 43-VC-2 *(Continued)*

(C) The mobilized flap is advanced into the anal canal, thus closing the radial defect of the anoderm and internal sphincter muscle. Interrupted 2-0 or 3-0 polyglycolic acid sutures are used to hold the diamond flap in place.

(D) The external wounds can generally be closed without tension, resulting in a tennis racquet–shaped incision. This is accomplished with polyglycolic acid suture.

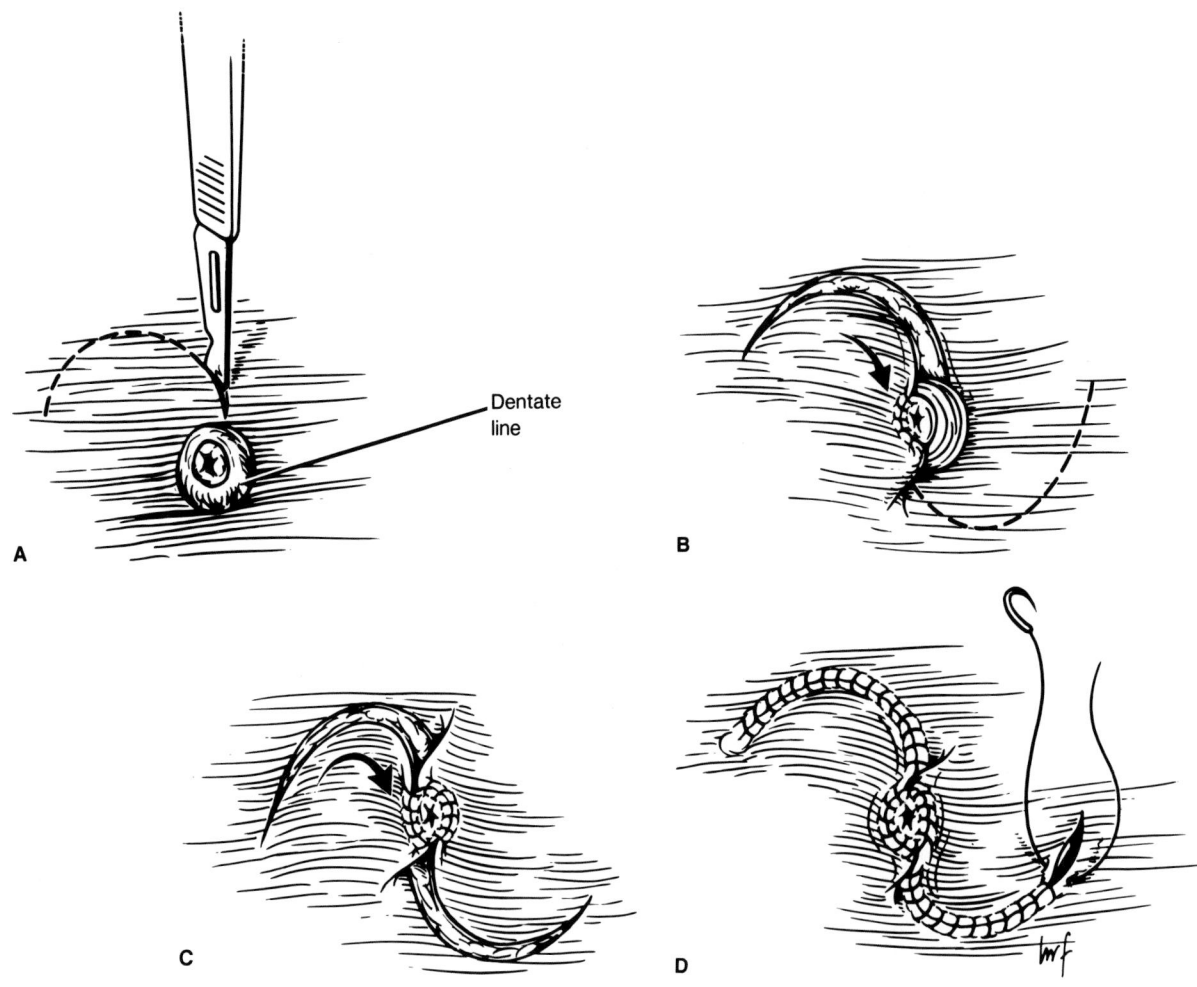

Dentate line

Figure 43-VC-3

S Flap Anoplasty

(A) With the patient in a prone jackknife position, the anoderm or mucosal ectropion, along with any stricture, has been excised to the level of the dentate line, thus exposing the internal sphincter muscle. An internal open sphincterotomy may be performed if necessary. A curved C flap is outlined on the buttocks skin posteriorly and incised. The flap is mobilized by deep undercutting.

(B) The mobilized flap is rotated into the anal canal by suturing to the dentate line with 2-0 or 3-0 polyglycolic acid sutures. If the defect is circumferential, a second C flap is constructed anteriorly. The combination of the two C flaps creates an S incision.

(C) Both flaps are rotated into the anal canal and sutured to the dentate line. This covers the circumferential defect created by excision of the anoderm.

(D) The large external wounds are closed completely when possible, using interrupted sutures or staples. For large flaps, it is advisable to close the subcutaneous portion over a closed-suction drain. If there is excess tension on the most lateral aspects of the flaps, the wounds can be left open to heal secondarily.

D. Surgery for Anal Fistulas

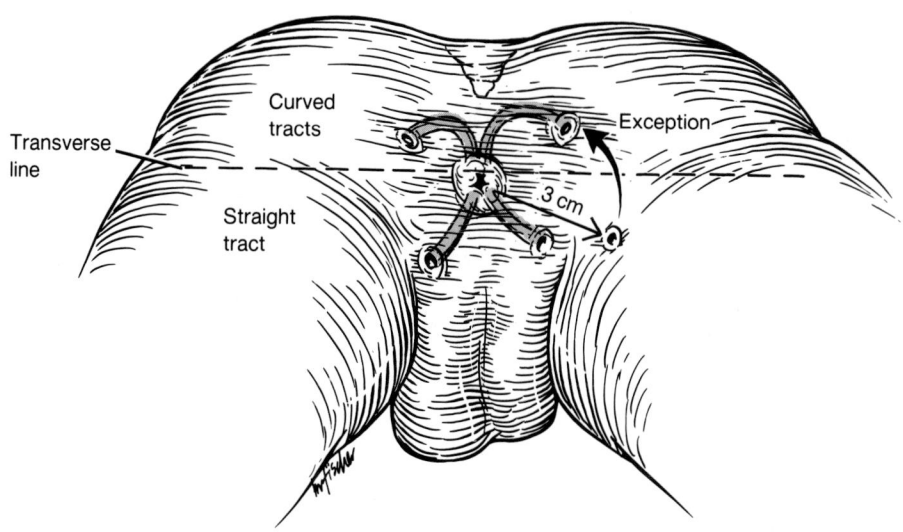

Figure 43-VD-1

Fistula-in-Ano

The number, location, and relation to the anal canal of external openings from chronic fistulas often reveal the cause of the fistula, the type of fistula (intersphincteric, transsphincteric, or more complex), and the origin of the fistula. Multiple external fistulas are highly suggestive of perianal Crohn's disease. External openings adjacent to the anal margin suggest an intersphincteric fistula, but external openings more distant from the anal margin suggest the possibility of a transsphincteric fistula. The greater the distance of the external opening from the anal margin, the greater is the probability that there is an associated, complicated upward extension of the basic fistula. The Goodsall rule suggests that if there is an opening posterior to the transverse anal line, the fistula probably originates from the posterior midline crypt. If the external opening is anterior to the transverse anal line, the fistula probably originates from the crypt directly in line with the external opening. External openings adjacent to the transverse anal line are exceptions to the rule and can track in any of a number of directions.

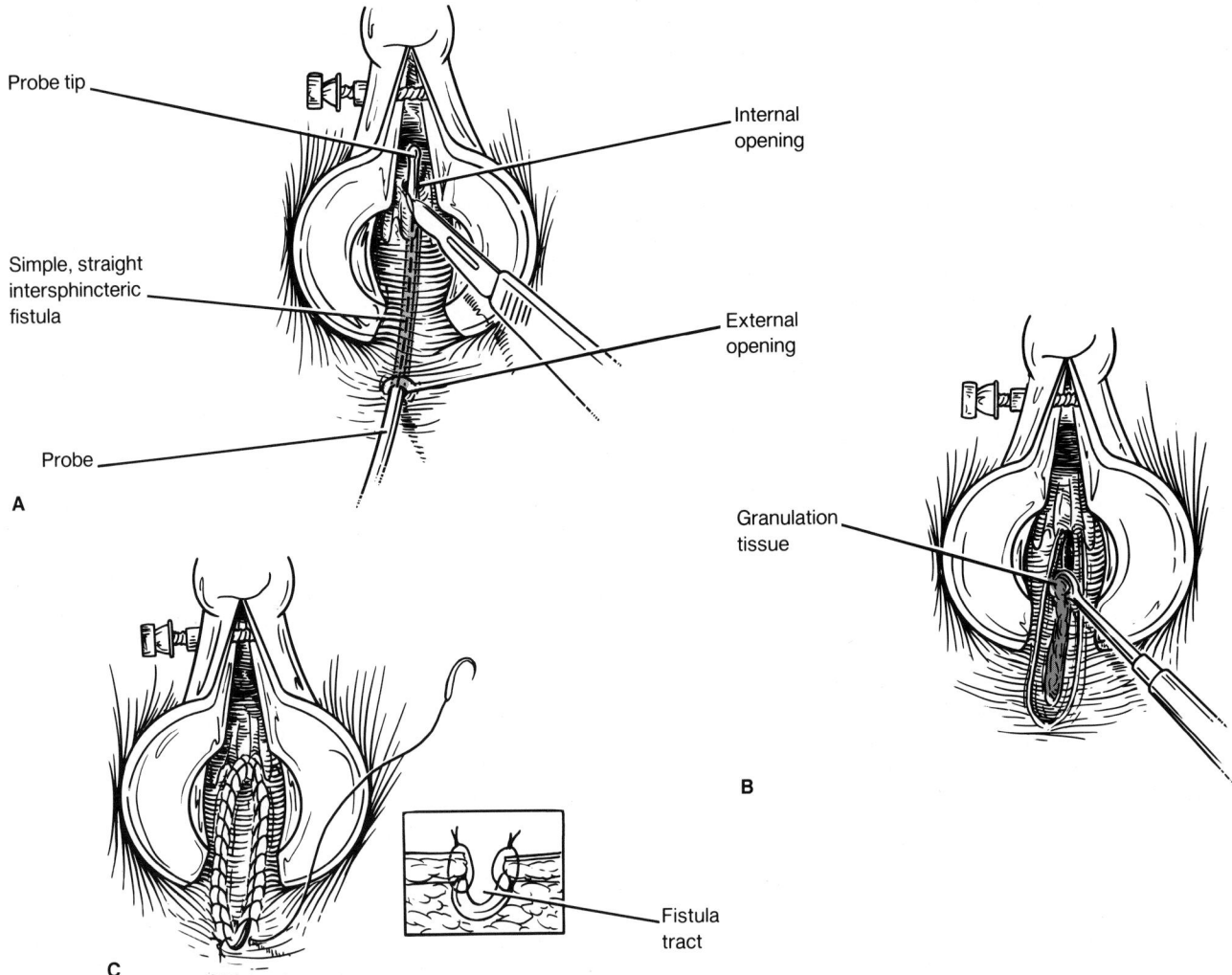

Figure 43-VD-2

Intersphincteric Fistulotomy

(A) Fistula surgery is preferably performed with the patient in a prone jackknife position under a local, regional, or general anesthetic. An anal bivalve speculum is inserted into the anal canal to exclude other pathology and search for the internal opening. If the internal opening is not initially apparent, a probe is gently inserted through the external opening. An intersphincteric fistula has been demonstrated by passing the probe from the external opening into the internal opening at the dentate line. A fistulotomy is performed by incising the mucosa, submucosa, and internal sphincter muscle overlying the probe. If the surgeon has difficulty identifying the internal opening, it is best not to force the probe. Instead, the fistulotomy is begun at the external opening and extended internally after the granulation tissue at the base of the fistula. Usually, this makes the internal opening apparent.

(B) After the initial fistulotomy, the excess granulation tissue along the base of the fistula is débrided with a curette. The external opening is often surrounded by an area of induration and can be excised sharply. The internal opening can similarly be excised by a small back cut at the level of the anal crypt.

(C) After achieving hemostasis with use of electrocautery, the fistula wound is marsupialized with a 3-0 absorbable suture. The cut edges are sewn down to the fibrous base of the fistula, which is left in place and not excised. This ensures hemostasis along the cut edges and decreases the size of the open wound, which heals secondarily with minimal discomfort to the patient. A fistulotomy is preferred over fistulectomy, which produces a much larger wound.

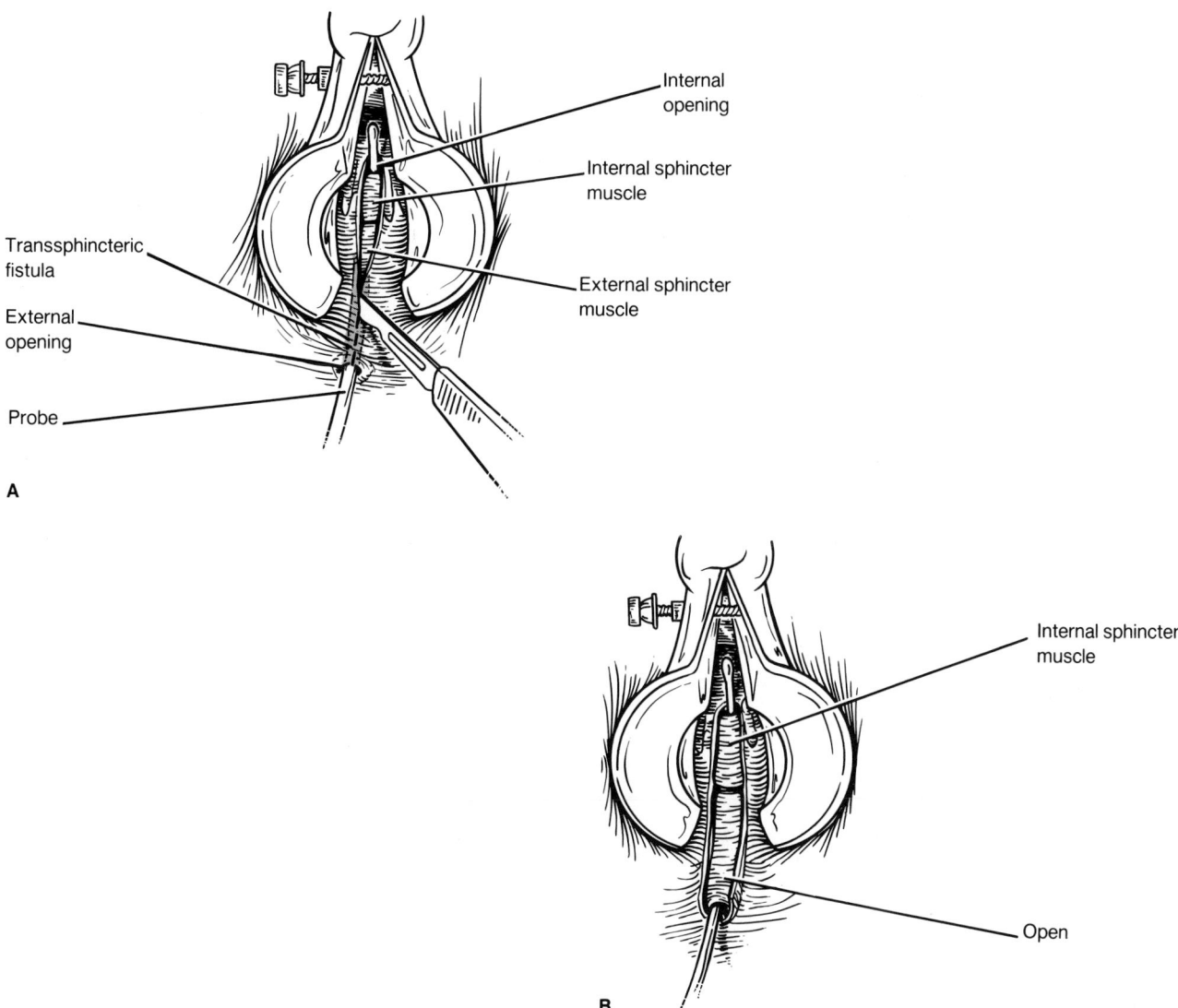

Figure 43-VD-3

Treatment of Transsphincteric Fistula

(A) An uncomplicated transsphincteric fistula has been demonstrated by passing the probe from the external opening into the internal opening. The mucosa, submucosa, and anoderm overlying the muscle are first incised to allow the surgeon to assess the degree of sphincter muscle involved in the transsphincteric fistula.

(B) Most uncomplicated transsphincteric fistulas cross the external sphincter muscle distally, and thus a lay-open technique results in division of only the distal portion of the external sphincter and the distal half of the internal sphincter. In most patients, this does not result in significant disturbance of continence. Anterior transsphincteric fistulas in women or transsphincteric fistulas in patients with preexisting partial anal incontinence, diarrheal conditions, or the elderly must be treated more conservatively.

(Continued)

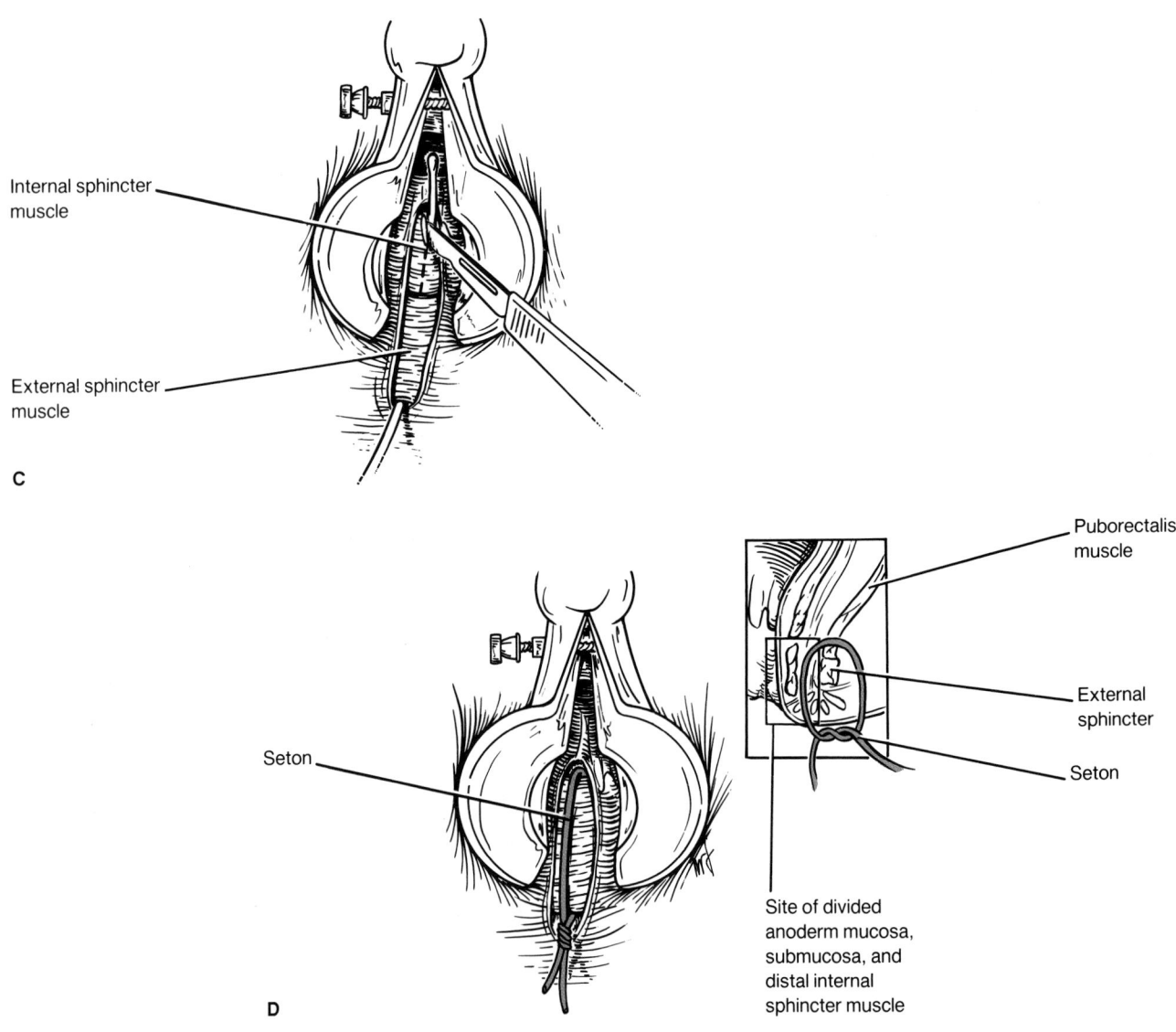

Figure 43-VD-3 *(Continued)*

(C) It is best to divide the distal internal sphincter muscle and reassess to determine how much external sphincter muscle is involved. If the transsphincteric fistula crosses proximally, incontinence results from division of the external sphincter muscle, and an alternative to the lay-open fistulotomy must be used.

(D) One option for management of a deep transsphincteric fistula is to place a nonabsorbable suture through the track to encircle the external sphincter muscle involved in the fistula. This acts as a drain to allow the rest of the wound to heal around the seton. The seton can then serve as a guide to the surgeon performing a second-stage fistulotomy. Alternatively, the seton can be used to "walk through" the external sphincter muscle, dividing a few fibers at a time and allowing fibrosis and scarring to occur on the opposite side of the seton until the seton finally is all the way through the sphincter muscle. This technique prevents the muscle from separating as a wide gap.

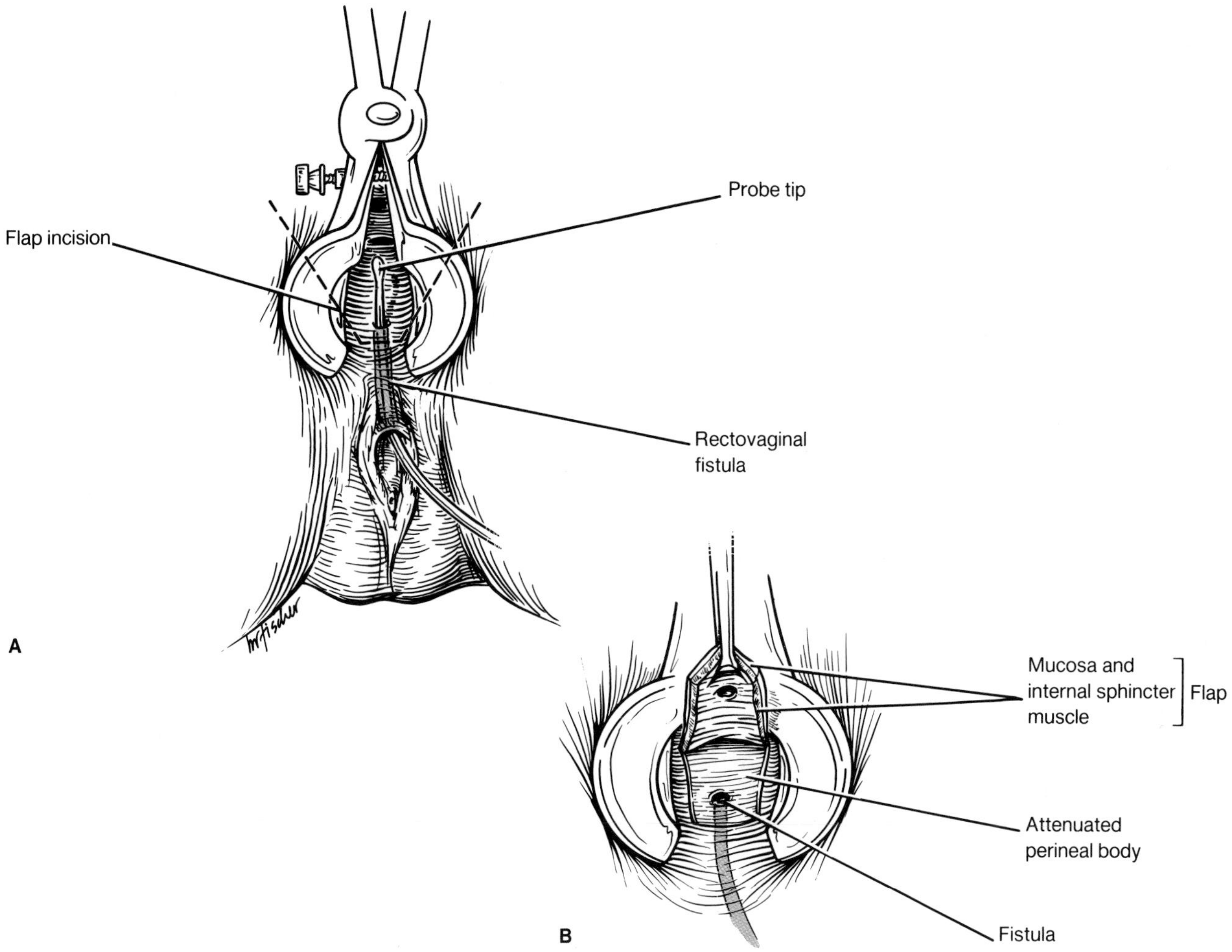

Figure 43-VD-4

Treatment of Rectovaginal Fistula

(A) Distal rectal vaginal fistulas not directly involving the anal sphincter mechanism can be treated with an endorectal flap advancement technique. Most such fistulas are due to birthing injuries. Many heal spontaneously over a period of several months after the labor and delivery. It is essential that local tissues are as close to normal with resolution of all sepsis before undertaking operative repair. With the patient in the prone jackknife position under a general or regional block anesthetic, a bivalve anoscope is used to expose the distal anal canal. The rectal vaginal fistula is identified by passing a probe through the vagina and through the fistula, entering the distal anal canal cephalad to the anal sphincter. A rectal flap around the fistula is outlined so that the base of the flap is about two times the width of the apex of the flap, thus ensuring adequate blood supply.

(B) The flap, consisting of mucosa, submucosa, and internal sphincter muscle, is elevated from the apex to the base. This exposes an attenuated perineal body surrounding the fistula into the vagina.

(Continued)

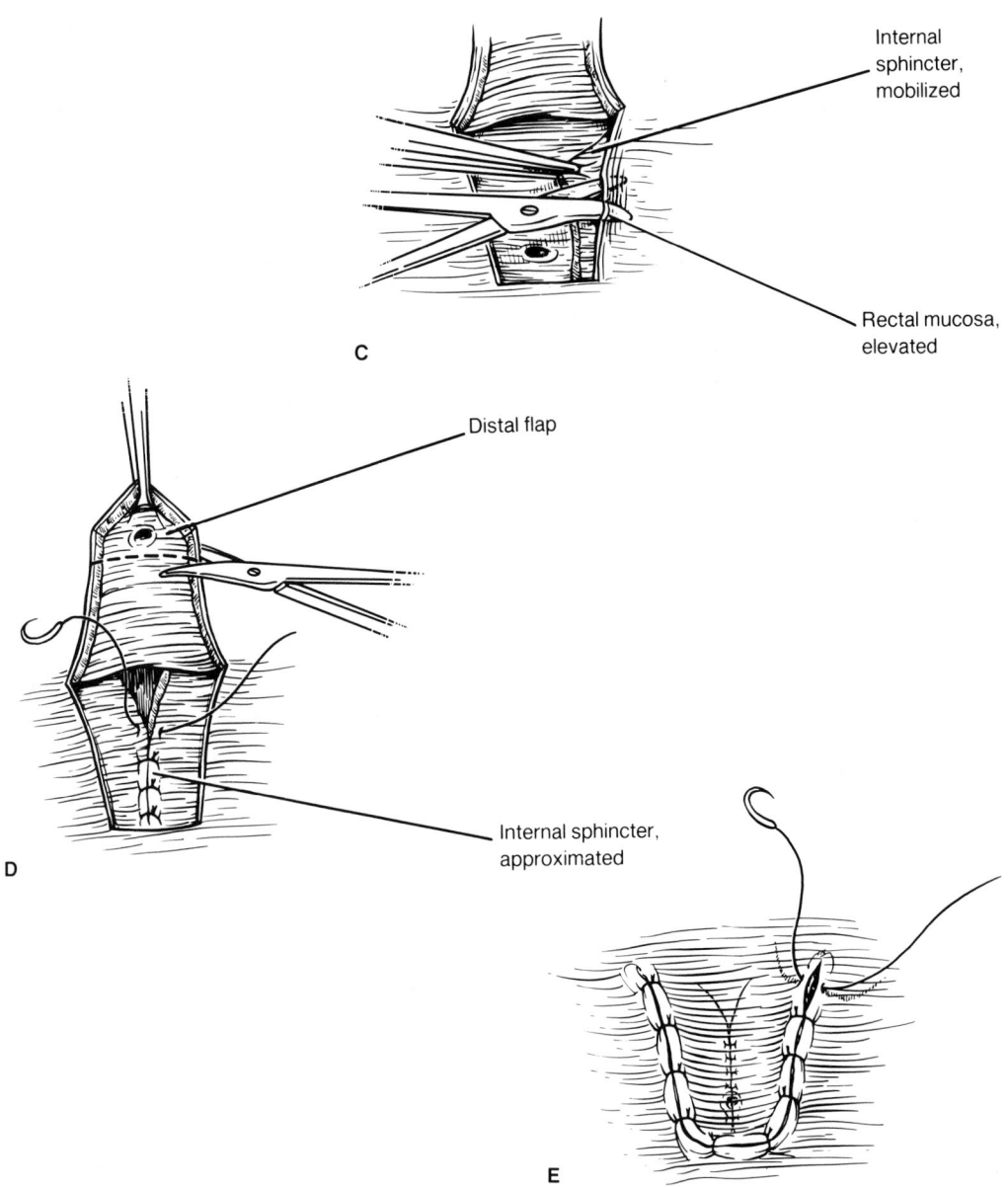

Figure 43-VD-4 *(Continued)*

(C) The cut edge of the circular muscle is grasped and retracted medially while the over-lying mucosa and submucosa are elevated laterally. Sufficient mobilization is necessary to allow the sphincter muscle to be approximated in the midline without tension.

(D) The perineal body and rectal vaginal septum are then reconstructed by placing multiple 2-0 polyglycolic acid sutures through the cut edge of the circular muscle. The sutures are tied serially to achieve a tension-free muscle approximation.

(E) After ensuring perfect hemostasis, the previously mobilized flap is sutured in place with 3-0 interrupted polyglycolic acid sutures along the sides and apex. Excess flap, in-cluding the site of the original fistula, is excised. This restores normal anal canal anatomy and obliterates the site of the fistula with two levels of well-vascularized muscle-containing tissue. The vaginal mucosa is left open for drainage.

E. Surgery for Rectal Procidentia

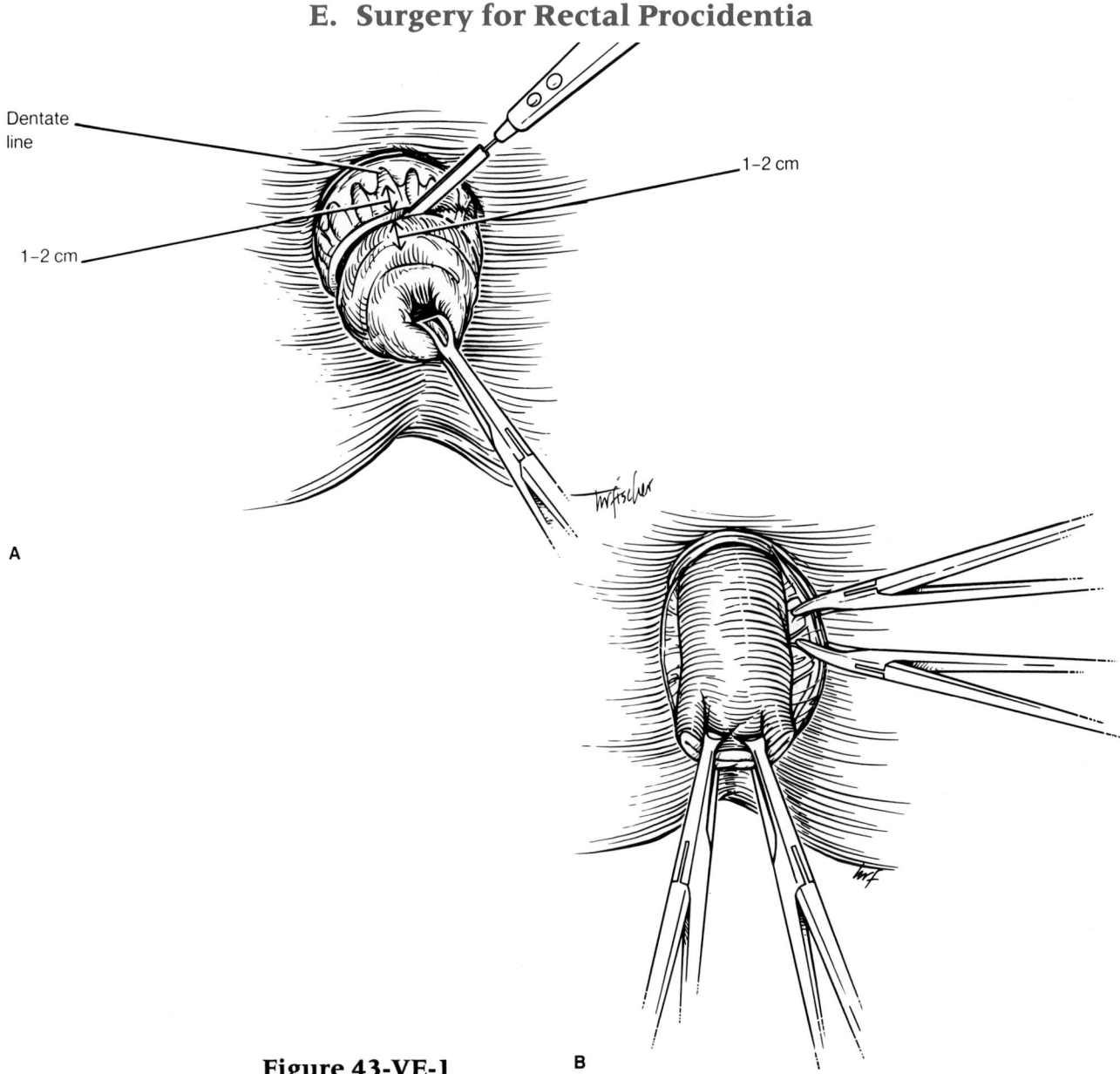

Figure 43-VE-1

Perineal Rectosigmoidectomy

(A) The patient has undergone a mechanical bowel preparation. Either lithotomy or prone jackknife position is used, and the operation is performed under local, regional block, or general anesthetic. The rectum is grasped and prolapsed out beyond the anal verge, as demonstrated. A circumferential incision through all layers of the outer rectal wall is made 1 to 2 cm proximal to the dentate line. This length allows an easy anastomosis to be performed but is not so long as to allow postoperative protrusion of redundant tissue.

(B) The mesorectum and mesenteric vessels supplying the prolapsed segment of bowel are clamped, divided, and tied with 2-0 absorbable suture. The peritoneum is exposed anteriorly and opened. All redundancy can be eliminated by traction on the prolapsing segment and mesenteric division until a moderate degree of tension exists.

(Continued)

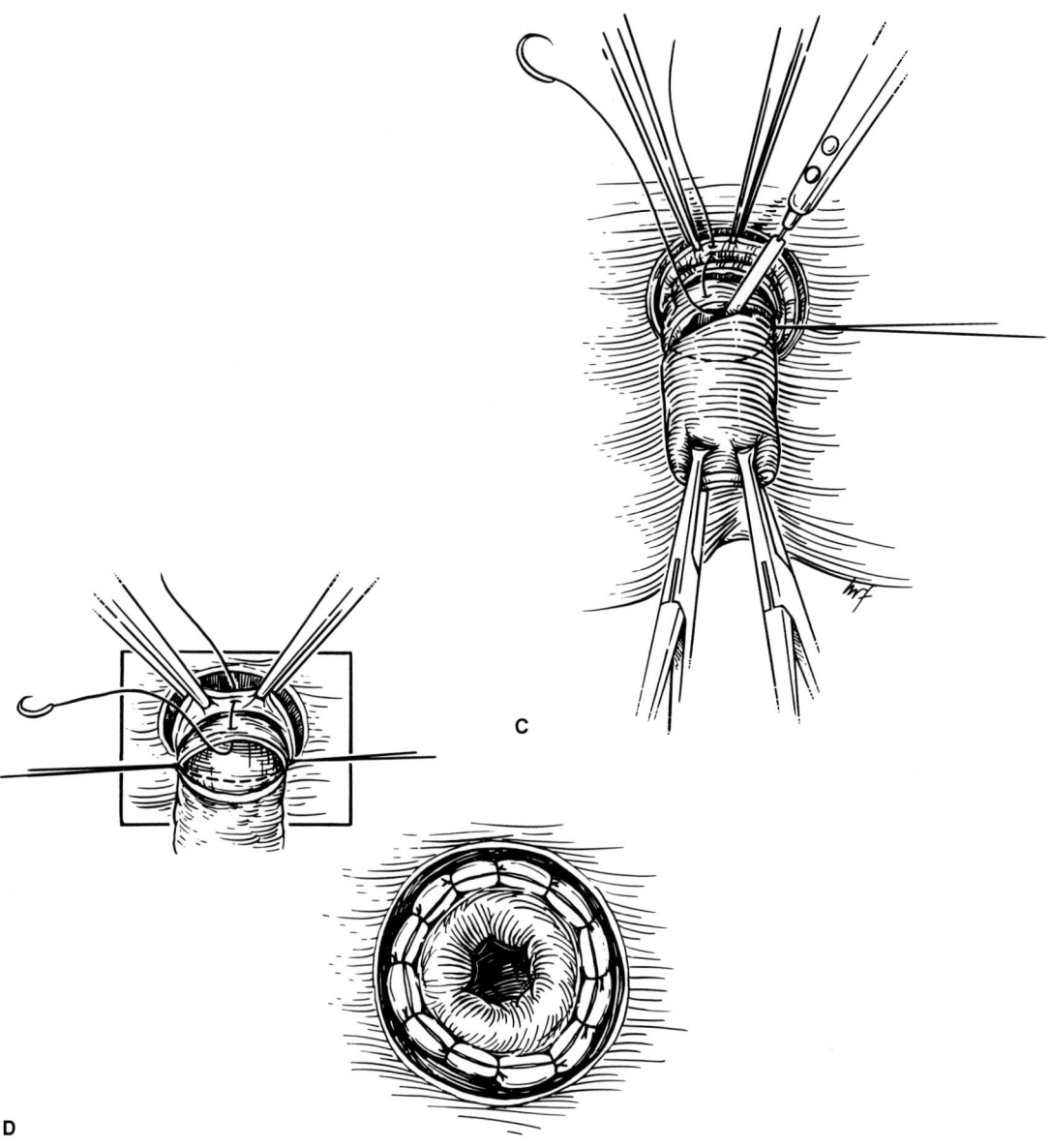

Figure 43-VE-1 *(Continued)*

(C) If there is no associated anal incontinence, the inner tube of bowel is divided and a coloanal anastomosis with 2-0 absorbable sutures is performed. If the patient has associated anal incontinence and a wide levator hiatus, a levatoroplasty is performed before resecting the prolapsed segment of bowel. The levator ani muscles are approximated anterior and posterior to the rectum with interrupted 3-0 permanent monofilament sutures. The surgeon must take care not to narrow the hiatus to the point that obstruction occurs. An index finger should be able to fit into the anal canal without difficulty.

(D) The coloanal anastomosis is completed with 12 to 16 interrupted 2-0 and 3-0 polyglycolic acid sutures. The slightly everted anastomosis is reduced.

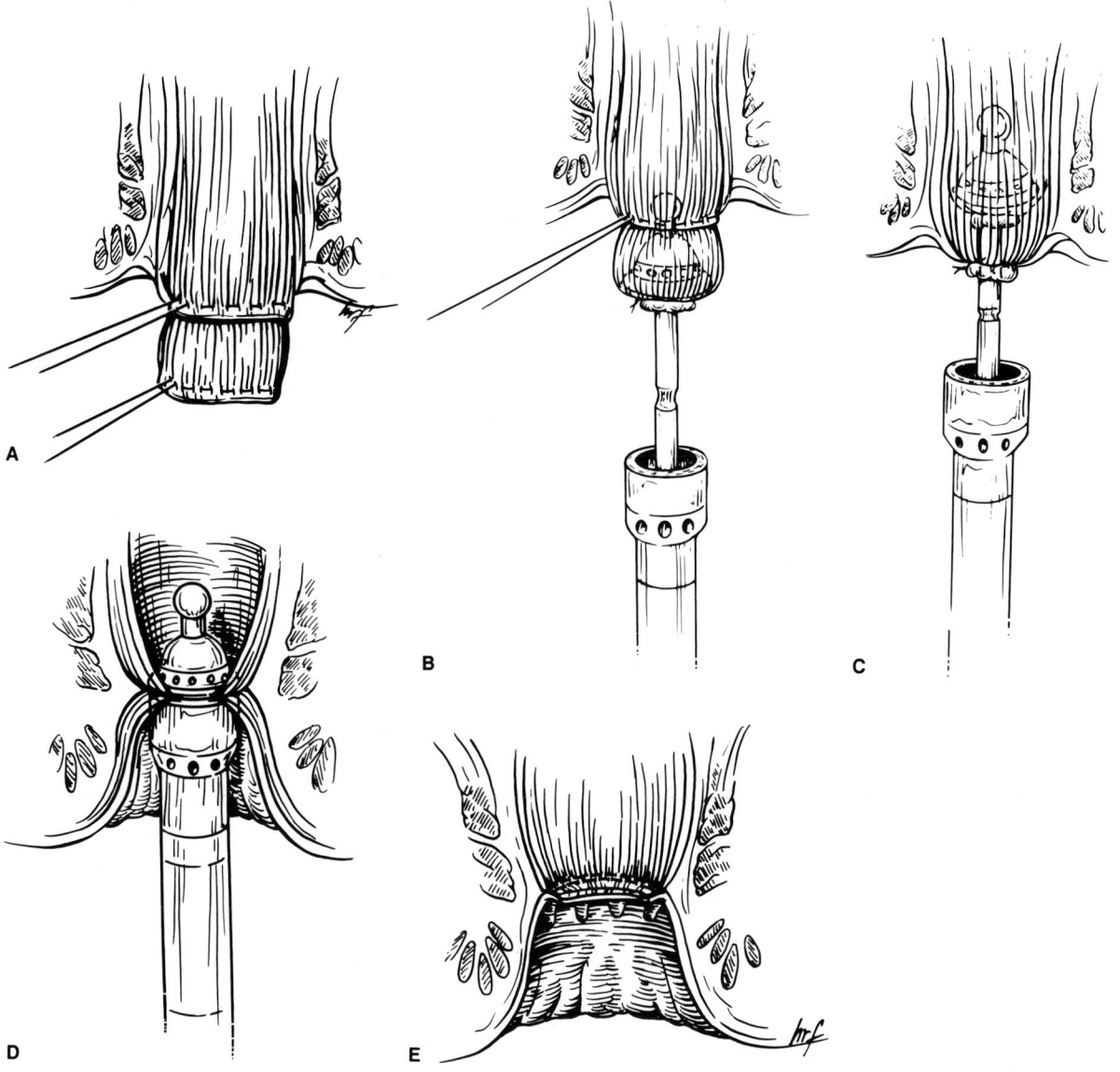

Figure 43-VE-2

Stapled Technique

(A) An alternative technique for performing the anastomosis is to place two concentric pursestring sutures on the two cut edges of bowel.

(B) The circular stapler is inserted, and the pursestring of the inner ring of bowel is tied around the anvil to the rod.

(C) The stapler is then inserted into the anal canal, and the pursestring of the distal segment of bowel is tied around the rod.

(D) The stapler is then closed and fired, thus creating an intra–anal canal end-to-end stapled anastomosis.

(E) The completed anastomosis is located just proximal to the dentate line.

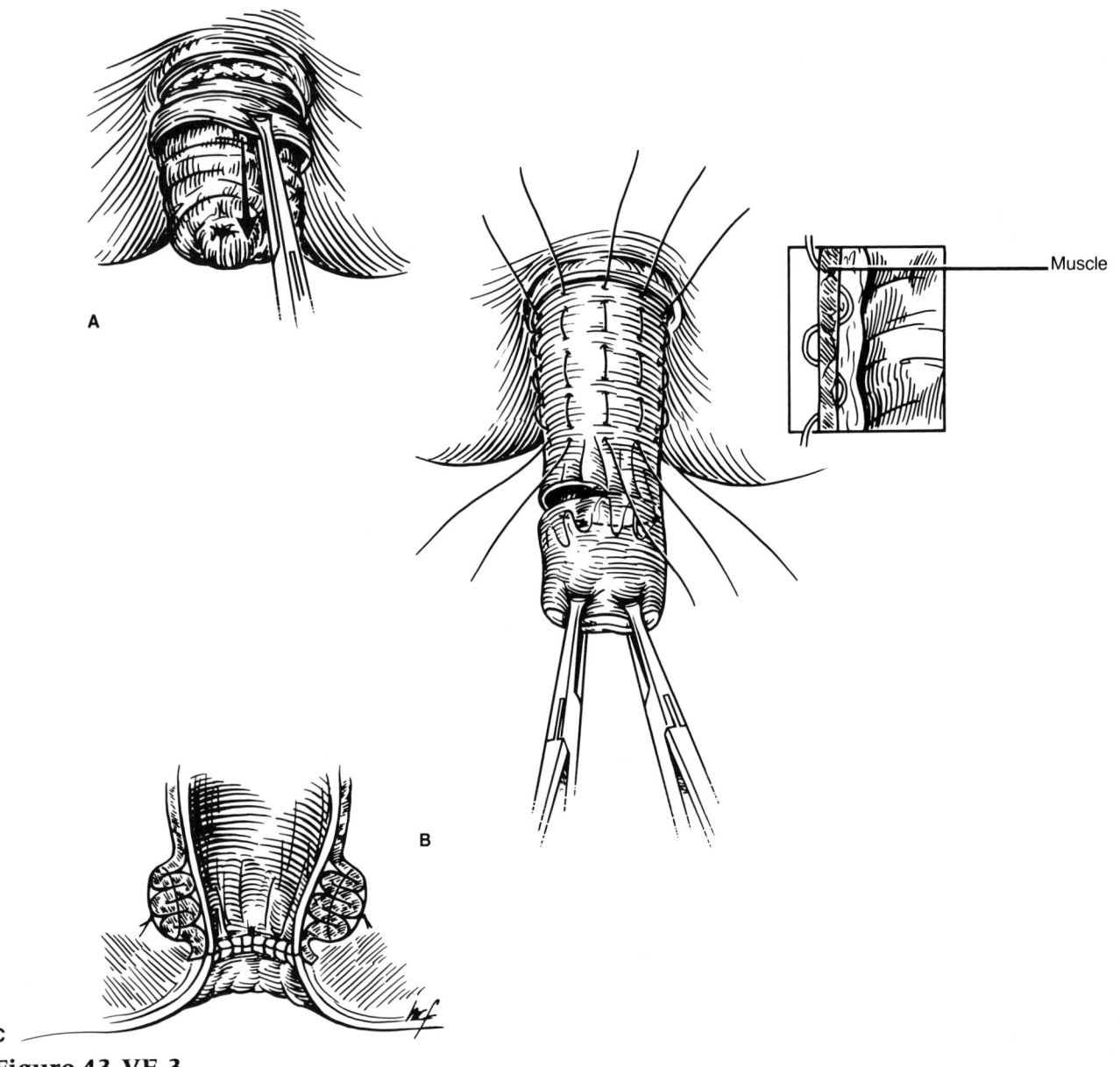

Muscle

Figure 43-VE-3

Delorme Procedure

(A) The Delorme procedure is an alternative perineal operation for patients with procidentia of the rectum. The prolapse is exposed by grasping the rectum and pulling distally.
A circumferential mucosal and submucosal incision is made 1 cm proximal to the dentate
line. The mucosa and submucosa of the prolapsed rectum are stripped from the underlying muscular tissue circumferentially.

(B) Multiple interrupted 2-0 polyglycolic acid sutures are placed along the muscular cuff
in the fashion shown to imbricate the muscularis. About six to eight sutures are used to
incorporate the bowel wall circumferentially.

(C) The sutures are serially tied, thus achieving an accordion-like reefing up of the muscularis of the anal canal. The mucosal defect is approximated with 3-0 interrupted sutures
of polyglycolic acid, thus effecting a coloanal anastomosis.

F. Sphincteroplasty and Levatoroplasty

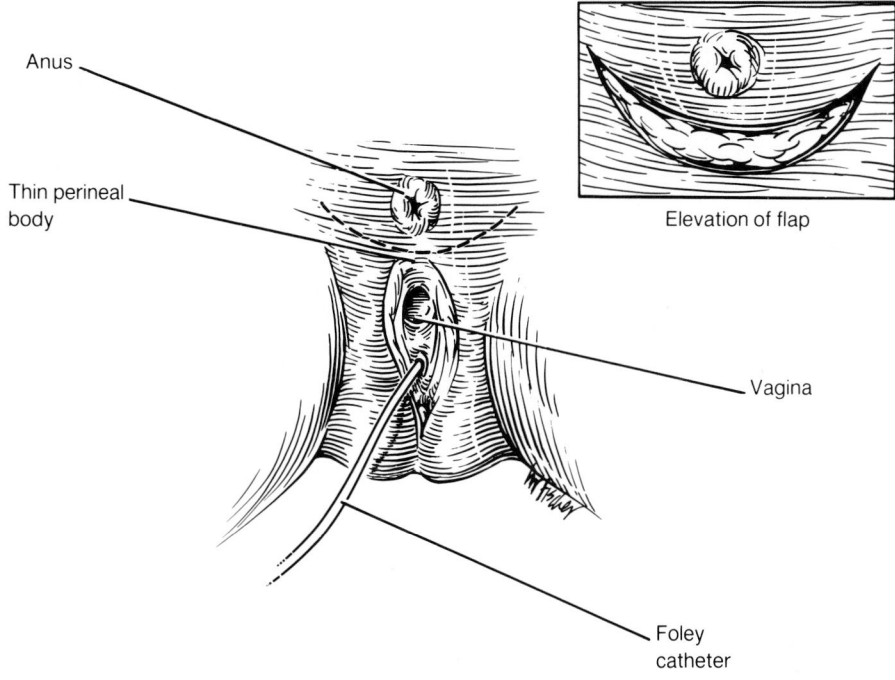

Elevation of flap

Anus

Thin perineal body

Vagina

Foley catheter

Figure 43-VF-1

Incision

Women who have birthing injuries resulting in anal incontinence generally have an anterior sphincter defect and a thin perineal body. The patient is prepared for operative repair by undergoing a full mechanical preparation, a general anesthetic, and placement in the prone jackknife position with a Foley catheter in the bladder. A curvilinear incision is made anterior to the anus, encompassing about 180 degrees.

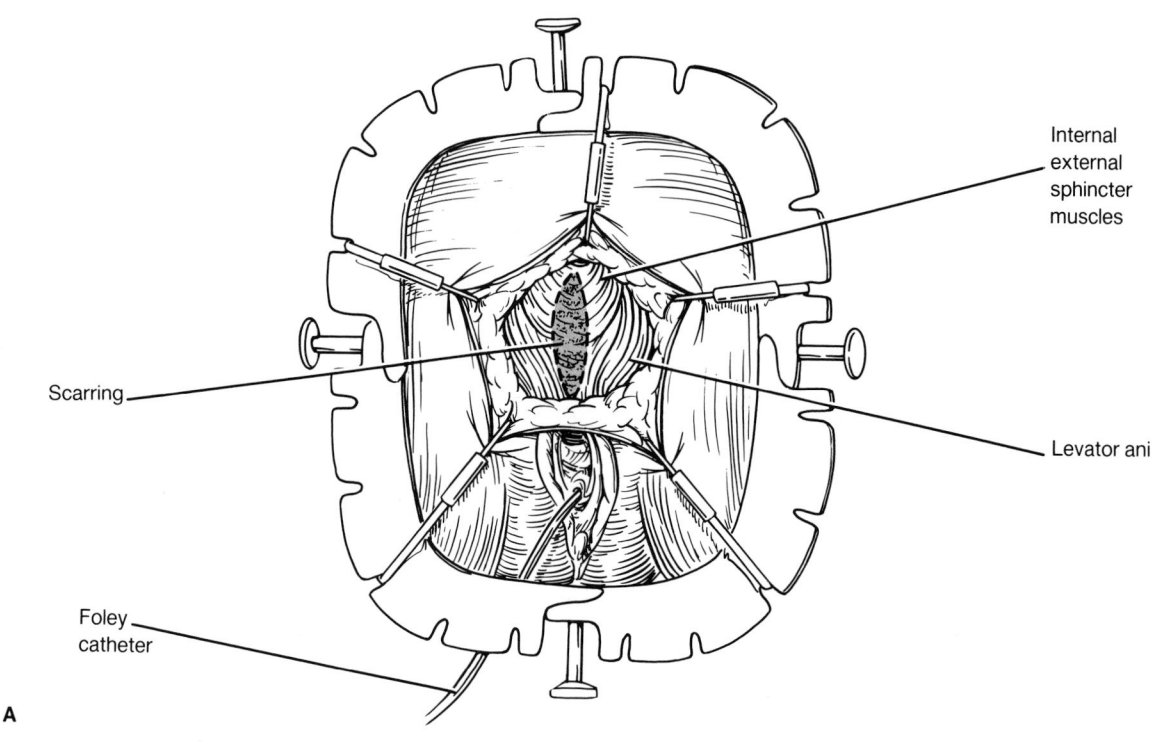

Internal
external
sphincter
muscles

Scarring

Levator ani

Foley
catheter

A

Figure 43-VF-2

Procedure

(**A**) A self-retaining retractor is used to efface the anus. The intact sphincter muscles are mobilized laterally on each side in the ischiorectal fossa. The dissection is continued anteriorly to expose and define the sphincter defect in the anterior midline.

(**B**) The anterior rectal wall is mobilized and retracted posteriorly. The external sphincter muscles are defined by mobilization laterally. In many injuries, the defect involves more than just the distal sphincter muscle and extends cephalad into the levator mechanism. The dissection must extend proximal to the injury. Sufficient mobilization of the sphincter is necessary to accomplish a tension-free repair.

(**C**) After achieving perfect hemostasis, an anterior levatoroplasty is performed using 3-0 nonabsorbable monofilament interrupted sutures.

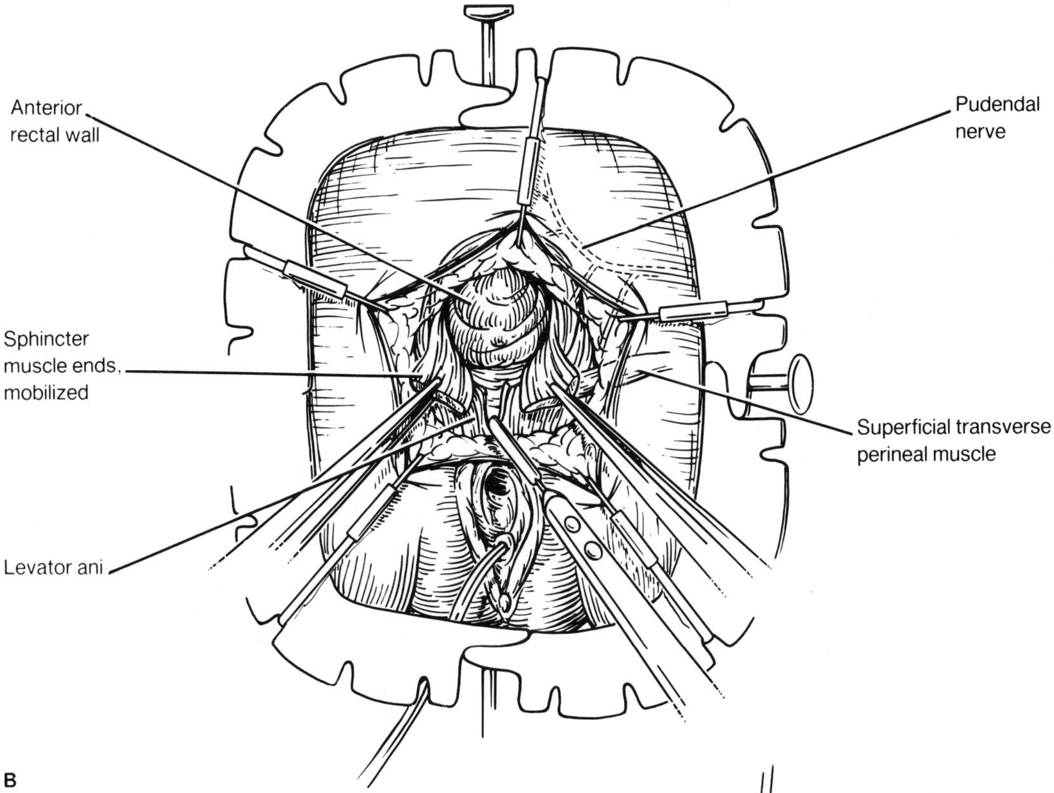

Anterior
rectal wall

Pudendal
nerve

Sphincter
muscle ends,
mobilized

Superficial transverse
perineal muscle

Levator ani

B

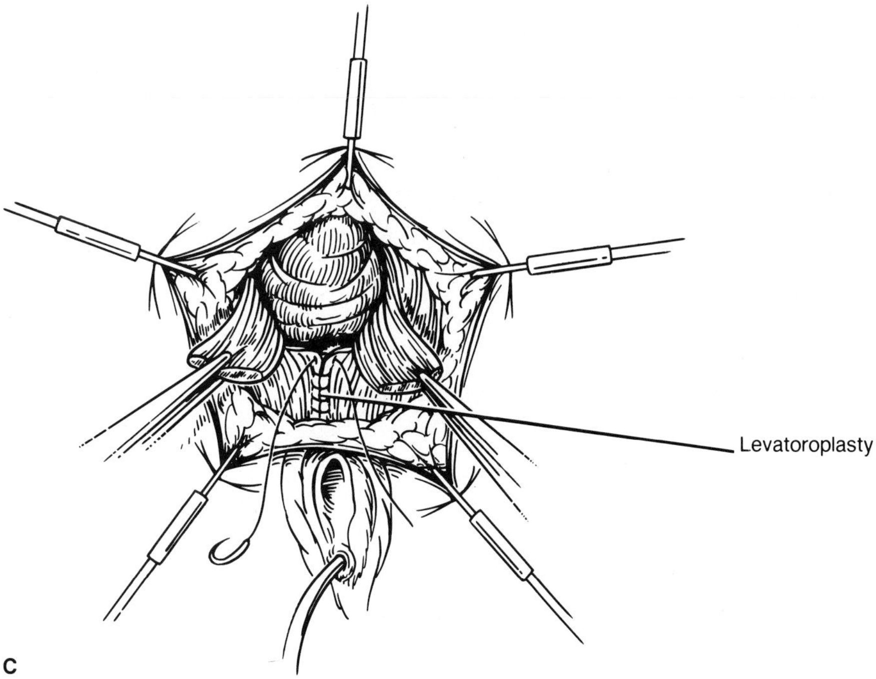

C

Levatoroplasty

Figure 43-VF-2 *(Continued)*

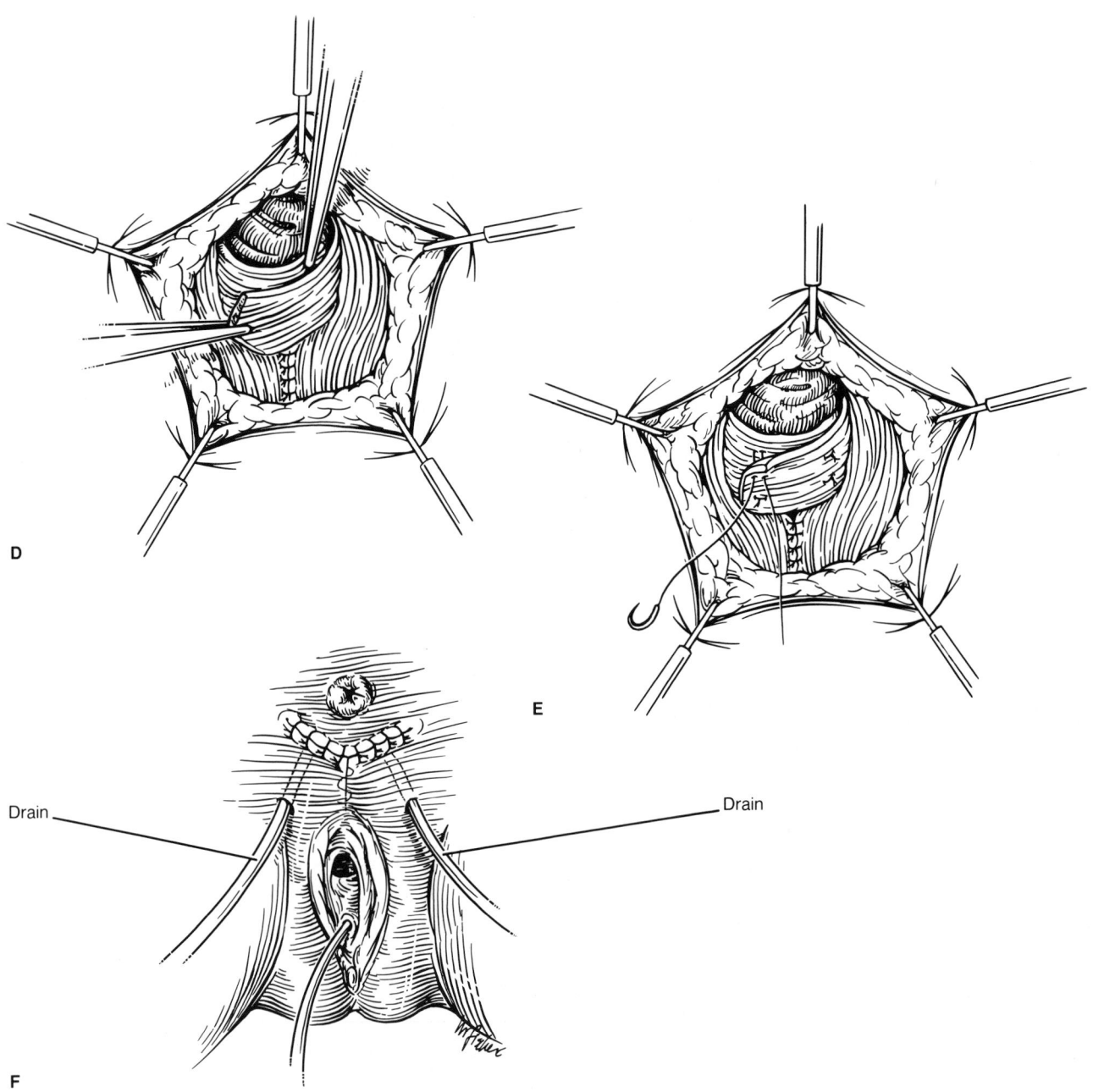

D

E

Drain _____   _____ Drain

F

Figure 43-VF-2 *(Continued)*

(D) The external sphincter repair is accomplished as an overlapping sphincteroplasty. Sufficient mobilization is necessary to achieve a tension-free repair.

(E) Multiple interrupted horizontal mattress sutures of 2-0 polyglycolic acid are first placed and then serially tied to hold the overlap in place.

(F) The skin defect is closed in a Y fashion with interrupted 3-0 absorbable sutures. Because of the increased distance between vagina and anus as a result of the repair and posterior relocation of the anus, the vertical limb of the Y closure is often several centimeters long. Quarter-inch Penrose drains exit through the skin closure from the depths of the wound and are removed in 24 to 48 hours.

G. Surgery for Abscess

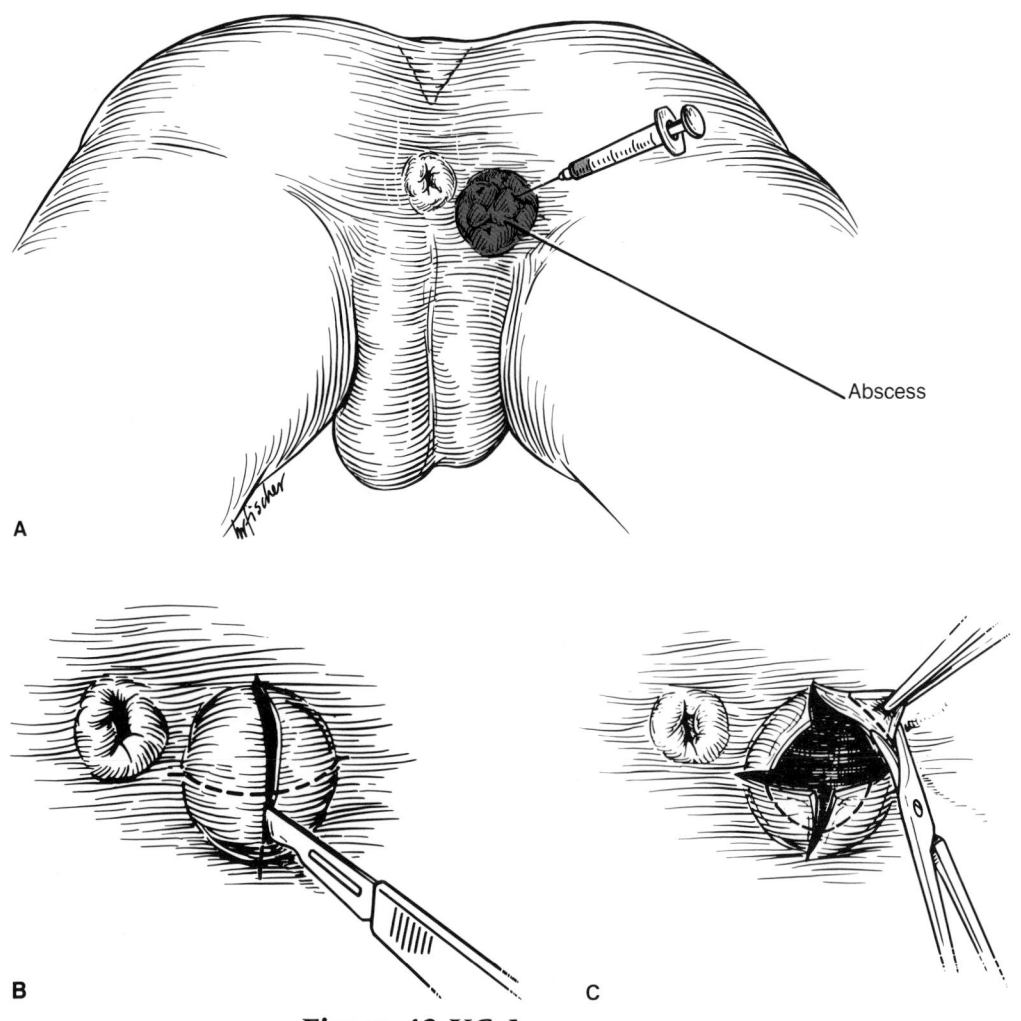

Figure 43-VG-1

Ischiorectal and Perianal Abscess

(A) Ischiorectal and perianal abscesses present in an acute fashion with patients complaining of severe perianal pain and swelling sometimes associated with fever. Most of these abscesses can be drained under a local anesthetic. A 30-gauge needle is used to inject the local anesthetic slowly into the skin overlying the abscess, which is usually obvious on clinical examination.

(B) Once anesthetized, the abscess is drained by making a cruciate incision.

(C) After drainage of the abscess, the skin edges are trimmed, thus leaving a circular defect. This allows adequate drainage from the depths of the abscess cavity without requiring uncomfortable packing of the wound.

(Continued)

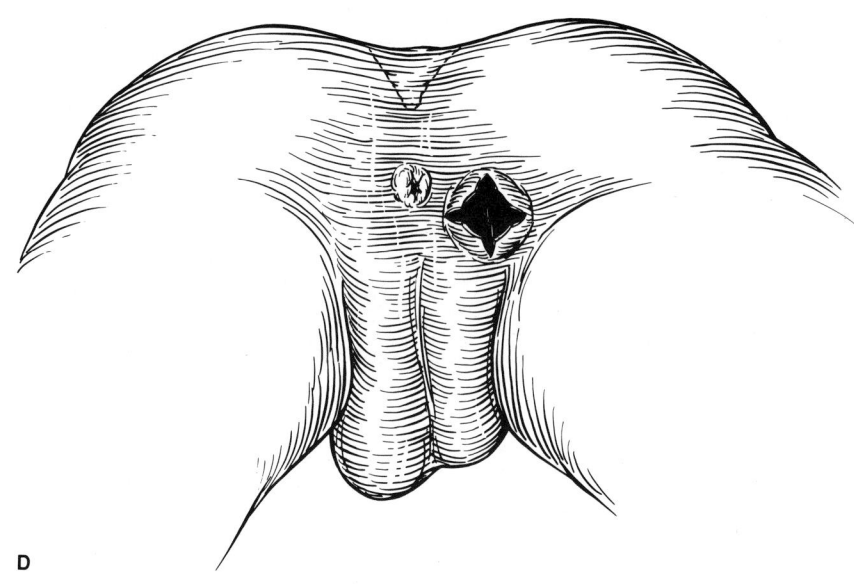

D

Figure 43-VG-1 *(Continued)*

(D) A soft dressing is applied externally to soak up drainage, but the wound is otherwise left open to heal secondarily. If there is an underlying fistula, drainage persists or abscesses recur. Subsequent fistulotomy would then be necessary.

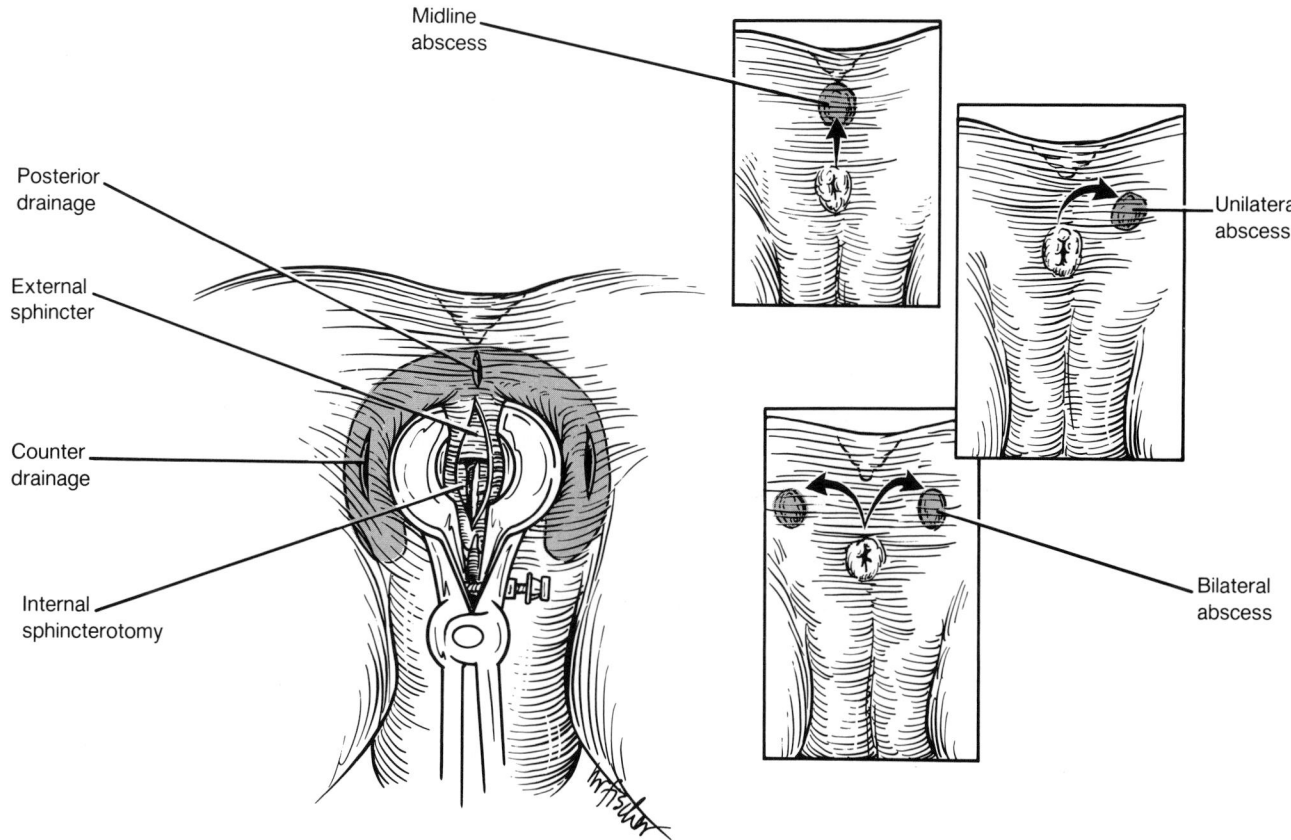

Figure 43-VG-2

Intersphincteric and Horseshoe Abscess

An intersphincteric abscess often presents with a sensation of pain high up in the anal canal without any obvious findings on external examination. This type of abscess requires examination and drainage under a general or block anesthetic. A small abscess may be noted by palpation or by observing a small amount of pus draining internally at the dentate line in the posterior midline. With the patient in the prone position, a bivalve anoscope is inserted. An incision is made through the posterior midline mucosa, submucosa, and internal sphincter muscle, thus allowing drainage of the intersphincteric abscess. If there is an associated horseshoe abscess, counter drainage can be made unilaterally or bilaterally as necessary. Sometimes, for a deep postanal space abscess, posterior drainage externally is also necessary.

H. Transanal Excision of Rectal Neoplasms

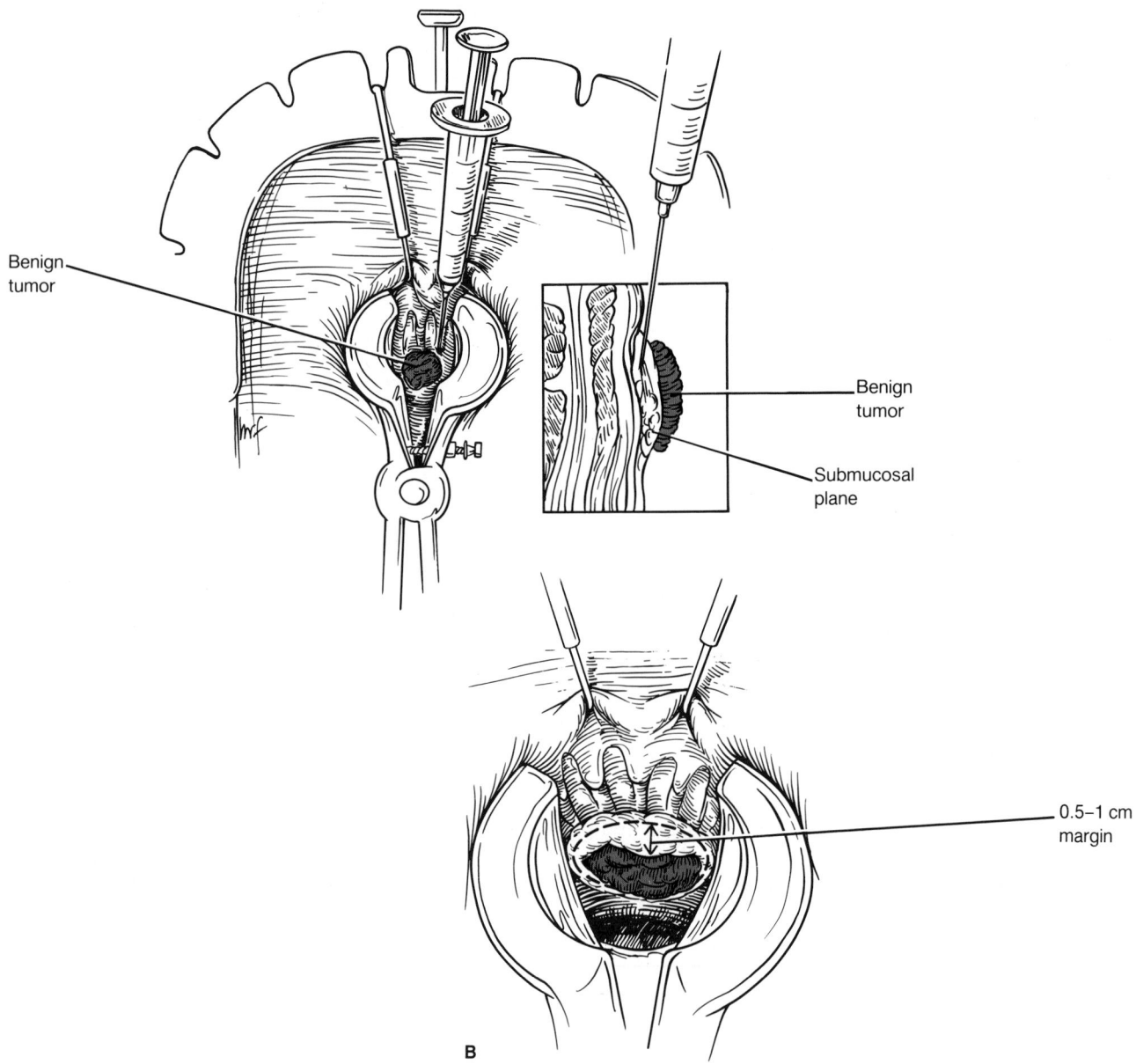

Figure 43-VH-1

Procedure

(A) Benign lesions of the anal canal and rectum can often be excised using a transanal approach. A self-retaining retractor is used to efface the anal canal and rectum. Dilute saline with epinephrine solution is injected into the submucosal plane beneath the lesion to elevate it from the underlying muscle.

(B) Electrocautery is used to make an incision about 1 cm distal to the tumor.

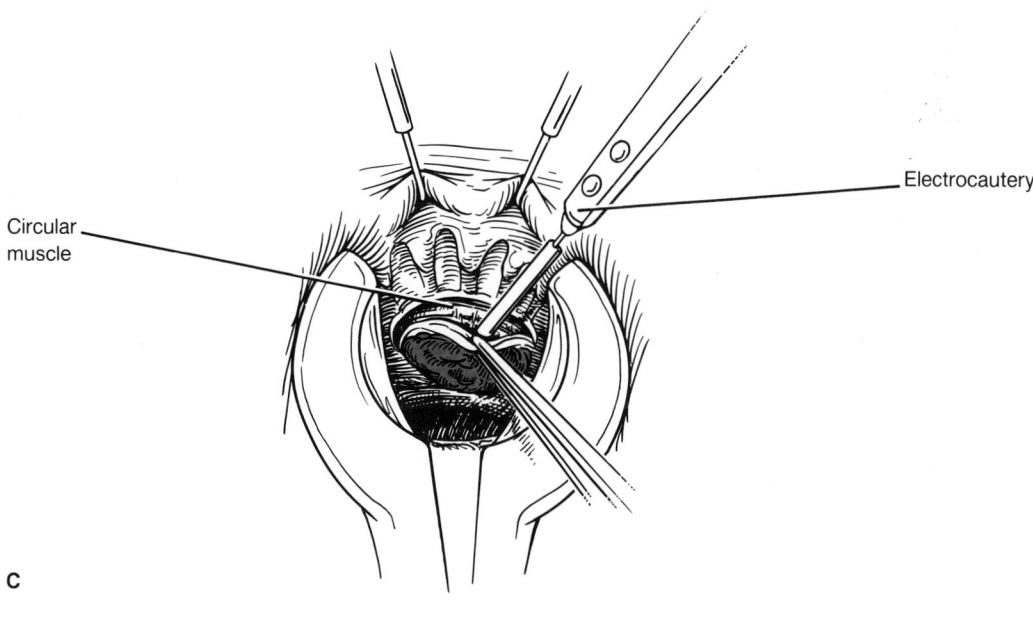

Circular muscle

Electrocautery

C

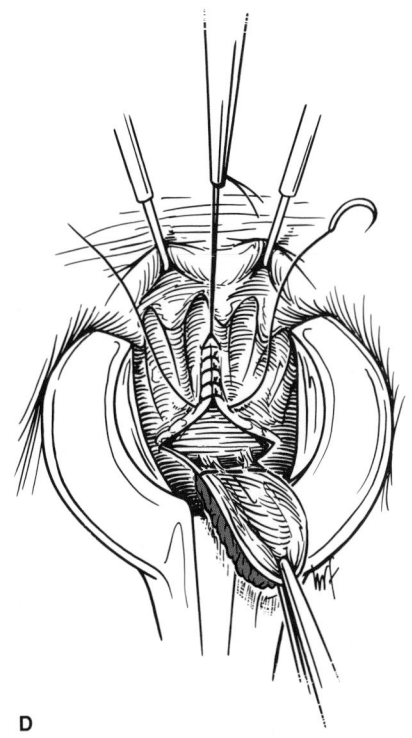

D

Figure 43-VH-1 *(Continued)*

(C) Using electrocautery, the lesion is mobilized from the underlying circular muscle, dissecting in a cephalad direction, maintaining a margin of at least 0.5 to 1 cm from the edge of the tumor.

(D) As the excision is taking place, the mucosa and submucosa are reapproximated with 2-0 interrupted absorbable polyglycolic acid sutures, which can be used for traction purposes. The disc excision of the tumor is removed intact and pinned out in an oriented fashion for pathology assessment.

(Continued)

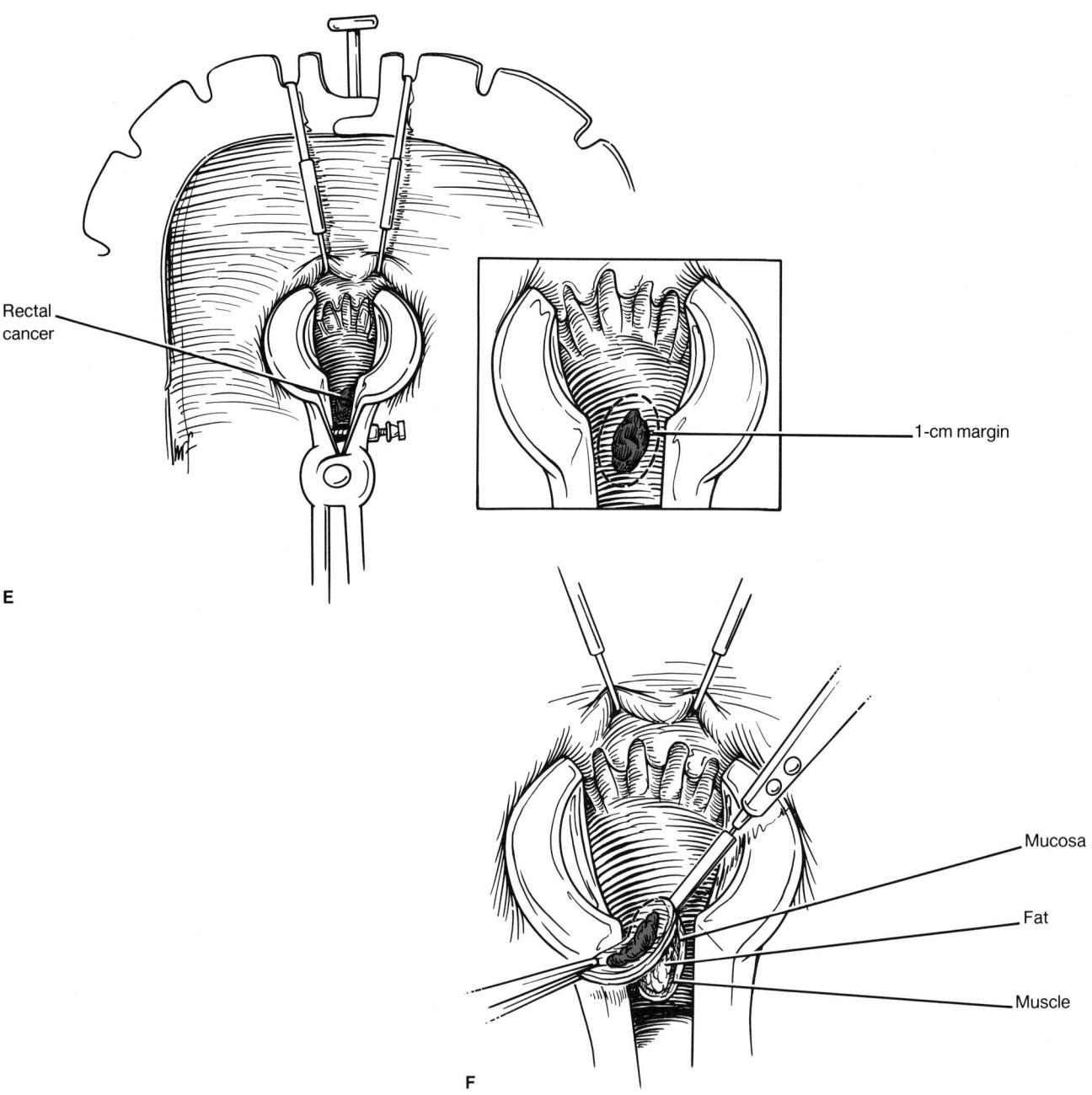

Rectal cancer

1-cm margin

E

Mucosa

Fat

Muscle

F

Figure 43-VH-1 *(Continued)*

(E) A similar dissection technique is used for highly selected malignancies of the distal anorectum. It is essential to have at least a 1-cm gross margin around such malignant lesions.

(F) A full-thickness excision is performed for known cancers of the distal anorectum.

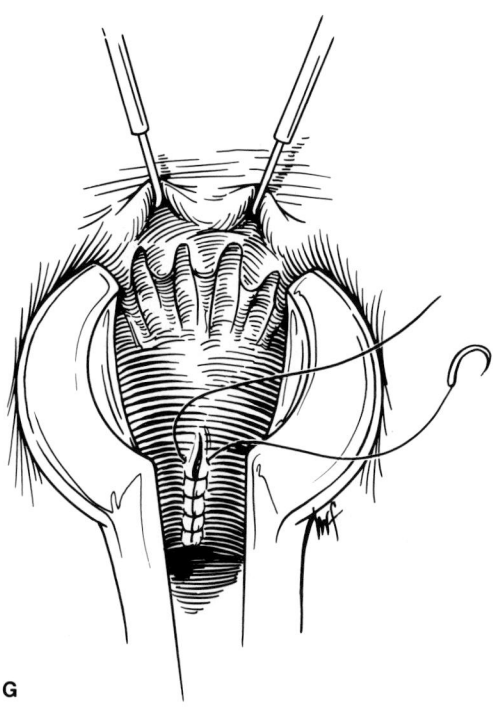

G

Figure 43-VH-1 *(Continued)*

(G) The repair is performed with multiple interrupted 2-0 polyglycolic acid sutures.

Index

Page numbers followed by *f* indicate figures; *t* represents tabular material; *CF* designates color figures; **bold face** numerals refer to atlas chapters.